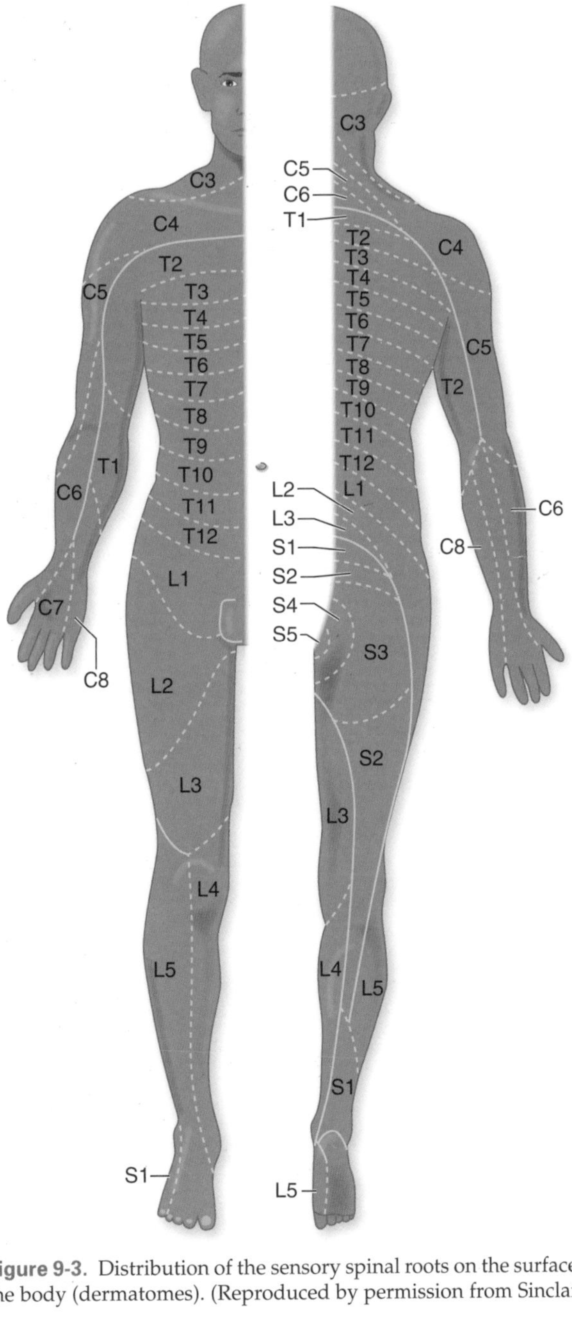

Figure 9-3. Distribution of the sensory spinal roots on the surface of the body (dermatomes). (Reproduced by permission from Sinclair.)

Adams and Victor's

PRINCIPLES OF NEUROLOGY

TENTH EDITION

NOTICE

Adams and Victor's

PRINCIPLES OF NEUROLOGY

TENTH EDITION

Allan H. Ropper, MD

Professor of Neurology
Harvard Medical School
Raymond D. Adams Master Clinician
Executive Vice Chair of Neurology
Brigham and Women's Hospital
Boston, Massachusetts

Martin A. Samuels, MD

Miriam Sydney Joseph Professor of Neurology
Harvard Medical School
Chair, Department of Neurology
Brigham and Women's Hospital
Boston, Massachusetts

Joshua P. Klein, MD, PhD

Assistant Professor of Neurology and Radiology
Harvard Medical School
Chief, Division of Hospital Neurology
Brigham and Women's Hospital
Boston, Massachusetts

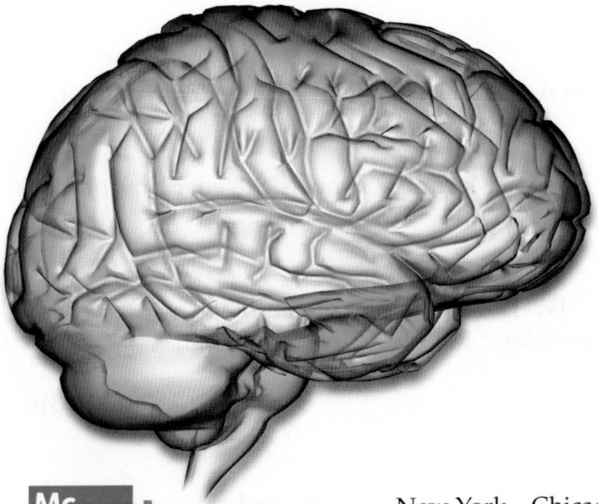

Mc Graw Hill Education | Medical

New York Chicago San Francisco Athens London Madrid
Mexico City Milan New Delhi Singapore Sydney Toronto

Adams and Victor's Principles of Neurology, Tenth Edition

3 4 5 6 7 8 9 0 DSS/DSS 19 18 17 16

ISBN 978-0-07-179479-4
MHID 0-07-179479-4

This book was set in Palatino by Cenveo® Publisher Services.
The editors were Anne M. Sydor and Kim J. Davis.
The production supervisor was Catherine H. Saggese.
Project management was provided by Sapna Rastogi of Cenveo Publisher Services.
The cover designer was Thomas De Pierro.
RR Donnelley/China was printer and binder.

This book is printed on acid-free paper.

Library of Congress Cataloging-in-Publication Data

Ropper, Allan H., author.
Adams and Victor's principles of neurology / Allan H. Ropper, Martin A. Samuels, Joshua P. Klein.—Tenth edition.
p. ; cm.
Principles of neurology
Preceded by Adams and Victor's principles of neurology / Allan H. Ropper, Martin A. Samuels. 9th ed. c2009.
Includes bibliographical references and index.
ISBN 978-0-07-179479-4 (hardcover : alk. paper)
ISBN 0-07-179479-4 (hardcover : alk. paper)
I. Samuels, Martin A., author. II. Klein, Joshua, author. III. Title. IV. Title: Principles of neurology.
[DNLM: 1. Nervous System Diseases. 2. Mental Disorders. 3. Neurologic Manifestations. WL 140]
RC346
616.8—dc23

2013048318

Contents

Preface

As the rest of medicine changes, so does neurology. Neurologic diagnosis and treatment has been so vastly altered by modern neuroimaging, molecular biology, and genetics that the original authors of this book, Raymond D Adams and Maurice Victor, would barely recognize the practices of today. Secular interest in neurologic diseases is also expanding because of the large number of problems of the brain, spinal cord, nerves, and muscles that arise with aging and from the treatment and control of other, non-neurologic, diseases. Whereas cancer and heart disease had occupied foremost positions in the minds of individuals within developed societies, Alzheimer, Parkinson, and related diseases are central to the modern conversation about the quality of life. Moreover, the desire to understand the workings of the brain and to gain insights into human behavior has become a preoccupation of the public. At the same time, the manner in which information, both accurate and otherwise, is transmitted about the nervous system and neurologic diseases has changed. Access to information about diseases, accepted treatments, and clinical symptoms and signs, ubiquitously clutters the Internet. Physicians now less frequently seek a comprehensive understanding of a disease or class of diseases, "the whole story" if you will, but instead favor rapid access to single answers to a clinical problem.

For many reasons, particularly the last of these regarding the nature of medical information, writing a textbook on neurology has become a complex enterprise. We have even asked ourselves if there is a role for a textbook in the modern era, especially one written by only three authors. Yet, in identifying the characteristics of the capable clinician, one who is equipped to help patients and play a role in society to the fullest extent possible, we continuously return to the need for careful clinical analysis that is combined with a deep knowledge of disease. These are still the basis for high-quality practice and teaching. Even if the current goals of efficiency and economy in medicine are to be met, neurology is so complex that the confident implementation of a plan of diagnostic or therapeutic action quickly finds itself beyond algorithms, flow charts, and guidelines. The goal of our textbook therefore is to provide neurologic knowledge in an assembled way that transcends facts and information and to present this knowledge in a context that cannot be attained by disembodied details. While the biological bases of neurologic diseases are being discovered rapidly, the major contribution of the clinical neurologist remains, as it is for the whole of medicine: a synthesis of knowing how to listen to the patient, where to find the salient neurologic signs, and what to acquire from laboratory tests and imaging.

There is always a risk of such a book being simply archival. But the dynamic nature of modern neurology requires more than ever a type of integration among knowledge of clinical neurosciences, traditional neurology, and the expanding scientific literature on disease mechanisms. Only a text that has been thoughtfully constructed for the educated neurologist can fulfill this need and we hope that we have done so in this edition. Furthermore, in appropriate conformity to the methods by which physicians obtain information, McGraw-Hill has made an investment in their Access Medicine website that will highlight our book as well as several other neurology texts. Combined with these books will be sophisticated search functions, teaching curricula for students and residents, and, hopefully in the future, a form of interaction with us, the authors. Another inception has been the addition of color figures and photographs to this edition in order to make the visual material more accessible and appropriate for the web version.

To these ends, we offer the current 10th edition of *Principles of Neurology* to meet the needs of the seasoned as well as the aspiring neurologist, neurosurgeon, internist, psychiatrist, pediatrician, emergency physician, physiatrist, and all clinicians who have need of a comprehensive discussion on neurologic problems. We begin with an explanation of the functioning of the nervous system as it pertains to neurologic disease in the first part of the book, followed by detailed descriptions of the clinical aspects of neurology in its great diversity. In all matters, we have put the patient and relief of suffering from neurologic disease in a central place. The book is meant to be practical without being prescriptive and readable without being too exhaustive. When there is a digression, it has been purposely structured to complete a picture of a particular disease. We have also retained historical aspects of many diseases that are central to the understanding of the specialty and its place in medicine.

By taking an inclusive and yet sensibly chosen clinical approach, we do not eschew or criticize the modern movement to homogenize medicine in order to attain uniformity of practice. We ourselves have witnessed over 35 years the unappealing aspects of idiosyncratic practices, which were based on limited basic information and on a superficial understanding of neurology. Nonetheless, the complexity of neurologic diseases, especially now, puts the practitioner in a position of choosing among many options for diagnosis and treatment that are equivalent, or for which the results are uncertain. Clinical trials abound in neurology and set a direction for clinical practice in large populations, but are difficult to apply to individual patients. The need for a coherent method of clinical work is one reason we have retained authorship rather than editorial management that characterizes many textbooks in other areas of medicine. Limited authorship permits a uniform style of writing and level of exposition across subject matter and chapter headings.

It also allows us to judiciously include our own experiences and opinions when we feel there is something more to say than is evident in published articles. Our comments should be taken as advisory and we have no doubt that our colleagues in practice will develop their own views based on the body of information provided in the book and what is available from many outside sources. To the extent that some of the views we express in the book may be perceived as having a "Boston-centric" outlook, we appeal to the reader's forbearance. We have neither a proprietary formula for success in neurology nor the answers to many of the big clinical questions. If there is a stylistic aspect that comes through in the book, we hope it is still that neurology must be taken one patient at a time.

We gratefully acknowledge on the following pages several experts in particular fields of neurology whose help was invaluable in revising this edition. We sought their guidance because of the high regard we have for their clinical skills and experience. If there are concerns regarding specific comments in the book, they are our responsibility.

With this edition, we introduce our colleague Joshua P. Klein, MD, PhD, the chief of the Division of Hospital Neurology in the Department of Neurology at Brigham and Women's Hospital. Dr. Klein is dually trained in neurology and neuroradiology. He brings a wealth of perspective on imaging and has been a powerful partner in moving the book toward a more modern idiom that recognizes the centrality of neuroimaging in practice. It is a privilege to have him join us to bring the book through the beginning of the current century.

Allan H. Ropper, MD
Martin A. Samuels, MD
Joshua P. Klein, MD, PhD

Acknowledgments

The authors gratefully acknowledge the colleagues listed below who gave considerably of their time to assist us with sections of the book. Any oversights in the content of the book are our responsibility. Updating this 10th edition of *Principles of Neurology* would not have been possible without these expert physicians and we extend to them our sincere thanks.

Dr. Philip Smith
Chapter 16 "Epilepsy and Other Seizure Disorders"
Department of Neurology, University Hospital of Wales; Professor of Neurology, Cardiff University School of Medicine, Cardiff, Wales, United Kingdom

Dr. Marc Hommel
Chapter 34 "Cerebrovascular Diseases"
Professor of Neurology, University Hospital of Grenoble, Grenoble, France

Dr. James Maguire
Chapter 32 "Infections of the Nervous System (Bacterial, Fungal, Spirochetal, Parasitic) and Sarcoidosis" and Chapter 33 "Viral Infections of the Nervous System, Chronic Meningitis, and Prion Diseases"
Department of Medicine, Division of Infectious Diseases, Brigham and Women's Hospital; Professor of Medicine, Harvard Medical School Boston, Massachusetts

Dr. Sashank Prasad
Chapter 13 "Disturbances of Vision" and Chapter 14 "Disorders of Ocular Movement and Pupillary Function"
Department of Neurology, Brigham and Women's Hospital; Assistant Professor of Neurology, Harvard Medical School, Boston, Massachusetts

Dr. Jeffrey Liou
Chapter 18 "Faintness and Syncope" and Chapter 26 "Disorders of the Autonomic Nervous System, Respiration, and Swallowing"
Department of Neurology, Brigham and Women's Hospital; Assistant Professor of Neurology, Harvard Medical School, Boston, Massachusetts

Dr. James Stankiewicz
Chapter 36 "Multiple Sclerosis and Allied Demyelinating Diseases"
Clerkship Director and Clinical Director, Partners Multiple Sclerosis Center, Department of Neurology, Brigham and Women's Hospital; Assistant Professor of Neurology, Harvard Medical School, Boston, Massachusetts

Dr. Anthony Amato
Chapter 46 "Diseases of the Peripheral Nerves" and Chapter 48 "Diseases of Muscle"
Chief, Neuromuscular Division and Vice-Chairman, Department of Neurology, Brigham and Women's Hospital; Assistant Professor of Neurology, Harvard Medical School, Boston, Massachusetts

Dr. Mel Feany
Chapter 39 "Degenerative Diseases of the Nervous System"
Associate Pathologist and Neuropathologist, Department of Pathology, Brigham and Women's Hospital; Professor of Pathology, Harvard Medical School, Boston, Massachusetts

Dr. Inderneel Sahai
Chapter 37 "Inherited Metabolic Diseases of the Nervous System"
Department of Pediatrics
Metabolic Disorders Unit
Massachusetts General Hospital for Children and New England Newborn Screening Program

Dr. Joseph B. Martin
Chapter 27 "The Hypothalamus and Neuroendocrine Disorders"
Department of Neurology, Brigham and Women's Hospital; Professor of Neurology, Harvard Medical School, Dean Emeritus, Harvard Medical School, Boston, Massachusetts

PART 1

THE CLINICAL METHOD OF NEUROLOGY

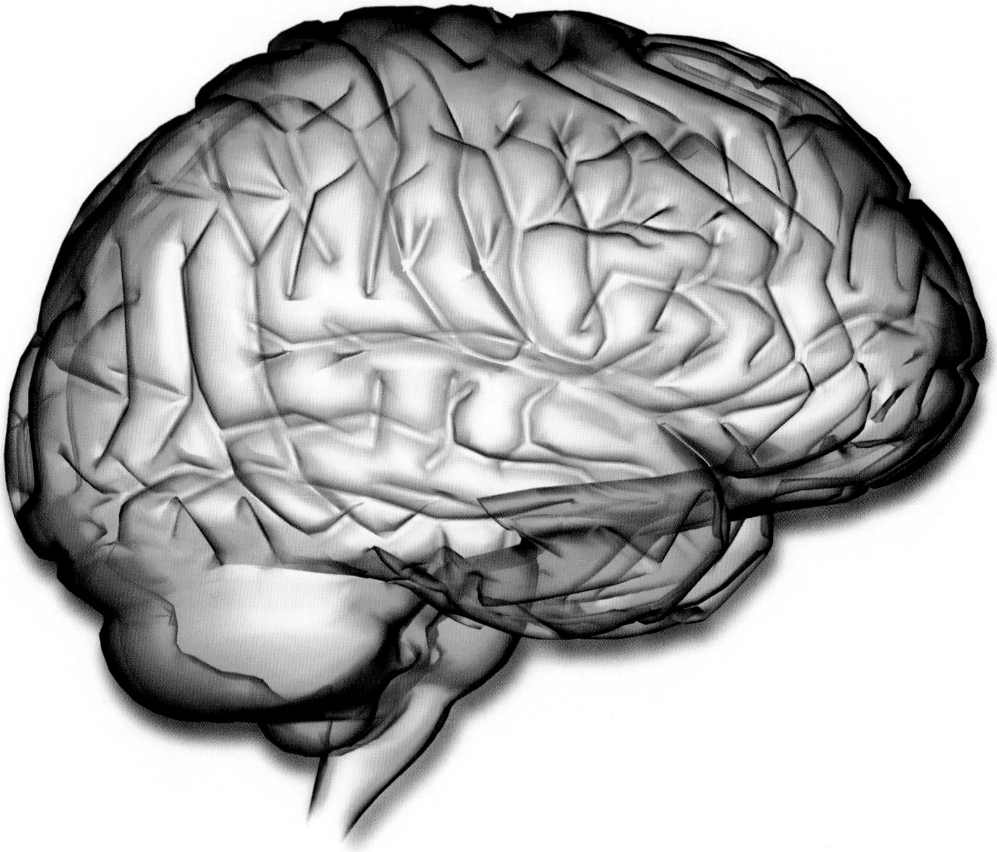

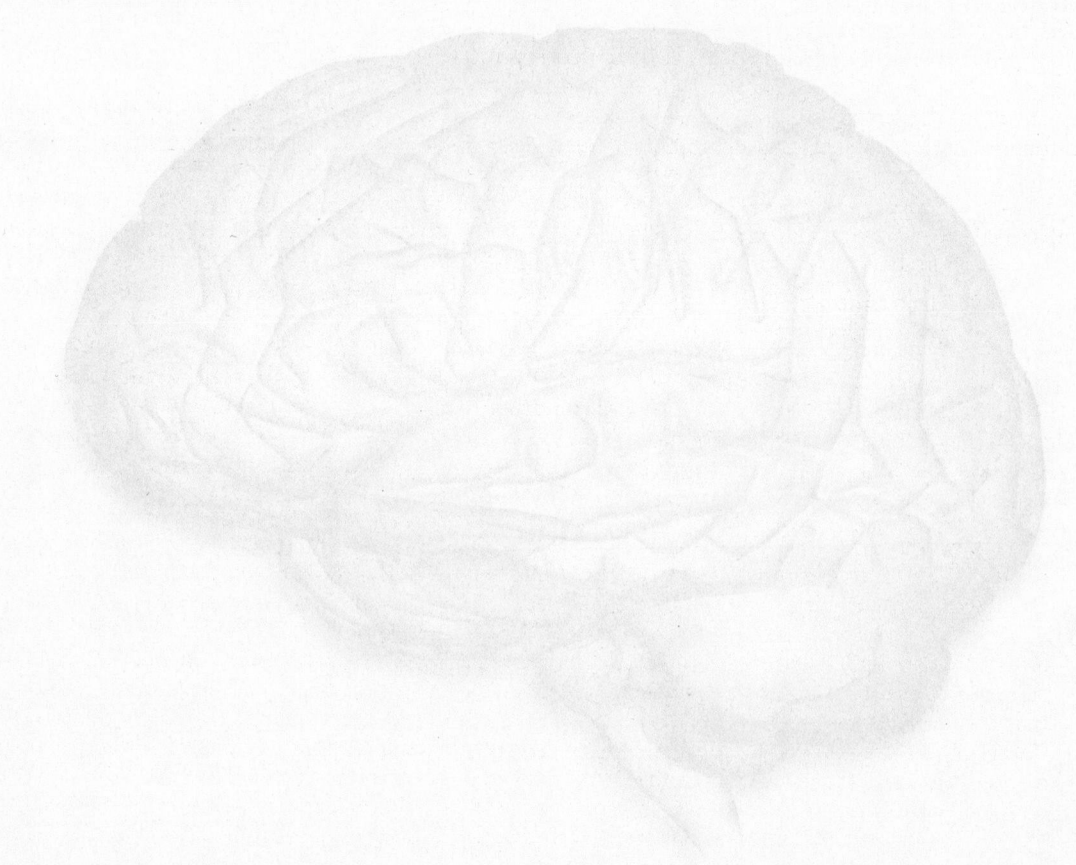

1

Approach to the Patient with Neurologic Disease

Neurology is regarded by many as one of the most difficult and exacting medical specialties. Students and residents who come to a neurology service for the first time may be intimidated by the complexity of the nervous system through their brief contact with neuroanatomy, neurophysiology, and neuropathology. The ritual they then witness of putting the patient through a series of maneuvers designed to evoke certain mysterious signs is hardly reassuring. In fact, the examination appears to conceal the intellectual processes by which neurologic diagnosis is made. Moreover, the students have had little or no experience with the many special tests used in neurologic diagnosis—such as lumbar puncture, EMG (electromyography), EEG (electroencephalography), CT (computed tomography), MRI (magnetic resonance imaging), and other imaging procedures—nor do they know how to interpret the results of such tests. Neurology textbooks only confirm their fears as they read the detailed accounts of the many unusual diseases of the nervous system.

The authors believe that many of the difficulties in comprehending neurology can be overcome by adhering to the basic principles of the clinical method. Even the experienced neurologist faced with a complex clinical problem depends on this basic approach.

The importance of the clinical method stands out more clearly in the study of neurologic disease than in certain other fields of medicine. In most cases, it consists of an orderly series of steps:

1. The symptoms and signs are secured with as much confidence as possible by history and physical examination.
2. The symptoms and physical signs considered relevant to the problem at hand are interpreted in terms of physiology and anatomy—i.e., one identifies the disorder(s) of function and the anatomic structure(s) that are implicated.
3. These analyses permit the physician to localize the disease process, i.e., to name the part or parts of the nervous system involved. This is the *anatomic*, or *topographic* diagnosis, which often allows the recognition of a characteristic clustering of symptoms and signs, constituting a syndrome. This step is called *syndromic diagnosis* and is sometimes conducted in parallel with anatomic diagnosis.
4. Expert diagnosticians often make successively more accurate estimates of the likely diagnosis, utilizing pieces of the history and findings on the examination to either further refine or exclude specific diseases. Flexibility of thought must be practiced so as to avoid the common pitfall of retaining an initially incorrect impression and selectively ignoring data that would bring it into question. It is perhaps not surprising that the method of successive estimations works well in that evidence from neuroscience reveals that this is the mechanism that the nervous system uses to process information.
5. From the anatomic or syndromic diagnosis and other specific medical data—particularly the mode of onset and speed of evolution of the illness, the involvement of nonneurologic organ systems, the relevant past and family medical histories, and the laboratory findings—one deduces the *pathologic diagnosis* and, when the mechanism and causation of the disease can be determined, the *etiologic diagnosis*. This may include the rapidly increasing number of molecular and genetic etiologies if they have been determined for a particular disorder.
6. Finally, the physician should assess the degree of disability and determine whether it is temporary or permanent (*functional diagnosis*); this is important in managing the patient's illness and judging the potential for restoration of function.

In recent decades, many of these steps have been eclipsed by imaging methods that allow precise localization of a lesion and furthermore often characterize the etiology of disease. Many of the elaborate parts of the examination that were intended to localize lesions are no longer necessary in daily clinical work. Nonetheless, insufficient appreciation of the history and examination and the resulting overdependence on imaging leads to diagnostic errors and has other detrimental consequences. A clinical approach is usually more efficient and far more economical than is resorting to scans. The loss of the personal impact by the physician that is created by listening to a story and observing responses to various maneuvers is regrettable. Images are also replete with spurious or unrelated findings, which elicit unnecessary further testing and needless worry on the part of the patient.

All of these steps are undertaken in the service of effective treatment, an ever-increasing prospect in neurology. As is emphasized repeatedly in later chapters, there is always a premium in the diagnostic process on the discovery of treatable diseases. Even when specific treatment is not available, accurate diagnosis may in its own right function as a therapy, as uncertainty about the cause of a neurologic illness may be more troubling to the patient than the disease itself.

Of course, the solution to a clinical problem need not always be schematized in this way. The clinical method offers a much wider choice in the order and manner by which information is collected and interpreted. In fact, in some cases, adherence to a formal scheme is not necessary at all. In relation to syndromic diagnosis, the clinical picture of Parkinson disease, for example, is usually so characteristic that the nature of the illness is at once apparent. In other cases it is not necessary to carry the clinical analysis beyond the stage of the anatomic diagnosis, which, in itself, may virtually indicate the cause of a disease. For example, when vertigo, cerebellar ataxia, unilateral Horner syndrome, paralysis of a vocal cord, and analgesia of the face occur with acute onset, the cause is an occlusion of the vertebral artery, because all the involved structures lie in the lateral medulla, within the territory of this artery. Thus, the anatomic diagnosis determines and limits the etiologic possibilities. If the signs point to disease of the peripheral nerves, it is usually not necessary to consider the causes of disease of the spinal cord. Some signs themselves are almost specific—e.g., opsoclonus for paraneoplastic cerebellar degeneration and Argyll Robertson pupils for neurosyphilitic or diabetic oculomotor neuropathy. Nonetheless, one is cautious in calling any single sign pathognomonic as exceptions are found regularly.

Ascertaining the cause of a clinical syndrome (etiologic diagnosis) requires knowledge of an entirely different order. Here one must be conversant with the clinical details, including the speed of onset, course, laboratory and imaging characteristics, and natural history of a multiplicity of diseases. Many of these facts are well known and form the substance of later chapters. When confronted with a constellation of clinical features that do not lend themselves to a simple or sequential analysis, one resorts to considering the broad classical division of diseases in all branches of medicine, as summarized in Table 1-1.

Table 1-1

THE MAJOR CATEGORIES OF NEUROLOGIC DISEASE

Infectious
Genetic–congenital
Traumatic
Degenerative
Vascular
Toxic
Metabolic
Inherited
Acquired
Neoplastic
Inflammatory–immune
Psychogenic
Iatrogenic

Irrespective of the intellectual process that one utilizes in solving a particular clinical problem, the fundamental steps in diagnosis always involve the accurate elicitation of symptoms and signs and their correct interpretation in terms of disordered function of the nervous system. Most often when there is uncertainty or disagreement as to diagnosis, it is found later that the symptoms or signs were incorrectly interpreted in the first place. Thus, if a complaint of dizziness is identified as vertigo instead of light-headedness or if partial continuous epilepsy is mistaken for a tremor or choreoathetosis, then the clinical method is derailed from the beginning. Repeated examinations may be necessary to establish the fundamental clinical findings beyond doubt. Hence the aphorism: A second examination is the most helpful diagnostic test in a difficult neurologic case.

PREVALENCE AND INCIDENCE OF NEUROLOGIC DISEASE

To offer the physician the broadest perspective on the relative frequency of neurologic diseases, estimates of their approximate prevalence in the United States, taken from several sources, including the NIH, are given in Table 1-2. Donaghy and colleagues have provided a similar but more extensive listing of the incidence of various neurologic diseases that are likely to be seen by a general physician practicing in the United Kingdom. They note stroke as far and away the most commonly

Table 1-2

RELATIVE PREVALENCE OF THE MAJOR NEUROLOGIC DISORDERS IN THE UNITED STATES

	INDIVIDUALS AFFECTED
Degenerative diseases	
Amyotrophic lateral sclerosis	5×10^4
Huntington disease	5×10^4
Parkinson disease	5×10^6
Alzheimer disease	5×10^6
Macular degeneration	5×10^7
Autoimmune neurologic diseases	
Multiple sclerosis	4×10^5
Stroke, all types	5×10^6
Central nervous system trauma	
Head	2×10^6
Spinal cord	2.5×10^5
Metabolic	
Diabetic retinopathy	2×10^6
Headache	3×10^7
Epilepsy	3×10^6
Back pain	5×10^7
Peripheral neuropathy	
Total	2.5×10^7
Inherited	1×10^4
Diabetic neuropathy	2×10^6
Mental retardation	
Severe	1×10^6
Moderate	1×10^7
Schizophrenia	3×10^6
Manic depressive illness	3×10^6

Table 1-3

APPROXIMATE ORDER OF INCIDENCE AND PREVALENCE OF NEUROLOGIC CONDITIONS IN A GENERAL PRACTICE IN THE UNITED KINGDOM

INCIDENCE IN GENERAL PRACTICE	PREVALENCE IN THE COMMUNITY
Stroke (all types)	Migraine
Carpal tunnel syndrome	Chronic tension headache
Epilepsy	Stroke
Bell's palsy	Alzheimer disease
Essential tremor	Epilepsy
Parkinson disease	Essential tremor
Brain tumor	Multiple sclerosis
Multiple sclerosis	Chronic fatigue syndrome
Giant cell arteritis	Parkinson disease
Migraine	Unexplained motor symptoms
Unexplained motor symptoms	Neurofibromatosis
Trigeminal neuralgia	Myasthenia gravis

Source: Adapted from Donaghy and colleagues: *Brain's Diseases of the Nervous System.*

encountered condition; those that follow in frequency are listed in Table 1-3. More focused surveys, such as the one conducted by Hirtz and colleagues, give similar rates of prevalence, with migraine, epilepsy, and multiple sclerosis being the most common neurologic disease in the general population (121, 7.1, and 0.9 per 1,000 persons in a year); stroke, traumatic brain injury, and spinal injury occurring in 183, 101, and 4.5 per 100,000 per year; and Alzheimer disease, Parkinson disease, and amyotrophic lateral sclerosis (ALS) among older individuals at rates of 67, 9.5, and 1.6 per 100,000 yearly. Data such as these assist in guiding societal resources to the cure of various conditions, but they are somewhat less helpful in leading the physician to the correct diagnosis except insofar as they emphasize the oft-stated dictum that "common conditions occur commonly" and therefore should be considered a priori to be more likely diagnoses (see further discussion under "Shortcomings of the Clinical Method").

TAKING THE HISTORY

In neurology, perhaps more than any other specialty, the physician is dependent upon the cooperation of the patient for a reliable history, especially for a description of those symptoms that are unaccompanied by observable signs of disease. If the symptoms are in the sensory sphere, only the patient can tell what he sees, hears, or feels. The first step in the clinical encounter is to enlist the patient's trust and cooperation and make him realize the importance of the history and examination procedure.

The practice of making notes at the bedside or in the office is recommended. Of course, no matter how reliable the history appears to be, verification of the patient's account by a knowledgeable and objective informant is always desirable.

The following points about taking the neurologic history deserve further comment:

1. Special care must be taken to avoid suggesting to the patient the symptoms that one seeks. Errors and inconsistencies in the recorded history are as often the fault of the physician as of the patient. The patient should be discouraged from framing his symptom(s) in terms of a diagnosis that he may have heard; rather, he should be urged to give a description of the symptom—being asked, for example, to choose a word that best describes his pain and to describe precisely what he means by a particular term such as dizziness, imbalance, or vertigo. The patient who is given to highly circumstantial and rambling accounts can be kept on the subject of his illness by directive questions that draw out essential points.
2. The setting in which the illness occurred, its mode of onset and evolution, and its course are of paramount importance. One must attempt to learn precisely how each symptom began and progressed. Often the nature of the disease process can be decided from these data alone, such as in stroke. If such information cannot be supplied by the patient or his family, it may be necessary to judge the course of the illness by what the patient was able to do at different times (e.g., how far he could walk, when he could no longer negotiate stairs or carry on his usual work) or by changes in the clinical findings between successive examinations.
3. In general, one tends to be careless in estimating the mental capacities of patients. Attempts are sometimes made to take histories from patients who are cognitively impaired or so confused that they have no idea why they are in a doctor's office or a hospital. Asking the patient to give his own interpretation of the possible meaning of symptoms may sometimes expose unnatural concern, anxiety, suspiciousness, or even delusional thinking. Young physicians and students also have a natural tendency to "normalize" the patient, often collaborating with a hopeful family in the misperception that no real problem exists. This attempt at sympathy does not serve the patient and may delay the diagnosis of a potentially treatable disease.

THE NEUROLOGIC EXAMINATION

The neurologic examination begins with observations of the patient while the history is being obtained. The manner in which the patient tells the story of his illness may betray confusion or incoherence in thinking, impairment of memory or judgment, or difficulty in comprehending or expressing ideas. A common error is to pass lightly over inconsistencies in history and inaccuracies about dates and symptoms, only to discover later that these flaws in memory were the essential features of the illness. A more extensive examination of attention, memory, cognitive ability, and language is undertaken if the history or the manner in which it is given indicates the problem lies in those spheres. Otherwise, asking the date and place, repeating words, and simple arithmetic are adequate screening procedures.

One then proceeds from an examination of the cranial nerves including the optic discs, neck, and trunk to the testing of motor, reflex, and sensory functions of the upper and lower limbs. This is followed by an assessment of the function of sphincters and the autonomic nervous system if appropriate and testing for meningeal irritation by examining the suppleness of the neck and spine. Gait and station (standing position) are observed before or after the rest of the examination.

When an abnormal finding is detected, whether cognitive, motor, or sensory, it becomes necessary to analyze the problem in a more elaborate fashion. Details of these sensitive examinations are addressed in appropriate chapters of the book (motor: Chaps. 3, 4, and 5; sensory: Chaps. 8 and 9; and cognitive and language disorders: Chaps. 22 and 23) and cursorily, below.

The neurologic examination is ideally performed and recorded in a relatively uniform manner in order to avoid omissions and facilitate the subsequent analysis of records. Some variation in the order of examination from physician to physician is understandable, but each examiner should establish a consistent pattern. Even when it is impractical to perform the examination in the customary way, as in patients who are unable to cooperate because of age or cognitive deficiency, it is good practice to record the findings in an accustomed and sequential fashion. If certain portions are not performed, this omission should be stated so that those reading the description at a later time are not left wondering whether an abnormality was not previously detected. Some aspects of the complete examination that were performed routinely by neurologists in former years are now infrequently included because they provide limited or duplicative information—among these are tests of olfaction and superficial reflexes but each finding may have a place in special circumstances or to corroborate another sign.

The thoroughness of the neurologic examination must also be governed by the type of clinical problem presented by the patient. To spend a half hour or more testing cerebral, cerebellar, cranial nerve, and sensorimotor function in a patient seeking treatment for a simple compression palsy of an ulnar nerve is pointless and uneconomical. The examination must also be modified according to the condition of the patient. Obviously, many parts of the examination cannot be carried out in a comatose patient; also, infants and small children, as well as patients with psychiatric disease, must be examined in special ways.

Portions of the general physical examination that may be particularly informative in the patient with neurologic disease should be included. For example, examination of the heart rate and blood pressure, as well as carotid and cardiac auscultation, are essential in a patient with stroke. Likewise, the skin can reveal a number of conditions that pertain to congenital, metabolic, and infectious causes of neurologic disease.

EXAMINING PATIENTS WHO PRESENT WITH NEUROLOGIC SYMPTOMS

Numerous guides to the examination of the nervous system are available (see the references at the end of this chapter). For a full account of these methods, the reader is referred to several of the monographs on the subject, including those of Bickerstaff and Spillane, Campbell (DeJong's Neurological Examination), and of the staff members of the Mayo Clinic, each of which approaches the subject from a somewhat different point of view. An inordinately large number of tests of neurologic function have been devised, and it is not proposed to review all of them here. Some are described in subsequent chapters dealing with disorders of mentation, cranial nerves, and motor, sensory, and autonomic functions. Many tests are of doubtful value or are repetitions of simpler tests and thus should not be taught to students of neurology. Merely to perform all of them on one patient would require several hours and, in most instances, would not make the examiner any the wiser. The danger with all clinical tests is to regard them as indicators of a particular disease rather than as ways of uncovering disordered functioning of the nervous system. The following approaches are relatively simple and provide the most useful information.

Testing of Higher Cortical Functions

These functions are tested in detail if the patient's history or behavior has provided a reason to suspect some defect. Broadly speaking, the mental status examination has two main components, although the separation is somewhat artificial: the psychiatric aspects, which incorporate affect, mood, and normality of thought processes and content, and the cognitive aspects, which include the level of consciousness, awareness (attention), language, memory, visuospatial, and other executive abilities.

Questions are first directed toward determining the patient's orientation in time and place and insight into his current medical problem. Attention, speed of response, ability to give relevant answers to simple questions, and the capacity for sustained and coherent mental effort all lend themselves to straightforward observation. There are many useful bedside tests of attention, concentration, memory, and clarity of thinking including repetition of a series of digits in forward and reverse order, serial subtraction of 3s or 7s from 100, and recall of three items of information or a short story after an interval of 3 min. More detailed examination procedures appear in Chaps. 20, 21, 22, and 23. The patient's account of his recent illness, dates of hospitalization, and day-to-day recollection of recent incidents are excellent tests of memory; the narration of the illness and the patient's choice of words (vocabulary) and syntax provide information about language ability and coherence of thinking.

If there is any suggestion of a speech or language disorder, the nature of the patient's spontaneous speech should be noted. In addition, the accuracy of reading, writing, and spelling, executing spoken commands, repeating words and phrases spoken by the examiner, naming objects and parts of objects, and solving simple logical problems should be assessed.

The ability to carry out commanded tasks (praxis) has great salience in the evaluation of several aspects of cortical function. Bisecting a line, drawing a clock or the floor plan of one's home or a map of one's country, and copying figures are useful tests of visuospatial perception and are indicated in cases of suspected cerebral disease. The testing of language, cognition, and other aspects of higher cerebral function are considered in Chaps. 21, 22, and 23.

Testing of Cranial Nerves

The function of the cranial nerves must be investigated more fully in patients who have neurologic symptoms than in those who do not. If one suspects a lesion in the anterior cranial fossa, the sense of smell should be tested in each nostril; then it should be determined whether odors can be discriminated. Visual fields can be outlined by confrontation testing, ideally by testing each eye separately. If an abnormality is suspected, it should be checked on a perimeter and scotomas sought on the tangent screen or, more accurately, by computerized perimetry. Pupil size and reactivity to light, direct, consensual, and during convergence, the position of the eyelids, and the range of ocular movements should next be observed. Details of these tests and their interpretations are given in Chaps. 12, 13, and 14.

Sensation over the face is tested with a pin and wisp of cotton. Also, the presence or absence of the corneal reflexes, direct and consensually, may be determined.

Facial movements should be observed as the patient speaks and smiles, for a slight weakness may be more evident in these circumstances than on movements to command.

The auditory meati and tympanic membranes should be inspected with an otoscope. A high-frequency (512 Hz) tuning fork held next to the ear and on the mastoid discloses hearing loss and distinguishes middle-ear (conductive) from neural deafness. Audiograms and other special tests of auditory and vestibular function are needed if there is any suspicion of disease of the vestibulocochlear nerve or of the cochlear and labyrinthine end organs (see Chap. 15). The vocal cords must be inspected with special instruments in cases of suspected medullary or vagus nerve disease, especially when there is hoarseness. Voluntary pharyngeal elevation and elicited reflexes are meaningful if there is an asymmetrical response; bilateral absence of the gag reflex is seldom significant. Inspection of the tongue, both protruded and at rest, is helpful; atrophy and fasciculations may be seen and weakness detected. Slight deviation of the protruded tongue as a solitary finding can usually be disregarded, but a major deviation represents under action of the hypoglossal nerve and muscle on that side. The pronunciation of words should be noted. The jaw jerk and the snout, buccal, and sucking reflexes should be sought, particularly if there is a question of dysphagia, dysarthria, or dysphonia.

Testing of Motor Function

In the assessment of motor function, the most informative aspects are observations of the speed and strength of movements and of muscle bulk, tone, and coordination and these are considered in the context of the state of tendon reflexes. The maintenance of the supinated arms against gravity is a useful test; the weak arm, tiring first, soon begins to sag, or, in the case of a corticospinal lesion, to resume the more natural pronated position ("pronator drift"). The strength of the legs can be similarly tested with the patient prone and the knees flexed and observing downward drift of the weakened leg. In the supine position at rest, weakness due to an upper motor neuron lesion causes external rotation of the hip.

It is essential to have the limbs exposed and to inspect them for atrophy and fasciculations. Abnormalities of movement and posture as well as tremors may be revealed by observing the limbs at rest and in motion (see Chaps. 4, 5, and 6). This is accomplished by watching the patient maintain the arms outstretched in the prone and supine positions; perform simple tasks, such as alternately touching his nose and the examiner's finger; make rapid alternating movements that necessitate sudden acceleration and deceleration and changes in direction, such as tapping one hand on the other while alternating pronation and supination of the forearm; rapidly touch the thumb to each fingertip; and accomplish simple tasks such as buttoning clothes, opening a safety pin, or handling common tools. Estimates of the strength of leg muscles with the patient in bed are often unreliable; there may seem to be little or no weakness even though the patient cannot arise from a chair or from a kneeling position without help. Running the heel down the front of the shin, alternately touching the examiner's finger with the toe and the opposite knee with the heel, and rhythmically tapping the heel on the shin are the only tests of coordination that need be carried out in bed.

Testing of Reflexes

Testing of the biceps, triceps, supinator-brachioradialis, patellar, Achilles, and cutaneous abdominal and plantar reflexes permits an adequate sampling of reflex activity of the spinal cord. Elicitation of muscle stretch (tendon) reflexes requires that the involved muscles be relaxed; underactive or barely elicitable reflexes can be facilitated by voluntary contraction of other muscles (Jendrassik maneuver).

The plantar response poses some difficulty because several different reactions besides the Babinski response can be evoked by stimulating the sole of the foot along its outer border from heel to toes. These are (1) the normal quick, high-level avoidance response that causes the foot and leg to withdraw; (2) the pathologic slower, spinal flexor nocifensive (protective) reflex (flexion of knee and hip and dorsiflexion of toes and foot, "triple flexion"). Dorsiflexion of the large toe and fanning of the other toes as part of the latter reflex is the well-known Babinski sign (see Chap. 3); (3) plantar grasp reflexes; and (4) support reactions in infants. Avoidance and withdrawal responses interfere with the interpretation of the Babinski sign and can sometimes be overcome by utilizing one of several alternative stimuli (e.g., squeezing the calf or Achilles tendon, flicking the fourth toe, downward scraping of the shin, lifting the straight leg, and others) or by having the patient scrape his own sole. An absence of the superficial cutaneous reflexes of the abdominal, cremasteric, and other muscles are useful ancillary tests for detecting corticospinal lesions, particularly when unilateral.

Testing of Sensory Function

Because this part of the examination is attainable only through the subjective responses of the patient, it requires considerable patient cooperation. For the same reason, it is subject to overinterpretation and suggestibility. Usually, sensory testing is reserved for the end of the examination and, if the findings are to be reliable, should not be prolonged for more than a few minutes. Each test should be explained briefly; too much discussion with a meticulous, introspective patient encourages the reporting of meaningless minor variations of stimulus intensity.

It is not necessary to examine all areas of the skin surface. A quick survey of the face, neck, arms, trunk, and legs with a pin takes only a few seconds. Usually one is seeking differences between the two sides of the body (it is better to ask whether stimuli on opposite sides of the body feel the same than to ask if they feel different), a level below which sensation is lost, or a zone of relative or absolute analgesia (loss of pain sensibility) or anesthesia (loss of touch sensibility). Regions of sensory deficit can then be tested more carefully and mapped. Moving the stimulus from an area of diminished sensation into a normal area is recommended because it enhances the perception of a difference. The finding of a zone of heightened sensation ("hyperesthesia") calls attention to a disturbance of superficial sensation.

The sense of vibration may be tested by comparing the thresholds at which the patient and examiner lose perception at comparable bony prominences. We suggest recording the number of seconds for which the examiner appreciates vibration at the malleolus, toe, or finger after the patient reports that the fork has stopped buzzing.

Variations in sensory findings from one examination to another reflect differences in technique of examination as well as inconsistencies in the responses of the patient. Sensory testing is considered in greater detail in Chaps. 8 and 9.

Testing of Gait and Stance

The examination is completed by observing the patient arise from a chair, stand and walk. An abnormality of stance or gait may be the most prominent or only neurologic abnormality, as in certain cases of cerebellar or frontal lobe disorder; and an impairment of posture and highly automatic adaptive movements in walking may provide the most definite diagnostic clues in the early stages of diseases such as Parkinson disease. Having the patient walk tandem or on the sides of the soles may bring out a lack of balance or dystonic postures in the hands and trunk. Hopping or standing on one foot may also betray a lack of balance or weakness. Standing with feet together and eyes closed will bring out disequilibrium due to sensory loss (Romberg test) that is usually attributable to a disorder of the large diameter sensory fibers in the nerves and posterior columns of the spinal cord. Disorders of gait are discussed in Chap. 7.

TESTING THE PATIENT WHO DOES NOT HAVE NEUROLOGIC SYMPTOMS (THE SCREENING NEUROLOGICAL EXAMINATION)

In this situation, brevity is desirable but any test that is undertaken should be done carefully and recorded. Accurate recording of negative data may be useful in relation to some future illness that requires examination. As indicated in Table 1-4, the patient's orientation, insight, judgment, and the integrity of language function are readily assessed in the course of taking the history. With respect to the cranial nerves, the size of the pupils and their reaction to light, ocular movements, visual and auditory acuity, and movements of the face, palate, and tongue should be tested. Observing the bare outstretched arms for atrophy, weakness ("pronator drift"), tremor, or abnormal movements; checking the strength of hand grip and dorsiflexion at the wrist; inquiring about sensory disturbances; and eliciting the biceps, brachioradialis, and triceps reflexes are usually sufficient for the upper limbs. Inspection of the legs while the feet, toes, knees, and hips are actively flexed and extended; elicitation of the patellar, Achilles, and plantar reflexes; testing of vibration and position sense in the fingers and toes; and assessment of coordination by having the patient alternately touch his nose and the examiner's finger and run his heel up and down the front of the opposite leg, and observation of walking complete the essential parts of the neurologic examination.

This entire procedure adds only a few minutes to the physical examination but the routine performance of these few simple tests provides clues to the presence of disease of which the patient is not aware. For example,

Table 1-4

BRIEF NEUROLOGIC EXAMINATION IN THE GENERAL MEDICAL OR SURGICAL PATIENT (PERFORMED IN 5 MIN OR LESS)

1. Orientation, insight into illness, language assessed during taking of the history
2. Size of pupils, reaction to light, visual and auditory acuity
3. Movement of eyes, face, tongue
4. Examination of the outstretched hands for atrophy, pronating or downward drift, tremor, power of grip, and wrist dorsiflexion
5. Biceps, supinator, and triceps tendon reflexes
6. Inspection of the legs during active flexion and extension of the hips, knees, and feet
7. Patellar, Achilles, and plantar reflexes
8. Vibration sensibility in the fingers and toes
9. Finger-to-nose and heel-to-shin testing of coordination
10. Gait

the finding of absent Achilles reflexes and diminished vibratory sense in the feet and legs alerts the physician to the possibility of diabetic or nutritional neuropathy, even when the patient does not report symptoms.

THE COMATOSE PATIENT

Although subject to obvious limitations, careful examination of the stuporous or comatose patient yields considerable information concerning the function of the nervous system. It is remarkable that, with the exception of cognitive function, almost all parts of the nervous system, including the cranial nerves, can be evaluated in the comatose patient. The demonstration of signs of focal cerebral or brainstem disease or of meningeal irritation is useful in the differential diagnosis of diseases that cause stupor and coma. The adaptation of the neurologic examination to the comatose patient is described in Chap. 17.

THE PSYCHIATRIC PATIENT

One is compelled in the examination of psychiatric patients to rely less on the cooperation of the patient and to be unusually critical of their statements and opinions. The depressed patient, for example, may perceive impaired memory or weakness when actually there is neither amnesia nor reduced power, or the sociopath or hysteric may feign paralysis. The opposite is as often true: Psychotic patients may make accurate observations of their symptoms, only to have them ignored because of their mental state. It is well to keep in mind that patients with even the most extreme psychiatric disease are subject to all of the neurologic conditions typical of others their age.

If the patient will speak and cooperate even to a slight degree, much may be learned about the functional integrity of different parts of the nervous system. By the manner in which the patient expresses ideas and responds to spoken or written requests, it is possible to determine whether there are hallucinations or delusions, defective memory, or other recognizable symptoms of brain disease merely by watching and listening to the patient. Ocular movements and visual fields can be tested with fair accuracy by observing the patient's response to a moving stimulus or threat in the visual fields. Cranial nerve, motor, and reflex functions are tested in the usual manner, but it must be remembered that the neurologic examination is never complete unless the patient will speak and cooperate in testing. On occasion, mute and resistive patients judged to be psychotic prove to have some widespread cerebral disease such as hypoxic or hypoglycemic encephalopathy, a brain tumor, a vascular lesion, or extensive demyelinative lesions.

INFANTS AND SMALL CHILDREN

The reader is referred to the special methods of examination described by Andrè-Thomas and colleagues, Volpe and the staff members of the Mayo Clinic, which are listed in the references and described in Chap. 28. Many of these volumes address the developmental aspects of the child's nervous system, and although some signs may be difficult to obtain because of the age of the patient, they still stand as the best explications of the child's neurologic examination.

THE GENERAL MEDICAL EXAMINATION

The general medical examination often reveals evidence of an underlying systemic disease that has secondarily affected the nervous system. In fact, many of the most serious neurologic problems are of this type. Two common examples will suffice: adenopathy or a lung infiltrate implicates neoplasia or sarcoidosis as the cause of multiple cranial nerve palsies, and the presence of low-grade fever, anemia, a heart murmur, and splenomegaly in a patient with unexplained stroke points to a diagnosis of bacterial endocarditis with embolic occlusion of cerebral arteries. The examination of a patient with stroke is incomplete without a search for hypertension, carotid bruits, heart murmurs, and irregular heart rhythm.

IMPORTANCE OF A WORKING KNOWLEDGE OF NEUROANATOMY, NEUROPHYSIOLOGY, MOLECULAR GENETICS, NEUROIMAGING AND NEUROPATHOLOGY

Once the technique of obtaining reliable clinical data is mastered, students and residents may find themselves handicapped in the interpretation of the findings by a lack of knowledge of the basic sciences of neurology. For this reason, each of the later chapters dealing with the motor system, sensation, special senses, consciousness, memory, and language is introduced by a review of the anatomic and physiologic facts that are necessary for understanding the associated clinical disorders.

At a minimum, physicians should know the anatomy of the corticospinal tract; motor unit (anterior horn cell, nerve, and muscle); basal ganglionic and cerebellar motor connections; main sensory pathways; cranial nerves; hypothalamus and pituitary; reticular formation of brainstem and thalamus; limbic system; areas of cerebral cortex and their major connections; visual, auditory, and autonomic systems; and cerebrospinal fluid pathways. A working knowledge of neurophysiology should include an understanding of neural excitability and nerve impulse propagation, neuromuscular transmission, and contractile process of muscle; spinal reflex activity; central neurotransmission; processes of neuronal excitation, inhibition, and release; and cortical activation and seizure production. The genetics and molecular biology of neurologic disease have assumed increasing importance in the past few decades. The practitioner should be familiar with the terminology of mendelian and mitochondrial genetics and the main aberrations in the genetic code that give rise to neurologic disease.

The wide availability of imaging offers the possibility of localization and etiologic diagnosis with limited input from the traditional clinical method. At a minimum, the educated neurologist must therefore be very familiar with the optimal imaging technique to disclose each of the multitudes of clinical diseases encountered in practice, the imaging appearance of each, and the risk and pitfalls of imaging.

From a practical diagnostic and therapeutic point of view, we believe the neurologist is helped by a knowledge of pathologic anatomy—i.e., the neuropathologic changes that are produced by disease processes such as infarction, hemorrhage, demyelination, physical trauma, compression, inflammation, neoplasm, and infection, to name the more common ones. Experience with the gross and microscopic appearances of these disease processes greatly enhances one's ability to explain their clinical effects. The ability to visualize the abnormalities of disease on nerve and muscle, brain and spinal cord, meninges, and blood vessels gives one a strong sense of which clinical features to expect of a particular disease and which features are untenable or inconsistent with a particular diagnosis. An additional advantage of being exposed to neuropathology is, of course, that the clinician is able to intelligently evaluate pathologic changes and reports of material obtained by biopsy. For many conditions there is a parallel representation of neuropathology through various imaging techniques. This allows the clinician to deduce the pathology from the imaging appearance.

From the foregoing description of the clinical method, it is evident that the use of laboratory aids, including imaging in the diagnosis of diseases of the nervous system is ideally preceded by rigorous clinical examination. As in all of medicine, laboratory study can be planned intelligently only on the basis of clinical information. To reverse this process is wasteful of medical resources and prone to the discovery of irrelevant information, and in some cases can expose a patient to unnecessary risk.

In the prevention of neurologic disease, however, the clinical method in itself is inadequate; thus, of necessity, one resorts to two other approaches, namely, the use of genetic information and laboratory screening tests. Biochemical screening tests are applicable to an entire population and permit the identification of neurologic diseases in individuals, mainly infants and children, who have yet to show their first symptom; in some diseases, treatment can be instituted before the nervous system has suffered damage. Similarly in adults, screening for atherosclerosis and its underlying metabolic causes is profitable in certain populations as a way of preventing stroke. Genetic information enables the neurologist to arrive at the diagnosis of certain illnesses and to identify patients and relatives at risk of developing certain diseases.

The laboratory methods that are available for neurologic diagnosis are discussed in the next chapter and in Chap. 45, on clinical electrophysiology. The relevant principles of genetic and laboratory screening methods for the prediction of disease are presented in the discussion of the disease to which they are applicable.

SHORTCOMINGS OF THE CLINICAL METHOD

If one adheres to the clinical method, neurologic diagnosis is greatly simplified. In most cases one can reach an anatomic diagnosis. However, even after the most assiduous application of the clinical method and laboratory procedures, there are numerous patients whose diseases elude diagnosis. In such circumstances we have often been aided by the following perspectives:

As mentioned earlier, when the main sign has been misinterpreted—if a tremor has been taken for ataxia or fatigue for weakness—the clinical method is derailed from the start. Focus the clinical analysis on the principal symptom and signs and avoid being distracted by minor signs and uncertain clinical data.

As the lessons of cognitive psychology have been applied to error analysis in medical diagnosis, several heuristics (rules of thumb) have been identified as both necessary to the diagnostic process and as major pitfalls for the unwary clinician. The advantage of awareness of these heuristics is the opportunity to incorporate corrective strategies when shortcuts are employed. Investigators such as Redelmeier have given the following categories of cognitive mistakes that are common in arriving at a diagnosis:

- The framing effect reflects excessive weighting of specific initial data in the presentation of the problem.
- Anchoring heuristic, in which an initial impression cannot be subsequently adjusted to incorporate new data.
- Availability heuristic, in which experience with recent cases has an undue impact on the diagnosis of the case at hand.
- Representative heuristic refers to the lack of appreciation of the frequency of disease in the population under consideration, a restatement of Bayes theorem.
- Blind obedience, in which there is undue deference to authority or to the results of a laboratory test.

With our colleague Vickery, we have reviewed the workings of these heuristics in neurological diagnosis. Common to all of these cognitive errors is the tendency to come to early closure in diagnosis. Often this is the result of premature fixation on some item in the history or examination, closing the mind to alternative diagnostic considerations (the anchoring effect). The first diagnostic formulation should be regarded as only a testable hypothesis, subject to modification when new items of information are secured (anchoring heuristic). Should the disease be in a stage of transition, time will allow the full picture to emerge and the diagnosis to be clarified.

When several of the main features of a disease in its typical form are lacking, an alternative diagnosis should always be entertained. In general, however, one is more likely to encounter rare manifestations of common diseases than the typical manifestations of rare diseases (a paraphrasing of the representative heuristic).

It is advantageous to base diagnosis on clinical experience with the dominant symptoms and signs and not on statistical analyses of the frequency of clinical phenomena. Nonetheless, implicit in all diagnostic methods is an assessment of the likely causes of a sign or syndrome in the context of the patient's broad demographic characteristics including their sex, age, race, ethnicity, and the geographical circumstances. Moreover, as mentioned earlier, neurologists place a premium on finding treatable illnesses, even if the odds do not favor its presence.

As pointed out by Chimowitz, students tend to err in failing to recognize a disease they have not seen, and experienced clinicians may fail to appreciate a rare variant of a common disease. There is no doubt that some clinicians are more adept than others at solving difficult clinical problems. Their talent is not intuitive, as sometimes is presumed, but is attributable to having paid close attention to the details of their experience with many diseases and having catalogued them for future reference. The unusual case is recorded in memory and can be resurrected when another one like it is encountered. To achieve expert performance in all areas, cognitive, musical, and athletic, a prolonged period of focused attention to the subject and to personal experience is required.

THERAPEUTICS IN NEUROLOGY

Among medical specialties, neurology has traditionally occupied a somewhat anomalous position, in the past being thought of by many as little more than an intellectual exercise concerned with making diagnoses of untreatable diseases. This view of our profession is fallacious, as we have pointed out in a recent review of 200 years of neurological progress (Ropper). There are a growing number of diseases, many medical and others surgical, for which specific therapy is now available; through advances in neuroscience, their number is steadily increasing. Among the most sweeping changes, now that many infectious diseases of the nervous system are being addressed, have been entirely novel medications for stroke, multiple sclerosis, Parkinson disease, migraine, neuropathy, brain tumor and epilepsy. These therapies and the dosages, timing, and manner of administration of particular drugs are considered in later chapters in relation to the description of individual diseases. The neurologist must also be familiar with the proper application of surgical treatment when it is an integral part of the amelioration or cure of disease, as it is for brain tumor, degenerative and neoplastic diseases of the spine, cerebral aneurysm, extracranial arterial stenosis, and some congenital disease of the brain and spinal cord.

There are, in addition, many diseases in which neurologic function can be restored to a varying degree by appropriate rehabilitation measures or by the judicious use of therapeutic agents. Claims for the effectiveness of a particular therapy based on statistical analysis of large-scale clinical studies must be treated circumspectly. Was the study well conceived as reflected in a clearly stated hypothesis and outcome criteria; was there adherence to the plans for randomization and admission of cases into the study; were the statistical methods appropriate; and were the controls truly comparable? It has been our experience that the original results must be accepted with caution and it is prudent to wait until further studies confirm the benefits that have been claimed.

There are, of course, many instances in which evidence is not available or is not applicable to difficult individual therapeutic decisions. This is in part true because small albeit statistically significant effects may be of little consequence when applied to an individual patient. It goes without saying that data derived from trials must be used in the context of a patient's overall physical and mental condition and age. Furthermore, for many neurologic conditions there is, at the moment, inadequate evidence on which to base treatment. Here, the patient requires a skilled physician to make judgments based on partial or insufficient data. Even deciding actively to wait before committing to an intervention displays wisdom and adheres to the dictum, "first, do no harm". Even when no effective treatment is possible, neurologic diagnosis is more than an intellectual pastime. The first step in the scientific study of any disease process is its identification in the living patient.

In closing this introductory chapter, a comment regarding the extraordinary burden of diseases of the nervous system throughout the world is appropriate. It is not just that conditions such as brain and spinal cord trauma, stroke, epilepsy, mental retardation, mental diseases, and dementia are ubiquitous and account for the majority of illness, second only in some parts of the world to infectious disease, but that these are highly disabling and often chronic in nature, altering in a fundamental way the lives of the affected individuals. Furthermore, more so than in other fields, the promise of cure or amelioration by new techniques such as molecular biology, genetic therapy, and brain–computer interfaces has excited vast interest, for which reason aspects of the current scientific insights are included in appropriate sections.

References

André-Thomas, Chesni Y, Dargassies St-Anne S: *The Neurological Examination of the Infant*. London, National Spastics Society, 1960.

Campbell WW: *DeJong's The Neurological Examination*, 6th ed. Philadelphia, Lippincott Williams & Wilkins, 2005.

Chimowitz MI, Logigian EL, Caplan LP: The accuracy of bedside neurological diagnoses. *Ann Neurol* 28:78,1990.

DeMyer WE: *Technique of the Neurologic Examination: A Programmed Text*, 4th ed. New York, McGraw-Hill, 1994.

Donaghy M, Compston A, Rossor M, Warlow C: *Clinical diagnosis, in Brain's Diseases of the Nervous System*, 11th ed. Oxford, UK, Oxford University Press, 2001, pp 11–60.

Hirtz D, Thurman DJ, Gwinn-Hardy K, et al: How common are the "common" neurologic disorders? *Neurology* 68:326, 2007.

Holmes G: *Introduction to Clinical Neurology*, 3rd ed. Revised by Bryan Matthews. Baltimore, Williams & Wilkins, 1968.

Mayo Clinic Examinations in Neurology, 7th ed. St. Louis, Mosby-Year Book, 1998.

Redelmeier DA: Improving patient care. The cognitive psychology of missed diagnoses. *Ann Intern Med* 142:115; 2005.

Ropper AH: Two centuries of neurology and psychiatry in the Journal. *New Engl J Med* 367:58, 2012.

Spillane JA: *Bickerstaff's Neurological Examination in Clinical Practice*, 6th ed. Oxford, Blackwell Scientific, 1996.

Vickery B, Samuels MA, Ropper AH: How neurologists think: A cognitive psychology perspective on missed diagnoses. *Ann Neurol* 67:425, 2010.

Volpe JJ: *Neurology of the Newborn*, 5th ed. Philadelphia, Saunders, 2008.

2

Imaging, Electrophysiologic, and Laboratory Techniques for Neurologic Diagnosis

The analysis and interpretation of data elicited by a careful history and examination may prove to be adequate for diagnosis. Special laboratory examinations then do no more than corroborate the clinical impression. However, it happens more often that the nature of the disease is not discerned by "case study" alone; the diagnostic possibilities may be reduced to two or three, but the correct one is uncertain. Under these circumstances, one resorts to ancillary examinations. The aim of the neurologist is to arrive at a final diagnosis by artful analysis of the clinical data aided by the least number of laboratory procedures.

Only a few decades ago, the only laboratory tests available to the neurologist were examination of a sample of cerebrospinal fluid, radiography of the skull and spinal column, contrast myelography, pneumoencephalography, and electroencephalography. The physician's armamentarium has been expanded to include a multitude of neuroimaging modalities, biochemical, and genetic methods. Some of these new methods give the impression of such accuracy that there is a temptation to substitute them for a careful, detailed history and physical examination. Reflecting the limitations of laboratory diagnosis, in a carefully examined series of 86 consecutively hospitalized neurologic patients reported by Chimowitz and colleagues, laboratory findings (including MRI) clarified the clinical diagnosis in 40 patients but failed to do so in the remaining 46. Moreover, it is common in practice for ancillary testing to reveal abnormalities that are of no significance to the problem at hand. Consequently, the physician should always judge the relevance and significance of laboratory data only in the context of clinical findings. Hence the neurologist must be familiar with all laboratory procedures relevant to neurologic disease, their reliability, and their hazards.

What follows is a description of laboratory procedures that have application to a diversity of neurologic diseases. Procedures that are pertinent to a particular symptom complex or category of disease—e.g., audiography to study deafness; electronystagmography (ENG) in cases of vertigo; electromyography (EMG) and nerve conduction studies, as well as nerve and muscle biopsy, where there is neuromuscular disease—are presented in the chapters devoted to these disorders.

LUMBAR PUNCTURE AND EXAMINATION OF CEREBROSPINAL FLUID

The information yielded by examination of the cerebrospinal fluid (CSF) is crucial in the diagnosis of certain neurologic diseases, particularly infectious and inflammatory conditions, subarachnoid hemorrhage, and processes that alter intracranial pressure. Combinations of findings, or formulas, in the CSF generally denote particular classes of disease; these are summarized in Table 2-1.

Indications for Lumbar Puncture

1. To obtain pressure measurements and procure a sample of the CSF for cellular, cytologic, chemical, and bacteriologic examination.
2. To aid in therapy by the administration of spinal anesthetics and occasionally, antibiotics or antitumor agents, or by reduction of CSF pressure.
3. To inject a radiopaque substance, as in myelography, or a radioactive agent, as in radionuclide cisternography.

Lumbar puncture (LP) carries some risks if the CSF pressure is very high (evidenced mainly by headache and papilledema), for it increases the possibility of a fatal cerebellar or transtentorial herniation. The risk is considerable when papilledema is the result of an intracranial mass, but it is much lower in patients with subarachnoid hemorrhage, in hydrocephalus with communication between all the ventricles, or with pseudotumor cerebri, conditions in which repeated LPs may at times be employed as a therapeutic measure. Asymmetric lesions, particularly those near the tentorium or foramen magnum carry a greater risk of herniation precipitated by lumbar puncture. In patients with purulent meningitis, there is also a small risk of herniation, but this is far outweighed by the need for a definitive diagnosis and the institution of appropriate treatment at the earliest moment. With this last exception, LP should generally be preceded by CT or MRI whenever an elevation of intracranial pressure is suspected. If radiologic procedures

Table 2-1

CHARACTERISTIC CSF FORMULAS

CONDITION	CELLS	PROTEIN	GLUCOSE	OTHER FEATURES
Bacterial infection	WBC >50/mm^3, often greatly increased	100–250 mg%	20–50 mg%; usually lower than half of blood glucose level	Gram stain shows organisms; pressure increased
Viral, fungal, spirochetal infection	WBC 10–100/mm^3	50–200 mg%	Normal or slightly reduced	Special culture techniques required; pressure normal or slightly increased
Tuberculous infection	WBC >25/mm^3	100–1,000 mg%	<50, often markedly reduced	Special culture techniques and PCR may be needed to detect organisms
Subarachnoid hemorrhage	RBC >500/mm^3; slight increase in WBC	60–150 mg%	Normal; slightly reduced later	Must be distinguished from traumatic lumbar puncture by presence of xanthochromia of spun sample; greatly increased pressure
Cerebral hemorrhage, trauma	RBC 50–200/mm^3; higher if ventricular rupture of blood	50–150 mg%	Normal	Pressure may be elevated
Ischemic stroke	Normal or few WBC	Normal	Normal	Normal pressure unless brain swelling
Multiple sclerosis	Normal or few WBC	Normal or slightly increased	Normal	Increased IgG fraction and oligoclonal bands
Meningeal cancer	WBC 10–100/mm^3	Usually elevated	Normal or depressed	Neoplastic cells in CSF; elevation of certain protein markers (e.g., β_2-microglobulin)

IgG, immunoglobulin G; PCR, polymerase chain reaction; RBC, red blood cells; WBC, white blood cells.

disclose a mass lesion that is causing displacement of brain tissue toward the tentorial opening or the foramen magnum (the presence of a mass alone is of less concern) and if it is considered essential to have the information yielded by CSF examination, the LP may be performed—with certain precautions. If the pressure proves to be very high—over 400 mm H_2O—one should obtain the smallest necessary sample of fluid and then, according to the suspected disease and patient's condition, administer mannitol or another hyperosmolar agent and ideally, to observe a fall in pressure on the manometer. Dexamethasone or an equivalent corticosteroid may generally also be given in an initial intravenous dose of 10 mg, followed by doses of 4 to 6 mg every 6 h in order to produce a sustained reduction in intracranial pressure. Corticosteroids are particularly useful in situations in which the increased intracranial pressure is caused by vasogenic cerebral edema (e.g., tumor-associated edema).

Cisternal (foramen magnum) puncture and lateral cervical subarachnoid puncture, although safe in the hands of an expert, are too hazardous to entrust to those without experience and do not circumvent the problem of increased intracranial pressure. LP is preferred except in obvious instances of spinal block requiring a sample of cisternal fluid or for myelography above the lesion.

Technique of Lumbar Puncture

Experience teaches the importance of meticulous technique and proper positioning of the patient. LP should be done under locally sterile conditions. Xylocaine is injected in and beneath the skin, which should render the procedure almost painless. Warming of the analgesic by rolling the vial between the palms seems to diminish the burning sensation that accompanies cutaneous infiltration. The patient is positioned on his side, preferably on the left side for right-handed physicians, with hips and knees flexed, and the head as close to the knees as comfort permits. The patient's hips should be vertical, the back aligned near the edge of the bed, and a pillow placed under the ear. The puncture is usually easiest to perform at the L3-L4 interspace, which corresponds in many individuals to the axial plane of the iliac crests, or at the interspace above or below. In infants and young children, in whom the spinal cord may extend to the level of the L3-L4 interspace, lower levels should be used. Experienced anesthesiologists have suggested that the smallest possible needle be used and that the bevel be oriented in the longitudinal plane of the dural fibers (see below regarding atraumatic needles). It is usually possible to appreciate a palpable "give" as the needle approaches the dura, followed by a subtle "pop" on puncturing the arachnoid membrane. At this point, the trocar should be removed slowly from the needle to avoid sucking a nerve rootlet into the lumen and causing radicular pain. Sciatic pain during the insertion of the needle indicates that it is placed too far laterally. If the flow of CSF slows, the patient's head can be elevated slowly. Occasionally, one resorts to gentle aspiration with a small-bore syringe to overcome the resistance of proteinaceous and viscous CSF. Failure to enter the lumbar subarachnoid space after two or three trials usually can be overcome by performing the puncture with the patient in the sitting position and then helping him to lie on one side for pressure measurements and fluid removal. The "dry tap" is more often the result of an improperly placed needle than of obliteration of the subarachnoid space by a compressive lesion of the cauda equina or by adhesive arachnoiditis. In an obese patient, in whom palpable spinal landmarks cannot be appreciated, or after several unsuccessful attempts in any patient, fluoroscopy can be employed to position the needle.

LP has few serious complications. The most common is headache, estimated to occur in one-third of patients, but in severe form in far fewer. Prolonged or severe post-lumbar puncture headache is usually seen in patients with a history of migraine. The pain is presumably the result of a reduction of CSF pressure from leakage of fluid at the puncture site and tugging on cerebral and dural vessels as the patient assumes the erect posture. Although neither recumbency nor oral fluid administration after LP has been shown to prevent headache, they are often implemented nonetheless. Strupp and colleagues have found that the use of an atraumatic needle almost halved the incidence of headache. Curiously, headaches are twice as frequent after diagnostic LP as they are after spinal anesthesia. Patients who are prone to frequent headaches before LP reportedly have higher rates of headache afterwards, which accords with our experience. Severe headache can be associated with vomiting and mild neck stiffness. Unilateral or bilateral sixth nerve or other cranial nerve palsies occur rarely after lumbar puncture, even at times without headache and rare cases of hearing loss or facial palsy have been reported. The syndrome of low CSF pressure, its treatment by "blood patch," and other complications of lumbar puncture are considered further in Chap. 30.

Bleeding into the spinal meningeal or epidural spaces after lumbar puncture can occur in patients who are taking anticoagulants (generally with an international normalized ratio [INR] >1.4), have low platelet counts (<50,000/mm^3), or impaired platelet function (alcoholism, uremia). Treatment is by reversal of the coagulopathy and, in some cases, surgical evacuation of the clot. Purulent meningitis and disc space infections rarely complicate LP as the result of imperfect sterile technique, and the introduction of particulate matter (e.g., talc) or irritant carriers of injected drugs can produce a sterile meningitis.

Examination Procedures For CSF

Once the subarachnoid space has been entered, the pressure and fluctuations with respiration of the CSF are determined, (see below) and samples of fluid are obtained. The gross appearance of the fluid is noted, after which the CSF, in separate tubes, can be examined for (1) number and type of cells and presence of microorganisms by direct observation; (2) protein and glucose content; (3) tumor cells (cytology); (4) presence of oligoclonal bands or content of gamma globulin and other protein fractions, and serologic tests; (5) pigments, lactate, LDH, and substances elaborated by some tumors (e.g., β_2 microglobulin); and (6) bacteria and fungi (by culture), cryptococcal antigen, mycobacteria, the DNA of herpesvirus, cytomegalovirus and other organisms (by polymerase chain reaction), markers or certain infections (e.g., 14-3-3 protein), and viral isolation.

Pressure

With the patient in the lateral decubitus position, the CSF pressure is measured by a manometer attached to the needle in the subarachnoid space. In the normal adult, the opening pressure varies from 100 to 180 mm H_2O, or 8 to 14 mm Hg. In children, the pressure is in the range of 30 to 60 mm H_2O. A pressure above 200 mm H_2O with the patient relaxed and legs straightened reflects increased intracranial pressure. In an adult, a pressure of 50 mm H_2O or below indicates intracranial hypotension, generally caused by leakage of spinal fluid or systemic dehydration. When measured with the needle in the lumbar sac and the patient in a sitting position, the fluid in the manometer rises to the level of the cisterna magna (pressure is approximately double that obtained in the recumbent position). It fails to reach the level of the ventricles because the latter are in a closed system under slight negative pressure, whereas the fluid in the manometer is influenced by atmospheric pressure. Normally, with the needle properly placed in the subarachnoid space, the fluid in the manometer oscillates through a few millimeters in response to the pulse and respiration and rises promptly with coughing, straining, and with jugular vein or abdominal compression. An apparent low pressure can also be the result of a needle aperture that is not fully within the subarachnoid space; this is evidenced by the lack of expected fluctuations in pressure with these maneuvers.

The presence of a spinal subarachnoid block was in the past confirmed by jugular venous compression (Queckenstedt test, which tests for a rapid rise in CSF pressure within a few seconds after application of the pressure on the vein). The maneuver risks worsening of a spinal block or of raised intracranial pressure and is of historical interest.

Gross Appearance and Pigments

Normally, the CSF is clear and colorless. Minor degrees of color change are best detected by comparing test tubes of CSF and water against a white background (by daylight rather than by fluorescent illumination) or by looking down into the tubes from above. (A microhematocrit tube is too narrow for this purpose.) The presence of red blood cells imparts a hazy or ground-glass appearance; at least 200 red blood cells (RBCs) per cubic millimeter (mm^3) must be present to detect this change. The presence of 1,000 to 6,000 RBCs per cubic millimeter imparts a hazy pink to red color, depending on the amount of blood; centrifugation of the fluid or allowing it to stand causes sedimentation of the RBCs. Several hundred or more white blood cells (WBCs) in the fluid (pleocytosis) may cause a slight opaque haziness.

A traumatic tap, in which blood from the epidural venous plexus has been introduced into the spinal fluid, may seriously confuse the diagnosis if it is incorrectly interpreted to indicate a preexistent subarachnoid hemorrhage. To distinguish between these two types of "bloody taps," two or three serial samples of fluid should be taken at the time of the LP. With a traumatic tap, there is usually a decreasing number of RBCs in the subsequent tubes. Also with a traumatic tap, the CSF pressure is usually normal, and if a large amount of blood is mixed with the fluid, it will clot or form fibrinous webs. These are not seen with preexistent hemorrhage because the blood has been greatly diluted with CSF and defibrinated by enzymes in the CSF. In subarachnoid hemorrhage, the RBCs begin to hemolyze within a few hours, imparting a pink-red discoloration (erythrochromia) to the supernatant fluid; if the spinal fluid is sampled more than a day following the hemorrhage, the fluid will have become yellow-brown (xanthochromia). Prompt centrifugation of bloody fluid from a traumatic tap will yield a colorless supernatant; only with large amounts of venous blood (RBC more than 100,000/mm^3) will the supernatant fluid be faintly xanthochromic due to contamination with serum bilirubin and lipochromes.

The fluid from a traumatic tap should contain one or two WBCs per 1,000 RBCs assuming that the hematocrit is normal, but in reality this ratio varies widely. With subarachnoid hemorrhage, the proportion of WBCs rises as RBCs hemolyze, sometimes reaching a level of several hundred per cubic millimeter; but the vagaries of this reaction are such that it, too, cannot be relied upon to distinguish traumatic from preexistent bleeding. The same can be said for crenation of RBCs, which occurs in both types of bleeding.

Why red corpuscles undergo rapid hemolysis in the CSF is not clear. It is surely not because of osmotic differences, as the osmolarity of plasma and CSF is essentially the same. Fishman suggested that the low protein content of CSF disequilibrates the red cell membrane in some way.

The pigments that discolor the CSF following subarachnoid hemorrhage are oxyhemoglobin, bilirubin, and methemoglobin. In pure form, these pigments are colored red (orange to orange-yellow with dilution), canary yellow, and brown, respectively. Oxyhemoglobin appears within several hours of hemorrhage, becomes maximal in approximately 36 h, and diminishes over a 7- to 9-day period. Bilirubin begins to appear in 2 to 3 days and increases in amount as the oxyhemoglobin decreases. Methemoglobin appears when blood is loculated or encysted and isolated from the flow of CSF. Spectrophotometric techniques can be used to distinguish the various hemoglobin breakdown products and thus determine the approximate time of bleeding.

Not all xanthochromia of the CSF is caused by hemolysis of RBCs. With severe jaundice, both conjugated and unconjugated bilirubin diffuse into the CSF. The quantity of bilirubin in the CSF ranges from one-tenth to one-hundredth that in the serum. Elevation of CSF protein from any cause results in a faint opacity and xanthochromia, more or less in proportion to the albumin-bound fraction of bilirubin. Only at protein levels greater than 150 mg/100 mL does the coloration become visible to the naked eye. Hypercarotenemia and hemoglobinemia (through hemoglobin breakdown products, particularly oxyhemoglobin) also impart a yellow tint to the CSF, as do blood clots in the subdural or epidural space of the cranium or spinal column. Myoglobin does not enter the CSF because a low renal threshold for this pigment permits rapid clearing from the blood.

Cellularity

During the first month of life, the CSF may contain a small number of mononuclear cells. Beyond this period, the CSF is normally nearly acellular (i.e., fewer than 5 lymphocytes or other mononuclear cells per cubic millimeter). An elevation of WBCs in the CSF always signifies a reactive process to bacteria or other infectious agents, blood, chemical substances, an immunologic inflammation, a neoplasm, or vasculitis. The WBCs can be counted in an ordinary counting chamber, but their identification requires centrifugation of the fluid and a Wright stain of the sediment or the use of a Millipore filter, cell fixation, and staining. One can then recognize and count differentially neutrophilic and eosinophilic leukocytes (the latter being prominent in Hodgkin disease, some parasitic infections, neurosyphilis, and cholesterol emboli), lymphocytes, plasma cells, mononuclear cells, arachnoid lining cells, macrophages, and tumor cells. Bacteria, fungi, and fragments of echinococci and cysticerci can also be seen in cell-stained or Gram-stained preparations. An India ink preparation is useful in distinguishing between lymphocytes and cryptococci or *Candida*. Acid-fast bacilli will be found in appropriately stained samples. The monographs of den Hartog-Jager and the article of Bigner are older but still excellent references on CSF cytology. Special cell separation and immunostaining techniques permit the recognition of leukemia and lymphoma cell markers, glial fibrillary acidic protein, and other special cellular elements and antigens. These and other specific methods for the examination of cells in the CSF are discussed in the appropriate chapters.

Proteins

In contrast to the high protein content of blood (5,500 to 8,000 mg/dL), that of the lumbar spinal fluid is 45 to 50 mg/dL or less in the adult. The protein content of CSF from the basal cisterns is 10 to 25 mg/dL and that from the ventricles is 5 to 15 mg/dL. This gradient may reflect the fact that CSF proteins leak from the blood plasma through capillary tight junctions, which form the blood–brain and blood–CSF barrier. The spinal fluid is an ultrafiltrate of blood made by the choroid plexus in the lateral and the fourth ventricles in a manner that is analogous to the formation of urine by the glomerulus. The amount of protein in the CSF would then be proportional to the length of time it is in contact with the blood–CSF barrier. Thus shortly after it is formed in the ventricles, the protein is low. More caudally in the basal cisterns, the protein is higher and in the lumbar subarachnoid space it is highest of all. In children, the protein concentration is somewhat lower at each level (<20 mg/dL in the lumbar subarachnoid space). Levels higher than normal indicate a pathologic process in or near the ependyma or meninges—in either the brain, spinal cord, or nerve roots—although the cause of modest elevations of the CSF protein, in the range of 75 mg/dL, frequently remains obscure.

As one would expect, bleeding into the ventricles or subarachnoid space results in spillage not only of RBCs but of serum proteins. If the serum protein concentrations are normal, the CSF protein should increase by about 1 mg per 1,000 RBCs provided that the same tube of CSF is used in determining the cell count and protein content. (The same holds for a traumatic puncture that allows seepage of venous blood into the CSF at the puncture site.) However, in the case of subarachnoid hemorrhage, caused by the irritating effect of hemolyzed RBC upon the leptomeninges, the CSF protein may be increased by many times this ratio.

The protein content of the CSF in bacterial meningitis, in which choroidal and meningeal perfusion are increased, often reaches 500 mg/dL or more. Viral infections induce a less intense and mainly lymphocytic reaction and a lesser elevation of protein—usually 50 to 100 mg/dL but sometimes up to 200 mg/dL; in some instances of viral meningitis and encephalitis the protein content is normal. Paraventricular tumors, by reducing the blood–CSF barrier, often raise the total protein to over 100 mg/dL. Protein values as high as 500 mg/dL are found in exceptional cases of the Guillain-Barré syndrome and chronic inflammatory demyelinating polyneuropathy. Values in the lumbar CSF of 1,000 mg/dL or more usually indicate a block to CSF flow; the fluid is then deeply yellow and clots readily because of the presence of fibrinogen; a combination called Froin syndrome. Partial CSF blocks by ruptured discs or tumor may elevate the protein to 100 to 200 mg/dL. Low CSF protein values are sometimes found in meningismus (a febrile illness with signs of meningeal irritation but normal CSF), in hyperthyroidism, or in conditions that produce low CSF pressure (e.g., after a recent LP as indicated in Chap. 30).

The quantitative partition of CSF proteins by electrophoretic and immunochemical methods demonstrate the presence of most of the serum proteins with a molecular weight of less than 150 to 200 kDa. The protein fractions that have been identified electrophoretically are prealbumin and albumin as well as $alpha_1$, $alpha_2$, $beta_1$, $beta_2$, and gamma globulin fraction, the last of these being accounted for mainly by immunoglobulins (the major immunoglobulin in normal CSF is IgG). The gamma globulin fraction in CSF is approximately 70 percent of that in serum. Table 2-2 gives the quantitative values of the different fractions. Immunoelectrophoretic methods have also demonstrated the presence of glycoproteins, ceruloplasmin, hemopexin, beta-amyloid and tau proteins. Large molecules—such as fibrinogen, IgM, and lipoproteins—are mostly excluded from the CSF unless generated there.

There are other notable differences between the protein fractions of CSF and plasma. The CSF always contains a prealbumin fraction and the plasma does not. Although derived from plasma, this fraction, for an unknown reason, concentrates in the CSF, and its level is greater in ventricular than in lumbar CSF, perhaps because of its concentration by choroidal cells. Also, tau (also identified as $beta_2$-transferrin) is detected only in the CSF and not in other fluids; its concentration is also higher in the ventricular than in the spinal fluid. The concentration of tau protein and in particular the ratio of tau to beta-amyloid, has found use in the diagnosis of Alzheimer disease, as discussed in Chap. 39. At present only a few of these proteins are known to be associated with specific diseases of the nervous system. The most important is IgG, which may exceed 12 percent of the total CSF protein in diseases such as multiple sclerosis, neurosyphilis, subacute sclerosing panencephalitis and other chronic viral meningoencephalitides. The serum IgG is not correspondingly increased, which means that this immune globulin originates in (or perhaps is preferentially transported into) the nervous system. However, an elevation of serum gamma globulin—as occurs in cirrhosis, sarcoidosis, myxedema, and multiple myeloma—will be accompanied by a rise in the CSF globulin. Therefore, in patients with an elevated CSF gamma globulin, it is necessary to determine the electrophoretic pattern of the serum proteins as well. Certain qualitative changes in the CSF immunoglobulin pattern, particularly the demonstration of several discrete (oligoclonal) electrophoretic "bands", each representing a specific immune globulin, and the ratio of IgG to total protein, are of special diagnostic importance in multiple sclerosis, as discussed in Chap. 36.

The albumin fraction of the CSF increases in a wide variety of central nervous system (CNS) and craniospinal nerve root diseases that increase the permeability of the blood–CSF barrier, but no specific clinical correlations can be drawn. Certain enzymes that originate in the brain, especially the brain-derived fraction of creatine kinase (CK-BB) but also enolase and neopterin, are found in the CSF after stroke, global ischemic hypoxia, or trauma, and have been used as markers of brain damage

Table 2-2

AVERAGE VALUES OF CONSTITUENTS OF NORMAL CSF AND SERUM

	CEREBROSPINAL FLUID	SERUM
Osmolarity	295 mOsm/L	295 mOsm/L
Sodium	138.0 mEq/L	138.0 mEq/L
Potassium	2.8 mEq/L	4.1 mEq/L
Calcium	2.1 mEq/L	4.8 mEq/L
Magnesium	2.3 mEq/L	1.9 mEq/L
Chloride	119 mEq/L	101.0 mEq/L
Bicarbonate	23.0 mEq/L	23.0 mEq/L
Carbon dioxide tension	48 mm Hg	38 mm Hg (arterial)
pH	7.31–7.33	7.41 (arterial)
Nonprotein nitrogen	19.0 mg/dL	27.0 mg/dL
Ammonia	30.0 g/dL	70.0 g/dL
Uric acid	0.24 mg/dL	5.5 mg/dL
Urea	4.7 mmol/L	5.4 mmol/L
Creatinine	1.1 mg/dL	1.8 mg/dL
Phosphorus	1.6 mg/dL	4.0 mg/dL
Total lipid	1.5 mg/dL	750.0 mg/dL
Total cholesterol	0.4 mg/dL	180.0 mg/dL
Cholesterol esters	0.3 mg/dL	126.0 mg/dL
Glucose	60 mg/dL	90.0 mg/dL
Lactate	1.6 mEq/L	1.0 mEq/L
Total protein	15–50 mg/dL	6.5–8.4 g/100 dL
Prealbumin	1–7%	Trace
Albumin	49–73%	56%
$Alpha_1$ globulin	3–7%	4%
$Alpha_2$ globulin	6–13%	10%
Beta globulin ($beta_1$ plus tau)	9–19%	12%
Gamma globulin	3–12%	14%

Source: Reproduced by permission from Fishman.

in experimental work. Other special markers such as elevation of the 14-3-3 protein, which has some diagnostic significance in prion disease, β_2-microglobulin in meningeal lymphomatosis, neuron specific enolase in traumatic and other severe brain injuries, and alpha fetoprotein in embryonal tumors of the brain, may be useful in specialized circumstances.

Glucose

The CSF glucose concentration is normally in the range of 45 to 80 mg/dL, i.e., about two-thirds of that in the blood (0.6 to 0.7 of serum concentrations). Higher levels parallel the blood glucose in this proportion; but with marked hyperglycemia, the ratio of CSF to blood glucose is reduced (0.5 to 0.6). With extremely low serum glucose, the ratio becomes higher, approximating 0.85. In general, CSF glucose values below 35 mg/dL are abnormal. After the intravenous injection of glucose, 2 to 4 h are required to reach equilibrium with the CSF; a similar delay follows the lowering of blood glucose. For these reasons, samples of CSF and blood for glucose determinations should ideally be drawn simultaneously in the fasting state or the serum should be obtained a few hours before the puncture but (this is often not practical). Low values of CSF glucose (hypoglycorrhachia) in the presence of pleocytosis usually indicate bacterial, tuberculous, or fungal meningitis, although similar reductions are observed in some patients with widespread neoplastic infiltration of the meninges and occasionally with sarcoidosis, subarachnoid hemorrhage (usually in the first week) and in chemically induced inflammation.

For a long time it was assumed that in meningitis the bacteria lowered the CSF glucose by their active metabolism, but the fact that the glucose remains at a subnormal level for 1 to 2 wk after effective treatment of the meningitis suggests that another mechanism is operative. Theoretically at least, an inhibition of the entry of glucose into the CSF, because of an impairment of the membrane transfer system, can be implicated. As a rule, viral infections of the meninges and brain do not lower the CSF glucose, although low glucose values have been reported in a small number of patients with mumps meningoencephalitis, and rarely in patients with herpes simplex and zoster infections. The almost invariable rise of CSF lactate in purulent meningitis probably suggests that some of the glucose is undergoing anaerobic glycolysis by polymorphonuclear leukocytes and by cells of the meninges and adjacent brain tissue.

Serologic and Virologic Tests

CSF testing for cryptococcal surface antigen has become widely available as a rapid method if this infection is suspected. On occasion, a false-positive reaction is obtained in the presence of high titers of rheumatoid factor or antitreponemal antibodies, but otherwise the test is diagnostically more dependable than the formerly used India ink preparation. The nontreponemal antibody tests of the blood—Venereal Disease Research Laboratories (VDRL) slide flocculation test and rapid plasma reagin (RPR) agglutination test—can also be performed on the CSF. When positive, these tests are usually diagnostic of neurosyphilis, but false-positive reactions may occur with collagen diseases, malaria, and yaws, or with contamination of the CSF by seropositive blood. Tests that depend on the use of treponemal antigens, including the Treponema pallidum immobilization test and the fluorescent treponemal antibody test, are more specific and assist in the interpretation of false-positive RPR and VDRL reactions. The value of CSF examinations in the diagnosis and treatment of neurosyphilis is discussed in Chap. 32, but testing of CSF for treponemal antibodies is no longer routine. Serologic tests for the Lyme spirochete are useful in circumstances of suspected infection of the central nervous system with this agent.

The utility of serum serologic tests for viruses is limited by the time required to obtain results, but they are useful in determining retrospectively the source of meningitis or encephalitis. More rapid tests that use the polymerase chain reaction (PCR) in CSF, which amplifies viral DNA fragments, are now widely available for diagnosis, particularly for herpesviruses, cytomegalovirus, and JC virus. These tests are most useful in the first week of infection, when the virus is being reproduced and its genomic material is most prevalent; after this time, serologic techniques for viral infection are more sensitive. Amplification of DNA by PCR is particularly useful in the rapid detection of tubercle bacilli in the CSF, the conventional culture of which takes several weeks at best., tests for the detection of 14-3-3- protein that reflects the presence of prion agents in the spinal fluid are available and may aid in the diagnosis of the spongiform encephalopathies, but the results have been erratic (Chap. 33).

Changes in Solutes and Other Components

The average osmolality of the CSF (295 mOsm/L) is identical to that of plasma. As the osmolality of the plasma is increased by the intravenous injection of hypertonic solutions such as mannitol or urea, there is a delay of up to several hours in the rise of osmolality of the CSF. It is during this period that the hyperosmolality of the blood maximally dehydrates the brain and decreases the volume of CSF. Table 2-2 lists the CSF and serum levels of sodium, potassium, calcium, and magnesium. Neurologic disease does not alter the CSF concentrations of these constituents in any characteristic way. The low CSF concentration of chloride that occurs in bacterial meningitis is not specific but a reflection of hypochloremia and, to a slight degree, of a greatly elevated CSF protein. Acid–base balance in the CSF is of interest in relation to metabolic acidosis and alkalosis but pH is not routinely measured. Normally, the pH of the CSF is approximately 7.31—i.e., somewhat lower than that of arterial blood, which is 7.41. The Pco_2 in the CSF is in the range of 45 to 49 mm Hg—i.e., higher than in arterial blood (about 40 mm Hg). The bicarbonate levels of the two fluids are about the same, 23 mEq/L. The pH of the CSF is precisely regulated, and it tends to remain relatively unchanged even in the face of severe systemic acidosis and alkalosis. Acid–base changes in the lumbar CSF do not necessarily reflect the presence of similar changes in the brain, nor are the CSF data as accurate an index of the systemic changes as direct measurements of arterial blood gases.

The ammonia content of the CSF is one-third to one-half that of the arterial blood; it is increased in hepatic encephalopathy, the inherited hyperammonemias, and the Reye syndrome; the concentration corresponds roughly with the severity of the encephalopathy. The uric acid content of CSF is approximately 5 percent of that in serum and varies with changes in the serum level (high in gout, uremia, and meningitis, and low in Wilson disease). The urea concentration in the CSF is slightly lower than that in the serum; in uremia, it rises in parallel with that in the blood. An intravenous injection of urea raises the blood level immediately and the CSF level more slowly, exerting an osmotic dehydrating effect on the central nervous tissues and CSF. All 24 amino acids have been isolated from the CSF. The concentration of amino acids in the CSF is approximately one-third that in plasma. Elevations of glutamine are found in all of the portosystemic encephalopathies including hepatic coma and the Reye syndrome. Concentrations of phenylalanine, histidine, valine, leucine, isoleucine, tyrosine, and homocystine are increased in the corresponding aminoacidurias.

Many of the enzymes found in serum are known to rise in CSF under conditions of disease, usually in relation to a rise in the CSF protein. None of the enzyme changes has proved to be a specific indicator of neurologic disease with the possible exception of lactic dehydrogenase, especially isoenzymes 4 and 5, which are derived from granulocytes and are elevated in bacterial meningitis but not in aseptic or viral meningitis. Lactic dehydrogenase is also elevated in cases of meningeal tumor infiltration, particularly lymphoma, as is carcinoembryonic antigen; the latter, however, is not elevated in bacterial, viral, or fungal meningitis. As to lipids, the quantities in CSF are small and their measurement is difficult.

The catabolites of the catecholamines can be measured in the CSF. Homovanillic acid (HVA), the major catabolite of dopamine, and 5-hydroxyindoleacetic acid (5-HIAA), the major catabolite of serotonin, are normally present in the spinal fluid; both are five or six times higher in the ventricular than the lumbar CSF. The levels of both catabolites are reduced in patients with idiopathic and drug-induced parkinsonism.

IMAGING TECHNIQUES OF THE SKULL, BRAIN, AND SPINE

A century ago, Harvey Cushing introduced the use of plain x-ray films of the cranium as part of the study of the neurologic patient, but it is has become evident that the yield of useful information from this procedure is relatively small. Even in patients with head injury, where radiography of the skull would seem to be an optimal method of examination, a fracture is found in only 1 of 16 cases, at a cost of thousands of dollars per fracture and a small risk from radiation exposure. Nevertheless plain skull films do demonstrate fractures, changes in contour of the skull, bony erosions and hyperostoses, infection in paranasal sinuses and mastoids, and changes in the basal foramina. Plain films of the spine are able to demonstrate destructive lesions resulting from degenerative processes as well neoplastic, dysplastic, and infectious diseases. It also detects, fracture dislocations, spondylolistheses, and spinal instability, utilizing images acquired during flexion and extension maneuvers.

Refinements of radiographic techniques have greatly increased the yield of valuable information but without question the most important advances in neuroradiology have come about with the development of CT and MRI.

Computed Tomography

In this procedure, x-radiation is attenuated as it passes successively through the scalp, skull, CSF, cerebral gray and white matter, and blood vessels. The intensity of the exiting radiation relative to the incident radiation is measured, the data are integrated, and two-dimensional images are reconstructed by computer. This major achievement in methodology, attributed to Hounsfield and others, permitted the technologic advance from plain radiographs of the skull to reconstructed images of the cranium and its contents in any plane. The differing densities of bone, CSF, blood, and gray and white matter are distinguishable in the resulting picture with great clarity. One can see hemorrhage, infarcted, contused and edematous brain, abscess, and tumor tissue and also the precise size and position of the ventricles and midline structures. The radiation exposure is not significantly greater than that from plain skull films and comparable to a chest x-ray.

As illustrated in Fig. 2-1A-D, in transverse (axial) section of the brain, one sees the cortex and underlying subcortical white matter , the caudate and lenticular nuclei and the internal capsules and thalami. The position and width of all the major sulci and fissures can be measured, and the optic nerves and medial and lateral rectus muscles stand out clearly in the posterior parts of the orbit. The brainstem, cerebellum, and spinal cord are easily visible in the scan at appropriate levels. The scans are also useful in imaging parts of the body that surround peripheral nerves and plexuses, thereby demonstrating tumors, inflammatory lesions, and hematomas that involve these nerves. Intravenous administration of radio-opaque contrast can be used with CT to visualize regions where the blood-brain barrier has been disrupted from tumors, demyelination and infection.

In imaging of the head, CT has a number of advantages over MRI, the most important being safety when metal may be present in the body and the clarity of blood from the moment of bleeding. Other advantages are its lower cost, broader availability, larger aperture of the machine that reduces patient claustrophobia, shorter examination time, and equivalent or superior visualization of calcium, fat, and bone, particularly of the skull base and vertebrae (Fig. 1*D*). If constant monitoring and use of life support equipment is required during the imaging procedure, it is accomplished more readily by CT than by MRI. Recent advances in CT technology have greatly increased the speed of the scanning procedure and have

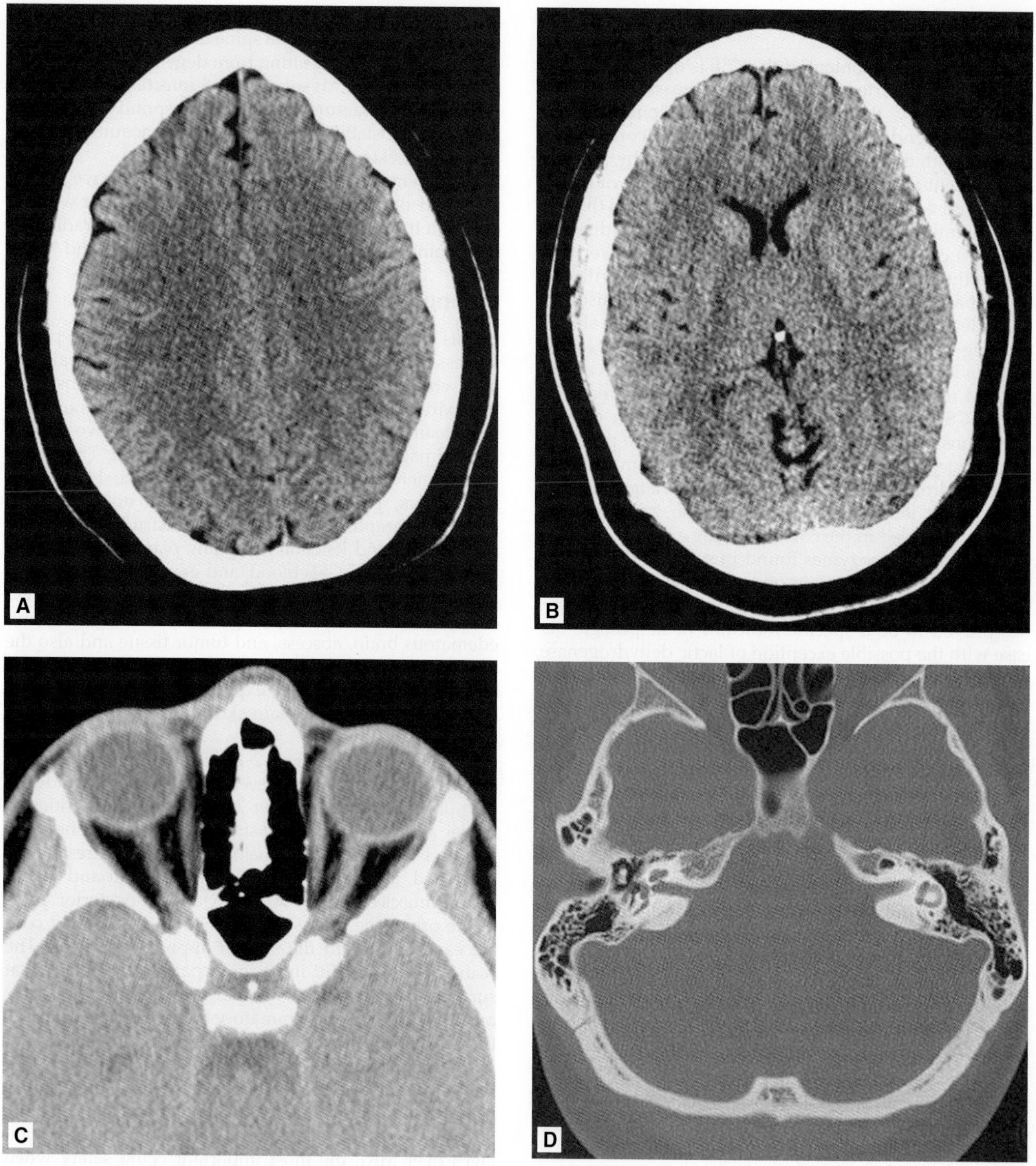

Figure 2-1. Normal axial CT scans of the brain, orbits, and skull base from a young healthy man. *A.* Image through the cerebral hemispheres at the level of the corona radiata. The dense bone of the calvarium is white, and fat-containing subcutaneous tissue is dark. Gray matter appears denser than white matter due to its lower lipid content. *B.* Image at the level of the lenticular nuclei. The caudate and lenticular nuclei are denser than the adjacent internal capsule. CSF within the frontal horns of the lateral ventricles as well as surrounding the slightly calcified pineal body appears dark. *C.* Image through the mid-orbits. The sclera appears as a dense band surrounding the globe. The bright optic nerves are surrounded by dark orbital fat. The medial and lateral rectus muscles lie along the orbital walls and have a fusiform shape. Air within the nasopharynx and paranasal sinuses appears dark. *D.* Image at skull base clearly shows the aerated mastoid air cells as well as the internal auditory canals and inner ear structures.

also made possible the visualization, with great clarity, of the cerebral vasculature (CT angiography; see further on).

CT Contrast Myelography

By injecting 5 to 25 mL of a water-soluble radiopaque contrast through an LP needle and then placing the patient in the Trendelenberg position, the entire spinal subarachnoid space can be visualized with radiography and fluoroscopy (Fig. 2-2*A-F*). The procedure is almost as harmless as the LP except for cases of complete spinal block, in which high concentrations of contrast near the block can cause pain and regional myoclonus. Iophendylate (Pantopaque), a formerly used fat-soluble dye, is still approved by the FDA but is now employed only in special circumstances (visualizing the upper level of a spinal canal lesion that completely obstructs the flow of water soluble dye). If iophendylate is left in the subarachnoid space, particularly in the presence of blood or inflammatory exudate, it may incite arachnoiditis of the spinal cord and brain.

CT of the vertebral column provides structural images of the spinal canal and intervertebral foramina in three planes. Herniated lumbar and cervical discs, cervical spondylotic bars and bony spurs encroaching on the spinal cord or roots, and spinal cord tumors can be visualized with clarity. MRI provides even sharper visualization of the spinal canal and its contents as well as the vertebrae and intervertebral discs (Fig. 2-2*D-F*); consequently, it has largely supplanted contrast myelography.

Limitations and Safety of CT

The risks of contrast infusion include allergic reactions and nephropathy, which is most often transient and reversible, but can be more severe in patients with underlying renal dysfunction. Intravenous contrast in generally withheld if the glomerular filtration rate (GFR) is less than 30 mL/min/1.73 m^2; with GFR of 30-60, hydration and discontinuation of potentially nephrotoxic medications precedes the administration of contrast, particularly nonsteroidal anti-inflammatory agents, cisplatin containing chemotherapy and aminoglycosides. Infusion is also avoided if there has been exposure to contrast in the previous 72 h.

The primary risk of CT is radiation exposure, and overexposure can have clinical consequences ranging from relatively benign alopecia to leukomalacia and neoplasia. The interested reader should refer to FDA guidelines. Given the need for repeated CT examinations in certain patients, tracking of total radiation exposure is recommended. CT should not be performed during pregnancy unless the mother's health is at imminent risk (i.e., following trauma). The potential harm to a fetus from radiation depends on gestational age and total absorbed dose. It is noteworthy that the fetal radiation dose from maternal cranial CT is lower than from maternal pelvic CT.

Magnetic Resonance Imaging

MRI also provides images in any plane, but it has the great advantage over CT in using nonionizing energy and providing higher resolution views, and improved contrast between different structures within the nervous system. For visualization of most neurologic lesions, MRI is the preferred procedure.

MRI is accomplished by placing the patient within a powerful magnetic field, causing certain endogenous isotopes (atoms) within the tissues and CSF to be aligned in the longitudinal orientation of the magnetic field. Application of a brief (few milliseconds) radiofrequency (RF) pulse into the field changes the axis of alignment of the atoms. When the RF pulse ceases, the atoms return to their original alignment and the RF energy that was absorbed is then emitted by the isotopes, producing a magnetic signal that is detected by receiver coils. To create contrasting tissue images from these signals, the RF pulse must be repeated many times (a pulse sequence), the signals being measured after the application of each pulse. The scanner stores the signals as a matrix of data, which is subjected to computer analysis and from which two-dimensional images are reconstructed.

Nuclear magnetic resonance can be detected from several endogenous isotopes, but current technology uses mainly signals derived from hydrogen atoms because hydrogen is the most abundant element in tissue and yields the strongest magnetic signal. The image is essentially a map of the hydrogen content of tissue, therefore reflecting largely the water concentration, but influenced also by the physical and chemical environment of the hydrogen atoms. The terms T1- and T2-weighting refer to the time constants for proton relaxation; these may be altered to highlight certain features of tissue structure. In T1-weighted images, CSF appears dark and gray matter is hypointense to white matter. In T2-weighted images, CSF appears bright, and gray matter is hyperintense to white matter. Lesions within the white matter, such as the demyelination of multiple sclerosis, are more easily seen on T2-weighted images, appearing hyperintense against normal white matter (Table 2-3).

Because of the high degree of contrast between white and gray matter, one can identify, on both T1- and T2-weighted images, all discrete nuclear structures (Fig. 2-3*A-D*). Lesions near the skull base and within the posterior fossa, in particular, are seen with greater clarity on MRI compared to CT, unmarred by signals from adjacent skeletal structures. Each of the products of disintegrated RBCs—oxyhemoglobin, deoxyhemoglobin, methemoglobin, and hemosiderin—can be recognized, enabling one to approximate the age of hemorrhages and to follow their resolution, as discussed in Chaps. 34 and 35. Gradient-echo (GRE), or susceptibility weighted imaging (SWI), is especially sensitive to blood and its breakdown products that appear hypointense. These sequences can reveal lobar microhemorrhages as seen in cerebral amyloid angiopathy.

MRI of the spine provides clear images of the vertebral bodies, intervertebral discs, spinal cord, and cauda equina (Fig. 2-2*D-F*). Abnormalities such as syringomyelia, herniated discs, tumors, epidural or subdural hemorrhages, areas of demyelination, and abscesses are well delineated.

Additional radiofrequency pulses can be applied to T1- and T2-weighted images in order to selectively suppress signal from fluid or fat. The FLAIR (fluid attenuated inversion recovery) sequence is a T2-weighted sequence

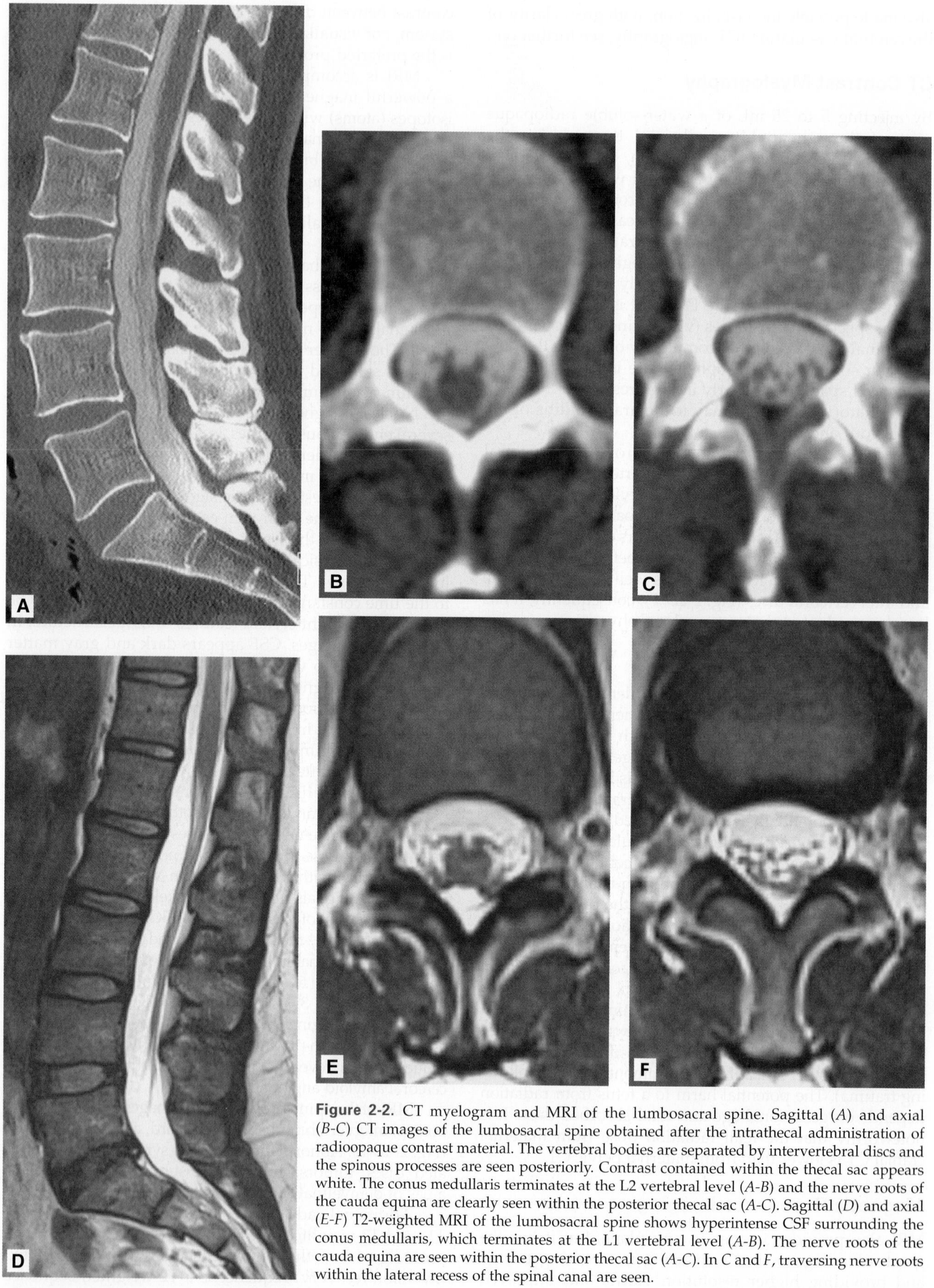

Figure 2-2. CT myelogram and MRI of the lumbosacral spine. Sagittal (*A*) and axial (*B-C*) CT images of the lumbosacral spine obtained after the intrathecal administration of radioopaque contrast material. The vertebral bodies are separated by intervertebral discs and the spinous processes are seen posteriorly. Contrast contained within the thecal sac appears white. The conus medullaris terminates at the L2 vertebral level (*A-B*) and the nerve roots of the cauda equina are clearly seen within the posterior thecal sac (*A-C*). Sagittal (*D*) and axial (*E-F*) T2-weighted MRI of the lumbosacral spine shows hyperintense CSF surrounding the conus medullaris, which terminates at the L1 vertebral level (*A-B*). The nerve roots of the cauda equina are seen within the posterior thecal sac (*A-C*). In *C* and *F*, traversing nerve roots within the lateral recess of the spinal canal are seen.

Table 2-3

CT AND MRI IMAGING CHARACTERISTICS OF VARIOUS TISSUES

TISSUE	CT GRAY SCALE	MRI T1 SIGNAL	MRI T2 SIGNAL
Brain	Gray	Gray	Gray
Air	Black	Black	Black
CSF	Black	Black	White
Fat	Black	White	Black
Calcium	White	Black	Black
Bone	Very white	Black	Black
Extravasated blood	White	White	Black
Inflammation	Contrast enhancing	Gray, gadolinium enhancing	White
Edema	Dark gray	Gray	White
Tumor	Gray or white and contrast enhancing	Gray or white and gadolinium enhancing	White

in which the bright signal of fluid is suppressed. This is a particularly useful sequence for visualizing lesions located near CSF compartments. Fat-suppression, which can be applied to T1 or T2 sequences, can be used to demonstrate inflammation of the optic nerve, visualize pathologic inflammation within the vertebral bodies, and show thrombus within the false lumen of a cervical dissection.

Diffusion-weighted imaging (DWI) is a technique that measures the free diffusion of water molecules within tissue. Preferential movement of water molecules along a particular direction, for example, parallel to white matter tracts, is referred to as anisotropy (i.e., nonisotropic movement). Many abnormal processes can produce anisotropy as well. In acute ischemic stroke, failure of the sodium-potassium ATPase pump leads to cellular swelling and reduced intercellular space, thus limiting the free movement of water and producing hyperintensity on DWI. This imaging technique reveals the abnormalities of ischemic stroke earlier than standard T1- or T2-weighted MRI, or CT. Pus-filled abscesses and hypercellular tumors can also show DWI hyperintensity, reflecting the limitation of free diffusion of water in these lesions.

Because of the relationship between DWI and T2 signal intensity, true restricted diffusion, appearing hyperintense on the DWI sequence in acute infarction, instead is *hypointense* on a related sequence termed apparent diffusion coefficient, or ADC. If the hyperintense DWI signal is also *hyperintense* on ADC, then diffusion is termed facilitated rather than restricted. This phenomenon is seen when the free movement of water within a tissue becomes more isotropic, as with vasogenic edema. Therefore, the interpretation of DWI signal hyperintensity must be gauged in the context of the ADC signal in the same region.

The administration of gadolinium, a paramagnetic agent that accelerates the process of proton relaxation during the T1 sequence of MRI, permits even sharper definition and highlights regions surrounding many types of lesions where the blood–brain barrier has been disrupted in the brain, spinal cord, or nerve roots.

Limitations and Safety of MRI

The degree of cooperation in holding still that is required to perform MRI limits its use in young children and in the cognitively impaired. Some form of sedation is required in these individuals and most hospitals have services to safely accomplish conscious sedation for this purpose. Studying a patient who requires a ventilator is also difficult but manageable by using either manual ventilation or nonferromagnetic ventilators (Barnett et al).

The main dangers in the use of MRI are torque, dislodgement or heating of metal clips on blood vessels, of dental devices and other ferromagnetic objects, and of small metal fragments in the orbit, the last of these often acquired unnoticed by operators of machine tools. For this reason it is wise, in appropriate patients, to obtain plain radiographs of the orbits so as to detect metal in these regions. Corneal metal fragments can be removed by an ophthalmic surgeon if an MRI is necessary. The presence of a cardiac pacemaker, defibrillator, or implanted stimulator in the brain or spinal cord is an absolute contraindication to the use of MRI as the magnetic field induces unwanted currents in the device and the wires exiting from it. However, many new implantable medical devices have been developed that do not distort the magnetic field. Most of the newer, weakly ferromagnetic prosthetic heart valves, joint prostheses, intravascular access ports, aneurysm clips, and ventricular shunts and adjustable valves do not represent an untoward risk for magnetic imaging although shunt valves may require resetting. An extensive list of devices that have been tested for their ferromagnetic susceptibility and their safety in the MRI machine can be found at www.mrisafety.com. MRI entails some risk in these situations unless there is direct knowledge of the type of material contained in the device. It should be noted that devices or materials that are deemed safe for 1.0 or 1.5 Tesla scanners may not be compatible with higher magnetic field strength scanners.

Because of the development of cataracts in the fetuses of animals exposed to MRI, there has been hesitation in performing MRI in pregnant patients, especially in the first trimester. However, current data indicate that imaging may be performed provided that the study is medically indicated. In a study of 1,000 pregnant MRI technicians who entered the magnetic field frequently (the magnet remains on between procedures), no adverse effects on the fetus could be discerned (Kanal et al).

In recent years, an additional risk of nephrogenic systemic fibrosis, a severe cutaneous sclerosing disease, has been linked to the administration of gadolinium. Most instances occur in patients with preexisting renal failure, for which reason it has become common to obtain BUN and creatinine measurements before administering gadolinium. The problem had not been appreciated previously in part because of its rarity (the frequency has not been well established) and because of a delay in the appearance of sclerosis in the kidney, of several days to two months.

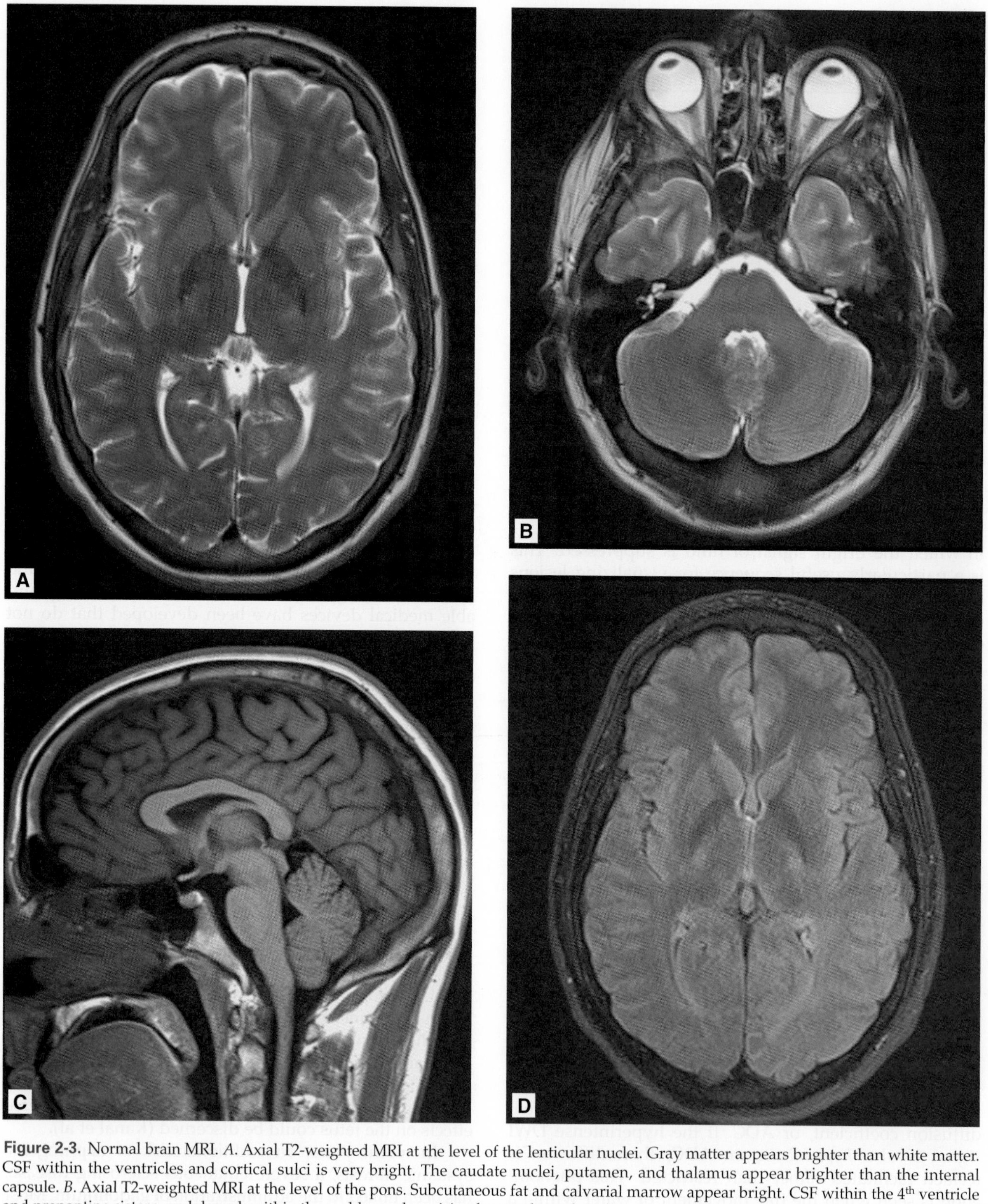

Figure 2-3. Normal brain MRI. *A*. Axial T2-weighted MRI at the level of the lenticular nuclei. Gray matter appears brighter than white matter. CSF within the ventricles and cortical sulci is very bright. The caudate nuclei, putamen, and thalamus appear brighter than the internal capsule. *B*. Axial T2-weighted MRI at the level of the pons. Subcutaneous fat and calvarial marrow appear bright. CSF within the 4th ventricle and prepontine cistern, endolymph within the cochlea and semicircular canals, and ocular vitreous fluid appears very bright. Signal is absent (i.e., a "flow void") within the basilar artery. *C*. Midline sagittal T1-weighted MRI of the brain. Note that white matter appears brighter than gray matter and the corpus callosum is well defined. The pons, medulla, and cervicomedullary junction are well delineated, and the pituitary gland is demonstrated with a normal posterior pituitary bright spot. The cerebral aqueduct is seen between the ventral midbrain and the tectum. The clivus and upper cervical vertebrae are noted as well. *D*. Axial T2-weighted fluid attenuated inversion recovery (FLAIR) MRI of the brain at the same level as in *A*. Note that the hyperintense fluid signal from CSF is now suppressed, and the differentiation between brighter gray matter and darker white matter is accentuated.

Many types of MRI image artifacts are known, most having to do with technical aspects of the electronic characteristics of the magnetic field or of the mechanics involved in the imaging procedure (for details, see Morelli). Among the most common and problematic are CSF flow artifacts in the thoracic spinal cord, giving the impression of an intradural mass; distortions of the appearance of structures at the base of the brain from ferromagnetic dental appliances; and lines across the entire image induced by vascular pulsations and patient movement.

The increasing use of MRI and the sensitivity of current machines and computer algorithms have had the unintended effect of revealing a large number of unimportant findings that create undue worry and often trigger a neurologic consultation. However, a surprising number of incidental brain lesions of consequence are also exposed. For example, a large survey of asymptomatic adults who were being followed in the "Rotterdam Study" is in accord with several prior studies in which cerebral aneurysms were found in approximately 2 percent, meningiomas in 1 percent, and a smaller but not insignificant number of vestibular schwannomas and pituitary tumors; the meningiomas, but not the aneurysms, increased in frequency with age. One percent had the Chiari type I malformation, and a similar number had arachnoid cysts. In addition, seven percent of adults older than age 45 years had occult strokes, mostly lacunar. Because this survey was performed without gadolinium infusion, it might be expected that even more small lesions could be revealed (Vernooij et al).

Special Imaging Techniques

Perfusion Imaging

This imaging modality is a contrast-based technique that can be performed with both CT and MRI. Images are rapidly and serially acquired as the contrast transits through the vasculature and parenchyma. A time-intensity curve is produced, from which measurements of cerebral blood flow, cerebral blood volume, and transit time can be derived. Perfusion imaging has provided a means of detecting regions of ischemic tissue, and to monitor the elevated blood volume in certain brain tumors.

Magnetic Resonance Spectroscopy

The tissue concentrations of a variety of cellular metabolites can be determined with the technique of magnetic resonance spectroscopy (MRS). Among these substances, *N*-acetyl aspartate (NAA) is a marker of neuronal integrity, and is decreased in both destructive lesions and in circumstances in which there is a reduction in the density of neurons (e.g., edema or glioma that increases the distance between neurons). Choline (Cho), a marker of membrane turnover, is elevated in some rapidly dividing tumors. Therefore, compared to normal white matter, the spectrogram of a glioma characteristically shows decreased NAA and increased Cho.

Diffusion Tractography

A technique related to DWI, termed diffusion tensor imaging (DTI) integrates measurements of directional anisotropy to reconstruct fiber tracts in the brain (tractography). This modality detects damage to, or displacement of white matter tracts because of trauma, vascular injury, or tumor, in extraordinary detail. Tractography is also occasionally used in surgical planning to localize critical white matter tracts avoid their inadvertent transection during operations.

Functional Imaging

In the last two decades, several remarkable techniques of functional imaging has been introduced to study activation of regions of cerebral cortex during activities, both mental and physical, carried out by test subjects. The MRI based technique shows the difference between oxy- and deoxy-hemoglobin, reflecting brain oxygen extraction, in two or three dimensions. This blood oxygen level-dependent (BOLD) signal can be extracted from MRI data and used as a surrogate for local cerebral metabolic activity. This technique has also been used in pre-surgical planning in order to avoid damage to eloquent cortex, and in epilepsy to help localize seizure foci.

Positron emission tomography (PET) produces images that reflect the regional concentration of systemically administered radioactive compounds. Positron-emitting isotopes (mainly ^{11}C, ^{18}F, and ^{15}O) are produced in a cyclotron or linear accelerator, injected into the patient, and incorporated into biologically active compounds in the body. The concentration of these tracers in various parts of the brain is determined by an array of radiation detectors and tomographic images are constructed by techniques similar to those used in CT and MRI.

Local patterns of cerebral blood flow, oxygen uptake, and glucose utilization can be measured by PET, and the procedure has proved to be of value in grading primary brain tumors, distinguishing tumor tissue from radiation necrosis, localizing epileptic foci, and, in differentiating types of degenerative diseases. The technique has been applied to specially labeled ligands of beta-amyloid, producing images of the deposition of this protein in Alzheimer disease. No doubt this approach will become increasingly important in the study of degenerative diseases and their response to treatment. The ability of the technique to quantitate neurotransmitters and their receptors also promises to be of importance in the study of Parkinson disease and other degenerative conditions. However, this technology is costly and does not always add to the certainty of diagnosis.

Single-photon emission computed tomography (SPECT), a technique which has evolved from PET, uses isotopes that do not require a cyclotron for their production. Radioligands (usually containing iodine) are incorporated into biologically active compounds, which, as they decay, emit only a single photon. This procedure allows the study of regional cerebral blood flow under conditions of cerebral ischemia and regional degenerative diseases of the cortex or during increased tissue metabolism (e.g., seizures and actively growing tumors). Once injected, the isotope localizes rapidly in the brain, with regional absorption proportional to blood flow, and is then stable for an hour or more. It is thus possible, for example, to inject the isotope at the time of a seizure, while the patient is undergoing video and electroencephalographic monitoring, and to scan the patient later. The limited anatomic resolution provided by SPECT has reduced its clinical usefulness, but it is more widely availability than other functional imaging techniques. PET and SPECT techniques that use I^{123} labeled dopamine, have been recently introduced and offer the possibility of imaging striatal dopamine and assisting in the diagnosis of Parkinson disease (see Chap. 39).

Angiography

This technique has evolved over the past century to the point where it is a safe and valuable method for the diagnosis of aneurysms, vascular malformations, narrowed or occluded arteries and veins, arterial dissections, and angiitis. Since the advent of CT and MRI, the use of angiography has practically been limited to the diagnosis of these vascular disorders, and refinements in the former two techniques (magnetic resonance angiography [MRA] and computed tomography angiography [CTA] described further on) promise to reduce or replace conventional x-ray angiography. However, new endovascular procedures for the ablation of aneurysms, arteriovenous malformations, and vascular tumors still may require the incorporation of conventional angiography. Following local anesthesia, a needle is placed in the femoral or brachial artery; a cannula is then threaded through the needle and along the aorta and the arterial branches to be visualized. In this way, a contrast agent is injected to visualize the arch of the aorta, the origins of the carotid and vertebral systems, and the extensions of these systems through the neck and into the cranial cavity and the vasculature in and surrounding the spinal cord. Experienced arteriographers can visualize the cerebral and spinal cord arteries down to about 0.1 mm in lumen diameter (under optimal conditions) and small veins of comparable size.With current refinements of radiologic technique that use digital computer processing it is possible to produce images of the major cervical and intracranial arteries with relatively small amounts of contrast medium introduced through smaller catheters than those used previously.

Angiography is not altogether without risk. High concentrations of the injected contrast may induce vascular spasm and occlusion, and clots may form on the catheter tip and embolize the artery. Overall morbidity from the procedure is approximately 2.5 percent, mainly in the form of worsening of a preexistent vascular lesion or from complications at the site of artery puncture. Occasionally, a cerebral or systemic ischemic lesion is produced, probably the result of either particulate atheromatous material dislodged by the catheter, thrombus formation at or near the catheter tip, or less often, by dissection of the artery by the catheter. The patient may be left hemiplegic, quadriplegic, or blind; for these reasons the procedure should not be undertaken unless it is deemed necessary to obtain a clear diagnosis or in anticipation of surgery that requires a definition of the location of the vessels. A cervical myelopathy is a rare but disastrous complication of vertebral artery contrast injection; the problem is heralded by pain in the back of the neck immediately after injection. Progressive cord ischemia from an ill-defined vascular process ensues over the following hours. This same complication may occur at other levels of the cord following visceral or spinal angiography.

Magnetic Resonance and Computed Tomographic Angiography

These are noninvasive techniques for visualizing the intracranial and cervical arteries. They can reliably detect intracranial vascular lesions and extracranial arterial stenosis and are supplanting conventional angiography. They approach the radiographic resolution of invasive angiography, but do not engender the risk of selective arterial catheterization (Fig. 2-4). Visualization of the cerebral veins is also possible by CT (Fig. 2-4*D*).

CT angiography requires contrast administration. In comparison, MR angiography can be performed without contrast, using the "time-of-flight" technique. This data can be reconstructed into an image that reflects flow-related enhancement. The signal obtained from time-of-flight MRA represents flow through the lumen of a vessel, rather than the configuration as obtained by contrast opacification. The use of these and other methods for the investigation of carotid artery disease is discussed further below and in Chap. 34, on cerebral vascular disease.

Ultrasonography

In recent years this technique has been refined to the point where it has become a principal methodology for clinical study of the fetal and neonatal brain and an important ancillary test for evaluating the cerebral vessels in adults. The instrument for this application consists of a transducer capable of converting electrical energy to ultrasound waves of a frequency ranging from 5 to 20 kHz. These are transmitted through the intact skull into the brain. Different tissues have specific acoustic impedances and send echoes back to the transducer, which displays them as waves of variable height or as points of light of varying intensity. In this way, one can obtain images in the neonate of choroid plexuses, ventricles, and central nuclear masses. Usually several coronal and parasagittal views are obtained by placing the transducer over open fontanelles or the child's thin calvarium. Intracerebral and subdural hemorrhages, mass lesions, and congenital defects can readily be visualized.

Similar instruments are used to insonate the basal vessels of the circle of Willis ("transcranial Doppler"), the cervical carotid and vertebral arteries, and the temporal arteries for the study of cerebrovascular disease. Their greatest use is in detecting and estimating the degree of stenosis of the origin of the internal carotid artery. In addition to providing an acoustic image of the vascular structures, the Doppler frequency shift caused by flowing red blood cells creates a display of velocities at each site in a vessel. The two techniques combined have been called "carotid duplex"; they allow an accurate localization of the locus of maximal stenosis as reflected by the highest rates of flow and turbulence. The display scale for the

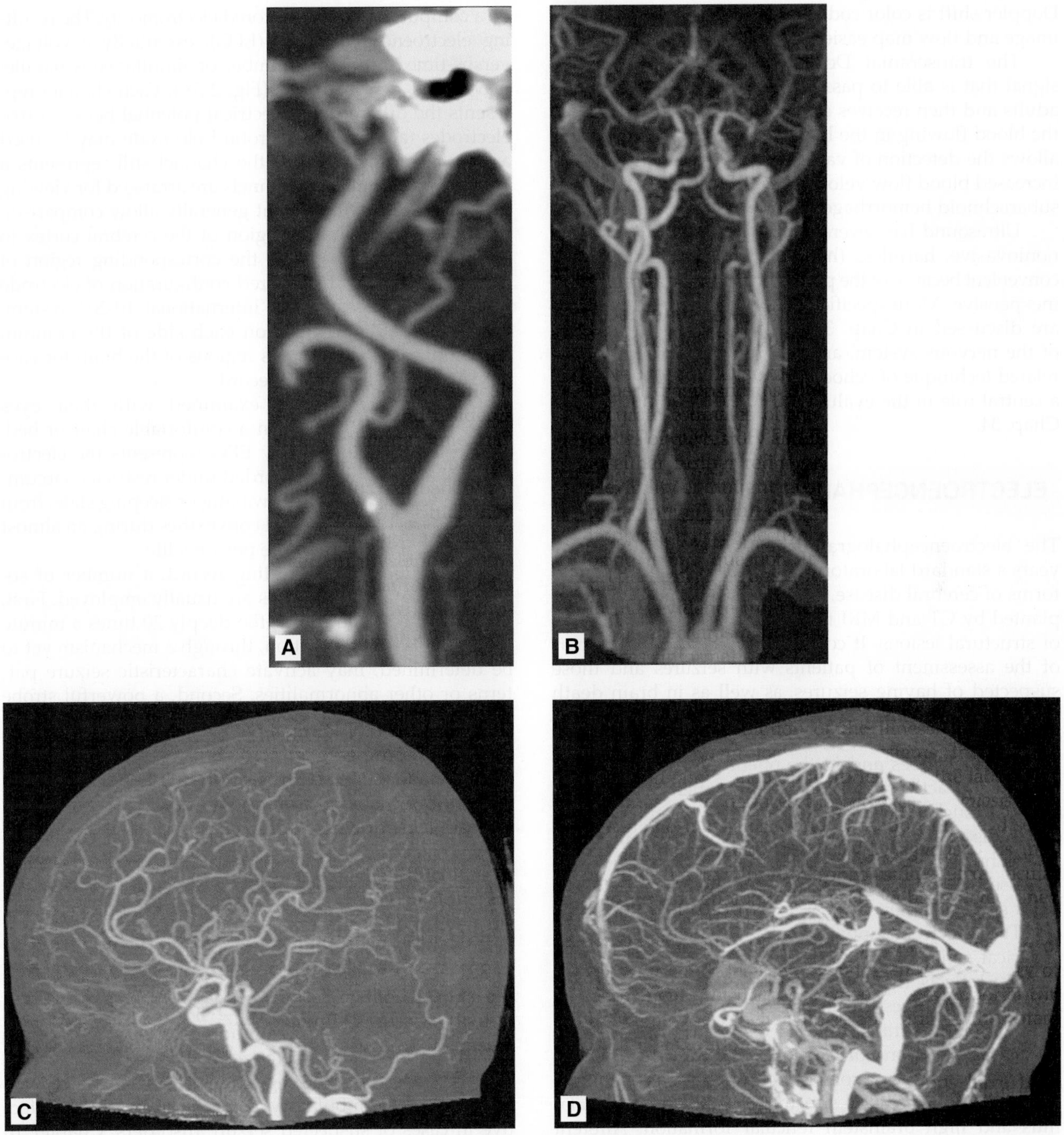

Figure 2-4. Intracranial and cervical angiography. *A.* Oblique CT angiogram of the neck showing the carotid bifurcation and the cervical segments of the internal and external carotid arteries. Note the slightly dilated carotid bulb at the initial segment of the internal carotid artery. A small focus of calcified atherosclerosis is noted near the origin of the external carotid artery. Note that the external carotid artery has multiple branches within the neck. *B.* Coronal MR angiogram of the neck showing the aortic arch, the origins and cervical courses of the carotid and vertebral arteries, and the vertebrobasilar junction. The sigmoid sinuses and internal jugular veins are faintly visible. *C-D.* Midline sagittal dynamic CT angiography of the head. Bony and soft tissue structures as well as brain parenchyma have been digitally subtracted. The image C was acquired during the arterial phase; the carotid and basilar termini and the anterior cerebral arteries are enhanced. Venous phase imaging shows enhancement of the superior and inferior sagittal sinuses, straight sinus, vein of Galen, internal cerebral veins, basal veins of Rosenthal, and the transverse and sigmoid sinuses.

Doppler shift is color coded so as to make the insonated image and flow map easier to view and interpret.

The transcranial Doppler uses a 2-MHz pulsed signal that is able to pass through the calvarial bone in adults and then receives a frequency-shifted signal from the blood flowing in the lumen of the basal vessels. This allows the detection of vascular stenoses and the greatly increased blood flow velocity caused by vasospasm from subarachnoid hemorrhage.

Ultrasound has several advantages, notably that it is noninvasive, harmless (hence can be used repeatedly), convenient because of the portability of the instrument, and inexpensive. More specific applications of this technique are discussed in Chap. 38, on developmental diseases of the nervous system, and in Chap. 34, on stroke. The related technique of echocardiography has also assumed a central role in the evaluation of stroke, as indicated in Chap. 34.

ELECTROENCEPHALOGRAPHY (EEG)

The electroencephalographic examination, for many years a standard laboratory procedure in the study of all forms of cerebral disease, has to a large extent been supplanted by CT and MRI for the purposes of localization of structural lesions. It continues to be an essential part of the assessment of patients with seizures and those suspected of having seizures, as well as in brain death and for the study of sleep (polysomnography). It is also used in evaluating the cerebral effects of many systemic metabolic diseases and in the operating room to monitor cerebral activity in anesthetized patients. For a few diseases, such as subacute spongiform encephalopathy (prion disease), it is a useful confirmatory laboratory test. The technique is described here in some detail, as its general use in neurology cannot suitably be assigned to any other single chapter.

The electroencephalograph records spontaneous electrical activity generated in the cerebral cortex. This activity reflects the electrical currents that flow in the extracellular spaces of the brain that are the summated effects of innumerable excitatory and inhibitory synaptic potentials upon cortical neurons. This spontaneous activity of cortical neurons is highly influenced and synchronized by subcortical structures, particularly the thalamus and high brainstem reticular formation. Afferent impulses from these deep structures are probably responsible for entraining cortical neurons to produce characteristic rhythmic brain-wave patterns, such as alpha rhythm and sleep spindles (see further on).

Electrodes, which are silver or silver-silver chloride discs 0.5 cm in diameter, are attached to the scalp by means of a conductive paste. The electroencephalograph has 8 to 32 or more amplifying units capable of recording from many areas of the scalp at the same time. The amplified brain rhythms are seen as waveforms of brain activity in the frequency range of 0.5 to 30 Hz (cycles per second) on a standard display of that runs at 3 cm/s. In the past, the amplified signals were recorded by a bank of pens but now, a digital format of the rhythms is displayed on a computer screen and stored electronically. The resulting electroencephalogram (EEG), essentially a voltage-versus-time graph, is a number of simultaneous parallel wavy lines, or "channels" (Fig. 2-5*A*). Each channel represents the difference in electrical potential between two electrodes (a common or ground electrode may be used as one recording site, but the channel still represents a bipolar recording). The channels are arranged for viewing into standard montages that generally allow comparison of the activity from one region of the cerebral cortex to others, and particularly to the corresponding region of the opposite side. The favored configuration of electrode pairs, or montage, is the "International 10-20" system, which uses 10 electrodes on each side of the cranium and emphasizes contiguous regions of the brain for ease of visual inspection of the record.

Patients are usually examined with their eyes closed and while relaxed in a comfortable chair or bed. Consequently, the ordinary EEG represents the electrocerebral activity that is recorded under restricted circumstances, usually during the waking or sleeping state, from several parts of the cerebral convexities during an almost infinitesimal segment of the person's life.

In addition to the resting record, a number of so-called activating procedures are usually employed. First, the patient is asked to breathe deeply 20 times a minute for 3 min. Hyperventilation, through a mechanism yet to be determined, may activate characteristic seizure patterns or other abnormalities. Second, a powerful strobe light is placed about 15 inches from the patient's eyes and flashed at frequencies of 1 to 20 per second with the patient's eyes open and closed. In a healthy subject, the occipital EEG leads show waves corresponding to each flash of light (photic driving, Fig. 2-5*B*).

The EEG is recorded after the patient is allowed to fall asleep naturally or occasionally, following the administration of sedative drugs. The drowsy state and the transition to and from deeper stages of sleep can reveal abnormalities.

Many abnormalities associated with sleep are more evident with long-term continuous EEG monitoring (hours to days) as described in Chap. 19. EEG activity can be synchronized with videographically recorded seizure activity in order to characterize the nature of the seizure. EEGs recorded by small digital devices or telemetry from freely moving ambulatory patients are similarly effective in cases of suspected seizure disorders. Chapter 16 discusses these techniques in detail. Chapter 19 contains information on the use of EEG to analyze disorders of sleep (polysomnography).

Certain preparations are necessary if electroencephalography is to be most useful. The patient should not be sedated (except as noted above) and should not have been without food for a long time, for both sedative drugs and relative hypoglycemia may modify the normal EEG pattern and should avoid caffeine if a sleep EEG study is planned. When dealing with patients who are suspected of having epilepsy and are already being treated for it, most physicians prefer to record the EEG while the patient continues to receive antiepileptic medications. During inpatient monitoring, these drugs are

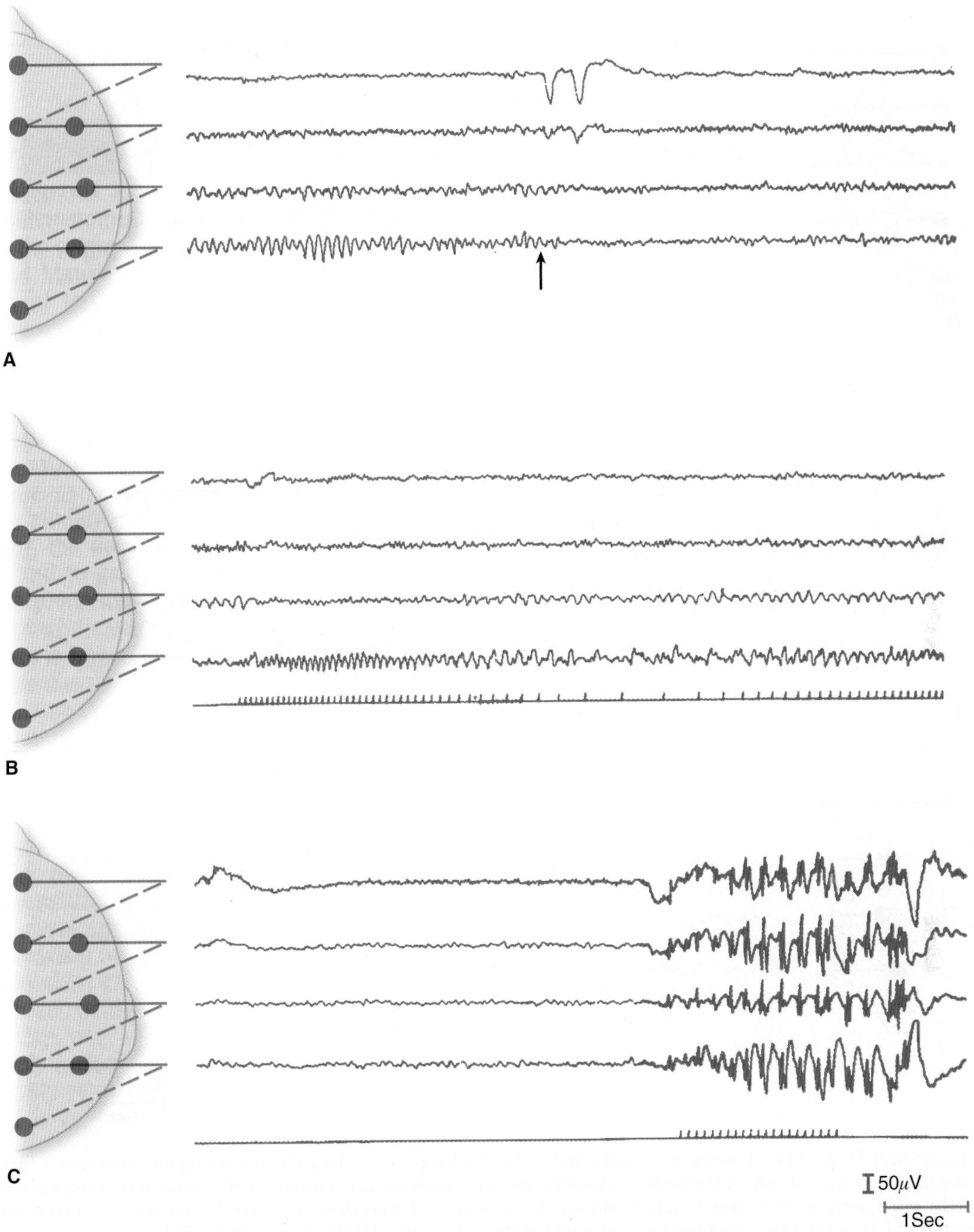

Figure 2-5. *A.* Normal alpha (8 to 12 per second) activity is present posteriorly (bottom channel). The top channel contains a large blink artifact. Note the striking reduction of the alpha rhythm with eye opening (arrow). *B.* Photic driving. During stroboscopic stimulation of a normal subject, a visually evoked response is seen posteriorly after each flash of light (signaled on the bottom channel). *C.* Stroboscopic stimulation at 14 flashes per second (bottom channel) has produced a photoparoxysmal response in this epileptic patient, evidenced by the abnormal spike and slow-wave activity toward the end of the period of stimulation. *(continued)*

often withdrawn for a day or two in order to increase the likelihood of recording a seizure discharge but this requires careful clinical monitoring.

The proper interpretation of EEGs involves the recognition of several characteristic normal and abnormal patterns and background rhythms (in accordance with the age of the patient), the detection of asymmetries and periodic changes in rhythm, and, importantly, the differentiation of artifacts from genuine abnormalities.

Normal EEG Patterns

The normal record in adults shows slightly asymmetrical 8- to 12-per-second 50-mV sinusoidal *alpha waves* in both

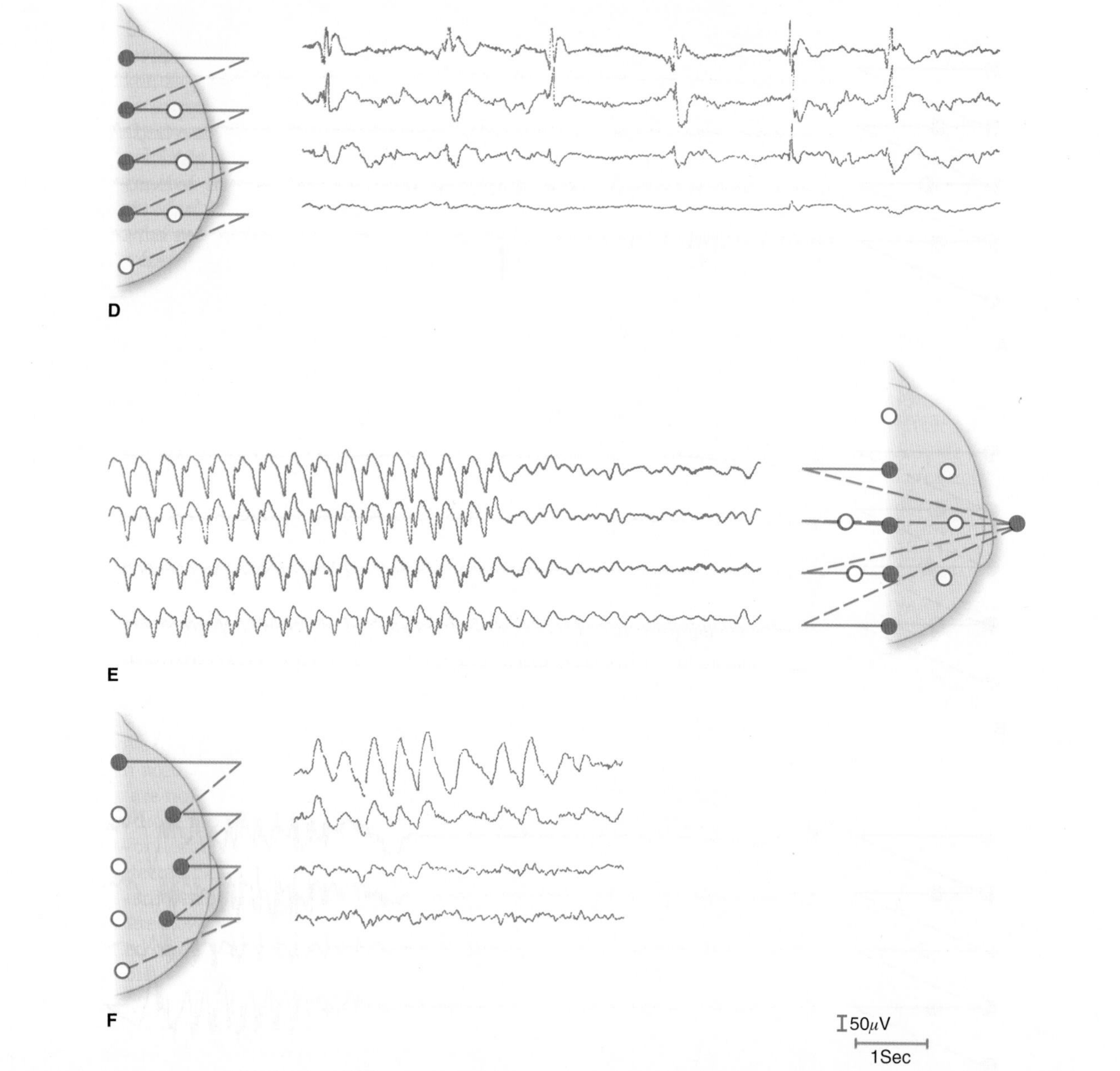

Figure 2-5. (*Continued*) *D*. An EEG showing focal spike-and-wave discharges over the right frontal region (channels 1 to 3). There were convulsive movements of the left side of the body. *E*. Absence seizures, showing generalized 3-per-second spike-and-wave discharge. The abnormal activity ends abruptly and normal background activity appears. *F*. Large, slow, irregular delta waves are seen in the right frontal region (channels 1 and 2). In this case a glioblastoma was found in the right cerebral hemisphere, but the EEG picture does not differ basically from that produced by a stroke, abscess, or contusion. (*continued*)

occipital and posterior parietal regions. These waves wax and wane in amplitude spontaneously and are attenuated or suppressed completely with eye opening or mental activity (see Fig. 2-5*A*). In contrast, the frequency of the alpha rhythm is almost invariant for an individual patient, although the rate slows with aging. Waves faster than 12 Hz and of lower amplitude (10 to 20 mV), called *beta waves*, are normally recorded from the frontal regions symmetrically. If benzodiazepines or other sedating drugs have been administered, an increase in the fast frequencies is typically observed. When the normal subject falls asleep, the alpha rhythm slows symmetrically and characteristic waveforms consisting of vertex sharp waves and sleep spindles appear (see Fig. 19-1). A small amount of theta (4- to 7-Hz) activity may normally be present over the temporal regions, somewhat more so in persons older than 60 years of age. Delta (1- to 3-Hz) activity is not present in the normal waking adult.

The presence of a photic driving a response indicates that some of the visual pathways are preserved. Spread of

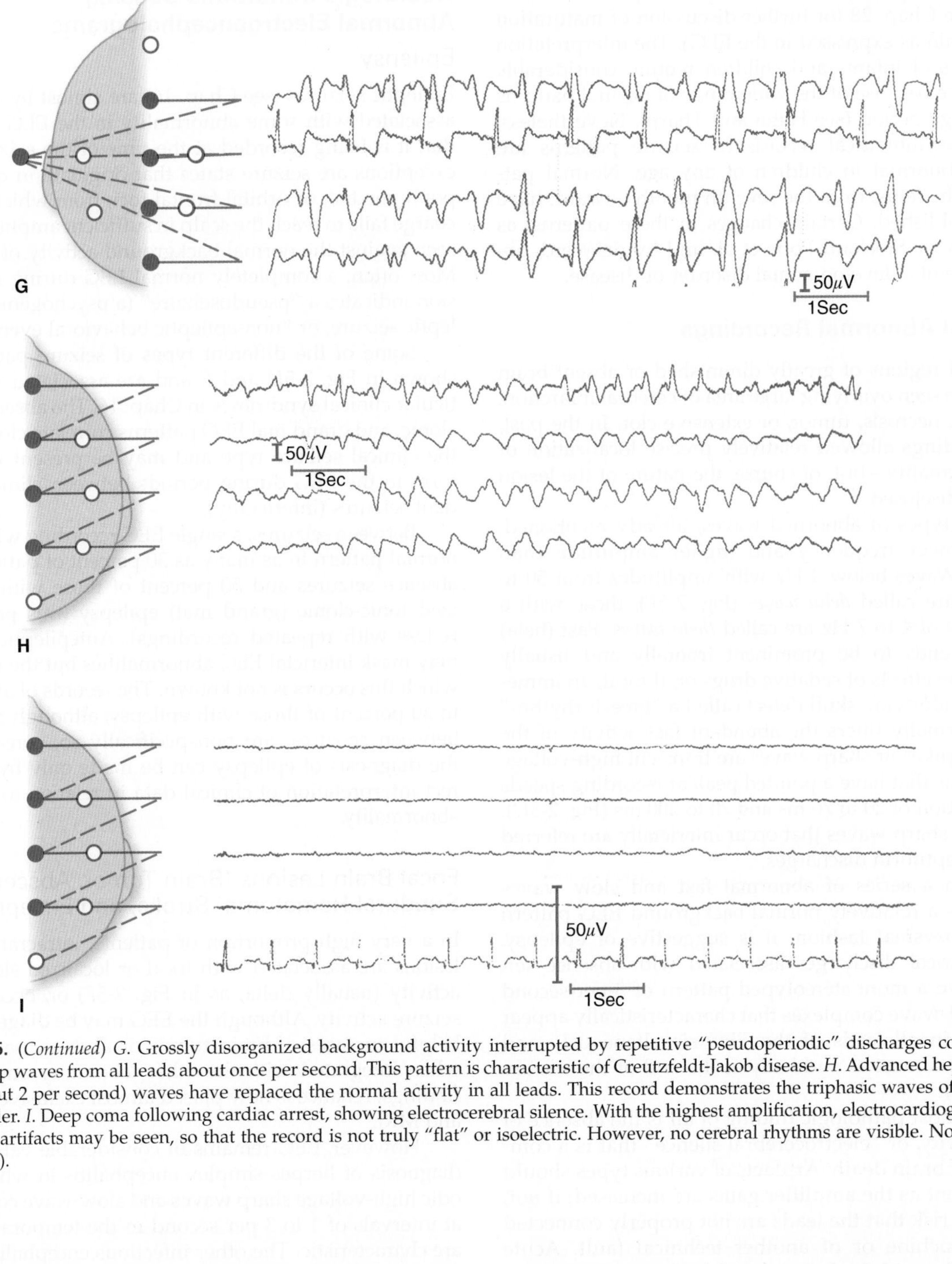

Figure 2-5. (*Continued*) *G*. Grossly disorganized background activity interrupted by repetitive "pseudoperiodic" discharges consisting of large, sharp waves from all leads about once per second. This pattern is characteristic of Creutzfeldt-Jakob disease. *H*. Advanced hepatic coma. Slow (about 2 per second) waves have replaced the normal activity in all leads. This record demonstrates the triphasic waves often seen in this disorder. *I*. Deep coma following cardiac arrest, showing electrocerebral silence. With the highest amplification, electrocardiogram (ECG) and other artifacts may be seen, so that the record is not truly "flat" or isoelectric. However, no cerebral rhythms are visible. Note the ECG (channel 5).

the occipital response induced by photic stimulation, with the production of abnormal sharp or paroxysmal waves, provides evidence of abnormal cortical excitability (Fig. 2-5*B* and *C*). Seizure patterns may be produced during this type of EEG testing, accompanied by gross myoclonic jerks of the face, neck, and limbs (photomyoclonic response), by electrographic seizure activity that outlasts the photic stimulation (photoparoxysmal response), or by or a convulsion (photoconvulsive response). Such effects occur with some regularity during periods of withdrawal from alcohol and other sedative drugs.

Children and adolescents are more sensitive than adults to all the activating procedures mentioned. It is customary for children to develop delta waves (3 to 4 Hz) during the middle and latter parts of a period of hyperventilation. This EEG activity, referred to as "breakdown," or "buildup," disappears soon after hyperventilation has stopped. The frequency of the dominant rhythms in infants is normally about 3 Hz, and they are very irregular. With maturation, there is a gradual increase in frequency and regularity of these occipital rhythms; an alpha rhythm appears by age 6 years and the adult frequency is reached by the age of 10 to 12 years (see Chap. 28 for further discussion of maturation of the brain as expressed in the EEG). The interpretation of records of infants and children require considerable experience because of the wide range of normal patterns at each age period (see Hahn and Tharp). Nevertheless, grossly asymmetrical records or seizure patterns are clearly abnormal in children of any age. Normal patterns in the fetus, from the seventh month onward, have been established. Certain changes in these patterns, as described by Stockard-Pope et al. and by deWeerd, are indicative of a developmental disorder or disease.

Types of Abnormal Recordings

Localized regions of greatly diminished or absent brain waves are seen overlying large area of cerebral infarction, traumatic necrosis, tumor, or extensive clot. In the past, these findings allowed relatively precise localization of the abnormality—but, of course, the nature of the lesion was not disclosed.

Two types of abnormal waves, already mentioned, are of lower frequency and higher amplitude than normal. Waves below 4 Hz with amplitudes from 50 to 350 mV are called *delta waves* (Fig. 2-5*F*); those with a frequency of 4 to 7 Hz are called *theta waves*. Fast (beta) activity tends to be prominent frontally and usually reflects the effects of sedative drugs or, if focal, an immediately underlying skull defect called a "breech rhythm" (bone normally filters the abundant fast activity of the cortex). Spikes or sharp waves are transient high-voltage waveforms that have a pointed peak at recording speeds and duration of 20 to 70 ms and 70 to 200 ms (Fig. 2-5*D*). Spikes or sharp waves that occur interictally are referred to as epileptiform discharges.

When a series of abnormal fast and slow waves interrupts a relatively normal background EEG pattern in a paroxysmal fashion, it is suggestive of epilepsy. The electrical discharges associated with absence seizures have a more stereotyped pattern of 3-per-second spike-and-wave complexes that characteristically appear abruptly in all leads of the EEG simultaneously and disappear almost as suddenly at the end of the seizure (Fig. 2-5*E*).

The most pathologic finding of all is the absence of EEG activity, or "electrocerebral silence" that is a component of brain death. Artifacts of various types should be apparent as the amplifier gains are increased; if not, there is a risk that the leads are not properly connected to the machine or of another technical fault. Acute intoxication with high levels of drugs such as barbiturates can transiently produce this sort of isoelectric EEG (Fig. 2-5I). In the absence of nervous system depressants or extreme degrees of hypothermia, a record that is isoelectric (<2 uV except for artifacts) over all parts of the head is almost always a result of profound cerebral hypoxia or ischemia or of trauma and raised intracranial pressure. Such a patient—without EEG activity, brainstem reflexes, and spontaneous respiratory or muscular activity of any kind—is said to be brain dead as discussed further in Chapter 17.

Neurologic Conditions Causing Abnormal Electroencephalograms

Epilepsy

Epileptic seizures (see Chap. 16) are almost by definition associated with some abnormality in the EEG provided that it is being recorded at the time of the seizure. Rare exceptions are seizure states that originate in deep temporal, medial, or orbital frontal foci, from which the discharge fails to reach the scalp in sufficient amplitude to be seen against the normal background activity of the EEG. Most often, a completely normal EEG during a convulsion indicates a "pseudoseizure" (a psychogenic nonepileptic seizure, or "non-epileptic behavioral event").

Some of the different types of seizure patterns are shown in Fig. 2-5*D* and *E* and are associated with particular clinical syndromes in Chap. 16. The absence, myoclonic, and grand mal EEG patterns correlate closely with the clinical seizure type and may be present in milder form in the EEG during periods between clinically evident seizures (interictally).

Between seizures, a single EEG recording will show a normal pattern in as many as 30 percent of patients with absence seizures and 50 percent of those with generalized tonic-clonic (grand mal) epilepsy (this percentage is less with repeated recordings). Antepileptic therapy may mask interictal EEG abnormalities but the degree to which this occurs is not known. The records of another 30 to 40 percent of those with epilepsy, although abnormal between seizures, are nonspecifically so; consequently, the diagnosis of epilepsy can be made only by the correct interpretation of clinical data in relation to the EEG abnormality.

Focal Brain Lesions (Brain Tumor, Abscess, Subdural Hematoma, Stroke, and Encephalitis)

In a very high proportion of patients, intracranial mass lesions are associated with focal or localized slow-wave activity (usually delta, as in Fig. 2-5*F*) or, occasionally, seizure activity. Although the EEG may be diagnostically helpful in cases of brain tumor or abscess, particularly when integrated with the other laboratory and clinical findings, reliance is now placed almost exclusively on CT and MRI.

However, EEG remains of considerable value in the diagnosis of herpes simplex encephalitis in which periodic high-voltage sharp waves and slow-wave complexes at intervals of 1 to 3 per second in the temporal regions are characteristic. The other infectious encephalitides are often associated with sharp or spike activity, particularly if there have been seizures. Figure 2-5*G* shows the characteristic pattern of almost periodic sharp waves seen in Creutzfeldt-Jakob disease.

The EEG is now little used in the differential diagnosis of stroke, except to distinguish a transient ischemic attack from a seizure. In the past, one practical value was in the ability to differentiate an acute ischemic lesion in the distribution of the middle cerebral artery, which produces a large area of slowing, from lacunar infarction deep in the cerebrum or brainstem, in which the surface EEG is usually normal despite prominent clinical abnormalities. After 3 to 6 months, in roughly 50 percent of patients with infarction in the territory of the middle cerebral artery, the focal EEG slowing becomes normal. Perhaps half these patients will have had normal EEGs even in the week or two following the stroke. A persistent abnormality is generally associated with a poor prognosis for further recovery. Large lesions of the diencephalon or midbrain produce bilaterally synchronous slow waves, but those of the pons and medulla (i.e., below the mesencephalon) are usually associated with a normal or near-normal EEG pattern despite catastrophic clinical changes.

A brief episode of cerebral concussion in animals is accompanied by a transitory disturbance in the EEG, but in humans this is usually no longer evident by the time a recording can be made. Large cerebral contusions produce focal EEG slowing similar to those described for cerebral infarction. Sharp waves or spikes sometimes emerge as the focal slow-wave abnormality resolves and may precede the occurrence of posttraumatic epilepsy; serial EEGs may be of prognostic value in this regard. During syncope, the EEG is slowed and of reduced amplitude even to the point of becoming "flat." Upon recovery, a number of patterns have been described as discussed further in Chap. 18.

Diseases that Cause Coma and States of Impaired Consciousness

The EEG is abnormal in almost all conditions in which there is impairment of the level of consciousness. There is, for example, a fairly close correspondence between the severity of acute anoxic damage from cardiac arrest and the degree of EEG slowing. The mildest forms are associated with generalized theta activity, intermediate forms with widespread delta waves and the loss of normal background activity, and the most severe forms with "burst suppression," in which brief isoelectric periods are followed by high-voltage sharp and irregular delta activity. The latter pattern usually progresses to the electrocerebral silence of brain death, a condition discussed earlier.

The term alpha coma refers to a unique EEG pattern in which an apparent alpha activity in the 8- to 12-Hz range is distributed widely over the hemispheres rather than in its normal location posteriorly. When analyzed carefully, this background activity, unlike the normal monorhythmic alpha, is found to vary slightly in frequency. This is usually a transitional pattern after global anoxia; less often, alpha coma occurs with large acute pontine lesions. With severe hypothyroidism, the brain waves are normal in configuration but usually of decreased amplitude and frequency.

In altered states of alertness, the more profound the depression of consciousness, in general, the more abnormal and slower the EEG rhythms. In states of deep stupor or coma, the slow (delta) waves are bilateral and of high amplitude and tend to be more conspicuous over the frontal regions (Fig. 2-5*H*). This pertains in such differing conditions as acute meningitis or encephalitis and disorders that severely alter blood gases, glucose, electrolytes, and water balance; uremia; diabetic coma; and impairment of consciousness accompanying the large cerebral lesions discussed above. In hepatic coma, the degree of abnormality in the EEG corresponds roughly to the degree of confusion, stupor, or coma. Characteristic of hepatic coma are paroxysms of bilaterally synchronous large, sharp "triphasic waves" (Fig. 2-5*H*), although such waveforms may also be seen with less regularity in encephalopathies related to renal or pulmonary failure and with acute hydrocephalus (intermittent biphasic frontal slowing is more typical of hydrocephalus).

An EEG may also be of help in the diagnosis of coma that is due to ongoing seizures ("nonconvulsive status epilepticus") or, when the pertinent history is not available and there was an unobserved convulsion. It may also point to an otherwise unexpected cause of coma, such as hepatic encephalopathy, intoxication with barbiturates or other sedative-hypnotic drugs, the effects of diffuse anoxia–ischemia, catatonia, or hysteria (in which the EEG is normal).

Diffuse Degenerative Diseases

Alzheimer disease and other degenerative diseases that cause serious impairment of cerebrocortical function are accompanied by relatively slight degrees of diffuse slow-wave abnormality in the theta (4- to 7-Hz) range; many recordings are normal in the early and midstages of illness. More rapidly progressive disorders—such as subacute sclerosing panencephalitis (SSPE), Creutzfeldt-Jakob disease, and to a lesser extent the cerebral lipidoses—often have, in addition, very characteristic and almost pathognomonic EEG changes consisting of periodic bursts of high-amplitude sharp waves, usually bisynchronous and symmetrical (Fig. 2-5*G*). In a negative sense, a normal EEG in a patient who is profoundly apathetic is a point in favor of the diagnosis of hysteria, catatonia, or schizophrenia (see below).

Other Diseases of the Cerebrum

Many disorders of the brain cause little or no alteration in the EEG. Multiple sclerosis and other demyelinating diseases are examples, although as many as 50 percent of patients with advanced disease will have an abnormal record of nonspecific type (mild focal or diffuse slowing). Delirium tremens and Wernicke-Korsakoff disease, despite the dramatic nature of the clinical picture, cause little or no change in the EEG. Interestingly, the psychoses (bipolar disorders or schizophrenia), intoxication with hallucinogenic drugs such as lysergic acid diethylamide (LSD), and the majority of cases of mental retardation are associated either with no modification of the normal record or with only minor nonspecific abnormalities unless seizures are present.

Clinical Significance of Minor Electroencephalogram Abnormalities

The gross EEG abnormalities discussed above are by themselves clearly abnormal, and any formulation of the patient's clinical state should attempt to account for them. Lesser degrees of abnormality form a continuum between the undoubtedly abnormal and the completely normal and are of correspondingly less significance. Findings such as 14- and 6-per-second positive spikes or small sharp waves during sleep, scattered 5- or 6-per-second slowing, minor voltage asymmetries, and persistence of "breakdown" for a few minutes after hyperventilation are interpreted as normal variants or borderline abnormalities. Whereas borderline deviations in an otherwise entirely normal person have no clinical significance, the same minimal EEG findings associated with particular clinical signs and symptoms become important. The significance of a normal or "negative" EEG in certain patients suspected of having a cerebral lesion was discussed above.

As a general clinical principle, the results of the EEG, like those of the EMG and electrocardiogram, are meaningful only in relation to the illnesses under consideration and the clinical state of the patient at the time the recordings were made.

EVOKED POTENTIALS

The stimulation of sense organs or peripheral nerves evokes an electrical response in the corresponding cortical receptive areas and in a number of subcortical relay stations. However, one cannot place a recording electrode near the nuclear relay stations, nor can one detect tiny potentials of only a few microvolts among the much larger background activity in the EEG. The use of computerized averaging methods, introduced by Dawson in 1954, has provided a means of overcoming these problems. Initially, emphasis was on the study of late waves (over 75 ms after the stimulus) because they are of high amplitude and easy to record. However, there is more clinical utility in recording the much smaller, short-latency waveforms, which are received at each nuclear relay within the main sensory systems. These waveforms are maximized by the computer to a point where their latency and voltage can easily be measured. One of the most remarkable properties of evoked potentials is their resistance to anesthesia, sedative drugs, and—in comparison with EEG activity—even damage of the cerebral hemispheres. This permits their use for monitoring the integrity of cerebral pathways in situations that render the EEG useless.

The interpretation of evoked potentials (visual, auditory, and somatosensory) is based on the prolongation of the latencies of the waveforms after the stimulus, the interwave latencies, and asymmetries in timing. Norms for latencies have been established, but it is advisable to confirm these in each laboratory. Typically 2.5 or 3 standard deviations above the mean latency for any measurement is taken as the definition of abnormality (Table 2-4). The amplitudes of the waves are less informative for clinical work.

Table 2-4

MAIN SENSORY EVOKED POTENTIAL LATENCIES FROM STIMULUS, MILLISECONDS[a]

TYPE OF EVOKED POTENTIAL	MEAN	UPPER LIMIT (MEAN + 3 SD)
PSVER (*70-min check size*)		
P100 absolute latency	104	118
Intereye difference	2	8
BAER (*60 dBSL, 10/s monaural stimuli*)		
Interwave latency		
I–III	2.1	2.6
III–V	1.9	2.4
I–V	4.0	4.7
Interside difference for most latencies	0.1	0.4
SEP—median nerve (*wrist stimulation*)		
Absolute latency		
Erb's point	9.7	12.0
P/N 13 (cervicomedullary)	13.5	16.3
N 19/P 21 (cortical)	19.0	22.1
Interwave latency		
Erb's-P/N 13	3.8	5.2
P/N 13–N 19	5.5	6.8
Interside difference		
P/N 13–N 19	0.3	1.1
SEP—tibial nerve (*ankle stimulation; Fz-Cz recording; 165-cm height; absolute latencies are shorter for stimulation at the knee*)		
Absolute latency		
Lumbar point (cauda equina)	20	25
N/P 37 (cortex)	36	42.5
Interwave latency		
Lumbar–N/P 37	16.4	21.6
Interside difference		
Lumbar–N/P 37	0.7	1.9

[a]Norms must be verified in each laboratory; in most instances they are sensitive to the technique and stimulus used and height of the patient in the cases of limb stimulation.

BAER, brainstem auditory evoked response; PSVER, pattern shift visual evoked response; SSEP, somatosensory evoked response.

Visual Evoked Potentials (VER, VEP)

For many years it had been known that a light stimulus flashing on the retina evokes a discernible waveform over the occipital lobes. In the EEG, such responses to fast rates of stimulation are referred to as the occipital driving response (Fig. 2-5 *B* and *C*). It also was appreciated decades ago that a visual evoked response is produced by the sudden change of a viewed checkerboard pattern. These responses, produced by rapidly reversing the pattern of black and white squares, are easier to detect and to measure than are flash responses and are more consistent in waveform from one individual to another. The pattern shift stimulus applied first to one eye and then to the other, can demonstrate conduction delays in the visual pathways of patients who have had disease of the optic nerve—even when there are no residual signs of reduced visual acuity, visual field abnormalities, alterations of the optic nerve head, or changes in pupillary reflexes. Furthermore, the presence of a normal visual evoked response belies blindness from a lesion in the anterior visual pathways and their projections to the occipital cortex. Figure 2-6 illustrates the normal pattern shift visual evoked response (PSVER) and two types of delayed

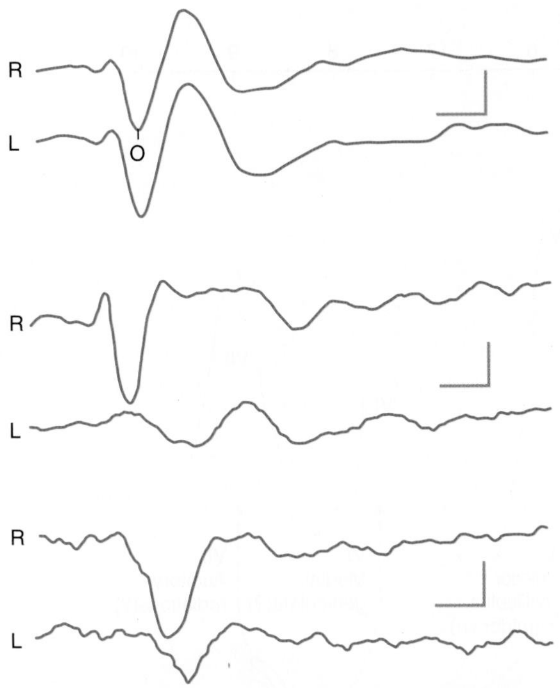

Figure 2-6. Pattern-shift visual evoked responses (PSVERs). Latency measured to first major positive peak (termed P100 because of its latency from the stimulus of approximate 100 msec) and marked by "o." Upper two tracings: These, from the right and left eyes, are normal. Middle tracings: PSVER from the right eye is normal but the latency of the response from the left eye is prolonged and its duration is increased. Lower tracings: PSVER from both eyes show abnormally prolonged latencies, somewhat greater on the left than on the right. Calibration: 50 ms, 2.5 mV.

responses. Reductions in the amplitude and duration of PSVER usually accompany prolonged latencies but are difficult to quantify.

The expected latency for the positive polarity, by convention a downward deflection, PSVER is near 100 ms (thus the term P100 has also been used to designate the waveform); an absolute latency from the stimulus longer than 118 ms or a difference in latencies of greater than 9 ms between the two eyes signifies involvement of one optic nerve (Table 2-4). Bilateral prolongation of latencies, demonstrated by separate stimulation of each eye, can be caused by lesions in both optic nerves, the optic chiasm, or the visual pathways posterior to the chiasm.

As indicated above, PSVER is especially valuable in proving the existence of active or residual disease of an optic nerve. Patients with previous optic neuritis will have abnormal latencies. Furthermore, similar prolongations of PSVER are found in about one-third of multiple sclerosis patients who have had no history or clinical evidence of optic nerve involvement. This acquires significance in that the finding of abnormal PSVER in a patient with a clinically apparent demyelinating lesion elsewhere in the CNS may usually be taken as evidence of multiple sclerosis, as discussed in Chap. 36.

A compressive lesion of an optic nerve will have the same effect as a primarily demyelinating one. Many other diseases of the optic nerves—including toxic and nutritional amblyopias, ischemic optic neuropathy, and the Leber type of hereditary optic neuropathy—show abnormalities of the PSVER. Glaucoma and other diseases involving structures anterior to the retinal ganglion cells, if severe enough to affect the optic nerve, may also produce increased latencies. Impaired visual acuity has little effect on the latency but does correlate well with the amplitude of the PSVER (a property that is exploited in some computerized testing for visual acuity). The use of these tests in detecting psychogenic blindness has already been mentioned. By presenting the pattern-shift stimulus to one hemifield, it is possible to isolate a lesion to an optic tract or radiation, or one occipital lobe, but with much less precision than that provided by the usual monocular testing.

Brainstem Auditory Evoked Potentials

The effects of auditory stimuli can be studied in the same way as visual ones by a procedure called brainstem auditory evoked responses, or potentials (BAERs, or BAEPs). Between 1,000 and 2,000 clicks, delivered first to one ear and then to the other, are recorded through scalp electrodes and superimposed on each other by computer and thereby maximized. A series of seven waves appears at the scalp within 10 ms after each stimulus. On the basis of depth recordings and the study of lesions produced in cats as well as pathologic studies of the brainstem in disease, it has been suggested that each of the first five waves is generated by a specific brainstem structure, as indicated in Fig. 2-7, but this has not been established with precision in humans. The generators of waves VI and VII in particular are uncertain. The presence of wave I and its absolute latency test the integrity of the auditory nerve.

Clinical interpretations of BAERs are based mainly on latency measurements from the stimulus and interwave latencies. The most important are the interwave latencies between I and III, and III and V (see Table 2-4). A lesion that affects one of the auditory nuclear relay stations or its immediate connections manifests itself by a delay in the appearance or an absence of all subsequent waves; in other words, the nuclei behave as if they are connected in series. These effects are more pronounced on the side of the stimulated ear than contralaterally. This is difficult to understand, as a majority of the cochlear-superior olivary-lateral lemniscal-medial geniculate fibers cross to the opposite side. It is also surprising that a lesion of one relay station would allow impulses, even though delayed, to continue their ascent and be recordable in the cerebral cortex.

BAEPs are a particularly sensitive means of detecting lesions of the eighth cranial nerve (vestibular schwannoma and other tumors of the cerebellopontine angle) and of the auditory pathways of the brainstem. Almost one-half of patients with definite multiple sclerosis and a lesser number with a possible or probable diagnosis of this disease will show abnormalities of the BAEPs, (usually a prolongation of interwave latencies I to III or III to V), even in the absence of clinical symptoms

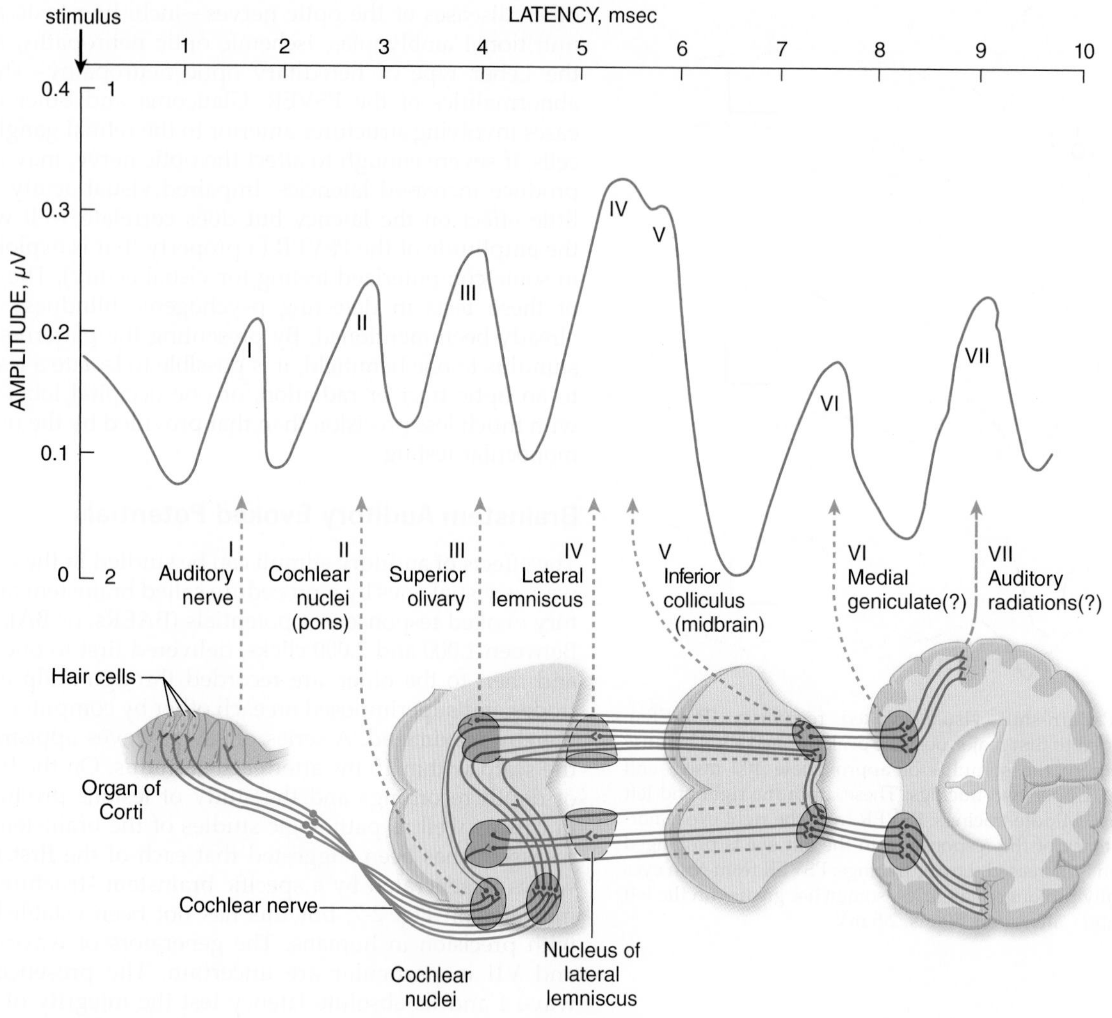

Figure 2-7. Short-latency brainstem auditory evoked responses (BAERs). Diagram of the proposed electrophysiologic–anatomic correlations in human subjects. Waves I through V are the ones measured in clinical practice.

and signs of brainstem disease. The BAEPs are also useful in assessing hearing in infants who have been exposed to ototoxic drugs, in young children who cannot cooperate with audiometry, and in those with psychogenic or feigned deafness.

Somatosensory Evoked Potentials (SSEP)

The technique consists of applying 5-per-second painless transcutaneous electrical stimuli to the median, peroneal, or tibial nerves and recording the evoked potentials (for the upper limb) sequentially as they pass the brachial plexus over the Erb point above the clavicle, over the C2 vertebra, and over the opposite parietal cortex, and (for the lower limb) over the lumbar roots of the cauda equina, the nuclei over the cervical spine, and the opposite parietal cortex. The impulses generated in large touch fibers by 500 or more stimuli and averaged by computer can be traced through the corresponding peripheral nerves, spinal roots, and posterior columns to the cuneate and gracile nuclei in the lower medulla, through the medial lemniscus to the contralateral thalamus, and thence to the sensory cortex of the parietal lobe. Delay between the stimulus site and the Erb point or the lumbar spine indicates peripheral nerve disease; delay from the Erb point (or lumbar spine) to C2 implies an abnormality in the appropriate nerve roots or, more frequently, in the posterior columns; the presence of lesions in the medial lemniscus and thalamoparietal pathway can be inferred from delays of subsequent waves recorded from the parietal cortex (Fig. 2-8). The normal waveforms are designated by the symbols P (positive) and N (negative), with a number indicating the interval of time in milliseconds from stimulus to recording (e.g., N11, N13, P13, P22, etc.). As shorthand for the polarity and approximate latency, the summated wave that is recorded at the cervicomedullary junction is termed N/P13, and the cortical potential from median nerve stimulation seen in two contiguous waves of opposite polarity is called N19–P22.

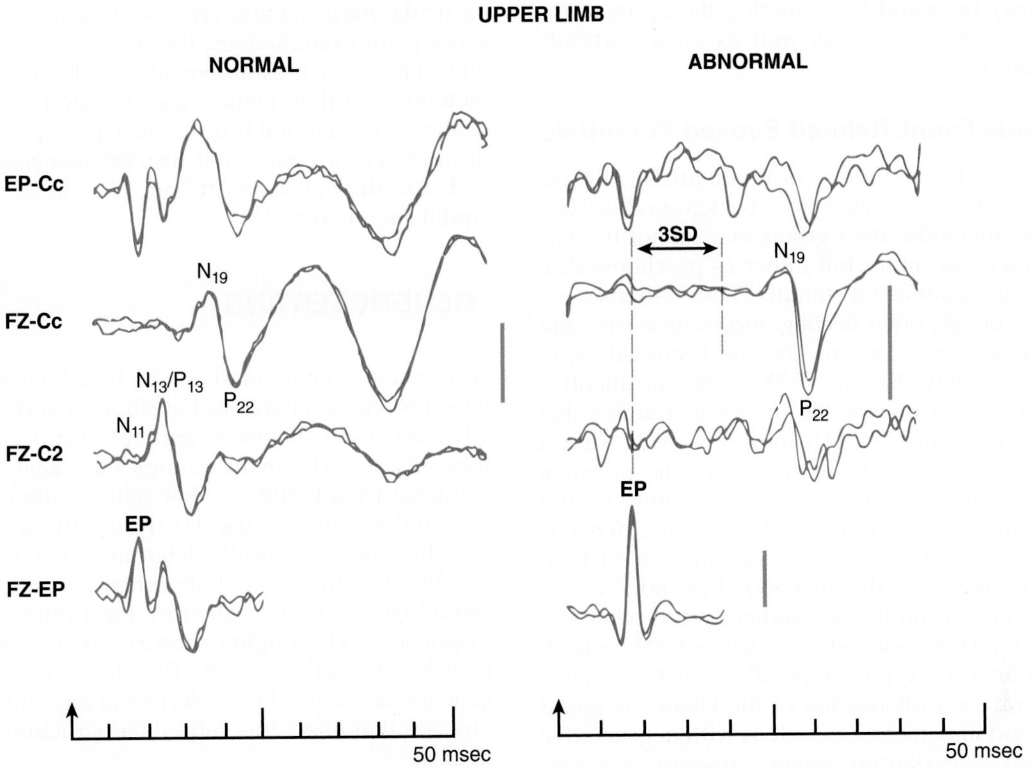

Figure 2-8. Short-latency SEPs produced by stimulation of the median nerve at the wrist. The set of responses shown at left is from a normal subject; the set at right is from a patient with multiple sclerosis who had no sensory symptoms or signs. In the patient, note the preservation of the brachial–plexus component (EP), the absence of the cervical cord (N11) and lower-medullary components (N/P13), and the latency of the thalamocortical components (N19 and P22), prolonged above the normal mean +3 SD for the interval from the brachial plexus potential. Unilateral stimulation occurred at a frequency of 5 per second. Each trace is the averaged response to 1,024 stimuli; the superimposed trace represents a repetition to demonstrate waveform consistency. Recording electrode locations are as follows: FZ, midfrontal; EP, the Erb point (the shoulder); C2, the middle back of the neck over the C2 cervical vertebra; and Cc, the scalp overlying the sensoriparietal cortex contralateral to the stimulated limb. Relative negativity at the second electrode caused an upward trace deflection. Amplitude calibration marks denote 2 mV. (Reproduced by permission from Chiappa and Ropper.)

The corresponding cortical wave after tibial or peroneal nerve stimulation is called N/P37.

For purposes of clinical interpretation, the generators of the SEP waves are assumed to be linked in series, so that an interwave prolongation in latency indicates a conduction defect between the generators of the two peaks involved (Chiappa and Ropper). Normal values are shown in Table 2-4. Recordings with pathologically verified lesions at these levels are to be found in the monograph by Chiappa. This test has been most helpful in establishing the existence of lesions in spinal roots, posterior columns, and brainstem in disorders such as the ruptured lumbar and cervical discs, multiple sclerosis, and lumbar and cervical spondylosis when the clinical data are uncertain. The cerebral counterpart also pertains—namely, that obliteration of the cortical waves (assuming that all preceding waves are unaltered) reflects profound damage to the somatosensory pathways in the hemisphere or to the cortex itself. For example, the bilateral absence of cortical somatosensory waves after cardiac arrest is a powerful predictor of a poor clinical outcome; the persistent absence of a cortical potential on one side after stroke usually indicates such profound damage that only a limited clinical recovery is to be expected.

Evoked potential techniques have also been used in the experimental study of olfactory and trigeminal sensation (see Chap. 12).

Magnetic Stimulation of the Motor System

It is possible, by using single-pulse high-amplitude magnetic stimulation, to directly activate the motor cortex (transcranial magnetic stimulation) and cervical spine segments, and to detect delays or lack of conduction in descending motor pathways. This technique, introduced by Marsden and associates, painlessly stimulates only the largest motor neurons (presumably Betz cells) and the fastest-conducting axons. Cervical magnetic stimulation is believed to activate the anterior roots. The difference in time between the motor cortical and cervical activation of hand or forearm muscles reflects the conduction velocity of the cortical–cervical cord motor neurons. The technique has been used to understand the organization, function, and recovery of the motor cortex and the pathophysiology of stroke, multiple sclerosis, and amyotrophic lateral sclerosis. Although the degree of functional deficit does not precisely correlate with the degree of electrophysiologic change, one expects that refinements of this technique may be useful in evaluating the status of the corticospinal motor system as well as other cortically based functions.

Endogenous Event-Related Evoked Potentials

Among the very late brain electrical potentials (>100-ms latency) that can be extracted from background activity by computer methods, are a group that cannot be classified as sensory or motor but rather as psychophysical responses to environmental stimuli. These responses are of very low voltage, often fleeting and inconsistent, and of unknown anatomic origin. The most studied types occur approximately 300 ms (P300) after an attentive subject identifies an unexpected or novel stimulus that has been inserted into a regular train of stimuli. Almost any stimulus modality can be used and the potential occurs even when a stimulus has been omitted from a regular pattern. The amplitude of the response depends on the difficulty of the task and has an inverse relationship to the frequency of the unexpected or "odd" event; the latency depends on the task difficulty and other features of testing. There is therefore no single P300; instead, there are numerous types, depending on the experimental paradigm. Prolongation of the latency is found with aging and in dementia as well as with degenerative diseases such as Parkinson disease, progressive supranuclear palsy, and Huntington chorea. The amplitude is reduced in schizophrenia and depression. The potential has been interpreted by some as a reflection of the subject's orienting behavior or attention and by others, including Donchin, who discovered the phenomenon, as related to an updating of the brain's representation of the environment. The P300 remains a curiosity for the clinical neurologist because abnormalities are detected only when large groups are compared to normal individuals, and the technique is not as standardized as the conventional evoked potentials. A review of the subject can be found in sections by Altenmüller and Gerloff and by Polich in the Niedermeyer and Lopes DaSilva text on electroencephalography.

ELECTROMYOGRAPHY AND NERVE CONDUCTION STUDIES

These are discussed in Chap. 45.

PSYCHOMETRY, PERIMETRY, AUDIOMETRY, AND TESTS OF LABYRINTHINE FUNCTION

These methods are used in defining and quantitating the nature of the psychologic or sensory deficits produced by disease of the nervous system. They are performed most often to obtain confirmation of a disorder of function in particular parts of the nervous system or to quantitate, by subsequent examinations, the progression of the underlying illness such as a dementia. A description of these methods and their clinical uses is found in the chapters dealing with cerebral function (Chap. 22), developmental disorders of the cerebrum (Chap. 28), dementia (Chap. 21), and disorders of vision (Chap. 13) and of hearing and equilibrium (Chap. 15).

GENETIC TESTING

Numerous genetic markers of heredofamilial disease have become available to the clinician and have greatly advanced both diagnosis and categorization of neurologic disease. The main examples are analyses of DNA extracted from blood or other cells for the identification of mutations (e.g., muscular dystrophy, spinocerebellar atrophies, and genetically determined polyneuropathies, and the quantification of abnormally long repetitions of certain trinucleotide sequences, most often used for the diagnosis of Huntington chorea). The use of these tests is elaborated in Chap. 39. The study of mitochondrial genetics has allowed the detection of an entire category of diseases that affect this subcellular structure, as detailed in Chap. 37.

BIOPSY OF MUSCLE, NERVE, SKIN, TEMPORAL ARTERY, BRAIN, AND OTHER TISSUE

The application of light, phase, and electron microscopy to the study of these tissues may be highly informative. The findings are discussed in Chaps. 37 (skin and conjunctivum in the diagnosis of metabolic storage diseases), 45 (muscle), and 46 (nerve). Temporal artery biopsy is indicated when giant cell arteritis is suspected (Chap. 34). Brain biopsy, aside from its main use in the direct sampling of a suspected neoplasm, may be diagnostic in cases of granulomatous angiitis, some forms of encephalitis, infectious abscesses. Biopsy of the pachymeninges or leptomeninges may disclose vasculitis, sarcoidosis, other granulomatous infiltrations, or an obscure infection, but its sensitivity is low. This is usually performed in concert with a biopsy of the underlying brain. Biopsy is now generally avoided in cases of suspected prion disease because of the risk of transmitting the causative agent. Abdominal fat pad biopsy is used in the diagnosis of amyloidosis.

In choosing to perform a biopsy in any of these clinical situations, the paramount issue is the likelihood of establishing a definitive diagnosis—one that would permit successful treatment or otherwise enhance the management of the disease.

References

Altenmüller EO, Münte TF, Gerloff C: *Neurocognitive function and the EEG*, in Niedermeyer E, Lopes DaSilva F (eds): *Electroencephalography: Basic Principles, Clinical Applications, and Related Fields*, 5th ed. Philadelphia, Lippincott Williams & Wilkins, 2005, pp 661–682.

American Electroencephalographic Society: Guidelines in electroencephalography, evoked potentials, and polysomnography. *J Clin Neurophysiol* 11:1–147, 1994.

Barnett GH, Ropper AH, Johnson KA: Physiological support and monitoring of critically ill patients during magnetic resonance imaging. *J Neurosurg* 68:246, 1988.

Barrows LJ, Hunter FT, Banker BQ: The nature and clinical significance of pigments in the cerebrospinal fluid. *Brain* 78:59, 1955.

Bigner SH: Cerebrospinal fluid (CSF) cytology: Current status and diagnostic applications. *J Neuropathol Exp Neurol* 51:235, 1992.

Blume WT, Kaibaro, Masato: *Atlas of Pediatric Electroencephalography*, 2nd ed. New York, Raven Press, 1999.

Chiappa KH, Ropper AH: Evoked potentials in clinical medicine. *N Engl J Med* 306:1140, 1205, 1982.

Chimowitz MI, Logigian EL, Caplan LR: The accuracy of bedside neurological diagnoses. *Ann Neurol* 28:78, 1990.

Ebersole JA, Pedley TA (eds): *Current Practice of Clinical EEG*, 3rd ed. Philadelphia, Lippincott Williams & Wilkins, 2003.

Dawson GD: A summation technique for the detection of small evoked potentials. *Electroencephalogr Clin Neurophysiol* 6:65, 1954.

Den Hartog-Jager WA: *Color Atlas of CSF Cytopathology*. New York, Elsevier-North Holland, 1980.

DeWeerd AW: *Atlas of EEG in the First Months of Life*. New York, Elsevier, 1995.

Filler AG, Kliot M, Howe FA, et al: Application of magnetic resonance in the evaluation of patients with peripheral nerve pathology. *J Neurosurg* 85:299, 1996.

Fishman RA: *Cerebrospinal Fluid in Diseases of the Nervous System*, 2nd ed. Philadelphia, Saunders, 1992.

Goldenshohn ES, Wolf S, Koszer S, Legatt A (eds): *EEG Interpretation*, 2nd ed. New York, Futura, 1999.

Greenberg JO (ed): *Neuroimaging: A Companion to Adams and Victor's Principles of Neurology*, 2nd ed. New York, McGraw-Hill, 1999.

Hahn JS, Tharp BR: Neonatal and pediatric electroencephalography, in Aminoff MJ (ed): *Electrodiagnosis in Clinical Neurology*, 4th ed. New York, Churchill Livingstone, 1999, pp 81–128.

Horowitz AL: *MRI Physics for Radiologists*, 2nd ed. New York, Springer, 1992.

Hughes JR: *EEG in Clinical Practice*, 2nd ed. Woburn, MA, Butterworth, 1994.

Huk WN, Gademann G, Friedman G: *MRI of Central Nervous System Diseases*. Berlin, Springer-Verlag, 1990.

Kanal E, Gillen J, Evans JA, et al: Survey of reproductive health among female MR workers. *Radiology* 187:395, 1993.

Latchaw RE (ed): *MRI and CT Imaging of the Head, Neck, and Spine*, 2nd ed. St. Louis, Mosby-Year Book, 1991.

Marsden CD, Merton PA, Morton HB: Direct electrical stimulation of corticospinal pathways through the intact scalp and in human subjects. *Adv Neurol* 39:387, 1983.

Modic MT, Masaryk TJ, Ross JS, et al: *Magnetic Resonance Imaging of the Spine*, 2nd ed. St. Louis, Mosby-Year Book, 1994.

Morelli JN, Runge VM, Ai F, et al: An image-based approach to understanding the physics of MR artifacts. *RadioGraphics* 31:849, 2011.

Polich J: P300 in clinical applications, in Niedermeyer E, Lopes DaSilva F (eds): *Electroencephalography: Basic Principles, Clinical Applications, and Related Fields*, 4th ed. Baltimore, Williams & Wilkins, 1999, pp 1073–1091.

Scher MS, Painter MJ: Electroencephalographic diagnosis of neonatal seizures, in Wasterlain CG, Vert P (eds): *Neonatal Seizures*. New York, Raven Press, 1990.

Shellock FG: *Reference Manual for Magnetic Safety*. CRC, Boca Raton, 2002.

Stockard-Pope JE, Werner SS, Bickford RG: *Atlas of Neonatal Electroencephalography*, 2nd ed. New York, Raven Press, 1992.

Strupp M, Schueler O, Straube A, et al: "Atraumatic" Sprotte needle reduces the incidence of post-lumbar puncture headache. *Neurology* 57:2310, 2001.

Vernooij MW, Ikran MA, Tanghe HL, et al: Incidental findings on brain MRI in the general population. *N Engl J Med* 357: 1821, 2007.

PART 2

CARDINAL MANIFESTATIONS OF NEUROLOGIC DISEASE

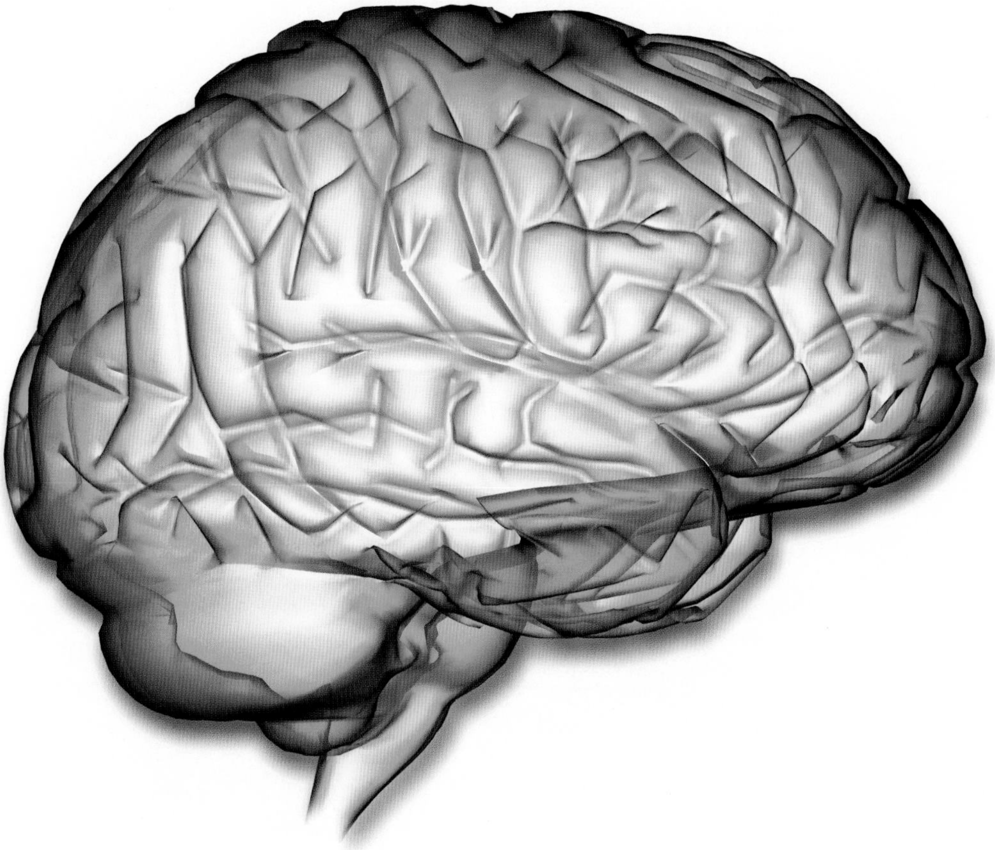

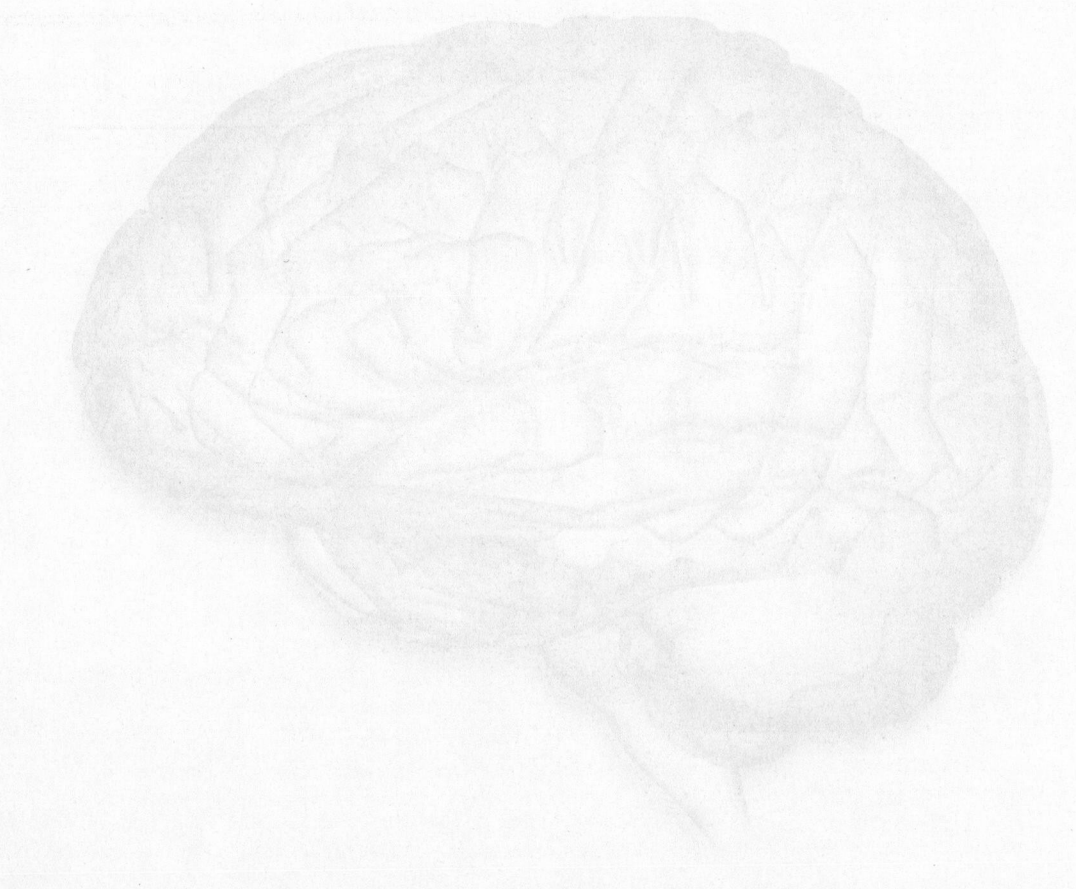

SECTION 1

Disorders of Motility

The control of motor function, to which much of the human nervous system is committed, is accomplished through the integrated action of a vast array of segmental and suprasegmental motor neurons. As originally conceived by Hughlings Jackson in 1858, purely on the basis of clinical observations, the motor system is organized hierarchically in three levels, each higher level controlling the one below. It was Jackson's concept that the spinal and brainstem neurons represent the lowest, simplest, and most highly organized motor centers; that the motor neurons of the posterior frontal region represent a more complex and less closely organized second motor center; and that the prefrontal parts of the cerebrum are the third and highest motor center. This scheme is still regarded as being essentially correct, although Jackson failed to recognize the importance of the parietal lobe and basal ganglia in motor control.

Since Jackson's time, physiologists, and more recently, experts in functional imaging, have repeatedly analyzed these three levels of motor organization and found them to be valid but to have remarkably complex relationships. Motor and sensory systems, although separated for practical clinical purposes, are not independent entities but are closely integrated. Without sensory feedback, motor control is ineffective. And at the higher cortical levels of motor control, motivation, planning, and other frontal lobe activities that subserve volitional movement are preceded and modulated by activity in the parietal sensory cortex.

Motor activities include not only those that alter the position of a limb or other part of the body (isotonic contraction) but also those that stabilize posture (isometric contraction). Movements that are performed slowly are called *ramp movements*. Very rapid movements, which are too fast for sensory control, are called *ballistic*. Physiologic studies, cast in their simplest terms, indicate that the following parts of the nervous system are engaged primarily in the control of movement and, in the course of disease, yield a number of characteristic derangements.

1. *The large motor neurons in the anterior horns of the spinal cord and the motor nuclei of the brainstem*. The axons of these nerve cells comprise the anterior spinal roots, the spinal nerves, and the cranial nerves, and they innervate the skeletal muscles. These nerve cells and their axons constitute the *lower motor neurons*, complete lesions of which result in a loss of all movement—voluntary, automatic, postural, and reflex. The lower motor neurons are the *final common pathway* by which all neural impulses are transmitted to muscle.
2. *The motor neurons in the frontal cortex adjacent to the rolandic fissure* (motor strip) connect with the spinal motor neurons by a system of fibers known, because of the shape of its fasciculus in the medulla, as the *pyramidal tract*. Because the motor fibers that extend from the cerebral cortex to the spinal cord are not confined to the pyramidal

tract, they are more accurately designated as *the corticospinal tract*, or, alternatively, as *the upper motor neurons*, to distinguish them from the lower motor neurons.

3. *Several brainstem nuclei that project to the spinal cord, notably the pontine and medullary reticular nuclei, vestibular nuclei, and red nuclei*. These nuclei and their descending fibers subserve the neural mechanisms of posture and movement, particularly when movement is highly automatic and repetitive. Certain of these brainstem nuclei are influenced by the motor or premotor regions of the cortex, e.g., via corticoreticulospinal relays.
4. *Two subcortical systems, the basal ganglia (striatum, pallidum, and related structures, including the substantia nigra and subthalamic nucleus)* and the *cerebellum*. Each of these systems plays an important role in the control of muscle tone, posture, and coordination.

These are the subjects of the following chapters.

3

Motor Paralysis

Definitions

Paralysis means loss of voluntary movement as a result of interruption of one of the motor pathways at any point from the cerebrum to the muscle fiber. A lesser degree of paralysis is spoken of as paresis. The word plegia comes from a Greek word meaning "to strike," and the word palsy is from an old French word that has the same meaning as paralysis. One generally uses paralysis or plegia for severe or complete loss of motor function and paresis for partial loss.

THE LOWER MOTOR NEURON

Anatomic and Physiologic Considerations

Each spinal and cranial motor nerve cell, through the extensive arborization of the terminal part of its efferent fiber, comes into contact with only a few or up to 1,000 or more muscle fibers; together, the nerve cell, its axons, and the muscle fibers they subserve constitute the *motor unit*. All variations in the force, range, rate, and type of movement are determined by the number and size of motor units called into action and the frequency and sequence of firing of each motor unit. Weak movements involve relatively few small motor units; powerful movements recruit many more units that accumulate to an increasing size.

Within a few days after interruption of a motor nerve, the individual denervated muscle fibers begin to contract spontaneously. This isolated activity of individual muscle fibers is called *fibrillation*. Inability of the isolated fiber to maintain a stable membrane potential is the likely explanation. Fibrillation is so fine that it cannot be seen through the intact skin, but it can be recorded as a small, repetitive, short-duration potential in the electromyogram (EMG) (Chap. 45). When a motor neuron becomes diseased, it may manifest increased irritability, i.e., the axon is unstable and capable of spontaneous impulse generation, and all the muscle fibers that it controls may discharge sporadically, in isolation from other units. The result of contraction of one or several such motor units is a visible twitch of a muscle fascicle, or *fasciculation*, which appears in the EMG as a large spontaneous muscle action potential. Simultaneous or sequential spontaneous contractions of multiple motor units cause a rippling of muscle, a condition known as *myokymia*. If the motor neuron is destroyed, all the muscle fibers that it innervates undergo profound atrophy—termed denervation atrophy.

The motor nerve fibers of each ventral root intermingle with those of neighboring roots to form plexuses, and then the named peripheral nerves. Although the muscles are innervated roughly according to segments of the spinal cord, each large muscle is supplied by two or more roots. In contrast, a single peripheral nerve usually provides the complete motor innervation of a muscle or group of muscles. For this reason, paralysis caused by disease of the anterior horn cells or anterior roots has a different topographic pattern than paralysis following interruption of a peripheral nerve. These patterns follow the distribution shown in Table 46-1. For example, section of the L5 motor root causes paralysis of the extensors of the foot with a foot drop and weakness of inversion of the foot, whereas a lesion of the peroneal nerve also causes foot drop but does not affect the invertors of the foot that are also supplied by L5 but via the tibial nerve.

All motor activity, even the most elementary reflex type, requires the synchronous activity of many muscles. Analysis of a relatively simple movement, such as clenching the fist, conveys some idea of the complexity of the underlying neuromuscular arrangements. In this act the primary movement is a contraction of the flexor muscles of the fingers, the flexor digitorum sublimis and profundus, the flexor pollicis longus and brevis, and the abductor pollicis brevis. In the terminology of Beevor, these muscles act as agonists, or prime movers. For flexion to be smooth and forceful, the extensor muscles (antagonists) must relax at the same rate as the flexors contract (reciprocal innervation, or Sherrington law). The muscles that flex the fingers also flex the wrist. If it is desired that only the fingers flex, the extensors of the wrist must be brought into play to prevent its flexion; they are synergists. During this action of the hand, appropriate flexor and extensor muscles stabilize the wrist, elbow, and shoulder; muscles that accomplish this serve as fixators. The coordination of agonists, antagonists, synergists, and fixators is effected mainly by segmental spinal reflexes under the guidance of proprioceptive sensory stimuli. In general, the more delicate the movement, the more precise must be the coordination between agonist and antagonist muscles.

All voluntary ballistic (phasic) movements towards a target are accomplished by the activation of ensembles of motor neurons, large ones supplying large motor units and small ones, small motor units. The smaller ones are more efficiently activated by sensory afferents from muscle spindles, more tonically active, and more readily recruited in reflex activities, postural maintenance, walking, and running. The large motor units participate mainly in phasic movements, which are characterized by an initial burst of activity in the agonist muscles, then a burst in the antagonists, followed by a third smaller burst in the agonists. The strength of the initial agonist burst determines the speed and distance of the movement, but there is always the same triphasic pattern of agonist, antagonist, and agonist activity (Hallett et al). The basal ganglia and cerebellum set the pattern and timing of the muscle action in any projected motor performance. These points are discussed further in Chaps. 4 and 5.

Unlike the phasic movements just described, certain basic motor activities do not involve reciprocal innervation. In support of the body in an upright posture, when the legs must act as rigid pillars, and in shivering, agonists and antagonists contract simultaneously. Locomotion requires that the extensor pattern of reflex standing be inhibited and that the coordinated pattern of alternating stepping movements be substituted; the latter is accomplished by multisegmental spinal and brainstem reflexes, the so-called locomotor centers. Suprasegmental control of the axial and proximal limb musculature (antigravity postural mechanisms) is mediated primarily by the reticulospinal and vestibulospinal tracts and manipulatory movements of the distal extremity muscles, by the rubrospinal and corticospinal tracts. These aspects of motor function are elaborated further on.

Muscle stretch (tendon) reflex activity and muscle tone depend on the status of the large motor neurons of the anterior horn (the alpha motor neurons), the muscle spindles and their afferent fibers, and the small anterior horn cells (gamma neurons), whose axons terminate on the small intrafusal muscle fibers within the spindles. Each anterior horn cell has on its surface membrane approximately 10,000 receptive synaptic terminals. Some of these terminals are excitatory, others inhibitory; in combination, they determine the activity of the neuron. Beta motor neurons effect cocontraction of both spindle and nonspindle fibers, but the physiologic significance of this innervation is not fully understood. Some of the gamma motor neurons are tonically active at rest, keeping the intrafusal (nuclear chain) muscle fibers taut and sensitive to active and passive changes in muscle length.

A tap on a tendon stretches or perhaps causes vibration of the spindle and activates its nuclear bag fibers. Afferent projections from these fibers synapse directly with alpha motor neurons in the same and adjacent spinal segments; these neurons, in turn, send impulses to the skeletal muscle fibers, resulting in the familiar monosynaptic muscle contraction or monophasic (myotatic) stretch reflex, commonly referred to as the tendon reflex or "tendon jerk" (Fig. 3-1), more correctly called the muscle stretch or proprioceptive reflex. All this occurs within 25 ms of sudden stretch. The alpha neurons of antagonist muscles are simultaneously inhibited but through disynaptic rather than monosynaptic connections. This is accomplished in part by inhibitory interneurons (*reciprocal inhibition*), which also receive input from descending pathways. Renshaw cells also participate by providing negative feedback through inhibitory synapses of alpha motor neurons (*recurrent inhibition*).

Thus the setting of the spindle fibers and the state of excitability of the alpha and gamma neurons (influenced greatly by descending fiber systems) determine the level of activity of the tendon reflexes and muscle tone (the responsiveness of muscle to stretch). Other mechanisms, of an inhibitory nature, involve the Golgi tendon organs, for which the stimulus is tension produced by active contraction of muscle. These encapsulated receptors, which lie in the tendinous and aponeurotic insertions of muscle, activate afferent fibers that end on internuncial cells, which, in turn, project to alpha motor neurons, thus forming a disynaptic reflex arc. Golgi tendon receptors are silent in relaxed muscle and during passive stretch; they serve, together with muscle spindles, to monitor or calibrate the length and force of muscle contraction under different conditions. They also play a role in naturally occurring limb movements, particularly in locomotion.

The alpha motor neurons of the medial parts of the anterior horn supply trunk or axial muscles, and neurons of the lateral parts supply the appendicular muscles. The largest neurons, in Rexed layer IX (see Fig. 8-1*B*), innervate large muscles with large motor units. Smaller anterior horn cells innervate small muscles and control more delicate movements, particularly those in the fingers and hand. Both groups of alpha neurons receive projections from neurons in the intermediate Rexed layers (V to VIII) and from propriospinal neurons in the fasciculi proprii of adjacent spinal segments (see Fig. 8-1*B*). All the facilitatory and inhibitory influences supplied by cutaneous and proprioceptive afferent and descending suprasegmental neurons are coordinated at segmental levels. For further details the reader may consult Burke and Lance and also Davidoff (1992).

There is considerable information concerning the pharmacology of motor neurons. The large neurons of the anterior horns of the spinal cord contain high concentrations of choline acetyltransferase and use acetylcholine as their transmitter at the neuromuscular junction. The main neurotransmitters of the descending corticospinal tract, in so far as can be determined in humans, are aspartate and glutamate. Glycine is the neurotransmitter released by Renshaw cells, which are responsible for recurrent inhibition, and by interneurons that mediate reciprocal inhibition during reflex action. Gamma-aminobutyric acid (GABA) serves as the inhibitory neurotransmitter of interneurons in the posterior horn. L-glutamate and L-aspartate are released by primary afferent terminals and interneurons and act specifically on excitatory amino acid receptors. There are also descending cholinergic,

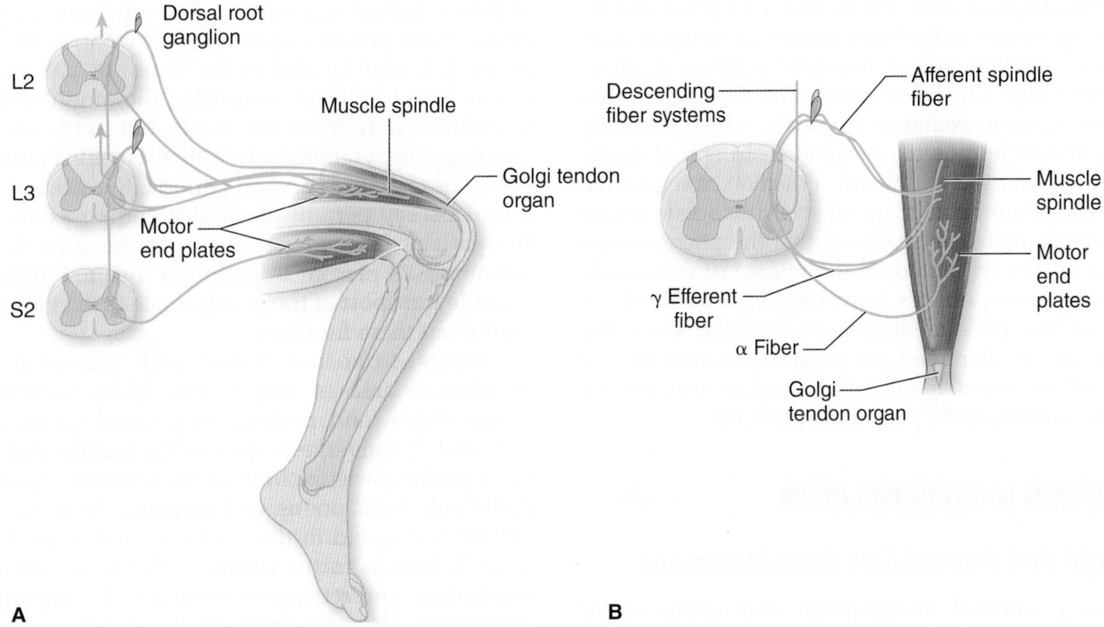

Figure 3-1. *A*. Patellar tendon reflex. Sensory fibers of the femoral nerve (spinal segments L2 and L3) mediate this myotatic reflex. The principal receptors are the muscle spindles, which respond to brisk stretching of the muscle effected by tapping the patellar tendon. Afferent fibers from muscle spindles are shown entering only the L3 spinal segment, while afferent fibers from the Golgi tendon organ are shown entering only the L2 spinal segment. In this monosynaptic reflex, afferent fibers entering spinal segments L2 and L3 and efferent fibers issuing from the anterior horn cells of these and lower levels complete the reflex arc. Motor fibers shown leaving the S2 spinal segment and passing to the hamstring muscles demonstrate the disynaptic pathway by which inhibitory influences are exerted upon an antagonistic muscle group during the reflex. *B*. The gamma loop is illustrated. Gamma efferent fibers (γ) pass to the polar portions of the muscle spindle. Contractions of the intrafusal fibers in the polar parts of the spindle stretch the nuclear bag region and thus cause an afferent impulse to be conducted centrally. The afferent fibers from the spindle synapse with many alpha motor neurons. Because the alpha motor neurons innervate extrafusal muscle fibers, excitation of the alpha motor neurons by spindle afferents causes a cocontraction of the muscle. In this way, both gamma and alpha fibers can simultaneously activate muscle contraction. Both alpha and gamma motor neurons are influenced by descending fiber systems from supraspinal levels. (Adapted by permission from Carpenter MB, Sutin J: *Human Neuroanatomy*, 8th ed. Baltimore, Williams & Wilkins, 1983.)

adrenergic, and dopaminergic axons, which play a less-well-defined role in reflex functions.

Paralysis Due to Lesions of the Lower Motor Neurons

If all, or practically all, peripheral motor fibers supplying a muscle are interrupted, the voluntary, postural, and reflex movements of that muscle are abolished. The muscle becomes lax and soft and does not resist passive stretching, a condition known as flaccidity. Muscle tone—the slight resistance that normal relaxed muscle offers to passive movement—is reduced (hypotonia or atonia). The denervated muscle undergoes extreme atrophy, being reduced to 20 or 30 percent of its original bulk within 3 to 4 months. The reaction of the muscle to sudden stretch, as by tapping its tendon, is lost (areflexia). Damage restricted to only a portion of the motor fibers supplying the muscle results in partial paralysis, or paresis, and a proportionate diminution in the force and speed of contraction. The atrophy will be less and the tendon reflex reduced instead of lost. The electrodiagnosis of denervation depends upon finding fibrillations, fasciculations, and other abnormalities on needle electrode examination. However, some of these abnormalities do not appear until several days or a week or two after nerve injury (see Chap. 45).

Lower motor neuron (infranuclear) paralysis is the direct result of loss of function or destruction of anterior horn cells or their axons in anterior roots and nerves. The signs and symptoms vary according to the location of the lesion. In any individual case, the most important clinical question is whether sensory changes coexist. The combination of a flaccid, areflexic paralysis and sensory changes usually indicates involvement of mixed motor and sensory nerves or of both anterior and posterior roots. If sensory changes are absent, the lesion must be situated in the anterior gray matter of the spinal cord, in the anterior roots, in a purely motor branch of a peripheral nerve, or in motor axons alone (or in the muscle itself). At times it may be impossible to distinguish between nuclear (spinal) and anterior root (radicular) lesions.

Preserved and often heightened tendon reflexes and spasticity in muscles weakened by lesions of the corticospinal systems attest to the integrity of the spinal segments below the level of the lesion. However, acute and profound spinal cord lesions and, to a lesser extent, corticospinal lesions in the brainstem and cerebrum, may temporarily abolish spinal myotatic reflexes ("spinal shock"; see Chap. 44). This is caused by the interruption of descending tonic excitatory impulses, which normally maintain a sufficient level of excitation in spinal motor neurons to permit the peripheral activation of segmental reflexes. The attenuation of spinal shock by opiate antagonists, such as naloxone, suggests that the phenomenon is at least in part mediated by the release of previously stored endogenous opiates from the distal terminals of neurons in the periaqueductal gray matter. Once the stored opiates are depleted, the presynaptic inhibition of motor neurons ceases, heralding the end of spinal shock and the beginning of the period of spasticity.

THE UPPER MOTOR NEURON

Anatomic and Physiologic Considerations

The terms pyramidal, corticospinal, and upper motor neuron are often used interchangeably, although they are not altogether synonymous. The pyramidal tract, strictly speaking, designates only those fibers that course longitudinally in the pyramid of the medulla oblongata. Of all the fiber bundles in the brain, the pyramidal tract has been known for the longest time, the first accurate description having been given by Türck in 1851. It descends from the cerebral cortex; traverses the subcortical white matter (corona radiata), internal capsule, cerebral peduncle, basis pontis (ventral pons), and pyramid of the upper medulla; decussates in the lower medulla; and continues its caudal course in the lateral funiculus (column) of the spinal cord—hence the alternative name *corticospinal tract*. This is the only *direct* long-fiber connection between the cerebral cortex and the spinal cord (Fig. 3-2). The *indirect* pathways through which the cortex influences spinal motor neurons are the rubrospinal, reticulospinal, vestibulospinal, and tectospinal; these tracts do not run in the pyramid. All of these pathways, direct and indirect, are embraced by the term *upper motor neuron* or supranuclear, meaning above the anterior horn cells.

A major source of confusion about the pyramidal tract stems from the traditional view, formulated at the turn of the 20th century, that it originates entirely from the large motor cells of Betz in the fifth layer of the precentral convolution (the primary motor cortex, or area 4 of Brodmann[1]) (Figs. 3-3 and 22-1). However, there are only some 25,000 to 35,000 Betz cells, whereas the medullary pyramid contains about 1 million axons (Lassek). Thus the pyramidal tract contains many fibers that arise from cortical neurons other than Betz cells, particularly in Brodmann areas 4 and 6 (the frontal cortex immediately rostral to area 4, including the medial portion of the superior frontal gyrus, i.e., the supplementary motor area); in the primary somatosensory cortex (Brodmann areas 3, 1, and 2); and in the superior parietal lobule (areas 5 and 7). Data concerning the origin of the pyramidal tract in humans are scanty, but in the monkey, by counting the pyramidal axons that remained after cortical excisions and long survival periods, Russell and DeMyer found that 40 percent of the descending axons arose in the parietal lobe, 31 percent in motor area 4, and the remaining 29 percent in premotor area 6. Studies of retrograde transport of tracer substance in the monkey have confirmed these findings.

Fibers from the motor and premotor cortices (Brodmann areas 4 and 6, Fig. 22-1), supplementary motor cortex, and portions of parietal cortex (areas 1, 3, 5, and 7) converge in the corona radiata and descend through the posterior limb of the internal capsule, basis pedunculi, basis pontis, and medulla. As the corticospinal tracts descend in the cerebrum and brainstem, they send collaterals to the striatum, thalamus, red nucleus, cerebellum, and reticular formations. Accompanying the corticospinal tracts in the brainstem are the corticobulbar tracts, which are distributed to motor nuclei of the cranial nerves ipsilaterally and contralaterally (Fig. 3-2). It has been possible to trace the direct projection of axons of cortical neurons to the trigeminal, facial, ambiguus, and hypoglossal nuclei (Iwatsubo et al). No axons were seen to terminate directly in the oculomotor, trochlear, abducens, or vagal nuclei. Insofar as the corticobulbar and corticospinal fibers have a similar origin and the motor nuclei of the brainstem are the homologues of the motor neurons of the spinal cord, the term *upper motor neurons* may suitably be applied to both these systems of fibers.

The corticospinal tracts decussate at the lower end of the medulla, although some of their fibers may cross above this level. The fibers destined for the upper limb neurons cross first (more rostrally). The proportion of crossed and uncrossed fibers varies to some extent from one person to another. About 75 to 80 percent of the fibers cross and the remaining fibers descend ipsilaterally, mostly in the uncrossed ventral corticospinal tract. In exceptional cases, these tracts cross completely; equally rarely, they remain uncrossed. These variations are probably of functional significance in determining the amount of neurologic deficit that results from a unilateral lesion such as capsular infarction. A few well-studied cases are found, such as the one described by Terakawa and colleagues, of acute stroke of the cerebral hemisphere causing hemiplegia on the same side. Also, Yakovlev found 3 instances of completely uncrossed pyramids among 130 autopsies of mentally retarded neonates but considering the maldevelopment of these brains, the finding may not be surprising.

The corticospinal tract is phylogenetically relatively new, being found only in mammals, which probably accounts for its variability between individuals as compared to the older vestibulospinal, rubrospinal and reticulospinalparapyramidal systems, which are invariant among persons. Uncrossed fibers in the corticospinal tract account for mirror movements that are seen during efforts at fine motor tasks, particularly in children, and

[1]Numbered areas in this and subsequent chapters refer to Brodmann areas of the cerebral cortex that are discussed in Chap. 23. "Layers" refer to the six neuronal layers of the cerebral cortex, also shown in detail in Chap. 23, on Cerebral Localization.

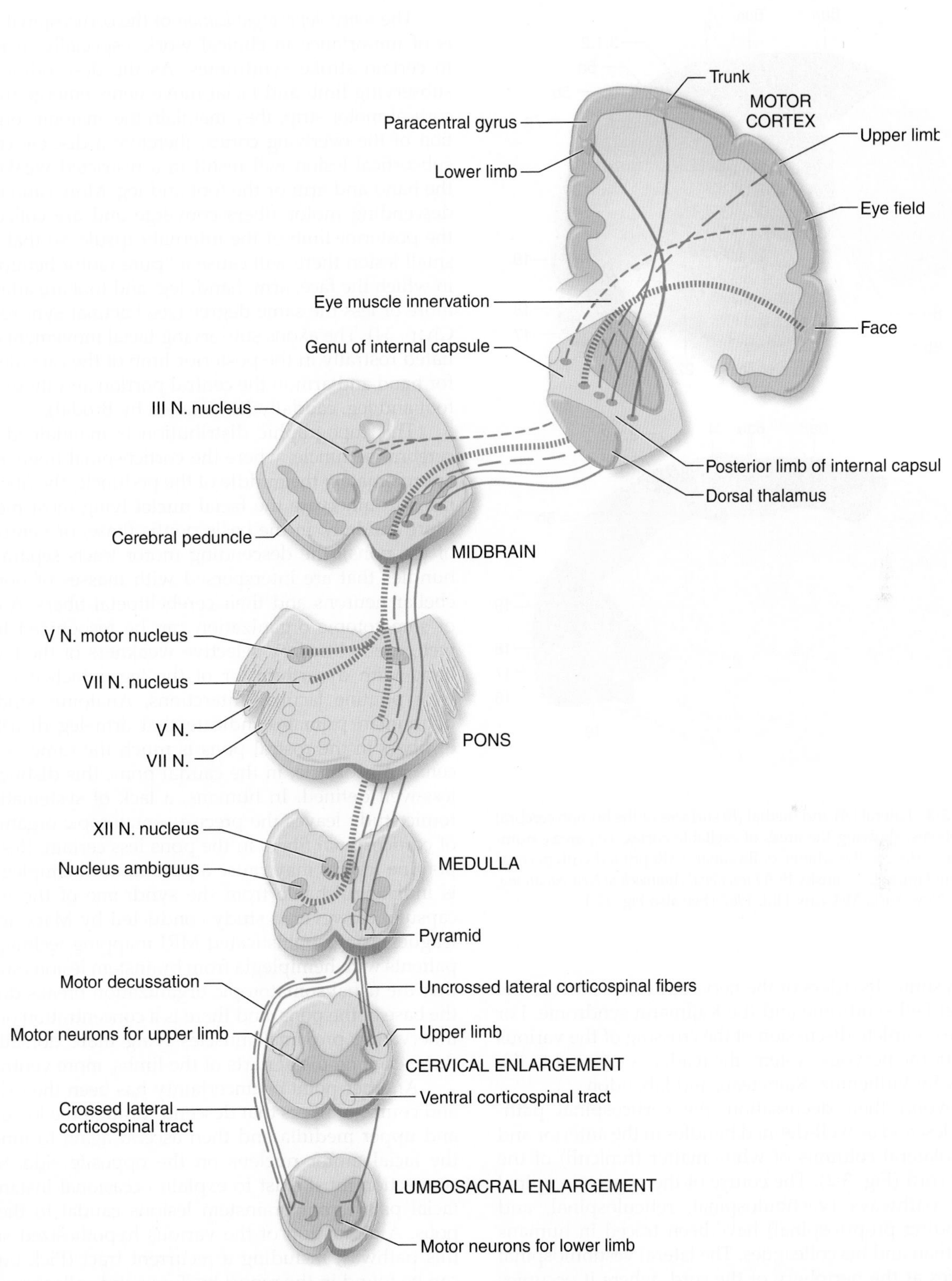

Figure 3-2. Corticospinal and corticobulbar tracts. The various lines indicate the trajectories of these pathways, from their origin in particular parts of the cerebral cortex to their nuclei of termination.

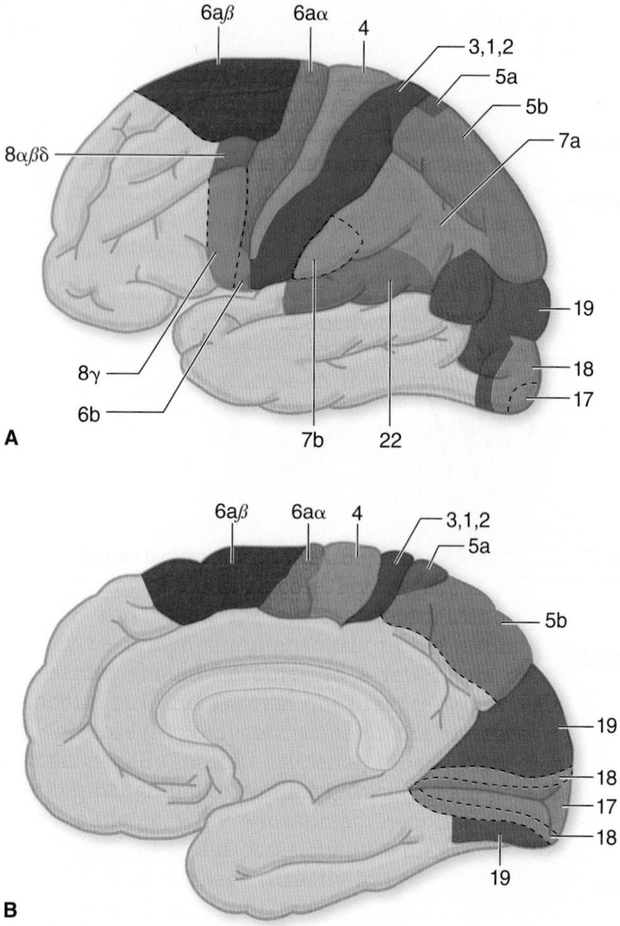

Figure 3-3. Lateral (*A*) and medial (*B*) surfaces of the human cerebral hemispheres, showing the areas of excitable cortex, i.e., areas, numbered according to the scheme of Brodmann. (Reprinted with permission from House EL, Pansky B: *A Functional Approach to Neuroanatomy*, 2nd ed. New York, McGraw-Hill, 1967.) See also Fig. 22-1.

also in some disorders of the nervous system such as the Klippel-Feil syndrome and the Kallmann syndrome. For a more complete discussion of the crossing of the various tracts of the nervous system, the reader is referred to the review by Vulliemoz, Raineteau, and Jabaudon.

Beyond their decussation, the corticospinal pathways descend as well-defined bundles in the anterior and posterolateral columns of white matter (funiculi) of the spinal cord (Fig. 3-2). The course of the noncorticospinal motor pathways (vestibulospinal, reticulospinal, and descending propriospinal) have been traced in humans by Nathan and his colleagues. The lateral vestibulospinal tract lies at the periphery of the cord, where it occupies the most anterolateral portion of the anterior funiculus. The medial vestibulospinal fibers mingle with those of the medial longitudinal fasciculus. Reticulospinal fibers are less compact; they descend bilaterally, and most of them come to lie just anterior to the lateral corticospinal tract. The descending propriospinal pathway consists of a series of short fibers (one or two segments long) lying next to the gray matter.

The *somatotopic organization* of the corticospinal system is of importance in clinical work, especially in relation to certain stroke syndromes. As the descending axons subserving limb and facial movements emerge from the cortical motor strip, they maintain the anatomic organization of the overlying cortex; therefore a discrete cortical–subcortical lesion will result in a restricted weakness of the hand and arm or the foot and leg. More caudally, the descending motor fibers converge and are collected in the posterior limb of the internal capsule, so that even a small lesion there will cause a "pure motor hemiplegia," in which the face, arm, hand, leg, and foot are affected to more or less the same degree (see Lacunar syndromes in Chap. 34). The axons subserving facial movement are situated rostrally in the posterior limb of the capsule, those for hand and arm in the central portion and those for the foot and leg, caudally (as detailed by Brodal).

This topographic distribution is maintained in the cerebral peduncle, where the corticospinal fibers occupy approximately the middle of the peduncle, the fibers destined to innervate the facial nuclei lying most medially. More caudally, in the basis pontis (base, or ventral part of the pons), the descending motor tracts separate into bundles that are interspersed with masses of pontocerebellar neurons and their cerebellipetal fibers. A degree of somatotopic organization can be recognized here as well, exemplified by selective weakness of the face and hand with dysarthria, or of the leg, which may occur with pontine lacunar infarctions. Anatomic studies in nonhuman primates indicate that arm–leg distribution of fibers in the rostral pons is much the same as in the cerebral peduncle; in the caudal pons, this distinction is less-well defined. In humans, a lack of systematic anatomic study leaves the precise somatotopic organization of corticospinal fibers in the pons less certain. Restricted pontine lesions may cause a pure motor hemiplegia that is indistinguishable from the syndrome of the internal capsule. However, a study conducted by Marx and colleagues using sophisticated MRI mapping techniques of patients with hemiplegia from brainstem lesions suggests that the usual somatotopic organization breaks down in the base of the pons, and there is a concentration of fibers innervating proximal muscles lying more dorsally and those exciting distal parts of the limbs, more ventrally.

Another point of uncertainty has been the existence and course of fibers that descend through the lower pons and upper medulla and then ascend again to innervate the facial motor nucleus on the opposite side. Such a connection must exist to explain occasional instances of facial palsy from brainstem lesions caudal to the midpons. A discussion of the various hypothesized sites of this pathway, including a recurrent tract (Pick bundle), can be found in the report by Terao and colleagues. They conclude from imaging studies that corticobulbar fibers destined for the facial nucleus descend in the ventromedial pons to the level of the upper medulla, where they decussate and then ascend again; but there is considerable variation between individuals in this configuration.

The descending pontine bundles, now devoid of their corticopontine fibers, reunite to form the medullary pyramid. The brachial–crural pattern may persist in the pyramids and is certainly reconstituted in the lateral columns of the spinal cord (Fig. 8-3), but it should be emphasized that the topographic separation of motor fibers at cervical, thoracic, lumbar, and sacral levels is not as discrete as usually shown in schematic diagrams of the spinal cord.

The corticospinal tracts and other upper motor neurons terminate mainly in relation to nerve cells in the intermediate zone of spinal gray matter (internuncial neurons), from which motor impulses are then transmitted to the anterior horn cells. Only 10 to 20 percent of corticospinal fibers (presumably the thick, rapidly conducting axons derived from Betz cells) establish direct synaptic connections with the large motor neurons of the anterior horns.

Motor, Premotor, and Supplementary Motor Cortices and Cerebral Control of Movement

The *motor area of the cerebral cortex* is defined physiologically as the region of electrically excitable cortex from which isolated movements can be evoked by stimuli of minimal intensity. The muscle groups of the contralateral face, arm, trunk, and leg are represented in the primary motor cortex (area 4 in Fig. 3-3), those of the face being in the most inferior part of the precentralgyrus on the lateral surface of the cerebral hemisphere and those of the leg in the paracentral lobule on the medial surface of the cerebral hemisphere. The parts of the body capable of the most delicate movements have, in general, the largest cortical representation, as displayed in the motor homunculus ("little man," a term first suggested by Wilder Penfield) shown in Fig. 3-4.

Area 6, the *premotor area*, is also electrically excitable but requires more intense stimuli than area 4 to evoke movements. Stimulation of its caudal aspect (area 6a) produces responses that are similar to those elicited from area 4. These responses are probably produced by transmission of impulses from all of area 6a to area 4 (as they cannot be obtained after ablation of area 4). Stimulation of the rostral premotor area (area 6a) elicits more general movement patterns, predominantly of proximal limb musculature. The latter movements are effected via pathways other than those derived from area 4 (hence, "parapyramidal"). Very strong stimuli elicit movements from a wide area of premotor frontal and parietal cortex, and the same movements may be obtained from several widely separated points. From this it may be assumed, as Ash and Georgopoulus point out, that the premotor cortex includes several anatomically distinct subregions with different afferent and efferent connections. In general, it may be said that the motor–premotor cortex is capable of synthesizing agonist actions into an almost infinite variety of finely graded, highly differentiated patterns. These are directed by visual (area 7) and tactile (area 5) sensory information and supported by appropriate postural mechanisms.

The *supplementary motor area* is the most anterior portion of area 6 on the medial surface of the cerebral hemisphere (area 6a in Fig. 3-3*B*). Stimulation of this area may induce relatively gross ipsilateral or contralateral movements, bilateral tonic contractions of the limbs, contraversive movements of the head and eyes with tonic contraction of the contralateral arm, and sometimes inhibition of voluntary motor activity and vocal arrest.

Precisely how the motor cortex controls movements is still a controversial matter. The traditional view, based on the interpretations of Hughlings Jackson and of Sherrington, has been that the motor cortex is organized not in terms of individual muscles but of movements, i.e., the coordinated contraction of groups of muscles. Jackson visualized a widely overlapping representation of muscle

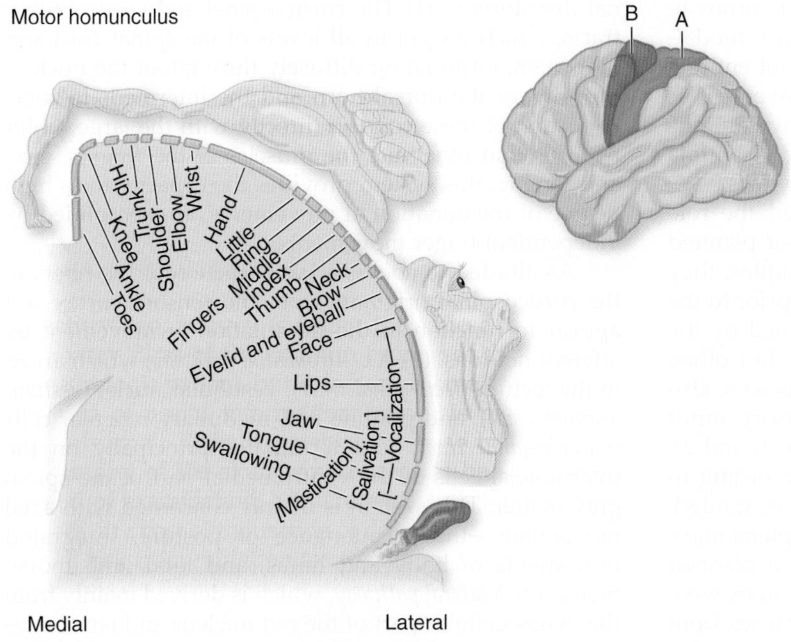

Figure 3-4. The representation of body parts in the motor cortex, commonly called the motor homunculus. The large area of cortex devoted to motor control of the hand, lips, and face is evident. B in the smaller diagram represents the motor cortex; A is the sensory cortex.

groups in the cerebral cortex on the basis of his observation that a patient could recover the use of a limb following destruction of the limb area as defined by cortical stimulation. This view was supported by Sherrington's observations that stimulation of the cortical surface activated not solitary muscles but a combination of muscles, and always in a reciprocal fashion—i.e., in a manner that maintained the expected relationship between agonists and antagonists. He also noted the inconstancy of stimulatory effects; the stimulation of a given cortical point that initiated flexion of a part on one occasion might initiate extension on another.

These interpretations must be viewed with circumspection, as must all observations based on the electrical stimulation of the surface of the cortex. It has been shown that to stimulate motor cells from the surface, the electric current has to penetrate the cortex to layer V, where these neurons are located, inevitably activating a large number of other cortical neurons. The elegant experiments of Asanuma and of Evarts and his colleagues, who stimulated the depths of the cortex with microelectrodes, demonstrated the existence of discrete zones of efferent neurons that control the contraction of individual muscles; moreover, the continued stimulation of a given efferent zone often facilitated rather than inhibited the contraction of the antagonists. These investigators have also shown that cells in the efferent zone receive afferent impulses from the particular muscle to which the efferent neurons project. When the effects of many stimulations at various depths were correlated with the exact sites of each penetration, cells that projected to a particular pool of spinal motor neurons were found to be arranged in radially aligned columns approximately 1 mm in diameter.

The columnar arrangement of cells in the sensorimotor cortex had been appreciated for many years; the wealth of radial interconnections between the cells in these columns led Lorente de Nó to suggest that these "vertical chains" of cells were the elementary functional units of the cortex. This notion received strong support from Mountcastle's observations that all the neurons in a column receive impulses of the same sensory modality, from the same part of the body. It is still not entirely clear whether the columns contribute to a movement as units or whether individual cells within many columns are selectively activated. Both Henneman and Asanuma summarized the evidence for these disparate views.

Evarts and his colleagues also elucidated the role of cortical motor neurons in sensory evoked or planned movement. Using single-cell recording techniques, they showed that pyramidal cells fire about 60 ms prior to the onset of a movement, in a sequence determined by the required pattern and force of the movement. But other, more complex properties of the pyramidal cells were also noted. Some of them received a somatosensory input transcortically from the parietal lobe (areas 3, 1, and 2), which could be turned on or off or gated according to whether the movement was to be controlled, i.e., guided, by sensory input. Many neurons of the supplementary and premotor cortices were activated before a planned movement. Thus pyramidal (area 4) motor neurons were prepared for the oncoming activation by impulses from the parietal, prefrontal, premotor, and auditory and visual areas of the cortex. This preparatory "set signal" could occur in the absence of any activity in the spinal cord and muscles. The source of the activation signal was found to be mainly in the supplementary motor cortex, which appears to be under the direct influence of the "readiness stimuli" (*Bereitschaft* potential) reaching it from the prefrontal areas for planned movements and from the posterior parietal cortex for motor activities initiated by sensory perceptions. There are also fibers that reach the motor area from the limbic system, presumably subserving motivation and attention. Roland has used functional cerebral blood flow measurements to follow these neural events.

Thus the prefrontal cortex, supplementary motor cortex, premotor cortex, and motor cortex are all responsive to afferent stimuli and are involved prior to, and in coordinated fashion with, a complex movement. As remarked later on, the striatopallidum and cerebellum, which project to these cortical areas, are also activated prior to or concurrently with the discharge of corticospinal neurons (see Thach and Montgomery for a critical review of the physiologic data).

Termination of the Corticospinal and Other Descending Motor Tracts

This has been studied in the monkey by interrupting the descending motor pathways in the medulla and more rostral parts of the brainstem and tracing the distribution of the degenerating elements in the spinal gray matter. On the basis of such experiments and other physiologic data, Lawrence and Kuypers proposed that the functional organization of the descending cortical and subcortical pathways is determined more by their patterns of termination and the motor capacities of the internuncial neurons upon which they terminate than by the location of their cells of origin. Three groups of motor fibers were distinguished according to their differential terminal distribution: (1) The corticospinal and corticobulbar tracts, which project to all levels of the spinal cord and brainstem, terminating diffusely throughout the nucleus proprius of the dorsal horn and the intermediate zone. A portion of these connect directly with the large motor neurons that innervate the muscles of the fingers, face, and tongue; this system provides the capacity for a high degree of fractionation of movements, as exemplified by independent finger movements.

As alluded to above, a large fraction of the fibers in the corticospinal originate from the sensory cortex and appear to function in the modulation of movement by afferent neurons. (2) A *ventromedial pathway*, which arises in the tectum (*tectospinal tract*), vestibular nuclei (*vestibulospinal tract*), and pontine and medullary reticular cells (*reticulospinal tract*) and terminates principally on the internuncial cells of the ventromedial part of the spinal gray matter. This system is mainly concerned with axial movements—the maintenance of posture, integrated movements of body and limbs, and total limb movements. (3) A *lateral pathway*, which is derived mainly from the magnocellular part of the red nucleus and terminates in the dorsal and lateral parts of the internuncial zone. This pathway adds to the capacity for independent use of the extremities, especially of the hands.

Reference has already been made to the corticomesencephalic, corticopontine, and corticomedullary fiber systems that project onto the reticulospinal, vestibulospinal, rubrospinal, and tectospinal nuclei. These control stability of the head (via labyrinthine reflexes) and of the neck and body in relation to the head (tonic neck reflexes) as well as postures of the body in relation to limb movements. Lesions in these systems are less well understood than those of the corticospinal system. They cause no paralysis of muscles but result in the liberation of unusual postures (e.g., hemiplegic dystonia), heightened tonic neck and labyrinthine reflexes, and decerebrate rigidity. In a strict sense these are all "extrapyramidal," as discussed in the next two chapters.

Paralysis Caused by Lesions of the Upper Motor Neurons

The corticospinal pathway may be interrupted by a lesion at any point along its course—at the level of the cerebral cortex, subcortical white matter, internal capsule, brainstem, or spinal cord. Usually, when hemiplegia is severe and permanent as a consequence of disease, much more than the long, direct corticospinal pathway is involved. In the cerebral white matter (corona radiata) and internal capsule, the corticospinal fibers are intermingled with corticostriate, corticothalamic, corticorubral, corticopontine, cortico-olivary, and corticoreticular fibers. It is noteworthy that thalamocortical fibers, which are a vital link in an ascending fiber system from the basal ganglia and cerebellum, also pass through the internal capsule and cerebral white matter. Thus lesions in these parts can simultaneously affect both corticospinal and extrapyramidal systems. Attribution of a capsular hemiplegia solely to a lesion of the corticospinal or pyramidal pathway is therefore not entirely correct. The term *upper motor neuron (supranuclear) paralysis*, which recognizes the involvement of several descending fiber systems that influence and modify the lower motor neuron, is more appropriate.

In primates, lesions limited to area 4 of Brodmann, the motor cortex, cause mainly hypotonia and weakness of the distal limb muscles. Lesions of the premotor cortex (area 6) result in weakness, spasticity, and increased stretch reflexes (Fulton). Lesions of the supplementary motor cortex lead to involuntary grasping. Resection of cortical areas 4 and 6 and subcortical white matter in monkeys causes complete and permanent paralysis and spasticity (Laplane et al). These clinical effects have not been as clearly defined in humans.

The one place where corticospinal fibers are entirely isolated is the pyramidal tract in the medulla. In humans, there are a few documented cases of a lesion more or less confined to this location. The result of such lesions has been an initial flaccid hemiplegia (with sparing of the face), from which there is considerable recovery. Similarly in monkeys—as was shown by Tower in 1940 and subsequently by Lawrence and Kuypers and by Gilman and Marco—interruption of both pyramidal tracts results in a hypotonic paralysis; ultimately, these animals regain a wide range of movements, although slowness of all movements and loss of individual finger movements remain as permanent deficits. Also, the cerebral peduncle had in the past been sectioned in patients in an effort to abolish involuntary movements (Bucy et al). In some of these patients, a slight degree of weakness or only a Babinski sign was produced but no spasticity developed. These observations indicate that a pure pyramidal tract lesion does not result in spasticity. Furthermore, to reiterate a previous comment, control over a wide range of voluntary movements depends at least in part on nonpyramidal motor pathways. Animal experiments suggest that the corticoreticulospinal pathways are particularly important in this respect, because their fibers are arranged somatotopically and influence stretch reflexes. Further studies of human disease, possibly using diffusion tensor imaging techniques, are necessary to settle problems related to volitional movement and spasticity.

The distribution of the paralysis caused by upper motor neuron (supranuclear) lesions varies with the locale of the lesion, but certain features are characteristic of all of them. A group of muscles is always involved, never individual muscles, and if any movement is possible, the proper relationships between agonists, antagonists, synergists, and fixators are preserved. On careful inspection, the paralysis never involves all the muscles on one side of the body, even in the severest forms of hemiplegia. Movements that are invariably bilateral—such as those of the eyes, jaw, pharynx, upper face, larynx, neck, thorax, diaphragm, and abdomen—are affected little or not at all. This occurs because these muscles are bilaterally innervated; i.e., stimulation of either the right or left motor cortex results in contraction of these muscles on both sides of the body. Upper motor neuron paralysis is rarely complete for any long period of time; in this respect it differs from the absolute paralysis that results from destruction of anterior horn cells or interruption of their axons.

Upper motor neuron lesions are characterized further by certain peculiarities of retained movement. There is decreased voluntary drive on spinal motor neurons (fewer motor units are recruitable and their firing rates are slower), resulting in a slowness of movement. There is also an increased degree of co-contraction of antagonistic muscles, reflected in a decreased rate of rapid alternating movements. These abnormalities probably account for the greater sense of effort and the manifest fatigability in effecting voluntary movement of the weakened muscles. Another phenomenon is the activation of paralyzed muscles as parts of certain automatisms (synkinesias). For example, the paralyzed arm may move suddenly during yawning and stretching. Attempts by the patient to move the hemiplegic limbs may also result in a variety of associated movements. Thus, flexion of the arm may result in involuntary pronation and flexion of the leg or in dorsiflexion and eversion of the foot. Also, volitional movements of the paretic limb often evoke imitative (mirror) movements in the normal one or vice versa. Mirror movements are also a feature of Parkinson disease and of lesions in the upper cervical spinal cord. In some patients, as they recover from hemiplegia, a variety of movement abnormalities emerge, such as tremor, athetosis, and chorea on the affected side. These are expressions of damage to basal ganglionic and thalamic structures and are discussed in Chap. 4.

If the upper motor neurons are interrupted above the level of the facial nucleus in the pons, hand and arm muscles are affected most severely and the leg muscles to a lesser extent; of the cranial musculature, only muscles of the tongue and lower part of the face are involved to any significant degree. Because Broadbent was the first to call attention to this distribution of facial paralysis that relatively spares the forehead muscles, it is referred to as "Broadbent's law." The precise course taken by fibers that innervate the facial nucleus is still somewhat uncertain; however, the majority crosses in the mid-pons to innervate the contralateral facial nerve nucleus. Some fibers may descend to the upper medulla and then ascend recurrently to the pons, (Pick's bundle accounting for the mild facial weakness that is seen with lesions of the lower pons and upper medulla.

At lower levels, such as the cervical cord, complete, acute, and bilateral lesions of the upper motor neurons not only cause a paralysis of voluntary movement but also temporarily abolish the spinal reflexes of segments below the lesion. This is the condition referred to earlier as *spinal shock*, a state of acute flaccid paralysis that is replaced later by *spasticity*. A comparable state of areflexia and hypotonia may occur with acute cerebral lesions but is less sharply defined than is the spinal state. With some acute cerebral lesions, spasticity and paralysis develop together; in others, especially with parietal lesions, the limbs remain flaccid but reflexes are retained.

Spasticity, Hyperreflexia, and the Babinski Sign

The identifying characteristics of paralysis from an upper motor neuron lesion are a predilection for involvement of certain muscle groups, a specific pattern of response of muscles to passive stretch (where resistance increases linearly in relation to velocity of stretch, and a manifest exaggeration of tendon reflexes. The antigravity muscles—the flexors of the arms and the extensors of the legs—are predominantly affected. The arm tends to assume a flexed and pronated position and the leg an extended and adducted one, indicating that certain spinal neurons are reflexly more active than others. At rest, with the muscles shortened to midposition, they are flaccid to palpation and electromyographically silent. If the arm is extended or the leg flexed very slowly, there may be little or no change in muscle tone. By contrast, if the muscles are briskly stretched, the limb moves freely for a very short distance (free interval), beyond which there is an abrupt catch and then a rapidly increasing muscular resistance up to a point; then, as passive extension of the arm or flexion of the leg continues, the resistance melts away. This velocity dependent tone constitutes the "clasp-knife" phenomenon of spasticity. With the limb in the extended or flexed position, a new passive movement may not encounter the same sequence; this entire pattern of response constitutes the lengthening and shortening reaction. Thus, the essential feature of spasticity is a velocity-dependent increase in the resistance of muscles to a passive stretch stimulus.

Although a clasp-knife relaxation following peak resistance is highly characteristic of cerebral hemiplegia, it is by no means found consistently. At times, a form of velocity-independent hypertonia is found that is termed rigidity and is more characteristic of basal ganglia lesions as discussed in Chap. 4.

Clinicians have known for some time that there is not a constant relationship between spasticity and weakness. Severe weakness may be associated with only the mildest signs of spasticity; in contrast, the most extreme degrees of spasticity, observed in certain patients with cervical spinal cord disease, may seem disproportionate to the extent of weakness, signifying that these two states depend on separate mechanisms. Indeed, the selective blocking of small gamma neurons abolishes spasticity as well as hyperactive segmental tendon reflexes but to leave power unchanged.

The heightened stretch reflexes (tendon jerks) of the spastic state may be a "release" phenomenon—the result of interruption of descending inhibitory pathways, but this appears to be only a partial explanation. Animal experiments have demonstrated that this aspect of the spastic state is also mediated through spindle efferents (increased tonic activity of gamma motor neurons) and, centrally, through reticulospinal and vestibulospinal pathways that act on alpha motor neurons. The clasp-knife phenomenon appears to derive at least partly from a lesion (or presumably a change in central control) of a specific portion of the reticulospinal system.

P. Brown, in a discussion of the pathophysiology of spasticity, emphasized the importance of two systems of fibers: (1) the dorsal reticulospinal tract, which has inhibitory effects on stretch reflexes; and (2) the medial reticulospinal and vestibulospinal tracts, which together facilitate extensor tone. He postulated that in cerebral and capsular lesions, cortical inhibition is reduced, resulting in spastic hemiplegia. In spinal cord lesions that involve the corticospinal tract, the dorsal reticulospinal tract is usually involved as well. If the latter tract is spared, only paresis, loss of support reflexes, and possibly release of flexor reflexes (Babinski phenomenon) occur. Pantano and colleagues suggested that primary involvement of the lenticular nucleus of the basal ganglia and thalamus is the feature that determines the persistence of flaccidity after stroke, but the anatomic and physiologic evidence for this view is insecure.

The most sensitive indications of an upper motor neuron lesion are the signs described by Babinski in 1896 (the great toe sign) and 1903 (the toe abduction, or fan sign). In modern parlance, the toe and fan signs have generally been conflated and termed the Babinski sign. Numerous monographs and articles have been written about the sign: a quite comprehensive one, by van Gijn, and an elegant but more arcane one by Fulton and Keller.

As Babinski himself indicated, a movement resembling the Babinski sign is present in normal infants (see Phiilipon and Poirer), but it disappears and its persistence or emergence in late infancy and childhood or later in life is an invariable indicator of a lesion at some level of the corticospinal tract. In its essential form, the sign consists of extension of the large toe and extension and fanning of the other toes during and immediately after stroking the lateral plantar surface of the foot. The stimulus is applied along the dorsum of the foot from the lateral heel and sweeping upward and across the ball of the foot. The stimulus must be firm but not necessarily painful. Several dozen surrogate responses (with numerous eponyms) have been described over the years, most utilizing alternative sites and types of stimulation, but all have the same significance as the Babinski response.

Clinical and electrophysiologic observations indicate that the extension movement of the toe is a component of a larger synergistic flexion or shortening reflex of the leg—i.e., toe extension when viewed from a physiologic perspective is a flexor protective (nocifensive, or defensive) response. The most characteristic of these is the "triple flexion response", in which the hip, thigh and ankle flex (dorsiflex) slowly, following an appropriate stimulus. These *spinal flexion reflexes*, of which the Babinski sign is the most characteristic, are common accompaniments to—but not essential components of—spasticity. They are present because of disinhibition or release of motor programs of spinal origin. Important characteristics of these responses are their capacity to be induced by weak superficial stimuli (such as a series of pinpricks) and their tendency to persist for a few moments after the stimulation ceases. With incomplete suprasegmental lesions, the response may be fractionated; for example, the hip and knee may flex but the foot may not dorsiflex, or vice versa.

The hyperreflexic state that characterizes spasticity may take the form of *clonus*, a series of rhythmic involuntary muscular contractions occurring at a frequency of 5 to 7 Hz in response to an abruptly applied and sustained stretch stimulus. It is usually designated in terms of the part of the limb to which the stimulus is applied (e.g., patella, ankle). The frequency is constant within 1 Hz and is not appreciably modified by altering peripheral or central nervous system activities. Clonus requires an appropriate degree of muscle relaxation, integrity of the spinal stretch reflex mechanisms, sustained hyperexcitability of alpha and gamma motor neurons (suprasegmental effects), and synchronization of the contraction–relaxation cycle of muscle spindles.

The cutaneomuscular abdominal and cremasteric reflexes ("cutaneous, or superficial reflexes") are elicited by rapid, gentle stroking of the skin overlying these muscles, and are usually abolished when the upper motor neuron is damaged. These were referred to as reflexes before the end of the nineteenth century, which leads to some confusion in interpreting the older clinical literature.

Spread, or *radiation of reflexes*, is regularly associated with spasticity, although the latter phenomenon may be observed to a slight degree in normal persons with brisk tendon reflexes. Tapping of the radial periosteum, for example, may elicit a reflex contraction not only of the brachioradialis but also of the biceps, triceps, or finger flexors. This spread of reflex activity is probably not the result of radiation of impulses in the spinal cord, but a result of the propagation of a vibration wave from bone to muscle, stimulating the excitable muscle spindles in its path (Lance). Other manifestations of the hyperreflexic state, are the Hoffmann sign and the crossed adductor reflex of the thigh muscles. Also, reflexes may be "inverted," as in the case of a lesion of the fifth or sixth cervical segment; here the biceps and brachioradialis reflexes are abolished and only the triceps and finger flexors, whose reflex arcs are intact, respond to a tap over the distal radius.

With bilateral cerebral lesions, exaggerated stretch reflexes may be elicited in cranial as well as limb and trunk muscles because of interruption of the corticobulbar pathways. These are seen as easily triggered masseter contractions in response to a brisk downward tap on the chin ("jaw jerk") and brisk contractions of the orbicularis oris muscles in response to tapping the philtrum or corners of the mouth. In advanced cases, weakness or paralysis or slowness of voluntary movements of the face, tongue, larynx, and pharynx are added (bulbar spasticity or "pseudobulbar" palsy; see also Chap. 25).

The many investigations of the biochemical changes that underlie spasticity and the mechanisms of action of antispasticity drugs have been reviewed by Davidoff. Because glutamic acid is the neurotransmitter of the corticospinal tracts, one would expect its action on inhibitory interneurons to be lost. As mentioned earlier, GABA and glycine are the major inhibitory transmitters in the spinal cord; GABA functions as a presynaptic inhibitor, suppressing sensory signals from muscle and cutaneous receptors. Baclofen, a derivative of GABA, as well as diazepam and progabide, are thought to act by reducing the release of excitatory transmitters from the presynaptic terminals of primary afferent terminals. Actually, none of these agents is entirely satisfactory in the treatment of spasticity when administered orally; the administration of baclofen intrathecally at times has a more beneficial effect. Glycine is the transmitter released by inhibitory interneurons and is measurably reduced in quantity, uptake, and turnover in the spastic animal. There is some evidence that the oral administration of glycine reduces experimentally induced spasticity, but its value in patients is uncertain. Interruption of descending noradrenergic, dopaminergic, and serotonergic fibers is undoubtedly involved in the genesis of spasticity, although the exact mode of action of these neurotransmitters on the various components of spinal reflex arcs remains to be defined.

Table 3-1 summarizes the main attributes of upper motor neuron lesions and contrasts them with those of the lower motor neuron discussed above.

Motor Disturbances Caused by Lesions of the Parietal Lobe

As indicated earlier in this section, a significant portion of the pyramidal tract originates in neurons of the parietal cortex. Also, the parietal lobes are important sources of visual and tactile information necessary for the control of movement. Pause and colleagues have described the motor disturbances caused by lesions of the parietal

Table 3-1

DIFFERENCES BETWEEN UPPER AND LOWER MOTOR NEURON PARALYSIS

UPPER MOTOR NEURON OR SUPRANUCLEAR PARALYSIS	LOWER MOTOR NEURON OR NUCLEAR-INFRANUCLEAR PARALYSIS
Muscles affected in groups; never individual muscles	Individual muscles may be affected
Atrophy slight and the result of disuse	Atrophy pronounced; up to 70% of total bulk
Spasticity with hyperactivity of the tendon reflexes and extensor plantar reflex (Babinski sign)	Flaccidity and hypotonia of affected muscles with loss of tendon reflexes
	Plantar reflex, if present, is of normal flexor type
Fasciculations absent	Fasciculations may be present
Normal nerve conduction studies; no denervation potentials in EMG	Abnormal nerve conduction studies; denervation potentials (fibrillations, fasciculations, positive sharp waves) in EMG

cortex. The patient is unable to maintain stable postures of the outstretched hand when his eyes are closed and cannot exert a steady contraction. Exploratory movements and manipulation of small objects are impaired, and the speed of tapping is diminished. Posterior parietal lesions (involving areas 5 and 7 in Fig. 3-3) are more detrimental in this respect than anterior ones (areas 1, 3, and 5), but both regions are affected in patients with the most severe deficits.

APRAXIA AND OTHER NONPARALYTIC DISORDERS OF MOTOR FUNCTION

All that has been said about the cortical and spinal control of the motor system gives one only a limited idea of human motility. Viewed objectively, the conscious and sentient human organism is continuously active—fidgeting, adjusting posture and position, sitting, standing, walking, running, speaking, manipulating tools, or performing the intricate sequences of movements involved in athletic or musical skills. Some of these activities are relatively simple, automatic, and stereotyped. Others have been learned and mastered through intense conscious effort and with long practice have become habitual—i.e., reduced to an automatic level—a process not at all understood physiologically. Still others are complex and voluntary, parts of a carefully formulated plan, and demand continuous attention and thought. What is more remarkable, one can be occupied in several of these variably conscious and habitual activities simultaneously, such as driving through heavy traffic while dialing a cellular phone (not endorsed) and engaging in animated conversation. Moreover, when an obstacle prevents a particular sequence of movements from accomplishing its goal, a new sequence can be undertaken automatically for the same purpose.

The term *apraxia* denotes a disorder in which an attentive patient loses the ability to execute previously learned activities in the absence of weakness, ataxia, sensory loss, or extrapyramidal derangement that would be adequate to explain the deficit. All of the elements of the activity may be demonstrated in circumstances other than in response to the command to execute the activity or gesture. This was the meaning given to apraxia by Liepmann, who introduced the term in 1900.

Apraxia has been divided into three types: ideational, ideomotor, and limb-kinetic. They are described in greater detail in Chap. 23 but a brief account is provided here because of their intimate involvement with motor activity. Any explanation of apraxia requires an appreciation of the interplay between cortical areas that create highly complex motor behaviors.

On the basis of studies of large numbers of patients with lesions of different parts of the brain, it appears that the initiating and planning of complex activities, conceptualizing their purpose, and continuously modifying the components of a motor sequence are directed by the frontal lobes. Lesions of the frontal lobes have the effect of reducing the impulse to think, speak, and act (i.e., abulia, or reduced "cortical tone," to use Luria's expression), and a complex activity will not be initiated or sustained long enough to permit its completion. However, clinical and functional imaging data indicate that planned or commanded action is normally first conceptualized not in the frontal lobe, where the impulse to action arises, but in the parietal lobe of the language-dominant hemisphere, where visual, auditory, and somesthetic information is integrated. The formation of ensembles of skilled movements, which Liepmann called a "space-time plan," depends on the integrity of the dominant parietal lobe; if this part of the brain is damaged, complex patterns of movement cannot be activated at all or the movements are awkward and inappropriate.

The failure to conceive or formulate an action to command, was referred to by Liepmann as *ideational apraxia*. Sensory areas 5 and 7 in the dominant parietal lobe, the supplementary and premotor cortices of both cerebral hemispheres and their integral connections are involved collectively to accomplish these actions. In *ideomotor apraxia*, the patient may know and remember the planned action, but because these areas or their connections are interrupted, he cannot actually execute it with either hand. Certain tasks are said to differentiate ideomotor from ideational apraxia, as discussed further on, but the distinction may be quite subtle. Nonetheless, ideational apraxia has been said to be characterized by difficulty in "what to do," whereas ideomotor apraxia is a block in "how to do" as a result of an inability to transmit the gesture to executive motor centers.

A third disorder, opaque to many neurologists, is *limb-kinetic apraxia* (or *kinetic-limb apraxia*). It is an ill-defined clumsiness and maladroitness that is the result of an inability to fluidly connect or to isolate individual movements of the hand and arm as described by Kleist. In the originally conceived form, a hand displays awkwardness that is disproportionate to weakness or sensory loss, yet gestures and complex movements can be accomplished, unlike the case in ideomotor apraxia. Central to the disorder is a breakdown of fine fractionated finger movements for which reason the nature of limb kinetic apraxia and its differentiation from a mild corticospinal disorder has been elusive enough that many neurologists do not view it as a true apraxia.

The term limb-kinetic apraxia has also been applied to cases of paralysis that obscures the apraxia on one side but causes a breakdown of fine finger movements on the opposite side. This is more properly termed "*sympathetic apraxia*". In particular, in a right-handed person, a lesion in the left frontal lobe that includes Broca's area, the left motor cortex, and the deep underlying white matter may cause left-limb apraxia. Clinically, there is a nonfluent aphasia, a right hemiparesis, and clumsiness of the nonparalyzed left hand.

These high-order abnormalities of learned movement patterns have several unique features. Seldom are they evident to the patient himself and therefore they are not sources of complaint, even if they disrupt daily activities such as dressing. Or, if the patient appreciates them, he has difficulty describing the problem except in narrow terms of the activity that is impaired, such as using a phone or dressing. For this reason they are also often overlooked by the examining physician. Obviously, if the patient is confused or aphasic, spoken or written requests to perform an act will not be understood and one must find ways of persuading him to imitate the movements of the examiner. Moreover, the patient must be able to recognize and name the articles that he attempts to manipulate.

In practical terms, the lesion responsible for ideomotor apraxia, which affects both hands, usually resides in the left parietal region. Kertesz and colleagues provided evidence that the lesions responsible for aphasia and apraxia are different, although the two conditions are frequently associated because of their origin in the left hemisphere. The exact location of the parietal lesion, whether in the supramarginal gyrus or in the superior parietal lobe (areas 5 and 7) and whether subcortical or cortical, has been variable. Although the majority of ideational and ideomotor apraxias occur with lesions in the left cerebral hemisphere, the right hemisphere retains some of these capacities. A small number of apraxic patients have right hemisphere damage. This also explains the preservation of most praxis skills in the left hand following callosal lesions. Geschwind accepted Liepmann's proposition that a lesion of a subcortical tract (presumably the arcuate fasciculus) can disconnect the parietal from the left frontal cortex, accounting for the ideomotor apraxia of the right limbs. The apraxia in the left limb is the consequence of a functional disconnection of the left and right premotor association cortices. These conceptualizations, while possibly valid, are of more theoretic than practical significance and depend heavily on the disconnection model discussed in Chap. 23. An alternative view is that there is not an actual disconnection of the two frontal lobes as much as there is a failure of the left to activate the right frontal lobe because the right does not receive instructions from the damaged left parietal lobe. It is the dominant parietal lobe that still embodies the property of praxis.

Of a somewhat different nature is an oral-buccal-lingual apraxia, which is probably the most commonly observed of all apraxias in practice. It may occur with lesions that undercut the left supramarginalgyrus or the left motor association cortex and may or may not be associated with the apraxia of the limbs described above. Such patients are unable to carry out facial movements on command (lick the lips, blow out a match, etc.) although they may do better when asked to imitate the examiner or when confronted with a lighted match. With lesions that are restricted to the facial area of the left motor cortex, the apraxia will be limited to the facial musculature bilaterally and may be associated with a verbal apraxia or cortical dysarthria (namely, Broca's aphasia, see Chap. 22).

So-called apraxia of gait is considered in Chap. 7, but strictly speaking, this not an apraxia as walking is not a learned act. The terms dressing apraxia and constructional apraxia are used to describe special manifestations of nondominant parietal lobe disease, in contrast to the above-described forms of apraxia that result from lesions on the dominant side. Although dressing apraxia in many ways resembles an ideomotor apraxia, it probably has a basis in a form of sensory extinction and a loss of appreciation of extrapersonal space. These issues are discussed further in Chap. 23.

Testing for apraxia is carried out in several ways. First, one observes the actions of the patient as he engages in simulated tasks as dressing, washing, shaving, and using eating utensils. Second, the patient is asked to carry out familiar symbolic acts—wave goodbye, salute the flag, shake a fist as though angry, or blow a kiss. If he fails, he is asked to imitate such acts made by the examiner. Finally, he is asked to show how he would hammer a nail, brush his teeth, take a comb out of his pocket and comb his hair, or to execute a more complex act, such as lighting and smoking a cigarette or opening a bottle of soda, pouring some into a glass, and drinking it. These actions, involving more complex sequences, are said to be tests of ideational apraxia; the simpler and familiar acts are considered tests of ideomotor apraxia. To perform these tasks in the absence of the tool or utensil is always more demanding because the patient must mentally formulate a plan of action rather than engage in a habitual motor sequence. The patient may fail to carry out a commanded or suggested activity (e.g., to take a pen out of his pocket), yet a few minutes later he may perform the same motor sequence automatically.

Children with cerebral diseases that retard mental development are often unable to learn the sequences of movement required in hopping, jumping over a barrier, hitting or kicking a ball, or dancing. They suffer a *developmental motor apraxia*. Certain tests quantitate failure in these age-linked motor skills (see Chap. 28).

In the authors' opinion, the time-honored division of apraxia into ideational, ideomotor, and kinetic types is not entirely satisfactory because of the difficulty separating them in practice. We have sometimes been unable to confidently separate ideomotor from ideational apraxia. The patient with a severe ideomotor apraxia nearly always has difficulty at the ideational level and, in any case, similarly situated left parietal lesions give rise to both types. Furthermore, in view of the complexity of the motor system, we have frequently been uncertain whether the clumsiness or ineptitude of a hand in performing a motor skill represents a kinetic apraxia or some other subtle fault in hand control by the corticospinal or one of the other parallel motor systems.

A related but poorly understood disorder of movement has been termed the *alien hand*. In the absence of volition, the hand and arm undertake complex and seemingly purposeful movements such as reaching into a pocket or handbag, placing the hand behind the head, tugging on the opposite hand or other body part, and rebuttoning the shirt immediately after it has been unbuttoned by the other hand. These activities may occur even during sleep. The patient is aware of the movements but has the sense that the actions are beyond his control and there is often an impression that the hand is estranged, as if commanded by an external agent (although the limb is recognized as one's own—there is no anosognosia); a grasp reflex and a tendency to grope are usually present. Most instances arise as a result of infarction in the territory of the opposite anterior cerebral artery, including the corpus callosum. When the callosum is involved, Feinberg and colleagues find that there frequently appears to be a conflict between the actions of the hands, the normal one sometimes even restraining the alien one. Damage in the left supplementary motor area from any cause, as well as from the degenerative disease called corticobasal ganglionic degeneration (corticobasal-ganglionic syndromes), are associated with a similar alien hand syndrome. A third form that results from a stroke in the posterior cerebral artery territory with associated sensory loss has also been observed by Ay and colleagues.

A possibly related phenomenon has been described by Lhermitte as "utilization behavior," in which the patient obligatorily seizes and uses objects in the surrounding environment. It is associated with extensive bilateral frontal lobe damage and has been likened, unsatisfactorily in our view, to a bilateral alien hand phenomenon.

Finally, it should be remarked again that the complexity of motor activity is almost beyond imagination. Reference was made earlier to the reciprocal innervation involved in an act as simple as making a fist. Scratching one's shoulder has been estimated to recruit about 75 muscles. But what must be involved in playing a piano concerto? Over a century ago Hughlings Jackson commented that "There are, we shall say, over thirty muscles in the hand; these are represented in the nervous centers in thousands of different combinations, that is, as very many movements; it is just as many chords, musical expressions, and tunes can be made out of a few notes." The execution of these complex movements, many of them learned and habitual, is made possible by the cooperative activities of not just the motor and sensory cortices but integrally of the basal ganglia, cerebellum, and reticular formation of the brainstem. All are continuously integrated and controlled by feedback mechanisms from the sensory and spinal motor neurons. These points, already touched upon in this chapter, are elaborated in the following three chapters.

A historical perspective that outlines the development of these concepts is given by Faglioni and Basso and an authoritative review of the subject of apraxia can be found in the chapter by Heilman and Gonzalez-Rothi.

PATTERNS OF PARALYSIS AND THEIR DIAGNOSIS

The diagnostic considerations in cases of paralysis can be simplified by using the following subdivision, based on the location and distribution of the muscle weakness:

1. *Monoplegia* refers to weakness or paralysis of all the muscles of one leg or arm. This term is not applied to paralysis of isolated muscles or groups of muscles supplied by a single nerve or motor root.
2. *Hemiplegia*, the commonest form of paralysis, involves the arm, the leg, and sometimes the face on one side of the body. With rare exceptions, mentioned further on, hemiplegia is attributable to a lesion of the corticospinal system on the side opposite to the paralysis.
3. *Paraplegia* indicates weakness or paralysis of both legs. It is most often the result of diseases of the thoracic spinal cord, cauda equina, or peripheral nerves, and rarely, both medial frontal cortices.
4. *Quadriplegia* (tetraplegia) denotes weakness or paralysis of all four extremities. It may result from disease of the peripheral nerves, muscles, or myoneural junctions; gray matter of the spinal cord; or the upper motor neurons bilaterally in the cervical cord, brainstem, or cerebrum. Diplegia is a special form of quadriplegia in which the legs are affected more than the arms. Triplegia occurs most often as a transitional condition in the development of, or partial recovery from, tetraplegia.
5. Isolated paralysis of one or more muscle groups due to disease of muscle, anterior horn cells, or nerve roots.
6. Nonparalytic disorders of movement (e.g., apraxia, ataxia).
7. Hysterical paralysis.

Monoplegia

The examination of patients who complain of weakness of one limb often discloses an asymptomatic weakness of another, and the condition is actually a hemiparesis or paraparesis. Or, instead of weakness of all the muscles in a limb, only isolated groups are found to be affected. Ataxia, sensory disturbances, or reluctance to move the limb because of pain should not be misinterpreted as weakness. Parkinsonism may give rise to the same error, as can rigidity or bradykinesia of other causation or a mechanical limitation because of arthritis and bursitis. The presence or absence of atrophy of muscles in a monoplegic limb is of particular diagnostic help, as indicated below.

Monoplegia without Muscular Atrophy

This is most often caused by a lesion of the cerebral cortex or the spinal cord (where it causes a monoplegia of the leg). Infrequently it results from a restricted subcortical lesion that selectively interrupts the motor pathways to one limb. A cerebral vascular lesion is the most common cause; a circumscribed tumor or abscess may have the same effect. A small cortical lesion may exceptionally paralyze half the hand or even just the thumb. Multiple sclerosis and spinal cord tumor, early in their course, may cause weakness of one limb, usually the leg. Monoplegia caused by a lesion of the upper motor neuron is usually accompanied by spasticity, increased reflexes, and an extensor plantar reflex (Babinski sign). In acute diseases of the lower motor neurons, the tendon reflexes are reduced or abolished, but atrophy may not appear for several weeks. Hence, before reaching an anatomic diagnosis, one must take into account the mode of onset and duration of the disease.

Monoplegia with Muscular Atrophy

This is more frequent than monoplegia without muscular atrophy. Long-continued disuse of one limb may lead to atrophy, but it is usually of lesser degree than atrophy caused by lower motor neuron disease (denervation atrophy). In disuse atrophy, the tendon reflexes are retained and nerve conduction studies are normal. With denervation of muscles, there may be visible fasciculations and reduced or abolished tendon reflexes in addition to paralysis. If the limb is partially denervated, the EMG shows reduced numbers of motor unit potentials (often of large size) as well as fasciculations and fibrillations. The location of the lesion (in nerves, spinal roots, or spinal cord) can usually be determined by the pattern of weakness, by the associated neurologic symptoms and signs, and by special tests—MRI of the spine, examination of the cerebrospinal fluid (CSF), and electrical studies of nerve and muscle.

A complete atrophic brachial monoplegia is uncommon; more often, only parts of a limb are affected. When present in an infant, it suggests brachial plexus trauma from birth; in a child, poliomyelitis or other viral infection of the spinal cord; and in an adult, syringomyelia, amyotrophic lateral sclerosis, or a brachial plexus lesion. Atrophic crural (leg) monoplegia is more frequent than atrophic brachial monoplegia and may be caused by any lesion of the thoracic cord—i.e., trauma, tumor, myelitis, multiple sclerosis, late radiation effect, etc. These disorders rarely cause severe atrophy. A prolapsed intervertebral disc and several varieties of mononeuropathy almost never paralyze all or most of the muscles of a limb. The effects of a centrally prolapsed disc or other compressive lesion of the cauda equina are rarely confined to one leg. However, a unilateral retroperitoneal tumor or hematoma may paralyze one leg by compressing the lumbosacral plexus. The mode of onset and temporal course differentiate these diseases.

Hemiplegia

This is the most frequent form of paralysis. With rare exceptions (a few unusual cases of poliomyelitis or motor neuron disease), this pattern of paralysis is a result of involvement of the corticospinal pathways.

The site or level of the lesion—i.e., cerebral cortex, corona radiata, capsule, brainstem, or spinal cord—can usually be deduced from the associated neurologic findings. Diseases localized to the cerebral cortex, cerebral white matter (corona radiata), and internal capsule usually manifest themselves by weakness or paralysis of the leg, arm, and lower face on the opposite side. The occurrence of seizures or the presence of a language disorder (aphasia), a loss of discriminative sensation (e.g., astereognosis, impairment of tactile localization), anosognosia, or a homonymous visual field defect suggests a contralateral cortical or subcortical location.

Damage to the corticospinal and corticobulbar tracts in the upper portion of the brainstem also causes paralysis of the face, arm, and leg of the opposite side (see Fig. 3-2). The lesion in the brainstem may be localized by the presence of a cranial nerve palsy or other segmental abnormality on the same side as the lesion (opposite the hemiplegia). With midbrain lesions there is a third nerve palsy (Weber syndrome), in low pontine lesions, an ipsilateral abducens or facial palsy is combined with a contralateral weakness or paralysis of the arm and leg (Millard-Gubler syndrome). Lesions in the medulla affect the tongue and sometimes the pharynx and larynx on one side and the arm and leg on the other. These "crossed paralyses," characteristic of brainstem lesions, are described further in Chap. 34.

Even lower in the medulla, a unilateral infarct in the pyramid causes a flaccid paralysis of the contralateral arm and leg, with sparing of the face and tongue. Some motor function may be retained, as in the case described by Ropper and colleagues; interestingly, in this case and in others previously reported, there was considerable recovery of voluntary power even though the pyramid was almost completely destroyed.

Rarely, an ipsilateral hemiplegia may be caused by a lesion in the lateral column of the cervical spinal cord. In the spinal cord, however, the pathologic process is more often larger and induces bilateral signs. A homolateral paralysis that spares the face, if combined with a loss of vibratory and position sense on the same side and a contralateral loss of pain and temperature, signifies disease of one side of the spinal cord (Brown-Séquard syndrome, as discussed in Chap. 44).

As indicated above, muscle atrophy that follows upper motor neuron lesions never reaches the proportions seen in diseases of the lower motor neuron. The atrophy in the former cases is mainly a consequence of disuse.

When the motor cortex and adjacent parts of the parietal lobe are damaged in infancy or childhood, normal development of the muscles, as well as the skeletal system in the affected limbs, is retarded. The limbs and even the trunk are smaller on one side than on the other. This does not happen if the paralysis occurs after puberty, by which time the greater part of skeletal growth has been attained. In hemiplegia caused by spinal cord lesions, muscles at the level of the lesion may atrophy as a result of damage to anterior horn cells or ventral roots.

In the causation of hemiplegia, ischemic and hemorrhagic vascular diseases of the cerebrum and brainstem exceed all others in frequency. Trauma (brain contusion, epidural and subdural hemorrhage) ranks second. Other important causes, less acute in onset, are, in order of frequency, brain tumor, demyelinating disease, brain abscess, and the vascular complications of meningitis and encephalitis. Most of these diseases can be recognized by their mode of evolution and characteristic imaging, which are presented in the chapters on specific neurologic diseases. Alternating transitory hemiparesis may be the result of a special type of migraine (see discussion in Chap. 10). From time to time, hysteria is found to be the cause of a hemiplegia, as discussed further on.

Paraplegia

Paralysis of both lower extremities may occur with diseases of the spinal cord, nerve roots, or, less often, the peripheral nerves. If the onset is acute, it may be difficult to distinguish spinal from neuropathic paralysis because of the element of spinal shock, which results in flaccidity and abolition of reflexes. In acute spinal cord diseases with involvement of corticospinal tracts, the paralysis or weakness affects all muscles below a given level; if the white matter is extensively damaged, sensory loss below a circumferential level on the trunk is conjoined (loss of pain and temperature sense because of spinothalamic tract damage, and loss of vibratory and position sense from posterior column involvement). Also in bilateral disease of the spinal cord, the bladder and bowel and their sphincters are usually affected. These abnormalities may be the result of an intrinsic lesion of the cord or an extrinsic mass that narrows the spinal canal and compresses the cord.

In peripheral nerve diseases, motor loss tends to involve the distal muscles of the legs more than the proximal ones (exceptions are certain varieties of the Guillain-Barré syndrome and some types of diabetic neuropathy and porphyria); sphincteric function is usually spared or impaired only transiently. Sensory loss, if present, is also more prominent in the distal segments of the limbs, and the degree of loss is often more for one modality than another.

For clinical purposes, it is helpful to separate the acute paraplegias from the chronic ones and to divide the latter into two groups: those beginning in adult life and those occurring in infancy.

The most common cause of *acute paraplegia* (or *quadriplegia* if the cervical cord is involved) is spinal cord trauma, usually associated with fracture–dislocation of the spine. Less-common causes are hematomyelia because of a vascular malformation, or a malformation that causes ischemia by an obscure mechanism, and infarction of the cord as a result of occlusion of the anterior spinal artery or, more often, to occlusion of segmental branches of the aorta because of dissecting aneurysm or atheroma, vasculitis, or nucleus pulposus embolism. Epidural or subdural hemorrhage from a hemorrhagic diathesis or warfarin therapy cause an acute or subacute paraplegia; in a few instances the bleeding follows a lumbar puncture. A special syndrome occurs in older men where chronic lumbar pain is followed after some months or years by the rapid development of paraplegia. This is caused by an arteriovenous fistula in the overlying dura of the lumbar region. Closure of the vascular shunt may lead to rapid reversal of paraplegia—a treatable form of paraplegia.

Paraplegia or quadriplegia that develops more slowly, subacutely over a period of hours or days is caused by postinfectious myelitis, demyelinating or necrotizing myelopathy, or epidural abscess or tumor with spinal cord compression. Paralytic poliomyelitis and acute Guillain-Barré syndrome—the former a purely motor disorder with mild meningitis, the latter predominantly motor but often with sensory disturbances—must be distinguished from the acute and subacute myelopathies and from each other.

In adult life, multiple sclerosis and tumor account for most cases of *chronic spinal paraplegia*, but a wide variety of extrinsic and intrinsic processes may produce the same effect: protruded cervical disc and cervical spondylosis (often with a congenitally narrow canal), epidural abscess and other infections (tuberculous, fungal, and other granulomatous diseases, HIV and HTLV-1), syphilitic meningomyelitis, motor system disease, subacute combined degeneration (vitamin B12 deficiency and copper deficiency), syringomyelia, epidural lipomatosis, neuromyelitis optica, and degenerative disease of the lateral and posterior columns. (See Chap. 44 for discussion of these spinal cord diseases.)

In *pediatric practice*, delay in starting to walk and difficulty in walking are common problems. These conditions may indicate a systemic disease (such as rickets), mental retardation, or, more commonly, a muscular or neurologic process. Congenital cerebral disease because of periventricular leukomalacia accounts for a majority of cases of infantile diplegia (weakness predominantly of the legs, with minimal weakness of the arms). Present at birth, it becomes manifest in the first months of life and may appear to progress, but actually the progression is only apparent, being exposed as the motor system develops; later there may seem to be slow improvement as a result of the normal maturation processes of childhood. These disorders fall under the heading of cerebral palsy, as discussed in Chap. 38. Congenital malformation or birth injuries of the spinal cord are other possibilities. Friedreich ataxia and familial paraplegia, muscular dystrophy, tumor, and the chronic varieties of polyneuropathy tend to appear later, during childhood and adolescence, and are slowly progressive causes of leg weakness and walking disorder. Transverse (usually demyelinative) myelitis is another cause of acute paraplegia in childhood.

Quadriplegia (Tetraplegia)

All that has been said about the spinal causes of paraplegia applies to quadriplegia, the lesion being in the cervical rather than the thoracic or lumbar segments of the spinal cord. If the lesion is situated in the low cervical segments and involves the anterior half of the spinal cord, as typified by the syndrome resulting from occlusion of the anterior spinal artery, there is a level on the trunk, below which pinprick and thermal sense is lost but there is retained vibration, deep sensation and joint position sense (anterior spinal artery syndrome). In all these processes, the paralysis of the arms may be flaccid and areflexic in type and that of the legs, spastic. If there is pain, it is usually in the neck and shoulders and there is numbness of the hands; elements of ataxia from posterior column lesions may accompany the paraparesis. Compression of the C1 and C2 spinal cord segments is caused by dislocation of the odontoid process. Rheumatoid arthritis and Morquio disease are other causes of compression of the upper cervical cord special note; in the latter, there is pronounced dural thickening.

A progressive syndrome of monoparesis, biparesis, usually of the arms, and then triparesis involving the leg on the side of the last affected arm ("around the clock" pattern) is caused by tumors and a variety of other compressive lesions in the region of the foramen magnum and high cervical cord. This is putatively explained by the pattern of corticospinal fiber decussation at the cervicomedullary junction. Bilateral infarction of the medullary pyramids from occlusion of the vertebral arteries or their anterior spinal branches is a rare cause of quadriplegia. Repeated strokes affecting both hemispheres may lead to bilateral hemiplegia, usually accompanied by pseudobulbar palsy (see Chap. 23 on spastic dysarthria and Chap. 25 on pseudobulbar laughing and crying). In infants and young children, aside from developmental abnormalities and anoxia of birth, certain metabolic cerebral diseases (metachromatic and other forms of leukoencephalopathy, lipid storage disease) may be responsible for a quadriparesis or quadriplegia, but always with psychomotor compromise.

Triplegia

Paralysis that remains confined to three limbs is observed only rarely; more often the fourth limb is weak or hyperreflexic, and the syndrome is really an incomplete tetraplegia. As indicated earlier, this pattern of involvement is important, because it may signify an evolving lesion of the upper cervical cord or cervicomedullary junction. A meningioma of the foramen magnum, for example, may begin with spastic weakness of one limb, followed by sequential involvement of the other limbs in the above noted "around-the-clock" pattern. There are usually bilateral Babinski signs early in the process, but there may be few sensory findings. We have also seen this pattern in patients with multiple sclerosis and other intrinsic inflammatory and neoplastic lesions. These same diseases may produce triplegia (or triparesis) by a combination of paraplegia from a thoracic spinal cord lesion and a separate unilateral lesion in the cervical cord or higher that results in a hemiparesis.

Paralysis of Isolated Muscle Groups

This pattern usually indicates a lesion of one or more peripheral nerves or of several adjacent spinal roots. The diagnosis of an individual peripheral nerve lesion is made on the basis of weakness or paralysis of a particular muscle or group of muscles and impairment or loss of sensation in the distribution of the nerve. Complete or extensive interruption of a peripheral nerve is followed by atrophy of the muscles it innervates and by loss of tendon reflexes of the involved muscles; abnormalities of vasomotor and sudomotor functions and trophic changes in the skin, nails, and subcutaneous tissue may occur if the condition has been chronic.

Detailed knowledge of the motor and sensory innervation of the peripheral nerve in question is needed for a diagnosis. It is impractical to memorize the precise sensorimotor distribution of each peripheral nerve and special manuals, such as *Aids to the Examination of the Peripheral Nervous System*, should be consulted (see also Table 46-1). Electromyography and nerve conduction studies are of great value for localization and to determine if the axon has been damaged or the process affects mainly myelin.

If there is no evidence of upper or lower motor neuron disease but certain movements are nonetheless imperfectly performed, one should look for a disorder of position sense or cerebellar coordination or for rigidity with abnormalities of posture and movement due to disease of the basal ganglia (Chap. 4). In the absence of these disorders, the possibility of an apraxic disorder should be investigated by the methods outlined earlier.

Psychogenic (Hysterical) Paralysis

Psychogenic paralysis may involve one arm or leg, both legs, or all of one side of the body. Tendon reflexes are of normal amplitude, there is no Babinski sign, and atrophy is lacking, features that distinguish it from chronic lower motor neuron disease. Diagnostic difficulty arises only in certain acute cases of upper motor neuron disease that lack the usual changes in reflexes and muscle tone. Sometimes there is loss of sensation in the paralyzed parts and loss of sight, hearing, and smell on the paralyzed side—a pattern of sensory changes that cannot be explained on the basis of organic disease of the nervous system. When the hysterical patient is asked to move the affected limbs, the movements tend to be slow, hesitant, and jerky, often with contraction of agonist and antagonist muscles simultaneously and intermittently ("give-way" weakness). Lack of effort is usually obvious, despite facial and other expressions to the contrary. Power of contraction improves with encouragement and the weakness is inconsistent; some movements are performed tentatively and moments later another movement involving the same muscles is performed naturally.

The Hoover sign and the trunk–thigh sign of Babinski are helpful in distinguishing hysterical from organic hemiplegia. To elicit the Hoover sign, the examiner places both hands under the heels of the recumbent patient, who is asked to press the heels down forcefully. Downward pressure will be felt from the nonparalyzed leg. The examiner then removes his hand from under the nonparalyzed leg, places it on top of the nonparalyzed one, and asks the patient to raise that leg. The sign is manifest in true hemiplegia, by the absence of downward pressure by the paralyzed leg. In psychogenic weakness, the heel of the supposedly paralyzed leg may press down on the examiner's hand. Or, more useful in our experience, the normal leg fails to demonstrate downward pressure when the hysteric is asked to elevate the supposedly paralyzed one, thereby indicating a lack of voluntary effort (i.e., normally, the good leg is fixated and pressed downward in order to raise the opposite leg). In a similar maneuver, the examiner tells the patient that he is testing the normal limb, while asking the patient to try to push the knees together. In hysterical weakness, the apparently paralyzed limb adducts with normal power. One can take advantage of midline motor actions in the upper extremity by asking the patient to push his hands together and telling him that the normal side is being tested. In hysterical weakness, there is adduction movement of the supposedly paralyzed limb.

To carry out the Babinski trunk–thigh test, the examiner asks the recumbent patient to sit up while keeping his arms crossed in front of his chest. In the patient with organic hemiplegia from an upper motor neuron lesion, there is an involuntary flexion of the paretic lower limb; in paraplegia, both limbs are flexed as the trunk is flexed; in hysterical hemiplegia, only the normal leg may be flexed; and in hysterical paraplegia, neither leg is flexed. Patients with apparently paralyzed legs who are seated on a rolling desk chair may propel themselves by pedaling along the floor (a sign attributed to Blocq by Okun and colleagues).

Muscular Paralysis and Spasm Unattended by Visible Changes in Nerve or Muscle

A discussion of motor paralysis would be incomplete without some reference to diseases in which muscle weakness may be profound but there are no overt structural changes in motor nerve cells or nerve fibers. Almost any disease of the neuromuscular junction and many diseases of muscle cause this combination. This group comprises myasthenia gravis, inflammatory myopathies, the muscular dystrophies, and myotonia congenita (Thomsen disease), familial periodic paralysis, disorders of potassium, sodium, calcium, and magnesium metabolism, botulism, black widow spider bite, stiff-man syndrome, and the thyroid and other endocrine myopathies. In these diseases, each with a fairly distinctive clinical picture, the abnormality is essentially physiological, biochemical; their investigation requires EMG, special biochemical and histochemical tests, and electron microscopic study. These subjects are discussed in the sections on muscle disease later in this book.

References

Aids to the Examination of the Peripheral Nervous System. London, BallièreTindall/Saunders, 1986.

Asanuma H: Cerebral cortical control of movement. *Physiologist* 16:143, 1973.

Asanuma H: The pyramidal tract, in Brooks VB (ed): *Handbook of Physiology*. Sec 1: The Nervous System. Vol 2: Motor Control, Part 2. Bethesda, MD, American Physiological Society, 1981, pp 702–733.

Ash J, Georgopoulos AP: Mechanisms of motor control, in Asbury AK, McKhann GM, McDonald WI, et al (eds): *Diseases of the Nervous System*, 3rd ed. Cambridge, Cambridge University Press, 2002, pp 447–460.

Ay H, Buonanno FS, Price BH, et al: Sensory alien hand syndrome. *J Neurol Neurosurg Psychiatry* 65:366, 1998.

Babinski J: De l'abduction des orteils (signe l'éventail). *Rev Neurol* 10:782,1903.

Babinski J : Sur le réflexe cutané plaintaire dans certains affections organiques deusysteme nerveux cebtral. *Rev Neurol* 4:415, 1896.

Brodal P: *The Central Nervous System: Structure and Function*, 5th ed. New York, Oxford University Press, 1992.

Brown P: Pathophysiology of spasticity. *J Neurol Neurosurg Psychiatry* 57:773, 1994.

Bucy PC, Keplinger JE, Siqueira EB: Destruction of the pyramidal tract in man. *J Neurosurg* 21:285, 1964.

Burke D, Lance JW: Myotatic unit and its disorders, in Asbury AK, McKhann GM, McDonald WI (eds): *Diseases of the Nervous System: Clinical Neurobiology*, 2nd ed. Philadelphia, Saunders, 1992, pp 270–284.

Davidoff RA: Antispasticity drugs: Mechanisms of action. *Ann Neurol* 17:107, 1985.

Davidoff RA: Skeletal muscle tone and the misunderstood stretch reflex. *Neurology* 42:951, 1992.

Denny-Brown D: *The Cerebral Control of Movement*. Springfield, IL, Charles C Thomas, 1966.

Denny-Brown D: The nature of apraxia. *J NervMent Dis* 12:9, 1958.

Evarts EV, Shinoda Y, Wise SP: *Neurophysiological Approaches to Higher Brain Functions*. New York, Wiley, 1984.

Faglioni PR, Basso A: Historical perspectives on neuroanatomical correlates of limb apraxia, in Roy EA (ed): *Neuropsychological Studies of Apraxia and Related Disorders*. Amsterdam, North Holland, 1985, pp 3–44.

Feinberg TE, Schindler RJ, Flanagan NG, Haber LD: Two alien hand syndromes. *Neurology* 42:19, 1992.

Fulton JF: *Physiology of the Nervous System*. New York, Oxford University Press, 1938, chap 20.

Fulton JF, Keller AD: *The Sign of Babinski. A Study in the Evolution of Cortical Dominance in Primates*. Charles C Thomas, Springfield, 1932.

Geschwind N: The apraxias: Neural mechanisms of disorders of learned movement. *Am Sci* 63:188, 1975.

Gilman S, Marco LA: Effects of medullary pyramidotomy in the monkey. *Brain* 94:495, 515, 1971.

Hallett M, Shahani BT, Young RR: EMG analysis of stereotyped voluntary movements in man. *J Neurol Neurosurg Psychiatry* 38:1154, 1975.

Heilman KM, Gonzalez-Rothi LJ: Apraxia, in Heilman KM, Valenstein E (eds): *Clinical Neuropsychology*, 4th ed. New York, Oxford University Press, 2003, pp 215–235.

Heilman KM, Vlanestein E: *Clinical Neuropsychology*, 4th ed. Oxford, Oxford University Press, 2003.

Henneman E: Organization of the spinal cord and its reflexes, in Mountcastle VB (ed): *Medical Physiology*, 14th ed. Vol 1. St. Louis, Mosby, 1980, pp 762–786.

Iwatsubo T, Kuzuhara S, Kanemitsu A, et al: Corticofugal projections to the motor nuclei of the brain stem and spinal cord in humans. *Neurology* 40:309, 1990.

Kertesz A, Ferro JM, Shewan CM: Apraxia and aphasia: The functional anatomical basis for their dissociation. *Neurology* 34:40, 1984.

Kleist K: Leitunsgaphasie (Nachtsprechaphasie). In Bonhoffer K (ed): *Handbuch der artzilichen Erhahrungen im Welktriege*. 1914/1918. Barth, Leipzig, 1934. pp 725–737.

Lance JW: The control of muscle tone, reflexes and movement: Robert Wartenburg Lecture. *Neurology* 30:1303, 1980.

Laplane D, Talairach J, Meininger V, et al: Motor consequences of motor area ablations in man. *J Neurol Sci* 31:29, 1977.

Lassek AM: *The Pyramidal Tract*. Springfield, IL, Charles C Thomas, 1954.

Lawrence DG, Kuypers HGJM: The functional organization of the motor system in the monkey. *Brain* 91:1, 15, 1968.

Lhermitte F: "Utilization behaviour" and its relation to lesions of the frontal lobes. *Brain* 106:237, 1983.

Liepmann H: Das Krankheitsbild der Apraxie (motorische Asymbolie auf Grund eines Falles von einseitiger Apraxie). *Monatsschr Psychiatr Neurol* 8:15, 102, 182, 1900.

Lorente de Nó R: Cerebral cortex: Architecture, intracortical connections, motor projections, in Fulton JF (ed): *Physiology of the Nervous System*, 3rd ed. New York, Oxford University Press, 1949, pp 288–330.

Luria AR: The Working Brain: *An Introduction to Neuropsychology*. New York, Basic Books, 1973.

Marx JJ, Ianetti GD, Thöme F, et al: Somatotopic organization of the corticospinal tract in the human brainstem: A MRI-based mapping analysis. *Ann Neurol* 57:824, 2005.

Mountcastle VB: Central nervous mechanisms in sensation, in Mountcastle VB (ed): *Medical Physiology*, 14th ed. Vol 1: Part 5. St. Louis, Mosby, 1980, pp 327–605.

Nathan PW, Smith M, Deacon P: Vestibulospinal, reticulospinal and descending propriospinal nerve fibers in man. *Brain* 119:1809, 1996.

Nyberg-Hansen R, Rinvik E: Some comments on the pyramidal tract with special reference to its individual variations in man. *Acta Neurol Scand* 39:1, 1963.

Okun MS, Rodriquez RL, Foote KD, et al: The "chair test" to aid in the diagnosis of psychogenic gait disorders. *The Neurologist* 13:87, 2007.

Pantano P, Formisano R, Ricci M, et al: Prolonged muscular flaccidity after stroke. Morphological and functional brain alterations. *Brain* 118:1329, 1995.

Pause M, Kunesch F, Binkofski F, Freund H-J: Sensorimotor disturbances in patients with lesions of the parietal cortex. *Brain* 112:1599, 1989.

Phillipon J, Porier J: *Joseph Babinski: A biography*. Oxford University Press, 2009, p 221.

Roland PE: Organization of motor control by the normal human brain. *Hum Neurobiol* 2:205, 1984.

Ropper AH, Fisher CM, Kleinman GM: Pyramidal infarction in the medulla: A cause of pure motor hemiplegia sparing the face. *Neurology* 29:91, 1979.

Russell JR, DeMyer W: The quantitative cortical origin of pyramidal axons of Macaca rhesus, with some remarks on the slow rate of axolysis. *Neurology* 11:96, 1961.

Terao S, Miura N, Takeda A, et al: Course and distribution of facial corticobulbar tract fibers in the lower brainstem. *J Neurol Neurosurg Psychiatry* 69:262, 2000.

Terakawa H, Abe K, Nakamura M, et al: Ipsilateral hemiparesis after putaminal hemorrhage due to uncrossed pyramidal tract. *Neurology* 54:1801, 2000.

Thach WT Jr, Montgomery EB Jr: Motor system, in Pearlman AL, Collins RC (eds): *Neurobiology of Disease*. New York, Oxford University Press, 1990, pp 168–196.

Tower SS: Pyramidal lesion in the monkey. *Brain* 63:36, 1940.

Van Gijn J: *The Babinski Sign. A Centenarary*. Universitiet Utrecht. Utrecht, 1996.

Vulliemoz S, Raineteau O, Jabaudon D. Reaching beyond the midline: why are human brains cross wired? *Lancet Neurol* 2005; 4: 87–99.

4

Abnormalities of Movement and Posture Caused by Disease of the Basal Ganglia

In this chapter, disorders of the automatic, static, postural, and other less-modifiable motor activities of the nervous system are discussed. They are an expression of what has come to be called the extrapyramidal motor system, meaning—according to S.A.K. Wilson, who introduced this term—the motor structures of the basal ganglia and certain related thalamic and brainstem nuclei.

The activities of the basal ganglia and the cerebellum are blended with and modulate the corticospinal system and the postural influence of the extrapyramidal system is indispensable to voluntary corticospinal movements. This close association of the basal ganglia and corticospinal systems becomes evident in the course of many forms of neurologic disease. In many aberrant motor patterns, one sees evidence not only of the activity of the basal ganglia but also of labyrinthine, tonic neck, and other postural reflexes that are mediated through nonpyramidal, bulbospinal and other brainstem motor systems. Observations such as these have blurred the original distinctions between pyramidal and extrapyramidal motor systems. Nevertheless, this division remains a useful concept in clinical work because it compels a distinction among several motor syndromes—one that is characterized by a loss of volitional movement accompanied by spasticity—the corticospinal syndrome; a second by bradykinesia, rigidity, and tremor without loss of voluntary movement—the hypokinetic basal ganglionic syndrome; a third by involuntary movements (choreoathetosis and dystonia)—the hyperkinetic basal ganglionic syndrome; and yet another by incoordination (ataxia)—the cerebellar syndrome. Table 4-1 summarizes the main clinical differences between corticospinal and extrapyramidal syndromes.

THE STRIATOPALLIDONIGRAL SYSTEM (BASAL GANGLIA)

Anatomic Considerations

As an anatomic entity, the basal ganglia have no precise definition. Principally they include the caudate nucleus and the lentiform (lenticular, from its lens-like shape) nucleus with its two subdivisions—the putamen and globus pallidus. Insofar as the caudate nucleus and putamen are really a continuous structure (separated only incompletely by fibers of the internal capsule) and are cytologically and functionally distinct from the pallidum, it is more meaningful to divide these nuclear masses into the striatum (or neostriatum), comprising the caudate nucleus and putamen, and the paleostriatum or pallidum, which has a medial (internal) and a lateral (external) portion. The putamen and pallidum lie on the lateral aspect of the internal capsule, which separates them from the caudate nucleus, thalamus, subthalamic nucleus, and substantia nigra on its medial side (Figs. 4-1 and 4-2). By virtue of their close connections with the caudate and lenticular nuclei, the subthalamic nucleus (nucleus of Luys) and the substantia nigra are included as parts of the basal ganglia. The claustrum and amygdaloid nuclear complex, because of their largely different connections and functions, are usually excluded.

For reasons indicated further on, some physiologists have expanded the list of basal ganglionic structures to include the red nucleus, the intralaminar thalamic nuclei, and the reticular formations of the upper brainstem. These structures receive direct cortical projections and give rise to rubrospinal and reticulospinal tracts that run parallel to the corticospinal (pyramidal) ones; hence they also were once referred to as extrapyramidal. However, these nonpyramidal linkages are structurally independent of the major extrapyramidal circuits and are better termed parapyramidal systems. As the final links in this circuit—the premotor and supplementary motor cortices—ultimately project onto the motor cortex, they are more aptly referred to as prepyramidal (Thach and Montgomery).

Earlier views of basal ganglionic organization emphasized serial connectivity and the funneling of efferent projections to the ventrolateral thalamus and thence to the motor cortex (Fig. 4-3). This concept was based largely on the experimental work of Whittier and Mettler and of Carpenter, in the late 1940s. These investigators demonstrated, in monkeys, that a characteristic movement disorder, which they termed choreoid dyskinesia, could be brought about in the limbs of one side of the body by a lesion localized to the opposite subthalamic nucleus. They also showed that for such a lesion to provoke dyskinesia, the adjacent pallidum and

Table 4-1

CLINICAL DIFFERENCES BETWEEN CORTICOSPINAL AND EXTRAPYRAMIDAL SYNDROMES

	CORTICOSPINAL	EXTRAPYRAMIDAL
Character of the alteration of muscle tone	Clasp-knife effect (spasticity)	Plastic, equal throughout passive movement (rigidity), or intermittent (cogwheel rigidity)
Distribution of hypertonus	Flexors of arms, extensors of legs	Generalized but predominates in flexors of limbs and of trunk
Involuntary movements	Absent	Presence of tremor, chorea, athetosis, dystonia
Tendon reflexes	Increased	Normal or slightly increased
Babinski sign	Present	Absent
Paralysis of voluntary movement	Present	Absent or slight

pallidofugal fibers had to be preserved; that is, a second lesion—placed in the medial segment of the pallidum, in the fasciculus lenticularis, or in the ventrolateral thalamus—abolished the dyskinesia. This experimental hyperkinesia could also be abolished by interruption of the lateral corticospinal tract but not by sectioning of the other motor or sensory pathways in the spinal cord. These observations were interpreted to mean that the subthalamic nucleus exerts an inhibitory or regulating influence on the globus pallidus and ventral thalamus. Removal of this influence by selective destruction of the subthalamic nucleus is expressed physiologically by an irregular activity that is now identified as chorea, presumably arising from the intact pallidum and conveyed to the ventrolateral thalamic nuclei, thence by thalamocortical fibers to the ipsilateral premotor cortex, and from there, to the motor cortex, all in a serial manner.

New observations have made it apparent that there are instead, a number of parallel circuits as detailed further on. However, a general principle that has withstood the test of time is the central role of the ventrolateral and ventroanterior nuclei of the thalamus. Together, these nuclei form a vital link, not only from the basal ganglia but also from the cerebellum, to the motor and premotor cortex. Thus, both basal ganglionic and cerebellar influences are brought to bear, via thalamocortical fibers, on the corticospinal system and on other descending pathways from the cortex. Direct descending pathways from the basal ganglia to the spinal cord are relatively insignificant.

The foregoing view of basal ganglionic organization has been broadened considerably as a result of newer anatomic, physiologic, and pharmacologic data (see reviews of Gombart and colleagues, of DeLong,

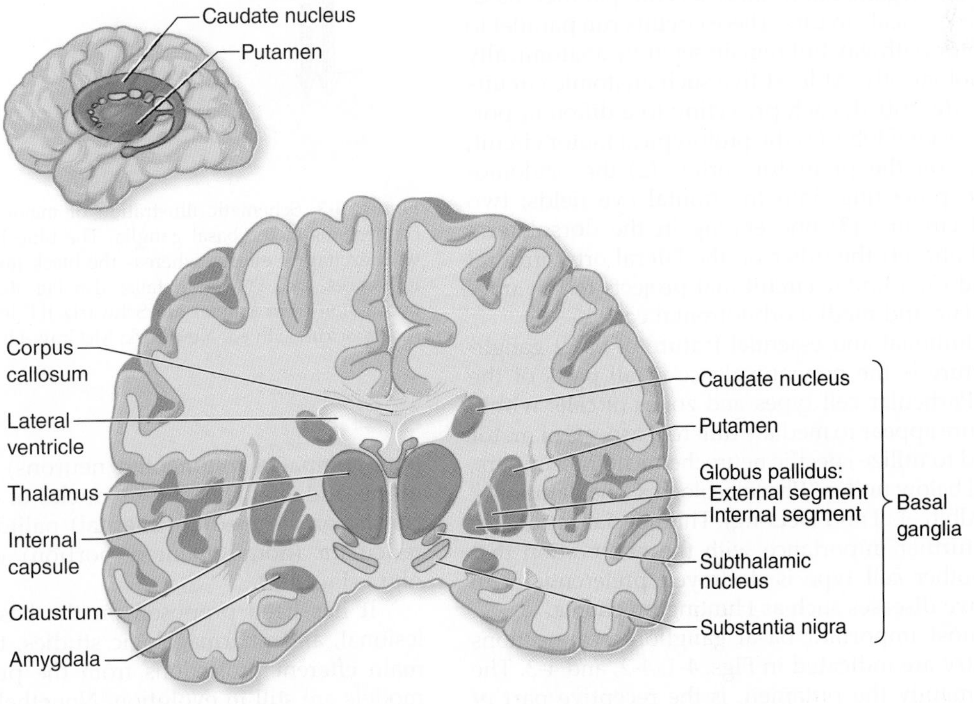

Figure 4-1. Overview of the components of the basal ganglia in coronal view. The main nuclei of the basal ganglia are represented in blue, as labeled on the right.

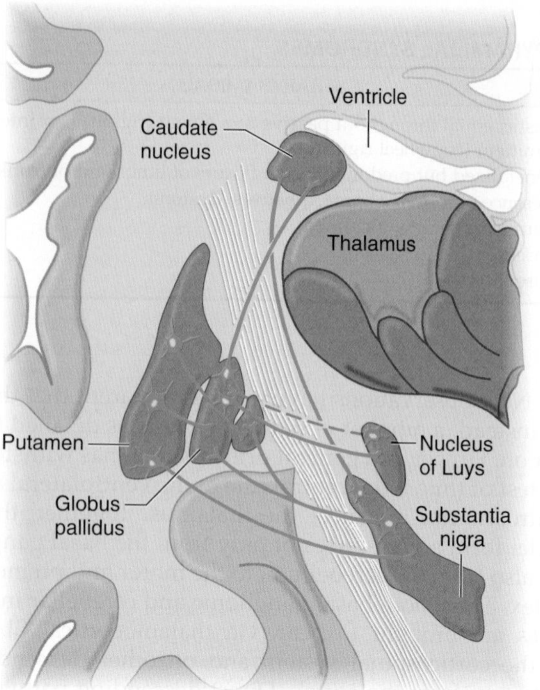

Figure 4-2. Diagram of the basal ganglia in the coronal plane, illustrating the main interconnections (see text for details). The pallidothalamic connections are illustrated in Fig. 4-3.

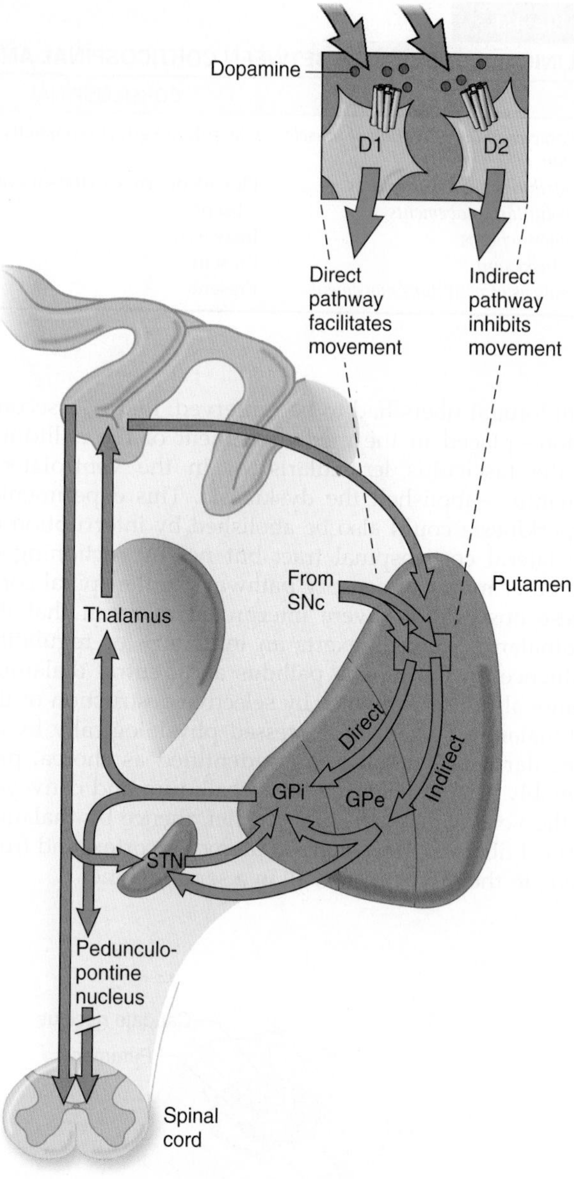

Figure 4-3. Schematic illustration of major efferent and afferent connections of the basal ganglia. The blue lines indicate neurons with excitatory effects, whereas the black lines indicate inhibitory influences. (See text for details; also Fig. 4-2.) (Reproduced with permission from Kandel ER, Schwartz JH, Jessell TM: *Principles of Neural Science*, 5th ed. New York: McGraw-Hill, 2013.)

and of Penney and Young). Whereas earlier concepts emphasized the serial connectivity of the basal ganglionic structures as mentioned earlier, current evidence indicates an organization into several parallel basal ganglionic–cortical circuits. These circuits run parallel to the premotor pathway but remain separate anatomically and physiologically. At least five such anatomic circuits have been described, each projecting to a different portion of the frontal lobe: (1) the prototypical motor circuit, converging on the premotor cortex; (2) the oculomotor circuit, projecting onto the frontal eye fields; two prefrontal circuits: (3) one ending in the dorsolateral prefrontal and (4) the other on the lateral orbitofrontal cortex; and (5) a limbic circuit that projects to the anterior cingulate and medial orbitofrontal cortex.

An additional and essential feature of basal ganglionic structure is the nonequivalence of all parts of the striatum. Particular cell types and zones of cells within this structure appear to mediate different aspects of motor control and to utilize specific neurochemical transmitters, as detailed below under "Pharmacologic Considerations" (see also Albin et al and DeLong). This specialization has taken on further importance with the observation that one or another cell type is destroyed preferentially in degenerative diseases such as Huntington chorea.

The most important basal ganglionic connections and circuitry are indicated in Figs. 4-1, 4-2, and 4-3. The striatum, mainly the putamen, is the receptive part of the basal ganglia, receiving topographically organized fibers from all parts of the cerebral cortex and from the pars compacta (pigmented neurons) of the substantia nigra, and that the output nuclei of the basal ganglia consist of the medial (internal) pallidum and the pars reticulata (nonpigmented portion) of the substantia nigra (Fig. 4-3).

It has been proposed on the basis of physiologic, lesional, and pharmacologic studies, that there are two main efferent projections from the putamen; but these models are still in evolution. Nonetheless, there are reasons to conceptualize 1) a *direct* efferent system from the putamen to the medial (internal) pallidum and then to the substantia nigra, particularly to the pars reticulata, and 2) an *indirect* system originating in the putamen that traverses the lateral (external) pallidum and continues to the subthalamic nucleus, with which it has strong reciprocal connections.

In most ways, the subthalamic nucleus and lateral pallidum operate as a single functional unit, (at least in terms of the effects of lesions in those locations on parkinsonian symptoms and the neurotransmitters involved. The medial pallidum and reticular part of the substantia nigra can be viewed in a similar unitary way, sharing the same input and output patterns. Within the indirect pathway, an internal loop is created by projections from the subthalamic nucleus to the medial segment of the pallidum and pars reticulata. A second offshoot of the indirect pathway consists of projections from the lateral pallidum to the medial pallidonigral output nuclei. A complete account of this intricate connectivity cannot be given, but the main themes outlined here seem valid.

From the internal pallidum, two bundles of fibers reach the thalamus—the ansa lenticularis and the fasciculus lenticularis. The ansa sweeps around the internal capsule; the fasciculus traverses the internal capsule in a number of small fascicles and then continues medially and caudally to join the ansa in the prerubral field. Both of these fiber bundles join the thalamic fasciculus, which then contains not only the pallidothalamic projections but also mesothalamic, rubrothalamic, and dentatothalamic ones. These projections are directed to separate targets in the ventrolateral nucleus of the thalamus and to a lesser extent in the ventral anterior and intralaminar thalamic nuclei. The centromedian nucleus of the intralaminar group projects back to the putamen and, via the parafascicular nucleus, to the caudate. A major projection from the ventral thalamic nuclei to the ipsilateral premotor cortex completes the large cortical–striatal–pallidal–thalamic–cortical motor loop, with conservation of the somatotopic arrangement of motor fibers, again emphasizing the nexus of motor control at the thalamic nuclei.

Physiologic Considerations

In simplest physiologic terms, Denny-Brown and Yanagisawa, who studied the effects of ablation of individual extrapyramidal structures in monkeys, concluded that the basal ganglia function as a kind of clearinghouse where, during an intended or projected movement, one set of activities is facilitated and all other unnecessary ones are suppressed. They used the analogy of the basal ganglia as a brake or switch, the tonic inhibitory ("brake") action preventing target structures from generating unwanted motor activity and the "switch" function referring to the capacity of the basal ganglia to select which of many available motor programs will be active at any given time. Still other theoretical constructs focus on the role of the basal ganglia in the initiation, sequencing, and modulation of motor activity ("motor programming"). Also, it appears that the basal ganglia participate in the constant priming of the motor system, enabling the rapid execution of motor acts without premeditation—e.g., hitting a baseball. In most ways, these conceptualizations restate the same notions of balance and selectivity imparted to all motor actions by the basal ganglia.

Physiologic evidence indicates that a balanced functional architecture, one excitatory and the other inhibitory, is operative within the individual circuits. The *direct* striatomedial pallidonigral pathway is activated by glutaminergic projections from the sensorimotor cortex and by dopaminergic nigral (pars compacta)–striatal projections. Activation of this direct pathway inhibits the medial pallidum, which, in turn, disinhibits the ventrolateral and ventroanterior nuclei of the thalamus. As a consequence, thalamocortical drive is enhanced and cortically initiated movements are facilitated. The *indirect* circuit arises from putaminal neurons that contain gamma-aminobutyric acid (GABA) and smaller amounts of enkephalin. These striatal projections have an inhibitory effect on the lateral pallidum, which, in turn, disinhibits the subthalamic nucleus through GABA release, providing subthalamic drive to the medial pallidum and substantia nigra pars reticulata. The net effect is thalamic inhibition that reduces thalamocortical input to the precentral motor fields and impedes voluntary movement. These complex anatomic and physiologic relationships have been summarized in numerous schematic diagrams similar to Fig. 4-4 and those by Lang and Lozano and by Standaert and Young.

Restated, the current view is that enhanced conduction through the indirect pathway leads to hypokinesia by increasing pallidothalamic inhibition, whereas enhanced conduction through the direct pathway results in hyperkinesia by reducing pallidothalamic inhibition. The direct pathway has been conceived by Marsden and Obeso as facilitating cortically initiated movements and the indirect pathway as suppressing potentially conflicting and unwanted motor patterns. In Parkinson disease, e.g., loss of dopaminergic input from the substantia nigra diminishes activity in the direct pathway and increases activity in the indirect pathway; the net effect is to increase inhibition of the thalamic nuclei and to reduce excitation of the cortical motor system.

Further insight into these systems and into the mechanism of Parkinson disease has come from the discovery that the parkinsonian syndrome is reproduced in humans and primates by the toxin 1-methyl-4-phenyl-1,2,3,6-tetrahydropyridine (MPTP). This toxin was discovered accidentally in drug addicts who self-administered an analogue of meperidine. The toxin binds with high affinity to monoamine oxidase (MAO), an extraneural enzyme that transforms it to pyridinium, a toxic metabolite that is bound by melanin in the dopaminergic nigral neurons in sufficient quantities to destroy the cells, probably by interfering with mitochondrial function. In monkeys made parkinsonian by the administration of MPTP, electrophysiologic studies have shown increased activity in the medial globus pallidus and decreased activity in the lateral globus pallidus, as predicted from the above described models. This comes about because of the differential loss of activity of dopaminergic striatal neurons that project to each of these parts of the pallidum. The end result is increased inhibition of thalamocortical neurons. It is, however, difficult to explain why medial pallidal

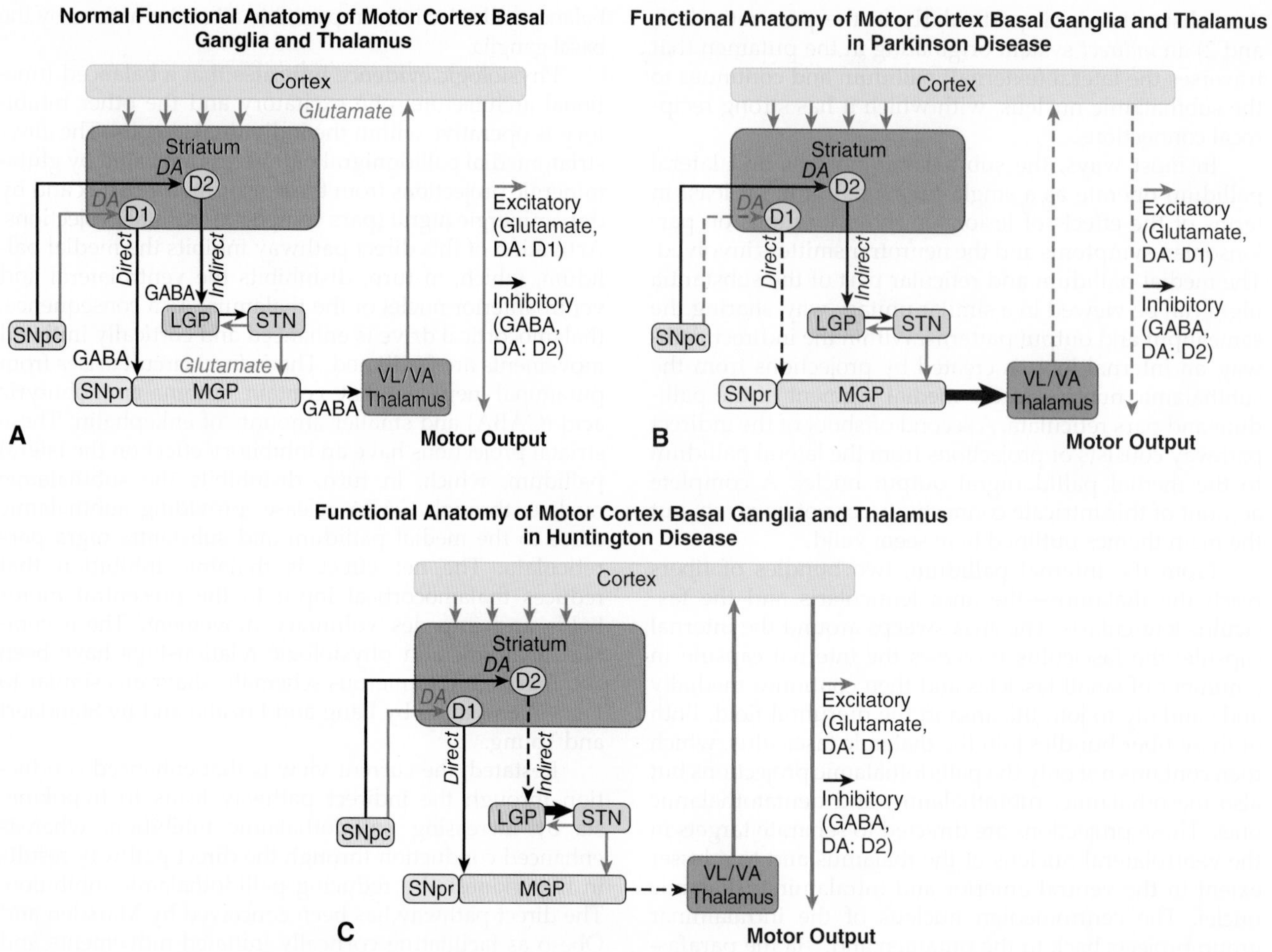

Figure 4-4. *A.* Schematic diagram of the main neurotransmitter pathways and their effects in the cortical–basal ganglia–thalamic circuits. The blue lines indicate neurons with excitatory effects; the black lines indicate inhibitory influences. The internal (medial) segment of the globus pallidus (MGP) and the zona reticulata of the substantia nigra (SNpr) are believed to act as one entity that projects via GABA-containing neurons to the thalamus (ventrolateral and ventroanterior nuclei) and to the pedunculopontine nuclei (not shown). Dopaminergic neurons (DA) arising in the pars compacta of the substantia nigra (SNpc) have an excitatory influence on the direct striatopallidal fibers (via D1 receptors) and an inhibitory effect on the indirect striatopallidal fibers (via D2 receptors) that project to the external (lateral) pallidum (LGP) and subthalamic nucleus (STN). Dotted lines in the subsequent figures denote a reduction in activity of the pathway. (See text.) *B.* Corresponding physiologic state as conceptualized in Parkinson disease, in which hypokinesia is the main finding as a result of reduced dopamine input from the substantia nigra and pars compacta to the striatum via the direct pathway, which results in withdrawal of inhibitory activity of the globus pallidus and, in turn, increased inhibitory drive on the thalamic nuclei, which reduces input to the cortical motor system. *C.* Schematic diagram of the theorized mechanism in Huntington disease, a hyperkinetic movement disorder resulting from reduced inhibition by the striatum within the indirect pathway, overdriving of the subthalamic nucleus, and causing excess activity in thalamocortical circuits. (See text.)

lesions do not regularly cause parkinsonism. Perhaps it is because the subtle imbalance between the medial and lateral pallidal circuits that exists in Parkinson disease is not reproduced. This subtlety may also explain why crude lesions, such as infarcts, hemorrhages, and tumors, rarely produce the complete parkinsonian syndrome of tremor, bradykinesia, and rigidity. Indeed, striking improvements in parkinsonian symptoms are obtained, paradoxically, by placing lesions in the medial pallidum (pallidotomy) as discussed in Chap. 39.

It is likely that the static model of inhibitory and excitatory pathways and the parsing of a direct and an indirect pathway, as useful as it is as a mnemonic, does not account well for the dynamic activities of the basal ganglia. In particular, the electrical activity of the neurons in these systems oscillate and influence the frequency of oscillations in other parts of the system, as well as bringing individual cells closer to firing. Another deficiency of currently conceived models is that they do not account for the tremor of Parkinson disease. To further complicate matters, the various subtypes of dopamine receptors act in both excitatory and inhibitory ways under different circumstances depending on their location as discussed below.

The manner in which excessive or reduced activity of various components of the basal ganglia gives rise to hypokinetic and hyperkinetic movement disorders is discussed further on, under "Symptoms of Basal Ganglia Disease."

Pharmacologic Considerations

A series of pharmacologic observations have considerably enhanced our understanding of basal ganglionic function and led to a rational treatment of Parkinson disease and other extrapyramidal syndromes. Whereas physiologists had for years failed to discover the functions of the basal ganglia by stimulation and crude ablation experiments, clinicians became aware that certain drugs, such as reserpine and the phenothiazines, could produce extrapyramidal syndromes (e.g., parkinsonism, choreoathetosis, dystonia). These observations stimulated the study of central nervous system (CNS) transmitter substances in general. The current view is that the integrated basal ganglionic control of movement can be best understood by considering, in the context of the anatomy described above, the physiologic effects of neurotransmitters that convey the signals between cortex, striatum, globus pallidus, subthalamic nucleus, substantia nigra, and thalamus.

The most important neurotransmitter substances from the point of view of basal ganglionic function are glutamate, GABA, dopamine, acetylcholine, and serotonin. Figure 4-4 summarizes their roles. A more complete account of this subject may be found in the reviews of Penney and Young, of Alexander and Crutcher, and of Rao.

The following is what is known with a fair degree of certainty. Glutamate is the neurotransmitter of the excitatory projections from the cortex to the striatum and of the excitatory neurons of the subthalamic nucleus. GABA is the inhibitory neurotransmitter of striatal, pallidal, and substantia nigra (pars reticulata) projection neurons.

Acetylcholine (ACh), long established as the neurotransmitter at the neuromuscular junction and the autonomic ganglia, is also physiologically active in the basal ganglia. The highest concentration of ACh, as well as of the enzymes necessary for its synthesis and degradation (choline acetyl transferase and acetylcholinesterase), is in the striatum. Acetylcholine is synthesized and released by the large but sparse (Golgi type 2) nonspiny striatal neurons. It has a mixed but mainly excitatory effect on the more numerous spiny neurons within the putamen that constitute the main origin of the direct and indirect pathways described above. It is likely that the effectiveness of atropinic agents—which have been used empirically for many years in the treatment of Parkinson disease and dystonia—depends on their capacity to antagonize ACh at sites within the basal ganglia and in projections from the pedunculopontine nuclei. Acetylcholine also appears to act on the presynaptic membrane of striatal cells and to influence their release of neurotransmitters, as discussed below. In addition, the basal ganglia contain other biologically active substances—substance P, enkephalin, cholecystokinin, somatostatin, and neuropeptide Y—which enhance or diminish the effects of other neurotransmitters, i.e., they act as neuromodulators.

Of the catecholamines, dopamine has the most pervasive role but its influence can be excitatory or inhibitory depending on the site of action and the subtype of dopamine receptor. Disturbances of dopamine signaling are essential abnormalities of several CNS disorders including parkinsonism, schizophrenia, attention deficit hyperactivity disorder, and drug abuse. Within the basal ganglia, the areas richest in dopamine are the substantia nigra, where it is synthesized in the nerve cell bodies of the pars compacta, and the termination of these fibers in the striatum. In the most simplified models, stimulation of the dopaminergic neurons of the substantia nigra induces a specific response in the striatum—namely, an inhibitory effect on the already low firing rate of neostriatal neurons. However, the effects of dopamine have proved even more difficult to resolve, in large part because there are now five known types of postsynaptic dopamine receptors (D1 to D5), each with a particular anatomic distribution and pharmacologic action. This heterogeneity is exemplified in the excitatory effect of dopamine on the small spiny neurons of the putamen and an inhibitory effect on others.

The five types of dopamine receptors are found in differing concentration throughout various parts of the brain, each displaying differing affinities for dopamine itself and for various drugs and other agents (Table 4-2; also see Jenner). The D1 and D2 receptors are highly concentrated in the striatum and are the ones most often implicated in diseases of the basal ganglia; D3 in the nucleus accumbens, D4 in the frontal cortex and certain limbic structures, and D5 in the hippocampus. In the striatum, the effects of dopamine act as a class of "D1-like" (D1 and D5 subtypes) and "D2-like" (D2, D3, and D4 subtypes) receptors. Activation of the D1 class stimulates adenyl cyclase, whereas D2 receptor binding inhibits this enzyme. Whether dopamine functions in an excitatory or inhibitory manner at a particular synapse is determined by the local receptor. As mentioned earlier, excitatory D1 receptors predominate on the small spiny putaminal neurons that are the origin of the direct striatopallidal output pathway, whereas D2 receptors mediate the inhibitory influence of dopamine on the indirect striatopallidal output, as indicated in Fig. 4-4.

Some of the clinical and pharmacologic effects of dopamine are made clear by considering both the anatomic sites of various receptors and their physiologic effects. For example, it appears that drug-induced parkinsonian syndromes and tardive dyskinesias (described further on) are prone to occur when drugs are administered that competitively bind to the D2 receptor, but that the newer antipsychosis drugs, which produce fewer of these effects, have a stronger affinity for the D4 receptor. However, the situation is actually far more complex, in part because of the synergistic activities of D1 and D2 receptors, each potentiating the other at some sites of convergence, and the presence on the presynaptic terminals of nigrostriatal neurons of D2 receptors, which inhibit dopamine synthesis and release.

Even these details do not capture the intricacy of neural transmission in the basal ganglia. In contrast to the almost instantaneous actions of glutamate and its antagonist, GABA, at synapses, the monoamines have more protracted effects, lasting for seconds or as long as several hours. Dopamine and related neurotransmitters have a slower influence through the "second messenger" cyclic adenosine monophosphate (cAMP), which, in

Table 4-2

PROPERTIES AND LOCALIZATION OF DOPAMINE RECEPTORS

	CLASSES OF DOPAMINERGIC RECEPTORS				
	D1	**D2**	**D3**	**D4**	**D5**
Within basal ganglia					
Striatum	+[a]	+[b]	+	+	+
Lateral GP		+		+	
Subthalamic nucleus	+	+	+		
Medial GP/SN pars reticulata	+				
SN pars compacta	+	+	+		
Outside basal ganglia					
Nucleus accumbens	+		+		
Frontal cortex	+			+	
Limbic structures				+	
Hippocampus				+	
Hypothalamus			+		+
Olfactory tubercle			+		
Pituitary	+				
Brainstem				+	
Drug affinities					
Dopamine	++	+++	++++	N/A	N/A
Bromocriptine	—	++	++	N/A	N/A
Pergolide	+	++++	+++	N/A	N/A
Ropinirole	0	+++	++++	N/A	N/A
Pramipexole	0	+++	++++	N/A	N/A

[a]Acts through direct striatal projection neurons.
[b]Acts through indirect striatal projection neurons.
GP, globus pallidus; SN, substantia nigra.

turn, controls the phosphorylation or dephosphorylation of numerous intraneuronal proteins. These intracellular effects have been summarized by Greengard.

The effects of certain drugs, some no longer in use, are also best comprehended by understanding the manner in which they alter neurotransmitter function. Several drugs—namely reserpine, the phenothiazines, and the butyrophenones (notably haloperidol)—induce prominent parkinsonian syndromes in humans. Reserpine, for example, depletes the striatum and other parts of the brain of dopamine; haloperidol and the phenothiazines work by a different mechanism, probably by blocking dopamine receptors within the striatum.

The basic validity of the physiologic-pharmacologic model outlined here is supported by the observation that excess doses of L-dopa or of a direct-acting dopamine receptor agonist lead to excessive motor activity. Furthermore, the therapeutic effects of the main drugs used in the treatment of Parkinson disease are understandable in the context of neurotransmitter function. To correct the basic dopamine deficiency from a loss of nigral cells that underlies Parkinson disease, attempts were at first made to administer dopamine directly. However, dopamine as such cannot cross the blood–brain barrier and therefore has no therapeutic effect. But its immediate precursor, L-dopa, does cross the blood–barrier and is effective in decreasing the symptoms of Parkinson disease as well as of the above-described MPTP-induced parkinsonism. This effect is enhanced by the addition of an inhibitor of dopadecarboxylase, an important enzyme in the catabolism of dopamine. The addition of an enzyme inhibitor of this type (carbidopa or benserazide) to L-dopa results in an increase of dopamine concentration in the brain, while sparing other organs from exposure to high levels of the drug. Similarly, drugs that inhibit catechol *O*-methyltransferase (COMT), another enzyme that metabolizes dopamine, prolong the effects of administered L-dopa.

Because of the pharmacologic effects of ACh and dopamine, it was originally postulated by Ehringer and Hornykiewicz (the latter originated the idea) that a functional equilibrium exists in the striatum between the excitatory activity of ACh and the inhibitory activity of dopamine. In Parkinson disease, the decreased release of dopamine by the substantia nigra onto the striatum disinhibits neurons that synthesize ACh, resulting in a predominance of cholinergic activity—a notion supported by the observation that parkinsonian symptoms are aggravated by centrally acting cholinergic drugs and improved by anticholinergic drugs. According to this theory, administration of anticholinergic drugs restores the ratio between dopamine and ACh, with the new equilibrium being set at a lower-than-normal level because the striatal levels of dopamine are low to begin with. This view has been validated in clinical practice in that one observes a beneficial effect on parkinsonian symptoms after the administration of anticholinergic agents. The use of drugs that enhance dopamine synthesis or its release, or that directly stimulate dopaminergic receptors in the striatum (e.g., pramipexole), represents another more direct method of treating Parkinson disease as outlined in Chap. 39.

The Pathology of Basal Ganglionic Disease

The extrapyramidal motor syndrome as we know it today was first delineated on clinical grounds and so named by S.A.K. Wilson in 1912. In the disease that now bears his name and that he called hepatolenticular degeneration, the most striking abnormality was a bilaterally symmetrical degeneration of the putamen, sometimes to the point of cavitation. To these lesions Wilson correctly attributed the characteristic symptoms of rigidity and tremor. Shortly thereafter, van Woerkom described a similar clinical syndrome in a patient with acquired liver disease (Wilson's cases were familial), the most prominent lesions again consisting of foci of neuronal degeneration in the striatum. Clinicopathologic studies of Huntington chorea—beginning with those of Meynert (1871) and followed by those of Jelgersma (1908) and Alzheimer (1911)—related the excessive movements and rigidity characteristic of the disease to a loss of nerve cells in the striatum. In 1920, Oskar and Cecile Vogt gave a detailed account of the neuropathologic changes in several patients who had been afflicted with choreoathetosis since early infancy; the changes, which they described as a "status fibrosus" or "status dysmyelinatus," were confined to the caudate and lenticular nuclei. Surprisingly, it was not until 1919 that Tretiakoff demonstrated the underlying cell loss of the substantia nigra in cases of what was then called paralysis agitans and is now known as Parkinson disease. Finally, a series of observations, culminating with those of J. Purdon Martin and later of Mitchell and colleagues, related hemiballismus to lesions in the subthalamic nucleus of Luys and its immediate connections. While these observations have been invaluable, it has become apparent from clinical work that none of the relationships between anatomic loci and movement disorders are exclusive and the same movement disorder can result from lesions at one of several sites.

Another broad perspective on the result of focal damage in the basal ganglia was afforded by Bhatia and Marsden, who reviewed some 240 cases in which there were lesions in the caudate, putamen, and globus pallidus associated with movement abnormalities. Dystonia occurred in 36 percent, chorea in 8 percent, parkinsonism in only 6 percent, and dystonia-parkinsonism in 3 percent. Bilateral lesions of the lenticular nuclei resulted in parkinsonism in 19 percent and dystonia-parkinsonism in 6 percent. It is also notable that a common associated behavioral abnormality was abulia (apathy and loss of initiative, spontaneous thought, and emotional responsivity), in those with caudate lesions. The deficiencies of this type of case analysis (i.e., the crudeness of computed tomography studies and obtained without regard to the temporal aspects of the clinical disorder), conceded by the authors, are obvious. We find it surprising that choreoathetosis was not more frequent. Needed are detailed anatomic (postmortem) studies of cases in which the disturbances of function were stable for many months or years. However, restating the comments above, there is no consistent association between any type of movement disorder and a particular location in the basal ganglia.

As a prelude to the next section, Table 4-3 summarizes the clinicopathologic correlations of extrapyramidal movement disorders that are accepted by most neurologists; it must be emphasized, however, that there is still some uncertainty as to the finer details.

SYMPTOMS OF BASAL GANGLIA DISEASE

In broad terms, all motor disorders consist of functional deficits (or negative symptoms) and conversely, excessive motor activity (positive symptoms), the latter being ascribed to the release or disinhibition of the activity of undamaged parts of the motor system. When diseases of the basal ganglia are analyzed along these lines, bradykinesia, hypokinesia, and loss of normal postural reflexes

Table 4-3
CLINICOPATHOLOGIC CORRELATIONS OF EXTRAPYRAMIDAL MOVEMENT DISORDERS

SYMPTOMS	PRINCIPAL LOCATION OF MORBID ANATOMY
Unilateral plastic rigidity with rest tremor (Parkinson disease)	Contralateral substantia nigra plus (?) other mesencephalic structures
Unilatral hemiballismus and hemichorea	Contralateral subthalamic nucleus of Luys or luysial–pallidal connections
Chronic chorea of Huntington type	Caudate nucleus and putamen
Athetosis and dystonia	Contralateral striatum (pathology of dystonia musculorum deformans unknown)
Cerebellar incoordination, intention tremor, and hypotonia	Ipsilateral cerebellar hemisphere; ipsilateral middle or inferior cerebellar peduncle; brachium conjunctivum (ipsilateral if below decussation, contralateral if above)
Decerebrate rigidity, i.e., extension of arms and legs, opisthotonos	Usually bilateral in tegmentum of upper brainstem at level of red nucleus or between red and vestibular nuclei
Palatal and facial myoclonus (rhythmic)	Ipsilateral central tegmental tract with denervation of inferior olivary nucleus and nucleus ambiguus
Diffuse myoclonus	Neuronal degeneration, usually diffuse or predominating in cerebral or cerebellar cortex and dentate nuclei

stand out as the primary negative symptoms, and tremor, rigidity, and the involuntary dyskinetic movements of chorea, athetosis, ballismus and dystonia, as the positive ones. Disorders of phonation, articulation, and locomotion due to basal ganglia disease are more difficult to classify. In some instances this group of disorders is clearly a consequence of rigidity and postural disorders, whereas in others, where rigidity is slight or negligible, they seem to represent primary deficiencies. Psychological stress and anxiety generally worsen the abnormal movements in extrapyramidal syndromes, just as relaxation improves them.

Hypokinesia and Bradykinesia

The terms hypokinesia and akinesia (the extreme form of hypokinesia) refer to a reduction in the spontaneous movements of an affected part and a failure to engage it freely in the natural actions of the body. In contrast to what occurs in paralysis (the primary symptom of corticospinal tract lesions), strength is not significantly diminished. Also, hypokinesia is unlike apraxia, in which a lesion erases the memory of the pattern of movements necessary for an intended act, leaving other actions intact. Hypokinesia is expressed most clearly in the parkinsonian patient where it takes the form of an extreme underactivity ("poverty") of movement. The frequent automatic, habitual movements observed in the normal individual—such as putting the hand to the face, folding the arms, or crossing the legs—are absent or greatly reduced. In looking to one side, the eyes move, but not the head. In arising from a chair, there is a failure to make the usual small preliminary adjustments, such as pulling the feet back, putting the hands on the arms of the chair, and so forth. Blinking is infrequent. Saliva is not swallowed as quickly as it is produced, and drooling results. The face lacks expressive mobility ("masked facies," or hypomimia). Speech is rapid, mumbling (or "cluttered"), and monotonic, and the voice is soft.

Bradykinesia, which connotes slowness rather than lack of movement, is another aspect of the same physiologic difficulty. Not only is the parkinsonian patient slightly "slow off the mark" (displaying a longer-than-normal interval between a command and the first contraction of muscle—i.e., increased reaction time), but the velocity of movement, or the time from onset to completion of movement, is slower than normal. Hallett distinguishes between akinesia and bradykinesia, equating akinesia with a prolonged reaction time and bradykinesia with a prolonged time of execution, but he has noted that if bradykinesia is severe, it results in akinesia. This is apparently not the result of slowness in formulating the plan of movement, which nonetheless seems at times to be another component of the parkinsonian syndromes. For a time, bradykinesia was attributed to the frequently associated rigidity, which could reasonably hamper all movements, but the limitation of this explanation became apparent when it was discovered that an appropriately placed stereotactic lesion in a patient with Parkinson disease may abolish rigidity while leaving the hypokinesia unaltered. Thus it appears that apart from their contribution to the maintenance of posture, the basal ganglia provide an essential element for the performance of the large variety of voluntary and semiautomatic actions required for the full repertoire of natural human motility.

Hallett and Khoshbin, in an analysis of ballistic (rapid) movements in the parkinsonian patient, found that the normal triphasic sequence of agonist–antagonist–agonist activation, as described in the next chapter, is intact but lacks the amplitude (number of activated motor units) to complete the movement. Several smaller triphasic sequences are then needed, which slow the movement. The patient experiences these phenomena as not only slowness but also a perceived weakness. That cells in the basal ganglia participate in the initiation of movement is also evident from the fact that the firing rates in these neurons increase before movement is detected clinically.

In terms of pathologic anatomy and physiology, bradykinesia may be caused by any process or drug that interrupts some component of the cortico-striato-pallido-thalamic circuit. Clinical examples include reduced dopaminergic input from the substantia nigra to the striatum, as in Parkinson disease; dopamine receptor blockade by neuroleptic drugs; extensive degeneration of striatal neurons, as in striatonigral degeneration and the rigid form of Huntington chorea; and destruction of the medial pallidum, as in Wilson diseases.

As illustrated in Fig. 4-4*B*, which gives a schematic representation of the hypokinetic state of Parkinson disease, changes in the cortico-striato-pallido-thalamic circuit (in this case mainly the direct striatopallidal pathway) can be interpreted in terms of altered neurochemical and resultant physiologic connectivity within the basal ganglia. The reciprocal situation, enhanced motor activity, is summarized in the analogous diagram for Huntington disease (Fig. 4-4C), in which a reduction in the activity of the indirect striatopallidal pathway leads to enhanced excitatory motor drive in the thalamocortical motor pathway.

A number of other disorders of voluntary movement may also be observed in patients with diseases of the basal ganglia. A persistent voluntary contraction of hand muscles, as in holding a pencil, may fail to be inhibited, so that there is interference with the next willed movement. This has been termed tonic innervation, or blocking, and may be brought out by asking the patient to repetitively open and close a fist or tap a finger. Attempts to perform an alternating sequence of movements may be blocked at one point, or there may be a tendency for the voluntary movement to adopt the frequency of a coexistent tremor (entrainment).

Disorders of Postural Fixation, Equilibrium, and Righting

These deficits are also demonstrated most clearly in the parkinsonian patient. The prevailing posture is one of involuntary flexion of the trunk and limbs and of the neck. Anticipatory and compensatory righting reflexes are also manifestly impaired. This occurs early in the course of progressive supranuclear palsy and later in

Parkinson disease. The inability of the patient to make appropriate postural adjustments to tilting or falling and his inability to move from the reclining to the standing position are closely related phenomena. A gentle push on the patient's sternum or a tug on the shoulders may cause a fall or start a series of small corrective steps that the patient cannot control (festination). These postural abnormalities are not attributable to weakness or to defects in proprioceptive, labyrinthine, or visual function, the principal forces that control the normal posture of the head and trunk.

Rigidity and Alterations in Muscle Tone

In the form of altered muscle tone known as rigidity, the muscles are continuously or intermittently firm and tense. Although brief periods of electromyographic silence can be obtained in selected muscles by persistent attempts to relax the limb, there is obviously a low threshold for involuntary sustained muscle contraction, and this is present during most of the waking state, even when the patient appears quiet and relaxed. In contrast to spasticity, the increased resistance on passive movement that characterizes rigidity is not preceded by an initial "free interval" and has an even or uniform quality throughout the range of movement of the limb, like that experienced in bending a lead pipe or pulling a strand of toffee. The contrasting terms clasp-knife for spasticity and lead-pipe for rigidity have been applied to the examiner's physical perception on attempting to smoothly manipulate the patient's limb through an arc of movement. Moreover, the rigidity of extrapyramidal disorder is not velocity-dependent, as it is in spasticity. The tendon reflexes are not enhanced in the rigid limb as they are in spasticity and, when released, the limb does not resume its original position, as happens in spasticity.

Rigidity usually involves both flexor and extensor muscle groups, but it tends to be more prominent in muscles that maintain a flexed posture, i.e., in the flexor muscles of trunk and limbs. It appears to be somewhat greater in the large muscle groups, but this may be merely a matter of muscle mass. Certainly the small muscles of the face and tongue and even those of the larynx are often affected by rigidity. Concordant with the physical examination, in the electromyographic tracing, motor-unit activity is more continuous in rigidity than in spasticity, persisting even after apparent relaxation.

A special feature that may accompany rigidity, first noted by Negro in 1901, is the cogwheel phenomenon. When the hypertonic muscle is passively stretched, e.g., when the hand is dorsiflexed, one encounters a rhythmically interrupted, ratchet-like resistance. Many believe that this phenomenon represents an underlying tremor that, if not manifestly present, emerges faintly during manipulation. In that case it would not be a fundamental property of rigidity and would be found in many tremulous states. However, numerous instances of severe tremor with minimally perceptible cogwheeling, and the opposite, suggest to us on clinical grounds that the phenomenon may be more complex.

Rigidity is a prominent feature of many basal ganglionic diseases, such as Parkinson disease, Wilson disease, striatonigral degeneration (multiple system atrophy), progressive supranuclear palsy, dystonia musculorum deformans (all discussed in Chap. 39), exposure to neuroleptic drugs, and mineralization of the basal ganglia (Fahr disease). Rigidity is characteristically variable in severity at different times; in some patients with involuntary movements, particularly in those with chorea or dystonia, the limbs may actually be intermittently or persistently hypotonic.

Another distinctive type of variable resistance to passive movement is one in which the patient seems unable to relax a group of muscles on request. When the limb muscles are passively stretched, the patient appears to actively resist the movement (gegenhalten, paratonia, or oppositional resistance). Natural relaxation normally requires concentration on the part of the patient. If there is inattentiveness—as happens with diseases of the frontal lobes, dementia, or other confusional states—this type of oppositional resistance may raise a question of parkinsonian rigidity. This is not a manifestation of basal ganglia disorder per se but may indicate that the connections of the basal ganglia to the frontal lobes are impaired. A similar difficulty in relaxation is observed normally in small children. Also not to be mistaken for rigidity or paratonia is the "waxy flexibility" displayed by the psychotic-catatonic patient when a limb placed in a suspended position is maintained for minutes in the identical posture (flexibilitas cerea, see Chap. 53).

Involuntary Movements (Chorea, Athetosis, Ballismus, Dystonia)

In deference to usual practice, these symptoms are described as though each represented a discrete clinical phenomenon, readily distinguishable from the others. In reality, they usually occur together or blend imperceptibly into each other and have many points of clinical similarity. There are reasons to believe that they have a common anatomic and physiologic basis although distinct sites in the brain have been tentatively implicated for each. One must be mindful that chorea, athetosis, and dystonia are symptoms and are not to be equated with disease entities that happen to incorporate one of these terms in their names (e.g., Huntington chorea, dystonia musculorum deformans). Here the discussion is limited to the symptoms. The diseases of which these symptoms are a part are considered mainly in Chap. 39.

Somewhat more ambiguous but in common clinical use is the term dyskinesia. It encompasses all the active movement phenomena that are a consequence of disease of the basal ganglia, usually implying an element of dystonia, but it has also been used to refer more specifically to the undifferentiated excessive movements that are induced in Parkinson patients at the peak of L-dopa effect and to numerous dystonic and athetotic movements that may follow the use of neuroleptic drugs ("tardive dyskinesias") that are discussed in Chaps. 6 and 43.

Chorea

Derived from the Greek word meaning "dance," chorea refers to involuntary arrhythmic movements of a forcible, rapid, jerky type. These movements may be simple or quite elaborate and of variable distribution. Although the movements are purposeless, the patient may incorporate them into a deliberate act, as if to make them less noticeable. When superimposed on voluntary actions, they may assume an exaggerated and bizarre character. Grimacing and peculiar respiratory sounds may be other expressions of the disorder. Usually the movements are discrete, but if very numerous, they become confluent and then resemble athetosis, as described below. In moments when the involuntary movements are held in abeyance, volitional movements of normal strength are possible; but they also tend to be excessively quick and poorly sustained. The limbs are often slack or hypotonic and because of this, the knee jerks tend to be pendular; in other words, with the patient sitting on the edge of the examining table and the foot free of the floor, the leg swings back and forth several times in response to a tap on the patellar tendon, rather than once or twice, as it does normally. A choreic movement may be superimposed on the reflex movement, checking it in flight, so to speak, and giving rise to the "hung-up" reflex.

The hypotonia in chorea as well as the pendular reflexes may suggest a disturbance of cerebellar function. Lacking, however, are "intention" tremor and true incoordination or ataxia. In some circumstances, it may be necessary to distinguish chorea from myoclonus. Chorea differs from myoclonus mainly with respect to the speed of the movements; the myoclonic jerk is much faster and may involve single muscles or part of a muscle as well as groups of muscles. Failure to appreciate these differences often results in an incorrect diagnosis.

Table 4-4 lists diseases characterized mainly by chorea. It is a major feature of Huntington disease, in which the movements tend more typically to be choreoathetotic. There may be subtle additional ataxia of gait, as noted by Breedveld and colleagues. Not infrequently, chorea has its onset in late life without the other identifying features of Huntington disease. It is then referred to as senile chorea, a term that is hardly helpful in understanding the process. Its relation to Huntington chorea in any individual case is settled by genetic testing. A number of less common degenerative conditions are associated with chorea, among them dentatorubropallidoluysian atrophy and a form of chorea associated with acanthocytosis of red blood cells. Also, there is an inherited form of chorea of childhood onset without dementia that has been referred to as benign hereditary chorea. These are discussed in Chap. 39.

Typical choreic movements are the dominant feature of Sydenham chorea and of the variety of that disease associated with pregnancy (chorea gravidarum), disorders that are strongly linked through some immune mechanism to streptococcal infection. Striatal abnormalities, usually transient and rarely persistent, have been demonstrated by MRI; (Emery and Vieco). It is perhaps not surprising that antibodies directed against cells of the basal ganglia have been detected in both acute and late Sydenham chorea (Church et al). Following from the connection to streptococcal infection and the detection of these antibodies, it has been suggested in recent years that the spectrum of poststreptococcal disorders can be extended to tic and obsessive-compulsive behavior in children. In these cases the neurologic problems are said to arise suddenly, subside, and return with future streptococcal infections, as discussed in Chap. 6. This seems unlikely to explain chorea in adults. There have been instances of paraneoplastic chorea associated in a very few cases with lung cancer and anti-CRMP or anti-Hu antibodies of the type described in Chap. 31, as reported by O'Toole and colleagues.

Table 4-4

DISEASES CHARACTERIZED BY CHOREA

Inherited disorders
Huntington disease
Benign hereditary chorea
Neuroacanthocytosis
Dentatorubropallidoluysian atrophy
Wilson disease
Immune mediated chorea
Sydenham chorea
Chorea gravidarum
Lupus erythematosus
Antiphospholipid antibodies
Paraneoplastic, often with other movements
Drug-induced chorea
Neuroleptics (phenothiazines, haloperidol, metoclopramide, and others)
Oral contraceptives
Phenytoin (occasionally other antiepileptic drugs)
Excess dosages of L-dopa and dopamine agonist medications
Cocaine
Chorea symptomatic of systemic disease
Thyrotoxicosis
Polycythemia vera
Hyperosmolar, nonketotic hyperglycemia
Toxoplasmosis in AIDS
Hemichorea
Stroke
Tumor
Vascular malformation

The chronic administration of phenothiazine drugs or haloperidol (or an idiosyncratic reaction to these drugs) is a common cause of extrapyramidal movement disorders of all types, including chorea; these may become manifest during use of the drug or in a delayed "tardive" fashion, as already mentioned. The newer antipsychosis drugs (the atypical neuroleptics) have been far less frequently associated with the problems. Excess dopamine administration in advanced Parkinson disease is perhaps the most common cause of a choreiform dyskinesia in practice, but the movements tend to be more complex and continuous than those seen in chorea.

The use of oral contraceptives sometimes elicits chorea in an otherwise healthy young woman, but many such patients have underlying systemic lupus erythematosus and antiphospholipid antibodies. Whether the chorea (usually unilateral) is the result of a small infarction (as suggested by a mild hemiparesis on the affected side) or is an immunologic condition is not settled. The reemergence of chorea in these circumstances as steroids are withdrawn or birth control pills are introduced suggests a more complex process than simply a small, deep infarction—perhaps something akin to Sydenham chorea. Also, only about one-third of cases involve a stroke, and some have demonstrated hypermetabolism of the basal ganglia, as in Sydenham chorea. A connection between hemichorea and the antiphospholipid syndrome alone, without lupus, is more tenuous.

The use of phenytoin or other anticonvulsant drugs may cause chorea in sensitive individuals. A transitory chorea may occur in the course of an acute metabolic derangement, mainly with hyperosmolar hyperglycemia, hypoglycemia, or hyponatremia, and with the inhalation of crack cocaine.

Rarely, chorea complicates hyperthyroidism, polycythemia vera, lupus erythematosus or some forms of cerebral arteritis. AIDS has emerged as a cause of a few cases of subacute progressive movement disorders that are initially asymmetrical. The usual associations in AIDS have been with focal lesions in or near basal ganglionic structures such as toxoplasmosis, progressive multifocal leukoencephalopathy, and lymphoma, but a number of instances of chorea are not explained by any of these focal lesions. A paraneoplastic variety may combine several aspects of chorea with athetosis, ballismus, or dystonia; inflammatory lesions are found in the striatum (Chap. 31).

Chorea may be limited to one side of the body (hemichorea). When the involuntary movements involve proximal limb muscles and are of wide range and flinging in nature, the condition is called hemiballismus (see further on). A cerebral infarction is the usual cause. A number of rare paroxysmal kinesigenic disorders, discussed later in this chapter, may have a choreic component.

The review by Piccolo and colleagues puts the frequency of the various causes of chorea in perspective. Of consecutive neurologic admissions to two general hospitals they identified 23 cases of chorea, of which 5 were drug-induced, 5 were AIDS-related, and 6 were caused by stroke. Sydenham chorea and arteritis were each found in 1 case. In 4 cases no cause could be determined, and 1 case proved to be Huntington disease.

The precise anatomic basis of chorea is often uncertain or at least inconsistent. In Huntington chorea, there are obvious lesions in the caudate nucleus and putamen. Yet one often observes vascular lesions in these parts without chorea. The localization of lesions in Sydenham chorea and other choreic diseases has not been determined beyond a generalized disturbance in the striatum, which is evident on some imaging studies. It is of interest that in instances of chorea related to acute metabolic disturbances, there are sometimes small infarctions in the basal ganglia or metabolic changes in the lenticular nucleus, as shown by imaging studies. One suspects from their close clinical similarity that chorea and hemiballismus relate to disorders of the same system of neurons; however, the subthalamic nucleus, the region typically implicated in ballismus, is affected only slightly in Huntington chorea and, on the other hand, transient chorea or ballismus arises from infarctions in any part of the striatum on the side opposite to the movement, particularly in the caudate.

Athetosis

This term stems from a Greek word meaning "unfixed" or "changeable." The condition is characterized by an inability to sustain the fingers and toes, tongue, or any other part of the body in one position. The maintained posture is interrupted by relatively slow, sinuous, purposeless movements that have a tendency to flow into one another. As a rule, the abnormal movements are most pronounced in the digits and hands, face, tongue, and throat, but no group of muscles is spared. One can detect as the basic patterns of movement an alternation between extension–pronation and flexion–supination of the arm and between flexion and extension of the fingers, the flexed and adducted thumb being trapped by the flexed fingers as the hand closes. Other characteristic movements are eversion–inversion of the foot, retraction and pursing of the lips, twisting of the neck and torso, and alternate wrinkling and relaxation of the forehead or forceful opening and closing of the eyelids. The movements appear to be slower than those of chorea, but all gradations between the two are seen; in some cases, it is impossible to distinguish between them, hence the term choreoathetosis. An apt description could be of a moving dystonia (see below). Discrete voluntary movements of the hand are executed more slowly than normal, and attempts to perform them may result in a cocontraction of antagonistic muscles and a spread (overflow) of contraction to muscles not normally required in the movement (intention spasm). The overflow appears related to a failure of the striatum to suppress the activity of unwanted muscle groups. Some forms of athetosis occur only during the performance of projected movement (intention or action athetosis). In other forms, the spasms appear to occur spontaneously, i.e., they are involuntary and, if persistent, give rise to more or less fixed dystonic postures.

Athetosis may affect all four limbs or may be unilateral, especially in children who have suffered a hemiplegia at some previous time (posthemiplegic athetosis). Many athetotic patients exhibit variable degrees of rigidity and motor deficit as a result of associated corticospinal tract disease; these may account for the slower quality of athetosis compared to chorea. In other patients with generalized choreoathetosis, as pointed out above, the limbs may be intermittently hypotonic.

The combination of athetosis and chorea of all four limbs is a cardinal feature of Huntington disease and of a state known as double athetosis, which begins in childhood. Athetosis appearing in the first years of life is usually the result of a congenital or postnatal condition such as hypoxia (cerebral palsy) or, rarely, kernicterus. Postmortem examinations in some of the cases have disclosed a unique pathologic change of probable hypoxic etiology, status marmoratus, in the striatum (Chap. 38). In other cases, of probable kernicteric (hyperbilirubinemic) etiology, there has been a loss of nerve cells and myelinated fibers—a status dysmyelinatus—in the same regions. In adults, athetosis may occur as an episodic or persistent disorder in hepatic encephalopathy, as a manifestation of chronic intoxication with phenothiazines or haloperidol, and as a feature of certain degenerative diseases, most notably Huntington chorea but also Wilson disease, Leigh disease, and other mitochondrial disease variants; less frequently athetosis may be seen with Niemann-Pick (type C) disease, Kufs disease, neuroacanthocytosis, and ataxia telangiectasia. It may also occur as an effect of excessive L-dopa in the treatment of Parkinson disease, in which case it appears to be caused by a decrease in the activity of the subthalamic nucleus and the medial segment of the globus pallidus (Mitchell et al). Athetosis, usually in combination with chorea, may occur rarely in patients with AIDS and in those taking anticonvulsants. Localized forms of athetosis may occasionally follow vascular lesions of the lenticular nucleus or thalamus, as in the cases described by Dooling and Adams.

Ballismus

This term designates an uncontrollable, poorly patterned flinging movement of an entire limb. As remarked earlier, it is closely related to chorea and athetosis, indicated by the frequent coexistence of these movement abnormalities and the tendency for ballismus to blend into a less-obtrusive choreoathetosis of the distal parts of the affected limb. Ballistic movements are usually unilateral (hemiballismus) and the result of an acute lesion of or near the contralateral subthalamic nucleus or immediately surrounding structures (infarction or hemorrhage, rarely a demyelinative or other lesion). Rarely, a transitory form is linked to a subdural hematoma or thalamic or parietal lesion. The flinging movements may be almost continuous or intermittent, occurring several times a minute, and of such dramatic appearance that it is not unusual for them to be regarded as hysterical in nature.

Bilateral ballismus is infrequent and usually asymmetrical; here a metabolic disturbance, particularly nonketotic hyperosmolar coma, is the usual cause. In combination with choreoathetosis, a paraneoplastic process is another rare cause. When ballismus persists for weeks on end, as it often did before effective treatment became available, the continuous forceful movements resulted in exhaustion and even death. In most cases, medication with haloperidol or phenothiazine suppresses the violent movements. In extreme cases, stereotactic lesions or implanted stimulating electrodes placed in the ventrolateral thalamus and zona incerta have proved effective (Krauss and Mundinger).

Dystonia (See Chap. 6 for a discussion of focal dystonias.)

Dystonia is an unnatural spasmodic movement of posture that puts the limb in a twisted posture. It is often patterned, repetitive or tremulous and can be initiated or worsened by attempted movement. There is unwanted overflow contraction of adjacent muscles and a central feature is involuntary cocontraction of agonist and antagonist muscles.

Dystonia may take the form of an overextension or overflexion of the hand, inversion of the foot, lateral flexion or retroflexion of the head, torsion of the spine with arching and twisting of the back, forceful closure of the eyes, or a fixed grimace (Fig. 4-5; see also Fig. 6-2).

Dystonia, like athetosis, may vary considerably in severity and may show striking fluctuations in individual patients. In its early stages it may be interpreted as an annoying mannerism or hysteria, and only later, in the face of persisting postural abnormality, lack of the usual psychologic features of hysteria, and the emerging character of the illness, is the correct diagnosis made. Dystonia may be limited to the facial, cervical, or trunk muscles or to those of one limb, and it may cease when the body is in repose and during sleep. Severe instances result in grotesque movements and distorted positions of the body; sometimes the whole musculature seems to be thrown into spasm by an effort to move an arm or to speak.

Causes of Generalized Dystonia Generalized dystonia is seen in its most pronounced form as an uncommon heritable disease, dystonia musculorum deformans, which is associated with a mutation in the DYT gene. It was in relation to this disease that Oppenheim and Vogt in 1911 introduced the term dystonia. Dystonia also occurs as a manifestation of many other diseases, each of which is characteristic of a certain age group. These include "double athetosis" caused by hypoxic damage to the fetal or neonatal brain, kernicterus, pantothenate kinase-associated neurodegeneration (formerly Hallevorden-Spatz disease), Huntington disease, Wilson disease, lysosomal storage diseases, striatopallidodentatal calcification (sometimes caused by hypoparathyroidism), thyroid disease, and exposure to neuroleptic drugs, as discussed below.

Widespread torsion spasm (another term for dystonia) may also be a prominent feature of certain rare heredodegenerative disorders, such as familial striatal necrosis with affection of the optic nerves and other parts of the nervous system (Marsden et al, Novotny et al). A distinct subset of patients with an idiopathic dystonia (described by Nygaard et al and discussed in Chap. 39) responds to extremely small doses of L-dopa. The disease is familial, usually autosomal dominant, and the dystonia-athetosis may be combined with elements of parkinsonism. Marked diurnal fluctuation of symptoms is characteristic with the movement disorder worsening as the day wears on and improving with sleep. This process has a number of names, including L-dopa–responsive dystonia and Segawa disease, for which specific causative mutations have been discovered. Another rare hereditary dystonia that has its onset in adolescence or early adulthood is of interest because of the rapid evolution, at times within an hour but more often over days, of severe dystonic spasms, dysarthria, dysphagia, and postural instability with bradykinesia, which may follow (Dobyns et al). A few cases have followed a febrile episode. The disorder is termed rapid-onset dystonia-parkinsonism. It is our understanding that the features of rapid-onset dystonia-parkinsonism are also mild and not responsive to L-dopa. Chapter 39 discusses these hereditary forms of dystonia.

A frequent cause of acute generalized dystonic reactions, more so in the past, has been from exposure to the

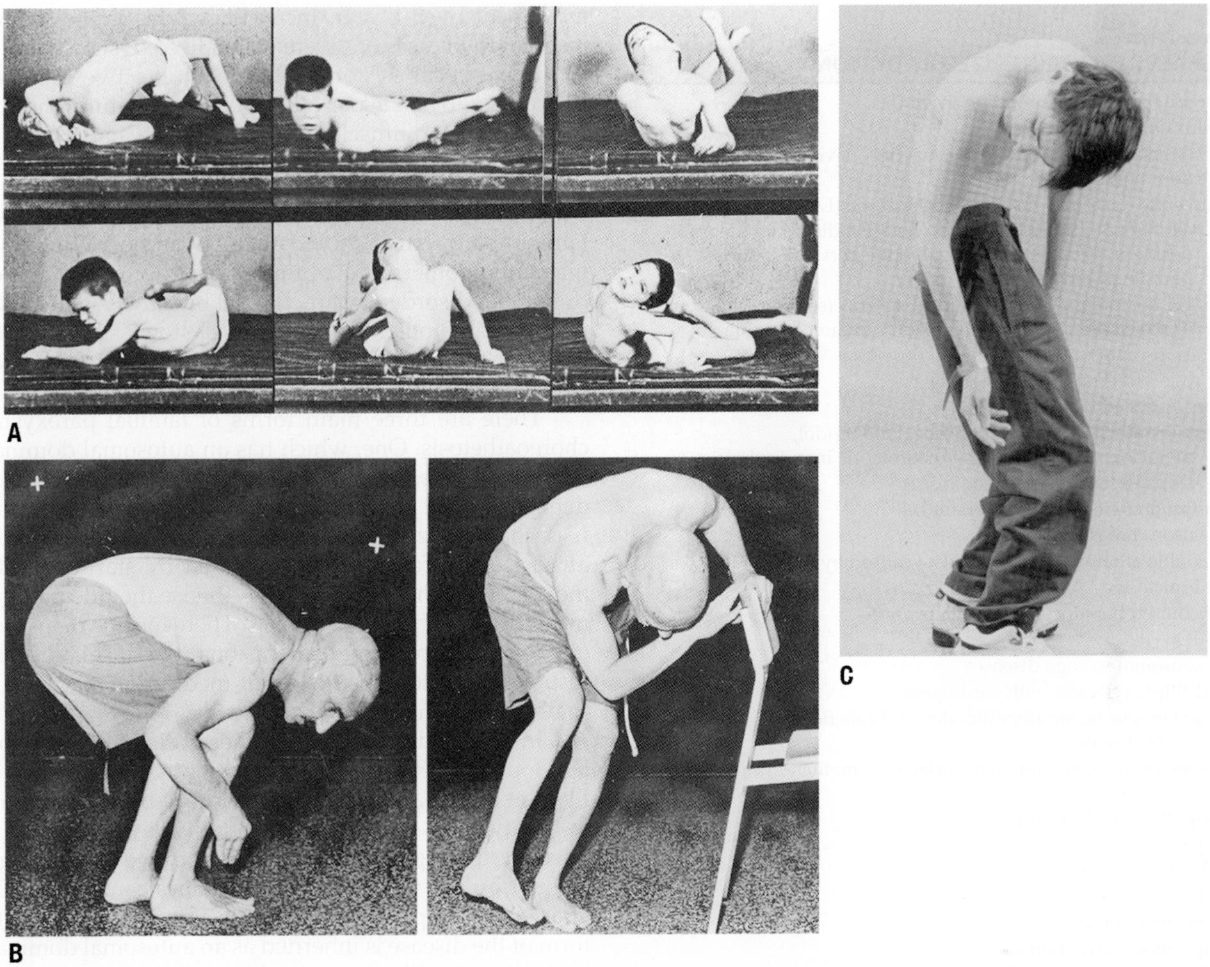

Figure 4-5. *A.* Characteristic dystonic deformities in a young boy with dystonia musculorum deformans. *B.* Sporadic instance of severe axial dystonia with onset in adult life. *C.* Incapacitating postural deformity in a young man with dystonia. (Photos courtesy of Dr. I.S. Cooper and Dr. Joseph M. Waltz.)

class of neuroleptic drugs—phenothiazines, butyrophenones, or metoclopramide—and even with the newer agents such as olanzapine, which has the advantage of producing these side effects less frequently than the others. A characteristic, almost diagnostic, example of the drug-induced dystonias consists of retrocollis (forced extension of the neck), arching of the back, internal rotation of the arms, and extension of the elbows and wrists—together simulating opisthotonos. These reactions respond to some extent to diphenhydramine or benztropine given two or three times over 24 to 48 h. L-Dopa, calcium channel blockers, and a number of anticonvulsants and anxiolytics are among a long list of other medications that may on occasion induce dystonia, the various causes of which are listed in Table 4-5. The acute dystonic drug reactions are idiosyncratic and now, probably as common as the "tardive dyskinesias" that had followed long-standing use or the withdrawal of a medication.

Finally, a peculiar and dramatic spasm of a limb or the entire body may be seen in patients with multiple sclerosis. The movements have aspects of dystonia and may be provoked by hyperventilation but they may not be, strictly speaking, dystonic. They are most likely to occur in patients with large demyelinative lesions of the cervical spinal cord.

Restricted or fragmentary forms of dystonia are the types most commonly encountered in clinical practice. Characteristically the spasms involve only the orbicularis oculi and face or mandibular muscles (blepharospasm-oromandibular dystonia), tongue, cervical muscles (torticollis), hand (writer's cramp), or foot. There may be an associated tremor, or tremor may be the only manifestation of an early dystonia. These are described in Chaps. 6 and 39.

Hemidystonia represents an unusual form of acquired movement that, in our experience, is rarely pure. In an analysis of 33 of their own cases and 157 previously published ones, Chuang and colleagues found stroke, mainly in the contralateral putamen, to be most often responsible. Traumatic and perinatal damage accounted for several cases and a large proportion had no lesions found by imaging tests. In the former, there was a delay of several years between the injury and the start of the movements; these authors also commented on the resistance of this syndrome to drug treatment.

Table 4-5

DISEASES CHARACTERIZED BY DYSTONIA

Hereditary and degenerative dystonias
- Huntington chorea
- Dystonia musculorum deformans (recessive and autosomal dominant forms)
- Juvenile dystonia—Parkinson syndrome (L-dopa–responsive)
- Dystonia with other heredodegenerative disorders (neural deafness, striatal necrosis with optic nerve affection, paraplegic amyotrophy)
- Focal dystonias and occupational spasms (see Chap. 6), some of which are allied with hereditary torsion dystonia
- Parkinson disease (occasional)
- Progressive supranuclear palsy

Drug-induced dystonias
- Acute and chronic phenothiazine, haloperidol, metoclopramide, and other neuroleptic intoxications
- L-Dopa excess in Parkinson disease

Symptomatic (secondary) dystonias
- Wilson disease
- Double athetosis (cerebral palsy) caused by cerebral hypoxia
- Kernicterus
- Acquired hepatocerebral degeneration
- AIDS
- Lysosomal storage diseases
- Multiple sclerosis with cord lesion
- Paraneoplastic striatopallidodentatal calcification (Fahr disease)
- Toxic necrosis of lenticular nuclei (e.g., methanol) can be delayed

Idiopathic focal dystonias
- Spasmodic torticollis
- Blepharospasm
- Hemifacial spasm
- Oromandibular dystonia
- Spasmodic dysphonia
- Writer's cramp and other occupational spasms

Treatment

Numerous drugs have been used to treat idiopathic chronic generalized dystonia, with a notable lack of success. However, Fahn has reported beneficial effects (more so in children than in adults) with the anticholinergic agents, trihexyphenidyl, benztropine, and ethopropazine given in massive amounts—which are achieved by increasing the dosage very gradually. The drug-induced tardive dyskinesias require specialized treatment, as described in Chaps. 6 and 42. Reinstitution of the offending drug or anticholinergic agents is often tried. Tetrabenazine, a centrally active monoamine-depleting agent, is effective but not readily available. The acute dystonic drug reactions are treated as noted above.

Stereotactic surgery on the pallidum and ventrolateral thalamus, a treatment introduced by Cooper in the middle of the last century, had reported generally positive but unpredictable results. In recent years there has been a renewed interest in a derivative of this form of treatment, deep brain stimulation (see Chap. 39). In a controlled trial, Vidailhet and colleagues demonstrated the effectiveness of this approach by stimulating the posteroventral globus pallidus bilaterally. Their patients had an average improvement of 50 percent on most scores of dystonic movement over 1 year. Increasingly, this is the method resorted to in cases of severe generalized dystonia.

In the focal dystonias, the most effective treatment has proved to be the periodic injection of botulinum toxin into the affected muscles as discussed in Chap. 6.

Paroxysmal Choreoathetosis and Dystonia

Under the names paroxysmal kinesigenic dyskinesia, familial paroxysmal choreoathetosis, and periodic dystonia, among others, are a number of uncommon sporadic or familial disorders characterized by paroxysmal attacks of choreoathetotic movements or dystonic spasms of the limbs and trunk. Both children and young adults are affected.

There are three main forms of familial paroxysmal choreoathetosis. One, which has an autosomal dominant (less often recessive) pattern of inheritance and a tendency to affect males, begins in adolescence or earlier. It is characterized by numerous brief (several minutes) attacks of choreoathetosis provoked by startle, sudden movement, or hyperventilation—hence the title paroxysmal kinesigenic choreoathetosis. There may be many dozens of attacks per day or occasional ones. This disorder responds well to anticonvulsant medication, particularly to phenytoin and carbamazepine.

In a second type, such as those originally described by Mount and Reback and subsequently by Lance and by Plant et al, the attacks take the form of persistent (5 min to 4 h) dystonic spasms and reportedly have been precipitated by the ingestion of alcohol or coffee or by fatigue but not by movement per se (nonkinesigenic type). The attacks may be predominantly one-sided or bilateral. This form of the disease is inherited as an autosomal dominant trait; a few families have displayed diplopia and spasticity and others have shown a familial tendency to infantile convulsions. Each of these types has a different causative gene. Attacks may occur every several days or be separated by years. A favorable response to benzodiazepines (clonazepam) has been reported, even when the drug is given on alternate days (Kurlan and Shoulson).

A third type, formerly thought to be a variant of the Mount-Reback type mentioned above, is precipitated by prolonged exercise. In addition to a response to benzodiazepines, it has the unique characteristic of improving with acetazolamide.

More common than these familial dyskinesias are sporadic cases and those secondary to focal brain lesions, such as the ones reported by Demirkirian and Jankovic. They classify the acquired paroxysmal dyskinesias according to the duration of each attack and the event or activity that precipitates the abnormal movements (kinesigenic, nonkinesigenic, exertional, or hypnagogic). As with the familial cases, the acquired kinesigenically induced movements often improve with anticonvulsants; others respond better to clonazepam.

Some intermittent dyskinesias are an expression of a neurologic or metabolic disease. They may follow injuries such as stroke, trauma, encephalitis, perinatal anoxia, multiple sclerosis, hypoparathyroidism, or thyrotoxicosis, and particularly, nonketotic hyperosmolarity. The most severe instances in our experience have been related to multiple sclerosis (tetanoid spasms), and, in the setting of HIV infection, as a result of toxoplasmosis, lymphoma, or presumed encephalitis caused by the retrovirus itself. These patients were relatively unresponsive to medications. Also, it should be recalled that oculogyric crises and other nonepileptic spasms have occurred episodically in patients with postencephalitic parkinsonism; these phenomena are now rarely seen with acute and chronic phenothiazine intoxication and with Niemann-Pick disease (type C).

The Identity of Chorea, Athetosis, and Dystonia

It may be evident from the foregoing descriptions that the distinctions between chorea, athetosis, and dystonia are probably not fundamental. Even their most prominent differences—the discreteness and rapidity of choreic movements and the slowness of athetotic ones—are more apparent than real. As pointed out by S.A. Kinnier Wilson, involuntary movements may follow one another in such rapid succession that they become confluent and therefore appear to be slow. In practice, one finds that the patient with relatively slow movements also shows discrete, rapid ones, and vice versa, and that many patients with chorea and athetosis also exhibit a persistent disorder of movement and posture that is essentially dystonic.

In a similar way, no meaningful distinction except one of degree can be made between chorea, athetosis, and ballismus. Particularly forceful movements of large amplitude (ballismus) are observed in some cases of Sydenham and Huntington chorea which, according to traditional teaching, exemplify pure forms of chorea and athetosis. The close relationship between these involuntary movements is illustrated by the patient with hemiballismus who, upon recovery, shows only choreoathetotic flexion–extension movements.

A role for the basal ganglia in cognitive function and abnormal behavior is hinted at provocatively in Parkinson disease, progressive supranuclear palsy, Tourette syndrome, and other processes, as summarized by Ring and Serra-Mestres. Slowness in thinking (bradyphrenia) in some of these disorders was alluded to earlier, but is inconsistent. Again, it would be an oversimplification to assign primary importance to the presence of depression, dementia, psychosis, and other disturbances in disease of the basal ganglia or to view changes in these structures as proximate causes of obsessive-compulsive and other behavioral disorders, but rather some role as part of a larger circuitry is likely. All that can be stated is that the basal ganglia modulate complex behavior, but the precise nature of their effect is not known at this time.

References

Albin RL, Young AB, Penney JB: The functional anatomy of basal ganglia disorders. *Trends Neurosci* 12:366, 1989.

Alexander GE, Crutcher MD: Functional architecture of basal ganglia circuits: Neural substrates of parallel processing. *Trends Neurosci* 13:266, 1990.

Alexander GE, DeLong MR: Macrostimulation of the primate neostriatum. *J Neurophysiol* 53:1417, 1433, 1985.

Bergman H, Wichmann T, DeLong MR: Reversal of experimental parkinsonism by lesions of the subthalamic nucleus. *Science* 249:1436, 1990.

Bhatia KP, Marsden CD: The behavioral and motor consequence of focal lesions of the basal ganglia in man. *Brain* 117:859, 1994.

Breedveld GJ, Percy AK, MacDonald ME, et al: Clinical and genetic heterogeneity in benign hereditary chorea. *Neurology* 59:579, 2002.

Brooks VB: *The Neural Basis of Motor Control*. New York, Oxford University Press, 1986.

Carpenter MB: Brainstem and infratentorial neuraxis in experimental dyskinesia. *Arch Neurol* 5:504, 1961.

Carpenter MB: Anatomy of the corpus striatum and brainstem integrating systems, in Brooks VB (ed): *Handbook of Physiology*. Sec 1: The Nervous System. Vol 2: Motor Control, part 2. Bethesda, MD, American Physiological Society, 1981, pp 947–995.

Carpenter MB, Whittier JR, Mettler FA: Analysis of choreoid hyperkinesia in the rhesus monkey: Surgical and pharmacological analysis of hyperkinesia resulting from lesions of the subthalamic nucleus of Luys. *J Comp Neurol* 92:293, 1950.

Ceballos-Baumann AO, Passingham RE, et al: Motor reorganization in acquired hemidystonia. *Ann Neurol* 37:746, 1995.

Chuang C, Fahn S, Frucht SJ: The natural history and treatment of acquired hemidystonia: Report of 33 cases and review of the literature. *J Neurol Neurosurg Psychiatry* 72:59, 2002.

Church AJ, Cardoso F, Dale RC, et al: Anti-basal ganglia antibodies in acute and persistent Sydenham chorea. *Neurology* 59:227, 2002.

Cooper IS: *Involuntary Movement Disorders*. New York, Hoeber-Harper, 1969.

DeLong MR: Primate models of movement disorders of basal ganglia origin. *Trends Neurosci* 13:281, 1990.

Demirkirian M, Jankovic J: Paroxysmal dyskinesias: Clinical features and classification. *Ann Neurol* 38:571, 1995.

Denny-Brown D, Yanagisawa N: The role of the basal ganglia in the initiation of movement, in Yahr MD (ed): *The Basal Ganglia*. New York, Raven Press, 1976, pp 115–148.

Dobyns WB, Ozelius LJ, Kramer PL, et al: Rapid-onset dystonia-parkinsonism. *Neurology* 43:2596, 1993.

Dooling EC, Adams RD: The pathological anatomy of post-hemiplegic athetosis. *Brain* 98:29, 1975.

Ehringer H, Hornykiewicz O: Vertielung von Noradrealin und Dopamin (3-hydroxytyramin) im Gehirn des Menschen und ihr Verhalten bei Erkrangungen des extrapyramidalen Systems. *Klin Wochenshr* 38:1236, 1960.

Emery SE, Vieco PT: Sydenham chorea: Magnetic resonance imaging reveals permanent basal ganglia injury. *Neurology* 48:531, 1997.

Fahn S: High-dosage anticholinergic therapy in dystonia. *Neurology* 33:1255, 1985.

Gombart L, Soares J, Alexander GE: Functional anatomy of the basal ganglia and motor systems, in Watts RL, Koller WC (eds): *Movement Disorders*, 2nd ed. New York, McGraw-Hill, 2004, pp 87–100.

Greengard P: The neurobiology of slow synaptic transmission. *Science* 294:1024, 2001.

Hallett M: Clinical neurophysiology of akinesia. Rev Neurol 146:585, 1990.

Hallett M, Khoshbin S: A physiological mechanism of bradykinesia. *Brain* 103:301, 1980.

Hudgins RL, Corbin KB: An uncommon seizure disorder: Familial paroxysmal choreoathetosis. *Brain* 91:199, 1968.

Jankovic J, Tolosa ES (eds): *Parkinson's Disease and Movement Disorders*, 3rd ed. Baltimore, Lippincott Williams & Wilkins, 1998.

Jenner P: Pharmacology of dopamine agonists in the treatment of Parkinson's disease. *Neurology* 58:S1–S8, 2002.

Krauss JK, Mundinger F: Functional stereotactic surgery for hemiballism. *J Neurosurg* 58:278, 1996.

Kurlan R, Shoulson I: Familial paroxysmal dystonic choreoathetosis and response to alternate-day oxazepam therapy. *Ann Neurol* 13:456, 1983.

Lance JW: Familial paroxysmal dystonic choreoathetosis and its differentiation from related syndromes. *Ann Neurol* 2:285, 1977.

Lang EA, Lozano AM: Parkinson's disease: Second of two parts. *N Engl J Med* 339:1130, 1998.

Marsden CD, Obeso JA: The functions of the basal ganglia and the paradox of stereotaxic surgery in Parkinson's disease. *Brain* 117:877, 1994.

Marsden CD, Lang AE, Quinn NP, et al: Familial dystonia and visual failure with striatal CT lucencies. *J Neurol Neurosurg Psychiatry* 49:500, 1986.

Martin JP: *Papers on Hemiballismus and the Basal Ganglia*. London, National Hospital Centenary, 1960.

Martin JP: *The Basal Ganglia and Posture*. Philadelphia, Lippincott, 1967.

Mitchell IJ, Boyce S, Sambrook MA, et al: A 2-deoxyglucose study of the effects of dopamine agonists on the parkinsonian primate brain. *Brain* 115:809, 1992.

Mount LA, Reback S: Familial paroxysmal choreoathetosis: Preliminary report on a hitherto undescribed clinical syndrome. *Arch Neurol Psychiatry* 44:841, 1940.

Novotny EJ Jr, Dorfman LN, Louis A, et al: A neurodegenerative disorder with generalized dystonia: A new mitochondriopathy? *Neurology* 35(Suppl 1):273, 1985.

Nygaard TG, Trugman JM, Yebenes JG: Dopa-responsive dystonia: The spectrum of clinical manifestations in a large North American family. *Neurology* 40:66, 1990.

O'Toole O, Lennon VA, Ahlskog JE, et al: Autoimmune chorea in adults. *Neurology* 80:1133, 2013.

Penney JB, Young AB: Biochemical and functional organization of the basal ganglia, in Jankovic J, Tolosa ES (eds): *Parkinson's Disease and Movement Disorders*, 3rd ed. Baltimore, Lippincott Williams & Wilkins, 1998, pp 1–13.

Piccolo I, Sterzi R, Thiella G, et al: Sporadic choreas: Analysis of a general hospital series. *Eur Neurol* 41:143, 1999.

Plant GT, Williams AC, Earl CJ, Marsden CD: Familial paroxysmal dystonia induced by exercise. *J Neurol Neurosurg Psychiatry* 47:275, 1984.

Rao J: Functional neurochemistry of the basal ganglia, in Watts RL, Koller WC: *Movement Disorders*, 2nd ed. New York, McGraw-Hill, 2004, pp 113–130.

Ring HA, Serra-Mestres J: Neuropsychiatry of the basal ganglia. *J Neurol Neurosurg Psychiatry* 72:12, 2002.

Segawa M, Hosaka A, Miyagawa F, et al: Hereditary progressive dystonia with marked diurnal fluctuation. *Adv Neurol* 14:215, 1976.

Standaert DG, Young AB: Treatment of central nervous system degenerative disorders, in *Goodman & Gilman's The Pharmacological Basis of Therapeutics*, 10th ed. New York, McGraw Hill, 2001, pp. 549–568.

Thach WT Jr, Montgomery EB Jr: Motor system, in Pearlman AL, Collins RC (eds): *Neurobiology of Disease*. New York, Oxford University Press, 1992, pp 168–196.

Van Woerkom W: La cirrhose hepatique avec alterations dans les centres nerveux evoluant chez des sujets d'age moyen. *Nouv Iconogr Saltpêtrière* 7:41, 1914.

Vernino S, Tuite P, Adler CH, et al: Paraneoplastic chorea associated with CRMP-5 neuronal antibody and lung carcinoma. *Ann Neurol* 51:25, 2002.

Vidailhet M, Vercueil L, Hoeto J-L, et al: Bilateral deep-brain stimulation of the globus pallidus in primary generalized dystonia. *N Engl J Med* 352:459, 2005.

Watts RL, Koller WC (eds): *Movement Disorders: Neurologic Principles and Practice*, 2nd ed. New York, McGraw-Hill, 2004.

Whittier JR, Mettler FA: Studies on the subthalamus of the rhesus monkey. *J Comp Neurol* 90:281, 319, 1949.

Wichmann T, DeLong M: Physiology of the basal ganglia and pathophysiology of movement disorders of basal ganglia origin, in Watts RL, Koller WC (eds): *Movement Disorders: Neurologic Principles and Practice*, 2nd ed. New York, McGraw-Hill, 2004, pp 101–112.

Wilson SAK: Disorders of motility and of muscle tone, with special reference to corpus striatum: The Croonian Lectures. *Lancet* 2:1, 53, 169, 215, 1925.

Wooten GF, Lopes MBS, Harris WO, et al: Pallidoluysian atrophy: Dystonia and basal ganglia functional anatomy. *Neurology* 43:1764, 1993.

Young AB, Penney JB: Biochemical and functional organization of the basal ganglia, in Jankovic J, Tolosa ES (eds): *Parkinson's Disease and Movement Disorders*, 3rd ed. Baltimore, Lippincott Williams & Wilkins, 1998, pp 1–11.

Zeman W: Pathology of the torsion dystonias (dystonia musculorum deformans). *Neurology* 20:79, 1970.

5

Ataxia and Disorders of Cerebellar Function

The cerebellum is responsible for the coordination of movements, especially skilled voluntary ones, the control of posture and gait, and the regulation of muscular tone. In addition, the cerebellum may play a role in the modulation of the emotional state and some aspects of cognition. The mechanisms by which these functions are accomplished have been the subject of intense investigation by anatomists and physiologists. Their studies have yielded a mass of data, testimony to the complexity of the organization of the cerebellum and its afferent and efferent connections. A coherent picture of cerebellar function is now emerging, although it is not yet possible, with a few exceptions, to relate each of the symptoms of cerebellar disease to a derangement of a discrete anatomic or functional unit of the cerebellum.

Knowledge of cerebellar function has been derived mainly from the study of natural and experimental ablative lesions and to a lesser extent from stimulation of the cerebellum, which actually produces little in the way of movement or alterations of induced movement. Furthermore, none of the motor activities of the cerebellum reaches conscious kinesthetic perception; its main role, a critical one, is to assist in the modulation of willed movements that are generated in the cerebral hemispheres. The following discussion of cerebellar structure and function has, of necessity, been simplified; a fuller account can be found in the writings of Jansen and Brodal, of Gilman, and of Thach and colleagues.

ANATOMIC AND PHYSIOLOGIC CONSIDERATIONS

Early studies of the comparative anatomy and fiber connections of the cerebellum led to its subdivision into three parts (Fig. 5-1): (1) The flocculonodular lobe, located inferiorly, which is phylogenetically the oldest portion of the cerebellum and is much the same in all animals (hence archicerebellum). It is separated from the main mass of the cerebellum, or corpus cerebelli, by the posterolateral fissure. (2) The anterior lobe, or paleocerebellum, which is the portion rostral to the primary fissure. In lower animals, the anterior lobe constitutes most of the cerebellum, but in humans it is relatively small, consisting of the anterosuperior vermis and the contiguous paravermian cortex. (3) The posterior lobe, or neocerebellum, consisting of the middle divisions of the vermis and their large lateral extensions. The major portion of the human cerebellar hemispheres falls into this, the largest, subdivision.

This anatomic subdivision corresponds roughly with the distribution of cerebellar function based on the arrangement of its afferent fiber connections. The flocculonodular lobe receives special proprioceptive impulses from the vestibular nuclei and is therefore also referred to as the vestibulocerebellum; it is concerned essentially with equilibrium. The anterior vermis and part of the posterior vermis are referred to as the spinocerebellum, since projections to these parts derive to a large extent from the proprioceptors of muscles and tendons in the limbs and are conveyed to the cerebellum in the dorsal spinocerebellar tract (from the lower limbs) and the ventral spinocerebellar tract (upper limbs). The main influence of the spinocerebellum appears to be on posture and muscle tone. The neocerebellum derives its afferent fibers indirectly from the cerebral cortex via the pontine nuclei and brachium pontis, hence the designation pontocerebellum. This portion of the cerebellum is concerned primarily with the coordination of skilled movements that are initiated at a cerebral cortical level. It is now appreciated that certain portions of the cerebellar hemispheres are also involved to some extent in tactual, visual, auditory, and even visceral functions.

Largely on the basis of ablation experiments in animals, three characteristic physiologic patterns corresponding to these major divisions of the cerebellum have been delineated. These constellations find some similarities in the clinical syndromes that are observed when various parts of the cerebellum are damaged and special terminology is applied to the corresponding clinical findings in patients. Lesions of the nodulus and flocculus have been associated with a disturbance of equilibrium and frequently with nystagmus; individual movements of the limbs are not affected. Anterior lobe ablation in primates results in increased shortening and lengthening reactions, somewhat increased tendon reflexes, and

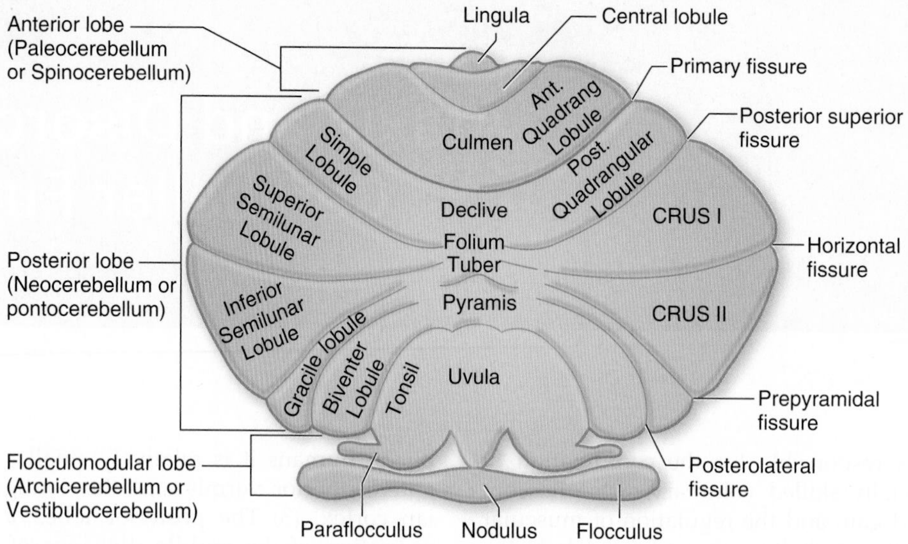

Figure 5-1. Diagram of the cerebellum, illustrating the major fissures, lobes, and lobules and the major phylogenetic divisions (left labels).

an exaggeration of the postural reflexes, particularly the "positive supporting reflex," in animals, which consists of extension of the limb in response to light pressure on the foot pad. Ablation of a cerebellar hemisphere in cats and dogs yields inconsistent results, but in monkeys it causes hypotonia and clumsiness of the ipsilateral limbs; if the dentate nucleus is included in the hemispheric ablation, these abnormalities are more enduring and the limbs also show an ataxic, or "intention" tremor.

The studies of Chambers and Sprague and of Jansen and Brodal have demonstrated that in respect to both its afferent and efferent projections, the cerebellum is organized into longitudinal (sagittal) rather than transverse zones. There are three longitudinal zones—the vermian, paravermian or intermediate, and lateral—and there seems to be considerable overlap from one to another. Chambers and Sprague, on the basis of their investigations in cats, concluded that the vermian zone coordinates movements of the eyes and body with respect to gravity and movement of the head in space. The intermediate zone, which receives both peripheral and central projections (from motor cortex), influences postural tone and also individual movements of the ipsilateral limbs. The lateral zone is concerned mainly with coordination of movements of the ipsilateral limbs but is also involved in other functions.

The efferent fibers of the cerebellar cortex, which consist essentially of the axons of Purkinje cells, project onto the deep cerebellar nuclei (see below). The projections from Purkinje cells are inhibitory whereas those from the nuclei are excitatory on other parts of the motor nervous system. According to the scheme of Jansen and Brodal, cells of the vermis project mainly to the fastigial nucleus; those of the intermediate zone, to the globose and emboliform nuclei (that are combined in humans as the interpositus nucleus); and those of the lateral zone, to the dentate nucleus.

The deep cerebellar nuclei, in turn, project to the cerebral cortex and certain brainstem nuclei via two main pathways: fibers from the dentate, emboliform, and globose nuclei form the superior cerebellar peduncle, enter the upper pontine tegmentum as the brachium conjunctivum, decussate at the level of the inferior colliculus, and ascend to the ventrolateral nucleus of the thalamus and, to a lesser extent, to the intralaminar thalamic nuclei (Fig. 5-2). Some of the ascending fibers, soon after their decussation, synapse in the red nucleus, but most of them traverse this nucleus without terminating, and pass on to the thalamus. Ventral thalamic nuclear groups that receive these ascending efferent fibers project to the supplementary motor cortex of that side. Since the pathway from the cerebellar nuclei to the thalamus and then on to the motor cortex is crossed, and the connection from the motor cortex through the corticospinal is again crossed, the effects of a lesion in one cerebellar hemisphere are manifest by signs on the ipsilateral side of the body.

One special pathway forms a loop, called the Guillain-Mollaret triangle that is of clinical interest. A small group of fibers of the superior cerebellar peduncle, following their decussation, descend in the ventromedial tegmentum of the brainstem via the central tegmental fasciculus and terminate in the reticulotegmental and paramedian reticular nuclei of the pons and inferior olivary nuclei of the medulla. These nuclei, in turn, project via the inferior cerebellar peduncle back to the cerebellum, mainly the anterior lobe, thus completing a cerebellar–reticular–cerebellar feedback system (Fig. 5-3). Several clinical syndromes result from lesions in the loop, notably palatal myoclonus, one of the few disorders of involuntary movement that continues during sleep.

The fastigial nucleus sends fibers to the vestibular nuclei of both sides and, to a lesser extent, to other nuclei

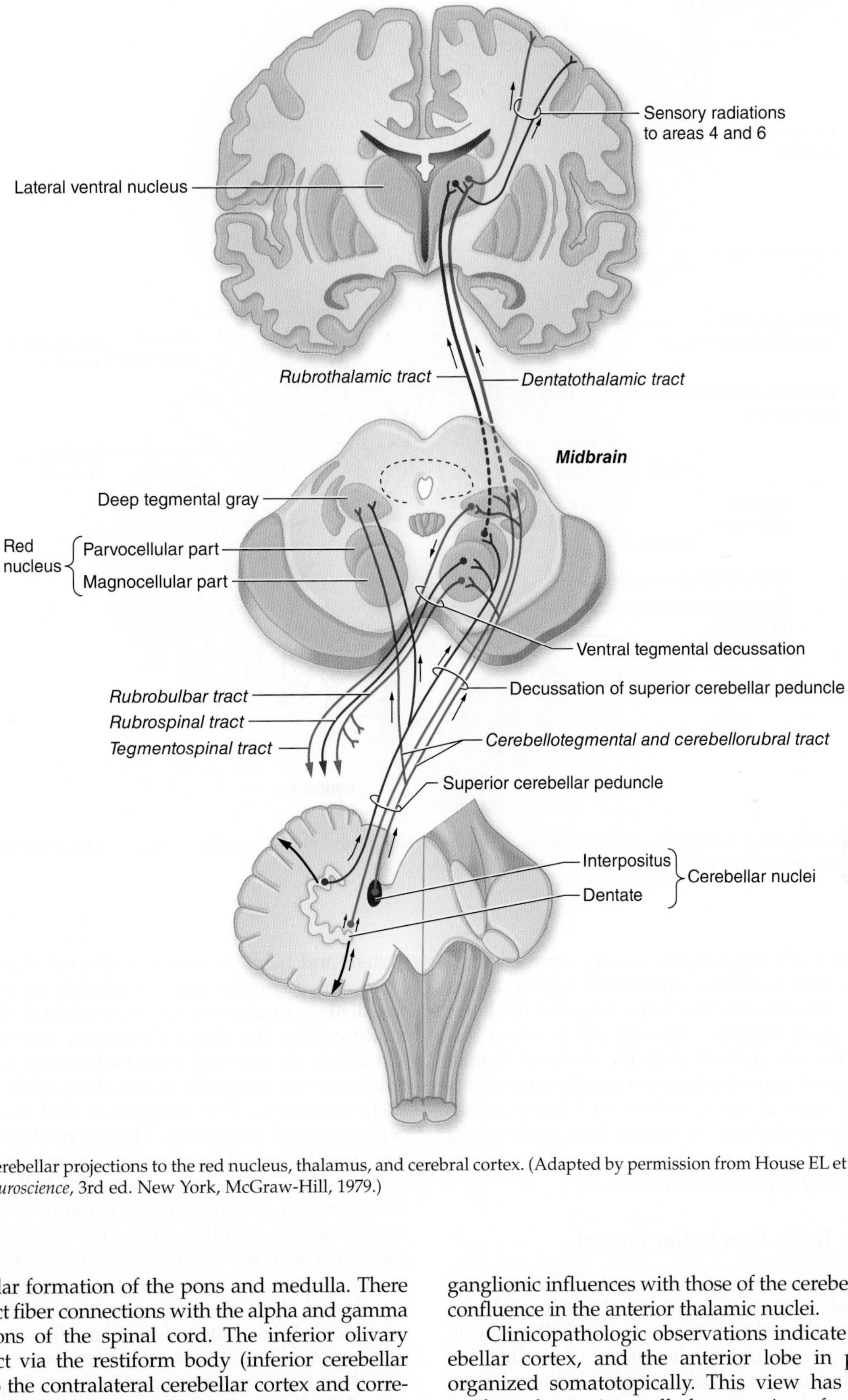

Figure 5-2. Cerebellar projections to the red nucleus, thalamus, and cerebral cortex. (Adapted by permission from House EL et al: *A Systematic Approach to Neuroscience*, 3rd ed. New York, McGraw-Hill, 1979.)

of the reticular formation of the pons and medulla. There are also direct fiber connections with the alpha and gamma motor neurons of the spinal cord. The inferior olivary nuclei project via the restiform body (inferior cerebellar peduncle) to the contralateral cerebellar cortex and corresponding parts of the deep cerebellar nuclei. Thus the cerebellum influences motor activity through its connections with the motor cortex and brainstem nuclei and their descending motor pathways. Chapter 4 details the integration of basal ganglionic influences with those of the cerebellum by their confluence in the anterior thalamic nuclei.

Clinicopathologic observations indicate that the cerebellar cortex, and the anterior lobe in particular, is organized somatotopically. This view has been amply confirmed experimentally by mapping of evoked potentials from the cerebellar cortex elicited by a variety of sensory stimuli, and an analysis of the subtle motor effects produced by stimulation of specific parts of the

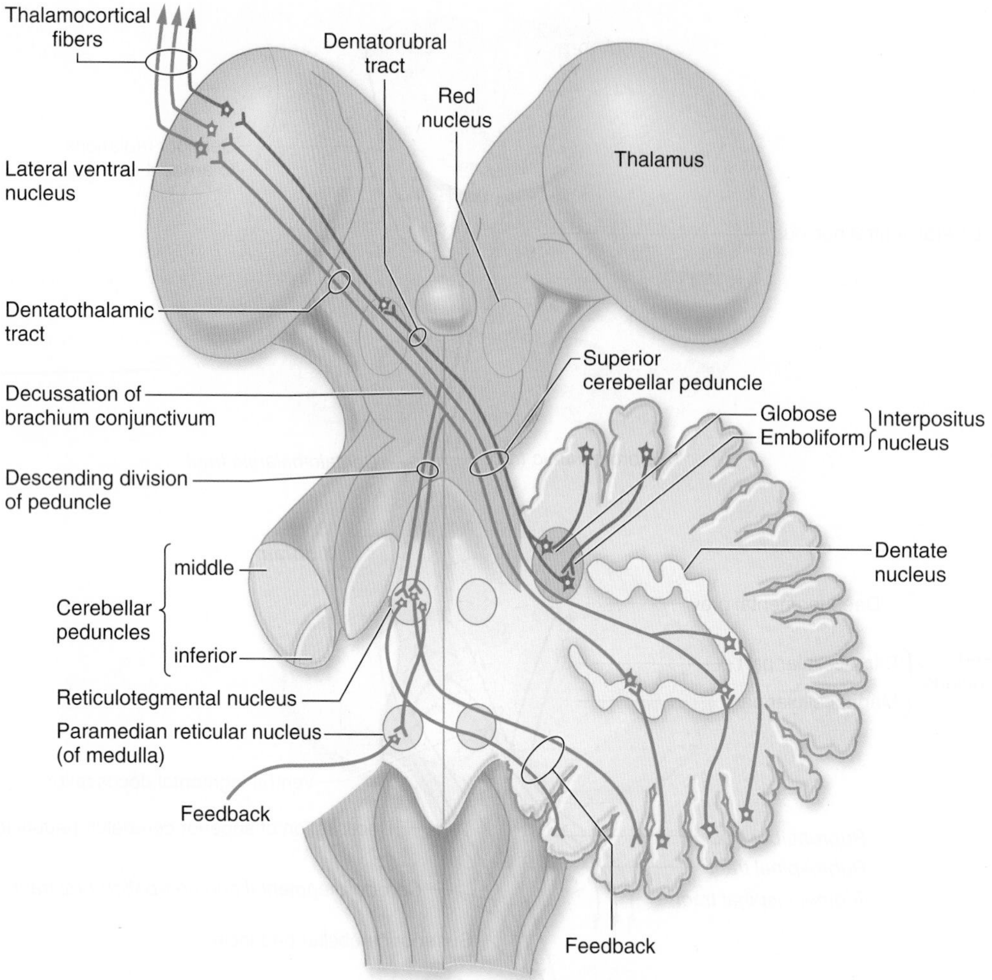

Figure 5-3. Dentatothalamic and dentatorubrothalamic projections via the superior cerebellar peduncle. The "feedback" circuit via the reticular nuclei and reticulocerebellar fibers is also shown (Mollaret triangle).

cerebellar cortex. The topographic sensory representation of body parts based on these experimental observations is assumed to be similar to the motor map but the latter is probably not as distinct. The similarity between this scheme and the one derived from the study of human disease becomes apparent when one considers the results of cerebellar lesions discussed further on. Diffuse degenerations of the cerebellum, of course, have widespread effects, including motor, articulatory, gait and eye movements, and subtle behavioral influences.

Role of the Deep Cerebellar Nuclei

The physiologic studies of Allen and Tsukahara and of Thach and colleagues have greatly increased our knowledge of the role of the deep cerebellar nuclei. These investigators studied the effects of cooling the deep nuclei during a projected movement in the macaque monkey. Their observations, coupled with established anatomic data, permit the following conclusions. The dentate nucleus receives information from the premotor and supplementary motor cortices via the pontocerebellar system and helps to initiate volitional movements. The latter are accomplished via efferent projections from the dentate nucleus to the ventrolateral thalamus and motor cortex. The dentatal neurons were shown to fire just before the onset of volitional movements, and inactivation of the dentatal neurons delayed the initiation of such movements. The interpositus nucleus also receives cerebrocortical projections via the pontocerebellar system; in addition, it receives spinocerebellar projections via the intermediate zone of the cerebellar cortex. The latter projections convey information from Golgi tendon organs, muscle spindles, cutaneous afferents, and spinal cord interneurons involved in movement. The interpositus nucleus fires in relation to a movement once it has started. Also, the prepositus nucleus appears to be responsible for making volitional oscillations (alternating movements). Its cells fire in tandem with these actions, and their regularity and amplitude are impaired when these cells are inactivated. In addition, Thach has pointed out that the nucleus interpositus normally damps physiologic tremor; he has suggested that this may play a part in the genesis of so-called intention tremor described further on. The fastigial nucleus controls antigravity and other muscle synergies in standing and walking; ablation of this nucleus greatly impairs these motor activities.

Neuronal Organization of the Cerebellar Cortex

Coordinated and fluid movements of the limbs and trunk result from a neuronal organization in the cerebellum that permits an ongoing and almost instantaneous comparison between desired and actual movements while the movements are being carried out. An enormous number of neurons are committed to these tasks, as attested by the fact that the cerebellum contributes only 10 percent to the total weight and volume of the brain but contains half of the brain's neurons. Also, it has been estimated that there are 40 times more afferent axons than efferent axons in the various cerebellar pathways—a reflection of the enormous amount of incoming (sensory) information that is required for the control of motor function.

The cerebellar cortex is configured as a stereotyped three-layered structure containing five types of neurons (Fig. 5-4). In its relatively regular geometry, it is similar to the columnar architecture of the cerebral cortex, but it differs in the greater degree of intracortical feedback between neurons and the convergent nature of input fibers. The outermost "molecular" layer of the cerebellum contains two types of inhibitory neurons, the stellate cells and the basket cells. They are interspersed among the dendrites of the Purkinje cells, the cell bodies of which lie in the underlying layer. The Purkinje cell axons constitute the main output of the cerebellum, which is directed at the deep cerebellar and vestibular nuclei described above. Purkinje cells are likewise entirely inhibitory and utilize the neurotransmitter gamma-aminobutyric acid (GABA). The innermost "granular" layer contains an enormous number of densely packed granule cells and a few larger Golgi interneurons. Axons of the granule cells travel long distances as "parallel fibers," which are oriented along the long axis of the folia and form excitatory synapses with Purkinje cells. Each Purkinje cell is influenced by as many as a million granule cells to produce a single electrical "simple spike."

The predominant afferent input to the cerebellum is via the mossy fibers, which are the axons of the spinocerebellar tracts and the projections from pontine, vestibular, and reticular nuclei. They enter through all three cerebellar peduncles, mainly the middle (pontine input) and inferior (vestibulocerebellar) ones. Mossy fibers ramify in the granule layer and excite Golgi and granule neurons through special synapses termed cerebellar glomeruli. The other main afferent input is via the climbing fibers, which originate in the inferior olivary nuclei (olives) and communicate somatosensory, visual, and cerebral cortical signals (Figs. 5-4 and 5-5). The climbing fibers, so named because of their vine-like configuration around Purkinje cells and their axons, preserve a topographic arrangement from olivary neuronal groups; a similar topographic arrangement is maintained in the Purkinje cell projections. The climbing fibers have specific excitatory effects on Purkinje cells that result in prolonged "complex spike" depolarizations. The firing of stellate and basket cells is facilitated by the same parallel fibers that excite Purkinje cells, and these smaller cells, in turn, inhibit the Purkinje cells. These reciprocal relationships form the feedback loops that permit the exquisitely delicate inhibitory smoothing of limb movements that are lost when the organ is damaged.

The uniform cortical structure of the cerebellum can reasonably lead to the conjecture that the organ has similar effects on all parts of the cerebrum to which it has projections (cortex, basal ganglia, thalamus, etc.). It would follow that the activities of these cerebral structures (motor, cognitive, sensory) may be modulated in similar ways by cerebellar activity.

Neurochemical Considerations

A number of biochemical considerations are of interest. Four of the five cell types of the cerebellar cortex (Purkinje, stellate, basket, Golgi) are inhibitory; the granule cells are an exception and are excitatory. Afferent fibers to the cerebellum are of three types, two of which have been mentioned above: (1) Mossy fibers, which are the main afferent input to the cerebellum, utilize aspartate. (2) Climbing fibers, which are the axons of cells in the inferior olivary nucleus and project to the Purkinje cells of the opposite cerebellar hemisphere. The neurotransmitter of the climbing fibers is probably glutamate, which acts on amino-3-hydroxy-5-methyl-4-isoxazole propionic acid (AMPA) receptors. (3) Aminergic fibers, which project through the superior cerebellar peduncle and terminate on the Purkinje and granule cells in all parts of the cerebellar cortex. They are of two types: dopaminergic fibers, which arise in the ventral mesencephalic tegmentum and project to the interpositus and dentate nuclei and to the granule and Purkinje cells throughout the cortex, and serotonergic neurons, which are located in the raphe nuclei of the brainstem and project diffusely to the granule cell and molecular layer. The granule cell axons elaborate the excitatory transmitter glutamate. All the inhibitory cerebellar cortical neurons appear to utilize GABA. The neurotransmitters of the deep nuclei have not been fully elucidated.

CLINICAL FEATURES OF CEREBELLAR DISEASE

Two eminent neurologists, Joseph Babinski and Gordon Holmes, were the first to cogently analyze the disturbances of movement and posture that result from lesions of the human cerebellum. For Babinski, the essential function of the cerebellum was the orchestration of muscle synergies in the performance of voluntary movement. A loss or impairment of this function—i.e., asynergia or dyssynergia—resulted in irregularity or fragmentation of the normal motor sequences involved in any given act. This deficit, most apparent in the execution of rapidly alternating movements, was referred to by Babinski as dys- or adiadochokinesis, as discussed below in the description of ataxia. He also pointed out that this was

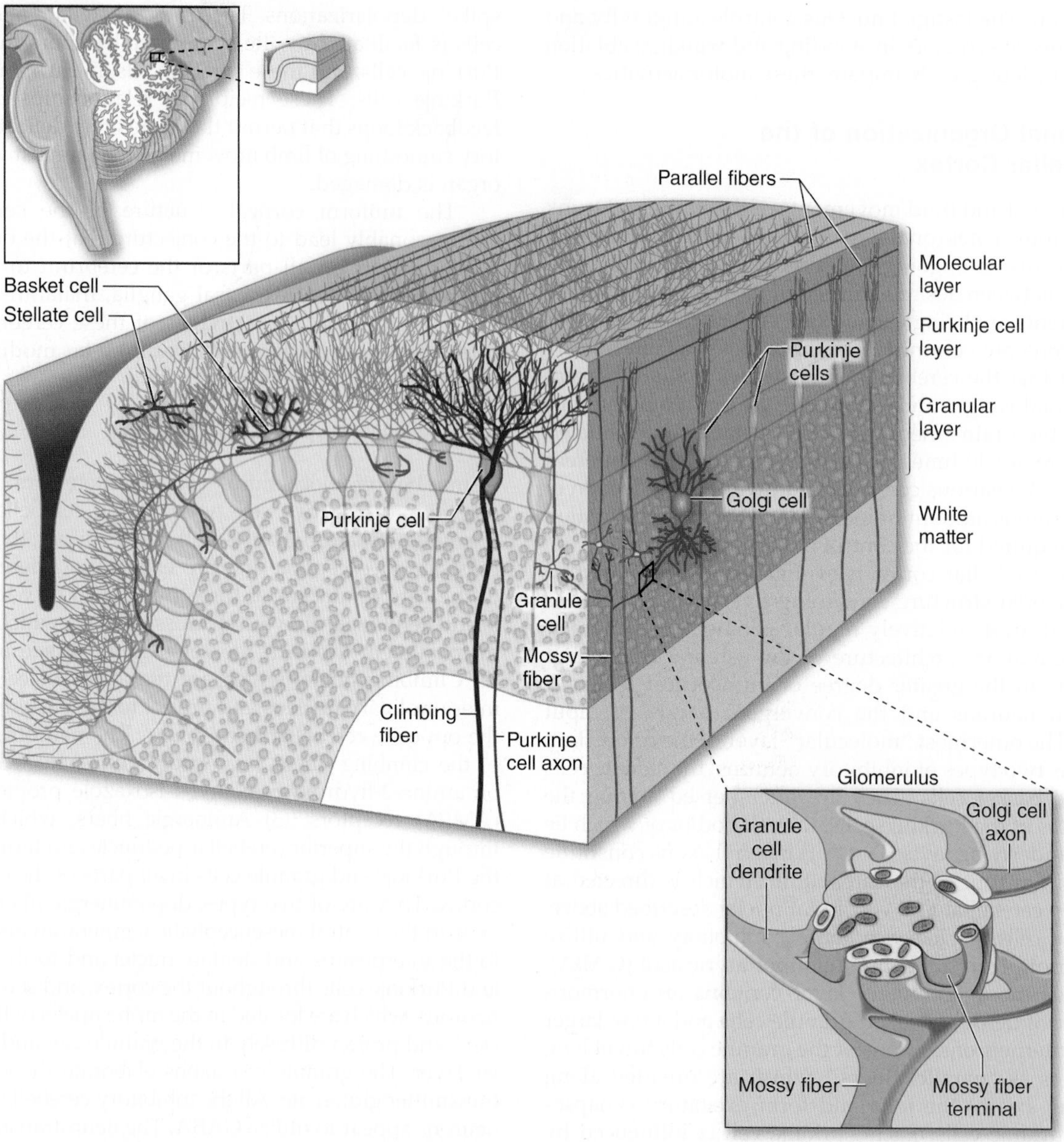

Figure 5-4. Anatomic organization of the cerebellar cortex in a longitudinal and transverse section of a folium. Shown are the relationships between (a) climbing fibers and Purkinje cells, (b) mossy fibers and both granule cells and Golgi cells, and (c) the parallel fibers that course longitudinally and connect these three main cell types. (Reproduced with permission from Kandel ER, Schwartz JH, Jessel TM: *Principles of Neural Science*, 5th ed. New York, McGraw-Hill, 2013.)

accompanied by certain maladjustments of stance and by catalepsy (perseveration of a posture), features that have not been as appreciated by modern observers.

Holmes summarized the effects of cerebellar disease as being in the acceleration and deceleration of movement. He characterized the effects in a more fundamental way than had Babinski, describing them as defects in the *rate, range, and force* of movement, resulting in an undershooting or overshooting of the target. He used the term decomposition to describe the fragmentation of a smooth movement into a series of irregular, jerky components. In Holmes' view, probably incorrectly, these abnormalities were attributable to an underlying hypotonia. The terminal ("intention") tremor, and the inability to check the displacement of an outstretched limb, both of which he elegantly described, he attributed to this latter defect (see further on). Gilman and colleagues have provided evidence that more than hypotonia is involved in the tremor of cerebellar incoordination. They found that deafferentation of the forelimb of a monkey resulted in dysmetria and kinetic tremor; subsequent cerebellar ablation significantly increased both the dysmetria and tremor, indicating the presence of a mechanism as yet unidentified in addition to depression of the fusimotor efferent–spindle afferent circuit.

Parts of the hypotheses of both Babinski and Holmes have been sustained by modern physiologic and clinical

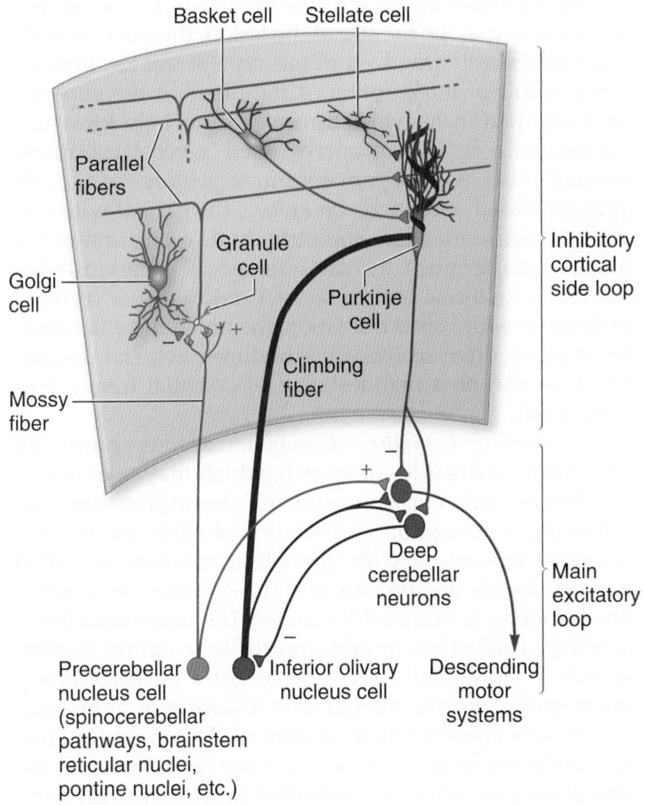

Figure 5-5. The physiologic organization of cerebellar circuitry. The main output of the deep cerebellar nuclei is excitatory and is transmitted through mossy and climbing fibers. This "main loop" is modulated by an inhibitory cortical loop, which is effected by Purkinje cell output but indirectly includes the other main cell types through their connections with Purkinje cells. Recurrent pathways between the deep nuclei and cortical cells via mossy and climbing fibers complete the cerebellar servomechanism for motor control. (Adapted, with permission, from Raymond JL, Lisberger SG, Mauk DM: The cerebellum: a neuronal learning machine? *Science* 272:1126-1131.)

studies. In an analysis of rapid (ballistic) movements, Hallett and colleagues have demonstrated that with cerebellar lesions, there is a prolongation of the interval between the commanded act and the onset of movement. More prominently, there is a derangement of the normal ballistic triphasic agonist–antagonist–agonist motor sequence, referred to in Chaps. 3 and 4. The agonist burst may be too long or too short, or it may continue into the antagonist burst, resulting in excessive agonist–antagonist cocontraction at the onset of movement. These findings may explain what was described by Babinski and Holmes as asynergia, decomposition of movement, and certainly explain dysmetria. Diener and Dichgans confirmed these fundamental abnormalities in the timing and amplitude of reciprocal inhibition and of cocontraction of agonist–antagonist muscles and remarked that these were particularly evident in pluriarticular movements.

The symptoms produced in animals by ablation of discrete anatomic or functional zones of the cerebellum bear only an imperfect relationship to the symptoms of cerebellar disease in humans. This is understandable for several reasons. Most of the lesions that occur in humans do not respect the boundaries established by experimental anatomists. Even with lesions that are more or less confined to discrete functional zones (e.g., flocculonodular lobe, anterior lobe), it is difficult to identify the resultant clinical syndromes with those produced by ablation of analogous zones in cats, dogs, and even monkeys, indicating that the functional organization of these parts varies from species to species.

Clinical observations affirm what was stated above—that lesions of the cerebellum in humans give rise to the following abnormalities: (1) incoordination (ataxia) of volitional movement; (2) a characteristic tremor ("intention", or ataxic tremor, by which is meant a side-to-side oscillation as movement approaches a target), described in detail in Chap. 6; (3) disorders of equilibrium and gait; and (4) diminished muscle tone, particularly with acute lesions. Dysarthria, a common feature of cerebellar disease, is probably predicated on a similar incoordination of the muscles of articulation. In addition, the stability of conjugate eye movements is affected, giving rise to nystagmus.

Extensive lesions of one cerebellar hemisphere, especially of the anterior lobe, cause mild hypotonia, postural abnormalities, ataxia, and a mild weakness of the ipsilateral arm and leg perceived by the patient. Lesions of the deep nuclei and cerebellar peduncles have the same effects as extensive hemispheral lesions. If the lesion involves a limited portion of the cerebellar cortex and subcortical white matter, there may be surprisingly little disturbance of function, or the abnormality may be greatly attenuated with the passage of time. For example, a congenital developmental defect or an early life sclerotic cortical atrophy of half of the cerebellum may produce no clinical abnormalities. Lesions involving the superior cerebellar peduncle or the dentate nucleus cause the most severe and enduring cerebellar symptoms, which manifest mostly as ataxia in the ipsilateral limbs. Disorders of stance and gait depend more on vermian than on hemispheral or peduncular involvement. Damage in the inferior cerebellum causes vestibulocerebellar symptoms—namely, dizziness, vertigo, vomiting, and nystagmus—in varying proportions. These symptoms often share with disturbances of the vestibular system the feature of worsening with changes in head position.

Ataxic Incoordination

The most prominent manifestations of cerebellar disease, namely, the abnormalities of intended (volitional) movement, are classified under the general heading of cerebellar incoordination or ataxia. Following Babinski, the terms dyssynergia, dysmetria, and dysdiadochokinesis came into common usage to describe cerebellar abnormalities of movement. Holmes's characterization of abnormalities in the rate, range, and force of movement is less confusing, as becomes apparent from an analysis of even simple movements. These abnormalities are brought out by standard neurologic tests, finger-to-nose and toe-to-finger movement, running the heel down the opposite shin, or tracing a square in the air with a hand or foot. In performing these tests, the patient should be asked to move the limb to the target accurately and rapidly.

The speed of initiating movement is slowed somewhat in cerebellar disease. In a detailed electrophysiologic analysis of this defect mentioned earlier, Hallett and colleagues noted, in both slow and fast movements, that the initial agonist burst was prolonged and the peak force of the agonist contraction was reduced. Also, there is irregularity and slowing of the movement itself, in both acceleration and deceleration. These abnormalities are particularly prominent as the finger or toe approaches its target. All of the foregoing defects in volitional movement are evident in acts that require alternation or rapid change in direction of movement, such as pronation–supination of the forearm or successive touching of each fingertip to the thumb. The normal rhythm of these movements is interrupted by irregularities of force and speed. Even a simple movement may be fragmented ("decomposition" of movement), each component being effected with greater or lesser force than is required. These movement abnormalities together impart a highly characteristic clumsiness to the cerebellar syndromes, an appearance that is not simulated by the weakness of upper or lower motor neuron disorders or by diseases of the basal ganglia.

Normally, deceleration of movement is smooth and accurate, even if sharp changes in the direction of a limb are demanded, as in following a moving target. With cerebellar disease, the velocity and force of the movement are not checked in the normal manner. The excursion of the limb may be arrested prematurely, and the target is then reached by a series of jerky movements. Or the limb overshoots the mark (hypermetria) because of delayed activation and diminished contraction of antagonist muscles; then the error is corrected by a series of secondary movements in which the finger or toe sways around the target before coming to rest, or moves from side to side a few times on the target itself. This side-to-side movement of the finger as it approaches its mark tends to assume a rhythmic quality; it has traditionally been referred to as intention tremor, or ataxic tremor. The tremor is mainly perpendicular to the trajectory of movement and mostly in the horizontal plane (the reason for the latter is not known). The term "intention" as applied to cerebellar tremor, while embedded in neurologic parlance, does not fully capture the necessity for the limb to be in action rather than for the patient to "intend" a movement for the tremor to be manifest. "Action tremor," however, has been used for an entirely different category of oscillations, as discussed in Chap. 6 so that simply "ataxic tremor" or "goal directed action tremor" may be preferable terms.

In addition to intention tremor, there may be a coarse, irregular, wide-range tremor that may be present in a position of repose and enhanced whenever the patient activates limb muscles, either to sustain a posture or to effect a movement. It is elicited by having the patient hold the arms out to the sides with elbows bent ("wing-beating tremor"). Holmes called it rubral tremor, and although the red nucleus may be the site of the lesion, the nucleus itself is not necessarily involved in this type of tremor. Instead, it is a result of interruption of the fibers of the superior cerebellar peduncle, which traverse the nucleus, for which reason it may be more properly called "cerebellar outflow tremor." Also, with certain sustained postures (e.g., with arms extended and hands on knees), the patient with cerebellar disease may develop a rhythmic oscillation of the fingers having much the same tempo as a parkinsonian tremor. A rhythmic tremor of the head or upper trunk (3 to 4 per second) called titubation, mainly in the anteroposterior plane, often accompanies midline cerebellar disease, but may also be a manifestation of essential tremor (see further on).

Cerebellar dysarthria Cerebellar lesions commonly give rise to a disorder of speech, which may take one of two forms, either a slow, slurring dysarthria, like that following interruption of the corticobulbar tracts, or a scanning dysarthria with variable intonation, so called because words are broken up into syllables, as when a line of poetry is scanned for meter. The latter disorder is uniquely cerebellar; in addition to its scanning quality, speech is slow, and each syllable, after an involuntary interruption, may be uttered with less force or more force ("explosive speech") than is natural. Urban and associates deduced from cases of cerebellar infarction that the articulatory muscles are controlled from the rostral paravermian area of the anterior lobe, and this area is affected in most cases with dysarthria.

Cerebellar eye movement abnormalities Ocular movement may be altered as a result of cerebellar disease, specifically if vestibular connections are involved. Patients with cerebellar lesions are unable to hold eccentric positions of gaze, resulting in a special type of nystagmus and the need to make rapid repetitive saccades to look eccentrically. Conjugate voluntary gaze can be accomplished only by a series of jerky movements. Smooth pursuit movements are slower than normal and require that the patient make small "catch-up" saccades in an attempt to keep the moving target near the fovea. On attempted refixation to a target, the eyes overshoot the target and then oscillate through several corrective cycles until precise fixation is attained. It will be recognized that these nystagmoid abnormalities, as well as those of speech, resemble the abnormalities of volitional ataxic movements of the limbs. Currently it is considered that nystagmus caused by cerebellar disease depends on lesions of the vestibulocerebellum (Thach and Montgomery). Skew deviation (vertical displacement of one eye), vertical nystagmus, ocular flutter, and ocular myoclonus (opsoclonus) may also be the result of cerebellar disease; these abnormalities and other effects of cerebellar lesions on ocular movement are discussed in Chap. 14.

Disorders of equilibrium and gait

The patient with cerebellar disease has variable degrees of difficulty in standing and walking, as described more fully in Chap. 7. Standing with feet together may be impossible or maintained only briefly before the patient pitches to one side or backward. Closing the eyes may worsen this difficulty slightly, but the Romberg sign (which signifies impaired proprioceptive input) is absent if the patient is allowed to steady himself before closing his eyes. In walking, the patient's steps are uneven and placement of the foot is misaligned, resulting in unexpected lurching.

Data from patients in whom accurate clinicoanatomic correlations can be made, indicate that the disequilibrium syndrome, with normal movements of the limbs, corresponds more closely with lesions of the anterior vermis than with those of the flocculus and nodulus. This conclusion is based in part on the study of a highly stereotyped form of cerebellar degeneration in alcoholics (Chap. 42). In such patients the cerebellar disturbance is often limited to one of stance and gait, in which case the pathologic changes are restricted to the anterior parts of the superior vermis. In more severely affected patients, in whom there is also incoordination of individual movements of the limbs, the changes are found to extend laterally from the vermis, involving the anterior portions of the anterior lobes (in patients with ataxia of the legs) and the more posterior portions of the anterior lobes (in patients whose arms are affected).

Similar clinicopathologic relationships pertain in patients with familial forms of pure cerebellar cortical degeneration. In both the alcoholic and familial degenerative cases, despite a serious disturbance of stance and gait, the flocculonodular lobe may be spared completely. In other diseases, however, involvement of the posterior vermis and its connections with the pontine and mesencephalic reticular formations has caused abnormalities of ocular movement in addition to a gait disorder (see Chap. 14).

Thus the evidence that flocculonodular lesions in humans cause a disturbance of equilibrium is not conclusive. It rests on the observation that with certain tumors of childhood, namely, medulloblastomas, there may be an unsteadiness of stance and gait but no tremor or incoordination of the limbs. Insofar as these tumors are thought to originate from cell rests in the posterior medullary velum, at the base of the nodulus, it has been inferred that the disturbance of equilibrium results from involvement of this portion of the cerebellum. However, the validity of this deduction remains to be proved. By the time such tumors are imaged or viewed at operation or autopsy, they have spread beyond the confines of the nodulus, and strict clinicopathologic correlations are not possible.

The point to be made is that midline anterior cerebellar lesions may produce solely a disorder of stance and gait, i.e., nystagmus, dysarthria, and limb ataxia are absent, so that the entire problem may be missed if the patient is not observed while standing and walking.

Hypotonia

This refers to a decrease in the normal resistance that is offered by muscles to passive manipulation (e.g., flexion and extension of a limb); it is the least evident of the cerebellar abnormalities but may explain certain clinical features not otherwise derived from the above deficits. It is related to a depression of gamma and alpha motor neuron activity, as discussed in Chap. 3. Experimentally, in cats and monkeys, acute cerebellar lesions and hypotonia are associated with a depression of fusimotor efferent and spindle afferent activity. With the passage of time, fusimotor activity is restored as hypotonia disappears (Gilman et al). As indicated earlier, Holmes believed that hypotonia was a fundamental defect in cerebellar disease, accounting not only for the defects in postural fixation (see below) but also for certain elements of ataxia and the tremor.

Hypotonia is much more apparent with acute than with chronic lesions and may be demonstrated in a number of ways. A conventional test for hypotonia is to tap the wrists of the outstretched arms, in which case the affected limb (or both limbs in diffuse cerebellar disease) will be displaced through a wider range than normal and may oscillate; this is the result of a failure of the hypotonic muscles to fixate the arm at the shoulder. When an affected limb is shaken, the flapping movements of the hand are of wider excursion than normal. If the patient places his elbows on the table with the arms flexed and the hands are allowed to hang limply, the hand of the hypotonic limb will sag. If the standing patient is rotated briefly to and fro at the shoulders, the hypotonic arm will be seen to continue to swing after the other has come to rest. Babinski also was impressed with gross alterations of posture, apparently related to hypotonia. These take the form of passive extension of the neck and involuntary bending of the knees, which are apparent when the patient is lifted from a bed or chair or upon first standing, or slumping of the shoulder on the affected side.

Failure to check a movement is a closely related phenomenon. Thus, after strongly flexing one arm against a resistance that is suddenly released, the patient may be unable to check the flexion movement, to the point where the arm may strike the face. This is the result of a delay in contraction of the triceps muscle, which ordinarily would arrest overflexion of the arm. This abnormality, incorrectly referred to as Holmes' rebound phenomenon, is more appropriately designated as an impairment of the check reflex. Stewart and Holmes, who first described this test, made the point that when resistance to flexion is suddenly removed, the normal limb moves only a short distance in flexion and then recoils very briefly in the opposite direction; in this sense, rebound of the limb is actually deficient in cerebellar disease.

Patients with these various abnormalities of tone may show little or no impairment of motor power, indicating that the maintenance of posture involves more than the voluntary contraction of muscles. It is noteworthy that the signs of cerebellar dysfunction (dysmetria, clumsiness, tremor) are absent in the hypotonic muscles of peripheral nerve disease—indicating that the cerebellum exerts a unique modulating effect on movement that is not explained by loss of tone.

Other Symptoms of Cerebellar Disease

It has been stated by some authors, not in accord with our experience, that there is a slight loss of muscular power and fatigability of muscle with acute cerebellar lesions. Insofar as these symptoms cannot be explained by other disturbances of motor function, they may be regarded as primary manifestations of cerebellar disease, but they are never severe or persistent and are of little clinical importance; anything approaching a hemiparesis in distribution or severity is not attributable to cerebellar disease.

Myoclonic movements—i.e., brief (50- to 100-ms), random contractions of muscles or groups of muscles—are, in some disease processes, combined with cerebellar ataxia. When multiple myoclonic jerks mar a volitional movement, they may be mistaken for an ataxic tremor. Action myoclonus may be the principal residual sign of hypoxic encephalopathy, as described in the discussion of postanoxic intention, or action myoclonus, in Chap. 40, and it has been proposed that this condition has a cerebellar origin. Myoclonus is described more fully in Chap. 6, where it is pointed out that it more often has its origin in diseases of the cerebral cortex.

More recently uncovered is the participation of the cerebellum in certain aspects of cognitive function and behavior (see the reviews by Leiner et al and by Schmahmann and Sherman). These authors and others have described a wide range of subtle alterations of memory and cognition, language function, and behavior in patients with disease apparently limited to the cerebellum (as determined by CT and MRI imaging). It is true that cerebellar lesions interfere with the establishment of conditioned reflexes and perhaps some deterioration in certain learning tasks as detected by specialized tests. However, it is not entirely clear if there is a uniform clinical pathologic syndrome in which a distinctive cognitive–behavioral deficit or group of deficits are related to a cerebellar disease or individual lesions. It seems to the current authors that recent investigations into the cerebral influences of the cerebellum are accurate and novel contributions to neurology, but at the same time, the changes referred to are subtle and often inapparent in the bedside neurologic examination. Rarely, as in a patient under our care, a fairly obvious aphasia from a prior insult to the cerebrum can be unmasked by an acute cerebellar lesion, such as a stroke. Slowly developing cerebellar disorders, such as tumors, do not appear to demonstrate this phenomenon.

Differential Diagnosis of Ataxia

In the diagnosis of disorders characterized by generalized cerebellar ataxia (affecting limbs, gait, and speech), the mode of onset, rate of development, and degree of permanence of the ataxia are of particular importance, as summarized in Table 5-1. Each of the major causes is discussed in an appropriate chapter. In adults, paraneoplastic and demyelinating cases account for the largest proportion of cases of subacute onset, and hereditary forms are the usual cause of very slowly progressive and chronic ones, particularly if gait is predominantly affected. The last category of genetic ataxias constitutes a large and heterogeneous group for which the mutation has been established in many cases; they are described in Chap. 39.

Unilateral ataxia without accompanying signs is most often caused by infarction or tumor in the ipsilateral cerebellar hemisphere or by demyelinating disease affecting cerebellar connections to the brainstem.

Table 5-1

DIAGNOSIS OF CEREBELLAR ATAXIA

MODE OF DEVELOPMENT	CAUSES
Acute-transitory	Intoxication with alcohol, lithium, barbiturate, phenytoin or other antiepileptics (associated with dysarthria, nystagmus; Chaps. 42 and 43) Diamox-responsive episodic ataxia (Chap. 37) Childhood hyperammonemias (Chap. 37)
Acute and usually reversible	Postinfectious, with inflammatory changes in CSF (Chap. 36) Viral cerebellar encephalitis (Chap. 33) Myxedema
Acute-enduring	Extreme hyperthermia with coma at onset (Chap. 17) Intoxication with mercury compounds or toluene (glue sniffing; spray painting; Chap. 43) Postanoxic with intention myoclonus Adulterated heroin ("chasing the dragon")
Subacute (over weeks)	Brain tumors such as medulloblastoma, astrocytoma, hemangioblastoma metastasis (usually with headache and papilledema; Chap. 31) Alcoholic–nutritional (Chaps. 41 and 42) Paraneoplastic cerebellar degeneration (Chap. 31) Creutzfeldt-Jakob (prion) disease (Chap. 33) Cerebellar abscess (Chap. 32) Whipple disease (characteristically with myoclonus and oculomasticatory movements) Sprue (gluten enteropathy) Multiple sclerosis
Chronic (months to years)	Friedreich ataxia and other spinocerebellar degenerations; other hereditary cerebellar degenerations (olivopontocerebellar degenerations; cerebellar cortical degenerations [Chap. 39]) Adult form of fragile X premutation syndrome (Chaps. 38 and 39) Hereditary metabolic diseases, often with myoclonus (Chap. 37) Childhood ataxias, including ataxia telangiectasia, cerebellar agenesis

The ataxia of severe sensory neuropathy and of posterior column or posterior spinal root disease (sensory ataxia) simulates cerebellar ataxia; presumably this is a result of involvement of the large peripheral spinocerebellar afferent fibers. Tabes dorsalis and sensory ganglionopathy are prime examples of this type of disorder. However, there should seldom be difficulty in separating the two if one takes note of the loss of distal joint position sense, absence of associated cerebellar signs such as dysarthria or nystagmus, loss of tendon reflexes, and the corrective effects of vision on sensory ataxia. In peripheral neuropathy and in spinal cord disease with ataxia, the Romberg sign is invariably present, reflecting a parallel dysfunction of large afferent fibers in the posterior columns; this sign is not found in lesions of the cerebellar hemispheres except that the patient may initially sway with eyes open and a bit more with eyes closed. A cerebellar type of tremor reaches an extreme form in the large-fiber polyneuropathy related to antibodies against myelin-associated glycoprotein but the features are closer to an enhanced action tremor, as discussed in the next chapter and in Chap. 46. In the Miller Fisher syndrome, which is considered to be a version of acute Guillain-Barré polyneuropathy, sensation is intact or affected only slightly and the severe ataxia and intention tremor are presumably a result of a highly selective peripheral disorder of spinocerebellar nerve fibers. Disorders of these same fibers in the spinocerebellar tracts of the cord may produce the same sensory-ataxic effects; subacute compressive lesions such as thoracic meningioma or demyelinating lesions are the usual causes. Again, there is a prominent Romberg sign. Occasionally, a cerebellar-like tremor in one limb results from a lesion in the dorsolateral cord that interrupts afferent fibers, presumably those directed to the spinocerebellar tracts.

Vertiginous ataxia is almost solely an ataxia of gait and is distinguished by the obvious complaint of vertigo and listing to one side, past pointing, and torsional-rotatory nystagmus, as discussed in Chap. 15. The nonvertiginous ataxia of gait caused by vestibular paresis (e.g., streptomycin toxicity) has special qualities, which are described in Chap. 7. Vertigo and cerebellar ataxia may be concurrent, as in some patients with a paraneoplastic disease and in those with infarction of the lateral medulla and inferior cerebellum. An unusual and transient ataxia of the contralateral limbs occurs acutely after infarction or hemorrhage in the anterior thalamus (thalamic ataxia); in addition to characteristic signs of thalamic damage, there may be an accompanying unilateral asterixis. Finally, a lesion of the superior parietal lobule (areas 5 and 7 of Brodmann) rarely results in a similar ataxia of the contralateral limbs.

References

Allen GI, Tsukahara N: Cerebrocerebellar communication systems. *Physiol Rev* 54:957, 1974.

Babinski J: De l'asynergie cerebelleuse. *Rev Neurol* 7:806, 1899.

Chambers WW, Sprague JM: Functional localization in the cerebellum: I. Organization in longitudinal cortico-nuclear zones and their contribution to the control of posture, both extrapyramidal and pyramidal. *J Comp Neurol* 103:104, 1955.

Chambers WW, Sprague JM: Functional localization in the cerebellum: II. Somatotopic organization in cortex and nuclei. *Arch Neurol Psychiatry* 74:653, 1955.

Diener HC, Dichgans J: Pathophysiology of cerebellar ataxia. *Mov Disord* 7:95, 1992.

Evarts EV, Thach WT: Motor mechanism of the CNS: Cerebrocerebellar interrelations. *Annu Rev Physiol* 31:451, 1969.

Gilman S: Cerebellar control of movement. *Ann Neurol* 35:3, 1994.

Gilman S, Bloedel J, Lechtenberg R: *Disorders of the Cerebellum.* Philadelphia, Davis, 1980, pp 159–177.

Hallett M, Berardelli A, Matheson J, et al: Physiological analysis of simple rapid movement in patients with cerebellar deficits. *J Neurol Neurosurg Psychiatry* 54:124, 1991

Hallett M, Shahani BT, Young RR: EMG analysis of patients with cerebellar deficits. *J Neurol Neurosurg Psychiatry* 38:1163, 1975.

Holmes G: The cerebellum of man: Hughlings Jackson Lecture. *Brain* 62:1, 1939.

Jansen J, Brodal A: *Aspects of Cerebellar Anatomy.* Oslo, Johan Grundt Tanum Forlag, 1954.

Kandel ER, Schwartz JH, Jessel TM (eds): *Principles of Neural Science*, 4th ed. New York, McGraw-Hill, 2000.

Leiner HC, Leiner AL, Dow RS: Does the cerebellum contribute to mental skills? *Behav Neurosci* 100:443, 1986

Schmahmann JD, Sherman JC: The cerebellar cognitive affective syndrome. *Brain* 121:561, 1998.

Sprague JM, Chambers WW: Control of posture by reticular formation and cerebellum in the intact, anesthetized and unanesthetized and in the decerebrated cat. *Am J Physiol* 176:52, 1954.

Stewart TG, Holmes G: Symptomatology of cerebellar tumors: A study of forty cases. *Brain* 27:522, 1904.

Thach WT Jr, Goodkin HP, Keating JG: The cerebellum and the adaptive coordination of movement. *Annu Rev Neurosci* 150:403, 1992.

Thach WT Jr, Montgomery EB Jr: Motor system, in Pearlman AL, Collins RC (eds): *Neurobiology of Disease.* New York, Oxford University Press, 1992, pp 168–196.

Urban PP, Marx J, Hunsche S, et al: Cerebellar speech representation. *Arch Neurol* 60:965, 2003.

6

Tremor, Myoclonus, Focal Dystonias, and Tics

The subject of tremor is considered at this point because of its association with diseases of the basal ganglia and cerebellum. In addition, a group of miscellaneous movement disorders—myoclonus, facial and cervical dyskinesias, focal limb dystonias, and tics—is described in this chapter. These disorders are largely involuntary in nature and can be quite disabling but they have an uncertain pathologic basis, as alluded to in Chap. 4, and an indefinite relationship to the extrapyramidal motor disorders or to other standard categories of neurologic disease. They are brought together here mainly for convenience of exposition.

TREMOR

Tremor may be defined as involuntary rhythmic oscillatory movement produced by alternating or irregularly synchronous contractions of reciprocally innervated muscles. Its rhythmic quality distinguishes tremor from other involuntary movements, and its oscillatory nature distinguishes it from myoclonus and asterixis.

Physiologic Tremor

A normal, or physiologic, tremor is embedded in the motor system. It is present in all contracting muscle groups and persists throughout the waking state and even in certain phases of sleep. The movement is so fine that it can barely be seen by the naked eye, and then only if the fingers are firmly outstretched; in most instances special instruments are required for its detection though asking the patient to aim a laser pointer at a distant target will often expose it. It ranges in frequency between 8 and 13 Hz, the dominant rate being 10 Hz in adulthood and somewhat less in childhood and old age. Several hypotheses have been proposed to explain physiologic tremor, a traditional one being that it reflects the passive vibration of body tissues produced by mechanical activity of cardiac origin, but this cannot be the whole explanation. As Marsden has pointed out, several additional factors—such as spindle input, the unfused grouped firing rates of motor neurons, and the natural resonating frequencies and inertia of the muscles and other structures—are probably of greater importance. Certain abnormal tremors, namely, the metabolic varieties of postural or action tremor and at least one type of familial tremor, are considered by some to be variants or exaggerations of physiologic tremor—i.e., "enhanced physiologic tremor," as discussed further on.

The following types of tremors, the clinical features of which are summarized in Fig. 6-1 and Table 6-1, are encountered most frequently in clinical practice. In clinical analysis they are usually distinguishable on the basis of (1) relation to movement and posture, (2) frequency, (3) the pattern of activity of opposing (agonist-antagonist pairs) muscles, i.e., synchronous or alternating, and (4) affected body parts. Such a classification also differentiates tremors from a large array of nontremorous movements, such as fasciculations, sensory ataxia, myoclonus, asterixis, epilepsia partialis continua, clonus, and rigor (shivering).

Action Tremors

Action tremors are evident during use of the affected body part, as opposed to tremor that is apparent in a position of rest or repose. Action tremors can be conveniently divided into two categories: goal directed action tremor of the ataxic type related to cerebellar disorders (discussed in Chap. 5) and postural tremors, which are either the enhanced physiologic variety or essential tremor (Fig. 6-1). A postural tremor occurs with the limbs and trunk actively maintained in certain positions (such as holding the arms outstretched) and may persist throughout active movement. More particularly, the tremor is absent when the limbs are relaxed but becomes evident when the muscles are activated. The tremor is accentuated as greater precision of movement is demanded, but it does not approach the degree of augmentation seen with cerebellar intention tremor. Most cases of action tremor are characterized by relatively rhythmic bursts of grouped motor neuron discharges that occur not quite synchronously in opposing muscle groups as shown in Fig. 6-2. Slight inequalities in the strength and timing of contraction of opposing muscle groups account for the tremor. In contrast, rest (parkinsonian) tremor, is characterized by alternating activity in agonist and antagonist muscles.

Enhanced Physiologic Tremor

The type of action tremor that seems merely to be an exaggeration of the above-described physiologic tremor,

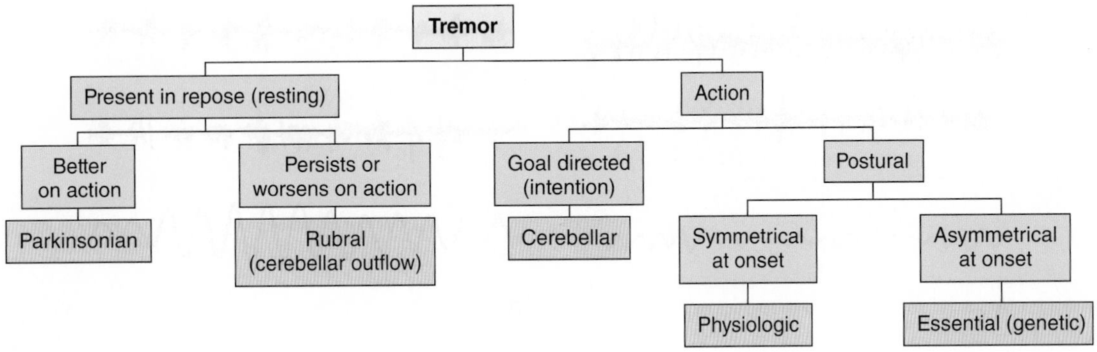

Figure 6-1. Tremor branch diagram.

can be brought out in most normal persons. It has the same fast frequency as physiologic tremor (about 10 Hz; Fig. 6-2) but with greater amplitude. Such a tremor, best elicited by holding the arms outstretched with fingers spread apart, is characteristic of intense fright and anxiety (hyperadrenergic states), certain metabolic disturbances (hyperthyroidism, hypercortisolism, hypoglycemia), pheochromocytoma, intense physical exertion, withdrawal from alcohol and other sedative drugs, and the toxic effects of several drugs—lithium, nicotinic acid, xanthines (coffee, tea, aminophylline), cocaine, methylphenidate, other stimulant drugs and corticosteroids. Young and colleagues have determined that the enhancement of physiologic tremor that occurs in metabolic and toxic states is not a function of the central nervous system but is instead a consequence of stimulation of muscular beta-adrenergic receptors by increased levels of circulating catecholamines.

A special type of postural action tremor, closely related to the enhanced physiologic tremor, occurs as the most prominent feature of the early stages of alcohol withdrawal. Withdrawal of other sedative drugs (benzodiazepines, barbiturates) following a sustained period of use produces much the same effect. LeFebvre-D'Amour and colleagues have described two tremors of slightly different frequency, one of which is indistinguishable from essential tremor (see below). Either of these may occur as the individual emerges from a relatively short period of intoxication ("morning shakes"). A number of alcoholics, on recovery from the withdrawal state, exhibit

Table 6-1
MAIN TYPES OF TREMOR

TYPE OF TREMOR	FREQUENCY, HZ	PREDOMINANT LOCATION	ENHANCING AGENTS	ATTENUATING AGENTS
Physiologic (enhanced)	8–13	Hands	Epinephrine, β-adrenergics	Alcohol, β-adrenergic antagonists
Parkinson (rest)	3–5	Hands and forearms, fingers, feet, lips, tongue	Emotional stress	L-Dopa, anticholinergics
Cerebellar (intention, ataxic, "rubral")	2–4	Limbs, trunk, head	Emotional stress	—
Postural, or action	5–8	Hands	Anxiety, fright, β-adrenergics, alcohol withdrawal, xanthines, lithium, exercise, fatigue	β-Adrenergic antagonists in some cases
Essential (familial, senile)	4–8	Hands, head, vocal cords	Same as above	Alcohol, propanolol, primidone
Alternate beat	3.5–6	Hands, head	Same as above	Clonazepam, alcohol, β-adrenergic antagonists
Orthostatic	4–8, irregular	Legs	Quiet standing	Repose, walking, clonazepam, valproate
Tremor of neuropathy	4–7	Hands	—	—
Palatal tremor	60–100/min	Palate, sometimes facial, pharyngeal, proximal limb muscles	—	Clonazepam, valproate
Dystonic	Irregular	Concordant with focal dystonia	—	Local botulinum toxin, gestes

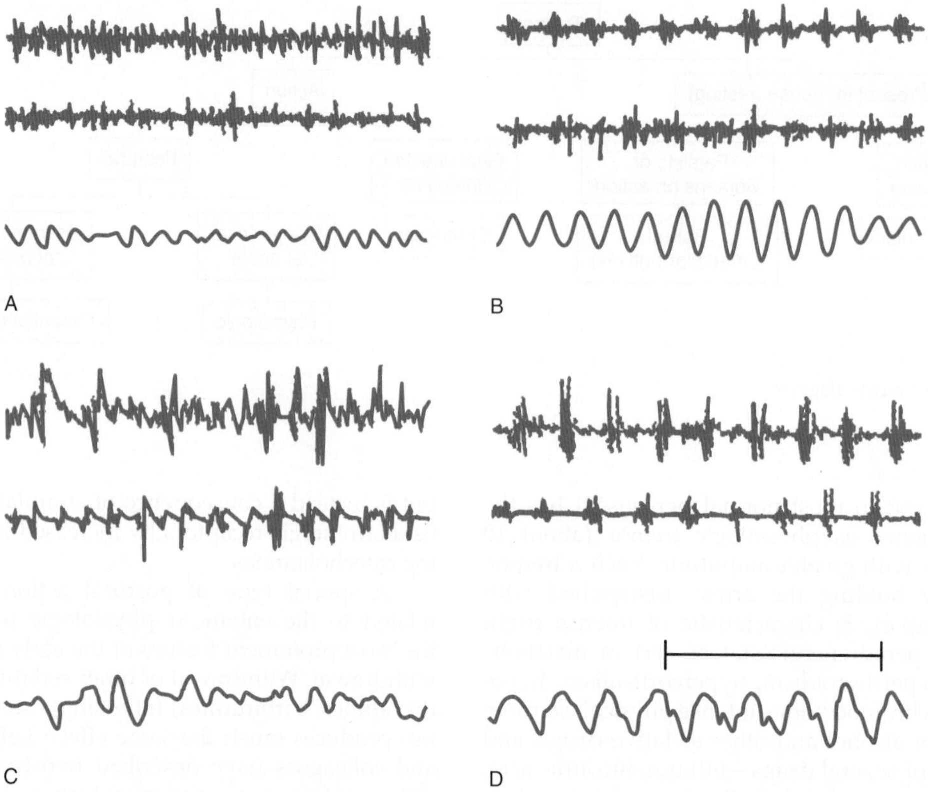

Figure 6-2. Types of tremor. In each, the lowest trace is an accelerometric recording from the outstretched hand; the upper two traces are surface EMG from the wrist extensor (upper) and flexor (middle) muscle groups. *A.* A physiologic tremor; there is no evidence of synchronization of EMG activity. *B.* Essential (familial) tremor; the movements are very regular and EMG bursts occur simultaneously in antagonistic muscle groups. *C.* Neuropathic tremor; movements are irregular and EMG bursts vary in timing between the two groups. *D.* Parkinsonian ("rest") tremor; EMG bursts alternate between antagonistic muscle groups. Calibration is 1 s. (Courtesy of Dr. Robert R. Young.)

a persistent tremor of essential (familial) type, described below. The mechanisms involved in alcohol withdrawal symptoms are discussed further in Chap. 42.

Essential (Familial, Hereditary) Tremor

This, the commonest type of tremor, is of lower frequency (4 to 8 Hz) than physiologic tremor and is unassociated with other neurologic changes; thus it is called "essential." It is usually at the lower end of this frequency range and of variable amplitude. Aside from its rate the identifying feature is its appearance or marked enhancement with attempts to maintain a static limb posture. Like most tremors, essential tremor is worsened by emotion, exercise, and fatigue. One infrequent type of essential tremor is faster than the usual essential tremor and of the same frequency (6 to 8 Hz) as enhanced physiologic tremor. Essential tremor may increase in severity to a point where the patient's handwriting becomes illegible and he cannot bring a spoon or glass to his lips without spilling its contents. Eventually, all tasks that require manual dexterity become difficult or impossible. The pathophysiology of this tremor and its treatment are discussed further on.

Typical essential tremor very often occurs in several members of a family, for which reason it has been called familial or hereditary essential tremor. Inheritance is in an autosomal dominant pattern with high penetrance. The idiopathic and familial types cannot be distinguished on the basis of their physiologic and pharmacologic properties and probably should not be considered as separate entities. This condition has been referred to as "benign essential tremor," but this is hardly so in many patients in whom it worsens with age and greatly interferes with normal activities.

Essential tremor most often makes its appearance late in the second decade, but it may begin in childhood and then persist. A second peak of increased incidence occurs in adults older than 35 years of age. Both sexes are affected. It is a relatively common disorder, with an estimated prevalence of 415 per 100,000 persons older than the age of 40 years (Haerer et al). As described by Elble, the tremor frequency diminishes slightly with age while its amplitude increases.

The tremor practically always begins in the arms and is usually almost symmetrical; in approximately 15 percent of patients, however, it may appear first in the dominant hand. A severe isolated arm or leg tremor should suggest another disease (Parkinson disease or focal dystonia, as described further on).

The tremor may remain limited to the upper limbs or a side-to-side or nodding movement of the head; tremor of the chin may be added or may occur independently. In certain cases of essential tremor, there is involvement of the jaw, lips, tongue, and larynx, the latter imparting a severe quaver to the voice (voice tremor). Infrequently, the tremor of the head or voice precedes that of the hands. The head tremor is also postural in nature and disappears when the head is supported. It has also been noted that the limb and head tremors tend to be muted when the patient walks. In some of our patients whose tremor remained isolated to the head for a decade or more, there has been little if any progression to the arms and almost no increase of the amplitude of movement.

The lower limbs are usually spared or only minimally affected. In the large series of familial tremor cases by Bain and colleagues, solitary jaw or head tremor was not found but we have observed isolated head tremor, as noted. Most patients with essential tremor will have identified the amplifying effects of anxiety and the ameliorating effects of alcohol on their tremor. We have also observed the tremor to become greatly exaggerated during emergence from anesthesia in a few patients.

Electromyographic studies reveal that the tremor is generated by more or less rhythmic and almost simultaneous bursts of activity in pairs of agonist and antagonist muscles (Fig. 6-2*B*). Less often, especially in the tremors at the lower range of frequency, the activity in agonist and antagonist muscles alternates ("alternate beat tremor"), a feature more characteristic of Parkinson disease, which the tremor then superficially resembles (see below). Tremor of either pattern may be disabling, but the less common, slower, alternate-beat tremor tends to be of higher amplitude, is more of a handicap, and is usually more resistant to treatment.

Treatment of Essential Tremor

A curious fact about essential tremor of the typical (non–alternate-beat) type is that it can be suppressed by a small amount of alcohol in more than 75 percent of patients; but once the effects of the alcohol have worn off, the tremor returns and may even worsen for a time. Of more therapeutic interest, essential tremor is inhibited by the beta-adrenergic antagonist propranolol (between 80 and 200 mg per day in divided doses or as a sustained-release preparation) taken orally over a long period of time. Often it takes several days or weeks for the effect to be evident. The benefit is variable and often incomplete; most studies indicate that 50 to 70 percent of patients have some symptomatic relief but may complain of side effects such as fatigue, erectile dysfunction, and bronchospasm.

The mechanism and site of action of beta-blocking agents is not known with certainty. It is blockade of the beta-2 adrenergic receptor that most closely aligned with reduction of the tremor. Several but not all of the other beta-blocking drugs are similarly effective to propranolol; metoprolol and nadolol, which are better tolerated than propranolol, are the ones most extensively studied, but they have yielded less consistent results than propranolol. The relative merits of different drugs in this class are discussed by Louis and by Koller et al (2000). Young and associates have shown that neither propranolol nor ethanol, when injected intraarterially into a limb, decreases the amplitude of essential tremor. These findings, and the delay in action of medications, suggest that their therapeutic effect is due less to blockade of the peripheral beta-adrenergic receptors than to their action on structures within the central nervous system. This is in contrast to the earlier mentioned muscle receptor-mediated effect of adrenergic compounds in physiologic tremor. It is possible that this ambiguity regarding the action of beta-blocking drugs is the result of their effect on physiological tremor that is superimposed on essential tremor.

The barbiturate drug primidone has also been effective in controlling essential tremor and may be tried in patients who do not respond to or cannot tolerate beta-blocking medications, but many patients cannot tolerate the side effects of drowsiness, nausea, and slight ataxia. Treatment should be initiated at 25 mg per day and increased slowly to 75 mg per day in order to minimize these effects. Gabapentin, topiramate (see Connor), mirtazipine, a variety of benzodiazepines and a large number of other drugs have been used with variable success, but at the moment should probably be considered second-line therapies; these alternatives are discussed by Louis. Amantadine also has a modest effect on tremor and may be used as an adjunct.

The alternate-beat, slow, high-amplitude, kinetic-predominant type of essential tremor is more difficult to suppress but has reportedly responded to clonazepam (Biary and Koller); in our experience, however, this approach has not been as successful. Alcohol and primidone have also had less effect than they do in typical essential tremor. Indeed, the tremor has often been resistant to most attempts at suppression, for which reason surgical approaches are now being used (see further on).

Injections of botulinum toxin into a portion of a limb can reduce the severity of essential tremor locally, but the accompanying weakness of arm and hand muscles often proves unacceptable to the patient. The same medication injected into the vocal cords can suppress severe voice tremor as described in a series of cases by Adler and colleagues as well as by others, but caution must be exercised to avoid paralyzing the cords. Doses as low as 1 U of toxin injected into each cord may be effective, with a latency of several days. The long-term repeated use of this treatment has not been adequately studied for essential-type limb or voice tremor.

In resistant cases of essential tremor of the fast or slow variety, stimulation by electrodes implanted in the ventral medial nucleus thalamus or the internal segment of the globus pallidus (of the same type used to treat Parkinson disease) has produced a durable response over many years; details can be found in the small study reported by Sydow and colleagues.

Tremor of Polyneuropathy

Adams and coworkers described a disabling action tremor in patients with chronic demyelinating and paraproteinemic polyneuropathies. It is a particularly prominent feature of the polyneuropathy caused by immunoglobulin M

(IgM) antibodies to myelin-associated glycoprotein (MAG) as mentioned in the preceding chapter. The movements simulate a coarse essential, or ataxic, tremor and typically worsen if the patient is asked to hold his finger near a target. The EMG pattern is more irregular than that in essential (familial) tremor (Fig. 6-2*C*). Pedersen and colleagues have found it to vary greatly in amplitude with considerable side-to-side oscillation, which is induced by co-contracting muscle activity; they also found little suppression of the tremor with loading of the limb, unlike most other organic tremors. It is hypothesized that there is a disturbance of muscle spindle afferents.

Some cases of acute or chronic inflammatory neuropathy or ganglionopathy may be marked by a similar and prominent ataxic tremor and a faster action tremor. A special type of Guillain-Barré syndrome (Fisher variant) is characterized by a tremor that is indistinguishable from ataxia. Also, the inherited disease, peroneal muscular atrophy (Charcot-Marie-Tooth disease), may be associated with tremor of the essential type but the two may be coincident rather than directly related; this combination of symptoms was the basis on which Roussy and Levy incorrectly set it apart as a distinct disease. Chapter 46 discusses these polyneuropathies.

True action tremors are seen in a number of other clinical settings. A coarse action tremor, sometimes combined with myoclonus, accompanies various types of meningoencephalitis (e.g., in the past it was quite common with syphilitic general paresis) and certain intoxications (methyl bromide and bismuth).

Parkinsonian (Repose, Rest) Tremor

This is a coarse, rhythmic tremor with a frequency of 3 to 5 Hz. Electromyographically, it is characterized by bursts of activity that alternate between opposing muscle groups. The tremor is most often localized in one or both hands and forearms and less frequently in the feet, jaw, lips, or tongue (Fig. 6-2*D*). It occurs when the limb is in an attitude of repose and is suppressed or diminished by willed movement, at least momentarily, only to reassert itself once the limb assumes a new position. Even though it is termed a "resting" tremor, maintaining the arm in an attitude of repose requires a certain degree of muscular contraction, albeit slight. If the tremulous hand is completely relaxed, as it is when the arm is fully supported at the wrist and elbow, the tremor usually disappears; however, the patient rarely achieves this state. Usually he maintains a state of slight tonic contraction of the trunk and proximal muscles of the limbs. Under conditions of complete rest, i.e., in all except the lightest phases of sleep, the tremor disappears, as do most abnormal tremors except various forms of myoclonus.

Parkinsonian tremor is "alternating" in the sense that it takes the form of flexion–extension or abduction–adduction of the fingers or the hand; pronation–supination of the hand and forearm is also a common presentation. Flexion–extension of the fingers in combination with adduction–abduction of the thumb yields the characteristic "pill-rolling" tremor of Parkinson disease. It continues and may worsen while the patient walks, unlike essential tremor; indeed, it may first become apparent to the patient during walking. When the legs are affected, the tremor takes the form of a flexion–extension movement of the foot, sometimes the knee. In the jaw and lips, it is seen as up-and-down and pursing movements, respectively. The eyelids, if they are closed lightly, tend to flutter rhythmically (blepharoclonus), and the tongue, when protruded, may move in and out of the mouth at about the same tempo as the tremor elsewhere.

The cogwheel effect, a ratchet-like interruption perceived by the examiner on passive movement of an extremitiy (the Negro sign). It is said by many authors to be no more than a palpable tremor superimposed on rigidity and as such, is not specific for Parkinson disease although it is most prominent in that condition. This explanation is called into question by the numerous cases in which Parkinson patients display minimal or no resting tremor but nonetheless have the cogwheel phenomenon as mentioned in Chap. 4. Cogwheeling can be brought out by having the patient engage the opposite limb, such as tracing circles in the air; this Froment sign, was originally described in essential tremor.

The parkinsonian tremor frequency is surprisingly constant over long periods, but the amplitude is variable. Emotional stress augments the amplitude and may add to the effects of an enhanced physiologic or essential tremor. With advance of the disease, increasing rigidity of the limbs obscures or reduces it. It is curious how little the tremor interferes with voluntary movement; for example, it is possible for a tremulous patient to raise a full glass of water to his lips and drain its contents without spilling a drop; this is not always the case with "benign" essential tremor, as already emphasized.

Almost always in Parkinson disease, the tremor is asymmetric and at the outset may be entirely unilateral. The tremor of postencephalitic parkinsonism (which is now virtually extinct) often had greater amplitude and involved proximal muscles. In neither disease is there a close correspondence between the degree of tremor and the degree of rigidity or akinesia. A bilateral parkinsonian type of tremor may also be seen in elderly persons without akinesia, rigidity, or mask-like facies. In some of these patients, the tremor is followed years later by the other manifestations of Parkinson disease, but in others it is not, the tremor remaining unchanged for decades or progressing very slowly, unaffected by anti-Parkinson drugs. This probably equates with the earlier mentioned alternate-beat type of essential tremor. Patients with the familial (wilsonian) or acquired form of hepatocerebral degeneration may also show a tremor of parkinsonian type, usually mixed with ataxic tremor and other extrapyramidal motor abnormalities. An alternating tremor may be seen in toxic-drug induced parkinsonism but it is relatively symmetric and tends not to be a prominent feature.

Parkinsonian tremor is suppressed to some extent by the anticholinergic drugs benztropine, trihexyphenidyl, and other anticholinergic drugs such as ethopropazine, a phenothizine derivative; it is also suppressed less consistently but sometimes impressively by L-dopa and dopaminergic agonist drugs, which are the mainstays of treatment for Parkinson disease as discussed in Chap. 39.

The situation is made more difficult because a parkinsonian tremor is often associated with an additional tremor of faster frequency; the latter is of essential type and responds better to beta-blocking drugs than to anti-Parkinson medications. Stereotactic lesions or electrical stimulation in the basal ventrolateral nucleus of the thalamus diminishes or abolishes tremor contralaterally; other stimulation sites such as the internal segment of the globus pallidus and the subthalamic nucleus are also effective but possibly to a lesser degree. Chapter 39 discusses treatment of Parkinson disease in greater detail.

Intention (Ataxic, Cerebellar, Goal Directed Action) Tremor

As discussed in Chap. 5, the word intention is ambiguous in this context because the tremor itself is not intentional and occurs not when the patient intends to make a movement but only during the most demanding phases of active performance. In this sense it is a kinetic or action tremor, but the latter term has connotations of the essential tremor to neurologists, as described earlier. The term ataxic is a suitable substitute for intention, because this tremor is always combined with cerebellar ataxia and adds to it, as described in Chap. 5. Its salient feature is that it requires for its full expression the performance of an exacting, precise, projected movement. The tremor is absent when the limbs are inactive and during the first part of a voluntary movement but as the action continues and fine adjustments of the movement are demanded (e.g., in touching the tip of the nose or the examiner's finger), an irregular, more or less rhythmic (2- to 4-Hz) interruption of forward progression with side-to-side oscillation appears and may continue for several beats after the target has been reached. Unlike essential and parkinsonian tremors, the oscillations occur in more than one plane but are mainly horizontal and perpendicular to the trajectory of movement. The tremor and ataxia may seriously interfere with the patient's performance of skilled acts. In some patients there is a rhythmic oscillation of the head on the trunk (titubation), or of the trunk itself, at approximately the same rate. As already indicated, this type of tremor points to disease of the cerebellum or its connections, particularly via the superior cerebellar peduncle, but certain peripheral nerve diseases may occasionally simulate it.

There is another, higher amplitude tremor associated with cerebellar ataxia, in which every movement, even lifting the arm slightly or maintaining a static posture with the arms held out to the side, results in a wide-ranging, rhythmic 2- to 5-Hz "wing-beating" movement, sometimes of sufficient force to throw the patient off balance. In such cases, the lesion is usually in the midbrain, involving the rostral projections of the dentatorubrothalamic fibers and the medial part of the ventral tegmental reticular nucleus. Because of the location of the lesion in the region of the red nucleus, Holmes originally called this a rubral tremor. However, experimental evidence in monkeys indicates that the tremor is produced not by a lesion of the red nucleus per se but by interruption of dentatothalamic fibers that traverse this nucleus—i.e., the cerebellar efferent fibers that form the superior cerebellar peduncle and brachium conjunctivum (Carpenter). This type of tremor is seen most often in patients with multiple sclerosis and Wilson disease, occasionally with vascular and other lesions of the tegmentum of the midbrain and subthalamus, and rarely as an effect of antipsychosis medications. Beta-adrenergic blocking agents, anticholinergic drugs, and L-dopa have little therapeutic effect. It is abolished by a surgical or ischemic lesion in the opposite ventrolateral nucleus of the thalamus. Thalamic stimulation may be particularly helpful in severe cases that are the result of demyelinating lesions in the cerebellar peduncles.

Chapter 5 and the section further on, "Pathophysiology of Tremor," discuss the mechanisms involved in the production of intention, or ataxic tremor.

Geniospasm

This is a strongly familial episodic tremor disorder of the chin and lower lip that begins in childhood and may worsen with age. Psychic stress and concentration are known to precipitate the movements, which are described by Danek as "trembling." Rare instances involve other facial muscles. The disorder must be distinguished from a similar tremor of the chin that is part of essential tremor, facial myokymia or fasciculations, and palatal tremor. The disorder results from a mutation on chromosome 9.

Primary Orthostatic Tremor (See also Chap. 7)

This is a rare but striking tremor isolated to the legs that is remarkable by its occurrence only during quiet standing and its cessation almost immediately on walking. It is difficult to classify and more relevant to disorders of gait than it is to tremors of other types. The frequency of the tremor has been recorded as approximately 14 to 16 Hz, making it difficult to observe and more easily palpable. Nonetheless, it may produce considerable disability as the patient attempts to stabilize himself in response to the tremulousness. An important accompanying feature is the sensation of severe imbalance, which causes the patient to assume a widened stance while standing; these patients are unable to walk a straight line (tandem gait). We have observed prominent tonic contraction of the legs during standing, seemingly in an attempt to overcome imbalance (see Heilman; and Thompson, Rothwell, Day et al). The arms are affected little or not at all. Often the first step or two when the patient begins to walk are halting, but thereafter, the gait is entirely normal. Because falls are infrequent, the condition is often attributed to hysteria. Tremulousness is not present when the patient is seated or reclining, but in the latter positions it can be evoked by strong contraction of the leg muscles against resistance.

Electromyographic recordings demonstrate rhythmic cocontraction of the gastrocnemius and anterior tibialis muscles. Although some authors, such as Wee and colleagues, have classified the disorder as a type of essential tremor, most of its characteristics suggest otherwise. Sharott and coworkers consider it an exaggerated physiologic tremor in response to imbalance; others have found an intrinsic rhythm at approximately 16 Hz generated by the damaged spinal cord in patients with myelopathy, suggesting a spinal origin for the tremor.

Some cases have responded to the administration of clonazepam, gabapentin, primidone, or sodium valproate alone or in combination but it often proves difficult to treat. A few intractable cases have been treated with an implanted spinal cord stimulator (Krauss et al, 2005).

Dystonic Tremor

Tremors may be an incipient feature of dystonia. When the underlying dystonic posturing is not overt, the tremor may be ascribed to the essential variety or to hysteria. Dystonic tremor is focal, superimposed, for example on torticollis, or it may be evident in a dystonic hand. The movement is not entirely rhythmic, sometimes jerky, and often intermittent. These cases are discussed further on in the section on focal dystonia. In addition, a fair number of patients with dystonia have an essential tremor.

Psychogenic Tremor

Tremor may be a quite dramatic manifestation of hysteria. It simulates many types of organic tremor, thereby causing difficulty in diagnosis. Psychogenic tremors are usually restricted to a single limb, often in the dominant hand; they are gross in nature, are less regular than the common static or action tremors, and diminish in amplitude or disappear if the patient is distracted as, for example, when asked to make a complex movement with the opposite hand. If the examiner restrains the affected hand and arm, the tremor may move to a more proximal part of the limb or to another part of the body ("chasing the tremor"). Other useful features in identifying hysterical tremor are exaggeration of the tremor by loading the limb—e.g., by having the patient hold a book or other heavy object—which reduces almost all other tremors with exception of those produced by polyneuropathy. Hysterical tremor persists in repose and during movement and is less subject than nonhysterical tremors to the modifying influences of posture and willed movement. Tremors of this type often acquire the frequency of a willed movement in a different limb. This can be brought out by asking the patient to rhythmically tap with the unaffected limb.

Tremors of Complex Type

Not all tremors correspond exactly with those described above and several of them may coexist. There is frequently a variation in one or more of the particulars from the typical pattern, or one type of tremor may show a feature ordinarily considered characteristic of another. In some parkinsonian patients, for example, the tremor is accentuated rather than dampened by active movement; in others, the tremor may be very mild or absent in repose and become obvious only with movement of the limbs. As mentioned above, a patient with a typical parkinsonian tremor may, in addition, show a fine essential tremor of the outstretched hands and occasionally even an element of ataxic tremor as well. In a similar way, essential or familial tremor may, in its advanced stages, assume the aspects of a cerebellar tremor. Further examples include patients with essential or familial tremor or with cerebellar degeneration who display a rhythmic parkinsonian tremor in relation to sustained postures.

Pathophysiology of Tremor

In patients with tremor of either the parkinsonian, postural, or intention type, Narabayashi has recorded rhythmic burst discharges of unitary cellular activity in the nucleus intermedius ventralis of the thalamus (as well as in the medial pallidum and subthalamic nucleus) synchronous with the beat of the tremor. Neurons that exhibit the synchronous bursts are arranged somatotopically and respond to kinesthetic impulses from the muscles and joints involved in the tremor. A stereotaxic lesion in this region of the thalamus abolishes the tremor. The effectiveness of a thalamic lesion may be a result of interruption of pallidothalamic and dentatothalamic projections or, more likely, of projections from the ventrolateral thalamus to the premotor cortex, as the impulses responsible for tremor are ultimately transmitted by the lateral corticospinal tract. Some of what is known about the physiology of specific tremors is noted in the following paragraphs.

Essential Tremor

To date, only a few cases of essential tremor have been examined postmortem, and these have disclosed no consistent lesion to which the tremor could indisputably be attributed (Herskovits and Blackwood; Cerosimo and Koller). A singular case of a 90-year-old woman studied by Louis and colleagues, demonstrated more extensive cerebellar cortical and dentate nucleus cell loss and reactive changes than had been previously recognized.

The question of the existence and locus of a generator for essential tremor as opposed to the unbalancing of a feedback loop system is unresolved. As indicated by McAuley, various studies that demonstrate rhythmic activity in the cortex corresponding to the tremor activity are more suggestive of a common source elsewhere than of a primary generator in the cortex. Based on electrophysiologic recordings in patients, two likely origins of oscillatory activity are the olivocerebellar circuits and the thalamus. Whether a particular structure possesses an intrinsic rhythmicity or, as currently favored, the tremor is an expression of reciprocal oscillations in circuits of the dentato–brainstem–cerebellar or thalamic–tegmental systems is not at all clear. Studies of blood flow in patients with essential tremor by Colebatch and coworkers affirm that the cerebellum is rhythmically activated; on this basis they argue that there is a release of an oscillatory mechanism in the olivocerebellar pathway. Dubinsky and Hallett demonstrated that the inferior olives also become hypermetabolic when essential tremor is activated, but this has been questioned by Wills and colleagues who recorded increased blood flow in the cerebellum and red nuclei, but not in the olive. These proposed mechanisms are reviewed by Elble and serve to emphasize the points made here.

Although this disorder is familial, a single genetic site has not yet been established; several candidate polymorphisms are promising.

Parkinsonian Tremor

The anatomic basis of parkinsonian tremor is not known. In Parkinson disease, the visible lesions predominate in the substantia nigra, and this was true also of the postencephalitic form of the disease. In animals, however, experimental lesions confined to the substantia nigra do not result in tremor; neither do lesions in the striatopallidum. Moreover, not all patients with lesions of the substantia nigra have tremor; in some there is only bradykinesia and rigidity. In a group of patients poisoned with the toxin MPTP (1-methyl-4-phenyl-1,2,3,6-tetrahydropyridine), a meperidine analogue that destroys the neurons of the substantia nigra pars compacta (see Chaps. 4 and 39), only half developed a tremor, which had more of the characteristics of a proximal action or postural tremor than of a rest tremor as discussed by Burns and colleagues. In all likelihood, these inconsistencies reflect the complex influence of dopamine on a number of basal ganglionic structures outlined in Chap. 4.

Ward and others have produced a Parkinson-like tremor in monkeys by placing a lesion in the ventromedial tegmentum of the midbrain, just caudal to the red nucleus and dorsal to the substantia nigra. He postulated that interruption of the descending fibers at this site liberates an oscillating mechanism in the lower brainstem; this presumably involves limb innervation via the reticulospinal pathway. Alternative possibilities are that the lesion in the ventromedial tegmentum interrupts the brachium conjunctivum, or a tegmental-thalamic projection, or the descending limb of the superior cerebellar peduncle, which functions as a link in a dentatoreticular-cerebellar feedback mechanism, a hypothesis similar to the one proposed for essential tremor (see Fig. 5-3). The differential effect of drugs on tremor and bradykinesia suggest that they must have separate mechanisms.

Ataxic Tremor (See also Chap. 5)

This has been produced in monkeys by inactivating the deep cerebellar nuclei or by sectioning the superior cerebellar peduncle or the brachium conjunctivum below its decussation. A lesion of the nucleus interpositus or dentate nucleus causes an ipsilateral tremor of ataxic type, as one might expect, associated with other manifestations of cerebellar ataxia. In addition, such a lesion gives rise to a "simple tremor," which is the term that Carpenter applied to a "resting" or parkinsonian tremor. He found that the latter was most prominent during the early postoperative period and was less enduring than ataxic tremor. Nevertheless, the concurrence of the two types of tremor and the fact that both can be abolished by ablation of the contralateral ventrolateral thalamic nucleus suggest that they have related neural mechanisms, at least in monkeys.

Palatal Tremor ("Palatal Myoclonus")

This is a rare disorder consisting of rapid, rhythmic, involuntary movements of the soft palate. For many years it was considered to be a form of uniphasic myoclonus (hence the terms palatal myoclonus and palatal nystagmus). Because of the persistent rhythmicity, it is now classified as a tremor. There are two forms of this movement, according to Deuschl and colleagues. One is essential palatal tremor that reflects the rhythmic activation of the tensor veli palatini muscles; it has no known pathologic basis. The palatal movement may impart a repetitive audible click, which ceases during sleep. The second, more common form is a symptomatic palatal tremor caused by a diverse group of brainstem lesions that interrupt the central tegmental tract(s); these columns contain descending fibers from midbrain nuclei to the inferior olivary complex (a component of the Guillain-Mollaret triangle described below and in Chap. 5 and Fig. 5-3). The frequency of the tremor varies greatly and is 26 to 420 cycles per minute in the essential form and 107 to 164 cycles per minute in the symptomatic form.

Symptomatic palatal tremor, in contrast to the essential type and all other tremors, persists during sleep and is sometimes associated with ocular myoclonus that is synchronized with the palatal movements. In some cases, the pharynx as well as the facial and extraocular muscles (pendular or convergence nystagmus), diaphragm, vocal cords, and even the muscles of the neck and shoulders partake of the persistent rhythmic movements. A similar phenomenon, in which contraction of the masseters occurs concurrently with pendular ocular convergence, has been observed in Whipple disease (oculomasticatory myorhythmia).

Magnetic resonance imaging (MRI) reveals no lesions to account for essential palatal tremor; in the symptomatic form, however, there are tegmental brainstem lesions and conspicuous enlargement of the inferior olivary nucleus unilaterally or bilaterally. With unilateral palatal tremor, it is the contralateral olive that becomes enlarged. It has been proposed that the lesions in the symptomatic form interrupt the circuit (dentate nucleus–brachium conjunctivum–red nucleus-central tegmental tract–olivary nucleus–dentate nucleus) that Lapresle and Ben Hamida called the triangle of Guillain-Mollaret (Fig. 5-3). The lesions have been vascular, neoplastic, especially demyelinating, or traumatic, and have been found mainly in midbrain or pontine portions of the central tegmental fasciculus.

The physiologic basis of palatal tremor remains conjectural. Matsuo and Ajax postulated a denervation hypersensitivity of the inferior olivary nucleus and its dentate connections, but others have suggested that the critical event is denervation not of the olive but of the nucleus ambiguus and the dorsolateral reticular formation adjacent to it. Dubinsky and colleagues have suggested that palatal tremor may be based on the same mechanism as postural tremor—i.e., presumably

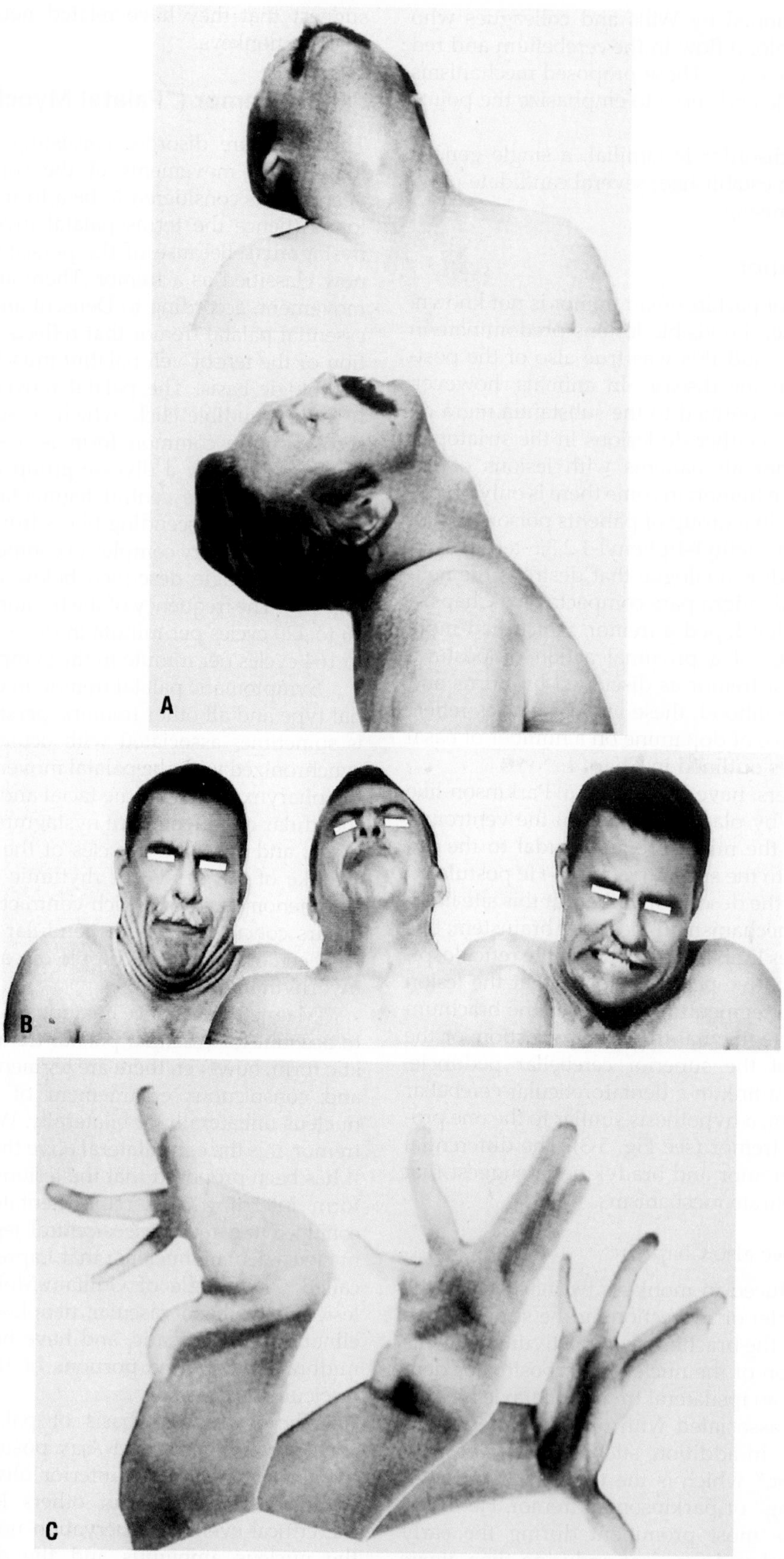

Figure 6-3. Dystonic movement disorders. *A.* Young man with severe spasmodic retrocollis. Note hypertrophy of sternocleidomastoid muscles. *B.* Meige syndrome of severe blepharospasm and facial-cervical dystonia. *C.* Characteristic athetoid-dystonic deformities of the hand in a patient with tardive dyskinesia. (Photographs courtesy of Dr. Joseph M. Waltz.)

a disinhibition of the olive and a rhythmic coupling of neurons in the olive induced by a lesion of the dentato-olivary pathway.

The use of drugs in treating this movement disorder has met with variable success. Clonazepam (0.25 to 0.5 mg/d, increasing gradually to 3.0 to 6.0 mg/d), sodium valproate (250 mg/d, increasing to 1,000 mg/d), and gabapentin (up to 2,100 mg) have suppressed the movement in some cases, particularly the last of these drugs, which reportedly has had a dramatic effect in some patients. Also, tetrabenazine and haloperidol have been helpful on occasion. Selective injection of the palatal muscles with botulinum toxin, while technically demanding, affords modest relief; it is particularly helpful in eliminating the annoying ear clicking.

ASTERIXIS

The movement disorder known as asterixis was described by Adams and Foley in patients with hepatic encephalopathy but it occurs with a variety of systemic metabolic disorders. It consists of arrhythmic lapses of sustained posture that allow gravity or the inherent elasticity of muscles to produce a movement, which the patient then corrects, sometimes with overshoot. Later, Leavitt and Tyler and then Young and Shahani demonstrated that the initial interruption or lapse in posture is associated with EMG silence for a period of 35 to 200 ms. By interlocking EMG and electroencephalogram (EEG) recordings, Ugawa et al found that a sharp wave, probably generated in the motor cortex, immediately precedes the period of EMG silence. This confirmed that asterixis differs physiologically from both tremor and myoclonus, with which it was formerly confused; it has incorrectly been referred to as a "negative tremor."

Asterixis is most readily evoked by asking the patient to hold his arms outstretched with hands dorsiflexed or to dorsiflex the hands and extend the fingers while resting the forearms on the bed or the arms of a chair. Flexion movements of the hands may then occur arrhythmically once or several times a minute. The same lapses in sustained muscle contraction can be provoked in any muscle group—including, for example, the protruded tongue, the closed eyelids, or the flexed trunk muscles. Sometimes, asterixis can be elicited best by asking the patient to place his hand flat on a table and raise the index finger.

This sign was first observed in patients with hepatic encephalopathy but was later noted with hypercapnia, uremia, and other metabolic and toxic encephalopathies. Asterixis may also be evoked by phenytoin and other anticonvulsants, usually indicating that these drugs are present in excessive concentrations. Similar rapid lapsing movements of the head or arms sometimes appear during drowsiness in normal persons ("nodding off").

Unilateral asterixis occurs in an arm and leg on the side opposite an anterior thalamic infarction or small hemorrhage, after stereotaxic thalamotomy, and with an upper midbrain lesion, usually as a transient phenomenon after stroke. In two series, Kim and coworkers and Montalban and colleagues, came to a similar conclusion, namely that unilateral asterixis is usually attributable to an acute thalamic stroke on the contralateral side, but there was an interesting variety of other localizations including the frontal lobe (anterior cerebral artery infarction), midbrain, and cerebellum in a few cases each. Our experience is limited to those arising from thalamic and overlying parietal lesions. Many drugs may unmask unilateral asterixis that has its basis in an underlying lesion of the anterior thalamus.

CLONUS, MYOCLONUS, AND POLYMYOCLONUS

The terms clonus (or clonic), myoclonus (or myoclonic), and polymyoclonus have been used, perhaps indiscriminately, to designate rhythmic or arrhythmic series of brief, shock-like muscular contractions associated with disease of the central nervous system. Clonus refers to a series of rhythmic, monophasic (i.e., unidirectional) contractions and relaxations of a group of muscles, differing in this way from tremors, which are always diphasic or bidirectional. Myoclonus specifies the very rapid, shock-like contractions of a group of muscles, irregular in rhythm and amplitude, and, with few exceptions, asynchronous and asymmetrical in distribution. If such contractions occur singly or are repeated in a restricted group of muscles, such as those of an arm or leg, the phenomenon is termed segmental myoclonus, whereas widespread, lightning-like, arrhythmic repeated contractions are referred to as polymyoclonus. The discussion that follows makes evident that each of the three phenomena has a distinctive pathophysiology and clinical implications.

Reference has already been made in Chap. 3 to the clonus that appears in relation to spasticity and heightened tendon reflexes in diseases affecting the corticospinal tract. It is most easily elicited by forcefully dorsiflexing the ankle; a series of rhythmic jerks of small to moderate amplitude result.

A common and benign example of myoclonus, familiar to many persons, is the "sleep-start" that consists of a jerking of the body, particularly the torso, while falling asleep or occasionally, just prior to waking (see Chap. 18). This movement will be vigorous enough to cause tongue biting and be mistaken for a convulsion.

Epilepsia partialis continua is a special type of rhythmic epileptic activity in which one group of muscles—usually of the face, arm, or leg—is continuously (day and night) involved in a series of rhythmic monophasic contractions. These may continue for weeks, months, or years. In most cases there is a corresponding EEG abnormality. The disorder appears to be cerebral in origin, but in most cases its precise anatomic and physiologic basis cannot be determined (see Chap. 16 for further discussion).

Focal and Regional Myoclonus

Patients with idiopathic epilepsy may complain of a localized myoclonic jerk or a short burst of myoclonic jerks, occurring particularly on awakening and on the day or two preceding a major generalized seizure, after which these movements cease. One-sided or focal myoclonic jerks are the dominant feature of a particular form of childhood epilepsy—so-called benign epilepsy with rolandic spikes (Chap. 16). Diffuse myoclonic jerks are the main—or sometimes only—manifestation of a fairly common seizure disorder with distinctive EEG features called juvenile myoclonic epilepsy; this diagnosis is suggested by an onset of myoclonus or single seizures during adolescence and myoclonus or lapses in upright posture, usually occurring in the morning, that become prominent with sleep deprivation and several hours after alcohol consumption. Myoclonus may be associated with atypical petit mal and akinetic seizures in the Lennox-Gastaut syndrome (absence or petit mal variants); the patient often falls during the brief lapse of postural mechanisms that follows a single myoclonic contraction. Similarly, in the West syndrome of infantile spasms, the arms and trunk are suddenly flexed or extended in a single massive myoclonic jerk ("jackknife" or "salaam" seizures); mental regression occurs in 80 to 90 percent of these cases, even when the seizures are successfully treated with adrenocorticotropic hormone (ACTH). These types of special "myoclonic epilepsies" are discussed further below and in Chap. 16 in relation to epilepsy.

Focal simple myoclonus is also one of the notable features of degenerative neurologic conditions, particularly corticobasal ganglionic degeneration; it is generally seen in a limb that is made rigid by this process.

Diffuse Myoclonus (Polymyoclonus)

Under the title paramyoclonus multiplex, Friedreich, in 1881, described a sporadic instance of widespread muscle jerking in an adult. It was probably in the course of this description that the term myoclonus was used for the first time. Muscles were involved diffusely, particularly those of the lower face and proximal segments of the limbs, and the myoclonus persisted for many years, being absent only during sleep. No other neurologic abnormalities accompanied the movement abnormality. The nature and pathologic basis of this disorder were never determined.

Over the years, the term paramyoclonus multiplex, or polymyoclonus has been applied to all varieties of myoclonic disorder (and other motor phenomena as well), to the point where it has nearly lost its specific connotation. Polymyoclonus may occur in pure or "essential" form as a benign, often familial, nonprogressive disease or as part of a more complex progressive syndrome that may prove disabling and fatal. More importantly, there are several acquired forms that are associated with various neurologic diseases as discussed below.

Essential (Familial; hereditary; genetic) Myoclonus

Symptoms may begin at any period of life but usually appear first in childhood and are of unknown etiology. An autosomal dominant mode of inheritance is evident in some families. The myoclonus takes the form of irregular twitches of one or another part of the body, involving groups of muscles, single muscles, or even a portion of a muscle. As a result, an arm may suddenly flex, the head may jerk backward or forward, or the trunk may curve or straighten. The face, neck, jaw, tongue, ocular muscles, and diaphragm may twitch. According to Wilson, even fascicles of the platysma may twitch. Some muscle contractions cause no visible displacement of a limb. In this and other forms of myoclonus, the muscle contraction is brief (20 to 50 ms)—i.e., faster than that of chorea, with which it may be confused. The speed of the myoclonic contraction is the same whether it involves a part of a muscle, a whole muscle, or a group of muscles. Some of the patients register little complaint, accepting the constant intrusions of motor activity with stoicism; they generally lead relatively normal, active lives. Seizures, dementia, and other neurologic deficits are notably absent. Occasionally there is hint of a mild cerebellar ataxia and, in one family studied by R.D. Adams, essential tremor was present as well, both in family members with polymyoclonus and in those without. Both the tremor and myoclonus were dramatically suppressed by the ingestion of alcohol. Similar families have been observed by Marsden and colleagues. In a Mayo Clinic series reported by Aigner and Mulder, 19 of 94 cases of polymyoclonus were of this "essential" type.

Several of the sleep-related syndromes that involve repetitive leg movements include an element of myoclonus. In a few patients, mainly older ones with severe "restless legs syndrome," the myoclonus and dyskinesias may become troublesome in the daytime as well. These patients march in place and rock their bodies during sleep (Walters et al). These disorders are discussed in Chap. 19.

Myoclonic Epilepsy (See also Myoclonic Seizures in Chap. 16)

Myoclonic epilepsy constitutes an important syndrome of multiple etiologies. A relatively benign idiopathic form, juvenile myoclonic epilepsy, has been mentioned and is discussed extensively in Chap. 16. A more serious type of myoclonic epilepsy, which in the beginning may be marked by polymyoclonus as an isolated phenomenon, is eventually associated with dementia and other signs of progressive neurologic disease (familial variety of Unverricht and Lundborg). An outstanding feature of the latter is a remarkable sensitivity of the myoclonus to stimuli of all sorts. If a limb is passively or actively displaced, the resulting myoclonic jerk may lead, through a series of progressively larger and more or less synchronous jerks, to a generalized convulsive seizure. In late childhood this type of stimulus-sensitive myoclonus is usually a manifestation of the juvenile form of lipid storage disease, which, in addition to myoclonus, is characterized by seizures, retinal degeneration, dementia, rigidity, pseudobulbar paralysis, and, in the late stages, by quadriplegia in flexion.

Another form of stimulus-sensitive (reflex) myoclonus, inherited as an autosomal recessive trait, begins in late childhood or adolescence and is associated with neuronal inclusions (Lafora bodies thus Lafora-body disease) in the cerebral and cerebellar cortex and in brainstem nuclei. In yet another familial type (described under the title of Baltic myoclonus by Eldridge and associates), autopsy has disclosed a loss of Purkinje cells but no inclusion bodies. Unlike Lafora-body disease, the Baltic variety of myoclonic epilepsy has a favorable prognosis, particularly if the seizures are treated with valproic acid.

Under the title of cherry-red-spot myoclonus syndrome, Rapin and associates have drawn attention to a familial (autosomal recessive) form of diffuse, incapacitating intention myoclonus associated with visual loss and ataxia. This disorder develops insidiously in adolescence. The earliest sign is a cherry-red spot in the macula that may fade in the chronic stages of the illness. The intellect is relatively unimpaired. The specific enzyme defect appears to be a deficiency of lysosomal alpha-neuroaminidase (sialidase), resulting in the excretion of large amounts of sialylated oligosaccharides in the urine. This has been referred to as type 1 sialidosis to distinguish it from a second type, in which patients are of short stature (as a result of chondrodystrophy) and often have a deficiency of beta-galactosidase in tissues and body fluids. In patients with sialidosis, a mucopolysaccharide-like material is stored in liver cells, but neurons show only a nonspecific accumulation of lipofuscin. A similar clinical syndrome of myoclonic epilepsy is seen in a variant form of neuroaxonal dystrophy and in the late childhood–early adult neuronopathic form of Gaucher disease, in which it is associated with supranuclear gaze palsies and cerebellar ataxia (Chap. 37).

Diffuse Myoclonus with Acquired Neurologic Disease

The clinical settings in which one observes widespread random myoclonic jerks as a transient or persistent phenomenon in adults include structural diseases such as viral encephalitis, Creutzfeldt-Jakob disease, general paresis, advanced Alzheimer and Lewy-body disease, and corticobasal ganglionic degeneration (the degenerative types are discussed in Chap. 39), occasionally in Wilson disease, and more often with acquired metabolic disorders (prototypically uremic and anoxic encephalopathy) and certain drug intoxications, notably with haloperidol, lithium, and amphetamines; Table 6-2 lists these and others. A subacute encephalopathy with diffuse myoclonus may occur in association with the autoantibodies that are characteristically a component of Hashimoto thyroiditis and also in Whipple disease (both are discussed in Chap. 40). An acute onset of polymyoclonus with confusion occurs with lithium intoxication; once ingestion is discontinued, there is improvement (slowly over days to weeks) and the myoclonus is replaced by diffuse action tremors, which later subside. Diffuse, severe myoclonus may be a prominent feature of early tetanus and strychnine poisoning.

Polymyoclonus that occurs in the acute stages of anoxic encephalopathy should be distinguished from postanoxic action or intention myoclonus that emerges with recovery from cardiac arrest or asphyxiation (it is discussed below and in Chap. 40). The factor common to all these disorders is the presence of diffuse neuronal disease.

Table 6-2
CAUSES OF GENERALIZED AND REGIONAL MYOCLONUS

Epileptic forms (myoclonic epilepsies)
Unverricht-Lundborg disease
Lafora-body disease
Baltic myoclonus
Benign epilepsy with rolandic spikes
Juvenile myoclonic epilepsy
Infantile spasms (West syndrome)
Cherry-red-spot myoclonus (sialidase deficiency)
Myoclonus epilepsy with ragged red fibers (MERRF)
Ceroid lipofuscinosis (Kufs disease)
Tay-Sachs disease
Epilepsia partialis continua
Essential and heredofamilial forms
Myoclonic dementias
Creutzfeldt-Jakob disease
Subacute sclerosing panencephalitis
Familial progressive poliodystrophy
Alzheimer, Lewy-body, and Wilson diseases (occasional in late stages)
Whipple disease of the central nervous system
Corticobasal ganglionic degeneration
Dentatorubropallidoluysian atrophy
AIDS dementia
Myoclonus with cerebellar disease (myoclonic ataxia)
Opsoclonus-myoclonus syndrome (paraneoplastic [anti-Ri], neuroblastoma, post- and parainfectious)
Postanoxic myoclonus (Lance Adams type)
Ramsay-Hunt dyssynergia cerebellaris myoclonica
Metabolic, immune, and toxic disorders
Cerebral hypoxia (acute and severe)
Uremia
Hashimoto thyroiditis
Lithium intoxication
Haloperidol and sometimes phenothiazine intoxication
Hepatic encephalopathy (rare)
Cyclosporine toxicity
Nicotinic acid deficiency encephalopathy
Tetanus
Other drug toxicities
Focal and spinal forms of myoclonus
Herpes zoster myelitis
Other unspecified viral myelitis
Multiple sclerosis
Traumatic spinal cord injury
Arteriovenous malformation of spinal cord
Subacute myoclonic spinal neuronitis
Paraneoplastic spinal myoclonus

Myoclonus in association with signs of cerebellar incoordination, including opsoclonus (rapid, irregular, but predominantly conjugate movements of the eyes in all planes as described in Chap. 14) is another syndrome of both children and adults. Most cases run a chronic course, waxing and waning in severity. Many of the childhood cases are associated with occult neuroblastoma, and some have responded to the administration of corticosteroids. In adults, a similar syndrome has been described as a remote effect of carcinoma (mainly of lung, breast, and ovary as discussed at length in Chap. 31), but it also occurs at all ages as a self-limited manifestation of a benign postinfectious (possibly viral) illness as described by Baringer and colleagues.

As mentioned above, diffuse myoclonus is a prominent and often early feature of the prion transmissible illness Creutzfeldt-Jakob disease, characterized by rapidly progressive dementia, disturbances of gait and coordination, and all manner of mental and visual aberrations (see Chap. 33). Initially the jerks are random but late in the disease they may attain an almost rhythmic and symmetric character. In addition there is an exaggerated startle response, and violent myoclonus may be elicited by tactile, auditory, or visual stimuli in advanced stages of the disease. In this condition too, there is a progressive destruction of neurons, mainly but not exclusively in the cerebral and cerebellar cortices, and a striking degree of gliosis. In addition to parenchymal destruction, the cortical tissue shows a fine-meshed vacuolation, hence the designation subacute spongiform encephalopathy.

In yet another group of myoclonic dementias, the most prominent associated abnormality is a progressive deterioration of intellect. Like the myoclonic epilepsies, the myoclonic dementias may be sporadic or familial and may affect both children and adults. A rare childhood type is subacute sclerosing panencephalitis (SSPE), which is an acquired subacute or chronic (occasionally remitting) disease related to a latent infection with the measles virus (Chap. 33).

Intention or Action (Postanoxic) Myoclonus

This type of myoclonus was described by Lance and Adams in a group of patients who were recovering from hypoxic encephalopathy. When the patient is relaxed, the limb and other skeletal muscles are quiet (except in the most severe cases); only seldom does the myoclonus appear during slow, smooth (ramp) movements. Fast (ballistic) movements, however, especially when directed to a target, as in touching the examiner's finger, elicit a series of irregular myoclonic jerks that differ in speed and rhythmicity from intention tremor. For this reason it was called intention or action myoclonus. Only the limb that is moving is involved; hence it is a localized, stimulus-evoked myoclonus. Speech may be fragmented by the myoclonic jerks, and a syllable or word may be almost compulsively repeated, as in palilalia.

Action myoclonus is almost always associated with cerebellar ataxia. The pathologic anatomy has not been entirely ascertained. Lance and Adams found the irregular discharges to be transmitted via the corticospinal tracts, preceded in some cases by a discharge from the motor cortex. Chadwick and coworkers postulated a reticular loop reflex mechanism, while Hallett and colleagues (1977) found that a cortical reflex mechanism was operative in some cases and a reticular reflex mechanism in others. Whether these are two aspects of one mechanism could not be decided.

Barbiturates and valproic acid have been helpful in some cases. Several clinical trials and case reports have suggested that the antiepileptic levitiracetam may be useful (Krauss et al, 2001). The use of 5-hydroxytryptophan alone or in combination with tryptophan or other drugs had been recommended in the past (van Woert et al). A combination of several of these medications is usually required to make the patient functional.

Spinal or Segmental Myoclonus (See also Subacute Spinal Neuronitis in Chap. 44)

The notion that monophasic-restricted myoclonus always emanates from the cerebral cortex, cerebellum, or brainstem cannot be sustained, as there are forms that are traceable to a purely spinal cause. The problem takes the form of an almost continuous arrhythmic jerking of a restricted group of muscles, often on one side of the body. Such a subacute spinal myoclonus of obscure origin was described many years ago by Campbell and Garland, and similar cases continue to be cited in the literature. We have seen several in which myoclonus was isolated to the musculature of the abdominal or thoracic wall on one side or to the legs; only rarely were we able to establish a cause, and the spinal fluid has been normal. This form has been referred to as "propriospinal" when it involves repetitive flexion or extension myoclonus of the torso that is aggravated by stretching or action.

Examples of myelitis with irregular and strictly segmental myoclonic jerks (either rhythmic or arrhythmic) have been reported in humans and have been induced in animals by the Newcastle virus. Many such myelitic cases involve the legs or a few muscles of one leg. In our experience, this type of myoclonus has occurred following zoster myelitis, postinfectious transverse myelitis, and rarely with multiple sclerosis, epidural cord compression, or after traumatic spinal injury. A paraneoplastic form has also been described, usually associated with breast cancer (Chap. 31). When highly ionic contrast media was in the past used for myelography, painful spasms and myoclonus sometimes occurred in segments where the dye was concentrated by a block to the flow of spinal fluid.

Treatment is difficult and one resorts to a combination of antiepileptic drugs and benzodiazepines, just as in cerebral myoclonus. The glycine inhibitor levetiracetam reportedly has been successful when other drugs have failed (Keswani et al).

Pathophysiology of Polymyoclonus

It seems logical to assume that myoclonus is caused by abnormal discharges of aggregates of motor neurons or interneurons because of the directly enhanced excitability of these cells or the removal of some inhibitory mechanism. Sensory relationships are a prominent feature of polymyoclonus, particularly those related to metabolic disorders, and will eventually shed some light on the mechanism. Flickering light, a loud sound, or an unexpected tactile stimulus to some part of the body initiates a jerk so quickly and consistently that it must utilize a direct sensorimotor pathway or the mechanism involved in the startle reaction. Repeated stimuli may recruit a series of incremental myoclonic jerks that culminate in a generalized convulsion, as often happens in the familial myoclonic syndrome of Unverricht-Lundborg. However, evidence implicating cortical hyperexcitability in myoclonus is only indirect, being based mainly on the finding that the cortical components of the somatosensory evoked potential are exceedingly large and that in some instances, the myoclonic jerks have a strict time relationship ("time-locked") to preceding spikes in the contralateral rolandic area (Marsden et al; Brown et al). Conversely, it is just as likely that these potentials originate from subcortical structures that project both to the descending motor pathways and upward to the cortex. In humans, the indication is that postanoxic action myoclonus has its basis in reflex hyperactivity of the reticular formation and that the only consistent damage is in the cerebellum rather than in the cerebral cortex (see above, under "Intention or Action Myoclonus"). As already noted, several types of myoclonus are closely coupled with cerebellar cortical degenerations.

Pathologic examinations have been of little help in determining the essential sites of this unstable neuronal discharge because in most cases, the neuronal disease is so diffuse. Nonetheless, the most restricted lesions associated with myoclonus are located in the cerebellar cortex, dentate nuclei, and pretectal region. A removal of the modulating influence of the cerebellum on the thalamocortical system of neurons has been postulated as a mechanism, but it is uncertain whether the disinhibited motor activity is then expressed through corticospinal or reticulospinal pathways. For example, pentylenetetrazol (Metrazol) injections evoke myoclonus in the limbs of animals, and the myoclonus persists after transection of corticospinal and other descending tracts until the lower brainstem (medullary reticular) structures are destroyed.

PATHOLOGIC STARTLE SYNDROMES

To some degree, everyone startles or jumps in reaction to a totally unanticipated, potentially threatening stimulus. This normal startle reflex is probably a protective reaction, being seen also in animals, and its purpose seemingly is to prepare the organism for escape. By pathologic startle we refer to a greatly exaggerated startle reflex and to a group of other stimulus-induced disorders of which startle is a predominant part. In most ways, startle cannot be separated from myoclonus (simplex) except for its generalized nature and a striking evocation by various stimuli. Any stimulus—most often an auditory one but also a flash of light, a tap on the neck, back, or nose, or even the presence of someone behind the patient—can normally evince a sudden contraction of the orbicularis, neck, and spinal musculature and even the legs. However, in the abnormal startle response that occurs in the diseases discussed below, the contraction is of greater amplitude and is more widespread, with less tendency to habituate. There may be a jump and occasionally an involuntary shout and fall to the ground.

Aside from exaggerated forms of the normal startle reflex, the commonest isolated syndrome is so-called startle disease, also referred to as hyperexplexia or hyperekplexia (see Gastaut and Villeneuve). This is a familial disease (e.g., the "jumping Frenchmen of Maine," and others, as described further on). The subject has been reviewed by Wilkins and colleagues and by Ryan and associates. The most common mutation is in the 1-subunit of the inhibitory glycine receptor GLRA1 (Shiang et al) but other glycine receptor related genes have been implicated in other cases.

As pointed out by Suhren and associates and by Kurczynski, the condition is transmitted in some families as an autosomal dominant trait. In the proband described by Kurczynski, affected infants were persistently hypertonic and hyperreflexic (up to 2 to 4 years of age) and had nocturnal and sometimes diurnal generalized myoclonic jerks, all of which subsided with maturation.

Later in life, excessive startle must be distinguished from epileptic seizures, which may begin with a startle or massive myoclonic jerk (startle epilepsy) and from the multiple tic disorder, Gilles de la Tourette syndrome, of which startle may be a prominent manifestation (Chap. 4). With idiopathic startle disease, even with a fall, there is no loss of consciousness, and the manifestations of tic and other neurologic abnormalities are absent.

An auditory startle response may be a manifestation of other neurologic diseases. It is a prominent feature of Tay-Sachs disease, SSPE, and of some cases of the "stiff-man syndrome." Auditory, visual, and somatic startle reactions are also conspicuous in some of the lipid storage diseases and, as mentioned, in Creutzfeldt-Jakob disease.

The mechanism of the startle response has been a matter of speculation. In animals, the origin of the phenomenon has been localized in the pontine reticular nuclei, with transmission to the lower brainstem and spinal motor neurons via the reticulospinal tracts. During the startle, the EEG may show a vertex or frontal spike–slow-wave complex, followed by a general desynchronization of the cortical rhythms; between startles the EEG is normal. Some authors have postulated a disinhibition of certain brainstem centers. Others, on the basis of testing by somatosensory evoked potentials, have suggested that hyperactive long-loop reflexes constitute the physiologic basis of startle disease (Markand et al). Wilkins and coworkers consider hyperexplexia to be an independent phenomenon (different from the normal startle reflex) and to fall within the spectrum of stimulus-sensitive myoclonic disorders. Presumably, the altered glycine receptor in startle disease is the source of some form of hyperexcitability in one or another of the motor or reticular alerting systems.

The nature of the phenomenon displayed by the "jumping Frenchmen of Maine" has been disputed. The syndrome was described originally by James Beard, in 1868 among small pockets of French-speaking lumberjacks in northern Maine. The subjects displayed a greatly exaggerated response to minimal stimuli, to which there was no adaptation. The reaction consisted of jumping, raising the arms, screaming, and flailing of limbs, sometimes with echolalia, echopraxia, and a forced obedience to commands, even if this entailed a risk of serious injury. A similar syndrome in Malaysia and Indonesia is known as latah and in Siberia as myriachit. This syndrome has been framed in psychologic terms as conditioned responses (Saint-Hilaire et al) or as culturally determined behavior (Simons). Possibly some of the complex secondary phenomena can be explained in this way, but the stereotyped onset with an uncontrollable startle and the familial occurrence in our view attest to a clear biologic basis for all these syndromes.

Treatment

Clonazepam controls the startle disorders to varying degrees. Levetiracetam has reportedly been helpful in some patients. Also, the act of flexing the neck and bringing the arms close to the torso may reduce the intensity of an attack (Vigevano maneuver).

SPASMODIC TORTICOLLIS AND OTHER FOCAL DYSTONIAS

The focal or segmental dystonias, in contrast to the generalized dystonic disorders described in Chap. 4, are intermittent, brief or prolonged spasms or contractions of a group of adjacent muscles that places the body part in a forced and unnatural position. When limited to the neck muscles, the most common type of focal dystonia, the spasms may be more pronounced on one side, with rotation and partial extension of the head (idiopathic cervical dystonia, or torticollis), or the posterior or anterior neck muscles may be involved predominantly and the head becomes hyperextended (retrocollic spasm, or retrocollis) or inclined forward (procollic spasm, or anterocollis). Other dystonias restricted to craniocervical muscle groups are spasms of the orbicularis oculi, causing forced closure of the eyelids (blepharospasm) and contraction of the muscles of the mouth and jaw, which may cause forceful opening or closure of the jaw and retraction or pursing of the lips (oromandibular dystonia). With the latter condition, the tongue may undergo forceful involuntary protrusion; the throat and neck muscles may be thrown into violent spasm when the patient attempts to speak or the facial muscles may contract in a grimace; the laryngeal muscles may be involved, imparting a high-pitched, strained quality to the voice (spasmodic dysphonia). More often, spasmodic dysphonia (sometimes incorrectly termed "spastic" dysphonia) occurs as an isolated phenomenon (Chap. 23).

Of the large number of focal dystonias seen in the movement disorder clinic of Columbia Presbyterian Hospital, 44 percent were classified as torticollis, 26 percent as spasmodic dysphonia, 14 percent as blepharospasm, 10 percent as focal dystonia of the right hand and arm (writer's cramp), and 3 percent as oromandibular dystonia.

These movement disorders are involuntary and cannot be inhibited, thereby differing from habit spasms or tics. At one time, torticollis was thought to be a type of psychological disorder but all now agree that it is a localized form of dystonia. As discussed in Chap. 4, it is characteristic of these spasms and of similar focal dystonias that occur in the hands or feet to display a simultaneous activation of agonist and antagonist muscles (co-contraction), to have a tendency for the spasm to spread to adjacent muscle groups that are not normally activated in the movement (overflow), and to include an arrhythmic intermixed tremor; but these features tend not to be as prominent in most focal dystonias as in the generalized varieties (described in Chap. 4). The tremor in particular may cause difficulty in diagnosis if the slight degree of underlying dystonia is not appreciated by careful observation and by palpation of the involved muscles.

Any of the typical forms of restricted dystonia may represent a tardive dyskinesia; i.e., they complicate treatment with neuroleptic drugs (see further on in "Drug-Induced Tardive Dyskinesias" and "Treatment"). Also, restricted dystonias of the hand or foot often emerge as components of a number of degenerative diseases—Parkinson disease, corticobasal ganglionic degeneration, and progressive supranuclear palsy (all described in Chap. 39). These dystonias may also occur in metabolic diseases such as Wilson disease and nonwilsonian hepatolenticular degeneration. Rarely, a focal dystonia emerges transiently after a stroke that involves the striatopallidal system, mainly the internal segment of the pallidum or the thalamus, but the varied locations of these infarctions makes it difficult to draw conclusions about the mechanism of dystonia. Several such cases that fall into the category of symptomatic or secondary dystonias are described by Krystkowiak and colleagues and by Munchau and colleagues. Janavs and Aminoff have summarized several types that are caused by acquired systemic disorders, including hypoxia, infections such as AIDS, drugs, and autoantibodies, including from systemic lupus erythematosus.

The pathogenesis of the idiopathic focal dystonias is uncertain, although there is evidence that some of them, like the generalized dystonias, are genetically determined. Authoritative commentators, including Marsden, classed the apparently idiopathic adult-onset focal dystonias with the category of genetically determined generalized torsion dystonia. This view is based on several lines of evidence: the recognition that each of the focal dystonias may appear as an early component of generalized syndrome in children, the occurrence of focal and segmental dystonias in family members of these children, as well as a tendency of the dystonia in some adult patients to spread to other body parts. Perhaps the most compelling observation in this regard has been the finding that there are families in which the only manifestation of the DYT1 mutation (the gene associated with generalized torsion dystonia) is a late-onset writer's cramp or other focal dystonia. Whether this explains most or even many of the cases of adult onset focal dystonia is unclear but it does emphasize the phenotypic variability associated with the DYT1 mutation. The genetics of primary torsion dystonia is more complex than portrayed here, and is reviewed in Chap. 39.

It is noteworthy that no consistent pathologic changes have been demonstrated in any of the idiopathic or genetically determined dystonias. Most physiologists cast the disorder in terms of reduced cortical inhibition of unwanted muscle contractions, as summarized by Berardelli and colleagues. Specific physiologic changes in the cortical areas that are pertinent to the dystonias associated with overuse of certain body parts (occupational dystonias) are described below.

Spasmodic Torticollis (Idiopathic Cervical Dystonia)

This, the most frequent form of restricted dystonia, is localized to the neck muscles. It usually begins in early to middle adult life (peak incidence in the fifth decade), is somewhat more common in women, as a subtle tilting or turning of the head and tends to worsen slowly (Fig. 6-3*A*). With the exception of the finding of DYT1 gene abnormality in a few patients, it is idiopathic. The quality of the neck and head movements varies; they may be deliberate and smooth or jerky but most often cause a persistent deviation of the head to one side. Sometimes brief bursts of myoclonic twitching or a slightly irregular, high-frequency tremor accompanies deviation of the head, possibly representing an effort to overcome the contraction of the neck muscles; however, the tremor tends to beat in the direction of the dystonic movement. At times the tremor is far more dominant than is the dystonia, causing difficulty in diagnosis. The spasms are often worse when the patient stands or walks and are characteristically reduced or abolished by a contactual stimulus, such as placing a hand on the chin or neck or exerting mild but steady counterpressure on the side of the deviation or sometimes on the opposite side, or bringing the occiput in contact with the back of a high chair. These maneuvers, termed gestes, become less effective as the disease progresses. In many cases, the spasms are reduced when the patient lies down. In chronic cases, as the dystonic position typically becomes increasingly fixed in position, the affected muscles undergo hypertrophy. Pain in the contracting muscles is a common complaint, especially if there is associated cervical arthropathy.

The most prominently affected muscles are the sternocleidomastoid, levator scapulae, and trapezius. EMG studies also show sustained or intermittent activity in the posterior cervical muscles on both sides of the neck. The levator spasm lifts the affected shoulder slightly, and tautness in this muscle is sometimes the earliest feature. As a general observation, we have been impressed with information gained from palpating the muscles of the neck and shoulder in order to establish which muscles are the predominant causes of the spasm and to direct treatment to them as noted further on. In most patients the spasms remain confined to the neck muscles and persist in unmodified form, but in some the spasms spread, involving muscles of the shoulder girdle and back or the face and limbs. The distinction between these patterns is not fundamental. About 15 percent of patients with torticollis also have oral, mandibular, or hand dystonia, 10 percent have blepharospasm, and a similarly small number have a family history of dystonia or tremor (Chan et al). As already noted, no neuropathologic changes have been found in the single case studies reported by Tarlov and by Zweig and colleagues.

Spasmodic torticollis is resistant to treatment with L-dopa and other antiparkinsonian agents, although occasionally they give slight relief. They are, however, effective in those few instances in which dystonia is a prelude to Parkinson disease. In a few of our patients (four or five of several dozens), the condition disappeared without therapy, an occurrence observed in 10 to 20 percent in the series of Dauer et al. In their experience, remissions usually occurred during the first few years after onset in patients whose disease began relatively early in life; however, nearly all these patients relapsed within 5 years.

Treatment

The periodic (every 3 to 6 months) injection of small amounts of botulinum toxin directly into several sites in the affected muscles is by far the most effective form of treatment. The injections are best guided by palpation of muscles in spasm and by EMG analysis to determine which of the tonically contracted muscles are most responsible for the aberrant postures. All but 10 percent of patients with torticollis have had some degree of relief from symptoms with this treatment. Adverse effects (excessive weakness of injected muscles, local pain, and dysphagia—the latter from a systemic effect of the toxin) are usually mild and transitory. Five to 10 percent of patients eventually become resistant to repeated injections because of the development of neutralizing antibodies to the toxin (Dauer et al). Trihexyphenidyl or benzotropine, in high doses, may allow some amelioration but they are difficult to tolerate.

In the past decade, the use of deep brain stimulation has found some success in the treatment of idiopathic cervical dystonia. The internal segments of the globus pallidus and the subthalamic nuclei have been used as targets. This approach is certainly preferable to the former use of ablative lesions in these areas and in the thalami. In the most severe cases and those refractory to treatment with botulinum toxin, a combined sectioning of the spinal accessory nerve and of the first three cervical motor roots bilaterally has been successful in reducing spasm of the muscles without totally paralyzing them. Considerable relief has been achieved for as long as 6 years in one-third to one-half of cases treated in this way (Krauss et al; Ford et al).

Blepharospasm

Patients in mid and late adult life, predominantly women, may present with the complaint of inability to keep their eyes open that is a manifestation of involuntary closure of the eyelids. Any attempt to look at a person or object is associated with a persistent tonic, symmetric spasm of the eyelids (see Fig. 6-3*B*). During conversation, the patient struggles to overcome the spasms and is distracted by them. All customary activities are hampered to a varying extent. Reading and watching television are impossible at some times but surprisingly easy at others. Jankovic and Orman in a survey of 250 such patients found that 75 percent progressed in severity over the years to the point, in about 15 percent of cases, of making the patients functionally blind. Some instances of blepharospasm are a component of the Meige syndrome that includes jaw spasms (see next section). Blepharospasm may also be a result of drug induced tardive dyskinesia.

One's first inclination is to think of this disorder as photophobia or a response to an ocular irritation, and, indeed, the patient may state that bright light is annoying (ocular inflammation, especially of the iris, may produce severe reflex blepharospasm). However, the spasms persist in dim light and even after anesthesia of the corneas. Extraocular movements are normal. Blepharospasm may occur as an isolated phenomenon, but just as often it is combined with oromandibular spasms and sometimes with spasmodic dysphonia, torticollis, and other dystonic fragments. With the exception of a depressive reaction in some patients, psychiatric symptoms are lacking, and the use of psychotherapy, biofeedback, acupuncture, behavior modification therapy, and hypnosis has generally failed to cure the spasms. No neuropathologic lesion or neurochemical profile has been established in any of these disorders (Marsden et al; see also Hallett). A genetic basis is possible although few cases seem to be inherited.

Treatment

The most effective treatment consists of the injection of botulinum toxin into several sites in the orbicularis oculi and adjacent facial muscles. The benefit lasts for 3 to 6 months and repeated cycles of treatment are usually required. There appear to be few adverse systemic effects because of the low doses used. In the treatment of blepharospasm, a variety of antiparkinsonian, anticholinergic, and tranquilizing medications may be tried, but one should not be optimistic about the chances of success. A few of our patients have had temporary and partial relief from L-dopa and we have found it useful to conduct a brief trial in most patients. Sometimes the blepharospasm disappears spontaneously (in 13 percent of the cases in the series of Jankovic and Orman). Thermolytic destruction of part of the fibers in the branches of the facial nerves that innervate the orbicularis oculi muscles is reserved for the most resistant and disabling cases.

Other Causes of Blepharospasm

There are several clinical settings other than the one described above in which blepharospasm or a condition that simulates it, may be observed. In the days following cerebral infarction or hemorrhage, the stimulus of lifting the patient's eyelids may lead to strong involuntary closure of the lids. Reflex blepharospasm, as Fisher has called this phenomenon, takes liberty with the term as it more in the character of an apraxia of opening of the lids. It is more commonly associated with a left than a right hemiplegia. A homolateral blepharospasm has also been observed with a small thalamomesencephalic infarct. In patients with Parkinson disease, progressive supranuclear palsy, or Wilson disease and with other lesions in the rostral brainstem, light closure of the eyelids may induce blepharospasm and an inability to open the eyelids voluntarily.

We have seen an instance of blepharospasm as part of paraneoplastic midbrain encephalitis, and there have been several reports of it with autoimmune disease such as systemic lupus but the mechanism in these cases is as obscure as for the idiopathic variety. Also among our patients have been two with myasthenia gravis and blepharospasm of the type described by Roberts and colleagues, but we have been unable to ascertain if this represented a second disturbance or simply an exaggerated response to keeping the lids open. Finally, eye closure with fluttering of the lids in patients with a high degree of suggestibility is usually indicative of a psychological disorder. Blepharospasm induced by pain from ocular conditions such as iritis and rosacea of the eyelids has already been mentioned.

Lingual, Facial, and Oromandibular Spasms

These special varieties of involuntary movements also appear in later adult life, with a peak age of onset in the sixth decade. Women are affected more frequently than men. The most common type is characterized by forceful opening of the jaw, retraction of the lips, spasm of the platysma, and protrusion of the tongue; or the jaw may be clamped shut and the lips may purse (Fig. 6-3*B*). Other patterns include lateral jaw deviation and bruxism. Common terms for this condition are Meige syndrome, after the French neurologist who gave an early description of it, and Brueghel syndrome, because of the similarity of the grotesque grimace to that of a subject in a Brueghel painting called De Gaper. Difficulty in speaking and swallowing (spastic or spasmodic dysphonia) and blepharospasm are also frequently conjoined, and occasionally patients with these disorders develop torticollis or dystonia of the trunk and limbs. A number have tremor of affected muscles or of the hands as well. All these prolonged, forceful spasms of facial, tongue, and neck muscles have followed the administration of phenothiazine and butyrophenone drugs. More often, however, the dyskinetic disorder induced by neuroleptics is somewhat different, consisting of choreoathetotic chewing, lip smacking, and licking movements (tardive orofacial dyskinesia, rabbit-mouth syndrome; see later).

Very few cases of the Meige syndrome have been studied neuropathologically. In most of them no lesions were found. In one patient there were foci of neuronal loss in the striatum (Altrocchi and Forno); another patient showed a loss of nerve cells and the presence of Lewy bodies in the substantia nigra and related nuclei (Kulisevsky et al); both are of uncertain significance.

A form of focal dystonia that affects only the jaw muscles has been described (masticatory spasm of Romberg); a similar dystonia may be a component of orofacial and generalized dystonias. In the cases described by Thompson and colleagues, the problem began with brief periods of spasm of the pterygoid or masseter muscle on one side. Early on, the differential diagnosis includes bruxism, hemifacial spasm, the odd rhythmic jaw movements associated with Whipple disease, and tetanus. As the illness progresses, forced opening of the mouth and lateral deviation of the jaw may last for days and adventitious lingual movements may be added. A form that occurs with hemifacial atrophy has been described by Kaufman. An intermittent spasm that is confined to one side of the face (hemifacial spasm) is not, strictly speaking, a dystonia and is considered with disorders of the facial nerve in Chap. 47.

Treatment

As with the other focal and regional dystonias, much greater success has been obtained with injections of botulinum toxin into the masseter, temporal, and medial pterygoid muscles. High doses of benztropine and related anticholinergic drugs may be helpful, but are not as good as botulinum toxin treatment. Many other drugs have been used in the treatment of these craniocervical spasms, but none has effected a cure.

Writer's Cramp, Musician's Spasm, and Other Task-Specific Dystonias

Occupational cramps or spasms are included here because the prevailing opinion is that they are an acquired form of restricted or focal "task-specific" dystonias. Men and women are equally affected, most often between the ages of 20 and 50 years. In the most common form, writer's cramp, the patient observes, upon attempting to write, that all the muscles of the thumb and fingers either go into spasm or are inhibited by a feeling of stiffness and pain or hampered in some other inexplicable way. The spasm may be painful and can spread into the forearm or even the upper arm and shoulder. Sometimes the spasm fragments into a tremor that interferes with the execution of fluid, cursive movements. Immediately upon cessation of writing, the spasm disappears. At all other times and in the execution of grosser movements, the hand is normal, and there are no other neurologic abnormalities. Many patients learn to write in new ways or to use the other hand, though that, too, may become involved. A few of our younger patients have developed spasmodic torticollis at a later date.

The performance of other highly skilled motor acts, such as playing the piano or fingering the violin, may acquire a similar highly task-dependent spasm ("musician's cramp", now commonly called "musician's dystonia") or in the past, telegrapher's palsy. The "loss of lip" in trombonists and other instrumentalists represents an analogous phenomenon, seen only in experienced musicians. In each case a delicate motor skill, perfected by years of practice and performed almost automatically, suddenly comes to require a conscious and labored effort for its execution. Discrete movements are impaired by a spreading recruitment of unneeded muscles (intention spasm). Once developed, the disability persists in varying degrees of severity, even after long periods of inactivity of the affected part.

In monkeys, Byl and colleagues found that sustained, rapid, and repetitive highly stereotypical movements greatly expand the area of cortical representation of sensory information from the hand. These authors hypothesized that degradation of sensory feedback to the motor cortex was responsible for excessive and persistent motor activity, including dystonia. A similar enlargement of the area of cortical response to magnetic stimulation has also been found by a number of investigators in patients with writer's cramp and the volume of gray matter was decreased in the sensorimotor cortex, thalamus, and cerebellum corresponding to the affected hand in the report by Delmaire and coworkers. Berardelli et al have reviewed other theories pertaining to the physiology of the focal dystonias.

Treatment

A high degree of success has been obtained by injections of botulinum toxin into specifically involved muscles, such as those of the hand and forearm in cases of writer's cramp (Cohen et al; Rivest et al), and this is now the most widely used form of therapy. The best results are obtained by guiding the injection from both palpation and EMG detection of the specific muscles that are active in the dystonic posture.

Transcutaneous electrical stimulation (TENS) of the forearm in 20-minute sessions has a modest effect according to a study by Tinazzi and colleagues. It had been claimed that the patient can be helped by a deconditioning procedure that delivers an electric shock whenever the spasm occurs or by biofeedback, but these forms of treatment have not been rigorously tested and have been largely abandoned in favor of botulinum treatments.

Drug-Induced Tardive (Delayed) Dyskinesias

(See also Chap. 43)

Dyskinesia is a broadly encompassing term that is applied to many hyperkinetic involuntary movements including those taking the conventional forms of dystonia, chorea, athetosis, and tremor and the less well-defined ones that are produced by L-dopa therapy in Parkinson disease. When modified by the adjective tardive, it refers specifically to movements induced by the use of neuroleptic drugs, often, but not always phenothiazines, which are delayed in onset from the initiation of drug therapy and persist after the drugs are withdrawn. These movements are distinguished from acute dystonic reactions that occur in the first few days of exposure to medications, are aborted by anticholinergic drugs, and do not persist (see Chap. 53).

Tardive dyskinesias are intermittent or persistent and not subject to the will of the patient. The facial, lingual, eyelid, and bulbar muscles are most often involved but neck, shoulder, and spine muscles with arching of the back may be implicated in individual cases as noted below. There may be added blepharospasm and truncal, hand, or neck movements and akathisia of the legs, but these are not nearly so prominent as the orofacial and lingual dyskinesias.

Longer exposure is more likely to cause the movements. If the drug is discontinued immediately after the movements appear, the problem may not persist. The problem is easily recognized and familiar to all physicians who treat psychiatric patients. Oromandibular spasm and blepharospasm (Meige syndrome) and Huntington disease may cause difficulty in diagnosis.

In addition to the typical neuroleptic drugs, less familiar ones such as metoclopramide, pimozide, amoxapine, and clebopride, some of which are used for disorders other than psychosis, and newer agents such as risperidone may also be causative. Less often, the movements arise soon after cessation of one of these same drugs.

There are a number of other drug-induced tardive movement syndromes, mainly varieties of dystonias, some of which have been mentioned earlier, and akathisia (see further on). Often they begin focally in the neck and spread over time to the limbs. One highly characteristic pattern combines retrocollis, backwards arching of the trunk, internal rotation of the arms, extension of the elbows, and flexion of the wrists simulating an opisthotonic posture. Other patients may have both orofacial and cervical dyskinesias. Many patients report that the dystonia abates during walking and other activities, quite unlike idiopathic torsion dystonia. These drug-induced dyskinesias are viewed as the result of changes in the concentration of dopamine receptors, five of which are currently known, as discussed in Chap. 4. Blockade and subsequent unmasking of the D2 receptor have been specifically linked to the development of the tardive syndromes.

Treatment

Little has been found to be consistently effective. If the movements follow withdrawal of one of the offending drugs, reinstitution of the medication in small doses often reduces the dyskinesias but may have the undesired side effects of causing parkinsonism and drowsiness. For this reason most clinicians who are experienced in this field avoid using the offending drugs if possible and choose to use the newer atypical neuroleptic drugs for the treatment of the underlying psychiatric condition. The newer "atypical" neuroleptic drugs have less of a propensity to cause tardive dyskinesia. The movements tend to lessen over a period of months or years and mild cases abate on their own or leave little residual effect; rarely have the symptoms worsened.

Dopamine and noradrenergic-depleting drugs such as reserpine and tetrabenazine have also been successful if used carefully but the more effective of the two, tetrabenazine, is difficult to obtain in the U.S. The dystonias also respond to anticholinergic drugs (trihexyphenidyl 2.5 mg once or twice daily, increased by small increments weekly up to 12.5 mg) if high enough doses can be tolerated.

Further discussion of the side effects of the antipsychosis drugs is found in Chaps. 43 and 53.

TICS AND HABIT SPASMS

When idle, adults often display a wide variety of fidgeting types of small amplitude movement, gestures, and mannerisms. They are slower and more complex than tics and spasms. Others, throughout their lives are given to odder and more intrusive but benign habitual movements. These range from simple, highly idiosyncratic mannerisms (e.g., of the lips and tongue) to repetitive actions such as sniffing, clearing the throat, protruding the chin, or blinking whenever these individuals become tense. Stereotypy and irresistibility are the main identifying features of these phenomena. The patient admits to making the movements and feels compelled to do so in order to relieve perceived tension. Such movements can be suppressed for a short time by an effort of will, but they reappear as soon as the subject's attention is diverted. In certain cases the tics become so ingrained that the person is unaware of them and seems unable to control them. An interesting feature of many tics is that they correspond to coordinated acts that normally serve some purpose to the organism. It is only their incessant repetition when uncalled for that marks them as habit spasms or tics. The condition varies widely in its expression from a single isolated movement (e.g., blinking, sniffing, throat clearing, tongue clicking, or stretching the neck) to a complex of movements.

Children between 5 and 10 years of age are especially likely to develop these habit spasms. These consist of blinking, hitching up one shoulder, sniffing, throat clearing, jerking the head or eyes to one side, grimacing, etc. If ignored, such spasms seldom persist for longer than a few weeks or months and tend to diminish on their own. In adults, relief of nervous tension by sedative or tranquilizing drugs may be helpful, but the disposition to tics persists. A putative relationship to streptococcal infection is discussed below.

Special types of rocking, head bobbing, hand waving (in autism) or hand wringing (typical of Rett syndrome), and other movements, particularly self-stimulating movements, are disorders of motility unique to the developmentally delayed child or adult. These "rhythmias" have no known pathologic anatomy in the basal ganglia or elsewhere in the brain. Apparently they represent a persistence of some of the rhythmic, repetitive movements of normal infants. In some cases of impaired vision and photic epilepsy, eye rubbing or moving the fingers rhythmically across the field of vision is observed, especially again in developmentally delayed children.

Gilles de la Tourette Syndrome

Multiple tics—sniffing, snorting, involuntary vocalization, and troublesome compulsive and aggressive impulses—constitute the rarest and most severe tic syndrome—Gilles de la Tourette syndrome (his complete surname). The problem begins in childhood, in boys three times more often than in girls, usually as a simple tic. As the condition progresses, new tics are added to the repertoire. It is the multiplicity of tics and the combination of motor and vocal tics that distinguish the disorder from the more benign, restricted tic disorders.

Vocal tics, usually loud and irritating in pitch, are characteristic. Some patients display repetitive and annoying motor behavior, such as jumping, squatting, or turning in a circle. Other common types of repetitive behavior include the touching of other persons and repeating one's own words (palilalia) and the words or movements of others. Explosive and involuntary cursing and the compulsive utterance of obscenities (coprolalia) are the most dramatic manifestations. Interestingly, the latter phenomena are uncommon in Japanese patients, whose decorous culture and language contain few obscenities. The full repertoire of tics and compulsions comprised by Gilles de la Tourette syndrome has been described by Tolosa and Bayes and in the reviews by Jankovic and by Leckman, which are recommended.

Stone and Jankovic have noted the occurrence of persistent blepharospasm, torticollis, and other dystonic fragments in a small number of patients. Isometric contractions of isolated muscle groups (tonic tics) may also occur. As in other tic disorders, there is a premonitory sensation of tightness, discomfort or paresthesia, or a psychic sensation or urge that is relieved by the movement. A fair proportion stutter or display a mild dysfluency of speech. So-called soft neurologic signs are noted in half of the patients. Feinberg and associates have described four patients with arrhythmic myoclonus and vocalization, but it is not clear whether these symptoms represent an unusual variant of the disease or a new syndrome. A degree of cyclicality of symptoms has been noted by several authors; tics tend to happen in groups over minutes or hours and they are clustered over weeks and months. This gives the appearance of a waxing and waning process.

The course of the illness is unpredictable. In half of adolescents the tics subside spontaneously by early adulthood and those that persist become milder with time. Others undergo long remissions only to have tics recur, but in other patients the motor disorder persists throughout life. This variability emphasizes the difficulty in separating transient habit spasms from the Gilles de la Tourette chronic multiple tic syndrome. Isolated and mild but lifelong motor tics probably represent a variant of Tourette syndrome insofar as they display the same predominantly male heredofamilial pattern and similar responses to medication.

An attention-deficit hyperactivity disorder (see Chap. 28), obsessive-compulsive traits, or both are said to be evident at some time in the course of the illness, and these interfere to a greater degree than do the tics with progress in school. Poor control of temper, impulsiveness, self-injurious behavior, and certain sociopathic traits are seen in a few but by no means all affected children. Evidence of "organic" impairment by psychologic tests was found in 40 to 60 percent of patients in the series reported by Shapiro and colleagues, but intelligence did not deteriorate. Nonspecific abnormalities of the EEG have occurred in more than half of the patients but are not consistent enough to be considered a feature of the disease.

In one-third of the cases reported by Shapiro and colleagues, isolated tics were observed in other members of the family. Several other studies have reported a familial clustering of cases in which the pattern of transmission appears to be autosomal dominant with incomplete penetrance (Pauls and Leckman) but this has been disputed and several predisposing genes have been found by linkage analysis. In any biologic explanation, the marked predominance of males must be accounted for. At the moment, Tourette syndrome cannot be attributed to a single genetic locus. Nonetheless, support for a primary genetic nature of Tourette syndrome derives from twin studies, which have revealed higher concordance rates in monozygotic twin pairs than in dizygotic pairs. An ethnic bias (Ashkenazi Jews) has been reported, ranging from 19 to 62 percent in several series, but this has not been borne out in equally large series in areas that do not have a high proportion of this ethnic population (Lees et al).

As to causation, little is known. There is no consistent association with infection, trauma, or other disease except the putative connection to streptococcal infections discussed further on. Hyperactive children who have been treated with stimulants appear to be at increased risk of developing or exacerbating tics (Price et al) but a causal relationship has not been established beyond doubt (see comments regarding treatment below). MRI has shown no uniform abnormalities; functional imaging has demonstrated numerous but inconsistent abnormalities. Histopathologic changes have not been discerned in the few brains examined by the usual methods. However, Singer and coworkers (1991), who analyzed pre- and postsynaptic dopamine markers in postmortem striatal tissue, found a significant alteration of dopamine uptake mechanisms; more recently, Wolf and colleagues have found that differences in D2 dopamine receptor binding in the head of the caudate nucleus reflected differences in the phenotypic severity of Gilles de la Tourette syndrome. These observations, coupled with the facts that L-dopa exacerbates the symptoms of the syndrome and that haloperidol, which blocks dopamine (particularly D2) receptors, is an effective treatment, support a dopaminergic abnormality in the basal ganglia, more specifically in the caudate. In this respect, instances of compulsive behavior in relation to lesions in the head of the caudate nucleus and its projections from orbitofrontal and cingulate cortices may be pertinent.

PANDAS syndrome

Using the model of Sydenham chorea, a recent line of investigation has implicated streptococcal infection in the genesis of abruptly appearing Tourette syndrome and of less-generalized tics in children. This association has been extended by some authors to explain obsessive-compulsive behavior of sudden and unexplained onset. These putative poststreptococcal disorders were summarized by Swedo and colleagues under the acronym PANDAS (pediatric autoimmune neuropsychiatric disorders with streptococcal infection). In a few cases there has been a relapsing course that is similar to that seen in Sydenham chorea. Two health database studies have suggested a modest association between tic disorder, obsessive-compulsive disorder and streptococcal infection. These observations taken together are intriguing but not confirmed and several groups have been unable to differentiate patients with PANDAS and Gilles de la Tourette syndrome from controls on the basis of epidemiologic factors or serum autoantibodies to streptococcus (Singer et al, 2005 and Schrag and coworders).

Treatment

Two classes of drugs are used in treatment. The alpha2-adrenergic agonists clonidine and guanfacine have been useful in several studies, but not in others. These are not as potent as treatment with neuroleptic drugs, but their side effects are far less severe and they are recommended as the first treatment. The newer drug, guanfacine has the advantage over clonidine of daily dosing and less sedating effect.

The initial dose is 0.5 to 1 mg given at bedtime and gradually increased as needed to a total dose of 4 mg. Clonidine is started as a bedtime dose of 0.05 mg and increased every several days by 0.05 mg until a total dose of about 0.1 mg three times daily; guanfacine is given as 1 mg at bedtime and increased by 1 mg monthly, up to 3 mg if needed. The neuroleptics haloperidol, pimozide, sulpiride, and tiapride have proved to be effective therapeutic agents but should be used only in severely affected patients and usually after the adrenergic agents have been tried. Haloperidol is instituted in small doses (0.25 mg initially, increasing the dosage gradually to 2 to 10 mg daily). The addition of benztropine mesylate (0.5 mg daily) at the outset of treatment may help to prevent the adverse motor effects of haloperidol. Pimozide, which has a more specific antidopaminergic action than haloperidol, may be more effective than haloperidol; it should be given in small amounts (0.5 mg daily) to begin with and increased gradually to 8 to 9 mg daily. The atypical neuroleptics, such as risperidone, have also been used with some success. The potent agent tetrabenazine, a drug that depletes monoamines and blocks dopamine receptors, may be useful if high doses can be tolerated. Further details of the use of these drugs can be found in the review by Leckman.

Another interesting approach has been to inject botulinum toxin in muscles affected by prominent focal tics, including the vocal ones as described by Scott and colleagues; curiously, this treatment is said to relieve the premonitory sensory urge. Kurlan and associates noted a lessening of tics after treatment with naltrexone, 50 mg daily. According to a trial conducted by the Tourette's Syndrome Study Group, the hyperactivity component of the Tourette syndrome can be treated safely with methylphenidate or clonidine without fear of worsening the tics. Deep brain stimulation shows promise in the treatment of drug resistant cases.

Isolated or limited motor tics in males, generally an inherited trait, is often greatly aided by clonazepam.

Akathisia

This term was coined by Haskovec in 1904 to describe an inner feeling of restlessness, an inability to sit still, and a compulsion to move about. When sitting, the patient constantly shifts his body and legs, crosses and uncrosses his legs, and swings the free leg. Running in place and persistent pacing are also characteristic. This abnormality of movement is most prominent in the lower extremities and may not be accompanied, at least in mild forms of akathisia, by perceptible rigidity or other neurologic abnormalities. In its advanced form, patients complain of difficulty in concentration, distracted, no doubt, by the constant urge to move.

First noted in patients with Parkinson disease and what is now known to be Alzheimer disease, akathisia is now observed most often in patients receiving neuroleptic drugs (Chap. 43). However, this disorder may be observed in psychiatric patients who are receiving no medication and in some unmedicated patients with Parkinson disease; it can also be induced in normal individuals by the administration of neuroleptic drugs or L-dopa.

The main diagnostic considerations are an agitated depression, particularly in patients already on neuroleptic medications, and the "restless legs" syndrome—a sleep disorder that may be evident during wakefulness in severe cases (Chap. 19). Patients with the restless leg syndrome describe a crawling or drawing sensation in the legs rather than an inner restlessness, although both disorders create an irresistible desire for movement. At times these distinctions are blurred. Many of the medications used for the restless legs syndrome, such as clonazepam, may be tried, or treatment can be directed to the akathisia by selecting a less potent neuroleptic (if it is the suspected cause) or by using an anticholinergic medication, amantadine, or—perhaps the more effective and best tolerated—beta-adrenergic–blocking drugs.

References

Adams RD, Foley JM: The neurological disorder associated with liver disease. *Res Publ Assoc Nerv Ment Dis* 32:198, 1953.

Adams RD, Shahani B, Young RR: Tremor in association with polyneuropathy. *Trans Am Neurol Assoc* 97:44, 1972.

Adler CH, Bansberg SF, Hentz JG, et al: Botulinum toxin type A for treating voice tremor. *Arch Neurol* 61:1416, 2004.

Aigner BR, Mulder DW: Myoclonus: Clinical significance and an approach to classification. *Arch Neurol* 2:600, 1960.

Altrocchi PH, Forno LS: Spontaneous oral-facial dyskinesia: Neuropathology of a case. *Neurology* 33:802, 1983.

Bain PG, Findley LJ, Thompson PD, et al: A study of hereditary essential tremor. *Brain* 117:805, 1994.

Baringer JR, Sweeney VP, Winkler GF: An acute syndrome of ocular oscillations and truncal myoclonus. *Brain* 91: 473, 1968.

Berardelli A, Rothwell JC, Hallett M, et al: The pathophysiology of primary dystonia. *Brain* 121:1195, 1998.

Biary N, Koller W: Kinetic-predominant essential tremor: Successful treatment with clonazepam. *Neurol* 37:471, 1987.

Brown P, Ridding MC, Werhaus KJ, et al: Abnormalities of the balance between inhibition and excitation in the motor cortex of patients with cortical myoclonus. *Brain* 119:309, 1996.

Burns RS, Lewitt PA, Ebert MH, et al: The classical syndrome of striatal dopamine deficiency: Parkinsonism induced by MPTP. *N Engl J Med* 312:1418, 1985.

Byl NN, Merzenich MM, Jenkins WM: A primate genesis model of focal dystonia and repetitive strain injury: I. Learning-induced differentiation of the representation of the hand in the primary somatosensory cortex in adult monkey. *Neurology* 47:508, 1996.

Campbell AMG, Garland H: Subacute myoclonic spinal neuronitis. *J Neurol Neurosurg Psychiatry* 19:268, 1956.

Carpenter MB: Functional relationships between the red nucleus and the brachium conjunctivum: Physiologic study of lesions of the red nucleus in monkeys with degenerated superior cerebellar brachia. *Neurology* 7:427, 1957.

Cerosimo M, Koller WC: Essential tremor, in Watts RL, Koller WC (eds): *Movement Disorders*, 2nd ed. New York, McGraw-Hill, 2004, pp 431–458.

Chadwick D, Hallett M, Harris R, et al: Clinical, biochemical, and physiological features distinguishing myoclonus responsive to 5-hydroxy-tryptophan, tryptophan with a monoamine oxidase inhibitor, and clonazepam. *Brain* 100:455, 1977.

Chan J, Brin MF, Fahn S: Idiopathic cervical dystonia: Clinical characteristics. *Mov Disord* 6:119, 1991.

Cohen LG, Hallett M, Geller BD, Hochberg F: Treatment of focal dystonias of the hand with botulinum toxin injections. *J Neurol Neurosurg Psychiatry* 52:355, 1989.

Colebatch JG, Findley LJ, Frakowiak RSJ, et al: Preliminary report: Activation of the cerebellum in essential tremor. *Lancet* 336:1028, 1990.

Connor GS: A double-blind placebo-controlled trial of topiramate for essential tremor. *Neurology* 59:132, 2002.

Danek A: Geniospasm: Hereditary chin trembling. *Mov Disord* 8:335, 1993.

Dauer WT, Burke RE, Greene P, Fahn S: Current concepts on the clinical features, aetiology, and management of idiopathic cervical dystonia. *Brain* 121:547, 1998.

Delmaire C, Vidailhet M, Elbaz A, et al: Structural abnormalities in the cerebellum and sensorimotor circuit in writer's cramp. *Neurology* 69:376, 2007.

Deuschl G, Toro C, Valls-Sole J, et al: Symptomatic and essential palatal tremor. Clinical, physiological and MRI analysis. *Brain* 117:775, 1994.

Dubinsky R, Hallett M: Glucose hypermetabolism of the inferior olive in patients with essential tremor. *Ann Neurol* 22:118, 1987.

Dubinsky R, Hallett M, DiChiro G, et al: Increased glucose metabolism in the medulla of patients with palatal myoclonus. *Neurology* 41:557, 1991.

Elble RJ: Origins of tremor. *Lancet* 355:1113, 2000.

Elble RJ: Essential tremor frequency decreases with age. *Neurology* 55:1427, 2000.

Eldridge R, Iivanainen M, Stern R, et al: "Baltic" myoclonus epilepsy: Hereditary disorders of childhood made worse by phenytoin. *Lancet* 2:838, 1983.

Feinberg TE, Shapiro AK, Shapiro E: Paroxysmal myoclonic dystonia with vocalisations: New entity or variant of pre-existing syndromes? *J Neurol Neurosurg Psychiatry* 49:52, 1986.

Fisher CM: Reflex blepharospasm. *Neurology* 13:77, 1963.

Ford B, Louis ED, Greene P, Fahn S: Outcome of selective ramisectomy for botulinum toxin resistant torticollis. *J Neurol Neurosurg Psychiatry* 65:472, 1998.

Gastaut R, Villeneuve A: A startle disease or hyperekplexia. *J Neurol Sci* 5:523, 1967.

Haerer AF, Anderson DW, Schoenberg BS: Prevalence of essential tremor. *Arch Neurol* 39:750, 1982.

Hallett M: Blepharospasm: Report of a workshop. *Neurology* 46:1213, 1996.

Hallett M, Chadwick P, Marsden CD: Ballistic movement overflow myoclonus: A form of essential myoclonus. *Brain* 100:299, 1977.

Hallett M, Chadwick D, Marsden CD: Cortical reflex myoclonus. *Neurology* 29:1107, 1979.

Hallett M, Chadwick D, Adams J, et al: Reticular reflex myoclonus: A physiological type of human post-hypoxic myoclonus. *J Neurol Neurosurg Psychiatry* 40:253, 1977.

Heilman KH: Orthostatic tremor. *Arch Neurol* 41:880, 1984.

Herskovits E, Blackwood W: Essential (familial, hereditary) tremor: A case report. *J Neurol Neurosurg Psychiatry* 32:509, 1969.

Hunt JR: Dyssynergia cerebellaris myoclonica—primary atrophy of the dentate system: A contribution to the pathology and symptomatology of the cerebellum. *Brain* 44:490, 1921.

Janavs JL, Aminoff MJ: Dystonia and chorea in acquired systemic disorders. *J Neurol Neurosurg Psychiatry* 65:436, 1998.

Jankovic J: Tourette's syndrome. *N Engl J Med* 345:1184, 2001

Jankovic J, Brin MF: Therapeutic uses of botulinum toxin. *N Engl J Med* 324:1186, 1991.

Jankovic J, Orman J: Blepharospasm: Demographic and clinical survey of 250 patients. *Ann Ophthalmol* 16:371, 1984.

Kaufman MD: Masticatory spasm in hemifacial atrophy. *Ann Neurol* 7:585, 1980.

Keswani SC, Kossoff EH, Krauss GK: Amelioration of spinal myoclonus with levetiracetam. *J Neurol Neurosurg Psychiatry* 73: 456, 2002.

Kim JS: Asterixis after unilateral stroke: Lesion location of 30 patients. *Neurology* 56:533, 2001.

Koller WC, Hristova A, Brin M: Pharmacologic treatment of essential tremor. *Neurology* 54(Suppl 4):30, 2000.

Krauss JK, Toups EG, Jankovic J, Grossman RG: Symptomatic and functional outcome of surgical treatment of cervical dystonia. *J Neurol Neurosurg Psychiatry* 63:642, 1997.

Krauss GL, Bergin A, Kramer RE, et al: Suppression of posthypoxic and post-encephalitic myoclonus with levetiracetam. *Neurology* 56:411, 2001.

Krauss JK, Weigel R, Blahak C, et al: Chronic spinal cord stimulation in medically intractable orthostatic tremor. *J Neurol Neurosurg Psychaitr* 77:1013, 2005.

Krystkowiak P, Martinat P, Defebvre L, et al: Dystonia after striatopallidal and thalamic stroke: Clinicoradiological correlations and pathophysiological mechanisms. *J Neurol Neurosurg Psychiatry* 65:703, 1998.

Kulisevsky J, Marti MJ, Ferrer I, Tolosa E: Meige syndrome: Neuropathology of a case. *Mov Disord* 3:170, 1988.

Kurczynski TW: Hyperexplexia. *Arch Neurol* 40:246, 1983.

Kurlan R, Majumdar L, Deeley C, et al: A controlled trial of propoxyphene and naltrexone in patients with Tourette's syndrome. *Ann Neurol* 30:19, 1991.

Lance JW, Adams RD: The syndrome of intention or action myoclonus as a sequel to hypoxic encephalopathy. *Brain* 87:111, 1963.

Lapresle J, Ben Hamida M: The dentato-olivary pathway. *Arch Neurol* 22:135, 1970.

Leckman JF: Tourette's syndrome. *Lancet* 360:1577, 2002.

Lees AS, Robertson M, Trimble MR, Murray HMF: A clinical study of Gilles de la Tourette syndrome in the United Kingdom. *J Neurol Neurosurg Psychiatry* 47:1, 1984.

LeFebvre-D'Amour M, Shahani BT, Young RR: Tremor in alcoholic patients, in Desmedt JE (ed): *Physiological Tremor and Clonus*. Basel, Karger, 1978, pp 160–164.

Louis ED: Essential tremor. *N Engl J Med* 346:709, 2001.

Louis ED, Vonsattel JP, Honig LS, et al: Essential tremor associated with pathologic changes in the cerebellum. *Arch Neurol* 63:1189, 2006.

Markand ON, Garg BP, Weaver DD: Familial startle disease (hyperexplexia). *Arch Neurol* 41:71, 1984.

Marsden CD: Blepharospasm-oromandibular dystonia syndrome (Brueghel's syndrome). *J Neurol Neurosurg Psychiatry* 39:1204, 1976.

Marsden CD: The problem of adult-onset idiopathic torsion dystonia and other isolated dyskinesias in adult life (including blepharospasm, oromandibular dystonia, dystonic writers cramp, and torticollis, or axial dystonia). *Adv Neurol* 14:259, 1976.

Marsden CD, Hallett M, Fahn S: The nosology and pathophysiology of myoclonus, in Marsden CD, Fahn S (eds): *Movement Disorders*. Oxford, Butterworth, 1982, pp 196–248.

Matsuo F, Ajax ET: Palatal myoclonus and denervation supersensitivity in the central nervous system. *Ann Neurol* 5:72, 1979.

McAuley JH: Does essential tremor originate in the cerebral cortex? *Lancet* 357:492, 2001.

Moe PG, Nellhaus G: Infantile polymyoclonia–opsoclonus syndrome and neural crest tumors. *Neurology* 20:756, 1970.

Montalban RJ, Pujedas F, Alvarez-Sabib J, et al: Asterixis associated with anatomic cerebral lesions: A study of 45 cases. *Acta Neurol Scand* 91:377, 1995.

Munchau A, Mathen D, Cox T, et al: Unilateral lesions of the globus pallidus: Report of four patients presenting with focal or segmental dystonia. *J Neurol Neurosurg Psychiatry* 69:494, 2000.

Narabayashi H: Surgical approach to tremor, in Marsden CD, Fahn S (eds): *Movement Disorders*. Oxford, Butterworth, 1982, pp 292–299.

Pauls DL, Leckman JF: The inheritance of Gilles de la Tourette's syndrome and associated behaviors: Evidence for autosomal dominant transmission. *N Engl J Med* 315:993, 1986.

Pedersen SF, Pullman SL, Latov N, et al: Physiologic tremor analysis of patients with anti-myelin associated glycoprotein associated neuropathy and tremor. *Muscle Nerve* 20:38, 1997.

Price RA, Leckman JF, Pauls DL, et al: Gilles de la Tourette's syndrome: Tics and central nervous stimulants in twins and nontwins. *Neurology* 36:232, 1986.

Rapin I, Goldfischer S, Katzman R, et al: The cherry-red spot–myoclonus syndrome. *Ann Neurol* 3:234, 1978.

Rivest J, Lees AJ, Marsden CD: Writer's cramp: Treatment with botulinum toxin injections. *Mov Disord* 6:55, 1991.

Roberts ME, Steiger MJ, Hart IK: Presentation of myasthenia gravis mimicking blepharospasm. *Neurology* 58:150, 2002.

Ryan SG, Sherman SL, Terry JC, et al: Startle disease, or hyperekplexia: Response to clonazepam and assignment of the gene (STHE) to chromosome 5q by linkage analysis. *Ann Neurol* 31:663, 1992.

Saint-Hilaire M-H, Saint-Hilaire J-M, Granger L: Jumping Frenchmen of Maine. *Neurology* 36:1269, 1986.

Schrag A, Gilbert R, Giovannoni G, et al: Streptococcal infection, Tourette syndrome, and OCD. *Neurology* 73:1256, 2009.

Scott BL, Jankovic J, Donovan DT: Botulinum toxin injections into vocal cord in the treatment of malignant coprolalia associated with Tourette's syndrome. *Mov Disord* 11:431, 1996.

Shapiro AK, Shapiro ES, Bruun RD, et al: Gilles de la Tourette's syndrome: Summary of clinical experience with 250 patients and suggested nomenclature for tic syndromes. *Adv Neurol* 14:277–283, 1976.

Sharott A, Marsden J, Brown P: Primary orthostatic tremor is an exaggeration of a physiologic tremor in response to instability. *Mov Disord* 18:195, 2003.

Sheehy MP, Marsden CD: Writer's cramp—a focal dystonia. *Brain* 105:461, 1982.

Shiang R, Ryan SG, Zhu Z, et al: Mutations in the alpha 1-subunit of the inhibitory glycine receptor causes the dominant neurologic disorder hyperexplexia. *Nat Genet* 5:351, 1993.

Simons RC: The resolution of the latah paradox. *J Nerv Ment Dis* 168:195, 1980.

Singer HS, Hahn I-H, Moran TH: Abnormal dopamine uptake sites in postmortem striatum from patients with Tourette's syndrome. *Ann Neurol* 30:558, 1991.

Singer HS, Hong JJ, Yoon DY, et al: Serum autoantibodies do not differentiate PANDAS and Tourette syndrome from controls. *Neurology* 65:1701, 2005.

Stone LA, Jankovic J: The coexistence of tics and dystonia. *Arch Neurol* 48:862, 1991.

Suhren D, Bruyn GW, Tuyman JA: Hyperexplexia, a hereditary startle syndrome. *J Neurol Sci* 3:577, 1966.

Sutton GG, Mayer RF: Focal reflex myoclonus. *J Neurol Neurosurg Psychiatry* 37:207, 1974.

Swanson PD, Luttrell CN, Magladery JW: Myoclonus: A report of 67 cases and review of the literature. Medicine (Baltimore) 41:339, 1962.

Swedo SE, Rappaport JL, Cheslow DL, et al: High prevalence of obsessive-compulsive symptoms in patients with Sydenham chorea. *Am J Psychiatry* 146:246, 1989.

Sydow O, Thobois S, Alexch F, et al: Multicentre European study of thalamic stimulation in essential tremor: a six-year follow up. *J Neurol Neurosurg Psychiatry* 74:1387, 2003.

Tarlov E: On the problem of spasmodic torticollis in man. *J Neurol Neurosurg Psychiatry* 33:457, 1970.

Thompson PD, Obeso JA, Delgado G, et al: Focal dystonia of the jaw and the differential diagnosis of unilateral jaw and masticatory spasm. *J Neurol Neurosurg Psychiatry* 49:651, 1986.

Thompson PD, Rothwell JC, Day BL, et al: The physiology of orthostatic tremor. *Arch Neurol* 43:584, 1986.

Tinazzi M, Farina S, Bhatia K, et al: TENS for the treatment of writer's cramp: A randomized, placebo-controlled study. *Neurology* 64:1946, 2005.

Tolosa ES, Bayes A: Tics and Tourette's syndrome, in Jankovic J, Tolosa ES (eds): *Parkinson's Disease and Movement Disorders*, 4th ed. Baltimore, Lippincott Williams & Wilkins, 2002, pp 491–512.

Leavitt S, Tyler HR: Studies in asterixis Part I. *Arch Neurol* 10:360, 1964.

Tourette's Syndrome Study Group: Treatment of ADHD in children with tics. A randomized controlled trial. *Neurology* 58:527, 2002.

Ugawa Y, Genba K, Shimpo T, Mannen T: Onset and offset of electromyographic (EMG) silence in asterixis. *J Neurol Neurosurg Psychiatry* 53:260, 1990.

Van Woert MH, Rosenbaum D, Howieson J, et al. Long-term therapy of myoclonus and other neurologic disorders with l-5-hydroxytryptophan and carbidopa. *N Engl J Med* 296:70, 1977.

Walters AS, Hening WA, Chokroverty S: Frequent occurrence of myoclonus while awake and at rest, body rocking and marching in place in a subpopulation of patients with restless legs syndrome. *Acta Neurol Scand* 77:418, 1988.

Ward AAR: The function of the basal ganglia, in Vinken PJ, Bruyn GW (eds): *Handbook of Clinical Neurology*. Vol 6: Basal Ganglia. Amsterdam, North-Holland, 1968, pp 90–115.

Watson CW, Denny-Brown DE: Myoclonus epilepsy as a symptom of diffuse neuronal disease. *Arch Neurol Psychiatry* 70:151, 1953.

Wee AS, Subramony SH, Currier RD: "Orthostatic tremor" in familial-essential tremor. *Neurology* 36:1241, 1986.

Wilkins DE, Hallett M, Wess MM: Audiogenic startle reflex of man and its relationship to startle syndromes. *Brain* 109:561, 1986.

Wills AJ, Jenkins IH, Thompson PD: Red nuclear and cerebellar but no olivary activation associated with essential tremor: A positron emission tomographic study. *Ann Neurol* 36:636, 1994.

Wilson SAK: *Neurology*. London, Edward Arnold, 1940.

Wolf SS, Jones DW, Knable MB, et al: Tourette syndrome: Prediction of phenotypic variation in monozygotic twins by caudate nucleus D2 receptor binding. *Science* 273:1225, 1996.

Young RR, Growdon JH, Shahani BT: Beta-adrenergic mechanisms in action tremor. *N Engl J Med* 293:950, 1975.

Young RR, Shahani BT: Asterixis: one type of negative myoclonus. *Adv Neurol* 43:137, 1986.

Zweig RM, Jankel WR, Whitehouse PJ, et al: Brainstem pathology in dystonia. *Neurology* 36(Suppl 1):74, 1986.

7

Disorders of Stance and Gait

Certain disorders of motor and sensory function manifest themselves most clearly as impairments of upright stance and locomotion; their evaluation depends on knowledge of the neural mechanisms underlying the peculiarly human function of standing and bipedal walking. The analysis of stance, carriage, and gait is a rewarding exercise; with some experience, the examiner can sometimes reach a neurologic diagnosis merely by noting the manner in which the patient enters the office. Considering the frequency of falls that result from gait disorders and their consequences, such as hip fracture, and the resultant need for hospital and nursing home care, this is an important subject for all physicians. The substantial dimensions of the social and economic problem of falls and the elderly have been described by Tinetti and Williams.

NORMAL GAIT

Obviously, gait varies considerably from one person to another and it is a commonplace observation that a person may be identified by the sound of his footsteps, notably the pace and the lightness or heaviness of tread. The manner of walking and the carriage of the body may even provide clues to an individual's personality and occupation. Sherlock Holmes expressed pride in his talent for reading such clues. It is said that Charcot could often make the correct diagnosis, even before seeing the patient, based on the sound of patient walking down the hallway on the way to the examining room. Furthermore, the gaits of men and women differ, a woman's steps being quicker and shorter. The changes in stance and gait that accompany aging—the slightly stooped posture and slow, stiff tread as described in Chap. 29, on aging—are so familiar that they are not perceived as abnormalities.

The normal gait seldom attracts attention but it should be observed with care if slight deviations from normal are to be appreciated. The body is erect, the head is straight, and the arms hang loosely and gracefully at the sides, each moving rhythmically forward with the opposite leg. The feet are slightly externally rotated, the steps are approximately equal, and the medial malleoli almost touch as each foot passes the other. The medial edges of the heels, as they strike the ground with each step, lie almost along a straight line. As each leg moves forward, there is coordinated flexion of the hip and knee, dorsiflexion of the foot, and a barely perceptible elevation of the hip, so that the foot clears the ground. Also, with each step, the thorax advances slightly on the side opposite the swinging lower limb. The heel strikes the ground first, and inspection of the shoes will show that this part is most subject to wear.

The normal gait cycle, defined as the period between successive points at which the heel of the same foot strikes the ground, is illustrated in Fig. 7-1, based on the studies of Murray and coworkers, and of Olsson. In this figure, the cycle is initiated by the heel strike of the right foot. The stance phase, during which the foot is in contact with the ground, occupies 60 to 65 percent of the cycle. The swing phase begins when the right toes leave the ground. For 20 to 25 percent of the walking cycle, both feet are in contact with the ground (double-limb support). In later life, when the steps shorten and the cadence (the rhythm and number of steps per minute) decreases, the proportion of double-limb support increases (see further on). Surface electromyograms show an alternating pattern of activity in the legs, predominating in the flexors during the swing phase and in the extensors during the stance phase.

When analyzed in greater detail, the requirements for locomotion in an upright, bipedal position may be reduced to the following elements: (1) antigravity support of the body, (2) stepping, (3) the maintenance of equilibrium, and (4) a means of propulsion. Locomotion is impaired in the course of neurologic disease when one or more of these mechanical principles are prevented from operating normally.

The muscles of greatest importance in maintaining the erect posture are the erector spinae and the extensors of the hips and knees. The upright support of the body is provided by righting and antigravity reflexes, which allow a person to arise from a lying or sitting position to an upright bipedal stance and to maintain firm extension of the knees, hips, and back, modifiable by the position of the head and neck. These postural reflexes depend on the afferent vestibular, somatosensory (proprioceptive and tactile), and visual impulses, which are integrated in the spinal cord, brainstem, and basal ganglia. Transection of the neuraxis between the red and vestibular nuclei leads to exaggeration of these antigravity reflexes—decerebrate rigidity.

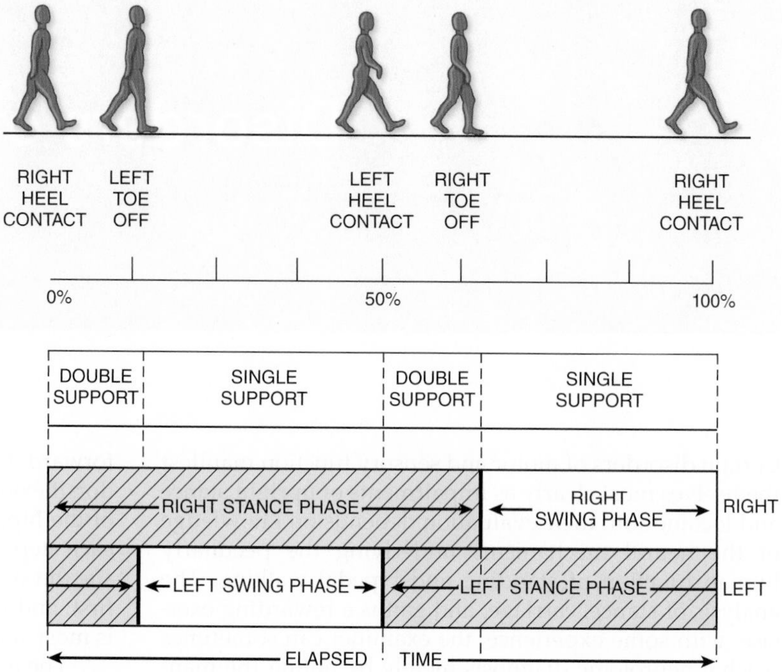

Figure 7-1. The normal gait cycle, based on the studies of Olsson and of Murray et al. See text for details.

Stepping, the second element, is a basic movement pattern present at birth and integrated at the spinal midbrain and diencephalic levels. It is elicited by contact of the sole with a flat surface and a shifting of the center of gravity—first laterally onto one foot, allowing the other to be raised, and then forward, allowing the body to move onto the advancing foot. Rhythmic stepping movements can be initiated and sustained in decerebrate or "spinal" cats and dogs. This is accomplished through the activity of interneurons that are organized as rhythmic "locomotor generators," akin to the pattern generators that permit the rhythmic movement of wings or fins. There is no clear evidence for a similar system of locomotor control in monkeys or humans, in whom the spinal mechanisms for walking cannot function independently of vaguely organized higher command centers. The latter are located in the posterior subthalamic region, caudal midbrain tegmentum, and pontine reticular formation; they control the spinal gait mechanisms through the reticulospinal, vestibulospinal, and tectospinal pathways in the ventral cord (see Eidelberg and colleagues and Lawrence and Kuypers). In the human, the brainstem locomotor regions are also activated by frontal cortical areas.

The frontal lobe is absolutely integral to initiating and engaging the gait cycle. The presence of a true "gait center" in the cerebrum is uncertain, although frontal lesions can devastate gait as discussed further on. Most often, it has been the supplementary motor areas relating to the legs (superior frontal gyri on both sides) that are implicated as pointed out by Della Sala and colleagues but Benson and coworkers have emphasized that the frontal periventricular areas are disproportionately involved when subcortical vascular disease compromises walking. The gait disorder of frontal lobe disease has a number of special characteristics including difficulty with starting to walk, short steps, widened base, difficulty lifting the feet off the floor (the magnetic gait) and a tendency to fall backwards (retropulsion). In all likelihood, the medial frontal lobes embody automatic programs for walking that are intimately tied to adjacent networks in the striatum.

Equilibrium involves the maintenance of balance in relation to gravity and to the direction of movement in order to retain a vertical posture. The center of gravity during the continuously unstable equilibrium that prevails in walking must shift within narrow limits from side to side and forward as the weight is borne first on one foot, then on the other. This is accomplished through the activity of highly sensitive postural and righting reflexes that have both peripheral (stretch reflexes) and central (vestibulocerebellar reflexes) components. These reflexes are activated within 100 ms of each shift in the support surface and require reliable afferent information from the visual, vestibular, and proprioceptive systems.

Propulsion is provided by leaning forward and slightly to one side and permitting the body to fall a certain distance before being checked by the support of the leg. Here, both forward and alternating lateral movements must occur. But in running, where at one moment both feet are off the ground, a forward drive or thrust by the trailing leg is also required.

ABNORMAL GAITS

General Comments

Because normal body posture and locomotion require intact vestibular function, proprioception, and vision (we see where we are going and adjust our steps), the effects of deficits in these senses are worth noting. A blind person—or a normal one who is blindfolded or walks in the dark—moves cautiously, with arms slightly forward to avoid collisions, and shortens his step slightly on a smooth surface; with shortening of the step, there is less rocking of the body and the gait is unnaturally stiff and cautious.

Patients with a chronic vestibulopathy show unsteadiness in standing and walking, often without widening their base, and an inability to descend stairs without holding onto the banister. They complain of a particular type of imbalance, usually with movement but at times when standing still—a sensation that may be likened to being on the deck of a rolling ship. Running and turning quickly are even more impaired, with lurching in all directions. The patient has great difficulty in focusing his vision on a fixed target when he is moving or on a moving target when he is either stationary or moving. When the body is in motion or the head is moved suddenly, objects in the environment may appear momentarily blurred or actually jiggle up and down or from side to side (oscillopsia). Driving a car or reading on a train is difficult or impossible; even when walking, the patient may need to stop in order to read a sign. These abnormalities indicate a loss of stabilization of ocular fixation by the vestibular system during body movements (the vestibular-ocular reflex, or VOR). An elderly person has difficulty compensating for these abnormalities. Proof that the gait of such persons with vestibulopathy is dependent on visual clues comes from their performance blindfolded or in the dark, when their unsteadiness and staggering increase to the point of falling. When standing with eyes closed, they sway more than normal but generally do not fall over (i.e., they do not have a Romberg sign, as described below). The diagnosis is confirmed by testing labyrinthine function (caloric and rotational testing, electronystagmography, and posture platform testing).

Chronic disorders of vestibular function in relation to gait disorders are most often the result of prolonged administration of aminoglycoside antibiotics or other toxic medications, which destroy the hair cells of the vestibular labyrinth. Vestibular suppressants, such as meclizine and similar medications, mostly anticholinergic and antihistaminic that are available over the counter, can lead to decreased function of the vestibular system, with a persistent gait disorder, if used for more than a few weeks. This also occurs in some patients in the late stages of Ménière disease and, infrequently, for no definable reason. The literature is replete with references to a "multimodal" gait disorder in the elderly that is the result of an ostensible aging of the vestibular organ, together with impaired proprioceptive function caused by distal neuropathy in the elderly, and impaired vision.

A loss of proprioception—as occurs in patients with severe large-fiber polyneuropathy, posterior nerve root lesions (e.g., tabes dorsalis, lumbosacral compression), or interruption of the posterior columns in the spinal cord (multiple sclerosis, vitamin B12 deficiency, spondylotic or tumor compression)—abolishes or seriously impairs the capacity for independent locomotion. After years of training, such patients still have difficulty in initiating gait and in forward propulsion. As J. Purdon Martin illustrated, they hold their hands slightly in front of the body, bend the body and head forward, walk with a wide base and irregular, uneven steps, but still rock the body. If they are tilted to one side, they fail to compensate for their abnormal posture. If they fall, they cannot rise without help; they are sometimes unable to crawl or to get into an "all fours" posture. They have difficulty in getting up from a chair. When standing, if instructed to close their eyes, they sway markedly and fall (Romberg sign); this sign is the clearest indication that the origin of the problem is a loss of proprioceptive sensibility.

With lesions of the basal ganglia, both in monkeys and in humans, the posture of the body and the postural responses to perturbations in equilibrium are faulty. There is difficulty in taking the first step; once it is taken, and in extreme cases, the body pitches forward and a fall can be prevented only by catch-up stepping (propulsive festination). Similarly, a step backward may induce a series of quickening steps in that direction (retropulsive fesitnation). Corrective righting reflexes are clearly faulty when the patient is pushed off balance (Denny-Brown). These abnormalities are elaborated further on, under "Parkinsonian and Festinating Gait."

Pain in the hips or knees can lead to a disorder (antalgic gait) that can be challenging to distinguish from neurological causes of gait problems. Slowness of the swing phase and reduction in the amount of time spent with the painful limb in contact with the ground may be clues to recognizing rheumatological and orthopedic causes of a gait disorder.

Examination of the Patient with Abnormal Gait

When confronted with a disorder of gait, the examiner must observe the patient's stance and the dominant positions of the legs, trunk, and arms, and their interrelationship. It is good practice to watch patients as they walk into the examining room, when they are apt to walk more naturally than during the performance of commanded tasks. They should be asked to stand with feet together and head erect, with eyes open and then closed. A normal person can stand with feet together and eyes closed while moving the head from side to side, a test that blocks both visual and vestibular cues and induces certain compensatory trunk and leg movements that depend solely on proprioceptive afferent mechanisms (Ropper). As already mentioned, the Romberg sign—marked swaying or falling with the eyes closed but not with the eyes open—usually indicates a loss of postural sense, not of cerebellar function, although with vestibular or cerebellar disease there may be an exaggeration of swaying. Swaying due to of nervousness may be overcome by asking the patient to touch the tip of his nose alternately with the forefinger of one hand and then the other.

Next, the patient should be asked to walk, noting in particular any hesitation in starting and negotiating

Table 7-1

FEATURES OF GAIT ABNORMALITIES

	CADENCE	STEP LENGTH	BASE	OTHER ASSOCIATED SIGNS
Cerebellar	Irregular	Slightly short	Wide	Erratic shifting of weight and step
Sensory ataxic (tabetic)	Normal	Short	Slightly wide	Excessive force in step resulting in stamping of feet; Romberg sign
Steppage	Normal	Normal	Normal	Overlifting and slapping of feet
Plegic	Slow	Short	Narrow	Circumduction and scraping of affected leg(s)
Dystonic	Slow	Normal	Erratic	Twisting athetoid movements interrupt walking
Parkinsonian-festinating	Slow until festination	Short	Normal	Quickening step, forward leaning, shuffling, may have trouble with gait initiation
Waddling-myopathic	Normal	Normal	Slightly wide	Overlifting of hip(s)
Toppling	Slow until fall	Short	Widened (protective)	Sudden loss of balance
Normal pressure hydrocephalus	Slow	Short	Slightly wide	Numerous problems with axial body movement
Frontal lobe	Slow	Greatly shortened	Slightly wide (protective)	Difficulty starting and stopping; tendency for feet to "stick" to floor
Aging and marche à petit pas	Slow	Slightly shortened	Slightly widened	Cautious, slight forward lean

turns, width of base, length of stride, foot clearance, arm swing, and cadence. A tendency to veer to one side, as occurs with unilateral cerebellar or vestibular disease, can be brought out by having the patient walk around a chair. When the affected side is toward the chair, the patient tends to walk into it; when it is away from the chair, there is a veering outward in ever-widening circles. More delicate tests of gait are walking a straight line heel to toe ("tandem walking test"), walking backward, and having the patient arise quickly from a chair, walk briskly, stop and turn suddenly, walk back, and sit down again. Turning the patient three full revolutions with eyes open, first right and then left, each time followed by asking the patient to walk naturally, allows the examiner to stress the vestibular apparatus and to compare the two sides. The patient affected by a vestibular or cerebellar process will veer to the side of a lesion. Marching in place with eyes closed (Unterberger, or Fukada stepping tests) also reveals a rotation in the yaw plane (rotation around the vertical axis), indicating an asymmetrical disorder in the plane of the horizontal semicircular ducts or their connections.

It is instructive to observe the patient's postural reaction to a sudden push or tug backward at the shoulders and forward or to the side. With postural instability of any type there is a delay or inadequacy of corrective actions. Finally, the patient may be asked to hop on one leg and to jog. If all these tests can be successfully executed, it may be assumed that any difficulty in locomotion is not because of impairment of a proprioceptive, labyrinthine-vestibular, basal ganglionic, or cerebellar mechanism. Detailed musculoskeletal and neurologic examination is then necessary to determine which of several other disturbances of function is responsible for the patient's disorder of gait.

The following types of abnormal gait (Table 7-1) are so distinctive that, with practice, they can be recognized at a glance and interpreted correctly.

Cerebellar Gait

The main features are a wide base (separation of legs), unsteadiness, irregularity of steps, and lateral veering. Steps are uncertain, some are shorter and others longer than intended, and the patient may compensate for these abnormalities by shortening his steps or even keeping both feet on the ground simultaneously, which creates the appearance of shuffling. Cerebellar gait is often referred to as "reeling" or "drunken," but these terms are not correct and are characteristic instead of intoxication and of certain types of labyrinthine disease, as explained further on.

With cerebellar ataxia, the unsteadiness and irregular swaying of the trunk are prominent when the patient arises from a chair or turns suddenly while walking and may be most evident when he has to stop walking abruptly and sit down; it may be necessary to grasp the chair for support. Cerebellar ataxia may be so severe that the patient cannot sit without swaying or assistance. If it is less severe, standing with feet together and head erect is difficult. In its mildest form, the ataxia is best demonstrated only by having the patient walk a line heel to toe; after a step or two, he loses his balance and finds it necessary to place one foot to the side to avoid falling.

As already emphasized, the patient with cerebellar ataxia who sways perceptibly when standing with feet together and eyes open will sway somewhat more with eyes closed. This slight increase in swaying may lead misattribution to a cerebellar sign of what is simply loss of proprioceptive input to the cerebellum. By contrast, removal of visual clues from a patient with proprioceptive loss causes a marked increase in swaying or falling (the Romberg sign). Thus, the defect in cerebellar disease is primarily in the coordination of the sensory input from proprioceptive, labyrinthine, and visual information with reflex movements, particularly those that are required to make rapid adjustments to changes in posture and position. This integrative deficiency is also reflected in the stepping test, in which the patient is asked to march on the spot with eyes closed as already mentioned. Those with vestibular and sometimes unilateral cerebellar disease have difficulty remaining stable and have a tendency to turn to the left or right or to move forward (occasionally backward) after 5 or 10 steps.

Cerebellar abnormalities of stance and gait are usually accompanied by signs of cerebellar incoordination of the legs, but they need not be. The presence of the latter signs depends on involvement of the cerebellar hemispheres as distinct from the anterosuperior (vermian) midline structures that dominate in the control of gait as described in Chap. 5. If the cerebellar lesions are bilateral, there is often titubation (tremor) of the head and trunk.

Cerebellar gait is seen most commonly in patients with multiple sclerosis, cerebellar tumors (particularly those affecting the vermis—e.g., medulloblastoma), stroke (ischemic and hemorrhage) paraneoplastic cerebellar syndrome, and prominently, in the cerebellar degenerations. Walking without the support of a cane or the arm of a companion brings out a certain stiffness of the legs and firmness of the muscles. The latter abnormality may be analogous to positive supporting reactions observed in cats and dogs following ablation of the anterior vermis; such animals react to pressure on the foot pad with an extensor thrust of the leg.

Reeling Gait of Intoxication

This is characteristic of inebriation with alcohol, sedative drugs, and antiepileptic drugs. The drunken patient totters, reels, tips forward and then backward, appearing each moment to be on the verge of losing his balance and falling. Control over the trunk and legs are greatly impaired. The steps are irregular and uncertain. Such patients appear indifferent to the quality of their performance, but under certain circumstances they can momentarily correct the defect. As indicated above, the adjectives drunken and reeling are used frequently to describe the gait of cerebellar disease, but the similarities between them are only superficial. The severely intoxicated patient reels or sways in many different directions and seemingly makes little or no effort to correct the staggering by watching his legs or the ground, as occurs in cerebellar or sensory ataxia. Also, the variability of the drunken gait is noteworthy. Despite wide excursions of the body and deviation from the line of march, the drunken patient may, for short distances, be able to walk on a narrow base and maintain his balance. In contrast, the patient with cerebellar gait has great difficulty in correcting his balance if he sways or lurches too far to one side. Milder degrees of the drunken gait more closely resemble the gait disorder that follows loss of labyrinthine function (see earlier discussion).

Gait of Sensory Ataxia

This disorder is caused by an impairment of joint position or muscular kinesthetic sense resulting from interruption of afferent nerve fibers in the peripheral nerves, posterior roots, sensory ganglia, posterior columns of the spinal cords, or medial lemnisci, and occasionally from a lesion of both parietal lobes. Whatever the location of the lesion, its effect is to deprive the patient of knowledge of the position of his limbs and, more relevant to gait, to interfere with a large amount of afferent proprioceptive and related information that does not attain conscious perception. A sense of imbalance is usually present but these patients do not describe dizziness. They are aware that the trouble is in the legs and not in the head, that foot placement is awkward, and that the ability to recover quickly from a misstep is impaired. The resulting disorder is characterized by varying degrees of difficulty in standing and walking; in advanced cases, there is a complete failure of locomotion, although muscular power is retained.

The principal features of sensory-ataxic gait are the brusqueness of movement of the legs and stamping of the feet as the foot is forcibly brought down onto the floor (apparently to detect the location of the foot as a substitute for proprioception). The feet are placed far apart to correct the instability, and patients carefully watch both the ground and their legs. As they step out, their legs are flung abruptly forward and outward, in irregular steps of variable length and height. The body is held in a slightly flexed position, and some of the weight is supported on the cane that the severely ataxic patient usually carries. To use Ramsay Hunt's characterization, the patient with this gait disorder is recognized by his "stamp and stick." The most specific feature is that the ataxia is markedly exaggerated when the patient is deprived of visual cues, as in walking in the dark. Such patients, when asked to stand with feet together and eyes closed, show greatly increased swaying and usually, the fully expressed Romberg sign with falling off to one side. It is said that in cases of sensory ataxia, the shoes do not show wear in any one place because the entire sole strikes the ground at once. Examination usually discloses a loss of position sense in the feet and legs and usually of vibratory sense as well. The peripheral or central location of the sensory lesions can be further determined by the state of the tendon reflexes.

Formerly, a disordered gait of this type was observed most frequently with tabes dorsalis, hence the term tabetic gait; but it is also seen in Friedreich ataxia and related forms of spinocerebellar degeneration, subacute combined degeneration of the spinal cord (vitamin B12 deficiency), a large number of sensory polyneuropathies, and those cases of multiple sclerosis or compression of the spinal cord (spondylosis and meningioma are the common causes) in which the posterior columns are involved.

Steppage or Equine Gait (Foot-Drop Gait)

This gait pattern is caused by paralysis of the pretibial and peroneal muscles, with resultant inability to dorsiflex the foot (foot drop). The steps are regular and even, but the advancing foot hangs with the toes pointing toward the ground. In its purest form it is the result of peroneal nerve or fifth lumbar root damage. Walking is accomplished by excessive flexion at the hip, the leg being lifted abnormally high in order for the foot to clear the ground. There is a slapping noise as the foot strikes the floor. Thus there is a superficial similarity to the tabetic gait, especially in cases of severe polyneuropathy, where the features of steppage and sensory ataxia may be combined. However, patients with steppage gait alone are not troubled by a perception of imbalance; they fall from tripping on carpet edges and curbstones.

Foot drop may be unilateral or bilateral and occurs in diseases that affect the peripheral nerves of the legs or motor neurons in the spinal cord, such as chronic acquired neuropathies (diabetic, inflammatory, toxic, and nutritional), Charcot-Marie-Tooth disease (peroneal muscular atrophy), progressive spinal muscular atrophy, and poliomyelitis. It may also be observed in certain types of muscular dystrophy in which the distal musculature of the limbs is involved.

A particular disorder of gait, also of peripheral origin and resembling steppage gait, may be observed in patients with painful dysesthesias of the soles of the feet. Because of the exquisite pain evoked by tactile stimulation of the feet, the patient treads gingerly, as though walking barefoot on hot sand or pavement, with the feet rotated in such a way as to limit contact with their most painful portions. The usual cause is one of the painful peripheral neuropathies (most often alcoholic-nutritional but also toxic and amyloid types), causalgia, or erythromelalgia.

Hemiplegic and Paraplegic (Spastic) Gaits

The patient with hemiplegia or hemiparesis holds the affected leg stiffly and does not flex it freely at the hip, knee, and ankle. The leg tends to rotate outward to describe a semicircle, first away from and then toward the trunk (circumduction). The foot scrapes the floor, contact being made by the toe and outer sole of the foot. One can recognize a spastic gait by the sound of slow, rhythmic scuffing of the foot and wearing of the medial toe of the shoe. The arm on the affected side is weak and stiff to a variable degree; it is carried in a flexed position and does not swing naturally. In the hemiparetic child, the arm tends to abduct as he steps forward. This type of gait disorder is most often a sequela of stroke or trauma but may result from any condition that damages the corticospinal pathway on one side.

The spastic paraplegic or paraparetic gait is, in effect, a bilateral hemiplegic gait. Each leg is advanced slowly and stiffly, with restricted motion at the hips and knees. The legs are extended or slightly bent at the knees and the thighs may be strongly adducted, causing the legs almost to cross as the patient walks (scissor-like gait). The steps are regular and short and the patient advances only with great effort as though wading waist-deep in water. The defect is in stiffness of the stepping mechanism and in propulsion, not in support or equilibrium.

A spastic paraparetic gait is the major manifestation of cerebral diplegia (Little disease, a type of cerebral palsy), the result of anoxic or other damage to the brain in the perinatal period. This disorder of gait is also seen in a variety of chronic spinal cord diseases involving the dorsolateral and ventral tracts, most often multiple sclerosis, but also including syringomyelia, any type of chronic meningomyelitis, subacute combined system disease of both the pernicious anemia and nonpernicious anemia types, spinal cord compression or traumatic injury, adrenomyeloneuropathy, and familial forms of spastic paraplegia. Frequently in these diseases, the effects of posterior column disease are added, giving rise to a mixed gait disturbance—a spinal spastic ataxia, characteristic of multiple sclerosis and certain spinal cord degenerations such as Friedreich ataxia.

Parkinsonian and Festinating Gait

Diminished or absent arm swing, forward bent torso, short or shuffling steps, turning en bloc, hesitation in starting to walk, shuffling, or "freezing" when encountering doorways or other obstacles are the features of the parkinsonian gait. When they are joined to the typical tremor, unblinking and mask-like facial expression, general attitude of flexion, and poverty of movement, there can be little doubt as to the diagnosis. The arms are carried slightly flexed and ahead of the body and do not swing. The legs are stiff and bent at the knees and hips. The steps are short, and the feet barely clear the ground as the patient shuffles along.

Once walking has started, the upper part of the body advances ahead of the lower part, and the patient is impelled to take increasingly short and rapid steps as though trying to catch up to his center of gravity. The steps become more and more rapid, and the patient could easily break into a trot and collide with an obstacle or fall if not assisted. The term *festination* derives from the Latin *festinare*, "to hasten," and appropriately describes the involuntary acceleration or hastening that characterizes the gait of patients with Parkinson disease. Festination may be apparent when the patient is walking forward or backward. The defects are in rocking the body from side to side, so that the feet can clear the floor, and in moving the legs quickly enough to overtake the center of gravity. The problem is compounded by the inadequacy of postural support reflexes, demonstrable in the standing patient by falling in response to a push against the sternum or a tug backward on the shoulder. A normal person readily retains his stability or adjusts to modest displacement of the trunk with a single step, but the parkinsonian patient may lean backward with the upper torso and then stagger or fall unless someone stands by to prevent it.

Quite often, one encounters an elderly patient with only the instability and freezing components of the parkinsonian gait disorder, so-called *lower-half parkinsonism*. Usually, this is not a manifestation of idiopathic Parkinson disease although a few patients are responsive to L-dopa for a brief period. It may be an early manifestation of progressive supranuclear palsy, a basal ganglionic degeneration, normal pressure hydrocephalus, or widespread subcortical vascular damage as discussed further on in this chapter, but it also occurs as a virtually isolated phenomenon that progresses independently of other movement disorders or of dementia. The basis is then probably a particular isolated frontal lobe degeneration (see further on). Within a few years, as pointed out by Factor and colleagues in their two papers, the patient is usually reduced to a chair-bound state.

Other very unusual gaits are sometimes observed in Parkinson disease and were particularly prominent in the postencephalitic form, which is now practically extinct. For example, such a patient may be unable to take a step forward or does so only after he takes a few hops or one or two steps backward (aptly mimicked by the Monty Python troupe in their skit, "Ministry of Silly Walks"). Or walking may be initiated by a series of short steps or a series of steps of increasing size. Occasionally such a patient may run better than he walks or walk backward better than forward. Often, walking so preoccupies the patient that talking simultaneously is impossible for him and he must stop to answer a question.

Choreoathetotic and Dystonic Gaits

Diseases characterized by involuntary movements and dystonic postures seriously affect gait. In fact, a disturbance of gait may be the initial and dominant manifestation of such diseases, and the testing of gait often brings out abnormalities of movement of the limbs and posture that are otherwise not conspicuous.

As the patient with congenital athetosis or Huntington chorea stands or walks, there is a continuous play of irregular movements affecting the face, neck, hands, and, in the advanced stages, the large proximal joints and trunk. The position of the arms and upper parts of the body varies with each step, at times giving the impression of a puppet. There are jerks of the head, grimacing, squirming and twisting movements of the trunk and limbs, and peculiar respiratory noises. One arm may be thrust aloft and the other held behind the body, with wrist and fingers undergoing alternate non-rhythmic flexion and extension, supination and pronation. The head may incline in one direction or the other, the lips alternately retract and purse, and the tongue intermittently protrudes from the mouth. The legs advance slowly and awkwardly, the result of superimposed involuntary movements and postures. Sometimes the foot is plantarflexed at the ankle and the weight is carried on the toes; or the foot may be dorsiflexed or inverted. An involuntary movement may cause the leg to be suspended in the air momentarily, imparting a lilting or waltzing character to the gait, or it may twist the trunk so violently that the patient may fall.

In dystonia musculorum deformans and focal dystonias, the first symptom may be a limp caused by inversion or plantarflexion of the foot or a distortion of the pelvis as discussed in Chap. 4. One leg may be rigidly extended or one shoulder elevated, and the trunk may assume a position of exaggerated flexion, lordosis, or scoliosis. Because of the muscle spasms that deform the body in this manner, the patient may have to walk with knees flexed. The gait may seem normal as the first steps are taken, the abnormal postures asserting themselves as the patient continues to walk. Prominence of the buttocks owing to a lumbar lordosis, combined with flexion of one or both legs at the hip, gives rise to the so-called dromedary gait of Oppenheim. In the more advanced stages, walking becomes impossible owing to torsion of the trunk or the continuous flexion of the legs.

Stiff-person syndrome, an unusual nondystonic disorder causing severe axial muscle spasm, imparts a characteristic appearance of stiffness of the legs and buttock muscles, slow propulsion, and lumbar lordosis; there is sometimes a mild superimposed ataxic disturbance of gait (see Chap. 50). Another unusual disorder affecting the body position during walking is camptocormia, a severe forward bending of the trunk at the waist that is symptomatic of either a dystonia, Parkinson disease, or one of several muscle diseases that focally weaken the extensors of the spine. Kyphosis because of spinal deformities does the same and all of these conditions cause the patient to walk while looking at the ground beneath the feet, but they rarely cause falling.

Chapter 4 more fully describes the general features of the gaits of choreoathetosis and dystonia.

Waddling (Gluteal, or Trendelenburg) Gait

This gait is characteristic of the gluteal muscle weakness that is seen in the progressive muscular dystrophies, but it occurs as well in chronic forms of spinal muscular atrophy, in certain inflammatory myopathies, lumbosacral nerve root compression, and with congenital dislocation of the hips.

In normal walking, as weight is placed alternately on each leg, the hip is fixated by the gluteal muscles, particularly the gluteus medius, allowing for a slight rise of the opposite hip and tilt of the trunk to the weight-bearing side. With weakness of the glutei, however, there is a failure to stabilize the weight-bearing hip, causing it to bulge outward and the opposite side of the pelvis to drop, with inclination of the trunk to that side. The alternation in lateral trunk movements results in the roll or waddle. With unilateral gluteal weakness, often the result of damage to the first sacral nerve root, tilting and dropping of the pelvis ("pelvic ptosis") is apparent on only one side as the patient overlifts the leg when walking.

In several of the muscular dystrophies, an accentuation of lumbar lordosis is often seen. Also, childhood cases may be complicated by muscular contractures, leading to an equinovarus position of the foot, so that the waddle is combined with walking on the toes ("toe walking").

Toppling Gait

Toppling, meaning tottering and falling, occurs with brainstem and cerebellar lesions, especially in the older person following a stroke. It is a frequent feature of the lateral medullary syndrome, in which falling occurs to the side of the infarction. In patients with vestibular neuronitis, falling also occurs to the same side as the lesion. With midbrain strokes, the falls tend to be backward. In patients with progressive supranuclear palsy (discussed in Chap. 39), where dystonia of the neck is combined with paralysis of vertical gaze and pseudobulbar features, unexplained falling is often an early and prominent feature. The falls of progressive supranuclear palsy may derive from such a disorder of the righting mechanism. In the advanced stages of Parkinson disease, falling of a similar type may be a serious problem, but it is more surprising how relatively infrequently it occurs. In addition, the gait is uncertain and hesitant—features that are enhanced, no doubt, by the hazard of falling unpredictably. The cause of the toppling phenomenon is unclear; it does not have its basis in weakness, ataxia, or loss of deep sensation. It appears to be a disorder of balance that is occasioned by precipitant action or the wrong placement of a foot and by a failure of the righting reflexes. Slowness of motor response is another factor.

In a related defect caused by a vestibular disorder, the patient may describe a sense of being pushed (pulsion) rather than of imbalance. It is most fully manifest in the lateral medullary syndrome. In midbrain disease, including progressive supranuclear palsy, a remarkable feature is the lack of appreciation of a sense of imbalance.

Primary Orthostatic Tremor

This unusual fast tremor of the legs may devastate gait. As discussed in Chap. 6, it is present only when the patient stands or exerts force with the legs while seated. The tremor ceases upon walking. In reaction to a perception of severe imbalance, which is characteristic of the disorder, the patient assumes a widened and often stiff-legged stance.

Gait Disorder in Normal-Pressure Hydrocephalus (See also Chap. 30)

Progressive difficulty in walking is typically the initial and most prominent symptom of normal-pressure hydrocephalus (NPH), a disorder of cerebrospinal fluid (CSF) circulation. However, the gait disturbance in NPH has few specific features. Certainly it cannot be categorized as an ataxic or spastic gait or what has been described as an "apraxic" gait; nor does it have more than a superficial resemblance to the parkinsonian gait. Its main features—slowed cadence, widened base and short steps—are the natural compensations observed in patients with all manner of gait disorders. Patients with the gait disorder of NPH may complain of a sense of imbalance or vague dizziness, but most have difficulty in articulating the exact problem. Like most patients with disorders of frontal lobe function, they are better able to carry out the motions of stepping while supine or sitting but have difficulty in taking steps when upright or attempting to walk. If these patients are observed as they get on and off an examining table and in and out of bed, they display poor management of the entire axial musculature, moving their bodies without shifting the center of gravity or adjusting their limbs appropriately. Changes in posture, even rolling over in bed, are made en bloc. The erect posture is assumed in an awkward manner—with hips and knees only slightly flexed and stiff and a delay in swinging the legs over the side of the bed.

Tone in the leg muscles of the NPH patient is often slightly increased, with a tendency to cocontraction of flexor and extensor muscle groups. Walking is perceptibly slower than normal, the body is held stiffly, arm swing is diminished, and there is a tendency to fall backward—features that are reminiscent of Parkinson disease, although the lack of arm swing and the stooped posture are more prominent in Parkinson disease than in NPH and, of course, the other major features of Parkinson disease are lacking. We have been impressed that NPH causes parkinsonian shuffling only when the hydrocephalus is very advanced.

As with the related "frontal gait," described below, patients with NPH often have difficulty initiating gait and have short steps that are helped by marching to a cadence or in step with the examiner. In patients with untreated NPH, one observes a progressive deterioration of stance and gait—from an inability to walk to an inability to stand, sit, and rise from or turn over in bed. There is no hint of ataxia but a study of the mechanics of the gait in NPH by Stolze and colleagues described a widened base and slight outward rotation of the feet. Also distinguishing the gait of NPH from that of Parkinson disease in their study was a response in the latter to acoustic and visual cues for cadence. Sudarsky and Simon quantified these defects by means of high-speed cameras and computer analysis. They reported a reduction in height of step, an increase in sway, and a decrease in rotation of the pelvis and counter-rotation of the torso.

Frontal Lobe Disorders of Gait

Standing and walking may be severely disturbed by diseases that affect the frontal lobes, particularly their medial parts and their connections with the basal ganglia. This disorder is sometimes spoken of as a frontal lobe as an "apraxia of gait" among numerous other labels, because the difficulty in walking cannot be accounted for by weakness, loss of sensation, cerebellar incoordination, or basal ganglionic abnormality. Whether the gait disorder should be designated as an apraxia, in the sense of the original concept of the loss of ability to perform a learned act, is questionable, as walking is instinctual and not learned. Patients with so-called apraxia of gait do not have apraxia of individual limbs, particularly of the lower limbs; conversely, patients with apraxia of the limbs usually walk normally. More likely, the frontal gait disorder represents a loss of integration, at the cortical and basal ganglionic levels, of the essential elements of stance and locomotion that are acquired in infancy and often lost in old age.

Patients typically assume a posture of slight flexion with the feet placed farther apart than normal. They advance slowly, with small, shuffling, hesitant steps. At times they halt, unable to advance without great effort, although they do much better with a little assistance or with exhortation to walk in step with the examiner or to a marching cadence. Walking and turning are accomplished by a series of tiny, uncertain steps that are made with one foot, the other foot being planted on the floor as a pivot.

"Lower-half" Parkinson has been applied to the pattern as mentioned earlier but the cause is rarely idiopathic Parkinson disease. The term "marche à petit pas" is used when the cause is vascular damage to the frontal white matter. There is a need to seek support from a companion's arm or nearby furniture. The initiation of walking becomes progressively more difficult; in advanced cases, the patient makes only feeble, abortive stepping movements in place, unable to move his feet and legs forward; eventually, the patient can make no stepping movements whatsoever, as though his feet were glued to the floor. These late phenomena have been referred to as "magnetic feet" and the difficulty initiating gait as "slipping clutch" syndrome (Denny-Brown) or "gait ignition failure" (Atchison et al). In some patients, difficulty in the initiation of gait may be an early and apparently isolated phenomenon but invariably, with the passage of time, the other features of the frontal lobe gait disorder become evident. Finally, as in untreated NPH, these patients become unable to stand or even to sit; without support, they fall helplessly backward or to one side.

Until the late stages of the process, these patients, while seated or supine are able to make complex movements with their legs, such as drawing imaginary figures or pedaling a bicycle and, quite remarkably, to simulate the motions of walking, all at a time when their gait is seriously impaired. Eventually, however, all movements of the legs become slow and awkward, and the limbs, when passively moved, offer variable counterresistance (paratonia or gegenhalten). As with Parkinson disease, difficulty in turning over in bed may eventually become impossible.

These advanced motor disabilities are usually associated with dementia, but the gait and mental disorders need not evolve in parallel. Thus, some patients with Alzheimer disease may show a serious degree of dementia for several years before a gait disorder becomes apparent; in other conditions, such as NPH and Binswanger disease, the opposite pertains. Or both the dementia and gait disorder may progress more or less together. Grasping, groping, hyperactive tendon reflexes and Babinski signs may or may not be present. The end result in some cases is a "cerebral paraplegia in flexion" (Yakovlev's term), in which the patient lies curled up in bed, immobile and mute, with the limbs fixed by contractures in an attitude of flexion.

On the basis of bilateral but isolated frontal lobe infarction in the territory of the anterior cerebral artery (medial frontal lobes), the existence of a "gait center" has been proposed as mentioned in the introduction (see Della Sala). In the most severe and localized instance of complete gait failure from a frontal lobe stroke we have observed, the lesion was situated in the left pericallosal, medial supplementary motor area. Benson and colleagues have reported in an analysis of MRIs from a selected group of stroke patients, that specific periventricular frontal and occipitoparietal ischemic lesions in the deep white matter are associated with deterioration of gait. Isolated pontine ischemic changes were associated with gait disequilibrium in another study by Kwa and colleagues for the Amsterdam Vascular Medicine Group. The clinical validity of all of these observations in regard to localization is uncertain but generally converges on the notion that ischemic damage at any of the aforementioned sites in the white matter can alter walking.

In addition to NPH and Alzheimer disease, the causes of the frontal lobe gait disorder include large neoplasms (meningioma, infiltrating glioma—gliomatosis cerebri), subcortical arteriosclerotic encephalopathy (Binswanger disease; see Thompson and Marsden), frontotemporal lobar degeneration (formerly Pick disease), and frontal lobe damage from trauma, stroke, or the residual of a ruptured anterior communicating aneurysm.

Gait of the Aged

An alteration of gait unrelated to overt cerebral disease is an almost universal accompaniment of aging and probably a variant of frontal lobe gait deterioration (Fig. 7-2). Lost with aging are speed, balance, and many of the quick and graceful adaptive movements that characterize the gait of younger individuals. The main objective characteristics are a slightly stooped posture, varying degrees of slowness and stiffness of walking, shortening of the stride, slight widening of the base, and a tendency to turn *en bloc*. The shortening of stride and widening of the base provide the support that enables the elderly individual to more confidently maintain his balance, but they result in a somewhat guarded gait, like that of a person walking on a slippery surface or in the dark.

Also lacking to a varying degree in the elderly is the ability to make the rapid compensatory postural changes ("rescue responses") that are necessary to cushion or prevent a fall. A slight misstep, a failure to elevate the foot sufficiently, or tipping of the center of gravity to one side often cannot be corrected—features no doubt

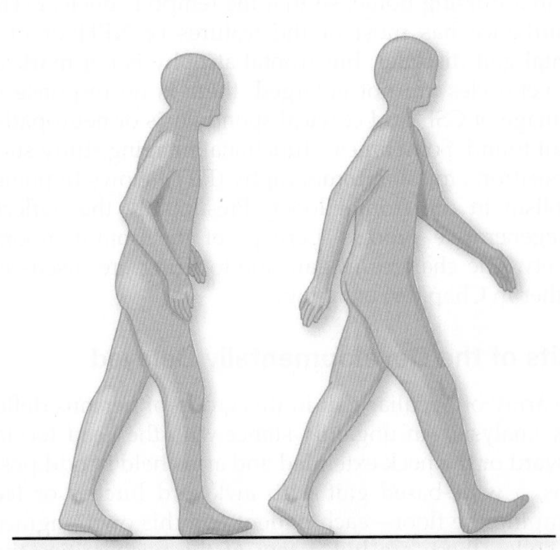

Figure 7-2. Diagram illustrating the changes in posture and gait that accompany aging ("senile gait"). With aging (figure on left), there occurs a decrease in the length of stride, excursion of the hip, elevation of the toes of the forward foot and the heel of the rear foot, shoulder flexion on forward arm swing, and elbow extension on backward swing. (Redrawn by permission from Murray et al.)

that account for the frequency of falls and fear of falling among the elderly. Most persons with this type of gait disturbance are aware of impaired balance and their need for caution to avoid falls (the "cautious gait"; see Nutt et al). As such, this gait lacks specificity, being combined with a general adaptive or defensive pattern of walking. Added to this, as long recognized by orthopedic specialists, knee buckling that is attributable to quadriceps weakness from osteoarthritis contributes to the problem, as discussed by Felson and colleagues. Furthermore, osteoarthritis, the almost inevitable accompaniment of aging, contributes to the disruption of gait as a result of pain and a reduced range of motion and is a component of many gait disorders.

The nature of the elderly gait disorder is not fully understood. It may simply represent a mild degree of cerebral neuronal loss, attributable to aging itself, which in a severe (pathologic) form is the frontal lobe disorder of gait discussed above. Inadequate proprioception, slowness in making corrective postural responses, diminished vestibular function, and weakness of pelvic and thigh muscles are probably contributing factors, as are degenerative joint changes of the spine, hips, and knees. However, Baloh and colleagues have found that changes in sensory function do not correlate well with deterioration in gait. Fisher remarked on the similarity of the senile gait to that of NPH and suggested that hydrocephalus underlies the gait disorder of many elderly.

We prefer to emphasize here the common and particularly vexing problem encountered so often in practice of an elderly person with gait disturbance but minimal dementia. Factor and colleagues identify this as a primary freezing gait disorder of many etiologies and it conforms to "lower-half Parkinson" pattern as discussed earlier. Walking deteriorates over a period of months or years in an elderly individual, sometimes while residing in a nursing home, so that the tempo is unclear. The disturbance has most of the features of NPH or of a frontal gait disorder; but frontal atrophy is not marked, the ventricles are not enlarged, there is no response to drainage of CSF, and cervical spondylosis or neuropathy is not found. Sometimes a functional imaging study such as positron emission tomography (PET) shows hypometabolism in the frontal lobes. Presumably this reflects a degenerative process, perhaps of the frontotemporal variety. The changes in gait due to aging are discussed further in Chap. 29, on aging.

Gaits of the Developmentally Delayed

The array of peculiar gait in this group of persons defies easy analysis. An ungainly stance with the head too far forward or the neck extended and arms held in odd positions, a wide-based gait with awkward lurches or feet stomping the floor—each patient with his own ungraceful style—these are but a few of the peculiarities that meet the eye. One tries in vain to relate them to a disorder of proprioception, cerebellar deficit, or pyramidal or extrapyramidal disease.

The only plausible explanation that comes to mind is that these variants of gait are based on a lag in the natural developmental sequence of the cerebral and spinal mechanisms involved in bipedal locomotion, posture, and righting. The acquisition of the refinements of locomotion—such as running, hopping, jumping, dancing, balancing on one foot, kicking a ball—is age-linked; i.e., each has its average age of acquisition. There are wide individual variations. The rhythmic rocking movements and hand clapping, odd mannerisms, waving of the arms, tremors, and other stereotyped patterns mentioned in Chap. 28, make gait even more maladroit. The Lincoln-Oseretsky scale is an attempt to quantitate these maturational delays in the locomotor sphere (see Chap. 28).

Hysterical Gait (See also Chap. 51)

This may take one of several forms, many well described by Keane. There may be a hysterical monoplegia, hemiplegia, or paraplegia. In walking, the patient may hesitate and advance the leg in a grossly ataxic or tremulous manner. Typically, patients with a hysterical paralysis of the leg do not lift the foot from the floor while walking; instead, they tend to drag the leg as a useless member or push it ahead of them as though it were on a skate. In hysterical hemiparesis, the characteristic circumduction seen in *bona fide* spastic paresis of the leg is absent, as are hemiparetic postures, hyperactive tendon reflexes, and Babinski sign. The hysterical paraplegic cannot very well drag both legs and usually depends on canes or crutches or remains helpless in bed or in a wheelchair; after months or longer of immobilization, the muscles may be flaccid or rigid from shortening, with development of contractures. The hysterical gait may take other dramatic forms. Some patients look as though they are walking on stilts, others assume extreme dystonic postures, and still others lurch wildly in all directions without falling, actually demonstrating by their gyrations a normal ability to make rapid and appropriate postural adjustments. The hysterical gait disorder may be accompanied by similarly exaggerated movements of the arms, as though to impress the observer with the great effort required to walk and maintain balance. Baik and Lang have emphasized the high frequency of coincident psychogenic movement and gait disorders in their speciality clinic. Leg movements in bed may be unimpaired or the patient may display a Hoover sign (described in Chap 3), which belies genuine leg weakness. Some of the patients exhibit additional abnormalities of the voice and visual fields, tremors, and asthenic weakness of muscle contraction.

Astasia-abasia—a term used to describe a psychogenic gait disorder in which patients, although unable to either stand or walk, display more or less normal use of their legs while in bed and have an otherwise normal neurologic examination and body carriage. When such patients are placed on their feet, they may take a few steps and then become unable to advance their legs; they lurch in all directions and crumple to the floor if not assisted.

On the other hand, one should not assume that a patient who manifests a disorder of gait or inability to walk but no other neurologic abnormality is necessarily suffering from hysteria. Lesions that are restricted to the anterosuperior cerebellar vermis may cause an ataxia or severe instability that becomes manifest only when the patient attempts to stand and walk; this is also true of very advanced NPH, frontal lobe disease, and various intoxications such as with alcohol or antiepileptic medications. Cases of severe peripheral neuropathy, particularly if there is prominent sensory loss, may also greatly impair the ability to stand or walk, and the unusual condition of orthostatic leg tremor (see Chap. 6) that may produce buckling of the legs when the patient stands for some period of time, a situation often mistaken for hysteria.

Rehabilitative Measures

Once the gait abnormality has stabilized, i.e., neither progressive nor regressive, one should explore the possibility of rehabilitation by a combination of medical therapy and other corrective measures. The antispasticity agents baclofen and tizanidine are somewhat helpful when stiffness of the limbs exceeds weakness. They may reduce spasticity of the legs, but sometimes at the expense of exposing, to a greater degree than before, a loss of muscle power—the net effect being to the patient's disadvantage. In extreme cases, a subarachnoid pump infusion of baclofen may be effective for spasticity.

Hypofunction of the labyrinths, as in drug-induced or idiopathic vestibulopathy, has greatly challenged physiatrists. Balance training and the more effective use of postural correction and vision have helped some of these patients to be more steady and better able to function (see Baloh and Honrubia). Vestibular sedatives (e.g. meclizine) should be discontinued. Exercises to strengthen leg muscles can be beneficial in many circumstances, as can weight loss. Likewise, gait ataxia from proprioceptive defects can probably be corrected to some extent by careful attention to visual control and proper placement of the feet. Ventricular shunting in idiopathic hydrocephalus has restored locomotion in patients with this syndrome. Once dementia becomes conjoined with any of the gait disorders that occur in advanced age or with frontal lobe disease, rehabilitation stands less chance of success, since the ability to attend to small changes in terrain and posture is lost. Progression from the use of a cane, to a pronged cane, and finally to a four-posted walker allows patients with all types of gait disorders to maintain some mobility. The optimal use of these orthoses is best directed by experienced physical therapists and physiatrists.

Gait training with encouragement has been a useful maneuver to improve psychogenic gait disorders but some prove resistant.

References

Atchison PR, Thompson PD, Frackowiak RS, Marsden CD: The syndrome of gait ignition failure: A report of six cases. *Mov Disord* 8:285, 1993.

Baik JS, Lang AE: Gait abnormalities in psychogenic movement disorders. *Mov Disord* 22:395, 2007.

Baloh RW, Honrubia V: *Clinical Neurophysiology of the Vestibular System*, 3rd ed. Oxford, Oxford University Press, 2001.

Baloh RW, Ying SH, Jacobson KM: A longitudinal study of gait and balance in older people. *Arch Neurol* 60:835, 2003.

Baloh RW, Yue Q, Socotch TM, Jacobson KM. White matter lesions and disequilibrium in older people: I. Case control comparison. *Arch Neurol* 52:970, 1995.

Baezner H, Oster M, Henning O, et al: Amantadine increases gait steadiness in frontal gait disorder due to subcortical vascular encephalopathy: A double-blind randomized placebo-controlled trial based on quantitative gait analysis. *Cerebrovasc Dis* 11:231, 2001.

Benson RR, Guttman CR, Wei S, et al: Older people with impaired mobility have specific loci of periventricular abnormality on MRI. *Neurology* 58:46, 2002.

Denny-Brown D: *The Basal Ganglia and Their Relation to Disorders of Movement*. Oxford, Oxford University Press, 1962.

Della Sala S, Francescani S, Spinnler H: Gait apraxia after bilateral supplementary motor area lesion. *J Neurol Neurosurg Psychiatry* 72:77, 2002.

Eidelberg E, Walden JG, Nguyen LH: Locomotor control in macaque monkeys. *Brain* 104:647, 1981.

Factor SA, Higgins DS, Qian J: Primary freezing gait: A syndrome with many causes. *Neurology* 66:411, 2006.

Factor SA, Jennings DL, Molho ES, et al: The natural history of the syndrome of primary progressive freezing gait. *Arch Neurol* 59:1778, 2002.

Felson DT, Niu J, McClennan C, et al: Knee buckling: prevalence, risk factors, and associated limitations in function. *Ann Intern Med* 147:534, 2007.

Fife TD, Baloh RW: Disequilibrium of unknown cause in older people. *Ann Neurol* 34:694, 1993.

Fisher CM: Hydrocephalus as a cause of disturbances of gait in the elderly. *Neurology* 32:1358, 1982.

Keane JR: Hysterical gait disorders. *Neurology* 39:586, 1989.

Kwa VI, Zaal LH, Verbeeten B, et al: Disequilibrium in patients with atherosclerosis. Relevance of pontine ischemic rarefaction. *Neurology* 51:570, 1998.

Lawrence DG, Kuypers HGSM: The functional organization of the motor system in the monkey: II. The effects of lesions of the descending brainstem pathways. *Brain* 91:15, 1968.

Martin JP: The basal ganglia and locomotion. *Ann R Coll Surg Engl* 32:219, 1963.

Masdeu JP, Sudarsky L, Wolfson L (eds): *Gait Disorders of Aging*. Philadelphia, Lippincott-Raven, 1997.

Meyer JS, Barron D: Apraxia of gait: A clinico-physiologic study. *Brain* 83:261, 1960.

Murray MP, Kory RC, Clarkson BH: Walking patterns in healthy old men. *J Gerontol* 24:169, 1969.

Mutt JG, Marsden CD, Thompson PD: Human walking and higher-level gait disorders, particularly in the elderly. *Neurology* 43:268, 1993.

Olsson E: Gait analysis in hip and knee surgery. *Scand J Rehabil Med Suppl* 15:1, 1986.

Ropper AH: Refined Romberg test. *Can J Neurol Sci* 12:282, 1985.

Stolze H, Kuhtz-Buschbeck JP, Drucke H, et al: Comparative analysis of the gait disorder of normal pressure hydrocephalus and Parkinson's disease. *J Neurol Neurosurg Psychiatry* 70:289, 2001.

Sudarsky L: Geriatrics: Gait disorders in the elderly. *N Engl J Med* 322:1441, 1990.
Sudarsky L, Simon S: Gait disorder in late-life hydrocephalus. *Arch Neurol* 44:263, 1987.
Thompson PD, Marsden CD: Gait disorder of subcortical arteriosclerotic encephalopathy: Binswanger's disease. *Mov Disord* 2:1, 1987.
Tinetti ME, Williams CS: Falls, injuries due to falls, and the risk of admission to a nursing home. *N Engl J Med* 337:1279, 1997.
Verghese J, Lipton RB, Hall CB, et al: Abnormality of gait as a predictor of non-Alzheimer dementia. *N Engl J Med* 347:1761, 2002.
Yakovlev PI: Paraplegia in flexion of cerebral origin. *J Neuropathol Exp Neurol* 13:267, 1954.

SECTION 2

Pain and Other Disorders of Somatic Sensation, Headache, and Backache

8

Pain

Pain is an important sign of illness, and it stands preeminent among all the sensory experiences by which humans judge the existence of disease within themselves. Indeed, pain is the most common medical symptom. Relatively few diseases do not have a painful phase and in many, pain is a characteristic without which diagnosis must be in doubt.

The painful experiences pose manifold problems in virtually every field of medicine; physicians must therefore be prepared to recognize disease in patients who have felt only the first rumblings of discomfort, before other symptoms and signs have appeared. Even more problematic are patients who seek treatment for pain that appears to have little or no structural basis; further inquiry may disclose that fear of serious disease, worry, or depression has aggravated some relatively minor ache or that the complaint of pain has become the means of seeking attention, drugs or monetary compensation. They must also cope with the "difficult" pain patients in whom no amount of investigation brings to light either medical or psychiatric illness. Finally, the physician must be prepared to manage patients who require relief from intractable pain caused by established and incurable disease. To deal intelligently with pain problems requires familiarity with the anatomy of sensory pathways and the sensory supply of body segments as well as insight into the psychological factors that influence the perception of and reaction to pain.

The ambiguity with which the term pain is used is responsible for some of our difficulty in understanding it. One aspect, the easier to comprehend, is the transmission of impulses along certain pathways in response to potentially tissue-damaging stimuli, i.e., nociception. Far more abstruse is its quality as a mental state intimately linked to emotion, i.e., the quality of anguish or suffering—"a passion of the soul," in the words of Aristotle—which defies definition and quantification. This duality (nociception and suffering) is of practical importance for certain drugs or surgical procedures, such as cingulotomy, may reduce the patient's reaction to painful stimuli, leaving awareness of the sensation largely intact. Alternatively, interruption of certain neural pathways may abolish all sensation in an affected part but the symptom of pain may persist (i.e., denervation dysesthesia or anesthesia dolorosa), even in an amputated limb ("phantom pain"). Finally, unlike most sensory modalities—which are aroused by a specific stimulus such as touch-pressure, heat, or cold—pain can be evoked by any one of these stimuli if it is intense enough.

It is apparent to us that in highly specialized medical centers, and often even in "pain centers," few physicians are capable of handling difficult and unusual pain problems in any comprehensive way. In fact, it is to the neurologist that other physicians regularly turn for help with these matters. Although much has been learned about the anatomy of pain pathways, their physiologic mechanisms, and which structures to ablate in order to produce analgesia, relatively little is known about which patients should be subjected to these destructive operations or how to manage their pain by medical means. The practice of pain medicine challenges every thoughtful physician, for it demands a high degree of skill in medicine, neurology, and psychiatry.

ANATOMY AND PHYSIOLOGY OF PAIN

Historical Perspective

For more than a century, views on the nature of pain sensation have been dominated by two major theories. One, the *specificity theory*, was from the beginning associated with the name of von Frey. He asserted that the skin consisted of a mosaic of discrete sensory spots and that each spot, when stimulated, gave rise to one sensation—either pain, pressure, warmth, or cold; in his view, each of these sensations had a distinctive end organ in the skin and each stimulus-specific end organ was connected by its own private pathway to the brain. A second theory was that of Goldscheider, who abandoned his own earlier discovery of pain spots to argue that they simply represented pressure spots, a sufficiently intense stimulation of which could produce pain. According to the latter theory, there were no distinctive pain receptors, and the sensation of pain was the result of the summation of impulses excited by pressure or thermal stimuli applied to the skin. Originally called the intensivity theory, it later became known as the *pattern* or *summation theory*.

In an effort to conciliate the pattern and specificity theories, Head and colleagues, in 1905, formulated a novel concept of pain sensation, based on observations that followed his purposeful division of the cutaneous branch of the radial nerve in his own forearm. The zone of impaired sensation contained an innermost area in which superficial sensation was completely abolished. This was surrounded by a narrower ("intermediate") zone, in which pain sensation was preserved but poorly localized; extreme degrees of temperature were recognized in the intermediate zone but perception of touch, lesser differences of temperature, and two-point discrimination were abolished. To explain these findings, Head postulated the existence of two systems of cutaneous receptors and conducting fibers: (1) an ancient *protopathic* system, subserving pain and extreme differences in temperature and yielding ungraded, diffuse impressions of an all-or-none type; and (2) a more recently evolved *epicritic* system, which mediated touch, two-point discrimination, and lesser differences in temperature, as well as localized pain. The pain and hyperesthesia that follow damage to a peripheral nerve were attributed to a loss of inhibition that was normally exerted by the epicritic upon the protopathic system. This theory was used for many years to explain the sensory alterations that occur with both peripheral and central (thalamic) lesions. It lost credibility for several reasons but mainly because Head's original observations and deductions upon which they were based could not be confirmed (see Trotter and Davies; also Walshe). Nevertheless, both fast and slow forms of pain conduction were later corroborated (see below).

A later refinement of the pattern and specificity concepts of pain was made in 1965 when Melzack and Wall articulated their "gate-control" theory. They observed, in decerebrate and spinal cats, that peripheral stimulation of large myelinated fibers produced a negative dorsal root potential and that stimulation of small unmyelinated C (pain) fibers caused a positive dorsal root potential. They postulated that these potentials, which were a reflection of presynaptic inhibition or excitation, modulated the activity of secondary transmitting neurons (T cells) in the dorsal horn and that this modulation was mediated through inhibitory (I) cells. The essence of this theory was that the large-diameter fibers excited the I cells, which, in turn, caused a presynaptic inhibition of the T cells; conversely, the small pain afferents inhibited the I cells, leaving the T cells in an excitatory state. Melzack and Wall emphasized that pain impulses from the dorsal horn must also be under the control of a descending system of fibers from the brainstem, thalamus, and limbic lobes.

At first the gate-control mechanisms seemed to offer an explanation of the pain of ruptured disc and of certain chronic neuropathies (particularly those with large fiber out-fall) and attempts were made to relieve pain by subjecting the peripheral nerves and dorsal columns (presumably their large myelinated fibers) to sustained transcutaneous electrical stimulation. Such selective stimulation would theoretically "close" the gate. In some clinical situations these procedures have indeed given relief from pain, but not necessarily as a result of stimulation of large myelinated fibers alone (see Taub and Campbell). But in a number of other instances relating to pain in large- and small-fiber neuropathies, the clinical behavior has been quite out of keeping with what one would expect on the basis of the gate-control mechanism. As with preceding theories, flaws have been exposed in the physiologic observations on which the theory is based. These and other aspects of the gate-control theory of pain have been critically reviewed by Nathan.

During the last few decades there has been a significant accrual of information on cutaneous sensibility, demanding modification of earlier anatomic–physiologic and clinical concepts. Interestingly, much of this information is still best described and rationalized in the general framework of the oldest theory, that of specificity, as is evident from the ensuing discussion on pain and that on other forms of cutaneous sensibility in the next chapter.

Pain Receptors and Peripheral Afferent Pathways

In terms of peripheral pain mechanisms, there is indeed a high degree, though not absolute, specificity in the von Frey sense. In keeping with distinctions between nerve types, the sensory (and motor) fibers have been classified according to their size and function (Table 8-1). It is now well established that two types of afferent fibers in the distal axons of primary sensory neurons respond maximally to nociceptive (i.e., potentially tissue-damaging) stimuli. One type is the very fine, unmyelinated, slowly conducting C fiber (0.3 to 1.1μ in diameter); the other is the thinly myelinated, more rapidly conducting A-δ fiber (2 to 5μ in diameter). The peripheral terminations of both of these primary pain afferents or receptors are the free, profusely branched nerve endings in the skin and other organs; these are covered by Schwann cells but contain little or no myelin.

There is considerable evidence, based on their response characteristics, that a degree of subspecialization exists within these freely branching, nonencapsulated endings and their small-fiber afferents. Three categories of free endings or receptors are recognized: mechanoreceptors, thermoreceptors, and polymodal nociceptors. Each ending transduces stimulus energy into an action potential in the distal nerve membranes. The first two types of receptors are activated by innocuous mechanical and thermal stimulation, respectively; the mechanoeffects are transmitted by both A-δ and C fibers and the thermal effects mostly by C fibers. The majority of C fibers are polymodal and are most effectively excited by noxious or tissue-damaging stimuli, but they can respond to both mechanical and thermal stimuli and to chemical mediators such as those associated with inflammation. Moreover, certain A-δ fibers respond to light touch, temperature, and pressure as well as to pain stimuli and are capable of discharging in proportion to the intensity of the stimulus. The stimulation of single fibers by intraneural electrodes indicates that they can also convey information concerning the nature and location of the stimulus. These observations on the polymodal functions of A-δ and C fibers would explain the earlier observations of Lele and Weddell that modes of sensation other than pain can be evoked from structures such as the cornea, which is innervated solely by free nerve endings.

Table 8-1

CLASSIFICATION AND FUNCTION OF SENSORY PERIPHERAL NERVE FIBER TYPES AND SYMPTOMS ASSOCIATED WITH INTRINSIC DYSFUNCTION OF EACH TYPE

FIBER TYPE	ALTERNATIVE DESIGNATION	FIBER DIAMETER	CONDUCTION VELOCITY (m/s)	FUNCTION AND SYMPTOMS OF DYSFUNCTION
A-α and -β Large, heavily myelinated	II	5–20	30–70	Touch, pressure
A-γ	Ia	3–6	15–30	Spindle afferents
A-δ Small, thinly myelinated	III	2–5	12–30	Pain and temperature, soma touch (sharp, lancinating, prickly pain)
B	1–3	3–15		
C Small, unmyelinated; polymodal	IV	0.3–1.1	0.5–2	Slow pain and temperature (dull, burning, poorly localized pain)

The manner in which painful stimuli are translated into electrical depolarizations in nerve endings is beginning to be understood. A number of specialized molecules, when activated by noxious stimuli, open cationic channels in membranes of the nerve ending. Opening of these channels, in turn, activates voltage-gated sodium channels and generates an action potential in the sensory axon. Mannion and Woolf have summarized the regulation and activation of these receptor molecules.

The peripheral afferent pain fibers of both A-δ and C types have their cell bodies in the dorsal root ganglia; central extensions of these nerve cells project, via the dorsal root, to the dorsal horn of the spinal cord (or, in the case of cranial pain afferents, to the spinal trigeminal nucleus, the medullary analogue of the dorsal horn). The pain afferents occupy mainly the lateral part of the root entry zone. Within the spinal cord, many of the thinnest fibers (C fibers) form a discrete bundle, the tract of Lissauer (Fig. 8-1*A*). That the tract of Lissauer is predominantly a pain pathway is shown (in animals) by the ipsilateral segmental analgesia that results from its transection but it contains deep sensory or propriospinal fibers as well. Although it is customary to speak of a lateral and medial division of the posterior root (the former contains small pain fibers and the latter, large myelinated fibers), the separation into discrete functional bundles is not complete, and in humans the two groups of fibers cannot be differentially interrupted by selective rhizotomy.

Dermatomic Distribution of Pain Fibers

(See Fig. 9.1) Each sensory unit (the sensory nerve cell in the dorsal root ganglion, its central and peripheral extensions, and cutaneous and visceral endings) has a unique topography that is maintained throughout the sensory system from the periphery to the sensory cortex. The discrete segmental distribution of the sensory units permits the construction of sensory maps, so useful to clinicians (see Fig. 9-1). This aspect of sensory anatomy is elaborated in the next chapter, which includes maps of the sensory dermatomes and cutaneous nerves. However, as a means of quick orientation to the topography of peripheral pain pathways, it is useful to remember that the facial structures and anterior cranium lie in the fields of the trigeminal nerves; the back of the head, second cervical; the neck, third cervical; the epaulet area, fourth cervical; the deltoid area, fifth cervical; the radial forearm and thumb, sixth cervical; the index and middle fingers, seventh cervical; the little finger and ulnar border of hand and forearm, eighth cervical–first thoracic; the nipple, fifth thoracic; the umbilicus, tenth thoracic; the groin, first lumbar; the medial side of the knee, third lumbar; the great toe, fifth lumbar; the little toe, first sacral; the back of the thigh, second sacral; and the genitoanal zones, third, fourth, and fifth sacral segments. The distribution of pain fibers from deep structures, although not fully corresponding to those from the skin, also follows a segmental pattern. The first to fourth thoracic nerve roots are the important sensory pathways for the heart and lungs; the sixth to eighth thoracic, for the upper abdominal organs; and the lower thoracic and upper lumbar, for the lower abdominal viscera. These areas of projection from visceral structures roughly correspond to the areas of adjacent root innervation, with some exceptions because of routing of sensory nerves to organs that migrate with development.

Neurologically relevant maps of pain projection from the bones, ligaments, and adjacent musculoskeletal structures have been termed *sclerotomes*; they differ slightly in their distribution from the dermatomes. A further discussion of referred pain and a figure comparing sclerotomes and dermatomes is given later in the chapter.

The Dorsal Horn

The afferent pain fibers, after traversing the tract of Lissauer, terminate in the posterior gray matter or dorsal horn, predominantly in the marginal zone. Most of the fibers terminate within the segment of their entry into the cord; some extend ipsilaterally to one or two adjacent rostral and caudal segments; and some project, via the

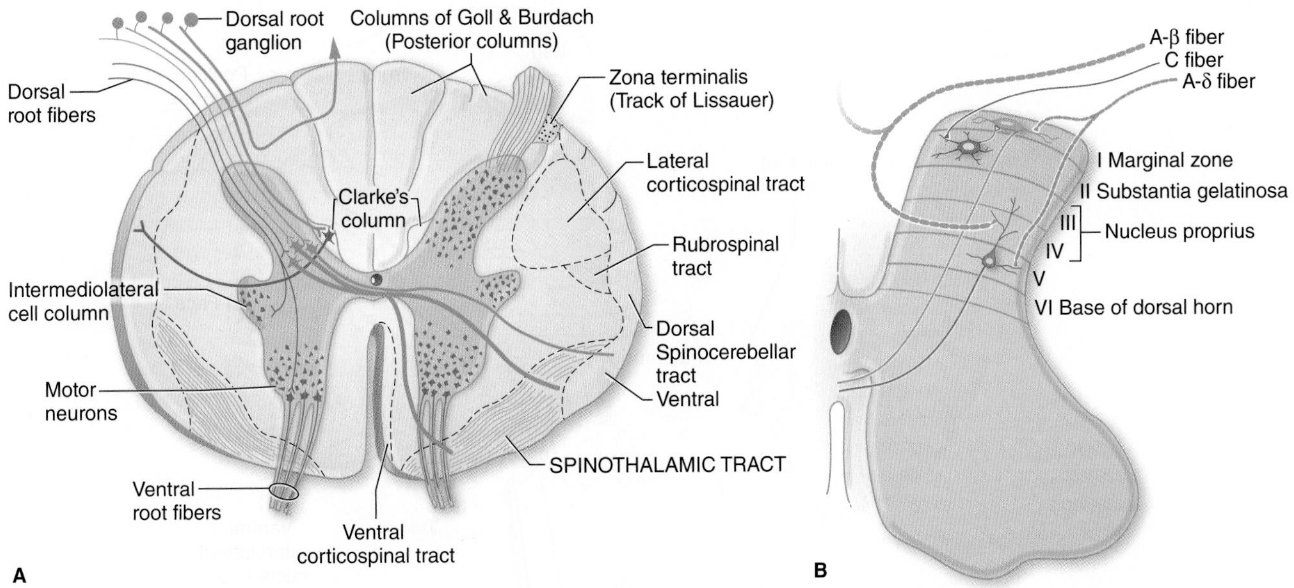

Figure 8-1. *A*. Spinal cord in transverse section illustrating the course of the afferent fibers and the major ascending pathways. Fast-conducting pain fibers are not confined to the spinothalamic tract but are scattered diffusely in the anterolateral funiculus (see also Fig. 8-3). (Adapted from Martin JH: *Neuroanatomy: Text and Atlas*. New York, McGraw-Hill, 2003, with permission.) *B*. Transverse section through a cervical segment of the spinal cord illustrating the subdivision of the gray matter into laminae according to Rexed and the entry and termination of the main sensory fibers. (Adapted from Fields HL: *Pain*. New York, McGraw-Hill, 1987, with permission.)

anterior commissure, to the contralateral dorsal horn. The cytoarchitectonic studies of Rexed in the cat (the same organization pertains in primates and probably in humans) have shown that second-order neurons, the sites of synapse of afferent sensory fibers in the dorsal horn, are arranged in a series of six layers or laminae (Fig. 8-1*B*). Thinly myelinated (A-δ) fibers terminate principally in lamina I of Rexed (marginal cell layer of Waldeyer) and also in the outermost part of lamina II; some A-δ pain fibers penetrate the dorsal gray matter and terminate in the lateral part of lamina V. Unmyelinated (C) fibers terminate in lamina II (substantia gelatinosa). Yet other cells that respond to painful cutaneous stimulation are located in ventral horn laminae VII and VIII. The latter neurons are responsive to descending impulses from brainstem nuclei as well as segmental sensory impulses. From these cells of termination, second-order axons connect with ventral and lateral horn cells in the same and adjacent spinal segments and subserve both somatic and autonomic reflexes. The main bundle of secondary neurons subserving pain sensation projects contralaterally (and to a lesser extent ipsilaterally) to higher levels; this constitutes the *spinothalamic tract*, discussed below.

A number of important observations have been made concerning the mode of transmission and modulation of pain impulses in the dorsal horn and brainstem. Excitatory amino acids (glutamate, aspartate) and nucleotides such as adenosine triphosphate (ATP) are the putative transmitters at terminals of primary A-δ sensory afferents. Also, A-δ pain afferents, when stimulated, release several neuromodulators that play a role in the transmission of pain sensation. Slower neurotransmission by C neurons involves other substances, of which the most important is the 11-amino-acid peptide known as substance P ("P" for powder extracted from animal tissue and urine by von Euler in 1931). In animals, substance P excites nociceptive dorsal root ganglion and dorsal horn neurons; furthermore, destruction of substance P fibers produces analgesia. In patients with the rare condition of congenital neuropathy and insensitivity to pain, there is a marked depletion of dorsal horn substance P.

A large body of evidence indicates that opiates are important modulators of pain impulses as they are relayed through the dorsal horn and through nuclei in the medulla and midbrain. Thus, opiates have been noted to decrease substance P; at the same time, flexor spinal reflexes, which are evoked by segmental pain, are reduced. Opiate receptors of three types are found on both presynaptic primary afferent terminals and postsynaptic dendrites of small neurons in lamina II. Moreover, lamina II neurons, when activated, release enkephalins, endorphins, and dynorphins—all of which are endogenous, morphine-like peptides that bind specifically to opiate receptors and inhibit pain transmission at the dorsal horn level. The subject of pain modulation by opiates and endogenous morphine-like substances is elaborated further on.

Spinal Afferent Tracts for Pain

The (Anterolateral, or Lateral) Spinothalamic Tract

As indicated above, axons of secondary neurons that sub-serve pain sensation originate in laminae I, II, V, VII, and VIII of the spinal gray matter. The principal bundle of these axons decussates in the anterior spinal commissure and ascends in the anterolateral fasciculus of the opposite side of the cord as the *spinothalamic tract* to terminate in brainstem and thalamic structures (Fig. 8-2).

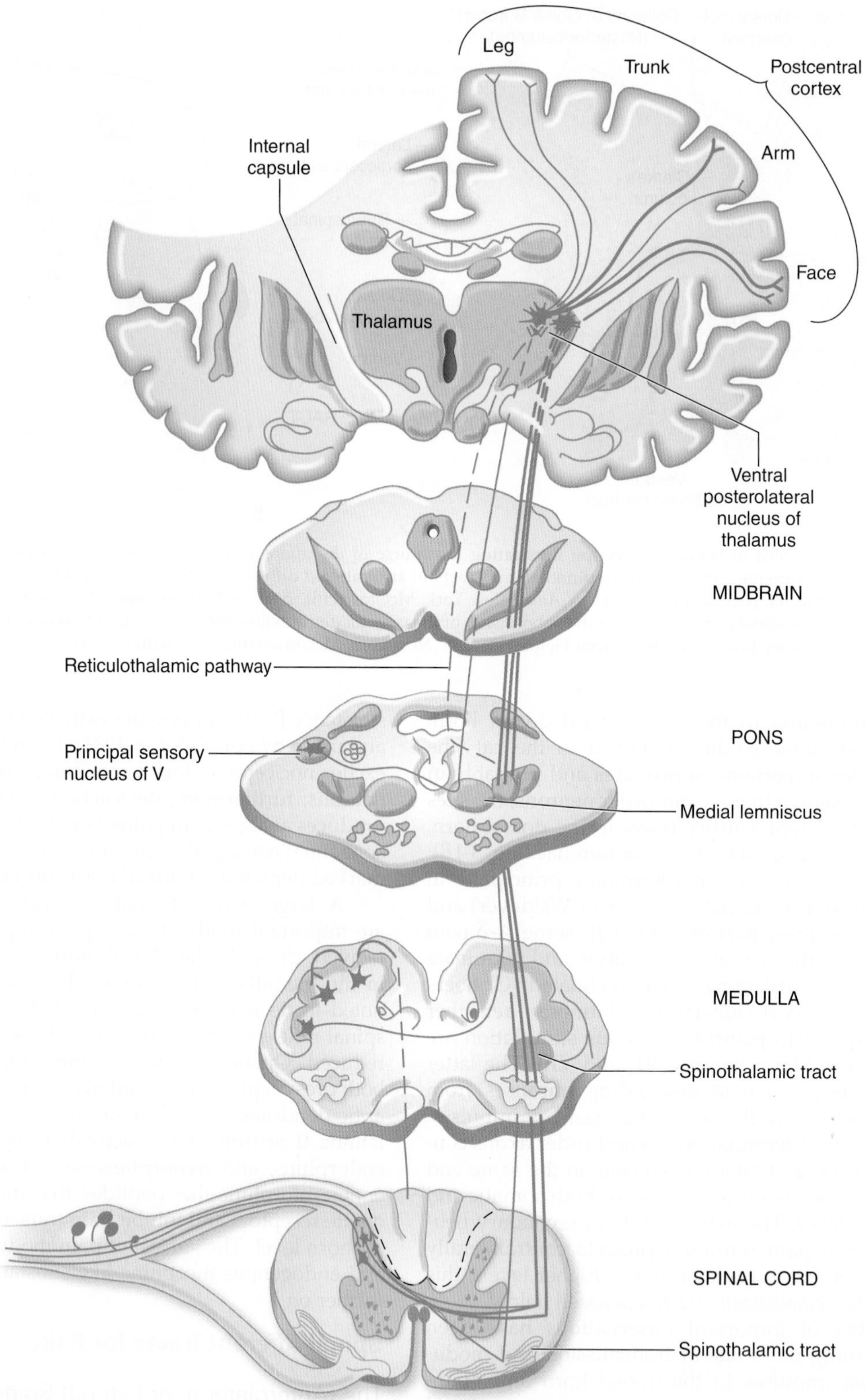

Figure 8-2. The spinothalamic tract (pain, thermal sense) is shown. In the bottom section, the fibers that form the spinothalamic tract cross over two or three segment rostral to their entry into the cord, not at the same level as depicted. Offshoots from the ascending anterolateral fasciculus (spinothalamic tract) to nuclei in the medulla, pons, and mesencephalon and nuclear terminations of the tract are indicated. The cortical representation of sensation is shown grossly; it is shown more explicitly in Fig. 9-5 and discussed in Chap. 9. The lemniscal (posterior column) system is shown in Fig. 9-4.

It is of clinical consequence that the axons carrying pain impulses from each dermatome decussate one to three segments rostral to the level of root entry. For this reason, a discrete lesion of the lateral spinal cord creates a loss of pain and thermal sensation of the *contralateral* trunk, the dermatomal level of which is *two to three segments below that of the spinal cord lesion*. As the ascending fibers cross the cord, they are added to the inner side of the spinothalamic tract (the principal afferent pathway of the anterolateral fasciculus), so that the longest fibers from the sacral segments come to lie most superficially and fibers from successively more rostral levels occupy progressively deeper positions (Fig. 8-3). This somatotopic arrangement is of importance to the neurosurgeon performing an operation for pain relief, insofar as the depth to which the funiculus is cut will govern the level of analgesia that is achieved; for the neurologist, it provides an explanation of the pattern of "sacral sparing" of pain and thermal sensation created by centrally placed lesions of the spinal cord. The termination of this tract, mainly in the thalamus, is described further on.

Other Spinocerebral Afferent Tracts

In addition to the anterolateral spinothalamic tract—a fast-conducting pathway that projects directly to the thalamus—the anterolateral fasciculus of the cord contains several more slowly conducting, medially placed systems of fibers. One such group of fibers projects directly to the reticular core of the medulla and midbrain and then to the medial and intralaminar nuclei of the thalamus; these fibers are referred to as the *spinoreticulothalamic* or *paleospinothalamic* pathway. At the level of the medulla, these fibers synapse in the nucleus gigantocellularis; more rostrally, they connect with nuclei of the parabrachial region, midbrain reticular formation, periaqueductal gray matter, and hypothalamus. A second, more medially placed pathway in the anterolateral cord ascends to the brainstem reticular core via a series of short interneuronal links. It is not clear whether these spinoreticular fibers are collaterals of the spinothalamic tracts, as Cajal originally stated, or whether they represent an independent system, as more recent data seem to indicate. Probably both statements are correct. There is also a third, direct spinohypothalamic pathway in the anterolateral fasciculus.

The conduction of diffuse, poorly localized pain arising from deep and visceral structures (gut, periosteum, peritoneum) has been ascribed to these slow-conducting, indirect pathways. Melzack and Casey have proposed that this fiber system (which they refer to as *paramedian*), with its diffuse projection via brainstem and thalamus to the limbic and frontal lobes, subserves the affective aspects of pain, i.e., the unpleasant feelings engendered by pain. It is evident that these spinoreticulothalamic pathways continue to evoke the psychic experience of pain even when the direct spinothalamic pathways have been interrupted. However, it is the direct spinothalamic pathway, which projects to the ventroposterolateral (VPL) nucleus of the thalamus and thence to discrete areas of the sensory cortex, that subserves the *sensory-discriminative* aspects of pain, i.e., the processes that underlie the localization, quality, and possibly the intensity of the noxious stimulus. Also, the pathways for *visceral pain* from the esophagus, stomach, small bowel, and

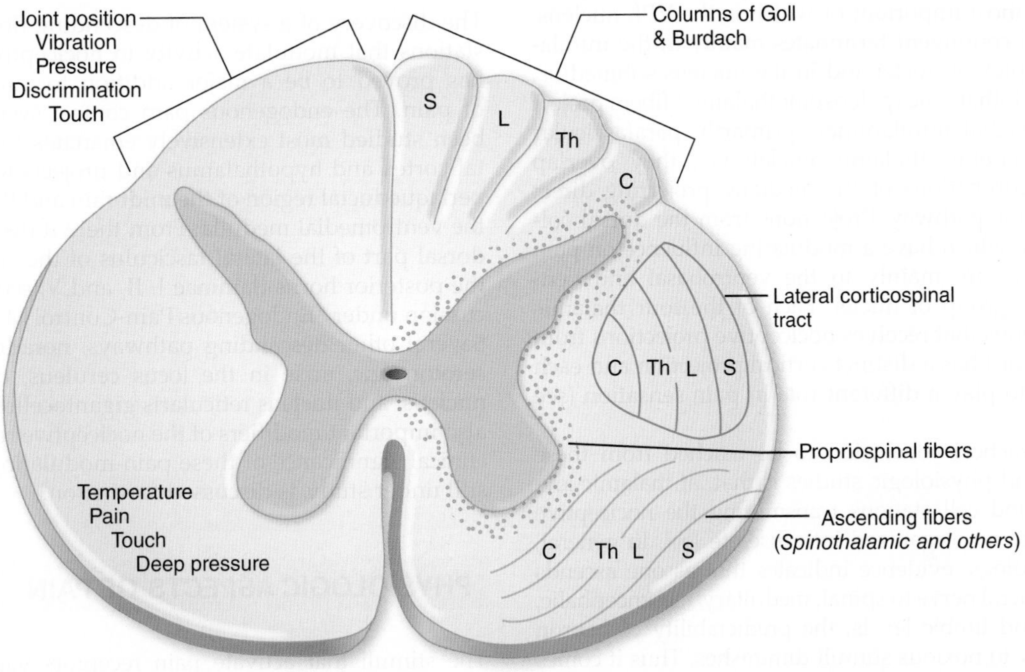

Figure 8-3. Spinal cord showing the segmental and laminated arrangement of nerve fibers within major tracts. On the left side are indicated the "sensory modalities" that appear to be mediated by the two main ascending pathways. *C*, cervical; *L*, lumbar; *S*, sacral; *Th*, thoracic. (Adapted by permission from Brodal A: *Neurological Anatomy*, 3rd ed. New York, Oxford University Press, 1981.)

proximal colon are carried largely in the vagus nerve and terminate in the nucleus of the solitary tract (nucleus tractus solitarius [NTS]) before projecting to the thalamus, as described below. Other abdominal viscera still activate the NTS when the vagus is severed in animals, probably transmitting impulses through the splanchnic plexus.

It should be emphasized that the foregoing data concerning the cells of termination of cutaneous nociceptive stimuli and the cells of origin of ascending spinal afferent pathways have all been obtained from studies in animals (including monkeys). In humans, the specific cells of origin of the direct spinothalamic tract fibers have not been fully identified. Information about this pathway in humans has been derived from the study of postmortem material and from the examination of patients subjected to anterolateral cordotomy for intractable pain. What can be stated of clinical importance is that unilateral section of the anterolateral funiculus produces a relatively complete loss of pain and thermal sense on the opposite side of the body, extending to a level two or three segments below the lesion as noted earlier. After a variable period of time, pain sensibility usually returns, probably being conducted by pathways that lie outside the anterolateral quadrants of the spinal cord that gradually increase their capacity to conduct pain impulses. One of these is a longitudinal polysynaptic bundle of small myelinated fibers in the center of the dorsal horn (the dorsal intracornual tract); another consists of axons of lamina I cells that travel in the dorsal part of the lateral funiculus.

Thalamic Terminus of Pain Fibers

The direct spinothalamic fibers separate into two bundles as they approach the thalamus. The lateral division terminates in the ventrobasal and posterior groups of nuclei, the most important of which is the VPL nucleus. The medial contingent terminates mainly in the intralaminar complex of nuclei and in the nucleus submedius. Spinoreticulothalamic (paleospinothalamic) fibers project onto the medial intralaminar (primarily parafascicular and centrolateral) thalamic nuclei; i.e., they overlap with the terminations of the medially projecting direct spinothalamic pathway. Projections from the dorsal column nuclei, which have a modulating influence on pain transmission, are mainly to the ventrobasal and ventroposterior group of nuclei. Each of the four thalamic nuclear groups that receives nociceptive projections from the spinal cord has a distinct cortical projection and each is thought to play a different role in pain sensation (see below).

One practical conclusion to be reached from these anatomic and physiologic studies is that, at thalamic levels, fibers and cell stations transmitting the nociceptive impulses are not organized into discrete loci. In general, neurophysiologic evidence indicates that as one ascends from peripheral nerve to spinal, medullary, mesencephalic, thalamic, and limbic levels, the predictability of neuron responsivity to noxious stimuli diminishes. Thus it comes as no surprise that neurosurgical lesions that interrupt afferent pathways at progressively higher levels of the brainstem and thalamus become decreasingly successful.

Thalamocortical Projections

The ventrobasal thalamic complex and the ventroposterior group of nuclei project to two main cortical areas: the primary sensory (postcentral) cortex (a small number terminate in the precentral cortex) and the upper bank of the sylvian fissure. These cortical projections are described more fully in Chap. 9 but it can be stated here that they are concerned mainly with the reception of tactile and proprioceptive stimuli and with all discriminative sensory functions, including pain. The extent to which either cortical area is activated by thermal and painful stimuli is uncertain. Certainly, stimulation of these (or any other) cortical areas in a normal, alert human being does not produce pain. The intralaminar nuclei, which also project to the hypothalamus, amygdaloid nuclei, and limbic cortex, probably mediate the arousal and affective aspects of pain and autonomic responses.

The thalamic projection to the primary sensory cortex that is distributed mainly along the postcentral gyrus of the anterior parietal lobe is shown in Fig. 9-5 (the "sensory homunculus"). The cortical representation allows for accurate localization of the site of origin of a painful stimulus but the notion that thalamic projections terminate solely in this region is an oversimplification.

Thalamic and cerebral cortical localization of *visceral sensation* is not well known. However, cerebral evoked potentials and increased cerebral blood flow (by positron emission tomography [PET] studies) have been demonstrated in the thalamus and pre- and postcentral gyri of patients undergoing rectal balloon distention (Silverman et al; Rothstein et al).

Descending Pain-Modulating Systems

The discovery of a system of descending fibers and way stations that modulate activity in nociceptive pathways has proved to be a major addition to our knowledge of pain. The endogenous pain control system that has been studied most extensively emanates from the frontal cortex and hypothalamus and projects to cells in the periaqueductal region of the midbrain and then passes to the ventromedial medulla. From there it descends in the dorsal part of the lateral fasciculus of the spinal cord to the posterior horns (laminae I, II, and V; see further discussion under "Endogenous Pain-Control Mechanisms"). Several other descending pathways, noradrenergic and serotonergic, arise in the locus ceruleus, dorsal raphe nucleus, and nucleus reticularis gigantocellularis and are also important modifiers of the nociceptive response. The clinical significance of these pain-modulating pathways, still under study, is discussed further on.

PHYSIOLOGIC ASPECTS OF PAIN

The stimuli that activate pain receptors vary from one tissue to another. The adequate stimulus for skin is one that has the potential to injure tissue, i.e., pricking, cutting, crushing, burning, and freezing. These stimuli are ineffective when applied to the stomach and intestine, where pain is produced by an engorged or inflamed mucosa, distention or spasm of smooth muscle, and traction on the mesenteric attachment. In skeletal muscle, pain is caused by ischemia (the basis of intermittent claudication), necrosis, hemorrhage, and injection of irritating solutions as well as by injuries of connective tissue sheaths. Prolonged contraction of skeletal muscle evokes an aching type of pain. Ischemia is also the most important cause of pain in cardiac muscle. Joints are insensitive to pricking, cutting, and cautery, but pain can be produced in the synovial membrane by inflammation and by exposure to hypertonic saline. The stretching and tearing of ligaments around a joint can evoke severe pain. Injuries to the periosteum give rise to pain but probably not to other sensations. Blood vessels are a source of pain when pierced by a needle or involved in an inflammatory process. Distention of arteries or veins, as occurs with thrombotic or embolic occlusion, may be sources of pain; other mechanisms of headache relate to traction on arteries or inflammation of the meningeal structures by which they are supported. (The subject of headache and its origins is taken up in Chap. 10.) Pain from intraneural lesions probably arises from the sheaths of the nerves. Nerve root(s) and sensory ganglia, when compressed (e.g., by a ruptured disc), give rise to pain.

With damage to tissue, there is a release of proteolytic enzymes, which act locally on tissue proteins to liberate substances that excite peripheral nociceptors. These pain-producing substances—which include histamine, prostaglandins, serotonin, and similar polypeptides, as well as potassium ions—elicit pain when they are injected intraarterially or applied to the base of a blister. Other pain-producing substances such as kinins are released from sensory nerve endings or are carried there by the circulation. Local vascular permeability is also increased by these substances.

In addition, direct stimulation of nociceptors releases polypeptide mediators that enhance pain perception. The best studied of these is substance P, which is released from the nerve endings of C fibers in the skin during peripheral nerve stimulation. It causes erythema by dilating cutaneous vessels and edema by releasing histamine from mast cells; it also acts as a chemoattractant for leukocytes. This reaction, called *neurogenic inflammation* by White and Helme, is mediated by antidromic action potentials from the small nerve cells in the spinal ganglia and is the basis of the axon reflex of Lewis; the reflex is abolished in peripheral nerve diseases and can be studied electrophysiologically as an aid to clinical localization.

Perception of Pain

The *threshold for perception of pain*, i.e., the lowest intensity of a stimulus recognized as pain, is approximately the same in all persons. Inflammation lowers the threshold for perception of pain by a process called *sensitization*. This process, termed allodynia, allows ordinarily innocuous stimuli to produce pain in sensitized tissues. The pain threshold is, of course, raised by local anesthetics and by certain lesions of the nervous system as well as by centrally acting analgesic drugs. Mechanisms other than lowering or raising the pain threshold are important as well. Placebos reduce pain in about one-third of the groups of patients in which such effects have been recorded. Acupuncture at sites anatomically remote from painful operative fields also reduces the pain in some individuals. Distraction and suggestion, by turning attention away from the painful part, reduce the awareness of and response to pain but not the threshold for its perception. Strong emotion (fear or rage) suppresses pain, presumably by activation of the above-described descending noradrenergic system. The experience of pain appears to be lessened in manic states and enhanced in depression. Anxious patients in general have the same pain threshold as normal subjects but their reaction may be excessive or abnormal. The pain thresholds of frontal lobotomized subjects are also unchanged but they react to painful stimuli only briefly or casually if at all.

The conscious awareness or perception of pain occurs only when pain impulses reach the thalamocortical level. The precise roles of the thalamus and cortical sensory areas in this mental process are not fully understood. It was believed that the recognition of a noxious stimulus as such is a function of the thalamus and that the parietal cortex is necessary for appreciation of the intensity, localization, and other discriminatory aspects of sensation. This traditional separation of sensation (in this instance, awareness of pain) and perception (awareness of the nature of the painful stimulus) has evolved to the view that sensation, perception, and the various conscious and unconscious responses to a pain stimulus comprise an indivisible process. That the cerebral cortex governs the patient's reaction to pain cannot be doubted. It is also likely that the cortex can suppress or otherwise modify the perception of pain in the same way that corticofugal projections from the sensory cortex modify the rostral transmission of other sensory impulses from thalamic and dorsal column nuclei. It has been shown that central transmission in the spinothalamic tract can be inhibited by stimulation of the sensorimotor areas of the cerebral cortex, and, as indicated above, a number of descending fiber systems have been traced to the dorsal horn laminae from which this tract originates.

The functional imaging studies by Wager and coworkers has given insights into the ensemble of brain regions that are activated by painful stimuli. In addition to the expected thalamic and parietal sensory regions, the hypothalamus, and both insular and cingulate cortices, are prominently involved, in proportion to the intensity of the stimulus. These investigators have sought to develop an imaging "pain signature" that could, in the future, objectify the pain response. Moreover, physical pain in their experiments could be differentiated from social and emotional pain. Whether this reductionist approach to pain will find clinical use is discussed by Jaillard and Ropper.

Endogenous Pain-Control Mechanisms

An important contribution to our understanding of pain has been the discovery of a neuronal analgesia system that can be activated by the administration of opiates or by naturally occurring brain substances that share the properties of opiates. This endogenous system was first demonstrated by Reynolds, who found that stimulation of the ventrolateral periaqueductal gray matter in the rat produced a profound analgesia without altering behavior or motor activity. Subsequently, stimulation of other discrete sites in the medial and caudal regions of the diencephalon and rostral bulbar nuclei (notably raphe magnus and paragigantocellularis) was shown to have the same effect. Under the influence of such electrical stimulation, the animal could be operated on without anesthesia and move around in an undisturbed manner despite the administration of noxious stimuli. Investigation disclosed that the effect of stimulation-produced analgesia (SPA) is inhibition of the neurons of laminae I, II, and V of the dorsal horn, i.e., the neurons that are activated by noxious stimuli. In human subjects, stimulation of the midbrain periaqueductal gray matter through stereotactically implanted electrodes has also produced a state of analgesia, though not consistently. Other sites in which electrical stimulation is effective in suppressing nociceptive responses are the rostroventral medulla (nucleus raphe magnus and adjacent reticular formation) and the dorsolateral pontine tegmentum. These effects are relayed to the dorsal horn gray matter via a pathway in the dorsolateral funiculus of the spinal cord. Ascending pathways from the dorsal horn, conveying noxious somatic impulses, are also important in activating the modulatory network.

Opiates also act pre- and postsynaptically on the neurons of laminae I and V of the dorsal horn, suppressing afferent pain impulses from both the A-δ and C fibers. Furthermore, these effects can be reversed by the opioid antagonist naloxone. Interestingly, naloxone can reduce some forms of stimulation-produced analgesia. Levine and colleagues have demonstrated that not only does naloxone enhance clinical pain, but it also interferes with the pain relief produced by placebos. These observations suggest that the heretofore mysterious beneficial effects of placebos (and perhaps of acupuncture) may be a result of activation of an endogenous system that shuts off pain through the release of pain-relieving endogenous opioids, or *endorphins* (see below). Prolonged pain and fear are the most powerful activators of this endogenous opioid-mediated modulating system. The same system is probably operative under a variety of other stressful conditions; for example, some soldiers, wounded in battle, require little or no analgesic medication ("stress-induced analgesia"). The opiates also act at several loci in the brainstem, at sites corresponding with those producing analgesia when stimulated electrically and generally conforming to areas in which neurons with endorphin receptors are localized.

Soon after the discovery of specific opiate receptors in the central nervous system (CNS), several naturally occurring peptides, which proved to have a potent analgesic effect and to bind specifically to opiate receptors, were identified. These endogenous, morphine-like compounds are generically referred to as *endorphins*, meaning "the morphines within." The most widely studied are β-endorphin, a peptide sequence of the pituitary hormone β-lipotropin, and two other peptides, *enkephalin* and *dynorphin*. They are found in greatest concentration in relation to opiate receptors in the midbrain. At the level of the spinal cord, exclusively enkephalin receptors are found. Figure 8-4 illustrates a theoretical construct of the roles of enkephalin (and substance P) at the point of entry of pain fibers into the spinal cord. A subgroup of dorsal horn interneurons that are in contact with spinothalamic tract neurons also contains enkephalin.

Thus it appears that the central effects of a painful condition are determined by many ascending and descending systems using a variety of transmitters. A deficiency in a particular region would explain persistent or excessive pain. Some aspects of opiate addiction and also the discomfort that follows withdrawal of the drug

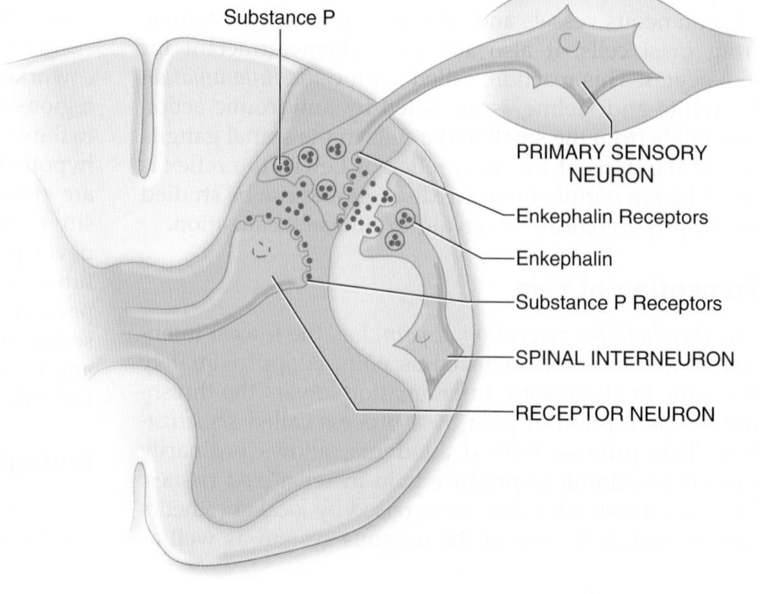

Figure 8-4. Mechanism of action of enkephalin (endorphin) and morphine in the transmission of pain impulses from the periphery to the CNS. Spinal interneurons containing enkephalin synapse with the terminals of pain fibers and inhibit the release of the presumptive transmitter, substance P. As a result, the receptor neuron in the dorsal horn receives less excitatory (pain) impulses and transmits fewer pain impulses to the brain. Morphine binds to unoccupied enkephalin receptors, mimicking the pain-suppressing effects of the endogenous opiate enkephalin.

might conceivably be accounted for in this way. Indeed, it is known that some of these peptides not only relieve pain but suppress withdrawal symptoms.

Finally it should be noted that the descending pain-control systems contain noradrenergic and serotonergic, as well as opiate, connections. A descending norepinephrine-containing pathway, as mentioned, has been traced from the locus ceruleus in the dorsolateral pons to the spinal cord, and its activation blocks spinal nociceptive neurons. The rostroventral medulla contains a large number of serotonergic neurons from which descending fibers inhibit dorsal horn cells concerned with pain transmission, perhaps providing a rationale for the use of certain antidepression medications that are serotonin agonists in patients with chronic pain.

CLINICAL AND PSYCHOLOGIC ASPECTS OF PAIN

Terminology (Table 8-2)

Several terms, related to the experience of altered sensations and pain, are often used interchangeably but each has specific meaning. *Hyperesthesia* is a general term for heightened cutaneous sensitivity. The term *hyperalgesia* refers to an increased sensitivity and a lowered threshold to painful stimuli. Inflammation and burns of the skin are common causes of hyperalgesia. The term *hypalgesia*, or *hypoalgesia*, refers to the opposite state—i.e., a decreased sensitivity and a raised threshold to painful stimuli. A demonstrable reduction in pain perception (i.e., an elevated threshold) associated with an increased reaction to the stimulus once it is perceived, is sometimes referred to as *hyperpathia* (subtly different from hyperalgesia). In this circumstance there is an excessive reaction to all stimuli, even those (such as light touch) that normally do not evoke pain, a symptom termed *allodynia*.

Table 8-2

NOMENCLATURE IN THE DESCRIPTION OF PAIN AND ABNORMAL SENSATION (SEE ALSO TABLE 9-1)

Dysesthesia: Any abnormal sensation described as unpleasant by the patient
Hyperalgesia: Exaggerated pain response from a normally painful stimulus; usually includes aspects of summation with repeated stimulus of constant intensity and aftersensation
Hyperpathia: Abnormally painful and exaggerated reaction to a painful stimulus; related to hyperalgesia
Hyperesthesia (hypesthesia): Exaggerated perception of touch stimulus
Allodynia: Abnormal perception of pain from a normally nonpainful mechanical or thermal stimulus; usually has elements of delay in perception and of aftersensation
Hypoalgesia (hypalgesia): Decreased sensitivity and raised threshold to painful stimuli
Anesthesia: Reduced perception of all sensation, mainly touch
Pallanesthesia: Loss of perception of vibration
Analgesia: Loss of perception of pain stimulus
Paresthesia: Spontaneous positive, prickling sensation that is not unpleasant; usually described as "pins and needles"
Causalgia: Burning pain in the distribution of one or more peripheral nerves

The elicited allodynic pain may have unusual features, outlasting the stimulus and being diffuse, modifiable by fatigue and emotion, and often being mixed with other sensations. The mechanism of these abnormalities is not clear but both hyperpathia and allodynia are common features of neuropathic or neurogenic pain, such as the pain generated by peripheral neuropathy. These features are also exemplified by causalgia, a type of burning pain that results from interruption of a peripheral nerve (see "Causalgia and Reflex Sympathetic Dystrophy").

Skin Pain and Deep Sensibility

As indicated earlier, the nerve endings in each tissue are activated by different mechanisms, and the pain that results is characterized by its quality, locale, and temporal attributes. *Skin pain* is of two types: a pricking pain, evoked immediately on penetration of the skin by a needle point, or a stinging or burning pain that follows in a second or two. Together they constitute the "double response" of Lewis. Both types of dermal pain can be localized with precision. Compression of nerves by the application of a tourniquet to a limb abolishes pricking pain before burning pain because large fibers are more susceptible to pressure. The first (fast) pain is transmitted by the larger (A-δ) fibers and the second (slow) pain, which is somewhat more diffuse and longer lasting, by the thinner, unmyelinated C fibers.

Deep pain from visceral and skeletomuscular structures is usually aching in quality; if intense, it may be sharp and penetrating (knife-like). Occasionally visceral derangements cause a burning type of pain, as in the "heartburn" of esophageal irritation and rarely in angina pectoris. The pain is felt as being deep to the body surface. It is diffuse and poorly localized, and the margins of the painful zone are not well delineated, presumably because of the relative paucity of nerve endings in viscera. Visceral pain produces two additional sensations. First, there is tenderness at remote superficial sites ("referred hyperalgesia") and, second, an enhanced pain sensitivity in the same and in nearby organs ("visceral hyperalgesia"). This is a restatement of Head's early observations, discussed above, and the referred "Head zones," where somatic and visceral sensibility overlap as discussed below. The concept of visceral hyperalgesia has received considerable attention in a number of pain syndromes in reference to the transition from acute to chronic pain, particularly in headache.

Referred Pain

The localization of deep pain of visceral origin raises a number of problems. Deep pain has indefinite boundaries and its location is distant from the visceral structure involved. It tends to be referred not to the skin overlying the viscera of origin but to other areas innervated by the same spinal segment (or segments). This pain, projected to some fixed site at a distance from the source, is called *referred pain*. The ostensible explanation for the site of referral is that small-caliber pain afferents from deep structures project to a wide range of lamina V neurons in the dorsal horn, as do cutaneous afferents. The convergence of deep and cutaneous afferents on the same dorsal horn cells, coupled with the fact that cutaneous afferents are far more numerous than visceral afferents and have direct connections with the thalamus, is probably responsible for the phenomenon.

Because the nociceptive receptors and nerves of any given visceral or skeletal structure may project upon the dorsal horns of several adjacent spinal or brainstem segments, the pain from these structures may be fairly widely distributed. For example, afferent pain fibers from cardiac structures, distributed through segments T1 to T4, may be projected to the inner side of the arm and the ulnar border of the hand and arm (T1 and T2) as well as the precordium (T3 and T4). Once this pool of sensory neurons in the dorsal horns of the spinal cord is activated, additional noxious stimuli may heighten the activity in the whole sensory field ipsilaterally and, to a lesser extent, contralaterally.

The regions of projection of pain that originate in the bones and adjacent ligamentous structures have been called by Kellgren, "sclerotomes." His maps of pain referral patterns were established from studies of the injection of hypertonic saline into muscle and interspinous ligaments. Although dermatomes and sclerotomes overlap, the patterns are slightly different as shown in Fig. 8-5, which is taken from Inman and Saunders. These sclerotomatous projections are useful to neurologists in analyzing the origins of unusual pains of the cranium, spine, and limbs (see Chaps. 10 and 11).

Another peculiarity of localization is *aberrant reference*, explained by an alteration of the physiologic status of the pools of neurons in adjacent segments of the spinal cord. For example, cervical arthritis or gallbladder disease, causing low-grade discomfort by constantly activating their particular segmental neurons, may induce a shift of cardiac pain cephalad or caudad from its usual locale. Once it becomes chronic, any pain may spread quite widely in a vertical direction on one side of the body. On the other hand, painful stimuli arising from a distant site exert an inhibitory effect on segmental nociceptive flexion reflexes in the leg, as demonstrated by DeBroucker and colleagues. Yet another clinical peculiarity of segmental pain is the reduction in power of muscle contraction that it may cause (reflex paralysis, or algesic weakness).

Chronic Pain

One of the most perplexing issues in the study of pain is the manner in which chronic pain syndromes arise. Several theories have been offered, none of which satisfactorily accounts for all the clinically observed phenomena. One hypothesis proposes that in an injured nerve, the unmyelinated sprouts of A-δ and C fibers become capable of spontaneous ectopic excitation and afterdischarge and are susceptible to ephaptic activation. A second proposal derives from the observation that these injured nerves are also sensitive to locally applied or intravenously administered catecholamines because of an overabundance of adrenergic receptors on the regenerating fibers. Either this mechanism or ephapse (nerve-to-nerve cross-activation) is thought to be the basis of causalgia (persistent burning and aching pain in the territory of a partially injured nerve and beyond) and its associated reflex sympathetic dystrophy; either would explain the relief afforded in these conditions by sympathetic block. This subject is discussed in greater detail in relation to peripheral nerve injuries (see "Peripheral Nerve Pain" and Chap. 46).

Central sensory structures, e.g., sensory neurons in the dorsal horns of the spinal cord or thalamus, if chronically bombarded with pain impulses, may become autonomously overactive (being maintained in this state perhaps by excitatory amino acids) and may remain so even after the peripheral pathways have been interrupted. Peripheral nerve lesions have been shown to induce enduring derangements of central (spinal cord) processing (Fruhstorfer and Lindblom). For example, avulsion of nerves or nerve roots may cause chronic pain even in analgesic zones (anesthesia dolorosa or "deafferentation pain"). In experimentally deafferented animals, neurons of lamina V begin to discharge irregularly in the absence of stimulation. Later the abnormal discharge subsides in the spinal cord but can still be recorded in the thalamus. Consequently, painful states such as causalgia, spinal cord pain, and phantom pain are not abolished simply by cutting spinal nerves or spinal tracts.

Certainly none of these phenomena can adequately explain the entire story of chronic pain. It is likely that structural changes in the spinal cord, of the type alluded to above, are able to produce persistent stimulation of pain pathways. Indo and colleagues review the molecular changes in the spinal cord that may give rise to persistence of pain after the cessation of an injurious episode. It is an open question whether the early treatment of pain may prevent the cascade of biochemical events that allows for both spread and persistence of pain in conditions such as causalgia, but it has been the experience of most clinical pain experts that preemptive treatment of certain painful conditions (e.g., herpes zoster) may reduce the risk of a chronic pain syndrome.

Pain has several other singular attributes. It does not appear to be subject to negative adaptation—i.e., pain may persist as long as the stimulus is operative—whereas other somatic stimuli, if applied continuously, soon cease to be perceived. Furthermore, prolonged stimulation of pain receptors sensitizes them, so that they become responsive to even low grades of stimulation, even to touch (allodynia).

The Emotional Reaction to Pain

Another remarkable characteristic of pain is the strong feeling or affect with which it is endowed, nearly always unpleasant. Since pain embodies this element, psychologic conditions assume great importance in all persistent painful states. It is of interest that despite this strong affective aspect of pain, it is difficult to recall precisely, or to reexperience from memory, a previously experienced acute pain. Also, the patient's tolerance of pain and capacity to experience it without verbalization are influenced by culture and personality. Some individuals—by virtue of training, habit, and phlegmatic temperament—remain stoic in the face of pain, and others react in an opposite fashion. In other words, there are inherent variations among individuals that determine the limbic system's response to pain. In this regard, it is important to emphasize that pain may be the presenting or predominant symptom in a depressive illness (Chap. 52). Price reviews this subject of the affective dimension of

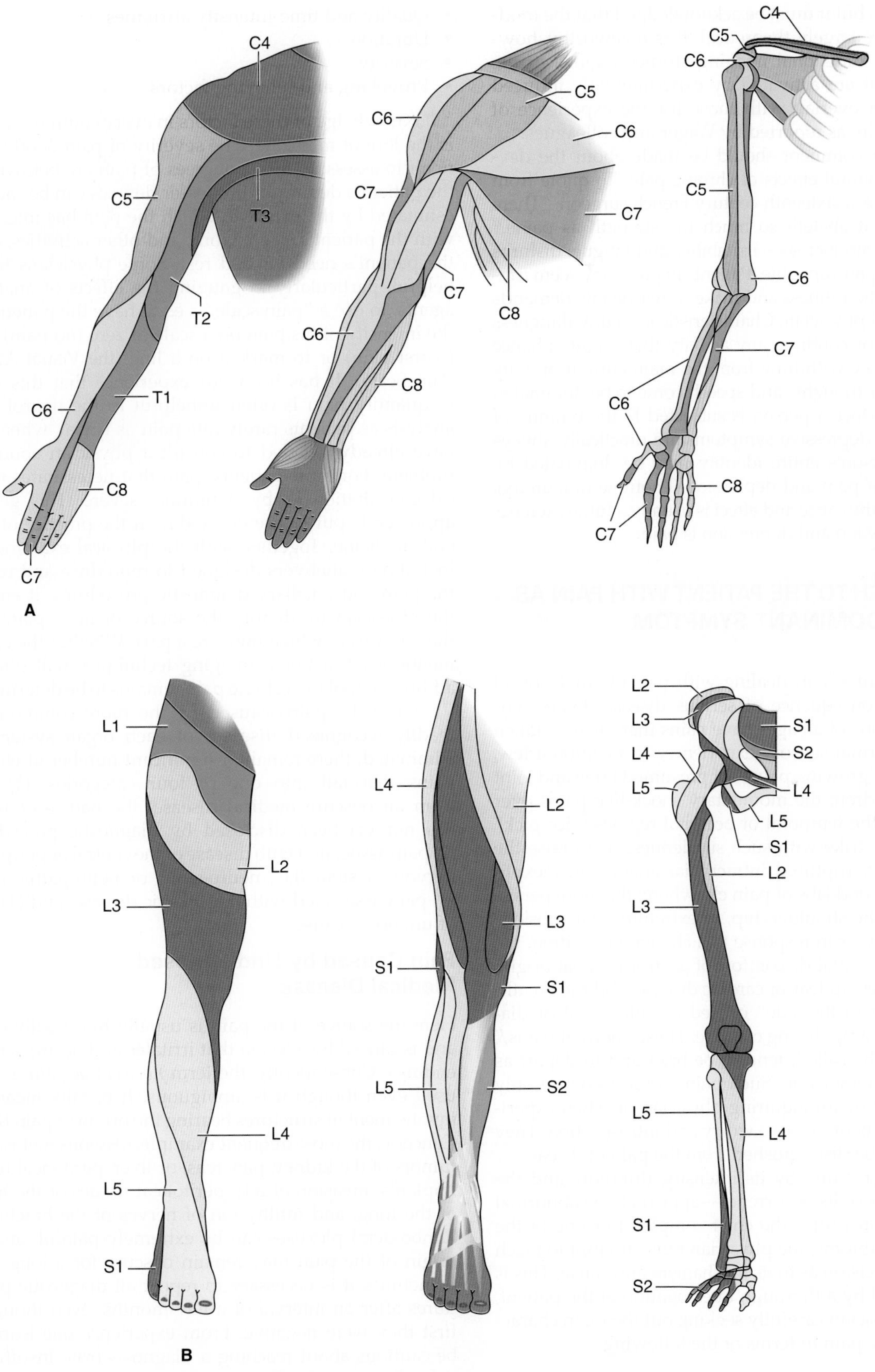

Figure 8-5. Sclerotome maps taken from Inman and Saunders with permission. The projections of pain from osteal and periosteal structures such as ligaments were established by the injection of hypertonic saline or formic acid into the upper extremity (*A*) and lower extremity (*B*) and can also be found in the articles of Kellgren. They may be compared to the dermatomal maps shown in Figs. 9-1 through 9-3.

pain in detail, but it must be acknowledged that the models offered are largely theoretical. It is noteworthy, however, that on functional imaging studies regions of the cerebrum that are activated by experimentally induced physical pain overlap with those for the experience of emotional pain, as reported by Wager and colleagues.

Finally, a comment should be made about the devastating behavioral effects of chronic pain. To quote from Ambroïse Paré, a sixteenth-century French surgeon, "There is nothing that abateth so much the strength as paine." Continuous pain increases irritability and fatigue, disturbs sleep, and impairs appetite. Patients in pain may seem irrational about their illness and make unreasonable demands on family and physician. Characteristic is an unwillingness to engage in or continue any activity that might enhance their pain. They withdraw from the main current of daily affairs as their thoughts and speech come to be dominated by the pain. Once a person is subjected to the tyranny of chronic pain, depressive symptoms are practically always added. A person's entire identity may be dominated by the mixture of pain and depression (l'homme doloureux). Determining the cause and effect is usually a futile exercise. Pain is depression and depression is pain.

APPROACH TO THE PATIENT WITH PAIN AS THE PREDOMINANT SYMPTOM

One learns quickly in dealing with patients that not all pain is the consequence of serious disease. Every day, healthy persons of all ages have pains that must be taken as part of normal sensory experience. To mention a few, there are the "growing pains" of presumed bone and joint origin of children; the momentary shock-like pains over an eye or in the temporal or occipital regions ("ice-pick" pain), which strike with such suddenness as to raise the suspicion of a ruptured intracranial aneurysm; inexplicable split-second jabs of pain elsewhere; the more persistent ache in the shoulder, hip, or extremity that subsides spontaneously or in response to a change in position; the fluctuant precordial discomfort of gastrointestinal origin, which conjures up fear of cardiac disease; and the breathtaking "stitch in the side" caused by intercostal or diaphragmatic cramp during exercise. These "normal pains," as they may be called, tend to be brief and to depart as obscurely as they came. Such pains come to notice only when elicited by an inquiring physician or when experienced by a patient given to worry and introspection. They must always be distinguished from the pain of disease.

Whenever pain—by its intensity, duration, and the circumstances of its occurrence—appears to be abnormal or when it constitutes the chief complaint or one of the principal symptoms, the physician must attempt to reach a tentative decision as to its mechanism and cause. This is accomplished by a thorough interrogation of the patient, with the physician carefully seeking out the main characteristics of the pain in terms of the following:

- Location
- Mode and time of onset
- Associated features, e.g., nausea, muscle spasm
- Quality and time-intensity attributes
- Duration
- Severity
- Provoking and relieving factors

Knowledge of these factors in every common disease is the lore of medicine. The severity of pain is often difficult to assess. Extreme degrees of pain are betrayed by the patient's demeanor but lesser degrees can be roughly estimated by the extent to which the pain has interfered with the patient's sleep, work, and other activities, or by the patient's need for bed rest. Some physicians find it helpful, particularly in gauging the effects of analgesic agents, to use a "pain scale," i.e., to have the patient rate the intensity of his pain on a scale of zero (no pain) to 10 (worst pain) or to mark it on a line (the Visual Analog Pain Scale). It has been our experience that this effort to quantify pain is often unhelpful to the neurological analysis as patients rarely rate pain as trivial, when they have already decided to consult a physician about the problem. For most patients, pain that necessitates medical consultation is, by definition, severe. This general approach is put to use every day in the practice of general medicine. Together with the physical examination, including maneuvers designed to reproduce and relieve the pain and ancillary diagnostic procedures, it enables the physician to identify the source of most pains and the diseases of which they are a part. Whether the earlier mentioned functional imaging techniques will offer an additional tool to evaluate pain remains to be determined.

Once the pains caused by the more common and readily recognized diseases of each organ system are eliminated, there remain a significant number of chronic pains that fall into one of four categories: (1) pain from an obscure medical disease, the nature of which has not yet been disclosed by diagnostic procedures; (2) pain associated with disease of the central or peripheral nervous system (i.e., neurogenic, or neuropathic pain); (3) pain associated with psychiatric disease; and (4) pain of unknown cause.

Pain Caused by Undiagnosed Medical Disease

Here the source of the pain is usually in a bodily organ and is caused by a lesion that irritates and destroys nerve endings. Consequently, the term *nociceptive pain* is often used even though it is ambiguous. It usually means an involvement of structures bearing the origin of pain fibers. Cancer is the most frequent example. Osseous metastases, tumors of the kidney, pancreas, or liver, peritoneal tumor implants, invasion of retroperitoneal tissues or the hilum of the lung, and infiltration of nerves of the brachial or lumbosacral plexuses can be extremely painful, and the origin of the pain may remain obscure for a long time. Sometimes it is necessary to repeat all diagnostic procedures after an interval of a few months, even though at first they were negative. From experience one learns to be cautious about reaching a diagnosis from insufficient data. Treatment in the meantime is directed to the relief of pain, at the same time instilling in the patient a need to cooperate with a program of expectant observation.

Neurogenic, or Neuropathic Pain

These terms are generally used interchangeably to designate pain that arises from direct stimulation of nervous tissue itself, central or peripheral, exclusive of pain as a consequence of stimulation of C fibers by lesions of other bodily structures (i.e., the nociceptive pain described above). This category comprises a variety of disorders involving single and multiple nerves, notably trigeminal neuralgia and those caused by herpes zoster, diabetes, and trauma; neuromas and neurofibromas, a number of polyneuropathies of diverse type; root irritation, e.g., from a prolapsed disc; spinal arachnoiditis and spinal cord injuries; the thalamic pain syndrome of Dejerine-Roussy; and, rarely, parietal lobe infarction such as the ones described by Schmahmann and Leifer. As a rule, lesions of the cerebral cortex and white matter are associated not with pain but with hypalgesia. Schott (1995) reviewed the clinical features that characterize central pain. Particular diseases giving rise to neuropathic pain are considered in their appropriate chapters but the following remarks are of a general nature, applicable to all of the painful states that compose this group.

The sensations that characterize neuropathic pain vary and are often multiple—burning, gnawing, aching, and shooting or lancinating qualities are described. There is an almost invariable association with one or more of the symptoms of hyperesthesia, hyperalgesia, allodynia, and hyperpathia (see above). The abnormal sensations coexist in many cases with a sensory deficit and local autonomic dysfunction. Furthermore, the pain generally responds poorly to treatment, including the administration of opioid medications.

Peripheral Nerve Pain

Painful states that fall into this category are in most cases related to disease of the peripheral nerves, and it is to pain from this source that the term *neuropathic* is more strictly applicable. Pain states of peripheral nerve origin far outnumber those caused by spinal cord, brainstem, thalamic, and cerebral disease. Although the pain is localized to a sensory territory supplied by a nerve, plexus or nerve root, it often radiates to adjacent areas. Sometimes the onset of pain is immediate on receipt of injury; more often it appears at some point during the evolution or recession of the disorder. The disease of the nerve may be obvious, expressed by the usual sensory, motor, reflex, and autonomic changes, or these changes may be undetectable by standard tests. In the latter case, the term *neuralgia* is used.

The postulated mechanisms of peripheral nerve pain are diverse and differ from those of central diseases. Some of the major ideas were mentioned in the earlier section on chronic pain. One mechanism is denervation hypersensitivity, first described by Walter Cannon. He noted that when a group of neurons is deprived of its natural innervation, they become hyperactive. Others point to a reduced density of certain types of fibers in nerves supplying a causalgic zone as the basis of the burning pain but the comparison of the density of nerves from painful and nonpainful neuropathies has not proved to be consistently different. For example, Dyck and colleagues, in a study of painful versus nonpainful axonal neuropathies, concluded that there was no difference between them in terms of the type of fiber degeneration. Also, the occurrence of ectopic impulse generation all along the surface of injured axons and the possibility of ephaptic activation of unsheathed axons seem applicable particularly to some causalgic states. Stimulation of the nervi nervorum of larger nerves by an expanding intraneural lesion or a vascular change was postulated by Asbury and Fields as the mechanism of nerve trunk pain. The sprouting of adrenergic sympathetic axons in response to nerve injury has already been mentioned and is an ostensible explanation for the abolition of causalgic pain by sympathetic blockade. This has given rise to the term *sympathetically sustained pain* for some cases of causalgia, as discussed below.

Regenerating axonal sprouts, as in a neuroma, are also hypersensitive to mechanical stimuli. On a molecular level, it has been shown that voltage-gated sodium channels accumulate at the site of a neuroma and all along the axon after nerve injury, and that this gives rise to ectopic and spontaneous activity of the sensory nerve cell and its axon. Such firing has been demonstrated in humans after nerve injury. This mechanism is concordant with the relief of neurogenic pain by sodium channel-blocking anti-epileptic drugs. Spontaneous activity in nociceptive C fibers is thought to give rise to burning pain; firing of large myelinated A fibers is believed to produce dysesthetic pain induced by tactile stimuli. The abnormal response to stimulation is also influenced by sensitization of central pain pathways, probably in the dorsal horns of the spinal cord, as outlined in the review by Woolf and Mannion. Hyperalgesia and allodynia are thought to result from such a spinal cord mechanism. Several observations have been made regarding the neurochemical mechanisms that might underlie these changes but none provides a consistent explanation. Possibly more than one of these mechanisms is operative in a given peripheral nerve disease.

Evidence that the sodium channel can generate neural pain is given by the extraordinary disease "paroxysmal extreme pain disorder" also known as "familial rectal pain syndrome." Here, a mutation of the sodium channel gene, *SCN9A*, leads to the early onset of paroxysmal autonomic changes and attacks of excruciating deep burning pain in the rectum, eye, or jaw, or diffusely, as described by Fertleman and coworkers. Similar but more diffuse painful states such as erythromelalgia and paroxysmal extreme pain disorder are being uncovered that are predicated on similar voltage-gated sodium channel mutations and more impressively, by the congenital absence of the ability to experience pain due to a loss of function mutation in a sodium channel gene and a mutation in the tyrosine kinase receptor gene. Fischer and Waxman provide a summary of the mutations in the sodium channel gene and their clinical presentations.

Causalgia and Reflex Sympathetic Dystrophy (Complex Regional Pain Syndrome)

Causalgia is the name that Weir Mitchell applied to a rare (except in time of war) type of peripheral neuralgia consequent upon trauma, with partial interruption of the median or ulnar nerve and, less often, the sciatic or peroneal nerve (see also "Chronic Pain" further on and discussion in Chap. 46). It is characterized by persistent, severe pain in the hand or foot, most pronounced in the digits, palm of the hand, or sole. The pain has a burning quality and frequently radiates beyond the territory of the injured nerve. The painful parts are exquisitely sensitive to contact, so the patient cannot bear the pressure of clothing or drafts of air; even ambient heat, cold, noise, or emotional stimuli intensify the causalgic symptoms. The affected extremity is kept protected and immobile, often wrapped in a cloth moistened with cool water. Sudomotor, vasomotor, and, later, trophic abnormalities are usual accompaniments of the pain. The skin of the affected part is moist and warm or cool and soon becomes shiny and smooth, at times scaly, devoid of hair, and discolored.

A number of theories have been proposed to explain the causalgic syndrome. For many years it was attributed to a short-circuiting of impulses, the result of an artificial connection between efferent sympathetic and somatic afferent pain fibers at the point of the nerve injury. The demonstration that causalgic pain could be abolished by depletion of neurotransmitters at sympathetic adrenergic endings shifted the presumed site of sympathetic-afferent interaction to the nerve terminals and suggested that the abnormal cross-excitation is chemical rather than electrical in nature. Another possible explanation is that an abnormal adrenergic sensitivity develops in injured nociceptors and that circulating or locally secreted sympathetic neurotransmitters trigger the painful afferent activity. Another theory holds that a sustained period of bombardment by sensory pain impulses from one region results in the sensitization of central sensory structures. "True causalgia" of this type can be counted on to respond favorably, if only temporarily, to procaine block of the appropriate sympathetic ganglia and, for a longer time, to regional sympathectomy. Prolonged cooling and the intravenous injection of guanethidine, a sympathetic-blocking drug, into the affected limb (with the venous return blocked for several minutes) may alleviate the pain for days or longer. Epidural infusions, particularly of analgesics or ketamine, intravenous infusion of bisphosphonates, and spinal cord stimulators are other forms of treatment (see Kemler et al). The roles of the central and sympathetic nervous systems in causalgic pain have been critically reviewed by Schott and by Schwartzman and McLellan.

Increasingly, reflex sympathetic dystrophy has been reported after limb and bone injury but in the absence of evident damage to adjacent nerves. Oaklander and Fields have speculated that this is due to an induced small fiber neuropathy; limited confirmation of this notion is given by those authors.

Recent investigations have begun to define the molecular changes that occur in sensory neurons and the spinal cord in cases of chronic pain of this type. Alterations in *N*-methyl-D-aspartate (NMDA) receptors, induction of cyclooxygenase and prostaglandin synthesis, and changes in gabanergic inhibition in the dorsal horns are all implicated (Woolf).

The term *causalgia* is, in our view, best reserved for the syndrome described above—i.e., persistent burning pain and local abnormalities of autonomic innervation from trauma to a major nerve in an extremity. Some neurologists use "causalgia" to describe only the burning feature of pain due to partial nerve injury. Others have applied the term to a wide range of conditions that are characterized by persistent burning pain but have only an inconstant association with sudomotor, vasomotor, and trophic changes and an unpredictable response to sympathetic blockade. These latter states, which have been described under a plethora of terms (e.g., complex regional pain syndrome type 2, Sudeck atrophy of bone, minor causalgia, shoulder–hand syndrome, algodystrophy, or algoneurodystrophy), may follow non-traumatic lesions of the peripheral nerves or even lesions of the CNS ("mimocausalgia").

We have no explanation for the so-called causalgia–dystonia syndrome (Bhatia et al) in which a fixed dystonic posture is engrafted on a site of causalgic pain. The clinical features of both the causalgic and dystonic elements of the syndrome have been somewhat unusual in the cases reported. The degree of injury was often trivial or nonexistent and no signs of a neuropathic lesion were evident. Remarkably, both the causalgia and dystonia spread from their initial sites to widely disparate parts of the limbs and body. The syndrome did not respond to any form of treatment, although some patients recovered spontaneously. Another interesting type of causalgia and reflex sympathetic dystrophy follows deep venous thrombosis in a leg and had in the literature been recorded as "algodystrophy." It may be similar to the left shoulder and hand changes that come on months after a myocardial infarction ("shoulder–hand syndrome").

The treatment of reflex sympathetic dystrophy is largely unsatisfactory, although a certain degree of improvement can be expected if treatment is started early and the limb is mobilized. The options for treatment are discussed further on.

Central Neurogenic Pain

There are several configurations of central lesions that damage the sensory system and produce severe pain. Deafferentation of secondary neurons in the posterior horns or of sensory ganglion cells that terminate on them may cause the deafferented cells to become continuously active and, if stimulated by a microelectrode, to reproduce pain. In the patient whose spinal cord has been transected, there may be intolerable pain in regions below the level of the lesion. It may be exacerbated or provoked by movement, fatigue, or emotion and projected to areas disconnected from suprasegmental structures (akin to the phantom pain in the missing part of an amputated limb). Here, and in the rare cases of intractable pain with lateral medullary or pontine lesions, loss of the descending inhibitory systems seems a likely explanation. This may also explain the pain of the Dejerine-Roussy *thalamic syndrome* described in Chap. 9. Altered sensitivity and hyperactivity of central neurons are alternative possibilities.

Further details concerning the subject of neuropathic pain can be found in the older but still informative writings of Scadding and of Woolf and Mannion.

Pain in Association with Psychiatric Diseases

It is not unusual for patients with depression to have pain as a dominant symptom. As emphasized previously, most patients with chronic pain of all types are depressed. Wells and colleagues, in a survey of a large number of depressed and chronic pain patients, have corroborated this clinical impression. Fields has elaborated a theoretical explanation of the overlap of pain and depression. In such cases, one is faced with an extremely difficult clinical problem—that of determining whether a depressive state is primary or secondary. Complaints of weakness and fatigue, depression, anxiety, insomnia, nervousness, irritability, palpitations, etc., are woven into the clinical syndrome, attesting to the prominence of a psychiatric disorder. In some instances the diagnostic criteria for depression cited in Chap. 52 provide some insight, but in others it is impossible to make this determination and may not be necessary as depression and pain are so often coincident. Empiric treatment with antidepressant medication or, failing this, with electroconvulsive therapy is one way out of the dilemma.

Intractable pain may also be the leading symptom of both somatization and conversion reactions. Experienced physicians are familiar with the patient who has undergone multiple surgical procedures to address painful complaints (so-called Briquet disease). The recognition and management of this group of disorders are discussed in Chap. 51.

The desire for compensation (e.g. workman's compensation, disability status) is usually colored by persistent complaints of headaches, neck pain (whiplash injuries), low back pain, and other painful conditions. The question of ruptured disc is often raised, and laminectomy and spinal fusion may be performed (sometimes more than once) on the basis of dubious radiologic findings. Long delay in the settlement of litigation, allegedly to determine the seriousness of the injury, only enhances the symptoms and prolongs the disability. The medical and legal professions have no certain approach to such problems and often work at cross-purposes. We have found that a frank, objective appraisal of the injury, an assessment of any psychiatric problem, and encouragement to settle the legal claims as quickly as possible work in the best interests of all concerned. Although hypersuggestibility and relief of pain by placebos may reinforce the physician's belief that there is a prominent factor of hysteria or malingering (see Chap. 51), such data are difficult to interpret.

The possibility of drug addiction as a motivation for visiting the physician and reporting severe pain should be addressed. It is impossible to assess pain in addicted individuals, for their complaints are woven into their need for medication. Temperament and mood should be evaluated carefully; the physician must remember that the depressed patient often denies feeling dysphoric and may even occasionally smile. The use of alcohol to self-medicate for pain usually indicates a depressive illness or lifelong alcohol dependence. When no medical, neurologic, or psychiatric disease can be established, one may be resigned to managing the painful state by the use of nonnarcotic medications and periodic clinical reevaluations. Such a course, though not altogether satisfactory, is preferable to prescribing excessive opioids or subjecting the patient to ablative surgery.

Chronic Pain of Indeterminate Cause

Pain in the thorax, abdomen, flank, back, face, head, or other part that cannot be traced to any visceral abnormality can create challenging clinical problems. In most cases, obscure neurologic sources, such as a spinal cord tumor and neuroma, have been excluded by repeated examinations and imaging procedures. A psychiatric disorder to which the patient's symptoms and behavior might be attributed cannot be discerned. Yet the patient complains continuously of pain, is disabled, and spends a great deal of effort and resources seeking medical aid.

In such a circumstance, some physicians and surgeons, rather than concede their helplessness, may resort to extreme measures, such as exploratory thoracotomy, laparotomy, or laminectomy. Or they may injudiciously attempt to alleviate the pain and avoid drug addiction by severing roots and spinal tracts, often with the result that the pain moves to an adjacent segment or to the other side of the body.

This type of patient benefits from being seen more than once by the physician. All the medical facts should be reviewed and the clinical and laboratory examinations repeated if some time has elapsed since they were last done. Tumors in the hilum of the lung or mediastinum; in the retropharyngeal, retroperitoneal, and paravertebral spaces; or in the uterus, testicle, kidney, or prostate pose a special difficulty in diagnosis, often being undetected for many months. More than once, we have seen a patient for months before a kidney or pancreatic tumor became apparent. Neurofibroma causing pain in an unusual site, such as one side of the rectum or vagina, is another type of tumor that may defy diagnosis for a long time. Truly neurogenic pain is almost invariably accompanied by alterations in cutaneous sensation and other neurologic signs, the finding of which facilitates diagnosis; however, the appearance of the neurologic signs may be delayed—for example, in brachial neuritis.

Because of the complexity and difficulty in diagnosis and treatment of chronic pain, most medical centers have found it advisable to establish pain clinics. Here a staff of internists, anesthesiologists, neurologists, neurosurgeons, and psychiatrists can review each patient in terms of drug dependence, neurologic disease, and psychiatric problems. Success is achieved by treating each aspect of chronic pain, and addressing the individual's problem rather than treating it generically with emphasis on increasing the patient's tolerance of pain by means of biofeedback, meditation, and related techniques; by using special analgesic procedures (discussed later in the chapter); by establishing a regimen of pain medication that does not lead to a rebound exaggeration of pain between doses; and by controlling depressive illness.

Rare and Unusual Disturbances of Pain Perception

Lesions of the parietooccipital regions of one cerebral hemisphere sometimes have peculiar effects on the patient's capacity to feel and react to pain. Under the title of *pain hemiagnosia*, Hecaen and Ajuriaguerra described several cases of left-sided paralysis from a right parietal lesion, which, at the same time, rendered the patient hypersensitive to noxious stimuli. When pinched on the affected side, the patient, after a delay, became agitated, moaned, and seemed distressed but made no effort to fend off the painful stimulus with the other hand or to withdraw from it. In contrast, if the good side was pinched, the patient reacted normally and moved the normal hand at once to the site of the stimulus to remove it. The motor responses seemed no longer to be guided by sensory information from one side of the body.

There are also two varieties of rare individuals who from birth are totally indifferent to pain coupled with anhidrosis ("congenital insensitivity to pain") or are incapable of feeling pain ("universal analgesia"). The former have been found by Indo and colleagues to have a mutation in the a neural tyrosine kinase receptor, a nerve growth factor receptor; those in the second group suffer from either a congenital lack of pain neurons in dorsal root ganglia, or to a mutation in the sodium channel discussed earlier. A similar loss of pain sensibility is encountered in the Riley-Day syndrome (congenital dysautonomia, see Chap. 26).

The phenomenon of *asymbolia for pain* is another rare and unusual condition wherein the patient, although capable of distinguishing the different types of pain stimuli from one another and from touch, is said to make none of the usual emotional, motor, or verbal responses to pain. The patient seems totally unaware of the painful or hurtful nature of stimuli delivered to any part of the body, whether on one side or the other. The current interpretation of asymbolia for pain is that it represents a particular type of agnosia (analgognosia) or apractagnosia (see Chap. 22), in which the person loses his ability to adapt his emotional, motor, and verbal actions to the consciousness of a nociceptive impression. Pre-frontal lobe lesions from stroke, trauma, tumor, or in former times frontal lobotomy, can produce a version of this syndrome.

Treatment of Intractable Pain

Once the nature of the patient's pain and underlying disease has been determined, therapy must include some type of pain control. Initially, of course, attention is directed to the underlying disease with the idea of eliminating the source of the pain by appropriate medical, surgical, or radiotherapeutic measures. When the primary disease is not treatable, the physician should, if time and the circumstances permit, attempt to use the milder measures for pain relief first—for example, non-narcotic analgesics and antidepressants or anti-epileptic drugs before resorting to narcotics, local nerve blocks or contemplating surgical approaches for pain relief. Not all situations allow this graduated approach, and large doses of narcotics may be required early in the course of illness—for example, to treat the pain of visceral and bone cancer. The same measured strategy is appropriate in the treatment of neuropathic pain and of pain of unclear origin except that one generally stops short of ablative procedures that irrevocably damage nerves or parts of the central nervous system.

The field of pain relief has been changed by the introduction of analgesic procedures that block nerves, alter neural conduction, or administer conventional medications in new ways. These have become the province of pain clinics and hospital pain services usually led by departments of anesthesiology. In addition, a number of special procedures or unique medications are highly effective for pain relief but are unique to specific situations. These include certain forms of headache and limb pain (temporal arteritis and polymyalgia rheumatica treated with corticosteroids, or migraine relief with "triptan" drugs); trigeminal neuralgia, which may be relieved by microvascular decompression of a branch of the basilar artery or by controlled damage of the gasserian ganglion; and painful dystonic disorders that are relieved by the injection of botulinum toxin. Special procedures that have been devised to treat various forms of spinal back pain fall into the same category. The following discussion provides some guidance for the physician who is asked to undertake or participate in the treatment of chronic pain or of neuropathic pain.

Narcotics (Opioids and Opiates)

A useful way in which to undertake the management of chronic pain that affects several parts of the body, as in the patient with metastases, is with codeine or oxycodone taken together with aspirin, acetaminophen, or another nonsteroidal antiinflammatory drug (NSAID), or tramadol. The analgesic effects of these types of drugs are additive, which is not the case when narcotics are combined with diazepam or phenothiazine. Antidepressants and antiepileptic drugs, as discussed further on, may have a beneficial effect on pain even in the absence of overt depression. This is true particularly in cases of neuropathic pain (painful polyneuropathy and some types of radicular pain). Sometimes these non-narcotic agents may, in themselves or in combination with these treatment modalities, be sufficient to control the patient's pain and the use of narcotics can then be kept in reserve.

Should the foregoing measures prove to be ineffective, one must turn to narcotic agents. Methadone and levorphanol are sometimes useful drugs with which to begin, because of their effectiveness by mouth and the relatively slow development of tolerance. Some pain clinics prefer the use of shorter-acting drugs such as oxycodone, given more frequently through the day. The oral route should be used whenever possible, as it is more comfortable for the patient than the parenteral route. Also, the oral route is associated with fewer side effects except for nausea and vomiting, which tend to be worse than with parenteral administration. Should the latter become necessary, one must be aware of the ratios of oral-to-parenteral dosages required to produce

Table 8-3

DRUGS FOR THE MANAGEMENT OF CHRONIC PAIN

GENERIC NAME	ORAL DOSE, mg	INTERVAL	COMMENTS
Nonopioid analgesics			
Aspirin	650	q4h	Enteric-coated preparations available
Acetaminophen	650	q4h	Side effects uncommon
Ibuprofen	400	q4–6h	
Naproxen	250–500	q12h	Delayed effects may be due to long half-life
Ketorolac	10–20	q4–6h	Useful postoperatively and for weaning from narcotics. Can be used intramuscularly
Trisalicylate	1,000–1,500	q12h	Fewer gastrointestinal or platelet effects than aspirin
Indomethacin	25–50	q8h	Gastrointestinal side effects common
Tramadol	50	q6h	Potent nonnarcotic with similar side effects but less respiratory depression
Narcotic analgesics			
Codeine	30–60	q4h	Nausea common
Oxycodone	—	5–10 q4–6h	Usually available combined with acetaminophen or aspirin
Morphine	10 q4h	60 q4h	
Morphine, sustained release	—	90 q12h	Oral slow-release preparation
Hydromorphone	1–2 q4h	2–4 q4h	Shorter acting than morphine sulfate
Levorphanol	2 q6–8h	4 q6–8h	Longer acting than morphine sulfate; absorbed well orally
Methadone	10 q6–8h	20 q6–8h	Delayed sedation because of long half-life
Meperidine	75–100 q3–4h	300 q4h	Poorly absorbed orally; normeperidine is a toxic metabolite
Fentanyl	25 to 100 μg	apply q72h	Parenteral and transcutaneous ("patch") use
Antiepileptic and related drugs			
Phenytoin	100	q6–8h	Side effects of drowsiness, ataxia, nystagmus
Carbamazepine	200–300	q6h	
Gabapentin	300–2,700	q8h	
Pregabalin	25–100	q8h	
Special Agents			
Mexiletine	150–200	q4–6h	Heart block
Ketamine	—	10–25 μg/kg/h IV	Dysphoria, confusion

equivalent analgesia. The main medications used in the treatment of pain are summarized in Table 8-3.

If oral medication fails to control the pain, the parenteral administration of codeine or more potent opioids becomes necessary. One may begin with methadone, dihydromorphine (Dilaudid), or levorphanol, given at intervals of 4 to 6 h because of their relatively long duration of action (particularly in comparison to meperidine). Alternatively, one may first resort to the use of transdermal patches of drugs such as fentanyl, which provide relief for 24 to 72 h and which we have found particularly useful in the treatment of pain from brachial or lumbosacral plexus invasion by tumor and of painful neuropathies such as those caused by diabetes and systemic amyloidosis. Long-acting morphine preparations are useful alternatives.

Should long-continued injections of opiates become necessary, the optimal dose for the relief of pain should be established and the drug then given at regular intervals around the clock, rather than "as needed." The administration of morphine (and other narcotics) in this way represents a laudable shift in attitude among physicians. For many years it was widely believed that the drug should be given in the smallest possible doses, spaced as far apart as possible, and repeated only when severe pain reasserted itself. It has become clear that this approach results in unnecessary discomfort and, in the end, the need to use larger doses. Most physicians now realize that the fear of creating narcotic dependence and the expected phenomenon of increasing tolerance must be balanced against the overriding need to relieve pain. The most pernicious aspect of addiction, that of compulsive drug-seeking behavior with its attendant sociopathic behaviors, occurs only rarely in this setting and usually in patients with a previous history of addiction or alcoholism, with depression as the primary problem, or with certain characterologic disorders that have been loosely referred to as "addiction proneness." Even in patients with severe acute or postoperative pain, the best results are obtained by allowing the patient to determine the dose and frequency of intravenous medication, a method known as patient-controlled analgesia (PCA). Again, the danger of producing addiction is minimal.

Guidelines for the use of orally and parenterally administered opioids for cancer-related pain are contained in the article of Cherny and Foley and in the publication of the U.S. Department of Health and Human Services, which unfortunately, is no longer easily obtained.

The approach outlined above conforms to our understanding about pain-control mechanisms. Aspirin and other NSAIDs are believed to prevent the activation of nociceptors by inhibiting the synthesis of prostaglandins in skin, joints, viscera, and other structures in the peripheral nervous system. Morphine and meperidine given orally, parenterally, or intrathecally presumably produce analgesia by acting as "false" neurotransmitters at opiate receptor sites in the posterior horns of the spinal cord—sites that are normally activated by endogenous opioid peptides. The separate sites of action of NSAIDs and opioids provide an explanation for the therapeutic usefulness of combining these drugs. Opioids not only act directly on the central pain-conducting sensory systems but also exert a powerful action on the affective component of pain.

Supplemental Medications for the Treatment of Pain

Tricyclic antidepressants, especially the methylated forms (imipramine, amitriptyline, and doxepin), block serotonin reuptake and thus enhance the action of this neurotransmitter at synapses and putatively facilitate the action of the intrinsic opiate analgesic system. As a general rule, relief is afforded with tricyclic antidepressants in the equivalent dose range of 75 to 125 mg daily of amitriptyline, but little benefit accrues with higher amounts. The specific serotonin reuptake inhibitors (SSRI) antidepressants seem not to be as effective for the treatment of chronic neuropathic pain (see review by McQuay and colleagues) but these agents have not yet been extensively investigated in this clinical condition.

Antiepileptic drugs (AEDs) have a beneficial effect on many central and peripheral neuropathic pain syndromes but are generally less effective for causalgic pain caused by partial injury of a peripheral nerve. The mode of action of phenytoin, carbamazepine, gabapentin, levetiracetam, and other AEDs in suppressing the lancinating pains of tic douloureux and certain polyneuropathies, as well as pain after spinal cord injury and myelitis, is not fully understood, but they are widely used. Their action has been attributed to the blocking of sodium channels on axons, thereby reducing the evoked and spontaneous activity in nerve fibers. The full explanation is certainly more complex and related to separate central and peripheral sites, as summarized by Jensen. Often, large doses must be utilized—for example, more than 2,400 mg per day for gabapentin for full effect—but the soporific and ataxic effects may be poorly tolerated.

Most often a combination of medications is used for the treatment of intractable chronic pain. A common combination is the addition of gabapentin to an opioid such as morphine, and perhaps not surprisingly, this was superior to either drug alone in a crossover trial in patients with postherpetic neuralgia and diabetic neuropathy conducted by Gilron and colleagues but at the expense of side effects and lower tolerated doses of both drugs.

Table 8-3 summarizes the main analgesics (nonnarcotic and narcotic), antiepileptics, and antidepressant drugs in the management of chronic pain.

Treatment of Cancer Pain

If the patient is ridden with neoplastic disease and will not live longer than a few weeks or months and has widespread pain, surgical measures are usually not advisable. Pain from widespread osseous metastases, even in patients with hormone-insensitive tumors, may be relieved by radiation therapy or by hypophysectomy. If these are not feasible, opioid medications are required and are effective, but they must be prescribed in adequate doses. Many patients prefer transdermal fentanyl to oral or intravenous agents. Usually, nerve section is not a satisfactory way of relieving restricted pain of the trunk and limbs because the overlap of adjacent nerves prevents complete denervation. Other procedures to be considered are the regional delivery of narcotic analogues, such as fentanyl or ketamine by means of an external pump and a catheter that is implanted percutaneously in the epidural space in proximity to the dorsal nerve roots of the affected region; this device can be used safely at home.

Treatment of Neuropathic Pain

The treatment of pain induced by nerve root or intrinsic peripheral nerve disease is a challenge for the neurologist and employs several techniques that are generally administered by an anesthesiologist. One usually resorts first to one of the antiepileptic drugs discussed earlier and listed in Table 8-3. The next simplest treatments are topical; if the pain is regional and has a predominantly burning quality, capsaicin cream can be applied locally, care being taken to avoid contact with the eyes and mouth. The irritative effect of this chemical, which releases substance P, seems in some cases to mute the pain. We have also had success with several concoctions of "eutectic" mixtures of local anesthetic (EMLA) creams or the simpler lidocaine gel with ketorolac, gabapentin, and other medications; these are applied directly to the affected area, usually the feet, in the morning and evening. Concoctions such as topical Ketamine mixed in soy lecithin to produce a gel with drug concentration of 5 mg/ml, have been reportedly useful in treating post herpetic neuralgia according to Quan and associates in a small randomized trial. Aspirin mixed with chloroform in cold cream is said to be very effective in the topical treatment of post herpetic neuralgia, as suggested by King (see Chap. 10). These preparations may provide considerable relief in postherpetic neuralgia and some painful peripheral neuropathies, but they are totally ineffective in others.

Several types of spinal injections, including epidural, root, and facet blocks, have long been used for the treatment of pain. Injections of epidural corticosteroids or mixtures of analgesics and steroids are helpful in selected cases of lumbar or thoracic nerve root pain, and occasionally in painful peripheral neuropathy, but precise criteria for the use of this measure are not well established. Several studies do not support a beneficial effect but there is little doubt, in our view, that quite a few patients are helped, if only for several days or weeks (see Chap. 11). Nerve root blocks with lidocaine or with longer-acting local anesthetics are sometimes helpful in establishing the precise source of radicular pain. Their main therapeutic use in our experience has been for thoracic radiculitis from shingles, chest wall pain after thoracotomy, and diabetic radiculopathy. Similar local injections are used in the treatment of occipital neuralgia. Injection of analgesic compounds into and around facet joints and the extension of this procedure, radiofrequency ablation of the small nerves that innervate the joint, are as controversial as epidural injections, with most studies failing to find a consistent benefit. Despite these drawbacks, we have found both of these approaches very useful when pain can be traced to a derangement of these joints, as discussed in Chap. 11.

The intravenous infusion of lidocaine has a brief beneficial effect on many types of pain, including neuropathic varieties, localized headaches, trigeminal neuralgia, and other facial pains; it is said to be useful in predicting the response to longer-acting agents such as mexiletine, its oral analogue, although this relationship has been erratic in our experience (see Table 8-3). Mexiletine is given in an initial dose of 150 mg per day and slowly increased to a maximum of 300 mg three times daily; it should be used very cautiously in patients with heart block and has fallen very much out of favor in many centers, partly due to cardiac conduction abnormalities during and after the infusion.

Reducing sympathetic activity within somatic nerves by direct injection of the sympathetic ganglia in affected regions of the body (stellate ganglion for arm pain and lumbar ganglia for leg pain) has met with mixed success in neuropathic pain, including that of causalgia and reflex sympathetic dystrophy. A variant of this technique uses regional intravenous infusion of a sympathetic-blocking drug (bretylium, guanethidine, reserpine) into a limb that is isolated from the systemic circulation by the use of a tourniquet. This is known as a "Bier block," after the developer of regional anesthesia for single-limb surgery. These techniques, as well as the administration of clonidine by several routes and the intravenous infusion of the adrenergic blocker phentolamine, is predicated on the concept of "sympathetically sustained pain," meaning pain that is mediated by the interaction of sympathetic and pain nerve fibers or by the sprouting of adrenergic axons in partially damaged nerves. These forms of treatment have been under study for many decades and have given variable results but the most consistent responses to regional sympathetic blockade are obtained in cases of true causalgia resulting from partial injury of a single nerve.

A number of other treatments have proven successful in some patients with reflex sympathetic dystrophy and other neuropathic pains but the clinician should be cautious about their chances of success over the long run. A novel one of these has been the use of bisphosphonates (pamidronate, alendronate), which have been beneficial in painful disorders of bone, such as Paget disease and metastatic bone lesions. It is theorized that this class of drug reverses the bone loss consequent to reflex sympathetic dystrophy but how this relates to pain control is unclear (Schott, 1997). Electrical stimulation of the posterior columns of the spinal cord by an implanted device, as discussed below, has become popular. Another treatment of last resort is the intravenous or epidural infusion of drugs such as ketamine; sometimes this has a lasting effect on causalgic pain.

The approaches enumerated here are usually undertaken in sequence; a combination of drugs—such as gabapentin, narcotics, and clonidine—in addition to anesthetic techniques—is usually required. The ongoing attention and support of the neurologist often becomes the patient's mainstay. Further references can be found in the thorough review by Katz.

Ablative Surgery in the Control of Pain

It is our considered opinion that a program of medical therapy should always precede ablative surgical measures. Only when a variety of analgesic medications (including opioids) and only when certain practical measures, such as regional analgesia or anesthesia, have completely failed, should one turn to neurosurgical procedures. Also, one should be very cautious in suggesting a procedure of last resort for pain that has no established cause as, for example, limb pain that has been incorrectly identified as causalgic because of a burning component but where there has been no nerve injury.

The least-destructive procedure consists of surgical exploration for a neuroma if a prior injury or operation may have partially sectioned a peripheral nerve. Magnetic resonance imaging of the region should be performed first and will demonstrate most such lesions, but we are uncertain if all small neuromas are visualized, and it is this ambiguity that justifies exploration. Another nondestructive procedure is implantation of a spinal electrical stimulator, usually adjacent to the posterior columns. This procedure, in which there is now a resurgence of interest, has afforded only incomplete relief in our patients and may be difficult to maintain in place. However Kemler and colleagues found a sustained reduction in pain intensity and an improved quality of life in patients with intractable reflex sympathetic dystrophy, even after 2 years in a randomized trial. It is clear that careful selection of patients is the best assurance of a good outcome. We can add from experience with our patients that a temporary trial of the stimulator is advisable before committing to its permanent use. The ill-advised use of nerve section and dorsal rhizotomy as definitive measures for the relief of regional pain was discussed above under "Treatment of Intractable Pain."

Spinothalamic tractotomy, in which the anterior half of the spinal cord on one side is sectioned at an upper thoracic level, effectively relieves pain in the opposite leg and lower trunk. This may be done as an open operation or as a transcutaneous procedure in which a radiofrequency lesion is produced by an electrode. The analgesia and thermoanesthesia may last a year or longer, after which the level of analgesia tends to descend and the pain tends to return. Bilateral tractotomy is also feasible but with greater risk of loss of sphincteric control and, at higher levels, of respiratory paralysis. Motor power is nearly always spared because of the position of the corticospinal tract in the posterior part of the lateral funiculus.

Pain in the arm, shoulder, and neck is more difficult to relieve surgically. High cervical transcutaneous cordotomy has been used successfully, with achievement of analgesia up to the chin. Commissural myelotomy by longitudinal incision of the anterior or posterior commissure of the spinal cord over many segments has also been performed, with variable success. Dorsal root entry zone (DREZ) lesions may relieve pain in the distribution of one or two nerve roots. Lateral medullary tractotomy is another possibility but must be carried almost to the mid-line to relieve cervical pain. The risks of this latter procedure and also of lateral mesencephalic tractotomy (which may actually produce pain) are so great that neurosurgeons have abandoned these operations.

Stereotactic surgery on the thalamus for one-sided chronic pain is still used in a few centers and the results have been instructive. Lesions placed in the ventroposterior nucleus are said to diminish pain and thermal sensation over the contralateral side of the body while leaving the patient with all the misery or affective experience of pain; lesions in the intralaminar or parafascicular-centromedian nuclei relieve the painful state without altering sensation (Mark). Because these procedures have not yielded predictable benefits to the patient, they are now seldom used. The same unpredictability pertains to cortical ablations. Patients in whom a severe depression of mood is associated with a chronic pain syndrome have been subjected to bilateral stereotactic cingulotomy or the equivalent—subcaudate tractotomy. A considerable degree of success has been claimed for these operations but the results are difficult to evaluate. Orbito-frontal leukotomy has been discarded because of the personality change that it produces.

Non-Medical Methods for the Treatment of Pain

Included under this heading are certain techniques such as biofeedback, meditation, imagery, acupuncture, spinal manipulation, as well as transcutaneous electrical stimulation. Among the most intriguing treatments has been mirror therapy in which the patient is instructed to perform movements in the painful arm while watching the same moves in a mirror, made by the unaffected arm. The majority of patients in one blinded trial benefitted in terms of pain and mobility, but this study by Cacchio and coworkers included only patients with strokes and paretic limbs, not those with peripheral nerve injury. Each of these may be of value in the context of a comprehensive pain management program, usually conducted in a pain clinic as a means of providing relief from pain and suffering, reducing anxiety, and diverting the patient's attention, even if only temporarily, from the painful body part. Attempts to quantify the benefits of these techniques—judged usually by a reduction of drug dosage—have given mixed or negative results. Nevertheless, it is unwise for physicians to dismiss these methods, as well-motivated and apparently psychologically stable persons have reported subjective improvement with one or another of these methods and in the final analysis, this is what really matters. Conventional psychotherapy in combination with the use of medication and, at times, electroconvulsive therapy can be of benefit in the treatment of associated depressive symptoms, as discussed above (under "Pain in Association with Psychiatric Diseases") but it should not otherwise be expected to change the experience of pain.

Whatever treatment is undertaken, medical, procedural or surgical, the objective should be to allow and encourage increased use and mobilization of the affected limb or part, as success at this is most closely associated with relief of pain and reduced suffering.

References

Amit Z, Galina ZH: Stress-induced analgesia: Adaptive pain suppression. *Physiol Rev* 66:1091, 1986.

Asbury AK, Fields HL: Pain due to peripheral nerve damage: An hypothesis. *Neurology* 34:1587, 1984.

Bhatia KP, Bhatt MH, Marsden CD: The causalgia-dystonia syndrome. *Brain* 116:843, 1993.

Cacchio A, DeBlasis E, Neconzione S, et al: Mirror therapy for chronic complex regional pain syndromes type I and stroke. *New Engl J Med* 361:634, 2009.

Cherny NI, Foley KM: Nonopioid and opioid analgesic pharmacotherapy of cancer pain. *Hematol Oncol Clin North Am* 10:79, 1996.

Cline MA, Ochoa J, Torebjork HE: Chronic hyperalgesia and skin warming caused by sensitized C nociceptors. *Brain* 112:621, 1989.

DeBroucker TH, Cesaro P, Willer JC, LeBars D: Diffuse noxious inhibitory controls in man: Involvement of the spino-reticular tract. *Brain* 113:1223, 1990.

Dyck PJ, Lambert EH, O'Brien PC: Pain in peripheral neuropathy related to rate and kind of fiber degeneration. *Neurology* 26:466, 1976.

Fertleman CR, Ferrie CD, Aicardi J, et al: Paroxysmal extreme pain disorder (previously familial rectal pain syndrome). *Neurology* 69:586, 2007.

Fields HL (ed): *Pain Syndromes in Neurology*. Oxford, Butterworth, 1990.

Fields HL: Depression and pain: A neurobiological model. *Neuropsychiatry Neuropsychol Behav Neurol* 4:83, 1991.

Fields HL: *Pain*. New York, McGraw-Hill, 1987.

Fields HL, Heinricher MM, Mason P: Neurotransmitters in nociceptive modulatory circuits. *Annu Rev Neurosci* 14:219, 1991.

Fields HL, Levine JD: Placebo analgesia—a role for endorphins? *Trends Neurosci* 7:271, 1984.

Fischer TZ, Waxman SG. *Ann N Y Acad Sci* 1184:196, 2010.

Friehs GM, Schröttner O, Pendl G: Evidence for segregated pain and temperature conduction within the spinothalamic tract. *J Neurosurg* 83:8, 1995.

Fruhstorfer H, Lindblom U: Sensibility abnormalities in neuralgic patients studied by thermal and tactile pulse stimulation, in von Euler C (ed): *Somatosensory Mechanisms. Wenner-Grenn International Symposium Series.* New York, Plenum Press, 1984, pp 353–361.

Gilron I, Bailey JM, Tu D: Morphine, gabapentin, or their combination for neuropathic pain. *N Engl J Med* 352:1324, 2005.

Goldscheider A: *Ueber den Schmerz in Physiologischer und Klinischer Hinsicht*. Berlin, Hirschwald, 1884.

Head H, Rivers WHR, Sherren J: The afferent nervous system from a new aspect. *Brain* 28:99, 1905.

Hecaen H, Ajuriaguerra J: Asymbolie è la douleur, ètude anatomo-clinique. *Rev Neurol* 83:300, 1950.

Hughes J, Smith TW, Kosterlitz HW, et al: Identification of two related pentapeptides from the brain with potent opiate agonist activity. *Nature* 258:577, 1975.

Indo Y, Tsurata M, Hayashida Y, et al: Mutations in the TRK/NGF receptor gene in patients with congenital insensitivity to pain and anhidrosis. *Nat Genet* 13:458, 1996.

Inman VT, Saunders JB: Referred pain from skeletal structures. *J Nerv Ment Dis* 99:660, 1944.

Jaillard A, Ropper AH: Pain, heat and emotion with functional MRI. *New Engl J Med* 368:1447, 2013.

Jensen TS: Anticonvulsants in neuropathic pain: Rationale and clinical evidence. *Eur J Pain* 6(Suppl A):61, 2002.

Katz N: Role of invasive procedures in chronic pain management. *Semin Neurol* 14:225, 1994.

Kellgren JH: On the distribution of pain arising from deep somatic structures with charts of segmental pain areas. *Clin Sci* 4: 35, 1939.

Kemler MA, Henrica CW, Barendse G, et al: The effect of spinal cord stimulation in patients with chronic reflex sympathetic dystrophy: Two years' follow-up of the randomized controlled trial. *Ann Neurol* 55:13, 2004.

King RB: Topical aspirin in chloroform and the relief of pain due to herpes zoster and postherpetic neuralgia. *Arch Neurol* 50:1046, 1993.

Lele PP, Weddell G: The relationship between neurohistology and corneal sensibility. *Brain* 79:119, 1956.

Levine JD, Gordon NC, Fields HL: The mechanism of placebo analgesia. *Lancet* 2:654, 1978.

Light AR, Perl ER: Peripheral sensory systems, in Dyck PJ, Thomas PK, Lambert EH, Bunge R (eds): *Peripheral Neuropathy*, 3rd ed. Philadelphia, Saunders, 1993, pp 149–165.

Mannion RJ, Woolf CJ: Peripheral nociception and genesis of persistent pain, in Asbury AK, McKhann GM, McDonald WI, Goadsby PJ, McArthur JC (eds): *Diseases of the Nervous System*. 3rd edition, Cambridge, Cambridge University Press, 2002, pp 873–878.

Mark VH: Stereotactic surgery for the relief of pain, in White JC, Sweet WH (eds): *Pain and the Neurosurgeon*. Springfield, IL, Charles C Thomas, 1969, pp 843–887.

McQuay HJ, Tramer M, Nye BA, et al: A systematic review of antidepressants in neuropathic pain. *Pain* 68:217, 1996.

Melzack R, Casey KL: Localized temperature changes evoked in the brain by somatic stimulation. *Exp Neurol* 17:276, 1967.

Melzack R, Wall PD: Pain mechanism: A new theory. *Science* 150:971, 1965.

Mountcastle VB: Central nervous mechanisms in sensation, in Mountcastle VB (ed): *Medical Physiology*, 14th ed. Vol 1, Part 5. St Louis, Mosby, 1980, pp 327–605.

Nathan PW: The gate-control theory of pain: A critical review. *Brain* 99:123, 1976.

Oaklander AL, Fields HL: Is reflex sympathetic dystrophy/complex regional pain syndrome type I a small-fiber neuropathy? *Ann Neurol* 65:629, 2009.

Price DD: Psychological and neural mechanisms of the affective dimension of pain. *Science* 288:1769, 2000.

Quan D, Wellish M, Gilden DH: Topical Ketamine treatment of post-herpetic neuralgia. *Neurology* 60: 1391, 2003.

Rexed B: A cytotectonic atlas of the spinal cord in the cat. *J Comp Neurol* 100:297, 1954.

Reynolds DV: Surgery in the rat during electrical analgesia induced by focal brain stimulation. *Science* 164:444, 1969.

Rothstein RD, Stecker M, Reivich M, et al: Use of positron emission tomography and evoked potentials in the detection of cortical afferents from the gastrointestinal tract. *Am J Gastroenterol* 91:2372, 1996.

Scadding JW: Neuropathic pain, in Asbury AK, McKhann GM, McDonald WI (eds): *Diseases of the Nervous System: Clinical Neurobiology*, 2nd ed. Philadelphia, Saunders, 1992, pp 858–872.

Schmahmann JD, Leifer D: Parietal pseudothalamic pain syndrome: Clinical features and anatomic correlates. *Arch Neurol* 49:1032, 1992.

Schott GD: From thalamic syndrome to central poststroke pain. *J Neurol Neurosurg Psychiatry* 61:560, 1996.

Schott GD: Bisphosphonates for pain relief in reflex sympathetic dystrophy. *Lancet* 350:1117, 1997.

Schott GD: Mechanisms of causalgia and related clinical conditions. *Brain* 109:717, 1986.

Schott GD: Reflex sympathetic dystrophy. *J Neurol Neurosurg Psychiatry* 71:291, 2001.

Schwartzman RJ, McLellan TL: Reflex sympathetic dystrophy: A review. *Arch Neurol* 44:555, 1987.

Silverman DH, Munakata JA, Ennes H, et al: Regional cerebral activity in normal and pathological perception of visceral pain. *Gastroenterology* 112:64, 1997.

Sinclair D: *Mechanisms of Cutaneous Sensation*. Oxford, Oxford University Press, 1981.

Snyder SH: Opiate receptors in the brain. *N Engl J Med* 296:266, 1977.

Taub A, Campbell JN: Percutaneous local electrical analgesia: Peripheral mechanisms, in *Advances in Neurology*. Vol 4: *Pain*. New York, Raven Press, 1974, pp 727–732.

Trotter W, Davies HM: Experimental studies in the innervation of the skin. *J Physiol* 38:134, 1909.

U.S. Department of Health and Human Services: *Management of Cancer Pain: Clinical Practice Guideline Number 9*. AHCPR Publications No. 94-0592 and 94-0593, Rockville, Public Health Service, Agency for Health Care Policy and Research, March 1994.

Von Euler US, Gaddum JH: An unidentified depressor substance in certain tissue extracts. *J Physiol* 70:74, 1931.

Von Frey M: Untersuchungen Über die Sinnesfunctionen der menschlichen Haut: I. Druckempfindung und Schmerz. *Königl Sächs Ges Wiss Math Phys Kl* 23:175, 1896.

Wager, TD, Atlas LY, Lindquist MA, et al: An fMRI-based neurologic signature of physical pain. *New Engl J Med* 368:1388, 2013.

Wall PD, Melzack R (eds): *Textbook of Pain*, 4th ed. New York, Churchill Livingstone, 1999.

Walshe FMR: The anatomy and physiology of cutaneous sensibility. A critical review. *Brain* 65:48, 1942.

Weddell G: The anatomy of cutaneous sensibility. *Br Med Bull* 3:167, 1945.

Wells KB, Stewart A, Hays RD, et al: The functioning and well-being of depressed patients. *JAMA* 262:914, 1989.

White D, Helme RD: Release of substance P from peripheral nerve terminals following electrical stimulation of sciatic nerve. *Brain Res* 336:27, 1985.

Woolf CJ: Pain: Moving from symptom control toward mechanism-specific pharmacologic management. *Ann Intern Med* 140:441, 2004.

Woolf CJ, Mannion RJ: Neuropathic pain: Aetiology, symptoms, mechanisms, and management. *Lancet* 353:1959, 1999.

Yaksh TL, Hammond DL: Peripheral and central substrates involved in the rostrad transmission of nociceptive information. *Pain* 13:1, 1982.

9

Other Somatic Sensation

Sensory and motor functions are interdependent, as was dramatically illustrated by the early animal experiments of Claude Bernard and Charles Sherrington, in which practically all effective movement of a limb was abolished by eliminating only its sensory innervation (sectioning of posterior roots). Interruption of other sensory pathways and destruction of the parietal cortex also has profound effects on motility. To a large extent, human motor activity depends on a constant influx of sensory impulses (most of them not consciously perceived). Sensory motor integration is therefore necessary for normal nervous system function but disease may affect motor or sensory functions independently. There may be loss or impairment of sensory function, and this can represent the principal manifestation of neurologic disease.

This chapter deals with general somatic sensation, i.e., afferent impulses that arise in the skin, muscles, or joints. One form of somatic sensation—pain—was discussed in Chap. 8. Because of its overriding clinical importance, pain has been accorded a chapter of its own, but that chapter and this chapter are of one piece. The special senses—vision, hearing, taste, and smell—are considered in the next section (Chaps. 12 to 15), and visceral sensation, most of which does not reach consciousness, is considered with the disorders of the autonomic nervous system (Chap. 26).

ANATOMIC AND PHYSIOLOGIC CONSIDERATIONS

An understanding of sensory disorders depends upon knowledge of functional anatomy. It is necessary to be familiar with the sensory receptors in the skin and deeper structures, the distribution of the peripheral nerves and roots, and the pathways by which sensory impulses are conveyed from the periphery and through the spinal cord and brainstem to the thalamus and cerebral cortex. These aspects of sensory anatomy and physiology were touched upon in Chap. 8 in relation to the perception of pain and are elaborated upon here to include all forms of somatic sensation. An appropriate starting point is Fig. 9-1 that shows the cutaneous distribution of the peripheral nerves.

All sensation depends on impulses that are excited by stimulation of receptors and conveyed to the central nervous system by afferent (sensory) fibers. Sensory receptors are of two general types: those in the skin, mediating superficial sensation (*exteroceptors*), and those in the deeper somatic structures (*proprioceptors*). Skin receptors are particularly numerous and transduce four types of sensory experience: warmth, cold, touch, and pain; these are conventionally referred to as *sensations* or *senses*, e.g., tactile sensation or sense of touch. Proprioceptors inform us of the position of our body or parts of our body; of the force, direction, and range of movement of the joints (kinesthetic sense); and a sense of pressure, both painful and painless. Histologically, a wide variety of sensory receptors have been described, varying from simple, free dendrite terminals to highly branched and encapsulated structures, the latter bearing the names of the anatomists who first described them (see below). These are called "dendrites" because the direction of flow of physiologic activity and of sensory information from these structures in the periphery is toward the cell body.

Mechanisms of Cutaneous Sensation

As indicated in the preceding chapter, it had been thought that each of the primary modalities of cutaneous sensation is subserved by a morphologically distinct end organ, each with its separate peripheral nerve fibers. According to this formulation, postulated by von Frey, each type of end organ was thought to respond only to a particular type of stimulus and to subserve a specific modality of sensation: Meissner corpuscles (named after Georg Meissner), touch; Merkel discs (named after Friedrich Sigmund Merkel), pressure; Ruffini plumes (names after Angelo Ruffini), warmth and skin stretch; Krause end bulbs (named after Wilhelm Krause), cold; Pacini (pacinian) corpuscles (named after Filippo Pacini), vibration and tickle; and for pain, nerve endings that not associated with transducer ("free nerve endings"). The last of these are also termed "naked" because they are surrounded by Schwann cells but are not myelinated (Fig. 9-2).

This *specificity theory*, as it came to be called, has held up best in respect to the peripheral mechanisms for pain, insofar as certain primary afferent fibers, namely the

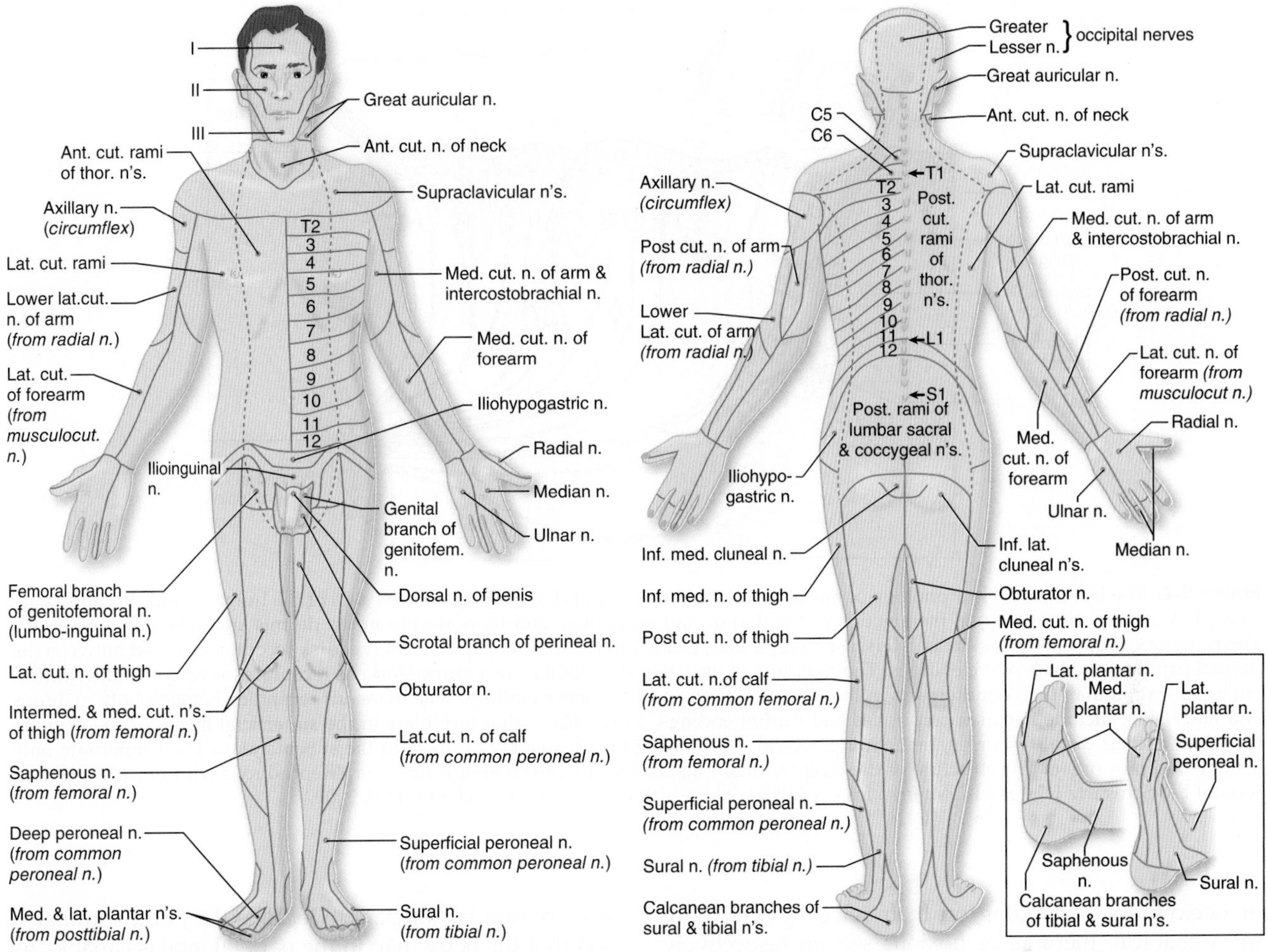

Figure 9-1. The cutaneous fields of peripheral nerves. (Reproduced by permission from Haymaker W, Woodhall B: *Peripheral Nerve Injuries*, 2nd ed. Philadelphia, Saunders, 1953.)

C and A-δ fibers and their free nerve ending receptors, respond maximally to noxious stimuli. Even these freely branching receptor endings and their pain fibers convey considerable non-noxious information; that is, their specificity as pain fibers is not absolute (Chap. 8). Nor has it been possible to ascribe a specific function to each of the many other types of receptors. Thus, Merkel discs and Meissner corpuscles within nerve plexuses around the hair follicles, and free nerve endings can all be activated by moving or stationary tactile stimuli. Conversely, a single type of receptor seems capable of generating more than one sensory modality. Lele and Weddell found that with appropriate stimulation of the cornea, each of the four primary modalities of somatic sensibility (touch, warmth, cold, pain) could be recognized, even though the cornea contains only fine, free nerve endings. In the outer ear, which is also sensitive to these four modalities, only two types of receptors—freely ending and perifollicular—are present. The lack of organized receptors—e.g., the end bulbs of Krause and Ruffini—in the cornea and ear makes it evident that these types of receptors are not essential for the recognition of cold and warmth as von Frey and other early anatomists had postulated.

Particularly instructive have been the observations of Kibler and Nathan, who studied the responses of warm and cold spots to different stimuli. (Warm and cold spots are those small areas of skin that respond most consistently to thermal stimuli with a sensation of warmth or cold.) They found that a cold stimulus applied to a warm spot gave rise to a sensation of cold and that a noxious stimulus applied to a warm or cold spot gave rise only to a painful sensation; they also noted that mechanical stimulation of these spots gave rise to a sensation of touch or pressure. These observations indicate that cutaneous receptors, some not easily distinguishable from one another on morphologic grounds, are probably endowed with only a relative degree of specificity, in the sense that each responds *preferentially* (i.e., has a lower threshold) to one particular form of stimulation. However, among the freely branching nociceptors there is some degree of specialization, as discussed in Chap. 8. Such end organs can then be classed as mechanoreceptors, thermoreceptors,

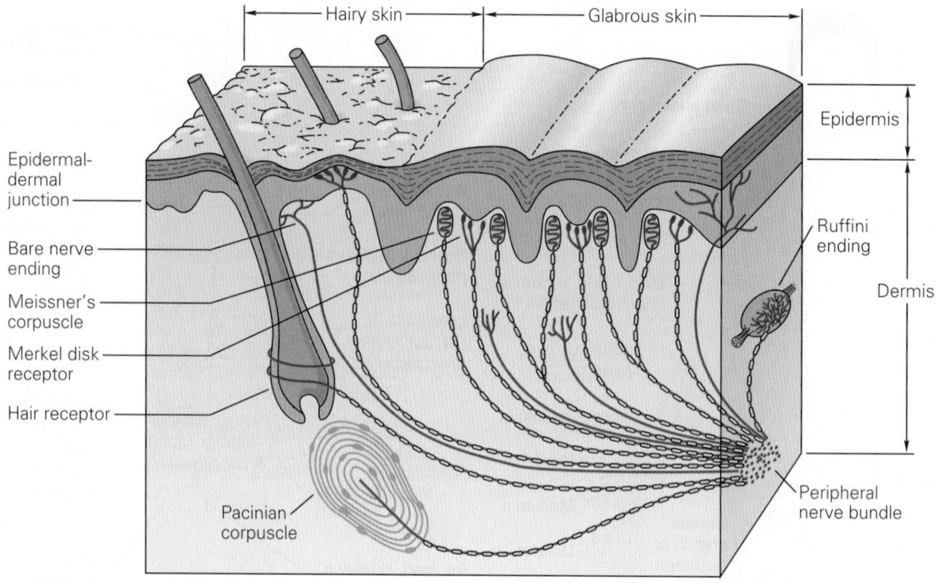

Figure 9-2. The location and morphology of mechanoreceptors in hairy and hairless (glabrous) skin of the human hand. Receptors are located in the superficial skin, at the junction of the dermis and epidermis, and more deeply in the dermis and subcutaneous tissue. The receptors of the glabrous skin are Meissner's corpuscles, located in the dermal papillae; Merkel disk receptors, located between the dermal papillae; and bare nerve endings. The receptors of the hairy skin are hair receptors, Merkel's receptors (having a slightly different organization than their counterparts in the glabrous skin), and bare nerve endings. Subcutaneous receptors, beneath both glabrous and hairy skin, include Pacinian corpuscles and Ruffini endings. Nerve fibers that terminate in the superficial layers of the skin are branched at their distal terminals, innervating several nearby receptor organs; nerve fibers in the subcutaneous layer innervate only a single receptor organ. The structure of the receptor organ determines its physiological function. (Reproduced with permission from Kandel ER, Schwartz JH, Jessell TM: *Principles of Neural Science*, 4th ed. New York: McGraw-Hill, 2000.)

or nociceptors, depending on their selective sensitivity to mechanical, thermal, or noxious stimuli respectively (Sinclair; Light and Perl).

Physiologic studies have shown that the *quality* of sensation depends on the type of nerve fiber that is activated. Different diseases therefore evoke a variety of sensory symptoms. Microstimulation of single sensory fibers in a peripheral nerve of an awake human subject arouses different sensations, depending on which fibers are stimulated and not on the frequency of stimulation. On the other hand, the frequency of stimulation governs the *intensity* of sensation, as does the number of sensory units that are stimulated. Stated somewhat differently, afferent impulse frequency (*temporal summation*) is encoded by the brain in terms of magnitude or intensity of sensation. In addition, as the intensity of stimulation increases, more sensory units are activated (*spatial summation*).

Localization of a stimulus was formerly thought to depend on the simultaneous activation of overlapping sensory units. Tower defined a peripheral sensory unit as a dorsal root ganglion cell, its central and distal processes, and all the sensory endings in the territory supplied by those distal processes (the receptive field of the sensory cell). In the very sensitive pulp of the finger, where the error of localization is less than 1 mm, there are 240 overlapping, low-threshold mechanoreceptors per square centimeter. Highly refined physiologic techniques have demonstrated that activation of even a single sensory unit is sufficient to localize the point stimulated and that the body map in the parietal lobe is capable, by its modular columnar organization, of encoding such refined topographic information. Also, each point in the skin that is stimulated may involve more than one type of receptor. To gain access to its receptor, a stimulus must pass through the skin and possess sufficient energy to transduce, i.e., depolarize, the nerve ending.

Not only does the threshold of stimulation vary but the nerve impulse that is generated is a graded one, not an all-or-none phenomenon like an action potential in nerve. This poorly understood peripheral generator potential determines the freqsuency of impulses in the nerve and to what degree it is sustained or fades out (i.e., adapts to the stimulus or fatigues). However, the mechanism by which a stimulus is translated into a sensory experience, i.e., is encoded, is now partially understood. Special molecules transduce physical alterations by opening cationic channels. As mentioned in Chap. 8, these changes lead to the opening of voltage-gated sodium channels, which generates an action potential. It is probably fair to say that each type of specialized ending has a membrane structure that facilitates the transduction process for a particular type of stimulus. In general, the encapsulated endings, which are more highly myelinated, are of low-threshold type, variably adaptable to continued stimulation (Meissner and pacinian corpuscles are rapidly adapting; Merkel discs and Ruffini endings are slowly adapting) and are connected to large sensory fibers (see Lindblom and Ochoa). The pacinian receptors are the most deeply situated (Fig. 9-1).

Sensory Pathways

Sensory Nerves

Fibers that mediate superficial sensation are located in cutaneous sensory or mixed sensorimotor nerves. In cutaneous nerves, unmyelinated pain and autonomic fibers exceed myelinated fibers by a ratio of 3 or 4:1. The myelinated fibers are of two types: small, lightly myelinated, A-δ fibers for pain and cold, as discussed in Chap. 8, and larger, faster-conducting A-α fibers for touch and pressure. Nonmyelinated autonomic fibers are efferent (postganglionic) and innervate piloerector muscles, sweat glands, and blood vessels. The differing conduction velocities of the fibers of these are discussed in Chap. 45.

A single cutaneous (touch, pain, and temperature) type of afferent fiber connects to several receptors, all of one type, which are irregularly distributed in the skin and account for sensory spots. Stimuli from a given spot are therefore conveyed by two or more fibers. The proprioceptive fibers subserve pressure sense and, with endings in articular structures, the sense of position and movement; they enable one to discriminate the form, size, texture, and weight of objects. Sensations of tickle, itch, and wetness are believed to arise from combinations of several types of receptors.

Itch is a distinctive sensation that can be separated on clinical and neurophysiologic grounds from touch and from pain. Two aspects are recognized: a brief primary localized itch at the site of stimulus or injury, and a subsequent more diffuse sensation that is greatly intensified by gentle touch. Itch sensation is transmitted by specific C fibers, not by touch mechanisms, for regions of analgesia no longer can be stimulated to itch but areas anesthesia retain this sensation. There is, however, no specialized peripheral itch receptor, the sensation depending instead on the spinal connections to itch pathways. Several forebrain regions are activated by itch, i.e., there is no central "itch center." From the perspective of neurologic diseases, the main cause of itch is postherpetic neuralgia, but cases of paroxysmal itch of central origin are known to be caused by multiple sclerosis. The pathophysiology of itching has been discussed by Greaves and Wall and is reviewed further by Yosipovitch and colleagues.

Spinal Roots

All the sensory neurons have their cell bodies in the dorsal root ganglia. The peripheral extensions of these cells constitute the sensory nerves; the central projections of these same cells form the posterior (dorsal) roots and enter the spinal cord. Each dorsal root contains all the fibers from skin, muscles, connective tissue, ligaments, tendons, joints, bones, and viscera that lie within the distribution of a single body segment (somite). This segmental innervation has been amply demonstrated in humans and animals by observing the effects of lesions that involve one or two spinal nerves, such as (1) herpes zoster, which also causes visible vesicles in the corresponding area of skin; (2) the effects of a prolapsed intervertebral disc, which causes hypalgesia in a single root zone; and (3) surgical section of several roots on each side of an intact root (method of remaining sensibility). Maps of the dermatomes derived from these several types of data are shown in Figs. 9-3 and 9-4. It should be noted that there is considerable overlap from one dermatomal segment to the other, more so for touch than for pain. By contrast, there is less overlap between adjacent

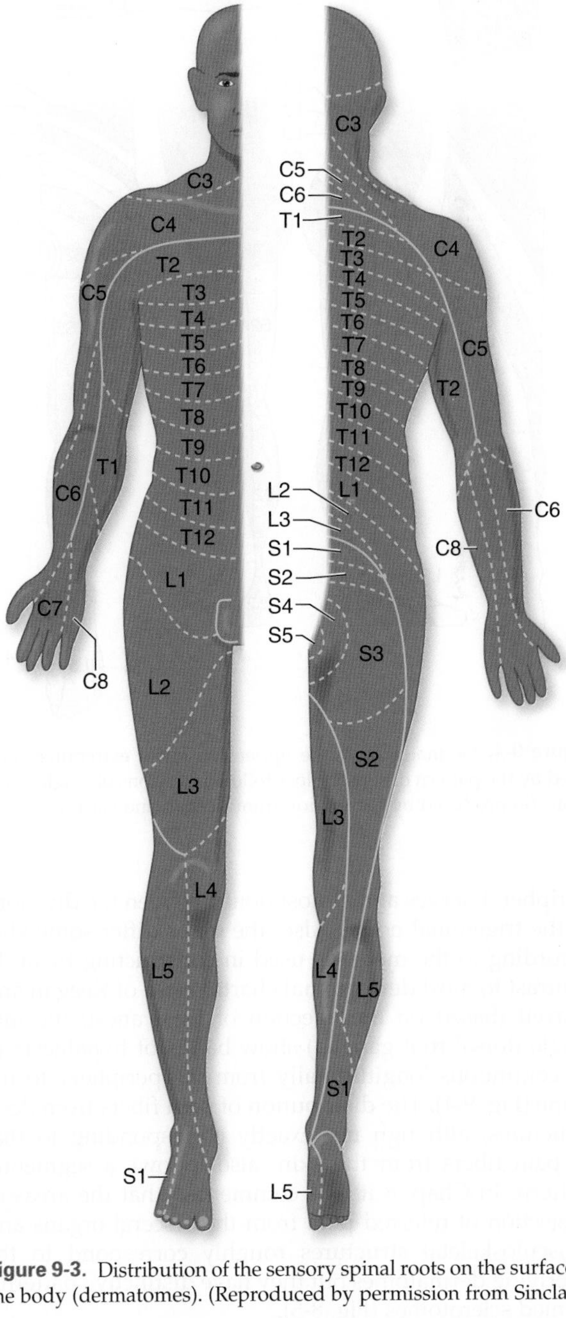

Figure 9-3. Distribution of the sensory spinal roots on the surface of the body (dermatomes). (Reproduced by permission from Sinclair.)

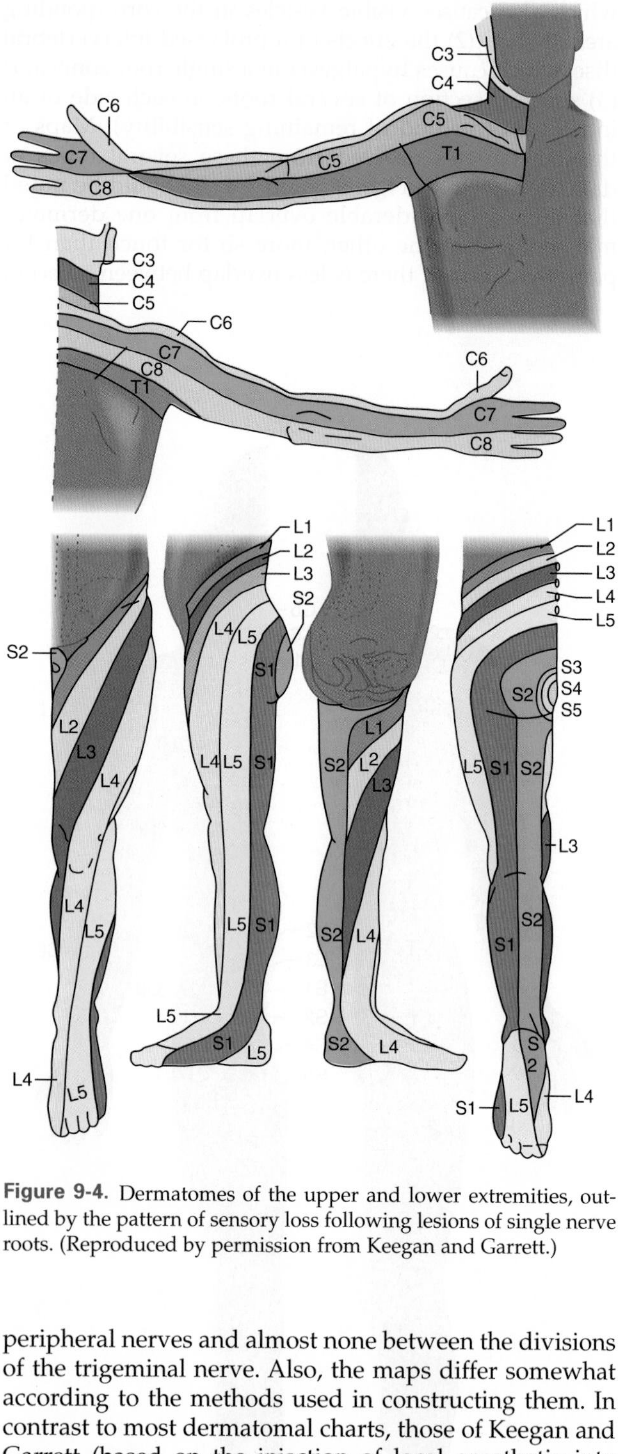

Figure 9-4. Dermatomes of the upper and lower extremities, outlined by the pattern of sensory loss following lesions of single nerve roots. (Reproduced by permission from Keegan and Garrett.)

peripheral nerves and almost none between the divisions of the trigeminal nerve. Also, the maps differ somewhat according to the methods used in constructing them. In contrast to most dermatomal charts, those of Keegan and Garrett (based on the injection of local anesthetic into single dorsal root ganglia) show bands of hypalgesia to be continuous longitudinally from the periphery to the spine (Fig. 9-4). The distribution of pain fibers from deep structures, although not exactly corresponding to that of pain fibers from the skin, also follows a segmental pattern. In Chap. 8 it was commented that the areas of projection of referred pain from the visceral organs and musculoskeletal structures roughly correspond to the overlying dermatomes but they have distinctive patterns, termed sclerotomes (Fig. 8-5).

Posterior Root Entry Zone, Dorsal Horns and Posterior Columns

In the dorsal roots, the sensory fibers are first rearranged according to function. Large and heavily myelinated fibers enter the cord just medial to the dorsal horn and divide into ascending and descending branches. The descending fibers and some of the ascending ones enter the gray matter of the dorsal horn within a few segments of their entrance and synapse with nerve cells in the posterior horns as well as with large ventral horn cells that subserve segmental reflexes. Some of the ascending fibers run uninterruptedly in the dorsal columns of the *same side of the spinal cord*, terminating in the gracile and cuneate nuclei in the upper cervical spinal cord and medulla (Fig. 9-5). The central axons of the primary sensory neurons are joined in the posterior columns by other secondary neurons whose cell bodies lie in the posterior horns of the spinal cord (see below). The fibers in the posterior columns assume a medial position as new fibers from each successively higher root are added laterally, thereby creating somatotopic laminations (see Fig. 8-3).

Of the long ascending posterior column fibers, which are activated by mechanical stimuli of skin and subcutaneous tissues and by movement of joints, only about 25 percent (from the lumbar region) reach the gracile nuclei at the upper cervical cord. The remaining fibers send collaterals to, or terminate in, the dorsal horns of the spinal cord, at least in the cat (Davidoff). An estimated 20 percent of ascending fibers originate from cells in Rexed layers IV and V of the posterior horns (see Fig. 8-1) and convey impulses from low-threshold mechanoreceptors that are sensitive to hair movement, skin pressure, or noxious stimuli. There are also descending fibers in the posterior columns, including fibers from cells in the dorsal column nuclei.

The posterior columns contain a portion of the fibers for the sense of touch as well as the fibers mediating the senses of touch-pressure, vibration, direction of movement and position of joints, and stereoesthesia—recognition of surface texture, shape, numbers, and figures written on the skin and two-point discrimination—all of which depend on patterns of touch-pressure (see Fig. 8-2). The nerve cells of the nuclei gracilis and cuneatus and accessory cuneate nuclei give rise to a secondary afferent path, which crosses the midline in the medulla and ascends as the medial lemniscus to the posterior thalamus. However, the fiber pathways in the posterior columns are not the sole mediators of proprioception in the spinal cord (see "Posterior [Dorsal] Column Syndrome" further on).

In addition to the well-defined posterior column pathways, there are cells in the more loosely structured "reticular" part of the dorsal column that receive secondary ascending fibers from the dorsal horns of the spinal cord and from ascending fibers in the posterolateral columns. These dorsal column fibers project to brainstem nuclei, cerebellum, and thalamic nuclei. Many other cells of the dorsal horn nuclei are interneurons, with both excitatory and inhibitory effects on local reflexes or on the primary ascending neurons. They are also under the influence of the sensorimotor cortex. Some act on descending corticospinal motor neurons. The functions

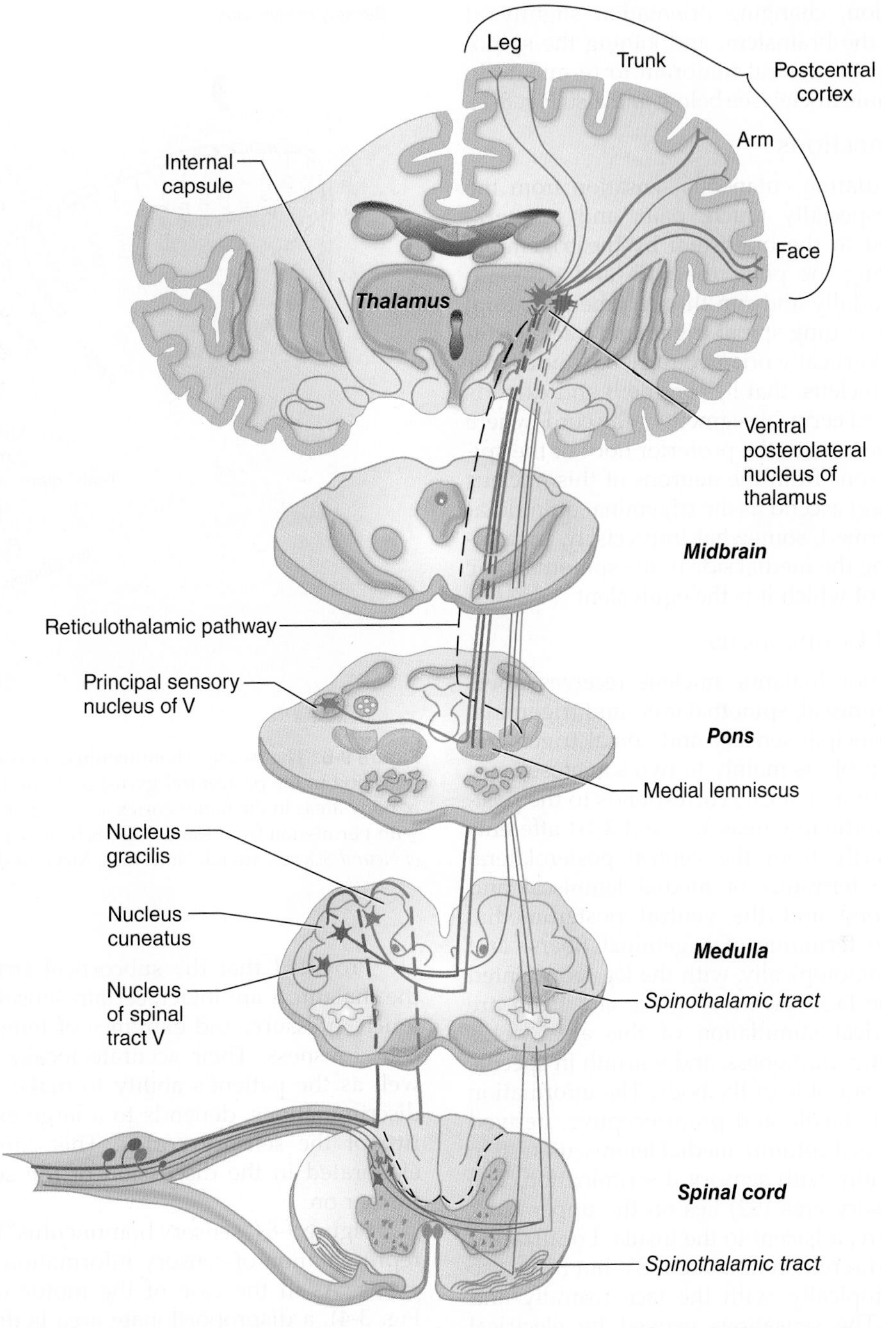

Figure 9-5. The main somatosensory pathways emphasizing the posterior column–lemniscal system (*thicker tract lines*). See Fig. 8-2 for comparison with the spinothalamic system.

of many of the extrathalamic projections of dorsal column cells are unknown (Davidoff).

Thinly myelinated or unmyelinated fibers, subserving mainly pain sensibility, but some sensitive to touch and pressure, enter the cord on the lateral aspect of the dorsal horn and synapse with dorsal horn cells, mainly within a segment or two of their point of entry into the cord. The dorsal horn cells, in turn, give rise to secondary sensory fibers, some of which may ascend ipsilaterally but most of which decussate and ascend in the spinothalamic tracts, as described in Chap. 8 (see Figs. 8-1 and 8-2). Observations based on surgical interruption of the anterolateral funiculus indicate that fibers mediating touch and deep pressure occupy the ventromedial part (anterior spinothalamic tract). Also as remarked in Chap. 8, an ascending tract of secondary sensory axons lies in or medial to the descending corticospinal system.

After the posterior columns terminate in the gracile and cuneate nuclei of the rostral cervical cord and medulla, synapses are made with fibers that cross the midline and ascend to form the medial lemniscal tracts in the brainstem. The lemniscal system is situated in a paramedian position, changing orientation slightly at different levels of the brainstem, and joining the spinothalamic system in the rostral midbrain to terminate in the posterior thalamic nuclei (see below and also Fig. 8-2).

Trigeminal Connections

The pathways mediating cutaneous sensation from the face and head—especially touch, pain, and temperature—are conveyed to the brainstem by the trigeminal nerve. After entering the pons, the pain and temperature fibers turn caudally and run through the ipsilateral medulla as the descending spinal trigeminal tract, terminating in the long, vertically oriented nucleus caudalis, or spinal trigeminal nucleus, that lies beside it and extends to the second or third cervical segment of the cord, where it becomes continuous with the posterior horn of the spinal gray matter. Axons from the neurons of this nucleus cross the midline and ascend as the trigeminal quintothalamic tract (also termed, somewhat imprecisely, trigeminal lemniscus) along the medial side of the spinothalamic tract (see Fig. 8-2), of which it is the equivalent.

Thalamocortical Connections

The ventral posterior thalamic nucleus receives fibers from the medial lemniscal, spinothalamic, and trigeminal (fibers from the principal sensory and spinal trigeminal nuclei) tracts, and projects mainly to two somatosensory cortical areas. The first area (S1) corresponds to the postcentral cortex or Brodmann areas 3, 1, and 2. S1 afferents are derived primarily from the ventral posterolateral nucleus (VPL, the terminus of medial lemniscal and spinothalamic fibers) and the ventral posteromedial nucleus (VPM, the terminus of trigeminal fibers) and are distributed somatotopically, with the leg represented uppermost and the face lowermost (face and hand are juxtaposed). Electrical stimulation of this area yields sensations of tingling, numbness, and warmth in specific regions on the *opposite* side of the body. The information transmitted to S1 is tactile and proprioceptive, derived mainly from the dorsal column–medial lemniscus system and concerned mainly with sensory discrimination. The second somatosensory area (S2) lies on the upper bank of the sylvian fissure, adjacent to the insula. Localization of function is less discrete in S2 than in S1, but S2 is also organized somatotopically, with the face rostrally and the leg caudally. The sensations evoked by electrical stimulation of S2 are much the same as those of S1 but, in distinction to the latter, may be felt bilaterally. Of note is the failure of cortical stimulation to evoke pain sensation.

Undoubtedly, the perception of sensory stimuli involves more of the cerebral cortex than the two discrete areas described above. Some sensory fibers probably project to the precentral gyrus and others to the superior parietal lobule. Moreover, S1 and S2 are not purely sensory in function; motor effects can be obtained by stimulating them electrically. It has been shown that sensory neurons in VPL, cuneate and gracile nuclei, and sensory neurons in the dorsal horns of the spinal cord all receive descending as well as ascending cortical projections. This reciprocal arrangement probably influences movement and the transmission and interpretation of pain, as discussed in Chap. 8.

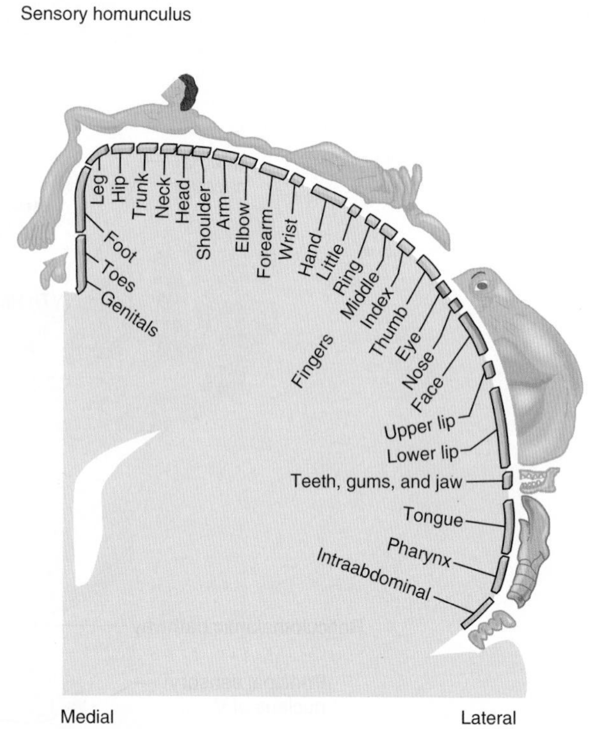

Figure 9-6. The "sensory homunculus," or cortical representation of sensation in the postcentral gyrus; compare this to the distribution of body areas in the motor cortex as shown in Fig. 3-4. (Reproduced with permission from Kandel ER, Schwartz JH, Jessel TM: *Principle of Neural Science*, 4th ed. New York, McGraw-Hill, 2000.)

Provided that the subcortical structures, especially the thalamus, are intact, certain sensations such as pain, touch, pressure, and extremes of temperature can reach consciousness. Their accurate localization, however, as well as the patient's ability to make other fine sensory discriminations, depends to a large extent on the integrity of the sensory cortex. This clinical distinction is elaborated in the discussion of the sensory syndromes further on.

Figure 9-6 ("sensory homunculus") shows the cortical representation of sensory information in the postcentral gyrus. As in the case of the motor representation (see Fig. 3-4), a disproportionate area is devoted to localization in the fingers, lips, and face.

From this brief account of the various channels of sensory information, one must conclude that at every level there is the possibility of feedback control from higher levels. Most external and some internal stimuli are highly complex and induce activity in more than one sensory system. In every system there is sufficient redundancy to allow lesser-used systems to compensate partially for the deficits incurred by disease.

EXAMINATION OF SENSATION

Most neurologists would agree that sensory testing is the most difficult part of the neurologic examination. For one thing, test procedures are relatively crude and are unlike those natural modes of stimulation with which the patient is familiar. It is also fair to say that few diagnoses are made solely on the basis of the sensory examination; more often the exercise serves to complement the motor examination. Quite often, no objective sensory loss can be demonstrated despite symptoms that suggest the presence of such an abnormality. Only rarely does the opposite pertain, i.e., one discovers a sensory deficit when there has been no complaint of sensory symptoms. Sensory symptoms in the nature of paresthesia or dysesthesia may be generated along axons of nerves not sufficiently diseased to impair or reduce sensory function; in the latter instance, loss of function may have been so mild and gradual as to pass unnoticed. Always there is some difficulty in evaluating the response to sensory stimuli, as it depends on the patient's interpretation of sensory experiences. This, in turn, will depend on the patient's general awareness and responsiveness and ability to cooperate, as well as degree of suggestibility. Children, by virtue of their simple and direct responses, are often better witnesses than more sophisticated individuals who are likely to analyze their feelings minutely and report small and insignificant differences in stimulus intensity.

General Considerations

Before proceeding to sensory testing, the physician should question patients about their symptoms; this, too, poses particular problems. Patients may be confronted with derangements of sensation that are unlike anything they have previously experienced, and they have limited terms to describe what they feel. They may say that a limb feels "numb" and "dead" when in fact they mean that it is weak. Occasionally a loss of sensation is discovered almost accidentally, e.g., by a lack of pain on touching an object hot enough to blister the skin or unawareness of articles of clothing and other objects in contact with the skin. More often, disease induces new and unnatural sensory experiences such as a band of tightness, a feeling of the feet being encased in cement, lancinating pains, an unnatural feeling when stroking the skin, a sensation as if walking on pebbles, and so on.

If nerves, sensory roots, or spinal tracts are damaged or partially interrupted, the patient may complain of tingling or prickling feelings ("like Novocain" or like the feelings in a limb that has "fallen asleep," the common colloquialism for nerve compression), cramp-like sensations, or burning or cutting pain occurring either spontaneously or in response to stimulation.

Experimental data support the view that partially damaged touch, pressure, thermal, and pain fibers become hyperexcitable and generate ectopic impulses along their course, either spontaneously or in response to a natural volley of stimulus-evoked impulses (Ochoa and Torebjork). These abnormal sensations are experienced as *paresthesias*, or *dysesthesias* if they are severe and distressing, as noted in Table 8-2. Another positive sensory symptom is *allodynia*, referring to a phenomenon in which one type of stimulus evokes another type of sensation—e.g., touch may induce pain.

Table 9-1

ORIGIN OF ABERRANT SENSATIONS

SYMPTOMS	STRUCTURES AFFECTED
Paresthesia, tingling, buzzing	Large fibers (in nerve or posterior columns)
Burning, heat, cold	Small fibers
Prickling pain	Combined small- and large-fiber
Pseudocramp	A type of paresthesia, probably related to large-fiber dysfunction
Band tightness	Lemniscal system of cord
Lancinating pain	Small-fiber neuropathy and radiculopathy
Hyperalgesia	Partial peripheral nerve damage

The clinical description of a sensation may divulge the particular sensory fibers involved (Table 9-1). It is known that stimulation of touch fibers gives rise to a sensation of tingling and buzzing; of muscle proprioceptors, to pseudocramp (the sensation of cramping without actual muscle contraction); of thermal fibers, to heat (including burning) and coldness; and of A-δ fibers, to prickling and pain. Paresthesia arising from ectopic discharges in large sensory fibers can be induced by nerve compression, hypocalcemia, hypomagnesemia, certain medications (niacin foremost among them), and diverse diseases of nerves. Band-like sensations on a limb or the trunk are the result of dysfunction in large sensory fibers, either in the periphery or their continuation in the posterior columns. Certain sensory symptoms suggest an anatomic location of nerve disease; for example, lancinating pains that radiate to the back or neck implicate root or, less often, sensory ganglion disease.

The presence of persistent paresthesiae incriminates a lesion involving sensory pathways in nerves, spinal cord, or higher structures. Most often, the large fibers in the peripheral nerves or posterior columns are involved. Evanescent paresthesia, of course, is usually of no significance. Every person has had the experience of resting a limb on the ulnar, sciatic, or peroneal nerve and having the extremity "fall asleep." This is because of compressive interruption of axonal transport and not of ischemia of the nerves or other components of the limb as is commonly assumed. The hyperventilation of anxiety may cause paresthesia of the lips and hands (sometimes unilateral) from diminution of CO_2 and thereby of ionized calcium; tetany may also occur, with carpopedal spasms. However, these sensory experiences are transient and should not be confused with the persistent, albeit frequently fluctuating, paresthesia of structural disease of the nervous system. Severe acral and peripheral paresthesias with perversion of hot and cold sensations are characteristic of certain neurotoxic shellfish poisonings (*ciguatera*) and some toxins, such as mercury.

Also worth comment are vibratory paresthesias, which we have encountered in only a handful of patients. One articulate physician described the sensation as a high-amplitude, low-frequency "buzz" that was distinctly different from the more common prickling paresthesia, burning, numbness, etc. We have the impression that these sensations are almost always a manifestation of central sensory disease, in one case probably attributable to the posterior columns and in another to cerebral disease. Beyond this, little is known about this symptom.

Effect of Age on Sensory Function

A matter of importance in the testing of sensation is the progressive impairment of sensory perception that occurs with advancing age. This requires that sensory thresholds, particularly in the feet and legs, be assessed in relation to age standards. The effect of aging is most evident in relation to vibratory sense, but proprioception, the perception of touch, and fast pain are also diminished with age. Sweating and vasomotor reflexes are reduced as well. These changes, which are discussed further in Chap. 29, are probably caused by neuronal loss in dorsal root ganglia and are reflected in a progressive depletion of fibers in the posterior columns. Receptors in the skin and special sense organs (taste, smell) also wither with age.

Terminology of Sensory Signs and Symptoms (See also Table 8-2)

A few additional terms require definition, as they are encountered in discussions of sensation. Some of these, relating to pain sensation, were mentioned in Chap. 8. *Anesthesia* refers to a complete loss and *hypesthesia* to a partial loss of all forms of sensation. Loss or impairment of specific cutaneous sensations may be indicated by an appropriate prefix or suffix, e.g., *thermoanesthesia* or *thermohypesthesia(loss and reduction in temperature sense)*, *analgesia* (loss of pain sense), *hypalgesia* (reduction in pain sensibility), *tactile anesthesia*, and *pallanesthesia, or apallesthesia* (loss of vibratory sense). The term *hyperesthesia*, as explained in Chap. 8, refers to an increased sensitivity to various stimuli and is usually used with respect to cutaneous sensation. It implies a heightened activity of the sensory apparatus. Under certain conditions (e.g., sunburn), there does appear to be an enhanced sensitivity of cutaneous receptors, but usually the presence of hyperesthesia betrays an underlying sensory defect. Careful testing will demonstrate an elevated threshold to tactile, painful, or thermal stimuli; but once the stimulus is perceived, it may have a severely painful or unpleasant quality (*hyperpathia*). Some clinicians use this last term to denote an exaggerated response to a painful stimulus (hyperalgesia which is subtly different from hyperpathia, denotes an abnormally painful reaction to a painful stimulus; Table 8-2). In *alloesthesia*, or *allesthesia*, a tactile or painful stimulus delivered on the side of hemisensory loss is experienced in a corresponding area of the opposite side or at a distant site on the same side. This phenomenon is observed most frequently with right-sided putaminal lesions (usually hemorrhage) and with anterolateral lesions of the cervical spinal cord; it presumably depends on the existence of an uncrossed ipsilateral spinothalamic pathway (see the original studies of Ray and Wolff).

Testing of Sensory Function

The detail with which sensation is tested is determined by the clinical situation. If the patient has no sensory complaints, it is sufficient to test vibration and position sense in the fingers and toes and the perception of pinprick over the extremities, and to determine whether the findings are the same in symmetrical parts of the body. A rough survey of this sort occasionally detects sensory defects of which the patient was unaware. More thorough testing is in order if the patient has complaints referable to the sensory system or if one finds localized atrophy or weakness, ataxia, trophic changes of joints, or painless ulcers.

A few other general rules are useful. It is easier for a patient to perceive the boundary of an abnormal area of sensation if the examiner proceeds from an area of reduced sensation toward the normal area. One should not press the sensory examination in the presence of fatigue, for an inattentive patient is a poor witness. Also, the examiner must avoid suggesting symptoms to the patient. After explaining in the simplest terms what is required, the examiner interposes as few questions and remarks as possible. Patients should generally not be asked, "Do you feel that?" each time they are touched; they are simply told to say "yes" or "sharp" every time they are touched or feel pain. Repetitive pinpricks within a small area of skin should be avoided, as this will make inapparent a subtle hypalgesia, because of the phenomenon of temporal summation as discussed earlier. In patients who may be overinterpreting slight changes in pinprick, differentiating between warm and cold is often more informative than differentiating between "sharp" and "dull." The patient should not directly observe the part under examination. A cooperative patient may, if asked to use a pin or his fingertips, outline an analgesic or anesthetic area or determine whether there is a graduated loss of sensation in the distal parts of a leg or arm. Finally, the findings of the sensory examination should be accurately recorded in narrative or on a chart by shading affected regions on a preprinted figure of the body or a sketch of a hand, foot, face, or limb.

Described below are the usual bedside methods of testing sensory function. These tests are sufficient for most clinical purposes. For clinical investigation and research into the physiology of pain, which require the detection of threshold values and quantification of sensory impairment, a wide range of instruments are available. Their use has been described by Dyck and colleagues (see also Lindblom and Ochoa and Bertelsmann et al).

Testing of Tactile Sensation

This is usually done with a wisp of cotton or light touch of a finger. The patient is first acquainted with the stimulus by applying it to a normal part of the body. Then, with eyes closed, he is asked to indicate if the sensation feels "natural" or to say "yes" each time various other parts are touched. A patient who is simulating sensory loss may say no in response to a tactile stimulus. Cornified areas of skin, such as the soles and palms, will require a heavier stimulus than other areas and the hair-clad parts a lighter one because of the numerous nerve endings around the follicles. Patients will be more sensitive to a moving stimulus of any kind than to a stationary one. The deft application of the examiner's or the patient's roving fingertips is a useful refinement and aids in demarcating an area of tactile loss, as Trotter and Davies originally showed.

More precise testing is possible by using a von Frey hair. By this method, a stimulus of constant strength can be applied and the threshold for tactile sensation determined by measuring the force required to bend a hair of known length. Spurious areas of hypesthesia may arise when a series of contactual stimuli lead to a decrement of sensation, either through adaptation of the end organ or because the initial sensation outlasts the stimulus and seems to spread.

Testing of Pain Perception

This is most efficiently assessed by pinprick, although it may be evoked by a variety of noxious stimuli. Patients must understand that they are to report the feeling of sharpness, not simply the feeling of contact or pressure of the pinpoint. If pinpricks are applied rapidly in one area, their effect may be summated and a heightened perception of pain may result; therefore they should be delivered about one per second and not over the same spot. Small differences in intensity can be discounted. An effective approach is to ask the patient to compare the pin sensation in two areas on a scale of 1 to 10; a report of "8 or 9" as compared to "10" is usually insignificant.

It is almost impossible, using an ordinary pin, to apply each stimulus with equal intensity. A pinwheel (Wartenberg wheel) is sometimes more effective because it allows the application of a more constant pressure, but risk of transmission of blood-borne infection from patient to patient has made this method outdated. This difficulty can be overcome to some extent by the use of an algesimeter, which delivers stimuli of constant intensity. Quantification of small-fiber sensation can be better assessed in the clinical laboratory by the use of thermal stimuli delivered by a computerized device as described below.

If an area of diminished or absent touch or pain sensation is encountered, its boundaries should be demarcated to determine whether it has a segmental or peripheral nerve distribution or is lost below a certain level on the trunk. As mentioned, such areas are best delineated by proceeding from the region of impaired sensation toward the normal. The changes may be confirmed by dragging a pin lightly over the parts in question. Areas of reduced pinprick sensation can be profitably corroborated by the thermal sense examination.

Testing of Deep-Pressure Pain

One can estimate the perception of this modality simply by lightly pinching or pressing deeply on the tendons, muscles, or bony prominences. Pain can often be elicited by heavy pressure even when superficial sensation is diminished; conversely, in some diseases, such as tabetic neurosyphilis, loss of deep-pressure pain may be more striking than loss of superficial pain. This uncomfortable examination can be omitted in routine neurological cases.

Testing of Thermal Sense

A quick but rough way to assess thermal loss (or to corroborate a previously found zone of hypalgesia) is to warm one side of a tuning fork by rubbing it briskly against the palm and apply its alternate sides to the patient's skin and asking the patient which side is colder (or warmer). This suffices for most bedside examinations.

If more careful examination is required, the skin should first be exposed to room air for a brief time before the examination. The test objects should be large, ideally two stoppered test tubes containing hot (45°C/113°F) and cold (20°C/68°F) tap water with thermometers that extend into the water through the flask stoppers. Extreme degrees of heat and cold may be employed first to delineate roughly an area of thermal sensory impairment. The side of each tube is applied successively to the skin for a few seconds and the patient is asked to report whether the flask feels "less hot" or "less cold" in comparison to a normal part. The qualitative change can then be quantitated as far as possible by recording the differences in temperature that the patient is able to recognize as the difference in temperature between the two tubes is gradually reduced. A normal person can detect a difference of 1°C (1.8°F) or even less in the range of 28°C (82.4°F) to 32°C (89.6°F); in the warm range, differences between 35°C (95°F) and 40°C (104°F) can be recognized, and in the cold range, between 10°C (50°F) and 20°C (68°F). If the temperature of the test object is below 10°C (50°F) or above 50°C (122°F), sensations of cold or heat become confused with pain. This technique has been largely supplanted by commercially manufactured electronic devices that can present a series of slightly differing thermal stimuli in sequence to a probe placed on the finger or toe. Special algorithms are used for the order and magnitude of temperature change and to determine whether the patient's reports are consistent and valid. The results are reported in the form of a "just noticeable difference" (JND) between temperatures or intensities of pain.

Testing of Proprioceptive Sense

Awareness of the position and movements of our limbs, fingers, and toes is derived from receptors in the muscles, tendons (Golgi tendon organs, according to Roland and Ladegaard-Pederson) and joints and is probably facilitated by the activation of skin receptors (Moberg). The two modalities comprising proprioception, i.e., sense of movement and of position, are usually both impaired, although clinical situations do arise in which perception of the position of a limb or digits is lost while that of passive and active movement (kinesthesia) of these parts is retained. The opposite occurs but is infrequent.

Abnormalities of position sense may be disclosed in several ways. When the patient has his arms outstretched and eyes closed, the affected arm will wander from its original position; if the patient's fingers are spread apart, they may undergo a series of changing postures ("piano-playing" movements, or pseudoathetosis); in attempting to touch the tip of his nose with his index finger, the patient may miss the target repeatedly, but the performance is corrected when the eyes are open.

Perception of passive movement is first tested in the fingers and toes as the defect, when present, is reflected maximally in these parts. It is important to grasp the digit at the sides, perpendicular to the plane of movement; otherwise the pressure applied by the examiner may allow the patient to identify the direction of movement. This applies as well to testing of the more proximal segments of the limb. The patient should be instructed to report each movement as being "up" or "down" from the previous position (directional kinesthesia). It is useful to demonstrate the test with a large and easily identified movement, but once the idea is clear to the patient, the smallest detectable changes should be determined. The part being tested should be moved rapidly. Normally, a very slight degree of movement is appreciated in the digits (as little as 1 degree of an arc). The test should be repeated enough times to eliminate chance (50 percent of responses). Defective perception of passive movement is judged by comparison with a normal limb or, if perception is bilaterally defective, on the basis of what the examiner has learned through experience to be normal. Slight impairment may be disclosed by a slowness of response or, if the digit is displaced very slowly, by an unawareness or uncertainty that movement has occurred; or, after the digit has been displaced in the same direction several times, the patient may misjudge the first movement in the opposite direction; or, after the examiner has moved the toe, the patient may make a number of small voluntary movements of the toe in an apparent attempt to determine its position or the direction of the movement. Inattentiveness will also cause some of these errors.

The lack of position sense in the legs can also be demonstrated by displacing the limb from its original position and having the patient, with eyes closed, place the other leg in the same position or point to the great toe. If proprioception if abnormal in axial structures, the patient will be unable to maintain his balance with feet together and eyes closed (*Romberg sign*). This test is often interpreted imprecisely. In the Romberg position, even a normal person whose eyes are closed will sway slightly, and the patient who lacks balance because of cerebellar ataxia or some other motor disorder will sway considerably more if his visual cues are removed. Only a marked discrepancy in balance with eyes open and with eyes closed qualifies as a Romberg sign. The most certain indication of abnormality is the need to step to the side or backward to avoid falling. Mild degrees of unsteadiness in an anxious or suggestible patient may be overcome by diverting his attention, e.g., by having him touch the index finger of each hand alternately to his nose while standing with eyes closed or by following the examiner's finger with his eyes. Patients with authentic proprioceptive problems will sway when there gaze is diverted from the ground and then become more unsteady when the eyes are closed. Patient with factitious unsteadiness, usually will remain stable when they look at the ceiling or a distant object and then become very unsteady when the eyes are closed. It is important to remember that any defect in proprioception (e.g. peripheral neuropathy, myelopathy or vestibulopathy) will lead to a Romberg sign even though the sign, described by Moritz Romberg, was meant to diagnose tabes dorsalis.

Testing of Vibratory Sense

This is a composite sensation comprising touch and rapid alterations of deep-pressure sense. The only cutaneous structure capable of registering such stimuli of this frequency is the rapidly adapting pacinian corpuscle. The conduction of vibratory sense depends on both cutaneous and deep afferent fibers that are carried in the muscle spindle afferent fibers and ascend mainly in the dorsal columns of the cord. Consequently, it is rarely affected by lesions of single nerves but will be disturbed in patients with disease of multiple peripheral nerves, dorsal columns, medial lemniscus, and thalamus. Vibration and position sense are usually impaired in similar conditions, although one of them (most often vibration sense) may be affected disproportionately. With advancing age, vibration is the sensation most commonly diminished, especially at the toes and ankles (see further on).

Vibration sense is tested by placing a tuning fork with a low rate and long duration of vibration (generally 128 Hz) over the bony prominences, making sure that the patient responds to the vibration, not simply to the pressure of the fork, and that he is not trying to listen to it. As with thermal and pain testing, there are mechanical devices that quantitate vibration sense. Quantitative tuning forks with a 0-8 scale are available but it is sufficient for most clinical purposes to compare the point tested with a normal part of the patient or the examiner. The examiner may detect the vibration after it ceases for the patient by holding a finger under the distal interphalangeal joint, the handle of the tuning fork being placed on the dorsal aspect of the joint. Or the vibrating fork is allowed to run down until the moment that vibration is no longer perceived, at which point the fork is transferred quickly to the corresponding part of the examiner and the time to extinction is noted. There is a small degree of accommodation to the vibration stimulus, so that slight asymmetries detected by rapid shifting from a body part on one side to the other should be interpreted accordingly. The perception of vibration at the patella after it has disappeared at the ankle or at the anterior iliac spine after it has disappeared at the knee is indicative of a length-dependent peripheral neuropathy. The approximate level of pinprick loss from a spinal cord lesion can be corroborated by testing vibratory sensation over the iliac crests and successive dorsal vertebral spines.

Testing of Discriminative (Parietal Lobe Cortical) Sensation

Damage to the parietal lobe sensory cortex or to the thalamocortical projections results in a particular type of disturbance—namely, an inability to make sensory discriminations and to integrate spatial and temporal sensory information (see further under "Sensory Loss Caused by Lesions of the Parietal Lobe" and Chap. 22). Lesions in these structures usually disturb complex sensory perception but leave the primary modalities (touch, pain, temperature, and vibration sense) relatively little affected. The integrity of discriminative sensory functions can be assessed only if it is first established that the primary sensory modalities on which they depend (mainly touch) are largely normal. If a cerebral lesion is suspected, discriminative function should be tested further in the following ways.

Two-Point Discrimination

The ability to distinguish two points from one is tested by using a compass, the points of which should be blunt and applied simultaneously and painlessly. The distance at which such stimuli can be recognized as a distinct pair varies but is roughly 1 mm at the tip of the tongue, 2 to 3 mm on the lips, 3 to 5 mm at the fingertips, 8 to 15 mm on the palm, 20 to 30 mm on the dorsal hands and feet, and 4 to 7 cm on the trunk. It is characteristic of the patient with a lesion of the sensory cortex to mistake two points for one, although occasionally the opposite occurs.

Cutaneous Localization and Figure Writing (Graphesthesia)

Localization of cutaneous tactile or painful stimuli is tested by touching various points on the body and asking the patient to place the tip of his index finger on the point stimulated or on the corresponding point of the examiner's limb. Recognition of numbers or letters traced on the skin (these should be larger than 4 cm on the palm) with a pencil or similar object or the direction of a line drawn across the skin also depends on localization of tactile stimuli. Normally, traced numbers as small as 1 cm can be detected on the pulp of the finger if drawn with a pencil. According to Wall and Noordenbos, these are also the most useful and simple tests of posterior column function.

Appreciation of Texture, Size, and Shape

Appreciation of texture depends mainly on cutaneous impressions, but recognition of the shapes and sizes of objects is based on sensory experience from deeper receptors as well. Inability to recognize shape and form is frequently a manifestation of cortical disease, but a similar clinical defect will occur if tracts that transmit proprioceptive and tactile sensation are interrupted by lesions of the spinal cord and brainstem (and, of course, of the peripheral nerves). This type of sensory defect is called *stereoanesthesia* (see further on, under "Posterior [Dorsal] Column Syndrome") and is distinguished from *astereognosis*, which connotes an inability to identify an object by palpation, even though the primary sense data (touch, pain, temperature, and vibration) are intact. In practice, pure astereognosis is rarely encountered, and the term is employed when the impairment of superficial and vibratory sensation in the hands seems to be of insufficient severity to account for the defect in tactile object identification. Defined in this way, astereognosis is either right- or left-sided and, with the qualifications mentioned below, is the product of a lesion in the opposite hemisphere, involving the sensory cortex, particularly S2 or the thalamoparietal projections.

The traditional doctrine that somatic sensation is represented only in the contralateral parietal lobe is not absolute. Beginning with the report by Oppenheim in 1906, there have been sporadic patients who showed bilateral astereognosis or loss of tactile sensation as a result of an apparently unilateral cerebral lesion. The correctness of these observations was corroborated by Semmes and colleagues, who tested a large series of patients with traumatic lesions involving either the right or left cerebral hemisphere. They found that the impairment of sensation (particularly discriminative sensation) following right- and left-sided lesions was not strictly comparable; the left hand as well as the right tended to be impaired by injury to the left sensorimotor region, whereas only the left hand tended to be affected by injury to the right sensorimotor region. These observations, with minor qualifications, were also confirmed by Carmon and by Corkin and associates, who investigated the sensory effects of cortical excisions in patients with focal epilepsy. Thus it appears that certain somatosensory functions in some patients are mediated not only by the contralateral hemisphere but also by the ipsilateral one, although the contribution of the former is undoubtedly the more significant.

The traditional concept of left hemispheric dominance in respect to tactile perception has been questioned by Carmon and Benton, who found that the right hemisphere is particularly important in perceiving the direction of tactile stimuli. Also, Corkin and associates observed that patients with lesions of the right hemisphere show a consistently greater failure of tactile-maze learning than those with left-sided lesions, pointing to a relative dominance of the right hemisphere in the mediation of tactile performance involving a spatial component. Certainly the phenomenon of sensory inattention or extinction is more prominent with lesions of the right as opposed to the left parietal lobe and is most informative if the primary and secondary sensory cortical areas are spared. These matters are considered further on in this chapter and in Chap. 22.

Finally, there is a distinction between astereognosis and tactile agnosia. Some authors (e.g., Caselli) have defined tactile agnosia as a strictly unilateral disorder, right or left, in which the impairment of tactile object recognition is unencumbered by a disturbance of the primary sensory modalities. Such a disorder would be designated by others as a pure form of astereognosis (see above). In our view, *tactile agnosia* is a disturbance in which a one-sided lesion lying posterior to the postcentral gyrus of the *dominant* parietal lobe results in an inability to recognize an object by touch in *both* hands. According to this view, tactile agnosia is a disorder of apperception of stimuli and of translating them into symbols, akin to the defect in naming parts of the body, visualizing a plan or a route, or understanding the meaning of the printed or spoken word (visual or auditory verbal agnosia). These and other agnosias are discussed in Chap. 22.

SENSORY SYNDROMES

Sensory Changes Caused by Interruption of a Single Peripheral Nerve

In these cases, the distribution of sensory loss will vary, depending on whether the nerve involved is predominantly muscular, cutaneous, or mixed. Following division of a *cutaneous nerve*, the area of sensory loss is always less than its anatomic distribution because of overlap from adjacent nerves. That the area of tactile loss is greater than that for pain relates both to a lack of collateralization (regeneration) from adjacent tactile fibers (in contrast to rapid collateral regeneration of pain fibers) and to a greater overlap of pain sensory units. If a large area of skin is involved, the sensory defect characteristically consists of a central portion in which all forms of cutaneous sensation are lost, surrounded by a zone of partial loss, which becomes less marked as one proceeds from the center to the periphery. Perceptions of deep pressure and passive movement are intact because these modalities are mediated by nerve fibers from subcutaneous structures and joints. Along the margin of the hypesthetic zone, the skin becomes excessively sensitive (hyperesthetic); light contact may be felt as smarting and mildly painful, more so as one proceeds from the periphery of the area to its center. According to Weddell, the dysesthesias are attributable to the greater sensitivity of collateral regenerating fibers that have made their way from surrounding healthy pain fibers into the denervated region.

Particular types of lesions have differing effects on sensory nerve fibers, as discussed earlier, but they are nearly always to some extent multimodal. *Compression* of a nerve ablates mainly the function of large touch and pressure fibers and leaves the function of small pain, thermal, and autonomic fibers intact; procaine and ischemia have the opposite effect. The tourniquet test is instructive in this respect. A sphygmomanometer cuff is applied above the elbow, inflated to a point well above the systolic pressure, and maintained there for as long as 30 min. (This is not particularly painful if the patient does not contract the forearm and hand muscles.) Paresthesiae appears within a few minutes, followed by sensory loss—first of touch and vibration, then of cold, fast pain, heat, and slow pain, in that order and spreading centripetally. Physiologic studies have confirmed the theory of Lewis and colleagues that compression blocks the function of nerve fibers in order of their size. Release of the cuff results in postcompression paresthesia, which has been shown to arise from spontaneous activity that is generated along the myelinated nerve fibers from ectopic sites at a distance from the compression. Within seconds of releasing the cuff, other changes appear—the cold, blanched hand becomes red and hot and there is an array of tingling, stinging, cramplike sensations that reach maximum intensity in 90 to 120 s and slowly fade (Lewis et al). Sensory function is recovered in an order inverse to that in which it was lost. Similar spontaneous and ectopic discharges probably explain the paresthetic symptoms early in the acute demyelinating neuropathies, even before the appearance of sensory loss or numbness. It is worth emphasizing that these features of compression are not because of nerve ischemia, as commonly stated; instead, they result from reversible physiologic changes in the myelin and underlying axon.

Certain maneuvers for the provocation of positive sensory phenomena—for example, the *Tinel sign* of tingling upon percussion of a regenerating peripheral nerve and the *Phalen sign* of paresthesia in the territory of the median nerve on wrist flexion—typify the susceptibility of a damaged nerve to pressure. In the case of a severed nerve, regeneration from the proximal end begins within days. The thin, regenerating sprouts are unusually sensitive to mechanical stimulation, which produces tingling, or the Tinel sign.

Sensory Changes Caused by Involvement of Multiple Nerves (Polyneuropathy) (Table 9-2)

In most instances of polyneuropathy, the sensory changes are accompanied by varying degrees of motor and reflex loss. Usually the sensory impairment is bilaterally symmetrical. Because in most types of polyneuropathy the longest and largest fibers are the most affected, sensory loss is most severe over the feet and legs and, if the upper limbs are affected, over the hands. The term *glove-and-stocking*, employed to describe the distribution of sensory loss of polyneuropathy, draws attention to the predominantly distal pattern of involvement but fails to indicate that the change from normal to impaired sensation is characteristically gradual. (In psychogenic sensory loss, by contrast, the border between normal and absent sensation is usually sharply defined.) The abdomen, thorax, and face are spared except in the most severe cases, in which sensory changes may be found over the anterior thoracoabdominal escutcheon and around the mouth.

Table 9-2

EXAMINATION FEATURES OF THE PERIPHERAL AND SPINAL CORD SENSORY SYNDROMES

Polyneuropathy
- Symmetrical distal sensory loss
- Sensory loss may affect one modality preferentially
- Areflexia or hyporeflexia
- Weakness, if present, symmetrical

Polyradiculopathy
- Asymmetrical sensory and motor loss
- Proximal and distal parts of limb differentially affected
- Reflex loss limited to region of affected root(s)

Ganglionopathy
- Implicates all sensory modalities
- Proximal body parts affected
- Ataxia

Tabetic syndrome
- Prominent loss of vibratory and position sense in feet
- Romberg sign
- Secondary (Charcot) joint deformities
- Areflexia

Myelopathy
- Complete transverse lesion: loss of all sensory modalities below level of lesion
- Syringomyelia: loss of pain and thermal sense with preservation of touch and joint position/vibration over restricted region of neck, cape, arms, hands
- Anterior spinal artery syndrome: loss of pain sense with preservation of vibration and joint position below level of lesion
- Posterior column: same as tabetic but reflexes preserved
- Hemicord (Brown-Séquard): loss of pain sense opposite to the lesion and beginning several levels below it; loss of vibration and joint position sense on the side of the lesion and below it

(See Fig. 9-7 and also Chap. 46.)

When the neuropathy is primarily demyelinating rather than axonal, paresthesia is an early feature. It is reported in the distal territories of nerves; when short nerves (e.g., the trigeminal) are involved, the paresthesia appears in proximal body parts, such as the perioral region.

The sensory loss of polyneuropathy usually involves all modalities of sensation, and—although it is difficult to equate the degrees of impairment of pain, touch, temperature, vibration, and position senses—one modality may be impaired disproportionately to the others. This clinical feature is explained by the fact that particular diseases of the peripheral nerves selectively damage sensory fibers of different size. For example, degeneration or demyelination of the large fibers that subserve kinesthetic sense causes a loss of vibratory and position sense and relative sparing of pain, temperature, and, to some degree, tactile perception. When extreme, such a polyneuropathy results in pseudoathetoid movements of the outstretched fingers or toes; it may also result in a sensory ataxia because of affection of the large-diameter nerves destined for the spinocerebellar tracts.

By contrast, involvement of the small-caliber myelinated and unmyelinated axons affects pain, temperature, and autonomic sensation, with preservation of proprioceptive, vibration, and tactile sense—producing a syndrome called "pseudosyringomyelia," because it simulates the dissociated pain from tactile sensory loss that is seen in this disease of the spinal cord (see further on, under "Sensory Spinal Cord Syndromes"). Prolonged analgesia may lead to trophic ulcers and Charcot joints. These patterns of sensory loss, as well as those produced by the plexopathies and mononeuritis multiplex, are discussed further in Chap. 46.

Sensory Changes from Involvement of Nerve Roots (Radiculopathy) (Figs. 9-1, 9-2, and 9-3 and Table 9-2)

The surface innervation of the sensory nerve roots serves as one of the most useful and dependable guides to localization in neurology and the main dermatomes are known to all physicians. Because of considerable overlap from adjacent roots, division of a single sensory root does not produce complete loss of sensation in any area of skin. However, compression of a single sensory cervical or lumbar root (e.g., by a herniated intervertebral disc) can cause a segmental impairment of cutaneous sensation. When two or more contiguous roots have been completely divided, a zone of sensory loss can be demonstrated; this is surrounded by a narrow zone of partial loss in which a raised threshold accompanied by excessive sensitivity may or may not be evident. For reasons not altogether clear, partial sensory loss from root lesions is easier to demonstrate by the use of a painful stimulus than by a tactile or pressure stimulus.

Disease of the nerve roots frequently gives rise to "shooting" (lancinating) pains and burning sensations that project down the course of their sensory nerves. The common examples are sciatica, from lower lumbar or upper sacral root compression, and sharp pain radiating from the shoulder and down the upper arm, from cervical disc protrusion.

When multiple roots are affected (*polyradiculopathy*) by an infiltrative, inflammatory, or compressive process, the syndrome is more complex and must be differentiated from polyneuropathy. The distinguishing features of a polyradiculopathy, aside from pain, are asymmetrical muscle weakness that involves both proximal and distal parts differentially in each limb and a pattern of sensory loss that is consistent with affection of several roots, not necessarily contiguous ones. Details are found in Chap. 46.

Sensory Changes from Involvement of Sensory Ganglia (Sensory Neuronopathy, Ganglionopathy) (Table 9-2)

Widespread disease of the dorsal root ganglia produces many of the same sensory defects as disease of the posterior nerve roots, but it is unique in that proximal areas of the body also show pronounced sensory loss; the face, oral mucosa, scalp, trunk, and genitalia may be sites of hypesthesia and hypalgesia. Proprioception is diminished or lost in distal and, to some extent, proximal body parts, giving rise also to ataxic movements, often quite severe, and to pseudoathetosis. Tendon reflexes are lost. Sometimes there are additional features of dysautonomia, but strength is entirely spared. Recognition of this unusual pattern of pansensory loss is of considerable diagnostic importance, because it raises for consideration a number of underlying diseases that might otherwise be overlooked; these diseases are discussed in Chap. 46. The main causes of this syndrome are paraneoplastic, connective tissue disease, particularly Sjögren syndrome, toxic exposure, and idiopathic inflammation.

Tabetic Syndrome

The tabetic syndrome may be considered a type of polyradiculopathy or ganglionopathy, but it is often considered with diseases of the spinal cord because it produces wallerian degeneration of posterior columns. It results from damage to the large proprioceptive and other fibers of the posterior lumbosacral (and sometimes cervical) roots. It was in the past typically caused by neurosyphilis but also by diabetes mellitus, and other diseases that involve the posterior roots or dorsal root ganglia. Numbness or paresthesia and "lightning" or lancinating pains are frequent complaints; areflexia, abnormalities of gait (gait of sensory ataxia), and hypotonia without significant muscle weakness are found on examination. The sensory loss may involve only vibration and position senses in the lower extremities, but loss or impairment of superficial or deep pain sense or of touch may appear in severe cases. In this case, loss of deep tendon reflexes distinguishes the sensory root syndrome from a lesion in the posterior columns. The feet and legs are most affected in tabes, much less often the arms and trunk. The Romberg sign is prominent. Frequently, atonicity of the bladder with retention of urine and trophic joint changes (Charcot joints) and crises of abdominal ("gastric") pains are associated.

Cases of congenital absence of all cutaneous sensation resulting from the lack of development of small sensory ganglion cells may produce the tabetic syndrome; this is discussed in Chap. 8. A similar but partial defect may be found in the Riley-Day syndrome (Chap. 26). There are also forms of hereditary polyneuropathy that cause universal insensitivity.

Sensory Spinal Cord Syndromes (Fig. 9-7)

See also Chap. 44.

Complete Spinal Sensory Syndrome

With a complete transverse disruption of the spinal cord, the most striking loss is of power; most characteristic, however, is a loss of all forms of sensation below a level that corresponds to the lesion. There may be a narrow zone of hyperesthesia at the upper margin of the anesthetic zone. Loss of pain, temperature, and touch sensation begins one or two segments below the level of the lesion; vibratory and position senses have less-discrete levels but they can be detected by careful examination. The sensory (and motor) loss in spinal cord lesions that involve both gray and white matter is expressed in patterns corresponding to bodily segments or dermatomes. These are shown in Figs. 9-3 and 9-4 and are most obvious on the trunk, where each intercostal nerve has a transverse distribution.

Also, it is important to remember that during the subacute evolution of a transverse spinal cord lesion, there may be a discrepancy between the level of the lesion and that of the sensory loss, the latter ascending as the lesion progresses. This can be understood if one conceives of a lesion as evolving from the periphery to the center of the cord, affecting first the outermost fibers carrying pain and temperature sensation from the legs. Conversely, a lesion advancing from the center of the cord will affect these modalities in the reverse order, in a pattern of *sacral sparing*, meaning that sensation is preserved over the buttocks and anal region but is absent over the trunk and legs.

Hemisection of the Spinal Cord (Brown-Séquard Syndrome)

Disease may be confined to or predominate on one side of the spinal cord; pain and thermal sensation are affected on the opposite side of the body, and proprioceptive sensation is affected on the same side as the lesion. Although rarely present in its entirety, a partial Brown-Séquard syndrome is common in practice. The loss of pain and temperature sensation begins one or two segments below the lesion. An associated spastic motor paralysis on the side of the lesion completes the syndrome (Fig. 9-7). Tactile sensation is not greatly affected, as the fibers from one side of the body are distributed in tracts (posterior columns, anterior and lateral spinothalamic) on both sides of the cord.

Syringomyelic Syndrome (Lesion of the Central Gray Matter)

Because fibers conducting pain and temperature sensation cross the cord in the anterior commissure, a lesion of considerable vertical extent in this location characteristically abolishes these modalities on one or both sides over several segments (dermatomes) but spares tactile sensation (Fig. 9-7). This type of *dissociated sensory loss* usually occurs in a segmental distribution, and because the lesion frequently involves other parts of the gray matter, varying degrees of segmental amyotrophy and reflex loss are usually present as well. If the lesion has spread to the white matter, corticospinal, spinothalamic, and posterior column signs will be conjoined. The most common cause of such a lesion in the cervical region is the centrally situated developmental syringomyelia; less-common causes are intramedullary tumor, trauma, and hemorrhage. A *pseudosyringomyelic* syndrome was mentioned earlier in relation to small-fiber neuropathies that simulate syringomyelia.

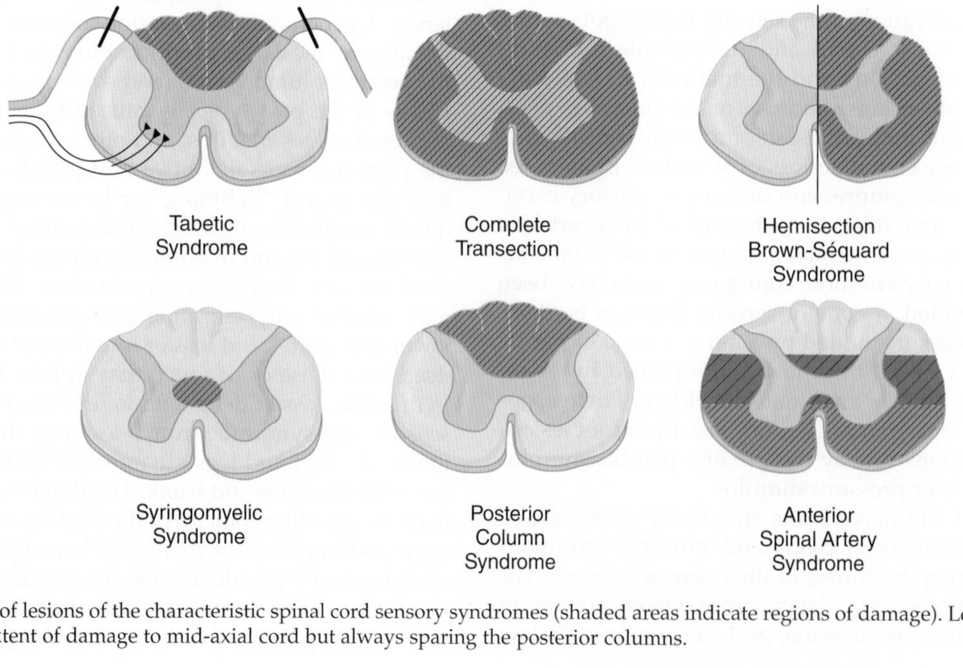

Figure 9-7. Sites of lesions of the characteristic spinal cord sensory syndromes (shaded areas indicate regions of damage). Lower right figure shows variable extent of damage to mid-axial cord but always sparing the posterior columns.

Posterior (Dorsal) Column Syndrome

Paresthesias in the form of tingling and pins-and-needles sensations or girdle- and band-like sensations are common complaints with posterior column disease. In some cases there may be the additional feature of a diffuse, burning, unpleasant sensation in response to pinprick. Loss of vibratory and position sense occurs below the level of the lesion, but the perception of pain and temperature is affected relatively little or not at all. Because posterior column lesions are caused by the interruption of central projections of the dorsal root ganglia cells, they may be difficult to distinguish from a process that affects large fibers in sensory roots (tabetic syndrome); however, the tendon reflexes are spared in the former and eliminated in tabes. In some diseases that involve the dorsal columns, vibratory sensation may be involved predominantly, whereas in others position sense is more affected.

With complete posterior column lesions, only a few of which have been verified by postmortem examinations, not only is the patient deprived of knowledge of movement and position of parts of the body below the lesion but all types of sensory discrimination are impaired (see Nathan et al for a review of the subject). If the lesion is in the high cervical region, there is clumsiness in the palpation of objects and an inability to recognize the qualities of objects by touch, even though touch-pressure sensation is relatively intact. Stereoanesthesia is also expressed by impaired graphesthesia and tactile localization. There may be unusual disturbances of touch and pressure, manifesting as lability of threshold, persistence of sensation after removal of the stimulus, and sometimes tactile and postural hallucinations. Nathan and colleagues confirmed this counterintuitive observation that lesions of the posterior columns cause only slight defects in touch and pressure sensation and that lesions of the anterolateral spinothalamic tracts also cause minimal or no defects in these modalities. This is not easily reconciled with clinical observations of patients with lesions in the posterior columns. However, a combined lesion in both pathways causes a total loss of tactile and pressure sensibility below the lesion.

The loss of sensory functions that follows a posterior column lesion—such as impaired two-point discrimination; figure writing; detection of size, shape, weight, and texture of objects; and ability to detect the direction and speed of a moving stimulus on the skin—may simulate a parietal "cortical" lesion, but differs in that vibratory sense is also lost in spinal cord syndromes. In several cases on record, interruption of the posterior columns by surgical incision or other type of injury did not cause a permanent loss of the sensory modalities thought to be subserved by these pathways (Cook and Browder, Wall and Noordenbos). Because postmortem studies of these cases were not performed, it is possible that some of the posterior column fibers had been spared. Also, it should be realized that not all proprioceptive fibers ascend to the gracile and cuneate nuclei; some proprioceptive fibers leave the posterior columns in the lumbar region and synapse with secondary neurons in the spinal gray matter and ascend in the ipsilateral posterolateral funiculus. Only cutaneous fibers continue to the gracile and cuneate nuclei.

The usual causes of the posterior column syndrome are multiple sclerosis, vitamin B_{12} deficiency, copper deficiency, tabes dorsalis, and HIV and human T-lymphotropic virus (HTLV) type 1 infection.

Anterior Myelopathy (Anterior Spinal Artery Syndrome)

With infarction of the spinal cord in the territory of supply of the anterior spinal artery or with other lesions that affect the ventral portion of the cord predominantly, as in some cases of myelitis, one finds a loss of pain and temperature sensation below the level of the lesion but with relative or absolute sparing of proprioceptive sensation. Because the corticospinal tracts and the ventral gray matter also lie within the area of distribution of the anterior spinal artery, spastic paralysis is a prominent feature (Fig. 9-7).

Disturbances of Sensation from Lesions of the Brainstem

A characteristic feature of medullary lesions is the occurrence, in many instances, of a crossed sensory disturbance, i.e., a loss of pain and temperature sensation on one side of the face and on the opposite side of the body. This is accounted for by involvement of the descending spinal trigeminal tract or its nucleus and the crossed lateral spinothalamic tract on one side of the brainstem and is nearly always caused by a lateral medullary infarction (Wallenberg syndrome). In the upper medulla, pons, and midbrain, the crossed trigeminothalamic and lateral spinothalamic tracts run together; a lesion at these levels causes loss of pain and temperature sense on the opposite half of the face and body. There are no tactile paresthesias, only thermal or painful dysesthesias. In the upper brainstem, the spinothalamic tract and the medial lemniscus become confluent, so that an appropriately placed lesion causes a contralateral loss of all superficial and deep sensation. Cranial nerve palsies, cerebellar ataxia, and motor paralysis are almost invariably associated, as indicated in the discussion of strokes in this region (Chap. 34). In other words, a lesion in the brainstem at any level is unlikely to cause an isolated sensory disturbance.

Hemisensory Loss Caused by a Lesion of the Thalamus (Syndrome of Dejerine-Roussy)

Involvement of the VPL and VPM nuclei of the thalamus, usually because of a vascular lesion, causes loss or diminution of all forms of sensation on the opposite side of the body. Position sense is affected more frequently than any other sensory function and is usually, but not always, more profoundly reduced than loss of touch and pinprick. With partial recovery of sensation, or with an acute but incomplete lesion, spontaneous pain or discomfort (thalamic pain), sometimes of the most distressing type, may appear on the affected side of the body and any stimulus may then have a diffuse, unpleasant, lingering quality (anterior and proximal syndromes). Thermal—especially cold—stimuli, emotional disturbance, loud sounds, and even certain types of music may aggravate the painful state. In spite of this overresponse to stimuli, the patient usually shows an elevated pain threshold, i.e., a stronger stimulus than normal is necessary to produce a sensation of pain (hypalgesia with hyperpathia). The same type of pain syndrome may occasionally accompany lesions of the white matter of the parietal lobe, the medial lemniscus, or even the posterior columns of the spinal cord.

It should be pointed out that a symptomatic hemisensory syndrome, usually with few objective changes, occurs frequently without manifest evidence of thalamic or spinal cord damage. This particularly occurs in young women, as pointed out by Toth. A number of our patients with this benign condition have had migraine, and one, as in Toth's series, had the antiphospholipid syndrome, but the connections between all these entities is tenuous and many cases are considered to be psychogenic.

Sensory Loss Caused by Lesions of the Parietal Lobe

In the anterior parietal lobe syndrome (Verger-Dejerine syndrome), there are disturbances mainly of discriminative sensory functions of the opposite arm, leg, and side of the face without impairment of the primary modalities of sensation (unless the lesion is extensive and deep). Loss of position sense and sense of movement, impaired ability to localize touch and pain stimuli (topagnosia), widening of two-point threshold, and astereognosis are the most prominent findings, as described earlier in this chapter and in Chap. 22, "Clinical Effects of Parietal Lobe Lesions."

Another characteristic manifestation of parietal lobe lesions is *sensory inattention, extinction*, or *neglect*. In response to bilateral simultaneous testing of symmetrical parts, using either tactile or painful stimuli, the patient may acknowledge only the stimulus on the sound side; or, if the face and hand or foot on the affected side is touched or pricked, only the stimulus to the face may be noticed. Apparently cranial structures command more attention than other less richly innervated parts. Yet each stimulus, when applied separately to each side or to each part of the affected side, is properly perceived and localized. In the case of sensory neglect, the patient ignores one side of the body and extrapersonal space contralateral to the parietal lesion, which is usually in the nondominant hemisphere. Left parietal lesions may also cause (right) sensory neglect, but less frequently and less profoundly. Sensory neglect or extinction, which may also occur occasionally with posterior column and medial lemniscus lesions, may be detected in persons who disclaim any sensory symptoms. These phenomena and other features of parietal lobe lesions are considered further in Chap. 22.

Yet another parietal lobe syndrome, Dejerine-Mouzon, is featured by a severe impairment of the primary modalities of sensation (pain, thermal, tactile, and vibratory sense) over half of the body. Motor paralysis is variable; with partial recovery, there may be a clumsiness that resembles cerebellar ataxia. Because the sensory disorder simulates that caused by a thalamic lesion, it was called *pseudothalamic* by Foix and coworkers. Hyperpathia, much like that of the Dejerine-Roussy syndrome (see above), has also been observed in patients with cortical–subcortical parietal lesions. The pseudothalamic syndrome was related by Foix and colleagues to a sylvian infarct; Bogousslavsky and associates traced it to a parietal infarct caused by occlusion of the ascending parietal branch of the middle cerebral artery. In each of the aforementioned parietal lobe syndromes, if the dominant hemisphere is involved, there may be an aphasia, a bimanual tactile agnosia, or a Gerstmann syndrome; with nondominant lesions, there may be anosognosia (see Chap. 22).

Often with parietal lesions, the patient's responses to sensory stimuli are variable. A common mistake, as emphasized by Critchley, is to attribute this abnormality to hysteria (see also below). A lesion confined to only a part of the parietal cortex (the best examples have been caused by glancing bullet or shrapnel wounds of the skull) may result in a circumscribed loss of superficial sensation in an opposite limb, mimicking a root or peripheral nerve lesion.

Sensory Loss Due to Suggestibility and Hysteria (See also Chap. 51)

The possibility of suggesting sensory loss to a patient is a very real one, as has already been indicated. Hysterical patients may complain of a complete hemianesthesia—sometimes with the overtly hysterical findings of reduced hearing, sight, smell, and taste on one side—as well as impaired vibration sense over only half the skull and sternum, most of these being anatomic impossibilities. A frequently used test to disclose this feature is performed by placing a vibrating tuning fork on each side adjacent to the middle of the forehead. The transmission of vibration through the bone assures that loss of sensation on one side of the midline is not possible. Anesthesia of an entire limb or a sharply defined sensory loss over part of a limb, not conforming to the distribution of a root or cutaneous nerve, may also be observed. The diagnosis of hysterical hemianesthesia is best made by eliciting the other relevant symptoms of hysteria or, if this is not possible, by noting the discrepancies between the sensory loss displayed by the patient and that which occurs as part of the known, anatomically verified sensory syndromes.

Sometimes, in a patient with no other neurologic abnormality or in one with a definite neurologic syndrome, one is dismayed by sensory findings that are completely inexplicable and discordant. In such cases, one must try to reason through to the diagnosis by disregarding the sensory findings or approach the finding as revealing a second disorder such as a neurofibroma of a nerve root.

Laboratory Diagnosis of Somatosensory Syndromes

Affirmation of the clinical sensory syndromes is often possible by the application of electrophysiologic testing. Slowing and reduced amplitude of sensory nerve conduction is found with lesions of nerve, but only if the lesion lies distal to (or within) the sensory ganglion. Severe sensory loss in a neuropathic pattern with preserved sensory nerve action potentials therefore indicates a radiculopathy. Loss or slowing of the H reflex and F responses corroborates the presence of lesions in proximal parts of nerves, plexuses, and roots. By the use of somatosensory evoked potentials, it is possible to demonstrate slowing of conduction in the peripheral nerves or roots, in the pathways from spinal cord to a point in the lower medulla, in the medial lemniscus to the thalamus, and in the pathway from the thalamus to the cerebral cortex. In the context of regional sensory loss, evoked potentials find their greatest utility in demonstrating root disease when sensory nerve conduction studies are normal; otherwise, they are used most frequently to support the diagnosis of multiple sclerosis, in which case there may or may not be corresponding sensory features. (See Chap. 2 for discussion of evoked potential testing.)

In practice, it is seldom necessary to examine all modalities of sensation and perception. With single peripheral nerve lesions, touch and pinprick testing are the most informative. With spinal cord disease, pinprick and thermal stimuli are most revealing of lateral column lesions; testing the senses of vibration, position, and movement, and particularly the sense of direction of a dermal stimulus, reliably indicates posterior column lesions. Touch is the least useful. In brainstem lesions, all modes of sensation, including touch, may be affected, and this applies in general to thalamic lesions. Thus, one is guided in the selection of tests by the suspected locale of the disease.

References

Bertelsmann FW, Heimans JJ, Weber EJM, et al: Thermal discrimination thresholds in normal subjects and in patients with diabetic neuropathy. *J Neurol Neurosurg Psychiatry* 48:686, 1985.

Bogousslavsky J, Assal G, Regli F: Aphasie afferente motrice et hemi-syndrome sensitif droite. *Rev Neurol* 138:649, 1982.

Brodal A: The somatic afferent pathways, in Brodal A: *Neurological Anatomy*, 3rd ed. New York, Oxford University Press, 1981, pp 46–147.

Carmon A: Disturbances of tactile sensitivity in patients with unilateral cerebral lesions. *Cortex* 7:83, 1971.

Carmon A, Benton AL: Tactile perception of direction and number in patients with unilateral cerebral disease. *Neurology* 19:525, 1969.

Caselli RJ: Rediscovering tactile agnosia. *Mayo Clin Proc* 66:129, 1991.

Cook AW, Browder EJ: Function of the posterior column. *Trans Am Neurol Assoc* 89:193, 1964.

Corkin S, Milner B, Rasmussen T: Tactually guided maze learning in man: Effects of unilateral cortical excision and bilateral hippocampal lesions. *Neuropsychologia* 3:339, 1965.

Corkin S, Milner B, Rasmussen T: Effects of different cortical excisions on sensory thresholds in man. *Trans Am Neurol Assoc* 89:112, 1964.

Critchley M: *The Parietal Lobes*. London, Arnold, 1953.

Davidoff RA: The dorsal columns. *Neurology* 39:1377, 1989.

Dyck PJ, Karnes J, O'Brien PC, Zimmerman IR: Detection thresholds of cutaneous sensation in humans, in Dyck PJ, Thomas PK, et al (eds): *Peripheral Neuropathy*, 3rd ed. Philadelphia, Saunders, 1993, pp 706–728.

Foix C, Chavany JA, Levy M: Syndrome pseudothalamique d'origine parietale. *Rev Neurol* 35:68, 1965.

Greaves MS, Wall PD: Pathophysiology of itching. *Lancet* 348:938, 1996.

Keegan JJ, Garrett FD: The segmental distribution of the cutaneous nerves in the limbs of man. *Anat Rec* 102:409, 1948.

Kibler RF, Nathan PW: A note on warm and cold spots. *Neurology* 10:874, 1960.

Lele PP, Weddell G: The relationship between neurohistology and corneal sensibility. *Brain* 79:119, 1956.

Lewis T, Pickering GW, Rothschild P: Centrifugal paralysis arising out of arrested blood flow to the limb, including notes on a form of tingling. *Heart* 16:1, 1931.

Light AR, Perl ER: Peripheral sensory systems, in Dyck PJ, Thomas PK, et al (eds): *Peripheral Neuropathy*, 3rd ed. Philadelphia, Saunders, 1993, pp 149–165.

Lindblom U, Ochoa J: Somatosensory function and dysfunction, in Asbury AK, McKhann GM, McDonald IW (eds): *Diseases of the Nervous System*, 2nd ed. Philadelphia, Saunders, 1992, pp 213–228.

Loh L, Nathan PW: Painful peripheral states and sympathetic blocks. *J Neurol Neurosurg Psychiatry* 41:664, 1978.

Mackel R: Human cutaneous mechanoreceptors during regeneration: Physiology and interpretation. *Ann Neurol* 18:165, 1985.

Mayo Clinic: *Examinations in Neurology*, 7th ed. St. Louis, Mosby, 1998.

Moberg E: The role of cutaneous afferents in position sense, kinaesthesia and motor function of the hand. *Brain* 106:1, 1983.

Mountcastle VG: Central nervous mechanisms in sensation, in Mountcastle VB (ed): *Medical Physiology*, 14th ed. Vol 1. Part 5. St. Louis, Mosby, 1980, pp 327–605.

Nathan PW, Smith MC, Cook AW: Sensory effects in man of lesions in the posterior columns and of some other afferent pathways. *Brain* 109:1003, 1986.

Ochoa JL, Torebjork HE: Paraesthesiae from ectopic impulse generation in human sensory nerves. *Brain* 103:835, 1980.

Ray BS, Wolff HG: Studies on pain: Spread of pain: Evidence on site of spread within the neuraxis of effects of painful stimulation. *Arch Neurol Psychiatry* 53:257, 1945.

Roland PE, Ladegaard-Pederson H: A quantitative analysis of sensations of tension and of kinaesthesia in man. *Brain* 100:671, 1977.

Semmes J, Weinstein S, Ghent L, Teuber H-L: *Somatosensory Changes after Penetrating Brain Wounds in Man*. Cambridge, MA, Harvard University Press, 1960.

Sinclair D: *Mechanisms of Cutaneous Sensation*. Oxford, UK, Oxford University Press, 1981.

Torebjork HE, Vallbo AB, Ochoa JL: Intraneural micro-stimulation in man: Its relation to specificity of tactile sensations. *Brain* 110:1509, 1987.

Toth C: Hemisensory syndrome is associated with a low diagnostic yield and a nearly uniform benign prognosis. *J Neurol Neurosurg Psychiatry* 74:1113, 2003.

Tower SS: Unit for sensory reception in the cornea. *J Neurophysiol* 3:486, 1940.

Trotter W, Davies HM: Experimental studies in the innervation of the skin. *J Physiol* 38:134, 1909.

Wall PD, Noordenbos W: Sensory functions which remain in man after complete transection of dorsal columns. *Brain* 100: 641, 1977.

Weddell G: The multiple innervation of sensory spots in the skin. *J Anat* 75:441, 1941.

Yosipovitch G, Greaves MW, Schmetz M: Itch. *Lancet* 361:690, 2003.

10

Headache and Other Craniofacial Pains

Of all the painful states that afflict humans, headache is undoubtedly the most frequent and rivals backache as the most common reason for seeking medical help. In fact, there are so many cases of headache that special headache clinics have been established in many medical centers. In addition to its frequency in general practice, many headaches are caused by general medical rather than neurologic diseases, and the subject is the legitimate concern of the general physician. Yet there is always the question of intracranial disease, so that it is difficult to approach the subject without a knowledge of neurologic medicine.

Why so many pains are centered in the head is a question of some interest. Several explanations come to mind. For one thing, the face and scalp are more richly supplied with pain receptors than many other parts of the body, perhaps to protect the precious contents of the skull. Also, the nasal and oral passages, the eye, and the ear—all delicate and highly sensitive structures—reside here and must be protected; when affected by disease, each is capable of inducing pain in its own way. Finally, there is greater concern about what happens to the head than to other parts of the body, since the former houses the brain, and headache frequently raises the specter of brain tumor or other cerebral disease.

Semantically, the term *headache* encompasses all aches and pains located in the head, but in practice, its application is restricted to discomfort in the region of the cranial vault. Facial, lingual, and pharyngeal pains are put aside as something different and are discussed separately in the latter part of this chapter and in Chap. 47, on the cranial nerves.

GENERAL CONSIDERATIONS

In the introductory chapter on pain, reference was made to the necessity, in dealing with any painful state, of determining its quality, severity, location, duration, and time course as well as the conditions that produce, exacerbate, or relieve it. In the case of headache, a detailed history following these lines will determine the diagnosis more often than will the physical examination or imaging. Although the examination is unlikely to be revealing, a few aspects are worth emphasis. Auscultation of the skull may disclose a bruit (with large arteriovenous malformations), and palpation may disclose the tender, hardened or elevated arteries of temporal arteritis, sensitive areas overlying a cranial metastasis, an inflamed paranasal sinus, or a tender occipital nerve, examination of neck flexion may reveal meningitis; however, apart from such special instances, examination of the head itself, although necessary, seldom discloses the diagnosis.

As to the *quality* of cephalic pain, the patient's description may or may not be helpful. When asked to compare the pain to some other sensory experience, the patient may allude to tightness, aching, pressure, bursting, sharpness, or stabbing. The most important information to be obtained is whether the headache is pulsatile, but one must keep in mind that patients sometimes use the word *throbbing* to refer to a waxing and waning of the headache without any relation to the pulse, or simply use the term to transmit the severity of pain, whereas authentic pulsatile throbbing, is characteristic of migraine.

Similarly, statements about *the intensity of the pain* must be accepted with caution, as they reflect as much the patient's temperament, attitudes and customary ways of experiencing and reacting to pain as its true severity. A better index of severity is the degree to which the pain has incapacitated the patient, especially if he is not prone to illness. A severe migraine attack seldom allows the migraineur to perform the day's work. Another rough index of the severity of headache is its propensity to awaken the patient from sleep or to prevent sleep. The most intense cranial pains are those associated with meningitis and subarachnoid hemorrhage, which have grave implications, and with migraine, cluster headache, or tic douloureux, which do not.

Data regarding the *location* of a headache are apt to be more informative. Migraine headache is unilateral in two-thirds of attacks and is commonly associated with nausea, vomiting, and sensitivity to light, sound, and smells. Inflammation of an extracranial artery causes pain localized to the site of the vessel. Lesions of the paranasal sinuses, teeth, eyes, and upper cervical vertebrae induce a less sharply localized pain but still one that is referred to a certain region, usually the forehead or maxilla or around the eyes. Intracranial lesions in the posterior fossa generally cause pain in the occipitonuchal region and usually are homolateral if the lesion is one-sided. Supratentorial lesions induce frontotemporal pain, or approximate the site of the lesion. Localization, however, may also be deceiving. Pain in the frontal regions may be caused by such diverse lesions and mechanisms as glaucoma, sinusitis, thrombosis of the vertebral or basilar artery, pressure on the tentorium, and increased intracranial pressure. Similarly, ear pain may signify disease of the ear itself, but as often, it is referred from other regions, such as the throat, cervical muscles, spine, or structures in the posterior fossa. Periorbital and supraorbital pain, while usually indicative of local disease, may reflect dissection of the cervical portion of the internal carotid artery. Headaches localized to the vertex or biparietal regions are infrequent and should raise the suspicion of sphenoid or ethmoid sinus disease or thrombosis of the superior sagittal venous sinus.

The *mode of onset,* the *variation of the pain over time,* and *duration* of the headache, with respect both to a single attack and to the profile of the headache over a period of years, are also useful data. At one extreme, the headache of subarachnoid hemorrhage (caused by a ruptured aneurysm) occurs as an abrupt attack that attains its maximal severity in a matter of seconds or minutes, or, in the case of meningitis, it may come on more gradually, over several hours or days. Simulating the rapid onset, severe headache of subarachnoid hemorrhage are a group of "thunderclap headaches" of diverse causes but principally cerebral venous thrombosis and vasospasm syndromes. Brief sharp pain, lasting a few seconds, in the eyeball (ophthalmodynia) or cranium ("ice-pick" pain) and "ice-cream headache" caused by pharyngeal cooling is more common in migraineurs, with or without the characteristic headache, but otherwise cannot be interpreted and is significant only by reason of its benignity.

Migraine of the classic type usually has its onset in the early morning hours or in the daytime, reaches its peak of severity typically over several to 30 min, and lasts, unless treated, for 4 to 24 h, occasionally for as long as 72 h or more. Often, it is terminated by sleep. A migrainous patient having several attacks per week usually proves to have a combination of migraine and tension headaches, an analgesic "rebound headache," or, rarely, some unexpected intracranial lesion. By contrast, the occurrence of unbearably severe unilateral orbitotemporal pain coming on within an hour or two after falling asleep or at predictable times during the day and recurring nightly or daily for a period of several weeks to months is typical of cluster headache; usually an individual attack of "cluster" dissipates in 30 to 45 min but some blend into more prolonged migraine. The headache of intracranial tumor may appear at any time of the day or night; it will interrupt sleep, vary in intensity, and last a few minutes to hours as the tumor raises intracranial pressure. With posterior fossa masses, the headache tends to be worse in the morning, on awakening. Tension headaches, described further on, may persist with varying intensity for weeks to months or even longer; when such headaches are protracted, there is usually an associated depressive illness. In general, headaches that have recurred regularly for many years prove to be migraine or tension in type.

The more or less constant *relationship of headache to certain biologic events and also to certain precipitating or aggravating (or relieving) factors* can be of great significance in diagnosis. Headaches that occur regularly in the premenstrual period are usually generalized and mild in degree, but attacks of migraine may also occur at this time (catamenial migraine). Headaches that have their origin in cervical spine disease are most typically intense after a period of inactivity, such as a night's sleep, and the first movements of the neck are stiff and painful. Headache, or more often face ache, from infection of the nasal sinuses may appear, with clock-like regularity, upon awakening or in midmorning and is characteristically worsened by stooping and changes in atmospheric pressure; there is associated midfrontal or maxillary tenderness. On the other hand, the regular recurrence of migraine headache is often misdiagnosed as chronic sinusitis. Eyestrain headaches, of course, follow prolonged use of the eyes, as after long-sustained periods of reading, or exposure to the glare of video displays, but the pain is transient. In certain individuals, alcohol, intense exercise (such as weight lifting), stooping, straining, coughing, and sexual intercourse are known to initiate a special type of bursting headache, lasting a few seconds to minutes. If a headache is made worse by sudden movement or by coughing or straining, an intracranial source is tentatively suggested. Migraine often occurs several hours or a day following a period of intense activity and stress ("weekend", or "letdown" migraine). Some patients have discovered that their migraine is relieved momentarily by gentle compression of the carotid or superficial temporal artery on the painful side, and others report that the carotid near the angle of the jaw is tender during the headache. Pain that is noticed when the scalp is stroked in combing or fixing the hair (allodynia) is common in migraine but could be a symptom of inflammation of the temporal arteries (temporal arteritis).

Pain-Sensitive Cranial Structures

Our understanding of headache has been augmented by observations made during operations on the brain (Ray and Wolff). These observations have informed us that only certain cranial structures are sensitive to noxious stimuli: (1) skin, subcutaneous tissue, muscles, extracranial arteries, and external periosteum of the skull; (2) the delicate structures of the eye, ear, nasal cavities, and paranasal sinuses; (3) intracranial venous sinuses and their large tributaries because they are intradural; (4) parts of the dura at the base of the brain and the arteries within the dura, particularly the proximal parts of the anterior and middle cerebral arteries and the intracranial segment of the internal carotid artery; (5) the middle meningeal and superficial temporal arteries; and (6) the first three cervical nerves and cranial nerves as they pass through the dura. Interestingly, pain is practically the only sensation produced by stimulation of these structures; the pain arises in the walls of blood vessels containing pain fibers (the nature of vascular pain is discussed further on). Much of the pia-arachnoid, the parenchyma of the brain, and the ependyma and choroid plexuses lack sensitivity.

The reference sites of pain from the aforementioned structures are important in understanding the genesis of cranial pain. Pain that arises from distention of the middle meningeal artery is projected to the back of the eye and temporal area. Pain from the intracranial segment of the internal carotid artery and proximal parts of the middle and anterior cerebral arteries is felt in the eye and orbitotemporal regions. The pathways whereby cephalic sensory stimuli are transmitted to the central nervous system (CNS) are the trigeminal nerves, particularly their first and, to some extent, second divisions, which convey impulses from the forehead, orbit, anterior and middle fossae of the skull, and the upper surface of the tentorium. The sphenopalatine branches of the facial nerve convey impulses from the nasoorbital region. The ninth and tenth cranial nerves and the first three cervical nerves transmit impulses from the inferior surface of the tentorium and all of the posterior fossa. Sympathetic fibers from the three cervical ganglia and parasympathetic fibers from the sphenopalatine and otic ganglia are mixed with the trigeminal and other sensory fibers. The tentorium roughly demarcates the trigeminal from the cervical–vagal–glossopharyngeal innervation zones. The central sensory connections, which ascend through the brainstem or the cervical spinal cord and brainstem to the thalamus, are described in Chaps. 8 and 9.

To summarize, pain from supratentorial structures is referred to the anterior two-thirds of the head, i.e., to the territory of sensory supply of the first and second divisions of the trigeminal nerve; pain from infratentorial structures is referred to the vertex and back of the head and neck predominantly by the second cervical roots. Trigeminal and cervical sensory inputs converge on the second order neurons at the C2 level, permitting pain from the neck and occipital regions to be referred to the forehead, and vice versa. The seventh, ninth, and tenth cranial nerves refer pain to the nasoorbital region, ear, and throat. There may be local tenderness of the scalp at the site of the referred pain. Dental or temporomandibular joint pain impulses are carried by the second and third divisions of the trigeminal nerve. With the exception of the cervical portion of the internal carotid artery, from which pain is referred to the eyebrow and supraorbital region, and the upper cervical spine, from which pain may be referred to the occiput, pain because of disease in extracranial parts of the body is not referred to the head. There are, however, rare instances of angina pectoris that may produce discomfort at the cranial vertex or adjacent sites and, of course, in the jaw.

Mechanisms of Cranial Pain

The studies of Ray and Wolff demonstrated that relatively few mechanisms are operative in the genesis of cranial pain. More specifically, *intracranial mass lesions* cause headache only if they deform, displace, or exert traction on vessels and dural structures at the base of the brain, and this may happen long before intracranial pressure rises. In fact, artificially raising the intraspinal and intracranial pressure by the subarachnoid or intraventricular injection of sterile saline solution does not consistently result in headache. This has been interpreted to mean that raised intracranial pressure does not cause headache—a questionable conclusion when one considers the relief of headache in some patients that follows lumbar puncture and lowering of the cerebrospinal fluid (CSF) pressure, particularly after subarachnoid hemorrhage. Actually, most patients with high intracranial pressure complain of bioccipital and bifrontal headaches that fluctuate in severity, probably because of traction on vessels or dura.

Dilatation of intracranial or extracranial arteries (and possibly sensitization of these vessels), of whatever cause, is likely to produce headache. The headaches that follow seizures and ingestion of alcohol are probably all caused by cerebral vasodilatation. Nitroglycerin, nitrites in cured meats ("hot-dog headache"), and monosodium glutamate in Chinese food may cause headache by the same mechanism. It is possible that the throbbing or steady headache that accompanies febrile illnesses has a vascular origin as well; it is likely that the increased pulsation of meningeal vessels activates pain-sensitive structures within their walls or around the base of the brain. Febrile headache may be generalized or predominate in the frontal or occipital regions and is relieved on one side by carotid or superficial temporal artery compression and on both sides by jugular vein compression. Like migraine, it is also increased by shaking the head. Certain systemic infectious agents, enumerated further on, have a tendency to cause severe headache.

A similar mechanism may be operative in the severe, bilateral, throbbing headaches associated with extremely rapid rises in blood pressure, as occurs with pheochromocytoma, malignant hypertension, sexual activity, and in patients being treated with monoamine oxidase inhibitors. Mild to moderate degrees of chronic hypertension, however, do not cause headaches despite a popular notion to the contrary. So-called cough and exertional headaches may also have their basis in the distention of intracranial vessels.

For many years, following the investigations of Harold Wolff, the headache of migraine was attributed to dilatation of the extracranial arteries. Now, it appears that this is not a constant relationship and that the headache is of complex intracranial as much as extracranial origin, perhaps related to the sensitization of blood vessels and their surrounding structures. Activation of the trigeminovascular system (the trigeminal nerves and the blood vessels they supply), leading to an inflammatory response that is generated by local neural mechanisms, "neurogenic inflammation," has also been assigned a role in migraine headache. These and other theories of causation are summarized by Cutrer and discussed further on in this chapter in the section on migraine.

With regard to cerebrovascular diseases causing head pain, the extracranial temporal and occipital arteries, when involved in giant cell arteritis (cranial or "temporal" arteritis), give rise to severe, persistent headache, at first localized on the scalp and then more diffuse. Most strokes caused by vascular occlusion do not cause head pain. However, with occlusion or dissection of the vertebral artery, there may be pain in the upper neck or postauricular area; basilar artery thrombosis causes pain to be projected to the occiput and sometimes to the forehead; and the ipsilateral eye and brow, and the forehead above it are the most common sites of projected pain from dissection of the carotid artery and occlusion of the stem of the middle cerebral arteries. Expanding or ruptured intracranial aneurysms of the posterior communicating or distal internal carotid arteries very often cause pain projected to the eye.

Infection or blockage of paranasal sinuses is accompanied by pain over the affected maxillary or frontal sinuses. Usually it is associated with tenderness of the skin and cranium in the same distribution. Pain from the ethmoid and sphenoid sinuses is localized deep in the midline behind the root of the nose or occasionally at the vertex (especially with disease of the sphenoid sinus). The mechanism in these cases involves changes in pressure and irritation of pain-sensitive sinus walls.

With frontal and ethmoidal sinusitis, the pain tends to be worse on awakening and gradually subsides when the patient is upright; the opposite pertains with maxillary and sphenoidal sinusitis. These relationships are believed to disclose their mechanism; pain is ascribed to filling of the sinuses and its relief to their emptying, induced by the dependent position of the ostia. Bending over intensifies the pain by causing changes in pressure, as does blowing the nose and air travel, especially on descent, when the relative pressure in the blocked sinus rises. Sympathomimetic drugs, such as phenylephrine hydrochloride, which reduce swelling and congestion, tend to relieve the pain. However, the pain may persist after all purulent secretions have disappeared, probably because of blockage of the orifice by boggy membranes and absorption of air from the blocked sinus, so called *vacuum sinus headaches.*

Headache of ocular origin, located as a rule in the orbit, forehead, or temple, is of the steady, aching type and tends to follow prolonged use of the eyes in close work. The main faults are hypermetropia and astigmatism (rarely myopia), which result in sustained contraction of extraocular as well as frontal, temporal, and even occipital muscles. In the uncommon and overemphasized circumstance of a refractive error causing headache, correction rapidly ameliorates the headache. Traction on the extraocular muscles or the iris during eye surgery will evoke pain. Patients who develop diplopia from neurologic causes or are forced to use one eye because the other has been occluded by a patch often complain of frontal headache. Another mechanism is involved in *iridocyclitis* and in *acute angle closure glaucoma,* in which raised intraocular pressure causes steady, aching pain in the region of the eye, radiating to the forehead. When acute angle closure glaucoma causes headache, the sclera is invariably red. Dilating the pupil risks precipitating angle closure glaucoma, a situation that can be reversed by the administration of pilocarpine 1 percent drops.

Headaches that accompany disease of ligaments, muscles, and apophysial joints in the upper part of the cervical spine are referred to the occiput and nape of the neck on the same side and sometimes to the temple and forehead. These headaches have been reproduced by the injection of hypertonic saline solution into the affected ligaments, muscles, and facet joints and are comparable to the regions of sclerotogenous referred pain that is discussed in Chap. 8. Such pains are especially frequent in late life because of the prevalence of degenerative changes in the cervical spine and tend also to occur after whiplash injuries or other forms of sudden flexion, extension, or torsion of the head on the neck. If the pain is arthritic in origin, the first movements after the individual has been still for some hours are stiff and painful. The pain of fibromyalgia, a controversial entity, is characterized by tender areas near the cranial insertion of cervical and other muscles. There are no pathologic data as to the nature of these vaguely palpable and tender regions, and it is uncertain whether the pain actually arises in them. They may represent only the deep tenderness felt in the region of referred pain or the involuntary secondary protective spasm of muscles. Massage of muscles, heat, and injection of the tender spots with local anesthetic has unpredictable effects but relieves the pain in some cases. Unilateral occipital headache is often misinterpreted as occipital neuralgia (see further on).

The headache of meningeal irritation (usually due to infection or hemorrhage) is typically acute in onset, usually severe, generalized, deep seated, constant, and associated with stiffness of the neck, particularly on forward bending. It has been ascribed to increased intracranial pressure; indeed, the withdrawal of CSF may afford some relief. However, dilatation and inflammation of meningeal vessels and the chemical irritation of pain receptors in the large vessels and meninges by endogenous chemical agents, particularly serotonin and plasma kinins, are probably more important factors in the production of pain and spasm of the neck extensors. In the chemically induced meningitis from rupture of an epidermoid cyst, for example, the spinal fluid pressure is usually normal, but the headache is severe. Meningeal irritation or inflammation may also be chronic and have as its main feature a concurrently ongoing headache.

A distinctive type of headache is produced by subarachnoid hemorrhage; it is very intense and very sudden in onset and is usually associated with vomiting and neck stiffness. It is not uncommon for the rupture of an aneurysm that gives rise to subarachnoid hemorrhage to be precipitated by exertion, even of minor degree. Other causes of what has been called "thunderclap headache" discussed further on simulate this disease (see Chap. 34). Among them is a type of diffuse cerebrovascular spasm that may be spontaneous, the result of sympathomimetic drugs, and extracranial vascular dissection of the carotid or vertebral arteries. Another cause is cerebral venous thrombosis.

Lumbar puncture (LP) or spontaneous low CSF pressure headache, as elaborated in Chap. 2, is characterized by a steady occipitonuchal and frontal pain coming on within a few minutes after arising from a recumbent position (orthostatic headache) and is relieved within a minute or two by lying down. Its cause is a persistent leakage of CSF into the lumbar tissues through the needle track, or a tear of the meninges that may be spontaneous or induced by spinal trauma. The CSF pressure is low (often zero in the lateral decubitus position), and installation of an epidural "blood patch" relieves the headache. Usually this type of headache is increased by compression of the jugular veins but is unaffected by digital obliteration of the carotid artery. It is likely that, in the upright position, a low intraspinal and negative intracranial pressure permits caudal displacement of the brain, with traction on dural attachments and dural sinuses. Pannullo and colleagues, with MRI, have demonstrated this downward displacement of the cranial contents. "Spontaneous" low-pressure headache may follow a cough, sneeze, strain, or athletic injury, sometimes as a result of rupture of the arachnoid sleeve along a nerve root (see "Spontaneous Intracranial Hypotension" in Chap. 30). Less frequently, LP is complicated by severe stiffness of the neck and pain over the back of the neck and occiput (see "Lumbar Puncture Headache" in Chap. 2); a second spinal tap in some instances discloses slight pleocytosis but no decrease in glucose—a sterile meningitis. This benign reaction must be distinguished from the rare occurrence of meningitis caused by introduction of bacteria through a rent in the meninges that has allowed both escape of spinal fluid and ingress of bacteria.

Headaches that are aggravated by lying down or lying on one side occur with acute and chronic subdural hematoma and with some brain masses, particularly those in the posterior fossa. The headache of subdural hematoma, when it occurs, is dull and unilateral, perceived over most of the affected side of the head. The global and nuchal headaches of idiopathic intracranial hypertension (pseudotumor cerebri) are also generally worse in the supine position (Chap. 31). In all these states of raised intracranial pressure, headaches are typically worse in the early morning hours after a long period of recumbency. Further on, we discuss the relative infrequency of headache as a result of brain tumor.

Exertional headaches are usually benign, but they are sometimes related to pheochromocytoma, arteriovenous malformation, or other intracranial lesions, in addition to the aforementioned subarachnoid hemorrhage from ruptured aneurysm. The same applies to headaches induced by stooping, most of which are benign or, at worst, are accounted for by sinus infection but there are exceptions and subdural hematoma is a known cause (see further on).

PRINCIPAL VARIETIES OF HEADACHE

The clinician's first goal when confronted with a patient with cranial pain is to determine if the headache is primary or secondary. The main primary headache syndromes are migraine, tension-type headache, cluster headache, or one of the trigeminal–sympathetic migraine variants of migraine or cluster. These tend to be chronic, recurrent, and unattended by other symptoms and signs of neurologic disease. Familiarity with the variety of symptoms, temporal profiles, and accompanying features of the primary headache disorders, and the proclivity for most of them to be familial, assist in identifying them from the patient's description. There should be little difficulty in recognizing the secondary headaches of diseases such as glaucoma, purulent sinusitis, subarachnoid hemorrhage, and bacterial or viral meningitis provided that these sources of headache are kept in mind. A fuller account of these types of "secondary" headache syndromes is given in later chapters of the book, where the underlying diseases are described. All other headaches that by their localization, quality of pain, and precipitating characteristics do not conform to one of the primary types should be suspected of being symptomatic of a cranial, cervical, or systemic disorder. Nonetheless, in many instances no such underlying cause will be found after investigation.

The following broad categories of headaches should be considered (Table 10-1). In general, the classification of these headaches and other types of craniofacial pain follow the plan outlined by the International Headache Society (see Olesen and http://ihs-classification.org/en/).

Migraine

Migraine is a highly prevalent and largely familial disorder characterized by periodic, commonly unilateral, often pulsatile headaches that begin in childhood, adolescence, or early adult life and recur with diminishing frequency during advancing years.

Two closely related clinical syndromes have been identified, the first called *migraine with aura* and the second, *migraine without aura* (terminology of the International Headache Society). For many years, the first syndrome was referred to as *classic* or *neurologic* migraine and the second as *common* migraine. The ratio of classic to common migraine is 1:5. Either type may be preceded by vague premonitory changes in mood and appetite. *Migraine with aura* is ushered in by a disturbance of nervous function, most often visual, followed in a few minutes to hours by hemicranial (or, in about one-third of cases, bilateral) headache, nausea, and sometimes vomiting, all of which last for hours or as long as a day or more. Migraine without aura is characterized by an unheralded onset over minutes or longer of increasing hemicranial headache or, less often, by generalized headache with or without nausea and vomiting, which then follows the same temporal pattern as the migraine with aura. Sensitivity to light, noise, and often smells (photophobia, phono- or sonophobia, and osmophobia) attends both types, and intensification with movement of the head is common. If the pain is severe, the patient prefers to lie down in a quiet, darkened room and tries to sleep. The *hemicranial* and the *throbbing* (pulsating) aspects of migraine are its most characteristic features in comparison to other headache types. Each patient displays a proclivity for the pain to affect one side or the other of the cranium, but not exclusively, so that some bouts are on the other side.

The heritable nature of classic migraine is apparent from its occurrence in several members of the family of the same and successive generations in 60 to 80 percent of cases; the familial frequency of common migraine is slightly lower. Twin and sibling studies have not revealed

Table 10-1

COMMON TYPES OF HEADACHE

TYPE	SITE	AGE AND SEX	CLINICAL CHARACTERISTICS	DIURNAL PATTERN	LIFE PROFILE	PROVOKING FACTORS	ASSOCIATED FEATURES	TREATMENT
Migraine without aura (common migraine)	Frontotemporal	Adolescents, young to middle-aged adults, sometimes children, more common in women	Throbbing (pulsatile); worse behind one eye or ear	Upon awakening or later in day	Irregular intervals, weeks to months	Bright light, noise, tension, alcohol	Nausea and vomiting in some cases	Triptans, ergotamine, nonsteroidal anti-inflammatory agents
	Uni- or bilateral		Becomes dull ache and generalized	Duration: 4–24 h in most cases, sometimes longer	Tends to decrease in middle age and during pregnancy	Relieved by darkness and sleep		Propranolol or amitriptyline for prevention
			Scalp sensitive					
Migraine with aura (neurologic migraine)	Same as above	Same as above	Same as above	Same as above	Same as above	Same as above	Scintillating lights, visual loss, and scotomas	Same as above
			Family history frequent				Unilateral paresthesias, weakness, dysphasia, vertigo, rarely confusion	
Cluster (histamine headache, migrainous neuralgia)	Orbitotemporal	Adolescent and adult males (90%)	Intense, nonthrobbing	Usually nocturnal, 1–2 h after falling asleep	Nightly or daily for several weeks to months	Alcohol in some	Lacrimation	O_2, sumatriptan, ergotamine before anticipated attack
	Unilateral			Occasionally diurnal	Recurrence after many months or years		Stuffed nostril	Corticosteroids, verapamil, valproate, and lithium in recalcitrant cases
							Rhinorrhea	
							Injected conjunctivum	
							Ptosis	
Tension headaches	Generalized	Mainly adults, both sexes, more common in women	Pressure (nonthrobbing), tightness, aching	Continuous, variable intensity, for days, weeks, or months	One or more periods of months to years	Fatigue and nervous strain	Depression, worry, anxiety	Antianxiety and antidepressant drugs

(Continued)

Table 10-1

COMMON TYPES OF HEADACHE (*CONTINUED*)

TYPE	SITE	AGE AND SEX	CLINICAL CHARACTERISTICS	DIURNAL PATTERN	LIFE PROFILE	PROVOKING FACTORS	ASSOCIATED FEATURES	TREATMENT
Meningeal irritation (meningitis, subarachnoid hemorrhage)	Generalized, or bioccipital, or bifrontal	Any age, both sexes	Intense, steady deep pain, may be worse in neck	Rapid evolution—minutes to hours	Single episode	None	Neck stiff on forward bending	For meningitis or bleeding (see text)
							Kernig and Brudzinski signs	
Brain tumor	Unilateral or generalized	Any age, both sexes	Variable intensity	Lasts minutes to hours; worse in early A.M., increasing severity	Once in a lifetime: weeks to months	None	Papilledema	Corticosteroids
			May awaken patient			Sometimes position	Vomiting	Mannitol
			Steady pain				Impaired mentation	Treatment of tumor
							Seizures	
							Focal signs	
Temporal arteritis	Unilateral or bilateral, usually temporal	Older than 50 years, either sex	Throbbing, then persistent aching and burning, arteries thickened and tender	Intermittent, then continuous	Persists for weeks to months	None	Loss of vision	Corticosteroids
							Polymyalgia rheumatica	
							Fever, weight loss, increased sedimentation rate, jaw claudication	

a consistent mendelian pattern in either the classic or common form. Certain special forms of migraine, such as familial hemiplegic migraine, appear to be monogenic disorders but the role of these genes, most of which code for ion channels, in classic and common migraine is speculative.

Migraine, with or without aura, is a remarkably common condition. A study by Stewart and colleagues in the United States showed differences in the prevalence of migraine between individuals of white, African, and Asian origin of approximately 20, 16, and 9 percent, respectively, among women, and 9, 7, and 4 percent for men (see also Lipton et al). One-third of migraineurs have more than three attacks monthly if untreated and many require bed rest or severe curtailment of daily activities. Migraine may have its onset in childhood but usually begins in adolescence or young adulthood; in more than 80 percent of patients, the onset is before 30 years of age, and the physician should be cautious in attributing headaches that appear for the first time after this age to migraine, although there are exceptions.

In younger women, the headaches often tend to occur during the premenstrual period; in approximately 15 percent of such migraineurs, the attacks are exclusively perimenstrual (also termed "catamenial migraine"). *Menstrual migraine,* discussed further on, had been considered to be solely related to the withdrawal of estradiol (based on the work of Somerville). It is now acknowledged that the influence of sex hormones on headache is more complex. Migraine tends to cease during the second and third trimesters of pregnancy in 75 to 80 percent of women, and in others they continue at a reduced frequency; less often, attacks of migraine or the associated neurologic symptoms first appear during pregnancy, usually in the first trimester.

Although migraine commonly diminishes in severity and frequency with age, it may actually worsen in some postmenopausal women, and estrogen therapy may either increase or, paradoxically, diminish the incidence of headaches. The use of birth control pills is associated with an increased frequency and severity of migraine and in rare instances has resulted in a permanent neurologic deficit (see further on and Chap 34).

Some patients link their attacks to certain dietary items—particularly chocolate, cheese, fatty foods, oranges, tomatoes, and onions—but these connections have proved invalid in controlled trials and, except in the occasional persuasive instance, they seem to us to be overrated. Some of these foods are rich in tyramine, which has been incriminated as a provocative factor in migraine. Alcohol, particularly red wine or port, regularly provokes an attack in some persons; in others, headaches are fairly consistently induced by exposure to glare or other strong sensory stimuli, sudden jarring of the head ("footballer's migraine"), or by rapid changes in barometric pressure. A common trigger is excess caffeine intake or withdrawal of caffeine.

Migraine with aura frequently has its onset soon after awakening, but it may occur at any time of day. During the preceding day or so, there may have been mild changes in mood (sometimes a surge of energy or a feeling of well-being), hunger or anorexia, drowsiness, or frequent yawning. Then, abruptly, there is a disturbance of vision consisting usually of unformed flashes of white, or silver, or, rarely, of multicolored lights (photopsia). This may be followed by an enlarging blind spot with a shimmering edge (*scintillating scotoma*), or formations of dazzling zigzag lines (arranged like the battlements of a castle, hence the term *fortification spectra,* or *teichopsia*). Other patients complain instead of blurred or shimmering or cloudy vision, as though they were looking through thick or smoked glass or the wavy distortions produced by heat rising from asphalt. These luminous hallucinations move slowly across the visual field for several minutes and may leave an island of visual loss in their wake (scotoma); the latter is usually homonymous (involving corresponding parts of the field of vision of each eye), pointing to its origin in the visual cortex. Patients often attribute these visual symptoms to one eye rather than to parts of both fields. Ophthalmologic abnormalities of retinal and optic nerve vessels have been described in some cases but are not typical.

Other focal neurologic symptoms, much less common than visual ones, include numbness and tingling of the lips, face, and hand (on one or both sides); slight confusion of thinking; weakness of an arm or leg; mild aphasia or dysarthria, dizziness, and uncertainty of gait or drowsiness. Only one or a few neurologic phenomena are present in any given patient and they tend to occur in more or less the same combination in each attack. If weakness or paresthetic numbness spreads from one part of the body to another, or if one neurologic symptom follows another, this occurs relatively slowly over a period of minutes (not over seconds, as in a seizure, or simultaneously in all affected parts as in a transient ischemic attack).

The visual or neurologic symptoms usually last for less than 30 min, sometimes longer. As they recede, a unilateral dull pain develops of slowly increasing intensity that progresses to a throbbing headache (usually but not always on the side of the cerebral disturbance). At the peak of the pain, within minutes to an hour, the patient may be forced to lie down and to shun light (photophobia) and noise (phonophobia). Light is irritating and may be painful to the globes, or it is perceived as overly bright (dazzle) and strong odors are disagreeable. Nausea and, less often, vomiting may occur. The headache lasts for hours and sometimes for a day or even longer and is always the most unpleasant feature of the illness. The temporal scalp vessels may be tender and the headache is worsened by strain or jarring of the body or head. Pressure on the scalp vessels or carotid artery may momentarily reduce the pain and releasing pressure accentuates it.

Between attacks, the migrainous patient is normal. In the past, it was believed that a migrainous personality existed, characterized by tenseness, rigidity of attitudes and thinking, meticulousness, and perfectionism. Further analyses, however, have not established a particular personality type in the migraineur. A relationship of migraine to epilepsy in general is also tenuous; however, the incidence of seizures is slightly higher in migrainous patients and their relatives than in the general population, and there are syndromes that encompass both disorders.

Some patients note that their attacks of migraine tend to occur during the "let-down period," after many days of hard work or tension. There is an overrepresentation of motion sickness or a vague instability of vision or accommodation, sensitivity to striped patterns, fainting, and of fleeting sensory symptoms on one side of the body in migraineurs. Moreover, as appreciated by Graham, migraine has a lifetime profile and is a familial disease that includes some or many of the following: colic in infancy, motion sickness, episodic abdominal pain, fainting, alcohol sensitivity, exercise-induced headaches, "sinus headaches," "tension headaches," and menstrual headaches. These are fairly dependable markers of the disease, and their absence in the patient or family members should at least cause the consideration of alternative explanations for cranial pain.

Migraine Variants

Much variation occurs in migraine. The headache may be exceptionally severe and abrupt in onset ("crash migraine" or "thunderclap headache"), raising the specter of subarachnoid hemorrhage. Careful questioning in these cases sometimes reveals that the headache did not truly attain its peak rapidly but evolved over several minutes. Nonetheless, the distinction of this type of "thunderclap headache" from subarachnoid hemorrhage can be made only by examination of the CSF and imaging of the brain (see further on, under "Special Varieties of Headache").

A headache may at times precede or accompany, rather than follow, the neurologic abnormalities of migraine with aura. Although typically hemicranial (the French word *migraine* is said to be derived from *megrim*, which, in turn, is from the Latin *hemicrania,* and its corrupted forms *hemigranea* and *migranea*), the pain may be frontal, temporal, or, quite often, generalized.

Any two of the three principal components—neurologic abnormality, headache, and gastrointestinal upset—may be absent. With advancing age, for example, there is a tendency for the headache and nausea to become less severe, finally leaving only the neurologic abnormality, which itself recurs with decreasing frequency. This is also subject to great variation. One common configuration is a full-blown visual aura without subsequent headache (migraine without headache, or migraine dissocié). Visual disturbances differ in detail from patient to patient; numbness and tingling of the lips and the fingers of one hand are probably next in frequency, followed by transient dysphasia or a thickness of speech and hemiparesis as mentioned earlier. Rarely, there is sudden but transient blindness or a hemianopia at the onset of a migraine attack, accompanied by only a mild headache.

Basilar Migraine

A less-common form of the migraine syndrome with prominent brainstem symptoms was described by Bickerstaff. The patients, usually children with a family history of migraine, first develop visual phenomena like those of typical migraine except that they occupy much or the whole of both visual fields (temporary cortical blindness may occur). There may be associated vertigo, staggering, incoordination of the limbs, dysarthria, and tingling in both hands and feet, and sometimes around both sides of the mouth. These symptoms last 10 to 30 min and are followed by headache, which is usually occipital. Some patients, at the stage when the headache would have been likely to begin, may faint, and others become confused or stuporous, a state that may persist for several hours or longer. Exceptionally, there is an alarming period of coma or quadriplegia. The symptoms closely resemble those caused by ischemia in the territory of the basilar-posterior cerebral arteries—hence the name *basilar artery* or *vertebrobasilar migraine*. Subsequent studies have indicated that basilar migraine, although more common in children and adolescents, affects men and women more or less equally over a wide age range, and that the condition is not always benign and transient.

Ophthalmoplegic and Retinal Migraine

The ophthalmoplegic migraines are recurrent unilateral headaches associated with weakness of extraocular muscles. A transient third-nerve palsy with ptosis, with or without involvement of the pupil, is the usual picture; rarely, the sixth nerve is affected. This disorder is more common in children. The ocular paresis often outlasts the headache by days or weeks; after many attacks, a slight mydriasis and, rarely, ophthalmoparesis may remain permanently.

In some cases of uniocular visual disturbance with scotoma, the retinal arterioles have been reported to be attenuated and, rarely, there are retinal hemorrhages as described by Berger and colleagues. More often, there are no funduscopic changes. Such events are referred to as *retinal migraine*, or, more accurately, *ocular migraine*, as either the retinal or the ciliary circulation may be involved. However, in adults the syndrome of headache, unilateral ophthalmoparesis, and loss of vision may have more serious causes, including temporal (cranial) arteritis.

Migraine following Head Injury

Cranial trauma of almost any degree may precipitate a migraine headache in persons prone to the condition. A particularly troublesome migraine variant occurs in a child or adolescent who, after a trivial or mild head injury, may lose vision, suffer severe headache or be plunged into a state of confusion, with belligerent and irrational behavior that lasts for hours or several days before clearing. In yet another variant, there is an abrupt onset of either one-sided paralysis or aphasia after virtually every minor head injury (we have seen this condition several times in college athletes) but without visual symptoms and little or no headache. Although a family history of migraine is frequent in such cases, there has been no history of hemiplegia in other family members.

Migraine in Young Children

This may present special difficulties in diagnosis, as a young child's capacity for accurate description is limited.

Instead of complaining of headache, the child appears limp and pale and complains of abdominal pain; vomiting is more frequent than in the adult, and there may be slight fever. Recurrent attacks were referred to in the past by pediatricians as the "periodic syndrome." Another variant in the child is episodic vertigo and staggering (paroxysmal disequilibrium) followed by headache, probably a type of basilar migraine (see Watson and Steele). Also, there are puzzling patients with bouts of fever or transient disturbances in mood ("psychic equivalents") and abdominal pain (*abdominal migraine*), that had been attributed to migraine but are dubious entities at best. We have seen several infants and young children who have had attacks of hemiplegia (without headache), first on one side then the other, every few weeks. Recovery was complete, and arteriography in one child, after more than 70 attacks, was normal. Alternating hemiplegia of childhood may terminate in a dystonic state. The relationship of this condition to familial hemiplegic migraine (see below) remains uncertain. The only advantage of considering such attacks as migrainous is that it may protect some patients from unnecessary diagnostic procedures and surgical intervention; but, by the same token, it may delay appropriate investigation and treatment.

Familial Hemiplegic Migraine

In a related disorder, known as *hemiplegic migraine*, a condition mostly of infants and children (rarely adults), there are episodes of unilateral paralysis that may long outlast the headache. Several families have been described in which this condition is the result of a mutation in an ion channel (*familial hemiplegic migraine; alternating hemiplegia of childhood*). Of the known loci, which together account for approximately 50 percent of cases, the most common one is in the gene coding for the P/Q-type calcium channel α subunit (CACNA1A). A second locus is in the gene for the Na^+/K^+-adenosine triphosphatase (ATPase) channel and a rarer subtype is caused by mutations in a sodium channel α-subunit gene, *SCNA1*. These do not account for all cases, indicating that there are other mutations that will inevitably be discovered. It is reasonable to surmise that many of the nonfamilial cases of hemiplegic migraine are also caused by these mutations. By their nature, these channelopathies would be expected to have clinical and genetic overlap with other neurologic diseases. Indeed, there are shared traits between some of the genetic forms of familial hemiplegic migraine and both episodic and degenerative cerebellar diseases (Goadsby, 2007). Ducros and colleagues have found a variety of other neurologic features in these families, including persistent cerebellar ataxia and nystagmus in 20 percent; others had attacks of coma and hemiplegia from which they recovered.

Complicating the situation is the undoubted existence of sporadic migraine with transient hemiplegia that has no familial trait. Neurologic symptoms lasting more than an hour or so should prompt investigation for alternative causes, but none may be found. Instances of hemiplegic migraine may account for some of the inexplicable strokes in young women and older adults of both sexes, as discussed below.

Transient Ischemic Attacks and Stroke with Migraine (See also Chap. 34.)

Attacks of migraine, instead of beginning in childhood, may have their onset later in life, and Fisher provided support for the hypothesis that some of the transient aphasic, hemianesthetic, or hemiplegic attacks of later life may be of migrainous origin ("transient migrainous accompaniment").

Rarely, migrainous neurologic symptoms, instead of being transitory, leave a prolonged or even permanent deficit (e.g., homonymous hemianopia), indicative of an ischemic stroke. This has been called *complicated migraine* and a small number of these prove to be *migrainous infarctions*. Platelet aggregation, edema of the arterial wall, increased coagulability, dehydration from vomiting, and intense, prolonged spasms of vessels have all been implicated (on rather uncertain grounds) in the pathogenesis of arterial occlusion and strokes that complicate migraine (Rascol et al).

The reported incidence of this complication has varied. At the Mayo Clinic, in a group of 4,874 patients ages 50 years or younger with a diagnosis of migraine, migraine equivalent, or vascular headache, 20 patients had migraine-associated infarctions (Broderick and Swanson). Caplan described 7 patients in whom attacks of migraine were complicated by strokes in the vertebrobasilar territory. A more recent study by Wolf and colleagues collected 17 instances of stroke and migraine. Most had a prolonged aura, either visual, sensory or aphasic and over two-thirds of the strokes, demonstrated by diffusion restriction on MRI, were in the posterior circulation territory and occurred in younger women. There is, nonetheless, a paucity of useful pathology by which to interpret the mechanism of migraine-associated stroke. The uncertain but potential role of antimigraine medications in producing stroke is discussed further on in the section on treatment. Estrogen medications have also been implicated in stroke in some women migraineurs.

In children and young adults with the mitochondrial disease MELAS (mitochondrial myopathy, encephalopathy, lactic acidosis, and stroke-like episodes) and in adults with the rare cerebral vasculopathy CADASIL (cerebral autosomal dominant arteriopathy with subcortical infarcts and leukoencephalopathy), migraine may be a prominent feature. Chap. 34 addresses these issues further.

The special problem of focal cerebral disorders associated with segmental or diffuse vasospasm, including the form that follows treatment with the "triptan" (serotonin agonist) drugs and Call-Fleming syndrome, is discussed further on in the section on treatment and under "Diffuse and Focal Cerebral Vasospasm" in Chap. 34.

A separate set of observations, mainly epidemiologic, pertain to the risk of mundane strokes in women with both migraine and cardiovascular disease later in life, and the related issue of imaging changes in migraineurs that are suggestive of small ischemic lesions. Regarding the last problem, a number of cross-sectional population studies, such as the ones by Kurth and colleagues, Scher et al, and Kruit and coworkers, indicated that MRI changes in both the deep and subcortical white matter were more frequent in women migraine patients who experienced auras than in those without auras and in the general population. A high frequency of migraine headaches was also associated in some studies with an increased number of white matter lesions. Some series have emphasized lesions in the cerebellar white matter.

In contrast, a meta-analysis of case control and cohort studies conducted by Schurks and colleagues were unable to demonstrate an increased risk for cardiovascular events. Other investigators, again depending on various population databases and few patient level studies, have come to the opposite conclusion (Bigal et al) and suggested that all cause mortality is increased in migraine patients (Gudmundsson et al).

The implications of the ubiquitous small white matter lesions in MRI that are now familiar to neurologists are unclear. Several studies indicate that migraineurs with these changes have no greater cognitive decline over time than those in the general population. The lesions are a frequent cause for neurological consultation, sometimes with the question of multiple sclerosis having been raised. We tend to underemphasize these lesions and the risk of stroke in discussion with patients but point out that the usual stroke risk factors, smoking, hypertension, hyperlipidemia, and cardiac rhythm abnormalities should be attended to assiduously.

The issue of oral contraceptives as a risk for stroke is a more complicated matter that has not been resolved. All that can be said at the moment is that this factor did not appear to be consistent in the above discussed epidemiologic surveys, and it is the population of young women who are likely to have both exposures. The pills are not interdicted in migraineurs but perhaps lower estrogen compounds are advisable as formulations with high estrogen concentrations have been associated with clotting in the venous circulation.

Patent foramen ovale and migraine Finally, there has long been discussion of an association between migraine and patent foramen ovale. A few physicians continue to favor a causal role and have advocated closure of the foramen in an attempt to alleviate migraine. Migraine with aura has been especially associated with an open foramen. However, the largest cross-sectional (Rundek et al) and case-control (Garg et al) studies have not affirmed these associations and the issue, while still under discussion, has been of waning interest.

Status Migrainosus

In some individuals, migraine attacks, for unaccountable reasons, may increase in frequency for several months. As many as three or four attacks may occur each week, leaving the scalp on one side continuously tender. An even more difficult clinical problem is posed by migraine that lapses into a condition of daily or virtually severe continuous headache (*status migrainosus*). The pain is initially unilateral, later more generalized, more or less throbbing, but with a constant superimposed ache and is disabling; vomiting or nausea is common at the outset but abates. Almost without exception, there is a preceding history compatible with migraine; in fact, the absence of prior headaches should raise concern about a more serious cause. Status migrainosus sometimes follows a head injury or a viral infection, but most cases have no explanation. Relief is sought by increasing the intake of ergot or serotonin agonist preparations or even opiates, often to an alarming degree, but with only temporary relief, serving at times to perpetuate the condition through a rebound mechanism.

In the diagnosis of such cases, the possibility should be considered that migraine has been combined with tension headache (migraine-tension or mixed-pattern headache) or transformed to so-called analgesia-rebound headache, or ergotamine, or serotonin agonist-dependency headache, as described by Taimi and colleagues. Narcotic addiction is another consideration. Although not generally popular, it is our practice to admit such patients to the hospital, discontinue all narcotic medications, and administer intravenous hydration, corticosteroids, one of the serotonin agonist medications, or dihydroergotamine intravenous infusion in selected patients (see further on for details of treatment). When admission is not possible or practical, the same therapeutic plan may be pursued in an ambulatory infusion center.

Migraine with CSF Pleocytosis (HaNDL)

An intriguing problem arises in the patient with migraine who is found to have a lymphocytic pleocytosis in the spinal fluid. Most of these cases in our experience have turned out to be simply instances of aseptic meningitis that have precipitated migraine in susceptible individuals. In others, a few cells are found in the spinal fluid during an attack of migraine without obvious explanation; probably a minor cellular reaction of 3 to 10 white blood cells (WBCs)/mL can be ignored if there is no fever or meningismus.

A more extensive syndrome was originally described by Bartleson, Swanson, and Whisnant under the title "A migrainous syndrome with cerebrospinal fluid pleocytosis". A series reported by Gomez-Aranda and colleagues gave the syndrome the name, "Pseudomigraine with Temporary Neurological Symptoms and Lymphocytic Pleocytosis", also called HaNDL (Headache with Neurological Deficits and CSF Lymphocytosis) by Berg and Williams, together describing what is probably yet another migraine variant. Gomez-Aranda's series comprised 50 adolescents and young adults, predominantly males, who developed several separate episodes of transient neurologic deficits lasting hours, accompanied by migraine-like headaches, sometimes with slight fever but no stiff neck. One-quarter of this group had a history of past migraine and a similar number had a viral-like illness within 3 weeks of the neurologic problem. The CSF contained from 10 to 760 lymphocytes per cubic millimeter, and the total protein was elevated. The transient neurologic deficits were mainly sensorimotor and aphasic; only 6 patients had visual symptoms. The patients were asymptomatic between attacks and in none did the entire illness persist beyond 7 weeks.

The causation and pathophysiology of this syndrome and its relation to migraine are obscure. We have observed several cases, all in otherwise healthy middle-aged men, none related to the use of nonsteroidal medications, which may cause an aseptic meningeal reaction, and we found corticosteroids to be helpful. The distinction between this syndrome and the recurrent aseptic meningitis of Mollaret and other chronic meningitic syndromes as well as cerebral vasospasm or vasculitis is difficult (see "Chronic Persistent and Recurrent Meningitis" in Chap. 32).

Cause and Pathogenesis of Migraine

So far, it has not been possible to determine from the many clinical observations and investigations, a unifying theory as to the cause and pathogenesis of migraine. Tension and other emotional states, which are claimed by some migraineurs to precede their attacks, are so inconsistent as to be no more than potential aggravating factors. Clearly, an underlying genetic factor is implicated, although it is expressed in a recognizable mendelian pattern in only a small number of families (see above). The puzzle is how this genetic predisposition is translated periodically into a regional neurologic deficit, unilateral headache, or both. For many years, our thinking about the pathogenesis of migraine was dominated by the views of Harold Wolff and others—that the headache was caused by the distention and excessive pulsation of branches of the external carotid artery. Certainly, the throbbing, pulsating quality of the headache and its relief by compression of the common carotid artery supported this view, as did the early observation of Graham and Wolff that the headache and amplitude of pulsation of the extracranial arteries diminished after the intravenous administration of ergotamine.

The importance of vascular factors continues to be emphasized by more recent findings but not in the way envisaged by Wolff. For example, in a group of 11 patients with classic migraine, Olsen and colleagues, using the xenon inhalation method, noted a regional reduction in cerebral circulation spreading forward from the occipital region during the period when neurologic symptoms appear. They concluded that the reduction in blood flow was consistent with the cortical spreading depression syndrome described below. In a subsequent study, Woods and colleagues described a patient who, during positron emission tomography (PET), fortuitously had an attack of common migraine with blurred vision. Sophisticated measurements showed a reduction in blood flow that started in the occipital cortex and spread slowly forward on both sides, in a manner much like that of the spreading cortical depression of Leão (see below) and Cutter and colleagues, using perfusion-weighted MRI, corroborated the finding of diminished occipital cerebral blood flow during the aura. However, a study using single-photon emission computed tomography (SPECT) in 20 patients during and after attacks of migraine without aura disclosed no focal changes of cerebral blood flow; also, no changes occurred after treatment of the attacks with 6 mg of subcutaneous sumatriptan (Ferrari et al, 1995).

In reference to the extracranial vessels, Iversen and associates, by means of ultrasonography, documented a dilatation of the superior temporal artery on the side of the migraine during the headache period. The same dilatation in the middle cerebral arteries has been inferred from observations with transcranial Doppler insonation. The complication of cerebral infarction is also in keeping with a vascular hypothesis, but it involves only a tiny proportion of migraineurs. The vascular hypothesis must be regarded as uncertain, but, clearly, there is frequently a reduction in posterior cortical blood flow during an aura. What is not established is whether the blood flow changes are fundamental or simply the result in a reduction in cortical activity. The original opinion expressed by Wolff that a vascular element is responsible for the cranial pain of migraine is also unconfirmed.

The relationship between the vascular changes and evolving neurologic symptoms of migraine are noteworthy. Lashley, who plotted his own visual aura, calculated that the cortical impairment progressed at a rate of 2 to 3 mm/min over the surface of the brain. Similarly, during the aura, there is a regional reduction in blood flow, as noted above. It begins in one occipital lobe and extends forward slowly (2.2 mm/min) as a wave of "spreading oligemia" that does not respect arterial boundaries (Lauritzen and Olesen). Both of these events are intriguingly similar to the above-mentioned phenomenon of "spreading cortical depression," first observed by Leão in experimental animals. He demonstrated that a noxious stimulus applied to the rat cortex was followed by vasoconstriction and slowly spreading waves of inhibition of the electrical activity of cortical neurons, moving at a rate of approximately 3 mm/min. Lauritzen and Olesen attribute both the aura and spreading oligemia to the spreading cortical depression, and considerable work since then has corroborated this idea. These observations, however, apply only to the aura.

An alternative, but not necessarily exclusive hypothesis links the aura and the painful phase of migraine through a neural mechanism originating in the trigeminal nerve as proposed by Moskowitz. This is based on the innervation of extracranial and intracranial vessels by small unmyelinated fibers of the trigeminal nerve that subserve both pain and autonomic functions (the "trigeminovascular" complex). This model provides an explanation for migraine pain in the trigeminal ganglion. Activation of these fibers releases substance P, calcitonin gene-related peptide (CGRP), and other peptides into the vessel wall, which serves to sensitize the trigeminal system to the pulsatility of cranial vessels, and to increase their permeability, thereby promoting an inflammatory response. The small molecules released from nerve endings adjacent to the cortex would then incite spreading depression in this model. Against this hypothesis is the occurrence of headache as often as not on the side opposite the side of generation of the aura and the lack of clinical effect of drugs that work in this experimental model. Most likely, both neural and vascular mechanisms are operative and they interact.

In part to address the action of the serotonin agonist drugs on migraine (see below), a body of evidence has been assembled that serotonin (5-HT) acts as a humoral mediator in the neural and vascular components of migraine headache. Serotonin is discharged from platelets at the onset of headache and the headache is reduced by the injection of 5-HT. This led to the development by Humphrey of sumatriptan, which acted selectively on 5-HT1B/D receptors so as to reduce side effects. This was the forerunner of the large group of "triptans." More recently, nitric oxide generated by endothelial cells has been implicated as the cause of the pain of migraine headache, but the reason for its release and the relationship to changes in blood flow is unclear.

Blau and Dexter and Drummond and Lance are confident that the presence or absence of headache does not depend solely on extracranial vascular factors. These authors point to their findings that occlusion of blood flow through the scalp or common carotid circulation fails to alleviate the pain of migraine in one-third to one-half the patients. Lance (1998) has suggested that the trigeminal pathways are in a state of persistent hyperexcitability in the migraine patient and that they discharge periodically, perhaps in response to hypothalamic stimulus acting on the endogenous pain control pathways. This is in keeping with current theories regarding the trigeminovascular complex discussed above, as well as with evolving ideas on central sensitization to pain because of repeated noxious stimulation from one body region that may produce a type of centrally mediated allodynia. The role of alternative factors in migraine has been reviewed by Lance and Goadsby and in a pictorial representation by Goadsby and colleagues.

The foregoing observations leave a number of questions unanswered. Is one to conclude that migraine with and without aura are different diseases, involving extracranial arteries in one instance and intracranial ones in another? Is the circulatory change the primary cause of headache, or is it a secondary or coincidental phenomenon? Is diminished neuronal activity (spreading depression) the primary cause of neurologic symptoms (it seems so) and headache (unclear), and is the diminished regional blood flow secondary to reduced metabolic demand? Why are the posterior portions of the brain (visual auras) so often implicated (perhaps because of richer trigeminal innervation of the posterior vessels)? The neural mechanisms that underlie these changes and precisely what is altered by the genetic predisposition to migraine are unresolved. No final reconciliation of all these data is possible and migraine remains incompletely explained.

Diagnosis

Migraine with aura should occasion no difficulty in diagnosis if a proper history is obtained. Most often, the symptoms begin as "positive," i.e., scintillation, paresthesia, as opposed to the later "negative" scotoma, numbness, aphasia, or paresis. The difficulties come from a lack of awareness that a progressively unfolding neurologic syndrome may be migrainous in origin and may occur without headache. Furthermore, recurrent migraine headaches take many forms, some of which may prove difficult to distinguish from the other common types of headache, and it is not generally recognized that migraine headaches need not be severe or disabling. Some of these problems merit elaboration because of their practical importance.

The neurologic part of the migraine syndrome may resemble a transient ischemic attack, focal epilepsy, the clinical effects of a slowly evolving hemorrhage from an arteriovenous malformation, or a thrombotic or embolic stroke. It is the pace of the neurologic symptoms of migraine that distinguish it from epilepsy and most cases of stroke. Furthermore, the positive rather than ablative nature of the symptoms assists in distinguishing it from the usual stroke syndromes.

Ophthalmoplegic migraine may suggest a carotid-cavernous or supraclinoid aneurysm. Transient monocular blindness from carotid stenosis is infrequent in the age group affected most by migraine, but the antiphospholipid syndrome, which has some ill-defined relationship to migraine, does cause episodic unilateral visual loss in this group and should be sought as the explanation for transient monocular blindness with or without headache. The invariant occurrence of migraine on the same side of the head increases the likelihood of an underlying arteriovenous malformation (AVM) or other structural lesion. R.D. Adams, who studied more than 1,200 patients with AVM, also found that the headaches, which occurred in more than 30 percent of these individuals, usually did not include the other features of either migraine or cluster headache. However, in about 5 percent, the headaches were associated with visual aura, making them indistinguishable from neurologic migraine. In most, the AVM was in the occipital region and on the side of the headache. Approximately half of the patients with AVM and migraine had a family history of migraine. It is unclear to us if AVM can be regarded as an acknowledged cause of recurrent migraine-like headache. It is, of course, possible that given the ubiquity of migraine in the population, that the association is coincidental.

Treatment of Migraine

This topic may be divided into two parts—control of the individual acute attack, and prevention that includes both medications and lifestyle modifications. The time to initiate treatment of an attack is during the neurologic (visual) prodrome or at the very onset of the headache (see below). If the headaches are mild, the patient may already have learned that aspirin, acetaminophen, or another nonsteroidal anti-inflammatory drug (NSAID) will suffice to control the pain. Insofar as a good response may be obtained from one type of NSAID and not another, it may be advisable to try two or three preparations in several successive attacks of headache and to use moderately high doses if necessary. Some of our colleagues state that reliable patients can be given small amounts of codeine or oxycodone, usually combined with aspirin or acetaminophen, for limited periods. The combination of aspirin or acetaminophen, caffeine, and butalbital, although popular with some patients, is usually incompletely effective if the headache is severe and is also capable of causing drug dependence. Numerous other medications have proved effective and each has had a period of popularity among neurologists and patients.

For severe attacks of migraine headache, sumatriptan or one of the other serotonin agonist "triptans" in this class (e.g., zolmitriptan, rizatriptan, naratriptan, almotriptan, eletriptan, and frovatriptan), or the ergot alkaloids, ergotamine tartrate, and particularly dihydroergotamine (DHE), are the most effective forms of treatment and are best administered early in the attack, ideally just after an aura or at the onset of headache.

Patients with waning visual auras should be advised to wait to self-administer subcutaneous serotonin agonists until the headache begins. Clinical experience and the study by Bates and colleagues suggests that the triptans are ineffective in preventing headache if given during the aura; they are albeit, safe (see below). In contrast, the slower acting nasal spray or oral formulations are often ineffective if given too long after the start of headache and patients have learned to administer them during the aura and, again, this seems safe.

A single 6-mg dose of sumatriptan or its equivalent, given subcutaneously, is an effective and well-tolerated treatment for migraine attacks. When successful, it eliminates or reduces the accompanying symptoms of nausea, vomiting, photophobia, and phonophobia. An advantage of the serotonin agonist drugs, aside from their relative safety, is the ease of self-administration using prepackaged injection kits, thus avoiding frequent and inconvenient visits to the emergency department. For example, sumatriptan can also be given orally in a 25- or 50-mg tablet and as a nasal spray (20 mg per spray), zolmitriptan in a 2.5- or 5-mg tablet, and rizatriptan in a 5- or 10-mg dose tablet, repeated, if needed, in 2 h. For these oral preparations, latency for headache relief is longer than with subcutaneous injection or inhalation. If one serotonin agonist is found to be ineffective, another drug or an alternative route of administration, such as intranasal, may be tried. These medications are summarized in Table 10-2.

A large and often cited meta-analysis of the available drugs in 53 separate trials conducted by Ferrari and colleagues (2001) found modest differences in overall efficacy between drugs. Loder has given a tabulated comparison of the main drugs for migraine and a review of their use in routine situations. Others in this class are sure to be developed in the future and subtle, but usually clinically minor, differences between them undoubtedly will be highlighted. Sumatriptan is available as a nasal spray, which is useful in patients with nausea and vomiting. The response rate after 2 h is similar to that of the orally administered drug, and the nasal spray acts more rapidly.

Ergotamine is an equally effective agent, but its peripheral and coronary vasoconstricting side effects have reduced its use. This is an alpha-adrenergic agonist with strong serotonin receptor affinity and vasoconstrictive action. The drug is taken as an uncoated 1- to 2-mg tablet of ergotamine tartrate, held under the tongue until dissolved (or swallowed), or in combination with caffeine. Repeat use is not advisable as it may lead to prolonged or daily headache. A single oral dose of promethazine 50 mg, or of metoclopramide 20 mg, given with the ergotamine, relaxes the patient and allays the potential nausea and vomiting from ergotamine. Patients in whom vomiting prevents oral administration may be given ergotamine by rectal suppository or DHE by nasal spray or inhaler (one puff at onset and another at 30 min) or can learn to give themselves a subcutaneous injection of DHE (usual dosage, 1 mg). Caffeine, 100 mg, is thought, on slim evidence, to potentiate the effects of ergotamine and other medications for migraine. When ergotamine is administered early in the attack, the headache will be abolished or reduced in severity and duration in 70 to 75 percent of patients.

An important problem pertains to the magnitude of risk of stroke from serotonin agonists in patients with prolonged visual aura or other neurologic symptoms that persist during the period of headache, or focal neurologic symptoms that are possibly attributable to migraine because of a past history of migraine with or without aura. As a matter of course, serotonin agonists and ergots are generally avoided if there is an ongoing and prolonged aura of any type, including visual, but particularly with hemiparesis, aphasia, or features such as vertigo, drowsiness, or diplopia, referable to the basilar artery. Not all experts agree with this proscription and some small series, among them 13 patients reported by Klapper and colleagues, have found triptans safe to use if a headache with neurologic signs has commenced, but this issue has not been resolved. As previously noted, although this class of drugs may not be helpful during the visual aura, they also seem to do no harm (see Bates et al).

Table 10-2

TRIPTANS FOR ORAL USE

TRIPTANS	TABLET SIZES, MG	OPTIMUM DOSES, MG	MAXIMUM SINGLE DOSES, MG	MAXIMUM DAILY DOSES, MG
Almotriptan	6.25 and 12.5	12.5	12.5	25
Eletriptan	20 and 40	20	40	80
Frovatriptan	2.5	2.5	2.5	7.5
Naratriptan	1 and 2.5	2.5	2.5	5
Rizatriptan	5 and 10	10[a]	10[a]	30[a]
Zolmitriptan	2.5 and 5	2.5	5	10
Sumatriptan*	25, 50, and 100	50	100	200

*Also available as 20 mg nasal spray and 6 mg subcutaneous injection.

Ergot drugs and triptans are contraindicated in symptomatic and asymptomatic coronary artery disease and poorly controlled hypertension. Rare cases of severe but reversible cerebral vasospasm have been reported after the use of ergotamine or a serotonin agonist drug, but most of these patients in fact had not had neurologic features as part of their initial headache syndrome. Of particular danger, however, is the often unnoticed, concurrent use of other sympathomimetic drugs such as phenylpropanolamine as in one of the cases described by Singhal and colleagues and by Meschia and associates (see discussion of Call-Fleming syndrome, "Diffuse Vasoconstriction," "Diffuse and Focal Cerebral Vasospasm" in Chap. 34). Cerebral hemorrhage is another rare complication of serotonin agonist use that possibly relates to hypertension induced by triptans or ergots.

For severely ill patients who arrive in the emergency department or physician's office, having failed to obtain relief from a prolonged headache with the above medications, Raskin (1986) has found metoclopramide 10 mg IV, followed by DHE 0.5 to 1 mg IV every 8 h for 2 days, to be effective. We also use this approach in cases of status migrainosus. The administration of intravenous DHE can be combined with a lidocaine infusion. The potential success of metoclopramide alone should not be dismissed, as we and others have occasionally found that the headache abates after this initial injection. The sympathomimetic drug isometheptene combined with a sedative, and acetaminophen (Midrin) has been useful for some patients and probably acts in a similar way to ergotamine and sumatriptan. A wide array of other drugs including almost all of the conventional nonsteroidal anti-inflammatory medications has been recommended as adjunctive therapy, e.g., prochlorperazine, chlorpromazine, ketorolac, and intranasal lidocaine. Each of these drugs, given alone, is effective in alleviating the headache in about half of patients, emphasizing the need for blinded placebo-controlled trials for any new drug that is introduced for the treatment of headache.

Intravenous and oral corticosteroids have been found anecdotally to be useful in refractory cases and as a means of terminating migraine status, but they should not be given continuously. In a randomized trial of intravenous dexamethasone 10 mg in an emergency department setting, Friedman et al found no benefit. As an alternative to steroids and more commonly used non-steroidal agents, Weatherall and colleagues used intravenous aspirin (lysine acetylsalicylate, 1 g, repeated up to five times) with reasonably good effect in inpatient management of migraine and other headache disorders. We have determined that this agent is difficult to obtain from hospital pharmacies.

If, in an individual attack, all of the foregoing measures fail, it is probably best to resort briefly to narcotics, which usually give the patient a restful, pain-free sleep. Halfway measures at this point are usually futile. However, the use of narcotics as the mainstay of acute or prophylactic therapy is to be avoided. As mentioned above, if the pain does not abate in 12 to 24 h, corticosteroids in any of several regimens may be added and continued for several days.

Based on the action of certain peptides in the trigeminovascular complex, novel antagonists of CGRP have been used with some success (Olesen et al). Drugs of this type as well as inducible nitric oxide synthase (iNOS) inhibitors and receptor blockers that work by a different mechanism than do the serotonin agonists may be alternatives in the future. So far, these have not been effective as prophylactic drugs but are currently being studied for acute treatment of migraine.

Preventive Treatment

In individuals with frequent migrainous attacks, efforts at prevention are worthwhile. The survey by Lipton and colleagues, found approximately one-fourth of patients were appropriate for some form of prophylactic treatment on the basis of the frequency and severity of their headaches, usually more than one severe episode per week. The most effective agents have been beta-adrenergic blockers, certain antiepileptic drugs, and tricyclic antidepressants. Often, comorbidities such as depression, hypertension, epilepsy or coronary artery disease guide the choice among these three classes of drugs. Some headache specialists have expressed the opinion that amitryptiline may be more effective than the others if headaches are very frequent and that propranolol is more effective if severity of headaches is the prime concern.

Considerable success has been obtained with propranolol, beginning with 10 to 20 mg two to three times daily and increasing the dosage gradually to as much as 240 mg daily, probably best given as a long-acting preparation in the higher dosage ranges. Under-dosing is a major reason for ineffectiveness. If propranolol is unsuccessful or not tolerated, one of the other beta blockers, specifically those that lack agonist properties—atenolol (40 to 160 mg/d), timolol (20 to 40 mg/d), or metoprolol (100 to 200 mg/d)—may prove to be effective. In patients who do not respond to these drugs over a period of 4 to 6 weeks, valproic acid 250 mg taken three to four times daily, other antiepileptic drug such as topiramate, or amitriptyline, 25 to 125 mg nightly may be tried. The newer antidepressants (e.g., specific serotonin reuptake inhibitors) are not as effective and may even cause headache in our experience. Calcium channel blockers (e.g., verapamil, 320 to 480 mg/d; nifedipine, 90 to 360 mg/d) are also reportedly effective in decreasing the frequency and severity of migraine attacks in some patients, but there is typically a lag of several weeks before benefit is attained and our success with them has been limited. Isometheptene (Midrin) as already mentioned; indomethacin, 150 to 200 mg/d; and cyproheptadine (Periactin), 4 to 16 mg/nightly are found to be helpful in some patients and may be particularly useful in preventing predictable attacks of perimenstrual migraine. A typical experience is for one of these medications to reduce the number and severity of headaches for several months and then to become less effective, whereupon an increase in the dosage, if tolerated, may help; or one of the many alternatives can be tried. The newest putative treatment for chronic or frequently repeating headaches, both migraine and tension, is the injection of botulinum toxin (Botox) into sensitive temporalis and other cranial muscles. Elimination of headaches for 2 to 4 months has been reported—a claim that justifies further study. Whether these injections are of value during an acute attack is uncertain. Surgical decompression of sensory nerves in the scalp and related techniques have also been advocated but require rigorous study.

Methysergide (Sansert), an ergot derivative that was more widely used in the past, in doses of 2 to 6 mg daily for several weeks or months is effective in the prevention of migraine. Retroperitoneal and pulmonary fibrosis are rare but serious complications that can be avoided by discontinuing the medication for 3 to 4 weeks after every 5-month course of treatment. Its use has virtually ceased.

Some patients allege that certain items of food induce attacks (chocolate, peanuts, hot dogs, smoked meats, oranges, and red wine are the ones most commonly mentioned), and it is obvious enough that they should avoid these foods if possible. Limiting caffeinated beverages may be helpful. In certain cases, the correction of a refractive error, an elimination diet, or behavioral modification is said to have reduced the frequency and severity of migraine and of tension headaches. However, the methods of study and the results have been so poorly controlled that it is difficult to evaluate them. All experienced physicians appreciate the importance of helping patients rearrange their schedules with a view to controlling tensions and hard-driving lifestyles. There is no single program to accomplish this. Psychotherapy has not been helpful, or at least one can say that there is no evidence of its value. The claims for sustained improvement of migraine with chiropractic manipulation are similarly unsubstantiated and do not accord with our experience. Meditation, acupuncture, and biofeedback techniques all have their advocates, but again, the results, while not to be entirely discounted, are uninterpretable.

Indomethacin Responsive Headaches

This is a group of relatively uncommon syndromes that may be allied with migraine but respond very well and specifically to indomethacin both acutely and as prophylaxis, so much so that some authors have defined a category of *indomethacin-responsive headaches*. These include orgasmic migraine, chronic paroxysmal hemicrania (see further on), hemicrania continua, exertional headache, hypnic headache, brief head pains (jabs and jolts and "ice-pick" headaches), and some instances of premenstrual migraine. These are summarized in Table 10-3.

Table 10-3

INDOMETHACIN RESPONSIVE HEADACHES

Valsalva related headaches
- Primary headache associated with sexual activity*
- Primary exertional (exercise induced, weight lifters) headache*
- Primary cough headache

Trigeminal-autonomic cephalgias
- Chronic paroxysmal hemicrania
- Episodic paroxysmal hemicrania
- Hemicrania continua*

SUNCT (short-lasting unilateral neuralgiform attacks with conjunctival injection and tearing)

Stabbing headaches
- "Jabs and jolts"
- Idiopathic stabbing (ice pick) headache

*These headache syndromes may improve with drugs other than Indomethacin.

Cluster Headache

This type of headache has been described in the past under a variety of names, including *paroxysmal nocturnal cephalalgia*, *migrainous neuralgia*, *histamine cephalalgia* (Horton's headache), and others. Kunkle and colleagues, who were impressed with the characteristic temporal "cluster pattern" of the attacks, coined the term in current use—*cluster headache*. This headache pattern occurs predominantly in adult men (age range: 20 to 50 years; male-to-female ratio approximately 5:1) and is characterized by a severe consistent unilateral orbital localization. The pain is felt deep in and around the eye, is very intense and nonthrobbing as a rule, and often radiates into the forehead, temple, and cheek—less often to the ear, occiput, and neck. Its denominative feature is the nightly recurrence, between 1 and 2 h after the onset of sleep, or several times during the night for several or more consecutive days; thus "cluster". Less often, it occurs during the day or early evening, unattended by aura or vomiting. The headache has been called the "alarm clock headache" because it may recur with remarkable regularity each night for periods extending as long as many weeks, followed thereafter by complete freedom for many months or even years. However, in approximately 10 percent of patients, the headache becomes chronic, persisting over days, months, or even years.

There are several associated vasomotor phenomena by which cluster headache can be identified: a blocked nostril, rhinorrhea, injected conjunctivum, lacrimation, miosis, and a flush and edema of the cheek, all lasting on average for 45 min (range: 15 to 180 min). Some of our patients, when alerted to the sign, also report a slight ptosis on the side of the orbital pain; in a few, the ptosis has become permanent after repeated attacks. The homolateral temporal artery may become prominent and tender during an attack, and the skin over the scalp and face may be hyperalgesic.

Most patients arise from bed during an attack and sit in a chair and rock or pace the floor, holding a hand to the side of the head. The pain of a given attack may leave as rapidly as it began or may fade away gradually. Almost always the same orbit is involved during a cluster of headaches as well as in recurring bouts. During the period of freedom from pain, alcohol, which commonly precipitates headaches during a cluster, no longer has the capacity to do so. The picture of cluster headache, including the patient's nocturnal behavior in response to it, is usually so characteristic that it cannot be confused with any other disease, although those unfamiliar with it may entertain a diagnosis of migraine, trigeminal neuralgia, carotid aneurysm, or temporal arteritis.

A somewhat similar syndrome is produced by the *Tolosa-Hunt syndrome* of eye pain and ocular motor paralysis caused by dural granuloma at the orbital apex (see further on) and the *paratrigeminal syndrome of Raeder*, which consists of paroxysms of pain somewhat like that of tic douloureux in the distribution of the ophthalmic and maxillary divisions of the fifth nerve, in association with unilateral Horner syndrome (ptosis and miosis but with preservation of facial sweating). Loss of sensation in a trigeminal nerve distribution and mild weakness of muscles innervated by the fifth nerve are often added. Raeder syndrome is now recognized as a heterogeneous syndrome, some cases being cluster and others caused by a structural lesion in or near the carotid siphon.

Trigeminal Autonomic Cephalgias (Cluster Variants)

Cases of paroxysmal pain behind the eye or nose or in the upper jaw or temple—associated with blocking of the nostril or lacrimation and described in the past under the titles of *sphenopalatine* (Sluder), *petrosal*, *vidian*, and *ciliary neuralgia* (Charlin or Harris)—probably represent variants of cluster headache. A similar head pain may occasionally be confined to the lower facial, postauricular, or occipital areas. Ekbom distinguished yet another "lower cluster headache" syndrome with infraorbital radiation of the pain, an ipsilateral partial Horner syndrome, and ipsilateral hyperhidrosis. There is no evidence to support the separation of these neuralgias as distinct entities, and they have collectively been called *trigeminal autonomic cephalgias*. They are important, however, because of the high frequency of underlying intracranial lesions. Favier and colleagues collected 4 of their own cases and 27 from the literature to emphasize the range of underlying diseases, including intracranial aneurysms, peritentorial or parasellar meningiomas, or other tumors and nasopharyngeal cancers surrounding the carotid artery. We have encountered a case of Wegener granulomatosis of the soft palate that presented as a paroxysmal trigeminal autonomic neuralgia. The headache syndrome disappeared with cyclophosphamide treatment of the underlying granulomatous disorder.

Chronic paroxysmal hemicrania was the name given by Sjaastad and Dale to a rapidly repetitive unilateral form of headache that resembles cluster headache in many respects but has several distinctive features. These are of much shorter duration (2 to 45 min) than cluster and usually affect the temporoorbital region of one side, accompanied by conjunctival hyperemia, rhinorrhea, and in some cases a partial Horner syndrome. Even periorbital ecchymosis may accompany a severe attack. Unlike cluster headache, however, the paroxysms occur many times each day, recur daily for long periods (the patient of Price and Posner had an average of 16 attacks daily for more than 40 years), and, most important, respond dramatically to the administration of indomethacin, 25 to 50 mg tid. Unlike cluster headache, chronic paroxysmal hemicrania is more common in women than in men (ratio of 3:1).

The acronym SUNCT (short-lasting unilateral neuralgiform attacks with conjunctival injection and tearing) has been applied to an episodic condition with attacks of even briefer duration, but otherwise similar to paroxysmal hemicrania in which the supraorbital or temporal pain lasts up to 4 min or so and frequent; it does not usually respond to indomethacin.

A similar hemicrania but without autonomic features, may be symptomatic of lesions near the cavernous sinus (mainly pituitary adenoma) or in the posterior fossa, but most cases are idiopathic. The typical episode of pain lasts approximately 20 min. Also known is a recurrent nocturnal headache in elderly individuals ("hypnic headache"), as described further on.

The relationship of cluster headache and all of its variants to migraine remains conjectural. No doubt the headaches in some persons have some of the characteristics of both, hence the terms *migrainous neuralgia* and *cluster migraine* (Kudrow). Lance and others, however, have pointed out differences that seem important to us: flushing of the face on the side of a cluster headache and pallor in migraine; increased intraocular pressure in cluster headache, normal pressure in migraine; increased skin temperature over the forehead, temple, and cheek in cluster headache, decreased temperature in migraine; and notable distinctions in sex distribution, age of onset, rhythmicity, and other clinical features, but prominently by differences among them in response to specific treatments. Cluster may be triggered in sensitive patients by the use of nitroglycerin and, as mentioned, by alcohol.

The cause and mechanism of the cluster headache syndrome are unknown. Gardner and coworkers originally postulated a paroxysmal parasympathetic discharge mediated through the greater superficial petrosal nerve and sphenopalatine ganglion. These authors obtained inconsistent results by cutting the nerve, but others (Kittrelle et al) reported that application of cocaine or lidocaine to the region of the sphenopalatine fossa (via the nostril) consistently aborts attacks of cluster headache. Capsaicin, applied over the affected region of the forehead and scalp, may have the same effect. Stimulation of the ganglion is said to reproduce the syndrome. Kunkle, on the basis of a large personal experience, concluded that the pain arises from the internal carotid artery, in the canal through which it ascends in the petrous portion of the temporal bone. In the course of an arteriogram, during which a patient with cluster headaches fortuitously developed an attack, Ekbom and Greitz noted a narrowing of the artery that was interpreted as being caused by swelling of the arterial wall, which, in turn, compromised the pericarotid sympathetic plexus and caused the Horner syndrome. This remains to be confirmed.

The cyclic nature of the attacks has been linked to a hypothalamic mechanism that governs the circadian rhythm. At the onset of the headache, the region of the suprachiasmatic nucleus appears to be active on PET (May et al). Hypothalamic activation has also been found in migraine, SUNCT, chronic paroxysmal hemicrania, and hemicrania continua. Moreover, stimulation of the hypothalamus has proved effective, although highly experimental, in stopping chronic cluster headache and SUNCT (see Leone et al and Bartsch et al).

Much was made in the past of the fact that cluster headaches could be reproduced by the intravenous injection of 0.1 mg histamine, but the effect was probably nonspecific. Goadsby has reviewed the pathophysiology of the cluster headache syndrome.

Treatment of Cluster Headache

Inhalation of 100 percent oxygen via mask for 10 to 15 min at the onset of cluster headache may abort the attack, but this is not always practical. Termination of a cycle of cluster can also be achieved with verapamil, starting with 80 mg qid and increasing the dose over days, but electrocardiogram (ECG) monitoring is recommended in the older individual. The usual nocturnal attacks of cluster headache can be treated with a single anticipatory dose of ergotamine at bedtime (2 mg orally) or with possibly lesser efficacy, an equivalent dose of serotonin agonist. Intranasal lidocaine or sumatriptan (or zolmitriptan as for migraine, see above) can also be used to abort an acute attack. In other patients, ergotamine given once or twice during the day, before an attack of pain is expected, has been helpful.

With regard to prevention of cluster headache, if ergotamine and sumatriptan are ineffective or become ineffective in subsequent bouts, many headache experts prefer to use verapamil, up to 480 mg per day. Ekbom introduced lithium therapy for cluster headache (600 mg, up to 900 mg daily), and Kudrow has confirmed its efficacy in chronic cases. Lithium and verapamil may be given together, but lithium toxicity is a frequent problem. A course of prednisone, beginning with 75 mg daily for 3 days and then reducing the dose at 3-day intervals, has been beneficial in many patients. Usually, it can be decided within a week if any one of these medications is effective. In brief, no method is effective in all cases, but the best initial approach probably involves the use of one of the triptan compounds. Rare cases of intractable cluster headache, in which the syndrome persists for weeks or longer without remission, have been treated by partial section of the trigeminal nerve, as described by Jarrar and colleagues, but these ablative measures are now always a last resort, especially when hypothalamic stimulation has been shown to be possibly effective, as mentioned earlier.

Tension Headache

This, said to be the most common variety of headache, is usually bilateral, with occipitonuchal, temporal, or frontal predominance, or diffuse extension over the top of the cranium. The pain is usually described as dull and aching, but questioning often uncovers other sensations, such as fullness, tightness, or pressure (as though the head were surrounded by a band or clamped in a vise) or a feeling that the head is swollen and may burst. On these sensations, waves of aching pain are superimposed. These may be interpreted as paroxysmal or throbbing and, if the pain is slightly more on one side, the headache may suggest a migraine without aura. However, absent in tension headache are the persistent throbbing quality, nausea, photophobia, phonophobia, and clear lateralization of migraine. Nor do most tension headaches seriously interfere with daily activities, as migraine does. The onset is more gradual than that of migraine, and the headache, once established, may persist with only mild fluctuations for days, weeks, months, or even years. In fact, this is the only type of headache that exhibits the peculiarity of being present throughout the day, day after day, for long periods of time for which the term *chronic tension-type headache* is used. There is often self-acknowledged anxiety and depression, as noted below. Although sleep is usually undisturbed, the headache develops soon after awakening, and the common analgesic remedies have limited effect if the pain is of more than mild to moderate severity.

The incidence of tension headache is certainly greater than that of migraine. However, most patients treat tension headaches themselves and do not seek medical advice. Like migraine, tension headaches are more common in women than in men. Unlike migraine, they infrequently begin in childhood or adolescence but are more likely to arise in middle age and to coincide with anxiety, fatigue, and depression in the trying times of life. In the large series reported by Lance and Curran, about one-third of patients with persistent tension headaches had readily recognized symptoms of depression. They carried out a controlled and blinded trial that demonstrated benefit from amitriptyline even in those patients who were not depressed. In our experience, chronic anxiety or depression of varying degrees of severity is present in the majority of patients with protracted headaches. Migraine and traumatic headaches may, of course, be complicated by tension headache, which, because of its persistence, often arouses fears of a brain tumor or other intracranial disease. However, as Patten points out, not more than one or two patients out of every thousand with tension headaches will be found to harbor an intracranial tumor, and its discovery has been most often incidental (see further on).

In a substantial group of patients with chronic daily headache, the pain, when severe, develops a pulsating quality, to which the term *tension-migraine* or *tension-vascular* headache has been applied (Lance and Curran). Observations such as these have tended to blur the sharp distinctions between migrainous and tension headaches in some cases.

For many years, it was thought that tension headaches were a result of excessive contraction of craniocervical muscles and an associated constriction of the scalp arteries. However, it is not clear that either of these mechanisms contributes to the genesis of tension headache, at least in its chronic form. In most patients with tension headache, the craniocervical muscles are quite relaxed (by palpation) and show no evidence of persistent contraction when measured by surface electromyographic (EMG) recordings. Anderson and Frank found no difference in the degree of muscle contraction between migraine and tension headache. However, using an ingenious laser device, Sakai and associates have reported that the pericranial and trapezius muscles are hardened in patients with tension headaches. Recently, nitric oxide has been implicated in the genesis of tension-type headaches, specifically by creating a central sensitization to sensory stimulation from cranial structures. The strongest support for this concept comes from several reports that an inhibitor of nitric oxide reduces muscle hardness and pain in patients with chronic tension headache (Ashina et al). At present, these are interesting but speculative ideas.

Treatment of Tension Headache

Simple analgesics, such as aspirin or acetaminophen or other NSAIDs, may be helpful, if only for brief periods. Persistent or frequent tension headaches respond best to the cautious use of one of several drugs that relieve anxiety or depression such as amitriptyline given as a single dose at night, especially when symptoms of these conditions are present. Stronger analgesic medication should be avoided. Raskin reports success with calcium channel blockers, phenelzine, and cyproheptadine. Ergotamine and propranolol are ineffective unless there are symptoms of both migraine and tension headache. Some patients respond to ancillary measures such as massage, meditation, and biofeedback techniques. Relaxation techniques may be helpful in teaching patients how to deal with underlying anxiety and stress. Gradual withdrawal of daily doses of analgesics, ergotamines, or triptan medications is an important aspect of treating chronic daily headache.

Headaches in the Elderly

In several surveys, headache with onset in the elderly age period was found to be a prominent problem in as many as 1 of 6 persons, and more often to have serious import than headache in a younger population. In a series reported by Pascual and Berciano, more than 40 percent were classified as having tension headaches (women more than men), and there was a wide variety of diseases in the others (posttraumatic headaches, cerebrovascular disease, intracranial tumors, cranial arteritis, severe hypertension). Cough-induced headaches and cluster headaches were present in some of the men. New-onset migraine in this age group was a rarity.

Raskin described a headache syndrome in older patients that shares with cluster headache a nocturnal occurrence (*hypnic headache*). It also may occur with daytime naps. However, it differs in being bilateral and unaccompanied by lacrimation and rhinorrhea. He has successfully treated a number of his patients with 300 mg of lithium carbonate or 75 mg of sustained-release indomethacin at bedtime. The nosologic position of this hypnic headache syndrome is undetermined.

Despite these considerations, the most treacherous and neglected cause of headache in the elderly is temporal (cranial) arteritis with or without polymyalgia rheumatica, as discussed further on.

Headache and Other Craniofacial Pain with Psychiatric Disease

The most common cause of generalized persistent headache, both in adolescents and adults, is probably mild depression or anxiety in one of its several forms. A small group of older patients has delusional symptoms involving pain and physical distortion of cranial structures. As the psychiatric symptoms subside, the headaches usually disappear. Odd cephalic pains, e.g., a sensation of having a nail driven into the head (*clavus hystericus*), may occur in hysteria or psychosis and raise perplexing problems in diagnosis. The bizarre character of these pains, their persistence in the face of every known therapy, the absence of other signs of disease, and the presence of other manifestations of psychiatric disease provide the basis for correct diagnosis. Older children and adolescents sometimes have peculiar behavioral reactions to headache: screaming, looking dazed, clutching the head with an agonized look. Usually, migraine is the underlying disorder in these cases, the additional manifestations responding to therapeutic support and suggestion.

Posttraumatic Headache

Severe, chronic, continuous, or intermittent headaches lasting several days or weeks appear as the cardinal symptom of several posttraumatic syndromes, separable in each instance from the headache that immediately follows head injury (i.e., scalp laceration and cerebral contusion with blood in the CSF or increased intracranial pressure).

The *headache of chronic subdural hematoma* is deep seated, dull, steady, mainly unilateral and may be accompanied or followed by drowsiness, confusion, and fluctuating hemiparesis. In more *acute subdural hematomas*, we have been impressed with the positional worsening of pain in some patients after lying down or leaning the head to one side. Tentorial hematomas produce the additional feature of pain in the eye. The head injury that gives rise to a subdural hematoma may have been minor, as described in Chap. 35, and forgotten by the patient and family. Typically, the headache increases in frequency and severity over several weeks or months. Patients who have received anticoagulation are particularly at risk. Diagnosis is established by CT or MRI.

Chronic headache is certainly a prominent feature of the postconcussion syndrome, comprising dizziness, fatigability, insomnia, nervousness, irritability, and inability to concentrate (a syndrome that we have also called *posttraumatic nervous instability*). This type of headache and associated symptoms, which resemble the tension headache syndrome, are described fully in Chap. 35, "Craniocerebral Trauma." The International Headache Society has classified persistence in this context as headache for longer than 3 months after injury. The patient with postconcussion syndrome requires supportive therapy in the form of repeated reassurance and explanations of the benign nature of the symptoms, a program of increasing physical activity, and the use of drugs that allay anxiety and depression. The early settlement of litigation, which is often an issue, works to the patient's advantage.

Tenderness and aching pain sharply localized to the scar of a long previous scalp laceration or surgical incision represent in a different problem and raise the question of a traumatic neuralgia or neuroma. Tender scars from scalp lacerations may be treated by repeated subcutaneous injections of local anesthetics, such as 5 mL of 1 percent procaine, which also acts as a diagnostic test.

With *whiplash injuries* of the neck, there may be unilateral or bilateral retroauricular or occipital pain, probably as a result of stretching or tearing of ligaments and muscles at the occipitonuchal junction or of a worsening of a preexisting cervical arthropathy. Much less frequently, cervical intervertebral discs and nerve roots are involved. However, it is questionable if chronic headache and vague neuropsychiatric symptoms can be attributed to whiplash (see Maleson).

One should also be alert to headache as a sign of carotid artery dissection after head or neck injury.

Headaches of Brain Tumor

It remains a popular notion that headache is a significant symptom in many patients with brain tumor, but it is actually infrequent, particularly as the heralding symptom of a tumor in an adult. While headache is sometimes stated to occur in one-third of brain tumor cases, this is certainly the result of the high frequency of cranial imaging in headache patients. Headache probably only arises if the tumor displaces major cerebral vessels or blocks the flow of CSF, but we have seen exceptions. The pain has no specific features; it tends to be deep seated, usually nonthrobbing (occasionally throbbing), and is described as aching or bursting. However, a major change in the pattern of an accustomed headache syndrome should raise suspicion of a structural lesion in the cranium. Physical activity and changes in position of the head may provoke pain, whereas rest sometimes diminishes it. Nocturnal awakening because of pain occurs in only a small proportion of brain tumor patients and is by no means diagnostic. Most headaches that awaken people at night are cluster-like headaches, hypnic headaches in the elderly, or those caused by caffeine withdrawal. Unexpected forceful (projectile) vomiting may punctuate brain tumor headache in its later stages, particularly in children, or occur early if the mass is in the posterior fossa.

If unilateral, the headache is nearly always on the same side as the tumor. Pain from supratentorial tumors is felt anterior to the interauricular circumference of the skull; from posterior fossa tumors, it is felt behind this line. Bifrontal and bioccipital headaches from tumor coming on after unilateral headaches probably signify the development of increased intracranial pressure or hydrocephalus.

Having stated that headache is not to be equated with brain tumor, one cannot help but be impressed with its frequency as a manifestation of *colloid cysts*, and we have several times stumbled on the correct diagnosis when an odd, unexplained bilateral headache led to brain imaging. The mechanism of headache in cases of colloid cyst, if such a relationship is valid, is not simply one of blocking the flow of CSF at the foramina of Monro, as it is not predicated on the development of hydrocephalus. Additionally, Harris described headaches of paroxysmal type with intra- and periventricular brain tumors, and many others have commented on the same type of headache with parenchymal tumors. These are severe headaches that reach their peak intensity in a few seconds, last for several minutes or as long as an hour, and then subside quickly. When they are associated with vomiting, transient blindness, leg weakness causing "drop attacks," and loss of consciousness, there is a possibility of brain tumor with greatly elevated intracranial pressure. With respect to its onset, this headache almost resembles that of subarachnoid hemorrhage, but the latter is far longer-lasting and even more abrupt in onset. In its entirety, this paroxysmal headache is most typical of the aforementioned colloid cyst of the third ventricle, but it can occur with other tumors as well, including craniopharyngiomas, pinealomas, and cerebellar masses.

Headaches of Temporal Arteritis (Giant Cell Arteritis) (See also Chap. 34)

This type of inflammatory disease of cranial arteries is an important cause of headache in older persons. All of our patients have been older than 55 years of age, most of them older than age 65. From a state of normal health, the patient develops an increasingly intense throbbing or nonthrobbing headache, often with superimposed sharp, stabbing pains. In a few patients the headache has had an almost explosive onset. The pain is usually unilateral, sometimes bilateral, and often localized to the site of the affected arteries in the scalp. The pain persists to some degree throughout the day and is particularly severe at night. It lasts for many months if untreated. The superficial temporal and other scalp arteries are frequently thickened and tender and without pulsation. Jaw claudication and ischemic nodules on the scalp, with ulceration of the overlying skin, have been described in severe cases.

Many of the patients feel generally unwell and have lost weight; some have a low-grade fever and anemia. Usually the sedimentation rate is greatly elevated (>50 mm/h and typically >75 mm/h) but elevation of the C-reactive protein (CRP) level is a more sensitive indicator of this inflammatory condition and is particularly helpful when the sedimentation rate is only mildly elevated. A few patients have a peripheral neutrophilic leukocytosis. As many as 50 percent of patients have generalized aching of proximal limb muscles, reflecting the presence of polymyalgia rheumatica (see Chap. 48, "Polymyalgia Rheumatica").

The importance of early diagnosis relates to the threat of blindness from thrombosis of the ophthalmic or posterior ciliary arteries. This may be preceded by several episodes of amaurosis fugax (transient monocular blindness). Ophthalmoplegia may also occur but is less frequent, and its cause, whether neural or muscular, is not settled. Masticatory claudication is a specific but not particularly sensitive symptom of cranial arteritis. The large intracranial vessels are occasionally affected, thereby causing stroke. Once vision is lost, it is seldom recoverable. For this reason, *the earliest suspicion* of cranial arteritis should lead to the administration of corticosteroids and then to biopsy of the appropriate scalp artery. Microscopic examination discloses an intense granulomatous or "giant cell" arteritis. If biopsy on one side fails to clarify the situation and there are sound clinical reasons for suspecting the diagnosis, the other side should be sampled. Arteriography of the external carotid artery branches is probably the most sensitive test but is seldom used, because of its relatively higher risk. Ultrasonographic examination of the temporal arteries may display a dark halo and irregularly thickened vessel walls. This technique has not yet been incorporated into the routine evaluation because its sensitivity has not been established; our own experience suggests that it may miss cases, but it could be useful in choosing the site for biopsy of the temporal artery.

Treatment

The administration of prednisone, 45 to 60 mg/d in single or divided doses over a period of several weeks, is indicated in all cases, with gradual reduction to 10 to 20 mg/d and maintenance at this dosage for several months or years, if necessary, to prevent relapse. The headache can be expected to improve within a day or two of beginning treatment; failure to do so brings the diagnosis into question. When the sedimentation rate or CRP is elevated, its return to normal, usually over months, is a reliable index of therapeutic response. Whether symptoms or the blood tests are a better guide to reducing the steroid dose is unclear, one should probably be cautious in lowering the medication if the erythrocyte sedimentation rate (ESR) and CRP remain high.

Headaches of Pseudotumor Cerebri (Benign or Idiopathic Intracranial Hypertension

(See Chap. 30)

The headache of pseudotumor cerebri assumes a variety of forms. Most typical is a feeling of occipital pressure that is greatly worsened by lying down, but many patients have—in addition, or only—headaches of migraine or tension type. Indeed, some of them respond to medications such as propranolol and ergot compounds. None of the proposed mechanisms for pain in pseudotumor cerebri seems to be adequate as an explanation, particularly the idea that cerebral vessels are displaced or compressed, as neither has been demonstrated. It is worth noting that facial pain may also be a feature of the illness, albeit rare. Chapter 30 has a more complete description of the clinical features and treatment.

After successful treatment for pseudotumor, some patients have persistent headaches that have the flavor of migraine.

SPECIAL VARIETIES OF HEADACHE

Low-Pressure and Spinal Puncture Headache

These are commonly known to neurologists, as noted earlier in this chapter. It occurs after lumbar punctures in approximately 5 percent of cases. The headache is associated with the greatly reduced pressure of the CSF compartment and probably caused by vertical traction or cranial blood vessels. Assuming the supine position almost immediately relieves the cranial pain and eliminates vomiting, but a blood-patch procedure may be required in persistent cases. In a limited number of cases, success has been obtained by the use of intravenous caffeine injections. The condition and its treatment are discussed in Chap. 30 "Lumbar Puncture Headache" and "Spontaneous Intracranial Hypotension."

Menstrual (Catamenial) Migraine and Other Headaches Linked to the Hormonal Cycle

The relation of headache to a drop in estradiol levels during the late luteal phase was mentioned in "Migraine" above. There it was also indicated that the mechanism is probably more complex. In practice, factors such as sleep deprivation are at least as important in triggering perimenstrual headaches. Premenstrual headache, taking the form of migraine or a combined tension-migraine headache, usually responds to the administration of an NSAID begun 3 days before the anticipated onset of the menstrual period; oral sumatriptan (25 to 50 mg qid) and zolmitriptan (2.5 to 5 mg bid) are also equally effective. Manipulation of the hormonal cycle with danazol (a testosterone derivative) or estradiol has also been effective but is rarely necessary.

The management of migraine during pregnancy poses special problems because one wants to restrict exposure of the fetus to medications. It can be stated that beta-adrenergic compounds and tricyclic antidepressants may be used safely in the small proportion of women whose headaches persist or intensify during pregnancy. From a limited registry of patients who were given sumatriptan during pregnancy, and from several small trials summarized by Fox and colleagues, no teratogenic effects or adverse effects on pregnancy arose, but serotonin agonist drugs should be used advisedly until their safety is further confirmed. For those women who use antiepileptic drugs as a means of headache prevention, it is recommended that the drugs be stopped prior to pregnancy or as soon as it is known that pregnancy has begun.

Cough and Exertional Headache

A patient may complain of very severe, transient cranial pain on coughing, sneezing, laughing heartily, lifting heavy objects, stooping, and straining at stool. Pain is usually felt in the front of the head, sometimes occipitally, and may be unilateral or bilateral. As a rule, it follows the initiating action within a second or two and lasts a few seconds to a few minutes. The pain is often described as having a bursting quality and may be of such severity as to cause the patient to cradle his head in his hands, thereby simulating the headache of acute subarachnoid hemorrhage.

Most often this syndrome is a benign idiopathic state that recurs over a period of several months to a year or two and then disappears. Many decades ago, Symonds emphasized the benignity of the condition. In a report of 103 patients followed for 3 years or longer, Rooke found that additional symptoms of neurologic disease developed in only 10. The cause and mechanism have not been determined. During the headache, the CSF pressure is normal. Bilateral jugular compression may induce an attack, possibly because of traction on the walls of large veins and dural sinuses. In a few instances, we have observed this type of headache after lumbar puncture or after a hemorrhage from an arteriovenous malformation.

Patients with cough or strain headache will only occasionally be found to have serious intracranial disease; when present, it has been traced to lesions of the posterior fossa and foramen magnum, arteriovenous malformation, subdural hematoma, Chiari malformation, basilar impression, or tumor. It may be necessary, therefore, to supplement the neurologic examination by appropriate CT and MRI. Far more common, of course, are the temporal and maxillary pains that are caused by dental or sinus disease, which may also be worsened by coughing.

All manner of headache has been attributed to Chiari type 1 malformation (with tonsils descended at least 3 mm below the lip of the foramen magnum) with little justification. However, some instances of exertional and Valsalva-induced suboccipital pain can be attributed to this disease. Some patients report radiating pain across the base of the neck and shoulders with straining and headache. In the survey by Pascual and colleagues of 50 patients with Chiari type 1 malformations, the incidence of migraine and tension-type headache was found to be appropriate to the population at large and only the degree of tonsillar descent correlated with the presence of exertional headache. It follows that suboccipital decompressive operations should be undertaken only selectively. Chiari malformation is discussed further in Chap. 38.

A special variant of exertional headache is "weight-lifter's headache." It occurs either as a single event or repeatedly over a period of several months, but each episode of headache may last many hours or days, again raising the suspicion of subarachnoid hemorrhage. The pain begins immediately or within minutes of heavy lifting. If the pain resolves in an hour or less and there is no meningismus or sign of bleeding on the CT, we have foregone lumbar puncture and angiography but have suggested that weight lifting not be resumed for several weeks. Athletes and runners in general seem to suffer exertional headaches quite often in our experience, and the episodes usually have migrainous features.

Indomethacin is usually effective in controlling exertional headaches; this has been confirmed in controlled trials. Useful alternatives are NSAIDs, ergot preparations, and propranolol. In a few of our patients, lumbar puncture appeared to immediately resolve the problem in some inexplicable way.

Headaches Related to Sexual Activity

Lance (1976) described 21 cases of this type of headache, 16 in males and 5 in females. The headache took one of two forms: one in which pain typical of tension headache developed as sexual excitement increased, and another in which a severe, throbbing, "explosive" headache occurred at the time of orgasm and persisted for several minutes or hours (orgasmic headache). The latter headaches were of such abruptness and severity as to suggest a ruptured aneurysm but the neurologic examination was negative in every instance, as was arteriography in 7 patients who were subjected to this procedure. In 18 patients who were followed for a period of 2 to 7 years, no other neurologic symptoms developed. Characteristically, the headache occurred on several consecutive occasions and then disappeared. In cases of repeated coital headache, indomethacin has been effective. Of course, so-called orgasmic headache is not always benign; a hypertensive hemorrhage, rupture of an aneurysm or vascular malformation, carotid artery dissection, or myocardial infarction may occur during the exertion of sexual intercourse. While there is no authoritative direction, it is justified to perform a spinal tap if a sexual-related headache is the first occurrence of headache in a patient's history.

Thunderclap Headache

The headache of subarachnoid hemorrhage caused by rupture of a berry aneurysm is among the most abrupt and dramatic of cranial pains (see Chap. 34). There are several reports regarding such pains as a "warning leak" of rupture and even reports suggesting that acute severe headaches occur as a consequence of unruptured aneurysms (although subsequent studies suggest that this is infrequent). It was in relation to an exceptional case of this nature that the term *thunderclap* was introduced by Day and Raskin. Patients in our services have offered colorful descriptions, such as "being kicked in the back of the head." Thunderclap headache, as pointed out by Dodick, has also been a symptom of pituitary apoplexy, cerebral venous thrombosis, cervical arterial dissection, non-aneurysmal perimesencephalic hemorrhage, or hypertensive crisis (Table 10-4). To this list we would add diffuse idiopathic arterial spasm (Call-Fleming syndrome; see "Diffuse and Focal Cerebral Vasospasm" in Chap. 34) and cerebral vasospasm as the result of the administration of sympathomimetic or serotonergic drugs, including cocaine and the triptan group of medications for the treatment of migraine. Recurrent thunderclap pain may be particularly indicative of multifocal or diffuse vasospasm, as pointed out by Chen and colleagues, who found this vasculopathy in 39 percent of their patients with recurrent thunderclap pain.

Table 10-4

CAUSES OF THUNDERCLAP HEADACHE
Migraine
Subarachnoid hemorrhage
Cerebral venous thrombosis
Diffuse cerebral vasospasm (Call-Fleming syndrome)
Accelerated hypertension
Pituitary apoplexy
Cocaine and adrenergically active drugs
Perimesencephalic non-aneurysmal subarachnoid hemorrhage

Nevertheless, in a large proportion of patients with thunderclap headache the pain is indistinguishable from that caused by subarachnoid hemorrhage, even to the extent of being accompanied by vomiting and acute hypertension. The diagnosis is clarified after lumbar puncture and cerebral imaging exclude bleeding and aneurysm, and the pain resolves in hours or less. Most cases turn out to be idiopathic. Wijdicks and colleagues confirmed that thunderclap headache is usually a benign condition; among 71 patients followed for more than 3 years they found no serious cerebrovascular lesions. For this reason, these idiopathic thunderclap headaches have been presumed to be a form of migraine ("crash migraine"). This opinion is based in part on a history of preceding or of subsequent headaches and migrainous episodes in affected individuals; however, in our experience not all of such patients have had migraine in the past. There is a notable tendency for thunderclap headaches to recur.

Erythrocyanotic Headache

An intense, generalized, throbbing headache may occur in conjunction with flushing of the face and hands and numbness of the fingers (erythromelalgia). Episodes tend to be present on awakening from sound sleep. This condition, called erythrocyanotic, has been reported in a number of unusual settings: (1) in mastocytosis (infiltration of tissues by mast cells, which elaborate histamine, heparin, and serotonin); (2) with carcinoid tumors; (3) with serotonin-secreting tumors; (4) with some tumors of the pancreatic islets; and (5) with pheochromocytoma. Seventy-five percent of patients with pheochromocytoma reportedly have vascular-type headaches coincident with paroxysms of hypertension and release of catecholamines (Lance and Hinterberger) but the flushing phenomenon has been rare in our experience.

Headache Related to Medical Diseases

A cardinal feature of meningitis of varied causes is headache. When accompanied by fever and stiff neck, the diagnosis is almost assured. However, severe headache may occur with a number of infectious illnesses caused by banal viral infections, by organisms such as *Mycoplasma,* and particularly by influenza. There is often accompanying neck pain and slight stiffness. The suspicion of meningitis is raised, even subarachnoid hemorrhage, but there is no reaction in the CSF ("meningism"). The mild aseptic meningitis that accompanies HIV seroconversion may also be accompanied by headache.

Approximately 50 percent of patients with hypertension complain of headache, but the relationship of one to the other is not clear. Minor elevations of blood pressure may be a result rather than the cause of tension headaches. Severe (accelerated) hypertension, with diastolic pressures of more than 120 mm Hg, is regularly associated with headache, and measures that reduce the blood pressure relieve it. In preeclampsia, the headaches occur at lower levels of blood pressure. Abrupt elevations of blood pressure, as occur in patients who take monoamine oxidase inhibitors and then ingest tyramine-containing food, can cause headaches that are abrupt and severe enough to simulate subarachnoid hemorrhage. However, it is the individual with moderately severe hypertension and frequent severe headaches that typically confronts the practitioner. In some of these patients, the headaches are of the common migrainous or tension type, but in others, they defy classification. According to Wolff, the mechanism of the hypertensive headache is similar to that of migraine. The headaches, however, bear no clear relation to even modest peaks in blood pressure. The acute headache of pheochromocytoma correlates with the rate of increase of blood pressure rather than its absolute value. Curiously, headaches that occur toward the end of renal dialysis or soon after its completion are associated with a fall in blood pressure (as well as a decrease in blood sodium levels and osmolality).

Headaches frequently follow a seizure, having been recorded in half of one large series of epileptic patients analyzed in a Great Britain study but the pain is infrequently severe. In migraineurs, the postictal headache may reproduce a typical migraine attack. Experienced physicians are aware of many other conditions in which headache may be a principal symptom. These include fevers of any cause, carbon monoxide exposure, chronic lung disease with hypercapnia (headaches often nocturnal or early morning), sleep apnea, hypothyroidism, Cushing disease, withdrawal from corticosteroid medication or alcohol, mountain (altitude) sickness, exposure to nitrates, occasionally in adrenal insufficiency, and acute anemia with hemoglobin below 10 g.

No attempt is made here to discuss the symptomatic treatment of headache that may accompany these many medical conditions. Obviously, the guiding principle is to address the underlying disease.

Headache Related to Diseases of the Cervical Spine

Headaches that accompany diseases of the upper cervical spine are well recognized, but their mechanism is obscure and their frequency possibly overestimated. Recent writings have focused on a wide range of causative lesions, such as zygapophyseal (facet) arthropathy, C2 dorsal root entrapment, calcified ligamentum flavum, hypertrophied posterior longitudinal ligament, and rheumatoid arthritis of the atlantoaxial region. As summarized by Bogduk and Govind, the most credible evidence for this group of disorders comes from systematic injection of anesthetics into cervical structures and effecting complete relief of headache. Even this is not uniformly successful in patients whose cranial pain has been attributed to a cervicogenic mechanism. CT and MRI have divulged a number of these abnormalities. One special variety is discussed further below, under "Third Occipital Nerve' Headache," and further in Chap. 11.

OTHER CRANIOFACIAL PAINS
(See Chap. 47)

Trigeminal Neuralgia (Tic Douloureux)

This is a common disorder of middle age and later life, consisting of paroxysms of intense, stabbing pain in the distribution of the mandibular and maxillary divisions (rarely the ophthalmic division) of the fifth cranial nerve. The pain seldom lasts more than a few seconds or rarely a minute or two, but it is often so intense that the patient winces involuntarily; hence the term *tic*. It is uncertain whether the tic is reflexive or quasivoluntary. The paroxysms recur frequently, both day and night, for several weeks or months at a time. Another characteristic feature is the initiation of a jab or a series of jabs of pain by stimulation of certain areas of the face, lips, or gums, as in shaving or brushing the teeth, or by movement of these parts in chewing, talking, or yawning, or even by a breeze—the so-called trigger factors. Sensory or motor loss in the distribution of the fifth nerve cannot be demonstrated, though there are minor exceptions to this rule. In addition to the paroxysmal pain, some patients complain of a more or less continuous discomfort, itching, or sensitivity of restricted areas of the face, features regarded as atypical even though not infrequent.

In studying the relationship between stimuli applied to the trigger zones and the paroxysms of pain, touch and possibly tickle are more likely to be precipitants rather painful or thermal stimulus. Usually a spatial and temporal summation of impulses is necessary to trigger a paroxysm of pain, which is followed by a refractory period of up to 2 or 3 min.

The *diagnosis* of tic douloureux must rest on the strict clinical criteria enumerated above, so that the condition can be distinguished from other forms of facial and cephalic neuralgia and pain arising from diseases of the jaw, teeth, or sinuses. Most cases of trigeminal neuralgia are without obvious cause (idiopathic), in contrast to *symptomatic trigeminal neuralgia*, in which paroxysmal facial pain is because of involvement of the fifth nerve by some other disease: multiple sclerosis (may be bilateral), aneurysm of the basilar artery, or tumor (acoustic or trigeminal schwannoma, meningioma, epidermoid) in the cerebellopontine angle. Each of the forms of symptomatic trigeminal neuralgia may give rise only to pain in the distribution of the trigeminal nerve, or it may produce a loss of sensation as well.

Vascular loop as a cause of trigeminal neuralgia It has also become apparent that a proportion of ostensibly idiopathic cases are caused by compression of the trigeminal roots by a small tortuous branch of the basilar artery, as originally pointed out by Dandy and brought to greater attention by Jannetta, who has observed it frequently and has relieved the pain by surgical decompression of the trigeminal root. In this procedure, the offending small vessel is removed from contact with the proximal portion of the nerve (see below). Others have declared a vascular compressive causation to be infrequent, but modern imaging has increasingly revealed a putative association. This and other disorders of the fifth nerve, some of which give rise to facial pain, are discussed in Chap. 47.

Treatment Carbamazepine is effective in 70 to 80 percent of patients, but half become tolerant over a period of several years. Other antiepileptic drugs such as phenytoin (300 to 400 mg/d), valproic acid (800 to 1,200 mg/d), clonazepam (2 to 6 mg/d), gabapentin (300 to 900 mg/d or more), pregabalin (150 to 300 mg/d), and carbamazepine (600 to 1,200 mg/d), alone or in combination, suppress or shorten the duration and severity of the attacks in most patients for varying times. Baclofen may be useful in patients who cannot tolerate carbamazepine or gabapentin, but it is most effective as an adjunct to one of the anticonvulsant drugs. Capsaicin applied locally to the trigger zones or the topical instillation in the eye of an anesthetic has been helpful in some patients. By temporizing and using these drugs, one may permit a spontaneous remission to occur in perhaps 1 in 5 patients over a year or two.

Most of the patients with intractable pain, however, come to vascular surgery or a surgical form of root destruction. The procedure of vascular decompression, popularized by Jannetta, which requires a posterior fossa craniotomy but leaves no sensory loss, has been the most popular. Barker and colleagues reported that 70 percent of 1,185 patients were relieved of pain by repositioning a small branch of the basilar artery that was found to compress the fifth nerve, and this benefit persisted with a recurrence rate of less than 1 percent annually for 10 years. It is not clear if conventional or CT arteriography is useful in identifying an aberrant blood vessel prior to surgery but most neurosurgeons obtain these studies before committing a patient to surgery.

A procedure used more in the past, was stereotactically controlled thermocoagulation of the trigeminal roots (Sweet and Wepsic). The therapeutic efficacy of the two surgical approaches is roughly equivalent; in recent years, there has been a preference for microvascular decompression on the basis of its sparing of sensation, especially late in the course of the illness (Fields). Gamma Knife and other forms of focused radiation are emerging as less intrusive alternatives to destroying the ganglion, but its full effect is not evident for months. In practice, an antiepileptic medication is often required for some period of time after any of these procedures, and it must be reinstituted when symptoms reoccur, as they often do in our experience.

Glossopharyngeal Neuralgia

This syndrome is much less common than trigeminal neuralgia but resembles the latter in many respects. The pain is intense and paroxysmal; it originates in the throat, approximately in the tonsillar fossa, and is provoked most commonly by swallowing but also by talking, chewing, yawning, laughing, etc. The pain may be localized in the ear or radiate from the throat to the ear, implicating the auricular branch of the vagus nerve. For this reason, White and Sweet suggested the term *vagoglossopharyngeal neuralgia*. This is the main craniofacial neuralgia that may be accompanied by bradycardia and even by syncope, presumably because of the triggering of cardioinhibitory reflexes by afferent vagal pain impulses. There is no demonstrable sensory or motor deficit.

Rarely, tumors, including carcinoma, lymphoma or epithelioma of the oropharyngeal-infracranial region or peritonsillar abscess may give rise to pain that is clinically indistinguishable from glossopharyngeal neuralgia.

Treatment For idiopathic glossopharyngeal neuralgia, a trial of carbamazepine, gabapentin, pregabalin, or baclofen may be useful. If these are unsuccessful, the conventional surgical procedure had been to interrupt the glossopharyngeal nerve and upper rootlets of the vagus nerve near the medulla but recent observations suggest that a vascular decompression procedure similar to the one used for tic and directed to a small vascular loop under the ninth nerve relieves the pain in a proportion of patients.

Acute Herpes Zoster and Postherpetic Neuralgia

Neuralgia associated with a vesicular eruption caused by the herpes zoster virus may affect cranial as well as peripheral nerves. Two syndromes are frequent: herpes zoster auricularis and herpes zoster ophthalmicus. Both may be exceedingly painful in the acute phase of the infection. In the auricular form, herpes of the external auditory meatus and pinna and sometimes of the palate and occipital region—with or without deafness, tinnitus, and vertigo—is combined with facial paralysis. This syndrome, since its original description by Ramsay Hunt, has been known as geniculate herpes, and also Ramsay-Hunt syndrome (see also Chap. 47). However, it has never been clear to us how there is a connection between the geniculate ganglion and the skin of the external ear canal and tympanic membrane and a careful pathologic study of the ganglion by Denny-Brown and Adams in one case showed no lesion there. The facial nerve, however, was heavily infiltrated with inflammatory cells, at least explaining the facial palsy.

The more common pain and herpetic eruption caused by herpes zoster infection of the gasserian ganglion are practically always limited to the first division (herpes zoster ophthalmicus). Ordinarily, the rash appears within 4 to 5 days or less after the onset of the pain, thereby making the clinical diagnosis difficult; however, treatment should be instituted (see below) based on the clinical likelihood of zoster infection. If the eruption does not appear, some cause other than herpes zoster will almost invariably declare itself; nevertheless, a few cases have been reported in which the characteristic location of pain with serologic evidence of herpes zoster infection was not accompanied by skin lesions.

The acute discomfort associated with the herpetic eruption usually subsides after several days or weeks, or it may linger for several months. It is mostly in the elderly that the pain becomes chronic and intractable. Usually it is described as a constant burning, with superimposed waves of stabbing pain, and the skin in the territory of the preceding eruption is exquisitely sensitive to the slightest tactile stimuli, even though the threshold of pain and thermal perception is elevated. This unremitting *postherpetic neuralgia* of long duration represents one of the most difficult pain problems with which the physician must deal. Some relief may be provided by application of capsaicin cream, use of a mechanical or electrical cutaneous stimulator, or administration of one of the antiepileptic drugs.

Treatment Treatment with acyclovir, along the lines indicated in Chap. 33, will shorten the period of eruption and pain, but the drug does not prevent its persistence as a chronic pain.

Antidepressants such as amitriptyline and fluoxetine are helpful in some patients, and Bowsher has suggested, on the basis of a small placebo-controlled trial, that treatment with amitriptyline during the early acute phase may prevent persistent pain. The use of preemptive measures, such as gabapentin or pregabalin administered at the outset, may be effective but a properly performed clinical trial is lacking. The addition of amitriptyline 75 mg at bedtime has proved to be a useful measure. Probably equivalent results are obtained by a combination of valproic acid and an antidepressant, as reported by Raftery. King has reported that two 325-mg aspirin tablets crushed and mixed with cold cream or chloroform (15 mL) and spread over the painful zone on the face or trunk relieved the pain for several hours in most patients with postzoster neuralgia. Ketamine cream has been suggested as an alternative. Extensive trigeminal rhizotomy or other destructive procedures should be avoided, as these surgical measures are not for long successful and may lead to a superimposed diffuse refractory dysesthetic component on the original neuralgia (anesthesia dolorosa).

Trochlear Headache

Under the heading of "primary trochlear headache," Yanguela and colleagues have described a periorbital pain that emanates from the superomedial orbit in the region of the trochlea (the pulley of the superior oblique muscle). Most of their patients were women. The pain was worsened by adduction and (paradoxically for the superior oblique) upgaze of the globe on the affected side, in the direction of action of the superior oblique muscle. The authors describe a diagnostic method of examination that begins by having the patient look downward so that the trochlea can be palpated and compressed; the patient then looks upward, eliciting or exaggerating the pain, while the examiner continues compression. Injection of the trochlea with corticosteroids relieved the pain in almost all of these patients. The authors made a distinction between primary trochlear headache and "trochleitis," which seems to us an ambiguous difference. There is no limitation of ocular movement or autonomic change and imaging of the orbit is normal. This syndrome, with which we have no experience, brings to mind the entity of the Brown syndrome of trochlear entrapment with diplopia and pain (Chap. 13). The above authors were also of the opinion that the trochlea may be a trigger point for migraine.

Otalgia

Pain localized in and around one ear is occasionally a primary complaint. It is commonly the incipient symptom of Bell's palsy but there are a number of different causes and mechanisms. During neurosurgical operations in awake patients, stimulation of cranial nerves V, VII, IX, and X causes ear pain, yet interruption of these nerves usually causes no or limited demonstrable loss of sensation in the ear canal or the ear itself (superficial sensation in this region is supplied by the great auricular nerve, which is derived from the C2 and C3 roots). The neurosurgical literature cites examples of otalgia that were relieved by section of the nervus intermedius (sensory part of VII) or of nerves IX and X. In otalgic cases, one is prompted to search for a nasopharyngeal tumor, vertebral artery aneurysm or to anticipate an outbreak of zoster. Formerly, lateral sinus thrombosis was a common cause in children. When these possibilities are eliminated by appropriate studies, there always remain examples of primary idiopathic otalgia, lower cluster headache, and glossopharyngeal neuralgia. Some patients with migraine have pain centered in the ear region and occiput, but we have never observed a trigeminal neuralgia in which the ear was the predominant site of pain. Occasionally, temporomandibular joint disease is the cause (see below).

Occipital Neuralgia

Paroxysmal pain may occasionally occur in the distribution of the greater or lesser occipital nerves (suboccipital, occipital, and posterior parietal areas). While tenderness may be localized to the region where these nerves cross the superior nuchal line, there is only questionable evidence of an occipital nerve lesion at this site. The finding of hypesthesia in the distribution of the occipital nerves makes the possibility of an entrapment neuropathy more convincing. Carbamazepine or gabapentin may provide some relief. Blocking the nerves with lidocaine may abolish the pain and encourage attempts to section one or more occipital nerves or the second or third cervical dorsal root, but the results have rarely been successful, and several such patients who had these procedures were later referred to us with disabling anesthesia dolorosa. We have advised repeated injections of local anesthetic agents and the use of steroids, traction, local heat, and analgesic and anti-inflammatory drugs. The pain at times may be difficult to distinguish from that arising in the upper three cervical facet joints, one type of which is discussed below. The approach of treating migraine by injection of the occipital nerves is controversial.

"Third Occipital Nerve" Headache

This condition, a unilateral occipital and suboccipital ache, may be a prominent symptom in patients with neck pain, particularly after neck injuries (a prevalence of 27 percent, according to Lord et al). Bogduk and Marsland attribute it to a degenerative or traumatic arthropathy involving the C2 and C3 apophysial joints with impingement on the "third occipital nerve" (a branch of the C3 dorsal ramus that crosses the dorsolateral aspect of the apophysial [facet] joint). Elimination of the neck pain and headache by percutaneous blocking of the third occipital nerve near the facet joint under fluoroscopic control is diagnostic and temporarily therapeutic. More sustained relief (weeks to months) has been obtained by radiofrequency coagulation of the nerve or steroid injections in and around the joint. NSAIDs also provide some relief.

Carotidynia and Extracranial Artery Dissection

Carotidynia was coined by Temple Fay in 1927 to designate a special type of cervicofacial pain that could be elicited by pressure on the common carotid arteries of patients with atypical facial neuralgia. Compression of the artery in the neck in these patients, or mild electrical stimulation at or near the bifurcation, produced a dull ache that was referred to the ipsilateral face, ear, jaws, and teeth or down the neck. This type of carotid sensitivity occurs as part of cranial (giant cell) arteritis and of the rare condition known as Takayasu arteritis (Chap. 34), and during attacks of migraine or cluster headache. It has also been described with displacement of the carotid artery by tumor and dissecting aneurysm of its wall; among these causes, the last is of greatest concern. The idiopathic variety of carotidynia may have to do with a swelling or inflammation of the tissue surrounding the carotid bifurcation, a change that has been demonstrated on MRI by Burton and colleagues, but the problem has been seen most frequently in migraineurs.

Roseman has described a variant of carotidynia that has a predilection for young adults. This syndrome takes the form of recurrent, self-limited attacks of pain and tenderness at the carotid bifurcation lasting a week or two. During the attack, aggravation of the pain by head movement, chewing, and swallowing is characteristic. This condition is treated with simple analgesics. Yet another possible variety of carotidynia appears at any stage of adult life and recurs in attacks lasting minutes to hours in association with throbbing headaches indistinguishable from common migraine (Raskin and Prusiner). This form responds favorably to the administration of ergotamine, methysergide, and other drugs that are effective in the treatment of migraine.

Although most pain of carotid or vertebral artery dissection is localized to the site of injury in the anterior or posterior neck, Arnold and colleagues have emphasized the frequency with which headache, and not neck pain, was the sole feature. Some had a paroxysmal ("thunderclap") onset but most had throbbing and progressive pain over days, sometimes bilaterally. The combination of focal neck pain and localized headache over an eye is particularly suggestive and, of course, if there are corresponding symptoms of fluctuating or static regional brain ischemia, Horner syndrome, or lower cranial nerve palsies, the diagnosis is likely.

Temporomandibular Joint Pain (Costen Syndrome)

This is a form of craniofacial pain from dysfunction of one temporomandibular joint. Malocclusion because of ill-fitting dentures or loss of molar teeth on one side with alteration of the normal bite may lead to distortion of and ultimately degenerative changes in the joint and to pain in front of the ear, with radiation to the temple and over the face (see Guralnick et al). Most patients, according to Scrivani and colleagues report deviation of the mandible to the affected side on jaw opening and clicking noises emanating from the joint. Locking of the jaw in either the open or closed position is another feature. The diagnosis is supported by the findings of tenderness over the joint, crepitus on opening the mouth, and limitation of jaw opening. The favored diagnostic maneuver involves palpating the joint from its posterior aspect by placing a finger in the external auditory meatus and pressing forward. The diagnosis can be made with some confidence only if this entirely reproduces the patient's pain. CT and plain films are rarely helpful, but effusions have been shown in the joints by MRI. Management consists of careful adjustment of the bite by a dental specialist. Small doses of amitryptiline at bedtime may be helpful. In our experience, most of the putative diagnoses of Costen syndrome that reach the neurologist have been erroneous, and the number of headaches and facial pains that are attributed to "temporomandibular joint dysfunction" is excessive, especially if judged by the response to treatment. The temporomandibular joint may also be the source of pain when involved with rheumatoid arthritis and other connective tissue diseases.

Facial Pain of Dental or Sinus Origin

Maxillary and mandibular discomfort is a common effect of nerve irritation from deep caries, abscess, dental pulp degeneration, or periodontal disease. The pain of dental nerve origin is usually most severe at night, slightly pulsating, and often associated with local tenderness at the root of the tooth in response to heat, cold, or pressure. The diagnosis can be confirmed by infiltrating the base of the tooth with lidocaine, and the pain is eradicated by proper dental management.

Trigeminal neuritis following dental extractions or oral surgery is another vexing problem. There may be sensory loss in the tongue or lower lip and weakness of the masseter or pterygoid muscle.

Sometimes the onset of "atypical facial pain" (see below) can be dated to a dental procedure such as tooth extraction, and, as usually happens, neither the dentist nor the neurologist is able to find a source for the pain or any malfunction of the trigeminal nerve. Roberts and coworkers, as well as Ratner and associates, have pointed out that residual microabscesses and subacute bone infection account for some of these cases. They isolated the affected region by using local anesthetic blocks, curetted the bone, and administered antibiotics, following which the pain resolved. The removed bone fragments showed vascular and inflammatory changes and infection with oral bacterial flora, but there was no control material.

Facial Pain of Uncertain Origin (Idiopathic, "Atypical" Facial Pain)

There remains—after all the aforementioned facial pain syndromes a fair number of patients with pain in the face for which no cause can be found. These patients are most often young women, who describe the pain as constant and unbearably severe, deep in the face, or at the angle of cheek and nose, and unresponsive to all varieties of analgesic medication. Because of the failure to identify an organic basis for the pain, one is tempted to attribute it to psychologic or emotional factors. Depression of varying severity is found in some. Some such patients, with or without depression, respond to tricyclic antidepressants and selective serotonin reuptake inhibitors (SSRI) medications. Differentiated from this group is the condition of trigeminal neuropathy with facial numbness, described in Chap. 47.

Facial pain of the "atypical type," like other chronic pain of indeterminate cause, requires close observation of the patient, looking for lesions such as nasopharyngeal carcinoma or apical lung carcinoma to declare themselves. The pain should be managed by the conservative methods outlined in the preceding chapter and not by destructive surgery. Antidepressants may be helpful, especially if the patient displays obsessive characteristics in relation to the pain; some European neurologists favor clomipramine for various facial and scalp pains.

Other Rare Types of Facial Pain

Neuralgia may arise in the terminal branches of the trigeminal, ciliary, nasociliary, and supraorbital nerves; some of which have already been mentioned. Some of these are vague entities at best and merely descriptive terms given to pains localized around the eye and nose. The Tolosa-Hunt syndrome of pain behind the eye and granulomatous involvement of some combination of cranial nerves III, IV, VI, and ophthalmic V, responsive to steroids, is discussed in Chap. 47.

A kind of *reflex sympathetic dystrophy of the face* is postulated as another rare form of persistent facial pain that may follow dental surgery or penetrating injuries to the face. It is characterized by severe burning pain and hyperpathia in response to all types of stimuli. Sudomotor, vasomotor, and trophic changes are lacking, unlike causalgia that affects the limbs. Nevertheless, this form of facial pain is said to respond to repeated blockade or resection of the stellate ganglion.

Under the title of *neck–tongue syndrome*, Lance and Anthony have described the occurrence of a sharp pain and tingling in the upper neck or occiput with numbness of the ipsilateral half of the tongue on sudden rotation of the neck. They attribute the syndrome to stretching of the C2 ventral ramus, which contains proprioceptive fibers from the tongue; these fibers run from the lingual nerve to the hypoglossal nerve and thence to the second cervical root.

A problem that has gone by the self-evident name *burning mouth syndrome (stomatodynia)* occurs mainly in middle-aged and older women, as commented in Chap. 12.

The tongue or other oral sites may be most affected or the entire oral mucosa may burn. A few patients are found to have diabetes, vitamin B_{12} deficiency, or Sjögren syndrome as possible causes. A hint to the last diagnosis is the inability to feel food in the mouth. The oral mucosa is normal when inspected, and no one treatment has been consistently effective, but gabapentin combined with antidepressants or clonazepam may be tried (see the review by Grushka et al). One of our patients with a limited form of this condition, which affected only the upper palate and gums, benefited from dental nerve blocks with lidocaine.

References

Anderson CD, Frank RD: Migraine and tension headache: Is there a physiological difference? *Headache* 21:63, 1981.

Arnold M, Cumurcivc R, Stapf C, et al: Pain as the only symptom of cervical artery dissection. *J Neurol Neurosurg Psychiatry* 77:1021, 2006.

Ashina M, Lassin LH, Bendsten L, et al: Effect of inhibition of nitric oxide synthetase on chronic tension type headache: A randomised crossover trial. *Lancet* 353:287, 1999.

Barker FG, Jannetta PJ, Bissonette DJ, et al: The long-term outcome of microvascular decompression for trigeminal neuralgia. *N Engl J Med* 334:1077, 1996.

Bartsch T, Pirsker MO, Rasche D, et al: Hypothalamic deep brain stimulation for cluster headache: experience from a new multicentre series. *Cephalalgia* 28:285, 2008.

Bates D, Ashford E, Dawson R, et al: Subcutaneous sumatriptan during the migraine aura: Sumatriptan Aura Study Group. *Neurology* 44:1587, 1994.

Berg MJ, Williams LS: The transient syndrome of headache with neurologic deficits and CSF lymphocytosis. *Neurology;* 45:1648-1654, 1995.

Bickerstaff ER: Basilar artery migraine. *Lancet* 1:15, 1961.

Bigal, ME, Kurth T, Santanello N, et al: Migraine and cardiovascular disease/A population-based study. *Neurology* 74:628-735, 2010.

Blau JN, Dexter SL: The site of pain origin during migraine attacks. *Cephalalgia* 1:143, 1981.

Bogduk N, Govind J: Cervicogenic headache: an assessment of the evidence on clinical diagnosis, invasive tests, and treatment. *Lancet Neuro* 8:959, 2009.

Bogduk N, Marsland A: On the concept of third occipital headache. *J Neurol Neurosurg Psychiatry* 49:775, 1986.

Bowsher D: The effects of pre-emptive treatment of postherpetic neuralgia with amitriptyline: A randomized, double-blind, placebo-controlled trial. *J Pain Symptom Manage* 13:327, 1997.

Broderick JP, Swanson JW: Migraine-related strokes. *Arch Neurol* 44:868, 1987.

Burger SK, Saul RF, Selhorst JB, et al: Transient monocular blindness caused by vasospasm. *N Engl J Med* 325:870, 1991.

Burton BS, Syms MJ, Peterman GW, Burgess LP: MR imaging of patients with carotidynia. *AJNR Am J Neuroradiol* 21:766, 2000.

Caplan LR: Migraine and vertebrobasilar ischemia. *Neurology* 41:55, 1991.

Chen SP, Fuh JL, Lirng JF, et al: Recurrent thunderclap headache and benign CNS angiopathy. *Neurology* 67:2164, 2006.

Cole AJ, Aube M: Migraine with vasospasm and delayed intracerebral hemorrhage. *Arch Neurol* 47:53, 1990.

Cutrer FM: Pain-sensitive cranial structures: Chemical anatomy, in Silberstein SD, Lipton RD, Dalessio DJ (eds): *Wolff's Headache and Other Head Pain*, 7th ed. Oxford, UK, Oxford University Press, 2001, pp 50–56.

Cutter FM, Sorensen AG, Weisskoff RM, et al: Perfusion-weighted imaging defects during spontaneous migraine aura. *Ann Neurol* 43:25, 1998.

Dandy WE: Concerning the cause of trigeminal neuralgia. *Am J Surg* 24:447, 1934.

Day JW, Raskin NH: Thunderclap headache symptomatic of unruptured cerebral aneurysm. *Lancet* 2:1247, 1986.

Dodick DW: Thunderclap headache. *J Neurol Neurosurg Psychiatry* 72:6, 2002.

Drummond PD, Lance JW: Contribution of the extracranial circulation to the pathophysiology of headache, in Olesen J, Edvinsson L (eds): *Basic Mechanisms of Headache*. Amsterdam, Elsevier, 1988, pp 321–330.

Ducros A, Denier C, Joutel A, et al: The clinical spectrum of familial hemiplegic hemianopic migraine associated with mutations in a neuronal calcium channel. *N Engl J Med* 345:17, 2001.

Ekbom K: cited by Kudrow L (see below).

Ekbom K, Greitz T: Carotid angiography in cluster headache. *Acta Radiol Diagn (Stockh)* 10:177, 1970.

Favier I, van Vilet JA, Roon KI, et al: Trigeminal autonomic cephalgias due to structural lesions. *Arch Neurol* 64:25, 2007.

Ferrari MD, Haan J, Blokland JAK, et al: Cerebral blood flow during migraine attacks without aura and effect of sumatriptan. *Arch Neurol* 52:135, 1995.

Ferrari MD, Roon KI, Lipton RB, et al. Oral triptans (serotonin 5-HT1B/1D agonists) in acute migraine treatment: a meta-analysis of 53 trials. *Lancet* 358:1668, 2001.

Fields HL: Treatment of trigeminal neuralgia. *N Engl J Med* 334: 1125, 1996.

Fisher CM: Late-life migraine accompaniments—further experience. *Stroke* 17:1033, 1986.

Fox AW, Chambers CD, Anderson PO, et al: Evidence-based assessment of pregnancy outcome after sumatriptan exposure. *Headache* 42:8, 2002.

Friedman BW, Greenwald P, Bania TC, et al: Randomized trial of IV dexamethasone for acute migraine in the emergency department. *Neurology* 69:2038, 2007.

Gardner WJ, Stowell A, Dutlinger R: Resection of the greater superficial petrosal nerve in the treatment of unilateral headache. *J Neurosurg* 4:105, 1947.

Garg P, Servoss SJ, Wu JC, et al: Lack of association between migraine headache and patent foramen ovale: Results of a case-control study. *Circulation* 121:1406-1412, 2010.

Goadsby PJ: Pathophysiology of cluster headache; A trigeminal autonomic cephalgia. *Lancet Neurol* 1:37, 2002.

Goadsby PJ: Recent advances in understanding migraine mechanisms, molecules and therapeutics. *Trends Mol Med* 13:39, 2007.

Gomez-Aranda F, Cañadillas F, Marti-Masso JF, et al: Pseudomigraine with temporary neurological symptoms and lymphocytic pleocytosis: A report of 50 cases. *Brain* 120:1105, 1997.

Graham JR. Migraine. Clinical aspects, in, Vinkin PJ, Bruyn GW (eds): *Handbook of Clinical Neurology*. Vol. 5, *Headaches and Cranial Neuralgias*. Amsterdam, North-Holland Publishing Company, 1968, pp 45–58.

Graham JR, Wolff HG: Mechanism of migraine headache and action of ergotamine tartrate. *Arch Neurol Psychiatry* 39:737, 1938.

Grushka M, Epstein JB, Gorski M: Burning mouth syndrome. *Am Fam Physician* 65:615, 2002.

Gudmundsson LS, Scher AI, Aspelund T, et al: Migraine with aura and risk of cardiovascular and all cause mortality in men and women: prospective cohort study. *BMJ* 341:c3966, 2010.
Guralnick W, Kaban LB, Merrill RG: Temporomandibular-joint afflictions. *N Engl J Med* 299:123, 1978.
Harris N: Paroxysmal and postural headaches from intra-ventricular cysts and tumours. *Lancet* 2:654, 1944.
Iversen HK, Nielsen TH, Olesen J: Arterial responses during migraine headache. *Lancet* 336:837, 1990.
Jannetta PJ: Structural mechanisms of trigeminal neuralgia: Arterial compression of the trigeminal nerve at the pons in patients with trigeminal neuralgia. *J Neurosurg* 26:159, 1967.
Jarrar RG, Black DF, Dodick DW, et al: Outcome of trigeminal nerve section in the treatment of chronic cluster headache. *Neurology* 60:1360, 2003.
King RB: Topical aspirin in chloroform and the relief of pain due to herpes zoster and postherpetic neuralgia. *Arch Neurol* 50:1046, 1993.
Kittrelle JP, Grouse DS, Seybold ME: Cluster headache. *Arch Neurol* 42:496, 1985.
Klapper J, Mathew N, Nett R: Triptans in the treatment of basilar migraine and migraine with prolonged aura. *Headache* 41:981, 2001.
Kruit MC, van Buchem, MA, Hofman PAM, et al: Migraine as a risk factor for subclinical brain lesions. *JAMA* 291:427, 2004.
Kruit MC, van Buchem, MA, Launer LJ, et al: Migraine is associated with an increased risk of deep white matter lesions, subclinical posterior circulation infarcts and brain iron accumulation: The population-based MRI CAMERA study. *Cephalagia* 30(2): 129, 2010.
Kudrow L: *Cluster Headache: Mechanisms and Management*. Oxford, UK, Oxford University Press, 1980.
Kunkle EC: Clues in the tempos of cluster headache. *Headache* 22:158, 1982.
Kunkle EC, Pfeiffer JB Jr, Wilhoit WM, Lamrick LW Jr: Recurrent brief headaches in cluster pattern. *N C Med J* 15:510, 1954.
Kurth T, Mohamed S, Maillard P, et al: Headache, migraine, and structural brain lesions and function: population based epidemiology of vascular ageing-MRI study. *BMJ* 342:7357, 2011.
Lance JW: Headaches related to sexual activity. *J Neurol Neurosurg Psychiatry* 39:1226, 1976.
Lance JW, Goadsby PJ. *Mechanism and Management of Headache*, 7th ed. Philadelphia, Elsevier, 2005.
Lance JW, Anthony M: Neck-tongue syndrome on sudden turning of the head. *J Neurol Neurosurg Psychiatry* 43:97, 1980.
Lance JW, Curran DA: Treatment of chronic tension headache. *Lancet* 1:1236, 1964.
Lance JW, Hinterberger H: Symptoms of pheochromocytoma, with particular reference to headache, correlated with catecholamine production. *Arch Neurol* 33:281, 1976.
Lashley KS: Pattern of cerebral integration indicated by the scotomas of migraine. *Arch Neurol Psychiatry* 46:331, 1941.
Lauritzen M, Olesen J: Regional cerebral blood flow during migraine attacks by xenon 133 inhalation and emission tomography. *Brain* 107:447, 1984.
Leão AAP: Spreading depression of activity in cerebral cortex. *J Neurophysiol* 7:359, 1944.
Leone M, Franzini A, Broggi G, et al: Hypothalamic stimulation for intractable cluster headache. *Neurology* 67:150, 2006.
Lipton RB, Bigal ME, Diamond M, et al: Migraine prevalence, disease burden, and the need for preventive therapy. *Neurology* 68:343, 2007.
Loder E: Triptan therapy in migraine. *New Engl J Med* 363:63, 2010.
Lord SM, Barnsley L, Wallis BJ, Bogduk N: Third occipital nerve headache: A prevalence study. *J Neurol Neurosurg Psychiatry* 57:1187, 1994.
May A, Bahra A, Büchel C, et al: Hypothalamic activation in cluster headache attacks. *Lancet* 352:275, 1998.
Malleson A: *Whiplash and Other Useful Illnesses*. Montreal, McGill-Queen's University Press, 2002.
Meschia JF, Malkoff MD, Biller J: Reversible segmental cerebral artery spasm and cerebral infarction: Possible association with excessive use of sumatriptan and Midrin. *Arch Neurol* 55:712, 1998.
Moskowitz MA: Neurogenic inflammation in the pathophysiology and treatment of migraine. *Neurology* 43(Suppl 3):S16, 1993.
Olesen J: Headache Classification Committee of the International Headache Society: Classification and diagnostic criteria for headache disorders, cranial neuralgia, and facial pain. *Cephalalgia* 8(Suppl 7):1, 1988.
Olesen J: The ischemic hypothesis of migraine. *Arch Neurol* 44:321, 1987.
Olesen J, Diener H-C, Husstedt IW, et al: Calcitonin gene-related peptide receptor antagonist BIBN 4096 BS for the acute treatment of migraine. *N Engl J Med* 350:1104, 2004.
Olsen TS, Friberg L, Lassen NA: Ischemia may be the primary cause of the neurologic defects in classic migraine. *Arch Neurol* 44:156, 1987.
Pannullo SC, Reich JB, Krol G, et al: MRI changes in intracranial hypotension. *Neurology* 43:919, 1993.
Pascual J, Oterino A, Berciano J: Headache in type 1 Chiari malformation. *Neurology* 42:1519, 1992.
Pascual J, Berciano J: Experience with headaches that start in elderly people. *J Neurol Neurosurg Psychiatry* 57:1255, 1994.
Patten J: *Neurological Differential Diagnosis*. London, Harold Starke, 1977.
Price RW, Posner JB: Chronic paroxysmal hemicrania: A disabling headache syndrome responding to indomethacin. *Ann Neurol* 3:183, 1978.
Raftery H: The management of postherpetic pain using sodium valproate and amitriptyline. *Ir Med J* 72:399, 1979.
Rascol A, Cambier J, Guiraud B, et al: Accidents ischemiques cerebraux au cours de crises migraineuses. *Rev Neurol* 135:867, 1980.
Raskin NH: Repetitive intravenous dihydroergotamine as therapy for intractable migraine. *Neurology* 36:995, 1986.
Raskin NH: Serotonin receptors and headache. *N Engl J Med* 325:353, 1991.
Raskin NH: The hypnic headache syndrome. *Headache* 28:534, 1988.
Raskin NH, Prusiner S: Carotidynia. *Neurology* 27:43, 1977.
Ratner EJ, Person P, Kleinman JD, et al: Jawbone cavities and trigeminal and atypical facial neuralgias. *Oral Surg Oral Med Oral Pathol* 48:3, 1979.
Ray BS, Wolff HG: Experimental studies on headache: Pain sensitive structures of the head and their significance in headache. *Arch Surg* 41:813, 1940.
Roberts AM, Person P, Chandra NB, Hori JM: Further observations on dental parameters of trigeminal and atypical facial pain. *Oral Surg Oral Med Oral Pathol* 58:121, 1984.
Rooke ED: Benign exertional headache. *Med Clin North Am* 52:801, 1968.
Roseman DM: Carotidynia. *Arch Otolaryngol* 85:103, 1967.
Rundek T, Elkind MSV, DiTullio MR, et al: Patent foramen ovale and migraine: A cross-sectional study from the Northern Manhattan study (NOMAS). *Circulation* 118:1419-1424, 2008.
Sakai F, Ebihara S, Akiyama M, Horikawa M: Pericranial muscle hardness in tension-type headache: A non-invasive measurement method and its clinical application. *Brain* 118:523, 1995.
Scher AI, Gudmundsson LS, Sigurdsson S, et al: Migraine headache in middle age and late-life brain infarcts. *JAMA* 301(24):2563, 2009.
Schüks M, Rist PM, Bigal ME, et al: Migraine and cardiovascular disease: systematic review and meta-analysis. *BMJ* 339:b3914, 2009.

Scrivani SJ, Keith DA, Kaban LB: Temporomandibular disorders. *New Engl J Med* 359:2693, 2008.

Singhal AB, Caviness VS, Begleiter MD, et al: Cerebral vasoconstriction and stroke after use of serotonergic drugs. *Neurology* 58:130, 2002.

Sjaastad O, Dale I: A new (?) clinical headache entity "chronic paroxysmal hemicrania." *Acta Neurol Scand* 54:140, 1976.

Somerville BW: The role of estradiol withdrawal in the etiology of menstrual migraine. *Neurology* 22:355, 1972.

Stewart WF, Lipton RB, Liberman J: Variation in migraine prevalence by race. *Neurology* 47:52, 1996.

Subcutaneous Sumatriptan International Study Group: Treatment of migraine attacks with sumatriptan. *N Engl J Med* 325:316, 1991.

Sweet WH: The treatment of trigeminal neuralgia (tic douloureux). *N Engl J Med* 315:174, 1986.

Sweet WH, Wepsic JG: Controlled thermocoagulation of trigeminal ganglion and rootlets for differential destruction of pain fibers. *J Neurosurg* 40:143, 1974.

Symonds CP: Cough headache. *Brain* 79:557, 1956.

Taimi C, Navez M, Perrin A-M, Laurent B: Cephales induites par abus des traitements symptomatique antalgiques et antimigraineux. *Rev Neurol* 157:1221, 2001.

Watson P, Steele JC: Paroxysmal dysequilibrium in the migraine syndrome of childhood. *Arch Otolaryngol* 99:177, 1974.

Weatherall MW, Telzerow AJ, Cittadini E, et al: Intravenous aspirin (lysine acetylsalicylate) in the inpatient management of headache. *Neurology* 75:1098, 2010.

Welch KMA: Migraine: A behavioral disorder. *Arch Neurol* 44:323, 1987.

White JC, Sweet WH: *Pain and the Neurosurgeon*. Springfield, IL, Charles C Thomas, 1969, p 265.

Wijdicks EF, Kerkhoff H, Van Gijn J: Long-term follow up of 71 patients with thunderclap headache mimicking subarachnoid hemorrhage. *Lancet* 2:68, 1988.

Wolf ME, Szabo K, Griebe M, et al: Clinical and MRI characteristics of acute migrainous infarction. *Neurology* 76:1191, 2011.

Wolff HG: *Headache and Other Head Pain*, 2nd ed. New York, Oxford University Press, 1963.

Woods RP, Iacoboni M, Mazziotta JC: Bilateral spreading cerebral hypoperfusion during spontaneous migraine headache. *N Engl J Med* 331:1690, 1994.

Yanguela J, Sanchez-del-Rio M, Bueno A, et al: Primary trochlear headache. A new cephalgia generated and modulated on the trochlear region. *Neurology* 62:1134, 2004.

Ziegler DK, Hurwitz A, Hassanein RS, et al: Migraine prophylaxis: A comparison of propranolol and amitriptyline. *Arch Neurol* 44:486, 1987.

11

Pain in the Back, Neck, and Extremities

We include an extensive chapter on this subject in recognition of the fact that back pain is among the most frequent of medical complaints. Up to 80 percent of adults have low back pain at some time in their lives and, according to Kelsey and White, an even larger percentage will be found at autopsy to have degenerative spine disease. One task of the neurologist is to determine whether a disease of the spine has compressed the spinal cord or the spinal roots. To do this effectively, a clear understanding of the structures involved and some knowledge of orthopedics and rheumatology is necessary.

Pains in the lower part of the spine and legs are caused by somewhat different types of disease than those in the neck, shoulder, and arms; therefore, these two categories are considered separately.

PAIN IN THE LOWER BACK AND LIMBS

The lower parts of the spine and pelvis, with their massive muscular attachments, are relatively inaccessible to palpation and inspection. Although some physical signs and imaging studies are helpful, diagnosis often depends on the patient's description of the pain and his behavior in different positions and during the execution of certain maneuvers. Seasoned clinicians appreciate the need for a systematic inquiry and method of examination, the descriptions of which are preceded here by a brief consideration of the anatomy and physiology of the spine.

Anatomy and Physiology of the Lower Part of the Back

The bony spine is a complex structure, roughly divisible into an anterior and a posterior part. The anterior component consists of the cylindrical vertebral bodies, articulated by the intervertebral discs and held together by the anterior and posterior longitudinal ligaments. The posterior elements are more delicate and extend from the vertebral bodies as pedicles and laminae, which encircle the *spinal canal*. Large transverse and spinous processes project laterally and posteriorly, respectively, and serve as the origins and insertions of the muscles that support and protect the spinal column. The bony processes are also held together by sturdy ligaments, the most important being the ligamentum flavum, which runs along the ventral surfaces of the laminae. The posterior longitudinal ligament lies opposite it—on the dorsal surfaces of the vertebral bodies. These two ligaments define the posterior and anterior margins of the spinal canal, respectively.

The posterior parts of the vertebrae articulate with one another at the diarthrodial *facet joints* (also called apophysial or zygapophysial joints), each of which is composed of the inferior facet of the vertebra above and the superior facet of the one below. Figure 11-1 illustrates these anatomic features. The configuration and orientation of the facet joints differs in the cervical, thoracic and lumbosacral parts of the spine. The facet and sacroiliac joints, which are covered by synovia, the compressible intervertebral discs, and the collagenous and elastic ligaments, permit a limited degree of flexion, extension, rotation, and lateral motion of the spine.

The stability of the spine depends on the integrity of the vertebral bodies, pedicles and intervertebral discs and on two types of supporting structures, ligamentous (passive) and muscular (active). Although the ligamentous structures are quite strong, neither they nor the vertebral body–disc complexes have sufficient integral strength alone to resist the enormous forces that may act on the spinal column. Consequently, the stability of the lower back is also largely dependent on the voluntary and reflex activity of the paraspinal, sacrospinalis, abdominal, gluteus maximus, and hamstring muscles.

The vertebral and paravertebral structures derive their innervation from the meningeal branches of the spinal nerves (also known as recurrent meningeal or sinuvertebral nerves). These meningeal branches spring from the posterior divisions of the spinal nerves just distal to the dorsal root ganglia, reenter the spinal canal through the intervertebral foramina, and supply pain fibers to the intraspinal ligaments, periosteum of bone, outer layers of the annulus fibrosus (which enclose the disc), and the capsule of the articular facets. Coppes and associates have found A-δ and C pain fibers extending into the inner layers of the annulus, and even into the nucleus pulposus.

Although the spinal cord itself is insensitive, many of the conditions that affect it produce pain by involving these adjacent structures. For example, the sensory fibers from the lumbosacral and sacroiliac joints enter the spinal cord via the fifth lumbar and first sacral roots. Motor

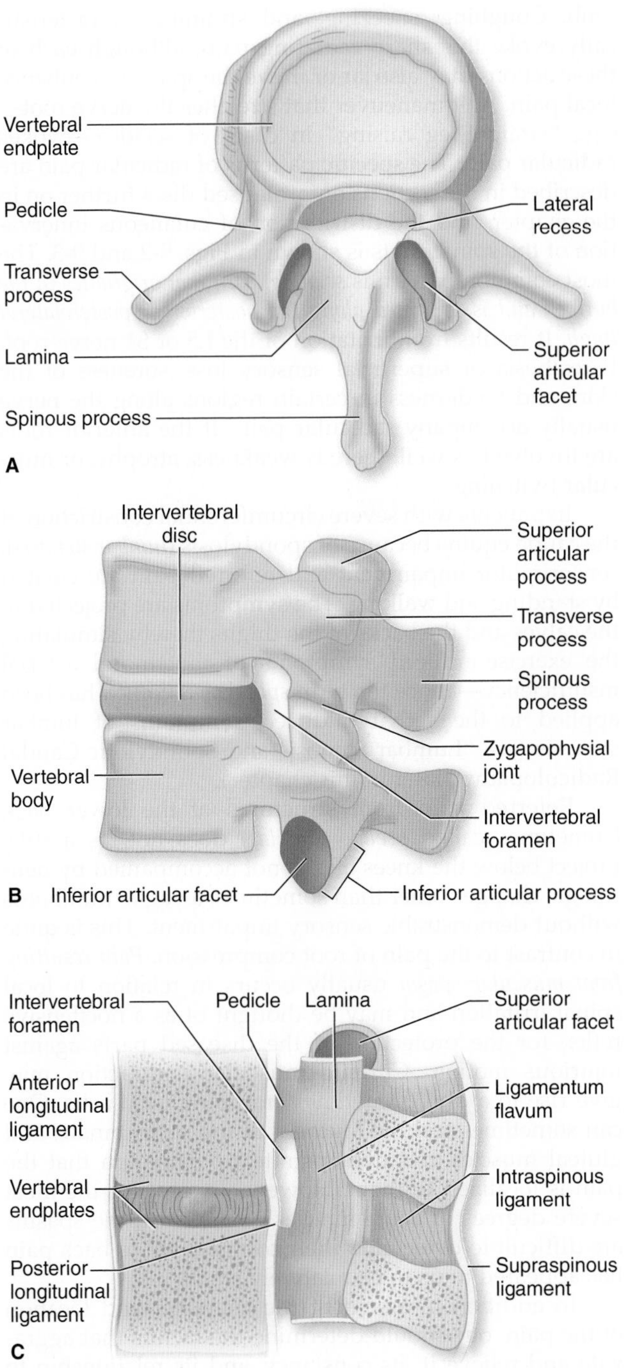

Figure 11-1. *A.* The lumbar vertebrae viewed from above from *B.* the side and *C.* mid-sagittally. *A* and *B* show the bony structures and their relationships to the disc space, facet joints and intervertebral foramina. *C* demonstrates in a cutaway mid-sagittal view, the main ligamentous structures of the spine in relation to the bones and discs. The ligaments and articulations are critical to the mechanical integrity of the spinal column.

fibers exit through the corresponding anterior roots and form the efferent limb of segmental reflexes.

The spinal roots in the lumbar region, after exiting from the spinal cord, course downward in the subarachnoid space of the spinal canal and are gradually displaced laterally until they angulate and exit at the intervertebral foramina. Prior to entering the proximal foraminal canal, the spinal root lies in a shallow furrow along the inner surface of the pedicle, the *lateral recess*. The lumbar nerve roots traverse this lateral recess one level superior to their exit through the foramen. The lateral recess is a common site of entrapment of the traversing root by posterolaterally herniated disc material and bony overgrowth.

The parts of the back that possess the greatest freedom of movement, and hence are most frequently subject to injury, are the lumbar, lumbosacral, and cervical. In addition to bending, twisting, and other voluntary movements, many actions of the spine are reflexive in nature and are the basis of erect posture.

Aging Changes in Spinal Structures

Degeneration in the intervertebral discs and ligaments is a consequence of aging and the succession of inevitable minor traumas to the spine. Deposition of collagen and elastin and alterations of glycosaminoglycans combine to decrease the water content of the nucleus pulposus; concomitantly, the cartilaginous endplate becomes less vascular (Hassler). The dehydrated disc thins out and becomes more fragile. Similar changes occur in the annulus of the disc, which frays to an increasing degree with the passage of time, permitting the nucleus pulposus to bulge and, sometimes with injury to the surrounding annulus, to extrude. This process can be observed by MRI, which shows a gradual reduction in the high T2 signal of the nucleus pulposus with the passage of time. In women who had MRI for gynecologic reasons, Powell and coworkers found an increasing frequency of lumbar disc degeneration and bulging, approaching 70 percent by the fiftieth year. Jensen and colleagues recorded similar abnormalities with aging in asymptomatic men and women (see further on).

The problem of degenerative spinal disease has been conceptualized as a series of events having its genesis in shrinkage of the disc that subsequently alters the alignment of the articular facets and vertebral bodies, leading to facet arthropathy and bony spur formation. These reactive changes contribute to stenosis of the spinal canal and directly compromise the lateral recesses of the canal and the intervertebral foramina, where they impinge on nerve roots. Osteoporosis, especially in older women, is a further important cause of vertebral flattening or collapse, additionally narrowing the spinal canal. All of these changes may further conspire to weaken ligaments and allow slippage of one vertebral body on adjacent ones, termed spondylolisthesis.

General Clinical Features of Low Back Pain

Types of Low Back Pain

Of the several symptoms of spinal disease (pain, stiffness, limitation of movement, and deformity), pain is foremost. Four types of pain may be distinguished: local, referred, radicular, and that arising from secondary muscular spasm. These several types of pain can often be discerned from the patient's description; reliance is placed mainly on the character of the pain, its location, and conditions that modify it.

Local pain is caused by any pathologic process that impinges on structures containing sensory endings, including the periosteum of the vertebral body, capsule of apophysial joints, annulus fibrosus, and ligaments. Destruction of the nucleus pulposus alone produces little or no pain but the annulus is innervated with small nerve fibers and, when subject to disruption, may produce considerable pain. This pain is steady and aching, but it may be intermittent and sharp, and, although not well circumscribed, is felt in or near the affected part of the spine. Pathologic change arising in spinal structures may also evoke discomfort in regions that share common innervation and thereby vaguely simulate the pain of radicular disease. These areas of projection may be considered similarly to the referred pain of the "sclerotomes" discussed in Chap. 8 and just below.

Referred pain in reference to the spine is of two types: one that is projected from the spine to viscera and other structures lying within the territory of the lumbar and upper sacral dermatomes, and another that is projected from pelvic and abdominal viscera to the spine. Pain caused by disease of the upper part of the lumbar spine may be referred to the medial flank, lateral hip, groin, and anterior thigh (sclerotomes; see Chap. 8). This has been attributed to irritation of the superior cluneal nerves, which are derived from the posterior divisions of the first three lumbar spinal nerves and innervate the superior portions of the buttocks. Pain from the lower part of the lumbar spine is usually referred to the lower buttocks and posterior thighs and is a result of irritation of lower spinal nerves, which activate the same pool of intraspinal neurons as the nerves that innervate the posterior thighs. Pain of this type is usually diffuse and has a deep, aching quality, but it tends at times to be more superficially projected. In general, the intensity of the referred pain parallels that of the local pain. Maneuvers that alter local pain have a similar effect on referred pain. McCall and colleagues and Kellgren have verified these areas of reference by the injection of hypertonic saline into the facet joints and the "sclerotomes" they determined are discussed in Chap. 8. But, as Sinclair and coworkers have pointed out, the sites of reference are inexact and cannot be relied on for precise anatomic localization.

In contrast to the movement-altered referred pain that originates in the spine, pain from visceral diseases felt within the abdomen, flanks, or lumbar region, is modified by the state of activity of the viscera and sometimes by assuming an upright or supine posture. In other words, its character and temporal relationships have little relationship to movement of the back.

Radicular or *"root" pain* has some of the characteristics of referred pain but differs in its greater intensity, distal radiation, circumscription to the territory of a root, and factors that excite it. The mechanism is stretching, irritation, or compression of a spinal root within or central to the intervertebral foramen. The pain is sharp, often intense, and usually superimposed on the dull ache of referred pain; it nearly always radiates from a paracentral position near the spine to some part of the lower limb. Coughing, sneezing, and straining characteristically evoke this sharp radiating pain, although each of these actions may also jar or move the spine and enhance local pain. Any maneuver that stretches the nerve root—e.g., "straight-leg raising" in cases of sciatica—evokes radicular pain. The specific patterns of radicular pain are described in the sections on prolapsed discs further on in the chapter, and the distribution of cutaneous innervation of the spinal roots is shown in Figs. 9-2 and 9-3. The most common pattern is *sciatica, pain that originates in the buttock and is projected along the posterior or posterolateral thigh.* It results from irritation of the L5 or S1 nerve root. Paresthesia or superficial sensory loss, soreness of the skin, and tenderness in certain regions along the nerve usually accompany radicular pain. If the anterior roots are involved as well, there is weakness, atrophy, or muscular twitching.

In patients with severe circumferential constriction of the cauda equina because of spondylosis (*lumbar stenosis*), sensorimotor impairment and referred pain are elicited by standing and walking. The symptoms are projected to the calves and the backs of the thighs thereby simulating the exercise-induced symptoms of iliofemoral arterial insufficiency—hence the term *spinal claudication* has been applied to the activity-induced symptoms of lumbar stenosis (see "Lumbar Stenosis and Spondylotic Caudal Radiculopathy" later in this chapter).

Referred pain from structures of the lower back (sometimes called *pseudoradicular*) does not, as a rule, project below the knees and is not accompanied by neurologic changes other than sometimes a vague numbness without demonstrable sensory impairment. This is quite in contrast to the pain of root compression. *Pain resulting from muscular spasm* usually occurs in relation to local spinal irritation and may be thought of as a nocifensive reflex for the protection of the diseased parts against injurious motion. Chronic muscular contraction may give rise to a dull, sometimes cramping local ache. One can sometimes feel the tautness of the sacrospinalis and gluteal muscles and demonstrate by palpation that the pain is localized to them. However, except for the most severe degrees of acute injuries of the back, the spasms are difficult to detect and their contribution to back pain has appeared to us to be relatively small.

In addition to assessing the character and location of the pain, one should determine the factors that aggravate and relieve it, its constancy, and its relationship to activity and to rest, posture, forward bending, coughing, sneezing, and straining. Frequently, the most important lead comes from knowledge of the mode of onset and the circumstances that initiated the pain. Inasmuch as many painful conditions of the back are the result of injuries incurred during work or in automobile accidents, the possibility of exaggeration or prolongation of pain for purposes of compensation must always be kept in mind.

Examination of the Lower Back

The main goals of the examination of the back are to differentiate pain that is caused by nerve root compression from those of musculoskeletal strains, metastatic spinal tumor, and infectious and inflammatory diseases of the spine and hips.

Some information may be gained by inspection of the back, buttocks, and lower limbs in various positions. The normal spine shows a thoracic kyphosis and lumbar lordosis in the sagittal plane, which in some individuals may be exaggerated. In the coronal plane, the spine is normally straight or shows a slight curvature, particularly in women. One should observe the spine for excessive curvature, a list, flattening of the normal lumbar lordosis, presence of a gibbus (a sharp, kyphotic angulation usually indicative of a fracture), pelvic tilt or obliquity (Trendelenburg sign), and asymmetry of the paravertebral or gluteal musculature. A sagging gluteal fold suggests involvement of the S1 root. In sciatica one may observe a flexed posture of the affected leg, presumably to reduce tension on the irritated nerve root. Or, patients in whom a free fragment of lumbar disc material has migrated posterolaterally may be unable to lie down and extend the spine.

The next step in the examination is observation of the spine, hips, and legs during certain motions. No advantage accrues from determining how much pain the patient can tolerate. More important is to determine when and under what conditions the pain begins or worsens. Observation of the patient's gait may disclose a subtle limp, a pelvic tilt, a shortening of step, or a stiffness of bearing—indicative of a disinclination to bear weight on a painful leg—the "antalgic gait". Analysis of this type of gait is covered in greater detail in Chap. 7. One looks for limitation of motion while the patient is standing, sitting, and reclining. When standing, the motion of forward bending normally produces flattening and reversal of the lumbar lordotic curve and exaggeration of the thoracic curve. With lesions of the lumbosacral region that involve the posterior ligaments, articular facets, or sacrospinalis muscles and with ruptured lumbar discs, protective reflexes prevent flexion, which stretches these structures ("splinting"). As a consequence, the sacrospinalis muscles remain taut and prevent motion in the lumbar part of the spine. Forward bending then occurs at the hips and at the thoracolumbar junction; also, the patient bends in such a way as to avoid tensing the hamstring muscles and putting undue leverage on the pelvis. In the presence of degenerative disc disease, straightening up from a flexed position is performed only with difficulty.

Lateral bending is usually less revealing than forward bending but, in unilateral ligamentous or muscular strain, bending to the opposite side aggravates the pain by stretching the damaged tissues. With unilateral sciatica, the patient lists to one side and strongly resists bending to the opposite side, and the preferred posture in standing is with the leg slightly flexed at the hip and knee. When the herniated disc lies lateral to the nerve root and displaces it medially, tension on the root is reduced and pain is relieved by bending the trunk to the side opposite the lesion; with herniation medial to the root, tension is reduced by inclining the trunk to the side of the lesion.

In the sitting position, flexion of the hips can be performed more easily, even to the point of bringing the knees in contact with the chest. The reason for this is that knee flexion relaxes tightened hamstring muscles and relieves the stretch on the sciatic nerve. This feature may also be evident in instances of lumbar disc disease, making the maneuver less sensitive than others.

Examination with the patient in the reclining position yields much the same information as in the standing and sitting positions. With lumbosacral disc lesions and sciatica, passive lumbar flexion causes little pain and is not limited as long as the hamstrings are relaxed, and there is no stretching of the sciatic nerve. Thus, with the knees flexed to 90 degrees, sitting up from the reclining position is unimpeded and not painful; with knees extended, there is pain and limited motion (Kraus-Weber test). With vertebral disease, passive flexion of the hips is free, whereas flexion of the lumbar spine may be impeded and painful.

Among the most helpful signs in detecting nerve root compression is passive *straight-leg raising* (possible up to almost 90 degrees in normal individuals) with the patient supine. This places the sciatic nerve and its roots under tension, thereby producing radicular, radiating pain from the buttock through the posterior thigh. This maneuver is the usual way in which compression of the L5 or S1 nerve root is detected (Lasègue sign), however, it may also cause an anterior rotation of the pelvis around a transverse axis, increasing stress on the lumbosacral joint and causing milder radiating pain if this joint is arthritic or otherwise diseased. *Straight raising of the opposite leg* ("crossed straight-leg raising," Fajersztajn sign) may cause sciatica on the opposite side and is a more specific sign of prolapsed disc than is the Lasègue sign. Several of the many derivatives of the straight-leg raising sign are discussed in the section on lumbar disc disease. Asking the seated patient to extend the leg so that the sole of the foot can be inspected is a way of checking for a feigned Lasègue sign.

A patient with lumbosacral strain or disc disease (except in the acute phase or if the disc fragment has migrated laterally) can usually extend the spine with little or no aggravation of pain. If there is an active inflammatory process or fracture of the vertebral body or posterior elements, hyperextension may be markedly limited. In disease of the upper lumbar roots, hyperextension of the leg with the patient prone is the motion that is most limited and reproduces pain; however, in some cases of lower lumbar disc disease with thickening of the ligamentum flavum, this movement is also painful.

Maneuvers in the *lateral decubitus position* yield less information but are useful in eliciting joint disease. In cases of sacroiliac joint disease, abduction of the upside leg against resistance reproduces pain in the sacroiliac region, sometimes with radiation of the pain to the buttock, posterior thigh, and symphysis pubis. Hyperextension of the upside leg with the downside leg flexed is another test for sacroiliac disease. Rotation and abduction of the leg evoke pain in a diseased hip joint and with *trochanteric bursitis*. A helpful indicator of *hip disease* is the Patrick test: with the patient supine, the heel of the offending leg is placed on the opposite knee, and pain is evoked by depressing the flexed leg and externally rotating the hip.

Gentle palpation and percussion of the spine are the last steps in the examination. It is preferable to first palpate the regions that are the least likely to evoke pain. The examiner should know what structures are being palpated (Fig. 11-2). Localized tenderness is seldom pronounced in disease of the spine because the involved structures are so deep. Nevertheless, tenderness over a spinous process or jarring by gentle percussion may indicate the presence of deeper, local spinal inflammation (as in disc space infection), pathologic fracture, metastasis, epidural abscess, or a disc lesion.

Tenderness over the interspinous ligaments or over the region of the articular facets between the fifth lumbar and first sacral vertebrae is consistent with lumbosacral disc disease (Fig. 11-2, sites *2* and *3*). Tenderness in this region and in the sacroiliac joints is also a frequent manifestation of ankylosing spondylitis. Arthritic changes at a facet may cause the same tenderness. Tenderness over the costovertebral angle often indicates genitourinary disease, adrenal disease, or an injury to the transverse process of the first or second lumbar vertebra (Fig. 11-2, site *1*).

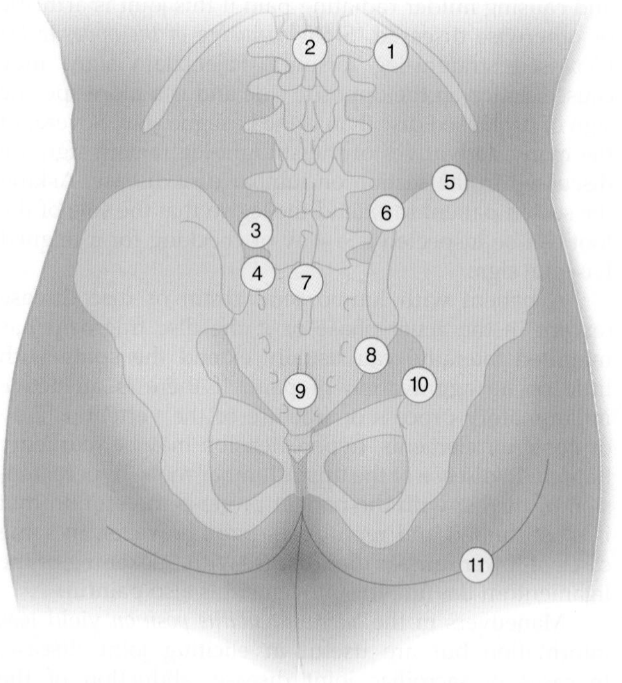

Figure 11-2. (*1*) Costovertebral angle. (*2*) Spinous process and interspinous ligament. (*3*) Region of articular facet (fifth lumbar to first sacral). (*4*) Dorsum of sacrum. (*5*) Region of iliac crest. (*6*) Iliolumbar angle. (*7*) Spinous processes of fifth lumbar and first sacral vertebrae (tenderness = faulty posture or occasionally spina bifida occulta). (*8*) Region between posterior superior and posteroinferior spines. Sacroiliac ligaments (tenderness = sacroiliac sprain, often tender, with fifth lumbar or first sacral disc). (*9*) Sacrococcygeal junction (tenderness = sacrococcygeal injury; i.e., sprain or fracture). (*10*) Region of sacrosciatic notch (tenderness = fourth or fifth lumbar disc rupture and sacroiliac sprain). (*11*) Sciatic nerve trunk (tenderness = ruptured lumbar disc or sciatic nerve lesion).

Tenderness on palpation of the paraspinal muscles may signify a strain of muscle attachments or injury to the underlying transverse processes of the lumbar vertebrae. Focal pain in the same parasagittal line along the thoracic spine points to inflammation of the costotransverse articulation between spine and rib (*costotransversitis*). Other sites of tenderness and the structures implicated by disease are shown in the figure.

In palpating the spinous processes, it is important to note any deviation in the lateral plane (this may be indicative of fracture or arthritis) or in the anteroposterior plane. A "step-off" forward displacement of the spinous process and exaggerated lordosis are important clues to the presence of *spondylolisthesis* (see further on).

Many of the processes discussed above can coexist, especially in the older individual, who may have hip and lumbar spine osteoarthropathy. This makes the interpretation of various signs difficult unless the symptoms are first analyzed properly.

On completion of the examination of the back and legs, one turns to a search for motor, reflex, and sensory changes in the lower extremities (see "Herniation of Lumbar Intervertebral Discs," further on in this chapter).

Diagnostic Procedures

Depending on the circumstances, these may include a blood count, erythrocyte sedimentation rate, and C-reactive protein (especially helpful in screening for spinal osteomyelitis, epidural abscess, or myeloma). Other useful blood tests are calcium, alkaline phosphatase, and prostate-specific antigen (if one suspects metastatic carcinoma of the prostate); a serum protein immunoelectrophoresis (myeloma proteins); in special cases, a tuberculin test or serologic test for *Brucella*; a test for rheumatoid factor; and human leukocyte antigen (HLA) typing (for ankylosing spondylitis), all in the appropriate settings.

Radiographs of the lumbar spine may be useful in the routine evaluation of low back pain and sciatica and can be performed with the patient in flexed and extended positions in the anteroposterior, lateral, and oblique planes. Readily demonstrable in plain films are narrowing of the intervertebral disc spaces, bony facetal or vertebral overgrowth, displacement of vertebral bodies (spondylolisthesis), and an unsuspected infiltration of bone by cancer. However, in cases of suspected disc herniation or tumor infiltration of the spinal canal, one generally proceeds directly to MRI. Administration of gadolinium at the time of MRI enhances regions of inflammation and tumor but is not particularly helpful in cases of degenerative and disc disease of the spine. T2-weighted MRI performed with elimination of the hyperintense signal of fat ("fat suppression", i.e., the short T1 inversion recovery or "STIR" sequence), allows inflammation and edema to be visualized in the bone marrow and paravertebral soft tissues that normally contain fat. The current generation of MRI scanners has largely replaced conventional myelography for the examination of spinal disease but the latter, when combined with CT, provides detailed information about the dural sleeves that surround the spinal roots as occur with arachnoiditis, disclosing subtle truncations caused by laterally situated disc herniations and at times revealing surface abnormalities of the spinal cord, such as arteriovenous malformations. When metallic devices such as a pacemaker preclude the performance of MRI, CT myelography remains very useful for diagnosis.

Nerve conduction studies and electromyography (EMG) are particularly helpful in suspected root and nerve diseases as indicated further on in the discussion of spinal nerve root disease. However, as for all the aforementioned tests, they must be interpreted in the context of the history and clinical examination; otherwise they are subject to over interpretation.

Conditions Giving Rise to Pain in the Lower Back

Congenital Anomalies of the Lumbar Spine

Anatomic variations of the spine are frequent and, though rarely themselves the source of pain and functional derangement, they may predispose an individual to discogenic and spondylotic complications by virtue of altering the mechanics and alignment of the vertebrae or size of the spinal canal.

A common anomaly is fusion of the fifth lumbar vertebral body to the sacrum ("sacralization") or, conversely, separation of the first sacral segment, giving rise to 6, rather than the usual 5 lumbar vertebrae ("lumbarization"). However, neither of these is consistently associated with any type of back derangement. Another less-common finding is a lack of fusion of the laminae of one or several of the lumbar vertebrae or of the sacrum (spina bifida). Occasionally, a subcutaneous mass, hypertrichosis, or hyperpigmentation in the lumbar or sacral area overlying the bony separation betrays the condition, but in most patients it remains occult until it is disclosed radiologically. The anomaly may be accompanied by malformation of vertebral joints and usually induces pain only when aggravated by injury. The neurologic aspects of defective fusion of the spine (dysraphism) are discussed in Chap. 38, with developmental abnormalities of the nervous system.

Many other congenital variants affect the lower lumbar vertebrae: asymmetrical facet joints, abnormalities of the transverse processes, are seen occasionally in patients with low back symptoms, but apparently with no greater frequency than in asymptomatic individuals. *Spondylolysis* consists of a congenital and probably genetic bony defect in the pars interarticularis (the segment at the junction of pedicle and lamina) of the lower lumbar vertebrae. It is remarkably common, affecting approximately 5 percent of the North American population and mainly a disease of children (peak incidence between 5 and 7 years of age). The defect assumes importance in that it predisposes to subtle fracture of the pars articularis, sometimes precipitated by slight trauma but often in the absence of an appreciated injury. In some young individuals, it is unilateral and may cause unilateral lumbar aching back pain that is accentuated by hyperextension and twisting. In the usual bilateral form, small fractures at the pars interarticularis allow the vertebral body, pedicles, and superior articular facets to move anteriorly, leaving the posterior elements behind. This leads to an anterior displacement of one vertebral body in relation to the adjacent one, *spondylolisthesis*. Considerable dull, aching back pain can result.

The main cause of spondylolisthesis in older adults is degenerative arthritic disease of the spine as discussed further on. Patients with progressive vertebral displacement and neurologic deficits require surgery. Reduction of displaced vertebral bodies before fusion and direct repair of pars defects are possible in special cases. Back pain is relieved in the majority of cases.

Traumatic Disorders of the Low Back

These constitute by far the most frequent causes of low back pain. In severe acute injuries from direct impact the examiner must be careful to avoid further damage and movements should be kept to a minimum until an approximate diagnosis has been made. If the patient complains of pain in the back and cannot move the legs, the spine may have been fractured and the cord or cauda equina compressed or crushed. (See Chap. 44 for further discussion of spinal cord injury.) Lesser degrees of injury, such as sprains and strains, are ubiquitous and can be handled with less caution because they do not involve compression of neural structures or displacement of spinal elements.

Acute Sprains and Strains The terms *lumbosacral strain*, *sprain*, and *derangement* are used loosely, and it is probably not possible to differentiate them. Furthermore, what was formerly referred to as "sacroiliac strain" or "sprain" is now known to be caused by, in some instances, disc disease. The term *acute low back strain* may be preferable for minor, self-limiting injuries that are usually associated with lifting heavy loads when the back is in a mechanically disadvantaged position, or there may have been a fall, prolonged uncomfortable postures such as in air travel or car rides, or sudden unexpected motion, as may occur in an auto accident.

Nonetheless, the discomfort of acute low back strain can be severe, and the patient may assume unusual postures related to spasm of the lower lumbar and sacrospinalis muscles. The pain is usually confined to the lower part of the back, in the midline, across the posterior waist, or just to one side of the spine. The diagnosis of lumbosacral strain is dependent on the biomechanics of the injury or activity that precipitated the pain. The injured structures are identified by the localization of the pain, the finding of localized tenderness, augmentation of pain by postural changes—e.g., bending forward, twisting, or standing up from a sitting position, and by the absence of signs of radicular involvement. In more than 80 percent of cases of acute low back strain of this type, the pain resolves in a matter of several days or a week, even with no specific treatment.

Sacroiliac joint and ligamentous strain is the most likely diagnosis when there is tenderness over the sacroiliac joint and pain radiating to the buttock and posterior thigh, but this always needs to be distinguished from the sciatica of a herniated intervertebral disc (see further on).

Strain is characteristically worsened by abduction of the thigh against resistance and may produce pain that is also felt in the symphysis pubis or groin.

Treatment of Acute Low Back Strain The pain of muscular and ligamentous strains is usually self-limiting, responding to simple measures in a relatively short period of time. The basic principle of therapy in both disorders is to avoid reinjury and reduce the discomfort of painful parts. As a result of several studies that have failed to demonstrate a benefit of bed rest, the recent practice has been to mobilize patients as soon as they are able and to prescribe exercises designed to stretch and strengthen trunk (especially abdominal) muscles, overcome faulty posture, and increase the mobility of the spinal joints. Despite this approach, the authors can affirm from personal experience that some injuries produce such discomfort that arising from a bed or chair is simply not possible in the early days after injury (see Vroomen et al). Lying on the side with knees and hips flexed, or supine with a pillow under the knees favor relief of pain. With strains of the sacrospinalis muscles and sacroiliac ligaments, the optimal position is hyperextension, which is effected by having the patient lie with a small pillow under the lumbar portion of the spine or by lying prone. Local physical measures—such as application of ice in the acute phase and, later, heat diathermy and massage—often relieve pain temporarily. Nonsteroidal antiinflammatory drugs (NSAIDs) may be given liberally during the first few days. Muscle relaxants (e.g., cyclobenzaprine, carisoprodol, metaxalone, and the diazepams) serve mainly to make bed rest more tolerable but have little primary effect. Traction, formerly a popular treatment, is infrequently used. When weight bearing is resumed, discomfort may be diminished by a light lumbosacral support, but many orthopedists refrain from prescribing this aid.

Spinal manipulation—practiced by chiropractors, osteopaths, and others—has always been a contentious matter partly because of unrealistic therapeutic claims made in treating diseases other than low back derangements. A type of slow muscle stretching and joint distraction (axial traction on a joint) administered by physiatrists and physical therapists is quite similar. It must be recognized that many patients seek chiropractic manipulation for back complaints, often before seeing a physician, and may not disclose this information. When the supporting elements of the spine (pedicles, facets, and ligaments) are not disrupted, chiropractic manipulation of the lumbar spine has provided acute relief to a number of our patients with low back strain or facet pain. At issue is the durability of the effect, particularly the need for repeated spinal adjustments. One randomized British trial has shown manipulation to be faster than analgesics and bed rest in returning patients to work after minor back injury (Meade et al). Some trials have corroborated this finding (Hadler et al), whereas others have not, or, often, the results have been ambiguous. In the study by Cherkin and colleagues comparing chiropractic, physical therapy (McKenzie method), and simple instruction to the patient from a booklet, manipulation yielded a slightly better outcome at the end of a month. Despite several hypotheses offered by practitioners of spinal manipulation, the mechanism of pain relief is not known. The cracking sound created by rapid distraction of the facet joints (and attributed to gas coming out of solution in the joint fluid) seems not to be necessary for pain relief. It is unlikely that mundane low back pain represents minor subluxation, as claimed by chiropractors. In the authors' clinical experience, chronic low back pain, discussed below, has been less successfully treated by manipulative procedures than has acute pain, but there are some patients who testify to improvement in their clinical state and admittedly, the medical profession has little to offer in most cases of chronic low back pain. The results for acute and chronic back pain with another popular approach, acupuncture, have been even more uncertain, most studies showing it to be no more effective than a sham treatment (Tudler et al). It should be emphasized, however, that the chronic use of NSAIDs or narcotic analgesics is hazardous and is not an appealing alternative.

Chronic and Recurrent Low Back Syndrome Often the symptoms of low back strain are recurrent and more chronic in nature, being regularly exacerbated by bending or lifting, suggesting that postural, muscular, and arthritic factors play a role. This is the most common syndrome seen in spine clinics, more often in men than in women.

Insidiously, or after some unusual activity, raising the question of trauma, especially if it happens in the workplace, the patient develops aching pain in the low back, increased by certain movements and attended by stiffness. The pain may additionally have a restricted radiation into the buttocks and posterior thigh, thereby simulating root compression. There are no motor, sensory, or reflex abnormalities. Radiographs and imaging procedures usually reveal some combination of osteoarthropathy, changes in vertebral discs, osteoarthritic changes in apophysial joints, and sometimes osteoporosis or slight spondylosis, or they may be entirely normal. Treatment with short-duration bed rest, analgesics, and physiotherapy, as outlined for acute strains, helps to relieve the symptoms, and the majority of patients recover within a few weeks, only to have a recurrence of similar pains in the future. Recurrent attacks are typical of degenerative spine disease that affects the vertebrae and facet joints. Usually, the origin of the pain cannot be assigned with certainty to spinal, joint, or muscular injury, but direct percussion tenderness of one vertebral segment always raises concern of metastatic disease as noted above. Quite often, changing the firmness of the mattress (in either direction) is helpful. Compensation relating to injuries at work or to an accident and related legal matters often add to the disability, but there are, of course, many legitimate injuries that occur in these circumstances.

Vertebral Fractures Fractures of lumbar vertebral bodies are usually the result of flexion injuries. Such trauma may occur in a fall or jump from a height (if the patient lands on his feet, the calcanei may also be fractured) or as a result of an auto accident or other violent injury. If the injury is severe, it may cause a fracture dislocation, a "burst" fracture of one or more vertebral bodies, or an asymmetrical fracture of a pedicle, lamina, or spinous process; most often, however, there is asymmetrical loss of height of a vertebral body (wedge *compression fracture*), which may be extremely painful at the onset. When compression or other fractures occur with minimal trauma (or spontaneously), the bone has presumably been weakened by some pathologic process. Most of the time, particularly in older individuals, osteoporosis is the cause of such an event, but there are many other causes, including osteomalacia, hyperparathyroidism, prolonged use of corticosteroids, myeloma, metastatic carcinoma, and a number of other conditions that are destructive of bone. Spasm of the lower lumbar muscles, limitation of all movements of the lumbar section of the spine, and the radiographic appearance of the damaged lumbar portion (with or without neurologic abnormalities) are the basis of clinical diagnosis. The pain is usually immediate, although occasionally it may be delayed for days.

A fractured transverse process, which is almost always associated with high-impact rotary injury of the spine and causes tearing of the paravertebral muscles and a local hematoma, produces deep tenderness at the site of the injury and limitation of all movements that stretch the lumbar muscles. The imaging findings, particularly MRI, confirm the diagnosis. In some circumstances, tears of the paravertebral musculature may be associated with extensive bleeding into the retroperitoneal space; this produces paraspinal or groin pain and proximal leg weakness with loss of the patellar reflex on the affected side. There may be a delayed subcutaneous hematoma in the flanks (Grey-Turner sign).

A problem not easily classified but having a distinctive clinical profile that should be known to neurologists is that of an osteoid osteoma. These benign tumors characteristically cause severe nocturnal pain located in one region of the parasagittal spine that awakens the patient from a peaceful sleep; also typical is complete relief after aspirin or small doses of other NSAIDs. MRI or CT is required to detect the lesion, as it may not be evident on plain radiographs of the spine. The typical appearance is a well-demarcated lytic lesion surrounded by a rim of bony sclerosis.

TREATMENT OF VERTEBRAL COMPRESSION FRACTURE For the mundane thoracic and lumbar fracture associated with osteoporosis, bed rest, and analgesics are usually adequate. In the past two decades several mechanical approaches to reducing pain have been investigated. The injection of various materials directly into the fracture site within the vertebral body (vertebroplasty) attained popularity because of reports of marked pain relief. Several large trials have addressed the use of vertebroplasty and given conflicting results. The best conducted of these, with a placebo control groups (see Buchbinder et al and Kallmes et al) concluded that there was no durable benefit, however, these two studies included patients with fractures up to a year old. Having witnessed a few patients with almost immediate and remarkable relief of severe pain, we are uncertain of the best course but acknowledge that this is probably not an effective treatment for the majority of patients. Further discussion can be found in the review by Ensrud and Schousboe.

Herniation of Lumbar Intervertebral Discs
(Table 11-1)

This condition is a major cause of severe and chronic or recurrent low back and leg pain. It occurs mainly during the third and fourth decades of life when the nucleus pulposus is still gelatinous. The disc between the fifth lumbar or first sacral vertebrae (L5-S1) is most often involved, and, with decreasing frequency, that between the fourth and fifth (L4-L5), third and fourth (L3-L4), second and third (L2-L3), and—quite infrequently—the first and second (L1-L2) lumbar vertebrae. Relatively rare but well described in the thoracic portion of the spine, disc disease is again frequent in the cervical spine at the fifth and sixth and the sixth and seventh cervical vertebrae (see further on).

The cause of a herniated lumbar disc in any individual case is often not identifiable and flexion injury is often imputed, but a considerable proportion of patients do not recall an inciting episode. Degeneration of the annulus and the posterior longitudinal ligaments, and changes nuclei pulposis itself may have taken place silently or have been manifest by mild, recurrent lumbar ache. A sneeze, lurch, or other trivial movement may then cause the nucleus pulposus to prolapse, pushing the frayed and weakened annulus posteriorly. Fragments of the nucleus pulposus protrude through rents in the annulus, usually to one side or the other (sometimes in the midline), where they impinge on one or more nerve roots and cause the characteristic sciatic or other radicular pains and neurologic signs. In more severe cases of disc disease, a small piece of the nucleus may be entirely extruded as a "free fragment", sometimes called a sequestered disc fragment, and be mobile enough to affect a root at an adjacent level or to give rise to unusual precipitating features of radicular pain. Large protrusions cause pain by compressing the adjacent root against the articular apophysis or lamina. The protruded material may become reduced in size over time, presumably from desiccation, but often there is continued chronic irritation of the root or a discarthrosis with posterior osteophyte formation.

The Clinical Syndrome of Lumbar Disc Herniation The fully developed syndrome of the common prolapsed intervertebral lower lumbar disc consists of (1) pain in the sacroiliac region, radiating into the buttock, thigh, and the calf, a symptom broadly termed *sciatica*; (2) a stiff or unnatural spinal posture; and often (3) some combination of paresthesia, weakness, and reflex impairment.

The pain of herniated intervertebral disc varies in severity from a mild aching discomfort to severe knifelike stabs that radiate the length of the leg and are superimposed on a constant intense ache. Sciatic pain is usually perceived by the patient as originating deep in the buttock and radiating to the posterolateral thigh; it may progress to the calf and ankle—to the medial malleolus (L4), lateral malleolus (L5), or heel (S1); however, distal radiation to the foot is less frequent. There are variations in the sciatic syndrome. Abortive forms may produce aching discomfort

Table 11-1

FEATURES OF THE MAIN ROOT-COMPRESSIVE SYNDROMES DUE TO CERVICAL AND LUMBAR DISC HERNIATION*

INTERVERTEBRAL DISC SPACE	ROOT AFFECTED	PAIN REFERRAL	WEAKNESS	REFLEX CHANGE	ADDITIONAL FEATURES
C4-C5	C5	Shoulder, trapezius	Supra- and infraspinatus deltoid, slight biceps weakness	Slightly diminished biceps jerk	
C5-C6	C6	Trapezius ridge and tip of shoulder, radiation to anterior upper arm, thumb, and index finger	Biceps, brachioradialis, extensor carpi radialis	Diminished biceps and supinator jerk	Tenderness over spine or scapula and suprascapular region; paresthesias in thumb and index finger
C6-C7	C7	Shoulder, axilla, posterolateral arm, elbow, and middle finger	Triceps, wrist extensors	Diminished or absent triceps jerk	Tenderness over medial scapula and supraclavicular region or triceps. May complain of paresthesias in most of the fingers
C7-T1	C8	Medial forearm	Intrinsic hand muscles	Slight or no decrease in triceps jerk	Mimics ulnar palsy
L2-L3	L3	Anterior thigh, over knee	Thigh adductor, quadriceps	Absent or diminished knee jerk	
L3-L4	L4	Anterolateral thigh, medial foreleg	Anterior tibial, sometimes with partial foot drop	Diminished or normal knee jerk	
L4-L5	L5	Posterolateral gluteal sciatica; lateral thigh, anterolateral foreleg, dorsal foot, lateral malleolus and great or second and third toe	Extensor hallucis longus and extensor digitorum brevis; some weakness of anterior tibialis, sometimes with foot drop	Unaffected (except posterior tibial)	Pain with straight-leg raising and variant tests; tenderness over fourth lumbar lateral process and lateral gluteal region
L5-S1	S1	Midgluteal sciatica; posterior thigh, posterolateral leg, lateral foot, heel, or lateral toes	Plantar-flexor and hamstring weakness	Absent or diminished ankle jerk	Pain with straight-leg raising and variant tests; tenderness over lumbosacral (L5-S1) joint and sciatic notch; discomfort walking on heels

*For pattern of sensory loss, see dermatomal diagram in Figs. 9-3 and 9-4.

only in the lower buttock or proximal thigh and occasionally only in the lower hamstring or upper calf. With the most severe pain, the patient is forced to stay in bed, avoiding the slightest movement; a cough, sneeze, or strain is intolerable. The most comfortable position may be lying on the back with legs flexed at the knees and hips and the shoulders raised on pillows to obliterate the lumbar lordosis. For some patients, a lateral decubitus position is more comfortable. Free fragments of disc that find their way to a lateral and posterior position in the spinal canal may produce the opposite situation, one whereby the patient is unable to extend the spine and lie supine. Sitting and standing up from a sitting position may be particularly painful. It is surprising to patients that a lumbar disc protrusion may cause little or no back pain. If there is back discomfort, it tends to be just paraspinal on the side of sciatica and mainly in the acute stages.

In cases of root compression, pain is also characteristically provoked by pressure along the course of the sciatic nerve at the classic points of Valleix (sciatic notch, retrotrochanteric gutter, posterior surface of thigh, and head of fibula). Pressure at one point may cause radiation of pain and tingling down the leg. Elongation of the nerve root by straight-leg raising or by flexing the leg at the hip and extending it at the knee (Lasègue maneuver as discussed earlier) is the most consistent of all pain-provoking signs. During straight-leg raising, the patient can distinguish between the discomfort of ordinary tautness of the hamstring and the sharper, less-familiar root pain, particularly when asked to compare the experience with that on the normal side. Many variations of the Lasègue maneuver have been described (with numerous eponyms), the most useful of which is accentuation of the pain by dorsiflexion of the foot (Bragard sign) or of the great toe (Sicard sign). The Lasègue maneuver with the healthy leg may evoke sciatic pain on the contralateral side), but usually of lesser degree (Fajersztajn sign). However, this "crossed straight-leg-raising sign" is highly indicative of a ruptured disc as the cause of sciatica (56 of 58 cases in the series of Hudgkins). With the patient standing, forward bending of the trunk may induce reflexive flexion of the knee on the affected side

(Neri sign). Sciatica may be provoked by forced flexion of the head and neck, coughing, or pressure on both jugular veins, all of which increase intraspinal pressure (Naffziger sign). Marked inconsistencies in response to these tests raise the suspicion of psychologic factors or of referred muscular pain.

An antalgic posture, referred to as *sciatic scoliosis,* is maintained by reflex contraction of the paraspinal muscles, which can be both seen and palpated. In walking, the knee is slightly flexed, and weight bearing on the painful leg is brief and cautious on the ball of the foot, giving a limp. It is particularly painful for the patient to go up and down stairs.

The signs of more severe spinal root compression are impairment of sensation, loss or diminution of tendon reflexes, and muscle weakness, as summarized in Table 11-1.

Generally, disc herniation compresses the root on one side, at the level just below the herniation (see below). Hypotonia may be evident on inspection and palpation of the buttock and calf. In a few patients, foot drop (L5 root) or weakness of plantar flexion (S1 root) is a main feature of disc protrusion, and some of these patients have little associated pain. The reflex changes noted below have little relationship to the severity of the pain or sensory loss. Furthermore, compression of the fourth, or sometimes fifth, lumbar root may occur without any change in the tendon reflexes. Bilaterality of symptoms and signs is rare, as is sphincteric paralysis, but they occur with large central protrusions that compress the cauda equina. The cerebrospinal fluid (CSF) protein is often elevated with disc rupture, more predictably with central rupture and then, usually in the range of 55 to 85 mg/dL, sometimes higher.

As emphasized earlier, herniations of the intervertebral lumbar discs occur most often between the fifth lumbar and first sacral vertebrae (compressing the traversing S1 or exiting L5 root; Fig. 11-3) and between the fourth and fifth lumbar vertebrae (compressing the traversing L5 or exiting L4 root).

Lesions of the fifth lumbar root (L5) produce pain in the region of the hip and posterolateral thigh (i.e., sciatica) and, in more than half such cases, lateral calf (to the lateral malleolus), and less often, the dorsal surface of the foot and the first or second and third toes. Pain is elicited by the straight-leg raising test or one of its variants, and protective nocifensive reflexes come into play, limiting further elevation of the leg. Paresthesia may be felt in the entire territory or only in its distal parts. The tenderness is in the lateral gluteal region and near the head of the femur. Weakness, if present, involves the extensors of the big toe and foot and the foot invertors (a distinguishing feature of foot drop originating in peroneal nerve damage). The ankle jerk may be diminished (more often it is normal), but the knee jerk is hardly ever altered.

With *lesions of the first sacral root (S1),* the pain is felt in the midgluteal region, mid-posterior part of the thigh, posterior region of the calf to the heel, outer plantar surface of the foot, and fourth and fifth toes. Tenderness is most pronounced over the midgluteal region. Paresthesia and sensory loss are mainly in the lower part of the leg and outer toes, and weakness, if present, involves the plantar flexor muscles of the foot and toes, abductors of the toes, and hamstring muscles. The Achilles reflex is diminished or absent in the majority of cases. In fact, loss of the Achilles reflex may be the only objective sign. Walking on the toes is more difficult and uncomfortable than walking on the heels because of weakness of the plantar flexors.

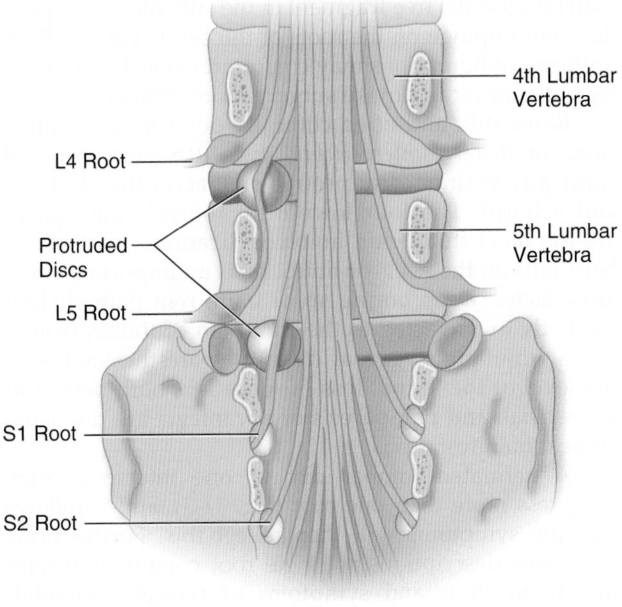

Figure 11-3. Mechanisms of compression of the fifth lumbar and first sacral roots by herniated lumbosacral discs. A lateral disc protrusion at the L4-L5 level usually involves the fifth lumbar root and spares the fourth; a protrusion at L5-S1 involves the first sacral root and spares the fifth lumbar root. Note that a more medially placed disc protrusion at the L4-L5 level (cross-hatched) may involve the fifth lumbar root as well as the first (or second and third) sacral root.

The less-frequent lesions of the *third (L3) and fourth (L4) lumbar roots* give rise to pain in the anterior part of the thigh and knee and anteromedial part of the leg (fourth lumbar), with corresponding sensory impairment in these dermatomal distributions. The knee jerk is diminished or abolished with compression of either root. Third lumbar (L3) motor root lesions may weaken the quadriceps, thigh adductor, and iliopsoas; L4 root lesions weaken the anterior tibial innervated muscles, sometimes with a mild foot drop. First lumbar (L1) root pain is projected to the groin, and L2, to the lateral hip.

Some patients have a distinctive syndrome associated with extreme lateral disc protrusions, particularly those situated within the proximal portion of the intervertebral spinal foramina. Unremitting radicular pain without back pain and a tendency to worsen with extension of the back and torsion toward the side of the herniation are characteristic. Also, in rare instances of lumbar *intradural* disc rupture, there may not be sciatic pain because the free fragment in the subarachnoid space does not impinge on the roots of the cauda equina. Both of these configurations may confound clinical and radiologic diagnosis and make surgery more difficult.

Rarer still, and often clinically obscure, are protrusions of *thoracic intervertebral discs* (0.5 percent of all surgically verified disc protrusions, according to Love and Schorn). The four lowermost thoracic interspaces are the most frequently involved. Trauma, particularly hard falls on the heels or buttocks, is an important causative factor. Deep boring spine pain; root pain circling the body or projected to the abdomen or thorax (sometimes simulating visceral disease); paresthesias below the level of the lesion; loss of sensation; both deep and superficial; and paraparesis or paraplegia are the usual clinical manifestations.

A herniated lumbar disc at one interspace may compress more than one root (Fig. 11-3), and it follows that the symptoms will then reflect this. Furthermore, the above descriptions of single root compression refer mainly to signs and symptoms of typical posterolateral disc protrusion. Very large *central disc protrusions* may compress the entire cauda equina with a dramatic syndrome that includes intense low back and bilateral sciatic pain, incomplete paraparesis, loss of both ankle jerks, and, most characteristic, varying degrees of urinary retention and incontinence. This circumstance demands surgical attention.

Anomalies of the lumbosacral roots may lead to errors in localization (see descriptions by Postacchini et al). The combined rupture of two or more discs occurs occasionally and complicates the clinical picture. When both the L5 and S1 roots are compressed by a large herniated disc, the signs of the S1 lesion usually predominate.

Herniation may occur directly into the adjacent vertebral body, giving rise to a Schmorl nodule. In such cases there are no signs of nerve root involvement although back pain may be present, sometimes recurrent and referred to the thigh. Most often, these well-circumscribed rounded radiographic densities adjacent to the endplate of the vertebral body are found incidentally on CT or MRI.

Diagnosis When all components of the lumbar disc syndrome are present, the diagnosis can be made with reasonable confidence. With persistent symptoms, many neurologists prefer to corroborate their clinical impression with MRI of the lumbar spine (Fig. 11-4). In the absence of neurological deficits, imaging generally need not be undertaken until the pain has persisted for several weeks (see Chou and colleagues). This, of course, may not be necessary if the pain is manageable and surgery is not contemplated (see further on). MRI is favored over CT because of the advantages of the distinction that can be made between disc material, annulus, nerves and bones and the clarity of their anatomic relationships. MRI also excludes disc herniations at other sites or an unsuspected tumor. As indicated earlier, in cases in which MRI is not

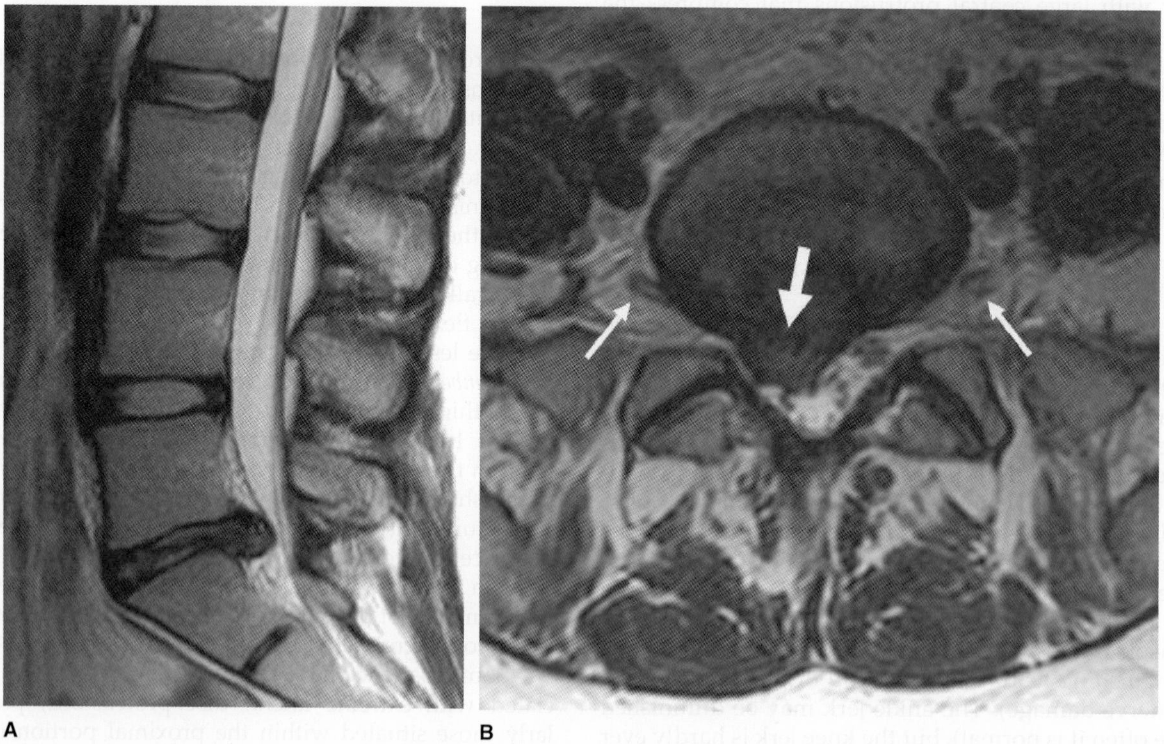

Figure 11-4. Lumbar disc herniation as shown by T2-weighted MRI. ***A.*** Sagittal view of a large herniated nucleus pulposus at L5-S1. The posteriorly protruding disc material indents and elevates the anterior thecal sac and narrows the spinal canal. The extruded material has the same signal characteristics of the parent disc. The disc space at this level is narrowed and the disc is less hyperintense than normal because of desiccation and the extruded component. ***B.*** Axial view showing the focal right paracentral posterior disc herniation (large arrow) protruding into the canal and compressing the traversing nerve root (the right S1 nerve root) at this level. The exiting L5 roots above are not affected and can be seen laterally to the disc (small arrows).

possible or it has been unrevealing, we often turn to CT or CT with myelography for a refined definition of the root sleeves and use the EMG to corroborate subtle findings.

The needle EMG study is abnormal, showing fibrillation potentials in denervated muscles after 1 or 2 weeks, but it may remain normal in 10 percent of cases according to Leyshon and colleagues. Loss or marked asymmetry of the H reflex is another useful indication of S1 radiculopathy, but this simply corroborates the loss of an Achilles reflex. The finding of denervation potentials in the paraspinal muscles (indicating root rather than peripheral nerve lesions) and in muscles that conform to a root distribution is also helpful, but again, some weeks must have elapsed from the onset of root pain for these findings to be present. We emphasize that, while useful information is to be gained from EMG, it is required in only a limited proportion of cases and often provides mainly corroborating data. It is more helpful when the diagnosis is uncertain. An entirely normal study should lead to reconsideration of the diagnosis, particularly if surgery was planned for relief of a compressive radiculopathy.

Many disc abnormalities observed on MRI and loosely referred to as "herniation" are incidental findings, unrelated to the patient's symptoms, or are simply bulges of the annulus. Jensen and colleagues, in an MRI study of the lumbar spine in 98 asymptomatic adults, found that in more than half, there was a symmetrical extension of a disc (or discs) beyond the margins of the interspace (*bulging*). In 27 percent, there was a focal or asymmetrical extension of the disc beyond the margin of the interspace (*protrusion*), and in only 1 percent was there more extreme extension of the disc (*extrusion or sequestration*). These findings emphasize the importance of using precise terms in describing the imaging abnormalities and evaluating them strictly in the context of the patient's symptoms.

Treatment of Ruptured Lumbar Disc

In the treatment of an *acute or chronic rupture of a lumbar disc*, many patients have found it nearly impossible to participate in physical activities and to assume certain positions that cause pain. However, the time-honored tenet of prolonged bed rest has been questioned by the results of several randomized studies (Vroomen et al). It would appear that the main benefit is simply that time has passed and the expected resolution of pain has taken its course in many patients. Traction is probably of little value. Analgesic medications, either NSAIDs or opioids, may be required for a few days. In a few patients with severe sciatica we have been impressed with the temporary relief afforded by administration of oral dexamethasone (4 mg every 8 h) for several days, although this approach has not been studied systematically and several of our colleagues decry it. The treatment of nerve root compression with repeated epidural injections of corticosteroids has enjoyed periods of popularity, but controlled studies have failed to confirm sustained efficacy (White et al; Cuckler et al), and it is not without complications including the rare but widely publicized outbreak of fungal meningitis from contaminated steroids. As with many similar studies, Carette and colleagues (1997) found only short-term improvement with epidural steroid injection and the ultimate need for surgery was not altered. Nevertheless, some pain specialists have not discarded this form of treatment in view of success in selected patients, even if short-lived.

Surgical Treatment of Lumbar Disc Disease An indication for emergency surgery is an acute compression of the cauda equina by massive disc extrusion, causing bilateral sensorimotor loss and sphincteric paralysis. Although not the recommended course, it should be pointed out that there have been instances in which even a dramatic syndrome of cauda equina compression had resolved spontaneously after several weeks.

If the pain and neurologic findings have not subsided in response to conservative management or the patient has suffered frequent disabling acute episodes, surgical treatment must be considered. Useful information regarding surgery and its timing can be ascertained from a randomized trial conducted by Peul and colleagues and from the Spine Patients Outcomes Research Trial (SPORT) conducted by Weinstein and coworkers (2006). In the first study, a large proportion of patients assigned to treatment with physical therapy and pain medications had enough pain that they required surgery within several months. In addition, patients assigned initially to surgery by microdiscectomy had considerably faster relief of back and sciatic pain, but at the end of a year, both groups had minimal disability and similar degrees of minor pain. The implications of this study are that avoiding surgery initially does not have adverse consequences but if more rapid pain relief and mobilization are the aims, surgery is preferable. In the second cited study there was even greater crossover between conservative and surgically assigned groups and there was a slightly more favorable outcome in those who underwent early surgery.

The surgical procedure most often indicated for lumbar disc disease is one of the variants of a hemilaminectomy with excision of the disc fragment introduced almost a century ago by Mixter and Barr. Questions relating to the relative merits of limited ("microscopic"), or minimally invasive excision of the lamina are often raised by patients and no clear answer can be given except that individual surgeons excel at one or another technique and the outcomes are similar. Eighty-five to 90 percent of cases with sciatic pain because of L4-L5 or L5-S1 disc ruptures are relieved by operation, are home in days or less, and are resuming activities within weeks. Rerupture occurs in approximately 5 percent of operated cases according to Shannon and Paul. Spinal fusion of the involved segments is indicated in cases in which there is instability, usually related to extensive or prior surgery or to an anatomic abnormality.

The features that are predictive of better outcome from decompressive surgery are a clearly delineated radicular leg pain, in contrast to general back pain alone, younger age, an identifiable precipitating event for the back and sciatic pain, clinical features that are restricted to compression of a single nerve root, and the absence of chronic or frequently recurrent back pain. Curiously, Barzouhi and colleagues found that the presence or absence of disc herniation in the MRI a year after operation had little relationship to the persistence of sciatica.

Other Causes of Sciatica and Low Back Pain

An increasing experience with lumbar back pain and sciatica has impressed the authors with the large number of such cases that have no clear cause. At one time, all these cases were classified as sciatic neuritis or "sacroiliac strain." After Mixter and Barr popularized the concept of herniated disc, all sciatica and lumbar pains were ascribed to this condition. Operations became somewhat indiscriminately practiced, not only for frank disc protrusion but also for "hard discs" (unruptured) and related pathologies of the spine. In large referral centers, the surgical results became decreasingly satisfactory until recently, as many patients were being seen with unrelieved postlaminectomy pain as with unoperated ruptured discs. This is no longer the case as selection of patients has been refined.

Other cases of chronic sciatic pain are due to one of a number of pathologic entities. Entrapment of lumbar roots may be the consequence not only of disc rupture but also of spondylotic spurs with *stenosis of the lateral recess*, cysts of the synovium derived from degenerative disease of the facet joint, hypertrophy of facets, and, rarely, arachnoiditis. Lateral recess stenosis in particular may be a cause of sciatica not relieved by conventional disc surgery (see below, under "Lumbar Stenosis"). Synovial cysts arising from a facet joint are not uncommon, and even very small ones may be situated in the proximal portion of the foramen, thereby causing sciatica. If pain is intractable, surgical removal of the cyst is indicated. Another surprising finding in the course of imaging the spinal canal is a cyst-like dilatation of the perineurial sheath (Tarlov cysts). One or more sacral roots may be involved at points where they penetrate the dura and may be associated with radicular symptoms. There are reports of relief from opening the cysts and freeing the roots, but the results seem more uncertain to us. Sciatica that is temporally linked to the premenstrual period is usually a result of endometriosis involving the nerve at the sciatic notch ("catamenial sciatica"). We have also observed cases of sciatica that occurred with each pregnancy, presumably from uterine traction on the nerve.

The notion of a pyriformis (piriformis) syndrome, so named by Kopell and Thompson, has arisen as a cause of otherwise unexplained buttock pain or vague sciatica. The muscle overlies or, in a small proportion, embeds the peroneal trunk of the sciatic nerve. Hypertrophy, spasm, or simply the anatomic variation in which the nerve is entrapped in the tendinous origin of the muscle have all putatively caused local and some degree of sciatic pain. Sciatica in these cases is elicited by stretching the muscle through flexion, adduction, and internal rotation of the hip. The validity of this syndrome is uncertain and it has been the subject of polemical discussions in the literature. EMG data are ambiguous but reportedly show distal denervation, sparing more proximally innervated muscles. Our practice would be to avoid surgery in such cases, but to endorse physical therapy.

Compression of the cauda equina by epidural masses, as described further on, most often begins with back pain or sciatica. The sciatic nerve or the plexus from which it originates may be directly implicated in tumor (lymphoma, neurofibrosarcoma).

Several *inflammatory diseases of the cauda equina* produce back pain and *bilateral sciatica* and may be mistaken for the more usual types of cauda equina compression; cytomegalovirus infection in AIDS patients, Lyme disease (Bannwarth syndrome), herpetic infection (Elsberg syndrome), and neoplastic meningitis at times behave in this fashion. In all of these, the CSF shows a pleocytosis. The Guillain-Barré syndrome may also produce misleading back and radicular pain before weakness is apparent. The caudal roots in these diseases usually enhance with gadolinium on MRI.

An unusual *lumbosacral plexus neuritis (Wartenberg plexitis)* is a unilateral (occasionally bilateral) disorder akin to brachial neuritis, which may cause sciatica, as does occasionally nerve infarction or damage from diabetes, herpes zoster, parvovirus, or a retroperitoneal mass (see Chap. 46).

Again, if one sees enough of these cases, the cause of a number of them, particularly those with bilateral burning along the sciatic nerve, cannot be determined.

Lumbar Spinal Canal Stenosis ("Lumbar Stenosis" and Neurogenic Claudication)

The term spondylosis is often applied to a general constellation of bone, joint and ligamentous changes that narrow the spinal canal and neural foramina. In the lumbar region, these osteoarthritic and related degenerative changes lead to compression of one or more lumbar and sacral roots because of narrowing of the spinal canal. The problem is more likely to occur if there is a congenitally narrow canal. The roots are typically compressed between the posterior surface of the vertebral body anteriorly, the facet joint laterally, and the ligamentum flavum posteriorly. Lateral recess stenosis and foraminal stenosis are common effects of spondylosis (as mentioned above in relation to disc disease) and either or both may be the main cause of individual root compression.

The usual features of lumbar stenosis are of fluctuating aching and sharp pain in the low back, buttock and sciatic distribution, occasionally including femoral areas, and generally elicited by prolonged sitting, standing, or walking and relieved by rest. Some patients have virtually constant pain in these areas but still have relief with rest in one or another body position.

In the distinctive syndrome of "neurogenic claudication", standing or walking causes a gradual onset of numbness and weakness of the legs, usually with asymmetrical sciatic, calf, or buttock discomfort that forces the patient to sit down. When the condition is more severe, the patient gains relief by squatting or lying with the legs flexed at the hips and knees, or in a forward leaning position with the hips and knees slightly flexed, as if in a bicyclists position. Often the numbness begins in one leg, spreads to the other, and ascends as standing or walking continues. The ankle tendon reflexes may disappear after walking a distance, only to return on flexing the spine. Pain in the low back and glutei is variable. Disturbances of micturition and impotence are infrequent unless there has been an additional more acute disc herniation. In some patients with lumbar stenosis, neurologic symptoms persist without relation to body position. The process is distinguished from vascular claudication of the legs by its appearance in the standing position, the prominence of numbness in some cases, and, of course, by the preservation of distal leg pulses and loss of ankle reflexes in the neurogenic variety.

This "claudication of the cauda equina" was described by van Gelderen in 1948, and it was shown by Verbiest to not be caused by ischemia but by encroachment on the cauda by hypertrophied joints, thickened ligaments, and protrusions of disc material on a developmentally shallow canal. A subluxation may contribute to the stenosis in the anteroposterior dimension. Later, the canal is also narrowed from side to side (reduced interpedicular distance).

A prominent feature of many cases of the degenerative spinal disorder is displacement and malalignment of one vertebral body in relation to the adjacent one, or spondylolisthesis. This may cause little difficulty at first but eventually the patient complains of limitation of motion and pain in the low back radiating into the thighs. In the extreme case, examination discloses tenderness near the segment that has "slipped" anteriorly (most often L5, occasionally L4 in middle-aged women) or a palpable "step" of the spinous process forward and shortening of the trunk with protrusion of the lower abdomen (anterior shift of L5 on S1, *spondyloptosis*). Compression of the corresponding spinal roots by the displaced vertebrae causes paresthesia and sensory loss, muscle weakness, and diminished reflexes. These neurologic features, however, tend not to be severe. When *spondylolisthesis* is unstable, new symptoms may appear abruptly in the form of a foot drop, urinary retention, or overflow incontinence. The spinal instability is evidenced on conventional radiographs by a change in the diameter of the spinal canal as the patient moves between the flexed and extended position of the back.

A striking syndrome that has been attached to lumbar stenosis consists of *painful legs–moving toes*, described by Spillane. There is burning leg pain and continuous and complex rhythmic movements of the toes, as the name implies. Symptoms may begin on one side but become bilateral. Lumbar nerve root compression, most often from lumbar stenosis, or other types of peripheral damage underlie most cases.

Treatment of Lumbar Stenosis Decompression of the spinal canal relieves the symptoms of lumbar stenosis in a considerable proportion of cases, but the results have been inconsistent. Patients must be chosen carefully for surgery, and success is likely if the clinical features conform to the typical syndrome, mainly pain that altered in various positions and at least partially relieved by rest, with definite evidence of root compression by imaging. In perhaps the most careful, controlled trial comparing surgery to conservative treatment for lumbar spinal stenosis, pain and overall function at 2 years was several-fold better in those who had operations (Weinstein et al, 2008). However, interpretation was hampered by a large number of patients who crossed over between arms of the study. Issues pertaining to the methodology of operation, the need for fusion of the lumbar spine to limit mobility, and various forms of "instrumentation" are of great interest, but are best discussed in textbooks of neurosurgery and orthopedics.

Insofar as lumbar stenosis is a cauda equina syndrome, its differential diagnosis is also considered in Chap. 44.

Atherosclerosis of the Distal Aorta (Vascular Claudication)

Atherosclerosis of large and medium-sized arteries often leads to symptoms that are induced by exercise (intermittent claudication) but may also occur at rest (ischemic rest pain) as already mentioned. The diabetic patient is especially susceptible. The muscle pain that is brought on by exercise and promptly relieved by rest most frequently involves the calf and thigh muscles. If the atherosclerotic narrowing or occlusion implicates the aorta and iliac arteries, it may also cause hip and buttock claudication and impotence in the male (Leriche syndrome). Ischemic rest pain—and sometimes attendant ulceration and gangrene—is usually localized to the foot and toes; it is the consequence of multiple sites of vascular occlusion. Pain at rest is characteristically worse at night and totally or partially relieved by dependency.

The examination of such patients will reveal a loss of one or more peripheral pulses, trophic changes in the skin and nails (in advanced cases), and the presence of bruits over or distal to sites of narrowing. The ankle reflexes are often diminished. The similarities to a claudicatory syndrome of lumbar spine stenosis have already been discussed.

Degenerative Osteoarthritis, or Osteoarthropathy

Independent of stenosis of the lumbar canal is chronic and recurring back pain caused by degenerative arthritic disease. It occurs in later life and may involve all or any part of the spine but is most prevalent in the cervical and lumbar regions. The pain is described as a stiffness that is centered in the affected part of the spine. It is increased initially by movement and is associated with limitation of motion but is often worse on arising in the morning. In contrast to the spinal claudicatory syndrome, warming up and progressive mobilization make the pain better. There is a notable absence of systemic symptoms such as fatigue, malaise, or fever, and, more importantly, *there are limited or no features of radicular compression*. Some patients complain of vague and intermittent pains in the upper or posterior legs, but sciatica is not a component and the straight-leg raising tests do not elicit pain. The sitting position is usually comfortable, although stiffness and discomfort are accentuated when the erect posture is resumed.

The severity of the symptoms often bears little relation to the radiologic changes; pain may be present despite minimal radiographic findings; conversely, marked osteophytic overgrowth with spur formation, ridging, bridging of vertebrae, narrowing of disc spaces, subluxation of posterior joints on flexion, and air in the disc spaces can be seen in both symptomatic and asymptomatic persons.

Facet Syndrome

This syndrome has been somewhat clarified in recent years, but its definition and nature remain imprecise. In the typical instance, osteoarthritic degeneration of the facet joint gives rise to a focal parasagittal lumbar back pain, with tenderness over the joint (Fig. 11-2, location 3) but without signs of root compression. The pain can be severe, worse at night, and prevent sleep if no comfortable position can be found. Nonsteroidal drugs are helpful. The diagnosis is confirmed when the pain is relieved for a variable period by injection of the joint with local anesthetic.

Often one is uncertain whether it was the analgesic effect on the joint or the infiltration of the region around the nerve root that relieved the pain. Two controlled studies have provided evidence of the inefficacy, both in the short and long term, of corticosteroid injections into the facet joints (Carette et al, 1991; Lilius et al). Notwithstanding these reports, we have found the injection of analgesics and steroids in and around the facet to be a useful temporizing measure in some patients. Some patients have discovered that they may obtain temporary relief from facet pain by forcefully twisting or stretching the back and creating an audible pop at the affected joint, comparable to chiropractic manipulation. Over time, they acquire a laxity of the supporting structures of the joint, which may actually perpetuate the problem.

If the diagnosis is established by local injection, pain centers offer radiofrequency ablation of the small recurrent sensory nerves that innervate the joint as a means of permanent relief. This has met with some success but has not been studied systematically.

Some writers have used the term facet syndrome to describe a painful state from facetal hypertrophy that gives rise to a lumbar monoradiculopathy indistinguishable from that caused by a ruptured disc or spondylosis. Reynolds and coworkers have documented such cases. At operation, the spinal root is compressed against the floor of the intervertebral canal by overgrowth of an inferior or superior facet. Foraminotomy and facetectomy, after exploration of the root from the dural sac to the pedicle, have relieved the pain in many operated cases.

Lumbar Adhesive Arachnoiditis

This is a somewhat vague entity in which the arachnoid membrane is thickened and opaque in the vicinity of the cauda equina. The term is also applied to thickening of the arachnoidal sheaths around roots (normal roots have essentially no epineurium). According to one review, lumbar arachnoiditis is rare, having been seen in only 80 of 7,600 myelograms, and it should virtually vanish as the use of MRI and water-soluble dyes for myelography take precedence. The usual clinical features are intractable low-back and leg pain and paresthesia, all positionally sensitive, in combination with neurologic abnormalities referable to lumbar spinal roots. In our few patients, multiple previous myelograms with lipid contrast agent (a problem of the past), disc rupture, operative procedures, infections, and subarachnoid bleeding have been causal. Some cases have followed spinal anesthesia and even epidural anesthesia by a period of months or years. The presumption is that the dura had been breached, and often, there were clinical signs of aseptic meningitis soon after the procedure. In the absence of such an acute reaction, the later diagnosis of arachnoiditis rests on less-certain grounds.

The MRI shows eccentrically thickened meninges in the spinal canal with arachnoid adhesions and collections of CSF that displace nerve roots (Fig. 11-5). Abnormalities are even more striking on CT myelographic studies in which the contrast is broken up and fails to outline the roots. Treatment is unsatisfactory. Lysis of adhesions under an operating microscope and administration of intrathecal steroids have been of limited value, although some experienced surgeons claim otherwise. Epidural injection of steroids is occasionally helpful according to some of our orthopedic surgeon colleagues.

Ankylosing Spondylitis

This disorder, referred to in the past as *rheumatoid spondylitis* and as *von Bechterew* or *Marie-Strümpell arthritis*, affects young adult males predominantly. Approximately 95 percent of patients with ankylosing spondylitis are marked by the histocompatibility antigen HLA-B27 (which is present in only 7 percent of nonaffected persons of European extraction). Pain, usually centered in the low back, is the main early complaint. Often it radiates to the back of the thighs and groin. At first, the symptoms are vague (tired back, "catches" up and down the back, sore back), and the diagnosis may be overlooked for many years. Although the pain is recurrent, limitation of movement is constant and progressive and comes to dominate the clinical picture. Early in the course of disease there is only "morning stiffness" or an increase in stiffness after periods of inactivity similar to lumbar osteoarthritis but unusual for the affected age group. In advanced stages, a cauda equina compression syndrome may complicate ankylosing spondylitis, the result apparently of an inflammatory reaction and proliferation of connective tissue (Matthews). Limitation of chest expansion, tenderness over the sternum, decreased motion and tendency to progressive flexion of the hips, and the characteristic immobility and flexion deformity of the spine ("poker spine") may be present early in the course of the disease.

The radiologic hallmarks are destruction and subsequent obliteration of the sacroiliac joints, followed by bony bridging of the vertebral bodies to produce the characteristic "bamboo spine." When this change becomes apparent, the pain usually subsides, but the patient by then has little motion of the back and neck. An unusual additional feature, almost unique to this condition but not present in all cases, is an extreme dilatation of the lumbar thecal sac. Ankylosing spondylitis may also

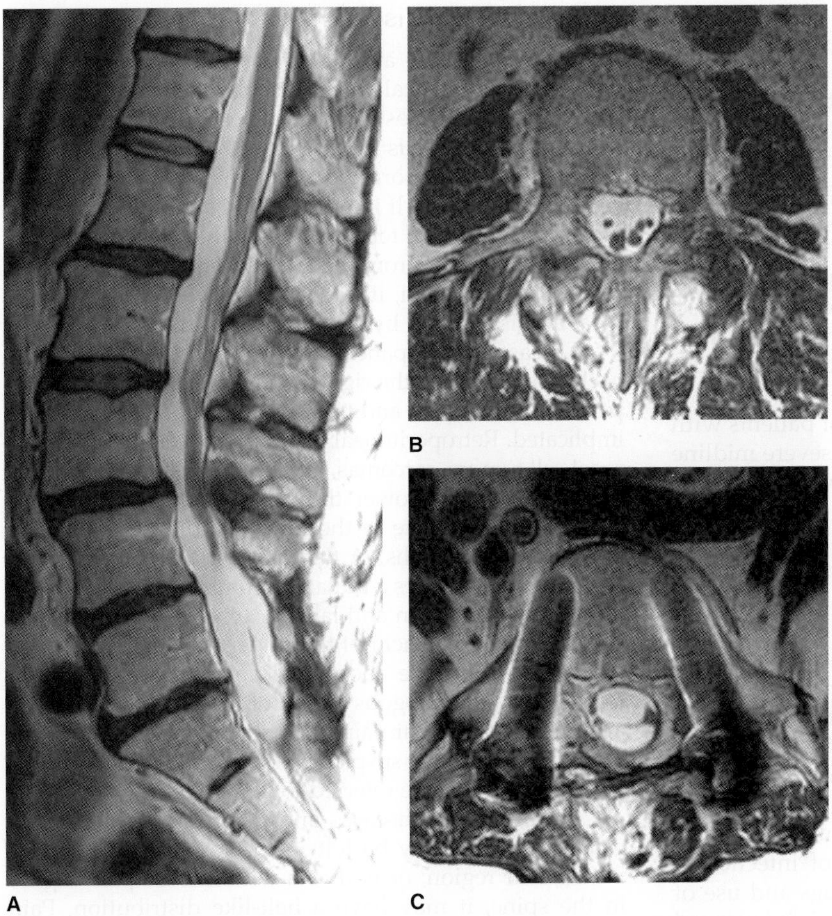

Figure 11-5. Lumbosacral MRI of a patient with lymphoma, with radiation-induced arachnoiditis causing severe back pain and leg weakness. ***A.*** Sagittal T2-weighted MRI showing clumping of the nerve roots of the cauda equina. ***B.*** Axial T2-weighted image at the L3 vertebral level showing clumping of the nerve roots. ***C.*** Axial T2-weighted image at the L5 vertebral level showing lateral displacement of nerve roots by acquired arachnoid cysts. There are bilateral metallic pedicle screws.

be accompanied by the Reiter syndrome, psoriasis, and inflammatory diseases of the intestine (see also Chap. 44). The great risk in this disease is fracture dislocation of the spine from relatively minor trauma, particularly flexion-extension injuries.

Occasionally, ankylosing spondylitis is complicated by destructive vertebral lesions. This complication should be suspected whenever the pain returns after a period of quiescence or becomes localized. The cause of these lesions is not known, but they may represent a response to nonunion of fractures, taking the form of an excessive production of fibrous inflammatory tissue. When it is severe, ankylosing spondylitis may involve both hips, greatly accentuating the back deformity and disability.

Rheumatoid arthritis of the spine may be confined to the cervical region and creates risk of fracture–dislocation; it is considered further on in this chapter.

Neoplastic and Infectious Diseases of the Spine
(See also Chap. 44)

Metastatic carcinoma (breast, bronchus, prostate, thyroid, kidney, stomach, uterus), multiple myeloma, and lymphoma are the common malignant tumors that involve the spine. The primary lesion may be small and asymptomatic, and the first manifestation of the tumor may be pain in the back caused by metastatic deposits. The pain is constant and dull; it is often unrelieved by rest and is generally worse at night, interrupting sleep. Radicular pain may be added if the metastasis extends laterally. A fracture of a vertebral body in an otherwise healthy young or middle-aged person should alert the physician to the possibility of an underlying metastasis. At the time of onset of the back pain, there may be no radiographic changes on plain radiographs; when such changes do appear, they usually take the form of destructive lesions in one or several vertebral bodies with little or no involvement of the disc space, even in the face of a compression fracture. However, the changes are evident on CT and MRI or radioactive isotope scan, including PET, and demonstrate areas of osteoblastic activity caused by neoplastic or inflammatory disease.

Infection of the vertebral column, *osteomyelitis*, is usually caused by staphylococci and less often by coliforms and mycobacteria. The patient complains of subacute or chronic pain in the back, which is exacerbated by movement but not materially relieved by rest. Motion becomes limited, and there is percussion-induced tenderness over the spine in the involved segments and pain with jarring of the spine, as occurs when the heels strike the floor. Often these patients are afebrile and do not have a leukocytosis. The erythrocyte sedimentation rate and C-reactive protein are elevated as a rule. Highly characteristic is the demonstration by CT scanning and MRI of involvement of both the vertebral body and the adjacent intervertebral disc, and *the finding of a breached disc space with involvement of two adjacent vertebral bodies* is one of the features that differentiates infectious from neoplastic diseases of the spine. A paravertebral mass is often found, indicating an abscess, which may, in the case of tuberculosis, drain spontaneously at sites quite remote from the vertebral column. In the postoperative setting or following trauma, a disc infection can occur by direct microbial seeding. It should be remembered that the intervertebral disc is an avascular structure, and therefore blood-borne pathogens first infect the bone and then secondarily spread to the adjacent disc. This is not the case in the neonatal period when the discs are directly perfused, for which reason neonates are subject to hematogenously seeded discitis.

We have also encountered a number of patients with bacterial endocarditis who complained of severe midline thoracic and lumbar back pain but had no evident infection of the spine.

Tuberculous spinal infection and the resultant kyphotic deformity (Pott disease) represent a special condition that is common in developing countries (see Chaps. 32 and 44).

Spinal Epidural Abscess Special emphasis is placed on this condition, which usually necessitates urgent surgical treatment. Failure to properly identify this lesion has led to paraplegia or death from sepsis. Most often this is caused by staphylococcal infection, which is carried in the bloodstream from a septic focus (e.g., furuncle) or is introduced into the epidural space from an osteomyelitic lesion. Another important avenue of infection is the intravenous self-administration of drugs and use of contaminated needles. Rarely, the infection is introduced in the course of a lumbar puncture, epidural injection, or laminectomy for disc excision. In some instances, the source of an epidural abscess cannot be ascertained. The main symptoms are low-grade fever, leukocytosis, and persistent and severe localized pain that are intensified by percussion and pressure over the vertebral spines. Additionally, the pain may acquire radicular radiation. These symptoms usually require investigation by MRI or CT myelography and surgical intervention, preferably before the signs of paraplegia, sphincter dysfunction, and sensory loss become manifest. Small abscesses and granulomas that are the residua of previous and partially treated abscesses can be sometimes treated successfully with antibiotics alone as discussed further on.

Intraspinal Hemorrhage (See Chap. 44)

Sudden, excruciating midline back pain (*le coup de poignard* or "the strike of the dagger")—often with rapidly evolving paraparesis, urinary retention, and numbness of the legs—may announce the occurrence of subarachnoid, subdural, or epidural bleeding. The most common causes of such an event are a coagulopathy (mainly from warfarin), and a spinal arteriovenous malformation (AVM), as discussed in Chap. 44. Spinal arterial aneurysms are much less common underlying lesions. It should be mentioned that focal back pain of comparable intensity may mark the onset of acute myelitis, spinal cord infarction, compression fracture, and occasionally, Guillain-Barré syndrome.

Back Pain from Visceral Disease

Peptic ulcer disease and carcinoma of the stomach and pancreas most typically induce pain in the epigastrium. However, if the posterior stomach wall is involved, particularly if there is retroperitoneal extension, the pain may be felt in the thoracic spine, centrally or to one side, or in both locations. If intense, it may seem to encircle the body. The back pain tends to reflect the temporal characteristics of the pain from the affected organ; e.g., if caused by gastric ulceration, it appears about two hours after a meal and is relieved by food and antacids.

Diseases of the pancreas are apt to cause pain in the back, being more to the right of the spine if the head of the pancreas is involved and to the left if the body and tail are implicated. Retroperitoneal neoplasms—e.g., lymphomas, renal cell tumors, sarcomas, and other malignancies—may evoke pain in the lower thoracic or lumbar spine with a tendency to radiate to the lower part of the abdomen, groins, anterior thighs, or flank. A tumor in the iliopsoas region often produces a unilateral lumbar ache with radiation toward the groin and labia or testicle; there may also be signs of involvement of the upper lumbar spinal roots. An aneurysm of the abdominal aorta may induce pain localized to an analogous region of the spine. The sudden appearance of lumbar pain in a patient receiving anticoagulants should arouse suspicion of retroperitoneal bleeding; this pain may also be referred to the groin.

Inflammatory diseases and neoplasms of the colon cause pain that may be felt in the lower abdomen, the midlumbar region, or both. As with intense pain higher in the spine, it may have a belt-like distribution. Pain from a lesion in the transverse colon or first part of the descending colon may be central or left-sided; its level of reference is to the second and third lumbar vertebrae. If the sigmoid colon is implicated, the pain is lower in the upper sacral spine and anteriorly in the suprapubic region or left lower quadrant of the abdomen. Retroperitoneal appendicitis may have an odd referral of pain to the low flank and back.

Gynecologic disorders often manifest themselves by back pain, and their diagnosis may prove difficult. Thorough abdominal palpation, as well as vaginal and rectal examination by an experienced physician, supplemented by ultrasonography and CT scanning or MRI, usually discloses the source of pain. The uterosacral ligaments are a pelvic source of chronic back pain. Endometriosis or carcinoma of the uterus (body or cervix) may invade these structures, causing pain localized to the sacrum either centrally or more to one side. In endometriosis, the pain begins premenstrually and often merges with menstrual pain, which also may be felt in the sacral region. Rarely, cyclic engorgement of ectopic endometrial tissue may give rise to sciatica and other radicular pain. Changes in posture may also evoke pain here when a fibroma of the uterus pulls on the uterosacral ligaments. Low back pain with radiation into one or both thighs is a common phenomenon during the last weeks of pregnancy.

The pain of neoplastic infiltration of pelvic nerve plexuses may be projected to the low back and is continuous, becoming progressively more severe; it tends to be more intense at night and may have a burning quality.

The primary lesion can be inconspicuous and may be overlooked on pelvic examination.

Coccydynia

This is the name applied to pain localized to the coccyx, the three or four small vestigial bones at the lower-most part of the sacrum. The trauma of childbirth, a fall on the buttocks, avascular necrosis, a neurofibroma or glomus tumor, or one of a variety of other rare tumors and anal disorders, and, of course, pilonidal cyst, can sometimes be established as the cause of pain in this region. Far more often, the source remains obscure. In the past, patients in this latter group were indiscriminately subjected to coccygectomy, but more recent studies have demonstrated that most cases respond favorably to injections of local anesthetic and methylprednisolone or to manipulation of the coccyx under anesthesia (Wray et al).

Obscure Types of Low Back Pain and the Question of Psychiatric Disease

Even after careful examination, there remains a sizable group of patients in whom no basis for the back pain can be found. Two categories can be recognized: one with postural back pain and pain after injury, and another with psychiatric illness, but there are always cases where the diagnosis remains obscure.

Low back pain may be a major symptom in patients with hysteria, malingering, anxiety, depression, and hypochondriasis as well as in many persons whose symptoms do not conform to any of these psychiatric illnesses. It is good practice to assume that pain in the back in such patients may signify disease of the spine or adjacent structures, and this should always be carefully sought. However, even when some organic factors are found, the pain may be exaggerated, prolonged, or woven into a pattern of invalidism because of coexistent primary or secondary factors. This is especially true when there is the possibility of secondary gain (notably workers' compensation or settlement of personal injury claims). Patients seeking compensation for protracted low back pain without obvious structural disease tend, after a time, to become suspicious, uncooperative, and hostile toward their physicians or anyone who might question the authenticity of their illness. One notes in them a tendency to describe their pain vaguely and a preference to discuss the degree of their disability and their mistreatment at the hands of the medical profession. The description of the pain may vary considerably from one examination to another. Often also, the region(s) in which pain is experienced and its radiation are nonphysiologic, and the condition fails to respond to rest and inactivity. These features and a negative examination of the back should lead one to suspect a psychologic factor. A few patients, usually frank malingerers, adopt bizarre gaits and attitudes, such as walking with the trunk flexed at almost a right angle (camptocormia), and are unable to straighten up. Or the patient may be unable to bend forward even a few degrees, despite the absence of muscle spasm, and may wince at the slightest pressure, even over the sacrum, which is seldom a site of tenderness unless there is pelvic disease.

The depressed and anxious patient with back pain represents a troublesome problem. The disability seems excessive for the degree of spinal malfunction. Anxiety and depression may become important components of the back syndrome, and the patient may ruminate about an undiagnosed cancer or other serious illness. In these circumstances, common and minor back ailments—e.g., those caused by osteoarthritis and postural ache—are enhanced and rendered intolerable. Such patients are still subjected to unnecessary surgical procedures. It is not clear if one can depend on the diagnostic features of a response to drugs that alleviate depression.

Failed Back Syndrome

Surely among the most difficult patients to manage are those with chronic low back pain who have already had one or more laminectomies and sometimes a fusion without substantial relief. In one perhaps dated but large series of patients operated on for proven disc herniation, 25 percent were left with troublesome symptoms and 10 percent required further surgery (Weir and Jacobs). In such patients our practice has been to repeat the MRI or CT myelography. In a small number it will be found that the disc has reruptured, or that there is unaddressed lateral recess stenosis, that a disc has ruptured at another level, or that there is there is increased spondylolisthesis with flexion or extension. It may happen that the surgeon did not remove all the herniated disc tissue, in which case another operation to remove the remainder will usually be successful. EMG and nerve conduction studies, searching for evidence of a radiculopathy, are also helpful. If there is evidence of a radiculopathy but no disc material, or only scar tissue is seen on MRI, one cannot know whether the pain is because of injury from the initial rupture or is the aftermath of surgery. Various explanations are then invoked—radiculitis, lateral recess syndrome, facet syndrome, unstable spine, and lumbar arachnoiditis, each described earlier in this chapter (see reviews by Quiles et al and by Long).

Transcutaneous stimulators, posterior column stimulators, intrathecal injections of analgesics, and epidural steroid injections have seldom helped for long in our experience, but we have seen striking exceptions, especially with epidural pumps that administer analgesics. At present, the best that can be offered the patient is weight reduction (in appropriate individuals), stretching and progressive exercise to strengthen abdominal and back muscles, as well as mild nonnarcotic analgesics and antidepressant drugs. A trial of massage and other types of physiotherapy or a limited course of spinal chiropractic manipulation is reasonable.

PAIN IN THE NECK, SHOULDER, AND ARM

General Considerations

It is useful to distinguish three major categories of painful disease of the neck and arms—that originating in the *cervical spine*, in the *brachial plexus*, and in the *shoulder*.

Although the distribution of pain from each of these sources may overlap, the patient can usually indicate its site of origin. Pain arising from the *cervical part of the spine* is felt in the neck or back of the head and is projected to the shoulder and upper arm; it is evoked or enhanced by certain movements or positions of the neck and is accompanied by limitation of motion of the neck and by tenderness to palpation over the cervical spine.

Pain of brachial plexus origin is experienced in the supraclavicular region, or in the axilla and around the shoulder; it may be worsened by certain maneuvers and positions of the arm and neck (extreme rotation). A palpable abnormality above the clavicle may disclose the cause of the plexopathy (aneurysm of the subclavian artery, tumor, and cervical rib). The combination of circulatory abnormalities and signs referable to the medial cord of the brachial plexus is characteristic of the *thoracic outlet syndrome,* described further on.

Pain localized to the shoulder region, worsened by motion, and associated with tenderness and limitation of movement, especially internal and external rotation and abduction, points to a tendonitis, subacromial bursitis, or tear of the rotator cuff or labrum of the shoulder joint, which is made up of the tendons of the muscles surrounding the shoulder joint. The term *bursitis* is often used loosely to designate the first three of these disorders. Shoulder pain, like spine and plexus pain, may radiate vaguely into the arm and rarely into the hand, but sensorimotor and reflex changes—which always indicate disease of nerve roots, plexus, or nerves—are absent. Shoulder pain of this type is very common in middle and late adult life. It may arise spontaneously or after unusual or vigorous use of the arm. Local tenderness over the greater tuberosity of the humerus is characteristic. Plain radiographs of the shoulder may be normal or show a calcium deposit in the supraspinatus tendon or subacromial bursa. MRI is able to demonstrate more subtle abnormalities, such as muscle and tendon tears of the rotator cuff or a labral tear of the joint capsule. In most patients the pain subsides gradually with immobilization and analgesics followed by a program of increasing shoulder mobilization. If it does not, the injection of small amounts of corticosteroids into the bursa, or the site of major pain indicated by passive shoulder movement in the case of rotator cuff injuries, is often temporarily effective and allows the patient to mobilize the shoulder. The more extreme problem of the "frozen shoulder" is addressed further on.

Osteoarthritis and osteophytic spur formation of the cervical spine may cause pain that radiates into the back of the head, shoulders, and arm on one or both sides. Coincident compression of nerve roots is manifest by paresthesia, sensory loss, weakness and atrophy, and tendon reflex changes in the arms and hands. Should bony ridges form in the spinal canal, as described in detail in Chap. 44 (*cervical spondylosis*), the spinal cord may be compressed, with resulting spastic weakness, ataxia, and loss of vibratory and position sense in the legs. The bony changes are evident on plain films but are better seen by CT and MRI. There may be difficulty in distinguishing cervical spondylosis with root and spinal cord compression from a disc (see further on) or from a primary neurologic disease (syringomyelia, amyotrophic lateral sclerosis, or tumor) with an unrelated cervical osteoarthritis. Here the MRI is of particular value in revealing compression of the spinal cord, but this study is prone to over interpretation when a bony ridge barely comes into contact with the cord but does not deform it or extends laterally to the proximal foramen but does not compress the nerve root (see "Cervical Spondylosis with Myelopathy" in Chap. 44).

Spinal *rheumatoid arthritis* may be restricted to or include the cervical zygapophysial (facet) joints and the atlantoaxial articulation. The usual manifestations are pain, stiffness, and limitation of motion in the neck and pain in the back of the head. In contrast to ankylosing spondylitis, rheumatoid arthritis is rarely confined to the spine. Because of evident disease of other joints, the diagnosis is relatively easy to make, but significant involvement of the cervical spine may be overlooked. In the advanced stages, one or several of the vertebrae may become displaced anteriorly, or a synovitis of the atlantoaxial joint may damage the transverse ligament of the atlas, resulting in forward displacement of the atlas on the axis, i.e., atlantoaxial subluxation. In either instance, serious and even life-threatening compression of the spinal cord may occur gradually or suddenly. Cautiously performed lateral radiographs in flexion and extension are useful in visualizing atlantoaxial dislocation or subluxation of the lower segments. Occipital headache and neck pain related to degenerative changes in the upper cervical facets is discussed with other cranial pains in "'Third Occipital Nerve' Headache" in Chap. 10.

Traumatic and Whiplash Injury

Injury to ligaments and muscles as a result of forcible extension and flexion of the neck can create a number of difficult clinical problems. The injury ranges from a minor sprain of muscles and ligaments to severe tearing of these structures, to avulsion of muscle and tendon from vertebral body, and even to vertebral and intervertebral disc damage. The latter lesions can be seen with MRI and, if severe, can result in root or spinal cord compression or, occasionally, in cartilaginous embolization leading to infarction of the spinal cord (see "Fibrocartilaginous Embolism" in Chap. 44). If there is preexisting cervical osteoarthritis, there may be considerable pain, and in extreme cases, cord compression.

However, the more ubiquitous and milder degrees of whiplash injury without the above described structural injuries are so often complicated by psychologic and compensation factors leading to prolonged disability that the syndrome has become a vexing issue without clear medical definition and it occupies a disproportionate amount of time on the part of physicians, compensation boards, and courts (see LaRocca for a review and especially the book by Malleson for an interesting discussion of the sociology and psychology of this subject). We have no doubt that authentic traumatic neck injuries exist, even at times from minor trauma, but we are in accord with these authors that the high frequency of putative whiplash injury is sustained by societal and legal structures.

Cervical Disc Herniation (See Table 11-1)

A common cause of neck, shoulder, and arm pain is disc herniation in the mid and lower cervical region; the process is comparable to disc herniation in the lumbar region but gives rise, of course, to a different set of symptoms (Table 11-1). The problem appears most often without a clear and immediate cause, but it may develop after trauma, which may be major or minor (from sudden hyperextension of the neck, falls, diving accidents, and forceful manipulations). The roots most commonly involved are the seventh (in 70 percent of cases) and the sixth (in 20 percent of cases); fifth- and eighth-root compression makes up the remaining 10 percent (Yoss et al).

When the protruded disc lies between the sixth and seventh vertebrae, there is involvement of the *seventh cervical root* as outlined in Table 11-1 and shown in Figure 11-6 A and B. The pain is then in the region of the shoulder blade, or spine of the scapula, and posterolateral upper arm; it may project to the elbow and dorsal forearm, index and middle fingers, or all the fingers. Occasionally discomfort is felt in the pectoral or axillary region. Tenderness is most pronounced over the medial aspect of the shoulder blade opposite the third to fourth thoracic spinous processes and in the supraclavicular area and triceps region. Paresthesia and sensory loss are most evident in the lateral index and middle fingers. Weakness involves the extensors of the forearm and sometimes of the wrist; occasionally the handgrip is weak as well; the triceps may be weak and the triceps reflex is usually diminished or absent; the biceps and supinator reflexes are preserved.

With a laterally situated disc herniation between the fifth and sixth cervical vertebrae, the symptoms and signs are referred to the *sixth cervical root*. The full syndrome is characterized by pain at the trapezius ridge and tip

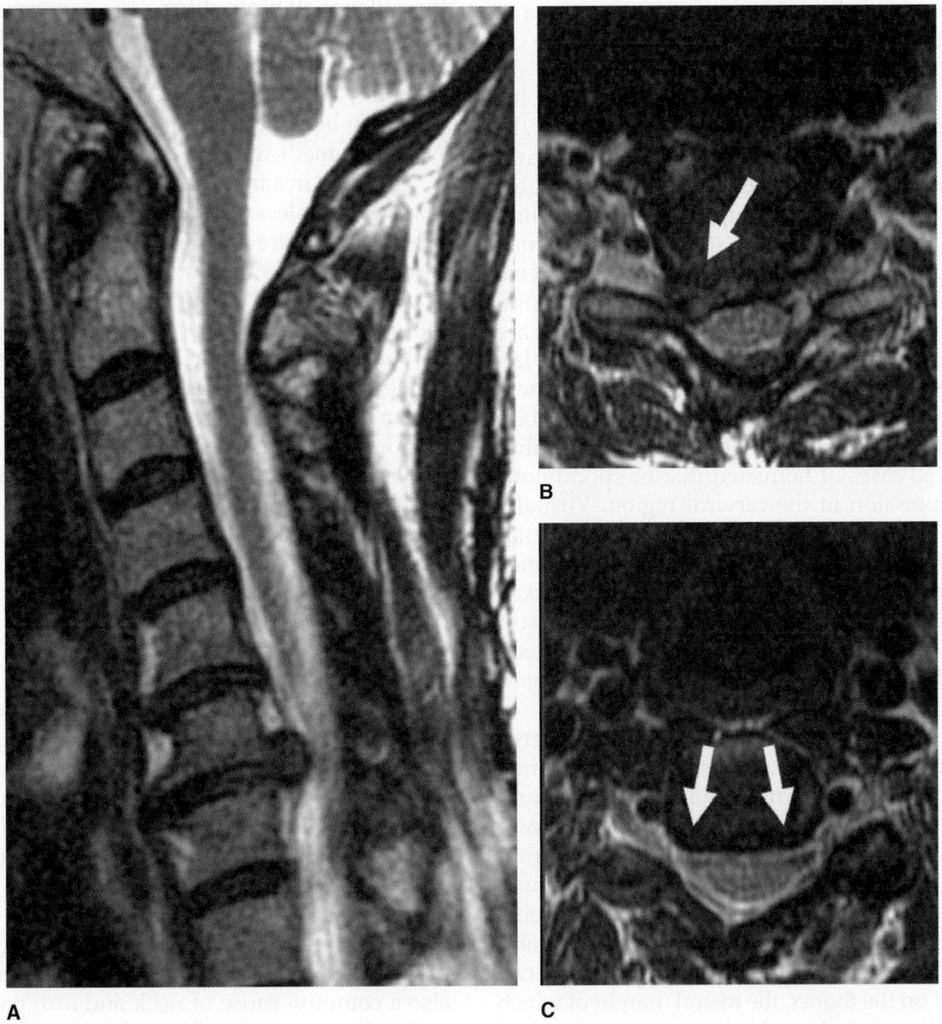

Figure 11-6. Cervical disc herniation as visualized with T2-weighted MRI. *A.* Parasagittal view of a large posterior disc extrusion at C6-C7. Smaller broad-based posterior disc bulges are seen at C4-C5 and C5-C6. *B.* Axial view of the large right posterolateral disc extrusion shown in (*A*) at C6-C7 (arrow) causing severe narrowing of the right neural foramen and compression of the exiting C7 nerve root. *C.* By way of contrast, an axial view of the broad-based posterior disc bulge at C4-C5 (arrows) causes only minimal narrowing of the spinal canal and no compression of the spinal cord.

of the shoulder, with radiation into the anterior-upper part of the arm, radial forearm, often the thumb, and sometimes the index finger as well. There may also be paresthesia and sensory impairment in the same regions; tenderness in the area above the spine of the scapula and in the supraclavicular and biceps regions; weakness in flexion of the forearm (biceps) and in contraction of the deltoid when sustaining arm abduction; and diminished or absent biceps and supinator reflexes (the triceps reflex is retained or sometimes has the appearance of being slightly exaggerated because of flaccidity of the biceps).

The *fifth cervical root* syndrome, produced by disc herniation between the fourth and fifth vertebral bodies, is characterized by pain in the shoulder and trapezius region and by supra- and infraspinatus weakness, manifest by an inability to abduct the arm and rotate it externally with the shoulder adducted (weakness of the supra- and infraspinatus muscles). There may be a slight degree of weakness of the biceps and a corresponding reduction in the reflex, but these are inconsistent findings. A small patch of diminished sensation commonly overlies the deltoid muscle.

Compression of the *eighth cervical root* at (C7-T1 disc) may mimic ulnar nerve palsy. The pain is along the medial side of the forearm and the sensory loss is in the distribution of the medial cutaneous nerve of the forearm and of the ulnar nerve in the hand. The weakness largely involves the intrinsic muscles supplied by the ulnar nerve (see "Ulnar Nerve" in Chap. 46). The reflexes may be unaffected but the triceps jerk is often slightly reduced.

These cervical disc syndromes are usually incomplete in that only one or several of the typical findings are present. Particularly noteworthy is the occurrence, in laterally placed cervical disc rupture, of isolated weakness without pain, especially with discs at the fifth and sixth levels. Friis and coworkers have described the distribution of pain in 250 cases of herniated disc or spondylotic nerve root compression in the cervical region. Virtually every patient with pain, irrespective of the particular root(s) involved, *showed a limitation in the range of motion of the neck and aggravation of pain with movement (particularly hyperextension)*. Coughing, sneezing, and downward pressure on the head in the hyperextended position usually exacerbated the pain, and manual traction of the neck tended to relieve it.

Unlike herniated lumbar discs, cervical ones, if large and centrally situated, result in compression of the spinal cord. The centrally situated disc is often painless, and the cord syndrome may simulate multiple sclerosis or a degenerative neurologic disease. Bilateral hand numbness, paresthesia, or similar altered sensation is common. Failure to consider a protruded cervical disc in patients with obscure symptoms in the legs, including stiffness and falling, is a common error. A vague sensory change can often be detected on the thorax, the rostral margin of which is several dermatomes below the level of compression. The diagnosis and the level of disc protrusion can be confirmed by MRI or (Fig. 11-6) by CT myelography. Nerve conduction studies, F responses, and EMG are helpful in confirming the level of root compression and distinguishing pain of radicular origin from that originating in the brachial plexus or in individual nerves of the arm (see "Brachial Neuritis" in Chap. 46).

Management of Herniated Cervical Disc

If pain alone is the problem, conservative measures should be instituted before turning to surgical removal of the disc. If there are signs of a rapidly or subacutely progressing myelopathy (i.e., leg and arm weakness, hyperreflexia in the legs, gait ataxia, sphincteric dysfunction) or intractable and persistent pain from radiculopathy, surgery is generally undertaken.

Treatment

In the case of cervical disc with radicular pain, a close-fitting foam collar is sometimes beneficial but many of our colleagues disagree on this point. The collar should be fitted so that minimal flexion and extension of the neck are allowed, but it must remain comfortable enough to encourage consistent use. The patient is advised to wear the collar at all times during the day, especially while riding in a car, unless this becomes completely impractical. Of even more uncertain value, and theoretically entailing a small risk, traction with a halter around the occiput and chin may be of some benefit in cervical disc syndromes. Analgesic medication may be required for many days.

In most instances the radicular pain subsides over a few weeks or less. Intractable cases may require surgery, especially if there is substantial weakness in the muscles corresponding to the affected root. Mild weakness alone is not recognized as an indication for surgery, and in those few cases where weakness alone has occurred, without pain, the same conservative measures outlined above should be implemented. However, there has never been a clear definition of the threshold of forearm, shoulder, or hand weakness that justifies surgery or might be irreversible if surgical decompression is not undertaken. Most often the surgeon tackles this problem through an anterior approach (transdiscally), which leaves the posterior elements intact and allows for retained stability of the spine.

Cervical Spondylosis (See also Chap. 44)

This is a chronic degenerative disease of the mid-and lower cervical spine that narrows the spinal canal and intervertebral foramina, causing compressive injury of the spinal cord and roots. The problem of central disc protrusion with overlying calcification, discussed above, often contributes as the main component of the narrowing of the canal. Hypertrophy of the facet joints and ligamentous buckling are added. Because the main effects of cervical spondylosis are on the cord, this process is discussed in detail in Chap. 44 but cervical spondylosis is also a common cause of neck and arm pain, as described earlier. If minor signs of spinal cord and root involvement are present, a collar to limit movement of the head and neck may halt the progression and lead to improvement. Decompressive laminectomy or anterior excision of single spondylotic spurs with or without fusion are reserved for instances of advancing neurologic symptoms or intractable pain as discussed in Chap. 44. As with lumbar stenosis, success is not assured with surgery, but almost invariably, progression of symptoms is prevented.

Epidural Lipomatosis and Extramedullary Hematopoiesis

The first of these is a regularly encountered disorder that results from proliferation of fat in the spinal epidural space, most often dorsally in the thoracic region. It may cause a compressive myelopathy but is as often found incidentally on MRI. In current practice, corticosteroid administration is the most frequent cause. Similarly, the second process is from proliferation of bone marrow because of failure of hematopoiesis in the normal regions of the bone marrow.

These subjects are discussed further in Chap. 44.

Thoracic Outlet Syndromes

A number of anatomic anomalies occur in the lateral cervical region. These may, under certain circumstances, compress the brachial plexus, the subclavian artery, and the subclavian vein, causing muscle weakness and wasting, pain, and vascular abnormalities in the hand and arm. The condition is undoubtedly diagnosed more often than is justified, and the term has been applied ambiguously to a number of conditions, some of which are almost certainly nonexistent, comparable to the piriformis syndrome in the buttock.

The most frequent of the abnormalities that cause neural compression and are encompassed by the term *thoracic outlet syndrome* are an anomalous incomplete cervical rib, with a sharp fascial band passing from its tip to the first rib; a taut fibrous band passing from an elongated and down-curving transverse process of C7 to the first rib; less often, a complete cervical rib, which articulates with the first rib; and anomalies of the position and insertion of the anterior and medial scalene muscles. Thus, the sites of potential neurovascular compression extend all the way from the intervertebral foramina and superior mediastinum to the axilla. Depending on the postulated abnormality and mechanism of symptom production, the terms *cervical rib*, *anterior scalene*, *costoclavicular*, and *neurovascular compression* have been applied. In addition, a *droopy shoulder syndrome* has been identified that purportedly stretches the brachial plexus and gives rise to similar symptoms; a majority of the patients have been young women with asthenic body habitus.

Variations in regional anatomy could explain these postulated mechanisms, but to this day there is not full agreement about the validity of anterior scalene and costoclavicular syndromes. An anomalous cervical rib, which arises from the seventh cervical vertebra and extends laterally between the anterior and medial scalene muscles and then under the brachial plexus and subclavian artery to attach to the first rib, obviously disturbs the anatomic relationships of these structures and may compress them (Fig. 11-7). However, as an estimated 1 percent of the population has cervical ribs, usually on both sides, and only about 10 percent of these persons have neurologic or vascular symptoms (almost always one-sided), other factors must be operative.

The anterior and middle scalene muscles, which flex and rotate the neck, are both inserted into the first rib so that the subclavian artery and vein and the brachial plexus must pass between them. Hence abnormalities of insertion and hypertrophy of these muscles were once thought to be causes of the syndrome but sectioning them (scalenectomy) has so rarely altered the symptoms that this mechanism is no longer given credence.

Three neurovascular syndromes are associated with a rudimentary and not fully ossified cervical rib (rarely with a complete cervical rib): subclavian venous or arterial compression and a brachial plexopathy. In all three forms, shoulder and arm pain is prominent. The discomfort is of the aching type and is felt in the posterior hemithorax, pectoral region, and upper arm. These syndromes sometimes coexist, but more often each occurs independently.

Compression or spontaneous thrombosis of the subclavian vein is a rare occurrence causing a dusky discoloration, venous distention, and edema of the arm. The vein may become thrombosed after prolonged exercise (Paget-Schrötter syndrome) or in cases of a clotting diathesis in cancer patients.

Compression of the subclavian artery, which results in ischemia of the limb, may be complicated by digital gangrene and retrograde embolization, also is a rare entity. A unilateral Raynaud phenomenon, brittle nails, and ulceration of the fingertips are important diagnostic findings. A supraclavicular bruit is suggestive but not in itself diagnostic of subclavian artery compression.

The conventional tests for vascular compression—obliteration of the pulse when the patient, seated and with the arm extended, takes and holds a full breath, tilts the head back, and turns it to the affected side (Adson test) or abducts and externally rotates the arm and braces the shoulders and turns the head to either side (Wright maneuver)—are not entirely reliable. Sometimes these maneuvers fail to obliterate the radial pulse in cases of proved compression; contrariwise, these tests may be positive in normal persons. Nevertheless, a positive test only on the symptomatic side (with reproduction of the patient's symptoms) is suggestive of the diagnosis of arterial compression and, by implication, some form of thoracic outlet syndrome. Plethysmographic recording of the radial pulse and ultrasound of the vessel add to the accuracy of these positional tests.

A primarily neurologic problem may characterize the thoracic outlet syndrome. There is slight wasting and weakness of the hypothenar, interosseous, adductor pollicis, and deep flexor muscles of the fourth and fifth fingers (i.e., the muscles innervated by the lower trunk of the brachial plexus and ulnar nerve). Weakness of the flexor muscles of the forearm may be present in advanced cases. Tendon reflexes are usually preserved. In addition, most patients complain of an intermittent aching of the arm, particularly of the ulnar side, and about half of them complain also of numbness and tingling along the ulnar border of the forearm and hand. A loss of superficial sensation in these areas is variable. It may be possible

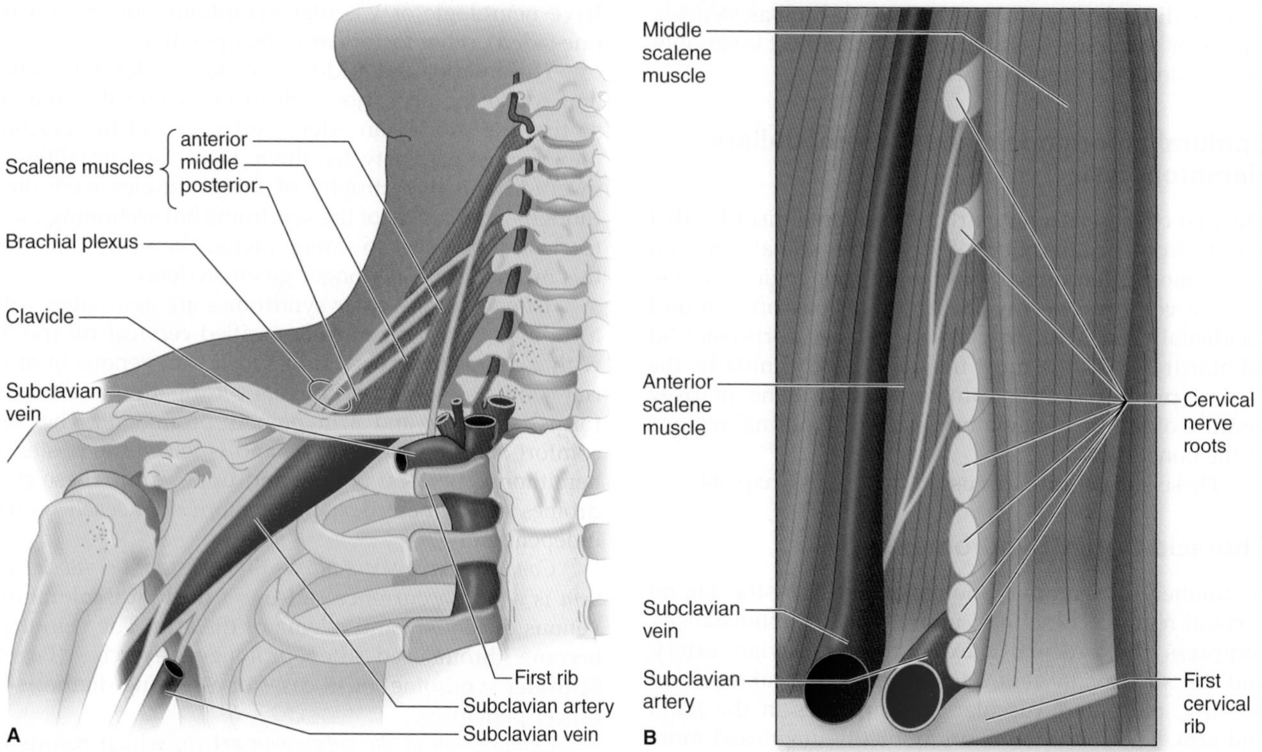

Figure 11-7. Course of the brachial plexus and subclavian artery between the anterior scalene and middle scalene muscles as seen from coronal oblique (*A*) and sagittal oblique (*B*) perspectives. Dilatation of the subclavian artery just distal to the anterior scalene muscle is illustrated in (*A*). Immediately distal to the anterior and middle scalene muscles is another potential area of constriction, between the clavicle and the first rib. With extension of the neck and turning of the chin to the affected side (Adson maneuver), the tension on the anterior scalene muscle is increased and the subclavian artery compressed, resulting in a supraclavicular bruit and obliteration of the radial pulse.

to reproduce the sensory symptoms by firm pressure backwards on the scalenus muscle just above the clavicle, or more typically by downward and dorsal traction on the arm. Vascular features are often absent or minimal in patients with the neurologic form of the syndrome.

In patients with neurologic signs, nerve conduction studies usually disclose reduced amplitude of the ulnar sensory potentials. There may be decreased amplitude of the median motor evoked potentials as well, a mild but uniform slowing of the median motor conduction velocity, and a prolongation of the F-wave latency. Needle examination of affected hand muscles reveals large-amplitude motor units, suggesting collateral reinnervation. Somatosensory evoked potentials may be a useful adjunct to the conventional nerve conduction and EMG studies (Yiannikas and Walsh). Brachial artery MR angiography is usually reserved for patients with a suspected arterial occlusion, an aneurysm, or an obvious cervical rib. The place of venography in the diagnostic workup is uncertain, for a number of otherwise normal individuals can occlude the subclavian vein by fully abducting the arm.

In the authors' experience, unambiguous instances of thoracic outlet syndrome are not common. This has also been the experience of Wilbourn, whose review of this subject is recommended. One should be skeptical of the diagnosis unless the clinical and EMG features enumerated above are present. Common mistakes are to confuse the thoracic outlet syndrome with carpal tunnel syndrome, ulnar neuropathy or entrapment at the elbow, or cervical radiculopathy caused by arthritis or disc disease. Brachial neuritis may have a similar presentation. Imaging studies and careful nerve conduction and EMG studies may be necessary to exclude all of these disorders.

Treatment

A conservative approach is advisable. If the main symptoms are pain and paresthesia, Leffert suggested the use of local heat, analgesics, muscle relaxants, and an assiduous program of special exercises to strengthen the shoulder muscles. A full range of neck motions is then practiced. On such a regimen, some patients experience a relief of symptoms after 2 to 3 weeks. Instruction by a physical therapist is invaluable.

Only if pain is severe and persistent and is clearly associated with the vascular or neurogenic features of the syndrome is surgery indicated. The usual approach is through the supraclavicular space, with cutting of fibrous bands and excision of the rudimentary rib. In cases of venous or minor arterial forms of the syndrome, some thoracic surgeons favor the excision of a segment of the first rib through the axilla. Pain is often relieved, but the sensorimotor defects improve only slightly. Sectioning of the scalenus muscle is not endorsed because, as already noted, the role of muscle in causing thoracic outlet syndrome has been questioned.

Other Painful Conditions Originating in the Neck, Brachial Plexus, and Shoulder

The brachial plexus is an important source of shoulder and arm pain. The main disorders are brachial neuritis and metastatic infiltration and radiation damage to the plexus. Chapter 46 discusses these disorders in detail.

Metastases to the cervical region of the spine are less common than to other parts of the vertebral column. They are, however, frequently painful and may cause root compression. Posterior extension of the tumor from the vertebral bodies or compression fractures may lead to the rapid development of quadriplegia. Infiltration of the brachial plexus from tumor or sarcoid can produce similar syndromes.

The Pancoast tumor, usually a squamous cell carcinoma in the superior sulcus of the lung, may implicate the lower cervical and upper thoracic (T1 and T2) spinal nerves as they exit the spine. In these cases, a Horner syndrome, numbness of the inner side of the arm and hand, and weakness of all muscles of the hand and of the triceps muscle are combined with pain beneath the upper scapula and in the arm. The neurologic abnormalities may occur long before the tumor becomes visible radiographically.

Shoulder injuries (the common rotator cuff injury, or tear), subacromial or subdeltoid bursitis, periarthritis or capsulitis (frozen shoulder), tendonitis, and arthritis may develop in patients who are otherwise well, but these conditions also occur as complications of hemiplegia. The pain tends to be severe and extends toward the neck and down the arm into the hand. The dorsum of the hand may tingle without other signs of nerve involvement. Immobility of an arm following myocardial infarction may be associated with pain in the shoulder and arm and with vasomotor changes and secondary arthropathy of the hand joints (shoulder-hand syndrome); after a time, osteoporosis and atrophy of cutaneous and subcutaneous structures occur (Sudeck atrophy or Sudeck-Leriche syndrome). Similar changes may occur in the foot and leg, or all articular structures on the side of a hemiplegia, or in association with the painful lesions described in the first part of this chapter. The neurologist should know that these complications can be prevented by proper exercises and relieved by cooling of the affected limb.

Vasomotor, sudomotor, and trophic changes in the skin, with atrophy of the soft tissues and decalcification of bone, may follow the prolonged immobilization and disuse of an arm (i.e., frozen shoulder syndrome) or leg for whatever reason.

Medial and lateral epicondylitis (tennis elbow) are readily diagnosed by demonstrating tenderness over the affected parts and an aggravation of pain on certain movements of the wrist. We have observed entrapment of the ulnar nerve in some cases of medial epicondylitis. Certain diabetic men seem to be prone to traumatizing their ulnar nerves at the elbow with various motions such as those of tennis.

The pain of the carpal tunnel syndrome often extends into the forearm and sometimes into the anterior biceps region and may be mistaken for disease of the shoulder or neck. Similarly, involvement of the ulnar, radial, or median nerves may be mistaken for brachial plexus or root lesions. EMG and nerve conduction studies resolves this. (this common disorder is discussed in Chap. 46).

Polymyalgia Rheumatica (See also Chaps. 10 and 34)

This syndrome is observed in middle-aged and elderly persons and is characterized by severe pain, aching, and stiffness in the proximal muscles of the limbs and a markedly elevated erythrocyte sedimentation rate and C-reactive protein level. The shoulders are most affected, but half of these patients have hip or neck pain as well. Constitutional symptoms (loss of weight, fever, and anemia) and articular swelling are less consistent manifestations. Many physicians have drawn attention to the high incidence of depression, but as is typical of chronic disease, it is difficult to know whether this is a cause or an effect. A few patients have pitting edema of the hands or feet, as illustrated in the review by Salvarini and colleagues; others have knee or wrist arthritis or carpal tunnel syndrome. Arthroscopy and MRI suggest that the pain originates in a synovitis or, sometimes more accurately, a bursitis, and in an inflammation of periarticular structures. The fundamental cause is not known.

Activity of the disease in a given patient correlates with elevation of the sedimentation rate, almost always above 40 mm/h and typically higher than 70 mm/h (and corresponding elevation of C-reactive protein); unlike the case in polymyositis, with which it is confused, creatine kinase levels are normal. In many patients, polymyalgia rheumatica is associated with the headache of giant cell (temporal, or cranial) arteritis as discussed in Chap. 10. The precise concordance of these two allied conditions is not known but there is not a high frequency of overlap. The arteritis may affect one or both optic nerves; blindness is the main risk of the disease, as discussed in detail in Chap. 13.

Treatment This disorder is self-limiting, lasting 6 months to 2 years, and responds dramatically to corticosteroid therapy, although this may have to be continued in low dosage for several months or a year or longer. We begin treatment with 20 mg of prednisone if there is no evidence of temporal arteritis (which requires higher doses). The absence of improvement in a day or two should bring the diagnosis into question. The degree of hip and shoulder pain is the best guide to the duration of steroid therapy and the rate at which the drug is withdrawn, usually in very small increments every 2 weeks. The sedimentation rate or C-reactive protein can be used as an additional guide, but neither alone is adequate to alter the medication schedule.

Reflex Sympathetic Dystrophy and Causalgia (See Chap. 8)

This painful response to injury of the shoulder, arm, or leg, is usually the result of an incomplete nerve injury. It consists of protracted pain, characteristically described as "burning," together with cyanosis or pallor, swelling, coldness, pain on passive motion, osteoporosis, and marked sensitivity of the affected part to tactile stimulation. The condition has been variously described under such terms as *Sudeck atrophy*, *posttraumatic osteoporosis* (in which case the bone scan may show increased local uptake of radioactive nuclide), and the related *shoulder-hand syndrome*. The current term is *complex regional pain syndrome*. When the pain syndrome occurs in isolation, it is referred to as *causalgia*. Pharmacologic or surgical sympathectomy appears to relieve the symptoms in some patients. In others with a hypersensitivity of both C-fiber receptors and postganglionic sympathetic fibers, it is not helpful. Chapter 8 discusses this subject further.

Neuroma Formation after Nerve Injury

Persistent and often incapacitating pain and dysesthesias may follow any type of injury that leads to partial or complete interruption of a nerve, with subsequent *neuroma formation* or *intraneural scarring*—fracture, contusion of the limbs, compression from prolonged lying on the arm while intoxicated, severing of sensory nerves in the course of surgical operations or biopsy of nerve, or incomplete regeneration after nerve suture. It is stated that the regenerated nerves in these cases contain a preponderance of unmyelinated C fibers and a reduced number of A-δ fibers; this imbalance is presumably related to the genesis of painful dysesthesias. These cases are best managed by complete excision of the neuromas with end-to-end suture of healthy nerve, but not all cases lend themselves to this procedure.

Another special type of neuroma is the one that forms at the end of a nerve severed at amputation (stump neuroma). Pain from this source is occasionally abolished by relatively simple procedures such as injection of lidocaine, resection of the distal neuroma, proximal neurotomy, or resection of the regional sympathetic ganglia. More common in clinical practice is the mundane, but painful, Morton neuroma, usually found on the plantar nerve between the third and fourth metatarsal bones (third interspace). Pain on compression of the forefoot is the characteristic Mulder sign. The Morton neuroma is visualized by MRI but those due to partial nerve injury are more difficult to reveal by imaging. Gadolinium infusion may be required and even then, differentiation from surrounding scar is problematic.

Erythromelalgia

This rare disorder of the microvasculature produces a burning pain and bright red color skin change, usually in the toes and forefoot and sometimes in the hands, precipitated by changes in ambient temperature. Since its first description by Weir Mitchell in 1878, many articles have been written about it, and recently the cause of a primary familial form was traced to a mutation in a component of a voltage-gated sodium channel. Each patient has a temperature threshold above which symptoms appear and the feet become bright red, warm, and painful. The afflicted patient rarely wears stockings or regular shoes because these tend to bring out the symptoms. The pain is relieved by walking on a cold surface or soaking the feet in cold water and by rest and elevation of the legs. The peripheral pulses are intact, and there are no motor, sensory, or reflex changes. The review by Layzer is recommended.

Most cases are idiopathic, some familial and inherited as a dominant trait. There are secondary forms of the disease, the most important one being that associated with essential thrombocythemia (up to 25 percent of patients may have erythromelalgia as the first symptom) but also with other myeloproliferative disorders such as polycythemia vera and with collagen vascular diseases, including thrombotic thrombocytopenic purpura (TTP), during the use of calcium channel blockers and certain dopaminergic agonists such as pergolide and bromocriptine, and with occlusive vascular diseases. Some instances arise as a result of a painful polyneuropathy that predominantly affects the small sensory fibers; more often in these latter conditions, the redness and warmth are constant and the result of damage to sympathetic nerve fibers; see Chap. 46. These symptomatic forms have led some experts to question whether erythromelalgia is a type of neuropathy or is a vasculopathy (Davis et al).

The familial form of erythromelalgia has been traced to a mutation in a voltage-gated sodium channel (NaV 1.7) that is selectively expressed in dorsal root ganglia nociceptive neurons. In addition to its inherent value in explaining the manifestations of this disease, the discovery of this channelopathy has evinced interest in novel ways to treat pain by manipulating sodium channels.

Treatment According to Abbott and to Mitts and others, aspirin is useful in the treatment of paroxysms of secondary erythromelalgia and of some primary cases as well; others had recommended methysergide, which has fallen out of use because of retroperitoneal and cardiac valvular fibrosis. Even small doses of aspirin provide relief within an hour, lasting for several days, a feature that is diagnostic. Sano and colleagues report that cyclosporine was of great benefit in a case of familial erythromelalgia that had not responded to other medications.

A similar condition, restricted in topography to the region of an acquired single nerve or skin injury, has been described by Ochoa under the term *ABC syndrome* (angry, backfiring C-nociceptors). Episodes of pain and cutaneous vasodilatation were induced by mechanical or thermal stimulation and relieved by cooling. There may be persistent hyperalgesia over the affected area. Lance has suggested that a similar mechanism is operative in the "red ear syndrome" as a result of irritation of the third cervical root.

Myofascial Pain Syndrome and Fibromyalgia

A confusing problem in the differential diagnosis of neck and limb pain is posed by the patient with pains that are clearly musculoskeletal in origin but are not attributable to a disease of the spine, articular structures, or nerves. The pain is localized to certain vague points in skeletal muscles, particularly the large muscles of the neck and shoulder girdle, arms, and thighs. We have been unable to corroborate the ill-defined tender nodules or cords (trigger points) that have been reported as an essential element of this illness. Excision of such nodules has not revealed any sign of inflammation or other disease process. The currently fashionable terms *myofascial pain syndrome*, *fibromyalgia*, and *fibrositis* have been attached to the syndrome, depending on the particular interest or personal bias of the physician. Many of the patients are middle-aged women, who also have the equally vague and vexing chronic fatigue syndrome. Some relief is afforded by local anesthetic injections, administration of local coolants, stretching of underlying muscles ("spray and stretch"), massage, etc., but the results in any given individual are unpredictable and the status of the disorder is not settled. Certain serotonin reuptake inhibitors, generally used to treat depression, are currently favored as treatment by many pain specialists and rheumatologists.

References

Abbott KH, Mitts MG: Reflex neurovascular syndromes, in Vinken PJ, Bruyn GW (eds): *Handbook of Clinical Neurology*, vol 8. Amsterdam, North-Holland, 1970, pp 321–356.

Buchbinder R, Osborne RH, Ebeling PR, et al: A randomized trial of vertebroplasty for painful osteoporotic vertebral fractures. New Engl J Med 361:557, 2009.

Barzouhi A, Vieggeert-Lankamp CL, Njeholt L, et al: Magnetic resonance imaging in follow-up assessment of sciatica. *New Engl J Med* 368:999,2013.

Carette S, Leclaire R, Marcoux S, et al: Epidural corticosteroid injections for sciatica due to herniated nucleus pulposus. *N Engl J Med* 336:1634, 1997.

Carette S, Marcoux S, Truchon R, et al: A controlled trial of corticosteroid injections into facet joints for chronic low back pain. *N Engl J Med* 325:1002, 1991.

Cherkin DC, Devo RA, Battiè M: A comparison of physical therapy, chiropractic manipulation, and provision of an educational booklet for the treatment of patients with low back pain. *N Engl J Med* 339:1021, 1998.

Chou R, Qaseem A, Snow V, et al. Diagnosis and treatment of low back pain: a joint clinical practice guideline from the American College of Physicians and the American Pain Society. *Ann Intern Med* 147:478, 2007.

Collier B: Treatment for lumbar sciatic pain in posterior articular lumbar joint syndrome. *Anaesthesia* 34:202, 1979.

Coppes MH, Marani E, Thomeer RTWM: Innervation of annulus fibrosus in low back pain. *Lancet* 1:189, 1990.

Cuckler JM, Bernini PA, Wiesel SW, et al: The use of epidural steroids in the treatment of lumbar radicular pain. *J Bone Joint Surg Am* 67:63, 1985.

Davis MD, Sandroni P, Rooke TW, Law PA: Erythromelalgia: Vasculopathy, neuropathy, or both. *Arch Dermatol* 139:1337, 2003.

Epstein NE, Epstein JA, Carras R, Hyman RA: Far lateral lumbar disc herniations and associated structural abnormalities: An evaluation in 60 patients of the comparative value of CT, MRI and myelo-CT in diagnosis and management. *Spine* 15:534, 1990.

Ensrud Schousboe JT: Clinical practice. Vertebral fractures. *N Engl J Med* 364:1634, 2011.

Evans BA, Stevens JC, Dyck PJ: Lumbosacral plexus neuropathy. *Neurology* 31:1327, 1981.

Finneson BE: *Low Back Pain*, 2nd ed. Philadelphia, Lippincott, 1981.

Friis ML, Bulliksen GC, Rasmussen P: Distribution of pain with nerve root compression. *Acta Neurochir (Wien)* 39:241, 1977.

Hadler NM, Curtis P, Gillings DB: A benefit of spinal manipulation as adjunctive therapy for acute low-back pain: A stratified controlled trial. *Spine* 12:703, 1987.

Hagen KD, Hilde G, Jamtveldt G, Winnem MF: The Cochrane review of bed rest for acute low back pain. *Spine* 25:2932, 2000.

Hassler O: The human intervertebral disc: A micro-angiographical study on its vascular supply at various ages. *Acta Orthop Scand* 40:765, 1970.

Hudgkins WR: The crossed straight leg raising sign (of Fajersztajn). *N Engl J Med* 297:1127, 1977.

Jensen MC, Brant-Zawadzki MN, Obuchowski N, et al: Magnetic resonance imaging of the lumbar spine in people without back pain. *N Engl J Med* 331:69, 1994.

Kallmes DF, Comstock BA, Heagarty PJ, et al: A randomized trial of vertebroplasty for osteoporotic spinal fractures. *New Engl J Med* 361:569, 2009.

Kellgren JH: On the distribution of pain arising from deep somatic structures with charts of segmental pain areas. *Clin Sci* 4:35, 1939.

Kelsey JL, White AA: Epidemiology and impact of low back pain. *Spine* 5:133, 1980.

Kopell HP, Thompson WA: *Peripheral Entrapment Neuropathies*. Baltimore, Williams & Wilkins, 1963.

Kristoff FV, Odom GL: Ruptured intervertebral disc in the cervical region. *Arch Surg* 54:287, 1947.

Lance JW: The red ear syndrome. *Neurology* 47:617, 1996.

LaRocca H: Acceleration injuries of the neck. *Clin Neurosurg* 25:209, 1978.

Layzer RB: Hot feet: Erythromelalgia and related disorders. *J Child Neurol* 16:199, 2001.

Leffert RD: Thoracic outlet syndrome, in Omer G, Springer M (eds): *Management of Peripheral Nerve Injuries*. Philadelphia, Saunders, 1980.

Leyshon A, Kirwan EO, Parry CB: Electrical studies in the diagnosis of compression of the lumbar root. *J Bone Joint Surg Br* 63B:71, 1981.

Lilius G, Laasonen EM, Myllynen P, et al: Lumbar facet joint syndrome: A randomized clinical trial. *J Bone Joint Surg Br* 71:681, 1989.

Long DM: Low-back pain, in Johnson RT, Griffin JW (eds): *Current Therapy in Neurologic Disease*, 5th ed. St. Louis, Mosby, 1997, pp 71–76.

Lord SM, Barnsley L, Wallis BJ, et al: Percutaneous radio-frequency neurotomy for chronic cervical zygapophyseal joint pain. *N Engl J Med* 335:1721, 1996.

Love JG, Schorn VG: Thoracic-disc protrusions. *JAMA* 191:627, 1965.

Matthews WB: The neurological complications of ankylosing spondylitis. *J Neurol Sci* 6:561, 1968.

Malleson A: *Whiplash and Other Useful Illnesses*. Montreal, McGill-Queen's University Press, 2002.

McCall IW, Park WM, O'Brian JP: Induced pain referral from posterior lumbar elements in normal subjects. *Spine* 4:441, 1979.

Meade TW, Dyer S, Browne W, et al: Low back pain of mechanical origin: Randomised comparison of chiropractic and hospital out-patient treatment. *BMJ* 300:1431, 1990.

Michiels JJ, Van Joost TH, Vuzevski VD: Idiopathic erythromelalgia: A congenital disorder. *J Am Acad Dermatol* 21:1128, 1989.

Mikhael MA, Ciric I, Tarkington JA, et al: Neurologic evaluation of lateral recess syndrome. *Radiology* 140:97, 1981.

Mixter WJ, Barr JS: Rupture of the intervertebral disc with involvement of the spinal canal. *N Engl J Med* 211:210, 1934.

Ochoa JL: Pain mechanisms and neuropathy. *Curr Opin Neurol* 7:407, 1994.

Peul WC, van Houweilingen HC, van den Hout WB, et al: Surgery versus prolonged conservative treatment for sciatica. *N Engl J Med* 356:356, 2007.

Postacchini F, Urso S, Ferro L: Lumbosacral nerve-root anomalies. *J Bone Joint Surg Am* 64A:721, 1982.

Powell MC, Szypryt P, Wilson M, et al: Prevalence of lumbar disc degeneration observed by magnetic resonance in symptomless women. *Lancet* 2:1366, 1986.

Quiles M, Marchisello PJ, Tsairis R: Lumbar adhesive arachnoiditis: Etiologic and pathologic aspects. *Spine* 3:45, 1978.

Reynolds AF, Weinstein PR, Wachter RD: Lumbar monoradiculopathy due to unilateral facet hypertrophy. *Neurosurgery* 10:480, 1982.

Salvarini C, Cantini F, Boiardi L, Hunder GG: Polymyalgia rheumatica and giant-cell arteritis. *N Engl J Med* 347: 261, 2002.

Sano S, Itami S, Yoshikawa K: Treatment of primary erythromelalgia with cyclosporine. *N Engl J Med* 349:816, 2003.

Shannon N, Paul EA: L4/5, L5/S1 disc protrusions: Analysis of 323 cases operated on over 12 years. *J Neurol Neurosurg Psychiatry* 42: 804, 1979.

Sinclair DC, Feindel WH, Weddell G, et al: The intervertebral ligaments as a source of segmental pain. *J Bone Joint Surg* 30B:515, 1948.

Tarlov IM: Perineurial cysts of the spinal nerve roots. *Arch Neurol Psychiatry* 40:1067, 1938.

Tudler MW, Cherkin DC, Berman B, et al: Acupuncture for low back pain. *Cochrane Database Syst Rev* 2:CD001351, 2000.

van Gelderen C: Ein orthotisches (lordotisches) Kaudasyndrom. *Acta Psychiatr Neurol Scand* 23:57, 1948.

Verbiest H: A radicular syndrome from developmental narrowing of the lumbar vertebral canal. *J Bone Joint Surg Br* 36B: 230, 1954.

Vroomen P, DeKrom M, Wilmink JT, et al: Lack of effectiveness of bed rest for sciatica. *N Engl J Med* 340:418, 1999.

Weinstein JN: Balancing science and informed decisions about vertebroplasty. New Engl J Med 361:619, 2009.

Weinstein JN, Tosteson TD, Lurie JD, et al: Surgical versus nonsurgical treatment for lumbar spinal stenosis. *N Engl J Med* 358:794, 2008.

Weinstein JN, Tosteson TD, Lurie JD, et al: Surgical vs nonoperative treatment for lumbar disk herniation. The spine patients outcomes research trial (SPORT): a randomized trial. *JAMA* 296: 2441, 2006.

Weir BKA, Jacobs GA: Reoperation rate following lumbar discectomy. *Spine* 5:366, 1980.

White AH, Derby R, Wynne G: Epidural injections for the diagnosis and treatment of low-back pain. *Spine* 5:78, 1980.

Wilbourn AJ: The thoracic outlet syndrome is overdiagnosed. *Arch Neurol* 47:328, 1990.

Wilbourn AJ: Thoracic outlet syndromes: Plea for conservatism. *Neurosurg Clin N Am* 2:235, 1991.

Wray CC, Easom S, Hoskinson J: Coccydynia: Aetiology and treatment. *J Bone Joint Surg Br* 73B:335, 1991.

Yiannikas C, Walsh JC: Somatosensory evoked responses in the diagnosis of the thoracic outlet syndrome. *J Neurol Neurosurg Psychiatry* 46:234, 1983.

Yoss RE, Corbin KB, MacCarty CS, Love JG: Significance of symptoms and signs in localization of involved root in cervical disc protrusion. *Neurology* 7:673, 1957.

SECTION 3

Disorders of the Special Senses

The four chapters in this section are concerned with the clinical aspects of the highly specialized functions of taste and smell, vision, hearing, and the sense of balance. These special senses and the cranial nerves that subserve them represent the most finely developed parts of the sensory nervous system. Dysfunctions of the eye and ear are, of course, the domain of the ophthalmologist and otorhinolaryngologist, but they also are of great interest to the neurologist. Some defects in the special sensory apparatus reflect the presence of systemic disease and others represent the initial or leading manifestation of neurologic disease. In keeping with the general scheme of this text, the disorders of the special senses and of ocular movement are discussed in a particular sequence: first, certain facts of anatomic and physiologic importance, followed by cardinal clinical manifestations of disease, and then the syndromes of which these manifestations are a part.

12

Disorders of Smell and Taste

The sensations of smell (olfaction) and taste (gustation) are suitably considered together. Physiologically, these modalities share the singular attribute of responding primarily to chemical stimuli; i.e., the end organs that mediate olfaction and gustation are chemoreceptors. Also, taste and smell are interdependent clinically, as the appreciation of the flavor of food and drink depends to a large extent on their aroma, and an abnormality of one of these senses is frequently misinterpreted as an abnormality of the other. In comparison to sight and hearing, taste and smell play a less critical role in the life of the individual. However, chemical stimuli in communication between humans are probably very important for some functions that have not been fully explored. Pheromones (*pherein*, "to carry"; *hormon*, "exciting"), that is, odorants exuded from the body as well as perfumes, play a part in sexual attraction; noxious body odors repel. In certain vertebrates the olfactory system is remarkably well developed, rivaling the sensitivity of the visual system, but even humans, in whom the sense of smell is relatively weak, have the capacity to discriminate between as many as 10,000 different odorants (Reed).

Disorders of taste and smell can be persistently unpleasant, but only rarely is the loss of either of these modalities a serious handicap. Nevertheless, as all foods and inhalants pass through the mouth and nose, these two senses serve to detect noxious odors (e.g., smoke) and to avoid tainted food and potential poisons. The loss of these senses could then have serious consequences. Also, because a loss of taste and smell may signify a number of intracranial, neurodegenerative, and systemic disorders, they assume clinical importance.

OLFACTORY SENSE

Anatomic and Physiologic Considerations

Nerve fibers subserving the sense of smell have their cells of origin in the mucous membrane of the upper and posterior parts of the nasal cavity (superior turbinates and nasal septum). The entire olfactory mucosa covers an area of about 2.5 cm^2 and contains three cell types: the olfactory or receptor cells, which number between 6 and 10 million in each nasal cavity; sustentacular or supporting cells, which maintain the electrolyte (particularly K) levels in the extracellular milieu; and basal cells, which are stem cells and the source of both the olfactory and sustentacular cells during regeneration. The olfactory cells are actually bipolar neurons. Each of these cells has a peripheral process (the olfactory rod) from which project 10 to 30 fine hairs, or cilia. These hair-like processes, which lack motility, are the sites of olfactory receptors.

The central processes of these cells, or *olfactory fila*, are very fine (0.2 mm in diameter) unmyelinated fibers that converge to form small fascicles enwrapped by Schwann cells that pass through openings in the cribriform plate of the ethmoid bone into the olfactory bulb (Fig. 12-1). Collectively, the central processes of the olfactory receptor cells constitute the *first cranial (olfactory) nerve*. Notably, this is the only site in the body where neurons are in direct contact with the external environment. The epithelial surface is covered by a layer of mucus, which is secreted by tubuloalveolar cells (Bowman glands) and within which there are immunoglobulins A and M, lactoferrin, and lysoenzyme as well as odorant-binding proteins. These molecules are thought to prevent the intracranial entry of pathogens via the olfactory pathway (Kimmelman).

In the olfactory bulb, the receptor-cell axons synapse with granule cells and mitral cells (so-called because they are triangular, like a bishop's miter), the dendrites of which form brush-like terminals or olfactory glomeruli (Fig. 12-1). Smaller "tufted" cells in the olfactory bulb also contribute dendrites to the glomerulus. Approximately 15,000 olfactory-cell axons converge on a single glomerulus. This high degree of convergence is thought to account for an integration of afferent information. The mitral and tufted cells are excitatory; the granule cells—along with centrifugal fibers from the olfactory nuclei, locus ceruleus, and piriform cortex—inhibit mitral cell activity. Presumably, interaction between these excitatory and inhibitory neurons provides the basis for the special physiologic aspects of olfaction.

The axons of the mitral and tufted cells form the olfactory tract, which courses along the olfactory groove of the cribriform plate to the cerebrum. Lying caudal to the olfactory bulbs are groups of cells that constitute the anterior olfactory nucleus (Fig. 12-1). Dendrites of these cells synapse with fibers of the olfactory tract, while their

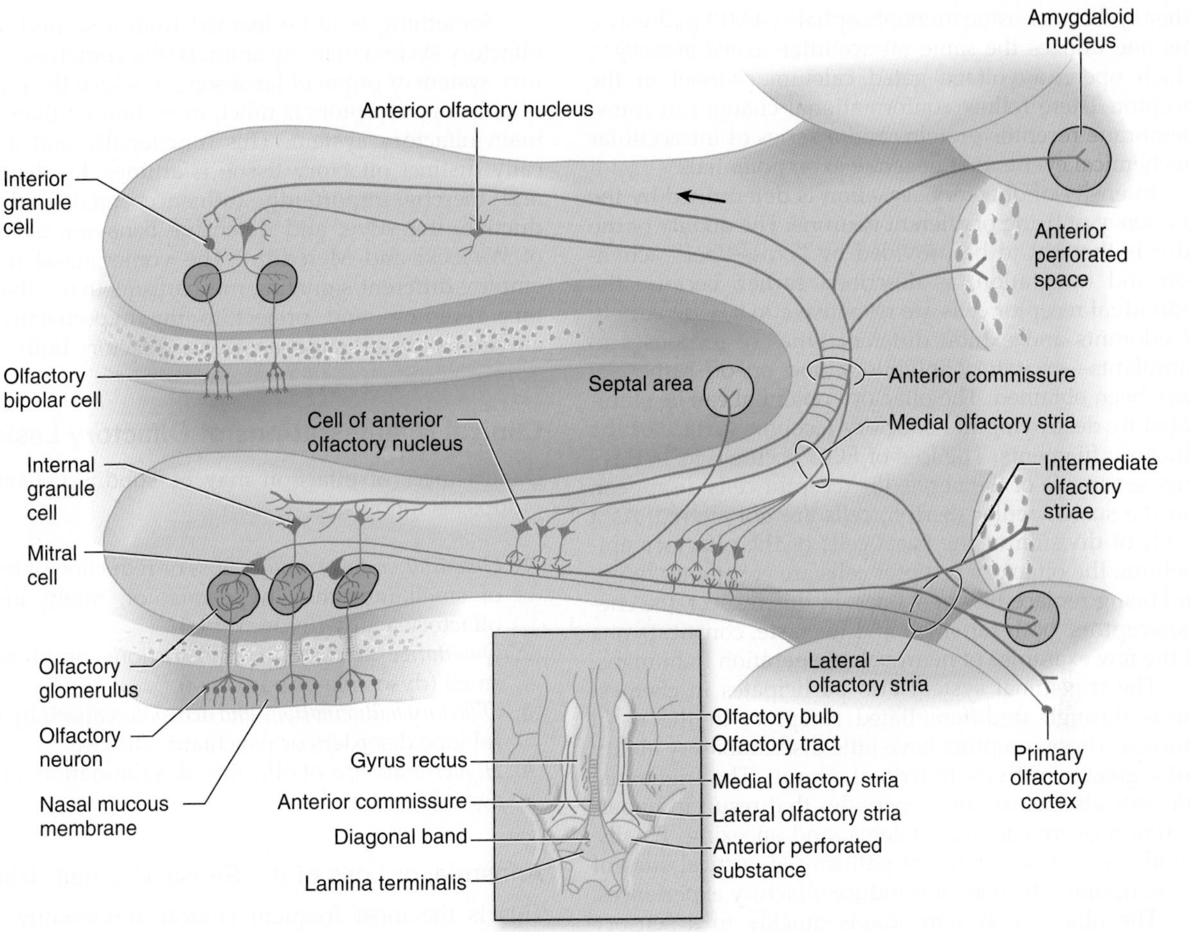

Figure 12-1. Diagram illustrating the relationships between the olfactory receptors in the nasal mucosa and neurons in the olfactory bulb and tract. Cells of the anterior olfactory nucleus are found in scattered groups caudal to the olfactory bulb. Cells of the anterior olfactory nucleus make immediate connections with the olfactory tract. They project centrally via the medial olfactory stria and to contralateral olfactory structures via the anterior commissure. *Inset:* diagram of the olfactory structures on the inferior surface of the brain (see text for details).

axons project to the olfactory nucleus and bulb of the opposite side; these neurons are thought to function as a reinforcing mechanism for olfactory impulses.

Posteriorly, the olfactory tract divides into medial and lateral olfactory striae. The medial stria contains fibers from the anterior olfactory nucleus; these pass to the opposite side via the anterior commissure. Fibers in the lateral stria originate in the olfactory bulb, give off collaterals to the anterior perforated substance, and terminate in the medial and cortical nuclei of the amygdaloid complex and the prepiriform area (also referred to as the lateral olfactory gyrus). The latter represents the *primary olfactory cortex*, which in humans occupies a restricted area on the anterior end of the parahippocampal gyrus and uncus (area 34 of Brodmann; see Figs. 22-1 and 22-2). Thus olfactory impulses reach the cerebral cortex without a relay through the thalamus; in this respect also, olfaction is unique among sensory systems. From the prepiriform cortex, fibers project to the neighboring entorhinal cortex (area 28 of Brodmann) and the medial dorsal nucleus of the thalamus; the amygdaloid nuclei connect with the hypothalamus and septal nuclei. The role of these latter structures in olfaction is not well understood, but presumably they subserve reflexes related to eating and sexual function. As with all sensory systems, feedback regulation occurs at every point in the afferent olfactory pathway.

In quiet breathing, little of the air entering the nostril reaches the olfactory mucosa; sniffing carries the air into the olfactory crypt, which contains the olfactory receptors. To be perceived as an odor, an inhaled substance must be volatile—i.e., spread in the air as very small particles—and soluble in water. Molecules provoking the same odor seem to be related by their shape than by their chemical quality. When a jet of scented vapor is directed to the sensory epithelium, as by sniffing, a slow negative potential shift called the *electroolfactogram* (EOG) can be recorded from an electrode placed on the mucosa. The conductance changes that underlie this receptor potential are induced by molecules of odorous material dissolved in the mucus overlying the receptor.

The transduction of odorant stimuli to electrical signals is mediated in part by a guanosine triphosphate (GTP)-dependent adenylyl cyclase ("G protein"). Like other cyclic adenosine monophosphate (AMP) pathways, this one utilizes the same intracellular *second messenger*, which opens a voltage gated calcium channel in the receptor. There follow conformational changes in transmembrane receptor proteins and a series of intracellular biochemical events that generate axon potentials.

Intensity of olfactory sensation is determined by the frequency of firing of afferent neurons. The quality of the odor is thought to be provided by "cross-fiber" activation and integration, as described earlier, because the individual receptor cells are responsive to a wide variety of odorants and exhibit different types of responses to stimulants—excitatory, inhibitory, and on–off responses have been obtained. The olfactory potential can be eliminated by destroying the olfactory receptor surface or the olfactory filaments. The loss of EOG occurs 8 to 16 days after severance of the nerve; the receptor cells disappear, but the sustentacular (Sertoli) cells are not altered. As a result of division of the basal cells of the olfactory epithelium, the olfactory receptor cells are constantly dying and being replaced by new ones. In this respect, the chemoreceptors, both for smell and for taste, constitute one of the few examples of neuronal regeneration in humans.

The trigeminal system also participates in chemesthesis through undifferentiated receptors in the nasal mucosa. These receptors have little discriminatory ability but a great sensitivity to irritant stimuli. The trigeminal afferents also release neuropeptides that result in hypersecretion of mucus, local edema, and sneezing. Finally, stimulation of the olfactory pathway at cortical sites of the temporal lobe may also induce olfactory experiences.

The olfactory system adapts quickly to a sensory stimulus, and for sensation to be sustained, there must be repeated stimulation. The olfactory sense differs from other senses in yet another way. It is common experience that an aroma can restore long-forgotten memories of complex experiences. That olfactory and emotional stimuli are strongly linked is not surprising in view of their common roots in the limbic system. Yet, paradoxically, the ability to recall an odor is negligible in comparison with the ability to recall sounds and sights. As Vladimir Nabokov has remarked, "Memory can restore to life everything except smells." It is also interesting that dreams do not embody olfactory experiences.

The remarkable evolutionary role of olfactory receptors can be appreciated by the fact that about 2 percent of the human genome exists to express unique odorant receptors (over 500 distinct genes). The wide diversity of these transmembrane proteins permits subtle differentiation of thousands of different odorant molecules, as delineated by Young and Trask and the genetic basis for which Buck and Axel were awarded a Nobel Prize.

This specificity for molecules is encoded neuroanatomically. Different odorant molecules activate specific olfactory receptors. Each olfactory neuron expresses only one allele of one receptor gene. Moreover, each olfactory glomerulus receives inputs from neurons expressing only one type of odorant receptor. In this way, each of the glomeruli is attuned to a distinct type of odorant stimulus. Presumably, this encoding is preserved in the olfactory cortex.

Something is to be learned from a second, distinct olfactory system in many animals (the vomeronasal olfactory system or organ of Jacobson), in which the repertoire of olfactory receptors is much more limited than in their main olfactory system. This functionally and anatomically distinct olfactory tissue is attuned to pheromones and thereby importantly influences menstrual, reproductive, ingestive, and defensive behavior (see review of Wysocki and Meredith). The vomeronasal receptors employ different signaling mechanisms than other olfactory receptors and project to the hypothalamus and amygdala via a distinct accessory olfactory bulb.

Clinical Manifestations of Olfactory Lesions

Disturbances of olfaction may be subdivided into four groups, as follows:

1. *Quantitative abnormalities:* loss or reduction of the sense of smell (anosmia, hyposmia) or, rarely, increased olfactory acuity (hyperosmia)
2. *Qualitative abnormalities:* distortions or illusions of smell (dysosmia or parosmia)
3. *Olfactory hallucinations and delusions* caused by temporal lobe disorders or psychiatric disease
4. *Higher-order loss* of olfactory discrimination (olfactory agnosia)

Anosmia, or Loss of the Sense of Smell (Table 12-1)

This is the most frequent clinical abnormality and, if unilateral, usually is not recognized by the patient. Unilateral anosmia can sometimes be demonstrated in the hysterical patient on the side of anesthesia, blindness, or deafness. Bilateral anosmia, on the other hand, is a common complaint, and the patient is usually convinced that the sense of taste has been lost as well (*ageusia*). This calls attention to the fact that taste depends largely on the volatile particles in foods and beverages, which reach the olfactory receptors through the nasopharynx, and that the perception of flavor is a combination of smell, taste, and tactile sensation. This can be proved by demonstrating that patients with anosmia but without a complaint of ageusia are able to distinguish the elementary taste sensations on the tongue (sweet, sour, bitter, and salty). The olfactory defect can be verified readily enough by presenting a series of nonirritating olfactory stimuli (vanilla, peanut butter, coffee, tobacco) and asking the patient to sniff once and identify them. If the odors can be detected and described, even if they cannot be named, it may be assumed that the olfactory nerves are relatively intact (humans can distinguish many more odors than they can identify by name). If they cannot be detected, there is an olfactory defect. Ammonia and similar pungent substances are unsuitable stimuli because they do not test the sense of smell but have a primary irritating effect on the mucosal-free nerve endings of the trigeminal nerves.

The value of testing smell in one nostril at a time has been questioned, for example by Welge-Luessen and colleagues, who studied olfactory groove meningiomas.

Table 12-1

MAIN CAUSES OF ANOSMIA

Nasal
Smoking
Chronic rhinitis (allergic, atrophic, cocaine, infectious—herpes, influenza)
Overuse of nasal vasoconstrictors
Olfactory epithelium
Head injury with tearing of olfactory filaments
Cranial surgery
Subarachnoid hemorrhage, meningitis
Toxic (organic solvents, certain antibiotics—aminoglycosides, tetracyclines, corticosteroids, methotrexate, opiates, L-dopa)
Metabolic (thiamine and B12 deficiency, adrenal and thyroid deficiency, cirrhosis, renal failure, menses)
Wegener granulomatosis
Compressive and infiltrative lesions (craniopharyngioma, meningioma, aneurysm, meningoencephalocele)
Central
Degenerative diseases (Parkinson, Alzheimer, Huntington)
Temporal lobe epilepsy
Malingering and hysteria

They found, contrary to expectations, that this test was not sensitive to the presence of a unilateral lesion, ostensibly because of mixing of air in the nasopharynx. Nonetheless, other experience suggests that rapidly sniffing through one nostril does briefly allow segregation of each side of the nasal cavities and can detect unilateral lesions.

A more elaborate scratch-and-sniff test has been developed and standardized by Doty and colleagues (University of Pennsylvania Smell Identification Test). In this test the patient attempts to identify 40 microencapsulated odorants, and olfactory performance is compared with that of age- and sex-matched normal individuals. Unique features of this test are a means for detecting malingering and amenability to self-administration. Air-dilution olfactory detection is an even more refined way of determining thresholds of sensation and of demonstrating normal olfactory perception in the absence of odor identification. The use of olfactory evoked potentials is being investigated in some electrophysiology laboratories, but their reliability is uncertain. These last two refined techniques are essentially research tools and are not used in neurologic practice.

The loss of smell usually falls into one of three categories: *nasal* (in which odorants do not reach the olfactory receptors), *olfactory neuroepithelial* (caused by destruction of receptors or their axon filaments), and *central* (olfactory pathway lesions).

Viewed from another perspective, in an analysis of 4,000 cases of anosmia from specialized clinics, Hendriks found that the three most common diagnoses were viral infection of the upper respiratory tracts (the largest group), nasal or paranasal sinus disease, and head injury.

Regarding the nasal diseases responsible for bilateral hyposmia or anosmia, the most frequent are those in which hypertrophy and hyperemia of the nasal mucosa prevent olfactory stimuli from reaching the receptor cells. Heavy smoking is probably the most frequent cause of hyposmia in clinical practice. Chronic atrophic rhinitis; sinusitis of allergic, vasomotor, or infective types; nasal polyposis; and overuse of topical vasoconstrictors are other common causes. Biopsies of the olfactory mucosa in cases of allergic rhinitis have shown that the sensory epithelial cells are still present, but their cilia are deformed and shortened and are buried under other mucosal cells. Influenza, herpes simplex, and hepatitis virus infections may be followed by hyposmia or anosmia caused by destruction of receptor cells; if the basal cells are also destroyed, this may be permanent. These cells may also be affected as a result of atrophic rhinitis and local radiation therapy or by a rare type of tumor (*esthesioneuroblastoma*) that originates in the olfactory epithelium. There is also a group of uncommon diseases in which the primary receptor neurons are congenitally absent or hypoplastic and lack cilia. One of these is the Kallmann syndrome of congenital anosmia and hypogonadotropic hypogonadism. A similar disorder occurs in Turner syndrome and in albinos because of an ill-defined congenital structural defect.

Anosmia that follows head injury is most often a result of tearing of the delicate filaments of the receptor cells as they pass through the cribriform plate, especially if the injury is severe enough to cause fracture. The damage may be unilateral or bilateral. With closed head injury, complete anosmia is relatively infrequent (6 percent of Sumner's series of 584 cases), but lesser degrees are common in our experience. Some recovery of olfaction occurs in about one-third of cases over a period of several days to months. Beyond 6 to 12 months, recovery is negligible. Cranial surgery, subarachnoid hemorrhage, and chronic meningeal inflammation may have similar effects.

In some of the cases of traumatic anosmia, there is also a loss of taste (ageusia). Ferrier, who first described traumatic ageusia in 1876, noted that there was always anosmia as well—an observation subsequently corroborated by Sumner. Often, the ageusia also clears within a few weeks. A bilateral traumatic lesion near the frontal operculum and paralimbic region, where olfactory and gustatory receptive zones are in close proximity, would best explain this concurrence, but this has not been proven. As stated earlier, the interruption of olfactory filaments alone would explain a reduction in the ability to perceive the subtleties of specific flavors, but not ageusia.

Olfactory acuity varies throughout the menstrual cycle, possibly through the imputed vomeronasal system in humans, and may be disordered during pregnancy. Nutritional and metabolic diseases such as thiamine deficiency (Wernicke disease), vitamin A deficiency, adrenal and perhaps thyroid insufficiency, cirrhosis, and chronic renal failure may give rise to anosmia, all as a result of sensorineural dysfunction. A large number of toxic agents—the more common ones being organic solvents (benzene), metals including platinum-containing chemotherapies, dusts, cocaine, corticosteroids, methotrexate, aminoglycoside antibiotics, tetracyclines, opiates, and L-dopa—can damage the olfactory epithelium (Doty et al). Alcoholics with Korsakoff psychosis also have a defect in odor discrimination (Mair et al). In this disorder, anosmia is presumably caused by degeneration of neurons in the higher-order olfactory systems involving the medial thalamic nuclei.

Anosmia has been found in some patients with temporal lobe epilepsy and particularly in such patients who had been subjected to anterior temporal lobectomy. In these conditions, Andy and coworkers have found impairment in discriminating the quality of odors and in matching odors with test objects seen or felt.

As with other sensory modalities, olfaction (and taste) is diminished with aging (presbyosmia). The receptor cell population is depleted, and if the loss is regional, neuroepithelium is slowly replaced with respiratory epithelium (which is normally present in the nasal cavity and serves to filter, humidify, and warm incoming air). Neurons of the olfactory bulb may also be reduced as part of the aging process.

Bilateral anosmia has been a manifestation of *malingering*, now that it has been recognized as a compensable disability. The fact that true anosmics will complain inordinately of a loss of taste (but show normal taste sensation) may help to separate them from malingerers. If it were to be perfected, testing of olfactory evoked potentials would be of use here.

The nasal epithelium or the olfactory nerves themselves may be affected in Wegener granulomatosis and by craniopharyngioma, respectively. A meningioma of the olfactory groove may implicate the olfactory bulb and tract and may extend posteriorly to involve the optic nerve, sometimes with optic atrophy; if combined with papilledema on the opposite side, these abnormalities are known as the Foster Kennedy syndrome (see Chap. 13). A large aneurysm of the anterior cerebral or anterior communicating artery may produce a similar constellation. With tumors confined to one side, the anosmia may be strictly unilateral, in which case it will not be reported by the patient but will be found on examination. The limitations of testing each side of the nose separately have been mentioned earlier. These defects in the sense of smell are attributable to lesions of either the receptor cells and their axons or the olfactory bulbs, and current test methods do not distinguish between lesions in these two localities. In some cases of increased intracranial pressure, olfactory sense has been impaired without evidence of lesions in the olfactory bulbs.

The term *specific anosmia* has been applied to an unusual olfactory phenomenon in which a person with normal olfactory acuity for most substances encounters a particular compound or class of compounds that is odorless to him, although obvious to others. In a sense, this is a condition of "smell blindness," analogous to color blindness. The basis of this disorder is unclear, although there is evidence that specific anosmia for musky and uriniferous odors is inherited as an autosomal recessive trait (see Amoore).

Whether a true *hyperosmia* exists is a matter of conjecture, but it is so frequently reported by migraineurs that the problem seems worthy of attention. Anxious, highly introspective individuals may complain of being unduly sensitive to odors, but there is no proof of an actual change in their threshold of perception of odors. This issue comes into play in institutions with large numbers of persons who claim to be "chemosensitive" to certain odors and induce a ban on these substances. The validity of this claim is in doubt.

Olfaction in Neurodegenerative Disease Hyman and colleagues have emphasized the many earlier observations of an early neuronal degeneration in the olfactory region of the hippocampus in cases of Alzheimer disease, Lewy body, and Parkinson disease. Moreover, a large proportion of patients with other degenerative diseases of the brain have anosmia or hyposmia. A number of theories have been proposed to explain the initial loss of smell, the most relevant of which is based on the finding that the earliest neuropathologic changes of many neurodegenerative processes begin in olfactory structures and then appears serially in neighboring structures, only later reaching the parts of the brain that produces the characteristic neurologic features of these diseases. The implication from these findings, originating with Braak and Braak, has been that Lewy bodies in particular are caused by a pathogen that enters through the peripheral olfactory system and proceeds centrally through the medial temporal lobe. Prions have been suggested as a candidate agent because of their ability to alter protein folding and to transfer this property in a sequentially topographic manner. The studies relating to olfaction in Parkinson disease have been reviewed by Doty, Braak and colleagues. and Benarroch. It should be emphasized to patients, however, that the reverse is not the case; i.e., the majority of individuals with hyposmia do not have a generalized neurodegenerative disease.

Dysosmia or Parosmia

These terms refer to distortions of odor perception where an odor is present. Parosmia may occur with local nasopharyngeal conditions such as infection of the nasal sinuses and upper respiratory infections. In some instances, the abnormal tissue itself may be the source of unpleasant odors; in others, where partial injuries of the olfactory bulbs have occurred, parosmia is in the nature of an olfactory illusion. Parosmia may also be a troublesome symptom in persons with depressive and psychotic illnesses, who may report that every article of food has an extremely unpleasant odor (cacosmia). Sensations of disagreeable taste are often associated (cacogeusia). Nothing is known of the basis of this state; there is usually no loss of discriminative sensation.

The treatment of parosmia is difficult. The use of neuroleptic or antiepileptic drugs has given unpredictable results. Claims for the efficacy of zinc and vitamins have not been verified (and there is a risk that zinc administration may interfere with the absorption of copper). Some reports indicate that repeated anesthetization of the nasal mucosa reduces or abolishes the parosmic disturbance. In many cases, the disorder subsides spontaneously. Minor degrees of parosmia are not necessarily abnormal, for unpleasant odors have a way of lingering for several hours and of being reawakened by other olfactory stimuli, as every pathologist knows.

Olfactory Hallucinations

The report of an odor without stimulus, olfactory hallucination, is always of central origin. The patient perceives an odor that no one else can detect (phantosmia). Most often this a manifestation of temporal lobe seizures ("uncinate fits"), in which circumstances the olfactory hallucinations are brief and accompanied or followed by an alteration of consciousness and other manifestations of epilepsy (see Chap. 16 on epilepsy).

If the patient is convinced of the presence of what is in fact a hallucination and also gives it personal origin, the symptom assumes the status of a delusion (a fixed false belief). The combination of olfactory hallucinations and delusions of this type signifies a psychiatric illness. Zilstorff wrote informatively on this subject. There is often a complaint of a large array of odors, most of them noxious and seemingly emanating from the patient (intrinsic hallucinations); in others, they are attributed to an external source (extrinsic hallucinations). Both types vary in intensity and are remarkable with respect to their persistence. They may be combined with gustatory hallucinations. According to Pryse-Phillips, who took note of the psychiatric illness in a series of 137 patients with olfactory hallucinations, most were associated with endogenous depression or schizophrenia. In schizophrenia, the olfactory stimulus is usually interpreted as arising externally, and as being induced by someone for the purpose of upsetting the patient. In depression, the perception is of the stimulus being intrinsic. The patient may go to great lengths to rid himself of the perceived odor, the usual ones being excessive washing and use of deodorants; the condition may lead to social withdrawal. There is reason to believe that the amygdaloid group of nuclei is the source of the hallucinations, as stereotactic lesions here have reportedly ameliorated both the olfactory hallucinations and the psychiatric disorder (see Chitanondh).

Olfactory hallucinations and delusions may occur in conjunction with Alzheimer dementia, but one should also consider the possibility of a late-life depression.

Loss of Olfactory Discrimination (Olfactory Agnosia)

Finally, one must consider a disorder in which the primary perceptual aspects of olfaction (detection of odors, adaptation to odors, and recognition of different intensities of the same odor) are intact, but the capacity to distinguish between odors and their recognition by quality is impaired or lost. In the writings on this subject, this deficit is usually referred to as a disorder of olfactory discrimination. In dealing with other sense modalities, however, the inability to identify and name a perceived sensation would be called an *agnosia*. To recognize this deficit requires special testing, such as matching to sample, the identification and naming of a variety of scents, and determining whether two odors are identical or different.

Such an alteration of olfactory function has been shown to characterize patients with the alcoholic form of Korsakoff psychosis; this impairment is not attributable to impaired olfactory acuity or to failure of learning and memory (Mair et al). As indicated above, the olfactory disorder in the alcoholic Korsakoff patient is most likely caused by lesions in the medial dorsal nucleus of the thalamus; several observations in animals indicate that this nucleus and its connections with the orbitofrontal cortex give rise to deficits in odor discrimination (Mair et al; Slotnick and Kaneko). Eichenbaum and associates demonstrated a similar impairment of olfactory capacities in a patient who had undergone extensive bilateral medial temporal lobe resections. The operation was believed to have eliminated a substantial portion of the olfactory afferents to the frontal cortex and thalamus, although there was no anatomic verification of this. In patients with stereotactic or surgical amygdalotomies, Andy and coworkers noted a similar reduction in odor discrimination. Thus it appears that both portions of the higher olfactory pathways (medial temporal lobes, and medial dorsal nuclei) are necessary for the discrimination and identification of odors.

GUSTATORY SENSE

Anatomic and Physiologic Considerations

The sensory receptors for taste (taste buds) are distributed over the surface of the tongue and, in smaller numbers, over the soft palate, pharynx, larynx, and esophagus. Mainly they are located in the epithelium along the lateral surfaces of the circumvallate and foliate papillae and to a lesser extent on the surface of the fungiform papillae. The taste buds are round or oval structures, each composed of up to 200 vertically oriented receptor cells arranged like the staves of a barrel. The superficial portion of the bud is marked by a small opening, the taste pore or pit, which opens onto the mucosal surface. The tips of the sensory cells project through the pore as a number of filiform microvilli ("taste hairs"). Fine, unmyelinated sensory fibers penetrate the base of the taste bud and synapse directly with the sensory taste cells, which have no axons.

The taste receptors are activated by chemical substances in solution and transmit their activity along the sensory nerves to the brainstem. There are four primary and readily tested taste sensations that have been long known: salty, sweet, bitter, and sour; recently a fifth, *umani,* signifying a savory taste—the taste of glutamate, aspartate, and certain ribonucleotides—has been added. The full range of taste sensations is much broader, consisting of combinations of these elementary gustatory sensations. Older notions of a "tongue map," which implied the existence of specific areas sub-serving one or another taste, are incorrect. Any one taste bud is capable of responding to a number of sapid substances, but it is always preferentially sensitive to one type of stimulus. In other words, the receptors are only relatively specific. The sensitivity of these receptors is remarkable: as little as 0.05 mg/dL of quinine sulfate will arouse a bitter taste when applied to the base of the tongue.

A G-protein transduction system (gustducin), similar to the one for olfaction, has been found to be operative in signaling taste sensations in the tongue receptors. A discussion of this system can be found in the commentary by Brand.

The receptor cells of the taste buds have a brief life cycle (about 10 days), being replaced constantly by mitotic division of adjacent basal epithelial cells. The number of taste buds, not large to begin with, is gradually reduced with age; also, changes occur in the taste cell membranes, with impaired function of ion channels and receptors (Mistretta). Gustatory (and olfactory) acuity diminishes with age (everything begins to taste and smell the same). According to Schiffman, taste thresholds for salt, sweeteners, and amino acids are 2 to 2.5 times higher in the elderly than in the young. The reduction in the acuity of taste and smell with aging may lead to a distortion of food habits (e.g., excessive use of salt and other condiments) and contribute to the anorexia and weight loss of elderly persons.

Richter has explored the biologic role of taste in normal nutrition. Animals made deficient in sodium, calcium, certain vitamins, proteins, etc., will automatically select the correct foods, on the basis of their taste, to compensate for their deficiency. Interesting genetic polymorphisms in the receptor for sweet substances in rats have been found to underlie differences in the proclivity to ingest sweet substances, and a similar system has been proposed in humans (Chaudhari and Kinnamon).

Neural Innervation of the Tongue

Sensory impulses for taste arise from several sites in the oropharynx and are transmitted to the medulla via several cranial nerves (V, VII, IX, and X). The main pathway arises on the *anterior two-thirds of the tongue;* these taste fibers first run in the lingual nerve (a major branch of the mandibular-trigeminal [V] cranial nerve). After coursing within the lingual nerve for a short distance, the taste fibers diverge to enter the chorda tympani (a branch of the seventh nerve); thence they pass through the pars intermedia and geniculate ganglion of the seventh nerve to the rostral part of the nucleus of the tractus solitarius in the posterolateral medulla, where all taste afferents converge (see below and Fig. 47-3).

From the *posterior one-third of the tongue,* soft palate, and palatal arches, the sensory taste fibers are conveyed via the glossopharyngeal (IX) nerve and ganglion nodosum to the nucleus of the tractus solitarius. Taste fibers from the extreme dorsal part of the tongue and the few that arise from taste buds on the pharynx and larynx run in the vagus nerve. The *gustatory nucleus* is situated in the rostral and lateral parts of the nucleus tractus solitarius, which receive the special afferent (taste) fibers from the facial and glossopharyngeal nerves. Probably both sides of the tongue are represented in this nucleus.

Fibers from the palatal taste buds pass through the pterygopalatine ganglion and greater superficial petrosal nerve, join the facial nerve at the level of the geniculate ganglion, and proceed to the nucleus of the solitary tract (see Fig. 47-3). Possibly, some taste fibers from the tongue may also reach the brainstem via the mandibular division of the trigeminal nerve. The presence of this alternative pathway probably accounts for reported instances of unilateral taste loss that have followed section of the root of the trigeminal nerve and instances in which no loss of taste has occurred with section of the chorda tympani.

The second sensory neuron for taste has been difficult to track. Neurons from the gustatory segment of the nucleus solitarius project to adjacent nuclei (e.g., dorsal motor nucleus of the vagus, ambiguus, salivatorius superior and inferior, trigeminal, and facial nerves), which serve viscerovisceral and viscerosomatic reflex functions, but those concerned with the conscious recognition of taste are currently considered to form an ascending pathway to a pontine parabrachial nucleus. From the latter, two ascending pathways have been traced (in animals). One is the solitariothalamic lemniscus to the ventroposteromedial nucleus of the thalamus. A second passes to the ventral parts of the forebrain, to parts of the hypothalamus (which probably influences autonomic function), and to other basal forebrain limbic areas in or near the uncus of the temporal lobe. Other ascending fibers lie near the medial lemniscus and are both crossed and uncrossed. Experiments in animals indicate that taste impulses from the thalamus project to the tongue–face area of the postrolandic sensory cortex. This is probably the end station of gustatory projections in humans as well, insofar as gustatory hallucinations have been produced by electrical stimulation of the parietal and/or rolandic opercula (Hausser-Hauw and Bancaud). Penfield and Faulk evoked distinct taste sensations by stimulating the anterior insula.

Clinical Manifestations of Disorders of Taste

Testing of Taste Sensation

Unilateral gustatory impairment can be identified by withdrawing the tongue with a gauze sponge and using a moistened applicator to place a few crystals of salt, sugar, lemon (sour), and quinine (bitter) on discrete parts of the tongue; the tongue is then wiped clean and the subject is asked to report what he had sensed. One use of such testing is to corroborate the existence of Bell palsy by comparing taste sensation on each side of the anterior tongue (see Chap. 47). A stimulus that has been used as a surrogate for sour sensation is a low-voltage direct current, the electrodes of which can be accurately placed on the tongue surface. If the taste loss is bilateral, mouthwashes with a dilute solution of sucrose, sodium chloride, citric acid, and quinine may be used. After swishing, the test fluid is spit out and the mouth rinsed with water. The patient indicates whether he had tasted a substance and is asked to identify it. Special types of apparatus (electrogustometers) have been devised for the measurement of taste intensity and for determining the detection and recognition thresholds of taste and olfactory stimuli (Krarup; Henkin et al), but these are beyond the needs of the usual clinical examination.

Causes of Loss of Taste

Apart from the loss of taste sensation that accompanies normal aging, smoking is probably the most common cause of impairment of taste sensation. Extreme drying of the tongue from any cause may lead to temporary loss or reduction of the sense of taste (*ageusia* or *hypogeusia*), as saliva is essential for normal taste function. Saliva acts as a solvent for chemical substances in food and for conveying them to taste receptors. Dryness of the mouth (xerostomia) from inadequate saliva, as occurs in Sjögren syndrome; hyperviscosity of saliva, as in cystic fibrosis; irradiation of head and neck; and pandysautonomia all interfere with taste. Also, in familial dysautonomia (Riley-Day syndrome), the number of circumvallate and fungiform papillae is reduced, accounting for a diminished ability to taste sweet and salty foods. If unilateral, ageusia is seldom the source of complaint. Taste is frequently lost over the anterior two-thirds of one side of the tongue in cases of mundane Bell palsy, as indicated above and in Chap. 47.

A permanent decrease in the acuity of taste and smell (hypogeusia and hyposmia), sometimes associated with perversions of these sensory functions (dysgeusia and dysosmia), may follow influenza-like illnesses. These abnormalities have been associated with pathologic changes in the taste buds as well as in the nasal mucous membranes. In a group of 143 patients who presented with hypogeusia and hyposmia, 87 were of this postinfluenzal type, as determined by Henkin and colleagues; the remainder developed their symptoms in association with scleroderma, acute hepatitis, viral encephalitis, myxedema, adrenal insufficiency, malignancy, deficiency of vitamins B and A, and the administration of a wide variety of drugs. Also, according to Schiffman, more than 250 drugs have been implicated in the alteration of taste sensation, making it necessary to consider virtually all drugs as a cause of taste loss. Lipid-lowering drugs, antihistamines, antimicrobials, antineoplastics, bronchodilators, antidepressants, and antiepileptics are the main offenders, but little is known about the mechanisms by which drugs induce these effects. More obvious is altered taste because of nasally and orally administered inhalant drugs, including the "triptans" for migraine and a variety of antiallergy and antiasthmatic medications.

Distortions of taste and loss of taste are sources of complaint in patients with certain local malignant tumors. Oropharyngeal tumors may, of course, abolish taste by invading the chorda tympani or lingual nerves and basal skull. Malnutrition because of neoplasm or radiation therapy may also cause ageusia. Some patients with certain cancers remark on a reduced perception for bitter foods, and some who have been radiated for breast cancer or sublingual or oropharyngeal tumors find sour foods intolerable. The loss of taste from radiation of the oropharynx is usually recovered within a few weeks or months; the reduced turnover of taste buds caused by radiation therapy usually recovers.

An interesting syndrome of *idiopathic hypogeusia*—in which decreased taste acuity is associated with dysgeusia, hyposmia, and dysosmia—has been described by Henkin, Schechter and colleagues. Food has an unpleasant taste and aroma, to the point of being revolting (cacogeusia and cacosmia); the persistence of these symptoms may lead to a loss of weight, anxiety, and depression.

Unilateral lesions of the medulla oblongata have not been reported to cause ageusia, perhaps because the nucleus of the tractus solitarius is usually outside the zone of infarction or because there is representation from both sides of the tongue in each nucleus. Unilateral thalamic and parietal lobe lesions, however, have both been associated with contralateral impairment of taste sensation in rare cases.

As indicated above, a gustatory aura occasionally marks the beginning of a seizure originating in the frontoparietal (suprasylvian) cortex or in the uncal region. Gustatory hallucinations are much less frequent than olfactory ones. Nevertheless, gustatory sensations were reported in 30 of 718 cases of intractable epilepsy (Hausser-Hauw and Bancaud). During surgery, these investigators produced an aura of disagreeable taste by electrical stimulation of the parietal and frontal opercula, and also by stimulation of the hippocampus and amygdala (uncinate seizures). In their view, the low-threshold seizure focus for taste in the temporal lobe is secondary to functional disorganization of the opercular gustatory cortex by the seizure. Gustatory hallucinations were more frequent with right-hemisphere lesions, and in half of the cases, the gustatory aura was followed by a convulsion.

Zinc supplements are contained in over-the-counter and complementary medical products aimed at improving smell and appetite and for the treatment of incipient colds. We have had no opportunity to confirm the often-cited benefits of zinc on any of these conditions, and the supporting evidence is sparse, however, the continued administration of zinc in high doses has been associated with the development of copper deficiency and a myeloneuropathy (see Chap. 38).

Burning Mouth Syndrome Another poorly defined disorder is the *burning mouth syndrome*, which occurs mainly in postmenopausal women and is characterized by persistent, severe intraoral pain (particularly of the tongue). We have seen what we believe to be fragmentary forms of the syndrome in which pain and burning are isolated to the alveolar ridge or gingival mucosa. The oral mucosa appears normal and some patients may report a diminution of taste sensation. A small number of such patients prove to have diabetes, Sjögren syndrome, or vitamins B_2 or B_{12} deficiency (causing glossitis), but in most no systemic illness or local abnormality can be found. Many such patients that we have encountered appeared to have a depressive illness, but they responded only inconsistently to administration of antidepressants. A few patients have this oral complaint as a component of a small fiber neuropathy or ganglionopathy (see Chap. 46). Clonazepam may be useful, and capsaicin has been tried with uncertain results. This disorder is also commented on in Chap. 10.

References

Amoore JE: Specific anosmias, in Getchell TV, Bartoshuk LM, Doty RL, Snow JB (eds): *Smell and Taste in Health and Disease*. New York, Raven Press, 1991, pp 655–664.

Andy OJ, Jurko MF, Hughes JR: The amygdala in relation to olfaction. *Confin Neurol* 37:215, 1975.

Benarroch EE: Olfactory system. Functional organization and involvement in neurodegenerative disease. *Neurology* 75:1104, 2010.

Brand JG: Within reach of an end to unnecessary bitterness. *Lancet* 356:1371, 2000.

Buck LB: Smell and taste: The chemical senses, in Kandel ER, Schwartz JH, Jessel TM (eds): *Principles of Neural Science*, 4th ed. New York, McGraw-Hill, 2000, pp 625–647.

Braak H, Ghebremedhin E, Rub U, et al: Stages of development of Parkinson's disease-related pathology. *Cell Tissue Res* 318:121, 2004.

Chitanondh H: Stereotaxic amygdalotomy in the treatment of olfactory seizures and psychiatric disorders with olfactory hallucinations. *Confin Neurol* 27:181, 1966.

Chaudhari N, Kinnamon SC: Molecular basis of the sweet tooth? *Lancet* 358:210, 2001.

Doty RL: Olfactory dysfunction in neurodegenerative disorders, in Getchell TV, Bartoshuk LM, Doty RL, Snow JB (eds): *Smell and Taste in Health and Disease*. New York, Raven Press, 1991, pp 735–751.

Doty RL, Shaman P, Applebaum SL: Smell identification ability: Changes with age. *Science* 226:1441, 1984.

Doty RL, Shaman P, Dann M: Development of University of Pennsylvania Smell Identification Test. *Physiol Behav* 32:489, 1984.

Eichenbaum H, Morton TH, Potter H, Corkin S: Selective olfactory deficits in case H.M. *Brain* 106:459, 1983.

Getchell TV, Bartoshuk LM, Doty RL, Snow JB Jr (eds): *Smell and Taste in Health and Disease*. New York, Raven Press, 1991.

Hausser-Hauw C, Bancaud J: Gustatory hallucinations in epileptic seizures. *Brain* 110:339, 1987.

Hendriks AP: Olfactory dysfunction. *Rhinology* 4:229, 1988.

Henkin RI, Gill JR Jr, Bartter FC: Studies on taste thresholds in normal man and in patients with adrenal cortical insufficiency: The effect of adrenocorticosteroids. *J Clin Invest* 42:727, 1963.

Henkin RI, Larson AL, Powell RD: Hypogeusia, dysgeusia, hyposmia and dysosmia following influenza-like infection. *Ann Otol Rhinol Laryngol* 84:672, 1975.

Henkin RI, Schechter PJ, Hoye R, Mattern CFT: Idiopathic hypogeusia with dysgeusia, hyposmia, and dysosmia: A new syndrome. *JAMA* 217:434, 1971.

Hyman BT, van Hoesen GW, Damasio AR: Alzheimer disease: Cell specific pathology isolates the hippocampal formation. *Science* 225:1168, 1984.

Kimmelman CP: Clinical review of olfaction. *Am J Otolaryngol* 14:227, 1993.

Krarup B: Electrogustometry: A method for clinical taste examinations. *Acta Otolaryngol* 69:294, 1958.

Mair R, Capra C, McEntee WJ, Engen T: Odor discrimination and memory in Korsakoff's psychosis. *J Exp Psychol* 6:445, 1980.

Mistretta CM: Aging effects on anatomy and neurophysiology of taste and smell. *Gerontology* 3:131, 1984.

Penfield W, Faulk ME: The insula: Further observations on its function. *Brain* 78:445, 1955.

Pryse-Phillips W: Disturbances in the sense of smell in psychiatric patients. *Proc R Soc Med* 68:26, 1975

Quinn NP, Rossor MN, Marsden CD: Olfactory threshold in Parkinson's disease. *J Neurol Neurosurg Psychiatry* 50:88, 1987

Reed RR: The molecular basis of sensitivity and specificity in olfaction. *Semin Cell Biol* 5:33, 1994.

Richter CP: Total self-regulatory functions in animals and human beings. *Harvey Lect* 38:63, 1942–1943.

Schiffman SS: Drugs influencing taste and smell perception, in Getchell TV, Bartoshuk LM, Doty RL, Snow RL (eds): *Smell and Taste in Health and Disease*. New York, Raven Press, 1991, pp 845–850.

Schiffman SS: Taste and smell losses in normal aging and disease. *JAMA* 276:1357, 1997.

Slotnick BM, Kaneko N: Role of mediodorsal thalamic nucleus in olfactory discrimination learning in rats. *Science* 214:91, 1981.

Sumner D: Disturbances of the senses of smell and taste after head injuries, in Vinken PJ, Bruyn GW (eds): *Handbook of Clinical Neurology*. Vol 24. Amsterdam, North-Holland, 1975, pp 1–25.

Sumner D: Post-traumatic ageusia. *Brain* 90:187, 1967.

Welge-Luessen A, Temmel A, Quint C, et al: Olfactory function in patients with olfactory groove meningiomas. *J Neurol Neurosurg Psychiatry* 70:218, 2001.

Wysocki CJ, Meredith H: The vomeronasal system, in Finger TE, Silver WL (eds): *Neurobiology of Taste and Smell*. New York, Wiley, 1987, pp 125–150.

Young JM, Trask BJ. The sense of smell: Genomics of vertebrate odorant receptors. *Hum Mol Genet* 11:1153, 2002.

Zilstorff W: Parosmia. *J Laryngol Otol* 80:1102, 1966.

13

Disturbances of Vision

The importance of the visual system is attested by the magnitude of its representation in the central nervous system (CNS). A large part of the cerebrum is committed to vision, including the visual control of movement and the perception of printed words, and the form and color of objects. The optic nerve, which is a CNS structure, contains more than a million fibers (compared to 50,000 in the auditory nerve). The visual system also has special significance in that study of this system has greatly advanced our knowledge of both the organization of all sensory neuronal systems and the relation of perception to cognition. Indeed, we know more about vision than about any other sensory function. Furthermore, the eyes, because of their diverse composition of epithelial, vascular, neural, and pigmentary tissues, are virtually a medical microcosm, susceptible to many diseases, and its tissues are available for inspection through a transparent medium.

Impairment of visual function, expressed as defects in acuity and alterations of visual fields, obviously stands as the most important symptom of eye disease. A number of terms are commonly used to describe visual loss. *Amaurosis* is a general term that refers to partial or complete loss of sight. *Amblyopia* refers to any monocular deficit in vision that occurs in the presence of normal ocular structures. A major cause of amblyopia is the suppression by the brain of vision from one eye during early childhood caused by either strabismus, anisometropia (a significant difference in refractive error), or by media opacities. *Nyctalopia* is the term for poor twilight or night vision and is associated with extreme myopia, cataracts, vitamin A deficiency, retinitis pigmentosa, and, often, color blindness. There are also a number of positive visual symptoms (phosphenes, migrainous scintillations, visual illusions, and hallucinations), but they are generally less significant than symptoms of visual loss. Irritation, redness, photophobia, pain, diplopia and strabismus, changes in pupillary size, and drooping or closure of the eyelids are other major ocular symptoms and signs. Impairment of vision may be unilateral or bilateral, sudden or gradual, episodic or enduring.

The common causes of failing eyesight vary with age. In infancy, congenital defects, retinopathy of prematurity, severe myopia, hypoplasia of the optic nerve, optic pits, and coloboma are the main causes. In childhood and adolescence, nearsightedness or myopia, and amblyopia as a result of strabismus are the usual causes (see Chap. 14), although a pigmentary retinopathy or a retinal, optic nerve, or suprasellar tumor may also begin at this age. In middle age, usually beginning in the fifth decade, a progressive loss of accommodation (presbyopia) is almost invariable (at this age, half or more of the amplitude of accommodative power is lost and must be replaced by plus lenses). Still later in life, cataracts, glaucoma, retinal vascular occlusion and detachments, macular degeneration, and tumor, unilateral or bilateral, are the most frequent causes of visual impairment.

As a rule, *episodic visual loss* in early adult life, often hemianopic, is the result of migraine. The other important cause of transient (weeks) monocular visual loss in this age period is optic neuritis, often a harbinger of multiple sclerosis. Amaurosis in the child or young adult may also be caused by systemic lupus erythematosus and the related antiphospholipid syndrome, or by migraine, or there may be no discernible cause. Later in life, transient monocular blindness, or *amaurosis fugax*, lasting minutes to hours is more common; it is caused by vascular disease, particularly stenosis of the ipsilateral carotid artery. Table 13-1 lists the main causes of episodic monocular visual loss. Of course, at any age, diseases of the retina and of other components of the ocular apparatus are important causes of *progressive visual loss*, and the problem may at first be transient.

APPROACH TO THE PROBLEM OF VISUAL LOSS

In the investigation of a disturbance of vision, one inquires as to what the patient means when he claims that he cannot see properly, for the disturbance in question may vary from near- or farsightedness to diplopia, partial syncope, dizziness, or a hemianopia. Fortunately, the patient's statement can be checked by the measurement of visual acuity, which is the single most important part of the ocular examination. Inspection of the refractive media and the optic fundi—especially the macular region—the testing of pupillary reflexes, color vision, and the plotting of visual fields complete this part of the

Table 13-1

CAUSES OF EPISODIC VISUAL LOSS

Adolescence and young adulthood
Migraine
Optic neuritis
Papilledema
Antiphospholipid antibody syndrome and systemic lupus erythematosus
Early tumor compression of the optic nerve
Takayasu aortic arteritis
Viral neuroretinitis
Idiopathic
Adulthood
Carotid stenosis or dissection
Embolism to the retina
Intrinsic central retinal artery atherosclerotic disease
Temporal arteritis (generally over age 55)
Glaucoma
Papilledema

examination. Examination of the eye movements is also essential, particularly if amblyopia predicated on an early life strabismus is suspected, as discussed in Chap. 14.

In the measurement of distance visual acuity the *Snellen chart*, which contains letters (or numbers or pictures) arranged in rows of decreasing size, is used (Fig. 13-1*A*). Each eye is tested separately and, if glasses are required, glasses for distance, not reading glasses, should be worn. The letter at the top of the chart subtends 5 min of an arc at a distance of 200 ft (or roughly 60 m). The patient follows rows of letters that can normally be read at lesser distances. Acuity is reported as a nonmathematical fraction that represents the patient's ability compared to that of a person with normal distance vision. Thus, if the patient can read only the top letter, which would be normally be visible at 200 feet, the acuity is expressed as 20/200, or if the distance is measured in meters rather than feet, as 6/60. If the patient's eyesight is normal, the visual acuity will equal 20/20, or 6/6, corresponding to the eighth line on most charts. Many persons, especially during youth, can read at 20 ft the line that can normally be read at 15 ft from the chart (20/15) and hence have better than "normal" vision.

For bedside testing, a "near card" or newsprint held 14 in from the eyes can be used, and the results expressed in a distance equivalent as if a distance chart had been used (Fig. 13-1*B*). Here, the Jaeger system is used (J1 is "normal" vision, corresponding to the line 20/25 on a Snellen chart, J5 to 20/50, J10 to 20/100, J16 to 20/200, and so on). In young children, acuity can be estimated by having them mimic the examiner's finger movements at varying distances or having them recognize and pick up objects of different sizes from varying distances. The Teller acuity cards test a child's preference (and hence

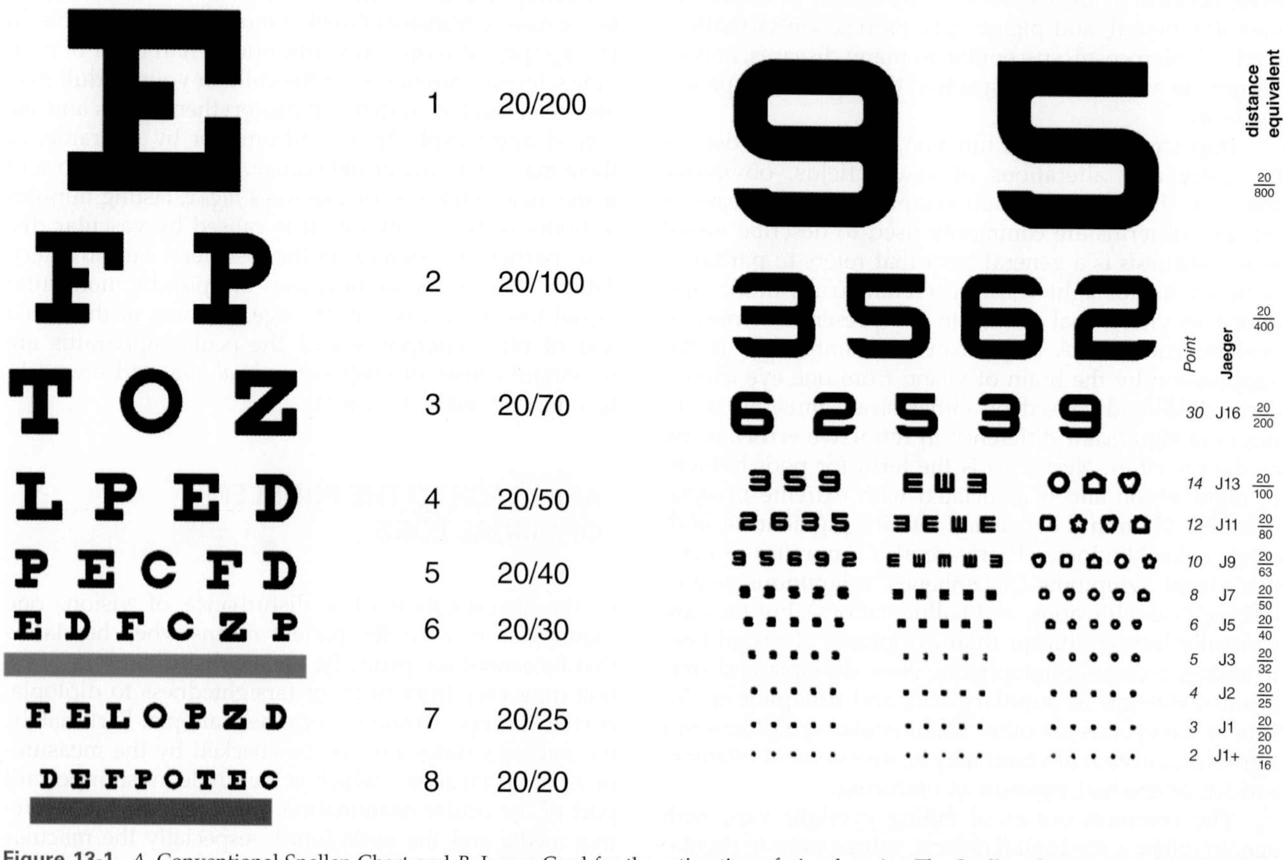

Figure 13-1. *A*. Conventional Snellen Chart and *B*. Jaeger Card for the estimation of visual acuity. The Snellen chart is placed 20 feet from the subject. The Jaeger card is used at 16 inches from the subject's eyes and approximates Snellen acuity if convergence and accommodation are normal.

ability) to view cards with increasingly fine stripes. In most jurisdictions, a corrected acuity of 20/40 or better in one eye is required to obtain and retain a driver's license.

If the visual acuity (with glasses) is less than 20/20, either the refractive error has not been properly corrected or there is some other reason for diminished acuity. The possibility of a nonrefractive error can usually be ruled out if the patient can read the 20/20 line (not the near card) through a pinhole in a cardboard held in front of the eye. The pinhole permits a narrow shaft of light to fall on the fovea (the area of greatest visual acuity) without distortion by the curvature of the lens; this eliminates the eye's optical system, thereby testing the macula alone, and should give an acuity of 20/20 if the structures of the ocular media (cornea, lens, aqueous and vitreous humors) are clear.

Light entering the eye is focused by the biconvex lens onto the outer layer of the retina. Consequently, the cornea, fluid of the anterior chamber, lens, vitreous, and retina itself must be transparent. The clarity of these media can be determined ophthalmoscopically, and a complete examination requires that the pupil be dilated to at least 6 mm in diameter. This is accomplished by instilling two drops of 2.5 percent phenylephrine and/or 0.5 to 1.0 percent tropicamide in each eye after the visual acuity has been measured, the pupillary response recorded, and the intraocular pressure estimated. In elderly persons, lower concentrations of these mydriatics should be used. The mydriatic action of phenylephrine lasts for 3 to 6 h. Rarely, an *attack of angle-closure glaucoma* (manifesting itself by diminished vision, ocular pain, nausea, and vomiting) may be precipitated by pharmacologic pupillary dilatation; this requires the administration of pilocarpine to the eye and the immediate attention of an ophthalmologist. It is advisable to have access to pilocarpine if the pupils are to be dilated.

By looking through a high-plus lens of the direct ophthalmoscope from a distance of 6 to 12 in, the examiner can visualize opacities in the refractive media; by adjusting the lenses from a high-plus to a zero or minus setting, it is possible to "depth-focus" from the cornea to the retina. Depending on the refractive error of the examiner, lenticular opacities are best seen within the range of +20 to +12. The retina comes into focus with +1 to -1 lenses. The illuminated pupil appears as a red circular structure (red reflex), the color being provided by blood in the capillaries of the choroid layer. If all the refractile media are clear, reduced vision that is uncorrectable by glasses is caused by a defect in the macula, the optic nerve, or parts of the brain with which they are connected. The main limit of direct ophthalmoscopy is its inability to visualize lesions in the retina that lie anterior to the equator of the globe; these are seen only by the indirect method.

NONNEUROLOGIC CAUSES OF REDUCED VISION

It is hardly possible within the confines of this chapter to describe all the causes of opacification of the refractive media. Those with the most important medical or neurologic implications are briefly commented upon. Although changes in the refractive media do not involve neural tissue primarily, certain ones assume importance because they are associated with neurologic disease and provide clues to its presence.

In the *cornea*, the most common abnormality that reduces vision is scarring caused by trauma and infection. Ulceration and subsequent fibrosis may occur following recurrent herpes simplex, herpes zoster, and trachomatous infections of the cornea, or with certain mucocutaneous-ocular syndromes (Stevens-Johnson, Reiter). Hypercalcemia secondary to sarcoidosis, hyperparathyroidism, and vitamin D intoxication or milk-alkali syndrome may give rise to precipitates of calcium phosphate and carbonate beneath the corneal epithelium, primarily in a plane corresponding to the interpalpebral fissure—so-called band keratopathy. Other causes of corneal opacity include chronic uveitis, interstitial keratitis, corneal edema, lattice corneal dystrophy (amyloid deposition), and long-standing glaucoma. Polysaccharides are deposited in the corneas in some of the mucopolysaccharidoses (see Chap. 37), and copper is deposited in the Descemet membrane in hepatolenticular degeneration (Kayser-Fleischer ring). Crystal deposits may be observed in multiple myeloma and cryoglobulinemia. The corneas are also diffusely clouded in certain lysosomal storage diseases (see Chap. 37). Arcus senilis occurring at an early age (because of hyperlipidemia), sometimes combined with yellow lipid deposits in the eyelids and periorbital skin (xanthelasma), serves as a marker of atheromatous vascular disease.

In the *anterior chamber* of the eye, a common problem is impediment to the outflow of aqueous fluid, associated with excavation of the optic disc and visual loss, i.e., *glaucoma*. In more than 90 percent of cases (of the open-angle type), the cause of this syndrome is unknown and a genetic factor is suspected. The drainage channels in this type appear normal. In approximately 5 percent of cases, the angle between iris and the peripheral cornea is narrow and blocked when the pupil is dilated (angle-closure glaucoma). In the remaining cases, the condition is a result of some disease process that blocks outflow channels—inflammatory debris of uveitis, red blood cells from hemorrhage in the anterior chamber (hyphema), new formation of vessels and connective tissue on the surface of the iris (rubeosis iridis), a relatively infrequent complication of ocular ischemia secondary to diabetes mellitus, retinal vein occlusion, or carotid artery occlusion. The visual loss is gradual in open-angle glaucoma and the eye looks normal, unlike the red, painful eye of angle-closure glaucoma that was described above in reference to pharmacologic dilation of the pupil to facilitate fundoscopy. However, some cases of open-angle glaucoma may progress to rapid loss of vision.

Intraocular pressures that are persistently above 20 mm Hg may damage the optic nerve over time. This may be manifest first as an arcuate defect in the upper or lower nasal field or as a paracentral field defect, which, if untreated, may proceed to blindness. The classic finding in glaucoma is the *Bjerrum field defect*, consisting of an arcuate scotoma extending from the blind spot and sweeping around the macula to end in a horizontal line at the nasal equator. Other characteristic glaucomatous field patterns are winged extensions from the blind spot (Seidel scotoma) and a narrowing of the superior nasal quadrant that may progress to a horizontal edge, corresponding to the horizontal raphe of the retina (nasal step). The damage is at the optic nerve head, the optic disc appearing excavated and any pallor that is present extends only to the rim of the disc and not beyond, thus distinguishing it from other optic neuropathies. Elongation of the optic cup in the vertical axis is typical. It is now appreciated that elevated intraocular pressure is only a concurrent finding and a risk factor for glaucoma and that optic damage may be seen in patients with near normal pressure. This represents a major revision of the previous view that pressure was the elemental cause of damage in glaucoma.

In the *lens*, cataract formation is the most common and mundane abnormality. The cause of the common type in the elderly is unknown. The "sugar cataract" of diabetes mellitus is the result of sustained high levels of blood glucose, which is changed in the lens to sorbitol, the accumulation of which leads to a high osmotic gradient with swelling and disruption of the lens fibers. Galactosemia is a much rarer cause, but the mechanism of cataract formation is similar, i.e., the accumulation of dulcitol in the lens. In hypoparathyroidism, lowering of the concentration of calcium in the aqueous humor is in some way responsible for the opacification of newly forming superficial lens fibers. Prolonged high doses of corticosteroids, as well as radiation therapy, induce lenticular opacities in some patients. Down syndrome and oculocerebrorenal syndrome (see Chap. 38), spinocerebellar ataxia with oligophrenia (see Chap. 39), and certain dermatologic syndromes (atopic dermatitis, congenital ichthyosis, incontinentia pigmenti) are also accompanied by lenticular opacities. Myotonic dystrophy (see Chap. 48) and, rarely, Wilson disease (see Chap. 37) are associated with special types of cataract. Subluxation of the lens, the result of weakening of its zonular ligaments, occurs in syphilis, Marfan syndrome (upward displacement), and homocystinuria (downward displacement).

In the *vitreous humor*, hemorrhage may occur from rupture of a ciliary or retinal vessel. On ophthalmoscopic examination, the hemorrhage appears as a diffuse haziness of part or all of the vitreous or, if the blood is between the retina and the vitreous and displaces the latter rather than mixing with it, takes the form of a sharply defined clot. The common cause is rupture of newly formed vessels of proliferative retinopathy in patients with diabetes mellitus, but there are many others including orbital or cranial trauma, rupture of an intracranial aneurysm or arteriovenous malformation with high intracranial pressure, retinal vein occlusion, sickle cell disease, age-related macular degeneration (ARMD), and retinal tears, in which the hemorrhage breaks through the internal limiting membrane of the retina. The most common vitreous opacities are benign "floaters" caused by the condensation of vitreous collagen fibers, which appear as darting gray flecks or threads with changes in the position of the eyes; they may be annoying or even alarming until the person stops looking for them.

A sudden burst of flashing lights associated with an increase in floaters may mark the onset of retinal detachment. Patients complaining of bright flashes and spots in vision should be examined with the indirect ophthalmoscope to rule out tears, holes, or detachments of the vitreous or retina. Another common occurrence with advancing age is shrinkage of the vitreous humor and retraction from the retina, causing persistent streaks of light, usually in the periphery of the visual field. These phosphenes, also known as *Moore lightning streaks*, had been thought to be quite benign, but they may at times, indicate incipient retinal or vitreous tears or detachment, and their first appearance requires prompt evaluation by an ophthalmologist. They are most prominent on movement of the globe, on closure of the eyelids, at the moment of accommodation, with saccadic eye movements, and with sudden exposure to dark. The vitreous may also be infiltrated by lymphoma originating in the brain; biopsy by planar vitrectomy may be used to establish the diagnosis in those rare instances where the lymphoma is restricted to the eye; its presence can be inferred when there is vitreous cellular infiltration and also a brain lymphoma.

The term *uveitis* refers to an infective or noninfective inflammatory disease that affects any of the uveal structures (iris, ciliary body, and choroid). According to Bienfang and colleagues, uveitis accounts for 10 percent of all cases of legal blindness in the United States. Infective causes of posterior uveitis (choroidal) are toxoplasmal and cytomegalic inclusion disease, occurring mainly in patients with AIDS and other forms of reduced immune function. Noninfective autoimmune types are also common in the adult. The inflammation may be in the anterior part of the eye or in the posterior part, behind the iris and extending to the retina and choroid. Anterior uveitis is sometimes linked to ankylosing spondylitis and the human leukocyte antigen (HLA) B-27 marker, sarcoidosis, and recurrent meningitis (Vogt-Koyanagi-Harada disease); the posterior forms are associated with sarcoidosis, Behçet disease, and lymphoma.

Retinal diseases, particularly ARMD and diabetic retinopathy, are a more common cause of blindness than are neurologic diseases, as discussed further on, under "Other Diseases of the Retina."

NEUROLOGIC CAUSES OF REDUCED VISION

Certain anatomic and physiologic facts are required for an interpretation of the neurologic lesions that affect vision. Visual stimuli entering the eye traverse the inner layers of the retina to reach its outer (posterior) layer, which contains two classes of photoreceptor cells: the flask-shaped cones and the slender rods. The photoreceptors rest on a single layer of pigmented epithelial cells, which form the outermost surface of the retina. The rods and cones and pigmentary epithelium receive their blood supply from the capillaries of the choroid and, to a smaller extent, from the retinal arterioles. The rod cells contain rhodopsin, a conjugated protein in which the chromophore group is a carotenoid akin to vitamin A. The rods function in the perception of visual stimuli in subdued light (twilight or scotopic vision), and the cones are responsible for color discrimination and the perception of stimuli in bright light (photopic vision). Most of the cones are concentrated in the macular region, particularly in its central part, the *fovea*, and are responsible for the highest level of visual acuity. Traquair described the rapid fall-off of acuity as the distance from the fovea increases as "an island of vision in a sea of blindness." Specialized pigments in the rods and cones absorb light energy and transform it into electrical signals, which are transmitted to the bipolar cells of the retina and then, in turn, to the superficially (anteriorly) placed neurons, or ganglion cells (Fig. 13-2). There are no ganglion cells in the fovea.

The axons of the retinal ganglion cells, as they stream across the inner surface of the retina, pursue an arcuate course. Being unmyelinated, they are not visible, although fluorescein retinography shows a trace of their outlines; an experienced examiner, using a bright light and deep green filter, can visualize them through direct ophthalmoscopy. The axons of ganglion cells are collected in the optic discs and then pass uninterruptedly through the *optic nerves*, *optic chiasm*, and *optic tracts* to synapse in the lateral geniculate nuclei, the superior colliculi, the midbrain pretectum and the suprachiasmatic nucleus of the hypothalamus (Figs. 13-2 and 13-3). The fibers derived from macular cells form a discrete bundle that first occupies the temporal side of the disc and optic nerve and then assumes a more central position within the nerve (papillomacular bundle). These fibers are of smaller caliber than the peripheral optic nerve fibers and appear to be especially sensitive to toxic and metabolic injury. Damage to the papillomacular bundle produces the "cecocentral" scotoma (extending from fixation to the blind spot). It is important to keep in mind that the retinal ganglion cells and their axon extensions are, properly speaking, an exteriorized part of the brain and that their pathologic reactions are the same as in other parts of the CNS.

In the optic chiasm, the fibers derived from the nasal half of each retina decussate and continue in the optic tract with the uncrossed temporal fibers of the other eye (Figs. 13-3 and 13-4). Thus, interruption of the left optic tract causes a right hemianopic defect in each eye, i.e., a homonymous (left nasal and right temporal) field defect (Fig. 13-3*D*). In partial tract lesions, the visual defects in the

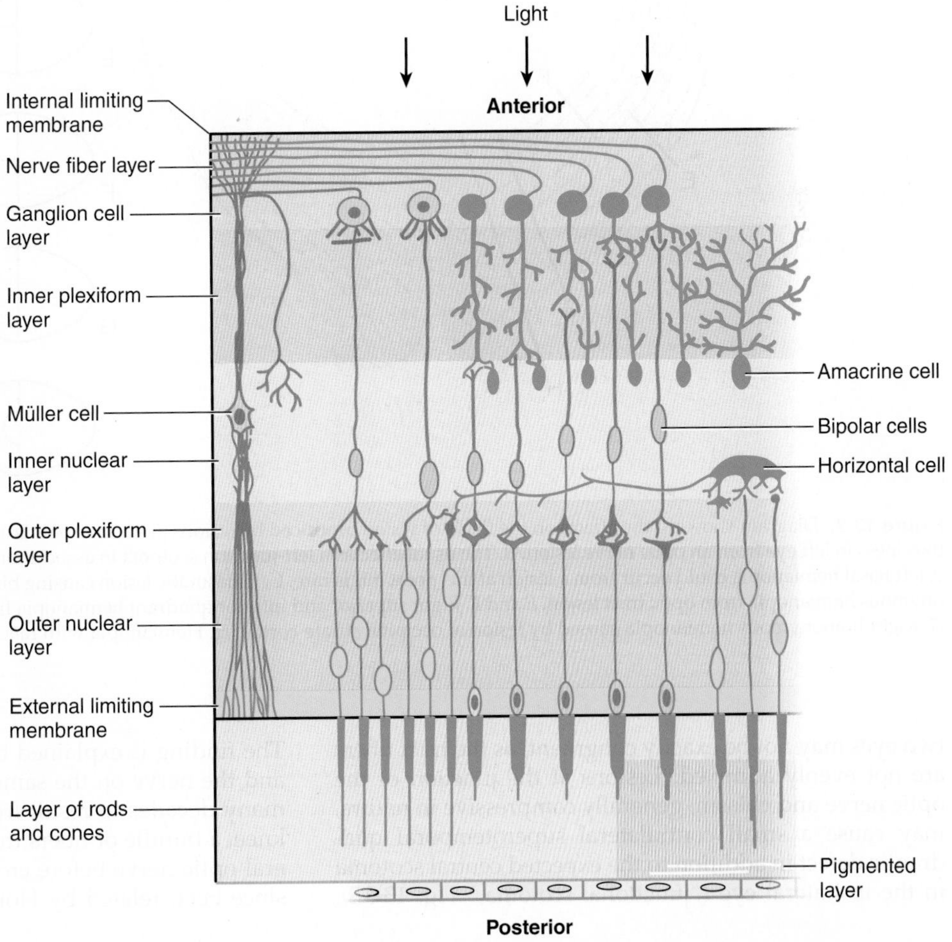

Figure 13-2. Diagram of the cellular elements of the retina. Light entering the eye anteriorly passes through the full thickness of the retina to reach the rods and cones (first system of retinal neurons). Impulses arising in these cells are transmitted by the bipolar cells (second system of retinal neurons) to the ganglion cell layer. The third system of visual neurons consists of the ganglion cells and their axons, which run uninterruptedly through the optic nerve, chiasm, and optic tracts, synapsing with cells in the lateral geniculate body. (Courtesy of Dr. E.M. Chester.)

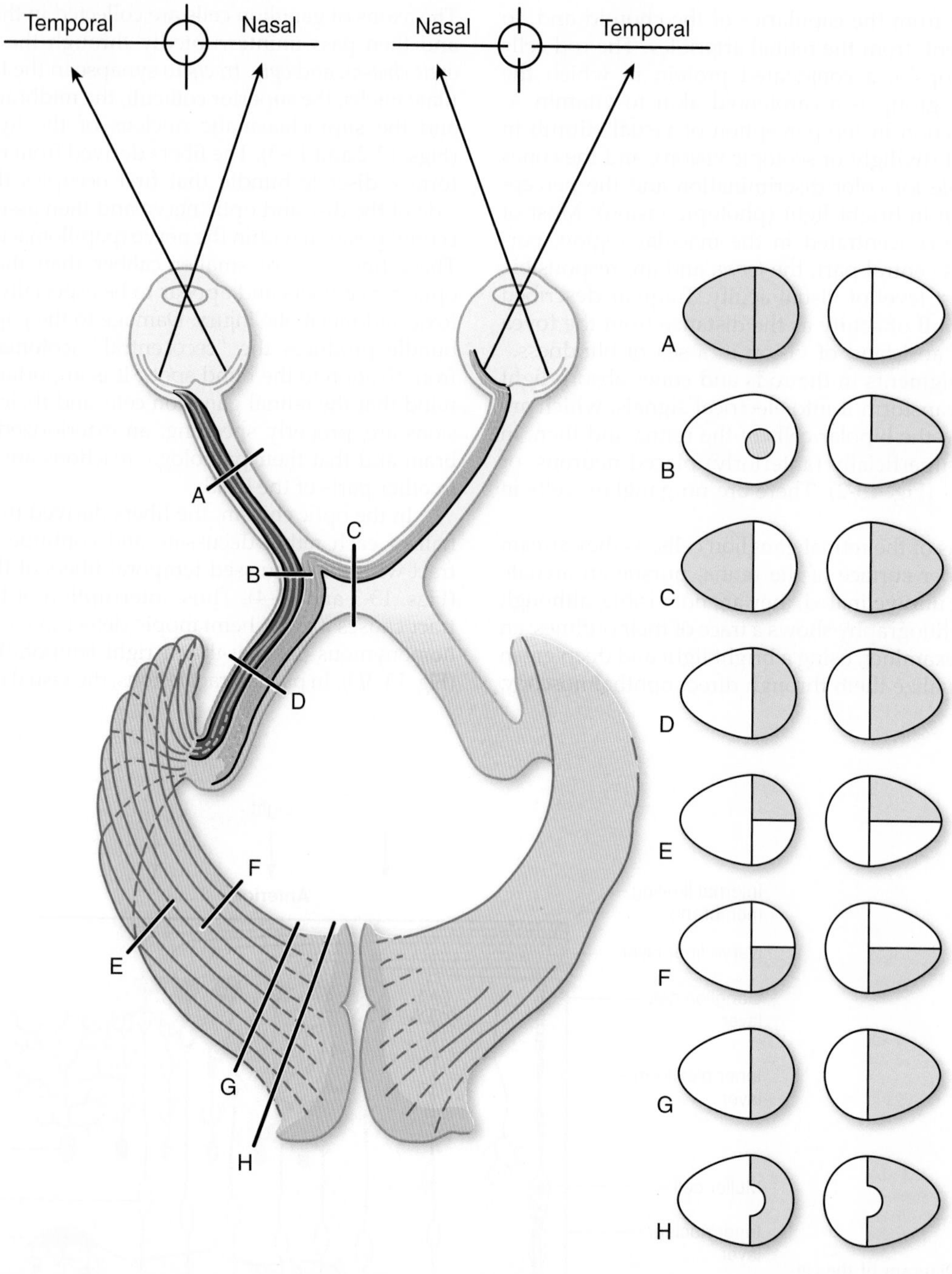

Figure 13-3. Diagram showing the effects on the fields of vision produced by lesions at various points along the optic pathway. *A*. Complete blindness in left eye from an optic nerve lesion. *B*. The usual effect is a left-junction scotoma in association with a right upper quadrantanopia. A left nasal hemianopia could occur from a lesion at this point but is rare. *C*. Chiasmatic lesion causing bitemporal hemianopia. *D*. Right homonymous hemianopia from optic tract lesion. *E* and *F*. Right superior and inferior quadrant hemianopia from interruption of visual radiations. *G*. Right homonymous hemianopia caused by lesion of occipital striate cortex. *H*. Hemianopia with macular sparing.

two eyes may not be exactly congruent, as the tract fibers are not evenly admixed. Lesions at the junction of the optic nerve and chiasm, generally compressive in nature, may cause a small contralateral superotemporal quadrantic defect in addition to the expected central scotoma in the ipsilateral eye ("junctional scotoma," Fig. 13-3*B*). The finding is explained by the compression of the tract and the nerve on the same side. It had been thought for many decades to result from compression of Wilbrand's knee, a bundle of fibers that turn back into the contralateral optic nerve before crossing in the chiasm, but it has since been related by Horton that the very existence of

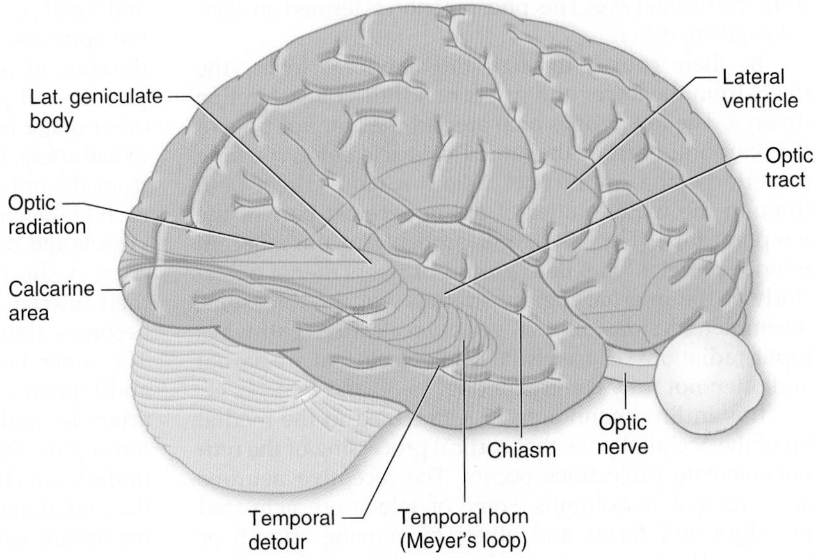

Figure 13-4. The geniculocalcarine projection, showing the detour of lower fibers around the temporal horn. Note that a very small proportion of the pathway traverses the parietal lobe.

the bundle is merely an artifact of fixation in experimental material. We are uncertain if the explanation of this particular configuration of visual field abnormality has a better explanation than the existence of Wilbrand's knee and are reluctant to discard it.

The optic chiasm lies just above the pituitary gland and also forms part of the anterior wall of the third ventricle; hence the crossing fibers may be compressed from below by a pituitary tumor, a meningioma of the tuberculum sellae, or an aneurysm, and from above by a dilated third ventricle or craniopharyngioma. The resulting field defect is bitemporal ("bitemporal hemianopia"; Fig. 13-3C); if the lesion has an anterior extension to the junction with one optic nerve there is a loss of full-field vision in that eye and a partial loss in the other ("functional scotoma"). Optic tract lesions, in comparison with chiasmatic and optic nerve lesions, are relatively rare and cause a full contralateral hemianopia. In albinism, there is an abnormality of chiasmatic decussation, in which a majority of the fibers cross to the other side. How this relates to the global albinic defect in pigmented epithelium is not known.

Approximately 80 percent of the fibers of the optic tract terminate in the lateral geniculate body, a thalamic nucleus, and synapse with the six laminae of its neurons. Three of these laminae (1, 4, 6), which constitute the large dorsal nucleus, receive crossed (nasal) fibers from the contralateral eye, and three (2, 3, 5) receive uncrossed (temporal) fibers from the ipsilateral eye. Selective occlusion of either component of the dual blood supply to the lateral geniculate, consisting of the anterior and posterior choroidal arteries, is infrequent but when it does occur, produces a characteristic "multiple sectoral field defect"; a quadruple sectoranopia, meaning homonymous sectoral defects in the upper and lower quadrants of both eyes due to occlusion of the anterior choroidal artery, and two horizontal sectoranopias with occlusion of the posterior (lateral) choroidal artery. The geniculate cells project to the visual (striate) cortex of the occipital lobe, also called area 17 (Brodmann classification) or V1 (Figs. 13-4 and 13-5).

Other optic tract fibers terminate in the pretectum and innervate both Edinger-Westphal nuclei, which subserve pupillary constriction and accommodation (see Fig. 14-8). A small group of fibers terminate in the suprachiasmatic nuclei in animals and presumably also in humans. These anatomic details explain several useful clinical signs. If there is a lesion in one optic nerve, a light stimulus to the affected eye will have no effect on the pupil of either eye, although the ipsilateral pupil will still constrict consensually, i.e., in response to a light stimulus

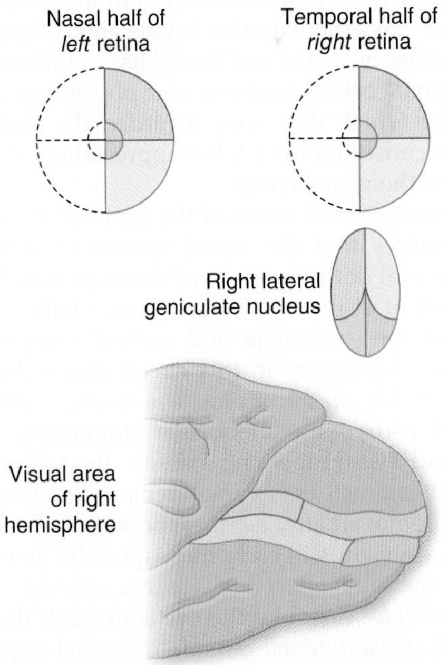

Figure 13-5. Diagrammatic depiction of the retinal projections, showing the disproportionately large representation of the macula in the lateral geniculate nucleus and visual (striate) cortex. (Redrawn by permission from Barr ML, Kiernan J: *The Human Nervous System*, 4th ed. Philadelphia, Lippincott, 1983.)

from the normal eye. This phenomenon is termed an *afferent pupillary defect*.

In their course through the temporal lobes, the fibers from the lower and upper quadrants of each retina diverge. The lower ones arch around the anterior pole of the temporal horn of the lateral ventricle before turning posteriorly; the upper ones follow a more direct path through the white matter of the uppermost part of the temporal lobe (Fig. 13-4), and probably of the adjacent interior parietal lobe. Both groups of fibers merge posteriorly at the internal sagittal stratum. For these reasons, incomplete lesions of the geniculocalcarine pathways (optic radiations) cause visual field defects that are partial and often not fully congruent (Fig. 13-3*E* and *F*).

It is in Brodmann area 17, embedded in the medial lip of the occipital pole, that cortical processing of the retinogeniculate projections occurs. The receptive neurons are arranged in columns, some of which are activated by edges and forms and others by moving stimuli or by color. The neurons for each eye are grouped together and have concentric, center-surround receptive fields. The deep neurons of area 17 project to the secondary and tertiary visual areas of the occipitotemporal cortex of the same and opposite cerebral hemispheres and also to other multisensory parietal and temporal cortices. Several of these extrastriate connections are just now being identified. Separate visual systems are utilized in the perception of motion, color, stereopsis, contour, and depth perception. Conceptually, the flow of secondary visual processing can be divided into a ventral stream, which carries predominantly spatial information to the parietal lobe ("the where") and a dorsal stream, which carries shape and color information to the temporal lobe ("the what") as articulated by Levine and colleagues. The classic studies of Hubel and Wiesel have elucidated much of this visual cortical anatomy and physiology and their papers, for which they were awarded the Nobel Prize, should be consulted for a fuller appreciation of the organization of the visual cortex.

The *normal development* of the connections described above requires that the visual system be activated at each of several critical periods of development. The early deprivation of vision in one eye causes a failure of development of the geniculate and cortical receptive fields of that eye. Moreover, in this circumstance the cortical receptive fields of the seeing eye become abnormally large and usurps the monocular dominance columns of the blind eye (Hubel and Wiesel). In children with a congenital cataract, the eye will remain amblyopic if the opacity is removed after a critical period of development. A severe strabismus in early life, especially an esotropia, will have the same effect (*amblyopia ex anopsia*).

The *vascular supply* of the eye is through the *ophthalmic branch of the internal carotid artery* that supplies the retina, posterior (uveal) coats of the eye, and optic nerve head. This artery gives origin to the posterior ciliary arteries; the latter form a rich circumferential plexus of vessels (arterial circle of Zinn-Haller) located deep to the lamina cribrosa. The lamina cribrosa is a sieve-like scleral (dural) structure through which the axons of the central and nasal part of the disc run. This arterial circle supplies the optic disc and adjacent part of the distal optic nerve, the choroid, and the ciliary body; it anastomoses with the pial arterial plexus that surrounds the optic nerve. The other major branch of the ophthalmic artery is the *central retinal artery*. It supplies the inner retinal layers and issues from the optic disc, where it divides into four branches, each of which supplies a quadrant of the retina; it is these vessels and their branches that are visible by ophthalmoscopy. A short distance from the disc, these vessels lose their internal elastic lamina and the media (muscularis) becomes thin; they are properly classed as arterioles. The inner layers of the retina, including the ganglion and bipolar cells, receive their blood supply from these arterioles and their capillaries, whereas the deeper photoreceptor elements and the fovea are nourished by the underlying choroidal vascular bed, by diffusion through the retinal pigmented cells and the semipermeable Bruch membrane upon which they rest. In up to a third of the population, a small cilioretinal artery may arise from either the choroidal circulation or from the circle of Zinn-Haller and supply the macula. In the case of a central retinal artery occlusion, the presence of this cilioretinal artery leads to the preservation of central acuity.

Abnormalities of the Retina

As indicated above, the thin (100- to 350-mm) retinal sheet and the optic nerve head, into which all visual information flows, are exteriorized parts of the CNS and the only part of the nervous system that can be inspected directly. A common limitation in the funduscopic examination in cases of visual loss is failure to carefully inspect the macular zone (which is located 3 to 4 mm lateral to the optic disc and provides for 95 percent of visual acuity). There are variations in the appearance of the normal macula and optic disc, and these may prove difficult to distinguish from disease. A normal macula may be called abnormal because of a slight aberration of the retinal pigment epithelium, a few drusen, or a deep optic cup (see further on). With experience, the examiner can visualize the unmyelinated nerve-fiber layer of the retina by using bright-green (red-free) illumination. This is most often helpful in detecting demyelinative lesions of the optic nerve, which produce a loss of discrete bundles of the radially arranged and arching bundles of retinal fibers as they converge to the disc.

The absence of receptive elements in the optic disc accounts for the normal blind spot. The normal optic disc varies in color, being paler in infants and in blond individuals. The ganglion cell axons normally acquire their myelin sheaths after penetration of the lamina cribrosa, but they sometimes do so in their intraretinal course, as they approach the disc. These myelinated fibers adjacent to the disc appear as white patches with fine-feathered edges and are a normal variant, not to be confused with exudates.

In evaluating *the retinal vessels*, one must remember that these are arterioles and not arteries. Since the walls of retinal arterioles are transparent, what is observed with the ophthalmoscope is a column of blood within them.

The central light streak of normal arterioles is thought to represent the reflection of light as it strikes the interface of the column of blood and the concave vascular wall. In *arteriolosclerosis* (usually coexistent with hypertension), the lumina of the vessels are segmentally narrowed because of fibrous tissue replacement of the media and thickening of the basement membrane. Straightening of the arterioles and venous compression by arterioles are other signs of hypertension and arteriolosclerosis. In this circumstance the vein is compressed by the thickened arteriole within the adventitial envelope shared by both vessels at the site of crossing. Progressive arteriolar disease, to the point of occlusion of the lumen, results in a narrow, white ("silver-wire") vessel with no visible blood column. This change is associated most often with severe hypertension but may follow other types of occlusion of the central retinal artery or its branches (see descriptions and retinal illustrations further on). Sheathing of the venules, probably representing focal leakage of cells from the vessels, is reportedly observed in up to 25 percent of patients with the optic neuritis of multiple sclerosis, but we have only rarely been able to detect it. Arterial and venule sheathing are also seen in leukemia, sarcoid, Behçet disease, and other forms of vasculitis.

In *malignant, or accelerated, hypertension* there are, in addition to swelling of the optic nerve head and the retinal arteriolar changes noted above, a number of extravascular lesions: the so-called soft exudates or cotton-wool patches, sharply marginated and glistening "hard" exudates, and retinal hemorrhages. In many patients who show these retinal changes, analogous lesions are found in the brain (necrotizing arteriolitis and microinfarcts) and underlie hypertensive encephalopathy.

Microaneurysms of retinal vessels appear as small, discrete red dots and are located in largest number in the paracentral region. They are most often a sign of diabetes mellitus, sometimes appearing before the usual clinical manifestations of that disease. The use of the red-free (green) light on the ophthalmoscope helps to pick out microaneurysms from the background. Microscopically, the aneurysms take the form of small (20- to 90-mm) saccular outpouchings from the walls of capillaries, venules, or arterioles. The vessels of origin of the aneurysms are invariably abnormal, being either acellular branches of occluded vessels or themselves occluded by fat or fibrin.

The ophthalmoscopic appearance of *retinal hemorrhage* is determined by the structure of the particular tissue in which it occurs. In the superficial layer of the retina, they are linear or flame-shaped ("splinter" hemorrhages) because of their confinement by the horizontally coursing nerve fibers in that layer. These hemorrhages usually overlie and obscure the retinal vessels. Round or oval ("dot-and-blot") hemorrhages lie behind the vessels, in the outer plexiform layer of the retina (synaptic layer between bipolar cells and nuclei of rods and cones—Fig. 13-2); in this layer, blood accumulates in the form of a cylinder between vertically oriented nerve fibers and appears round or oval when viewed end-on with the ophthalmoscope. Rupture of arterioles on the inner surface of the retina—as occurs with ruptured intracranial saccular aneurysms, arteriovenous malformations, and other conditions causing sudden severe elevation of intracranial pressure—permits the accumulation of a sharply outlined lake of blood between the internal limiting membrane of the retina and the vitreous or hyaloid membrane (the condensed gel at the periphery of the vitreous body); this is the subhyaloid or preretinal hemorrhage, termed *Terson syndrome*. Either the small superficial or deep retinal hemorrhage may show a central or eccentric pale (Roth) spot, which is caused by an accumulation of white blood cells, fibrin, histiocytes, or amorphous material between the vessel and the hemorrhage. This lesion is said to be characteristic of bacterial endocarditis, but it is also seen in leukemia and occasionally in embolic retinopathy caused by carotid disease.

Cotton-wool patches, or soft exudates, like splinter hemorrhages, overlie and tend to obscure the retinal blood vessels. These patches, even large ones, rarely cause serious disturbances of vision unless they involve the macula. Soft exudates are in reality infarcts of the nerve-fiber layer, caused by occlusion of precapillary arterioles; they are composed of clusters of ovoid structures called *cytoid bodies*, representing the terminal swellings of interrupted axons. *Hard exudates* appear as punctate white or yellow bodies; they lie in the outer plexiform layer, behind the retinal vessels, like the punctate hemorrhages. If present in the macular region, they are arranged in lines radiating toward the fovea (*macular star*). Hard exudates consist of lipid and other serum precipitants as a result of abnormal vascular permeability of a type that is not completely understood. They are observed most often in cases of diabetes mellitus and chronic hypertension.

Drusen in the retina (colloid bodies) appear ophthalmoscopically as pale yellow spots and are difficult to distinguish from hard exudates except when they occur alone; as a rule, hard exudates are accompanied by other funduscopic abnormalities. Although retinal drusen may be a benign finding, in many cases they reflect an ARMD and their accumulation in the macula eventually leads to significant visual loss. The source of retinal drusen is uncertain, but they may result from chronic inflammation generated by degeneration of the retinal pigment epithelium. *Hyaline bodies* located on or near the optic disc, are also referred to as drusen but must be distinguished from those occurring peripherally. In contrast to peripheral retinal drusen, drusen of the optic discs are probably mineralized residues of dead axons and can be seen on CT in some cases. Their main significance for neurologists is that drusen that are buried under the disc ("buried drusen") are often associated with anomalous elevation of the disc that can be mistaken for papilledema (see further on) but they are for the most part, benign.

The periphery of the retina may harbor a hemangioblastoma, which may appear during adolescence, before the more characteristic cerebellar lesion. A large retinal artery may be seen leading to it and there may be a large draining vein. Occasionally, retinal examination discloses the presence of a vascular malformation that may be coextensive with a much larger malformation of the optic nerve and basilar portions of the brain.

Ischemic Lesions of the Retina

Transient monocular blindness Transient ischemic attacks of visual loss involving all or part of the field of vision of one eye are referred to as *amaurosis fugax* or *transient monocular blindness (TMB)*. They are common manifestations of atherosclerotic carotid stenosis but have other causes. An altitudinal horizontal border, or "shade", is often, but not invariably, an aspect of the visual loss. The shade may rise or fall at the onset or cessation of the spell and occasionally remains throughout the episode. Fortuitous inspection of the retina during an attack may show segments of arteries that are filled with white material that migrate distally over many minutes. There can be stagnation of arterial and venous blood flow, which returns within seconds or minutes as vision is restored (Fisher). One interpretation of these observations is that an embolus had occurred to the central retinal artery and had broken up and moved distally. Fisher went on to discredit the theory of the time that transient monocular blindness was due to vasospasm of the retinal arteries.

One or dozens of attacks may precede infarction of a cerebral hemisphere, or as often, they may abate without adverse consequence. In one series of 80 patients followed by Marshall and Meadows for 4 years, in an era prior to modern treatment of atherosclerosis, 16 percent developed permanent unilateral blindness, a completed hemispheral stroke, or both. Chapter 34 discusses this subject further.

Occlusion of the internal carotid artery usually causes no disturbance of vision whatsoever, provided that there are adequate anastomotic branches from the external carotid artery or other sources to the ophthalmic artery. Occasionally, occlusion of the proximal internal carotid artery is marked by an episode of transient monocular blindness on the same side, just as a hemispheral transient ischemic attack may indicate recent acute carotid occlusion. Chronic carotid occlusion with inadequate collateralization is associated with an ischemic oculopathy, which may predominantly affect the anterior or posterior segment or both. In this case, insufficient circulation to the anterior segment of the globe is manifest by scleral vascular congestion, cloudiness of the cornea, anterior chamber flare, and low intraocular pressure, or sometimes high intraocular pressure if neovascularization of the iris (rubeosis iridis) occurs and compromises the outflow of aqueous humor. Ischemia of the posterior segment of the eye is manifest by circulatory changes in the optic nerve or by venous stasis. Other signs of carotid disease may be present, for example, a local bruit over the carotid bifurcation.

Central retinal artery occlusion Most often, ischemia of the retina can be traced to occlusion of the central retinal artery or its branches by thrombi or emboli—*central retinal artery occlusion* (abbreviated CRAO). Occlusion is attended by sudden painless blindness. The retina becomes opaque and has a gray-yellow appearance; the arterioles are narrowed, with segmentation of columns of blood and a cherry-red appearance of the fovea (Fig. 13-6). With occlusions of smaller branches of the central retinal artery by emboli, one may be able to see the occluding material. Most frequently observed are Hollenhorst plaques—glistening, white-yellow atheromatous particles (Fig. 13-7) seen in 40 of 70 cases of retinal embolism in the series of Arruga and Sanders but are as often an asymptomatic manifestation of carotid or aortic atherosclerosis. The particles may alternatively have the appearance white calcium from calcified aortic or mitral valves or atheroma of the great vessels, and red or white fibrin-platelet emboli from a number of sources, mostly undefined, or perhaps from the heart or its valves. Emboli to retinal artery branches may be difficult to see without fluorescein retinography; furthermore, most of these emboli soon disappear. Central retinal artery occlusion also occurs as a consequence of giant cell arteritis; patients who are in their 50s or older should be screened for this condition.

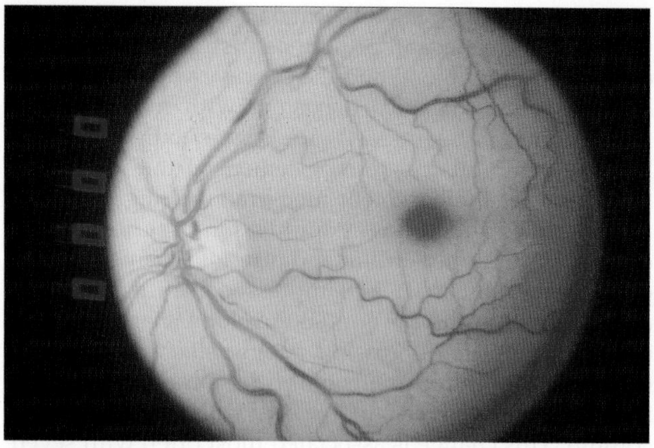

Figure 13-6. Appearance of the fundus in central retinal artery occlusion. In addition to the paucity of blood flow in retinal vessels, the retina has a creamy gray appearance, and there is a "cherry-red spot" at the fovea. (Courtesy of Dr. Shirley Wray.)

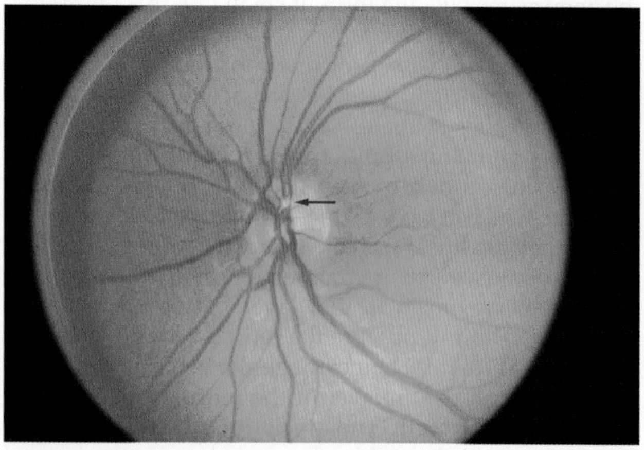

Figure 13-7. Glistening "Hollenhorst plaque" occlusion of a superior retinal artery branch (*arrow*). These occlusions represent atheromatous particles or, less often, platelet-fibrin emboli. Some are asymptomatic and others are associated with segmental visual loss or are seen after central retinal artery occlusion. (Courtesy of Dr. Shirley Wray.)

It has become routine in some centers to treat acute central retinal artery occlusion in an urgent manner with a number of methods in the hope that the embolus or thrombus will be propelled into more distal vessels. These treatments are generally aimed at lowering intraocular pressure (acetazolamide, inhalation of carbon dioxide; paracentesis of the anterior chamber, ballottement), to dilate the vessels, and reestablish flow. We can only offer the impression that these procedures have often not been successful, but some case series have suggested that local thrombolysis with intraarterial agents may be useful. A multicenter controlled trial of thrombolysis (Eagle Study cited under Schumacher and colleagues) was halted early because of safety concerns so this is not likely to remain an option for treatment.

Retinal venous occlusion Because the central retinal artery and vein share a common adventitial sheath, atheromatous plaques in the artery are said to be associated with *thrombosis of the retinal vein*. This results in a spectacular display of retinal lesions that differs from the picture of central retinal artery occlusion. The veins are engorged and tortuous, and there are multiple diffuse "dot-and-blot" and streaky linear retinal hemorrhages (Fig. 13-8). Retinal vein thrombosis is observed most frequently with diabetes mellitus, hypertension, and leukemia; less frequently with sickle cell disease; and rarely with multiple myeloma, and Waldenstrom macroglobulinemia in relation to the hyperviscosity that these two diseases cause. Sometimes, no associated systemic disease can be identified, in which case the possibility of an orbital mass (e.g., optic nerve glioma) should always be considered. In retinal vein thrombosis, visual loss is variable and there may be recovery of useful vision. In cases where macular edema ensues, recovery may be enhanced by laser photocoagulation.

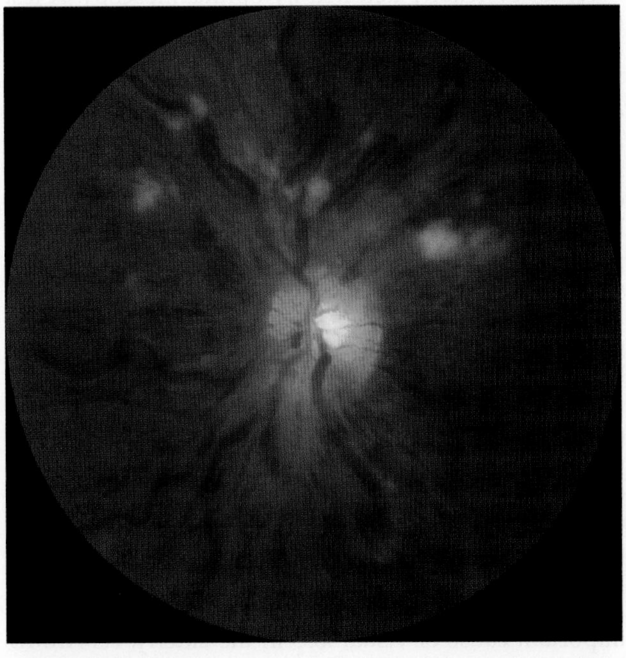

Figure 13-8. Occlusion of the central retinal vein with suffusion of the veins, swelling of the disc, and florid retinal hemorrhages. (Courtesy of Dr. Shirley Wray.)

Other causes of transient monocular blindness In addition to the typical ischemic cause of this syndrome, transitory retinal ischemia is observed occasionally as a manifestation of migraine; it has also occurred in polycythemia, hyperglobulinemia, antiphospholipid syndrome, hyperviscosity of any type, and sickle cell anemia. In younger persons, transient monocular blindness is relatively uncommon and the cause is often not immediately apparent. Ischemia related to the antiphospholipid antibody or "retinal migraine" is presumed to be responsible for many cases. Rarely, vasospasm of the central retinal artery may be implicated as a cause of transient monocular blindness, in which case the episodes may cease with the introduction of a calcium channel blocker, as reported by Winterkorn and colleagues.

A common and critical cause of sudden monocular blindness, especially in elderly persons, is *anterior ischemic optic neuropathy (AION), essentially an infarction of the nerve head*. It is caused by disease of posterior ciliary vessels that supply the optic nerve and is considered further on in the discussion of diseases of the optic nerve. The retinal vessels in this condition usually have a normal appearance, but the disc is swollen. The arteritic form of this process is discussed in more detail in Chap. 34, but most cases are related to occlusion of small vessels as occurs typically in diabetes.

In summary, *sudden, painless, monocular loss of vision* should raise the question of either retinal ischemia, caused by occlusive disease of the central retinal artery or vein, or of ischemic optic neuropathy from disease of the ciliary vessels. Detachment of the retina, and macular and vitreous hemorrhages are relatively obvious causes as noted below.

Other Diseases of the Retina

Aside from vascular lesions, tears and detachments of the retina may impair vision acutely. The most common form of detachment is an intraretinal one caused by separation of the pigment epithelium layer from the sensory retina with fluid accumulation through a tear or hole in the retina. In so-called traction detachment—observed in cases of premature birth or proliferative retinopathy secondary to diabetes or other vascular disease—contracting fibrous tissue pulls the retina from the choroid.

Serous retinopathy, a cause of monocular visual disturbance in young or middle-aged males, may be associated with the use of corticosteroids. The entire perimacular zone is elevated by edema fluid. The condition may arise acutely or slowly. Metamorphopsia (distortion of vision) in one eye is a common presentation, but acuity is not much impaired. The optic disc remains normal. The retinal change (leakage of vascular fluid into the subretinal space) causes a loss of visualization of the detail of the choroid and is demonstrated by fluorescein angiography or by optical coherence tomography (OCT). The condition tends to resolve over several months and is treated by laser to seal the sites of leakage.

Chorioretinitis, generally the result of an infectious process, may cause difficulty in diagnosis. In many patients the initial diagnosis had been retrobulbar neuritis. One cannot depend upon the appearance of a macular star (see above) for diagnosis.

A large number of patients with HIV-AIDS develop retinal lesions of various types. Infarcts of the nerve-fiber layer (cotton-wool patches), hemorrhages, and perivascular sheathing are the usual findings. Toxoplasmosis is the most common infective lesion, followed in frequency by cytomegalovirus (CMV), but histoplasmosis, *Pneumocystis carinii*, herpes zoster, syphilis, and tuberculosis are well documented. CMV may cause a particularly severe necrotizing retinitis and permanent impairment of vision. Both the retina and choroid may be involved by these diseases, in which case the ophthalmoscopic picture is characteristic, showing the destruction of the "punched-out" lesions that exposes the whitish sclera, and deposits of black pigment. The choroid may also be the site of viral and noninfective inflammatory reactions, often in association with painful recurrent iridocyclitis and lacrimal inflammation.

Degenerations of the retina are important causes of chronic progressive visual loss. The retinal degenerations assume several forms and many are associated with progressive conditions of the brain or other organs. The most frequent in youth and middle age is *retinitis pigmentosa*, a hereditary disease of the outer photoreceptor layer and subjacent pigment epithelium. The retina is thin, and there are fine deposits of black pigment in the shape of bone corpuscles, more in the periphery; later the optic discs become pale. The disorder is marked by constriction of the visual fields with relative sparing of central vision ("gun-barrel" vision), metamorphopsia (distorted vision), delayed recovery from glare, and nyctalopia (reduced twilight vision). The causes of retinitis pigmentosa and related retinal degenerations are diverse, too numerous to list here. Furthermore, the condition has been linked to deficits in more than 75 different genes. In one form of isolated retinitis pigmentosa, which follows an autosomal dominant pattern of inheritance, the gene for rhodopsin (a combination of vitamin A and the rod-cell protein opsin) produces a defective opsin, resulting in a diminution of rhodopsin, diminished response to light, and eventual degeneration of the rod cells (Dryja et al). Retinitis pigmentosa is associated with the Laurence-Moon-Biedl syndrome, with certain mitochondrial diseases (Kearns-Sayre syndrome, Chap. 38), and with a number of degenerative and metabolic diseases (e.g., Refsum disease) of the nervous system. Another early life hereditary retinal degeneration, characterized by massive central retinal lesions, is the autosomal recessive Stargardt form of juvenile tapetoretinal degeneration. Like retinitis pigmentosa, Stargardt disease may be accompanied by progressive spastic paraparesis or ataxia. *Nonpigmentary retinal degeneration* is a familiar feature of a number of rare syndromes and diseases, such as neuronal ceroid lipofuscinosis, Bassen-Kornzweig disease, Batten-Mayou disease, and others (see Chap. 37).

Medications have emerged as a cause of retinal damage. Phenothiazine derivatives, less often used in practice than they had been, may conjugate with the melanin of the pigment layer, resulting in degeneration of the outer layers of the retina and a characteristic "bull's-eye retinopathy" observed by fluorescein angiography. If these drugs are administered in high dosages for protracted periods, the patient should be tested for defects in visual fields and color vision. Among drugs used to treat neurologic disease, the antiepileptic drug *vigabatrin* is notable for causing retinal degeneration and a concentric restriction of the visual fields in almost half of exposed patients. Elevated levels of gamma-aminobutyric acid (GABA) in the retina are presumably the cause of toxicity. High-dose tamoxifen has caused toxicity in the retina, characterized by the deposition of refractile opacities and in more severe cases, by macular edema.

A cancer-associated retinopathy (CAR) has been described in patients with an oat-cell carcinoma of the lung as a paraneoplastic illness (see Chap. 31). The typical presentation is of positive visual phenomenon and rapid bilateral visual loss. Antibodies against the recoverin protein, which modulates rhodopsin kinase, have been demonstrated in the serum of affected patients (Grunwald et al; Kornguth et al; Jacobson et al). More recently, a melanoma-associated retinopathy (MAR) that affects only rods has been described. These paraneoplastic processes are further described in Chap. 31.

Certain lysosomal diseases of infancy and early childhood are characterized by an abnormal accumulation of undegraded proteins, polysaccharides, and lipids in cerebral neurons, as well as in the macula and other parts of the retina (hence the terms *storage diseases* and *cerebromacular degenerations*). Corneal clouding, cherry-red spot and graying of the retina, and later optic atrophy are the observed ocular abnormalities. Chapter 37 discusses these diseases.

In some of these retinal diseases, minimal changes in the pigment epithelium or other layers of the retina may not be readily detected by ophthalmoscopy. A test to expose such subtle retinal changes is to estimate the time required for recovery of visual acuity following light stimulation (macular photostress test). The test is conducted by shining a strong light through the pupil of an affected eye for 10 s and measuring the time necessary for the acuity to return to the pretest level (normally 50 s or less). With macular lesions, recovery time is prolonged, but with lesions of the optic nerve, it is not affected. This phenomenon may also be observed in the eye on the side of a carotid occlusion, in essence, an ischemic retinopathy. Retinal diseases reduce or abolish the electrical activity generated by the outer layers of the retina, and this can be measured by the electroretinogram (ERG). Fluorescein retinography and various new imaging tests are now essential for proper diagnosis of retinal disease. OCT uses reflected light to construct a high-resolution two-dimensional image of the retinal layers; it is able to demonstrate with remarkable resolution retinal edema, tears, macular holes, and the thinning of the retinal nerve-fiber layer that follows optic neuropathy.

Age-Related Macular Degeneration This is the most important cause of visual loss in the elderly. As ARMD begins to disturb vision, the straight lines on the Amsler grid are observed by the patient to be distorted. Examination discloses a central scotoma, and an alteration of the retina around the macula. Central vision is at first distorted, then gradually diminishes, impairing reading, but these patients can still get about because of retained peripheral vision. The two most common types of macular degeneration are an atrophic "dry" type, which is a true pigmentary degeneration associated with retinal drusen, of unknown cause but with a genetic component, and an exudative "wet" type, which is the result of choroidal neovascularization that results in secondary macular damage. The wet form is amenable to laser treatment and to the injection into the orbit of ranibizumab or similar antiangiogenic monoclonal antibodies against vascular endothelial growth factor. Progression of the dry form may be slightly reduced by the use of antioxidants and zinc. The pathophysiology and treatment of ARMD have been reviewed by DeJong.

Diabetic Retinopathy Although not strictly speaking a problem taken up by neurologists, this is such an important cause of reduced vision and blindness that the basic facts should be known to all physicians. The earliest changes are of microaneurysms, and tiny intraretinal hemorrhages; these are present in almost all diabetics who have had type 1 disease for more than 20 years. Cotton-wool spots and small hemorrhages appear as the retina becomes ischemic. Subsequently, there is a more threatening proliferative retinopathy that consists of the formation of new blood vessels, and consequent leakage of proteins and blood. The proliferative feature occurs in half of type 1 diabetics, and 10 percent of those who have had type 2 disease for 15 to 20 years. The new vessels can grow into the vitreous, and hemorrhages from them may cause traction on the retina, which results in detachment. Visual loss may also be the result of macular edema. Reabsorption of the edema leads to the deposition of lipid "hard exudates." The maintenance of glucose control reduces the frequency and severity of retinopathy but does not prevent it. Locally elevated levels of vascular endothelial growth factor have been shown to be the involved in the pathophysiology of diabetic retinal neovascularization, and recent studies show that improvement in neovascular leakage can be obtained, at least in the short term, with intravitreal injections of the antivascular endothelial growth factor (anti-VEGF) antibody, bevacizumab. The review of the subject by David and colleagues is recommended.

Papilledema and Raised Intracranial Pressure

Of the various abnormalities of the optic disc, *papilledema* or *optic disc swelling* has the greatest neurologic implication, for it signifies the presence of increased intracranial pressure. The term papilledema has come to mean disc swelling due to raised intracranial pressure although there are other causes of a similar funduscopic appearance. It must be made clear, however, that an ophthalmoscopic appearance identical to that of papilledema can be produced by infarction of the optic nerve head (the "papillopathy" of anterior ischemic optic neuropathy) and by inflammatory changes in the intraorbital portion of the optic nerve ("papillitis", a form of optic neuritis). Certain clinical and funduscopic findings, listed in Table 13-2 and described below, assist in distinguishing between these processes, although all share the basic feature of conspicuous optic disc swelling.

In its mildest form, papilledema appears as slight elevation of the disc and blurring of the disc margins, especially of the superior and inferior aspects, and a mild fullness of the veins in the disc. Subtle disc elevation

Table 13-2

CAUSES OF OPTIC DISC SWELLING

OPHTHALMIC ABNORMALITY	UNDERLYING CAUSE	VISUAL LOSS	ASSOCIATED SYMPTOMS	PUPILS
Papilledema	Increased intracranial pressure	None or transient blurring; constriction of visual fields and enlargement of blind spot; findings almost always binocular	Headache; signs of intracranial mass	Normal unless succeeded by optic atrophy
Anterior ischemic optic neuropathy	Infarction of disc and intraorbital optic nerve due to atherosclerosis or temporal arteritis	Acute visual loss, monocular (usually); may be an altitudinal defect	Headache with temporal arteritis	Afferent pupillary defect
Optic neuritis[a] ("papillitis")	Inflammatory changes in disc and intraorbital part of optic nerve—usually due to MS, sometimes to ADEM	Rapidly progressive visual loss; usually monocular	Tender globe, pain on ocular movement	Afferent pupillary defect
Hyaline bodies[b] (drusen)	Congenital, familial	Usually none but may be slowly progressive Enlargement of blind spot or arcuate inferior nasal defect	Usually none; rarely transient visual obscurations	Normal

MS, multiple sclerosis; ADEM, acute disseminated encephalomyelitis.
[a]Optic neuritis affecting the retrobulbar portion of the nerve shows no funduscopic changes.
[b]May be mistaken for papilledema (pseudopapilledema).

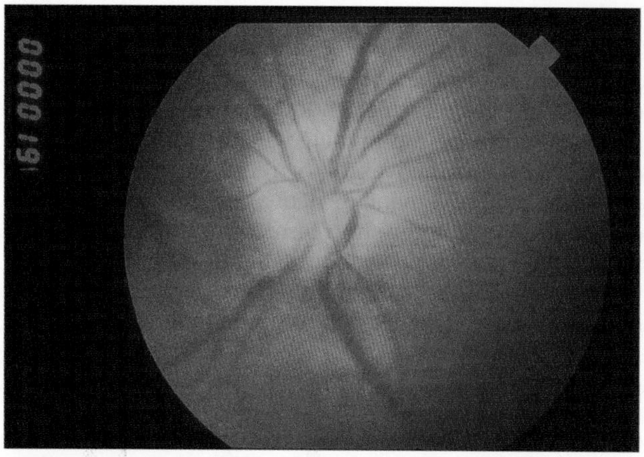

Figure 13-9. Mild papilledema with hyperemia of the disc and slight blurring of the disc margins. (Courtesy of Dr. Shirley Wray.)

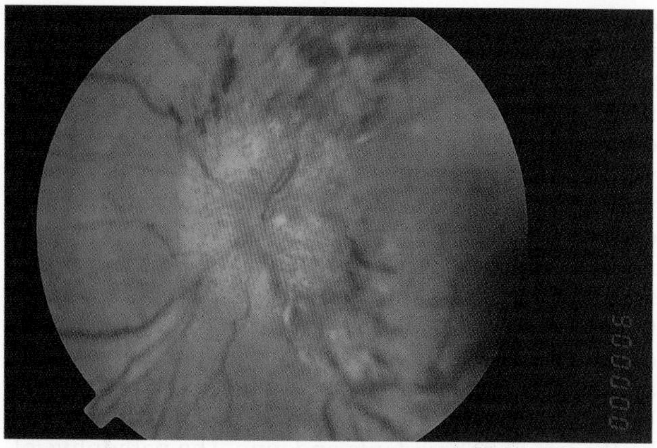

Figure 13-10. Fully developed papilledema. The main characteristics are marked swelling and enlargement of the disc, vascular engorgement, obscuration of small vessels at the disc margin as a result of nerve-fiber edema, and white "cotton-wool spots" that represent superficial infarcts of the nerve-fiber layer. (Courtesy of Dr. Shirley Wray.)

is also indicated by a loss of definition of the vessels overlying the disc as they approach the disc margin from the periphery; this appearance is produced by edema in the adjacent retina. Because many normal individuals, especially those with hypermetropia, have ill-defined disc margins, the early stage of papilledema may be difficult to detect (Fig. 13-9). Pulsations of the retinal veins, best seen where the veins turn to enter the disc, will have disappeared by the time intracranial pressure is raised, but this finding is not specific, as venous pulsations are not present in a proportion of normal individuals in the seated position. On the other hand, the presence of spontaneous venous pulsations is a reliable indicator of an intracranial pressure below 200 mm H_2O, and thus usually excludes papilledema (Levin). Fluorescein angiography, red-free fundus photos (which highlight the retinal nerve fibers), and newer imaging techniques alluded to above (ocular coherence tomography) are helpful in detecting early edema of the optic discs.

More severe degrees of papilledema appear as further elevation, or "mushrooming" of the entire disc and surrounding retina. There is subtle or overt edema and obscuration of vessels at the disc margins and, in some instances, peripapillary hemorrhages (Fig. 13-10). When advanced as a result of raised intracranial pressure, papilledema is almost always bilateral although it may asymmetric. Purely unilateral edema of the optic disc is indicative of a perioptic meningioma or other tumor involving the optic nerve, but it can sometimes occur at an early stage of increased intracranial pressure. As the papilledema becomes chronic, elevation of the disc margin becomes less prominent and pallor of the optic nerve head, representing a dropout of nerve fibers (atrophy), becomes more evident (Fig. 13-11). Varying degrees of secondary optic atrophy remain in the wake of papilledema that has persisted for more than several days or weeks, leaving the disc pale, gliotic, and shrunken. Constriction in one quadrant of the nasal portion of the visual field is an early sign of the loss of nerve fibers from optic atrophy.

Acute papilledema, while it may enlarge the blind spot slightly, does not greatly affect visual acuity (except transiently during spontaneous waves of increased intracranial pressure). Therefore, acute optic disc swelling in a patient with severely reduced vision cannot be attributed to papilledema; instead, intraorbital optic neuritis (papillitis) or infarction of the nerve head (ischemic optic neuropathy) must be present. Chronic or recurrent papilledema may result in optic atrophy and cause a reduction in visual acuity by that mechanism.

The examiner is also aided by the fact that *papilledema due to raised intracranial pressure is generally bilateral*, although, as mentioned earlier, the degree of disc swelling may not be symmetrical. In contrast, papillitis and infarction of the nerve head affect one eye, but there are exceptions to both of these statements. The pupillary reaction to light is muted only with infarction and optic neuritis, not with acute papilledema (once secondary optic atrophy supervenes, the loss of afferent light reaction is indeed observed). The occurrence of papilledema on one side

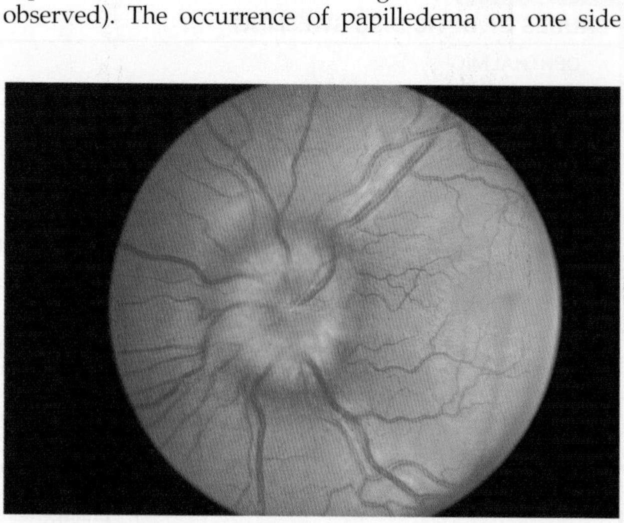

Figure 13-11. Chronic papilledema with beginning optic atrophy, in which the disc stands out like a champagne cork. The hemorrhages and exudates have been absorbed, leaving a glistening residue around the disc. (Courtesy of Dr. Shirley Wray.)

and optic atrophy on the other is referred to as the Foster Kennedy syndrome; it is typically caused by a frontal lobe tumor or an olfactory meningioma on the side of the atrophic disc. In its complete form, which is seen only rarely, there is also anosmia on the side of the optic atrophy. Another cause of the same funduscopic appearance has been called the "pseudo-Foster Kennedy syndrome," which occurs when papillitis in one eye occurs years after an optic neuropathy of the opposite one.

Although, as mentioned, the term papilledema is generally reserved for disc swelling from raised intracranial pressure, an identical appearance caused by infarction of the nerve head is characterized by extension of the swelling beyond the nerve head, as described below. The papilledema of increased pressure is associated with peripapillary hemorrhages whereas these are uncommon with infarction of the nerve. Often these distinctions cannot be made on the basis of the funduscopic appearance alone, in which case the most reliable distinguishing feature is again the presence or absence of visual loss (Table 13-2). Papilledema caused by increased intracranial pressure cannot be distinguished from combined edema of the optic nerve and retina, which typifies malignant hypertension.

Chronic papilledema, as occurs in pseudotumor cerebri (see Chap. 31), presents a special problem in diagnosis, and represents a risk for permanent reduction in visual acuity from secondary optic atrophy. In addition to testing visual acuity at regular intervals, our colleagues advise serial evaluation of the visual fields as constriction of the nasal field, detectable by automated perimetry and tangent screen testing, is an early and ominous optic atrophy.

The essential element in the pathogenesis of papilledema is an increase in pressure in the sheaths surrounding the optic nerves, which communicate directly with the subarachnoid space of the brain. This was demonstrated convincingly by Hayreh (1964), who produced bilateral chronic papilledema in monkeys by inflating balloons in the subarachnoid space and then opening the sheath of one optic nerve; the papilledema promptly subsided on the operated side but not on the opposite side. The appearance of the swollen disc, however, has also been ascribed to a blockage of axoplasmic flow in the optic nerve fibers (Minckler et al; Tso and Hayreh). It was found that compression of the optic nerve by elevated cerebrospinal fluid (CSF) pressure resulted in swelling of axons behind the optic nerve head and leakage of their contents into the extracellular spaces of the disc. In our opinion, the block in axoplasmic flow alone could not account for the marked congestion of vessels and hemorrhages that accompany papilledema and a component of vascular congestion is likely.

The mechanism of papilledema that on rare occasions accompanies spinal tumors, particularly oligodendrogliomas, and the Guillain-Barré syndrome is not entirely clear. Usually the CSF protein is more than 1,000 mg/100 mL, but this cannot be the entire or only explanation, as instances occur in which the protein concentration is only slightly elevated (also the concentration of protein in the ventricular and cerebral subarachnoid spaces is considerably lower than in the lumbar sac, where it is usually sampled; see Chap. 30). In other diseases that at times give rise to papilledema—e.g., chronic lung disease with hypercapnia, cancer with meningeal infiltration, or dural arteriovenous malformation—the mechanism is most often one of a generalized increase of intracranial pressure. Other causes of papilledema are cyanotic congenital heart disease, and other forms of polycythemia, hypocalcemia though an obscure mechanism, and POEMS (polyneuropathy, organomegaly, endocrinopathy, monoclonal gammopathy, and skin changes; see Chap. 46).

Diseases of the Optic Nerves

The optic nerves, which constitute the axonic projections of the retinal ganglion cells to the lateral geniculate bodies and superior colliculi can be inspected in the optic nerve head. Observable changes in the optic disc are therefore of particular importance. They may reflect the presence of raised intracranial pressure as already described; optic neuritis ("papillitis"); infarction of the optic nerve head; congenital defects of the optic nerves (optic pits and colobomas); hypoplasia and atrophy of the optic nerves; and glaucoma. Illustrations of these and other abnormalities of the disc and ocular fundus can be found in the atlas by E.M. Chester and in the text by Biousse and Newman. In general, optic neuropathies are distinguished from other causes of visual loss by a predominance of loss of color vision and by the presence of an afferent pupillary defect.

Table 13-3 lists the main causes of optic neuropathy, which are discussed in the following portions of this chapter.

Optic Neuritis (Papillitis; Retrobulbar Neuritis) (See Chap. 36)

This inflammatory process causes unilateral acute impairment of vision that may appear in one or both eyes, either simultaneously or successively. It develops in a number of clinical settings, but has a special relationship to multiple sclerosis. The most common situation is one in which an adolescent or young adult woman has a rapid diminution of vision in one eye as though a veil had covered the eye, sometimes progressing within hours or days to complete blindness.

The optic disc and retina may appear normal, in which case the condition is of the more common retrobulbar variety, but if the inflammation is near the nerve head, there is swelling of the disc, i.e., papillitis (Fig. 13-12). The disc margins are then seen to be elevated, blurred, and, rarely, surrounded by hemorrhages. As indicated above, papillitis is associated with marked impairment of vision and a central scotoma that encompasses the blind spot (cecocentral), thus distinguishing it from the acute papilledema of increased intracranial pressure. Pain on movement and tenderness on pressure of the globe, and a difference between the two eyes in the perception of brightness of light are other common, but not invariable findings (Table 13-2). The pupil on the affected side has a muted constriction response to direct light. In the following days and weeks, the patient may report an increase in blurring of vision with exertion or with exposure to heat (Uhthoff phenomenon). In papillitis, but not retrobulbar neuritis, examination may disclose haziness of the

Table 13-3

CAUSES OF UNILATERAL AND BILATERAL OPTIC NEUROPATHY

I.	Demyelinative (optic neuritis)
	Multiple sclerosis
	Postinfectious and viral neuroretinitis
II.	Ischemic
	Arteriosclerotic (usually in-situ occlusion; occasionally carotid artery disease)
	Granulomatous (giant cell) arteritis
	Syphilitic arteritis
III.	Parainfectious
	Cavernous sinus thrombosis
	Paranasal sinus infection
IV.	Toxins and drugs
	Methanol
	Ethambutol
	Chloroquine
	Streptomycin
	Chlorpropamide
	Chloramphenicol
	Tiagabine
	Linezolid
	Infliximab
	Sildenafil
	Ergot compounds
V.	Deficiency states
	Vitamin B_{12}
	Thiamine or possibly several B vitamins ("tobacco-alcohol" amblyopia)
	Epidemic nutritional types (Cuban, Jamaican)
VI.	Heredofamilial and developmental
	Dominant juvenile optic atrophy
	Leber optic atrophy
	Developmental failure of disc or papillomacular bundle
	Progressive hyaline body encroachment
VII.	Compressive and infiltrative
	Meningioma of sphenoid wing or olfactory groove
	Metastasis to optic nerve or chiasm
	Glioma of optic nerve (neurofibromatosis type I)
	Optic atrophy following long-standing papilledema
	Pituitary tumor and apoplexy
	Thyroid ophthalmopathy
	Sarcoidosis
	Giant aneurysms
	Lymphoma
	Wegener granulomatosis
VIII.	Radiation-induced optic neuropathy

vitreous that causes difficulty in visualizing the retina. Inflammatory sheathing of the retinal veins, as described by Rucker, is known to occur but has been uncommon in our patients. In extreme cases, edema may suffuse from the disc to cause a rippling in the adjacent retina. However, as just noted, most cases of optic neuritis are retrobulbar, and little is seen when examining the optic nerve head. In approximately 10 percent of cases, both eyes are involved, either simultaneously or in rapid succession.

Sometimes, no cause can be found for optic neuropathy, but a first bout of multiple sclerosis is always suspected, as discussed in Chap. 36. After several weeks to months, there is spontaneous recovery; vision returns to normal in more than two-thirds of cases. Recovery of

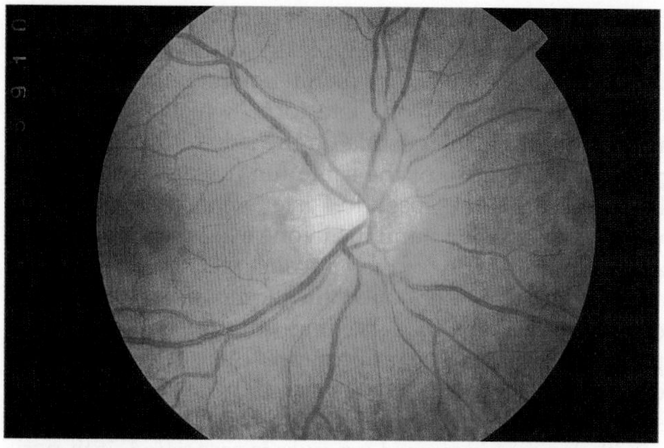

Figure 13-12. Acute optic neuritis in a patient with multiple sclerosis. The disc is swollen from an inflammatory process near the nerve head (papillitis), and the patient is virtually blind in the affected eye.

vision occurs spontaneously, or may be hastened by the intravenous administration of high doses of corticosteroids. In one frequently cited study, the oral administration of these drugs increased the frequency of a relapse of optic neuritis so that intravenous agents are used instead (see "Treatment of Optic Neuritis" in Chap. 36). Diminution of brightness, dyschromatopsia, or a scotoma may remain; rarely, the patient is left blind.

As time progresses, more than half of adults with optic neuritis will develop other symptoms and signs of multiple sclerosis, usually within 5 years, and probably even more do so when they are observed for longer periods. Conversely, in approximately 15 percent of patients with multiple sclerosis, the history discloses that retrobulbar neuritis was the first symptom. A proportion of patients with acute optic neuritis are found at the time of an acute attack to have characteristic features of multiple sclerosis on MRI of the cerebrum and spine.

Postinfectious demyelinating disease is a possible cause in some cases that do not later show signs of multiple sclerosis. Less is known about children with retrobulbar neuropathy, in whom the disorder is more often bilateral and frequently related to a preceding viral infection ("neuroretinitis," see below). Their prognosis is better than that of adults. Formerly, optic neuritis was often attributed to paranasal sinus disease, but this condition rarely affects vision and with a few exceptions, the association is tenuous, as discussed further on. Optic neuritis is a main component of neuromyelitis optica (Devic disease; see Chap. 36); the prognosis for recovery is generally poorer than for optic neuritis in multiple sclerosis, but there are many exceptions.

Despite the return of visual acuity in the majority of patients with optic neuritis, a degree of optic atrophy almost always results. The disc then appears shrunken and pale, particularly in its temporal half (temporal pallor), and the pallor extends beyond the margins of the disc into the peripapillary retinal nerve fibers. The pattern-shift visual evoked potential becomes delayed; as a result, this test is a highly sensitive indicator of previous, even asymptomatic, episodes of optic neuritis.

The treatment of optic neuritis is taken up with multiple sclerosis in Chap. 36.

Leber hereditary optic neuropathy, a maternally inherited mitochondrial disorder, is an infrequent but important cause of blindness in children and younger adults because it may simulate the more common inflammatory optic neuropathies, even at times causing a relatively abrupt onset of visual loss followed by some degree of recovery (see "Hereditary Optic Atrophy of Leber" in Chap. 37). The visual field defect typically takes the form of a cecocentral scotoma. Certain nutritional and toxic states may do the same, as well as sarcoidosis and the numerous other causes of optic neuropathy discussed further on.

Neuroretinitis is a rare post- or parainfectious process seen mostly in children and young adults, sometimes in association with exposure to the *Bartonella henselae* bacteria the cause of cat scratch fever. Papillitis is accompanied by macular edema and exudates situated radially in the Henle layer, producing a "macular star" appearance.

Ischemic Optic Neuropathy (Anterior, AION and Posterior, PION)

In persons older than 50 years of age, *ischemic infarction of the optic nerve head* is the most common cause of a persistent monocular loss of vision (Fig. 13-13). The onset is abrupt and painless, but on occasion the visual loss is progressive for several days. The field defect is often altitudinal and involves the area of central fixation, accounting for a severe loss of acuity. Swelling of the optic disc, extending for a short distance beyond the disc margin, and associated small, flame-shaped hemorrhages, is typical; less often, if the infarction is situated behind the optic nerve head, the disc appears entirely normal. The retina and retinal vessels are not affected, as they are in cases of embolic occlusion of the central retinal artery. AION may also complicate intraocular surgery. As the disc edema subsides, optic atrophy becomes evident. The second eye may be similarly affected at a later date, particularly in those patients with hypertension and diabetes mellitus. Usually, there are no premonitory symptoms or episodes of transient visual loss.

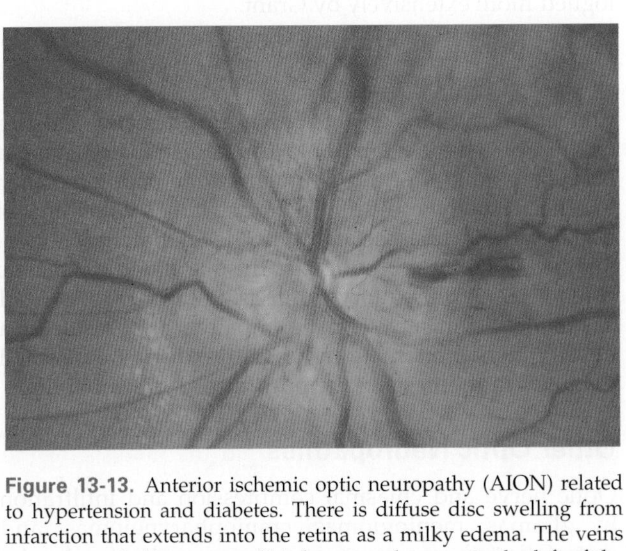

Figure 13-13. Anterior ischemic optic neuropathy (AION) related to hypertension and diabetes. There is diffuse disc swelling from infarction that extends into the retina as a milky edema. The veins are engorged. "Cotton-wool" infarcts can be seen to the left of the disc and a "flame" hemorrhage extends from the right disc margin.

Despite these distinctive features, ischemic optic neuropathy can sometimes be difficult to differentiate from optic neuritis, as pointed out by Rizzo and Lessell. This proves particularly problematic when visual loss evolves over days, the disc is swollen, and pain accompanies the ischemic condition. However, the age of the patient and nature of the field defect (central in optic neuritis in contrast to sometimes altitudinal in ischemic neuropathy) further serve to clarify the situation. Furthermore, arteritic and non-arteritic forms of ischemic optic neuropathy are distinguished, the former being the result of temporal (giant cell) arteritis.

As to the pathogenesis of non-arteritic ischemic optic neuropathy, the usual (anterior) form has been attributed by Hayreh to ischemia in the posterior ciliary artery circulation and more specifically to occlusion of the branches of the peripapillary choroidal arterial system. A small cup-to-disc ratio is reportedly a risk factor. Infarction of the posterior portions of the optic nerve(s) is uncommon (posterior ischemic optic neuropathy, PION). Most cases of either type occur on a background of hypertensive vascular disease and diabetes, but not necessarily in relation to carotid artery atherosclerotic stenosis, which in our experience has accounted for only a few cases (see below).

A relationship has been observed between ischemic optic neuropathy and the use of nitric oxide inhibitors, such as sildenafil, for erectile dysfunction. The visual loss has occurred within 24 h of taking the drug and is usually unilateral. According to Pomeranz and colleagues, all affected patients have had risk factors for vascular disease such as hypertension, diabetes, or hyperlipidemia, but there have been exceptions, and these risk factors are likely to be present in older men who are also likely to use the drug. There may be complete recovery or persistent blindness. Massive blood loss or intraoperative hypotension, particularly in association with the use of cardiac surgery with a bypass pump, may also produce visual loss, and ischemic infarction of the retina and optic nerve.

A remarkable unilateral or bilateral optic neuropathy, which we have observed and which is also presumably ischemic in nature, occurs after prolonged laminectomy operations that are performed with the patient in the prone position. Obese individuals and those with small optic cups are seemingly at risk for this complication. Some recovery is possible after many weeks but most patients remain blind from infarction of the optic nerve heads. Blood loss of greater than 1 L, and surgery longer than 6 hours seem to be common to most cases. The reported cases have been summarized from a registry by Lee and coworkers.

Temporal, or *giant cell, arteritis* is another important cause of AION or PION (see also Chap. 10 on the related headache and Chap. 34 for a discussion of cerebrovascular disease in association with giant cell arteritis). Fleeting premonitory symptoms of visual loss (amaurosis fugax) may precede infarction of the nerve. Infarction caused by cranial arteritis may affect both optic nerves in close succession and, less often, ocular motor function. Temporal arteritis less often presents with the picture of central retinal artery occlusion or posterior ischemic optic neuropathy (in which ischemic injury to the optic nerve is not accompanied by acute changes in the appearance of the disc).

The condition called "orbital pseudotumor", essentially an inflammatory condition of all the orbital contents, is discussed in Chap. 14 on oculomotor disorders but is mentioned here because optic neuropathy and visual loss can be a component of the syndrome.

Systemic lupus erythematosus, diabetes, sarcoidosis, neurosyphilis, and AIDS rarely give rise to optic neuropathies.

Optic Neuropathy Caused by Acute Cavernous and Paranasal Sinus Disease

A number of disease processes adjacent to the orbit and optic nerve can cause blindness, usually with signs of compression or infarction of the optic and oculomotor nerves. They are seen far less frequently than are ischemic optic neuropathy and optic neuritis. Septic cavernous sinus thrombosis (see "Cavernous Sinus Thrombosis" in Chap. 34), for example, may be accompanied by blindness of one eye or both eyes asymmetrically. In our experience with 4 such patients, the visual loss appeared days after the characteristic chemosis and oculomotor palsies of the venous sinus occlusion. The mechanism of visual loss, sometimes without swelling of the optic nerve head, is unclear but most likely relates to retrobulbar ischemia of the nerve.

Similarly, optic and oculomotor disorders may rarely complicate ethmoid or sphenoid sinus infections. Severe diabetes with mucormycosis or other invasive fungal or bacterial infection is the usual setting for these complications. Although the formerly held notion that uncomplicated sinus disease is a cause of optic neuropathy is no longer tenable, there are still a few instances in which such an association occurs but the nature of the visual loss remains unclear. Slavin and Glaser described a case of loss of vision from a sphenoethmoidal sinusitis with cellulitis at the orbital apex. Visual symptoms in these exceptional circumstances can occur prior to overt signs of local inflammation. An otherwise benign sphenoidal mucocele may cause a compressive optic neuropathy, usually with accompanying ophthalmoparesis and slight proptosis.

Toxic and Nutritional Optic Neuropathies (Table 13-3)

Simultaneous impairment of vision in the two eyes, with central or centrocecal scotomas, is often caused not by a demyelinative process but also by toxic or nutritional processes. The latter condition is observed most often in the chronically alcoholic or malnourished patient. Impairment of visual acuity evolves over several days or a week or two, and examination discloses bilateral, roughly symmetrical central or centrocecal scotomas, the peripheral fields being intact. With appropriate treatment (nutritious diet and vitamins B) instituted soon after the onset of amblyopia, complete recovery is possible. If treatment is delayed, patients are left with varying degrees of permanent defect in central vision and pallor of the temporal portions of the optic discs. This disorder has been referred to as "tobacco-alcohol amblyopia," the implication being that it is caused by the toxic effects of tobacco or alcohol or both. In fact, the problem is one of nutritional deficiency and is more properly designated as *deficiency amblyopia* or *nutritional optic neuropathy* (see Chap. 41). The same disorder may be seen under conditions of severe dietary deprivation (see Chap. 41) and in patients with vitamin B_{12} deficiency.

A subacute optic neuropathy of possible toxic origin was described in Jamaican natives. It was characterized by bilaterally symmetrical central visual loss and had additional features of nerve deafness, ataxia, and spasticity in some cases. A similar condition is described periodically in other Caribbean countries, two decades ago in Cuba, where an optic neuropathy of epidemic proportions was associated with a sensory polyneuropathy. A nutritional etiology, possibly contributed to by tobacco use (putatively cigars in the Cuban epidemic), was the likely cause of these outbreaks (see Sadun et al and The Cuba Neuropathy Field Investigation Team report). A putative role of exposure to cyanide, either from smoking or consumption of cassava, has been a feature of some of these epidemics.

Impairment of vision because of *methyl alcohol intoxication* (methanol) is abrupt in onset and characterized by large symmetrical central scotomas as well as symptoms of acidosis. Treatment is directed mainly to correction of the acidosis and possibly, the administration of fomepizole. The same may occur with ethylene glycol ingestion. The subacute development of central field defects is attributable to other toxins and to the chronic administration of certain therapeutic agents, notably halogenated hydroxyquinolines (clioquinol), chloramphenicol, ethambutol, linezolid, isoniazid, streptomycin, chlorpropamide (Diabinese), infliximab, and various ergot preparations. The main drugs reported to have a toxic effect on the optic nerves are listed in Table 13-3 and have been catalogued more extensively by Grant.

Developmental Abnormalities of the Optic Nerve

Congenital cavitary defects because of defective closure of the optic fissure may be a cause of impaired vision because of failure of development of the papillomacular bundle. Usually the optic pit or a larger coloboma is unilateral and unassociated with developmental abnormalities of the brain (optic disc dysplasia and dysplastic coloboma). A hereditary form is known (Brown and Tasman). Vision may also be impaired as a result of a developmental anomaly in which the discs are of small diameter (hypoplasia of the optic disc, or micropapilla).

Other Optic Neuropathies

Optic nerve and chiasmal compression and infiltration by gliomas, meningiomas, craniopharyngiomas, and metastatic tumors may cause scotomas and optic atrophy (see Chap. 31). Pituitary tumors characteristically cause bitemporal hemianopia, but very large adenomas, in particular if there is pituitary apoplexy (involutional bleeding into the pituitary), can cause blindness in one or both eyes (see "Pituitary Apoplexy" in Chap. 31). Infiltration of an optic nerve may occur in sarcoidosis (see Fig. 32-4, *bottom panel*), granulomatosis with polyangiitis (formerly Wegener granulomatosis), and with certain neoplasms, notably leukemia and lymphoma.

Of particular importance is the optic nerve glioma that occurs in 15 percent of patients with type I von Recklinghausen neurofibromatosis. Usually, it develops in children, often before the fourth year, causing a mass within the orbit and progressive loss of vision. If the eye is blind, the recommended therapy is surgical removal to prevent extension into the optic chiasm and hypothalamus. If vision is retained, radiation and chemotherapy are the recommended forms of treatment. Although most such gliomas are of low grade, a rare malignant form (glioblastoma) has been described in adults.

Thyroid ophthalmopathy with orbital edema, exophthalmos, and usually, swelling of extraocular muscles is an occasional cause of optic nerve compression.

Radiation-induced damage of the optic nerves and chiasm has been well documented. In a series of 219 patients at the M.D. Anderson Cancer Center who received radiotherapy for carcinomas of the nasal or paranasal region, retinopathy occurred in 7, optic neuropathy with blindness in 8, and chiasmatic damage with bilateral visual impairment in 1. These complications followed the use of more than 50 Gy (5,000 rad) of radiation (see Jiang et al). Radiation-induced optic neuropathy is typically delayed, occurring at an average of 18 months after radiation exposure, and is often accompanied by enhancement of the nerve on MRI. This is also addressed in Chap. 31.

In the case of pseudotumor cerebri, the visual loss may be unexpectedly abrupt, appearing in a day or less, and even sequentially in both eyes. This seems to happen most often in patients with constitutionally small optic nerves, no optic cup of the nerve head and, presumably, a small aperture of the lamina cribrosa. Such explosive visual loss in pseudotumor cerebri may respond to urgent optic nerve fenestration, but this approach is controversial, as discussed in "Pseudotumor Cerebri" in Chap. 30.

NEUROLOGY OF THE CENTRAL VISUAL PATHWAYS

From the retina there is a point-to-point projection to the lateral geniculate nucleus and from there, to the calcarine cortex of the occipital lobe. Thus the visual cortex receives a spatial pattern of stimulation that corresponds with the retinal image of the visual field. Visual impairments caused by lesions of the central pathways usually involve only a part of the fields, and a plotting of the fields provides fairly specific information as to the site of the lesion.

For purposes of description of the visual fields, each retina and macula are divided into a temporal and nasal half by a vertical line passing through the fovea. A horizontal line represented roughly by the junction of the superior and inferior retinal vascular arcades also passes through the fovea and divides each half of the retina and macula into upper and lower quadrants. Visual field defects are always described from the patient's view (nasal, temporal, superior, inferior) rather than of the retinal defect or the examiner's perspective. The retinal image of an object in the visual field is inverted and reversed from right to left, like the image on the film of a camera. Thus the left visual field of each eye is represented in the opposite half of each retina, with the upper part of the field represented in the lower part of the retina (Fig. 13-3). Figure 13-5 illustrates the retinal projections to the geniculate nuclei and occipital cortex.

Testing for Abnormalities of the Visual Fields

Figure 13-3 illustrates the visual field defects caused by lesions of the retina, optic nerve and tract, lateral geniculate body, geniculocalcarine pathway, and striate cortex of the occipital lobe. In the alert, cooperative patient, the visual fields can be plotted fairly accurately at the bedside. With one of the patient's eyes covered and the other fixed on the corresponding eye of the examiner (patient's right with examiner's left), a target—such as a moving finger, a cotton pledget, or a white disc mounted on a stick—is brought from the periphery toward the center of the visual field (confrontational testing). With the target at an equal distance between the eye of the examiner and that of the patient, the fields of the patient and examiner are then compared. Similarly, the patient's blind spot can be aligned with the examiner's, and its size determined by moving a small target outward from the blind spot until it is seen. Central and paracentral defects in the field can be outlined the same way. For reasons not known, red-green test objects are more sensitive than white ones in detecting defects of the visual pathways.

It should be emphasized that movement of the visual target provides the coarsest stimulus to the retina, so that a perception of its motion may be preserved while a stationary target of the same size may not be seen. In other words, moving targets are less useful than static ones in confrontational testing of visual fields. Finger counting and comparison of color intensity of a red object or the clarity of the examiner's hand from quadrant to quadrant are simple confrontation tests that will disclose most field defects. Glaser recommends presenting the examiner's hands simultaneously, one on each side of the vertical meridian; the hand in the hemianopic field appears blurred or darker than the other. Similarly, a scotoma may be defined by asking the patient to report changes in color or brightness of a red test object as it is moved toward or away from the point of fixation. Similarly, a central scotoma may be identified by having the patient fix with one eye on the examiner's nose, on which the examiner places the index finger of one hand or a white-headed pin and has the patient compare it for brightness, clarity, and color with a finger or pin held in the periphery.

We continue to teach that these confrontation techniques are reasonably sensitive for routine clinical work if performed carefully, but we are chastened by the article from Pandit and colleagues, who found false-negative findings in 42 percent of patients tested with quadrant finger counting, using static automated perimetry as a standard. If any defect is found or suspected by confrontational testing, the fields should be charted and scotomas outlined on a tangent screen or perimeter. Accurate computer-assisted perimetry is now available in most ophthalmology clinics. Although the commonly used automated techniques encompass only the central visual field, this is adequate to detect most clinically important changes.

The method of testing by double simultaneous stimulation may elicit defects in the central processing of vision that are undetected by conventional perimetry. Movement of one finger in all parts of each temporal field may disclose no abnormality, but if movement is simultaneous in analogous parts of both temporal fields, the patient with a parietal lobe lesion, especially on the right, may perceive only the one in the normal right hemifield. In young children or uncooperative patients, the integrity of the fields may be roughly estimated by observing whether the patient is attracted to objects in the peripheral field or blinks in response to sudden threatening gestures in half of the visual field.

A type of abnormality disclosed by visual field examination is *concentric constriction*. This may be a result of severe papilledema, in which case it is usually accompanied by an enlargement of the blind spot. A progressive constriction of the visual fields, at first unilateral and later bilateral, associated with pallor of the optic discs (optic atrophy), should suggest a chronic meningeal process involving the optic nerves (syphilis, cryptococcosis, sarcoidosis, lymphoma). Long-standing, untreated glaucoma and retinitis pigmentosa are other causes of concentric constriction. Marked constriction of the visual fields of unvarying degree, regardless of the distance of the visual stimulus from the eye ("gun-barrel" or "tunnel" vision), however, is a sign of hysteria. With organic disease, the constricted visual field naturally enlarges as the distance between the patient and the test object increases.

A regional constriction of the field, especially in a nasal quadrant, usually signifies early optic atrophy, as mentioned earlier; it is the first sign that chronic papilledema is threatening the patient's vision.

Prechiasmal Lesions

Lesions of the macula, retina, or optic nerve cause a *scotoma* (an island of impaired vision surrounded by normal vision) rather than a defect that extends to the periphery of one visual field ("field cut"). Scotomas are named according to their position (central, cecocentral) or their shape (ring, arcuate). A small scotoma that is situated in the macular part of the visual field may seriously impair visual acuity.

Scotomas are the main features of optic neuropathy, the main causes of which were discussed earlier and are listed in Table 13-3. Demyelinatng disease (optic neuritis), Leber hereditary optic atrophy, toxins and nutritional deficiencies, and vascular disease (ischemic optic neuropathy or occlusion of a branch of the retinal artery) are the main ones. Orbital or retroorbital tumors and infectious or granulomatous processes (e.g., sarcoidosis, retinal toxoplasmosis in AIDS) are other common causes. In the elderly, there may be compression of the optic nerve by a dolichoectatic aneurysm of the carotid, ophthalmic, or basilar arteries.

As discussed earlier, certain toxic and malnutritional states are characterized by more or less symmetrical bilateral central scotomas (involving the fixation point), or cecocentral ones (involving both the fixation point and the blind spot). The cecocentral scotoma, which tends to have an arcuate border, represents a lesion that is predominantly in the distribution of the papillomacular bundle. However, the presence of this visual field abnormality does not establish whether the primary defect is in the cells of the origin of the bundle, i.e., the retinal ganglion cells, or in their fibers. Demyelinating disease is characterized by unilateral or asymmetrical bilateral scotomas. Vascular lesions that take the form of retinal hemorrhages or infarctions of the nerve-fiber layer (cotton-wool patches) give rise to unilateral scotomas; occlusion of the central retinal artery or its branches causes infarction of the retina and, as a rule, a loss of central vision, while occlusion of a branch of the retinal artery may cause an altitudinal defect. As pointed out earlier, AION causes sudden monocular blindness, or an altitudinal field defect. Since the optic nerve also contains the afferent fibers for the pupillary light reflex, extensive lesions of the nerve will cause an afferent pupillary defect, which was mentioned earlier and is considered further in Chap. 14.

Lesions of the Chiasm, Optic Tract, and Geniculocalcarine Pathway

Hemianopia (hemianopsia) means blindness in half of the visual field. *Bitemporal hemianopia* indicates a lesion of the decussating fibers of the optic chiasm and is caused most often by the suprasellar extension of a tumor of the pituitary gland (Fig. 13-3C). It may also be the result, at this same site, of a craniopharyngioma, a saccular aneurysm or dolichoectatic artery of the anterior circle of Willis, and a meningioma of the tuberculum sellae; less often, it may be a result of sarcoidosis, metastatic carcinoma, ectopic pinealoma or dysgerminoma, Hand-Schüller-Christian disease, or hydrocephalus with dilatation and downward herniation of the anterior part of the third ventricle (Corbett). In some instances a tumor pushing upward presses the medial parts of the optic nerves, just anterior to the chiasm, against the anterior cerebral arteries. Chiasmal syndromes from causes other than pituitary adenoma are usually associated with unilateral optic disc atrophy, a relative afferent pupillary defect and a greater defect in the inferior field.

Heteronymous field defects, i.e., scotomas or field defects that differ in the two eyes, are a sign of involvement of the optic chiasm or the adjoining optic nerves or tracts; they are caused by craniopharyngiomas, or other suprasellar tumors and, rarely, by mucoceles, angiomas, giant carotid aneurysms, and opticochiasmic arachnoiditis.

The visual field pattern created by a lesion in the optic nerve as it joins the chiasm typically includes a scotomatous defect on the affected side coupled with a contralateral superior quadrantanopia ("junctional field defect"). As noted previously, the latter is caused by interruption of nasal retinal fibers from the contralateral optic nerve. This was originally attributed to fibers projecting into the base of the affected optic nerve but there is now evidence against the existence of this structure as mentioned earlier, and discussed in the reference by Horton. Variations in the pattern of visual loss from chiasmal lesions are frequent, in part accounted for by the location of the chiasm in an individual patient—a postfixed chiasm making unilateral eye findings more common.

Homonymous hemianopia (a loss of vision in corresponding halves of the visual fields) signifies a lesion of the visual pathway behind the chiasm and, if complete, gives no more information than that. *Incomplete homonymous hemianopia* has more localizing value. As a rule, if the field defects in the two eyes are identical (congruous), the lesion is likely to be in the calcarine cortex and subcortical white matter of the occipital lobe; if they are *incongruous*, the visual fibers in the optic tract or in the parietal or temporal lobe are more likely to be implicated. Absolute congruity of field defects is actually infrequent, even with occipital lesions.

The lower fibers of the geniculocalcarine pathway (from the inferior retinas) swing in a wide arc over the temporal horn of the lateral ventricle and then proceed posteriorly to join the upper fibers of the pathway on their way to the calcarine cortex (Fig. 13-3). This arc of fibers is known variously as the Flechsig, Meyer, or Archambault loop, and a lesion that interrupts these fibers will produce a *superior homonymous quadrantanopia* (contralateral upper temporal and ipsilateral upper nasal quadrants; Fig. 13-3*E*), or in incomplete cases, a homonymous superior wedge defect respecting the vertical meridian. This clinical effect was first described by Harvey Cushing, so that his name also was in the past applied to the loop of temporal visual fibers. Parietal lobe lesions are said to affect the inferior quadrants of the visual fields more than the superior ones, but this is difficult to document; with a lesion of the right parietal lobe, the patient ignores the left half of space; with a left parietal lesion, the patient is often aphasic. As to the localizing value of *quadrantic defects*, the report of Jacobson is of interest; he found, in reviewing the imaging studies of 41 patients with inferior quadrantanopia and 30 with superior quadrantanopia, that in 76 percent of the former and 83 percent of the latter the lesions were confined to the occipital lobe.

If the entire optic tract or calcarine cortex on one side is destroyed, the homonymous hemianopia is complete. But often that part of the field subserved by the macula is spared, i.e., there is a 5- to 10-degree island of vision around the fixation point on the side of the hemianopia (sparing of fixation, or *macular sparing*). With infarction of the occipital lobe as a result of occlusion of the posterior cerebral artery, the macular region, represented in the most posterior part of the striate cortex, may be spared by virtue of collateral circulation from branches of the middle cerebral artery. With other types of destructive lesions, this effect is not seen. Incomplete lesions of the optic tract and radiation also usually spare central (macular) vision. Nonvascular lesions of both occipital poles result in bilateral central scotomas; if all the calcarine cortex or all the subcortical geniculocalcarine fibers on both sides are completely destroyed, the bilateral hemianopias cause cerebral, or *"cortical,"* blindness (see below and Chap. 22).

An *altitudinal defect* is one that is confined by a horizontal border and crosses the vertical meridian. *Homonymous altitudinal hemianopia* is usually caused by lesions of both occipital lobes below or above the calcarine sulcus, and rarely to a lesion of the optic chiasm or nerves. Just as with the contralateral representation of the visual fields in respect to the vertical meridian, the representation of the upper visual field is in the bank of neurons below the calcarine fissure and vice versa. The most common cause of this rare phenomenon is still occlusion of both posterior cerebral arteries. Herniation of the occipital lobe over the tentorial margin can produce a homonymous superior altitudinal defect by selectively compressing the inferior branches of the posterior cerebral arteries. A monocular altitudinal hemianopia, by contrast, is almost invariably an ischemic optic neuropathy that arises from occlusion of the posterior ciliary vessels.

In certain instances of homonymous hemianopia, the patient is capable of some visual perception in the hemianopic fields, a circumstance that permits the study of the vulnerability of different visual functions. Colored targets may be detected in the hemianopic fields, whereas achromatic ones cannot. But even in seemingly complete hemianopic defects, in which the patient admits to being blind, it has been shown that he may still react to visual stimuli when forced-choice techniques are used. Blythe and coworkers found that 20 percent of their patients with no ability to discriminate patterns in the hemianopic field nonetheless could still reach accurately and look at a moving light in the "blind" field. This type of residual visual function has been called "blindsight" by Weiskrantz and colleagues. These residual visual functions are generally attributed to the preserved function of retinocollicular or geniculoprestriate cortical connections, but in some cases, they may be a result of sparing of small islands of calcarine neurons. In yet other instances of complete homonymous hemianopia, the patient may be little disabled by visual field loss (Benton et al; Meienberg). This is because of preservation of vision in a small monocular part of the visual field known as the *temporal crescent*. The latter is a peripheral unpaired portion of the visual field, between 60 and 100 degrees from the fixation point, and is represented in the most anterior part of the visual striate cortex. In particular, the temporal crescent is sensitive to moving stimuli, allowing the patient to avoid collisions with people and objects. The tendency for patients with occipital lesions to have greater sensitivity for kinetic stimuli than for static ones was described by Riddoch in 1917.

Blindness in the Hysterical or Malingering Patient

Hysterical, or *psychogenic blindness,* is described in Chap. 51, along with other features of hysteria, but a few comments are in order here. Feigned or hysterical visual loss is usually detected by attending to the patient's activities when he thinks he is unobserved, and it can be confirmed by a number of simple tests. Complete feigned blindness is disproved by observing the normal ocular jerk movements in response to a rotating optokinetic drum or strip, or by noting that the patient's eyes follow their own image in a mirror that is moved in front of them. The hysterical nature of *total monocular blindness* is apparent from the presence of a normal direct pupillary response to light. An optokinetic response in the nonseeing eye (with the good eye covered) is an even more convincing test. The visual evoked potential from the allegedly blind eye is also normal. Hysterical monocular loss may also be revealed by the use of red-green glasses and an acuity chart with red and green letters, where each eye can only see letters with the color of its lens. The patient cannot tell which letters should be visible to them, and the intact acuity in the involved eye is soon exposed. *Hysterical homonymous hemianopia* is rare and is displayed mostly by practiced malingerers; all manner of field defects are common in this population (Keane). The uniformly constricted tubular field defect of hysteria has already been mentioned. Star- and spiral-shaped visual fields are also indicative of psychogenic visual loss.

Cerebral Forms of Blindness and Visual Agnosia (See also Chap. 22)

The ability to recognize visually presented objects and words depends on the integrity not only of the visual pathways and primary visual area of the cerebral cortex (area 17 of Brodmann) but also of those cortical areas that lie just anterior to area 17 (areas 18 and 19 of the occipital lobe and area 39—the angular gyrus of the dominant hemisphere). Blindness that is the result of destruction of both visual and adjacent regions of the occipital lobes is termed *cortical* or *cerebral blindness*. Another remarkable condition exists in which the patient denies or is oblivious to blindness despite overt manifestations of the defect (Anton syndrome).

In distinction to these forms of blindness, there is a less-common category of visual impairment in which the patient cannot understand the meaning of what he sees, i.e., *visual agnosia*. Primary visual perception is more or less intact, and the patient may accurately describe the shape, color, and size of objects and draw copies of them. Despite this, he cannot identify the objects unless he hears, smells, tastes, or palpates them. The failure of visual recognition of words alone is called *visual verbal agnosia,* or *alexia*. Visual-object agnosia rarely occurs as an isolated finding: as a rule, it is combined with visual verbal agnosia, homonymous hemianopia, or both. These abnormalities arise from lesions of the dominant occipital cortex and adjacent temporal and parietal cortex (angular gyrus) or from a lesion of the left calcarine cortex combined with one that interrupts the fibers crossing from the right occipital lobe (see Fig. 22-6). In the latter case, fibers responsible for writing are spared, and the patient remains with a syndrome of alexia without agraphia.

Failure to understand the meaning of an entire picture even though some of its parts are recognized is referred to as *simultanagnosia*, and is found in bilateral lesions of the occipital–parietal junction. When combined with deficits in visual control of eye and hand movements (optic ataxia and ocular apraxia), the resulting condition is referred to as Balint syndrome. A failure to recognize familiar faces is called *prosopagnosia* and typically results from occipital–temporal lesions. These and other variants of visual agnosia (including visual neglect) and their pathologic bases are dealt with more fully in Chap. 22.

Other cerebral disturbances of vision include various types of distortion in which images seem to recede into the distance (teleopsia), appear too small (micropsia), or, less frequently, seem too large (macropsia). If such distortions are perceived with only one eye, a local retinal lesion should be suspected. If perceived with both eyes, they usually signify disease of the temporal lobes, in which case the visual disturbances tend to occur in attacks and are accompanied by other manifestations of temporal lobe seizures (see Chap. 16). Palinopsia, a persistence of repetitive afterimages, similar to the appearance of a celluloid movie strip, occurs with right parietooccipital lesions; it has been a consequence of seizures in the cases we have encountered, but instances associated with static disorders (tumor, infarction) have been described as well. Patients describe the images as "trailing" or "echoing." With parietal lobe lesions, objects may appear to be askew or even turned upside down. More often, lesions of the vestibular nucleus or its immediate connections produce the illusion that objects are tilted or turned upside down (tortopsia), or that straight lines are curved. Presumably this is the result of a mismatch between the visual image and the otolithic, or vestibular input to the visual system.

Abnormalities of Color Vision

Normal color vision depends on the integrity of cone cells, which are most numerous in the macular region. When activated, they convey information to special columns of cells in the striate cortex. Three different cone pigments with optimal sensitivities to blue, green, and orange-yellow wavelengths are said to characterize these cells; presumably each cone possesses only one of these pigments. Transmission to higher centers for the perception of color is effected by neurons and axons that encode at least two pairs of complementary colors: red-green in one system and yellow-blue in the other. In the optic nerves and tracts, the fibers for color are of small caliber and seem to be preferentially sensitive to certain noxious agents and to pressure. The geniculostriate fibers for color are separate from fibers that convey information about form and brightness, but course alongside them; hence, there may be a homonymous color hemianopia (hemiachromatopsia). The visual fields for blue-yellow are smaller than those for white light, and the red and green fields are smaller than those for blue-yellow.

Diseases may affect color vision by abolishing it completely (*achromatopsia*) or partially by quantitatively reducing one or more of the three attributes of color—brightness, hue, and saturation. Or, only one of the complementary pairs of colors may be lost, usually red-green. The disorder may be congenital and hereditary or acquired. The most common form, and the one to which the term *color blindness* is usually applied, is a male sex-linked inability to see red and green while normal visual acuity is retained. The main problem arises in relation to traffic lights, but patients learn to use the position of the light as a guide. Several other genetic abnormalities of cone pigments and their phototransduction have been identified as causes of achromatopsia. The defect cannot be seen by inspecting the retina. A failure of the cones to develop or a degeneration of cones may cause a loss of color vision, but in these conditions visual acuity is often diminished, a central scotoma may be present, and, although the macula also appears to be normal ophthalmoscopically, fluorescein angiography shows the pigment epithelium to be defective. Whereas congenital color vision defects are usually protan (red) or detan (green), leaving yellow-blue color vision intact, most acquired lesions affect all colors, at times disparately. Lesions of the optic nerves usually affect red-green more than blue-yellow; the opposite is true of retinal lesions. An exception is a rare, dominantly inherited, optic atrophy, in which the scotoma mapped by a large blue target is larger than that for red.

Damasio has drawn attention to a group of acquired deficits of color perception with preservation of form vision, the result of focal damage (usually infarction) of the visual association cortex, and subjacent white matter. Color vision may be lost in a quadrant, half of the visual field, or the entire field. The latter, or full-field achromatopsia, is the result of bilateral occipitotemporal lesions involving the fusiform and lingual gyri, a localization that accounts for its frequent association with visual agnosia (especially prosopagnosia), and some degree of visual field defect. A lesion restricted to the inferior part of the right occipitotemporal region, sparing both the optic radiations and striate cortex, causes the purest form of achromatopsia (left hemiachromatopsia). With a similar left-sided lesion, alexia may be associated with the right hemiachromatopsia.

Other Visual Disorders

In addition to the losses of perception of form, movement, and color, lesions of the visual system may also give rise to a variety of positive sensory visual experiences. The simplest of these are called phosphenes, i.e., flashes of light and colored spots in the absence of luminous stimuli. Mechanical pressure on the normal eyeball may induce them at the retinal level, as every child discovers. Or they may occur with disease of the visual system at many different sites. As mentioned earlier, elderly patients commonly complain of flashes of light in the peripheral field of one eye, most evident in the dark (*Moore lightning streaks*); these are related to vitreous tags that rest on the retinal equator, and may be quite benign, or may be residual evidence of retinal detachment. Cancer associated retinopathy is frequently associated with photopsias prior to visual loss. Retinal toxicity from digitalis causes chromatopsia with a characteristic "yellowish vision" and may also cause photopsias. In patients with migraine, activation of nerve cells in the occipital lobe, gives rise to the bright zigzag lines of a fortification spectrum. Stimulation of the cortical terminations of the visual pathways accounts for the simple or unformed visual hallucinations in epilepsy. Formed or complex visual hallucinations (of people, animals, landscapes) are observed in a variety of conditions, notably in old age when vision fails (Charles Bonnet syndrome, discussed in "Visual Hallucinations" in Chap. 22), in the withdrawal state following chronic intoxication with alcohol and other sedative-hypnotic drugs (see Chaps. 42 and 43), in Alzheimer disease, and in infarcts of the occipitoparietal or occipitotemporal regions (release hallucinations) or the diencephalon ("peduncular hallucinosis"). These disorders are also discussed in Chap. 22.

Occasionally, patients in whom a hemianopia is evident only when tested by double simultaneous stimulation (a component of visual neglect) may displace an image to the non-affected half field (*visual allesthesia*), or a visual image may persist for minutes to hours or reappear episodically, after the exciting stimulus has been removed (*palinopsia* or *paliopsia* mentioned earlier); the latter disorder also occurs in defective but not blind homonymous fields of vision. *Polyopia*, the perception of multiple images when a single stimulus is presented, is said to be associated predominantly with right occipital lesions and can occur with either eye. Usually there is one primary and a number of secondary images, and their relationships may be constant or changing. Bender and Krieger, who described several such patients, attributed the polyopia to unstable fixation. When this is monocular, there is either a defect in the lens or, more often, hysteria. *Oscillopsia*, or illusory movement of the environment, is a perception caused by nystagmus and occurs mainly with lesions of the labyrinthine-vestibular apparatus; it is described with disorders of ocular movement. A rare idiopathic myokymia of one superior oblique muscle may produce a monocular oscillopsia (see "Fourth Nerve Palsy" in Chap. 14).

Chapter 22 further discusses the clinical effects and syndromes that result from occipital lobe lesions.

Amblyopia Because of Early Life Strabismus (Amblyopia Ex Anopsia)

As noted in the introductory part of this chapter, the generic term "amblyopia" has been adopted for a special circumstance in which a normal eye fails to acquire its potential visual acuity because images are not properly projected onto the fovea during a formative period of cerebral development. It is a disorder, as in the quip by van Noorden and Campos, "in which the patient sees nothing and the doctor sees nothing." The period of risk is during the first 7 years but is greatest in the earlier part of this epoch, and the visual loss may still be rectifiable beyond the time.

The degradation of vision and disuse of the fovea may be the result of a number of processes, most often misaligned ocular axes (strabismus) and also including unequal refractive errors (anisometropia; discussed in Chap. 14). These conditions are the most common sources of visual disturbance in children. The uncorrected condition also accounts for an estimated 3 percent of monocular visual loss in adults. By convention, the diagnosis of amblyopia requires that a loss of 2 lines or more between eyes be observed on the Snellen chart.

The developmental deficiency in the occipital cortex that gives rise to amblyopia has been extensively studied in animals and humans; a discussion of the subject can be found in numerous texts including the one by van Noorden and Campos. Neurologists should be aware that screening children for the disorder is highly valuable even if treatment is not always successful. The correction of refractive errors, cataract, and other correctible ocular problems are attended to first. Attempts are then made to force the utilization of the disadvantaged eye in preference to the normal one; patching and atropine drops are the typical methods to accomplish this. Other techniques of management and a summary of clinical trials of each can be found in the review by Holmes and Clarke. Chapter 14 discusses the problem of strabismus and the latent phorias that create confusion in the neurologic examination.

References

Arruga J, Sanders M: Ophthalmologic findings in 70 patients with evidence of retinal embolism. *Ophthalmology* 89:1336, 1982.

Bender MB, Krieger HP: Visual function in perimetric blind fields. *Arch Neurol Psychiatry* 65:72, 1951.

Benton S, Levy I, Swash M: Vision in the temporal crescent in occipital infarction. *Brain* 103:83, 1980.

Bienfang DC, Kelly LD, Nicholson DH, et al: Ophthalmology. *N Engl J Med* 323:956, 1990.

Biousse V, Newman NJ: *Neuro-Ophthalmology Illustrated*. Thieme, New York, 2009.

Blythe IM, Kennard C, Ruddock KH: Residual vision in patients with retrogeniculate lesions of the visual pathways. *Brain* 110:887, 1987.

Brown GC, Tasman WS: *Congenital Anomalies of the Optic Disc*. New York, Grune & Stratton, 1983.

Chester EM: *The Ocular Fundus in Systemic Disease*. Chicago, Year Book, 1973.

Corbett JJ: Neuro-ophthalmologic complications of hydrocephalus and shunting procedures. *Semin Neurol* 6:111, 1986.

Damasio AR: Disorder of complex visual processing: Agnosia, achromatopsia, Balint's syndrome and related difficulties of orientation and construction, in Mesulam M-M (ed): *Principles of Behavioral Neurology*. Philadelphia, Davis, 1985, pp 259–288.

D'Amico DJ: Disease of the retina. *N Engl J Med* 331:95, 1994.

Antonetti DA, Klein R, Gardner TW: Diabetic Retinopathy. *N Engl J Med* 366:1227, 2012.

DeJong PT: Age-related macular degeneration. *N Engl J Med* 355:1474, 2006.

Digre KB, Kurcan FJ, Branch DW, et al: Amaurosis fugax associated with antiphospholipid antibodies. *Ann Neurol* 25:228, 1989.

Dryja TP, McGee TL, Reichel E, et al: A point mutation of the rhodopsin gene in one form of retinitis pigmentosa. *Nature* 343:364, 1990.

Fisher CM: Observations on the fundus in transient monocular blindness. *Neurology* 9:333, 1959.

Grant WM: *Toxicology of the Eye*. Springfield, IL, Charles C Thomas, 1986.

Grunwald GB, Klein R, Simmonds MA, Kornguth SE: Autoimmune basis for visual paraneoplastic syndrome in patients with small cell lung carcinoma. *Lancet* 1:658, 1985.

Hayreh SS: Anterior ischemic optic neuropathy. *Arch Neurol* 38:675, 1981.

Hayreh SS: Blood supply of the optic nerve head and its role in optic atrophy, glaucoma, and oedema of the optic disc. *Br J Ophthalmol* 53:721, 1969.

Hayreh SS: Pathogenesis of oedema of the optic disc (papilloedema). *Br J Ophthalmol* 48:522, 1964.

Holmes JM, Clarke MP: Amblyopia. *Lancet* 367:1343, 2006.

Horton JC: Wilbrand's knee of the primate optic chiasm is an artefact of monocular enucleation. *Trans Am Ophthalmol Soc* 95:579, 1997.

Hubel DH, Wiesel TN: Functional architecture of macaque monkey visual cortex. *Proc R Soc Lond B Biol Sci* 198:1, 1977.

Jacobson DM: The localizing value of a quadrantanopia. *Arch Neurol* 54:401, 1997.

Jacobson DM, Thurkill CE, Tipping SJ: A clinical triad to diagnose paraneoplastic retinopathy. *Ann Neurol* 28:162, 1990.

Jiang GL, Tucker SL, Guttenberger R, et al: Radiation-induced injury to the visual pathway. *Radiother Oncol* 30:17, 1994.

Keane JR: Patterns of hysterical hemianopia. *Neurology* 51:1230, 1998.

Kornguth SE, Klein R, Appen R, Choate J: The occurrence of anti-retinal ganglion cell antibodies in patients with small cell carcinoma of the lung. *Cancer* 50:1289, 1982.

Lee LA, Roth S, Cheney FW, et al: The American Society of Anesthesiologists Postoperative Visual Loss Registry: Analysis of 93 spine surgery cases with postoperative visual loss. *Anesthesiology* 105:652, 2006.

Levin BE: The clinical significance of spontaneous pulsations of the retinal vein. *Arch Neurol* 35:37, 1978.

Levine DN, Warach J, Farrah M: Two visual systems in mental imagery: Dissociation of "what" and "where" in imagery disorders due to bilateral posterior cerebral lesions. *Neurology* 35:1010, 1985.

Marshall J, Meadows S: The natural history of amaurosis fugax. *Brain* 91:419, 1968.

Meienberg O: Sparing of the temporal crescent in homonymous hemianopia and its significance for visual orientation. *Neuroophthalmology* 2:129, 1981.

Minckler DS, Tso MOM, Zimmerman LE: A light microscopic autoradiographic study of axoplasmic transport in the optic nerve head during ocular hypotony, increased intraocular pressure, and papilledema. *Am J Ophthalmol* 82:741, 1976.

Newman NJ: Optic neuropathy. *Neurology* 46:315, 1996.

Pandit RJ, Gales K, Griffiths PG: Effectiveness of testing of visual fields by confrontation. *Lancet* 358:1339, 2001.

Pearlman AJ: Visual system, in Pearlman AL, Collins RC (eds): *Neurobiology of Disease*. New York, Oxford University Press, 1990, pp 124–148.

Pomeranz HD, Smith KH, Hart WM, Egan RA: Nonarteritic ischemic optic neuropathy developing soon after use of sildenafil (Viagra): a report of seven cases. *J Neuroophthalmol* 25:9, 2005.

Rizzo JF, Lessell S: Optic neuritis and ischemic optic neuropathy. *Arch Ophthalmol* 109:1668, 1999.

Rucker CW: Sheathing of retinal venus in multiple sclerosis. *Mayo Clin Proc* 47:335, 1972.

Sadun RA, Martone JF, Muci-Mendoza R, et al: Epidemic optic neuropathy in Cuba: Eye findings. *Arch Ophthalmol* 112:691, 1994.

Savino PJ, Paris M, Schatz NJ, et al: Optic tract syndrome. *Arch Ophthalmol* 96:656, 1978.

Schumacher M, Schmidt D, Jurklies B, et al: Central retinal artery occlusion: local intra-arterial fibrinolysis versus conservative treatment, a multicenter randomized trial. *Ophthalmology* 117:1367, 2010.

Slavin M, Glaser JS: Acute severe irreversible visual loss with sphenoethmoiditis-posterior orbital cellulitis. *Arch Ophthalmol* 105:345, 1987.

Smith JL, Hoyt WP, Susac JO: Optic fundus in acute Leber's optic atrophy. *Arch Ophthalmol* 90:349, 1973.

The Cuba Neuropathy Field Investigation Team: Epidemic optic neuropathy in Cuba—clinical characteristics and risk factors. *N Engl J Med* 333:1176, 1995.

Traquair HM. *An Introduction to Clinical Perimetry*. St. Louis, CV Mosby, 1948.

Tso MOM, Hayreh SS: Optic disc edema in raised intracranial pressure: III. A pathologic study of experimental papilledema. *Arch Ophthalmol* 95:1448, 1977.

Tso MOM, Hayreh SS: Optic disc edema in raised intracranial pressure: IV: Axoplasmic transport in experimental papilledema, *Arch Ophthalmol* 95:1458, 1977.

Van Noorden GK, Campos E: *Binocular Vision and Ocular Motility*, 6th ed. St. Louis, Mosby, 2002.

Weiskrantz L, Warrington EK, Sanders MD, Marshall J: Visual capacity in the hemianopic field following a restricted occipital ablation. *Brain* 97:709, 1974.

Winterkorn J, Kupersmith MJ, Wirtschafter JD, Forman S: Treatment of vasospastic amaurosis fugax with calcium-channel blockers. *N Engl J Med* 329:396, 1993.

Wray SH: Neuro-ophthalmologic diseases, in Rosenberg RN (ed): *Comprehensive Neurology*, 2nd ed. New York, Wiley-Liss, 1998, pp 561–594.

Wray SH: Visual aspects of extracranial carotid artery disease, in Bernstein EF (ed): *Amaurosis Fugax*. New York, Springer-Verlag, 1988, pp 72–80.

Young LHY, Appen RE: Ischemic oculopathy. *Arch Neurol* 38:358, 1981.

14

Disorders of Ocular Movement and Pupillary Function

Ocular movement and vision are virtually inseparable. A moving object evokes movement of the eyes and almost simultaneously arouses attention and initiates the perceptive process. To look searchingly, i.e., to peer, requires stable fixation of the visual image on the center of the two retinas. One might say that the ocular muscles are at the service of vision.

Abnormalities of ocular movement are of three basic types. One category can be traced to a lesion of the extraocular muscles themselves, the neuromuscular junction, or to the cranial nerves that supply them (*nuclear* or *infranuclear palsy*). The second type is a derangement in the highly specialized neural mechanisms that enable the eyes to move together (*supranuclear* and *internuclear palsies*). This distinction, in keeping with the general concept of upper and lower motor neuron paralysis, hardly portrays the complexity of the neural mechanisms governing ocular motility. Perhaps more common but not primarily neurologic is a third group of disorders, *strabismus*, in which there is a congenital imbalance of the yoked muscles of extraocular movement that may lead to a developmental reduction in monocular vision (amblyopia), as discussed at the end of the previous chapter. Knowledge of the anatomic basis of normal movement is essential to an understanding of abnormal movement.

SUPRANUCLEAR CONTROL OF EYE MOVEMENT

Anatomic and Physiologic Considerations

In no aspect of human anatomy and physiology is the sensory guidance of muscle activity more instructively revealed than in the neural control of coordinated ocular movement. Moreover, the entirely predictable and "hardwired" nature of the central and peripheral oculomotor apparatus allows for a very precise localization of lesions within these pathways. To focus the eyes voluntarily, to stabilize objects for scrutiny when one is moving, to bring into sharp focus near and far objects—all require the perfect coordination of six sets of extraocular muscles and three sets of intrinsic muscles (ciliary muscles, sphincters, and dilators of the iris). The neural mechanisms that govern these functions reside mainly in the midbrain and pons but are greatly influenced by centers in the medulla, cerebellum, basal ganglia, and the frontal, parietal, and occipital lobes of the brain. Most of the nuclear structures and pathways concerned with fixation and stable ocular movements are now known and much has been learned of their physiology both from clinical-pathologic correlations in humans and from experiments in monkeys.

Accurate binocular vision is actually achieved by the associated action of all the ocular muscles. The symmetrical and synchronous movement of the eyes is termed *conjugate movement* or *gaze* (*conjugate* meaning yoked or joined together). The simultaneous movement of the eyes in different directions, as in convergence, is termed *dysconjugate* or *disjunctive*. These two forms of normal ocular movements are also referred to as *versions* (versional) and *vergence*, respectively. *Vergence movements* have two components—fusional and accommodative. The fusional movements are *convergence* and *divergence*, which maintain binocular single vision and depth perception (stereopsis); they are necessary at all times to ensure that visual images fall on corresponding parts of the retinas. *Convergent movements* are brought into action when one looks at a near object. The eyes turn inward and at the same time the pupils constrict and the ciliary muscles relax to thicken the lens and allow near vision (the accommodative-near reflex, or triad). Divergence, albeit slight, is required for distant vision.

Rapid voluntary conjugate movements of the eyes to the opposite side are initiated in area 8 of the frontal lobe (see Fig. 22-1) and relayed to the pons. These quick movements are termed *saccadic* (peak velocity may exceed 700 degrees per second). Their purpose is to rapidly change ocular fixation and bring images of new objects of interest onto the foveae. Saccades are so rapid that there is no subjective awareness of movement during the change in eye position, essentially, a momentary blindness. Saccadic movements can be elicited by instructing an individual to look to the right or left (commanded saccades), or to move the eyes to a target (refixation saccades). These two movements are sometimes differently affected in neurologic disease. Saccades may also be elicited reflexively, as when a sudden sound or the appearance of an object in the peripheral field of vision attracts attention and triggers an automatic movement of the eyes in the direction of the stimulus. Saccadic latency, the interval between the appearance of a target and the initiation of a saccade, is approximately 200 ms.

The neurophysiologic pattern of pontine neurons that produces a saccade has been characterized as "pulse-step" in type. This refers to the sudden increase in neuronal firing (the pulse) that is necessary to overcome the inertia and viscous drag of the eyes and move them into their new position; it is followed by a return to a new baseline firing level (the step), which maintains the eyes in their new position by tonic contraction of the extraocular muscles (*gaze holding*).

Saccades are distinguished from the slower and smoother *pursuit* or *following movements*, for which the major stimulus is a moving target. The function of pursuit movements is to stabilize the image of a moving object on the foveae, and thus to maintain a continuous clear image of the object as the object changes position ("smooth tracking"). Unlike saccades, pursuit movements to each side are generated in the *ipsilateral* parietooccipital cortex, with modulation by the ipsilateral cerebellum, especially the vestibulocerebellum (flocculus and nodulus). Another portion of the cerebellum, the posterior vermis, also influences saccadic movements (see further on).

When following a moving target, as the visual image slips off the foveae, the firing rate of the governing motor neurons increases in proportion to the speed of the target, so that eye velocity matches target velocity. If the eyes fall behind the target, supplementary catch-up saccades are required for refixation. The pursuit movement is then not smooth, but becomes jerky ("saccadic" pursuit). A lesion of one cerebral hemisphere may cause pursuit movements to that side to break up into saccades. Diseases of the basal ganglia are also a common cause of a disruption of normally smooth pursuit into a ratchet-like saccadic pursuit in all directions.

If a series of visual targets enters the visual field, as when one is watching trees from a moving car or the stripes on a rotating drum, involuntary repeated quick saccades refocus the eyes centrally; the resulting cycles of pursuit and refixation are termed *optokinetic nystagmus*. This phenomenon is used as a bedside test, the main value of which is in revealing a lesion of the ipsilateral posterior parietal lobe. It may also be found that a frontal lobe lesion eliminates the quick nystagmoid refixation phase away from the side of the lesion, thereby causing the eyes to continue to follow the target until it is out of view. This optokinetic phenomenon is described more fully further on, in the section on nystagmus.

Vestibular influences are of particular importance in stabilizing images on the retina during head and body movement. By means of the *vestibuloocular reflex* (VOR), a prompt short latency movement of the eyes is produced that is equal and opposite to movement of the head. During sustained rotation of the head, the VOR is supplemented by the optokinetic system, which enables one to maintain compensatory eye movements for a more prolonged period. If the VOR is lost, as occurs with disease of the vestibular apparatus or eighth nerve, the slightest movements of the head, especially those occurring during locomotion, cause a movement of images across the retina large enough to impair vision. A unilateral loss of the VOR strongly implicates a disease of the vestibular apparatus on the side toward the rotation of the head. When objects are tracked using both eye and head movements, the VOR must be suppressed, otherwise the eyes would remain fixed in space; to accomplish this, the smooth pursuit signals cancel the unwanted vestibular ones (Leigh and Zee). It follows that the inability to suppress the VOR, while viewing a target as the patient is rotated, is indicative of a defect of supranuclear pursuit.

Horizontal Gaze

Saccades

As already mentioned, the signals for volitional horizontal gaze saccades originate in the eye field of the opposite frontal lobe (area 8 of Brodmann, see Fig. 22-1) and are modulated by the adjacent supplementary motor eye field and by the posterior visual cortical areas. Leichnetz traced the cortical-to-pontine pathways for saccadic horizontal gaze in the monkey. These fibers traverse the internal capsule and separate at the level of the rostral diencephalon into two bundles, the first being a primary ventral "capsular–peduncular" bundle, which descends through the most medial part of the cerebral peduncle. This more ventral pathway undergoes a partial decussation in the low midbrain, at the level of the trochlear nucleus, and terminates mainly in the vaguely defined paramedian pontine reticular formation (PPRF) of the opposite side, neurons of which, in turn, project to the adjacent sixth nerve nucleus (Fig. 14-1). A second, more dorsal "transthalamic" bundle is predominantly uncrossed and courses through the internal medullary lamina and paralaminar parts of the thalamus to terminate diffusely in the pretectum, superior colliculus, and periaqueductal gray matter. An off-shoot of these fibers (the prefrontal oculomotor bundle) projects to the rostral part of the oculomotor nucleus and to the ipsilateral rostral interstitial nucleus of the medial longitudinal fasciculus (riMLF) and to the interstitial nucleus of Cajal (INC), which are involved in vertical eye movements, as discussed in the next section.

Pursuit

The pathways for smooth pursuit movements are less well defined. One probably originates in the posterior parietal cortex and the adjacent temporal, and anterior occipital cortex (area MT of the monkey) and descends to the ipsilateral dorsolateral pontine nuclei. Also contributing to smooth pursuit movements are projections from the frontal eye fields to the ipsilateral dorsolateral pontine nuclei. The latter, in turn, project to the flocculus and dorsal vermis of the cerebellum, which provide stability for the pursuit movements. However, for the purposes of clinical work, lesions of the posterior parietal cortex are the ones known to impair pursuit toward the damaged side. Part of the frontal eye fields have been shown experimentally to participate in pursuit eye movements, but the influence of this area on pursuit is far less than that of the parietal lobes and is insignificant clinically.

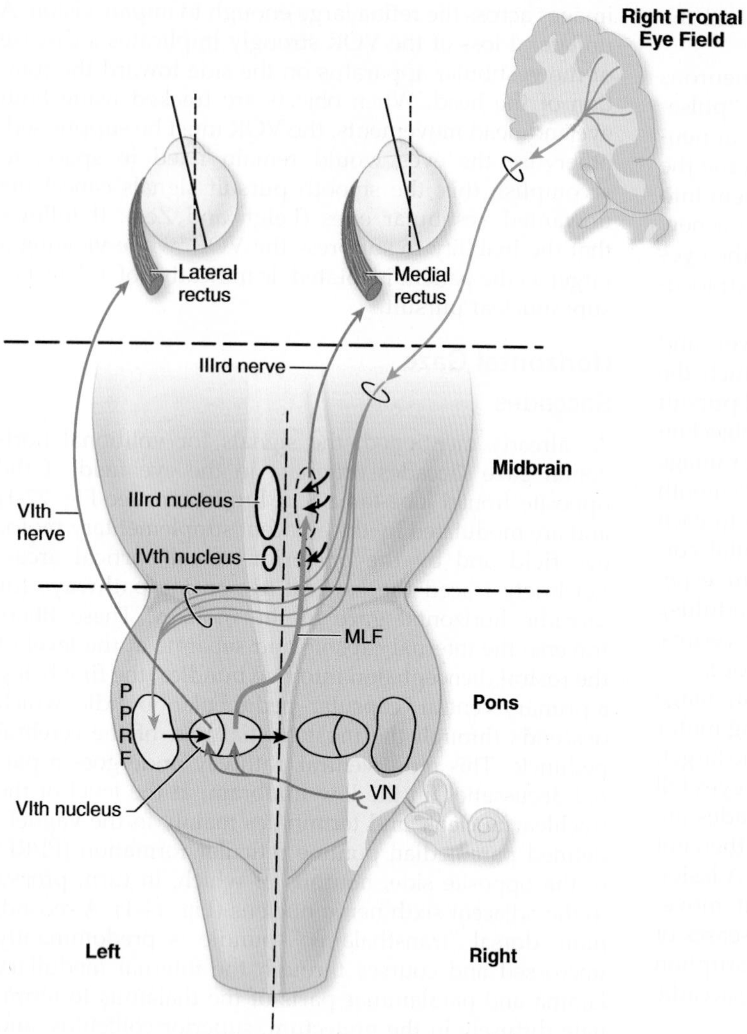

Figure 14-1. The supranuclear pathways subserving saccadic horizontal gaze to the left. The pathway originates in the right frontal cortex, descends in the internal capsule, decussates at the level of the rostral pons, and descends to synapse in the left pontine paramedian reticular formation (PPRF). Further connections with the ipsilateral sixth nerve nucleus and contralateral medial longitudinal fasciculus are also indicated. Cranial nerve nuclei III and IV are labeled on left; nucleus of VI and vestibular nuclei (*VN*) are labeled on right. The right MLF (green line) is labelled between the 3rd and 6th nerves on that side. *LR*, lateral rectus; *MLF*, medial longitudinal fasciculus; *MR*, medial rectus.

Brainstem (Internuclear) Pathways and Oculomotor Nuclei

Conventionally, the term *ocular motor nuclei* refers to the nuclei of the third, fourth, and sixth cranial nerves; the term *oculomotor nucleus* refers to the third nerve nucleus alone. Ultimately, all the pathways mediating saccadic and pursuit movements in the horizontal plane, as well as for vestibular and optokinetic movements, converge on the pontine tegmental center for horizontal gaze, the PPRF. Also required for horizontal versional movements are the nuclei prepositus hypoglossi and their commissure, the abducens and medial vestibular nuclei, and pathways in the pontine and tegmentum of the brainstem that interconnect the oculomotor nuclei (Fig. 14-1).

The PPRF and the prepositus and medial vestibular nuclei are conceptualized as a "neural integrator" and relay station for horizontal saccade pathways. It is further considered that the PPRF projects to the sixth nerve nucleus to command horizontal eye movement. However, it is understood from animal experiments that supranuclear neural signals that encode smooth pursuit, and vestibular and optokinetic movements bypass the PPRF and project independently to the abducens nuclei (Hanson et al).

The fiber bundle connecting the third and sixth nerve nuclei, and connecting both these nuclei with the vestibular nuclei lies in the medial tegmentum of the brainstem; this pathway is the *medial longitudinal fasciculus* (MLF). The fibers of the MLF emanating from the sixth nerve nucleus cross in the pons and ascend to the contralateral medial rectus subnucleus of the third nerve. In this way, the abduction of one eye is yoked to adduction of the opposite one to produce conjugate horizontal gaze as described just below.

The abducens nucleus contains two groups of neurons, each with distinctive morphologic and physiologic properties: (1) the intranuclear abducens motor neurons, which innervate the ipsilateral lateral rectus muscle, and (2) abducens internuclear neurons, which project via the contralateral MLF to the medial rectus neurons of the opposite oculomotor nucleus. Conjugate lateral gaze is accomplished by the simultaneous activation of the ipsilateral lateral rectus, and the contralateral medial rectus, again, the latter through fibers that run in the medial portion of the MLF. Interruption of the MLF results in a discrete impairment or loss of adduction of the eye ipsilateral to the lesion, a sign referred to as *internuclear ophthalmoplegia*, the details of which are discussed further on (Fig. 14-1).

Two other ascending pathways between the pontine centers and the mesencephalic reticular formation have been traced: one traverses the central tegmental tract and terminates in the pretectum, in the nucleus of the posterior commissure; the other is a bundle separate from the MLF that passes around the nuclei of Cajal and Darkschewitsch to the riMLF. These nuclei are involved more in vertical gaze and are described below. In addition, each vestibular nucleus projects onto the abducens nucleus, and the MLF of the opposite side. This pathway is considered to generate the slow phase of the VOR.

Although direct projections from the frontal eye fields that bypass the PPRF and innervate the oculomotor nuclei, as described above, undoubtedly exist, indirect projections are more important in the voluntary control of conjugate eye movements. According to Leigh and Zee, a more accurate view of these various voluntary influences is one of a hierarchy of cell stations and parallel pathways that do not project directly to oculomotor nuclei but to adjacent *premotor* or *burst neurons*, which discharge at high frequencies immediately preceding a saccade. The premotor or burst neurons for horizontal saccades lie within the PPRF and those for vertical saccades in the riMLF (see below). Yet a third class of neurons (omnipause cells), lying in the midline of the pons, is involved in the inhibition of unwanted saccadic discharges. Nonetheless, in clinical work, the circuit that comprises in sequence (1) frontal lobe eye fields, (2) contralateral pontine PPRF, (3) abducens nucleus, (4) MLF, and (5) opposite oculomotor nucleus makes understandable a number of highly characteristic defects of horizontal ocular motion, as detailed in the remainder of the chapter.

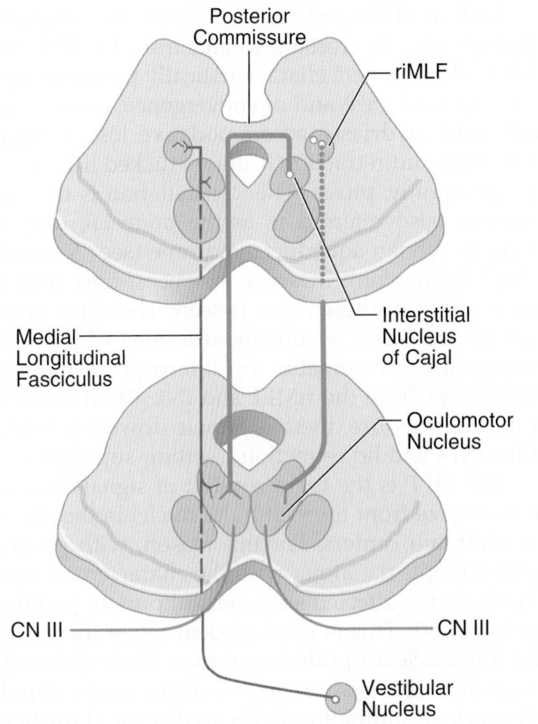

Figure 14-2. Pathways for the control of vertical eye movements. The main structures are the interstitial nucleus of Cajal (INC), the rostral interstitial nucleus of the medial longitudinal fasciculus (riMLF), and the subnuclei of the third nerve, all located in the dorsal midbrain. Voluntary vertical movements are initiated by the simultaneous activity of both frontal cortical eye fields. The riMLF serves as the generator of vertical saccades and the INC acts tonically to hold eccentric vertical gaze. The INC and riMLF connect with their contralateral nuclei via the posterior commissure, where fibers are subject to damage. Projections for upgaze cross through the commissure before descending to innervate the third nerve nucleus, while those for downgaze may travel directly to the third nerve, thus accounting for the frequency of selective upgaze palsies (see text). The MLF carries signals from the vestibular nuclei, mainly ipsilaterally, to stabilize the eyes in the vertical plane (VOR) and maintain tonic vertical position.

Vertical Gaze

In contrast to horizontal gaze, which is generated by unilateral aggregates of cerebral and pontine neurons, vertical eye movements, with few exceptions, are under bilateral control of the cerebral cortex and upper brainstem. The groups of nerve cells and fibers that govern upward and downward gaze, as well as torsional saccades, are situated in the pretectal areas of the midbrain and involve three integrated structures—the riMLF, the INC, and the nucleus and fibers of the posterior commissure (Fig. 14-2).

The *riMLF* lies at the junction of the midbrain and thalamus, at the rostral end of the medial longitudinal fasciculus, just dorsomedial to the rostral pole of the red nucleus. It functions as the "premotor" nucleus with "burst cells" for the production of fast (saccadic) vertical versional and torsional movements. Input to the riMLF arises both from the PPRF and the vestibular nuclei. Each riMLF projects mainly ipsilaterally to the oculomotor and trochlear nuclei, but each riMLF is also connected to its counterpart by fibers that traverse the posterior commissure. Bilateral lesions of the riMLF or of their interconnections in the posterior commissure are more common than unilateral ones, and cause a loss either of downward saccades or of all vertical saccades.

The *INC* is a small collection of cells that lies just caudal to the riMLF on each side. Each nucleus projects to the motor neurons of the opposite elevator muscles (superior rectus and inferior oblique) by fibers that cross through the posterior commissure, and it projects ipsilaterally and directly to the depressor muscles (inferior rectus and superior oblique). The functional role of the INC appears to be in holding eccentric vertical gaze, especially after a saccade; it is also integral to the vestibuloocular reflex. Lesions of the INC produce a vertical gaze-evoked and torsional nystagmus, and an ocular tilt reaction and probably slow all conjugate eye movements, mainly vertical ones.

Lesions of the *posterior commissure* are common; they interrupt signals crossing to and from the INC and the riMLF. A lesion here characteristically produces a paralysis of upward gaze and of convergence, often associated with mild mydriasis, accommodative loss, convergence nystagmus, lid retraction (Collier "tucked lid" sign), and, less commonly, ptosis. This constellation is the *Parinaud syndrome,* also referred to as the pretectal, dorsal midbrain, or sylvian aqueduct syndrome (see "Vertical Gaze Palsy" further on). In some instances, only a restricted combination of these signs is seen. The same syndrome may be produced by unilateral lesions of the posterior commissure, presumably by interrupting bidirectional connections from the riMLF and INC. With acute lesions of the commissure, there is a tonic downward deviation of the eyes and lid retraction ("setting-sun sign").

The MLF is the main conduit of signals that control vertical gaze from the vestibular nuclei in the medulla to the midbrain centers. For this reason, with internuclear ophthalmoplegia, along with the characteristic adductor paresis on the affected side, vertical pursuit and the VOR are impaired. This is most evident when there are bilateral internuclear ophthalmoplegias. Vertical deviation of the ipsilateral eye (*skew*) may be seen in cases of unilateral internuclear ophthalmoplegia, as discussed further on.

Vestibulocerebellar Influences on Eye Movements

There are important vestibulocerebellar influences on both smooth pursuit and saccadic movements (see also Chap. 5). The flocculus and posterior vermis of the cerebellum receive abundant sensory projections from proprioceptors of the cervical musculature (responsive to head velocity), the retinas (sensitive to target velocity), proprioceptors of eye muscles (eye position and eye velocity), auditory and tactile receptors, and the superior colliculi and PPRF. Cerebellar efferents concerned with ocular movement project onto the vestibular nuclei, and the latter, in turn, influence gaze mechanisms through several projection systems: one, for horizontal movements, consists of direct projections from the vestibular nuclei to the contralateral sixth nerve nucleus; another, for vertical movements, projects via the contralateral MLF to third and fourth nerve nuclei (Figs. 14-1 and 14-2).

Lesions of the flocculus and posterior vermis are consistently associated with deficits in smooth pursuit movements and an inability to suppress the vestibuloocular reflex by fixation (Baloh et al). Floccular lesions are also an important cause of downbeat nystagmus. As indicated in Chap. 5, patients with cerebellar (floccular) lesions are unable to hold eccentric positions of gaze and must make repeated saccades to look at a target that is away from the neutral position (*gaze-paretic nystagmus,* a term also applied to nystagmus arising from a lesion in the PPRF). This phenomenon is explained by the fact that with acute, one-sided lesions of the vestibulocerebellum, the inhibitory discharges of the Purkinje cells onto the ipsilateral medial vestibular nucleus are removed, and the eyes deviate away from the lesion. When gaze to the side of the lesion is attempted, the eyes drift back to the midline, and fixation can be corrected only by a saccadic jerk. The head and neck may also turn away from the lesion (the occiput toward the lesion and the face away). In addition, the vestibuloocular reflexes, which coordinate eye movements with head movements, are improperly adjusted (Thach and Montgomery). The interested reader can find further details concerning cerebellar influences on ocular movements in the monograph by Leigh and Zee and the review by Lewis and Zee.

Testing of Conjugate Gaze

It is apparent from the foregoing remarks that there is considerable clinical information to be obtained from an analysis of ocular movements. To fully examine the eye movements, the patient should be asked to look quickly to each side as well as up and down (saccades) and to follow a moving target (pursuit of a light, the examiner's finger, or an optokinetic drum). A patient with stupor and coma can be examined by passively turning the head or by irrigating the external auditory canals; these are vestibular stimuli to reflex eye movement as discussed in Chap. 17.

Most individuals make accurate saccades to a target. Alterations of saccadic movements, particularly overshooting of the eyes (*hypermetria*), are characteristic of a cerebellar lesion. *Slowness of saccadic movements* is mainly the result of disease of the basal ganglia such as Huntington and Wilson diseases, ataxia-telangiectasia, progressive supranuclear palsy, olivopontocerebellar degeneration, and certain lipid storage diseases. Lesions involving the PPRF may also be accompanied by slow saccadic movements to the affected side. Hypometric, slow saccades occurring only in the adducting eye indicate an incomplete internuclear ophthalmoparesis caused by a lesion of the ipsilateral MLF. When the earliest sign of a progressive eye movement disorder is slow saccades in the vertical plane, the likely diagnosis is progressive supranuclear palsy, but the same sign may occur in Parkinson disease and several less common processes that affect the basal ganglia, as discussed further on under "Vertical Gaze Palsy." Slow up-and-down saccades are also found in Niemann-Pick disease type C.

Yet another saccadic disorder takes the form of an *inability to initiate voluntary movements,* either vertically or horizontally. This abnormality may be congenital in nature, as in the ocular "apraxia" of childhood (Cogan syndrome, see below) and in ataxia-telangiectasia; an acquired difficulty in the initiation of saccadic movements may be seen in patients with Huntington disease or with a lesion of the contralateral frontal lobe or ipsilateral pontine tegmentum. The most common explanation for the inability to move the eyes is hysteria, a circumstance that can be exposed by noting the patient will follow his own eyes in a mirror.

In addition to abnormalities of the saccades themselves, saccadic latency or reaction time (the interval between the impulse to move and movement) is prolonged in Huntington chorea and Parkinson disease. Saccadic latency is also increased in corticobasal ganglionic degeneration (see Chap. 39), in which case it seems to correspond to the degree of motor apraxia. The obligate need to initiate eye movements with a blink is often a subtle sign of disordered supranuclear control of conjugate movements that is evident in these same diseases and in other processes including frontal lobe lesions.

Fragmentation of smooth pursuit movement, a frequent neuroophthalmic finding, is a jerky irregularity of tracking that has been called "saccadic pursuit". Two broad categories of disorders give rise to this phenomenon; a vestibulocerebellar and an extrapyramidal type. The former is commonly the result of sedative drug intoxication—with barbiturates, diazepam, and others as well as from a lesion of the vestibulocerebellar apparatus. In both, there is gaze directed nystagmus that seemingly interrupts pursuit movements as well. It is possible that sedatives cause this disturbance by affecting this same system.

A similar-appearing phenomenon, but one that does not manifest nystagmus, nicely called *"cogwheel eye movements"*, is seen in certain extrapyramidal diseases such as Parkinson disease, Huntington disease, and progressive supranuclear palsy. In these diseases there is a ratchet-like impairment of smooth pursuit movements in association with slow, hypometric saccades ("saccadic pursuit"). Indeed, according to Vidailhet and colleagues, smooth pursuit movements are impaired in all types of basal ganglionic degenerations.

Asymmetrical impairment of smooth pursuit movements is indicative of a parietal or a frontal lobe lesion. Pursuit is impaired *toward the side of a parietal lesion and away from a frontal lesion*, as described earlier. This is not a common clinical phenomenon unless elicited by optokinetic testing as explained further on.

Vestibuloocular Reflex (VOR) Testing

This refers to involuntary conjugate eye movements that are contraversive to head turning and is manifest in unresponsive patients. Stimulation of the labyrinths by caloric or electrical activation elicits an identical phenomenon and can be performed in awake patients as well, as described in Chap. 17 on Coma.

Optic Fixation Reflex

The ability to *suppress* the VOR by visual fixation can provide considerable information and may be tested in various ways depending on the clinical need. One such test in the cooperative patient is performed by requesting that the patient fixate on a distant target and rapidly turning the head to one side by 5 to 10 degrees and (see "Tests of Labyrinthine Function" in Chap. 15). Slippage of fixation (impaired vestibuloocular reflex) is appreciated by observing a small corrective saccade in the direction opposite head turning. An alternative is to rotate the patient in a chair while he fixates on the thumb of his outstretched hand. There should be no loss of fixation at moderate rotational speeds; nystagmus during this maneuver is an abnormal sign. Zee has described yet another means of testing the VOR in which the examiner observes the optic nerve head while the patient rotates the head back and forth at a rate of one to two cycles per second. If the VOR is impaired, the optic nerve head appears to oscillate. Normally, movement of the head at this rate does not cause blurring of vision because of the rapidity with which the VOR accomplishes compensatory eye movements. As a result of inability to suppress the VOR, the patient experiences a feeling of instability.

Testing the Near Response (Accommodative Triad)

Combined convergence and accommodative movements are tested by asking the patient to look at his thumbnail, the examiner's finger, or object as it is brought toward the eyes. However, these fusional movements are frequently impaired in the elderly and in confused or inattentive patients and should not be interpreted as the result of disease in the ocular motor pathways. Otherwise, the absence or impairment of these movements should suggest a lesion in the rostral midbrain as a component of the Parinaud syndrome. *Convergence spasms* and *retraction nystagmus* may accompany paralysis of vertical gaze from a dorsal midbrain lesion. But when such convergent spasms occur alone, they are characteristic of hysteria, in which full horizontal movement can usually be obtained if each eye is tested separately. Also, cycloplegic eye drops will abolish accommodation and pupillary miosis.

Impairment of Conjugate Gaze

Horizontal Gaze Palsy

Strictly speaking, gaze palsy refers to a complete loss of both saccadic and pursuit movements to one side. Gaze paresis would then refer to an incomplete loss of the same capacity. Operationally, a distinction is made between supranuclear disorders of gaze that can be overcome by intense stimuli, and certain nuclear lesions that cause an insurmountable loss of gaze to one side that cannot be overcome except by physically moving the globes (forced ductions).

As a rule, the horizontal gaze palsies of cerebral and pontine origin are readily distinguished by the side of an accompanying hemiparesis. When there is a tonic deviation of the eyes ipsilateral to a cerebral lesion, this relationship is expressed as *"the eyes look toward the lesion and away from the hemiparesis."* The opposite pertains to brainstem gaze palsies, that is, gaze is impaired toward the side opposite the lesion, and if there is gaze deviation, the eyes are turned toward a hemiparesis. Palsies of pontine origin need not have an accompanying hemiparesis but are associated with other signs of pontine disease, particularly peripheral facial palsies and internuclear ophthalmoplegia on the same side as the paralysis of gaze. Pontine gaze palsies tend to be longer lasting than those of cerebral origin. Also, in the case of a cerebral lesion (but not a pontine lesion), the eyes turn to the paralyzed side if they are fixated on the target, and the head is rotated passively to the opposite side (i.e., by utilizing the VOR).

Cerebral Origin An acute lesion of one frontal lobe, such as an infarct, usually causes impersistence or paresis of contralateral gaze (more so than an actual palsy of gaze), and the eyes may for a limited time turn involuntarily toward the side of the cerebral lesion. In most cases of acute frontal lobe damage, the gaze palsy is incomplete and temporary, lasting for a week or less. Almost invariably, it is accompanied by hemiparesis. Forced closure of the eyelids may cause the eyes to move paradoxically to the side of the hemiparesis rather than upward (the latter being the Bell phenomenon), as would be expected. Similarly, during sleep, the eyes may also deviate conjugately away from the side of the lesion toward the side of the hemiplegia. As indicated above, pursuit movements away from the side of the lesion tend to be fragmented or lost. Posterior parietal lesions reduce pursuit movements but do not cause gaze palsy.

With bilateral frontal lesions, the patient may be unable to turn his eyes voluntarily in any direction but retains fixation and following movements. Occasionally, a deep cerebral lesion, particularly a thalamic hemorrhage extending into the midbrain, will cause the eyes to deviate conjugately to the side opposite the lesion ("wrong-way" gaze); the basis for this anomalous phenomenon is not established, but interference with descending oculomotor tracts in the midbrain has been postulated by Tijssen. It should be emphasized that cerebral gaze paralysis is not attended by strabismus or diplopia, i.e., the eyes always move conjugately. The usual causes of gaze paresis are vascular occlusion with infarction, hemorrhage, and abscess or tumor of the frontal lobe.

A seizure originating in the frontal lobe may also drive the eyes to the opposite side. When the eyes are driven contralaterally from the cerebral focus they may not return to the midline, giving the impression of gaze palsy. Also, in the postictal period, the eyes may reside in the opposite direction, ipsilaterally to the seizure focus.

Brainstem Origin The most common source of a nuclear-infranuclear gaze palsy is a lesion in the pontine horizontal gaze complex (PPRF; also involving the abducens nucleus), which causes ipsilateral gaze palsy and deviation of the eyes to the opposite side (Table 14-1). A unilateral lesion in the rostral midbrain tegmentum, by interrupting the cerebral pathways for horizontal conjugate gaze before their decussation, will also cause a paresis of gaze to the opposite side. Vestibulocerebellar lesions can cause yet another disorder of conjugate gaze that simulates a gaze palsy in which the eyes are forced, or driven to one side in a manner termed "pulsion" that prevents voluntary movement to the other side.

Table 14-1

DISEASES EXHIBITING UPGAZE OR VERTICAL GAZE PALSY

Midbrain infarction and hemorrhage
Tumor in the region of the dorsal midbrain (e.g., pinealoma)
Advanced hydrocephalus with enlargement of third ventricle
Progressive supranuclear palsy
Parkinson disease
Lewy body disease
Cortical basal ganglionic degeneration
Whipple disease
Metabolic diseases of childhood (Niemann-Pick type C, Gaucher, Tay-Sachs)
Any cause of bilateral internuclear ophthalmoplegia (e.g., multiple sclerosis)

Vertical Gaze Palsy

Midbrain lesions affecting the pretectum and the region of the posterior commissure interfere with conjugate movements in the vertical plane. Paralysis of vertical gaze is a prominent feature of the *Parinaud* or *dorsal midbrain syndrome* described earlier. Upward gaze in general is affected far more frequently than downward gaze because, as already explained, some of the fibers subserving upgaze cross rostrally and posteriorly between the riMLF and INC and are subject to interruption before descending to the oculomotor nuclei, whereas the pathways for downgaze apparently project directly downward to oculomotor nuclei from the two controlling centers.

The range of upward gaze is frequently restricted by extraneous factors, such as drowsiness, increased intracranial pressure, and particularly, aging. In a patient who cannot elevate the eyes voluntarily, the presence of reflex upward deviation of the eyes in response to flexion of the head ("doll's-head maneuver") or to voluntary forceful closure of the eyelids (*Bell phenomenon*) indicates that the nuclear and infranuclear mechanisms for upward gaze are intact and that the defect is supranuclear. However, useful this rule may be, in some instances of disease of the peripheral neuromuscular apparatus—such as Guillain-Barré syndrome and myasthenia gravis—in which voluntary upgaze may be limited, the strong stimulus of eye closure may cause upward deviation, whereas voluntary attempts at upgaze are unsuccessful, thereby spuriously suggesting a lesion of the upper brainstem. In addition, approximately 15 percent of normal adults do not show a Bell phenomenon; in others, deviation of the eyes is paradoxically downward.

In patients who during life had shown an isolated palsy of downward gaze, autopsy has disclosed bilateral lesions of the rostral midbrain tegmentum (just medial and dorsal to the red nuclei). An unusual case, described by Bogousslavsky and colleagues, suggests that a paralysis of vertical gaze may follow a strictly unilateral infarction that comprises the posterior commissure, riMLF, and INC. Hommel and Bogousslavsky have summarized the location of strokes that cause monocular and binocular vertical gaze palsies.

Several *degenerative* and related processes exhibit selective or prominent upgaze or vertical gaze palsies, as mentioned earlier (Table 14-1). In progressive supranuclear palsy, a highly characteristic feature is a selective paralysis of vertical gaze, with the more specific feature being downward paralysis beginning with impairment of saccades and later, restriction of all vertical movements. Parkinson and Lewy-body diseases (see Chap. 39), corticobasal ganglionic degeneration (see Chap. 39), and Whipple disease of the brain (see Chap. 40) may also produce vertical gaze palsies as these diseases progress.

Other Supranuclear Disorders of Gaze

The *ocular tilt reaction*, in which skew deviation (unilateral vertical separation of the eyes, discussed further on) is combined with ocular torsion and head tilt, is attributed to an imbalance of otolithic-ocular and otolithic-colic reflexes. In lesions involving the vestibular nuclei, as occurs in lateral medullary infarction, the eye is lower on the side of the lesion. With lesions of the MLF or INC, which can also cause skew and an ocular tilt reaction, the eye is higher on the side of the lesion.

Another unusual disturbance of gaze is the *oculogyric crisis*, or *spasm*, which consists of a tonic spasm of conjugate deviation of the eyes, usually upward and less frequently, laterally or downward. Recurrent attacks, sometimes associated with spasms of the neck, mouth, and tongue muscles and lasting from a few seconds to an hour or two, were pathognomonic of postencephalitic parkinsonism in the past. Now this phenomenon is observed as an acute reaction in patients being given phenothiazine and related neuroleptic drugs and in Niemann-Pick disease. The pathogenesis of these ocular spasms is not known. In the drug-induced form, upward deviation of the eyes is often associated with a report by the patient of peculiar obsessional thoughts; the entire syndrome can be terminated by the administration of an anticholinergic medication such as benztropine.

Congenital oculomotor "apraxia" (Cogan syndrome) is a congential disorder characterized by unusual eye and head movements that are obligately tied together during attempts to change the position of the eyes. The patient is unable to make normal voluntary horizontal saccades when the head is stationary. If the head is free to move and the patient is asked to look at an object to either side, the head is thrust to one side and the eyes turn in the opposite direction; the head overshoots the target, and the eyes, as they return to the central position, fixate on the target. Both voluntary saccades and the quick phase of vestibular nystagmus are defective. The pathologic anatomy is not understood but the condition abates over time. This same phenomenon is also seen in ataxia-telangiectasia (Louis-Bar disease, Chap. 37) and with agenesis of the corpus callosum, in which both horizontal and vertical saccades may be affected.

NUCLEAR AND INFRANUCLEAR DISORDERS OF EYE MOVEMENT

Anatomic Considerations

The third (oculomotor), fourth (trochlear), and sixth (abducens) cranial nerves innervate the extrinsic muscles of the eye. Because their actions are closely integrated and many diseases involve all of them at once, they are suitably considered together.

The *oculomotor (third-nerve)* nuclei consist of several paired groups of motor nerve cells adjacent to the midline, and ventral to the aqueduct of Sylvius at the level of the superior colliculi. A centrally located group of cells that innervate the pupillary sphincters and ciliary bodies (muscles of accommodation) is situated dorsally in the Edinger-Westphal nucleus that subserves pupillary reactions to light and the near vision response; this is the parasympathetic portion of the oculomotor nucleus. Ventral to this nuclear group are cells that mediate the actions of the levator of the eyelid, superior and inferior recti, inferior oblique, and medial rectus, in this dorsal–ventral order. This functional arrangement has been determined in cats and monkeys by extirpating individual extrinsic ocular muscles and observing the retrograde cellular changes (Warwick). Subsequent studies using radioactive tracer techniques have shown that medial rectus neurons occupy three disparate locations within the oculomotor nucleus rather than being confined to its ventral tip (Büttner-Ennever and Akert). These experiments also indicated that the medial and inferior recti, and the inferior oblique are innervated strictly ipsilaterally from the oculomotor nuclei, whereas the superior rectus receives only crossed fibers, and the levator palpebrae superioris (lid elevators) has bilateral innervations. Whether this precise arrangement is reproduced in humans is not known. Vergence movements are under the control of medial rectus neurons and not, as was once supposed, by an unpaired medial group of cells (nucleus of Perlia).

The fibers of the third-nerve nucleus course ventrally in the midbrain, crossing the medial longitudinal fasciculus, red nucleus, substantia nigra, and medial part of the cerebral peduncle successively. Lesions involving these structures therefore interrupt oculomotor fibers in their intramedullary (fascicular) course and give rise to several crossed syndromes of hemiplegia and ocular palsy. With regard to the oculomotor subnuclei, schematic arrangements of their projections have been derived from various sources, mainly experimental but some clinical, and are shown in the figure from Ksiazek and colleagues (Fig. 14-3). The emerging fibers can be considered as situated in medial, lateral and rostro-caudal groups, with

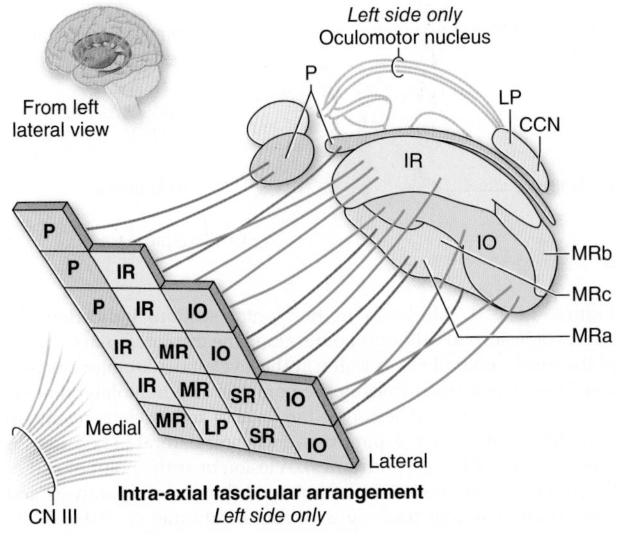

Figure 14-3. Topographic arrangement of oculomotor fascicular fibers in the mesencephalon. P, pupil; SR, superior rectus; IR, inferior rectus; MR, medial rectus; IO, inferior oblique; LP, levator palpebrae; CCN, central caudal nucleus. (From Ksiazek SM, Slamovits TL, Rosen CE, et al: Fascicular arrangement in partial oculomotor paresis. Am J Ophthalmol 118: 97, 1994.)

the pupillary fibers occupying the rostro-medial aspect. This location of axons destined for the pupil continues through the third nerve. This information becomes useful in recognizing that combined pupillary and inferior and medial rectus palsies on one side may be the result of a fascicular lesion of the oculomotor nerve.

The *sixth nerve (abducens)* arises at the level of the lower pons from a paired group of cells in the floor of the fourth ventricle, adjacent to the midline. The intrapontine portion of the facial nerve loops around the sixth-nerve nucleus before it turns anterolaterally to make its exit; a lesion in this locality therefore causes a homolateral paralysis of the lateral rectus and facial muscles. It is important to note that the efferent fibers of the oculomotor and abducens nuclei have a considerable intramedullary extent, i.e., their fascicular portions (Fig. 14-4*A* and *B*).

The cells of origin of the *trochlear nerves* are just caudal to those of the oculomotor nerves in the lower midbrain. Unlike the third and sixth nerves, the fourth nerve emerges from the dorsal surface of the lower midbrain and then courses posteriorly (dorsally) and decussates a short distance from its origin, just caudal to the inferior colliculi.

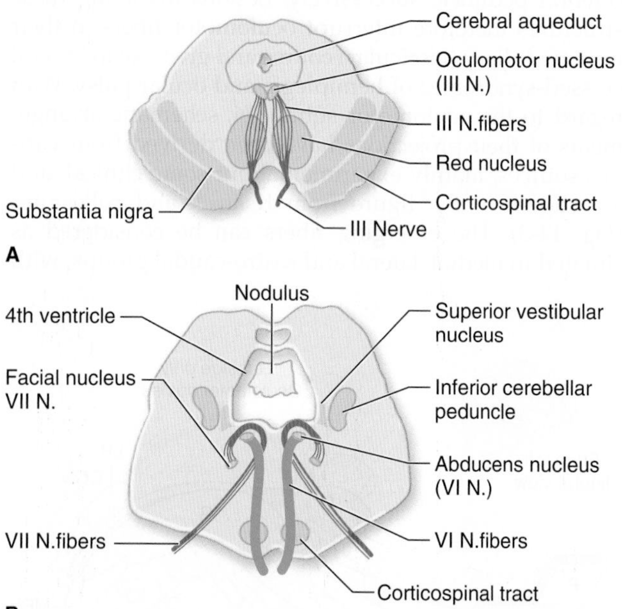

Figure 14-4. *A.* Midbrain in horizontal section, indicating the effects of lesions at different points along the intramedullary course of the third-nerve fibers. A lesion at the level of oculomotor nucleus results in homolateral third-nerve paralysis and homolateral anesthesia of the cornea. A lesion at the level of red nucleus results in homolateral third-nerve paralysis and contralateral ataxic tremor (Benedikt and Claude syndromes). A lesion near the point of exit of third-nerve fibers results in homolateral third-nerve paralysis and crossed corticospinal tract signs (Weber syndrome; see Table 47-2). *B.* Brainstem at the level of the sixth-nerve nuclei, indicating effects of lesions at different loci. A lesion at the level of the nucleus results in homolateral sixth- and seventh-nerve paralyses with varying degrees of nystagmus and weakness of conjugate gaze to the homolateral side. A lesion at the level of corticospinal tract results in homolateral sixth-nerve paralysis and crossed hemiplegia (Millard-Gubler syndrome).

The nerves proceed circumferentially and ventrally around the midbrain toward the entry of the nerve into the posterior cavernous sinus. Each nucleus therefore innervates the *contralateral* superior oblique muscle. The long extraaxial course and the position of the nerves adjacent to the brainstem is a putative explanation for the common complication of fourth-nerve palsy in head injury (see Chap. 35). The superior oblique muscle forms a tendon that passes through a pulley structure (the trochlea) and attaches to the upper aspect of the globe. When the eye is adducted, the muscle exerts an upward pull, but being attached to the globe behind the axis of rotation, it causes depression and intorsion of the eye; in abduction, it thereby pulls the ocular meridian toward the nose, thereby causing intorsion (i.e., clockwise in the right eye and counterclockwise in the left from the examiner's perspective).

The oculomotor nerve, soon after it emerges from the brainstem, passes between the superior cerebellar and posterior cerebral arteries. The nerve (and sometimes the posterior cerebral artery) may be compressed at this point by herniation of the uncal gyrus of the temporal lobe through the tentorial opening (see Chap. 17). The sixth nerve, after leaving the brainstem, sweeps upward along the clivus and then runs alongside the third and fourth cranial nerves; together they course anteriorly, pierce the dura just lateral to the posterior clinoid process, and run in the lateral wall of the cavernous sinus, where they are closely applied to the internal carotid artery and first and second divisions of the fifth nerve (Fig. 14-5 and "Cavernous Sinus Thrombosis" in Chap. 34).

When infraclinoid retrocavernous compressive lesions, such as aneurysms and tumors, affect the oculomotor nerve, they tend to also involve all three divisions of the trigeminal nerve. In the posterior portion of the cavernous sinus, the first and second trigeminal divisions are involved along with the oculomotor nerves; in the anterior portion, only the ophthalmic division of the trigeminal nerve is affected.

Just posterior and superior to the cavernous sinus, the oculomotor nerve crosses the terminal portion of the internal carotid artery at its junction with the posterior communicating artery. An aneurysm at this site frequently damages the third nerve; this serves to localize the site of compression or bleeding.

Together with the first division of the fifth nerve, the third, fourth, and sixth nerves enter the orbit through the superior orbital fissure. The oculomotor nerve, as it enters the orbit, divides into superior and inferior branches, although a functional separation of nerve bundles occurs well before this anatomic bifurcation. The superior branch supplies the superior rectus and the voluntary (striated) part of the levator palpebrae (the involuntary part is under the control of sympathetic fibers of Müller); the inferior branch supplies the pupillary and ciliary muscles and all the other extrinsic ocular muscles except, of course, two—the superior oblique and the lateral rectus which are innervated by the trochlear and abducens nerves, respectively. *Superior branch lesions* of the oculomotor nerve caused by an aneurysm or more commonly by diabetes, result in ptosis and uniocular upgaze paresis.

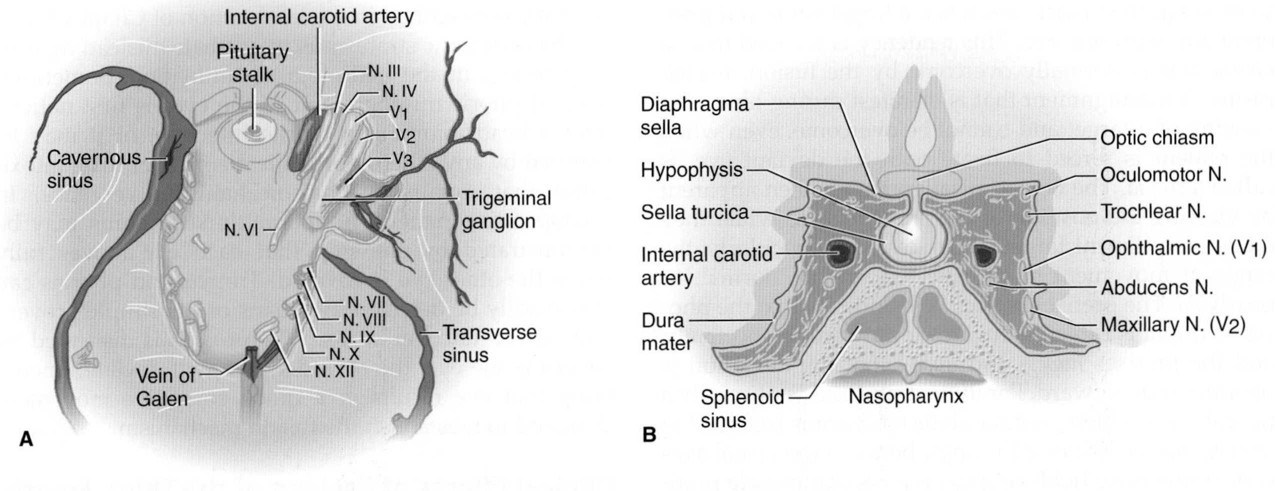

Figure 14-5. (See also Fig. 34-29.) The cavernous sinus and its relation to the cranial nerves. *A*. Base of the skull; the cavernous sinus has been removed on the right. *B*. The cavernous sinus and its contents viewed in the coronal plane.

Diplopia and Strabismus

Under normal conditions, all the extraocular muscles participate in every movement of the eyes; for proper movement, the contraction of any muscle requires relaxation of its antagonist. Clinically, however, an eye movement can be thought of in terms of the one muscle that is predominantly responsible for an agonist movement in that direction, e.g., outward movement of the eye requires the action of the lateral rectus; inward movement, action of the medial rectus. The action of the superior and inferior recti and the oblique muscles varies according to the position of the eye. When the eye is turned outward, the elevator is the superior rectus and the depressor is the inferior rectus. When the eye is turned inward, the elevator and depressor are the inferior and superior oblique muscles, respectively. The actions of the ocular muscles in different positions of gaze are illustrated in Fig. 14-6 and Table 14-2.

The term *binocular diplopia* refers to the symptom of double vision caused by a misalignment of the visual axes of the two eyes. With very few exceptions, in order to experience diplopia there must be some vision in both eyes. Put another way, covering one eye usually obliterates double vision. If the visual axes are separated by a significant amount, the individual may suppress the image from one eye and not experience diplopia. There is a form of *monocular diplopia* that is due to lenticular or retinal disease and is also a manifestation of hysteria.

Strabismus, strictly speaking, refers to a muscle imbalance that results in misalignment of the visual axes, but the term is used most often by neurologists to describe a congenital variety of misalignment. Strabismus may be caused by weakness of an individual eye muscle (*paralytic strabismus*) or by an imbalance of muscular tone, presumably because of a faulty "central" mechanism that normally maintains a proper angle between the two visual axes (*nonparalytic* or *pediatric strabismus*, see below).

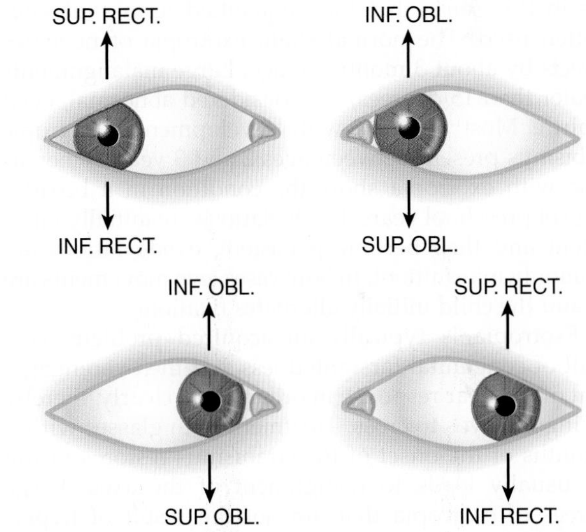

Figure 14-6. Muscles chiefly responsible for vertical movements of the eyes in different positions of gaze. (Adapted by permission from Cogan DG: *Neurology of the Ocular Muscles*, 2nd ed. Springfield, IL, Charles C Thomas, 1956.)

Table 14-2

ACTIONS OF THE EXTRAOCULAR MUSCLES

MUSCLE	PRIMARY ACTION	SECONDARY ACTION	OCULOMOTOR NERVE
Medial rectus	Adduction	—	III
Lateral rectus	Abduction	—	VI
Superior rectus	Elevation	Intorsion	III
Inferior rectus	Depression	Extorsion	III
Superior oblique	Intorsion	Depression	IV
Inferior oblique	Extorsion	Elevation	III

(See also Fig. 14-5.)

Almost everyone has a slight tendency to strabismus, i.e., to misalign the visual axes when a target is viewed preferentially with one eye. This tendency is referred to as a *phoria* and is normally overcome by the fusion mechanisms. A misalignment that is manifest during binocular viewing of a target and cannot be overcome, even when the patient is forced to fixate with the deviant eye, is called a *tropia*. The ocular misalignment is then apparent by viewing the position of the patient's eyes while they fixate on a distant target. When tested monocularly, the range of movement in the affected eye are normal, or nearly so. The prefixes *eso-* and *exo-* indicate that the phoria or tropia is directed inward or outward, respectively, and the prefixes *hyper-* and *hypo-*, that the deviation is upward or downward. Paralytic strabismus is primarily a neurologic problem; nonparalytic strabismus (referred to as *comitant strabismus* if the angle between the visual axes is the same in all fields of gaze) is an ocular muscle problem that is managed by ophthalmologists, although it is associated with a number of congenital cerebral diseases and forms of developmental delay.

Pediatric Nonparalytic Strabismus

It is in this sense that the unqualified term *strabismus* is often used. The normal slight exotropia of neonates corrects by about 3 months of age. Large malalignments (greater than 15 degrees) are considered abnormal, even at birth. Most children with developmental esotropic strabismus present between ages 2 and 3 years, whereas those with exotropia show the condition in a broader range of preschool years. Esodeviations are initially intermittent and then become persistent; exodeviations are commonly intermittent. In both cases, eye movements are full and the child initially alternates fixation.

Esotropia is typically an acquired problem as a result of congenital farsightedness and the overengagement of the near response in order to see clearly, thereby driving the eyes to cross. Treatment with glasses within 6 months of the onset of the strabismus restores vision and usually leads to realignment of the axes. Large degrees of esotropia that are not the result of hypermetropia (farsightedness) are best treated by surgical realignment.

In contrast, persistent exotropic strabismus in a child is usually associated with a developmental delay, often as a component of a recognizable mental retardation syndrome, as detailed in Chap. 38, or with ocular pathology. It does, however, occur in neurologically normal children. If mild, intermittent exotropia is initially treated by one of a number of nonsurgical means such as patching and visual exercises to stimulate convergence; surgical correction is reserved for unresponsive cases. Donohue has written an informative review of the subject.

Once binocular fusion is established, usually by 6 months of age, any type of ocular muscle imbalance will cause diplopia, as images then fall on disparate or noncorresponding parts of the two functionally active retinas. After a time, however, the child eliminates the diplopia by suppressing the image from one eye. After another variable period, the suppression becomes permanent, and the individual retains diminished visual acuity in that eye, the result of prolonged disuse (*amblyopia ex anopsia*), as described in the last portion of Chap. 13.

Nonparalytic strabismus may create misleading ocular findings in the neurologic examination. Sometimes a slight phoric misalignment of the eyes is first noticed after a head injury or a febrile infection, or it may be exposed by any other neurologic disorder or drug intoxication that impairs fusional mechanisms (vergence). In a cooperative patient, nonparalytic strabismus may be demonstrated by showing that each eye moves fully when the other eye is covered. Tropias and phorias can also readily be detected by means of the simple "cover" and "cover–uncover" tests. When fusion is disrupted by covering one eye, the occluded eye will deviate; uncovering that eye results in a quick corrective movement designed to reestablish the fusion mechanism.

Clinical Effects of Lesions of the Third, Fourth, and Sixth Ocular Nerves

Third (Oculomotor) Nerve

A complete *third nerve lesion* causes ptosis, or drooping of the upper eyelid (as the levator palpebrae is supplied mainly by this nerve), and an inability to rotate the eye upward, downward, or inward. This corresponds to the weaknesses of the medial, superior, and inferior recti and the inferior oblique muscles. The remaining actions of the fourth and sixth nerves give rise to a position of the eye described by the mnemonic "down and out." The patient experiences diplopia in which the image from the affected eye is projected upward and medially. In addition, one finds a dilated, light-nonreactive pupil (iridoplegia), and paralysis of accommodation (cycloplegia) because of interruption of the parasympathetic fibers in the third nerve. However, the extrinsic and intrinsic (papillary) eye muscles may be affected separately in certain diseases. For example, infarction of the central portion of the oculomotor nerve, as occurs in diabetic ophthalmoplegia, typically spares the pupil, as the parasympathetic preganglionic pupilloconstrictor fibers lie near the surface. Conversely, compressive lesions of the nerve usually dilate the pupil as an early manifestation. After injury, regeneration of the third-nerve fibers may be aberrant, in which case some of the fibers that originally moved the eye in a particular direction now reach another muscle or the iris; in the latter instance the pupil, which is unreactive to light, may constrict when the eye is turned up and in.

Fourth (Trochlear) Nerve

A lesion of the *fourth nerve*, which innervates the superior oblique muscle, is the most common cause of isolated symptomatic vertical diplopia. Although oculomotor palsy was a more common cause of vertical diplopia in Keane's 1975 series, as stated earlier, in instances where this is the sole complaint, trochlear palsy (and brainstem lesions) have predominated in our material. Paralysis of the superior oblique muscle results in weakness of downward movement of the affected eye, most marked when the eye is turned inward (Fig. 14-7*E*), so that the patient complains of special difficulty in reading or going down stairs. The affected eye tends *to deviate slightly upward when the patient*

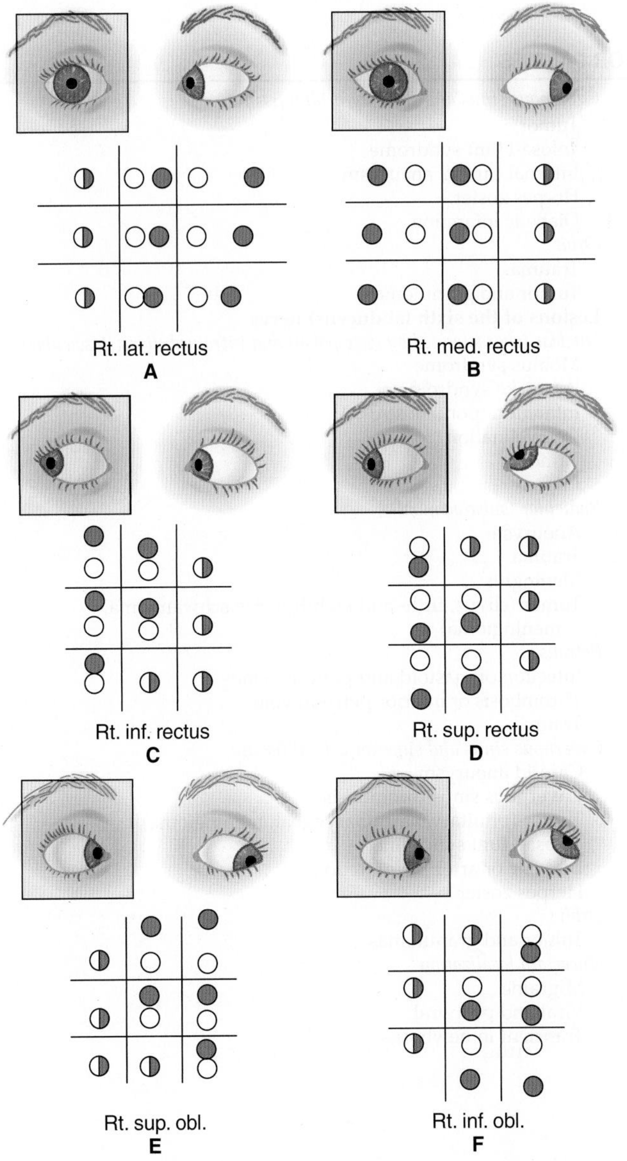

Figure 14-7. Diplopia fields with individual muscle paralysis. *The red glass is in front of the right eye, and the fields are projected as the patient sees the images (see text). A.* Paralysis of right lateral rectus. Characteristic: right eye does not move to the right. Field: horizontal homonymous diplopia increasing on looking to the right. *B.* Paralysis of right medial rectus. Characteristic: right eye does not move to the left. Field: horizontal crossed diplopia increasing on looking to the left. *C.* Paralysis of right inferior rectus. Characteristic: right eye does not move downward when eyes are turned to the right. Field: vertical diplopia (image of right eye lowermost) increasing on looking to the right and down. *D.* Paralysis of right superior rectus. Characteristic: right eye does not move upward when eyes are turned to the right. Field: vertical diplopia (image of right eye uppermost) increasing on looking to the right and up. *E.* Paralysis of right superior oblique. Characteristic: right eye does not move downward when eyes are turned to the left. Field: vertical diplopia (image of right eye lower-most) increasing on looking to left and down. *F.* Paralysis of right inferior oblique. Characteristic: right eye does not move upward when eyes are turned to the left. Field: vertical diplopia (image of right eye uppermost) increasing on looking to left and up. (Adapted by permission from Cogan DG: *Neurology of the Ocular Muscles*, 2nd ed. Springfield, IL, Charles C Thomas, 1956.)

looks straight ahead. This defect may be overlooked in the presence of a third-nerve palsy if the examiner fails to note the absence of an expected intorsion as the patient tries to move the paretic eye downward. Head tilting to the opposite shoulder (Bielschowsky sign) is especially characteristic of fourth-nerve lesions; this maneuver causes a compensatory intorsion of the unaffected eye and ameliorates the double vision. Lesions affecting the trochlear nucleus (rather than the nerve itself) will cause paresis of the contralateral superior oblique muscle; here, the patient will tilt their head toward the side of the lesion to ameliorate the diplopia.

Bilateral trochlear palsies, as may occur after head trauma, give a characteristic alternating hyperdeviation depending on the direction of gaze (unilateral traumatic trochlear paresis is still the more common finding with head injury). A useful review of the approach to vertical diplopia is given by Palla and Straumann.

Sixth (Abducens) Nerve

Lesions of the *sixth nerve* result in a paralysis of the abducens muscle and a resultant weakness of lateral or outward movement leading to a crossing of the visual axes. The affected eye *deviates medially,* i.e., in the direction of the opposing muscle. Diplopia is experienced as horizontal separation that is greatest at a distance form the patient and the image of the affected eye is projected outward. Fig 14-7A). With incomplete sixth-nerve palsies, turning the head toward the side of the paretic muscle overcomes the diplopia.

Many causes of oculomotor palsies and of *combined palsies,* which are discussed in a later section, are listed in Table 14-3 and are illustrated in Fig. 14-7 and below.

The Analysis of Diplopia

Almost all instances of diplopia (i.e., seeing a single object as double) are the result of an acquired paralysis or paresis of one or more extraocular muscles. The signs of the oculomotor palsies, as described above, are manifest in various degrees of completeness. With complete palsies, the affected muscle can often be surmised from the resting dysconjugate positions of the globes. With incomplete paresis, noting the relative positions of the corneal light reflections and having the patient perform common versional movements will usually disclose the faulty muscle(s) *as the eyes are turned into the field of action of the paretic muscle.* The muscle weakness may be so slight, however, that no strabismus or defect in ocular movement is obvious, yet the patient experiences diplopia. It is then necessary to use the patient's report of the relative positions of the images of the two eyes. Certain precautions should be taken in testing: one is cognizance of the above-mentioned absence of diplopia when the visual axes are widely separated and, the object or light used for testing should not be obscured by the patient's nose.

Two rules are applied sequentially to identify the affected ocular muscle in the analysis of diplopia:

1. The *direction in which the images are maximally separated indicates the action of the pair of muscles at fault.*

Table 14-3

MAIN CAUSES OF INDIVIDUAL AND COMBINED OCULOMOTOR PALSIES

Lesions of the third (oculomotor) nerve
Nuclear and intramedullary (fascicular)
Infarction (midbrain stroke)
Demyelination
Tumor
Trauma
Wernicke disease
Radicular (subarachnoid space and tentorial edge)
Aneurysm (posterior communicating or basilar)
Meningitis (infectious, neoplastic, granulomatous)
Diabetic infarction
Tumor
Raised intracranial pressure (shift and herniation of medial temporal lobe, hydrocephalus, pseudotumor cerebri)
Cavernous sinus and superior orbital fissure
Diabetic infarction of nerve
Aneurysm of internal carotid artery
Carotid-cavernous fistula
Cavernous thrombosis (septic and bland)
Tumor (pituitary, meningioma, nasopharyngeal carcinoma, metastasis)
Pituitary apoplexy
Sphenoid sinusitis and mucocele
Herpes zoster
Tolosa-Hunt syndrome
Orbit
Trauma
Fungal infection (mucormycosis, etc.)
Tumor and granuloma
Orbital pseudotumor
Uncertain localization
Migraine
Postinfectious cranial mono- and polyneuropathy
Lesions of the fourth (trochlear) nerve
Nuclear and intramedullary (fascicular)
Midbrain hemorrhage and infarction
Tumor
Arteriovenous malformation
Demyelination
Radicular (subarachnoid space)
Traumatic
Tumor (pineal, meningioma, metastasis, etc.)
Hydrocephalus
Pseudotumor cerebri and other causes of increased intracranial pressure
Meningitis (infectious, neoplastic, granulomatous)
Cavernous sinus and superior orbital fissure
Tumor
Tolosa-Hunt syndrome
Internal carotid aneurysm
Herpes zoster
Diabetic infarction
Orbit
Trauma
Tumor and granuloma
Lesions of the sixth (abducens) nerve
Nuclear (characterized by gaze palsy) and intramedullary (fascicular)
Möbius syndrome
Wernicke syndrome
Infarction (pontine stroke)
Demyelination
Tumor
Lupus
Radicular (subarachnoid)
Aneurysm
Trauma
Meningitis
Tumor (clivus, fifth- and eighth-nerve schwannoma, meningioma)
Petrous
Infection of mastoid and petrous bone
Thrombosis of inferior petrosal vein
Trauma
Cavernous sinus and superior orbital fissure
Carotid aneurysm
Cavernous sinus thrombosis
Tumor (pituitary, nasopharyngeal, meningioma)
Tolosa-Hunt syndrome
Diabetic or arteritic infarction
Herpes zoster
Orbit
Tumor and granulomas
Uncertain localization
Migraine
Viral and postviral
Transient in newborns

Source: Adapted by permission from Leigh and Zee.

For example, if the greatest horizontal separation is in looking to the right, either the right abductor (lateral rectus) or the left adductor (medial rectus) muscle is weak; if maximal when gazing to the left, the left lateral rectus and right medial rectus are implicated (Fig. 14-6*A* and *B*). As a corollary, if the separation is mainly horizontal, the paresis will be found in one of the horizontally acting recti (a small vertical disparity should be disregarded); if the separation is mainly vertical, the paresis will be found in the remaining vertically acting muscles, and a small horizontal deviation should be disregarded.

2. *The second step in analysis identifies which of the two implicated muscles is responsible for the diplopia. The image projected farther from the center is attributable to the eye with the paretic muscle.*

The simplest maneuver for the analysis of diplopia consists of asking the patient to follow an object or light into the six cardinal positions of gaze. When the position of maximal separation of images is identified, one eye is covered and the patient is asked to identify which image disappears. The *red-glass* test is an enhancement of this technique. A red glass is placed in front of the patient's right eye (the choice of the right eye is arbitrary, but if the test is always done in the same way, interpretation is simplified). The patient is then asked to look at a flashlight (held at a distance of 1 m), to turn the eyes sequentially to the six cardinal points in the visual fields, and to indicate the positions of the red and white images and the relative distances between them. The positions of the two images are plotted as the patient indicates them to the examiner (i.e., from the patient's perspective;

Fig. 14-7). This allows the identification of both the field of maximal separation and the eye responsible for the eccentric image. If the white image on right lateral gaze is to the right of the red (i.e., the image from the left eye is projected outward), then the left medial rectus muscle is weak.

If the maximum vertical separation of images occurs on looking downward and to the *left* and the white image is projected farther down than the red, the paretic muscle is the left inferior rectus; if the red image (from the right eye) is lower than the white, the paretic muscle is the right superior oblique. As already mentioned, correction of vertical diplopia by a tilting of the head implicates the superior oblique muscle of the opposite side (or the ipsilateral trochlear nucleus). Separation of images on looking up and to the right or left will similarly distinguish paresis of the inferior oblique and superior rectus muscles. Most patients are attentive enough to open and close each eye and determine the source of the image thrown most outward in the field of maximal separation.

In the widely reproduced diagram analyzing diplopia from Cogan's 1956 book, we have noted the curiosity that the fields are shown from the perspective of the examiner rather than of the patient, as is the convention (and as incorrectly stated in the original legend). We have taken the liberty of repairing this reversal and showing the fields from the patient's perspective in Fig. 14-7.

There are several alternative methods for studying the relative positions of the images of the two eyes. One, a refinement of the red-glass test, is the *Maddox rod*, in which the occluder consists of a transparent red lens with series of parallel cylindrical bars that transform a point source of light into a red line perpendicular to the cylinder axes. The position of the red line is easily compared by the patient with the position of a white point source of light seen with the other eye. Another technique, the *alternate cover test*, requires less cooperation than the red-glass test and is, therefore, a passive maneuver that is more useful in the examination of children and inattentive patients. It does, however, require sufficient visual function to permit central fixation with each eye. The test consists of rapidly alternating an occluder or the examiner's hand from one eye to another and observing the deviations from and return to the point of fixation, as described earlier in the chapter in the discussion of tropias and phorias. Measuring the prismatic correction in each field of gaze with a prism bar allows the quantification of deviation and provides a method to follow diplopia over time.

The more sophisticated Lancaster test uses red/green glasses and a red and green bar of laser light projected on a screen to accomplish essentially the same result but has the advantage of reflecting the actual position and torsion of each eye. Detailed descriptions of the Maddox rod and alternate cover tests, which are the ones favored by neuroophthalmologists, can be found in the monographs of Leigh and Zee and of Glaser. In all these tests the examiner is aided by committing to memory the cardinal actions of the ocular muscles shown in Fig. 14-6 and Table 14-2.

Other Forms of Diplopia

The red-glass and other similar tests are most useful when a single muscle is responsible for the diplopia. If testing suggests that more than one muscle is involved, myasthenia gravis and thyroid ophthalmopathy are likely causes as they affect several muscles of ocular motility. Palsy of the oculomotor nerve causes a similar circumstance.

Monocular diplopia occurs most commonly in relation to diseases of the cornea and lens rather than the retina; usually the images are overlapping or superimposed rather than discrete. In most cases, monocular diplopia can be traced to a lenticular distortion or displacement but in some, no abnormality can be found and it is usually attributable to hysteria. Monocular diplopia has been reported in association with cerebral disease (Safran et al), but this must be a rare occurrence. Occasionally, patients with homonymous scotomas caused by a lesion of the occipital lobe will see multiple images (polyopia) in the defective field of vision, particularly when the target is moving.

Rarely, the acute onset of *convergence paralysis* gives rise to diplopia and blurred vision at all near points; most cases are a result of head injury, some to encephalitis or multiple sclerosis. Many instances of convergence paralysis do not have a demonstrable neurologic basis; they are caused by hysteria or remain unexplained. The ill-defined entity of *divergence paralysis* causes diplopia at a distance because of crossing of the visual axes; in such patients images fuse only at a near position. This disorder, the basis of which is unknown and for which there is no common lesion, is difficult to distinguish from mild bilateral sixth-nerve palsies and from convergence spasm, which is common in malingerers and hysterics. A special type of divergence paralysis is seen regularly with strokes in the rostral midbrain; these display an asymmetrical incompleteness of ocular abduction on both sides (*pseudosixth palsy*). Based on scant clinical data, a center for active divergence has been postulated to reside in the rostral midbrain tegmentum.

Causes of Individual Third-, Fourth-, and Sixth-Nerve Palsies (Table 14-3)

Ocular palsies may have a central cause—i.e., a lesion of the nucleus or the intramedullary (fascicular) portion of the cranial nerve—but more often they are peripheral. Weakness of ocular muscles because of a lesion in the brainstem is usually accompanied by involvement of other cranial nerves and by signs referable to the "crossed" brainstem syndromes of a cranial nerve palsy on one side and a hemiparesis on the opposite side (see Table 34-3 and Chap. 47). Peripheral lesions, which may or may not be solitary, have a great variety of causes.

In the series reported by Rucker (1958, 1966), who analyzed 2,000 cases of paralysis of the oculomotor nerves, the most common sources of individual ocular motor palsies were tumors at the base of the brain or skull (primary, metastatic, meningeal carcinomatosis), head trauma, ischemic infarction of a nerve (generally associated with diabetes), and aneurysms of the circle of Willis, in that order. The sixth nerve was affected in about half of the cases; third-nerve palsies were about half as common; and the fourth nerve was involved in less than 10 percent of cases. In 1,000 unselected cases reported subsequently by Rush and Younge, trauma was a more frequent cause than neoplasm and the frequency of aneurysm-related cases was fewer than in the aforementioned series; otherwise the findings were similar. Less-common causes of paralysis of the oculomotor nerves, but nonetheless seen by most practitioners, include variants of Guillain-Barré syndrome, herpes zoster, giant cell arteritis, ophthalmoplegic migraine, carcinomatous or lymphomatous meningitis, and the granulomatous disease sarcoidosis and Tolosa-Hunt syndrome, as well as fungal, tuberculous, syphilitic, and other forms of mainly chronic meningitis. *Myasthenia gravis*, discussed in Chap. 49, must always be considered in cases of ocular muscle palsy, particularly if several muscles are involved and if fluctuating ptosis is a prominent feature. Thyroid ophthalmopathy, discussed further on, presents in a similar fashion but without ptosis and is less common than myasthenia. Actually, in the above mentioned series, no cause could be assigned in 20 to 30 percent, although more cases are now being resolved with MRI.

Sixth-Nerve Palsy

Infarction of the sixth nerve is a common cause of sixth-nerve palsy in diabetics, in which case there is usually pain near the lateral canthus of the eye at the onset. An idiopathic form that occurs in the absence of diabetes—possibly atherosclerotic—is also well known. Isolated sixth nerve palsy with global headache, and more specifically when the sign is bilateral, sometimes proves to be caused by raised intracranial pressure from an intracranial neoplasm. In children, the most common tumor involving the sixth nerve is a pontine glioma; in adults, it is tumor arising from the nasopharynx. As the abducens nerve passes near the apex of the petrous bone it is in close relation to the trigeminal nerve. Both may be implicated by inflammatory or infectious lesions of the petrous (apex petrositis), manifest by facial pain and diplopia (Gradenigo syndrome). Among the causes of this syndrome is osteomyelitis of the petrous bone. Fractures at the base of the skull and petroclival tumors may have a similar effect, and sometimes head injury alone is the only assignable cause. Even in the absence of a fracture, fourth-nerve palsy is a more common complication of closed cranial injury (as noted below).

As mentioned, unilateral or bilateral abducens weakness may be a nonspecific sign of increased intracranial pressure from any source—including brain tumor, meningitis, and pseudotumor cerebri; rarely, it may appear after lumbar puncture, epidural injections, or insertion of a ventricular shunt. The type of bilateral weakness of ocular abduction that arises with infarction of the rostral mid-brain (pseudosixth) was described above. Occasionally, the nerve is compressed by a congenitally persistent trigeminal artery. A congenital form of bilateral abducens palsy is associated with bilateral facial paralysis (Mobius syndrome) as discussed in Chap. 38. Patients with the Duane retraction syndrome (absent sixth nerve) usually do not have diplopia and are aware of the retraction problem but an examiner may note a defect in unilateral abduction (this entity is discussed further on).

Fourth-Nerve Palsy

The fourth nerve is particularly vulnerable to head trauma (this was the cause in 43 percent of 323 cases of trochlear nerve lesions collected by Wray from the literature). The reason for this vulnerability has been speculated to be the long, crossed course of the nerves. A fair number of cases remain idiopathic even after careful investigation. The fourth and sixth nerves are practically never involved by aneurysm. This reflects the relative infrequency of carotid artery aneurysms in the infraclinoid portion of the cavernous sinus, where they could impinge on the sixth nerve. (In contrast, supraclinoid aneurysms commonly involve the third nerve.) Herpes zoster ophthalmicus may affect any of the oculomotor nerves but particularly the trochlear, which shares a common sheath with the ophthalmic division of the trigeminal nerve. Diabetic infarction of the fourth nerve occurs, but far less frequently than infarction of the third or sixth nerves. Trochlear-nerve palsy may also be a false localizing sign in cases of increased intracranial pressure, but again, not nearly as often as abducens palsy. Entrapment of the superior oblique tendon is a rare cause (Brown syndrome) in which, in addition to diplopia, there is focal pain at the superomedial corner of the orbit; hence it may be mistaken for the Tolosa-Hunt syndrome, discussed further on. Trochlear-nerve palsies have been described in patients with lupus erythematosus and with Sjögren syndrome, but their basic pathology is not known. Some cases of fourth-nerve palsy are idiopathic and most of these resolve.

Superior oblique myokymia is an unusual but easily identifiable movement disorder, characterized by recurrent episodes of vertical diplopia, monocular blurring of vision, and a tremulous sensation in the affected eye; in this way it simulates a palsy. The globe is observed to make small arrhythmic torsional movements, especially when viewed with an ophthalmoscope. The problem is usually benign and responds to carbamazepine but rare instances presage pontine glioma or demyelinating disease. Compression of the fourth nerve by a small looped branch of the basilar artery has been suggested as the cause of the idiopathic variety, analogous to several other better documented vascular compression syndromes affecting cranial nerves. This notion is supported by findings on MRI reported by Yousry and colleagues.

Third-Nerve Palsy

The third nerve is commonly compressed by aneurysm, tumor, or temporal lobe herniation. In a series of 206 cases of third-nerve palsy collected by Wray and Taylor, neoplastic diseases accounted for 25 percent and aneurysms for 18 percent. Of the neoplasms, 25 percent were parasellar meningiomas and 4 percent were pituitary adenomas. The palsy is usually chronic, progressive, and painless. As emphasized earlier, enlargement of the pupil is a sign of extramedullary third nerve compression because of the peripheral location in the nerve of the pupilloconstrictor fibers. By contrast, infarction of the nerve in diabetics usually spares the pupil, as the damage is situated in the central portion of the nerve. The oculomotor palsy that complicates diabetes (the cause in 11 percent in the Wray and Taylor series) develops over a few hours and is accompanied by pain, usually severe, in the forehead and around the eye. The prognosis for recovery (as in other nonprogressive lesions of the oculomotor nerves) is usually good because of the potential of the nerve to regenerate. Infarction of the third nerve occurs in nondiabetics as well.

In chronic compressive lesions of the third nerve (distal carotid, basilar, or, most commonly, posterior communicating artery aneurysm; pituitary tumor, meningioma, cholesteatoma) the pupil is almost always affected by way of dilatation or reduced light response. However, the chronicity of the lesion may permit aberrant nerve regeneration. This is manifest by pupillary constriction on adduction of the eye or by retraction of the upper lid on downward gaze or adduction.

Rarely, children or young adults have one or more attacks of ocular palsy in conjunction with an otherwise typical migraine (ophthalmoplegic migraine). The muscles (both extrinsic and intrinsic) innervated by the oculomotor or less commonly, by the abducens nerve, are affected. Possibly, spasm of the vessels supplying these nerves or compression by edematous arteries causes a transitory ischemic paralysis but these are speculations. Arteriograms done after the onset of the palsy usually disclose no abnormality. The oculomotor palsy of migraine tends to recover; after repeated attacks, however, there may be permanent partial paresis.

Painful Ophthalmoplegia, Tolosa-Hunt Syndrome, Cavernous Sinus Syndrome, and Orbital Pseudotumor (Table 14-4)

Some of the diseases discussed above are associated with a degree of pain, often over the site of an affected nerve

Table 14-4

CAUSES OF PAINFUL OPHTHALMOPLEGIA

Vascular
- Intracavernous carotid artery aneurysm
- Posterior communicating or posterior cerebral artery aneurysm
- Cavernous sinus thrombosis (septic and aseptic)
- Carotid-cavernous fistula
- Diabetic oculomotor mononeuroapthy
- Temporal arteritis
- Ophthalmoplegic migraine

Neoplastic
- Pituitary adenoma
- Pituitary apoplexy
- Pericavernous meningioma
- Metastatic nodules to dura of cavernous sinus
- Giant-cell tumor of orbital bone
- Nasopharyngeal tumor invading cavernous sinus or orbit

Inflammatory and infectious
- Tolosa-Hunt syndrome
- Orbital pseudotumor
- Sinusitis
- Mucocele
- Herpes zoster
- Mucormycosis
- Sarcoidosis

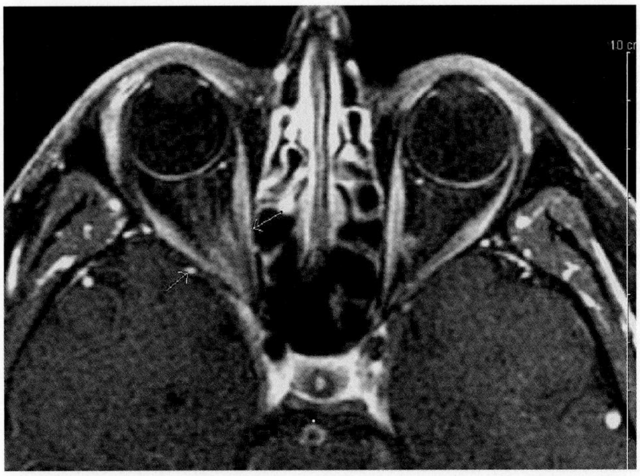

Figure 14-8. MRI of orbital pseudotumor showing swelling of the extraocular muscles and adjacent orbital contents. A "streaming" appearance of the fat as shown in the right orbit is characteristic. This patient was responsive to corticosteroids.

or muscle or in the immediately surrounding area. But the development over days or longer of a *painful unilateral ophthalmoplegia* constitutes a special syndrome that is usually traceable to an aneurysm, tumor, or inflammatory and granulomatous process in the anterior portion of the cavernous sinus or the adjacent superior orbital fissure. The idiopathic granulomatous painful condition has been termed *Tolosa-Hunt syndrome*; a similar but more extensive process is known as *orbital pseudotumor*. Although there is little pathologic material on which to base an understanding of these two diseases, they appear to be related orbital inflammations.

Orbital pseudotumor causes an inflammatory enlargement of the extraocular muscles, which often also encompasses the globe and other orbital contents accompanied by injection of the conjunctiva and lid and slight proptosis (Fig. 14-8). The Tolosa-Hunt syndrome lacks these features but is occasionally associated with additional signs of cavernous sinus disease, particularly sensory loss in the periorbital branches of the trigeminal nerve. In pseudotumor of the orbit, a single muscle or several may be involved and there is a tendency to relapse and later to involve the opposite globe. Visual loss from compression of the optic nerve is a rare complication of either condition. Associations with connective tissue disease have been reported in orbital pseudotumor but most cases in our experience have occurred in isolation. Ultrasonography examination or CT scans of the orbit show enlargement of the orbital contents in pseudotumor, mainly the muscles, similar to the findings in thyroid ophthalmopathy (which is not, however, painful unless there is secondary corneal ulceration).

The inflammatory changes of Tolosa-Hunt syndrome are limited to the superior orbital fissure and can sometimes be detected by MRI; coronal views taken after gadolinium infusion show the lesion to best advantage. However, sarcoidosis, lymphomatous infiltration, and a small meningioma may produce similar radiographic findings and granulomatous (temporal) arteritis rarely causes ophthalmoplegia. The sedimentation rate in our patients with orbital pseudotumor or Tolosa-Hunt syndrome has varied but it has been moderately elevated in reported cases, sometimes accompanied by a leukocytosis at the onset of symptoms. Sarcoidosis also can infiltrate the posterior orbit or cavernous sinus and cause a single or multiple unilateral nerve ophthalmoparesis as discussed in Chaps. 13 and 47.

Treatment

Both the Tolosa-Hunt syndrome and orbital pseudotumor are treated with corticosteroids. A marked response with reduction in pain and improved ophthalmoplegia in 1 or 2 days is confirmatory of the diagnosis; however, as pointed out in the review by Kline and Hoyt, tumors of the parasellar region that cause ophthalmoplegia may also respond, albeit not to the same extent. In both diseases, we have generally given prednisone 60 mg and tapered the medication slowly; although there are no data to guide the proper treatment, corticosteroids should be continued for several weeks or longer. The absence of a response to steroids should cause reconsideration of the diagnosis of Tolosa-Hunt syndrome.

Cavernous sinus syndrome In the *cavernous sinus syndrome*, involvement of the oculomotor nerve on one or both sides is accompanied by periorbital pain and chemosis (Fig. 14-5*B*). In a series of 151 such cases reported by Keane, the third nerve (typically with pupillary abnormalities) and sixth nerve were affected in almost all and the fourth nerve in one-third; complete ophthalmoplegia, usually unilateral, was present in 28 percent. Sensory loss in the distribution of the ophthalmic division of the trigeminal nerve was often added, a finding that is helpful in the differentiation of cavernous sinus disease from other causes of orbital edema and ocular muscle weakness.

Trauma and neoplastic invasion are the most frequent causes of the cavernous sinus syndrome. Thrombophlebitis, intracavernous carotid aneurysm or fistula, fungal infection, meningioma, and pituitary tumor or hemorrhage account for a smaller proportion (see "Septic Cavernous Sinus Thrombophlebitis" and "Cavernous Sinus Thrombosis" in Chaps. 10 and 34). A dural arteriovenous fistula is another rare cause. Chapter 34 discusses this process more fully with other disorders of the cerebral venous sinuses; the optic neuropathy that sometimes accompanies the syndrome is noted in Chap. 13.

The other important considerations in older patients with painful ophthalmoplegia are *temporal arteritis* as mentioned above (see Chap. 10) and *thyroid ophthalmopathy* (although pain tends not to be prominent in the latter), which are discussed further on.

Acute Ophthalmoplegia (Table 14-5)

When a total or nearly complete loss of eye movements of both eyes evolves within a day or days, it raises a limited number of diagnostic possibilities. Keane, who analyzed 60 such cases, found the responsible lesion to lie within the brainstem in 18 (usually infarction and less often Wernicke disease), in the cranial nerves in 26 (Guillain-Barré syndrome or tuberculous meningitis), within the cavernous sinus in 8 (tumors or infection), and at the myoneural junction in 8 (myasthenia gravis and botulism). Our experience has tended toward the Guillain-Barré syndrome, as did Keane's later series (2007), and, somewhat less frequently in our material, myasthenia. The ophthalmoplegic form of Guillain-Barré syndrome is almost always associated with circulating antibodies to GQ1b ganglioside (see Chap. 46). There may be an accompanying paralysis of the dilator and constrictor of the pupil ("internal ophthalmoplegia") that is not seen in myasthenia.

Table 14-5

CAUSES OF COMPLETE OPHTHALMOPLEGIA (ACUTE SYNDROMES ARE NOTED BY AN ASTERISK)

Brainstem lesions
Wernicke disease*
Pontine infarction*
Infiltrating glioma
Acute disseminated encephalomyelitis and multiple sclerosis
Cranial nerve lesions
Guillain-Barré syndrome*
Neoplastic meningitis
Granulomatous meningitis (tuberculous, sarcoid)
Cavernous sinus thrombosis
Tolosa-Hunt syndrome
Orbital pseudotumor*
Neuromuscular junction syndromes
Myasthenia gravis*
Thyroid ophthalmopathy
Lambert-Eaton syndrome
Botulism*
Congenital myasthenic syndromes ("slow-channel" disease)
Muscle disease
Progressive external ophthalmoplegia (mitochondrial and dystrophic types)
Oculopharyngeal dystrophy
Congenital polymyopathies (myotubular, nemaline rod, central core)

Unilateral complete ophthalmoplegia has an even more limited list of causes, largely related to local disease in the orbit and cavernous sinus, mainly infectious, neoplastic, or thrombotic and most of which have already been mentioned.

Chronic and Progressive Bilateral Ophthalmoplegia

This is most often caused by an ocular myopathy (the mitochondrial disorder known as progressive external ophthalmoplegia), a restricted muscular dystrophy, thyroid ophthalmopathy (see below and Chap. 48), and, sometimes, myasthenia gravis or Lambert-Eaton syndrome. We have encountered instances of the Lambert-Eaton myasthenic syndrome that caused an almost complete ophthalmoplegia (but not as an initial sign, as it may be in myasthenia) and a patient with paraneoplastic brainstem encephalitis similar to the case reported by Crino and colleagues, but both of these are certainly rare as causes of complete loss of eye movements. Among the group of congenital myopathies, most of which are named for the morphologic characteristic of the affected limb musculature. A few of these—such as the central core, myotubular, and nemaline types, as well as the slow channel congenital myasthenic syndrome—may cause a generalized ophthalmoparesis (see Chap. 48). Among the chronic conditions, progressive supranuclear palsy may ultimately produce complete ophthalmoplegia, after first affecting vertical gaze. Thyroid ophthalmopathy as a cause of chronic ophthalmoparesis is discussed below.

The *Duane retraction syndrome* (so-called because of the retraction of the globe and narrowing of the palpebral fissure that is elicited by attempted adduction) occurs when the lateral rectus branches are aberrantly innervated by the third nerve. Cocontraction of the medial and lateral recti results in retraction of the globe in all directions of ocular movement.

Mechanical-Restrictive Ophthalmoparesis Including Thyroid Ophthalmopathy

Several causes of a *pseudoparalysis of ocular muscles* that are due to mechanical restriction of the ocular muscles are distinguished from the neuromuscular and brainstem diseases discussed above. Processes that infiltrate the orbit, such as lymphoma, carcinoma and granulomatosis may limit the range of motion of individual or all the ocular muscles. In *thyroid disease*, a swollen and tight inferior or superior rectus muscle may limit upward and downward gaze; less frequently, involvement of the medial rectus limits abduction. The frequency of involvement of the ocular muscles is given by Wiersinga and colleagues as inferior rectus 60 percent; medical rectus 50 percent; and superior rectus 40 percent. In most instances of thyroid ophthalmopathy, diagnosis is clear as there is an associated proptosis, but in the absence of the latter sign, and particularly if the ocular muscles are affected on one side predominantly, there may be difficulty. The extraocular muscle enlargement can be demonstrated by CT scans and ultrasonography. This disorder is discussed further in Chap. 48. In a significant number of cases, 10 percent according to Bahn and Heufelder, there are no signs of hyperthyroidism. However, most of these patients have laboratory evidence of thyroid autoimmune disease.

The mechanical restriction of motion is confirmed by *forced duction tests* in which the eye is physically pulled or pushed over by the examiner. In the past, the insertions of the extraocular muscles were anesthetized and grasped by toothed forceps and attempts to move the globe are palpably restricted; more often, a cotton swab applied to the sclera is used to manipulate the globe.

Mixed Gaze and Ocular Muscle Paralysis

We have already considered two types of neural paralysis of the extraocular muscles: paralysis of conjugate movements (gaze) and paralysis of individual ocular muscles. Here we discuss a third, more complex one—namely, mixed gaze and ocular muscle paralysis. The mixed type is always a sign of an intrapontine or mesencephalic lesion that may be caused by a wide variety of pathologic changes.

Internuclear Ophthalmoplegia and Other Pontine Gaze Palsies

These abnormalities have been mentioned previously because they are components of numerous tegmental brainstem syndromes affecting both horizontal and vertical gaze. A lesion of the lower pons in or near the sixth-nerve nucleus causes an ipsilateral paralysis of the lateral rectus muscle and a failure of adduction of the opposite eye, which is manifest simply as a gaze palsy to the side of the lesion. As already indicated, a presumed pontine center accomplishes horizontal conjugate gaze by simultaneously innervating the ipsilateral lateral rectus (via the abducens neurons) and the contralateral medial rectus via fibers that originate in the internuclear neurons of the abducens nucleus and cross at the level of the nucleus to traverse the MLF of the opposite side (Fig. 14-1).

With a complete lesion of the left MLF, the left ipsilateral eye fails to adduct when the patient looks to the right; this condition is referred to as *internuclear ophthalmoplegia* (INO; reciprocally, with a lesion of the right MLF, the right eye fails to adduct when the patient looks to the left—namely, *right internuclear ophthalmoplegia*). Quite often, rather than a complete paralysis of adduction, there are only slowed adducting saccades in the affected eye while its opposite quickly arrives at its fully abducted position. This can be brought out by having the patient make large side-to-side refixation movements between two targets or by observing the slowed corrective saccades induced by optokinetic stimulation. Typically, the affected eye at rest does not lie in an abducted position, but there are exceptions and in most cases the absence of exotropia most dependably differentiates INO from a partial third-nerve palsy with weakness of the medial rectus muscle. The exception is the WEBINO syndrome noted below. The two medial longitudinal fasciculi lie close together, each being situated adjacent to the midline, so that they are frequently affected together, yielding a bilateral internuclear ophthalmoplegia; this condition should be suspected when the predominant ocular finding is bilateral paresis of adduction.

A second component of INO is a nystagmus that is limited to, or most prominent in, the opposite (abducting) eye. The intensity of nystagmus varies greatly from case to case. Several explanations have been offered to account for this dissociated nystagmus, all of them speculative. The favored one invokes the Hering law in which activated pairs of yoked muscles receive equal and simultaneous innervation; because of an adaptive increase in innervation of the weak adductor there is a commensurate increase in innervation to the strong abductor (manifest as nystagmus). Whatever the afferent stimulus for this over-drive, it is probably proprioceptive (i.e., not visual), because occlusion of the affected eye does not suppress the nystagmus. The MLF also contains axons that originate in the vestibular nuclei and govern vertical eye position, for which reason an INO may also cause a skew (vertical deviation of one eye) or monocular vertical nystagmus with impairment of vertical fixation and pursuit (bilaterally with bilateral INO).

Lesions involving the MLF in the high midbrain cause a loss of convergence and an exotropia because of proximity to the medial rectus subnucleus. When the lesion is bilateral, both eyes are slightly abducted, giving rise to a "wall-eyed INO", or WEBINO. Abducting nystagmus tends to be slight in this mesencephalic type. More commonly, the MLF is involved by a lesion in the pons and convergence is spared and the globes are orthotopic, but there is sometimes an additional slight degree of horizontal gaze or sixth-nerve palsy as a result of disturbance of adjacent horizontal gaze centers. There may be yet another rare syndrome that has gone by the term "posterior INO of Lutz" (INO of abduction, in which the MLF is not involved); the lesion is proposed to be between the PPRF and the sixth nerve nucleus and the abduction paresis can be overcome by vestibular stimulation. The terms "anterior" and "posterior" INO have also been applied to these topographic syndromes but their meaning has been taken differently by various authors thus making them less useful.

The main cause of *unilateral INO* is a small paramedian pontine infarction. Other common lesions are lateral medullary infarction (where skew deviation is often a component), a demyelinating plaque of multiple sclerosis (more common as a cause of bilateral INO, as noted below), lupus erythematosus, and infiltrative tumors of the brainstem and fourth ventricular region. Occasionally, an INO is an unexplained finding after mild head injury or with subdural hematoma or hydrocephalus. Some of the more unusual causes are given in the experience of Keane (2005). Infarction and multiple sclerosis remained the most common in his series but trauma, transtentorial herniation, tumor, infection and hemorrhage were alternatives, the point being that a quarter were from unconventional processes. In addition, adductor weakness from myasthenia gravis can simulate an INO, even to the point of showing nystagmus in the abducting eye.

Bilateral INO is most often the result of a demyelinating lesion (multiple sclerosis) in the posterior part of the midpontine tegmentum. Pontine myelinolysis, pontine infarction from basilar artery occlusion, Wernicke disease, or infiltrating tumors are other causes. Brainstem damage following compression by a large cerebral mass has on occasion produced the syndrome.

An ipsilateral gaze palsy is the simplest oculomotor disturbance that results from a lesion in the paramedian tegmentum. More complex is the *one-and-a-half syndrome that* involves the pontine center for gaze plus the adjacent ipsilateral MLF on one side that combines an INO and a horizontal gaze palsy on the same side. It is usually of vascular or, less often, demyelinative cause. The gaze palsy is, of course, on the side of the lesion and the eyes are deviated contrawise. As a result, one eye lies fixed in the midline for all horizontal movements; the other eye makes only abducting movements and may be engaged in horizontal nystagmus in the direction of abduction (see Fisher; also Wall and Wray). Unlike the situation of an INO alone, the mobile eye rests abducted because of the gaze palsy, a sign that has been termed "paralytic pontine exotropia." In some cases the patient is able to adduct the eye ("nonparalytic exotropia," a condition which has other causes).

An incomplete version of the bilateral INO displays only bilateral nystagmus on gaze in one direction (due to paresis of gaze) and nystagmus only in the abducting eye with gaze directed to the other side (due to the lesion in the MLF on the same side). This has been summarized the mnemonic of nystagmus in both eyes looking toward the pontine lesion and in one eye looking away from the lesion.

Caplan has summarized the features of mixed oculomotor defects that occur with thrombotic occlusion of the upper part of the basilar artery ("top of the basilar" syndromes). These include upgaze or complete vertical gaze palsy and so-called pseudoabducens palsy, mentioned earlier. The latter is characterized by bilateral incomplete esotropia that simulates bilateral sixth nerve paresis (pseudoabducens palsy) but appears to be a type of sustained convergence or a paresis of divergence; it can be overcome by vestibular stimulation.

Skew Deviation *Skew deviation* is a disorder in which there is vertical deviation of one eye above the other that is caused by an imbalance of the vestibular inputs to the oculomotor system. The patient may complain of similar degrees of diplopia in all fields of gaze (comitant), or diplopia may vary with different directions of gaze. In either case, the patient complains of vertical diplopia. A noncomitant vertical deviation of the eyes, most pronounced when the affected eye is adducted and turned down, is characteristic of fourth-nerve palsy, described further on. Skew deviation does not have precise localizing value and is associated with a variety of lesions of the cerebellum and the brainstem, particularly those involving the MLF. With skew deviation due to cerebellar disease, the eye on the side of the lesion usually rests lower (in a ratio of 2:1 in Keane's series), but sometimes it is higher than the other eye. The corresponding image, of course, rests higher in the first instance and lower with the latter, which is most often a component of an INO.

The hypertropic eye has been known to alternate with the direction of gaze ("alternating skew") and has also been seen with the condition known as *periodic alternating nystagmus*. A cerebellar or other posterior fossa lesion is the usual cause. A mechanism for this sign has been proposed based on otolithic influences on cerebellar centers. Ford and coworkers have described a rare form of skew deviation caused by a monocular palsy of elevation stemming from a lesion immediately rostral to the ipsilateral oculomotor nucleus; a lesion of upgaze efferents from the ipsilateral riMLF was postulated but an abnormality of the vertical gaze holding mechanism related to the function of the INC is an alternative explanation.

Among the most unusual of the complex ocular disturbances is a subjective tilting of the entire visual field that may produce any angle of divergence but most often creates an illusion of environmental tilting of 45 to 90 degrees (*tortopia*) or of 180-degree vision (*upside-down vision*). Objects normally on the floor, such as chairs and tables, are perceived to be on the wall or ceiling. Although this symptom may arise as a result of a lesion of the parietal lobe or in the otolithic (utricular) apparatus, it has most often been associated in our experience with an internuclear ophthalmoplegia and slight skew deviation. Presumably the vestibular-otolithic nucleus or its connections in the MLF that maintain the vertical position of the ipsilateral eye are impaired. Lateral medullary infarction has been a common cause; other cases may be migrainous (Ropper, 1983). Ocular lateropulsion, in which the eyes are driven to one side and the patient feels pushed or pulled in the same direction, is another component in some cases of lateral medullary infarction as discussed in Chap. 34.

Nystagmus

Nystagmus refers to involuntary rhythmic movements of the eyes and is of two general types. In the more common *jerk nystagmus*, the movements alternate between a slow component and a fast corrective component, or jerk, in the opposite direction. In *pendular nystagmus*, the oscillations are roughly equal in rate in both directions, although on lateral gaze the pendular type may be converted to the jerk type with the fast component to the side of gaze. Nystagmus reflects an imbalance in one or more of the systems that maintain stability of gaze. The causes may therefore be viewed as originating in (1) structures that maintain steadiness of gaze in the primary position; (2) the system for holding eccentric gaze—the so-called neural integrator; or (3) the VOR system, which maintains foveal fixation of images as the head moves. For the purposes of clinical work, however, certain types of nystagmus are identified as corresponding to lesions in specific structures within each of these systems, and it is this approach that we take in the following pages. One classification considers nystagmus as the result of a disturbance in the vestibular apparatus or its brainstem nuclei, the cerebellum, or a number of specific regions of the brainstem such as the MLF.

In testing for nystagmus, the eyes should be examined first in the central position and then during upward, downward, and lateral movements. *Jerk nystagmus* is the more common type. It may be horizontal or vertical and is elicited particularly on ocular movement in these planes, or it may be rotatory and, rarely, retractory or vergent. By custom the direction of the nystagmus is designated according to the direction of the fast component (referred to as "beating" to that side). There are several varieties of jerk nystagmus. Some occur spontaneously; others are readily induced in normal persons by drugs or by labyrinthine or visual stimulation.

Drug intoxication is certainly the most frequent cause of nystagmus. Alcohol, barbiturates, other sedative-hypnotic drugs, phenytoin, and other antiepileptic drugs are the common ones. This form of nystagmus is most prominent on deviation of the eyes in the horizontal plane, but occasionally it also may appear in the vertical plane. For no known reason, it may occasionally be asymmetrical in the two eyes.

Oscillopsia is the symptom of illusory movement of the environment in which stationary objects seem to move back and forth, up and down, or from side to side. It may be caused by ocular flutter (a cerebellar sign as discussed later) or coarse nystagmus of any type. With lesions of the labyrinths (as in aminoglycoside toxicity), the symptom of oscillopsia is only provoked by motion—e.g., walking or riding in an automobile—and indicates an impaired ability of the vestibular system to stabilize ocular fixation during body movement (i.e., impaired VOR function). In these circumstances, cursory examination of the eyes may disclose no abnormalities; however, if the patient's head is rotated slowly from side to side or moved rapidly in one direction while attempting to fixate a target, impairment of smooth eye movements and their replacement by saccadic or nystagmoid movements is evoked (see Chap. 15 for further discussion of these tests). If episodic and involving only one eye, oscillopsia is usually caused by myokymia of an ocular muscle (usually the superior oblique).

Nystagmus of Labyrinthine Origin (See also Chap. 15)

This is predominantly a horizontal or vertical unidirectional jerk nystagmus, often with a slight torsional component, that is evident when the eyes are close to the central position and changes minimally with the direction of gaze. It is more prominent when visual fixation is eliminated (conversely, it is suppressed by fixation). The observation of suppression with visual fixation is facilitated by the use of Frenzel lenses, but most instances are evident without elaborate apparatus. Vestibular nystagmus of peripheral (labyrinthine) origin beats in most cases away from the side of the lesion and increases as the eyes are turned in the direction of the quick phase (the Alexander law). In contrast, as noted below, nystagmus of brainstem and cerebellar origin is most apparent when the patient fixates upon and follows a moving target and the direction of nystagmus changes with the direction of gaze. Labyrinthine-vestibular nystagmus is horizontal, vertical, or oblique, and that of purely labyrinthine origin characteristically has an additional torsional component. Tinnitus and hearing loss are often associated with disease of the peripheral labyrinthine mechanism; also, vertigo, nausea, vomiting, and staggering may accompany disease of any part of the labyrinthine-vestibular apparatus or its central connections. These points are elaborated in Chap. 15. As a characteristic example, the intense nystagmus of benign positional vertigo (described fully in Chap. 15) is evoked by moving from the sitting to the supine position, with the head turned to one side. In this condition, nystagmus of vertical-torsional type and vertigo develop a few seconds after changing head position and persist for another 10 to 15 s. When the patient sits up, the nystagmus changes to beat in the opposite direction.

In many normal individuals, a few irregular jerks are observed when the eyes are moved far to one side ("nystagmoid" jerks), but the movements cease once lateral fixation is attained. A fine rhythmic nystagmus may also occur normally in extreme lateral gaze, beyond the range of binocular vision; but it is bilateral and disappears as the eyes move a few degrees toward the midline. These latter movements are probably analogous to the tremulousness of skeletal muscles when maximally contracted.

Nystagmus Caused by Brainstem and Cerebellar Disease

Brainstem lesions often cause a coarse, unidirectional, *gaze-dependent nystagmus*, which may be horizontal or vertical, meaning that the nystagmus is exaggerated when the eyes sustain an eccentric position of gaze; vertical nystagmus, for example, is brought out usually on upward gaze, less often downward. Unlike the vestibular nystagmus discussed above, the central type usually also changes direction depending on the direction of gaze. The presence of bidirectional vertical nystagmus usually indicates disease in the pontomedullary or mesencephalic tegmentum. Vertigo is less common or less intense than with labyrinthine nystagmus, but signs of disease of other nuclear structures and tracts in the brainstem are frequent.

Spontaneous *upbeat nystagmus* is observed frequently in patients with demyelinating or vascular disease, tumors, or Wernicke disease. There is still uncertainty about the anatomic basis of coarse upbeat nystagmus. According to some authors, it has been associated with lesions of the anterior cerebellar vermis or another cerebellar site. Kato and associates cite cases with a lesion at the pontomedullary junction involving the nucleus prepositus hypoglossi, which receives vestibular connections and projects to all brainstem and cerebellar regions concerned with oculomotor functions. Bilateral internuclear ophthalmoplegia is also a cause.

Downbeat nystagmus, which is always of central origin, is characteristic of lesions in the medullary–cervical region such as syringobulbia, Chiari malformation, basilar invagination, and demyelinating plaques. It has also been seen with Wernicke disease and may be an initial sign of either paraneoplastic brainstem encephalitis or cerebellar degeneration with opsoclonus. Downbeat nystagmus, usually in association with oscillopsia, has also been observed in patients with lithium intoxication or with profound magnesium depletion (Saul and Selhorst). Halmagyi and coworkers, who studied 62 patients with downbeat nystagmus, found that half were associated with the Chiari malformation and various forms of cerebellar degeneration; in most of the remainder, the cause could not be determined. Cases associated with antibodies against glutamic acid decarboxylase (GAD), a substance that has a documented relationship to the stiff man syndrome have been reported by Antonini and colleagues and by other groups. Whether this antibody explains the idiopathic cases of downbeat nystagmus is not known.

Nystagmus of several types—including gaze-evoked nystagmus, downbeat nystagmus, and "rebound nystagmus" (gaze-evoked nystagmus that changes direction with refixation to the primary position)—occurs with cerebellar disease, particularly with lesions of the vestibulocerebellum or with brainstem lesions that involve the nucleus prepositus hypoglossi and the medial vestibular nucleus. Characteristic of cerebellar disease are several closely related disorders of saccadic movement that appear as nystagmus (opsoclonus, flutter, dysmetria) described below. Tumors situated in the cerebellopontine angle may cause a coarse bilateral horizontal nystagmus that is higher amplitude to the side of the lesion.

Nystagmus that occurs only in the abducting eye is referred to as *dissociated nystagmus* and is a common sign of internuclear ophthalmoplegia, as discussed earlier.

Infantile (Congenital, Pendular) Nystagmus

This is found in a variety of conditions in which central vision is lost early in life, such as albinism and various other diseases of the retina and refractive media. Occasionally it is observed as a congenital abnormality, even without poor vision. The defect is postulated to be an instability of smooth pursuit or gaze-holding mechanisms. The nystagmus is always binocular and in one plane; i.e., it will remain horizontal even during vertical movement. It is mainly pendular (sinusoidal) except in extremes of gaze, when it comes to resemble jerk nystagmus. Head oscillation may accompany the nystagmus and is probably compensatory. With eye movement recordings it displays a feature unique among nystagmus, an exponentially increasing velocity of the slow phase.

Indications as to the congenital nature of nystagmus are that it remains horizontal in all directions of gaze; it is suppressed during convergence and may be associated with odd head positions or with head oscillations and with strabismus. Also characteristic is a paradoxical response to optokinetic testing (see below), in which the quick phase is in the same direction as the drum rotation.

The related condition of *latent nystagmus* is the result of a lack of normal development of stereoscopic vision and may be detected by noting that the nystagmus changes direction when the eyes are alternately covered. In a few individuals who later in life lose vision in one eye, the latent nystagmus becomes a *manifest latent nystagmus*.

In addition, severe visual loss or blindness of acquired type that eliminates the ability to accurately direct gaze, even in adulthood, produces nystagmus of pendular or jerk variety. Both horizontal and vertical components are evident and the characteristic feature is a fluctuation over several seconds of observation in the dominant direction of beating. We have seen this sign a number of times in patients who became blind from severe optic neuritis few years back. The formerly common syndrome of "miner's nystagmus" is an associated condition that occurs in patients who have worked for many years in comparative darkness. The oscillations of the eyes are usually very rapid, increase on upward gaze, and may be associated with compensatory oscillations of the head.

Spasmus nutans, a specific type of pendular nystagmus of infancy, is accompanied by head nodding, and occasionally by wry positions of the neck. Most cases begin between the fourth and twelfth months of life, never after the third year. The nystagmus may be horizontal, vertical, or rotatory; it is usually more pronounced in one eye than the other (or limited to one eye) and can be intensified by immobilizing or straightening the head. Most infants recover within a few months or years. Most cases are idiopathic, but symptoms like those of spasmus nutans betray the presence of a perichiasmal or third ventricular tumor (see also seesaw nystagmus below in "Other Types of Nystagmus"); rare cases accompany childhood retinal diseases. Although there is no direct connection to this syndrome, the rare condition of bobble-head doll syndrome, consisting of rhythmic head movements caused by lesions in or adjacent to the third ventricle as described in Chap 30.

Acquired forms of pendular nystagmus may occur with adult leukodystrophies (see Chap. 37), multiple sclerosis (see Chap. 36), toluene intoxication, and in the oculomasticatory myorhythmia of Whipple disease, in which the nystagmus is conjoined to rhythmic jaw movements (see Chap. 32).

Other Types of Nystagmus

Convergence nystagmus has already been alluded to in several contexts—it refers to a rhythmic oscillation in which a slow abduction of both eyes is followed by a quick movement of adduction, usually accompanied by quick rhythmic retraction movements of the eyes (*nystagmus retractorius, retraction nystagmus*) and by one or more features of the Parinaud–dorsal midbrain syndrome discussed earlier in the chapter. There may also be rhythmic movements of the eyelids or a maintained spasm of convergence, best brought out on attempted elevation of the eyes on command or downward rotation of an OKN drum (see below for discussion of optokinetic nystagmus, OKN). These unusual phenomena all point to a lesion of the upper midbrain tegmentum and are usually manifestations of vascular disease, traumatic damage, or tumor, notably pinealoma that compresses this region.

Seesaw nystagmus is a torsional-vertical oscillation in which the intorting eye moves up and the opposite (extorting) eye moves down, then both move in the reverse direction. It is occasionally observed in conjunction with chiasmatic bitemporal hemianopia caused by sellar or parasellar masses and after pituitary surgery. Spasmus nutans has some similarities, as mentioned above, and alternating skew may be a related phenomenon.

Periodic alternating nystagmus is a remarkable horizontal jerking that periodically (every 90 seconds or so) changes direction, interposed with a brief neutral period during which the eyes show no nystagmus, or jerk downward. Alternating nystagmus is seen with lesions in the lower brainstem but has also been reported with Creutzfeldt-Jakob disease, hepatic encephalopathy, lesions of the cerebellar nodulus, carcinomatous meningitis, anti-GAD antibodies, and varied other processes. A congenital form is associated with albinism. It differs from *ping-pong gaze*, which is a saccadic variant with a more rapid alternating of gaze from side to side and usually the result of bilateral cerebral strokes.

So-called *palatal nystagmus*, which is really a tremor, is caused by a lesion of the central tegmental tract and may be accompanied by a convergence–retraction nystagmus that has the same beat as the palatal and pharyngeal muscles, as discussed in Chap. 4.

Optokinetic Nystagmus

When one is watching a moving object (e.g., the passing landscape from a train window, a rotating drum with vertical stripes, or a strip of cloth with similar stripes), a rhythmic jerk nystagmus, *optokinetic nystagmus* (OKN), normally appears. This phenomenon is explained by a slow component of nystagmus that represents an involuntary pursuit movement to the limit of comfortable conjugate gaze followed by a quick saccadic movement in the opposite direction in order to fixate the next new target that is entering the visual field. With unilateral lesions of the parietal region, the slow pursuit phase of the OKN may be lost or diminished when the stimulus—e.g., the striped OKN drum—is moving *toward the side of the lesion*, whereas rotation of the drum to the opposite side elicits a normal response. (A prominent neurologist of our acquaintance in past days correctly made the diagnosis of parietal lobe abscess on the basis of fever and absent pursuit to the side of the lesion.) It is remarkable that patients with hemianopia caused by an occipital lobe lesion show a normal optokinetic response. The loss of the pursuit phase with a parietal lesion is presumably because of interruption of efferent pathways from the parietal cortex to the brainstem centers for conjugate gaze. On the other hand, frontal lobe lesions allow the eyes to tonically follow in the direction of the target but with little or no fast-phase correction in the direction opposite the lesion. In recent years, however, it has been suggested from primate experiments that there is a subcortical relay station for OKN in the geniculate nucleus of the optic tract contralateral to the slow phase of nystagmus.

An important additional fact about OKN is that the ability to evoke it in all directions proves that the patient is not blind. Each eye can be tested separately to exclude monocular blindness. Thus the test is of particular value in the examination of hysterical patients and malingerers who claim that they cannot see, and of neonates and infants (a nascent OKN is established within hours after birth and becomes more easily elicitable over the first few months of life).

Caloric-induced nystagmus *Labyrinthine stimulation*—e.g., irrigation of the external auditory canal with warm or cold water, or "caloric testing"—produces a marked nystagmus. Cold water induces a slow tonic deviation of the eyes toward the irrigated ear and a compensatory nystagmus in the opposite direction; warm water does the reverse. Thus the acronym taught to generations of medical students: COWS, or "cold opposite, warm same," to refer to the direction of the fast phase of the induced nystagmus. The slow tonic component reflects impulses originating in the semicircular canals, and the fast component is a corrective movement. Chapter 15 discusses the production of nystagmus by labyrinthine stimulation and other features of vestibular nystagmus.

Other Spontaneous Ocular Movements

Roving conjugate eye movements are characteristic of light coma. Slow horizontal ocular deviations that shift every few seconds from side to side (*ping-pong gaze*) is a form of roving eye movement that occurs with bihemispheric infarctions or sometimes with posterior fossa lesions. Fisher has noted a similar slower, side-to-side pendular oscillation of the eyes ("windshield-wiper eyes"). This phenomenon has been associated with bilateral hemispheric lesions that have presumably released a brainstem pacemaker.

Ocular bobbing is a term coined by Fisher to describe a distinctive spontaneous fast downward jerk of the eyes followed by a slow upward drift to the midposition. It is observed in comatose patients in whom horizontal eye movements have been obliterated by large destructive lesions of the pons, less often of the cerebellum. The movements may be disconjugate in the vertical plane, especially if there is an associated third-nerve palsy on one side.

Other spontaneous vertical eye movements have been given a variety of confusing names: *atypical bobbing, inverse bobbing, reverse bobbing*, and *ocular dipping*. For the most part, they are observed in coma of metabolic or anoxic origin and in the context of preserved horizontal eye movements (in distinction to ocular bobbing). *Ocular dipping* is the term we have used to describe an arrhythmic slow conjugate downward movement followed in several seconds by a more rapid upward movement; it occurs spontaneously but may at times be elicited by moving the limbs or neck. Anoxic encephalopathy has been the most common cause, but a few cases have followed drug overdose (Ropper, 1981).

Oculogyric crisis, formerly associated with postencephalitic parkinsonism, is now most often caused by phenothiazine drugs, as discussed earlier.

Saccadic Intrusions (Opsoclonus and Ocular Dysmetria)

This group of phasic or repetitive eye movements is distinguished from nystagmus in that the first movement is a fast saccade, in contrast to jerk nystagmus, where by definition the movement starts with a slow phase. *Opsoclonus* is the term applied to rapid, conjugate oscillations of the eyes in horizontal, rotatory, and vertical directions, made worse by voluntary movement or the need to fixate the eyes. These movements are continuous and chaotic, without an intersaccadic pause (hence the colorful term *saccadomania*), and are almost unique among disorders of ocular movement in that they persist in sleep. As indicated in Chap. 6, they are sometimes part of a widespread myoclonus associated with parainfectious disease, occasionally with AIDS, poststreptococcal infection, West Nile virus encephalitis, and rickettsial infections, but most characteristically as a paraneoplastic manifestation with severe ataxia ("Paraneoplastic Cerebellar Degeneration" discussed in Chap. 31). Opsoclonus may also be observed in patients who are intoxicated with antidepressants, anticonvulsants, organophosphates, cocaine, lithium, thallium, and haloperidol; in the nonketotic hyperosmolar state; and in cerebral Whipple disease, where the eye movements are coupled with rhythmic jaw movements (oculomasticatory myorhythmia). A childhood form, associated with limb ataxia and myoclonus that is responsive to adrenocorticotropic hormone (ACTH), may persist for years without explanation, as in the "dancing eyes" of children (Kinsbourne syndrome). However, a distant (paraneoplastic) effect of neuroblastoma remains the main consideration in children with this ocular disorder. There is also a self-limited benign form in neonates. Similar movements have been produced in monkeys by creating bilateral lesions in the pretectum.

Ocular dysmetria, the analogue of limb dysmetria, consists of an overshoot or undershoot of the eyes on attempted fixation followed by several cycles of oscillation of diminishing amplitude until fixation is attained. The dysmetria may occur on eccentric fixation or on refixation to the primary position of gaze. It probably reflects dysfunction of the anterosuperior vermis and underlying deep cerebellar nuclei.

Ocular flutter refers to occasional bursts of very rapid horizontal oscillations around the point of fixation; this abnormality is also associated with cerebellar disease. Flutter at the end of a saccade, called *flutter dysmetria ("fish-tail nystagmus")* has the appearance of dysmetria, but careful analysis indicates that it is probably a different phenomenon. Whereas the inaccurate saccades of ataxia are separated by normal brief pause (intersaccadic interval), flutter dysmetria consists of consecutive saccades without an intersaccadic interval (Zee and Robinson). Nonetheless, all those movements have the same implication of cerebellar cortical disease.

Opsoclonus, ocular dysmetria, and flutter-like oscillations may occur together, or a patient may show only one or two of these ocular tremors, either simultaneously or in sequence. One hypothesis relates opsoclonus and ocular flutter to a disorder of the saccadic "pause neurons" (see above), but their exact anatomic basis has not been elucidated. Some normal individuals can voluntarily induce flutter.

An eye movement difficult to classify is ocular neuromyotonia that is found after radiation that includes the field of the ocular motor nerves (and less characteristically from vascular or tumor compression). There is intermittent contraction of one or more ocular muscles that may cause paroxysmal diplopia. The similar syndrome of superior oblique myokymia was discussed in an earlier section of the chapter.

Disorders of the Eyelids and Blinking

A consideration of oculomotor disorders would be incomplete without reference to the eyelids and blinking. In the normal individual, the eyelids on both sides are at the same level with respect to the limbus of the cornea and there is a variable prominence of the eyes, depending on the width of the palpebral fissure. The function of the lids is to protect the delicate corneal surfaces against injury and the retinae against glare; this is done by blinking and lacrimation. Eyelid movement is normally coordinated with ocular movement—the upper lids elevate when looking up and descend when looking down. Turning the eyes quickly to the side is sometimes attended by a single blink, which is necessarily brief so as not to interfere with vision. When the blink duration is prolonged, it is indicative of an abnormally intense effort required to initiate the saccade; usually this is because of frontal lobe or basal ganglionic disease.

Closure and opening of the eyelids is accomplished through the reciprocal action of the levator palpebrae and orbicularis oculi muscles. Relaxation of the levator and contraction of the orbicularis effect closure; the reverse action of these muscles effects opening of the closed eyelids. Opening of the lids is aided by the tonic innervation of the superior tarsal (Müller) muscle, which is innervated by sympathetic fibers. The levator is innervated by the oculomotor nerve, and the orbicularis by the facial nerve. The trigeminal nerves provide sensation to the eyelids and are also the afferent limbs of corneal and palpebral reflexes. Central mechanisms for the control of blinking, in addition to the reflexive brainstem connections between the third-, fifth-, and seventh-nerve nuclei, include slower and polysynaptic circuits of the cerebrum, basal ganglia, and hypothalamus. Voluntary lid closure is initiated through frontobasal ganglionic connections.

The eyelids are kept open by the tonic contraction of the levator muscles, which overcomes the elastic properties of the periorbital muscles. The eyelids close during sleep and certain altered states of consciousness as a result of relaxation of the levator muscles. Facial paralysis causes the closure to be incomplete.

Blinking occurs irregularly at a rate of 12 to 20 times a minute, the frequency varying with the state of concentration and with emotion. The natural stimuli for the blink reflex (blinking is always bilateral) are corneal contact (corneal reflex), a tap on the brow or around the eye, visual threat, an unexpected loud sound, and, as indicated above, turning of the eyes to one side. There is normally a rapid adaptation of blink to visual and auditory stimuli but not to corneal stimulation.

Electromyography of the orbicularis oculi reveals two components of the blink response, an early and late one, features that are readily corroborated by clinical observation. The early response consists of only a slight movement of the upper lids; the immediately following response is more forceful and approximates the upper and lower lids. Whereas the early part of the blink reflex is beyond volitional control, the second part can be inhibited voluntarily.

Blepharospasm, an excessive and forceful closure of the lids, is a common disorder that is seen in isolation or as part of a number of dyskinesias and drug-induced movement disorders. Extremes of this condition may result in functional blindness. Increased blink frequency is a subtle part of the same condition but also occurs with corneal irritation. The opposite sign, reduced frequency of blinking (<10/min), is characteristic of progressive supranuclear palsy and Parkinson disease. In these cases, adaptation to repeated supraorbital tapping at a rate of about 1/s is impaired; therefore the patient continues to blink with each tap on the forehead or glabella, referred to as the glabellar, or *Myerson sign*.

A lesion of the oculomotor nerve, by paralyzing the levator muscle, causes *ptosis*, i.e., drooping of the upper eyelid. A lesion of the facial nerve, as in Bell palsy, results in an inability to close the eyelids because of weakness of orbicularis oculi, retraction of the upper lid (as a result of the unopposed action of the levator), and loss of the blink reflex on the affected side. In some instances of Bell palsy, even after nearly full recovery of facial movements, blink frequency and amplitude may be reduced on the previously paralyzed side. A trigeminal nerve lesion on one side, by reducing corneal sensation, interferes with the blink reflex on both sides, whereas Bell palsy does not abolish the contralateral blink. Aberrant regeneration of the third nerve after an injury may result in a condition wherein the upper lid retracts on lateral or downward gaze (pseudo-von Graefe sign). Aberrant regeneration of the facial nerve after Bell palsy has an opposite effect—closure of the lid with jaw movements or speaking (one of the Marcus Gunn phenomena, the other being an afferent pupillary defect to light). There is also a congenital and sometimes hereditary anomaly in which a ptotic eyelid retracts momentarily when the mouth is opened or the jaw is moved to one side. In other cases, inhibition of the levator muscle and ptosis occurs with opening of the mouth ("inverse Marcus Gunn phenomenon," or Marin Amat syndrome).

A useful clinical rule is that a combined paralysis of the levator, and orbicularis oculi muscles (i.e., the muscles that open and close the lids) indicates a myopathic disease such as myasthenia gravis or myotonic dystrophy. This is because the third and seventh cranial nerves are rarely affected together in peripheral nerve or brainstem disease. An infrequent but overlooked cause of unilateral static ptosis is a dehiscence of the tarsal muscle attachment; it can be identified by the loss of the upper lid fold just below the brow.

Bilateral ptosis is a characteristic feature of certain muscular dystrophies and of myasthenia gravis; congenital ptosis and progressive sagging of the upper lids in the elderly are other common forms as well botulism whether naturally acquired of after botulinum toxin treatments. An effective way of demonstrating that mild ostensibly unilateral ptosis is in fact bilateral is to lift the ptotic side and observe that the opposite lid promptly droops. This reflects the enhanced effort required to maintain patency of the lids. Unilateral ptosis is a notable feature of third-nerve lesions (see above) and of sympathetic paralysis, namely, the Horner syndrome. It may be accompanied by an overaction (compensation) of the frontalis and the contralateral levator palpebrae muscles. In patients with myasthenia, Cogan has described a "lid twitch" phenomenon, in which there is a transient retraction of the upper lid when the patient moves visual fixation from the down position to straight ahead. Brief fluttering of the lid margins upon moving the eyes vertically is also characteristic of myasthenia.

The opposite of ptosis, i.e., *retraction of the upper lids*, with a staring expression (Collier sign) is observed with orbital tumors and in thyroid disease, the latter also being the most common cause of unilateral and bilateral proptosis. A staring appearance alone is observed in Parkinson disease, progressive supranuclear palsy, and hydrocephalus in young children, in which there may be downturning of the eyes ("sunset sign"), and paralysis of upward gaze. Retraction of the eyelids may also be part of a dorsal midbrain syndrome and is accompanied by a light-near pupillary dissociation; it is not accompanied by a lid lag (von Graefe sign) on downward gaze, in distinction to what is observed in thyroid ophthalmopathy. Slight lid retraction has been observed in a few patients with hepatic cirrhosis, Cushing disease, chronic steroid myopathy, and hyperkalemic periodic paralysis. Lid retraction can be a reaction to ptosis on the other side; this is clarified by lifting the ptotic lid manually, and observing the disappearance of contralateral retraction as mentioned above.

Myotonic dystrophy features ptosis as a component of the myopathic facies. In myotonia congenita, forceful closure of the eyelids may induce a strong aftercontraction. In certain extrapyramidal diseases, particularly progressive supranuclear palsy, and Parkinson disease, even gentle lid closure may elicit blepharoclonus and blepharospasm on attempted opening of the lids; or there may be a delay in the opening of the tightly closed eyelids. Acute right parietal or bifrontal lesions often produce a peculiar disinclination to open the eyelids, even to the point of offering active resistance to forced opening. The closed lids give the false impression of diminished alertness and has incorrectly been called an apraxia of lid opening.

THE PUPILS

The testing of pupillary size and reactivity, which can be accomplished by the use of a flashlight and simple gauge (we favor the circular laminated card—the *Iowa pupil gauge*), yields important, often vital clinical information. Essential, of course, is the proper interpretation of pupillary reactions, and this requires some knowledge of their underlying neural mechanisms.

The diameter of the pupil is determined by the balance of innervation between the constricting sphincter and radially arranged dilator muscles of the iris, the sphincter muscle playing the major role in the light response. The *pupilloconstrictor (parasympathetic)* fibers arise in the Edinger-Westphal nucleus in the high mid-brain, join the third cranial (oculomotor) nerve, and synapse in the ciliary ganglion, which lies in the posterior part of the orbit. The postganglionic fibers then enter the globe via the short ciliary nerves; approximately 3 percent of the fibers innervate the sphincter pupillae and 97 percent the ciliary body, which is primarily responsible for accommodative constriction of the pupil. The sphincter of the pupil comprises 50 motor units, according to Corbett and Thompson.

The *pupillodilator (sympathetic)* fibers arise in the posterolateral part of the hypothalamus and descend, uncrossed, in the lateral tegmentum of the midbrain, pons, medulla, and cervical spinal cord to the eighth cervical, and first and second thoracic segments, where they synapse with lateral horn neurons. The latter give rise to preganglionic fibers, most of which leave the cord by the second ventral thoracic root and proceed through the stellate ganglion to synapse in the superior cervical ganglion. The postganglionic fibers course along the internal carotid artery and traverse the cavernous sinus, where they join the first division of the trigeminal nerve, finally reaching the eye as the long ciliary nerve that innervates the dilator muscle of the iris. Some of the postganglionic sympathetic fibers also innervate the sweat glands and arterioles of the face, and Müller's muscle in the eyelid.

The Pupillary Light Reflex

The most common stimulus for pupillary constriction is exposure of the retina to light. Reflex pupillary constriction is also part of the act of convergence and accommodation for near objects (near synkinesis).

The pathway for the pupillary light reflex consists of three parts (Fig. 14-9). There is an *afferent limb*, fibers of which originate in the retinal receptor cells, pass through the bipolar cells, and synapse with the retinal ganglion cells; axons of these cells run in the optic nerve and in the ipsilateral tract. The light reflex fibers leave the optic tract just rostral to the lateral geniculate body and enter the high mid-brain, where they synapse in the pretectal nucleus. The *special intercalated neurons*, which pass ventrally to the ipsilateral Edinger-Westphal nucleus and, via fibers that cross in the posterior commissure, go on to the contralateral Edinger-Westphal nucleus (labeled "pretecto-oculomotor" tract in Fig. 14-9). The effector arm of the reflex consists of an *efferent two-neuron pathway from the Edinger-Westphal nucleus* that synapses in the ciliary ganglion, from which the short ciliary nerves innervate the sphincter to cause pupillary constriction.

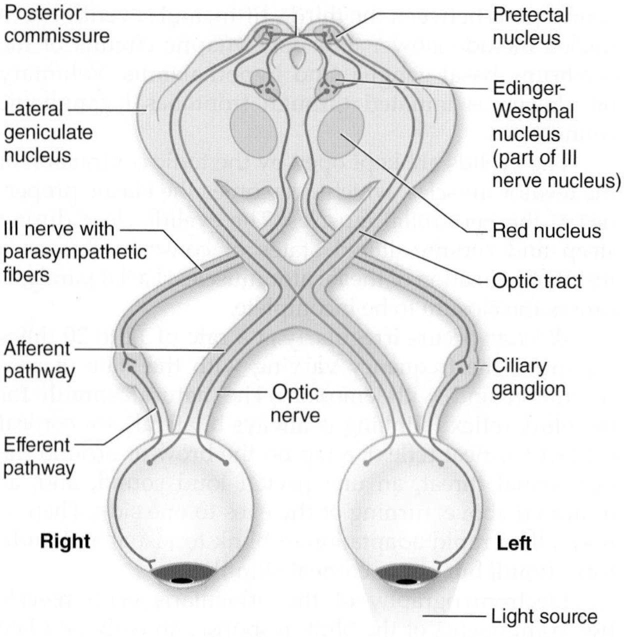

Figure 14-9. Diagram of the pathways subserving the pupillary light reflex. (Redrawn with permission from Bradford CA [ed]: *Basic Ophthalmology*, 7th Edition. San Francisco, American Academy of Ophthalmology, 1975.)

Alterations of the Pupils

The pupils tend to be large in children and small in the aged, sometimes markedly miotic but still reactive (senile miosis). An asymmetry of the pupils of 0.3 to 0.5 mm is found in 20 percent or more of normal individuals. A lesion that destroys only a small number of nerve cells in the Edinger-Westphal nucleus or ciliary ganglion will cause paralysis of a sector or sectors of the iris and deform the pupil to a pear or elliptical shape.

Normally the pupil constricts under a bright light (direct reflex), and the other unexposed pupil also constricts (consensual reflex). With complete or nearly complete interruption of the optic nerve, the pupil will fail to react to direct light stimulation; however, the pupil of the blind eye will still show a consensual reflex, i.e., it will constrict with illumination of the healthy eye.

Contrariwise, lack of direct and consensual light reflex with retention of the consensual reflex in the opposite eye places the lesion in the efferent limb of the reflex arc, i.e., in the homolateral oculomotor nerve or its nucleus. A lesion of the afferent limb of the light reflex pathway will not affect the near responses of the pupil, and lesions of the visual pathway caudal to the point where the light reflex fibers leave the optic tract will not alter the pupillary light reflex (Fig. 14-9).

Following initial constriction, the pupil may normally dilate slightly in spite of a light shining steadily in one or both eyes. Slowness of response along with failure to sustain pupillary constriction, or "pupillary escape," is sometimes referred to as the *Marcus Gunn pupillary sign*; a mild degree of it may be observed in normal persons, but it is far more prominent in cases of damage to the retina or optic nerve. The unilateral inadequacy of pupillary response may be used to expose mild degrees of retrobulbar optic neuropathy. This relative "afferent pupillary defect" is tested always in a dimly lighted room with the patient fixating on a distant target. If a light is shifted quickly from the normal to the impaired eye, the direct light stimulus is no longer sufficient to maintain the previously evoked consensual pupillary constriction and both pupils dilate. A variant of this maneuver is the "swinging-flashlight test," in which each pupil is alternately exposed to light at 3-s intervals and the pupil on the side of an optic neuropathy displays a paradoxical dilatation just as the light is brought to it.

Hippus, a rapid fluctuation in pupillary size, is common in metabolic encephalopathy but otherwise has no particular significance and is occasionally seen in normal persons. To distinguish hippus from the Marcus Gunn afferent pupillary defect one carefully observes the first movement of the pupil as the light is repeatedly moved to the affected eye; in hippus, half of the initial responses will be dilation and half, constriction, whereas in a deafferented pupil all the initial movements are dilation.

Horner Syndrome

Interruption of the sympathetic fibers results in miosis and ptosis (because of paralysis of the pupillary dilator muscle and of Müller muscle, respectively). The lesion may be central, between the hypothalamus and the points of exit of sympathetic fibers from the spinal cord (C8 to T3, mainly T2), or peripheral, in the cervical sympathetic chain, superior cervical ganglion, or along the carotid artery. A congenital form caused by perinatal injury, usually of the sympathetic chain in the neck is seen regularly in our clinics (Fig. 14-10). A hereditary form of the Horner syndrome (autosomal dominant) is also known, usually but not always associated with a congenital absence of pigment in the affected iris (heterochromia iridis) (Hageman et al).

To the ophthalmic findings may be added loss of sweating on the same side of the face and redness of the conjunctiva. The entire complex is called the *Horner syndrome*, *Bernard-Horner syndrome*, or oculosympathetic palsy. The pupillary change may be subtle and may require covering the eyes or dimming the room lights to observe the lack of expected mydriasis on one side.

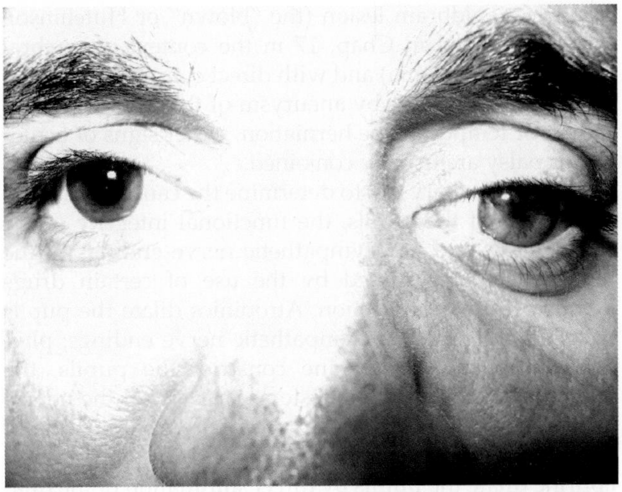

Figure 14-10. Congenital Horner syndrome on the patient's left. In addition to the miosis and ptosis, the patient's left iris is gray in color and the right, brown.

Most cases are caused by peripheral interruption of the sympathetic chain but the same effect may be produced by ipsilateral lesions of the sympathetic tract in the medulla or cervical cord. The pattern of sweating may be helpful in localizing the lesion in the following manner: With lesions at the level of the common carotid artery, loss of sweating involves the entire side of the face. With lesions distal to the carotid bifurcation, loss of sweating is not found or is confined to the medial aspect of the forehead and side of the nose (Morris et al). Retraction of the eyeball (enophthalmos), considered a component of the syndrome, is probably an illusion created by narrowing of the palpebral fissure.

Bilateral Horner syndrome is a rare occurrence; usually it is found in autonomic neuropathies and in high cervical cord transection. Although difficult to appreciate, bilateral miosis may be detected (using pupillometry or direct observation) by noting a lag in the redilation of the initially small pupils when light is withdrawn (Smith and Smith, 1999).

Stimulation or irritation of the sympathetic fibers, a rare phenomenon, has the opposite effect, i.e., lid retraction, dilatation of the pupil, and apparent proptosis. Use is made of this phenomenon in the testing of the *ciliospinal pupillary reflex*, which is evoked by pinching the neck (afferent, C2, C3) and effecting pupillary enlargement through cervical efferent sympathetic fibers.

Extreme bilateral constriction of the pupils (miosis) is commonly observed with pontine lesions, presumably because of interruption of the pupillodilator fibers but the mechanism is not entirely clear. Narcotic ingestion is the most common cause of bilateral miosis in clinical practice except in the elderly, who often acquire small pupils, particularly if medication drops for glaucoma are being used.

Interruption of the parasympathetic fibers causes an abnormal dilatation of the pupils (mydriasis), often with loss of pupillary light reflex; in cases of coma, this is the result of a midbrain lesion (the "blown" or Hutchinson pupil, described in Chap. 17 in the context of cerebral masses causing coma) and with direct compression of the oculomotor nerve, as by aneurysm of the circle of Willis, tumor, or temporal lobe herniation. Other signs of oculomotor palsy are usually conjoined.

As an ancillary test to determine the cause of changes in the size of the pupils, the functional integrity of the sympathetic and parasympathetic nerve endings in the iris may be determined by the use of certain drugs detailed in the next section. Atropinics dilate the pupils by paralyzing the parasympathetic nerve endings; physostigmine and pilocarpine constrict the pupils, the former by inhibiting cholinesterase activity at the neuromuscular junction and the latter by direct stimulation of the sphincter muscle of the iris. Epinephrine and phenylephrine dilate the pupils by direct stimulation of the dilator muscle. Cocaine dilates the pupils by preventing the reabsorption of norepinephrine into the nerve endings. Morphine and other narcotics act centrally to constrict the pupils. More recently, the alpha-agonist drug, apraclonidine, has been shown to reliably reverse the anisocoria of Horner syndrome and has become the preferred drug for testing. One drop (0.5 percent solution) is placed in each eye, the eyes are kept closed for 1 min and the drops are repeated 5 min later. Enlargement of the miosis with the affected pupil becoming larger than the unaffected one 30 to 45 min after instillation is definite evidence of a Horner syndrome. Ptosis is also reduced, sometimes to a remarkable extent. It was originally developed as a treatment for glaucoma (Koc et al).

In *diabetes mellitus*, where autonomic spinal and cranial nerves are often involved, the pupils are affected in the majority of cases. They are smaller than would be expected for age because of involvement of pupillodilator sympathetic fibers, and mydriasis is excessive upon instillation of sympathomimetic drugs. The light reflex, mediated by parasympathetic fibers (which are also damaged), is reduced, usually to a greater degree than constriction on accommodation (Smith and Smith, 1987). Some of these abnormalities require special methods for their demonstration.

Argyll Robertson Pupil (Table 14-6)

In almost all the forms of late syphilis, particularly tabes dorsalis, the pupils are bilaterally small, irregular, and unequal; they fail to react to light, although they do constrict on accommodation (light-near dissociation) and do not dilate properly in response to mydriatic drugs. Atrophy of the iris is associated in some cases. This is known as the *Argyll Robertson pupil*. The exact locality of the lesion is not certain but it is generally believed to be in the tectum of the midbrain proximal to the oculomotor nuclei where the descending pupillodilator fibers are in close proximity to the light reflex fibers (Fig. 14-9). This putatively explains the sparing of the afferent accommodative pathways from the retina to the Edinger-Westphal nuclei. The possibility of a partial third-nerve lesion extending to the ciliary ganglion seems as plausible to us. A similar pupillary abnormality has been observed in the meningoradiculitis of Lyme disease and in diabetes. A dissociation of the light reflex from the accommodation-convergence reaction is also sometimes observed with a variety of midbrain lesions—e.g., pinealoma, multiple sclerosis; in these diseases, miosis, irregularity of pupils, and failure to respond to a mydriatic are usually not present. S.A.K. Wilson referred to this condition as the *Argyll Robertson pupillary phenomenon*.

Adie Tonic Pupil (Holmes-Adie Syndrome)

(Table 14-6)

Another interesting pupillary abnormality is the tonic reaction, also referred to as the *Adie pupil*. This syndrome is caused by a degeneration of the ciliary ganglia and the postganglionic parasympathetic fibers that normally constrict the pupil and effect accommodation. The patient may complain of unilateral blurring of vision or photophobia or may have noticed that one pupil is larger than the other. The affected pupil is slightly enlarged in ambient light and the reaction to light is absent at the outset of the syndrome or greatly reduced if tested in the customary manner, although the pupil will slowly constrict with prolonged bright light stimulation. Characteristically, there is a light-near dissociation, i.e., like the Argyll Robertson pupil, the Adie pupil responds better to near (accommodation) than it does to light. The most characteristic feature is that once the pupil has constricted, it tends to remain tonically constricted and redilates very slowly (the "tonic' aspect of the syndrome). Once dilated, the pupil remains in this state for many seconds, up to a minute or longer. Light and near paralysis of a segment or segments of the pupillary sphincter is also characteristic of the syndrome; this segmental irregularity can be seen with the high plus lenses of an ophthalmoscope. The affected pupil constricts promptly in response to the common miotic drugs and is unusually sensitive to a 0.1 percent solution of pilocarpine,

Table 14-6

CHARACTERISTICS OF ARGYLL ROBERTSON AND ADIE PUPILS

	SIZE AND SIDE	LIGHT REACTION	ACCOMMODATIVE REACTION	SPECIAL FEATURES
Argyll Robertson pupil	Small, irregular, asymmetrical	No	Yes	Syphilitic, but also diabetic
Adie tonic pupil	Initially fixed, later enlarged to medium size; bilateral	No or poor; only with sustained bright light	Yes, with tonic reaction	Tonic contraction to prolonged accommodation; associated areflexia

a concentration that has only minimal effect on a normal pupil (due to denervation supersensitivity).

The tonic pupil usually appears during the third or fourth decade of life and is much more common in women than in men; it may be associated with absence of knee or ankle jerks (*Holmes-Adie syndrome*) and hence be mistaken for tabes dorsalis. From all available data, it represents a special form of mild inherited polyneuropathy. There is a familial tendency to the syndrome, in some cases associated with a mutation in the myelin protein zero (MP0) gene that is implicated in one of the less-common forms of Charcot-Marie-Tooth inherited polyneuropathy (see Chap. 46).

An acquired type of tonic pupil has also been associated, sometimes on uncertain grounds, with diabetes, viral infection, and trauma. We have observed it in migraine and following recovery from the Guillain-Barré syndrome.

Springing Pupil

Mention should be made of this rare pupillary phenomenon characterized by transient episodes of unilateral mydriasis for which no cause can be found (the *springing pupil*). Episodes of mydriasis, which are more common in women, last for minutes to days and may recur at random intervals. Oculomotor palsies and ptosis are notably lacking, but sometimes the pupil is distorted during the attack. Some patients complain of blurred vision and head pain on the side of the mydriasis, suggesting an atypical ophthalmoplegic migraine. In children, following a minor or major seizure, one pupil may remain dilated for a protracted period of time. The main consideration in an awake patient is that the cornea has inadvertently (or purposefully) been exposed to mydriatic solutions, among them vasopressor agents used in cardiac resuscitation.

Differential Diagnosis of Anisocoria

(Figure 14-11)

In regard to pupillary disorders, there are two main issues with which the neurologist has to contend. One is the problem of unequal pupils (anisocoria), and determining whether this abnormality is derived from sympathetic or parasympathetic denervation. The second problem is the relative afferent pupillary defect, and how to recognize it; this was discussed earlier.

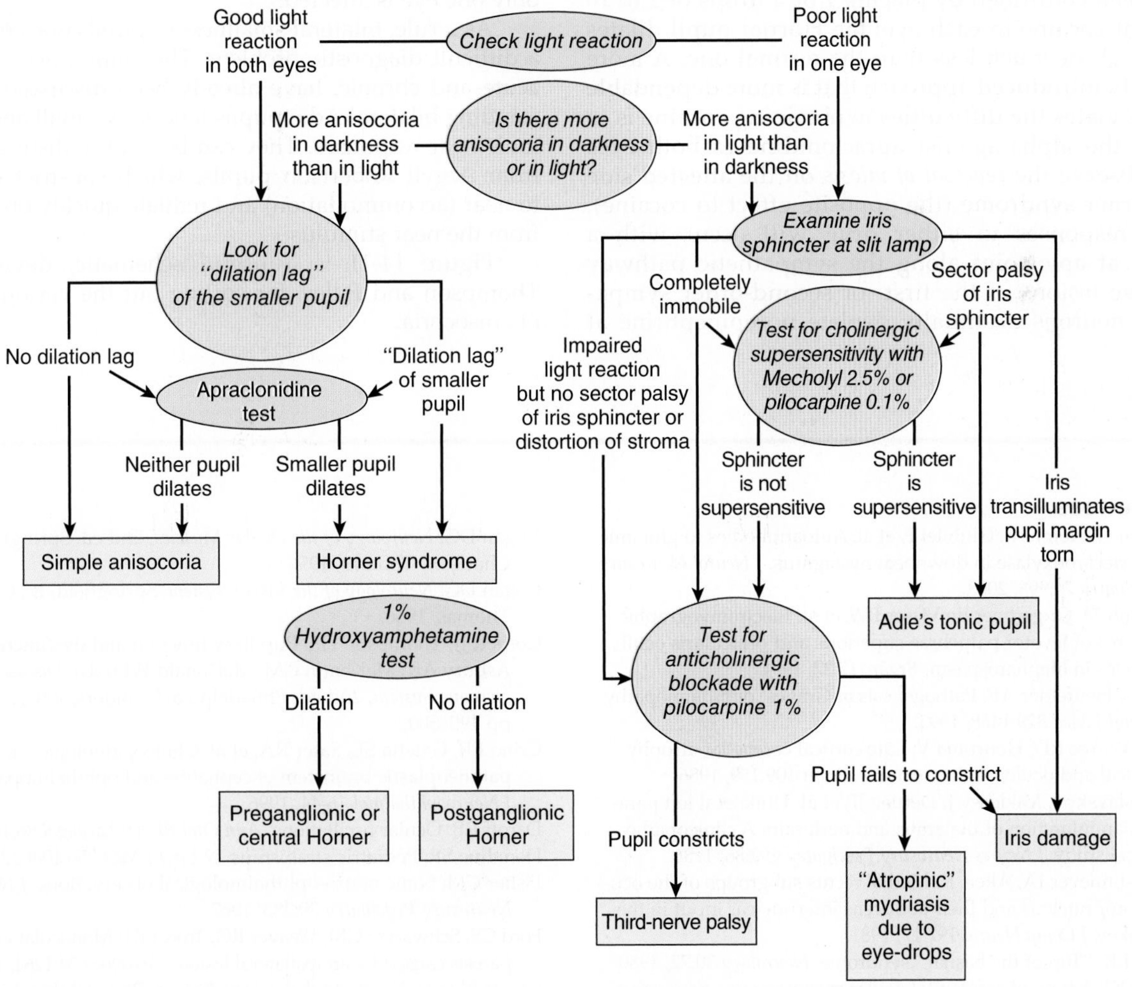

Figure 14-11. A schematic approach for sorting out the nature of anisocoria. (Adapted by permission from Thompson and Pilley.)

In dealing with anisocoria, 20 percent of normal persons show an inequality of 0.3 to 0.5 mm or more in pupillary diameter. This is "simple," or *physiologic, anisocoria*, and it may be a source of confusion in patients with small pupils. Its main characteristic is that the same degree of asymmetry in size is maintained in low, ambient, and bright light conditions. It is also variable from day to day and even from hour to hour, and often will have disappeared at the time of a second examination (Loewenfeld; Lam et al).

The first step in the analysis of pupillary asymmetry is to determine which of the pupils is abnormal. An abnormal larger pupil can be identified by a reduced direct and consensual light reaction. If the smaller pupil is causing asymmetry, it will fail to enlarge in response to shading both eyes or reducing ambient light. More simply stated, *light exaggerates the anisocoria caused by a third-nerve lesion, and darkness accentuates the anisocoria in the case of a Horner syndrome.*

A *persistently small pupil* always raises the question of a Horner syndrome, a diagnosis that may be difficult if the ptosis is slight. In darkness, the Horner pupil dilates more slowly and to a lesser degree than the normal one because it lacks the pull of the dilator muscle (dilation lag). The diagnosis in the past had been confirmed by placing 1 or 2 drops of 2 to 10 percent cocaine in each eye; the Horner pupil dilates not at all or much less than the normal one. A more recently introduced approach that is more dependable and obviates the difficulties in obtaining cocaine is to apply the alpha-agonist apraclonidine to both eyes and observe the *reversal of miosis* on the affected side of Horner syndrome (the opposite effect to cocaine). Such responses to either drug will occur with a lesion at any point along the sympathetic pathway because lesions of the first- or second-order sympathetic neurons eventually deplete norepinephrine at the synapses with third-order neurons. The reduction of neurotransmitter at the nerve endings in the ciliary dilator muscle greatly reduces the reuptake blocking effects of cocaine. If the subsequent (24 h after cocaine) application of the adrenergic mydriatic hydroxyamphetamine (1 percent) has no effect, the lesion can be localized to the postganglionic portion of the pathway as this drug releases any norepinephrine that may remain in the third-order neuron. Localization of the lesion to the central or preganglionic parts of the sympathetic pathway depends upon the associated symptoms and signs (see Chap. 26).

A variety of lesions, some of them purely ocular, such as uveitis, may also give rise to a *dilated pupil.*

Drug-induced iridoplegia is another cause of anisocoria. Not infrequently, particularly among nurses and pharmacists, a mydriatic fixed pupil is the result of accidental or deliberate application of an atropinic or sympathomimetic drug. We have observed this in house officers after they had participated in resuscitation from a cardiac arrest and been inadvertently sprayed with a sympathomimetic drug. Failure of 1 percent pilocarpine drops to contract the pupil provides proof that the iris sphincter has been blocked by atropine or some other anticholinergic agent. This is particularly the case when only one eye is affected.

As a rule, bilateral smallness of pupils does not pose a difficult diagnostic problem. The clinical associations, acute and chronic, have already been discussed. Longstanding bilateral Adie pupils tend to be small and show tonic near responses. They can be readily distinguished from Argyll Robertson pupils, which constrict quickly to near (accommodation) and redilate quickly on release from the near stimulus.

Figure 14-11 is a useful schematic, devised by Thompson and Pilley, for sorting out the various types of anisocoria.

References

Antonini G, Nemni R, Giubilei F, et al: Autoantibodies to glutamic acid decarboxylase in downbeat nystagmus. *J Neurol Neurosurg Psychiatry* 74:998, 2003.

Aramideh M, Ongerboer de Visser BW, et al: Electromyographic features of levator palpebrae superioris and orbicularis oculi muscles in blepharospasm. *Brain* 117:27, 1994.

Bahn RS, Heufelder AE: Pathogenesis of Graves' ophthalmopathy. *N Engl J Med* 329:1468, 1993.

Baloh RW, Yee RD, Honrubia V: Late cortical cerebellar atrophy: Clinical and oculographic features. *Brain* 109:159, 1986.

Bogousslavsky J, Miklossy J, Deruaz JP, et al: Unilateral left paramedian infarction of thalamus and midbrain: A clinicopathological study. *J Neurol Neurosurg Psychiatry* 49:686, 1986.

Büttner-Ennever JA, Akert K: Medial rectus subgroups of the oculomotor nucleus and their abducens internuclear input in the monkey. *J Comp Neurol* 197:17, 1981.

Caplan LR: "Top of the basilar" syndrome. *Neurology* 30:72, 1980.

Cogan DG: A type of congenital ocular motor apraxia presenting jerky head movements. *Am J Ophthalmol* 36:433, 1953.

Cogan DG: *Neurology of the Ocular Muscles*, 2nd ed. Springfield, IL, Charles C Thomas, 1956.

Cogan DG: *Neurology of the Visual System*. Springfield, IL, Charles C Thomas, 1966.

Corbett JJ, Thompson HS: Pupillary function and dysfunction, in Asbury AK, McKhann GM, McDonald WI (eds): *Diseases of the Nervous System*, 2nd ed. Philadelphia, Saunders, 1992, pp 490–500.

Crino PR, Galetta SL, Sater RA, et al: Clinicopathologic study of paraneoplastic brainstem encephalitis and ophthalmoparesis. *J Neuroophthalmol* 16:44, 1996.

Daroff RB: Ocular oscillations. *Ann Otol Rhinol Laryngol* 86:102, 1977.

Donahue SP: Pediatric strabismus. *N Engl J Med* 356:1040, 2007.

Fisher CM: Some neuro-ophthalmological observations. *J Neurol Neurosurg Psychiatry* 30:383, 1967.

Ford CS, Schwartze GM, Weaver RG, Troost BT: Monocular elevation paresis caused by an ipsilateral lesion. *Neurology* 34:1264, 1984.

Glaser JS (ed): *Neuro-ophthalmology*, 3rd ed. Philadelphia, Lippincott Williams & Wilkins, 1999.

Guy JR, Schatz NJ Paraneoplastic downbeating nystagmus. A sign of occult malignancy. *J Clin Neuroophthalmol* 8:269, 1988.

Hageman G, Ippel PF, Nijenhuis F: Autosomal dominant congenital Horner syndrome in a Dutch family. *J Neurol Neurosurg Psychiatry* 55:28, 1992.

Halmagyi GM, Rudge P, Griesty M, Sanders MD: Downbeating nystagmus. *Arch Neurol* 40:777, 1983.

Hanson MR, Hamid MA, Tomsak RL, et al: Selective saccadic palsy caused by pontine lesions: Clinical, physiological and pathological correlations. *Ann Neurol* 20:209, 1986.

Hommel M, Bogousslavsky J: The spectrum of vertical gaze palsy following unilateral brainstem stroke. *Neurology* 41:1229, 1991.

Hotson R: Cerebellar control of fixation eye movements. *Neurology* 32:31, 1982.

Jacobs L, Anderson PJ, Bender MG: The lesions producing paralysis of downward but not upward gaze. *Arch Neurol* 28:319, 1973.

Kato I, Nakamura T, Watanabe J, et al: Primary posterior upbeat nystagmus: Localizing value. *Arch Neurol* 42:819, 1985.

Keane JR: Acute bilateral ophthalmoplegia: 60 cases. *Neurology* 36:279, 1986.

Keane JR: Cavernous sinus syndrome: Analysis of 151 cases. *Arch Neurol* 53:967, 1996.

Keane JR: Ocular skew deviation. *Arch Neurol* 32:185, 1975.

Keane JR: Internuclear ophthalmoplegia. Unusual causes in 114 of 410 patients. *Arch Neurol* 62:714, 2005.

Keane JR: Bilateral ocular paralysis. Analysis of 31 inpatients. *Arch Neurol* 64:178, 2007.

Kline IB, Hoyt WF: The Tolosa-Hunt syndrome. *J Neurol Neurosurg Psychiatry* 71:577, 2001.

Koc F, Kavuncu S, Kansu T, et al: The sensitivity and specificity of 0.5% apraclonidine in the diagnosis of oculosympathetic paralysis. *Br J Ophthalmol* 89:1442, 2005.

Kompf D, Pasik T, Pasik P, Bender MB: Downward gaze in monkeys: Stimulation and lesion studies. *Brain* 102:527, 1979.

Lam BL, Thompson HS, Corbett JJ: The prevalence of simple anisocoria. *Am J Ophthalmol* 104:69, 1987.

Leichnetz GR: The prefrontal cortico-oculomotor trajectories in the monkey. *J Neurol Sci* 49:387, 1981.

Leigh RJ, Zee DS: *The Neurology of Eye Movements*, 2nd ed. Philadelphia, Davis, 1991.

Lewis RF, Zee DS: Ocular motor disorders associated with cerebellar lesions: Pathophysiology and topical localization. *Rev Neurol* 149:665, 1993.

Loewenfeld IE: "Simple, central" anisocoria: A common condition seldom recognized. *Trans Am Acad Ophthalmol Otolaryngol* 83:832, 1977.

Morris JGL, Lee J, Lim CL: Facial sweating in Horner's syndrome. *Brain* 107:751, 1984.

Palla A, Straumann D: Neurological evaluation of acute vertical diplopia. *Schweiz Arch Neurol Psychiatr* 153:180, 2002.

Ranalli PJ, Sharpe JA, Fletcher WA: Palsy of upward and downward saccadic, pursuit, and vestibular movements with a unilateral midbrain lesion: Pathophysiologic correlations. *Neurology* 38:114, 1988.

Ropper AH: Ocular dipping in anoxic coma. *Arch Neurol* 38:297, 1981.

Ropper AH: Illusion of tilting of the visual environment. *J Clin Neuroophthalmol* 3:147, 1983.

Rucker CW: Paralysis of the third, fourth, and sixth cranial nerves. *Am J Ophthalmol* 46:787, 1958.

Rucker CW: The causes of paralysis of the third, fourth and sixth cranial nerves. *Am J Ophthalmol* 61:1293, 1966.

Rush JA, Younge BR: Paralysis of cranial nerves III, IV, and VI: Cause and prognosis in 1000 cases. *Arch Ophthalmol* 99:76, 1981.

Safran AB, Kline LB, Glaser JS, Daroff RB: Television-induced formed visual hallucinations and cerebral diplopia. *Br J Ophthalmol* 65:707, 1981.

Saul RF, Selhorst JB: Downbeat nystagmus with magnesium depletion. *Arch Neurol* 38:650, 1981.

Smith AS, Smith SC: Assessment of pupillary function in diabetic neuropathy, in Dyck PJ, Thomas PK, Asbury AK, et al (eds): *Diabetic Neuropathy*. Philadelphia, Saunders, 1987, pp 134–139.

Smith SA, Smith SE: Bilateral Horner's syndrome: Detection and occurrence. *J Neurol Neurosurg Psychiatry* 66:48, 1999.

Thach WT, Montgomery EB: Motor system, in Pearlman AL, Collins RC (eds): *Neurobiology of Disease*. New York, Oxford University Press, 1990, pp 168–196.

Thompson HS: Diagnosing Horner's syndrome. *Trans Am Acad Ophthalmol Otolaryngol* 83:OP840, 1977.

Thompson HS, Pilley SFJ: Unequal pupils: A flow chart for sorting out the anisocorias. *Surv Ophthalmol* 21:45, 1976.

Tijssen CC: Contralateral conjugate eye deviation in acute supratentorial lesions. *Stroke* 25:215, 1994.

Vidailhet M, Rivaud S, Gouider-Khouja N, et al: Eye movements in parkinsonian syndromes. *Ann Neurol* 35:420, 1994.

Von Noorden GK: *Van Noorden-Maumenee's Atlas of Strabismus*, 3rd ed. St. Louis, Mosby, 1977.

Wall M, Wray SH: The one-and-a-half syndrome—a unilateral disorder of the pontine tegmentum: A study of 20 cases and review of the literature. *Neurology* 33:971, 1983.

Warwick R: Representation of the extraocular muscles in the oculomotor nuclei of the monkey. *J Comp Neurol* 98:449, 1953.

Warwick R: The so-called nucleus of convergence. *Brain* 78:92, 1955.

White OB, St Cyr JA, Sharpe JA: Ocular motor deficits in Parkinson's disease. *Brain* 106:555, 571, 1983.

Wiersinga WM, Smit T, van der Gaag R, et al: Clinical presentation of Grave's ophthalmopathy. *Ophthalmic Res* 21:73, 1989.

Wray SH: Neuro-ophthalmologic diseases, in Rosenberg RN (ed): *Comprehensive Neurology*. New York, Raven Press, 1991, pp 659–697.

Wray SH, Taylor J: Third nerve palsy: A review of 206 cases. Unpublished data, quoted in Wray SH (above).

Yousry I, Dieterich M, Naidich TP, et al: Superior oblique myokymia: Magnetic resonance imaging support for the neurovascular compression hypothesis. *Ann Neurol* 51:361, 2002.

Zee DS: Ophthalmoscopy in examination of patients with vestibular disorders. *Ann Neurol* 3:373, 1978.

Zee DS, Robinson DA: A hypothetical explanation of saccadic oscillations. *Ann Neurol* 5:405, 1979.

Zee DS, Yee RD, Cogan DG, et al: Ocular motor abnormalities in hereditary cerebellar ataxia. *Brain* 99:207, 1976.

15

Deafness, Dizziness, and Disorders of Equilibrium

Sounds alert us to danger; spoken words are the universal means of communication; music is one of our most exalted aesthetic pleasures. The loss of hearing excludes the individual from much of what is happening, and adjustment to this deprivation imposes profound challenge. Prevention of deafness is a goal toward which medicine strives. Likewise, vestibular function ensures one's ability to stand steadily, stabilize eye position during head movement, and move about gracefully. Hence an understanding of the functions of the eighth cranial nerves and their derangements by disease is as much the concern of the neurologist as the otologist. As a general rule, the association of vertigo and deafness signifies a disease of the end organs for hearing and vestibular function, or of the eighth nerve. The precise locus of the disease is determined by tests of labyrinthine and auditory function, described further on, and by findings on neurologic examination and imaging studies that implicate the primary and secondary connections of the eighth cranial nerve.

ANATOMIC AND PHYSIOLOGIC CONSIDERATIONS

The vestibulocochlear, or eighth, cranial nerve has two separate components: the cochlear nerve, which subserves hearing, and the vestibular nerve, which is concerned with equilibrium (balance) and orientation of the body and eyes to the surrounding world. The acoustic division has its cell bodies in the spiral ganglion of the cochlea. This ganglion is composed of bipolar cells, the peripheral processes of which convey auditory impulses from the specialized neuroepithelium of the inner ear, the spiral organ of Corti. This is the end organ of hearing, wherein sound is transduced into nerve impulses. It consists of approximately 15,000 neuroepithelial (hair) cells that rest on the basilar membrane, which extends along the entire 2.5 turns of the cochlea. Projecting from the inner surface of each hair cell are approximately 60 very fine filaments, or stereocilia, which are embedded in the tectorial membrane, a gelatinous structure overlying the organ of Corti (Fig. 15-1). Sound causes the basilar membrane to vibrate; upward displacement of the basilar membrane bends the relatively fixed stereocilia and provides a stimulus adequate for activating the hair cells. The stimulus is then transmitted to the sensory fibers of the cochlear nerve, which end synaptically at the base of each hair cell.

Each afferent auditory fiber and the hair cell with which it is connected have a minimum threshold at one frequency ("characteristic" or "best" frequency). The basilar membrane vibrates at different frequencies throughout its length, according to the frequency of the sound stimulus. In this way, the fibers of the cochlear nerve respond to the full range of audible sound and can differentiate and resolve complexes of sounds.

The inner hair cells, numbering about 3,500, are of particular importance, because they synapse with approximately 90 percent of the 30,000 afferent cochlear neurons. The central processes of the primary auditory neurons constitute the cochlear division of the eighth cranial nerve. In addition, the nerve contains approximately 500 efferent fibers, which arise from the superior olivary nuclei (80 percent from the contralateral nucleus and 20 percent from the ipsilateral one) and synapse with the afferent neurons from the hair cells (Rasmussen). The function of this efferent pathway is not clear. It is thought to play some part in the auditory processing generated in the ear itself, possibly to enhance the sharpness of sound perception by a feedback mechanism. The eighth nerve also contains adrenergic postganglionic fibers that are derived from the cervical autonomic chain and innervate the cochlea and labyrinth. Their function has been the subject of investigation.

The semicircular ducts, utricle, and saccule, collectively comprising the vestibular apparatus, contain the sense organs for the detection of angular and linear acceleration. They are filled with an intracellular fluid, endolymph, and are surrounded by cerebrospinal fluid (perilymph) within excavated spaces of the temporal bone, the semicircular canals. The latter term, canal, is used interchangeably with the proper description, ducts, to describe the vestibular apparatus.

The vestibular division of the eighth nerve arises from cells in the vestibular, or Scarpa ganglion, which is situated in the internal auditory meatus. This ganglion is also composed of bipolar cells, the peripheral processes of which terminate in hair cells of the specialized sensory

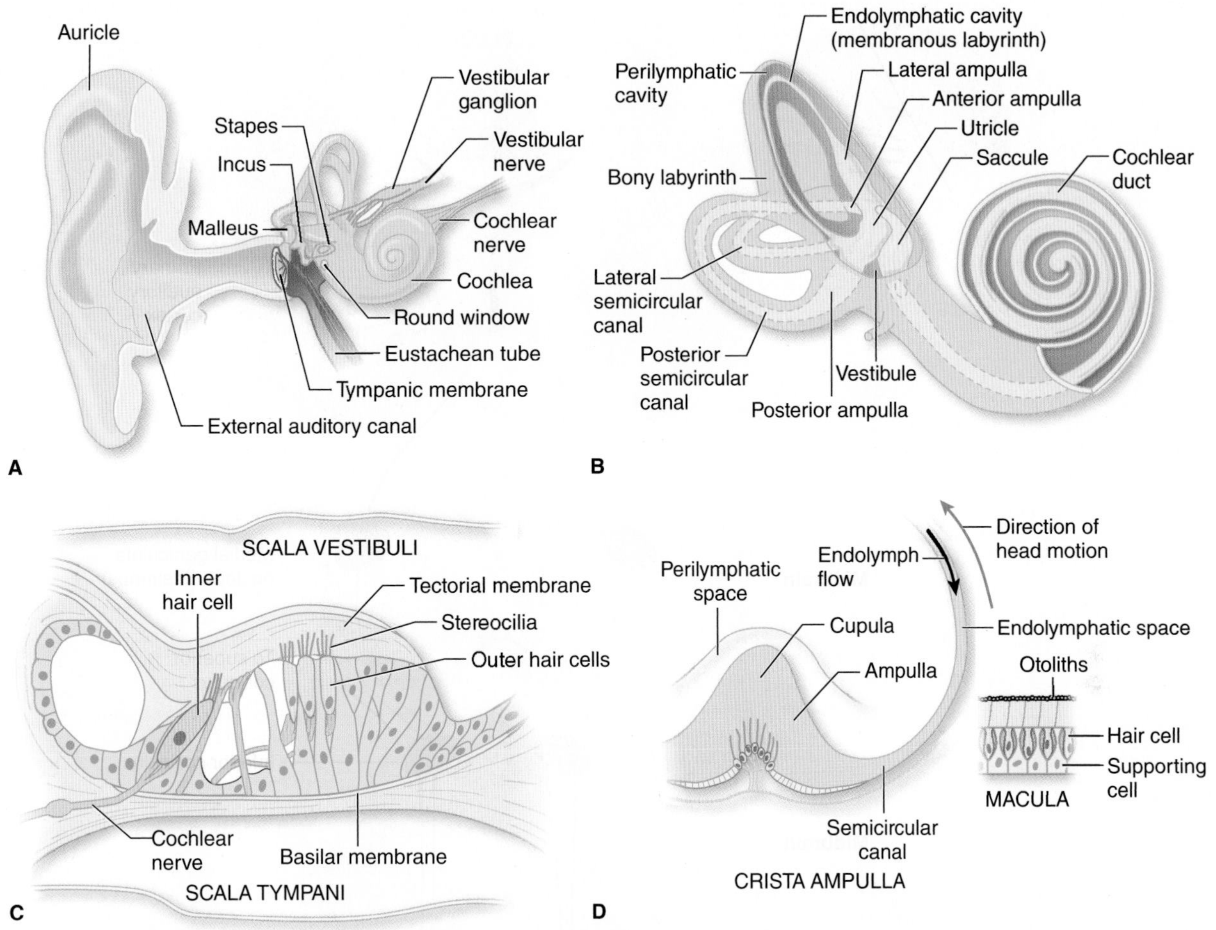

Figure 15-1. The auditory and vestibular systems. *A*. The right ear, viewed from the front, showing the external ear and auditory canal, the middle ear and its ossicles, and the inner ear. *B*. The main parts of the right inner ear, viewed from the front. The *perilymph* is located between the wall of the bony labyrinth and the membranous labyrinth. In the cochlea, the perilymphatic space takes the form of two coiled tubes—the *scala vestibuli* and *scala tympani*. The *endolymph* is located within the membranous labyrinth, which includes the three semicircular canals, utricle, and saccule. *C*. The *organ of Corti*. This is the end organ of hearing; it consists of a single row of inner hair cells and three rows of outer hair cells. The stereocilia of the hair cells are embedded in the tectorial membrane. *D*. Diagram of a crista ampulla, the specialized sensory epithelium of a semicircular canal. The crista senses the displacement of endolymph during head rotation. The direction of head rotation is indicated by the *large arrow*, and endolymph flow by the *small arrow*. The *macula* is the locus of the sensory epithelium in the utricle and saccule. Note that the tips of the hair cells are in contact with the otoliths (calcareous material), which are embedded in a gelatinous mass called the *cupula*.

epithelium of the labyrinthine apparatus. The sensory epithelium is located on hillocks (cristae) in the dilated openings or ampullae of the semicircular ducts, where they are called the *cristae ampullaris*, and in the utricle and saccule, where they are called *maculae acusticae*. The hair cells of the maculae are covered by the *otolithic membrane*, or *otolith*, which is composed of calcium carbonate crystals embedded in a gelatinous matrix. The sensory cells of the cristae are covered by a sail-shaped gelatinous mass called a *cupula* (Fig. 15-1). The labyrinthine semicircular ducts transduce angular acceleration of the head, and the otoliths transduce linear acceleration, including the effects of gravity.

The central fibers from the cells of the spiral and vestibular ganglia travel in a common trunk, the eighth cranial nerve, which enters the cranial cavity through the internal auditory meatus (accompanied by the facial and intermediate nerves). They traverse the cerebellopontine angle and enter the lateral brainstem at the junction of the pons and medulla. Here the cochlear and vestibular fibers become separated. The cochlear fibers bifurcate and terminate almost at once in the dorsal and ventral cochlear nuclei. The fibers from each cochlear nucleus pursue separate crossing and ascending pathways; they pass to both inferior colliculi (mainly to the opposite side) via the lateral lemnisci. Secondary acoustic fibers project via the trapezoid body and lateral lemniscus to the medial geniculate bodies, a special component of the thalamic sensory system (Fig. 15-2). Some fibers terminate in the trapezoid body and superior olivary complex and sub-serve such reflex functions as auditory attention, sound localization, auditory startle, and oculopostural orientation to sound.

Both excitatory and inhibitory neurons are located at every level of these pathways. At all levels there are

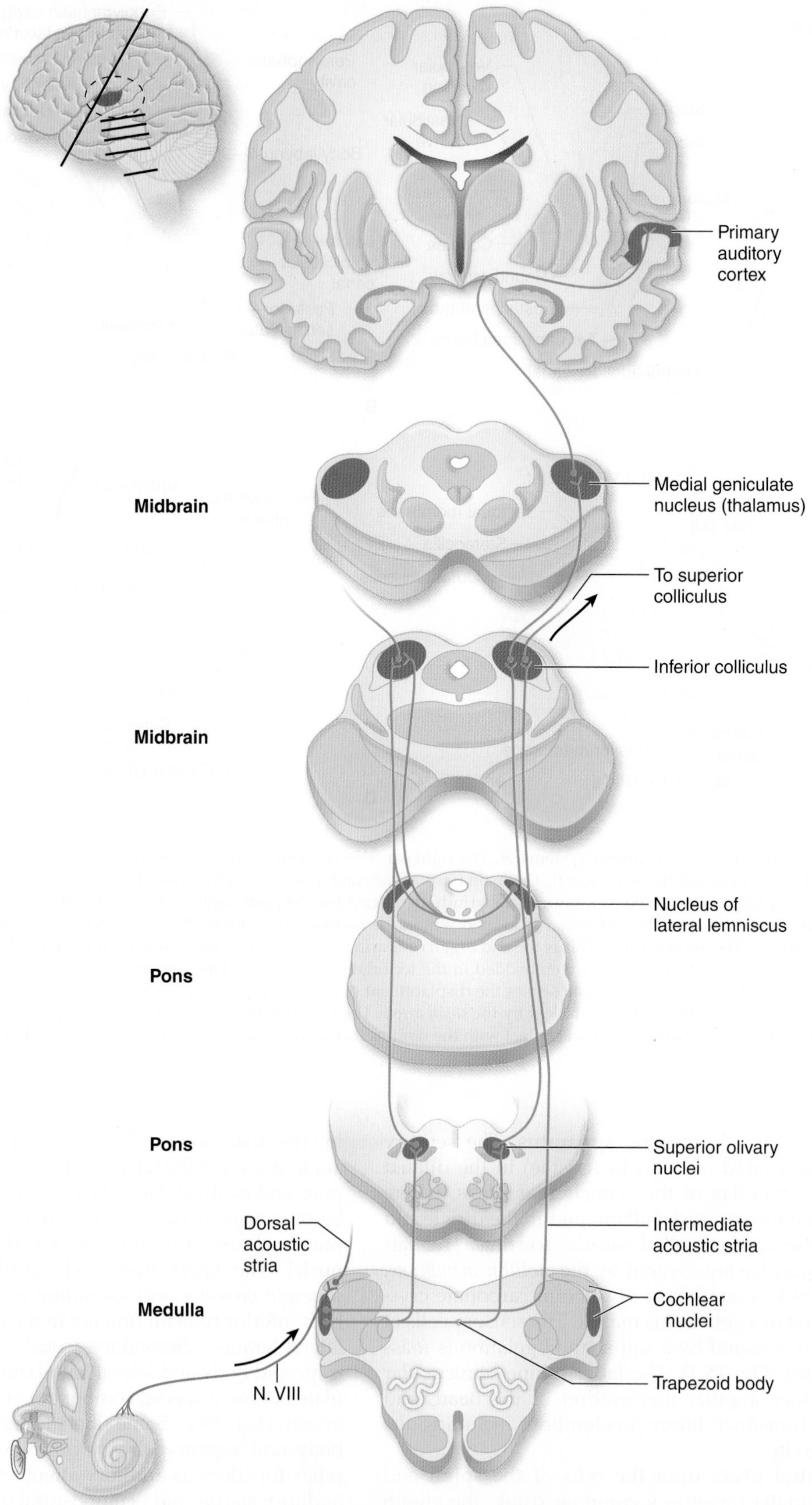

Figure 15-2. The ascending auditory pathways. The lower part of the diagram is a horizontal section through the upper medulla. (Reproduced with permission from Noback CR: *The Human Nervous System*, 3rd ed. New York, McGraw-Hill, 1981.)

strong commissural connections through which auditory signals come to be represented bilaterally in the cerebrum. From the medial geniculate bodies, fibers project to the cortex via the auditory radiations—relatively compact bundles that course ventrolaterally through the posterior parts of the putamen before dispersing and ending in the *transverse gyri of Heschl* and other auditory cortical areas (Tanaka et al).

The auditory cortical field comprises the superior temporal gyrus and the upper bank of the sylvian fissure (Brodmann area 41; see Fig. 22-1), or *primary auditory cortex*, and the surrounding secondary and tertiary cortices in the adjacent temporal lobe. The latter are of particular importance in the interpretation of sound (Celesia) including spoken language. Bilateral temporal lobe lesions involving the geniculocortical fasciculi result in cortical deafness, although such lesions are rare. Unilateral cortical lesions do not affect hearing, but defects in function such as dichotic listening can be detected by specialized tests. At several levels of these ascending fiber systems, there is feedback to lower structures.

The vestibular fibers of the eighth nerve terminate in the four vestibular nuclei: superior (Bechterew), lateral (Deiters), medial (triangular, or Schwalbe), and inferior (spinal, or descending). In addition, some of the fibers from the semicircular canals project directly to the cerebellum via the juxtarestiform body and terminate in the flocculonodular lobe and adjacent vermian cortex (consequently, these structures are called the "vestibulocerebellum," as noted in Chap. 5). Efferent fibers from this portion of the cerebellar cortex, in turn, project ipsilaterally to the vestibular nuclei and to the fastigial nucleus; fibers from the fastigial nucleus project back to the contralateral vestibular nuclei, again via the juxtarestiform body. Thus each side of the cerebellum exerts an influence on the vestibular nuclei of both sides (Fig. 15-3; see also Chap. 5).

The lateral and medial vestibular nuclei also have important connections with the spinal cord, mainly via the uncrossed lateral vestibulospinal tract and the crossed and uncrossed medial vestibulospinal tracts (Fig. 15-4). Presumably, vestibular effects on posture are mediated via these pathways—the axial muscles being acted upon

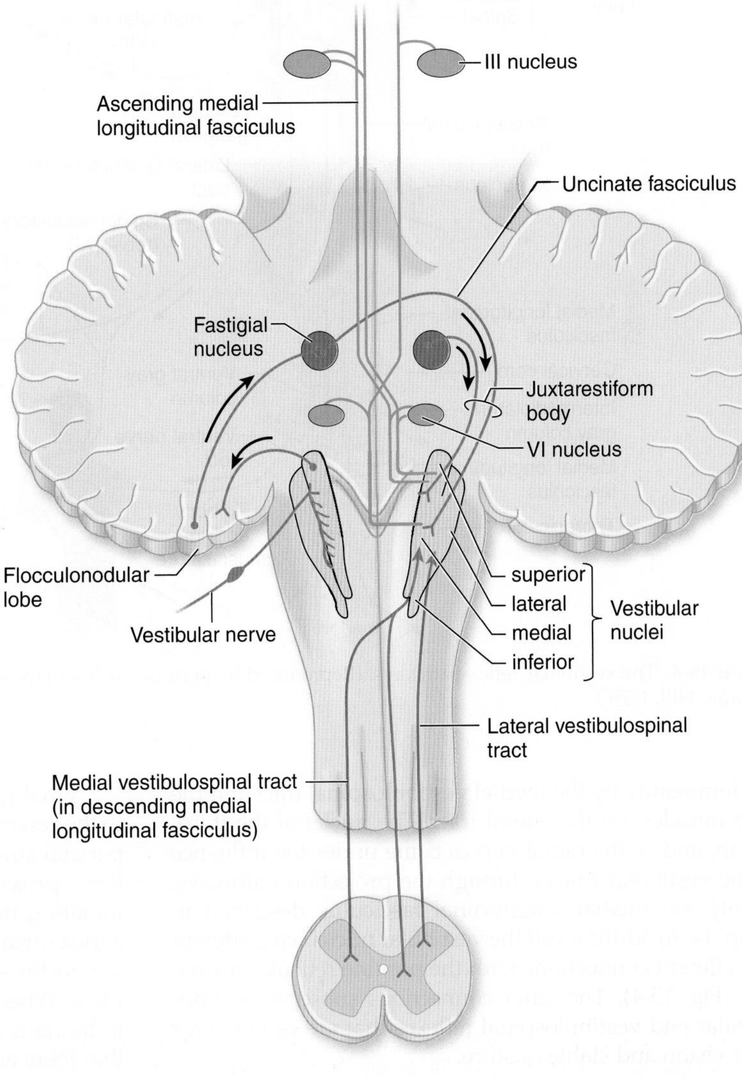

Figure 15-3. A simplified diagram of the vestibulocerebellar and vestibulospinal pathways and connections between vestibular and ocular motor nuclei. The medial longitudinal fasciculi (*blue lines*) are the main pathways for ascending vestibular impulses. (See text and also Fig. 14-1.)

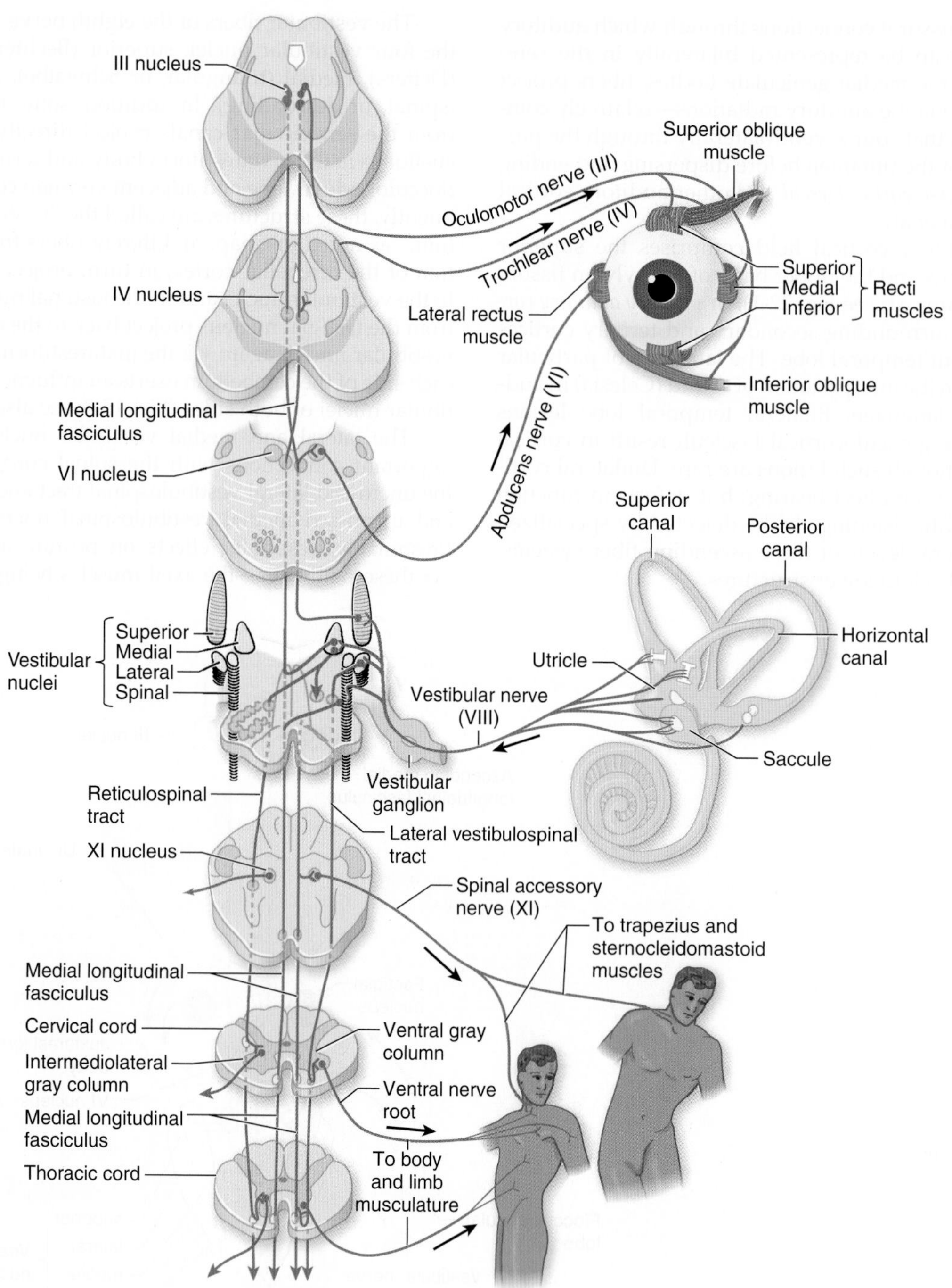

Figure 15-4. The vestibular reflex pathways. (Reproduced by permission from House EL: *A Systematic Approach to Neuroscience*. New York, McGraw-Hill, 1979.)

predominantly by the medial vestibulospinal tract and the limb muscles, by the lateral tract. The nuclei of the third, fourth, and sixth cranial nerves come under the influence of the vestibular nuclei through the projection pathways, mainly the medial longitudinal fasciculus described in Chap. 14. In addition, all the vestibular nuclei have afferent and efferent connections with the pontine reticular formation (Fig. 15-4). The latter connections subserve vestibuloocular and vestibulospinal reflexes that are essential for clear vision and stable posture.

Finally, there are projections from the vestibular nuclei to the cerebral cortex, specifically to the regions of the intraparietal sulcus and superior sylvian gyrus. In the monkey, these projections are almost exclusively contralateral, terminating near the "face area" of the first somatosensory cortex (area 2 of Brodmann). Lesions in the posterior insula impair the sense of verticality, body orientation, and movement. Whether the vestibular nuclei project to the thalamus in humans is not entirely settled; most anatomists indicate that there are no such direct connections.

These brief remarks convey some notion of the complexity of the anatomic and functional organization of the vestibular system (for a full discussion, see the monographs of Brodal and of Baloh and Honrubia). In view of the proximity of cochlear and vestibular elements, it is understandable that acoustic and vestibular functions are often affected together in the course of disease although each may also be affected separately.

DEAFNESS, TINNITUS, AND OTHER DISORDERS OF AUDITORY PERCEPTION

Deafness

Figures from a National Health Survey (National Institute on Deafness and Other Communication Disorders) indicated that approximately 28 million Americans of all ages had a significant degree of deafness and that 2 million were profoundly deaf. More than one-third of persons older than age 75 years were handicapped to some extent by hearing loss.

Deafness is of three general types: (1) *conductive deafness*, caused by a defect in the mechanism by which sound is transformed (amplified) and conducted to the cochlea. These are disorders of the external or middle ear—obstruction of the external auditory canal by atresia or cerumen, thickening of the tympanic membrane from infection or trauma, chronic otitis media, otosclerosis (the main cause of deafness in early adult life), and obstruction of the eustachian tube. (2) *Sensorineural deafness* (also called, imprecisely, *nerve deafness*), which is caused by disease of the cochlea or of the cochlear division of the eighth cranial nerve. Although cochlear and eighth nerve causes of deafness have conventionally been combined in one (sensorineural) category, the neurologist recognizes that the symptoms and causes of the two are quite different and that it is more practical to think of them as cochlear (end organ) and retrocochlear (nerve) deafness. (3) *Central deafness*, caused by lesions of the cochlear nuclei and their connections with the primary auditory receptive areas in the temporal lobes. For example, complete tone deafness, which is probably inherited as an autosomal dominant trait, is a central disorder.

The two peripheral forms of deafness—conductive and sensorineural deafness—must be distinguished from each other, because important remedial measures are available, particularly for the former. In differentiating them, the tuning-fork tests are often of value. When a vibrating fork, preferably of 512-Hz frequency, is held about 2.5 cm from the ear (test for air conduction), sound waves can be appreciated only as they are transmitted through the middle ear; they will be reduced with disease in this location. When the vibrating fork is applied to the skull (test for bone conduction), the sound waves are conveyed directly to the cochlea, without intervention of the sound-transmission apparatus of the middle ear, and will therefore not be reduced or lost in outer or middle ear disease. Normally air conduction is better than bone conduction, and the sound transmitted though the air is appreciated for about twice as long as that passing through the bone.

These principles form the basis for several simple tests of auditory function. In the *Weber test*, the vibrating fork is applied to the forehead in the midline (or to a central incisor). A normal person hears the bone-conducted sound equally in both ears. In nerve deafness, the sound is localized to the normal ear for the reasons noted above; in conductive deafness, the sound is perceived as louder in the affected ear because interference from ambient sounds is muted on the affected side. In the *Rinne test*, the fork is applied to the mastoid process. At the moment the patient indicates that the sound ceases, the fork is held at the auditory meatus. In middle ear deafness, the sound cannot be heard by air conduction after bone conduction has ceased (abnormal Rinne test). In nerve deafness, the reverse may be true (normal Rinne test), but more saliently, both air and bone conduction are quantitatively decreased. The *Schwabach test* consists of comparing the patient's bone conduction with that of the normal examiner.

In general, early sensorineural deafness is characterized by a partial loss of perception of high-pitched sounds and conductive deafness by a partial loss of low-pitched sounds. This can be ascertained by the use of tuning forks of different frequencies but most accurately by the use of an audiometer and the construction of an audiogram, which reveals the entire range of hearing at a glance. The audiogram is the one essential test in the evaluation of hearing loss and the point of departure for subsequent diagnostic evaluation. A ticking watch (infrequently found on doctor's wrists or pockets any longer) or rubbing the patient's hair together near the ear can be used as a surrogate test of gross hearing for the bedside, but these maneuvers emit mostly high-frequency noise and will not detect low-frequency conductive loss.

A cochlear type of hearing loss can be recognized by the presence of the symptoms of recruitment and diplacusis. *Recruitment* refers to a heightened perception of loudness once the threshold for hearing has been exceeded; thus the patient's retort "You don't have to shout" when the examiner raises his voice (see below). *Diplacusis* refers to a defect in frequency discrimination that is manifest by a lack of clarity of spoken syllables or by the perception that music is out of tune and unpleasant (described by patients as a "mushiness" of sounds).

Because each cochlear nucleus is connected with the cortex of both temporal lobes, hearing is unaffected by unilateral cerebral lesions as already mentioned. Deafness caused by brainstem lesions is observed only rarely, as a massive lesion is required to interrupt both the crossed and uncrossed projections from the cochlear nuclei—so massive, as a rule, that other neurologic abnormalities usually make the testing of hearing impossible.

Special Audiologic Procedures

A number of special tests prove to be helpful in distinguishing cochlear from retrocochlear (nerve) lesions. Although an absolute distinction cannot be made on the basis of any one test, the results taken together (particularly loudness recruitment and threshold tone decay) make it possible to predict the site of the lesion with considerable accuracy. These tests, usually carried out by an otologist or audiologist, include the following:

1. *Loudness recruitment.* This phenomenon, mentioned above, is thought to depend on the selective destruction of low-intensity elements subserved by the external hair cells of the organ of Corti. The high-intensity elements are preserved, so that loudness is appreciated only at high intensities. In testing for loudness recruitment, the difference in hearing between the two ears is estimated and the loudness of the pure-tone stimulus of a given frequency delivered to each ear is then increased by regular increments. In *nonrecruiting deafness* (characteristic of a nerve lesion), the original difference in hearing persists in all comparisons of loudness, since both high- and low-intensity fibers are affected. In *recruiting deafness* (which occurs with a lesion in the organ of Corti—e.g., Ménière disease), the more affected ear gains in loudness and may finally be equal to the better one. In bilateral disease, recruitment is assessed by the intensity of the stimulus that causes discomfort, about 100 dB (decibels) in normal persons.
2. *Speech discrimination.* This consists of presenting the patient with a list of 50 phonetically balanced monosyllabic words (e.g., *thin, sin*) at suprathreshold levels. The speech-discrimination score is the percentage of the 50 words correctly repeated by the patient. Marked reduction (less than 30 percent) in the speech-discrimination scores is characteristic of eighth nerve (retrocochlear) lesions.
3. *Audiometry.* Continuous and interrupted tones are presented at various frequencies. Tracings are made, measuring the increments by which the patient must increase the volume in order to continue to hear the continuous and interrupted tones just above threshold. Clinically, analysis has shown that there are four basic configurations, referred to as types I to IV Békésy audiograms. Type III or IV usually indicate the presence of a retrocochlear lesion, the type II response points to a lesion of the cochlea itself, and type I is considered normal. Related tests, such as threshold tone decay and the short increment sensitivity index, were formerly used to a greater extent than they are currently; therefore, we have not described them here.
4. *Brainstem auditory evoked potentials, or response, See Chap. 2* (BAEP, or BAER). This method provides very refined information as to the integrity of primary and secondary auditory pathways from the cochlea to the superior colliculus. It has the advantage of being accurate in uncooperative and even comatose patients as well as infants who cannot cooperate with audiometry. It is of some value in detecting small acoustic and vestibular schwannomas; in localizing brainstem lesions such as those caused by demyelination; in corroborating the state of brain death, in which all waves, except occasionally the eighth nerve (wave I), responses are abolished; and in assessing sensorineural damage in neonates who have had meningitis or been exposed to ototoxic medications.
5. The *acoustic-stapedial reflex* can be used as a measure of conduction in the auditory (and the facial) nerve. This reflex normally protects the cochleas from excessively loud sound. When sound of intensity greater than 70 to 90 dB above threshold hearing reaches the inner ear, the stapedius muscles on both sides contract reflexively, relaxing the tympanum and offering impedance to further sound. It may be tested by insufflating the external auditory canal with pressured air and measuring the change in pressure that follows immediately after a loud sound. The response is muted in patients with conductive hearing loss because of the mechanical restriction of ossicular movement, but otherwise the test is sensitive to cochlear and acoustic nerve lesions.

Tinnitus

This is the other major manifestation of cochlear and auditory disease. Tinnitus aurium literally means "ringing of the ears" (Latin tinnire, "to ring or jingle") and refers to sounds originating in the ear, although they need not be ringing in character. Buzzing, humming, whistling, roaring, hissing, clicking, chirping, or pulse-like sounds are also reported. Some otologists use the term tinnitus cerebri to distinguish other head noises from those that arise in the ear, but the term tinnitus when used without qualification refers to tinnitus aurium.

Tinnitus is a remarkably common symptom, affecting more than 37 million Americans, according to Marion and Cevette. It may be defined as any sensation of sound for which there is no source outside the individual. Two basic types are recognized, *tonal* and *nontonal* (nonvibratory and vibratory, in the terminology of Fowler). The tonal type is by far the more common and is what is meant when the unqualified term *tinnitus* is used. It is also called *subjective tinnitus*, because it can be heard only by the patient. The nontonal form is sometimes *objective*, in the sense that under certain conditions the tinnitus can be heard by the examiner as well as by the patient. In either case, whether tinnitus is produced in the inner ear or in some other part of the head and neck, sensory auditory neurons must be stimulated, for only the auditory neural pathways can transmit an impulse that will be perceived as sound.

According to a large survey conducted by Stouffer and Tyler, about one-third of patients report that persistent tinnitus is unilateral; the others experience it bilaterally or with a lateralized predominance. Many more patients have brief episodes of tinnitus and are concerned enough to bring the symptom to the attention of a physician; some are produced by loud noises or by the ingestion of common drugs, such as aspirin but most such cases are transient and innocuous.

Nontonal and Pulsatile Tinnitus

These head noises are mechanical in origin and are conducted to the inner ear through the various hard or soft structures or the fluid or gaseous media of the body.

They are not caused by a primary dysfunction of the auditory neural mechanism but have their origin in the contraction of muscles of the eustachian tube, middle ear (stapedius, tensor tympani), palate (palatal myoclonus), or pharynx (muscles of deglutition), or in vascular structures near the ear. One of the common forms of subjective tinnitus is a self-audible bruit, the source of which is the turbulent flow of blood in the large vessels of the neck or in an arteriovenous malformation or glomus jugulare tumor. The sound is pulsatile and appreciated by the patient as emanating from one side of the cranium, but it is only sometimes detectable by the examiner.

Other noteworthy causes of pulsatile tinnitus are pseudotumor cerebri or raised intracranial pressure of any type, in which the noise is attributed to a pressure gradient between the cranial and cervical venous structures and the resulting venous turbulence; thyroid enlargement with increased venous blood flow. Other causes include intracranial aneurysm; aortic stenosis; and vascular tumors of the skull, such as histiocytosis X. In the case of a vascular tumor or a large arteriovenous malformation, the examiner may hear the bruit over the mastoid process. Obliteration of the sound by gentle compression of the jugular vein on the symptomatic side is a useful indicator of a venous origin. It has been suggested that diseases that raise the cardiac output markedly (such as severe anemia) may cause pulsatile tinnitus. A flow-related carotid bruit—originating from fibromuscular dysplasia, atherosclerotic stenosis, carotid dissection, and enhanced blood flow in a vessel contralateral to a carotid occlusion—has also been incriminated. However, carotid artery stenosis is infrequently causes a self-audible bruit. The same holds for diseases of the vertebral artery. In 100 consecutive cases of pulsatile tinnitus collected by Sismanis and Smoker, the most common causes were intracranial hypertension, glomus tumors, and carotid disease. One must be cautious in overinterpreting this symptom, because normal persons can hear their pulse when lying with one ear on a pillow, and introspective individuals may become excessively worried about it. We have suggested that normal variations in the size and location of the jugular bulb may explain some benign cases (Adler and Ropper).

Another type of tinnitus is the rhythmic clicking of palatal myoclonus caused by intermittent contraction of the tensor tympani or stapedius muscles, termed *middle ear myoclonus* as discussed in Chap. 6 with other forms of tremor. This process has been treated with a variety of medications, including diazepam or, in extremely annoying cases, by section of the offending muscles (Badia et al). Clicking noises caused by palatal myoclonus have also been successfully treated by the injection of botulinum toxin into the soft palatal tissues (Jamieson et al).

Tonal Tinnitus

This is the common persistent form of tinnitus that arises in the middle or inner ear and is associated in a proportion of patients with cochlear damage. For this reason, the first step in analysis after the clinical examination is an audiogram. Under ideal acoustic circumstances (in a soundproof room having an ambient noise level of 18 dB or less), slight tinnitus is present in 80 to 90 percent of adults ("physiologic tinnitus"). The ambient noise level in ordinary living conditions usually exceeds 35 dB and is of sufficient intensity to mask physiologic tinnitus. Tinnitus because of disease of the middle ear and auditory neural mechanisms may also be masked by environmental noise and hence becomes troublesome only in quiet surroundings—at night, in the country, etc.

Most often, subjective tinnitus signifies a disorder of the tympanic membrane, ossicles of the middle ear, inner ear, or eighth nerve. As already remarked, a majority of patients who complain of persistent tinnitus have some degree of deafness as well. Tinnitus that is localized to one ear and is described as having a tonal character (such as a ringing, bell-like, or like a high and steady musical tone) is particularly likely to be associated with impairment of cochlear or neural function. Tinnitus associated with sensorineural hearing loss of high frequency is often described as "chirping," and that of low frequency as "whooshing" or blowing (Marion and Cevette). Tinnitus as a result of middle ear disease (e.g., otosclerosis) tends to be more constant than the tinnitus of sensorineural disorders; it is of variable intensity and lower pitch and is characterized by clicks, pops, and rushing sounds.

As remarked above, the pitch of tinnitus associated with a conductive hearing loss is generally of low frequency (median frequency of 490 Hz, with a range of 90 to 1,450 Hz). That which accompanies sensorineural loss is higher (median frequency of 3,900 Hz, with a range of 545 to 7,500 Hz). This rule does not apply to Ménière disease, in which the tinnitus is usually described as a low-pitched whoosh, buzz, or roar (median frequency of 320 Hz, with a range of 90 to 900 Hz), thus resembling the tinnitus that accompanies a conductive rather than a sensorineural hearing loss (Nodar and Graham). The tinnitus of Ménière disease often fluctuates in intensity, like the hearing loss.

The mechanism of tonal tinnitus has not been established although a number of theories have been postulated. One supposition attributes tinnitus to an overactivity or disinhibition of hair cells adjacent to a part of the cochlea that has been injured. Another postulates a decoupling of hair cells from the tectorial membrane. Yet a third theory is based on the finding of an abnormal discharge pattern of afferent neurons, attributed to ephaptic transmission between nerve fibers that have been damaged by vascular compression (Møller).

Treatment

Relief of unilateral tinnitus in certain selected cases has reportedly been achieved by vascular decompression of the eighth nerve in a manner comparable to hemifacial spasm, superior oblique myokymia, and some cases of trigeminal neuralgia (Jannetta). However, for most forms of tinnitus, there is little effective treatment (see the review by Lockwood et al). Many patients become reconciled to its presence once the benign nature of the disorder is explained to them. It is possible to fit some patients with a special audiologic instrument, like a hearing aid, that masks the tinnitus by delivering a sound of like pitch and intensity. Patients who are likely to benefit can be identified during the audiogram by noting improvement in tinnitus with the application of superimposed tones. Also, a hearing aid that improves audition may suppress or diminish tinnitus. Antiepileptic drugs and tocainide hydrochloride have been suggested as treatments, but have not been helpful in our experience. Some success in reducing the symptom has been achieved with small doses of amitriptyline at night. In extreme circumstances some groups have experimented with implanted stimulators on the temporal cortex.

If bilateral tinnitus is the basis of persistent complaints, one often discovers that the patient is anxious or depressed, in which case a careful history will reveal the other features of these disorders. Treatment then must be directed to the psychiatric symptoms. In their review, Lockwood and colleagues suggest that all patients with undifferentiated tinnitus be protected from loud sounds and ototoxic drugs (the main ones being aminoglycoside antibiotics, certain loop diuretics, neurotoxic chemotherapies such as cisplatin, and perhaps high doses of aspirin). The American Tinnitus Association website may be helpful to some patients as a source of reassurance (*http://www.ata.org*).

Tinnitus that is unilateral, pulsatile, or fluctuating and associated with vertigo should be investigated by appropriate neurologic and audiologic studies.

Other Disorders of Auditory Perception

On occasion, pontine lesions may be accompanied by complex auditory illusions, sometimes with the qualities of true hallucinations (pontine auditory hallucinosis) as in the patients, one of whom was ours, described by Cascino and Adams. These consist of alternating musical tones, like those of an organ; a jumble of sound, like a symphony orchestra tuning up; or siren-like or buzzing sounds, like a swarm of bees. These auditory sense disturbances are more complex than neurosensory tinnitus but less formed than temporal lobe hallucinations. They are usually associated with impairment of hearing in one or both ears and other neurologic signs related to the pontine lesion. An unpleasant degree of hyperacusis in the contralateral ear has also been reported with upper pontine tegmental lesions. BAEPs reveal intact cochlear, auditory nerve, and cochlear nuclear responses. As in the case of peduncular visual hallucinosis, patients realize that the sounds are unreal, i.e., they have insight into their illusory nature.

Another well-recognized but inexplicable type of auditory hallucinosis occurs in elderly patients with long-standing neurosensory deafness. All day long, or for several hours at a time, they hear songs, symphonies, choral music, or familiar or unfamiliar melodies interrupted only by other ambient noise, sleep, or conversations that engage their attention. The "choice" of music has been referable, not surprisingly, to the individual's earlier life. Our patients, like those reported by Hammeke and colleagues, have been neither depressed nor demented, and antiepileptic and neuroleptic drugs have had no effect. Activation of the right auditory cortex on single-photon emission tomography (SPECT) and magnetoencephalography has been reported in such a case by Kasai and colleagues. The problem may be analogous to the one of Charles Bonnet syndrome, in which elderly individuals with failing vision experience rich visual hallucinations. We find it puzzling that pontine lesions are implicated in some cases, as mentioned above.

Complex auditory hallucinations may occur as part of temporal lobe seizures arising from a variety of temporal lobe lesions. Conversely, seizures may be induced by musical sounds as well as by other auditory stimuli. These topics are discussed in Chaps. 16 and 22. Paracusis, a condition in which a sound, tune, or a voice is repeated for several seconds, is also a cerebral auditory phenomenon, similar in a sense to the visual phenomenon of palinopsia. The precise anatomy is unknown. The auditory hallucinations of schizophrenia have been extensively studied in relation to activity of the temporal lobes, as discussed in Chap. 53.

Middle Ear Deafness

The common causes are otosclerosis, otitis media, and trauma. Of the various types of progressive conductive deafness, otosclerosis is the most frequent, being the cause of about half the cases of bilateral (but not necessarily symmetrical) deafness that have their onset in early adult life, usually in the second or third decade. A predilection to otosclerosis is transmitted as an autosomal dominant trait with variable penetrance. Pathologically, it is characterized by an overgrowth of labyrinthine capsular bone around the oval window, leading to progressive fixation of the stapes. The remarkable advances in microotologic surgery designed to mobilize or replace the stapes and to reconstruct the ossicular chain, have greatly altered the prognosis in this disease; significant improvement in hearing can now be achieved in the majority of patients.

The use of antibiotic drugs has markedly reduced the incidence of purulent otitis media, both the acute and chronic forms, which in former years were common causes of conductive hearing loss in children. Repeated attacks of serous otitis media are, however, still an important cause of this type of deafness.

Fractures of the temporal bone, particularly those in the long axis of the petrous pyramid, may damage middle ear structures; frequently there is bleeding into the middle ear as well, and a ruptured tympanic membrane. Transverse fractures through the petrous pyramid are more likely to damage both the cochlear–labyrinthine structures and the facial nerve. Other diseases of the temporal bone—such as Paget disease, fibrous dysplasia, and osteopetrosis—may impair hearing by compression of the cochlear nerve. It should be noted that rupture of the tympanic membrane, as for example from blast injury does not cause much hearing loss; in the case of a blast, the cause of reduced hearing is cochlear damage.

Sensorineural Deafness

This has many causes. The common high-frequency sensorineural type of hearing loss in the aged (presbycusis) is probably a result of neuronal degeneration, i.e., progressive loss of spiral ganglion neurons (Suga and Lindsay). Explosions or intense, sustained noise in certain industrial settings or from gun blasts or even rock music may result in a high-tone sensorineural hearing loss from cochlear damage. Certain antimicrobial drugs (namely, the aminoglycoside group and vancomycin) damage cochlear hair cells and, after prolonged use, can result in severe hearing loss. If these drugs have been used to treat bacterial meningitis, it may be difficult to determine whether the antibiotic or the infection is the cause. A variety of other commonly used drugs are ototoxic, including certain neurotoxic cancer chemotherapies, especially platinum containing drugs, usually in a dose-dependent fashion (see Nadol). Quinine and acetylsalicylic acid may impair sensorineural function transiently.

The cochlea of a neonate may have been damaged in utero by rubella in the pregnant mother. Mumps, acute purulent meningitis (particularly from *Pneumococcus* and *Haemophilus*), or chronic infection spreading from the middle to the inner ear may cause nerve deafness in childhood. The meningeal infection spreads along the cochlear aqueduct, a structure that connects the cerebrospinal fluid (CSF) space with the perilymph of the cochlea. Measles vaccination, *Mycoplasma pneumoniae* infection, and scarlet fever have been associated with acute deafness, with or without vestibular symptoms. It is uncertain whether the deafness in these cases is due to direct infection of the cochlea or represents an autoimmune reaction directed to the inner ear. Also, the inner ear contains melanocytes, and their involvement in Vogt-Koyanagi-Harada disease adds dysacusis, tinnitus, and sensorineural deafness to the usual manifestations of vitiligo of the eyebrows, poliosis (depigmented forelock of hair), iritis, retinal depigmentation, and recurrent meningitis. Meningeal hemosiderosis, a rare process that results from repeated bouts of subarachnoid hemorrhage, also causes eighth nerve damage and deafness, presumably as a toxic effect of iron deposition in the meninges adjacent to the nerve. Cases of acute sensorineural hearing loss or reduced acuity have occurred following CSF drainage or lumbar puncture, likely either the result of traction on the cochlear nerve due to pressure gradients, or endolymphatic hydrops (see further on) through a patent cochlear aqueduct. Most cases are transient.

Episodic deafness in one ear, even without vertigo, proves in most instances to be the result of *Ménière disease* (see further on).

Otologists have described a progressive sensorineural type of hearing loss as a late manifestation of congenital syphilis, sometimes occurring despite prior treatment with adequate doses of penicillin. It has been claimed that the long-term administration of steroids may be useful in such cases. The pathologic basis of the hearing loss has not been determined and the causal relationship to congenital syphilis remains to be established.

The *auditory* nerve may be involved by tumors of the cerebellopontine angle or by mycotic, lymphomatous, carcinomatous, tuberculous, Listeria, melioidosis, or other types of chronic meningitis and rarely, in sarcoidosis. Lymphomatous meningitis has a particular predilection to cause unilateral hearing loss; we have seen several such cases in which no other cranial nerves were infiltrated. Carcinomatous meningitis may do the same but almost always in the context of other cranial and spinal nerve palsies (see Chap. 31). Of the solid tumors, the ones that involve the auditory nerve most frequently are schwannomas, neurofibromas, meningiomas, dermoids, and metastatic carcinoma. In neurofibromatosis type II, the involvement by vestibular and acoustic schwannomas is typically bilateral as discussed in Chap. 37. Unilateral deafness may also result from demyelinative plaques, infarction, or tumor involving the cochlear nerve fibers or nuclei in the brainstem. Rarely, deafness is the result of bilateral lesions of the temporal lobes (Chap. 22). The condition called *pure word deafness*, a type of aphasia, is also caused by left temporal lobe disease; despite normal pure-tone perception and audiometry and normal brainstem auditory evoked potentials, spoken words cannot be understood. This condition is discussed in Chap. 23.

Sudden idiopathic hearing loss

Of equal concern to neurologists is the onset in an adult of sudden and permanent unilateral hearing loss without vertigo and lacking all the other features of Ménière disease. Little is known about the pathogenesis of this (idiopathic) syndrome. A vascular causation (occlusion of the cochlear artery or presumed arterial spasm in the course of migraine) has been postulated, on uncertain grounds. We do not know how to interpret the findings of DeFelice and colleagues as well as others, who report that the posterior communicating arteries are absent in a disproportionate number of patients with sudden hearing loss. A few cases are due to complicated herpes zoster and mumps parotitis, but aside from these there is no proven relationship to the usual viral respiratory infections. An immune-mediated cause may also be operative in some patients, a hypothesis that has led some neurologists and otologists to treat such patients with a brief course of orally administered corticosteroids. In a prospective report of the natural history of 88 cases of acute sensorineural hearing loss, two-thirds recovered their hearing completely within a few days or a week or two (Mattox and Simmons). In the remaining patients, recovery was much slower and often incomplete; in this latter group, the hearing loss was predominantly for high tones and in some cases was associated with varying degrees of vertigo and hypoactive caloric responses.

The same problem has been reported to follow cardiopulmonary bypass surgery and has been ascribed, without confirmation, to microemboli. Less often, such an event follows general anesthesia for nonotologic surgery (Evan et al); the pathogenesis is obscure. None of the currently popular therapeutic agents—such as histamine, calcium channel blockers, anticoagulants, inhalation of carbogen (30 percent carbon dioxide), and corticosteroids—seems to clearly affect the outcome of sudden unilateral or bilateral deafness without vertigo. Nonetheless, as mentioned, corticosteroids are often prescribed, based on the uncertain theory that this illness is analogous to an immune form of vestibular neuritis.

Hereditary Deafness (Table 15-1)

A large number of *genetically determined syndromes* that feature a neural or conductive type of deafness—some

Table 15-1

REPRESENTATIVE GENETIC FORMS OF HEARING LOSS

DESIGNATION	INHERITANCE	GENE DEFECT	TYPE OF HEARING LOSS	ASSOCIATED DEFECTS	FREQUENCY
I. Nonsyndromic					
DFN A	AD	GJB2 (connexin), MYO7, USH, SLC26A4, and allelic variants of these genes; GJB2 accounts for half of cases in most populations (AD)	Progressive sensorineural	Same loci as cause syndromic hearing loss such as Usher and Pendred syndromes, as noted below; 80% of hereditary deafness from recessive gene	Accounts for half of nonsyndromic recessive deafness (connexin)
DFN B	AR (most common)	—	—	—	—
DFN X	X-linked	—	—	—	—
Familial otosclerosis	AD with reduced penetrance	COLIA1	Conductive	—	—
II. Syndromic					
Waardenburg	AD	PAX3 and some due to SOX, WSIV (transcription factors)	Variable sensorineural	Dystopic canthi, heterochromia, iritis, poliosis	Most common dominant syndromic hearing loss; accounts for 3% of childhood hearing loss
Type I	—		—		
Type II	—	—	—	Same as type I but no dystopia	—
Type III	—	—	—	Upper limb defects	—
Type IV	—	EDN (receptors in endothelin pathways)	—	Pigmentary defects and Hirschsprung disease	—
Branchio-oto-renal syndrome	AD	EYA1 in half (transcription factor involved in development of inner ear and kidney)	Conductive (75%), sensorineural and mixed	Second most common dominant form of hearing loss. Brachial cleft cysts, cleft palate, malformations of external ear and of kidney	2%
Stickler	AD	STL 1–3	Progressive sensorineural hearing loss	Cleft palate, epiphyseal dysplasia; severe myopia and retinal detachment in types 1 and 3	—
Neurofibromatosis type 2	AD	NF 2	Acoustic neuromas	Evident on MRI; proclivity to other tumors	—
Usher	AR	USH genes (unconventional myosin and adhesion molecules)	Severe congenital sensorineural hearing loss, vestibular dysfunction; retinitis pigmentosa	Most common recessive types; retinitis pigmentosa after first decade; type 1 has abnormal vestibular function	3–6%
Type I					
Type II	—	—	Moderate to severe hearing loss, late retinitis	—	—

Type III	—	—	Progressive hearing loss and variable retinitis	—	—
Pendred	AR	SLC13A4 in half (same mutation causes nonsyndromic hearing loss)	Profound congenital sensorineural hearing loss; abnormal bony labyrinth (Mondini dysplasia)	Euthyroid goiter	4%
Jervell and Lange-Nielsen	AR	KVQT, KCNE (delayed potassium rectifier inner ear)	Congenital deafness	Prolonged QT interval on ECG; syncope, sudden death	<1%
Refsum	AR	—	Progressive sensorineural deafness	Retinitis pigmentosa, sensory polyneuropathy; elevated phytanic acid	—
Alport	X-linked	X-linked in 85% but also autosomal dominant and recessive forms (basement membrane formation in cochlea, eye, and kidney)	Progressive sensorineural hearing loss	Glomerulonephritis and renal failure	1%
Mohr-Tranebjerg	X-linked	TIMMBA (a translocation protein from cyutopsol to mitochondria)	Progressive childhood deafness	Visual disability, dystonia, mild retardation	—
Kearns-Sayre	Mitochondrial	MTRNT 1at 3243 site and MTTS 1 of mitochondrial genome	Late-onset progressive sensorineural hearing loss	Diabetes, other features typically associated with mitochondrial mutations—see Chap. 37	—
Bartter IV	—	BSND; Cl^- channel	Congenital, severe	Salt wasting	—

AD, autosomal dominant; AR, autosomal recessive.

congenital and others having their onset in childhood or early adult life—have come to light (see articles by Tekin et al and Gorlin et al). The majority of cases of congenital deafness are inherited as an autosomal recessive trait with no other syndromic features. In most of the remainder, inheritance is autosomal dominant in type and in a small number, it is sex linked.

The singular genetic advance in this field has been the identification in recessive nonsyndromic deafness of a mutation of the connexin-26 gene on chromosome 13 (designated GJB2). This mutation is found in half of recessive familial cases of pure deafness; what is more striking is that the same gene abnormality occurs in 37 percent of cases of sporadic congenital deafness, almost certainly from a spontaneous mutation (Estivill et al and Morell et al). The connexin protein is a component of gap junctions and the mutation is theorized to interfere with the recycling of potassium from the cochlear hair cells to the endolymph. As a result of the human genome project, more than 20 other gene loci have been detected that may be related to congenital deafness syndromes; these have been summarized by Tekin and colleagues, but none, except the one for connexin, accounts for more than a very small proportion of cases. These unattached, nonsyndromic types of congenital deafness are denominated by genes in a family called DFN (for DeaFNess); for example, the connexin mutation is in DFNB1. The mutations in this gene can be recessive, dominant or X-linked. The genetic errors involve either cytoskeletal or structural proteins of the organ of Corti or the ion channel apparatus.

It is remarkable that deafness is a component of over 400 more complex different genetic syndromes (e.g., Waardenburg, branchio-oto-renal, Stickler, Pendred, Usher, Alport, Bartter, among many others listed in the table and those omitted because of their rarity). Among these, the finding of a mutation in a gene called PAX3 in the Waardenburg syndrome in the early 1990s began a flood of other gene defects underlying the many disorders that had been described on clinical grounds over the previous century. The mutations that give rise to some of these diseases, particularly the Usher syndrome, may also cause nonsyndromic congenital deafness. The syndromic forms of genetic deafness have been classified largely on the basis of their associated defects: retinitis pigmentosa, malformations of the external ear; integumentary abnormalities such as hyperkeratosis, hyperplasia or scantiness of eyebrows, albinism, large hyperpigmented or hypopigmented areas, ocular abnormalities such as hypertelorism, severe myopia, optic atrophy, and congenital and juvenile cataracts, cerebellar ataxia, myoclonus, and mental deficiency; skeletal abnormalities; and renal, thyroid, or cardiac abnormalities. Deafness is also a feature of several mitochondrial disorders, particularly the Kearns-Sayre syndrome and occasionally the MELAS (mitochondrial myopathy, encephalopathy, lactic acidosis, and stroke-like episodes) syndrome. The Wolfram syndrome, of which sensorineural deafness is a major feature, can have either a nuclear or mitochondrial genetic origin. Table 15-1 summarizes this and the other main hereditary syndromes. Chinnery et al have summarized the mitochondrial causes of deafness. Chapters 37 and 39 discuss further the association of neurosensory deafness with degenerative and developmental neurologic disease.

Differing from the degenerations is a group of acoustic aplasias. Four types of inner ear aplasia have been described: (1) *Michel defect*, a complete absence of the otic capsule and eighth nerve; (2) *Mondini defect*, an incomplete development of the bony and membranous labyrinths and the spiral ganglion; (3) *Scheibe defect*, a membranous cochleosaccular dysplasia with atrophy of the vestibular and cochlear nerves; and (4) rare chromosomal aberrations (trisomies) characterized by abnormality of the end organ and absence of the spiral ganglion.

Hysterical Deafness

It is possible to distinguish hysterical and feigned deafness from that caused by structural disease in several ways. In the case of bilateral deafness, the distinction can be made by observing a blink (cochleo-orbicular reflex) or an alteration in skin sweating (psychogalvanic skin reflex) in response to loud sound. Unilateral hysterical deafness may be detected by an audiometer, with both ears connected, or by whispering into the bell of a stethoscope attached to the patient's ears, closing first one and then the other tube without the patient's knowledge. The elicitation of the first two waves of the brainstem auditory evoked potentials provides indisputable evidence that sounds are reaching the receptive auditory structures and that the patient should be capable of hearing sounds. A brief episode of deafness with fully preserved consciousness may rarely be caused by seizure activity in one temporal lobe (epileptic suppression of hearing).

DIZZINESS AND VERTIGO

Dizziness and other sensations of imbalance are, along with headache, back pain, and fatigue, among the most frequent complaints in medicine (Kroenke and Mangelsdorff). The significance of these complaints varies greatly. For the most part they are benign, but there is always the possibility that they signal an important neurologic disorder. Diagnosis of the underlying disease demands that the complaint of dizziness be analyzed correctly—the nature of the disturbance of function being determined first and then its anatomic localization. This approach to neurologic diagnosis is invaluable in the patient whose main complaint is dizziness.

The term *dizziness* is applied by the patient to a number of different sensory and psychic experiences—a feeling of rotation or whirling as well as nonrotatory swaying, weakness, faintness, light-headedness, or unsteadiness. Blurring of vision, feelings of unreality, syncope, and even petit mal or other seizure phenomena may be called "dizzy spells." These experiences fall into four categories: (1) vertigo, a physical sensation of motion of self or the environment; (2) near syncope, a sensation of faintness; (3) disequilibrium, a disorder of imbalance of stance or gait; and (4) ill-defined light-headedness, or "giddiness," a symptom that often accompanies anxiety. Hence, close questioning of the patient as to how he is using the term *dizziness* is a necessary first step in clinical work.

Physiologic Considerations

Several mechanisms are responsible for the maintenance of a balanced posture and for awareness of the position of the body in relation to its surroundings and to gravity. Continuous afferent impulses from the eyes, labyrinths, muscles, and joints inform us of the position of different parts of the body. In response to these impulses, the adaptive movements necessary to maintain equilibrium are carried out. Normally, we are unaware of these adjustments because they operate largely at a reflex level. The most important of the afferent impulses are the following.

1. *Visual information* from the retinae and possibly proprioceptive impulses from the ocular muscles, enable us to judge the distance of objects from the body. This information is coordinated with sensory information from the labyrinths and neck (see below) to stabilize gaze during movements of the head and body.
2. *Impulses from the labyrinths,* which function as highly specialized spatial proprioceptors and register changes in the velocity of motion (either acceleration or deceleration) and position of the body in relation to the gravitational vertical. The cristae of the three semicircular canals sense angular acceleration of the head in the three planes of roll, pitch and yaw, and the maculae of the saccule and utricle sense linear acceleration and gravitational pull. In each of these structures, displacement of sensory hair cells is the effective stimulus. In the semicircular ducts, this is accomplished by movement of the endolymphatic fluid, which, in turn, is induced by rotation of the head. In the utricle and saccule, the hairs are displaced by the movement of the otoliths in response to gravity, thus generating a force that displaces the otoliths. This end organ is a force transducer that converts the generated force into neural impulses that are conducted down the vestibular nerve to the vestibular nuclei. In either case (angular and linear acceleration), the force causes depolarization of the nerve terminals and initiation of impulses in the vestibular nerve, with the production of two main reflex responses: the vestibuloocular, which stabilizes the eyes, and the vestibulospinal, which stabilizes the position of the head and body.
3. *Impulses from the proprioceptors* of the joints and muscles are essential to all reflex, postural, and volitional movements. Those from the neck are of special importance in relating the position of the head to the rest of the body. The sense organs listed above are connected with the cerebellum and pathways in the brainstem, particularly the vestibular nuclei and, via the medial longitudinal fasciculi, with the ocular motor nuclei. These cerebellar and brainstem structures are the important coordinators of the sensory data and provide for postural adjustments and the maintenance of equilibrium. They are the basis of the mechanisms whereby the perceptions of one's self (the body schema) and one's surroundings (the environmental schema) are matched. Accordingly, any disease that disrupts these neural mechanisms may give rise to vertigo and disequilibrium. The interdependence of the two schemata (self and environment) is ascribed to the fact that the various sense organs—retinal, labyrinthine, and proprioceptive—are usually activated simultaneously by any body movement.

One element of the sense of stable equilibrium derives from the ability to match visual and positional information during motion. Through reflex mechanisms, we come to see objects as stationary, while we are moving (mainly the ocular fixation reflex) and moving objects as having motion when we are either moving or stationary (vestibuloocular reflex). At times, especially when our own sensory information is incomplete, we mistake movement of our surroundings for movements of our own body. A well-known example is the feeling of movement that one experiences in a stationary train when a neighboring train is moving.

A factor that influences equilibrium is the effect of aging on all the afferent structures that subserve stability. The elderly may lose their balance on extending the neck, and their peripheral sensory afferents are often impaired, as are the protective postural mechanisms, making falls more frequent. A destructive lesion of one or both labyrinths may leave an elderly person permanently unbalanced, whereas a younger person largely compensates for the loss.

Clinical Characteristics of Vertigo

A careful history and physical examination usually afford the basis for separating true vertigo from the dizziness caused by near syncope, gait disorder, and anxiety. Any illusion or hallucination of motion in any plane qualifies as vertigo. The recognition of vertigo is usually not difficult when the patient states that objects in the environment have spun around or moved rhythmically in one direction or that a sensation of whirling of the head and body was experienced. A distinction is sometimes drawn between subjective vertigo, meaning a sense of turning of one's body, and objective vertigo, an illusion of movement of the environment, but its significance is limited.

Often, however, the patient is not so explicit and a number of related experiences may be described. The feeling may be described as to-and-fro or up-and-down movement of the body, usually of the head, or the patient may compare the feeling to that imparted by the pitch and roll of a ship. Or the floor or walls may seem to tilt or to sink or rise up. In walking, the patient may have felt unsteady and veered to one side, or may have had a sensation of leaning or being pulled to the ground or to one side or another (pulsion or static tilt), as though being drawn by a strong magnet. This feeling is particularly characteristic of vertigo. Oscillopsia, a rhythmic, jerking, illusory movement of the environment, is another effect of vestibular disorder, especially if induced by movement of the head. Observant patients may actually note this rhythmic movement of the environment due to nystagmus.

Some patients may be able to identify their symptoms only when asked to compare them with the feeling of movement they experience when they come to a halt after rapid rotation. If the patient is unobservant or imprecise in descriptions, a helpful tactic is to provoke a number of dissimilar sensations by rapid rotation, or by asking the patient to stoop for a minute and straighten up; having him stand relaxed for 3 min and checking his blood pressure for orthostatic effect; and, particularly, having him hyperventilate for 3 min. Should the patient be unable to distinguish among these several types of induced dizziness or to ascertain the similarity of one of the types to his own condition, the history is probably too inaccurate for purposes of diagnosis.

When the patient's symptoms are mild or poorly described, small items of the history—a desire to keep still and a disinclination to stoop or walk during an attack, a tendency to list to one side, an aggravation of symptoms by turning over in bed or closing his eyes, a sense of imbalance when making a quick turn on foot or in a car, and a preference for one position of the body or head—help to identify them as vertigo. At the other end of the scale are attacks of such abruptness and severity as to virtually throw the patient to the ground. Independently occurring vertiginous attacks of the usual variety mark these falling episodes as part of Ménière disease (see further on). On the other hand, a dizzy sensation that is not made worse markedly by vigorous shaking of the head is unlikely to relate to vertigo, particularly that type due to peripheral vestibular disease.

All but the mildest forms of vertigo are accompanied by some degree of nausea, vomiting, pallor, perspiration, and some difficulty with walking. The patient may simply be disinclined to walk or may walk unsteadily and veer to one side, or he may be unable to walk at all if the vertigo is intense. Forced to lie down, the patient realizes that one position, usually on one side with eyes closed, reduces the vertigo and nausea, and that the slightest motion of the head aggravates them. One common form of vertigo, benign positional vertigo (see further on), occurs with the repositioning that accompanies lying down, sitting up, turning, or looking upwards. The source of the gait ataxia associated with vertigo (vertiginous ataxia) is recognized by the patient as being "in the head," not in the control of the legs and trunk. It is noteworthy that the coordination of individual movements of the limbs is not impaired in these circumstances—a point of difference from most instances of cerebellar disease. Loss of consciousness as part of a vertiginous attack nearly always signifies another type of disorder (seizure or faint).

Nonvertiginous Types of Dizziness

It is important to distinguish vertigo from the more common complaints for which the term dizziness is used by patients. These include the feeling of impending fainting (near syncope), a disorder of gait (disequilibrium), and an ill-defined feeling of lightheadedness. Many patients in the last category who initially complain of dizziness will, on closer questioning, describe his symptoms as a "distant feeling," "walking on air," "inability to focus," or some other unnatural sensation in the head. These sensory experiences are particularly common in states characterized by anxiety or panic attacks—often, but not always, with depression.

This constellation of nonvertiginous symptoms has been loosely referred to as "phobic," "functional," and "psychogenic" vertigo. Every clinician encounters numerous such patients. In Brandt's (1996) extensive experience, phobic vertigo (his term) was second only to benign positional vertigo (described below) as a cause of consultation in his dizziness clinic. He relates the disorder to anxiety and panic spells, but finds that it exists more often as an independent entity that is subject to improvement after careful explanation and reassurance. We agree with Furman and Jacobs that the term *psychiatric dizziness*, if used at all, should be restricted to dizziness that occurs as part of a recognized psychiatric syndrome, notably extreme anxiety disorder. Often, there is a component of avoidance of crowds, open spaces and tight circumstances. There seems to be little point in signifying the nonvertiginous symptoms with separate designations based on the settings in which they commonly occur ("supermarket syndrome," "motorist disorientation syndrome," "phobic postural vertigo," "street neurosis") but they do emphasize the psychogenic nature and may facilitate recognition of the syndrome. Furman and Jacobs have related anxiety-type dizziness to minor degrees of vestibular dysfunction, but we have not found it possible to determine whether there is a genuine labyrinthine disorder in all of these patients.

Oculomotor disorders, such as ophthalmoplegia with diplopia, may be a source of spatial disorientation and brief sensations of vertigo, mild nausea, and staggering. These symptoms are maximal when the patient looks in the direction of action of the paralyzed muscle; it is attributable to the receipt of two conflicting visual images. Some normal persons may experience such symptoms for brief periods when first adjusting to bifocal glasses.

In a peculiar symptom called the *Tullio phenomenon*, a loud sound, or yawning, produces a brief sensation of vertigo or tilting of the environment. Some patients with this symptom are found to have an absence or thinning of the bony roof of the superior semicircular canal, which can be detected by thin (1 mm) slice CT. This disorder, which is a form of perilymphatic fistula, is caused by a spontaneous or traumatic dehiscence of the bone of the superior canal. Occasionally, patients with Ménière disease report this symptom.

Other causes of dizziness are more difficult for the physician and patient to define. In severe anemic states, particularly pernicious anemia, and in aortic stenosis, easy fatigability and languor may be attended by lightheadedness, related particularly to postural change and exertion. In the emphysematous patient, physical effort may be associated with weakness and peculiar cephalic sensations, and violent paroxysms of coughing may lead to giddiness and even fainting (tussive syncope) because of impaired venous return to the heart. The dizziness that often accompanies acute hypertension is difficult to evaluate; sometimes it is an expression of anxiety, or it may conceivably be the result of an unstable adjustment of cerebral blood flow. It is doubtful that chronic hypertension causes dizziness, although many of the medications for its treatment certainly can cause the symptom.

Postural nonvertiginous dizziness is another state in which inadequate vasomotor reflexes prevent a constant cerebral circulation; it is notably frequent in persons with orthostatic hypotension of any cause, for example, in those taking antihypertensive drugs, as well as in patients with a polyneuropathy that has an autonomic component. Such persons, on rising abruptly from a recumbent or sitting position, experience a swaying type of dizziness, dimming of vision, and spots before the eyes that last for several seconds. The patient is forced to stand still and steady himself by holding onto a nearby object. Occasionally, a syncopal attack may occur at this time (see Chap. 18). Hypoglycemia gives rise to yet another form of dizziness, marked by a sense of hunger and attended by trembling, sweating, and other autonomic symptoms. Drug intoxication—particularly with alcohol, sedatives, and antiepileptic drugs—may induce a nonspecific dizziness and, at advanced stages of intoxication, true vertigo.

In practice, it may nonetheless be difficult to separate these types of dizziness from vertigo, for there may, or may not be, feelings of rotation, impulsion, up-and-down movement, oscillopsia, or other disturbance of motion. The ancillary symptoms of true vertigo—namely, nausea, vomiting, tinnitus and deafness, staggering, and the relief obtained by sitting or lying still—are also absent. Furthermore, it is not an uncommon circumstance to find more than one type of dizziness in an individual who is carefully tested.

The Neurologic and Otologic Causes of Vertigo

The fact that vertigo may constitute the aura of an epileptic seizure supports the view that this symptom may have a cerebrocortical origin. Indeed, electrical stimulation of the cerebral cortex in an unanesthetized patient, either of the posterolateral aspects of the temporal lobe or the inferior parietal lobule adjacent to the sylvian fissure, may evoke intense vertigo. The occurrence of vertigo as the initial symptom of a seizure is, however, infrequent. In such cases, a sensation of movement—either of the body away from the side of the lesion or of the environment in the opposite direction—lasts for a few seconds before being submerged in other seizure activity. Vertiginous epilepsy of this type should be differentiated from vestibulogenic seizures, in which an excessive vestibular discharge serves as the stimulus for a seizure. The latter is a rare form of reflex epilepsy, in which tests that induce vertigo may provoke the seizure (see Chap. 16).

The issue of *migraine* as a cause of vertigo has occasioned much discussion. Several authoritative clinicians attribute many instances of otherwise unexplained dizziness and vertigo to migraine with aura, but it is not entirely clear whether they are referring to an attack of basilar migraine, usually in children (migrainous vertigo), or to episodes of vague disequilibrium or vertigo at various times in migraineurs, which has been more typical in our experience. A survey by Neuhauser and colleagues found that 7 to 9 percent of patients had conventional migrainous symptoms during or before a vertiginous attack, and in half of those the vertigo was regularly associated with migraine. This number is certainly higher than in most practices, but it does support the idea that migraine can cause vertigo as discussed further on.

Lesions of the cerebellum produce vertigo depending on which part of this structure is involved. Large, destructive processes in the cerebellar hemispheres and vermis, such as cerebellar hemorrhage may, or at times may not, cause vertigo. However, strokes in the territory of the medial branch of the posterior inferior cerebellar artery (which arises distal to the branches to the medulla, and therefore does not involve the lateral medulla) causes intense vertigo and vomiting that is *indistinguishable from that caused by labyrinthine disorder*. In two such pathologically studied cases, a large zone of infarction extended to the midline and involved the flocculonodular lobe (Duncan et al). Falling in these cases was toward the side of the lesion; nystagmus was present on gaze to each side but was more prominent on gaze to the side of the infarct. These findings have been confirmed by CT and MRI (Amarenco et al). Early in the course of an acute attack of vertigo, when it may be difficult to assess the gait and the quality of nystagmus, it may be necessary to exclude a cerebellar infarct or hemorrhage by use of imaging procedures.

Labyrinthine disease, on the other hand, causes predominantly unidirectional nystagmus to the side opposite the impaired labyrinth and swaying or falling toward the involved side—i.e., the direction of the nystagmus is opposite to that of the falling and past pointing (the latter referring to overshooting a target by the patient's finger with eyes closed, as originally described by Bárány [1921]). Ataxia and dysarthria are, of course, typical of many forms of cerebellar disease but may be minimal or absent in cerebellar hemorrhage and some infarctions as well as being lacking in all forms of vestibular disease.

The topic of vertigo with fluctuating ischemia in the territory of the basilar and vertebral arteries (transient ischemic attack [TIA]) and the problem of subclavian steal syndrome are discussed further on under "Vertigo of Brainstem Origin" and in Chap. 34. Also common in practice is vertigo caused by the demyelinating lesions of multiple sclerosis, as noted in the later section.

Biemond and DeJong described a kind of nystagmus and vertigo originating in the upper cervical roots and the muscles and ligaments that they innervate (so-called cervical vertigo). Spasm of the cervical muscles, trauma to the neck, and irritation of the upper cervical sensory roots were said to produce asymmetrical spinovestibular stimulation and thus to evoke nystagmus, prolonged vertigo, and disequilibrium. Toole and Tucker demonstrated a reduced flow through these vessels (in cadavers) when the head was rotated or hyperextended. In our view, the existence of "cervical vertigo," or at least these interpretations of it, is open to question. However, we acknowledge having encountered patients with cervical dystonia who describe something akin to vertigo, and this may speak to a relationship between cervical proprioceptors and vertigo.

Causes of vertigo other than Ménière disease that originate in the vestibular nerve are discussed further on.

In summary, for all practical purposes, vertigo indicates a disorder of the vestibular end organs, the vestibular division of the eighth nerve, or the vestibular nuclei in the brainstem and their immediate connections, including the inferior cerebellum. Although lesions of the cerebral cortex, eyes, and perhaps the cervical muscles may give rise to vertigo, they are not common sources of the symptom, and vertigo is rarely the dominant manifestation of disease in these structures. The clinical problem resolves by deciding which portion of the labyrinthine–vestibular apparatus is involved. Usually this determination can be made on the basis of the form of the vertiginous attack, the nature of the ancillary symptoms and signs, and tests of labyrinthine function. These tests are described below, followed by a description of the common labyrinthine–vestibular syndromes.

Tests of Labyrinthine Function

The most rudimentary test of labyrinthine function is simply to have the patient shake his head from side-to-side in an attempt to elicit symptoms that simulate the dizziness that has been described and to observe the degree of postural instability during this maneuver. Falling and marked intensification of the dizziness is almost always an indication of labyrinthine disease. Also, nystagmus may be evoked, indicating a vestibular instability. More informative in identifying a diseased labyrinth is the "rapid head impulse" test, which is conducted by asking the patient to fixate on a target and then for the examiner to rotate the patient's head quickly by 10 degrees (an explanation must be given to encourage the patient to relax the neck muscles and remain focused on the fixation point). The eyes are observed for a slippage from the target; this is most evident by a quick saccadic return to the point of focus. Ocular instability is observed when the patient turns his head toward the side of the affected labyrinth. This use of the vestibuloocular reflex is said by Halmagyi and Crener to be among the most dependable bedside tests of labyrinthine function.

Maneuvers designed to elicit positional vertigo by rapidly changing from a seated to a supine position with the head turned to one side bring about vertigo in a number of conditions but are specifically intended to detect benign positional vertigo and are described further on.

A number of other interesting but less validated tests that bring out instabilities in station and gait may be used to supplement the conventional tests for vestibular dysfunction. The Unterberger maneuver requires the patient to march in place with eyes closed and arms outstretched. Normally, less than 15 degrees or so of rotation is displayed; asymmetry of labyrinthine function is manifest as excessive rotation away from the diseased side. A related test involves having the patient walk around a chair with eyes closed; an increasing or decreasing radius is indicative of an imbalance between the two sides of the labyrinthine apparatus. Both of these tests, however, often show abnormalities with cerebellar disease as well, in which the patient veers to the affected side. The sensitivity of maneuvers such as these has been questioned. We can only comment that they seem in our experience to demonstrate vestibulocerebellar lesions.

Vestibular (labyrinthine) stimulation can also be produced by rotating the patient in a Bárány chair or any type of swivel chair. The patient is asked not to fixate or is defocused with Frenzel lenses during rotation to avoid the effects of optokinetic nystagmus. The normal response is nystagmus in the direction opposite to rotation. In contrast, if the patient is asked to focus on his own thumb in an outstretched arm, there should be no nystagmus if the rotational velocity is slow; the ability to suppress this vestibuloocular response reflects the integrity of the vestibular organ and nerve on the side toward the direction of rotation. Electronystagmography (ENG) provides a more refined method of detecting disordered labyrinthine function because it permits the accurate recording of eye movements without visual fixation. ENG is usually coupled with caloric stimulation or with modern devices for rotational testing that allow precise control of the velocity, acceleration, and extent of rotation beyond what can be done with a traditional chair.

Irrigation of the ear canal alternately with cold and warm water (caloric testing) may be used to disclose a reduction in labyrinthine function in the form of an impairment or loss of thermally induced nystagmus on the involved side. Caloric testing is accomplished by having the patient lay supine on the examining table with the head tilted forward 30 degrees to bring the horizontal semicircular canal into a vertical plane, the position of maximal sensitivity of this canal to thermal stimuli. Each external auditory canal is irrigated for 30 s, first with water at 30°C (86°F) and then at 44°C (111.2°F), with a pause of at least 5 min between each irrigation. In normal persons, cold water induces a slight tonic deviation of the eyes to the side being irrigated, followed, after a latent period of about 20 s, by nystagmus to the opposite side (direction of the fast phase). Warm water induces nystagmus to the irrigated side. (As noted in Chap. 14, this is the basis for the mnemonic COWS: cold opposite, warm same, referring to the direction of fast phase of the nystagmus.) In normal subjects, the nystagmus usually persists for 90 to 120 s, although the range is considerably larger. Nausea and symptoms of excessive reflex vagal activity may occur in sensitive individuals.

Simultaneous irrigation of both canals with cold water causes a tonic downward deviation of the eyes with nystagmus (quick component) upward. Bilateral irrigation with warm water yields a tonic upward movement and nystagmus in the opposite direction ("cold upward, warm down, referring again to the fast phase of nystagmus; "CUWD"). Caloric testing will reliably answer whether the vestibular end organs react, and comparison of the responses from the two ears will indicate which one is paretic. Recording of eye movements during the test allows quantification of these responses.

Galvanic stimulation of the labyrinths is effective but offers no particular advantage over caloric stimulation.

Ménière Disease and Other Forms of Labyrinthine Vertigo

Labyrinthine disorders are the most common causes of true vertigo. Ménière disease is characterized by paroxysmal attacks of vertigo associated with fluctuating tinnitus and deafness. One or the other of the latter two symptoms may be absent during the initial attacks of vertigo, but invariably they assert themselves as the disease progresses and increase in severity during acute attacks. Ménière disease affects the sexes about equally and has its onset most frequently in the fifth decade of life, although it may begin earlier or later. Cases of Ménière disease usually occurs as a sporadic trait, but hereditary forms, both autosomal dominant and recessive, have been described (see reviews by Konigsmark). The main pathologic changes consist of an increase in the volume of endolymph and distention of the endolymphatic system (endolymphatic hydrops). It had been speculated several decades ago that the paroxysmal attacks of vertigo are related to ruptures of the membranous labyrinth and release of potassium-containing endolymph into the perilymph, changes that have a paralyzing effect on vestibular nerve fibers and lead to degeneration of the delicate cochlear hair cells (Friedmann). An immune pathogenesis has also been proposed, based tentatively on the presence of circulating antibodies putatively against heat shock protein in some patients.

In typical Ménière disease, the attacks of vertigo are abrupt and last for several minutes to an hour or longer. The vertigo is unmistakably whirling or rotational and usually so severe that the patient cannot stand or walk. Varying degrees of nausea and vomiting, low-pitched tinnitus, a feeling of fullness in one ear and a diminution in hearing are practically always associated. Nystagmus is present during the acute attack; it is horizontal in type, usually with a rotary component and with the slow phase to the side of the affected ear. On attempting to touch a target with the eyes closed, there is past pointing as well as a tendency to fall toward the affected ear when standing or walking. The patient prefers to lie with the faulty ear uppermost and is disinclined to look toward the normal side, which exaggerates the nystagmus and dizziness. As the attack subsides, hearing improves, as does the sensation of fullness in the ear; with further attacks, however, there is a progressive increase in deafness.

The attacks vary considerably in frequency and severity. They may recur several times weekly for many weeks on end, or there may be remissions of several years' duration. Frequently recurring attacks may give rise to a mild chronic state of disequilibrium and a reluctance to move the head or to turn quickly. With milder forms of the disease, the patient may complain more of head discomfort and of difficulty in concentrating than of vertigo and then may be considered to signify anxiety. Symptoms of anxiety are common in patients with Ménière disease, particularly in those with frequent severe attacks.

A small proportion of patients with Ménière disease experience sudden, violent falling attacks. These episodes have been referred to by the quaint name "otolithic catastrophe of Tumarkin" who attributed them to deformation of the otolithic membrane of the utricle and saccule. Patients characteristically describe a sensation of being pushed or knocked to the ground without warning, or there may be a sudden movement or tilt of the environment just before the fall. Consciousness is not lost, and vertigo of the usual type and its accompaniments are not part of the falling attack, although some patients become aware of these symptoms after falling. The attacks may occur early or late in the course of the disease. Typically, several attacks occur over a period of a year or less and remit spontaneously (Baloh et al). An initial attack must be distinguished from other types of drop attacks, but the occurrence of the more typical vertiginous attacks of Ménière disease, with deafness and tinnitus, clarifies the diagnosis.

The hearing loss in Ménière disease usually precedes the first attack of vertigo but it may appear later. Episodic deafness without vertigo has been called *cochlear Ménière syndrome*. As already mentioned, with recurrent attacks, there is a saltatory progressive unilateral hearing loss (in most series only 10 percent of cases involve both ears, but Baloh places the figure closer to 30 percent). Early in the disease, deafness affects mainly the low tones and fluctuates in severity; actually, tones below 500 Hz are affected early on, and this loss is not evident to the patient. Without measurable fluctuations in pure-tone audiometric thresholds, the diagnosis is left uncertain. Later the fluctuations cease and high tones are affected. Speech discrimination is relatively preserved. The attacks of vertigo usually cease when the hearing loss is complete but there may be an interval of months or longer before this occurs. Audiometry reveals a sensorineural type of deafness, with air and bone conduction equally depressed. Provided that deafness is not complete, loudness recruitment can be demonstrated in the involved ear (see earlier).

Treatment

During an acute attack of Ménière disease, rest in bed is effective treatment, as the patient can usually find a position in which vertigo is minimal. The antihistaminic agents—cyclizine, meclizine, or transdermal scopolamine—are useful in the more protracted cases. Promethazine is an effective vestibular suppressant, as is trimethobenzamide (given in 200-mg suppositories), which also suppresses nausea and vomiting. For many years, a low-salt diet in combination with ammonium chloride or potassium and diuretics has been used in the treatment of Ménière disease, but the value of this regimen has never been established. The same is true for dehydrating agents such as oral glycerol and more recently introduced calcium channel blockers. Mild sedative drugs may help the anxious patient between attacks. The administration of corticosteroids was at one time popular but they have never been proven effective; transtympanic irrigation with dexamethasone is still practiced by some otologists but neither of these approaches is currently popular.

If the attacks are very frequent and disabling, permanent relief can be obtained by surgical means. Destruction of the labyrinth should be considered only in patients with strictly unilateral disease and who have reached the point of complete or nearly complete loss of hearing. In patients with bilateral disease or significant retention of hearing, the vestibular portion of the eighth nerve can be sectioned. Currently, an endolymphatic–subarachnoid shunt is the operation favored by some surgeons, and selective destruction of the vestibule by a cryogenic probe or transtympanic injection of gentamicin is favored by others. Decompression of the eighth cranial nerve, by separating it from an adjacent vessel, as suggested by Janetta, is still a controversial measure and probably better suited to the treatment of sustained and disabling but unexplained vertigo, rather than the treatment of Ménière disease. The decision to undertake any surgical procedure must be tempered by the fact that a majority of the patients, who are middle-aged, stabilize spontaneously in a few years.

Benign Paroxysmal Positional Vertigo (BPPV)

This disorder of labyrinthine function is more frequent than Ménière disease and—while it does not have the same implications in the long-term, an acute attack can be quite disabling. It is characterized by *paroxysmal vertigo* and nystagmus that occur *only with the assumption of certain positions of the head*, particularly lying down or rolling over in bed, bending over and straightening up, or tilting the head backward. It is common for the patient to report that the paroxysm of vertigo began in the middle of the night or early morning, presumably while shifting position during sleep and rapidly making one ear dependent, on rolling over to get out of bed, or to turn off an alarm. Brandt (1994) prefers the descriptive adjective *positioning vertigo* to *positional vertigo*, insofar as the symptoms are induced not by a particular head position but only by rapid changes in head position. This disorder was first described by Bárány (1921) but Dix and Hallpike emphasized its benign nature and were responsible for its further characterization, particularly the discrete positional movements that provoke it. Individual episodes last for less than a minute, but these may recur periodically for several days or for many months—rarely for years. As a rule, examination discloses no abnormalities of hearing or other identifiable lesions in the ear or elsewhere. A thorough summary of the condition has been given by Furman and Cass.

The diagnosis of this disorder is settled at the bedside by moving the patient from the sitting position to recumbency, with the head tilted 30 to 40 degrees over the end of the table and 30 to 45 degrees to one side, as originally described by Dix and Hallpike (Fig. 15-5). This need not be done abruptly but should occur in one smooth motion over a few seconds or less. After a latency of a few seconds, this maneuver provokes a paroxysm of vertigo; the patient may become frightened and grasp the examiner or the table or struggle to sit up. The dysfunctional ear is the one that is downward when vertigo is elicited. We cannot refute the contention made by von Brevern and colleagues that the right labyrinth is more often responsible. The vertigo is accompanied by oscillopsia and nystagmus with the rapid components away from the affected (dependent) ear. The nystagmus is predominantly torsional with an additional vertical component in the eye opposite the affected ear according to Baloh and colleagues. The induced vertigo and nystagmus last no more than 30 to 40 s and usually less than 15 s. *Changing from a recumbent to a sitting position reverses the direction of vertigo and nystagmus* (position-changing nystagmus), and this is perhaps the most certain sign that the disorder originates in the labyrinth. With repetition of the maneuver, vertigo and nystagmus become less apparent, and after three or four trials, they can no longer be elicited (referred to as "fatigue"); they can be reproduced in their original severity only after a protracted period of rest. The head-hanging maneuver does not always evoke vertigo and nystagmus in patients whose histories are otherwise consistent with the diagnosis of benign paroxysmal vertigo; therefore Froehling and coworkers do not insist on it for diagnosis if the history is compatible but without the sign, we are uncertain how to confirm the diagnosis. It may still be appropriate to prescribe the corrective exercises as a trial.

Such attacks of vertigo may come and go for years, particularly in the elderly, and require no treatment. At the other end of the scale is the rare patient with positional vertigo of such persistence and severity as to require surgical intervention.

Baloh and colleagues, in their study of 240 cases of benign positional vertigo, found that 17 percent had their onset within several days or weeks after cerebral trauma and 15 percent after presumed viral neurolabyrinthitis. The significance of these preceding events is unclear, insofar as they did not appear to influence the clinical symptoms or course of the disorder. The provocative suggestion has been made on the basis of small epidemiologic studies such as the one by Jeong and colleagues that osteoporosis is associated with an increased frequency of the disorder.

Sudden changes in position, particularly of the head, may induce vertigo and nystagmus or cause a worsening of these symptoms in patients with all types of vestibular–labyrinthine disease, including Ménière disease and the types associated with vertebrobasilar stroke, trauma, and posterior fossa tumors. However, only if the paroxysm has the special characteristics noted above—namely, elicitation by change in head position, latency of onset, brevity, reversal of direction of nystagmus on sitting up, fatigability with repetition of the test, and the presence of distressing subjective symptoms of vertigo or its recurrence for months or years without other symptoms—can it be regarded as "benign paroxysmal" in type.

Schuknecht is credited with demonstrating that benign positional vertigo was caused by cupulolithiasis, in which otolithic crystals become detached and attach themselves to the cupula of the posterior semicircular canal. It is now generally believed that the debris, probably detached from the otolith, forms a free-floating clot in the endolymph of the canal (canalolithiasis) and gravitates to the most dependent part of the canal during changes in the position of the head (see Brandt et al).

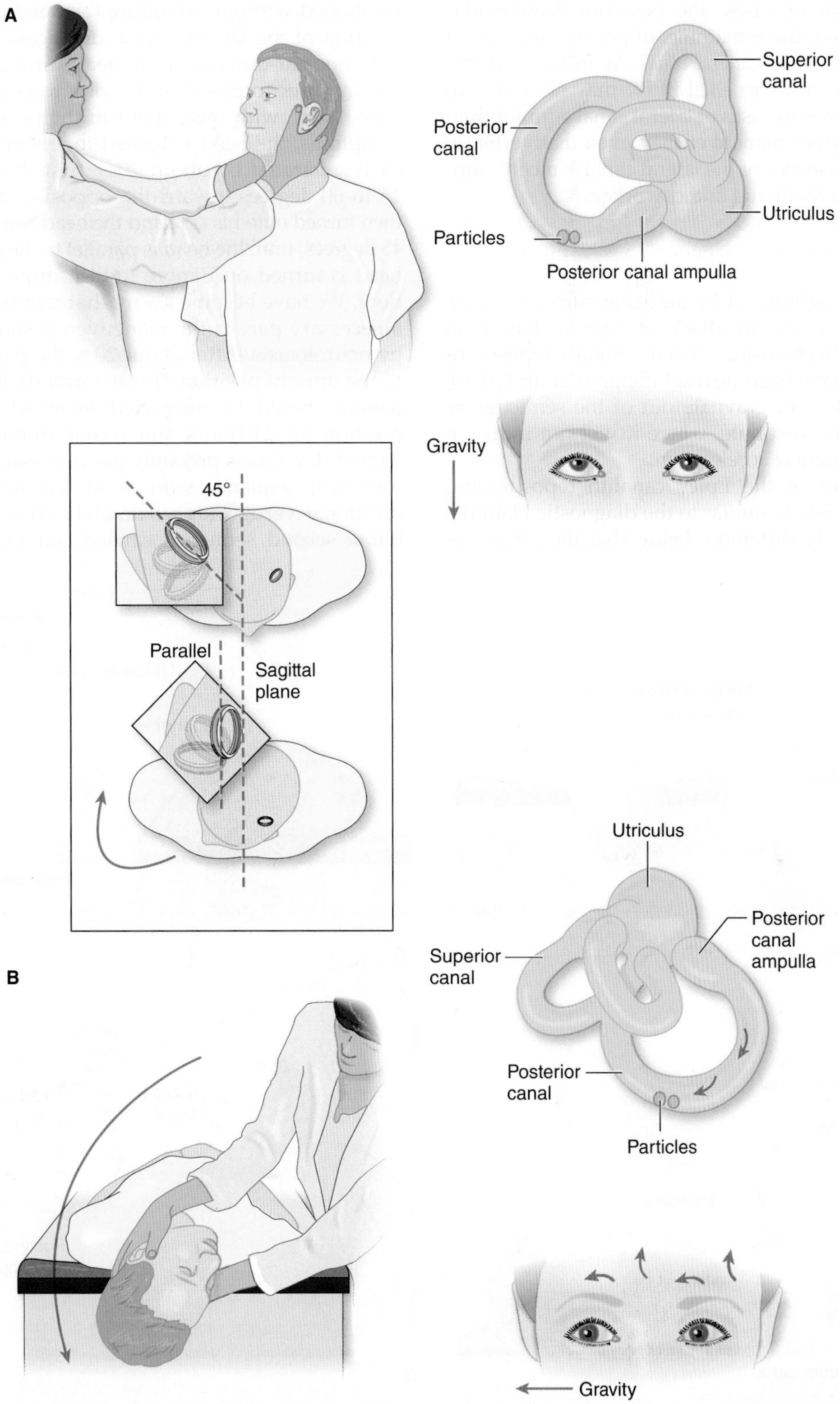

Figure 15-5. Dix-Hallpike maneuver to elicit benign positional vertigo (originating in the right ear). *A.* The maneuver begins with the patient seated and the head turned to one side at 45 degrees, which aligns the right posterior semicircular canal with the sagittal plane of the head. *B.* The patient is then helped to recline rapidly so that the head hangs over the edge of the table, still turned 45 degrees from the midline. Within several seconds, this elicits vertigo and nystagmus that is right beating with a rotary (counterclockwise) component. An important feature of this type of "peripheral" vertigo is a change in the direction of nystagmus when the patient sits up again with his head still rotated. If no nystagmus is elicited, the maneuver is repeated after a pause of 30 s, with the head turned to the left. Treatment with the canalith repositioning maneuver is shown in Fig. 15-6.

In 90 percent of cases, the posterior semicircular canal is implicated; the remaining 10 percent are caused by cupulolithiasis in the *lateral canal*. As mentioned, the conventional maneuver to elicit BPPV may not only fail to induce symptoms in cases of lateral canal cupulolithiasis but the corrective maneuver may even inadvertently produce it. The disorder of the lateral canal is nicely summarized by De la Meilleure and coworkers.

Treatment

The debris is thought to act by inducing currents on the cupula and triggering an attack of vertigo. Based on this presumed mechanism, several canalith repositioning maneuvers have been devised (Semont et al; Epley), allowing the debris to gravitate out of the semicircular canal and into the vestibule, where it will not induce a current during angular acceleration.

The first part of the Epley canalith repositioning maneuver (Fig. 15-6) is similar to the diagnostic Hallpike maneuver, the only difference being that the patient is positioned without extending the head into the hanging position of the Dix-Hall-pike diagnostic maneuver, first with one ear down and the head turned, then the other ear, in order to establish the side responsible for symptoms. Next, with the patient in the position that causes symptoms, the head is turned in a series of three steps, each separated by about 20 s: first the head is turned 45 to 60 degrees toward the opposite ear; the patient is then turned onto his side and the head turned an additional 45 degrees, until the head is parallel to the ground; then the head is turned once more until it more nearly faces the floor. We have become aware that this last step, which is a necessary part of the maneuver, is sometimes omitted by neurologists. After about 20 s, the patient is returned to the upright position. It was formerly believed that the patient should be instructed to avoid the head-down position for 24 hours, but recent studies have demonstrated that this is probably not necessary. Often a single treatment sequence suffices to terminate a period of positional vertigo (approximately 80 percent respond), but a second sequence carried out immediately after

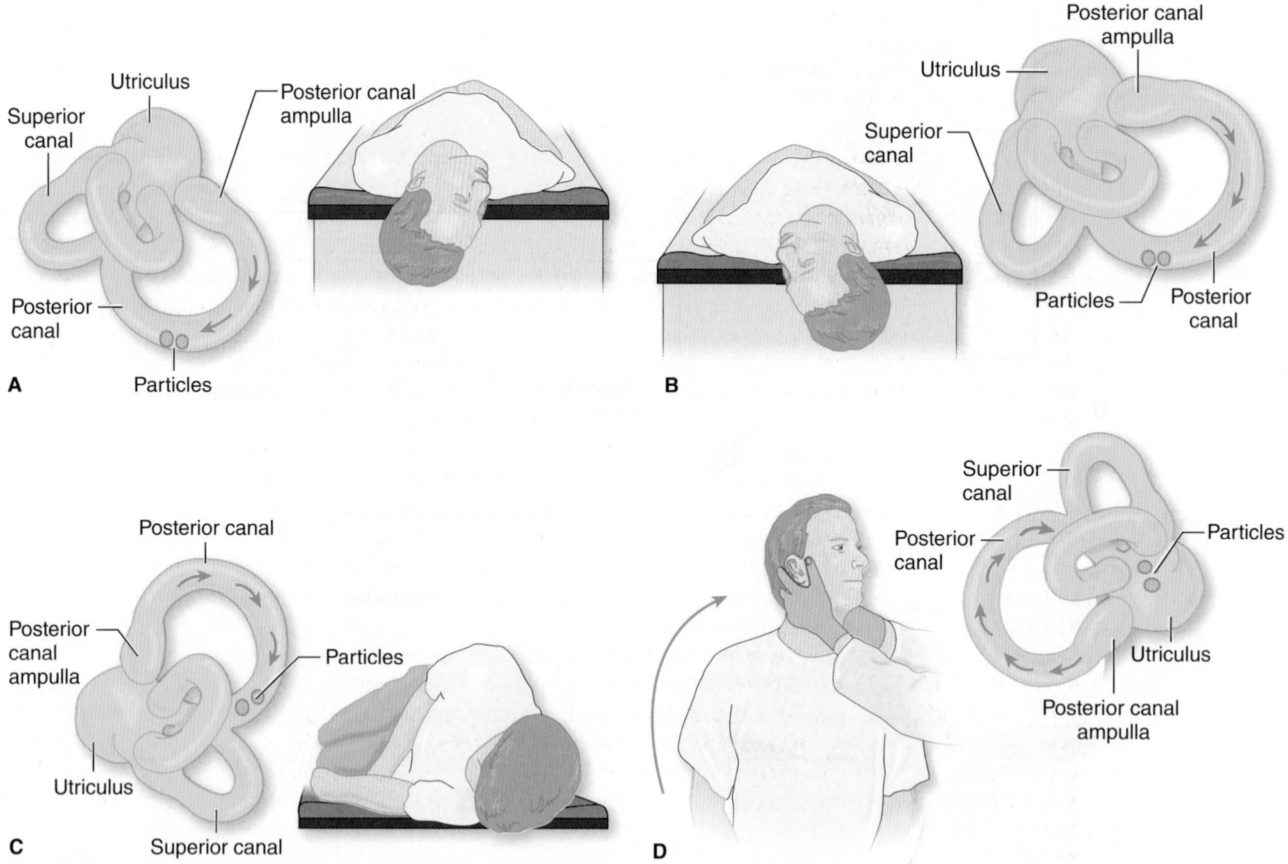

Figure 15-6. Bedside maneuver for the treatment of a patient with benign paroxysmal positional vertigo affecting the right ear. The presumed position of the debris within the labyrinth during the maneuver is shown on each panel. The maneuver is a four-step procedure. First, a Dix–Hallpike test is performed with the patient's head rotated 45 degrees toward the (affected) right ear and the neck slightly extended with the chin pointed slightly upward. *A*. This position results in the patient's head hanging to the right. *B*. Once the vertigo and nystagmus provoked by this maneuver cease, the patient's head is rotated about the rostral–caudal body axis until the left ear is down. *C*. Then the head and body are further rotated until the head is almost facing down. The vertex of the head is kept tilted upward throughout the rotation. The patient should be kept in the final, face down position for about 10 to 15 s. *D*. With the head kept turned toward the left shoulder, the patient is brought into the seated position.

the first probably gains another small group who derive benefit. Additional treatments carried out in the same session are said to add no further benefit. In recalcitrant cases, our otolaryngology colleagues have applied a large vibrator to the temporal bone while the Epley maneuver was being performed, after which the episodes ceased; presumably this mobilizes the crystals and aids in moving them out of the canal. An incompletely implemented Epley maneuver risks converting the usual posterior semicircular canal cupulolithiasis to one involving the lateral canal, which may be more difficult to treat.

Patients who fail to respond to the Epley maneuver may respond to variations of repositioning such as the Semont maneuver (the patient begins in a sitting position with the head turned 45 degrees to one side, then drops laterally to a side lying position on the opposite ear, followed by a brisk swing of the body to drop the opposite side lying position) or the similar Brandt-Daroff exercises (sitting, to side lying, to sitting, performed repeatedly).

Positional vertigo caused by lateral canalolithiasis causes a purely horizontal nystagmus rather than the torsional and vertical type described above. In this case, another repositioning maneuver that involves rolling from one side to the other is used to liberate and reposition the otolithic debris.

It is important to reiterate that in some patients with positional vertigo, the disorder is neither benign nor paroxysmal. Jannetta and colleagues have described a group of patients in whom symptoms of vertigo and disequilibrium were almost constant (even in the upright position) and disabling and unresponsive to habituation and other medical therapy (*disabling positional vertigo*). They attributed this disorder to cross-compression of the root entry zone of the eighth cranial nerve by an adjacent blood vessel and have reported that decompression of the nerve provides lasting relief of symptoms.

Toxic and Idiopathic Bilateral Vestibulopathy

The common and serious ototoxic effects of the aminoglycoside antibiotics have already been mentioned—both on the cochlear hair cells, with loss of hearing and independently, on the vestibular labyrinths. Prolonged exposure to these agents produces a bilateral vestibulopathy without vertigo. Instead, there tends to be a disequilibrium associated with oscillopsia. The symptoms are especially troublesome when the patient moves. Often the disequilibrium is not discovered until a bedbound patient tries to walk.

Less-well appreciated is the occurrence of a slowly progressive vestibulopathy for which no cause can be discerned. The disorder affects men and women alike, with onset in middle or late adult life with the main abnormalities being unsteadiness of gait, which is worse in the dark or with eyes closed, and oscillopsia, which occurs with head movements and is particularly noticeable when walking. Vertigo and hearing loss are absent, as are other neurologic abnormalities. Bilateral vestibular loss can be documented with caloric and rotational testing. Baloh and colleagues, in a report of 22 patients with idiopathic vestibulopathy of this type, found that a significant proportion (9 of 22 cases) had a prior history of prolonged episodes of vertigo consistent with the diagnosis of bilateral sequential vestibular neuritis (see below).

Vestibular Neuritis (Neuronitis)

This was the term applied originally by Dix and Hallpike to a distinctive disturbance of vestibular function, characterized clinically by a paroxysmal and usually a prolonged single attack of vertigo and by a conspicuous absence of tinnitus and deafness. The entity is, however, more nebulous than most discussions indicate.

This disorder occurs mainly in young to middle-aged adults (children and older individuals also may be affected), without preference for either sex. The patient frequently gives a history of an antecedent upper respiratory infection of nonspecific type, but it is not clear whether this is requisite for the diagnosis. Usually, the onset of vertigo is fairly abrupt, although some patients describe a prodromal period of several hours or days in which they felt "top-heavy" or "off balance." Persistence of the symptoms for a day or more differentiates the process from Ménière disease. The vertigo is severe as a rule and is associated with nausea, vomiting, and the need to remain immobile.

Nystagmus (quick component) and a sense of body motion are to the opposite side, whereas falling and past pointing are to the side of the affected labyrinth. In some patients, the caloric responses are abnormal bilaterally, and in some, the vertigo may recur, affecting the same or the other ear. Auditory function is normal. Examination discloses vestibular paresis on one side, i.e., an absent or diminished response to caloric stimulation of the horizontal semicircular canal. If the patient will tolerate small head movements, the previously described rapid-head-impulse test of Halmagyi and Cremer is one of the best means of demonstrating absent function of one lateral semicircular canal.

Although the symptoms can be quite disabling for a short period, vestibular neuritis is an ostensibly benign disorder. The severe vertigo and associated symptoms subside in a matter of several days, but lesser degrees of these symptoms, made worse by rapid movements of the head, may persist for months. The caloric responses are gradually restored to normal as well. In some patients, there has been a recurrence months or years later, as already mentioned.

The portion of the vestibular pathway that is primarily affected in this disease is thought to be the superior part of the vestibular nerve trunk, which was observed to show degenerative changes by Schuknecht and Kitamura. Earlier, Dix and Hallpike had reasoned that the lesion was located central to the labyrinth, as hearing is spared and vestibular function usually returns to normal. They used the term *vestibular neuritis* because of the uncertainty of more precise localization within the peripheral vestibular pathway. The cause of vestibular neuritis is still uncertain, but many authorities have attributed it to a viral infection of the vestibular nerve, analogous to Bell's palsy, and from time to time, enhancement of the eighth nerve or the membranous labyrinth is seen after gadolinium administration on MRI. For want of more specific etiologic or pathologic data, many neurologists prefer the term *vestibular neuropathy* or *neuritis* or *acute unilateral peripheral vestibulopathy*. It is likely that the conditions described under the terms *epidemic vertigo, epidemic labyrinthitis,* and *acute labyrinthitis* or *neurolabyrinthitis* refer to the same process. Certainly, herpes zoster oticus causes this syndrome (as well as affecting the seventh nerve); this characterizes the Ramsay Hunt syndrome described in Chaps. 10 and 47.

During the acute stage, antihistamine drugs, promethazine, clonazepam, and scopolamine may be helpful in reducing the symptoms. Vestibular exercises are recommended by Baloh (2003) in his review of the subject. One clinical trial has demonstrated a more rapid recovery with the use of methylprednisolone, 100 mg orally, tapered over 3 weeks; valacyclovir did not have this effect (Strupp et al).

Other Causes of Vertigo of Vestibular Nerve Origin

Vertigo may occur with diseases that involve the eighth nerve in the petrous bone or at the cerebellopontine angle. Aside from vestibular neuritis, discussed above, the two most common causes of vertigo of eighth nerve origin are probably an acoustic or vestibular schwannoma and vascular irritation or compression by a small branch of the basilar artery. The frequency of the vascular compression syndrome as a cause of otherwise undifferentiated vertigo is not known (see earlier).

Regarding vestibular schwannoma, vertigo is rarely the initial symptom; the usual sequence is deafness affecting the high-frequency tones initially, followed some months or years later by mild chronic imbalance rather than vertigo and by impaired caloric responses, and then, if untreated, by additional cranial nerve palsies (the seventh, fifth, and tenth nerves), ipsilateral ataxia of limbs, and headache. Variations in the sequence of development of symptoms are frequent, and probably many vestibular schwannomas discovered in the process of an evaluation for vertigo are incidental; i.e., almost 1 percent of the general population harbors small tumors. In the diagnosis of vestibular and acoustic schwannoma, MRI and BAEP are the most important ancillary examinations. Bilateral vestibular/acoustic Schwannomas are almost always a manifestation of neurofibromatosis type 2.

Labyrinthine infarction can be a component of the stroke syndrome from occlusion of the anterior inferior cerebellar artery (AICA). In the complete syndrome there is hearing loss, cerebellar ataxia, and sometimes "screaming tinnitus" or lesser degrees of tonal tinnitus. Also reported is a clinical syndrome of unknown nature consisting of a single abrupt attack of severe vertigo, nausea, and vomiting without tinnitus or hearing loss but with permanent ablation of labyrinthine function on one side. It has been suggested that this syndrome is a result of occlusion of the labyrinthine division of the internal auditory artery, but so far, anatomic confirmation has not been obtained. Labyrinthine hemorrhage has been demonstrated by MRI in some of these patients; others are attributed, speculatively, to viral infection.

Basser described a particular form of paroxysmal vertigo that occurs in childhood. The attacks occur in a setting of good health and are of sudden onset and brief duration. Pallor, sweating, and immobility are prominent manifestations; occasionally, vomiting and nystagmus occur. No relation to posture or movement has been observed. The attacks are recurrent but tend to cease spontaneously after a period of several months or years. The outstanding abnormality is demonstrated by caloric testing, which shows impairment or loss of vestibular function, bilaterally or unilaterally, frequently persisting after the attacks have ceased. Cochlear function is unimpaired. The pathologic basis of this disorder has not been determined, and a suggested connection with migraine is tenuous. The special case of basilar artery migraine is discussed below.

Cogan has described an infrequent syndrome in young adults in which a *nonsyphilitic interstitial keratitis* is associated with vertigo, tinnitus, nystagmus, and rapidly progressive deafness. The prognosis for vision is good, but the deafness and loss of vestibular function are usually permanent. The cause and pathogenesis of this syndrome are unknown, although approximately half of the patients later develop aortic insufficiency or a systemic vasculitis that resembles polyarteritis nodosa. These vascular complications proved fatal in 7 of 78 cases reviewed by Vollertsen and colleagues.

There are many other causes of aural vertigo, such as purulent labyrinthitis complicating mastoiditis or meningitis; serous labyrinthitis caused by infection of the middle ear; "toxic labyrinthitis" caused by intoxication with alcohol, quinine, or salicylates; motion sickness; and hemorrhage into the inner ear. Bárány (1911) was the first to draw attention to the nystagmus and positional vertigo, worse on closing the eyes that occurs at a certain level of intoxication with alcohol and lasts a few hours. Such an episode of alcohol-induced vertigo tends to last longer than a vertiginous attack of Ménière disease, but in other respects, the symptoms (excepting tinnitus) are similar.

Vertigo with varying degrees of spontaneous or positional nystagmus and reduced vestibular responses is a frequent complication of *cranial trauma*. Vertigo, often of the nonrotatory, to-and-fro type, may follow cerebral concussion or whiplash injury, in which the head has not been impacted. Brandt has attributed this syndrome to a loosening or dislodgement of the otoconia in the otoliths. The vertigo in these circumstances usually improves in a few days or weeks and is rarely accompanied by impairment of hearing—in distinction to the vertigo that follows fractures of the temporal bones (as described earlier in this chapter in the discussion of deafness). Dizziness is also a prominent complaint as part of the syndrome of a postconcussion syndrome as described in Chap. 35, but usually this proves to be ill-defined giddiness rather than true vertigo.

There is, nonetheless, a type of vestibular concussion accompanying closed head trauma that may leave the patient with imbalance or positional vertigo. Otolaryngologists are familiar with a syndrome resulting from a perilymph fistula after traumatic injury. The trauma may be minor, even forceful coughing, sneezing, or lifting; some cases are a result of chronic ear infection or cholesteatoma. Disruption of the oval or round windows causes a leak of perilymph into the middle ear. Vertigo and nystagmus can be induced by pressure in the external ear canal (the fistula test). If enough perilymph migrates to the middle ear, a conductive hearing loss may also be detected. Superior canal dehiscence, in which loud sounds induce brief vertigo and nystagmus (Tullio phenomenon) is another result of perilymphatic fistula, as discussed earlier. A perilymph fistula may be pronounced enough to also cause low pressure of the spinal fluid with the characteristic enhancement of the dura on MRI.

Vertigo of Brainstem Origin

Reference was made above to the occurrence of vertigo and nystagmus with lower and upper brainstem lesions. In these cases, vestibular nuclei and their connections are implicated. Auditory function is nearly always spared, because the vestibular and cochlear fibers diverge upon entering the brainstem at the junction of the medulla and pons. The vertigo of brainstem origin, as well as the accompanying nausea, vomiting, nystagmus, and disequilibrium, is generally more protracted but less severe than with labyrinthine lesions, but one can think of exceptions to this statement. Nevertheless, with brainstem lesions, one often observes marked nystagmus without the slightest degree of vertigo—which does not happen with labyrinthine disease. The nystagmus of brainstem origin may be uni- or bidirectional, purely horizontal, vertical or rotary, and is characteristically worsened by attempted visual fixation. In contrast, nystagmus of labyrinthine origin is unidirectional, usually with a rotary component, and past pointing and falling are in the direction of the slow phase; purely vertical nystagmus does not occur, and a purely horizontal nystagmus without a rotary component is unusual. Furthermore, labyrinthine nystagmus is inhibited by visual fixation and reverses direction with changes in the position of the head; nystagmus of brainstem origin generally displays none of these features. Either may have a positional- or movement-induced worsening, but this finding is more prominent in labyrinthine disease. Table 15-2 summarizes these findings.

The central localization of vertigo is confirmed mainly by finding signs of involvement of other structures within the brainstem (cranial nerves, sensory and motor tracts, etc.). The mode of onset, duration, and other features of the clinical picture depend on the nature of the causative disease, which may be vascular, demyelinative, or neoplastic.

Table 15-2

DIFFERENTIATION OF PERIPHERAL FROM CENTRAL NYSTAGMUS (SEE TEXT)

	PERIPHERAL	CENTRAL
Vertigo and nausea	Pronounced	Mild
Direction of nystagmus	• Mixed torsional-vertical • Mixed torsional-horizontal • May be pure horizontal	• Pure horizontal • Pure vertical • Pure torsional
Influence of gaze	Does not change direction with gaze	Direction changes with gaze
Visual fixation	Inhibits nystagmus	Does not affect nystagmus
Latency following repositioning maneuver	Up to 20 s	Brief
Direction changing with reversal of head position	Present and characteristic	Absent
Hearing loss/ tinnitus	Variably present	Absent
Signs of brainstem or cerebellar disease	Absent	Generally present

Vertigo is a prominent symptom of ischemic attacks and of brainstem infarction occurring in the territory of the vertebrobasilar arteries, particularly the Wallenberg syndrome of lateral medullary infarction.

On the other hand, our colleague C.M. Fisher had pointed out that vertigo as the *sole* manifestation of brainstem ischemia from basilar arterial disease is rare. Unless other symptoms and signs of a brainstem disorder appear contemporaneously or soon after the vertigo, one can usually postulate an aural origin and nearly always exclude vascular disease of the brainstem. However, we have encountered rare patients with repeated brief attacks of vertigo that later proved to be caused by basilar artery stenosis, but in whom only a few episodes were associated with signs of brainstem disease such as dysarthria, facial numbness, or diplopia. In other words, frequent and sudden episodes of vertigo lasting a minute or so may infrequently be related to transient brainstem ischemia.

Vertigo of cerebellar origin is exceptional in this respect in that it may rarely be the sole manifestation of cerebellar infarction or hemorrhage, as described earlier in the introductory sections of the chapter and in Chap. 34. It follows that isolated vertigo may be the result of occlusion of the posterior inferior cerebellar artery or its parent vertebral artery although most often, there are additional features related to damage to the lateral medulla. In instances of isolated vertigo, one seeks confirmation that there are no features pointing to a central origin or conversely, if there are signs such as nystagmus in more than one direction of gaze with a single position of the head, or vertical nystagmus, there is concern for ischemia of the brainstem. The nystagmus and ataxia of gait (more of a propelling, or pulsion, to one side) that accompany acute cerebellar lesions are toward the same side (the side of the lesion), while in acute vestibulopathies, nystagmus beats away from the side of the lesion and pulsion is still toward the affected side.

Multiple sclerosis may be the explanation of persistent vertigo in an adolescent or young adult, sometimes with little or no nystagmus.

The relationship of migraine to vertigo was mentioned earlier. This refers to otherwise mundane migraine in which the vertigo is perhaps an aura, or to episodes of paroxysmal vertigo in adults that are considered to be migraine equivalents. In addition, attacks of vertigo followed by an intense unilateral and often suboccipital headache and vomiting are the characteristic features of *basilar artery migraine*. The prodromal visual symptoms take the form of blindness or of photopsia that occupies all of the visual fields. Between headaches, tests of cochlear and vestibular function in these patients are normal. Some authorities have stated that most cases of recurrent vertigo without hearing loss over many years can be attributed to migraine and not to Ménière disease. An instructive series of such cases has been published by Dieterich and Brandt.

Finally, mention should be made of a *familial vestibulocerebellar syndrome*, beginning in childhood or early adult life and characterized by recurrent episodes of vertigo and imbalance. Diplopia and dysarthria complicate some attacks, which seem to be precipitated by extreme exertion and emotion. Repeated attacks are followed by a mild, persistent ataxia, mainly of the trunk. This disorder was first described by Farmer and Mustian and more recently by Baloh and Winder, who have pointed out that both the episodic vertigo and ataxia are markedly reduced or abolished by the administration of acetazolamide. This process is most likely related to the inherited acetazolamide-responsive ataxic channelopathy syndrome described in Chap. 5. A form that is kinesigenic, i.e., brought on by activity, has a similar appearance.

In summary, the nature of the nystagmus, instability of the eyes during the head impulse test, and the other features of the neurologic examination allow a distinction to be made between central and peripheral cases of vertigo. Associated hearing loss favors a vestibular cause of vertigo. Tables 15-2 and 15-3 summarize the features of the various vertiginous syndromes.

Table 15-3

VERTIGINOUS SYNDROMES WITH LESIONS OF DIFFERENT PARTS OF THE VESTIBULAR SYSTEM

SYNDROME	NEUROLOGIC FINDINGS	DISORDERS OF EQUILIBRIUM	TYPE OF NYSTAGMUS[a]	HEARING	LABORATORY EXAM
Labyrinths (postural vertigo, trauma, Ménière disease, aminoglycoside toxicity, labyrinthitis)	None	Ipsilateral past pointing and lateral propulsion to side of lesion	Horizontal or rotary to side opposite lesion, positional and position changing, fatigable	Normal or conduction or neurosensory deafness with recruitment	Vestibular paresis by caloric testing, directional preponderance
Vestibular nerve and ganglia (vestibular neuronitis, herpes zoster)	Auditory eighth and seventh cranial nerve abnormalities; abnormal head impulse test to affected side	Ipsilateral past pointing and lateral propulsion to side of lesion	Unidirectional positional	Sometimes sensorineural deafness, without recruitment (vestibulolabyrinthitis)	Imaging may be normal or abnormal Vestibular paresis on caloric testing Directional preponderance
Cerebellopontine angle (acoustic neuroma, glomus and other tumors)	Ipsilateral fifth, seventh, ninth, tenth cranial nerves, cerebellar ataxia Increased intracranial pressure (late)	Ataxia and falling ipsilaterally	Gaze-paretic, positional, coarser to side of lesion	Sensorineural deafness without recruitment	Imgaing abnormal Vestibular paresis on caloric testing BAEPs abnormal Increased CSF protein
Brainstem and cerebellum (infarcts, tumors, viral infections)	Multiple cranial nerves, brainstem tract signs, cerebellar ataxia	Ataxia present with eyes open	Coarse horizontal and vertical, gaze-paretic	Usually normal	Hyperactive labyrinths or directional preponderance on caloric testing Imaging, and BAEPs abnormal in most cases
Higher (cerebral) connections	Aphasia, visual field, hemimotor, hemisensory, and other cerebral abnormalities, seizures	No change	Usually absent	Normal	No change in caloric responses Imaging and electroencephalogram may be abnormal

[a]See text and Chap. 14 for description of types of nystagmus.

References

Adler JR, Ropper AH: Self-audible venous bruits and high jugular bulb. *Arch Neurol* 43:257, 1986.

Amarenco P, Roullet E, Hommel M, et al: Infarction in the territory of the medial branch of the posterior inferior cerebellar artery. *J Neurol Neurosurg Psychiatry* 53:731, 1990.

Badia L, Parikh A, Bookes GB: Management of middle ear myoclonus. *J Laryngol Otol* 108:380, 1994.

Baloh RW: *Clinical Neurotology*. London, Baillière Tindall, 1994.

Baloh RW: Vertigo. *Lancet* 352:1841, 1998.

Baloh RW: Vestibular neuronitis. *N Engl J Med* 348:1027, 2003.

Baloh RW, Honrubia V: *Clinical Neurophysiology of the Vestibular System*, 2nd ed. Philadelphia, Davis, 1990.

Baloh RW, Honrubia V, Jacobson K: Benign positional vertigo: Clinical and oculographic features in 240 cases. *Neurology* 37:371, 1987.

Baloh RW, Jacobson K, Honrubia V: Idiopathic bilateral vestibulopathy. *Neurology* 39:272, 1989.

Baloh RW, Jacobson K, Wilson T: Drop attacks with Ménière's syndrome. *Ann Neurol* 28:384, 1990.

Baloh RW, Winder A: Acetazolamide responsive vestibulocerebellar syndrome. Clinical and oculographic features. *Neurology* 41:429, 1991.

Bárány R: Experimentelle Alkohol-intoxication. *Monatsschr Ohrenheilk* 45:959, 1911.

Bárány R: Diagnose von Krankheitserscheinungen im Bereiche des Otolithenapparatus. *Acta Otolaryngol* 2:234, 1921.

Basser LS: Benign paroxysmal vertigo of childhood. A variety of vestibular neuronitis. *Brain* 87:141, 1964.

Biemond A, DeJong JMBV: On cervical nystagmus and related disorders. *Brain* 92:437, 1969.

Brandt T: Phobic postural vertigo. *Neurology* 46:1515, 1996.

Brandt T: Man in motion: Historical and clinical aspects of vestibular function—a review. *Brain* 114:2159, 1991.

Brandt T, Steddin S, Daroff RB: Therapy for benign paroxysmal positioning vertigo, revisited. *Neurology* 44:796, 1994.

Brodal A: The cranial nerves, in *Neurological Anatomy*, 3rd ed. New York, Oxford University Press, 1981, pp 448–577.

Cascino G, Adams RD: Brainstem auditory hallucinosis. *Neurology* 36:1042, 1986.

Celesia GG: Organization of auditory cortical areas in man. *Brain* 99:403, 1976.

Chinnery PF, Elliott C, Green GR, et al: The spectrum of hearing loss due to mitochondrial DNA defects. *Brain* 123:82, 2000.

Cogan DG: Syndrome of nonsyphilitic interstitial keratitis and vestibuloauditory symptoms. *Arch Ophthalmol* 34:144, 1945.

DeFelice C, DeCapua B, Tassi R, et al: Non-functioning posterior communicating arteries of circle of Willis in idiopathic sudden hearing loss. *Lancet* 356:1237, 2000.

De la Meilleure G, Dehaene I, Depondt M, et al. Benign paroxysmal positional vertigo of the horizontal canal. *J neurol Neurosurg Psychiatr* 60:68,1991.

DeRidder D, DeMulder G, Verstraeten E, et al: Primary and secondary auditory cortex stimulation for intractable tinnitus. *ORL J Otorhinolarygol Res* 68:48, 2006.

Dieterich M, Brandt T: Episodic vertigo related to migraine (90 cases): Vestibular migraine? *J Neurol* 246:883, 1999.

Dix M, Hallpike C: Pathology, symptomatology and diagnosis of certain disorders of the vestibular system. *Proc R Soc Med* 45:341, 1952.

Duncan GW, Parker SW, Fisher CM: Acute cerebellar infarction in the PICA territory. *Arch Neurol* 32:364, 1975.

Epley JM: The canalith repositioning procedure for treatment of benign paroxysmal positional vertigo. *Otolaryngol Head Neck Surg* 107:399, 1992.

Estivill X, Fortina P, Surrey S, et al: Connexin-26 mutations in sporadic and inherited sensorineural deafness. *Lancet* 351:394, 1998.

Evan KE, Tavill MA, Goldberg AN, Siverstein H: Sudden sensorineural hearing loss after general anesthesia for nonotologic surgery. *Laryngoscope* 107:747, 1997.

Farmer TW, Mustian VM: Vestibulocerebellar ataxia. *Arch Neurol* 8:471, 1963.

Fetterman BL, Luxford WM, Saunders JE: Sudden bilateral sensorineural hearing loss. *Laryngoscope* 106:1347, 1996.

Fowler EP: Head noises in normal and in disordered ears. *Arch Otolaryngol* 39:498, 1944.

Friedmann I: Ultrastructure of ear in normal and diseased states, in Hinchcliffe R, Harrison D (eds): *Scientific Foundations of Otolaryngology*. London, Heinemann, 1976, pp 202–211.

Froehling DA, Silverstein MD, Mohr DN, et al: Benign positional vertigo: Incidence and prognosis in a population-based study in Olmsted County, Minnesota. *Mayo Clin Proc* 16:596, 1991.

Furman JM, Cass SP: Benign paroxysmal positional vertigo. *N Engl J Med* 341:1591, 1999.

Furman JM, Jacob RG: Psychiatric dizziness. *Neurology* 48:1161, 1997.

Gorlin RS, Pindborg JJ, Cohen MM Jr: *Syndromes of the Head and Neck*. New York, McGraw-Hill, 1976.

Graham JT, Newby HA: Acoustical characteristics of tinnitus. *Arch Otolaryngol* 75:162, 1962.

Halmagyi GM, Cremer PD: Assessment and treatment of dizziness. *J Neurol Neurosurg Psychiatry* 68:129, 2000.

Hammeke TA, McQuillen MP, Cohen BA: Musical hallucinations associated with acquired deafness. *J Neurol Neurosurg Psychiatry* 46:570, 1983.

Hotson JR, Baloh RW: Acute vestibular syndrome. *N Engl J Med* 339:680, 1998.

Jamieson DRS, Mann C, O'Reilly B, Thomas AM: Ear click in palatal tremor caused by activity of the levator veli palatini. *Neurology* 46:1168, 1996.

Jannetta PJ: Neurovascular decompression in cranial nerve and systemic disease. *Am J Surg* 192:518, 1980.

Jannetta PJ, M MB, Moller AR: Disabling positional vertigo. *N Engl J Med* 310:1700, 1984.

Jeong SH, Choi SH, Kim JY, et al. Osteopenia and osteoporosis in idiopathic benign positional vertigo. *Neurology* 24:1069-76. 2009.

Kasai K, Asada T, Yumoto M, et al: Evidence for functional abnormality in the right auditory cortex during musical hallucinosis. *Lancet* 354:1703, 1999.

Konigsmark BW: Hereditary deafness in man. *N Engl J Med* 281:713, 774, 827, 1969.

Konigsmark BW: Hereditary diseases of the nervous system with hearing loss, in Vinken PJ, Bruyn GW (eds): *Handbook of Clinical Neurology*. Vol 22. Amsterdam, North-Holland, 1975, pp 499–526.

Konigsmark BW: Hereditary progressive cochleovestibular atrophies, in Vinken PJ, Bruyn GW (eds): *Handbook of Clinical Neurology*. Vol 22. Amsterdam, North-Holland, 1975, pp 481–497.

Kroenke K, Mangelsdorff AD: Common symptoms in ambulatory care: Incidence, evaluation, therapy, and outcome. *Am J Med* 86:262, 1989.

Leigh RJ, Zee DS: *The Neurology of Eye Movements*, 2nd ed. Philadelphia, Davis, 1991.

Lockwood AH, Salvi RJ, Burkard RF: Tinnitus. *N Engl J Med* 347:904, 2002.

Marion MS, Cevette MJ: Tinnitus. *Mayo Clin Proc* 66:614, 1991.

Mattox DE, Simmons FB: Natural history of sudden sensorineural hearing loss. *Ann Otol Rhinol Laryngol* 86:463, 1977.

Møller AR: Pathophysiology of tinnitus. *Ann Otol Rhinol Laryngol* 93:39, 1984.

Morell RJ, Kim HJ, Hood LJ, et al: Mutations in the connexin 26 gene (GJB2) among Ashkenazi Jews with nonsyndromic recessive deafness. *N Engl J Med* 339:1500, 1998.

Nadol JB Jr: Hearing loss. *N Engl J Med* 329:1092, 1993.

National Institute on Deafness and Other Communication Disorders: *A Report of the Task Force on the National Strategic Research Plan*. Bethesda, MD, National Institutes of Health, 1989.

Neuhauser H, Leopold M, van Brevern M, et al: The interpretation of migraine, vertigo and migrainous vertigo. *Neurology* 56:436, 2001.

Nodar RH, Graham JT: An investigation of frequency characteristics of tinnitus associated with Ménière's disease. *Arch Otolaryngol* 82:28, 1965.

Page J: Audiologic tests in the differential diagnosis of vertigo. *Otolaryngol Clin North Am* 6:53, 1973.

Proctor CA, Proctor B: Understanding hereditary nerve deafness. *Arch Otolaryngol* 85:23, 1967.

Rasmussen GI: An efferent cochlear bundle. *Anat Rec* 82:441, 1942.

Rudge P: *Clinical Neuro-Otology*. Edinburgh, Churchill-Livingstone, 1983.

Schuknecht HF: Cupulolithiasis. *Arch Otolaryngol Head Neck Surg* 90:765, 1969.

Schuknecht HF, Kitamura K: Vestibular neuronitis. *Ann Otol Rhinol Laryngol* 90:1, 1981.

Semont A, Freyss G, Vitte E: Curing the BPPV with a liberatory maneuver. *Adv Otorhinolaryngol* 42:290, 1988.

Sismanis A, Smoker WR: Pulsatile tinnitus: Recent advances in diagnosis. *Laryngoscope* 104:681, 1994.

Stouffer JL, Tyler RS: Characterization of tinnitus by tinnitus patients. *J Speech Hear Disord* 55:439, 1990.

Strupp M, Zingler VC, Anbusow V, et al: Methylprednisolone, valacyclovir, or the combination for vestibular neuritis. *N Engl J Med* 351:354, 2004.

Suga S, Lindsay JR: Histopathological observations of presbyacusis. *Ann Otol Rhinol Laryngol* 85:169, 1976.

Tanaka Y, Kamo T, Yoshida M, Yamadori A: So-called cortical deafness. *Brain* 114:2385, 1991.

Tekin M, Arnos KS, Pandy A: Advances in hereditary deafness. *Lancet* 358:1082, 2001.

Toole JF, Tucker H: Influence of head position upon cerebral circulation. *Arch Neurol* 2:616, 1960.

Tumarkin A: The otolithic catastrophe: A new syndrome. *Br Med J* 1:175, 1936.

Vollertsen RS, McDonald TJ, Younge BR, et al: Cogan's syndrome: 18 cases and a review of the literature. *Mayo Clin Proc* 61:344, 1986.

von Brevern M, Seelig T, Neuhauser H, et al: Benign positional vertigo predominantly affects the night labyrinth. *J Neurol Neurosurg Psychiatry* 75:1487, 2004.

Epilepsy and Disorders of Consciousness

SECTION 4

16

Epilepsy and Other Seizure Disorders

The prevalence and importance of epilepsy, i.e., recurrent cerebral cortical seizures, can hardly be overstated. From the epidemiologic studies of Hauser and colleagues, one may extrapolate an incidence of approximately 2 million individuals in the United States who are subject to epilepsy and predict about 44 new cases per 100,000 persons each year. These figures are exclusive of patients in whom seizures transiently complicate febrile and other illnesses or injuries. It has also been estimated that slightly less than 1 percent of persons in the United States will have epilepsy by the age of 20 years (Hauser and Annegers). Over two-thirds of all epileptic seizures begin in childhood (most in the first year of life), and this is the period when seizures assume the widest array of forms. In the practice of pediatric neurology, epilepsy is one of the most common disorders, and the chronicity of childhood forms adds to their importance. The incidence increases again after age 60 years. For all these reasons, physicians should know something of the nature of seizure disorders and their treatment. It is notable that, in striking contrast to the many treatments available for epilepsy, as pointed out by J. Engel, 80 to 90 percent of persons with epilepsy in the developing world never receive medical attention.

In 1870, Hughlings Jackson, the eminent British neurologist, postulated that seizures were due to "an excessive and disorderly discharge of cerebral nervous tissue on muscles." The discharge may result in an almost instantaneous loss of consciousness, alteration of perception or impairment of psychic function, convulsive movements, disturbance of sensation, or some combination thereof.

Terminologic difficulty arises from the diversity of the clinical manifestations of seizures. The term *convulsion*, referring as it does to an intense paroxysm of involuntary repetitive muscular contractions, is inappropriate for a disorder that may consist only of an alteration of sensation or consciousness. *Seizure* is preferable as a generic term, because it embraces all paroxysmal electrical discharges of the brain, and also because it lends itself to qualification. The term *motor* or *convulsive seizure*, therefore, is not tautologic, and one may likewise speak of a *sensory seizure* or *psychic seizure*. The word *epilepsy* is derived from Greek words meaning "to seize upon" or a "taking hold of." Our predecessors referred to it as the "falling sickness" or the "falling evil." Although a useful medical term to denote recurrent seizures, the words *epilepsy* and *epileptic* may still have unpleasant connotations and should be used advisedly in dealing with patients. There is also a curious, but common entity of "nonconvulsive seizure" that may impair consciousness, but not manifest any abnormal bodily movement. This represents an important and potentially treatable form of a confusional state.

A first solitary seizure or brief outburst of seizures may occur during the course of many medical illnesses. It indicates that the cerebral cortex has been affected by disease, either primarily or secondarily. If prolonged or repeated every few minutes, the condition termed *status epilepticus*, may threaten life. Equally important, a seizure or a series of seizures may be the manifestation of an ongoing neurologic disease that requires special diagnostic, and therapeutic measures. Status epilepticus may be of the nonconvulsive type, and continuously impair consciousness and is difficult to detect clinically because of the absence of characteristic movements.

A more common and less-grave circumstance is for a seizure to be but one in an extensive series recurring over a long period of time, with most of the attacks being more or less similar in type. In this instance, they may be the result of an inactive lesion that remains as a scar in the cerebral cortex. The original disease may have passed unnoticed, or perhaps had occurred in utero, at birth, in infancy, or in parts of the brain inaccessible for examination or too immature to manifest signs. The increasingly refined techniques of MRI now also reveal small zones of developmental cortical dysplasia and hippocampal sclerosis, both of which tend to be epileptogenic. Patients with such long-standing but subtle lesions probably make up a large portion of those with recurrent seizures. If there is no underlying lesion, the condition is classified as idiopathic or primary, but in the modern era, this is come to be almost synonymous with a genetic cause. In this category, there are a large number of important types of epilepsy for which no pathologic basis has been established, and for which there is no apparent underlying cause except perhaps a genetic one. Included here are special hereditary forms including types of generalized tonic-clonic (grand mal), and "absence" seizure states as suggested in classifications many years ago by Lennox and Forster. Persistent seizures, whether idiopathic or not, can secondarily damage cortical tissue by several mechanisms that may include excitotoxicity and, in the setting of prolonged tonic seizures, systemic hypoxia.

CLASSIFICATION OF SEIZURES AND EPILEPSIES

Seizures have been grouped in several ways: according to their presumed etiology, i.e., idiopathic (primary) or symptomatic (secondary); their site of origin; their clinical form (generalized or focal); their frequency (isolated, cyclic, or repetitive, or the closely spaced sequence of status epilepticus); or by special electrophysiologic correlates. A distinction must be made between the classification of *seizures* (the clinical manifestations of epilepsy: generalized tonic clonic (grand mal), absence (petit mal), myoclonic, partial, and others), and the classification of the *epilepsies*, or *epileptic syndromes*, which are specific diseases, most of which may manifest several seizure types. These are discussed later in the chapter. A further distinction is made by clinical and EEG features. This approach allows for the reasonable predictability of response to specific medications and to some extent, in prognosis. Basically, this classification divides seizures into two types—*focal (formerly termed partial)*, in which a focal or localized onset can be discerned clinically or by EEG, and *generalized*, in which the seizures appear to begin bilaterally.

Generalized seizures are of two types—*convulsive* and *nonconvulsive*. (This dichotomy is not part of the main classification, but it is fundamental.) The common convulsive type is the *tonic-clonic (grand mal) seizure*. Less common is a purely tonic, purely clonic, or clonic-tonic-clonic generalized seizure. The typical nonconvulsive generalized seizure is the brief lapse of consciousness or absence (*petit mal*); included also under this heading are minor motor phenomena such as brief myoclonic, atonic, or tonic seizures.

The classification followed here was first proposed by Gastaut in 1970 and has been refined repeatedly by the Commission on Classification and Terminology of the International League Against Epilepsy. This nomenclature, based mainly on the clinical form of the seizure, and its electroencephalographic (EEG) features, has been adopted worldwide and is generally referred to as the "International Classification". A modified version of it is reproduced in Table 16-1.

It is also useful clinically, and etiologically to separate epilepsies that originate as truly generalized electrical discharges in the brain from those that spread secondarily from a focus to become generalized. The *primary generalized epilepsies* are a group of somewhat diverse, age-dependent phenotypes that are characterized by generalized 2.5- to 4-Hz bifrontally predominant spikes or polyspike-and-slow-wave discharges that arise without underlying structural abnormalities. In most instances, these individuals have normal intelligence. What is most significant is that a genetic component underlies many of these disorders. By contrast, epilepsies manifesting as

Table 16-1

INTERNATIONAL CLASSIFICATION OF EPILEPTIC SEIZURES

I. Generalized seizures (bilaterally symmetrical and without focal onset)
  A. Tonic, clonic, or tonic-clonic (grand mal)
  B. Absence (petit mal)
    1. typical
    2. atypical
    3. special features
      a. eyelid myoclonia
      b. myoclonic absence
  C. Clonic
  D. Tonic
  E. Atonic
  F. Myoclonic including atonic and tonic types
II. Focal (formerly "partial"); characterized by main feature(s). See Table 16-2
  A. Simple (*without* loss of consciousness or alteration in psychic function)
    1. Aura; somatosensory or special sensory (visual, auditory, olfactory, gustatory, vertiginous)
    2. Motor
    3. Autonomic
    4. Awareness retained (formerly ("simple") or impaired (formerly "complex")
III. Unclassifiable; cannot be characterized as focal, generalized or both, including epileptic spasms

Table 16-2

COMMON FOCAL SEIZURE PATTERNS

CLINICAL TYPE	LOCALIZATION
Somatic motor	
Jacksonian (focal motor)	Prerolandic gyrus
Masticatory, salivation, speech arrest	Amygdaloid nuclei, opercular
Simple contraversive	Frontal
Head and eye turning associated with arm movement or athetoid-dystonic postures	Supplementary motor cortex
Somatic and special sensory (auras)	
Somatosensory	Contralateral postrolandic
Unformed images, lights, patterns	Occipital
Auditory	Heschl gyri
Vertiginous	Superior temporal
Olfactory	Mesial temporal
Gustatory	Insula
Visceral: autonomic	Insular-orbital-frontal cortex
Focal seizure with altered consciousness	
Formed hallucinations	Temporal neocortex or amygdaloid–hippocampal complex
Illusions	—
Dyscognitive experiences (déjà vu, dreamy states, depersonalization)	—
Affective states (fear, depression, or elation)	Temporal
Automatism (ictal and postictal)	Temporal and frontal
Staring	Frontal cortex, amygdaloid–hippocampal complex, reticular–cortical system

Source: Modified by permission from Penfield and Jasper.

seizures that begin locally and may evolve into generalized tonic-clonic seizures, termed *secondarily generalized tonic clonic seizures* (termed bilateral convulsive in Fig. 16-1), generally have no such genetic component and are usually the result of underlying brain disease, either acquired or a result of congenital malformations or metabolic defects. Quite often, the initial focal phase is not appreciated, leading to misdiagnosis. An increasing frequency and severity of this group of disorders with age reflects the accumulation of focal cerebral damage from trauma, strokes, and other damage.

Focal seizures are further classified according to their additional features such as a specific subjective experience (*aura*), motor, autonomic, and most importantly, whether awareness or consciousness is disturbed; the latter was formerly called *partial complex seizure*. A prominent component of such seizures is a dyscognitive state. In reality, an aura represents the initial phase of a focal seizure; in some instances, it may constitute the entire epileptic attack.

The classification of seizures and of the epilepsies is constantly being modified. In an older but still useful version, the so-called syndromic classification (*Epilepsia* 30:389, 1989), an attempt had been made to incorporate all of the seizure types and epileptic syndromes and to categorize them not only as partial and generalized but also according to their age of onset, their primary (generalized) or secondary nature, the evidence of cortical loci of the epileptogenic lesions, and the many clinical settings in which they occur. This classification is semantically difficult and, in our view, too complicated for general clinical application; it has been replaced with current classifications already mentioned. Because many epileptic syndromes share overlapping features, it is often not possible to fit a newly diagnosed case of epilepsy into a specific category in this new classification. The Commission is continuously engaged in revision of terminology and classification in the field of epilepsy.

We begin our discussion with a practical approximation of the most recent classification that was given in 2010 (see Berg and colleagues) and is shown in Fig. 16-1, followed by consideration of a number of well-defined epilepsies and epileptic syndromes.

It is also useful to view the various types of seizures and epilepsies in the context of the age at which they occur. A proposed current classification based on the age of onset of the seizure disorder is shown in Fig. 16-2, and the distribution of the seizure types for each age epoch, obtained and aggregated from several sources is shown in Fig. 16-3. There has also been substantial progress in defining the molecular basis of familial and hereditary epilepsies over the last decade; it is likely that these insights will lead to modification of both the clinical classifications and management of the epilepsies.

GENERALIZED SEIZURES

Generalized Tonic-Clonic Seizures (Grand Mal)

In the common primary type of seizure, most often a convulsion starts with little or no warning. Sometimes the patient senses the approach of a seizure by several subjective phenomena (*prodrome*) even prior to an epileptic aura, which represents a focal seizure. For some hours, the patient may feel apathetic, depressed, irritable, or,

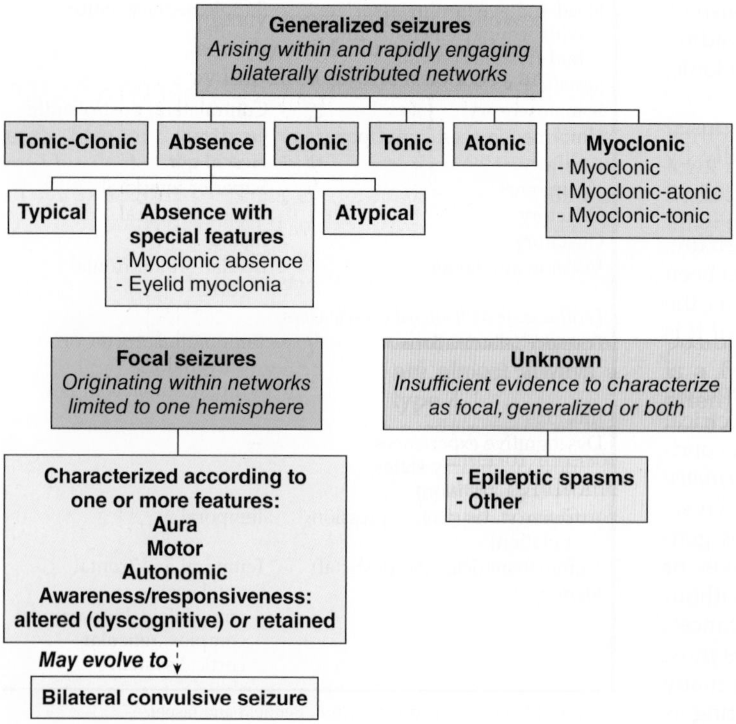

Figure 16-1. ILAE proposal for revised terminology for organization of seizures and epilepsies 2010 classification of seizures. (From http://www.ilae.org/Visitors/Centre/ctf/documents/ILAEHandoutV10_000.pdf/.)

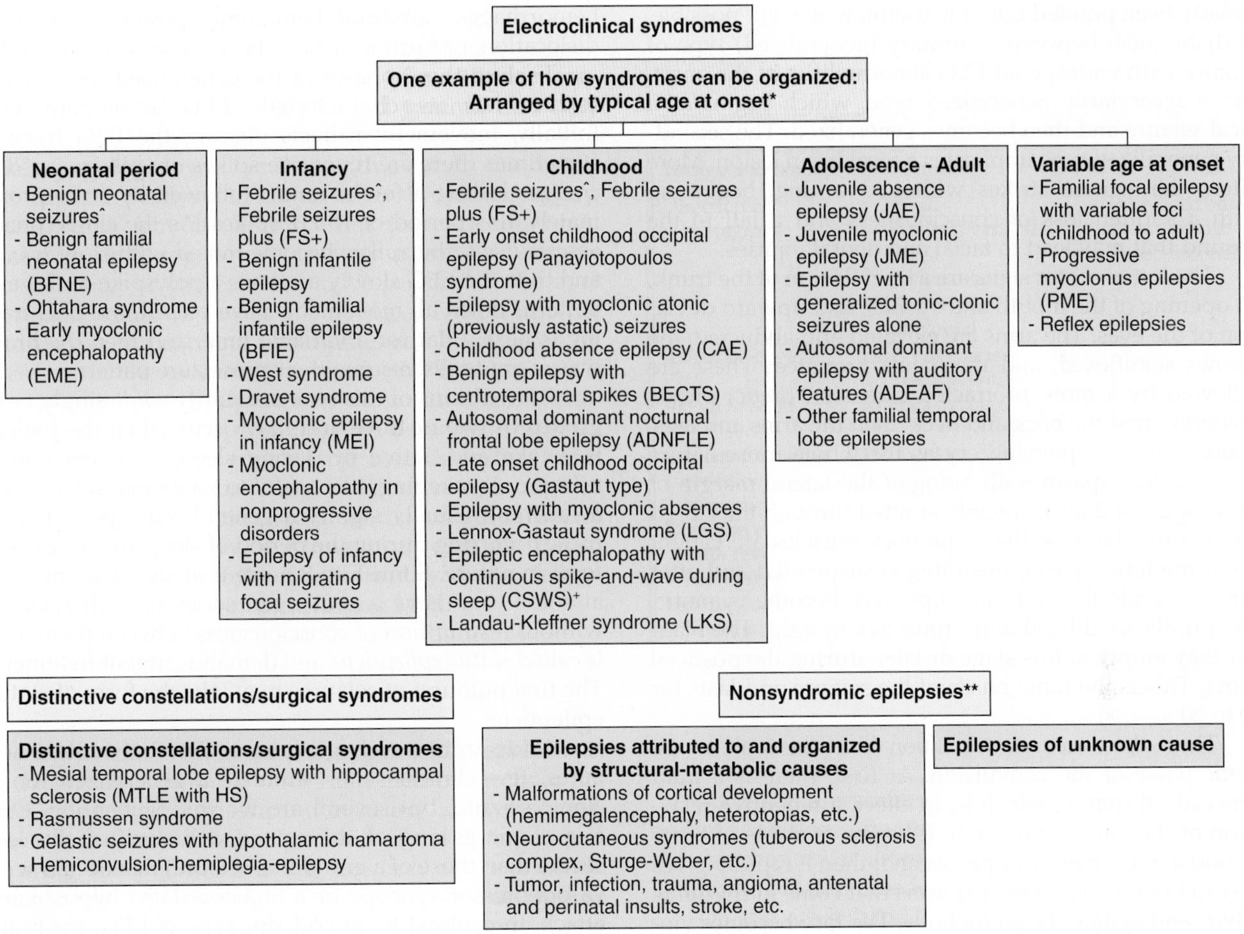
Electroclinical syndromes
One example of how syndromes can be organized: Arranged by typical age at onset*
Neonatal period
- Benign neonatal seizures^
- Benign familial neonatal epilepsy (BFNE)
- Ohtahara syndrome
- Early myoclonic encephalopathy (EME)
Infancy
- Febrile seizures^, Febrile seizures plus (FS+)
- Benign infantile epilepsy
- Benign familial infantile epilepsy (BFIE)
- West syndrome
- Dravet syndrome
- Myoclonic epilepsy in infancy (MEI)
- Myoclonic encephalopathy in nonprogressive disorders
- Epilepsy of infancy with migrating focal seizures
Childhood
- Febrile seizures^, Febrile seizures plus (FS+)
- Early onset childhood occipital epilepsy (Panayiotopoulos syndrome)
- Epilepsy with myoclonic atonic (previously astatic) seizures
- Childhood absence epilepsy (CAE)
- Benign epilepsy with centrotemporal spikes (BECTS)
- Autosomal dominant nocturnal frontal lobe epilepsy (ADNFLE)
- Late onset childhood occipital epilepsy (Gastaut type)
- Epilepsy with myoclonic absences
- Lennox-Gastaut syndrome (LGS)
- Epileptic encephalopathy with continuous spike-and-wave during sleep (CSWS)+
- Landau-Kleffner syndrome (LKS)
Adolescence - Adult
- Juvenile absence epilepsy (JAE)
- Juvenile myoclonic epilepsy (JME)
- Epilepsy with generalized tonic-clonic seizures alone
- Autosomal dominant epilepsy with auditory features (ADEAF)
- Other familial temporal lobe epilepsies
Variable age at onset
- Familial focal epilepsy with variable foci (childhood to adult)
- Progressive myoclonus epilepsies (PME)
- Reflex epilepsies
Distinctive constellations/surgical syndromes
Nonsyndromic epilepsies**
Distinctive constellations/surgical syndromes
- Mesial temporal lobe epilepsy with hippocampal sclerosis (MTLE with HS)
- Rasmussen syndrome
- Gelastic seizures with hypothalamic hamartoma
- Hemiconvulsion-hemiplegia-epilepsy
Epilepsies attributed to and organized by structural-metabolic causes
- Malformations of cortical development (hemimegalencephaly, heterotopias, etc.)
- Neurocutaneous syndromes (tuberous sclerosis complex, Sturge-Weber, etc.)
- Tumor, infection, trauma, angioma, antenatal and perinatal insults, stroke, etc.
Epilepsies of unknown cause

Figure 16-2. ILAE proposal for revised terminology for organization of seizures and epilepsies 2010 electroclinical syndromes and other epilepsies grouped by specificity of diagnosis. (From http://www.ilae.org/Visitors/Centre/ctf/documents/ILAEHandoutV10_000.pdf.)

rarely, the opposite—ecstatic. In a patient with generalized epilepsy (juvenile myoclonic epilepsy being one typical type), one or more myoclonic jerks of the trunk or limbs on awakening may herald a seizure later in the day. Abdominal pains or cramps, a sinking, rising, or gripping feeling in the epigastrium, pallor or redness of the face, throbbing headache, constipation, or diarrhea have been given prodromal status, but they do not occur consistently enough to be predictive of an oncoming seizure.

In more than half of cases of generalized seizure, there is some type of movement for a few seconds before consciousness is lost (turning of the head and eyes or whole body or intermittent jerking of a limb), although the patient often fails to form a memory of this and such information is obtained only from an observer. As has

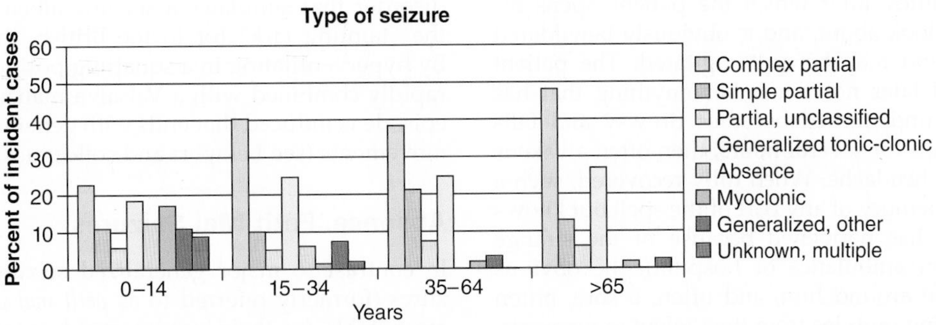

Figure 16-3. The distribution of the main types of epilepsy by age. The overrepresentation of absence and myoclonic seizures in childhood and of complex partial seizures in older individuals is evident. (Adapted from Hauser and Annegers and the texts of Engel and of Pedley.)

already been pointed out, it is useful, whenever possible, to distinguish between a primary (generalized) type of seizure with widespread EEG abnormalities at the onset, and a secondarily generalized type, which begins as a focal seizure and then becomes generalized. The secondary generalized type implicates a focal brain lesion. More often, the seizure strikes without warning, beginning with a sudden loss of consciousness and a fall to the ground that may lead to facial and dental injuries.

The initial motor signs are a brief flexion of the trunk, an opening of the mouth and eyelids, and upward deviation of the eyes. The arms are elevated and abducted, the elbows semiflexed, and the hands pronated. These are followed by a more protracted extension (*tonic*) phase, involving first the back and neck, then the arms and legs. There may be a piercing cry as the whole musculature is seized in a spasm with biting of the lateral margin of the tongue, and air is forcibly emitted through the closed vocal cords. Because the respiratory muscles are caught up in the tonic spasm, breathing is suspended and after some seconds the skin and lips may become cyanotic. The pupils are dilated and unreactive to light. The bladder may empty at this stage or later, during the postictal coma. This is the tonic phase of the seizure and lasts for 10 to 20 s.

There then occurs a transition from the tonic to the *clonic phase* of the convulsion. At first, there is a mild generalized tremor, which is, in effect, a repetitive relaxation of the tonic contraction. It begins at a rate of 8 per second and coarsens to 4 per second; then it rapidly gives way to brief, violent flexor spasms that come in rhythmic salvos and agitate the entire body. The face becomes violaceous and contorted by a series of grimaces. Autonomic signs are prominent: the pulse is rapid, blood pressure is elevated, pupils are dilated, and salivation and sweating are prominent; bladder pressure may increase sixfold during this phase. The clonic jerks decrease in amplitude and frequency over a period of about 30 s. The patient remains apneic until the end of the clonic phase, which is often marked by a deep inspiration. Instead of the whole dramatic sequence described above, the seizures may be abbreviated or limited in scope by anticonvulsive medications.

In the terminal phase of the seizure, all movements have ended and the patient is motionless and limp in a deep coma. The pupils now begin to contract to light. Breathing may be quiet or stertorous. This state persists for several minutes, after which the patient opens his eyes, begins to look about, and is obviously bewildered and confused and may be quite agitated. The patient may speak and later not remember anything that has been said and undisturbed becomes drowsy and falls asleep, sometimes for several hours, then often awakens with a pulsatile headache. When fully recovered, such a patient has no memory of any part of the spell but knows that something has happened because of the strange surroundings (in ambulance or hospital), the obvious concern of those around him, and often, a sore, bitten tongue and aching muscles from the violent movements. The contractions, if violent enough, may crush a vertebral body or result in a serious injury; a fracture, periorbital hemorrhages, subdural hematoma, posterior shoulder dislocation, or burn may have been sustained in the fall.

Each of these phases of the generalized tonic-clonic seizure has its characteristic EEG accompaniment. Initially, movement artifacts obscure the EEG tracing; sometimes there are repetitive spikes or spike-wave discharges lasting a few seconds, followed by an approximately 10-s period of 10-Hz spikes. As the clonic phase asserts itself, the spikes become mixed with slow waves and then the EEG slowly assumes a polyspike-and-wave pattern. When all movements have ceased, the EEG tracing is nearly flat for a variable time, and then the brain waves gradually resume their preseizure pattern.

Convulsions of this type ordinarily come singly or in groups of two or three and may occur when the patient is awake and active or during sleep, or when falling asleep or awakening. It is useful to know that seizures on awakening usually signify a generalized type, whereas those occurring during the period of sleep are more often focal in nature. Some 5 to 8 percent of such patients will at some time have a prolonged series of such seizures without resumption of consciousness between them; this is called *status epilepticus* and demands urgent treatment. The first outburst of seizures may take the form of status epilepticus.

Aside from psychogenic episodes that imitate seizures, few clinical states simulate a generalized tonic-clonic seizure, but several are worthy of mention. One is a clonic jerking of the extended limbs (usually less severe than those of a grand mal seizure) that occurs with vasodepressor syncope or a Stokes-Adams hypotensive attack. In contrast to an epileptic type of EEG, the brain waves are slow in frequency and low in amplitude during the jerking movements. A rarer phenomenon that may be indistinguishable from a generalized convulsion occurs as part of the syndrome of basilar artery occlusion. This presumably has its basis in ischemia of the corticospinal tracts in the pons (Ropper); a similar ischemic mechanism in the cortex has been invoked for "limb-shaking TIAs" (transient ischemic attacks), in which there are clonic movements of one limb or one side of the body during an episode of cerebral ischemia. Clonic limb movements occur immediately after a traumatic concussion and an observer who arrives at this moment will be unable to determine if the inciting event was a seizure or a collision. In infants, a breath-holding spell may closely simulate the tonic phase of a generalized seizure. Another disorder that simulates a seizure, albeit self-induced, is the "fainting lark" (or in the British, the 'mess trick)." By hyperventilating in a squatting position and standing rapidly combined with a Valsalva maneuver, a syncopal episode is induced that ends with generalized convulsive movements (see Lempert and colleagues).

Absence, Petit Mal Seizures

In contrast to major generalized seizures, absence seizures (formerly referred to as *petit mal* or *pyknoepilepsy*) are notable for their brevity, rapid onset and cessation, and frequency and the paucity of motor activity. Indeed, they may be so brief that the patients themselves are sometimes not aware of them; to an onlooker, they resemble a moment of absentmindedness or daydreaming. The attack, coming without warning, consists of a sudden interruption of consciousness, for which the French word *absence* ("not present," "not in attendance") has been retained. The patient stares and briefly stops talking or ceases to respond. Only about 10 percent of such patients are completely motionless during the attack; in the remainder, one observes a brief burst of fine clonic (myoclonic) movements of the eyelids, facial muscles, or fingers or small synchronous movements of both arms, all at a rate of 3 per second. This rate corresponds to that of the EEG abnormality, which takes the form of a generalized 3-per-second spike-and-wave pattern (Fig. 2-3*E*). Absence seizures are said to be "typical" if they have a rapid onset and offset, typical three per second spike and wave, and complete loss of awareness.

Minor automatisms—in the form of lip-smacking, chewing, and fumbling movements of the fingers—are common during an attack but may be subtle. Postural tone may be slightly decreased or increased, and occasionally there is a mild vasomotor disorder. As a rule, such patients do not fall; they may even continue complex acts such as walking or riding a bicycle. After 2 to 10 s, occasionally longer, the patient reestablishes full contact with the environment and resumes his preseizure activity. Only a loss of the thread of conversation or the place in reading betrays the occurrence of the momentary "blank" period (the absence). In many such patients, voluntary hyperventilation for 2 to 3 min is an effective way of inducing absence attacks.

Typical absence seizures constitute the most characteristic epilepsy of childhood ("childhood absence"); rarely do the seizures begin before 4 years of age or after puberty. Another attribute is their great frequency (hence, the old term *pykno*, meaning "compact" or "dense"). As many as several hundred may occur in a single day, sometimes in bursts at certain consistent times of the day. They produce periods of inattention and may appear in the classroom when the child is sitting quietly rather than participating actively in his lessons. If frequent, they disturb attention and thinking to the point that the child's performance in school is impaired. Less frequently, such attacks may last for hours with no interval of normal mental activity between them—so-called *absence* or *petit mal status*. Absence epilepsy of adolescent onset ("juvenile absence") does not have the very high seizure frequency of the childhood type. Cases of absence status have also been described in adults with frontal lobe epilepsy (see below). In contrast to childhood absence seizures, the disorder may last well into adulthood and be punctuated by generalized tonic-clonic seizures or a burst of seizures. Akinesia (motionlessness) is not unique to any seizure type.

The typical absence, with or without myoclonic jerks, rarely causes the patient to fall. Absence should be considered a separate entity because of its relative benignity. It may be the only type of seizure during childhood. The attacks tend to diminish in frequency in adolescence and then often disappear, only to be replaced in many instances by major generalized seizures. About one-third of children with absence attacks will, in addition, display symmetrical or asymmetrical myoclonic jerks without loss of consciousness, and about half will at some time have major generalized (tonic-clonic) convulsions.

Absence Variants

Distinguished from typical absence seizures are variants in which the loss of consciousness is less complete or in which myoclonus is prominent, and others in which the EEG abnormalities are less regularly of a 3-per-second spike-and-wave type (they may occur at the rate of 2 to 2.5 per second or take the form of irregular 4- to 6-Hz polyspike-and-wave complexes). *Atypical absence* is a term that was introduced to describe long runs of slow spike-and-wave activity, usually with no apparent loss of consciousness. External stimuli, such as asking the patient to answer a question or to count, interrupt the run of abnormal EEG activity. The current classification (Fig. 16-1) separates the disorder into groups that are identified as typical, atypical, and having special features, namely, myoclonic jerks or eyelid myoclonus.

Lennox-Gastaut Syndrome

In sharp contrast to the typical absence epilepsies, is a form that has its onset between 2 and 6 years of age and is characterized by atonic, or astatic, seizures (i.e., falling attacks), often succeeded by various combinations of minor motor, tonic-clonic, and partial seizures and by progressive intellectual impairment in association with a distinctive, slow (1- to 2-Hz) spike-and-wave EEG pattern. This is the *Lennox-Gastaut syndrome*. Often it is preceded in earlier life by infantile spasms, a characteristic high-amplitude chaotic EEG picture ("hypsarrhythmia"), and an arrest in mental development, a triad sometimes referred to as the *West syndrome* (see further on). The early onset of atonic seizures with abrupt falls, injuries, and associated abnormalities nearly always has a grave implication—namely, the presence of serious neurologic disease. Prematurity, perinatal injury and metabolic diseases of infancy are the most common underlying conditions. This is essentially a form of symptomatic generalized epilepsy, in contrast to the foregoing idiopathic types such as typical absence epilepsy (petit mal). The Lennox-Gastaut syndrome may persist into adult life and is one of the most difficult forms of epilepsy to treat.

Myoclonic Seizures

The phenomenon of myoclonus was discussed in Chap. 6, where the relationship to seizures was emphasized. Characterized by a brusque, brief, muscular contraction, some myoclonic jerks may be so small as to involve only one muscle or part of a muscle; others are so large as to displace a limb on one or both sides of the body or the entire trunk musculature. Many are brief, lasting 50 to 100 ms; they may occur intermittently and unpredictably or present as a single jerk or a brief salvo.

As mentioned earlier, a series of several small, rhythmic myoclonic jerks may appear with varying frequency as part of atypical absence seizures, and as isolated events in patients with generalized clonic-tonic-clonic or tonic-clonic seizures. As a rule, seizure-associated myoclonus, when occurring in isolation, is relatively benign and usually responds well to medication. In contrast, there are diseases in which myoclonus is progressive in severity or very frequent. These disorders have their onset in childhood and raise the suspicion of entities such as the myoclonus-opsoclonus-ataxia syndrome, lithium or other drug toxicity or, if lasting a few weeks, subacute sclerosing panencephalitis. Chronic progressive polymyoclonus with dementia characterizes the group of juvenile lipidosis, Lafora-type familial myoclonic epilepsy, certain mitochondrial disorders, and other chronic familial degenerative diseases of undefined type (paramyoclonus multiplex of Friedreich) as noted in Table 16-3.

The large number of adult diseases causative of myoclonus and seizure disorders are discussed in Chaps. 33, 37, and 39. Myoclonus as a phenomenon is described in Chap. 6.

Juvenile Myoclonic Epilepsy

This is the most common form of idiopathic generalized epilepsy in older children and young adults. It begins in adolescence, typically around age 15 years, with a range that essentially spans all of the teenage years. The patient comes to attention because of a generalized tonic-clonic seizure, often upon awakening or because of myoclonic jerks in the morning that involve the entire body; sometimes absence seizures are prominent. The family reports that the patient has occasional myoclonic jerks of the arm and upper trunk that is brought out with fatigue, early stages of sleep, or alcohol ingestion. A few patients in our experience have had only the myoclonic phenomena and rare absence or tonic-clonic seizures that persisted unnoticed for years. The EEG shows characteristic bursts of 4- to 6-Hz irregular polyspike activity. A linkage has been established to chromosome 6 in some cases of this illness, and in some other forms of juvenile-onset epilepsy, and several are the result of mutations in ion channel genes.

The disorder does not impair intelligence and tends not to be progressive, for which reason it has been called "benign", but a proclivity to infrequent seizures usually continues throughout life. A report by Bakan and colleagues has indicated that, over an average of two decades, the majority of patients have long seizure-free periods and a great reduction in myoclonic seizures. Valproic acid in particular and some other antiepileptic drugs are highly effective in eliminating the seizures and myoclonus but they should be continued indefinitely as discontinuation of medication is associated with a high rate of relapse. Owing to the potential teratogenicity of valproate, women of childbearing age are often given levitiracetam or lamotrigine, acknowledging that they may not be as effective as the first choice of drug.

FOCAL SEIZURES

As indicated earlier, the International Classification divides all seizures into two types—generalized, in which the clinical and EEG manifestations indicate bilateral and diffuse cerebral cortical involvement from the onset, and focal, in which the seizure is often the product of a demonstrable focal lesion or EEG abnormality in some part of the cerebral cortex. Partial seizures vary with the locale of the lesion and are conventionally qualified based their specific clinical characteristics and on whether consciousness is retained or impaired. Focal seizures with sensory or motor features at the onset most often arise from foci in the sensorimotor cortex. Those with impairment of consciousness, which occurs in many forms, most often have their focus in the limbic and autonomic areas or in the temporal lobe, but a frontal localization is also known. Table 16-2, on a previous page, lists the common sites of the lesions and the types of seizures to which they give rise.

Relatively few focal seizures can be localized precisely from clinical data alone. However, when combined with scalp and intracranial EEG recording and MRI, the localization is reasonably accurate.

Frontal Lobe Seizures (Focal Motor and Jacksonian Seizures)

Focal or partial motor seizures are attributable to a discharging lesion of the frontal lobe. The most common type, originating in the supplementary motor area, takes the form of a turning movement of the head and eyes to the side opposite the irritative focus, often associated with a tonic extension of limbs, also on the side contralateral to the affected hemisphere. This may constitute the entire seizure, or it may be followed by generalized clonic movements. The extension of the limbs may occur just before or simultaneously with loss of consciousness but a lesion in one frontal lobe may give rise to a major generalized convulsion without an initial turning of the head and eyes. It has been postulated that in both types of seizures, the one with and the one without turning movements, there is an immediate spread of the discharge from the frontal lobe to integrating centers in the thalamic or high midbrain reticular formation, accounting for the loss of consciousness.

The frontal lobe, being so large, can give rise to numerous forms of seizure. In addition to the typical Jacksonian type described above, there are adversive, speech arrest, frontal, absence types, and a number of unusual disorders related to discharges from the supplementary motor area including hyperkinetic and postural tonic varieties. In practice, it is often difficult to distinguish such seizures from parasomnic (sleep related) events (see Chap. 18).

Jacksonian seizures begin with forceful, sustained deviation of the head and eyes, and sometimes of the entire body, are referred to as *versive* or *adversive*. Because the turning movements are usually to the side opposite the irritative focus (sometimes to the same side), *contraversive* and *ipsiversive*, respectively, might be preferable terms. Nonforceful, unsustained, or seemingly random lateral head movements during the ictus do not have localizing value. The same is true for the head and eye turning that occurs at the end of the generalized tonic-clonic phase of seizures (Wylie et al). Contraversive deviation of only the head and eyes can

Table 16-3

MONOGENIC EPILEPTIC DISORDERS

	GENE	PROTEIN INVOLVED
Channelopathies		
Sodium channels		
Familial generalized seizures with febrile seizures "plus"; see text	SCN1A,B, ($GABA_A$)	Sodium channel subunits; less often, GABA receptor
Benign familial neonatal convulsions	SCN2A	Sodium channel subunits
Dravet syndrome (severe myoclonic epilepsy of infancy)	SCN1A	Sodium channel α-subunit
Potassium channels		
Benign infantile epilepsy	KCNQ2,3	Potassium channel subunits
Episodic ataxia type 1 with partial epilepsy	KCNA1	
Ligand-gated channels		
Autosomal dominant nocturnal frontal seizures	CHRNA 2,4	Nicotinic acetylcholine receptor subunits
Familial generalized and febrile seizures	GABRG2	$GABA_A$ receptor subunit
Juvenile myoclonic epilepsy	GABRA1 (CACNB4)	$GABA_A$ receptor subunit; less often, calcium channel subunit
Glucose transporter-1 deficiency	SLC2A1	GLUT1 (responsive to ketogenic diet)
Calcium channels		
Episodic ataxia type 2 with spike-wave seizures	CACNA1A	Calcium channel subunit
Malformations of cortical development		
Holoprosencephaly, generalized epilepsy	SHH, PTCH, ZIC2, SIX3, TGIF	Sonic hedgehog, SHH receptor, transcription factors
Schizencephaly, generalized epilepsy	EMX2	Homeodomain protein
Tuberous sclerosis, generalized epilepsy	TSC1, 2	Hamartin, tuberin
Lissencephaly, generalized epilepsy	LIS1	Platelet-activating factor acid hydrolase
Double-cortex syndrome, generalized epilepsy	DCX	Doublecortin
Heterotopia, focal epilepsy	FLN1	Filamin1
Fukuyama muscular dystrophy, lissencephaly, generalized epilepsy	FCMD	Fukutin
Walker-Warburg syndrome, generalized epilepsy	POMT1	*O*-mannosyl transferase
Muscle-eye-brain disease, generalized epilepsy	MEB	Glycosyltransferase, PMGnT1
Angelman syndrome: myoclonic, tonic-clonic, atonic seizures	UBE3A	Ubiquitin-protein ligase
Progressive myoclonic epilepsies (PME)		
Unverricht-Lundborg disease with PME	EPM1	Cystatin B
Lafora body disease with PME	EPM2A	Laforin, protein tyrosine phosphatase
Myoclonic epilepsy with ragged red fibers	tRNAlys	Mitochondrial lysine tRNA
Dentatorubro-pallidoluysian atrophy with PME	DRPLA	Atrophin-1
Gaucher disease	PSAP	*β*-Glucocerebrosidase
Sialidosis type I	NEU1	Sialidase
Ceroid lipofuscinosis (CLN) and PME	CLN	CLN2, CLN3, CLN5, CLN6 also cause generalized, atonic and atypical absence seizures
Mixed seizure types		
Lipoid proteinosis and temporal lobe epilepsy	ECM1	Extracellular matrix protein 1
Autosomal dominant lateral temporal lobe epilepsy	LGI1	Leucine-rich glioma inactivated protein
CLN8; progressive nonmyoclonic epilepsy with retardation	CLN8	Membrane protein in endoplasmic reticulum
Pyridoxine deficiency	ALDH7A1	Antiquitin (ATQ-1)

be induced most consistently by electrical stimulation of the superolateral frontal region (area 8), just anterior to area 6 (see Figs. 22-1 and 22-2). In seizures of temporal lobe origin, early in the seizure, there may be head turning ipsilaterally followed by forceful, contraversive head (and body) turning. These head and body movements, if they occur, are preceded by quiet staring or automatisms.

The *Jacksonian motor seizure* may also begin with a tonic contraction of the fingers of one hand, the face on one side, or the muscles of one foot. This transforms into clonic movements in these parts in a fashion analogous to that in a generalized clonic-tonic-clonic convulsion. Sometimes a series of clonic movements of increasing frequency build up to a tonic contraction. The movements spread ("march") from the part first affected to other muscles on the same side of the body. In this typical Jacksonian form, the seizure spreads from the hand, up the arm, to the face, and down the leg; or if the first movement is in the foot, the seizure marches up the leg, down the arm, and to the face, usually in a matter of 20 to 30 s. Interestingly, spontaneously occurring focal motor seizures, e.g., those beginning in the toes or fingers, may sometimes be arrested (inhibited) by applying a ligature above the affected part or, in the case of focal sensory seizures, by applying a vigorous sensory stimulus ahead of the advancing sensory aura. Rarely, the first muscular contraction is in the abdomen, thorax, or neck. In some cases, the one-sided seizure activity is followed by turning of the head and eyes to the convulsing side, occasionally to the opposite side, and then by a generalized seizure with loss of consciousness. Consciousness is not lost if the sensorimotor symptoms remain confined to one side.

Following convulsions that have a prominent focal motor signature, there may be a transient paralysis of the affected limbs. This "Todd's paralysis" persists for minutes or at times for hours after the seizure, usually in proportion to the duration of the convulsion. Continued focal paralysis beyond this time usually indicates the presence of a focal brain lesion as the underlying cause of the seizure or persisting seizures in a nonconvulsive form. A similar Todd phenomenon is found in cases of focal epilepsy that involve the language, somesthetic, or visual areas; here the persistent deficit corresponds to the region of brain affected.

The high incidence of focal motor epilepsy that originates with movements in the face, hands, and toes is probably related to the disproportionately large cortical representation of these parts. The disease process or focus of excitation is usually in or near the rolandic (motor) cortex, i.e., area 4 of Brodmann (Figs. 3-3 and 22-2); in some cases, and especially if there is a sensory accompaniment, it has been found in the postrolandic convolution. Lesions confined to the motor cortex are reported to assume the form of clonic contractions, and those confined to the premotor cortex (area 6), tonic contractions of the contralateral arm, face, neck, or all of one side of the body. Tonic elevation and extension of the contralateral arm ("fencing posture") and choreoathetotic and dystonic postures have been associated with high medial frontal lesions (area 8 and supplementary motor cortex), as have complex, bizarre, and flailing movements of a contralateral limb, but this always raises the suspicion of hysterical seizure. Perspiration and piloerection occur occasionally in parts of the body involved in a focal motor seizure, suggesting that these autonomic functions have a cortical representation in or adjacent to the rolandic area. Focal motor and Jacksonian seizures have essentially the same localizing significance.

Seizure discharges arising from the cortical language areas may give rise to a brief aphasic disturbance (*ictal aphasia*) and ejaculation of a word or, more frequently, a vocal arrest. Ictal aphasia is usually succeeded by other focal or generalized seizure activity but may occur in isolation, without loss of consciousness, in which case it can later be described by the patient. Postictal aphasia is more common than ictal aphasia, which typically takes the form of complete speech arrest. Verbalization at the onset of a seizure has no consistent lateralizing significance and, paradoxically, is usually associated with an origin in the nondominant hemisphere. These disturbances should be distinguished from the stereotyped repetition of words or phrases or the garbled speech that characterizes some complex partial seizures or the postictal confusional state and, of course, Wernicke aphasia.

Somatosensory, Visual, and Other Types of Sensory Seizures

Somatosensory seizures, either focal or "marching" to other parts of the body on one side, are nearly always indicative of a focus in or near the postrolandic convolution of the opposite cerebral hemisphere. Penfield and Kristiansen found the seizure focus in the postcentral or precentral convolution in 49 of 55 such cases. The sensory disorder is usually described as numbness, tingling, or a "pins-and-needles" feeling and occasionally as a sensation of crawling (formication), electricity, or movement of the part. Pain and thermal sensations may occur but are exceedingly rare. In the majority of cases, the onset of the sensory seizure is in the lips, fingers, or toes, and the spread to adjacent parts of the body follows a pattern determined by sensory arrangements in the postcentral (postrolandic) convolution of the parietal lobe. If the sensory symptoms are localized to the head, the focus is in or adjacent to the lowest part of the convolution, near the sylvian fissure; if the symptoms are in the leg or foot, the upper part of the convolution, near the superior sagittal sinus or on the medial surface of the hemisphere, is involved.

Olfactory hallucinations, perhaps the most important of the sensory seizures because they signify a particular localization, are associated with disease of the inferior and medial parts of the temporal lobe, usually in the region of the parahippocampal convolution or the uncus (hence Jackson's term *uncinate seizures* [see also Chap. 12]). Usually the perceived odor is exteriorized, i.e., projected to someplace in the environment, and is described as disagreeable or foul, though otherwise unidentifiable. *Gustatory hallucinations* also have been recorded in proven cases of temporal lobe disease and less often with lesions of the insula and parietal operculum; salivation and a sensation of thirst may be associated. Electrical stimulation in the depths of the sylvian fissure, extending into the insular region, has produced peculiar sensations of taste.

Visual seizures are relatively rare but also have localizing significance. Lesions in or near the striate cortex of the occipital lobe usually produce elemental visual sensations of darkness or sparks and flashes of light, which may be stationary or moving and colorless or colored. According to Gowers, red is the most frequently reported color, followed by blue, green, and yellow. These images may be referred to the visual field on the side opposite of the lesion or may appear straight ahead. If they occur on one side of the visual field, patients perceive that only one eye is affected (the one opposite the lesion), probably because most persons are aware of only the temporal half of a homonymous field defect. Curiously, a seizure arising in one occipital lobe may cause momentary blindness in both fields. It has been noted that lesions on the lateral surface of the occipital lobe (Brodmann areas 18 and 19) are likely to cause a sensation of twinkling or pulsating lights. More complex or formed visual hallucinations are usually caused by a focus in the posterior part of the temporal lobe, near its junction with the occipital lobe, and may be associated with auditory hallucinations. The localizing value of visual auras has been confirmed by Bien and colleagues in a group of 20 surgically treated patients with intractable seizures. They found that elementary visual hallucinations and visual loss were typical of occipital lobe epilepsy but could also occur with seizure foci in the anteromedial temporal and occipitotemporal regions.

Auditory hallucinations are infrequent as an initial manifestation of a seizure and usually represent a psychotic disorder or one of several more benign conditions. Occasionally, a patient with a focus in one superior temporal convolution will report a buzzing or roaring in the ears. A human voice, sometimes repeating unrecognizable words, or the sound of music has been noted a few times with lesions in the more posterior part of one temporal lobe. Some people with epilepsy and a strong family history of seizures with auditory auras, may have normal imaging but turn out to have mutations in the LGI1 gene.

Vertiginous sensations of a type suggesting a vestibular origin may on rare occasions be the first symptom of a seizure. The lesion is usually located in the superoposterior temporal region or the junction between parietal and temporal lobes. In one of the cases reported by Penfield and Jasper, a sensation of vertigo was evoked by stimulating the cortex at the junction of the parietal and occipital lobes. Occasionally with a temporal focus, the vertigo is followed by an auditory sensation. Giddiness, or light-headedness, is a frequent prelude to a seizure, but this symptom, as discussed in Chap. 15, has so many different connotations that it is of little diagnostic value.

Vague and often indefinable *visceral sensations* arising in the thorax, epigastrium, and abdomen are among the most frequent of auras, as already indicated. Most often they have a temporal lobe origin, although in several such cases the seizure discharge has been localized to the upper bank of the sylvian fissure, in the upper or middle frontal gyrus, or in the medial frontal area near the cingulate gyrus. Palpitation and acceleration of the heart rate at the beginning of the attack have also been related mainly to a temporal lobe focus.

Focal Seizures Characterized by Altered Awareness or Responsiveness (Formerly Termed Complex Partial Seizures, Psychomotor Seizures, Temporal Lobe Seizures)

These differ from the major generalized and absence seizures discussed above in that (1) they signify a focal onset in the temporal lobe as reflected by an aura that may be a hallucination or perceptual illusion, and (2) instead of a complete loss of control of thought and action, there is a period of altered behavior and consciousness, for which the patient is later found to be amnesic.

Although it is difficult to enumerate all the psychic experiences that may occur during these types of seizures, they may be categorized into a somewhat arbitrary hierarchy of illusions, hallucinations, depersonalization states, and affective experiences. Sensory illusions, or distortions of ongoing perceptions, are the most common. Objects or persons in the environment may shrink or recede into the distance, or they may enlarge (micropsia and macropsia), or perseverate as the head is moved (palinopsia). Tilting of the visual environment has been reported. Hallucinations are most often visual or auditory, consisting of formed or unformed visual images, sounds, and voices; less frequently, they may be olfactory (usually unpleasant, unidentifiable sensations of smell), gustatory, or vertiginous. Among the altered psychic states are a feeling of intense perception of familiarity in an unfamiliar circumstance or place (déjà vu) or, conversely, of strangeness or unfamiliarity (jamais vu) in a previously known place or circumstance. There may be the experience of autoscopy, a type of depersonalization, or dream-like state in which the patient views himself as an external observer. Fragments of certain old memories or scenes may insert themselves into the patient's mind and recur with striking clarity, or there may be an abrupt interruption of memory. (See Gloor for a more detailed description of the experiential phenomena of temporal lobe epilepsy.) Associated epigastric and abdominal sensations have been alluded to above and likely have their origin in autonomic and limbic structures.

Emotional experiences as a result of seizure, while less common, may be dramatic—fear, sadness, loneliness, anger, happiness, and sexual excitement have all been recorded. Fear and anxiety are the most common affective experiences, while occasionally the patient describes a feeling of rage or intense anger as part of a complex partial seizure. Ictal fear has no apparent connection to objective experience and is generally not related to the situation in which the patient finds himself during the seizure.

Each of these subjective psychic states may constitute the entire seizure or some combination may occur and immediately precedes a period of altered awareness. These "auras" represent electrical seizures as already mentioned and have the same localizing significance as motor convulsions do for the frontal cortex.

The motor components of a focal temporal lobe or limbic seizure, if they occur, arise during the later phase of the seizure and take the form of *automatisms* such as lip-smacking, chewing or swallowing movements, salivation, fumbling of the hands, or shuffling of the feet. Patients may walk around in a daze or act inappropriately (undressing in public, speaking incoherently, etc.). Certain complex acts that were initiated before the loss of consciousness—such as walking, chewing food, turning the pages of a book, or even driving—may continue. However, when asked a specific question or given a command, the patients are obviously out of contact with their surroundings. There may be no response at all, or the patient may look toward the examiner in a perplexed way or utter a few stereotyped phrases. The patient may walk repetitively in small circles (*volvular epilepsy*), run (*epilepsia procursiva*), or simply wander aimlessly, either as an ictal or postictal phenomenon (*poriomania*). These forms of seizure, according to some epileptologists, are actually more common with frontal lobe than with temporal lobe foci of origin.

In a very small number of patients with temporal lobe seizures (7 of 123 patients studied by Ebner et al), some degree of responsiveness (to simple questions and motor commands) is preserved in the presence of prominent automatisms such as lip-smacking and swallowing. Interestingly, in this small group of partially responsive patients, the seizures originate in the right temporal lobe.

The patient, in a confused and irritable state, may resist or strike out at the examiner. These types of behaviors, which occur in a limited number of patients with temporal lobe or frontal seizures, usually take the form of nondirected oppositional resistance to restraint. These behaviors manifest during a period of automatic behavior (so called because the patient presumably acts like an automaton) or, more often, in the postictal period. Unprovoked assault or outbursts of intense rage or blind fury are very unusual; Currie and associates found such outbursts in only 16 of 666 patients (2.4 percent) with temporal lobe epilepsy. Penfield once commented that he had never observed a rage state as a result of temporal lobe stimulation. It is exceedingly unlikely that an organized violent act requiring several sequential steps in its performance, such as obtaining a weapon and using it in a directed manner, could represent a temporal lobe seizure.

Rarely, laughter may be the most striking feature of a seizure (*gelastic epilepsy*). A particular combination of gelastic seizures and precocious puberty has been traced to a hamartoma of the hypothalamus. Crying, on the other hand, is very infrequent as a component of seizure and usually indicates a psychogenically induced episode.

Dystonic stiffness of the arm and leg contralateral to the seizure focus is found to be an accompaniment of temporal lobe seizures (more often this is from the supplementary motor of the frontal than the temporal lobes).

The patient with temporal lobe seizures may exhibit only one of the foregoing manifestations of seizure activity or various combinations. In a series of 414 patients studied by Lennox, 43 percent displayed some of the motor changes; 32 percent, automatic behavior; and 25 percent, alterations in psychic function. Because of the frequent concurrence of these symptom complexes, he referred to them as the *psycho-motor triad*. Probably the clinical pattern varies with the precise locality of the lesion and the direction and extent of spread of the electrical discharge.

After the attack, the patient usually has no memory or only fragments of recall for what was said or done. Any type of complex partial seizures may proceed to other forms of secondary generalized seizures. The tendency to generalization holds true for all types of partial or focal epilepsy.

Temporal lobe seizures are not peculiar to any period of life, but they do show an increased incidence in adolescence and the adult years and have an uncertain relationship to febrile seizures. The topic of febrile seizures is broader than this association suggests; it is taken up in a later section of the chapter. Neonatal convulsions, head trauma, and various other non-progressive perinatal neurologic disorders are other antecedents that place a child at risk of developing complex partial seizures (Rocca et al). Two-thirds of patients with temporal lobe seizures also have generalized tonic-clonic seizures or have had them in early childhood, and it has been theorized that the generalized seizures may have led to secondary excitotoxic damage to the hippocampal portions of the temporal lobes. In the latter cases, carefully performed and quantitated MRI in the coronal plane may disclose a loss of volume in the hippocampi and adjacent gyri on one or both sides—i.e., *medial temporal sclerosis* (Fig. 16-4).

Temporal lobe seizures are highly variable in duration. Behavioral automatisms rarely last longer than a minute or two, although postictal confusion and amnesia may persist for a considerably longer time. Some consist only of a momentary change in facial expression and a blank spell, resembling an absence. Almost always, however, temporal lobe events are characterized by distinct ictal and postictal phases, whereas patients with absence attacks usually have an instantaneous return of full consciousness following the ictus.

Postictal behavior after temporal lobe seizures is often accompanied by widespread or focal slowing in the EEG. Prolonged disorientation for time and place suggests a right-sided source. Automatisms in the postictal period have no lateralizing connotation (Devinsky et al). However, postictal posturing and paresis of an arm (*Todd's paralysis*) or an aphasic difficulty are helpful in determining the side of the lesion (Cascino). Postictal nose wiping, which is reported on video recording to occur in half of patients with temporal lobe seizures, is carried out by the hand ipsilateral to the seizure focus according to Leutzmezer and colleagues, but we are in no position to confirm this.

Amnesic Seizures (Transient Epileptic Amnesia)

Rarely, recurrent attacks of transient amnesia are the only manifestations of temporal lobe epilepsy, although it is unclear whether the amnesia in such patients represents an ictal or postictal phenomenon. These attacks of pure amnesia have been referred to as *transient epileptic amnesia* (TEA; Palmini et al; Zeman et al). If the patient functions at a fairly high level during the attack, as may happen, there is a resemblance to transient global amnesia (described in Chap. 20). However, in contrast to transient global amnesia, the relative brevity and frequency of the amnesic spells, their tendency to occur on awakening, the impaired performance on complex cognitive tasks, and the absence of repetitive stereotyped questions help to make the distinction.

Behavioral and Psychiatric Disorders with Epilepsy

Some comments are in order concerning the issues of *behavioral* and *psychiatric disorders* in patients who have seizures. Data as to prevalence of these disorders have been

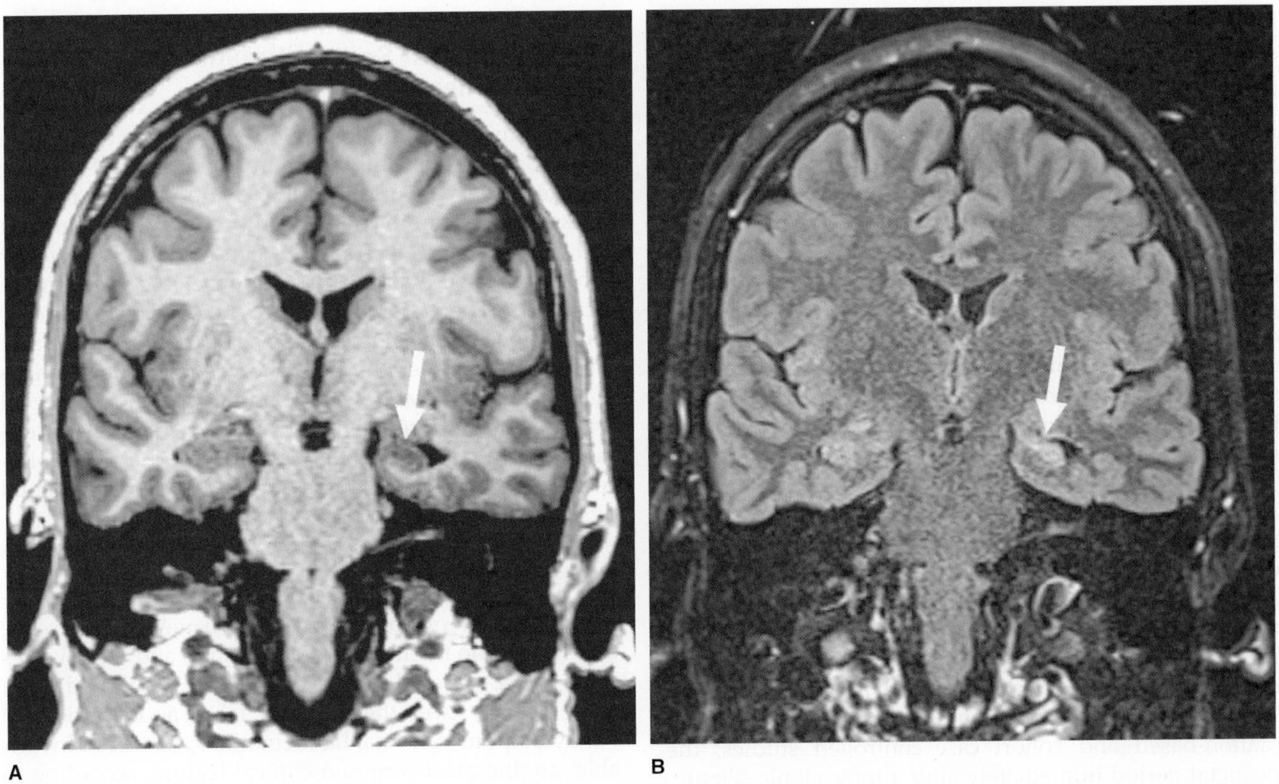

Figure 16-4. Medial temporal sclerosis. *A.* T1-weighted MRI in the coronal plane, showing reduced volume of the left hippocampus (*shown by arrow*) and secondary enlargement of the adjacent temporal horn of the lateral ventricle. *B.* Coronal T2-FLAIR image showing abnormal hyperintense signal within the left hippocampus (*shown by arrow*).

derived mainly from studies of selected groups of patients attending university hospitals and other specialty clinics that tend to treat the most difficult and complicated cases. In one such study (Victoroff), approximately one-third of epileptic patients had a history of major depressive illness, and an equal number had symptoms of anxiety disorder; psychotic symptoms were found in 10 percent. Similar figures, also from a university-based epilepsy center, have been reported by Blumer et al. It must be emphasized that these remarkably high rates of psychiatric morbidity do not reflect the prevalence in the entire population of patients with epilepsy. Epidemiologic studies provide only limited evidence of an association with psychosis in the overall population of epileptics (see Trimble and Schmitz and the review by Trimble for a critical discussion of this subject). Furthermore, it should be borne in mind that many chronic medical conditions are associated with psychiatric reactions. On the other hand, the unpredictability and stigma of the epileptic disorders may contribute to depression and anxiety.

The postictal state in patients with temporal lobe epilepsy rarely incorporates a protracted *paranoid-delusional* or *amnesic psychosis* lasting for days or weeks. The EEG during this period may show no seizure discharge, although this does not exclude repeated seizures in temporal lobe structures that are remote from the recording electrodes. This disorder, virtually indistinguishable from psychosis, may also present in the interictal period.

It had been observed that some patients with temporal lobe seizures may exhibit a number of personal peculiarities. It was stated that they are slow and rigid in their thinking, verbose, circumstantial and tedious in conversation, inclined to mysticism, and preoccupied with rather naive religious and philosophical ideas. Obsessionalism, humorless sobriety, emotionality (mood swings, sadness, and anger), and a tendency to paranoia are other frequently described traits. Diminished sexual interest and potency in men and menstrual problems in women, not readily attributable to antiepileptic drugs, are common among patients with complex partial seizures of temporal lobe origin. Geschwind proposed that a triad of behavioral abnormalities—hyposexuality, hypergraphia, and hyperreligiosity—constitutes a characteristic syndrome.

Bear and Fedio suggested that certain personality traits were more common with *right* temporal lesions, and that anger, paranoia, and cosmologic or religious conceptualizing are more characteristic of *left* temporal lesions. However, Rodin and Schmaltz found no features that would distinguish foci on either side and they found no behavioral changes that would distinguish patients with temporal lobe epilepsy from other groups of epileptics. The problem of personality disturbances in epilepsy has not been clarified and modern clinicians no longer identify these traits as parts so the epileptic syndrome, having in the past been imputed to these patients by societal and medical biases (see review by Trimble).

Sudden Unexplained Death in Epilepsy (SUDEP)

In the past few decades, sudden death has been emphasized as an underappreciated problem in the epileptic population. Certainly, the mortality in individuals with epilepsy is increased ostensibly from accidents, suicide, and the underlying cause of seizures. However, the main contributor to the increased mortality rate in healthy people with epilepsy is unexpected death outside of circumstances such as drowning, trauma from a fall, myocardial infarction, and automobile accidents during the seizure. It is to this group that the acronym "SUDEP" has been applied. Surprisingly, unexpected death is predominantly an issue of adulthood more than of childhood. The rate of unexpected death increases with the duration and severity of epilepsy and several population studies suggest that the rate may be as high as 9% lifetime incidence but others cite a much lower figure. Most patients affected have a history of generalized tonic-clonic seizures and die in bed. In children, those with treatment resistant epilepsy, developmental delay and several syndromes such as tuberous sclerosis are at particular risk.

Several factors have emerged as risks from population-based and cohort case controlled studies; the postictal period immediately after a tonic clonic seizure, increasing seizure frequency (including three generalized seizures in the preceding year), lack of successful treatment (i.e., patients not in remission as documented in a 40 year follow up of childhood epilepsy by Sillanpää and Shinnar), or subtherapeutic levels of antiepileptic drugs, the period of early adulthood, long-standing epilepsy, and mental retardation.

Most instances of SUDEP occur when the patient is unattended or during sleep. Although respiratory difficulty and cardiac changes including asystole and ventricular arrhythmias are known to occur during and immediately after seizures, none of these has been a consistent factor and usually, the precise mechanism of death has been difficult to determine. A postictal "shutdown" of brainstem activity resulting in hypercapnia or hypoxemia has been suggested.

One approach to preventing sudden death is adequate treatment with antiepileptic drugs. The risk of sudden death is as high as 20 times greater for untreated patients. Some specialists in the field of epilepsy have suggested that an open conversation be undertaken about the problem with patients and their families. More often, neurologists raise the issue only in high risk patients or when specifically asked. A review of this subject has been provided by Devinsky.

SPECIAL EPILEPTIC SYNDROMES

There remain to be considered several epileptic syndromes and other seizure states that cannot be readily classified with the usual types of generalized or partial seizures.

Benign Epilepsy of Childhood with Centrotemporal Spikes (Rolandic Epilepsy, Sylvian Epilepsy)

This common focal motor epilepsy is unique among the focal epilepsies of childhood in that it is self-limiting despite a very abnormal EEG pattern. It is usually transmitted in families as an autosomal dominant trait and begins between 5 and 9 years of age. It typically announces itself by a nocturnal tonic-clonic seizure with focal onset. Thereafter, the seizures take the form of clonic contractions of one side of the face, less often of one arm or leg, and the interictal EEG shows high-voltage spikes in the contralateral lower rolandic or centrotemporal area. Seizures are readily controlled by a single anticonvulsant drug and gradually disappear during adolescence. The relation of this syndrome to developmental dyslexia is unsettled.

Epilepsy with Occipital Spikes

A similar type of epilepsy, usually benign in the sense that there is no intellectual deterioration and the seizures often cease in adolescence, has been associated with spike activity over the occipital lobes as identified by Panayiotopoulos. Visual hallucinations, while not invariable, are the most common clinical feature, according to the review by Taylor and colleagues; sensations of movements of the eyes, tinnitus, or vertigo are also reported in cases of occipital epilepsy. These authors point out symptomatic causes of the syndrome, mainly cortical heterotopias. In both of these types of childhood epilepsy the observation that spikes are greatly accentuated by sleep is a useful diagnostic sign.

Infantile Spasms (West Syndrome)

This term is applied to a special and particularly dramatic form of epilepsy of infancy and early childhood. West, in the mid-nineteenth century, described the condition in his son in great detail. This disorder, which in most cases appears during the first year of life, is characterized by recurrent, single or brief episodes of gross flexion movements of the trunk and limbs and, less frequently, by extension movements (hence the alternative terms *infantile spasms* or *salaam* or *jackknife seizures*). Most but not all patients with this disorder show major EEG abnormalities consisting of continuous multifocal spikes and slow waves of large amplitude. However, this pattern, named by Gibbs and Gibbs as *hypsarrhythmia* ("mountainous" dysrhythmia), is not specific for infantile spasms, being frequently associated with other developmental or acquired abnormalities of the brain. As the child matures, the seizures diminish and usually disappear by the fourth to fifth year. If MRI and CT scans are more or less normal, the usual pathologic findings according to Jellinger are cortical dysgeneses. Both the seizures and the EEG abnormalities may respond dramatically to treatment with adrenocorticotropic hormone (ACTH), corticosteroids, or the benzodiazepine drugs, of which clonazepam is probably the most widely used. A type of West syndrome that is caused by tuberous sclerosis also responds dramatically to gamma-aminobutyric acid (GABA)-inhibiting drugs such as vigabatrin, as noted below. However, most patients, even those who were apparently normal when the seizures appeared, are left mentally impaired. Infantile spasms may later progress to the *Lennox-Gastaut syndrome*, a seizure disorder of early childhood of graver prognosis as discussed in a previous section.

Febrile Seizures

The well-known uncomplicated *febrile seizure*, specific to infants and children between 6 months and 5 years of age (peak incidence ages 9 to 20 months) and with a strong inherited tendency, is generally regarded as a benign condition. It usually takes the form of a single, generalized motor seizure occurring as the patient's core temperature rises or reaches its peak. Seldom does the seizure last longer than a few minutes and by the time an EEG can be obtained, there is no abnormality and recovery is complete. The temperature is usually above 38°C (100.4°F). Any viral or bacterial illness, or, rarely, an immunization, may be the precipitant of the fever; herpesvirus 6 is one of the common precipitants, probably because of its tendency to cause high fever. Prophylactic antiepileptic drugs have not been found to be helpful in preventing febrile seizures. Except for a presumed genetic relationship with benign epilepsy of childhood (Luders et al), which in itself is transient in nature, these patients' risk of developing epilepsy in later life is only slightly greater than that of the general population. In some families, such as those studied by Nabbout and colleagues, febrile seizures alone, without generalized epilepsy, have been associated with a particular gene by linkage analysis. Presumably, when the gene products are identified, some insight into the nature of defects that lower the seizure threshold will be forthcoming.

This benign type of febrile seizure should not be confused with more serious illnesses in which a febrile acute encephalitic or encephalopathic state causes focal or prolonged seizures, generalized or focal EEG abnormalities, and repeated episodes of febrile convulsions during a febrile illness (*complicated febrile seizures*). In these cases, these seizures may recur not only with infections but also at other times. When patients with both types are combined together under the rubric of *febrile convulsions*, it is not surprising that a high percentage are complicated by later atypical petit mal, atonic, and astatic spells followed by tonic seizures, mental retardation, and partial complex epilepsy. In a study of 67 patients with medial temporal lobe epilepsy by French and colleagues, 70 percent had a history of complicated febrile seizures during the first 5 years of life, although many did not again develop seizures until their teens. Bacterial meningitis was an important risk factor; head and birth trauma were less-common factors. Epidemiologic studies have substantiated this clinical point of view. Annegers and colleagues observed a cohort of 687 children for an average of 18 years after their initial febrile convulsion. Overall, these children had a five-fold excess of unprovoked seizures in later life. Among the children with simple febrile convulsions, the risk was only 2.4 percent. By contrast, children with what Annegers and colleagues called complex febrile convulsions (focal, prolonged, or repeated episodes of febrile seizures) had a greatly increased risk—8, 17, or 49 percent, depending on the association of one, two, or three of the complicating features.

Reflex Epilepsies

It has been appreciated for a long time that seizures can be evoked in certain individuals by a discrete physiologic or psychologic stimulus. The term *reflex epilepsy* is reserved for this small subgroup. Forster classified these seizures in accordance with their evocative stimuli into five types: (1) *visual*—flickering light, visual patterns, and specific colors (especially red), leading to rapid blinking or eye closure; (2) *auditory*—sudden unexpected noise (startle), specific sounds, musical themes, and voices; (3) *somatosensory*—either a brisk unexpected tap or sudden movement after sitting or lying still, or a prolonged tactile or thermal stimulus to a certain part of the body; (4) *writing* or *reading* of words or numbers; and (5) *eating*.

Visually induced seizures are by far the most common type. The seizures are usually myoclonic but may be generalized and triggered by the photic stimulation of television or an EEG examination or by the photic or pattern stimulation of video games. In other types of reflex epilepsy, the evoked seizure may be focal (beginning often in the part of the body that was stimulated) or generalized and may take the form of one or a series of myoclonic jerks or of an absence or tonic-clonic seizure. Seizures induced by reading, voices, or eating are most often of the complex partial type; seizures induced by music are usually myoclonic, simple, or complex partial. A few such instances of reflex epilepsy have been caused by focal cerebral disease, particularly occipital lesions.

Clonazepam, valproate, carbamazepine, and phenytoin (as well as many of the new antiepileptic drugs) are all effective in controlling individual instances of reflex epilepsy. Some patients learn to avert the seizure by undertaking a mental task, e.g., thinking about some distracting subject, counting, etc., or by initiating some type of physical activity. Forster has demonstrated that in certain types of reflex epilepsy, the repeated presentation of the stimulus may eventually render the trigger innocuous but this requires a great deal of time and reinforcement, which limits its therapeutic value.

Epilepsia Partialis Continua

This is a special type of focal motor epilepsy characterized by persistent rhythmic clonic movements of one muscle group—usually of the face, arm, or leg—which are repeated at fairly regular intervals every few seconds and continue for hours, days, weeks, or months without spreading to other parts of the body. Thus epilepsia partialis continua is, in effect, a highly restricted and very persistent focal motor status epilepticus. The distal muscles of the leg and arm, especially the flexors of the hand and fingers, are affected more frequently than the proximal ones. In the face, the recurrent contractions involve either the corner of the mouth or one or both eyelids. Occasionally, isolated muscles of the neck or trunk are affected on one side. The clonic activity may be accentuated by active or passive movement of the involved muscles and may be reduced in severity but not abolished during sleep.

First described by Kozhevnikov in patients with Russian spring-summer encephalitis, these ongoing partial seizures may be induced by a variety of acute or chronic cerebral lesions. In some cases the underlying disease is not apparent (this has applied to most of the cases in our experience), and the clonic movements may be mistaken for some type of slow tremor or extrapyramidal movement disorder. Most patients with epilepsia partialis continua show focal EEG abnormalities, either repetitive slow-wave abnormalities or sharp waves or spikes over the central areas of the contralateral hemisphere. In some cases, the spike activity can be related precisely in location and time to the clonic movements (Thomas et al). In the series collected by Obeso and colleagues, there were various combinations of epilepsia partialis continua and cutaneous reflex myoclonus (cortical myoclonus occurring only in response to a variety of afferent stimuli).

As would be expected, a wide range of causative lesions has been implicated—developmental anomalies, encephalitis, demyelinative diseases, tumors, metabolic abnormalities, particularly hyperosmolarity, and degenerative diseases; but in many instances, as already emphasized, the underlying cause is not found even after extensive investigation. Epilepsia partialis continua is particularly common in patients with the rare condition, Rasmussen encephalitis (see further on).

Whether cortical or subcortical mechanisms are responsible for epilepsia partialis continua is an unresolved question. The electrophysiologic evidence adduced by Thomas and colleagues favors a cortical origin; the pathologic evidence is less definite. In each of eight cases in which the brain was examined postmortem, they found some degree of involvement of the motor cortex or adjacent cortical area contralateral to the affected limbs. However, all but one of these patients also had some involvement of deeper structures on the same side as the cortical lesion, on the opposite side, or on both sides.

Rasmussen Syndrome

In rare cases, a lesion, usually identified by MRI and confirmed by biopsy, and in some cases by special autoantibodies, takes the form of a chronic focal encephalitis. In 1958, Rasmussen described three children in whom the clinical problem consisted of intractable focal epilepsy in association with a progressive hemiparesis. The cerebral cortex disclosed a mild meningeal infiltration of inflammatory cells and an encephalitic process marked by neuronal destruction, gliosis, neuronophagia, some degree of tissue necrosis, and perivascular cuffing. Many additional cases were soon uncovered and Rasmussen was able to summarize the natural history of 48 personally observed patients (see the often cited monograph by Andermann).

An expanded view of the syndrome has added several interesting features. The affected children are typically ages 3 to 15 years, more girls than boys. Half of them have epilepsia partialis continua. The progression of the disease leads to hemiplegia or other deficits and focal brain atrophy in most cases. The neuropathology of five fully examined cases has revealed extensive destruction of the cortex and white matter with intense gliosis and lingering inflammatory reactions.

The CSF shows a pleocytosis and sometimes oligoclonal bands but these are not uniform findings. Focal cortical and subcortical lesions are usually visualized by MRI and are bilateral in some cases. The finding of antibodies to glutamate receptors (GluR3) in a proportion of patients with Rasmussen encephalitis has raised interest in an immune causation (see review by Antel and Rasmussen). An autoimmune hypothesis has been supported by the findings of Twyman and colleagues that these antibodies cause seizures in rabbits and lead to the release of the neurotoxin kainate in cell cultures. However, Wendl's group and others have found these antibodies in many types of focal epilepsy and have questioned their specificity.

The unrelenting course of the disease had in the past defied medical therapy. In some patients the process eventually burns out, but in those with continuous focal epilepsy the seizures continued despite all antiepileptic drugs. The use of high doses of corticosteroids, when started within the first year of the disease, proved beneficial in 5 of the 8 patients treated by Chinchilla and colleagues. Repeated plasma exchanges and immune globulin have also been tried, but the results are difficult to interpret. When the disease is extensive and unilateral, neurosurgeons have resorted to partial hemispherectomy.

PSYCHOGENIC NONEPILEPTIC SEIZURES (PNES, PSEUDOSEIZURES)

These common episodes, which simulate convulsive or nonconvulsive seizures, are not the result of an abnormal neuronal discharge. They have been termed psychogenic non-epileptic seizures (PNES) and comprise a heterogeneous group of disorders that are easily mistaken for epileptic spells. Moreover, they comprise a large proportion of treatment resistant epilepsy and often are treated with multiple antiepileptic drugs, to which they are unresponsive. It has been estimated that 70% of people diagnosed with PNES have been previously diagnosed and treated for epilepsy. In large series, non-epileptic seizures comprise 4% of cases of transient loss of consciousness, 20% of referrals to specialist epilepsy services, and 50% of apparent status epilepticus. It should be emphasized that patients with true epileptic seizures can exhibit psychogenic ones as well, making the distinction between the two particularly difficult. It is this population that proves most vexing (and common) in specialty epilepsy services.

Our current conceptualization is that the condition arises as a behavioral response to underlying emotional or psychological distress. Episodes may be derived from traumatic experiences in early life, particularly physical, sexual, and mental abuse during childhood. Many experts consider them to be allied with hysteria (*Briquet disease, conversion disorder*, as discussed in Chap. 51) or malingering. Recent studies suggest that a conversion-hysterical disorder accounts for most cases, even in males, and that malingering is rare but this has certainly not been our experience.

Three broad categories of psychogenic states seem to generate pseudoseizures: (1) panic disorder that is itself common in people with epilepsy; (2) dissociative disorders, in which convulsions are typically prolonged, resembling generalized tonic-clonic seizures, or alternatively, swooning as in a faint or presyncopal spell, or blank spells that closely simulate absence seizure; and (3) malingering, the deliberate feigning of seizures to avoid certain situations, e.g., imprisonment.

Usually, the unconventional motor display in the course of a nonepileptic seizure is sufficient to identify it as such: completely asynchronous thrashing of the limbs and repeated side-to-side movements of the head; striking out at a person who is trying to restrain the patient; hand-biting, kicking, trembling, and quivering; pelvic thrusting and opisthotonic arching postures; and screaming or talking during the ictus. It is helpful to observe that the eyes are kept quietly or forcefully closed in pseudoseizure whereas the lids are open or show clonic movement in epilepsy. Psychogenic spells are likely if attacks are prolonged (many minutes, even hours), if there is rapid breathing (whereas apnea is typical during and after a seizure), or if there is tearfulness after an episode. Pseudoseizures tend to occur in the presence of observers, to be precipitated by emotional factors. With few exceptions, tongue-biting, incontinence, hurtful falls, or postictal confusion are lacking but if the tongue is bitten in a pseudoseizure it is usually the front, compared to the lateral tongue injury that is characteristic of an epileptic attack. Incontinence does not assist in making a clear distinction from epileptic seizures.

Another clue to non-epileptic seizures in our experience has been highly resistant epilepsy in an individual with normal intellect and normal brain imaging. Often in these persons in particular, there has been a background of unexplained medical problems, previous psychological problems (depression, panic disorder, overdose, self harm, addiction), and a life story that includes intense emotional trauma. Prolonged *fugue states* usually prove to be manifestations of hysteria or a psychopathy, even in a known epileptic.

The serum creatine kinase levels are normal after nonepileptic seizures; this may be helpful in distinguishing them from epilepsy. Where doubt remains, a recording of the ictal or postictal EEG or the prolonged combined video and EEG recording of an attack may settle the issue.

THE NATURE OF THE DISCHARGING LESION IN EPILEPSY

Physiologically, the epileptic seizure has been defined as a sudden alteration of central nervous system (CNS) function resulting from a paroxysmal high-frequency or synchronous low-frequency, high-voltage electrical discharge. This discharge arises from an assemblage of excitable neurons in any part of the cerebral cortex and possibly in secondarily involved subcortical structures as well. Of course, there need not be a visible lesion in the brain. In the proper circumstances, a seizure discharge can be initiated in an entirely normal cerebral cortex, as when the cortex is activated by ingestion of drugs, or by withdrawal from alcohol or other sedative drugs. A special mechanism that ostensibly creates a secondary seizure focus, "kindling," is the result of repeated stimulation with subconvulsive electrical pulses from an established focus elsewhere; it is known to occur in animal models but is a controversial entity in humans.

Viewed from a larger physiologic perspective, seizures require three conditions: (1) a population of pathologically excitable neurons; (2) an increase in excitatory, mainly glutaminergic, activity through recurrent connections in order to spread the discharge; and (3) a reduction in the activity of the normally inhibitory GABAergic projections. Each of these has been challenged but is supported by considerable data and together they serve as a reasonable model, as noted below. Understanding of the initial discharges and their spread has been advanced by the identification of several rare forms of familial epilepsy that are the result of mutations in sodium, potassium, acetylcholine receptor, or GABA channels on neurons. These are discussed further on under "Role of Genetics."

Just why the neurons in or near a focal cortical lesion discharge spontaneously and synchronously is not fully understood. Some of the electrical properties of a cortical epileptogenic focus suggest that its neurons have been deafferented. Neurons in these circumstances are hyperexcitable, and they may chronically remain in a state of partial depolarization, able to fire irregularly at rates as high as 700 to 1,000 per second. The cytoplasmic membranes of such cells have an increased ionic permeability, which renders them susceptible to activation by hyperthermia, hypoxia, hypoglycemia, hypocalcemia, and hyponatremia, as well as by repeated sensory (e.g., photic) stimulation and during certain phases of sleep (where *hypersynchrony* of neurons occurs).

As an example, epileptic foci induced in the animal cortex by the application of penicillin are characterized by spontaneous interictal discharges, during which the neurons of the discharging focus exhibit large, calcium-mediated paroxysmal depolarizations (depolarizing shifts), followed by prolonged afterhyperpolarizations. The latter are caused in part by calcium-dependent potassium currents, but enhanced synaptic inhibition also plays a role. The depolarizing shifts occur synchronously in the penicillin focus and summate to produce surface-recorded interictal EEG spikes; the afterpolarizations correspond to the slow wave of the EEG spike-and-wave complex (see Engel). The neurons surrounding an epileptogenic focus are hyperpolarized and release inhibitory GABA. The spread of seizures depends on factors that activate neurons in the focus or inhibit those surrounding it. Beyond this, the precise mechanism that governs the transition from a circumscribed interictal discharge to a widespread seizure state is not understood.

Biochemical studies of neurons from a seizure focus have not greatly clarified the problem. Levels of extracellular potassium are elevated in glial scars near epileptic foci, and a defect in voltage-sensitive calcium channels has also been postulated. Epileptic foci are known to be sensitive to acetylcholine and to be slower in binding and removing it than is normal cerebral cortex. A deficiency of the inhibitory neurotransmitter GABA, increased glycine, decreased taurine, and either decreased or increased glutamic acid have been variously reported in excised human epileptogenic tissue, but whether these changes are the cause or result of seizure activity has not been determined. The interpretation of reported abnormalities of GABA, biogenic amines, and acetylcholine in the cerebrospinal fluid (CSF) of epileptic patients poses great difficulties.

Concurrent EEG recordings from an epileptogenic cortical focus and subcortical, thalamic, and brainstem centers in the animal model have enabled investigators to construct a sequence of electrical and clinical events that characterize an evolving focal seizure. Firing of the involved neurons in the cortical focus is reflected in the EEG as a series of periodic spike discharges, which increase progressively in amplitude and frequency. Once the intensity of the seizure discharge exceeds a certain point, it overcomes the inhibitory influence of surrounding neurons and spreads to neighboring cortical regions via short corticocortical synaptic connections. If the abnormal discharge remains confined to the cortical focus and the immediate surrounding cortex, there are probably no clinical symptoms or signs of seizure, and the EEG abnormality that persists during the interseizure period reflects this restricted type of abnormal cortical activity.

A provocative finding, based on sophisticated mathematical analysis of EEG tracings, indicates that subtle electrographic changes arise several minutes before the ictal discharge (see LeVan Quyen et al). This suggests that seizures could be triggered either by a change in central thalamic rhythm generators or a subtle alteration in the electrical activity in the region of a focal lesion. Of interest are the findings of Litt and colleagues that in a small number of patients there are prolonged bursts of seizure-like activity detected by sophisticated techniques even days before the onset of temporal lobe seizures. Their proposal is that these events cause a cascade of electrophysiologic changes that very gradually culminate in a seizure.

If unchecked, cortical excitation spreads to the adjacent cortex and to the contralateral cortex via interhemispheric pathways, and also to anatomically and functionally related pathways in subcortical nuclei (particularly the basal ganglionic, thalamic, and brainstem reticular nuclei). It is at this time that the clinical manifestations of the seizure begin. The excitatory activity from the subcortical nuclei is conceived to feed back to the original focus and to other parts of the cerebrum, a mechanism that serves to amplify their excitatory activity and to give rise to the characteristic high-voltage polyspike discharge in the EEG. The spread of excitation to the subcortical, thalamic, and brainstem centers corresponds to the tonic phase of the seizure and to loss of consciousness as well as to the signs of autonomic nervous system overactivity (salivation, mydriasis, tachycardia, increased blood pressure). Breathing may be arrested, but usually for only a few seconds. The development of unconsciousness and the generalized tonic contraction of muscles are reflected in the EEG by a diffuse high-voltage discharge pattern appearing simultaneously over the entire cortex.

Soon after the spread of excitation, a diencephalic inhibition begins and intermittently interrupts the seizure discharge, changing it from the persistent tonic phase to the intermittent bursts of the clonic phase. In the surface EEG, a transition occurs from a continuous polyspike to a spike-and-wave pattern. The intermittent clonic bursts become decreasingly frequent and finally cease altogether, leaving in their wake an "exhaustion" (paralysis) of the neurons of the epileptogenic focus and a regional increase in permeability of the blood–brain barrier and regional edema in magnetic resonance images. An excess of these inhibitory mechanisms and metabolic exhaustion are thought to be the basis of *Todd's postepileptic paralysis* and of postictal stupor, sensory loss, aphasia, hemianopia, headache, and diffuse slow waves in the EEG. Plum and associates observed a two- to threefold increase in glucose utilization during seizure discharges and suggested that the paralysis that follows might be a result of neuronal depletion of glucose and an increase in lactic acid. However, inhibition of epileptogenic neurons may occur in the absence of neuronal exhaustion. The exact roles played by each of these factors in postictal paralysis of function are not settled.

Insights to absence seizures have been obtained from animal models of bilaterally synchronous 3-per-second high-voltage spike-and-wave discharges. The spike-and-wave complex, which represents brief excitation followed by slow-wave inhibition, is the type of EEG pattern that characterizes the clonic (inhibitory) phase of the focal motor or grand mal seizure. By contrast, this strong element of inhibition is present diffusely throughout an "absence" attack, a feature that perhaps accounts for the failure of excitation to spread to lower brainstem and spinal structures (tonic-clonic movements do not occur). However, the absence seizure can also at times activate the mechanism for rhythmic myoclonus, probably at an upper brainstem level.

Current physiologic data indicate that the characteristic EEG patterns of generalized forms of epilepsy are generated entirely in the neocortex but are enhanced by the synchronizing influences of subcortical structures. The generalization of the clinical and electrical manifestations depends upon activation of a deep, centrally located physiologic mechanism, which, as outlined in Chap. 17, includes the midbrain reticular formation and its diencephalic extension, the intralaminar and nonspecific thalamic projection systems (originally referred to by Penfield as the "centrencephalon"). There is little evidence, however, that seizure activity originates in these deep structures; thus the term *centrencephalic* has been replaced by *corticoreticular epilepsy*.

Of theoretical importance is the observation that a seizure focus may establish, via commissural connections, a persistent secondary focus in the corresponding cortical area of the opposite hemisphere (*mirror focus*). The nature of this phenomenon is obscure; it may be similar to the "kindling" phenomenon mentioned earlier in animals, where a repeated nonconvulsive electrical stimulation of normal cortex induces a permanent epileptic focus. No morphologic change is visible in the mirror focus, at least by light microscopy. The mirror focus may be a source of confusion when trying to identify the side of the primary discharging lesion by EEG. However, there is only limited evidence that mirror foci of the kindling phenomenon produce seizures in humans (see Goldensohn).

Severe seizures may be accompanied by a systemic lactic acidosis with a fall in arterial pH, reduction in arterial oxygen saturation, and rise in Pco_2. These effects are secondary to the respiratory arrest and excessive muscular activity. If prolonged, they may cause hypoxic-ischemic damage to remote areas in the cerebrum, basal ganglia, and cerebellum. In paralyzed and artificially ventilated subjects receiving electroconvulsive therapy, these changes are less marked and the oxygen tension in cerebral venous blood may actually rise. Heart rate, blood pressure, and particularly CSF pressure rise briskly during an ECT-induced seizure. According to Plum and colleagues, the rise in blood pressure evoked by a seizure usually causes a sufficient increase in cerebral blood flow to meet the increased metabolic needs of the brain.

EEG AND LABORATORY TESTING IN EPILEPSY

The origins of EEG activity of an epileptic focus and the generalization of seizures are discussed in Chap. 2 and earlier in this chapter. The EEG provides confirmation of Hughlings Jackson's concept of epilepsy—that it represents a recurrent, sudden, excessive discharge of cortical neurons. The EEG is the most sensitive, indeed indispensable, tool for the diagnosis of epilepsy; but like other ancillary tests, it must be used in conjunction with clinical data. In patients with idiopathic generalized seizures, and in a high proportion of their relatives, interictal spike-and-wave abnormalities without any clinical seizure activity are common, especially if the EEG is repeated several times or taken over long periods. By contrast, a proportion of epileptic patients have a perfectly normal interictal EEG. Using standard methods of scalp recording, the EEG may even be normal during the experiential aura of a simple or complex partial seizure. Furthermore, interpretation of EEG abnormalities must take into account that a small number of healthy persons (approximately 2 to 3 percent) show paroxysmal EEG abnormalities.

A single EEG tracing obtained during the interictal state is abnormal to some degree in 30 to 50 percent of epileptic patients; this figure rises to 60 to 70 percent if patients are subjected to several recordings. Many EEG patterns are possible in seizures. One consistent observation, however, has been that the region of earliest spike activity corresponds best to the epileptogenic focus, a rule that has come to guide epilepsy surgery. The postseizure or postictal state also has an EEG correlate, taking the form of random generalized slow waves after generalized seizures and focal slowing following partial seizures. With clinical recovery, the EEG returns to normal or to the preseizure state.

A higher yield of abnormalities and a more precise definition of seizure types can be obtained by the use of several special EEG procedures, as described in Chap. 2. Here it is restated that activating procedures such as hyperventilation, photic stroboscopic stimulation, and sleep increase the yield of EEG recordings. EEG recording during sleep is particularly helpful because focal abnormalities, particularly in the temporal lobes, may become prominent in slow-wave and stage II sleep. Sphenoidal leads have been used to detect inferomedial temporal seizure activity, but they are uncomfortable and probably add little more information than can be obtained by the placement of additional subtemporal scalp electrodes. Nasopharyngeal electrode recordings are too contaminated by artifact to be clinically useful.

Beyond dependably identifying artifacts in the EEG recording, one of the main challenges for the electroencephalographer is to differentiate between normal patterns that simulate seizures and true epileptic or interictal discharges. These paroxysmal but ostensibly normal patterns appear mostly during sleep, each with a highly characteristic morphology. These include small sharp spikes, "14 and 6" polyspike activity, lambda and posterior occipital mu rhythm, and occipital sharp transients. These are pictured in most standard textbooks on the subject of EEG and discussed in Chap 2.

Several methods of *long-term EEG monitoring* are now in common use and are of particular value in the investigation of patients with surgically removable epileptogenic foci and of non-epileptic spells. The most common of these makes use of telemetry systems, in which the patient is attached to the EEG machine by cable or radio transmitter without unduly limiting freedom of movement. The telemetry system is joined to an audiovisual recording system, making it possible to record seizure phenomena (even at night, under dim infrared light) and to synchronize them with the EEG abnormalities. An alternative is the use of a small digital recording device that is attached to a miniature EEG machine worn by the patient at home and at work ("ambulatory EEG"). The patient is instructed to push a button if he experiences an "event," which can later be correlated with EEG activity.

Other Laboratory Abnormalities Associated with Seizures

MRI is the most useful tool for the detection of structural abnormalities underlying epilepsy. Medial temporal sclerosis, heterotopias and other disorders of neuronal migration, glial scars, and porencephaly can be clearly visualized.

After a seizure, particularly one with a focal component, MRI sometimes discloses subtle focal cortical swelling and signal change in the FLAIR (fluid-attenuated inversion recovery) and diffusion-weighted sequences, or, if a contrast agent is administered, an ill-defined cortical blush may be visible on MRI. There is an approximate relationship between the duration of seizure activity and the intensity and extent of these secondary changes. Likewise, angiography or perfusion imaging performed soon after a seizure may show a focal area of enhanced blood flow or elevated blood volume. All of these imaging abnormalities are thought to reflect transient disruption of the blood–brain barrier, and they rarely persist for more than a day or two. Less-well understood is the findings on MRI of increased T2 signal or restricted diffusion in the hippocampi after a prolonged seizure or status epilepticus. In some cases, a thalamic or cerebellar signal change is seen on MRI after a seizure; these may also persist for days. There are also imaging changes in the white matter, particularly the splenium of the corpus callosum that may occur soon after the withdrawal of certain antiepileptic medications as discussed in the later section on the use of these drugs and by Gürtler and colleagues).

The CSF after a seizure occasionally contains a small number of white blood cells (rarely up to 50/mm^3, but more often in the range of 10/mm^3) in about 15 percent of patients. A slight increase in protein is also possible. Like the imaging abnormalities these findings may lead to spurious conclusions about the presence of an active intracranial lesion, particularly if polymorphonuclear leukocytes predominate; a larger pleocytosis should always be construed as a sign of inflammatory or infectious disease.

Systemic (lactic) acidosis is a common result of convulsive seizures, and it is not unusual for the serum pH to reach levels near or below 7 if taken immediately after a convulsion. Of more practical value is the fact that almost all generalized convulsions produce a rise in serum creatine kinase activity that persists for hours, a finding that could be used to greater advantage in emergency departments to assist in distinguishing seizures from fainting. Of course, extensive muscle injury from a fall or prolonged compression during a period of unconsciousness can produce the same abnormality.

Concentrations of serum prolactin, like those of other hypothalamic hormones, rise for 10 to 20 min after all types of generalized seizures, including complex partial types, but not in absence or myoclonic types. An elevation may help differentiate a psychogenic seizure from a genuine one; however, serum prolactin may also be slightly elevated after a syncopal episode. Testing is facilitated by collecting capillary blood from the finger on filter paper for analysis (Fisher et al). There is also a postictal rise in ACTH and serum cortisol, but these changes have a longer latency and briefer duration. If elevations in these hormonal levels are used as diagnostic tests, one must have information about normal baseline levels, diurnal variations, and the effects of concurrent medications. Changes in body temperature, which are said to sometimes precede a seizure, may reflect hypothalamic changes but are far less consistent and difficult to use in clinical work.

PATHOLOGY OF EPILEPSY

In most autopsied cases of primary generalized epilepsy of the genetic variety, the CNS is grossly and microscopically normal. MRI, which has been used as a surrogate for pathology, has not improved matters much except to expose some cortical heterotopias that had been previously difficult to detect, and to highlight the frequency of gliosis in the medial temporal lobes. Not surprisingly, there are also no visible lesions in the seizure states complicating drug intoxication and withdrawal, transient hyper- and hyponatremia, and hyper- and hypoglycemia, which presumably represent derangements at the cellular level.

In contrast, symptomatic epilepsies have definable lesions. These include zones of neuronal loss and gliosis (scars) or other lesions such as heterotopia, dysgenic cortex, hamartoma, vascular malformation, porencephaly, and tumor. Vascular malformations, hamartomas, ganglioneuromas and related dysembryoplastic neuroectodermal tumors (DNET), which are important causes of drug resistant epilepsy, and low-grade astrocytomas were less frequent; again, in a small number, no abnormalities could be found. Certainly the focal epilepsies are associated with the highest incidence of structural abnormalities, although in certain cases no morphologic change is visible. With reference to the focal epilepsies, it has not been possible to determine which component of the lesion is responsible for the seizures. Gliosis, fibrosis, vascularization, and meningocerebral cicatrix have all been incriminated, but they are found in nonepileptic foci as well. The Scheibels' Golgi studies of neurons from epileptic foci in the temporal lobe showed distortions of dendrites, loss of dendritic spines, and disorientation of neurons near the scars, but these findings have dubious status because they were not usually compared with similar nonepileptic lesions. Once a gliotic focus of whatever cause becomes epileptogenic, it may remain so throughout the patient's lifetime.

Medial Temporal Sclerosis

In several series of cases of temporal lobe excisions in prior decades, such as the often cited one described by Falconer, a specific pattern of neuronal loss with gliosis (sclerosis) in the hippocampal and amygdaloid region was found in the majority, and this abnormality is being increasingly recognized with MRI, as already noted (*medial temporal sclerosis*; Fig. 16-4). The associated histologic finding is loss of neurons in the CA1 segment (Sommer sector) of the pyramidal cell layer of the hippocampus, often unilateral, extending into contiguous regions of both the pyramidal layer and the underlying dentate gyrus. It is still undetermined whether this neuronal loss is primary or secondary and, if the latter, whether it was incurred at birth or happened later as the consequence of recurrent seizures.

However, early life head trauma, infections, and a variety of less-common perturbations may also cause the ensemble of neuron loss and mild gliosis of medial temporal sclerosis. The cessation of seizures in many patients following surgical resection of the medial temporal lobe favors the first interpretation that the pathologic change is primary in most cases (see further on under "Surgical Treatment of Epilepsy"). Attesting to the uncertainty of cause or effect are numerous surgical series that favor one view or the other (see editorial by Sutula and Pitkänen).

Role of Genetics

Most primary epilepsies have a genetic basis and, as in many other diseases such as diabetes and atherosclerosis, the mode of inheritance is complex, i.e., some are likely to be polygenic but increasingly, single mutations are being found. That a genetic factor is operative in the primary generalized epilepsies is suggested by a familial incidence in 5 to 10 percent of such patients and, in certain families, the inheritance of a seizure disorder through specific genes (Gourfinkel-An et al). The importance of genetic factors in the primary epilepsies is also underscored by evidence from twin studies; in six major series, the overall concordance rate was 60 percent for monozygotic twins and 13 percent for dizygotic pairs.

Of course, epilepsy is a component of many genetic syndromes that are defined by their dysmorphic appearance or neurocutaneous disorder with or without mental retardation. What we consider here are the few idiopathic seizure disorders that are inherited by a simple (mendelian) pattern. These include a subgroup of benign neonatal familial convulsions inherited as an autosomal dominant trait (Leppert et al), and a similar disorder of infantile onset and a benign myoclonic epilepsy of childhood (autosomal recessive). Particularly informative are a special group of epileptic disorders in which monogenic genetic defects are related to abnormalities of ion channels or neurotransmitter receptors (Table 16-3). These were mentioned earlier in the discussion of the physiology of seizures and despite their rarity they suggest that idiopathic epilepsy may be caused by a disruption in the function of these same channels.

The consequences of almost all of these mutations are to enhance overall neuronal excitability. Examples include autosomal dominant nocturnal frontal lobe epilepsy, which may present as a partial seizure (in which the offending mutations are in subunits of the nicotinic acetylcholine receptor subunit); "generalized epilepsy with febrile seizures plus" (subunits of a neuronal sodium channel associated with various combinations of uncomplicated febrile seizures, febrile seizures persisting beyond childhood, generalized, absence, myoclonic, atonic, and complex partial seizures.); benign familial neonatal convulsions (two different potassium channels); and forms of juvenile myoclonic epilepsy and childhood absence epilepsy (subunits of the brain $GABA_A$ receptor).

Some of these are summarized in Table 16-3, and their number will almost certainly expand in the next few years. As with numerous other genetic neurologic disorders, a single mutation may produce different epilepsy and seizure types, and a single type may be the result of one of several different mutations. Also notable is the low penetrance of some monogenic epileptic disorders, particularly the autosomal dominant one associated with nocturnal frontal seizures.

Another group of epilepsies with mendelian inheritance has been ascribed to genetic defects that do not implicate ion channels. Most of these are primarily myoclonic disorders in which the epilepsy is one component. Two forms of progressive myoclonic epilepsy, Unverricht-Lundborg disease and Lafora body disease, are the result, respectively, of mutations in genes encoding cystatin B and tyrosine phosphatase. To these inherited forms of epilepsy may be added diseases such as tuberous sclerosis and ceroid lipofuscinosis (Chap. 37), which have a strong proclivity to cause seizures and genetically determined heterotopias such as FLN1 (this and other developmental aberrations are discussed in Chap. 38).

A more complex genetic element is also identified in several childhood seizure disorders—absence epilepsy with 3-per-second spike-and-wave discharges and benign epilepsy of childhood with centrotemporal spikes—both of which are transmitted as autosomal dominant traits with incomplete penetrance or perhaps in a more complicated manner. In the partial, or focal, epilepsies the role of heredity is not nearly so clear. Yet in numerous studies there has been a greater-than-expected incidence of seizures, EEG abnormalities, or both among first-degree relatives. Among the familial cortical epilepsies, both a temporal and frontal lobe type, are inherited in a polygenic fashion or in an autosomal dominant pattern. Undoubtedly also inherited, is the tendency to develop simple febrile convulsions, though the mode of inheritance is uncertain.

CLINICAL APPROACH TO EPILEPSY

The physician faced with a patient who seeks advice about an episodic disorder of nervous function must determine first, whether the episode in question is a seizure. In the diagnosis of epilepsy, history is the key; in most adult cases the physical examination is relatively unrevealing. The examination in infants and children is of greater value, as the finding of dysmorphic and cutaneous abnormalities allow the diagnosis of a number of highly characteristic cerebral diseases that give rise to epilepsy.

Paramount in establishing that there has been a seizure is a description from a witness. A detailed account of the event is required and in particular, the type and duration of bodily movements, level of alertness and responsiveness during and immediately after the episode, skin color and breathing, and incontinence. If a witness is not available, then a telephone call to observers and family may give more information than does sophisticated laboratory testing. From the patient, information can be obtained regarding tongue biting, incontinence, and recollection of the event of the immediately preceding epoch. If the patient is able to provide information, previous events that may have been misinterpreted as other than a seizure, for example, brief losses of consciousness, myoclonic jerks, rumpled bedsheets with incontinence, unexplained falls with injury and so forth, may hint at preceding seizures. The family history, developmental milestones, neonatal events and the circumstances of birth are useful additional aspects of the evaluation of epilepsy.

The conditions most likely to simulate an epileptic seizure are psychogenic nonepileptic seizures and other paroxysmal events such as panic attack and syncope but also, unexplained falls (drop attacks), transient ischemic attacks, particularly those associated with limb shaking, sleepwalking and rapid eye movement (REM) sleep behavior disorder, subarachnoid hemorrhage, migraine, hypoglycemia, cataplexy, paroxysmal ataxia and choreoathetosis, and transient global amnesia. In emergency departments it is often difficult to differentiate the postictal effects of an unwitnessed seizure from the confusion and amnesia following cerebral concussion.

The clinical differences between a seizure and a *syncopal attack* are considered in Chapter 18; there it was emphasized that no single criterion stands inviolate. Particularly emphasized because of their potential gravity are episodes of cardiac syncope from a serious arrhythmia, especially ventricular tachycardia. Cardiac arrhythmias may present as episodes of unheralded loss of consciousness, sometimes with associated convulsive movements that simulate epileptic disorders and the failure to pursue the diagnosis of arrhythmia may have important consequences. Palpitations, previous myocardial infarction, EKG abnormalities, valvular disease, and thoracic trauma may direct attention to the proper diagnosis.

Absence attacks may be difficult to identify because of their brevity. Helpful maneuvers are to have the patient hyperventilate to evoke an attack or to observe the patient counting aloud for several minutes. Those with frequent absence attacks will pause or skip one or two numbers. The diagnosis of temporal lobe epilepsy is similarly difficult. These attacks are so variable and so often induce disturbances of behavior and psychic function—rather than overt interruptions or loss of consciousness—that they may be mistaken for temper tantrums in children, drug ingestion, hysteria, panic attacks, or acute psychosis. These seizures may include verbalizations that cannot be remembered, walking aimlessly, repetitive olfactory and gustatory hallucinations, stereotyped hand movements or automatism such as lip smacking. The nature of the patient's report of a psychic experience is often helpful in distinguishing seizures from psychogenic events. In the former, patients attempt to focus with great effort on the description of the experience, although the term "indescribable" is often included in the report, whereas vague and imprecise descriptions of "something being wrong" or resorting to a friend or family member to describe the event usually implicates a psychogenic seizure. We place emphasis on amnesia for the events of at least part of the seizure as an important criterion for the diagnosis of temporal lobe epilepsy.

Migraine may be mistaken for a seizure. One feature of the focal neurologic disorder of typical migraine is particularly helpful—namely, the pace of the sequence of cerebral malfunction over a period of minutes rather than seconds, as in focal epilepsy. Even this criterion may fail occasionally, especially if both migraine and partial seizures are joined, e.g., as expressions of a vascular malformation of the brain.

Identification of a TIA and its separation from focal epilepsy are aided by considering that most paroxysmal vascular disorders are characterized by loss of function that can be attributed to one area of the cortex such as paralysis, blindness, diplopia, or aphasia. If the ischemic attack is marked by an evolution of symptoms, they tend to develop more slowly than those of a seizure. The patient's age and presence of vascular risk factors, evidence of disease of the heart and carotid arteries, and the lack of disorder of consciousness or amnesia may be supportive of the diagnosis of vascular disease. However, a "limb-shaking" TIA and convulsive phenomena at the outset of basilar artery occlusion may be nearly impossible to distinguish from epilepsy.

Regarding the distinction of seizures from odd disorders such as cataplexy, paroxysmal ataxia or choreoathetosis, transient global amnesia, it is sufficient to be aware of the diagnostic features for each of these conditions. Hysterical fugues can cause substantial difficulty in diagnosis. They may be recognized by the loss of personal identity and by episodes that are longer that typical or seizures, sometimes up to a few days. REM sleep behavior disorder tend to occur later in the sleep cycle, as they require REM, whereas frontal epileptic seizures with violent motions or acts that might be mistaken for REM sleep behavior disorder, can occur at any time of the night and tend to be briefer than the sleep disorder. *Drop attacks* (falling to the ground without loss of consciousness as discussed in Chap. 7) remain an enigma. In most cases, it has not been possible to substantiate an association with circulatory disturbances of the vertebrobasilar system and seldom have we observed drop attacks to be an expression of atonic or myoclonic epilepsy.

Several laboratory studies are usually included in the initial diagnostic evaluation—complete blood count (CBC), blood chemistries, EKG, EEG, and imaging study of the brain, preferably MRI. CT scanning gives limited information on major problems that may underlie epilepsy but MRI is vastly superior in detecting the various structural causes of epilepsy. Nonetheless, CT may be the only feasible study when MRI is not available or in emergency circumstances. If blood is tested after the episode in question, elevation in creatine kinase (persistent for hours) and formerly, elevation of prolactin (for up to 10 min) may occur after an unwitnessed convulsive seizure but the test is not specific enough to be useful in general practice. Other forms of testing—e.g., cardiac stress tests, Holter monitor, tilt-table testing, long-term patient-activated cardiac monitors, and sleep studies—are sometimes indicated in order to exclude some of the nonepileptic disorders listed earlier. Some patients may need prolonged EEG monitoring, either in the hospital or with portable equipment at home. In all forms of epilepsy, prolonged EEG and video monitoring in a hospital unit may prove diagnostic.

Seizures in Each Age Period

(Table 16-4 and Fig. 16-5)

Having concluded that the neurologic disturbance under consideration is one of seizure, the next issue is to identify its type. Indeed, in most cases this determines the nature of treatment. Because there are so many seizure types, especially in childhood and adolescence, each one tending to predominate in a certain age period, a clinical advantage accrues to considering seizures from just this point of view. A broader approach includes consideration of the neurologic and EEG findings, the response to drugs, etiology, and prognosis.

Table 16-4

CAUSES OF RECURRENT SEIZURES IN DIFFERENT AGE GROUPS

AGE OF ONSET	PROBABLE CAUSE[a]
Neonatal	Congenital maldevelopment, birth injury, anoxia, metabolic disorders (hypocalcemia, hypoglycemia, vitamin B6 deficiency, biotinidase deficiency, phenylketonuria, and others)
Infancy (1–6 months)	As above; infantile spasms (West syndrome)
Early childhood (6 months–3 years)	Infantile spasms, febrile convulsions, birth injury and anoxia, infections, trauma, metabolic disorders, cortical dysgenesis, accidental drug poisoning
Childhood (3–10 years)	Perinatal anoxia, injury at birth or later, infections, thrombosis of cerebral arteries or veins, metabolic disorders, cortical malformations, Lennox-Gastaut syndrome, "idiopathic," probably inherited, epilepsy (Rolandic epilepsy)
Adolescence (10–18 years)	Idiopathic epilepsy, including genetically transmitted types, juvenile myoclonic epilepsy, trauma, drugs
Early adulthood (18–25 years)	Idiopathic epilepsy, trauma, neoplasm, withdrawal from alcohol or other sedative drugs
Middle age (35–60 years)	Trauma, neoplasm, vascular disease, alcohol or other drug withdrawal
Late life (older than 60 years)	Vascular disease (usually postinfarction), tumor, abscess, degenerative disease, trauma

[a]Meningitis or encephalitis and their complications may be a cause of seizures at any age. This is true also of severe metabolic disturbances. In tropical and subtropical countries, parasitic infection of the CNS is a common cause.
(See also Fig. 16-5.)

Figure 16-5 displays the frequency of each seizure type and the main causes of seizures by age group. These data are assembled from various sources and are approximate, but they highlight several points of clinical importance.

Neonatal Seizures

The neonatologist is often confronted by an infant who begins to convulse in the first days of life. In most instances, the seizures are fragmentary—an abrupt movement or posturing of a limb, stiffening of the body, rolling up of the eyes, a pause in respirations, lip-smacking, chewing, or bicycling movements of the legs. Even the experienced observer may have difficulty at times in distinguishing seizure activity from the normal movements of the neonate. If manifest seizures are frequent and stereotyped, the diagnosis is less difficult. The seizures correlate with focal or multifocal cortical discharges; however, as is the case with most EEG changes in neonates, these are poorly formed and less distinct than seizure discharges in later life. Presumably the immaturity of the cerebrum prevents the development of a fully organized seizure pattern, and the incomplete corticocortical myelination prevents bihemispheric spread. The EEG is nonetheless helpful in diagnosis. For example, periods of EEG suppression may alternate with sharp or slow waves, or there may be discontinuous theta activity that represents electrographic seizure activity. Conversely, electrical seizure activity in the neonate may be unattended by clinical manifestations.

An early onset of myoclonic jerks, either fragmentary or massive, with an EEG pattern of alternating suppression and complex bursts of activity is particularly ominous. Ohtahara described another unfavorable form of neonatal seizure evolving in infancy into infantile spasms (West syndrome) and Lennox-Gastaut syndrome and leaving in its wake severe brain damage. Most reported patients have been left developmentally delayed.

Neonatal seizures occurring within 24 to 48 h of a difficult birth are usually indicative of severe cerebral damage, usually anoxic, either antenatal or parturitional. Such infants often succumb, and about half of the survivors are seriously handicapped. *Seizures having their onset several days or weeks after birth* are more often an expression of acquired or hereditary metabolic disease. In the latter group, hypoglycemia is the most frequent cause; another, hypocalcemia with tetany, has become infrequent. A hereditary form of pyridoxine deficiency is a rare cause, sometimes also inducing seizures in utero and characteristically responding promptly to massive doses (100 mg) of vitamin B_6 given intravenously. Biotinidase deficiency is a rare but correctable cause. Nonketotic hyperglycemia, maple syrup urine disease, as well as other metabolic disorders may lead to seizures in the first week or two of life and are expressive of a more diffuse encephalopathy.

In contrast, benign forms of neonatal seizures have also been identified. Plouin described a form of benign neonatal clonic convulsions beginning on days 2 and 3, up to day 7, ("fifth day seizures") in which there were no specific EEG changes. The seizures then remit and have a

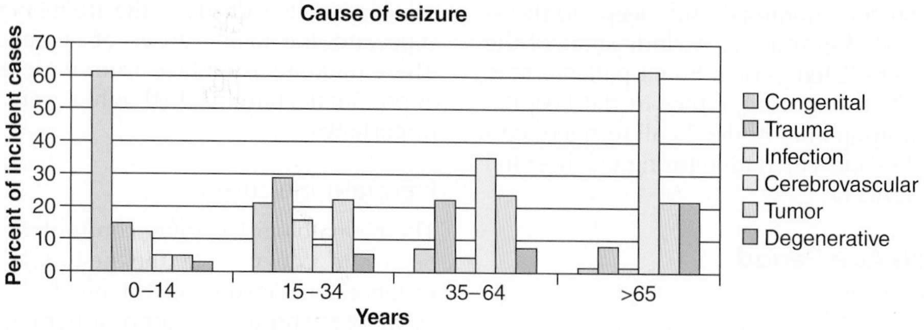

Figure 16-5. Distribution of the main causes of epilepsy at different ages. Evident is the prevalence of congenital causes in childhood and the emergence of cerebrovascular disease in older patients. (Adapted from several sources including Hauser and Annegers and the texts of Engel and of Pedley.)

good prognosis. The inheritance is autosomal dominant. There are other nonfamilial cases with onset on days 4 to 6, wherein the partial seizures may even increase to status epilepticus; the EEG consists of discontinuous theta activity. In both these groups, the outlook for normal development is good and seizures seldom recur later in life. There are also benign forms of polymyoclonus without seizures or EEG abnormality in this age period. Some occur only with slow-wave sleep or feeding. They disappear after a few months and require no treatment. A form of benign nocturnal myoclonus in the neonate is also well known.

Infantile Epilepsies

Neonatal seizures may continue into the infantile period, or seizures may begin in an infant who seemed to be normal up to the time of the first convulsive attack. While the most common type of convulsion is the febrile seizure, not strictly a type of epilepsy, the most characteristic epilepsy at this age is the massive sudden myoclonic jerk of head and arms leading to flexion or, less often, to extension of the body (*infantile spasms*, salaam spasms). This form, which characterizes the West syndrome as described earlier, has many underlying causes. The same seizure type occurs in infants with tuberous sclerosis (diagnosed in infancy by the presence of hypopigmentated macules, or "ash-leaf spots"), phenylketonuria, or Sturge-Weber angiomatosis, but most often it is associated with other diseases beginning in this age period. Some instances of infantile spasms may be due to a metabolic encephalopathy of unknown type or, a cortical dysgenesis (Jellinger). West syndrome is characterized by an EEG picture of large bilateral slow waves and multifocal spikes (*hypsarrhythmia*).

The recently clarified Dravet syndrome, which includes myoclonic and focal seizures, occurs in this age group but has become relevant to adult practice as patients are recognized with resistant epilepsy and learning disability or developmental delay. It the past the epilepsy and developmental delay were attributed to a febrile illness or vaccination in infancy but it has become clear that the syndrome has a genetic underpinning and a resultant abnormality of a sodium channel protein (SCN1A) and the manifestations have simply been bought forward by the initial neonatal event.

When myoclonus begins in infancy with fever and unilateral or bilateral clonic seizures or with focal seizures followed by focal neurologic abnormalities, there is a likelihood of developmental delay. The latter types are sometimes referred to as *complicated febrile seizures*, but, as indicated above, they must be distinguished from the benign familial febrile seizure syndrome discussed earlier in the chapter. Infantile spasms cease by the end of the second year and are replaced by focal and secondarily generalized seizures. They do not respond well to the usual antiepileptic medications. While myoclonic activity with seizures in this age group raises concern of a serious condition, there is a common benign form that has a heritable component and does not lead to developmental delay.

Seizures Presenting in Early Childhood

A number of focal epilepsies may appear for the first time during this age period and carry a good prognosis, i.e., the neurologic and intellectual capacities remain relatively unimpaired and seizures may cease in adolescence. These disorders begin between 3 and 13 years of age and there is often a familial predisposition. Most are marked by distinctive focal spike activity that is accentuated by sleep (see above, in reference to benign childhood epilepsy with centrotemporal or occipital spikes). Several of these have been discussed earlier under the Special Epileptic Syndromes. In one form, benign childhood epilepsy with centrotemporal spikes, unilateral tonic or clonic contractions of the face and limbs recur repeatedly with or without paresthesia; anarthria may follow the seizure. There are central and temporal spikes in the EEG interictally. Less commonly, the focus originates in an occipital lobe with EEG spiking on eye closure. An acquired aphasia characterizes another disorder that was described by Landau and Kleffner to mark the beginning of an illness in which there are partial or generalized motor seizures and multifocal spike or spike-and-wave discharges in the EEG and deterioration of language function.

Among the generalized epilepsies, childhood absence epilepsy arises in children of this age, as described earlier as well. As in any age group, there are structural causes of seizures that include medial temporal sclerosis, described in several places in this chapter, tumor and arteriovenous malformation.

The convulsive state in this age group may present around the age of 4 years as a focal myoclonus with or without astatic seizures, atypical absence, or generalized tonic-clonic seizures. The EEG, repeated if initially normal, is most helpful in diagnosis; it reveals a paroxysmal 2- to 2.5-per-second spike-and-wave pattern on a background of predominant 4- to 7-Hz slow waves. Many of these cases qualify as the Lennox-Gastaut syndrome, are difficult to treat, and are likely to be associated with developmental delay. At this age, perhaps more than any other, the first burst of seizures may take the form of status epilepticus and, if not successfully controlled, may end fatally.

In contrast to the Lennox-Gastaut group, the more typical absence, with its regularly recurring 3-per-second spike-and-wave EEG abnormality, also begins in this age period (rarely before age 4 years) and carries a good prognosis. This seizure disorder responds well to medications, as indicated further on. Its features are fully described in "Absence Variants." The special case of Rasmussen encephalitis and intractable seizures has already been discussed under the Special Epileptic Syndromes.

Seizures in Later Childhood and Adolescence

These represent a common problem in practice but present a special difficulty because this is the age at which syncope and psychogenic seizures begin to occur and alcohol and drug abuse may begin. Here, we face the frequent issue relating to the nature and management of the first seizure in an otherwise normal young person. As in other age groups, the history often discloses the likely cause of seizures, as for example, in young person has been sleep deprived or imbibing alcohol or one of many abused drugs and has a first seizure. A search for a cause is necessary by MRI, EKG, and EEG but these tests infrequently disclose hippocampal sclerosis, cortical heterotopia, tumor, infection, or a vascular malformation and the epilepsy, if there are certain characteristic other features such as myoclonic jerks or more than one seizure, is then classified as idiopathic and genetic. If there has only been a single event and no clinical or EEG features to corroborate epilepsy, the diagnosis must remain uncertain. However, the type of seizure that first brings the child or adolescent to medical attention is most likely to be a generalized tonic-clonic convulsion and often marks the beginning of idiopathic generalized epilepsy or juvenile myoclonic epilepsy, as described an earlier section. As described there the latter syndrome is identified by intermittent myoclonic jerks when the patient is tired or after the ingestion of alcohol. Seizures are usually grand mal but a few have had a history of absence. The EEG shows a characteristic polyspike pattern, about one-third with a photomyoclonic response, and treatment with certain anticonvulsants is very successful at suppressing seizures and myoclonus.

In a case where there had been some type of seizure at an earlier period, one should suspect a developmental disorder, parturitional hypoxic-ischemic encephalopathy (birth injury), or one of the hereditary metabolic diseases.

When the seizures are an expression of a long-standing epileptic focus or foci that is associated with developmental delay or scholastic failure, the diagnostic and therapeutic problem becomes much more demanding. Some patients of this group will eventually fall into the category of epilepsy with complex partial seizures. In this age period in particular, as the adolescent strives for independence, the social disruption caused by seizures are likely to take a toll on the relationships and educational progress of the emerging adult.

In the special group of younger individuals with *long-standing seizures*, nearly half have temporal lobe epilepsy. Huttenlocher and Hapke, in a follow-up study of 145 infants and children with intractable epilepsy, found that the majority had borderline or subnormal intelligence.

Opinion is divided on whether treatment is required for the older child or adolescent who comes to medical attention because of a first seizure that appears to be idiopathic. When such cases have been left untreated, such as in the series reported by Hesdorfer and colleagues, the risk of another seizure over 10 years was 13 percent unless the first episode was status epilepticus, in which case the risk was 41 percent. Age, sex, and the circumstances of the seizure (withdrawal from drugs or alcohol, myoclonic episodes, family history) all figure into the risk. Attention to what had in the past been called "hygiene" can be all that is required until the problem has ceased or clarified itself as an epileptic disorder, namely regularizing sleep and minimizing alcohol and stimulants.

Seizures Due to Underlying Medical Disease

Several diseases announce themselves by an acute convulsion. Here we focus on generalized medical disorders as causes of single and episodic seizures, in contrast to structural lesions of the brain that cause focal or generalized epilepsy.

Withdrawal Seizures

The possibility of abstinence seizures in patients who abuse alcohol, barbiturates, or benzodiazepine and related sedative drugs must be considered when seizures occur for the first time in adult life or in adolescence. Suspicion is raised by the stigmata of alcohol abuse or a history of prolonged anxiety and depression requiring sedative drugs. Also, sleep disturbance, tremulousness, disorientation, illusions, and hallucinations can be associated with the convulsive phase of the illness. Seizures in this setting may occur singly, but as often, in a brief flurry, the entire convulsive period lasting for several hours and rarely for a day or longer, during which time the patient may display twitchiness or myoclonus and be unduly sensitive to photic stimulation. Chapter 42 discusses alcohol and other drug-related seizures in detail.

Infections and Inflammatory-immune Conditions

An outburst of seizures is also a prominent feature of all varieties of *bacterial meningitis*, more so in children than in adults. Fever, headache, and stiff neck provide the clues to diagnosis, and lumbar puncture yields the salient data. Myoclonic jerking and seizures may appear early in acute *herpes simplex encephalitis* and other forms of viral, treponemal, and parasitic encephalitis, including those derived from HIV infection, both directly and indirectly such as toxoplasmosis and brain lymphoma; and in subacute sclerosing panencephalitis. In tropical countries, cysticercosis and tuberculous granulomas of the brain are very common causes of epilepsy. Seizure(s) without fever or stiff neck may be the initial manifestation of syphilitic meningitis, a fact worth noting as this process reemerges in AIDS patients.

A special case of autoimmune encephalitides may cause seizures as, for example, those caused by the anti-NMDA receptor antibody that is associated with ovarian and other teratomas and other paraneoplastic conditions such as the antibody syndrome directed at the voltage-gated potassium channel complex (see Chap. 31).

Seizures in Metabolic Encephalopathy

Uremia has a strong convulsive tendency. Of interest is the relation of seizures to the development of acute anuric renal failure, generally from acute tubular necrosis but occasionally due to glomerular disease. Total anuria may be tolerated for several days without the appearance of neurologic signs, and then there is an abrupt onset of twitching, trembling, myoclonic jerks, and brief generalized motor seizures; acute hypertension probably plays a role. The entire motor constellation, one of the most dramatic in medicine, lasts several days until the patient sinks into terminal coma or recovers by dialysis. When this *twitch-convulsive syndrome* accompanies lupus erythematosus, seizures of undetermined cause, or generalized neoplasia, one should suspect its basis in renal failure.

Other *acute metabolic illnesses and electrolytic disorders* complicated by generalized and multifocal motor seizures are hyponatremia and its opposite, the hypernatremic, hyperglycemic and other hyperosmolar states, thyrotoxic storm, porphyria, hypoglycemia, hypomagnesemia, and hypocalcemia. In all these cases, *rapidly evolving electrolyte abnormalities are more likely to cause seizures than those occurring gradually.* For this reason it is not possible to assign absolute levels of sodium, blood urea nitrogen (BUN), osmolarity, or glucose concentrations above or below which seizures are likely to occur. Lead (in children) and mercury (in children and adults) are the most frequent of the metallic poisons that cause convulsions. The presence of these heavy metals in culturally based homeopathic treatments should not be overlooked.

In most cases of seizures caused by metabolic and withdrawal states, treatment with antiepileptic drugs is not necessary as long as the underlying disturbance is rectified. Indeed, antiepileptic drugs are usually ineffective in halting the seizures if the metabolic disorder persists.

Generalized seizures, with or without twitching, occur in the advanced stages of many other illnesses, such as *hypertensive encephalopathy*, the posterior reversible encephalopathy syndrome from causes other than hypertension (PRES as discussed in Chap. 34), sepsis—especially gram-negative septicemia with shock—hepatic stupor, and intractable congestive heart failure. Usually, seizures in these circumstances can be traced to an associated metabolic abnormality and are revealed by appropriate studies of the blood. Seizures are a central feature of the eclamptic syndrome as discussed in a separate section below.

Medications as a Cause of Seizures

A large number of medications are capable of causing seizures, usually when toxic blood levels are attained. The antibiotic imipenem and excessive doses of other penicillin congeners and linezolid may be responsible, particularly if renal failure leads to drug accumulation. Cefepime, a fourth-generation cephalosporin, widely used for the treatment of gram-negative sepsis, can result in status epilepticus, if given in excessive dosage (Dixit et al). The tricyclic antidepressants, bupropion, and lithium may cause seizures, particularly in the presence of a structural brain lesion. Lidocaine and aminophylline are known to induce an unheralded single convulsion if administered too quickly or in excessive doses. The use of the analgesic tramadol has also been associated with seizures. Curiously, the anesthetic propofol, which is discussed further on as a potent anticonvulsant in the treatment of status epilepticus, has caused marked myoclonic phenomena in some patients and, rarely, seizures. These may occur during induction or emergence from anesthesia or as a delayed effect (Walder et al).

The list of medications that at one time or another have been associated with a convulsion is long and, if no other explanation for a single seizure is evident, the physician is advised to look up in standard references the side effects of the drugs being administered to the patient. In a few of our otherwise healthy adult patients, extreme *sleep deprivation* coupled with ingestion of large doses of antibiotics or adrenergic medications or other remedies that are used indiscriminately for the symptomatic relief of colds has been the only plausible explanation for a single or doublet seizure.

Global Arrest of Circulation

Cardiac arrest, suffocation or respiratory failure, carbon monoxide poisoning, or other causes of *hypoxic encephalopathy* tend to induce diffuse myoclonic jerking and generalized seizures as cardiac function resumes. The myoclonic-convulsive phase of this condition may last only a few hours or days, in association with coma, stupor, and confusion; or it may persist indefinitely as an intention myoclonus state (Lance-Adams syndrome).

Cerebrovascular Diseases

Convulsive seizures are quite uncommon in the acute or evolving phases of an arterial stroke. The ischemic convulsive phenomena of a "limb-shaking TIA" and a burst of generalized clonic motor activity during basilar artery occlusion have been mentioned earlier, but are uncommon and are not epileptic phenomena. Only exceptionally will acute embolic infarction of the brain cause a focal seizure at the onset. Otherwise, a new seizure should not be attributed to an acute arterial occlusion in the cerebrum.

However, embolic infarcts involving the cortex become epileptogenic in fewer than 10 percent of cases and only after an interval of several months or longer. It has been stated in texts that thrombotic infarcts involving the cortex are almost never convulsive at their onset but any distinction in seizure frequency between stroke types seems to us to be based on limited data. Lacunar infarction, being deep and not involving the cortical surface, of course, does not produce convulsions.

In contrast, *cortical venous thrombosis* with underlying ischemia and infarction acts as a highly epileptogenic lesion (see Chap. 34). The same is true for hypertensive encephalopathy (including the above mentioned reversible posterior encephalopathy and eclampsia) and thrombotic thrombocytopenic purpura (TTP), which has a strong tendency to cause nonconvulsive status epilepticus. The rupture of a saccular aneurysm is sometimes marked by one or two generalized convulsions that are not epileptic in nature and are probably predicated on the arrest of cerebral circulation. Deep cerebral hemorrhages, spontaneous or traumatic, also occasionally become sources of recurrent focal seizures.

The use of anticonvulsants as prophylaxis for seizures after a typical cortical stroke of embolic or thrombotic type or cerebral hemorrhage is not necessary. The rate of such seizures has been estimated to be 3 percent or less in the first year. This subject is addressed further in Chap. 34.

Seizures with Acute Head Injury

It is not uncommon for severe concussion to be attended by brief convulsive movements (see Chap. 35). The appearance is in most cases of clonic twitching but may include a momentary tonic phase. Rarely, a prolonged clonic convulsion occurs. The nature of this event, whether originating in the reticular formation as a component of concussion, or from some disruption of cortical activity, is not clear. Almost invariably in our experience, the EEG recorded hours or a day later is normal, and imaging studies are likewise normal or show a small contusion. There is little to guide one in treatment of these patients; we tend to give a course of antiepileptic medications for several weeks but it is not established if this is the correct approach. Aside from penetrating brain trauma, the risk of delayed seizures is low. Further details on this subject can be found in Chap. 35.

Seizures during Pregnancy

Here one contends with two problems: one, the woman with epilepsy who becomes pregnant; the other, the woman who has her first seizure during pregnancy. According to the extensive EURAP study, about two-thirds of epileptic women who become pregnant have no change in seizure frequency or severity (the majority remain seizure free); the remainder are evenly split between those in whom the frequency increases and in an equal number, it lessens. In a large cohort of such women, there was a slight increase in the number of stillbirths and a doubling in the expected incidence of developmental delay and nonfebrile seizures in their offspring (see later).

Issues regarding a coagulopathy in the fetus exposed to phenobarbital (now infrequently used for adult seizure disorders) and certain of the other drugs are well known to obstetricians and pediatric specialists and are treated with the oral administration of vitamin K, 20 mg/d during the eighth month or 10 mg IV 4 h before birth and 1 mg IM to the neonate. The conventional anticonvulsants also seem to be safe for the baby during breast-feeding in that only small amounts are excreted in lactated milk. For example, carbamazepine in human milk is found to be 40 percent of the mother's serum concentration which results in a neonatal blood level that is below the conventionally detectable amount. Phenytoin is excreted at 15 percent of maternal serum concentration, and valproate, being highly protein bound, is virtually absent in breast milk. No adverse effects have been attributed to these small amounts of drug.

The special issue of the teratogenicity of antiepileptic drugs is addressed further on.

Seizures with Eclampsia (See also Chap. 34.)

This syndrome appears during the last trimester of pregnancy or soon after delivery and may announce itself by hypertension and convulsions; the latter are generalized and tend to occur in clusters. The standard practice is to induce labor or perform a cesarean section and manage the seizures as one would manage those of hypertensive encephalopathy (of which this is one type). The administration of magnesium sulfate continues to be the favored treatment by obstetricians for the prevention of eclamptic seizures; two randomized trials have reestablished its value in preventing seizures in preeclamptic women (Lucas et al) and in avoiding a second convulsion once one had occurred (Eclampsia Trial Collaborative Group). Magnesium sulfate, 10 g IM, followed by 5 g every 4 h, proved comparable to standard doses of phenytoin as prophylaxis for seizures. Our colleagues use a regimen of 4 g IV over 5 to 10 min followed by a maintenance dose of 5 g every 4 h IM or 1 to 2 g/h IV. In nontoxic gestational epilepsy, approximately 25 percent of patients are found to have some disease (neoplastic, vascular, or traumatic) that will persist.

Epilepsy in Late Adult Life

Seizures in this age group present special problems in diagnosis. Often, these individuals live alone so there is no witness to the event, they have multiple medical problems, they may have cognitive difficulty that impedes an accurate history, multiple medications are almost the rule, and cerebral imaging is likely to show abnormalities that may not be referable to the problem at hand.

Nonetheless, Hauser and Kurland reported an increase in the incidence of seizures as the population ages—from 11.9 per 100,000 in the 40- to 60-year-old age group to 82 per 100,000 in those 60 years of age or older. It is possible that these are overestimates due to the complicating factors alluded to in the paragraph above. A person in the latter age group who begins to have seizures of either partial or generalized type is always to be suspected of harboring a primary or secondary tumor or a past cerebral infarct that had not declared itself clinically.

Recent published series suggesting that the majority of seizures in this age group are caused by infarction and a small number by tumor are not in accord with our experience. For example, according to Sung and Chu, previous infarcts are by far the most common lesions underlying status epilepticus in late adult life, but our experience has been that old trauma is considerably more common. Probably the nature of the population in a given clinic determines the relative frequency of underlying causes. In any case, cerebral imaging usually settles the issue.

However, many apparent seizures in this age group are the result of a primary cardiac event, particularly an arrhythmia such as ventricular tachycardia. Therefore, a 12 lead EKG and further monitoring of heart rhythm are important ancillary tests if the episode remains unexplained.

Cortical and subcortical lesions, the result of previous traumatic contusions, are a particularly important cause of seizures among older alcoholics; the lesions are revealed by brain imaging and are typically located in the anterior frontal and temporal lobes. Brain abscess and other inflammatory and infectious illnesses remain common causes of adult seizures in tropical regions. In the elderly, seizures as a result of Alzheimer and other degenerative diseases occur in up to 10 percent of cases, but are not a source of diagnostic challenge; nonetheless, these patients are subject to falls, subdural hematoma, and all other illnesses of old age, such as cancer, that affect the brain.

In the common case of an adult with a first unexplained seizure, it has been our practice not to administer an antiepileptic medication unless there is an underlying structural lesion or an abnormality on a single EEG or with prolonged monitoring and to reevaluate the situation in 6 to 12 months. Usually, a second MRI and EEG are performed to exclude focal abnormalities that were not appreciated during the initial evaluation, but often these studies are again unrevealing. This approach has been prompted by data such as those of Hauser and colleagues, who found that about one-third of patients with a single unprovoked seizure will have another seizure within 5 years; the risk is even greater if there is a history of seizures in a sibling, a complex febrile convulsion in childhood, or a spike-and-wave abnormality in the EEG. Moreover, the risk of recurrence is greatest in the first 24 months. In patients with two or three unexplained seizures, a far higher proportion, about 75 percent, have further seizures in the subsequent 4 years.

TREATMENT OF EPILEPSY

The treatment of epilepsy of all types can be divided into four parts: the use of antiepileptic drugs, the surgical excision of epileptic foci and other surgical measures, the removal of causative and precipitating factors, and the regulation of physical and mental activity.

Antiepileptic Drugs—General Principles

The goal of drug treatment is to create a seizure-free state if possible and with the fewest side effects. In the past, a few seizures a year had been considered adequate control but with the bevy of newer medications it is advisable to aspire to the goal of eliminating seizures. On the other hand, it is an error to make the patients so mentally dulled as to interfere with function at work or school. The choice and dose of medication depends on many factors including sex, age, other medications being used by the individual, and renal or hepatic dysfunction or other medical conditions and psychiatric that might be favorably influenced by a particular agent. As a general rule, starting in the lower dose range and attempting to provide twice daily or daily administration are favored.

In approximately 70 percent of all patients with epilepsy, the seizures are controlled completely or almost completely by medications; in an additional 20 to 25 percent, the attacks are significantly reduced in number and severity. Table 16-5 lists the most commonly used drugs along with their dosages, effective blood levels, and serum half-lives. Because of the long half-lives of phenytoin, phenobarbital, and ethosuximide, these drugs need be taken only once daily, preferably at bedtime. Valproate and carbamazepine have shorter half-lives, and their administration should be spaced during the day. It is useful to be familiar with the serum protein-binding characteristics of antiepileptic drugs and the interactions among these drugs, and between antiepileptic and other drugs.

Certain drugs are somewhat more effective in one type of seizure than in another, and it is necessary to use the proper drugs in optimum dosages for different circumstances. Initially, only one drug should be used and the dosage increased until sustained therapeutic levels have been attained. If the first drug does not control seizures, a different one should be tried, but frequent shifting of drugs is not advisable; each should be given an adequate trial before another is substituted. A general approach to the choice of drug in certain common forms of epilepsy is given in Tables 16-6 for adults and 16-7 for children, but it must be noted that there are a number of drugs that may be appropriate in each circumstance.

It is difficult to give definitive guidance on combining medications for refractory seizures. Several general principles are, however, worth noting. First, it is sensible to avoid drugs combinations with similar putative mechanisms because their side effects may be additive, for example, the addition of lamotrigine to carbamazepine or of phenytoin to carbamazepine may not be ideal but at the same time, it should be mentioned that the mechanism of action has little influence on clinical effectiveness. Second, the clinician should be aware of known interactions through metabolic pathways such as valproate combined with either lamotrigine or phenobarbital as they share the cytochrome P450 degradation pathway. Third, although it is appropriate to use drugs that are known to be effective for the class of seizures under treatment, it is often necessary to extend the choices beyond these restrictions.

The therapeutic dose for any given patient must be determined, to some extent by clinical effect, guided by measurement of serum levels, as described below. Inquiry regarding seizure control and drug side effects is more valuable than adjustment of medication based solely on drug concentrations. Blood for

Table 16-5

COMMON ANTIEPILEPTIC DRUGS

GENERIC NAME	TRADE NAME	USUAL DOSAGE: CHILDREN, MG/KG	USUAL DOSAGE: ADULTS, MG/D	PRINCIPAL THERAPEUTIC INDICATIONS	SERUM HALF-LIFE, H	EFFECTIVE BLOOD LEVEL,[a] µG/ML
Major antiepileptic used as monotherapy						
Valproic acid	Depakote	30–60	1,000–3,000	Generalized tonic-clonic, partial, absence, myoclonic	6–15	50–100
Phenytoin	Dilantin	4–7	300–400	Generalized tonic-clonic, partial, absence, myoclonic	12–36	10–20
Carbamazepine	Tegretol	20–30	600–1,200[b]	Generalized tonic-clonic, partial	14–25	4–12
Oxcarbazepine	Trileptal	10–40	900–2,400	Partial	1–5	—
Phenobarbital	Luminal	3–5 (8 for infants)	90–200	Generalized tonic-clonic, partial	40–120	15–40
Lamotrigine	Lamictal	0.5	300–500	Generalized, partial	15–60	2–7
Levetiracetam	Keppra	20–60	500–3,000[b]	Partial, myoclonic	6–8	—
Adjuvant and special-use anticonvulsants						
Topiramate	Topamax	—	400	Generalized tonic-clonic, atypical absence, myoclonic, partial	20–30	—
Lacosamide	Vimpat					
Zonisamide	Zonegren					
Primidone	Mysoline	10–25	750–1,500[b]	Generalized tonic-clonic, partial	6–18	5–12
Ethosuximide	Zarontin	20–40	750–1,500	Absence	20–60	50–100
Methsuximide	Celontin	10–20	500–1,000	Absence	28–50	40–100
ACTH	—	40–60 Units daily	—	Infantile spasms	—	—
Clonazepam	Klonopin	0.01–0.2	2–10	Absence, myoclonus	18–50	0.01–0.07
Anticonvulsants for status epilepticus *(initial loading or continuous infusion doses shown)*[c]—phenytoin and phenobarbital used in doses higher than shown above						
Diazepam	Valium	0.15–2	2–20	Status epilepticus	—	—
Lorazepam	Ativan	0.03–0.22	2–20	Status epilepticus	—	—
Midazolam	Versed	—	0.1–0.4 mg/kg/h	Status epilepticus	—	—
Propofol	Diprivan	2.5–3.5	2–8 mg/kg/h	Status epilepticus	—	—
Fosphenytoin	Cerebyx	30–50 mg	1,000–1,500	Status epilepticus	—	10–20

[a]Average trough values.
[b]May require slow dose escalation.
[c]Administered intravenously.

serum levels is ideally drawn in the morning before breakfast, before the first ingestion of anticonvulsants ("trough levels"), a practice that introduces consistency in measurement. Not uncommonly, a drug is discarded as being ineffective when a slight increase in dosage would have led to suppression of attacks. On the other hand, drug levels can be helpful in detecting non-compliance or poor absorption in instances of inadequate seizure control. The management of seizures is facilitated by having patients chart their daily medication and the number, time, and circumstances of each episode. Some patients find it helpful to use a dispenser that is filled with medications with sufficient pills to last the week. This indicates to the patient whether a dose had been missed and whether the supply of medications is running low.

Table 16-5 indicates the effective serum levels for each of the commonly used antiepileptic drugs. In general, higher serum concentrations of drugs are necessary

Table 16-6

CHOICES OF ANTIEPILEPTIC DRUGS BY TYPE OF ADULT SEIZURE DISORDER

SEIZURE TYPE	INITIAL CHOICE	SECOND LINE
Generalized tonic-clonic	Valproate, phenytoin	Lamotrigine, levitiracetam, carbamazepine, oxcarbazepine
Myoclonic	Valproate	Topiramate, levetiracetam, zonisamide
Focal (with or without secondary generalized)	Carbamazepine, phenytoin	Valproate, lamotrigine, oxcarbazepine, levitiracetam, lacosamide,
Absence	Valproate	Ethosuximide
Status epilepticus	Diazepines	Phenytoin, fosphenytoin, propofol, levetiracetam

Table 16-7

CHOICES OF ANTIEPILEPTIC DRUGS IN CHILDHOOD SEIZURE DISORDERS

SEIZURE TYPE	INITIAL CHOICE	SECOND	THIRD
Generalized tonic-clonic	Valproate, carbamazepine	Lamotrigine, oxcarbazepine	Phenytoin
Myoclonic	Valproate, levetiracetam	Lamotrigine	Phenobarbital, clobazam
Absence	Valproate	Topiramate, levetiracetam, ethosuximide	Lamotrigine
Focal	Carbamazepine, phenytoin	Valproate, levetiracetam, oxcarbazepine	Lamotrigine, vigabatrin, topiramate
Infantile spasms	ACTH, vigabatrin,	Valproate	Lamotrigine
Lennox-Gastaut	Valproate	Topiramate, lamotrigine	Levetiracetam

for the control of focal seizures than for generalized ones. The usual blood level assay is of the total concentration of the drug; this is not a precise reflection of the amount of drug entering the brain, because—in the case of the most widely used anticonvulsants—the large proportion of drug is bound to albumin and does not penetrate nervous tissue. Also, in patients who are malnourished or chronically ill or who have a constitutional reduction in proteins, there may be intoxication at low total serum levels. Certain antiepileptic drugs also have active metabolites that are not measured by methods ordinarily used to determine serum concentrations but nonetheless produce toxicity. This is particularly true for the epoxide of carbamazepine. The situation may be further complicated by interactions between one anticonvulsant and the metabolites of another, as, for example, the inhibition of epoxide hydrolase by valproic acid, leading to toxicity through the buildup of carbamazepine epoxide. In circumstances of unexplained toxicity in the face of conventionally obtained serum levels that are normal, measurement may be undertaken of the levels of free drug and the concentration of active metabolites by chromatographic techniques.

The use of saliva for measurement of free drug levels has merit but has not been adopted frequently in practice. The measurements correlate with free drug levels. It has the advantage of allowing the patient to collect a sample before breakfast and avoid venipuncture.

Finally, the pharmacokinetics of each drug plays a role in toxicity and the serum level that is achieved with each alteration in the dose. This is particularly true of phenytoin, which, as the result of saturation of liver enzymatic capacity, has nonlinear kinetics once serum concentration exceeds 10 mg/mL. For this reason, a typical increase in dose from 300 to 400 mg daily results in a disproportionate elevation of the serum level and toxic side effects. Elevations in drug concentrations are also accompanied by prolongation of the serum half-life, which increases the time to reach a steady-state concentration of phenytoin after dosage adjustments. Contrariwise, carbamazepine is known to induce its own metabolism, so that doses adequate to control seizures at the outset of therapy are no longer effective several weeks later.

Antiepileptic Drug Interactions

Antiepileptic drugs have manifold interactions with each other and with a wide variety of other drugs. Although many such interactions are known, only a few are of clinical significance and most pertain to older generations of medications, requiring adjustment of drug dosages (see Kutt). Among interactions between anticonvulsant drugs, valproate often leads to accumulation of active phenytoin and of phenobarbital by displacing them from serum proteins, as well as slightly elevating serum total levels. Agents that alter the concentrations of antiepileptic medications are chloramphenicol, which causes the accumulation of phenytoin and phenobarbital, and erythromycin, which causes the accumulation of carbamazepine. Antacids reduce the blood phenytoin concentration, whereas histamine blockers used to reduce gastric acid output do the opposite. Salicylates reduce the total plasma levels of anticonvulsant drugs but elevate the free fraction by displacing the drug from its protein carrier. More importantly, warfarin levels are decreased by the addition of phenobarbital or carbamazepine and may be increased by phenytoin although, with this last drug there may be unexpected alterations of the international normalized ratio (INR) in either direction. Enzyme-inducing drugs such as phenytoin, carbamazepine, and barbiturates can greatly increase the chance of breakthrough menstrual bleeding in women taking oral contraceptives and may lead to failure of contraceptive medications, and adjustments in the amount of estradiol must be made. These interactions are emphasized further below under the discussions of each agent.

Hepatic function greatly affects antiepileptic drug concentrations, since most of these drugs are metabolized in the liver. Serum levels must be checked more frequently than usual if there is liver failure, and with hypoalbuminemia it is advisable to obtain free drug levels for reasons just mentioned. Renal function has an indirect effect on the concentrations of the commonly used antiepileptics, but some newer agents, such as levetiracetam, gabapentin, and pregabalin, are excreted through the kidneys and require dosage adjustment in cases of renal failure. The main renal effects have to do with alterations in protein binding that are induced by uremia. In end-stage renal failure, serum levels are not an accurate guide to therapy and the goal should be to attain adequate free concentrations of, for example, 1 to 2 mg/mL. In addition, uremia causes the accumulation of phenytoin metabolites, which are measured with the parent drug by enzyme-multiplied immunoassay techniques. In patients who are being dialyzed, total blood levels of phenytoin tend to be low because of decreased protein binding; in this situation it is also necessary to track free (unbound) phenytoin levels. Because dialysis removes phenobarbital and ethosuximide, dosage of these drugs may have to be increased. Decreased phenytoin levels are also known to occur during viral illnesses, and supplementary doses are occasionally necessary.

Teratogenic Effects of Antiepileptic Medications

Because it is essential to prevent convulsions in the pregnant epileptic woman, anticonvulsant medication should not be discontinued or arbitrarily reduced, particularly if there have been recent convulsions. The conventional drugs (phenytoin, carbamazepine, phenobarbital, valproate, lamotrigine) are all tolerated in pregnancy. Plasma levels of most of these drugs, both the free and protein-bound fractions, fall slightly in pregnancy and are cleared more rapidly from the blood. The main practical issues pertains to the potential teratogenicity of most of the drugs with valproate having slightly more risk than the others, and a slight reduction in IQ in children born of mothers who had been exposed to valproate during pregnancy.

The most common teratogenic effects have been cleft lip and cleft palate, but infrequently also a subtle facial dysmorphism ("fetal anticonvulsant syndrome"), similar to the fetal alcohol syndrome. The risks are highest with valproate. In general, the risk of major congenital defects is low; it increases to 4 to 5 percent in women taking anticonvulsant drugs during pregnancy, in comparison to 2 to 3 percent in the overall population of pregnant women. These statistics are essentially confirmed in the large study by Holmes and colleagues, conducted among several Boston hospitals. When all types of malformations were included, both major and minor, 20 percent of infants born to mothers who took anticonvulsants during pregnancy showed abnormalities, compared to 9 percent of mothers who had not taken medications. These authors identified "midface hypoplasia" (shortened nose, philtrum, or inner canthal distance) and finger hypoplasia as characteristic of anticonvulsant exposure; these changes were found in 13 and 8 percent of exposed infants, respectively. However, it should be emphasized that in large surveys, major malformations have occurred in only 5 percent of infants exposed to antiepileptic drugs. The infants born of a group of women with epilepsy who had not taken anticonvulsants during pregnancy showed an overall rate of dysmorphic features comparable to that in control infants, but there was still a 2 to 3 percent rate of facial and finger hypoplasia. This risk is shared more or less equally by all the major anticonvulsants again, with concern that valproate is associated with a higher rate. Aggregating eight databases, Jetnik and colleagues found a number of malformations of the nervous and somatic systems to be increased in comparison to other antiepileptic drugs.

Of equal or greater concern has been the findings by Meador and colleagues that in utero exposure to valproate was associated with lower IQs (by 9 points) compared to lamotrigine in children at the age of 4. It is not clear if the effect persists after this age. Children who had been exposed to phenytoin or to carbamazepine also had slightly lower IQs but this difference was ostensibly accounted for by lower maternal IQ. Some studies, including the one by Meador and colleagues (2011) suggest that folate may have an ameliorating effect on this detrimental effect at age 3, whereas there is an uncertain benefit in preventing fetal malformations.

The risk of neural tube defects is also slightly increased by anticonvulsants during pregnancy, and greatest for the use of valproate. It had been considered to be reduced by giving folate before pregnancy has begun (it is not clear if this is true for valproate), but epilepsy experts avoid the use of valproate during pregnancy altogether. These risks are greater in women taking more than one anticonvulsant, so that monotherapy is a desirable goal. Furthermore, the risk is disproportionately increased in families with a history of these defects. Some of the newer anticonvulsants should probably be used cautiously until greater experience has been obtained. As each new anticonvulsant has been introduced over the years, there has usually been a tentative claim of reduced teratogenic effects, often proven later to be incorrect. Claims have been made of safety in this regard for lamotrigine, causing many specialists to change from the more conventional drugs to this one in women who anticipate becoming pregnant, but lamotrigine levels tend to fall precipitously during pregnancy. A report by Cunningham and colleagues using registry information suggests that the incidence of major birth defects in the fetuses exposed to lamotrigine during the first trimester is just under 3 percent, similar to risk estimates for the general population but also close to the 3 to 4 percent risk derived from most registries of women on anticonvulsants. Polytherapy with lamotrigine and valproate raised the estimate of risk to 12 percent.

If a woman with seizure disorder has been off epilepsy medications for a time before getting pregnant and seizes during the pregnancy, the best choice of medication currently may be phenytoin for its advantage in rapid seizure control, or levetiracetam. Exposure of the fetus late in gestation poses few teratogenic risks. If a woman discovers she is pregnant while on an antiepileptic drug, changing medications is unlikely to reduce the chances of birth defects, even for valproate, but this drug retains the risk of lower IQ in the child. The special case of eclamptic seizures is managed by infusion of magnesium. Epileptic women of childbearing age should be advised that higher doses of the estradiol component of birth control agents are required or they may be exposed to the issues of becoming pregnant while antiepileptic medications.

Skin Eruptions from Antiepileptic Drugs

Rashes are the most frequent idiosyncratic reactions to the drugs used to treat epilepsy. The aromatic compounds (phenytoin, carbamazepine, phenobarbital, primidone, and lamotrigine) are the ones most often responsible. Furthermore, *there is a high degree of cross-reactivity within this group*, particularly between phenytoin, carbamazepine, and phenobarbital, and, possibly, lamotrigine. The problem arises most often in the first month of use. The typical eruption is maculopapular, mainly on the trunk; it usually resolves within days of discontinuing the medication. More severe rashes may develop, sometimes taking the form of erythema multiforme and Stevens-Johnson syndrome, or even toxic epidermal necrolysis, especially with lamotrigine.

Certain polymorphisms in HLA genes (HLA-B*1502) have been associated with an increased risk of these types of severe skin reactions, particularly those of Asian ancestry but probably also in Caucasians, in whom this genotype is rare. Another allele HLA-A* 3101 may be associated with skin eruptions in Caucasians (McCormack et al), but it (HLA-B 1502) does not seem reasonable at this time to screen non-Asian patients for such an infrequent complication. Another rare systemic hypersensitivity syndrome associated with the use of antiepileptic medications is one of high fever, rash, lymphadenopathy, and pharyngitis. Eosinophilia and hepatitis (or nephritis) may follow.

If any of these reactions require that one of the aromatic drugs be replaced, valproate, gabapentin, topiramate, or levetiracetam are reasonable substitutes, depending, of course, on the nature of the seizures.

Discontinuation of Anticonvulsants

Withdrawal of anticonvulsant drugs may be undertaken in patients who have been free of seizures for a prolonged period. There are few firm rules to guide the physician in this decision. One plan, applicable to most forms of epilepsy, is to obtain an EEG whenever withdrawal of medication is contemplated. We have taken the approach that if the tracing is abnormal by way of showing paroxysmal activity, it is generally better to continue treatment. However, a normal EEG may not be helpful in making the decision to discontinue medications. A prospective study by Callaghan and colleagues showed that in patients who had been seizure-free during 2 years of treatment with a single drug, one-third relapsed after discontinuation of the drug, and this relapse rate was much the same in adults and children and whether the drug was reduced over a period of weeks or months. The relapse rate was lower in patients with absence and generalized-onset seizures than in patients with focal seizures. Another study by Specchio and colleagues gave results similar to those of the large Medical Research Council Antiepileptic Drug Withdrawal Study—namely, that after 2 years on a single anticonvulsant during which no seizures had occurred, the rate of relapse was 40 percent 2.5 years later and 50 percent at 5 years after discontinuation; this compared to a seizure recurrence rate of 20 percent for patients remaining on medication. Other epileptologists have suggested that a longer seizure-free period is associated with a lesser rate of relapse.

Often in practice, the suggestion to stop medications after a lengthy seizure free period comes form the patient, for example if pregnancy is planned or there are untoward side effects but otherwise, the change is never risk free and therefore is infrequently impelled by the physician. Decisions regarding the cessation of medication are also tempered by patient's desire to continue driving and their concern that another seizure may prevent a return to driving.

Patients with juvenile myoclonic epilepsy, even those with long seizure-free periods, should probably continue medication life-long, but there have been no thorough studies to support this dictum. In young women with this disorder who plan or a likely to become pregnant, changing from valproate to levetiracetam may be sensible. The appropriate duration of treatment for postinfarction epilepsy has not been studied, and most neurologists continue to use one drug indefinitely. Interestingly, epilepsy caused by military brain wounds tends to wane in frequency or to disappear in 20 to 30 years, thereafter no longer requiring treatment (Caveness). In contrast, childhood uncomplicated absence seizures do not require lifelong treatment.

A curious and unexplained lesion in the splenium of the corpus callosum has been detected in patients who have had their antiepileptic drug(s) withdrawn in the previous few days. A review of 16 patients by Gürtler and colleagues did not find a clinical correlate for this change. A broad range of drugs was implicated and the lesion was most prominent on FLAIR MRI.

Specific Drugs in the Treatment of Seizures

General Comments

Phenytoin, carbamazepine, levetiracetam, and *valproate* are representative antiepileptic drugs and are more or less equally effective in the treatment of both generalized and partial seizures (see Table 16-5 for typical initial dosages). Valproate is probably less effective in the treatment of complex partial seizures. The first two of these drugs putatively act by blocking sodium channels, thus preventing abnormal neuronal firing and seizure spread. Lamotrigine is emerging as a popular alternative for partial seizures with a different side effect profile from the other three.

Because carbamazepine (or the related oxcarbazepine) and levetiracetam have somewhat fewer side effects, one or the other is preferred as the initial drug by many neurologists, though phenytoin and valproate have very similar therapeutic and side-effect profiles. Carbamazepine and valproate are probably preferable to phenytoin for epileptic children because they do not coarsen facial features and do not produce gum hypertrophy or breast enlargement. In many cases, phenytoin or carbamazepine alone will control the seizures. If not, the use of valproate (which facilitates GABA activity) alone, or the combined use of phenytoin and carbamazepine, produces better control. In others, the addition of valproate to carbamazepine may prove effective. Because of the high incidence of myoclonic epilepsy in adolescence, it has been our practice to use valproate as the first drug in this age group. Weight gain, menstrual irregularities (see below) during the period of initiation of valproate, and its teratogenic effects may also figure into the decision regarding the choice of initial drug for otherwise uncomplicated seizures in young women.

Most of the commonly used antiepileptic drugs cause, to varying degrees, a decrease in bone density and an increased risk of fracture from osteoporosis in older patients, particularly in women. Several mechanisms are probably active, among them, induction of the cytochrome P450 system, which enzymatically degrades vitamin D.

No specific recommendations have been offered to counteract this effect of bone loss, but we have advised patients to take calcium supplements or one of the bisphosphonates if there is no contraindication, or to check bone density at regular intervals.

Finally, several reports and meta analyses over the past decades have suggested that antiepileptic drugs might increase the incidence of suicide, both in individuals with epilepsy and psychiatric patients. The issue may never be entirely resolved because of confounding factors but a patient level-analysis performed by Arana and colleagues showed no such relationship in epilepsy once underlying depression was accounted for.

Phenytoin Oral, intramuscular, and intravenous forms are available. Rash, fever, lymphadenopathy, eosinophilia and other blood dyscrasias, and polyarteritis are manifestations of idiosyncratic *phenytoin hypersensitivity*; their occurrence calls for discontinuation of the medication. *Overdose with phenytoin* causes ataxia, diplopia, and stupor. The prolonged use of phenytoin often leads to hirsutism (mainly in young girls), hypertrophy of gums, and coarsening of facial features in children. A clinical trial conducted by Arya and colleagues suggests that folate supplementation may prevent gingival hyperplasia in children. Chronic phenytoin use over several decades may occasionally be associated with peripheral neuropathy and probably with a form of cerebellar degeneration (Lindvall and Nilsson); it is not clear if these are strictly dose-related effects or idiosyncratic reactions. An antifolate effect on blood and interference with vitamin K metabolism have also been reported, for which reason pregnant women taking phenytoin (and in fact most other antiepileptic drugs) should be given folate supplementation and vitamin K before delivery and the newborn infant also should receive vitamin K to prevent bleeding. Phenytoin should not be used together with disulfiram (Antabuse), chloramphenicol, sulfamethizole, phenylbutazone, or cyclophosphamide, and the use of either phenobarbital or phenytoin is not advisable in patients receiving warfarin (Coumadin) because of the undesirable interactions already described. Choreoathetosis is a rare idiosyncratic side effect. Fosphenytoin for intramuscular and intravenous administration allows somewhat faster attainment of serum levels and may have minor advantages in special circumstances, especially the availability of the IM route. Intravenous phenytoin and fosphenytoin are discussed further in the section on status epilepticus.

Carbamazepine This drug causes many of the same side effects as phenytoin, but to a slightly lesser degree. Mild leukopenia is common, and there have been rare instances of pancytopenia, hyponatremia (inappropriate antidiuretic hormone [ADH]), and, rarely, diabetes insipidus as idiosyncratic reactions. It is advisable therefore, that a complete blood count be done before or soon after treatment is instituted and that counts are rechecked regularly. *Oxcarbazepine*, a more recently introduced analogue of carbamazepine, has fewer of these side effects than the parent drug, especially marrow toxicity, but its long-term therapeutic value is not as well established. Hyponatremia has been reported in 3 percent of patients taking oxcarbazepine. Should drowsiness or increased seizure frequency occur, this complication should be suspected.

Valproate All preparations of this drug are occasionally hepatotoxic, an adverse effect that is usually (but not invariably) limited to children 2 years of age and younger. The use of valproate with hepatic enzyme-inducing drugs increases the risk of liver toxicity. However, mild elevations of serum ammonia and mild impairments of liver function tests in an adult do not require discontinuation of the drug. An increasingly emphasized problem with valproate has been weight gain during the first months of therapy. In one study there was an average addition of 5.8 kg, and even more in those disposed to obesity. In addition, menstrual irregularities and polycystic ovarian syndrome may appear in young women taking the drug, perhaps as a consequence of the aforementioned weight gain. Pancreatitis is a rare but important complication of valproate. Tremor and slight bradykinesias have been seen and they vaguely simulate parkinsonism. The major issues, however, pertain to its use in pregnancy as discussed earlier.

An intravenous form of valproate is available and may be useful in status epilepticus. The maximum recommended rate of administration is 3 mg/kg per min.

Phenobarbital Introduced as an antiepileptic drug in 1912, phenobarbital is still highly effective, but because of its toxic effects—drowsiness and mental dullness, nystagmus, and staggering, as well as the availability of better alternatives—it is seldom used in adults. The adverse effects of *primidone* are much the same. Both drugs may provoke behavioral problems in developmentally delayed children and they are still used to advantage as an adjunctive anticonvulsant and as primary therapy in infantile seizures.

Lamotrigine *Lamotrigine* closely resembles phenytoin in its antiseizure activity but has different features relating to toxicity. It functions by selectively blocking the slow sodium channel, thereby preventing the release of the excitatory transmitters glutamate and aspartate. It is effective as a first-line and adjunctive drug for generalized and focal seizures, and may be an alternative to valproate in young women because it does not provoke weight gain and ovarian problems. The main limitation to its use has been a serious rash in approximately 1 percent of patients, requiring discontinuation of the drug, and lesser dermatologic eruptions in 12 percent. It should be pointed out that some registries have reported considerably lower rates of these complications. The slow introduction of the medication may reduce the incidence of drug eruptions (see below). Rare cases of reversible chorea have been reported, especially with the concurrent use of phenytoin. Combined use with valproate greatly increases the serum level of lamotrigine.

Levetiracetam This is a relatively novel drug with uncertain mechanism that has been useful in the treatment of both partial and generalized seizures. The agent affects the SV2A synaptic vesicle protein, but how this relates to its antiepileptic properties is still being investigated. It is well tolerated if initiated slowly, but produces considerable sleepiness and dizziness otherwise and if used at high doses. It also may produce irritability and depression.

A major advantage is that there are no important interactions with other antiepileptic drugs for which reason it is often chosen as a first-line agent in patients who have organ failure and require numerous medications, as well as those receiving hepatically-metabolized chemotherapeutics.

Other Antiepileptic Drugs Two other drugs, *gabapentin* and *vigabatrin*, were synthesized specifically to enhance the intrinsic inhibitory system of GABA in the brain. Gabapentin is chemically similar to GABA, but its anticonvulsant mechanism is not known; it has an apparent effect on calcium channels. It is moderately effective in partial and secondary generalized seizures and has the advantage of not being metabolized by the liver. Vigabatrin inhibits GABA transaminase. Vigabatrin is no longer used in adults because of the side effect or retinal damage. *Tiagabine* is considered to be an inhibitor of GABA reuptake.

Topiramate, has much the same mode of action and probably a broader effectiveness as tiagabine. It will rarely cause serious dermatologic side effects, especially if used with valproate, and appears to induce renal stones in 1.5 percent of patients. Angle-closure glaucoma has also been reported as a complication. A minor problem has been the development of hyperchloremic metabolic acidosis.

Lacosamide, a potent drug for seizures that have a focal onset and generalize or remain focal, is currently used currently mainly as an adjunctive therapy. Like levetiracetam, its mechanism of action is not entirely known but it has been shown to modulate voltage-gated sodium channel activity. The main but infrequent side effects are headache and diplopia. The drug may prolong the P-R interval and worsen heart failure.

Ethosuximide and valproate are equally effective for the treatment of absence seizures, the former having fewer cognitive side effects according to a study by Glauser and colleagues. It is good practice, so as to avoid excessive sleepiness, to begin with a single dose of 250 mg of ethosuximide per day and to increase it every week until the optimum therapeutic effect is achieved. *Methsuximide* (Celontin) is useful in individual cases where ethosuximide and valproate have failed. In patients with benign absence attacks that are associated with photosensitivity, myoclonus, and clonic-tonic-clonic seizures (including juvenile myoclonic epilepsy), valproate is the drug of choice. Valproate is particularly useful in children who have both absence and grand mal attacks, as the use of this drug alone often permits the control of both types of seizures. The concurrent use of valproate and clonazepam has been known to produce absence status.

Zonisamide, similar to topiramate, seems to be useful for myoclonic epilepsy but its main use is currently as an adjuvant in al epilepsy. It is not a sodium channel blocker and can be taken in parallel with carbamazepine. Some clinicians have found it to produce fewer cognitive side effects than topiramate.

Treatment of Seizures in the Neonate and Young Child

This specialized area of neonatal seizures is discussed by Fenichel and by Volpe and in children by Guerrini. In general, phenobarbital has been preferred for seizure control in infancy. Probably the form of epilepsy that is most difficult to treat is the childhood *Lennox-Gastaut* syndrome. Some of these patients have as many as 50 or more seizures per day, and there may be no effective combination of anticonvulsant medications. Valproic acid (900 to 2,400 mg/d) will reduce the frequency of spells in approximately half the cases. The newer drugs—lamotrigine, topiramate, vigabatrin—are each effective in approximately 25 percent of cases. Clonazepam also has had limited success. In the special case of Dravet syndrome, a disorder of the sodium channel, antiepileptic drugs that block that same channel are avoided.

In the treatment of infantile spasms, ACTH or adrenal corticosteroids had been used, but vigabatrin is now found to be as effective, including in patients with underlying tuberous sclerosis (see Elterman et al).

Status Epilepticus

Recurrent generalized convulsions at a frequency that precludes regaining of consciousness in the interval between seizures (convulsive status) constitutes the most serious problem in epilepsy, with an overall mortality of 20 to 30 percent, according to Towne and colleagues, but probably lower in recent years. Some patients who die of epilepsy do so because of uncontrolled seizures of this type, complicated by the effects of the underlying illness or an injury sustained as a result of a convulsion. Rising temperature, acidosis, hypotension, and renal failure from myoglobinuria is a sequence of life-threatening events that may be encountered in cases of convulsive status epilepticus. Prolonged convulsive status (for longer than 30 min) also carries a risk of serious neurologic sequelae ("epileptic encephalopathy"). The MRI during and for days after a bout of status epilepticus may show signal abnormalities in the region of a focal seizure or in the hippocampi, most often reversible, but we have had several such patients who awakened and were left in a permanent amnesic state. The MRI changes are most evident on FLAIR and diffusion-weighted sequences. With regard to acute medical complications, from time to time a case of neurogenic pulmonary edema is encountered during or just after the convulsions, and some patients may become extremely hypertensive, making it difficult to distinguish the syndrome from hypertensive encephalopathy.

The etiologies of status epilepticus vary among age groups but all the fundamental causes of seizures are able to produce the syndrome. The most recalcitrant cases we have encountered in adults have been associated with viral or paraneoplastic encephalitis, old traumatic injury, and epilepsy with severe mental retardation. Stroke and brain tumor have, in contrast, been infrequent causes.

Treatment of Convulsive Status Epilepticus
(Table 16-8)

The many regimens that have been proposed for the treatment of status epilepticus attest to the fact that no one of them is altogether satisfactory and none is clearly superior (Treiman et al).

We have had the most success with the following program: When the patient is first seen, an initial

Table 16-8

APPROACH TO THE TREATMENT OF STATUS EPILEPTICUS IN ADULTS

Initial assessment
Ensure adequate ventilation, oxygenation, blood pressure
Intubate if necessary, based on low oxygen saturation and labored breathing
Insert intravenous line
Administer glucose and thiamine in appropriate circumstances
Send toxic screen
Assess quickly for cranial and cervical injury if onset of seizures is unwitnessed
Immediate suppression of convulsions
Lorazepam or diazepam, 2 to 4 mg/min IV to a total dose of 10 to 15 mg with blood pressure monitoring when higher rates or doses are used
Initiation or reloading with anticonvulsants
Phenytoin 15–20 mg/kg IV at 25–50 mg/min in normal saline or fosphenytoin at 50 to 75 mg/min
General anesthetic doses of medication for persistent status epilepticus
Midazolam 0.2 mg/kg loading dose followed by infusion at 0.1 to 0.4 mg/kg/h or propofol 2 mg/kg/h
Further treatment if convulsions or electrographic seizures persist after several hours
May add valproate or phenobarbital 10 mg/min to total dose of 20 mg/kg as additional anticonvulsants intravenously, or carbamazepine or levetiracetam by nasogastric tube if there is gastric and bowel activity
Consider neuromuscular paralysis with EEG monitoring if convulsions persist
Pentobarbital 10 mg/kg/h
Inhalational anesthetics (isoflurane)

assessment of cardiorespiratory function is made and an oral airway established. A large-bore intravenous line is inserted; blood is drawn for glucose, BUN, electrolytes, and a metabolic and drug screen. A normal saline infusion is begun and a bolus of glucose is given (with thiamine if malnutrition and alcoholism are potential factors). To rapidly suppress the seizures, we have used diazepam intravenously at a rate of about 2 mg/min until the seizures stop or a total of 20 mg has been given; alternatively, lorazepam, 0.1 mg/kg given by intravenous push at a rate not to exceed 2 mg/min, is now favored, being marginally more effective than diazepam because of its clinically longer duration of action (see Table 16-8).

Immediately thereafter, a loading dose (20 mg/kg) of phenytoin is administered by vein at a rate of less than 50 mg/min. More rapid administration risks hypotension and heart block; consequently, it is recommended that the blood pressure and electrocardiogram be monitored during the infusion. Phenytoin must be given through a freely running line with normal saline (it precipitates in other fluids) and should not be injected intramuscularly. A study by Treiman and colleagues has demonstrated the superiority of using lorazepam instead of phenytoin as the first drug to control status, but this is not surprising considering the longer latency of onset of phenytoin.

In the field, emergency medical technicians can administer lorazepam drug or midazolam. Attesting to the benefit of rapidly treating seizures, Silbergleit and colleagues have shown that intramuscular administration is slightly superior to the intravenous route simply because of the delay in inserting an intravenous line. Alldredge and colleagues showed that diazepines can be administered by paramedical workers in nursing homes with good effect in status epilepticus, terminating the seizures in about half of cases.

Nonetheless, a long-acting antiepileptic such as phenytoin must be given immediately after a diazepine has controlled the initial seizures. An alternative is the water-soluble drug fosphenytoin, which is administered in the same dose equivalents as phenytoin but can be injected at twice the maximum rate. Moreover, it can be given intramuscularly in cases where venous access is difficult. However, the delay in hepatic conversion of fosphenytoin to active phenytoin makes the latency of clinical effect approximately the same for both drugs.

In an epileptic patient known to be taking seizure medications chronically but in whom the serum level of drug is unknown, it is probably best to administer the full-recommended dose of phenytoin. If it can be established that the serum phenytoin is above 10 mg/mL, a lower loading dose may be advisable. If seizures continue, an additional 5 mg/kg is indicated. If this fails to suppress the seizures and status has persisted for 20 to 30 min, an endotracheal tube should be inserted and O_2 administered.

Having emphasized the dangers of this syndrome, at each stage of treatment it is worthwhile considering if a refractory convulsive episode is of psychogenic, nonepileptic nature. The reader is referred to the previous section on this subject.

Several approaches have been suggested to control status epilepticus that persists after these efforts. At this stage we have resorted to the approach suggested by Kumar and Bleck of giving high doses of midazolam (0.2 mg/kg loading dose followed by an infusion of 0.1 to 0.4 mg/kg/h as determined by clinical and EEG monitoring). If seizures continue, the dose can be raised as blood pressure permits. We have used in excess of 20 mg/h because of a diminishing effect over days. This regimen of midazolam and phenytoin may be maintained for several days without major ill effect in previously healthy patients. Propofol given in a bolus of 2 mg/kg and then as an intravenous drip of 2 to 8 mg/kg/h is an effective alternative to midazolam, but after 24 h the drug behaves like a high dose of barbiturate and there may be hypotension. Prolonged use of propofol may precipitate hypertriglyceridemia-associated pancreatitis or a fatal shock and acidosis ("propofol syndrome").

Valproate and levetiracetam are available as intravenous preparations, making them suitable for administration in status, but their role in this circumstance has not been extensively studied. Another dependable approach is infusion of either pentobarbital, starting with 5 mg/kg, or phenobarbital, at a rate of 100 mg/min until the seizures stop or a total dose of 20 mg/kg is reached; a long period of stupor must be anticipated after. Hypotension often limits the continued use of the barbiturates, but Parviainen and colleagues were able to manage this problem by fluid infusions, dopamine, and neosynephrine.

If none of these measures controls the seizures, a more aggressive approach is taken to subdue all brain electrical activity by the use of general anesthesia. The preferred medications for this purpose have been pentobarbital or propofol, which, despite their moderate efficacy as primary anticonvulsants, are easier to manage than the alternative inhalational anesthetic agents. An initial intravenous dose of 5 mg/kg pentobarbital or 2 mg/kg propofol is given slowly to induce an EEG burst-suppression pattern, which is then maintained by the administration of pentobarbital, 0.5 to 2 mg/kg/h, or propofol, up to 10 mg/kg/h. Every 12 to 24 h, the rate of infusion is slowed to determine whether the seizures have stopped. The experience of Lowenstein and colleagues, like our own, is that most instances of status epilepticus that cannot be controlled with the combination of standard anticonvulsants and midazolam will respond to high doses of barbiturates or to propofol, but that these infusions cause hypotension and cannot be carried out for long periods.

Should the seizures continue, either clinically or electrographically, despite all these medications, one is justified in the assumption that the convulsive tendency is so strong that it cannot be checked by reasonable quantities of medications. However, a few patients in this predicament have survived and awakened, even at times with minimal neurologic damage depending on the underlying cause.

The volatile anesthetic agent isoflurane has also been used in these circumstances with good effect, as we have reported (Ropper et al), but the continuous administration of inhalational anesthetic agents is impractical in most critical care units. Halothane has been relatively ineffective as an anticonvulsant, but ether, although impractical, has in the past been effective in some. In the end, in patients with truly intractable status, one usually depends on phenytoin, phenobarbital (smaller doses in infants and children than are shown in Table 16-8), and on measures that safeguard the patient's vital functions. Ketamine infusions have been a last resort, in combination with a midazolam infusion. A few times over the years, we have also resorted to inducing ketosis in adults by manipulating the nutrition given through a nasogastric tube.

A word is added here concerning neuromuscular paralysis and continuous EEG monitoring in status epilepticus. With failure of aggressive anticonvulsant and anesthetic treatment, there may be a temptation to paralyze all muscular activity, an effect easily attained with drugs such as pancuronium, while neglecting the underlying seizures. The use of neuromuscular blocking drugs without a concomitant attempt to suppress seizure activity is inadvisable. If such measures are undertaken, continuous or frequent intermittent EEG monitoring is essential; this may also be also helpful in the early stages of status epilepticus in that it guides the dosages of anticonvulsants required to suppress the seizures.

In the related but less-serious condition of *acute repetitive seizures*, in which the patient awakens between convulsions, a diazepam gel, which is well absorbed if given rectally, is available and has been found useful in institutional and home care of epileptic patients, although it is quite expensive. A similar effect has been attained by the nasal or buccal (transmucosal) administration of midazolam, which is absorbed from these sites (5 mg/mL, 0.2 mg/kg nasally; 2 mL to 10 mg buccally). Midazolam may be preferred among the diazepines for transmucosal use because it produces somewhat less respiratory depression than the others in the class and has been more effective at controlling seizures according to a study by McIntyre and colleagues. Still, only half were controlled. These approaches have found their main use in children with frequent seizures who live in supervised environments, where a nurse or parent is available to administer the medication.

Absence status should be managed by intravenous lorazepam, valproic acid, or both, followed by ethosuximide. Nonconvulsive generalized status is treated along the lines of grand mal status, usually stopping short of using anesthetic agents (see Meierkord). In the case of epilepsia partialis continua, typically a difficult condition to control, a balance must be found between stopping the phenomenon and the risk of overuse of medications that can produce stupor. The patient must be involved by way of determining how troubling the movements are to him.

Surgical Treatment of Epilepsy

The surgical excision of epileptic foci that have not responded to intensive and prolonged medical therapy is being used with increasing effectiveness in a growing number of specialized epilepsy units. At these centers, it has been estimated that approximately 25 percent of all patients with epilepsy are candidates for surgical therapy and more than half of these may benefit from extirpation of the epileptic cortical focus. With increasing experience and standardized approaches, especially in patients with temporal lobe epilepsy, it has been suggested that many patients are waiting too long before the surgical option. A perspective that may promote surgery in even more patients is the observation that approximately 60 percent of patients with focal seizures will respond to a conventional anticonvulsant, but that among the remainder, few will respond to the addition of a second or third drug.

However, considerable effort, time and technology are required to determine the site of epileptic discharge and the method of safe removal of the cortical tissue. To locate the discharging focus requires a careful analysis of clinical, imaging, and EEG findings, often including those obtained by long-term video/EEG monitoring and, sometimes, intracranial EEG recording by means of intraparenchymal depth electrodes, subdural strip electrodes, and subdural grids. Recently, functional imaging, magnetoencephalography, and specialized EEG analysis have been introduced to supplement these methods.

The most favorable candidates for surgery are those with focal seizures that induce altered consciousness and a unilateral temporal lobe focus, in whom rates of cure and significant improvement approach 90 percent in some series but overall, are probably closer to 50 percent after 5 years. A randomized trial conducted by Wiebe and colleagues gave representative results after temporal lobectomy of 58 percent of 40 carefully studied patients remaining seizure-free after 1 year, in contrast to 8 percent on medication alone. Furthermore, as reported by Yoon and colleagues, among those patients who remain free of seizures for 1 year after surgery, more than half are still free of seizures after 10 years and most of the remainder had one or fewer episodes per year. It should be emphasized that most of the patients who underwent surgery in these studies still required anticonvulsant medication. Excision of cortical tissue that contains a structural lesion outside of the temporal lobe accomplishes complete seizure-free states in approximately 50 percent. Taking all seizure types together, only approximately 10 percent of patients obtain no improvement at all and less than 5 percent are worse. The matter of resection of areas of focal cortical dysplasias in children is a highly specialized area. It has been indicated that the histologic features of the dysplasia are important determinants of the success of surgery (Fauser et al).

Other surgical procedures of value in highly selected cases are sectioning of the corpus callosum, which is for the most part palliative, and hemispherectomy, which may be curative in special circumstances. The most encouraging results with callosotomy have been obtained in the control of intractable partial and secondarily generalized seizures, particularly when atonic drop attacks are the most disabling seizure type. Removal of the entire cortex of one hemisphere, in addition to the amygdala and hippocampus, has been of value in children, as well as in some adults with severe and extensive unilateral cerebral disease and intractable contralateral motor seizures and hemiplegia. Rasmussen encephalitis, Sturge-Weber disease, and large porencephalic cysts at times fall into this category. Surgical, focused radiation, or endovascular reduction of arteriovenous malformations may reduce the frequency of seizures, but the results in this regard are somewhat unpredictable (see Chap. 34).

Vagal Nerve Stimulation

This technique has found some favor in cases of intractable partial and secondarily generalizing seizures. A pacemaker-like device is implanted in the anterior chest wall and stimulating electrodes are connected to the vagus at the left carotid bifurcation. The procedure is well tolerated except for hoarseness in some cases. Several trials have demonstrated an average of 25 percent reduction in seizure frequency among patients who were resistant to all manner of anticonvulsant drugs (see Chadwick for a discussion of clinical trials). The mechanism by which vagal stimulation produces its effects is unclear, and its role in the management of seizures is still being defined. Stimulation of the cerebellum and of other sites in the brain has also been used in the control of seizures, with no clear evidence of success. They must currently be considered to be experimental.

Ketogenic Diet

Since the 1920s, interest in this form of seizure control has varied, being revived periodically in centers caring for many children with intractable epilepsy. Despite the absence of controlled studies showing its efficacy or an agreed upon hypothesis for its mechanism, several trials in the first half of the twentieth century, and again more recently, demonstrated a reduction in seizures in half of the patients, including handicapped children with severe and sometimes intractable episodes. The diet is used mainly in children between the ages of 1 and 10 years. The regimen is initiated during hospitalization by starvation for a day or two in order to induce ketosis, followed by a diet in which 80 to 90 percent of the calories are derived from fat (Vining). The difficulties in making such a diet palatable leads to its abandonment by about one-third of children and their families.

A summary of experience from the numerous trials of the ketogenic diet can be found in the review by Lefevre and Aronson and in the report of its use in 58 children by Kinsman and colleagues. They both concluded that the diet is effective in refractory cases of epilepsy in childhood, reducing seizure frequency in two-thirds of children and allowing a reduction in the amount of anticonvulsant medication in many. It has also been commented that some benefit persists even after the diet has been stopped. Nephrolithiasis is a complication in somewhat less than 10 percent of children, and this risk is particularly high if topiramate is being used.

Keotgenic diet is the main treatment for children with GLUT1 deficiency syndrome, as discussed earlier.

Safety and Regulation of Physical and Mental Activity

Driving and Epilepsy

A person with incompletely controlled epilepsy should not be allowed to drive an automobile. Only a few states in the United States and most provinces of Canada mandate that physicians report patients with seizures under their care to the state motor vehicle bureau. Nonetheless, physicians should counsel such a patient regarding the obvious danger to himself and others if a seizure should occur while driving (the same holds for the risks of swimming unattended). What few data are available suggest that accidents caused directly by a seizure are rare and, in any case, 15 percent have been the result of a first episode of seizure that could not have been anticipated. In some states where a driver's license has been suspended on the occurrence of a seizure, there is usually some provision for its reinstatement—such as a physician's declaration that the patient is under medical care and has been seizure-free for some period of time (usually 6 months or 1 to 2 years). The Epilepsy Foundation website can be consulted for updated information regarding restrictions on driving, and this serves as an excellent general resource for patients and their families (*http://www.efa.org*).

General Health Hygiene

The most important factors in seizure breakthrough, next to the abandonment of medication or a natural reduction of serum levels of medication, are loss of sleep and abuse of alcohol or other drugs. The need for moderation in the use of alcohol must be stressed, as well as the need to maintain regular hours of sleep. Advice to collegians about moderating alcohol is particularly important.

With proper safeguards, even potentially more dangerous sports, such as swimming, may be permitted. However, operating unguarded machinery, climbing ladders, or taking baths behind locked doors are not advisable; such a person should swim only in the company of a good swimmer. There is concern about epileptic mothers bathing their infants without additional safety guards.

Psychosocial difficulties are common and must be identified and addressed early. The stigma of epilepsy remains an issue in society. Advice and reassurance to attempt to pursue a normal life will aid in preventing or overcoming any feelings of inferiority and self-consciousness of many younger patients with epilepsy. However, the situation is rarely so simple and patients and their families may benefit from more extensive counseling.

References

Alldrege BK, Gelb AM, Isaacs SM, et al: A comparison of lorazepam, diazepam, and placebo for the treatment of out-of-hospital status epilepticus. *N Engl J Med* 345:631, 2001.

Andermann F (ed): *Chronic Encephalitis and Epilepsy: Rasmussen Syndrome*. Boston, Butterworth-Heinemann, 1991.

Annegers JF, Hauser WA, Shirts SB, Kurland LT: Factors prognostic of unprovoked seizures after febrile convulsions. *N Engl J Med* 316:493.1987.

Antel JP, Rasmussen T: Rasmussen's encephalitis and the new hat. *Neurology* 46:9, 1996.

Arana A, Wentworth CE, Ayuso-Mateos JL, Arellano FM: Suicide-related events in patients treated with antiepileptic drugs. *N Engl J Med* 363:542, 2010.

Arya R, Gulati S, Kabra M, et al: Folic acid supplementation prevents phenytoin-induced gingival overgrowth in children. *Neurology* 76:1338, 2011.

Baykan B, Altindag EA, Bebek N, et al: Myoclonic seizures subside in the fourth decade in juvenile myoclonic epilepsy. *Neurology* 70:2123, 2008.

Bear DM, Fedio P: Quantitative analysis of interictal behavior in temporal lobe epilepsy. *Arch Neurol* 34:454, 1977.

Berg AT et al. Revised terminology and concepts for organization of seizures and epilepsies: report of the ILAE Commission on Classification and Terminology, 2005-2009. *Epilepsia* 51:676, 2010.

Bien CG, Benninger FO, Urbach H, et al: Localizing value of epileptic visual auras. *Brain* 123:244, 2000.

Bleck TP: Intensive care unit management of patients with status epilepticus. *Epilepsia* 48 (Suppl 8):59, 2007.

Blumer D, Montouris G, Hermann B: Psychiatric morbidity in seizure patients on a neurodiagnostic monitoring unit. *J Neuropsychiatry Clin Neurosci* 7:445, 1995.

Callaghan N, Garrett A, Goggin T: Withdrawal of anticonvulsant drugs in patients free of seizures for two years. *N Engl J Med* 318:942, 1988.

Cascino GD: Intractable partial epilepsy: Evaluation and treatment. *Mayo Clin Proc* 65:1578, 1990.

Caveness WF: Onset and cessation of fits following craniocerebral trauma. *J Neurosurg* 20:570, 1963.

Chadwick D: Vagal nerve stimulation for epilepsy. *Lancet* 357:1726, 2001.

Chinchilla D, Dulac O, Roban O, et al: Reappraisal of Rasmussen syndrome with special emphasis on treatment with high dose steroids. *J Neurol Neurosurg Psychiatry* 57:1325, 1994.

Cole AJ, Andermann F, Taylor L, et al: The Landau-Kleffner syndrome of acquired epileptic aphasia: Unusual clinical outcome, surgical experiences, and absence of encephalitis. *Neurology* 38:31, 1988.

Commission on Classification and Terminology of the International League Against Epilepsy: Proposal for revised clinical and electroencephalographic classification of epileptic seizures. *Epilepsia* 22:489, 1981.

Commission on Classification and Terminology of the International League Against Epilepsy: Classification of epilepsy and epileptic syndromes. *Epilepsia* 30:389, 1989.

Cunningham M, Tennis P, et al: Lamotrigine and the risk of malformations in pregnancy. *Neurology* 64:955, 2005.

Currie S, Heathfield KWG, Henson RA, Scott DF: Clinical course and prognosis of temporal lobe epilepsy. *Brain* 94:173, 1971.

Daly DD, Pedley TA: *Current Practice of Clinical Electroencephalography*, 2nd ed. New York, Raven Press, 1990.

Delgado-Escueta AV, Greenberg DA, Treiman L, et al: Mapping the gene for juvenile myoclonic epilepsy. *Epilepsia* 30:S8, 1989.

Delgado-Escueta AV, Ganesh S, Yamakawa K: Advances in the genetics of progressive myoclonus epilepsy. *Am J Med Genet* 106:129, 2002.

Devinsky O: Sudden unexpected death in epilepsy. *N Engl J Med* 365:1801, 2011.

Devinsky O, Kelley K, Yacubian EM, et al: Postictal behavior: A clinical and subdural electroencephalographic study. *Arch Neurol* 51:254, 1994.

Dixit S, Kurle P, Buyan-Dent L, Sheth RD: Status epilepticus associated with cefepime. *Neurology* 54:2153, 2000.

Eadie MJ, Tyrer JH: *Anticonvulsant Therapy: Pharmacological Basis and Practice*, 3rd ed. New York, Churchill Livingstone, 1989.

Ebner A, Dinner DS, Noachtar S, Luders H: Automatisms with preserved responsiveness: A lateralizing sign in psychomotor seizures. *Neurology* 45:61, 1995.

Eclampsia Trial Collaborative Group: Which anticonvulsant for women with eclampsia? Evidence from the Collaborative Eclampsia Trial. *Lancet* 345:1455, 1995.

Elterman RD, Shields WD, Mansfield KA, et al: Randomized trial of vigabatrin in patients with infantile spasms. *Neurology* 57:1416, 2001.

Engel J Jr: Surgery for epilepsy. *N Engl J Med* 334:647, 1996.

Engel J Jr, Pedley TA: *Epilepsy: A Comprehensive Textbook*. Philadelphia, Davis, 1998.

EURAP Study Group, The. Seizure control and treatment in pregnancy. *Neurology* 66:354, 2006.

Falconer MA: Genetic and related aetiological factors in temporal lobe epilepsy: A review. *Epilepsia* 12:13, 1971–1972.

Fauser S, Bast T, Altenmüller DM, et al: Factors influencing surgical outcome in patients with focal cortical dysplasia. *J Neurol Neurosurg Psychiatry* 79:103, 2008.

Fenichel GM: *Neonatal Neurology*, 3rd ed. Philadelphia, Saunders, 1990.

Fisher RS, Chan DW, Bare M, Lesser RP: Capillary prolactin measurements for diagnosis of seizures. *Ann Neurol* 29:187, 1991.

Forster FM: *Reflex Epilepsy, Behavioral Therapy, and Conditional Reflexes*. Springfield, IL, Charles C Thomas, 1977.

French JA, Williamson PD, Thadani VM, et al: Characteristics of medial temporal lobe epilepsy: I. Results of history and physical examination. *Ann Neurol* 34:774, 1993.

Gastaut H, Aguglia U, Tinuper P: Benign versive or circling epilepsy with bilateral 3-cps spike and wave discharges in late childhood. *Ann Neurol* 9:301, 1986.
Gastaut H, Gastaut JL: Computerized transverse axial tomography in epilepsy. *Epilepsia* 47:325, 1978.
Geschwind N: Interictal behavioral changes in epilepsy. *Epilepsia* 24(Suppl):523, 1983.
Glauser TA, Craan A, Shinnar S, et al: Ethosuximide, valproic acid, and lamotrigine in childhood absence epilepsy. *N Engl J Med* 362:790, 2010.
Gloor P: Experiential phenomena of temporal lobe epilepsy: Facts and hypothesis. *Brain* 113:1673, 1990.
Goldensohn E: The relevance of secondary epileptogenesis to the treatment of epilepsy: Kindling and the mirror focus. *Epilepsia* 25(Suppl 2):156, 1984.
Gourfinkel-An I, Baulac S, Nabbout R, et al. Monogenic idiopathic epilepsies. *Lancet Neurol* 3:209, 2004.
Gowers WR: *Epilepsy and Other Chronic Convulsive Diseases: Their Causes, Symptoms and Treatment*. New York, Dover, 1964 (originally published in 1885; reprinted as volume 1 in The American Academy of Neurology reprint series).
Gürtler S, Ebner A, Tuxhorn I, et al: Transient lesion in the splenium of the corpus callosum and antiepileptic drug withdrawal. *Neurology*. Oct 11;65(7):1032,2005.
Guerrini R: Epilepsy in children. *Lancet* 367:499, 2006.
Gürtler S, Ebner A, Tuxhorn I, et al: Transient lesion in the splenium of the corpus callosum and antiepileptic drug withdrawal. *Neurology* 65:1032, 2005.
Hauser WA, Annegers JF: Epidemiology of epilepsy, in Laidlaw JP, Richens A, Chadwick D (eds): *Textbook of Epilepsy*, 4th ed. New York, Churchill Livingstone, 1992, pp 23–45.
Hauser WA, Annegers JF: Incidence of epilepsy and unprovoked seizures in Rochester, Minnesota, 1935–1984. *Epilepsia* 34:453, 1993.
Hauser WA, Kurland LT: The epidemiology of epilepsy in Rochester, Minnesota, 1935–1967. *Epilepsia* 16:1, 1975.
Hauser WA, Rich SS, Lee JR, et al: Risk of recurrent seizures after two unprovoked seizures. *N Engl J Med* 338:429, 1998.
Hesdorfer DC, Logroscina G, Cascino G, et al: Risk of unprovoked seizure after acute symptomatic seizure: Effect of status epilepticus. *Ann Neurol* 44:908, 1998.
Holmes LB, Harvey EA, Coull BA, et al: The teratogenicity of anticonvulsants. *N Engl J Med* 344:1132, 2001.
Huttenlocher PR, Hapke RJ: A follow-up study of intractable seizures in childhood. *Ann Neurol* 28:699, 1990.
Jellinger K: Neuropathologic aspects of infantile spasms. *Brain Dev* 9:349, 1987.
Jetnik J, Loane MA, Dolk H, et al: Valproic acid monotherapy in pregnancy and major congenital malformations. *N Eng J Med* 362:285, 2010.
Kinsman SL, Vining EP, Quaskey SA, et al: Efficacy of the ketogenic diet for intractable seizure disorders. *Epilepsia* 33:1132, 1992.
Kumar A, Bleck TP: Intravenous midazolam for the treatment of status epilepticus. *Crit Care Med* 20:438, 1992.
Kutt H: Interactions between anticonvulsants and other commonly prescribed drugs. *Epilepsia* 25(Suppl 2):188, 1984.
Landau WM, Kleffner FR: Syndrome of acquired aphasia with convulsive disorder in children. *Neurology* 7:523, 1957.
Lefevre F, Aronson N: Ketogenic diet for the treatment of refractory epilepsy in children: A systematic review of efficacy. *Pediatrics* 105:46, 2000.
Lempert T, Bauer M, Schmidt D: Syncope: A videometric analysis of 56 episodes of transient cerebral hypoxia. *Ann Neurol* 36:233, 1994.
Lennox MA: Febrile convulsions in childhood. *Am J Dis Child* 78:868, 1949.
Lennox W, Lennox MA: *Epilepsy and Related Disorders*. Boston, Little, Brown, 1960.
Leppert M, Anderson VE, Quattelbaum T, et al: Benign familial neonatal convulsions linked to genetic markers on chromosome 20. *Nature* 337:647, 1989.
Leutzmezer F, Serles W, Lehner J, et al: Postictal nose wiping: A lateralizing sign in temporal lobe complex partial seizures. *Neurology* 51:1175, 1998.
LeVan Quyen M, Martinerie J, Navarro V, et al: Anticipation of epileptic seizures from standard EEG recordings. *Lancet* 357:189, 2001.
Lindvall O, Nilsson B: Cerebellar atrophy following phenytoin intoxication. *Ann Neurol* 16:258, 1984.
Litt B, Esteller R, Echauz J, et al: Epileptic seizures may begin hours in advance of clinical onset: A report of five patients. *Neuron* 30:51, 2001.
Lowenstein DH, Aldredge BK: Status epilepticus. *N Engl J Med* 338:970, 1998.
Lucas MJ, Leveno KJ, Cunningham FG: A comparison of magnesium sulfate with phenytoin for the prevention of eclampsia. *N Engl J Med* 333:201, 1995.
Luders H, Lesser RP, Dimmer DS, Morris HH III: Benign focal epilepsy of childhood, in Luders H, Lesser RP (eds): *Epilepsy: Electro-clinical Syndromes*. London, Springer-Verlag, 1987, pp 303–346.
Mattson RH, Cramer JA, Collins JF, et al: Comparison of carbamazepine, phenobarbital, phenytoin, and primidone in partial and secondarily generalized tonic-clonic seizures. *N Engl J Med* 313:145, 1985.
McCormack M, Alfirevic A, Bourgeois S, et al: HLA-A*3101 and carbamazepine-induced hypersensitivity reactions in Europeans. *N Engl J Med* 354:12, 2011.
McIntyre J, Robertson S, Norris E, et al: Safety and efficacy of buccal midazolam versus rectal diazepam for emergency treatment of seizures in children: a randomised controlled trial. *Lancet* 366:205, 2005.
Meador KJ, Baker GA, Browning N, et al: Cognitive function at 3 years of age after fetal exposure to antiepileptic drugs. *N Eng J Med* 360:1597, 2009.
Medical Research Council Antiepileptic Drug Withdrawal Study Group. Randomised study of antiepileptic drug withdrawal in patients in remission. *Lancet* 337:1175, 1991.
Meierkord H, Holtkamp M. Non-convulsive status epilepticus in adults: clinical forms and treatment. *Lancet Neurology* 6:329, 2007.
Messouak O, Yayaoui M, Benabdeljalil M, et al: La maladie de Lafora a revelation tardive. *Rev Neurol* 158:74, 2002.
Nabbout R, Prud'homme J, Herman A, et al: A locus for simple pure febrile seizures maps to chromosome 6q22-24. *Brain* 125:2668, 2002.
Niedermeyer E: *The Epilepsies: Diagnosis and Management*. Baltimore, Urban and Schwarzenberg, 1990.
Obeso JA, Rothwell JC, Marsden CD: The spectrum of cortical myoclonus. *Brain* 108:193, 1985.
Ohtahara S: Seizure disorders in infancy and childhood. *Brain Dev* 6:509, 1984.
Palmini AL, Gloor P, Jones-Gotman M: Pure amnestic seizures in temporal lobe epilepsy. *Brain* 115:749, 1992.
Panayiotopoulos CP: Early-onset benign childhood occipital seizure susceptibility syndrome: A syndrome to recognize. *Epilepsia* 40:621, 1999.
Parviainen I, Usaro A, Kalviainen R, et al: High-dose thiopental in the treatment of refractory status epilepticus in intensive care unit. *Neurology* 59:1249, 2002.
Pedley TA: Discontinuing antiepileptic drugs. *N Engl J Med* 318:982, 1988.
Pedley TA (ed): *Epilepsy: A Comprehensive Textbook*. Philadelphia, Lippincott-Raven, 1998.
Penfield W, Jasper HH: *Epilepsy and Functional Anatomy of the Human Brain*. Boston, Little, Brown, 1954.

Penfield W, Kristiansen K: *Epileptic Seizure Patterns*. Springfield, IL, Charles C Thomas, 1951.
Penry JK, Porter RJ, Dreifuss FE: Simultaneous recording of absence seizures with video tape and electroencephalography. *Brain* 98:427, 1975.
Plouin P: Benign neonatal convulsions (familial and nonfamilial), in Roger J, Drevet C, Bureau M, et al (eds): *Epileptic Syndromes in Infancy, Childhood, and Adolescence*. London, John Libbey Eurotext, 1985, pp 2–9.
Plum F, Howse DC, Duffy TE: Metabolic effects of seizures. *Res Publ Assoc Res Nerv Ment Dis* 53:141, 1974.
Porter RJ: *Epilepsy: 100 Elementary Principles*, 2nd ed. Philadelphia, Saunders, 1989.
Rasmussen T: Further observations on the syndrome of chronic encephalitis and epilepsy. *Appl Neurophysiol* 41:1, 1978.
Rasmussen T, Olszewski J, Lloyd-Smith D: Focal seizures due to chronic localized encephalitis. *Neurology* 8:435, 1958.
Rivera R, Segnini M, Baltodano A, et al: Midazolam in the treatment of status epilepticus in children. *Crit Care Med* 21:991, 1993.
Rocca WA, Sharbrough FW, Hauser WA, et al: Risk factors for complex partial seizures: A population-based case-control study. *Ann Neurol* 21:22, 1987.
Rodin E, Schmaltz S: The Bear-Fedio personality inventory and temporal lobe epilepsy. *Neurology* 34:591, 1984.
Ropper AH: "Convulsions" in basilar artery disease. *Neurology* 38:1500, 1988.
Ropper AH, Kofke A, Bromfield E, Kennedy S: Comparison of isoflurane, halothane and nitrous oxide in status epilepticus. *Ann Neurol* 19:98, 1986.
Salanova V, Andermann F, Rasmussen T, et al: Parietal lobe epilepsy. Clinical manifestations and outcome in 82 patients treated surgically between 1929 and 1988. *Brain* 118:607, 1995.
Scheibel ME, Scheibel AB: Hippocampal pathology in temporal lobe epilepsy: A Golgi survey, in Brazier MAB (ed): *Epilepsy: Its Phenomena in Man*. New York, Academic Press, 1973, pp 315–357.
Schomer DL: Partial epilepsy. *N Engl J Med* 309:536, 1983.
Silbergleit R, Durkalski V, Lowenstein D, et al: Intramuscular therapy for prehospital status epilepticus. *N Engl J Med* 366:591, 2012.
Sillanpää M, Shinnar S: Long-term mortality in childhood onset epilepsy. *N Engl J Med* 363:252, 2010.
Specchio LM, Tramacere L, LaNeve A, Beghi E: Discontinuing anti-epileptic drugs in patients who are seizure-free on monotherapy. *J Neurol Neurosurg Psychiatry* 72:22, 2002.
Sung C, Chu N: Status epilepticus in the elderly: Aetiology, seizure type and outcome. *Acta Neurol Scand* 80:51, 1989.
Sutula TP, Pitkänen A: More evidence for seizure-induced neuron loss. Is hippocampal sclerosis both cause and effect of epilepsy? *Neurology* 57:169, 2001.
Taylor I, Scheffer IE, Berkovic SF: Occipital epilepsies: Identification of specific and newly recognized syndromes. *Brain* 126:753, 2003.
Thomas JE, Regan TJ, Klass DW: Epilepsia partialis continua: A review of 32 cases. *Arch Neurol* 34:266, 1977.
Todt H: The late prognosis of epilepsy in childhood: Results of a prospective follow-up study. *Epilepsia* 25:137, 1984.
Towne AR, McGee FE, Mercer EL, et al: Mortality in a community-based status epilepticus study. *Neurology* 40(Suppl 1):229, 1990.
Treiman DM, Meyers PD, Walton NY, et al: A comparison of four treatments for generalized status epilepticus. *N Engl J Med* 339:792, 1998.
Trimble MR: Personality disturbance in epilepsy. *Neurology* 33:1332, 1983.
Twyman RE, Gahring LC, Spiess J, Rogers SW: Glutamate receptor antibodies activate a subset of receptors and reveal an agonist binding site. *Neuron* 14:755, 1995.
Victoroff J: DSM-III-R psychiatric diagnoses in candidates for epilepsy surgery: Lifetime prevalence. *Neuropsychiatry Neuropsychol Behav Neurol* 7:87, 1994.
Vining EP: The ketogenic diet. *Adv Exp Med Biol* 497:225, 2002.
Volpe JJ: *Neurology of the Newborn*, 4th ed. Philadelphia, Saunders, 2001.
Walder B, Tramer MR, Seeck M: Seizure-like phenomena and propofol. A systematic review. *Neurology* 58:1327, 2002.
Wendl H, Bien CG, Bernasconi P, et al: GluR3 antibodies: Prevalence in focal epilepsy but not specific for Rasmussen's encephalitis. *Neurology* 57:1511, 2001.
Wiebe S, Blume WT, Girvin JP, et al: A randomized, controlled trial of surgery for temporal-lobe epilepsy. *N Engl J Med* 345:311, 2001.
Wylie E, Luders H, Morris HH, et al: The lateralizing significance of versive head and eye movements during epileptic seizures. *Neurology* 36:606, 1212, 1986.
Yoon HH, Kwon HL, Mattson RH: Long-term seizure outcome in patients initially seizure-free after resective epilepsy surgery. *Neurology* 61:445, 2003.
Zeman AZ, Boniface SJ, Hodges JR: Transient epileptic amnesia: A description of the clinical and neuropsychological features in 10 cases and a review of the literature. *J Neurol Neurosurg Psychiatry* 64:435, 1998.

17

Coma and Related Disorders of Consciousness

In hospital and emergency neurology, the clinical analysis of unresponsive and comatose patients becomes a practical necessity. There is always an urgent need to determine the underlying disease and the direction in which it is evolving in order to protect the brain against more serious or irreversible damage. When called upon, the physician must therefore be prepared to implement a rapid, systematic investigation of the comatose patient and prompt therapeutic and diagnostic action that allows little time for deliberate, leisurely investigation.

Some idea of the dimensions of the problem of coma can be obtained from published statistics. Eighty years ago, in two large municipal hospitals, it was estimated that 3 percent of all admissions to the emergency wards were for diseases that had caused coma. Alcoholism, cerebral trauma, and cerebrovascular diseases were the most common, accounting for 82 percent of the comatose patients admitted to the Boston City Hospital (Solomon and Aring). Epilepsy, drug intoxication, diabetes, and severe infections were the other major causes for admission. It is perhaps surprising to learn that more contemporary figures from large city hospitals are much the same; they emphasize that the common conditions underlying coma are relatively invariant in general medical practice. For example, in the series collected by Plum and Posner (Table 17-1), only 25 percent proved to have cerebrovascular disease, and in only 6 percent was coma the consequence of trauma. Indeed, all intracranial masses and their secondary effects—such as tumors, abscesses, hemorrhages, and infarcts—made up less than one-third of the coma-producing diseases. A majority was the result of exogenous (drug overdose) and endogenous (metabolic) intoxications and hypoxia. Subarachnoid hemorrhage, meningitis, and encephalitis accounted for another 5 percent of the total. Thus, intoxication, stroke, and cranial trauma stand as the "big three" of coma-producing conditions. Equally common in some series, although obvious and usually transient, is the coma that follows seizures or resuscitation from cardiac arrest.

The terms *consciousness, confusion, stupor, unconsciousness*, and *coma* have been endowed with so many different meanings that it is almost impossible to avoid ambiguity in their usage. They are not strictly medical terms but are also literary, philosophic, and psychologic ones. The word *consciousness* is the most difficult of all. William James remarked that everyone knows what consciousness is until he attempts to define it. To the psychologist, consciousness denotes a state of continuous awareness of one's self and environment. Knowledge of self includes all "feelings, attitudes and emotions, impulses, volitions, and the active or striving aspects of conduct"; in short, a near continuous self-awareness of a person's mental functioning, particularly of cognitive processes and their relation to memories and experience. These can be judged only by the individual's verbal account of his introspections and indirectly, by his actions.

Physicians, being more practical and objective for the most part, give greater credence to the patient's behavior and reactions to overt stimuli than to what the patient says. For this reason, they use the term *consciousness* in its broadest operational meaning—namely, the state of awareness of self and environment, and responsiveness to external stimulation and inner need. This narrow definition has an advantage in that *unconsciousness* has the opposite meaning: a state of unawareness of self and environment or a suspension of those mental activities by which people are made aware of themselves and their environment, coupled always with a diminished responsiveness to environmental stimuli.

Arousal, or the level of consciousness, refers to the appearance of being *awake* as displayed by the facial muscles, eye opening, fixity of gaze, and body posture, i.e., wakefulness. A clear distinction is made in medicine between the *level* of consciousness and the *content* of consciousness, the latter reflecting the quality and coherence of thought and behavior. For neurological purposes, the loss of normal arousal is by far the more important and dramatic aspect of disordered consciousness and the one identified by laypersons and physicians as being the central feature of coma.

Much more could be said about the history of our ideas concerning consciousness, and the theoretical problems with regard to its definition. There has been an ongoing polemic among philosophers of mind as to whether it will ever be possible to understand mind and consciousness in terms of reductionist physical entities, such as cellular and molecular neural systems. Although it serves little practical purpose to review these subjects in detail here, we note that contemporary investigations indicate that one constructive approach is to define the

Table 17-1

FINAL DIAGNOSIS IN 500 PATIENTS ADMITTED TO HOSPITAL WITH "COMA OF UNKNOWN ETIOLOGY"

Metabolic and other diffuse disorders		326 (65%)
Drug poisoning	149	
Anoxia or ischemia	87	
Hepatic encephalopathy	17	
Encephalomyelitis and encephalitis	14	
Subarachnoid hemorrhage	13	
Endocrine disorders (including diabetes)	12	
Acid–base disorders	12	
Temperature regulation	9	
Uremic encephalopathy	8	
Pulmonary disease	3	
Nutritional	1	
Nonspecific metabolic coma	1	
Supratentorial mass lesions		101 (20%)
Intracerebral hematoma	44	
Subdural hematoma	26	
Cerebral infarct	9	
Brain tumor	7	
Brain abscess	6	
Epidural hematoma	4	
Thalamic infarct	2	
Pituitary apoplexy	2	
Closed head injury	1	
Subtentorial lesions		65 (13%)
Brainstem infarct	40	
Pontine hemorrhage	11	
Cerebellar hemorrhage	5	
Cerebellar tumor	3	
Cerebellar infarct	2	
Brainstem demyelination	1	
Cerebellar abscess	1	
Posterior fossa subdural hemorrhage	1	
Basilar migraine	1	
Psychiatric disorders		8 (2%)

Note: Listed here are only those patients in whom the initial diagnosis was uncertain, and a final diagnosis was established. Thus, obvious poisonings and closed head injuries are underrepresented.
Source: Adapted from Plum and Posner.

neurobiologic correlates of those elements of consciousness that are subject to observation by behavioral, electrical, and particularly imaging methods. Importantly, these controversies are informed in neurology by analyses of unusual neurologic disorders, such as those that disturb perception and consciousness of perception (phantom limb, "blindsight," etc.). The interested reader is referred to the discussions of consciousness by Crick and Koch, Plum and Posner, Young, and Zeman listed in the references.

STATES OF NORMAL AND IMPAIRED CONSCIOUSNESS

The following definitions are of service to clinicians and provide a convenient terminology for describing the states of awareness and responsiveness of patients.

Normal Consciousness

This is the condition of the normal person when awake. In this state the individual is fully responsive to a thought or perception and indicates by his behavior and speech the same awareness of self and environment as that of the examiner. There is attention to, and interaction with, the immediate surroundings. This normal state may fluctuate during the day from one of keen alertness or deep concentration with a marked constriction of the field of attention to one of mild general inattentiveness, but even in the latter circumstances, the normal individual can be brought immediately to a state of full alertness and function.

Confusion

The term *confusion* lacks precision, but in general it denotes an inability to think with customary speed, clarity, and coherence. Almost all states of confusion are marked by some degree of inattentiveness and disorientation. In this condition the patient does not take into account all elements of his immediate environment. This state also implies a degree of imperceptiveness and distractibility, referred to traditionally as "clouding of the sensorium." Here, one difficulty is to define *thinking*, a term that refers variably to problem solving or to coherence of ideas. Confusion results most often from a process that influences the brain globally, such as a toxic or metabolic disturbance or a dementia. In addition, any condition that causes drowsiness or stupor, including the natural state that comes from sleep deprivation, results in some degradation of mental performance and the emergence of inattentiveness and a state of confusion. In this way, confusion, which exists along the axis of *content* of consciousness, is linked to alertness and the *level* of consciousness.

A confusional state can also accompany focal cerebral disease in various locations, particularly in the right hemisphere, or result from disorders that disturb mainly language, memory, or visuospatial orientation, but a distinction is made between these isolated disruptions in mental function and the global confusional state. They represent special states that are analyzed differently, matters discussed further in Chaps. 20 and 23.

The mildest degree of confusion may be so slight that it can be overlooked unless the examiner searches for deviations from the patient's normal behavior and ability to carry on a coherent conversation. The patient may even be roughly oriented as to time and place, with only occasional irrelevant remarks betraying a lack of clarity and slowness of thinking. Their responses are inconsistent, attention span is reduced, and they are unable to stay on one topic, together suggesting a fundamental flaw in attention. Usually, they are disoriented and distractible, at the mercy of every stimulus. Sequences of movement may reveal impersistence and poor planning.

Severely confused and inattentive persons are unable to do more than carry out the simplest commands, and these only inconsistently and in brief sequence. Speech may be limited to a few words or phrases; or the opposite pertains—namely, some confused individuals are voluble. They give the appearance of being unaware of much that goes on around them, are disoriented in time and place, do not grasp their immediate situation or the predicament of their own confusion, and may misidentify people or objects. These illusions may lead to fear or agitation. Occasionally, hallucinatory, illusionary, or delusional experiences impart a psychotic cast to the clinical picture, obscuring the deficit in attention.

Many events that involve the confused patient leave no trace in memory; in fact, the capacity to recall events of the past hours or days is one of the most delicate tests of mental clarity. Another is the use of "working memory," which requires the temporary storage of the solution of one task for use in the next. A deficit in working memory, which is such a common feature of the confusional states, can be demonstrated by tests of serial subtraction, and the spelling of words (or repeating a phone number) forward and then backward. Careful analysis will show these defects to be tied to inattention and impaired perception or registration of information rather than to a fault in retentive memory. These phenomena that betray inattention are the central features of most confusional states. As already stated, the observed behavior of a confused person transcends inattention alone. It may incorporate elements of clouded interpretation of internal and external experience, and an inability to integrate and attach symbolic meaning to experience (apperception). The degree of confusion often varies from one time of day to another. It tends to be least pronounced in the morning and increases as the day wears on, peaking in the early evening hours ("sundowning") when the patient is fatigued, and environmental cues are not as clear.

In some medical writings, particularly in the psychiatric literature, the terms *delirium* and *confusion* are used interchangeably, the former connoting nothing more than a nondescript confusional state. However, in the syndrome of delirium tremens (observed most often but not exclusively in alcoholics), the vivid hallucinations; extreme agitation; trembling, startling easily, and convulsion; and the signs of overactivity of the autonomic nervous system suggest to us that the term *delirium* should be retained for this type of highly distinctive confusional syndrome (elaborated in Chap. 20).

As commented earlier in the discussion of the term "confusion," a relationship between the level of consciousness and disordered thinking or, content of consciousness, is evident as patients pass through states of inattention, drowsiness, confusion, stupor, and coma.

Drowsiness and Stupor

In these states, mental, speech, and physical activity are reduced. *Drowsiness* denotes an inability to sustain a wakeful state without the application of external stimuli. Furthermore, in distinction to stupor discussed later, alertness is sustained spontaneously for at least some brief period, without the further neccessity of stimuli. As a rule, some degree of inattentiveness and mild confusion are coupled with drowsiness, both improving with arousal. The patient still shifts positions somewhat naturally and without prompting. The lids droop; there may be snoring, the jaw and limb muscles are slack, and the limbs are relaxed. This state is indistinguishable from light sleep, sometimes with, slow arousal elicited by speaking to the patient or applying a tactile stimulus.

Stupor describes a state in which the patient can be roused only by vigorous and repeated stimuli and in which arousal cannot be sustained without repeated stimulation. Responses to spoken commands are either absent, curtailed, or slow and inadequate. Restless or stereotyped motor activity is common, and there is a reduction or elimination of the natural shifting of body positions. When left unstimulated, these patients quickly drift back into a deep sleep-like state. The eyes move outward and upward, a feature that is shared with sleep (see further on). Tendon and plantar reflexes, and the breathing pattern may or may not be altered, depending on how the underlying disease has affected the nervous system. In psychiatry, the term *stupor* has been used in a second sense—to denote an uncommon condition in which the perception of sensory stimuli is presumably normal but activity is suspended and motor activity is profoundly diminished (catatonia, or catatonic stupor).

However, these states, including coma, exist in a continuum, and an alternative practical method of making distinctions between them was given by Fisher, who suggested that a verbal command is required to overcome drowsiness whereas a noxious stimulus is required to overcome stupor. This allows for further gradations in the level of consciousness based on the intensity of stimulation that is necessary to produce arousal. Also encompassed in this continuum is the observation that stuporous and drowsy patients may not always be aroused to a fully awake state.

Coma

The patient who is incapable of being aroused by external stimuli or inner need, is in a state of coma. There are variations in the degree of coma, and the findings and signs depend on the underlying cause of the disorder. In its deepest stages, no meaningful or purposeful reaction of any kind is obtainable and corneal, pupillary, pharyngeal responses are diminished. In lighter stages, sometimes referred to by the ambiguous terms *semicoma or obtundation*, most of the above reflexes can be elicited, and the plantar reflexes may be either flexor or extensor (Babinski sign). As mentioned, the depth of coma and stupor may be gauged by the response to externally applied stimuli and is most useful in assessing the direction in which the disease is evolving, particularly when compared in serial examinations.

Relationship of Sleep to Coma

Persons in sleep give little evidence of being aware of themselves or their environment; in this respect, they are unconscious. Sleep shares a number of other features with the pathologic states of drowsiness, stupor, and coma. These include yawning, closure of the eyelids, cessation of blinking and reduction in swallowing, upward deviation or divergence or roving movements of the eyes, loss of muscular tone, decrease or loss of tendon reflexes, and even the presence of Babinski signs and irregular respirations, sometimes Cheyne-Stokes in type. Upon being awakened from deep sleep, a normal person may be confused for a few moments, as every physician knows from personal experience. Nevertheless, sleeping persons may still respond to unaccustomed stimuli and are capable of some mental activity in the form of dreams that leave traces of memory, thus differing from stupor or coma. The most important difference, of course, is that persons in sleep, when stimulated, can be roused to normal and persistent consciousness. There are important physiologic differences as well. Cerebral oxygen uptake does not decrease during sleep, as it usually does in coma. Recordable electrical activity—electroencephalographic (EEG) and cerebral evoked responses—and spontaneous motor activity differ in the two states, as indicated later in this chapter and in Chap. 19. The anatomic and physiologic bases for these differences are only partly known.

THE VEGETATIVE AND MINIMALLY CONSCIOUS STATES, LOCKED-IN SYNDROME, AND AKINETIC MUTISM

Vegetative State

With increasing refinements in the treatment of severe systemic diseases and cerebral injury, larger numbers of patients, who formerly would have died, have survived for indefinite periods without regaining any meaningful mental function. For the first week or two after the cerebral injury, these patients are in a state of deep coma. Then they begin to open their eyes, at first in response to painful stimuli, and later spontaneously and for increasingly prolonged periods. The patient may blink in response to threat or to light and intermittently the eyes move from side to side, seemingly following objects or fixating momentarily on the physician or a family member and giving the erroneous impression of recognition. Respiration may quicken in response to stimulation, and certain automatisms—such as swallowing, bruxism, grimacing, grunting, and moaning—may be observed (Zeman). However, the patient remains unresponsive and, for the most part, unconscious, does not speak, and shows no signs of awareness of the environment or inner need; motor activity is limited to primitive postural and reflex movements of the limbs. There is loss of sphincter control. There may be arousal or wakefulness in alternating cycles as reflected in partial eye opening, but the patient regains neither awareness nor purposeful behavior. These features define the *vegetative* state. One sign of the vegetative state is a lack of *consistent* visual following of objects; brief observation of ocular movements is subject to misinterpretation, and repeated examinations are required. These perspectives have been altered by the findings of some conscious activity that can be detected by functional imaging in relation to certain commands and verbal cues such as the individual's name as detailed below.

This state is characterized by one of a number of EEG abnormalities. There may be predominantly low-amplitude delta-frequency background activity, burst suppression, widespread alpha and theta activity, an alpha coma pattern, and sleep spindles, all of which have been described in this syndrome, as summarized by Hansotia (see Chap. 2). One important feature is a lack of—or minimal change in—the background EEG activity during and after stimulating the patient.

In the initial days and weeks, this syndrome of unconscious awakening has been referred to as the vegetative state and, if lasting 3 months after nontraumatic and 12 months after traumatic injury, the syndrome has been termed the *persistent vegetative state* (PVS; Jennett and Plum). These terms have gained wide acceptance and apply to this clinical appearance whatever the underlying cause.

The most common pathologic bases of this state are diffuse cerebral injury as a result of closed head trauma, widespread necrosis of the cortex after cardiac arrest, and thalamic necrosis from a number of causes. Most often, the prominent pathologic changes are in the thalamic and subthalamic nuclei, as in the widely known Quinlan case (Kinney et al) rather than solely in the cortex; this holds for postanoxic as well as traumatic cases. A review by J.H. Adams and colleagues found these thalamic changes, but attributed them to secondary degeneration from white matter and cortical lesions. However, in several of our cases the thalamic damage stood almost alone as the cause of persistent "awake coma." In traumatic cases, the pathologic findings are often of diffuse subcortical white matter degeneration (described as *diffuse axonal injury*), prominent thalamic degeneration, and ischemic damage in the cortex. Taken together, these anatomic findings suggest the concept that PVS is a state in which the cortex is either diffusely injured or effectively disconnected and isolated from the thalamus, or the thalamic nuclei are destroyed. In either the traumatic or anoxic types of PVS, atrophy of the cerebral white matter may lead to ventricular enlargement and thinning of the corpus callosum.

The vegetative state or the minimally conscious state described further on, may also be the terminal phase of progressive cortical degenerative processes such as Alzheimer and Creutzfeldt-Jakob disease (where the pathologic changes may include the thalamus).

In all these clinical states, the profound and widespread dysfunction of the cerebrum is reflected by extreme reductions in cerebral blood flow and metabolism, measured with positron emission tomography (PET) and other techniques. On the basis of PET studies in a patient with carbon monoxide poisoning, Laureys and colleagues observed that the main difference between the vegetative state and the later recovered state was the degree of hypometabolism in the parietal lobe association areas. Anatomic changes in this same cortical region have been implicated in the transition from minimally conscious to a more awake state. The finding in this PET study that noxious somatosensory stimulation fails to activate the association cortices is consistent with the concept that large regions of cortex are isolated from thalamic input or that the critical parietal interpretive areas are isolated from the rest of the cortex.

Of practical value is the observation that the CT and MRI may show progressive and profound cerebral atrophy in cases of vegetative state. In the absence of this atrophy after several months or more, it may be unwise to offer a pessimistic prognosis. One patient with clinical features of the traumatic vegetative state but lacking cerebral atrophy on imaging studies regained normal cognitive ability after a year, although he remained paralyzed (R. Cranford, personal communication).

These observations notwithstanding, there is little doubt that the neuroanatomic and neurophysiologic basis of the vegetative state will prove to be complex or at least separable into categories defined by the locus of brain damage. In particular, a striking observation has been made by Owen and colleagues in a 23-year-old woman who had been vegetative for 5 months after a head injury (thus not strictly speaking a "persistent" vegetative state). They observed localized cortical activity in the middle and superior temporal gyri in response to the presentation of spoken sentences that was comparable to the brain activity in normal individuals. Di and colleagues have similarly demonstrated brain activation only to the patient's own name and not to other names in vegetative patients. These data suggest that some forms of mental processing can go on during a vegetative state but it is not clear if this situation is representative nor does it provide information about self-awareness, a requisite for consciousness. The most compelling demonstration of cognitive processing in vegetative and minimally conscious patients has been provided by Monti and colleagues as displayed by functional MRI. Five of their 54 patients, all with traumatic brain injury but none after anoxic ischemic damage, could on command, willfully modulate focal brain activity by playing tennis (frontal lobe activation) or mentally navigating a familiar place such as their home (temporal lobe activation). In one patient, this activity could be used as a means of communication.

At a minimum, these demonstrations emphasize the care that must be taken in establishing diagnoses of PVS and minimally conscious states. Whether these findings with functional imaging simply reflect preserved islands of function in severe brain injury that were not examinable clinically or whether they require an entire rethinking of the neurologic examination that determines the state of consciousness cannot yet be stated (see editorial by Ropper, 2010).

An additional observation of some consequence is the finding of purported axonal growth over time in a patient with traumatic brain injury who had been in a minimally conscious state (see below) for 19 years and then began to speak and comprehend, while remaining virtually quadriplegic. Voss and colleagues, using sophisticated MRI diffusion tensor imaging, have shown axonal sprouting in the posterior parietal and midline cerebellar regions. They compared the results of tensor imaging to a patient who had been in a minimally conscious state for 6 years without improvement and to 20 normal individuals. Their findings are subject to several interpretations, but axonal growth in the parietal lobes offers a potential explanation for the few instances in which recovery from severe injury does occur. When combined with the findings of Laureys and colleagues, a case can be made for the posterior parietal regions as necessary for integrated consciousness. This further raise the possibility that certain islands of limited awareness may be dissociated from global brain function.

Additional terms that have been used to describe this syndrome of preserved autonomic and respiratory function without cognition include *apallic syndrome* and *neocortical death*. A position paper has codified the features of the PVS and suggests dropping a number of related ambiguous terms, although some, such as *akinetic mutism*, discussed further on, have a more specific neurologic meaning and are still useful (see Multi-Society Task Force on PVS).

It is difficult to predict which comatose patients will later fall permanently into the vegetative or minimally conscious categories (see Chap. 40). Plum and Posner reported that of 45 patients with signs of the vegetative state at 1 week after onset, 13 had awakened and 5 of these had satisfactory outcomes. After being vegetative for close to 2 weeks, only 1 recovered to a level of moderate disability; after 2 weeks, the prognosis was uniformly poor. Larger studies by Higashi and colleagues have given similar results. As a rough guide to prognosis specifically in head injury, Braakman and colleagues found that among a large group of comatose patients, 59 percent regained consciousness within 6 h, but of those in a vegetative state at 3 months, none became independent. At no time before 3 or 6 months was it possible to distinguish patients who would remain in a vegetative state from those who would die. Further comments regarding recovery are made in the next section on the minimally conscious state.

A study by the Multi-Society Task Force on PVS concluded that the outcome from a vegetative state is better in traumatic as compared to nontraumatic cases. J.H. Adams and coworkers have proposed that this reflects differences in the state of thalamic neurons in the two situations. They suggested that after acute hypoxia, neurons subjected to ischemic necrosis are liable to be permanently lost; by contrast, in trauma, the loss of thalamic neurons is more frequently secondary to transsynaptic degeneration following diffuse axonal injury, allowing a greater potential for recovery. Many of these ideas are speculative.

Minimally Conscious State

The vegetative state blends into a less severe but still profound dementia that has been termed the "minimally conscious state," wherein the patient is capable of some rudimentary behavior such as following a simple command, gesturing, or producing single words or brief phrases, always in an inconsistent way from one examination to another (see Giacino et al). Here, there is preservation of the ability to carry out basic motor behaviors that demonstrate a degree of awareness, at least at some times. The minimally conscious state is found as either a transitional or permanent condition and is sometimes difficult to separate from akinetic mutism discussed further on. Any notion of such a patient's self-awareness is purely conjectural, but there may be an impressive array of behaviors and activation of associative cortex that suggest at least some relationship to processing of external information beyond a rudimentary level (see discussion by Bernat). The causes and pathologic changes underlying the minimally conscious state are identical to those of the vegetative state, including the frequent finding of thalamic and multiple cerebral lesions, and the distinction between them is one of degree.

It is useful to maintain a critical view of reports of remarkable recuperation after months or years of prolonged coma or the vegetative state. When the details of such cases become known, it is evident that recovery might reasonably have been expected. There are, however, numerous reported instances of partial recovery in patients—particularly children and young adults—who display vegetative features for several weeks or, as Andrews and Childs and Mercer describe, even several months after injury. Such observations cast doubt on unqualified claims of success with certain therapies, such as sensory stimulation. Nevertheless, the occurrence of very late recovery in adults must be acknowledged (see Andrews; Higashi et al; and Rosenberg et al, 1977) and a relation of awakening to the recovery of connections to the parietal lobes has already been mentioned. Cases of improvement from the "minimally conscious state" are more plausible than those from the vegetative state. More recent reports, for example by Estraneo and colleagues and by Luaté and coworkers, may be more instructive but still not entirely directive. In contrast to the notion that late recovery is exceptional, the first case series of 50 consecutive patients in a PVS for a year, 10 showed late improvement an average of 2 years later, but all were severely impaired. In the second series, none of the 12 vegetative patients improved at 5 years but 13 of 39 MCS cases emerged to consciousness with severe disability.Of course, the assignation of a poor prognosis by the application of these terms to an individual patient often leads to the withdrawal of care, and the self-fulfilling poor prognosis. This is a much discussed problem that has not been satisfactorily but it emphasizes that simply labeling patients with certain diagnoses has implications for accurately assessing the natural history of some diseases.

Among the interesting recent therapeutic observations, one observation has come from Schiff and colleagues, who were able to improve function by stimulating the medial (interlaminar) thalamic nuclei through implanted electrodes in a patient who had been initially vegetative and made a natural transition to a minimally conscious state after traumatic brain injury. Longer periods of eye opening and increased responses to execute commands, such as bringing a cup to his mouth, were observed, including, for the first time since his injury, intelligible verbalization. The authors point out that this individual had preserved language cortex and connections between thalamus and cortex. Whether this remarkable result is generalizable is not known.

It cannot go without comment that the degree of disability that families find acceptable varies greatly and leads to difficult decisions regarding the continuation of medical care. The knowledgeable, sympathetic, and flexible physician is in the best position to offer perspective and guide these matters as discussed at the end of this chapter.

Locked-in Syndrome

The states of coma described above and the vegetative state must be distinguished from a syndrome in which there is little or no disturbance of consciousness, but only an inability of the patient to respond adequately. The latter is referred to as the *locked-in syndrome* or the *deefferented state*. The term *pseudocoma* as a synonym for this state is best avoided, because it is used by some physicians to connote the unconsciousness of the hysteric or malingerer, the dissociative state, or catatonia. The locked-in syndrome is most often caused by a lesion of the ventral pons (basis pontis) as a result of occlusion of the basilar artery. Such an infarction spares both the somatosensory pathways, and the ascending neuronal systems responsible for arousal and wakefulness, as well as certain midbrain elements that allow the eyelids to be raised in wakefulness; the lesion essentially interrupts the corticobulbar and corticospinal pathways, depriving the patient of speech and the capacity to respond in any way except by vertical gaze and blinking. Severe motor neuropathy (e.g., Guillain-Barré syndrome), pontine myelinolysis, or periodic paralysis may have a similar effect.

Akinetic Mutism

One could logically refer to the locked-in state as *akinetic mutism* insofar as the patient is akinetic (motionless) and mute, but this is not the sense in which the term was originally used by Cairns and colleagues, who described a patient who appeared to be awake but was unresponsive (actually their patient was able to answer in whispered monosyllables). Following each of several drainings of a third ventricular cyst, the patient would become aware and responsive but would have no memory for any of the events that had taken place when she was in the akinetic mute state. This state of apparent vigilance in an imperceptive and unresponsive patient has been referred to by French authors as *coma vigile*, but the same term has been applied to the vegetative state.

The term *akinetic mutism* has been applied to yet another group of patients who are silent and inert as a result of bilateral lesions usually of the anterior parts of the frontal lobes, leaving intact the motor and sensory pathways; the patient is profoundly apathetic, lacking to an extreme degree the psychic drive or impulse to action (abulia). However, the abulic patient, unlike Cairns' patient, registers most of what is happening about him and is intensely stimulated, may speak normally, relating events observed in the recent and distant past.

Catatonia

The patient with *catatonia* appears unresponsive, in a state that simulates stupor, light coma, or akinetic mutism. There are no signs of structural brain disease, such as pupillary or reflex abnormalities. Oculocephalic responses are preserved, as in the awake state—i.e., the eyes move concurrently as the head is turned. There is usually resistance to eye opening, and some patients display a waxy flexibility of passive limb movement that gives the examiner a feeling of bending a wax rod (*flexibilitas cerea*); there is also the retention for a long period of seemingly uncomfortable limb postures (*catalepsy*). Peculiar motor mannerisms or repetitive motions, seen in a number of these patients, may give the impression of seizures; choreiform jerking has also been reported, but the latter sign should also suggest the possibility of seizure activity. The EEG shows normal posterior alpha activity that is attenuated by stimulation. Catatonia is discussed further in Chaps. 20 and 53.

Because there is considerable imprecision in the use of terms by which various states of reduced consciousness are designated, the physician would be better advised to supplement designations such as *coma* and *akinetic mutism* by simple descriptions indicating whether the patient appears awake or asleep, drowsy or alert, aware or unaware of his surroundings, and responsive or unresponsive to a variety of stimuli. This requires that the patient be observed more frequently or over a longer period than the several minutes usually devoted to this portion of the neurologic examination. The aforementioned findings of apparent limited responsiveness reflected with functional imaging only further emphasizes the care with which these clinical diagnoses should be determined.

BRAIN DEATH

In the late 1950s, European neurologists called attention to a state of coma in which the brain was irreversibly damaged and had ceased to function, but pulmonary and cardiac function could still be maintained by artificial means. Mollaret and Goulon referred to this condition as *coma dépassé* (a state beyond coma). A Harvard Medical School committee, in 1968, called it *brain death* and established a set of clinical criteria by which it could be recognized (Beecher et al). R.D. Adams, who was a member of the committee, defined the state as one of complete unresponsiveness to all modes of stimulation, arrest of respiration, and absence of all EEG activity for 24 h. The concept that a person is dead if the brain is dead and that death of the brain may precede the cessation of cardiac function has posed a number of important ethical, legal, and social problems, as well as medical ones. All aspects of brain death have since been the subject of close study by several professional committees, which for the most part have confirmed the 1968 guidelines for determining that the brain is dead. The American Academy of neurology published guidelines on this subject in 1995 and affirmed them with some refinements in 2010. The monograph by Wijdicks is a thorough modern source on the subject of brain death and also addresses the subject from an international perspective.

The philosophical underpinnings of the equating of brain death to death, giving it the same status as cessation of cardiorespiratory death, a utilitarian approach, are complex.

The ethical and moral dimensions of brain death are complex and subject to differing interpretations in various societies, religions, and cultures. One justification for equating brain death with somatic death is the general inevitability of cardiorespiratory failure in patients who fulfill the standard criteria. This tenet has exceptions, the most striking of which is a well-studied case of 20-year survival in a boy who had meningitis reported by Reptinger and colleagues, and other cases of long survival have been described with varying degrees of documentation. These have been collected by Shewmon who makes the further point that the arguments equating brain death with death on the basis of the brain's role in creating "somatic unity" are weakened by the existence of such cases as well as by delivery of live babies from brain-dead mothers. In the end, these philosophical concerns matter but the operational state called brain death serves both patients and society well and is compatible with most of the world's religions.

The central considerations in the diagnosis of brain death are (1) absence of all cerebral functions; (2) absence of all brainstem functions, including spontaneous respiration; and (3) irreversibility of the state. Following from the last of these criteria, it is necessary to demonstrate an irrefutable cause of the underlying catastrophic brain damage (e.g., trauma, cardiac arrest, cerebral hemorrhage) and to exclude reversible causes such as drug overdose and extreme hypothermia.

In the diagnosis of brain death, the absence of cerebral function is demonstrated by the presence of deep coma and total lack of spontaneous movement and of motor and vocal responses to all visual, auditory, and cutaneous stimulation. Spinal reflexes may persist, and the toes often flex slowly in response to plantar stimulation; but a well-developed Babinski sign is unusual in our experience (although its presence does not exclude the diagnosis of brain death). Extensor or flexor posturing is seen from time to time as a transitional phenomenon just before or after brain death becomes evident, and the status of these movements in the diagnosis is ambiguous, but the physician should proceed cautiously in declaring a patient dead in the presence of posturing and should consider conducting the examination again at a later time.

The absence of brainstem function is judged by the loss of spontaneous eye movements, midposition of the eyes, and lack of response to oculocephalic and caloric (oculovestibular) testing; the presence of dilated or midposition fixed pupils (not smaller than 3 mm); paralysis of bulbar musculature (no facial movement or gag, cough, corneal, or sucking reflexes); an absence of motor and autonomic responses to noxious stimuli; and absence of respiratory movements. The clinical findings should show complete absence of brain function, not an approximation that might be reflected, e.g., by small or poorly reactive pupils, slight eye deviation with oculovestibular stimulation, posturing of the limbs, as mentioned earlier.

As a demonstration of destruction of the medulla, it has become customary to perform an "apnea test" to demonstrate unresponsiveness of the medullary centers to a high carbon dioxide tension. This test is conducted by first employing preoxygenation for several minutes with high inspired oxygen tension, the purpose of which is to displace nitrogen from the alveoli and create a reservoir of oxygen that will diffuse along a gradient into the pulmonary circulation. The patient can then be disconnected from the respirator for several minutes during which time 100 percent oxygen is being delivered by cannula or ventilator that has its pumping mechanism turned off; this allows the arterial Pco_2 to rise to 50 to 60 mm Hg (typically, CO_2 rises approximately 2.5 mm Hg per minute at normal body temperature—slower if the patient is hypothermic). The hypercarbia serves both as a stimulus to breathing and a confirmation that spontaneous ventilation has failed. If no breathing is observed and examination of the blood gases shows that an adequate level of Pco_2 has been attained, the presence of this component of brain death is corroborated. Several sets of formal criteria have chosen a level of CO_2 of 60 mm Hg (7.98 kPa [kilopascals]) as adequate to stimulate the medulla, even under circumstances in which it has been badly damaged. In our experience, patients who have a severely damaged brainstem but nonetheless breathe, have done so at a Pco_2 well below 50 mm Hg, but there are exceptions in which higher levels were required as a stimulus.

The risks of apnea testing are minimal, as discussed in the American Academy of Neurology's 2010 document, but hypotension, hypoxemia, cardiac arrhythmias, and barotrauma may occasionally occur. In patients who cannot tolerate the test for more than a brief period, initially raising the CO_2 rapidly by insufflation of this gas has been suggested, but this approach has not been studied extensively. Delivering oxygen during the test with a low tidal volume and a ventilator rate of 1 to 2 breaths per minute or by continuous positive airway pressure may ameliorate hypoxia and resultant hypotension to allow apnea to continue for a period long enough to reach the target Pco_2, but this technique has also not been adequately studied.

Most, but not all, brain-dead patients have diabetes insipidus. The absence of this syndrome in some cases reflects the imprecision of clinical signs in detecting a total loss of brain function. Other ancillary bedside tests may be conducted. Among the ones we use from time to time is the inability to produce tachycardia in response to the injection of atropine; this reflects the loss of innervation of the heart by the medullary vagal neurons.

The authors have observed a number of dramatic spontaneous movements when severe hypoxia is attained upon terminal disconnection from the ventilator for several minutes. These include opisthotonos with chest expansion that simulates a breath, elevation of the arms and crossing them in front of the chest or neck (termed the Lazarus sign by Ropper, 1984), head-turning, shoulder-shrugging, and variants of these posturing-like movements. For this reason the advice that the family not be in attendance immediately after mechanical ventilation has been discontinued.

The EEG provides confirmation of cerebral death, and many institutions prefer this corroboration by the demonstration of electrocerebral silence ("flat" or, more accurately, isoelectric EEG, shown first by Schwab). However, most U.S. institutions do not require an EEG for the confirmation of death. Electrocerebral silence is considered to be present if there is no electrical potential of more than 2 mV during a 30-min recording except for artifacts created by the ventilator, electrocardiograph, and surrounding electrical devices; the absence of these artifacts suggests a technical problem with the recording.

There are cases on record in which a patient with an isoelectric EEG has had preserved brainstem reflexes so that cerebral unresponsiveness and a flat EEG do not alone signify brain death; both may also occur and may be reversible in states of profound hypothermia or intoxication with sedative-hypnotic drugs and immediately following cardiac arrest. Therefore, it has been recommended that the diagnosis of brain death not be entertained until several hours have passed from the time of initial observation. If the examination is performed at least approximately 6 h after the precipitating event, and there is prima facie evidence of overwhelming brain injury from trauma, or massive cerebral hemorrhage (the most common conditions causing brain death), there is no need for serial testing. If cardiac arrest was the antecedent event, or the cause of neurologic damage is unclear, or drug or alcohol intoxication could reasonably have played a role in suppressing the brainstem reflexes, it is advisable to wait about 24 h before repeating the testing and pronouncing the patient dead. Toxicologic screening of the serum or urine is requisite in the latter circumstances.

The impact of any requirement to perform a second brain death examination at some interval such as 6 hours has been studied by Lustbader and coworkers. Their extensive survey in New York State, where a second examination had been recommended by a panel, was instructive; of 1,311 adult and pediatric cases, none who were found to be brain dead regained brainstem function on a second test that was performed about 18 hours later. However, 12 percent had cardiac arrest and in others, consent for organ donation was withheld during the time between examinations. Several authoritative authors have argued against a second test on this basis.

Because evoked potentials show variable abnormalities in brain-dead patients, they are not of primary value in the diagnosis. Some centers use nuclide brain scanning or cerebral angiography to demonstrate an absence of blood flow to the brain, equating this with brain death; but there are technical pitfalls in the use of these methods, and it is preferable to establish the diagnosis of death primarily on clinical grounds. The specificity of radionuclide scanning is close to 100 percent but there is a self-referential aspect to this statement as the clinical diagnosis has been used as a gold standard. An additional problem arises in the observation that the sensitivity may be only about 75 percent (Joffe et al). Others take the view that demonstrating absent cerebral blood flow equates with brain death. False-negative tests are possible if a small amount of filling of the intracranial vertebral arteries or nuclide uptake in the inferior cerebellum is revealed. The same can be said for transcranial Doppler sonography, which in brain death shows a to-and-fro, *pendelfluss* blood-flow pattern in the basal vessels.

The main difficulties that arise in relation to brain death are not the technical ones, but those involving the sensitive conversations with the family of the patient and, to some extent, with other medical professionals. These tasks often fall to the neurologist. It is best not to embark on clinical or EEG testing for brain death unless there is a clear intention on the part of the physician to remove the ventilator or follow through with organ donation at the end of the process. The nature of testing for brain death and its intended outcome should be explained to the family in plain language. The family's desires regarding organ transplantation should be sought after adequate time has passed for them to absorb the shock of the circumstances. Neurologists must, of course, resist pressures from diverse sources that might lead them to the premature designation of a declaration of brain death. To avoid the appearance of conflict of motivations, most centers have a separate team, often from an organ bank, to address the issues of organ transplantation after brain death has been established. The complex matter of a family's desire to maintain ventilation and other medical support in a brain-dead relative is best addressed with kind consideration and counseling by clergy, ethics ("optimal care") committees, and hospital staff so as to avoid confrontation. Time often allows such situations to be defused.

At the same time, it should be clarified that while brain death is an operational state that allows transplantation to proceed, and mandates withdrawal of ventilation and blood pressure support, patients with overwhelming brain injuries need not fulfill these absolute criteria in order for medical support to be withdrawn.

A task force for the determination of *brain death in children* has recommended the adoption of essentially the same criteria as for adults. However, the great difficulty in evaluating the status of nervous function in relation to perinatal insults, has led them to suggest that the determination not be made before the seventh postnatal day and that the period of observation should be extended to 48 h. As with adults, the possibility of reversible brain dysfunction from toxins, drugs, hypothermia, and hypotension must always be considered.

THE ELECTROENCEPHALOGRAM AND DISTURBANCES OF CONSCIOUSNESS

The EEG provides one of the most delicate confirmations of the fact that states of impaired consciousness are expressions of neurophysiologic changes in the cerebrum. Some change of brain electrical activity occurs in all disturbances of consciousness except for the milder degrees of confusion, delirium tremens, and in catatonia. These alterations usually consist of a disorganization of the EEG background pattern, including disappearance of the normal alpha rhythm and replacement by random slow waves of low to moderate voltage in the initial stages of confusion and drowsiness; a more regular pattern of slow, 2- to 3-per-second waves of high voltage occurs in stupor; slow low-voltage waves or intermittent suppression of organized electrical activity in the deep coma of hypoxia and ischemia; and, ultimately, a complete absence of electrical activity in brain death.

In some deeply comatose patients, the EEG may transiently show diffuse and variable alpha (8- to 12-Hz) activity, which may be mistaken for the physiologic alpha rhythm. However, this pattern (alpha coma), unlike normal alpha, is not limited to the posterior cerebral regions, is not monorhythmic like normal alpha activity, and displays no reactivity to sensory stimuli. Alpha coma is usually associated with pontine or diffuse cortical lesions and has a poor prognosis (see Iragui and McCutchen). A rarer EEG abnormality is "spindle coma," in which sleep spindles dominate the record (see "Disorders of Sleep Related to Neurologic Disease" in Chap. 19).

The EEG accurately reflects the depth of certain metabolic comas, particularly those caused by hepatic or renal failure. In these conditions, the slow waves become higher in amplitude as coma deepens, ultimately assuming a high-voltage rhythmic delta pattern and a triphasic configuration. Not all cerebral disorders that cause confusion, stupor, and coma have the same effects on the EEG. In cases of intoxication with sedatives, exemplified by barbiturates and diazepines, fast (beta) activity initially replaces normal rhythms. Coma in which myoclonus or twitching is a major clinical feature may show frequent sharp waves or a sharpness of the background slowing of the EEG. A relatively normal EEG in delirium tremens has already been commented on. The differences in EEG changes among metabolic derangements probably represent biologic distinctions at the neuronal level that have not yet been elucidated (see also Chap. 2).

THE ANATOMY AND NEUROPHYSIOLOGY OF ALERTNESS AND COMA

Our current understanding of the anatomy and physiology of alertness comes largely from the elegant experiments of Bremer and of Moruzzi and Magoun in the 1930s and 1940s. Observing cats in whom he had sectioned the brainstem between the pons and midbrain and at the level of the lower medulla, Bremer found that the rostral section caused a sleep-like state and "synchronized" EEG rhythms that were characteristic of sleep; animals with the lower section remained awake with appropriate "desynchronized" EEG rhythms. He interpreted this to mean, in large part correctly, that a constant stream of sensory stimuli, provided by trigeminal and spinal sources, was required to maintain the awake state. More recently, a system of "nonspecific" projections from the thalamus to all cortical regions, independent of any specific sensory nucleus has been demonstrated. A critical refinement of this concept resulted from the observation by Moruzzi and Magoun that electrical stimulation of the medial midbrain tegmentum and adjacent areas just above this level caused a lightly anesthetized animal to become suddenly alert and its EEG to change correspondingly, i.e., to become "desynchronized," in a manner identical to normal arousal by sensory stimuli. The sites at which stimulation led to arousal consisted of a series of points extending from the nonspecific medial thalamic nuclei down through the caudal midbrain. These loci were situated along the loosely organized core of neurons that anatomists refer to as the reticular system or formation.

The anatomic studies of the Scheibels have described widespread innervation of the reticular formation by multiple bifurcating and collateral axons of the ascending sensory systems, implying that this area is maintained in a tonically active state by ascending sensory stimulation. Because this region, especially the medial thalamus, projects widely to the cerebral hemispheres, the concept arose of a reticular activating system (RAS) that maintained the alert state and the inactivation or destruction of which led to an unarousable state. In this way, despite a number of experimental inconsistencies (see Steriade), the paramedian upper brainstem tegmentum and lower diencephalon came to be conceived as the locus of the arousal system of the brain.

The anatomic boundaries of the upper brainstem RAS are somewhat indistinct. The neurons of this system are interspersed throughout the paramedian regions of the upper (rostral) pontine and midbrain tegmentum; at the thalamic level, the RAS includes the functionally related posterior paramedian, parafascicular, and medial portions of the centromedian and adjacent intralaminar nuclei. In the brainstem, nuclei of the reticular formation receive collaterals from the spinothalamic and trigeminal–thalamic pathways and project not just to the sensory cortex of the parietal lobe, as do the thalamic relay nuclei for somatic sensation, but to the whole of the cerebral cortex. Thus, it would seem that sensory stimulation has a double effect—it conveys information to the brain from somatic structures and the environment and also activates those parts of the nervous system on which the maintenance of consciousness depends. The cerebral cortex not only receives impulses from the ascending RAS but also modulates this incoming information via corticofugal projections to the reticular formation. Although the physiology of the RAS is far more complicated than this simple formulation would suggest, it nevertheless, as a working idea, retains a great deal of clinical credibility, and makes comprehensible some of the neuropathologic observations noted further on, as well as the effects of deep brain stimulation to improve function in minimally conscious patients (see further on).

The presence of alpha rhythm with the eyes closed is a marker for wakefulness, but its representation at the cortical surface is not required for wakefulness as it is obliterated in cases of bilateral occipital infarction. It is, of course, possible that deep nuclei are still projecting the rhythm to other parts of the cerebrum to maintain wakefulness. Although for many years it has been taught that arousal causes a desynchronization of brainwave activity (in distinction to the synchronized activity of sleep), it has become apparent that during wakefulness, there is a widespread low-voltage fast rhythm (a gamma rhythm that has a frequency of 30 to 60 Hz). This activity, coordinated by the thalamus, has been theorized to synchronize cortical activity and to account perhaps for the unification of modular aspects of experience (color, shape, motion) that are processed in different cortical regions. In this way, the rhythm is said to "bind" various aspects of a sensory experience or memory. This fast and widespread electrographic activity is not appreciated with the usual EEG surface recordings but it can be extracted by sophisticated mathematical transformations. Using such electrophysiologic methods, Meador and colleagues have shown that the gamma rhythm can be detected over the primary somatosensory cortex after an electrical stimulus on the contralateral hand is perceived, but not if the patient fails to perceive it. The clinical relevance of the rhythm is uncertain but it has elicited interest because it may give insight into several intriguing questions about conscious experience.

METABOLIC MECHANISMS THAT DISTURB CONSCIOUSNESS

In a number of diseases that disturb consciousness, there is direct interference with the metabolic activities of the nerve cells in the cerebral cortex and the central nuclei of the brain. Hypoxia, global ischemia, hypoglycemia, hyper- and hypoosmolar states, acidosis, alkalosis, hypokalemia, hyperammonemia, hypercalcemia, hypercarbia, drug intoxication, and severe vitamin deficiencies are well-known examples (see Chap. 40 and Table 40-1). In general, the loss of consciousness in these conditions parallels the reduction in cerebral metabolism. For example, in the case of global ischemia, in which oxygen and glucose are removed from the brain, an acute drop in cerebral blood flow (CBF) to 25 mL/min/100 g brain tissue from its normal 55 mL/min/100 g causes slowing of the EEG and syncope or impaired consciousness; a drop in CBF below 12 to 15 mL/min/100 g causes electrocerebral silence, coma, and cessation of most neuronal metabolic and synaptic functions. Lower levels of ischemia are tolerated if acquired more slowly, but neurons cannot survive when flow is reduced below 8 to 10 mL/min/100 g. Oxygen consumption of 2 mg/min/100 g (approximately half of normal) is incompatible with an alert state. In other types of metabolic encephalopathy, or with widespread anatomic damage to the hemispheres, blood flow may stay near normal while metabolism is greatly reduced. An exception to these statements is the coma that arises from seizures, in which metabolism and blood flow are greatly increased. Extremes of body temperature (above 41°C [105.8°F] or below 30°C [86F°]) also induce coma through a nonspecific effect on the metabolic activity of neurons. Some of these metabolic changes are probably epiphenomena, reflecting in each particular encephalopathy a specific type of dysfunction in neurons and their supporting cells. Again, for most metabolic alterations, the rate of change is equivalently important to the absolute level in causing a change in consciousness.

The endogenous metabolic toxin(s) that are responsible for coma cannot always be identified. In diabetes, acetone bodies (acetoacetic acid, β-hydroxybutyric acid, and acetone) are present in high concentration; in uremia, there is probably an accumulation of dialyzable small molecular toxins, notably phenolic derivatives of the aromatic amino acids. In hepatic coma, elevation of blood NH_3 (ammonia) to 5 to 6 times normal levels corresponds roughly to the level of coma. Lactic acidosis may affect the brain by lowering arterial blood pH to less than 7.0. The impairment of consciousness that accompanies pulmonary insufficiency is related mainly to hypercapnia. This is not to say that the toxic effects of these molecules has been confirmed or is well understood, as noted below. In acute hyponatremia (Na <120 mEq/L) of whatever cause, neuronal dysfunction is probably a result of the intracellular movement of water, leading to neuronal swelling and loss of potassium chloride from the cells. The mode of action of bacterial toxins is not fully understood.

Drugs such as general anesthetics, which are addressed more fully in a later section, alcohol, opiates, barbiturates, phenytoin, antidepressants, and benzodiazepines induce coma by their direct effects on neuronal membranes in the cerebrum and RAS or on neurotransmitters and their receptors. Others, such as methyl alcohol and ethylene glycol, both act directly and by producing a metabolic acidosis. Although the coma of toxic and metabolic diseases usually evolves through stages of drowsiness, confusion, and stupor (and the reverse sequence occurs during emergence from coma), each disease imparts its own characteristic clinical features.

The sudden and excessive neuronal discharge that characterizes an epileptic seizure is another common mechanism of coma. Focal seizure activity has little effect on consciousness until it spreads from one side of the brain (and the body if there is a convulsion) to the other. Coma then ensues, presumably because the extension of the seizure discharge to deep central neuronal structures paralyzes their function. In other types of seizures, in which consciousness is interrupted from the very beginning, a diencephalic origin has been postulated (centrencephalic seizures of Penfield, as discussed in Chap. 16), but this idea has been contentious for decades.

Concussion exemplifies yet another special pathophysiologic mechanism of coma. In closed head injury, it has been shown that at the moment of the concussive injury there is an enormous increase in intracranial pressure, on the order of 200 to 700 lb/in^2, lasting a few thousandths of a second. The vibration set up in the skull and transmitted to the brain was for many years thought to be the basis of the abrupt paralysis of nervous function that characterizes concussive head injury (commotio cerebri). While not excluding this mechanism, it is more likely that the sudden swirling motion of the brain induced by the acceleration or deceleration from blow to the head produces a rotation (torque) of the cerebral hemispheres around the axis of the upper brainstem. Disruption of the function of neurons in some unknown way from the mechanical deformation is the proximate cause of loss of consciousness. These same physical forces, when extreme, cause multiple shearing lesions or hemorrhages in the diencephalon and upper brainstem. Chapter 35 fully discusses the subject of concussion.

Yet another unique form of coma is that produced by inhalation anesthetics. The effects of general anesthesia had for many years been attributed to changes in the physical chemistry of neuronal membranes. More recently, it has been recognized that interactions with ligand-gated ion channels, particularly gamma-aminobutyric acid (GABA)-A receptors and alterations in neurotransmitter function are a more likely mechanism of anesthesia-induced unconsciousness. An extensive summary of what is known about the metabolic neurochemistry of anesthetics has been given by Campagna and colleagues and by Brown and coworkers; it emphasizes the changes in neurotransmitter function rather than alterations in membrane fluidity but still cannot give a unified theory of the effects of these agents, partly because different classes of drug act at different sites. Inhalation anesthetics are unusual among coma-producing drugs in respect to the sequence of inhibitory and excitatory effects that they produce at different concentrations. During anesthesia, sufficient inhibition of brainstem activity can be attained to eliminate the pupillary responses and the corneal reflex. Both return to normal by the time the patient is able to speak. Sustained clonus, exaggerated tendon reflexes, and Babinski signs are common during the process of arousal. Rosenberg and associates systematically studied these findings. Preexisting focal cerebral deficits from strokes often worsen transiently with the administration of anesthetics, as is true to a lesser extent with other sedatives, metabolic encephalopathies, and hyperthermia.

RECURRING STUPOR AND COMA

Aside from repeated drug overdose, recurring episodes of stupor are usually a result of the recurrence of an underlying biochemical derangement, hepatic failure being the most common. A similar condition of periodic hyperammonemic coma in children and adults can come about from urea cycle enzyme defects, such as ornithine transcarbamylase deficiency. These are discussed in Chap. 37.

Under the title of *idiopathic recurring stupor*, a rare condition has been described in adult men who displayed a prolonged state of deep sleepiness lasting from hours to days intermittently over a period of many years. Despite the impression of a sleep disorder related to narcolepsy, the EEG showed widespread fast (beta) activity, and both the stupor and EEG changes were promptly reversed by flumazenil, a benzodiazepine receptor antagonist. During the bouts, a 100 fold increase of circulating endozepine-4, an ostensibly naturally occurring diazepine agonist, was present in the serum and spinal fluid. Subsequently, the authors of the original reports (Lugaresi et al) found, by the use of more advanced techniques, that intoxication with lorazepam may have accounted for at least some of the cases. Although such cases in which diazepine antagonists reverse episodes of recurrent coma continue to be reported (Huberfeld et al), the status of this entity is ambiguous. The vigilance-producing drug, modafinil, has also been effective in one report (Scott and Ahmed).

A peculiar form of transient unresponsiveness in elderly individuals has been pointed out by Haimovic and Beresford. It accounted for 2 percent of hospitalized patients referred to them for coma. The EEG and other evaluations gave no explanation but their 5 patients had various systemic illnesses. It may recur but appears to be benign. Our patients had no systemic illness with this disorder and were men in their eighth decade who lacked Babinski signs, pupillary abnormalities and, for the most part, eye movement limitations (one had disproportionately better horizontal than vertical gaze with oculocephalic testing). Patients with advanced Parkinson disease will occasionally display episodic unresponsiveness with eyes open.

It is unclear to us whether migraine can cause a similar syndrome, as suggested in the study of familial hemiplegic migraine by Fitzsimmons and Wolfenden. Basilar migraine may exceptionally cause transient stupor and coma. Catatonic stupor and Kleine-Levin syndrome of periodic hypersomnolence and behavioral changes (Chap. 19) also need to be considered.

PATHOLOGIC ANATOMY OF COMA

Coma is produced by 1 of 2 broad problems: The first is clearly morphologic, consisting either of a discrete structural lesion in the upper brainstem and lower diencephalon (which may be primary or secondary to compression) or of more widespread destructive changes throughout the hemispheres. The second is metabolic or submicroscopic, resulting in suppression of neuronal activity in the cerebrum and reticular activating system. The clinical examination in coma is designed to separate these mechanisms and to gauge the depth of brain dysfunction.

With regard to visible lesions, the study of a large number of human cases in which coma preceded death by several days has disclosed 3 types of lesions, each of which directly or indirectly damage the function of the RAS or its projections to the cortices. In the *first type*, a large mass in the cerebral hemisphere—chiefly a tumor; abscess; massive edematous infarct; intracerebral, subarachnoid, subdural, or epidural hemorrhage, or obstructive hydrocephalus—is demonstrable. The mass in or surrounding the hemisphere usually involves only a portion of the cortex and white matter, leaving much of the cerebrum intact. These mass lesions cause coma by secondary compression of the midbrain and subthalamic region of the RAS. Either lateral displacement or compression of these structures by herniation of the temporal lobe into the tentorial opening may be the proximate cause of compression (see below and also Chap. 31). Likewise, a cerebellar lesion may compress the adjacent upper brainstem reticular region by displacing it forward and upward. A detailed clinical record will show the coma to have coincided with these displacements and herniations as discussed further on.

In the *second configuration*, which occurs less frequently than the first, a destructive lesion is located within the thalamus or midbrain, in which case the neurons of the RAS are damaged directly. This pathoanatomic pattern characterizes brainstem stroke from basilar artery occlusion, thalamic and upper brainstem hemorrhages, as well as some forms of traumatic damage.

In the *third type of structural damage*, there is widespread bilateral damage to the cortex and cerebral white matter, the result of traumatic damage (contusions, diffuse axonal injury), bilateral infarcts or hemorrhages, encephalitis, meningitis, hypoxia, or global ischemia. The coma in these cases results from interruption of thalamocortical impulses or from generalized destruction of cortical neurons. It is only if the cerebral lesions are bilateral and extensive that the consciousness impaired. Many of the diseases in this category also cause severe thalamic damage of the type mentioned earlier; the thalamic damage may contribute to the coma.

Thus, the pathologic changes found in cases of coma are compatible with physiologic deductions—namely that the state of coma correlates with lesions of the diencephalic cortical-activating system of neurons. Small and discrete lesions restricted to the upper dorsal brainstem and lower midline thalami are sufficient to produce coma. A study by Parvizi and Damasio, on the basis of 9 cases of restricted dorsal bilateral pontine lesions, has suggested that damage at a site caudal to the midbrain lesion may cause coma. This view may expand our conceptions of the areas of the reticular system that are necessary for arousal, but further study is justified. One conceptual explanation for this configuration would be the disruption of noradrenergic input from the locus coeruleus to the reticular system.

In the largest group of cases of coma, no structural lesion is revealed by any technique of conventional pathology. Instead, a metabolic or toxic abnormality or generalized electrical discharge (seizure) causes neuronal failure at a subcellular or molecular level.

PATHOANATOMY OF BRAIN DISPLACEMENT AND HERNIATIONS (See Also Chap. 31)

As pointed out above, large, destructive, and space-consuming lesions of the cerebrum, such as hemorrhage, tumor, abscess, or infarction with brain swelling, impair consciousness mostly indirectly by lateral and downward displacement of the subthalamic–upper brainstem structures and herniation of the medial part of the temporal lobe (uncus, hippocampus) into the opening in the tentorium. One consequence of lateral displacement is that the upper midbrain, particularly the cerebral peduncle, is pushed against the opposite free edge of the tentorium (the resulting creasing of the lateral edge of the peduncle is called the *Kernohan notch* or, more properly, the *Kernohan-Woltman phenomenon*). This causes weakness and a Babinski sign ipsilateral to the hemispheral lesion and later, extensor posturing on that side. The ipsilateral posterior cerebral artery and rarely the cisternal segment of the ipsilateral oculomotor nerve may also be compressed at the edge of the tentorium, leading to infarction of the ipsilateral occipital lobe in the former, and ophthalmoparesis with pupillary enlargement in the latter.

It follows from the foregoing discussion that unilateral destructive lesions of the hemispheres, such as infarcts or hemorrhages, do not usually cause coma unless they create some degree of mass effect, which secondarily compresses the upper brainstem. There are exceptions in which patients with massive strokes affecting the territory of the internal carotid artery are drowsy and inattentive from the onset, even before brain swelling occurs. More often they are simply apathetic with a tendency to keep their eyes closed, a state that may be misinterpreted as stupor.

The term *herniation* refers to the dislocation of a portion of the cerebral or cerebellar hemisphere from its normal position to an adjacent compartment that is bounded by dural folds, a phenomenon that is evident both at the autopsy table and by imaging of the brain. Thus, herniations are termed *transfalcine* (across the falx) or *transtentorial* (through the tentorial aperture) or are named by the structure that is displaced—*cerebellar, uncal*, etc. Figure 17-1 and Table 17-2 illustrate these displacements between dural compartments. Plum and Posner, following from earlier observations by McNealy and Plum, divided the transtentorial brainstem displacements into two groups: one a central herniation syndrome with downward displacement and midline compression of the upper brainstem, and the other a unilateral insinuation of the medial temporal lobe, including the uncal gyrus, into the tentorial opening and compression of the midbrain from the sides.

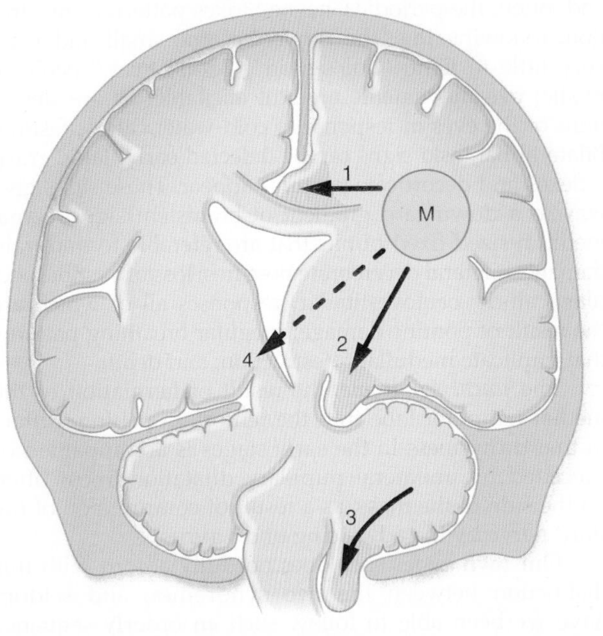

Figure 17-1. Schematic depiction of brain herniations between dural compartments. Transfalcial (*1*), transtentorial uncal-parahippocampal (2), cerebellar tonsillar (*3*), and horizontal (*4*), causing Kernohan-Woltman notch phenomenon. Herniations are shown in pink. M = mass.

According to these authors, the *central syndrome* takes the form of a rostral–caudal deterioration of brainstem function: there is first confusion, apathy, and drowsiness,

Table 17-2

CLINICOPATHOLOGIC FEATURES OF TEMPORAL LOBE–TRANSTENTORIAL HERNIATION

PATHOLOGIC CHANGE	MECHANISM	CLINICAL DISORDERS
Injury to outer fibers of ipsilateral oculomotor nerve	Strangulation of nerve between herniating tissue and medial petroclinoid ligament; stretching of nerve over clivus from lateral displacement of midbrain; entrapment of nerve between posterior cerebral and superior cerebellar arteries from downward displacement of midbrain	Pupillary dilatation (Hutchinson pupil), ophthalmoplegia later
Creasing of contralateral cerebral peduncle (Kernohan notch)	Pressure of laterally displaced midbrain against sharp edge of tentorium	Hemiplegia ipsilateral to herniation (*false localizing sign*) and bilateral corticospinal tract signs
Lateral flattening of midbrain, and zones of necrosis and secondary hemorrhages in tegmentum and base of subthalamus, midbrain, and upper pons (Duret hemorrhages)	Crushing of midbrain between herniating temporal lobe and opposite leaf of tentorium and vascular occlusion (hemorrhages around arterioles and veins)	Cheyne-Stokes respirations; stupor; coma; bipyramidal signs; decerebration; dilated, fixed pupils and alterations of gaze (facilitated oculocephalic reflex movement giving way to loss of all response to head movement and labyrinthine stimulation)
Unilateral or bilateral infarction (hemorrhagic) of occipital lobes	Compression of posterior cerebral artery against the tentorium by herniating temporal lobe	Usually none detectable during coma; hemianopia (unilateral or bilateral) with recovery
Rising intracranial pressure and hydrocephalus	Lateral flattening of aqueduct and third ventricle and blockage of perimesencephalic subarachnoid space	Increasing coma, rising blood pressure, bradycardia (Cushing response)

and, often, the periodic Cheyne-Stokes pattern of respiration; following this, the pupils become small and react very little to light; "doll's-head" ("doll's-eyes," oculocephalic) eye movements are still elicitable, as are deviations of the eyes in response to cold-water caloric testing. Bilateral Babinski signs can be detected early; later, grasp reflexes and decorticate postures appear. These signs give way to a downward gradient of brainstem signs: coma; medium-sized fixed pupils that are referable to midbrain damage; bilateral decerebrate postures; loss of vestibuloocular (caloric, oculovestibular) responses all of which are the result of pontine damage; irregular breathing patterns that implicate medullary destruction; and death.

The *uncal syndrome*, the result of herniation of the medial temporal lobe into the tentorial opening, differs in that drowsiness in the early stages is accompanied or preceded by unilateral pupillary dilatation, most often on the side of the mass, as a result of compression of the third nerve by the advancing uncal gyrus.

Our own experience does not fully accord with this distinction between the two syndromes, and seldom have we been able to follow such an orderly sequence of neural dysfunction from the diencephalic to the medullary level but we do not promote this as a contrary view to the herniation syndromes. With lateral shift and uncal herniation, one sometimes observes smallness of the pupils, rather than ipsilateral pupillary dilatation, as drowsiness develops. Or, infrequently, the contralateral pupil may dilate before the ipsilateral one. Nor is it clear that the dilatation of one pupil is always due to compression of the oculomotor nerve by the herniated uncus. As often in pathologic material, the third nerve is stretched and angulated over the clivus or compressed under the descended posterior cerebral artery. Involvement of the third nerve nucleus or its fibers of exit within the midbrain may be responsible for the dilatation of the opposite pupil, the usual occurrence after the pupil on the side of the mass has become fixed (Ropper, 1990).

In our serial study of 12 patients with brain swelling and lateral diencephalic–mesencephalic shifts caused by hemispheral infarcts, 4 initially had no ipsilateral pupillary enlargement; in 1 patient, the pupillary enlargement was contralateral; in 3 patients, the pupils were symmetrical when drowsiness gave way to stupor or coma (Ropper and Shafran). Cyclic Cheyne-Stokes breathing was an early sign of deterioration. In one patient, the first motor sign was an ipsilateral decerebrate rigidity rather than decorticate posturing; most of the patients had bilateral Babinski signs by the time they became stuporous. The appearance of a Babinski sign on the nonhemiparetic side has been a dependable sentinel of secondary brain tissue shift at the tentorial opening.

The important elements of secondary compression of the upper brainstem may occur in some cases entirely above the plane of the tentorium. With acute masses, a 3- to 5-mm horizontal displacement of the pineal calcification is associated with drowsiness; 5 to 8 mm, with stupor; and greater than 8 or 9 mm, with coma (Ropper, 1986). Shift of the septum pellucidum less dependably predicts the level of consciousness. The degree of vertical tissue distortion differs between cases. Pleasure and colleagues described a syndrome of low cerebrospinal fluid (CSF) pressure causing a purely downward herniation and stupor that was corrected by the infusion of fluid into the spinal canal. Others, notably Reich and colleagues, have found evidence for vertical shift to be more compelling than for horizontal displacement.

In any case, the location as well as the size of a mass determines the degree of brain distortion and displacement of crucial structures in the diencephalon and upper midbrain. Andrews and colleagues have pointed out that frontal and occipital hemorrhages are less likely to displace deep structures and to cause coma than are clots of equivalent size in the parietal or temporal lobes. Nor is it surprising that slowly enlarging masses, such as brain tumors, cause massive shifts of brain tissue, yet result in few clinical changes. In other words, all of the above comments must take into consideration the rate of evolution of a mass and its location and relationship to vital structures that maintain arousal.

The resulting neural dysfunction of deep structures resulting from compression is probably due to ischemia but this issue has not been well studied and it is possible that mechanical distortion of neurons or glia may contribute.

CLINICAL APPROACH TO THE COMATOSE PATIENT

Many times the primary disorder underlying coma is perfectly obvious, as with severe cranial trauma. All too often, however, the comatose patient is brought to the hospital and little pertinent medical information is available. The need for efficiency in reaching a diagnosis and providing appropriate acute care demands that the physician have a methodical approach that addresses the common and treatable causes of coma. When the comatose patient is first seen, the patient's airway is cleared and blood pressure is restored; if trauma has occurred, one must check for bleeding from a wound or ruptured organ (e.g., spleen or liver). With hypotension, placement of a central venous line and administration of fluids and pressor agents, oxygen, blood, or glucose solutions (preferably after blood is drawn for glucose determinations and thiamine is administered) take precedence over diagnostic procedures. If respirations are shallow or labored, or if there is emesis with a threat of aspiration, tracheal intubation and mechanical ventilation are instituted. An oropharyngeal airway is usually adequate in a comatose patient who is breathing normally. Deeply comatose patients with shallow respirations require endotracheal intubation. The patient with a head injury may also have suffered a fracture of the cervical vertebrae, in which case caution must be exercised in moving the head and neck as well as in intubation lest the spinal cord be inadvertently damaged. These matters are discussed in detail further on, under "Management of the Acutely Comatose Patient."

An inquiry is then made as to how the patient was found and their previous health, whether there was a history of diabetes, a head injury, a convulsion, alcohol or drug use, or a prior episode of coma or attempted suicide, and the circumstances in which the person was found. Persons who accompany the comatose patient to the hospital should be encouraged to remain until they have been questioned.

In assessing confusion, stupor, or coma in an already hospitalized patient, it is most instructive to review the patient's medications carefully. A large number of compounds may reduce alertness to the point of profound somnolence or stupor, particularly if there are underlying medical problems (e.g., a liver failure). Prominent in lists of iatrogenic drug intoxications are anesthetics, sedatives, antiepileptic drugs, opiates, certain antibiotics, antidepressants, and antipsychosis compounds. Chronic administration of nitroprusside for hypertension can induce stupor from cyanide toxicity. From an initial survey, many of the common causes of coma, such as severe head injury, alcoholism or other forms of drug intoxication, and hypertensive brain hemorrhage, are readily recognized.

General Examination

Alterations in vital signs (temperature, heart rate, respiratory rate, and blood pressure) are important aids in diagnosis. *Fever* is most often the result of a systemic infection such as pneumonia or bacterial meningitis or viral encephalitis. An excessively high body temperature (42°C [107.6°F] or 43°C [109.4°F]) associated with dry skin should arouse suspicion of heat stroke or intoxication by a drug with anticholinergic activity. Fever should not be too easily ascribed to a brain lesion that has disturbed the temperature-regulating center, so-called central fever, which is a rare occurrence. Hypothermia is observed in patients with alcohol or barbiturate intoxication, drowning, exposure to cold, peripheral circulatory failure, advanced tuberculous meningitis, and myxedema.

Slow breathing points to opiate or barbiturate intoxication and occasionally to hypothyroidism, whereas deep, rapid breathing (Kussmaul respiration) should suggest the presence of pneumonia, diabetic or uremic acidosis, pulmonary edema, or the less-common occurrence of an intracranial disease that causes central neurogenic hyperventilation. Diseases that elevate intracranial pressure or damage the brain often cause slow, irregular, or cyclic Cheyne-Stokes respiration. The various disordered patterns of breathing and their clinical significance are described further on. *Vomiting* at the outset of sudden coma, particularly if combined with pronounced hypertension, is characteristic of cerebral hemorrhage within the hemispheres, brainstem, cerebellum, or subarachnoid spaces. Marked *hypertension* is observed in patients with cerebral hemorrhage and in hypertensive encephalopathy and in children with markedly elevated intracranial pressure. *Hypotension* is the usual finding in states of depressed consciousness because of diabetes, alcohol or barbiturate intoxication, internal hemorrhage, myocardial infarction, dissecting aortic aneurysm, septicemia, Addison disease, or massive brain trauma. The *heart rate*, if exceptionally slow, suggests heart block from medications such as tricyclic antidepressants or anticonvulsants, or if combined with periodic breathing and hypertension, an increase in intracranial pressure.

Inspection of the skin may yield valuable information. Cyanosis of the lips and nail beds signifies inadequate oxygenation. Cherry-red coloration is typical of carbon monoxide poisoning. Multiple bruises (particularly a bruise or boggy area in the scalp), bleeding, CSF leakage from an ear or the nose, or periorbital hemorrhage greatly raises the likelihood of cranial fracture and intracranial trauma or of a severe coagulopathy causing intracranial bleeding. Telangiectases and hyperemia of the face and conjunctivae are the common stigmata of alcoholism; myxedema imparts a characteristic puffiness of the face, and hypopituitarism an equally characteristic sallow complexion. Marked pallor suggests internal hemorrhage. A macular-hemorrhagic rash indicates the possibility of meningococcal infection, staphylococcal endocarditis, typhus, or Rocky Mountain spotted fever. Excessive sweating suggests hypoglycemia or shock, and excessively dry skin, diabetic acidosis, or uremia. Large blisters, sometimes bloody, may form over pressure points such as the buttocks if the patient has been motionless for a time; this sign is particularly characteristic of the deeply unresponsive and prolonged motionless state of acute sedation, alcohol and opiate intoxication. Thrombotic thrombocytopenic purpura (TTP), disseminated intravascular coagulation, and fat embolism may cause diffuse petechiae or purpura; the last of these are often aggregated in the anterior axillary folds.

The *odor of the breath* may provide a clue to the etiology of coma. Alcohol is easily recognized. The spoiled-fruit odor of diabetic ketoacidotic coma, the uriniferous odor of uremia, the musky and slightly fecal fetor of hepatic coma, and the burnt almond odor of cyanide poisoning are distinctive enough to be identified by physicians who possess a keen sense of smell. The distinctive odor of melena is a sign of rapid gastrointestinal bleeding.

Neurologic Examination of the Stuporous or Comatose Patient

Although limited in some ways in comparison to the examination of the alert patient, the neurologic examination of the comatose patient is relatively simple. Watching the patient for a few moments often yields considerable information. The predominant postures of the limbs and body; the presence or absence of spontaneous movements on one side; the position of the head and eyes; and the rate, depth, and rhythm of respiration each give substantial information. The state of responsiveness is then estimated by noting the patient's reaction to calling his name, to simple commands, or to noxious stimuli such as tickling the nares, supraorbital or sternal pressure, pinching the side of the neck or inner parts of the arms or thighs, or applying pressure to the knuckles. By gradually increasing the strength of these stimuli, one can roughly estimate both the degree of unresponsiveness and changes from hour to hour. Vocalization may persist in stupor and is the first response to be lost as coma appears. Grimacing and deft avoidance movements of stimulated parts of the body are preserved in stupor; their presence substantiates the integrity of corticobulbar and corticospinal tracts. Yawning and spontaneous shifting of body positions indicate a minimal degree of unresponsiveness. These signs have been elegantly summarized by Fisher based on his own observations. The widely adopted Glasgow Coma Scale, constructed originally as a quick and simple means of quantitating the responsiveness of patients with cerebral trauma, can be used in the grading of other acute coma-producing diseases as mentioned earlier in this chapter (see also Chap. 35). Several other scales such as the "FOUR Score" (Wijdicks et al 2005) have been devised and are used in various units.

It is usually possible to determine whether coma is associated with meningeal irritation. In all but the deepest stages of coma, meningeal irritation from either bacterial meningitis or subarachnoid hemorrhage will cause resistance to the initial excursion of passive flexion of the neck but not to extension, turning, or tilting of the head. Meningismus is a fairly specific but somewhat insensitive sign of meningeal irritation as commented in Chap. 1. Resistance to movement of the neck in all directions may be part of generalized muscular rigidity or dystonia (as in phenothiazine intoxication) or indicate disease of the cervical spine. In the infant, bulging of the anterior fontanel is at times a more reliable sign of meningitis than is a stiff neck. A temporal lobe or cerebellar herniation or decerebrate rigidity may also create resistance to passive flexion of the neck and be confused with meningeal irritation.

A coma-causing lesion in a cerebral hemisphere can be detected by careful observation of spontaneous movements, responses to stimulation, prevailing postures, and by examination of the cranial nerves. *Hemiplegia* is revealed by a lack of restless movements of the limbs on one side and by inadequate protective movements in response to painful stimuli. The weakened limbs are usually slack and, if lifted from the bed, they "fall flail." The hemiplegic leg lies in a position of external rotation (this may also be caused by a fractured femur), and the affected thigh appears wider and flatter than the nonhemiplegic one. In expiration, the cheek and lips puff out on the paralyzed side of the face. A lesion in one cerebral hemisphere causes the eyes to be turned away from the paralyzed side (toward the lesion, as described below); the opposite occurs with brainstem lesions. In most cases, a hemiplegia and an accompanying Babinski sign are indicative of a contralateral hemispheral lesion; but with lateral mass effect and compression of the opposite cerebral peduncle against the tentorium, extensor posturing, a Babinski sign, and weakness of arm and leg may appear ipsilateral to the lesion (the earlier-mentioned Kernohan-Woltman sign). A moan or grimace may be provoked by painful stimuli applied to one side but not to the other, reflecting hemianesthesia. During grimacing in response to stimuli, facial weakness may be noted.

Of the various indicators of brainstem function, the most useful are pupillary size and reactivity, ocular movements, oculovestibular reflexes and, to a lesser extent, the pattern of breathing. These functions, like consciousness itself, are dependent on the integrity of structures in the midbrain and rostral pons.

Pupillary Reactions

These are of great diagnostic importance in the comatose patient. A unilaterally enlarged pupil is an early indicator of stretching or compression of the third nerve and reflects the presence of an overlying ipsilateral hemispheral mass as described earlier in the section on herniations. A loss of light reaction usually precedes enlargement of the pupil. As a transitional phenomenon, the pupil may become oval or pear-shaped or appear to be off center (corectopia) because of a differential loss of innervation of a portion of the pupillary sphincter. The light-unreactive pupil continues to enlarge to a size of 6 to 9 mm diameter and is soon joined by a slight outward deviation of the eye. In unusual instances, the pupil contralateral to the mass may enlarge first; this has reportedly been the case in 10 percent of subdural hematomas but has been far less frequent in our experience. As midbrain displacement continues, both pupils dilate and become unreactive to light, probably as a result of compression of the oculomotor nuclei in the rostral midbrain (Ropper, 1990). The last step in the evolution of brainstem compression tends to be a slight reduction in pupillary size on both sides, to 5 mm or smaller. Normal pupillary size, shape, and light reflexes indicate integrity of midbrain structures and direct attention to a cause of coma other than a mass.

Pontine tegmental lesions cause extremely miotic pupils (<1 mm in diameter) with barely perceptible reaction to strong light; this is characteristic of the early phase of pontine hemorrhage. The ipsilateral pupillary dilatation from pinching the side of the neck (the ciliospinal reflex) is usually lost in brainstem lesions. The Horner syndrome (miosis, ptosis, and reduced facial sweating) may be observed ipsilateral to a lesion of the brainstem or hypothalamus or as a sign of dissection of the internal carotid artery.

With coma caused by drug intoxications and intrinsic metabolic disorders, pupillary reactions are usually spared, but there are notable exceptions. Serum concentrations of opiates that are high enough to cause coma have as a consistent sign pinpoint pupils, with constriction to light that may be so slight that it is detectable only with a magnifying glass. High-dose barbiturates may act similarly, but the pupillary diameter tends to be 1 mm or more. Systemic poisoning with atropine or with drugs that have atropinic qualities, especially the tricyclic antidepressants, is characterized by wide dilatation and fixity of the pupils. Hippus, or fluctuating pupillary size, is occasionally characteristic of metabolic encephalopathy.

Movements of Eyes and Eyelids and Corneal Responses

These are altered in a variety of ways in coma. In light coma of metabolic origin, the eyes rove conjugately from side to side in seemingly random fashion, sometimes resting briefly in an eccentric position. These movements disappear as coma deepens, and the eyes then remain motionless and slightly exotropic.

A lateral and slight downward deviation of one eye suggests the presence of a third-nerve palsy, and a medial deviation, a sixth-nerve palsy. There is persistent conjugate deviation of the eyes to one side—away from the side of the paralysis with a large cerebral lesion (looking toward the lesion) and toward the side of the paralysis with a unilateral pontine lesion (looking away from the lesion). "Wrong-way eyes" a paradoxical conjugate deviation to the side opposite the lesion may sometimes occur with thalamic and upper brainstem lesions. During a focal seizure the eyes turn or jerk toward the convulsing side (opposite to the irritative focus). The globes turn down and inward (looking at the nose) with hematomas or ischemic lesions of the thalamus and upper midbrain (a variant of Parinaud syndrome). Retraction and convergence nystagmus and "ocular bobbing," described in Chap. 14, occur with lesions in the tegmentum of the mid-brain and pons, respectively. "Ocular dipping," in which the eyes move down slowly and return rapidly to the meridian, is observed with coma caused by anoxia and drug intoxications; horizontal eye movements are preserved with ocular dipping but obliterated in cases of ocular bobbing as a result of destruction of pontine gaze centers. Coma-producing structural lesions of the brainstem abolish most if not all conjugate ocular movements, whereas metabolic disorders generally do not (except for instances of deep hepatic coma and antiepileptic drug overdose).

Oculocephalic reflexes (doll's-eye movements) are elicited by turning or tilting the head. The response in coma of metabolic origin or that caused by bihemispheric structural lesions consists of conjugate movement of the eyes in the opposite direction. Elicitation of these ocular reflexes in a comatose patient provides two pieces of information: (1) evidence of unimpeded function of the midbrain and pontine tegmental structures that integrate ocular movements and of the oculomotor nerves, and (2) loss of the cortical inhibition that normally holds these movements in check. In other words, the presence of unimpaired reflex eye movements implies that coma is not caused by compression or destruction of the upper midbrain. There must instead be widespread cerebral dysfunction, such as occurs after anoxia or with metabolic–toxic suppression of cortical neuronal activity. It must be conceded, however, that sedative or anticonvulsant intoxication profound enough to cause coma may obliterate the brainstem mechanisms for oculocephalic reactions and, in extreme cases, even the vestibular-ocular (caloric) responses as noted below.

Asymmetry of the elicited eye movements remains a dependable sign of focal brainstem disease. In instances of coma caused by a large mass in one cerebral hemisphere that secondarily compresses the upper brainstem, the oculocephalic reflexes are usually present, but the movement of the eye on the side of the mass may be impeded in adduction as a result of a compressive third-nerve paresis.

Irrigation of one ear with 10 mL of cold water (or room-temperature water if the patient is arousable) causes slow conjugate deviation of the eyes toward the irrigated ear, followed in a few seconds by compensatory nystagmus (fast component away from the stimulated side). This is the *oculovestibular,* or *caloric* test. The ears are irrigated separately several minutes apart. In comatose patients, the fast "corrective" phase of nystagmus is lost and the eyes are tonically deflected to the side irrigated with cold water or away from the side irrigated with warm water; this position may be held for 2 to 3 min. Brainstem lesions disrupt these vestibuloocular reflexes; if one eye abducts and the other fails to adduct, one can conclude that the medial longitudinal fasciculus has been interrupted (an internuclear ophthalmoplegia on the side of adductor paralysis). Abducens palsy is indicated by an esotropic resting position and a lack of outward deviation of one eye with the reflex maneuvers. The complete absence of ocular movement in response to oculovestibular testing indicates a severe disruption of brainstem tegmental systems in the pons or midbrain or, as already mentioned, a profound overdose of sedative, anesthetic, or anticonvulsant drugs.

A reduction in the frequency and eventual loss of spontaneous blinking, then a loss of response to touching the eyelashes, and, finally, a lack of response to corneal touch (the corneal reflex afferent limb travels in the trigeminal nerve and efferent limb, facial nerve) are among the most dependable signs of deepening coma. A marked asymmetry in corneal responses indicates either an acute lesion of the opposite hemisphere or, less often, an ipsilateral lesion in the brainstem.

Spontaneous Limb Movements

Restless movements of both arms and both legs and grasping and picking movements signify that the corticospinal tracts are more or less intact. Oppositional resistance to passive movement (paratonic rigidity), complex avoidance movements, and discrete protective movements have the same meaning; especially if they are bilateral and they suggest the coma is not deep. Abduction movements (away from the midline) to escape a noxious stimulus have the same significance and differentiate a motor response from posturing, described below. Focal motor epilepsy indicates that the corticospinal pathway to the convulsing side is intact. With massive destruction of a cerebral hemisphere, as occurs in hypertensive hemorrhage or internal carotid–middle cerebral artery occlusion, seizure activity may be manifest solely in the ipsilateral limbs, the contralateral limbs being prevented from participating by the hemiplegia. Elaborate forms of semivoluntary movement may be manifest on the nonhemiparetic side in patients with extensive disease in one hemisphere; they probably represent some type of disinhibition of cortical and subcortical movement patterns. Choreic, athetotic, or hemiballistic movements indicate a disorder of the basal ganglionic and subthalamic structures, just as they do in the alert patient, but are not helpful in localizing the cause of coma.

Posturing in the Comatose Patient

An abnormal posture of some consequence is *decerebrate rigidity*, which in its fully developed form consists of opisthotonos, clenching of the jaws, and stiff extension of the limbs, with internal rotation of the arms and plantar flexion of the feet (see Chap. 3). It is most often manifest as brief tonic extension of the limbs. This postural pattern was first described by Sherrington, who produced it in cats and monkeys by transecting the brainstem at the intercollicular level. Decerebrate posture was noted in animals to be ipsilateral to a one-sided lesion, hence not a result of involvement of the corticospinal tracts; the opposite is true in humans. A precise anatomic correlation between posturing and the level of the lesion is rarely possible in patients who develop stereotyped extensor posturing as it arises in a variety of settings—with midbrain compression caused by a hemispheral mass; with cerebellar or other posterior fossa lesions; in certain metabolic disorders such as anoxia and hypoglycemia; and, rarely, with hepatic coma and profound drug or alcohol intoxication. Patients with an acute lesion of one cerebral hemisphere may show a similar type of extensor posturing of the contralateral and sometimes ipsilateral limbs, and this may coexist with the ability to make purposeful movements of the same limb. Extensor postures, unilateral or bilateral, occur spontaneously, but more often they are in response to manipulation of the limbs or a tactile or noxious stimulus. Another related pattern consists of extensor posturing of an arm and leg on one side, and flexion and abduction of the opposite arm.

In some patients with the extensor postural changes the lesion is clearly in the cerebral white matter or basal ganglia, which is difficult to reconcile with the classic physiologic explanation for decerebrate posturing. Decerebrate posturing, either in experimental preparations or in humans, is usually not a persistent state. Hence the term *decerebrate state*, as suggested by Feldman, is preferable to *decerebrate rigidity*, which implies a fixed, tonic extensor attitude.

Decorticate posturing, usually, with arm or arms in flexion and adduction and leg(s) extended, signifies lesions at a more rostral level of the nervous system—in the cerebral white matter or internal capsule and thalamus. Bilateral decorticate rigidity is essentially a bilateral spastic hemiplegia. Diagonal postures, e.g., flexion of one arm and extension of the opposite arm and leg, usually indicate a supratentorial lesion. Forceful extensor postures of the arms and weak flexor responses of the legs are usually seen with lesions at about the level of the vestibular nuclei. Lesions below this level lead to flaccidity and abolition of all postures and movements. If preceded by decorticate or decerebrate postures, the coma is profound and usually progresses to brain death.

Only in the most advanced forms of intoxication and metabolic coma, as might occur with anoxic necrosis of neurons throughout the entire brain, are coughing, swallowing, hiccoughing, and spontaneous respiration all abolished. Further, the tendon and plantar reflexes may give little indication of what is happening. Tendon reflexes are preserved until the late stages of coma that is due to metabolic disturbances and intoxications. In coma caused by a large cerebral infarct or hemorrhage, the tendon reflexes may be normal or only reduced on the hemiplegic side and the plantar reflexes may initially be absent before becoming extensor. Plantar flexor responses, succeeding extensor responses, signify either a return to normalcy or, in the context of deepening coma, a transition to brain death.

Patterns of Breathing

Massive supratentorial lesions, bilateral deep-seated cerebral lesions, and mild metabolic disturbances give rise to altered patterns of breathing, particularly periods of waxing and waning hyperpnea alternating with a shorter period of apnea (*Cheyne-Stokes respiration*). This phenomenon has been attributed, on uncertain grounds, to isolation of the brainstem respiratory centers from the cerebrum, rendering them more sensitive than usual to carbon dioxide (hyperventilation drive). It is postulated that as a result of overbreathing, the blood carbon dioxide drops below the concentration required to stimulate the centers, and breathing gradually stops. Carbon dioxide then reaccumulates until it exceeds the respiratory threshold, and the cycle then repeats itself. Alternatively, the periodicity has been attributed to the stimulating effect of a low arterial Po_2 on a depressed respiratory center. In either case, the presence of Cheyne-Stokes breathing signifies bilateral dysfunction of cerebral structures, usually deep in the hemispheres or diencephalon, usually from intoxication or a metabolic derangement or occasionally, from bilateral structural lesions such as subdural hematomas. In itself, Cheyne-Stokes breathing is not a grave sign. It may occur during sleep in elderly individuals and can be a manifestation of a variety of cardio-pulmonary disorders in awake patients. Only when it gives way to more irregular respiratory patterns that reflect structural damage of the brainstem is the patient in imminent danger, as discussed below.

A number of other aberrant breathing rhythms occur from brainstem lesions (these are reviewed in Chap. 26), but few are specifically localizing. The more conspicuous respiratory arrhythmias are associated with lesions below the level of the reticular-activating system and are therefore found in the late stages of brainstem compression or with destructive brainstem lesions such as infarction, hemorrhage, or infiltrating tumor.

Lesions of the lower midbrain-upper pontine tegmentum, either primary or secondary to transtentorial herniation, may give rise to *central neurogenic hyperventilation* (CNH). This disorder is characterized by an increase in the rate and depth of respiration to an extent that produces advanced respiratory alkalosis. The pattern must be distinguished from compensatory overbreathing caused by systemic acidosis, particularly diabetic ketoacidosis (Kussmaul breathing). In addition, mild degrees of hyperventilation are common after a number of acute neurologic events, notably head injury. The neurologic basis of central neurogenic hyperventilation is uncertain. It is theorized to represent a release of the reflex mechanisms for respiratory control in the lower brainstem. It has been observed with tumors of the medulla, lower pons, and midbrain. However, North and Jennett, in a study of respiratory abnormalities in neurosurgical patients, found no consistent correlation between tachypnea and the site of the lesion. As noteworthy, primary brain lymphoma without brainstem involvement has emerged as a curious cause of central hyperventilation, of which we have seen several examples (Pauzner et al).

Low pontine lesions, usually caused by basilar artery occlusion, sometimes cause *apneustic breathing* (a pause of 2 to 3 s in full inspiration) or so-called short-cycle Cheyne-Stokes respiration, in which a few rapid deep breaths alternate with apneic cycles. With lesions of the dorsomedial part of the medulla, the rhythm of breathing is chaotic, being irregularly interrupted and each breath varying in rate and depth (*Biot breathing;* also called "ataxia of breathing"). This pattern progresses to one of intermittent prolonged inspiratory gasps that are recognized by all physicians as agonal in nature, and finally to apnea. In fact, respiratory arrest is the mode of death of most patients with serious central nervous system (CNS) disease.

Probably all of these erratic patterns of breathing are interrelated in some manner. Webber and Speck have shown that apnea, Biot breathing, and gasping could be produced in the same animal with lesions in the dorsolateral pontine tegmentum by altering the depth of anesthesia. As pointed out by Fisher and by Plum and Posner, when certain supratentorial lesions progress to the point of temporal lobe and cerebellar herniation, one may observe a succession of respiratory patterns (Cheyne-Stokes, then hyperventilation, then Biot breathing), indicating an extension of the functional disorder from upper to lower brainstem; but again, such a sequence is not always observed. Rapidly evolving lesions of the posterior fossa, mainly masses in the cerebellum, more often cause sudden respiratory arrest without any of the aforementioned abnormalities of breathing as intermediaries; presumably apnea results from fulminant medullary compression by the cerebellar tonsils.

Clinical Signs of Increased Intracranial Pressure

A history of headache before the onset of coma, vomiting, severe hypertension beyond the patient's static level, unexplained bradycardia, and subhyaloid retinal hemorrhages (Terson syndrome) are immediate clues to the presence of increased intracranial pressure, usually from one of the types of intracranial hemorrhage. Papilledema develops within 12 to 24 h in cases of brain trauma and hemorrhage, and if it is apparent when coma supervenes, it usually signifies brain tumor or abscess, i.e., a lesion of longer duration. Increased intracranial pressure produces coma by impeding global cerebral blood flow; but this occurs only at extremely high levels of pressure. Increased pressure within one compartment displaces central structures and produces a series of "false localizing" signs because of lateral distortion of deep brain tissue and herniations, as noted in the earlier discussion of this type. However, the absence of papilledema does not exclude the presence of increased intracranial pressure, particularly in the elderly.

Acute Hydrocephalus

The syndrome of acute hydrocephalus, most often from subarachnoid hemorrhage or from obstruction of the ventricular system by a tumor in the posterior fossa, induces a state of abulia (slowed responsivity), followed by stupor, and then coma with bilateral Babinski signs. The pupils are small and the tone in the legs is increased or there may be extensor posturing. The signs of hydrocephalus may be accompanied by headache and systemic hypertension, mediated through raised intracranial pressure. Chapter 30 discusses this subject further.

Laboratory Procedures for the Diagnosis of Coma

Unless the cause of coma is established at once by history and physical examination, it becomes necessary to carry out a number of laboratory procedures. In patients with signs of raised intracranial pressure or indications of brain displacements, CT scan or MRI should be obtained as the primary procedure. As discussed in Chap. 2, lumbar puncture, although carrying a small risk of promoting further herniation, is nevertheless necessary in some instances to exclude bacterial meningitis or encephalitis. If poisoning or drug overdosage is suspected, aspiration and analysis of the gastric contents are sometimes helpful, but greater reliance should be placed on chromatographic analysis of the blood and urine ("toxic screen"). Accurate means are available for measuring the blood concentrations of most antiepileptic drugs, opiates, diazepines, barbiturates, alcohol, and a wide range of other toxic substances. These screening procedures vary widely between hospitals and certain toxins must be specifically sought. A specimen of urine is obtained by catheter for determination of specific gravity and for glucose, acetone, and protein content. Proteinuria may also be found for 2 or 3 days after a subarachnoid hemorrhage or with high fever. Urine of high specific gravity, glycosuria, and acetonuria occurs almost invariably in diabetic coma; but transient glycosuria and hyperglycemia may be precipitated solely by a massive cerebral lesion. Blood counts should be obtained and in malarial districts, a blood smear should be examined for parasites. Neutrophilic leukocytosis occurs in bacterial infections and mild elevations of the white blood cell counts also with brain hemorrhage and infarction, although rarely exceeding 12,000/mm^3. Venous blood should be examined for the concentrations of glucose, urea, carbon dioxide, bicarbonate, ammonia, sodium, potassium, chloride, calcium, and AST (aspartate serum transaminase); analysis of blood gases and carboxyhemoglobin should be obtained in appropriate cases of anoxia or exposure to carbon monoxide by smoke inhalation or faulty heating systems.

It should be kept in mind that disorders of water and sodium balance, reflected in hyper- or hyponatremia, may be the result of cerebral disease (excess antidiuretic hormone [ADH] secretion, diabetes insipidus, atrial natriuretic factor release), as well as being the proximate cause of coma.

An EEG may be highly informative if no adequate explanation for coma is forthcoming from the initial examinations. At times, this is the only way to reveal nonconvulsive status epilepticus as the cause of stupor.

Classification of Coma and Differential Diagnosis (See also Table 17-3)

The demonstration of focal brain disease by hemiparesis, and meningeal irritation with abnormalities of the CSF serve to divide the diseases that cause coma into three classes, as follows:

I. Diseases that cause no focal or lateralizing neurologic signs, usually with normal brainstem functions. CT scan and cellular content of the CSF are normal.
   A. Exogenous intoxications: alcohols, barbiturates and other sedative drugs, opiates (Chaps. 42 and 43)

Table 17-3

IMPORTANT POINTS IN THE DIFFERENTIAL DIAGNOSIS OF THE COMMON CAUSES OF COMA

GENERAL GROUP	SPECIFIC DISORDER	IMPORTANT CLINICAL FINDINGS	IMPORTANT LABORATORY FINDINGS	REMARKS
Coma *with* focal or lateralizing signs	Cerebral hemorrhage	Hemiplegia, hypertension, cyclic breathing, specific ocular signs (See Chaps. 14 and 33)	Hyperdense blood on CT	Sudden onset, often with headache, vomiting; history of chronic hypertension; late pupillary enlargement
	Basilar artery occlusion (thrombotic or embolic)	Extensor posturing and bilateral Babinski signs; early loss of oculocephalic responses; ocular bobbing	Hyperdense basilar artery (acute thrombosis) on CT; reduced diffusivity and T2 hyperintensity (on MRI) in brainstem and PCA territory; normal cerebrospinal fluid (CSF)	Onset subacute (thrombosis), or sudden (rostral basilar embolism)
	Territorial infarction in internal carotid territory	Hemiplegia, unilateral unresponsive, or enlarged pupil	Extensive edema, loss of gray-white matter differentiation, sulcal and ventricular effacement, subfalcine and uncal herniation	Coma preceded by drowsiness for several days after stroke
	Subdural hematoma	Slow or cyclic respiration, rising blood pressure, hemiparesis, unilateral enlarged pupil	Hyperdense blood on CT; CSF xanthochromic with relatively low protein	Signs or history of trauma, headache, confusion, progressive drowsiness
	Trauma	Signs of cranial and facial injury	CT and MRI show contusions, hemorrhages, and other injuries; CSF may be bloody	Unstable blood pressure, associated systemic injuries
	Brain abscess	Neurologic signs depending on location	Rim-enhancing mass with surrounding edema	Systemic infection or neurosurgical procedure, fever
	Hypertensive encephalopathy; eclampsia	Blood pressure >210/110 mm Hg (lower in eclampsia and in children), headache, seizures, hypertensive retinal changes	Posterior predominant hypodensity on CT and T2 hyperintensity on MRI affecting gray matter and subcortical white matter; CSF pressure elevated	Acute or subacute evolution, use of aminophylline or catecholamine medications
	Thrombotic thrombocytopenic purpura (TTP)	Petechiae, seizures shifting focal signs	Multiple small cortical infarctions and/or microhemorrhages; thrombocytopenia	Similar to fat embolism; multifocal microvasculopathy
Coma *without* focal or lateralizing signs, *with* signs of meningeal irritation	Meningitis and encephalitis	Stiff neck, Kernig sign, fever, headache	Possible cerebral edema; meningeal enhancement; pleocytosis, increased protein, low glucose in CSF	Subacute or acute onset
	Subarachnoid hemorrhage	Stertorous breathing, hypertension, stiff neck, Kernig sign	Cisternal and sulcal blood; bloody or xanthochromic CSF under increased pressure	Sudden onset with severe headache
Coma *without* focal neurologic signs or meningeal irritation; CT scan and CSF normal	Alcohol intoxication	Hypothermia, hypotension, flushed skin, alcohol breath	Elevated blood alcohol	May be combined with head injury, infection, or hepatic failure
	Sedative intoxication	Hypothermia, hypotension	Drug in urine and blood; electroencephalogram (EEG) often shows fast activity	History of intake of drug; suicide attempt
	Opioid intoxication	Slow respiration, cyanosis, constricted pupils		Administration of naloxone causes awakening and withdrawal signs
	Carbon monoxide intoxication	Cherry-red skin	Reduced diffusivity in globus pallidi; Carboxyhemoglobin	Pallidal necrosis

Global ischemia–anoxia	Rigidity, decerebrate postures, fever, seizures, myoclonus	Reduced diffusivity and edema in cerebral and cerebellar cortex and deep nuclei; CSF normal; EEG may be isoelectric or show high-voltage delta	Abrupt onset following cardiopulmonary arrest; damage permanent if anoxia exceeds 3–5 min
Hypoglycemia	Same as in anoxia	Low blood and CSF glucose	Characteristic slow evolution through stages of nervousness, hunger, sweating, flushed face; then pallor, shallow respirations, and seizures
Diabetic coma	Signs of extracellular fluid deficit, hyperventilation with Kussmaul respiration, "fruity" breath	Glycosuria, hyperglycemia, acidosis; reduced serum bicarbonate; ketonemia and ketonuria, or hyperosmolarity	History of polyuria, polydipsia, weight loss, or diabetes
Uremia	Hypertension; sallow, dry skin, uriniferous breath, twitch-convulsive syndrome	Protein and casts in urine; elevated blood urea nitrogen and serum creatinine; anemia, acidosis, hypocalcemia	Progressive apathy, confusion, and asterixis precede coma
Hepatic coma	Jaundice, ascites, and other signs of portal hypertension; asterixis	T1 hyperintensity from manganese deposition in globus pallidi and other structures; Elevated blood NH_3 levels; CSF yellow (bilirubin) with normal or slightly elevated protein	Onset over a few days or after paracentesis or hemorrhage from varices; confusion, stupor, asterixis, and characteristic EEG changes precede coma
Hypercapnia	Papilledema, diffuse myoclonus, asterixis	Increased CSF pressure; Pco_2 may exceed 75 mm Hg; EEG theta and delta activity	Advanced pulmonary disease; profound coma and brain damage uncommon
Severe infections (septic shock); heat stroke	Extreme hyperthermia, rapid respiration	Vary according to cause	Evidence of a specific infection or exposure to extreme heat
Seizures	Episodic disturbance of behavior or convulsive movements	In status epilepticus, reduced diffusivity on MRI in the involved cortex; characteristic EEG changes	History of previous attacks

B. Endogenous metabolic disturbances: anoxia, diabetic acidosis, uremia, hepatic failure, nonketotic hyperosmolar hyperglycemia, hypo- and hypernatremia, hypoglycemia, addisonian crisis, profound nutritional deficiency, carbon monoxide poisoning, thyroid states, hypercalcemia (Chaps. 40 and 41)
C. Severe systemic infections: pneumonia, peritonitis, typhoid fever, malaria, septicemia, Waterhouse-Friderichsen syndrome
D. Circulatory collapse (shock) from any cause
E. Postseizure states and convulsive and nonconvulsive status epilepticus (Chap. 16)
F. Hypertensive encephalopathy and eclampsia (Chap. 34)
G. Hyperthermia and hypothermia (Chap. 40)
H. Concussion (Chap. 35)
I. Acute hydrocephalus (Chap. 30)
J. Late stages of certain degenerative diseases and Creutzfeldt-Jakob disease

II. Diseases that cause meningeal irritation and an excess of white blood cells (WBCs) or red blood cells (RBCs) in the CSF, usually without focal or lateralizing cerebral or brainstem signs. CT scanning or MRI (which preferably should precede lumbar puncture) may be normal or abnormal.
A. Subarachnoid hemorrhage from ruptured aneurysm, arteriovenous malformation, and cerebral trauma (Chaps. 34 and 35)
B. Acute bacterial meningitis (Chap. 32)
C. Viral meningoencephalitis (Chap. 33)
D. Neoplastic meningeal infiltration (Chap. 31)
E. Parasitic meningitis (Chap. 32)
F. Pituitary apoplexy (Chap. 31)

III. Diseases that cause focal brainstem or lateralizing cerebral signs, with or without changes in the CSF. CT scan and MRI are abnormal.
A. Hemispheral hemorrhage or massive cerebral infarction (Chap. 34)
B. Brainstem infarction caused by basilar artery thrombosis or embolism (Chap. 34)
C. Brain abscess, subdural empyema, herpes encephalitis (Chap. 32)
D. Epidural and subdural hemorrhage and brain contusion (Chap. 35)
E. Brain tumor (Chap. 31)
F. Cerebellar and pontine hemorrhage (Chap. 34)
G. Miscellaneous: cortical vein thrombosis, focal embolic infarction caused by bacterial endocarditis, acute disseminated (postinfectious) encephalomyelitis, intravascular lymphoma, TTP, diffuse fat embolism, and others

Problems in Differential Diagnosis of Coma (Table 17-3)

Using the clinical criteria outlined above, one can usually ascertain whether a given case of coma falls into one of these three categories. Concerning the group without focal or lateralizing or meningeal signs (which includes most of the metabolic encephalopathies, intoxications, concussion, and postseizure states), it must be kept in mind that residua from previous neurologic disease may confuse the clinical picture. Thus, an earlier hemiparesis from vascular disease or trauma may reassert itself in the course of uremic or hepatic coma with hypotension, hypoglycemia, diabetic acidosis, or following a seizure. In hypertensive encephalopathy, focal signs may also be present. Occasionally, for no understandable reason, one leg may seem to move less, one plantar reflex may be extensor, or seizures may be predominantly or entirely unilateral in a metabolic coma, particularly in the hyperglycemic–hyperosmolar states. Babinski signs and extensor rigidity, conventionally considered to be indicators of structural disease, do sometimes occur in profound intoxications with a number of agents or with hepatic encephalopathy.

The diagnosis of concussion or of postictal coma depends on observation of the precipitating event or indirect evidence, as discussed in Chap. 35. Usually, a convulsive seizure is marked by a bitten tongue, urinary incontinence, and an elevated creatine kinase–skeletal muscle fraction; it may be followed by another seizure or burst of seizures. The presence of small clonic or myoclonic convulsive movements of a hand or foot or fluttering of the eyelids or eyes requires that an EEG be performed to determine whether status epilepticus is the cause of coma. This state, nonconvulsive status epilepticus, described in Chap. 16, must be considered in the diagnosis of unexplained coma, especially in known epileptics (Table 17-3).

With respect to the second group in the above classification with signs primarily of meningeal irritation (head retraction, stiffness of neck on forward bending, Kernig and Brudzinski signs), bacterial meningitis and subarachnoid hemorrhage are the usual causes. However, if the coma is profound, stiff neck may be absent in both infants and adults. In such cases the spinal fluid must be examined in order to establish the diagnosis. In most cases of bacterial meningitis, the CSF pressure is elevated but is not exceptionally high (usually < 400 mm H_2O). However, in cases associated with brain swelling, the CSF pressure is greatly elevated; the pupils become fixed and dilated, and there may be signs of compression of the brainstem with arrest of respiration. Patients in coma from ruptured aneurysms also have high CSF pressure; the CSF is overtly bloody and the blood is invariably visible in the CT scan throughout the basal cisterns and ventricles if the bleeding has been severe enough to cause coma.

In the third group of patients, it is the focality of sensorimotor signs and the abnormal pupillary and ocular reflexes, postural states, and breathing patterns that provide the clues to serious structural lesions in the cerebral hemispheres and their pressure effects upon segmental brainstem functions. As the brainstem features become more prominent, they may obscure earlier signs of cerebral disease.

It is worth emphasizing once more that profound hepatic, hypoglycemic, hyperglycemic, and hypoxic states may resemble the coma due to a brainstem lesion in that asymmetrical motor signs, focal seizures, and decerebrate postures arise and deep coma from drug intoxication may obliterate reflex eye movements. Conversely, *certain structural lesions of the cerebral hemispheres are so diffuse as to produce a picture that simulates a metabolic disturbance*; TTP, fat embolism, vasculitis, intravascular lymphoma, acute disseminated encephalomyelitis, and the late effects of global ischemia–anoxia are examples of such states. At other times, they cause a diffuse encephalopathy with superimposed focal signs.

Unilateral cerebral infarction because of anterior, middle, or posterior cerebral artery occlusion produces no more than drowsiness, as a rule; however, with massive unilateral infarction as a result of carotid artery occlusion, coma can occur if extensive brain edema and secondary tissue shift develop. There are exceptional cases wherein stupor results from massive infarction of the dominant (left) hemisphere. Edema of a degree serious enough to compress the brainstem and cause coma seldom develops before 12 or 24 h. Rapidly evolving hydrocephalus causes smallness of the pupils, rapid respiration, extensor rigidity of the legs, Babinski signs, and sometimes a loss of eye movements.

Of course, diagnosis has as its prime purpose the direction of therapy. The treatable causes of coma are drug and alcohol intoxications, shock from infection, cardiac failure, or systemic bleeding, uremia, epidural and subdural hematomas, brain abscess, bacterial and fungal meningitis, diabetic acidosis or hyperosmolar state, hypoglycemia, hypo- or hypernatremia, hepatic coma, hypercalcemia, uremia, status epilepticus, Wernicke disease, Hashimoto encephalopathy, and hypertensive encephalopathy. Also treatable to a varying degree are cerebellar hemorrhages, which can be removed successfully; edema from massive stroke, which may be ameliorated by hemicraniectomy; and hydrocephalus from any cause, which may respond to ventricular drainage.

Management of the Acutely Comatose Patient

Seriously impaired states of consciousness, regardless of their cause, are often fatal not only because they represent an advanced stage of many diseases but also because they add their own particular burdens to the primary disease. The physician's main objective, of course, is to find the cause of the coma and to treat it appropriately. It often happens, however, that the disease process is one for which there is no specific therapy; or, as in hypoxia or hypoglycemia, the acute, irreversible effects have already occurred before the patient comes to the attention of the physician. Again, the problem may be highly complex, for the disturbance may be attributable not to a single cause but to several factors acting in unison, no one of which could account for the total clinical picture. In certain circumstances two processes contribute to depressing consciousness, particularly head injury combined with drug or alcohol intoxication. In lieu of specific therapy, supportive measures must be used; indeed, the patient's chances of surviving the original disease often depend on the effectiveness of these general medical measures.

The successful management of the insensate patient requires the services of a well-coordinated team of nurses and a physician. Necessary treatments must be instituted rapidly, even before all the diagnostic steps have been completed; diagnosis and treatment may have to proceed concurrently. The following is a brief outline of the principles involved in the treatment of such patients. The details of management of shock, fluid and electrolyte imbalance, and other complications that threaten the comatose patient (pneumonia, urinary tract infections, deep venous thrombosis, etc.) can be found in *Harrison's Principles of Internal Medicine*.

1. Shallow and irregular respirations, stertorous breathing (indicating obstruction to inspiration), and cyanosis require the establishment of a clear airway and delivery of oxygen. The patient should initially be placed in a lateral position so that secretions and vomitus do not enter the tracheobronchial tree. Secretions and vomitus should be removed by suctioning as soon as they accumulate; otherwise they will lead to atelectasis and bronchopneumonia. Arterial blood gases should be measured and further observed by monitoring of oxygen saturation. A patient's inability to protect against aspiration and the presence of either hypoxia or hypoventilation dictate the use of endotracheal intubation and a positive-pressure respirator.
2. The management of shock, if present, takes precedence over all other diagnostic and therapeutic measures.
3. Concurrently, an intravenous line is established and blood samples are drawn for determination of glucose, intoxicating drugs, and electrolytes and for tests of liver and kidney function. Naloxone, 0.5 mg, should be given intravenously if a narcotic overdose is a possibility. Hypoglycemia that has produced stupor or coma requires the infusion of glucose, usually 25 to 50 mL of a 50 percent solution followed by a 5 percent infusion; this must be supplemented with thiamine. A urine sample is obtained for drug and glucose testing. If the diagnosis is uncertain, both naloxone and the glucose-thiamine combination should be administered.
4. With the development of elevated intracranial pressure from a mass lesion, mannitol, 25 to 50 g in a 20 percent solution, should be given intravenously over 10 to 20 min and hyperventilation instituted if deterioration occurs, as judged by pupillary enlargement or deepening coma. Repeated CT scanning allows the physician to follow the size of the lesion and degree of localized edema and to detect displacements of cerebral tissue. With massive cerebral lesions, it may be appropriate to place a pressure-measuring device in the cranium of selected patients (see Chap. 35 for details of intracranial pressure monitoring and treatment).
5. A lumbar puncture should be performed if meningitis or subarachnoid hemorrhage is suspected on the basis of headache and meningismus (and fever in the case of infectious meningitis), keeping in mind the risks of this procedure and the means of dealing with them. A CT scan may have disclosed a primary

subarachnoid hemorrhage, in which case lumbar puncture is not necessary. In the case of meningitis, broad-spectrum antibiotics that penetrate the meninges should be instituted immediately, independent of the timing of the lumbar puncture. The choice of drug is then determined by the principles set forth in Chap. 32. If CSF pressure is greatly elevated when measured from a lumbar puncture that has been performed to diagnose bacterial meningitis, it has been recommended that the stylette should be left in the lumen of the needle, as little CSF should be withdrawn as is necessary for diagnostic purposes, and mannitol or hypertonic saline should be administered to lower the pressure.

6. Convulsions should be controlled by measures outlined in Chap. 16, usually by intravenous diazepines.
7. As indicated earlier, gastric aspiration and lavage with normal saline may be diagnostically and therapeutically useful in some instances of coma due to drug ingestion. Salicylates, opiates, and anticholinergic drugs (tricyclic antidepressants, phenothiazines, scopolamine), all of which induce gastric atony, may be recovered many hours after ingestion. Caustic materials should not be lavaged because of the danger of gastrointestinal perforation. The administration of activated charcoal is indicated in certain drug poisonings. Measures to prevent gastric hemorrhage and excessive gastric acid secretion are usually advisable.
8. The temperature-regulating mechanisms may be disturbed and extreme hypothermia or hyperthermia should be corrected. In severe hyperthermia, evaporative-cooling measures are indicated in addition to antipyretics.
9. The bladder should not be permitted to become distended; if the patient does not void, decompression should be carried out with an indwelling catheter. Needless to say, the patient should not be permitted to lie in a wet or soiled bed.
10. Diseases of the CNS may disrupt the control of water, glucose, and sodium. The unconscious patient can no longer adjust the intake of food and fluids by hunger and thirst. Both salt-losing and salt-retaining syndromes have been described with brain disease (see Chap. 27). Water intoxication and severe hyponatremia may of themselves prove damaging. If coma is prolonged, the insertion of a nasogastric tube will ease the problems of feeding the patient and maintaining fluid and electrolyte balance. It is quite acceptable to leave the tube in place for long periods. Otherwise, approximately 35 mL/kg of isotonic fluid should be administered per 24 h (5 percent dextrose in 0.45 percent saline with potassium supplementation unless there is brain edema, in which case the use of hypertonic normal saline is indicated).
11. Aspiration pneumonia is avoided by prevention of vomiting (gastric tube and endotracheal intubation), proper positioning of the patient, and restriction of oral fluids. Should aspiration pneumonia occur, it requires treatment with appropriate antibiotics and aggressive pulmonary physical therapy. Oral decontamination with chlorhexidine is advised to reduce the incidence of ventilator-associated pneumonia.
12. Leg vein thrombosis, a common occurrence in comatose and hemiplegic patients, often does not manifest itself by obvious clinical signs. An attempt may be made to prevent it by the subcutaneous administration of heparin, 5,000 U q12h, or of low-molecular-weight heparin, and by the use of intermittent pneumatic compression boots. There are few absolute contraindications to the prophylactic use of low-dose anticoagulants such as heparin and enoxaparin.
13. If the patient is capable of moving, suitable restraints should be used to prevent him from falling out of bed and to avert self-injury from convulsions.
14. Regular conjunctival lubrication and oral cleansing should be instituted.

Prognosis of Coma (See also "Prognosis of Hypoxic-Ischemic Brain Injury" in Chap. 40.)

As a general rule, recovery from coma of metabolic and toxic causes is far better than from anoxic coma, with head injury occupying an intermediate prognostic position. Most patients who are initially comatose as a result of a stroke will die; subarachnoid hemorrhage in which coma is a result of hydrocephalus is an exception and those cases in which brain shift is relieved by craniectomy are also exceptions. In regard to all forms of coma, but particularly after cardiac arrest, if there are no pupillary, corneal, or oculovestibular responses within 1 day of the onset of coma, the chances of regaining independent function are practically nil (Levy et al). Other signs that predict a poor outcome are absence of corneal reflexes, eye-opening responses, atonia of the limbs at 1 and 3 days after the onset of coma, and absence of the cortical component of the somatosensory-evoked responses on both sides (see Booth et al for an analysis of prior studies and consult Chap. 40 for further details). It is the unfortunate survivor from this latter group who may remain in a vegetative state for months or years, breathing without aid and with preserved hypothalamo-pituitary functions. The frequency of vegetative state after head injury and the negligible chances of improvement if the condition persists for several months have already been discussed, and a discussion of the outcome of anoxic–ischemic coma can be found in Chap. 40. The novel perspectives that have been introduced by demonstrating residual and willful cognitive activity in survivors of traumatic brain injury have been discussed in an earlier section.

In all other cases, the nature of the underlying disease determines outcome; the reader should refer to the appropriate sections of this book for details.

References

Adams JH, Graham DI, Jennet B: The neuropathology of the vegetative state after an acute brain insult. *Brain* 125:1327, 2000.

Andrews BT, Chiles BW, Olsen WL, et al: The effects of intracerebral hematoma location on the risk of brainstem compression and outcome. *J Neurosurg* 69:518, 1988.

Andrews K: Recovery of patients after four months or more in the persistent vegetative state. *BMJ* 306:1597, 1993.

Beecher HK, Adams RD, Sweet WH: A definition of irreversible coma: Report of the Committee of Harvard Medical School to examine the definition of brain death. *JAMA* 205:85, 1968.

Bernat JL: Chronic disorders of consciousness. *Lancet* 367:1181, 2006.

Booth CM, Boone RH, Tomlinson G, Detsky AS: Is this patient dead, vegetative, or severely impaired? *JAMA* 291:870, 2004.

Braakman R, Jennett WB, Minderhound JM: Prognosis of the post-traumatic vegetative state. *Acta Neurochir (Wien)* 95:49, 1988.

Bremer F: L'activité cerebralé au cours du sommeil et de la narcose. *Bull Acad R Soc Belg* 2:68, 1937.

Brown N, Lydic R, Schiff ND: General anesthesia, sleep, and coma. *N Engl J Med* 363:2638, 2010.

Cairns H, Oldfield RC, Pennybacker JB, et al: Akinetic mutism with an epidermoid cyst of the third ventricle. *Brain* 64:273, 1941.

Campagna JA, Miller KW, Forman SA: Mechanisms of actions of inhaled anesthetics. *N Engl J Med* 348:2210, 2003.

Childs NL, Mercer WN: Late improvement in consciousness after post-traumatic vegetative state. *N Engl J Med* 334:24, 1996.

Crick FA, Koch C. Framework for consciousness. *Nat Neurosci* 6:119, 2003.

Di HB, Yu SM, Wend XC, et al: Cerebral response to patient's own name in the vegetative and minimally conscious states. *Neurology* 68:895, 2007.

Estraneo A, Moretta P, Loreto V, et al: Late recovery after traumatic, anoxic, or hemorrhagic long-lasting vegetative state. *Neurology* 75:239, 2010.

Feldman MH: The decerebrate state in the primate: I. Studies in monkeys. *Arch Neurol* 25:501, 1971.

Feldman MH, Sahrmann S: The decerebrate state in the primate: II. Studies in man. *Arch Neurol* 25:517, 1971.

Fisher CM: The neurological examination of the comatose patient. *Acta Neurol Scand* 45 (Suppl 36):1, 1969.

Fitzsimmons RB, Wolfenden WH: Migraine coma: Meningitic migraine with cerebral oedema associated with a new form of autosomal dominant cerebellar ataxia. *Brain* 108:555, 1985.

Frederiks JAM: Consciousness, in Vinken PJ, Bruyn GW (eds): *Disorders of Higher Nervous Function: Handbook of Clinical Neurology*. Vol 4. Amsterdam, North-Holland, 1969, p 48.

Giacino JT, Ashwal S, Childs N, et al: The minimally conscious state. Definition and diagnostic criteria. *Neurology* 58:349, 2002.

Guidelines for the detection of brain death in children. *Ann Neurol* 21:616, 1987.

Haimovic IC, Beresford HR: Transient unresponsiveness in the elderly. Report of five cases. *Arch Neurol* 49:35, 1992.

Hansotia PL: Persistent vegetative state: Review and report of electrodiagnostic studies in eight cases. *Arch Neurol* 42:1048, 1985.

Higashi K, Sakata Y, Hatano M, et al: Epidemiologic studies on patients with a persistent vegetative state. *J Neurol Neurosurg Psychiatry* 40:876, 1977.

Huberfeld G, Dupont S, Hazemann P, et al: Stupeur recurrente idiopathique ches un patient: Imputabilite benzodiazepines endogenes ou exogenes? *Rev Neurol* 158:824, 2002.

Iragui VJ, McCutchen CB: Physiologic and prognostic significance of "alpha coma." *J Neurol Neurosurg Psychiatry* 46:632, 1983.

Jennett B, Plum F: Persistent vegetative state after brain damage. *Lancet* 1:734, 1972.

Joffe AR, Lequier L, Cave D: Specificity of radionuclide brain blood flow testing in brain death – Case report and review. *J Int Care Med* 25:53, 2010.

Kernohan JW, Woltman HW: Incisura of the crus due to contralateral brain tumor. *Arch Neurol Psychiatry* 21:274, 1929.

Kinney HC, Korein J, Panigraphy A, et al: Neuropathological findings in the brain of Karen Ann Quinlan—the role of thalamus in the persistent vegetative state. *N Engl J Med* 330:1469, 1994.

Laureys S, Lemaire C, Maquet P, et al: Cerebral metabolism during vegetative state and after recovery of consciousness. *J Neurol Neurosurg Psychiatry* 67:121, 1999.

Levy DE, Bates D, Caronna JJ: Prognosis in nontraumatic coma. *Ann Intern Med* 94:293, 1981.

Luaté J, Maucort-Boulch D, Tell L, et al: Long-term outcomes of chronic minimally conscious and vegetative states. *Neurology* 75:246, 2010.

Lugaresi E, Montagna P, Tinuper P, et al: Suspected covert lorazepam administration misdiagnosed as recurrent endozepine stupor. *Brain* 121:2201, 1998.

Lustbader D, O'Hara D, Wijdicks EF, et al: Second brain death examination may negatively affect organ donation. *Neurology* 76:119, 2011.

Magnus R: Some results of studies in the physiology of posture. *Lancet* 2:531, 585, 1926.

McNealy DE, Plum FP: Brainstem dysfunction with supratentorial mass lesions. *Arch Neurol* 7:10, 1962.

Meador KJ, Ray PG, Echauz JR, et al: Gamma coherence and conscious perception. *Neurology* 59:847, 2002.

Mollaret P, Goulon M: Le coma dépassé. *Rev Neurol* 101:3, 1959.

Monti MM, Vanhaudenhuyse A, Coleman M, et al: Willful modulation of brain activity in disorders of consciousness. *New Engl J Med* 362:579, 2010.

Moruzzi G, Magoun H: Brain stem reticular formation and activation of EEG. *Electroencephalogr Clin Neurophysiol* 1:455, 1949.

Multi-Society Task Force on PVS. Medical aspects of the persistent vegetative state: Parts I and II. *N Engl J Med* 330:1499, 1572, 1994.

North JB, Jennett B: Abnormal breathing patterns associated with acute brain damage. *Arch Neurol* 32:338, 1974.

Owen AM, Coleman MR, Boly M, et al: Detecting awareness in the vegetative state. *Science* 313:1402, 2006.

Parvisi J, Damasio JR: Neuroanatomical correlates of brainstem coma. *Brain* 126:1524, 2003.

Pauzner R, Mouallem M, Sadeh M, et al: High incidence of primary cerebral lymphoma in tumor-induced central neurogenic hyper-ventilation. *Arch Neurol* 46:510, 1989.

Pleasure SJ, Abosch A, Friedman J, et al: Spontaneous intracranial hypotension resulting in stupor caused by diencephalic compression. *Neurology* 50:1854, 1998.

Plum F: Coma and related global disturbances of the human conscious state, in Peters A (ed): *Cerebral Cortex*. Vol 9. New York, Plenum Press, 1991, pp 359–425.

Plum F, Posner JB: *Diagnosis of Stupor and Coma*, 3rd ed. Philadelphia, Davis, 1980.

Rees G, Kreiman G, Koch C. Neural correlates of consciousness in humans. *Nat Rev Neurosci* 3:261, 2002.

Reich JB, Sierra J, Camp W, et al: Magnetic resonance imaging measurement and clinical changes accompanying transtentorial and foramen magnum brain herniation. *Ann Neurol* 33:159, 1993.

Reptinger S, Fitzgibbons WP, Omojoia MF, et al: Long survival following bacterial meningitis associated brain destruction. *J Child Neurol* 21:591, 2006.

Ropper AH: Unusual spontaneous movements in brain-dead patients. *Neurology* 34:1089, 1984.

Ropper AH: Lateral displacement of the brain and level of consciousness in patients with an acute hemispheral mass. *N Engl J Med* 314:953, 1986.

Ropper AH: The opposite pupil in herniation. *Neurology* 40:1707, 1990.

Ropper AH: Cogito ergo sum by MRI. *New Engl J Med* 362:648, 2010.

Ropper AH, Shafran B: Brain edema after stroke: Clinical syndrome and intracranial pressure. *Arch Neurol* 41:26, 1984.

Rosenberg GA, Johnson SF, Brenner RP: Recovery of cognition after prolonged vegetative state. *Ann Neurol* 2:167, 1977.

Rosenberg H, Clofine R, Bialik O: Neurologic changes during awakening from anesthesia. *Anesthesiology* 54:125, 1981.

Scheibel AB: On detailed connections of the medullary and pontine reticular formation. *Anat Rec* 109:345, 1951.

Schiff ND, Giacino JT, Kalmar K, et al: Behavioural improvement with thalamic stimulation after severe traumatic brain injury. *Nature* 448:600, 2007.

Scott S, Ahmed I: Modafinil in endozepine stupor. A case report. *Can J Neurol Sci* 31:409, 2004.

Sherrington CS: Decerebrate rigidity and reflex coordination of movements. *J Physiol* 22:319, 1898.

Shewmon DA: Chronic "brain death": Meta-analysis and conceptual consequences. *Neurology* 51:1538, 1998.

Solomon P, Aring CD: Causes of coma in patients entering a general hospital. *Am J Med Sci* 188:805, 1934.

Steriade M: Arousal: Revisiting the reticular activating system. *Science* 272:225, 1996.

Voss HU, Ulug AM, Dyke JP, et al: Possible axonal regrowth in late recovery from the minimally conscious state. *J Clin Invest* 116:2005, 2006.

Webber CL Jr, Speck DF: Experimental Biot periodic breathing in cats: Effects of changes in PiO_2 and $PiCO_2$. *Respir Physiol* 46:327, 1981.

Wijdicks EFM: *Brain Death.* Lippincott Williams & Wilkins, Philadelphia, 2001.

Wijdicks EFM, Bamlet WR, Maramattom BV, et al: Validation of a new coma scale: The FOUR score. *Ann Neurol* 58:585, 2005.

Young GB: Consciousness, in Young GB, Ropper AH, Bolton CG: *Coma and Impaired Consciousness: A Clinical Perspective.* New York, McGraw Hill, 1998, pp 3–38.

Zeman A: Persistent vegetative state. *Lancet* 350:795, 1997.

Zeman A: Consciousness. *Brain* 124:1263, 2001.

18

Faintness and Syncope

The term *syncope* (Greek: *synkope*) literally means a "cessation," a "cutting short," or "pause." Medically, it refers to an episodic loss of consciousness and postural tone and an inability to stand because of a diminished flow of blood to the brain. It is synonymous in everyday language with *fainting*. *Feeling faint* and a *feeling of faintness* are also commonly used terms to describe the loss of strength and other symptoms that characterize the impending or incomplete fainting spell. This latter state is referred to as *presyncope*. Relatively abrupt onset, brief duration, and spontaneous and complete recovery not requiring specific resuscitative measures are other typical features.

Faintness and syncope are among the most common of all medical problems. Practically every adult has experienced some presyncopal symptoms, if not a fully developed syncopal attack, or has observed such attacks in others. Description of these symptoms, as with other predominantly subjective states, is often ambiguous. The patient may refer to the experience as light-headedness, dizziness, a "drunk feeling," a weak spell, or, if consciousness was lost, a "blackout." Careful questioning may be necessary to ascertain the exact meaning the patient has given to these words. In many instances the nature of the symptoms is clarified by the fact that they include a sensation of faintness and then a momentary loss of consciousness, which is easily recognized as a faint, or syncope. This sequence also informs us that under certain conditions any difference between faintness and syncope is only one of degree. These symptoms must be clearly set apart from certain types of epilepsy, the other major cause of episodic unconsciousness, and from disorders such as cataplexy, transient ischemic attacks (TIAs), "drop attacks," and vertigo, which are also characterized by episodic attacks of generalized weakness or inability to stand upright, but not by a loss of consciousness.

CAUSES OF EPISODIC FAINTNESS AND SYNCOPE

From a clinical perspective, syncope is essentially of three main types, all ultimately causing hypotension and each of which may lead to a temporary reduction in the flow of blood to the brain. The first, reflex withdrawal of vascular sympathetic tone (vasodepressor effect), triggered by centrally mediated inhibition of the normal tonic sympathetic influences, is often associated with excessive vagal effect and bradycardia (vagal effect). The type associated with bradycardia is called *vasovagal syncope*, a special form of neurogenic, or *neurocardiogenic syncope*, by which is meant the withdrawal of sympathetic tone through a reflex neural mechanism. Neurocardiogenic syncope usually signifies that the inciting stimulus originates in neural receptors within the heart. Each may cause the common faint, the clinical details of which are described later.

The second is a failure of sympathetic innervation of blood vessels and of autonomically activated compensatory responses (reflex tachycardia and vasoconstriction), which occurs with assumption of the upright body position and leads to pooling of blood in the lower parts of the body—causing *orthostatic hypotension* and syncope. Typically, in individuals with these first two forms of syncope, there is no evidence of underlying cardiac disease.

Syncope of a third type is caused by a primary diminished cardiac output because of disease of the heart itself as in the Stokes-Adams bradyarrhythmia attack, severe aortic or subaortic stenosis, or ischemic heart disease. Greatly reduced blood volume from dehydration or blood loss usually causes only near syncope, but complete loss of consciousness may certainly occur in severe circumstances.

As a rough guide to the relative frequency of the various causes of syncope, the large amount of information from the Framingham Heart Study accumulated by Soteriades and colleagues can be taken as representative: the leading cause was vasovagal, a cardiac cause was established in about 10 percent; and orthostatic hypotension in another 10 percent. Also, 7 percent of cases were attributed to medications, mainly those that interfered with sympathetic tone, and remaining 40 percent could not be categorized.

The three main types of syncope as well as several others that cannot readily be classified within these categories can be further subdivided by their pathophysiologic mechanism, as follows:

I. Neurogenic vasodepressor reactions
   A. Elicited by *extrinsic signals* to the medulla from baroreceptors
      1. Vasodepressor (vasovagal)
      2. Neurocardiogenic

3. Carotid sinus hypersensitivity
4. Vagoglossopharyngeal
5. Severe pain, especially if arising in a viscera (bowel, ovary, testicle, etc.)

B. Coupled with diminished venous return to the heart
1. Micturitional
2. Tussive
3. Valsalva, straining, breathholding, weight lifting
4. Postprandial

C. Intrinsic and extrinsic psychic stimuli
1. Fear, anxiety (presyncope is more common)
2. Sight of blood
3. Hysterical

II. Failure of sympathetic nervous system innervation (postural–orthostatic hypotension)

A. Peripheral nervous system autonomic failure (peripheral neuropathy, autonomic neuropathy
1. Diabetes
2. Pandysautonomia
3. Guillain-Barré syndrome
4. Amyloid neuropathy
5. Surgical sympathectomy
6. Antihypertensive medications and other blockers of vascular sympathetic innervation and presynaptic alpha agonsits
7. Pheochromocytoma

B. Central nervous system (CNS) autonomic failure
1. Primary autonomic failure (idiopathic orthostatic hypotension)
2. Multiple system atrophy (parkinsonism, ataxia, orthostatic hypotension)
3. Lewy-body and Parkinson diseases
4. Spinal cord trauma, infarction, and necrosis
5. Centrally acting antihypertensive and other medications

III. Reduced cardiac output or inadequate intravascular volume (hypovolemia)

A. Reduced cardiac output
1. Cardiac arrhythmias
   a. Bradyarrhythmias
      i. Atrioventricular (AV) block (second and third degree) with Stokes-Adams attacks
      ii. Ventricular asystole
      iii. Sinus bradycardia, sinoatrial block, sinus arrest, sick sinus syndrome
   b. Tachyarrhythmias
      i. Episodic ventricular tachycardia
      ii. Supraventricular tachycardia (infrequently causes syncope)
2. Myocardial: angina, infarction, or severe congestive heart failure with reduced cardiac output
3. Obstruction to left ventricular or aortic outflow: aortic stenosis, hypertrophic subaortic stenosis, Takayasu arteritis
4. Obstruction to pulmonary flow: pulmonic stenosis, tetralogy of Fallot, primary pulmonary hypertension, pulmonary embolism
5. Pericardial tamponade

B. Inadequate intravascular volume (hemorrhage); dehydration

IV. Other causes of episodic faintness and syncope

A. Hypoxia
B. Severe anemia
C. Diminished CO_2 as a result of hyperventilation (faintness common, syncope rare)
D. Hypoglycemia (faintness frequent, syncope rare)
E. Anxiety (panic) attacks
F. Environmental overheating

This list of conditions causing faintness and syncope is deceptively long and involved, but the usual types are reducible to a few well-established mechanisms. So as not to obscure these mechanisms by too many details, only the varieties of fainting commonly encountered in clinical practice and those of particular neurologic interest are discussed below.

CLINICAL FEATURES OF SYNCOPE

The Common Faint (Vasodepressor Syncope)

This is the common faint, seen mainly in young individuals. A familial predisposition is well known (Mathias et al). The evocative factors are usually strong emotion, physical injury—particularly to viscera (testicles, gut)—or other factors (see below). As described earlier, the vasodilatation of adrenergically innervated "resistance vessels" is postulated to lead to a reduction in peripheral vascular resistance, but cardiac output fails to exhibit the compensatory rise that normally occurs in hypotension. Some physiologic studies suggest that the dilatation of intramuscular vessels, innervated by beta-adrenergic fibers, may be more important than dilatation of the splanchnic ones.

Skin vessels, in contrast, are constricted. Vagal stimulation may be superimposed either as a primary or a reactive phenomenon (hence the term *vasovagal*) causing bradycardia and leading possibly to a slight further drop in blood pressure. Other vagal effects are perspiration, increased peristaltic activity, nausea, and salivation. However, bradycardia probably contributes little to the hypotension and syncope. The term *vasovagal* was used originally by Thomas Lewis. As Lewis himself pointed out, atropine, "while raising the pulse rate up to and beyond normal levels during the attack, leaves the blood pressure below normal and the patient still pale and not fully conscious."

The vasodepressor faint occurs (1) in normal health under the influence of strong emotion, particularly in some susceptible individuals (sight of blood or an accident) or in conditions that favor peripheral vasodilatation, e.g., hot, crowded rooms ("heat syncope"), especially if the person is hungry or tired or has had alcoholic drinks; (2) during a painful illness or after bodily injury (especially of the abdomen or genitalia), as a consequence of fright, pain, and other factors (where pain is involved, the vagal element tends to be more prominent in the genesis of the faint); and (3) during exercise in some sensitive persons (see further on).

The clinical manifestations of fainting attacks vary to some extent, depending on their mechanisms and the settings in which they occur. The most common types of faint—namely, *vasodepressor* and *vasovagal syncope*, conform more or less to the following pattern. In these types, which are taken in this section as one characteristic manifestation, the patient is usually in the upright position at the beginning of the attack, either sitting or standing. Certain subjective symptoms, the prodrome, mark the onset of the faint. The person feels queasy, is assailed by a sense of giddiness and apprehension, may sway, and sometimes develops a headache. What is most noticeable at the beginning of the attack is pallor or an ashen-gray color of the face; often the face and body become bathed in cool perspiration. Salivation, epigastric distress, nausea, and sometimes vomiting may accompany these symptoms, and the patient tries to suppress them by yawning, sighing, or breathing deeply. Vision may dim or close in concentrically, the ears may ring, and it may be impossible to think clearly ("grayout"). This serves to introduce the common faint that is known to all physicians and most laypersons.

The duration of the prodromal symptoms is variable from a few minutes to only a few seconds. If, during the prodromal period, the person is able to lie down promptly, the attack may be averted before complete loss of consciousness occurs; otherwise, consciousness is lost and the patient falls to the ground. The more or less deliberate onset of this type of syncope enables patients to lie down or at least to protect themselves as they slump. A hurtful fall is exceptional in the young, although an elderly person may be injured.

The depth and duration of unconsciousness vary. Sometimes the person is not completely oblivious to his surroundings; he may still hear voices or see the blurred outlines of people. More often there is a complete lack of awareness and responsiveness. The patient lies motionless, with skeletal muscles fully relaxed. Sphincteric control is maintained in nearly all cases. The pupils are dilated. The pulse is thin and slow or cannot be felt; or they may be tachycardic, the systolic blood pressure is reduced (to 60 mm Hg or less as a rule), and breathing may be almost imperceptible. It is the brief period of hypotension and cerebral hypoperfusion that is the unifying feature of the various forms of syncope. The depressed vital functions, striking facial pallor, and unconsciousness almost simulate death.

Once the patient is horizontal, the flow of blood to the brain is restored. The strength of the pulse soon improves and color begins to return to the face. Breathing becomes quicker and deeper. Then the eyelids flutter and consciousness is quickly regained. However, should unconsciousness persist for 15 to 20 s, convulsive movements may occur. The term *convulsive syncope* has been used to describe this phenomenon, but it has also been used for an authentic seizure caused by a prolonged period of brain hypoxia. These movements, which are often mistaken for a seizure, usually take the form of brief, mild, clonic jerks of the limbs and trunk and twitchings of the face or a tonic extension of the trunk and clenching of the jaw. Occasionally, the extensor rigidity and jerking flexor movements are more severe, but very rarely is there urinary incontinence or biting of the tongue, features that characterize a generalized tonic-clonic convulsion.

Gastaut and Fischer-Williams used the oculocardiac inhibitory reflex to study the pattern of electroencephalographic (EEG) changes in syncope. They found that the heightened vagal discharge produced by compression of the eyeballs (oculovagal reflex, a cause of syncope in acute glaucoma) could produce brief periods of cardiac arrest and syncope. This effect was produced in 20 of 100 patients who had a history of syncopal attacks. These investigators found that after a 7- to 13-s period of cardiac arrest, there was a loss of consciousness, pallor, and muscle relaxation and changes in EEG activity. Toward the end of this period, runs of bilaterally synchronous theta and delta waves appeared in the EEG, predominantly in the frontal lobes; in some patients there were one or more myoclonic jerks, synchronous with the slow waves. If the hypotension persisted beyond 14 or 15 s, the EEG became flat. This period of electrical silence lasted for 10 to 20 s and was sometimes accompanied by a generalized tonic spasm with incontinence. Following the spasm, heartbeats and large-amplitude delta waves reappeared, and after another 20 to 30 s, the EEG reverted to normal. It is noteworthy that rhythmic clonic seizures or epileptiform EEG activity was not observed at any time during the periods of cardiac arrest, syncope, and tonic spasm.

From the moment that consciousness is regained, there is a correct perception of the environment. Confusion, headache, and drowsiness, the common sequelae of a convulsive seizure, do not follow a syncopal attack. Nevertheless, the patient often feels weak and groggy after a vasodepressor faint and, by arising too soon, may precipitate another faint.

The clinical features of *cardiac* and *carotid sinus syncope* are in some ways the same as those described above except that the onset may be absolutely abrupt, without any warning symptoms, and is independent of the patient being in an upright posture. The clinical particulars of these and other forms of syncope are described further on.

Neurogenic Syncope

This term refers to all forms of syncope that result directly from the vascular effects of neural signals coming from the central nervous system. In essence, all the types of syncope in this category are "vasovagal," meaning a combination of vasodepressor and vagal effects in varying proportions; the only differences are in the stimuli that elicit the reflex response.

A number of stimuli, mostly from the viscera but some of psychologic or emotional origin, are capable of eliciting this response, which consists of a reduction or loss of sympathetic vascular tone coupled with a heightened vagal activity. The nucleus of the tractus solitarius (NTS) in the medulla integrates these afferent stimuli and normal baroreceptor signals with the efferent sympathetic mechanisms that maintain vascular tone (see further on and Chap. 26).

Several lines of study suggest that there are disturbances of both sympathetic control of vascular tone and also of the responsiveness of baroreceptors in neurogenic syncope, but the precise mechanisms are unclear. By the use of microneurography, Wallin and Sundlof have demonstrated an increase in sympathetic outflow in peripheral nerves just prior to syncope, as would be expected; however, this activity then ceases at the onset of fainting. Unmyelinated (postganglionic sympathetic) fibers cease firing during vasovagal fainting at a point when the blood pressure falls below 80/40 mm Hg and the pulse, below 60. This would signify that there is an initial attempt to compensate for the falling blood pressure, following which there is a centrally mediated withdrawal of sympathetic activity. Which one of these mechanisms (perhaps both) is responsible for syncope is not clear. More recently, Bechir and colleagues showed that muscle sympathetic activity as assessed using microneurography is increased in the resting state in patients with orthostatic hypotension and, importantly, does not increase further with venous pooling (induced by lower-body negative pressure). Moreover, in the same patients, the response of the cardiac baroreceptors to pooling was significantly diminished. These data are only partially in agreement with those of Wallin and Sundlof, and they are not in accord with an initial increase in sympathetic activity prior to syncope.

There is agreement that peripheral vascular resistance is greatly reduced just prior to and at the onset of fainting. This drop in resistance has been attributed to an initial adrenergic discharge that, at high levels, causes a vasodilatation (rather than constriction) in intramuscular blood vessels. High levels of epinephrine and the vasodilating effects of nitric oxide acting on vascular endothelium, as well as greatly augmented levels of circulating acetylcholine during syncope, also have been invoked as additional or intermediary factors, but all remain speculative. In the current view, the drop in blood pressure is the result of a transient but excessive activity of sympathetic nerves that paradoxically leads to vascular dilatation in muscle and viscera from an imbalance between beta-adrenergic and alpha-adrenergic activity peripherally.

It has been further suggested, on the basis of reasonable but inconclusive physiologic evidence, that the early sympathotonic attempt to maintain blood pressure leads to overly vigorous contractions of the cardiac chambers and that this, in turn, acts as the afferent stimulus for withdrawal of sympathetic tone in common fainting (see "Neurocardiogenic Syncope," later).

Also of interest are abnormalities in the response to hypocarbia of patients who are prone to syncope. Norcliffe-Kaufmann and colleagues recorded a greater-than-normal reduction in cerebral blood flow velocity (gauged by transcranial Doppler) and an excessively reduced vascular resistance in the forearm in response to hypocarbia, and the opposite reactions to hypercarbia. They relate the degree of these changes to variations in orthostatic tolerance among patients and suggest that the two aforementioned changes relate to decreased cerebral blood flow that may engender syncope.

Neurocardiogenic Syncope

This entity, a component or perhaps a subtype of vasodepressor syncope, has received attention as a cause of otherwise unexplained fainting in healthy and athletic children and young adults. As mentioned earlier, it may be the final precipitant in the common vasodepressor faint, and the term is used synonymously with *vasovagal* or *vasodepressor syncope* by some authors.

Oberg and Thoren were the first to observe that the left ventricle itself can be the source of neurally mediated syncope in much the same way as the carotid sinus when stimulated, produces vasodilatation and bradycardia. During acute blood loss in cats, they noted a paradoxical bradycardia that was preceded by increased afferent activity in autonomic fibers arising from the ventricles of the heart, a reaction that could be eliminated by sectioning these nerves. This concept of the heart as the afferent source of vasodepressor reflexes had been suggested earlier by Bezold, as well as by Jarisch and Zoterman, and came to be known as the *Bezold-Jarisch reflex*. The inferoposterior wall of the left ventricle is the site of most of the subendocardial mechanoreceptors that are responsible for the afferent impulses to the nucleus tractus solitarius.

For this mechanism to become active, very vigorous cardiac contractions must occur in the presence of deficient filling of the cardiac chambers (hence "neurocardiogenic"). In the simple faint, an initial burst of sympathetic activity is thought to precipitate physiologic circumstances of excessive cardiac contraction. Echocardiographic findings of a diminished ventricular chamber size and vigorous contractions just prior to syncope support this notion (the "empty-heart syndrome"). The remaining baroreceptors in the aorta may be responsible for the increased afferent activity.

According to Kaufmann, a proclivity to primary neurocardiogenic syncope can be identified by the finding of delayed fainting when the patient is placed at a 60-degree upright position on a tilt table. After approximately 10 min of upright posture, the blood pressure drops below 100 mm Hg; soon thereafter, the patient complains of dizziness and sweating and subsequently faints. In contrast, patients with primary sympathetic failure will faint soon after upward tilting. Half of patients with unexplained syncope display a delayed tilt-table reaction, but it is also seen in 5 percent of controls (see "Tilt-Table Testing" further on). The value of isoproterenol as a cardiac stimulant and peripheral vasodilator to enhance the effect of upright posture and expose neurocardiogenic syncope during the tilt-table test is controversial.

Exercise-Induced Syncope

Aerobic exercise, particularly running, is known to induce fainting in some persons, a trait that may become apparent in late childhood or later and may be familial. There is nausea as well as other presyncopal symptoms; the faint can be avoided by discontinuing exercise or not exceeding a threshold of effort set by the patient himself. Such persons do not seem unduly sensitive to nonaerobic exercise and have no recognizable electrocardiographic or structural heart problems. They have a predilection to faint with prolonged tilt-table testing and with isoproterenol infusion, suggesting that this represents a form of neurocardiogenic syncope. For this reason, these patients may benefit from beta-adrenergic-blocking drugs if given under careful supervision. As discussed further on, exercise can also precipitate syncope in patients with a number of underlying cardiac conditions (myocardial ischemia, long QT syndrome, aortic outflow obstruction, cardiomyopathy, structural chamber anomalies, exercise-induced ventricular tachycardia, and, less often, supraventricular tachycardias).

Athletes who faint unpredictably during exercise pose a particularly difficult problem. Obviously those found to have serious heart disease should give up competitive sports, but the majority has no demonstrable cardiac abnormality. Subjecting these patients to intense exercise and other testing sometimes fails to elicit the faints, but many have varying degrees of hypotension when subjected to prolonged head-up tilt, again suggesting that the cause of fainting is essentially neurocardiogenic (see above). Implanted cardiac pacemakers are not curative in these vasodepressor faints, as the main deficiency is in vascular resistance. Unless the results of tilt-table testing are unequivocal and reproducible, it is best to consider the more serious causes of exercise-induced syncope and to treat the patient appropriately.

Carotid Sinus Syncope

The carotid sinus is normally sensitive to stretch and gives rise to sensory impulses carried via the nerve of Hering, a tributary of the glossopharyngeal nerve, to the medulla. Massage of one of the carotid sinuses or of both alternately, particularly in elderly persons, causes (1) a reflex cardiac slowing (sinus bradycardia, sinus arrest, or even atrioventricular block)—the *vagal type* of response, or (2) a fall of arterial pressure without cardiac slowing—the *vasodepressor type* of response. Another ("central") type of carotid sinus syncope was in the past ascribed to cerebral arteriolar constriction, but such an entity has never been validated.

Faintness or syncope because of carotid sinus sensitivity reportedly has been initiated by turning of the head to one side while wearing a tight collar or even by shaving over the region of the sinus. However, the absence of a history of such an association does not exclude the diagnosis. The attack nearly always occurs when the patient is upright, usually standing. The onset is sudden, often with falling. Small convulsive movements occur quite frequently in both the vagal and vasodepressor types of carotid sinus syncope. The period of unconsciousness in carotid sinus syncope seldom lasts longer than 30 s, and the sensorium is immediately clear when consciousness is regained. The majority of the reported cases have been in men.

In some circumstances, it is important to avoid compression of the carotid artery as an evocative test, particularly if a carotid bruit is heard over either carotid vessel. Moreover, carotid sinus compression for syncope testing should be conducted in controlled circumstances.

A number of other types of purely reflexive cardiac slowing can be traced to direct irritation of the vagus nerves (from esophageal diverticula, mediastinal tumors, gallbladder stones, carotid sinus disease, bronchoscopy, and needling of body cavities). Here, the reflex bradycardia is more often of sinoatrial than atrioventricular type. Weiss and Ferris called such faints *vagovagal*.

Through a similar mechanism, tumors or lymph node enlargements at the base of the skull or in the neck that impinge on the carotid artery, as well as postradiation fibrosis, are capable of causing dramatic syncopal attacks, sometimes preceded by unilateral head or neck pain. Often the episodes are unpredictable, but some patients find that turning the head stimulates an attack. The mechanism in one of our patients with cervical adenopathy was primarily a vasodepressor response; patients with prominent bradycardia have generally had tumors that directly surrounded or infiltrated the glossopharyngeal and vagus nerves (Frank et al; see also MacDonald et al). If the tumor can be safely removed from the carotid region, the syncope often abates; in many cases, however, intracranial section of the ninth and upper rootlets of the tenth nerves on the side of the mass is necessary.

Syncope in Association With Glossopharyngeal Neuralgia

Glossopharyngeal neuralgia typically begins in the sixth decade with paroxysms of pain localized to the base of the tongue, pharynx or larynx, tonsillar area, or an ear (see discussion in Chaps. 10 and 47). In only a small proportion of cases (estimated at 2 percent) are the paroxysms of pain complicated by syncope. Always the sequence is pain, then bradycardia, and, finally, syncope. Presumably the pain gives rise to a massive volley of afferent impulses along the ninth cranial nerve, activating the medullary vasomotor centers via collateral fibers from the nucleus of the tractus solitarius. An increase in parasympathetic (vagal) activity slows the heart. Wallin and colleagues demonstrated that, in addition to bradycardia, there is an element of hypotension caused by inhibition of peripheral sympathetic activity. Here, the effects of the bradycardia exceed those of the vasodepressor hypotension, sometimes to the point of asystole, reflecting the opposite relationship from that seen in most other types of syncope.

The medical treatment of this type of syncope parallels that of trigeminal neuralgia (which is associated in approximately 10 percent of cases, usually on the same side). Antiepileptic drugs and baclofen are helpful in reducing both the pain and syncope in some patients. Intracranial vascular decompression procedures involving small branches of the basilar artery that impinge on the ninth nerve are said to be useful, but such patients have not been extensively studied. Conventional surgical treatment, which consists of sectioning the ninth cranial nerve and upper rootlets of the tenth, has proved to be effective in intractable cases.

The same mechanism is probably operative in so-called *deglutitional syncope*, in which consciousness is lost during or immediately after a forceful swallow. The administration of anticholinergic drugs (propantheline 15 mg tid) has abolished these attacks (Levin and Posner).

Micturition Syncope

This infrequent condition is usually seen in men, sometimes in young adults but more often in the elderly, who arise from bed at night to urinate. The syncope occurs at the end of micturition or soon thereafter, and the loss of consciousness is abrupt, with rapid and complete recovery. Several factors are probably operative. A full bladder causes reflex vasoconstriction; as the bladder empties, this gives way to vasodilatation, which, combined with an element of postural hypotension, might be sufficient to cause fainting in some individuals. Vagally mediated bradycardia and, in some cases, a mild Valsalva effect may also be factors, and alcohol ingestion, hunger, fatigue, and upper respiratory infection are common predisposing factors. Moreover, the use of alpha-adrenergic blockers for bladder outlet obstruction in men may contribute to the situation. In some instances, especially in the elderly, the nocturnal faint has caused serious head injury.

Tussive and Valsalva Syncope

Syncope as a result of a severe paroxysm of coughing was first described by Charcot in 1876. Affected patients are usually heavyset males who smoke and have chronic bronchitis. Occasionally, the problem occurs in children, particularly following paroxysmal coughing spells of pertussis and laryngitis. After sustained hard coughing, the patient suddenly becomes weak and may lose consciousness momentarily. This is mainly attributable to the greatly elevated intrathoracic pressure, which interferes with venous return to the heart. Increased cerebrospinal fluid (CSF) pressure and diminished Pco_2, with resultant cerebral vasoconstriction, are possibly contributing factors.

Powerful efforts to exhale against a closed glottis (as occurs in tussive syncope) are referred to as the *Valsalva maneuver*. The unconsciousness that results from *breathholding spells* in infants is probably based on this mechanism as well; the so-called pallid attacks in infants probably represent reflex vasodepression. Also, the loss of consciousness that occurs during competitive weight lifting ("weight lifters' blackout") is mainly the effect of a Valsalva maneuver, added to which are the effects of vascular dilatation produced by squatting and hyperventilation. Lesser degrees of this phenomenon (faintness and light-headedness) often follow other kinds of strenuous activity, such as unrestrained laughing, straining at stool, heavy lifting, underwater diving, or effortful trumpet playing. Rarely, a brief faint may occur in each of these circumstances.

Syncope may occur occasionally in the course of prostatic or rectal examination, but there is only pallor and bradycardia unless the patient stands immediately (prostatic syncope). A Valsalva effect and reflex vagal stimulation appear to be contributing factors. *Postprandial hypotension* may occasionally lead to syncope in elderly persons, in whom impaired baroreflex function cannot compensate for pooling of blood in splanchnic vessels.

Sympathetic Nervous System Failure

Orthostatic Hypotension

This type of syncope is the result of orthostatic loss of blood pressure. It affects persons whose adrenergic innervation to the blood vessels is defective or, of course, those who are hypovolemic. The patient with autonomic failure, on assuming an upright position, shows a steady decline in blood pressure that begins almost immediately and, if not checked, declines to a level at which the cerebral circulation cannot be supported. This rapid effect and the slow decline in pressure are quite different from the situation in neurocardiogenic syncope, in which there is a delayed but then rapid onset of hypotension.

These conditions are easily understood if one keeps in mind that, on assuming the erect posture, the pooling of blood in the lower parts of the body is normally prevented by (1) reflex arteriolar and arterial constriction, through alpha- and beta-adrenergic effector mechanisms; (2) reflex acceleration of the heart by means of aortic and carotid reflexes, as described earlier; and (3) muscular activity, which improves venous return. Lipsitz has pointed out that aging is associated with a progressive impairment of these compensatory mechanisms, thus rendering the older person especially vulnerable to syncope. However, even in some younger persons, after the blood pressure has fallen slightly and stabilized at a lower level, the compensatory reflexes may also fail suddenly, with a precipitant drop in blood pressure.

With few exceptions (see Chap. 26), peripheral autonomic failure includes an element of vagal dysfunction that precludes the development of a compensatory tachycardia because vagal tone has already been maximally reduced, and also contrary to what happens in vasodepressor syncope, there tend to be no autonomic responses such as pallor, sweating, nausea, or release of norepinephrine.

Postural syncope occurs under a wide variety of clinical conditions: (1) in otherwise normal individuals who, in certain circumstances, experience an excess centrally mediated sympathetic discharge, as described earlier under vasodepressor syncope, or the simple faint; (2) as part of a chronic, probably degenerative central nervous system syndrome known as idiopathic orthostatic hypotension or primary autonomic insufficiency and with a variety of central nervous system degenerations of the basal ganglia that have autonomic failure as a parallel pathology (multiple system atrophy, Parkinson disease, Lewy-body disease); (3) after a period of prolonged illness with recumbency, especially in elderly individuals with poor muscle tone; (4) in association with diseases of the peripheral nerves that involve autonomic nerve fibers—diabetes, tabes dorsalis, amyloidosis, Guillain-Barré syndrome, a primary idiopathic autonomic neuropathy, pandysautonomia, and several other polyneuropathies, all of which interrupt vasomotor reflexes; (5) in patients receiving L-dopa, dopamine agonists, antihypertensive agents, and certain sedative and antidepressant drugs; (6) in spinal cord transection above the T6 level, particularly in the acute stage; (7) in patients with hypovolemia, (8) in pheochromocytoma, in which repeated exposure to catecholamines leads to desensitization of alpha receptors on resistance blood vessels.

The diagnosis of orthostatic hypotension from autonomic failure is established by measuring the blood pressure in the supine and then in the standing position and noting a substantial drop accompanied by symptoms of dizziness or syncope. It should be emphasized that the *bedside testing of orthostatic blood pressure is best performed by having the patient stand quickly and taking readings immediately and again at 1 min and at 3 min*, rather than using the lying-sitting-standing sequence.

Orthostatic hypotension involves the failure to maintain blood pressure in the upright posture. The maintenance of blood pressure during various levels of activity and with postural changes depends on pressure-sensitive receptors (baroreceptors) in the aortic arch and carotid sinus and mechanoreceptors in the walls of the heart. These receptors, which are the sensory nerve endings of the glossopharyngeal and vagus nerves, send afferent impulses to the vasomotor centers in the medulla, more specifically the NTS. Axons from the NTS project to the reticular formation of the ventrolateral medulla, which in turn, sends fibers to the intermediolateral cell column of the spinal cord, thereby controlling vasomotor tone in skeletal muscles, skin, and the splanchnic bed. A diminution of sensory impulses from baroreceptors increases the flow of excitatory signals, which raise the blood pressure and cardiac output, thus restoring cerebral perfusion. This subject is discussed further in relation to the regulation of blood pressure in Chap. 26.

Postural Orthostatic Tachycardia Syndrome

As described by Low and colleagues, postural orthostatic tachycardia syndrome (POTS) consists of intolerance of the standing position accompanied by tachycardia up to 120 beats per minute or more, but *without* orthostatic hypotension. Dyspnea, fatigue, and tremulousness and a complaint of "dizziness" accompany the assumption of an upright posture, and the same constellation of symptoms may be brought out by upright tilting. There is a frequent association with longer term fatigue and with exercise intolerance. The situation is comparable to orthostatic intolerance in the chronic fatigue and postviral syndromes, with which POTS shares many features. An impairment of cerebral autoregulation has been hypothesized; others consider the condition to be a limited form of dysautonomia. The component of the syndrome that simulates anxiety makes it difficult in some cases to differentiate the anticipation of symptoms from a genuine form of autonomic dysfunction.

Goldstein and associates compared a cohort of POTS patients with a group that experienced recurrent postural near-syncope and found that in the former group there was increased myocardial epinephrine release from intact cardiac sympathetic nerves. The basis for this is not known, although the researchers did exclude the possibility of defects in the cardiac norepinephrine transporter membrane and in norepinephrine synthesis.

Primary Autonomic Insufficiency (Idiopathic Orthostatic Hypotension)

This presents in two forms. In one, there is a selective degeneration of neurons in the sympathetic ganglia with denervation of smooth muscle vasculature and adrenal glands. The pathology has not been fully delineated, but lesions in other parts of the nervous system are not evident. In the second type, there is a degeneration of preganglionic neurons in the lateral columns of gray matter in the spinal cord, leaving postganglionic neurons isolated from spinal control. The latter lesion is often associated with degeneration of other systems of neurons in the CNS, particularly the basal ganglia but also the cerebellum. These processes are subsumed under the term *multiple system atrophy*, as discussed in Chap. 39. Parkinson disease and Lewy-body dementia may be associated with the same type of central loss of sympathetic neurons, but orthostatic hypotension and a variety of other features of autonomic insufficiency are early, more pronounced, and progressive in multiple system atrophy than in the other diseases named. Most of the dopaminergic drugs used in the treatment of Parkinson disease can exaggerate the hypotension. There are cases in which neuronal degeneration is limited to the sympathetic neurons of the intermediolateral cell columns—the Shy-Drager syndrome. All of these forms of degenerative disease have their onset in adult life, and the associated hypotension and syncope are usually part of a more widespread autonomic dysfunction that includes other features such as a fixed cardiac rate, vocal cord paralysis, a loss of sweating in the lower parts of the body, redness of the digits, atonicity of the bladder, constipation, and impotence.

Syncope of Cardiac Origin

This is caused by a sudden reduction in cardiac output, usually because of an arrhythmia. Normally, a heart rate as low as 35 to 40 beats per min or as high as 150 beats per min is well tolerated, especially if the patient is recumbent. Changes in heart rate beyond these extremes impair cardiac output and may lead to syncope. Upright posture, anemia, and coronary, myocardial, and valvular disease all render the individual more susceptible to these alterations in heart rate and rhythm. Detailed discussions of the various valvular and myocardial abnormalities and arrhythmias that may compromise cardiac output and lead to syncope are to be found in the articles by Lipsitz, and by Kapoor and colleagues.

Cardiac syncope occurs most frequently in patients with *complete atrioventricular block* and a heart rate of 40 beats or less per minute (Stokes-Adams attacks, or Adams-Stokes-Morgagni syndrome). The block may be persistent or intermittent; it is often preceded by fascicular or second-degree heart block. Ventricular arrest of 4 to 8 s, if the patient is upright, is enough to cause syncope; if the patient is supine, the asystole must last 12 to 15 s. After asystole of 12 s, according to Engel, the patient turns pale and becomes momentarily weak or may lose consciousness without warning; this may occur regardless of the position of the body. If the duration of cerebral ischemia exceeds 15 to 20 s, there are a few clonic jerks. With still longer asystole, the clonic jerks merge with tonic spasms and stertorous respirations and the ashen-gray pallor gives way to cyanosis, incontinence, fixed pupils, and bilateral Babinski signs. As heart action resumes, the face and neck become flushed. The report of this sequence of signs by a dependable observer helps to distinguish syncope from epilepsy. In cases of even more prolonged asystole (4 to 5 min), or if the patient is trapped in an upright or seated position for briefer periods, there may be cerebral injury caused by a combination of hypoxia and ischemia. Coma may persist or may be replaced by confusion and other neurologic signs. Focal ischemic changes, often irreversible, may then be traced to the fields of occluded atherosclerotic cerebral arteries or the border zones between the areas of supply of major arteries. Cardiac faints of the Stokes-Adams type may recur several times a day. The heart block is usually intermittent at first, and between attacks the electrocardiogram (ECG) may show only evidence of heart disease. A continuous ECG using a Holter monitor or telemetry is then needed to demonstrate the arrhythmia (see further on).

Less easily recognized are faintness and syncope caused by *dysfunction of the sinus node*, and manifested by marked sinus bradycardia, sinoatrial block, or sinus arrest ("sick sinus syndrome"). The nodal block results in prolonged atrial asystole. Supraventricular tachycardia or atrial fibrillation may occur, alternating with sinus bradycardia (bradycardia–tachycardia syndrome).

Tachyarrhythmias alone are less likely to produce syncope. Certainly, intermittent ventricular fibrillation can cause fainting, and supraventricular tachycardias with rapid ventricular responses (usually over 180 beats per minute) cause syncope when sustained, predominantly in patients who are upright at the time. The *long QT syndrome* is a rare familial condition in which syncope and ventricular arrhythmias are prone to occur. Mutations in at least six different genes encoding cardiac sodium and potassium channels cause this syndrome. Another inherited syndrome with right bundle branch block and ST-segment elevation in the right precordial leads is known to cause syncope and even sudden death (Brugada syndrome). Some patients with mitral valve prolapse seem disposed to syncope and presyncope and an inordinate number are also said to have panic attacks but these associations, like others with mitral valve prolapse, have never been adequately settled.

Aortic stenosis or *subaortic stenosis* from cardiomyopathy often sets the stage for exertional syncope, because cardiac output cannot keep pace with the demands of exercise. Primary pulmonary hypertension and obstruction of right ventricular outflow (pulmonic valvular or infundibular stenosis) or intracardiac tumors may also be associated with exertional syncope. Syncope may also be a manifestation of large pulmonary embolism. Vagal overactivity may be a factor contributing to the syncope in these conditions as well as in the syncope that may accompany acute aortic outflow obstruction. Tetralogy of Fallot is the congenital cardiac malformation that most often leads to syncope. Other cardiac causes are listed in the classification given at the opening of this chapter.

Syncope Associated With Cerebrovascular Disease

It is now widely appreciated that syncope is not a manifestation of conventional cerebrovascular disease (see further on for discussion and the problem of "drop attacks" that do not have loss of consciousness as a feature). Specifically, syncope does not occur as a manifestation of TIAs that are confined to the territory of the internal carotid arteries and it is rare, if ever, that pure syncopal attacks occur with vertebrobasilar ischemia (see further on). Cases of syncope that do occur are usually associated with multiple occlusions of the large arteries in the thorax or neck. The main examples are found in patients with the aortic-arch syndrome (Takayasu disease) in which the brachiocephalic, common carotid, and vertebral arteries have become narrowed. Physical activity may then critically reduce blood flow to the upper part of the brainstem, causing abrupt loss of consciousness. Stenosis or occlusion of vertebral arteries and the "subclavian steal syndrome" are other examples of cerebrovascular diseases that may cause syncope under the special circumstance of overuse of an arm (see Chap. 34). Fainting also occurs occasionally in patients with congenital anomalies of the upper cervical spine (Klippel-Feil syndrome) or cervical spondylosis, in which the vertebral circulation is compromised. Head turning may then cause vertigo, nausea and vomiting, visual scotomas and, finally, unconsciousness.

Cerebral Hemorrhage and Syncope

The onset of a subarachnoid hemorrhage may be signaled by a syncopal episode, often with transient apnea. Because the bleeding is arterial, there is a momentary cessation of cerebral circulation as the levels of intracranial pressure and blood pressure approach one another. Unless there has been vomiting, a complaint of headache immediately preceding the syncope, or the discovery of severe hypertension or stiff neck when the patient awakens, the diagnosis may not be suspected until a CT scan or lumbar puncture is performed.

An associated problem, with which we have had numerous unsatisfactory encounters, is posed by the patient who falls suddenly forward, striking the head without apparent cause, has headache, and is found to have bifrontal hematomas and subarachnoid blood on CT. These cases highlight the difficulty of distinguishing a primary aneurysmal subarachnoid hemorrhage from an accidental fall or syncope with secondary frontal brain contusions; in almost every case, we have felt obliged to perform some form of cerebral angiography to exclude an anterior communicating artery aneurysm, but we have rarely found one.

Fainting in Hysteria

Hysterical fainting is rather frequent and usually occurs under dramatic circumstances (Chap. 51). The evident lack of change in pulse, blood pressure, or color of the skin or any outward display of anxiety distinguishes it from the vasodepressor faint. Irregular jerking movements and generalized spasms without loss of consciousness or change in the EEG are typical features (Linzer et al, 1992). The diagnosis is based on these negative findings in a person who exhibits the general personality and behavioral characteristics of hysteria. Several interesting instances of mass faintness and syncope of hysterical type have been described—for example, in school marching bands (R.J. Levine).

Syncope of Unknown Cause

Finally, after careful evaluation of patients with syncope and the exclusion of the many forms of the condition described earlier, there remains a significant proportion (one-third to one-half, according to Kapoor and 40 percent in the earlier-noted Framingham Heart Study) in which a cause for the syncope cannot be ascertained. The question of whether a single positive tilt-table test signifies that a prior episode of syncope was neurocardiogenic is not resolved; this obviously has a bearing on the proportion of cases that remain without a diagnosis. If the episodes are repetitive and erratically spaced, a cardiac arrhythmia, intraventricular conduction defect, or seizure should be sought by use of prolonged cardiac rhythm monitoring and conduction studies as well as long-term EEG recordings.

DIFFERENTIAL DIAGNOSIS

Anxiety Attacks and the Hyperventilation Syndrome

These are probably the most important diagnostic considerations in unexplained faintness without syncope. The light-headedness of anxiety and hyperventilation are frequently described as a feeling of faintness, but a loss of consciousness does not follow (see Linzer et al, 1990). Such symptoms are not accompanied by facial pallor or relieved by recumbency. The diagnosis is made on the basis of the associated symptoms, the absence of laboratory and tilt-table abnormalities, and the finding that part of the attack can be reproduced by having the patient hyperventilate. The symptoms produced in this way mimic the persistent or episodic dizziness that accompanies anxiety and panic states (Chap. 15). When anxiety attacks are combined with a Valsalva effect or prolonged standing, fainting may occur. The relationship of anxiety-panic to the previously described postural orthostatic tachycardia syndrome is uncertain.

Hypoglycemia

In diabetics and nondiabetics, hypoglycemia may be an obscure cause of episodic weakness and very rarely of syncope. With progressive lowering of blood glucose, the clinical picture is one of hunger, trembling, flushed facies, sweating, confusion, and, finally, after many minutes, seizures and coma. The diagnosis depends largely on the history, the documentation of reduced blood glucose during an attack, and reproduction of the patient's spontaneous attacks by an injection of insulin or hypoglycemia-inducing drugs (or ingestion of a high-carbohydrate meal in the case of reactive hypoglycemia).

Acute Blood Loss

Acute hemorrhage, usually within the gastrointestinal tract, is a cause of weakness, faintness, or even unconsciousness when the patient stands suddenly. The cause (gastric or duodenal ulcer is the most common) may remain inevident until the passage of black stools.

Drop Attacks

This term has been applied to falling spells that occur without warning and *without* loss of consciousness or postictal symptoms. The patient, usually elderly, suddenly falls down while walking or standing, rarely while stooping. The knees inexplicably buckle. There is no dizziness or impairment of consciousness, and the fall is usually forward, with scuffing of the knees and sometimes the nose. The patient, unless obese, is able to right himself and to rise immediately and go his way, quite embarrassed. There may be several attacks during a period of a few weeks and none thereafter. The interval EEGs and ECGs are normal. One potential mechanism is a lapse of tone in leg muscles during the silent phase of an unnoticed myoclonic or axterixis jerk. Primary orthostatic tremor (see Chap. 4) has a similar appearance. Drop attacks also occur in acute hydrocephalus, and with the Chiari amlformation, and these patients, although conscious, may not be able to arise for several hours. Rare instances of Ménière disease, in which the patient is suddenly thrown to the ground ("otolithic catastrophe of Tumarkin," see "Ménière Disease and Other Forms of Labyrinthine Vertigo" in Chap. 15) may be mistaken for a syncopal or drop attack, but only briefly, until vertigo becomes prominent.

Drop attacks as defined above are usually without an identifiable mechanism, requiring no treatment if cardiologic studies are normal. On uncertain grounds, they are often attributed to brainstem ischemia. In only about one-quarter of such cases, according to Meissner and coworkers, can an association be made with cardiovascular or cerebrovascular disease to which treatment should be directed.

Orthopedic surgeons and rheumatologists are familiar with knee-buckling attacks, which they attribute to arthritic or tendinous disorders of the knee. Painful impulses arising in and around the knee could result in brief reflex silence of the antigravity muscles (primarily the quadriceps), producing a phenomenon akin to asterixis. Greenwood and Hopkins long ago proposed this mechanism. Although brief periods of silence have been recorded in the quadriceps muscles of patients with drop attacks, the reflex mechanism and its relationship to knee pain is speculative. This problem is also taken up in Chap. 7.

Seizures and Syncope

In epilepsy, whether major or minor, the arrest in consciousness is almost instantaneous and, as revealed by the EEG, is accompanied by a paroxysm of electrical activity occurring simultaneously in all of the cerebral cortex and thalamus. There are a number of important clinical distinctions between epileptic and syncopal attacks. The epileptic attack may occur day or night, regardless of the position of the patient; syncope rarely appears when the patient is recumbent, the only common exception being the Stokes-Adams attack. The patient's color usually does not change at the onset of an epileptic attack; pallor is an early and almost invariable finding in most types of syncope except those caused by chronic orthostatic hypotension or hysteria, and it precedes unconsciousness. If an aura is present, it rarely lasts longer than a few seconds before consciousness is abolished. The onset of syncope is usually more gradual, and the prodromal symptoms are quite distinctive and different from those of seizures. In general, injury from falling is more frequent in epilepsy than in syncope, because protective reflexes are instantaneously abolished in the former. (Nevertheless, cardiogenic syncope is an important cause of hurtful falls, especially in the elderly.) The return of consciousness is slow in epilepsy, prompt in syncope; mental confusion, headache, and drowsiness are common sequelae of seizures, and physical weakness with clear sensorium, of syncope (a brief period of grogginess may follow vasodepressor syncope). Biting of the tongue is well known, albeit not always present in convulsion; it is exceptional in syncope. Repeated spells of unconsciousness in a young person at a rate of several per day or month are much more suggestive of epilepsy than of syncope.

Tonic spasm of muscles with upturning of the eyes is a prominent and often initial feature of epilepsy, but also occurs in the course of a faint and cannot be depended upon to make the distinction between the 2 processes. Urinary incontinence is a frequent occurrence in epilepsy, but it need not occur during an epileptic attack and may occasionally occur with syncope, so that it also cannot be used as a means of separating the disorders.

The EEG may be helpful in differentiating syncope from epilepsy. In the interval between epileptic seizures, the EEG, particularly if repeated once or twice, shows some degree of abnormality in 50 to 75 percent of cases, whereas it should be normal between syncopal attacks. Sometimes one must resort to continuous EEG monitoring by tape recording or telemetry to clarify the situation (this can be combined with continuous ECG recording). Another useful laboratory marker of a seizure, especially if unwitnessed, is an elevation of the serum creatine kinase (CK) concentration; such a finding occurs only infrequently in the rare case of syncope associated with extensive muscle trauma. Elevated prolactin levels have not proved discriminating enough for routine use in separating seizure from syncope but remain useful in distinguishing both of these from other causes of loss of consciousness, particularly hysteria, in which such elevations do not occur.

No single criterion will absolutely differentiate epilepsy from syncope, but taken as a group and supplemented by the EEG, these criteria usually enable one to distinguish the 2 conditions.

Cardiovascular structures represented in the insular cortex may give rise to seizures that produce cardiac arrhythmias, leading in turn to syncope. As a rule, seizures arising from the left insula prolong the QT interval and increase sympathetic tone, thereby lowering the threshold for ventricular arrhythmia, whereas those arising from the right insula shorten the QT interval and increase parasympathetic tone, thereby increasing the risk of vagally mediated syncope. *Sympathetic storms* may arise from the brain in circumstances of generalized injury (e.g., trauma, subarachnoid hemorrhage, infarction, or intracerebral hemorrhages). When severe, this sympathetic hyperactivity can cause an acute left ventricular apical cardiomyopathy that causes syncope.

SPECIAL METHODS OF EXAMINATION

In patients who complain of recurrent faintness or syncope but do not have a spontaneous occurrence while under observation, an attempt to reproduce attacks may prove to be of great assistance in diagnosis. Here it is important to recall that normal persons can faint if made to squat and overbreathe and then to stand erect and hold their breath (especially if the Valsalva maneuver is added). Prolonged standing at attention in the heat often causes even well-conditioned soldiers to faint, as does compression of the chest and abdomen while holding one's breath, as in the parlor trick of adolescents ("fainting lark").

When an anxiety state is accompanied by faintness, the pattern of symptoms can often be reproduced by having the subject hyperventilate—that is, breathe rapidly and deeply for 2 to 3 min. This test may also be of therapeutic value, because the underlying anxiety tends to be lessened when the patient learns that the symptoms can be produced and alleviated at will simply by controlling breathing.

Most patients with tussive syncope cannot reproduce an attack by the Valsalva maneuver but can sometimes do so by voluntary coughing, if severe enough. Another useful procedure is to have the patient perform the Valsalva maneuver for more than 10 s (thus trapping blood behind closed valves in the veins) while the pulse and blood pressure are measured (see "Tests for Abnormalities of the Autonomic Nervous System" in Chap. 26).

In each of the aforementioned instances, the crucial point is not whether symptoms are produced but whether they reproduce the exact pattern of symptoms that occurs in the spontaneous attacks.

Other conditions in which the diagnosis is clarified by reproducing the attacks are carotid sinus hypersensitivity (massage of one or the other carotid sinus) and orthostatic hypotension (observations of pulse rate, blood pressure, and symptoms in the recumbent and standing positions or, even better, with the patient on a tilt table).

The measurement of beat-to-beat variation in heart rate is a simple but sensitive means of detecting vagal dysfunction, as described in Chap. 26 but its role in the evaluation of syncope has not been established.

Careful, continuous monitoring of the ECG in the hospital or by using a portable (Holter) recorder may determine whether an arrhythmia is responsible for the syncopal episode. A continuous cardiac loop ECG recorder (which continually records and erases cardiac rhythm) permits prolonged (a month or longer) ambulatory monitoring at reasonable cost. The diagnostic yield from loop recording is modestly greater than that from Holter monitoring (Linzer et al, 1990).

Tilt-Table Testing

Upright tilting on a tilt table may cause, within seconds, up to 20 or 25 mm Hg drop in systolic blood pressure and

5 to 10 mm Hg in diastolic pressure in normal individuals, usually with only minor symptoms. In response, the heart rate rises 5 to 15 beats per minute.

There are 2 types of abnormal response to upright tilting: (1) early hypotension (occurring within moments of tilting) that slowly progresses with continued upright posture; this signifies inadequate sympathetic tone and baroreceptor function; and (2) a delayed (up to several minutes) hypotension that appears abruptly at the end of that period and indicates a neurocardiogenic mechanism.

The normal response to a 60- to 80-degree head-up tilt after approximately 10 min is a transient drop in systolic blood pressure (5 to 15 mm Hg), a rise in diastolic pressure (5 to 10 mm Hg), and a rise in heart rate (10 to 15 beats per minute). Hypotension and fainting after tilting for this duration, a positive test, as already emphasized, is taken as a proclivity to neurocardiogenic fainting and at least an ostensible explanation for the problem. However, because it occurs in a proportion of individuals who have never fainted; it is not to be taken as incontrovertible evidence that a recent spell is explained by this mechanism. Although controversial, in some circumstances the infusion of the catecholamine isoproterenol (1 to 5 mcg/min for 30 min during head-up tilt) may be a more effective means of producing hypotension (and syncope) than the standard tilt test alone (Almquist et al; Waxman et al). While it brings out more cases of neurocardiogenic syncope, some of these are false positives.

TREATMENT OF SYNCOPE

Patients seen during the preliminary stages of fainting or after they have lost consciousness should be placed in a position that permits maximal cerebral blood flow, i.e., with head lowered between the knees if sitting, or, far preferably, in the supine position with legs elevated. All tight clothing and other constrictions should be loosened and the head and body positioned so that the tongue does not fall back into the throat and the possible aspiration of vomitus is avoided. Nothing should be given by mouth until the patient has regained consciousness. The patient should not be permitted to rise until the sense of physical weakness and the appearance of pallor have passed and he should be watched carefully for a few minutes after arising.

As a rule, the physician sees the patient after recovery from the faint and is asked to explain why it happened and how it can be prevented in the future. One should think first of those causes of fainting that constitute a therapeutic emergency. Among them are massive internal hemorrhage and myocardial infarction, and cardiac arrhythmias. In an elderly person, a sudden faint without obvious cause must always arouse the suspicion of a complete heart block or other cardiac arrhythmia.

The prevention of fainting depends on the mechanisms involved. In the usual vasodepressor faint of adolescents—which tends to occur in circumstances favoring vasodilatation (warm environment, hunger, fatigue, alcohol intoxication) and periods of emotional excitement—it is enough to advise the patient to avoid such circumstances and to maintain adequate hydration. In postural hypotension, patients should be cautioned against arising suddenly from bed. Instead, they should first exercise the legs for a few seconds, then sit on the edge of the bed and make sure they are not light-headed or dizzy before starting to walk. Standing for prolonged periods can sometimes be tolerated without fainting by crossing the legs forcefully. The same regimen suffices for cases of syncope from deconditioning. Alternatives should be found for medications that are conceivable causes of orthostasis. Beta-adrenergic blocking agents, diuretics, antidepressants, and sympatholytic antihypertensive drugs are the common culprits.

In the syndrome of chronic orthostatic hypotension, from central or peripheral sympathetic failure, special mineralocorticoid preparations—such as fludrocortisone acetate (Florinef) 0.05 to 0.4 mg/d in divided doses—and increased salt intake to expand blood volume are helpful. The alpha$_1$-agonist midodrine, beginning with 2.5 mg every 4 h and slowly increasing the dose to 5 mg every 4 to 6 h, has been used successfully in several studies, but this medication has the potential to worsen the situation and must be used with care. Domperidone may be helpful in patients with parkinsonism. Sleeping with the head posts of the bed elevated on wooden blocks 8 to 12 in high and wearing a snug elastic abdominal binder and elastic stockings are measures that often prove helpful. Tyramine and monoamine oxidase inhibitors have given limited relief in some cases of Shy-Drager syndrome, and beta blockers (propranolol or pindolol) and indomethacin (25 to 50 mg tid) in others. These and other approaches that have proved useful in treating orthostatic hypotension are reviewed by Mathias and Kimber. Anticholinesterase drugs such as pyridostigmine are entering a phase of popularity for the treatment of many forms of orthostatic hypotension (Singer and colleagues).

Neurally mediated syncope (neurocardiogenic or vasodepressor syncope), identified largely by the clinical circumstances and by tilt-table testing, may be prevented by the use of beta-adrenergic blocking agents. Our colleagues in cardiology have recently favored acebutolol 400 mg daily, in part because of its partial alpha-adrenergic activity, which raises baseline blood pressure, but atenolol 50 mg may be as effective. The anticholinergic agent disopyramide has also been used (Milstein et al). Several other drugs (e.g., ephedrine, metoclopramide, dihydroergotamine) have been variably successful in individual patients, but their utility as standard medications remains to be established; the beta-blocking agents are generally preferred.

The treatment of carotid sinus syncope involves, first of all, instructing the patient in measures that minimize the hazards of a fall (see below). A loose collar should be worn, and the patient should learn to turn his whole body, rather than the head alone, when looking to one side. Atropine or one of the sympathomimetic group of drugs may be used, respectively, in patients with pronounced bradycardia or hypotension during attacks. If atropine is not successful, and it is certainly not practical for any period of time, and the syncopal attacks are incapacitating, the insertion of a dual-chamber pacemaker should be considered. Radiation or surgical denervation of the carotid sinus had apparently yielded favorable results in some patients, but it is no longer practiced. Vagovagal attacks usually respond well to an anticholinergic agent (propantheline, 15 mg tid). Syncope arising from glossopharyngeal neuralgia tends to benefit from medications that reduce the incidence of episodes, such as gabapentin.

In the elderly person, a faint carries the additional hazard of a fracture or other trauma as a consequence of the fall. Therefore the patient subject to recurrent syncope should cover the bathroom floor and bathtub with mats and have as much of his home carpeted as is feasible. Especially important is the floor space between the bed and the bathroom, because this is the route along which faints in elderly persons most commonly occur. Outdoor walking should be on soft ground rather than hard surfaces, and the patient should avoid standing still for prolonged periods, which is more likely than walking to induce an attack. Padded hip protectors, now available as a commercial product, should be considered in elderly patients at risk of recurrent falls of any kind but evidence of their effectiveness in large populations is so far, lacking.

References

Abboud FM: Neurocardiogenic syncope. *N Engl J Med* 328:1117, 1993.

Almquist A, Goldenberg IF, Milstein S, et al: Provocation of bradycardia and hypotension by isoproterenol and upright posture in patients with unexplained syncope. *N Engl J Med* 320:346, 1989.

Bannister R, Mathias W (eds): *Autonomic Failure: A Textbook of Clinical Disorders of the Autonomic Nervous System*, 4th ed. New York, Oxford University Press, 1999.

Bechir M, Binggeli C, Corti R, et al: Dysfunctional baroreflex regulation of sympathetic nerve activity in patients with vasovagal syncope. *Circulation* 107:1620, 2003.

Compton D, Hill PM, Sinclair JD: Weight-lifters' blackout. *Lancet* 2:1234, 1973.

Engel GL: *Fainting*, 2nd ed. Springfield, IL, Charles C Thomas, 1962.

Frank JI, Ropper AH, Zuniga G: Vasodepressor carotid sinus syncope associated with a neck mass. *Neurology* 42:1194, 1992.

Gastaut H, Fischer-Williams M: Electro-encephalographic study of syncope: Its differentiation from epilepsy. *Lancet* 2:1018, 1957.

Goldstein DS, Holmes C, Frank SM, et al: Cardiac sympathetic dysautonomia in chronic orthostatic intolerance syndromes. *Circulation* 106:2358, 2002.

Greenwood R, Hopkins A: Landing from an unexpected fall and voluntary step. *Brain* 99:375, 1976.

Jarisch A, Zoterman Y: Depressor reflexes from the heart. *Acta Physiol Scand* 16:31, 1948.

Kapoor WN: Evaluation and management of the patient with syncope. *JAMA* 268:2553, 1992.

Kapoor WN, Karpf M, Maher Y, et al: Syncope of unknown origin. *JAMA* 247:2687, 1982.

Kaufmann H: Neurally mediated syncope: Pathogenesis, diagnosis, and treatment. *Neurology* 45(Suppl 5):S12, 1995.

Kontos HA, Richardson DW, Norvell JE: Norepinephrine depletion in idiopathic orthostatic hypotension. *Ann Intern Med* 82:336, 1975.

Levin B, Posner JB: Swallow syncope: Report of a case and review of the literature. *Neurology* 22:1086, 1972.

Levine RJ: Epidemic faintness and syncope in a school marching band. *JAMA* 238:2373, 1977.

Lewis T: A lecture on vasovagal syncope and the carotid sinus mechanism. *Br Med J* 1:873, 1932.

Linzer M, Pritchett ELC, Pontinen M, et al: Incremental diagnostic yield of loop electrocardiographic recorders in unexplained syncope. *Am J Cardiol* 66:214, 1990.

Linzer M, Varia I, Pontinen M, et al: Medically unexplained syncope: Relationship to psychiatric illness. *Am J Med* 92:185, 1992.

Lipsitz LA: Orthostatic hypotension in the elderly. *N Engl J Med* 321:952, 1989.

Low PA, Opfer-Gehrking TL, Textor SC, et al: Postural tachycardia syndrome (POTS). *Neurology* 45(Suppl 5):19, 1995.

MacDonald DR, Strong E, Nielsen S, Posner JB: Syncope from head and neck cancer. *J Neurooncol* 1:257, 1983.

Mark AL: The Bezold-Jarisch reflex revisited: Clinical implications of inhibitory reflexes originating in the heart. *J Am Coll Cardiol* 1:90, 1983.

Mathias CJ, Keguchi K, Bleasdale-Barr K, Kimber JR: Frequency of family history in vasovagal syncope. *Lancet* 352:33, 1998.

Mathias CJ, Kimber JR: Treatment of postural hypotension. *J Neurol Neurosurg Psychiatry* 65:285, 1998.

Meissner L, Wiebers DO, Swanson JW, O'Fallon WM: The natural history of drop attacks. *Neurology* 36:1029, 1986.

Milstein S, Buetikofer J, Dunnigan A, et al: Usefulness of disopyramide for prevention of upright tilt-induced hypotension-bradycardia. *Am J Cardiol* 65:1339, 1990.

Norcliffe-Kaufmann LJ, Kaufmann H, Hainsworth R: Enhanced vascular responses to hypocapnia in neurally medicated syncope. *Ann Neurol* 63:288, 2008.

Oberg B, Thoren P: Increased activity in left ventricular receptors during hemorrhage or occlusion of caval veins in the cat: A possible cause of the vasovagal reaction. *Acta Physiol Scand* 85:164, 1972.

Ross RT: *Syncope*. Philadelphia, Saunders, 1988.

Schoenberg BS, Kuglitsch JF, Karnes WE: Micturition syncope—not a single entity. *JAMA* 229:1631, 1974.

Shy GM, Drager GA: A neurological syndrome associated with orthostatic hypotension: A clinical-pathologic study. *Arch Neurol* 2:511, 1960.

Singer W, Sandroni P, Opfer-Gehrking TL, et al. "Pyridostigmine treatment trial in neurogenic orthostatic hypotension." *Archives of Neurology*, 63: 513, 2006.

Soteriades ES, Evans JC, Larson MG, et al: Incidence and prognosis of syncope. *N Engl J Med* 347:878, 2002.

Wallin BG: New aspects of sympathetic function in man, in Stälberg E, Young RR (eds): *Clinical Neurophysiology*. Oxford, Butterworth, 1981, pp 145–167.

Wallin BG, Sundlof G: Sympathetic outflow to muscles during vasovagal syncope. *J Auton Nerv Syst* 6:287, 1982.

Wallin BG, Westerberg CE, Sundlof G: Syncope induced by glossopharyngeal neuralgia: Sympathetic outflow to muscle. *Neurology* 34:522, 1984.

Waxman MB, Yao L, Cameron DA, et al: Isoproterenol induction of vasodepressor-type reaction in vasodepressor-prone persons. *Am J Cardiol* 63:58, 1989.

Weiss S, Capps RB, Ferris EB Jr, Munro D: Syncope and convulsions due to a hyperactive carotid sinus reflex: Diagnosis and treatment. *Arch Intern Med* 58:407, 1936.

Weiss S, Ferris EB Jr: Adams-Stokes syndrome with transient complete heart block of vagovagal reflex origin: Mechanism and treatment. *Arch Intern Med* 54:931, 1934.

19

Sleep and Its Abnormalities

Sleep, that familiar yet inexplicable condition of repose in which consciousness is in abeyance, is obviously not abnormal, yet it is appropriately considered in connection with abnormal phenomena because there are a number of interesting and common irregularities of sleep, some of which approach serious extremes. Furthermore, a number of neurological conditions have special types of sleep disruption as common features. The psychologic and physiologic benefits of sleep are of paramount importance, and it is increasingly recognized that disruption of sleep increases the risks for a number of medical diseases, including stroke, hypertension, and coronary disease. Everyone, of course, has had a great deal of personal experience with sleep, or lack of it, and has observed people in sleep, so it requires no special knowledge to understand something about this condition or to appreciate its importance to health and well-being.

Physicians are frequently consulted by patients who suffer from some derangement of sleep. Most often, the problem is one of sleeplessness, but sometimes it concerns excessive sleepiness or some peculiar phenomenon occurring in connection with sleep. Certain points concerning normal sleep and the sleep–wake mechanisms are worth reviewing, as familiarity with them is necessary for an understanding of disorders of sleep. A great deal of information about sleep and sleep abnormalities is now available as a result of the development of the subspecialty of sleep medicine, and the creation of centers for the diagnosis and treatment of sleep disorders.

Most disorders of sleep can be readily recognized if one attends closely to the patient's description of the disturbance. Only complex or odd cases or those requiring the documentation of apneic episodes or seizures, and other motor disorders during sleep, need study in special sleep laboratories.

PHYSIOLOGY OF SLEEP AND SLEEP–WAKE MECHANISMS

Sleep represents one of the basic 24-h (circadian) rhythms, traceable through all mammalian, avian, and reptilian species. The neural control of circadian rhythms is thought to reside in the ventral-anterior region of the hypothalamus, more specifically, in the suprachiasmatic nuclei. Lesions in these nuclei result in a disorganization of the sleep–wake cycles as well as of the rest–activity, temperature, and feeding rhythms. Chapter 27 describes the ancillary role of melatonin and the pineal body in modulating this cyclic activity. There is also an important dimension of a homeostatic drive to sleep as the day wears on. This modulates the circadian rhythm independent of light entrainment of the circadian rhythm and makes the workday possible.

Effects of Age

Observations of the human sleep–wake cycle show it to be closely age linked. The newborn baby sleeps from 16 to 20 h a day, and the child, 10 to 12 h. Total sleep time drops to 9 to 10 h by mid-adolescence and to about 7 to 7.5 h during young adulthood. A gradual decline to about 6.5 h develops in late adult life. However, there are wide individual differences in the length and depth of sleep, apparently as a result of genetic factors, early life conditioning, the amount of physical activity, and psychologic states.

The pattern of sleeping, which is adjusted to the 24-h day, also varies in the different epochs of life. The circadian rhythm, with predominance of daytime wakefulness and nighttime sleep, begins to appear only after the first few weeks of postnatal life of the full-term infant; as the child matures, the morning nap is omitted, then the afternoon nap; by the fourth or fifth year, sleep becomes consolidated into a single long nocturnal period. (Actually, a large part of the world's population continues to have an afternoon nap, or siesta, as a lifelong sleep–wake pattern.) Fragmentation of the sleep pattern begins in late adult life. Over ensuing years, night awakenings tend to increase in frequency, and the daytime waking period may be interrupted by episodic sleep lasting seconds to minutes (microsleep), as well as by longer naps. From about 35 years of age onward, women tend to sleep slightly more than men.

Stages of Sleep

Seminal contributions to our understanding of the physiology of sleep were made by Loomis and associates and by Aserinsky, Dement, and Kleitman through electroencephalographic analysis and clinical observation. As a result of their studies, five stages of sleep, representative of two alternating physiologic mechanisms, have been defined. In each stage, the electrical activity of the brain occurs in organized and recurring cycles, referred to as the *architecture of sleep*. As the electrophysiologic stages of sleep progress, sleep becomes deeper, meaning that arousal requires a more intense stimulus. These findings put to rest the antiquated ideas that sleep is a purely passive state and reflects fatigue and reduction in environmental stimuli.

Relaxed wakefulness with the eyes closed is accompanied in the electroencephalogram (EEG) by posterior alpha waves of 9 to 11 Hz (cycles per second) and intermixed low-voltage fast activity of mixed frequency. Except for the facial muscles, the electromyogram (EMG) is silent when the patient is sitting or lying quietly. With drowsiness, as the first stage of sleep sets in, the eyelids begin to droop, the eyes may rove slowly from side to side, and the pupils become smaller. As the early stage of sleep evolves, the muscles relax and the EEG pattern changes to one of progressively lower voltage and mixed frequency with a loss of alpha waves; this is associated with slow, rolling eye movements and is called *stage 1 sleep*. As this changes into *stage 2 sleep*, 0.5- to 2-s bursts of biparietal 12- to 14-Hz waves (sleep spindles) and intermittent high-amplitude, central-parietal sharp slow-wave complexes appear (vertex waves) (Fig. 19-1). The American Academy of Sleep Medicine (AASM) recommends the following staging: stage W (wakefulness), stage N1 (non-REM sleep, or NREM 1, formerly stage 1), stage N2 (NREM 2, formerly stage 2), stage N3 (NREM 3, combining former stages 3 and 4—or slow-wave sleep), and stage R (rapid eye movement [REM] sleep). The essential difference between this new nomenclature and the one formerly used by neurologists is that stage N3 now represents *slow-wave sleep*, replacing stage 3 and stage 4 sleep, composed of an increasing proportion of high-amplitude delta waves (0.75-μV, 0.5- to 2-Hz) in the EEG (Table 19-1). If the eyelids are raised gently, the globes are usually seen to be exotropic and the pupils are even smaller than before, but with retained responses to light. An additional stage of the sleep cycle, which follows the others intermittently throughout the night, is associated with further reduction in muscle tone except in the extraocular muscles and with bursts of rapid eye movement; thus the term *REM sleep* designates this stage. The EEG becomes desynchronized, i.e., it has a low-voltage, high-frequency discharge pattern. The first three stages of sleep are called *nonrapid eye movement (NREM) sleep* or *synchronized sleep*; the last stage, in addition to REM sleep, is variously designated as *fast-wave, nonsynchronized*, or *desynchronized sleep*. Figure 19-2 illustrates these features.

In the first portion of a typical night's sleep, the normal young and middle-aged adult passes successively through stages N1, N2, N3, and R (REM) sleep. After about 70 to 100 min, a large proportion of which consists

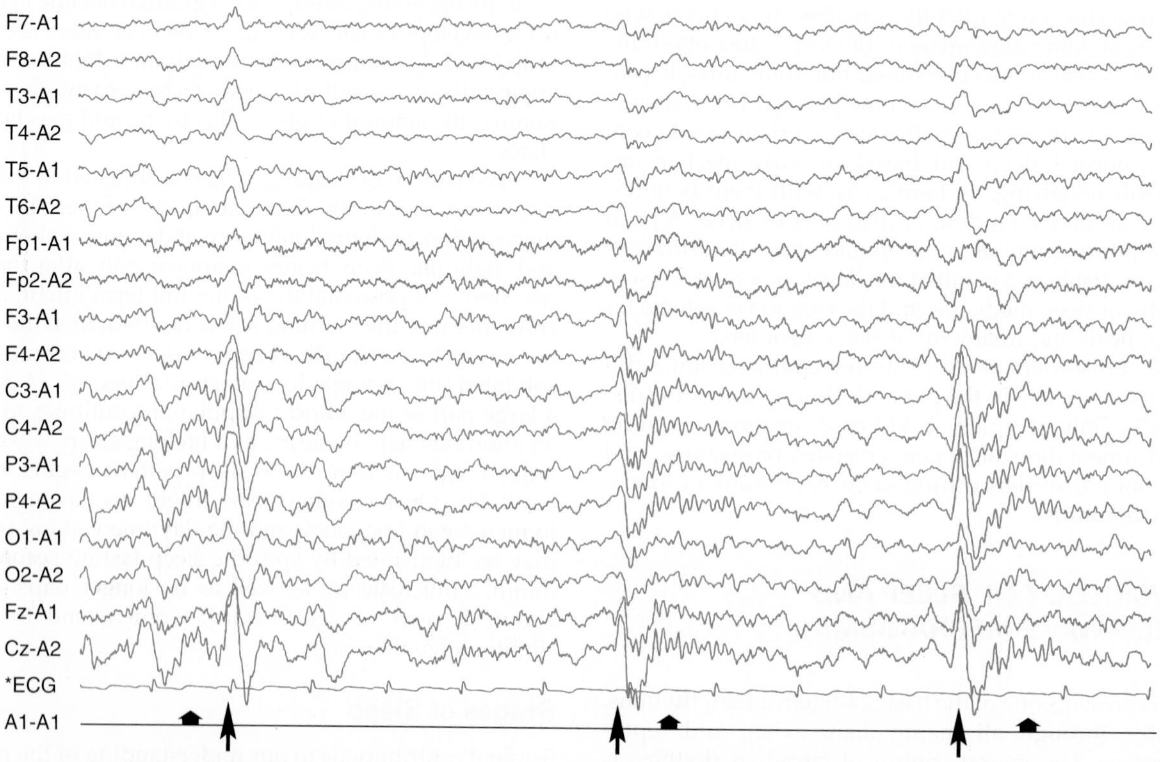

Figure 19-1. Conventional EEG (30 mm/s) of a young healthy woman in stage 2 (N2) sleep showing vertex waves (*large arrows*) and sleep spindles (*small arrows*), best seen in the central regions.

Table 19-1

AMERICAN ACADEMY OF SLEEP MEDICINE (AASM) SLEEP SCORING SYSTEM

AMERICAN ACADEMY OF SLEEP MEDICINE	FORMER NOMENCLATURE	EEG CHARACTERISTICS	BEHAVIORAL STATE
W	—	Posterior reactive alpha rhythm	Awake
N1	Stage 1	Diffuse theta and loss of alpha	Drowsy
N2	Stage 2	Sleep spindles and K complexes	Light sleep
N3	Stages 3 and 4	High-voltage theta and delta activity	Deep sleep
R	REM	Diffuse theta	Predominance of dreaming (see text)

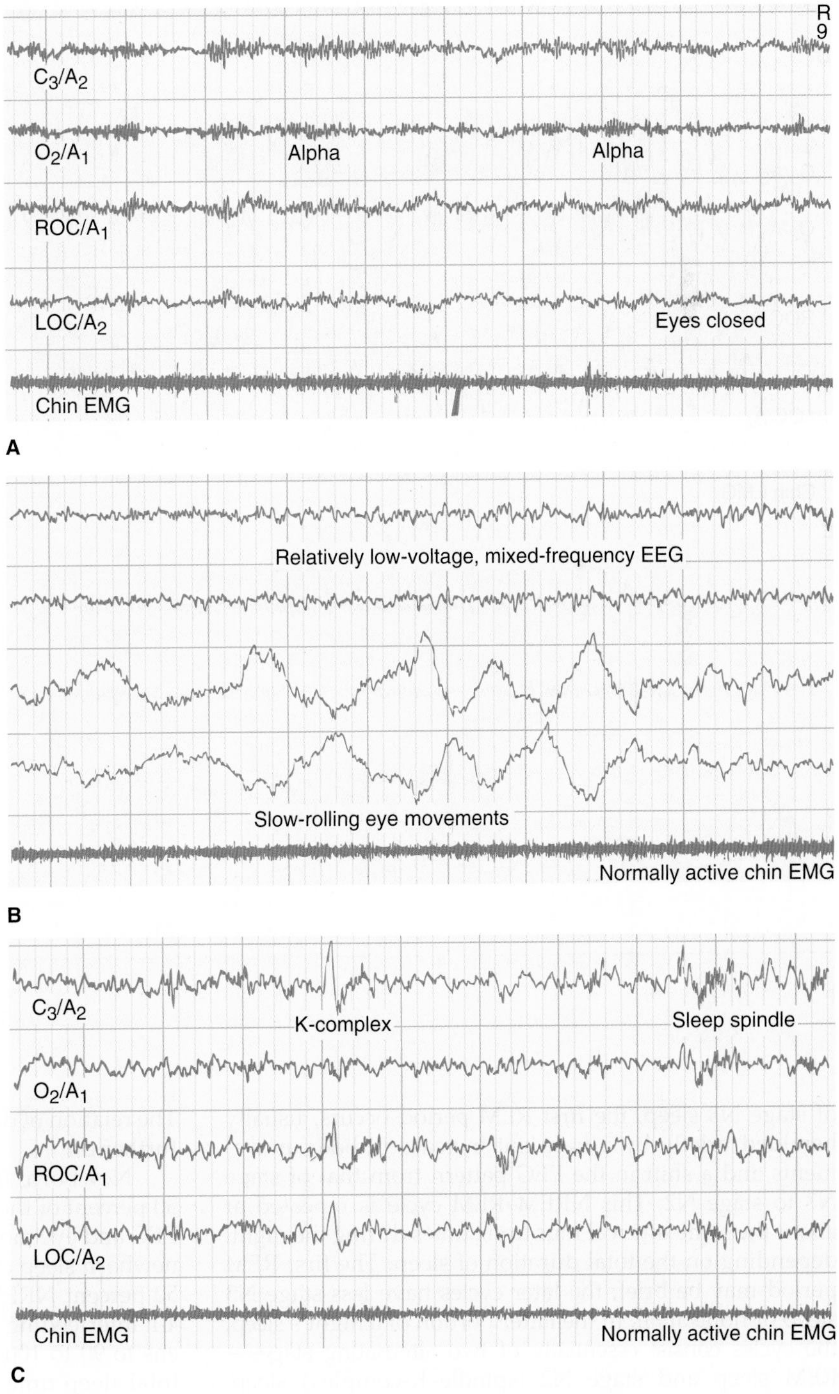

Figure 19-2. Representative polysomnographic recordings from adults in the awake state and various stages of sleep. Recordings are made at conventional sleep laboratory speed of 10 mm/s (i.e., at the paper speed of one-third standard clinical EEG recordings). *A. Upper tracings*: Awake state (with eyes closed). Alpha rhythms are prominent in EEG. Normally active chin EMG. *B. Middle tracings*: Stage 1 (N1) sleep. Onset of sleep is defined by the diminished amplitude of alpha waves in the occipital EEG channel ("flat" appearance). *C. Lower tracings*: Stage 2 (N2) sleep, characterized by appearance of high-amplitude single-complex (K) waves and bursts of 13- to 16-Hz waves (sleep spindles) on a background of low frequency. *D. Upper tracings*: Stage 3 (N3) sleep. Appearance of high-voltage slow (delta) waves. *E. Middle tracings*: Deepest stage of N3 sleep, with predominant delta-wave activity occupying 50 percent of a 30-s tracing. *F. Lower tracings*: Rapid eye movement (REM) sleep, characterized by episodes of REM and occasional muscle twitches in an otherwise flat chin EMG. *Technical Note*: Four sites from the same montage are illustrated in each recording: C_3/A_2, left central to right mastoid; O_2/A_1, right occipital to left mastoid; ROC/A_1, right outer canthus to left mastoid; LOC/A_2, left outer canthus to right mastoid. A chin EMG tracing is added to each recording. (Adapted with permission from Butkov N. *Atlas of Clinical Polysomnography*. Vol 1. Synapse Media, Medford, OR, 1996.)

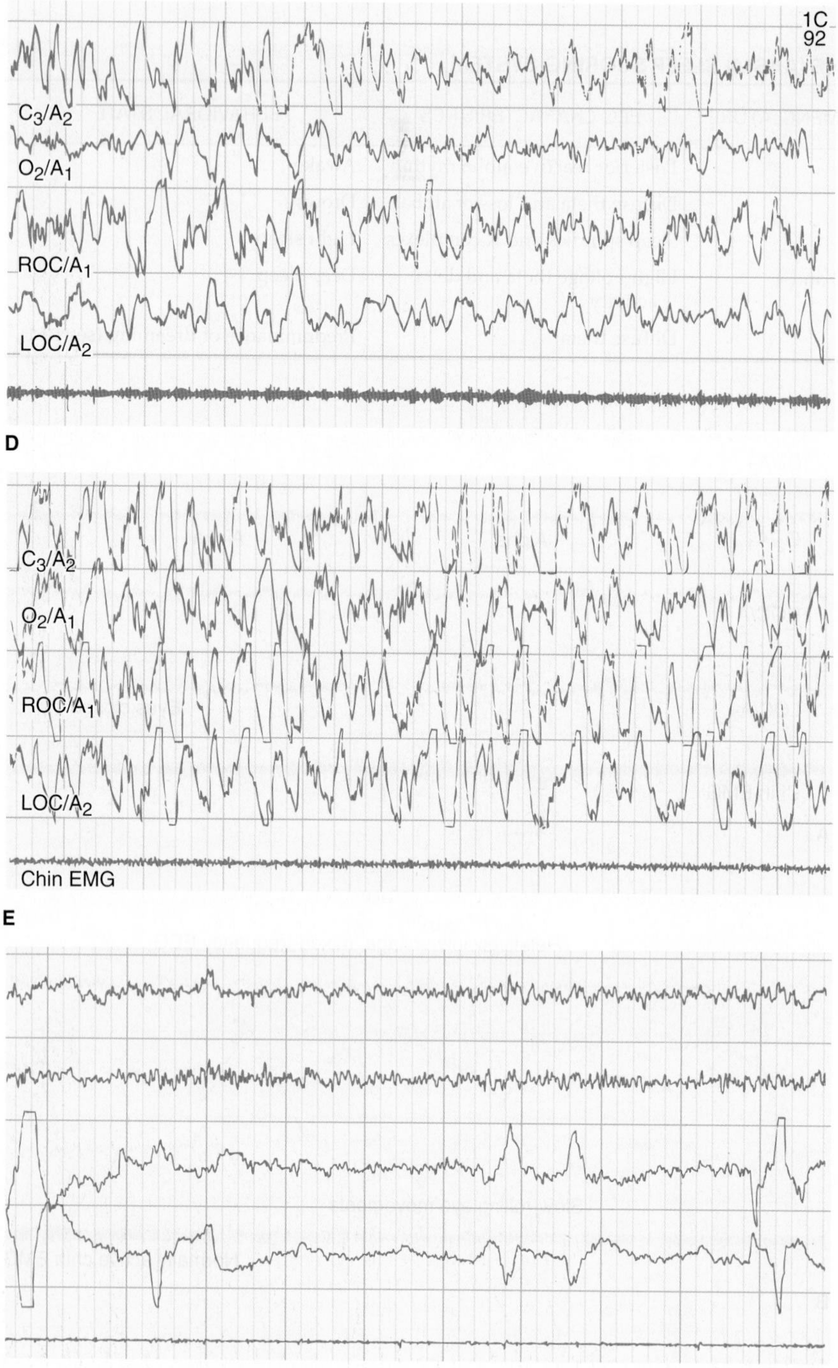

Figure 19-2. *(Continued)*

of stage N3 sleep, the first REM period occurs, usually heralded briefly by a transient increase in body movements and a shift in the EEG pattern from that of stage N3 to stage N2. This NREM–REM cycle is repeated at about the same interval four to six times during the night, depending on the total duration of sleep. The first REM period may be brief; the later cycles have less stage N3 sleep or none at all. In the latter portion of a night's sleep, the cycles consist essentially of two alternating stages—REM sleep and stage N2 (spindle–K-complex) sleep. The relation of dreaming to these sleep stages is described further on.

Newborn full-term infants spend approximately 50 percent of their sleep in the REM stage (although their EEG and eye movements differ from those of adults). The newborn sleep cycle lasts about 60 min (50 percent REM, 50 percent NREM, generally alternating through a 3- to 4-h interfeeding period); with age, the sleep cycle lengthens to 90 to 100 min. Approximately 20 to 25 percent of total sleep time in young adults is spent in REM sleep,

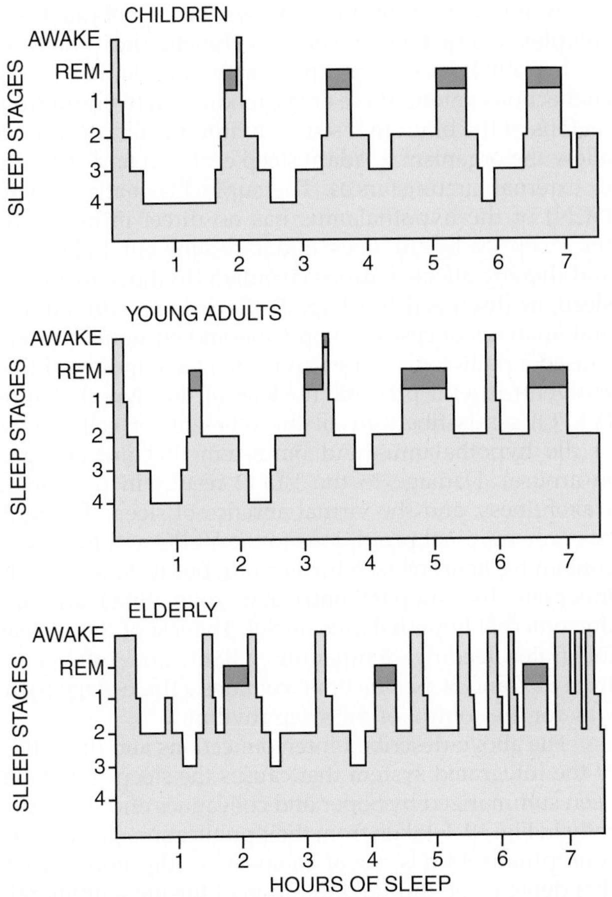

Figure 19-3. Sleep architecture, or sleep cycles. REM sleep (*darkened areas*) occurs cyclically throughout the night at intervals of approximately 90 min in all age groups. REM sleep shows little variation in the different age groups, whereas stage 4 sleep decreases with age. Stages 3 and 4 are now considered N3. (Redrawn by permission from Kales, Kales, and Soldatos.)

3 to 5 percent in stage N1, 50 to 60 percent in stage N2, and 10 to 20 percent in stage N3 combined. The amount of sleep in N3 decreases with age, and persons older than 70 years of age have virtually no very deep slow-wave sleep (Fig. 19-3). The 90- to 100-min cycle is fairly stable in any one person and is believed to continue to operate to a less-perceptible degree during wakefulness in relation to a number of other cyclic phenomena, such as core body temperature, gastric motility, hunger, urinary output, alertness, and capacity for cognitive activity.

Physiologic Changes and Dreaming in NREM and REM Sleep

A comparison of the physiologic changes in NREM and REM sleep is of interest. The change in the EEG pattern has already been indicated. Cortical neurons tend to discharge in synchronized bursts during NREM sleep and in nonsynchronized bursts during wakefulness. In REM sleep, the EEG pattern is generally asynchronous as well. Much of the night's complex visual dreaming has been found to occur in the REM period, with the qualifications noted below, and dreams are recalled most consistently if the subject is awakened during this time. It is important to point out, however, that dreaming activity is reported by subjects awakened from NREM sleep, although less consistently. Because the time spent in NREM is so much greater than that in REM, approximately 20 percent of dreaming occurs outside of REM periods but REM sleep nonetheless maintains a special relationship to dreaming.

Subjects are easily aroused from REM sleep, but arousing a person during stage N3 is more difficult; full arousal may take minutes or more, during which time the subject may be slightly disoriented and confused (for which reason, physicians called at night should, if possible, avoid making complex medical decisions during this brief period).

As mentioned above, tonic muscle activity is minimal during REM sleep, although small twitches in facial and digital muscles (hand and foot) can still be detected. Eye movements of REM sleep are conjugate and occur in all directions (horizontal more than vertical). They can be appreciated through the closed eyelids. Gross body movements occur every 15 min or so in all stages of sleep but are maximal in the transition between REM and NREM sleep, at which time the sleeping person changes position, usually from side to side (most people sleep on their sides).

On closer study, REM sleep has been found to have phasic and tonic components. In addition to the rapid eye movements, phasic phenomena include activation of the sympathetic nervous system with attendant alternate dilatation and constriction of the pupils and fluctuation of the blood pressure, heart rate, and respiration. The phasic activities are related to bursts of neuronal activity in the pontine, vestibular, and median raphe nuclei and are conducted through the corticobulbar and corticospinal tracts. In the nonphasic periods of REM sleep, alpha and gamma spinal neurons are inhibited, the H responses diminish (see Chap. 45), and the tendon and postural and flexor reflexes diminish or are abolished. This flaccidity and atonia, which are prominent in the abdominal, upper airway, and intercostal muscles, may compromise breathing during REM sleep and pose a threat to infants with respiratory difficulty and to adults who are obese or have respiratory difficulty as a result of kyphoscoliosis, muscular dystrophy, hypoplastic or otherwise compromised airways, and neuromuscular paralyses (see Guilleminault and Dement).

It has long been known that body temperature falls slightly during sleep; however, if sleep does not occur, there is still a drop in body temperature as part of the circadian (24-h) temperature pattern. This reduction in temperature is also independent of the 24-h recumbency–ambulatory cycle. During sleep, the decline in temperature occurs mainly during the NREM period, and the same is true of the heartbeat and respiration, both of which become slow and more regular in this period. Cerebral blood flow and oxygen consumption in muscle diminish during NREM sleep and increase during REM sleep. Also, cerebral blood flow and metabolism are markedly reduced across the entire brain during deep

NREM sleep; however, during REM sleep, metabolism and blood flow are restored to the levels of the waking state (Madsen and Vorstrup). Presumably, as a result of increased blood flow, intracranial pressure rises during REM sleep.

Urine excretion decreases during sleep and the absolute quantity of sodium and potassium that is eliminated also decreases; however, urine specific gravity and osmolality increase, presumably because of increased antidiuretic hormone excretion, and reabsorption of water. Parasympathetic outflow is activated periodically in REM sleep; sympathetic activity is suppressed. It has also been recognized that there is a drop in blood pressure and heart rate during slow-wave sleep and the loss of this dip, for example as a result of sleep apnea, has been associated with daytime hypertension and increased risk for cardiovascular events. As mentioned, in phasic REM sleep, there is an increase in sympathetic tone. Breathing is more irregular, and heart rate and blood pressure fluctuate. Penile erections appear periodically, usually during REM periods.

A number of endocrine changes also have a regular relationship to the sleep–wake cycle. During the first 2 h of sleep, there is a surge of growth hormone secretion, mainly during slow-wave sleep. In men, there tends to be a single peak, whereas women have a multiple episodes of increased secretion. This feature persists through middle and late adult life and then disappears. The secretion of cortisol and particularly of thyroid-stimulating hormone peaks at the onset of sleep. High concentrations of cortisol are also characteristically found on awakening. Melatonin, elaborated by the pineal gland, is produced at night and ceases upon retinal stimulation by sunlight (see Chap. 27). Prolactin secretion increases during the night in both men and women, the highest plasma concentrations being found soon after the onset of sleep. Secretion of prolactin is influenced by sleep stages. Circadian mechanisms and the stages of sleep alter testosterone secretion and are therefore disrupted by sleep disorders, especially in younger individuals. Also, an increased sleep-associated secretion of luteinizing hormone occurs in pubertal boys and girls.

Neurophysiology of Sleep and Dreaming

Hobson originally proposed that the basic oscillation of the sleep cycle is the result of reciprocal interaction of excitatory and inhibitory neurotransmitters. Single-cell recordings from the pontine reticular formation suggest that there are two interconnected neuronal populations whose levels of activity fluctuate periodically and reciprocally. During wakefulness, according to this conceptualization, the activity of aminergic (inhibitory) neurons is high; because of this inhibition, the activity of the cholinergic neurons is low. During NREM sleep, aminergic inhibition gradually declines and cholinergic excitation increases; REM sleep occurs when the shift is complete. It is likely that these monoaminergic neuronal circuits are modulated by input from hypocretin (also called orexin)-secreting neurons of the hypothalamus, but the details of this control system are not entirely known. Hypocretin, a peptide that assumes great importance in the pathophysiology of narcolepsy, is discussed further on.

A refinement of these views has elaborated the complex interaction of specially functioning nuclei in the hypothalamus, pons, and basal forebrain. Reciprocal connections among these areas, modulated by input from regions of the brain that sense environmental conditions, allow the organism to adapt sleep cycles to its needs and to external circumstances. The suprachiasmatic nucleus (SCN) of the hypothalamus has no direct influence on the sleep cycle but does integrate ambient light cues, and thereby affects various circadian rhythms, including sleep, as discussed in Chap. 27. Experiments in animals and analyses of cases of von Economo encephalitis (that caused a pathologic sleep syndrome) have indicated that the ventrolateral preoptic nucleus of the hypothalamus (VLPO) sends fibers to all the other major cell groups of the hypothalamus and brainstem that are engaged in arousal. Damage to the VLPO results in pathologic wakefulness, and the virtual absence of sleep. The SCN has only minimal projections to the VLPO and to orexin-containing neurons (see further on), but it does strongly innervate the subparaventricular zone (SPZ) and the dorsomedial hypothalamic nuclei. The last of these areas integrates feeding, temperature, light, and other cues from SPZ and SCN. The brain contains a three-stage pathway for the control of the sleep rhythm.

The above-described interconnections and the action of the integrated system that causes the sleep state have been summarized by Saper and colleagues and schematically in Fig. 19-4, taken from their publication. The current conceptualization is one of an unstable "flip-flop" switch that depends on mutual inhibition of the monoaminergic system and the VLPO. The state of the switch is indirectly stabilized by the orexin neurons. In this model, the awake state is maintained by monoaminergic activity (locus ceruleus, tuberomammillary nucleus [TMN], and the raphe nuclei) that inhibits the VLPO. Sleep occurs when the VLPO is activated, which reciprocally removes the tonic inhibitory action of the monoaminergic system. The orexin neurons act through the monoaminergic system as a stabilizing influence to prevent rapid transitions from one state to the other.

Apart from the overall diurnal sleep cycle, evidence from animal studies suggests that the physiologic mechanisms and transitions between NREM and REM sleep are governed by the pontine reticular formation and are influenced by acetylcholine. *Cholinergic neurons* are found in two major loci in the parabrachial region of the dorsolateral pontine tegmentum—in the pedunculopontine group of nuclei and the lateral dorsal tegmental group. The cholinergic cell groups project rostrally, but the precise anatomy of this projection system has not been defined. Cells from these groups make up parts of the ascending reticular activating system.

Despite the heuristic value of Hobson's reciprocal interaction hypothesis, some of its features remain controversial. Although it is generally agreed that cholinergic mechanisms selectively promote REM sleep, and its components—rapid eye movements, absence of activity in the antigravity muscles (i.e., atonia), and desynchronized EEG—the role of amines has been more difficult to establish. Thus, lesions of the locus ceruleus and raphe

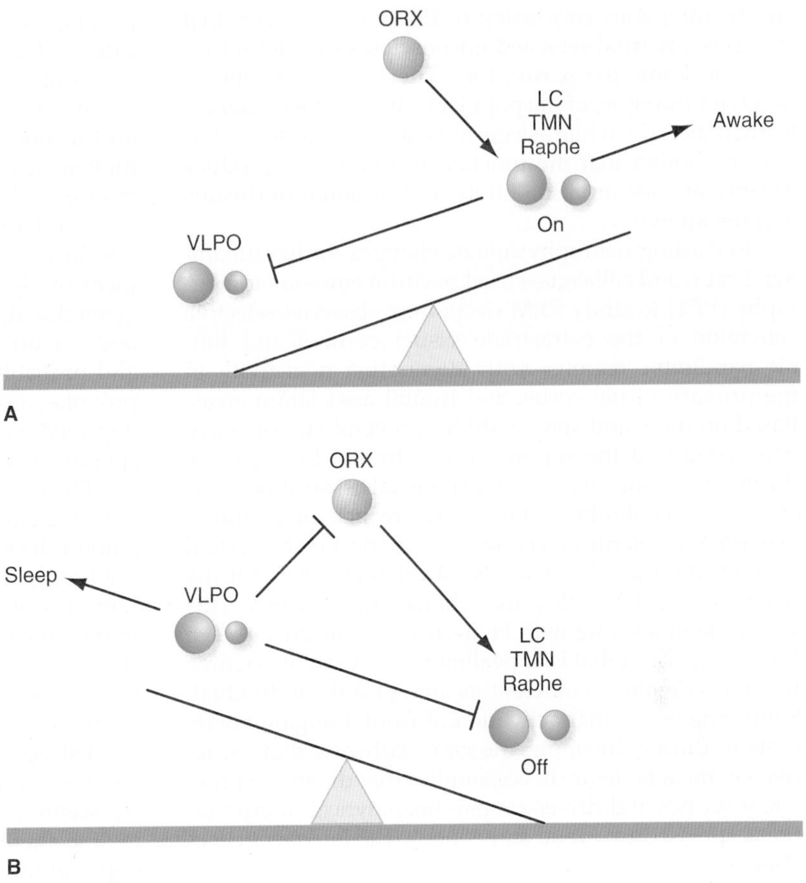

Figure 19-4. Schematic representation of the "flipflop" mechanism of transition between sleep and waking, which is determined by the state of activity of the ventrolateral preoptic nucleus (VLPO). *A.* During wakefulness, the monoaminergic nuclei (*LC*, locus ceruleus; *TMN*, tuberomammillary nucleus; raphe nuclei) inhibit the VLPO, thereby relieving the inhibition of the monoaminergic cells, and that of the orexin (*ORX*) neurons. Because the VLPO neurons do not have orexin receptors, orexin serves to reinforce the monoaminergic tone, rather than directly inhibiting the VLPO. *B.* During sleep, firing of VLPO neurons inhibits the monoaminergic cell groups, thereby relieving their own inhibition. This inhibits the orexin neurons, further preventing monoaminergic activation that might interrupt sleep. The mutual inhibition between the VLPO and the monoaminergic cell groups forms a flip-flop switch, which produces sharp transitions in state, but is relatively unstable. The addition of the orexin neurons stabilizes the switch. (Reproduced with permission from Saper, Scammell, and Lu.)

nuclei, which contain neurons rich in norepinephrine, do not greatly alter REM sleep. Nevertheless, a considerable body of pharmacologic data suggests that a decrease in monoamines causes an increase in REM activity and vice versa. Insofar as the bulk of cholinergic and aminergic neurons are found in the pedunculopontine group of nuclei, Shiromani and colleagues have suggested that interaction between these neurons occurs in the region of the pedunculopontine nuclei rather than in the medial pontine reticular formation, as suggested by Hobson and associates.

Solms (1995, 1996) and others have questioned the traditional view that dreaming and REM sleep are obligately or even closely connected and has presented an alternative model. Among patients with cerebral lesions that eliminate or disrupt REM sleep, he cites several cases in which dreaming was retained. Conversely, in 9 of his patients with basal forebrain (frontal) lesions, dreaming was lost, at least for a time, while REM periods remained undisturbed through the night. This same observation had been made in patients who had prefrontal leukotomies. Solms has proposed that the dopaminergic systems in the basal forebrain areas elicit or modulate dreaming. This view is supported by reports of diminished dreaming in patients being treated with dopaminergic blockers and the enhancement of dreaming reported by patients taking L-dopa or dopamine agonsits. Notable in this regard is the fact that major intracortical dopaminergic pathways originate in the frontal lobes.

In regard to the neurophysiology of the EEG and sleep rhythms, much has been gleaned from intracellular recordings in animals. As with the earlier-described anatomic and neurochemical data, the degree to which similar electrophysiologic changes are reflected in humans is not known. Most of the integrated rhythms of sleep that are recorded at the surface of the brain, including the background activity of slow-wave sleep and the faster and more synchronized sleep spindles and vertex waves, have their origins in the thalamus. Steriade and colleagues have performed a substantial amount of the modern work in this area and summarize it in their review. They make clear that these complex EEG rhythms, while apparent in nascent form in certain isolated neurons, are oscillations that arise from integrated ensembles of cells, with the thalamus as a nexus. It is evident that there is as yet no agreement concerning the integration of all these brainstem and thalamic–hypothalamic mechanisms in the production of sleep or of dreams.

The Function of Sleep and Dreams

These questions have been pondered endlessly by physiologists and psychiatrists (and philosophers). Parkes has reviewed the main theories—body restitution, facilitation of motor function, consolidation of learning and memory—and tends to agree with the ungrammatical but unambiguous conclusion of Popper and Eccles that "Sleep is a natural repeated unconsciousness that we do not even know the reason for." There is no convincing proof, for example, of the popular notion that we stabilize learned material while asleep, nor can one logically entertain the notion that the function of sleep is to produce dreams, at least until the utility and meaning of dreams become known.

Regarding neurophysiologic changes during dreaming, Braun and colleagues used positron emission tomography (PET) to study REM sleep; they observed selective activation of the extrastriate visual cortices and limbic–paralimbic regions, with attenuation of activity in the primary visual cortex and frontal association areas. Based on these and similar studies, several authors have speculated that the suppression of frontal lobe activity during dreaming, at a time when visual association areas and their paralimbic connections are activated, might explain the uncritical acceptance of the bizarre visual content, the disordered temporal relationships, and the heightened emotionality that characterize dreams. This would be in keeping with Hobson's view of dreams as a form of delirium that is appealing to us. As an alternative that links dreams to inherent meaning for the individual, Solms suggested that activation of frontal dopaminergic systems during dreaming, the same pathways that participate in most biologic drives, implies that dreams express latent wishes and drives—a psychoanalytical interpretation expressed by Freud in his book *The Interpretation of Dreams*.

The Effects of Sleep Deprivation

Deprived of sleep, experimental animals will die within a few weeks, no matter how well they are fed, watered, and housed (Rechtschaffen et al), but whether a similar degree of sleep deprivation leads to death in humans is unknown. Nevertheless, humans beings deprived of sleep do suffer a variety of very unpleasant symptoms quite distinct from the effects of the usual types of insomnia.

Despite many studies of the deleterious emotional and cognitive effects of sleeplessness, we still know little about them. If deprived of sleep (NREM and REM) for periods of 60 to 200 h, human beings experience increasing sleepiness, fatigue, irritability, and difficulty in concentration. Performance of skilled motor activities also deteriorates; if the tasks are of short duration and slow pace, the subject can manage them, but if speed and perseverance are demanded, he cannot. Self-care is neglected, incentive to work wanes, sustained thought and action are interrupted by lapses of attention, judgment is impaired, and the subject becomes decreasingly inclined to communicate. With sustained deprivation, sleepiness becomes increasingly more intense, momentary periods of sleep ("microsleep") become more intrusive, and the tendency to all types of accidents becomes more marked. Eventually, subjects fail to perceive inner and external experiences accurately and to maintain their orientation. Illusions and hallucinations, mainly visual and tactile ones, intrude into consciousness and become more persistent as the period of sleeplessness is prolonged. This may be a component of the decompensation of individuals with bipolar psychiatric disease, sometimes triggering manic episodes.

Neurologic signs of sleep deprivation include a mild and inconstant nystagmus, impairment of saccadic eye movements, loss of accommodation, exophoria, a slight tremor of the hands, ptosis of the eyelids, expressionless face, and thickness of speech, with mispronunciations, and incorrect choice of words. The EEG shows a decrement of alpha waves, and closing of the eyes no longer generates alpha activity. The seizure threshold is reduced, and seizure foci in the EEG may be activated. Rarely and probably only in predisposed persons, loss of sleep provokes a psychotic episode (2 to 3 percent of 350 sleep-deprived patients studied by Tyler); however, many sleep specialists dispute the production of psychosis.

During recovery from prolonged sleep deprivation, the amount of sleep obtained is never equal to the amount lost. This is probably a result of the intrusion of brief sleep periods during the waking state and represents a sizable amount of time if summated (it is virtually impossible to deprive a human being or animal totally of sleep). When falling asleep after a long period of deprivation, the subject rapidly enters N3 (NREM) sleep, which continues for several hours at the expense of N2 and REM sleep. But by the second recovery night, REM sleep rebounds and exceeds that of the predeprivation period. N3 seems to be the most important sleep stage in restoring the altered functions that result from prolonged sleep deprivation.

The effects of differential REM sleep deprivation are more difficult to interpret than the effects of total or near-total deprivation. Some subjects in whom REM sleep is prevented night after night show an increasing tendency to hyperactivity, emotional lability, and impulsivity—a state that has been compared to the heightened activity, excessive appetite, and hypersexuality of animals deprived of REM sleep. However, in humans, monoamine inhibitors are able to completely suppress REM sleep for months to years without obvious harm. Differential deprivation of NREM sleep (N3) leads, instead, to hyporesponsiveness and excessive daytime sleepiness as noted.

Because the need for sleep varies considerably from person to person, it is difficult to decide what constitutes sleep deprivation. Certain individuals apparently function well on 4 h or even less of sleep per 24-h period, and others, who sleep long hours, claim not to obtain maximum benefit from it.

SLEEP DISORDERS

Insomnia

The term *insomnia* signifies a chronic inability to sleep despite adequate opportunity to do so; it is used popularly to indicate any impairment in the duration, depth, or restorative properties of sleep. There may be difficulty in falling asleep or remaining asleep, awakening may come too early, or there may be a combination of these complaints. Precision as to what constitutes pathologic insomnia is impossible at the present time because of our uncertainty as to the exact amounts of sleep required, and the role of sleep in the economy of the human body. All that can be said is that some form of sleeplessness is a frequent complaint (20 to 40 percent of the population) and is more prominent in the elderly and in women. Only a small proportion of persons who perceive their sleep to be inadequate seek professional help or use sleeping pills, according to Mellinger and colleagues.

Two general classes of insomnia can be recognized—one in which there appears to be a primary abnormality of the normal sleep mechanism, and another in which the sleep disturbance is secondary to, or perhaps more accurately comorbid with, a medical or psychologic disorder. Polysomnographic studies have defined yet another subgroup who actually sleep enough, but who perceive their sleep time to be shortened or disrupted ("paradoxical insomnia").

Primary Insomnia

This term is reserved for the condition in which nocturnal sleep is disturbed for prolonged periods and none of the symptoms of anxiety, depression, pain, or other psychiatric or medical diseases can be invoked to explain the sleep disturbance. In some patients, like those described by Hauri and Olmstead, the disorder is lifelong. Unlike the rare individuals who seem to be satisfied with 4 h or even less of sleep a night, insomniacs suffer the effects of partial sleep deprivation and resort to medications, alcohol, and their lives come to revolve around sleep to such an extent that they have been called "sleep pedants" or "sleep hypochondriacs." Although statements on the quantity and quality of sleep given by insomniacs are often not to be taken as entirely valid, Rechtschaffen and Monroe have confirmed that most of them do, indeed, sleep for shorter periods, move and awaken more often, spend less time in N3 sleep than normal persons, and show a heightened physiologic arousal. Personality inventories have disclosed a high incidence of psychologic disturbances in this group, but whether these are cause or effect is not clear.

Furthermore, a category of "conditioned', or "psychophysiological" insomnia has been denominated, in which a situational trigger for insomnia has ceased, but the sleep disorder persists. Although insomniacs, regardless of the cause, tend to exaggerate the amount of sleep lost, primary insomnia should be recognized as an entity and not passed off as a neurotic quirk.

Secondary Insomnia

This common type of insomnia, which is often transitory, can be ascribed to pain or some other recognizable bodily disorder, such as drug or alcohol abuse or, most commonly, to anxiety, worry, or depression. Of the medical disorders conducive to abnormal wakefulness, certain ones stand out—pain in the joints or in the spine, abdominal discomfort from peptic ulcer and carcinoma, pulmonary and cardiovascular insufficiency, and the nocturia engendered by prostatism. The "restless legs" syndrome and periodic leg movements of sleep are not considered in this category and have their own physiology, phenomenology, and treatment.

Restless Legs Syndrome, Periodic Leg Movements of Sleep, and Related Disorders

The disorder known as the *restless legs syndrome* may regularly delay the onset of sleep and usually occurs in its early stages. Ekbom called it asthenia crurum paresthetica and also, anxietas tibiarum. This disorder is surprisingly prevalent, affecting more than 2 percent of the population. The patient may complain of unpleasant aching and drawing sensations in the calves and thighs, often associated with creeping or crawling feelings; other descriptions have included "worms," "internal itch," and "coldness," and the legs may feel tired, heavy, and weak. The symptoms are provoked by rest, and rapidly, but temporarily, relieved by moving the legs. An urge to move the legs can be suppressed voluntarily for a brief period but is ultimately irresistible. Moving the limbs alleviates the sensation briefly. It is interesting that a small proportion of patients have similar symptoms in the arms after many years of symptoms. There may be variants of nocturnal restlessness in other parts of the body such as the abdomen, as suggested by Pérez-Díaz and colleagues. Their patients described an unpleasant abdominal musculature restlessness that required movement for relief and was eliminated with dopamine agonists.

Fatigue worsens restless legs syndrome, and there is a tendency for it to be worse in warm weather. In a few patients, mainly older ones with a severe form of the nighttime disorder, these movements and an associated myoclonus spill over into wakefulness and are accompanied by restlessness, foot spasms, foot stamping, body rocking, and marching that are only partly under voluntary control. The daytime phenomena may require several medications used simultaneously for control.

The syndrome is idiopathic and persists for years. Iron-deficiency anemia and low ferritin levels are associated with the syndrome in many instances, as is thyroid disease, pregnancy, and certain drugs, such as antidepressants and antihistamines. Occasionally, it is a prelude to a peripheral neuropathy, particularly in relation to uremia. Also, reduced levels of iron in the cerebrospinal fluid (CSF) have been found with restless legs syndrome and with periodic limb movements of sleep (see below). The basis for this relationship is not well defined, but it makes it advisable to check for reduced iron stores and anemia in most patients. One hypothesis is that a disturbance of iron storage in the basal ganglia causes a decrement in dopamine binding by dopamine receptors and transporters, as has been described in studies using PET and single-photon emission tomography (SPECT) scans. Another potential relationship, unproved, is that iron is a cofactor for the enzyme, tyrosine hydroxylase, which is required to produce dopamine.

A closely related disturbance is *periodic leg movements of sleep*. Like the restless legs syndrome, it may result in sleep deprivation and daytime somnolence or, more often, in disturbance of a bed partner. However, the diagnosis of periodic leg movements depends on finding them during polysomnographic recordings, whereas restless leg syndrome is identified on clinical grounds. Originally described as "nocturnal myoclonus," periodic leg movements are slower than myoclonic jerks. They consist of a series of repetitive movements of the feet and legs occurring every 20 to 90 s for several minutes to an hour; mainly the anterior tibialis is involved, with dorsiflexion of the feet and big toes, sometimes followed by flexion of the hip and knee. The movements are similar to the triple-flexion (Babinski) response, which can be elicited in normal sleeping persons. These movements produce frequent microarousals or, if severe and periodic, full arousals. The patient, usually unaware of these sleep-related movements at the time they occur, is told of them by a bed mate or suspects their occurrence from the disarray of the bedclothes. Periodic leg movement is closely associated with the restless legs syndrome and many sleep specialists consider it an integral part of the syndrome, but it also occurs independently with narcolepsy, sleep apnea, following the use of tricyclic and serotonin reuptake inhibiting antidepressants, L-dopa, and withdrawal from anticonvulsants and sedative-hypnotic drugs. Approximately eighty percent of individuals with restless leg syndrome will display periodic leg movements, but the opposite is not the case, as only twenty to thirty percent of patients with periodic leg movements have restless leg syndrome.

A seminal genetic finding by Stefansson and colleagues derived from several populations, including the homogenous Icelandic, is that a nucleotide variant in a short segment of chromosome 6p is associated with periodic leg movements of sleep. This was found to hold in those with and without restless legs syndrome. If nothing else, as pointed out by the authors, this establishes that periodic limb movements are a distinct entity as defined in the era of genomics. The biologic significance and frequency in other populations of this variant is not yet known. Nonetheless, we continue to be impressed at the frequent cooccurrence of the two conditions and several shared underlying conditions such as iron deficiency, and treatments that are effective in both.

Treatment

A search for iron deficiency, and its correction if present, is indicated in almost all cases. A large number of symptomatic medications have proved helpful in the treatment of both the restless legs syndrome and periodic leg movements. As a first choice, many practitioners favor treatment with dopamine agonists such as pramipexole (0.25 to 0.75 mg) or ropinirole (0.5 to 1.5 mg), either one taken 1.5 to 2 h before bedtime. Long-acting combinations of L-dopa/carbidopa (12.5/50 or 25/100 mg dose) taken at bedtime have also been successful, but L-dopa, and sometimes the dopamine agonists, causes some patients to develop the movements earlier, i.e., in the daytime, which become more intense and spread to other body parts. A longer acting dopamine agonist, rotigotine patch is available to treat patients who have this augmentation phenomenon. The latter is also helpful for periodic leg movements.

A major problem, recently recognized, is one of "augmentation," or enhancement of the restless leg syndrome with the long-term use of this class of drugs. This is less prominent with some of the other numerous drugs that have been effective including gabapentin, pregabalin, clonazepam (0.5 to 2.0 mg), temazepam (30 mg), taken 30 min before retiring and extended release gabapentin which are available to minimize the augmentation phenomenon. Other drugs—e.g., baclofen, opioids, carbamazepine seem to be helpful in certain patients, but they are infrequently required. The lengthy list of medications that have been effective is given in Earley's review. It is sometimes useful to give a medication in 2 divided doses, the first early in the evening, and the second just before sleep or, in severe cases, during the night by setting an alarm clock before the anticipated time of symptoms.

Other Causes of Secondary Insomnia

Among the secondary insomnias, those caused by some type of *psychologic disturbance* are particularly common. Domestic or business worries may keep the patient's mind in turmoil (situational insomnia). A strange bed or unfamiliar surroundings may prevent drowsiness and sleep. Under these circumstances, the main difficulty is in falling asleep, with a tendency to sleep late in the morning. These facts emphasize that conditioning and environmental factors (social and learned) are normally involved in readying the mind and body for sleep.

Illnesses in which anxiety and fear are prominent symptoms also result in difficulty in falling asleep and in light, fitful, or intermittent sleep. Disturbing dreams are frequent in these situations and may awaken the patient. Exceptionally, a patient may even try to stay awake in order to avoid them. In contrast, *depressive illness* produces early morning waking and inability to return to sleep; the quantity of sleep is reduced, and nocturnal motility is increased. REM sleep in depression, although not always reduced, comes earlier in the night. If anxiety is combined with depression, there is a tendency for both the above patterns to be observed. Yet another common pattern of disturbed sleep can be discerned in individuals who are under great tension and worry or are overworked and tired out. These people sink into bed and sleep through sheer exhaustion, but they awaken early with their worries and are unable to get back to sleep.

Chronic and even short-term use of alcohol, barbiturates, and certain nonbarbiturate sedative-hypnotic drugs markedly reduces REM sleep as well as stages 3 and 4 of NREM sleep (N3). Following withdrawal of these drugs, there is a rapid and marked increase of REM sleep, sometimes with vivid dreams and nightmares. "Rebound insomnia," a worsening of sleep compared with pretreatment levels, has also been reported upon discontinuation of short-half-life benzodiazepine hypnotics, notably triazolam (Gillin et al) and including the newer sleep agents mentioned below. Furthermore, a form of drug-withdrawal or rebound insomnia may actually occur during the same night in which the drug is administered. The drug produces its hypnotic effect in the first half of the night and a worsening of sleep during the latter half of the night, as the effects of the drug wear off; the patient and the physician may be misled into thinking that these latter symptoms require more of the hypnotic drug or a different one. Alcohol taken in the evening acts in the same way. Rebound insomnia must be distinguished from the early morning awakening that accompanies anxiety and depressive states.

A wide variety of other pharmacologic agents may give rise to sporadic or persistent disturbances of sleep. Caffeine-containing beverages, corticosteroids, bronchodilators, central adrenergic-blocking agents, amphetamines, certain "activating" antidepressants such as fluoxetine, and cigarettes are the most common offenders. Others are listed in the extensive review of Kupfer and Reynolds.

Acroparesthesias, a predominantly nocturnal tingling and numbness of the fingers and palms caused by tight carpal ligaments (carpal tunnel syndrome), may awaken the patient at night (see further on, under "Sleep Palsies and Acroparesthesias"). *Cluster headaches* characteristically awaken the patient within 1 to 2 h after falling asleep (see Chap. 10 for a fuller discussion). In a few patients, cluster headaches occur only during or immediately after the REM period.

The sleep rhythm is totally deranged in acute confusional states and especially in delirium, and the patient may doze for only short periods, both day and night, the total amount and depth of sleep in a 24-h period being reduced. Frightening hallucinations may prevent sleep. The senile patient tends to catnap during the day and to remain alert for progressively longer periods during the night, until sleep is obtained in a series of short naps throughout the 24 h; the total amount of sleep may be increased or decreased.

Treatment of Insomnia

In general, a sedative-hypnotic drug for the management of insomnia should be prescribed only as a short-term aid during an illness or some unusual circumstance, i.e., for acute insomnia. For patients who have difficulty falling asleep, a quick-acting, fairly rapidly metabolized hypnotic is useful. The most commonly used medications are the benzodiazepine receptor agonists, which act on the gamma-aminobutyric acid (GABA)-A receptor complex. In the past, benzodiazepines were popular but these have been replaced by newer nonbenzodiazepine receptor agonists with shorter half-lives and fewer side effects (e.g., zolpidem, zaleplon, and eszopiclone). Patients who do not respond to these medications may be given an intermediate-duration benzodiazepine such as temazepam. Hypnotic use is inadvisable during pregnancy and should be used cautiously in patients with alcoholism or advanced renal, hepatic, or pulmonary disease, and should be avoided in patients with sleep apnea syndrome.

Melatonin (3 to 12 mg) has reportedly been as effective as the sedative-hypnotics and may cause fewer short-term side effects, but both of these statements are difficult to confirm. Melatonin has a short half-life, and it has only weak hypnotic effect. Therefore, for sleep rhythm disturbances, it is ideally taken three to four hours before sleep time. Amitriptyline (25 to 50 mg at bedtime) appears to be a sleep-enhancing drug even in those who are not anxious or depressed. Tolerance develops to the drug, and there are morning side effects so the drug may find its best use in patients who are taking it for alternative reasons such as headache or depression. Some practitioners indicate that it may also worsen restless leg or periodic leg movement disorders. When pain is a factor in insomnia, the sedative may be combined with a suitable analgesic. Nonprescription drugs containing diphenhydramine (Benadryl), valerian, or doxylamine, which are minimally or not at all effective in inducing sleep, may impair the quality of sleep and lead to drowsiness the following morning.

The chronic insomniac who has no other symptoms should be discouraged from using sedative drugs. The solution of this problem is rarely to be found in medication. One should search out and correct, if possible, any underlying situational or psychologic difficulty, using medication only as a temporary measure. Patients should be encouraged to regularize their daily schedules, including their bedtimes, and to be physically active during the day but to avoid strenuous physical and mental activity before bedtime. It has been suggested that illumination from broad-spectrum light (television) in the late evening is detrimental. Dietary excesses must be corrected, and all nonessential medications interdicted. Coffee and alcohol should be avoided at night, if not throughout the day. A number of simple behavioral modifications may be useful, such as using the bedroom only for sleeping, arising at the same time each morning regardless of the duration of sleep, avoiding daytime naps, and limiting the time spent in bed strictly to the duration of sleep. A helpful approach is to lessen the patient's concern about sleeplessness by pointing out that he will always get as much sleep as needed and that there is pleasure to be derived from staying awake and reading, or viewing a movie.

Disorders of Sleep Related to Neurologic Disease

Many neurologic conditions seriously derange the total amount and patterns of sleep (see Culebras). Lesions in the upper pons, near the locus ceruleus, are particularly prone to do so. Markand and Dyken have described the most substantial of these, pontine infarction with involvement of the tegmental raphe nuclei. The clinical abnormality took the form of diminished NREM sleep and near abolition of REM sleep lasting for weeks or months. Bilateral lacunar infarctions in the pontine tegmentum, demonstrable by MRI, also appear to be the basis of some instances of the so-called REM sleep behavior disorder (Culebras and Moore) described further on with the other parasomnias. Bilateral paramedian thalamic infarctions are a potent cause of hypersomnia, the result of disruption of both arousal mechanisms and NREM sleep (Bassetti et al).

Medullary lesions may affect sleep by altering automatic ventilation; the most extreme examples occur with bilateral tegmental lesions that may completely abolish breathing during sleep ("Ondine's curse," as described in Chap. 26). Lesser degrees of tegmental damage—as might occur with Chiari malformations, unilateral medullary infarction, syringobulbia, or poliomyelitis—may cause sleep apnea, and daytime drowsiness. Patients with large hemispheric strokes may also be left with daytime lethargy on the basis of inversion of sleep–wake rhythm. Certain instances of mesencephalic infarction that are characterized by vivid visual hallucinations (peduncular hallucinosis) may be associated with disruption of sleep.

von Economo encephalitis, now an extinct illness, was usually associated with a hypersomnolent state but caused persistent insomnia in some instances. The latter was related to a predominance of lesions in the anterior hypothalamus and basal frontal lobes, in distinction to hypersomnia, which was related to lesions mainly in dorsal hypothalamus and subthalamus. This subject and other forms of hypersomnia are elaborated further on under "Pathologic Excessive Sleep (Hypersomnia)."

A remarkable illness, termed *fatal familial insomnia*, was initially described by Lugaresi and colleagues. This disorder, with onset in middle age and a clinical course of 7 to 36 months, is characterized by a virtual incapacity to sleep and to generate EEG sleep patterns. The cerebral changes consist mainly of profound neuronal loss in the anterior or anteroventral, and mediodorsal thalamic nuclei. These cases apparently represent a usually familial form of prion disease similar to diseases that cause subacute spongiform encephalopathy and Gerstmann-Sträussler-Scheinker disease (see Chap. 33). Interestingly, the alcoholic form of the Korsakoff amnesic state, associated with less severe lesions in the same thalamic nuclei, is also characterized by a sleep disturbance, taking the form of an increased frequency of intermittent periods of wakefulness (Martin et al). When carefully sought, similar sleep–wake disturbances have been found in sporadic Creutzfeldt-Jakob-prion disease (Landolt et al).

Major *head injury* is an important cause of sleep disturbance. The abnormalities, which may persist for months or years, consist mainly of a decrease in stages 1 and 2 sleep, and less than the expected amounts of REM sleep and dreaming. Some patients in the persistent vegetative state show a cycle of changes in the EEG, progressing from a picture of abortive spindles and K complexes with cyclic alterations in respiration and pupil size to the acquisition of a more normally structured sleep activity. This sequence usually presages the change from a state of coma to one of minimally conscious state (Chap. 17). Organized sleep activity is absent in virtually all types of coma that are the result of anatomic damage to the brain. An exception, albeit a semantic one, occurs in the unusual condition known as "spindle coma," in which persistent coma, and the electrographic features of sleep coexist. This particular combination of events has been described after head trauma, and rarely, in association with profound metabolic encephalopathies. Despite what appears to be a genuine comatose state (not simply hypersomnolence) from a lesion of the reticular-activating system, the EEG displays frequent spindle activity and vertex waves, attesting to the integrity of thalamocortical pathways for sleep activity (see Nogueira de Melo et al).

Migraine, cluster headaches, and paroxysmal hemicrania all have been linked to certain sleep stages and are discussed in Chap. 10 in relation to other forms of "hypnic headaches." A variety of sleep disturbances may accompany brain tumors or follow surgical resection of an intracranial tumor. These include excessive daytime sleepiness, sleep apnea, and, rarely, nocturnal epilepsy. The location of the lesion, rather than the tumor type, is predictive of such a disturbance; thus, tumors affecting the hypothalamus, and pituitary are associated with excessive daytime drowsiness, whereas medullary lesions cause respiratory disturbances that may affect sleep (Rosen et al). A symptomatic form of narcolepsy is associated with tumors located adjacent to the third ventricle, and midbrain (see below). Schwartz and associates reported transient cataplexy (see further on) following surgery for a craniopharyngioma, but a delirious state has been more common in a few cases for which we have been consulted.

However, it is the disturbed sleep patterns in patients with Alzheimer disease, Huntington chorea, olivopontocerebellar degeneration, and progressive supranuclear palsy that have attracted the most attention by neurologists (Parkes). Dreaming is also absent in some of these conditions. The peculiarities of sleep in *Parkinson disease* have been extensively studied. Many patients in the early stages of the disease complain of fragmented and unrestful sleep, particularly in the early morning hours; some advanced cases have pathologic insomnia, and this is influenced also by medications used to treat the disease and by deep brain stimulation (see Chap. 39 for a discussion of the nonmotor effects of Parkinson disease). The loss of natural body movements and the alerting effects of L-dopa contribute to the insomnia. The directly acting dopaminergic agonist drugs used for the treatment of Parkinson disease may have the side effect of a pronounced and often rapid daytime sleepiness; however, a similar problem arises in some patients with advancing disease alone.

In striatonigral degeneration (multiple system atrophy), Lewy-body disease, and other parkinsonian syndromes, there is often a characteristic REM sleep disorder, in which the patient moves and speaks violently and aggressively during dreaming. This "REM sleep behavior disorder" does not reflect the personality of the patient or his behavior in the daytime. The majority of patients are able to recall their dream and report that it involved escaping or protecting another person from harm. In these degenerative conditions that affect the basal ganglia the sleep disturbances may precede other symptoms or be an essential part of the illness (see later in this chapter and Chap. 39).

Disorders of Sleep Associated with Changes in Circadian Rhythm

Sleep is also disturbed and diminished when the normal circadian rhythm of the sleep–wake cycle is exogenously altered. This is observed most often in shift workers, who periodically change their work schedule from day to night, and as a result of transmeridianal air travel—i.e., jet lag (Baker and Zee). Eastbound travelers fall asleep late and face an early sunrise. The consequent fatigue is a product of both sleep deprivation and a phase change required by changing time zones. A review of the subject can be found by Sack. One antidote is to reset one's watch on the plane and conform to the routine of the destination—i.e., to stay awake all day until the usual evening hour for sleep—and to take a short-acting sedative at bedtime. Melatonin is also used for this purpose, and a meta-analysis by Herxheimer and Petrie of four trials suggests it is slightly effective. These measures facilitate the resetting of the circadian rhythm. Westbound travelers face a late sunset and a long night's sleep and adjust more readily to resetting of the circadian rhythm than do those traveling east. Exposure to light during the extended day is helpful in entraining the sleep cycle; this adjustment is also accomplished more easily when traveling west than east. Shifting of the circadian rhythm in animals suggests that brief exposure to light at crucial times effectively resets the sleep–wake cycle; apparently, the period just before 4 A.M. is a nodal time for susceptibility to this phase change. The sleep problems caused by shift work are more complicated (see Monk).

The *delayed-sleep-phase syndrome* is a chronic inability to fall asleep and to arise at conventional clock times. Sleep onset is delayed until 3 to 6 A.M.; the subject then sleeps normally until 11 A.M. to 2 P.M. An imposed sleep period from 11 P.M. to 7 A.M. leads to a prolonged sleep latency and daytime sleepiness. By contrast, the *advanced-sleep-phase syndrome* is characterized by an early evening sleep onset (8 to 9 P.M.) and early morning awakening (3 to 5 A.M.). Simply delaying the onset of sleep usually fails to prevent early morning awakening. This pattern is not uncommon among healthy elderly persons (and also among college students), in whom it should probably not be defined as an insomnia syndrome. Still other persons show a completely *irregular sleep–wake pattern*; sleep consists of persistent but variable short or long naps throughout the night and day, with a nearly normal 24-h accumulation of sleep.

Parasomnic Disturbances and Isolated Sleep Symptoms

Although new classifications have rearranged the nosology of these phenomena, included under this title are several diverse disorders: somnolescent starts, sensory paroxysms, nocturnal paroxysmal dystonia, sleep paralysis, night terrors and nightmares, somnambulism, and REM sleep behavior disorder.

Somnolescent (Sleep, Hypnic, Myoclonic) Starts

As sleep comes on, certain motor centers may be excited to a burst of insubordinate activity. The result is a sudden "start" or myoclonic bodily jerk of large amplitude, which rouses the incipient sleeper. It may involve one or both legs or the trunk, less often, the arms. If the start occurs repeatedly during the process of falling asleep and is a nightly event, it may become a matter of great concern to the patient. The starts are more apt to occur in individuals in whom the sleep process develops slowly; they are especially frequent under conditions of tension and anxiety. Polysomnographic recordings have shown that these bodily jerks occur at the moment of falling asleep or during the early stages of sleep. Sometimes they appear as part of an arousal response to a faint external stimulus and are then associated with a frontal K complex in the EEG. These bodily jerks are not variants of epilepsy.

A small proportion of otherwise healthy infants exhibit rhythmic jerking of the hands, arms, and legs or abdomen, both at the onset and in the later stages of sleep (*benign neonatal myoclonus*). The movements begin in the first days of life and disappear within months. There may be a familial tendency toward these movements. Coulter and Allen differentiate this state from myoclonic epilepsy and neonatal seizures by the absence of EEG changes, and its occurrence only during sleep.

Sensory Sleep Paroxysms

Sensory centers may be disturbed in a similar way to the earlier-described sleep starts, either as an isolated phenomenon or in association with motor phenomena. The patient, dropping off to sleep, may be roused by a sensation that darts through the body, a sudden flash of light, or a sudden crashing sound or thunderclap of head pain—cephalgia fugax, or "the exploding head syndrome" (Pearce). Sometimes there is a sensation of being turned or lifted, and dashed to the ground; conceivably, these are sensory paroxysms involving the labyrinthine-vestibular mechanism. Though obvious causes for concern by patients, these sensory paroxysms are benign.

Nocturnal Frontal Lobe Epilepsy

Numerous forms of epilepsy become more prominent during sleep as noted in a later section and in Chap. 16 on epilepsy. However, one isolated seizure disorder is characterized by paroxysmal bursts of generalized choreoathetotic, ballistic, and dystonic movements occurring during NREM sleep (Lugaresi et al, 1986). Sometimes the patient appears awake and has a fearful or astonished expression, or there are repetitive utterances and an appearance of distress, similar to what is seen in night terrors, the main differential diagnosis discussed further on. The attacks may begin at any age, affect both sexes, and are usually nonfamilial. Two forms of this disorder have been recognized: in one, the attacks last 60 s or less; they may be diurnal as well as nocturnal; some patients in addition have epileptic seizures of the more usual type; and all respond to treatment with carbamazepine. The studies of Tinuper and coworkers, using prolonged video-EEG monitoring, indicate that these brief attacks of nocturnal paroxysmal dystonia may actually be epileptic seizures of frontal lobe origin. In a second and more rare type, the attacks are longer lasting (2 to 40 min). Ictal and interictal EEGs during wakefulness and sleep are normal, and these attacks do not respond to anticonvulsants of any type. Except for the lack of familial incidence and occurrence only during sleep, the disorder is very much the same as the "familial paroxysmal dystonic choreoathetosis" described by Lance (see "Paroxysmal Choreoathetosis and Dystonia" in Chap. 4).

Sleep Paralysis

Curious paralytic phenomena, referred to as *pre- and post-dormital paralyses*, may occur in the transition from the sleeping to the waking state. Sometimes in the morning and less frequently when falling asleep, otherwise healthy persons—though awake, conscious, and fully oriented—are seemingly unable to activate their muscles. Respiratory and diaphragmatic function and eye movements are usually unaffected, although a few patients have reported a sensation of being unable to breathe. They lie as though still asleep, with eyes closed, and may become quite frightened while engaged in a struggle for movement. They have the impression that if they could move one muscle, the paralysis would be dispelled instantly, and they would regain full power. It has been stated that the slightest stimulus, such as the touch of a hand or calling the patient's name, will abolish the paralysis. Sleep deprivation is a common precipitant to the syndrome.

Such attacks are also observed in patients with narcolepsy (discussed later in this chapter) and with the hypersomnia of the pickwickian syndrome and other forms of sleep apnea. Some cases are familial.

The weakness or paralysis is thought to be a dissociated form of the atonia of REM sleep. Usually, the attacks are brief (minutes or less); if they occur in isolation and only on rare occasions, they are of no special significance. If frequent, as in narcolepsy, they can be prevented by the use of tricyclic antidepressants, particularly clomipramine, which has serotonergic activity.

Night Terrors and Nightmares

The night terror (*pavor nocturnus*) is mainly a problem of childhood. It usually occurs soon after falling asleep, during stage 3 or 4 sleep. The child awakens abruptly in a state of intense fright, screaming or moaning, with marked tachycardia (150 to 170 beats/min) and deep, rapid respirations. Children with night terrors are often sleepwalkers as well, and both kinds of attack may occur simultaneously. The entire episode lasts only a minute or two, and in the morning the child recalls nothing of it or only a vague unpleasant dream. It has been suggested that night terrors and somnambulism represent impaired or partial arousal from deep sleep, as EEGs taken during such episodes show a waking type of mixed frequency and alpha pattern. Children with night terrors and somnambulism do not show an increased incidence of psychologic abnormalities and tend to outgrow these disorders. The persistence of such problems into adult life, however, has, in a small number of cases, been associated with psychopathology (Kales et al). It has been found that diazepam, which reduces the duration of the deep stages of sleep, will prevent night terrors. Selective serotonin reuptake inhibitors have also been used successfully, especially when night terrors are associated with sleepwalking. Frequent night terrors have reportedly been eliminated by having parents awaken the child for several successive nights, just prior to the usual time of the attack or at the first sign of restlessness and autonomic arousal (Lask).

Frightening dreams or nightmares are far more frequent than night terrors and affect children and adults alike. They occur during periods of normal REM sleep and are particularly prominent during periods of increased REM sleep (REM rebound) following the withdrawal of alcohol or other sedative-hypnotic drugs that had suppressed REM sleep chronically. Autonomic changes are slight or absent, and the content of the dreams can usually be recalled in considerable detail. Some of these dreams (e.g., the ones occurring in the alcohol-withdrawal period) are so vivid that the patient may later have difficulty in separating them from reality; indeed, they may merge with the hallucinations of delirium tremens. Nightmares are of little significance as isolated events. Fevers dispose to them, as do conditions such as indigestion and the reading of bloodcurdling stories or exposure to terrifying movies or television programs before bedtime (truly). Some patients report nightmares and extremely vivid dreams when first taking certain medications such as beta blockers and, particularly in our experience, L-dopa. We have also consulted on a few patients who complained of almost nightly nightmares and concurrent severe headaches, but without apparent depression or other psychiatric illness; the nature of their problem was obscure. Persistent nightmares may be a pressing medical complaint and are often accompanied by other behavioral disturbances or anxieties.

Childhood Somnambulism and Sleep Automatism

This condition occurs far more commonly in children (average age: 4 to 6 years) than in adults, and is often associated with nocturnal enuresis and night terrors, as indicated above. It is estimated that 15 percent of children have at least one episode of sleepwalking, and that 1 in 5 sleepwalkers has a family history of this disorder. Motor performance and responsiveness during the sleepwalking incident vary considerably. The most common behavioral abnormality is for a patient to sit up in bed or on the edge of the bed without actually walking. When walking about the house, he may turn on a light or perform some other familiar act. There may be no outward show of emotion, or the patient may be frightened (night terror), but the frenzied, aggressive behavior of some adult sleepwalkers, described below, is rare in the child. Usually the eyes are open, and such sleepwalkers are guided by vision, thus avoiding familiar objects; the sight of an unfamiliar object may awaken them. Sometimes they make no attempt to avoid obstacles and may injure themselves. If spoken to, they make no response; if told to return to bed, they may do so, but more often they must be led back. Sometimes they repeatedly mutter strange phrases or perform certain repetitive acts, such as pushing against a wall or turning a doorknob back and forth. The episode lasts for only a few minutes, and the following morning, they usually have no memory of it, or only a fragmentary recollection.

A popular belief is that the sleepwalker is acting out a dream. The observations of sleep laboratories are entirely at variance with this view, as somnambulism has been found to occur almost exclusively during deeper stages of NREM sleep (stage N3) and during the first third of the night when dreaming is least likely to occur. In fact, the entire nocturnal sleep pattern of such individuals does not differ from normal. Also, there is no evidence that somnambulism is a form of epilepsy. It is probably allied to talking in one's sleep, although the two conditions seldom occur together. Sleepwalking must be distinguished from fugue states and ambulatory automatisms of complex partial seizures discussed in Chap. 16.

The major consideration in the treatment of childhood somnambulism is to guard patients against injury by locking doors and windows, removing dangerous objects from the patients' usual routes of march, having them sleep on the ground floor, etc. Children usually outgrow this disorder; parents should be reassured on this score and disabused of the notion that somnambulism is a sign of psychiatric or any other disease.

Somnambulism in Adults

The onset of sleepwalking or night terrors for the first time in adult life is most unusual, and, in an occasional case, may suggest the presence of psychiatric disease or drug intoxication. Almost always, the adult sleepwalker has a history of sleepwalking as a child, although there may have been a period of freedom between the childhood episodes and their reemergence in the third and fourth decades. Adult somnambulism also occurs during N3 of NREM sleep, but unlike the childhood type, is not confined to the earlier part of the night. If one extends the category of somnambulism to all forms of nocturnal wandering, it seems to be remarkably common, with a lifetime prevalence of 29% of U.S. adults according to the survey by Ohayon and colleagues.

Somnambulism in the adult, as in the child, can be a purely passive event unaccompanied by fear or other signs of emotion. More frequently, however, the attack is characterized by frenzied or violent behavior associated with fear and tachycardia, like that of a night terror and sometimes with self-injury. Very rarely, crimes have reportedly been committed during sleepwalking, but the authors are skeptical that organized and planned sequential activity is possible. The finding of normal sleep patterns on polysomnography distinguishes these attacks from complex partial seizures. They can be eliminated or greatly reduced by the administration of clonazepam (0.5 to 1.0 mg) at bedtime. Some patients respond better to a combination of clonazepam and phenytoin or to flurazepam (Kavey et al).

An associated but unclassifiable disorder is "sleep eating" in which the individual seeks out mainly carbohydrates and is only aware of their actions on the following morning when they see the mess they have left. Also, in the provocatively named "sexomnia," the individual, male or female, engages in sexual activity, sometimes forcefully, and has no recollection of the events. The status of these syndromes as authentic parasomnias is unclear.

REM Sleep Behavior Disorder

This is a recognized parasomnic disorder, occurring in adult life, most commonly in older men without a history of childhood sleepwalking. It is characterized by attacks of vigorous, agitated, and often dangerous motor activity accompanied by vivid dreams (Mahowald and Schenck). The characteristic features are angry speech with shouting, violent activity with injury to self and bed mate, a very high arousal threshold, and the variable but sometimes detailed recall of a nightmare of being attacked and fighting back or attempting to flee. The episodes vary in frequency in affected individuals, occurring once every week or two or several times nightly. The episodes, which occur *exclusively during REM sleep*, usually in the second half of the night, are out of keeping with the patient's waking personality. Polysomnographic recordings during these episodes have disclosed augmented muscle tone but no seizure activity.

The rare appearance of this disorder with pontine infarctions has been mentioned earlier in the chapter. However, in a series of 93 cases of REM sleep behavior disorder reported by Olson and colleagues, more than half were associated with some other neurologic disorder, in particular Parkinson disease, multiple system atrophy, and Lewy-body dementia, but in other series, with a number of degenerative and varied neurologic conditions. A more systemic polysomnographic examination of 457 patients with Parkinson disease by Sixel-Döring and colleagues found REM sleep behavior disorder in 46%. Viewed from another perspective, Postuma and coworkers have reported that one-quarter of individuals with idiopathic REM sleep disorder later developed a neurodegenerative disorder, similar to or slightly lower than other series. These observations have led to the suggestion that this disorder is an early manifestation of a degenerative brain disease characterized by the deposition of alpha-synuclein in certain neuronal systems, as summarized by Boeve and associates.

The episodes can be suppressed by the administration of clonazepam in doses of 0.5 to 1.0 mg at bedtime and by melatonin, 3 to 12 mg. The advantage of the latter is that sleep apnea is not affected as it is with benzodiazepines. Discontinuation of medication, even after years of effective control, has resulted in relapse. Antidepressants are said to exacerbate the disorder with the possible exception of bupropion.

The patient and family should probably be advised about safety including removal of weapons, sharp objects and try to insure spousal safety by this and by means of sleeping in another room.

Nocturnal Epilepsy (See also Chap. 16)

It has long been known that seizures, both convulsive and nonconvulsive, often occur during sleep, especially in children. This is such a frequent occurrence that the practice of inducing sleep has been adopted as an activating EEG procedure to obtain confirmation of epilepsy. Seizures may occur soon after the onset of sleep or at any time during the night, but mainly in stages 1 and 2 of NREM sleep or, rarely, in REM sleep. They are also common during the first hour after awakening. On the other hand, deprivation of sleep may be conducive to a seizure.

Sleeping epileptic patients may attract attention to their seizures by a cry, violent motor activity, unusual but stereotyped actions, such as sitting up and crossing the arms over the chest, the adoption of a "fencing" posture, or labored breathing. After the tonic-clonic phase, patients become quiet and fall into a state resembling deep sleep, but they cannot be aroused from it for some minutes or longer. If the nocturnal seizure is unobserved, the only indication of it may be disheveled bedclothes, a few drops of blood on the pillow from a bitten tongue, wet bed linen from urinary incontinence, or sore muscles. Or the occurrence of a seizure may be disclosed only by confusion, muscle soreness, or headache, the common aftermaths of a major generalized seizure. Rarely, a patient may die in an epileptic seizure during sleep, sometimes from smothering in the bed clothes or aspirating vomitus or for some obscure reason (possibly respiratory or cardiac dysrhythmia). Epilepsy occasionally occurs in conjunction with night terrors and somnambulism; the question then arises whether the latter disorders represent postepileptic automatisms. Usually no such relationship is established. EEG studies during a nocturnal period of sleep are most helpful in such cases. Measurement of serum creatine kinase concentration in the hours following an event may distinguish seizure from night terrors, and the other described sleep-related motor behaviors.

Pathologic Excessive Sleep (Hypersomnia)

Encephalitis lethargica, or von Economo "epidemic encephalitis," the remarkable illness that appeared on the medical horizon as a pandemic following World War I, provided some of the most dramatic instances of pathologic somnolence. Protracted sleep lasting for days to weeks was such a prominent symptom of this disease that it was called *sleeping sickness* (a term also applied to African trypanosomiasis, as noted below). The patient appeared to be in a state of continuous sleep, or *somnosis*, and could be kept awake only by constant stimulation. Although the infective agent of von Economo disease was never isolated, the pathologic anatomy was fully disclosed by many excellent studies, all of which demonstrated a destruction of neurons in the midbrain, subthalamus, and hypothalamus. Patients who survived the acute phase of the illness often had difficulty in reestablishing their normal sleep–wake rhythm. As the somnolence disappeared, some patients exhibited a reversal of the normal pattern, tending to sleep by day, and stay awake at night; many of them also developed a parkinsonian syndrome months or years later. The hypersomnia was possibly related to destruction or functional paralysis of dopamine-rich neurons in the substantia nigra, resulting in overactivity of the raphe (serotonergic) neurons.

Hypersomnia is also a manifestation of *trypanosomiasis*, the common cause of *sleeping sickness* in Africa, and of other diseases localized to the mesencephalon, and the floor and walls of the third ventricle. Small tumors in this area have been associated with arterial hypotension, diabetes insipidus, hypo- or hyperthermia, and protracted somnolence lasting many weeks. Such patients can be aroused; but if left alone, they immediately fall asleep. Traumatic and vascular lesions and other diseases affecting the mesencephalon may have a similar effect.

Sleep drunkenness is the name given to a special form of hypersomnia, characterized by a failure of the patient to attain full alertness for a protracted period after awakening. Unsteadiness, drowsiness, disorientation, and automatic behavior are the main features. This disorder is usually associated with idiopathic hypersomnia, and sometimes with sleep apnea or other forms of sleep deprivation, but often no such connection can be discerned, in which case a motivational factor should be suspected.

An interesting type of transient unresponsiveness in elderly patients, as described by Haimovic and Beresford, has been in our experience akin to a deep sleep, but the EEG has not shown sleep patterns.

Kleine-Levin Syndrome

Kleine in 1925 and Levin in 1936 described an episodic disorder characterized by somnolence and overeating. For days or weeks, the patients, mostly adolescent boys, sleep 18 h or more a day, awakening only long enough to eat and attend to toilet needs. They appeared dull, often confused, and restless, and were sometimes troubled by hallucinations. In the series of 18 cases collected by Critchley, the age range was from puberty to 45 years. There may be a brief prodromal period of inertia and drowsiness. The duration of nocturnal sleep may be greatly prolonged, or, as in our patients referred to below, they may sleep for days on end. Food intake during and around the period of hypersomnia may exceed three times the normal (bulimia) and occurs almost compulsively during brief periods of semiwakefulness; to a variable extent, there are other behavioral changes such as social withdrawal, negativism, slowness of thinking, incoherence, inattentiveness, and disturbances of memory. The somnolence has been well studied by modern laboratory methods; except for the total duration of sleep, the individual components of the NREM and REM cycles are normal. Between episodes these patients are behaviorally and cognitively normal.

The basis of this condition has never been clarified. A psychogenic mechanism has been proposed, without foundation in our opinion. The syndrome usually disappears during adulthood, and there is limited pathologic material (see further discussion in the context of hypothalamic syndromes in Chap. 27). A series of 108 cases reviewed by Arnulf and colleagues frame the clinical features; a predominance of males, higher C-reactive protein than controls, and a history of early childhood developmental problems. There was no human leukocyte antigen (HLA) clustering, but children of Jewish heritage were overrepresented. We have cared for a sibling pair who had the illness into young adulthood (Katz and Ropper). The case reported by Carpenter and coworkers, in which an acute and chronic inflammation in the medial thalamus, but not the hypothalamus, was found, must be questioned as representative of the idiopathic adolescent condition. Their patient was a man 39 years of age who had episodes of diurnal drowsiness, hyperphagia (intermittently relieved by methylphenidate), and hypersexuality over a period of months. In some patients with this disorder, schizophrenic and sociopathic symptoms have been recorded between attacks, raising doubt as to whether all the reported cases are of the same type. We have seen variants of this syndrome manifesting themselves in drowsiness and extreme inactivity lasting for a few weeks, then with a complete return to normalcy. In two of our patients, the use of serotonergic antidepressants lengthened the interval between episodes.

No consistent change in the level of hypocretin (orexin) has been found in the spinal fluid, as occurs in narcolepsy (see further on), and the two disorders are distinct. In one typical case, there was pronounced hypoperfusion of the left medial temporal lobe both during and between attacks, but the interpretation of this finding is unclear (Portilla et al).

No treatment has been consistently effective (e.g., antidepressant drugs), but some of the stimulants that are used for the treatment of narcolepsy may be useful (see further on).

Finally, it should be mentioned that sleep laboratories now recognize a form of *idiopathic hypersomnia* in which there are repeated episodes of drowsiness throughout the day. This condition is discussed further on, in relation to the diagnosis of narcolepsy, with which it is most often confused.

A related disorder has been described of "menstrual related hypersomnia" that has a cyclic catamenial nature.

Sleep Apnea and Excessive Daytime Sleepiness

Excessive daytime sleepiness is a common complaint in general medical practice (Table 19-2). Certainly, the most frequent causes are inadequate sleep and the use of any one of the large variety of medications that are not prescribed primarily for their sedative effect. Abuse of alcohol and illicit drugs should also be included in this category. Most conditions associated with severe fatigue produce daytime sleepiness and a desire to nap. A notable medical cause is infectious mononucleosis but many other viral infections have the same effect. Certain chronic neurologic conditions can produce fatigue and sleepiness, multiple sclerosis being the outstanding example. Among general medical conditions, hypothyroidism and hypercapnia must always be considered when daytime sleepiness is a prominent feature. One must not overlook the possibility that excessive daytime drowsiness is the result of repeated episodes of sleep apnea, discussed below, or the disruption of nocturnal sleep by disorders such as the restless legs syndrome.

As mentioned above, REM sleep is characterized by irregular breathing, and this may include several brief periods of apnea up to 10 s in duration. Such apneas and those occurring at the onset of sleep are not in themselves considered to be pathologic. In some individuals, however, sleep-induced apneic periods are particularly frequent and prolonged (> 10 s) and such a condition is responsible for a variety of clinical disturbances in children and adults. This pathologic form of sleep apnea may be the result of a reduction of respiratory drive (so-called central apnea), an obstruction of the upper airway, or a combination of these two mechanisms.

Table 19-2

CAUSES OF DAYTIME SLEEPINESS

1. Medications (including many types of sedatives, tranquilizers, anticonvulsants, antihistaminics, antidepressants, β-adrenergic blockers, and atropinic drugs), L-dopa and dopaminergic agonists, abuse of alcohol and illicit drugs
2. Acute medical illness of the mononucleosis type, including mundane respiratory and gastrointestinal infections
3. Postsurgical, postconcussive, and postanesthetic states
4. Chronic neurologic diseases: multiple sclerosis, dementias
5. Depression
6. Metabolic derangements: hypothyroidism, Addison disease, severe diabetes
7. Encephalitic diseases
   A. Following viral encephalitis
   B. Trypanosomiasis
   C. Encephalitis lethargica (historical)
8. Lesions of the hypothalamus
   A. Kleine-Levin syndrome
   B. Hypothalamic tumor or granuloma
9. Sleep apnea syndromes; central and obstructive
10. Narcolepsy-cataplexy
11. Idiopathic hypersomnia

Sleep-Disordered Breathing

Obstructive Sleep Apnea Apnea of the *obstructive type* in which the posterior pharyngeal muscles collapse and narrow the upper airway is far more common than the central variety. Obstructive apnea is associated with obesity and also accompanies acromegaly, hypothyroidism or myxedema, micrognathia, and myotonic dystrophy. In children, more than in adults, adenotonsillar hypertrophy may be a factor. Instances occur as a result of neuromuscular diseases that weaken the posterior pharyngeal musculature; motor neuron disease is the most common example of this group. Obstructive sleep apnea is characterized by noisy snoring of a cyclic type. After a period of regular albeit noisy breathing, there occurs a waning of breathing efforts; then, despite repeated inspiratory efforts, airflow ceases. Following a prolonged period of apnea (10 to 30 s or even longer), the patient makes a series of progressively greater breathing efforts until breathing resumes, accompanied by very loud snorting sounds and a brief arousal.

Obstructive sleep apnea occurs during both REM and NREM sleep. The upper respiratory muscles (genioglossus, geniohyoid, tensor veli palatini, and medial pterygoid) normally contract just before the diaphragm contracts, resisting the collapse of the oropharynx. If the airway is obstructed or the muscles are weakened and then go slack, the negative intrathoracic pressure causes narrowing of this passage. Sedative medications, alcohol intoxication, excessive tiredness, a recent stroke, head trauma or other acute neurologic disease, and primary pulmonary disease may all exaggerate obstructive sleep apnea, particularly in the obese patient with a tendency to snore.

Hypoxia or perhaps other stimuli induce an arousal response, either a lightening of sleep or a very brief awakening, which is followed by an immediate resumption of breathing. The patient quickly falls asleep again and the sequence is repeated, several hundred times a night in severe cases, greatly disrupting the sleep pattern and reducing the total sleep time. Paradoxically, these patients are very difficult to rouse at all times during the night.

Obstructive sleep apnea is predominantly a disorder of overweight, middle-aged men and usually presents as *excessive daytime sleepiness*, a complaint that is sometimes mistaken for narcolepsy (see below). Other patients, usually those with the much-less-common central form of apnea, complain mainly of a disturbance of sleep at night, or insomnia, which may be incorrectly attributed to anxiety or depression. The occurrence of an obstructive sleep apnea is accompanied after a period of weeks or months by progressive hemoglobin oxygen desaturation, hypercapnia and hypoxia, a transient increase in systemic and pulmonary arterial pressures, and sinus bradycardia or other arrhythmias. Morning headache, inattentiveness, grogginess, and decline in school or work performance are other symptoms attributable to sleep apnea. Ultimately, systemic and pulmonary arterial hypertension, cor pulmonale, polycythemia, and heart failure may develop. When combined with obesity, these symptoms have been referred to as the "pickwickian syndrome," so named by Burwell and coworkers, who identified this clinical syndrome with that of the extraordinarily sleepy, red-faced, fat boy described by Dickens in *The Pickwick Papers*.

The full-blown syndrome of obstructive sleep apnea is readily recognized by the features of daytime sleepiness, loud snoring, and the typical habitus of affected individuals. However, in patients who complain only of excessive daytime sleepiness or insomnia, the diagnosis may be elusive and require all-night polysomnographic sleep monitoring.

Central Sleep Apnea This disorder has been observed in patients with a variety of severe and life-threatening lower brainstem lesions—bulbar poliomyelitis, lateral medullary infarction, spinal (high cervical) surgery, syringobulbia, brainstem encephalitis, as well as with striatonigral degeneration, Creutzfeldt-Jakob disease, anoxic encephalopathy, and olivopontocerebellar degeneration. When a unilateral lesion (e.g., infarction) of the medulla is the cause, there is almost always involvement of crossing fibers between respiratory nuclei (see discussion in Chap. 26).

In addition to these symptomatic forms of sleep apnea, there is a disorder referred to as *primary*, or *idiopathic, hypoventilation syndrome* ("Ondine's curse," as described in Chap. 26). This last term is now applied to many forms of total loss of automatic breathing, especially during sleep. Awakenings during the night are frequent, usually after an apneic period, and insomnia is a common complaint. Snoring is mild and intermittent. In the few autopsied cases of congenital central hypoventilation of childhood, Liu and colleagues found the external arcuate nuclei of the medulla to be absent, and the neuron population in the medullary respiratory areas to be depleted.

Complex sleep apnea, or "treatment emergent central sleep apnea," occurs most often in patients with cardiovascular conditions, particularly congestive heart failure, wherein, after sleep apnea is treated with positive airway pressure, central apnea emerges.

Treatment The approach is governed by the severity of symptoms and the predominant type of apnea, central or obstructive. In the treatment of *obstructive apnea*, continuous positive airway pressure (CPAP) or bilevel positive airway pressure (BIPAP) is the most useful measure. These therapies are delivered by a tight-fitting nasal mask that is worn at night and connected to a pressure-cycled ventilator that is triggered by the patient's breath. The increased airway pressure maintains patency of the naso- and oropharynx, thereby reducing the obstruction. A nasal device that passively resists nasal collapse by providing expiratory resistance is used by some specialists for mild sleep apnea. All of these approaches have a level of discomfort that is not tolerable to some patients.

Patients benefit from losing weight, lateral positioning during sleep, and avoidance of alcohol and other sedative drugs. Surgical correction of an upper airway defect may be helpful, but it is difficult to predict which patients will benefit. There are no clear guidelines for procedures such as uvulopalatopharyngoplasty and related surgeries or uvulectomy and tonsillectomy except in children. These may obliterate snoring more than it ameliorates the sleep apnea. Oral alignment devices that are produced by dentists, aimed at advancing the mandible, have been helpful to some patients, especially for those who cannot tolerate positive pressure.

Those few patients with the most severe hypersomnia and cardiopulmonary failure who cannot tolerate nocturnal positive pressure ventilation require tracheostomy and nocturnal respirator care. (See Parkes for a fuller account of therapeutic measures.) Some patients with non-obstructive apnea may also benefit from nighttime treatment with CPAP, but the results are far less consistent than with the obstructive type.

In *central apnea*, any underlying abnormality, such as congestive heart failure or nasal obstruction, should, of course, be treated insofar as possible. Where no underlying cause can be found, one of several medications—acetazolamide, medroxyprogesterone, protriptyline, and particularly clomipramine—may be helpful in the short run (Brownell et al). However, drug treatment has proven generally unsatisfactory. Low-flow oxygen may also be useful in reducing central sleep apnea.

Narcolepsy and Cataplexy

This clinical entity has long been known to the medical profession. Gélineau gave it the name *narcolepsy* in 1880, although several authors had described the recurring attacks of irresistible sleep even before that time. Gélineau had also mentioned that the sleep attacks were sometimes accompanied by falls ("astasias"), but it was Loewenfeld, in 1902, who first recognized the common association between the sleep attacks and the temporary paralysis of the somatic musculature during bouts of laughter, anger, and other emotional states; this was referred to as cataplectic inhibition by Henneberg (1916), and later as cataplexy by Adie (1926). The term *sleep paralysis*—used to designate the brief, episodic loss of voluntary movement that occurs during the period of falling asleep (hypnagogic, or predormital) or less often when awakening (hypnopompic, or postdormital)—was introduced by S.A. Kinnier Wilson in 1928. Actually, Weir Mitchell had described this latter disorder in 1876, under the title of *night palsy*.

Sometimes sleep paralysis is accompanied or just preceded by vivid and terrifying hallucinations (*hypnagogic hallucinations*), which may be visual, auditory, vestibular (a sense of motion), or somatic (a feeling that a limb or finger or other part of the body is enlarged or otherwise transformed). These four conditions—narcolepsy, cataplexy, hypnagogic paralysis, and hallucinations—constitute a clinical tetrad. Wilson has reviewed the historical aspects and early accounts of this subject. The most important observations regarding the pathophysiology of this process have been special relationship to a disordered pattern of REM sleep, and the more recent finding of abnormalities in hypothalamic substances that induce sleep, as discussed below.

Clinical Features

This syndrome is encountered regularly by neurologists; Daly and Yoss recorded about 100 new cases a year at the Mayo Clinic. Dement and colleagues have estimated the prevalence at 50 to 70 per 100,000 in the San Francisco and Los Angeles areas. Men and women are affected equally. Several papers have found an epidemiologic relationship to just preceding outbreaks of H1N1 pandemics and the vaccine (see Ham et al and Dauvilliers et al).

As a rule, narcolepsy has a gradual onset between the ages of 15 and 35 years; in fully 90 percent of narcoleptics, the condition is established by the 25th year of life. Narcolepsy is usually the first symptom, less often cataplexy, and rarely sleep paralysis. The essential disorder is one of frequent attacks of irresistible sleepiness. Several times a day, usually after meals or while sitting in class or in other boring or sedentary situations, the affected person is assailed by an uncontrollable desire to sleep. The eyes close, the muscles relax, breathing deepens slightly, and by all appearances, the individual is dozing. A noise, a touch, or even the cessation of the lecturer's voice is enough to awaken the patient. The periods of sleep rarely last longer than 15 min unless the patient is reclining, when he may continue to sleep for an hour or longer. At the conclusion of a nap, the patient feels somewhat refreshed. It should be emphasized that there are many narcoleptics who tend to be pervasively drowsy throughout the day. What distinguishes the typical narcoleptic sleep attacks from commonplace postprandial drowsiness and napping is the frequent occurrence of the former (two to six times every day as a rule), their irresistibility, and their occurrence in unusual situations, as while standing, eating, or carrying on a conversation. Blurring of vision, diplopia, and ptosis may attend the drowsiness and may bring the patient first to an ophthalmologist.

In addition to episodes of outright sleep, narcoleptics, like other very drowsy persons, may experience episodes of automatic behavior and amnesia. Initially the patient feels drowsy and may recall attempts to fight off the drowsiness, but gradually he loses track of events. The patient may continue to perform routine tasks automatically but does not respond appropriately to a new demand or answer complex questions. Often there is a sudden burst of words, without meaning or relevance to what was just said. Such an outburst may terminate the attack, for which there is complete or nearly complete amnesia. In many respects, the attacks resemble episodes of nocturnal sleepwalking. Such attacks of automatic behavior and amnesia are common, occurring in more than half of a large series of patients with narcolepsy-cataplexy (Guilleminault and Dement). Affected patients are frequently involved in driving accidents, even more frequently than epileptics.

Nocturnal sleep is often disrupted and reduced in amount. The number of hours in a 24-h day spent in sleep by the narcoleptic is no greater than that of a normal individual. Narcoleptics have an increased incidence of sleep apnea and periodic leg and body movements, but not of somnambulism.

Approximately 70 percent of narcoleptics first seeking help will report having some form of cataplexy, and about half of the remainder will develop cataplexy later in life. *Cataplexy* refers to a sudden loss of muscle tone brought on by strong emotion—that is, circumstances in which hearty laughter or, more rarely, excitement, surprise, anger, or intense athletic activity cause the patient's head to fall forward, the jaw to drop, the knees to buckle, even with sinking to the ground—all with perfect preservation of consciousness. Cataplectic attacks occur without provocation in perhaps 5 percent of cases. The attacks last only a few seconds or a minute or two and are of variable frequency and intensity. In most of our patients, they have appeared at intervals of a few days or weeks. Exceptionally, there are many attacks daily and even status cataplecticus, in which the atonia lasts for hours. This is more likely to happen at the beginning of the illness or upon discontinuing tricyclic medication.

Most attacks of cataplexy are partial (e.g., only a dropping of the jaw or "weakening of the knees"). Wilson found that the tendon reflexes were abolished during the attack. Pupillary reflexes are absent in some cases.

Rarely, cataplexy precedes the advent of sleep attacks, but usually it follows them, sometimes by many years. Sleep paralysis and hypnagogic hallucinations together are stated to occur in about half the patients. Of course, hypnagogic paralysis and hallucinations occur in otherwise normal persons, and normal children, especially when tickled, may laugh to the point of cataplexy. About 10 percent of persons with sleep attacks indistinguishable from those of narcolepsy have none of the associated phenomena ("independent narcolepsy"), and in these cases, REM periods are not found consistently at the onset of sleep (see further on).

Once established, narcolepsy and cataplexy usually continue for the remainder of the patient's life. The degree of sleepiness rarely lessens, although cataplexy, sleep paralysis, and hallucinations improve or disappear with age in about one-third of patients who have those features (Billiard and Cadilhac). No other condition is consistently associated with narcolepsy-cataplexy, and none develops later.

Cause and Pathogenesis

A familial component has been recognized for years; the risk of narcolepsy in a first-degree relative of an affected individual is 1 to 2 percent, more than 25 times that in the general population. As reviewed by Chabas and colleagues, important insights into the pathogenesis have come from studies of recessively inherited narcolepsy in three species of dogs, in which mutations have been identified in a gene encoding a receptor for the protein hypocretin (Lin et al). These studies implicate the peptide hypocretin in the control of sleep. The hypocretins were thought in the past to regulate feeding behavior and energy metabolism; indeed, they were also designated "orexins," from the Greek word for appetite. In mice, inactivation of two hypocretin receptors reproduces narcolepsy. In both humans and animals, hypocretin-containing neurons in the hypothalamus send projections widely through the brain and particularly to structures implicated in control of sleep as discussed earlier and shown in Fig. 19-4: the locus ceruleus (noradrenergic), the tuberomammillary nucleus (histaminergic), the raphe nucleus (serotonergic), and the ventral tegmental area (dopaminergic).

A number of compelling observations implicate hypocretin and its receptors in human narcolepsy. First, a narcoleptic patient has been described with a mutation in the gene encoding human hypocretin. Second, hypocretin-secreting neurons are depleted in the brains of human narcoleptics, and CSF hypocretin levels are reduced or absent in affected patients. In some studies, the absence of CSF hypocretin distinguished narcoleptic individuals from patients with other categories of sleep disorders.

Perhaps surprisingly, several lines of evidence suggest an autoimmune causation for narcolepsy. For example, it has long been known that there is an almost universal association with specific alleles of the histocompatibility antigen HLA-DQ (B1-0602) (Neely et al; Kramer et al). Therapeutic approaches to narcolepsy based on a presumed autoantibody have also been developed as noted below. Because the mode of inheritance of narcolepsy is not clearly mendelian (Kessler et al), it has been proposed that the disease reflects a genetic predisposition, possibly with a superimposed autoimmune reaction that impairs the function of hypocretin neuronal systems or damages the neurons that secrete the peptide.

Finally, the approximate similarities to the post infectious sleep states of von Economo encephalitis and, as provocatively, the aforementioned increased incidence of narcolepsy after outbreaks of H1N1 respiratory infection, or after administration of the vaccine, implicates an infectious or post infectious inflammatory cause, ostensibly affecting the hypothalamic nuclei (Dauvillers et al, 2010).

As mentioned earlier, a *secondary or symptomatic narcolepsy* syndrome on occasion results from cerebral trauma, multiple sclerosis, craniopharyngioma, or other tumors of the third ventricle or upper brainstem, head trauma, or a sarcoid granuloma within the hypothalamus (Servan et al).

Our understanding of narcolepsy was greatly advanced by the demonstration by Dement and his group that this disorder is associated with a reversal in the order of the two states of sleep, with REM rather than NREM sleep occurring at the onset of the sleep attacks. Not all the sleep episodes of the narcoleptic begin with REM sleep, but almost always a number of sleep attacks with such an onset can be identified in narcoleptic-cataplectic patients in the course of a polysomnographic sleep study. The hypnagogic hallucinations, cataplexy, and sleep-onset paralysis (caused by inhibition of anterior horn cells) all coincide with the REM period. These investigators have also shown that the night sleep pattern of patients with narcolepsy-cataplexy may begin with a REM period. This may occur in normal subjects, though infrequently and usually with severe sleep deprivation. Furthermore, the nocturnal sleep pattern is altered in narcoleptics, who have frequent body movements and transient awakenings and a decrease in sleep stage N3, as well as in total sleep duration. Another important finding in narcoleptics is that *sleep latency* (the interval between the point when an individual tries to sleep and the point of onset of EEG sleep patterns), measured repeatedly in diurnal nap situations, is greatly reduced. Thus, narcolepsy is not simply a matter of excessive diurnal sleepiness (essential daytime drowsiness) or even a disorder of REM sleep but a generalized disorganization of sleep–wake function.

Diagnosis

The greatest difficulty in diagnosis relates to the problem of separating narcolepsy from the daytime sleepiness of sedentary, obese adults who, if unoccupied, doze readily after meals, while watching television or in the theater. Many of these patients prove to have obstructive sleep apnea. Excessive daytime somnolence, easily mistaken for narcolepsy, may also attend heart failure, hypothyroidism, excessive use of soporific, other medications including antihistamines, use of alcohol, cerebral trauma, and certain brain tumors (e.g., craniopharyngioma; see Table 19-2). A more serious form of recurrent daytime sleepiness, referred to as *independent narcolepsy* or *essential narcolepsy*, is described further on. However, both of these forms of daytime drowsiness are isolated disturbances, lacking the other disturbances of sleep and motor activity that characterize the narcolepsy syndrome. The brief attacks of automatic behavior and amnesia of the narcoleptic must be distinguished from hysterical fugues and complex partial seizures.

Cataplexy must also be distinguished from syncope, drop attacks (Chap. 17), and atonic seizures; in atonic seizures, consciousness is temporarily abolished. The careful documentation of narcolepsy by laboratory techniques is imperative when the diagnosis is in doubt, in part because of the potential for abuse of stimulant drugs used for treatment. Overnight polysomnography followed by a standardized multiple sleep latency test, in which the patient is afforded opportunities for napping at 2-h intervals, permit the quantification of drowsiness and increase the probability of detecting short-latency REM activity (within 15 min from the onset of each sleep period). According to some investigators, a reduced level (below 110 pg/mL) of hypocretin in the spinal fluid is virtually diagnostic of narcolepsy in the proper clinical circumstances (see Mignot et al). We would comment, however, that it is not necessary to resort to any of these studies in clinically typical cases.

Treatment

No single therapy will control all the symptoms. Narcolepsy responds best to (1) strategically placed 15- to 20-min naps (during lunch hour, before or after dinner, etc.); (2) the use of stimulant drugs—modafinil, dextroamphetamine sulfate, or methylphenidate hydrochloride to heighten alertness; and (3) antidepressants (sertraline, venlafaxine, protriptyline, imipramine, or clomipramine) for control of cataplexy. All these drugs are potent suppressants of REM sleep. Monoamine oxidase (MAO) inhibitors also inhibit REM sleep and can be used if they are tolerated. Modafinil (200 mg daily, up to 600 mg in divided doses) may prove to be the safest of the stimulants (Fry), but experience with this agent is still being acquired. Methylphenidate, because of its prompt action and relative lack of side effects, is also widely used. It is usually given in doses of 10 to 20 mg tid on an empty stomach. Alternatively, amphetamine 5 to 10 mg may be given 3 to 5 times a day; this is ordinarily well tolerated and does not cause wakefulness at night. Pemoline, a potent stimulant (50 to 75 mg daily) is no longer available in the United States because of potential hepatic toxicity. The tricyclic antidepressants had been used to reduce cataplexy, but they have been overtaken by selective serotonin reuptake inhibitors such as sertraline and by norepinephrine reuptake inhibitors such as venlafaxine. Sodium oxybate, whose active agent is gamma-hydroxybutyrate, is also beneficial for cataplexy and narcolepsy in many individuals.

The combined use of these stimulant and tricyclic antidepressant drugs is often indicated. A problem with the stimulant drugs is the development of tolerance over a 6- to 12-month period, which requires the switching and periodic discontinuation of drugs. Excessive amounts of amphetamines may induce a schizophreniform psychosis. The stimulant drugs and the tricyclic antidepressants increase catecholamine levels; their chronic administration may produce hypertension.

An entirely different approach, based on a presumed autoimmune attack on hypothalamic neurons, has introduced immune globulin infusions in early cases of narcolepsy. This must still be considered preliminary but the results are interesting (see Dauvillers et al, 2004).

Narcoleptics must be warned of the dangers of falling asleep and lapses of consciousness while driving or during engagement in other activities that require constant alertness. The earliest feeling of drowsiness should prompt the patient to pull off the road and take a nap. Long-distance driving should probably be avoided completely.

Idiopathic Hypersomnia (Essential Narcolepsy; NREM Narcolepsy)

As has been indicated, recurrent daytime sleepiness may be the presenting symptom in a number of varied disorders other than narcolepsy. When chronic daytime sleepiness occurs repeatedly and persistently without known cause, it is classified as essential or idiopathic hypersomnolence. Roth distinguishes this state from narcolepsy on the basis of longer and unrefreshing daytime sleep periods, deep and undisturbed night sleep, difficulty in awakening in the morning or after a nap ("sleep drunkenness"), all of these occurring in the absence of REM-onset sleep and cataplexy. Admittedly, this condition proves difficult to distinguish from narcolepsy unless laboratory studies exclude the latter, and even then, there is overlap between the two syndromes (Bassetti and Aldrich). Treatment, however, is the same as that for narcolepsy. Idiopathic hypersomnia, as defined in this manner, proves to be a rare syndrome once narcolepsy, and all other causes of daytime sleepiness have been excluded.

Pathologic Wakefulness

This state, as remarked earlier, has been induced in animals by lesions in the tegmentum (median raphe nuclei) of the pons. Comparable states are known to occur in humans but are rare. Asomnia in hospital practice is a result of delirium of any type, including delirium tremens and drug-withdrawal states. Drug-induced psychoses and mania may induce a similar state. We have seen a number of patients with a delirious hyperalertness lasting a week or more after temporofrontal cerebral contusions or in association with a hypothalamic lymphoma. None of the various treatments we have tried has been successful in suppressing this state. It was transitory in the traumatic cases.

Additional Syndromes Occurring during Sleep

Sleep Palsies and Acroparesthesias

Several paresthetic disturbances, sometimes distressing in nature, may arise during sleep. Everyone is familiar with the phenomenon of an arm or leg "falling asleep." Immobility of the limbs and maintenance of uncomfortable postures, without any awareness of them, permit undue pressure to be applied on peripheral nerves (especially the ulnar, radial, and peroneal). Pressure of the nerve against the underlying bone may interfere with intraneural function in the compressed segment of nerve. Sustained pressure may result in a sensory and motor paralysis—sometimes referred to as *sleep or pressure palsy*. Usually, this condition lasts only a few hours or days, but if compression is prolonged recovery may be delayed. Deep sleep or a stupor, as in alcohol intoxication or anesthesia, renders patients especially liable to pressure palsies merely because they are not able to heed the discomfort of a sustained unnatural posture.

Acroparesthesias are frequent in adult women and are not unknown in men. The patient, after being asleep for a few hours, is awakened by numbness or a tingling, prickling, "pins-and-needles" feeling in the fingers, and hands. There are also aching, burning pains or tightness, and other unpleasant sensations. With vigorous rubbing or shaking of the hands or extension of the wrists, the paresthesia subsides within a few minutes, only to return later or upon first awakening in the morning. At first, there is a suspicion of having slept on an arm, but the frequent bilaterality of the symptoms and their occurrence regardless of the position of the arms dispels this notion. Usually the paresthesia is in the distribution of the median nerves, and almost invariably proves to be caused by carpal tunnel syndrome.

Bruxism

Nocturnal grinding of the teeth, sometimes diurnal as well, occurs at all ages and may be as distressing to the bystander as it is to the patient. It may also cause serious dental problems unless the teeth are protected in some way. There are many hypothetical explanations, all without proof. Stress is most often blamed, and claimants point to EMG studies that show the masseter and temporalis muscles to be excessively contracted. When present in the daytime, it may also represent a fragment of segmental dystonia or tardive dyskinesia.

Nocturnal Enuresis (See also Chap. 26)

Nocturnal bedwetting with daytime continence is a frequent disorder during childhood, which may persist into adult life. Approximately 1 of 10 children 4 to 14 years of age is affected, boys more frequently than girls (in a ratio of 4:3); even among adults (military recruits), the incidence is 1 to 3 percent. The incidence is much higher if one or both parents were enuretic. Although the condition was formerly thought to be psychogenic, the studies of Gastaut and Broughton revealed a peculiarity of bladder physiology. The intravesicular pressure periodically rises to much higher levels in the enuretic than in normal persons, and the functional bladder capacity of the enuretic is smaller than normal. This suggests a maturational failure of certain modulating nervous influences.

An enuretic episode is most likely to occur 3 to 4 h after sleep onset, and usually, but not necessarily, in stages 3 and 4 sleep. It is preceded by a burst of rhythmic delta waves associated with a general body movement. If the patient is awakened at this point, he does not report any dreams. Imipramine (10 to 75 mg at bedtime) has proved to be an effective agent in reducing the frequency of enuresis. A series of training exercises designed to increase the functional bladder capacity and sphincter tone may also be helpful. Sometimes all that is required is to proscribe fluid intake for several hours prior to sleep and to awaken the patient and have him empty his bladder about 3 h after going to sleep. One interesting patient, an elderly physician with lifelong enuresis, reported that he had finally obtained relief (after all other measures had failed) by using a nasal spray of an analogue of antidiuretic hormone (desmopressin) at bedtime. This has now been adopted for the treatment of intractable cases. Diseases of the urinary tract, diabetes mellitus or diabetes insipidus, epilepsy, sleep apnea syndrome, sickle cell anemia, and spinal cord or cauda equina disease must be excluded as causes of symptomatic enuresis.

Relation of Sleep to Medical Illnesses

The high incidence of thrombotic stroke that is apparent upon awakening, a phenomenon well known to neurologists, has been studied epidemiologically by Palomaki and colleagues. These authors have summarized the evidence for an association between snoring, sleep apnea, and an increased risk for stroke. As already mentioned, cluster headache and migraine have an intricate relationship to sleep, the former almost always occurring during or soon after the first REM period, and the latter often curtailed by a sound sleep.

Patients with coronary arteriosclerosis may show electrocardiogram (ECG) changes during REM sleep, and nocturnal angina has been recorded at this time. Snoring is strongly associated with chronic hypertension. Asthmatics frequently have their attacks at night, but not concomitantly with any specific stage of sleep; they do have a decreased amount of stage N3 sleep and frequent awakenings, however. Patients with hypothyroidism have shown a decrease of stages N3 sleep, and a return to a normal pattern when they become euthyroid. Demented patients generally exhibit reduced amounts of REM and slow-wave sleep, as do children with Down syndrome, phenylketonuria, and other forms of brain damage. Alcohol, barbiturates, and other sedative-hypnotic drugs that suppress REM sleep produce extraordinary excesses of REM during withdrawal periods. This may, in part, account for the hyperactivity and confusion, and perhaps the hallucinosis, seen in withdrawal states.

References

Aldrich MS: Diagnostic aspects of narcolepsy. *Neurology* 50(Suppl):S2, 1998.

Arnulf I, Lin L, Gadoth N, et al: Kleine-Levin syndrome: A systematic study of 108 patients. *Ann Neurol* 63:482, 2008.

Aserinsky E, Kleitman N: A motility cycle in sleeping infants as manifested by ocular and gross bodily activity. *J Appl Physiol* 8:11, 1955.

Baker SK, Zee PC: Circadian disorders of the sleep–wake cycle, in Keyger MH, Roth T, Dement WC (eds): *Principles and Practice of Sleep Medicine*, 3rd ed. Philadelphia, Saunders, 2000, pp 606–614.

Bassetti C, Aldrich MS: Idiopathic hypersomnia: A series of 42 patients. *Brain* 120:1423, 1997.

Bassetti C, Mathis J, Gugger M, et al: Hypersomnia following para-median thalamic stroke: A report of 12 patients. *Ann Neurol* 39:471, 1996.

Billiard M, Cadilhac J: Narcolepsy. *Rev Neurol (Paris)* 141:515, 1985.

Boeve BF, Silber MH, Saper CB, et al: Pathophysiology of REM sleep behaviour disorder and relevance to neurodegenerative disease. *Brain* 130:2770, 2007.

Braun AR, Balkin TJ, Wesenten NJ, et al: Dissociated pattern of activity in visual cortices and their projections during human rapid eye movement sleep. *Science* 279:91, 1998.

Brownell LG, West PR, Sweatman P, et al: Protriptyline in obstructive sleep apnea. *N Engl J Med* 307:1037, 1982.

Burwell CS, Robin ED, Whaley RD, Bickelmann AG: Extreme obesity associated with alveolar hypoventilation: A pickwickian syndrome. *Am J Med* 21:811, 1956.

Carpenter S, Yassa R, Ochs R: A pathologic basis for Kleine-Levin syndrome. *Arch Neurol* 39:25, 1982.

Chabas D, Taheri S, Renier C, Mignot E: The genetics of narcolepsy. *Annu Rev Genomics Hum Genet* 4:459, 2003.

Coulter DL, Allen RJ: Benign neonatal sleep myoclonus. *Arch Neurol* 39:192, 1982.

Critchley M: Periodic hypersomnia and megaphagia in adolescent males. *Brain* 85:627, 1962.

Culebras A, Moore JT: Magnetic resonance findings in REM sleep behavior disorder. *Neurology* 39:1519, 1989.

Daly D, Yoss R: Narcolepsy, in Vinken PJ, Bruyn GW (eds): *Handbook of Clinical Neurology*. Vol 15: The Epilepsies. Amsterdam, North-Holland, 1974, pp 836–852.

Dauvillers Y, Montplaisir J, Cochen V, et al: Post-H1N1 narcolepsy-cataplexy. *Sleep* 33:1428, 2010.

Dauvillers Y, Carlander B, Rivier F, et al: Successful management of cataplexy with intravenous immunoglobulins shortly after narcolepsy onset. *Ann Neurol* 56:905, 2004.

Dement WC, Carskadon MA, Ley R: The prevalence of narcolepsy. *Sleep Res* 2:147, 1973.

Dement WC, Kleitman N: Cyclic variations in EEG during sleep and their relation to eye movements, bodily motility and dreaming. *Electroencephalogr Clin Neurophysiol* 9:673, 1957.

Earley CJ: Restless legs syndrome. *N Engl J Med* 348:2103, 2003.

Ford DE, Kamerow DB: Epidemiologic study of sleep disturbances and psychiatric disorders. *JAMA* 262:1479, 1989.

Fry JM: Treatment modalities for narcolepsy. *Neurology* 50(Suppl):S43, 1998.

Gastaut H, Broughton R: A clinical and polygraphic study of episodic phenomena during sleep. *Recent Adv Biol Psychiatry* 7:197, 1965.

Gillin JC, Spinweber CL, Johnson LC: Rebound insomnia: A critical review. *J Clin Psychopharmacol* 9:161, 1989.

Guilleminault C, Dement WC: 235 cases of excessive daytime sleepiness: Diagnosis and tentative classification. *J Neurol Sci* 31:13, 1977.

Guilleminault C, Dement WC: *Sleep Apnea Syndromes*. New York, Liss, 1978.

Guilleminault C, Flagg W: Effect of baclofen on sleep-related periodic leg movements. *Ann Neurol* 15:234, 1984.

Haimovic IC, Berseford HR: Transient unresponsiveness in the elderly. Report of five cases. *Arch Neurol* 49:35, 1992.

Han F, Lin L, Warby SC, et al: Narcolepsy onset is seasonal and increased following the 2009 H1N1 pandemic in China. *Ann Neurol* 70:410, 2011.

Hauri P, Olmstead E: Childhood onset insomnia. *Sleep* 3:59, 1980.

Herxheimer A, Petrie KJ: Melatonin for the prevention and treatment of jet lag. *Cochrane Database Sys Rev* 2:2002: CB001520.

Hobson JA: Dreaming as delirium: A mental status analysis of our nightly madness. *Semin Neurol* 17:121, 1997.

Hobson JA, Lydic R, Baghdoyan H: Evolving concepts of sleep cycle generation: From brain centers to neuronal populations. *Behav Brain Sci* 9:371, 1986.

Kales A: Chronic hypnotic use: Ineffectiveness, drug-withdrawal insomnia and hypnotic drug dependence. *JAMA* 27:513, 1974.

Kales A, Cadieux RJ, Soldatos CR, et al: Narcolepsy-cataplexy: 1. Clinical and electrophysiologic characteristics. *Arch Neurol* 39:164, 1982.

Kales AL, Kales JD, Soldatos CR: Insomnia and other sleep disorders. *Med Clin North Am* 66:971, 1982.

Katz JD, Ropper AH: Familial Kleine-Levin syndrome: Two siblings with unusually long hypersomnic spells. *Arch Neurol* 59:1959, 2002.

Kavey NB, Whyte J, Resor SR Jr, Gidro-Frank S: Somnambulism in adults. *Neurology* 40:749, 1990.

Kessler S, Guilleminault C, Dement W: A family study of 50 REM narcoleptics. *Acta Neurol Scand* 50:503, 1974.

Kramer RE, Dinner DS, Braun WE, et al: HLA-DR2 and narcolepsy. *Arch Neurol* 44:853, 1987.

Krueger BR: Restless legs syndrome and periodic movements of sleep. *Mayo Clin Proc* 65:999, 1990.

Kryger MH, Roth T, Dement WC (eds): *Principles and Practice of Sleep Medicine*, 4th ed. Philadelphia, Saunders, 2005.

Kupfer DL, Reynolds CF: Management of insomnia. *N Engl J Med* 336:341, 1998.

Landolt HP, Glatzel M, Blättler T, et al: Sleep-wake disturbances in sporadic Creutzfeldt-Jakob disease. *Neurology* 66:1418, 2006.

Lask B: Novel and non-toxic treatment for night terrors. *BMJ* 297:592, 1988.

Lin L, Faraco J, Li R, Kadotani H, et al: The sleep disorder canine narcolepsy is caused by a mutation in the hypocretin (orexin) receptor 2 gene. *Cell* 98:365, 1999.

Liu HM, Loew JM, Hunt CE: Congenital central hypoventilation syndrome: A pathologic study of the neuromuscular system. *Neurology* 28:1013, 1978.

Loomis AL, Harvey EN, Hobart G: Cerebral states during sleep as studied by human brain potentials. *J Exp Psychol* 21:127, 1937.

Lugaresi E, Cirignorra F, Montagna P: Nocturnal paroxysmal dystonia. *J Neurol Neurosurg Psychiatry* 49:375, 1986.

Lugaresi E, Medori R, Montagna P, et al: Fatal familial insomnia and dysautonomia with selective degeneration of thalamic nuclei. *N Engl J Med* 315:997, 1986.

Madsen PL, Vorstrup S: Cerebral blood flow and metabolism during sleep. *Cerebrovasc Brain Metab Rev* 3:281, 1991.

Mahowald MW, Schenck CH: REM sleep parasomnias, in Kryger MH, Roth T, Dement WC (eds): *Principles and Practice of Sleep Medicine*, 4th ed. Philadelphia, Saunders, 2005, pp 897–916.

Markand OHN, Dyken ML: Sleep abnormalities in patients with brainstem lesions. *Neurology* 26:769, 1976.

Martin PR, Loewenstein RJ, Kaye WJ, et al: Sleep EEG in Korsakoff's psychosis and Alzheimer's disease. *Neurology* 36:411, 1986.

Mellinger GD, Balter MB, Uhlenhoth EH: Insomnia and its treatment: Prevalence and correlates. *Arch Gen Psychiatry* 42:225, 1985.

Mignot E, Lammers GJ, Ripley V, et al: The role of cerebrospinal fluid hypocretin measurement in the diagnosis of narcolepsy and other hypersomnias. *Arch Neurol* 59:1553, 2002.

Mitler MM: Toward an animal model of narcolepsy-cataplexy, in Guilleminault C, Dement WC, Passouant P (eds): *Narcolepsy*. New York, Spectrum, 1976, pp 387–409.

Monk TH: Shift work, in Kryger MH, Roth T, Dement WC (eds): *Principles and Practice of Sleep Medicine*, 3rd ed. Philadelphia, Saunders, 2000, pp 600–605.

Neely SE, Rosenberg RS, Spire JP, et al: HLA antigens in narcolepsy. *Neurology* 137:1858, 1987.

Nogueira De Melo A, Kraus GL, Niedermeyer E: Spindle coma: Observations and thoughts. *Clin Electroencephalogr* 21(Suppl 3): 151, 1990.

Ohayon MM, Mahowald MW, Dauvilliers W, et al: Prevalence and comorbidity of nocturnal wandering in the US adult general population. *Neurology* 78:1583, 2012.

Olson EJ, Boeve BF, Silber MH: Rapid eye movement sleep behavior disorder: Demographic, clinical, and laboratory findings in 93 cases. *Brain* 123:331, 2000.
Palomaki H, Partinen M, Erkinjuntti T, et al: Snoring, sleep apnea syndrome, and stroke. *Neurology* 42(Suppl 6):75, 1992.
Parkes JD: *Sleep and Its Disorders*. Philadelphia, Saunders, 1985.
Pearce JMS: Clinical features of the exploding head syndrome. *J Neurol Neurosurg Psychiatry* 52:907, 1989.
Pérez-Díaz H, Iranzo A, Rye DB, Santamaría J: Restless abdomen. A phenotypic variant of restless leg syndrome. *Neurology* 77:1283, 2011.
Popper KR, Eccles JC: *The Self and the Brain*. Berlin, Springer-Verlag, 1977.
Portilla P, Durand E, Chalvon A, et al: Hypoperfusion temporomésiale gauche en TEMP dans un syndrome de Kleine-Levin. *Rev Neurol* 158:593, 2002.
Postuma RB, Gagnon JF, Vendette M, et al: Quantifying the risk of neurodegeneration disease in idiopathic REM sleep behavior disorder. *Neurology* 72:1296, 2009.
Rechtschaffen A, Gilliland MA, Bergman BM, et al: Physiological correlates of prolonged sleep deprivation in rats. *Science* 221:182, 1983.
Rechtschaffen A, Monroe LJ: Laboratory studies of insomnia, in Kales A (ed): *Sleep: Physiology and Pathology—A Symposium*. Philadelphia, Lippincott, 1969, p 158.
Rosen GM, Bendel AE, Neglia JP, et al: Sleep in children with neoplasms of the central nervous system: Case review of 14 children: *Pediatrics* 112:46, 2003.
Roth B: *Narcolepsy and Hypersomnia*. Basel, Springer-Verlag, 1980.
Sack RL: Jet lag. *New Engl J Med* 362:440, 2010.
Saper CB, Scammell TE, Lu J: Hypothalamic regulation of sleep and circadian rhythm. *Nature* 437:1257, 2005.
Schwartz JW, Stakes WJ, Hobson JA: Transient cataplexy after removal of a craniopharyngioma. *Arch Neurol* 34:1372, 1984.
Servan J, Marchand F, Garma L, et al: Narcolepsie revelatrice d'une neurosarcoidose. *Rev Neurol (Paris)* 151:281, 1995.
Shiromani PJ, Armstrong DM, Berkowitz A, et al: Distribution of choline acetyltransferase immunoreactive somata in the feline brainstem: Implications for REM sleep generation. *Sleep* 11:1, 1988.
Sixel-Döring F, Trautmann E, Mollenhauer B, Trenkwalder C: Associated factors for REM sleep behavior disorder in Parkinson disease. *Neurology* 72:1048, 2011.
Solms M: *The Neuropsychology of Dreams: A Clinico-Anatomical Study*. London, Lawrence Erlbaum Associates, 1996.
Solms M: New findings on the neurological organization of dreaming: Implications for psychoanalysis. *Psychoanal Q* 64:43, 1995.
Steffansson H, Rye DB, Hicks A, et al: A genetic risk factor for periodic limb movements in sleep. *N Engl J Med* 357:639, 2007.
Steriade M, McCormick DA, Senjowski TJ: Thalamocortical oscillations in the sleeping and aroused brain. *Science* 262:679, 1993.
Tinuper P, Cerullo A, Cirignotta F, et al: Nocturnal paroxysmal dystonia with short lasting attacks: Three cases with evidence for an epileptic frontal lobe origin for seizures. *Epilepsia* 31:549, 1990.
Tyler DB: Psychological change during experimental sleep deprivation. *Dis Nerv Syst* 16:239, 1955.
Weitzman ED, Boyar RM, Kapen S, Hellman L: The relationship of sleep and sleep stages to neuroendocrine secretion and biological rhythms in man. *Recent Prog Horm Res* 31:399, 1975.
Wilson SAK: *Neurology*. London, Edward Arnold, 1940, pp 1545–1560.

Derangements of Intellect, Behavior, and Language Caused by Diffuse and Focal Cerebral Disease

SECTION 5

Physicians sooner or later discover, through clinical experience, the need for special competence in assessing the mental faculties of their patients. They must be able to observe with objectivity the patient's attention, intelligence, memory, judgment, mood, character, and other attributes of cognitive performance, and personality in much the same fashion as they observe the patient's movements, gait, and reflexes. The systematic examination of these intellectual and affective functions permits the physician to reach conclusions regarding the patient's mental status and its relationship to his illness. Without such data, there are likely to be errors in the diagnosis and treatment of the patient's neurologic, general medical, and psychiatric disease.

The content of this section will be more clearly understood if a few of the introductory remarks to the later section on psychiatric diseases are anticipated here. The main thesis of the neurologist is that mental and physical functions of the nervous system are simply two aspects of the same neural process. Mind and behavior both have their roots in the self-regulating, goal-seeking activities of the organism, the same ones that provide impulse to all forms of mammalian life. But the prodigious complexity of the human brain permits, to an extraordinary degree, the solving of difficult problems, the capacity for remembering past experiences, and casting them in a symbolic language that can be written and read, and the planning for events that have yet to take place. The constant but sometimes meandering internal verbal experience of this ideation during waking was aptly named "stream of thought" by William James. Somehow there emerges in the course of these complex cerebral functions a continuous awareness of one's self, and the operation of one's psychic processes. It is this continuous inner consciousness of one's self, of one's past experiences, and of ongoing cognitive activities that might be called *mind*. Whether this is an emergent property of various mental functions or simply their representation cannot be answered, but any separation of the mental from the observable behavioral aspects of cerebral function is probably illusory. Biologists and psychologists have reached this view by placing all known activities of the nervous system (growth, development, behavior, and mental function) on a continuum and noting the inherent purposiveness and creativity common to all of them. The physician is persuaded of the truth of this view through daily clinical experience, in which every possible aberration of behavior and intellect appears at some time or other as an expression of cerebral disease. Furthermore, in many brain diseases, one witnesses parallel disorders of the patient's behavior and a dissolution or distortion of the introspective awareness of his own mental capacities.

The reader will find that Chaps. 20 and 21 are concerned with common disturbances of the sensorium and of cognition, which stand as cardinal manifestations of cerebral diseases. The most frequent of these are delirium and other acute confusional states, as well as disorders of learning, memory, and other intellectual functions. A consideration of these abnormalities leads naturally to an examination of the symptoms that result from focal cerebral lesions, which are discussed in Chap. 22, and of derangements of language, which are discussed in Chap. 23. As emphasized in those chapters, even these disturbances fall between the readily localizable functions of the cerebrum and those that can be assigned only broadly to large regions or systems of the brain.

Because the psychiatric causes of disordered thinking and behavior have special qualities that make them separable from most of the conditions considered in the next several chapters, they are discussed in Chaps. 51 to 53 at the end of the book, rather than here.

20

Delirium and Other Acute Confusional States

The striking event in which a patient with previously intact mentality becomes acutely confused is observed almost daily on the medical, surgical, and emergency wards of a general hospital. Occurring, as it often does, during an infection with fever or in the course of a toxic or metabolic disorder (such as renal or hepatic failure) or as an effect of medication, drugs, or alcohol, it never fails to create grave problems for the physician, nursing personnel, and family. The physician has to cope with the problem of diagnosis, often without the advantage of a lucid history, and any program of therapy is constantly impeded by the patient's inattention, agitation, sleeplessness, and inability to cooperate. Nurses are burdened with the need to provide satisfactory care and a safe immediate environment for the patient, and at the same time, maintain a tranquil atmosphere for other patients. The family must be supported as it faces the frightening specter of a deranged mind with peculiar behaviors and all it signifies.

These difficulties are magnified when the patient arrives in the emergency ward, having behaved in some irrational way, and the clinical analysis must begin without knowledge of the patient's background and underlying medical illnesses. It is our view that such patients should be admitted to a general medical or neurologic ward. Transfer of the patient to a psychiatric service is undertaken only if the behavioral disorder proves impossible to manage on a general hospital service.

DEFINITION OF TERMS

The definition of normal and abnormal states of mind is difficult because the terms used to describe them have been given so many different meanings in both medical and non-medical writings. Compounding the difficulty is the fact that the pathophysiology of the confusional states and delirium is not fully understood, and the definitions depend to some extent on their clinical causes and relationships, with all the imprecision that this entails. The following nomenclature has proved useful to us and is employed in this and subsequent chapters.

Confusion is a general term *denoting the patient's incapacity to think with customary speed, clarity, and coherence.* Its most conspicuous attributes are impaired attention and power of concentration, disorientation—which may be manifest or is demonstrated only by direct questioning—an inability to properly register immediate events and to recall them later, a reduction in the amount and a disruption in the quality of all mental activity, including the normally constant inner ideation and sometimes, by the appearance of bewilderment. Thinking, speech, and the performance of goal-directed actions are impersistent or abruptly arrested by the intrusion of irrelevant thoughts or distracted by the slightest external stimulus. Reduced perceptiveness and accompanying visual and auditory illusions or hallucinations and paranoid delusions (psychosis) are variable features that may be appended to the picture.

These psychologic disturbances may appear in many contexts. Confusion, as defined in this way, is an essential ingredient of the state called *delirium* (discussed further on), in which agitation, hallucinations, and sometimes tremulousness accompany the confusional state. Also, as pointed out in Chap. 17, a confusional state may appear at any stage in the evolution and resolution of a number of diseases that lead to drowsiness, stupor, and coma—typically in the metabolic encephalopathies but also in diseases affecting those parts of the brain that maintain normal arousal.

Confusion is also a characteristic feature of the chronic syndrome of *dementia*, where it is the product of a progressive failure of cognition, language, memory, and other intellectual functions; there it is the long-standing and progressive nature of the mental confusion that differentiates dementia from the acute confusional and delirious states that carry quite different implications. Finally, intense emotional disturbances, of either *manic or depressive* type, may interfere with attentiveness and coherence of thinking and thereby produce an apparent confusional state.

Special restricted forms of what could be called confusion appear as a result of certain focal cerebral lesions, particularly of the frontal, parietal, and temporal lobe association areas. Then, instead of a global inattention and incoherence, there are specific and circumscribed syndromes, such as unilateral neglect of self or of the environment, inability to identify persons or objects, and sensorimotor defects as described in Chap. 22. Yet another special form of confusion arises as a result of disordered language function, which also alters the stream of thought; this aphasia is a consequence of lesions in the language areas of the left temporal lobe. These are considered separately in Chap. 23.

The many mental and behavioral aberrations that are seen in confused patients, and their occurrence in various combinations and clinical contexts, make it unlikely that all forms of confusion derive from a single elementary psychologic abnormality such as a disturbance of attention. While attention is near the core of confusion, phenomena as diverse as drowsiness and stupor, hallucinations and delusions, disorders of perception and registration, impersistence and perseveration, and so forth are not easily reduced to a disorder of one psychologic or physiologic mechanism. It seems more likely to us that a number of separable disorders of function are involved. Indeed, one view of the confusional state that we find attractive conceptualizes confusion as a loss of the integrative functions among all the elementary and localizable cerebral functions such as symbolic language, memory retrieval, and apperception (the interpretation of primary perceptions). All of these are included under the rubric of *the confusional state*, for want of a better term.

We reserve the term *delirium* to denote a special agitated type of confusional state. In addition to many of the negative elements of incoherent thinking mentioned above, delirium is characterized by a prominent disorder of perception; hallucinations and vivid dreams; a kaleidoscopic array of strange and absurd fantasies and delusions; inability to sleep; a tendency to twitch, tremble, and convulse; and intense fear or other emotional reactions. Delirium is distinguished not only by extreme inattentiveness but also by a state of heightened alertness—i.e., an increased readiness to respond to stimuli—and by overactivity of psychomotor and autonomic nervous system functions, sometimes striking in degree. Implicit in the term *delirium* are its nonmedical connotations as well—namely, intense agitation, or frenzied excitement, and trembling. This distinction between delirium and other acute confusional states is not universally accepted. Many authors attach no particular significance to the autonomic and psychomotor overactivity and the hallucinatory and dream-like features of delirium, or to the underactivity and somnolence that characterize most other confusional states. All such states are categorized together as we continue to find it useful to set delirium apart from other nondescript confusional states because the two conditions are manifestly different and tend to occur in different clinical contexts. Nevertheless, implicit in both designations is the idea of an acute, transient, and usually completely reversible disorder.

An impairment of memory is often included among the symptoms of delirium and other confusional states. Registration and recall are indeed greatly impaired in the states under discussion, but they are affected in proportion to the degree of inattention and the inability to register new material. The term *amnesia*, however, refers more precisely to an isolated loss of past memories as well as to an inability to form new ones, despite an alert state of mind and normal attentiveness. Amnesia further presupposes an ability of the patient to grasp the meaning of what is going on around him. The failure in the amnesic state is one of retention, recall, and reproduction and must be distinguished from states of drowsiness, acute confusion, and delirium, in which information and events seem never to have been adequately perceived and registered in the first place. In both a confusional state and in amnesia, the patient will be left with a permanent gap in memory for his acute illness.

In a similar way, the term *dementia* (literally, an undoing of the mind) denotes a deterioration of all intellectual or cognitive functions with little or no disturbance of consciousness or perception. Implied in dementia is the idea of a gradual degradation of mental powers in a person who formerly possessed a normal mind. *Amentia*, by contrast, indicates a congenital feeblemindedness more commonly referred to as *mental retardation*, or more properly, *developmental cognitive delay*. Dementia and amnesia are discussed more explicitly in Chap. 21.

OBSERVABLE ASPECTS OF BEHAVIOR AND INTELLECT IN CONFUSION, DELIRIUM, AMNESIA, AND DEMENTIA

The intellectual, emotional, and behavioral activities of the human organism are so complex and varied that one may question the feasibility of using derangements of these activities as reliable indicators of cerebral disease. Certainly they do not have the same tangibility and ease of anatomic and physiologic interpretation as sensory and motor paralysis or aphasia. Yet one observes patterns of disturbed higher cerebrocortical function with such regularity as to make them clinically useful in identifying certain diseases. Some of these disturbances gain specificity because they are combined in certain ways to form syndromes.

The components of mentation and behavior that lend themselves to bedside observation and examination are (1) the processes of attention; (2) perception and apperception (awareness and interpretation of sensory stimuli); (3) the capacity to memorize and recall events of the recent and distant past; (4) the ability to think and reason; (5) temperament, mood, and emotion; (6) initiative, impulse, and drive; (7) social behavior; and (8) insight. Of these, the first two are *sensory*, the third and fourth are *cognitive*, the fifth is *affective*, the sixth is *conative* or volitional, the seventh refers to the patient's relationships with those around him, and the last refers to the patient's capacity to assess his own functioning. Each component of behavior and intellect has its objective side, expressed in the behavioral responses produced by certain stimuli, and its subjective side, expressed in the thinking and feeling described by the patient in relation to the stimuli. Less accessible to the examiner, but nevertheless possible to study by questioning of the patient, are the memories, planning, and other psychic activities that continuously occupy the mind of an alert person. They, too, are disordered or quantitatively diminished by cerebral disease.

Disturbances of Attention

Critical to clear thinking is a process of maintaining awareness of one or a limited number of external stimuli or internal thoughts for a fixed period of time and to simultaneously disregard the numerous distracting sensations and ideas that constantly bombard the nervous system. Without this ability to focus or "pay attention" and have an "attention span," a coherent stream of thought or action is not possible. The undue interruption of these activities by the intrusion of other thoughts or actions is termed *inattention,* or *distractibility.* Two essential components are embodied in the attention mechanism: one, a continuous state of alertness that is normally present throughout waking life (and underlies self-awareness); the other, a process of selecting from the myriad sensations and thoughts those that are relevant to the immediate situation to the exclusion of others.

The confused patient may demonstrate inattention in almost every task undertaken. If the degree of confusion is slight, the patient may report a difficulty with concentration. If severe, there is a parallel lack of insight and the problem is evident by observing easy distractibility by ambient stimuli and by impersistence and perseveration in conversation and motor tasks. Restated, attention has such a pervasive effect on all other aspects of mental performance that it is often difficult to determine whether the confused patient also has primary disorders of memory, executive, or visuospatial function. Indeed, retentive memory may be severely reduced in confusional states. Furthermore, the ability to carry out a series of actions or mental operations wherein one is required to hold in memory the result of the previous operation ("working memory") is intimately tied to attention and is particularly prone to disruption in confusional states.

The general ability to persist in a motor or mental task emphasizes an executive side of attention, but here one encounters a problem because the term *attention* has been applied to a number of seemingly different mental activities. One can view attention as a separate and unique cerebral function or simply a way of referring to the persistence or impersistence of any activity. We would argue that the entire cerebrum participates in attentiveness and the frontal and perhaps the parietal lobes are responsible for directing its content, but that the thalamocortical system is in a special way responsible for its raw maintenance. Mesulam, who has thought substantially about this problem, considers the frontal and parietal lobes to be at the nexus of an "attentional matrix"; in his model, the prefrontal, parietal association, and limbic cortices direct and modulate attention in an executive manner. Certainly, the temporal lobes and other regions are involved as well.

Attention to a particular sensory modality requires the participation of the sensory cortex, which must simultaneously initiate the perceptive and apperceptive processes discussed later. What are called "modality" and "domain-specific" attentions (for example, face or object recognition) are more complex, and disorders of these functions result in unique types of inattention, such as agnosia and anosognosia (lack of recognition of a part of the body, as discussed in Chap. 22). These are not derived from the all-encompassing loss of attention that is part of general confusional states but can instead be viewed as highly restricted forms of disruption of insight.

Disturbances of Perception

The process of acquiring through the senses a knowledge of the world or, of one's self by cohering what is experienced into apperception, involves much more than the simple sensory process of being aware of the attributes of a stimulus. New visual stimuli, for example, activate the striate cortex and visual association areas, wherein are probably stored the coded past representations of these and similar classes of stimuli. Recognition involves the reactivation of this system by the same or similar stimuli at a later time. Essential elements in the perceptual process are the maintenance of attention, the selective focusing on a stimulus, elimination of all extraneous stimuli, and identification of the stimulus by recognizing its relationship to remembered experience.

The perception of stimuli undergoes predictable derangement in disease. Most often there is a reduction in the number of perceptions in a given unit of time and a failure to synthesize them properly and to relate them to the ongoing activities of the mind. Or, there may be inattentiveness and fluctuations of attention, distractibility (pertinent and irrelevant stimuli having equal value), and inability to concentrate and persist in an assigned task. This often leads to disorientation in time and place. Qualitative changes also appear, mainly in the form of sensory distortions, causing misinterpretations of environmental stimuli (illusions) and misidentifications of persons; these, at least in part, form the basis of hallucinatory experience in which the patient reports and reacts to environmental stimuli that are not evident to the examiner. There is an inability to perceive simultaneously all elements of a large complex of stimuli, a defect that has been termed "failure of subjective organization." These major disturbances in the perceptual sphere, traditionally referred to as "clouding of the sensorium," are characteristic of delirium, and other confusional states.

More specific partial losses of perception are manifest in the "neglect syndromes." The most dramatic examples are observed with right parietal lesions, which render a patient unaware of the left half of his body and the environment on the left side. There are numerous other examples of focal cerebral lesions that disturb or distort sensory perceptions, each subject to neurologic testing; these are discussed in Chap. 22. Their close connection to spatial experience makes them understandable as alterations of apperception in the spatial-sensory sphere.

Disturbances of Memory

The retention of learned information and experiences is involved in all mental activities. Memory may be arbitrarily subdivided into several parts: (1) registration; (2) fixation, mnemonic integration, and retention; (3) recognition and recall; and (4) reproduction. As stated above, there is a failure of learning and memory in patients with impaired perception and attention because the material to be learned was never registered and assimilated in the first place. In almost all circumstances, the formation of new memories and the ability to recall old ones are disturbed in tandem.

In the *Korsakoff amnesic syndrome*, newly presented material appears to be correctly registered but cannot be retained for more than a few minutes (*anterograde amnesia*, or failure of learning). In this syndrome, there is always an associated defect in the recall and reproduction of memories that had been formed several days, weeks, or even years before the onset of the illness (*retrograde amnesia*). The fabrication of stories, called *confabulation*, constitutes a third feature of the syndrome but is neither specific nor invariably present. Intact retention with failure of recall (retrograde amnesia without anterograde amnesia) when it is severe and extends to all events of past life and even personal identity, is usually a manifestation of hysteria or malingering. Certain other characteristic defects occur in almost all memory disorders, for example, the relative retention of older memories in preference to newer ones (Ribot's rule). Chapter 22 discusses this subject more fully.

Disturbances of Thinking

Thinking, the highest order of intellectual activity, remains the most elusive of all mental operations. If by thinking one means the selective ordering of symbols for learning, organizing information, and problem solving, as well as the capacity to reason and form sound judgments, then the working units of this type of mental activity are words and numbers. The substitution of words and numbers for the objects for which they stand (symbolization) is a fundamental part of the process. These symbols are formed into ideas or concepts, and the arrangement of new and remembered ideas into certain orders or relationships constitutes an intricate part of thought, presently beyond the scope of analysis. Reference is made further on to Luria's analysis of the steps involved in problem solving in connection with frontal lobe function, but actually, as he points out, the whole cerebrum is implicated in all forms of thinking. In a general way, one may examine thinking in terms of its speed and efficiency, ideational content, coherence and logical relationships of ideas, and the quantity and quality of associations to a given idea. Feelings and behaviors engendered by an idea are more in the realm of emotion and affect. Aphasic disturbances are uncommon in global confusional and delirious states, but Geschwind has emphasized misnaming as an important feature among the "nonaphasic disorders of speech" in these conditions. Spontaneous speech is normal, but there may be slight inaccuracies in repetition that are most likely the result of inattention rather than a focal cerebral lesion.

Disorders of thinking are quite prominent in delirium and other confusional states, in mania, dementia, and schizophrenia. In confusional states of all types, the organization of thought processes is disrupted, with fragmentation, repetition, and perseveration; this is spoken of as an "incoherence of thinking." Derangements of thinking may also take the form of a flight of ideas; patients move too facilely from one idea to another, and their associations are numerous, and loosely linked. This is a common feature of hypomanic and manic states, and of some schizophrenic psychoses. The opposite condition, poverty of ideas, is characteristic both of depressive illnesses, in which it is combined with gloomy thoughts, of schizophrenia, and of dementing diseases, in which it is part of a reduction of all inner psychic intellectual activity. This overall reduction in thought and action is the most prominent feature of diseases that damage the frontal lobes.

A related condition of slowed thought, or *bradyphrenia*, is comparable to the bradykinesia of extrapyramidal disorders. The two often coexist and the patient, for example with Parkinson's disease, can articulate that thinking is so slow as to be virtually blocked. The content of thought is not much altered, but it may be rendered almost useless when slowed to this degree. The outward manifestation of bradyphrenia is what one would expect, a delay in response and slowness in gathering one's thoughts to express ideas.

Thinking may be distorted in such a way that ideas are not checked against reality. When a false belief is maintained in spite of convincing evidence to the contrary, the patient is said to have a *delusion*. This abnormality is common to several illnesses, particularly bipolar, schizophrenic, and paranoid states, as well as the early stages of dementia. Often the story related by the patient has internal logic but is patently absurd. Psychotic patients may believe that ideas have been implanted in their minds by some outside agency, such as the internet, radio, television, or atomic energy; these thought control or "passivity feelings" are highly characteristic of schizophrenia, and sometimes of manic episodes. Also diagnostic of some forms of schizophrenia are distortions of logical thought, such as gaps in sequential thinking, intrusion of irrelevant ideas, and condensation of associations. Chapter 53 discusses these aspects of psychoses.

Disturbances of Emotion, Mood, and Affect

The emotional life of the patient is expressed in a variety of ways. It is widely appreciated that there are marked individual differences in basic temperament in the normal population; throughout their lives some persons are cheerful, gregarious, optimistic, and free from worry, whereas others are just the opposite. The state of emotionality, and changes that are uncharacteristic to the individual lend themselves to observation and have clinical significance. Furthermore, some inherent personality traits may precede the development of overt mental disease. For example, the volatile, cyclothymic person is said to be liable to bipolar disease, and the suspicious, withdrawn, introverted person to schizophrenia and paranoia, but there are frequent exceptions to these statements.

Strong, persistent emotional states, such as fear and anxiety, may occur as reactions to life situations and are accompanied by numerous derangements of visceral function. If excessive, prolonged, and disproportionate to the stimulus, they are usually manifestations of an anxiety state or depression. In depression, almost all stimuli also tend to enhance the somber mood of unhappiness. Affective displays that are excessively labile and poorly controlled or uninhibited are a common manifestation of many cerebral diseases, particularly those involving the corticopontine and corticobulbar pathways. This disorder constitutes part of the syndrome of spastic bulbar (pseudobulbar) palsy, as discussed in Chap. 25, but it may occur independently of any problem with brainstem function. Affect being the external appearance of emotional life, the pseudobulbar state is characterized by a relative disconnection between the patient's reported emotional feelings and the outward display, most often being in the same general direction, but excessive in appearance. Conversely, all emotional feeling and expression may be lacking, as in states of profound apathy or depression. Or excessive cheerfulness may be maintained in the face of serious, potentially fatal disease or other adversity—a pathologic *euphoria*. Finally, a patient's emotional responses may be inappropriate to the stimulus, e.g., a depressing or morbid thought may seem amusing and be attended by a smile, a bizarre affective state as in schizophrenia.

Temperament, mood, and other emotional experiences are evaluated by observing the patient's behavior and appearance while questioning him about his feelings. For these purposes, it is convenient to divide emotionality into *mood* and *affect*. By mood is meant the prevailing internal emotional state of an individual. By contrast, *affect* (or *feeling*) refers to the outward emotional reactions evoked by a thought or an environmental stimulus. As such, it is the observable aspect of emotion. Emotionality may only be inferred from a person's affect and any more accurate assessment of the emotional state is made largely by the patient's self-report. It may be cheerful and optimistic or gloomy and melancholic. The patient's language (e.g., the adjectives used), facial expression, attitude, posture, and speed of movement reflect prevailing mood. These distinctions are at times rather tenuous, but they are clinically valuable because pathologic processes may dissociate the two to an extreme degree, as mentioned above. Chapter 25 more fully discusses the emotional disturbances relating to neurologic disease and Chap. 52 addresses depression.

Disturbances of Impulse (Conation) and Activity

Reference was made in Chaps. 3 and 4 to weakness, akinesia, and bradykinesia as manifestations of corticospinal and extrapyramidal disease. Disorders of these parts of the motor system interfere with voluntary or automatic movements, much to the distress of the patient. But motility and activity can be impaired in more general ways in which the overall tone of the motor system is enhanced or diminished. One such disorder is a lack of *conation*, or *impulse*. These terms designate that the basic biologic urges, driving forces, or purposes by which every organism is motivated to achieve an endless series of objectives. Indeed, motor activity is ostensibly a necessary and satisfying objective in itself, for few individuals can remain still for long before they become fidgety or doodle, and the severely retarded apparently obtain gratification from certain rhythmic movements, such as rocking, head banging, and hand flapping. These are all presumed to be driven by mental impulses. As discussed in Chap. 6, tics and compulsions apparently also represent the fulfillment of some psychic urge.

It is our impression that a quantitative reduction in spontaneous activity, i.e., in the amount of activity per unit of time, is one of the most frequent manifestations of cerebral disease. An important aspect of this state, called *abulia* is the concomitant reduction and prominent delay in producing movement, speech, ideation, and emotional reaction (apathy). The terms bradyphrenia, and "psychomotor retardation," referred to above may be a related or perhaps identical phenomena. With certain cerebral diseases the disinclination to move and act may reach an extreme degree, to a point where a person who is wide awake and perceptive of the environment does not speak or move for weeks on end (akinetic mutism). Such patients seem indifferent to what is happening around them, and unconcerned about the consequences of their inactivity.

Abulia and akinetic mutism must be distinguished from two allied states, *catatonia* and the *psychomotor retardation* of depression. Kahlbaum, who first used the term *catatonia* in 1874, described it as a condition in which the patient sits or lies silent and motionless, with a staring countenance, completely without volition and without reaction to sensory impressions. Sometimes there is resistance to the examiner's efforts to move the patient, or the patient repeats certain movements or phrases hour after hour. If the limbs are moved passively, they may retain their new position for a prolonged period (*flexibilitas cerea*, or "waxy flexibility"), but more often there is no actual motor rigidity except that of voluntary resistance, termed *paratonia*. Profound depression or other psychosis is the usual cause of catatonia. The psychomotor retardation of depression and catatonia may be so profound that the patient makes no attempt to help himself in any way and ultimately starves unless fed with a nasogastric tube.

Less easy to understand is a form of "lethal catatonia," originally described by Stauder, in which the completely inert catatonic patient develops a high fever, collapses, and dies. In some respects, this state resembles the neuroleptic malignant syndrome, an idiosyncratic consequence of intoxication with neuroleptic drugs. In abulia, catatonia, and depression, the mind is usually sufficiently alert to record events and later to recount them, which differentiates these states from stupor. But this distinction is not always valid, for we have seen catatonic schizophrenic and greatly slowed depressive patients who could not recall what had happened during the period of illness.

Pathologic degrees of motor or mental restlessness and hyperactivity represent the opposite extreme from abulia. *Akathisia* refers to constant restless movements and inability to sit still; in some patients, this is a consequence of the prolonged use of phenothiazines, butyrophenones, newer antipsychosis drugs, and L-dopa, but it is also seen in agitated depressions. Hyperactivity-inattention disorders describe yet another form of excessive motor activity that usually accompanies an attention deficit syndrome of children, mostly boys (attention-deficit hyperactivity disorder [ADHD]). In the manic form of bipolar disease (and to a lesser extent in hypomania), continuous activity and insomnia are added to the flight of ideas and the euphoric (although somewhat irritable) mood. Following certain cerebral diseases, notably some forms of encephalitis and during recovery from traumatic lesions of the frontal lobes, the patient may remain in a state of constant uncontrollable and sometimes destructive activity. Kahn referred to this state as "organic drivenness."

Disorders of Social Behavior

Behavioral disturbances are common manifestations of all delirious–confusional states, particularly those of toxic–metabolic origin, but also those caused by more obvious structural disease of the brain. The patient may be completely indifferent to all persons around him, or the opposite, when any approach may excite anger and aggressive action. Family members may be treated with disrespect, regarded with suspicion, or falsely accused of harming the patient, stealing his possessions, or trying to poison him. The embarrassment consequent to urinating in public or soiling the bed may be absent and, particularly in men, there may be lewd behavior toward the opposite sex. In its most extreme form, usually seen in the later stages of dementing diseases, irascible behavior degenerates to kicking, screaming, biting, spitting, and an aversion to being touched, making it entirely impossible to approach the patient. These aspects of disordered mental function are the most alarming to the family and are difficult to manage in the hospital. Previously upstanding, socially appropriate, and abstemious persons may lose all regard for their actions and become profligate, gamblers, or alcoholics. In cases of damage to the frontal lobes, even beyond a neglect for social conventions, there is an indifference to others and to the consequences of the patient's actions on other members of society.

In contrast, docility and amiable social behavior characterize certain conditions such as Down and Williams syndromes, and social indifference and a lack of ability to interpret the emotional state of others are major features of autism (see "Delirium" later on).

Loss of Insight

The state of being aware of the nature and degree of one's deficits and their consequences becomes manifestly impaired or abolished in relation to many cerebral diseases, not just those of the frontal lobes. Lack of insight is a far more complex phenomenon than the operational definition given above suggests. In particular, there are many restricted forms of unawareness of gross neurologic deficits. These are the *agnosias*, discussed in Chap. 22. Patients with these diseases rarely seek advice or help for their illnesses; instead, the family usually brings the patient to the physician. And, after the diagnosis has been made, the loss of insight may be reflected in a lack of compliance with planned therapy. It follows that diseases that produce abnormalities of insight also reduce the patient's capacity to make accurate introspections concerning his psychic function.

CONFUSIONAL SYNDROMES

To summarize, the entire group of acute confusional and delirious states is characterized principally by an alteration of consciousness and by prominent disorders of attention and perception, which interfere with the speed, clarity, and coherence of thinking, the formation of memories, and the capacity for performance of self-directed and commanded activities. Three major clinical syndromes can be recognized. One is an *acute confusional state* in which there is manifest reduction in alertness and psychomotor activity. A second syndrome, already alluded to as a special form of confusion, *delirium*, is marked by overactivity, sleeplessness, tremulousness, and prominence of vivid hallucinations, sometimes with excessive sympathetic activity. These two illnesses tend to develop acutely, to have multiple causes and, except for a few cerebral diseases, to remit within a relatively short period of time of days to weeks, leaving the patient without residual damage. The third syndrome is one in which a confusional state occurs in persons with an underlying chronic cerebral disease, particularly a dementia. Such cerebral disease may be focal or diffuse. Dr. Raymond Adams had designated this disposition to a superimposed acute confusional state in the context of dementia as a *beclouded dementia* but the term, while very apt, seems not to have caught on.

From the neurologic perspective, the generic term *psychosis* applies to states of confusion in which elements of hallucinations, delusions, and disordered thinking comprise the prominent features. An important point to be made here is that psychoses typically leave the sensorium relatively unclouded and allow for normal attentions and high-level performance of many mental tasks. These syndromes and some aspects of psychotic confusion are elaborated below.

Characteristically, these abnormalities *fluctuate in severity*, typically being worse at night ("sundowning"). In the mildest form, the patient appears alert and may even pass for normal; only the failure to recollect and accurately reproduce happenings of the past few hours or days reveals the subtle inadequacy of his mental function. The more obviously confused patient spends much of his time in idleness, and what he does may be inappropriate and annoying to others. Only the more automatic acts and verbal responses are performed properly, but these may permit the examiner to obtain a number of relevant replies to questions about age, occupation, and residence. Orientation to the date, day of the week, and place is imprecise, often with the date being off by several days, the year being given as several years or one decade previous, or with the last two numbers transposed, e.g., 2015 given as 2051. Such patients may, before answering, repeat every question that is put to them, and their responses tend to be brief and mechanical. It is difficult or impossible for them to sustain a conversation. Their attention wanders and they constantly have to be brought back to the subject at hand. They may even fall asleep during the interview, and if left alone are observed to sleep more hours each day than is natural or to sleep at irregular intervals.

As the confusion deepens, conversation becomes more difficult, and at a certain stage these patients no longer notice or respond to much of what is happening around them. Questions may be answered with a single word or a short phrase, spoken in a soft tremulous voice or whisper, or the patient may be mute. Asterixis is a common accompaniment if a metabolic or toxic encephalopathy is responsible for the confusional state. In the most advanced stages of the illness, confusion gives way to stupor and, finally, to coma (see Chap. 17). With improvement in the underlying condition, they may pass again through the stages of stupor and confusion in the reverse order. All this informs us that at least one category of confusion is but a manifestation of the same disease processes that affect awakeness and alertness and, in their severest form, cause coma.

Etiology

Table 20-1 lists some of the many causes of this common type of confusional state. The most frequent in general practice are drug intoxications and endogenous metabolic encephalopathies, mainly electrolyte and water imbalance (hypo- and hypernatremia, hyperosmolarity), hypercalcemia, disorders of acid–base balance, renal and hepatic failure, hyper- and hypoglycemia, febrile and septic states ("septic encephalopathy" discussed further on), and chronic cardiac and pulmonary insufficiency.

Table 20-1

CLASSIFICATION OF DELIRIUM AND ACUTE CONFUSIONAL STATES

I. **Acute confusional states associated with psychomotor underactivity**
  A. Associated with a medical or surgical disease (no focal or lateralizing neurologic signs; cerebrospinal fluid [CSF] clear)
    1. Metabolic disorders (hepatic stupor, uremia, hypo- and hypernatremia, hypercalcemia, hypo- and hyperglycemia, hypoxia, hypercapnia, porphyria, and some endocrinopathies)
    2. Infectious illnesses (pneumonia, endocarditis, urosepsis, peritonitis, and other illnesses causing bacteremia and septicemia—septic encephalopathy)
    3. Congestive heart failure
    4. Postoperative and posttraumatic states
  B. Associated with drug intoxication (no focal or lateralizing signs; CSF clear): opiates, anticholinergics, barbiturates and other sedatives, trihexyphenidyl, corticosteroids, anticonvulsants, L-dopa, dopaminergic agonists, serotonergic antidepressants
  C. Associated with diseases of the nervous system (with focal or lateralizing neurologic signs or CSF changes)
    1. Cerebrovascular disease, tumor, abscess (especially of the right parietal, left temporal and occipital, and inferofrontal lobes)
    2. Subdural hematoma
    3. Meningitis
    4. Encephalitis
    5. Cerebral vasculitis (e.g., granulomatous, lupus)
    6. Hypertensive encephalopathy
    7. Postconvulsive state

II. **Delirium**
  A. In a medical or surgical illness (no focal or lateralizing neurologic signs; CSF usually clear)
    1. Pneumonia
    2. Septicemia and bacteremia (septic encephalopathy)
    3. Postoperative and postconcussive states
    4. Thyrotoxicosis and corticosteroid excess (exogenous or endogenous)
    5. Infectious fevers such as typhoid, malaria
  B. In neurologic disease that causes focal or lateralizing signs or changes in the CSF
    1. Vascular, neoplastic, or other diseases, particularly those involving the temporal lobes and upper part of the brainstem
    2. Concussion and contusion (traumatic delirium)
    3. Meningitis of acute purulent, fungal, tuberculous, and neoplastic types (Chap. 32)
    4. Encephalitis from viral (e.g., herpes simplex, infectious mononucleosis), bacterial (mycoplasma), and other causes (Chaps. 32 and 33)
    5. Subarachnoid hemorrhage
  C. Abstinence states, exogenous intoxications, and postconvulsive states (signs of other medical, surgical, and neurologic illnesses absent or coincidental)
    1. Withdrawal of alcohol (delirium tremens), barbiturates, and nonbarbiturate sedative drugs, following chronic intoxication (Chaps. 42 and 43)
    2. Drug intoxications: scopolamine, amphetamine, cocaine, and other drugs, particularly hallucinogens, phencyclidine, etc.
    3. Postconvulsive delirium

III. Psychosis, particularly with manic characteristics

IV. **Confusional states caused by focal cerebral lesions** (see Chap. 22)

V. **Beclouded dementia,** i.e., dementing or other brain disease in combination with infective fevers, drug reactions, trauma, heart failure, or other medical or surgical diseases

Diffuse or multifocal disease of the cerebral hemispheres is another class of transient or persisting confusional states. Concussion and seizures, especially petit mal or psychomotor status, and certain focal (e.g., right parietal and temporal) cerebral lesions may also be followed by a period of confusion. Focal lesions, most often infarctions but also hemorrhages, of the right cerebral hemisphere may evoke an acute confusional state. Such syndromes have been described with strokes mainly in the territory of the right middle cerebral artery (Mesulam et al; Caplan et al; Mori and Yamadori); usually the infarcts have involved the posterior parietal lobe or inferior frontostriatal regions, but they have also occurred with strokes in the territory of one posterior cerebral artery. A variety of more generalized or multifocal cerebral diseases may be associated with transient or persistent confusional states. Among these are meningitis, encephalitis, thrombotic thrombocytopenic purpura (TTP), disseminated intravascular coagulation, tumors, subdural hematoma, and cranial trauma.

A more restricted group of focal cerebral diseases, including drug and alcohol withdrawal and systemic infections cause delirium, as discussed below.

Pathophysiology of Confusional States

All that has been said on this subject in Chap. 17 regarding coma is applicable to at least one subgroup of the confusional states. In most cases, no consistent pathologic change is found because the abnormalities are metabolic and subcellular. As discussed in Chap. 2, the electroencephalogram (EEG) is almost invariably abnormal in even mild forms of this syndrome, in contrast to delirium, where the changes may be relatively minor. Bilateral high-voltage slow waves in the range of 2 to 4 per second (delta) or 5 to 7 per second (theta) are the usual findings with confusion. These changes surely reflect one aspect of the central problem—the diffuse impairment of the cerebral mechanisms governing alertness and attention and the property of coherence imparted by these functions. If only metaphorically, this mental incoherence and the disorganized thinking and behavior of the confusional states reflect the loss of integrated activity of all of the associative regions of the cortex as mentioned earlier in the chapter.

Delirium

This is best depicted in the patient undergoing withdrawal from alcohol after a sustained period of intoxication. The symptoms usually develop over a period of 2 or 3 d. The first indications are difficulty in concentration, restless irritability, increasing tremulousness, and insomnia. There may be momentary disorientation, an occasional inappropriate remark, or transient illusions or hallucinations.

These initial symptoms rapidly give way to a clinical picture that is one of the most colorful in medicine. The patient is inattentive and unable to perceive the elements of his situation. He may talk incessantly and incoherently, and look distressed and perplexed; his expression may be in keeping with vague notions of being annoyed or threatened by someone. From his manner and the content of speech, it is evident that he misinterprets the meaning of ordinary objects and sounds, misidentifies the people around him, and is experiencing vivid visual, auditory, and tactile hallucinations, often of a most unpleasant type. At first the patient can be brought into touch with reality and may identify the examiner and answer other questions correctly; but almost at once he relapses into a preoccupied, confused state, giving incorrect answers and being unable to think coherently. As the process evolves, the patient cannot shake off his hallucinations and is unable to make meaningful responses to the simplest questions and is profoundly distracted and disoriented. Sleep is impossible or occurs only in brief naps. Speech is reduced to unintelligible muttering.

The signs of overactivity of the autonomic nervous system, more than any others, distinguish delirium from other confusional states. Tremor of fast frequency and jerky restless movements are practically always present and may be violent. The face is flushed, the pupils are dilated, and the conjunctivae are injected; the pulse is rapid, blood pressure elevated, and the temperature may be raised. There is excessive sweating. Most of these signs are reflections of overactivity of the sympathetic nervous system.

The most certain indication of the subsidence of the attack is the occurrence of lucid intervals of increasing length and sound sleep. Recovery is usually complete. In retrospect, the patient has only a few vague memories of his illness or none at all. Single seizures may punctuate the syndrome at any time, including before its development.

Fragments of the full syndrome are common. Brief disorientation, isolated hallucinations, or restlessness with mild hypersympathetic features all occur in withdrawal states, febrile illnesses, and with various intoxications.

The brains of patients who have died in delirium tremens without associated disease or injury usually show no pathologic changes of significance. Intoxication with a number of medications, particularly those with atropinic effects, and certain abused drugs, such as the hallucinogens, causes a delirious state. Delirium may also occur in association with a number of recognizable cerebral diseases, such as viral (herpes) encephalitis or meningoencephalitis, Wernicke disease, cerebral trauma, cerebral hemorrhage after surgery for craniopharyngioma or other tumors in the same region, or multiple embolic strokes caused by subacute bacterial endocarditis, cholesterol or fat embolism, or following cardiac or other surgery. An unusual type arises in young women with ovarian teratomas and circulating antibodies against the NMDA receptor.

The topography of the lesions in most of the deliriums that are symptomatic of underlying destructive processes is of interest; they tend to be localized in the rostral midbrain and hypothalamus or in the temporal lobes, where they involve the reticular activating and limbic systems. Involvement of the hypothalamus perhaps accounts for the autonomic hyperactivity that characterizes delirium in some cases of cerebral disease and the autoantibody condition. That these are not the only sites implicated is emphasized by the observations that an acute agitated delirium has occurred, albeit infrequently, with lesions involving the fusiform and lingual gyri and the calcarine cortex (Horenstein et al); the hippocampal and lingual gyri (Medina et al); or the middle temporal gyrus (Mori and Yamadori).

Electrical stimulation studies of the human cerebral cortex during surgical exploration and studies by positron emission tomography (PET) have emphasized the importance of the temporal lobe in the genesis of complex visual, auditory, and olfactory hallucinations. Subthalamic and midbrain lesions may give rise to visual hallucinations that are not unpleasant and are accompanied by good insight ("peduncular hallucinosis" of Lhermitte). For reasons not easily explained, with pontine-midbrain lesions, there may be unformed auditory hallucinations.

The EEG in delirium may show symmetrical mild generalized slow activity in the range of 5 to 10 per second. In milder degrees of delirium, there is usually no abnormality at all; this is in stark contrast to the generalized slowing and disruption of EEG activity that accompany most other forms of confusion in proportion to the severity of the clinical state.

Analysis of the conditions conducive to delirium suggests several physiologic mechanisms. Alcohol and sedative drugs are known to have a strong depressant effect on certain regions of the central nervous system; presumably, the disinhibition and overactivity of these parts after withdrawal of the drug are the basis of delirium. Another mechanism is operative in the case of bacterial infections with sepsis and poisoning by certain drugs, such as atropine and scopolamine, in which visual hallucinations are a prominent feature. Here the delirious state probably results from the direct action of the toxin or chemical agent on the same parts of the brain. It has long been suggested that some persons are much more liable to delirium than others, but there is reason to doubt this. Many years ago, Wolff and Curran showed that randomly selected persons developed delirium if the causative mechanisms were strongly operative. This is not surprising, for any normal person may, under certain circumstances, experience phenomena akin to those of delirium. A healthy person can be induced to hallucinate by being isolated for several days in an environment free of sensory stimulation (sensory deprivation). A relationship of delirium to dream states has also been postulated; both are characterized by a loss of appreciation of time, a richness of visual imagery, indifference to inconsistencies, and "defective reality testing." Formulations in the field of dynamic psychiatry seem more reasonably to explain the topical content of delirium than its occurrence. Wolff and Curran, having observed the same content in repeated attacks of delirium from different causes, concluded that the content depends more on the age, gender, intellectual endowment, occupation, personality traits, and past experiences than on the cause of the delirium.

Confusional States and Delirium Induced by Medications (See also Chap. 43)

In considering the pathophysiology of delirium and confusion, it must be again emphasized that drug intoxication—predominantly with drugs prescribed by physicians—is among the most common causes in practice. The most distinctive syndromes are those from drugs that have direct or indirect anticholinergic properties. The delirium associated with these agents is centrally mediated but may be accompanied by peripheral anticholinergic manifestations. This point is critical in the differential assessment of agitated confusional states because other compounds, particularly serotonergic agents used to treat depression, also can produce delirium. Thus, in addition to confusion, toxic levels of anticholinergic compounds typically cause dry skin, dry mouth, diminished bowel motility, and urinary hesitancy, if not frank retention. (The clinical maxim that applies is "red as a beet, dry as a bone, blind as a bat, hot as a hare, and mad as a hatter." The last part of this mnemonic has been also attached to the dementia of mercury intoxication [see Mintzer and Burns].) By contrast, in the toxic serotonergic syndrome associated with excessive doses of the newer antidepressant drugs, salivation is normal, sweating is increased, and the gut is hyperactive; diarrhea is common. Moreover, the deep tendon reflexes may be exaggerated, and there may be clonus and myoclonus as described by Birmes and associates. Drugs with dopaminergic activity used in the treatment of Parkinson disease are notorious for the induction of confusion or delirium, but it appears that the underlying disease provides an important substrate. Allied compounds with sympathomimetic actions such as cocaine and phencyclidine produce a hallucinatory delirium and yet others with different pharmacologic properties such as glutaminergic activity may result in a variety of delirious fragments or pure hallucinosis. Another entity that arises in this context is the neuroleptic malignant syndrome, a state associated with an agitated confusion followed by stupor. However, the characteristic features in neuroleptic malignant syndrome (NMS) are progressive muscle rigidity and evidence of myonecrosis as indicated by elevations of the serum creatine kinase; usually there is in addition some elevation of body temperature. The clinical examination and a thorough history aid greatly in determining which category of drug is implicated.

Diffuse Cerebral and Dementing Disease Complicated by Confusional States

Physicians are all too familiar with the situation of an elderly patient who enters the hospital with a medical or surgical illness or begins a prescribed course of medication and displays a newly acquired mental confusion. Presumably, the liability to this state is determined by preexisting brain disease, most often Alzheimer disease but sometimes Parkinson disease, multiple small deep cerebral infarctions, or another dementing process, which may or may not have been obvious to the family before. All the clinical features that one observes in the acute confusional states may be present, but their severity varies greatly. Confusion may be reflected only in the patient's inability to relate the history of the illness sequentially, or it may be so severe that the patient is virtually non compos mentis.

Although almost any complicating illness may bring out a confusional state in an elderly person, the most common are febrile infectious diseases; trauma, notably concussive brain injuries; surgical operations, general anesthesia and pre- and postoperative medication; even small amounts of pain or sedative medications used for any cause; and congestive heart failure, chronic respiratory disease, and severe anemia, especially pernicious anemia. With regard to medications, those with atropinic effects have the highest tendency to cause confusion, but others, even seemingly innocuous ones, may do the same (e.g., histamine blockers used to reduce gastric acid, anticonvulsants, corticosteroids, and L-dopa as mentioned earlier and described in Chap. 39).

Very often, it is difficult to determine which of several possible factors is responsible for the patient's confusion, and often there may be more than one. In a cardiac patient, for example, fever, hypoxia or hypercarbia, one or more drugs, and electrolyte imbalance each may contribute.

Infectious and Postoperative Confusional States

In the instance of fever and confusion, particularly in the elderly person, the problem of "septic encephalopathy" is offered as an explanation, but it may simply be a rephrasing of the well-known problem of infection such as pneumonia leading to a global confusion or delirium. Young has called attention to the high frequency of this disorder in critically ill patients, 70 percent of their bacteremic patients, and its accompaniment by a polyneuropathy in a high proportion of cases. Paratonic rigidity of the limbs (an oppositional action on the patient's part that is proportioned to the effort of the examiner in moving the limbs) is an almost universal accompaniment; according to these authors, focal cerebral or cranial nerve signs are not encountered. All other potential causes of a confusional state must, of course, be excluded before attributing the state to an underlying infection. The EEG is slowed in approximation to the level of consciousness, but it shows mild changes even in the bacteremic patient who is fully alert. The spinal fluid is normal or has a slightly elevated protein concentration. While there is no doubt that young and healthy patients may become confused when affected with high fever and overwhelming infections such as pneumonia, most cases of septic encephalopathy are of the "beclouded dementia" type in the older patient. The point made by Young is that subtle degrees of confusion are ubiquitous with serious infections of many varieties. Among the most perplexing cases of this type have been healthy older persons we have observed who acquired an agitated delirium following spinal column infection after surgery. The delirium ceased within hours of drainage of an abscess. The older literature contains similar examples with closed space infection in other locations. The chapter by Young can be consulted for an exposition of the various theories of pathogenesis of this state. High fever itself (above 40.6°C [105°F]) is probably an adequate explanation for confusion in some cases. A similar global confusional state occurs in patients with severe burns (burn encephalopathy).

All that has been stated above is true of the patient with a nondescript *postoperative confusional state*, in which a number of factors, such as fever, infection, dehydration, and drug and anesthetic effects, are implicated. In a study of 1,218 postoperative patients by Moller and colleagues, older age was by far the most important factor associated with persistent confusion after an operation; but a number of other factors—including the duration of anesthesia, need for a second operation soon after the first, postoperative infection, and respiratory complications—were also predictive of mental difficulty in the days after the procedure. Unacknowledged alcoholism and withdrawal effects undoubtedly cause the same problem quite often on surgical services (see also "Stroke with Cardiac Surgery" in Chap. 34).

When such patients recover from the medical or surgical illness, they usually return to their premorbid state, though their shortcomings, now drawn to the attention of the family and physician, are far more obvious than before. For this reason, families will date the onset of a dementia to the time of the medical illness or surgical procedure, and continue to minimize the previous gradual decline in cognition. In other cases, however, the acute medical illness seemingly marks the beginning of a persistent decline in mental clarity that over time can be identified as a dementing illness. A related problem that has recently come under study is persistent cognitive loss after critical illness. The rates of this irreversible change are apparently high, up to one-quarter of severely ill patients in some series, but accurate estimates are difficult to obtain because of the lack of pre-illness psychometric testing.

Nonconvulsive status epilepticus

This problem has attracted increasing attention in the past decades as a cause of otherwise obscure confusional states. It is discussed in Chaps. 16 and 17, but here we only comment that the process may be portrayed clinically only because of small myoclonic twitches or eyelid fluttering. The only certain way to arrive at, or exclude the diagnosis is with EEG monitoring for more than the usual 30 minute recording if possible. One suspects nonconvulsive seizures particularly in known epileptics, septic patients, and in certain medical diseases such as TTP.

Schizophrenic or Bipolar Psychosis During a Medical or Surgical Illness

A small proportion of psychoses of schizophrenic or bipolar type first become manifest during an acute medical illness or following an operation or parturition and need to be distinguished from an acute confusional state. Rarely, a catatonic state will make its first appearance in these circumstances. A causal relationship between the psychosis and medical illness is sought but cannot be established. The psychosis may have preceded the medical illness but was not recognized. The diagnostic study of the psychiatric illness must then proceed along the lines suggested in Chaps. 52 and 53. Close observation will usually disclose a clear sensorium and relatively intact memory, features that permit differentiation from an acute confusional or delirious state or dementia.

CLASSIFICATION AND DIAGNOSIS OF ACUTE CONFUSIONAL STATES

The syndromes themselves and their main clinical causes are the only satisfactory basis for classification until such time as their actual causes and pathophysiology are discovered (Table 20-1).

The first step in diagnosis is to recognize that the patient is confused. This is obvious in most cases but, as pointed out earlier, the mildest forms, particularly when some other alteration of personality is prominent, may be overlooked. Sometimes, the patient's attention can be best engaged by whispering rather than shouting or using a conversational amplitude of voice. A subtle disorder of orientation may be betrayed by an incorrect response regarding dates (off by more than one day of the month or day of the week), or in misnaming the hospital. The ability to retain a span of digits forward (normally 7) and backward (normally 5), spelling a word such as *world* or *earth* forward and then backward, reciting the months of the year in their reverse order, and serial subtraction of 3's from 30 or 7's from 100 are useful bedside tests of the patient's capacity for attentiveness and sustained mental activity, though some of these presuppose that the patient is literate or has a knowledge of mathematics. Another is the efficiency in performing dual tasks such as tapping alternately with each hand while reading aloud. Memory of recent events is one of the most delicate tests of adequate mental function and is readily accomplished by having the patient relate the details of entry to the hospital; examinations undertaken in the previous days; naming the president, vice president; and summarizing major current events, as outlined in Chap. 21. Errors in performance should not be minimized or attributed to age, for they may presage serious upcoming problems during the hospitalization.

Once it is established that the patient is confused, the differential diagnosis must be made between an acute confusional state associated with psychomotor underactivity, delirium, a beclouded dementia, and a confusional state that complicates focal cerebral disease. This is done by taking into account the degree of the patient's alertness, wakefulness, psychomotor and hallucinatory activity, and disturbances of memory and impulse, as well as the presence or absence of asterixis or myoclonus or signs of overactivity of the autonomic nervous system and of generalized or focal cerebral disease. In the neurologic examination, particular attention should be given to the presence or absence of focal neurologic signs and to asterixis, myoclonus, and seizures.

In the chronically demented patient, there are usually a number of "frontal release" signs, such as picking at the bedsheets and clothes, grasping, groping, sucking, and paratonic rigidity of the limbs. However, some demented patients are as bewildered as those with confusional psychosis, and the two conditions are distinguishable only by differences in their mode of onset and chronicity. This suggests that the affected parts of the nervous system may be the same in both conditions.

At times, a left hemispheral lesion causing a mild Wernicke's aphasia resembles a confusional state in that the stream of speech and thought are incoherent. The prominence of paraphasias and neologisms in spontaneous speech, difficulties in auditory comprehension, and normal nonverbal behavior mark the disorder as aphasic in nature. However, a problem with naming may be more common in non-aphasic global confusional states, as alluded to earlier in the chapter and emphasized in a brief piece by Geschwind. Spontaneous speech in these circumstances is unaffected.

The distinction between an acute confusional state and dementia is difficult at times, particularly if the mode of onset and the course of the mental decline are not known. The patient with an acute confusional state is said to have a "clouded sensorium" (an ambiguous term referring to a symptom complex of inattention, disorientation, perhaps drowsiness, and an inclination to inaccurate perceptions and sometimes to hallucinations and delusions), whereas the patient with dementia usually has a clear sensorium.

As indicated earlier, schizophrenia and bipolar psychosis can usually be separated from the confusional states by the presence of a clear sensorium and relatively intact memory function.

Once a case has been appropriately classified, it is important to determine its clinical associations as outlined in Table 20-1.

A thorough medical and neurologic examination, CT or MRI, and—in cases with fever or with no other apparent cause—blood count, chest X-ray, and lumbar puncture should be performed. The medical, neurologic, and laboratory findings (including measurements of Na, Ca, CO_2, blood urea nitrogen [BUN], NH_3, calcium, glucose, PAO_2, PCO_2, "toxic screen") determine the underlying disease and its treatment, and they also give information concerning prognosis. An approach to the laboratory tests that are useful in revealing the common conditions that give rise to the confusional state when the cause is not self-evident from the history and physical examination is given in Table 20-2; but as always, the choice of tests is governed by the clinical circumstances.

Table 20-2

AN APPROACH TO THE LABORATORY EVALUATION OF THE ACUTELY CONFUSED PATIENT

I. Afebrile, no meningismus, and no focal neurologic signs
   A. Endogenous metabolic disorders: glucose, sodium, calcium, BUN, PAO_2, PCO_2, NH_3, T_4, and special tests in particular circumstances (for porphyria, Hashimoto thyroid disease, etc.)
   B. Exogenous toxic state: toxicologic screening of blood and urine
II. Febrile or signs of meningeal irritation
   A. Systemic infection: complete blood count, chest radiograph, urine analysis and culture, blood cultures, erythrocyte sedimentation rate
   B. Meningitis and encephalitis: lumbar puncture
III. Focal neurologic signs or seizures
   A. CT scan or MRI
   B. EEG

CARE OF THE DELIRIOUS AND CONFUSED PATIENT

These details are of the utmost importance. It has been estimated that 20 to 25 percent of medically ill hospital inpatients will experience some degree of confusion; moreover, elderly patients who are delirious have a significant level of mortality, variously estimated at 22 to 76 percent according to Weber and colleagues. Optimal care begins with the identification of individuals at risk for delirium, including those who have an underlying dementia, preexisting medical illnesses, or a history of alcoholism or serious depression. Furthermore, delirium is more common in males and, not surprisingly, is more likely when sensory function is already impaired (loss of vision and hearing) (Burns et al; Weber et al).

The primary effort is directed toward elimination of the underlying medical problem, particularly to discontinuing offending drugs or toxic agents. Other important objectives are to quiet the agitated patient and protect him from injury. A nurse, attendant, or member of the family should be with a seriously confused patient if this can be arranged. A room with adequate natural lighting will aid in creating a diurnal rhythm of activity and reduce "sundowning." It is often better to let an agitated patient walk about the room than to restrain him in bed, which may increase his fright or excitement and cause him to struggle to the point of exhaustion, collapse, or self-harm. The less-active patient can be kept in bed by side rails, wrist restraints, or a restraining sheet or vest. Sensitive explanations of these restraints to the family should be made in terms that emphasize the patient's health and safety. The fully awake but mildly confused patient should be permitted to sit up or walk about part of the day unless the primary disease contraindicates this.

All drugs that could possibly be responsible for the acute confusional state or delirium should be discontinued if this can be done safely. These include sedating, antianxiety, narcotic, anticholinergic, antispasticity, and corticosteroid medications, L-dopa, metoclopramide, and cimetidine, as well as antidepressants, antiarrhythmics, antiepileptics, and antibiotics. Despite the need to be sparing with medications in these circumstances, haloperidol, quetiapine, and risperidone are helpful in calming the severely agitated and hallucinating patient, but they too should be used in the lowest effective doses. An exception is alcohol or sedative withdrawal, in which chlordiazepoxide or other diazepines are favored by most physicians (see Chap. 42). In delirious patients, the purpose of sedation is to assure rest and sleep, avoid exhaustion, and facilitate nursing care, but one must be cautious in attempting to suppress delirium completely. Warm baths were also known in the past to be effective in quieting the delirious patient, but hospitals no longer have facilities for this valuable method of treatment.

It would seem obvious that attempts should be made to preempt the problem of confusion in the hospitalized elderly patient. Inouye and colleagues devised an intervention program that includes frequent reorientation to the surroundings with signs, verbal reminders, and a clock; mentally stimulating activities; ambulation several times a day or similar exercises when possible; and attention to providing visual and hearing aids in patients with these impairments. They recorded a 40 percent reduction in the frequency of a confusional illness in comparison to patients who did not receive this type of organized program. Preventive strategies of the type they outline are most important in the elderly, even those without overt dementia, but a routine plan is advisable so that nurses and ancillary staff are able to apply them consistently.

Finally, the physician should be aware of the benefit of many small therapeutic measures that allay fear and suspicion and reduce the tendency to hallucinations. The room should be kept dimly lighted at night, and, if possible, the patient should not be moved from one room to another. Every procedure should be explained to the patient, even such simple ones as the taking of blood pressure or temperature. It may be some consolation and also a source of professional satisfaction to remember that most confused and delirious patients recover if they receive competent medical and nursing care (and are almost always amnestic for the ordeal). The family may be reassured on this point but forewarned that improvement may take several days or weeks and that episodes of confusion may be exposing an underlying dementia. They must also understand that the patient's abnormal behavior is not willful but rather symptomatic of a transitory brain disease. (See also Chaps. 42 and 43 for specific aspects of management of delirium due to withdrawal of alcohol and other sedative-hypnotic drugs.)

References

Birmes P, Coppin D, Schmitt L, et al: Serotonin syndrome: A brief review. *CMAJ* 168:1439, 2003.

Burns A, Gallagley A, Byrne J. Delirium. *J Neurol Neurosurg Psychiatry* 75:362, 2004.

Caplan LR, Kelly M, Kase CS, et al: Mirror image of Wernicke's aphasia. *Neurology* 36:1015, 1986.

Engel GL, Romano J: Delirium: A syndrome of cerebral insufficiency. *J Chronic Dis* 9:260, 1959.

Geschwind N: Non-aphasic disorders of speech. *Int J Neurol* 4:207, 1964.

Horenstein S, Chamberlin W, Conomy T: Infarction of the fusiform and calcarine regions: Agitated delirium and hemianopia. *Trans Am Neurol Assoc* 92:85, 1967.

Inouye SK, Bogardus ST, Charpentier PA, et al: A multicomponent intervention to prevent delirium in hospitalized older patients. *N Engl J Med* 340:669, 1999.

Kahn E: *Psychopathic Personalities*. New Haven, CT, Yale University Press, 1931.

Lipowski ZJ: *Delirium: Acute Confusional States*. New York, Oxford University Press, 1990.

Medina JL, Rubino FA, Ross A: Agitated delirium caused by infarction of the hippocampal formation, fusiform and lingual gyri. *Neurology* 24:1181, 1974.

Mesulam MM: Attentional networks, confusional states, and neglect syndromes, in Mesulam MM (ed): *Principles of Behavioral and Cognitive Neurology*. Oxford, UK, Oxford University Press, 2000, pp 174–256.

Mesulam MM, Waxman SG, Geschwind N, et al: Acute confusional states with right middle cerebral infarctions. *J Neurol Neurosurg Psychiatry* 39:84, 1976.

Mintzer J, Burns A: Anticholinergic side effects of drugs in elderly people. *J R Soc Med* 93:457, 2000.

Moller JT, Cluitmans P, Rasmussen LS: Long-term postoperative cognitive dysfunction in the elderly: ISPOCD1 study. *Lancet* 351:857, 1998.

Mori E, Yamadori A: Acute confusional state and acute agitated delirium. *Arch Neurol* 44:1139, 1987.

Stauder HK: Die todliche Katatonie. *Arch Psychiatr Nervenkrankh* 102:614, 1934.

Weber JB, Coverdale JH, Kunik ME: Delirium: Current trends in prevention and treatment. *Intern Med J* 34:115, 2004.

Wolff HG, Curran D: Nature of delirium and allied states. *Arch Neurol Psychiatry* 33:1175, 1935.

Young GB: Other inflammatory disorders, in Young GB, Ropper AH, Bolton CF (eds): *Coma and Impaired Consciousness*. McGraw-Hill, New York, 1998, pp 271–303.

21

Dementia, the Amnesic Syndrome, and the Neurology of Intelligence and Memory

Increasingly, as the number of elderly in our population rises, the neurologist is consulted because an otherwise healthy person begins to fail mentally and loses his capacity to function effectively at work or in the home. This may indicate the development of a degenerative brain disease, a brain tumor, multiple strokes, chronic subdural hematomas, drug intoxication, chronic meningoencephalitis (such as caused by HIV or syphilis), normal-pressure hydrocephalus, or a depressive illness. Formerly, when there was little that could be done about these clinical states, no great premium was attached to diagnosis. But there are now effective means of treating several of these conditions, and in some instances, of restoring the patient to normal mental competence. Moreover, diagnostic technologies allow earlier recognition of the underlying pathologic process, thus improving the chances of recovery or of preventing the disease's progression.

The definitions of normal and abnormal states of mind were considered in Chap. 20, where it was pointed out that the term *dementia* denotes a persistent deterioration of intellectual or cognitive function with little or no disturbance of consciousness or perception. In current neurologic parlance, the term is used to designate a syndrome of failing memory and impairment of other intellectual functions as a result of chronic progressive degenerative disease of the brain. Such a definition may be too narrow. The term more accurately includes a number of closely related syndromes characterized not only by intellectual deterioration but also by certain behavioral abnormalities and changes in personality. Furthermore, dementia can be the result of a static encephalopathy such as head trauma or cerebral anoxia or of a progressive degenerative disease, but it differs from "encephalopathy" in its chronicity. Thus, it is not possible to determine if a confused, amnestic person is demented until some time has passed and the deficits have perished. Encephalopathies, by contrast, are largely reversible.

Beyond the need to properly define these terms, the two entities have different causes. There are several states of dementia of differing causes and mechanisms and that a degeneration of certain systems of cerebral neurons, albeit common, is only one of the many types. Thus, it is more correct to speak of the *dementias* or the *dementing diseases*.

To understand the phenomenon of intellectual deterioration, it is helpful to have some idea of how intellectual functions, particularly intelligence and memory, are normally organized and sustained, and the manner in which deficits in these functions relate to diffuse and focal cerebral lesions. The neurology of intelligence is considered in this chapter as a prelude to a discussion of the dementias and the neurology of memory.

INTELLIGENCE

Intelligence, or *intelligent behavior*, has been variously defined as a "general mental efficiency," as "innate cognitive ability," or as "the aggregate or global capacity of an individual to act purposefully, to think rationally, and to deal effectively with his environment" (Wechsler) in other words, the capacity to have ideas and reason about them. It is global because it characterizes an individual's behavior as a whole; it is an aggregate in the sense that it is composed of a number of independent and qualitatively distinguishable cognitive abilities. This topic should be of interest to neurologists because intelligence is disturbed by many disorders of the brain but cannot be easily attributed to any cerebral region or particular cognitive function. In the dementias and in developmental delays, intelligence is affected in a way that cannot be explained except by some global aspect of brain function.

As every educated person knows, intelligence has something to do with normal cerebral function. It is also apparent that the level of intelligence differs widely from one person to another, and members of certain families are exceptionally bright and intellectually accomplished, whereas members of other families are just the opposite. If properly motivated, intelligent children excel in school and score high on intelligence tests. Indeed, the first intelligence tests, devised by Binet and Simon in 1905, were for the purpose of predicting scholastic success. The term *intelligence quotient*, or *IQ*, was introduced by the German psychologist Stern and used by Terman in 1916 for the development of intelligence testing. It denotes the figure that is obtained by dividing the subject's mental age (as determined by the Binet-Simon scale) by his chronologic age (up to the 14th year) and multiplying the result by 100. The IQ correlates, but only broadly, with achievement in school and eventual success in professional work. IQ increases with age up to the 14th to 16th years and then remains stable, at least until late adult life. At any given age, a large sample of normal children attains test scores of a normal, or gaussian, distribution.

The original studies of pedigrees of highly intelligent and mentally less-able families, which revealed a striking concordance between parent and child, lent support to the idea that intelligence is to a large extent inherited. However, it became evident that the tests were also greatly influenced by the environment in which the child was reared. Moreover, tests were less reliable in identifying talented children who were not offered optimal opportunities. This led to the widespread belief that intelligence tests are only achievement tests and that environmental factors fostering high performance are the important factors determining intelligence.

Neither of these views is likely to be entirely correct. Studies of monozygotic and dizygotic twins raised in the same or different families have put the matter in a clearer light. Identical twins reared together or apart are more alike in intelligence than nonidentical twins brought up in the same home (see reviews of Willerman, of Shields, and of Slater and Cowie). A study of elderly twins by McClearn and colleagues has shed further light on the issue; even in twins who were older than 80 years of age, a substantial part (an estimated 62 percent) of cognitive performance could be accounted for by genetic traits. These findings suggest that life experience alters intelligence, but in only a limited way. There can be little doubt, therefore, that genetic endowment is the more important factor—a view that was championed by Piercy and more recently by Herrnstein and Murray. However, there is also evidence that early learning modifies the level of ability that is finally attained. The latter should be looked upon not as the sum of genetic and environmental factors but as the product of the two. More importantly, it is generally appreciated that nonscholastic achievement or success is governed by factors other than intellectual ones, such as curiosity, a readiness to learn, interest, persistence, sociability, and ambition or motivation—factors that vary considerably from person to person and are not measured by tests of intelligence.

As to the genetic mechanisms involved in the inheritance of intelligence, a limited amount is known. There is an excess of males with mental retardation, and there are several well-characterized syndromes in which the inheritance of mental retardation is X-linked as described in Chaps. 28 and 38. Also notable is the somewhat different patterns of subtest performance between males and females (males perform better on subtests of spatial ability and certain mathematical tasks). Males may be more likely to be affected by advantageous or aberrant genes on a single X chromosome, whereas females benefit from the mosaic provided by two X chromosomes. In some families, high intelligence segregates to certain individuals through an X-linked pattern. Further study will determine the validity of this view and its contribution to our understanding of what will certainly prove to be a polygenic inheritance of intellectual traits.

One would think that neurologic structure and function would correlate in some way with intelligence, but with the exception of the pathologically developmentally delayed (Chaps. 28 and 38), such an association has been difficult to document. Brain weight and the complexity of the convolutional pattern are not correlated with intelligence—despite popular notions to the contrary, including a widely criticized analysis of the brain of Albert Einstein. (In regard to Einstein's brain, Witelson and colleagues proposed that an enlarged inferior parietal lobule, a crossmodal association area, accounted for his visuospatial and mathematical genius, but this has been disputed.) Only laboratory measures of vigilance and facility of sensory registration (speed of motor responses/reaction time and rapid recognition of differences between lines, shapes, or pictures) have a definite but still modest correlation with IQ. However, it is of interest that morphometric features of the regions of the cortex that are presumed to underlie IQ and verbal skills, such as the frontal and language areas, show a heritable component when measured on high-resolution MRI scans in twins (see Thompson et al).

As to psychologic theories of intelligence, several have traditionally been held at different historical periods. One is the two-factor theory of Spearman, who noted that all the separate tests of cognitive abilities correlated with each other, suggesting that a general factor (*g factor*) enters into all performance. Because none of the correlations between subtests approached unity, he postulated that each test measures not only this general ability (commonly identified with intelligence) but also a subsidiary factors specific to the individual tests, which he designated the *s factors*. A second theory, the multifactorial theory of Thurstone, proposed that intelligence consists of a number of primary mental abilities, such as memory, verbal facility, numerical ability, visuospatial perception, and capacity for problem solving, all of them more or less equivalent. These primary abilities, although correlated, are not subordinate to a more general ability. For Eysenck, intelligence exists in three forms: biologic (the genetic component), social (development of the genetic component in relation to personal relationships), and a number of specific abilities subject to measurement by psychometric tests.

Thurstone's multifactorial theory of intelligence has been periodically resurrected, most recently by Gardner who recognizes six categories of high-order cerebral ability but restates them in more modern terms: linguistic (encompassing all language functions); musical (including composition and performance); logical–mathematical (the ideas and works of mathematicians); spatial (including artistic talent and the creation of visual impressions); bodily–kinesthetic (including dance and athletic performance); and the personal (consciousness of self and others in social interactions). He refers to each of these as *intelligences*, defined as the ability to solve problems or resolve difficulties and to be creative within the particular field. Several lines of evidence are marshaled in support of this parceling of separable skills and abilities: (1) each may be developed to an exceptionally high level in certain individuals, constituting virtuosity or genius; (2) each can be destroyed or spared in isolation as a consequence of a lesion in a certain part of the nervous system; (3) in certain individuals, i.e., in prodigies, special competence in one of these abilities is evident at an unusually early age; (4) in the autism spectrum, one or more of these abilities may be selectively spared or developed to an abnormally high degree (*idiot savant*). Each of these entities appears to have a genetic basis in so far as musical, artistic, mathematical, and athletic ability often runs in families, but their full development is influenced by environmental factors.

There are only limited data regarding the highest levels of intelligence identified as genius. Terman and Ogden's longitudinal study of 1,500 California school children who were initially tested in 1921 supported the idea that an extremely high IQ predicted future scholastic accomplishments (though not necessarily occupational and life success). On the other hand, most individuals recognized as geniuses have been especially skilled in one domain—such as painting, linguistics, music, chess, or mathematics—and such "domain genius" is not necessarily predicated on high IQ scores, although certain individuals display crossmodal superiorities—particularly in mathematics and music.

Chapter 28 discusses the developmental aspects of intelligence in detail. One of the leading theories has been that of Piaget, who proposed that this is accomplished in discrete stages related to age: sensorimotor, from 0 to 2 years; preconceptual thought, from 2 to 4 years; intuitive thought, from 4 to 7 years; concrete operations (conceptualization), from 7 to 11 years; and, finally, the period of "formal operations" (logical or abstract thought), from 11 years on. This scheme implies that the capacity for logical thought, developing as it does according to an orderly timetable, is coded in the genes. Surely, one can recognize these states of intellectual development in the child, but Piaget's theory has been criticized as being too anecdotal and lacking the quantitative validation that could be derived only from studies of a large normal population. Furthermore, it does not take into account an individual's special abilities, which do not usually develop and reach their maximum at the same time as the more general intellectual capacities.

One would suppose that in neurology, where one is exposed to so many diseases affecting the cerebrum, it might be possible to verify one of these several theories of intelligence and to determine the anatomy of this cognitive entity. Presumably, the g factor of intelligence would be maximally impaired, by diffuse lesions, in proportion to the mass of brain involved, an idea expressed by Lashley as the "mass-action principle." Indeed, according to Chapman and Wolff, there is a correlation between the volume of brain tissue lost and a general deficit of cerebral function. Others disagree, claiming that no universal psychologic deficit can be linked to lesions affecting particular parts of the brain. Probably the truth lies between these two divergent points of view. According to Tomlinson and colleagues, who studied the effects of vascular lesions in the aging brain, lesions that involve more than 50 mL of tissue cause some general reduction in performance, especially in speed and capacity to solve problems. Piercy, on the other hand, found correlations only between specific intellectual deficits and lesions of particular parts of the left and right hemispheres. These problems are discussed in Chap. 22. It is surprising that lesions of the frontal lobes, and particularly the prefrontal regions, which so profoundly disorder planning and "executive" functions, do not measurably affect IQ except in subtests specific to these skills.

The authors conclude from experience and from evidence provided by neurologic studies that intelligence is a combination of multiple primary abilities, each of which seems to be inherited and each of which has a separate but as yet poorly delineated anatomy. Yet we would disagree with both Thurstone and Gardner that these special abilities are of equivalent weight with regard to what is generally considered as "intelligence." When viewed in the light of the classics of literature, history, and science, we attach a disproportionate importance to some of them, namely linguistic and mathematical, and perhaps spatial–dimensional, abilities. These are integral to ideation and problem solving and are largely absent in the developmentally delayed and lost early in dementing diseases. To the extent that facility with general mental performance, that requiring the manipulation of abstract symbols and thoughts, marks an individual as "intelligent" and that these correlate with each other, we find Spearman's g factor to be a credible but not completely satisfying concept for intelligence.

Neurologic data certainly do not exclude the possibility of a general factor for intelligence—one that is unavoidably measured in many different tests of cerebral functions. It is expressed in thinking and abstract reasoning and is operative only if the connections between the frontal lobes and other parts of the brain are intact. Attention, drive, and motivation are noncognitive psychologic attributes of fundamental importance, the precise anatomy and physiology of which remain to be identified but are largely generated in the frontal and prefrontal region. It is also possible, if not likely, that the associative areas of the cerebrum are engaged in the apperception of sensory experiences and their manipulation in symbolic form. This applies equally to the ability to relate thoughts to each other and to stored concepts, but here, memory plays a central role. We view memory and capacity to learn as a separate cognitive entity, with its own neuroanatomic localizations. The interrelationships between some of these special abilities had been thoughtfully analyzed by Luria (see the section on frontal lobes in Chap. 22). An account of the subject of IQ and intelligence can also be found in the monograph by Mackintosh.

An even more complex problem arises in the neurologic analysis of the highest human achievement and the method of human advancement, namely creativity. In some ways, creativity is tied to special skills along the lines of Gardner's modality-based intelligence, particularly as it relates to artistic work, but the brain structures involved in aesthetics and abstraction are entirely obscure, as Zeki points out. Some insight is gained from the fact that intelligence and problem-solving ability are innately but only roughly tied to creativity and that there are congenital absences and deficiencies of appreciation of visual, artistic, or mathematical skills. The capacity to be creative may be inhibited by other functions of the brain, as exposed in the case described by Seeley and colleagues of a woman with frontotemporal dementia whose artistic abilities emerged as her facility with language deteriorated. But, as pointed out in the following chapter, traits such as creativity almost certainly do not reside in a particular lobe or structure of the brain and may depend on the overdevelopment of certain associative areas, as well as on frontal lobe drive and, of course, are fully manifest only by educational exposure.

THE NEUROLOGY OF DEMENTIA

Dementia is a syndrome consisting of a loss of several separable but overlapping intellectual abilities and presents in a number of different combinations. These constellations of intellectual deficits constitute the preeminent clinical abnormalities in several cerebral diseases and are sometimes virtually the only abnormalities. Table 21-1 lists the most common types of dementing diseases and their relative frequency.

What is noteworthy about the figures in this table is the apparently high level of accuracy of diagnosis. Rather consistently, postmortem examination confirms that the accuracy of the clinical diagnosis of Alzheimer disease is in excess of 80 percent when rigid research criteria are used (Table 21-2). Of course, the high frequency of this disease in the older population makes the likelihood of correct diagnosis higher. In most cases, the degenerative diseases can be differentiated by one or two characteristic clinical features, but these distinctions may be difficult to discern early in the disease process. In particular, a proportion of patients thought to have Alzheimer disease are found to have another type of degenerative cerebral atrophy, such as Lewy-body disease, progressive supranuclear palsy, Huntington disease, Parkinson disease, corticobasal degeneration, Pick disease, or one of the frontotemporal lobar degenerative diseases (all described in Chap. 39). Or such patients have one of a variety of other processes, such as multiinfarct dementia or hydrocephalus alone or in combination with one of the other disorders. Of special importance is the fact that approximately 10 percent of patients who are referred to a neurologic center with a question of dementia prove to have a potentially reversible psychiatric or metabolic disorder. Emphasized again are the group of nonprogressive dementias that are the lasting result of a monophasic injury to the brain and do not appear in Table 21-2.

In the following pages, we consider the prototypic dementing syndromes. They are observed most frequently with degenerative diseases of the brain (Chap. 39) and less often as part of other categories of disease (vascular, traumatic, infectious, demyelinating), which are considered in their appropriate chapters.

Table 21-2

NEUROPATHOLOGIC DIAGNOSES FOR 261 CASES WITH A CLINICAL DIAGNOSIS OF ALZHEIMER DISEASE: DATA FROM THE MASSACHUSETTS ADRC BRAIN REGISTRY, 1984–1993

NEUROPATHOLOGIC DIAGNOSIS	NUMBER OF CASES	PERCENT
Alzheimer disease	218	83.5
Parkinson and Alzheimer diseases	16	6.1
Lewy-body disease	8	3.1
Pick disease	6	2.3
Multiple infarcts	5	1.9
Binswanger disease	1	0.4
Corticobasal ganglionic degeneration	1	0.4
Mixed dementia	1	0.4
Other	5	1.9
Total	261	100

Source: Courtesy of Dr. John Growdon.

Table 21-1

THE COMMON TYPES OF DEMENTING DISEASES AND THEIR APPROXIMATE FREQUENCIES

DEMENTING DISEASE	RELATIVE FREQUENCY, %
Cerebral atrophy, mainly Alzheimer but including Lewy-body, Parkinson, frontotemporal, and Pick diseases	50
Multiinfarct dementia	10
Alcoholic dementia	7
Intracranial tumors	5
Normal-pressure hydrocephalus	5
Huntington chorea	2
Chronic drug intoxications	3
Miscellaneous diseases (hepatic failure; pernicious anemia; hypo- or hyperthyroidism; dementias with amyotrophic lateral sclerosis, amyloid angiopathy, neurosyphilis; Creutzfeldt–Jakob disease; multiple sclerosis; chronic epilepsy)	6
Cerebral trauma	2
AIDS dementia	2
Pseudodementias (depression, hypomania, schizophrenia, hysteria, undiagnosed)	8

Source: Adapted from Van Horn, from Mayeux et al, and from Cummings JL, Benson DF: Dementia: A Clinical Approach, 2nd ed. Boston, Butterworth, 1992.
(See also Table 21-2.)

Mild Cognitive Impairment and Early Dementia

It has become apparent that many individuals have memory complaints that are mild and do not interfere with daily functioning but are still disproportionate for the patient's age and education. It is often difficult to differentiate this less-intrusive problem, which may be a result of the normal process of aging, from dementia. The former condition has been called *mild cognitive impairment*, *age-associated memory impairment*, and, in the past, *benign senescent forgetfulness*, as discussed in Chap. 29. When other aspects of mental functioning are affected, terms such as *aging-associated cognitive decline* are used. Defining the boundaries of such a condition has proved problematic, and determining the risk of progression to a dementing illness that does interfere with daily function, even more so. There is a further problem introduced by the premise that highly intelligent individuals would have to decline considerably on intelligence and memory tests to be identified as being below certain age-adjusted norms. However, a notion has evolved in which Alzheimer disease and mild cognitive impairment exist in a spectrum (see Petersen), and one of the main values to identifying such patients in a presymptomatic period of Alzheimer disease is the potential for early institution of treatment.

In most studies, 10 to 20 percent per year of such affected patients with mild cognitive decline will be found to have later acquired Alzheimer disease. A number of factors have been identified as associated with a progression to a state of indisputable dementia. These include elevated blood pressure, changes in the cerebral white matter on MRI, abnormality of gait, and—perhaps not surprisingly—certain biologic markers that are connected to Alzheimer disease. Other factors for the development of dementia, particularly the level of prior education and maintenance of an active mental life, have been studied in relation to Alzheimer disease (C.F. Willis et al) and are discussed in that section of Chap. 39.

At the moment, the clinician must simply counsel caution and reassurance in advising patients with mild memory impairment, and exclude treatable causes. Nonetheless, if the symptoms are progressive or begin to interfere in any consistent way with other mental functions or with the performance of daily activities, a dementing illness is likely.

Dementia Caused By Degenerative Diseases

The earliest signs of dementia caused by degenerative disease may be so subtle as to escape the notice of the most discerning physician. An observant relative of the patient or an employer may become aware of a certain lack of initiative or lack of interest in work, a neglect of routine tasks, or an abandonment of pleasurable pursuits. Initially, these changes may be attributed to depression, fatigue, or boredom in retirement. More often, gradual development of forgetfulness is the most prominent early symptom. Proper names are no longer remembered and cannot be recalled with time, to a far greater extent than can be attributed to "mild cognitive impairment." Difficulty in balancing a checkbook and making change becomes evident. The purpose of an errand is forgotten, appointments are not kept, and recent conversations or social events have been overlooked. The patient may ask the same question repeatedly over the course of a day, having failed to retain the answers that were previously given.

Later, it becomes evident that the patient is easily distracted by every passing incident. He no longer finds it possible to think about or discuss a problem with customary clarity or to comprehend all aspects of complex situations. The ability to make proper deductions and inferences from given premises are greatly reduced. One feature of a situation or some relatively unimportant event may become a source of unreasonable concern or worry. Tasks that require several steps cannot be accomplished, and all but the simplest directions cannot be followed. The patient may get lost, even along habitual routes of travel. Day-to-day events are not recalled, and perseveration or impersistence in speech, action, and thought becomes evident.

In yet other instances, an early abnormality may be in the nature of emotional instability, taking the form of unreasonable outbursts of anger, easy tearfulness, or aggressiveness. A change in mood becomes apparent, deviating more toward depression than elation. Apathy is common. Some patients are irascible; a few are cheerful and facetious. The direction of the mood change is said to depend on the patient's previous personality rather than on the character of the disease, but one can think of glaring exceptions from clinical experience. Excessive lability of affect may also be observed—for example, easy fluctuation from laughter to tears on slight provocation.

A considerable group of patients come to the physician with physical complaints, the most common being dizziness, a vague mental "fogginess," and nondescript headaches. The patient's inability to give a coherent account of his symptoms bears witness to the presence of dementia. Sleep disturbances, especially insomnia, are prominent in some cases and a particular disorder relating to the acting out of dreams during REM sleep marks some of the degenerative dementia. Sometimes the mental failure is brought to light more dramatically by a severe confusional state attending a febrile illness, a concussive head injury, an operative procedure, or the administration of some new medicine, as discussed below and in Chap. 20. As noted there, the family almost uniformly, but mistakenly, dates an abrupt onset of dementia to the time of the intercurrent illness.

Loss of social graces and indifference to social customs may occur, but usually later in the course of illness. Judgment becomes impaired, early in some, late in others. At certain phases of the illness, suspiciousness or frank paranoia may develop. Although more typical of advanced cases, on occasion the first indication of an oncoming dementia is the expression of paranoia—for example, relating to being robbed by employees or to the infidelity of a spouse. When the patient's condition is probed by an examination, there are no signs of depression, hallucinations, or illogical ideas, but memory and problem solving are found to be deficient. The troublesome paranoid ideas then persist throughout the illness. Also more typical of late disease but an early feature of certain degenerative dementias, visual and auditory hallucinations, sometimes quite vivid in nature, may be added. Wandering, pacing, and other aimless activities are common in the intermediate stage of the illness, while other patients sit placidly for hours. By this point, these patients have little or no realization of the changes occurring within themselves; i.e., they lack insight into the problem.

As the condition progresses, all intellectual faculties become impaired; but in the most common degenerative diseases, memory is most affected. Deference to a spouse or child when the patient is unable to answer the examiner's questions is characteristic. Up to a certain point in the illness, memories of the distant past are relatively well retained at a time when more recently acquired information has been lost (Ribot's law). Eventually, patients also fail to retain remote memories, to recognize their relatives, and even to recall the names of their children.

Apraxias and agnosias are early and prominent in one special group of degenerative conditions, occurring only later in Alzheimer disease. These defects may alter the performance of the simplest tasks, such as preparing a meal, setting the table, or even using the telephone or a knife and fork, dressing, or walking. Or, language functions are impaired almost from the beginning of certain forms of dementia. Lost in these cases is the capacity to understand nuances of the spoken and written word, as are the suppleness and spontaneity of verbal expression. Vocabulary becomes restricted and conversation is rambling and repetitious. The patient gropes for proper names and common nouns and no longer formulates ideas with well-constructed phrases or sentences. Instead, there is a tendency to resort to clichés, stereotyped phrases, and exclamations, which hide the underlying defect during conversation. Paraphasias and difficulty in comprehending complex conversations become prominent. Subsequently, more severe degrees of aphasia, dysarthria, palilalia, and echolalia may be added to the clinical picture. As pointed out by Chapman and Wolff, there is loss also of the capacity to express feelings, to suppress impulses, and to tolerate frustration and restrictions.

However, several clinical variants of dementia in which memory is relatively spared have long been recognized, and in recent years three of them—frontotemporal dementia (Pick disease), primary progressive aphasia, and semantic dementia—have been subsumed under the summary term *frontotemporal lobar degeneration*. Several consensus statements on the clinical diagnostic criteria for these syndromes have been published, although not all writings on this subject are in agreement (see Morris).

The most common clinical syndrome in this group is characterized by features that would be expected of degeneration of the frontal lobes: early personality changes, particularly apathy or disinhibition, euphoria, perseveration in motor and cognitive tasks, ritualistic and repetitive behaviors, and laconic speech leading to mutism—all with relative preservation of memory, orientation, and visuospatial capability. With anterior temporal lobe involvement, hyperorality, excessive smoking, or overeating occur, and there may be added anxiety, depression, and anomia. Diminished capacity for abstraction, attention, planning, and problem solving may be observed as the degenerative process continues. These are subsumed under the term *disorders of "executive functions."* To these features in some patients is added a parkinsonian syndrome.

In the advanced stages of some dementias, restraining the patient leads to disagreeable behavior, petulance, agitation, shouting, and whining. Well known to physicians is nighttime confusion and inversion of the normal sleep pattern, as well as increased confusion and restlessness in the early evening ("sundowning"), as described in Chap. 20. Any febrile illness, drug intoxication, anesthesia, surgery, or metabolic upset is poorly tolerated, leading to severe confusion and even stupor—an indication of the precarious state of cerebral compensation.

It would be an error to think that the abnormalities in the degenerative dementing diseases are confined to the intellectual sphere. The patient's appearance and the physical examination yield highly informative data. The first impression is often revealing; the patient may be unkempt and unbathed. He may look bewildered, as though lost, or his expression may be vacant, and he does not maintain a lively interest or participate in the interview. There is a kind of psychic inertia. Movements may be slightly slow, sometimes suggesting an oncoming parkinsonian syndrome.

Sooner or later, gait is characteristically altered in many of the dementias (Chap. 7). Passive movements of the limbs encounter a fluctuating resistance or paratonia (gegenhalten). Mouthing movements and a number of abnormal reflexes—grasping and sucking (in response to visual as well as tactile stimuli), inability to inhibit blink on tapping the glabella, snout reflex (protrusion of the lips in response to perioral tapping), biting or jaw clamping (bulldog) reflex, corneomandibular reflex (jaw clenching when the cornea is touched), and palmomental reflex (retraction of one side of the mouth and chin caused by contraction of the mentalis muscle when the thenar eminence of the palm is stroked)—all occur with increasing frequency in the advanced stages of the dementia. Many of these abnormalities are considered to be motor disinhibitions that appear when the premotor areas of the brain are involved.

In the very later stages, physical deterioration is inexorable. Food intake, which may be increased at the onset of the illness, sometimes to the point of gluttony, is in the end reduced, with resulting emaciation. Finally, these patients remain in bed most of the time, oblivious of their surroundings, and succumb at this stage to pneumonia or some other intercurrent infection. Some patients, should they not die in this way, become virtually decorticate—totally unaware of their environment, unresponsive, mute, incontinent, and adopting a posture of flexion. They lie with their eyes open but do not look about. Food and drink are no longer requested but are swallowed if placed in the patient's mouth. The term *persistent vegetative state* is appropriately applied to these patients, although it was originally devised to describe patients in this inert state after cardiac arrest or head injury. Occasionally, diffuse choreoathetotic movements or random myoclonic jerking can be observed, and seizures occur in a few advanced cases. Pain or an uncomfortable posture goes unheeded. The course of the prototype of dementia, Alzheimer disease, extends for 5 to 10 years or more from the time that the memory defect becomes evident. The clinical course of advanced dementia has been studied by Mitchell and colleagues in nursing homes. Those who acquired pneumonia, a febrile episode or an eating disorder, not surprisingly, had high rates of mortality, approaching half, in the subsequent 6 months.

Naturally, every case does not follow the exact sequence outlined here. Often, a patient is brought to the physician because of an impaired facility with language. In other patients, impairment of memory with relatively intact reasoning power may be the dominant clinical feature in the first months or even years of the disease; or low impulsivity (apathy and abulia) may be the most conspicuous feature, resulting in obscuration of all the more specialized higher cerebral functions. Gait disorder, although usually a late development, may occur early, particularly in patients in whom the dementia is associated with or superimposed on frontal lobe degeneration, Parkinson disease, normal pressure hydrocephalus, cerebellar ataxia, or progressive supranuclear palsy. Insofar as the types of degenerative disease do not affect certain parts of the brain equally, it is not surprising that their symptomatology varies. Moreover, frank psychosis with delusions and hallucinations may be woven into the dementia and are particularly characteristic of certain diseases such as Lewy-body dementia. Chapter 39 discusses these variations and others more fully.

The aforementioned alterations of intellect and behavior are the direct consequence of neuronal loss in certain parts of the cerebrum. In other words, the symptoms are the primary manifestations of neurologic disease. However, some symptoms are secondary; i.e., they may represent the patient's reactions to his mental incapacity. For example, a demented person may seek solitude to hide his affliction and thus may appear to be asocial or apathetic. Again, excessive orderliness may be an attempt to compensate for failing memory; apprehension, gloom, and irritability may reflect a general dissatisfaction with a necessarily restricted life. According to Goldstein, who has written about these "catastrophic reactions," as he calls them, even patients in a state of fairly advanced deterioration are still capable of reacting to their illness and to persons who care for them.

In the early and intermediate stages of the illness, special neuropsychologic tests aid in the quantitation of some of these abnormalities, as indicated in the later part of this chapter.

Subcortical Dementia and Dementias Associated With Diseases of the Basal Ganglia

McHugh, who introduced the concept of subcortical dementia, pointed out that the cognitive decline of certain predominantly basal ganglionic diseases—such as progressive supranuclear palsy, Huntington chorea, and Parkinson disease—is different in several respects from the cortical dementia of Alzheimer disease. In addition to the obvious disorders of motility and involuntary movements, there are degrees of mild forgetfulness, slowed thought processes, lack of initiative, and depression of mood. Relatively spared, however, are vocabulary, naming, and praxis. By contrast, the "cortical dementias" (exemplified by Alzheimer disease) are distinguished by more severe disturbances of memory, language, and calculation, prominent signs of apraxia and agnosia, and impaired capacity for abstract thought.

The pathologic changes underlying the subcortical dementias predominate in the basal ganglia, thalamus, rostral brainstem nuclei, and mostly, in the ill-defined projections in the white matter from these regions to the cortex, particularly of the frontal lobes; however, it would be overly simplistic to attribute the dementia to changes in these areas. One of the problems with the concept of subcortical dementia is the name itself, implying as it does that symptoms of dementia are ascribed to lesions confined to subcortical structures. Anatomically, none of the neurodegenerative dementias is strictly cortical or subcortical. The attribution of dementia to subcortical gliosis, for example, has almost always proved to be incorrect; invariably there are cortical neuronal changes as well. In a similar way, the changes of Alzheimer disease may extend well beyond the cerebral cortex, involving the striatum, thalamus, and even cerebellum. Also, functionally, these lesions produce their effects by interrupting neural links to the frontal and other parts of the cerebral cortex. Similar ambiguity arises when one considers the dementias caused by Lewy-body disease (probably second in frequency only to Alzheimer disease) and by normal-pressure hydrocephalus; here there are parkinsonism and dementing features that could be construed as both cortical and subcortical in nature.

Certain authors, notably Mayeux and Stern and their colleagues as well as Tierney and coworkers, have been critical of the concept of subcortical dementia. They argue that the distinctions between cortical and subcortical dementias are not fundamental and that any differences between them are probably attributable to differences in the relative severity of the dementing processes. Nonetheless, a number of studies do indeed indicate that the constellations of cognitive impairments in the two groups of dementias differ along the lines indicated earlier (see Pillon et al). And, the clinical distinction between cortical and subcortical dementia based on a relative sparing of core cortical functions is very useful.

Pathogenesis of Dementia

Attempts to relate the impairment of general intellectual function to lesions in certain parts of the brain or a particular pathologic change have been largely unsuccessful. Lashley's concept of loss of intelligence in proportion to brain damage has already been mentioned. This is not to say that certain parts of the cognitive apparatus are not localizable. It is the integrated capacity to think that defies easy attribution to a part of the brain. Two types of difficulty have obstructed progress in this field. First, there is the problem of defining and analyzing the nature of the intellectual functions as already discussed. Second, the pathologic anatomy of the dementing diseases is often so diffuse and complex that it cannot be fully localized and quantitated.

As described in Chap. 22, certain portions of the intellectual ensemble are controlled by circumscribed regions of the cerebrum. Memory impairment, which is a central feature of some dementias, may occur with extensive disease in several different parts of the cerebrum, but the integrity of certain discrete parts of the diencephalon and inferomedial parts of the temporal lobes is fundamental to memory. In a similar way, impairment of language function is associated specifically with disease of the dominant cerebral hemisphere, particularly the perisylvian parts of the frontal, temporal, and parietal lobes. Loss of capacity for reading and calculation is related to lesions in the posterior part of the left (dominant) cerebral hemisphere; loss of use of tools and imitation of gestures (apraxias) is related to loss of tissue in the dominant parietal region. Impairment in drawing or constructing simple and complex figures with blocks, sticks, picture arrangements, etc., is observed with parietal lobe lesions, more often with right-sided (nondominant) than with left-sided ones. And problems with modulation of behavior and stability of personality are generally related to frontal lobe degeneration. Thus, the clinical picture resulting from cerebral disease depends in part on the extent of the lesion, i.e., the amount of cerebral tissue destroyed, and in part on the region of the brain that bears the brunt of the pathologic change.

Dementia of the degenerative types is related to obvious structural diseases of the cerebral cortex but the diencephalon and, as mentioned earlier, the basal ganglia are also implicated. Rarely, purely thalamic degenerations may be the basis of a dementia because of the integral relationship of the thalamus to the cerebral cortex, particularly as regards memory. Even when a particular disease disproportionately affects one part of the cerebrum, additional areas are often implicated and contribute to the mental decline. One such important example is found in Alzheimer disease, in which the main site of damage is in the hippocampus, but degeneration of the cholinergic nuclei of the basal frontal region, which project to the hippocampus, greatly augments the deterioration in memory function. Indeed, replacement of this lost cholinergic influence is one of the main approaches to the treatment of the disease.

Arteriosclerotic cerebrovascular disease, which pursues a different course than the neurodegenerative diseases, results in multiple foci of infarction throughout the thalami, basal ganglia, brainstem, and cerebrum, including the motor, sensory, and visual projection areas as well as the association areas. There is no evidence, however, that arteriosclerosis *per se,* without vascular occlusion and infarction, is a cause of progressive dementia as was thought in previous decades. Undoubtedly, the cumulative effects of recurrent strokes impair the intellect. Usually, but not always, the stroke-by-stroke advance of the disease is apparent in such patients (multi-infarct dementia). More uncertain in our opinion is the notion that a decline in mental function can be attributed to periventricular white matter changes (leukoaraiosis), which are observed on CT and MRI scans of many elderly patients and are presumed to be ischemic in nature (see review of van Gijn). Also, the construct that small strokes exaggerate or in some way biologically produce an Alzheimer neuropathologic process has been uncritically accepted in some quarters. The two processes do seem to coincide more often than chance. The special problem of arteriosclerotic or multi-infarct dementia is discussed in Chap. 34 on cerebrovascular disease.

The lesions of *severe cerebral trauma,* if they result in dementia, are found in the cerebral convolutions (mainly frontal and temporal poles), corpus callosum, and thalamus. In some cases, there is widespread degeneration of the deep cerebral hemispheres, because of a mechanical disruption of the deep white matter termed *axonal shearing.* Most traumatic lesions that produce dementia are quite extensive, making localization difficult. Our own experience suggests that the thalamic lesions are critical, but many authorities view the axonal shearing lesions as the primary cause of traumatic dementia. The special problem of chronic traumatic encephalopathy is addressed in Chap. 35.

Mechanisms other than the overt destruction of brain tissue may operate in some cases of dementia. *Chronic hydrocephalus,* regardless of cause, is often associated with a general impairment of mental function. Compression of the cerebral white matter is probably the main factor, but this has not been settled. The extrinsic compression of one or both of the cerebral hemispheres by *chronic subdural hematomas* may have the same effect. A *diffuse inflammatory process* is at least in part the basis of dementia in syphilis, cryptococcosis, other chronic meningitides, and viral infections such as HIV encephalitis, herpes simplex encephalitis, and subacute sclerosing panencephalitis; presumably, there is a loss of some neurons and an inflammatory derangement of function in the neurons that remain. The prion diseases (e.g., Creutzfeldt–Jakob disease) cause a diffuse loss of cortical neurons, replacement gliosis, and spongiform change and produce special patterns of cognitive dysfunction.

The adult forms of *leukodystrophy* (Chap. 37) also give rise to a dementing state, generally a "subcortical" syndrome with prominent frontal lobe features. Or extensive lesions in the white matter may be the result of advanced multiple sclerosis, progressive multifocal leukoencephalitis, or some of the vascular dementias already mentioned (Binswanger disease and CADASIL [cerebral autosomal dominant arteriopathy with subcortical infarcts and leukoencephalopathy]). Last, several of the metabolic and toxic disorders discussed in Chaps. 37, 40, and 43 may interfere with nervous function over a period of time and create a clinical picture similar, if not identical, to that of one of the dementias. One must suppose in those cases that the altered biochemical environment has affected neuronal function.

Classification of the Dementing Diseases

Conventionally, the dementing diseases have been classified according to cause if known, to the pathologic changes, or more recently, to a genetic mutation. Another, more practical approach, which follows logically from the method by which much of the subject matter is presented in this book, is to divide the diseases into three categories on the basis of the neurologic signs and associated clinical and laboratory signs of medical disease: (1) dementia with medical disease, (2) dementia that is accompanied by other prominent neurologic signs, and (3) dementia as the sole or predominant feature of the illness (Table 21-3). Once it has been determined that the patient suffers from a dementing illness, it must then be decided from

Table 21-3

BEDSIDE CLASSIFICATION OF THE DEMENTIAS

I. Diseases in which dementia is associated with clinical and laboratory signs of other medical diseases
   A. AIDS–HIV infection
   B. Endocrine disorders: hypothyroidism, Cushing syndrome, rarely hypopituitarism, Hashimoto encephalopathy
   C. Nutritional deficiency states: Wernicke–Korsakoff syndrome, subacute combined degeneration (vitamin B_{12} deficiency), pellagra
   D. Chronic meningoencephalitis: general paresis, meningovascular syphilis, cryptococcosis
   E. Hepatolenticular degeneration—familial (Wilson disease) and acquired
   F. Chronic drug and environmental intoxications (including CO poisoning)
   G. Prolonged hypoglycemia or hypoxia
   H. Paraneoplastic "limbic" encephalitis
   I. Heavy metal exposure: arsenic, bismuth, gold, manganese, mercury
   J. Dialysis dementia (now rare)

II. Diseases in which dementia is associated with other neurologic signs but not with obvious medical diseases
   A. Invariably associated with other neurologic signs
      1. Huntington chorea (choreoathetosis)
      2. Multiple sclerosis, Schilder disease, adrenal leukodystrophy, and related demyelinative diseases (spastic weakness, pseudobulbar palsy, blindness)
      3. Lipid-storage diseases (myoclonic seizures, blindness, spasticity, cerebellar ataxia)
      4. Myoclonic epilepsy (diffuse myoclonus, generalized seizures, cerebellar ataxia)
      5. Subacute spongiform encephalopathy; Creutzfeldt-Jakob disease; Gerstmann-Sträussler-Scheinker disease (prion, myoclonic dementias)
      6. Cerebrocerebellar degeneration (cerebellar ataxia)
      7. Cerebrobasal ganglionic degenerations (apraxia-rigidity)
      8. Dementia with spastic paraplegia
      9. Progressive supranuclear palsy (falls, vertical gaze palsy)
      10. Parkinson disease
      11. Amyotrophic lateral sclerosis (ALS) and ALS-Parkinson-dementia complex
      12. Other rare metabolic diseases, including polyglucosan disease and leukodystrophies
   B. Often associated with other neurologic signs
      1. Multiple thrombotic or embolic cerebral infarctions and Binswanger disease
      2. Brain tumor (primary or metastatic) or abscess
      3. Brain trauma, such as cerebral contusions, midbrain hemorrhages, chronic subdural hematoma
      4. Lewy-body disease (parkinsonian features)
      5. Communicating, normal-pressure, or obstructive hydrocephalus (usually with ataxia of gait)
      6. Progressive multifocal leukoencephalitis
      7. Marchiafava-Bignami disease (often with apraxia and other frontal lobe signs)
      8. Granulomatous and other vasculitides of the brain

III. Diseases in which dementia is usually the only evidence of neurologic or medical diseases
   A. Alzheimer disease
   B. Pick disease
   C. Some cases of AIDS
   D. Progressive aphasia syndromes
   E. Frontotemporal and "frontal lobe" dementias associated with tau deposition, Alzheimer change, or with no specific pathologic alteration
   F. Degenerative disease of unspecified type

Note: The special clinical features and morbid anatomy of these many dementing diseases are discussed in appropriate chapters throughout this book, particularly Chap. 39 on degenerative disorders, Chaps. 37 and 41 on metabolic and nutritional disturbances, and Chap. 33 on chronic infections.

the medical, neurologic, and ancillary data into which category the case fits. This classification may at first seem somewhat dated and not based on newer genetic and molecular models, but it is likely to be more useful to the student or physician who must confront the many diseases that cause dementia.

Differential Diagnosis

Although dementia per se does not indicate a particular disease, certain combinations of symptoms and neurologic signs are more or less characteristic and may aid in diagnosis. The age of the patient, the mode of onset of the dementia, its clinical course and time span, the associated neurologic signs, and the accessory laboratory data constitute the basis of differential diagnosis. It must be admitted, however, that some of the rarer types of degenerative brain disease are at present recognized mainly by pathologic examination or genetic testing. The correct diagnosis of treatable forms of dementia—subdural hematoma, certain brain tumors, chronic drug intoxication, normal-pressure hydrocephalus, HIV (reversible to some extent), neurosyphilis, cryptococcosis, pellagra, vitamin B_{12} and thiamine deficiency states, hypothyroidism, and other metabolic and endocrine disorders—is, of course, of greater practical importance than the diagnosis of the untreatable ones. Also important is the detection of a *depressive illness*, which may masquerade as dementia, and chronic intoxication with drugs or chemical agents, both of which are treatable.

The first task in dealing with this class of patients is to verify the presence of intellectual deterioration and personality change. *It may be necessary to examine the patient serially before one is confident of the clinical findings and their chronicity.* A mild aphasia from a focal brain lesion must not be mistaken for dementia. Aphasic patients appear uncertain of themselves, and their speech may be incoherent. Careful attention to the patient's language performance will lead to the correct diagnosis in most instances. It is a clinical truism that the abrupt onset of mental symptoms points to a delirium or other type of acute confusional state or to a stroke; inattention, perceptual disturbances, and often drowsiness are conjoined (Chap. 20). Also, progressive deafness or loss of sight in an elderly person may sometimes be misinterpreted as dementia.

There is always a tendency to assume that mental function is normal if a patient complains only of anxiety, fatigue, insomnia, or vague somatic symptoms, and to label the patient as anxious. This will be avoided if one keeps in mind that these disorders rarely have their onset in middle or late adult life.

Clues to the diagnosis of *depression* are the presence of frequent sighing, crying, loss of energy, psychomotor underactivity or its opposite, agitation with pacing, persecutory delusions, persistent hypochondriasis, and a history of depression in the past and in the family. Although depressed patients may complain of memory failure, scrutiny of their complaints will show that they can usually remember the details of their illness and that little or no qualitative change in other intellectual functions has taken place. Their difficulty is either a lack of energy and interest or preoccupation with personal worries and anxiety, which prevents the focusing of attention on anything except their own problems. Even during mental tests, their performance may be impaired by "emotional blocking," in much the same way as the worried student blocks during an examination ("experiential confusion"). When such patients are calmed by reassurance and encouraged to try harder, their mental function improves, indicating that intellectual deterioration has not occurred. Conversely, it is helpful to remember that demented patients rarely have sufficient insight to complain of mental deterioration; if they admit to poor memory, they do so without conviction or full appreciation of the degree of their disability. The physician must not rely on the patient's statements alone in gauging the efficiency of mental function and should seek corroboration from family members. Yet another problem is that of the impulsive, cantankerous, and quarrelsome patient who is a constant source of distress to employer and family. Such changes in personality and behavior (as, for example, in Huntington disease) may precede or mask early intellectual deterioration.

The neuropsychiatric symptoms associated with metabolic, endocrine, or toxic disorders (e.g., Cushing syndrome, vitamin B_{12} deficiency, hypercalcemia, uremia) may present difficulties in diagnosis because of the wide variety of clinical pictures by which they manifest themselves. Drowsiness or stupor and asterixis are the surest signs of a metabolic or drug-induced encephalopathy, but they are not always present. Psychosis with hallucinations and a great deal of fluctuation in behavior also bespeak an exogenously caused confusional state, with the exception that Lewy-body dementia also has these characteristics. Whenever any such metabolic or toxic disorder is suspected, a thorough review of the patient's medications is crucial. Medications with atropinic activity, for example, can produce an apparent dementia or worsen a structurally based dementia, as discussed in Chap. 20. Occupational exposure to toxins and heavy metals should also be explored, but this is an infrequent cause of dementia; therefore, slight or even moderately elevated levels of these chemicals in the blood should be interpreted cautiously. It is also useful to keep in mind that seizures are not a usual component of the degenerative dementias; when they are present, they generally do not appear until a very late stage.

Once it is decided that the patient suffers from a dementing condition, the next step is to determine by careful physical examination, whether there are other neurologic signs or indications of a particular medical disease. This enables the physician to place the case in one of the three aforementioned categories in the bedside classification (see above and Table 21-3).

Experienced neurologists recognize that certain leading neurologic features are indicative of particular degenerative dementias. For example, prominent and early parkinsonian signs such as bradykinesia, tremor, and shortened gait step are parts of the subcortical dementias of Lewy body and Parkinson diseases. Rigidity of the limbs and apraxia may have a similar clinical appearance but point to corticobasal degeneration as the cause of mental decline. An early aphasia or visuospatial difficulty that is manifest as either geographic confusion or difficulty with drawing, copying, and recognizing faces and objects are characteristic of a focal degeneration of the parietal or inferior temporal lobes. Involuntary movements such as choreoathetosis, dystonia, ataxia, and myoclonus are each signs of particular degenerative disorders that include Huntington disease, acquired and inherited hepatocerebral degenerations, and prion disorder, all of which are discussed in later chapter. Frequent falls and a disorder of vertical eye movements are the core components of progressive supranuclear palsy that often has an attendant dementia. In the nondegenerative categories of dementia, spasticity and Babinski signs are typical of vascular dementias.

Ancillary examinations—such as CT, MRI, electroencephalography (EEG), lumbar puncture, measurement of blood urea nitrogen, as well as serum concentrations of calcium and electrolytes, and liver function tests—should be carried out in appropriate cases. Brain MRI and CT are of major importance in objectifying hydrocephalus, lobar atrophy, cerebrovascular disease, tumor, and subdural hematoma. Testing for syphilis, vitamin B_{12} deficiency, and thyroid function is also done in many clinics almost as a matter of routine because the tests are simple and the dementias they cause are reversible. These are supplemented in individual circumstances by serologic testing for HIV infection, measurement of copper and ceruloplasmin levels (Wilson disease), heavy metal concentrations in urine or tissues, serum cortisol levels, and drug toxicology screening. The final step is to determine, from the total clinical picture, the particular disease within any one category.

THE AMNESIC SYNDROME (KORSAKOFF SYNDROME) (See also Chap. 41)

The terms listed above are used interchangeably to designate a unique disorder of cognitive function in which memory and learning are deranged almost in isolation from all other components of mentation and behavior. The amnesic state, as originally defined by Ribot, possesses two salient features that may vary in severity but are always conjoined: (1) an impaired ability to recall events and other information that had been firmly established before the onset of the illness (*retrograde amnesia*) and (2) an impaired ability to acquire new information, i.e., to learn or to form new memories (*anterograde amnesia*). This duality inspired the White Queen, one of Lewis Carroll's characters, to quip, "It's a poor sort of memory that works only backwards." In other words, the functions of memory and learning are inseparable. A third feature of the Korsakoff syndrome, contingent upon retrograde amnesia, is impaired temporal localization of past experience. Other cognitive functions, particularly the capacity for concentration, spatial organization, and visual and verbal abstraction, which depend little or not at all on memory, are usually not affected. Equally important in the definition of the *Korsakoff syndrome,* or *amnesic state* (these terms are preferable to the older term, *Korsakoff psychosis*), is this integrity of certain aspects of behavior and mental function.

In order to establish the presence of the Korsakoff syndrome, the patient must be awake, attentive, and responsive—capable of perceiving and understanding the written and spoken word, of making appropriate deductions from given premises, and of solving such problems as can be included within his forward memory span. These features are of particular diagnostic importance because they help to distinguish the Korsakoff amnesic state from a number of other disorders in which the basic defect is not in memory but in some other abnormality—e.g., impairment in attention and perception (as in the delirious, confused, or stuporous patient), in loss of personal identity (as in the hysterical patient), or in volition (as in the apathetic or abulic patient with frontal lobe disease or depression).

Immediate recall, a function of *working memory,* allows the patient with Korsakoff syndrome to repeat a string of digits, but this is more a measure of attention and registration. Remote memory is relatively less affected than recent memory (the Ribot rule, as discussed later).

Confabulation

The creative falsification of memory in an alert, responsive individual is often included in the definition of the Korsakoff amnesic state but is not a requisite for diagnosis. It can be provoked by questions as to the patient's recent activities. The replies may be recognized as partially remembered events and personal experiences that are inaccurately localized in the past and related with no regard to their proper temporal sequence. Less frequent in Korsakoff syndrome, but more dramatic, is a spontaneous recital of personal experiences, many of which are fantasies. These two forms of confabulation have been referred to as "momentary" and "fantastic". In the patients with the alcoholic Korsakoff syndrome studied by Victor and Adams, fantastic confabulation was observed mainly in the initial phase of the illness, in which it could be related to a state of profound general confusion. In the chronic, stable stage of the illness, confabulation was rarely elicitable irrespective of how broadly this symptom was defined. Confabulation therefore is not an obligate feature of the Korsakoff syndrome.

Neuropsychology of Memory

Memory function obeys certain neurologic laws. As memory fails, it first loses its hold on recent events. The extent in time of retrograde amnesia is generally proportionate to the magnitude of the underlying neurologic disorder. Early life memories are better preserved and often have been integrated into habitual responses; nevertheless, with natural aging, there is also a gradual loss of early life memories. In transitory amnesias (e.g., concussive head injury), memories are recovered in reverse order: first the remote and then the more recent. The enduring aspect of early life memories in contrast to more recently experienced and learned material, a restatement of the Ribot law, is apparent in both normal adults and in demented patients. As quoted by Kopelman, Ribot in 1882 stated: "The progressive destruction of memory follows a logical order—a law—it begins at the most recent recollections which, being rarely repeated and having no permanent associations, represent organization in its feeblest form."

In the further analysis of the Korsakoff amnesic syndrome, it is necessary to consider the proposition that memory is not a unitary function, but takes several forms. One practical classification that adheres broadly to current ideas in the field is shown in Fig. 21-1 and Table 21-4. An initial separation is made between the aforementioned immediate recall and the other types of memory. Short-term memory is exemplified by the common daily acts of hearing a phone number and retaining it to be able to walk across a room and dial the phone; or, performing a series of mental calculations that requires holding an intermediate sum briefly in mind; all the numbers are soon forgotten. Long–term memory can be viewed from the perspective the individual's awareness of the learning of new material (explicit memory), or not being conscious of the event of acquiring memory (implicit memory). Functions such the acquisition of physical skills (such as driving a car or playing tennis) are implicit memories termed procedural memory. Classic conditioning is considered another type of implicit memory.

Explicit memory subsumes what most persons consider to be memory and learning, that is, the ability to retain and recount events that were consciously experienced by

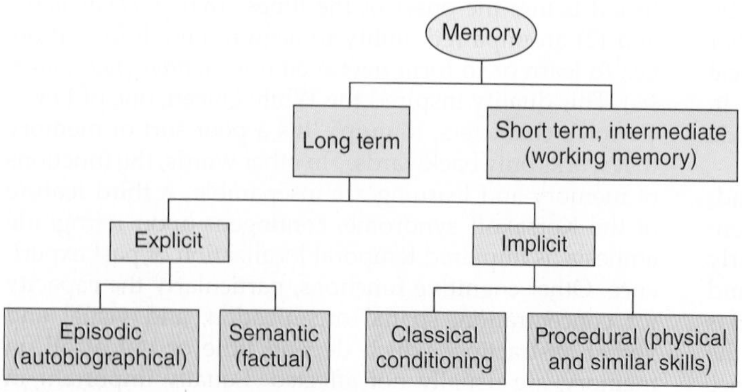

Figure 21-1. Schematic definitions of memory systems (see text). (From Budson and Price with permission.)

Table 21-4

NEUROPSYCHOLOGIC CATEGORIES OF MEMORY

			LONG-TERM MEMORY			
			EXPLICIT		IMPLICIT	
	IMMEDIATE RECALL	WORKING MEMORY	SEMANTIC	EPISODIC	PROCEDURAL	VISUAL
Function	Repetition	Short-term recall of objects, plans, names, sequencing	Recall for facts and their relationships	Recall for temporally organized events	Operational recall ("how to do")	Recall of visual representations
Conscious access	Yes	Yes	Yes	Yes	Usually	No
Anatomic regions involved	Perisylvian cortex of dominant hemisphere	Prefrontal cortex, medial temporal lobes, dorsomedial thalamus	Anterior, inferior temporal lobes; frontal lobes	Association cortex	Premotor and motor cortex, basal ganglia, cerebellum	Occipital lobes
Conditions that disturb memory	Agitation, confusion (impaired attention)	Wernicke–Korsakoff syndrome, herpes encephalitis, infarction of hippocampi, dorsomedial thalamus	AD, frontotemporal dementia, encephalitis, chronic toxins, tumors	Hippocampal infarction, alcoholic Korsakoff syndrome, AD and other CNS degenerative disorders, encephalitis, chronic toxic exposure, tumors	AD and other CNS degenerative disorders, encephalitis, chronic toxic exposure, tumors	AD, other CNS degenerative disorders, encephalitis, tumors

AD, Alzheimer disease; CNS, central nervous system.

the person, including the time and general circumstances of the acquisition (episodic, or autobiographical memory). *Semantic memory,* the learning of the nature of the environment and factual knowledge (such as the shape and color of a lion) is also a type of explicit memory but the event of acquiring the memory cannot be recalled. A patient with virtually no capacity to learn any newly presented information can nonetheless still acquire some simple manual and pattern-analyzing skills. Moreover, having acquired these skills, the patient may have no memory of the circumstances in which they were acquired. The learning of simple mechanical skills has been referred to as *procedural memory,* in distinction to learning new data information. Cohen and Squire have described this dichotomy as "knowing how" as opposed to "knowing that."

As confirmation of the separation of episodic from semantic memory functions, Gadian and colleagues have described young patients who showed severe impairments of episodic memory with relative preservation of semantic memory that was attributable to hypoxic-ischemic injury (bilateral hippocampal atrophy) sustained early in life. Here, again, the subject matter most relevant to amnesia involves episodic, or autobiographical, memory. The same occurs in early Alzheimer disease and herpes simplex encephalitis.

A pervasive problem with these terms is the lack of uniformity in defining the terms of memory. To Tulving, whose writings on this subject are recommended, the term *episodic* denotes a memory system for dating personal experiences and their temporal relationships; *semantic* memory is one's repository of perceptual and factual knowledge, which makes it possible to comprehend language and make inferences. This hardly constitutes a novel concept; Korsakoff himself clearly recognized that certain aspects of mental function (among them those now being defined as semantic memory) remain intact, despite the profound impairment of episodic memory. Damasio has introduced yet another set of terms—*generic* in place of semantic and *contextual* for episodic. To Damasio, generic memory denotes the basic properties of acquired information, such as its class membership and function; he makes the point that in the amnesic syndrome, this component of declarative memory remains intact and only the contextual component is impaired.

The full significance of these categorizations is still being explored. The categorical purity of semantic memory is open to question, as is the notion of a strict dichotomy between semantic and episodic memory. Most importantly, a separate anatomic basis for these systems of memory has not been clearly established (see below). Further interesting derivative issues regarding the neuropsychology of memory in relation to brain diseases can be found in the review by Kopelman. Among these is the degree to which a disparity between retrograde and anterograde memory can be detected in certain diseases. He also points out nicely the subtle distinctions between recall and memory by recognition.

Neuropsychologists have further subdivided memory and suggested that there are corresponding anatomic regions for specific categories (see Table 21-4). Some of these more complex subtypes have been alluded to above and others are simply restatements of the act of registration. Furthermore, it is not surprising that the participation of certain areas of the brain not primarily involved in memory function, particularly the language and visuospatial areas, is required for the performance of certain memory tasks. Among the special modules of memory, the notion of a *working memory* has both clinical and neuropsychologic credibility. This relates to the capacity to register and attend to a task, and there is little question that it is a measurable form of memory. Several regions of the brain must be active during tasks of working memory, including the hippocampi and dorsal thalamus, but lesions of the dorsolateral prefrontal cortex most specifically impair the skill. The original work of Goldman-Rakic may be referred to for discussion of the mechanisms that underlie working memory.

Finally, there are reasons, based mainly on the neuroanatomic and functional imaging studies discussed later, to view episodic memory for spatial and topographic information in a particular way. Certainly the recollection of personally experienced events can be dissociated to some degree from the memory of the topographic arrangement of the scene in which these memories were formed, but often these two elements are inextricably bound in one experience. More salient may be a disproportionate degradation of learned topographic and directional information compared to learned semantic material; such a dissociation can be found, but only in relative terms, in patients who have injuries to their right hippocampus, whereas semantic material is dependent more on the left hippocampus (see later).

Anatomic Basis of the Amnesic Syndrome

Two anatomic structures are of central importance in memory function: the diencephalon (specifically the medial portions of the dorsomedial and adjacent midline nuclei of the thalamus) and the hippocampal formations of the medial temporal lobes including their associated structures (dentate gyrus, hippocampus, parahippocampal gyrus, subiculum, and entorhinal cortex). Discrete bilateral lesions in these two main regions derange memory and learning disproportionate to all other cognitive functions, and even a unilateral lesion of these structures, especially of the dominant hemisphere, can produce a lesser degree of the same effect. The clinical–anatomic relationships that bear on this subject are discussed in detail by Aggleton and Saunders and in the monograph on Wernicke–Korsakoff syndrome by Victor et al.

While central to memory function, these are not the only regions engaged in the formation and retrieval of memory. A severe but less-enduring defect in memory is observed with damage of the anterior septal gray matter; a cluster of midline nuclei at the base of the frontal lobes, just below the interventricular septum and including the septal nucleus, nucleus accumbens, diagonal band of Broca; and paraventricular hypothalamic gray matter. The case of infarction of this region reported by Phillips and colleagues confirms the participation of this region in memory formation and retrieval. The amnesic syndrome, usually not permanent, that follows a ruptured anterior communicating aneurysm is a consequence of disruption of these nuclei. These septal nuclei have connections with the hippocampus through the precommissural fornix and with the amygdala through the diagonal band. Again, what is most remarkable about this basal frontal amnesic syndrome is its initial severity lasting for weeks to months and the potential for almost complete recovery.

Observations of human disease have confirmed the fundamental importance of the diencephalic–hippocampal structures in all memory function. The difficulty of evaluating memory function in monkeys has been largely overcome by use of the "delayed nonmatching-to-sample task," which is essentially a refined test of recognition memory and is impaired both in patients with the amnesic syndrome and in monkeys with lesions of the mediodorsal nuclei of the thalamus and inferomedial temporal cortical regions (Mishkin and Delacour). Using this method and several others that simulate a restricted form of human amnesia, Zola-Morgan and colleagues have shown that bilateral lesions of the hippocampal formation cause an enduring impairment of memory function. Lesions confined to the fornices or mammillary bodies and stereotaxic lesions of the amygdala that spared the adjacent cortical regions (entorhinal and perirhinal cortices) failed to produce a memory defect. However, lesions that were restricted to the perirhinal and entorhinal cortex (Brodmann areas 35 and 36) and the closely associated parahippocampal cortex did cause a persistent memory defect, presumably by interrupting the major afferent pathways conveying cortical information to the hippocampus. Lesions of the anteromedial parts of the diencephalon, which receive and send fibers to the amygdala and hippocampus, similarly abolished memory function.

A body of work using functional neuroimaging also addresses the anatomic mechanisms of memory function. It has been found that the hippocampal formations are consistently engaged during memory acquisition and retrieval tasks. In addition, Maguire's group found a differential activation of the right side during recall of topographic spatial information and the left side for autobiographical memory. Their clever use of London taxi drivers as subjects for imaging studies has further suggested that the volume of the right hippocampus is larger in subjects who have more experience navigating the arcane streets of London. An asymmetrical representation of certain modalities of memory is in keeping with limited clinicopathologic studies of patients who have undergone temporal lobectomy on one side.

These observations in aggregate confirm that integrity of the hippocampal formations and the medial-dorsal nuclei of the thalamus are essential for normal memory and learning. Interestingly, there are only sparse direct anatomic connections between these two regions. The importance assigned to the hippocampal formations and medial thalamic nuclei in memory function does not mean that the mechanisms governing this function are confined to these structures or that these parts of the brain form a "memory center." It informs us only that these are the sites where the smallest lesions have the most devastating effects on memory and learning. Normal memory function, as emphasized, involves many parts of the brain in addition to diencephalic–hippocampal structures. The aforementioned basal frontal nuclei that project to the hippocampi are an example.

It is also clear that particular lesions of the neocortex may cause impairment of specific forms of memory and learning. Thus, a lesion of the dominant temporal lobe impairs the ability to remember words (loss of explicit semantic memory), and a lesion of the inferior parietal lobule undermines the recognition of written or printed words as well as the ability to relearn them (alexia). The dominant parietal lobe is related to recollection of geometric figures and numbers; the nondominant parietal lobe, to visuospatial relations; the inferoposterior temporal lobes, to the recognition of faces; and the dominant posterofrontal region, to acquiring and remembering motor skills and their affective associations. Whether these are truly forms of memory, or whether these regions of cortex must be entrained in order to retrieve and "experience" the memory, is philosophical. Taken to its extremes, aphasia from a left temporal perisylvian lesion (Wernicke's aphasia) could be viewed as an amnesia for language, and parietal lesions that cause ideomotor apraxia could be taken to represent a loss of memory for these previously learned acts. What remains inviolate is that the integrity of both the hippocampal–thalamic system and the appropriate cortical region is required for memory as we refer to it in this chapter, but only the former is integrated into all modalities of learning and retrieval.

It is a remarkable feature of the Korsakoff amnesic state that no matter how severe the defect in memory may be, it is never complete. Certain past memories can be recalled, but imperfectly and with no regard for their normal temporal relationships, giving them a fictional quality and explaining many instances of confabulation. Another noteworthy fact is that long-standing social habits, automatic motor skills, and memory for words (language) and visual impressions (visual or pictorial attributes of persons, objects, and places) are unimpaired. Long periods of repetition and usage may have made these implicit or procedural memories virtually automatic; they no longer require the participation of the diencephalic–hippocampal structures that were necessary to learn them originally. All of this suggests that these special memories, or coded forms of them, through a process of relearning and habituation, come to be stored or filed in other regions of the brain; i.e., they acquire a separate and autonomous anatomy that may be regional, cellular, or subcellular.

Several fundamental questions concerning the amnesic syndrome remain unanswered. Not known is how a disease process, acting over a brief period of time, not only impairs all future learning but also wipes out portions of a vast reservoir of past memories that had been firmly established for many years before the onset of the illness. Most likely, it is not the memories themselves that are obliterated but the mechanism required to access them.

One of the most provocative new observations regarding memory has been the enhancement of performance by electrical stimulation of the entorhinal area in individuals with epilepsy. The study by Suthana and colleagues is one of several demonstrating this effect in an improved ability to retain topographic-spatial landmarks in a simulated exercise. At a minimum, these findings confirm the critical role of parahippocampal regions (perforant pathways) in forming and stabilizing memories, in these cases, the major source of afferent input to the hippocampus.

This begs the fascinating question of "what is *a* memory?" Current notions suggest that no single hippocampal neuron, for example, embodies a memory but that the connections between an ensemble of neurons in the medial temporal lobes and modality-specific neurons in the associative cortices are, in fact, the memory. Strengthening synaptic connections among this network serves to establish the memory. This may occur through long-term potentiation, as the work of Kandel has emphasized in experimental models. It is not clear if a hippocampal neuron is the trigger to the memory ensemble or the entirety of hippocampal system serves a generic role in cohering all memories. The cellular mechanisms involved in learning and the formation of memories are only beginning to be understood. Whether physiologic phenomena such as long-term potentiation or anatomic changes in the dendritic structure of neurons are at the center of memory storage is not known; certainly both are likely to be involved. The neurochemical systems that are activated during formation and recall of memory are also obscure. Kandel has provided a detailed review of information on this subject. The anatomic and physiologic mechanisms that govern immediate registration, which remains intact in even the most severely damaged patients with the Korsakoff amnesic syndrome has not been fully deciphered.

Other psychologic features of human memory that must be accounted for by any model purporting to explain this function are the importance of cueing in eliciting learned material and the imprecision of past memories, allowing for unwitting embellishment and false recollection, to the point of fabrication. The latter aspect has been a topic of considerable importance in children who have (or have not) been subjected to sexual abuse and in adults and children whose memories of past abuse have been suggested by the examiners (see Schacter).

The separate roles of the thalamus, the hippocampi, and the frontal lobes in memory and the differences in the nature of the amnesia resulting from damage at each site remain to be clarified. That isolated thalamic lesions, without implicating medial temporal areas, can cause a Korsakoff syndrome is evident from the experience with alcoholism and stroke. Graff-Radford and colleagues have found that with purely thalamic lesions, as appreciated by imaging studies, anterograde learning is more affected than retrograde recall; but comparing these functions quantitatively is difficult. Kopelman, in reviewing his own studies and those of others, concludes that the differences are subtle and pertain mostly to temporal ordering and the modality of information, which is degraded more with diencephalic–temporal lesions than with frontal lobe damage.

Each of the amnesic states listed in Table 21-5 is considered at an appropriate point in subsequent chapters of this book. The only exception is the striking syndrome of *transient global amnesia*, the nature of which is not certain.

Table 21-5

CLASSIFICATION OF THE AMNESIC STATES

I. Amnesic syndrome of sudden onset—usually with gradual but incomplete recovery
   A. Bilateral or left (dominant) hippocampal infarction because of atherosclerotic-thrombotic or embolic occlusion of the posterior cerebral arteries or their inferior temporal branches
   B. Bilateral or left (dominant) infarction of anteromedial thalamic nuclei
   C. Infarction of the basal forebrain due to occlusion of anterior cerebral–anterior communicating arteries
   D. Subarachnoid hemorrhage (usually rupture of anterior communicating artery aneurysm)
   E. Trauma to the diencephalic, inferomedial temporal, or orbitofrontal regions
   F. Cardiac arrest, carbon monoxide poisoning, and other hypoxic states (hippocampal damage)
   G. Following prolonged status epilepticus
   H. Following delirium tremens
II. Amnesia of sudden onset and short duration
   A. Temporal lobe seizures
   B. Postconcussive states
   C. Transient global amnesia
   D. Hysteria
III. Amnesic syndrome of subacute onset with varying degrees of recovery, usually leaving permanent residua
   A. Wernicke–Korsakoff syndrome
   B. Herpes simplex encephalitis
   C. Tuberculous and other forms of meningitis characterized by a granulomatous exudate at the base of the brain
IV. Slowly progressive amnesic states
   A. Tumors involving the floor and walls of the third ventricle and limbic cortical structures
   B. Alzheimer disease (early stage) and other degenerative disorders with disproportionate affection of the temporal lobes
   C. Paraneoplastic and other forms of immune "limbic" encephalitis

It cannot be included with any assurance with the epilepsies or the cerebrovascular diseases or any other category of disease and is therefore considered here.

TRANSIENT GLOBAL AMNESIA

This was the name applied by Fisher and Adams to a particular transient type of memory disorder that they observed in more than 20 middle-aged and elderly persons. The condition was characterized by an episode of amnesia and bewilderment lasting for several hours. The symptoms had their basis in an amnesia for events of the recent past coupled with an ongoing anterograde amnesia. During the attack, there is no impairment in the state of consciousness, no other sign of confusion, and no overt seizure activity; personal identification is intact, as are motor, sensory, and reflex functions. The patient's behavior is normal except for a very characteristic incessant, repetitive questioning about his immediate circumstances—usually of the identical question over and over at intervals of 20 to 60 seconds after a response to the query has been given by the examiner (e.g., "What am I doing here?"; "How did we get here?"). Unlike psychomotor epilepsy, the patient is alert, in contact with his surroundings, and capable of high-level intellectual activity and language function during the attack. As soon as the episode has ended, no abnormality of mental function is apparent except for a permanent gap in memory for the period of the attack itself and for a brief period (hours or days) preceding it. The patient may be left with a mild headache. Incomplete or mild attacks are infrequent, and they may be as brief as 1 h, but are typically longer. The condition is among the most curious in neurology and may be mistaken for a psychiatric episode.

Hodges and Ward have made detailed psychologic observations in 5 patients during an episode. The psychologic deficit, except for its transience, was much the same as that in a permanent amnesia syndrome. Personality, cognition involving high-level functioning, semantic language, and visuospatial discrimination were all preserved. So-called immediate memory—i.e., registration (see earlier)—was likewise operating normally, but memory was essentially obliterated. The duration of retrograde amnesia was highly variable, but characteristically it shrank after the attack, leaving a permanent retrograde gap of about 1 h. However, subtle impairment of new learning persisted for up to a week after the acute attack insofar as this defect could be detected by special testing.

In a survey conducted in the Rochester, Minnesota, area, transient global amnesia (TGA) occurred at an annual rate of 5.2 cases per 100,000 population. The recurrence of such attacks is not uncommon, having been noted in 66 of 277 older adults who were observed for an average period of 80 months (Miller et al) and in 16 of 74 patients followed for 7 to 210 months (Hinge et al). Hinge and colleagues estimate the mean annual recurrence rate to be so low (4.7 percent) that most patients are likely to experience only one attack. One of our patients had more than 50 attacks, but among all the rest (more than 100 cases), 5 was the maximum. It seems children are not susceptible to the condition; however, a 13-year-old and 16-year-old with migraine were reported to have had similar attacks during participation in sports (Tosi and Righetti).

No consistent antecedent events have been identified, but certain ones—such as a highly emotional experience like hearing of the death of a family member, pain, exposure to cold water, sexual activity, and mild head trauma—have been reported in some cases (Haas and Ross; Fisher). The similarity to postconcussive amnesia is notable; this is always a concern if the patient was not under observation at the onset of the attack. We have also seen several patients in whom the attacks appeared after minor diagnostic procedures such as colonoscopy, but the residual effects of sedation are suspect in some of these. Several cases have been reported in high-altitude climbers and have created difficulty in distinguishing TGA from altitude sickness.

One can conceive of TGA as a syndrome that has several non idiopathic causes. The main concern is a focal temporal lobe seizure that can simulate the syndrome. Transient ischemic attack involving the same posterior regions is another. Whether migrainous episodes can produce a clinical syndrome is uncertain, as noted later, but by far the largest number of cases are idiopathic after extensive evaluation.

The pathogenesis of idiopathic TGA has not been settled. It has been suggested that typical case represents an unusual form of temporal lobe epilepsy (transient epileptic amnesia [TEA]), but this seems an unlikely unifying hypothesis. A large number of patients have been studied with EEGs during an attack or shortly thereafter and have not shown seizure activity (Miller et al). Moreover, amnesic episodes caused by seizures are usually much briefer than those of TGA, and most or all temporal lobe seizures are associated with impairment of consciousness and an inability to interact fully with the social and physical environment. Using EEG and nasopharyngeal leads, Rowan and Protass found mesiotemporal spike discharges in 5 of 7 patients. Curiously, they attributed the discharges to ischemic lesions during drug-induced sleep. Palmini and coworkers cite exceptional cases of pure amnesic seizures in temporal lobe epilepsy, but even in their best examples, ictal and postictal function was not normal.

Transient global amnesia may be ischemic or perhaps migrainous in nature, though not atherosclerotic-thrombotic, but rarely (if ever) do the attacks progress to stroke. Regarding cerebrovascular disease and TGA, Hinge and associates and Hodges and Warlow, in a case-control study of 114 patients with TGA, found no evidence of an association with cerebrovascular disease; there was, however, a significantly increased history of migraine, as there was in the series of Miller and coworkers (14 percent) and of Caplan and colleagues. From indirect evidence of retrograde blood flow in the internal jugular arteries during the Valsalva maneuver (occasionally reported to precipitate an attack), Sander and colleagues and Chung and coworkers have suggested that venous congestion of the temporal lobes was operative. Other studies suggest that the draining veins in the neck lack valves in patients who have had TGA, which permits venous ischemia in the temporal lobes (Schreiber et al); rare cases associated with lateral sinus thrombosis also implicate derangements in venous blood flow in the genesis of TGA. None of these is definitive and they are mentioned here for completeness.

The most compelling cases for an ischemic basis of TGA, perhaps most relevant to migraine, come from Stillhard and colleagues, who demonstrated bitemporal hypoperfusion during an attack of TGA, and from Strupp and associates and Sedlaczek and colleagues, who demonstrated hippocampal and peri-hippocampal lesions (interpreted as cellular edema) with diffusion-weighted MRI, but only 2 days following an attack, not acutely. Like the clinical syndrome, the MRI findings are reversible (Fig. 21-2). The precipitation of identical attacks by vertebrobasilar and coronary angiography is also suggestive of an ischemic or migrainous causation.

A hypothesis generated by the authors of studies on delayed MRI lesions is of a mismatch between cerebral blood supply and demand in the limbic regions. This provides a potential explanation for the association of highly emotional events prior to an episode.

The benignity of transient global amnesia in most patients is noteworthy. Once the history and examination have excluded vertebrobasilar ischemia and temporal lobe epilepsy, no treatment is required other than an explanation of the nature of the attack and reassurance, although we often hospitalize such patients briefly to be certain that the episode clears without further incident. The diagnosis of TGA should not be accepted if there has been ataxia, vertigo, diplopia, or other visual complaints, or if there are deficits in cognition that extend beyond the limited retrograde and complete anterograde amnesia.

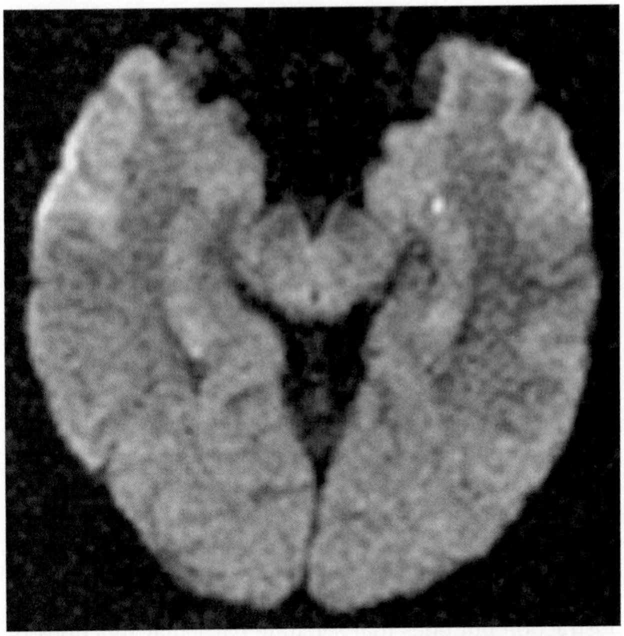

Figure 21-2: MRI showing a tiny area of restricted diffusion in the left hippocampus, 36 hours after an episode of transient global amnesia.

APPROACH TO THE PATIENT WITH DEMENTIA AND THE AMNESIC STATE

The physician presented with a patient suffering from dementia must adopt an examination technique designed to expose the intellectual defect fully. Abnormalities of posture, movement, sensation, and reflexes cannot be relied on to disclose the disease process. Suspicion of a dementing disease is aroused when the patient presents multiple complaints that seem totally unrelated to one another and to any known syndrome; when symptoms of irritability, nervousness, and anxiety are vaguely described and do not fit exactly into one of the major psychiatric syndromes; and when the patient is incoherent in describing the illness and the reasons for consulting a physician.

Three categories of data are useful for the recognition and differential diagnosis of dementing brain disease:

1. A reliable history of the illness and its impact on daily life
2. Findings on mental examination
3. Ancillary examinations: CT, MRI, functional imaging, sometimes lumbar puncture, EEG, and appropriate laboratory procedures, as described in Chap. 2

The history should always be supplemented by information obtained from a person other than the patient, because, through lack of insight, the patient will have limited and variable grasp of his illness or its gravity; indeed, he may be unaware even of his chief complaint. Special inquiry should be made about the patient's general behavior, capacity for work, personality changes, language, mood, special preoccupations and concerns, delusional ideas, hallucinatory experiences, personal habits and care in hygiene, and such faculties as memory and judgment.

The examination of the mental status should include some of the following general categories with suggested examples for testing as modified for each patient's circumstances. In addition, the mode of answering and solving problems gives invaluable information about the mental operations of the subject and must be incorporated into any analysis of cognition. A perplexed or slowed individual may ultimately perform adequately but nonetheless have seriously flawed cortical or subcortical function. Each of the tests below is necessarily an abstraction but ones that separate particular functions of the brain. As already emphasized, the patient must have normal, or nearly so, attentiveness to carry out these tasks and a deficiency in any one of them may disrupt the performance of others.

1. *Insight* (patient's replies to questions about the chief symptoms): What is your difficulty? Are you ill? When did your illness begin?
2. *Orientation* (knowledge of personal identity and present situation): What is your name, address, telephone number? What is your occupation? Are you married?
   a. *Place*: What is the name of the place where you are now (building, city, state)? How did you get here? What floor is it on? Where is the bathroom?
   b. *Time*: What is the date today (day of week and of month, year)? What time of the day is it? What meals have you had? When was the last holiday?
3. *Memory:*
   a. *Long-term*: Tell me the names of your children (or grandchildren) and their birth dates. When were you married? What was your mother's maiden name? What was the name of your first schoolteacher? What jobs have you held? These must be corroborated by a spouse or other family member. We also find it useful to quiz the patient about cultural icons of the past that are appropriate to his age. Most patients should be able to name the recent presidents in reverse order.
   b. *Recent past*: Tell me about your recent illness (compare with previous statements). What is my name (or the nurse's name)? When did you see me for the first time? What tests were done yesterday? What were the headlines of the newspaper today?
   c. *Immediate recall (attention, short-term working memory)*: Repeat these numbers after me (give series of 3, 4, 5, 6, 7, 8 digits at a speed of 1 per second). Now when I give a series of numbers, repeat them in reverse order. Cross out all the a's on a printed page; count forward and backward; say the months of the year forward and backward; spell *world* forward and then backward. Verbal trail making (reciting alternating letters of the alphabet and their ordinal place, i.e., A-1, B-2, C-3, D-…)
   d. *Memorization (learning)*: The patient is given three or four simple data (examiner's name, date, time of day, and a fruit, structure, or trait, such as honesty—we use "a red ball, Beacon Street, and an envelope") and is asked to repeat them after a minute; or is given a brief story containing several facts and is asked to recount the main facts as soon as the story is over. The capacity to reproduce them at intervals after committing them to memory is a test of *memory span*.
   e. Another test of memory and verbal fluency we have found useful is the generation of a list of objects in a category; ask the patient to give the names of animals, vegetables, or makes of cars, as many as come to mind in 30 s or so; most individuals can list at least 12 items in each category.
   f. *Visual facility*: Show the patient a picture of several objects; then ask him to name the objects.
4. *Capacity for calculation, construction, and abstraction:*
   a. *Calculation*: Test ability to add, subtract, multiply, and divide. Subtraction of serial 3s and 7s from 100 is a good test of calculation as well as of concentration.
   b. *Constructions*: Ask the patient to draw a clock and place the hands at 7:45, a map of the United States, a floor plan of her house; ask the patient to copy a cube and other figures.
   c. *Abstract thinking*: See if the patient can describe the similarities and differences between classes of objects (orange and apple, horse and dog, desk and bookcase, newspaper and radio) or explain a proverb or fable ("People who live in glass houses shouldn't throw stones"; "A stitch in time saves nine"; "A rolling stone gathers no moss"; "Idle hands are the devil's workshop").
5. *General behavior*: Attitudes, general bearing, evidence of hallucinosis, stream of coherent thought and attentiveness (ability to maintain a sequence of mental operations), mood, manner of dress, etc.
6. *Special tests of localized cerebral functions*: Grasping, sucking, aphasia battery, praxis with both hands, and corticosensory function.

To enlist the full cooperation of the patient, the physician must prepare him for questions of this type. Otherwise, the patient's first reaction will be one of embarrassment or anger because of the implication that his mind is unsound. It could be pointed out to the patient that some individuals are rather forgetful or have difficulty in concentrating, or that it is necessary to ask specific questions in order to form some impression about his degree of nervousness when being examined. Reassurance that these are not tests of intelligence or of sanity is helpful. If the patient is agitated, suspicious, or belligerent, intellectual functions must be inferred from his remarks and from information supplied by the family.

This type of mental status survey can be accomplished in about 10 min. In our experience, a high level of performance on all tests eliminates the possibility of dementia in almost all cases. It may fail to identify a dementing disease in an uncooperative patient and in a highly intelligent individual in the earliest stages of disease.

The question of whether to resort to formal psychologic tests is certain to arise. Such tests yield quantitative data of comparative value but cannot of themselves be used for diagnostic purposes. The Mini-Mental Status Examination (MMSE) devised by Folstein and coworkers (Table 21-6), and the Montreal Cognitive Assessment (MOCA) are popularly used. A score of 24 on the widely used "mini-mental" is considered normal and scores below 21 generally indicate cognitive impairment. Patients with lower levels of education and older age have lower normative scores, but even individuals in their eighties with a high school education score 23 or above if not demented (see Crum et al for age and education adjusted normal score). A number of other tests that measure the degree of dementia (carrying the names of their originators: Roth, Pfeiffer, Blessed, Mattis) rely essentially on the points mentioned above and a brief assessment of the patient's ability to accomplish the activities of daily living, which is lost in the later stages of disease.

Probably the Wechsler Adult Intelligence Scale (WAIS) is also accurate in detecting dementia. In this test, an index of deterioration is provided by the discrepancy between the vocabulary, picture-completion, and object-assembly tests as a group (these correlate well with premorbid intelligence and are relatively insensitive to dementing brain disease) and other measures of general performance, namely arithmetic, block-design, digit-span, and digit-symbol tests. The Wechsler Memory Scale estimates the degree of memory failure and can be used to distinguish the amnesic state from a more general dementia (discrepancy of more than 25 points between the WAIS and the memory scale). Questions that measure spatial and temporal orientation and memory are the key items in most of these abbreviated scales of dementia. All of the aforementioned clinical and psychologic tests, and several others as well, measure the same aspects of behavior and intellectual function. The WAIS, MOCA, and the MMSE of Folstein and associates are the most widely used clinically in our experience and serve the clinician well.

MANAGEMENT OF THE DEMENTED PATIENT

Dementia is a clinical state of the most serious nature. The physician can see the patient serially over a period of weeks, during which the appropriate laboratory tests (blood, cerebrospinal fluid analysis, and CT, MRI and functional imaging as discussed in Chap. 39) can be carried out. The management of demented patients in the

Table 21-6

"MINI-MENTAL" STATUS TEST OF FOLSTEIN, FOLSTEIN, AND McHUGH

TASK	INSTRUCTIONS	SCORING	
Date orientation	"Tell me the date?" Ask for omitted items.	One point each for year, season, date, day of week, and month	5
Place orientation	"Where are you?" Ask for omitted items.	One point each for state, county, town, building, and floor or room	5
Register three objects	Name three objects slowly and clearly. Ask the patient to repeat them.	One point for each item correctly repeated	3
Serial sevens	Ask the patient to count backwards from 100 by 7. Stop after 5 answers. (Or ask them to spell *world* backwards.)	One point for each correct answer (or letter)	5
Recall three objects	Ask the patient to recall the objects mentioned above.	One point for each item correctly remembered	3
Naming	Point to your watch and ask the patient "What is this?" Repeat with a pencil.	One point for each correct answer	2
Repeating a phrase	Ask the patient to say "no ifs, ands, or buts."	One point if successful on first try	1
Verbal commands	Give the patient a plain piece of paper and say "Take this paper in your right hand, fold it in half, and put it on the floor."	One point for each correct action	3
Written commands	Show the patient a piece of paper with CLOSE YOUR EYES printed on it.	One point if the patient's eyes close	1
Writing	Ask the patient to write a sentence.	One point if sentence has a subject, a verb, and makes sense	1
Drawing	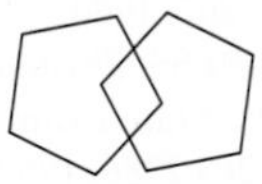 Ask the patient to copy a pair of intersecting pentagons onto a piece of paper.	One point if the figure has 10 corners and 2 intersecting lines	1
Scoring	**A score of 24 or above is considered normal.**		30

hospital may be relatively simple if they are quiet and cooperative. If the disorder of mental function is severe, it is helpful if a nurse, attendant, or member of the family can stay with the patient at all times.

The primary responsibility of the physician is to diagnose the treatable forms of dementia and to institute appropriate therapy. If it is established that the patient has an untreatable dementing brain disease and the diagnosis is sufficiently certain, a responsible member of the family should be informed of the medical facts and prognosis and assisted in the initiation of social and support services. In the past, it was considered that patients themselves need be told only that they have a condition for which they are to be given rest and treatment. Most physicians (and patients) find this too patronizing; certainly, in the current social environment, patients ask directly if they have Alzheimer disease. To this query we usually respond that they may, but that more time is required to be certain. Some intelligent patients have insisted on knowing the details and implications of this statement, and we have felt obliged to give as much useful information as required by them.

Reassurance that the physician will be available to help the patient and family manage the situation is of utmost value. Crises should be preempted by regular contact with a general physician. If the dementia is slight and circumstances are suitable, patients should remain at home for the first years, continuing to engage in those accustomed activities of which they are capable. They should be spared responsibility and guarded against injury that might result from imprudent action, such as leaving a stove turned on or driving and getting lost—or worse. If they are still at work, plans for occupational retirement should be carried out. In more advanced stages of the disease, when mental and physical enfeeblement become pronounced, a skilled nursing facility or supervised home care should be arranged.

The value of centrally acting cholinergic agents and glutamate antagonists in the treatment of Alzheimer disease is modest but clear and should be weighed against the need for blood testing and side effects. These medications, however, offer psychologic benefit to the patient and family; Chap. 39 discusses the use of these medications.

Undesirable restlessness, nocturnal wandering, and belligerency may be reduced by administration of one of the antipsychotic or benzodiazepine drugs (see Chaps. 20, 43, and 48). Although randomized trials of these drugs have failed to show benefit in extreme circumstances, partly as a result of poor tolerance, there are few other options. Emotional lability and paranoid tendencies may be managed by the judicious use of quetiapine, olanzapine, risperidone, or haloperidol. Some patients are helped by short-acting sedatives such as lorazepam without any worsening of the mental condition, but all these drugs must be given with caution and some may be particularly problematic in patients with combined parkinsonism and dementia syndromes.

Questions asked by the patient's family must be answered patiently and sensitively by the physician. Common questions are "Should I correct or argue with the patient?" (No.) Orientation as to date, circumstances, and planned appointments is, however, helpful in preparing the patient for the day's activities. "Can the patient be left alone?" "Must I be there constantly?" (Depends on specific circumstances and the severity of dementia.) "Should the patient manage his own money?" (Generally not.) "Will a change of environment or a trip help?" (Generally not; often the disruption in daily routine worsens behavior and orientation.) "Can he drive?" (Best to advise against driving in most instances.) "What shall we do about the patient's fears at night and his hallucinations?" (Medication under supervision may help.) "When is a nursing home appropriate?" "How will the condition worsen? What should the family expect, and when?" (Uncertain, but usually a 5- to 10-year course.) Many families have found the information on the Alzheimer Association website, *http://www.Alz.org*, helpful, but physician guidance is required to make the material applicable to individual circumstances.

Visiting nurses, social agencies, live-in healthcare aides, day care settings, and respite care to relieve families from the constant burden of caring for the patient should all be used to advantage. Some of the inevitable practical problems accompanying the dissolution of personal life caused by dementia can be ameliorated by judicious use of powers of attorney or guardianship and similar legal vehicles.

References

Aggleton JP, Saunders RC: The relationships between temporal lobe and diencephalic structures implicated in anterograde amnesia. *Memory* 5:49, 1997.

Alexander WP: Intelligence, concrete and abstract. *Br J Psychol* 1:1, 1935.

Budson AE, Price BH: Memory: Clinical disorders. *Encyclopedia of Life Sciences*. London, McMillan Ltd. Nature Publishing Group, 2001, p 1.

Caplan L, Chedru F, Lhermitte F, Mayman G: Transient global amnesia and migraine. *Neurology* 31:1167, 1981.

Chapman LF, Wolff HF: The cerebral hemispheres and the highest integrative functions. *Arch Neurol* 1:357, 1959.

Chung CP, Hsu HY, Chao AC, et al: Detection of intracranial venous reflux in patients of transient global amnesia. *Neurology* 66:1873, 2006.

Cohen NJ, Squire LR: Personal learning and retention of pattern-analyzing skill in amnesia: Dissociation of knowing how and knowing that. *Science* 210:207, 1980.

Crum RM, Anthony JC, Bassett SS, Folstein MF: Population-based norms for the Mini-Mental State Examination by age and educational level. *JAMA* 269:2386, 1993.

Eysenck HJ: Revolution in the theory and measurement of intelligence. *Eval Psicol* 1:99, 1985.

Fisher CM: Transient global amnesia: Precipitating activities and other observations. *Arch Neurol* 39:605, 1982.
Fisher CM, Adams RD: Transient global amnesia. *Acta Neurol Scand* 40(Suppl 9):1, 1964.
Folstein MF, Folstein SE, McHugh PR: "Mini-mental status": A practical method for grading the cognitive state of patients for the clinician. *J Psychiatr Res* 12:189, 1975.
Gadian DG, Aicardi J, Watkins KE, et al: Developmental amnesia associated with early hypoxic-ischaemic injury. *Brain* 123:499, 2000.
Gardner H: *Multiple Intelligences: The Theory in Practice*. New York, Basic Books, 1993.
Goldman-Rakic PS: Working memory and the mind. *Sci Am* 267:110, 1992.
Goldstein K: *The Organism: A Holistic Approach to Biology*. New York, American Book Company, 1939, pp 35–61.
Graff-Radford NR, Tranel D, van Hoesen GW, Brandt JP: Diencephalic amnesia. *Brain* 113:1, 1990.
Growdon JH, Rossor MN: *The Dementias*. Boston, Butterworth-Heinemann, 1998.
Haas DC, Ross GS: Transient global amnesia triggered by mild head trauma. *Brain* 109:251, 1986.
Herrnstein RJ, Murray C: *The Bell Curve: Intelligence and Class Structure in American Life*. New York, Free Press, 1994.
Hinge HH, Jensen TS, Kjaer M, et al: The prognosis of transient global amnesia. *Arch Neurol* 43:673, 1986.
Hodges JR, Ward CD: Observations during transient global amnesia: A behavioral and neuropsychological study of five cases. *Brain* 112:595, 1989.
Hodges JR, Warlow CP: The aetiology of transient global amnesia: A case-control study of 114 cases with prospective follow-up. *Brain* 113:639, 1990.
Kandel ER: Cellular mechanisms of learning and the biological basis of individuality, in Kandel ER, Schwartz JH, Jessel TM (eds): *Principles of Neural Science*, 4th ed. New York, McGraw-Hill, 2000, pp 1247–1279.
Kokmen E, Smith GE, Petersen RC, et al: The short test of mental status: Correlations with standardized psychometric testing. *Arch Neurol* 48:725, 1991.
Kopelman MD: Disorders of memory. *Brain* 125:2152, 2002.
Lashley KS: *Brain Mechanisms and Intelligence*. Chicago, University of Chicago Press, 1929.
Lund and Manchester Groups, The: Consensus statement: Clinical and neuropathological criteria for fronto-temporal dementia. *J Neurol Neurosurg Psychiatry* 57:416, 1994.
Mackintosh NJ: *IQ and Human Intelligence*. Oxford, Oxford University Press, 1998.
Maguire EA: Neuroimaging, memory and the human hippocampus. *Rev Neurol* 157:791, 2001.
Maguire EA, Frackowiak RSJ, Frith CD: Recalling routes around London: Activation of the right hippocampus in taxi drivers. *J Neurosci* 17:7013, 1997.
Mayeux R, Foster NL, Rossor MN, Whitehouse PJ: The clinical evaluation of patients with dementia, in Whitehouse PJ (ed): *Dementia*. Philadelphia, Davis, 1993, pp 92–129.
Mayeux R, Stern Y: Subcortical dementia. *Arch Neurol* 44:129, 1987.
McClearn GE, Johansson B, Berg S, et al: Substantial genetic influence on cognitive abilities in twins 80 or more years old. *Science* 276:1560, 1997.
McHugh PR: The basal ganglia: The region, the integration of its symptoms and implications for psychiatry and neurology, in Franks AJ, Ironside JW, Mindham RHS, et al (eds): *Function and Dysfunction in the Basal Ganglia*. New York, Manchester Press, 1990, pp 259–268.
McHugh PR, Folstein MF: Psychiatric syndromes of Huntington's chorea: A clinical and phenomenologic study, in Benson DF, Blumer D (eds): *Psychiatric Aspects of Neurologic Disease*. New York, Grune & Stratton, 1975, pp 267–286.
Miller JW, Peterson RC, Metter EJ, et al: Transient global amnesia: Clinical characteristics and prognosis. *Neurology* 37:733, 1987.
Miller JW, Yanagihara T, Peterson RC, Klass DW: Transient global amnesia and epilepsy. *Arch Neurol* 44:629, 1987.
Mishkin M: A memory system in the monkey. *Philos Trans R Soc Lond B Biol Sci* 298:85, 1982.
Mishkin M, Delacour J: An analysis of short-term visual memory in the monkey. *J Exp Psychol Anim Behav Proc* 1:326, 1975.
Mitchell SL, Teno JM, Kisly DK, et al: The clinical course of advanced dementia. *New Engl J Med* 361:1529, 2009.
Morris JC: Frontotemporal dementias, in Clark CM, Trojanowski JQ: *Neurodegenerative Dementias*. New York, McGraw-Hill, 2000, pp 279–290.
Neary D, Snowden JS, Gustafson L, et al: Frontotemporal lobar degeneration: A consensus on clinical diagnostic criteria. *Neurology* 51:1546, 1998.
Palmini AL, Gloor P, Jones-Gotman M: Pure amnestic seizures in temporal lobe epilepsy. *Brain* 115:749, 1992.
Petersen RC: Clinical practice. Mild cognitive impairment. *N Engl J Med* 364:2227, 2011.
Phillips S, Sangelang V, Sterns G: Basal forebrain infarction. *Arch Neurol* 44:1134, 1987.
Piaget J: *The Psychology of Intelligence*. London, Routledge & Kegan Paul, 1950.
Piercy M: Neurological aspects of intelligence, in Vinken PJ, Bruyn GW (eds): *Handbook of Clinical Neurology*. Vol 3: Disorders of Higher Nervous Activity. Amsterdam, North-Holland, 1969, pp 296–315.
Pillon B, DuBois B, Ploska A, Agid Y: Severity and specificity of cognitive impairment in Alzheimer's, Huntington's, and Parkinson's diseases and progressive supranuclear palsy. *Neurology* 41:634, 1991.
Ribot TH: *Diseases of Memory: An Essay in Positive Psychology*. New York, Appleton, 1882.
Rowan AJ, Protass LM: Transient global amnesia: Clinical and electroencephalographic findings in 10 cases. *Neurology* 29:869, 1979.
Sander D, Winbeck K, Eigen T, et al: Disturbance of venous flow patterns in patients with transient global amnesia. *Lancet* 356:1982, 2000.
Schacter DL: *Searching for Memory*. New York, Basic Books, 1996.
Schreiber SJ, Doepp F, Klingebiel R, Valdueza JM: Internal jugular vein valve incompetence and intracranial venous anatomy in transient global amnesia. *J Neurol Neurosurg Psychiatry* 76:509, 2005.
Sedlaczek O, Hirsch JG, Grips G, et al: Detection of delayed focal MR changes in the lateral hippocampus in transient global amnesia. *Neurology* 62:2165, 2004.
Seeley WW, Matthews BR, Crawford RK, et al: Unravelling Boléro: Progressive aphasia, transmodal creativity and the right posterior neocortex. *Brain*. 131:39, 2008.
Shields J: Heredity and psychological abnormality, in Eysenck HJ (ed): *Handbook of Abnormal Psychology*, 2nd ed. London, Pitman, 1973, pp 173–192.
Shields J: *Monozygotic Twins Brought Up Apart and Brought Up Together: An Investigation Into the Genetic and Environmental Causes of Variation in Personality*. Oxford, Oxford University Press, 1962.
Slater E, Cowie V: *The Genetics of Mental Disorders*. Oxford, Oxford University Press, 1971, pp 196-200.
Spearman CE: *The Abilities of Man*. London, Macmillan, 1927.
Stillhard G, Landis T, Schiess R, et al: Bitemporal hypoperfusion in transient global amnesia: 99m-Tc-HM-PAO SPECT and neuropsychological findings during and after an attack. *J Neurol Neurosurg Psychiatry* 53:339, 1990.

Strupp M, Ning R, Hua R, et al: Diffusion-weighted MRI in transient global amnesia: Elevated signal intensity in the left mesial temporal lobe in 7 of 10 patients. *Ann Neurol* 43:164, 1998.

Suthana N, Haneef Z, Stern J, et al: Memory enhancement and deep-brain stimulation of the entorhinal area. *New Engl J Med* 366:502, 2012.

Terman LM, Ogden MH: *The Gifted Group at Mid-life: Genetic Studies of Genius.* Vol IV. Stanford, CA, Stanford University Press, 1959.

Thompson PM, Cannon TD, Narr KL, et al: Genetic influences on brain structure. *Nat Neurosci* 4:1253, 2001.

Thurstone LL: *The Vectors of the Mind.* Chicago, University of Chicago Press, 1953.

Tierney MC, Snow WG, Reid DW, et al: Psychometric differentiation of dementia. *Arch Neurol* 44:720, 1987.

Tomlinson BE, Blessed G, Roth M: Observations on the brains of demented old people. *J Neurol Sci* 11:205, 1970.

Tosi L, Righetti CA: Transient global amnesia and migraine in young people. *Clin Neurol Neurosurg* 99:63, 1997.

Tulving E: Episodic memory: From mind to brain. *Annu Rev Psychol* 53:1, 2002.

Turner G: Intelligence and the X chromosome. *Lancet* 347:1814, 1996.

Van Gijn J: Leukoaraiosis and vascular dementia. *Neurology* 51(Suppl 3):83, 1998.

Van Horn G: Dementia. *Am J Med* 83:101, 1987.

Victor M, Adams RD, Collins GH: *The Wernicke-Korsakoff Syndrome*, 2nd ed. Philadelphia, Davis, 1989.

Victor M, Agamanolis D: Amnesia due to lesions confined to the hippocampus: A clinical-pathologic study. *J Cogn Neurosci* 2:246, 1990.

Wechsler D: *The Measurement of Adult Intelligence*, 3rd ed. Baltimore, Williams & Wilkins, 1944.

Willerman L: *The Psychology of Individual and Group Differences*. San Francisco, Freeman, 1978, pp 106–129.

Willis SL, Tennstedt SL, Marsike M, et al: Long-term effects of cognitive training on every day functional outcomes in older adults. *JAMA* 296:2805, 2006.

Witelson SF, Kigar DL, Harvey T: The exceptional brain of Albert Einstein. *Lancet* 353:219, 1999.

Zeki S: Artistic creativity and the brain. *Science* 293:51, 2001.

Zola-Morgan S, Squire LR, Amaral DG: Lesions of the amygdala that spare adjacent cortical regions do not impair memory or exacerbate the impairment following lesions of the hippocampal formation. *J Neurosci* 9:1922, 1989.

Zola-Morgan S, Squire LR, Amaral DG: Lesions of the hippocampal formation but not lesions of the fornix or the mammillary nuclei produce long-lasting memory impairment in monkeys. *J Neurosci* 9:898, 1989.

Zola-Morgan S, Squire LR, Amaral DG: Lesions of perirhinal and parahippocampal cortex that spare the amygdala and hippocampal formation produce severe memory impairment. *J Neurosci* 9:4355, 1989.

22

Neurologic Disorders Caused By Lesions in Specific Parts of the Cerebrum

The long-standing controversy about cerebral functions, whether they are diffusely represented in the cerebrum with all parts roughly equivalent, or localized to certain lobes or regions, has been resolved to the satisfaction of most neurologists. Clinicians have demonstrated beyond doubt that particular functions are assignable to certain cortical regions. For example, the pre- and postrolandic zones control motor and sensory activities, respectively, the striate occipital zones control visual perception, the superior temporal gyri are auditory, and so on. Beyond these broad correlations, however, there is a notable lack of precision in the cortical localization of most of the behavioral and mental operations described in Chaps. 20 and 21. In particular, of the higher order functions, such as attention, vigilance, apperception, and analytic and synthetic thinking, none has a precise and predictable anatomy; or, more accurately, the neural systems on which they depend are widely distributed among several regions.

One may inquire into what precisely is meant by *cerebral localization*. Does it refer to the physiologic function of a circumscribed group of neurons in the cerebral cortex, indicated clinically by a loss of that function when the neurons in question are destroyed? This is the way in which neurologists have assigned functions to particular areas of the cerebral cortex. However, from what we know of the rich connectivity of all parts of the specialized cortical centers, one must assume that this is only partly the case. Most who ponder this subject believe that the organization of cerebral function is based on discrete networks of closely interconnected afferent and efferent neurons in several regions of the brain. These ensembles must be linked by both regional and more widespread systems of fibers. This is especially apparent in the discussion of the anatomy of complex cognitive properties such as intelligence, as described in Chap. 21. Thus, many basic functions are anchored in one cortical region and a lesion there causes loss of a particular ability. But it is apparent from physiologic studies such as functional imaging and electromagnetic stimulation that widely distributed networks are engaged, which nonetheless encompasses the region that can be ablated and eliminate the function in question.

These aspects of cerebral localization—brought out so clearly in the writings of Wernicke, Déjerine, and Liepmann, have been elaborated by Luria (1966 and 1969) and the Russian school of physiologists and psychologists and extended by Geschwind (1965). In keeping with the model of interconnected networks, they viewed function not as the direct property of a particular, highly specialized region of the cerebrum but as the product of complex, diffusely distributed activity by which sensory stimuli are analyzed and integrated at various levels of the nervous system and then united, through a system of temporarily acquired connections, into a working mosaic adapted to accomplish a particular task. To some extent, this model has been corroborated by functional imaging studies, which show increased metabolic activity in several cortical regions during almost every form of human behavior, including willed motor acts, language tasks, and those coinciding with perceptive and apperceptive sensory experiences. Within such a functional system, the initial and final points (the task and the effect) remain unchanged, but the intermediate links (the means of performance of a given task) may be modified within wide limits and will never be exactly the same on two consecutive occasions. Thus, when a certain act is called for by a spoken command, the dominant temporal lobe must receive the message and transmit it to the premotor areas. Or it may be initiated by the intention of the individual, in which case the first measurable cerebral activity (a "readiness potential") occurs anterior to the premotor cortex. The motor cortex is also always under the dynamic control of the proprioceptive, visual, and vestibular systems. Thus, a lesion that affects any one of several elements in the act may cause loss of a skilled ability, either the motor centers themselves or their connections with the other elements.

Another theoretical scheme of cerebral function identifies cortices of similar overall structure and divides the cerebral mantle into three longitudinally oriented zones, the triune brain articulated by Paul Maclean. A central vegetative neuronal system (allocortex and hypothalamus) provides the mechanisms for all internal functions, the *milieu intérieur* of Bernard and Cannon. An outer zone, comprising the sensorimotor and association cortices and their projections, provides the mechanisms for perceiving the external world and interacting with it, and a region between them (limbic–paralimbic cortices) that provides the bridges that permit the adaptation of

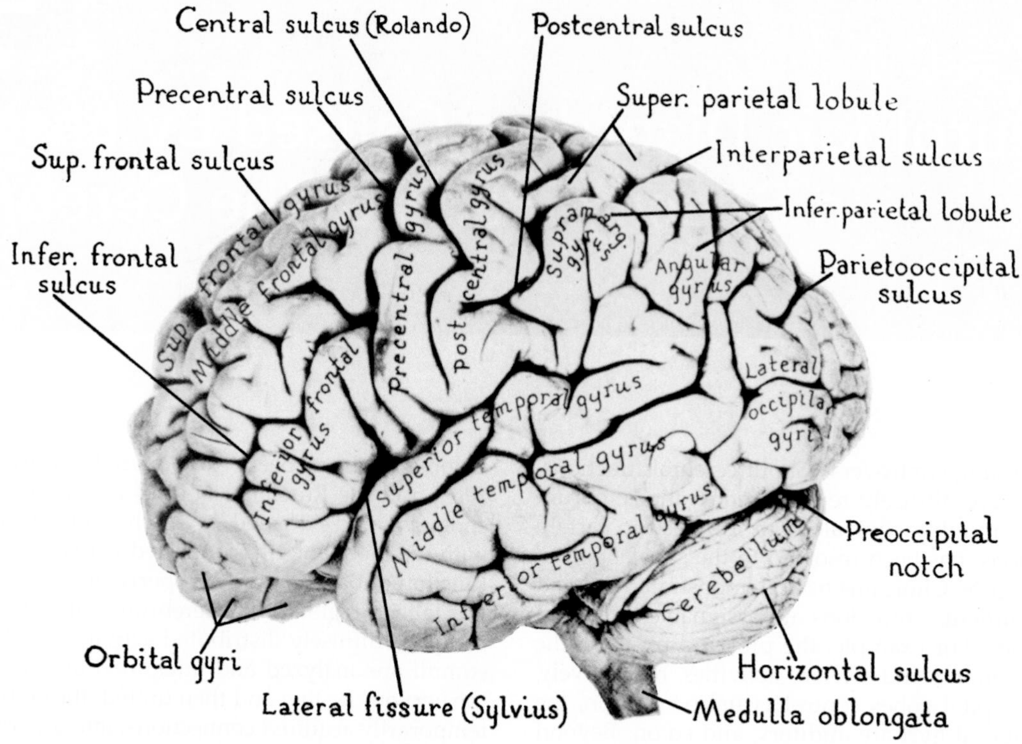

Figure 22-1. Photograph of the lateral surface of the human brain. (Reproduced by permission from Carpenter MB, Sutin J: *Human Neuroanatomy*, 8th ed. Baltimore, Williams & Wilkins, 1982.)

the organism's needs to the external environment. This ostensibly metaphoric concept of central nervous system function, first proposed by Broca, was elaborated by Yakovlev and has been adopted more recently by Benson and by Mesulam (1998). Such a model retains to a large degree the cytoarchitectural similarities among areas that serve similar functions (i.e., the scheme of Brodmann discussed further on) and also respects the sequence of brain maturation (myelination) of connecting pathways proposed by Flechsig (see Fig. 28-3). In this way, localization may be viewed as the product of genetic patterns of structure, which mature during development, and their synaptic formations, which permit the development of complex circuits during lifelong learning and experience.

It is worthwhile to point out that these broadened concepts of cerebral function, which apply to all mental activities, contradicts both the historical notion that there is a functional equivalence of all cerebral regions and also the more recently developed one that assumes strict localization of any given activity.

From these remarks, it follows that subdivision of the cerebrum into frontal, temporal, parietal, and occipital lobes is somewhat of an abstraction in terms of landmarks and cerebral function. Some of these delineations were made long before our first glimmer of knowledge about the function of the cerebrum. Even when neurohistologists began parceling the neocortex, they found that their areas did not fall neatly within zones bounded by sulci and fissures. Therefore, when the terms *frontal*, *parietal*, *temporal*, and *occipital* are used, it is largely to provide the clinician with familiar and manageable anatomic landmarks for localization (Fig. 22-1).

The current method of study of cortical activity is by functional imaging techniques (positron emission tomography [PET] and functional magnetic resonance imaging [fMRI]). Invariably, an ensemble of areas, a "network" of the variety described earlier, is activated to perform even seemingly simple tasks such as recalling a name, visualizing or identifying an object, or carrying out a commanded task. The fact that multiple areas of the cortex are entrained may seem at odds with the classic view of lesional neurology, but as already stated, the discrepancy is one of epistemology in that normal function does not equate with abnormal function as exposed by a focal lesion. A lesion in the cerebrum merely exposes the site at which damage results in the greatest loss of that particular function but does not reveal the much wider area that is essential for the full normal operation of that function. Imaging studies similarly demonstrate that certain regions of the cortex are necessary to fully conduct particular behaviors, but they are not sufficient for their enactment.

GENERAL ANATOMIC AND PHYSIOLOGIC CONSIDERATIONS OF CORTICAL FUNCTION

Pertinent to this subject are a number of morphologic and physiologic observations. Along strictly histologic lines, Brodmann distinguished 47 different areas of

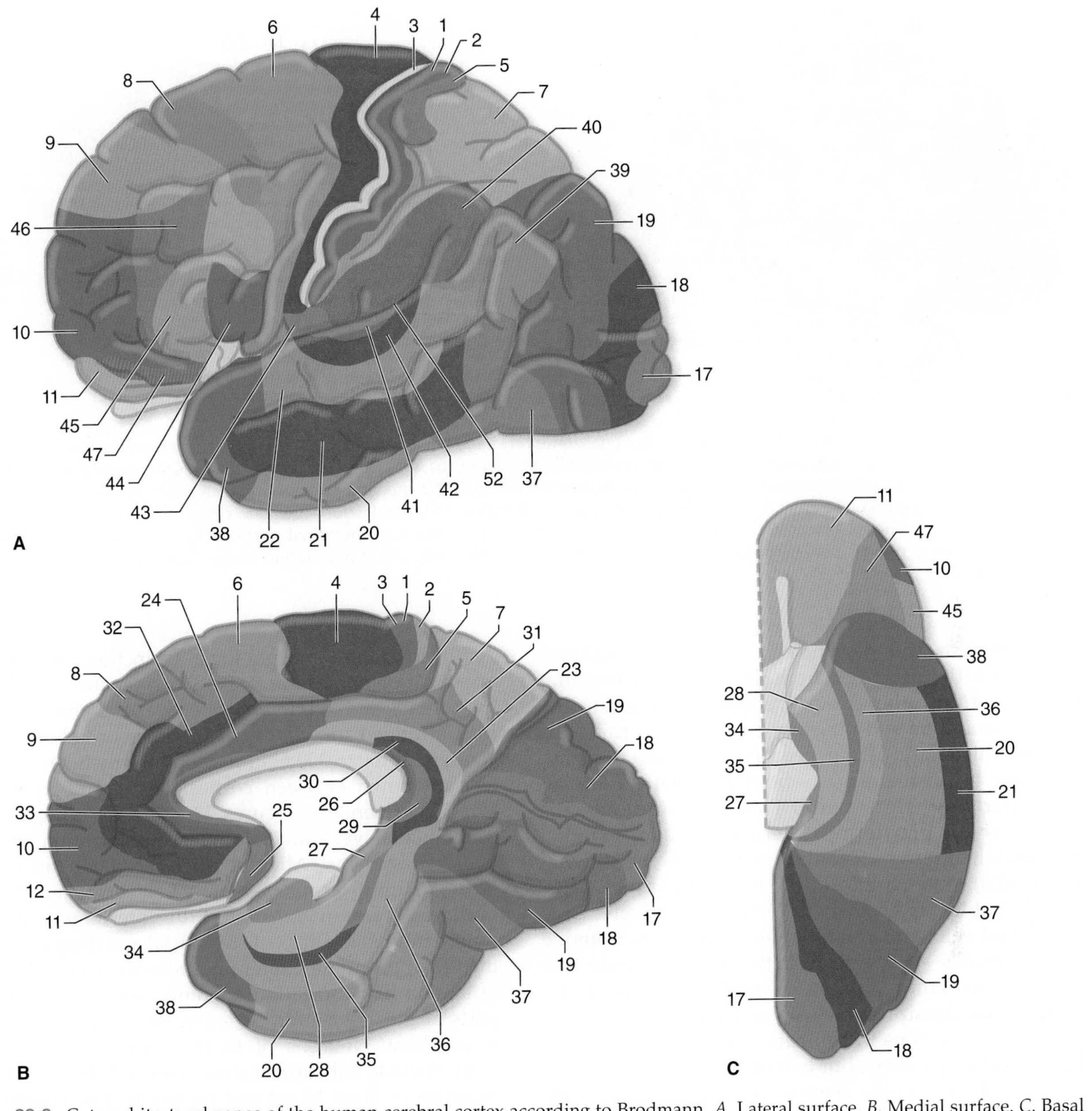

Figure 22-2. Cytoarchitectural zones of the human cerebral cortex according to Brodmann. *A*. Lateral surface. *B*. Medial surface. *C*. Basal inferior surface. The functional zones of the cortex are illustrated in Fig. 22-3.

cerebral cortex (Fig. 22-2), and von Economo identified more than twice that number. Although this parceling was severely criticized by Bailey and von Bonin (and the data upon which Brodmann based his system were never published), it is still used by physiologists and clinicians, who find that the Brodmann areas do indeed approximate certain functional zones of the cerebral cortex (Fig. 22-3). Also, the cortex has been shown to differ in its various parts by virtue of connections with other areas of the cortex and with the thalamic nuclei and other lower centers. Hence, one must regard the cortex as a heterogeneous array of many anatomic systems, each with highly organized intercortical and diencephalic connections.

The sheer size of the cortex is remarkable. Unfolded, it has a surface extent of about 4,000 cm^2, about the size of a full sheet of newsprint (right and left pages). Contained in the cortex are many billions of neurons (estimated at 10 to 30 billion) and five times this number of supporting glial cells. The intercellular synaptic connections number in the trillions. Because nerve cells look alike and presumably function alike, the remarkable diversity in human intelligence, store of knowledge, and behavior must depend on the potential for almost infinite variations in neuronal interconnectivity.

Most of the human cerebral cortex is phylogenetically recent, hence the term *neocortex*. It was also referred to as *isocortex* by Vogt because of its uniform

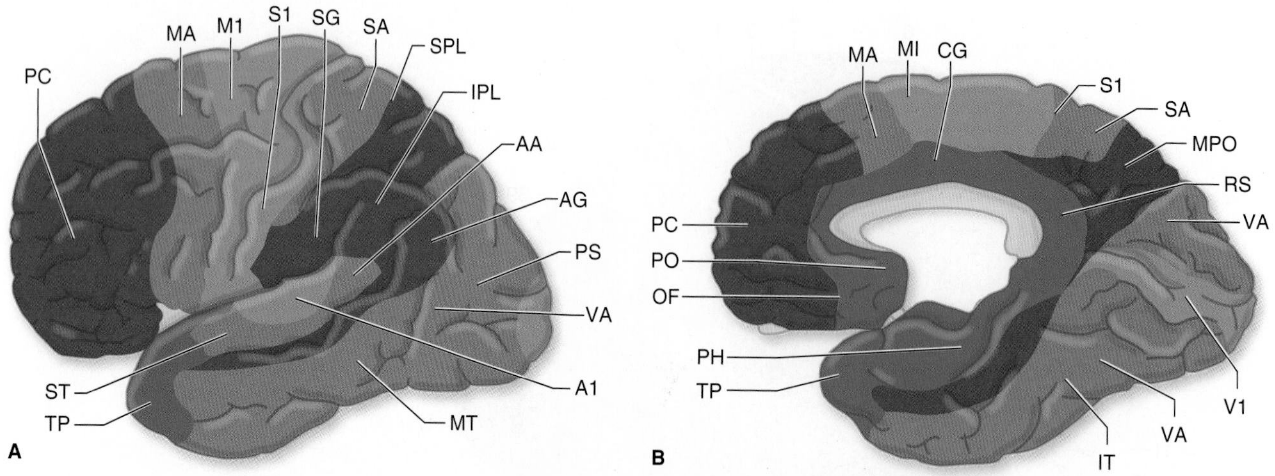

Figure 22-3. *A* and *B*. Approximate distribution of functional zones on lateral (*A*) and medial (*B*) aspects of the cerebral cortex. *Abbreviations:* A1, primary auditory cortex; AA, auditory association cortex; AG, angular gyrus; CG, cingulate cortex; IPL, inferior parietal lobule; IT, inferior temporal gyrus; M1, primary motor area; MA, motor association cortex; MPO, medial parietooccipital area; MT, middle temporal gyrus; OF, orbitofrontal region; PC, prefrontal cortex; PH, parahippocampal region; PO, parolfactory area; PS, peristriate cortex; RS, retrosplenial area; S1, primary somatosensory area; SA, somatosensory association cortex; SG, supramarginal gyrus; SPL, superior parietal lobule; ST, superior temporal gyrus; TP, temporopolar cortex; V1, primary visual cortex; VA, visual association cortex. (Redrawn by permission from M-M Mesulam.)

embryogenesis and morphology. These latter features distinguish the neocortex from the older and less uniform *allocortex* ("other cortex"), which comprises mainly the hippocampus and olfactory cortex. Concerning the detailed histology of the neocortex, six layers (laminae) can be distinguished—from the pial surface to the underlying white matter they are as follows: the molecular (or plexiform), external granular, external pyramidal, internal granular, ganglionic (or internal pyramidal), and multiform (or fusiform) layers (illustrated in Fig. 22-4). Two cell types—relatively large pyramidal cells and smaller, more numerous rounded (granular) cells—predominate in the neocortex, and variations in its lamination are largely determined by variations in the size and density of these neuronal types.

Many variations in lamination have been described by cortical mapmakers, but two main types of neocortex are recognized: (1) the *homotypical cortex*, in which the six-layered arrangement is readily discerned, and (2) the *heterotypical cortex*, in which the layers are less distinct. The association cortex—the large areas (75 percent of the surface) that are not obviously committed to primary motor or sensory functions—is generally of this latter type. Homotypical areas are characterized by either granular or agranular nerve cells. The precentral cortex (Brodmann areas 4 and 6, mainly motor region) is dominated by pyramidal rather than granular cells, especially in layer V (hence the term *agranular*). Agranular cortex is distinguished by a high density of large pyramidal neurons. In contrast, the primary sensory cortices, postcentral gyrus (areas 3, 1, 2), banks of the calcarine sulcus (area 17), and the transverse gyri of Heschl (areas 41 and 42), where layers II and IV are strongly developed for the receipt of afferent impulses, has been termed *granular cortex* because of the marked predominance of granular cells a preponderance of which are small neurons (Fig. 22-5).

Beyond these morphologic distinctions, the intrinsic organization of the neocortex follows a pattern elucidated by Lorente de Nó. He described vertical chains of neurons arranged in cylindrical modules or columns, each containing 100 to 300 neurons and heavily interconnected up and down between cortical layers and to a lesser extent, horizontally. Figures 22-4 and 22-5 illustrate the fundamental vertical (columnar) organization of these neuronal systems. Afferent fibers activated by various sensory stimuli terminate mainly in layers II and IV. Their impulses are then transmitted by internuncial neurons (interneurons) to adjacent superficial and deep layers and then to appropriate efferent neurons in layer V. Neurons of lamina III (association efferents) send axons to other parts of the association cortex in the same and opposite hemisphere. Neurons of layer V (projection efferents) send axons to subcortical structures and the spinal cord. Neurons of layer VI project mainly to the thalamus. In the macaque brain, each pyramidal neuron in layer V has about 60,000 synapses, and one afferent axon may synapse with dendrites of as many as 5,000 neurons; these figures convey some idea of the wealth and complexity of cortical connections. These columnar ensembles of neurons, on both the sensory and motor sides, function as the elementary working units of the cortex.

Whereas certain regions of the cerebrum are committed to special perceptual, motor, sensory, mnemonic, and linguistic activities, the underlying intricacy of the anatomy and psychophysical mechanisms in each region are just beginning to be envisioned. The lateral geniculate-occipital organization in relation to vision and recognition of form, stemming from the work of Hubel and Wiesel, may be taken as an example. In area 17, the polar region of the occipital lobe, there are discrete, highly specialized groups of neurons, each of which is activated in a small area of lamina 4 by spots of light or lines and transmitted

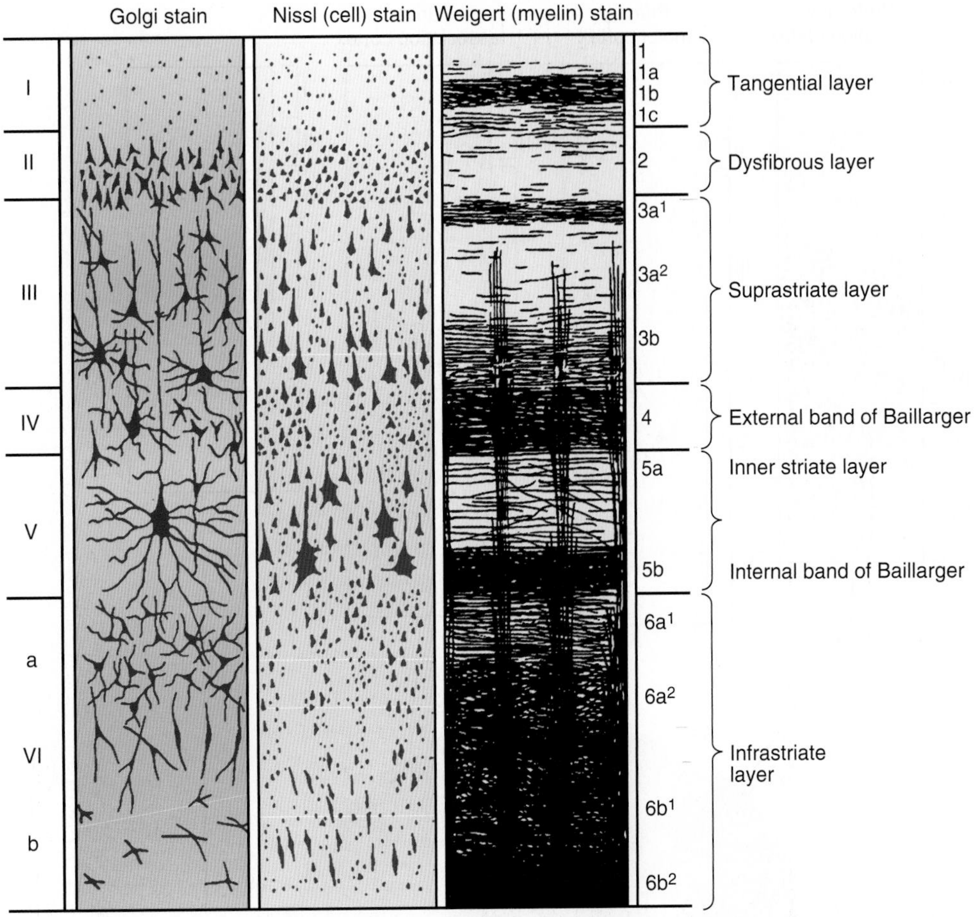

Figure 22-4. The basic cytoarchitecture of the cerebral cortex, adapted from Brodmann. The six basic cell layers are indicated on the left, and the fiber layers on the right (see text).

via particular cells in the lateral geniculate bodies; other groups of adjacent cortical neurons are essential for the perception of color. Lying between the main unimodal receptive areas for vision, audition, and somesthetic perception are zones of integration called *heteromodal* cortices. Here neurons respond to more than one sensory modality or neurons responsive to one sense are interspersed with neurons responsive to another.

The integration of cortical with subcortical structures is reflected in volitional or commanded movements. A simple movement of the hand, for example, requires activation of the premotor cortex (also called *accessory motor cortex*), which projects to the striatum and cerebellum and back to the motor cortex via a complex thalamic circuitry before the direct and indirect corticospinal pathways can activate certain combinations of spinal motor neurons, as described in Chaps. 3 and 4.

Interregional connections of the cerebrum are required for all natural sensorimotor functions; moreover, as indicated above, their destruction disinhibits or "releases" other areas. Denny-Brown referred to the latter as cortical tropisms. Thus, destruction of the premotor areas, leaving the precentral and parietal lobes intact, results in release of sensorimotor automatisms such as groping, grasping, and sucking. Parietal lesions result in complex avoidance movements to contactual stimuli. Temporal lesions lead to a visually activated reaction to every observed object and its oral exploration, and limbic sexual mechanisms are rendered hyperactive.

Another group of disorders known as *disconnection syndromes* depend not merely on involvement of certain cortical regions but more specifically on the interruption of inter- and intrahemispheric fiber tracts. Extensive white matter lesions may virtually isolate certain cortical zones and result in a functional state that is the equivalent of destruction of the overlying cortical region. Some of these disconnections are indicated schematically in Fig. 22-6; the usually involved fiber systems include the corpus callosum, anterior commissure, uncinate temporofrontal fasciculus, occipito- and temporoparietal tracts. An example is the isolation of the perisylvian language areas from the rest of the cortex, as occurs with anoxic–ischemic infarction of border zones between major cerebral arteries (see "Disconnection Syndromes" further on).

SYNDROMES CAUSED BY LESIONS OF THE FRONTAL LOBES

Anatomic and Physiologic Considerations

The frontal lobes lie anterior to the central or rolandic sulcus and superior to the sylvian fissure (see Fig. 22-1). They are larger in humans (30 percent of the cerebrum)

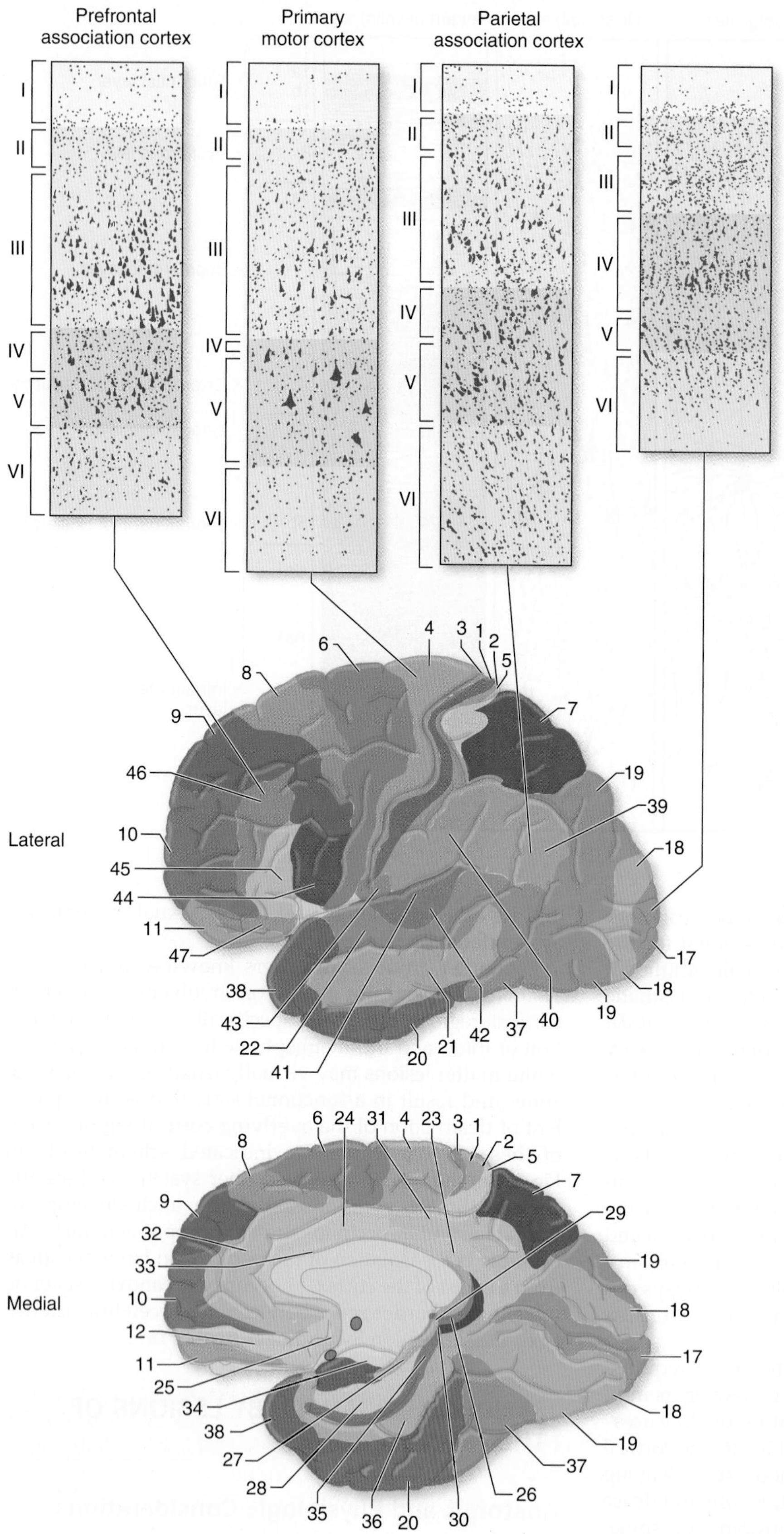

Figure 22-5. Four fundamental types of cerebral cortex and their distribution in the cerebrum. The primary visual cortex has a preponderance of small neurons; hence, it was historically called "granular." The primary motor cortex, by contrast, has relatively fewer small neurons and was described as "agranular." (Reproduced with permission from Kandel ER, Schwartz JH, Jessel TM: *Principles of Neural Science*, 4th ed. New York, McGraw-Hill, 2000.)

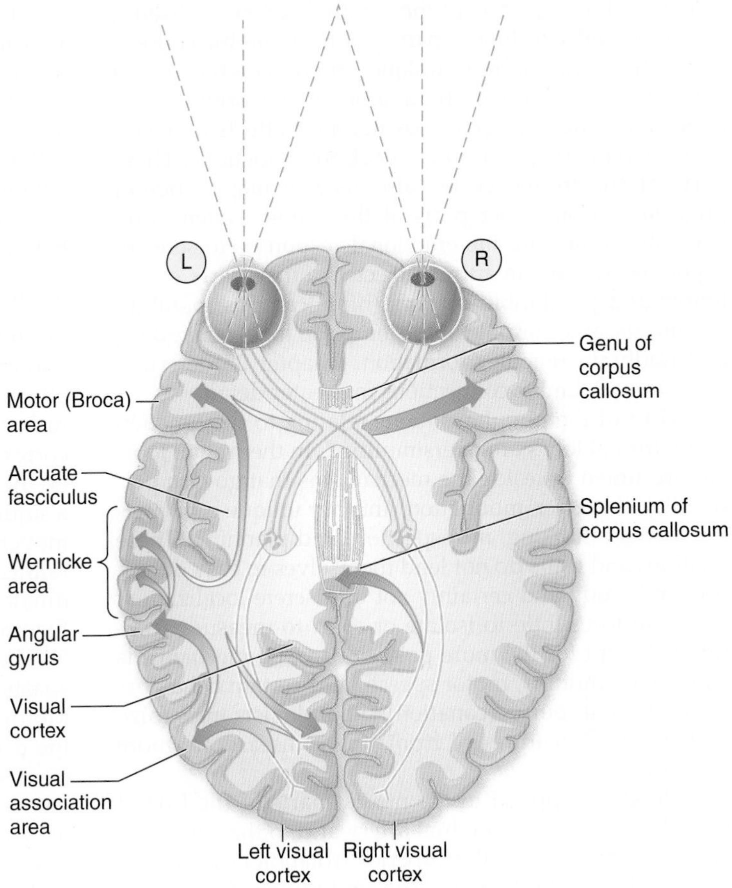

Figure 22-6. Connections involved in naming a seen object and in reading. The visual pattern is transferred from the visual cortex and association areas to the angular gyrus, which arouses the auditory pattern in the Wernicke area. The auditory pattern is transmitted to the Broca area through the arcuate fasciculus, where the articulatory form is aroused and transferred to the contiguous face area of the motor cortex. With destruction of the left visual cortex and splenium (or intervening white matter), the words perceived in the right visual cortex cannot cross over to the language areas and the patient cannot read.

than in any other primate (9 percent in the macaque). Several systems of neurons are located here, and they subserve different functions. Brodmann areas 4, 6, 8, and 44 relate specifically to motor activities. The *primary motor cortex*, i.e., area 4, is directly connected with somatosensory neurons of the anterior part of the postcentral gyrus as well as with other parietal areas, thalamic and red nuclei, and the reticular formation of the brainstem. The supplementary motor cortex, a portion of area 6, shares most of these connections. As pointed out in earlier chapters, all motor activity requires sensory guidance, and this comes from the somesthetic, visual, and auditory cortices and from the cerebellum via the ventral tier of thalamic nuclei.

Area 8 is concerned with turning the eyes and head contralaterally. Area 44 of the dominant hemisphere (Broca area) and the contiguous part of area 4 are "centers" of motor speech and related functions of the lips, tongue, larynx, and pharynx. Left-sided lesions cause a distinctive articulatory and language syndrome, and bilateral lesions in these areas cause paralysis of articulation, phonation, and deglutition. The medial-orbital gyri and anterior parts of the cingulate and insular gyri, which are the frontal components of the limbic system, take part in the control of respiration, blood pressure, peristalsis, and other autonomic functions. The most anterior parts of the frontal lobes (areas 9 to 12 and 45 to 47), sometimes referred to as the *prefrontal areas*, are particularly well developed in human beings but have imprecisely determined functions. They are not, strictly speaking, parts of the motor cortex in the sense that electrical stimulation evokes no direct movement (the prefrontal cortex is said to be inexcitable). Yet these areas are involved in the initiation of planned action and executive control of all mental operations, including emotional expression.

The frontal agranular cortex (areas 4 and 6) and more specifically, pyramidal cells of layer V of the pre- and postcentral convolutions provide most of the cerebral efferent motor system that forms the pyramidal, or corticospinal, tract (see Figs. 3-2 and 3-3). Another massive projection from these regions is the frontopontocerebellar tract. In addition, there are several parallel fiber systems that pass from frontal cortex to the caudate and putamen, subthalamic and red nuclei, brainstem reticular formation, substantia nigra, and inferior olive, as well as to the ventrolateral, mediodorsal, and dorsolateral nuclei of the thalamus. Areas 8 and 6 are connected with the ocular and other brainstem motor nuclei and with identical areas of the other cerebral hemisphere through the corpus callosum. A tract, the fronto-occipital fasciculus, connects the frontal with the occipital lobe and the uncinate bundle connects the orbital part of the frontal lobe with the temporal lobe.

The granular frontal cortex has a rich system of connections both with lower levels of the brain (medial and ventral nuclei and pulvinar of the thalamus) and with virtually all other parts of the cerebral cortex, including its limbic and paralimbic parts. As to its limbic connections, the frontal lobe is unique among cerebrocortical areas in that electrical stimulation of the orbitofrontal cortex and cingulate gyrus has manifest effects on respiratory, circulatory, and other vegetative functions. These parts of the frontal cortex also receive major afferent projections from other parts of the limbic system, presumably to mediate the emotional responses to sensory experiences; they, in turn, project to other parts of the limbic and paralimbic cortices (hippocampus, parahippocampus, anterior pole of the temporal lobe), amygdala, and midbrain reticular formation. Chapter 25 describes these frontal–limbic connections in greater detail.

Most of the popular notions relating to the function of the frontal lobes are oversimplified. In the frontal lobe, are presumed to reside the mechanisms that govern personality, character, motivation, and our unique capacities for abstract thinking, introspection, and planning. These qualities and traits do not lend themselves to easy definition and study and certainly not to discrete localization. Most are too subtle to isolate or even to measure accurately. Except for the more posterior frontal mechanisms subserving motility, motor speech, and certain behaviors relating to impulse (conation), neurologists recognize that the other features of frontal lobe disease are more abstruse.

Blood is supplied to the medial parts of the frontal lobes by the anterior cerebral artery and to the convexity and deep regions, by the superior (rolandic) division of the middle cerebral artery. The underlying deep white matter is supplied by a series of small penetrating arteries, called lenticulostriate vessels that originate directly from the initial portion (stem) of the middle cerebral artery, as detailed in Chap. 34.

Clinical Effects of Frontal Lobe Lesions

For descriptive purposes, the clinical effects of frontal lobe lesions can be grouped under the following categories: (1) motor abnormalities related to the prerolandic motor cortex; (2) speech and language disorders related to the dominant frontal lobe, which are described in the next chapter; (3) incontinence of bladder and bowel; (4) impairment of capacity for goal-directed sustained mental activity, and the ability to shift from one line of thought or action to another, i.e., aspects of attention manifest as impersistence and perseveration; (5) akinesia and lack of initiative and spontaneity (apathy and abulia); (6) changes in personality, particularly in mood and self-control (disinhibition of behavior); and (7) an abnormality of gait that has proved difficult to characterize (see also Chap. 7 on disorders of gait).

With regard to behavior and the frontal lobe, the anterior half of the brain is in a general sense committed to the planning, initiation, monitoring, and execution of all cerebral activity. This was aptly summarized by Luria (1966 and 1973) as "goal-directed behavior." Of necessity in such a scheme, there must also be inhibitory mechanisms that control or modulate behavior. Thus, aside from the overt abnormalities of motor, speech, and voluntary movement, lesions of the frontal lobes give rise to a loss of drive, impairment of consecutive planning, an inability to maintain serial relationships of events, and to shift easily from one mental activity to another. These are combined with sucking, grasping, and groping reflexes and other obligate behaviors. In the emotional sphere, frontal lobe lesions may cause anhedonia (lack of pleasure), apathy, loss of self-control, disinhibited social behavior, and euphoria, as described further on.

Motor Abnormalities

Voluntary movement involves the motor cortex in its entirety or at least large parts of it, and of the various effects of frontal lobe lesions, most is known about the motor abnormalities. Electrical stimulation of the motor cortex elicits contraction of corresponding muscle groups on the opposite side of the body; focal seizure activity has a similar effect. Stimulation of Brodmann area 4 produces movement of discrete muscle groups or, if sufficiently refined, of individual muscles. Repertoires of larger coordinated movements are evoked by stimulation of area 6, the premotor and supplementary motor cortices.

Lesions in the posterior part of the frontal lobe cause spastic paralysis of the contralateral face, arm, and leg. Motor impulses from the frontal lobe are conducted by the direct corticospinal tract and by tracts that descend from the motor, premotor, supplementary motor, and anterior parietal cortex to the spinal cord, either directly or via the red and reticular nuclei in the brainstem. Lesions of the more anterior and medial parts of the motor cortex result in less paralysis and more spasticity, as well as a release of sucking, groping, and grasping reflexes, the actual mechanisms for which probably reside in the parietal lobe and which, as conceptualized by Denny-Brown, are tropisms or automatisms that are normally inhibited by the frontal cortex. When the lesions of the motor parts of the frontal lobe are bilateral, there is a tetraparesis in which the weakness is not only more severe but also more extensive than in unilateral lesions, affecting both spinal and cranial muscles (pseudobulbar palsy).

Ablation of the right or left *supplementary motor areas* (the parts of area 6 that lie on the medial surfaces of the cerebral hemispheres) was found by Laplane and colleagues (1977b) to cause mutism, contralateral motor neglect, and impairment of bibrachial coordination. On the basis of blood flow studies, Roland and colleagues and Fuster suggest that an important function of the supplementary motor area is the ordering of motor tasks or the recall of memorized motor sequences, further evidence of the executive functions of the frontal lobes. Some insight into organization in supplementary motor cortex is given by seizures originating there; they give rise to curious postures such as a fencing position or flailing of the opposite arm.

Temporary paralysis of contralateral eye turning and sometimes of head turning follows a destructive lesion in area 8, on the dorsolateral aspect (convexity) of the cerebral cortex, often referred to as the frontal eye field (see Fig. 22-1). Seizure activity in this area causes a tonic deviation of the head and eyes to the opposite side.

Destruction of the Broca convolution (areas 44 and 45) and the adjacent insular and motor cortex of the dominant hemisphere result in a reduction or loss of motor speech, and of agraphia, and apraxia of the face, lips, and tongue, as described in Chap. 23.

The gait condition described by Bruns that is caused by a frontal lobe lesion was designated by him as an *ataxia of gait*; he made no reference to an ataxia of limb movements. This disorder is often also referred to now as an apraxia of gait, inappropriately in our opinion, because the term *apraxia* is best used to describe an inability to carry out a commanded or learned motor task, not an ingrained one (see Chap. 3). What is meant by these terms in application to gait has never been clearly specified, but broadly speaking, they signify a loss of the ability to use the lower limbs in the act of walking that cannot be explained by weakness, loss of sensation, or ataxia. The patient may retain these fundamental motor and sensory functions when examined in bed and can even make motions that simulate walking while seated or reclining. As detailed in Chap. 7, the resultant pattern is a slowed, slightly imbalanced, and short-stepped gait with the torso and legs not properly in phase when placed in motion, to which may be added the feature of "magnetic" gait, where one or both feet appear to be stuck to the ground as the body moves forward. Probably the basal ganglia and their connections to the frontal lobes are involved in these cases. The steps are shortened to a shuffle and balance is precarious; with further deterioration, the patient can no longer walk or even stand. *Cerebral paraplegia in flexion* is the most advanced stage; the affected individual lies curled up in bed, unable even to turn over (see Chap. 7 for further discussion).

Damage to the cortices anterior to areas 6 and 8, i.e., areas 9, 10, 45, and 46, the *prefrontal cortex*, and also the anterior cingulate gyri, has less easily defined effects on motor behavior. The prefrontal cortex is heteromodal and has strong reciprocal connections with the visual, auditory, and somatosensory cortices. Of these, the visuomotor relationships are the most powerful. These frontal areas as well as the supplementary motor areas are involved in the planning and initiation of sequences of movement, as indicated in Chap. 4. In the monkey, for example, when a visual signal evokes movement, some of the prefrontal neurons become active immediately preceding the motor response; other prefrontal neurons are activated if the response is to be delayed. With prefrontal lesions on one side or the other, a series of motor abnormalities occur, for example, slight grasping and groping responses, a tendency to imitate the examiner's gestures and to compulsively manipulate objects that are in front of the patient (imitation and utilization behavior described by Lhermitte [1983]), reduced and delayed motor and mental activity (abulia), motor perseveration or impersistence (with left and right hemispheric lesions, respectively), and paratonic rigidity on passive manipulation of the limbs (oppositional resistance, or gegenhalten).

Incontinence is another manifestation of frontal lobe disease. Right- or left-sided lesions involving the posterior part of the superior frontal gyrus, the anterior cingulate gyrus, and the intervening white matter result in a loss of control of micturition and defecation (Andrew and Nathan). There is no warning of fullness of the bladder or of the imminence of urination or bowel evacuation, and the patient is surprised at suddenly being wet or soiled. Less-complete forms of the syndrome are associated with frequency and urgency of urination during waking hours. The patient is embarrassed unless an element of indifference is added when the more anterior (nonmotor) parts of the frontal lobes are the sites of disease.

In the spheres of *speech and language*, a number of abnormalities other than Broca's aphasia appear in conjunction with disease of the frontal lobes: laconic speech, lack of spontaneity of speech, telegrammatic speech (agrammatism), loss of fluency, perseveration of speech, a tendency to whisper instead of speaking aloud, and dysarthria. These are more prominent with left-sided lesions and are fully described in Chap. 23.

Cognitive and Intellectual Changes

In general, when one speaks of cognitive and behavioral aspects of frontal lobe function, reference is made to the more anterior (prefrontal) parts rather than the motor and linguistic parts. These most recently developed parts of the human brain, called the "organ of civilization" by Halstead and repeated by Luria, have the most elusive functions.

The effects of lesions of the frontal lobes were nicely divulged by Harlow's famous case of Phineas Gage, published in 1868; it has been the subject of numerous monographs ever since. His patient was a capable foreman of a railroad gang who became irreverent, dissipated, irresponsible, and vacillating (he also confabulated freely) following an injury in which an explosion drove a large iron-tamping bar into his frontal lobes. In Harlow's words, "he was no longer Gage." Another similarly dramatic example was Dandy's patient (the subject of a monograph by Brickner), who underwent a bilateral frontal lobotomy during the removal of a meningioma. Feuchtwanger, in a clinical study of 200 cases of frontal lobe injury, was impressed most with the lack of initiative, changes in mood (euphoria), and inattentiveness, without intellectual and memory deficits. Rylander, in a classic monograph, described similar changes in patients with unilateral and bilateral frontal lobectomies (see later). Kleist (1934), under the heading of *alogia*, stressed the importance of loss of capacity for abstract thought, as shown in tests of analogies, proverbs, definitions, etc. In chimpanzees, Jacobsen observed that the removal of the premotor parts of the frontal lobes led to social indifference, tameness, placidity, forgetfulness, and difficulty in problem solving, findings that led Egas Moniz, in 1936, to perform prefrontal lobotomies on psychotic patients (see Damasio). This operation and its successor, prefrontal leukotomy (undercutting of the prefrontal white matter) reached their height of popularity in the 1940s and (tragically) provided the opportunity to study the effects of a wide range of frontal lobe lesions in a large number of patients.

The findings in patients who underwent frontal leukotomy have been the subject of endless controversy.

Some workers claimed that there were few or no discernible effects of the operation, even with bilateral lesions. Others insisted that if the proper tests were used, a series of predictable and diagnostic changes in cognition and behavior could be demonstrated. The arguments pro and con and the inadequacies of many of the studies, both in methods of testing and in anatomic verification of the lesions (the extent and location of the lesions varied considerably, and this influenced the clinical effects), have been well summarized by Walsh. Admittedly, in patients who underwent bilateral frontal lobotomy, there was little if any impairment of memory function or of cognitive function as measured by intelligence tests, and certainly no loss of alertness and orientation. And some patients who had been disabled by schizophrenia, anxious depression, obsessive–compulsive neurosis, or a chronic pain syndrome did improve with respect to their psychiatric and pain symptoms. However, many were left with changes in personality, much to the distress of their families. They were indifferent to the feelings of others; gave no thought to the effects of their conduct; were tactless, distractible, and socially inept; and were given to euphoria and emotional outbursts. El-Hai has written a fascinating historical account of the procedure in the United States and a portrait of its main proponent at the time, Dr. Walter Freeman. Although no longer undertaken, the procedure must be viewed in the context of the understanding of, and limited options for, psychiatric disease at that time.

Luria (1973) had another interesting conception of the role of the frontal lobes in intellectual activity. He postulated that problem solving of whatever type (perceptual, constructive, arithmetical, psycholinguistic, or logical, definable also as goal-related behavior) proceeds in four steps: (1) the specification of a problem (in other words, a goal is perceived and the conditions associated with it are set); (2) formulation of a plan of action or strategy, requiring that certain linguistic activities be initiated in orderly sequence; (3) execution, including implementation and control of the plan; and (4) checking or comparing the results against the original plan to see if it was adequate.

Obviously, such complex psychologic activity must implicate many parts of the cerebrum and will suffer to some extent from a lesion in any of the parts that contribute to the functional system. Luria found that when the frontal lobes are injured, there was not only a general psychomotor slowing and easy distractibility but also an erroneous analysis of the above-listed conditions of the problem. "The plan of action that is selected quickly loses its regulating influence on behavior as a whole and is replaced by a perseveration of one particular link of the motor act or by the influence of some connection established during the patient's past experience." Furthermore, there was a failure to distinguish the essential sequences in the analysis and to compare the final solution with the original conception of the problem. Plausible as this scheme appears, like Goldstein's "loss of the abstract attitude" (the patient thinks concretely, i.e., he reacts directly to the stimulus situation), such psychophysiologic analyses of the mental processes are highly theoretical, and the factors to which they refer are not easily measured.

Finally, a lesion that includes the frontal eye field may engender a type of reduced attention to the contralateral visual environment. This probably is the result of a defect in visually guided attention and it is seen only irregularly in clinical practice. The degree of neglect seen with a nondominant parietal lobe lesion is not observed with frontal lobe lesions, and it is difficult to differentiate the frontal defect from the simple impediment of being unable to direct gaze in one direction.

In modern parlance, the frontal lobe, particularly its prefrontal components, is said to exert an executive function, referring here to the overall control and sequencing of other cognitive functions. This allows for a type of self-monitoring that guides the selection of strategies to solve problems, the inhibition of incorrect responses, the ability to deal with change in focus and novelty in tasks, and probably to be able to generalize from experience. Indeed, all ability to adapt to changes in circumstance and to learn from experience requires this executive function. Unlike some of the psychic properties mentioned above, these are subject to measurement by testing and they are observable during the clinical examination as deterioration in problem solving, by repetitiousness and stereotypes, and by ineptitude in managing simple social situations. Probably, the trouble all individuals experience in maintaining a stream of thought when interrupted, a type of loss of attention, tests this function.

Other Alterations of Behavior and Personality

A lack of initiative and spontaneity is the most common effect of frontal lobe disease, and it is much easier to observe than to quantitate. With relatively mild forms of this disorder, patients exhibit an idleness of thought, speech, and action, and they lapse into this state without complaint. They are tolerant of most conditions in which they are placed, although they may act unreasonably for brief periods if irritated, seemingly unable to think through the consequences of their actions. They let members of the family answer questions and "do the talking," interjecting a remark only rarely and unpredictably. Questions directed to such patients may evoke only brief, unqualified answers. Once started on a task, they may persist in it ("stimulus bound"); i.e., they tend to perseverate. Fuster, in his studies of the prefrontal cortex, emphasizes the failure over time to maintain events in serial order (impairment of temporal grading) and to integrate new events and information with previously learned data. Placidity is a notable feature of the behavior. Worry, anxiety, self-concern, hypochondriasis, complaints of chronic pain, and depression are all reduced by frontal lobe disease, as they were to some extent by frontal lobotomy.

Extensive and bilateral frontal lobe disease is accompanied by a quantitative reduction in all psychomotor activity. The number of movements, spoken words, and thoughts per unit of time diminish. Milder degrees of this state, associated with only a delay in responses, are called *abulia* as described earlier. The most severe degrees take the form of *akinetic mutism* wherein a nonparalyzed patient, alert and capable of movement and speech, lies or sits motionless and silent for days or weeks on end. It has been attributed to bilateral lesions in the ventromedial frontal regions or frontal-diencephalic connections (but focal lesions in the upper midbrain do the same). Laplane found that the lack of motivation of the patient with bifrontal lesions and bipallidal lesions to be the same, although one would expect the latter to manifest more as a bradykinesia than as a bradyphrenia (slowness of thinking).

The opposite state, in a sense, is a behavioral disinhibition that in extreme form becomes a hyperactivity syndrome, or "organic drivenness," described by von Economo in children who had survived an attack of encephalitis lethargica. Disinhibition occurs largely with dorsolateral frontal lesions. In our patients, this syndrome has been produced most often by combined frontal and temporal lobe lesions, usually traumatic but also encephalitic, although exact clinicopathologic correlations could not be made. Such patients may also exhibit brief but intense involvement with some meaningless activity, such as sorting papers in an attic or hoarding objects or food. Possibly, compulsive behavior is related in some manner to this state and more particularly to lesions damaging the caudate-frontal connections. Combativeness and extreme insomnia or an otherwise disrupted sleep cycle are often part of the syndrome.

Pathological collecting behavior (hoarding) may be related to this type of drivenness and has been attributed to medial frontal lobe damage, including the cingulate gyri, by Anderson and colleagues based on a series of 13 patients. These patients, otherwise displaying mental clarity and despite negative personal and social consequences, collect massive amounts of useless items such as newspapers, junk mail, catalogs, food, clothing, and appliances, often encompassing several categories.

In addition to the disorders of initiative and spontaneity, frontal lobe lesions result in a number of other changes in personality and behavior. These, too, are easier to observe in the patient's natural environment than to measure by psychologic tests. It has been difficult to find a term for all these personality changes. Some patients, particularly those with inferofrontal lesions, feel compelled to make silly jokes that are inappropriate to the situation, *witzelsucht* or moria; they are socially uninhibited and lack awareness of their behavior. The patient is no longer the sensitive, compassionate, effective human being that he once was, having lost his usual ways of reacting with affection and consideration to family and friends. In more advanced instances, there is an almost complete disregard for social conventions and an interest only in immediate personal gratification. The patient at the same time seems to lose an appreciation of the motivations and thought processes of other sapient persons ("theory of mind"); this results in the inability to incorporate these factors into his responses. These changes, observed characteristically in lobotomized patients, came to be recognized as too great a price to pay for the loss of anxiety, pain, depression, and "tortured self-concern," hence the procedure became obsolete.

In general, the greatest cognitive-intellectual deficits relate to lesions in the dorsolateral parts of the prefrontal lobes and that the greatest personality, mood, and behavioral changes stem from lesions of the medial-orbital parts, although the two disorders often merge with one another. Benson (and Kleist and others before him) related the syndrome of apathy and lack of initiative to lesions in the dorsolateral frontal cortex, and a facetious, unguarded, and socially inappropriate state (see below) to orbital and medial frontal lesions. This distinction has held up only broadly in our experience. Some studies of penetrating brain injuries have reported an inconsistent but interesting relationship between left dorsal frontal lesions and anger with hostility, and right side orbitofrontal lesions, with anxiety and depression. Again, in clinical work, few lesions have this degree of localizability, making conclusions about emotional states somewhat uncertain.

Although the frontal lobes are the subject of a vast literature and endless speculation (see reviews of Stuss and Benson and of Damasio), a unified concept of their function has not emerged, probably because they are so large and include several heterogeneous systems. There is no doubt that the mind is greatly altered by disease of the prefrontal parts of the frontal lobes, but often it is difficult to say exactly how it is changed. Perhaps at present it is best to regard the frontal lobes as the part of the brain that quickly and effectively orients and drives the individual, with all the percepts and concepts formed from past life experiences, toward action that is projected into the future.

Psychologic tests of frontal lobe function These are of particular value in establishing the presence of frontal lobe disease and are generally constructed to detect the ability to persist in a task and the opposite, to switch mental focus on demand. They include the Wisconsin card-sorting test, the Stroop color-naming test, sequencing of pictures, "trail making" (a two-part test in which the patient draws lines, first connecting randomly arrayed numbers on a paper in order and then connecting numbers and letters that correspond in order), the verbal equivalent of trail making, and the "go-no-go" test, both of which are used regularly in the mental status examination (see below), and the three-step hand posture test of Luria. The alphabet-number verbal trailmaking test requires the patient to give each letter of the alphabet followed by the corresponding number (A-1, B-2, C-3, etc.). In the Luria test and its variants, the patient is, for example, asked to imitate, then reproduce, a sequence of three hand gestures, typically making a closed fist, holding the open hand on its side, and then opening an outstretched palm. Patients with frontal lesions on either or both sides have difficulty performing the test in correct sequence, often perseverating, balking, or making unwanted gestures. Luria suggested testing this with the sequence of arm thrusting forward, clenching the fist, and forming a ring with the first two fingers—derivatives of this test are now used. He also pointed out (1969) that the natural kinetic "melody," or smoothness of transition from one hand position to the next is disrupted and there is a tendency to perseverate. This has been termed "kinetic limb apraxia" by some behavioral neurologists.

It should be kept in mind that similar impairments of performance may occur with all manner of confusional and inattentive states so that no conclusion can be made if the patient is less than fully attentive. More complex mental acts that may be easily tested and betray frontal lobe disease but are less specific, in that they are also disordered by lesions in other brain regions, include serial subtraction ("working memory"), interpretation of proverbs, tests of rapid motor response, and others.

Effects of frontal lobe disease may be summarized as follows:

I. Effects of unilateral frontal disease, either left or right
   A. Contralateral spastic hemiplegia
   B. Contralateral gaze paresis
   C. Apathy and loss of initiative or its opposite, slight elevation of mood, increased talkativeness, tendency to joke inappropriately (*witzelsucht*), lack of tact, difficulty in adaptation
   D. If entirely prefrontal, no hemiplegia; but grasp and suck reflexes or instinctive grasping may be released
   E. Anosmia with involvement of orbital parts
II. Effects of right frontal disease
   A. Left hemiplegia
   B. Changes as in I.*B*, *C*, and *D*
III. Effects of left frontal disease
   A. Right hemiplegia
   B. Broca's aphasia with agraphia, with or without apraxia of the lips and tongue (see Chap. 23)
   C. Sympathetic apraxia of left hand (see "Apraxia" in Chap. 3)
   D. Changes as in I.*B*, *C*, and *D*
IV. Effects of bifrontal disease
   A. Bilateral hemiparesis
   B. Spastic bulbar (pseudobulbar) palsy
   C. If prefrontal, abulia or akinetic mutism, lack of ability to sustain attention and solve complex problems, rigidity of thinking, bland affect, social ineptitude, behavioral disinhibition, inability to anticipate, labile mood, and varying combinations of grasping, sucking, obligate imitative movements, utilization behavior
   D. Decomposition of gait and sphincter incontinence

SYNDROMES CAUSED BY LESIONS OF THE TEMPORAL LOBES

Anatomic and Physiologic Considerations

The sylvian fissure separates the superior surface of each temporal lobe from the frontal lobe and anterior parts of the parietal lobe. There is no natural anatomic boundary between the temporal lobe and the occipital or the parietal lobe but the angular gyrus serves as a landmark for the latter. Figure 22-1 indicates the boundaries of the temporal lobes. The inferior branch of the middle cerebral artery supplies blood to the convexity of the temporal lobe, and the temporal branch of the posterior cerebral artery supplies the medial and inferior aspects, including the hippocampus.

The temporal lobe includes the superior, middle, and inferior temporal, lateral occipitotemporal, fusiform, lingual, parahippocampal, and hippocampal convolutions and the transverse gyri of Heschl. The last of these constitutes the primary auditory receptive area and is located within the sylvian fissure. It has a tonotopic arrangement: fibers carrying high tones terminate in the medial portion of the gyrus and those carrying low tones, in the lateral and more rostral portions (Merzenich and Brugge). The planum temporale (area 22), an integral part of the auditory cortex, lies immediately posterior to the Heschl convolutions, on the superior surface of the temporal lobe. The left planum is larger in right-handed individuals. There are rich reciprocal connections between the medial geniculate bodies and the Heschl gyri. These gyri project to the unimodal association cortex of the superior temporal gyrus, which, in turn, projects to the paralimbic and limbic regions of the temporal lobe and to temporal and frontal heteromodal association cortices and the inferior parietal lobe. There is also a system of fibers that project back to the medial geniculate body and to lower auditory centers. The cortical receptive zone for labyrinthine impulses is less well demarcated than the one for hearing but is probably situated on the inferior bank of the sylvian fissure, just posterior to the auditory area. Least well delimited is the role of the medial parts of the temporal lobe in olfaction and gustatory perception, although seizure foci in the region of the uncus (uncinate seizure) often excite hallucinations of these senses.

The middle and inferior temporal gyri (areas 21 and 37) receive a massive contingent of fibers from the striate cortex (area 17) and the parastriate visual association areas (areas 18 and 19). These temporal visual areas make abundant connections with the medial limbic, rhinencephalic (olfactory), orbitofrontal, parietal, and occipital cortices, allowing for an intimate interconnection between the cortices subserving vision and hearing.

The superior part of the dominant temporal lobe is concerned with the acoustic or receptive aspects of language, as discussed in Chap. 23, which is devoted to this subject. The middle and inferior convolutions are sites of visual discriminations; they receive fiber systems from the striate and parastriate visual cortices and, in turn, project to the contralateral visual association cortex, the prefrontal heteromodal cortex, the superior temporal cortex, and the limbic and paralimbic cortex. Presumably, these systems subserve such functions as spatial orientation, estimation of depth and distance, stereoscopic vision, and hue perception. Similarly, the unimodal auditory cortex is closely connected with a series of auditory association areas in the superior temporal convolution, and the latter are connected with prefrontal and temporoparietal heteromodal areas and the limbic areas (see Mesulam, 1998). Most of these auditory connections have been worked out in the macaque but the limited number of well-studied lesions in patients suggests that they are also involved in complex verbal and nonverbal auditory discriminations in humans.

The most important functions of the hippocampus and other structures of the hippocampal formation (dentate gyrus, subiculum, entorhinal cortex, and parahippocampal gyrus) are learning and memory, already discussed in Chap. 21. There is an abundance of connections between the medial temporal lobe and the entire limbic system. For this reason, MacLean referred to these parts as the "visceral brain," and Williams, as the "emotional brain." Also included in this anatomic concept are the hippocampus, the amygdaloid nuclei, the fornices and limbic portions of the inferior and medial frontal regions, the cingulate cortices, and the septal and associated subcortical nuclei referred to as the limbic system (see Chap. 25).

Most of the temporal lobe cortex, including Heschl gyri, has nearly equally developed pyramidal and granular layers. In this respect, it resembles more the granular cortex of the frontal and prefrontal regions and inferior parts of the parietal lobes. Unlike the six-layered neocortex, the hippocampus and dentate gyrus are typical of the phylogenetically older three-layered allocortex.

A massive fiber system projects from the striate and parastriate zones of the occipital lobes to the inferior and medial parts of the temporal lobes. The temporal lobes are connected to one another through the anterior commissure and middle part of the corpus callosum; the inferior or uncinate fasciculus connects the anterior temporal and orbital frontal regions. The arcuate fasciculus connects the posterosuperior temporal lobe to the motor cortex and Broca area.

Physiologically, the temporal lobe is an integrator of "sensations, emotions, and behavior" in so far as it relates the organism's sensory experiences to emotional meaning thought it's proximity to the limbic system. Similar integrative mechanisms are operative in the parietal lobe, but only in the temporal lobe are they brought into close relationship to one's instinctive and emotional life. Self-awareness also requires a coherent and sequential stream of thought. Where the inner "stream of thought" (William James' term for constant thinking) is perceived is still an open question. Given the requirement that it be close to other integrated sensory experiences and that it incorporate the temporal lobe functions of both language and memory, a locus in the temporal lobes seems likely. Some hint of the role of the temporal lobe in our personal and emotional lives was suggested by Hughlings Jackson in the nineteenth century, derived from his insightful analysis of the psychic states accompanying temporal lobe seizures. Later, the observations of Penfield and his collaborators on the effects of stimulating the temporal lobes in the conscious patient undergoing surgical correction of epilepsy revealed something of its complex functions. The seminal writings on this subject include Williams' chapter on temporal lobe syndromes in the *Handbook of Clinical Neurology* and the monographs by Penfield and Rasmussen (*The Cerebral Cortex of Man*) and by Alajouanine and colleagues (*Les Grandes Activités du Lobe Temporale*).

Clinical Effects of Temporal Lobe Lesions

The symptoms that arise as a consequence of disease of the temporal lobes may be divided into disorders of: (1) special senses (visual, auditory, olfactory, and gustatory), (2), language, (3) memory and time perception, (4) emotion, and behavior. Of central importance also are the roles of the superior part of the dominant (usually left) temporal lobe in language and handedness. Several of these functions and their derangements are of such scope and importance that they are accorded separate chapters. Language is discussed in Chap. 23, memory in Chap. 21, and the neurology of emotion and behavior in Chap. 25; these subjects are omitted from further discussion here.

Visual Disorders

In Chap. 13 (on vision), it was pointed out that lesions of the white matter of the central and posterior parts of the temporal lobe characteristically involve the lower arching fibers of the geniculocalcarine pathway (Meyer loop). This results in an upper homonymous quadrantanopia, usually not perfectly congruent. However, there is considerable variability in the arrangement of visual fibers as they pass around the temporal horn of the lateral ventricle, accounting for the smallness of the field defect in some patients after temporal lobectomy or stroke and extension into the inferior field in others. Quadrantanopia from a dominant (left-sided) lesion is often combined with aphasia.

Bilateral lesions of the temporal lobes render a monkey psychically blind. It can see and pick up objects but does not recognize them until they are explored orally. Natural emotional reactions such as fear are lost. This syndrome, named for Klüver and Bucy, has been identified only in partial form in humans. Using special tests, lesser degrees of visual imperception were uncovered in patients by Milner (1971) and by McFie and colleagues. This syndrome is further discussed in Chap. 25.

Visual hallucinations of complex form, including ones of the patients himself (autoscopy), appear during temporal lobe seizures. Penfield was able to induce what he called "interpretive illusions" (altered impressions of the present) and to reactivate past experiences completely and vividly in association with their original emotions. Temporal lobe abnormalities may also distort visual perception; seen objects may appear too large (macropsia) or small (micropsia), too close or far away, or unreal. Some visual hallucinations have an auditory component: an imaginary figure may speak and move and, at the same time, arouse intense emotion in the patient. The entire experience may seem unnatural and unreal to the patient.

Cortical Deafness

Bilateral lesions of the transverse gyri of Heschl, while rare, are known to cause a central deafness. Henschen, in his extensive review of 1,337 cases of aphasia that had been reported up to 1922, found 9 in which these parts were destroyed by restricted vascular lesions, with resulting deafness. There are now many more cases of this type in the medical literature; lesions in other parts of the temporal lobes have no effect on hearing. These observations are the basis for the localization of the primary auditory receptive area in the cortex of the transverse gyri (chiefly the first) on the posterosuperior surface of the temporal lobe, deep within the sylvian fissure (areas 41 and 42). Subcortical lesions, which interrupt the fibers from both medial geniculate bodies to the transverse gyri, as in the two cases described by Tanaka and colleagues, have the same effect. With left-sided superotemporal lesions, there is usually an aphasia because of the proximity of the transverse gyri to the superotemporal association cortex. Hécaen has remarked that "cortically deaf" persons may seem to be unaware of their deafness, a state similar to that of blind persons who act as though they could see (the latter, called Anton syndrome is described further on).

For a long time, unilateral lesions of Heschl gyri were believed to have no effect on hearing; it has been found, however, that subtle deficits can be detected with careful testing. If very brief auditory stimuli are delivered, the threshold of sensation is elevated in the ear opposite the lesion. Also, while unilateral lesions do not diminish the perception of pure tones or clearly spoken words, the ear contralateral to a temporal lesion is less efficient if the conditions of hearing are rendered more difficult (binaural testing). For example, if words are slightly distorted (electronically filtered to alter consonants), they are heard less well in the ear contralateral to the lesion. In addition, the patient has more difficulty in equalizing the volume of sounds that are presented to both ears and in perceiving rapidly spoken numbers or different words presented to the two ears (dichotic listening). Few of these changes are evident by clinical examination.

Auditory Agnosia

Lesions of the secondary (unimodal association) zones of the auditory cortex—area 22 and part of area 21—have no effect on the perception of sounds and pure tones. However, the appreciation of complex combinations of sounds is severely impaired. This impairment, or auditory agnosia, takes several forms: inability to recognize sounds, different musical notes (amusia), or words and presumably each has a slightly different anatomic basis.

In *agnosia for sounds*, auditory sensations cannot be distinguished from one another. Such varied sounds as the tinkling of a bell, the rustling of paper, running water, and a siren all sound alike. The condition is usually associated with word deafness ("Pure Word Deafness" in Chap. 23 and below) or with amusia. Hécaen observed an agnosia for sounds alone in only two cases; one patient could identify only half of 26 familiar sounds, and the other could recognize no sound other than the ticking of a watch. Yet in both patients, the audiogram was normal, and neither had trouble understanding spoken words. In both, the lesion involved the right temporal lobe and the corpus callosum was intact.

Amusia proves to be more complicated, for the appreciation of music has several aspects: the recognition of a familiar melody and the ability to name it (musicality itself); the perception of pitch, timbre, and rhythm; and the ability to produce, read, and write music. There are many reports of musicians who became word-deaf with lesions of the dominant temporal lobe but retained their recognition of music and their skill in producing it. Others became agnosic for music but not for words, and still others were agnosic for both words and music. According to Segarra and Quadfasel, impaired recognition of music results from lesions in the middle temporal gyrus and not from lesions at the pole of the temporal lobe, as had been postulated by Henschen. Many other studies implicate the superior temporal gyrus in these deficits. A loss of the ability to perceive and produce rhythm may or may not be associated. In any case, the temporal lobe opposite that responsible for language (i.e., the right) is implicated in almost all cases.

That the appreciation of music is impaired by lesions of the nondominant temporal lobe finds support in Milner's studies of patients who had undergone temporal lobectomy. She found a lowering of the patient's appreciation of the duration of notes, timbre, intensity of sounds, and memory of melodies following right temporal lobectomy; these abilities were preserved in patients with left temporal lobectomies, regardless of whether Heschl gyri were included. Shankweiler had made similar observations, but in addition found that patients had difficulty in denominating a note or naming a melody following left temporal lobectomy.

More recent observations permit somewhat different interpretations. Tramo and Bharucha examined the mechanisms mediating the recognition and discrimination of timbre (the distinctive tonal quality produced by a particular musical instrument) in patients whose right and left hemispheres had been separated by callosotomy. They found that timbre could be recognized by *each* hemisphere, somewhat better by the left than by the right. Also, it was observed that lesions of the right auditory cortex impaired the recognition of melody (the temporal sequence of pitches) and of harmony (the sounding of simultaneous pitches). However, if words were added to the melody, then either a left- or right-sided lesion impaired its recognition (Samson and Zatorre). From functional imaging studies, it appears that the left inferior frontal region is activated by tasks that involve the identification of familiar music (Platel et al), as if this were a semantic test, but passively listening to melodies activates the right superior temporal and occipital regions (Zatorre et al).

By way of summary, Stewart and colleagues systematically reviewed the subject and were able to separate disorders of musical listening into the following categories: appreciation of pitch (including interval, pattern, and tonal structure), timbre, temporal structure, emotional content, and memory for music. The authors present clinical cases, mostly strokes that illustrate each defect. Taken together, these data suggest that the nondominant hemisphere is important for the recognition of harmony and melody (in the absence of words), but that the naming of musical scores and all the semantic (writing and reading) aspects of music require the integrity of the dominant temporal and probably the frontal lobes as well.

Word Deafness (Auditory Verbal Agnosia)

In essence, word deafness is a failure of the left temporal lobe function in decoding the acoustic signals of speech and converting them into understandable words. This is the essential element of Wernicke's aphasia and is discussed in Chap. 23. However, word deafness can occur by itself, without other features of Wernicke's aphasia. Other aspects of language such as reading, are not affected. The syndrome is sometimes seen as patients are improving from Wernicke's aphasia. Also, as mentioned earlier, verbal agnosia may be combined with agnosia for sounds and music, or the two may occur separately.

Auditory Illusions and Hallucinations
(See also Chap. 15)

Temporal lobe lesions that leave hearing intact may cause a hearing disorder in which sounds are perceived as being louder or less loud than normal. Sounds or words may seem strange or disagreeable, or they may seem to be repeated, a kind of sensory perseveration. If auditory hallucinations are also present, they may undergo similar alterations. Such paracusias may last indefinitely and, by changing timbre or tonality, alter musical appreciation as well.

With lesions of the temporal lobes, these may be elementary (murmurs, blowing, sound of running water or motors, whistles, clangs, sirens) or complex (musical themes, choruses, voices). Usually sounds and musical themes are heard more clearly than voices. Patients may recognize hallucinations for what they are, or they may be convinced that the voices are real and respond to them with intense emotion. Hearing may fade before or during the hallucination.

In temporal lobe epilepsy, the auditory hallucinations are known to occur alone or in combination with visual or gustatory hallucinations, visual distortions, dizziness, and aphasia. There may be hallucinations based on remembered experiences (experiential hallucinations, in the terminology of Penfield and Rasmussen).

The anatomy of lesions underlying auditory illusions and hallucinations, formerly the province of study by ablative lesions, is currently being studied using functional imaging techniques. In some instances, these sensory phenomena have been combined with auditory verbal (or nonverbal) agnosia; the superior and posterior parts of the dominant or both temporal lobes were then involved. Clinicoanatomic correlation is difficult in cases associated with tumors that distort the brain without completely destroying it and that also cause edema of the surrounding tissue. Moreover, it is often uncertain whether symptoms have been produced by destruction of tissue or by excitation, i.e., by way of seizure discharges. Elementary hallucinations have been reported with lesions of either temporal lobe, whereas the more complex auditory hallucinations and particularly polymodal ones (visual plus auditory) occur more often with left-sided lesions. It should also be noted that complex but unformed auditory hallucinations (e.g., the sound of an orchestra tuning up), as well as entire strains of music and singing, also occur, inexplicably, with lesions that appear to be restricted to the pons (*pontine auditory hallucinosis*, as noted in Chap. 15).

It is tempting to relate complex auditory hallucinations to disorders in the auditory association areas surrounding the Heschl gyri, but the available data do not clearly justify such an assumption. In schizophrenic patients, the areas activated during a period of active auditory hallucinosis include not only Heschl gyri but also the hippocampus and other widely distributed structures mainly in the dominant hemisphere (see Chap. 53).

Vestibular Disturbances

In the superior and posterior part of the temporal lobe (posterior to the primary auditory cortex), there is an area that responds to vestibular stimulation by establishing one's sense of verticality in relation to the environment. If this area is destroyed on one side, the only clinical effect may be a transient illusion that the environment is tipped on its side or is upside down; more often, there is only subtle change in eye movements on optokinetic stimulation. Epileptic activation of this area induces vertigo or a sense of disequilibrium. As pointed out in Chap. 15, pure vertiginous epilepsy does occur but is a rarity, and if vertigo precedes a seizure, it is usually momentary and quickly submerged in other components of the seizure.

Autoscopy and out-of-body experiences Recently, there has been interest in the cortical vestibular area and states of autoscopy (seeing one's self from an external perspective) and the associated but not identical "out-of-body experience" that has been reported by patients who have near-death episodes. Stimulation of this cortical area for the treatment of intractable tinnitus has elicited autoscopy (DeRidder et al) and seizures originating in the same or adjacent areas have produced out of body sensations. These observations suggest that one's mental perspective of corporeal place may be mediated by the cortex at the temporal-parietal junction. This is not surprising as the representation of extrapersonal space is found in the parietal lobes as described further on (see Blanke et al).

Disturbances of Time Perception

In a temporal lobe seizure originating on either side, time may seem to stand still or to pass with great speed. On recovery from such a seizure, the patient, having lost all sense of time, may repeatedly look at the clock. Assal and Bindschaedler have reported an extraordinary abnormality of time sense in which the patient invariably placed the day and date 3 days ahead of the actual ones. There had been aphasia from a left hemispheral stroke years before, but the impairment of time sense occurred only after a left temporal stroke that also produced cortical deafness.

Certainly, the most common disruptions of the sense of time occur as part of confusional states of any type. The usual tendency is for the patient to report the current date as an earlier one, much less often as a later one. Characteristically, in this situation, the responses vary from one examination to the next. The patient with a Korsakoff amnesic state is unable to place events in their proper time relationships, presumably because of failure of retentive memory, a function assignable to the medial temporal lobes.

Disturbances of Smell and Taste

(See also Chap. 12)

The central anatomy and physiology of these two senses in humans have been elusive. Brodal concluded that the hippocampus was not involved; however, seizure foci in the medial part of the temporal lobe (in the region of the uncus) often evoke olfactory hallucinations. This type of "uncinate fit," as originally pointed out by Jackson and Stewart, is often accompanied by a dreamy state, or, in the words of Penfield, an "intellectual aura." The central areas identified physiologically with olfaction are the posterior orbitofrontal, subcallosal, anterior temporal, and insular cortices, i.e., the areas that mediate numerous visceral functions.

In comparison, hallucinations of taste are less common. Stimulation of the posterior insular area elicited a sensation of taste along with disturbances of alimentary function (Penfield and Faulk). There are cases in which a lesion in the medial temporal lobe caused both gustatory and olfactory hallucinations. Sometimes the patient cannot decide whether he experienced an abnormal odor, taste, or both. The anatomy and physiology of smell and taste are discussed further in Chap. 12. Alterations or loss of taste and smell with temporal lobe lesions has not been adequately studied, and these do not appear to be common in clinical practice.

Other (Nonauditory) Temporal Lobe Syndromes

There is a large inferolateral expanse of temporal lobe that has only vaguely assignable integrative functions. With lesions in these parts of the dominant temporal lobe, a defect in the retrieval of words (*amnesic dysnomia*) has been frequently observed. Stimulation of the posterior parts of the first and second temporal convolutions of fully conscious epileptic patients can arouse complex memories and visual and auditory images, some with strong emotional content (Penfield and Roberts).

The loss of certain visual integrative abilities, particularly face recognition (prosopagnosia), is usually assigned to lesions of the inferior occipital lobes, as discussed further on, but the area implicated borders on the adjacent inferior temporal lobe as well.

Careful psychologic studies disclose a difference between the effects of dominant and nondominant partial (anterior) temporal lobectomy (Milner, 1971). With the former, there is dysnomia and impairment in the learning of material presented through the auditory sense; with the latter, there is impairment in the learning of visually presented material. In addition, about 20 percent of patients who have undergone temporal lobectomy, left or right, show a syndrome similar to that which results from lesions of the prefrontal regions. Perhaps more significant is the observation that the remainder of the cases show little or no defect in personality or behavior.

Disorders of Memory, Emotion, and Behavior

Finally, attention must be drawn to the central role of the temporal lobe, notably its hippocampal and limbic parts, in memory and learning and in the emotional life of the individual. As indicated earlier, these functions and their derangements have been accorded separate chapters. Memory is discussed in Chap. 21 and the neurology of emotion and behavior in Chap. 25.

To summarize, human temporal lobe syndromes include the following:

I. Effects of unilateral disease of the dominant temporal lobe
   A. Homonymous contralateral upper quadrantanopia
   B. Wernicke's aphasia (word deafness; auditory verbal agnosia)
   C. Dysnomia or amnesic aphasia
   D. Amusia (some types)
   E. Visual agnosia
   F. Occasionally, amnesic (Korsakoff) syndrome
II. Effects of unilateral disease of the nondominant temporal lobe
   A. Homonymous upper quadrantanopia
   B. Inability to judge spatial relationships in some cases
   C. Impairment in tests of visually presented nonverbal material
   D. Agnosia for sounds and some qualities of music
III. Effects of disease of either temporal lobe
   A. Auditory, visual, olfactory, and gustatory hallucinations
   B. "Dreamy" states with seizure (focal temporal lobe seizure)
   C. Emotional and behavioral changes
   D. Delirium-confusional states (usually nondominant)
   E. Disturbances of time perception
IV. Effects of bilateral disease
   A. Korsakoff amnesic defect (hippocampal formations)
   B. Apathy and placidity
   C. Klüver-Bucy syndrome: compulsion to attend to all visual stimuli, hyperorality, hypersexuality, blunted emotional reactivity; the full syndrome is rarely seen in humans

SYNDROMES CAUSED BY LESIONS OF THE PARIETAL LOBES

Anatomic and Physiologic Considerations

This part of the cerebrum, lying behind the central sulcus and above the sylvian fissure, is the least well demarcated (see Fig. 22-1). Its posterior boundary, where it merges with the occipital lobe, is obscure, as is part of the inferior-posterior boundary, where it merges with the temporal lobe. On its medial side, the parietooccipital sulcus marks the posterior border, which is completed by extending the line of the sulcus downward to the preoccipital notch on the inferior border of the hemisphere. Within the parietal lobe, there are two important sulci: the postcentral sulcus, which forms the posterior boundary of the somesthetic cortex, and the interparietal sulcus, which runs anteroposteriorly from the middle of the posterior central sulcus and separates the mass of the parietal lobe into superior and inferior lobules (see Fig. 22-1). The inferior parietal lobule is composed of the supramarginal gyrus (Brodmann area 40) and the angular gyrus (area 39). The superior parietal lobule is that remaining part of the lobe that is bounded below by interparietal sulcus, anteriorly by the postcentral sulcus, and extends onto the medial surface of the brain in Brodmann areas 5 and 7 (Fig. 22-2). The architecture of the postcentral convolution is typical of all primary receptive areas (homotypical granular cortex). The rest of the parietal lobe resembles the association cortex, both unimodal and heteromodal, of the frontal and temporal lobes.

The superior and inferior parietal lobules and adjacent parts of the temporal and occipital lobes are relatively much larger in humans than in any of the other primates and are relatively slow in attaining their fully functional state (beyond age 7 years). This area of heteromodal cortex has large fiber connections with the frontal, occipital, and temporal lobes of the same hemisphere and, through the middle part of the corpus callosum, with corresponding parts of the opposite hemisphere.

The *postcentral gyrus*, or *primary somatosensory cortex*, receives most of its afferent projections from the ventroposterior thalamic nucleus, which is the terminus of the ascending somatosensory pathways. The contralateral half of the body is represented somatotopically in this gyrus on the posterior bank of the rolandic sulcus. It has been shown in the macaque that spindle afferents project to area 3a, cutaneous afferents to areas 3b and 1, and joint afferents to area 2 (Kaas). Stimulation of the postcentral gyrus elicits a numb, tingling sensation and sense of movement. Penfield (1941) remarked that rarely are these tactile illusions accompanied by pain, warmth, or cold. Stimulation of the motor cortex may produce similar sensations, as do discharging seizure foci from these regions. The primary sensory cortex projects to the superior parietal lobule (area 5), which is the somatosensory association cortex. Some parts of areas 1, 3, and 5 (except the hand and foot representations) probably connect, via the corpus callosum, with the opposite somatosensory cortex. There is some uncertainty as to whether area 7 (which lies posterior to area 5) is unimodal somatosensory or heteromodal visual and somatosensory; certainly, it receives a large contingent of fibers from the occipital lobe.

In humans, electrical stimulation of the cortex of the superior and inferior parietal lobules evokes no specific motor or sensory effects. Overlapping here, however, are the integrative zones for vision, hearing, and somatic sensation, the supramodal integration of which is essential to our awareness of space and person and certain aspects of language and calculation (apperception), as described below.

The parietal lobe is supplied by the middle cerebral artery, the inferior and superior divisions supplying the inferior and superior lobules, respectively, although the demarcation between the areas of supply of these two divisions is quite variable.

Despite Critchley's pessimistic prediction that establishing a formula of normal parietal function would prove to be a "vain and meaningless pursuit," our concepts of the activities of this part of the brain have assumed some degree of order, in part from his own work. There is little reason to doubt that the anterior parietal cortex contains the mechanisms for tactile percepts. Discriminative tactile functions, listed below, are organized in the more posterior, secondary sensory areas. But the greater part of the parietal lobe functions as a center for integrating somatosensory with visual and auditory information in order to construct an awareness of one's own body (body schema) and its relation to extrapersonal space. Connections with the frontal and occipital lobes provide the necessary proprioceptive and visual information for movement of the body and manipulation of objects and for certain constructional activities (constructional apraxia). Impairment of these functions implicates the parietal lobes, more clearly the nondominant one (on the right).

The conceptual patterns on which complex voluntary motor acts are executed also depend on the integrity of the parietal lobes, particularly the dominant one. Defects in this region give rise to ideomotor apraxia, as discussed in Chap. 3 and further on. The understanding of spoken and written words is partly a function of the supramarginal and angular gyri of the dominant parietal lobe as elaborated in Chap. 23. The recognition and utilization of numbers, arithmetic principles, and calculation, which have important spatial attributes, are other functions integrated principally through these structures.

Clinical Effects of Parietal Lobe Lesions

Within the brain, perhaps no other territory surpasses the parietal lobes in the rich variety of clinical phenomena exposed under conditions of disease. Our current understanding of the effects of parietal lobe disease contrasts sharply with that of the late nineteenth century, when these lobes, in the textbooks of Oppenheim and Gowers, were considered to be "silent areas." However, some of the clinical manifestations of parietal lobe disease may be subtle, requiring special techniques for their elicitation.

Close to the core of the complex behavioral features that arise from lesions of the parietal lobes is the problem of *agnosia*. Allusion has already been made to agnosia in the discussion of lesions of the temporal lobes that affect language, and similar findings occur with lesions of the occipital lobe as discussed further on. In those contexts, agnosia refers to *a loss of recognition of an entity that cannot be attributed to a defect in the primary sensory modality*. The term *agnosia* extends to a loss of more complex integrated functions and mental symbolism as described below, a number of intriguing deficits arise. These syndromes expose properties of the parietal lobe that have implications regarding a map of the body schema and of external topographic space, of the ability to calculate, to differentiate left from right, to write words, and other problems discussed below. The fact that *apraxia*, an inability to carry out a commanded task despite the retention of motor and sensory function, may also arise from parietal lobe damage, and the relationship of the apraxias to language and to agnosias, exposes some of the most complicated issues in behavioral neurology. Some of the theoretical aspects of agnosia, particularly those related to the disturbances of visual processing, are discussed later in the chapter.

Cortical Sensory Syndromes

The effects of a parietal lobe lesion on somatic sensation were first described by Verger and then more completely by Déjerine, in his monograph *L'agnosie corticale*, and by Head and Holmes. The latter, in their important paper of 1911, noted the close interrelationships between the thalamus and the sensory cortex. Although difficult to study, it is apparent that a large lesion of the primary sensory cortex, or beneath it, results in a circumscribed loss or reduction in sensation on the opposite side of the body. When primary sensory perception is altered, analysis of more complex and integrative sensory function is rendered less accurate.

However, as pointed out in the discussion of the organization of the sensory systems in Chap. 9, the parietal postcentral cortical defect is essentially one of *sensory discrimination*, i.e., impairment of the ability to integrate and localize stimuli that is reflected by an inability to distinguish objects by their size, shape, weight, and texture (astereognosis); to recognize figures written on the skin (agraphesthesia); to distinguish between single and double contacts (impairment of two-point discrimination); and to detect the direction of movement of a tactile stimulus. This type of sensory defect is sometimes referred to as "cortical," although it can be produced just as well by lesions of the subcortical connections. Clinicoanatomic studies indicate that parietocortical lesions that spare the postcentral gyrus produce only transient somatosensory changes or none at all (Corkin et al; Carmon and Benton). In other words, the primary perception of pain, touch, pressure, vibratory stimuli, and thermal stimuli is relatively intact in lesions of the parietal cortex that does not involve the postcentral gyrus.

The question of bilateral sensory deficits as a result of lesions in only one postcentral convolution was raised by the studies of Semmes and of Corkin and their associates. In tests of pressure sensitivity, two-point discrimination, point localization, position sense, and tactile object recognition, they found bilateral disturbances in nearly half of their patients with unilateral lesions, but the deficits were always more severe contralaterally and mainly in the hand and therefore the ipsilateral effect is rarely evident in clinical work. These disturbances of discriminative sensation and the subject of tactile agnosia are discussed more fully in Chap. 9.

Déjerine and Mouzon described the sensory syndrome in which touch, pressure, pain, thermal, vibratory, and position sense are lost on one side of the body or in a limb. This syndrome, typically the result of a thalamic lesion and not of a parietal one, may nonetheless occur with large, acute lesions (infarcts, hemorrhages) in the central and subcortical white matter of the parietal lobe. In this case, the symptoms partially recede in time, leaving more subtle defects in sensory discrimination. Smaller lesions, particularly ones that result from a glancing blow to the skull or a small infarct or hemorrhage, may cause a defect in cutaneous–kinesthetic perception in a discrete part of a limb, e.g., the ulnar or radial half of the hand and forearm; these cerebral lesions may mimic a peripheral nerve or root lesion (Dodge and Meirowsky).

A *pseudothalamic pain syndrome* on the side deprived of sensation by a parietal lesion has been described (Biemond). In a series of 12 such patients described by Michel and colleagues, burning or constrictive pain, identical to the thalamic pain syndrome (described in Chap. 9), resulted from vascular lesions restricted to the cortex. The discomfort involved the entire half of the body or matched the region of cortical hypesthesia; in a few cases, the symptoms were paroxysmal.

Head and Holmes drew attention to a number of interesting points about patients with parietal sensory defects: the easy fatigability of their sensory perceptions; the inconsistency of responses to painful and tactile stimuli; the difficulty in distinguishing more than one contact at a time; the disregard of stimuli on the affected side when the healthy side is stimulated simultaneously (tactile inattention or extinction); the tendency of superficial pain sensations to outlast the stimulus and to be hyperpathic; and the occurrence of hallucinations of touch. Of these, the testing of sensory extinction by the presentation of two tactile stimuli simultaneously on both sides of the body has become a component of the routine neurologic examination for parietal lesions. In modern parlance, these are "cortical sensory" defects of extinction of double simultaneous stimulation—astereognosis and agraphesthesia.

With anterior parietal lobe lesions, there is sometimes an associated mild hemiparesis, as this portion of the parietal lobe contributes a considerable number of fibers to the corticospinal tract. Occasionally there is such a large degree of inability or disinclination to use the limb that it simulates a hemiplegia. More often, there is only a poverty of movement or a weak effort of the opposite side. The affected limbs, if involved with this apparent weakness, tend to remain hypotonic and the musculature may undergo slight atrophy of a degree possibly not explained entirely by inactivity alone. In some cases, as noted below, there is clumsiness in reaching for and grasping an object under visual guidance (optic ataxia), and exceptionally, at some phase in recovery from the hemisensory deficit, there is incoordination of movement and intention tremor of the contralateral arm and leg that closely simulates a cerebellar deficit (pseudocerebellar syndrome). While relatively rare, this type of ataxia is authenticated by our own case observations.

In instances of cortical sensory disturbance, the outstretched hand may display small random "searching" movements of the fingers that simulate playing a piano (pseudoathetosis); these are exaggerated when the eyes are closed. Fixed dystonic postures and asterixis have also been described after parietal lesions with sensory loss, but these are most often the result of thalamic damage.

Agnosia

A conceptual inability to recognize objects, persons, or sensory stimuli in the absence of a primary deficit in the sensory modality is termed *agnosia*, derived from the

Greek for lack of knowledge. It was included as a form of loss of insight as part of the confusional state in Chap. 20.

The idea that visual and tactile sensory information is synthesized into a body schema or image (perception of one's body and the relations of bodily parts to one another) was first formulated by Pick and elaborated by Brain. Long before their time, however, it was suggested that such information was the basis of our emerging awareness of ourselves, and philosophers had assumed that this comes about by the constant interplay between inherent percepts of ourselves and of the surrounding world.

The formation of the body schema is considered to be based on the constant influx and storage of sensations from our bodies as we move about; hence, motor activity is important in its development. A sense of extrapersonal space is central to this activity, and this also depends upon visual and labyrinthine stimulation. The mechanisms of these perceptions are best appreciated by studying their derangements in the course of neurologic disease of the parietal lobes.

Denny-Brown and Banker introduced the idea that the basic disturbance in all these defects is an inability to integrate a series of "spatial impressions"—tactile, kinesthetic, visual, vestibular, or auditory—a defect they referred to as *amorphosynthesis*. Examples of the loss of concept in their schema include finger agnosia, right-left confusion, acalculia, and all the apperceptive losses that attend damage of integrative sensory areas of the brain. The theoretical problem presented by agnosia is taken up in a later section.

Anosognosia and hemispatial neglect (Anton–Babinski syndrome) The observation that a patient with a dense hemiplegia, usually of the left side, may be indifferent to a paralysis, or is entirely unaware of it, was first made by Anton; later, Babinski named this disorder *anosognosia*. It expresses itself in several ways. For example, a lack of concern regarding paralysis was called *anosodiaphoria* by Babinski, an interesting term that is now little used. The term "denial" was introduced by Freud to explain the problem but is laden with psychic and psychoanalytical meaning and is less precise than "neglect."

With regard to parietal lobe disease, the term "anosognosia," using "anos," disease, is used to describe a group of disorders in which there is an unawareness of a deficit. While used most frequently to describe a lack of recognition, neglect, or indifference to a left sided paralysis or even to ownership of the limb, the term anosognosia is appropriate to denote the inability to perceive a number of deficits based on cerebral disease including blindness, hemianopia, deafness, and memory loss. Anosognosia is usually associated with a number of additional abnormalities. Often there is a blunted emotionality. The patient is inattentive and apathetic, and shows varying degrees of general confusion. There may be an indifference to performance failure, a feeling that something is missing, visual and tactile illusions when sensing the paralyzed part, hallucinations of movement, and allochiria (one-sided stimuli are felt on the other side).

The patient may act as if nothing were the matter. If asked to raise the paralyzed arm, he may raise the intact one or do nothing at all. If asked whether the paralyzed arm has been moved, the patient may say "yes." If the fact that the arm has not been moved is pointed out, the patient may admit that the arm is slightly weak. If told it is paralyzed, the patient may deny that this is so or offer an excuse: "My shoulder hurts." If asked why the paralysis went unnoticed, the response may be, "I'm not a doctor." Some patients report that they feel as though their left side had disappeared, and when shown the paralyzed arm, they deny it is theirs and assert that it belongs to someone else or even take hold of it and fling it aside. The mildest form of anosognosia is reflected by an imperfect and reduced appreciation of the degree of weakness. On the other extreme of the conceptual negation of paralysis are instances of self-mutilation of the paralyzed limb (apotemnophilia). It should be pointed out that the loss of body schema and the lack of appreciation of a left hemiplegia are separable, some patients displaying only one feature.

The lesion responsible for the various forms of one-sided anosognosia lies in the cortex and white matter of the superior parietal lobule. Rarely, a deep lesion of the ventrolateral thalamus and the juxtaposed white matter of the parietal lobe will produce a similar contralateral neglect. Unilateral asomatognosia is many times more frequent with right (nondominant) parietal lesions as with left-sided ones (seven times more often according to Hécaen). The apparent infrequency of right-sided agnosic symptoms with left parietal lesions is attributable in part, but not entirely, to their obscuration by an associated aphasia.

Another common group of parietal symptoms consists of neglect of one side of the body in dressing and grooming, recognition only on the intact side of bilaterally and simultaneously presented stimuli (*sensory extinction*) as mentioned above, deviation of head and eyes to the side of the lesion (transient), and torsion of the body in the same direction. The patient may fail to shave one side of the face, apply lipstick, or comb the hair only on one side.

Unilateral spatial neglect is brought out by having the patient bisect a line, draw a daisy or a clock, or name all the objects in the room. Homonymous hemianopia and varying degrees of hemiparesis may or may not be present and interfere with the interpretation of the lack of application on the left side of the drawing.

Clinical observations indicate that patients with right parietal lesions show variable but lesser elements of ipsilateral neglect in addition to the striking degree of contralateral neglect, suggesting that, *in respect to spatial attention, the right parietal lobe is truly dominant* (Weintraub and Mesulam). Damage of the superior parietal lobule, in addition to producing agnosias and apraxias, may interfere with voluntary movement of the opposite limbs, particularly the arm, as pointed out by Holmes. In reaching for a visually presented target in the contralateral visual field, and to a lesser extent in the ipsilateral field, the movement is misdirected and dysmetric (the distance to the target is misjudged).

Another subtle aspect of parietal lobe physiology revealed by human disease is the loss of exploratory and orienting behavior with the contralateral arm and even a tendency to avoid tactile stimuli. Mori and Yamadori call this *rejection behavior*. Denny-Brown and Chambers attributed the released grasping and exploring that follow frontal lobe lesions to a disinhibition of inherent parietal lobe automatisms but there is no way of confirming this. It is of interest that demented patients with prominent grasp reflexes tend not to grasp parts of their own bodies, but if there has been an additional parietal lesion, there is "self-grasping" of the forearm opposite the lesion (Ropper).

Conventional treatments for hemispatial neglect use prismatic glasses and training in visual exploration of the left side. Another approach demonstrates improvement by the application of vibratory stimulation to the right side of the neck, as reported by Karnath and colleagues, or of the ipsilateral labyrinth by caloric or electrical means (a similar treatment has been successful in some cases of dystonic torticollis, see Chap. 6). Based on the work of Ramachandran and colleagues, mirrors have been used to assist recovery of the side with agnosia. With a mirror in the right parasagittal plane, the patient observes the mirror image of their neglected hand and space and is induced to use that side more naturally. The larger problem is that these patients may not respond to rehabilitation if they lack an innate body schema.

Ideomotor and Ideational Apraxia
(See also Chap. 3)

As discussed extensively in Chap. 3, patients with parietal lesions of the *dominant* hemisphere who exhibit no defects in motor or sensory function, lose the ability to perform learned motor skills on command or by imitation. They can no longer use common implements and tools, either in relation to their bodies (e.g., brushing teeth, combing hair) or in relation to objects in the environment (e.g., a doorknob or hammer). The patient holds the implement awkwardly or seems at a loss to begin the act. It is as though the patient had forgotten the sequences of learned movements. The effects are bilateral. When defects of apraxia are intertwined with agnosic defects, the term *apractognosia* seems appropriate. A special type of visuospatial disorder, separable from neglect but also associated with lesions of the nondominant parietal lobe, is reflected in the patient's inability to reproduce geometric figures (*constructional apraxia*). A number of tests have been designed to elicit these disturbances, such as indicating the time by placement of the hands on a clock, drawing a map, copying a complex figure, reproducing stick-pattern constructions and block designs, making three-dimensional constructions, and constructing puzzles.

From the above descriptions, it is evident that the left and right parietal lobes function differently. The most obvious difference, of course, is that language and arithmetical functions are centered in the left hemisphere. It is hardly surprising, therefore, that verbally mediated spatial and praxic functions are more affected with left-sided than with right-sided lesions. This is ostensibly because language function, sited in the left hemisphere, is central to all cognitive functions. Hence cross-modal matching tasks (auditory–visual, visual–auditory, visual–tactile, tactile–visual, auditory–tactile, etc.) are most clearly impaired with lesions of the dominant hemisphere. Such patients can read and understand spoken words but cannot grasp the meaning of a sentence if it contains elements of relationship (e.g., "the mother's daughter" versus "the daughter's mother," "the father's brother's son," "Jane's complexion is lighter than Marjorie's but darker than her sister's"). There are similar difficulties with calculation. The recognition and naming of parts of the body and the distinction of right from left and up from down are learned, verbally mediated spatial concepts that are disturbed by lesions in the dominant parietal lobe.

Gerstmann Syndrome

This syndrome, caused by a left (dominant) inferior parietal lesion, provides the most striking example of what might be viewed as a bilaterally manifest agnosia (the previously mentioned asomatognosia of Denny-Brown and Banker). The characteristic tetrad of features is (i) inability to designate or name the different fingers of the two hands (finger agnosia), (ii) confusion of the right and left sides of the body, (iii) inability to calculate (acalculia), and (iv) inability to write (dysgraphia). One or more of these manifestations may be associated with word blindness (alexia) and homonymous hemianopia or a lower quadrantanopia. The lesion is in the left *inferior parietal lobule* (below the interparietal sulcus), particularly involving the angular gyrus or subjacent white matter of the left hemisphere.

There has been a dispute as to whether the four main elements of the Gerstmann syndrome have a common basis or only an association. Benton states that they occur together in a parietal lesion no more often than do constructional apraxia, alexia, and loss of visual memory and that every combination of these symptoms and those of the Gerstmann syndrome occurs with equal frequency in parietal lobe disease. Others, including the authors, tend to disagree and have the experience that right–left confusion, digital agnosia, agraphia, and acalculia have special significance, possibly being linked through a unitary defect in spatial orientation of fingers, body sides, and numbers. The relationship between the finger agnosia and the inability to enumerate is especially intriguing and relates to other arithmetic difficulties, discussed below. Attempts to clarify a common or fundamental source for all the elements of the Gerstmann syndrome by functional imaging have been difficult to comprehend. In healthy subjects, Rusconi and colleagues were unable to find a shared cortical substrate that could give rise to the features of the Gerstmann syndrome.

Dyscalculia has attracted little critical attention, perhaps because it occurs most often as a by-product of aphasia and an inability of the patient to appreciate numerical language. Primary dyscalculia is usually associated with the other elements of the Gerstmann syndrome. Computational difficulty may also be part of the more complex visuospatial abnormality of the nondominant parietal lobe; there is then difficulty in the placing of numbers in specific spatial relationships while calculating. In such cases, there is no difficulty in reading or writing the numbers or in describing the rules governing the calculation, but the computation cannot be accomplished correctly with pencil and paper. Hécaen has made a distinction between this type of *anarithmetia* and dyscalculia. In the latter, the process of calculation alone has been disturbed; in the former, there is an inability to manipulate numbers and to appreciate their ordinal relationships. Recognition and reproduction of numbers are intact in both. An analysis of how computation goes awry in each individual case is therefore required.

Visual Disorders With Parietal Lesions

A lesion deep to the inferior part of the parietal lobe, at its junction with the temporal lobe, involves the geniculocalcarine radiations and results in an incongruous homonymous hemianopia or an inferior quadrantanopia on the opposite side; but just as often, in practice, the defect is complete or almost complete and congruous. If the lesion is small and predominantly cortical, optokinetic nystagmus is usually retained; with deep lesions, it is abolished, with the target moving ipsilaterally (see Chap. 14).

Visual neglect is a typical feature of posterior parietal lesions on either side, more prominent with right-sided lesions. The problem that often arises is of distinguishing visual hemineglect (particularly of the left side) from a hemianopia. In its more severe forms the neglect is evident from casual observation of the patient's behavior or in drawings made by the patient that omit features on the left side; but here a more pervasive syndrome of *hemispatial neglect*, discussed earlier, may underlie the visual behavior. Occasionally, severe left-sided *visual neglect* results from a lesion in the right angular gyrus (see Mort et al). Visual neglect can also occur after focal lesions in the posterior medial temporal lobe (supplied by a branch of the posterior cerebral artery, in contrast to the middle cerebral artery supply of the angular gyrus of the inferior parietal lobule).

With posterior parietal lesions, as noted by Holmes and Horrax, there are deficits in localization of visual stimuli, inability to compare the sizes of objects, failure to avoid objects when walking, inability to count objects, disturbances in smooth-pursuit eye movements, and loss of stereoscopic vision. Cogan observed that the eyes may deviate away from the lesion upon forced lid closure, a "spasticity of conjugate gaze."

A common disorder of motor behavior of the eyelids is seen in many patients with large acute lesions of the right parietal lobe. Its mildest form is a disinclination to open the lids when the patient is spoken to. This gives the erroneous impression that the patient is drowsy or stuporous, but it will be found that a quick reply is given to whispered questions. In more severe cases, the lids are held shut and opening them is strongly resisted, to the point of making an examination of the pupils and fundi impossible.

Visual disorientation and disorders of extrapersonal space (topographic localization) Spatial orientation depends on the integration of visual, tactile, and kinesthetic perceptions, but there are instances in which the defect in visual perception predominates. Patients with this disorder are unable to orient themselves in an abstract spatial setting (*topographagnosia*). Such patients cannot draw the floor plan of their house, a map of their town, or of the United States and cannot describe a familiar route, as from home to work, for example, or find their way in familiar surroundings. In brief, such patients have lost topographic memory. This disorder is almost invariably caused by lesions in the white matter deep to the inferior and superior parietal lobules and it is separable from anosognosia as summarized by Levine and colleagues.

A clever mental experiment posed to patients by Bisiach and Luzzatti has suggested that the loss of attention to one side of the environment extends to, or perhaps is derived from, the mental representation of space. Their patient with a right parietal lesion was asked to describe from memory the buildings lining the Piazza del Duomo, first as if seen from one corner of the piazza and then from the opposite corner. In each instance, the description omitted the left side of the piazza from the observer's perspective.

An important and not infrequent disorder of visual agnosia, a disorder of visually directed reaching with the hand, difficulty directing gaze, and simultanagnosia, is given the name *Balint syndrome*. It is, strictly speaking, a bilateral disorder of the parietal lobes but we discuss it below for convenience in order to append it to the clinically similar entity of cortical blindness.

Auditory Neglect

This defect in appreciation of the left side of the environment is less apparent than is visual neglect, but it is no less striking when it occurs. Many patients with acute right parietal lesions are initially unresponsive to voices or noises on the left side, but the syndrome is rarely persistent. Special tests demonstrate a displacement of the direction of the perceived origin of sounds toward the right. This defect is separable from visual agnosia (see De Renzi et al); curiously, it may be worsened by the introduction of visual cues. Subtle differences between the allocation of spatial attention to sound (auditory neglect) and a distortion in its localization may be found in different cases, but the main lesion usually lies in the right superior lobule.

In summary, the effects of disease of the parietal lobes are as follows:

I. Effects of unilateral disease of the parietal lobe, right or left
   A. Corticosensory syndrome and sensory extinction (or total hemianesthesia with large acute lesions of white matter)
   B. Mild hemiparesis or poverty of movement (variable), poverty of movement, hemiataxia (seen only occasionally)
   C. Homonymous hemianopia or inferior quadrantanopia (incongruent or congruent) or visual inattention
   D. Abolition of optokinetic nystagmus with target moving toward side of the lesion
   E. Neglect of the opposite side of external space (more prominent with lesions of the right parietal lobe; see later)

II. Effects of unilateral disease of the dominant (left) parietal lobe (in right-handed and most left-handed patients); additional phenomena include
   A. Disorders of language (especially alexia)
   B. Gerstmann syndrome (dysgraphia, dyscalculia, finger agnosia, right–left confusion)
   C. Tactile agnosia (bimanual astereognosis)
   D. Bilateral ideomotor and ideational apraxia (see Chap. 3)
III. Effects of unilateral disease of the nondominant (right) parietal lobe
   A. Visuospatial disorders
   B. Topographic memory loss
   C. Anosognosia, dressing, and constructional apraxias (these disorders may occur with lesions of either hemisphere but are observed more frequently and are of greater severity with lesions of the nondominant one)
   D. Confusion
   E. Tendency to keep the eyes closed, resist lid opening, and blepharospasm
IV. Effects of bilateral disease of the parietal lobes
   A. Balint syndrome: visual-spatial imperception (simultagnosia), optic apraxia (difficulty directing gaze), and optic ataxia (difficulty reaching for objects)

With all these parietal syndromes, if the disease is sufficiently extensive, there may be a reduction in the capacity to think clearly as well as inattentiveness and slightly impaired memory.

It does seem reasonably certain that, in addition to the perception of somatosensory impulses that arrive in the postcentral gyrus, the parietal lobe participates in the integration of all sensory data, especially those that provide an awareness of one's body as well as a percept of one's surroundings and of the relation of one's body to extrapersonal space and of objects in the environment to each other. In this respect, the parietal lobe may be regarded as a special high-order sensory organ, the locus of transmodal intersensory, integration, particularly tactile and visual ones, which are the basis of our concepts of spatial relations. In this way, parietal lesions cause disorders of specific types of self-consciousness or self-awareness that are tied to sensory modalities. This is distinctly different from the distortions of perception caused by lesions of the temporal lobes.

Authoritative references on parietal function include Critchley's monograph on the parietal lobes and the chapter by Botez and Olivier in the *Handbook of Clinical Neurology*.

SYNDROMES CAUSED BY LESIONS OF THE OCCIPITAL LOBES

Anatomic and Physiologic Considerations

The occipital lobes are the termini of the geniculocalcarine pathways and are essential for visual perception and recognition. This part of the brain has a large medial surface and smaller lateral and inferior surfaces (see Fig. 22-1). The parietooccipital fissure creates a noticeable medial boundary with the parietal lobe, but laterally the occipital lobe merges with the parietal and temporal lobes. The large calcarine fissure courses in an anteroposterior direction from the pole of the occipital lobe to the splenium of the corpus callosum; area 17, the primary visual receptive cortex, lies on its banks (see Figs. 22-1 and 22-2). Area 17 is a typical homotypical cortex but is unique in that its fourth receptive layer is divided into two granular cell laminae by a greatly thickened band of myelinated fibers, the external band of Baillarger. This stripe, also called the *line* or *band of Gennari*, is grossly visible and has given this area its name, *striate cortex*. The largest part of area 17 is the terminus of the retinal macular fibers that arrive via the lateral geniculate (see Fig. 13-2). The parastriate cortex (areas 18 and 19) lacks the line of Gennari and resembles the granular unimodal association cortex of the rest of similar areas in the cerebrum. Area 17 contains cells that are activated by the homolateral geniculocalcarine pathway (corresponding, of course, exclusively to the contralateral visual field); these cells are interconnected and project also to cells in areas 18 and 19. The latter are connected with one another and with the angular gyri, lateral and medial temporal gyri, frontal motor areas, limbic and paralimbic areas, and corresponding areas of the opposite hemisphere through the posterior third (splenium) of the corpus callosum.

The occipital lobes are supplied almost exclusively by the posterior cerebral arteries and their branches, either directly in most individuals or through an embryologically persistent branch of the internal carotid arteries ("fetal" posterior cerebral artery). A small area of the occipital pole receives blood supply from the inferior division of the middle cerebral artery. This assumes importance in the clinical finding of "macular sparing," discussed in Chap. 13.

The connections among these several areas in the occipital lobe are complex, and the notion that area 17 is activated by the lateral geniculate neurons and that this activity is then transferred and elaborated in areas 18 and 19 is surely not complete. Actually, 4 or 5 occipital receptive fields are activated by lateral geniculate neurons, and fibers from area 17 project to approximately 20 other visual areas, of which only 5 are well identified. These extrastriate visual areas lie in the lingula and posterior regions of the occipital lobes. As Hubel and Wiesel have shown, the response patterns of neurons in both occipital lobes to edges and moving visual stimuli, to on-and-off effects of light, and to colors reflects this complexity. Hence form, location, color, and movement each have separate localizable hierarchical arrangements of neurons in series. The monographs of Polyak and of Miller contain detailed information about the anatomy and physiology of this part of the brain.

Beyond the effects on vision of lesions in the occipital lobes, monkeys with bilateral lesions in the temporal visual zones lose the ability to identify objects; with posterior parietal lesions, there is loss of ability to locate objects.

Clinical Effects of Occipital Lobe Lesions

Visual Field Defects

The most familiar clinical abnormality resulting from a lesion of one occipital lobe, a contralateral *homonymous hemianopia*, has already been discussed in Chap. 13. Extensive destruction abolishes all vision in the corresponding opposite half of each visual field. With a neoplastic lesion that eventually involves the entire striate region, the field defect may extend from the periphery toward the center, and loss of color vision (hemiachromatopsia) often precedes loss of black and white. Destruction of only part of the striate cortex on one side yields characteristic field defects that accurately indicate the loci of the lesion. A lesion confined to the pole of the occipital lobe results in a central hemianopic defect that splits the macula and leaves the peripheral fields intact. This observation indicates that half of each macula is unilaterally represented and that the maculae may be involved (split) in hemianopia. Bilateral lesions of the occipital poles, as in embolism of the posterior cerebral arteries, result in bilateral hemianopias and cortical blindness as detailed below. Unilateral quadrant defects and altitudinal field defects due to striate lesions indicate that the cortex on one side, above or below the calcarine fissure, is damaged. The cortex below the fissure is the terminus of fibers from the lower half of the retina; the resulting field defect is in the upper quadrant, and vice versa. Most bilateral altitudinal defects, either superior or inferior, are traceable to incomplete bilateral occipital lesions (cortex or terminal parts of geniculocalcarine pathways). Head and Holmes described several such delimited cases caused by gunshot wounds; embolic infarction is now the common cause.

As indicated in Chap. 13, the homonymous hemianopia that results from ablation of one occipital lobe is not absolute. In monkeys, visuospatial orientation and the capacity to reach for moving objects in the defective field are preserved (Denny-Brown and Chambers). In humans also, flashing light and moving objects can sometimes be seen in the blind field even without the patient's full awareness. Weiskrantz and colleagues have referred to these preserved functions as *blindisms* or *blindsight*. It is useful as a practical matter to note that the optokinetic responses are usually spared in hemianopic deficits of occipital origin.

Many of the complex behavioral defects involving visual function are caused by lesions at the junctions of the occipital and parietal or temporal lobes. They are discussed here with the occipital lobe syndromes for convenience but should be considered as transcending the largely arbitrary boundaries of these three lobes of the brain.

Cortical Blindness

With bilateral lesions of the occipital lobes (destruction of area 17 of both hemispheres), there is a loss of sight that can be conceptualized as bilateral hemianopia. The degree of blindness may be equivalent to that which follows severing of the optic nerves. The pupillary light reflexes are preserved because they depend upon visual fibers that terminate in the midbrain, but reflex closure of the eyelids to threat or bright light may, or may not, be preserved (see Fig. 14-9). No changes are detectable in the retinas. The eyes are still able to move through a full range and, if there is macular sparing as there usually is with vascular lesions, optokinetic nystagmus can be elicited. Visual imagination and visual imagery in dreams are preserved. With rare exceptions, no cortical potentials can be evoked in the occipital lobes by light flashes or pattern changes (visual evoked response), and the alpha rhythm is lost in the electroencephalogram (EEG; see Chap. 2).

Less-complete bilateral lesions leave the patient with varying degrees of visual perception. There may also be visual hallucinations of either elementary or complex types. The mode of recovery from cortical blindness has been studied carefully by Gloning and colleagues, who describe a regular progression from cortical blindness through visual agnosia and partially impaired perceptual function to recovery. Even with recovery, the patient may complain of visual fatigue (asthenopia) and difficulties in fixation and fusion.

The usual cause of cortical blindness is occlusion of the posterior cerebral arteries (most often embolic) or the equivalent, occlusion of the distal basilar artery. The above-mentioned macular sparing may leave the patient with an island of barely serviceable central vision. The infarct may also involve the mediotemporal regions or thalami, which share the posterior cerebral artery supply, with a resulting Korsakoff amnesic defect and a variety of other neurologic deficits referable to the high midbrain and diencephalon (drowsiness, akinetic mutism as described in Chap. 17).

Visual Anosognosia (Anton Syndrome)

The main characteristic of this disorder is the denial of blindness by a patient who obviously cannot see. These patients act as though they could see, and in attempting to walk, collide with objects, even to the point of injury. They may offer excuses for the difficulties—"I lost my glasses," "The light is dim"—or may only evince indifference to loss of sight. The lesions in cases of negation of blindness extend beyond the striate cortex to involve the visual association areas.

Rarely, the opposite condition arises: a patient is able to see small objects but claims to be blind. This individual walks about avoiding obstacles, picks up crumbs or pills from the table, and catches a small ball thrown from a distance. This simulates the condition of hysterical blindness (see further on).

Visual Illusions (Metamorphopsias)

These may present as distortions of form, size, movement, or color. In a group of 83 patients with visual perceptual abnormalities, Hécaen found that 71 fell under one of four headings: deformation of the image, change in size, illusion of movement, or a combination of all three. Illusions of these types have been reported with lesions confined to the occipital lobes but are more frequently caused by shared occipitoparietal or occipitotemporal lesions; consequently, they are also considered in earlier sections of this chapter as well as in Chaps. 13 and 16. The right hemisphere appears to be involved more often than the left. Illusions of movement occur more frequently with posterior temporal lesions or seizures, polyopia (one object appearing as two or more objects) more frequently with occipital lesions (it also occurs in hysteria), and palinopsia (perseveration of visual images, as in the frames of a celluloid film) with both posterior parietal and occipital lesions. Visual field defects are present in many of the cases. In all these conditions, the anatomic correlates are imprecise.

It is likely that an element of cortical vestibular disorder underlies the metamorphosis of parietooccipital lesions. The vestibular and proprioceptive systems are represented in the parietal lobes of each side and the lesions there are probably responsible for misperceptions of movement and spatial relations. The illusion of tilting of the environment or upside-down vision is known to occur with parietooccipital lesions, but occurs more often with abnormalities of the vestibular system.

Visual Hallucinations

These phenomena may be elementary or complex, and both types have sensory as well as cognitive aspects. Elementary (or unformed) hallucinations include flashes of light, colors, luminous points, stars, multiple lights (like candles), and geometric forms (circles, squares, and hexagons). They may be stationary or moving (zigzag, oscillations, vibrations, or pulsations). They are much the same as the effects that Penfield and Erickson obtained by stimulating the calcarine cortex in a conscious patient. Complex (formed) hallucinations include objects, persons, or animals and infrequently, more complete scenes that are indicative of lesions in the visual association areas or their connections with the temporal lobes. They may be of natural size, Lilliputian, or grossly enlarged. With hemianopia, they appear in the defective field or move from the intact field toward the hemianopic one. The patient may realize that the hallucinations are false experiences or may be convinced of their reality. Because the patient's response is usually in accord with the nature of the hallucination, he may react with fear to a threatening vision or casually if its content is benign.

The clinical setting for the occurrence of visual hallucinations varies. The simplest black-and-white moving scintillations are part of migraine. Others, some colored, occur as a seizure aura (see Chap. 16). Often, they are associated with a homonymous hemianopia, as already indicated. Frequently, they are part of a confusional state or delirium (see Chap. 20). Similar phenomena may occur as part of hypnagogic hallucinations in the narcolepsy–cataplexy syndrome. In the "peduncular hallucinosis" of Lhermitte (1932), the hallucinations are purely visual, appear natural in form and color, sometimes in pastels, move about as in an animated cartoon, and are considered by the patient to be unreal, abnormal phenomena (preserved insight). Ischemia in the territories of the posterior cerebral arteries is the usual cause. Lhermitte used the term peduncle to represent the midbrain as the source of the hallucinations was ischemia in the high mesencephalon, creating images that may be akin to those experienced in dreaming. The hallucinations as mentioned are purely visual; if hallucinations are polymodal, the lesion is always in the occipitotemporal parts of the cerebrum.

A special syndrome of ophthalmopathic hallucinations occurs in persons with reduced vision, as discussed in Chap. 13. A similar phenomenon in elderly patients with partially impaired vision has been called the *Charles Bonnet syndrome*, following his description of visual hallucinations in a "sane" person. The topic of senile hallucinosis has been reviewed by Gold and Rabin, and 60 such patients with Bonnet syndrome were reported in detail by Teunisse and colleagues. The latter authors found that 11 percent of older persons with reduced vision experienced these phenomena at one time or another. Further comments are to be found in Chap. 13.

It is usually the case that the lesions responsible for visual hallucinations are situated in the occipital lobe or posterior part of the temporal lobe and that elementary hallucinations have their origin in the occipital cortex, and complex ones in the temporal cortex. However, the opposite may pertain; in some cases, formed hallucinations are related to lesions of the occipital lobe and unformed ones to lesions of the temporal lobe, according to Weinberger and Grant. Also, as emphasized by these authors, lesions that give rise to visual hallucinations, simple or elaborate, need not be confined to central nervous system structures but may be caused by lesions at every level of the neurooptic apparatus (retina, optic nerve, chiasm, etc.).

The Visual Agnosias (See also Lesions of the Parietal Lobe and Temporal Lobe)

Several syndromes involving visual dysfunction are due to lesions that span the occipital lobe and either the adjacent temporal or parietal lobes. They have been divided conceptually and anatomically into a dorsal and a ventral stream of information processing, the former running from the occipital to the parietal lobe and the latter from the occipital to the temporal lobe. Those of the temporal lobe include visual object agnosia, prosopagnosia, alexia, and color agnosia. In this way, the ventral stream may be considered to represent the "what" of visual processing to identify objects. The parietal-occipital, or dorsal stream syndromes are visual simultanagnosia, Balint syndrome and the earlier mentioned topographagnosia, that reflect disorders of "where" in visual behavior.

Visual object agnosia This rare condition, first described by Lissauer in 1890, consists of a failure to name and indicate the use of a seen object by spoken or written word or by gesture. The patient cannot even determine the generic class of the object presented. Visual acuity is intact, the mind is clear, and the patient is not aphasic—conditions requisite for the diagnosis of agnosia. If the object is palpated, it is recognized at once, and it can also be identified by smell or sound if it has an odor or makes a noise. Moving the object or placing it in its customary surroundings facilitates recognition. In most reported instances of object agnosia, the patient retains normal visual acuity but cannot identify, match, or name objects presented in any part of the visual fields; if misnamed, the object is used in a fashion that reflects the incorrect perception. Amazingly, one encounters patients who have lost the capacity to recognize only one class of objects, e.g., animals or vegetables—suggesting that, in the human, stored information is grouped and classified in a way that is necessary for visual perception (we are unable to corroborate this from our own material). Lissauer conceived of visual object recognition as consisting of two distinct processes, the construction of a perceptual representation from vision (perception) and the mapping of this perceptual representation onto stored percepts or engrams of the object's functions and associations (apperception), and he proposed that impairment of either of these processes could give rise to a defect in visual object recognition.

As indicated in Chap. 13, visual object agnosia is usually associated with *visual verbal agnosia* (*alexia*) and homonymous hemianopia. *Prosopagnosia* (the inability to identify faces; see further on) is also present in most cases. The underlying lesions are usually bilateral, although McCarthy and Warrington have related a case with a restricted lesion of the left occipitotemporal region (by MRI). Two of our patients with visual object agnosia had an incomplete amnesic syndrome from a left-sided inferior occipital and mediotemporal infarction, reflecting a proximal occlusion of the posterior cerebral artery.

Prosopagnosia This term (from the Greek *prosopon*, "face," and *gnosis*, "knowledge") was introduced by Bodamer for a type of visual defect in which the patient cannot identify a familiar face by looking at either the person or a picture, even though he knows that a face is a face and can point out its features. Such patients also cannot learn to recognize new faces. They may also be unable to interpret the meaning of facial expressions or to judge the ages or distinguish the genders of faces. In identifying persons, the patient depends on other data, such as the presence and type of glasses or moustache, the type of gait, or sound of the voice. Similarly, species of animals and birds and specific models or types of cars cannot be distinguished from one another, but the patient can still recognize an animal, bird, or car as such. Other agnosias may be present in such cases (color agnosia, simultanagnosia) and there may be topographic disorientation, disturbances of body schema, and constructional or dressing apraxia. Visual field defects are nearly always present. Some neurologists have interpreted this condition as a simultanagnosia involving facial features. Another view is that the face, though satisfactorily perceived, cannot be matched to a memory store of faces. Levine has found a deficit in perception, characterized by insufficient feature analysis of all visual stimuli.

The small number of cases that have been studied anatomically and by CT scanning and MRI indicate that prosopagnosia is most often associated with bilateral lesions of the ventromedial occipitotemporal regions (Damasio et al) including the inferior occipital or midfusiform gyri, but there are exceptions that are attributable to unilateral damage, almost always on the right side. The notion that there is a "face area" in the fusiform gyrus is expressed uncritically in the literature and seems to be an oversimplification.

A variant of this disorder is characterized by specific difficulty with facial matching or discrimination from partial cues, such as portions of the face or a profile. The distinction between this deficit and the usual type of prosopagnosia rests on the use of tests that do not require memory of a specific face. This difficulty with facial matching and discrimination is more likely to be seen with lesions of the right than of the left posterior hemisphere.

Closely allied and often associated with prosopagnosia is a subtle syndrome of loss of environmental familiarity, in which the patient is unable to recognize familiar places. The patient may be able to describe a familiar environment from memory and locate it on a map, but he experiences no sense of familiarity and gets lost when faced with the actual landscape. In essence, this is an *environmental agnosia*. This syndrome is associated with right-sided, medial temporooccipital lesions, although in some patients, as in those with prosopagnosia, the lesions are bilateral (Landis et al).

Environmental agnosia can be distinguished from the visual disorientation and disorder of spatial (topographic) localization discussed earlier. Patients with the latter disorder are unable to orient themselves in an abstract spatial setting (*topographagnosia*, or loss of topographic memory). They cannot draw the floor plan of their house or a map of their town or the United States and cannot describe a familiar route, as from their home to their place of work, or find their way in familiar surroundings.

Visual agnosia for words (alexia without agraphia) See Chap. 23 and further on in this chapter in the discussion of alexia without agraphia, under the "Disconnection Syndromes."

Color agnosia Here one must distinguish several different aspects of identification of colors, such as the correct perception of color (the loss of which is called *color blindness*) or the naming of a color. The common form of retinal color blindness is congenital and is readily tested by the use of Ishihara plates. Acquired color blindness caused by a cerebral lesion, with retention of form vision, is referred to as *central achromatopsia*. Here the disturbance is one of hue discrimination; the patient cannot sort a series of colored wools according to hue (Holmgren test) and may complain that colors have lost their brightness or that everything looks gray. Achromatopsia is frequently associated with visual field defects and with prosopagnosia. Most often, the field defects are bilateral and tend to affect the upper quadrants. However, full-field achromatopsia may exist with retention of visual acuity and form vision. There may also be a hemi- or quadrant-achromatopsia without other abnormalities, although special testing is required to reveal this defect. These features, together with the usually associated prosopagnosia, point to involvement of the inferomedial, occipital, and temporal lobe(s) and the lower part of the striate cortex or optic radiation (Damasio et al, 1974a). The existence of a central achromatopsia is not surprising in view of the animal studies of Hubel, which identified sets of cells in areas 17 and 18 that are activated only by color stimuli.

A second group of patients with color agnosia have no difficulty with color perception (i.e., they can match seen colors), but they cannot reliably name them or point out colors in response to their names. They have a *color anomia*, of which there are at least two varieties. One is typically associated with pure word blindness, i.e., alexia without agraphia, and is best explained by a disconnection of the primary visual areas from the language areas (see further on). In the second variety, the patient fails not only in tasks that require the matching of a seen color with its spoken name but also in purely verbal tasks pertaining to color naming, such as naming the colors of common objects (e.g., grass, banana). This latter disorder is probably best regarded as a form of anomic aphasia, in which the aphasia is more or less restricted to the naming of colors (Meadows, 1974b). According to Damasio and associates, the lesion has involved the medial part of the left hemisphere at the junction of the occipital and temporal lobes, just below the splenium of the corpus callosum. All their patients also had a right homonymous hemianopia as a result of destruction of the left lateral geniculate body, optic radiation, or calcarine cortex.

Visual simultanagnosia This describes an inability to grasp the sense of the multiple components of a total visual scene despite retained ability to identify individual details. Wolpert pointed out that there was an inability to read all but the shortest words, spelled out letter by letter, and a failure to perceive simultaneously all the elements of a scene and to properly interpret the scene, which Wolpert called *simultanagnosia*. A cognitive defect of synthesis of the visual impressions was thought to be the basis of this condition. Some patients with this disorder have a right homonymous hemianopia; in others, the visual fields are full but there is one-sided extinction when tested with double simultaneous stimulation. This is an integral part of the Balint syndrome described below.

Through tachistoscopic testing, Kinsbourne and Warrington (1963) found that reducing the time of stimulus exposure permits single objects to be perceived, but not two objects. Rizzo and Robin proposed that the primary defect is in sustained attention to incoming visuospatial information. There is consistent localization. Nielsen has described it with a lesion of the inferolateral part of the dominant occipital lobe (area 18). In a patient who presented with an isolated "spelling dyslexia" and simultanagnosia, Kinsbourne and Warrington (1962) found the lesion to be localized within the inferior part of the left occipital lobe. In other instances, the lesions have been bilateral in the superior parts of the occipital association cortices.

Balint syndrome (See also Chap. 13.) In this not uncommon syndrome, the appreciation of a coherent and detailed visual world is disrupted and the patient perceives only disconnected individual parts of the scene, as in the visual simultanagnosia described earlier. While it is due to lesions that span the occipital and parietal lobes, it is presented here for ease of exposition. Balint, a Hungarian neurologist, was the first to recognize this constellation. The defect is noted when the patient describes a complex scene in a disjointed way, single objects being pointed out, others missed entirely, the relationships and context of parts of the picture remaining unappreciated. The entire syndrome consists of (1) a disorder of visual attention mainly to the periphery of the visual field, in which the totality of a scene is not perceived despite preservation of vision for individual elements (visual simultanagnosia as discussed earlier); (2) difficulty in grasping or touching an object under visual guidance, as though hand and eye were not coordinated (called by Balint *optic ataxia*); and (3) an inability to project gaze voluntarily into the peripheral field and to scan it despite the fact that eye movements are full (termed psychic paralysis of fixation of gaze by Balint, incorrectly called *optic apraxia*).

An essential feature of the Balint syndrome appears to be a failure to properly direct oculomotor function in the exploration of space. This psychic paralysis of gaze is apparent when the patient is unable to turn his eyes to fixate an object in the right or left visual field or to consistently follow a moving object. The pattern in which the patient scans a picture is haphazard and fails to encompass on entire areas. Normal individuals accomplish visual scanning in a fairly uniform manner beginning paracentrally and moving clockwise, then to the corners. Thus, the mechanism of simultanagnosia may be in part the result of this abnormality of eye movements as pointed out by Tyler.

Optic ataxia is detected when the patient reaches for an object, either spontaneously or in response to verbal command. To reach the object, the patient engages in a tactile search with the palm and fingers, presumably using somatosensory cues to compensate for a lack of visual information. The disorder may involve one or both hands and give the erroneous impression that the patient is blind. In contrast, movements that do not require visual guidance, such as those directed to the body or movements of the body itself, are performed naturally. The presence of visual inattention is tested by asking the patient to carry out tasks such as looking at a series of objects or connecting a series of dots by lines; often only one of a series of objects can be found, even though the visual fields seem to be full.

In almost all reported cases of the Balint syndrome, the lesions have been bilateral, mainly in the vascular border zones (areas 19 and 7) of the parietooccipital regions, although instances of optic ataxia alone have been described within a single visual field contralateral to a right or left parietooccipital lesion, and visual simultanagnosia, as noted earlier, has had variable localization. The neuropsychologic aspects of the syndrome and several interesting historical notes, including the attribution of original reporting to Inouye, can be found in the review by Rizzo and Vecera.

The effects of disease of the occipital lobes may be summarized as follows:

I. Effects of unilateral disease, either right or left
   A. Contralateral (congruent) homonymous hemianopia, which may be central (splitting the macula) or peripheral; also homonymous hemiachromatopsia
   B. Elementary (unformed) hallucinations—usually because of irritative lesions
II. Effects of left occipital disease
   A. Right homonymous hemianopia
   B. If deep white matter and splenium of corpus callosum is involved, alexia without agraphia
   C. Visual object agnosia
III. Effects of right occipital disease
   A. Left homonymous hemianopia
   B. With more extensive lesions, visual illusions (metamorphopsias) and hallucinations (more frequent with right-sided than left-sided lesions)
   C. Loss of topographic memory and visual orientation
IV. Bilateral occipital disease
   A. Cortical blindness bilateral hemianopias,
   B. Anton syndrome (visual anosognosia, denial of cortical blindness)
   C. Loss of perception of color (achromatopsia)
   D. Prosopagnosia (impaired face recognition, bilateral temporooccipital including fusiform gyrus)
   E. Balint syndrome (bilateral dorsal parietooccipital) (see description in text)

DISTURBANCES OF CONNECTIONS BETWEEN THE CEREBRAL HEMISPHERES AND DISCONNECTION SYNDROMES

A line of disagreement, as old as neurology itself, pertains to the relationship between the two cerebral hemispheres. Fechner, in 1860, speculated that since the two hemispheres, joined by the corpus callosum, were virtual mirror images of one another and functioned in totality in conscious life, separating them would result in two minds. William McDougall rejected this idea and is said to have offered to have his own brain divided by Charles Sherrington should he have an incurable disease. He died of cancer, but the callosotomy was considered unnecessary, for already there were indications from the work of Sperry and colleagues that when separated, the two hemispheres had different functions.

The practice of surgical sectioning of the corpus callosum for the control of epilepsy greatly stimulated interest in the special functions of the right cerebral hemisphere when isolated from the left. It is in the sphere of visuospatial perception that right hemispheral dominance is most convincing. Lesions of the right posterior cerebral region result in an inability to utilize information about spatial relationships in making perceptual judgments and in responding to objects in a spatial framework. This is manifest in constructing figures (constructional apraxia), in the spatial orientation of the patient in relation to the environment (topographic agnosia), in identifying faces (prosopagnosia), and in relating a scattering of visual stimuli to one another (simultanagnosia). Also, there are claims that the right hemisphere is more important than the left in visual imagery, attention, emotion (both in feeling and in the perception of emotion in others), and manual drawing (but not writing); in respect to these functions, however, the evidence is less firm. The idea that attention is a function of the right hemisphere derives from the neglect of left visual space and of somatic sensation in the anosognosic syndrome and also from the apathy that characterizes such patients. Certainly, the popular notion of the right hemisphere as "emotional" in contrast to the left one as "logical" has no basis in fact and represents a gross oversimplification of brain function and localization.

Similar issues arise, of course, in relation to handedness and language dominance in the left hemisphere as discussed in the following chapter. Here we comment only on how intriguing it is that praxis and linguistic skill are aligned on the same side of the brain, suggesting that an essential property of the dominant hemisphere is its ability to comprehend and manipulate symbolic representations of all types. At the same time, the colocalization of gnosis and visuospatial ability in the nondominant hemisphere has salience in that the two are so often interdependent in normal functioning.

Following the insightful clinical observations and anatomic studies of Wernicke, Déjerine, and Liepmann, the concept of disconnection of parts of one or both cerebral hemispheres as a cause of neurologic difficulty was introduced to neurologic thinking. In recent years, these ideas were resurrected and modernized by Geschwind (1965) and greatly extended by Sperry and by Gazzaniga. Geschwind called attention to several clinical syndromes resulting from interruption of the connections between the two cerebral hemispheres in the corpus callosum or between different parts of one hemisphere. Some of these are illustrated in Fig. 22-6.

When the entire corpus callosum is destroyed by tumor or surgical section, the language and perception areas of the left hemisphere are isolated from the right hemisphere. Patients with such lesions, if blindfolded, are unable to match an object held in one hand with that in the other. Objects placed in the right hand are named correctly, but not those in the left. Furthermore, if rapid presentation is used to avoid bilateral visual scanning, such patients cannot match an object seen in the right half of the visual field with one in the left half. They are also alexic in the left visual field, because the verbal symbols that are seen there and are projected to regions of the right hemisphere have no access to the language areas of the left hemisphere. If given a verbal command, such patients will execute it correctly with the right hand but not with the left; if asked to write from dictation with the left hand, they will produce only an illegible scrawl. Many remarkable conclusions regarding the nature of behavior and the special roles of each cerebral hemisphere have been drawn from clever observations of patients with callosal section. Extensive discussion of these neuropsychologic abnormalities cannot be undertaken here; suffice it to say that these are not features seen in patients with the usual neurologic diseases, but they are nonetheless of interest to neurologists and are discussed in the writings of Gazzaniga.

In most lesions confined to the posterior portion of the corpus callosum (splenium), only the visual part of the disconnection syndrome occurs. Cases of occlusion of the left posterior cerebral artery provide the best examples. Because infarction of the left occipital lobe causes a right homonymous hemianopia, all visual information needed for activating the speech areas of the left hemisphere must thereafter come from the right occipital lobe. The patient with a lesion of the splenium of the corpus callosum or the adjacent white matter cannot read or name colors because the visual information cannot reach the left language areas. There is, however, no difficulty in copying words; presumably, the visual information for activating the left motor area crosses the corpus callosum more anteriorly. Spontaneous writing and writing to dictation are also intact because the language areas, including the angular gyrus, Wernicke and Broca areas, and the left motor cortex, are intact and interconnected, but after a delay, the patient is unable to read what he has previously written (unless it was memorized). This is the syndrome of *alexia without agraphia* mentioned earlier.

Surprisingly, a lesion that is limited to the anterior third of the corpus callosum (or a surgical section of this part, as in patients with intractable epilepsy) does not result in an apraxia of the left hand. A section of the entire corpus callosum does result in such an apraxia, i.e., a failure of only the left hand to obey spoken commands, the right one performing normally, indicating that the fiber systems that connect the left to the right motor areas cross in the corpus callosum posterior to the genu (but anterior to the splenium). Object naming and matching of colors without naming them are also done without error. However, when blinded, the patient cannot name a finger touched on the left hand or use it to touch a designated part of the body.

Of interest to the authors is the fact that one sometimes encounters patients with a lesion in all or some part of the corpus callosum without being able to demonstrate any aspect of the aforementioned disconnection syndromes. Notable is the observation that in some patients with a congenital agenesis of the corpus callosum (a developmental abnormality), none of the interhemispheral disconnection syndromes can be found. One must suppose that in such patients, information is transferred by another route—perhaps the anterior or posterior commissure—or that dual dominance for language and praxis was established during early development. (See a review of this subject by Lassonde and Jeeves.)

In addition to *alexia without agraphia*, the following intrahemispheral disconnections have received the most attention. They are mentioned here only briefly and are considered in more detail in the following chapter.

1. *Conduction* (also called "central") *aphasia*. The patient has severely impaired repetition, but fluent and paraphasic speech and writing and relatively intact comprehension of spoken and written language. The Wernicke area in the temporal lobe is putatively separated from the Broca area, presumably by a lesion in the arcuate fasciculus or external capsule or subcortical white matter. However, most often the lesion is in the supramarginal gyrus, as discussed in Chap. 23.
2. *Sympathetic apraxia in Broca's aphasia*. By destroying the origin of the fibers that connect the left and right motor association cortices, a lesion in the more anterior parts of the corpus callosum or the subcortical white matter underlying Broca area and contiguous frontal cortex causes an apraxia of commanded movements of the left hand (see Chap. 3 and earlier discussion).
3. *Pure word deafness*. Although the patient is able to hear and identify nonverbal sounds, there is loss of ability to discriminate speech sounds, i.e., to comprehend spoken language. The patient's speech may be paraphasic, presumably because of the inability to monitor his own speech. This defect has been attributed to a subcortical lesion of the left temporal lobe, spanning the Wernicke area and interrupting also those auditory fibers that cross in the corpus callosum from the opposite side. Thus, there is a failure to activate the left auditory language area (Wernicke area). Bilateral lesions of the auditory cortex have the same effect (see Chap. 23).
4. Furthermore, all of the syndromes that span the occipital and either parietal or temporal lobes are, in effect intrahemispheral disconnections in the stream of visual information as discussed earlier.

SPECIAL NEUROPSYCHOLOGIC TESTS

In the study of focal cerebral disease, there are two complementary approaches: the clinical-neurologic and the neuropsychologic. The first consists of the observation and recording of qualitative changes in behavior and performance and the identification of syndromes from which one may deduce the locus and nature of certain diseases. The second consists of recording a patient's performance on a variety of psychologic tests that have been standardized in a large population of age-matched normal individuals. These tests provide data that can be graded and treated statistically. An example is the *deterioration index*, deduced from the difference in performance on subtest items of the Wechsler Adult Intelligence Scale that hold up well in cerebral diseases (vocabulary, information, picture completion, and object assembly) and those that undergo impairment (digit span, similarities, digit symbol, and block design). A criticism of this index and others is the implicit assumption that cerebrocortical activity is a unitary function. However, it cannot be denied that certain psychometric scales reveal disease in certain parts of the cerebrum more than in others. These tests allow comparison of the patient's deficits from one point in the course of an illness to another. Walsh has listed the ones that he finds most valuable. In addition to the Wechsler

Adult Intelligence Scale, Wechsler Memory Scale, and an aphasia screening test, he recommends the following for quantifying particular psychologic abilities and skills:

I. *Frontal lobe disorders*
   A. Milan Sorting Test, Halstead Category Test, and Wisconsin Card-Sorting Test as tests of ability to abstract and shift paradigms
   B. The Porteus Maze Test, Reitan Trail-Making Test, and the recognition of figures in the Figure of Rey as tests of planning, regulating, and checking programs of action
   C. Benton's Verbal Fluency Test for estimating verbal skill and verbal regulation of behavior
II. *Temporal lobe disorders*
   A. Figure of Rey, Benton Visual Retention Test, Illinois Nonverbal Sequential Memory Test, Recurring Nonsense Figures of Kimura, and Facial Recognition Test as modality-specific memory tests
   B. Milner's Maze Learning Task and Lhermitte-Signoret amnesic syndrome tests for general retentive memory
   C. Seashore Rhythm Test, Speech-Sound Perception Test from the Halstead-Reitan battery, Environmental Sounds Test, and Austin Meaningless Sounds Test as measures of auditory perception
III. *Parietal lobe disorders*
   A. Figure of Rey, Wechsler Block Design and Object Assembly, Benton Figure Copying Test, Halstead-Reitan Tactual Performance Test, and Fairfield Block Substitution Test as tests of constructional praxis
   B. Several mathematical and logicogrammatical tests as tests of spatial synthesis
   C. Crossmodal association tests as tests of suprasensory integration
   D. Benson-Barton Stick Test, Cattell's Pool Reflection Test, and Money's Road Map Test, as tests of spatial perception and memory
IV. *Occipital lobe disorders*
   A. Color naming, color form association, and visual memory, as tests of visual perception; recognition of faces of prominent people, map drawing

It is the authors' opinion that the data obtained from the above tests should be used to supplement clinical observations. Taken alone, they cannot be depended upon for the localization of cerebral lesions.

References

Alajouanine T, Aubrey M, Pialoux P: *Les Grandes Activités du Lobe Temporale*. Paris, Masson, 1955.

Anderson SW, Damasio H, Damasio AR: A neural basis for collecting behavior in humans. *Brain* 128:201, 2005.

Andrew J, Nathan PW: Lesions of the anterior frontal lobes and disturbances of micturition and defaecation. *Brain* 87:233, 1964.

Assal G, Bindschaedler C: Délire et trouble auditif d'origine corticale. *Rev Neurol* 146:249, 1990.

Bailey P, von Bonin G: *The Isocortex in Man*. Urbana, University of Illinois Press, 1951.

Balint R: Seelenlahmung des "Schauens" optische Ataxie, raumliche Storung der Aufmerksamkeit. *Monatsschr Psychiatr Neurol* 25:51, 1909.

Bay E: Disturbances of visual perception and their examination. *Brain* 76:515, 1953.

Benson DF: *The Neurology of Thinking*. New York, Oxford University Press, 1994.

Benson DF, Geschwind N: Psychiatric conditions associated with focal lesions of the central nervous system, in Arieti S, Reiser MF (eds): *American Handbook of Psychiatry*. Vol 4. New York, Basic Books, 1975, pp 208–243.

Benton AL: The fiction of Gerstmann's syndrome. *J Neurol Neurosurg Psychiatry* 24:176, 1961.

Biemond A: The conduction of pain above the level of the thalamus opticus. *Arch Neurol Psychiatry* 75:231, 1956.

Bisiach E, Luzzatti C: Unilateral neglect of representational space. *Cortex* 14:129, 1978.

Blanke O, Landis T, Spinelli L, et al: Out-of-body experience and autoscopy of neurological origin. *Brain* 127:243, 2004.

Blumer D, Benson DF: Personality changes with frontal and temporal lobe lesions, in Blumer D, Benson DF (eds): *Psychiatric Aspects of Neurologic Disease*. New York, Grune & Stratton, 1975, pp 151–170.

Bodamer J: Die Prosopagnosie. *Arch Psychiatr Nervenkr* 179:6, 1947.

Botez TH, Olivier M: Parietal lobe syndrome, in Vinken PJ, Bruyn GW, Klawans HL (eds): *Handbook of Clinical Neurology*. Vol. 45. Amsterdam, Elsevier, 1985, pp 63–85.

Brain R: Visual disorientation with special reference to lesions of the right hemisphere. *Brain* 64:244, 1941.

Brickner RM: *The Intellectual Functions of the Frontal Lobes*. New York, Macmillan, 1936.

Brodal A: The hippocampus and the sense of smell. *Brain* 70:179, 1947.

Brodmann B: Vergleichende Lokalisationslehre der Grosshirnrinde in ihren Prinzipien dargestellt auf Grund des Zellenbaues, Johann Ambrosius Barth Verlag, Leipzig, Germany, 1909.

Brown JW: Frontal lobe syndromes, in Vinken PJ, Bruyn GW, Klawans HL (eds): *Handbook of Clinical Neurology*. Vol 45. Amsterdam, Elsevier, 1985, pp 23–43.

Bruns L. Uber Sturugen des Gleichgewiches bei stimhimtumoren. *Dtsch Med Wochenschr* 18:138, 1892.

Carmon A: Sequenced motor performance in patients with unilateral cerebral lesions. *Neuropsychologia* 9:445, 1971.

Carmon A, Benton AL: Tactile perception of direction and number in patients with unilateral cerebral disease. *Neurology* 19:525, 1969.

Chapman LF, Wolff HF: The cerebral hemispheres and the highest integrative functions of man. *Arch Neurol* 1:357, 1959.

Cogan DG: *Neurology of Ocular Muscles*. Springfield, Charles C Thomas, 1948, p 103.

Corkin S, Milner B, Rasmussen T: Effects of different cortical excisions on sensory thresholds in man. *Trans Am Neurol Assoc* 89:112, 1964.

Critchley M: *The Parietal Lobes*. London, Arnold, 1953.

Damasio A, Yamada T, Damasio H, et al: Central achromatopsia: Behavioral, anatomic, and physiologic aspects. *Neurology* 30:1064, 1980.

Damasio AR: Egas Moniz, pioneer of angiography and leucotomy. *Mt Sinai J Med* 42:502, 1975.

Damasio AR: The frontal lobes, in Heilman KM, Valenstein E (eds): *Clinical Neuropsychology*, 3rd ed. New York, Oxford University Press, 1993, pp 409–459.

Damasio AR, Damasio H, van Hoesen GW: Prosopagnosia: Anatomic basis and behavioral mechanisms. *Neurology* 32:331, 1982.

Damasio AR, van Hoesen GW: Emotional disturbances associated with focal lesions of the limbic frontal lobe, in Heilman KM, Satz P (eds): *Neuropsychology of Human Emotion*. New York, Guilford Press, 1983, pp 85–110.

Déjerine J, Mouzon J: Un nouveau type de syndrome sensitif corticale observé dans un cas de monoplégie corticale dissociée. *Rev Neurol* 28:1265, 1914–1915.

Denny-Brown D: The frontal lobes and their functions, in Feiling A (ed): *Modern Trends in Neurology*. New York, Hoeber-Harper, 1951, pp 13–89.

Denny-Brown D, Banker B: Amorphosynthesis from left parietal lesion. *Arch Neurol Psychiatry* 71:302, 1954.

Denny-Brown D, Chambers RA: Physiologic aspects of visual perception: 1. Functional aspects of visual cortex. *Arch Neurol* 33:219, 1976.

Denny-Brown D, Meyer JS, Horenstein S: Significance of perceptual rivalry resulting from parietal lesions. *Brain* 75:433, 1952.

De Renzi E, Gentilini M, Barbieri C: Auditory neglect. *J Neurol Neurosurg Psychiatry* 52:613, 1989.

DeRidder D, Van Laere K, Dupont P, Menovsky T, Van de Heyning P: Visualizing out-of-body experience in the brain. *N Engl J Med* 357:1829, 2007.

Dodge PR, Meirowsky AM: Tangential wounds of skull and scalp. *J Neurosurg* 9:472, 1952.

El-Hai J: *The Lobotomist*. Hoboken, NJ, John Wiley & Sons, 2005.

Feuchtwanger E: Die Functionen des Stirnhirns. *Monogr Neurol Psychiatr* 38:194, 1923.

Flechsig P: *Anatomie der menschlichen Gehirns und Ruckenmarks auf myelogenetischer Grundlage*. Leipzig, Germany, Thieme, 1920.

Fuster JM: *The Prefrontal Cortex*, 2nd ed. New York, Raven Press, 1989.

Gassel MM: Occipital lobe syndromes (excluding hemianopia), in Vinken PJ, Bruyn GW (eds): *Handbook of Clinical Neurology*. Vol 2. New York, American Elsevier, 1969, pp 640–679.

Gazzaniga MS: Cerebral specialization and interhemispheric communication. *Brain* 123:1293, 2000.

Geschwind N: Disconnexion syndromes in animals and man. I. *Brain* 88:237, 585, 1965.

Geschwind N, Quadfasel FA, Segarra J: Isolation of the speech area. *Neuropsychologia* 6:327, 1968.

Gloning I, Gloning K, Haff H: *Neuropsychological Symptoms and Syndromes in Lesions of the Occipital Lobes and Adjacent Areas*. Paris, Gauthier-Villars, 1968.

Gold K, Rabin PV: Isolated visual hallucinations and the Charles Bonnet syndrome: A review of the literature and presentation of six cases. *Compr Psychiatry* 30:90, 1989.

Goldstein K: The significance of the frontal lobes for mental performance. *J Neurol Psychopathol* 17:27, 1936.

Halstead WC: *Brain and Intelligence*. Chicago, University of Chicago Press, 1947.

Harlow JM: Quoted in Denny-Brown D: The frontal lobes and their functions, in Feiling A (ed): *Modern Trends in Neurology*. New York, Hoeber-Harper, 1951, p 65.

Head H, Holmes G: Sensory disturbances from cerebral lesions. *Brain* 34:102, 1911.

Hécaen H: Clinical symptomatology in right and left hemispheric lesions, in Mountcastle VB (ed): *Interhemispheric Relations and Cerebral Dominance*. Baltimore, MD, Johns Hopkins University Press, 1962, pp 215–263.

Heilman KA, Valenstein E: *Clinical Neuropsychology*, 4th ed. New York, Oxford University Press, 2003.

Henschen SE: *Klinische und Anatomische Beitrage zur Pathologie des Gehirns*. Vols 5–7. Stockholm, Nordiska Bokhandeln, 1920–1922.

Holmes G: Disturbances of visual orientation. *Br J Ophthalmol* 2:449, 506, 1918.

Holmes G, Horrax G: Disturbances of spatial orientation and visual attention with loss of stereoscopic vision. *Arch Neurol Psychiatry* 1:385, 1919.

Hubel D: Exploration of the primary visual cortex. *Nature* 299:515, 1982.

Hubel DH, Wiesel TN: Receptive fields, binocular interaction and functional architecture in the cat's visual cortex. *J Physiol* 160:106, 1962.

Jackson JH, Stewart P: Epileptic attacks with a warning of crude sensation. *Brain* 22:534, 1899.

Jacobsen CF: Functions of frontal association in primates. *Arch Neurol Psychiatry* 33:558, 1935.

Kaas JH: What if anything is S1? Organization of the first somatosensory area of cortex. *Physiol Rev* 63:206, 1983.

Karnath HO, Christ K, Hartje W: Decrease of contralateral neglect by neck muscle vibration and spatial orientation of trunk midline. *Brain* 116:383, 1993.

Kinsbourne M, Warrington EK: A disorder of simultaneous form perception. *Brain* 85:461, 1962.

Kinsbourne M, Warrington EK: The localizing significance of limited simultaneous visual form perception. *Brain* 86:697, 1963.

Kleist K: *Gehirnpathologie*. Leipzig, Germany, Barth, 1934.

Kleist K: *Sensory Aphasia and Amusia: The Myeloarchitectonic Basis*. Tr. by Fish FJ, Stanton JB. Oxford, UK, Pergamon Press, 1962.

Klüver H, Bucy PC: An analysis of certain effects of bilateral temporal lobectomy in the rhesus monkey with special reference to psychic blindness. *J Psychol* 5:33, 1938.

Landis T, Cummings JL, Benson DF, Palmer EP: Loss of topographic familiarity: An environmental agnosia. *Arch Neurol* 43:132, 1986.

Laplane D: La perte d'auto-activation psychique. *Rev Neurol* 146:397, 1990.

Laplane D, Talairach J, Meininger V, et al: Clinical consequences of corticectomies involving supplementary motor area in man. *J Neurol Sci* 34:301, 1977b.

Laplane D, Talairach J, Meininger V, et al: Motor consequences of motor area ablations in man. *J Neurol Sci* 31:29, 1977a.

Lassonde M, Jeeves MA (eds): *Callosal Agenesis: A Natural Split Brain?* New York, Plenum Press, 1994.

Levine DN: Prosopagnosia and visual object agnosia. *Brain Lang* 5:341, 1978.

Levine DN, Calvanio R: A study of the visual defect in verbal alexia-simultanagnosia. *Brain* 101:65, 1978.

Levine DN, Warach J, Farrah M: Two visual systems in mental imagery: Dissociation of "what" and "where" in imagery disorders due to bilateral posterior cerebral lesions. *Neurology* 35:1010, 1985.

Lhermitte F: Human autonomy and the frontal lobes: II. Patient behavior in complex and social situations—the "environmental dependency syndrome." *Ann Neurol* 19:335, 1986.

Lhermitte F: Utilization behavior and its relation to lesions of the frontal lobes. *Brain* 106:237, 1983.

Lhermitte J: L'hallucinose pédonculaire. *Encephale*, 27, 422, 1932.

Lilly R, Cummings JL, Benson DF, Frankel M: The human Klüver-Bucy syndrome. *Neurology* 33:1141, 1983.

Luria AR: Frontal lobe syndromes, in Vinken PJ, Bruyn GW (eds): *Handbook of Clinical Neurology*. Vol 2. Amsterdam, North-Holland, 1969, pp 725–759.

Luria AR: *Higher Cortical Functions in Man*. New York, Basic Books, 1966.

Luria AR: *The Working Brain*. London, Allen Lane, 1973.
MacLean PD: Chemical and electrical stimulation of hippocampus in unrestrained animals: II. Behavioral findings. *Arch Neurol Psychiatry* 78:128, 1957.
Marlowe WB, Mancall EL, Thomas JJ: Complete Klüver-Bucy syndrome in man. *Cortex* 11:53, 1975.
McCarthy RA, Warrington EK: Visual associative agnosia: A clinico-anatomical study of a single case. *J Neurol Neurosurg Psychiatry* 49:1233, 1986.
McFie J, Piercy MF, Zangwill OL: Visual-spatial agnosia associated with lesions of the right cerebral hemisphere. *Brain* 73:167, 1950.
Meadows JC: The anatomical basis of prosopagnosia. *J Neurol Neurosurg Psychiatry* 37:489, 1974a.
Meadows JC: Disturbed perception of colors associated with localized cerebral lesions. *Brain* 97:615, 1974b.
Merzenich MM, Brugge JF: Representation of the cochlear partition on the superior temporal plane of the macaque monkey. *Brain Res* 50:275, 1973.
Mesulam M-M: From sensation to cognition. *Brain* 121:1013, 1998.
Mesulam M-M (ed): *Principles of Behavioral and Cognitive Neurology*. New York, Oxford University Press, 2000.
Michel D, Laurent B, Convers P, et al: Douleurs corticales: Etude clinique, electrophysiologique, et topographique de 12 cas. *Rev Neurol* 146:405, 1990.
Miller NR: *Walsh and Hoyt's Clinical Neuro-ophthalmology*, 4th ed. Vol 1. Baltimore, MD, Williams & Wilkins, 1982, pp 83–103.
Milner B: Psychological defects produced by temporal lobe excision. *Res Publ Assoc Res Nerv Ment Dis* 36:244, 1956.
Milner B: Interhemispheric differences in the localization of psychological processes in man. *Br Med Bull* 27:272, 1971.
Mori E, Yamadori A: Rejection behavior: A human analogue of the abnormal behavior of Denny-Brown and Chambers' monkey with bilateral parietal ablation. *J Neurol Neurosurg Psychiatry* 52:1260, 1989.
Mort DJ, Malhotra P, Mannan K, et al: The anatomy of visual neglect. *Brain* 126:1986, 2003.
Nielsen JM: *Agnosia, Apraxia, Aphasia: Their Value in Cerebral Localization*, 2nd ed. New York, Hoeber, 1946.
Obrador S: Temporal lobotomy. *J Neuropathol Exp Neurol* 6:185, 1947.
Papez JW: A proposed mechanism of emotion. *Arch Neurol Psychiatry* 38:725, 1937.
Penfield W, Erickson TC: *Epilepsy and Cerebral Localization*. Springfield, IL, Charles C Thomas, 1941.
Penfield W, Faulk ME: The insula: Further observations of its function. *Brain* 78:445, 1955.
Penfield W, Rasmussen TP: *The Cerebral Cortex of Man*. New York, Macmillan, 1950.
Penfield W, Roberts L: *Speech and Brain Mechanisms*. Princeton, NJ, Princeton University Press, 1956.
Phillips S, Sangalang V, Sterns G: Basal forebrain infarction: A clinicopathologic correlation. *Arch Neurol* 44:1134, 1987.
Platel H, Price C, Baron JC, et al: The structural components of music perception. A functional anatomical study. *Brain* 120:229, 1997.
Polyak SL: *The Vertebrate Visual System*. Chicago, University of Chicago Press, 1957.
Porter R, Lemon R: *Corticospinal Function and Voluntary Movement*. London, Oxford University Press, 1994.
Reitan RW: Psychological deficits resulting from cerebral deficits in man, in Warren JM, Akert K (eds): *The Frontal Granular Cortex and Behavior*. New York, McGraw-Hill, 1964, chap 14.
Rizzo M, Robin DA: Simultanagnosia: A defect of sustained attention yields insights on visual information processing. *Neurology* 40:447, 1990.
Rizzo M, Vecera SP: Psychoanatomical substrates of Balint's syndrome. *J Neurol Neurosurg Psychiatry* 72:162, 2002.
Roland PE, Larsen B, Lassen NA, Skinhoj E: Supplementary motor area and other cortical areas in organization of voluntary movements in man. *J Neurophysiol* 43:118, 1980.
Ropper AH: Self-grasping: A focal neurological sign. *Ann Neurol* 12:575, 1982.
Rusconi E, Pinel P, Eger E, et al: A disconnection account of Gerstmann syndrome functional neuroanatomy evidence. *Ann Neurol* 66:654, 2009.
Rylander G: Personality changes after operations on the frontal lobes. *Acta Psychiatr Scand Suppl* 20:1–327, 1939.
Samson S, Zatorre RJ: Recognition memory for text and melody of songs after unilateral temporal lobe lesion: Evidence for dual encoding. *J Exp Psychol Learn Mem Cogn* 17:793, 1991.
Segarra JM, Quadfasel FA: Destroyed temporal lobe tips: Preserved ability to sing. *Proc VII Internat Congr Neurol* 2:377, 1961.
Semmes J, Weinstein S, Ghent L, Teuber HL: *Somatosensory Changes After Penetrating Brain Wounds in Man*. Cambridge, MA, Harvard University Press, 1960.
Seyffarth H, Denny-Brown D: The grasp reflex and instinctive grasp reaction. *Brain* 71:109, 1948.
Shankweiler DP: Performance of brain-damaged patients on two tests of sound localization. *J Comp Physiol Psychol* 54:375, 1961.
Sperry RW, Gazzaniga MS, Bogen JE: The neocortical commissures: Syndrome of hemisphere disconnection, in Vinken PJ, Bruyn GW (eds): *Handbook of Clinical Neurology*, Vol 4. Amsterdam, North-Holland, 1969, pp 273–290.
Stewart L, Von Kriegstein K, Warren JD, et al: Music and the brain: Disorders of musical listening. *Brain* 129:2533, 2006.
Stuss DT, Benson DF: *The Frontal Lobes*. New York, Raven Press, 1986.
Tanaka Y, Kamo T, Yoshida M, Yamadori A: So-called cortical deafness, clinical, neurophysiological, and radiological observations. *Brain* 114:2385, 1991.
Teunisse RJ, Cruysberg JR, Hoefnagels WH, et al: Visual hallucinations in psychologically normal people: Charles Bonnet syndrome. *Lancet* 347:794, 1996.
Tramo MJ, Bharucha JJ: Musical priming by the right hemisphere post-callosotomy. *Neuropsychologia* 29:313, 1991.
Tyler HR: Abnormalities of perception with defective eye movements (Balint's syndrome). Cortex 4:154, 1968.
von Economo C: *Encephalitis Lethargica: Its Sequelae and Treatment*. London, Oxford University Press, 1931.
Walsh KW: *Neuropsychology: A Clinical Approach*, 3rd ed. New York, Churchill Livingstone, 1994.
Weinberger LM, Grant FC: Visual hallucinations and their neuro-optical correlates. *Arch Ophthalmol* 23:166, 1941.
Weintraub S, Mesulam M-M: Right cerebral dominance in spatial attention. *Arch Neurol* 44:621, 1987.
Weiskrantz L, Warrington EK, Saunders MD, et al: Visual capacity in the blind field following a restricted occipital ablation. *Brain* 97:709, 1974.
Williams W: Temporal lobe syndromes, in Vinken PJ, Bruyn GW (eds): *Handbook of Clinical Neurology*, Vol. 2. Amsterdam, North-Holland, 1969, pp 700–724.
Wolpert I: Die Simultanagnosie-Storung der Gesamtauffassung. *Z Gesamte Neurol Psychiatr* 93:397, 1924.
Yakovlev PI: Motility, behavior, and the brain: Stereodynamic organization and neural co-ordinates of behavior. *J Nerv Ment Dis* 107:313, 1948.
Zatorre RJ, Evans AC, Meyer E: Neural mechanisms underlying melodic perception and memory for pitch. *J Neurosci* 14:1908, 1994.

23

Disorders of Speech and Language

Speech and language functions are of fundamental human significance, both in social interaction and in private intellectual life. When they are disturbed as a consequence of brain disease, the functional loss exceeds in many ways all others in gravity—even blindness, deafness, and paralysis. The neurologist is concerned with all derangements of speech and language, including those of reading and writing because they are almost invariably manifestations of disease of the brain.

Viewed broadly, language is the means of symbolic representation of objects, actions, and events and, therefore, the mirror of all higher mental activity. The internal manipulation of these symbols constitutes thinking and their retention is the substance of memory. In a narrower context, language is the means whereby patients communicate their complaints and problems to the physician and at the same time, the medium for all delicate interpersonal transactions. Consequently, any disease process that interferes with speech or the understanding of spoken words touches the very core of the physician–patient relationship. Finally, the study of language disorders and the development of language (taken up in Chap. 28) serve to illuminate the relationship between psychologic functions and the anatomy and physiology of the brain.

GENERAL CONSIDERATIONS

It has been remarked that as human beings, we owe our commanding position in the animal world to two faculties: First, the ability to develop and employ verbal symbols as a background for our own ideation and as a means of transmitting thoughts, by spoken and written word, and second, the remarkable facility in the use of our hands. One curious and provocative fact is that both language and manual dexterity (as well as praxis) have evolved in relation to particular aggregates of neurons and pathways in one cerebral hemisphere (the dominant one). This is a departure from most other localized neurophysiologic activities, which are organized according to a contralateral or bilateral and symmetrical plan. The dominance of one hemisphere, usually the left, emerges in brain development together with speech and the preference for the right hand, especially its use for writing. It follows that a lack of development or loss of cerebral dominance as a result of disease deranges both these traits, causing aphasia and apraxia.

There is abundant evidence that higher animals are able to communicate with one another by vocalization and gesture. However, the content of their communication is their feeling or reaction of the moment. This emotional language, as it is called, was studied by Charles Darwin, who noted that it undergoes increasing differentiation in the animal kingdom. Only in the chimpanzee do the first semblances of propositional language become recognizable. Indeed, there are distinct differences between the human and chimp versions of a gene called *FOXP2,* which has been linked to the ability to produce language, as noted in Chap. 28 (also see Balter). Another genetic influence on language has been found by Somerville and colleagues, who studied the locus implicated by a deletion in Williams syndrome and found that a duplication at this site caused a severe delay in the acquisition of expressive speech (see Chap. 38 for a discussion of the skills that are affected in Williams syndrome).

Instinctive patterns of emotional expression are, of course, also observed in human beings. They are the earliest modes of expression to appear (in infancy) and may have been the original forms of speech in primitive human beings. Moreover, the utterances we use to express joy, anger, and fear are retained even after destruction of all the language areas in the dominant cerebral hemisphere. The neural arrangement for this paralinguistic form of communication (intonation, exclamations, facial expressions, eye movements, body gestures), which subserves emotional expression, is bilateral and symmetrical and does not depend solely on the cerebrum. The experiments of Cannon and Bard demonstrated that emotional expression is possible in animals even after removal of both cerebral hemispheres provided that the diencephalon, particularly its hypothalamic part, remains intact. In the human infant, emotional expression is well developed at a time when much of the cerebrum is still immature.

Propositional, or symbolic language differs from emotional language in several ways. Instead of communicating feelings, it is the means of transferring ideas from one person to another, and it requires the substitution of a series of sounds or marks for objects, persons, and concepts. This is the essence of language.

It is not instinctive but learned and is therefore subject to all the modifying social and cultural influences of the environment. However, the learning process becomes possible only after the nervous system has attained a certain degree of maturation. Mature language function involves the comprehension, formulation, and transmission of ideas and feelings by the use of conventionalized verbal symbols, sounds, and gestures and their sequential ordering according to accepted rules of grammar. Facility in symbolic language, which is acquired over a period of 15 to 20 years, depends on maturation of the nervous system and on education. Many attempts have been made to crystallize the essential difference between human language and that of the higher primates that are able to communicate. Such distinctions, of course, bear on the definitions of language-dependent function, such as thinking, analysis, synthesis, and creativity. Beyond simply the complexity and range of symbolic representation and grammar available to humans in comparison to animals, Chomsky has proposed that the ability to frame recursive ideas (ones that refer to themselves by embedded phrases, such as: "John's sister's house") underlies creativity in human language and an infinite variety of sentences. This has been challenged but is an interesting concept.

Although speech and language are closely interwoven functions, they are not synonymous. Language refers to the production and comprehension of words whereas speech refers to the articulatory and phonetic aspects of verbal expression. A derangement of language function is always a reflection of an abnormality of the brain and, more specifically of the dominant cerebral hemisphere. A disorder of speech may have a similar origin, but not necessarily; it may be a result of abnormalities in different parts of the brain or to extracerebral mechanisms.

The profound importance of language may not be fully appreciated unless one reflects on the proportion of our time devoted to purely verbal pursuits. *External speech*, or exophasia, by which is meant the expression of thought by spoken or written words and the comprehension of the spoken or written words of others, is an almost continuous activity when human beings gather together. This contrasts with *inner speech*, or endophasia, i.e., the silent processes of thought and the formulation in our minds of unuttered words on which thought depends. The latter is almost incessant during our preoccupations, as we think always with words. Thought and language are thus inseparable. In learning to think, the child talks aloud to himself and only later learns to suppress the vocalization. Even adults may mutter subconsciously when pondering a difficult proposition. As Gardiner has remarked, any abstract thought can be held in mind only by the words or mathematic symbols denoting it. It is virtually impossible to comprehend what is meant by the word *religion*, for example, without the controlling and limiting consciousness of the word itself. "Words have thus become an integral part of the mechanism of our thinking and remain for ourselves and for others the guardians of our thoughts" (quoted from Brain). This is the reasoning that persuaded Head, Wilson, Goldstein, and others that any comprehensive theory of language must include explanations in terms not only of cerebral anatomy and physiology but also of the psycholinguistic processes that are involved.

Disorders of speech and language may be broadly characterized under four headings;

1. Loss or impairment of the production or comprehension of spoken or written language because of an acquired lesion of the brain. This is the condition called *aphasia* or *dysphasia*.
2. Disturbances of speech and language with diseases that globally affect higher-order mental function, i.e., confusion, delirium, mental retardation, and dementia. Speech and language functions are seldom lost in these conditions but are deranged as part of a general impairment of perceptual and intellectual functions (Chap. 21). Common to this category are certain special disorders of speech, such as mutism as outlined by Geschwind in his article on the "non-aphasic disorders of speech" (1964) and extreme perseveration (*palilalia* and *echolalia*), in which the patient repeats, parrot-like, sounds, words, and phrases (see further on). The odd constructs of language and other disorders of verbal communication of schizophrenics and some autistic individuals, extending to the production of meaningless phrases, neologisms, or jargon, are probably best included in this category as well but they derive from a disorder of thought.
3. A defect in articulation with intact mental functions, and comprehension of spoken and written language and normal syntax (grammatical construction of sentences). This is a pure motor disorder of the muscles of articulation and may be a result of flaccid or spastic paralysis, rigidity, repetitive spasms (stuttering), or ataxia. The terms *dysarthria* and *anarthria* are applied to this category of speech disorder.
4. An alteration or loss of voice because of a disorder of the larynx or its innervation—*aphonia* or *dysphonia*. Articulation and language are unaffected.

Chapter 28 fully considers the important but separable category of developmental disorders of speech and language.

ANATOMY OF THE LANGUAGE FUNCTIONS

The conventional teaching, based on correlations between various disorders of language and damage to particular areas of the brain, postulates four main language areas, situated in most persons in the left cerebral hemisphere (Fig. 23-1). The entire language zone that encompasses these areas is perisylvian, i.e., it borders the sylvian fissure. Two language areas are receptive and two are executive, i.e., the latter are concerned with the production (output) of language. The main receptive area, subserving the perception of spoken and probably of internal language, occupies the posterosuperior temporal area (the posterior portion of area 22) and Heschl gyri (areas 41 and 42). The posterior part of area 22 in the planum temporale is referred to as *Wernicke area*. A second receptive

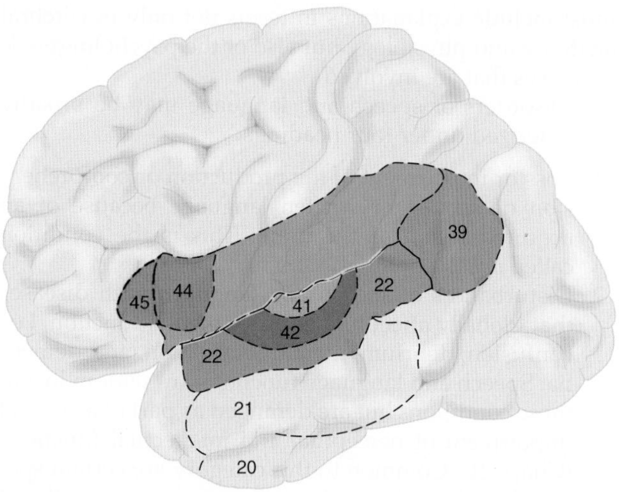

Figure 23-1. Diagram of the brain showing the classic language areas, numbered according to the scheme of Brodmann. The elaboration of speech and language probably depends on a much larger area of cerebrum, indicated roughly by all the shaded zones (see text). Note that areas 41 and 42, the primary auditory receptive areas, are shown on the lateral surface of the temporal lobe but extend to its superior surface, deep within the sylvian fissure.

area occupies the angular gyrus (area 39) in the inferior parietal lobule, anterior to the visual receptive areas. The supramarginal gyrus, which lies between these auditory and visual language "centers," and the inferior temporal region, just anterior to the visual association cortex, are probably part of the language apparatus as well. Here are located the integrative centers for cross-modal visual and auditory language functions.

The main executive, or output, region, situated at the posterior end of the inferior frontal convolution (Brodmann areas 44 and 45), is referred to as *Broca area* and is concerned with motor aspects of speech. In some models of language, visually perceived words are given expression in writing through a fourth language area, the so-called Exner writing area in the posterior part of the second frontal convolution. However, this latter concept is controversial in view of the fact that widely separated parts of the language zone may cause a disproportionate disorder of writing. In any case, there are two parallel systems for understanding the spoken word and producing speech and for the understanding of the written word and producing writing. They develop separately but are the integral components of the semantic system.

These sensory and motor language areas are intricately connected with one another by a rich network of nerve fibers, one large bundle of which, the arcuate fasciculus, passes through the isthmus of the temporal lobe and around the posterior end of the sylvian fissure; other connections may traverse the external capsule of the lenticular nucleus (subcortical white matter of the insula). Many additional corticocortical connections lead into the perisylvian zones and project from them to other parts of the brain. Of special importance for the production of speech are the short association fibers that join the Broca area with the lower rolandic cortex, which, in turn, innervates the muscles of the lips, tongue, pharynx, and larynx. The perisylvian language areas are also connected with the striatum and thalamus and with corresponding areas in the nondominant cerebral hemisphere through the corpus callosum and anterior commissure (see Fig. 22-6).

Having indicated the main regions involved with language, there remains considerable difference of opinion concerning the status of cortical language areas, and objection has been made to calling them "centers," for they do not represent histologically or circumscribed structures of constant function. Moreover, a neuroanatomist would not be able to distinguish the cortical language areas microscopically from the cerebral cortex that surrounds them.

Knowledge of the anatomy of language has come almost exclusively from the postmortem study of humans with focal brain diseases. Two major theories have emerged from these studies. One has subdivided the language zone into separate afferent (auditory and visual) receptive parts, connected by identifiable tracts to the executive (efferent–expressive) centers. Depending on the exact location of the lesions, a number of special syndromes are elicited. The other broad theory, advanced originally by Marie (he later claims to have changed his mind) and supported by Head, Wilson, Brain, and Goldstein, favored the idea of a single language mechanism, roughly localized in the opercular, or perisylvian region of the dominant cerebral hemisphere. The aphasia in any particular case was presumed to be a result of the summation of damage to input or output modalities relative to this central language zone. Undeniably, there is recognizable afferent and efferent localization within the perisylvian language area, as discussed above, but there is also an undifferentiated central integrative mass action, in which the degree of deficit is to a considerable extent influenced by the size of the lesion. In addition, a strict division of aphasias into expressive and receptive, while still a strong practical concept, is not fully borne out by clinical observation. Nevertheless, there are several localizable language functions in the perisylvian cortex.

Carl Wernicke more than any other person must be credited with the anatomic–psychologic scheme upon which many contemporary ideas of aphasia rest. Earlier, Paul Broca (1865), and, even before him, Dax (1836), made the fundamental observations that a lesion of the insula and the overlying operculum deprived a person of speech and such lesions were always in the left hemisphere. Wernicke's thesis was that there were two major anatomic loci for language: (1) an anterior locus, in the posterior part of the inferior frontal lobe (Broca's area), in which were contained the "memory images" of speech movements, and (2) the insular region and adjoining parts of the posterior perisylvian cortex, in which were contained the images of sounds. (Meynert had already shown that aphasia could occur with lesions in the temporal lobe, the Broca area being intact.) Wernicke believed that the fibers between these regions ran in the insula and mediated the reflex arc between the heard and spoken word. Later, Wernicke came to accept von Monakow's view that the connecting fibers ran around the posterior end of the sylvian fissure, in the arcuate fasciculus. Wernicke gave a comprehensive description of the receptive, or sensory, aphasia that now bears his name. The four main features he pointed out were (1) a disturbance of comprehension of spoken language and (2) of written language (alexia), (3) agraphia, and (4) fluent paraphasic speech. In Broca's aphasia, by contrast, comprehension was intact, but the patient was mute or employed only a few simple words. Wernicke also theorized that a lesion interrupting the connecting fibers between the two cortical speech areas would leave the patient's comprehension undisturbed but would prevent the intact sound images from exerting an influence on the choice of words. Wernicke proposed that this variety of aphasia be called *Leitungsaphasie*, or *conduction aphasia* (called *central aphasia* by Kurt Goldstein and *deep aphasia* by Martin and Saffran). Careful case analyses since the time of Broca and Wernicke have borne out these associations between a receptive (Wernicke) type of aphasia and lesions in the posterior perisylvian region and between a predominantly (Broca) motor aphasia and lesions in the posterior part of the inferior frontal lobe and the adjacent, insular, and opercular regions of the frontal cortex. We have certainly encountered cases that conform to the Wernicke model of conduction aphasia; the lesion in these cases may lie in the parietal operculum, involving the white matter deep to the supramarginal gyrus, where it presumably interrupts the arcuate fasciculus and posterior insular subcortex (the issue of conduction aphasia is discussed further on).

How these regions of the brain are organized into separable but interactive modules, resulting in the complex behavior of which we make daily use in interpersonal communication, is still being studied by linguists and cognitive neuropsychologists. They have dissected language into its most basic elements—phonemes (the smallest units of sound recognizable as language), morphemes (the smallest meaningful units of a word), graphemes, lexical and semantic elements (words and their meanings), and syntax (sentence structure). In general, as a restatement of the Wernicke-Broca scheme, *phonologic speech output difficulties are derived from left frontal lesions; semantic–comprehension difficulties are the result of left temporal lesions; and alexia and agraphia are associated with inferior parietal lesions*. These "modules" of language have been diagrammed by psycholinguists as a series of boxes and are connected to one another by arrows to indicate the flow of information and the manner in which they influence the spoken output of language. "Boxologies," as they are called, are consistent with current cognitive theory, which views language functions as the result of synchronized activity in vast neuronal networks made up of many cerebrocortical regions and their interconnecting pathways (Damasio and Damasio, 1989).

On the other hand, despite this level of theoretical sophistication, attempts to delineate the anatomy of speech and language disorders by means of conventional brain imaging techniques in aphasic patients have been somewhat disappointing. In early studies using CT, LeCours and Lhermitte were unable to establish a consistent correspondence between the type of aphasia and the location of the demonstrable lesion. Similarly, Willmes and Poeck, in a retrospective study of 221 aphasic patients, failed to find an unequivocal association between the type of aphasia and the CT localization of the lesion. These poor correlations are in part related to the timing and the crudity of the CT scan. MRI scans performed soon after a stroke show somewhat more consistent correlations between the type of language disturbance and the location of lesions in the perisylvian cortex, but lesions in identical locations may produce functionally different language disorders. Functional magnetic resonance imaging (fMRI), while subjects are engaged in language production and comprehension, provides an additional perspective for understanding the language process, but so far only the broadest rules of localization can be confirmed. Studies of blood flow and topographic physiology during the acts of reading and speaking, while generally affirming nineteenth-century models of language, have shown widespread activation of Wernicke and Broca areas, as well as of the supplementary motor area and areas of the opposite hemisphere (see Price).

Although localization of the lesion that produces aphasia is in most instances roughly predictable from the clinical deficit, there are wide variations. The inconsistency has several explanations, one being that the net effect of any lesion depends not only on its locus and extent but also on the degree of cerebral dominance, i.e., on the degree to which the nondominant hemisphere assumes language function after damage to the dominant one. According to this view, a left-sided lesion has less effect on language function if cerebral dominance is poorly established than if dominance is strong. In all likelihood, the variability between patients in lesion location and the characteristics of aphasia has to do with subtle differences in the organization of the language cortices. Another explanation invokes the poorly understood concept that individuals differ in the ways in which they acquire language as children. This is believed to play a role in making available alternative means for accomplishing language tasks when the method initially learned has been impaired through brain disease. The extent to which improvement of aphasia represents "recovery" of function or generation of new modes of response has not been settled.

CEREBRAL DOMINANCE AND ITS RELATION TO LANGUAGE AND HANDEDNESS

The functional supremacy of one cerebral hemisphere is fundamental to language function. There are many ways of determining that the left side of the brain is dominant: (1) by the loss of speech that occurs with disease in parts of the left hemisphere and its preservation with lesions involving corresponding parts of the right hemisphere;

(2) by preference for and greater facility in the use of the right hand, foot, and eye; (3) by the arrest of speech with a focal seizure or with electrical or magnetic stimulation of the anterior (left) language area; (4) by the injection of sodium amytal or an equivalent drug into the left internal carotid artery (the Wada test—a procedure that produces mutism for a minute or two, followed by misnaming, including perseveration and substitution; misreading; and paraphasic speech); (5) by dichotic listening, in which different words or phonemes are presented simultaneously to the two ears (yielding a right ear–left hemisphere advantage); (6) by observing increases in cerebral blood flow during language processing; and (7) by lateralization of speech and language functions following commissurotomy.

Language hemisphere dominance is ostensibly related to hand dominance, but this is more of a supposition than a statement. Approximately 90 to 95 percent of the general population is right-handed; i.e., they innately choose the right hand for intricate, complex acts and are more skillful with it. The preference is more complete in some persons than in others. Most individuals are neither completely right-handed nor completely left-handed but strongly favor one hand for more complicated tasks. The reason for hand preference is not fully understood. There is strong evidence of a hereditary factor but the mode of inheritance is uncertain. Learning is also a factor; many left-handed children are shifted at an early age to right (shifted sinistrals) because it had been a perceived handicap to be left-handed in a right-handed world. Most right-handed persons, when obliged to use only one eye (looking through a keyhole, gun sight, telescope, etc.), sight with the right eye, and it has been stated that eye preference coincides with hand preference. Even if true, this still does not account for hemispheral dominance. It is, however, noteworthy that handedness develops simultaneously with language. The most that can be said at present is that localization of language and a preference for one eye, hand, and foot, as well as praxis, are all manifestations of some fundamental, partly inherited tendency for hemispheric specialization.

There are slight but definite anatomic differences between the dominant and the nondominant cerebral hemispheres. Yakovlev and Rakic, in a study of infant brains, observed that the corticospinal tract coming from the left cerebral hemisphere contains more fibers and decussates higher than the tract from the right hemisphere. More pertinent to language, the *planum temporale*, the region on the superior surface of the temporal lobe posterior to Heschl gyri and extending to the posterior end of the sylvian fissure, is slightly larger on the left in 65 percent of brains and larger on the right in only 11 percent (Geschwind and Levitsky). LeMay and Culebras noted in cerebral angiograms that the left sylvian fissure is longer and more horizontal than the right and that there is a greater mass of cerebral tissue in the area of the left temporoparietal junction. CT scanning has shown the right occipital horn to be smaller than the left, indicative perhaps of a greater right-sided development of visuospatial connections. Also, subtle cytoarchitectonic asymmetries of the auditory cortex and posterior thalamus have been described; these and other biologic aspects of cerebral dominance have been reviewed by Geschwind and Galaburda particularly as they relate to developmental dyslexia (Chap. 28).

Left-handedness may result from disease of the left cerebral hemisphere in early life; this probably accounts for its higher incidence among the mentally retarded and brain injured. Presumably, the neural mechanisms for language then come to be represented during early development in the right cerebral hemisphere. Handedness and cerebral dominance may fail to develop in some individuals; this is particularly true in certain families. In these individuals, defects in reading as well as the faults of stuttering, mirror writing, and general clumsiness are frequent. In right-handed individuals, aphasia is almost invariably related to a left cerebral lesion; aphasia in such individuals as a result of purely right cerebral lesions ("crossed aphasia") is very rare, occurring in only 1 percent of cases (Joanette et al). Cerebral language dominance in ambidextrous and left-handed persons is not nearly so uniform. In a large series of left-handed patients with acquired aphasia, 60 percent had lesions confined to the left cerebral hemisphere (Goodglass and Quadfasel). Furthermore, in the relatively rare case of aphasia caused by a right cerebral lesion, the patient is nearly always left-handed and the language disorder is less severe and less enduring than in right-handed patients with comparable lesions in the left hemisphere (Gloning; Subirana). Taken together, these findings suggest a bilateral—albeit unequal—representation of language functions in non–right-handed patients. This has been affirmed by the Wada test; Milner and colleagues found evidence of bilateral speech representation in 32 (about 15 percent) of 212 consecutive left-handed patients.

The undoubted language capacities of the nondominant hemisphere have been documented by lesional neurology. In cases of congenital absence (or surgical section) of the corpus callosum, which permits the testing of each hemisphere, there has been virtually no demonstrable language function of the right hemisphere. However, Levine and Mohr found that the nondominant hemisphere retains a limited capacity to produce oral speech after extensive damage to the dominant hemisphere; their patient recovered the ability to sing, recite, curse, and utter one- or two-word phrases, all of which were completely abolished by a subsequent right hemisphere infarction. The fact that varying amounts of language function may remain after dominant hemispherectomy in adults with glioma also suggests a definite though limited capacity of the adult nondominant hemisphere for language production. Kinsbourne's observations of the effect of sodium amytal injections into the right-hemispheral arteries of patients who are aphasic from left-sided lesions make the same point.

Despite its minimal contribution to the purely linguistic or propositional aspects of language, the right hemisphere does have a role in the implicit communication of emotion through the subtleties of propositional language. These modulative aspects of language are subsumed under the term *prosody*, by which is meant the melody of speech, its intonation, inflection, and pauses, all of which have emotional overtones. The prosodic components of speech and the gestures that accompany them enhance the meaning of the spoken word and endow speech with its richness and vitality. The related issue of an individual's accent, which carries such a strong regional identity and is acquired early in life, may also have an anatomic basis, but one that remains obscure (see later comments on the "Foreign Accent Syndrome").

Many diseases and focal cerebral lesions mute or reduce the prosody of speech, the most dramatic examples being the hypophonic monotone of Parkinson disease and the effortful utterances of Broca's aphasia. Largely through the work of Ross, it has become apparent that prosody is also greatly disordered in patients with strokes involving portions of the nondominant hemisphere that mirror the language areas of the left hemisphere. In these cases, there is impairment both of comprehension and of production of the emotional content of speech and its accompanying gestures. A prospective study of middle cerebral artery infarctions by Darby corroborated this view: *aprosodia*, as it has come to be called, was present only in those patients with lesions in the territory of the inferior division of the right middle cerebral artery. The deficit was most prominent soon after the stroke and was not found with lacunar lesions. In our patients, using bedside tests, we have had difficulty in appreciating aprosodia as a result solely of right perisylvian lesions, and in most cases, the damage has been more widespread.

There has been recent interest in a role for the cerebellum in language function, based partly on observations in the Williams syndrome, in which mental retardation is associated with a preservation of language skills that is sometimes striking in degree (Chap. 38). In this disease, the cerebellum is spared in the face of greatly diminished volume of the cerebral hemispheres (see Leiner et al). Some studies of cerebral blood flow also implicate the cerebellum in various language functions; based on our clinical experience, however, we would judge any language deficits from cerebellar disease to be subtle or nonexistent. Dysarthria, of course, is common with cerebellar disease.

APPROACH TO THE PATIENT WITH LANGUAGE DISORDERS

In the investigation of aphasia, it is first necessary to inquire into the patient's native language, handedness, and previous level of literacy and education. It has been surmised that following the onset of aphasia, individuals who had been fluent in more than one language (polyglots) improved more quickly in their native language than in a subsequently acquired one (a derivative of the Ribot law of retained distant memory). This rule seems to hold if the patient is not truly fluent in the more recently acquired language or has not used it for a long time. More often, the language most used before the onset of the aphasia will recover first (Pitres law). Usually, if adequate testing is possible, more or less the same aphasic abnormalities are found in both the first and the more recently acquired language. Dementing illnesses such as Alzheimer disease, however, do cause increasing use of the first acquired language.

Many naturally left-handed children are trained to use the right hand for writing; therefore, in determining handedness, one must ask which hand is preferred for throwing a ball, threading a needle, sewing, or using a tennis racket or hammer, and which eye is used for sighting a target with a rifle or other instrument. It is important, before beginning the examination, to determine whether the patient is alert and can participate reliably in testing, as accurate assessment of language depends on these factors.

One should quickly ascertain whether the patient has other gross signs of a cerebral lesion such as hemiplegia, facial weakness, homonymous hemianopia, or cortical sensory loss. When a constellation of these major neurologic signs is present, the aphasic disorder is usually of the total (global) type. A right brachiofacial paralysis aligns with Broca's aphasia; in contrast, a restricted right hemianopia or quadrantanopia is a common accompaniment of Wernicke's aphasia, and hemiparesis is absent. Dyspraxia of limbs and speech musculature in response to spoken commands or to visual mimicry is generally associated with Broca's aphasia, but sometimes with Wernicke's aphasia. Homonymous hemianopia without motor weakness tends often to be linked to pure word blindness, to alexia with or without agraphia, and to anomic aphasia.

The bedside analysis of aphasic disorders that we find most useful entails the systematic testing of six aspects of language function: *conversational speech, comprehension, repetition, reading, writing,* and *naming*. Simply engaging the patient in conversation permits assessment of the motor aspects of speech (praxis and prosody), fluency, and language formulation. If the disability consists mainly of sparse, laborious, nonfluent speech, it suggests, of course, Broca's aphasia, and this possibility can be pursued further by tests of repeating from dictation and by special tests of praxis of the oropharyngeal muscles. Fluent but empty paraphasic speech with impaired comprehension is indicative of Wernicke's aphasia. Impaired comprehension but perfectly normal formulated speech and intact ability to read suggest the rare syndrome of pure word deafness.

When conversation discloses virtually no abnormalities, other tests may still be revealing. The most important of these are reading, writing, repetition, and naming. Reading aloud single letters, words, and text may disclose the dissociative syndrome of pure word blindness. Except for this syndrome and isolated mutism (aphemia; see earlier), writing is disturbed in all forms of aphasia. Literal and verbal paraphasic errors may appear in milder cases of Wernicke's aphasia as the patient reads aloud from a text or from words in the examiner's handwriting. Similar errors appear even more frequently when the patient is asked to explain the text, read aloud, or give an explanation in writing.

Testing the patient's ability to repeat spoken language is a simple and important maneuver in the evaluation of aphasic disorders. As with other tests of aphasia, it may be necessary to increase the complexity of the test from digits and simple words to complex words, phrases, and sentences to disclose the full disability. Defective repetition occurs in all the major forms of aphasia (Broca's, Wernicke's, and global) because of lesions in the perisylvian language areas. The patient may be unable to repeat what is said to him, despite relatively adequate comprehension—the hallmark of conduction aphasia. Contrariwise, normal repetition in an aphasic patient (transcortical aphasia) indicates that the perisylvian area is largely intact. In fact, the tendency to repeat may be excessive (echolalia). Preserved repetition is also characteristic of anomic aphasia and occurs occasionally with subcortical lesions. Disorders confined to naming, other language functions (reading, writing, spelling) being adequate, are diagnostic of amnesic, or anomic, aphasia and referable usually to lower temporal lobe lesions.

These deficits can be quantified by the use of any one of several examination procedures. Those of Goodglass and Kaplan (Boston Diagnostic Aphasia Examination [BDAE]) and of Kertesz (Western Aphasia Battery [WAB]) are the most widely used in the United States. The use of these procedures will enable one to predict the type and localization of the lesion in approximately two-thirds of the patients, which is not much better than detailed bedside examination. Using these tests, aphasia of the Broca, Wernicke, conduction, global, and anomic types accounted for 392 of 444 unselected cases studied by Benson.

CLINICAL VARIETIES OF APHASIA

In analyzing disorders of speech and language in the clinic or at the bedside, the first objective is to separate *dysarthria*, or slurred speech with preservation of language, from a genuine impairment in language function, *aphasia*. Here, we offer a practical approach to aphasia. Dysarthria is addressed in a later section. To recapitulate, the features of a language disorder that are used to advantage by the examiner in determining the type of aphasia are:

- natural sounding fluency, including normal cadence, the use of prepositions, and correct grammar;
- comprehension of language;
- the proper selection, use, and relationships between words;
- naming of displayed objects;
- the ability to repeat in comparison to spontaneous speech;
- reading; and
- writing

This type of systematic examination will enable one to decide whether a patient has a predominantly: (i) *motor* or *Broca's aphasia*, sometimes called "expressive," "anterior," or "nonfluent" aphasia; (ii) *sensory* or *Wernicke's aphasia*, referred to also as "receptive," "posterior," or "fluent" aphasia; (iii) a *total* or *global aphasia*, with loss of all or nearly all speech and language functions; (iv) *transcortical aphasia*, meaning a motor or sensory aphasia with preserved repetition; or (v) one of the *disconnection language syndromes*, such as conduction aphasia, word deafness (auditory verbal agnosia), and word blindness (visual verbal agnosia or alexia). In addition, there is a condition of mutism, or a complete absence of verbal output, but this syndrome does not permit one to predict the exact locus of the lesion. *Anomia* (also called *nominal* or *amnesic* aphasia, meaning loss of naming ability) and the impaired ability to communicate by writing (*agraphia*) are found to some degree in practically all types of aphasia. As for agraphia, it rarely exists alone. Table 23-1 summarizes these main aphasic syndromes, which are described below. Even though these descriptions are based largely on deficits from vascular occlusion, they serve well in most circumstances of focal brain disease that cause language disturbances.

Broca's Aphasia

Broca's aphasia conforms to a primary deficit in language output and speech production with relative preservation of comprehension. There is a wide range of variation in the severity of the motor speech deficit, from the mildest poverty of speech and minimal dysarthria with entirely intact comprehension and ability to write (so-called Broca area aphasia; "mini-, or baby-Broca"), to a complete loss of all means of lingual, phonetic, written, and gestural communication. Because the muscles that can no longer be used in speaking may still function in other acts, they are not paralyzed. The term *apraxia* has been imprecisely applied to this deficit in oro-buccal-lingual use (it does not represent the loss of a previously learned ability) but there are accompanying apractic deficits of the orofacial apparatus as noted below.

In the most advanced form of the syndrome, patients lose all power of speaking. Not a word can be uttered in conversation, in attempting to read aloud, or in trying to repeat words that are heard. One might suspect that in this mutism the lingual and phonatory apparatus is paralyzed, until patients are observed to have no difficulty chewing, swallowing, clearing the throat, crying or shouting, and even vocalizing without words. Occasionally, the words *yes* and *no* can be uttered, usually in the correct context. Or patients may repeat a few stereotyped utterances over and over again, as if compelled to do so, a disorder referred to as *monophasia* (Critchley), *recurring utterance* (Hughlings Jackson), *verbal stereotypy*, or verbal automatism. If speech is possible at all, certain habitual expressions, such as "hi," "fine, thank you," or "good morning," seem to be the easiest to elicit, and the words of well-known songs may be sung hesitantly, or counting by consecutive numbers may remain facile. When angered or excited, an expletive may be uttered, thus emphasizing the fundamental distinction between propositional and emotional speech. The patient recognizes

Table 23-1

THE MAIN APHASIC SYNDROMES

TYPE OF APHASIA	SPEECH	COMPREHENSION	REPETITION	ASSOCIATED SIGNS	LOCALIZATION[a]
Broca's	Nonfluent, effortful, agrammatical, paucity of output but transmits ideas	Relatively preserved	Impaired	Right arm and face weakness	Frontal suprasylvian
Wernicke's	Fluent, voluble, well articulated but lacking meaning	Greatly impaired	None	Hemi- or quadrantanopia, no paresis	Temporal, infrasylvian including angular and supramarginal gyri
Conduction	Fluent	Relatively preserved	None	Usually none	Supramarginal gyrus or insula
Global	Scant, nonfluent	Very impaired	None	Hemiplegia usual	Large perisylvian or separate frontal and temporal
Transcortical motor	Nonfluent	Good	Largely preserved	Variable	Anterior or superior to Broca's area
Transcortical sensory	Fluent	Impaired as Wernicke's	Largely preserved	Variable	Surrounding Wernicke's area
Pure word deafness	Mildly paraphasic or normal	Impaired	Impaired	None or quadrantanopia	Bilateral (or left) middle of superior temporal gyrus
Pure word blindness (and alexia without agraphia)	Normal but unable to read aloud	Normal	Normal	Right hemianopia; unable to read own writing	Calcarine and white matter or callosum (or angular gyrus)
Pure word mutism (aphemia)	Mute, but able to write	Normal	None	None	Region of Broca's area
Anomic aphasia	Isolated word-finding difficulty	Normal various sites	Normal	Variable	Deep temporal lobe

[a]Lesion in dominant (left) hemisphere unless noted.
Source: Adapted by permission from Damasio AR: Aphasia. *N Engl J Med* 326:531, 1992.

his verbal ineptitude and mistakes. Repeated failures in speech cause demonstrations of exasperation.

As a result of damage to the adjacent prerolandic motor area, the arm and lower part of the face are usually weak on the right side. The tongue may early on deviate away from the lesion, i.e., to the right, and be slow and awkward in rapid movements. For a time, despite the relative preservation of auditory comprehension and the ability to read, commands to purse, smack, or lick the lips, or to blow and whistle and make other purposeful orolingual and facial movements are poorly executed, which signifies that an apraxia has extended to certain acts involving the lips, tongue, and pharynx. In these circumstances, imitation of the examiner's actions is performed better than spontaneous execution of acts on command. Self-initiated actions and spontaneous emotional expressions of the face, by contrast, may be normal or better preserved. From imaging findings in patients with this type of speech, it is apparent that the coordination of orolingual movements that are responsible for articulation takes place in the left anterior insular cortex (see Dronkers) rather than primarily in the Broca area. Positron emission tomography (PET) shows activation of the insular region as well as of the lateral premotor cortex and the anterior pallidum during repetition of single words (Wise et al).

In the milder forms of Broca's aphasia and in the recovery phase of the severe form, patients are able to speak aloud to some degree, but the normal cadence and parsing of speech is choppy or lacking. Words are uttered slowly and laboriously, and enunciated poorly. Missing is the normal inflection, intonation, phrasing of words in a series, and pacing of word utterances. The overall impression is one of a *lack of fluency*, a term that has come to be almost synonymous with aphasias that derive from damage in and around the Broca area (nonfluent aphasia). This labored, uninflected speech stands in contrast to the fluent speech of Wernicke's aphasia described later, but there are exceptions in which nonfluency extends to Wernicke's aphasia.

Language is clearly affected in a restricted way in Broca's aphasia. Speech is sparse (10 to 15 words per minute as compared with the normal 100 to 115 words per minute) and consists mainly of nouns, transitive verbs, or important adjectives; phrase length is abbreviated and many of the small words (articles, prepositions, conjunctions) are omitted, giving the speech an abbreviated, telegraphic character (so-called agrammatism). The substantive content of the patient's language permits the crude communication of ideas, sometimes despite gross expressive difficulties. Repetition of the examiner's spoken language is as abnormal as the patient's own speech.

If a patient with nonfluent Broca's aphasia has no difficulty in repetition, the condition is termed *transcortical motor aphasia* (see further on). Furthermore, a true defect in language production is evidenced by impairment in the content of written words and sentences. Should the right hand be paralyzed, the patient cannot print with the left one, and if the right hand is spared, the patient fails as miserably in writing to dictation or replying to questions in written form. Letters are malformed and words misspelled. Although writing to dictation is impossible, letters and words can still be copied. The dysgraphia usually corresponds in degree to the severity of the spoken disturbance, but there are exceptions in which one is far more affected.

The comprehension of spoken and written language, though seemingly normal under casual conditions, is usually slightly defective in the full syndrome of Broca's aphasia and will break down under stringent testing, especially when novel or complicated material is introduced. The naming of objects and particularly parts of objects may be faulty in articulation, but the proper name can be chosen from a list. These are the most variable and controversial aspects of Broca's aphasia, as in some patients with a loss of motor speech and agraphia as a result of cerebral infarction, the understanding of spoken and written language may be normal. Mohr and colleagues (1978) have pointed out that in such patients an initial mutism is usually replaced by a rapidly improving dyspraxic and effortful articulation (a "mini-Broca's aphasia," in his terms), leading to complete recovery. The lesion in such cases is restricted to a zone in and immediately around the posterior part of the inferior frontal convolution (the latter being the Broca area per se). Mohr and colleagues (1978) have stressed the distinction between this relatively mild and restricted type of motor speech disorder and the more complex syndrome that is traditionally referred to as *Broca's aphasia*.

The lesion in the major form of Broca's aphasia subsumes a much larger area than the inferior frontal gyrus and includes the subjacent white matter and even the head of the caudate nucleus and putamen (Fig. 23-2), the anterior insula, and frontoparietal operculum. (The term *operculum* refers to the cortex that borders the sylvian fissure and covers or forms a lid over the insula, or island of Reil.) In other words, the lesion in the usual form of Broca's aphasia extends well beyond the so-called Broca area (Brodmann areas 44 and 45). Furthermore, persistence of Broca's aphasia is associated with the larger type of lesion illustrated in Fig. 23-2.

It is interesting historically that in one of Broca's original patients, whose expressive language had been limited to a few verbal stereotypes for 10 years before his death, inspection of the surface of the brain (the brain was never cut, although CT scans have since been made) disclosed an extensive lesion encompassing the left insula; the frontal, central, parietal operculum and included even part of the inferior parietal lobe posterior to the sylvian fissure. Wernicke area was spared, refuting a prediction made at the time by Marie. Inexplicably, Broca attributed the aphasic disorder to the lesion of the frontal operculum alone, and ignored the rest of the

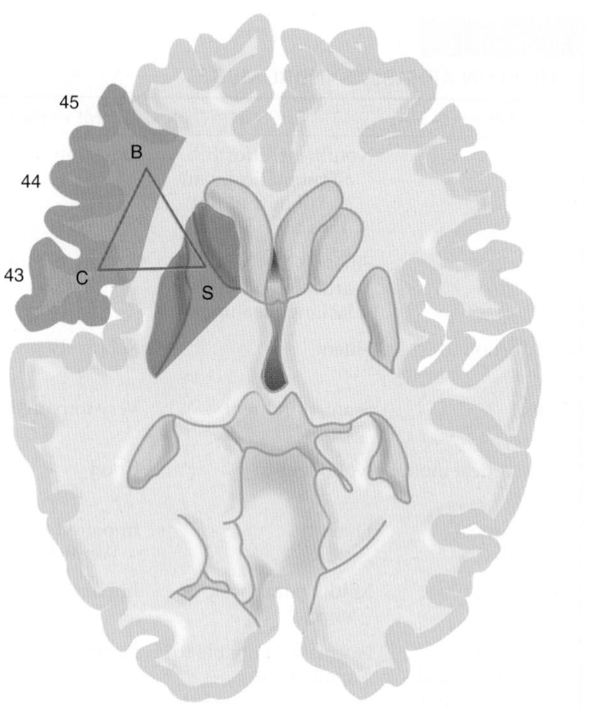

Figure 23-2. Cerebral structures concerned with language output and articulation. Broca's area; pre- and postcentral gyri; striatum. Areas 43, 44, and 45 are Brodmann cytoarchitectonic areas. A lesion in any one of the components of this output network (*B*, *C*, or *S*) can produce a mild and transient Broca's aphasia. Large lesions, damaging all three components, produce severe, persistent Broca's aphasia with sparse, labored, agrammatic speech but well-preserved comprehension. (Illustration courtesy of Dr. Andrew Kertesz.)

lesion, which he considered to be a later spreading effect of the stroke. Perhaps he was influenced by the prevailing opinion of the time (1861) that articulation was a function of the inferior parts of the frontal lobes. The fact that Broca's name later became attached to a discrete part of the inferior frontal cortex helped to entrench the idea that Broca's aphasia is equated with a lesion in the Broca's area. However, as pointed out earlier, a lesion confined only to this area gives rise to a relatively modest and transient motor speech disorder (Mohr et al) or to no disorder of speech at all (Goldstein).

Motor speech disorders, both severe Broca's aphasia and the more restricted and transient types, are most often a result of vascular lesions. Embolic stroke in the territory of the upper (rolandic, superior) division of the middle cerebral artery is the most frequent type and results in an abrupt onset of aphasia. Small strokes may give way to rapid improvement (hours to days); contrariwise, infarctions that extend beyond the central Broca region at times produce a more severe clinical syndrome than might be anticipated from the size of the lesion. It is these latter strokes, especially if the underlying frontal white matter is damaged, that tend to cause lasting speech difficulty. Because of the territory that is supplied by the superior branch of the middle cerebral artery, strokes that cause Broca's aphasia are usually associated with right-sided faciobrachial paresis (face, proximal arm, and hand) as described earlier, and sometimes with a left-sided manual-brachial apraxia (sympathetic apraxia as described in Chap. 3). Atherosclerotic thrombosis, primary or metastatic tumor, subcortical hypertensive, traumatic, or anticoagulant-induced hemorrhage, and seizure, should they involve the appropriate parts of the motor language cortex, may also declare themselves by a Broca's aphasia.

A closely related syndrome, *pure word mutism* (*aphemia*), causes the patient to be wordless (mute) but leaves inner speech intact and writing undisturbed. Anatomically, this is believed to be in the nature of a disconnection of the motor cortex (Broca area) for speech from lower centers and is described with the dissociative speech syndromes discussed further on in this chapter.

Wernicke's Aphasia

This syndrome comprises two main elements: (1) impairment in the comprehension of speech—basically an inability to perceive word elements, both spoken and written, and (2) a relatively fluent but paraphasic speech (further defined below). The first of these grossly affects the internal stream of conversation and its attendant manipulation of symbolic language and causes a restricted form of confusion. The defect in language is manifest further by a variable inability to repeat spoken and written words. The location of the lesion in cases of Wernicke's aphasia is the left superior lateral temporal lobe near the primary auditory cortex. The involvement of visual association areas or their separation from the primary visual cortices is a common accompaniment that is reflected in an inability to read (alexia).

In contrast to Broca's aphasia, the patient with Wernicke's aphasia usually talks volubly, gestures freely, and appears strangely unaware of his deficit. Speech is produced mostly without effort; the phrases and sentences appear to be of normal length and are properly intoned and articulated. These attributes, in the context of aphasic disturbances, are referred to as "fluency" of speech (i.e., Wernicke's is a fluent aphasia). Despite the fluency and normal prosody, the patient's speech is remarkably devoid of meaning. The patient with Wernicke's aphasia produces many nonsubstantive words, and the words themselves are often malformed or inappropriate, a disorder referred to as *paraphasia*. A phoneme (the minimal unit of sound recognizable as language) or a syllable may be substituted within a word (e.g., "The grass is greel"); this is called *literal paraphasia*. The substitution of one word for another ("The grass is blue") is termed *verbal paraphasia* or *semantic substitution* and is even more characteristic of Wernicke's aphasia. Neologisms, i.e., syllables or words that are not part of the language, may also appear ("The grass is grumps"). In its extreme, the fluent, paraphasic speech of Wernicke's aphasia may be entirely incomprehensible (gibberish or *jargon aphasia*). Fluency, however, is not an invariable feature of Wernicke's aphasia. In some patients speech may be hesitant, in which case the block tends to occur in the part of the phrase that contains the central communicative (predicative) item, such as a key noun, verb, or descriptive phrase. The patient with such a disorder conveys the impression of constantly searching for the correct word and of having difficulty in finding it. Wernicke's aphasia may also at times begin with complete mutism.

Although the motor apparatus required for the expression of language is intact, patients with severe Wernicke's aphasia have difficulty in functioning as social organisms because they are deprived of the main means of communication. They cannot understand fully what is said to them; a few simple commands may still be executed, but there is failure to carry out complex ones. They cannot read aloud or silently with comprehension, tell others what they want or think, or write spontaneously. Written letters are often combined into meaningless words, but there may be a scattering of correct words. In trying to designate an object that is seen or felt, they cannot find the name, even though they can sometimes repeat it from dictation; nor can they write from dictation the very words that they can copy. Copying performance is notably slow and laborious and conforms to the contours of the model, including the examiner's handwriting style. All these defects are present in varying degrees of severity and the mildest form consists of mild verbal and literal paraphasias and minimal difficulty with comprehension of grammatically complex material ("mini-Wernicke"). In general, the disturbances in reading, writing, naming, and repetition parallel the severity of impairment in comprehension. There are, however, exceptions in which either reading or the understanding of spoken language is disproportionately affected. Some aphasiologists thus speak of two Wernicke syndromes.

In terms of the idealized Broca-Wernicke schema, in Wernicke's aphasia the motor language areas are no longer under control of the auditory and visual areas. The disconnection of the motor speech areas from the auditory and visual ones accounts for the impairment of repetition and the inability to read aloud. Reading may remain fluent, but with the same paraphasic errors that mar conversational language. The occurrence of dyslexia (impaired visual perception of letters and words) with lesions of the Wernicke area is ostensibly explained by the fact that most individuals learn to read by transforming the printed word into the auditory form before it can gain access to the integrative centers in the posterior perisylvian region. Only in the congenitally deaf is there thought to be a direct pathway between the visual and central integrative language centers.

Wernicke's aphasia that is caused by stroke usually improves in time, sometimes to the point where the deficits can be detected only by asking the patient to repeat unfamiliar words, to name unusual objects or parts of objects, to spell difficult words, or to write complex self-generated sentences. A more favorable prognosis attends those forms in which some of the elements, e.g., reading, are only slightly impaired from the outset.

As discussed earlier, the term *Wernicke area* has been applied to the posterior part of area 22 in the most lateral part of the planum temporale. As a rule, in Wernicke's aphasia the lesion lies in the posterior perisylvian region (comprising posterosuperior temporal, supramarginal, angular, and posterior insular gyri) and is usually a result of embolic occlusion of the inferior (lower) division of the left middle cerebral artery. A hemorrhage confined to the subcortex of the temporoparietal region or involvement of this area by tumor, abscess, herpes encephalitis, or extension of a small putaminal or thalamic hemorrhage may have similar effects but a better prognosis. Any lesion that involves structures deep to the posterior temporal cortex, including stroke, will cause an associated right homonymous quadrant or hemianopia. Usually, there is no weakness of limbs or face for which reason the fluently aphasic patient may be misdiagnosed as psychotic or confused, especially if there is jargon aphasia. According to Kertesz and Benson, persistence of Wernicke's aphasia is related to a lesion that involves both the left supramarginal and angular gyri and therefore, elements of Gerstmann syndrome may be evident.

The posterior perisylvian region, therefore, appears to encompass a variety of language functions, and seemingly minor changes in the size and locale of the lesion are associated with important variations in the elements of Wernicke's aphasia or lead to *conduction aphasia, pure word blindness,* or to *pure word deafness* (see below). The interesting theoretical problem is whether all the deficits observed are indicative of a unitary language function that resides in the posterior perisylvian region or, instead, of a series of separate sensorimotor activities whose anatomic pathways happen to be crowded together in a small region of the brain. In view of the multiple ways in which language is learned and deteriorates in disease, the latter hypothesis seems more likely.

Global Aphasia

This syndrome is caused by destruction of a large part of the language zone, embracing both Broca and Wernicke areas and much of the territory between them. The cause is usually an occlusion of the proximal middle cerebral artery, but it may be the result of hemorrhage, tumor, abscess or other lesions, and transiently as a postictal effect. Almost invariably, in cases of global aphasia, there is a degree of right hemiplegia, hemianesthesia, and homonymous hemianopia.

All aspects of speech and language are affected. At most, the patient can say only a few words, usually some cliché or habitual phrase, and can imitate single sounds, or only emit a syllable, such as "ah," or cry, shout, or moan. Many are initially mute. They may understand a few words and phrases, but, because of rapid fatigue and verbal and motor perseveration—they characteristically fail to carry out a series of simple commands or to name a series of objects. They cannot read or write or repeat what is said to them. The patient may participate in common gestures of greeting, show modesty and avoidance reactions, and engage in self-help activities. With the passage of time, some degree of comprehension of language may return, and the clinical picture that is then most likely to emerge is closest to that of a severe Broca's aphasia.

Improvement frequently occurs when the underlying cause is cerebral trauma, compression from edema, ictal or postictal paralysis, or a transient metabolic derangement such as hypoglycemia or hyponatremia, which may also worsen the aphasia of an old lesion that had involved language areas.

TRANSCORTICAL AND CONDUCTION APHASIAS

These terms refer to disorders of language that result not from lesions of the cortical language areas themselves but from an apparent interruption of association pathways joining the primary receptive (sensory, auditory, and visual) areas to the language areas. Included also in this category are aphasias from lesions that separate the more strictly receptive parts of the language mechanism itself from the purely motor ones (conduction aphasia; see below) and to lesions that isolate the perisylvian language areas, separating them from the other parts of the cerebral cortex (*transcortical aphasias*).

The anatomic basis for most of these so-called disconnection syndromes is only partly defined. The theoretical concept is an interesting one and emphasizes the importance of afferent, intercortical, and efferent connections of the language mechanisms. However, the locale of the lesion that causes loss of a language function does not localize the language function itself, a warning enunciated long ago by Hughlings Jackson. Nevertheless, the language disorders described below occur with sufficient regularity and clinical uniformity to be almost as useful as the more common types of aphasia in localization and in revealing the complexity of language functions.

Conduction Aphasia

As indicated earlier, Wernicke theorized that certain clinical symptoms would follow a lesion that effectively separated the auditory and motor language areas without directly damaging either of them. Since then a number of well-studied cases have been described that conform to his proposed model of *Leitungsaphasie* (conduction aphasia), which is the name he gave it. The characteristic feature is severely impaired repetition of spoken language; the defect applies to both single words and nonwords. The second essential feature is reduced but still relatively preserved comprehension in comparison to Wernicke's aphasia. In other respects, the features of conduction aphasia resemble those of a mild Wernicke's aphasia. They share fluency and paraphasias in self-initiated speech, in repeating what is heard, and in reading aloud; writing is also similarly impaired. Dysarthria and dysprosody are usually lacking. Speech output is normal or somewhat reduced. As mentioned, comprehension is by no means perfect, but compared with one who has Wernicke's aphasia, the patient with conduction aphasia has relatively little difficulty in understanding words that are heard or seen and is aware of his deficit.

The lesion in the few autopsied cases has been located in the cortex and subcortical white matter in the upper bank of the left sylvian fissure, usually involving the supramarginal gyrus and occasionally the most posterior part of the superior temporal region. The reason for classifying this aphasia as a disconnection syndrome according to Damasio and Geschwind is that the Wernicke and Broca areas are spared, and the critical structure involved is the connection between them—the arcuate fasciculus. This fiber tract streams out of the temporal lobe, proceeding somewhat posteriorly, around the posterior end of the sylvian fissure; there it joins the superior longitudinal fasciculus, deep in the anteroinferior parietal region, and proceeds forward, deep to the suprasylvian operculum, to the motor association cortex, including the Broca and Exner areas (see Fig. 22-1). However, in most of the reported cases, including those described by the Damasios, the left auditory complex, insula, and supramarginal gyrus were also involved. In any case, the usual cause of conduction aphasia is an embolic occlusion of the ascending parietal or posterior temporal branch of the middle cerebral artery, but other forms of vascular disease, particularly small subcortical hemorrhage, neoplasm, or trauma in this region produce the same syndrome.

Transcortical Aphasias (Preservation of Repetition)

The identifying feature of these language disturbances is a preservation of the ability to repeat. Destruction of the vascular border zones between anterior, middle, and posterior cerebral arteries, usually as a result of prolonged hypotension, carbon monoxide poisoning, or other forms of anoxic–ischemic injury, may effectively isolate the intact motor and sensory language areas, all or in part, from the rest of the cortex of the same hemisphere. In the case reported by Assal and colleagues, for example, multiple infarcts had isolated all of the language area.

In *transcortical sensory aphasia* the patient suffers a deficit of auditory and visual word comprehension, making writing and reading impossible, in every way conforming to Wernicke's aphasia. Speech remains fluent, with marked paraphasia, anomia, and empty circumlocutions. However, unlike the deficit in Wernicke's and conduction aphasias, the ability to repeat the spoken word is preserved. This facility in repetition may be of extreme degree, taking the form of echoing, parrot-like, word, phrases, and songs that are heard (echolalia). In a series of 15 such patients, CT and isotope scans have uniformly disclosed a lesion in the posterior parietooccipital region, according to Kertesz and colleagues. In general, this disorder has a good prognosis.

Presumably, in transcortical sensory aphasia, as in Wernicke's aphasia, information cannot be transferred to the Wernicke area for conversion into word meaning. Paraphasia is thought to result from the reduced control of the motor language areas by the auditory and visual areas, though the direct connection between them, presumably the arcuate fasciculus, is preserved. Preservation of this direct connection is said to account for the ability to repeat.

In *transcortical motor aphasia,* the patient is unable to initiate conversational speech, producing only a few grunts or syllables as in Broca-type aphasia. Comprehension is relatively preserved, but *repetition is strikingly intact,* distinguishing this syndrome from pure word mutism. Transcortical motor aphasia occurs in two clinical contexts: (1) in a mild or partially recovered Broca's aphasia in which repetition remains superior to conversational speech (repeating and reading aloud are generally easier than self-generated speech) and (2) in states of abulia and akinetic mutism with frontal lobe damage. Several cases under our observation have resulted from infarctions in the watershed zone between the anterior and middle cerebral arteries after cardiac arrest or shock.

Pure Word Deafness

This uncommon disorder, a derivative of Wernicke's aphasia originally described by Lichtheim in 1885, is characterized by an impairment of auditory comprehension and repetition and an inability to write to dictation. Self-initiated utterances are usually correctly phrased. but sometimes paraphasic; spontaneous writing and the ability to comprehend written language are preserved, thus distinguishing this disorder from Wernicke's aphasia. Patients with pure word deafness may declare that they cannot hear, but shouting does not help, sometimes to their surprise. Audiometric testing and auditory evoked potentials disclose no hearing defect, and nonverbal sounds, such as a doorbell, can be heard without difficulty. The patient is forced to depend heavily on visual cues and frequently uses them well enough to understand most of what is said. However, tests that prevent the use of visual cues readily uncover the deficit. If able to describe the auditory experience, the patient says that words sound like a jumble of noises. As in the case of visual verbal agnosia (see below), the syndrome of pure auditory verbal agnosia is not pure, particularly at its onset, and paraphasic and other elements of Wernicke's aphasia may be detected (Buchman et al). At times, this syndrome is the result of resolution of a more typical Wernicke's aphasia, and it will be recognized that word deafness is an integral feature of all instances of Wernicke's aphasia. Conceptually, it has been thought of as an exclusive injury of the auditory processing system therefore allowing relative preservation of internal language.

In most recorded autopsy studies, the lesions have been bilateral, in the middle third of the superior temporal gyri, in a position to interrupt the connections between the primary auditory cortex in the transverse gyri of Heschl and the associated areas of the superoposterior cortex of the temporal lobe. In a few cases, unilateral lesions have been localized in this part of the dominant temporal lobe (see Chap. 22). Requirements of small size and superficiality of the lesion in the cortex and subcortical white matter are best fulfilled by an embolic occlusion of a small branch of the lower division of the middle cerebral artery.

Pure Word Blindness (Alexia Without Agraphia, Visual Verbal Agnosia)

The most striking feature of this syndrome is the retained capacity to write fluently, after which the patient cannot read what has been written (*alexia without agraphia*).

In fact, reading of any material is greatly impaired. When the patient with alexia also has difficulty in auditory comprehension and in repeating spoken words, the syndrome corresponds more closely to Wernicke's aphasia. In such cases, the individual loses the ability to understand written script, and, often, to name colors, i.e., to match a seen color to its spoken name, *visual verbal color anomia*. Such a person can no longer name or point on command to words, although he is sometimes able to read letters or numbers. However, understanding spoken language, repetition of what is heard, writing spontaneously and to dictation, and conversation are all intact. The ability to copy words is impaired but is better preserved than reading, and the patient may even be able to spell a word or to identify a word by having it spelled to him or by reading one letter at a time (letter-by-letter reading). In some cases, the patient manages to read single letters but not to join them together (*asyllabia*).

Autopsies of such cases have usually demonstrated a lesion that destroys the left visual cortex and underlying white matter, particularly the geniculocalcarine tract, as well as the callosal connections of the right visual cortex with the intact language areas of the dominant hemisphere (see "Disconnection Syndromes" in Chap. 22). In the case originally described by Déjerine in 1892, the disconnection occurred in the posterior part (splenium) of the corpus callosum, wherein lie the connections between the visual association areas of the two hemispheres (see Fig. 22-6). More often, the callosal pathways are interrupted in the forceps major or in the paraventricular region (Damasio and Damasio, 1983). In either event, the patient is blind in the right half of each visual field by virtue of the left occipital lesion, and visual information reaches only the right occipital lobe; however, this information cannot be transferred, via the callosal pathways to the language area of the left hemisphere.

A rare variant of this syndrome takes the form of *alexia without agraphia and without hemianopia*. A lesion deep in the white matter of the left occipital lobe, at its junction with the parietal lobe, interrupts the projections from the intact (right) visual cortex to the language areas, but spares the geniculocalcarine pathway (Greenblatt). This lesion, coupled with one in the splenium, prevents all visual information from reaching the language areas, including the angular gyrus, and Wernicke area.

In yet other cases, the lesion is confined to the angular gyrus or the subjacent white matter. In such cases also, a right homonymous hemianopia will be absent, but the *alexia may be combined with agraphia* and other elements of the Gerstmann syndrome, i.e., right-left confusion, acalculia, and finger agnosia (see "Gerstmann Syndrome," Chap. 22). This entire constellation of symptoms is sometimes referred to as the *syndrome of the angular gyrus*. Anomic aphasia may be added (see later).

Pure Word Mutism (Aphemia)

This syndrome was mentioned in the earlier discussion on Broca's aphasia. As a result of a vascular lesion or other type of localized injury of the dominant frontal lobe, the patient loses all capacity to speak while retaining perfectly the ability to write, to understand spoken words, to read silently with comprehension, and to repeat spoken words. Right facial and brachial paresis may be associated. From the time speech becomes audible, language may be syntactically complete, showing neither loss of vocabulary nor agrammatism; or there may be varying degrees of dysarthria (hence "cortical dysarthria"), anomia, and paraphasic substitutions, especially for consonants. The most notable feature of this type of speech disorder is its transience; within a few weeks or months, language is restored to normal. Bastian, Broca, and more recently other authors called this syndrome *aphemia*, a term that was used originally by Broca in another context to describe the severe motor aphasia that now carries his name. Probably the syndrome is closely allied to the "mini-Broca's aphasia" described earlier under "Broca's Aphasia."

The anatomic basis of pure word mutism has not been determined precisely. In a few postmortem cases, reference is made to a lesion in Broca area. Damasio and Geschwind have stated that the lesion is anterior and superior to this area. A well-studied case has been reported by LeCours and Lhermitte. Their patient uttered only a few sounds for 4 weeks, after which he recovered rapidly and completely. From the onset of the stroke, the patient showed no disturbance of comprehension of language or of writing. Autopsy disclosed an infarct that was confined to the cortex and subjacent white matter of the lowermost part of the precentral gyrus; the Broca's area, one gyrus forward, was completely spared. Other cases have involved mainly the Broca's area.

Anomic (Amnesic, Nominal) Aphasia

Some degree of word-finding difficulty is part of almost every type of language disorder, including that which occurs with the confusional states and dementia. In fact, without an element of anomia, a diagnosis of aphasia is usually incorrect. Only when this feature is the most notable aspect of language difficulty is the term *anomic aphasia* employed. In this condition, a relatively uncommon form of aphasia in pure form, the patient loses only the ability to name people and objects. There are pauses in speech, groping for words, circumlocution, and substitution of another word or phrase that is intended to convey the meaning. Perseveration may be prominent. Or the patient may simply fail to name a shown object, in contrast to the usual aphasic patient, who produces a paraphasic error. Less frequently used words give more trouble. When shown a series of common objects, the patient may tell of their use, or demonstrate the same, instead of giving their names. The difficulty applies not only to objects seen but also to the names of things heard or felt (as per Geschwind). In addition to displaying normal fluency of spontaneous speech and preserved comprehension and repetition, the patients we have seen with anomic aphasia have been surprisingly adept in spelling.

Beauvois and coworkers have described a form of bilateral tactile aphasia caused by a left parietooccipital lesion in which objects seen and verbally described could be named, but not those felt with either hand. Recall of the names of letters, digits, and other printed verbal material is almost invariably preserved, and immediate repetition of a spoken name is intact. That the deficit is principally one of naming is shown by the patient's correct use of the object and, usually, by an ability to point to the correct object on hearing or seeing the name and to choose the correct name from a list. The patient's understanding of what is heard or read is normal.

There is a tendency for patients with anomia to attribute their failure to forgetfulness or to give some other implausible excuse for the disability, suggesting that they are not completely aware of the nature of their difficulty, but some are aware of the defect. Of course, there are many more patients who fail not only to name objects but also to recognize the correct word when it is given to them. In such patients, the understanding of what is heard or read is not normal, i.e., the naming difficulty is but one symptom of another type of aphasic disorder.

Anomic aphasia has been associated with lesions in different parts of the language area, typically in the left temporal lobe. In these cases, the lesion has been deep to the posterior temporal lobe, particularly in the left thalamus, or in the middle temporal convolution, in a location to interrupt connections between sensory language areas and the hippocampal regions concerned with learning and memory. Mass lesions, such as a tumor, herpes encephalitis, or an abscess, are the most frequent causes; as these lesions enlarge, a contralateral upper quadrantic visual field defect or a Wernicke's aphasia is added. Occasionally, anomia appears with lesions caused by occlusion of the temporal branches of the posterior cerebral artery, and it is in these instances that we have seen the most pronounced cases of anomia, usually associated with a right hemianopia and alexia but normal writing ability. Anomia may be a prominent manifestation of transcortical motor aphasia (see later) and may be associated with the Gerstmann syndrome, in which case the lesions are found in the frontal lobe and angular gyrus, respectively.

An anomic type of aphasia is often an early sign of Alzheimer and Pick disease (minor degrees of it are common in old age) and is a principal feature of one type of degenerative lobar cerebral atrophy in the category of the primary progressive aphasias (see Chap. 39). Finally, anomic aphasia may be the only residual abnormality after partial recovery from Wernicke's, conduction, transcortical sensory, or (rarely) Broca's aphasia (Benson).

Foreign Accent Syndrome

This rare and somewhat amusing condition defies classification but is worthy of comment because it may be mistaken for hysteria or psychosis. An accent that is distinctly foreign but vague in actual region of origin replaces the patient's native speech pattern. The syndrome arises after a left-sided lesion, most often a stroke with a mild associated Broca's aphasia. Although the accent may be interpreted by the listener as compatible with German, Spanish, French, Asian, or another nationality, authoritative analysis indicates that the alterations are not specific to any genuine language and are simply attributed by the listener to a known foreign accent. The syndrome is also encountered as a transient phenomenon during recovery from stroke. The relation to disorders of prosody, which is produced by lesions of the nondominant hemisphere, is unclear. LeCours and Lhermitte made an analysis of the disorder based on the obligate use of diphthongs in certain languages; these were not properly pronounced in the foreign accent syndrome and made French listeners detect an English accent. An extensive examination of one case and references to additional ones can be found in the article by Kurowski and colleagues.

AGRAPHIA

Writing is, of course, an integral part of language function, but a less essential and universal component, for a segment of the world's population speaks but does not read or write. It might be supposed that all the rules of language derived from the study of aphasia would be applicable to agraphia. In large part, this is true. One must be able to formulate ideas in words and phrases in order to have something to write as well as to say; hence, disorders of writing, like disorders of speaking, reflect all the basic defects of language. But there is an obvious difference between these two expressive modes. In speech, only one final motor pathway coordinating the movements of lips, tongue, larynx, and respiratory muscles is available, whereas if the right hand is paralyzed, one can still write with the left one, or with a foot, and even with the mouth by holding a pencil between the teeth (a contrivance used by individuals whose arms are paralyzed by cervical root avulsion from motorcycle accidents). An accurate general statement is that written language is disordered similarly to spoken language in the Broca's and Wernicke's aphasias and in most of their derivatives. When comprehension is impaired, writing to dictation is often impossible. Paraphasias appear in the writings of aphasics much the same as they do in speech.

The writing of a word can be accomplished either by the direct lexical method of recalling its spelling or by sounding out its phonemes and transforming them into learned graphemes (motor images), i.e., the phonologic method. Some authors state that in agraphia there is a specific difficulty in transforming phonologic information, acquired through the auditory sense, into orthographic forms; others see it as a block between the visual form of phonemes, and the cursive movements of the hand (Basso et al). In support of the latter idea is the fact that reading and writing usually develop together and are long preceded by the development of speech as a means of communication.

Pure agraphia as the initial and sole disturbance of language function is a rarity, but such cases have been described as summarized by Rosati and de Bastiani. Pathologically verified cases are virtually nonexistent, but imaging sometimes discloses a lesion of the posterior perisylvian area. This is in keeping with the observation that a lesion in or near the angular gyrus will occasionally cause a disproportionate disorder of writing as part of the Gerstmann syndrome. As mentioned earlier in the chapter, the notion of specific center for writing in the posterior part of the second frontal convolution (the "Exner writing area") has been questioned (see Leischner). However, Croisile and associates do cite cases of dysgraphia in which a lesion (in the case they reported, a hematoma) was located in the centrum semiovale beneath the motor parts of the frontal cortex and direct electrical stimulation of the cortex rostral to the primary motor hand area disturbs handwriting without affecting other language or manual tasks according to Roux and colleagues, a veritable apraxia of writing.

Quite apart from these *aphasic agraphias*, in which spelling and grammatical errors abound, there are special forms of agraphia caused by abnormalities of spatial perception and praxis. Disturbances in the perception of spatial relationships underlie *constructional agraphia*. In this circumstance, letters and words are formed clearly enough but are wrongly arranged on the page. Words may be superimposed, reversed, written diagonally or in a haphazard arrangement, or from right to left; in the form associated with right parietal lesions, only the right half of the page is used. Usually one finds other constructional difficulties as well, such as inability to copy geometric figures or to make drawings of clocks, flowers, and maps, etc. This is a common feature of developmental dyslexia.

A third group of writing disorder may be called the *apraxic agraphias*. Here, language formulation is correct and the spatial arrangements of words are respected, but the hand has lost its skill in forming letters and words. Handwriting becomes a scrawl, losing all personal character. There may be an uncertainty as to how the pen should be held and applied to paper; apraxias (ideomotor and ideational) are present in the right hander. As a rule, other learned manual skills are simultaneously disordered. Speculations as to the basic fault here are discussed in Chap. 3, under "Apraxia and Other Nonparalytic Disorders of Motor Functions," and in Chap. 22, in relation to the functions of the frontal and parietal lobes.

In addition to the neurologic forms of agraphia, described above, psychologists have defined a group of *linguistic agraphias*, subdivided into phonologic, lexical, and semantic types. These linguistic models are based on loss of the ability to write (and to spell) particular classes of words. For example, the patient may be unable to spell pronounceable nonsense words, with preserved ability to spell real words (phonologic agraphia); or there may be preserved ability to write nonsense words but not irregular words, such as *island* (lexical agraphia); patients with semantic agraphia have difficulty incorporating the proper meaning into the written word, e.g., "the moon comes out at knight." For the most part, these linguistic agraphias have no well-established cerebral localization and only tenuous associations with the classic aphasias, for which reason this subject is of greater interest to linguists and psychologists than to neurologists.

The orthographic qualities of writing deteriorate in many motor disorders such as Parkinson disease, tremors, dystonias, and spasticity, but careful inspection shows that language content is normal.

Also worth brief comment is *mirror writing*, in which script runs in the opposite direction to normal with each letter also being reversed. Some normal individuals have an unusual facility to produce mirror writing, and it has been reported in developmentally delayed left-handed children. Those few instances in which mirror writing is acquired tend to be transient and incomplete with strokes in various parts of the left hemisphere, or rarely, the right hemisphere or bifrontal lesions (see the review by Schott).

SUBCORTICAL APHASIA (THALAMIC AND STRIATOCAPSULAR APHASIAS)

A lesion of the dominant thalamus, usually vascular and involving the posterior nuclei, may cause an aphasia, the clinical features of which are not entirely uniform. Typically, there is mutism initially and comprehension is impaired. During the early phases of recovery, spontaneous speech is reduced in amount and is dysfluent; less often, speech is fluent and paraphasic to the point of jargon. Reading and writing may or may not be affected. Characteristically, the patient's ability to repeat dictated words and phrases is preserved. This configuration has been termed "mixed transcortical aphasia," a syndrome originally described in bilateral border-zone infarctions or large left-frontal lesions. It may exist in isolation or in combination with the mixed transcortical aphasia. Complete recovery in a matter of weeks is the rule unless the underlying cause is a tumor. Anomia has also been described with ventrolateral thalamic lesions (Ojemann).

Aphasia has also been described frequently with dominant striatocapsular lesions, particularly if they extend laterally into the subcortical white matter of the temporal lobe and insula. The head of the caudate, anterior limb of the internal capsule, or the anterosuperior aspect of the putamen are the structures involved in different patients. The aphasia is characterized by nonfluent, dysarthric, paraphasic speech and varying degrees of difficulty with comprehension of language, naming, and repetition. The lesion is vascular as a rule, and a right hemiparesis is usually associated with it. In general, striatocapsular aphasia recovers more slowly and less completely than thalamic aphasia.

These two subcortical aphasias, thalamic and striatocapsular, resemble but are not identical to the Wernicke and Broca types of aphasia, respectively. For further discussion, the reader is directed to the articles of Naeser and of Alexander and their colleagues.

OTHER CEREBRAL DISORDERS OF LANGUAGE

The effects on speech and language of diffuse cerebral disorders, such as delirium tremens and Alzheimer disease, were mentioned in Chaps. 20 and 21. Pathologic changes in parts of the cerebrum other than the perisylvian regions may secondarily affect language function. The lesions that occur in the border zones between major cerebral arteries and effectively isolate perisylvian areas from other parts of the cerebrum fall into this category (transcortical aphasias, see previous pages). Other examples are the lesions in the mediorbital or superior and lateral parts of the frontal lobes, which impair all motor activity to the point of abulia or akinetic mutism. The mute patient, in contrast to the aphasic one, emits no sounds. If the patient is less severely hypokinetic, his speech tends to be laconic, with long pauses and an inability to sustain a monologue. Extensive occipital lesions will, of course, impair reading, but they also reduce the utilization of all visual and lexical stimuli. Deep cerebral lesions, by causing fluctuating states of inattention and disorientation, induce fragmentation of words and phrases and sometimes protracted, uncontrollable talking (logorrhea). The nonaphasic language disorders of the confusional states, emphasized by Geschwind, have already been mentioned.

Also common in global or multifocal cerebral diseases are defects in prosody, both expressive and receptive. These appear in numerous states that affect global cerebral function, such as Alzheimer disease as well as with lesions of the nondominant (right) perisylvian region, as noted in Chap. 22.

Severe developmental delay often results in failure to acquire even spoken language, as pointed out in Chaps. 28 and 38. If there is any language skill, it consists only of the understanding of a few simple spoken commands. The subject of developmental dyslexia is discussed in "Developmental Dyslexia" in Chap. 28.

Treatment of Aphasia

The sudden onset of aphasia would be expected to cause great apprehension, but except for cases of pure or almost pure motor disorders of speech, most patients show remarkably little concern. It appears at times that the very lesion that deprives them of speech also causes at least a partial loss of insight into their own disability. This reaches almost a ludicrous extreme in some cases of Wernicke's aphasia, in which the patient becomes indignant when others cannot understand his jargon. Nonetheless, as improvement occurs, many patients do become discouraged. Reassurance and a program of speech rehabilitation are the best ways of helping the patient at this stage.

Whether contemporary methods of speech therapy accomplish more than can be accounted for by spontaneous recovery is still uncertain. Most aphasic disorders are caused by vascular disease and trauma, and they are nearly always accompanied by some degree of spontaneous improvement in the days, weeks, and months that follow the stroke or accident. A Veterans Administration Cooperative Study (Wertz et al) has suggested that intensive therapy by a speech pathologist does hasten improvement. Also, Howard and colleagues have shown increased efficacy of word retrieval in a group of chronic stable aphasics treated by two different techniques. More studies of this type, which control for the effects of time, of the patient's motivation and the interest of family and therapist, are needed. In an interesting personal experiment by Wender, a classicist who had become aphasic, practice of Greek vocabulary and grammar led to recovery in that language, but there was little recovery of her facility with Latin, which was not similarly exercised.

The methods of language rehabilitation are specialized, and it is advisable to call in a person who has been trained in this field. However, inasmuch as a part of the benefit is also psychologic, an interested family member or schoolteacher can be of help if a speech therapist is not available in the community. Frustration, depression, and paranoia, which complicate some aphasias, may require psychiatric evaluation and treatment. The developmental language disorders of children pose special problems and are considered in Chap. 28.

In general, recovery from aphasia that is due to cerebral trauma is usually faster and more complete than that from aphasia because of stroke. The type of aphasia and particularly its initial severity (extent of the lesion) clearly influence recovery: global aphasia usually improves little, and the same is true of severe Broca's and Wernicke's aphasias (Kertesz and McCabe). Minimal or "mini" Broca's aphasia characterized by slightly effortful and halting speech, recovers quickly. The various dissociative speech syndromes and pure word mutism also tend to improve rapidly and often completely. In general, the outlook for recovery from any particular aphasia is more favorable in a left-handed person than in a right-handed one. Characteristically, in the course of recovery, a severe aphasia of one type may evolve into another type (global into severe Broca's; Wernicke's, transcortical, and conduction into anomic), which are patterns of recovery that may be attributed to the effects of therapy.

DISORDERS OF ARTICULATION AND PHONATION

The act of speaking involves a highly coordinated sequence of actions of the respiratory musculature, larynx, pharynx, palate, tongue, and lips. These structures are innervated by the vagal, hypoglossal, facial, and phrenic nerves, the nuclei of which are controlled by both motor cortices through the corticobulbar tracts. As with all movements, those involved in speaking are subject to extrapyramidal influences from the cerebellum and basal ganglia. The act of speaking requires that air be expired in regulated bursts and each expiration must be maintained long enough (by pressure mainly from the intercostal muscles) to permit the utterance of phrases and sentences. The current of expired air is then finely regulated by the activity of the various muscles engaged in speech.

Phonation, or the production of vocal sounds, is a function of the larynx, more particularly the vocal cords. The pitch of the speaking or singing voice depends upon the length and mass of the membranous parts of the vocal cords and can be varied by changing their tension; this is accomplished by means of the intrinsic laryngeal muscles, before any audible sound emerges. The controlled intratracheal pressure forces air past the glottis and separates the margins of the cords, setting up a series of vibrations and recoils. Sounds thus formed are modulated as they pass through the nasopharynx and mouth, which act as resonators. *Articulation* consists of contractions of the pharynx, palate, tongue, and lips, which interrupt or alter the vocal sounds. Vowels are of laryngeal origin, as are some consonants, but the latter are formed for the most part during articulation; the consonants *m*, *b*, and *p* are labial, *l* and *t* are lingual, and *nk* and *ng* are guttural (throat and soft palate).

Defective articulation (dysarthria) and phonation (dysphonia) are recognized at once by listening to the patient speak during ordinary conversation or read aloud. Contrived test phrases such as "Methodist Episcopal" or attempts at rapid repetition of lingual, labial, and guttural consonants (e.g., *la-la-la-la*, *me-me-me-me*, or *k-k-k-k*) bring out the particular abnormality. Disorders of phonation call for a precise analysis of the voice and its apparatus.

Dysarthria and Anarthria

In pure dysarthria or its most severe representation, anarthria, there is no abnormality of the cortical language mechanisms. The patient is able to understand perfectly what is heard and has no difficulty in reading and writing, although he may be unable to utter intelligible words. This is the strict meaning of being inarticulate. Defects in articulation may be subdivided into several types: lower motor neuron (neuromuscular); spastic (pseudobulbar); rigid (extrapyramidal); cerebellar-ataxic; and hypo- and hyperkinetic dysarthrias, each of which is taken up below.

Lower Motor Neuron and Neuromuscular Dysarthria

This pattern of speech is caused by weakness or paralysis of the articulatory muscles, the result usually of disease of the motor nuclei of the medulla and lower pons or their intramedullary or peripheral extensions (*lower motor neuron paralysis*). In advanced forms of this disorder, the shriveled tongue lies inert and fasciculating on the floor of the mouth, and the lips are lax and tremulous. Saliva constantly collects in the mouth because of dysphagia, and drooling is troublesome. Dysphonia, an alteration of the voice to a rasping monotone because of vocal cord paralysis, is often an additional feature. As this condition evolves, speech becomes slurred and progressively less distinct. There is special difficulty in the enunciation of vibratives, such as *r*, and as the paralysis becomes more complete, lingual and labial consonants are finally not pronounced at all. In the past, bilateral paralysis of the palate, causing nasality of speech, often occurred with diphtheria and poliomyelitis, but now it occurs most often with progressive bulbar palsy, a form of motor neuron disease (see "Progressive Bulbar Palsy," Chap. 39), and with certain other neuromuscular disorders, particularly myasthenia gravis. Bilateral paralysis of the lips, as occurs in the facial diplegia of the GuillainBarré syndrome or of Lyme disease, interferes with enunciation of labial consonants; *p* and *b* are slurred and sound more like *f* and *v*. Degrees of both of these abnormalities are also observed in myasthenia gravis, but there are usually additional features of palatal weakness and softening of guttural consonants and nasal air escape.

Spastic (Pseudobulbar) Dysarthria

Diseases that involve the corticobulbar tracts bilaterally, usually a result of vascular, demyelinating, or motor neuron disease (amyotrophic lateral sclerosis), result in the syndrome of spastic bulbar (pseudobulbar) palsy. The patient may have had a clinically inevident vascular lesion at some time in the past, affecting the corticobulbar fibers on one side; however, because the bulbar muscles on each side are innervated by both motor cortices, there may be little or no impairment in speech or swallowing until another stroke occurs involving the other corticobulbar tract at any level. Upon the second stroke, the patient immediately becomes dysphagic, dysphonic, and anarthric or dysarthric, often with paresis of the tongue and facial muscles. This condition, unlike bulbar paralysis from lower motor neuron involvement, entails no atrophy or fasciculations of the paralyzed muscles; instead, the jaw jerk and other facial reflexes usually become exaggerated, the palatal reflexes are retained or increased, and emotional control is impaired (spasmodic, crying, and laughing—the pseudobulbar affective state described in Chap. 25). Amyotrophic lateral sclerosis is a condition in which the signs of spastic and atrophic bulbar palsy are combined.

When the dominant frontal operculum is damaged, speech may be dysarthric, usually without pseudobulbar impairment in emotional control. In the beginning, with vascular lesions, the patient may be mute; but with recovery or in mild degrees of the same condition, speech is notably slow, thick, and indistinct, much like that of partial bulbar paralysis. The terms *cortical dysarthria* and *cortical anarthria*, among many others, have been applied to this disorder, which is more closely related to forms of Broca's aphasia than to the dysarthrias being considered in this section. Also, in many cases of partially recovered Broca's aphasia and in the "mini-Broca" syndrome, the patient is left with a dysarthria that may be difficult to distinguish from a pure articulatory defect. Careful testing of other language functions, especially writing reveals the aphasic aspect of the defect.

A severe dysarthria that is difficult to classify, but resembles that of cerebellar disease, may occur with a left hemiplegia, usually the result of capsular or right opercular infarction. It tends to improve over several weeks but initially may be so severe as to make speech incomprehensible (Ropper).

Rigid (Extrapyramidal) Dysarthria

In Parkinson and other extrapyramidal diseases associated with rigidity of muscles, one observes a rather different disturbance of articulation, characterized by rapid mumbling and cluttered utterance and slurring of words and syllables. The voice is low-pitched and monotonous, lacking both inflection and volume (hypophonia), and trailing off in volume at the ends of sentences. Words are spoken hastily and run together in a pattern that is almost the opposite of the slowed pattern of spastic dysarthria. In advanced cases, speech is whispered and almost unintelligible. It may happen that the patient finds it impossible to talk while walking but can speak better if standing still, sitting, or lying down. In the extrapyramidal disorder of progressive supranuclear palsy, the dysarthria and dysphonia tend instead to be spastic in nature.

With chorea and myoclonus, speech may also be affected in a highly characteristic way. Talking is loud, harsh, improperly stressed or accented, and poorly coordinated with breathing (*hyperkinetic dysarthria*). Unlike the defect of pseudobulbar palsy or Parkinson disease, chorea and myoclonus cause abrupt interruptions of the words by superimposition of involuntary inspirations and movements of bulbar muscles. The abnormality has been described as "hiccup speech," in that the breaks are unexpected, as in singultation. Accompanying grimacing and other movement abnormalities must sometimes be depended upon for diagnosis. The Tourette syndrome of multiple motor and vocal tics is characterized both by startling vocalizations (barking noises, squeals, shrieks, grunting, sniffing, snorting) and by speech disturbances, notably stuttering and the involuntary utterance of obscenities (coprolalia).

Elements of both corticobulbar (spastic) and extrapyramidal speech disturbances are combined in Wilson disease, acquired hepatocerebral degeneration, in Hallervorden-Spatz disease (PKAN, the new and preferable designation based on the kinase that is affected in the disease), and in the form of cerebral palsy called *double athetosis*. The speech is loud, slow, and labored; it is poorly coordinated with breathing and accompanied by facial contortions and athetotic excesses of tone in other muscles. In diffuse cerebral diseases such as syphilitic general paresis, slurred, tremulous speech is one of the cardinal signs.

Ataxic Dysarthria (See Chap. 5)

This condition is a component of acute and chronic cerebellar lesions. It may be observed in multiple sclerosis and various degenerative disorders involving the cerebellum, or as a sequela of anoxic encephalopathy or heat stroke. The principal features are slowness of speech, slurring, monotony, and unnatural separation of the syllables of words. The coordination of speech and respiration is erratic. There may not be enough breath to utter certain words or syllables, and others are expressed with greater force than intended (explosive speech). *Scanning dysarthria*, speaking metronomically as if scanning poetry for meter, is another distinctive cerebellar pattern and is most often a result of mesencephalic lesions involving the brachium conjunctivum. However, in some cases of cerebellar disease, especially if there is an element of spastic weakness of the tongue from corticobulbar involvement, there may be only a slurring dysarthria, and it is not possible to predict the anatomy of the lesions from analysis of speech alone. Myoclonic jerks involving the speech musculature may be superimposed on cerebellar ataxia in a number of diseases such as Creutzfeldt-Jakob prion infection and Lance-Adams postanoxic encephalopathy.

Acquired Stuttering

This abnormality, characterized by interruptions of the normal rhythm of speech by involuntary repetition and prolongation or arrest of uttered letters or syllables, is a common developmental disorder, discussed in Chap. 28. But as pointed out by Rosenbek and colleagues and by Helm and colleagues, it may appear in patients who are recovering from aphasic disorders and who had never stuttered in childhood. This form of acquired stuttering in adults has some different features from the developmental type in that the repetitions, prolongations, and blocks are not restricted to the initial syllables of words, stuttering occurs at equal frequency for grammatical as for substantive words, there is little adaptation with continued speaking, and is generally unaccompanied by grimacing or associated movements, as happens in some developmental types. These features are discussed in the review by Lundgren and colleagues. Stuttering differs from palilalia, in which there is repetition of a word or phrase with increasing rapidity, and from echolalia, in which there is an obligate repetition of words or phrases.

In many instances, acquired stuttering is transitory; if it is permanent, according to Helm and associates, bilateral cerebral lesions are present. Nevertheless, we have observed some cases in which only a left-sided, predominantly motor aphasia provided the background for acquired stuttering, and others in which stuttering was an early sign of cerebral glioma originating in the left parietal region. Benson also cites patients in whom stuttering accompanied fluent aphasia. The causative lesion in acquired stuttering may be subcortical and even, as in an exceptional case described by Ciabarra and colleagues, located in the pons. The treatment of Parkinson disease with L-dopa and, occasionally, an acquired cerebral lesion may reactivate developmental stuttering. The latter may explain the emergence of stuttering with oddly situated lesions, such as the aforementioned pontine infarct.

Aphonia and Dysphonia

A few points should be made concerning the fourth group of speech disorders, i.e., those that are a result of disturbances of phonation. In adolescence, there may be a persistence of the unstable "change of voice" normally seen in boys during puberty. As though by habit, the patient speaks part of the time in falsetto, and the condition may persist into adult life. Its basis is unknown. Probably the larynx is not masculinized, i.e., there is a failure in the spurt of growth (length) of the vocal cords that ordinarily occurs in pubertal boys. Voice training has been helpful.

Paresis of respiratory movements, as in myasthenia gravis, Guillain-Barré syndrome, and severe pulmonary disease, may affect the voice because insufficient air is provided for phonation. Also, disturbances in the rhythm of respiration may interfere with the fluency of speech. This is particularly noticeable in extrapyramidal diseases, where one may observe that the patient tries to talk during part of inspiration as noted earlier. Another common feature of the latter diseases is the reduction in volume of the voice (hypophonia) because of limited excursion of the breathing muscles—the patient is unable to shout or to speak above a whisper. Whispering speech is also a feature of advanced Parkinson disease, stupor, and occasionally concussive brain injury and frontal lobe lesions, but strong stimulation may make the voice audible.

With paresis of both vocal cords, the patient can speak only in whispers. Because the vocal cords normally separate during inspiration, their failure to do so when paralyzed may result in an inspiratory stridor. If one vocal cord is paralyzed as a result of involvement of the tenth cranial nerve by tumor, for example, the voice becomes hoarse, low-pitched, rasping, and somewhat nasal in quality. The pronunciation of certain consonants such as *b*, *p*, *n*, and *k* is followed by an escape of air into the nasal passages. The abnormality is sometimes less pronounced in recumbency and increased when the head is thrown forward. Prolonged tracheal intubation that causes pressure necrosis of the posterior cricoarytenoid cartilage and the underlying posterior branch of the laryngeal nerve is an increasingly common iatrogenic cause.

Various tremor disorders, but especially severe essential tremor, affect the voice by creating an oscillatory effect on the vocal cords (see Chap. 6 for a full discussion). An unusual form of this disease causes a vibrato voice tremor almost in isolation, but most cases occur in the context of severe generalized essential tremor. As noted below, the pitch of voice may increase and simulate spasmodic dysphonia. Only the most severe cases of Parkinson tremor impart a warbling to the voice but this appears to be from vibration of the body and chest.

Spasmodic ("Spastic") Dysphonia

This is a relatively common condition about which little is known. *Spasmodic dysphonia* is a better term than the still-appearing spastic dysphonia, as the adjective *spastic* suggests corticospinal involvement, whereas the disorder is probably of extrapyramidal origin. The authors, like most neurologists, have seen many patients, middle-aged or elderly men and women, otherwise healthy, who lose the ability to speak quietly and fluently. Any attempt to speak results in simultaneous contraction of the speech musculature, so that the patient's voice is strained and speaking requires an effort. The patient sounds as though he were trying to speak while being strangled. Shouting is easier than quiet speech, and whispering is unaltered. Other actions utilizing approximately the same muscles (swallowing and singing) are usually unimpeded.

Spasmodic dysphonia is usually relatively nonprogressive and occurs as an isolated phenomenon, but we have observed exceptions in which it occurs in various combinations with blepharospasm, spasmodic torticollis, writer's cramp, or some other type of segmental dystonia. The nature of spasmodic dysphonia is unclear. As a neurologic disorder, it may be akin to writer's cramp, i.e., a restricted dystonia (see Chap. 6). As mentioned just above, we have at times had difficulty differentiating a severe essential tremor of voice from spasmodic dysphonia. They may even coexist (fortunately, the treatments are similar). An anatomic basis for the condition has not been demonstrated, but careful neuropathologic studies have not been made.

Glottic spasm, as in tetanus, tetany, and certain hereditary metabolic diseases, results in crowing, stridulous phonation.

Treatment Speech therapists, observing such a patient strain to achieve vocalization, often assume that relief can be obtained by making the patient relax, and psychotherapists believed at first that a search of the patient's personal life around the time when the dysphonia began would enable the patient to understand the problem and regain a normal mode of speaking. But both these methods have failed without exception. Drugs useful in the treatment of Parkinson disease and other extrapyramidal diseases are practically never effective. Sectioning of one recurrent laryngeal nerve can be beneficial, but recurrence is to be expected. The most effective treatment, comparable to treatment of other segmental dystonias, consists of the injection of 5 to 20 U of botulinum toxin, under laryngoscopic guidance, into each thyroarytenoid or cricothyroid muscle. Relief lasts for several months. Hoarseness and raspiness of the voice is also a result of structural changes in the vocal cords, the result of cigarette smoking, acute or chronic laryngitis, polyps, and laryngeal edema after extubation.

References

Alexander MP, Benson DF: The aphasias and related disturbances, in Joynt RJ (ed): *Clinical Neurology*. Vol 1. New York, Lippincott, 1991, chap 10.

Alexander MP, Naeser MA, Palumbo CL: Correlation of subcortical CT lesion sites and aphasia profiles. *Brain* 110:961, 1987.

Assal G, Regli F, Thuillard A, et al: Syndrome de l'isolement de la zone du language. *Rev Neurol* 139:417, 1983.

Balter M: "Speech gene" tied to modern humans. *Science* 297:1105, 2002.

Basso A, Taborelli A, Vignolo LA: Dissociated disorders of reading and writing in aphasia. *J Neurol Neurosurg Psychiatry* 41:556, 1978.

Beauvois MF, Saillant B, Meininger V, Lhermitte F: Bilateral tactile aphasia: A tacto-verbal dysfunction. *Brain* 101:381, 1978.

Benson DF: *Aphasia, Alexia, and Agraphia*. New York, Churchill Livingstone, 1980.

Brain R: *Speech Disorders. Aphasia, Apraxia and Agnosia*. Oxford, Butterworth, 1967.

Broca P: Portée de la parole: Ramollisement chronique et destruction partielle du lobe anterieur gauche du cerveau. *Paris Bull Soc Anthropol* 2:219, 1861.

Buchman AS, Garron DC, Trost-Cardomone JE, et al: Word deafness: One hundred years later. *J Neurol Neurosurg Psychiatry* 49:489, 1986.

Ciabarra AM, Elkind MS, Roberts JK, Marshall RS: Subcortical infarction resulting in acquired stuttering. *J Neurol Neurosurg Psychiatry* 69:546, 2000.

Critchley M: Aphasiological nomenclature and definitions. *Cortex* 3:3, 1967.

Croisile B, Laurent B, Michel D, et al: Pure agraphia after a deep hemisphere haematoma. *J Neurol Neurosurg Psychiatry* 53:263, 1990.
Damasio AR: Aphasia. *N Engl J Med* 326:531, 1992.
Damasio AR, Damasio H: The anatomic basis of pure alexia. *Neurology* 33:1573, 1983.
Damasio AR, Geschwind N: Anatomical localization in clinical neuropsychology, in Vinken PJ, Bruyn GW, Klawans HL (eds): *Handbook of Clinical Neurology*. Vol 45. Amsterdam, Elsevier, 1985, pp 7–22.
Damasio H, Damasio AR: The anatomical basis of conduction aphasia. *Brain* 103:337, 1980.
Damasio H, Damasio AR: *Lesion Analysis in Neuropsychology*. New York, Oxford University Press, 1989.
Darby DG: Sensory aprosodia: A clinical clue to lesions of the inferior division of the right middle cerebral artery? *Neurology* 43:567, 1993.
Déjerine J: Contribution a l'étude anatomo-pathologique et clinique des differentes varietés de cécitéverbale. *Mem Soc Biol* 4:61, 1892.
Dronkers NF: A new brain region for coordinating speech articulation. *Nature* 384:159, 1996.
Gardiner AH: *The Theory of Speech and Language*. Westport, CT, Greenwood Press, 1979.
Geschwind N: Non-aphasic disorders of speech. *Int J Neurol* 4:207, 1964.
Geschwind N: Disconnection syndromes in animals and man. *Brain* 88:237, 585, 1965.
Geschwind N: The varieties of naming errors. *Cortex* 3:97, 1967.
Geschwind N: Wernicke's contribution to the study of aphasia. *Cortex* 3:449, 1967.
Geschwind N, Galaburda AM: *Cerebral Dominance: Biological Foundations*. Cambridge, MA, Harvard University Press, 1988.
Geschwind N, Levitsky W: Human brain: Left-right asymmetries in temporal speech region. *Science* 161:186, 1968.
Gloning K: Handedness and aphasia. *Neuropsychologia* 15:355, 1977.
Goldstein K: *Language and Language Disturbances*. New York, Grune & Stratton, 1948, pp 190–216.
Goodglass H, Kaplan E: *The Assessment of Aphasia and Related Disorders*. Philadelphia, Lea & Febiger, 1972.
Goodglass H, Quadfasel FA: Language laterality in left-handed aphasics. *Brain* 77:521, 1954.
Greenblatt SH: Alexia without agraphia or hemianopsia. *Brain* 96:307, 1973.
Head H: *Aphasias and Kindred Disorders*. Cambridge, UK, Cambridge University Press, 1926.
Helm NA, Butler RB, Benson DF: Acquired stuttering. *Neurology* 28:1159, 1978.
Howard D, Patterson K, Franklin S: Treatment of word retrieval deficits in aphasia: A comparison of two therapy methods. *Brain* 108:817, 1985.
Joanette Y, Puel JL, Nespoulosis A, et al: Aphasie croisee chez les droities. *Rev Neurol* 138:375, 1982.
Kertesz A: *Aphasia and Associated Disorders*. Needham Heights, MA, Allyn & Bacon, 1979.
Kertesz A: Clinical forms of aphasia. *Acta Neurochir (Wien)* 56(Suppl):52, 1993.
Kertesz A: *The Western Aphasia Battery*. New York, Grune & Stratton, 1982.
Kertesz A, Benson F: Neologistic jargon: A clinicopathologic study. *Cortex* 6:362, 1970.
Kertesz A, McCabe P: Recovery patterns and prognosis in aphasia. *Brain* 100:1, 1977.
Kertesz A, Sheppard A, Mackenzie R: Localization in transcortical sensory aphasia. *Arch Neurol* 39:475, 1982.
Kinsbourne M: *Hemispheric Disconnection and Cerebral Function*. Springfield, IL, Charles C Thomas, 1974.
Kohn & Weigert, 1874. English translation by Eggert GH: *Wernicke Works on Aphasia: A Source Book and Review*. The Hague, Mouton, 1977.
Kurowski KM, Blumstein SE, Alexander M: The foreign accent syndrome: A reconsideration. *Brain Lang* 54:1, 1996.
LeCours H, Lhermitte F: *Aphasiology*. Eastbourne, UK, Ballière-Tindall, 1989.
LeCours H, Lhermitte F: The pure form of the phonetic disintegration syndrome (pure anarthria). *Brain Lang* 3:88, 1976.
Leiner HC, Leiner SL, Dow RS: Cognitive and language functions of the human cerebellum. *Trends Neurosci* 16:444, 1993.
Leischner A: The agraphias, in Vinken PJ, Bruyn GW (eds): *Handbook of Clinical Neurology*. Vol 4: Disorders of Speech, Perception and Symbolic Behavior. Amsterdam, North-Holland, 1969, pp 141–180.
LeMay M, Culebras A: Human brain morphologic differences in the hemispheres demonstrable by carotid angiography. *N Engl J Med* 287:168, 1972.
Lesser RP, Lueders H, Dinner DS, et al: The location of speech and writing functions in the frontal language area. *Brain* 107:275, 1984.
Levine DN, Mohr JP: Language after bilateral cerebral infarctions: Role of the minor hemisphere in speech. *Neurology* 29:927, 1979.
Lundgren K, Helm-Estabrooks N, Klein R: Stuttering following acquired brain damage: A review of the literature. *J Neurolingustics* 23:447, 2010.
Martin N, Saffran EM: A computational account of deep dysphasia: Evidence from a single case study. *Brain Lang* 43:240, 1992.
Milner B, Branch C, Rasmussen T: Evidence for bilateral speech representation in some non-right-handers. *Trans Am Neurol Assoc* 91:306, 1966.
Mohr JP: Broca's area and Broca's aphasia, in Whitaker H, Whitaker H (eds): *Studies in Neurolinguistics*. Vol 1. New York, Academic Press, 1976, pp 201–235.
Mohr JP: The vascular basis of Wernicke aphasia. *Trans Am Neurol Assoc* 105:133, 1980.
Mohr JP, Pessin MS, Finkelstein S, et al: Broca aphasia: Pathologic and clinical. *Neurology* 28:311, 1978.
Naeser MA, Alexander MP, Helm-Estabrook N, et al: Aphasia with predominantly subcortical lesion sites. *Arch Neurol* 39:2, 1982.
Ojemann G: Cortical organization of language. *J Neurosci* 11:2281, 1991.
Price CJ: Functional-imaging studies of the 19th century neurological model of language. *Rev Neurol* 157:833, 2001.
Ropper AH: Severe dysarthria with right hemisphere stroke. *Neurology* 37:1061, 1987.
Rosati G, de Bastiani P: Pure agraphia: A discrete form of aphasia. *J Neurol Neurosurg Psychiatry* 42:266, 1979.
Rosenbek J, Messert B, Collins M, et al: Stuttering following brain damage. *Brain Lang* 6:82, 1975.
Ross ED: The aprosodias, in Feinberg TE, Farah MJ (eds): *Behavioral Neurology and Neuropsychology*. New York, McGraw-Hill, 1997, pp 699–717.
Roux FE, Dufor O, Giussani C, et al: The graphemic/motor frontal area. Exner's area revisited. *Ann Neurol* 66:537, 2009.
Schott GD: Mirror writing: Neurological reflections on an unusual phenomenon. *J Neurol Neurosurg Psychiatry* 78:5, 2007.
Somerville MJ, Mervis CB, Young EJ, et al: Severe expressive-language delay related to duplication of the Williams-Beuren locus. *N Engl J Med* 353:1694, 2005.
Subirana A: Handedness and cerebral dominance, in Vinken PJ, Bruyn GW (eds): *Handbook of Clinical Neurology*. Vol 4: Disorders of Speech, Perception and Symbolic Behavior. Amsterdam, North-Holland, 1969, pp 284–292.

Symonds C: Aphasia. *J Neurol Neurosurg Psychiatry* 16:1, 1953.
Wender D: Aphasic victim as investigator. *Arch Neurol* 46:91, 1989.
Wernicke C: Der *Aphasische Symptomkomplex*. Breslau, Germany, 1874.
Wertz RT, Weiss DG, Aten JL, et al: Comparison of clinic, home, and deferred language treatment for aphasia: A Veterans Administration Cooperative study. *Arch Neurol* 43:653, 1986.
Willmes K, Poeck K: To what extent can aphasic syndromes be localized? *Brain* 116:1527, 1993.
Wilson SAK: *Aphasia*. London, Kegan Paul, 1926.
Wise RJ, Greene J, Büchel C, Scott SK: Brain regions involved in articulation. *Lancet* 353:1057, 1999.
Yakovlev PI, Rakic P: Patterns of decussation of bulbar pyramids and distribution of pyramidal tracts on the two sides of the spinal cord. *Trans Am Neurol Assoc* 91:366, 1966.

SECTION 6

Disorders of Energy, Mood, and Autonomic and Endocrine Functions

24

Fatigue, Asthenia, Anxiety, and Depression

In this chapter, we consider the clinically related phenomena of lassitude, fatigue, nervousness, irritability, anxiety, and depression. These complaints form the core of a group of "symptom-based" disorders that are a large part of medical practice. Although more abstruse than paralysis, sensory loss, seizures, or aphasia, they are no less important, if for no other reason than their frequency. In an audit of one neurologic practice, anxiety and depressive reactions were the main diagnosis in 20 percent of patients, second only to the symptom of headache (Digon et al). Similarly, in two primary care clinics in Boston and Houston, fatigue was the prominent complaint in 21 and 24 percent of patients, respectively. Some of these symptoms represent only slight aberrations of function or a heightening or exaggeration of normal reactions to environmental stress or to medical and neurologic diseases; others are integral features of the diseases themselves; and still others represent disturbances of neuropsychiatric function that are components of the diseases described in Chaps. 51 through 53 on psychiatry.

FATIGUE AND ASTHENIA

Of the symptoms considered in this chapter, lassitude and fatigue are the most frequent, and the most vague. *Fatigue* refers to the universally familiar state of weariness or exhaustion resulting from physical or mental exertion. *Lassitude* has much the same meaning, although it connotes more of an inability or disinclination to be active, physically or mentally. More than half of all patients entering a general hospital register a complaint of fatigability or admit to it when questioned. During World War I, fatigue was such a prominent symptom in combat personnel as to be given a separate place in medical nosology, namely *combat fatigue*, a term that came to be applied to practically all acute psychiatric disorders occurring on the battlefield. In subsequent wars, it has become a key element of the posttraumatic stress disorders related to exposure to highly stressful circumstances. The common clinical antecedents and accompaniments of fatigue, its significance, and its physiologic and psychologic bases will be better understood if we first consider the effects of fatigue on the normal individual.

Effects of Fatigue on the Normal Person

Fatigue has three basic meanings: (1) biochemical and physiologic changes in muscles and a reduced capacity to generate force manifest as weakness, or asthenia; (2) a disorder in behavior, taking the form of a reduced output of work (*work decrement*) or a lack of endurance; and (3) a subjective feeling of tiredness and discomfort.

The *decreased productivity and capacity for work*, which is a direct consequence of fatigue, has been investigated by industrial psychologists. Their findings clearly demonstrate the importance of motivational factors on work output, whether the effort is of physical or mental type. Quite striking are individual constitutional differences in energy, which vary greatly, just as do differences in temperament. What should be emphasized is that *in the majority of persons complaining of fatigue, one does not find true muscle weakness*. This may be difficult to prove, for many such individuals are disinclined to exert full effort in tests of peak power of muscle contraction or in endurance of muscular activity.

The Clinical Significance of Fatigue

Patients experiencing lassitude and fatigue have a more or less characteristic way of expressing their symptoms. They say that they are "wiped, or burned out," "tired all the time," "weary," "exhausted," or "pooped out," or that they have "no pep," "no ambition," or "no interest." They manifest their condition by showing an indifference to the tasks at hand, by emphasizing how hard they are working, and how stressed they are by circumstances; they are inclined to sit around or lie down or to occupy themselves with trivial tasks. On closer analysis, one observes and hears that many such patients have difficulty in initiating activity and also in sustaining it; i.e., their endurance is diminished. This condition, of course, is the familiar aftermath of sleeplessness or prolonged mental or physical effort, and, under such circumstances, it is accepted as a normal physiologic reaction. When, however, similar symptoms appear without relation to such antecedents, they should be suspected of being the manifestations of disease.

The physician's task is initially to determine whether the patient is merely suffering from the common physical and mental effects of overwork. Overworked, overwrought people are observable everywhere in our society. In addition to fatigue, such persons frequently show irritability, restlessness, sleeplessness, and anxiety, sometimes to the point of panic attacks and a variety of somatic symptoms, particularly abdominal, thoracic, and cranial discomforts. Formerly, society accepted this state in responsible individuals and prescribed the obvious cure, a vacation. Even Charcot made time for regular "cures" during the year, in which he retired to a spa without family, colleagues, or the drain of work. Nowadays, the need to contain this type of stress, to which some individuals are more prone than others, has spawned an industry of meditation, yoga, and similar activities. Individuals with hobbies, nonwork interests, and athletic pursuits seem to be less subject to this problem. A common error in diagnosis, however, is to ascribe fatigue to overwork when actually it is a manifestation of anxiety or depression, as described below.

Fatigue as a Symptom of Psychiatric Illness

The majority of patients who seek medical help for unexplained chronic fatigue and lassitude are found to have some type of psychiatric illness. Formerly this state was called "neurasthenia," a term introduced by Beard, but because lassitude and fatigue rarely exist as isolated phenomena, the current practice is to label such cases according to the total clinical picture. The usual associated symptoms are anxiety, irritability, depression, insomnia, headaches, dizziness, difficulty in concentrating, reduced sexual drive, and loss (or sometimes increase) of appetite. In one series, 85 percent of persons admitted to a general hospital and seen in consultation by a psychiatrist for the chief complaint of chronic fatigue were diagnosed, finally, as having anxious depression or an anxiety state. In a subsequent study, Wessely and Powell found similarly that 72 percent of patients who presented to a neurologic center with unexplained chronic fatigue proved to have a psychiatric disorder, most often a depressive illness.

Several features are common to the psychiatric group with fatigue. Tests of peak muscle power on command, with the patient exerting full effort, reveal no weakness. The sense of fatigue may be worse in the morning. There is an inclination to lie down and rest, but sleep does not follow. The fatigue is worsened by mild exertion and relates more to some activities than to others. Inquiry may disclose that the symptom was first experienced in temporal relation to a grief reaction, a surgical procedure, physical trauma such as an automobile accident, or a medical illness such as myocardial infarction. The feeling of fatigue interferes with both mental and physical activities; the patient is easily worried, is "full of complaints," and finds it difficult to concentrate in attempting to solve a problem or to read a book, or in carrying on a complicated conversation. Also, sleep is disturbed, with a tendency to early morning waking, so that such persons are at their worst in the morning, both in spirit and in energy output. Their tendency is to improve as the day wears on, and they may even feel fairly normal by evening. It may be difficult to decide whether the fatigue is a primary manifestation of the disease or secondary to a lack of interest.

Among chronically fatigued individuals without medical disease, not all deviate enough from normal to justify the diagnosis of anxiety or depression. Many persons, because of circumstances beyond their control, have little motivation and much idle time. They are bored with the monotony of their routine. Such circumstances are conducive to fatigue, just as the opposite, a strong emotion or a new enterprise that excites optimism and enthusiasm, will dispel fatigue. Some persons are born with low impulse and energy and become more so at times of stress; they have a lifelong inability to exercise vigorously, to compete successfully, to work hard without exhaustion, to withstand illness or recover quickly from it, or to assume a dominant role in a social group—a "constitutional asthenia" (Kahn's term). Most of these traits are evident from childhood. These difficulties are not currently framed in these terms because they sound judgmental, but disorders of this type have been known since antiquity and only vary in name and social context in each era.

Fatigue in Neurologic Diseases

Not unexpectedly, fatigue and intolerance of exercise (i.e., fatigue with mild exertion) are prominent manifestations of myopathic disease. Even in myasthenia gravis, the muscles exhibiting fatigue are usually weak, however, in the resting state. In addition to myasthenia gravis, the classes of myopathy in which weakness, inability to sustain effort, and excessive fatigue are notable features include the muscular dystrophies, congenital myopathies, other disorders of neuromuscular transmission (Lambert-Eaton syndrome), toxic myopathies (e.g., from cholesterol-lowering drugs), some of the glycogen storage myopathies, and mitochondrial myopathies. One type of glycogen storage disease, McArdle phosphorylase deficiency, is exceptional in that fatigue and weakness are accompanied by pain and sometimes by cramps and contracture. The first contractions after rest are of near-normal strength, but after 20 to 30 contractions, there occurs a deep ache and an increasing firmness and shortening of the contracting muscles. Another such process, acid maltase deficiency, is at times associated with disproportionate weakness and fatigue of respiratory muscles, which leads to dyspnea and retention of carbon dioxide. The characteristics of these diseases are presented in the chapters on muscle disease. Further comments on muscular fatigue can be found in Chap. 48.

Fatigue of varying degree is also a regular feature of all diseases that are marked by denervation of muscle and loss of muscle fibers. Fatigue in these cases is a result of the excessive work imposed on the remaining intact muscle (overwork fatigue). This is most characteristic of amyotrophic lateral sclerosis and the postpolio syndrome, but it also occurs in patients who are recovering from Guillain-Barré syndrome and in those with chronic polyneuropathy.

Not surprisingly, many neurologic diseases that are characterized by incessant muscular activity or by difficulty engaging the muscles (Parkinson disease, cerebral palsy, Huntington disease, hemiballismus) also induce fatigue. Muscles partially paralyzed by a stroke feel tired and may cause an overall fatigue state. The distinguished neuroanatomist A. Brodal gave an interesting account of his own stroke and its effects on muscle power. Fatigue is often a major complaint of patients with multiple sclerosis; its cause is unknown, although the effect of cytokines circulating in the cerebrospinal fluid has been postulated. The depression that follows stroke or myocardial infarction frequently presents with the complaint of fatigue rather than other signs of mood disorder. Inordinate fatigue is a common complaint among patients with postconcussive syndrome (see Chap. 35). Severe fatigue that causes the patient consistently to go to bed right after dinner and makes all mental activity effortful should suggest an associated depression. These central fatigue states and their possible mechanisms, almost all speculative, have been discussed by Chaudhuri and Behan.

Many states of disordered autonomic function in which static or orthostatic hypotension are features, are associated with a fatigue state. Whether there is in addition a type of central autonomic (hypothalamic) fatigue, aside from the endocrine changes discussed below, is uncertain, but such an entity seems plausible and has been included in models of the illness currently called chronic fatigue syndrome.

Fatigue in Medical Diseases

A wide variety of *medications* and other therapeutic agents, particularly when first administered, sometimes induce fatigue. The main offenders in this respect are antihypertensive drugs, especially beta-adrenergic blocking agents, antiepileptics, antispasticity drugs, anxiolytics, chemotherapy and radiation therapy and, paradoxically, many antidepressant and antipsychotic drugs. Introduction of these medications in gradually escalating doses may obviate the problem, but just as often, an alternative medicine must be chosen. The administration of beta-interferon for the treatment of multiple sclerosis (and alpha-interferon for other diseases) induces fatigue of varying degree. Surgeons and nurses can testify to fatigue that comes with exposure to anesthetics in inadequately ventilated operating rooms. Similarly, fatigue and headache may result from exposure to carbon monoxide or natural gas in homes with furnaces in disrepair or from leaking gas pipes, but this is also a frequent delusion in anxious, depressed, or demented patients.

The *sleep apnea* syndrome is an important and often overlooked cause of fatigue and daytime drowsiness. In overweight men who snore loudly and need to nap frequently, testing for sleep apnea is indicated (this subject was taken up in Chap. 19). Correcting the obstructive apnea that underlies this condition leads to a dramatic reduction in fatigue. The same holds for patients who have neuromuscular diseases that affect the diaphragm and other respiratory muscles.

Acute or chronic infection is an important cause of fatigue. Everyone has at some time or other sensed the abrupt onset of exhaustion, a tired ache in the muscles, or an inexplicable listlessness, only to discover later that he was "coming down with the flu." Chronic infections such as hepatitis, tuberculosis, brucellosis, infectious mononucleosis, HIV, and bacterial endocarditis may not be evident immediately but should be suspected when fatigue is a new symptom and disproportionate to other symptoms such as mood change, nervousness, and anxiety. Whether a chronic form of Lyme disease is responsible for chronic fatigue, as often imputed, is uncertain at best. Often, fatigue begins with an obvious infection (such as influenza, hepatitis, or infectious mononucleosis), but persists for several weeks after the overt manifestations of infection have subsided; it may then be difficult to decide whether the fatigue represents the lingering effects of the infection or is due to psychologic-asthenic symptoms during convalescence. This difficult problem is discussed below. Patients with systemic lupus, Sjögren syndrome, or polymyalgia rheumatica may complain of severe fatigue; in the last of these, fatigue may be the initial and a profound symptom.

Metabolic and endocrine diseases of various types may cause inordinate degrees of lassitude and fatigue. Sometimes there is, in addition, a true muscular weakness. In Addison, Sheehan, and Simmonds diseases, fatigue may dominate the clinical picture. Aldosterone deficiency is another established cause of chronic fatigue. In persons with hypothyroidism with or without frank myxedema, lassitude and fatigue are frequent complaints, as are muscle aches and joint pains. Fatigue may also be present in patients with hyperthyroidism, but it is usually less troublesome than nervousness. Uncontrolled diabetes mellitus is accompanied by excessive fatigability, as are hyperparathyroidism, hypogonadism, and Cushing disease. Fatigue as a feature of vitamin B_{12} deficiency, as stated in many textbooks, has not been evident in the cases with mild deficiency that we have observed.

Reduced cardiac output and diminished pulmonary reserve are important causes of breathlessness and fatigue, which are brought out by mild exertion. Anemia, when severe, is another cause, probably predicated on a similar inadequacy of oxygen supply to tissues. Mild grades of anemia are usually asymptomatic, and tiredness is still far too often ascribed to it. An occult malignant tumor, e.g., pancreatic, hepatic, or gastric carcinoma, may announce itself by inordinate fatigue. In patients with metastatic carcinoma, and especially lymphoma, leukemia, or multiple myeloma, fatigue is a usual and prominent symptom. Uremia is accompanied by fatigue; the associated anemia may play a role. Any type of *nutritional deficiency* may, when severe, cause lassitude; in its early stages, this may be the chief complaint. Weight loss and a history of alcoholism and dietary inadequacy provide the clues to the nature of the illness.

Pregnancy causes fatigue, which may be profound in the later months. To some extent the underlying causes, including the work of carrying excess weight and an anemia, are obvious; but if excessive weight gain and hypertension are associated, preeclampsia should be suspected.

Postviral and Chronic Fatigue Syndromes

A particularly difficult problem arises in the patient who complains of severe fatigue for many months or even years after a bout of infectious mononucleosis or some other viral illness. This has been appropriately called the *postviral fatigue syndrome*. The majority of patients are women between 20 and 40 years of age, but there are undoubtedly young men with the same illness. A few such patients had been found to have unusually high titers of antibody to Epstein-Barr virus (EBV), which suggested a causal relationship and gave rise to terms such as the *chronic infectious mononucleosis* or *chronic EBV syndrome* (Straus et al). However, subsequent studies made it clear that a majority of patients with complaints of chronic fatigue have neither a clear-cut history of infectious mononucleosis nor serologic evidence of this or another infection (Straus; Holmes et al). In some of these patients, the fatigue state has allegedly been associated with obscure immunologic abnormalities similar to those attributed (spuriously) to silicone breast implants or minor trauma. The currently fashionable designation for these abstruse states of persistent fatigue is the *chronic fatigue syndrome*.

Some perspective is provided by the recognition that a malady of this precise nature, under many different names, has long pervaded postindustrial western society, as described by Shorter in an informative history of the chronic fatigue syndrome. The attribution of fatigue to viral or Lyme infection and to ill-defined immune dysfunction are only the latest in a long line of putative explanations. At various times, even in our recent memory, colitis and other forms of bowel dysfunction, spinal irritation, hypoglycemia, brucellosis, and chronic candidiasis, "multiple chemical sensitivity," retroviral infection, or environmental allergies, among others, have been proposed without basis as causes. Unfortunately, these spurious associations have only served to marginalize the disease and patients who suffer from it.

The current criteria for the diagnosis of chronic fatigue syndrome are the presence of persistent and disabling fatigue for at least 6 months, coupled with an arbitrary number (6 or 8) of persistent or recurrent somatic and neuropsychologic symptoms including low-grade fever, cervical or axillary lymphadenopathy, myalgias, migrating arthralgias, sore throat, forgetfulness, headaches, difficulties in concentration and thinking, irritability, and sleep disturbances (Holmes et al). A number of such patients in our experience have complained of paresthesias in the feet or hands. On close questioning, many of these sensations prove to be odd, particularly numbness in the bones or muscles or fluctuating patches of numbness or paresthesia on the chest, face, or nose. Unusual descriptions may be given if the patient is allowed adequate time to describe the symptoms. A few have reported blurred or "close to" double vision; in neither case are there physical findings to corroborate the sensory experiences.

There is a common association with the similarly obscure entity of *fibromyalgia*, consisting of neck, shoulder, and paraspinal pain and point tenderness, as described in Chaps. 11 and 48. Despite these complaints, the patient may look surprisingly well and the neurologic examination is normal. The term for this same entity, *myalgic encephalomyelitis*, is preferred in Great Britain and captures the association between the two syndromes.

Complaints of muscle weakness are also frequent among such patients, but Lloyd and coworkers, who studied their neuromuscular performance and compared them with control subjects, found no difference in maximal isometric strength or endurance in repetitive submaximal exercise and no change in intramuscular acidosis, serum creatine kinase (CK) levels, or depletion of energy substrates. These individuals share with depressed patients a subnormal response to cortical magnetic motor stimulation after exercise (Samii et al), which can be said to match their symptoms of reduced endurance but otherwise is difficult to interpret. In a small number of affected persons, a chronic but usually mild hypotension, elicited with tilt-table testing and reversed by mineralocorticoids, has been proposed as a cause of chronic fatigue (Rowe et al). Electromyography and nerve conduction studies are typically normal, as is the spinal fluid, but the electroencephalogram (EEG) may be mildly and nonspecifically slowed. Batteries of psychologic tests have disclosed variable impairments of cognitive function, misinterpreted by advocates of the "organic" nature of the syndrome as proof of some type of encephalopathy.

In a large group of patients who were studied 6 months after viral infections, Cope and colleagues found that none of the features of the original illness was predictive of the development of chronic fatigue; however, a previous history of fatigue or psychiatric problems, and an indefinite diagnosis were often associated with persistent disability. In one study of more than 1,000 patients who were observed for 6 months following an infective illness, the chronic fatigue syndrome was no more frequent than in the general population (Wessely et al). One thing is clear to the authors: that applying the label of *chronic fatigue syndrome* in susceptible individuals tends to perpetuate this state.

Having oriented the above discussion to imply that many cases of chronic fatigue have a psychologic, or asthenic basis, it should be emphasized that previously healthy individuals, for years after a severe febrile viral infection may have persistent fatigue; the best-characterized situation follows mononucleosis, but other febrile illnesses have been implicated as well. These cases, in our experience, have arisen suddenly, mostly in adolescents and young men, and less often women, who experience overwhelming fatigue during a well-documented and prolonged viral infection. They continue to take interest in activities in which they are able to participate, do not show anxiety or major depressive symptoms, and have the best prognosis, although complete recovery may take up to 3 to 5 years. Often these patients are able to define the date on which the illness began. The term *postviral fatigue state* is most appropriate for this group. Impressive in some of our cases have been severe headaches and orthostatic hypotension, with wide swings in blood pressure resulting in syncope as well as intermittent hypertension. Alcohol intolerance may develop. It would seem that the more ambiguous and less-severe cases of chronic fatigue, particularly those with fibromyalgia, may have a different basis, but this cannot be stated with certainty.

At the present time, the status of the chronic fatigue syndrome is undetermined. The possibility of an obscure metabolic or immunologic derangement secondary to a viral infection cannot be dismissed, as discussed by

Swartz, but the majority of cases lack such a history. Certainly, high levels of cytokines, such as occur after many types of illness and with cancer, and some of the numerous endocrine aberrations are capable of causing fatigue and lethargy. From a neurologic perspective, the hypothalamus is the structure most implicated by the loss of endurance and the presence of associated symptoms such as orthostatic intolerance, tachycardia and some of the endocrine changes enumerated later in the chapter. Treatment is discussed further on.

Differential Diagnosis of Fatigue

If one looks critically at patients who seek medical help because of incapacitating exhaustion, lassitude, and fatigability, it is evident that the most commonly overlooked diagnoses are anxiety and depression as described in Chap. 52. The correct conclusion can usually be reached by keeping these illnesses in mind as one elicits the history from patient and family. Difficulty arises when symptoms of the psychiatric illness are so inconspicuous as not to be appreciated; one comes then to suspect the diagnosis only by having eliminated the common medical causes. Repeated observation may bear out the existence of an anxiety state or gloomy mood. Reassurance in combination with a therapeutic trial of antidepressant drugs may suppress symptoms of which the patient was barely aware, thus clarifying the diagnosis. The best that can be done is to assist the patient in adjusting to the adverse circumstances that have brought him under medical surveillance.

In intractable cases, tuberculosis, brucellosis, Lyme disease, hepatitis, bacterial endocarditis, mycoplasmal pneumonia, HIV, EBV, cytomegalovirus (CMV), coxsackie B, and other viral infections, and malaria, hookworm, giardiasis, and other parasitic infections need to be considered in the differential diagnosis, and an inquiry made for their characteristic symptoms, signs, and when appropriate, laboratory findings; however, such infections are infrequently found. There should also be a search for anemia, renal failure, chronic inflammatory disease such as temporal arteritis and polymyalgia rheumatica (sedimentation rate); an endocrine survey (thyroid, calcium, and cortisol levels) and an evaluation for an occult tumor are also in order in obscure cases. It must be remembered that chronic intoxication with alcohol, barbiturates, or other sedative drugs, some of which are given to suppress nervousness or insomnia, may contribute to fatigability. The rapid and recent onset of fatigue should always suggest the presence of an infection, a disturbance in fluid balance, gastrointestinal bleeding, or rapidly developing circulatory failure of either peripheral or cardiac origin. The features that suggest sleep apnea have been mentioned above and are discussed further in Chap. 19.

Finally, it bears repeating that lassitude and fatigue must be distinguished from genuine muscular weakness. The demonstration of reduced power, reflex changes, fasciculations, and atrophy sets the case analysis along different lines, bringing up for particular consideration diseases of the peripheral nervous system or of the musculature. Rare, difficult-to-diagnose diseases that cause inexplicable muscle weakness and exercise intolerance are otherwise inevident hyperthyroidism, hyperparathyroidism, ossifying hemangiomas with hypophosphatemia, some of the periodic paralyses, hyperinsulinism, disorders of carbohydrate and lipid metabolism, and the mitochondrial myopathies, all of which are discussed in later chapters of the book on disease of muscle.

Treatment of Fatigue

It has been our impression that most patients with ongoing complaints of very low energy without a clearly preceding febrile infection from the outset and without one of the medical illnesses associated with fatigue, have elements of depression. They are probably best treated with gradually increasing exercise levels and perhaps with antidepressant medication, although this regimen has not always been successful. There are reports of success in treating these patients with mineralocorticoids (predicated on the above-mentioned orthostatic intolerance), estradiol patches, hypnosis, and a variety of other medical and nonmedical treatments. Cognitive and behavioral therapies have been summarized in the *Effective Health Care* report by Bagnall and colleagues from the National Health Service Centre for Reviews and Dissemination and in the extensive review by Chambers and colleagues, neither of which came to a firm conclusion about the effects of treatment, but acknowledged that cognitive behavioral therapy and graded exercise therapy may be of value. A few patients with chronic fatigue exhibit the psychologic disorder related to litigation ("compensation neurosis"). Noteworthy is the frequency with which a similar syndrome has become the basis of court action against employers or claims against the government, as in the "building-related illness" (formerly "sick-building syndrome"). As alluded to earlier, attribution of fatigue to Lyme disease and obscure infections or allergies should be made cautiously if there is no firm evidence.

NERVOUSNESS, ANXIETY, STRESS, AND IRRITABILITY

The world is full of nervous, tense, apprehensive, and worried people. The stresses of contemporary society are often blamed for their plight. The poet W.H. Auden referred to his era as "the age of anxiety," and little has changed since then. Medical historians have identified comparable periods of pervasive anxiety dating back to the time of Marcus Aurelius and Constantine, when societies were undergoing rapid and profound changes, and individuals were assailed by an overwhelming sense of insecurity, personal insignificance, and fear of the future (Rosen).

Like lassitude and fatigue, nervousness, irritability, and anxiety are among the most frequent symptoms encountered in office and hospital practice. A British survey found that more than 40 percent of the population, at one time or another, experienced symptoms of severe anxiety, and approximately 5 percent suffered from lifelong anxiety states (Lader). The vast amount of antianxiety medication and alcohol that is consumed in our society would tend to corroborate these figures. Of course, any person facing a challenging or threatening task for which he may feel unprepared and inadequate experiences some degree of nervousness and anxiety. Anxiety is then not abnormal, and the alertness and attentiveness that accompany it may actually improve performance up to a point. Barratt and White found that mildly anxious medical students performed better on examinations than those lacking in anxiety. As anxiety increases, so does the standard of performance, but only to a point, after which increasing anxiety causes a rapid decline in performance (Yerkes-Dodson law).

If worry or depression stands in clear relation to serious economic reverses or loss of a loved one, the symptom is also usually accepted as normal, but no less worthy of emotional support. Only when it is excessively intense or prolonged or when accompanying visceral derangements are prominent do anxiety and depression become matters of medical concern. Admittedly, the line that separates normal emotional reactions and pathologic ones is not sharp. Chapter 52 deals with these matters more fully.

Here we are concerned with *nervousness, irritability, stress, anxiety, and depression as symptoms*, together with current views of their origins and biologic significance.

Anxiety Reactions and Panic Attacks

There is no unanimity among psychiatrists as to whether symptoms of nervousness, irritability, anxiety, and fear comprise a single emotional reaction, varying only in its severity or duration, or a group of discrete reactions, each with distinctive clinical features. In some writings, anxiety is classified as a form of subacute or chronic fear but there is reason to question this assumption. Anxious patients, when frightened under experimental conditions, state that the fear reaction differs in being more overwhelming. The exceedingly frightened person is "frozen," unable to act or to think clearly, and his responses are automatic and sometimes irrational. The fear reaction is characterized by overactivity of both the sympathetic and parasympathetic nervous systems, and the parasympathetic effects (bradycardia, sphincteric relaxation) may predominate, unlike anxiety, in which sympathetic effects are the more prominent ones. Long ago, Cicero distinguished between an acute and transient attack of fear provoked by a specific stimulus (*angor*) and a protracted state of fearfulness (*anxietas*). This distinction was elaborated by Freud, who regarded fear as an appropriate response to a sudden, unexpected external threat and anxiety as a neurotic maladjustment.

Less readily distinguishable from anxiety is the complaint of *nervousness*. By this vague term, the layperson usually refers to a state of restlessness, inner tension, uneasiness, apprehension, irritability, or hyperexcitability. Unfortunately, the term may have a wide range of other connotations, such as a distressing hallucination or paranoid idea, a frankly hysterical outburst, or even tics or tremulousness. Obviously, a careful inquiry as to what the patient means in complaining of nervousness is always a necessary first step in the analysis.

Most often nervousness represents no more than a transient psychic and behavioral state in which the person is maximally challenged or threatened by difficult personal problems. Some persons claim to have been nervous throughout life or to be nervous periodically for no apparent reason. In these instances, the symptoms blend imperceptibly with those of anxiety disorder or depression, described below.

We use the term *anxiety* to denote an emotional state characterized by subjective feelings of nervousness, irritability, uneasy anticipation, and apprehension, often but by no means always with a definite topical content and the physiologic accompaniments of strong emotion, i.e., one or more of the symptoms of breathlessness, tightness in the chest, choking sensation, palpitation, increased muscular tension, dizziness, trembling, sweating, and flushing. The vasomotor and visceral accompaniments are mediated through the autonomic nervous system, particularly its sympathetic part, and involve also the thyroid and adrenal glands.

Panic Attacks

The symptoms of anxiety may be manifest either in acute episodes, each lasting several minutes or up to an hour, or as a protracted state that may last for weeks, months, or years. In the *panic attack*, the patient is suddenly overwhelmed by feelings of apprehension, or a fear that he may lose consciousness and die, have a heart attack or stroke, lose his reason or self-control, become insane, or commit some horrible crime. These experiences are accompanied by a series of physiologic reactions, mainly sympathoadrenal hyperactivity, resembling the "fight-or-flight" reaction. Breathlessness, a feeling of suffocation, dizziness, sweating, trembling, palpitation, and precordial or gastric distress are typical but not invariable physical accompaniments. As a persistent and less-severe state, the patient experiences fluctuating degrees of nervousness, palpitation or excessive cardiac impulse, shortness of breath, light-headedness, faintness, easy fatigue, and intolerance of physical exertion.

Attacks tend to occur during periods of relative calm and in nonthreatening circumstances. Usually, the apprehension and physical symptoms escalate over a period of minutes to an hour and then abate over 20 to 30 min, leaving the patient tired, weak, and perplexed. The dramatic symptoms of the panic attack have usually abated by the time the patient reaches a doctor's office or an emergency department, but the blood pressure may still be elevated, and there may be tachycardia. Otherwise, the patient looks remarkably collected. Often, discrete anxiety attacks and persistent states of anxiety merge with one another. The fear of further attacks leads many patients, particularly women, to become agoraphobic and homebound, fearing public places, especially if alone.

Because panic is a common disorder, affecting 2 to 4 percent of the population at some time in their lives as cited by Roy-Byrne and colleagues, and the symptoms mimic acute neurologic disease, the neurologist is often called upon to distinguish panic attacks from temporal lobe seizures or from vertiginous disorders. Except for the occasional inability of the patient to think or articulate clearly during a panic attack, the manifestations of epilepsy are quite different. Practically never is consciousness lost during a panic attack. If dizziness predominates in the attacks, there may be concern about vertebrobasilar ischemia or labyrinthine dysfunction (see Chap. 15). Vertigo from any cause is accompanied by many of the autonomic symptoms displayed during a panic attack, but careful questioning in the latter will elicit the characteristic apprehension, breathlessness, and palpitations, and the absence of ataxia or other neurologic signs.

Recurrent panic attacks and chronic anxiety have a familial aspect, with one-fifth of first-degree relatives affected and a high degree of concordance in monozygotic twins. The panic symptoms tend to be periodic, beginning in the patient's twenties; a later onset is more usually coupled with depression, treatment of which is discussed in Chap. 52. Most often, panic in younger persons is a component of a generalized anxiety disorder, but it may stand alone as the only mental symptom or be an opening feature of schizophrenia.

Persistent Anxiety and Anxious Depression

Episodic or sustained anxiety without a disorder of mood (i.e., without depression) is classified as *generalized anxiety disorder,* or formerly, *anxiety neurosis*. The term *neurocirculatory asthenia* (among many others) had been applied to the chronic form when accompanied by prominent fatigue and exercise intolerance, in which case it blends into the fatigue states discussed earlier. The symptoms of anxiety may, however, be part of several other psychiatric disorders; it may be combined with other somatic symptoms in hysteria and is the most prominent feature of *phobic disorder*. Symptoms of persistent anxiety with insomnia, lassitude, and fatigue should always raise the suspicion of a *depressive* illness, especially when they begin in middle adult life or beyond. Also, unexplained anxiety or panic attacks may sometimes herald the onset of a schizophrenic illness. As with fatigue, the symptoms of both anxiety and depression are prominent features of the postconcussion syndrome, and of *posttraumatic stress syndrome* (see Chap. 35). These disorders highlight the difficulty in separating generalized anxiety disorder as a unique psychiatric entity. When visceral symptoms predominate or the psychic counterparts of fear and apprehension are absent, the presence of thyrotoxicosis, Cushing disease, pheochromocytoma, hypoglycemia, and menopausal symptoms should be considered.

Posttraumatic Stress Disorder (PTSD)

This state has been alluded to previously in several contexts, but in the past decades it has come to have specific connotation and to stand as a separate disorder. An extremely stressful, or traumatic event that causes fear and helplessness, triggers a persistent psychological state in which the patient reexperiences the event, avoids reminders of it, and is in a constant state of hyperarousal. Current diagnostic criteria require that this condition persist for over a month, prior to that time the condition is termed "acute stress disorder." Even proponents of posttraumatic stress disorder (PTSD) as a separate medical condition acknowledge that there is considerable overlap with anxious depression, the critical difference being the existence of a triggering traumatic event. They make the point that the original event may not be initially articulated by the patient but symptoms such as palpitations, dyspnea, dysphoria, and unexplained pains and other physical symptoms may be prominent, just as in depression.

The biologic distinctions that have been made between anxious depression and PTSD include lower-than-normal cortisol levels, an attenuated increase of these levels in the immediate aftermath of the event, and an exaggerated suppression in response to dexamethasone. However, elevated circulating levels of norepinephrine and increased sensitivity of alpha$_2$-adrenergic receptors that are found in the posttraumatic syndrome are shared with all other anxiety states (Southwick et al). Many of these studies have been poorly controlled.

It is apparent that there is a wide range of human vulnerability to prolonged difficulties after traumatic events. In all probability, this parallels to some extent an endogenous susceptibility to PTSD. Examples of this are the elicitation of symptoms by events not even witnessed personally, such as national disasters that are shared by large populations but produce symptoms in only a very few individuals, and the wide variation of responses to witnessing death and destruction during wartime.

The authors' view is in agreement with the consensus that PTSD represents a special type of induced anxiety state with fairly stereotyped psychologic aspects, often with an accompanying depression and somatic symptoms. Separating it by highlighting the triggering event serves a useful nosologic purpose and draws attention to the need for treatment in individuals such as those returning from battle or after rape or violent attack.

Selective serotonin reuptake inhibitors have been suggested for initial treatment but the other classes of antidepression drugs are also effective. Limiting anxiolytics such as benzodiazepines is recommended, but there are few data on which to make these judgments. A sympathetic psychiatrist is helpful in reassuring affected individuals and giving them perspectives to cope with the trauma. The review by Yehuda is very informative on this subject and many of the comments above are taken from her summary. An emerging notion is that sedatives or narcotics administered immediately after the inciting event may reduce the incidence and severity of PTSD, for example in battlefield conditions.

Stress and Stress Syndromes

The psychologic phenomenon of *stress* is closely allied to nervousness, fatigue, and anxiety and all of them are pervasive features of modern life. In general terms, stress has been defined as a feeling of self-doubt about being able to cope with some situation over a period of time. The term *stress syndrome* refers to perturbations of behavior and accompanying physiologic changes that are ascribable to environmental challenges of such intensity and duration as to overwhelm the individual's adaptive capacity. The biologic effects of this phenomenon can be recognized in many species; chickens laying fewer eggs when moved to a new coop and cows giving less milk when put in a new barn, or monkeys going berserk when repeatedly frustrated by threats that they cannot control. Human beings forced to work under confined conditions and constant danger and cultural groups removed from their home and traditional way of life lose their coping skills and suffer anxiety and stress reactions.

Hans Selye, influenced by Pavlov's concepts of stress, produced lesions in the visceral organs by exposing animals to life-threatening stressors combined with corticosteroids. Cardiac contraction-band necrosis and the shallow hemorrhagic gastrointestinal tract lesion (Cushing ulcer) are two examples of such catecholamine-mediated organ damage that is precipitated by acutely stressful circumstances. The dramatic syndrome of ballooning of the left ventricular apex, or takotsubo-like cardiomyopathy (so-named for the shape of the Japanese octopus trapping pot), is a manifestation of catecholamine excess caused by acute stress.

There is also equivocal epidemiologic evidence that chronic stress in certain individuals, captured in the type A personality, raises the risk of cardiac disease, but the mechanism here, if it indeed exists, is likely to be through a physiologic intermediary such as systemic hypertension or perhaps inflammation that leads to atherosclerosis. Presumably, they have an increased output of "stress hormones" (cortisol and adrenaline).

Such psychologic disorders, bearing a direct relationship to environmental stressors, are among the most common occupational health problems. Stress syndromes are distinguished from anxiety disorders, in which the psychologic disturbance arises from within the individual and has no definite relationship to environmental stimuli. Whether certain individuals are by nature hyperresponsive to such stimuli is not known. The only therapeutic approach is to attempt to alter the patient's perception of stress—for example, with psychotherapy and meditation exercises—and to remove him, if possible, from recognizable environmental stressors. (See "Editorial" in references.)

Irritable Mood and Aggressive Behavior

The phenomenon of irritability, or an irritable mood, must be familiar to almost everyone, exposed as we are to all of the noise, niggling inconveniences, and annoyances of daily life. It is, nevertheless, a difficult symptom to interpret in the context of psychopathology. Freud used the term *Reisbarkeit* in a restricted sense to denote an undue sensitivity to noise—and considered it a manifestation of anxiety, but obviously, this symptom has a much broader connotation and significance. For one thing, some people are by nature irritable throughout life. Also, irritability is an almost expected reaction in overworked, overwrought individuals, who become irritable by force of circumstances. An irritable mood or feeling may be present without observed manifestations (inward irritability), or there may be an overt loss of control of temper, with irascible verbal and behavioral outbursts, provoked by trivial but frustrating events.

Irritability in the foregoing circumstances can hardly be considered a departure from normal. However, when it becomes a recurrent event in a person of normally placid temperament, it assumes significance, for it may then signify an ongoing anxiety state or depression. Irritability is also a common symptom of obsessive–compulsive disorders. Here the irritability tends to be directed inward, indicating perhaps a sense of frustration with personal disability (Snaith and Taylor). Depressed patients are frequently irritable; as a corollary, this symptom should always be sought in patients suspected of being depressed. The days preceding menses and the mother's common postnatal mood disorder are characterized by high levels of outwardly directed irritability. Short-temperedness and irritability are also common features of the manic state. The most extreme degrees of irritability, exemplified by repeated quarrelsome and assaultive behavior (irritable aggression), are rarely observed in anxiety disorders and endogenous depression but are usually the mark of sociopathy and conventional brain disease (in the past, general paresis). Such irritable aggression is also observed in some patients with Alzheimer disease and other types of dementia, particularly of the frontotemporal type, and following traumatic contusions or encephalitis of the temporal and frontal lobes.

Cause, Mechanism, and Biologic Significance of Nervousness and Anxiety

These have been the subjects of much biologic and psychologic speculation, and completely satisfactory explanations are not available. As noted above, some individuals go through life in a chronic state of low-grade anxiety, the impetus for which may or may not be apparent. Spontaneous episodes of anxiety demand another explanation. Some psychologists regard anxiety as anticipatory behavior, i.e., a state of uneasiness about something that may happen in the future. William McDougall spoke of it as "an emotional state arising when a continuing strong desire seems likely to miss its goal." The primary emotion, somewhat muted perhaps, may be one of fear, and its arousal under conditions that are not overtly threatening may be explained as a conditioned response to some recondite component of a formerly threatening stimulus. The James-Lange theory of emotion, which is dated but should not be dismissed, suggests that the dominant feature of the experience of anxiety is simply the physical experience of the associated autonomic discharge.

Infusions of lactic acid can make the symptoms of anxiety worse and, in susceptible individuals, may elicit a panic attack. The patient seems not to tolerate the work or exercise needed to build up stamina. The urinary excretion of epinephrine was found to be elevated in some patients with panic disorder; in others, there is an increased urinary excretion of norepinephrine and its metabolites. During periods of intense anxiety, aldosterone excretion is increased to 2 or 3 times normal.

There is evidence that corticosteroids and corticotropin-releasing hormone (CRH) have a role in the genesis of anxiety. A systemic release of corticosteroid accompanies all states of stress, and the administration of corticosteroids may give rise to anxiety and panic in some patients and to depression in others, suggesting a linkage between steroid stimulation of the limbic system activities that generate these states. In animal models, stress elicited by predators or electric shock as well as by withdrawal of alcohol and other drugs precipitates activity in CRH pathways (amygdala to hypothalamus, raphe nuclei, nucleus ceruleus, and other regions of the brainstem); blocking such activity by drugs or by destruction of the amygdala eliminates anxiety and fear-like behavior. Admittedly, the concepts of fear, stress, and anxiety are used interchangeably in these models, but repeated stimuli that produce fear and stress may eventually induce a state akin to anxiety, and the amygdala appears to be involved in the perpetuation of this anxiety state. The meaning of these effects, i.e., whether they are primary or secondary, is not certain, but it is evident that prolonged and diffuse anxiety is associated with certain biochemical abnormalities of the blood and probably of the brain.

In addition to the role of the amygdala, animal studies have related acute anxiety to a disturbance of function of the locus ceruleus and the septal and hippocampal areas, the principal norepinephrine-containing nuclei. The locus ceruleus is involved in rapid eye movement (REM) sleep and drugs such as the tricyclic antidepressants and monoamine oxidase inhibitors, which suppress REM sleep, also decrease anxiety. Certain of the serotonin receptors in the brain, different from those implicated in depression, have been related to anxiety. Other parts of the brain must also be involved; bifrontal orbital leukotomy diminishes anxiety, possibly by interrupting the medial forebrain connections with the limbic parts of the brain. Positron emission tomography (PET) studies in subjects who anticipate an electric shock show enhanced activity in the temporal lobes and insula, implicating these regions in the experience of acute anxiety (see also "Physiology of the Limbic System" in Chap. 25). Other credible studies have demonstrated a role for the anterior cingulate gyrus in eliciting many of the autonomic features (particularly increased heart rate) of excessive arousal and anxiety.

Several other alterations in neurotransmitter function have been implicated in the anxious state. The finding that a small proportion of the inherited personality trait of anxiety can be accounted for by one polymorphism of the serotonin transporter gene is provocative (Lesch et al) but requires confirmation.

DEPRESSIVE REACTIONS

There are few persons who do not at some time experience periods of severe discouragement and despair. As with nervousness, irritability, and anxiety, depression of mood that is appropriate to a given situation in life (e.g., grief reaction) is seldom the basis of medical concern. Persons in these situations tend to seek help only when their grief or unhappiness is persistent and beyond control. However, there are numerous instances in which the symptoms of depression assert themselves for reasons that are not apparent. Often the symptoms are interpreted as a medical illness, bringing the patient first to the internist or neurologist. Sometimes another disease is found (such as cancer, chronic hepatitis, or other infection or postinfectious asthenia) in which chronic fatigue is confused with depression; more often the opposite pertains, i.e., an endogenous depression is the essential problem even when there has been evidence earlier of a viral or bacterial infection.

From the patient and the family it is learned that the patient has been "feeling unwell," "low in spirits," "blue," "down," "unhappy," or "morbid." There has been a change in his emotional reactions of which the patient may not be fully aware. Activities that were formerly found pleasurable are no longer so. Often, however, change in mood is less conspicuous than reduction in psychic and physical energy, and it is in this type of patient that diagnosis is most difficult. A complaint of fatigue is almost invariable; not uncommonly, it is worse in the morning after a night of restless sleep. The patient complains of a "loss of energy," "weakness," "tiredness," "having no energy," that his job has become more difficult. His outlook is pessimistic. The patient is irritable and preoccupied with uncontrollable worry over trivialities. With excessive worry, the ability to think with accustomed efficiency is reduced; the patient complains that his mind is not functioning properly, and he is forgetful and unable to concentrate. If the patient is naturally of suspicious nature, paranoid tendencies may assert themselves.

Particularly troublesome may be the patient's tendency to *hypochondriasis*. Indeed, most cases formerly diagnosed as hypochondriasis are now regarded as depression with superimposed anxiety. Pain from whatever cause, a stiff joint, a toothache, fleeting chest or abdominal pains, muscle cramps, or other disturbances such as constipation, frequency of urination, insomnia, pruritus, burning tongue, or weight loss may lead to obsessive complaints. The patient passes from doctor to doctor, seeking relief from symptoms that would not trouble the normal person, and no amount of reassurance relieves his state of mind. The anxiety and depressed mood of these persons may be obscured by their preoccupation with visceral functions.

When the patient is examined, his facial expression is often plaintive, troubled, pained, or anguished. The patient's attitude and manner betray a prevailing mood of depression, hopelessness, and despondency. In other words, the affect, which is the outward expression of feeling, is consistent with the depressed mood. During the interview, the patient may be tearful and may cry openly. In some, there is a kind of immobility of the face that mimics parkinsonism, though others are restless and agitated (pacing, wringing their hands, etc.). Occasionally the patient will smile, but the smile impresses one as more a social gesture than a genuine expression of feeling.

The stream of speech is slow. Sighing is frequent. There may be long pauses between questions and answers. The latter are brief and may be monosyllabic. There is a paucity of ideas. The impediment extends to all topics of conversation and affects movement of the limbs as well. The most extreme forms of decreased motor activity, rarely seen in the office or clinic, border on muteness and stupor ("anergic depression"). Conversation is replete with pessimistic thoughts, fears, and expressions of unworthiness, inadequacy, inferiority, hopelessness, and sometimes guilt. In severe depressions, bizarre ideas and bodily delusions may be expressed ("blood drying up," "bowels are blocked with cement," "I am half dead").

Several theories have emerged concerning the cause of the pathologic depressive state, but none can be confirmed with confidence except for a heritable aspect. These views are elaborated on in Chap. 52.

It is the authors' belief that depressive states are among the most commonly overlooked diagnoses in clinical medicine. Part of the trouble is with the word itself, which implies being unhappy about something. Endogenous depression should be suspected in all states of chronic ill health, hypochondriasis, disability that exceeds the manifest signs of a medical disease, neurasthenia and ongoing fatigue, and chronic pain syndromes. Inasmuch as recovery is the rule, suicide is a tragedy for which the medical profession must sometimes share responsibility. In extreme circumstances, however, the patient is impelled to suicide and efforts on the part of the physician cannot be considered as a failure.

Depressive illnesses and theories of their causation and management are considered extensively in Chap. 52.

References

Bagnall AM, Hempel S, Chambers D, et al: *The treatment and management of chronic fatigue syndrome/myalgic encephalomyelitis in adults and children*. National Health Service Centre for Reviews and Dissemination. CRD Report; 35, 2007.

Barratt ES, White R: Impulsiveness and anxiety related to medical students' performance and attitudes. *J Med Educ* 44:604, 1969.

Beard J: Neurasthenia, or nervous exhaustion. *Boston Med Surg J* III:217, 1869.

Brodal A: Self-observations and neuro-anatomical considerations after a stroke. *Brain* 96:675, 1973.

Cassidy WL, Flanagan NB, Spellman M, Cohen ME: Clinical observations in manic depressive disease. *JAMA* 164:1535, 1953.

Chambers D, Bagnall AM, Hempell S, et al: Interventions for the treatment, management and rehabilitation of patients with chronic fatigue syndrome/myalgic encephalomyelitis: an updated systematic review. *J R Soc Med* 99:506, 2006.

Chaudhuri A, Behan PO: Fatigue in neurological disorders. *Lancet* 363:978, 2004.

Cope H, David A, Pelosi A, et al: Predictors of chronic "postviral" fatigue. *Lancet* 344:864, 1994.

Dawson DM, Sabin TD: *Chronic Fatigue Syndrome*. Boston, Little, Brown, 1993.

Digon A, Goicoechea A, Moraza MJ: A neurological audit in Vitoria, Spain. *J Neurol Neurosurg Psychiatry* 55:507, 1992.

Editorial: The essence of stress. *Lancet* 344:1713, 1994.

Freud S: On the grounds for detaching a particular syndrome from neurasthenia under the description "anxiety neurosis," in Strachey J (ed): *The Complete Psychological Works of Sigmund Freud*, standard edition. Vol 3. London, Hogarth Press, 1962, p 90.

Holmes GP, Kaplan JE, Glantz NM, et al: Chronic fatigue syndrome: A working case definition. *Ann Intern Med* 108:387, 1988.

Kahn E: *Psychopathic Personalities*. New Haven, CT, Yale University Press, 1931.

Lader M: The nature of clinical anxiety in modern society, in Spielberger CD, Sarason IG (eds): *Stress and Anxiety*. Vol 1. New York, Halsted, 1975, pp 3–26.

Lesch KP, Bengel D, Jeils A, et al: Association of anxiety-related traits with a polymorphism in the serotonin transporter gene regulatory system. *Science* 274:1527, 1996.

Lloyd AR, Gandevia SC, Hales JP: Muscle performance: Voluntary activation, twitch properties, and perceived effort in normal subjects and patients with chronic fatigue syndrome. *Brain* 114:85, 1991.

McDougall W: *Outlines of Abnormal Psychology*. New York, Scribners, 1926.

Rosen G: Emotions and sensibility in ages of anxiety: A comparative historical review. *Am J Psychiatry* 124:771, 1967.

Rowe PC, Bou-Holaigah I, Kan JS, et al: Is neurally mediated hypotension an unrecognized cause of chronic fatigue? *Lancet* 345:623, 1995.

Roy-Byrne P, Craske MG, Stein MB: Panic disorder. *Lancet* 368:1023, 2006.

Samii A, Wassermann EM, Ikoma K, et al: Decreased postexercise facilitation of motor evoked potentials in patients with chronic fatigue or depression. *Neurology* 47:1410, 1996.

Shorter E: *From Paralysis to Fatigue: A History of Psychosomatic Illness in the Modern Era*. New York, Free Press, 1992.

Snaith RP, Taylor CM: Irritability: Definition, assessment, and associated factors. *Br J Psychiatry* 147:127, 1985.

Southwick SM, Krystal JH, Morgan CA, et al: Abnormal noradrenergic function in post traumatic stress disorder. *Arch Gen Psychiatry* 50:266, 1993.

Straus SE: The chronic mononucleosis syndrome. *J Infect Dis* 157:405, 1988.

Straus SE, Dale JK, Tobi M, et al: Acyclovir treatment of the chronic fatigue syndrome. *N Engl J Med* 319:1692, 1988.

Swartz MN: The chronic fatigue syndrome—one entity or many? *N Engl J Med* 319:1726, 1988.

Wessely S, Chalder T, Hirsch S, et al: Postinfectious fatigue: Prospective cohort study in primary care. *Lancet* 345:1333, 1995.

Wessely S, Powell R: Fatigue syndromes: A comparison of chronic "postviral" fatigue with neuromuscular and affective disorders. *J Neurol Neurosurg Psychiatry* 52:940, 1989.

Wheeler EO, White PD, Reed EW, Cohen ME: Neurocirculatory asthenia (anxiety neurosis, effort syndrome, neurasthenia). *JAMA* 142:878, 1950.

Yehuda R: Post-traumatic stress disorder. *N Engl J Med* 346:108, 2002.

25

The Limbic Lobes and the Neurology of Emotion

The medical literature is replete with references to illnesses based on emotional disorders. Careful examination of clinical material discloses that diverse phenomena are being so classified: anxiety states, cycles of depression and mania, reactions to distressing life situations, psychosomatic diseases, and illnesses of obscure nature. Obviously, great license is being taken with the term *emotional*. Such ambiguity renders neurologic analysis difficult. Nevertheless, in certain clinical states patients appear to be excessively apathetic or elated under conditions that are not normally conducive to such displays of emotion. It is to these disturbances that the following remarks pertain. Emotion may be defined as any feeling state—for example, fear, anger, excitement, love, or hate—associated with certain types of bodily changes (mainly visceral and under control of the autonomic nervous system) and leading usually to an impulse to action or to a certain type of behavior. If the emotion is intense, there may ensue a disturbance of intellectual functions, that is, a disorganization of rational thought and a tendency toward a more automatic behavior of unmodulated, stereotyped character.

In its most easily recognized human form, emotion is initiated by a stimulus, real or imagined, the perception of which involves recognition, memory, and specific associations. The emotional state that is engendered is mirrored in a psychic experience, i.e., a *feeling*, which is purely subjective and known to others only through the patient's verbal expressions or by judging his behavioral reactions. This behavioral aspect, which is in part autonomous (hormonal–visceral) and in part somatic, shows itself in the patient's facial expression, bodily attitude, vocalizations, or directed voluntary activity, an observable display for which we use the term *affect*. In other words, the components of emotion appear to consist of (1) the perception of a stimulus, which may be internal (an idea) or external, (2) the feeling, (3) the autonomic–visceral changes, (4) the outward display (affect), and (5) the impulse to a certain type of activity. In many cases of neurologic disease, it is not possible to separate these components from one another, and to emphasize one of them does no more than indicate the particular bias of the examiner. Obviously, neural networks of both affective response and cognition are involved.

Anatomic Considerations

The occurrence of abnormal emotional reactions in the course of disease is associated with lesions that preferentially involve certain parts of the nervous system. These structures are grouped under the term *limbic* and are among the most complex and least understood parts of the nervous system. The Latin word *limbus* means "border" or "margin." Credit for introducing the term *limbic* to neurology is usually given to Broca, who used it to describe the ring of gray matter formed primarily by the cingulate and parahippocampal gyri that encircles the corpus callosum and underlying upper brainstem. Actually, Thomas Willis had pictured this region of the brain and referred to it as the *limbus* in 1664. Broca preferred his term, *le grand lobe limbique*, to *rhinencephalon*, which was the term then in vogue and referred more specifically to structures having an olfactory function. Neuroanatomists have extended the boundaries of the *limbic lobe* to include not only the cingulate and parahippocampal gyri but also the underlying hippocampal formation, the subcallosal gyrus, and the paraolfactory area. The terms *visceral brain* and *limbic system*, introduced by MacLean, have an even wider designation and more completely describe the structures involved in emotion and its expression; in addition to all parts of the limbic lobe, they include a number of associated subcortical nuclei such as those of the amygdaloid complex, septal region, preoptic area, hypothalamus, anterior thalamus, habenula, and central midbrain tegmentum, including the raphe nuclei and interpeduncular nucleus. The major structures that constitute the limbic system and their relationships are illustrated in Figs. 25-1 and 25-2.

The cytoarchitectonic arrangements of the limbic cortex clearly distinguish it from the surrounding neocortex. The latter, as stated in Chap. 22, differentiates into a characteristic six-layer structure (isocortex). In contrast, the inner part of the limbic cortex, the hippocampus, is composed of irregularly arranged aggregates of nerve cells that tend to be in a trilaminate configuration (archi- or allocortex). The cortex of the cingulate gyrus, which forms the outer ring of the limbic lobe, is transitional between neocortex and allocortex—hence, it is called mesocortex. The entorhinal cortex adjacent to the anterior hippocampus has a similar

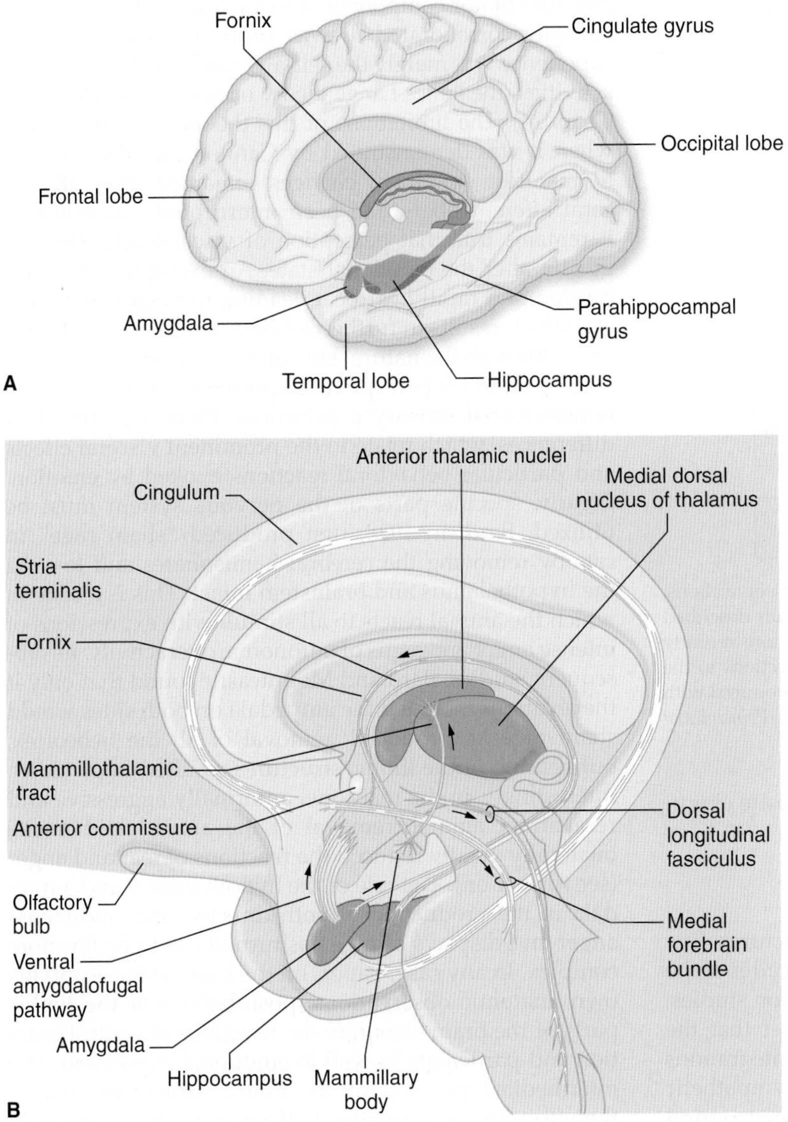

Figure 25-1. Sagittal diagram of the limbic system. *A.* Surface topography of the limbic system and associated prefrontal cortex. *B.* Connections of the limbic structures and their relation to the thalamus, hypothalamus, and midbrain tegmentum. The cortical parts of the limbic system, or limbic lobe, are interconnected by a septohypothalamic–mesencephalic bundle ending in the hippocampus, and the fornix, which runs from the hippocampus back to the mammillary bodies, and by tracts from the mammillary bodies to the thalamus and from the thalamus to the cingulate gyrus. The Papez circuit is the internal component of this system. See also Fig. 25-2 and the text. (Reproduced with permission from Kandel ER, Schwartz JH, Jessell TM: *Principles of Neural Science*, 4th ed. New York, McGraw-Hill, 2000.)

transitional architecture. Information from a wide array of cortical neurons is funneled into the dentate gyrus and then to the CA (cornu ammonis) pyramidal cells of the hippocampus. Output from the hippocampus is mainly from the pyramidal cells of the CA1 segment and subiculum, whose axons form the fibria and fornix. The amygdaloid complex, a subcortical nuclear component of the limbic system, also has a unique composition, consisting of several separable nuclei, each with connections to other limbic structures.

The connections between the orbitofrontal neocortex and limbic lobes, between the individual components of the limbic lobes, and between the limbic lobes and the hypothalamus and midbrain reflect their many functional relationships in regard to emotion. At the core of this system lies the medial forebrain bundle, a complex set of ascending and descending fibers that connect the orbitomesiofrontal cortex, septal nuclei, amygdala, and hippocampus rostrally, and certain nuclei in the midbrain and pons caudally. This system, of which the hypothalamus is the central part, was designated by Nauta as the *septohypothalamo–mesencephalic continuum*.

There are many other interrelationships among various parts of the limbic system, only a few of which can be indicated here. The best known of these is *Papez circuit*. It leads from the hippocampus, via the fornix, to the mammillary body and septal and preoptic regions (see Fig. 25-1). The mammillothalamic tract (bundle of Vicq d'Azyr) connects the mammillary nuclei with the anterior nuclei of the thalamus, which, in turn project to the cingulate gyrus and then, via the cingulum back to the hippocampus. The cingulum runs concentric to the curvature of the corpus callosum; it connects various parts of the limbic lobe to one another and projects to the striatum and to certain brainstem nuclei as well. Also, the cingulum receives fibers from the inferior parietal lobule and temporal lobe, which are multimodal association centers for the integration of visual, auditory, and

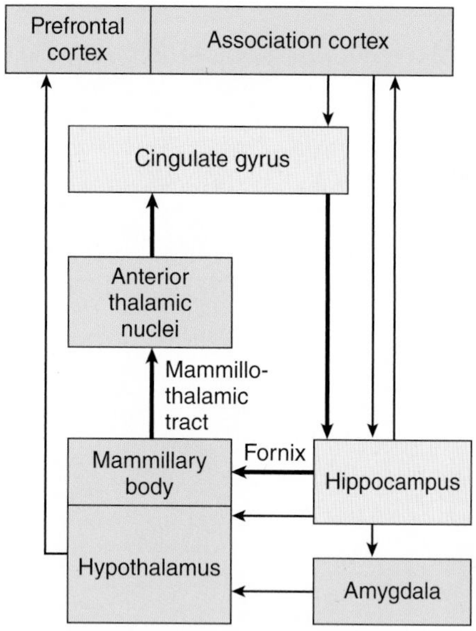

Figure 25-2. Schematic block diagram of the limbic connections. The internal connections (*bold lines*) represent the circuit described by Papez. The external connections (*thin lines*) are more recently described pathways. This figure also shows the connections to the amygdala and prefrontal and association cortices. (Reproduced with permission from Kandel ER, Schwartz JH, Jessell TM: *Principles of Neural Science*, 4th ed. New York, McGraw-Hill, 2000.)

tactile perceptions. It is connected to the opposite cingulum through the anterior corpus callosum.

Physiology of the Limbic System

The functional properties of the limbic structures first became known during the third and fourth decades of the twentieth century. From ablation and stimulation studies, Cannon, Bard, and others established the fact that the hypothalamus contains the suprasegmental integrations of the autonomic nervous system, both the sympathetic and parasympathetic parts. Soon after, anatomists found efferent pathways from the hypothalamus to the neural structures subserving parasympathetic and sympathetic reflexes. One such segmental reflex, involving the sympathetic innervation of the adrenal gland, served as the basis of Cannon's emergency theory of sympathoadrenal action, which for many years dominated thinking about the neurophysiology of acute emotion.

Following Cannon, Bard incorrectly localized the central regulatory apparatus for respiration, wakefulness, and sexual activity in the hypothalamus. Only later, the hypothalamus was found to contain neurosecretory cells, which control the secretion of the pituitary hormones; also within it are special sensory receptors for the regulation of hunger, thirst, body temperature, and levels of circulating electrolytes. Gradually the idea emerged of a hypothalamic–pituitary–autonomic system that is essential to both the basic homeostatic and emergency ("fight-or-flight") reactions of the organism. The functional anatomy of these autonomic and neuroendocrine systems is discussed in Chaps. 26 and 27.

The impression of the leading psychologists of the nineteenth century that autonomic reactions were the essential motor component of instinctual feeling has been partially corroborated. It was proposed that emotional experience was merely the self-awareness of these visceral activities (the James-Lange theory of emotion alluded to in Chap. 24). The limitations of this theory became evident when it was demonstrated by Cannon that the capacity to manifest emotional changes remained after all visceral afferent fibers had been interrupted. Nonetheless, it remains true that perception of visceral activities can greatly alter the emotional state. An example is the perception of a rapid heartbeat, leading to heightened anxiety, which results in further acceleration in the heart rate.

Although the natural stimuli for emotion involve the same neocortical perceptive–cognitive mechanisms, as do nonemotional sensory experiences, there are important differences, which relate to the prominent visceral effects and particular behavioral reactions evoked by emotion. Clearly, specific parts of the nervous system must be utilized. Bard, in 1928, first produced "sham rage" in cats by removing the cerebral hemispheres and leaving the hypothalamus and brainstem intact. This is a state in which the animal reacts to all stimuli with expressions of intense anger and signs of autonomic overactivity. In subsequent studies, Bard and Mountcastle found that only if the ablations included the amygdala on both sides would sham rage be produced; removal of all the neocortex, but sparing of the limbic structures resulted in placidity. Interestingly, in the macaque, a normally aggressive and recalcitrant animal, removal of the amygdaloid nuclei bilaterally greatly reduced the reactions of fear and anger (see further on). The role of the hypothalamus and amygdala in the production of both directed and undirected anger and displays of rage has turned out to be far more complex. In any case, Papez, on the basis of these and his own anatomic observations, postulated that the limbic parts of the brain elaborate the functions of central emotion and participate as well in emotional expression. The intermediate position of the limbic structures enables them to transmit neocortical effects from their outer side to the hypothalamus and midbrain on their inner side.

The role of the *cingulate gyrus* in the behavior of animals and humans has been the subject of much discussion. Stimulation is said to produce autonomic effects similar to the vegetative correlates of emotion (increase in heart rate and blood pressure, dilatation of pupils, piloerection, respiratory arrest, breathholding). More complex responses, such as fear, anxiety, or pleasure, have been reported during neurosurgical stimulative and ablative procedures, although these results are inconsistent. Bilateral cingulectomies performed in the past on psychotic and anxious patients result in an overall diminution of emotional reactions (Ballantine et al; Brown). Some investigators believe that the cingulate gyri are also involved in memory processing (functioning presumably in connection with the mediodorsal thalamic nuclei and mediotemporal lobes) and in exploratory behavior and visually focused attention. In humans, this system appears to be more efficient in the nondominant hemisphere. According to Bear, and as conceptualized by Baleydier and Mauguiere, the cingulate gyri serve dual functions in cognition and in emotional reactions.

Another aspect of limbic function has come to light with information about the neurotransmitters that interconnect the structures within the system. The concentration of norepinephrine is highest in the hypothalamus and next highest in the medial parts of the limbic system; at least 70 percent of this monoamine is concentrated in terminals of axons that arise in the medulla and in the locus ceruleus of the rostral pons. Axons of other ascending fibers, especially those originating in the reticular formation of the midbrain and terminating in the amygdala and septal nuclei as well as in lateral parts of the limbic lobe are rich in serotonin.

The axons of neurons in the ventral tegmental parts of the midbrain, which ascend in the medial forebrain bundle and the nigrostriatal pathway, contain a high content of dopamine. Perhaps this explains the observation that a severe depressive reaction may be produced by electrical stimulation of the substantia nigra with an aberrantly placed electrode for the treatment of Parkinson disease (see Chap. 39). The many structures listed above and their connections certainly constitute a unified functional system. The term *limbic system* is a simplification, particularly as the various parts differ widely in respect to their connections with the neocortex and central nuclei, their transmitters, and their effects when damaged. But it can be said that lesions in this system most consistently and specifically alter emotionality; thus it remains a useful concept.

EMOTIONAL DISTURBANCES DUE TO DISEASES INVOLVING LIMBIC STRUCTURES

Many of the foregoing ideas about the role of the limbic system have come from experimentation in laboratory animals. Only in relatively recent years have neurologists, primed with the knowledge of these studies, begun to relate emotional disturbances in patients with disease of limbic structures. These clinical observations, summarized in the following pages, form an interesting chapter in neurology. Table 25-1 lists the most readily recognized disturbances of emotion. The list is tentative, as our understanding of many of these states, particularly their pathologic basis, is incomplete. Only a small number of these derangements can be used as indicators of lesions and diseases in particular parts of the human brain. Taken in context, however, these disturbances are useful diagnostically. As knowledge of emotional disorders increases, an understanding of the functioning of limbic structures will undoubtedly bring together large segments of psychiatry and neurology.

Emotional Disturbances in Hallucinatory and Pain States

These are portrayed by the patient with a florid delirium. Threatened by imaginary figures and voices that seem real and inescapable, the patient trembles, struggles to escape, and displays the full picture of terror. The patient's affect, emotional reaction, and visceral and somatic motor responses are altogether appropriate to the content of hallucinations. We have seen a patient slash his wrists and another try to drown himself in response to hallucinatory voices that admonished them for their worthlessness and the shame they had brought on their families. But the abnormality in these circumstances is one of disordered perception and thinking, and we have no reason to believe that there is a fundamental derangement of the mechanisms for emotional expression.

Table 25-1

NEUROLOGY OF EMOTIONAL DISTURBANCES

I. Disturbances of emotionality because of:
A. Perceptual abnormalities (illusions and hallucinations)
B. Cognitive derangements (delusions)
II. Disinhibition of emotional expression
A. Emotional lability
B. Pathologic laughing and crying (psuedobulbar state)
III. Rage reactions and aggressivity
IV. Apathy and placidity
A. Klüver-Bucy syndrome
B. Other syndromes (frontal and thalamic)
V. Altered sexuality
VI. Endogenous fear, anxiety, depression, and euphoria

There also occurs a state, difficult to classify, of overwhelming emotionality in patients who are in severe, acute pain. The patient's attention can be captured only briefly, but within moments, there is a return to an extreme state of angst, groaning, and anger. We have encountered this with spinal subdural hemorrhage, subarachnoid hemorrhage, explosive migraine, trauma with multiple fractures, and intense pelvic, renal, or abdominal pain, all understandable as responses to extralimbic stimuli.

Disinhibition of Emotional Expression

Emotional Lability

It is a commonplace clinical experience that cerebral diseases of many types, seemingly without respect to location, weaken the mechanism of control of emotional expression. A patient whose cerebrum has been damaged, for example, by a series of vascular lesions, may suffer the humiliation of crying in public upon meeting an old friend or hearing the national anthem, or of displaying uncontrollable laughter in response to a mildly amusing remark or an attempt to tell a funny story. There may also be easy vacillation from one state to another, an *emotional lability* that has for more than a century been accepted as a sign of "organic brain disease." In this type of emotional disturbance, the response, while excessive, does not quite reach the degree of forced emotionality of the special form of lability described as pseudobulbar (see below); furthermore, it is appropriate to the stimulus and the affect is congruent with the visceral and motor components of the expression. The anatomic substrate is obscure. Perhaps lesions of the frontal lobes more than of other parts of the brain are conducive to this state, but the authors are unaware of a critical clinicoanatomic study that substantiates this impression. Emotional lability is a frequent accompaniment of diffuse cerebral diseases, such as Alzheimer disease, but these diseases involve the limbic cortex as well. Also under this heading might be included the tearfulness and facile mood that so often accompany chronic diseases of the nervous system, and the shallow facetiousness (*witzelsucht*) and behavioral disinhibition of the patient with frontal lobe disease.

Pseudobulbar (Spasmodic) Laughing and Crying

This form of disordered emotional expression, characterized by outbursts of involuntary, uncontrollable, and stereotyped laughing or crying, has been recognized since the late nineteenth century. Numerous references to these conditions (the *Zwangslachen* and *Zwangsweinen* noted by German neurologists and the *rire et pleurer spasmodiques* described by the French) can be found in the writings of Oppenheim, von Monakow, and Wilson (see Wilson for historical references). The term *emotional incontinence* applied by psychiatrists may be accurate but is a bit pejorative. Forced laughing or crying always has a pathologic basis in the brain, either diffuse or focal; hence, this stands as a syndrome of multiple causes. It may occur with degenerative and vascular diseases of the brain (Table 25-2) and no doubt is the direct result of them, but often the diffuse nature of the underlying disease precludes useful topographic analysis and clinicoanatomic correlation.

The best examples of pathologic laughing and crying are provided by multiple lacunar vascular disease and by amyotrophic lateral sclerosis, multiple sclerosis, and progressive supranuclear palsy, in each case the lesions being distributed bilaterally and generally involving the motor tracts, specifically, the corticobulbar motor system as discussed further on. They may also be part of the residue of the more widespread lesions of hypoxic–ischemic encephalopathy, Binswanger ischemic encephalopathy, cerebral trauma, infiltrative gliomas of the frontal lobe or pons, and infectious and noninfectious encephalitides. Typical in our experience is a sudden hemiplegia from a stroke that is engrafted upon a preexistent (and often clinically silent) lesion in the opposite hemisphere; this sets the stage for the pathologic displays of emotionality.

Table 25-2

CAUSES OF PSEUDOBULBAR AFFECTIVE DISPLAY

Bilateral strokes (lacunes in the cerebral hemispheres or pons) most often after several strokes in succession
Binswanger diffuse leukoencephalopathy (Chap. 34)
Amyotrophic lateral sclerosis with pseudobulbar palsy
Progressive supranuclear palsy
Multiple sclerosis with bilateral corticobulbar demyelinative lesions
Bilateral traumatic lesions of the hemispheres
Gliomatosis cerebri
Hypoxic–ischemic encephalopathy
Pontine myelinolysis
Wilson disease

In this state, there is sometimes a striking incongruity between the loss of voluntary movements of muscles innervated by the motor nuclei of the lower pons and medulla (inability to forcefully close the eyes, elevate and retract the corners of the mouth, open and close the mouth, chew, swallow, phonate, articulate, and move the tongue) and the preservation of movement of the same muscles in yawning, coughing, throat clearing, and spasmodic laughing or crying (i.e., in reflexive pontomedullary activities). This is the motor syndrome of *pseudobulbar palsy* for which reason the term *pseudobulbar affective state* has been applied to the emotional disorder.

On the slightest provocation and sometimes for no apparent reason, the patient is thrown into a stereotyped spasm of laughter that may last for moments or up to many minutes, to the point of exhaustion. Or, far more often, the opposite happens—the mere mention of the patient's family or the sight of the doctor provokes an uncontrollable spasm of crying or, more accurately stated, a caricature of crying. The severity of the emotional display and the ease with which it is provoked does not correspond with the severity of the pseudobulbar paralysis or with an exaggeration of the facial and masseter ("jaw jerk") tendon reflexes. In some patients with forced crying and laughing, there is little or no detectable weakness of facial and bulbar muscles; in others, forced laughing and crying are lacking despite a severe upper motor neuron weakness of these muscles. In certain diseases, such as progressive supranuclear palsy and central pontine myelinolysis, of which pseudobulbar palsy is a frequent manifestation, forced laughing and crying are less dramatic or absent. Consequently, the pathologic emotional state cannot be equated with pseudobulbar palsy even though the two usually occur together.

Is this state, whether one of involuntary laughing or of crying, activated by an appropriate stimulus? In other words, does the emotional response accurately reflect the patient's affect or feeling? There are no simple answers to these questions. One problem is to determine what constitutes an appropriate stimulus for the patient in question. Virtually always, the emotional response is set off by some stimulus or thought; but usually, it is trifling, or at least it appears so to the physician. Merely addressing the patient or making some casual remark in his presence may suffice. Oppenheim and others stated that these patients need not feel sad when crying or mirthful when laughing, and at least in some cases, this is in agreement with our experience. Other patients, however, do report a general congruence of affect and emotional experience (mood), but the amplitude of the response is nonetheless excessive.

Noteworthy are the stereotyped nature of the initial motor facial response, and the relatively undifferentiated nature of the emotional reaction. Laughter or crying may merge, one with the other. Poeck (1985) puts great emphasis on the latter point, but it does not seem surprising when one considers the closeness of these two forms of emotional expression, a phenomenon that is particularly evident in young children. More impressive to us is the fact that in some patients with pseudobulbar palsy, laughing and crying, or caricatures thereof, are the only available forms of emotional expression; intermediate phenomena, such as smiling and frowning, are lost. In other patients with pseudobulbar palsy, there are lesser degrees of forced laughing and crying, perhaps bridging the gap between this phenomenon, and the type of emotional lability discussed earlier.

Wilson, in his discussion of the anatomic basis and mechanism of forced laughing and crying, pointed out that both involve the same facial, vocal, and respiratory musculature and have similar visceral accompaniments (dilatation of facial vessels, secretion of tears, etc). Two major supranuclear pathways control the pontomedullary mechanisms of facial and other movements required in laughing and crying. One is the familiar corticobulbar pathway that runs from the motor cortex through the posterior limb of the internal capsule and controls volitional movements; the other is a more anterior pathway that descends just rostral to the genu of the internal capsule, and contains facilitatory and inhibitory fibers. Unilateral involvement of the anterior pathway leaves the opposite side of the face under volitional control but paretic during laughing, smiling, and crying (emotional facial paralysis); the opposite is observed with a unilateral lesion of the posterior pathway. Wilson's argument, based to some extent on clinicopathologic evidence, was that in pseudobulbar palsy, it was the descending motor pathways, which naturally inhibit the expression of the emotions, that were interrupted although he was uncertain of the exact level. Almost 40 years later, Poeck (1985), after reviewing all the published pathologic anatomy in 30 verified cases, was able to do no more than conclude that supranuclear motor pathways are always involved, with loss of a control mechanism somewhere in the brainstem between thalamus and medulla. However, this clinical state is observed in amyotrophic lateral sclerosis, where the corticobulbar tracts may be involved at a cortical and subcortical level. As mentioned earlier, the lesions are bilateral in practically all instances (Poeck, 1985). There have been reports of spasmodic laughter following unilateral striatocapsular infarction (Ceccaldi et al) and occasional cases after unilateral pontine infarction or arteriovenous malformation, but these were not verified pathologically.

Of interest is the beneficial effect on distressing pseudobulbar displays of drugs such as imipramine and fluoxetine (Schiffer et al). A study has also shown benefit from dextromethorphan combined with quinidine in the pseudobulbar state of amyotrophic lateral sclerosis (Brooks et al). In a few personally observed cases, both the emotional lability and pathologic laughter and crying were partially suppressed by these drugs; but in most others, there was no effect.

A rare but probably related syndrome is *le fou rire prodromique* (prodromal laughing madness) of Féré, in which uncontrollable laughter begins abruptly and is followed after several hours by hemiplegia. We have seen two such cases in which basilar artery occlusion evolved after a brief bout of such forced laughter. Martin cites examples where patients laughed themselves to death. Again, the pathologic anatomy is unsettled. Protracted laughing and (less often) crying may occur rarely as a manifestation of epileptic seizures, usually of focal temporal lobe type. Ictal laughter is usually without affect (mirthless laughter); Daly and Mulder referred to these as "gelastic" seizures. The concurrence of gelastic seizures and precocious puberty is characteristic of an underlying hamartoma (or other lesion) of the hypothalamus (see Chaps. 16 and 27).

Aggressiveness, Anger, Rage, and Violence

Aggressiveness is an integral part of social behavior. The emergence of this trait early in life enables the individual to secure a position in the family and later in an ever-widening social circle. Individual differences are noteworthy. Timidity, for example, is a persistent trait recognized in infancy (Kagan). Males tend to be more aggressive than females. The degree to which excessively aggressive behavior is tolerated varies in different cultures. In most civilized societies, tantrums, rage reactions, and outbursts of violence and destructiveness are not condoned and one of the principal objectives of child rearing and education is the suppression and sublimation of such behavior. The rate at which this developmental process proceeds varies from one individual to another. In some males and the cognitively impaired, it is not complete until 25 to 30 years of age; the deviant behavior results in *sociopathy* (see Chap. 28). Undoubtedly, from our own casual and others' more systematic observations, aggressiveness is an inherited tendency.

That seemingly groundless outbreaks of unbridled and disorganized rage may rarely represent the initial or main manifestation of disease is not fully appreciated. A patient with these symptoms may, with little provocation, change from a reasonable state to one of the wildest rage, with a blindly furious impulse to violence and destruction. In such states, the patient appears out of contact with reality and is impervious to all argument or pleading. There are examples also of a dissociation of affect and behavior in which the patient may spit, cry out, attack, or bite without seeming to be angry. This is especially true of the developmentally delayed.

All the human and animal data point to an origin of aggressiveness, anger, and rage in the temporal lobes and particularly in the amygdala. In humans, stimulation of the medial amygdaloid nuclei, through depth electrodes, evokes a display of anger, whereas stimulation of the lateral nuclei does not; destruction of the amygdaloid complex bilaterally reportedly reduces aggressiveness (Kiloh; Narabayashi et al). Lesions in the mediodorsal thalamic nuclei, which receive projections from the amygdaloid nuclei, render humans more placid and docile. In an unintended experiment in a patient with Parkinson disease, Bejjani and colleagues found that aggressive behavior could be induced by stimulation of the posteromedial hypothalamus. As with the comparable elicitation of depression from an aberrant electrode in the substantia nigra that was reported by the same group, it is not clear whether the effect was because of changes induced in adjacent neuronal pathways or if the physiologic response was the result of excitatory or inhibitory neuronal activity in the hypothalamus.

Sex hormones influence the activity of these temporal lobe circuits; testosterone promotes aggressiveness and estradiol suppresses it, suggesting an explanation for sex differences in the disposition to anger. Surprisingly, propranolol and lithium have benefited such patients more than haloperidol, other neuroleptics, or sedatives.

Animal studies have corroborated observations in humans. As mentioned in the introductory section, bilateral removal of the amygdaloid nuclei in the macaque greatly reduces the expressions of both fear and anger. Electrical stimulation in or near the amygdala of the unanesthetized cat yields a variety of motor and vegetative responses. One of these has been referred to as the *fear* or *flight* response, in which the animal appears frightened, and runs away and hides; another is the *anger* or *defense* reaction, characterized by growling, hissing, and piloerection. However, structures other than the amygdaloid nuclei are also involved in these reactions. Lesions in the ventromedial nuclei of the hypothalamus (which receive abundant input from the amygdaloid nuclei) have been shown to cause aggressive behavior, and bilateral ablation of Brodmann area 24 (rostral cingulate gyrus) has produced the opposite state—tameness and reduced aggressiveness—at least in some species.

Rage reactions of the intensity described above may be encountered in the following medical settings: (1) rarely as part of a temporal lobe seizure; (2) as an episodic reaction without recognizable seizures or other neurologic abnormality, as in certain sociopaths; (3) in the course of a recognizable acute neurologic disease; and (4) with the clouding of consciousness that accompanies a metabolic or toxic encephalopathy; (5) as a reaction to designed psychogenic drugs (dragonfly, K4, and others).

Rage in Temporal Lobe Seizures

(See also "Focal Seizures" in Chap. 16)

According to Gastaut and colleagues, a directed attack of uncontrollable rage may occur either as part of a seizure or as an interictal phenomenon. Some patients describe a gradual heightening of excitability for 2 to 3 days, either before or after a seizure, before bursting into a rage. Certainly, such attacks have been observed, but they are rare. A lesser degree of aggressive behavior as part of a temporal lobe seizure is not uncommon; it is usually part of the ictal or postictal behavioral automatism and tends to be brief in duration and poorly directed. Usually, the lesion is in the temporal lobe of the dominant hemisphere. Similarly, a feeling of rage or severe anger occurs but is relatively infrequent as an ictal emotion, much less common than feelings of fear, sadness, or pleasure (Williams reported only 17 cases of anger among 165 patients with ictal emotion). Geschwind emphasized the frequency of a profound deepening of all of the patient's emotional experiences in temporal lobe epilepsy.

Rage Attacks Without Seizure Activity

In some instances of this type, the patient had from early life been hot-headed, intolerant of frustration, and impulsive, exhibiting behavior that would be classified as sociopathic (Chap. 51). There are others, however, who, at certain periods of life, usually adolescence or early adulthood, begin to have episodes of wild, aggressive behavior. Alcohol or some other drug may trigger episodes. One suspects epilepsy, but there is no history of a recognizable seizure and no interruption of consciousness, which are so typical of focal temporal lobe epilepsy. We have been consulted from time to time on patients who report a proclivity to anger, cursing, and momentary unreasonableness in behavior that is acquired in adulthood. Most such individuals are remorseful afterwards and otherwise function at a high cognitive level. Each of these patients described a first-order relative with the same traits. In a very few such cases, in which aggression has resulted in serious injury to others (or homicide), depth electrodes placed in the amygdaloid nuclear complex have recorded what could be construed as seizure discharges. Attacks of excitement and various autonomic accompaniments have been aroused by stimulation of the same region, and the abnormal behavior has in some instances been relieved by ablation of the abnormally discharging structures. Mark and Ervin have documented a number of examples of this "dyscontrol syndrome," but we are doubtful that they are truly epileptic.

Violent Behavior in Acute or Chronic Neurologic Disease

One encounters patients in whom intense excitement, rage, and aggressiveness begin abruptly in association with an acute neurologic disease or in a phase of partial recovery. In most cases, the medial and anterior temporal lobes have been damaged. Serious head injury with protracted coma may be followed by personality changes consisting of aggressive outbursts, suspiciousness, poor judgment, indifference to the feelings of family, and variable degrees of cognitive impairment. Hemorrhagic leukoencephalitis, lobar hemorrhage, infarction, traumatic contusion, and herpes simplex encephalitis affecting the medial and orbital portions of the frontal lobes and anterior portions of the temporal lobes may have the same effect (Fig. 25-3). Fisher noted the occurrence of intense rage reactions as an aftermath of a dominant temporal lobe lesion that had caused a Wernicke type of aphasia. Cases of this type have also been reported with ruptured aneurysm of the circle of Willis and extension of a pituitary adenoma; references to these reports can be found in the articles of Poeck (1969) and of Pillieri.

Also of interest are the effects of slow-growing tumors of the temporal lobe. Malamud described outbursts of rage in association with temporal lobe gliomas. Other of his patients harboring such tumors had no rage reactions but exhibited a clinical picture superficially resembling schizophrenia. It is noteworthy that 8 of the 9 patients with temporal lobe glioma described by Malamud also had seizures. The anteromedial part of the left temporal lobe has been the site of the tumor in the majority of cases. Falconer and Serafetinides have described patients with rage reactions in whom there was a hamartoma or sclerotic focus in this region.

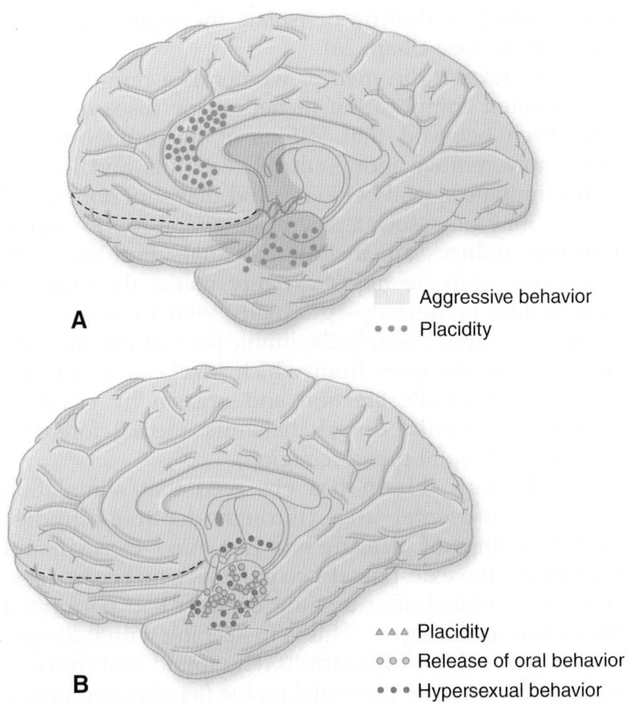

Figure 25-3. *A*. Localization of lesions that, in humans, can lead to aggressive behavior and placidity. *B*. Localization of lesions that, in humans, can lead to placidity, release of oral behavior, and hypersexuality. (From Poeck [1969].)

A special form of violent outburst during REM sleep is detailed in Chap. 19, on Sleep. This, REM sleep behavior disorder, is associated with certain degenerative brain diseases.

Aggressive Behavior in Acute Toxic–Metabolic Encephalopathies and Drug Intoxications

Here the patient is not in a clear-headed state and rage or aggression is superimposed on an encephalopathy of toxic or metabolic origin. The most dramatic examples in our experience have been during hypoglycemic reactions. When the patient is left alone, the aggressive behavior is undirected and disorganized, but anyone in the immediate neighborhood may be struck by the agitated individual. Attempts at physical restraint provoke an even more violent reaction.

A similar state may occur with phencyclidine and cocaine intoxication, and with other hallucinogens, accompanied by agitation and, usually, by hallucinosis. Perhaps the most berserk episodes we have encountered have been after ingestion of large amounts of designed street drugs such as the hallucinogen dragonfly and with cannabis derivatives such as K4 (Spice). These furious behaviors may last for hours or days and are resistant to large doses of haloperidol and benzodiazepines. We have found alpha-2 agonists such as dexmedetomidine to be effective. Outbursts of rage and violence with alcohol intoxication are somewhat different in nature: some instances represent a rare paradoxical or idiosyncratic reaction to alcohol (see Chap. 42); more typically alcohol appears to disinhibit an underlying sociopathic behavior pattern.

Placidity and Apathy

Animals normally indulge in and display highly energized, exploratory activity of their environment. Some of this activity is motivated by the drive for sexual satisfaction and procurement of food; in humans, it may be a matter of curiosity. These activities are governed by "expectancy circuits," involving nuclear groups in mesolimbic and mesocortical dopaminergic circuits connected with the diencephalon and mesencephalon via the medial forebrain bundles; lesions that interrupt these connections are said to abolish the expectancy reactions. Positron emission tomography (PET) studies correlate functional difficulty in the initiation of movements with impaired activation of the anterior cingulum, putamen, prefrontal cortex, and supplementary motor area (Playford et al).

A quantitative reduction in all activity is probably the most frequent of all psychobehavioral alterations in patients with cerebral disease, particularly in those with involvement of the anterior parts of the frontal lobes. There are fewer thoughts, fewer words uttered, and fewer movements per unit of time. That this is not a purely motor phenomenon is disclosed in conversation with the patient, who seems to perceive and think more slowly, to make fewer associations with a given idea, to initiate speech less frequently, and to exhibit less inquisitiveness and interest. This reduction in psychomotor activity is recognized as a striking personality change by the family.

Depending on how this state is viewed, it may be interpreted as a heightened threshold to stimulation, inattentiveness or inability to maintain an attentive attitude, impaired thinking, apathy, or lack of impulse (*abulia*). In a sense, all are correct, for each represents a different aspect of the reduced mental activity. Clinicoanatomic correlates are inexact, but bilateral lesions deep in the septal region (basal frontal, as sometimes occur with bleeding from an anterior communicating aneurysm) have resulted in the most striking lack of impulse, spontaneity, and conation (drive) (see Fig. 25-3). Impairment of learning and memory functions may be added. Typically, the patient is fully attentive, wide awake, and looks around. Upon recovery, memory is retained for all that happened. In this respect, abulia differs from stupor and hypersomnolence.

Patients who exhibit abulia are difficult to test because they respond slowly or not at all to every type of test. Yet on rare occasions, when intensely stimulated, they may speak and act normally. It is as though some energizing mechanism (possibly striatocortical), different from the reticular activating system of the upper brainstem, were impaired. Often, patients with severe abulia perform better with automatic or overlearned behaviors, such as talking on the telephone.

Quite apart from this abulic syndrome, which has already been discussed in relation to coma and to extensive lesions of the frontal lobes (Chaps. 17 and 22), there are lesser degrees in which a lively, sometimes volatile person has been rendered placid (hypobulic) by a disease of the nervous system.

Most often, the frontal lobe damage is bilateral, but sometimes on the left only, as discussed in Chap. 22.

Diseases as diverse as hydrocephalus, glioma, strokes, trauma, and encephalitis may be causative. Formerly, changes of this type were observed following bilateral prefrontal leukotomy. Barris and Schuman, and many others have documented states of extreme placidity with lesions of the anterior cingulate gyri. Unlike the case in depression, the mood is neutral; the patient is apathetic rather than depressed.

The subdued emotional behavior described earlier differs from that observed in the *Klüver-Bucy syndrome*, which results from total bilateral temporal lobectomy in adult rhesus monkeys (see also Chap. 22). While these animals were made rather placid and lacked the ability to recognize objects visually (they could not distinguish edible from inedible objects), they had a striking tendency to examine everything orally, were unusually alert and responsive to visual stimuli (they touched or mouthed every object within their visual fields), became hypersexual, and increased their food intake. This constellation of behavioral changes has been sought in human beings, for example, after removal of the temporal lobes but the complete picture has occurred only infrequently (Marlowe et al; Terzian and Dalle). Pillieri, and Poeck (1969) have collected cases that have come closest to reproducing the syndrome (see Fig. 25-3). Many human examples have occurred in conjunction with diffuse diseases (Alzheimer and Pick cerebral atrophies, meningoencephalitis because of toxoplasmosis, herpes simplex, and AIDS) and hence are of limited value for anatomic analysis. With bitemporal surgical ablations, placidity and enhanced oral behavior were the most frequent consequences; altered sexual behavior and visual agnosia were less frequent. In all patients who showed placidity and an amnesic state, the hippocampi and medial parts of the temporal lobe had been destroyed, but not the amygdaloid nuclei.

Reduced emotionality in humans, albeit one that is very restricted in scope, is associated with acute lesions in the right, or nondominant, parietal lobe. Not only is the patient indifferent to the paralysis but, as Bear points out, he is unconcerned about his other diseases as well as personal and family problems, is less able to interpret the emotional facial expressions of others, and is inattentive in general. There may be a lack of emotional inflection to speech (aprosodia) and an inability to interpret the emotional state of other individuals, as discussed in Chap. 23. Dimond and coworkers interpret this to mean that the right hemisphere is more involved in affective-emotional experience than the left, which is committed to language. Observations derived from the study of split-brain patients and from selective anesthetization of the cerebral hemispheres by intracarotid injection of amobarbital (Wada test) lend some support to this probably oversimplified view. Rarely, lesions of the left (dominant) hemisphere appear to induce the opposite effect, a frenzied excitement lasting for days or weeks.

Altered Sexuality

The normal pattern of sexual behavior in both males and females may be altered by cerebral disease quite apart from impairment due to obvious physical disability or to diseases that destroy or isolate the segmental reflex mechanisms (see Chap. 26).

Hypersexuality in men or women is a rare but well-documented complication of neurologic disease. It has long been believed that lesions of the orbital frontal lobes may remove moral-ethical restraints and lead to indiscriminate sexual behavior, and that superior frontal lesions may be associated with a general loss of initiative that reduces all, including sexual, impulsivity. In rare cases, extreme hypersexuality marks the onset of encephalitis or develops gradually with tumors of the temporal region. Possibly the limbic parts of the brain are disinhibited, the ones from which MacLean and Ploog could evoke penile erection and orgasm by electrical stimulation (medial dorsal thalamus, medial forebrain bundle, and septal preoptic region).

In humans, Heath has observed that stimulation of the ventroseptal area (through depth electrodes) evokes feelings of pleasure and lust. Also, Gorman and Cummings have described two patients who became sexually disinhibited after a shunt catheter had perforated the dorsal septal region. This is in keeping with the experience of Heath and Fitzjarrell, who found that infusion of acetylcholine into the septal region (as an experimental treatment for Parkinson disease) produced euphoria and orgasm, and with Heath's recordings from the septum of patients during sexual intercourse, showing greatly increased activity with spikes and slow waves. Perhaps these are examples of a true overdrive of libido, as contrasted with simple disinhibition of sexual behavior. However, we know of no case in which a stable lesion that caused abnormal sexual behavior has been studied carefully by sections of the critical parts of the brain.

In clinical practice, the most common cause of disinhibited sexual behavior, next to the aftermaths of head injury and cerebral hemorrhage, is the use of dopaminergic drugs in Parkinson disease. An intriguing effect of the administration of L-dopa in a few patients has been excessive or perverse sexual behavior, as in the cases described by Quinn and colleagues. Usually there are other manifestations of manic behavior. Primary mania may do the same.

Hyposexuality, meaning loss of libido, is most often the result of a depressive illness. However, certain medications, notably antihypertensive, antiepileptic, serotonergic antidepressant, and neuroleptic drugs may be responsible in individual patients. A variety of cerebral diseases may also have this effect, in parallel with a loss of interest and drive in a number of spheres.

Lesions that involve the tuberoinfundibular region of the hypothalamus are known to cause specific disturbances in sexual function. If such lesions are acquired early in life, pubertal changes are prevented from occurring; or, hamartomas of the hypothalamus, as in von Recklinghausen neurofibromatosis and tuberous sclerosis, may cause sexual precocity. Autonomic neuropathies and lesions involving the sacral parts of the parasympathetic system, the most common being prostatectomy, may abolish normal sexual performance but do not alter libido or orgasm.

Blumer and Walker have reviewed the literature on the association of epilepsy and abnormal sexual behavior. They note that sexual arousal, as an ictal phenomenon, is apt to occur in relation to temporal lobe seizures, particularly when the discharging focus is in the mediotemporal region. However, these authors also emphasize the high incidence of global hyposexuality in patients with temporal lobe epilepsy. Temporal lobectomy in such patients has sometimes been followed by a period of hypersexuality.

Acute Fear, Anxiety, Elation, and Euphoria

The phenomenon of acute fear and anxiety occurring as a prelude to or part of a seizure is familiar to every neurologist. Williams's study, already mentioned, is of particular interest; from a series of about 2,000 epileptics, he was able to cull 100 patients in whom an emotional experience was part of the seizure. Of the latter, 61 experienced feelings of fear and anxiety, and 21 experienced depression. Daly has made similar observations. These clinical data call to mind the effects that had been noted by Penfield and Jasper when they stimulated the upper, anterior, and inferior parts of the temporal lobe and cingulate gyrus during surgical procedures; frequently, the patient described feelings of strangeness, uneasiness, and fear. In most instances, consciousness was variably impaired at the same time, and some patients had hallucinatory experiences as well.

In these cortical stimulations, neuronal circuits subserving fear are coextensive with those of anger; both are thought to lie in the medial part of the temporal lobe and amygdala, as discussed earlier. Both in animals and in humans, electrical stimulation in this region can arouse each emotion, but the circuitry subserving fear appears to be located lateral to that of anger and rage. Destruction of the central part of the amygdaloid nuclear complex abolishes fear reactions. These nuclei are connected to the lateral hypothalamus and midbrain tegmentum, regions from which Monroe and Heath, as well as Nashold and associates, have been able to evoke feelings of fear and anxiety by electrical stimulation.

Depression is less frequent as an ictal emotion, although it occurs often enough as an interictal phenomenon (Benson et al). Of interest is the observation that lesions of the dominant hemisphere are more likely than nondominant ones to be attended by an immediate pervasive depression of mood, disproportionate to the degree of severity of physical disability (Robinson et al). We are inclined to the view that the onset of depression after a stroke is a reaction to disability, i.e., a reactive depression, akin to that which follows myocardial infarction (Chap. 52).

Odd mixtures of depression and anxiety are often associated with temporal lobe tumors and less often with tumors of the hypothalamus and third ventricle (see review by Alpers), and they sometimes occur at the onset of a degenerative disease, such as multiple system atrophy.

Elation and *euphoria* are less well documented as limbic phenomena, nor has this elevation in mood in some patients with multiple sclerosis ever been adequately explained. Feelings of pleasure and satisfaction as well as "stirring sensations" are unusual, but well-described emotional experiences in patients with temporal lobe seizures, and this type of affective response, like that of fear, has been elicited by stimulating several different parts of the temporal lobe (Penfield and Jasper). In states of hypomania and mania, every experience may be colored by feelings of delight and pleasure, and a sense of power, and the patient may remember these experiences after he has recovered.

Differential Diagnosis of Perturbations in Emotion and Affect

Aside from clinical observation, there are no reliable means of evaluating or quantifying the emotional disorders described earlier. Although neurologic medicine has done little more than describe and classify some of the clinical states dominated by emotional derangements, knowledge of this type is nonetheless of both theoretical and practical importance. In theory, it prepares one for the next step, of passing from a superficial to a deeper order of inquiry, where questions of pathogenesis and etiology can be broached. Practically, it provides certain clues that are useful in differential diagnosis. A number of particular neurologic possibilities must always be considered when one is confronted with one of the following clinical states.

Uninhibited Laughter and Crying and Emotional Lability

As indicated earlier, one may confidently assume that the syndrome of forced or spasmodic laughing and crying signifies cerebral disease, and, more specifically, bilateral disease of the corticobulbar tracts (see Table 25-2). Usually the motor and reflex changes of spastic bulbar (pseudobulbar) palsy (described in the discussion of "Spastic [Pseudobulbar] Dysarthria" in Chap. 23) are associated usually, but not always, with heightened facial and mandibular reflexes ("jaw jerk"), and often corticospinal tract signs in the limbs as well. Extreme emotional lability also indicates bilateral cerebral disease, although only the signs of unilateral disease may be apparent clinically. The most common pathologic bases for these clinical states are lacunar infarction or other cerebrovascular lesions, diffuse hypoxic-hypotensive encephalopathy, amyotrophic lateral sclerosis, and multiple sclerosis, as already indicated; but in a number of less-common processes, such as progressive supranuclear palsy and Wilson disease, it may be quite a prominent feature. Abrupt onset, of course, points to vascular disease.

Placidity and Apathy

These may be the earliest and most important signs of cerebral disease. Clinically, placidity and apathy must be distinguished from the akinesia or bradykinesia of Parkinson disease and the reduced mental activity of depressive illness. Here, Alzheimer disease, normal-pressure hydrocephalus, and frontal-corpus callosum tumors are the most common pathologic states underlying apathy and placidity, but these disturbances may complicate a variety of other frontal and temporal lesions, such as those occurring with demyelinating disease or as an aftermath of ruptured anterior communicating aneurysm.

Outbursts of Rage and Violence

Most often such an outburst is but another episode in a lifelong sequence of sociopathic behaviors (see Chap. 51).

More significance attaches to its abrupt appearance as a sudden departure from an individual's normal personality. If an outburst of rage accompanies a seizure, the rage should be viewed as the consequence of the disruptive effect of seizure activity on temporal lobe function; however, as indicated earlier, an outburst of uncontrolled rage and violence is only rarely a manifestation of temporal lobe epilepsy. Lesser degrees of poorly directed combative behavior as part of ictal or postictal automatism are more common. Rarely, rage and aggressivity are expressive of an acute neurologic disease that involves the mediotemporal and orbitofrontal regions, such as a glioma. We have several times observed such states in the course of a dementing disease and in a stable individual as a transient expression of an obscure encephalopathy.

Rage reactions with continuous violent activity must be distinguished from *mania*, in which there is flight of ideation to the point of incoherence, euphoric or irritable mood, and incessant psychomotor activity; from *organic drivenness*, in which continuous motor activity, accompanied by no clear ideation occurs, usually in a child, as an aftermath of encephalitis; and from extreme instances of *akathisia*, where incessant restless movements and pacing may occur in conjunction with extrapyramidal symptoms.

Extreme Fright and Agitation

Here the central problem must be clarified by determining whether the patient is delirious (clouding of consciousness, psychomotor overactivity, and hallucinations), deluded (schizophrenia), manic (overactive, flight of ideas), or experiencing an isolated panic attack (palpitation, trembling, feeling of suffocation). Rarely does panic prove to be an expression of temporal lobe epilepsy. In an adult without a characterologic trait of anxiety, an acute panic attack may signify the onset of a depressive illness or schizophrenia.

Bizarre Ideation Developing Over Weeks or Months

Although these symptoms are usually caused by a psychosis (schizophrenia or bipolar disease), one should consider a tumor, immune or paraneoplastic encephalitis, or other lesion of the temporal lobe, particularly when accompanied by temporal lobe seizures, aphasic symptoms, rotatory vertigo (rare), and quadrantic visual field defects. Such states have also been described in hypothalamic disease, suggested by somnolence, diabetes insipidus, visual field defects, and in hydrocephalus (see Chap. 27).

References

Alpers BJ: Personality and emotional disorders associated with hypothalamic lesions. *Res Publ Assoc Nerv Ment Dis* 20:725, 1939.

Angevine JB Jr, Cotman CW: *Principles of Neuroanatomy*. New York, Oxford University Press, 1981, pp 253–283.

Baleydier C, Mauguiere F: The duality of the cingulate gyrus in monkey. *Brain* 103:525, 1980.

Ballantine HT, Cassidy WL, Flanagan NB, et al: Stereotaxic anterior cingulotomy for neuropsychiatric illness and chronic pain. *J Neurosurg* 26:488, 1967.

Bard P: A diencephalic mechanism for the expression of rage with special reference to the sympathetic nervous system. *Am J Physiol* 84:490, 1928.

Bard P, Mountcastle VB: Some forebrain mechanisms involved in the expression of rage with special reference to suppression of angry behavior. *Assoc Res Nerv Ment Dis Proc* 27:362, 1947.

Barris RW, Schuman HR: Bilateral anterior cingulate gyrus lesions: Syndrome of the anterior cingulate gyri. *Neurology* 3:44, 1953.

Bear DM: Hemispheric specialization and the neurology of emotion. *Arch Neurol* 40:195, 1983.

Bejjani BP, Houeto JL, Hariz M, et al: Aggressive behavior induced by intraoperative stimulation in the triangle of Sano. *Neurology* 59:1425, 2002.

Benson DF, Mendez MF, Engel J, et al: Affective symptomatology in epilepsy. *Int J Neurol* 19–20:30, 1985–1986.

Blumer D, Walker AE: The neural basis of sexual behavior, in Benson F, Blumer D (eds): *Psychiatric Aspects of Neurologic Disease*. New York, Grune & Stratton, 1975, pp 199–217.

Brooks BR, Thisted SH, Appel WG, et al: Treatment of pseudobulbar affect in ALS with dextromethorphan/quinidine: A randomized trial. *Neurology* 63:1364, 2004.

Brown JW: Frontal lobe syndromes, in Vinken PJ, Bruyn GW, Klawans HL (eds): *Handbook of Clinical Neurology*. Vol 45. Amsterdam, Elsevier Science, 1984, pp 23–42.

Cannon WB: *Bodily Changes in Pain, Hunger and Fear*, 2nd ed. New York, Appleton, 1929.

Ceccaldi M, Poncet M, Milandre L, Rouyer C: Temporary forced laughter after unilateral strokes. *Eur Neurol* 34:36, 1994.

Daly DD: Ictal affect. *Am J Psychiatry* 115:97, 1958.

Daly DD, Mulder DW: Gelastic epilepsy. *Neurology* 7:189, 1957.

Damasio AR, Van Hoesen GW: The limbic system and the localization of herpes simplex encephalitis. *J Neurol Neurosurg Psychiatry* 48:297, 1985.

Dimond SJ, Farrington L, Johnson P: Differing emotional responses from right and left hemisphere. *Nature* 261:690, 1976.

Engel J Jr, Bandler R, Caldecott-Hazard S: Modification of emotional expression induced by clinical and experimental epileptic disturbances. *Int J Neurol* 19–20:21, 1985–1986.

Falconer MA, Serafetinides EA: A follow-up study of surgery in temporal lobe epilepsy. *J Neurol Neurosurg Psychiatry* 26:154, 1963.

Féré MC: Le fou rire prodromique. *Rev Neurol* 11:353, 1903.

Fisher CM: Anger associated with dysphasia. *Trans Am Neurol Assoc* 95:240, 1970.

Gastaut H, Morin G, Lefevre N: Etude de comportement des épileptiques psychomoteurs dans l'intervalle de leurs crises. *Ann Med Psychol (Paris)* 1:1, 1955.

Geschwind N: The clinical setting of aggression in temporal lobe epilepsy, in Field WS, Sweet WH (eds): *The Neurobiology of Violence*. St. Louis, MO, Warren H Green, 1975.

Gorman DG, Cummings JL: Hypersexuality following septal injury. *Arch Neurol* 49:308, 1992.

Heath RG: Pleasure and brain activity in man. *J Nerv Ment Dis* 154:3, 1972.

Heath RG, Fitzjarrell AT: Chemical stimulation to deep forebrain nuclei in parkinsonism and epilepsy. *Int J Neurol* 18:163, 1984.

Kagan J: *The Nature of the Child*. New York, Basic Books, 1984.

Kiloh LG: The treatment of anger and aggression and the modification of sex deviation, in Smith JS, Kiloh LG (eds): *Psychosurgery and Psychiatry*. Oxford, UK, Pergamon Press, 1977, pp 37–54.

Klüver H, Bucy PC: An analysis of certain effects of bilateral temporal lobectomy in the rhesus monkey with special reference to psychic blindness. *J Psychol* 5:33, 1938.

MacLean PD: Contrasting functions of limbic and neocortical systems of the brain and their relevance to psychophysiological aspects of medicine. *Am J Med* 25:611, 1958.

MacLean PD, Ploog DW: Cerebral representation of penile erection. *J Neurophysiol* 25:29, 1962.

Malamud N: Psychiatric disorder with intracranial tumors of limbic system. *Arch Neurol* 17:113, 1967.

Mark VH, Ervin FR: *Violence and the Brain*. New York, Harper & Row, 1970.

Marlowe WB, Mancall EL, Thomas JJ: Complete Klüver-Bucy syndrome in man. *Cortex* 11:53, 1975.

Martin JP: Fits of laughter (sham mirth) in organic cerebral disease. *Brain* 70:453, 1950.

Mesulam MM: Large-scale neurocognitive networks and distributed processing for attention, language and memory. *Ann Neurol* 28:596, 1990.

Monroe RR, Heath RC: Psychiatric observations on the patient group, in Heath RC (ed): *Studies in Schizophrenia*. Cambridge, MA, Harvard University Press, 1983, pp 345–383.

Narabayashi H, Nacao Y, Yoshida M, Nagahata M: Stereotaxic amygdalectomy for behavior disorders. *Arch Neurol* 9:1, 1963.

Nashold BS, Wilson WP, Slaughter DE: Sensations evoked by stimulation in the midbrain of man. *J Neurosurg* 30:14, 1969.

Nauta WJH: The central visceromotor system: A general survey, in Hockman CH (ed): *Limbic System Mechanisms and Autonomic Function*. Springfield, IL, Charles C Thomas, 1972, pp 21–33.

Papez JW: A proposed mechanism of emotion. *Arch Neurol Psychiatry* 38:725, 1937.

Penfield W, Jasper H: *Epilepsy and the Functional Anatomy of the Human Brain*. Boston, Little, Brown, 1954, pp 413–416.

Pillieri G: The Klüver-Bucy syndrome in man. *Psychiatr Neurol (Basel)* 152:65, 1966.

Playford ED, Jenkins LH, Passingham RE, et al: Impaired mesial frontal and putamen activation in Parkinson's disease: A positron emission tomography study. *Ann Neurol* 32:151, 1992.

Poeck K: Pathological laughter and crying, in Vinken PJ, Bruyn GW, Klawans HL (eds): *Handbook of Clinical Neurology*. Vol 45. Amsterdam, North-Holland, 1985, pp 219–225.

Poeck K: Pathophysiology of emotional disorders associated with brain damage, in Vinken PJ, Bruyn GW (eds): *Handbook of Clinical Neurology*. Vol 3: Disorders of Higher Nervous Activity. Amsterdam, North-Holland, 1969, pp 343–367.

Quinn ND, Toone B, Lang AE, et al: Dopa dose-dependent sexual deviation. *Br J Psychiatry* 142:296, 1983.

Robinson RG, Kubos KL, Starr LB, et al: Mood disorders in stroke patients: Importance of location of lesion. *Brain* 107:81, 1984.

Schiffer RB, Herndon RM, Rudick RA: Treatment of pathologic laughing and weeping with amitriptyline. *N Engl J Med* 312:1480, 1985.

Terzian H, Dalle G: Syndrome of Klüver-Bucy reproduced in man by bilateral removal of the temporal lobes. *Neurology* 5:373, 1955.

Williams D: The structure of emotions reflected in epileptic experiences. *Brain* 79:29, 1956.

Wilson SAK: Some problems in neurology. II: Pathological laughing and crying. *J Neurol Psychopathol* 16:299, 1924.

26

Disorders of the Autonomic Nervous System, Respiration, and Swallowing

The human internal environment is regulated in large measure by the integrated activity of the autonomic nervous system and endocrine glands. Their visceral and homeostatic functions, essential to life and survival, are involuntary. Why the forces of evolution favored this separation from volition is an interesting question. Claude Bernard expressed this idea in sardonic terms when he wrote, "nature thought it prudent to remove these important phenomena from the caprice of an ignorant will."

Although only few neurologic diseases exert their effects primarily or exclusively on the autonomic–neuroendocrine axis, there are numerous medical diseases that implicate this system in some way: hypertension, asthma, and certain dramatic disorders of cardiac conduction, to name some of the important ones. However, many general neurologic diseases involve the autonomic nervous system to a varying extent, giving rise to symptoms such as syncope, sphincteric dysfunction, pupillary abnormalities, erectile dysfunction, diaphoresis, cardiac dysrhythmias, and disorders of thermoregulation. Finally, in addition to their central role in visceral innervation, autonomic parts of the neuraxis and parts of the endocrine system are engaged in all emotional experience and its display, as discussed in Chap. 25.

Breathing is unusual among nervous system functions. Although continuous throughout life, it is not altogether automatic, being partly under volitional control. Current views of the central and peripheral control of breathing, and the ways in which it is altered by certain diseases are of considerable interest to neurologists, if for no other reason than respiratory failure is common in neurologic conditions such as coma, cervical spinal cord injury, and a large number of acute and chronic neuromuscular diseases. Many of these same comments pertain to the function of swallowing, which is largely automatic and continues at regular intervals even in sleep but is also initiated voluntarily. Furthermore, swallowing fails in ways similar to breathing as a consequence of neurologic diseases.

The autonomic, endocrine, and respiratory systems, although closely related, give rise to disparate clinical syndromes. This chapter deals more strictly with the autonomic nervous system and the neural mechanisms of respiration and swallowing, and the next chapter, with the hypothalamus and neuroendocrine disorders. The following discussion of anatomy and physiology serves as an introduction to both chapters.

Anatomic Considerations

The most remarkable feature of the autonomic nervous system is that a major part of it is located outside the brain and spinal cord, in proximity to the visceral structures that it innervates. This position alone seems to symbolize its relative independence from the cerebrospinal system. In distinction to the somatic neuromuscular system, where a single motor neuron bridges the gap between the central nervous system (CNS) and the effector organ, in the autonomic nervous system there are always two efferent neurons serving this function, one (preganglionic) arising from its nucleus in the brainstem or spinal cord and the other (postganglionic) arising from specialized nerve cells in peripheral ganglia. Figure 26-1 illustrates this fundamental anatomic feature.

The autonomic nervous system, from an anatomic point of view, is divided into two parts: the craniosacral, or parasympathetic, and the thoracolumbar, or sympathetic (Figs. 26-2 and 26-3). The systems differ architecturally in that the ganglion in the sympathetic nervous system is located in a contiguous and interconnected, longitudinal chain (sympathetic chain) paravertebrally, whereas the parasympathetic ganglia are distributed in proximity to the structures they innervate. Moreover, the main neurotransmitter of the postganglionic connection to the end organ is norepinephrine in the case of the sympathetic nerves and acetylcholine for parasympathetic innervation. There are exceptions with regard to the sympathetic innervation of sweat glands (sudomotor), which are cholinergic. The neurotransmitter between the pre- and postneurons throughout the autonomic nervous system, sympathetic and parasympathetic, is acetylcholine as reiterated further on. These synapses between pre- and postganglionic cholinergic nerves are not blocked by atropine (nicotinic) whereas the postganglionic impulses are blocked by atropine (muscarinic).

Functionally, the two parts are complementary in maintaining a balance in the tonic activities of many visceral structures and organs. This rigid separation into sympathetic and parasympathetic parts, although useful for purposes of exposition, is physiologically not absolute.

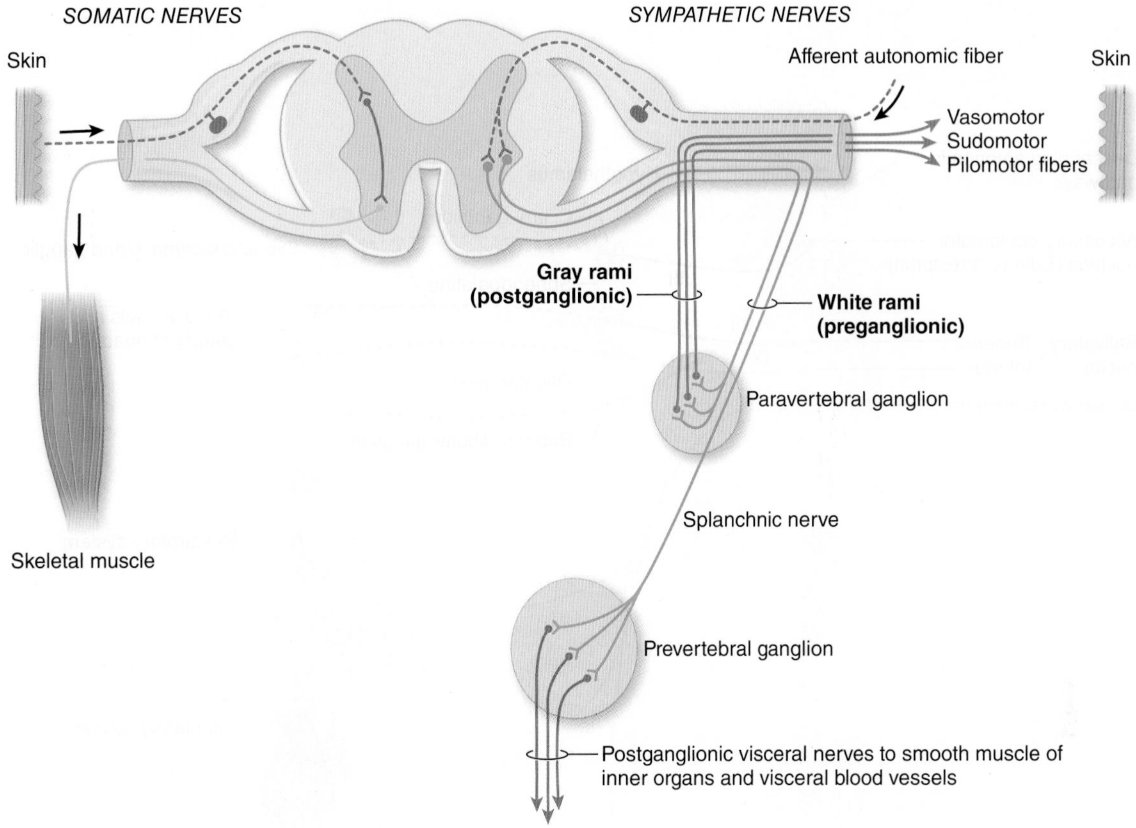

Figure 26-1. Sympathetic outflow from the spinal cord and the course and distribution of sympathetic fibers. The preganglionic fibers are in heavy lines; postganglionic fibers are in thin lines. (From Pick.)

From a neurologist's perspective, the two components are often affected together. Nonetheless, the notion of a balanced sympathetic and parasympathetic autonomic system has stood the test of time and remains a valid concept.

The Parasympathetic Nervous System
(See Fig. 26-2)

There are two divisions of the parasympathetic nervous system: cranial and sacral. The *cranial division* originates in the visceral nuclei of the midbrain, pons, and medulla. These nuclei include the Edinger-Westphal pupillary nucleus, superior and inferior salivatory nuclei, dorsal motor nucleus of the vagus, and adjacent reticular nuclei.

Axons (preganglionic fibers) of the visceral cranial nuclei course through the oculomotor, facial, glossopharyngeal, and vagus cranial nerves. The preganglionic fibers from the Edinger-Westphal nucleus traverse the oculomotor nerve and synapse in the ciliary ganglion in the orbit; axons of the ciliary ganglion cells innervate the ciliary muscle and pupillary sphincter (see Fig. 14-9).

The preganglionic fibers of the superior salivatory nucleus enter the facial nerve and, at a point near the geniculate ganglion, form the greater superficial petrosal nerve, through which they reach the sphenopalatine ganglion; postganglionic fibers from the cells of this ganglion innervate the lacrimal gland (see also Figs. 26-2 and 47-3). Other fibers originating in the salivatory nuclei are carried in the facial nerve and traverse the tympanic cavity as the chorda tympani to eventually join the submandibular ganglion. Cells of this ganglion innervate the submandibular and sublingual glands. Axons of the inferior salivatory nerve cells enter the glossopharyngeal nerve and reach the otic ganglion through the tympanic plexus and lesser superficial petrosal nerve; cells of the otic ganglion send fibers to the parotid gland.

Preganglionic fibers, derived from the dorsal motor nucleus of the vagus and adjacent visceral nuclei in the lateral reticular formation (mainly the nucleus ambiguus), enter the vagus nerve and terminate in ganglia situated in the walls of many thoracic and abdominal viscera. The ganglionic cells give rise to short postganglionic fibers that activate smooth muscle and glands of the pharynx, esophagus, and gastrointestinal tract (the vagal innervation of the colon is somewhat uncertain but considered to extend up to the descending colon) and of the heart, pancreas, liver, gallbladder, kidney, and ureter.

The *sacral part of the parasympathetic system* originates in the lateral horn cells of the second, third, and fourth sacral segments. Axons of these sacral neurons, constituting the preganglionic fibers, traverse the sacral spinal nerve roots of the cauda equina and synapse in ganglia that lie within the walls of the distal colon, bladder, and other pelvic organs. Thus, the sacral autonomic neurons, like the cranial ones, have long preganglionic and short postganglionic fibers, a feature that permits a circumscribed influence upon the target organ.

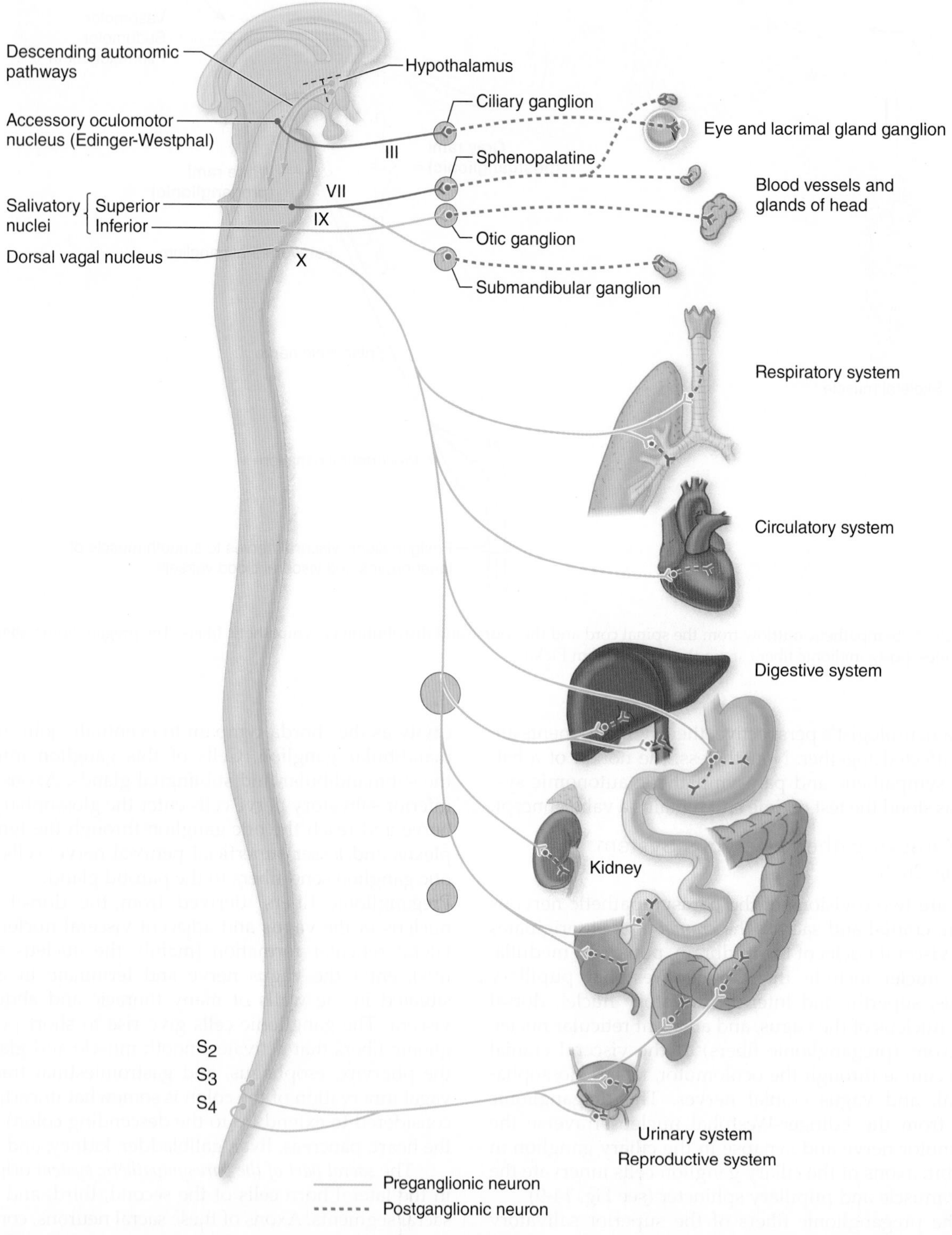

Figure 26-2. The parasympathetic (craniosacral) division of the autonomic nervous system. Preganglionic fibers extend from nuclei of the brainstem and sacral segments of the spinal cord to peripheral ganglia. Short postganglionic fibers extend from the ganglia to the effector organs. The lateral-posterior hypothalamus is part of the supranuclear mechanism for the regulation of parasympathetic activities. The frontal and limbic parts of the supranuclear regulatory apparatus are not indicated in the diagram (see text). (Reproduced by permission from Noback CL, Demarest R: *The Human Nervous System*, 3rd ed. New York, McGraw-Hill, 1981.)

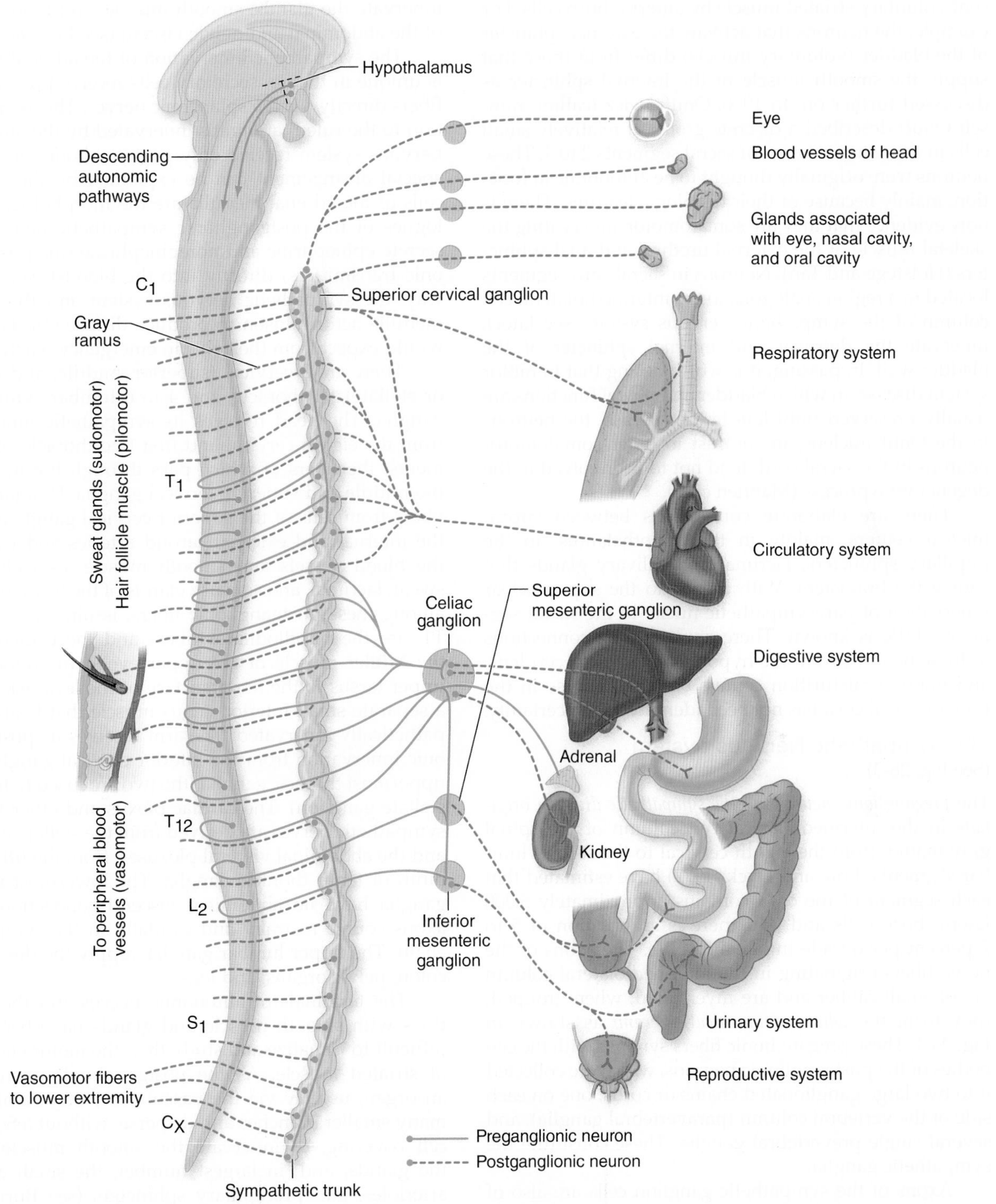

Figure 26-3. The sympathetic (thoracolumbar) division of the autonomic nervous system. Preganglionic fibers extend from the intermediolateral nucleus of the spinal cord to the peripheral autonomic ganglia, and postganglionic fibers extend from the peripheral ganglia to the effector organs, according to the scheme in Fig. 26-1. (Reproduced by permission from Noback CL, Demarest R: *The Human Nervous System*, 3rd ed. New York, McGraw-Hill, 1981.)

In organs containing smooth muscle that is innervated by parasympathetic fibers and therefore not under voluntary control, there is a parallel innervation of adjacent voluntary striated muscle by anterior horn cells. For example, the neurons that activate the external sphincter of the bladder (voluntary muscle) differ from those that supply the smooth muscle of the internal sphincter as discussed further on. In 1900, Onufrowicz (calling himself Onuf) described a discrete group of relatively small cells in the anterior horns of sacral segments 2 to 4. These neurons were originally thought to be autonomic in function, mainly because of their histologic features. There is now evidence that they are somatomotor, innervating the skeletal muscle of the external urethral and anal sphincters (Holstege and Tan). Neurons in sacral cord segments located in a region analogous to the intermediolateral cell column of the sympathetic nervous system (see later), innervate the detrusor and internal sphincter of the bladder wall. In passing, it is worth noting that in motor system disease, in which bladder and bowel functions are usually preserved until late in the disease, the neurons in the Onuf nucleus, in contrast to other somatomotor neurons in the sacral cord, tend not to be involved in the degenerative process (Mannen et al).

There are elaborate connections between supranuclear centers, mainly in the hypothalamus, to the pupillary sphincters, lacrimal and salivary glands that course the brainstem. With regard to the supranuclear innervation of parasympathetic nuclei in the sacral segments, little is known. There appear to be connections to these neurons from the hypothalamus, locus ceruleus, and pontine micturition centers but their course in the human spinal cord has not been identified with certainty.

The Sympathetic Nervous System
(See Fig. 26-3)

The *preganglionic neurons of the sympathetic division originate* in the intermediolateral cell column of the spinal gray matter, from the eighth cervical to the second lumbar segments. Low and Dyck (1977) have estimated that each segment of the cord contains approximately 5,000 lateral horn cells and that there is an attrition of 5 to 7 percent per decade in late adult life. The axons of the nerve fibers originating in the intermediolateral column are of small caliber and are myelinated; when grouped, they form the *white communicating rami* as shown in Fig. 26-1. These preganglionic fibers synapse with the cell bodies of the postganglionic neurons, which are collected into two large ganglionated chains or cords, one on each side of the vertebral column (paravertebral ganglia), and several single prevertebral ganglia. These constitute the sympathetic ganglia.

Axons of the sympathetic ganglion cells are also of small caliber but are unmyelinated. Most of the postganglionic fibers pass via *gray communicating rami* to their adjacent spinal nerves of T5 to L2; they supply blood vessels, sweat glands, and hair follicles, and also form plexuses that supply the heart, bronchi, kidneys, intestines, pancreas, bladder, and sex organs. The postganglionic fibers of the prevertebral ganglia (located in the retroperitoneal posterior abdomen rather than paravertebrally, along the sides of the spinal column) form the hypogastric, splanchnic, and mesenteric plexuses, which innervate the glands, smooth muscle, and blood vessels of the abdominal and pelvic viscera (see Fig. 26-3).

The sympathetic innervation of the adrenal medulla is unique in that its secretory cells receive preganglionic fibers directly, via the splanchnic nerves. This is an exception to the rule that organs innervated by the autonomic nervous system receive only postganglionic fibers. This special arrangement can be explained by the fact that cells of the adrenal medulla are the morphologic homologues of the postganglionic sympathetic neurons and secrete epinephrine and norepinephrine (the postganglionic transmitters) directly into the bloodstream. In this way, the sympathetic nervous system and the adrenal medulla act in unison to produce diffuse effects, as one would expect from their role in emergency reactions.

There are 3 cervical (superior, middle, and inferior, or stellate), 11 thoracic, and 4 to 6 lumbar sympathetic ganglia. The head receives its sympathetic innervation from the eighth cervical and first two thoracic cord segments, the fibers of which pass through the inferior to the middle and superior cervical ganglia. Postganglionic fibers from cells of the superior cervical ganglion follow the internal and external carotid arteries and innervate the blood vessels and smooth muscle, as well as the sweat, lacrimal, and salivary glands of the head. Included among these postganglionic fibers, issuing mainly from T1, are the pupillodilator fibers and those innervating the Müller muscle of the upper eyelid (it connects the upper tarsus to the undersurface of the levator); there is a separate small inferior tarsus muscle that is also sympathetically innervated. The arm receives its postganglionic innervation from the inferior cervical ganglion and uppermost thoracic ganglia (the two are fused to form the stellate ganglion). The cardiac plexus and other thoracic sympathetic nerves are derived from the stellate ganglion and the abdominal visceral plexuses, from the fifth to the ninth or tenth thoracic ganglia. The lowermost thoracic ganglia have no abdominal visceral connections; their axons course rostrally and caudally in the sympathetic chain. The upper lumbar ganglia supply the descending colon, pelvic organs, and legs.

The terminals of autonomic nerves and their junctions with smooth muscle and glands have been more difficult to visualize and study than the motor end plates of striated muscle. As the postganglionic axons enter an organ, usually via the vasculature, they ramify into many smaller branches and disperse, without a Schwann cell covering, to innervate the smooth muscle fibers, the glands, and, in largest number, the small arteries, arterioles, and precapillary sphincters (see Burnstock). Some of these terminals penetrate the smooth muscle of the arterioles; others remain in the adventitia. At the ends of the postganglionic fibers and in part along their course there are swellings that lie in close proximity to the sarcolemma or gland cell membrane; often the muscle fiber is grooved to accommodate these swellings. The axonal swellings contain synaptic vesicles, some clear and others with a dense granular core. The clear vesicles contain acetylcholine and those with a dense core contain catecholamines, particularly norepinephrine (Falck). This is well illustrated in the iris, where nerves to the dilator muscle (sympathetic) contain dense-core vesicles and those to the constrictor (parasympathetic) contain clear vesicles. A single nerve fiber innervates multiple smooth muscle and gland cells.

Visceral Afferents Somewhat arbitrarily, anatomists have declared the autonomic nervous system to be purely efferent motor and secretory in function. However, most autonomic nerves are mixed, also containing afferent fibers that convey sensory impulses from the viscera and blood vessels. The cell bodies of these sensory neurons lie in the posterior root sensory ganglia; some central axons of these ganglionic cells synapse with lateral horn cells of the spinal cord and subserve visceral reflexes; others synapse in the dorsal horn and convey or modulate impulses for conscious sensation. Secondary afferents carry sensory impulses to certain brainstem nuclei, particularly the nucleus tractus solitarius, as described later, and the thalamus via the lateral spinothalamic and polysynaptic pathways.

The Central Regulation of Visceral Function

Integration of autonomic function takes place at two levels, the brainstem and the cerebrum. In the brainstem, the main visceral afferent nucleus is the nucleus tractus solitarius (NTS). Cardiovascular, respiratory, and gastrointestinal afferents, carried in cranial nerves X and IX via the nodose and petrosal ganglia, terminate on specific subnuclei of the NTS. The caudal subnuclei are the primary receiving site for viscerosensory fibers; other less-well-defined areas receive baroreceptor and chemoreceptor information. The caudal NTS integrates these signals and projects to a number of critical areas in the hypothalamus, amygdala, and insular cortex, involved primarily in cardiovascular control, as well as to the pontine and medullary nuclei controlling respiratory rhythms. The NTS therefore serves a critical integratory function for both circulation and respiration, as described further on.

Perhaps the major advance in our understanding of the autonomic nervous system occurred with the elaboration of the autonomic regulating functions of the hypothalamus. Small, insignificant-appearing nuclei in the walls of the third ventricle and in buried parts of the limbic cortex have rich bidirectional connections with autonomic centers in various parts of the nervous system. As indicated in Chap. 25, the hypothalamus serves as the integrating mechanism of the autonomic nervous system and limbic system. The regulatory activity of the hypothalamus is accomplished in two ways, through direct pathways that descend to particular groups of cells in the brainstem and spinal cord, and through the pituitary and thence to other endocrine glands. The supranuclear regulatory apparatus of the hypothalamus includes three main cerebral structures: the frontal lobe cortex, the insular cortex, and the amygdaloid and adjacent nuclei.

The ventromedial prefrontal and cingulate cortices function as the highest levels of autonomic integration. Stimulation of one frontal lobe may evoke changes in temperature and sweating in the contralateral arm and leg; massive lesions here, which usually cause a hemiplegia, may modify the autonomic functions in the direction of either inhibition or facilitation. Lesions involving the posterior part of the superior frontal and anterior part of the cingulate gyri (usually bilateral, occasionally unilateral) result in loss of voluntary control of the bladder and bowel. Most likely a large contingent of these fibers terminates in the hypothalamus, which, in turn, sends fibers to the brainstem and spinal cord. The descending spinal pathways from the hypothalamus are believed to lie ventromedial to the corticospinal fibers.

The insular cortex receives projections from the NTS, the parabrachial nucleus of the pons, and the lateral hypothalamic nuclei. Direct stimulation of the insula produces cardiac arrhythmias and a number of other alterations in visceral function. The cingulate and hippocampal gyri and their associated subcortical structures (substantia innominata and the amygdaloid, septal, piriform, habenular, and midbrain tegmental nuclei) have been identified as important cerebral autonomic regulatory centers. Together they have been called the *visceral brain* (see Chap. 25). Of particular importance in autonomic regulation is the amygdala, the central nucleus of which is a major site of origin of projections to the hypothalamus and brainstem. The anatomy and the effects of stimulation and ablation of the amygdala have been discussed in Chap. 25, in relation to the neurology of emotion.

In addition to the aforementioned central relationships, it should be noted that important interactions between the autonomic nervous system and the endocrine glands occur at a peripheral level. The best-known example is in the adrenal medulla. A similar relationship pertains to the pineal gland, in which norepinephrine (NE) released from postganglionic fibers that end on pineal cells stimulates several enzymes involved in the biosynthesis of melatonin. Similarly, the juxtaglomerular apparatus of the kidney and the islets of Langerhans of the pancreas may function as neuroendocrine transducers insofar as they convert a neural stimulus (in these cases adrenergic) to an endocrine secretion (renin, glucagon, and insulin, respectively). The numerous autonomic–endocrine interactions are elaborated in the next chapter.

Finally, there is the essential role that the hypothalamus plays in the initiation and regulation of autonomic activity, both sympathetic and parasympathetic. Sympathetic responses are most readily obtained by stimulation of the posterior and lateral regions of the hypothalamus, and parasympathetic responses from the anterior regions. The descending sympathetic fibers are largely or totally uncrossed. According to Carmel, fibers from the caudal hypothalamus at first run in the prerubral field, dorsal and slightly rostral to the red nucleus, and then ventral to the ventrolateral thalamic nuclei; then they descend in the lateral tegmentum of the midbrain, pons, and medulla to synapse in the intermediolateral cell column of the spinal cord. In the medulla, the descending sympathetic pathway is located in the posterolateral retroolivary area, where it is frequently involved in lateral medullary infarctions. In the cervical cord, the fibers run in the posterior angle of the anterior horn (Nathan and Smith). According to the latter authors, some of the fibers supplying sudomotor neurons run outside this area but also remain ipsilateral. Jansen and colleagues, by the use of viral vectors in rodents, were able to label certain neurons of the hypothalamus and the ventral medulla that stimulated sympathetic activity in both the stellate ganglion and the adrenal gland. They hypothesized that this dual control underlies the fight-or-flight response, as described in Chap. 25. By contrast, the pathways of descending parasympathetic fibers are not well defined.

Afferent projections from the spinal cord to the hypothalamus have been demonstrated in animals and provide a potential route by which sensation from somatic and possibly visceral structures may influence autonomic responses.

Physiologic and Pharmacologic Considerations

The function of the autonomic nervous system in its regulation of the visceral organs is to a high degree independent of voluntary control and awareness. Furthermore, when the autonomic nerves are interrupted, these organs continue to function (the organism survives), but they are no longer as effective in maintaining homeostasis and adapting to the demands of changing internal conditions and external stresses.

Viscera have a double-nerve supply, sympathetic and parasympathetic and in general these two parts of the autonomic nervous system exert opposite effects. For example, the effects of the sympathetic nervous system on the heart are excitatory and those of the parasympathetic inhibitory. However, some structures—sweat glands, cutaneous blood vessels, and hair follicles—receive only sympathetic postganglionic fibers, and the adrenal gland, as indicated earlier, has only a preganglionic sympathetic innervation. Also, some parasympathetic neurons have been identified in sympathetic ganglia.

Neurohumoral Transmission

All autonomic functions are mediated through the release of chemical transmitters. The modern concept of neurohumoral transmission had its beginnings in the early decades of the twentieth century. In 1921, Loewi discovered that stimulation of the vagus nerve released a chemical substance (*Vagusstoff*) that slowed the heart. Later this substance was shown by Dale to be acetylcholine (ACh). Also, in 1920, Cannon reported that stimulation of the sympathetic trunk released an epinephrine-like substance, which increased the heart rate and blood pressure. He named this substance "sympathin," subsequently shown to be noradrenaline, or NE. Dale found that ACh had pharmacologic effects similar to those obtained by stimulation of parasympathetic nerves; he designated these effects as "parasympathomimetic." These observations placed neurochemical transmission on solid ground and laid the basis for the distinction between cholinergic and adrenergic transmission in the autonomic nervous system.

The most important of the autonomic neurotransmitters are ACh and NE. ACh is synthesized at the terminals of axons and stored in presynaptic vesicles until it is released by the arrival of nerve impulses. ACh is released at the terminals of all preganglionic fibers (in both the sympathetic and parasympathetic ganglia), as well as at the terminals of all postganglionic parasympathetic and a few special postganglionic sympathetic fibers, mainly those subserving sweat glands. Of course, ACh is also the chemical transmitter of nerve impulses to the skeletal muscle fibers. Parasympathetic postganglionic function is mediated by two distinct types of ACh receptors: *nicotinic* and *muscarinic*, so named by Dale because the choline-induced responses were similar either to those of nicotine or to those of the alkaloid, muscarine. The postganglionic parasympathetic receptors are located within the innervated organ and are muscarinic; i.e., they are antagonized by atropinic drugs. As already mentioned the receptors in ganglia, like those of skeletal muscle, are nicotinic; they are not blocked by atropine but are counteracted by other agents (e.g., tubocurarine).

It is likely that more than ACh is involved in nerve transmission at a ganglionic level. Many peptides—substance P, enkephalins, somatostatin, vasoactive intestinal peptide, adenosine triphosphate (ATP), and nitric oxide—have been identified in the autonomic ganglia, localizing in some cases to the same cell as ACh. (This negates "Dale's principle," or "law," which stipulates that one neuron elaborates only one neurotransmitter.) Particular neuronal firing rates appear to cause the preferential release of one or another of these substances. Most of the neuropeptides exert their postsynaptic effects through the G-protein transduction system, which uses adenyl cyclase or phospholipase C as an intermediary. The neuropeptides act as modulators of neural transmission, although their exact function in many cases remains to be determined.

With two exceptions, postganglionic sympathetic fibers release only NE at their terminals. The sweat glands and some blood vessels in muscle are innervated by postganglionic sympathetic fibers, but their terminals, as mentioned, release ACh. The NE that is discharged into the synaptic space activates specific *adrenergic receptors* on the postsynaptic membrane of target cells.

Adrenergic receptors are of two types, classified originally by Ahlquist as *alpha* and *beta*. In general, the alpha receptors mediate vasoconstriction, relaxation of the gut, and dilatation of the pupil; beta receptors mediate vasodilatation, especially in muscles, relaxation of the bronchi, and an increased rate and contractility of the heart. Each of these receptors is subdivided further into two types. Alpha_1 receptors are postsynaptic; alpha_2 receptors are situated on the presynaptic membrane and, when stimulated, *diminish the release of the transmitter*. Beta_1 receptors are, for all practical purposes, limited to the heart; their activation increases the heart rate and contractility. Beta_2 receptors, when stimulated, relax the smooth muscle of the bronchi and of most other sites, including the blood vessels of skeletal muscle. A comprehensive account of neurohumoral transmission and receptor function can be found in the monograph by Cooper and colleagues.

Discussed in the following pages are the ways in which the two divisions of the autonomic nervous system, acting in conjunction with the endocrine glands, maintain the homeostasis of the organism. As stated earlier, the integration of these two systems is achieved primarily in the hypothalamus. In addition, the endocrine glands are influenced by circulating catecholamines, and some of them are innervated by adrenergic fibers. Chapter 27 discusses further these autonomic–endocrine relations.

Regulation of Blood Pressure

As was indicated briefly in Chap. 18, blood pressure depends on the adequacy of intravascular blood volume, on systemic vascular resistance, and on the cardiac output. Both the autonomic and endocrine systems influence the muscular, cutaneous, and mesenteric (splanchnic) vascular beds, heart rate, and stroke volume of the heart. Together, these actions serve to maintain normal blood pressure and allow reflex maintenance of blood pressure with changes in body position. Two types of baroreceptors function as the afferent component of this reflex arc by sensing pressure gradients across the walls of large blood vessels. Those in the carotid sinus and aortic arch are sensitive to reductions in pulse pressure (the difference between systolic and diastolic blood pressure), while those in the right heart chambers and pulmonary vessels respond more to alterations in blood volume. The carotid sinus baroreceptors are rapidly responsive and capable of detecting beat-to-beat changes, in contrast to the aortic arch nerves, which have a longer response time and discriminate only the larger and more prolonged alterations in pressure.

The nerves arising from these receptors are small-caliber, thinly myelinated fibers that course in cranial nerves IX and X and terminate in the nucleus of the tractus solitarius (NTS). In response to increased stimulation of these receptors, vagal efferent activity is reduced, resulting in reflex cardioacceleration. This is accomplished through polysynaptic connections between the NTS and the dorsal motor nucleus of the vagus; it is from this structure that vagal neurons project to the sinoatrial node, atrioventricular node, and the muscle of the left ventricle. Thus, vagal activity results in reduction in heart rate and in the contractile force of the myocardium (negative inotropy). Increased systemic vascular resistance is mediated concurrently through parallel connections between the NTS and the medullary pressor areas that project to the intermediolateral cells of the midthoracic cord. The main sympathetic outflow from these thoracic segments is via the greater splanchnic nerve to the celiac ganglion, the postganglionic nerves of which project to the capacitance vessels of the gut. The splanchnic capacitance veins act as a reservoir for as much as 20 percent of the total blood volume, and interruption of the splanchnic nerves results in severe postural hypotension. After a high-carbohydrate meal there is a marked hyperemia of the gut and compensatory peripheral vasoconstriction in the muscles and skin. It has also been noted that the mesenteric vascular bed is responsive to the orthostatic redistribution of blood volume but not to mental stress.

The opposite response to the one described earlier, namely bradycardia and hypotension, results when vagal tone is enhanced and sympathetic tone reduced. This response can be triggered by baroreceptors, or it may arise from cerebral stimuli such as fear or sight of blood in susceptible individuals as well as from extreme pain, particularly arising in the viscera.

Two slower-acting humoral mechanisms regulate blood volume and complement the control of systemic vascular resistance. Pressure-sensitive renal juxtaglomerular cells release renin, which stimulates production of angiotensin and influences aldosterone production, both of which affect an increase of blood volume. Of lesser influence in the control of blood pressure is antidiuretic hormone, discussed in the next chapter; but the effects of this peptide become more important when autonomic failure forces a dependence on secondary mechanisms for the maintenance of blood pressure. In addition to its presence in autonomic ganglia, nitric oxide has been found to have an important local role in maintaining vascular tone, mainly by way of attenuating the response to sympathetic stimulation. The extent to which this latter function is under neural control is not clear.

Regulation of Bladder Function

The familiar functions of the bladder and lower urinary tract—the storage and intermittent evacuation of urine—are served by three structural components: the bladder itself, the main component of which is the large detrusor (transitional type) muscle; a functional internal sphincter composed of similar muscle; and the striated external sphincter or urogenital diaphragm. The sphincters assure continence; in the male, the internal sphincter also prevents the reflux of semen from the urethra during ejaculation. For micturition to occur, the sphincters must relax, allowing the detrusor to expel urine from the bladder into the urethra. This is accomplished by a complex mechanism involving mainly the parasympathetic nervous system (the sacral peripheral nerves derived from the second, third, and fourth sacral segments of the spinal cord and their somatic sensorimotor fibers) and, to a lesser extent, sympathetic fibers derived from the thorax. The vaguely localizable brainstem "micturition centers," with their spinal and suprasegmental connections, may contribute (Fig. 26-4).

The detrusor muscle receives motor innervation from nerve cells in the intermediolateral columns of gray matter, mainly from the third and also from the second and fourth sacral segments of the spinal cord (the "detrusor center"). These neurons give rise to preganglionic fibers that synapse in parasympathetic ganglia within the bladder wall. Short postganglionic fibers end on muscarinic acetylcholine receptors of the muscle fibers. There are also beta-adrenergic receptors in the dome of the bladder, which are activated by sympathetic fibers that arise in the intermediolateral nerve cells of T10, T11, and T12 segments. These preganglionic fibers pass via inferior splanchnic nerves to the inferior mesenteric ganglia (see Fig. 26-1); pre- and postganglionic sympathetic axons are conveyed by the hypogastric nerve to the pelvic plexus

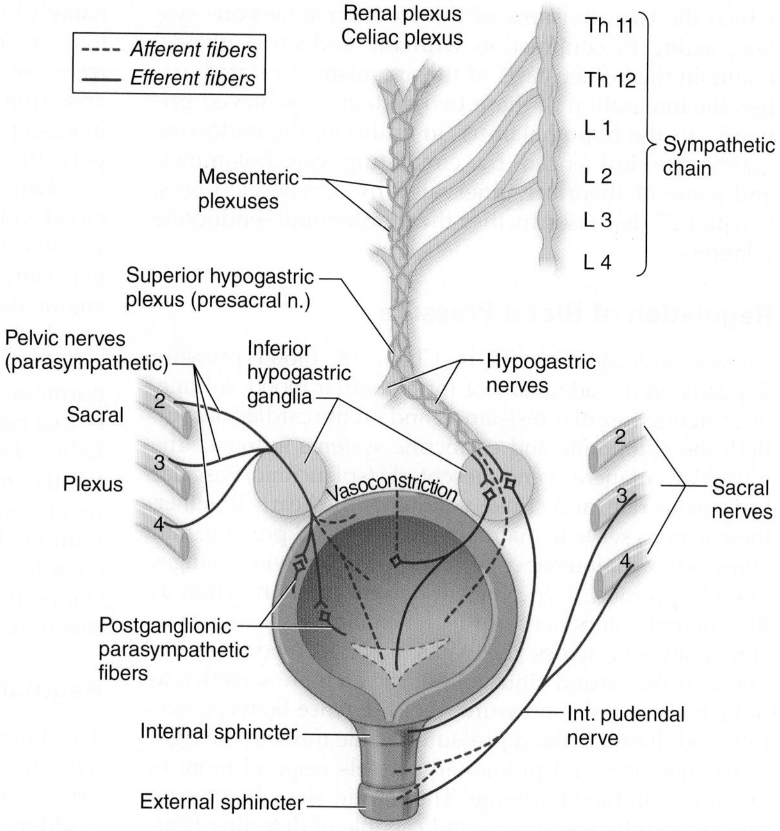

Figure 26-4. Innervation of the urinary bladder and its sphincters.

and the bladder dome. The internal sphincter and base of the bladder (trigone), consisting of smooth muscle, are also innervated to some extent by the sympathetic fibers of the hypogastric nerves; their receptors are mainly of alpha-adrenergic type, which makes it possible to therapeutically manipulate the function of the sphincter with adrenergically active drugs as well as the more commonly used cholinergic ones (see further on).

The external urethral and anal sphincters are composed of striated muscle fibers. Their innervation, via the pudendal nerves, is derived from a densely packed group of somatomotor neurons (nucleus of Onuf) in the anterolateral horns of sacral segments 2, 3, and 4. Cells in the ventrolateral part of Onuf's nucleus innervate the external urethral sphincter, and cells of the mediodorsal part innervate the anal sphincter. The muscle fibers of the sphincters respond to the nicotinic effects of ACh.

The pudendal nerves also contain afferent fibers coursing from the urethra and the external sphincter to the sacral segments of the spinal cord. These fibers convey impulses for reflex activities and, through connections with higher centers, for sensation. Some of these fibers probably course through the hypogastric plexus, as indicated by the fact that patients with complete transverse lesions of the cord as high as T12 may report vague sensations of urethral discomfort. The bladder is sensitive to pain and pressure; these senses are transmitted to higher centers along the sensory pathways described in Chaps. 8 and 9.

Unlike skeletal striated muscle, the detrusor, because of its postganglionic system, is capable of some contractions, although imperfect, after complete destruction of the sacral segments of the spinal cord. Isolation of the sacral cord centers (transverse lesions of the cord above the sacral levels) and their peripheral nerves permits contractions of the detrusor muscle, but they still do not empty the bladder completely; patients with such lesions usually develop dyssynergia of the detrusor and external sphincter muscles (see later), indicating that coordination of these muscles must occur at supraspinal levels (Blaivas). With acute transverse lesions of the upper cord, the function of sacral segments is abolished for several weeks in the same way as the motor neurons of skeletal muscles (the state of spinal shock).

The storage of urine and the efficient emptying of the bladder are possible only when the spinal segments, together with their afferent and efferent nerve fibers, are connected with the so-called micturition centers in the pontomesencephalic tegmentum. In experimental animals, this center (or centers) lies within or adjacent to the locus ceruleus. A medial region triggers micturition, while a lateral area seems more important for continence. These neurons receive afferent impulses from the sacral cord segments; their efferent fibers course downward via the reticulospinal tracts in the lateral funiculi of the spinal cord and activate cells in the nucleus of Onuf, as well as in the intermediolateral cell groups of the sacral segments (Holstege and Tan). In cats, the pontomesencephalic centers receive descending fibers from anteromedial parts of the frontal cortex, thalamus, hypothalamus, and cerebellum, but the brainstem centers and their descending pathways have not been precisely defined in humans. Other fibers from the motor cortex descend with the corticospinal fibers to the anterior horn cells of the sacral cord and innervate the external sphincter. According to Ruch, the descending pathways from the midbrain tegmentum are inhibitory and those from the pontine tegmentum and posterior hypothalamus are facilitatory. The pathway that descends with the corticospinal tract from the motor cortex is inhibitory. Thus the net effect of lesions in the brain and spinal cord on the micturition reflex, at least in animals, may be either inhibitory or facilitatory (DeGroat).

Almost all of this information has been inferred from animal experiments; there is little human pathologic material to corroborate the role of brainstem nuclei and cortex in bladder control. What information is available is reviewed extensively by Fowler, whose article is recommended. Also of interest here is the study by Blok and colleagues, who performed positron emission tomography (PET) studies in volunteer subjects during micturition. Increased blood flow was detected in the right pontine tegmentum, periaqueductal region, hypothalamus, and right inferior frontal cortex. When the bladder was full but subjects were prevented from voiding, increased activity was seen in the right ventral pontine tegmentum. The meaning of these lateralized findings is unclear, but the study supports the presumption that pontine centers are involved in the act of voiding.

The act of micturition is both reflex and voluntary. When the normal person desires to void, there is first a voluntary relaxation of the perineum, followed sequentially by an increased tension of the abdominal wall, a slow contraction of the detrusor, and an associated opening of the internal sphincter; finally, there is a relaxation of the external sphincter (Denny-Brown and Robertson). It is useful to think of the detrusor contraction as a spinal stretch reflex, subject to facilitation and inhibition from higher centers. Voluntary closure of the external sphincter and contraction of the perineal muscles cause the detrusor contraction to subside. The abdominal muscles have little role in initiating micturition except when the detrusor muscle is not functioning normally. The voluntary restraint of micturition is a cerebral affair and is mediated by fibers that arise in the frontal lobes (paracentral motor region), descend in the spinal cord just anterior and medial to the corticospinal tracts, and terminate on the cells of the anterior horns and intermediolateral cell columns of the sacral segments, as described earlier. The coordination of detrusor and external sphincteric function depends mainly on the descending pathway from the posited centers in the dorsolateral pontine tegmentum.

Regulation of Bowel Function

The colon and anal sphincters are obedient to the same principles that govern bladder function. Unique to the bowel, however, is an intrinsic enteric nervous system that originates in the myenteric (or Auerbach) plexus and the submucosal plexus (of Meissner), located in the gut wall. The first stimulates smooth muscle and the latter also regulates mucosal secretion and blood flow. This embedded system controls peristalsis largely independent of other autonomic influences but is highly responsive to local chemical and mechanical stimuli. As outlined in the thorough review by Benarroch that should be consulted by interested readers, acetylcholine is the dominant neurotransmitter in the enteric nerves but nitric oxide and numerous peptide transmitters are found in profusion.

Emergency and Alarm Reactions

Inasmuch as the autonomic nervous system and the adrenal glands were accepted for many years as the neural and humoral basis of all instinctive and emotional behavior. In states of chronic anxiety and acute panic reactions, depressive psychosis, mania, and schizophrenia, all of which are characterized by an altered emotionality, no consistent autonomic or endocrine dysfunction has been demonstrated except perhaps for diminished responses of growth hormone in panic disorders. The lack of cortisol suppressibilty by injection of adrenocorticotropic hormone (ACTH) had for some time also been considered to be a consistent aspect of depressive illnesses but that too, has not been entirely specific. This has been disappointing, as the emergency theory of sympathoadrenal action provided by Cannon was such a promising concept of the neurophysiology of acute emotion, and Selye had extended this theory so plausibly to explain all the reactions to stress in animals and humans.

According to these theories, strong emotion, such as anger or fear, excites the sympathetic nervous system and the adrenal cortex (via corticotropin-releasing factor [CRF] and ACTH), which are under direct neural and endocrine control. These sympathoadrenal reactions are brief and sustain the animal in "flight or fight" as discussed in Chap. 25. Animals deprived of adrenal cortex or human beings with Addison disease cannot tolerate stress because they are incapable of mobilizing both the adrenal medulla and adrenal cortex. Prolonged stress and production of ACTH activates all the adrenal hormones (glucocorticoids, mineralocorticoids, and adrenocorticoids) and has been studied extensively in relation to immune reactions and other systemic functions but with no consistent findings that are yet clinically applicable.

Tests for Abnormalities of the Autonomic Nervous System

With few exceptions, such as testing pupillary reactions and examination of the skin for abnormalities of color and sweating, the neurologist tends to be casual in evaluating the function of the autonomic nervous system. Nonetheless, several simple but informative tests can be used to confirm one's clinical impressions and to elicit abnormalities of autonomic function that may aid in diagnosis. For the detection of certain disease, it is almost imperative that blood pressure be evaluated to detect a drop with change in body position from lying or sitting, to standing. A combination of tests is usually necessary, because certain ones are particularly sensitive to abnormalities of sympathetic function and others to parasympathetic or baroreceptor afferent function. These are described later and are summarized in Table 26-1. A scheme for the examination of pupillary abnormalities was presented in Fig. 14-11.

Testing of Blood Pressure and Heart Rate

These are among the simplest and most important tests of autonomic function and most laboratories have automated techniques to quantitate them. McLeod and Tuck state that in changing from the recumbent to the standing position, a fall of more than 30 mm Hg systolic and 15 mm Hg diastolic is abnormal; others give figures of 20 and 10 mm Hg. They caution that the arm on which the cuff is placed must be held horizontally when standing, so that the decline in arm pressure will not be obscured by the added hydrostatic pressure. As emphasized in Chap. 18 on syncope, the determination of blood pressure in orthostatic testing is ideally done by having the patient remain supine for as long as it is practical before testing, and shifting from a supine to standing position, without the interposition of sitting. Moreover, blood pressure is most informative if measured immediately after standing and again at approximately 1 and 3 min. The expected response is a momentary and slight increase in pressure that is usually not detected with a manual blood pressure cuff, followed by a slight drop within seconds of standing, and then a slow recovery during the first minute. Persistent hypotension at 1 min indicates sympathetic adrenergic failure and the later measurement affirms this if blood pressure fails to recover or continues to decline (Fig. 26-5*A*).

The main cause of an orthostatic drop in blood pressure is, of course, hypovolemia. In the context of recurrent

Table 26-1

CLINICAL TESTS OF AUTONOMIC FUNCTION

TEST	NORMAL RESPONSE	MAIN PART OF REFLEX ARC TESTED
Noninvasive Bedside Tests		
Blood-pressure response to standing or vertical tilt	Fall in BP ≤30/15 mm Hg	Afferent and sympathetic efferent limbs
Heart rate response to standing	Increase 11–90 beats/min; 30:15 ratio ≥1.04	Vagal afferent and efferent limbs
Isometric exercise	Increase in diastolic BP, 15 mm Hg	Sympathetic efferent limb
Heart rate variation with respiration	Maximum-minimum heart rate ≥15 beats/min; E:I ratio 1.2[a]	Vagal afferent and efferent limbs
Valsalva ratio (see text)	≥1.4[a]	Afferent and efferent limbs
Sweat tests	Sweating over all body and limbs	Sympathetic efferent limb
Axon reflex	Local piloerection, sweating	Postganglionic sympathetic efferent fibers
Plasma noradrenaline level	Rises on tilting from horizontal to vertical	Sympathetic efferent limb
Plasma vasopressin level	Rise with induced hypotension	Afferent limb
Invasive Tests		
Valsalva maneuver (BP response with indwelling arterial catheter or continuous noninvasive BP measurement)	Phase I: Rise in BP Phase II: Gradual reduction of BP to plateau; tachycardia Phase III: Fall in BP Phase IV: Overshoot of BP, bradycardia[a]	Afferent and sympathetic efferent limbs
Baroreflex sensitivity	(1) Slowing of heart rate with induced rise of BP[a] (2) Steady-state responses to induced rise and fall of BP	(1) Parasympathetic afferent and efferent limbs (2) Afferent and efferent limbs
Infusion of pressor drugs	(1) Rise in BP (2) Slowing of heart rate	(1) Adrenergic receptors (2) Afferent and efferent parasympathetic limbs
Other Tests of Vasomotor Control		
Radiant heating of trunk	Increased hand blood flow	Sympathetic efferent limb
Immersion of hand in hot water	Increased blood flow of opposite hand	Sympathetic efferent limb
Cold pressor test	Reduced blood flow, rise in BP	Sympathetic efferent limb
Emotional stress	Increased BP	Sympathetic efferent limb
Tests of Pupillary Innervation		
4% cocaine	Pupil dilates	Sympathetic innervation
0.1% adrenaline	No response	Postganglionic sympathetic innervation
1% hydroxyamphetamine hydrobromide	Pupil dilates	Postganglionic sympathetic innervation
2.5% methacholine 0.125% pilocarpine	No response	Parasympathetic innervation
0.5% apraclonidine	Pupil dilates and ptosis resolves in Horner syndrome	Parasympathetic innervation

[a]Age-dependent response.

BP, blood pressure; E:I, expiration:inspiration.

Source: Reproduced by permission from McLeod and Tuck.

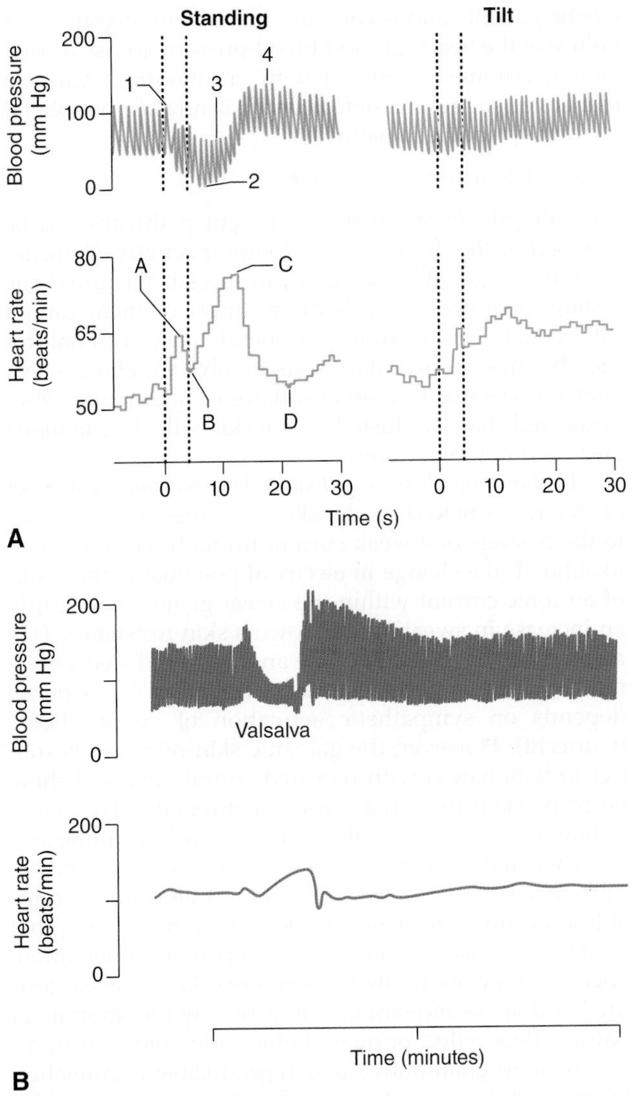

Figure 26-5. *A*. Blood pressure and heart rate changes elicited by standing and head-up tilt in a healthy individual. *B*. Blood pressure and heart rate changes elicited by Valsalva in a healthy individual. (With permission from Bannister R: *Autonomic Failure: A Textbook of Clinical Disorders of the Autonomic Nervous System*, 2nd ed. Oxford, Oxford University Press, 1988.)

fainting, however, an excessive drop reflects inadequate sympathetic vasoconstrictor activity. The use of a tilt table, as described in "Tilt-Table Testing" in Chap. 18 and further on, is an additional means of inducing orthostatic changes and also elicits reflex fainting in patients prone to syncope from an oversensitive cardiac reflex, i.e., one that produces vasodilatation (neurocardiogenic syncope). In response to the induced drop in blood pressure, the heart rate (under vagal control) normally increases. *The failure of the heart rate to rise in response to the drop in blood pressure with standing is the simplest bedside indicator of vagal nerve dysfunction.* Neurally mediated syncope may show one of three initial patterns with testing on a tilt table: a paroxysmal vasodepressor response alone, a combined bradycardic and hypotensive response, and solely bradycardia. The tilt table allows differentiation among these or, more often, clarifies the order in which the events occur.

In addition, the heart rate, after rising initially in response to upright standing posture (not with the tilt table), slows after about 15 beats to reach a stable rate by the thirtieth beat. The ratio of R-R intervals in the electrocardiogram (ECG), corresponding to the thirtieth and fifteenth beats (the 30:15 ratio), is an even more sensitive measure of the integrity of vagal inhibition of the sinus node. A ratio in adults under age 60 of less than 1.07 is usually abnormal, indicating a loss of vagal tone and the normal ratio is progressively higher for younger ages, for example, it is usually above 1.12 at age 30 and 1.1 at age 40.

Another simple procedure for quantitating purely vagal function consists of measuring the *variation in heart rate during deep breathing* (respiratory sinus arrhythmia). The ECG is recorded while the patient breathes at a regular rate of 6 breaths per minute. Normally, the heart rate varies by as many as 15 beats per minute or even more between expiration and inspiration; differences of less than 7 beats per minute for ages 60 to 69 and 9 for ages 50 to 59 may be abnormal.

A yet more accurate test of vagal function is the measurement of the ratio of the longest R-R interval during forceful slow expiration (standardized as constant blowing at a pressure of 40 mm Hg for 10 s) to the shortest R-R interval during inspiration, which allows the derivation of an expiration–inspiration (E:I) ratio. This is the best validated of all the heart-rate measurements, particularly as computerized methods can be used to display the spectrum of beat-to-beat ECG intervals during breathing. The results of these tests must always be compared with those obtained in normal individuals of the same age. Up to age 40 years, E:I ratios of less than 1.2 (signifying a variation of 20 percent) are abnormal. The ratio decreases with age, and markedly so beyond age 60 years (at which time it approaches 1.04 or less), as it does also in the presence of even mild diabetic neuropathy. Thus the test results must be interpreted cautiously in the elderly or in diabetic individuals. Similar ratios have been developed for heart-rate change during the Valsalva maneuver; the *Valsalva ratio*.

Computerized methods of *power spectral analysis* may be used to express the variance in heart rate as a function of the beat-to-beat interval. Several power peaks are appreciated: one related to the respiratory sinus arrhythmia and others that reflect baroreceptor and cardiac sympathetic activity. All of these tests of heart-rate variation are usually combined with measurement of heart rate and blood pressure during the Valsalva maneuver, as described below, and with the tilt-table test, as described in Chap. 18.

In the *Valsalva maneuver*, the subject exhales into a manometer or against a closed glottis for 10 to 15 s, creating a markedly positive intrathoracic pressure. The sharp reduction in venous return to the heart causes a drop in cardiac output and in blood pressure; the response on baroreceptors is to cause a reflex tachycardia and, to a lesser extent, peripheral vasoconstriction. With release of intrathoracic pressure, the venous return, stroke volume, and blood pressure rise to higher-than-normal levels; reflex parasympathetic influence then predominates and a bradycardia results (Fig. 26-5*B*). Failure of the heart rate to increase during the positive intrathoracic pressure phase of the Valsalva maneuver points to sympathetic dysfunction, and failure of the rate to slow during the period of blood pressure overshoot points to a parasympathetic disturbance. In patients with autonomic failure, the fall in blood pressure is not aborted during the last few seconds of increased intrathoracic pressure, and there is no overshoot of blood pressure when the breath is released. The Valsalva ratio, referring to the maximum heart rate generated by the maneuver to the lowest heart rate within 30 s of that peak, is another often-used measure in comprehensive autonomic testing.

Tests of Vasomotor Reactions

These generally test sympathetic cholinergic function. Measurement of the skin temperature is a rough but useful index of vasomotor function. Vasomotor paralysis results in vasodilatation of skin vessels and a rise in skin temperature; vasoconstriction lowers the temperature. With a skin thermometer, one may compare affected and normal areas under standard conditions. The normal skin temperature is 31°C (87.8°F) to 33°C (91.4°F) when the room temperature is 26°C (78.8°F) to 27°C (80.6°F). Vasoconstrictor tone may also be tested by measuring the reduction in skin temperature at a distant site before and after immersing one or both hands in cold water (see the discussion of the cold pressor test later).

The integrity of the sympathetic reflex arc, which includes baroreceptors in the aorta and carotid sinus, their afferent pathways, the vasomotor centers, and the sympathetic and parasympathetic outflow can be tested in a general way by combining the cold pressor test, grip test, mental arithmetic test, and Valsalva maneuver, as described below.

Vasoconstriction induces an elevation of the blood pressure. This is the basis of the *cold pressor test*. In normal persons, immersing one hand in ice water for 1 to 5 min raises the systolic pressure by 15 to 20 mm Hg and the diastolic pressure by 10 to 15 mm Hg. Similarly, the *sustained isometric contraction* of a group of muscles (e.g., those of the forearm in handgrip) for 5 min normally increases the heart rate and the systolic and diastolic pressures by at least 15 mm Hg. The response in both of these tests is reduced or absent with lesions of the sympathetic reflex arc, particularly of the efferent limb, but neither of these tests has been well quantitated or validated. The stress involved in doing *mental arithmetic* in noisy and distracting surroundings will also stimulate a mild but measurable increase in pulse rate and blood pressure. Obviously this response does not depend on the afferent limb of the sympathetic reflex arc and must be mediated by cortical–hypothalamic mechanisms.

If the response to the Valsalva maneuver is abnormal and the response to the cold pressor test is normal, the lesion is probably in the baroreceptors or their afferent nerves; such a defect has been found in diabetic and tabetic patients and is common in many neuropathies. A failure of the heart rate and blood pressure to rise during mental arithmetic coupled with an abnormal Valsalva maneuver suggests a defect in the central or peripheral efferent sympathetic pathways.

Tests of Sudomotor Function

The integrity of sympathetic efferent pathways can be assessed further by tests of sudomotor activity. There are several of these, all used mainly in specialized autonomic testing laboratories; furthermore, most of them cannot differentiate central from peripheral causes of anhidrosis. The most rudimentary tests involve weighing sweat after it is absorbed by small squares of filter paper. Also, powdered charcoal dusted on the skin will cling to moist areas and not to dry ones.

In the *sympathetic or galvanic skin-resistance* test, a set of electrodes placed on the skin measures the resistance to the passage of a weak current through the skin; in all likelihood, the change in electrical potential is the result of an ionic current within the sweat glands, not simply an increase in sweating that lowers skin resistance. This method can be used to outline an area of reduced sweating because of a peripheral nerve lesion, as the response depends on sympathetic activation of sweat glands (Gutrecht). However, the galvanic skin response is subject to habituation with repeated stimuli and will show no response if there is a sensory neuropathy. The starch iodine test or use of a color indicator such as quinizarin (gray when dry, purple when wet) and the more recently introduced plastic or silicone method are other acceptable procedures to delineate peripheral nerve or spinal cord lesions based on the loss of sympathetic innervation. Together they are termed "thermoregulatory sweat testing" and are semiquantitave and mainly topographic in nature. They reflect postganglionic sudomotor function.

A more quantitative and reproducible examination of postganglionic sudomotor function, termed QSART (quantitative sudomotor axon reflex test), has been developed and studied extensively by Low. It is essentially a test of distal sympathetic axonal integrity utilizing the local axon reflex. A 10 percent solution of acetylcholine is iontophoresed onto the skin using 2 mA for 5 min. Sweat output is recorded in the adjacent skin by sophisticated circular cells that detect the sweat water. The forearm, proximal leg, distal leg, and foot have been chosen as standardized recording sites. By this test, Low has been able to define patterns of absent or delayed sweating that signify postganglionic sympathetic failure in small-fiber neuropathies and excessive sweating or reduced latency in response, as is seen in reflex sympathetic dystrophy. This is the preferred method of studying sweating and the function of distal sympathetic fibers, but its technical complexity makes it available only in specially equipped laboratories.

Lacrimal Function

Tearing can be estimated roughly by inserting one end of a 5-mm-wide and 25-mm-long strip of thin filter paper into the lower conjunctival sac while the other end hangs over the edge of the lower lid (the Schirmer test). The tears wet the strip of filter paper, producing a moisture front. After 5 min, the moistened area extends for a length of approximately 15 mm in normal persons. An extent of less than 10 mm is suggestive of hypolacrima. This test is used mainly to detect the dry eyes (keratoconjunctivitis sicca) of the Sjögren syndrome, but it may also be helpful in fully studying various autonomic neuropathies.

Tests of Bladder, Gastrointestinal, and Penile Erectile Function

Bladder function is best assessed by the cystometrogram, which measures intravesicular pressure as a function of the volume of saline solution permitted to flow by gravity into the bladder. The rise of pressure as 500 mL of fluid is allowed to flow gradually into the bladder, the emptying contractions of the detrusor, and the volume at which the patient reports a sensation of bladder fullness can be recorded by a manometer. (A detailed account of cystometric techniques can be found in the monograph of Krane and Siroky.) A simple way of determining bladder atony (prostatic obstruction and overdistention having been excluded) is to measure the residual urine (by catheterization of the bladder) immediately after voluntary voiding or to estimate its volume by ultrasound imaging.

Disorders of gastrointestinal motility are readily demonstrated radiologically. In dysautonomic states, a barium swallow may disclose a number of abnormalities, including atonic dilatation of the esophagus, gastric atony and distention, delayed gastric emptying time, and a characteristic small bowel pattern consisting of an increase in frequency and amplitude of peristaltic waves and rapid intestinal transit. A barium enema may demonstrate colonic distention and a decrease in propulsive activity. Sophisticated manometric techniques are now available for the measurement of gastrointestinal motility (see Low et al).

Nocturnal penile tumescence is recorded in some sleep laboratories and may be used as an ancillary test of sacral autonomic (parasympathetic) innervation.

Pharmacologic Tests of Autonomic Function

After examining the pupils in ambient light, bright light, and low light to determine if one has lost sympathetic or parasympathetic innervation, pharmacologic tests can be used to refine diagnosis. Part of the rationale behind these special tests is the "Cannon law," or the phenomenon of denervation hypersensitivity, in which an effector organ, 2 to 3 wk after denervation, becomes hypersensitive to its particular neurotransmitter substance and related drugs. In clinical testing, an agent is instilled into both conjunctival sacs and the nonmiotic pupil is used as a control to compare the one suspect of being involved by Horner syndrome.

Relatively recently, the weak direct sympathetic agonist apraclonidine has been used most widely to demonstrate that miosis is due to sympathetic denervation of the pupil. It reverses miosis that is due to a central or a peripheral lesion and is easier to obtain then older agents. A positive test, reversal of miosis, depends on the denervation hypersensitivity that develops after several days or more of the presence of the Horner syndrome. If there is a negative result, no enlargement of the pupil, the miosis is probably physiologic. The drug has the additional advantage of often reversing the ptosis of Horner syndrome (see Chap. 14 and Fig. 14-10 for discussion). The drug may cause respiratory suppression in children and is avoided.

Once the presence of a genuine Horner syndrome has been established, it is possible to differentiate pre- from postganglionic (superior cervical ganglion) sympathetic denervation of the pupil by instilling 1 percent hydroxyamphetamine; its effect depends on the presence of existing norepinephrine in the end terminals of the nerves that innervate the iris. Failure to dilate indicates a postganglionic lesion.

Another test, now used mostly in children, in whom apraclonidine represents a risk, is the topical application into the conjunctival sac of a 4 to 10 percent cocaine solution that potentiates the effects of NE by preventing its reuptake. A normal response to cocaine consists of pupillary dilatation. In sympathetic denervation caused by lesions of the post- or preganglionic fibers, no change in pupillary size occurs because no transmitter substance is available and the cocaine has no substrate to potentiate. The reason for lack of response in chronic preganglionic lesions is presumed to be a depletion of NE in the postganglionic fibers. In cases of central sympathetic lesions, slight mydriasis may occur.

Cutaneous Flare Response

The intracutaneous injection of 0.05 mL of 1:1,000 histamine normally causes a 1-cm wheal after 5 to 10 min. This is surrounded by a narrow red areola, which in turn, is surrounded by an erythematous flare that extends 1 to 3 cm beyond the border of the wheal. A similar "triple response" follows the release of histamine into the skin as the result of a scratch. It can be elicited in sensitive individuals by scratching the skin (dermatographia).

The wheal and the deeply colored red areola are caused by the direct action of histamine on blood vessels in response to local injury, while the flare depends on the integrity of the axon reflex. This axon reflex is mediated by antidromic stimulation of small sensory C fibers that results in the release by the same fibers of various vasoactive substances such as bradykinin and substance P. Destruction of the dorsal root ganglion, but not the dorsal root, eliminates the flare. The flare component is influenced centrally through a yet unknown mechanism. In familial dysautonomia, the flare response to histamine and to scratch is absent. It may also be absent in peripheral neuropathies that involve sympathetic nerves (e.g., diabetes, alcoholic–nutritional disease, Guillain-Barré disease, amyloidosis, porphyria). The quantitative sudomotor response to topical acetylcholine, described earlier, is preferred for its sensitivity and accuracy but requires special equipment.

The dermatographic wheal and flare response may be lost below the level of a recent cord injury but returns over days or longer, comparable to recovery from spinal shock.

Pressor Infusion and Other Direct Cardiovascular Tests

While these are not parts of the routine laboratory evaluation of autonomic nervous system disease, they nonetheless present interesting physiologic information. The infusion of NE causes a rise in blood pressure, which is usually more pronounced for a given infusion rate in dysautonomic states than it is with normal subjects. In many instances, e.g., the Guillain-Barré syndrome, the excessive rise in blood pressure is thought to be more a result of inadequate muting of the hypertension by baroreceptors than it is a reflection of true denervation hypersensitivity, i.e., it reflects dysfunction of the afferent limb of the reflex arc. In patients with familial dysautonomia, the infusion of NE produces erythematous blotching of the skin, like that which may occur under emotional stress, probably representing an exaggerated response to endogenous NE.

The infusion of angiotensin II into patients with idiopathic orthostatic hypotension also causes an exaggerated blood pressure response. A similar response to methacholine and NE has been interpreted as a denervation hypersensitivity to neurotransmitter or related substances. A different mechanism must be invoked for the blood pressure response induced by angiotensin; perhaps it is caused by a defective baroreceptor function.

The integrity of autonomic innervation of the heart can be evaluated by the intramuscular injection of atropine, ephedrine, or neostigmine while the heart rate is monitored. Normally, the intramuscular injection of 0.8 mg of atropine causes tachycardia as a result of a parasympathetic block and a withdrawal of vagal tone. No such change occurs in cases of parasympathetic (vagal) denervation of the heart, the most common such conditions being diabetes and the Guillain-Barré syndrome and the most dramatic being the brain death state, in which there is no longer any tonic vagal activity to be ablated by atropine.

Laboratory methods are available for the measurement of NE and dopamine β-hydroxylase in the serum. Normally, when a person changes from a recumbent to a standing position, the serum NE level rises two- or threefold. In patients with central and peripheral autonomic failure, there is little or no elevation on standing or with exercise. The dopamine β-hydroxylase enzyme is deficient in patients with a rare form of sympathetic dysautonomia.

In summary, the noninvasive tests listed in Table 26-1 and described earlier are quite adequate for the clinical testing of autonomic function. Low has emphasized that the most informative tests are those that are quantitative and have been standardized and validated in patients with both mild and severe autonomic disturbances. At the bedside, the most convenient ones are measurement of orthostatic heart rate and blood pressure changes, blood pressure response to the Valsalva maneuver, estimation of heart-rate changes with deep breathing, pupillary responses to light and dark, and a rough estimate of sweating of the palms and soles and with lesions of the spinal cord, on the trunk. The results of these tests and the clinical situation will determine whether further testing is needed.

CLINICAL DISORDERS OF THE AUTONOMIC NERVOUS SYSTEM

Acute Autonomic Paralysis (Dysautonomic Polyneuropathy; Pure Pandysautonomia)

Since this condition was first reported by Young and colleagues in 1975, many more cases in both adults and children have been placed on record. Over a period of a week or a few weeks with or without a preceding systemic or respiratory infection, the patient develops some combination of anhidrosis, orthostatic hypotension, paralysis of pupillary reflexes, loss of lacrimation and salivation, erectile dysfunction, impaired bladder and bowel function (urinary retention, postprandial bloating, and ileus or constipation), and loss of certain pilomotor and vasomotor responses in the skin (flushing and heat intolerance). Fatigue, sometimes severe, is a prominent complaint in most patients, and abdominal pain and vomiting in others. A few develop sleep apnea or the syndrome of inappropriate secretion of antidiuretic hormone (SIADH), leading to hyponatremia. The cerebrospinal fluid (CSF) protein is normal or slightly increased.

Clinical and laboratory findings indicate that both the sympathetic and parasympathetic parts of the autonomic nervous system are affected, mainly at the postganglionic level. Somatosensory and motor nerve fibers appear to be spared or are affected to only a slight extent, although many patients complain of paresthesias, and tendon reflexes are frequently lost. In one of the patients described by Low and colleagues, there was physiologic and morphologic (sural biopsy) evidence of loss of small myelinated and unmyelinated somatic fibers and foci of epineurial mononuclear cells; in other cases, sural nerve fiber counts have been normal; and in an autopsied case, in which there had also been sensory loss, there was lymphocytic infiltration in sensory and autonomic nerves (Fagius et al). The original patient described by Young and colleagues and most of the other patients reported with pure dysautonomia are said to have recovered completely or almost so within several months, but many of our patients have been left with disordered gastrointestinal and sexual functions. In addition to an idiopathic form of autonomic paralysis, some cases are postinfectious, and there is a similar but rare paraneoplastic form (see Chap. 31 under "Paraneoplastic Sensory Neuronopathy"). Antibodies against ganglionic acetylcholine receptors have been found in half of idiopathic cases and one-quarter of paraneoplastic ones (Vernino et al).

Some children with this disease and a few adults have had a syndrome of predominantly cholinergic dysautonomia with pain and dysesthesias (Kirby et al); there is little or no postural hypotension and the course has been more chronic than that in cases of complete dysautonomia described earlier.

In view of the identical autonomic disturbances in the Guillain-Barré syndrome and the high incidence of minor degrees of weakness, reflex loss, CSF protein elevation, and especially paresthesias, it is likely that pure pandysautonomia is also an immune-mediated polyneuropathy affecting the autonomic fibers within peripheral nerves, in most ways comparable to the Guillain-Barré syndrome. The aforementioned autopsy findings reported by Fagius and coworkers support such a relationship. In animals, autonomic paralysis has been produced by injection of extracts of sympathetic ganglia and Freund's adjuvant (Appenzeller et al), similar to the experimental immune neuritis that is considered as an animal model of the Guillain-Barré syndrome.

An acquired form of orthostatic intolerance, referred to as *sympathotonic orthostatic hypotension* (Polinsky et al), may represent another variant or partial form of autonomic paralysis. In this syndrome, unlike the common forms of orthostatic hypotension (see later), the fall in blood pressure is accompanied by tachycardia. Hoeldtke and colleagues, who described 4 such patients, found that the vasomotor reflexes and NE production were normal; these investigators were inclined to attribute the disorder to a process affecting lower thoracic and lumbar sympathetic neurons. Its relationship to the entity of *postural orthostatic tachycardia syndrome* (POTS) discussed in Chap. 18 and to the orthostatic intolerance associated with the chronic fatigue syndrome is uncertain. Individual cases of POTS have been associated with mutations or epigenetic alterations in the norepinephrine transporter gene (Shannon and colleagues). Some instances of orthostatic intolerance appear as part of the asthenia–anxiety disorders in which the autonomic changes may represent sympathetic overactivity in susceptible individuals.

There are several reports of improvement of pandysautonomia after intravenous gamma globulin infusion, but these are difficult to judge as many patients improve spontaneously over the same time frame, usually many months. In addition, plasma exchange has been used with apparent benefit in a patient with antibodies against the ganglionic acetylcholine receptor (Schroeder et al).

Lambert-Eaton Myasthenic Syndrome One of the characteristic features of the fully developed Lambert-Eaton myasthenic syndrome, which is discussed in Chap. 53, is *dysautonomia*, characterized by dryness of the mouth, erectile dysfunction, difficulty in starting the urinary stream, and constipation. Presumably, circulating antibodies against the voltage-gated calcium channel interfere with the release of ACh at both muscarinic and nicotinic sites.

Idiopathic Orthostatic Hypotension; Pure Autonomic Failure (See also Chap. 18)

This clinical state is now known to be caused by at least two conditions. One is a degenerative disease of middle and late adult life, first described by Bradbury and Eggleston in 1925 and designated by them as *idiopathic orthostatic hypotension* and by subsequent authors, "primary autonomic failure." In this disorder, the lesions involve mainly the postganglionic sympathetic neurons (Petito and Black); the parasympathetic system is relatively spared and the CNS is uninvolved. In the second more common disorder that is now classified as a *multiple system atrophy*, described initially by Shy and Drager, the preganglionic lateral horn neurons of the thoracic spinal segments degenerate; these changes are responsible for the orthostatic hypotension. Later, signs of basal ganglionic or cerebellar disease or both are added as discussed later and in Chaps. 18 and 39 but a few cases remain as a pure autonomic failure. In both types of orthostatic hypotension, anhidrosis, erectile dysfunction and atonicity of the bladder may be conjoined, but orthostatic fainting is the main problem.

The clinical differentiation of these two types of orthostatic hypotension depends largely on the appearance, with time, of associated CNS signs as described later. The distinction between the sympathetic postganglionic and the central preganglionic types of disease is also based on pharmacologic and neurophysiologic evidence, but it must be emphasized that the results of these tests do not always conform to clinical expectations from the examination. Nonetheless, Cohen and associates, who studied the postganglionic sudomotor and vasomotor functions of 62 patients with IOH, found that the signs of postganglionic denervation were uncommon in patients classified as having the central type.

In the postganglionic type of autonomic failure, plasma levels of NE are subnormal while the patient is recumbent because of failure of the damaged nerve terminals to synthesize or release catecholamines. When the patient stands, the NE levels do not rise, as they do in a normal person. Also, in this type, there is denervation hypersensitivity to infused NE. In the central preganglionic (Shy-Drager) type, the resting NE levels in the plasma are normal but again, on standing, there is no rise, and the response to exogenously administered NE is normal. In both types, the plasma levels of dopamine β-hydroxylase, the enzyme that converts dopamine to NE, are subnormal (Ziegler et al). The use of these neurochemical tests in clinical practice is difficult and the data in the literature are inconsistent. Low's monograph should be consulted for procedural details.

Pathologic studies have disclosed the central type of autonomic failure to be somewhat heterogeneous. Oppenheimer, who collected all the reported central cases with complete autopsies, found that they fell into two groups: (1) that which was designated by Adams as *striatonigral degeneration* or, later, *Shy-Drager syndrome*, where autonomic failure was associated with a parkinsonian syndrome and often with the presence of cytoplasmic inclusions in sympathetic neurons, and (2) another with involvement of the striatum, cerebellum, pons, and medulla but without inclusions, formerly designated *olivopontocerebellar degeneration* (there are now reported to be glial and neuronal cytoplasmic inclusions in all these cases). Both conditions are now referred to as *multiple system atrophy*, the term introduced by Oppenheimer, the first type, MSA-P to denote the parkinsonism and the second type, MSA-C reflecting cerebellar degeneration as discussed in Chap. 39. If the process remains purely an autonomic failure, MSA-A is used.

In all forms of multiple system atrophy, the autonomic failure is attributable to degeneration of lateral horn cells of the thoracic cord. There is also a degeneration of nerve cells in the vagal nuclei as well as nuclei of the tractus solitarius, locus ceruleus, and sacral autonomic nuclei, accounting for laryngeal abductor weakness (laryngeal paralysis and stridor are features in some cases), incontinence, and erectile dysfunction. NE and dopamine are depleted in the hypothalamus (Spokes et al). The sympathetic ganglia have usually been normal. In Parkinson disease, where fainting is sometimes a problem, Lewy bodies are found in degenerating sympathetic ganglion cells but the medications used for treatment also exaggerate hypotension.

Treatment of orthostatic hypotension consists of having the patient sleep with the head of the bed elevated, administering the peripherally acting alpha agonist, midodrine starting at 2.5 mg q4h, slowly raising the dose to 5 mg q4h, taking the last dose before about 7 P.M. to void supine hypertension while asleep, and if that is not successful, the mineralocorticoid fludrocortisone acetate (Florinef) 0.1 mg twice daily. The latter should be used cautiously in patients with severe supine hypertension; its effect may take up to 2 wk to be manifest so rapid elevation of the dose is not advised. Fainting can sometimes be avoided by the countermaneuvers of having the patient tightly cross his legs upon standing and using elastic stockings that compress the veins of the legs and lower abdomen.

Peripheral Neuropathy With Secondary Orthostatic Hypotension

Impairment of autonomic function, of which orthostatic hypotension is the most serious feature, occurs as part of many acute and chronic peripheral neuropathies (e.g., diabetic, alcoholic–nutritional, amyloid, Guillain-Barré, heavy metal, toxic, and porphyric). Disease of the peripheral nervous system may affect the circulation in two ways: the nerves from baroreceptors may be affected, interrupting normal afferent homeostatic reflexes, or postganglionic efferent sympathetic fibers may be involved in their course in the spinal nerves. The severity of the autonomic failure need not parallel the degree of motor weakness. An additional feature of the acute dysautonomias is a tendency to develop hyponatremia, presumably as a result of dysfunction of afferent fibers from venous, right atrial, and aortic arch volume receptors; this elicits a release of antidiuretic hormone arginine vasopressin (AVP). These same stretch baroreceptors are implicated in the intermittent hypertension that sometimes complicates these acute neuropathies.

Of particular importance is the autonomic disorder that accompanies diabetic neuropathy. It presents as erectile dysfunction, constipation, or diarrhea (especially at night), hypotonia of the bladder, gastroparesis, and orthostatic hypotension, in some combination. Invariably, there are signs of a sensory polyneuropathy, consisting of a distal loss of vibratory and thermal-pain sensation and reduced or lost ankle reflexes; but again, the severity of affection of the two systems of nerve fibers may not be parallel. The pupils are often small and the amplitude of constriction to light is reduced (similar to Argyll Robertson pupils); this has been attributed to damage of cells in the ciliary ganglia. A curious syndrome or "insulin neuritis" has been described, in which, autonomic failure and painful sensory neuropathy arise at the time of rapid glycemic control (see Gibbons and Freeman).

Gastroparesis can be disabling, painful, and difficult to treat, for example in diabetic autonomic neuropathy. Camilleri has reviewed the subject and outlined the defect in gastric emptying that interrelates with glucose metabolism and an unexplained association with psychiatric symptoms. Management is by altering nutritional intake and with metoclopramide for mild cases and additional domperidone, prochlorperazine, and erythromycin in severe ones.

Another polyneuropathy with unusually prominent dysautonomia is that caused by amyloidosis. Extensive loss of pain and thermal sensation is usually present; other forms of sensation may also be reduced to a lesser degree. Motor function is much less altered. Sympathetic function is more affected than parasympathetic. Iridoplegia (pupillary paralysis) and disturbances of other smooth muscle and glandular functions are variable. Diabetic and amyloid polyneuropathy are further described in Chap. 46.

Both the primary and secondary types of orthostatic hypotension are also discussed in connection with syncope in Chap. 18.

Familial Autonomic Neuropathy in Infants and Children (Riley-Day Syndrome) and Other Inherited Dysautonomias (See also Chap. 46)

Riley-Day syndrome is a disease of children, inherited as an autosomal recessive trait. The main symptoms are postural hypotension and lability of blood pressure, faulty regulation of temperature, diminished hearing, hyperhidrosis, blotchiness of the skin, insensitivity to pain, emotional lability, and cyclic vomiting. The tendon reflexes are hypoactive, and mild slowing of motor nerve conduction velocities is common. There is denervation sensitivity of the pupils and other structures. The main pathologic feature is a deficiency of neurons in the superior cervical ganglia and in the lateral horns of the spinal cord. Also, according to Aguayo and to Dyck and their colleagues, the number of unmyelinated nerve fibers in the sural nerve is greatly decreased. It is likely that this disease represents a failure of embryologic migration or formation of the first- and second-order sympathetic neurons. It is now known that this defect is the result of a mutation in the gene (*IKBKAP*) that codes for a protein (IKAP) that is currently considered to be associated with transcription regulation (Anderson et al). This results in a decrease in the amount of functional protein in autonomic neurons.

Autonomic symptoms are also a prominent feature of the small-fiber neuropathy of Fabry disease (alpha-galactosidase deficiency) as a result of the accumulation of ceramide in hypothalamic and intermediolateral column neurons (see "Fabry Disease" in Chap. 46).

Another inherited form of peripheral dysautonomia is characterized by severe pain in the feet on exercise and an autosomal dominant pattern of inheritance (Robinson et al). Bending, crouching, and kneeling increase stabbing pains in the feet. There is no sweat response to intradermal injection of 1 percent ACh and no autonomic fibers were found in punch biopsies of the skin. Systemic amyloidosis is the other type of peripheral neuropathy that has prominent features of autonomic failure.

Autonomic Failure in the Elderly

(See also Chap. 29)

Orthostatic hypotension is prevalent in the elderly, so much so that norms of blood pressure and heart rate changes have been difficult to establish. Caird and coworkers reported that among individuals who were older than 65 years of age and living at home, 24 percent had a fall of systolic blood pressure on standing of 20 mm Hg; 9 percent had a fall of 30 mm Hg; and 5 percent had a fall of 40 mm Hg. An increased frequency of thermoregulatory impairment also has been documented. The elderly are also more liable to develop hypothermia and, when exposed to high ambient temperature, to hyperthermia. Loss of sweating of the lower parts of the body and increased sweating of the head and arms probably reflect a neuropathy or neuronopathy. The number of sensory ganglion cells decreases with age (Castro). Erectile dysfunction and incontinence also increase with age, but these, of course, may be the result of a number of processes besides autonomic failure and many of the medications used to treat ailments that come with aging, such as hypertension, prostatic hypertrophy, depression, and impotence, have autonomic effects and can cause orthostatic hypotension.

It is of interest that an idiopathic type of small fiber neuropathy that occurs predominantly in elderly women ("burning hands and feet" syndrome) has no associated autonomic features (see Chap. 46).

Horner (Oculosympathetic) and Stellate Ganglion Syndromes (See also Chap. 14)

Interruption of postganglionic sympathetic fibers at any point along the internal carotid arteries or a lesion of the superior cervical ganglion results in miosis, drooping of the eyelid, and abolition of sweating over one side of the face; this constellation is the Horner, or more properly, Bernard-Horner syndrome (see also "Horner Syndrome" in Chap. 14). The same syndrome in less-obvious form may be caused by interruption of the preganglionic fibers at any point between their origin in the intermediolateral cell column of the C8-T2 spinal segments and the superior cervical ganglion or by interruption of the descending, uncrossed hypothalamospinal pathway in the tegmentum of the brainstem or cervical cord. The common causes are neoplastic or inflammatory involvement of the cervical lymph nodes or proximal part of the brachial plexus, surgical and other types of trauma to cervical structures (e.g., jugular venous catheters), carotid artery dissection, syringomyelic or traumatic lesions of the first and second thoracic spinal segments, and infarcts or other lesions of the lateral part of the medulla (Wallenberg syndrome). There is also an idiopathic variety that is in some cases hereditary. If a Horner syndrome develops early in life, the iris on the affected side fails to become pigmented and remains blue or mottled gray-brown (heterochromia iridis; see Fig 14-10).

A lesion of the stellate ganglion, e.g., compression by a tumor arising from the superior sulcus of the lung (Pancoast tumor), produces the interesting combination of a Horner syndrome and paralysis of sympathetic reflexes in the limb (the hand and arm are dry and warm). With preganglionic lesions, facial flushing may develop on the side of the sympathetic disorder; this is brought on in some instances by exercise (harlequin effect). The combination of segmental anhidrosis and an Adie pupil is sometimes referred to as the *Ross syndrome*; it may be abrupt in onset and idiopathic, or it may follow a viral infection.

Keane has provided data as to the relative frequency of the lesions causing oculosympathetic (Horner) paralysis. In 100 successive cases, 63 were of central type caused by brainstem strokes, 21 were preganglionic from trauma or tumors of the neck, 13 were postganglionic from miscellaneous causes, and in 3 cases the localization could not be determined (see Chap. 14 for further discussion).

The pupillary disturbances associated with oculomotor nerve lesions, the Adie pupil, and other parasympathetic and pharmacologic testing for sympathetic abnormalities of pupillary function are considered fully in Chap. 14 and in Table 14-6 with the accompanying text. Apraclonidine, 0.5 percent, has become the favored drug for diagnostic testing as noted earlier.

Sympathetic and Parasympathetic Paralysis in Tetraplegia and Paraplegia

Lesions of the C4 or C5 segments of the spinal cord, if complete, will interrupt suprasegmental control of both the sympathetic and sacral parasympathetic nervous systems. Much the same effect is observed with lesions of the upper thoracic cord (above T6). Lower thoracic lesions leave much of the descending sympathetic outflow intact, only the descending sacral parasympathetic control being interrupted. Traumatic necrosis of the spinal cord is the usual cause of these states, but they also may be a result of infarction, certain forms of myelitis, radiations damage, and tumors.

As discussed in greater detail in Chap. 44, the initial effect of an acute cervical cord transection is abolition of all sensorimotor reflex, and autonomic functions of the isolated spinal cord. The autonomic changes include hypotension, loss of sweating and piloerection, paralytic ileus and gastric atony, and paralysis of the bladder. The flare component of the axon reflex may be lost. Plasma epinephrine and NE are reduced. This state, known as *spinal shock*, usually lasts for several weeks as described in Chap. 44. The basic mechanisms are not known, but changes in neurotransmitters (catecholamines, enkephalins, endorphins, substance P, and 5-hydroxytryptamine) and their inhibitory activities are considered to play a role. Naloxone mitigates some of the aspects of spinal shock; this may be, at least in part, the result of release of preformed endogenous opioids from the distal axons that are separated from their cells of origin in the periaqueductal gray region. Once these endogenous substances are exhausted, the phenomenon of spinal shock ends (see Chap. 44).

After spinal shock dissipates, reflex sympathetic and parasympathetic functions return because the afferent and efferent autonomic connections within the isolated segments of the spinal cord are intact, although no longer under the control of higher centers. With *cervical cord lesions*, there is a loss of the sympathetically mediated cardiovascular changes in response to stimuli reaching the medulla. However, cutaneous stimuli (pinprick or cold) in segments of the body below the transection will raise the blood pressure. However, a fall in blood pressure is not compensated by sympathetic vasoconstriction. Hence tetraplegics are almost obligatorily prone to orthostatic hypotension. Pinching the skin below the lesion causes gooseflesh in adjacent segments. Heating the body results in flushing and sweating over the face and neck, but not in the trunk and legs, because of the loss of connections from the hypothalamus. Bladder and bowel, including their sphincters, which are at first flaccid, become automatic as spinal reflex control returns. There may be reflex penile erection or priapism and even rarely ejaculation. With lesions in the upper thoracic cord, similar but lesser degrees of labile blood pressure are seen; in several of our patients with destructive myelitis, a viral infection of fever brought out episodes of a drop in blood pressure to approximately 80/60 mm Hg and a subsequent rapid rise to 190/110 mm Hg.

After a time, the tetraplegic patient may develop a *mass reflex* in which flexor spasms of the legs and involuntary emptying of the bladder are associated with a marked rise in blood pressure, bradycardia, and sweating and pilomotor reactions in parts below the cervical segments (*autonomic dysreflexia*). These reactions may also be evoked by pinprick, passive movement, contactual stimuli of the limbs and abdomen, and pressure on the bladder. An exaggerated vasopressor reaction also occurs in response to injected NE. In such attacks, the patient experiences paresthesias of the neck, shoulders, and arms; tightness in the chest and dyspnea; pupillary dilatation; pallor followed by flushing of the face; sensation of fullness in the head and ears; and a throbbing headache. Plasma NE and dopamine rise slowly during the autonomic discharge. When such an attack is severe and prolonged, electrocardiographic changes may appear, sometimes with evidence of myocardial injury that has been attributed to direct catecholamine toxicity or, alternatively, to myocardial ischemia caused by increased afterload or to coronary vasospasm. Seizures and visual defects have also been observed, related to cerebral dysautoregulation. Clonidine, up to 0.2 mg tid, has been useful in preventing the hypertensive crises.

Acute Autonomic Crises ("Sympathetic Storm")

Several toxic and pharmacologic agents such as cocaine and phenylpropanolamine are capable of producing abrupt overactivity of the sympathetic and parasympathetic nervous systems—severe hypertension and mydriasis coupled with signs of CNS excitation—sometimes including seizures. Tricyclic antidepressants in excessive doses are also known to produce autonomic effects, but in this case cholinergic blockade leads to dryness of the mouth, flushing, absent sweating, and mydriasis. The main concern with tricyclic antidepressant overdose is the development of a ventricular arrhythmia, also on an autonomic basis, presaged by prolongation of the QT interval on the ECG. Poisoning with organophosphate insecticides (e.g., Parathion), which have anticholinesterase effects, causes a combination of *parasympathetic overactivity* and motor paralysis (see discussion of poisonings in Chap. 43). A severe autonomic disturbance involving both postganglionic sympathetic and parasympathetic function is produced by ingestion of the rodenticide *N*-3-pyridylmethyl-*N'*-*p*-nitrophenylurea (PNU, Vacor). The exaggerated sympathetic state that accompanies tetanus—manifest by diaphoresis, mydriasis, and labile or sustained hypertension—has been attributed to circulating catecholamines.

Among the most dramatic syndromes of unopposed sympathetic-adrenal medullary hyperactivity occur in cases of severe head injury and with hypertensive cerebral hemorrhage. Three separate mechanisms of the hypersympathetic state are observed at different times after the injury or cerebral hemorrhage: an outpouring of adrenal catecholamines at the time of the ictus with acute hypertension and tachycardia; a brainstem-mediated vasopressor reaction (Cushing response, described later); and a later chronic phenomenon, consisting of episodes of extreme hypertension, profuse diaphoresis, and pupillary dilatation, usually arising during episodes of several minutes' duration of rigid extensor posturing (the "diencephalic autonomic seizures" of Penfield, described later and in Chap. 35 in relation to head injury). Most patients who exhibit such paroxysms are decorticate from traumatic lesions of the deep cerebral white matter or from acute hydrocephalus (the likely explanation of Penfield's cases); in any case, they are clearly not epileptic. These attacks may be the result of the removal of inhibitory influences on the hypothalamus, creating, in effect, a hypersensitive decorticated autonomic nervous system.

Regarding the acute sympathetic reaction, experimental evidence suggests that nuclei in the caudal medullary reticular formation (reticularis gigantocellularis and parvocellularis) can precipitate severe hypertensive reactions. These nuclear centers are tonically inhibited by the NTS, which receives afferent input from arterial baroreceptors and chemoreceptors. Bilateral lesions of the NTS therefore produce extreme elevations in blood pressure, and this abrupt rise plays a role in the genesis of "neurogenic" pulmonary edema. These sympathetically mediated effects are eliminated by sectioning of the cervical spinal cord and by alpha-adrenergic blockade.

The *Cushing response*, reflex, triad, or "reaction," as Cushing described it, occurs as a result of an abrupt increase in intracranial pressure. It consists of hypertension, bradycardia, and slow, irregular breathing elicited by the stimulation of mechanically sensitive regions in the paramedian caudal medulla (Hoff and Reis). Similar pressure-sensitive areas in the upper cervical spinal cord are also implicated in the Cushing response when intraspinal pressure is raised abruptly; a ventral medullary vasodepressor area that acts in the opposite manner has been found in animals. The proximate cause of the Cushing response is probably from mechanical distortion of the lower brainstem, either from a mass in the posterior fossa or, more often, from a large mass in one of the hemispheres or a subarachnoid hemorrhage that elevates the pressure within the fourth ventricle. Often, only the hypertensive component of the reaction occurs, with the systolic blood pressure reaching levels of 200 mm Hg, spuriously suggesting the presence of a pheochromocytoma or renal artery stenosis. The most severe instances of this type of centrally provoked hypertensive syndrome have occurred in children with cerebellar tumors who presented with headache and extreme systolic hypertension. Difficulty may arise in differentiating this response from hypertensive encephalopathy, especially from cases that derive from renovascular hypertension, which may likewise be accompanied by headache and papilledema. In differentiating these two, it is useful to note that primary hypertensive encephalopathy is associated with a tachycardia or normal heart rate and that systolic blood pressure levels above 210 mm Hg are attained only rarely in the Cushing response.

During episodes of intense sympathetic discharge of any type, there are *alterations in the ECG*, mainly in the ST segments and T waves; in extreme cases, evidence of myocardial damage can be observed. Both direct sympathetic innervation of the heart and the surge in circulating NE and cortisol are the cause of these findings. A similar hyperadrenergic mechanism has been proposed to explain sudden death from fright, asthma, status epilepticus, and cocaine overdose. Investigations by Schobel and colleagues had suggested that sustained sympathetic overactivity is responsible for the hypertension of *preeclampsia*, which may be considered in some ways as a dysautonomic state but this may be an oversimplification. Further information on these topics is contained in Chap. 35 and in the reviews by Samuels and Ropper.

A role has also been inferred for the ventrolateral medullary pressor centers in the maintenance of *essential hypertension*. Geiger and colleagues removed a looped branch of the posteroinferior cerebellar artery that had been apposed to the ventral surface of the medulla in 8 patients who had intractable essential hypertension; they found that 7 improved. Vascular decompression of cranial nerves has proved to be a credible therapeutic measure for hemifacial spasm and some cases of vertigo and trigeminal neuralgia, as discussed in Chap. 4, but the notion of vascular compression of the ventral medulla as a mechanism for typical essential hypertension requires confirmation before being accepted.

The Effects of Thoracolumbar Sympathectomy

Surgical resection of the thoracolumbar sympathetic trunk, widely used in the 1940s in the treatment of hypertension but now of historical interest, provided the clinician with the clearest examples of extensive injury to the peripheral sympathetic nervous system, though a similar defect had long been suspected in one type of primary orthostatic hypotension (see earlier). In general, bilateral thoracolumbar sympathectomy results in surprisingly few disturbances. Aside from loss of sweating over the denervated areas of the body, the most pronounced abnormality is an impairment of vasomotor reflexes. In the upright posture, faintness and syncope are frequent because of pooling of blood in the splanchnic bed and lower extremities. Although the blood pressure may fall steadily to shock levels, there is little or no pallor, nausea, vomiting, or sweating—the usual accompaniments of syncope. Bladder, bowel, and sexual function are preserved, though semen is sometimes ejaculated into the posterior urethra and bladder (retrograde ejaculation).

Raynaud Syndrome

This disorder, characterized by episodic, painful blanching of the fingers and presumably caused by digital artery spasm, was first described by Raynaud in 1862. The appearance is of a triphasic sequence of color change of pallor, cyanosis, and subsequent rubor of the affected fingers or toes, but about one-third of such patients have no cyanosis. The episodes are brought on by cold or emotional stress and are usually followed by redness on rewarming. Numbness, paresthesia, and burning often accompany the color changes. It is a disease of early onset, the mean age in idiopathic cases being 14 years; it occurs in a number of clinical settings.

Although most cases are idiopathic, in about half there is an associated connective tissue disease, scleroderma being the main one (Porter et al). In these patients, mostly women with the onset of digital symptoms after age 30 years, the Raynaud phenomenon may antedate the emergence of scleroderma or another rheumatologic autoimmune disorder by many years; such disease usually develops within 2 years. In a small group, predominantly men, the syndrome is induced by local trauma, such as prolonged sculling on a cold day, and particularly by vibratory injury incurred by the sustained use of a pneumatic drill or hammer (a syndrome well known in quarry workers). Obstructive arterial disease—as might occur with the thoracic outlet syndrome, vasospasm because of drugs (ergot, cytotoxic agents, cocaine), previous cold injury (frostbite), and circulating cryoglobulins—is a less-common cause. Still, in 64 of 219 patients studied by Porter and coworkers, the Raynaud syndrome was classified as idiopathic, and most of our cases have been of this type. Formerly, the idiopathic form was called *Raynaud disease*; the type with associated disease is known as *Raynaud phenomenon*. The presence of distorted and proliferative capillaries in the nail bed, visible with an ophthalmoscope, has been used as a bedside aid to reveal cases of connective tissue disease.

Other processes seen by neurologists, foremost among them carpal tunnel syndrome, also cause cold sensitivity in the fingers. Attacks of digital pain and color change from vasculitis, atherosclerotic vascular occlusion, and other causes of occlusive vascular disease only superficially resemble the Raynaud phenomenon; a search for cryoprecipitable proteins (cryoglobulins) is another cause and a search for these proteins in the blood is appropriate.

Irrespective of the associated disease, one of two mechanisms seems to be operative in the pathogenesis—either an arterial constriction or a decrease in the intraluminal pressure. The former, in purest form, is observed in young women on exposure to cold and aggravated by emotional stress; a decrease in intraluminal pressure is associated with arterial obstruction. Treatment is directed to the associated conditions and prevention of precipitating factors. Cervicothoracic sympathectomy has not proved to be an effective measure.

Treatment Avoidance of cold exposure is an obvious strategy, as almost all affected patients have discovered by the time they see the physician. Drugs that cause vasoconstriction are interdicted (ergots, sympathomimetics, clonidine, and serotonin receptor agonists). Calcium channel blockers are most effective, nifedipine being the most widely used, in doses of 30 to 60 mg per day. Other treatments are summarized in the review by Wigley.

Erythromelalgia, first described by S. Weir Mitchell, is a condition in which the feet and lower extremities become red and painful on exposure to warm temperatures for prolonged periods (see the section on this disease in Chap. 11, where the clinical and genetic aspects of this illness are described).

Disorders of Sweating

Hyperhidrosis results from overactivity of sudomotor nerve fibers under a variety of conditions. It may occur as an initial excitatory phase of certain peripheral neuropathies (e.g., because of arsenic or thallium) and be followed by anhidrosis; it is one aspect of the reflex sympathetic dystrophy pain syndromes (see Chap. 5). This is also observed as a localized effect in painful mononeuropathies (causalgia) and diffusely in a number of painful polyneuropathies ("burning foot" syndrome). A type of nonthermoregulatory hyperhidrosis may occur in spinal paraplegics, as mentioned earlier. Loss of sweating in one part of the body may require a compensatory increase in normal parts—for example, the excessive facial and upper truncal sweating that occurs in patients with transection of the high thoracic cord.

Localized hyperhidrosis may be a troublesome complaint in some patients. One variety, presumably of congenital origin, affects the palms. The social embarrassment of a "succulent hand" or a "dripping paw" is often intolerable. It is taken to be a sign of nervousness, although many persons with this condition disclaim all other anxiety symptoms. Cold, clammy hands are common in individuals with anxiety; indeed, this has been a useful sign in distinguishing an anxiety state from hyperthyroidism, in which the hands are also moist but warm. Extirpation of T2 and T3 sympathetic ganglia relieves the more severe cases of palmar sweating; a Horner syndrome does not develop if the T1 ganglion is left intact. In other cases, the hyperhidrosis affects mainly the feet or the axillae. Treatment with local injections of botulinum toxin has been useful and is now favored over ablative procedures.

Anhidrosis in restricted skin areas is a frequent and useful finding in peripheral nerve disease. It is caused by the interruption of the postganglionic sympathetic fibers, and its boundaries can be mapped by means of the sweat tests described earlier in the chapter. The loss of sweating corresponds to the area of sensory loss. In contrast, sweating is not affected in restricted spinal root disease because there is much intersegmental mixing of the preganglionic axons once they enter the sympathetic chain and there are no preganglionic autonomic fibers in the roots below L2.

A postinfectious anhidrosis syndrome has been described, sometimes accompanied by mild orthostatic hypotension. This process is probably a limited form of the "pure pandysautonomia" described earlier. Corticosteroids are said to be beneficial but the process is so infrequent that there are no dependable data.

Other rare but interesting disorders of sweating are *Ross syndrome*, of Adie pupil (see Chap. 14), areflexia and segmental anhidrosis with compensatory hyperhydrosis in other regions of the body, and idiopathic *pure sudomotor failure*, characterized by urticaria, generalized anhidrosis and elevated IgE; in this syndrome there is no sweating to thermoregulatory needs but preserved sweating with emotional stimuli.

Disturbances of Bladder Function

With regard to the neurologic diseases that cause bladder dysfunction, multiple sclerosis, usually with urinary urgency, is by far the most common. In Fowler's clinic, other spinal cord disorders accounted for 12 percent of cases, degenerative diseases (Parkinson disease and multiple system atrophy) for 14 percent, and frontal lobe lesions for 9 percent. These data and the physiologic principles elaborated earlier enable one to understand the effects of the following lesions on bladder function:

Complete Destruction of the Cord Below T12 This occurs with lesions of the conus, as from trauma, myelodysplasias, tumor, venous angioma, and necrotizing myelitis. The bladder is paralyzed for voluntary and reflex activity and there is no awareness of the state of fullness; voluntary initiation of micturition is impossible; the tonus of the detrusor muscle is abolished and the bladder distends as urine accumulates until there is overflow incontinence; voiding is possible only by the Credé maneuver, i.e., lower abdominal compression and abdominal straining. Usually the anal sphincter and colon are similarly affected, and there is "saddle" anesthesia and abolition of the bulbocavernosus and anal reflexes as well as the tendon reflexes in the legs. The cystometrogram shows low pressure and no emptying contractions.

Disease of the Sacral Motor Neurons in the Spinal Gray Matter, the Anterior Sacral Roots, or Peripheral Nerves Innervating the Bladder The typical causes of this configuration are lumbosacral meningomyelocele and the tethered cord syndrome, in effect, a lower motor neuron paralysis of the bladder. The disturbance of bladder function is the same as above, except that sacral and bladder sensation are intact. Other causes of cauda equina disease are compression by epidural tumor or disc, neoplastic meningitis, and radiculitis from herpes or cytomegalovirus (Elsberg syndrome). It is noteworthy that a hysterical patient can suppress motor function and suffer a similar distention of the bladder (see later).

Interruption of Sensory Afferent Fibers From the Bladder Diabetes and tabes dorsalis are typical causes, leaving the motor nerve fibers unaffected. This is a primary sensory bladder paralysis. The disturbance in function is the same as in the two processes earlier. Although a flaccid (atonic) paralysis of the bladder may be purely motor or sensory, as described earlier, in most clinical situations there is *interruption of both afferent and efferent innervation*, as in cauda equina compression or severe polyneuropathy. Neuropathies affecting mainly the small fibers are the ones usually implicated (diabetes, amyloid, etc.), but urinary retention also occurs in certain acute neuropathies such as Guillain-Barré syndrome.

Upper Spinal Cord Lesions, Above T12 Such lesions result in a *reflex neurogenic (spastic) bladder*. In addition to multiple sclerosis and traumatic and compressive myelopathies, which are the most common causes, myelitis, neuromyelitis optica, spondylosis, dural arteriovenous fistula, syringomyelia, and tropical spastic paraparesis may cause a bladder disturbance of this type. If the cord lesion is of sudden onset, the detrusor muscle suffers the effects of spinal shock. At this stage, urine accumulates and distends the bladder to the point of overflow. This overflow incontinence is the result of vesicular pressure exceeding the opening pressure of the sphincter in an areflexic bladder. As the effects of spinal shock subside, the detrusor usually becomes reflexively overactive, and because the patient is unable to inhibit the detrusor and control the external sphincter, urgency, precipitant micturition, and incontinence result. Incomplete lesions result in varying degrees of urgency in voiding. With slowly evolving processes involving the upper cord, such as multiple sclerosis, the bladder spasticity and urgency worsen with time and incontinence becomes more frequent. In addition, initiation of voluntary micturition is impaired and bladder capacity is reduced. Bladder sensation depends on the extent of involvement of sensory tracts. Bulbocavernosus and anal reflexes are preserved. The cystometrogram shows uninhibited contractions of the detrusor muscle in response to small volumes of fluid. Most puzzling to the authors have been cases of cervical cord injury in which reflex activity of the sacral mechanism does not return; the bladder remains hypotonic.

Stretch Injury of the Bladder Wall This occurs with anatomic obstruction at the bladder neck and occasionally with psyhcogenic retention of urine. Repeated overdistention of the bladder wall often results in varying degrees of decompensation of the detrusor muscle and permanent atonia or hypotonia, although the evidence for this mechanism is uncertain. The bladder wall becomes fibrotic and bladder capacity is greatly increased. Emptying contractions are inadequate, and there is a large residual volume even after the Credé maneuver (manual abdominal compression) and strong contraction of the abdominal muscles. As with motor and sensory paralyses, the patient is subject to cystitis, ureteral reflux, hydronephrosis and pyelonephritis, and calculus formation.

Nonpsychogenic Urinary Retention in Women Fowler has described a disorder of bladder function in women, in which there is impaired relaxation of the periurethral striated muscle, as recorded by EMG. The complex repetitive discharges that are characteristic of the disorder are similar to, but distinctive from those seen in myotonia and cannot be voluntarily simulated. Fowler has theorized that the disorder is an efferent denervation of the detrusor muscle, which is coincident with the clinical observation that bladder distention in these patients is usually painless. This disorder has been seen in association with polycystic ovarian syndrome. Most young women with painless dilation of the bladder are diagnosed as having a psychogenic cause. The existence of a *bona fide* organic disorder may reduce stigma and facilitate treatment in some such patients. Some patients have been successfully treated with a sacral nerve stimulator.

Frontal Lobe Incontinence There is a supranuclear type of hyperactivity of the detrusor that results in precipitant voiding. If the lesions are extensive enough in the frontal lobes, the patient, because of an abulic or confused mental state, may additionally be unconcerned by the subsequent incontinence. The bladder itself and the associated sphincter functions are normal as would be seen in a precontinent child. These types of frontal lobe incontinence are considered in the description of abnormalities consequent to frontal lobe damage in Chap. 22.

Brainstem Lesions Influencing Bladder Function As discussed earlier, a role for pontine centers in human micturition has been inferred from animal experiments. The existence of a well-delineated pontine nucleus for micturition is controversial (Barrington nucleus). MRI studies by Sakakibara and colleagues have documented isolated pontine lesions as a cause of several different types of micturition difficulties.

Therapy of Disordered Micturition

Several drugs have been used in the management of flaccid and spastic disturbances of bladder function. In the case of a flaccid paralysis, bethanechol (Urecholine) produces contraction of the detrusor by direct stimulation of its muscarinic cholinergic receptors. In spastic paralysis, the detrusor can be relaxed by propantheline (Pro-Banthine, 15 to 30 mg tid), which acts as a muscarinic antagonist, and by oxybutynin (Ditropan, 5 mg bid or tid), which acts directly on the smooth muscle and also has a muscarinic antagonist action. Atropine, which is mainly a muscarinic antagonist, only partially inhibits detrusor contraction.

More recently, alpha$_1$-sympathomimetic–blocking drugs such as terazosin, doxazosin, and tamsulosin have been used to relax the urinary sphincter and facilitate voiding. Their widest use has been in men with prostatic hypertrophy, but they may be beneficial in patients with dyssynergia of the sphincter (failure of the sphincter to open when the detrusor contracts) from neurologic disease. Several other drugs may be useful in the treatment of neurogenic bladder but can be used rationally only on the basis of sophisticated urodynamic investigations (Krane and Siroky).

Often the patient must resort to intermittent self-catheterization, which can be safely carried out with scrupulous attention to sterile technique (washing hands, disposable catheter, etc.). Some forms of chronic antibiotic therapy and acidification of urine with vitamin C (1,000 g/d) are practical aids, but their use has gone through cycles of popularity based on various studies with differing results. In selected paraplegic patients, the implantation of a sacral anterior root stimulator may prove to be helpful in emptying the bladder and achieving continence (Brindley et al).

Disturbances of Bowel Function

Ileus from spinal shock, reflex neurogenic colon, and sensory and motor paralysis are all recognized clinical entities. The colon, stomach, and small intestine may be hypotonic and distended and the anal sphincters lax, either from deafferentation, deefferentation, or both. The anal and, in the male, the bulbocavernosus reflex may be abolished. Defecation may be urgent and precipitant with higher spinal and cerebral lesions. Because the same spinal segments and nearly the same spinal tracts subserve bladder and bowel function, meningomyeloceles and other cauda equina and spinal cord diseases often cause so-called double incontinence. Fecal incontinence is less frequent than urinary incontinence, however, because the bowel is less-often filled and its content is usually solid.

Bowel dysmotility, mainly by way of ileus may be a prominent feature of immune neuropathies such as Guillain-Barré syndrome (see Chap. 46), pure pandysautonomia, and severe diabetic autonomic neuropathy discussed earlier. In a few cases of the latter, antibodies against the alpha subunit of the ganglionic acetylcholine receptor has been found by Vernino and colleagues. Systemic diseases may affect the colonic sphincters; examples are myotonic dystrophy and scleroderma, which may weaken the internal sphincter, and polymyositis and myasthenia gravis, which may impair the function of the external sphincter and allow bowel gas to escape (Schuster). The inability to control flatulence may be an early sign of skeletal muscle sphincteric weakness in myasthenia. Also, sphincteric damage may complicate hemorrhoidectomy.

In recent years there has been considerable interest in weakness of the muscles of the pelvic floor as a cause of double incontinence, especially in the female. Also, it has been suggested that paradoxical contraction of the puborectus and external anal sphincter may be a cause of severe constipation (anismus). Extreme degrees of descent of the pelvic floor are believed to injure the pudendal nerves, as reflected in prolonged terminal latencies in nerve conduction studies.

Many cases of ileus, even to the extent of megacolon, have a pharmacologic basis, being a result of the use of drugs that paralyze the parasympathetic system or narcotics that have a direct effect on the motility of gastrointestinal smooth muscle.

The serotonin receptor agonist cisapride had been used in partially restoring gastrointestinal motility in some cases of neurogenic ileus as, for example, the early stages of the Guillain-Barré syndrome and in pediatric bowel diseases. Because of ventricular arrhythmias and a few cases of sudden cardiac death, its administration is currently allowed only by experienced pediatric gastroenterologists.

Congenital Megacolon (Hirschsprung Disease)

This is a rare disease affecting mainly male infants and children. It is caused by a congenital absence of ganglion cells in the myenteric plexus. The internal anal sphincter and rectosigmoid are involved most often and are the parts affected in restricted forms of Hirschsprung disease (75 percent of cases), but the aganglionosis is sometimes more extensive. The aganglionic segment of the bowel is constricted and cannot relax, thus preventing propagation of peristaltic waves, which, in turn, produces retention of feces and massive distention of the colon above the aganglionic segment. Enterocolitis is the most serious complication and is associated with a high mortality. Some cases of megaloureter are attributed to a similar defect.

Hirschsprung disease in most cases has been traced to a mutation of the RET oncogene and perhaps to polymorphisms in other genes; the variability in clinical severity corresponds to polymorphisms in the responsible gene. Other genes, such as the one that codes for the endothelin receptor, are implicated in a small group with the disease. There are several other familial diseases that may manifest as an enteric neuropathy including an unusual mitochondrial disorder discussed in Chap. 37, Allgrove syndrome, and an entity termed familial visceral myopathy.

Disturbances of Sexual Function

Sexual function in the male, which is not infrequently affected in neurologic disease, may be divided into several parts: (1) sexual impulse, drive, or desire, referred to as *libido*, discussed in Chap. 25; (2) penile erection, enabling the act of sexual intercourse (potency); and (3) ejaculation of semen by the prostate through the urethra.

The arousal of libido in men and women may result from a variety of stimuli, some purely psychic. Neocortical influences referable to sex involve the limbic system and are transmitted to the hypothalamus and spinal centers. The suprasegmental pathways traverse the lateral funiculi of the spinal cord near the corticospinal tracts to reach sympathetic and parasympathetic segmental centers. Penile erection is effected through sacral parasympathetic motor neurons (S3 and S4), the nervi erigentes, and pudendal nerves. There is some evidence also that a sympathetic outflow from thoracolumbar segments (originating in T12-L1) via the inferior mesenteric and hypogastric plexuses can mediate psychogenic erections in patients with complete sacral cord destruction. Activation from these segmental centers opens vascular channels between arteriolar branches of the pudendal arteries and the vascular spaces of the corpora cavernosa and corpus spongiosum (erectile tissues), resulting in tumescence. Detumescence occurs when venous channels open widely. Ejaculation involves rhythmic contractions of the prostate, compressor (sphincter) urethrae, and bulbocavernosus and ischiocavernosus muscles, which

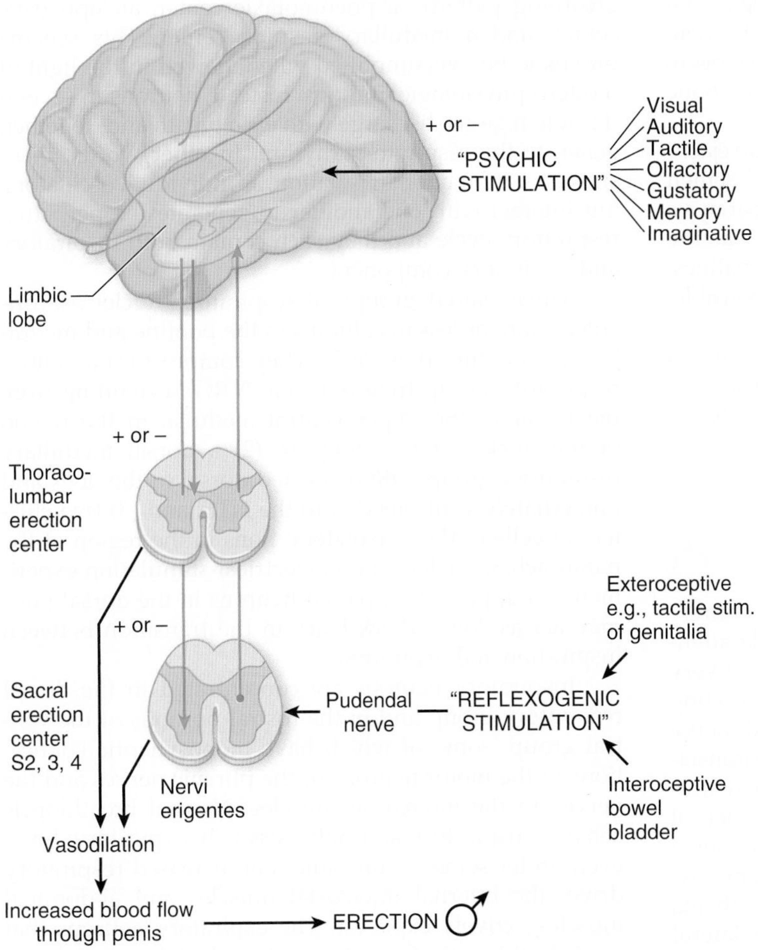

Figure 26-6. The pathways involved in human penile erection. See text for details. (Reproduced by permission from Weiss.)

are under the control of both the sympathetic and parasympathetic centers. Afferent segmental influences arise in the glans penis and reach parasympathetic centers at S3 and S4 (reflexogenic erections). Figure 26-6 shows the organization of this neural system and the locations of lesions that can abolish normal erectile function. Similar neural arrangements exist in females.

The different aspects of sexual function may be affected separately. Loss of libido may depend on both psychic and somatic factors. It may be complete, as in old age or in medical and endocrine diseases, or it may occur only in certain circumstances or in relation to certain situations. In the latter case, which is a result of psychologic factors, reflex penile erection during rapid eye movement (REM) sleep, and even emission of semen, may occur.

Sexual desire can be altered in the opposite direction, i.e., it may be excessive. This, too, is usually psychologic or psychiatric in origin, as in manic states, but sometimes it occurs with neurologic disease, such as encephalitis and tumors that affect the diencephalon, septal region, and temporal lobes; with the dementias; and as a result of certain medications such as L-dopa, as discussed in Chap. 25. In the instances of neurologic diseases with hypersexuality, there are usually other signs of disinhibited behavior as well.

On the other hand, sexual drive may be present but penile erection impossible to attain or sustain. The most common cause of erectile dysfunction is a depressive state. Prostatectomy is another, the result of damage to the parasympathetic nerves embedded in the capsule of the gland. It occurs also in patients who suffer disease of the sacral cord segments and their afferent and efferent connections (e.g., cord tumor, myelitis, tabes, and diabetic and many other polyneuropathies), in which case nocturnal erections are absent. The parasympathetic nerves cannot then be activated to cause tumescence of the corpora cavernosa and corpus spongiosum. The phosphodiesterase inhibitors such as sildenafil (Viagra) have proved to be useful in the treatment of erectile dysfunction in some patients with sexual dysfunction of neurologic cause. During sexual stimulation, it enhances the effect of local nitric oxide on the smooth muscle of the corpus cavernosum; this results in relaxation of the smooth muscle and inflow of blood. The high rate of success of this drug in patients with spinal cord injury indicates that segmental innervation is all that is required for reflexive erection in response to tactile stimulation of the penis.

Diseases of the spinal cord may abolish psychogenic erections but leave reflexive ones intact. In fact, the latter may become overactive, giving rise to sustained painful erections (*priapism*). This indicates that the segmental mechanism for penile erection is relatively intact. There are many other nonneurologic causes for priapism, among them are sickle cell anemia and other thrombotic states and perineal trauma.

Other sexual difficulties include the premature ejaculation of semen. After lumbar sympathectomy, the semen may be ejected back into the bladder because of paralysis of the periurethral muscle within the prostate, at the verumontanum (colliculus seminalis). Polyneuropathies, such as those caused by diabetes, may be responsible; acute or chronic prostatitis may have a similar effect.

Cerebral disorders of sexual function are discussed further in Chap. 25 (see section on "Altered Sexuality") and the development of sexual function, in Chap. 28.

NERVOUS SYSTEM CONTROL OF RESPIRATION

Considering that the act of breathing is directed entirely by the nervous system, it is surprising how little attention it has received other than from physiologists. Every component of breathing—the lifelong automatic cycling of inspiration, the transmission of coordinated nerve impulses to and from the respiratory muscles, the translation of systemic influences such as acidosis to the neuromuscular apparatus of the diaphragm—is under neural control. Moreover, respiratory failure is one of the most serious disturbances of neurologic function in comatose states and in neuromuscular diseases such as myasthenia gravis, Guillain-Barré syndrome, amyotrophic lateral sclerosis, muscular dystrophy, and poliomyelitis. Finally, death—or brain death—is now virtually defined in terms of the ability of the nervous system to sustain respiration, a reversion to ancient methods of determining the cessation of all vital forces. Neurologists should be familiar with the alterations of respiration caused by diseases in different parts of the nervous system, the effects of respiratory failure on the brain, and the rationale that underlies modern methods of treatment. A full understanding of respiration requires knowledge of the mechanical and physiologic workings of the lungs as organs of gas exchange; but here we limit our remarks to the nervous system control of breathing.

The Central Respiratory Motor Mechanisms

It has been known for more than a century that breathing is controlled mainly by the lower brainstem, and that each half of the brainstem is capable of producing an independent respiratory rhythm. In patients with poliomyelitis, for example, the occurrence of respiratory failure was associated with lesions in the ventrolateral tegmentum of the medulla (Feldman; Cohen). Until fairly recently, thinking on this subject was dominated by Lumsden's scheme of the breathing patterns that resulted from sectioning the brainstem of cats at various levels. He postulated the existence of several centers in the pontine tegmentum, each corresponding to an abnormal breathing pattern—a pneumotaxic center, an apneustic center, and a medullary gasping center. This scheme proves to be oversimplified when viewed in the light of modern physiologic findings. Instead, neurons in several discrete regions discharge with each breath and, together, generate the respiratory rhythm. In other words, these sites do not function in isolation, as individual oscillators, but interact with one another to generate the perpetual respiratory cycle and they each contain both inspiratory and expiratory components.

Three paired groups of respiratory nuclei are oriented more or less in columns in the pontine and medullary tegmentum (Fig. 26-7). They comprise (1) a ventral respiratory group (referred to as VRG), extending from the lower to the upper ventral medulla, in the region of the nucleus retroambiguus; (2) a dorsal medullary respiratory group (DRG), located dorsal to the obex and immediately ventromedial to the NTS; and (3) two clusters of cells in the dorsolateral pons in the region of the parabrachial nucleus. From electrical-stimulation experiments, it appears that paired neurons in the dorsal pons may act as "on–off" switches in the transition between inspiration and expiration.

Inspiratory neurons are concentrated in the dorsal respiratory group and in the rostral portions of the ventral group, some of which have monosynaptic connections to the motor neurons of the phrenic nerves and the nerves to the intercostal muscles. Normal breathing is actively inspiratory and only passively expiratory; however, under some circumstances of increased respiratory drive, the internal intercostal muscles and abdominal muscles actively expel air. The expiratory neurons that mediate this activity are concentrated in the caudal portions of the ventral respiratory group and in the most rostral parts of the dorsal group. On the basis of both neuroanatomic tracer and physiologic studies, it has been determined that these expiratory neurons project to spinal motor neurons and have an inhibitory influence on inspiratory neurons.

The pathway of descending fibers that arises in the inspiratory neurons and terminates on phrenic nerve motor neurons lies just lateral to the anterior horns of the upper cervical cord segments. When these tracts are damaged, automatic but not voluntary diaphragmatic movement is lost. As noted later, the fibers carrying voluntary motor impulses to the diaphragm course more dorsally in the cord. The phrenic motor neurons form a thin column in the medial parts of the ventral horns, extending from the third through fifth cervical cord segments. Damage to these neurons, of course, precludes both voluntary and automatic breathing.

As mentioned, the exact locus from which the breathing rhythm is generated, if there is such a site, is not known. The conventional understanding has been that the DRG was the dominant generator of the respiratory rhythm but the situation is certainly more complex. Animal experiments have focused attention instead on the rostral ventrolateral medulla (VRG). This region contains a group of neurons in the vicinity of the "Botzinger complex" (which itself contains neurons that fire mainly

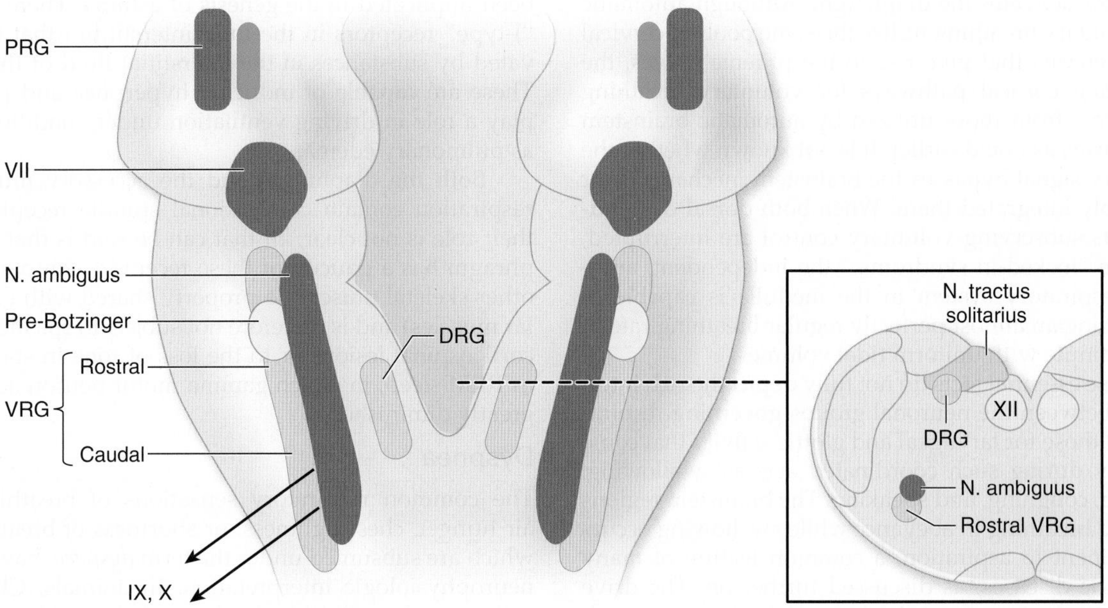

Figure 26-7. The location of the main centers of respiratory control in the brainstem as currently envisioned from animal experiments and limited human pathology. There are three paired groups of nuclei: (1) The dorsal respiratory group (*DRG*), containing mainly inspiratory neurons, located in the ventrolateral subnucleus of the nucleus of the tractus solitarius; (2) a ventral respiratory group (*VRG*), situated near the nucleus ambiguus and containing in its caudal part neurons that fire predominantly during expiration and in its rostral part neurons that are synchronous with inspiration—the latter structure merges rostrally with the Botzinger complex, which is located just behind the facial nucleus and contains neurons that are active mostly during expiration; and (3) a pontine pair of nuclei (*PRG*), one of which fires in the transition between inspiration and expiration and the other between expiration and inspiration. The intrinsic rhythmicity of the entire system probably depends on interactions between all these regions, but the "pre-Botzinger" area in the rostral ventromedial medulla may play a special role in generating the respiratory rhythm. (Adapted by permission from Duffin et al.)

during expiration). Cooling of this area or injection with neurotoxins in animals causes the respiratory rhythm to cease (see the review by Duffin et al). It has also been shown that the paired respiratory nuclei in the pons that are thought to act as switches between inspiration and expiration possess a degree of autonomous rhythmicity but their role in engendering cyclic breathing has not been clarified. Some workers are of the opinion that two or more sets of neurons in the VRG create a rhythm by their reciprocal activity or that oscillations arise within even larger networks (see Blessing for details).

There are also centers in the pons that do not generate respiratory rhythms but may, under extreme circumstances, greatly influence them. One pontine group, the "pneumotaxic center," modulates the response to hypoxia, hypocapnia, and lung inflation. In general, expiratory neurons are located laterally and inspiratory neurons medially in this center, but there is an additional group that lies between them and remains active during the transition between respiratory phases. Also found in the lower pons is a group of neurons that prevent unrestrained activity of the medullary inspiratory neurons ("apneustic center"). In addition to these ambiguities regarding a "center" for the generation of respiratory rhythm, there is the difficulty that the nuclei described earlier are not well defined in humans.

As to the effects of a unilateral brainstem lesion on ventilation, numerous cases of hypoventilation or total loss of automatic ventilation ("Ondine's curse"—see further on) have been recorded (Bogousslavsky and colleagues). We have observed several such remarkable cases as well, in most instances caused by a large lateral medullary infarction. If the neural oscillators on each side were totally independent, such a syndrome should not be possible. The likely explanation is that a unilateral lesion interrupts the connections between each of the paired groups of nuclei, which normally synchronize the two sides in the generation of rhythmic bursts of excitatory impulses to spinal motor neurons. It is of interest that in a case of a very delimited metastasis to the NTS there was no apparent impact on the breathing pattern until a terminal respiratory arrest (Rhodes and Wightman).

Voluntary Control of Breathing

During speech, swallowing, breathholding, or voluntary hyperventilation, the automaticity of the brainstem mechanisms of respiration is arrested in favor of reflexive or of conscious control of diaphragmatic contraction. The observations of Colebatch and coworkers, using PET scanning, indicate that voluntary control of breathing is associated with activity in the motor and premotor cortex. The experiments of Maskill and associates demonstrated that magnetic cortical stimulation of a region near the cranial vertex activates the diaphragm. Although automatic and voluntary breathing utilize the same pools of cervical motor neurons that give rise to the phrenic nerves, the descending cortical pathways for voluntary breathing are distinct from those utilized by automatic brainstem mechanisms as noted earlier. It is not known whether the voluntary signal bypasses the brainstem mechanisms or is possibly integrated there. When both dorsal descending tracts subserving voluntary control are interrupted, as in the "locked-in syndrome," the independent, automatic respiratory system in the medulla is capable of maintaining an almost perfectly regular breathing rate of 16 per minute with uniform tidal volumes.

These essential facts do not fully depict the rich interactions between the neuronal groups governing respiration and those for laryngeal and glottic activity that come into play during such coordinated acts as swallowing, sneezing, coughing, and speaking. The brainstem regions that hold breathing in abeyance while swallowing occurs are pertinent to aspiration, a common feature of many neurologic diseases, as discussed further on. The drive applied to these systems is damped in processes such as Parkinson disease, causing discoordination between breathing and swallowing, and may contribute to the problem of aspiration, as also discussed further on.

Afferent Respiratory Influences

A number of signals that modulate respiratory drive originate in chemoreceptors located in the carotid artery. These receptors are influenced both by changes in pH and by hypoxia. Chemoreceptor afferents pass along the carotid sinus nerves, which join the glossopharyngeal nerves and terminate in the NTS. Aortic body receptors, which are less important as detectors of hypoxia, send afferent volleys to the medulla through the aortic nerves, which join the vagus nerves. There are also chemoreceptors in the brainstem, but their precise location is uncertain. Their main locus is thought to be in the ventral medulla, but other areas that are responsive to changes in pH have been demonstrated in animals. What is clear is that these regions are sensitive not to the pH of CSF, as had been thought, but to the pH of the extracellular fluid of the medulla.

Numerous stretch receptors within smooth muscle cells of the airways also project via the vagus nerves to the NTS and influence the depth and duration of breathing. Afferent signals from these specialized nerve endings mediate the Hering-Breuer reflex, described in 1868—a shortened inspiration and decreased tidal volume triggered by excessive lung expansion. The Hering-Breuer mechanism seems not to be important at rest, as bilateral vagal section has no effect on the rate or depth of respiration. These aspects of afferent pulmonary modulation of breathing have been reviewed by Berger and colleagues. It is interesting, however, that patients with high spinal transections and inability to breathe can still sense changes in lung volume, attesting to a nonspinal afferent route to the brainstem from lung receptors, probably through the vagus nerves. In addition, there are receptors located between pulmonary epithelial cells that respond to irritants such as histamine and smoke. They have been implicated in the genesis of asthma. There are also "J-type" receptors in the lung interstitium that are activated by substances in the interstitial fluid of the lungs. These are capable of inducing hyperpnea and probably play a role in driving ventilation under conditions such as pulmonary edema.

Both the diaphragm and the accessory muscles of respiration contain conventional spindle receptors, but their role is not clear; all that can be said is that the diaphragm has a paucity of these receptors compared with other skeletal muscles (a property shared with extraocular muscles) and is therefore not subject to spasticity with corticospinal lesions or to the loss of tone in states such as REM sleep, in which gamma motor neuron activity is greatly diminished.

Dyspnea

The common respiratory sensations of breathlessness, air hunger, chest tightness, or shortness of breath, all of which are subsumed under the term *dyspnea*, have defied neurophysiologic interpretation. In animals, Chen and colleagues from Eldridge's laboratory have demonstrated that neurons in the thalamus and central midbrain tegmentum discharge in a graduated manner as respiratory drive is increased. These neurons are influenced greatly by afferent information from the chest wall, lung, and chemoreceptors and are postulated to be the thalamic representation of sensation from the thorax that is perceived at a cortical level as dyspnea. However, functional imaging studies indicate that various areas of the cerebrum are activated by dyspnea, mainly the insula and limbic regions.

Aberrant Respiratory Patterns

Many of the most interesting respiratory patterns observed in neurologic disease are found in comatose patients, and several of these patterns have been assigned localizing value, some of uncertain validity: *central neurogenic hyperventilation, apneusis, and ataxic breathing*. These are discussed in relation to the clinical signs of coma (see Chap. 17) and sleep apnea (see Chap. 19). Some of the most bizarre cadences of breathing—those in which unwanted breaths intrude on speech or those characterized by incoordination of laryngeal closure, diaphragmatic movement, or swallowing or by respiratory tics—have occurred in paraneoplastic brainstem encephalitis. Similar incoordinated patterns occur in certain extrapyramidal diseases. Patterns such as episodic tachypnea up to 100 breaths per minute and loss of voluntary control of breathing were, in the past, noteworthy features of postencephalitic parkinsonism.

In *Leeuwenhoek's disease*, named for the discoverer of the microscope who described and was afflicted with the problem, there is an almost continuous epigastric pulsation and dyspnea in association with rhythmic bursts of activity in the inspiratory muscles—a respiratory myoclonus akin to palatal myoclonus (Phillips and Eldridge). Two such cases in our clinical material followed influenza-like illnesses and resolved slowly over months. Another patient with similar movements intermittently causing gasping sounds gave us the impression of having a psychogenic disease.

Cheyne-Stokes breathing, the common and well-known waxing and waning type of cyclic ventilation reported by Cheyne in 1818 and later elaborated by Stokes, has for decades been ascribed to a prolongation of circulation time, as in congestive heart failure; but there are data that support a primary neural origin of the disorder, particularly the observation that it occurs most often in patients with deep hemispheral lesions of the cerebral hemispheres or advanced stages of metabolic encephalopathy. The level of consciousness in these circumstances parallels the respiratory pattern. During the apneic period the patient is less responsive. The onset of respiration is heralded by arousal, marked by eye opening and sometimes vocalization. At the peak of the hyperventilation phase, the patient is maximally awake. Consciousness then wanes followed by slowing of the respiratory rate and finally coma to complete a full cycle. The fact that the level of consciousness changes before the respiratory rate is altered implies that Cheyne-Stokes breathing is only one component of a cyclic autonomic brainstem phenomenon. (See Chap. 17 for further comments on the physiologic explanation for this pattern.)

Another striking aberration of ventilation is a loss of automatic respiration during sleep, with preserved voluntary breathing (*Ondine's curse*). The term stems from the German myth in which Ondine, a sea nymph, condemns her unfaithful lover to a loss of all movements and functions that do not require conscious will. Patients with this condition are compelled to remain awake lest they stop breathing, and they must have nighttime mechanical ventilation to survive. Presumably the underlying pathology is one that selectively interrupts the ventrolateral descending medullocervical pathways that subserve automatic breathing. The syndrome has been documented mostly in cases of unilateral and bilateral brainstem infarctions, hemorrhage, encephalitis (neoplastic or infectious—for example, due to *Listeria*), in Leigh syndrome (a destructive process in the lower brainstem of mitochondrial origin), and with traumatic Duret hemorrhages in the lower brainstem. The issue of a loss of automatic ventilation as a result of a unilateral brainstem lesion has been addressed earlier. A state in which there is complete loss of voluntary control of ventilation but preserved automatic monorhythmic breathing has also been described (Munschauer et al). Incomplete variants of this latter phenomenon are regularly observed in cases of brainstem infarction or severe demyelinating disease, and may be a component of the "locked-in state."

Often neglected is the dyspnea that patients experience with orthostatic hypotension (*orthostatic dyspnea*). In a questionnaire given to patients in an autonomic laboratory, Gibbons and Freeman reported that one-third had this symptom. They proposed that some form of mismatch between lung ventilation and perfusion was the cause.

The *congenital central hypoventilation syndrome* is thought to be an idiopathic version of the loss of automatic ventilation (see Shannon et al). This rare condition begins in infancy with apneas and sleep disturbances of varying severity or later in childhood with signs of chronic hypoxia leading to pulmonary hypertension. As mentioned in "Sleep Apnea and Excessive Daytime Sleepiness" in Chap. 19, several subtle changes in the arcuate nucleus of the medulla and a depletion of neurons in regions of the respiratory centers have been found in this condition, but further study is necessary.

Neurologic lesions that cause *hyperventilation* are diverse and widely located throughout the brain, not just in the brainstem. In clinical practice, episodes of hyperventilation are most often seen in anxiety and panic states. The traditional view of "central neurogenic hyperventilation" as a manifestation of a pontine lesion has been brought into question by the observation that it may occur as a sign of primary cerebral lymphoma, in which postmortem examination has failed to show involvement of the brainstem regions controlling respiration (Plum).

Hiccup (singultus) is a poorly understood phenomenon. It does not seem to serve any useful physiologic purpose, existing only as a nuisance, and is typically not associated with any particular disease. It may occur as a component of the lateral medullary syndrome (see Chap. 34) as in 7 of 51 cases studied by Park and colleagues, with masses in the posterior fossa or medulla, and occasionally with generalized elevation of intracranial pressure, brainstem encephalitis, or with metabolic encephalopathies such as uremia. Rarely, singultation may be provoked by medication, one possible offender in our experience being dexamethasone. Because the triggers of hiccup often seem to arise in epigastric organs adjacent to the diaphragm, it is considered to be a gastrointestinal reflex, more than a respiratory one. A physiologic study by Newsom Davis demonstrated that hiccup is the result of powerful contraction of the diaphragm and intercostal muscles, followed immediately by laryngeal closure. This results in little or no net movement of air. He concluded that the projections from the brainstem responsible for hiccup are independent of the pathways that mediate rhythmic breathing.

Within a single burst or run of hiccups, the frequency remains relatively constant, but at any one time it may range anywhere from 15 to 45 per minute. The contractions are most liable to occur during inspiration and they are inhibited by therapeutic elevation of arterial carbon dioxide (CO_2) tension. We cannot vouch for the innumerable home-brewed methods that are said to suppress hiccups (breathholding, induced fright, anesthetization, or stimulation of the external ear canal or concha, etc.), but where the neurologist is asked to help in an intractable case (usually in a male), baclofen is sometimes effective. Drugs that act to empty the stomach (e.g., metoclopramide) may work as well.

Disorders of Ventilation Caused by Neuromuscular Disease

Failure of ventilation in the neuromuscular diseases causes one of two symptom complexes: an acute one occurs in patients with rapidly evolving generalized weakness, such as Guillain-Barré syndrome and myasthenia gravis, and the other in patients with subacute or chronic diseases, such as motor neuron disease, myopathies (acid maltase, nemaline), and muscular dystrophy. The review by Polkey and colleagues provides a more extensive list of diseases that cause these problems. Patients in whom respiratory failure evolves in a matter of hours become anxious, tachycardic, and diaphoretic. They may display *paradoxical respiration*, in which the abdominal wall retracts during inspiration, owing to the failure of the diaphragm to contract, while the intercostal and accessory muscles create a negative intrathoracic pressure. Or, there is *respiratory alternans*, a pattern of diaphragmatic descent only on alternate breaths (this is more characteristic of airway obstruction). These signs appear in the acutely ill patient when the vital capacity has been reduced to approximately 10 percent of normal, or 500 mL in the average adult.

Patients with chronic but stable weakness of the respiratory muscles, demonstrate signs of CO_2 retention, such as daytime somnolence, headache upon awakening, nightmares, and, in extreme cases, papilledema. The accessory muscles of respiration are recruited in an attempt to maximize tidal volume, and there is a tendency for the patient to gulp or assume a rounded "fish mouth" appearance in an effort to inhale additional air. In general, patients with chronic respiratory difficulty tolerate lower tidal volumes without dyspnea than do patients with acute disease, and symptoms in the former may occur only at night, when respiratory drive is diminished and compensatory mechanisms for obtaining additional air are in abeyance.

Treatment of the two conditions differs. The chronic type of respiratory failure may require only nighttime support of ventilation, which can be provided by negative pressure devices such as a cuirass or preferably, by intermittent positive pressure applied by a tight-fitting mask over the nose (bilevel positive airway pressure [BIPAP] or continuous positive airway pressure [CPAP]). These measures may also be used temporarily in acute situations, but in many cases there will be need of a positive-pressure ventilator that provides a constant volume with each breath. This can be effected only through an endotracheal tube.

Typical ventilator settings in cases of acute mechanical respiratory failure, if there is no pneumonia, are for tidal volumes of 6 to 8 mL/kg, depending on the compliance of the lungs and the patient's comfort, at a ventilator rate between 4 and 12 breaths per minute, adjusted to the degree of respiratory failure. The tidal volume is kept relatively constant so as to prevent atelectasis, and only the rate is changed as the diaphragm becomes weaker or stronger. Decisions regarding the need for these mechanical devices are frequently difficult, particularly as patients with chronic neuromuscular illnesses often become dependent on a ventilator. Further details regarding the management of ventilation in acute neuromuscular weakness are given in the section on Guillain-Barré syndrome in Chap. 46.

The presence of oropharyngeal weakness as a result of the underlying neuromuscular disease may leave the patient's airway unprotected and require endotracheal intubation before mechanical ventilation becomes necessary. It is even difficult to decide when to remove an endotracheal tube in a patient with oropharyngeal weakness. Because the safety of the swallowing mechanism cannot be assessed with the tube in place, one must be prepared to reintubate the patient or to have a surgeon prepared to perform a tracheostomy after extubation, in the event that aspiration occurs.

We frequently encounter patients in whom the earliest feature of neuromuscular disease is *subacute respiratory failure*; this is manifest as dyspnea and exercise intolerance but *without other overt signs of neuromuscular disease*. Most such cases prove to be motor neuron disease, but rare instances of myasthenia gravis (especially the type associated with the MUSK autoantibody), acid maltase deficiency, polymyositis, nemaline myopathy, Lambert-Eaton syndrome, or chronic inflammatory demyelinating polyneuropathy may present in this way. The neurologist may be consulted in these cases after other physicians have found no evidence of intrinsic pulmonary disease. The spirometric flow-volume loop in cases of neuromuscular respiratory failure shows low airflow rates with diminished lung volumes that together simulate restrictive lung disease. Among such patients we have also found instances of isolated unilateral or *bilateral phrenic nerve paresis* that followed abdominal or cardiac surgery or an infectious illness. The least of these is probably a form of brachial neuritis (see Chap. 46 for a discussion of brachial neuritis).

Neuromuscular Respiratory Failure in Critically Ill Patients Neurologists increasingly are being called upon to determine if there is an underlying neuromuscular cause for respiratory failure in a critically ill patient. Malnutrition, hypophosphatemia (induced by hyperalimentation), and hypokalemia always need to be kept in mind as causes of muscular weakness. Aside from the acute neuromuscular diseases listed above, Bolton and colleagues have delineated a *critical illness polyneuropathy*, which accounts for as many as 40 percent of cases of an inability to wean a patient from the ventilation. Most of these patients have had an episode of sepsis or have multiple organ failure (see Chap. 46). The EMG demonstrates widespread denervation with relative sparing of sensory potentials. Less often, a *critical illness myopathy* occurs in relation to the administration of high-dose corticosteroids (see Chap. 51). This myopathy occurs mainly in patients who are receiving neuromuscular postsynaptic blocking drugs such as pancuronium simultaneously with high-dose steroids but corticosteroids alone have been implicated (see Chap. 51).

The Neurologic Basis of Swallowing

The act of swallowing, like breathing, continues periodically through waking and sleep, largely without conscious will or awareness. Swallowing occurs at a natural frequency of about once per minute while an individual is idle; it is suppressed during concentration and emotional excitement.

The fundamental role of swallowing is to move food from the mouth to the esophagus and thereby to begin the process of digestion, but it also serves to empty the oral cavity of saliva and prevent its entry into the respiratory tract. Because the oropharynx is a shared conduit for breathing and swallowing, obligatory reflexes exist to assure that breathing is held in abeyance during swallowing. Because of this relationship and the frequency with which dysphagia and aspiration complicate neurologic disease, the neural mechanisms that underlie swallowing are of considerable importance to the neurologist and are described here. The reader is also referred to other parts of this book for a discussion of derangements of swallowing consequent upon diseases of the lower cranial nerves (see Chap. 47), of muscle (see Chap. 48), and of the neuromuscular junction (see Chap. 53).

Anatomic and Physiologic Considerations

A highly coordinated sequence of muscle contractions is required to move a bolus of food smoothly and safely through the oropharynx. This programmed activity may be elicited voluntarily or by reflex movements that are triggered by sensory impulses from the posterior pharynx. Swallowing normally begins as the tongue, innervated by cranial nerve XII, sweeps food to the posterior oral cavity, and brings the bolus into contact with the posterior wall of the oropharynx. As the food passes the pillars of the fauces, tactile sensation, carried through nerves IX and X, reflexly triggers (1) the contraction of levator and tensor veli palatini muscles, which close the nasopharynx and prevent nasal regurgitation, followed by (2) the upward and forward movement of the arytenoid cartilages toward the epiglottis (observed as an upward displacement of the hyoid and thyroid cartilages), which closes the airway. With these movements, the epiglottis guides the food into the valleculae and into channels formed by the epiglottic folds and the pharyngeal walls. The airway is closed by sequential contractions of the arytenoid–epiglottic folds, and below them, the false cords, and then the true vocal cords, which seal the trachea.

All of these muscular contractions are effected largely by cranial nerve X (vagus). The palatopharyngeal muscles pull the pharynx up over the bolus and the stylopharyngeal muscles draw the sides of the pharynx outward (nerve IX). At the same time, the upward movement of the larynx opens the cricopharyngeal sphincter. A wave of peristalsis then begins in the pharynx, pushing the bolus through the sphincter into the esophagus. These muscles relax as soon as the bolus reaches the esophagus. The entire swallowing ensemble can be elicited by stimulation of the superior laryngeal nerve (this route is used in experimental studies.)

Reflex swallowing requires only medullary functioning and is retained in the vegetative and locked-in states as well as in normal and anencephalic neonates. The integrated sequence of muscle activity for swallowing is organized in a region of brainstem that roughly comprises a swallowing center, located in the region of the NTS, close to the respiratory centers. This juxtaposition ostensibly allows the refined coordination of swallowing with the cycle of breathing. Besides a programmed period of apnea, there is a slight forced exhalation after each swallow that further prevents aspiration. The studies of Jean, Kessler, and others (cited by Blessing), using microinjections of excitatory neurotransmitters, have localized the swallowing center in animals to a region adjacent to the termination of the superior laryngeal nerve. Unlike the generators of respiratory rhythm, the entire reflex apparatus for swallowing may be located in the NTS. There is, however, no direct connection between the NTS and the cranial nerve motor nuclei. Thus it is presumed that control must be exerted through premotor neurons located in adjacent reticular brainstem regions. There have been few comparable anatomic studies of the structures responsible for swallowing in humans. As to the cortical regions that are involved in swallowing, it appears from PET studies that the inferior precentral gyrus and the posterior inferior frontal gyrus are activated, and lesions in these parts of the brain give rise to the most profound cases of dysphagia.

Dysphagia and Aspiration

Weakness or incoordination of the swallowing apparatus is manifest as dysphagia and, at times, aspiration. The patient himself is often able to discriminate one of several types of defects: (1) difficulty initiating swallowing, which leaves solids stuck in the oropharynx; (2) nasal regurgitation of liquids; (3) frequent coughing and choking immediately after swallowing and a hoarse, "wet cough" following the ingestion of fluids; or (4) some combination of these. Extrapyramidal diseases, notably Parkinson disease, reduce the frequency of swallowing and cause an incoordination of breathing and swallowing, as noted later.

It is surprising how often the tongue and the muscles that cause palatal elevation appear on direct examination to act normally despite an obvious failure of coordinated swallowing. Similarly, the use of the gag reflex as a neurologic sign is quite limited, being most helpful when there is a medullary lesion or the lower cranial nerves are damaged. In our experience, palatal elevation in response to touching the posterior pharynx only demonstrates that cranial nerves IX and X and the local musculature are not entirely dysfunctional; in other words, the presence of the reflex does not assure the smooth coordination of the swallowing mechanism and, more importantly, does not obviate aspiration. Difficulties with swallowing may begin subtly and express themselves as weight loss or as a noticeable increase in the time required to eat a meal. Nodding or sideways head movements to assist the propulsion of the bolus, or the need to repeatedly wash food down with water, are other clues to the presence of dysphagia. Often, recurrent minor pneumonias are the only manifestation of intermittent ("silent") aspiration.

A defect in the initiation of swallowing is usually attributable to weakness of the tongue and may be a feature of myasthenia gravis, motor neuron disease or rarely, inflammatory disease of the muscle; it may be caused by palsies of the twelfth cranial nerve (metastases at the base of the skull or meningoradiculitis, carotid dissection), or to a number of other causes. In all these cases there is usually an associated dysarthria with difficulty pronouncing lingual sounds. The second type of dysphagia, associated with nasal regurgitation of liquids, indicates a failure of velopalatine closure and is characteristic of myasthenia gravis, tenth nerve palsy of any cause, or incoordination of swallowing because of bulbar or pseudobulbar palsy. A nasal pattern of speech with air escaping from the nose is a usual accompaniment.

Viewed from a physiologic perspective, the causes of aspiration fall into four main categories: (1) weakness of the pharyngeal musculature because of lesions of the vagus on one or both sides; (2) myopathy (polymyositis, myotonic and oculopharyngeal dystrophies) or neuromuscular disease (amyotrophic lateral sclerosis and myasthenia gravis); (3) a medullary lesion that affects the NTS or the cranial motor nuclei (lateral medullary infarction is the prototype)—but syringomyelia-syringobulbia and, rarely, multiple sclerosis, polio, and brainstem tumors may have the same effects; or (4) less-well-defined mechanisms of slowed or discoordinated swallowing arising from corticospinal disease (pseudobulbar palsy, hemispheral stroke) or from diseases of the basal ganglia (mainly Parkinson disease) that alter the timing of breathing and swallowing and permit the airway to remain open as food passes through the posterior pharynx. In the latter cases, a decreased frequency of swallowing also causes saliva to pool in the mouth (leading to drooling) and adds to the risk of aspiration.

Because of its frequency, the neurologist will encounter stroke in a cerebral hemisphere as a cause of discoordinated swallowing. The problem is most evident during the first few days after a hemispheral stroke on either side of the brain (Meadows). These effects last days or weeks and render the patient subject to pneumonia and fever. In the clinical and fluoroscopic study by Mann and colleagues, half of patients still had manifest abnormalities of swallowing 6 months after their strokes. For this reason, it has become customary for patients to have swallowing evaluations in the days after acute stroke. Some insight into the nature of swallowing dysfunction after stroke is provided by Hamdy and colleagues, who correlated the presence of dysphagia with a lesser degree of motor representation of pharyngeal muscles in the unaffected hemisphere, as assessed by magnetic stimulation of the cortex.

Pain on swallowing occurs under a different set of circumstances, the one of most neurologic interest being glossopharyngeal neuralgia as discussed in Chaps. 10 and 47.

Videofluoroscopy has become a useful tool in determining the presence of aspiration during swallowing and in differentiating the several types of dysphagia. The movement of the bolus by the tongue, the timing of reflex swallowing, and the closure of the pharyngeal and palatal openings are judged directly by observation of a bolus of food mixed with barium or of liquid barium alone. However, authorities in the field, such as Wiles, whose reviews are recommended (see also Hughes and Wiles), warn that unqualified dependence on videofluoroscopy is unwise. They remark that observation of the patient swallowing water and repeated observation of the patient while eating can be equally informative. Having the patient swallow water is a particularly effective test of laryngeal closure; the presence of coughing, wet hoarseness or breathlessness, and the need to swallow small volumes slowly are indicative of a high risk of aspiration.

Based on bedside observations and on videofluoroscopy studies, an experienced therapist can make recommendations regarding the safety of oral feeding, changes in the consistency and texture of the diet, postural adjustments, and the need to insert a tracheostomy or feeding tube.

Vomiting

Vomiting is a complex, sequential act that may be triggered by numerous external, gastrointestinal, and neural stimuli. The main central nervous system structure of interest in eliciting the vomiting reflex is the *area postrema*, which is located at the base of the fourth ventricle. The neurons within the area postrema are chemosensitive and are activated by circulating toxins, which have direct access to these neurons because of the absence of a blood–brain barrier. Axons from the area postrema project to the *nucleus of the solitary tract* (NTS), which is also a convergence point of input from the pharynx, larynx, and gastrointestinal tract. The NTS engages groups of neurons in the medulla, which coordinates the sequential elements of vomiting; there is no "vomiting center," as reviewed by Hornby. In addition to stimulation of the area postrema, vestibular, pharyngeal (gag reflex), and psychic stimuli can induce vomiting.

The final expulsion of gastric contents is effected through a combination of lowering of intrathoracic pressure by inspiration against a closed glottis and an increase in abdominal pressure during abdominal muscle contraction. Retroperistalsis begins in the small intestine and there is relaxation of the lower esophageal and pyloric sphincters; the stomach itself does not contract.

The vagus carries afferent information from the enteric system as well as conducting efferent signals from the NTS to the gastrointestinal structures. The neurons in the area postrema contain D2 dopamine, 5-HT3 serotonin, opioids, substance P, and acetylcholine receptors, as well as the aquaporin channel. This affords an explanation for the emetic properties of dopaminergic agents and the antiemetic activity of dopamine and serotonin antagonists. However, other potent antiemetics such as ondansetron, a 5-HT3 receptor antagonist, have their effect on vagal afferents.

Lesions near the area postrema, including tumors, hemorrhage, infarctions, and demyelination are the usual neurologic causes of vomiting. We have seen, and it has been reported in the literature, that vomiting may have a relation to the periventricular lesions of neuromyelitis optica due the enrichment of aquaporin-4 channels in this area (Iorio and colleagues). The mechanism of vomiting from raised intracranial pressure has not been fully explored but could be the result of transmission of pressure to the dorsal medulla.

Cyclic Vomiting Syndrome This syndrome of obscure cause is associated with abdominal migraine in children (see Chap. 10), and is a prominent component of Riley-Day dysautonomia. It is also well known as a factitious self-induced disorder, for example, in bulimia.

References

Aguayo AJ, Nair CPV, Bray GM: Peripheral nerve abnormalities in Riley-Day syndrome. *Arch Neurol* 24:106, 1971.

Ahlquist RP: A study of adrenotropic receptors. *Am J Physiol* 153:586, 1948.

Anderson SL, Coli R, Daly IW, et al: Familial dysautonomia is caused by a mutation in the IKAP gene. *Am J Hum Genet* 68:753, 2001.

Appenzeller O, Arnason BG, Adams RD: Experimental autonomic neuropathy: An immunologically induced disorder of reflex vasomotor function. *J Neurol Neurosurg Psychiatry* 28:510, 1965.

Benarroch EF: Enteric nervous system. Functional organization and neurologic implications. *Neurology* 69:1955, 2007.

Berger AJ, Mitchell JH, Severinghaus JW: Regulation of respiration. *N Engl J Med* 297:92, 1977.

Blaivas JG: The neurophysiology of micturition: A clinical study of 550 patients. *J Urol* 127:958, 1982.

Blessing WW: *The Lower Brainstem and Bodily Homeostasis*. New York, Oxford, 1997.

Blok BFM, Willemsen ATM, Holstege G: A PET study on brain control of micturition in humans. *Brain* 120:111, 1997.

Bogousslavsky J, Khurana R, Deruaz JP, et al: Respiratory failure and unilateral caudal brainstem infarction. *Ann Neurol* 28:668, 1990.

Bolton CF, Laverty DA, Brown JD, et al: Critically ill polyneuropathy: Electrophysiological studies and differentiation from Guillain-Barré syndrome. *J Neurol Neurosurg Psychiatry* 49:563, 1986.

Bradbury S, Eggleston C: Postural hypotension: A report of three cases. *Am Heart J* 1:73, 1925.

Brindley GS, Polkey CE, Rushton DN, Cardozo L: Sacral anterior root stimulation for bladder control in paraplegia: The first 50 cases. *J Neurol Neurosurg Psychiatry* 49:1104, 1986.

Burnstock G: Innervation of vascular smooth muscle: Histochemistry and electron microscopy. *Clin Exp Pharmacol Physiol* 2(Suppl):2, 1975.

Caird FI, Andrews GR, Kennedy RD: Effect of posture on blood pressure in the elderly. *Br Heart J* 35:527, 1973.

Camilerri M: Diabetic gastroparesis. *New Eng J Med* 356:820, 2007.

Cannon WB: *Bodily Changes in Pain, Hunger, Fear and Rage*, 2nd ed. New York, Appleton, 1920.

Carmel PW: Sympathetic deficits following thalamotomy. *Arch Neurol* 18:378, 1968.

Chen Z, Eldridge FL, Wagner PG: Respiratory-associated thalamic activity is related to level of respiratory drive. *Respir Physiol* 90:99, 1992.

Cohen J, Low P, Fealey R, et al: Somatic and autonomic function in progressive autonomic failure and multiple system atrophy. *Ann Neurol* 22:692, 1987.

Cohen MI: Neurogenesis of respiratory rhythm in the mammal. *Physiol Rev* 59:1105, 1979.

Colebatch JG, Adams L, Murphy K, et al: Regional cerebral blood flow during volitional breathing in man. *J Physiol* 443:91, 1991.

Cooper JR, Bloom FE, Roth RH: *The Biochemical Basis of Neuropharmacology*, 8th ed. New York, Oxford University Press, 2003.

de Castro F: Sensory ganglia of the cranial and spinal nerves: Normal and pathological, in Penfield W (ed): *Cytology of Cellular Pathology of the Nervous System*. New York, Hafner, 1965, pp 93–143.

DeGroat WC: Nervous control of urinary bladder of the cat. *Brain Res* 87:201, 1975.

Denny-Brown D, Robertson EG: On the physiology of micturition. *Brain* 56:149, 1933.

Denny-Brown D, Robertson EG: The state of the bladder and its sphincters in complete transverse lesions of the spinal cord and cauda equina. *Brain* 56:397, 1933.

Duffin J, Kazuhisa E, Lipski J: Breathing rhythm generation: Focus on the rostral ventrolateral medulla. *News Physiol Sci* 10:133, 1995.

Dyck PJ, Kawamer Y, Low PA, et al: The number and sizes of reconstituted peripheral, autonomic, sensory, and motor neurons in a case of dysautonomia. *J Neuropathol Exp Neurol* 37:741, 1978.

Fagius J, Westerber CE, Olson Y: Acute pandysautonomia and severe sensory deficit with poor recovery: A clinical, neurophysiological, and pathological case study. *J Neurol Neurosurg Psychiatry* 46:725, 1983.

Falck B: Observations on the possibilities of the cellular localization of monoamines by a fluorescence method. *Acta Physiol Scand* 56(Suppl):197, 1962.

Feldman JL: Neurophysiology of breathing in mammals, in Bloom FE (ed): *Handbook of Physiology*. Vol IV: The Nervous System. Bethesda, MD, American Physiological Society, 1986, pp 463–524.

Fowler CJ: Neurological disorders of micturition and their treatment. *Brain* 122:1213, 1999.

Fowler CJ, Christman TJ, Chapple CR, et al: Abnormal electromyographic activity of the urethral sphincter, voiding dysfunction and polycystic ovaries: A new syndrome? *BMJ* 1988:297, 1436.

Geiger H, Naraghi R, Schobel HP, et al: Decrease of blood pressure by ventrolateral medullary decompression in essential hypertension. *Lancet* 352:446, 1998.

Gibbons CH, Freeman R: Orhtostatic dyspnea: A neglected symptom of orthostatic hypotension. *Clin Auton Res* 15:40, 2005.

Gibbons CH, Freeman R: Treatment-induced diabetic neuropathy: A reversible painful autonomic neuropathy. *Ann Neurol* 67:534, 2010.

Gutrecht JA: Sympathetic skin response. *J Clin Neurophysiol* 11:519, 1994.

Hamdy S, Aziz Q, Rothwell JC, et al: Explaining oropharyngeal dysphagia after unilateral hemispheric stroke. *Lancet* 350:686, 1997.

Hoeldtke RD, Dworkin GE, Gaspar SR, Israel BC: Sympathotonic orthostatic hypotension: A report of 4 cases. *Neurology* 39:34, 1989.

Hoff JT, Reis DJ: Localization of regions mediating the Cushing response in CNS of cat. *Arch Neurol* 23:228, 1970.

Holstege G, Tan J: Supraspinal control of motor neurons innervating the striated muscles of the pelvic floor, including urethral and anal sphincters in the cat. *Brain* 110:1323, 1987.

Hornby PJ. Central neurocircuitry associated with emesis. *Am J Medicine* 111(8a):106s, 2001.

Hughes TA, Wiles CM: Neurogenic dysphagia: The role of the neurologist. *J Neurol Neurosurg Psychiatry* 64:569, 1998.

Iorio R, Lucchinetti CF, Lennon VA, et al: Intractable nausea and vomiting from autoantibodies against a brain water channel. *Clin Gastroenterol Hepatol* 11:240, 2013.

Iverson LL, Iverson SD, Bloom FE, Roth RH: *Introduction to Neuropsychopharmacology*. New York, Oxford University Press, 2009.

Jansen SP, Sguyen XV, Karpitsky V, et al: Central command neurons of the sympathetic nervous system: Basis of the fight-or-flight response. *Science* 270:644, 1995.

Keane JR: Oculosympathetic paresis: Analysis of 100 hospitalized patients. *Arch Neurol* 36:13, 1979.

Kirby R, Fowler CV, Gosling JA, et al: Bladder dysfunction in distal autonomic neuropathy of acute onset. *J Neurol Neurosurg Psychiatry* 48:762, 1985.

Krane RJ, Siroky MD (eds): *Clinical Neurourology*, 2nd ed. Boston, Little, Brown, 1991.
Lewis P: Familial orthostatic hypotension. *Brain* 87:719, 1964.
Low PA: *Clinical Autonomic Disorders*, 2nd ed. Philadelphia, Lippincott-Raven, 1997.
Low PA, Dyck PJ: Splanchnic preganglionic neurons in man: II. Morphometry of myelinated fibers of T7 ventral spinal root. *Acta Neuropathol* 40:219, 1977.
Low PA, Dyck PJ, Lambert EH: Acute panautonomic neuropathy. *Ann Neurol* 13:412, 1983.
Lumsden T: Observations on the respiratory centers. *J Physiol* 57:354, 1923.
Mann G, Hankey GJ, Cameron D: Swallowing function after stroke: Prognosis and prognostic factors at 6 months. *Stroke* 30:744, 1999.
Mannen T, Iwata M, Toyokura Y, Nagashima K: Preservation of a certain motoneuron group of the sacral cord in amyotrophic lateral sclerosis: Its clinical significance. *J Neurol Neurosurg Psychiatry* 40:464, 1977.
Maskill D, Murphy K, Mier A, et al: Motor cortical representation of the diaphragm in man. *J Physiol* 443:105, 1991.
McLeod JG, Tuck RR: Disorders of the autonomic nervous system. Part I: Pathophysiology and clinical features. Part II: Investigation and treatment. *Ann Neurol* 21:419, 519, 1987.
Meadows JC: Dysphagia in unilateral cerebral lesions. *J Neurol Neurosurg Psychiatry* 36:853, 1973.
Munschauer FE, Mador MJ, Ahuja A, Jacobs L: Selective paralysis of voluntary but not limbically influenced automatic respiration. *Arch Neurol* 48:1190, 1991.
Nathan PW, Smith MC: The location of descending fibers to sympathetic neurons supplying the eye and sudomotor neurons supplying the head and neck. *J Neurol Neurosurg Psychiatry* 49:187, 1986.
Newsom Davis J: An experimental study of hiccup. *Brain* 39:851, 1970.
Onufrowicz B: On the arrangement and function of cell groups of the sacral region of the spinal cord of man. *Arch Neurol Psychopathol* 3:387, 1900.
Oppenheimer D: Neuropathology of autonomic failure, in Bannister R (ed): *Autonomic Failure*, 2nd ed. New York, Oxford University Press, 1988, pp 451–463.
Park MH, Kim BJ, Koh SB, et al: Lesional location of lateral medullary infarction presenting hiccups (singultus). *J Neurol Neurosurg Psychiatr* 75:95, 2005.
Pasztor A, Pasztor E: Spinal vasomotor reflex and Cushing response. *Acta Neurochir (Wien)* 52:85, 1980.
Penfield W, Jasper H: *Epilepsy and the Functional Anatomy of the Human Brain*. Boston, Little, Brown, 1954, p 414.
Petito CK, Black IB: Ultrastructure and biochemistry of sympathetic ganglia in idiopathic orthostatic hypotension. *Ann Neurol* 4:6, 1978.
Phillips JR, Eldridge FL: Respiratory myoclonus (Leeuwenhoek's disease). *N Engl J Med* 289:1390, 1973.
Pick J: *The Autonomic Nervous System*. Philadelphia, Lippincott, 1970.
Plum F: Cerebral lymphoma and central hyperventilation. *Arch Neurol* 47:10, 1990.
Polinsky RJ: Neuropharmacological investigation of autonomic failure, in Mathias CJ, Bannister R (eds): *Autonomic Failure: A Textbook of Clinical Disorders of the Autonomic Nervous System*, 4th ed. New York, Oxford University Press, 1999, pp 334–358.
Polinsky RJ, Kopin IJ, Ebert MH, Weise V: Pharmacologic distinction of different orthostatic hypotension syndromes. *Neurology* 31:1, 1981.
Polkey MI, Lyall RA, Moxham J, Leigh PN: Respiratory aspects of neurological disease. *J Neurol Neurosurg Psychiatry* 66:5, 1999.
Porter JM, Rivers SP, Anderson CS, Baur GM: Evaluation and management of patients with Raynaud's syndrome. *Am J Surg* 142:183, 1981.
Rhodes RH, Wightman HR: Nucleus of the tractus solitarius metastasis: Relationships to respiratory arrest? *Can J Neurol Sci* 27:328, 2000.
Robinson B, Johnson R, Abernethy D, Holloway L: Familial distal dysautonomia. *J Neurol Neurosurg Psychiatry* 52:1281, 1989.
Ropper AH: Acute autonomic emergencies and autonomic storm, in Low PA (ed): *Clinical Autonomic Disorders*, 2nd ed. Boston, Little, Brown, 1997, pp 791–801.
Ropper AH, Wijdicks WFM, Truax BT: *Guillain-Barré Syndrome*. Philadelphia, Davis, 1991, pp 109–112.
Ruch T: The urinary bladder, in Ruch TC, Patton HD (eds): *Physiology and Biophysics*. Vol 2: Circulation, Respiration, and Fluid Balance. Philadelphia, Saunders, 1974, pp 525–546.
Sakakibara R, Hattori T, Yasuda K, et al: Micturitional disturbance and the pontine tegmental lesion: Urodynamic and MRI analyses of vascular cases. *J Neurol Sci* 141:105, 1996.
Samuels MA: The brain heart connection. *Circulation* 116:77, 2007.
Schobel HP, Fischer T, Heuszer K, et al: Preeclampsia—a state of sympathetic overactivity. *N Engl J Med* 335:1480, 1996.
Schroeder C, Vervino S, Birkenfeld A, et al: Plasma exchange for primary autoimmune autonomic failure. *N Engl J Med* 353:1585, 2005.
Schuster MM: Clinical significance of motor disturbances of the enterocolonic segment. *Am J Dig Dis* 11:320, 1966.
Selye H: The general adaptation syndrome and the diseases of adaptation. *J Clin Endocrinol Metab* 6:117, 1946.
Shannon DC, Marsland DW, Gould JB, et al: Central hypoventilation during quiet sleep in two infants. *Pediatrics* 57:342, 1976.
Shannon JR, Flatem, NL, Jordan J, et al: Orthostatic intolerance and tachycardia associated with norepinephrine-transporter deficiency. *N Engl J Med* 342:541, 2005.
Shy GM, Drager GA: A neurological syndrome associated with orthostatic hypotension: A clinical-pathologic study. *Arch Neurol* 2:511, 1960.
Spokes EGS, Bannister R, Oppenheimer DR: Multiple system atrophy with autonomic failure. *J Neurol Sci* 43:59, 1979.
Tansey EM: Chemical neurotransmission in the autonomic nervous system: Sir Henry Dale and acetylcholine. *Clin Auton Res* 1:63, 1991.
Thompson PD, Melmon KL: Clinical assessment of autonomic function. *Anesthesiology* 29:724, 1968.
Vernino S, Low PA, Fealey RD, et al: Autoantibodies to ganglionic acetylcholine receptors in autoimmune autonomic neuropathies. *N Engl J Med* 343:847, 2000.
Weiss HD: The physiology of human penile erection. *Ann Intern Med* 76:792, 1972.
Westfall TC, Westfall D: Neurotransmission: The autonomic and somatic motor nervous systems, in Hardman JG, Limbird LE (eds): *The Pharmacological Basis of Therapeutics*, 12th ed. New York, McGraw-Hill, 2011, pp 171–218.
Wigley FM: Raynaud's phenomenon. *N Engl J Med* 347:1001, 2002.
Wiles CM: Neurogenic dysphagia. *J Neurol Neurosurg Psychiatry* 54:1037, 1991.
Young RR, Asbury AK, Corbett JL, Adams RD: Pure pandysautonomia with recovery: Description and discussion of diagnostic criteria. *Brain* 98:613, 1975.
Ziegler MG, Lake R, Kopin IJ: The sympathetic nervous system defect in primary orthostatic hypotension. *N Engl J Med* 296:293, 1977.

27

The Hypothalamus and Neuroendocrine Disorders

The hypothalamus plays three roles in the actions of the nervous system. The first, as the "head ganglion" of the autonomic nervous system, was described in the preceding chapter; the second, as the circadian and seasonal clock for behavioral and sleep–wake functions, was considered in Chap. 19 on sleep; and the third, as the neural center of the endocrine system, is the subject of this chapter. In the hypothalamus, these systems are integrated with one another as well as with neocortical, limbic, and spinal influences. Together, they maintain homeostasis and participate in the substructure of emotion and affective behavior.

The expansion of knowledge of neuroendocrinology during the past few decades stands as one of the significant achievements in neurobiology. It has been learned that neurons, in addition to transmitting electrical impulses, can synthesize and secrete complex molecules locally and into the systemic circulation, and that these molecules are capable of activating or inhibiting endocrine, renal, and vascular cells at distant sites.

The concept of neurosecretion probably had its origins in the observations of Speidel, in 1919, who noted that some of the hypothalamic neurons had the morphologic characteristics of glandular cells. Their suggestion that such cells might secrete hormones into the bloodstream was so novel, however, that it was rejected by most biologists at the time. This seems surprising now that neurosecretion is viewed as a fundamental part of the science of endocrinology.

Following these early observations, it was found that peptides secreted by neurons in the central and peripheral nervous systems were also contained in glandular cells of the pancreas, intestines, and heart. This seminal observation was made in 1931 by Euler and Gaddum, who isolated a substance from the intestines that was capable of acting on smooth muscle and called it "P" (from powder). But it was not until some 35 years later that Leeman and her associates purified an 11-amnio-acid peptide that is now called substance P (see Aronin et al). Then followed the discovery of six hypothalamic mediators of anterior pituitary hormone secretion: TRH, and somatostatin 1973, GnRH, CRH, and GHRH. In the background was always dopamine that acted as an inhibitor of pituitary hormone secretion. Subsequently, a number of other neuropeptides including enkephalin, neuropeptide Y, orexin as discussed in Chap. 19.

THE HYPOTHALAMUS

Anatomic Features

The hypothalamus lies on each side of the third ventricle and is continuous across the floor of the ventricle. It is bounded posteriorly by the mammillary bodies, anteriorly by the optic chiasm and lamina terminalis, superiorly by the hypothalamic sulci, laterally by the optic tracts, and inferiorly by the hypophysis. It comprises three main nuclear groups: (1) the anterior group, which includes the preoptic, supraoptic, and paraventricular nuclei; (2) the middle group, which includes the tuberal, arcuate, ventromedial, and dorsomedial nuclei; and (3) the posterior group, comprising the mammillary and posterior hypothalamic nuclei.

Nauta and Haymaker have subdivided the hypothalamus sagittally. The *lateral part* lies lateral to the fornix; it is sparsely cellular and its cell groups are traversed by the medial forebrain bundle—which carries finely myelinated and unmyelinated ascending and descending fibers to and from the rostrally placed septal nuclei, substantia innominata, nucleus accumbens, amygdala, and piriform cortex—and the caudally placed tegmental reticular formation. The *medial hypothalamus* is rich in cells, some of which are the neurosecretory cells for pituitary regulation and visceral control. It contains two main efferent fiber systems—the mammillothalamic tract of Vicq d'Azyr (named for the physician to Louis XIV, a paramour of Marie Antoinette), which connects the mammillary nuclei with the anterior thalamic nucleus (which, in turn, projects to the cingulate gyrus), and the mammillotegmental tract. Additional structures of importance are the stria terminalis, which runs from the amygdala to the ventromedial hypothalamic nucleus, and the fornix, which connects the hippocampus to the mammillary body, septal nuclei, and periventricular parts of the hypothalamus. The lateral and medial parts of the hypothalamus are interconnected and their functions are integrated.

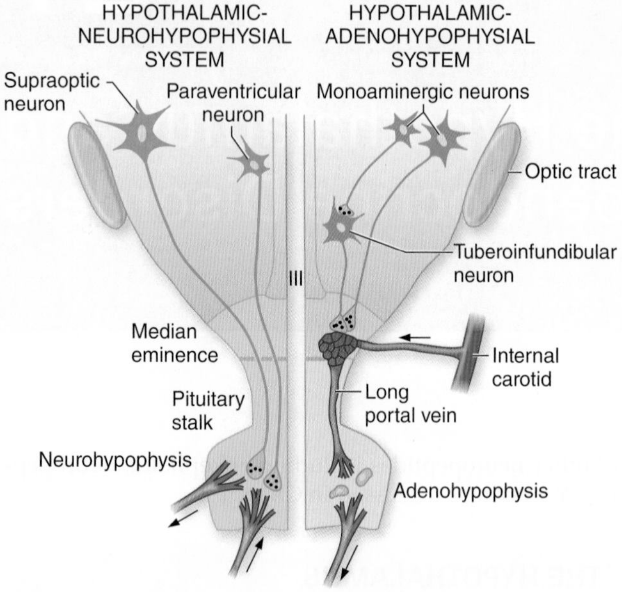

Figure 27-1. Diagram of the hypothalamic–pituitary axis. Indicated on the left is the hypothalamic–neurohypophyseal system, consisting of supraoptic and paraventricular neurons, axons of which terminate on blood vessels in the posterior pituitary (neurohypophysis). The hypothalamic–adenohypophyseal system is illustrated on the right. Tuberoinfundibular neurons, the source of the hypothalamic regulatory hormones, terminate on the capillary plexus in the median eminence. (Courtesy of Dr. J.B. Martin.)

The inferior surface of the hypothalamus bulges downward from the floor of the fourth ventricle; this region is known as the tuber cinereum. The infundibulum is a critical structure that arises from the tuber cinereum. The superior hypophyseal artery, derived from the internal carotid artery, forms a network of capillaries in the *median eminence*, the veins of which are the critical *portal system* (Fig. 27-1).

The median eminence assumes special importance because of the intimate relation of its cells to the vessels of the portal system that bathe the anterior lobe of the pituitary gland. The releasing hormones of the hypothalamus are delivered directly to their target cells in the anterior pituitary via the portal vessels extending through the stalk, thereby avoiding systemic dilution of these factors. In this way the portal system represents the interface between converging pathways from the brain and the pituitary. The tuberoinfundibular neurons of the arcuate nucleus and anterior periventricular nuclei synthesize most of the releasing factors described in Fig. 27-1.

The infundibulum extends into the pituitary stalk, which in turn, enters the neurohypophysis. The infundibulum is a structure that stands out because it contains the median eminence as well as the neurohypophyseal fibers, containing vasopressin and oxytocin, which course through the infundibulum on their way to the posterior pituitary. The main blood supply to the posterior pituitary is from the inferior hypophyseal artery that is a branch of the cavernous part of the internal carotid artery.

The abundant blood supply of the hypothalamus (from several feeding arteries) is of importance to neurosurgeons who attempt to obliterate aneurysms that derive from adjacent vessels. Many small radicles, arising, not just from the carotid arteries, but also the posterior and anterior communicating arteries as well as from the most proximal portions of the anterior and posterior cerebral arteries, form a network of such redundancy that infarction of the hypothalamus is infrequent. The venous drainage from the portal system is to the petrosal sinus, where hormone levels can be sampled.

Readers requiring a more extensive source of information on anatomic and other aspects of the hypothalamus are directed to the comprehensive material by Swaab in the two-volumes of the *Handbook of Clinical Neurology* devoted to this subject, and to the monograph by Martin and Reichlin.

The Hypothalamic-Releasing Hormones
(Table 27-1)

Thyrotropin-Releasing Hormone (TRH)

This was the first of the releasing hormones to be identified; its tripeptide structure was determined in 1968. The hormone is elaborated by the anterior periventricular, paraventricular, arcuate, ventromedial, and dorsomedial

Table 27-1
ANTERIOR PITUITARY HORMONES

HORMONE	TARGET GLAND	SECRETORY CELL DESIGNATION	AMINO ACIDS	NORMAL RANGE
Growth hormone (GH)	Liver, other organs	Somatotrope	191	<0.5 μg/L per 24 h
ACTH[a]	Adrenal	Coritcotrope	39	4–22 pg/L
Prolactin (PRL)	Breast, other tissues	Lactotrope	199	M <15 μg/L; F <20 μg/L
Thyroid-stimulating hormone (TSH)	Thyroid	Thyrotrope	211	0.1–0.5 mU/L
FSH and LH[b]	Ovary, testes	Gonadotrope	210; 201	M 5–20 IU/L; F 2–20 IU/L (basal level)

[a]Adrenocorticotropic hormone.
[b]Follicle-stimulating hormone (FSH) and luteinizing hormone (LH).
IU, international units.
For tests of pituitary sufficiency, see Table 31-4 and Melmed S, Jameson JL: Disorders of the anterior pituitary and hypothalamus, in Longo DL, Fauci AS, Kasper DL et al (eds): *Harrison's Principles of Internal Medicine,* 18th ed. New York, McGraw-Hill, 2012, Table 339-3, p. 2881.

neurons, but not by those of the posterior hypothalamic or thalamic nuclei. It stimulates the release of thyroid-stimulating hormone (TSH) from the pituitary gland. TSH, in turn, increases the activity of every step of the synthesis of thyroid hormone and stimulates the release of T_4 (thyroxine) and T_3 (triiodothyronine). Pituitary cells that release dopamine and somatostatin are also stimulated to a slight degree; the latter has an inhibitory effect on TSH. There is also an inhibitory feedback of T_3 on TSH and TRH. Actually, more than half of brain TRH is found outside the hypothalamus—in brainstem raphe nuclei, tractus solitarius, and the anterior and lateral horn cells of spinal cord—suggesting that TRH may function as a central regulator of the autonomic nervous system.

Growth Hormone-Releasing Hormone (GHRH)

This hormone and somatostatin (also known as growth hormone release-inhibiting hormone, or SRIH) are both secreted by specialized tuberoinfundibular neurons and released into the hypophyseal–portal circulation, by which they are carried to specific growth hormone (GH) secreting cells of the anterior pituitary gland (somatotropes). Immunohistochemical staining has shown the sources of GHRH and somatostatin to be neurons of the posterior part of the arcuate and ventromedian hypothalamic nuclei and other neurons of the median eminence and premammillary area. Somatostatin, a 14-amino-acid peptide, is produced more anteriorly by neurons in the periventricular area and small cell part of the paraventricular nucleus. The amygdala, hippocampus, and other limbic structures project to the arcuate nuclei via the medial corticohypothalamic tract (in the stria terminalis) and are believed to account for the sleep- and stress-induced fluctuations of GH and somatostatin. Also, it has been demonstrated that all 4 biogenic amines (dopamine, norepinephrine, epinephrine, and serotonin) influence GH regulation, as does acetylcholine, either by direct action on pituitary somatotropic cells or on hypothalamic regulatory neurons. TRH also increases GH from somatotropes. Many of the latter pituitary cells contain large eosinophilic granules, but others, previously identified incorrectly as chromophobe cells, also contain GH. Somatomedin C, a basic peptide that is synthesized in the liver, exerts feedback control of GH by inhibiting the pituitary somatotropes and stimulating the release of somatostatin. Growth hormone enhances skeletal growth by stimulating the proliferation of cartilage and growth of muscle. It also regulates lipolysis, stimulates the uptake of amino acids in cells, and has anti-insulin effects. The blood concentrations of GH fluctuate from 1 or 2 ng/mL to more than 60 ng/mL, being highest within the first hour or two after the onset of sleep.

Corticotropin-Releasing Hormone (CRH)

This hormone, a 14-amino-acid peptide, acts synergistically with vasopressin to release adrenocorticotropic hormone (ACTH) from basophilic cells in the pituitary. ACTH stimulates the synthesis and release of the hormones of the adrenal cortex, mainly glucocorticoids (cortisol or hydrocortisone) but also mineralocorticoids (aldosterone) and androcorticoids (converted in the tissues to testosterone). The neurons of origin of CRH lie in a particular part of the paraventricular nucleus, other cells of which form the paraventricular–supraopticohypophysial tract (neurohypophysis) and elaborate vasopressin, oxytocin, and several other substances (neurotensin, dynorphin, vasoactive intestinal peptide). These hypothalamic cells receive an extensive input from other regions of the nervous system, particularly via the noradrenergic pathways (from reticular neurons in the medulla and those of the locus ceruleus and tractus solitarius) and from many of the limbic structures. Presumably, these extrahypothalamic connections provide the mechanism by which stress and pain activate the secretion of ACTH and cortisol. CRH itself is widely distributed in the brain. There is feedback control of CRH and ACTH via glucocorticoid receptors in the hypothalamus and anterior lobe of the pituitary. Serotonin and acetylcholine enhance ACTH secretion, whereas the catecholamines are inhibitory.

Gonadotropin-Releasing Hormone (GnRH)

This 10-amino-acid peptide originates in the arcuate nucleus and is present in highest concentration near the median eminence. It effects the release of the two gonadotropic hormones—luteinizing hormone (LH) and follicle-stimulating hormone (FSH). The ovary and testis, by secreting a peptide called *inhibin*, are able to suppress FSH, as do gonadal steroids—i.e., estrogens. GnRH is under the influence of other neuronal systems, which are modulated by catecholamines, serotonin, acetylcholine, and dopamine. Puberty, menstruation, ovulation, lactation, and menopause are all related to the effects of GnRH, FSH, and LH on the ovaries, uterus, breasts, and testes. Normal levels of blood FSH are 2.5 to 4.9 ng/mL in prepuberty and 7.5 to 11 ng/mL in the adult; levels of blood LH are 2.8 to 9.6 ng/mL in prepuberty and 10 to 18 ng/mL in the adult.

Prolactin Inhibition (Dopamine)

Dopamine is released by neurons in the region of the arcuate nucleus and inhibits lactotrophic cells of the anterior pituitary. The hypothalamopituitary axis is responsive to sensory stimuli from the nipples, via pathways in the spinal cord and brainstem, accounting for the effect of suckling on milk production. Nipple stimulation is also an important influence on oxytocin secretion, as described later. The normal blood levels of prolactin are 5 to 25 ng/mL.

This inhibitory action of dopamine on prolactin secretion accounts for galactorrhea and reproductive disorders, which occur with tumors that compress the pituitary stalk. These interrupt the venous portal transport of dopamine from the hypothalamus to the dopamine-sensitive lactotrophs in the pituitary. This mechanism also explains galactorrhea following the administration of dopamine-blocking medications such as Haldol.

The Neurohypophysis: Vasopressin and Oxytocin

The oligopeptides *vasopressin* and *oxytocin* are elaborated by cells of the supraoptic and paraventricular nuclei and are transported, via their axons, through the stalk of the pituitary to its posterior lobe, where these substances are stored. Together, these elements constitute the neurohypophysis (posterior pituitary), which develops as an evagination of the floor of the third ventricle. Some of the vasopressin-containing nerve endings also terminate on cells of origin of the autonomic nervous system and on the capillary plexus of the hypophyseal portal circulation, through which they influence the secretion of CRH and GH. The delivery to the posterior pituitary of oxytocin and vasopressin is therefore through the nerve endings that originate in the hypothalamus and terminate in the neurohypophysis. There is some influence of anterior pituitary hormones. The peptide parts of vasopressin and oxytocin, whose chemical nature was determined by DuVigneaud, are almost identical, differing from one another by only two amino acids.

Vasopressin, acting on the V2 receptors in kidney tubules, serves as the antidiuretic hormone (ADH) and, complemented by thirst mechanisms, maintains the osmolality of the blood. Plasma osmolality modifies vasopressin secretion by acting directly on the supraoptic and paraventricular neurons or on separate osmoreceptors in the hypothalamus. The sensitivity of the vasopressin–ADH mechanism is demonstrated by the absence of antidiuretic effect when vasopressin is below 1 pg/mL and by maximal antidiuresis when plasma levels reach 5 pg/mL. If serum osmolality falls below 280 mOsm/L, the release of ADH is completely inhibited. This system is most effective in maintaining homeostasis when serum osmolality is relatively close to the normal range, between 280 and 295 mOsm/L.

Alterations in blood volume and pressure also affect vasopressin release through neural mechanisms that have their origin in baro- and mechanoreceptors of the aortic arch, carotid sinus, and right atrium. Afferent signals from these regions are conveyed in the vagus and glossopharyngeal nerves, which synapse in the nucleus of the tractus solitarius; the precise pathways to the hypothalamus have not been delineated, however. With severe hypotension, ADH release will continue even if there is a low serum osmolality, i.e., pressure predominates over osmolarity as a stimulus. Vasopressin secretion is also influenced by nonosmotic factors. Nausea, for example, is a potent stimulus, raising levels of the hormone 100-fold. Hypoglycemia has a less-profound effect. Drugs such as morphine, nicotine, alcohol, and certain chemotherapeutic agents (cyclophosphamide) also cause release of the stored peptide. Pain, emotional stress, and exercise have long been thought to cause release of vasopressin, but it is unclear whether this is a direct effect or is mediated through hypotension or nausea.

Oxytocin initiates uterine contraction and has milk-ejecting effects. Its release is stimulated by distention of the cervix, labor, breastfeeding, and estrogen. The effects of oxytocin are inhibited by alcohol.

In summary, it is apparent that the regulatory system of hypothalamic-releasing hormones is complex. The releasing factors have overlapping functions, and the hypothalamic nuclei act on many parts of the brain in addition to the pituitary. Conversely, many parts of the brain influence the hypothalamus through neural connections or modulate its activity and that of the pituitary gland through the action of neurotransmitters and modulators (catecholamines, acetylcholine, serotonin, and dopamine). There is feedback control between every part of the hypothalamus and the endocrine structures on which it acts. The factors that influence hypothalamic neurons have been reviewed in detail by Reichlin. Some of these relationships have been mentioned and others will emerge further on in this chapter and in later chapters, particularly as they relate to behavioral and psychiatric disorders.

Of particular significance is the role of the hypothalamus in the integration of the endocrine and autonomic nervous systems at both the peripheral and central levels. The best-known example of this interaction is in the adrenal medulla, as indicated in Chap. 26. Similarly, the juxtaglomerular apparatus of the kidney and the islets of Langerhans of the pancreas function as neuroendocrine transducers, in that they convert a neural stimulus (in these cases adrenergic) to an endocrine secretion (renin from the kidney and glucagon and insulin from the islet cells).

Role of the Hypothalamus in Sexual Development (See also Chap. 28)

The hypothalamus also plays a critical role in the development of human sexuality and its expression, a theme elaborated in the next chapter. The suprachiasmatic nucleus and the number of neurons it contains are considerably larger in men than in women, a dimorphism that becomes evident during postnatal development. The interstitial nucleus of the hypothalamus is reportedly smaller in the homosexual male, evidence perhaps that homosexuality has a recognizable morphologic basis (Levay). This biologic evidence has been sharply challenged (Byne). These issues are addressed further in the section on sexual development in Chap. 28. The intimate relationship of the hypothalamus with the development of sexual characteristics at all stages of life is shown by the appearance, in the infundibular area, of hypertrophic neurons that are rich in estrogen receptors; it has been proposed that some of the symptoms of menarche are timed and mediated by these hypothalamic neurons. With aging, and more so in Alzheimer disease, the neuronal population in this region decreases markedly; the sleep disturbances of senescence and some aspects of the "sundowning" syndrome (confusion and delirium occurring in the evening) have also been attributed to this cell loss.

Regulation of Sympathetic and Parasympathetic Activity

Finally, the central role of the hypothalamus in the regulation of both sympathetic and parasympathetic activities must be emphasized. This aspect of hypothalamic function is discussed in the preceding chapter.

The Pineal Gland and Melatonin

The pineal gland, or pineal body, is a small glandular structure (about 9 mm in diameter) that projects from the dorsal diencephalon and lies just posterior to the third ventricle. In the past, the pineal body figured prominently in philosophic and religious writings; for Descartes, it was the seat of the soul. When this idea was discredited, the pineal gland was relegated to the status of a vestigial organ. The identification of melatonin, the pineal hormone—followed by recognition of its role in maintaining biologic rhythms and the modulating effects on its secretion by the circadian light–dark cycle—revived scientific interest in the structure. Even though the hormone was found to have an indirect effect on several other neuroendocrine systems, neurologists took little interest in pineal function because ablation of the gland in humans, with attendant loss of most of its circulating melatonin, leads to few if any clinical changes.

It is the cyclic secretion of melatonin that appears to be the most important activity of the pineal gland. However, melatonin secretion is more accurately regarded as a linked manifestation of the circadian rhythm than as its controlling mechanism. The main cellular element of the gland, the pinealocyte, is thought to be derived from neural photoreceptors in lower vertebrates. The latter cells, structurally analogous to retinal cones, transduce light directly into neural impulses and are among the mechanisms for circadian entrainment of hormonal rhythms. In humans, the pineal no longer possesses the ability to transduce light directly. However, it does retain an input from photic stimuli and influences the circadian light–dark cycle through a pathway that originates in the retina, synapses in the suprachiasmatic nucleus, passes through descending sympathetic tracts to the intermediolateral cell columns and superior cervical ganglia, and then ascends to innervate noradrenergic terminals on the pinealocytes. Darkness elicits a release of norepinephrine from the photoreceptors, stimulating the synthesis and release of melatonin. During daylight the retinal photoreceptor cells are hyperpolarized, norepinephrine release is inhibited, and there is little melatonin production. The concentration of the hormone peaks between 2 and 4 A.M. and gradually falls thereafter. An approximate circadian rhythmicity to melatonin release is preserved in continuous darkness and, inexplicably, the blind maintain a light suppression of secretion. It is readily appreciated that, in humans, it is difficult to separate the changes that occur in the suprachiasmatic nucleus from those of the pineal gland.

Like other neuroendocrine cells, pinealocytes release peptides that are produced in the Golgi apparatus and packaged in secretory granules. Whether secretion is the main mechanism for melatonin release is unclear, as these cells can use an alternative ependymal type of vacuolar secretion. The entire gland is invested by a rich vasculature to receive the released peptide (in some mammals the blood flow per gram of pineal tissue is surpassed only by that of the kidney). The biochemistry and physiology of melatonin have been extensively reviewed by Brzezinski.

In humans, a regular feature of pineal pathology is the accumulation of calcareous deposits in structures termed *acervuli* ("brain sand"). These have a more complex composition than simply calcium; they are actually composed of carbonate-containing hydroxyapatite that is linked to calcium and other metals. A review of the mineralization of the pineal can be found in the text by Haymaker and Adams. These concretions are formed within vacuoles of pinealocytes and released into the extracellular space. The mineralization of the pineal body provides a convenient marker for its position in plain films and on various imaging studies.

It is of significance that pineal tumors do not secrete melatonin, but the loss of melatonin may be used as a marker for the completeness of surgical pinealectomy. Most interest in the past several years has centered on melatonin as a soporific agent and its potential to reset sleep rhythms. Its concentration in depressive illnesses, especially in the affected elderly, is also decreased. The subject of pineal tumors is discussed later and is contained in Chap. 31, with discussion of other brain tumors.

HYPOTHALAMIC SYNDROMES

Hypothalamic syndromes are of two distinct types (Martin and Reichlin). In one, all or many hypothalamic functions are disordered, often in combination with signs of disease in contiguous structures ("global hypothalamic syndromes," as described below). The second type is characterized by a selective loss of hypothalamic–hypophyseal function, attributable to a discrete lesion of the hypothalamus and often resulting in a deficiency or overproduction of a single hormone—*a partial hypothalamic syndrome.*

Global Hypothalamic Syndromes

A variety of lesions can invade and destroy all or a large part of the hypothalamus. These include sarcoid and other granulomatous diseases, an idiopathic inflammatory disease, and germ-cell and other tumors. The hypothalamus is involved in approximately 5 percent of cases of sarcoidosis, sometimes as the primary manifestation of the disease, but more often in combination with facial palsy and hilar lymphadenopathy. The lesion may be visible by MRI (see Fig. 32-2).

Tumors that involve the hypothalamopituitary axis include metastatic carcinoma, lymphoma, craniopharyngioma, and a variety of germ-cell tumors. The last category (reviewed by Jennings et al) includes germinomas, teratomas, embryonal carcinoma, and choriocarcinoma. They develop during childhood, tend to invade the posterior hypothalamus, and are accompanied in some instances by an increase in serum alpha-fetoprotein or the beta subunit of chorionic gonadotropin. A unique syndrome of gelastic epilepsy is caused by a hamartoma of the hypothalamus (see Chap. 16).

Among the inflammatory conditions, infundibuloneurohypophysitis, or *infundibulitis*, is a cryptogenic inflammation of the neurohypophysis and pituitary stalk, with thickening of these parts by infiltrates of lymphocytes (mainly T cells) and plasma cells (Imura et al). It is thought to be an autoimmune disorder. Histiocytosis X—a group of diseases comprising Letterer-Siwe disease, Hand-Schüller-Christian disease, and eosinophilic granuloma—implicates multiple organs, including the hypothalamus and neighboring structures and leptomeninges (often causing cells to appear in the cerebrospinal fluid [CSF]). These conditions of children pursue an indolent course. The cell type is a proliferating histiocyte. The obscure infiltrative and inflammatory condition, Erdheim-Chester disease, can also involve this region sometimes with proptosis, but is primarily a bone disease.

Partial Hypothalamic Syndromes

Diabetes Insipidus (DI)

This is a state of polyuria with dilute urine and polydipsia that results in the loss of action of antidiuretic hormone. As long ago as 1913, Farini of Venice and von den Velden of Dusseldorf (quoted by Martin and Reichlin) independently discovered that diabetes insipidus was associated with destructive lesions of the hypothalamus. They showed, moreover, that in patients with this disorder, the polyuria could be corrected by injections of extracts of the posterior pituitary. Ranson elucidated the anatomy of the neurohypophysis; the Scharrers traced the posterior pituitary secretion to granules in the cells of the supraoptic and paraventricular nuclei and followed their passage to axon terminals in the posterior lobe of the pituitary. As mentioned in the introductory section, DuVigneaud and colleagues determined the chemical structure of the two neurohypophyseal peptides, vasopressin and oxytocin, of which these granules were composed.

As already stated, the usual cause of DI is a lack of vasopressin (ADH) as a result of a lesion of the neurohypophysis. This leads to a reduction in its action in the kidneys, where it normally promotes the absorption of water. As a consequence, there is diuresis of low-osmolar urine (polyuria), reduction in blood volume, and increased thirst and drinking of water (polydipsia) in an attempt to maintain osmolality. A congenital abnormality of renal tubular epithelium or destruction of the epithelium has a similar effect—nephrogenic DI. DI is also of interest to the neurologist because of its association with lithium toxicity, which impairs renal tubular water absorption.

Among the established *causes of acquired DI*, the most important are brain tumors, infiltrative granulomatous diseases, head injury, and intracranial surgical trauma (which has become less frequent with the transsphenoidal approach to pituitary tumors). In a series of 135 cases of persistent DI reported by Moses and Stretten, 25 percent were idiopathic, 15 percent complicated primary brain tumors, 24 percent were postoperative (mostly after hypophysectomy or surgery for craniopharyngioma), 18 percent were caused by head trauma, and fewer than 10 percent were associated with intracranial histiocytosis, metastatic cancer, sarcoidosis, and ruptured aneurysm. Granulomatous infiltration of the base of the brain by sarcoid, eosinophilic granuloma, Letterer-Siwe disease, or Hand-Schüller-Christian disease, is a more frequent cause of DI in young patients. Of the primary tumors, glioma, hamartoma and craniopharyngioma, granular cell tumor (choristoma), large chromophobe adenomas, and pinealoma are notable. The primary tumors can present with DI alone, whereas the granulomatous infiltrating processes generally exhibit other systemic manifestations before polydipsia and polyuria appear. Metastatic tumors originating in the lung or breast or leukemic and lymphomatous infiltration may also cause DI, sometimes in conjunction with pituitary disturbances and impairment of vision. The mild global hypothalamic dysfunction that often follows brain irradiation for glioma may occasionally include DI as a feature. The most extreme cases of hypothalamic destruction occur in brain death, in which DI is a regular component, although it is not always evident at the time brainstem reflexes are lost.

Pituitary tumors are infrequently associated with DI unless they become massive and invade the stalk of the pituitary and the infundibulum. This anatomic relationship was substantiated in past years by surgical sections of the stalk for metastatic carcinoma and for retinitis proliferans, which result in DI only if the section is high enough to produce retrograde degeneration of supraoptic neurons.

Among the idiopathic forms of DI, there also exists a *congenital type of hypothalamic DI*, of which only a small number of familial cases have been described. The disorder is evident at an early age and persists throughout life owing to a developmental defect of the supraoptic and paraventricular nuclei and smallness of the posterior lobe of the pituitary. This defect has been related in some cases to a point mutation in the vasopressin-neurophysin-glycopeptide gene. It may be combined with other genetic disorders such as diabetes mellitus, optic atrophy, deafness (Wolfram syndrome), and Friedreich ataxia.

Acquired idiopathic DI may occur at any age, most often in childhood or early adult life and more often in males, and by definition has no apparent cause. Other signs of hypothalamic or pituitary disease are lacking in 80 percent of such patients, but steps must be taken to exclude other disease processes by repeating endocrine and radiologic studies periodically. In some cases of idiopathic DI, there are serum antibodies that react with the supraoptic neurons, raising the question of an autoimmune disorder. In a few such instances, postmortem examination has disclosed a decreased number of neurons in the supraoptic and paraventricular nuclei. Also, anorexia nervosa is often associated with mild DI.

Finally, it should be mentioned that certain drugs used in neurologic practice—for example, carbamazepine—may be the cause of reversible DI (excessive secretion of ADH is more common in relation to this drug) and, as mentioned, lithium regularly causes DI, even at times at the upper range of its therapeutic serum concentration.

In all these conditions, the severity and permanence of the DI are determined by the nature of the lesion. In cases of acute onset, three phases have been delineated: First, a severe DI lasting days; then, as the neurohypophysis degenerates, a reduction in severity of DI or even the opposite, hyponatremia from excessive hormone, as a result of the release of stored ADH and, finally, a persistent pattern, usually lifelong. The neurohypophyseal axons can regenerate, allowing for some degree of recovery even after years.

Diagnosis of Diabetes Insipidus This is always suggested by the passage of large quantities of dilute urine accompanied by polydipsia and polyuria lasting throughout the night. The thirst mechanism and drinking usually prevent dehydration and hypovolemia, but if the patient is stuporous or the thirst mechanism is inoperative, severe dehydration and hypernatremia can occur, leading to coma, seizures, and death. In an unresponsive patient careful measurement of fluid output and input are needed to expose the disorder.

A low urine osmolality and specific gravity are found in DI, in conjunction with high serum osmolality and sodium values. Osmotic dehydration as a cause of the polydipsia–polyuria syndrome, such as occurs with the glycosuria of diabetes mellitus must, of course, be excluded. A period of 6 to 8 h of dehydration increases urinary osmolality in a person with normal kidneys and neurohypophysis; it is this change in urine concentration that is most useful in the differential diagnosis of polyuria, particularly in distinguishing compulsive water drinkers from those with DI; in the latter group, urinary volume and serum electrolytes normalize with dehydration. Proof that the patient has a central cause of DI and not nephrogenic unresponsiveness to vasopressin is obtained by injecting 5 U of vasopressin (Pitressin) subcutaneously; this will diminish urine output and increase osmolality when there is a central cause of DI. Diagnosis is also aided by the radioimmunoassay for plasma ADH; ADH is usually reduced to less than 1.0 pg/mL in patients with central DI (normal: 1.4 to 2.7 pg/mL).

Treatment of Diabetes Insipidus Vasopressin tannate in oil, synthetic vasopressin nasal spray, and a long-acting analogue of arginine vasopressin (desmopressin [DDAVP]) administered by nasal insufflation (10 to 20 mg or 0.1 to 0.2 mL) are used to control chronic DI. The nasal form is generally preferred because of its long antidiuretic action and few side effects. In unconscious patients, aqueous vasopressin, 5 to 10 U given subcutaneously, is effective for 3 to 6 h; DDAVP, 1 to 4 mg subcutaneously, is effective for 12 to 24 h. These drugs must be given repeatedly, guided by urine output and osmolality (we have given these drugs intravenously in critical situations). The brief duration of action of the medication is advantageous in postoperative states and after head injury, for it allows the recognition of recovery of neurohypophyseal function and the avoidance of water intoxication. If a longer duration of treatment is anticipated, one uses vasopressin tannate in oil (2.5 U), the action of which persists for 24 to 72 h. In the unconscious patient, great care must be taken in the acute stages to replace the fluid lost in the urine, but not to the point of water intoxication. These problems can be avoided by matching the amount of intravenous fluids to the urinary volume and by evaluating serum and urine osmolalities every 8 to 12 h. This pertains even if a patient is receiving concurrent ADH analogues. For patients with partial preservation of ADH function, chlorpropamide, clofibrate, or carbamazepine can be used to stimulate release of the hormone.

Syndrome of Inappropriate Antidiuretic Hormone Secretion

As mentioned, blood volume and osmolality are normally maintained within narrow limits by the secretion of ADH and the thirst mechanism. A reduction in osmolality of even 1 percent stimulates osmoreceptors in the hypothalamus to decrease ADH and to suppress thirst and drinking; increased osmolality and reduced blood volume do the opposite. Normally, blood osmolality is about 282 mmol/kg and is maintained within a very narrow range. Release of ADH begins when osmolality reaches 287 mmol/kg (the "osmotic threshold"). At this point, plasma ADH levels are 2 pg/mL and increase rapidly as the osmolality rises. The response of ADH secretion to hyperosmolality is not the same for all plasma solutes; in contrast to hypernatremia, for example, hyperosmolality induced by elevations in urea nitrogen or endogenous glucose produce minimal or no elevations in ADH.

Derangement of this delicately regulated mechanism, taking the form of dilutional hyponatremia and water retention without edema, is observed under a variety of clinical circumstances in which the plasma ADH is above normal or inappropriately normal despite plasma hypoosmolality. The term *inappropriate secretion of antidiuretic hormone* (SIADH) was applied to this syndrome by Schwartz and Bartter because of its similarity to that produced in animals by the chronic administration of ADH. The same syndrome can arise from ectopic production of the hormone by tumor tissue. In such cases, the thirst mechanism is not inhibited by decreased osmolality, and continued drinking further increases blood volume and reduces its solute concentration; ADH levels are found to be persistently elevated. The physiologic hallmarks of this condition are a concentrated urine, usually with an osmolality above 300 mOsm/L, and low serum osmolality and sodium concentrations. Because of the dilutional effects, urea nitrogen and uric acid are reduced in the blood and serve as markers for excessive total body water. Tissue edema is not seen because sodium excretion in the urine is maintained by suppression of the renin–angiotensin system and by an increase in atrial natriuretic peptide secretion (see below).

SIADH is observed frequently with a variety of cerebral lesions (infarct, tumor, hemorrhage, meningitis, encephalitis) that do not involve the hypothalamus directly and with many types of local hypothalamic diseases (trauma, surgery, vascular lesions). In most cases, it tends to be a transient feature of the underlying illness. The acute dysautonomia of Guillain-Barré syndrome is a common neurologic cause of SIADH; it is ostensibly the result of the neuropathy affecting the afferent nerves from volume receptors in the right atrium and jugular veins. (Hyponatremia is particularly likely to occur in such patients on positive-pressure ventilation.) The increased thoracic pressure induced by positive-pressure ventilation promotes SIADH in susceptible patients. Acute porphyric episodes have the same effect. Neoplasms, particularly small cell tumors, and sometimes inflammatory lesions of the lung, may elaborate an ADH-like substance, and certain drugs—such as carbamazepine, chlorpromazine, chlorothiazide, chlorpropamide, clofibrate, nonsteroidal antiinflammatory agents, and vincristine—also stimulate ADH release and may lead to hyponatremia. In some cases, no cause or associated disease is apparent.

A fall in serum sodium to 125 mEq/L usually has few clinical effects, although signs of an associated neurologic disease, such as a previous stroke or a subdural hematoma, may worsen. Sodium levels of less than 120 mEq/L are attended by nausea and vomiting, inattentiveness, drowsiness, stupor, and generalized seizures. There may be asterixis. As is characteristic of most metabolic encephalopathies, the more rapid the decline of the serum sodium, the more likely there will be accompanying neurologic symptoms.

Treatment of SIADH The rapid restitution of serum sodium to normal or above-normal levels carries a risk of producing an osmotic demyelination (also called central pontine myelinolysis; see Chap. 40). Our usual procedure in patients with serum sodium concentrations of 117 to 125 mEq/L is to slowly correct the sodium concentration by restricting water to 400 to 800 mL/d and to verify the desired urinary loss of water by checking the patient's weight and serum sodium until it reaches approximately 130 mEq/L. If there is drowsiness, confusion, or seizures that cannot be confidently attributed to the underlying neurologic illness, or if the serum sodium is in the range of 100 to 115 mEq/L, isotonic or 3 percent NaCl should be infused over 3 to 4 h and furosemide 20 to 40 mg administered to prevent fluid overload. A safe clinical rule is to raise the serum sodium by no more than 12 mEq/L in the first 24 h and by no more than 20 mEq/L in 48 h so as to prevent myelinolysis.

Neurogenic (Cerebral) Salt Wasting (Nelson Syndrome)

A moderate reduction in the serum sodium concentration is a common finding in patients with acute intracranial diseases and postoperatively in neurosurgical patients. Originally it was described as a "cerebral salt-wasting" syndrome by Peters and colleagues and later was erroneously identified with the then newly described Schwartz-Bartter syndrome of SIADH. In recent years it has again come to be recognized as being a result of natriuresis and not of water retention caused by ADH secretion. As Nelson and colleagues demonstrated many years ago, neurosurgical patients with hyponatremia have a reduction in blood volume, suggesting sodium loss rather than water retention. This distinction has important clinical implications because the use of fluid restriction with the intention to treat SIADH can have disastrous results if a state of volume contraction exists from salt wasting.

One leading hypothesis concerning the mechanism of hyponatremia in these cases is secretion of another oligopeptide, atrial natriuretic factor (ANF) that is found mainly in the walls of the cardiac atria but also in neurons surrounding the third ventricle in the anteroventral hypothalamic region. Physiologically, ANF activity opposes that of ADH in the kidney tubules and also has a potent inhibitory effect on ADH release from the hypothalamus; i.e., it causes a natriuresis (see review by Samson). ANF, like some other neural peptides, is secreted in bursts, and the natriuresis is evident only if total urinary sodium content is measured over many hours or days.

The role of ANF in causing the hyponatremia that follows subarachnoid hemorrhage is controversial (see Wijdicks et al and Diringer et al for opposing views), but it is our experience that the hyponatremia in this condition is the result mainly of salt loss, not water retention. Because fluid restriction after subarachnoid hemorrhage may precipitate cerebral ischemia from vasospasm, the proper approach is to maintain normal intravascular volume with intravenous fluids and to correct hyponatremia by infusion of normal saline.

In addition to head trauma, salt wasting has also been reported with cerebral tumors, after pituitary surgery, and in the dysautonomia of Guillain-Barré syndrome, conditions that have also been associated at times with SIADH. As already stated, in each of these disorders, should the patient be hyponatremic, it is desirable to determine the intravascular volume and the urine sodium output before instituting treatment.

Other Disturbances of Antidiuretic Hormone and Thirst

Conditions have been described in which the osmoreceptor control of ADH and of thirst appear to be dissociated. As reported by Hayes and coworkers, one of our colleagues' patients repeatedly developed severe hypernatremia (levels as high as 180 to 190 mEq/L), at which time he became confused and stuporous. Although the patient was able to initiate a release of ADH, his thirst mechanism was nonfunctional. Only when the patient was compelled to drink water at regular intervals did his serum sodium fall. Robertson and others have described similar cases with abnormalities of thirst. These have been reported under the title of "central" or "essential" hypernatremia.

Pituitary Insufficiency

Loss of function of the anterior pituitary gland may result from disease of the pituitary itself or from hypothalamic disease. In either event, it leads to a number of clinical abnormalities, each predicated on the deficiency of one or more hormones that depend on the pituitary trophic factors described earlier. The condition of *panhypopituitarism* represents the more serious illness in that it requires supplementation with multiple hormones. Hypopituitarism may have its onset in childhood, either as an inherited process that affects individual or multiple hormones or as a secondary process caused by a destructive lesion of the pituitary or the hypothalamus from tumor, e.g., craniopharyngioma. Later in life the causes vary, but the most common are pituitary surgery, infarct of the gland from a rapidly growing adenoma (*pituitary apoplexy*, see "Pituitary Apoplexy" in Chap. 31), involutional changes that occur at the end of pregnancy (Sheehan syndrome), cranial irradiation for cerebral tumors other than those in the pituitary fossa, lymphocytic hypophysitis, and granulomatous and neoplastic invasion.

The clinical features of pituitary failure vary, but impairments of thyroid function tend to be more prominent than those of adrenal failure. The neurologic accompaniments of pituitary failure depend on the underlying cause; Lamberts and colleagues have reviewed the endocrinologic aspects and a detailed discussion can be found in *Harrison's Principles of Internal Medicine*.

Other Hypothalamic Syndromes

Apart from DI and SIADH, there are a variety of other special clinical phenomena resulting from disease of the hypothalamus. These usually occur not in isolation but in various combinations, comprising a number of rare, but well-characterized, syndromes.

Precocious Puberty

This term refers to the abnormally early onset of androgen secretion and spermatogenesis in boys and of estrogen secretion and cyclic ovarian secretion in girls. It is associated with the premature development of secondary sexual characteristics. The occurrence of precocious puberty always calls for a neurologic as well as an endocrine investigation. In the male, one searches for evidence of a teratoma of the pineal gland or mediastinum or an androgenic tumor of the testes or adrenals. In the female with early development of secondary sexual characteristics and menstruation, one seeks other evidence of hypothalamic disease, as well as an estrogen-secreting ovarian tumor.

A hamartoma of the hypothalamus (part of von Recklinghausen disease, or of polyostotic fibrous dysplasia of McCune-Albright syndrome) is a leading cause of precocious puberty in both boys and girls; in a number of such cases, so-called *gelastic seizures* have been conjoined (Breningstall, see "Complex Partial Seizures" in Chap. 16). Neurologic study entails CT and MRI imaging of the hypothalamus, ovaries, and adrenals.

Failure of Puberty

Several genetic conditions can lead to failure of puberty. *Kallman syndrome* is a type of hypogonadotropic hypogonadism that is associated with anosmia. GnRH-secreting neurons formed in the olfactory placode migrate across the cribriform plate into the olfactory bulb and ultimately reside in the hypothalamus. In Kallman syndrome, the olfactory bulb does not develop normally, leading to loss of hypothalamic control of FSH and LH release, and failure of puberty to initiate, as well as anosmia. Several causative X-linked and autosomal dominant gene mutations have been discovered.

Prader-Willi syndrome, discussed in Chap. 38, is associated with hypogonadism and incomplete sexual development along with other endocrine abnormalities affecting growth and satiety. The *Bardet-Biedl syndrome* is a heterogenous disorder affecting multiple organ systems. Variable growth retardation, obesity, and diabetes mellitus are seen, along with hypogonadism and anosmia. The causative mutations affect ciliary function at several sites.

Adiposogenital Dystrophy (Froehlich Syndrome)

Under this title, in 1901, Froehlich first described the association of obesity and gonadal underdevelopment. He related the disorder to a pituitary tumor. But a few years later, Erdheim recognized that the same syndrome could be a manifestation of a lesion (a suprasellar cyst in his case) involving or restricted to the hypothalamus. Later it was determined that obesity and hypogonadism could occur together or separately and were often combined with a loss of vision and unprovoked rage, aggression, or antisocial behavior. DI may be added. In some patients, the clinical state is characterized by abulia, apathy, and reduced verbal output. The usual causes of the Froehlich syndrome are craniopharyngioma, adamantinoma, and glioma, but many other tumors have been reported (pituitary adenoma, cholesteatoma, lipoma, meningioma, glioma, angiosarcoma, and chordoma). The condition bears clinical similarities to the Prader-Willi syndrome, in which hypothalamic abnormalities are not found, as discussed in Chap. 38.

Hypothalamic Disorders Associated With Alterations in Weight

Neuroanatomic studies have localized a satiety center in the ventromedial nucleus of the hypothalamus and an appetite center in the ventrolateral nucleus. Lesions in the lateral hypothalamus may result in a failure to eat and, in the neonate, failure to thrive; lesions in the medial hypothalamus may result in overeating and obesity. Bray and Gallagher, who analyzed 8 cases of the latter type, concluded that the critical lesion was bilateral destruction of the ventromedial regions of the hypothalamus. Most of the reported cases of this type have been caused by tumors, particularly craniopharyngioma, and some to trauma, inflammatory disease, and hydrocephalus (Suzuki et al). In a case that was subject to clinicopathologic correlation, Reeves and Plum found that a hamartoma had destroyed the medial eminence and the ventromedial nuclei bilaterally but spared the lateral hypothalamus. Hyperphagia and rage reactions were the main clinical features; the associated polydipsia and polyuria were due to extension of the tumor to the anterior hypothalamus. It is evident that in only a tiny fraction of people can obesity be traced to a hypothalamic lesion. Of overriding importance are genetic factors, such as the number of lipocytes that one inherits and their ability to store fat.

A disorder of infants has been described under the name *diencephalic syndrome*. Progressive and ultimately fatal emaciation (failure to thrive), despite normal or near-normal food intake, in an otherwise alert and cheerful infant is the main clinical feature. The lesion has usually proved to be a low-grade astrocytoma of the anterior hypothalamus or optic nerve (Burr et al).

Extrahypothalamic parts of the brain, if diseased, may also be associated with increased food-seeking behavior, food ingestion, and weight gain. Examples are involvement of limbic structures, as in the Klüver-Bucy syndrome and basal frontal lobe lesions leading to gluttony. Indeed, the primacy of hypothalamic lesions in causing pathologic weight gain has been challenged in a review of published cases by Uher and Treasure.

Anorexia Nervosa and Bulimia

The special syndromes called *anorexia nervosa* and *bulimia* have been difficult to classify and are mentioned in this chapter only because they are associated with alterations in several hypothalamic functions, including appetite, temperature control, and menstruation. In all likelihood, these alterations are not the result of a primary dysfunction of hypothalamic nuclei but are secondary to the extreme weight loss, which is the primary feature of the disease. However, a causal link between these idiopathic diseases and hypothalamic dysfunction has been suggested by the rare patients with an anorexia nervosa syndrome who were later found to have hypothalamic tumors (Bhanji and Mattingly; Berek et al; and Lewin et al).

Anorexia nervosa and bulimia are probably best regarded as disorders of behavior, in this case an obsession with thinness; consequently, they are discussed with the psychiatric disorders (see Chap. 51). But the developmental nature of the disease (arising in early adolescence), its virtual absence in men, and the hypothalamic alterations mentioned above do not allow the dismissal of a primary disorder of the brain's appetite centers.

Abnormalities of Growth

Presumably, in most instances of growth retardation, there is a deficiency of GHRH or of GH per se. In the *Prader-Willi syndrome* (obesity, hypogonadism, hypotonia, mental retardation, and short stature), Bray and Gallagher found the deficiency to be one of GHRH. In certain congenital and developmental diseases, the hypothalamus appears to be incapable of releasing GH. This appears to be the case in the de Morsier septooptic defect of the brain (median facial cleft, cavum septum pellucidum, optic defect), as Stewart and colleagues found an isolated deficiency of GH. In children with idiopathic hypopituitarism in whom stunting of growth is associated with other endocrine abnormalities, the deficiency is probably in the synthesis or release of GHRH. In some dwarfs (Laron dwarf, Seckel bird-headed dwarf), there are extremely high levels of circulating GH, suggesting either a defect in the GH molecule or an unresponsiveness of target organs. Many patients with the more severe forms of mental retardation are subnormal in height and weight, but the explanation for this has not been ascertained. It has not been reducible to changes in the level of GHRH or GH.

Of course, the vast majority of unusually short children who are otherwise healthy do not have a recognizable defect in GH or GHRH. Often their parents are short. The therapeutic use of GH in such children is a controversial matter. The hormone effects a spurt in growth during the first year of its administration, but whether it significantly influences growth in the long term is still under investigation. There is concern about the risk of transmitting prion or viral diseases through administration of the biologically derived hormone; this problem is obviated if a genetically produced hormone is used.

In *gigantism*, most of the reported cases have been caused by pituitary adenomas that secrete an excess of GH. This must occur prior to closure of the epiphyses. Hypersecretion of GH after closure of the epiphyses results in *acromegaly*. The notion of a purely hypothalamic form of gigantism or acromegaly (hypothalamic acromegaly) has been affirmed by Asa and associates, who described 6 patients with hypothalamic gangliocytomas that produced GHRH. The possibility of an ectopic source of GH must also be considered. The mentally retarded individuals with gigantism described by Sotos and coworkers were found to have no abnormalities of GHRH, GH, or somatomedin.

Disturbances of Temperature Regulation

Bilateral lesions in the anterior parts of the hypothalamus, specifically of temperature-sensitive neurons in the preoptic area, may result in *hyperthermia*. The heat-dissipating mechanisms of the body, notably vasodilatation and sweating, are impaired. This effect has followed operations or other trauma in the region of the floor of the third ventricle but we have seen it most often after massive rupture of an anterior communicating artery aneurysm. The temperature rises to 41°C (106°F) or higher and remains at that level until death some hours or days later, or it drops abruptly with recovery. Acetylsalicylic acid has little effect on central hyperthermia; the only way to control it is by active evaporative cooling of the body while administering sedation. A less-dramatic example of the loss of natural circadian temperature patterns is seen in patients with postoperative damage in the suprachiasmatic area (Cohen and Albers) and suprachiasmatic metastasis (Schwartz et al). These types of lesions are invariably associated with other disorders of intrinsic rhythmicity, including sleep and behavior. It should be emphasized, however, that instances of "central fever" are rare, and unexplained fever of moderate degree should not be attributed to an existing or putative brain lesion.

Hyperthermia is also part of the *malignant hyperthermia* syndrome, in which, in a limited number of cases, there is an inherited (autosomal dominant) susceptibility to develop hyperthermia and muscle rigidity in response to inhalation anesthetics and skeletal muscle relaxants ("Malignant Hyperthermia" in Chap. 50). In some of these instances, it has been found to be caused by a defective ryanodine receptor. Closely related is the *neuroleptic malignant syndrome*, which is the result of an idiosyncratic reaction to neuroleptic drugs ("Neuroleptic Malignant Syndrome" in Chap. 43). Wolff and colleagues have described a syndrome of *periodic hyperthermia*, associated with vomiting, hypertension, and weight loss and accompanied by an excessive excretion of glucocorticoids; the symptoms had no apparent explanation, although there was a symptomatic response to chlorpromazine.

Lesions in the posterior part of the hypothalamus have had a different effect; i.e., they often produce *hypothermia* (a persistent temperature of 35°C [95°F] or less) or *poikilothermia* (equilibration of body and environmental temperatures). The latter may pass unnoticed unless the patient's temperature is taken after lowering and raising the room temperature. Somnolence, confusion, and hypotension may be associated. *Spontaneous periodic hypothermia*, probably first described by Gowers, has been found in association with a cholesteatoma of the third ventricle (Penfield) and with agenesis of the corpus callosum (Noel et al). Episodically, there are symptoms of autonomic disturbance—salivation, nausea and vomiting, vasodilatation, sweating, lacrimation, and bradycardia; the rectal temperature may fall to 30°C (86°F), and seizures may occur. Penfield referred to these attacks incorrectly as "diencephalic epilepsy." Between attacks, which last a few minutes to an hour or two, neurologic abnormalities are usually not discernible and temperature regulation is normal.

Chronic hypothermia is a more familiar state than hyperthermia, being recorded in cases of severe hypothyroidism, hypoglycemia, and uremia; after prolonged immersion or exposure to cold; and in cases of intoxication with barbiturates, phenothiazines, or alcohol. It tends to be more frequent among elderly patients, who are often found to have an inadequate thermoregulatory mechanism.

Cardiovascular Disorders With Hypothalamic Lesions

Ranson demonstrated a number of autonomic effects upon stimulation of the hypothalamus; these effects as well as hypertension were recorded in Penfield's case of "diencephalic epilepsy." Since Byer and colleagues' description of large, upright T waves and prolonged QT intervals in patients with stroke, it has been appreciated that acute lesions of the brain—particularly subarachnoid hemorrhage and head trauma—may be accompanied by changes in the electrocardiogram (ECG) as well as by supraventricular tachycardia, ectopic ventricular beats, and ventricular fibrillation. Most of the same effects can be induced by very high levels of circulating norepinephrine and corticosteroids. Considering the numerous catastrophic lesions of the brain as well as extreme emotional states that can provoke arrhythmias and other changes in the ECG, the hypothalamus, with its limbic connections and ability to mount a massive sympathoadrenal discharge, is the likely source of these autonomic changes. Cropp and Manning found that the changes seen in the ECG, particularly "cerebral T waves" and other reversible repolarization abnormalities, could occur almost instantaneously (too quickly for attribution to circulating factors) during surgery for a cerebral aneurysm. Again, the hypothalamus is implicated, but as yet no direct evidence links this structure to direct cardiac control.

Gastric Hemorrhage

In experimental animals, lesions placed in or near the tuberal nuclei induce superficial erosions or ulcerations of the gastric mucosa in the absence of hyperacidity (Cushing ulcers). Gastric lesions of similar type are seen in patients with several types of acute intracranial disease (particularly subdural hematoma and other effects of head injury, cerebral hemorrhages, and tumors). In seeking causative lesions, as in patients dying with cardiac changes after head injury or subarachnoid hemorrhage, one searches in vain for a lesion in the various hypothalamic nuclei. A functional disorder in this region is nonetheless suspected.

"Neurogenic" Pulmonary Edema

Following the original observations by Maire and Patton in humans, numerous cases of massive and often fatal pulmonary edema have been described in relation to catastrophic intracranial lesions—head injury, subarachnoid and intracerebral hemorrhage, bacterial meningitis, and status epilepticus being the usual ones. A sudden elevation in intracranial pressure is involved in most cases, usually accompanied by a brief bout of extreme systemic hypertension but without obvious left ventricular failure—which is one reason the pulmonary edema has been attributed to a "neurogenic" rather than a cardiogenic cause. Also, it has been shown that experimental lesions in the caudal hypothalamus are capable of producing this type of pulmonary edema, but almost always with the interposed event of brief and extreme systemic hypertension.

Both the pulmonary edema and hypertensive response can be prevented by sympathetic blockade at any level, suggesting that the adrenergic discharge and the hypertension it causes are essential for the development of pulmonary edema. The rapid rise in vascular resistance and systemic blood pressure is similar to the pressor reaction obtained by destruction of the nucleus of the tractus solitarius, as described in Chap. 26, making understandable the few instances of neurogenic edema that have followed acute lesions in the medullary tegmentum (as was seen in one of our patients [Brown et al]). At issue is whether the hypothalamus exerts a direct sympathetic influence on the pulmonary vasculature, allowing a leakage of protein-rich edema fluid, or if the edema is the result of sudden and massive overloading of the pulmonary circulation by a shift of fluid from the systemic vasculature. The latter theory, essentially one of momentary right-heart failure, is currently favored but does not explain all aspects of the syndrome. Likewise, the role of circulating catecholamines and adrenal steroids has not been fully elucidated. These issues have been summarized in the text on neurologic intensive care by Ropper and colleagues.

Disorders of Consciousness and Personality

Since Ranson's experimental work in monkeys, it has been appreciated that acute lesions in the posterior and lateral parts of the hypothalamus may be associated with stupor, although it has always been difficult to determine the precise structures that were involved. One can be certain that permanent coma from small lesions in the caudal diencephalon (thalamus) may occur in the absence of any changes in the hypothalamus and, conversely, that chronic hypothalamic lesions may be accompanied by no more than drowsiness or confusion or no mental change at all. In one of our cases, involving an infundibuloma entirely confined to the hypothalamus, the patient lay for weeks in a state of torpor, drowsy and confused. His blood pressure was low, his body temperature was 34°C (93.2°F) to 35°C (95°F), and he had diabetes insipidus. When aroused, he was aggressive, like the patient of Reeves and Plum (see earlier).

Among the cases of acquired changes in personality and sleep patterns from ventral hypothalamic disease that we have seen, a few have been impressive because of a tendency to a hypomanic, hypervigilant state with insomnia, lasting days on end, and an impulsiveness and disinhibition suggestive of involvement of the frontal connections to the hypothalamus. In one recent case we examined following removal of a craniopharyngioma, a delirious, agitated state lasted 3 weeks during which the patient's attention could not be captured for even a moment. These and other cognitive disorders with hypothalamic lesions are difficult to interpret and are usually transient. Often the lesions are acute or postoperative and involve adjacent areas, making it impossible to attribute them to the hypothalamus alone.

Periodic Somnolence and Bulimia (Kleine-Levin Syndrome)

Kleine in 1925 and Levin in 1936 described an episodic disorder characterized by somnolence and overeating. For days or weeks, the patients, mostly adolescent boys, sleep 18 or more hours a day, waking only long enough to eat and attend to toilet needs. They appeared dull, often confused, and restless, and were sometimes troubled by hallucinations. The hypothalamus has been implicated on the basis of these symptoms, but without definite pathologic confirmation. We have had some experience with patients having this disorder; a further discussion can be found in "Kleine-Levin Syndrome" in Chap. 19.

Neuroendocrine Syndromes Related to the Adrenal Glands (See also Chap. 30)

Cushing Disease and Cushing Syndrome

The clinical features of Cushing disease, first described in Cushing's monograph in 1932, are familiar to everyone in medicine: truncal obesity with reddish purple cutaneous striae over the abdomen and other parts; dryness and pigmentation of the skin and fragility of skin vessels; excessive facial hair and baldness; cyanosis and mottling of the skin of the extremities; osteoporosis and thoracic kyphosis; proximal muscular weakness; hypertension; glycosuria; and a number of psychologic disturbances. Adrenal hyperplasia secondary to a basophil adenoma of the pituitary (*pituitary basophilia* was Cushing's term) was the established pathology in Cushing's cases. It is to the pituitary form of hyperadrenalism that the term *Cushing disease* has been applied. But the same combination of abnormalities may be associated with chronically increased production of cortisol from a primary adrenal tumor, ectopic production of ACTH by carcinoma of the lung or other carcinomas, and most commonly, with the prolonged administration of glucocorticoids (prednisone, methylprednisolone, or ACTH). For these latter conditions, all but the last being associated with secondary adrenal hyperplasia, the term *Cushing syndrome* is appropriate. Some components of the syndrome may be lacking or less conspicuous than in florid Cushing disease; diagnosis is then facilitated by measurements of ACTH and cortisol in the blood and urine. Cushing syndrome of ectopic type differs clinically from primary pituitary Cushing disease with respect to its more rapid development and greater degrees of proximal limb weakness, skin pigmentation, hypokalemia, hypertension, and glycosuria. Plasma concentrations of ACTH are usually above 20 pg/ml and may exceed 50 pg/ml in the ectopic type and are not suppressed by dexamethasone.

In Orth's review of 630 cases of Cushing syndrome of endogenous cause, 65 percent were caused by hyperpituitarism (Cushing disease), 12 percent by ectopic production of ACTH, 10 percent by an adrenal adenoma, and 8 percent by adrenal carcinoma.

In *Cushing disease*, either hyperplasia of pituitary cells or a better-defined basophil or chromophobe adenoma produces ACTH, which stimulates the adrenals. Unlike the usual pituitary tumors, the corticotroph (basophil) type are usually microadenomas (<1 cm) and enlarge the sella in only 20 percent of cases. However, it is now appreciated by MRI or high-resolution CT through the sella, that either micro- or macroadenomas are the cause in approximately 80 percent of cases, higher than in the aforementioned series by Orth and all studies prior to the inception of modern brain imaging. There are only a few cases in which a hypothalamic tumor such as a gangliocytoma has caused Cushing syndrome.

For *diagnostic purposes*, measurement of the excretion of cortisol over 24 h in the urine is the most expeditious test and superior to serum sampling because of fluctuations in the serum levels of ACTH. If a 24-h urine collection is not feasible, it is advisable to obtain two or three daily urine determinations, as the values may vary from day to day in Cushing syndrome and patients are frequently unable to save all their urine. The normal value for urinary excretion of cortisol is approximately 12 to 40 mg in 24 h, but some assays that measure additional metabolites of the hormone may allow normal values up to 100 mg. This should be followed by low- or high-dose dexamethasone suppression testing. A test using high doses of dexamethasone (2 mg every 6 h orally for 2 d, or a single dose of 8 mg at midnight) is the most dependable screening method for separating Cushing disease from ectopic secretion of ACTH. In the latter condition, the urinary excretion of cortisol is not suppressed by the administration of dexamethasone, whereas there is a reduction of 90 percent in urinary excretion in 60 to 70 percent of patients with Cushing disease.

Treatment is governed by the cause of the syndrome. A pituitary adenoma, if not extending out of the sella and encroaching on the optic chiasm (microadenoma), is ideally treated by transsphenoidal pituitary microsurgery, as discussed in Chap. 31. The alternative is focused proton beam or gamma radiation, but the long latency of response to these forms of treatment, 6 months or more, makes them less desirable. If such indirect methods of treatment are used, hypercortisolism may be suppressed in the interim by adrenal enzyme inhibitors such as ketoconazole, metapyrone, or aminoglutethimide. The rate of cure for pituitary microadenoma by transsphenoidal surgery approaches 80 percent, although operative complications—CSF leakage, transient diabetes insipidus, visual abnormalities, meningitis—occur in as many as 10 percent of patients. In approximately 20 percent of patients, removal of the tumor is incomplete and symptoms persist or recur. In such circumstances reoperation is often undertaken, with total excision of the gland and a consequent requirement for extensive hormone replacement in many cases. As an alternative, radiotherapy may be used after failed surgery. If there is an urgent need to suppress the effects of hypercortisolism, bilateral adrenalectomy is effective but has obvious limitations.

Depending on the functional status of the pituitary after any mode of successful treatment, replacement therapy may be needed for a variable period or for the patient's lifetime.

Adrenocortical Insufficiency (Addison Disease)

The classic form of adrenal insufficiency, described by Addison in the nineteenth century, is a result of primary disease of the adrenals. It is characterized by pigmentation of the skin and mucous membranes, nausea, vomiting, and weight loss, as well as muscle weakness, languor, and a tendency to faint. Since Addison's time, hypotension, hyperkalemia, hyponatremia, and low serum cortisol concentrations have come to be recognized as important laboratory features.

In the past, the most common cause of primary adrenal disease was tuberculosis. Now, most cases are designated as idiopathic and thought to represent an autoimmune disorder, often associated with Hashimoto thyroiditis and diabetes mellitus and rarely with other polyglandular autoimmune endocrine disorders. A less-frequent cause is a hereditary metabolic disease of the adrenals—in combination with a demyelinating disease of brain, spinal cord, and nerves and occurring predominantly in males (adrenoleukodystrophy; see Chap. 37). In primary adrenal disease, plasma concentrations of cortisol are low, in response to which the concentrations of ACTH rise. Adrenal insufficiency of whatever cause is a life-threatening condition; there is always a danger of collapse and even death, particularly during periods of infection, surgery, injury, and the like. Lifelong replacement therapy is usually required, with a glucocorticoid (cortisone, 25 to 50 mg, or prednisone, 7.5 to 15 mg daily) and a mineralocorticoid, such as fludrocortisone acetate (Florinef), 0.05 to 0.2 mg daily.

When adrenal insufficiency is secondary to disease of the pituitary, ACTH is low or absent and cortisol secretion is markedly reduced, but aldosterone levels are sustained. Hyperpigmentation is notably absent; it is the elevation of ACTH that causes melanoderma, such as occurs, for example, in patients subjected to bilateral adrenalectomy. Hypothalamic lesions, principally involving the paraventricular nuclei, may also cause adrenal insufficiency, but less frequently than do pituitary lesions.

References

Anderson AE: *Practical Comprehensive Treatment of Anorexia Nervosa and Bulimia*. Baltimore, Johns Hopkins University Press, 1985.

Aronin N, DiFiglea M, Leeman SE: Substance P, in Krieger DT, Brownstein NJ, Martin JB (eds): *Brain Peptides*. New York, Wiley, 1983, pp 783–804.

Asa SL, Scheithauer BW, Bilbau J, et al: A case of hypothalamic acromegaly: A clinico-pathologic study of 6 patients with hypothalamus gangliocytomas producing growth hormone releasing factor. *J Clin Endocrinol Metab* 58:796, 1984.

Berek K, Aichner F, Schmutzhard E, et al: Intracranial germ cell tumour mimicking anorexia nervosa. *Klin Wochenschr* 69:440, 1991.

Bhanji S, Mattingly D: *Medical Aspects of Anorexia Nervosa*. London, Wright, 1988.

Bray GA, Gallagher TF Jr: Manifestations of hypothalamic obesity in man: A comprehensive investigation of eight patients and a review of the literature. *Medicine (Baltimore)* 54:301, 1975.

Brazeau P, Vale W, Bargus R, et al: Hypothalamic polypeptide that inhibits the secretion of immunoreactive pituitary growth hormone. *Science* 179:77, 1973.

Breningstall GN: Gelastic seizures, precocious puberty and hypothalamic hamartoma. *Neurology* 35:1180, 1985.

Brown RH, Beyerl BD, Iseke R, Lavyne MH: Medulla oblongata edema associated with neurogenic pulmonary edema. *J Neurosurg* 64:494, 1986.

Brzezinski A: Melatonin in humans. *N Engl J Med* 336:186, 1997.

Burr IM, Slonim AE, Danish RK: Diencephalic syndrome revisited. *J Pediatr* 88:429, 1976.

Byer E, Ashman R, Toth LA: Electrocardiogram with large upright T-wave and long Q-T intervals. *Am Heart J* 33:796, 1947.

Byne W: The biological evidence challenged, in The Editors of Scientific American Magazine (eds): *The Scientific American Book of the Brain*. New York, Lyons Press, 1999, pp 181–194.

Carmel PW: Sympathetic deficits following thalamotomy. *Arch Neurol* 18:378, 1968.

Cavallo A: The pineal gland in human beings: Relevance to pediatrics. *J Pediatr* 123:843, 1993.

Cohen RA, Albers HE: Disruption of human circadian and cognitive regulation following a discrete hypothalamic lesion: A case study. *Neurology* 41:726, 1991.

Cropp CF, Manning GW: Electrocardiographic change simulating myocardial ischemia and infarction associated with spontaneous intracranial hemorrhage. *Circulation* 22:24, 1960.

Cushing H: Basophil adenomas of the pituitary body and their clinical manifestations (pituitary basophilia). *Bull Johns Hopkins Hosp* 50:137, 1932.

Diringer M, Ladenson PW, Stern BJ, et al: Plasma atrial natriuretic factor and subarachnoid hemorrhage. *Stroke* 19:1119, 1988.

DuVigneaud V: Hormones of the posterior pituitary gland: Oxytocin and vasopressin. *Harvey Lect* 50:1, 1954–1955.

Euler US, Gaddum JH: An unidentified depressor substance in certain tissue abstracts. *J Physiol* 612:74, 1931.

Erdheim J: Über Hypophysengangs Geschwülste und Hirn Cholesteatome. Sitzungs DK Akad d Wissensch. *Math Natur WC Wien* 113:537, 1904.

Froehlich A: Ein Fall von Tumor der Hypophysis cerebri ohne Akromegalie. *Wien Klin Wochenschr* 15:883, 1901.

Hayes R, McHugh PR, Williams H: Absence of thirst in hydrocephalus. *N Engl J Med* 269:277, 1963.

Haymaker W, Adams RD: The pineal gland, in *Histology and Histopathology of the Nervous System*. Springfield, IL, Charles C Thomas, 1982, pp 1801–2023.

Hughes IT, Smith W, Kosterlitz HW, et al: Identification of two related pentapeptides from the brain with potent opiate agonist activity. *Nature* 258:577, 1975.

Imura H, Nakoa K, Shimatsu A, et al: Lymphocytic infundibuloneurohypophysitis as a cause of central diabetes insipidus. *N Engl J Med* 329:683, 1993.

Jennings MT, Gelman R, Hochberg FH: Intracranial germ-cell tumors: Natural history and pathogenesis. *J Neurosurg* 63:155, 1985.

Lamberts SWJ, DeHerder WW, Van der Lely AJ: Pituitary insufficiency. *Lancet* 352:127, 1998.

Leeman SE, Mroz EA: Substance P. *Life Sci* 15:2033, 1974.

Levay S: A difference in the hypothalamic structure between heterosexual and homosexual men. *Science* 253:1034, 1991.

Lewin K, Mattingly D, Mills RR: Anorexia nervosa associated with hypothalamic tumour. *Br Med J* 2:629, 1972.

Martin JB, Reichlin S: *Clinical Neuroendocrinology*, 2nd ed. Philadelphia, Davis, 1987.

Mechanick JI, Hochberg FH, LaRocque A: Hypothalamic dysfunction following whole-brain radiation. *J Neurosurg* 65:490, 1986.

Moses AM, Stretten DHP: Disorders of the neurohypophysis, in Braunwald E, Fauci A, Kasper D, et al (eds): *Harrison's Principles of Internal Medicine*, 14th ed. New York, McGraw-Hill, 1998, p 1924.

Nauta WJH, Haymaker W: Hypothalamic nuclei and fiber connections, in Haymaker W, Anderson E, Nauta WJH (eds): *The Hypothalamus*. Springfield, IL, Charles C Thomas, 1969, pp 136–209.

Nelson PB, Seif SM, Maroon JC, Robinson AG: Hyponatremia in intracranial disease: Perhaps not the syndrome of inappropriate secretion of antidiuretic hormone (SIADH). *J Neurosurg* 55:938, 1981.

Noel P, Hubert JP, Ectors M, et al: Agenesis of the corpus callosum associated with relapsing hypothermia. *Brain* 96:359, 1973.

Orth DN: Cushing's syndrome. *N Engl J Med* 332:791, 1995.

Penfield W: Diencephalic autonomic epilepsy. *Arch Neurol Psychiatry* 22:358, 1929.

Peters JP, Welt LG, Sims EAH, et al: A salt wasting syndrome associated with cerebral disease. *Trans Assoc Am Physicians* 63:57, 1950.

Ranson SW: Somnolence caused by hypothalamic lesions in the monkey. *Arch Neurol Psychiatry* 41:1, 1939.

Reeves AG, Plum F: Hyperphagia, rage and dementia accompanying a ventromedial hypothalamic neoplasm. *Arch Neurol* 20:616, 1969.

Reichlin S: Neuroendocrinology, in Wilson JD, Foster DW (eds): *Williams Textbook of Endocrinology*, 8th ed. Philadelphia, Saunders, 1992, pp 135–219.

Robertson GL: Posterior pituitary, in Selig P, Baxter JD, Broadus AE, Frohman LA (eds): *Endocrinology and Metabolism*, 2nd ed. New York, McGraw-Hill, 1987, pp 338–385.

Ropper AH, Gress DR, Diringer MN, et al: Pulmonary aspects of neurological intensive care, cardiovascular aspects of neurological intensive care, in Ropper AH (ed): *Neurological and Neurosurgical Intensive Care*. Baltimore, Lippincott Williams & Wilkins, 2004, pp 52–104.

Samson WK: Atrial natriuretic factor and the central nervous system. *Endocrinol Metab Clin North Am* 16:145, 1987.

Scheithauer BW, Kovacs KT, Jariwala LK, et al: Anorexia nervosa: An immunohistochemical study of the pituitary gland. *Mayo Clin Proc* 63:23, 1988.

Schwartz WB, Bartter FC: The syndrome of inappropriate secretion of antidiuretic hormone. *Am J Med* 42:790, 1967.

Schwartz WJ, Busis NA, Hedley-Whyte T: A discrete lesion of the ventral hypothalamus and optic chiasm that disrupted the daily temperature rhythm. *J Neurol* 233:1, 1986.

Sotos JF, Dodge PR, Muirhead D, et al: Cerebral gigantism in childhood. *N Engl J Med* 271:109, 1964.

Speidel CC: Gland-cells of internal secretion in the spinal cord of the skates. *Papers from the Department of Marine Biology of the Carnegie Institution of Washington* 13:1–31, 1919.

Stewart C, Castro-Magana M, Sherman J, et al: Septo-optic dysplasia and median cleft face syndrome in a patient with isolated growth hormone deficiency and hyperprolactinemia. *Am J Dis Child* 137:484, 1983.

Suzuki N, Shinonaga M, Hirata K, et al: Hypothalamic obesity due to hydrocephalus caused by aqueductal stenosis. *J Neurol Neurosurg Psychiatry* 53:1102, 1990.

Swaab DF: The human hypothalamus: Basic and clinical aspects. Part I, Nuclei of the human hypothalamus; Part II, Neuropathology of the human hypothalamus and adjacent structures, in Aminoff MJ, Boller F, Swaab DF (eds): *Handbook of Clinical Neurology*, Volumes 79 and 80, series 3. Amsterdam, Elsevier, 2003.

Uher R, Treasure J: Brain lesions and eating disorders. *J Neurol Neurosurg Psychiatry* 76:852, 2005.

von Economo CJ: *Encephalitis Lethargica*. New York, Oxford University Press, 1930.

Wijdicks EF, Ropper AH, Hunnicutt EJ, et al: Atrial natriuretic factor and salt wasting after aneurysmal subarachnoid hemorrhage. *Stroke* 22:1519, 1991.

Wolff SM, Adler RC, Buskirk ER, et al: A syndrome of periodic hypothalamic discharge. *Am J Med* 36:956, 1964.

PART 3

GROWTH AND DEVELOPMENT OF THE NERVOUS SYSTEM AND THE NEUROLOGY OF AGING

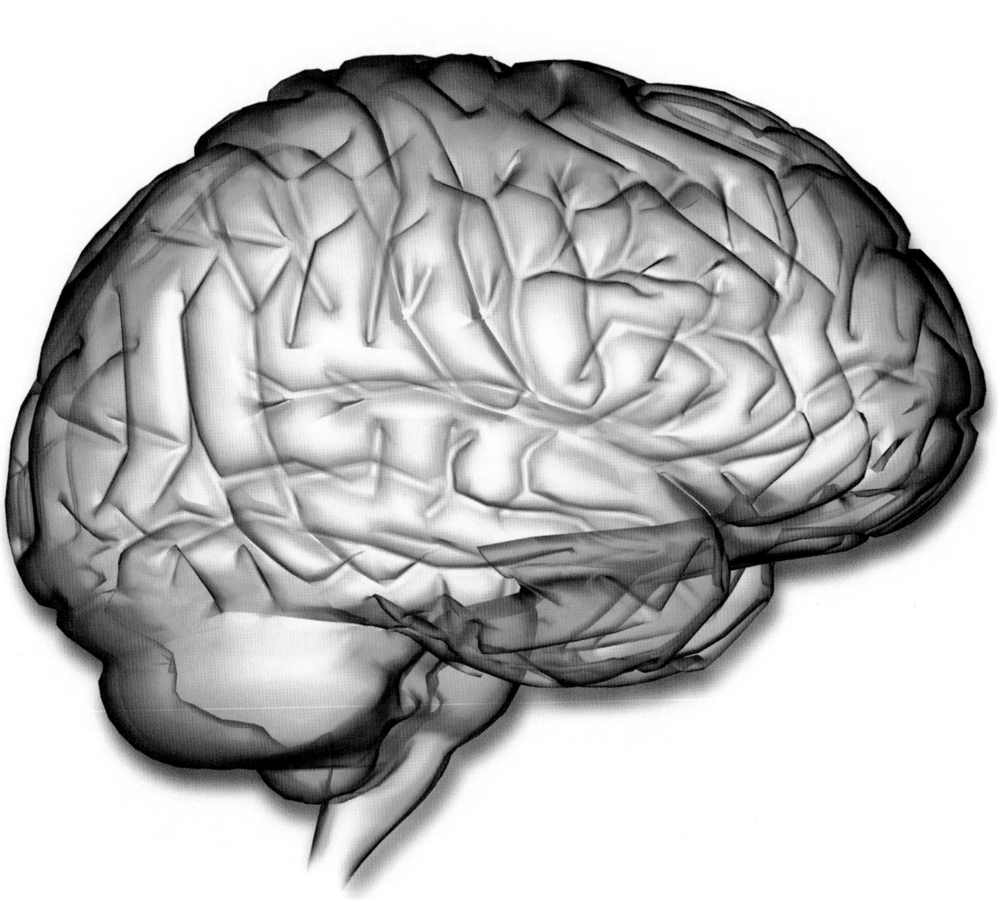

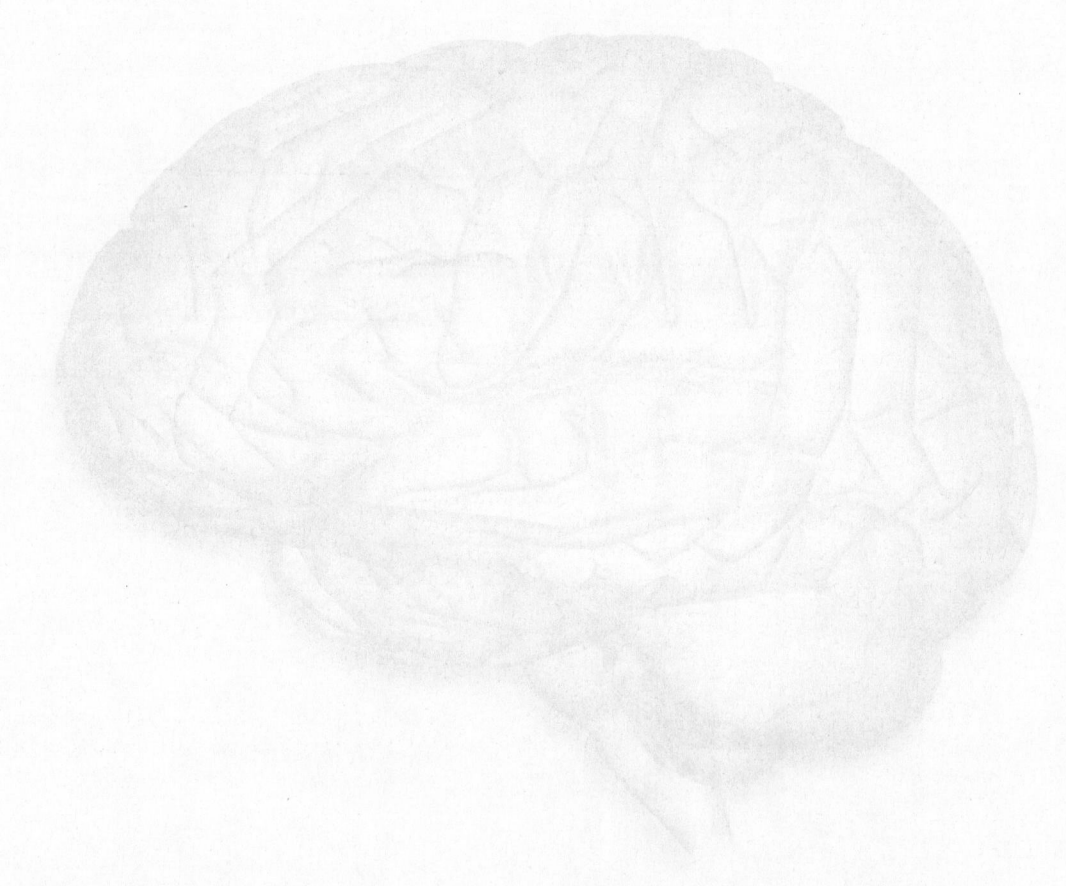

28

Normal Development and Deviations in Development of the Nervous System

In this chapter and the next one on aging, we consider the effects of growth, maturation, and aging on the nervous system. These are discussed in some detail because certain aspects of neurologic diseases are meaningful only when viewed against the background of these natural age-linked changes. Developmental diseases of the nervous system, e.g., malformations, genetic defects, and other forms of damage that are acquired in the intrauterine period of life, are considered in Chap. 38.

SEQUENCES OF NORMAL DEVELOPMENT

The establishment of a biologic timescale of human development requires observation of a large number of normal individuals of known ages and testing them for measurable items of behavior. Because of individual variations in the tempo of development, it is equally important to study the growth and development of any one individual over a prolonged period. If these observations are to be correlated with stages of neuroanatomic development, the clinical and morphologic data must be expressed in units that are comparable. Early in life, very precise age periods are difficult to ascertain because of the difficulty in fixing the time of conception. The average human gestational period is 40 weeks (280 days), but birth may occur with survival as early as about 24 or as late as 49 weeks (a time span of almost 5 months), and the extent of nervous system development varies accordingly.

After birth, any given item of behavior or structural differentiation must always have two reference points: (1) to a particular item of behavior that has already been achieved, and (2) to units of chronologic time or duration of life of the organism. The chronologic or biologic scale assumes special significance in early prenatal life. During that period development proceeds at such a rapid pace that small units of time weigh heavily and the organism appears to change literally day by day. In infancy, the tempo of development slows somewhat but is still very rapid in comparison with later childhood.

The neurologist will find it advantageous to organize knowledge of normal development and disease around the timetables for human growth and development listed in Tables 28-1 and 28-2. In addition, the last decade has brought startling advances in the understanding of the genetic and molecular control of neural development. That topic is considered in Chap. 38.

Neuroanatomic Bases of Normal Development

A large body of knowledge has accumulated concerning the functional and structural status of the nervous system during each successive period of life. This information is reviewed briefly in the following paragraphs and is summarized in Table 28-2. It must be kept in mind that development of the nervous system does not proceed stepwise, from one period to the next, but is continuous from conception to maturity. The sequences of development are much the same in all infants, although the rate may vary slightly. Any given behavioral function, in order to be expressed, must await the development of its neural substrate. Furthermore, at any given moment in development, several measurable functions appear in parallel, and it is often a dissociation between them that acquires clinical significance.

Embryonal and Fetal Periods

What we know of the nervous system in the germinal and embryonal periods has been derived from the study of a relatively small number of fetuses that have come into the hands of anatomists. Neuroblastic differentiation, migration, and neuronal multiplication are already well under way in the first 3 weeks of embryonic life. The control of each of these phases (and, later, of connectivity of neurons) is determined by the genome of the organism. Primitive cells destined to become neurons originate in, or close to, the neuroepithelium of the neural tube. These cells proliferate at an astonishingly rapid rate (250,000 per minute, according to Cowan) for a circumscribed period (several days to weeks). They become transformed into bipolar neuroblasts, which migrate in a series of waves toward the marginal layer of what is to become the cortex of the cerebral hemispheres. The first glial cells also appear very early and provide the scaffolding along which the neuroblasts move. Each step in the differentiation and migration of the neuroblasts proceeds in an orderly fashion, and one stage progresses to the next with remarkable precision. The process of neuronal migration

Table 28-1

TIMESCALE OF STAGES IN HUMAN GROWTH AND DEVELOPMENT

GROWTH PERIOD	APPROXIMATE AGE
Prenatal	From 0 to 280 days
Ovum	From 0 to 14 days
Embryo	From 14 days to 9 weeks
Fetus	From 9 weeks to birth
Premature infant	From 27 to 37 weeks
Birth	Average 280 days
Neonate	First 4 weeks after birth
Infancy	First year
Early childhood (preschool)	From 1 to 6 years
Later childhood (prepubertal)	From 6 to 10 years
Adolescence	Girls, 8 or 10 to 18 years
	Boys, 10 or 12 to 20 years
Puberty (average)	Girls, 13 years
	Boys, 15 years

Source: Reproduced by permission from Lowrey GH: *Growth and Development of Children,* 8th ed. Chicago, Year Book, 1986.

is largely completed by the end of the fifth fetal month but continues at a much slower rate up to 40 weeks of gestation, according to the classic studies of Conel and of Rabinowicz. Because the migration of most neurons involves postmitotic cells, the cerebral cortex by this time has presumably acquired its full complement of nerve cells, numbered in the many billions. This concept has been revised in recent years with the discovery that active stem cells in the adult brain generate neurons in the hippocampal formation and in the subventricular matrix zones, giving rise most evidently to olfactory neurons in the adult brain but possibly also to other nerve cells (see Kempermann and also Alvarez-Buylla and Garcia-Verdugo).

Table 28-2

TIMETABLE OF GROWTH AND NERVOUS SYSTEM DEVELOPMENT IN THE NORMAL EMBRYO AND FETUS

FETAL AGE, DAYS	SIZE (CROWN–RUMP LENGTH), MM	NERVOUS SYSTEM DEVELOPMENT
18	1.5	Neural groove and tube
21	3.0	Optic vesicles
26	3.0	Closure of anterior neuropore
27	3.3	Closure of posterior neuropore; ventral horn cells appear
31	4.3	Anterior and posterior roots
35	5.0	Five cerebral vesicles
42	13.0	Primordium of cerebellum
56	25.0	Differentiation of cerebral cortex and meninges
150	225.0	Primary cerebral fissures appear
180	230.0	Secondary cerebral sulci and first myelination appear in brain
8–9 months	240.0	Further myelination and growth of brain (see text)

Despite the almost universal acceptance of the presence of neuron genesis in the human brain, the methodology that demonstrates it is complex and has been questioned by authoritative individuals such as Rakic, whose perspective should be consulted for a complete portrait of the subject. Actually, we have little idea of the number of nerve cells in the cerebral and cerebellar cortices at different ages. Many more are formed than survive, as programmed cell death (apoptosis) constitutes an important component of development.

Within a few months of mid-fetal life, the cerebrum, which begins as a small bihemispheric organ with hardly a trace of surface indentation, evolves into a deeply sulcated structure. Every step in the folding of the surface to form fissures and sulci follows a temporal pattern of such precision as to permit a reasonably accurate estimation of fetal age by this criterion alone. The major sylvian, rolandic, and calcarine fissures take on the adult configuration during the fifth month of fetal life, the secondary sulci in the sixth and seventh months, and the tertiary sulci, which vary slightly in location from one individual to another, in the eighth and ninth months (see Fig. 28-1 and Table 28-2).

Concomitantly, subtle changes in neuronal organization are occurring in the cerebral cortex and central ganglionic masses. Involved here are the processes of synaptogenesis and axonal pathfinding. Neurons become more widely separated as differentiation proceeds, owing to an increase in the size and complexity of dendrites and axons and enlargement of synaptic surfaces (Fig. 28-2). The cytoarchitectural patterns that demarcate one part of the cerebral cortex from another (as described in Chap. 22) are already in evidence by the thirtieth week of fetal life and become definitive at 40 weeks and in succeeding months. As the maturational process of cortical neurons proceeds, the patterns of neuronal organization in different regions of the brain (motor, premotor, sensory, and striate cortices, Broca and Wernicke areas) continue to change.

Myelination provides another parallel index of development and maturation of the nervous system and is apparently related to the functional activity of the fiber systems. The timing and precision of these connecting pathways are no less precise and time locked than is neuronal development (see Flechsig's myelinogenic cycle as shown in Fig. 28-3). The acquisition of myelin sheaths by the spinal nerves and roots by the tenth week of fetal life is associated with the beginning of reflex motor activities. Segmental and intersegmental fiber systems in the spinal cord myelinate soon afterward, followed by ascending and descending fibers to and from the brainstem (reticulospinal, vestibulospinal). The acoustic and labyrinthine systems stand out with singular clarity in myelin-stained preparations by the twenty-eighth to thirtieth weeks, and the spinocerebellar and dentatorubral systems by the thirty-seventh week.

Neonatal Period and Infancy

After birth, the brain continues to grow dramatically. From an average weight of 375 to 400 g at birth (40 weeks), it reaches about 1,000 g by the end of the first postnatal year.

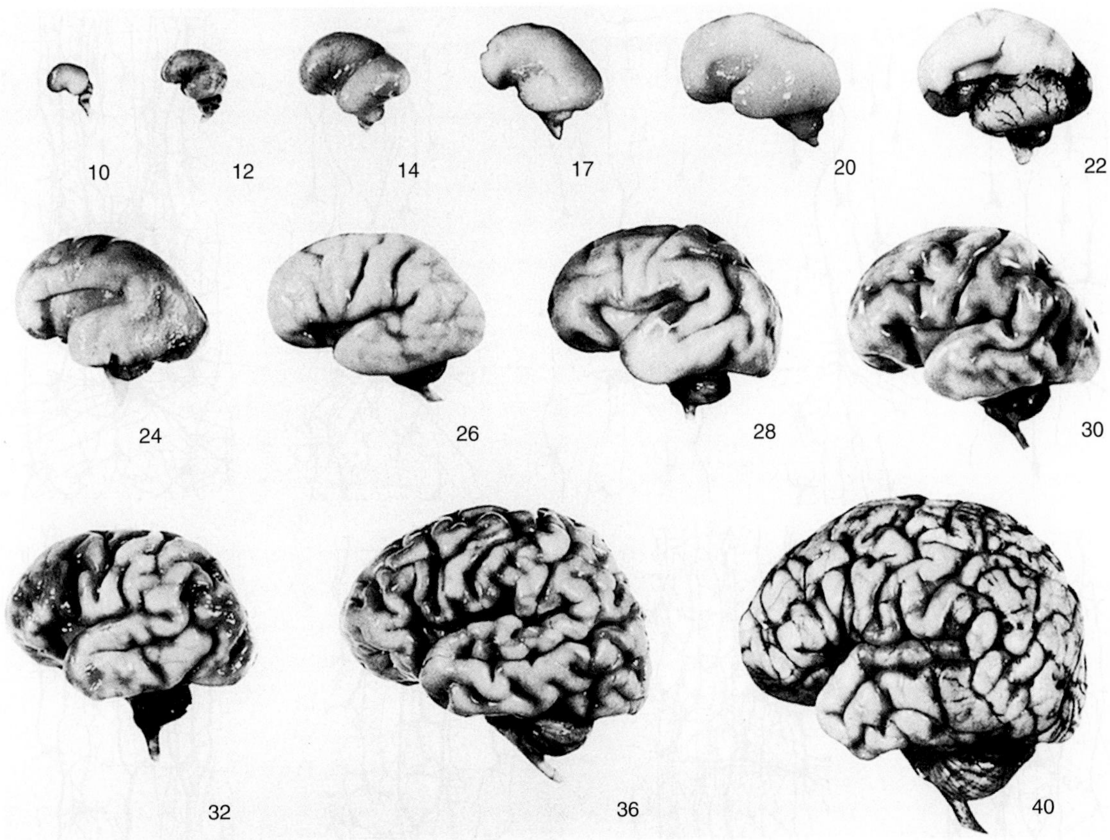

Figure 28-1. Lateral views of the fetal brain, from 10 to 40 weeks of gestational age. (Reproduced by permission from Feess-Higgins and Larroche.)

Glial cells (oligodendrocytes and astrocytes) derived from the matrix zones continue to divide and multiply during the first 6 months of postnatal life. The visual system begins to myelinate about the fortieth gestational week; its myelination cycle proceeds rapidly, being nearly complete a few months after birth. The corticospinal tracts are not fully myelinated until halfway through the second postnatal year. Most of the principal tracts are myelinated by the end of this period. In the cerebrum, the first myelin is seen at 40 weeks in the posterior frontal and parietal lobes, and the occipital lobes (geniculocalcarine tracts) myelinate soon thereafter. Myelination of the anterior frontal and temporal lobes occurs later, during the first year of postnatal life. By the end of the second year, myelination of the cerebrum is largely complete (see Fig. 28-3). These steps in myelination can be followed by MRI. Despite these careful anatomic observations, their correlation with developmental clinical and electroencephalographic data has not been precise.

Childhood, Puberty, and Adolescence

Growth of the brain continues, at a much slower rate than before, until 12 to 15 years, when the average adult weight of 1,230 to 1,275 g in females and 1,350 to 1,410 g in males is attained. Myelination also continues slowly during this period. Yakovlev and Lecours, who reexamined Flechsig's classic findings on the ontogeny of myelination (the term *Flechsig's myelinogenic cycle* is still used), traced the progressive myelination of the middle cerebellar peduncle, acoustic radiation, and bundle of Vicq d'Azyr (mammillothalamic tract) beyond the third postnatal year; the nonspecific thalamic radiations continued to myelinate beyond the seventh year and fibers of the reticular formation, great cerebral commissures, and intracortical association neurons to at least the tenth year and beyond (see Fig. 28-3). These investigators noted that there was an increasing complexity of fiber systems through late childhood and adolescence, and perhaps even into middle adult life. Similarly, in the extensive studies of Conel and Rabinowicz, depicting the cortical architecture at each year from mid-fetal life to the twentieth year, the dendritic arborizations and cortical interneuronal connections were observed to increase progressively in complexity; the "packing density" of neurons, i.e., the number of neurons in any given volume of tissue increases through the age of approximately 15 months and then decreases (see Fig. 28-2).

Interesting questions are whether neurons begin to function only when their axons have acquired a myelin sheath; whether myelination is under the control of the cell body, the axon, or both; and whether the usual myelin stains yield sufficient information as to the time of onset and degree of the myelination process. At best these correlations can be only approximate. It seems likely that systems of neurons begin to function before the first appearance of myelin, at least insofar as shown

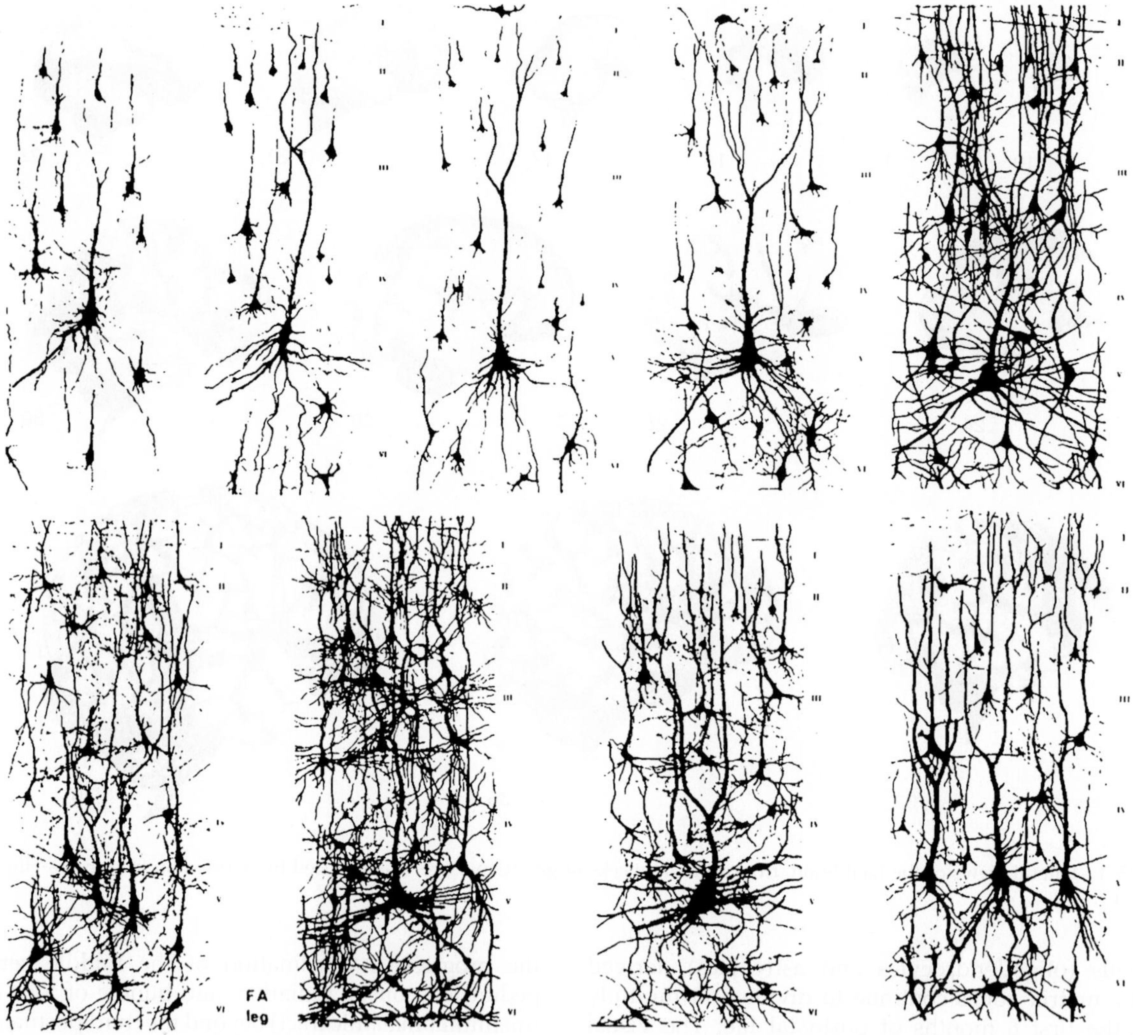

Figure 28-2. Cox-Golgi preparations of the leg area of the motor cortex (area 4). *Upper row, left to right:* 1 month premature (8 months gestation); newborn at term; 1 month; 3 months; and 6 months. *Lower row, left to right:* 15 months; 2 years; 4 years; 6 years. Apical dendrites of Betz cells have been shortened, all to the same degree, for the purposes of display. (Courtesy of T. Rabinowicz, University of Lausanne.)

in conventional myelin stains. These correlations will undoubtedly be restudied using more delicate measures of function and finer staining techniques, as well as the techniques of quantitative biochemistry and phase and electron microscopy.

Physiologic and Psychologic Development

Neural Development in the Fetus

The human fetus is capable of a complex series of reflex activities, some of which appear as early as 5 weeks of postconceptional age. Cutaneous and proprioceptive stimuli evoke slow, generalized, patterned movements of the head, trunk, and extremities. More discrete movements appear to differentiate from these generalized activities. Reflexes subserving blinking, sucking, grasping, and visceral functions, as well as tendon and plantar reflexes, are all elicitable in late fetal life. They seem to develop along with the myelination of peripheral nerves, spinal roots, spinal cord, and brainstem. By the twenty-fourth week of gestation, the neural apparatus is functioning sufficiently well to give the fetus some chance of survival should birth occur at this time. However, most infants fail to survive birth at this age, usually owing to an inadequacy of pulmonary function. Thereafter, the basic neural equipment matures so rapidly that, by the thirtieth week, postnatal viability is relatively common. It seems that nature prepares the fetus for the contingency of premature birth by hastening the establishment of vital functions necessary for extrauterine existence.

It is in the last trimester of pregnancy that a complete timetable of fetal movements, posture, and reflexes would be of the greatest value, for mainly during this period does the need for a full clinical evaluation arise. That there are recognizable differences between infants born in the sixth, seventh, eighth, and ninth months of fetal life has been documented by Saint-Anne Dargassies, who applied the neurologic tests earlier devised by André-Thomas and herself. Her observations document

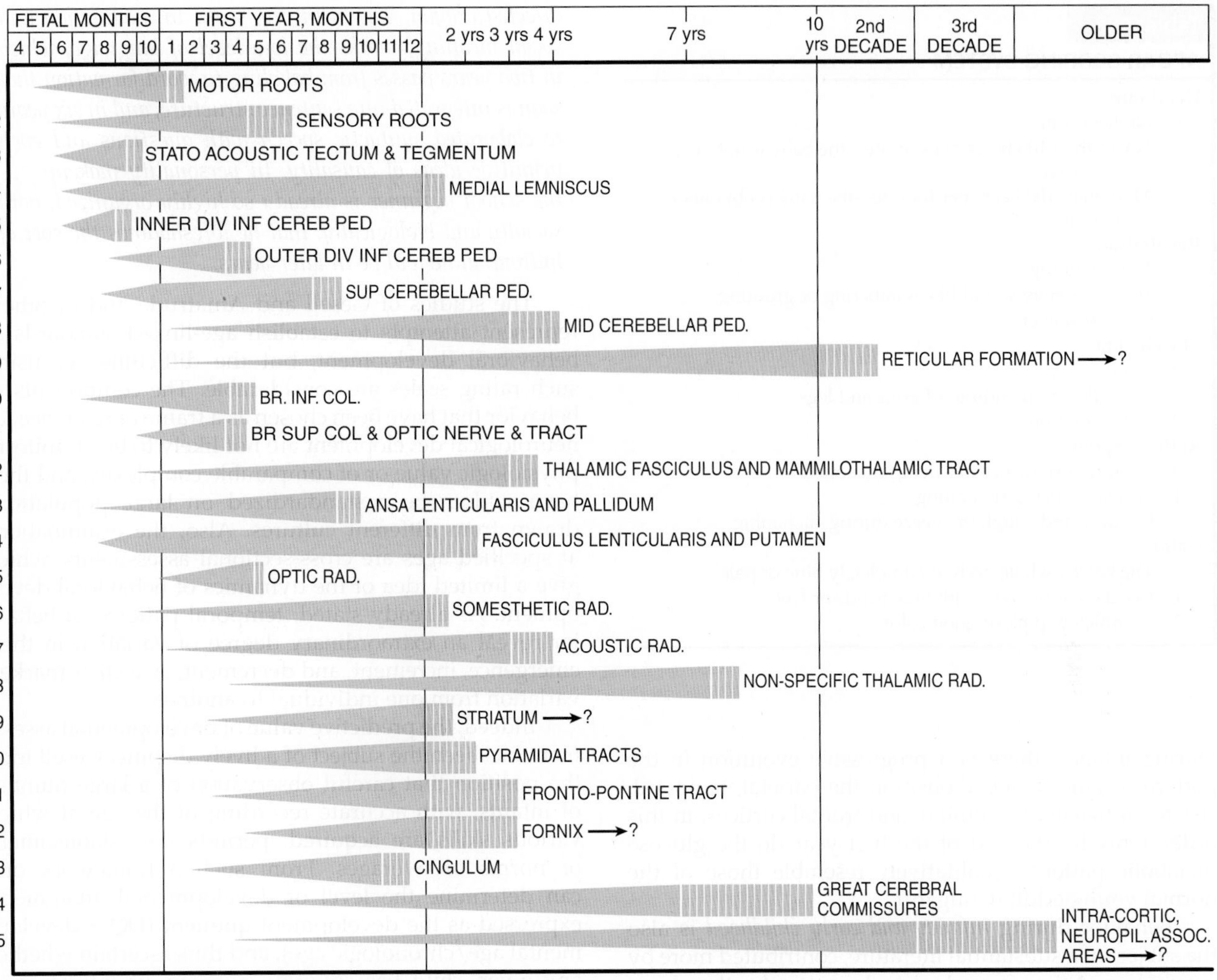

Figure 28-3. The myelogenetic chronology. (Reproduced from Yakovlev and Lecours.)

prevailing postures; control and attitude of head, neck, and limbs; muscle tonus; and grasp and sucking reflexes. These findings are of interest and may well be a means of determining exact age, but many more observations are needed with follow-up data on later development before they can be fully accepted. Part of the difficulty here is the variability of the premature infant's neurologic functions, which may change literally from hour to hour. Even at term there may be variability in neurologic functions from one day to the next. This variability reflects in part the effects of parturition and the effects of drugs given to the mother, as well as the inaccurate dating of conception and rapid developmental changes in the brain.

Development During the Neonatal Period, Infancy, and Early Childhood

At term, effective sucking, rooting, and grasping reactions are present. The infant is able to swallow and cry, and the startle reaction (e.g., Moro reflex, as described further on) can be evoked by loud sound and sudden extension of the neck. Support and steppage movements can be demonstrated by placing the infant on its feet, and incurvation of the trunk by stroking one side of the back. Also present at birth is the placing reaction, wherein the foot or hand, brought passively into contact with the edge of a table, is lifted automatically and placed on the flat surface. These neonatal automatisms depend essentially on the functioning of the spinal cord, brainstem, and possibly diencephalon and pallidum. The *Apgar score*, a universally used but somewhat imprecise index of the well-being of the newly born infant, is in reality a numerical rating of the adequacy of brainstem-spinal mechanisms (breathing, pulse, color of skin, tone, and responsivity) (Table 28-3).

Studies of local cerebral glucose metabolism by positron emission tomography (PET) have provided interesting information about the functional maturation of the brain. There are remarkable differences between the newborn and the mature individual. Neonatal values, adjusted for brain weight, are only one-third those of the adult; except for the primary sensorimotor cortex, they are confined to brainstem, cerebellum, and thalamus.

Table 28-3

APGAR SCORING SYSTEM

Heart rate	
0	No heart rate
1	Fewer than 100 beats per minute—the baby is not very responsive
2	More than 100 beats per minute—the baby is obviously vigorous
Respiration	
0	Not breathing
1	Weak cry; may sound like wimpering or grunting
2	Good strong cry
Muscle tone	
0	Limp
1	Some flexing (bending) of arms and legs
2	Active motion
Reflex response	
0	No response to airways being suctioned
1	Grimace during suctioning
2	Grimace and cough or sneeze during suctioning
Color	
0	The baby's whole body is completely blue or pale
1	Good color in body with blue hands or feet
2	Completely pink or good color

During infancy, there is a progressive evolution in the pattern of glucose metabolism in the parietal, temporal, striate, dorsolateral occipital, and frontal cortices, in this order. Only by the end of the first year do the glucose metabolic patterns qualitatively resemble those of the normal young adult (Chugani).

Behavior during *infancy and early childhood* is also the subject of a substantial literature, contributed more by psychologists than neurologists. In particular they have explored sensorimotor performance in the first year and language and social development in early childhood. In the first 6 years of life, the infant and young child traverse far more ground developmentally than they ever will again in a similar period. From the newborn state, when the infant demonstrates a few primitive feeding and postural reflexes, there are acquired, within a few months, smiling and head and hand–eye control; by 6 months, the ability to sit; by 10 months, the strength to stand; by 12 months, the muscle coordination required to walk; by 2 years, the ability to run; and by 6 years, mastery of the rudiments of a game of baseball or a musical skill. On the perceptual side, the neonate progresses, in less than 3 months, from a state in which ocular control is tentative and tonic deviation of the eyes occurs only in response to labyrinthine stimulation to one in which he is able to fixate on and follow an object. (This last corresponds to the development of the macula.) Later, the child is able to make fine discriminations of color, form, and size. Gesell has provided a graphic summation of the variety and developmental sweep of a child's behavior. He writes

> *At birth the child reflexly grasps the examiner's finger, with eyes crudely wandering or vacantly transfixed . . . and by the sixth year the child adaptively scans the perimeter of a square or triangle, reproducing each form with directed crayon. The birth cry, scant in modulation and social meaning, marks the low level of language, which in two years passes from babbling to word formation that soon is integrated into sentence structure, and in six years to elaborated syntactic speech with questions and even primitive ideas of causality. In personality makeup . . . the school beginner is already so highly organized, both socially and biologically, that he foreshadows the sort of individual he will be in later years.*

The studies of Gesell and Amatruda and of others represent attempts to establish age-linked standards of behavioral development, but the difficulties of using such rating scales are considerable. The components of behavior that have been chosen as a frame of reference for neurological development are not likely to be of uniform physiologic value or of comparable complexity, and they have seldom been standardized on large populations drawn from different cultures. Also, the examinations at specified ages are cross-sectional assessments, which give a limited idea of the dynamics of behavioral development. As already stated, temporal patterns of behavior reveal an extraordinary degree of variation in their emergence, increment, and decrement, as well as marked variation from one individual to another.

Indeed, the predictive value of developmental assessment has been the subject of a lively dispute. Gesell took the position that careful observation of a large number of infants, with accurate recording of the age at which various skills are acquired, permits the establishment of norms or averages. From such a framework one can determine the level of developmental attainment, expressed as the development quotient (DQ = developmental age/chronologic age), and thus ascertain whether any given child has superior, average, or inferior performance. Furthermore, after examining 10,000 infants over a period of 40 years, Gesell concluded that "attained growth is an indicator of past growth processes and a foreteller of growth yet to be achieved." In other words, the DQ predicts potential attainment.

The other position—taken by Anderson and others—is that developmental attainments are of no real value in predicting the level of intelligence but are measures of completely different functions. Illingworth and most clinicians, including the authors, have taken an intermediate position, that the developmental scale in early life is a useful source of information, but it must be combined with a full clinical assessment. When this is done, the clinician has a reasonably certain means of detecting delays in cognitive development and other forms of neurologic impairment.

The trajectory of rapid growth and maturation continues in late childhood and adolescence, although at a slower pace than before. Motor skills attain their maximal precision in the performances of athletes, artists, and musicians, whose peak development is at maturity (age 18 to 21 years). Intelligence and the capacity for reflective thought and the manipulation of mathematical symbols become possible for most individuals only in adolescence and later. Emotional control, precarious in the school age and all through adolescence, stabilizes in adulthood. We tend to think of all these phenomena as being achieved through the stresses of human relations, which are conditioned and habituated by the powerful influences of social approval. In this extensive and pervasive interaction between the individual and the environment, which is the preoccupation of the child psychiatrist, it is well to remember that the processes of extrinsic and intrinsic organization can be separated only for the purpose of analytic discussion. There is always interdependence between them.

Motor Development

As indicated earlier and in Table 28-4, the wide variety and seemingly random movements displayed by the healthy neonate are from birth, and certainly within days, firmly organized into reflexive-instinctual patterns called *automatisms*. The most testable of the automatisms are blinking in response to light, tonic deviation of the eyes in response to labyrinthine stimulation (turning of the head), prehensile and sucking movements of the lips in response to labial contact, swallowing, avoidance movements of the head and neck, startle reaction (Moro response, see further on) in response to loud noise or dropping of the head into an extended position, grasp reflexes, and support, stepping, and placing movements. This repertoire of movements, as mentioned earlier, depends on reflexes organized mainly at the spinal and brainstem levels. Only the placing reactions, ocular fixation, and following movements (the latter are established by the third month) are thought to depend on emerging cortical connections, but even this is debatable. In the neonatal period, when little of the cerebrum has begun to function, extensive cerebral lesions may cause little derangement of motor function and may pass unnoticed unless special methods of examination—sensory evoked potentials, electroencephalography (EEG), CT, and MRI—are used. Of clinically testable neurologic phenomena in the neonatal period, disturbances of ocular movement, seizures, tremulousness of the arms, impaired arousal reactions and muscular tone, all of which relate essentially to upper brainstem and diencephalic mechanisms, provide the most reliable clues to the presence of neurologic disease. Prechtl and associates have affirmed the importance of disturbances of these neurologic functions at this early age as predictors of delayed development.

During early infancy, the motor system undergoes a variety of differentiations as visual, auditory, and tactile motor mechanisms develop. Bodily postures are modified to accommodate these complex sensorimotor acquisitions. In the normal infant, these emerging motor differentiations follow a time schedule prescribed by the maturation of neural connections. Normalcy is expressed by the age at which each of these appears, as shown in Table 28-4. It is also evident from this table that reflex and instinctual motor activities are the most dependable means of evaluating early development. Moreover, in the normally developing infant, some of these activities disappear as others appear. For example, the grasp reflex, extension of the limbs without a flexor phase, Moro response, tonic neck reflexes, and crossed adduction in response to eliciting the knee jerk gradually become less prominent and are usually not elicitable by the sixth month. *The absence of these reflexes in the first few months of life and conversely, their persistence beyond this time indicate a defect in cerebral development*, as described in more detail further on, under "Delays in Motor Development." By contrast, neck-righting reflexes, support reactions, the Landau reaction (extending neck and legs when held prone), the parachute maneuver, and the pincer grasp, which are absent in the first 6 months, begin to appear by the seventh to eighth months and are present in all normal infants by the twelfth month.

Because many functions that are classified as "mental" at a later period of life have a different anatomic basis than motor functions, it is not surprising that early motor achievements do not correlate closely with childhood intelligence. The converse does not apply, however; delay in the acquisition of motor milestones often correlates with developmental delay. In other words, *most cognitively delayed children sit, stand, walk, and run at a later age than normal children*, and deviations from this rule occur mainly in special diseases such as autism.

In the period of early childhood, the reflexive-instinctual activities are no longer of help in evaluating cerebral development, and one must turn to the examination of language functions and learned sensory and motor skills, which are outlined in Tables 28-5 and 28-6.

Quite apart from the early stage of motor development, in later childhood and adolescence one observes a remarkable variation in levels of muscular activity, strength, and coordination. Motor acquisitions of later childhood such as hopping on one foot, kicking a ball, jumping over a line, walking gracefully, dancing, and certain skills in sports are linked to age but there is wide variability in the finesse with which they are performed. Ozeretzkii has combined these in a scale that putatively discloses arrests in motor development in the developmentally delayed. Also in later childhood, precocity in learning complex motor skills as well as skill in games and the development of an all-around interest in athletic activity becomes evident. By adolescence, high individual physical achievement is well recognized. At the other end of the spectrum are instances of motor underachievement, ineptitude, and intrinsic awkwardness; a member of this group will easily stand out and be designated as "an awkward child." Such awkwardness is to be clearly distinguished from the motor impairment associated with a number of cerebral diseases.

Sensory Development

Under normal circumstances, sensory development keeps pace with motor development, and at every age sensorimotor interactions are apparent. However, under conditions of disease, this generalization may not hold; i.e., motor development may remain relatively normal in the face of a sensory defect, or vice versa. The sense organs are fully formed at birth. The neonate is crudely aware of visual, auditory, tactile, and olfactory stimuli, which elicit only low-level reflex responses. Moreover, any stimulus-related response is only to the immediate situation; there is no evidence that previous experience

Table 28-4

NEUROLOGIC FUNCTIONS AND DISTURBANCES IN INFANCY AND EARLY CHILDHOOD

AGE	NORMAL FUNCTIONS	PATHOLOGIC SIGNS
Newborn period	Blinking, tonic deviation of eyes on turning head, sucking, rooting, swallowing, yawning, grasping, brief extension of neck in prone position, incurvation response, Moro response, flexion postures of limbs Biceps reflexes present and others variable; infantile type of flexor plantar reflex; stable temperature, respirations, and blood pressure; periods of sleep and arousal: vigorous cry	Lack of arousal (stupor or coma) High-pitched or weak cry Abnormal (incomplete or absent) Moro response Opisthotonus Flaccidity or hypertonia Convulsions Tremulous limbs Failure of tonic deviation of eyes on passive movement of head or of head and body
2–3 months	Supports head Smiles Makes vowel sounds Adopts tonic asymmetrical neck postures (tonic neck reflexes) Large range of movements of limbs, tendon reflexes usually present Fixates on and follows a dangling toy Suckles vigorously Period of sleep sharply differentiated from awake periods Support and stepping unelicitable Vertical suspension—legs flex, head up Optokinetic nystagmus elicitable	Absence of any or all of the normal functions Convulsions Hypotonia or hypertonia of neck and limbs Vertical suspension—legs extend and adduct
4 months	Good head support, minimal head lag Coos and chuckles Inspects hands Tone of limbs moderate or diminished Turns to sounds Rolls over from prone to supine Grasping, sucking, and tonic neck reflexes subservient to volition	Lack of head support Motor deficits Hypertonia Lack of social reactions Tonic neck reflexes present Strong Moro response Absence of symmetrical attitude
5–6 months	Babbles Reaches and grasps Vocalizes in social play Discriminates between family and strangers Moro and grasp reflexes disappear Tries to recover lost object Begins to sit; no head lag on pull to sit Positive support reaction Tonic neck reflexes gone Landau response (holds head above horizontal, arches back when held horizontally) Begins to grasp objects with one hand; holds bottle	Altered tone Obligatory postures Cannot sit or roll over Hypo- or hypertonia Persistent Moro and grasp Persistent tonic neck reflexes No Landau response
9 months	Creeps and pulls to stand; stands holding on Sits securely Babbles "Mama," "Dada," or equivalent Sociable; plays "pat-a-cake," seeks attention Drinks from cup Landau response present Parachute response present Grasps with thumb to forefinger	Fails to attain these motor, verbal, and social milestones Persistent automatisms and tonic neck reflexes or hypo- or hypertonia
12 months	Stands alone May walk, or walks if led Tries to feed self May say several single words, echoes sounds Plantar reflexes definitely flexor Throws objects	Failure to attain 12-month milestones Persistence of automatisms
15 months	Walks independently (9–16 months), falls easily Moves arms steadily Says several words; scribbles with crayon Requests by pointing Interest in sounds, music, pictures, and animal toys	Retardation in reaching milestones expected at this age Persistent abnormalities of tone and posture Sensory discriminations defective

(*continued*)

Table 28-4

NEUROLOGIC FUNCTIONS AND DISTURBANCES IN INFANCY AND EARLY CHILDHOOD (*CONTINUED*)

AGE	NORMAL FUNCTIONS	PATHOLOGIC SIGNS
18 months	Says at least 6 words Feeds self; uses spoon well May obey commands Runs stiffly; seats self in chair Hand dominance Throws ball Plays several nursery games Uses simple tools in imitation Removes shoes and stockings Points to two or three parts of body, common objects, and pictures in book	Cannot walk No words
24 months	Says 2- or 3-word sentences Scribbles Runs well; climbs stairs one at a time Bends over and picks up objects Kicks ball; turns knob Organized play Builds tower of 6 blocks Sometimes toilet trained	Retarded in all motor, linguistic, and social adaptive skills

Source: Reproduced by permission of the Gesell Institute of Child Development.

Table 28-5

DEVELOPMENTAL ACHIEVEMENTS OF THE NORMAL PRESCHOOL CHILD

AGE	OBSERVED ITEMS	USEFUL CLINICAL TESTS
2 years	Runs well Goes up and down stairs, 1 step at a time Climbs on furniture Opens doors Helps to undress Feeds well with spoon Puts 3 words together Listens to stories with pictures	Pencil-paper test: scribbles, imitates horizontal stroke Folds paper once Builds tower of 6 blocks
2.5 years	Jumps on both feet; walks on tiptoes if asked Knows full name; asks questions Refers to self as "I" Helps put away toys and clothes Names animals in book, knows 1 to 3 colors Can complete 3-piece form board	Pencil-paper test: copies horizontal and vertical line Builds tower of 8 blocks
3 years	Climbs stairs, alternating feet Talks constantly; recites nursery rhymes Rides tricycle Stands on one foot momentarily Plays simple games Helps in dressing Washes hands Identifies 5 colors	Builds 9-cube tower Builds bridge with 3 cubes Imitates circle and cross with pencil
4 years	Climbs well; hops and skips on one foot; throws ball overhand; kicks ball Cuts out pictures with scissors Counts 4 pennies Tells a story; plays with other children Goes to toilet alone	Copies cross and circle Builds gate with 5 cubes Builds a bridge from model Draws a human figure with 2 to 4 parts other than head Distinguishes short and long line
5 years	Skips Names 4 colors; counts 10 pennies Dresses and undresses Asks questions about meaning of words	Copies square and triangle Distinguishes heavier of 2 weights More detailed drawing of a human figure

Table 28-6

USEFUL PSYCHOMETRIC TESTS FOR EVALUATING LEARNING AND BEHAVIORAL DISABILITIES IN CHILDREN[a]

DEFICIT	TEST
Development	Denver Developmental Test; Vineland Social Maturity Test; Leiter International Performance Scale; Otis Group Intelligence Test
Achievement	Wide Range Achievement Test; Gates Primary Reading Test
Attentiveness	Dehoit Test of hearing aptitude
Calculation	Key Math Diagnostic Arithmetic Test
Vocabulary	Peabody Picture Vocabulary
Developmental Gerstmann syndrome (finger agnosia, right–left disorientation)	Finger Order Tests; Benton Right–Left Discrimination Test
Figure copying	Visual–Motor Integration Test
Visual memory	Benton Visual Retention Test
Error patterns	Boder Test of Reading–Spelling Patterns
Impulsiveness	Matching Familiar Figures Test

[a]For descriptions of individual tests, see Kinsbourne, 1995.

with the stimulus has influenced the response; i.e., that the newborn can learn and remember. The capacity to attend to a stimulus, to fixate on it for any period of time, also comes later. Indeed, the length of fixation time is a quantifiable index of perceptual development in infancy.

Information is available about the time at which the infant makes the first interpretable responses to each of the different modes of stimulation. The most nearly perfect senses in the newborn are those of touch and pain. A series of pinpricks cause distress, whereas an abrasion of the skin seems not to do so. The sense of touch clearly plays a role in feeding behavior. Newborn infants react vigorously to irritating odors such as ammonia and acetic acid, but discrimination between olfactory stimuli is not evident until much later. Sugar solutions initiate and maintain sucking from birth on, whereas quinine (bitter) solutions seldom do, and the latter stimulus elicits avoidance behavior. Hearing in the newborn is manifest within the first few postnatal days. Sharp, quick sounds elicit responsive blinking and sometimes startle. In some infants, the human voice appears to cause similar reactions by the second week. Strong light and objects held before the face evoke reactions in the neonate; later, visual searching is an integrating factor in most projected motor activities.

Sensation in the newborn infant must be judged largely by its motor reactions, so that sensory and motor developments seem to run in parallel but this may be partly artifactual. There are nonetheless discernible maturational stages that constitute sensory milestones, so to speak. This is most apparent in the visual system, which is more easily studied than the other senses. Sustained ocular fixation on an object is observable at term and even in some preterm infants; at these ages it is essentially a reflexive phototropic reaction. It has been observed that the neonate will consistently gaze at some stimuli more often than others, suggesting, according to Fantz, that there must already be some elements of perception and differentiation at this early stage. Voluntary fixation (i.e., following a moving object) is a later development. Horizontal following occurs at about 50 days; vertical following, at 55 days; and following an object that is moving in a circle, at 75 days. Preference for a colored stimulus over a gray one was recorded by Staples by the end of the third month. By 6 months the infant discriminates between colors, and saturated colors can be matched at 30 months. Perception of form, at least as judged by the length of time spent in looking at different visual presentations, is evident at 2 or 3 months of age (Fantz). At this time infants are attracted more to certain patterns than to colors. At 3 months, most infants have discovered their hands and spend considerable time watching their movements. The ages at which infants begin to observe color, size, shape, and numbers can be determined by means of the Terman-Merrill and Stutzman intelligence tests (see Gibson and Olum). Perception of size becomes increasingly accurate in the preschool years. An 18-month-old child discriminates among pictures of familiar animals and recognizes them equally well if they are upside down.

Visual discrimination is reflected in manual reactions, just as auditory discrimination is reflected in vocal responses. Much of early visual development (first year) involves peering at objects, judging their position, reaching for them, and seizing and manipulating them. The inseparability of sensory and motor functions is never more obvious. Sensory deprivation impedes not only the natural sequences of perceptual awareness of the child's surroundings but also the development of all motor activities. *Auditory discrimination*—reflected in vocalizations such as babbling and, later, in word formation—is discussed further on in connection with language development.

The Development of Intelligence

(See also Chap. 21)

The subject of intellectual endowment and the development and testing of intelligence were touched upon in Chap. 21. There it was pointed out that although intelligence is modifiable by training, practice, and schooling, it is much more a matter of native endowment and not simply a question of environment and providing the stimulus to learn, although these are clearly factors. It is evident early in life that some individuals have a superior intelligence; they also clearly maintain this differentiation all through life, and the opposite pertains in others.

Much of the uncertainty about the relative influence of heredity and environment relates to our imprecise views of what constitutes intelligence. The authors tend to agree with those who view intelligence as a general mental capability, embracing a number of primary abilities: the capacity to comprehend complex ideas, learn from experience, think abstractly, reason, plan, draw analogies, and solve problems. Thus intelligence includes a multiplicity of abilities, which probably accounts for a lack of consensus about its mechanism. Everyday experience teaches us that it is not always abstract tasks that suffer most when intelligence is impaired. Indeed, even abstraction is not likely to be a unitary function. Theoreticians, like Carl Spearman, believed that intelligence comprises a general (*g*), or core, factor and a series of special (*s*) factors. In contrast, Thurstone conceived of intelligence as a mosaic of factors such as drive and curiosity, verbal and arithmetic ability, memory, capacity for abstract thinking, practical skills in manipulating objects, geographic or spatial sense, and athletic and musical ability—each of which appears to be largely genetically determined. These and other theories concerning intellectual development in the child, such as those of Eysenck and of Gardner, and particularly those of Piaget, were considered briefly in Chap. 21, which may be read as an extension of this section.

The beginnings of the development of intelligence are difficult to discern. It is readily assessed at 8 to 9 months of life, when the infant begins to crawl and explore. Now, learning proceeds rapidly as adults attach names to objects and help the baby manipulate them. Gradually the child acquires verbal facility (learning what words mean), memory, color and spatial perception, a concept of number, and the practical use of tools, each at a particular time according to a schedule set largely by the maturational state of the brain. Nevertheless, in these early achievements individuals differ considerably, reflecting to some extent the influence of their parents and others around them. Also, the young child exhibits elementary modes of thinking but is highly suggestible and often incapable of separating imagination from reality.

Neurologists who need a quick and practical method of ascertaining whether an infant or preschool child is measuring up to normal standards for a particular age will find Table 28-4 useful. The main items are drawn from Gesell and Amatruda and from the Denver Developmental Test. In addition, a variety of intelligence tests have been designed to measure the child's special abilities and increasing success in learning in accordance with age (these are listed in Table 28-5). Starting at age 6 to 7 years, there is a steady improvement in intelligence scores that parallels chronologic age up to about age 13 years; thereafter the rate of advance diminishes. By age 16 to 17 years, performance reaches a plateau, but this is probably an artifact of the commonly used tests, which are designed to predict success in school. Only late in life do test scores begin to diminish, in a manner that is described in the next chapter on aging. Individuals with high or low IQs at 6 years of age tend to maintain their rank at 10, 15, and 20 years unless the early scores were impaired by anxiety, poor motivation, or a gross lack of opportunity to acquire the skills that are necessary to take such tests (language skill in particular). Even then, performance tasks, which largely eliminate verbal and mathematical skills, will disclose many individual differences.

The reliability of intelligence tests and their validity as predictive measures of scholastic, occupational, and economic success have been heatedly debated for many years. This aspect of the subject is discussed in the section on Intelligence in Chap. 21 and need not be repeated here. The most persuasive argument for these tests as an index of some type of native ability is that individuals drawn from a fairly homogeneous environment tend to maintain the same rating on the intelligence scale throughout their lives. While native endowment may set some limits on learning and achievement; opportunity, personality traits, and other factors clearly determine how nearly the individual's full potential is realized.

The Development of Language

Closely tied to the development of intelligence is the acquisition of language. Indeed, facility with language is one of the best indices of intelligence (Lenneberg). The acquisition of speech and language by the infant and child has been observed methodically by a number of eminent investigators, and their findings provide a background for the understanding of a number of derangements in the development of these functions (Ingram; Rutter and Martin).

Early verbalizations consist of *babbling*, *cooing*, and *lalling stages*, during which the infant, a few weeks old, emits a variety of cooing and then, at about 6 months, babbling sounds in the form of vowel–consonant (labial and nasoguttural) combinations. Later, babbling becomes interspersed with pauses, inflections, and intonations drawn from what the infant hears. At first this appears to be a purely self-initiated activity, being the same in normal and deaf infants. However, study of the latter shows that auditory modifications begin within a period of 2 to 3 months; without an auditory sense, babblers do not produce the variety of random sounds of the normal infant, nor do they begin to imitate the sounds made by the mother. Thus motor speech is stimulated and reinforced mainly by auditory sensations, which become linked to the kinesthetic ones arising from the speech musculature. It is not clear whether the capacity to hear and understand the spoken word precedes or follows the first motor speech. Perhaps it varies from one infant to another, but the dependence of motor speech development on hearing is undeniable. Comprehension seems to postdate the first verbal utterance of words in most infants.

Soon babbling merges with *echo speech*, in which short sounds are repeated parrot-like; gradually longer syllable groups are repeated correctly as the praxic function of the speech apparatus develops. As a general rule, the first recognizable words appear by the end of 12 months. Initially these are attached directly to persons and objects and then are used increasingly to designate objects. The word then becomes the symbol, and this substitution greatly facilitates speaking and later thinking about people and objects. Nouns are learned first, then verbs and other parts of speech. Exposure to and correction by parents and siblings gradually shapes vocal behavior, including the development of a distinctive and enduring accent, to conform to that of the social group in which the child is raised.

During the second year of life, the child begins to use word combinations. They form the propositions, which, according to Hughlings Jackson, are the essence of language (a notion in part echoed by modern linguists as noted in Chap. 23). On average, at 18 months the child can combine an average of 1.5 words; at 2 years, 2 words; at 2.5 years, 3 words; and at 3 years, 4 words. Pronunciation of words undergoes a similar progression; 90 percent of children can articulate all vowel sounds by the age of 3 years. At a slightly later age the consonants *p, b, m, h, w, d, n, t,* and *k* are enunciated; *ng* by the age of 4 years; *y, j, zh,* and *wh* by 5 to 6 years; and *f, l, v, sh, ch, s, v,* and *th* by 7 years. Girls tend to acquire articulatory facility earlier than boys. The vocabulary increases, so that at 18 months the child knows 6 to 20 words; by 24 months, 50 to 200 words; by 3 years, 200 to 400 words. By 4 years, the child is normally capable of telling stories, but with little distinction between fact and imagination. By 6 years, the average child knows several thousand words. Also by that age, children can indicate spatial and temporal relationships and start to inquire about causality. The understanding of spoken language always exceeds the child's speaking vocabulary; that is to say, most children understand more than they can say.

The next stage of language development is reading. Here there must be an association of graphic symbols with the auditory, visual, and kinesthetic images of words already acquired. Usually the written word is learned by associating it with the spoken word rather than with the seen object. The integrity of the superior gyrus of the temporal lobe (Wernicke area) and contiguous parietooccipital areas of the dominant hemisphere are essential to the establishment of these crossmodal associations. Writing is learned soon after reading, the audiovisual symbols of words being linked to cursive movements of the hand. The tradition of beginning grade school at 5 or 6 years is based not on an arbitrary decision but on the empirically determined age at which the nervous system of the average child is ready to learn and execute the tasks of reading, writing, and, soon thereafter, calculating.

Once language is fully acquired, it is integrated into all aspects of complex action and behavior. Movements of volitional type are activated by a spoken command or the individual's inner phrasing of an intended action. Every plan for the solution of a problem must be cast into language, and the final result is analyzed in verbal terms. Thinking and language are, therefore, inseparable.

Anthropologists see in all this a grander scheme wherein the individual recapitulates the language development of the human race. They point out that in primitive peoples, language consisted of gestures and the utterance of simple sounds expressing emotion and that, over periods of time, movements and sounds became the conventional signs and verbal symbols of objects. Later these sounds came to designate the abstract qualities of objects. Historically, signs and spoken language were the first means of human communication; graphic records appeared much later. Native Americans, for instance, never reached the level of syllabic written language. Writing commenced as pictorial representation and only much later in human evolution were alphabets devised. The reading and writing of words are comparatively late achievements. For further details concerning communicative and cognitive abilities and methods of assessment, the reader may consult the monograph by Minifie and Lloyd.

Sexual Development

The terms *sexual* and *sexuality* have several meanings in medical and nonmedical writings. The most obvious one relates to the functions of the male and female sexual organs through which procreation occurs and the survival of the species is assured as well as to behaviors that serve to attract the opposite sex and ultimately lead to mating. The terms refer also to a person's concern or preoccupation with sex or his erotic desires or activities. A more ambiguous meaning has been proposed by some psychologists, for whom the term is equated with all growth and development, the experience of pleasure, and survival.

Much of now discredited Freudian psychoanalytic theory centers on the sexual development of the child and, on the basis of questionable observations, espouses the view that repression of the sexual impulse and the psychic conflicts resulting therefrom are the main sources of neurosis and possibly psychosis.

The following are the main chronologic steps in sexual development, taken from the observations of Gesell and colleagues and itemized in de Ajuriaguerra's monograph. The timetable of menarche and other aspects of sexual development show considerable variation. If sexuality is not allowed natural expression, it often becomes a source of worry and preoccupation. Some 10 percent of the population fails to develop heterosexual orientation. Perverse derangements of psychosexual function are another matter entirely and are not addressed here.

Homosexuality

This denotes a preferential erotic attraction to members of the same sex. Most psychiatrists exclude from the definition of homosexuality those patterns of behavior that are not motivated by specific preferential desire, such as the incidental homosexuality of adolescents and the situational homosexuality of prisoners.

Figures on incidence are difficult to secure. According to the early reports of Kinsey and colleagues, approximately 4 percent of American males are exclusively homosexual and 8 percent have been "more or less exclusively homosexual for at least 3 years, sometime between the ages of 16 and 65." For females, the incidence is lower, perhaps half that for males. It was estimated, on the basis of the examination of large numbers of military personnel during World War II, that 1 to 2 percent of servicemen were exclusively or predominantly homosexual. More recent estimates, both in men and women, range from 1 to 5 percent (see LeVay and Hamer). These widely variable figures share a problem with all estimates derived from surveys and questionnaires: they cannot count people who do not wish to be counted.

The origins of homosexuality are obscure. The authors favor the hypothesis that differences or variations in genetic patterning of the nervous system (possibly of the hypothalamus) set the sexual predilection during early life. Several morphologic studies of the hypothalamus are significant in this regard. Swaab and Hofman have reported that the preoptic zone is three times larger in heterosexual males than it is in females, but it is about the same size in homosexual males as it is in females. As mentioned in Chap. 27, LeVay found that an aggregate of neurons in the suprachiasmatic nucleus of the hypothalamus is two to three times larger in heterosexual men than it is in women, and also two to three times larger in heterosexual than in homosexual men. If confirmed, these findings, which have been disputed by Byne and others, would support the view that homosexuality has a biologic basis. Genetic studies point in the same direction. Pooled data from 5 studies in men show that approximately 57 percent of identical twins (and 13 percent of brothers) of homosexual men are also homosexual. The figures for lesbians are much the same. In most studies, the inheritance pattern of male homosexuality comes from the maternal side, implicating a gene on the X chromosome (LeVay and Hamer) but to suggest there is a simple genetic connection is oversimplified.

Psychoanalytic explanations of homosexuality have never been substantiated. Attempts to demonstrate an endocrine basis for homosexuality have also failed. The most widely held current view is that homosexuality is not a mental or a personality disorder, though it may at times lead to secondary reactive disturbances. The studies of Kinsey and colleagues indicate that a homosexual orientation cannot be traced to a single social or psychologic root. Instead, as indicated above, homosexuality seems to arise from a deep-seated predisposition, biologic in origin and as ingrained as heterosexuality. The status of bisexuality is undetermined.

The Development of Personality and Social Adaptation (See also Chap. 51)

Personality, the most inclusive of all psychologic terms, encompasses the entirety of psychologic traits that distinguish one individual from every other. The notion that one's physical characteristics are determined by inheritance is a fundamental tenet of biology. One has but to observe the resemblances between parent and child to confirm this view. Just as no two persons are physically identical, not even monozygotic twins, so, too, do they differ in any other refined quality one chooses to measure, particularly those that determine behavior and modes of thinking. Strictly speaking, the normal person is an abstraction, just as is a typical example of any disease.

It is in nonphysical attributes that individuals display the greatest differences. Here reference is made to their variable place on a scale of energy, capacity for effective work, sensitivity, temperament, emotional responsivity, aggressivity or passivity, risk taking, ethical sense, flexibility, and tolerance to change and stress. The composite of these qualities constitutes the human personality or character. The current model of personality structure identifies 5 dimensions, which account for the covariation of most personality traits: (1) neuroticism versus emotional stability; (2) extraversion versus introversion; (3) openness to experience versus aversion to change; (4) agreeableness versus irascibility; and (5) conscientiousness versus unscrupulousness, and all five of these are heritable, as discussed in Chap. 51.

In the formation of personality, especially the part concerned with feeling and emotional sensitivity, basic temperament surely plays a large part. By nature, some children from the beginning seem to be happy, cheerful, and unconcerned about immediate frustrations; others are the opposite. By the third month of life, Birch and Belmont recognized individual differences in activity–passivity, regularity–irregularity, intensity of action, approach–withdrawal, adaptivity–unadaptivity, high–low threshold of response to stimulation, positive–negative mood, high–low selectivity, and high–low distractibility. Ratings at this early age were found to correlate with the results of examinations made at age 5 years. Kagan and Moss recognized the trait of timidity as early as 6 months of age and noted that it persists lifelong.

The more common aspects of personality, i.e., anxiety or serenity, timidity or boldness, the power of instinctual drives and need of satisfaction, sympathy for others, sensitivity to criticism, and degree of disorganization resulting from adverse circumstances, are presumed to be genetically determined. Identical twins raised apart are remarkably alike in these and many other personality traits (and have the same IQs, within a few points; Moser et al). Scarr and associates have also demonstrated the strong genetic influence on personality development. The related subject of the development of a moral sense that can be said to be part of an individual's personality has been subject to several competing theories. The interested reader is referred to Damon's summary of the topic.

Chapter 51 discusses disorders of personality and the genetic predisposition to certain personality traits further.

Social behavior, like other neurologic and psychologic functions in general, depends to a great extent on the development and maturation of the brain. Involved also are genetic and environmental factors, for one cannot adapt to society except in the presence of other people; i.e., social interaction is necessary for the emergence of many basic biologic traits. The roots of social behavior are traceable to certain instinctive patterns that are progressively elaborated by conditioned emotional reactions. In the long series of human interactions—first with parents, then with siblings and other children, and finally with a widening circle of individuals in the classroom and community, the capacity to cooperate, to subjugate one's own egocentric needs to those of the group, and to lead or be led appear as secondary modes of response (i.e., secondary to some of the basic impulses of anger, fear, self-protection, love, and pleasure). The sources of these social reactions are even more obscure than those of temperament, character, and intelligence.

In children, difficulty in social adaptation tends first to be manifest by an inability to take their places in a classroom. However, the greatest demands and frustrations in social development are likely to occur in late childhood and adolescence. The development of adult gonadal function and the further evolution of psychosexual impulses create a bewildering array of new challenges in social adaptation. These types of social adjustments continue as long as life continues. As social roles change, as intellectual and physical capacities first advance and later recede, new challenges demand new adaptations.

DELAYS AND FAILURES OF NORMAL NEUROLOGIC DEVELOPMENT

Delays in Motor Development

A delay in motor development is often accompanied by a delay in cognitive development, in which case both are parts of a developmental lag or immaturity of the entire cerebrum. The most severe forms of delayed motor development, those associated with spasticity and athetosis, are usually manifestations of prenatal and perinatal diseases of the brain subsumed under the term cerebral palsy; these are discussed in Chap. 38.

In assessing developmental abnormalities of the motor system in the neonate and young infant, the following maneuvers, which elicit certain postures and reflexive movements, are particularly useful:

1. The *Moro response* is the infant's reaction to startle and can be evoked by suddenly withdrawing support of the head and allowing the neck to extend. A loud noise, slapping the bed, or jerking one leg will have the same effect, causing an elevation and abduction of the arms followed by a clasping movement to the midline. This response is present in newborns and infants, it wanes after 2 months and is no longer elicitable after about 5 months of age, and its absence before that time or persistence afterwards indicates a disorder of the motor system. An absent or inadequate Moro response on one side is found in infants with hemiplegia, brachial plexus palsy, or a fractured clavicle. Persistence of the Moro response beyond 4 or 5 months of age is noted only in infants with severe neurologic defects.
2. The *tonic neck reflex* consisting of extension of the arm and leg on the side to which the head is passively turned and flexion of the opposite limbs, if obligatory and sustained, is a sign at any age of pyramidal or extrapyramidal motor abnormality. Barlow reports that he has obtained this reflex in 25 percent of developmentally delayed infants at 9 to 10 months of age. Fragments of the reflex, such as a brief extension of one arm, may be elicited in 60 percent of normal infants at 1 to 2 months of age and may be adopted spontaneously by the infant up to 6 months of age. As with the Moro response, persistence beyond this age represents a malfunction of the nervous system.
3. The *placing reaction* in which the foot or hand, brought into contact with the edge of a table, is lifted automatically and placed on the flat surface, is present in all normal newborns. Its absence or asymmetry in infants younger than 6 months of age indicates a motor abnormality.
4. In the *Landau maneuver*, the infant, if suspended horizontally in the prone position, will extend the neck and trunk and will break the trunk extension when the neck is passively flexed. This reaction is present by age 6 months; its delayed appearance in a hypotonic child is indicative of a faulty motor apparatus.
5. If an infant is held prone in the horizontal position and is then dropped toward the bed, an extension of the arms is evoked, as if to break the fall. This is known as the *parachute response* and is elicitable in most 9-month-old infants. If it is asymmetrical, it indicates a unilateral motor abnormality.

The detection of gross delays or abnormalities of motor development in the neonatal or early infantile period of life is aided little by tests of tendon and plantar reflexes. Arm reflexes are always rather difficult to obtain in infants, and a normal neonate may have a few beats of ankle clonus. The plantar response tends to be wavering and uncertain in pattern. However, a consistent extension of the great toe and fanning of the toes on stroking the side of the foot is abnormal at any age.

The early detection of cerebral palsy is hampered by the fact that the corticospinal tract is not fully myelinated until 18 months of age, allowing only quasivoluntary movements up to this time. For this reason, a *congenital hemiparesis* may not be evident until many months after birth. Even then it is manifest only by subtle signs, such as holding the hand in a fisted posture or clumsiness in reaching for objects and in transferring them from one hand to the other. Later, the leg is seen to be less active as the infant crawls, steps, and places the foot. Early hand dominance should always raise the suspicion of a motor defect on the opposite side. In the upper limb, the characteristic catch and yielding resistance of spasticity is most evident in passive abduction of the arm, extension of the elbow, dorsiflexion of the wrist, and supination of the forearm; in the leg, the change in tone is best detected by passive flexion of the knee. However, the time of appearance and degree of spasticity are variable from child to child. The stretch reflexes are hyperactive, and the plantar reflex may be extensor on the affected side. With bilateral hemiplegia, the same abnormalities are detectable, but there is a greater likelihood of pseudobulbar manifestations, with delayed, poorly enunciated speech.

Later, intelligence is likely to be impaired (in 40 percent of hemiplegias and 70 percent of bilateral hemiplegias). In *diparesis* or *diplegia*, hypotonia gives way to spasticity and the same delay in motor development except that it predominates in the legs. Aside from the hereditary spastic paraplegias, which may become evident in the second and third years, the common causes of weak spastic legs are prematurity and matrix hemorrhages. These various forms of cerebral palsy are described in Chap. 38.

Developmental motor delay and other abnormalities are present in a large proportion of infants with *hypotonia*. When the "floppy" infant is lifted and its limbs are passively manipulated, there is little muscle reactivity. In the supine position, the weakness and laxity result in a "frog-leg" posture, along with an increased mobility at the ankles and hips. Hypotonia, if generalized and accompanied by an absence of tendon reflexes, is most often a result of Werdnig-Hoffmann disease (an early life loss of anterior horn cells, a type of spinal muscular atrophy), although the range of possible diagnoses is large and includes diseases of muscle, nerve, and the central nervous system (see Chaps. 38 and 48). The other causes of this type of neonatal and infantile hypotonia include muscular dystrophies and congenital myopathies, maternal myasthenia gravis, polyneuropathies, Down syndrome, Prader-Willi syndrome, and spinal cord injuries, each of which is described in its appropriate chapter. Hypotonia that arises in utero may be accompanied by congenital fixed contractures of the joints, termed *arthrogryposis*, as discussed in Chap. 48.

Infants who will later manifest a central motor defect can sometimes be recognized by the briskness of their tendon reflexes and by the postures they assume when lifted. In the normal infant, the legs are flexed, slightly rotated externally, and associated with vigorous kicking movements. The hypotonic infant with a defect of the motor projection pathways may extend the legs or rotate them internally, with dorsiflexion of the feet and toes. Exceptionally, the legs are firmly flexed, but in either instance relatively few movements are made.

When hypotonia is a forerunner of an extrapyramidal motor disorder (so-called double athetosis, another type of cerebral palsy), the first hint of abnormality may be opisthotonic posturing of the head and neck. However, involuntary choreic movements usually do not appear in the upper limbs before 5 to 6 months of age and often are so slight as to be overlooked. They worsen as the infant matures and by 12 months assume a more athetotic character, often combined with tremor. Tone in the affected limbs is by then increased but may be interrupted during passive manipulation.

Hypotonia may also be a prelude to a cerebellar motor defect. The ataxia becomes apparent when the infant makes the first reaching movements. Tremulous, irregular movements of the trunk and head are seen when the infant attempts to sit without support. Still later, as the infant attempts to stand, there is unsteadiness of the entire body.

In distinction to the gross deficits in motor development described earlier, there is a distinct group of young children who exhibit only mild abnormalities of muscle tone, clumsiness or unusual postures or rhythmic movements of the hands, tremor, and ataxia ("fine motor deficit"), or "developmental coordination disorders." Such awkwardness in the somewhat older child is referred to as a "soft sign" and has been reviewed by Gubbay and colleagues in what they have called "the clumsy child." Like speech delay and dyslexia, fine motor deficits of this sort are more frequent in males. Tirosh found that intranatal problems were more prevalent among children with fine motor deficits (compared to those with gross motor deficits), as were minor physical anomalies and seizures.

Systemic diseases in infancy pose special problems in evaluation of the motor system. The achievement of motor milestones is delayed by illnesses such as congenital heart disease (especially cyanotic forms), cystic fibrosis, renal and hepatic diseases, infections, and surgical procedures. Under such conditions one does well to deal with the immediate illnesses and defer pronouncements about the status of cerebral function. The brain proves to be simultaneously affected in 25 percent of patients with serious forms of congenital heart disease and an even higher proportion of patients with rubella and coxsackie B viral infections. In a disease such as cystic fibrosis, where the brain is not affected, it is advisable to depend more on the analysis of language development than on assessment of motor function, because muscular activity may be generally enfeebled.

Delays in Sensory Development

Failure to see and to hear are the most important sensory defects affecting the infant and child. When *both* senses are affected, a severe cerebral defect is usually responsible; only at a later age, when the child is more testable, does it become apparent that the trouble is not with the peripheral sensory apparatus but with the central integrating mechanisms of the brain.

Failure of development of visual function is usually revealed by strabismus and by disorders of ocular movements, as described in Chap. 13. Any defect of the refractive apparatus or the acuity of the central visual pathways results in wandering, jerky movements of the eyes. The optic discs may be atrophic in such cases, but it should be pointed out that the discs in infants tend naturally to be paler than those of an older child. In congenital hypoplasia of the optic nerves, the nerve heads are extremely small. Defects in the retina and choroid are detectable by funduscopy. Faulty vision becomes increasingly apparent in older infants when the normal sequences of hand inspection and visuomanual coordination fail to emerge. Retention of pupillary light reflexes in a sightless child signifies a defect in the geniculocalcarine tracts or occipital lobes—conditions that may be confirmed by MRI and testing of visual evoked responses.

With respect to hearing, again there is the difficulty in evaluating this function in an infant. Normally, after a few weeks of life, alert parents notice that the child makes a brisk startle to loud noises and a response to other sounds. A tinkling bell brought from behind the infant usually results in hearkening or head turning and visual searching, but a lack of these responses warns only of the most severe hearing defects. The detection of slight degrees of deafness, enough to interfere with auditory learning, requires special testing. To make the problem even more difficult, both a peripheral and a central disorder may be present in some conditions, such as the now infrequent disorder of kernicterus. Brainstem auditory evoked responses are particularly helpful in confirming peripheral (cochlear and eighth nerve) abnormalities in the infant and young child. After the first few months, impaired hearing becomes more obvious and interferes with language development, as described further on. It is of interest that the identification and remediation of early (infants) hearing defects by screening leads to higher scores on language tests later in childhood but not improved speech, according to a study by Kennedy and colleagues.

RESTRICTED DEVELOPMENTAL ABNORMALITIES

A considerable portion of neuropediatric practice is committed to the diagnosis and management of children with learning disabilities. These problems usually come to light in the school-age child (hence the term *school dysfunction*), whose aptitude for classroom learning is poorer than the child's general intelligence. The medical referral may be from a parent, teacher, or psychologist. The clinician's objective is to determine by history and examination whether there is (1) a general congenital developmental abnormality impairing intelligence; (2) a specific deficit in reading, writing, arithmetic, or attention, any one of which may interfere with the child's ability to learn; (3) a primary sensory defect, particularly in audition; or (4) neither of these—for example, a behavior disorder or home situation that interferes with schooling.

Once diagnosis is achieved, the goal of management, undertaken in collaboration with psychologists and educators, is to fashion a program of remedial exercises that will maximize the child's skills to a point commensurate with his talent and aptitude, and restore his self-confidence.

Disorders in the Development of Speech and Language

In the pediatric age period and extending into adult life, one encounters an interesting assortment of developmental disorders of speech and language. Many patients with such disorders come from families in which similar speech defects, ambidexterity, and left-handedness are also frequent. Males predominate; in some series, male-to-female ratios as high as 10:1 have been reported.

Developmental disorders of speech and language are far more frequent than acquired disorders, e.g., aphasia. The former include developmental speech delay, congenital deafness with speech delay, developmental word deafness, dyslexia (special reading disability), cluttered speech, infantilisms of speech, and stuttering or stammering, and mechanical disorders such as cleft-palate speech. Often in these disorders, the various stages of language development described earlier are not attained at the usual age and may not be achieved even by adulthood. Disorders of this type, especially those restricted to the language areas of the cerebrum, are far more frequently a result of slowness in the normal processes of maturation than to an acquired disease. With the possible exception of developmental dyslexia (see further on), cerebral lesions have not been described in these cases, although it must be emphasized that only a small number of brains of such individuals have been thoroughly studied by proper methods.

In discussing the developmental disorders of speech and language, we have adopted a conventional classification. Not usually included in such a classification are the many mundane peculiarities of speech and language that are usually accepted without comment: lack of fluency, inability to speak uninterruptedly in complete sentences, and lack of proper intonation, inflection, and melody of speech (dysprosody).

Developmental Speech Delay

Fully two-thirds of children say their first words between 9 and 12 months of age and their first word combinations before their second birthday; when this does not happen, it becomes a matter of parental concern. Children who fail to reach these milestones at the stated times fall into two general categories. In one group there is no clear evidence of cognitive delay or impairment of neurologic or auditory function. In a second group, the speech delay has an overt pathologic basis.

The first group, comprising *otherwise normal children who talk late*, is the more puzzling. It is virtually impossible to predict whether such a child's speech will eventually be normal in all respects and just when this will occur. Prelanguage speech continues into the period when words and phrases should normally be used in propositional speech. The combinations of sounds are close to the standard of normal vowel–consonant combinations of the 1- to 2-year-old, and they may be strung together as if forming sentences. Yet, as time passes, the child may utter only a few understandable words, even by the third or fourth year. Three of 4 such patients will be boys and often one discovers a family history of delayed speech. When the child finally begins to talk, he may skip the early stages of spoken language and progress rapidly to speak in full sentences and to develop fluent speech and language in weeks or months. During the period of speech delay, the understanding of words and general intelligence develop normally, and communication by gestures may be remarkably facile. In such children, motor speech delay does not presage mental backwardness. (It is said that Albert Einstein did not speak until the age of 4 and lacked fluency at age 9.)

Nevertheless, the eventual acquisition of fluent speech is no guarantee of normalcy (Rutter and Martin). Many such children do have later educational difficulties, mainly because of dyslexia and dysgraphia, a combination that is sometimes inherited as an autosomal dominant trait, again more frequently in boys (see further on). In a smaller subgroup, articulation remains infantile and the content of speech is impoverished semantically and syntactically. Yet others, as they begin to speak, express themselves fluently, but with distortions, omissions, and cluttering of words, but such patients usually acquire normal speech patterns with development.

A second broad group of children with speech delay or slow speech development (no words by 18 months, no phrases by 30 months) comprises those in whom an overt pathologic basis is evident. In clinics where children of the latter type are studied systematically, 35 to 50 percent of cases occur in those with global developmental delay or "cerebral palsy." Hearing deficit explains many of the other cases, as discussed later, and a few represent what appears to be a specific lack of maturation of the motor speech areas or an acquired lesion in these parts. Only in this small, latter group is it appropriate to refer to the language disorder as aphasia, i.e., a derangement or loss of language caused by a cerebral lesion.

Aphasia, when it occurs as the result of an acquired lesion (vascular, traumatic) is essentially of the motor variety and typically lasts but a few months in the child. It may be accompanied by a right-sided hemiplegia. An interesting type of acquired aphasia, possibly encephalitic, has been described by Landau and Kleffner in association with seizures and bitemporal focal discharges in the EEG (see "Seizures Presenting in Early Childhood" in Chap. 16).

Congenital Deafness

Speech delay caused by congenital deafness, whether peripheral (loss of pure-tone acuity) or central (pure-tone threshold normal by audiogram), is a most important condition but may at first be difficult to discern. One suspects that faulty hearing is causal when there is a history of familial deaf mutism, congenital rubella, erythroblastosis fetalis, meningitis, chronic bilateral ear infections, or the administration of ototoxic drugs to the pregnant mother or newborn infant—the well-known antecedents of deafness. It is estimated that approximately 3 million American children have hearing defects; 0.1 percent of the school population are deaf and 1.5 percent are hard of hearing. The parents' attention may be drawn to a defect in hearing when the infant fails to heed loud noises, to turn the eyes to sound sources outside the immediate visual fields, and to react to music; but in other instances, it is the delay in speaking that calls attention to it.

As already mentioned, the deaf child makes the transition from crying to cooing and babbling at the usual age of 3 to 5 months. After the sixth month, however, the child becomes much quieter, and the usual repertoire of babbling sounds becomes stereotyped and unchanging, though still uttered with pleasant voice. A more conspicuous failure comes somewhat later, when babbling fails to give way to word formation. Should deafness develop within the first few years of life, the child gradually loses such speech as had been acquired but can be retaught by the lipreading method. Speech, however, is harsh, poorly modulated, and unpleasant, and accompanied by many peculiar squeals and snorting or grunting noises. Social and other acquisitions appear at the expected times in the congenitally deaf child, unlike in the developmentally delayed child. The deaf child seems eager to communicate and makes known all his needs by gesture or pantomime, often very cleverly. The deaf child may attract attention by vivid facial expressions, motions of the lips, nodding, or head shaking. The Leiter performance scale, which makes no use of sounds, will show that intelligence is normal. Deafness can be demonstrated at an early age by careful observation of the child's responses to sounds and by free-field audiometry, but the full range of hearing cannot be accurately tested before the age of 3 or 4 years. Recording of brainstem auditory evoked potentials and testing of the labyrinths, which are frequently unresponsive in deaf mutes, may be helpful. Early diagnosis is important so as to fit the child with a hearing aid and to begin appropriate language training.

In contrast to the child in whom deafness is the only abnormality, the developmentally delayed child generally talks little but may display a rich personality. Autistic children may also be mute; if they speak, echolalia is prominent and the personal "I" is avoided. Blind children of normal intelligence tend to speak slowly and fail to acquire imitative gestures.

Congenital Word Deafness

This disorder, also called *developmental receptive dysphasia*, *verbal auditory agnosia*, or *central deafness*, is rare and may be difficult to distinguish from peripheral deafness. Usually the parents have noted that the word-deaf child responds to loud noises and music, but obviously this does not assure perfect hearing, particularly for high tones. The word-deaf child does not understand what is said, and delay and distortion of speech are evident.

Presumably, the receptive auditory elements of the dominant temporal cortex fail to discriminate the complex acoustic patterns of words and to associate them with visual images of people and objects. Despite intact pure-tone hearing, the child does not seem to hear word patterns properly and fails to reproduce them in natural speech. In other ways the child may be bright, but more often this auditory imperception of words is associated with hyperactivity, inattentiveness, bizarre behavior, or other perceptual defects incident to focal brain damage, particularly of the temporal lobes. Word-deaf children may chatter incessantly and often adopt a language of their own design, which the parents come to understand. This peculiar type of speech is known as *idioglossia*. It is also observed in children with marked articulatory defects.

Speech rehabilitation of the bright word-deaf child follows along the same lines as that of the congenitally deaf one. Such a child learns to lip-read quickly and is very facile at acting out his or her own ideas.

Congenital Inarticulation

In this developmental defect the child seems unable to coordinate the vocal, articulatory, and respiratory musculature for the purpose of speaking. Again, boys are affected more often than girls, and there is often a family history of the disorder, although the data are not quite sufficient to establish the pattern of inheritance. The incidence is 1 in every 200 children. The motor, sensory, emotional, and social attainments correspond to the norms for age, although in a few cases, a minority in the authors' opinion, there has been some indication of cranial nerve abnormality in the first months of life (ptosis, facial asymmetry, strange neonatal cry, and altered phonation).

In children with congenital inarticulation, the prelanguage sounds are probably abnormal, but this aspect of the speech disorder has not been well studied. Babbling tends to be deficient, and, in the second year, in attempting to say something, the child makes noises that do not sound at all like language; in this way the child is unlike the late talker already described. Again, the understanding of language is entirely normal; the comprehension vocabulary is average for age, and the child can appreciate syntax, as indicated by correct responses to questions by nodding or shaking the head and by the execution of complex spoken commands. Usually such patients are shy but otherwise quick in responding, cheerful, and without other behavioral disorders. Some are bright, but a combination of congenital inarticulation and mild mental slowness is also not uncommon. If many of the spontaneous utterances are intelligible, speech correction should be attempted (by a trained therapist). However, if the child makes no sounds that resemble words, the therapeutic effort should be directed toward a modified school program, and speech rehabilitation usually waits until some words are acquired.

Studies of the cerebra of such patients are not available, and it is doubtful if they would show any abnormality by the usual techniques of neuropathologic examination. Occasionally, suspicion of a lesion is raised by focal changes in the EEG or a slight widening of the temporal horn of the left ventricle. All manner of delayed speech is often attributed to being "tongue-tied," i.e., a short lingual frenulum, but this idea now seems outdated. Also, psychologists have attributed incomplete development of speech to overprotectiveness or excessive pressure by the parents but these are certainly the result rather than the cause of the delay.

A fuller review of this subject can be found in the text *The Child with Delayed Speech*, edited by Rutter and Martin.

Stuttering and Stammering

These difficulties occur in an estimated 1 to 2 percent of the school population. Often the conditions disappear in late childhood and adolescence; by adulthood, only about 1 in 300 individuals suffer from a persistent stammer or stutter. Mild degrees are to some extent cultivated and permit a pause in speech for collecting one's thoughts, and stammering appears to be an affectation in certain social circles, as in the past among educated Englishmen (and some Americans).

Stammering and stuttering are difficult to classify. In some respects they belong to and are customarily included in the developmental language disorders, but they differ in being largely centered in articulation. There is no valid reason to distinguish between these two forms of the inarticulation, as they are intermingled, and the terms *stammer* and *stutter* are now used synonymously. Essentially they represent a disorder of rhythm—an involuntary, repetitive prolongation of speech because of an insuppressible *spasm of the articulatory muscles.* The spasm may be tonic and result in a complete blocking of speech (at one time referred to specifically as stammering) or clonic speech, i.e., a rapid series of spasms interrupting the emission of consonants, usually the first letter or syllable of a word (stuttering). Certain sounds, particularly *p* and *b*, offer greater difficulty than others; *paperboy* comes out *p-p-paper b-b-boy*. The problem is usually not apparent when single words are being spoken and dysfluency tends to be worse at the beginning of a sentence or an idea. The severity of the stutter is increased by excitement and stress, as when speaking before others, and is reduced when the stutterer is relaxed and alone or when singing in a chorus. When severe, the spasms may overflow into other groups of muscles, mainly of the face and neck and even of the arms. The muscles involved in stuttering show no fault in actions other than speaking, and all gnostic and semantic aspects of receptive language are intact.

Males are affected four times as often as females. The time of onset of stuttering is mainly at two periods in life: between 2 and 4 years of age, when speech and language are evolving, and between 6 and 8 years of age, when these functions extend to reciting and reading aloud in the classroom. However, there may be a later onset. Many afflicted children have an associated difficulty in reading and writing. If stuttering is mild, it tends to develop or to be present only during periods of emotional stress, and in 4 of 5 children it disappears entirely or almost so during adolescence or the early adult years (Andrews and Harris). If severe, it persists throughout life regardless of treatment but tends to improve as the patient grows older.

Theories of causation are legion, attesting to a lack of actual explanation. Slowness in developing hand and eye preference, ambidexterity, or an enforced change from left- to right-hand use have been popular explanations, of which Orton and Travis were leading advocates. According to their theory, stuttering results from a lack of the necessary degree of unilateral control in the synchronization of bilaterally innervated speech mechanisms. Fox and colleagues support a theory of failure of left hemisphere dominance. By performing PET studies while a subject was reading, they found that the auditory and motor areas of the right hemisphere are activated instead of those of the left hemisphere. However, these explanations probably apply to only a minority of stutterers (Hécaen and de Ajuriaguerra). It is of interest that stutterers activate the motor cortex prematurely when reading words aloud and, as noted by Sandak and Fiez, affected individuals seem to initiate motor programs before the articulatory code is prepared. Recently, several groups have reported subtle structural anomalies in the gray matter of the perisylvian region, but no common theme has emerged, and others are skeptical of these findings (see editorial by Packman and Onslow). It has been commented in the literature on this subject that speech production is a highly distributed system and that compensatory mechanisms used by stutterers may confound interpretation of functional imaging studies.

The disappearance of mild stuttering with maturation has been attributed incorrectly to all manner of treatment (hypnosis, progressive relaxation, speaking in rhythms, etc.) and used to bolster particular theories of causation. Because stuttering may reappear at times of emotional strain, a psychogenesis has been proposed, but—as pointed out by Orton and by Baker and colleagues—if there are any psychologic abnormalities in the stutterer, they are secondary rather than primary. We have observed that many stutterers, probably as a result of this impediment to free social interaction, do become increasingly fearful of talking and may become very self-conscious. By the time adolescence and adulthood are reached, emotional factors are so prominent that many physicians still mistake stuttering for a psychogenic disorder. Usually there is little or no evidence of any personality deviation before the onset of stuttering, and psychotherapy has not had a significant effect on the underlying defect. (The eminent Dr. Stanley Cobb undertook Jungian psychoanalysis for the condition according to R.D. Adams, with no benefit whatsoever.) A strong family history in many cases and male dominance point to a genetic origin, but the inheritance does not follow a readily discernible pattern.

Stuttering is not associated with any detectable weakness or ataxia of the speech musculature. The muscles of speech go into spasm *only* when called upon to perform the specific act of speaking. The spasms are not invoked by other actions (which may not be as complex or voluntary as speaking), differing in this way from an apraxia and the intention spasm of athetosis. Also, palilalia is a different condition in which a word or phrase, usually the last one in a sentence, is repeated many times with decreasing volume. We are inclined toward a tentative view that stuttering represents a special category of extrapyramidal dystonic movement disorder, much like writer's cramp.

Rarely, in adults as well as in children, stuttering may be acquired as a result of a lesion in the motor speech areas. A distinction has been drawn between developmental and acquired stuttering. The latter is said to interfere with the enunciation of any syllable of a word (not just the first), to favor involvement of grammatical and substantive words, and to be unaccompanied by anxiety and facial grimacing. Such distinctions are probably illusory. The reported lesion sites in acquired stuttering are so variable (right frontal, corpus striatum, left temporal, left parietal) as to be difficult to reconcile with proposed theories of developmental stuttering (see Fleet and Heilman).

Another form of acquired stuttering is more manifestly an expression of an extrapyramidal disorder. Here there occurs a prolonged repetition of syllables (vowel and consonant), which the patient cannot easily interrupt. The abnormality involves throat-clearing and other vocalizations, similar to what is seen in tic disorders.

Treatment The therapy of stuttering is difficult to evaluate and, on the whole, the therapy of speech-fluency disorders has been a frustrating effort. As remarked earlier, all these disturbances are modifiable by environmental circumstances. Thus a certain proportion of stutterers will become more fluent under certain conditions, such as reading aloud; others will stutter more severely at this time. Again, a majority of stutterers will be adversely affected by talking on the telephone; a minority are helped by this device. Some stutterers are more fluent under conditions of mild alcohol intoxication. Nearly every stutterer is fluent while singing. Schemes such as the encouragement of associated muscular movements ("penciling," etc.) and the adoption of a "theatrical" approach to speaking have been advocated. Common to all such efforts has been the difficulty of achieving carry-over into the natural speaking environment. Progressive relaxation, hypnosis, delayed auditory feedback, loud noise that masks speech sounds, and many other ancillary measures may help, but only temporarily. Canevini and colleagues have made the interesting observation that stuttering improved in an epileptic treated with levetiracetam, and Rosenberger has commented on other drug therapies.

Cluttering, or Cluttered Speech

This is another special developmental disorder. It is characterized by uncontrollable speed of speech, which results in truncated, dysrhythmic, and often incoherent utterances. Omissions of consonants, elisions, improper phrasing, and inadequate intonation occur. It is as though the child were too hurried to take the trouble to pronounce each word carefully and to compose sentences. Cluttering is frequently associated with other motor speech impediments. Speech therapy (elocutionary) and maturation may be attended by a restoration of more normal rhythms.

Other Articulatory Defects

Milder speech defects are common in preschool children, having an incidence of up to 15 percent. There are several varieties. One is *lisping*, in which the *s* sound is replaced by *th*, e.g., *thimple* for *simple*. Another common condition, *lallation*, or *dyslalia*, is characterized by multiple substitutions or omissions of consonants. Milder degrees consist of difficulty in pronouncing one or two consonants that give the impression of "baby talk" and are referred to as "infantilisms." For example, the letter *r* may be incorrectly pronounced, so that it sounds like *w* or *y*; *running a race* becomes *wunning a wace* or *yunning a yace*. In severe forms, speech may be almost unintelligible. The child seems to be unaware that his or her speech differs from that of others and is distressed at not being understood. More important is the fact that in more than 90 percent of cases, the articulatory abnormalities disappear by the age of 8 years, either spontaneously or in response to speech therapy. The latter is usually started if these conditions persist into the fifth year. Presumably the natural cycle of motor speech acquisition has only been delayed, not arrested. Such abnormalities, however, are more frequent among developmentally delayed children than in normal children; with cognitive defects in general, many consonants are persistently mispronounced.

Another disorder is a congenital form of spastic bulbar speech, described by Worster-Drought, in which words are spoken slowly, with stiff labial and lingual movements, hyperactive jaw and facial reflexes, and, sometimes, mild dysphagia and dysphonia. The limbs may be unaffected, in contrast to cerebral palsy.

The mechanical speech disorder resulting from *cleft palate* is easily recognized. Many of these patients also have a harelip; the two abnormalities together interfere with sucking and later in life with the enunciation of labial and guttural consonants. The voice has an unpleasant nasality; often, if the defect is severe, there is an audible escape of air through the nose.

The aforementioned developmental abnormalities of speech pattern are only sometimes associated with disturbances of higher-order language processing. Rapin and Allen have described a number of such disturbances. In one, which they call the "semantic pragmatic syndrome," a failure to comprehend complex phrases and sentences is combined with fluent speech and well-formed sentences lacking in content. The syndrome resembles Wernicke or transcortical sensory aphasia (Chap. 23). In another, "semantic retrieval-organization syndrome," a severe anomia blocks word finding in spontaneous speech. A mixed expressive–receptive disorder may also be seen as a developmental abnormality; it contains many of the elements of acquired Broca's aphasia (Chap. 23). Recently, a category of "specific language impairment" has been created to encompass all failures to acquire language competence despite normal intelligence.

The role of certain genes, particularly *FOXP2*, in the development of language is mentioned in Chap. 23. Here it is pointed out that there is an isolated developmental verbal dyspraxia that is caused by a point mutation in this gene but that other disorders, such as dyslexia, have not yielded clearly to genetic analysis as discussed below. However, Vernes and colleagues have found that *FOXP2* downregulates a gene (*CNTNAP2*) that encodes neurexin in the developing cortex. Polymorphisms of the gene are found in children with a number of specific but seemingly unrelated language deficits. They propose that this is a mechanistic link between different developmental language syndromes.

Developmental Dyslexia (Congenital Word Blindness)

This condition, first described by Hinshelwood in 1896, becomes manifest in an older child who is found to lack the aptitude for one or more of the specific skills necessary to derive meaning from the printed word. Also defined as a significant discrepancy between "measured intelligence" and "reading achievement" (Hynd et al), it has been found in 3 to 6 percent of all schoolchildren. There have been several excellent writings on the subject over the past century, to which the interested reader is referred for a detailed account (Orton; Critchley and Critchley; Rutter and Martin; Shaywitz; Rosenberger).

The main problem is an inability to read, spell, and to write words despite the ability to see and recognize letters. There is no loss of the ability to recognize the meaning of objects, pictures, and diagrams. According to Shaywitz, these children lack an awareness that words can be broken down into individual units of sound and that each segment of sound is represented by a letter or letters. This has been summarized as a problem in "phonologic processing," referring to the smallest unit of spoken language, the phoneme, and as a parallel inability of dyslexic individuals to appreciate a correspondence between phonemes and their written representation (graphemes). A defect in the decoding of acoustic signals is one postulated mechanism. In addition to the essential visuoperceptual defect, some individuals also manifest a failure of sequencing ability and altered cognitive processing of language. De Renzi and Luchelli have found a deficit of verbal and visual memory in some affected children as noted below.

Much of what has been learned about dyslexia applies to native speakers of English more than to those who speak Romance languages. English is more complex phonologically than most other languages; e.g., it uses 1,120 graphemes to represent 40 phonemes, in contrast to Italian, which uses 33 graphemes to represent 22 phonemes (see Paulesu et al). Children with native orthographic languages, such as Chinese and Japanese, apparently have a far lower incidence of dyslexia.

Often, before the child enters school, reading failure can be anticipated by a delay in attending to spoken words, difficulty with rhyming games, and speech characterized by frequent mispronunciations, hesitations, and dysfluency; or there may be a delay in learning to speak or in attaining clear articulation. In the early school years there are difficulties in copying, color naming, and formation of number concepts as well as the persistent reversal of letters. The child's writing reflects faulty perception of form and a kind of constructional and directional apraxia. Often, there is an associated vagueness about the serial order of letters in the alphabet and months in the year, as well as difficulty with numbers (acalculia) and an inability to spell and to read music. The complex of dyslexia, dyscalculia, finger agnosia, and right-left confusion is found in a small number of these children and is interpreted as a developmental form of the Gerstmann syndrome described in Chap. 22.

Lesser degrees of dyslexia are found in a large segment of the school population and are more common than the severe ones. Approximately 10 percent of schoolchildren in some surveys have some degree of this disability. The disorder is stable and persistent; however, as a result of effective methods of training, only a few children are unable to read at all after many years in school.

This form of language disorder, unattended by other neurologic signs, is strongly familial, in various series being almost in conformity with an autosomal dominant or sex-linked recessive pattern. Loci on chromosomes 6 and 15 have been implicated but not confirmed. There is also a higher incidence of left-handedness among these persons and members of their families. Shaywitz et al have suggested that the reported predominance of reading disabilities in boys (male-to-female ratios of 2:1 to 5:1) represents a bias in subject selection—many more boys than girls being identified because of associated hyperactivity and other behavioral problems; but to us this does not seem the entire explanation. Our casual clinical experience suggests that there is a genuine and substantial male preponderance. Nonetheless, an estimated 12 to 24 percent of dyslexic children will also have an attention-deficit hyperactivity disorder (ADHD) (see further on).

In the study of dyslexic and dysgraphic children, a number of other apparently congenital developmental abnormalities were documented, such as inadequate perception of space and form (poor performance on form boards and in tasks requiring construction); inadequate perception of size, distance, and temporal sequences and rhythms; and inability to imitate sequences of movements gracefully, as well as slight degrees of clumsiness and reduced proficiency in all motor tasks and games (the *clumsy child syndrome* as described by Gubbay et al and also by Denckla et al as mentioned earlier in the chapter under "Delays in Motor Development"). These disorders may also occur in brain-injured children; hence there may be considerable difficulty in separating simple delay or arrest in development from a pathologic process in the brain. However, in the majority of dyslexic children these additional features are absent or so subtle as to require special testing for their detection.

A few careful morphometric studies have provided insight into the basis of this disorder. Galaburda and associates have studied the brains of 4 males (ages 14 to 32 years) with developmental dyslexia. In each case there were anomalies of the cerebral cortex consisting of minor neuronal ectopias and architectonic dysplasias, located mainly in the perisylvian regions of the left hemisphere. More in conformity with imaging studies noted below, all of the brains were characterized by relative symmetry of the planum temporale, in distinction to the usual pattern of cerebral asymmetry that favors the planum temporale of the left side. Similar changes have been described in 3 women with developmental dyslexia (Humphreys et al). CT and MRI scanning of large numbers of dyslexic patients (as well as some patients with autism and developmental speech delay) have demonstrated an increased prevalence of relative symmetry (reversed or "atypical" asymmetry) of the temporal planes of the two hemispheres (Rosenberger; Hynd et al). It is important to note, however, that not all patients with developmental dyslexia show this anomalous anatomic asymmetry (Rumsey et al). In other studies, a number of variable alterations of cortical organization were found by Casanova and colleagues, most notably, in one case, an enlargement of the minicolumns in the temporal cortex. (A similar developmental change has been found in the brains of individuals with Down syndrome and with autism.)

Leonard and colleagues, using MRI, demonstrated several other gyral anomalies in dyslexic subjects: in the planum temporale and neighboring parietal operculum of both hemispheres, some gyri were missing and others were duplicated. In some dyslexic individuals, the visual evoked to rapid low-contrast stimuli are diminished. This abnormality has been related to a deficit of large neurons in the lateral geniculate bodies (see Livingstone et al).

Specific *spelling difficulty* probably represents another developmental language disorder, distinct from dyslexia.

Additional physiologic data from functional imaging studies support the presence of an abnormal temporoparietal cortex in dyslexics. These regions, particularly the posterior portion of the superior temporal, angular, and supramarginal gyri, are selectively activated during reading in normal individuals but not in dyslexics, who activate very restricted regions of the cerebral hemisphere, mainly the Broca area. In addition, they recruit other areas not normally activated during reading, such as the inferior frontal regions. It is noteworthy that Simos and coworkers were able to show that these aberrant patterns (using functional MRI) normalized after several weeks of intensive training. If nothing else, these findings validate the localization of the functional problem in the dominant temporoparietal area, and support the notion that developmental dyslexia is susceptible to improvement by proper training.

Treatment The steady practice (many hours per week) of a cooperative and motivated child by a skillful teacher over an extended period slowly overcomes the handicap and enables an otherwise intelligent child to read at grade level and to follow a regular program of education. The Orton phonologic method has been one of the most widely used over the years (for details, see Rosenberger). Secondary school and college students with reading deficits successfully resort to tape recorders, tutorial aids, and laptop computers that allow for review of material after classes.

Developmental Dysgraphia

Developmental writing disorders differ from dyslexia in having both linguistic and motor (orthographic) aspects. As indicated earlier, dysgraphias are present in many dyslexic children and may be combined with difficulty in calculation (so-called developmental Gerstmann syndrome). Two forms of dysgraphia have been distinguished. In one there is good spontaneous handwriting and formation of letters and spacing but miswriting of dictated words (*linguistic dysgraphia*). In the other, there are reversals of letters and letter order and poor alignment (*mechanical dysgraphia*). It is this latter type that seems to us to be the genuine, or at least the purer, dysgraphia.

Developmental Dyscalculia

This disorder, like dyslexia, usually becomes evident in the first few years of grade school, when the child is challenged by tasks of adding and subtracting and, later, multiplying and dividing. In some instances there is an evident disorder in the spatial arrangements of numbers that has been termed "anarithmetia" as noted in Chap. 22 (supposedly a right hemispheral fault). In others, there is a lexical–graphical abnormality (naming and reading the names of numbers) akin to aphasia.

Probably most of what has been said about the treatment of developmental dyslexia applies to *acalculia* and *agraphia*. The usual type of conventional classroom work does little to increase the child's proficiency in writing and arithmetic, but special tutoring and drills aid the student to some extent. All of these impairments may be associated with hyperactivity and attentional defects, as described below (Denckla et al).

Precocious Reading and Calculating

In direct contrast to the conditions discussed above, precocious reading and calculating abilities have also been identified. A 2- or 3-year old child may read with the skill of an average adult. Extraordinary facility with numbers (mathematical prodigies) and memorization ability (eidetic imagery) are comparable traits. One of these special abilities may be observed in a child with a mild form of autism (Asperger syndrome, see Chap. 38). Such children exhibit great skill in performing particular mathematical tricks but are unable to solve simple arithmetical problems or to understand the meaning of numbers ("idiot savant"). In the child with *Williams syndrome*, language and sometimes musical skills are not so much precocious as relatively normal in comparison to the overall mental deficiency, indicating that not all forms of cognitive delay impair language skills.

Congenital Amusia

One would expect that developmental deficiencies similar to those found for language would exist for music. This uncommon condition, commonly known as *tone deafness*, has only recently been studied. According to the careful studies of Ayotte and colleagues, there are deficits not only in appreciating pitch variation but also in music memorization, singing, and rhythmicity. These authors propose that the defect in pitch perception is at the root of the other abnormalities. What is also interesting is that amusia occurs without any difficulty in the processing of speech and language, specifically, prosody and prosodic interpretation are preserved. (See Chap. 22 for a discussion of the acquired defects of musical appreciation.)

Attention-Deficit Hyperactivity Disorder

A large portion of ambulatory pediatric neurology practice consists of children who are referred because of failure in school related to overactivity, impulsivity, and inattentiveness. The question often asked is whether they have an identifiable brain disease. According to Barlow, when a large number of such cases is analyzed, fully 85 percent prove to have no major signs of neurologic disease. Perhaps 5 percent are mentally subnormal and another 5 to 10 percent show some evidence of a minimal brain disorder. Many are clumsy. In the larger group without neurologic signs, the IQ is normal, although there are also cases of borderline intelligence. Boys are more often found to be hyperactive and inattentive than girls, just as they often have more trouble in learning to read and write. Dyslexia is frequently associated, as noted earlier. Girls with ADHD tend to have more trouble with numbers and arithmetic.

Human infants exhibit astonishing differences in amount of activity almost from the first days of life. Some babies are constantly on the move, wiry, and hard to hold; others are placid and slack as a sack of meal. Irwin, who studied motility in the neonate, found a difference of 290 times between the most and least active in terms of amount of movement per 24 h.

Once walking and running begin, children normally enter a period of extreme activity, more so than at any other period of life. The degree of activity, which varies widely from one child to another, seems not to be correlated with the age of achieving motor milestones or with motor skill at a later time.

Again, two groups of overactive children can be discerned early in life. In one, infants are constitutionally overactive from birth, sleeping less and feeding poorly; by the age of 2 years, the syndrome is obvious. In the other group, an inability to sit quietly only becomes apparent at the preschool age (4 to 6 years). Seldom do such children remain in one position for more than a few seconds, even when watching television. They are seen as fidgety, constantly in motion, and a bit wild in public places such as restaurants. Attention to any task cannot be sustained, hence the term *attention-deficit hyperactivity disorder*. As a rule, there is also an abnormal impulsivity and often an intolerance of all measures of restraint.

Currently, three clinical subsyndromes have been delineated: (1) combined hyperactivity, impulsivity, and inattention, which describes approximately 80 percent of affected children; (2) a predominantly inattentive syndrome; and (3) a small group that display only hyperactivity. It is also valuable to point out that a syndrome with most of the features of ADHD can be embedded in several forms of overarching cognitive and developmental delay, including in children with autistic traits. This takes on special significance in the exploration of a genetic basis for attention-deficit disorder, as noted below.

Once the child is in school, the attention deficit becomes a more troubling, practical problem. Now these children must sit still, watch and listen to the teacher when she speaks to another child, and not react to distracting stimuli. They cannot stay at their desks, take turns in reciting, be quiet, or control their impulsivity. The teacher finds it difficult to discipline them and the school often insists that the parents seek medical consultation for the child. A few are so hyperactive that they cannot attend regular classes. Their behavior verges on the "organic drivenness" that has been known to occur in children whose brains have been injured by encephalitis. In certain families, the disorder is probably inherited (Biederman et al). In about half the hyperactivity subsides gradually by puberty or soon thereafter, but in the remainder the symptoms persist in modified form into adulthood (Weiss et al).

It has also become clear that there are a large group of children who have difficulty sustaining concentration but do not manifest hyperactivity or behaviors that betray the attention deficit. It is presumed that they share a similar core problem with hyperkinetic children, and it has been observed that they may be helped in studying and school performance by the same stimulant drugs that are used for the treatment of more overt ADHD. A precise relationship between motor hyperactivity and the inability to concentrate and stay focused on a series of tasks has not been established. It would seem that these are but two aspects of the same fundamental disorder of drive and attention, but it is clear that there are individuals who have difficulty concentrating but who are not manifestly hyperactive. This becomes a particular issue in adults with ostensible ADHD who feel they have always had trouble focusing as discussed further on.

For a number of years there was a tendency to consider children with the hyperkinetic syndrome as having a form of minimal brain disease. "Soft neurologic signs" such as right–left confusion, mirror movements, minimal "choreic" instability of the hands, awkwardness, finger agnosia, tremor, and borderline hyperreflexia were said to be more frequent among them. The issue of mild developmental disorders of coordination constitutes its own subject independent of ADHD. The notion of this type of clumsiness has been known for over a century and was called *debilite motrice* by Dupre. The connection to ADHD, however, is evident in Annell's description (taken from the review by Kirby and Sugden) ". . . awkward in movements, poor at games, hopeless in dancing and gymnastics, a bad writer and defective in communication. He is inattentive, cannot sit still, leaves his shoelaces untied, does buttons wrongly, bumps into furniture, breaks glassware, slips off his chair, kicks his legs against the desk, and perhaps reads badly." Dyslexia is found in approximately 20 percent and a similar clumsiness is known to occur in many developmental disorders and forms of cognitive delay. These signs, however, are seen so often in normal children that their attribution to disease is invalid. Consequently, Schain and others substituted the term *minimal brain dysfunction*, which is no more accurate and simply restates the problem and, furthermore, may not be accurate in many cases.

Lacking altogether are clinicoanatomic and clinicopathologic correlative data, but some morphologic and physiologic data are available. In an MRI study of the brains of 10 children with ADHD, Hynd and colleagues found the width of the right frontal lobe to be smaller than normal; also fairly consistently, there was a reduction in the volume of the dorsolateral, cingulate, and striatal regions. Unlike dyslexics, in whom the planum temporale tends to be equal in the two hemispheres, the left planum was larger in the attention-deficit cases, just as it is in normals. Also, functional imaging studies have suggested that changes in the striatum underlie the inability of these children to block impulsive reactions and the improvement that is seen with methylphenidate. One would expect the prefrontal cortex to be implicated in such a disinhibitory syndrome but what data exist have been complex and difficult to interpret.

Another approach to understanding the process has been to study a strain of mice that have been genetically altered to eliminate a dopamine transporter gene. These animals display behavioral symptoms that are said to replicate those of ADHD in children and also to respond to stimulants, observations that implicate an abnormality of dopamine and serotonin. This idea is provocative because several genetic linkage studies have suggested an association between ADHD and a polymorphism of the gene that codes for the same dopamine transporter gene. Furthermore, copy number variations in genes that relate to development, a rich field for study in autism, give rise to global forms of cognitive delay that display prominent features of ADHD. Most of these are duplications or deletions that congregate on chromosomes 15 and 16.

Apart from the reports of parents and teachers and observation of the child, one is aided in the diagnosis of ADHD (and other learning disabilities) by psychometry. An observant psychologist, in performing intelligence tests, notes distractibility and difficulty in sustaining any activity. Erratic performance that is not the result of a defect in comprehension is also characteristic. The Vanderbilt Assessment Scale is a checklist that is completed with parents or teachers.

Treatment of ADHD The treatment of the hyperactive child can proceed reasonably only after medical and psychologic evaluations have clarified the context in which the hyperactivity occurs. If the child is hyperactive and inattentive mainly in school and less so in an unstructured environment, it may be that mild developmental delay or a specific cognitive deficiency or dyslexia, which prevents scholastic success, is a source of frustration and boredom. The child then turns to other activities that may happen to disturb the classroom. Or the hyperactive child may have failed to acquire self-control because of a disorganized home life, and the overactivity may be but one manifestation of anxiety or intolerance of constraint. Clearly problems such as these require a modification of the educational program.

For overactive children of normal intelligence who have failed to control their impulses, who at all times have boundless energy, require little sleep, exhibit a wriggling restlessness (the "choreiform syndrome" of Prechtl and Stemmer), and manifest incessant exploratory activity that repeatedly gets them into mischief, even to their own dismay, medical therapy is justified. Paradoxically, stimulants have a quieting effect on these children, whereas sedatives may do the opposite.

Methylphenidate is the drug most widely used and its use has been validated in several studies. Children weighing less than 30 kg are given 5 mg each morning on school days for 2 weeks, after which the dose can be raised to 5 mg morning and noon. Children weighing more than 30 kg can be given a single 20-mg sustained-release tablet each morning. If methylphenidate proves ineffective after several weeks or cannot be tolerated, dextroamphetamine 2.5 to 5 mg three times daily or a mixed amphetamine-dextroamphetamine are suitable substitutes. Atomoxetine, a norepinephrine inhibitor, is also effective and is not classified as a stimulant but has caused a few cases of liver failure. If these agents control the activity and improve school performance (they can be continued for a number of years), there is then no need to alter the child's school program. It is not clear if there should be a long-term concern about hypertension, but the blood pressure is not generally measured at frequent intervals. If stimulants are ineffective, tricyclic antidepressants, particularly desipramine, may be tried. Multiple medications should be generally avoided. Classroom behavioral conditioning techniques and psychotherapy may be needed for brief periods but are not as effective as medication. Remedial education is reserved for recalcitrant cases. Biederman and Faraone have summarized approaches to treatment.

Adult Attention-Deficit Disorder

Certainly this disease is a lifelong problem for a proportion of children, although it is just as clear that many "outgrow" the hyperactivity and attention deficit. Hill and Schoener estimate that there is a 50 percent decline in prevalence with each 5 years that pass. Other authorities state that the problem persists in 80 percent. In addition to the child with ADHD who grows to adulthood with persistent problems, there recently has emerged an emphasis on a group of adults who present for the first time with features of difficulty focusing or concentrating that they or their physicians attribute to ADHD. The hyperactivity component is generally absent and may not have occurred in childhood, making the validity of the diagnosis uncertain in adults who were not identified as having ADHD in childhood. A study by Kessler and colleagues suggests that 4.4 percent of adults in the United States have the disorder. European investigators use more restrictive criteria for diagnosis and find far lower frequencies in both children and adults, with consequentially far fewer prescriptions being written for stimulant drugs.

An approach to screening in adults has been given by McCann and Roy-Byrne. Most often these adults come to realize they have had a lifelong problem that is similar to the motor restlessness and wandering attention that led to the diagnosis of ADHD in their own children. The efficacy and safety of stimulant drugs in the adult group are not known with certainty, but this class of medications has been tried with some benefit according to many patients. Some data have emerged that the cardiovascular risks are greater in adults than in children; reports of anxiety and palpations, as well as elevations in blood pressure, are common among adults taking the medications.

Many such individuals are of above-average intelligence and have attained high degrees of professional success, perhaps as a result of strategies developed implicitly over the years, such as note taking, organizers, mental reminders to focus, etc. These same adjustments can be quite useful to others who are struggling with the disorder so that medication is not the only alternative to surmount the cognitive problem. In relation to persistent traits of ADHD from childhood, several psychiatrists have pointed out that there may be an increase in drug and alcohol dependence among adolescents with the disorder (Zametkin and Ernst) and a slight overrepresentation of tic disorders such as Gilles de la Tourette syndrome. Our general clinical experience suggests that these additional problems do not arise in the great majority of such children. Recent studies have been reassuring in this regard, but the concern regarding tics has remained.

Enuresis

Voluntary sphincteric control develops according to a predetermined time scale. Usually normal children stop soiling themselves before they can remain dry, and day control precedes night control. Some children are toilet trained by their second birthday, but many do not acquire full sphincteric control until the fourth year. Constant dribbling usually indicates spina bifida, another form of dysraphism, or a tethered cord, but in the boy, one must look also for obstruction of the bladder neck, and in the girl, for an ectopic ureter entering the vagina.

When a child 5 years of age or older wets the bed nearly every night and is dry by day, the child is said to have *nocturnal enuresis*. This condition afflicts approximately 10 percent of children between 4 and 14 years of age, boys more than girls, and continues in many cases to be a problem even into adolescence and adulthood. Although developmentally delayed children are notably late in acquiring sphincter control (some never do), the majority of enuretic individuals are normal in other respects.

The cause of this condition is disputed. Often there is a family history of the same complaint. Some psychiatrists have insisted that overzealous parents "pressure" the child until he develops a "complex" about his bedwetting; this is highly doubtful. The underlying condition is believed by most neurologists to be a delay in the maturation of higher control of spinal reflex centers during sleep. These and other abnormalities of bladder function in the enuretic child, as well as treatment, are also discussed Chap. 19 in relation to sleep.

Sociopathy

Extremes of egocentricity, lack of understanding of the feelings, needs, and actions of others, and an inability to judge one's own strengths and weaknesses stand as the central issues in a certain type of personality disorder. Such difficulties usually become manifest by adolescence. The complete detachment of the child with psychosis, the amorality of the constitutional sociopath, the major disturbances in thinking of the schizophrenic, and the mood swings of the bipolar also express themselves in many, if not most, instances by adolescence and sometimes by late childhood. Here one confronts a key problem in psychiatry—the extent to which sociopathy has its roots in genetically determined personality traits or in derangements in the affective and social life of the individual consequent to a harmful environment. The answers to these questions cannot be given with finality but most clinicians believe that genetic factors are more important than environmental ones. The discovery that unusually tall males with severe acne vulgaris and aggressive sociopathic behavior may have a karyotype of XYY chromosomes is an extreme but instructive example of a genetic relationship. The patients with Turner syndrome in whom competent social adaptation is linked closely to an X chromosome of paternal origin is another example. Furthermore, there is no critical evidence to show that deliberate alteration of the familial and social environmental measures now so popular have ever prevented sociopathy.

It is during the period of late childhood and adolescence, when the personality is evolving and least stable, that transient symptoms resembling the psychopathologic states of adult life are most frequent and difficult to interpret. Some of these disorders represent the early signs of schizophrenia or bipolar disease. Others are forerunners of sociopathy. But many of these traits have a way of disappearing as adult years are reached so that one can only surmise that they represented either a maturational delay in the attainment of mature social behavior or were expressions of adolescent turmoil, or what has been called "adolescent adjustment reaction."

Many issues that have been touched upon in the preceding discussion are considered more fully in the section on psychiatric disorders (particularly Chap. 51).

INTELLECTUAL AND DEVELOPMENTAL DISABILITY

(See also Chap. 38)

A symptom complex of incomplete development of global cognitive capacities and certain associated behavioral changes combines many of the developmental abnormalities already discussed. What has been called mental retardation and now, intellectual and developmental delay, stands as the single largest neuropsychiatric disorder in every industrialized society. In deference changed

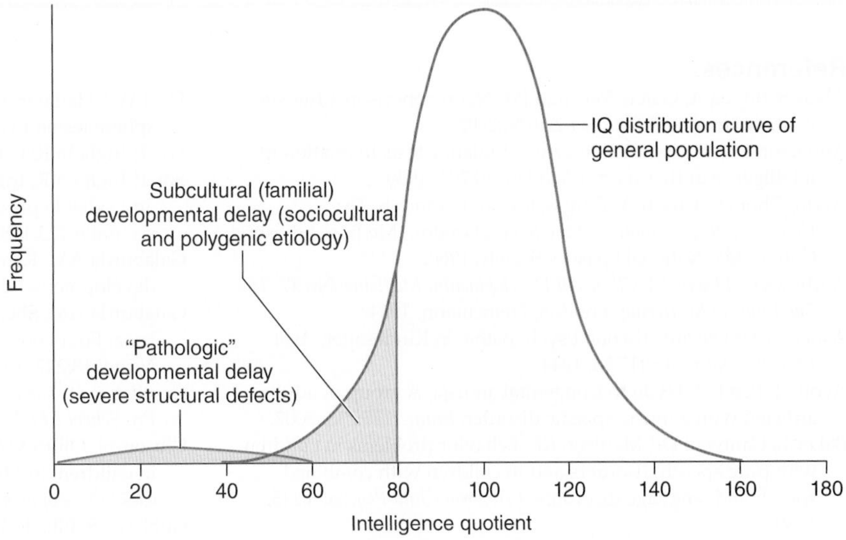

Figure 28-4. Gaussian or bell-shaped curve of intelligence and its skewing by the group of mentally retarded individuals with diseases of the brain. The shaded areas indicate the two groups of developmentally delayed. The hump representing the pathologically retarded is purely diagrammatic, illustrating its overlap with the subculturally delayed discussed in the text and in Chap. 38. When the population plotted is limited to "mental defectives," a truly bimodal distribution is seen, segregating the two groups of retarded.

attitudes towards the formerly used term "mental retardation," we employ alternatives in this text. The overall frequency of the problem cannot be stated precisely but rough estimates are that in children between 9 and 14 years of age, approximately 2 percent or slightly more will be unable to profit from conventional education or to adapt socially and, when grown, to live independently.

Using any one of a number of indices of social and cognitive delay, two somewhat overlapping groups are recognized: (1) the *mildly impaired* (IQ 45 to 70), and (2) the *severely impaired*, corresponding to an IQ below 45. The second group, called the *pathologically delayed*, makes up approximately 10 percent of the mental retardation population. The more mildly affected first group, includes a group of the *familial developmentally delayed*, is much larger.

Within the severely delayed there are gradations. Because of the objectionable implications of the previously used terms *idiot, imbecile,* and *moron,* the developmentally delayed can be grouped instead into four categories: (1) those with *profound deficiency*, incapable of self-care (IQ below 25); (2) those with *severe deficiency*, incapable of living an independent existence and essentially untrainable (IQ 25 to 39); (3) those with *moderate deficiency*, trainable to some extent (IQ 40 to 54); and (4) those with *mild deficiency*, who are impaired but trainable and to some extent educable. The above terms, while in common use, satisfy neither neurologists nor psychologists because of their generality, embracing as they do any lifelong global deficit in mental capacities. The terms convey no information of the particular type of intellectual impairment, their causes and mechanisms, or their anatomic and pathologic bases. Moreover, they express only one aspect of impaired mental function—the cognitive—and ignore the inadequate development of personality, social adaptation, and behavior. A more comprehensive view is provided by assessing the individual's adaptive abilities along the lines of conceptual, social, and practical skills that allow planning for maximizing independence and productivity.

When the brains of severely affected people are examined by conventional methods, gross lesions are found in approximately 90 percent of cases. Just as noteworthy is the fact that among the remaining 10 percent of the severely delayed, the brains are grossly and microscopically normal. Despite the recent discovery of many mutations that may give rise to a delay in cognitive development only a modest proportion of cases of those with milder deficiency can presently be traced to one of the congenital abnormalities of development that are described in Chap. 38 and the vast majority of the less-severely delayed also lack a recognizable tissue pathology and have not exhibited any of the conventional signs of cerebral disease.

In our view, a more acceptable view of the mildly affected group is that they represent the proportion of the population that is on the low end of the Gaussian curve of intelligence, i.e., they constitute the group that falls between 2 to 3 standard deviations (SD) below the mean (Fig. 28-4) and are the opposite in this respect to genius. Lewis was one of the first to call attention to this large group of mildly delayed individuals and he referred to them by the ambiguous term *subcultural*. The term *familial retardation* was in the past applied to this group, because in some of the families, members of the same and previous generations have reduced cognitive ability.

An important advance in the understanding of developmental delay has now emerged from careful genetic studies that have identified specific loci that at which deletions or duplications result in intellectual disability. Some of these express particular syndromes such as cognitive delay with autism or epilepsy; however, the same genetic changes can be found among individuals who have only autism or schizophrenia. While a unifying explanation for these disparate disorders has yet to be defined, they probably have subcellular and synaptic changes in common as summarized by Mefford, Batshaw, Hoffman in their review that is recommended to the reader.

Both the milder and more-severe forms of developmental delay that are associated with physical abnormalities and diseases of the brain, as well as nondysmorphic and genetic forms of delayed development are discussed in Chap. 38.

References

Alvarez-Buylla A, Garcia-Verdugo JM: Neurogenesis in adult subventricular zone. *J Neurosci* 22:629, 2002.
Anderson LD: The predictive value of infancy tests in relation to intelligence at five years. *Child Dev* 10:203, 1939.
André-Thomas, Chesni Y, Dargassies Saint-Annes S: *The Neurological Examination of the Infant*. London, Medical Advisory Committee, National Spastics Society, 1960.
Andrews G, Harris M: *Clinics in Developmental Medicine*: No 17. *The Syndrome of Stuttering*. London, Heinemann, 1964.
Asperger H: Die autistischen Psychopathie in Kindesalter. *Arch Psychiatr Nervenkr* 117:76, 1944.
Ayotte J, Peretz I, Hyde K: Congenital amusia. A group of adults afflicted with a music-specific disorder. *Brain* 1125:238, 2002.
Baker L, Cantwell DP, Mattison RE: Behavior problems in children with pure speech disorders and in children with combined speech and language disorders. *J Abnorm Child Psychol* 8:245, 1980.
Barlow C: *Mental Retardation and Related Disorders*. Philadelphia, Davis, 1978.
Bayley H: Comparisons of mental and motor test scores for age 1–15 months by sex, birth order, race, geographic location and education of parents. *Child Dev* 36:379, 1965.
Bender L: *A Visual-Motor Gestalt Test and Its Use*. New York, American Orthopsychiatric Association, 1938.
Benton AL: Right-left discrimination. *Pediatr Clin North Am* 15:747, 1968.
Benton AL: *Revised Visual Retention Test*. New York, Psychological Corporation, 1974.
Biederman J, Munir K, Knee D, et al: A family study of patients with attention deficit disorder and normal controls. *J Psychiatr Res* 20:263, 1986.
Biederman J, Faraone SV: Attention-deficit hyperactivity disorder. *Lancet* 366:237, 2005.
Birch HG, Belmont L: Auditory-visual integration in normal and retarded readers. *Am J Orthopsychiatry* 34:852, 1964.
Byne W: The biological evidence challenged: A scientific American article, in *The Scientific American Book of the Brain*. New York, Lyons Press, 1999, pp 181–194.
Canevini MP, Chifari R, Piazzini A: Improvement of a patient with stuttering on levetiracetam. *Neurology* 59:1288, 2002.
Capute AJ, Accardo PJ: *Developmental Disabilities in Infancy and Childhood*. Baltimore, MD, Brookes, 1996.
Casanova MF, Buxhoeveden DP, Cohen M, et al: Minicolumnar pathology in dyslexia. *Ann Neurol* 52:108, 2002.
Chugani HT: Functional brain imaging in pediatrics. *Pediatr Clin North Am* 39:777, 1992.
Conel J: *The Postnatal Development of the Human Cerebral Cortex*. Vols 1–8. Cambridge, MA, Harvard University Press, pp 1939–1967.
Cowan WM: The development of the brain. *Sci Am* 241:112, 1979.
Critchley M, Critchley EA: *Dyslexia Defined*. Springfield, IL, Charles C Thomas, 1978.
Damon W: The moral development of children. *Sci Am* 281:72, 1999.
De Ajuriaguerra J: *Manuel de psychiatrie de l'enfant*, 2nd ed. Paris, Masson, 1974.
Denckla MB, Rudel RG, Chapman C, et al: Motor proficiency in dyslexic children with and without attentional disorders. *Arch Neurol* 42:228, 1985.
De Renzi E, Luchelli F: Developmental dysmnesia in a poor reader. *Brain* 113:1337, 1990.
Fantz RL: The origin of form perception. *Sci Am* 204:66, 1961.
Feess-Higgins A, Larroche J-C: *Development of the Human Fetal Brain*. Paris, Masson, 1987.
Fleet WS, Heilman KM: Acquired stuttering from a right hemisphere lesion in a right hander. *Neurology* 35:1343, 1985.
Fox P, Ingham R: Commentary on stuttering. *Science* 270:1438, 1995.
Fox P, Ingham R, Ingham JC, et al: Brain correlates of stuttering and syllable production. A PET performance-correlation analysis. *Brain* 123:1985, 2000.
Galaburda AM, Kemper TL: Cytoarchitectonic abnormalities in developmental dyslexia: A case study. *Ann Neurol* 6:94, 1979.
Galaburda AM, Sherman CF, Rosen GD, et al: Developmental dyslexia: Four consecutive patients with cortical anomalies. *Ann Neurol* 18:222, 1985.
Gesell A (ed): *The First Five Years of Life: A Guide to the Study of the Pre-School Child*. New York, Harper & Row, 1940.
Gibson EJ, Olum V: Experimental methods of studying perception in children, in Mussen P (ed): *Handbook of Research Methods in Child Development*. New York, Wiley, 1960, pp 311–373.
Gubbay SS, Ellis E, Walter JN, Court SDM: Clumsy children: A study of apraxic and agnosic defects in 21 children. *Brain* 88:295, 1965.
Hécaen N, De Ajuriaguerra J: *Left-Handedness*. New York, Grune & Stratton, 1964.
Hill JC, Schoener EP: Age-dependent decline of attention deficit hyperactivity disorder. *Am J Psychiatry* 153:1143, 1996.
Hinshelwood J: A case of dyslexia—a peculiar form of word blindness. *Lancet* 2:1454, 1896.
Humphreys P, Kaufmann WE, Galaburda AM: Developmental dyslexia in women: Neuropathological findings in three patients. *Ann Neurol* 28:727, 1990.
Hynd GW, Semrud-Clikeman M, Lorys AR, et al: Brain morphology in developmental dyslexia and attention deficit disorder/hyper-activity. *Arch Neurol* 47:919, 1990.
Illingworth RS: *The Development of the Infant and Young Child, Normal and Abnormal*, 3rd ed. Edinburgh, Churchill Livingstone, 1966.
Ingram TTS: Developmental disorders of speech, in Vinken PJ, Bruyn W (eds): *Handbook of Clinical Neurology*. Vol 4: Disorders of Speech, Perception and Symbolic Behavior. Amsterdam, North-Holland, 1969, pp 407–442.
Irwin OC: Can infants have IQ's? *Psychol Rev* 49:69, 1942.
Kagan J, Moss HA: *Birth to Maturity: A Study of Psychological Development*. New York, Wiley, 1962.
Kanner I: Early infantile autism. *J Pediatr* 25:211, 1944.
Kempermann G: Why new neurons? Possible functions for adult hippocampal neurogenesis. *J Neurosci* 22:635, 2002.
Kennedy CR, McCann DC, Campbell MJ, et al: Language ability after early detection of permanent childhood hearing impairment. *N Engl J Med* 354:2131, 2006.
Kessler RC, Adler L, Barkley R, et al: The prevalence and correlates of adult ADHD in the Unites States: Results from the National Comorbidity Survey Replication. *Am J Psychiatry* 163:716, 2006.
Kinsbourne M: Developmental Gerstmann's syndrome: A disorder of sequencing. *Pediatr Clin North Am* 15:771, 1968.
Kinsbourne M: Disorders of mental development, in Menkes JH (ed): *Textbook of Child Neurology*, 5th ed. Baltimore, MD, Williams & Wilkins, 1995, pp 924–964.
Kinsey A, Pomeroy W, Martin C, Gebhard P: *Sexual Behavior in the Human Female*. Philadelphia, Saunders, 1948.
Kirby A, Sugden DA: Children with developmental coordination disorders. *J R Soc Med* 100:182, 2007.
Landau WM, Kleffner FR: Syndrome of acquired aphasia with convulsive disorder in children. *Neurology* 7:523, 1957.
Lenneberg EH: *Biological Foundations of Language*. New York, Wiley, 1967.

Leonard CM, Voeller KKS, Lombardino LJ, et al: Anomalous cerebral structure in dyslexia revealed with magnetic resonance imaging. *Arch Neurol* 50:461, 1993.

LeVay S: A difference in hypothalamic structure between heterosexual and homosexual men. *Science* 253:1034, 1991.

LeVay S, Hamer DH: Evidence for a biological influence in male homosexuality. *Sci Am* 270:44, 1994.

Lewis EO: Types of mental differences and their social significance. *J Ment Sci* 79:298, 1933.

Livingstone MS, Rosen GD, Drislane FW, Galaburda AM: Physiological and anatomical evidence for a magnocellular defect in developmental dyslexia. *Proc Natl Acad Sci U S A* 88:7943, 1991.

McCann BS, Roy-Byrne P: Screening and diagnostic utility of self-report attention deficit hyperactivity disorder scales in adults. *Compr Psychiatry* 45:175, 2004.

Mefford HC, Batshaw ML, Hoffman EP: Genomics, intellectual disability, and autism. *N Engl J Med* 366:733, 2012.

Minifie FD, Lloyd LL: *Communicative and Cognitive Abilities—Early Behavioral Assessment*. Baltimore, MD, University Park Press, 1978.

Orton ST: *Reading, Writing and Speech Problems in Children*. New York, Norton, 1937.

Ozeretzkii NI: Technique of investigating motor function, in Gurevich M, Ozeretzkii NI (eds): *Psychomotor Function*. Moscow, 1930. Quoted by Luria AR: *Higher Cortical Functions in Man*. New York, Basic Books, 1966.

Packman A, Onslow M: Searching for the cause of stuttering. *Lancet* 360:655, 2002.

Paulesu E, Demonent J-F, Fazia F, et al: Dyslexia; cultural diversity and biological unity. *Science* 291:2165, 2001.

Piaget J: *The Psychology of Intelligence*. London, Routledge & Kegan Paul, 1950.

Prechtl HFR: Prognostic value of neurological signs in the newborn. *Proc R Soc Med* 58:3, 1965.

Prechtl HFR, Beintema D: *The Neurological Examination of the Full Term Newborn Infant*. Little Club Clinics in Developmental Medicine, no 12. London, Heinemann, 1964.

Prechtl HFR, Stemmer CJ: The choreiform syndrome in children. *Dev Med Child Neurol* 4:119, 1962.

Rabinowicz T: The differential maturation of the cerebral cortex, in Falkner F, Tanner JM (eds): *Human Growth*. New York, Plenum Press, 1986.

Rakic P: Neurogenesis in adult primate neocortex: An evaluation of the evidence. *Nat Rev Neurosci* 3:55, 2002.

Rapin I, Allen DA: Developmental language disorders: Nosologic considerations, in Kirk U (ed): *Neuropsychology of Language, Reading and Spelling*. New York, Academic Press, 1983, pp 155–184.

Raven's Colored Progressive Matrices. New York, Psychological Corporation, 1947 and 1963.

Rosenberger PB: Morphological cerebral asymmetries and dyslexia, in Pavlidis GT (ed): *Perspectives on Dyslexia*. Vol 1. New York, Wiley, 1990, pp 93–107.

Rosenberger PB: Learning disorders, in Berg B (ed): *Principles of Child Neurology*. New York, McGraw-Hill, 1996, pp 335–369.

Rumsey JM, Donohue BC, Brady DR, et al: A magnetic resonance imaging study of planum temporale asymmetry in men with developmental dyslexia. *Arch Neurol* 54:1481, 1997.

Rutter M, Martin JAM (eds): *Clinics in Developmental Medicine*. No 43. The Child with Delayed Speech. London, Heinemann, 1972, pp 48–51.

Saint-Anne Dargassies S: *Neurological Development in the Full-Term and Premature Neonate*. New York, Excerpta Medica, 1977.

Sandak R, Fiez JA: Stuttering: A view from neuroimaging. *Lancet* 356:445, 2000.

Scarr S, Webber RA, Weinberg RA, Wittig MA: Personality resemblance among adolescents and their parents in biologically related and adoptive families. *Prog Clin Biol Res* 69:99, 1981.

Schain RJ: *Neurology of Childhood Learning Disorders*, 2nd ed. Baltimore, MD, Williams & Wilkins, 1977.

Shaywitz SE: Dyslexia. *N Engl J Med* 338:307, 1998.

Shaywitz SE, Shaywitz BA, Fletcher JM, et al: Prevalence of reading disabilities in boys and girls. *JAMA* 264:998, 1990.

Simos PG, Fletcher JM, Bergman G, et al: Dyslexia-specific brain deterioration profile becomes normal following remedial training. *Neurology* 58:1203, 2002.

Spearman C: *Psychology Down the Ages*. London, Macmillan, 1937.

Staples R: Responses of infants to color. *J Exp Psychol* 15:119, 1932.

Swaab DF, Hofman MA: An enlarged suprachiasmatic nucleus in homosexual men. *Brain Res* 537:141, 1990.

Thurstone LL: *The Vectors of the Mind*. Chicago, University of Chicago Press, 1953.

Tirosh E: Fine motor deficit: An etiologically distinct entity. *Pediatr Neurol* 10:213, 1994.

Travis LE: *Speech Therapy*. New York, Appleton-Century, 1931.

Turner G, Turner B, Collins E: X-linked mental retardation without physical abnormality: Renpenning's syndrome. *Dev Med Child Neurol* 13:71, 1971.

Vernes SC, Newbury DF, Abrahams BS, et al: A functional genetic link between distinct developmental language disorders. *N Engl J Med* 359:2337, 2008.

Weiss G, Hechtman L, Milroy T, Perlman T: Psychiatric status of hyperactives as adults: A controlled prospective 15-year follow-up of 63 hyperactive children. *J Am Acad Child Adolesc Psychiatry* 24:211, 1985.

Worster-Drought C: Congenital suprabulbar paresis. *J Laryngol Otol* 70:453, 1956.

Yakovlev PI, Lecours AR: The myelogenetic cycles of regional maturation of the brain, in Minkowski A (ed): *Regional Development of the Brain in Early Life*. Oxford, UK, Blackwell, 1967, pp 3–70.

Zametkin AJ, Ernst M: Problems in the management of attention-deficit hyperactivity disorder. *N Engl J Med* 340:40, 1999.

Zametkin AJ, Nordahl TE, Gross M, et al: Cerebral glucose metabolism in adults with hyperactivity of childhood onset. *N Engl J Med* 323:1361, 1990.

29

The Neurology of Aging

As indicated in the preceding chapter, standards of growth, development, and maturation provide a frame of reference against which every pathologic process in early life must be viewed. It has been less appreciated, however, that at the other end of the life cycle, neurologic deficits must be judged in a similar way, against a background of normal aging changes (senescence). The earliest of these changes begins long before the acknowledged period of senescence and continues throughout the remainder of life. Most authors use the terms *aging* and *senescence* interchangeably, but some draw a fine semantic distinction between the purely passive and chronologic process of aging and the composite of bodily changes that characterize this process (senescence).

Biologists have measured many of these changes. Table 29-1 gives estimates of the structural and functional decline that accompanies aging between ages 30 and 80 years. It appears that all structures and functions share in the aging process. Some persons withstand the onslaught of aging far better than others, and this constitutional resistance to the effects of aging seems to be familial. It can also be said that such changes are unrelated to Alzheimer disease and other degenerative diseases but that in general, the changes of aging reduce the capacity to recover from virtually any illness or trauma. An entity of "frailty" has been conceived to encompass the sum of breakdown in multiple organ systems as a result of aging. The review by Clegg and colleagues is recommended on this subject. With respect to the nervous system, it entails loss of muscle mass, strength and endurance, decreased appetite, unintentional weight loss, and reduced mobility and balance. A working definition of frailty has been given by Fried and is summarized in Table 29-2. In the past, this was referred to as "failure to thrive," a term adopted from pediatrics.

Effects of Aging on the Nervous System

Of all the age-related changes, those in the nervous system are of paramount importance. Actors portray old people as being feeble, idle, obstinate, given to reminiscing and having tremulous hands, quavering voices, stooped posture, and slow, shuffling steps. In so doing, they have selected some of the most obvious effects of aging on the nervous system. The lay observer, as well as the medical one, often speaks glibly of the changes of advanced age as a kind of second childhood. "Old men are boys again," said Aristophanes.

Critchley, in 1931 and 1934, drew attention to a number of neurologic abnormalities that he had observed in octogenarians and for which no cause could be discerned other than the effects of aging itself. Several reviews of this subject have appeared subsequently (see especially those of Jenkyn, of Benassi, and of Kokmen [1977] and their associates). The most consistent of the neurologic signs of aging are the following:

- *Neuroophthalmic signs:* progressive smallness of pupils, decreased reactions to light, and near farsightedness (hyperopia) as a result of impairment of accommodation (presbyopia), insufficiency of convergence, restricted range of upward conjugate gaze, frequent loss of the Bell phenomenon, diminished dark adaptation, and increased sensitivity to glare.
- *Progressive hearing loss* (presbycusis), especially for high tones, and commensurate decline in speech discrimination. Mainly these changes are a result of a diminution in the number of hair cells in the organ of Corti.
- *Diminution in the sense of smell* and, to a lesser extent, of taste (see Chap. 12).
- *Motor signs:* reduced speed and amount of motor activity, slowed reaction time, impairment of fine coordination and agility, reduced muscular power (legs more than arms and proximal muscles more than distal ones) and thinness of muscles (sarcopenia), particularly the dorsal interossei, thenar, and anterior tibial muscles. A progressive decrease in the number of anterior horn cells is partially responsible for these changes, as described further on.
- *Changes in tendon and frontal reflexes:* A depression of tendon reflexes at the ankles in comparison with those at the knees is observed frequently in persons older than 70 years of age, as is a loss of Achilles reflexes in those older than 80 years of age. The snout or palmomental reflexes, which can be detected in mild form in a small proportion of healthy adults, are frequent findings in the elderly (in as many as half of normal subjects older than 60 years of age, according to Olney). However, other so-called cortical release signs, such as suck and grasp reflexes, when prominent, are indicative of frontal lobe disease but sometimes are expected simply as a result of aging.
- *Impairment or loss of vibratory sense* in the toes and ankles. Proprioception, however, is impaired very

Table 29-1

PHYSIOLOGIC AND ANATOMIC DETERIORATION AT 80 YEARS OF AGE

	PERCENT DECREASE
Brain weight	10–15
Blood flow to brain	20
Speed of return of blood acidity to equilibrium after exercise	83
Cardiac output at rest	35
Number of glomeruli in kidney	44
Glomerular filtration rate	31
Number of fibers in nerves	37
Nerve conduction velocity	10
Number of taste buds	64
Maximum O_2 utilization with exercise	60
Maximum ventilation volume	47
Maximum breathing capacity	44
Power of hand grip	45
Maximum work rate	30
Basal metabolic rate	16
Body water content	18
Body weight (males)	12

Source: Adapted by permission from Shock.

little or not at all. Thresholds for the perception of cutaneous stimuli increase with age but require the use of refined methods of testing for their detection. These changes correlate with a loss of sensory fibers on sural nerve biopsy, reduced amplitude of sensory nerve action potentials, probably as a result of loss of dorsal root ganglion cells.

- The most obvious neurologic aging changes—those of *stance, posture, and gait*—are fully described in Chap. 7 and further on in this chapter.

Table 29-2

CRITERIA FOR FRAILTY (THE PRESENCE OF 3 OR MORE OF THE 5 FEATURES MAY BE USED TO DEFINE FRAILTY)

MEN		WOMEN	
1. *Weight loss*			
Greater than 10 lb or 5% of weight loss in the last year			
2. *15-ft walk time*			
Height ≤173 cm	≥7 s	Height ≤159 cm	≥7 s
Height >173 cm	≥6 s	Height >159 cm	≥6 s
3. *Grip strength (lb)*			
BMI ≤24	≤29	BMI ≤23	≤17
BMI 24.1–26	≤30	BMI 23.1–26	≤17.3
BMI 26.1–28	≤30	BMI 26.1–29	≤18
BMI >28	≤32	BMI >29	≤21
4. *Physical activity*			
<383 kcal/wk		<270 kcal/wk	
5. *Exhaustion*			
A score of 2 or 3 on either question on the CES-D			

BMI, body mass index; CES-D, Center for Epidemiologic Studies Depression Scale.
Source: Adapted from Fried.

Jenkyn and colleagues, based on their examinations of 2,029 individuals aged 50 to 93 years, have determined the incidence of certain common neurologic signs of aging. Notable again is the high frequency of snout and glabellar responses, but also limited downgaze and upgaze in approximately one-third of persons older than age 80 years. Table 29-3 summarizes these data.

With regard to the interesting population of the "oldest old," those older than 85 years of age, Kaye and colleagues reported that deficits in balance, olfaction, and visual pursuit are distinctly worse than in younger elderly persons. Also of interest is the observation by van Exel and colleagues that women in this age group perform better than men on cognitive tests.

Effects of Aging on Memory and Other Cognitive Functions

Probably the most detailed information as to the effects of age on the nervous system comes from the measurement of cognitive functions. In the course of standardization of the original Wechsler-Bellevue Intelligence Scale (1955), cross-sectional studies of large samples of the population indicated that there was a steady decline in cognitive function starting at 30 years of age and progressing into old age. Apparently all forms of cognitive function partake of this decline—although in general certain elements of the verbal scale (vocabulary, fund of information, and comprehension) withstand the effects of aging better than those of the performance scale (block design, reversal of digits, picture arrangement, object assembly, and the digit symbol task).

However, the concept of a linear regression of cognitive function with aging has had to be modified in the light of subsequent longitudinal studies. If the same individual is examined over a period of many years, there is virtually no decline in his performance, as measured by tests of verbal function, until 60 years of age. Beyond this age, verbal intelligence does decline, but very slowly—by an average of less than 5 percent through the seventh decade and by less than 10 percent through the eighth decade (Schaie and Hertzog). Also, in a series of 460 community-dwelling individuals (55 to 95 years of age) studied by Smith and coworkers (1992), there was no significant decline with age in verbal memory and in registration–attention; similar results were found by Peterson and colleagues in 161 normal, community-dwelling individuals 62 to 100 years of age. The most definite effects of age were in learning and memory and in problem solving—cognitive impairments probably attributable to a progressive reduction in the speed of processing information. The latter may be reflected in the slowing of event-related evoked potentials and by a number of special psychologic tests (see Verhaeghen et al).

As regards these cognitive functions, the ability to memorize, acquire, and retain new information, recall of names, and avoidance of distraction once set on a course of action, diminishes with advancing age, particularly in those older than 70 years of age. Moreover, memory function may be disturbed in this way despite the relative

Table 29-3

FREQUENCY OF NEUROLOGIC SIGNS IN UNCOMPLICATED AGING (IN PERCENT)

	AGE (YEARS)			
SIGN	65–69	70–74	75–79	>80
Glabellar sign (inability to inhibit blink)	10	15	27	37
Snout reflex	3	8	7	26
Limited upgaze	6	15	27	29
Limited downgaze	8	15	26	34
Abnormal visual tracking	8	18	22	32
Paratonic rigidity	6	10	12	21
Unable to recall 3 words	24	28	25	55
Unable to spell *world* backward	10	12	18	21

Source: Data from Jenkyn et al.

retention of other intellectual abilities. Characteristically, there is difficulty with recall of a name or the specific date of an experience ("episodic" memory) despite a preservation of memory for the experience itself or for the many features of a person whose name is momentarily elusive ("tip-of-the-tongue syndrome"). Also characteristic is an inconsistent retrieval of the lost name or information at a later date. It has been found, however, that if older persons are allowed to learn new material very well, until no errors are made, they forget this information at a rate similar to that of younger individuals.

Kral, who first wrote informatively on this type of memory disturbance 50 years ago, referred to it as *benign senescent forgetfulness*. He pointed out that such a memory disturbance, in distinction to that of Alzheimer disease, worsens very little or not at all over a period of many years and does not interfere significantly with the person's work performance or activities of daily living. Crook and coworkers have refined the diagnostic criteria for senescent forgetfulness and have proposed a new term—*age-associated memory impairment* (AAMI). The diagnostic criteria for AAMI include age of 50 years or older, a subjective sense of decline in memory, impaired performance on standard tests of memory function (at least one SD below the mean), and absence of any other signs of dementia. The current terminology is *minimal cognitive impairment*, but there has been increasing recognition that Kral's original notion of a benign condition may have been incorrect and that cognitive decline in later years may be a symptom of Alzheimer disease.

In judging the degree of cognitive decline, several abbreviated tests of mental status have been developed and are of practical value (Kokmen et al, 1991; Folstein et al) in that they can be administered in the office or at the bedside in 5 to 10 min. Repetition of spoken items, such as a series of digits, orientation as to place and time, capacity to learn and to retain several items, tests of arithmetic and calculation (concentration), and specific tests for memory (particularly tests of delayed recall or forgetfulness) distinguish the performance of normal aging persons from that of patients with Alzheimer disease (Larrabee et al). With regard to performance on the Mini-Mental Status Examination (see Table 21-6; Folstein et al), a study by Crum and associates of a large urban population indicates a median score of 19 to 20 for individuals older than age 80 years who have a fourth grade education and 27 for those with a college education (out of maximum score of 30).

The foregoing effects of age on mental abilities are extremely variable. Some 70-year-olds perform better on psychologic testing than some "normal" 20-year-olds. And a few individuals retain exceptional mental power and perform creative work until late life. Verdi, for example, composed *Otello* at the age of 73 and *Falstaff* at 79. Humboldt wrote the five volumes of his *Kosmos* between the ages of 76 and 89 years; Goethe produced the second part of *Faust* when he was more than 70 years old; Galileo, Laplace, and Sherrington continued to make scientific contributions in their eighth decades; and Picasso continued to paint in his nineties. It must be pointed out, however, that these accomplishments were essentially continuations of lines of endeavor that had been initiated in early adult life. Indeed, little that is new and original is started after the fortieth year. High intelligence, well-organized work habits, and sound judgment compensate for many of the progressive shortcomings of old age.

Personality Changes in the Aged

These are less-easily measured than cognitive functions, but certain trends are nevertheless observable and may seriously disturb the lives of aged persons and those around them. Many old people become more opinionated, repetitive, self-centered, and rigid and conservative in their thinking; the opposite qualities—undue pliancy, vacillation, and the uncritical acceptance of ideas—are observed in others. Often these changes can be recognized as exaggerations of lifelong personality traits. Elderly persons tend to become increasingly cautious; many of them seem to lack self-confidence and require a strong probability of success before undertaking certain tasks. These changes may impair their performance on psychologic testing. Kallman's studies of senescent monozygotic twins suggest that genetic factors are more important than environmental ones in molding these traits.

One of the weaknesses of studies of the aged has been the bias in selection of patients. Many of the reported observations have been made in cohorts of individuals residing in nursing homes. Studies of functionally intact old people of comparable age and living independently, such as those of Kokmen (1977) and of Benassi and their colleagues, reveal fewer deficits, consisting mainly of forgetfulness of names, smallness of pupils, restriction of convergence and upward conjugate gaze, diminished Achilles reflexes and vibratory sense in the feet, stooped posture, and impairments of balance, agility, and gait (as mentioned earlier and below).

Effects of Aging on Stance and Gait and Related Motor Impairments (See also Chap. 7)

These are among the most conspicuous manifestations of the aging process. Motor agility actually begins to decline in early adult life, even by the thirtieth year; it seems related to a gradual decrease in neuromuscular control as well as to changes in joints and other structures. The reality of this motor decrement is best appreciated by professional athletes who retire at age 35 or thereabout because their legs give out and cannot be restored to their maximal condition by training. They cannot run as well as younger athletes, even though the strength and coordination of their arms, when tested independently of other functions, are relatively preserved. More subtle and imperceptibly evolving changes in stance and gait are ubiquitous features of aging (see Chap. 7). Gradually the steps shorten, walking becomes slower, and there is a tendency to stoop. The older person becomes less confident and more cautious in walking and habitually touches the handrail in descending stairs, to prevent a misstep.

To be distinguished from the ubiquitous and subtle changes in gait of the "normal" older population is a more rapidly evolving and inordinate deterioration of gait that afflicts a small proportion of the aging population while they remain relatively competent in other ways. In all likelihood, this latter disorder represents an age-linked degenerative disease of the brain, as most instances of it are sooner or later accompanied by mental changes. The basis of this gait disorder is probably a combined frontal lobe–basal ganglionic degeneration, the anatomy of which has never been fully clarified, as discussed in "Frontal Lobe Disorder of Gait" in Chap. 7. However, in many of such patients we have observed, there is no disproportionate atrophy or reduction of blood flow in the frontal lobes, making the cause of the gait disorder obscure. It has also been postulated that age-related changes in the substantia nigra are the cause of the parkinsonian appearance of the gait of the aged, but it does not respond to L-dopa or to any other therapeutic measure. The main differential diagnostic consideration is *normal-pressure hydrocephalus*, correctable by a ventriculoperitoneal shunt, which accounts for the gait disorder of a sizable group of these elderly patients, as discussed in Chaps. 7 and 30. Parkinson disease is yet another potentially treatable cause of walking difficulty. Progressive supranuclear palsy is a degenerative process in which gait and stability are affected early and profoundly.

Urinary incontinence, defined as a state in which "involuntary loss of urine is a social or hygienic problem and is objectively demonstrated," is a common occurrence in the elderly (Wells and Diokno). Doubtless this complex of motor impairments is based on the aforementioned neuronal losses in the spinal cord, cerebellum, and cerebrum.

Falls in the Elderly

Among elderly persons without apparent neurologic disease, falls constitute a major health problem. Approximately 30 percent suffer one or more falls each year; this figure rises to 40 percent among those older than age 80 years and to more than 50 percent among elderly persons living in nursing homes. According to Tinetti and colleagues, 10 to 15 percent of falls in the elderly result in fractures and other serious injuries; they are reportedly an underlying cause of about 9,500 deaths annually in the United States.

Several factors, some mentioned earlier in regard to deterioration of gait, are responsible for the inordinately high rate of falling among older persons. Impairment of visual function and particularly of vestibular function with normal aging are important contributors. In a group of 34 elderly patients who were free of neurologic disease, postural hypotension, and leg deformities, Weiner and colleagues found a moderate or severe degree of postural reflex impairment in two-thirds. The failure to make rapid postural adjustments, which is a product of aging alone, accounts for the occurrence of falls in the course of usual activities such as walking, changing position, or descending stairs. Orthostatic hypotension, often because of antihypertensive agents and the use of sedative drugs, is another important cause of falling in the elderly.

Of course, falling is an even more prominent feature of certain age-related neurologic diseases: stroke, Parkinson disease, normal-pressure hydrocephalus, and progressive supranuclear palsy, among others.

Other Restricted Motor Abnormalities in the Aged

These are too numerous to be more than catalogued. They reflect the many ways in which the motor system can deteriorate. Compulsive, repetitive movements are the most frequent: mouthing movements, stereotyped grimacing, protrusion of the tongue, side-to-side or to-and-fro tremor of the head, odd vocalizations such as sniffing, snorting, and bleating. In some respects these disorders resemble tics (quasivoluntary movements to relieve tension), but careful observation shows that they are not really voluntary. Haloperidol and other drugs of this class have an unpredictable therapeutic effect, seeming at times to benefit the patient only by the superimposition of a drug-induced rigidity and are not recommended.

Old age is thought always to carry a liability to tremulousness, and indeed, one sees this association with some frequency. The head, chin, or hands tremble and the voice quavers, yet there is not the usual slowness and poverty of movement, facial impassivity, or flexed posture that would stamp the condition as parkinsonian. Some instances of tremor are clearly familial, having appeared or worsened only late in life. However, the relation of tremulousness to aging is sometimes open to doubt. Charcot, in a review of over 2,000 elderly inhabitants of the Salpêtrière Hospital, could find only about 30 with tremor. Some cases probably represent the exaggeration or emergence of essential tremor, but many cases cannot be explained on this basis.

Spastic or spasmodic dysphonia, a disorder of middle and late life characterized by spasm of all the throat muscles on attempted speech, is discussed in Chap. 6.

Morphologic and Physiologic Changes in the Aging Nervous System

These have never been fully established. From the third decade of life to the beginning of the tenth decade, the average decline in weight of the male brain is from 1,394 to 1,161 g, a loss of 233 g. The pace of this change, very gradual at first, accelerates during the sixth or seventh decades. The loss of brain weight, which correlates roughly with enlargement of the lateral ventricles and widening of the sulci, is presumably the result of neuronal degeneration and replacement gliosis. The counting of cerebrocortical neurons is fraught with technical difficulties, even with the use of computer-assisted automated techniques (see the critical review of neuron-counting studies by Coleman and Flood). Most studies, point to a depletion of the neuronal population in the neocortex, especially evident in the seventh, eighth, and ninth decades.

Cell loss in the limbic system (hippocampus, parahippocampal, and cingulate gyri) is of special interest in regard to memory. Ball, who measured the neuronal loss in the hippocampus, recorded a linear decrease of 27 percent between 45 and 95 years of age. Dam reported a similar degree of cell loss and replacement gliosis. These changes seem to proceed without relationship to Alzheimer neurofibrillary changes and senile plaques (Kemper). However, more recent morphologic work, summarized by Morrison and Hof, suggests that cerebral cell loss with aging is less pronounced than previously thought. Furthermore, as pointed out by Morrison, the hippocampus may have only minimal cell loss. Moreover, this is partially a result of neurogenesis in this region. Brain shrinkage is accounted for in part by the reduction in size of large neurons, not their disappearance. There is a more substantial reduction in neuronal number in the substantia nigra, locus ceruleus, and basal forebrain nuclei. It may be possible to differentiate normal aging from disease in the medial temporal lobe by distinguishing between cell loss in specific regions (see Small et al), but novel techniques are required.

Mueller and colleagues employed quantitative volumetric MRI techniques to examine a cohort of 46 nondemented elderly individuals. They found small, constant rates of loss of brain volume with aging. Moreover, the rates of volume loss in the last decades of life were no greater than in the immediately preceding decades, suggesting that large changes in brain volume in the elderly are attributable to the dementing diseases common to this age period. Rusinek and colleagues found that serial MRIs of elderly persons predict which individuals will develop disproportionate atrophy and dementia. In particular, hippocampal atrophy increases at the rate of less than 2 percent per year in healthy elderly people, in comparison to 4 to 8 percent a year in early Alzheimer disease. This longitudinal method of study is more sensitive than cross-sectional population studies.

Among lumbosacral anterior horn cells, sensory ganglion cells, and putaminal and Purkinje cells, neuronal loss amounts to at most 25 percent between youth and old age. Not all neuronal groups are equally susceptible. For example, the locus ceruleus and substantia nigra, as already commented, lose approximately 35 percent of their neurons, whereas the vestibular nuclei and inferior olives maintain a fairly constant number of cells throughout life. A very subtle loss, decade by decade, of the major systems of nerve cells and myelinated fibers of the spinal cord was demonstrated by Morrison. This accelerates after the age of 60 (Tomlinson and Irving).

As described earlier in normal aging, there is a gradual decline in memory and in some cognitive functions. In light of the studies just summarized, it is no longer considered that these changes can be ascribed simply to neuronal loss. Rather, they are probably caused, at least in part, by alterations in synaptic connectivity within critical cortical structures.

Scheibel and coworkers have described a loss of neuronal dendrites in the aging brain, particularly the horizontal dendrites of the third and fifth layers of the neocortex. However, the Golgi method, which was used in these studies, is difficult to interpret because of artifacts. The morphometric studies of Buell and Coleman showed that the surviving neurons actually exhibit expanded dendritic trees, suggesting that even aging neurons have the capacity to react to cell loss by developing new synapses. With advancing age, there is an increasing tendency for neuritic (amyloid and neurofibrillary) plaques to appear in the brains of nondemented individuals. At first the plaques appear in the hippocampus and parahippocampus, but later they become more widespread. These are loose aggregates of amorphous argentophilic material containing amyloid. They occur in increasing numbers with advancing age; by the end of the ninth decade of life, few brains are without them. However, as shown by Tomlinson and colleagues, relatively fewer plaques are present in the brains of mentally intact old people, in contrast to the large numbers in those with Alzheimer disease. Even more impressive is the correlation of neurofibrillary tangles and Alzheimer disease. Very few such tangles are found in the brains of mentally sound individuals, and those that are found are essentially confined to the hippocampus and adjacent entorhinal cortex. By contrast, neurofibrillary tangles are far more abundant and diffusely distributed in patients with Alzheimer disease.

The view is often expressed that neuritic plaques and Alzheimer type of neurofibrillary changes simply represent an acceleration of the natural aging process in the brain. Most investigators are more inclined to the idea that the plaques and neurofibrillary changes represent an *acquired age-linked disease*, analogous in this respect to certain cerebrovascular diseases or osteoarthritis. In support of this latter view are several observations.

First, *Homo sapiens* is the only animal species in which Alzheimer neurofibrillary changes and neuritic plaques are regularly found in the aging brain. A few plaque-like structures (but no neurofibrillary changes) have been seen occasionally in old dogs and monkeys but not in mice or rats. It seems unbiologic that human aging should differ from that of all other animal species. Second, some of the most severe forms of Alzheimer disease occur in middle adult life, long before old age. Third, these histopathologic changes in variable proportion occur in a number of other diseases unrelated to aging, such as dementia pugilistica ("punch-drunk" state), Down syndrome, postencephalitic Parkinson disease, and progressive supranuclear palsy. Fourth, neurofibrillary tangles can be reproduced in the experimental animal by such toxins as aluminum, vincristine, vinblastine, and colchicine. Finally, a small proportion of Alzheimer cases are definitely familial, as described in Chap. 39.

Virtually every molecular structure within the cell is subject to age-related biochemical modifications, such as the formation of carbonyl proteins, glycation of sugars, and oxidative changes in lipids. Some of these subcellular phenomena contribute to the aging process (see Mrak et al for details), as do the accumulation of mitochondrial DNA mutations and shortened lengths of the telomeres. Among the visible biochemical alterations is an increasing accumulation of lipofuscin granules in the cytoplasm of neurons, sometimes extreme in degree. Also, there is an age-related neuronal accumulation of iron and other pigment bodies. Granulovacuolar changes are a regular finding in aging hippocampi, regardless of the mental state of the individual. The accumulation of glycogen-containing concretions (corpora amylacea) around nerve roots and diffusely in the subpial space is yet another aging effect, which has no known clinical correlate.

Cerebral atherosclerosis is, of course, a frequent finding in the elderly, but it does not parallel aging with any degree of precision, being severe in some 30- to 40-year-old individuals and practically absent in some octogenarians. In the normotensive individual, it tends to occur in scattered, discrete plaques mostly in the aorta and cervical arteries (carotid bifurcation and higher segments), proximal middle cerebral arteries, and at the vertebrobasilar junction and basilar portions of the cerebral arterial system. In the hypertensive and diabetic, it is more diffuse and extends into finer branches of the cerebral and cerebellar arteries. One or more cerebral infarcts are found in approximately 25 percent of all individuals older than 70 years of age who were carefully examined postmortem. In addition to atherosclerotic disease, the basilar arteries become somewhat larger and more tortuous and opaque in the elderly.

Cerebral blood flow has been extensively investigated in the elderly population. Most studies show that flow declines with age and that the cerebral metabolic rate declines in parallel. There is also an age-related increase in cerebrovascular resistance. Declines in flow are somewhat greater in the cortex than in white matter and greater in prefrontal regions than in other parts of the hemispheres. Obrist demonstrated a 28 percent reduction in cerebral flow by age 80. It is noteworthy, however, that every cohort of elderly persons tested in this way contained a significant proportion in which cerebral blood flow was equivalent to that in young control subjects. In fact, in a group of 72-year-old men rigorously selected on the basis of freedom from disease, Sokoloff demonstrated that cerebral blood flow and oxygen consumption did not differ from those of normal men 22 years of age. Nevertheless, cerebral glucose metabolism was reduced in all the elderly subjects.

With advancing age there is a general tendency for the electroencephalogram (EEG) to show a slowing of the alpha rhythm, an increase in beta activity, a decline in the percentage of slow-wave sleep, and an increasing intrusion of theta rhythms, particularly over the temporal lobes, although there are large individual differences.

With respect to the neurotransmitters, it is generally agreed that the concentrations of acetylcholine, norepinephrine, and dopamine decline in the course of normal aging. Also, the concentration of gamma-aminobutyric acid (GABA) has been shown to decline with age, particularly in the frontal cortex (Spokes et al). Analyses of postmortem human and animal brains have failed to demonstrate a decline with age in the concentration of serotonin or its metabolites (McEntee and Crook). Accurate assessment of other neurotransmitters has been more difficult because of their marked lability in postmortem material. Data from experiments in rats suggest that the glutamate content of the brain and the number of *N*-methyl-D-aspartate (NMDA) receptors diminish with age, but the functional significance of this finding is unclear. Unlike the case in Alzheimer disease, normal aging is associated with only slight and inconsistent abnormalities of cholinergic innervation of the hippocampus and cortex. This is true also of the acetylcholine content and the activity of choline acetyltransferase (the synthesizing enzyme of acetylcholine) in these regions and the number of cholinergic neurons in the nucleus basalis of Meynert (substantia innominata) and other nuclei of the basal forebrain (Decker). Again, the significance of these changes is difficult to judge. They probably reflect the depletion of cells that occurs with aging. The topics of cholinergic and glutamatergic function in the aging brain have been critically reviewed by McEntee and Crook.

Aging Changes in Muscles and Nerves

With advancing age, skeletal muscles lose cells (fibers) and undergo a gradual reduction in their weight more or less parallel to that of the brain. Atrophy of muscles and diminution in peak power and endurance are clinical expressions of these changes. Many processes contribute to this age-dependent loss of lean muscle mass, described as *sarcopenia*. These include decreased physical activity; diminished appetite associated with loss of smell and elevated levels of cholecystokinin, a satiety hormone; other endocrine changes such as diminished levels of growth hormone and androgens; and (as in the brain) the accumulation of subcellular defects such as nuclear and mitochondrial DNA mutations alluded to earlier. Moreover, with aging, the slow loss of motor neurons contributes to a component of denervation atrophy. Our own observations, with Dr. R.D. Adams, of neuropathologic material indicate that the wasting involves several processes, some principally myopathic and others relating to disuse or denervation from loss of motor neurons. In this material, denervation atrophy of the gastrocnemius muscles was found in 80 percent of individuals older than 70 years of age. The lost muscle fibers are gradually replaced by endomysial connective tissue and fat cells. The surviving fibers are generally thinner than normal (possibly because of disuse atrophy), but some enlarge, resulting in a wider-than-normal range of fiber size. Groups of fibers all at the same stage of atrophy undoubtedly relate to loss of motor innervation. The reduction in conduction velocity and decrease in amplitude of motor nerve potentials and, to a greater extent, of sensory nerves in the aged may be taken as other indices of loss of motor and sensory axons. All these changes are more marked in the legs than elsewhere. However, when Roos and colleagues examined the contractile speed and firing rates of the quadriceps muscle in young men and compared them to those of men close to 80 years old, they found little difference despite a 50 percent reduction in the maximum voluntary contraction force developed by the muscle in the older men.

It has been repeatedly observed that age is an important prognostic factor in a large number of human diseases. This effect is very evident, for example, in the markedly slower and less-complete recovery from Guillain-Barré polyneuropathy in older age groups compared with younger ones. One presumes that the structural changes of aging in peripheral nerves limit the degree of myelin regeneration and lower the threshold for failure of electrical transmission.

GERONTOLOGIC NEUROLOGY

Gerontology is defined as the study of aging and *geriatrics* as the study of the disorders of aging, both of aging itself and of the age-related diseases. Geriatric neurology has emerged as a subspecialty focused on age-related disorders of the nervous system (see the review of the field by Stanton). In comparison to pediatric neurology, these disciplines have not aroused much interest, yet many neurologic patients seen in practice are elderly, especially if one includes those with vascular diseases of the brain. Furthermore, many of their diseases are preventable or therapeutically controllable such as hypertension, atrial fibrillation, and hypercholesterolemia as causes of stroke. Some of the age-related nutritional and endocrine disorders (e.g., vitamin B deficiencies, diabetes mellitus) and many of the common restricted involutional changes (e.g., presbyopia) can be corrected. And always, there is the need to counsel the elderly patient on matters pertaining to health and daily activities. This was appreciated even in the time of Cicero, who, in his *De Senectute*, urged the practice of moderation in exercise and giving due attention to the mind, which must be kept active or, like a lamp that is not supplied with oil, it will grow dim.

As medical science and public health measures have brought diseases of aging and other diseases under control, the number of elderly persons has increased and will continue to do so. The U.S. Census Bureau reported a 18.5% increase in persons 60 years and older (45.8 to 57.1 million) and a 9.0% increase in persons 70 years and older (25.5 to 27.8 million) between the years 2000 and 2010. As the number of elderly increases, the need to look after them will occupy an increasing amount of the energies of physicians and the resources of society at large.

References

Albert ML, Knoefel JE (eds): *Clinical Neurology of Aging*, 2nd ed. New York, Oxford University Press, 1994.

Albert MS: Memory decline: The boundary between aging and age-related disease. *Ann Neurol* 51:282, 2002.

Antel JP, Minuk J: Neuroimmunology of aging, in Albert ML, Knoefel JE (eds): *Clinical Neurology of Aging*, 2nd ed. New York, Oxford University Press, 1994, pp 121–135.

Ball MJ: Neuronal loss, neurofibrillary tangles and granulovacuolar degeneration in the hippocampus with aging and dementia. *Acta Neuropathol* 27:111, 1977.

Benassi G, D'Alessandro R, Gallassi R, et al: Neurological examination in subjects over 65 years: An epidemiological survey. *Neuroepidemiology* 9:27, 1990.

Blessed G, Tomlinson BE, Roth M: The association between quantitative measures of dementia and of senile change in the cerebral grey matter of elderly subjects. *Br J Psychiatry* 114:797, 1968.

Buell SJ, Coleman PD: Dendritic growth in the aged human brain and failure of growth in senile dementia. *Science* 206:854, 1979.

Clegg A: The frailty syndrome. *Clinical medicine* 11:72, 2011.

Coleman PD, Flood DG: Neuron numbers and dendritic extent in normal aging and Alzheimer's disease. *Neurobiol Aging* 8:521, 1987.

Comfort A: *The Biology of Senescence*, 3rd ed. New York, Elsevier, 1979.

Critchley M: The neurology of old age. *Lancet* 1:1221, 1931.

Critchley M: Neurologic changes in the aged. *J Chronic Dis* 3:459, 1956.

Crook T, Bartus RT, Ferris SH, et al: Age-associated memory impairment: Proposed diagnostic criteria and measures of clinical change—report of a National Institute of Mental Health Work Group. *Dev Neuropsychol* 2:261, 1986.

Crum RM, Anthony JC, Bassett SS, Folstein MF: Population-based norms for the mini-mental status examination by age and educational level. *JAMA* 18:2386, 1993.

Dam AM: The density of neurons in the human hippocampus. *Neuropathol Appl Neurobiol* 5:249, 1979.

Decker MW: The effects of aging on hippocampal and cortical projections of the forebrain cholinergic system. *Brain Res* 434:423, 1987.

Folstein MF, Folstein SE, McHugh PR: "Mini-mental state": A practical method for grading the cognitive state of patients for the clinician. *J Psychiatr Res* 12:189, 1975.

Fried LP: Frailty, in Cassel C, Liepzig R, Cohen H, et al (eds): *Geriatric Medicine*. New York, Springer-Verlag, 2003, pp 1067–1074.

Fries JF: Aging, natural death, and the compression of morbidity. *N Engl J Med* 303:130, 1980.

Fries JF, Crapo LM: *Vitality and Aging*. San Francisco, Freeman, 1981.

Hazzard WR, Blass JP, Ettinger WH, et al (eds): *Principles of Geriatric Medicine and Gerontology*, 4th ed. New York, McGraw-Hill, 1999.

Jenkyn LR, Reeves AG, Warren T, et al: Neurologic signs in senescence. *Arch Neurol* 42:1154, 1985.

Kallman FJ: Genetic factors in aging: Comparative and longitudinal observations on a senescent twin population, in Hoch PH, Zubin J (eds): *Psychopathology of Aging*. New York, Grune & Stratton, 1961.

Kaye JA, Oken BS, Howieson DB, et al: Neurologic evaluation of the optimally healthy oldest old. *Arch Neurol* 51:1205, 1994.

Kemper TL: Neuroanatomical and neuropathological changes during aging and dementia, in Albert ML, Knoefel JE (eds): *Clinical Neurology of Aging*, 2nd ed. New York, Oxford University Press, 1994, pp 3–67.

Kokmen E, Bossemeyer RW Jr, Barney J, Williams WJ: Neurologic manifestations of aging. *J Gerontol* 32:411, 1977.

Kokmen E, Smith GE, Petersen RC, et al: The short test of mental status: Correlations with standardized psychometric testing. *Arch Neurol* 48:725, 1991.

Kral VA: Senescent forgetfulness: Benign and malignant. *Can Med Assoc J* 86:257, 1962.

Larrabee GH, Levin HS, High WM: Senescent forgetfulness: A quantitative study. *Dev Neuropsychol* 2:373, 1986.

McEntee WJ, Crook TH: Serotonin, memory, and the aging brain. *Psychopharmacology (Berl)* 103:143, 1991.

Morrison JH, Hof RP: Life and death of neurons in the aging brain. *Science* 278:412, 1997.

Morrison LR: *The Effect of Advancing Age upon the Human Spinal Cord*. Cambridge, MA, Harvard University Press, 1959.

Mrak RE, Griffin ST, Graham DI: Aging-associated changes in human brain. *J Neuropathol Exp Neurol* 56:1269, 1997.

Mueller EA, Moore MM, Kerr DC, et al: Brain volume preserved in healthy elderly through the eleventh decade. *Neurology* 51:1555, 1998.

Obrist WD: Cerebral circulatory changes in normal aging and dementia, in Hoffmeister F, Muller C (eds): *Brain Function in Old Age*. Berlin, Springer-Verlag, 1979, pp 278–287.

Olney RK: The neurology of aging, in Aminoff MJ (ed): *Neurology and General Medicine*, 3rd ed. New York, Churchill Livingstone, 2001, pp 939–952.

Petersen RC, Smith GE, Kokmen E, et al. Memory function in normal aging. *Neurology* 42:396, 1992.

Poon LW: Differences in human memory with aging: Nature, causes, and clinical implications, in Birren JE, Schaie KW (eds): *Handbook of the Psychology of Aging*. New York, Van Nostrand Reinhold, 1985, pp 427–462.

Roos MR, Rice CL, Connelly DM, Vandervoort AA: Quadriceps muscle strength, contractile properties, and motor unit firing rates in young and old men. *Muscle Nerve* 22:1094, 1999.

Roth M, Tomlinson BE, Blessed G: Correlation between scores for dementia and counts of senile plaques in cerebral grey matter of elderly subjects. *Nature* 209:109, 1966.

Rusinek H, De Santi S, Frid D, et al: Regional brain atrophy rate predicts future cognitive decline: 6-year longitudinal MRI imaging study of normal aging. *Radiology* 229:691, 2003.

Schaie KW, Hertzog C: Fourteen-year cohort-sequential analyses of adult intellectual development. *Dev Psychol* 19:531, 1983.

Scheibel M, Lindsay RD, Tomiyasu U, Scheibel AB: Progressive dendritic changes in aging human cortex. *Exp Neurol* 47:392, 1975.

Shock MW: System integration, in Masoro EJ, Austad SN (eds): *Handbook of the Biology of Aging*. Amsterdam: Elsevier Academic Press, 2006.

Small SA, Tsai WY, DeLaPaz R, et al: Imaging hippocampal function across the human life span: Is memory decline normal or not? *Ann Neurol* 51:290, 2002.

Smith GE, Malec JF, Ivnik RJ: Validity of the construct of nonverbal memory: A factor-analytic study in a normal elderly sample. *J Clin Exp Neuropsychol* 14:211, 1992.

Sokoloff L: Effects of normal aging on cerebral circulation and energy metabolism, in Hoffmeister F, Muller C (eds): *Brain Function in Old Age*. Berlin, Springer-Verlag, 1979, pp 367–380.

Spokes EGS, Garrett NJ, Rossor MN, et al: Distribution of GABA in postmortem brain tissue from control, psychotic, and Huntington's chorea subjects. *J Neurol Sci* 48:303, 1980.

Stanton BR: The neurology of old age. *Clinical Medicine* 11:54, 2011.

Tinetti ME, Speechley M: Prevention of falls among the elderly. *N Engl J Med* 320:1055, 1989.

Tinetti ME, Speechley M, Ginter SF: Risk factors for falls among elderly persons living in the community. *N Engl J Med* 319:1701, 1988.

Tomlinson BE, Blessed G, Roth M: Observations on the brains of non-demented old people. *J Neurol Sci* 7:331, 1968.

Tomlinson BE, Blessed G, Roth M: Observations on the brains of demented old people. *J Neurol Sci* 11:205, 1970.

Tomlinson BE, Irving D: The numbers of limb motor neurons in the human lumbosacral spinal cord throughout life. *J Neurol Sci* 34:213, 1977.

Van Exel E, Gussekloo J, De Craen AJ, et al: Cognitive function in the oldest old: Women perform better than men. *J Neurol Neurosurg Psychiatry* 71:29, 2001.

Verhaeghen P, Marcoen A, Goossens L: Facts and fiction about memory aging: A quantitative integration of research findings. *J Gerontol* 48:157, 1993.

Weiner WJ, Nora LM, Glantz RH: Elderly inpatients: Postural reflex impairment. *Neurology* 34:945, 1984.

Wells TJ, Diokno AC: Urinary incontinence in the elderly. *Semin Neurol* 9:60, 1989.

PART 4

MAJOR CATEGORIES OF NEUROLOGIC DISEASE

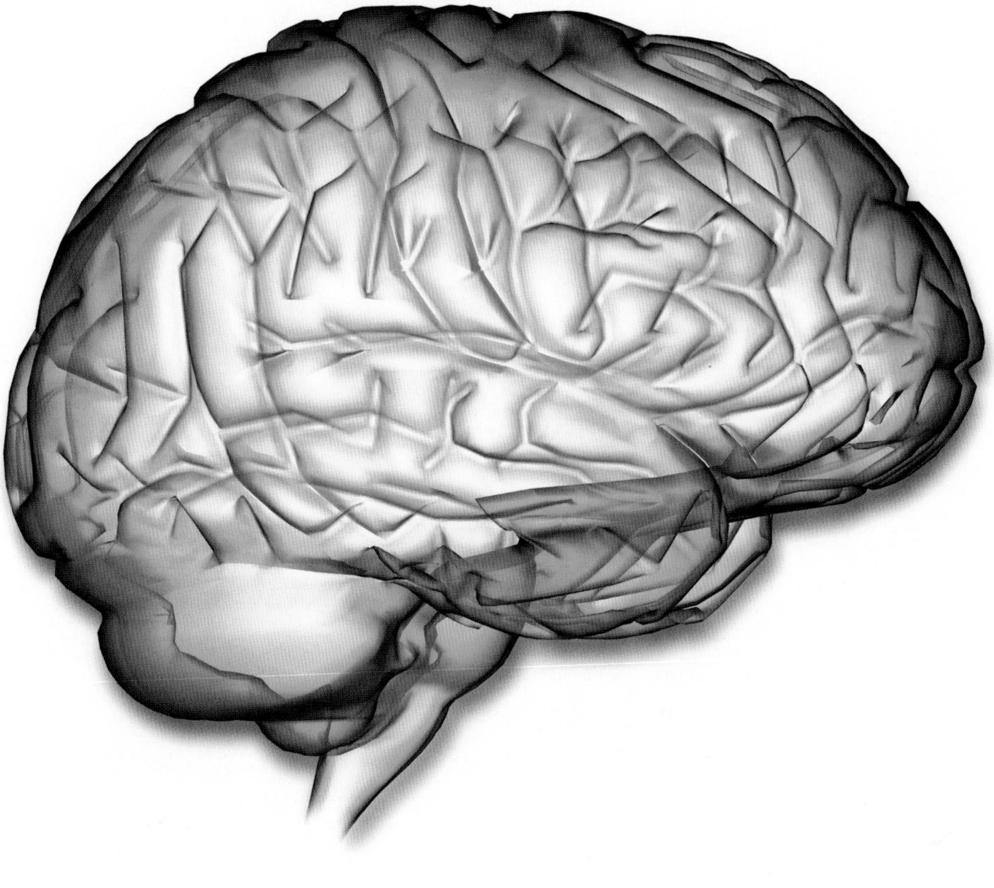

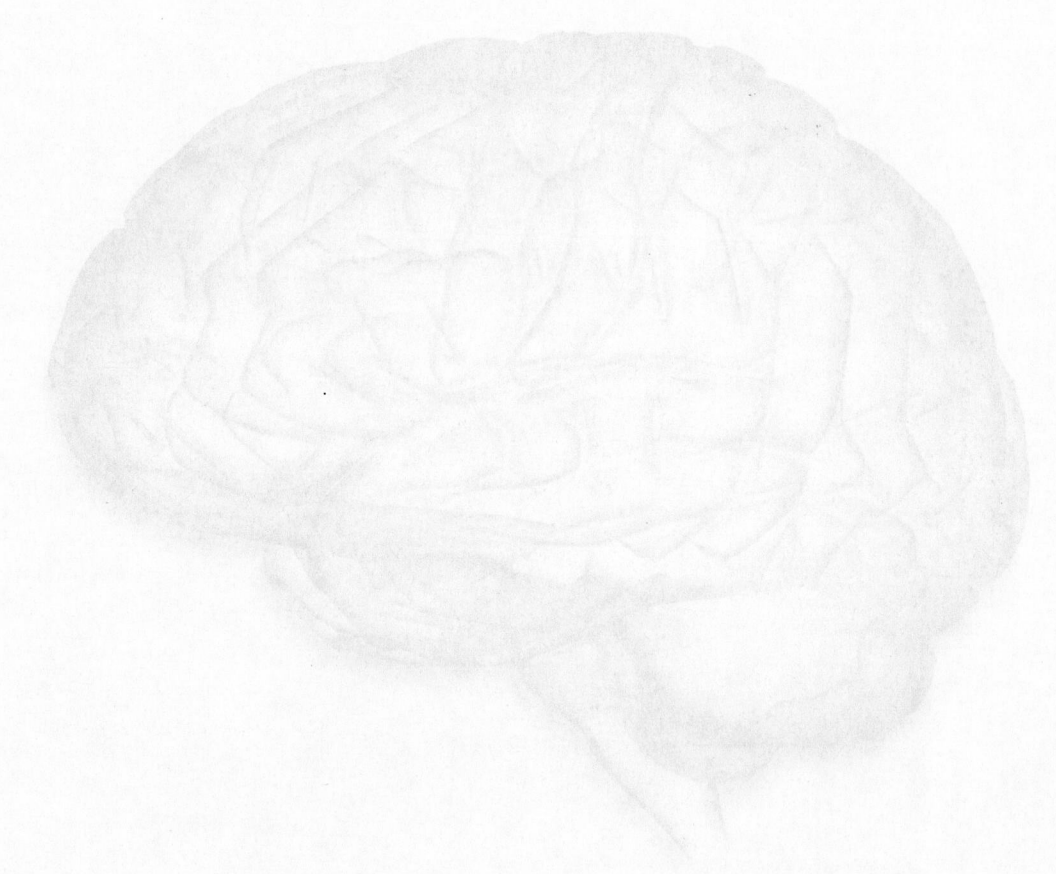

30

Disturbances of Cerebrospinal Fluid, Including Hydrocephalus, Pseudotumor Cerebri, and Low-Pressure Syndromes

In the chapters to follow, reference is made to the ways in which changes in the cerebrospinal fluid (CSF) reflect the basic pathologic processes in a variety of inflammatory and infectious, neoplastic, demyelinative, and degenerative diseases. The CSF alterations in these circumstances raise so many important problems that we consider it worthwhile to discuss in one place the mechanisms involved in the formation, circulation, and absorption of the CSF, particularly as they pertain to alterations of intracranial pressure (ICP). Considered in this chapter are hydrocephalus, pseudotumor cerebri, and syndromes produced by reduced pressure in the CSF compartment. Further information on the management of raised ICP as it pertains to traumatic brain injury, of which the CSF is an essential part, can be found in Chap. 35. Examination of the CSF as a diagnostic aid in neurology was discussed in Chap. 2, and the primary infectious and noninfectious inflammatory reactions of the pia-arachnoid (leptomeninges) and ependyma of the ventricles are considered in Chap. 32.

A few historical points call to mind that our understanding of the physiology, chemistry, and cytology of the CSF is the result of a technical innovation that was introduced a century ago. Although the lumbar puncture was introduced by Quincke in 1891, it was not until 1912 that Mestrezat made correlations between disease processes and the cellular and chemical changes in the CSF. In 1937, Merritt and Fremont-Smith published their monograph on CSF changes in a broad variety of disease. Our knowledge of CSF cytology has accumulated since the late 1950s, when membrane filtration techniques (particularly the cellulose ester or Millipore filter) were introduced. The studies of Dandy (1919) and of Weed (1935) provided the basis of our knowledge of CSF formation, circulation, and absorption. The important studies of Pappenheimer and of Ames and their colleagues followed, and then the monographs of Fishman and of Davson and coworkers, which are important modern contributions. (See Chap. 2 for references.) Recent inceptions in analyzing the lymphocytic cells and protein fractions in the CSF have expanded on modern technology that was developed in hematology.

PHYSIOLOGY OF THE CEREBROSPINAL FLUID

The primary function of the CSF appears to be a mechanical one; it serves as a kind of water jacket for the spinal cord and brain, protecting them from potentially injurious blows to the spinal column and skull and acute changes in venous pressure. Also, it provides the brain with buoyancy. As pointed out by Fishman, the 1,500-g brain, which has a water content of approximately 80 percent, weighs only 50 g when suspended in CSF, so the brain virtually floats in its CSF. Many of the physiologic mechanisms described below are committed to maintaining the relatively constant volume–pressure relationships of the CSF. In addition, because the brain and spinal cord have no lymphatic channels, the CSF, through its "sink action," serves to remove waste products of cerebral metabolism, the main ones being CO_2, lactate, and hydrogen ions. The composition of the CSF is maintained within narrow limits, despite major alterations in the blood; thus the other main function of CSF, along with the intercellular fluid of the brain, is to preserve a stable chemical environment for neurons, astrocytes, and myelinated fibers. There is no reason, however, to believe that the CSF is actively involved in the metabolism of the cells of the brain, and spinal cord.

In the adult, the average intracranial volume is 1,700 mL; the volume of the brain is from 1,200 to 1,400 mL, CSF volume ranges from 70 to 160 mL (mean: 104 mL), and that of blood is approximately 150 mL. In addition, the spinal subarachnoid space contains 10 to 25 mL of CSF. Thus, at most, the CSF occupies somewhat less than 10 percent of the intracranial and intraspinal spaces. The proportion of CSF in the ventricles, and cerebral cisternae and sulci in the subarachnoid spaces varies with age. These variations have been plotted in CT scans by Meese and coworkers; the distance between the caudate nuclei at the anterior horns gradually widens by approximately 1.0 to 1.5 cm, and the width of the third ventricle increases from 3 to 6 mm by age 60 years.

Formation of CSF

The introduction of the ventriculocisternal perfusion technique by Pappenheimer and colleagues made possible measurements of the rates of formation and absorption of the CSF. They established that the average rate of CSF formation is 21 to 22 mL/h (0.35 mL/min), or approximately 500 mL/d; thus the volume of CSF as a whole is renewed 4 or 5 times daily.

The choroid plexuses, located in the floor of the lateral, third, and fourth ventricles, are the main sites of CSF formation (some CSF is formed by the meninges even after the choroid plexuses are removed). The thin-walled vessels of the plexuses allow passive diffusion of substances from the blood plasma into the extracellular space surrounding choroid cells. The choroidal epithelial cells, like other secretory epithelia, contain organelles, indicating their capacity for an energy-dependent secretory function, i.e., "active transport." The blood vessels in the subependymal regions and the pia also contribute to the CSF, and some substances enter the CSF as readily from the meninges as from the choroid plexuses. Thus, electrolytes equilibrate with the CSF at all points in the ventricular and subarachnoid spaces, and the same is true of glucose. The transport of sodium, the main cation of the CSF, is accomplished by the action of a sodium-potassium-ion exchange pump at the apical surface of the choroid plexus cells, the energy for which is supplied by adenosine tri-phosphate (ATP); drugs that inhibit the ATP system therefore reduce CSF formation (Cutler and Spertell). Electrolytes enter the ventricles somewhat more readily than they enter the subarachnoid space (water does the opposite). It is also known that the penetration of certain drugs and metabolites into the CSF (and brain) is in direct relation to their lipid solubility. Ionized compounds, such as hexoses and amino acids, being relatively insoluble in lipids, enter the CSF slowly unless facilitated by a membrane transport system. This type of facilitated (carrier) diffusion is stereospecific; i.e., the carrier (a specific protein or proteolipid) binds only with a solute having a specific configuration, and conducts it across the membrane, where it is released into the CSF, and intercellular fluid.

Diffusion gradients appear to determine the entry of serum electrolytes and proteins into the CSF, and also the exchanges of CO_2. Water and sodium diffuse as readily from blood to CSF and intercellular spaces as in the reverse direction. This explains the rapid effects of intravenously injected hypotonic and hypertonic fluids. Studies using radioisotopic tracer techniques show that the various constituents of the CSF (see Table 2-2) are in dynamic equilibrium with the blood. Similarly, CSF in the ventricles and subarachnoid spaces is in equilibrium with the intercellular fluid of the brain, spinal cord, and olfactory and optic nerves. Certain structures that maintain this equilibrium are subsumed under the term *blood–brain barrier*, which is used to designate all of the interfaces between blood, brain, and CSF. The site of the barrier varies for the different plasma constituents. One is the endothelium of the choroidal and brain capillaries; another is the plasma membrane and adventitia (Rouget cells) of these vessels; a third is the pericapillary foot processes of astrocytes. Large molecules, such as albumin, are prevented from entry by the capillary endothelium, and this is the barrier also for such molecules as are bound to albumin, e.g., aniline dyes (trypan blue), bilirubin, and many drugs. Other smaller molecules are blocked from entering the brain by the capillary plasma membrane or astrocytes.

The substances formed in the nervous system during its metabolic activity diffuse rapidly into the CSF. Thus, the CSF has, as mentioned, a "sink action," to use Davson's term, by which the products of brain metabolism are removed into the bloodstream as CSF is absorbed.

CSF Circulation

Harvey Cushing aptly termed the CSF the "third circulation," comparable to that of blood and lymph. From its principal site of formation in the choroid plexus of the lateral ventricles, CSF flows downward sequentially through the third ventricle, aqueduct, fourth ventricle, and foramina of Magendie (medially) and Luschka (laterally) at the base of the medulla, to the perimedullary and perispinal subarachnoid spaces, thence around the brainstem and rostrally to the basal and ambient cisterns, through the tentorial aperture, and finally to the lateral and superior surfaces of the cerebral hemispheres, where most of it is absorbed (Fig. 30-1). The pressure in the CSF

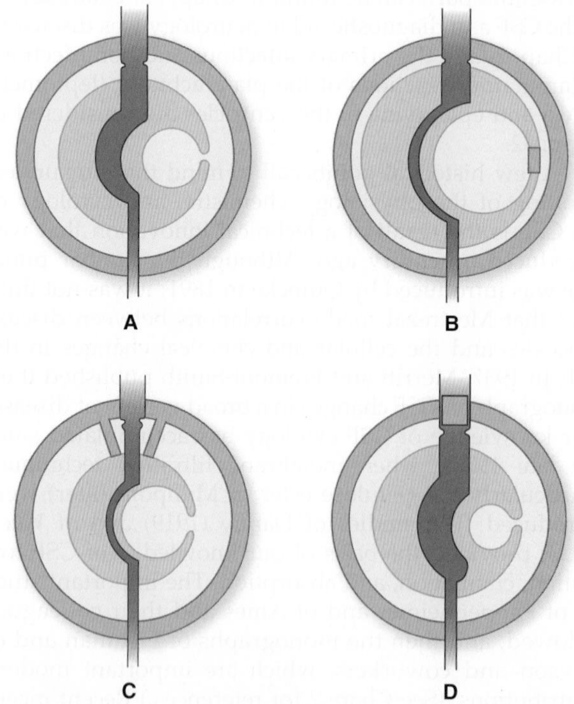

Figure 30-1. *A.* Schematic representation of the three components of the intracranial contents: the incompressible brain tissue (*orange*); the vascular system (*dark blue channel*); and the CSF (*light blue*). The red outer circle represents the intracranial compartment, which is fixed in size. *B.* With ventricular outflow obstruction. *C.* With obstruction at or near the points of outlet of the CSF. *D.* With obstruction of the venous outflow. (Redrawn with permission from Foley.)

compartment is highest in the ventricles and diminishes successively along the subarachnoid pathways. Arterial pulsations of the choroid plexuses help drive the fluid centrifugally from the ventricular system.

The spinal fluid is in contact everywhere with the extracellular fluid of the brain and spinal cord, but the extent of bulk flow of the CSF through the brain parenchyma is small under normal conditions. The periventricular tissue offer considerable resistance to the entrance of CSF and although the pressure difference between the ventricles and the subarachnoid spaces over the convexity of the hemispheres (transmantle pressure) is above zero, the open ventricular–foraminal–subarachnoid pathway directs the bulk of CSF flow in this direction. Only if this conduit is obstructed does the transmantle pressure rise, compressing the periventricular tissues and leading to ventricular enlargement, i.e., hydrocephalus, and transependymal flow of CSF.

CSF Absorption

Absorption of CSF is mainly through the arachnoid villi. These are microscopic excrescences of arachnoid membrane that penetrate the dura and protrude into the superior sagittal sinus and other venous structures. Multiple villi are aggregated in these locations to form the pacchionian granulations or bodies, some of them large enough to indent the inner table of the calvarium. These may increase in size with aging, and large ones (3.0 to 9.5 mm in diameter) may rarely herniate through bony defects and erode, providing a portal of entry to organisms from the ear that lead to meningitis (Samuels et al).

The arachnoid villi, most numerous on both sides of the superior sagittal sinus, are also present at the base of the brain and around the spinal cord roots and have been thought to act as functional valves that permit unidirectional "bulk flow" of CSF into the vascular lumen. However, electron microscope studies show that the arachnoid villi have a continuous membranous covering. This layer is extremely thin, and CSF passes through the villi at a linearly increasing rate as CSF pressures rise above 68 mm H_2O. This passive route is not the only manner in which CSF water and other contents are transported. Tripathi and Tripathi, in serial electron micrographs, found that the mesothelial cells of the arachnoid villus continually form giant cytoplasmic vacuoles that are capable of transcellular bulk transport. Certain substances, such as penicillin and organic acids and bases, are also absorbed by cells of the choroid plexus; the bidirectional action of these cells resembles that of the tubule cells of the kidneys. Some substances have been shown in pathologic specimens to pass between the ependymal cells of the ventricles and to enter subependymal capillaries and venules.

By infusing and withdrawing CSF under controlled circumstances, the resistance to CSF absorption and its rate of replacement can be calculated. The resistance to the passage of CSF into the venous system has been termed R_0 and can be expressed in terms similar to the Ohm law ($E = IR$): the voltage (E) reflects the difference in pressure between the CSF and the venous system ($P_{CSF} - P_V$), which drives CSF into the dural sinuses, and the equivalent of electrical current, termed I_f, represents the flow rate of CSF. In the steady state, this flow rate is equal to the rate of CSF production (0.3 mL/min). R_0, the resistance to absorption, which under normal circumstances is approximately 2.5, rises when there is a blockage in the CSF circulation. The equation for CSF pressure can therefore be expressed as $P_{CSF} - P_V = I_f \times R_0$; when rearranged, $P_{CSF} = P_V + I_f \times R_0$. Because the product of $I_f \times R_0$ is only 0.8 mm Hg, it can be appreciated that the main contribution to CSF pressure—as measured by spinal puncture—is the venous pressure, P_V. Restated, the intracranial pressure and CSF pressure, which are in equilibrium, are derived predominantly from transmitted vascular pressures and not from CSF outflow resistance. However, in pathologic conditions such as bacterial meningitis and subarachnoid hemorrhage, R_0 may rise to levels that impede CSF circulation, raise pressure.

Cerebrospinal Fluid Volume and Pressure

In the recumbent position, ICP and, consequently, CSF pressure are normally about 8 mm Hg or 110 mm H_2O (1 mm Hg equals 13.7 mm H_2O), with an upper limit of normal that is higher in children than in adults according to Huh and colleagues. As the head and trunk are progressively elevated, the weight of the column of CSF is added incrementally to the pressure in the lumbar subarachnoid space, and the intracranial CSF pressure drops correspondingly, so that it is close to zero in the standing position. As described above, the CSF pressure is in equilibrium with the capillary and prevenous vascular pressures, which are influenced mainly by circulatory changes that alter arteriolar tone. Elevations in systemic arterial pressure cause little or no increase of pressure at the capillary level because of cerebrovascular autoregulation, and hence, little increase in CSF pressure. Extremely low blood pressure (BP), in the range of a mean of 40 mm Hg, however, cannot be compensated for and correspondingly, lower the CSF pressure (which is, of course, zero when the heart stops).

In contrast to the limited effect caused by changes in arterial BP, increased venous pressure exerts an almost immediate effect on CSF pressure by increasing the volume of blood in the cerebral veins, venules, and dural sinuses. If the jugular veins are compressed, there is a rise of ICP that is transmitted to the lumbar subarachnoid space (unless there is a spinal subarachnoid block). This was the basis of the now little used Queckenstedt test, mentioned in Chap. 2. In the case of a spinal block, pressure on the abdominal wall, which affects the spinal veins below the point of subarachnoid block, will still increase the lumbar CSF pressure. The Valsalva maneuver, as well as coughing, sneezing, and straining, causes an increased intrathoracic pressure, which is transmitted to the jugular and then to the cerebral and spinal veins and directly to the CSF compartment through the intervertebral foramina. The jugular venous valves prevent unimpeded transmission of pressure to the cranial veins but this threshold can be exceeded if central and jugular venous pressures become greatly elevated. Mediastinal tumors, by obstructing the superior vena cava, have the same effect.

The inhalation or retention of CO_2 raises the blood Pco_2 and correspondingly decreases the pH of the CSF. By a mechanism that is not fully understood, this acidification of the CSF acts as a potent cerebral vasodilator, causing an increase in cerebral blood flow and blood volume, thus leading to intracranial hypertension. Hyperventilation, which reduces Pco_2, has the opposite effect; it increases the pH and the cerebral vascular resistance and thereby decreases CSF pressure; this maneuver of lowering the arterial CO_2 content by hyperventilation is used in the treatment of acutely raised ICP.

DISTURBANCES OF CEREBROSPINAL FLUID PRESSURE, VOLUME, AND CIRCULATION

Increased Intracranial Pressure

Physiologic Considerations

The intact cranium and vertebral canal, together with the relatively inelastic dura, form a rigid container, such that an increase in the volume of any of its contents—brain, blood, or CSF—will elevate the ICP. Furthermore, an increase in any one of these components must be at the expense of the other two, a relationship that is known as the Monro-Kellie doctrine. Small increments in brain volume do not immediately raise the ICP because of the countervailing buffering effect of displacement of CSF from the cranial cavity into the spinal canal. To a lesser extent, there is deformation of the brain and stretching of the infoldings of the relatively unyielding dura, specifically, the falx cerebri between the hemispheres and the tentorium between the hemispheres and cerebellum. Once these compensating measures have been exhausted, a mass within one dural compartment leads to displacement, or "herniation" of brain tissue from that compartment into an adjacent one. Any further increment in brain volume necessarily reduces the volume of intracranial blood contained in the veins and dural sinuses. Also, the CSF is formed more slowly in circumstances of raised ICP. These accommodative volume-pressure relationships occur concurrently and are subsumed under the term *intracranial elastance* (the change in ICP for a given change in intracranial volume, or its inverse, compliance). As the volume of brain, blood, or CSF continue to increase, the accommodative mechanisms fail and ICP rises exponentially, as in an idealized elastance curve. The normal curve begins its steep ascent at an ICP of approximately 25 mm Hg. After this point, small increments in intracranial volume result in marked elevations in ICP.

The numerical difference between ICP and mean BP within the cerebral vessels is termed *cerebral perfusion pressure* (CPP). Besides the aforementioned brain tissue shifts, which are discussed more fully in relation to their clinical signs in Chap. 17, elevation in ICP that approaches the level of mean systemic BP eventually causes a widespread reduction in cerebral blood flow. In its most severe form, this results in global ischemia and produces brain death. Lesser degrees of raised ICP and reduced cerebral perfusion cause correspondingly less severe, but still widespread, cerebral infarction that is similar to what arises after cardiac arrest. In all circumstances, not only the severity but also the duration of reduced cerebral perfusion, are the main determinants of the degree of cerebral damage. These are theoretical models that guide practice but are often found to be imprecise in clinical circumstances.

Lundberg has been credited with recording and analyzing intraventricular pressures over long periods of time in patients with brain tumors. He found ICP to be subject to periodic spontaneous fluctuations, of which he described three types of pressure waves, designated as A, B, and C. Only the A waves have proved to be separable from arterial and respiratory pulsations and are of clinical consequence. They consist of rhythmic wave-like elevations of ICP, up to 50 mm Hg, occurring every 15 to 30 min and lasting about 1 min, or of smaller but more protracted elevations. These *plateau waves*, as they have come to be known, coincide with an increase in intracranial blood volume, presumably as a result of a temporary failure of cerebrovascular autoregulation. Rosner and Becker have observed that plateau waves are sometimes preceded by a brief period of mild systemic hypotension. In their view, this slight hypotension induces cerebral vasodilatation in order to maintain normal blood flow. Upon recovery of the BP, the response in cerebrovascular tone is delayed, thereby allowing intracranial blood volume to accumulate in the dilated vascular bed, and raising ICP in the form of a plateau wave. In support of this explanation is the observation that a brief period of induced elevation of BP paradoxically restores the normal cerebrovascular tone and leads to an abrupt cessation of a plateau wave.

The high rates of mortality and morbidity of acute cerebral mass lesions is in part related to uncontrolled elevation in ICP. In a normal adult reclining with the head and trunk elevated to 45 degrees, the ICP is in the range of 2 to 5 mm Hg. Levels above 15 mm Hg that are considered abnormal are not in themselves hazardous; in fact, adequate cerebral perfusion can be maintained at an ICP of 40 mm Hg provided BP remains normal. A higher ICP or a lower BP may combine to reduce CPP and cause diffuse ischemic damage.

Causes of Raised ICP

In clinical practice, there are several mechanisms for elevated ICP:

1. *A cerebral or extracerebral mass* such as brain tumor; cerebral infarction with edema; traumatic contusion; parenchymal, subdural, or extradural hematoma; or abscess, all of which tend to be localized and deform the adjacent brain. The brain deformation is greatest locally, being compartmentalized to a varying degree by dural partitions.
2. *Generalized brain swelling*, as occurs in ischemic–anoxic states, acute hepatic failure, hypertensive

encephalopathy, hypercarbia, and the Reye hepatocerebral syndrome. In these disorders, the increase in pressure can reduce cerebral perfusion, but tissue shifts are minimal because the mass effect is uniformly distributed throughout the cranial contents.

3. An *increase in venous pressure* because of cerebral venous sinus thrombosis, heart failure, or obstruction of the superior mediastinal or jugular veins.
4. *Obstruction to the flow and absorption of CSF*. If the obstruction is within the ventricles or in the subarachnoid space at the base of the brain, *hydrocephalus* results. Extensive meningeal disease from any number of causes (infectious, carcinomatous, granulomatous, hemorrhagic) is another mechanism of blockage to CSF flow. If the block is confined to the absorptive sites adjacent to the cerebral convexities and superior sagittal sinus, the ventricles remain normal in size or enlarge only slightly, because the pressure over the convexities approximates the pressure within the lateral ventricles (see further on).
5. Any *process that expands the volume of CSF* (meningitis, subarachnoid hemorrhage) or increases CSF production (choroid plexus tumor). In this situation, there may be a pressure gradient between the cerebral and spinal compartments, resulting in hydrocephalus.

Clinical Features of Raised ICP (See also Chap. 17)

The clinical manifestations of increased ICP in children and adults are headache, nausea and vomiting, drowsiness, ocular palsies, and papilledema. Papilledema may result in periodic visual obscurations; if it is protracted, optic atrophy and blindness may follow (see Chap. 13 for further discussion of papilledema and optic nerve atrophy). The practice of monitoring ICP with a pressure device inserted into the cranial cavity has permitted approximate correlations to be made between clinical signs and the levels of ICP. However, the main neurologic signs of a large intracranial mass, pupillary dilatation, abducens palsies, drowsiness, and the Cushing response, as discussed below and in Chaps. 17 and 35, are caused by displacement of brain tissue, and therefore do not bear a strict relationship to ICP.

As a rule, patients with normal BP retain normal mental alertness with ICP of 25 to 40 mm Hg unless there is concurrent shift of brain tissue. Stated another way, coma generally cannot be attributed to elevated ICP alone. Only when ICP exceeds 40 to 50 mm Hg does cerebral blood flow diminish to a degree that results in loss of consciousness. Any further elevations are followed imminently by global ischemia and brain death. From our own observations, the brain shift and herniation that causes the pupil to dilate on the side of a mass lesion generally occurs at an ICP of 28 to 34 mm Hg. (Again, this is not a direct effect of the elevated ICP.) There are instances in which the dissociation between ICP and clinical signs is striking, for example, a mass in the medial temporal lobe that is contiguous to the third nerve will compress the nerve at a time when pressure is little raised, and slowly growing lesions, which raise ICP slowly and allow for compensation cause few clinical signs. Likewise, unilateral or bilateral abducens palsies do not have a uniform relationship to the degree of elevation of ICP. Rather, abducens palsies are most frequent when raised ICP is a result of diffusely distributed brain swelling, hydrocephalus, meningitic processes, or pseudotumor states.

The consequences of increased ICP take on special features *in infants and small children*, whose cranial sutures have not closed. The head enlarges and the eyes may bulge. Then the clinical problem involves differentiation from other types of enlargement of the head with or without hydrocephalus, such as constitutional macrocrania or an enlarged brain (megalencephaly; or hereditary metabolic diseases such as Krabbe disease, Alexander disease, Tay-Sachs disease, Canavan spongy degeneration of the brain), and from subdural hematoma or hygroma, neonatal ventricular hemorrhage, and various cysts and tumors.

Monitoring Intracranial Pressure

There is evidence, mainly from retrospective cohorts of patients with traumatic brain injury, that the outcome in patients with intracranial mass lesions is better if the ICP is maintained at levels well below those that compromise cerebral perfusion. An ICP below 15 or 20 mm Hg is often given as a therapeutic target, as the elastance curve becomes steep beyond this level and small increments in cerebral volume may cause large elevations in pressure. However, guiding treatment by the direct measurement of ICP has not yielded uniformly beneficial results, and—after several decades of popularity—the advantage of such devices over clinical and imaging signs of increasing mass effect, is not certain. Nonetheless, in a patient who cannot be examined because of induced paralysis or sedation, or who will be subjected to a procedure that risks further elevating ICP, monitoring seems sensible.

The problem in demonstrating an advantage to monitoring may partly be a matter of the level of ICP at which treatment is instituted and the proper selection of patients for treatment. Contributing to the decision to institute monitoring are the prospects of ameliorating the underlying lesion, the patient's age, and associated medical disease(s). Our practice has been to measure ICP with an indwelling fiberoptic monitor or intraventricular catheter in otherwise salvageable patients who are stuporous or comatose, and in whom a traumatic or other intracranial mass has caused either a shift of intracranial structures or severe generalized brain swelling. Published guidelines suggest that monitoring should be undertaken in patients with severe traumatic brain injury if they are over 40 years of age, and have a Glasgow Coma Score below 9 (see Chap 35). The monitor is generally placed on the same side as a mass lesion. Whether recent studies, such as the one by Chesnut and colleagues comparing monitoring to clinical and imaging in directing therapy, negate these guidelines is also uncertain.

The emergency management of raised ICP is considered in greater detail in Chaps. 34 and 35 where the subject is discussed in relation to stroke and cerebral trauma. A comprehensive review can be found in the monograph on intensive care (Ropper) listed in the references.

Hydrocephalus

This is a condition of ventricular enlargement as a result of an obstruction to the normal flow of CSF. The sites of obstruction may be at the third ventricle, aqueduct of Sylvius, at the medullary foramina (Luschka and Magendie), or in the basal or convexity subarachnoid spaces. Because of the obstruction, CSF accumulates within the ventricles under increasing pressure, enlarging the ventricles, and expanding the hemispheres. As stated earlier, in the infant or young child, the head increases in size because the expanding cerebral hemispheres separate the sutures of the cranial bones.

Regarding terminology, the term *hydrocephalus* (literally, "water brain") is frequently but incorrectly applied to any enlargement of the ventricles, even if consequent to cerebral atrophy, i.e., *hydrocephalus ex vacuo*, or to ventricular enlargement because of failure of development of the brain, a state known as *colpocephaly*. Reference to these conditions as hydrocephalic is so common that it is unlikely to change; the use of "tension hydrocephalus," although not widely adopted, separates enlargement caused by pressure from passive enlargement of the ventricles.

In 1914, Dandy and Blackfan introduced the also somewhat inaccurate but now well-established terms *communicating* and *noncommunicating (obstructive) hydrocephalus*. The concept of communicating hydrocephalus was based on the observations that dye injected into a lateral ventricle would diffuse readily downward into the lumbar subarachnoid space and that air injected into the lumbar subarachnoid space would pass into the ventricular system; in other words, the ventricles were in communication with the spinal subarachnoid space. If the lumbar spinal fluid remained colorless after the injection of dye, the hydrocephalus was assumed to be obstructive, or noncommunicating. In actuality, the distinction between these two types is not fundamental, because all forms of true hydrocephalus are obstructive at some level, and the obstruction is virtually never complete.

Pathogenesis of Hydrocephalus

There are several sites of predilection of obstruction to the flow of CSF. One foramen of Monro may be blocked by a tumor or by horizontal displacement of central brain structures from a large cerebral mass. This obstruction may cause expansion of the lateral ventricle or a portion of it. Tumors within the third ventricle (e.g., colloid cyst) block the egress of CSF from both foramina of Monro, leading to dilatation of both lateral ventricles. The aqueduct of Sylvius, narrow to begin with, may be occluded by a number of developmental or acquired lesions (genetically determined atresia or forking, perinatally acquired gliosis, ependymitis, hemorrhage, tumor), and lead to dilatation of the third and both lateral ventricles. If the obstruction is in the fourth ventricle, the dilatation includes the aqueduct. Other sites of obstruction of the CSF in the ventricular pathways are at the foramina of Luschka and Magendie (e.g., congenital failure of opening of the foramina, Dandy-Walker syndrome). More common is a blockage to flow of CSF in the subarachnoid space around the brainstem caused by inflammatory or fibrosing meningitis. This form of obstruction results in enlargement of the entire ventricular system, including the fourth ventricle. A useful adage, attributed to Ayer, is that the ventricle closest to the obstruction enlarges the most; meaning, for example, that occlusion of the basal CSF pathways causes a disproportionate enlargement of the fourth ventricle, and a mass within the fourth ventricle leads to a greater dilatation of the third than of the lateral ventricles.

Another potential site of obstruction is in the subarachnoid spaces over the cerebral convexities. A matter of considerable practical as well as theoretical interest is whether a meningeal obstruction at the site of the arachnoidal villi, or a blockage of the venous sinuses into which the CSF is absorbed, can result in hydrocephalus. Russell, in her extensive neuropathologic material and review of the world's literature, could not find a well-documented example of either of these suggested etiologies, and the same is true of the pathologic material collected by our colleague R.D. Adams. Moreover, experiments in animals in which all the draining veins had been occluded, tension hydrocephalus with enlarging lateral ventricles was produced in only a few cases. Yet Gilles and Davidson have stated that hydrocephalus in children may be the result of a congenital absence, or deficient number of arachnoidal villi, and Rosman and Shands have reported an instance that they attributed to increased intracranial venous pressure. Our hesitation in accepting such examples stems from the difficulty that the pathologist has in judging the patency of the basilar subarachnoid space. This is much more reliably visualized by radiologic than by neuropathologic means. Theoretically, as mentioned earlier, if the obstruction is high, near (or in) the superior sagittal sinus, the CSF should accumulate under pressure outside as well as inside the brain, and the ventricles should not enlarge at all or only slightly, and only after a prolonged period.

The rarely encountered radiologic picture of enlarged subarachnoid spaces over and between the cerebral hemispheres, coupled with modest enlargement of the lateral ventricles has been referred to as *external hydrocephalus*. Although such a condition does exist, many of the cases so designated have proved to be examples of subdural hygromas or arachnoid cysts. The condition is now seen somewhat more regularly after surgical hemicraniectomy if the bone is not replaced.

Processes such as subarachnoid hemorrhage, or cerebral hemorrhage or brain abscess that rupture into the ventricles and rapidly expand the volume of CSF produce the most dramatic forms of *acute hydrocephalus*. The obstruction of the CSF pathways may also be found within the ventricular system or at the basal meninges. The corresponding clinical syndrome is described below.

An increase in the rate of formation or decrease in the rate of absorption would be expected to cause an accumulation of CSF and increased ICP. The only reported examples of overproduction of CSF are papillomas of the choroid plexus, but even in this circumstance, there is usually an associated ventricular obstruction, either of the third or fourth ventricle or of one lateral ventricle.

Characteristically in these cases, there is both a generalized dilatation of the ventricular system and basal cisterns (possibly because of increased CSF volume), and an asymmetrical enlargement of the lateral ventricles caused by obstruction of one foramen of Monro.

Syndromes of Hydrocephalus

This process gives rise to various syndromes depending on the age of the patient and the rapidity of evolution. One type occurs very early in life, before fusion of the cranial sutures and causes enlargement of the head. If the cranial sutures have fused, the head remains normal in size and the ventricular enlargement may remain asymptomatic or cause gait, urinary and cognitive difficulties. A special form of the latter is arrested or compensated hydrocephalus of late adult life that is one of the causes of *normal-pressure hydrocephalus* that is addressed in Chap. 7 and extensively below.

Congenital or Infantile Hydrocephalus The cranial bones fuse by the end of the third year; for the head to enlarge, the tension hydrocephalus must develop before this time. It may begin in utero, but usually happens in the first few months of life. Even up to 5 years of age (and very rarely beyond this time), a marked increase of ICP, particularly if it evolves rapidly, may separate the newly formed sutures (diastasis). Tension hydrocephalus, even of mild degree, also molds the shape of the skull in early life, and in radiographs, the inner table is unevenly thinned, an appearance referred to as "beaten silver", or as convolutional or digital markings. The frontal skull regions are unusually prominent (bossed) and the skull tends to be brachiocephalic, except in the Dandy-Walker syndrome where, because of bossing of the occiput from enlargement of the posterior fossa, the head is dolichocephalic. With marked enlargement of the skull, the face looks relatively small and pinched, and the skin over the cranial bones is tight and thin, revealing prominent distended veins.

The usual causes of this disorder are (1) intraventricular matrix hemorrhages in premature infants, (2) fetal and neonatal infections, (3) type II Chiari malformation, (4) aqueductal atresia and stenosis, and (5) the Dandy-Walker syndrome.

In congenital hydrocephalus, the head usually enlarges rapidly and soon surpasses the ninety-seventh percentile. The anterior and posterior fontanels are tense even when the patient is in the upright position. The infant is fretful, feeds poorly, and may vomit frequently. With continued enlargement of the brain, torpor sets in and the infant appears languid, uninterested in his surroundings, and unable to sustain activity. Later it is noticed that the upper eyelids are retracted, and the eyes tend to turn down; there is paralysis of upward gaze, and the sclerae above the irises are visible. This is the "setting-sun sign" that has been incorrectly attributed to downward pressure of the frontal lobes on the roofs of the orbits. The fact that it disappears on shunting the lateral and third ventricles indicates that it is caused by hydrocephalic pressure on the mesencephalic tegmentum. Gradually, if left untreated, the infant adopts a posture of flexed arms and flexed or extended legs. Signs of corticospinal tract damage are usually elicitable. Movements are feeble, and sometimes the arms are tremulous. There is no papilledema, but later the optic discs become pale and vision is reduced.

If the hydrocephalus becomes arrested, the infant or child is usually developmentally delayed in motor function but often surprisingly verbal. The head may be so large that the child cannot hold it up and must remain in bed. If the head is only moderately enlarged, the child may be able to sit but not stand, or stand but not walk. If ambulatory, the child is clumsy. Acute exacerbations of hydrocephalus or a febrile illness may cause vomiting, stupor, or coma.

The special features of congenital hydrocephalus associated with the Chiari malformation, aqueductal atresia and stenosis, and the Dandy-Walker syndrome are discussed in Chap. 38. Also mentioned here is a rare condition termed "bobble head" syndrome that is caused by a suprachiasmatic arachnoid cyst or by third ventricular enlargement, as discussed in Chap. 31. These lesions cause the child's head to move forward and backward or side-to-side constantly or intermittently at about 2 to 3 Hz. There is no direct connection to another rhythmic head movement, spasmus nutans (listed in some books as "mutans"), or to seesaw nystagmus described in Chap. 14, but the location of the causative lesions, in and adjacent to the third ventricle, is similar in all of them.

Occult Childhood Hydrocephalus Here, the ventricular enlargement becomes evident only after the cranial sutures have closed (Fig. 30-2). The causes of obstruction to the flow of CSF are diverse, and although some are clearly congenital, symptoms may be delayed as late

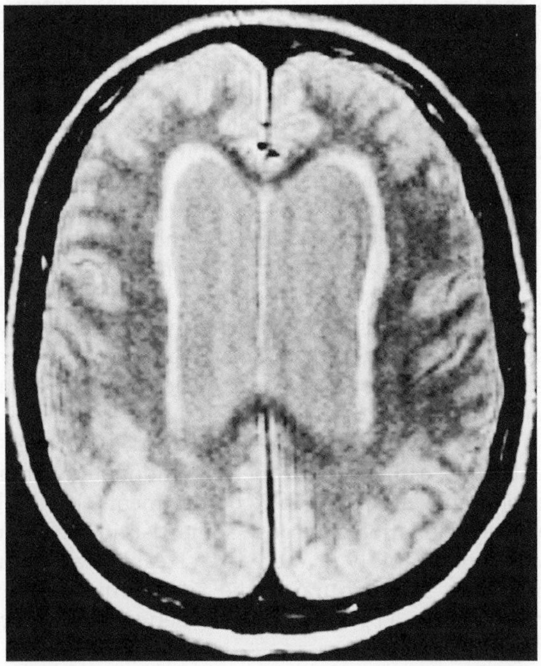

Figure 30-2. MRI of adult tension hydrocephalus from a congenital stenosis of the cerebral aqueduct. There is transependymal movement of water that appears as a T2 signal rimming the lateral ventricles. The third ventricle, but not the fourth, was enlarged.

as adolescence, or early adult life, or even later. In some instances, the condition gives rise to *normal-pressure hydrocephalus*, as discussed below and in Chap. 7. The clinical features of occult hydrocephalus and the course of the illness are quite variable. We have seen a few cases in adults in whom the gait disturbance from congenital aqueductal stenosis appeared abruptly enough to give the impression of a cerebellar or frontal stroke. For unexplained reasons, the symptoms of previously occult hydrocephalus may also appear abruptly after minor cranial trauma. A suck reflex and grasp reflexes of the hands and feet are variably present; plantar reflexes are sometimes extensor. Last, there may be urinary urgency leading to sphincteric incontinence, often without the patient's awareness.

Chapter 31 discusses occult hydrocephalus caused by intracranial tumor growth.

Acute Hydrocephalus Surprisingly, little has been written about this syndrome despite its frequency in clinical practice. It is seen most often following subarachnoid hemorrhage from a ruptured aneurysm, less often with bleeding from an arteriovenous malformation or from deep intracerebral hemorrhage that dissects into the ventricles; it may also occur as the result of obstruction of the CSF pathways in the fourth ventricle by a tumor or cerebellar–brainstem hemorrhage, or within the basal cisterns by neoplastic infiltration of the meninges, although this last process tends to evolve more subacutely. The patient complains of a headache of varying severity and often of visual obscuration, may vomit, and then becomes drowsy or stuporous over a period of minutes or hours. Bilateral Babinski signs are the rule, and in the advanced stages, which are associated with coma, there is increased tone in the lower limbs and extensor posturing. Early in the process, the pupils are normal in size and the eyes may rove horizontally; as the ventricles continue to enlarge, the pupils become miotic, the eyes then cease roving and assume an aligned position, or there may be bilateral abducens palsies and limitation of upward gaze. The speed with which hydrocephalus develops determines whether there is accompanying papilledema.

If this condition is left untreated, the pupils eventually dilate symmetrically, the eyes no longer respond to oculocephalic maneuvers, and the limbs become flaccid. Or, there is an unanticipated cardiac or respiratory arrest, even at an early stage of evolution of the hydrocephalus; this complication is seen particularly in children with masses, particularly at the foramen magnum, and may be presaged by brain compression at the level of the perimesencephalic cisterns, detectable by imaging studies.

Treatment is by drainage of CSF, usually effected by a ventricular catheter or, if there is undoubted communication between all the CSF compartments, by lumbar puncture. The latter may pose some risk if spinal fluid is withdrawn rapidly or there is a sizeable leak of fluid through the spinal dura at the site of the puncture, thereby creating a pressure gradient between the cerebral and spinal regions.

Neuropathologic Effects of Hydrocephalus

Ventricular expansion tends to be maximal in the frontal horns, explaining the hydrocephalic impairment of frontal lobe functions and of basal ganglionic–frontal motor and gait activity in most forms of hydrocephalus. The central white matter yields to pressure, while the cortical gray matter, thalami, basal ganglia, and brainstem structures remain relatively unaffected. There is an increase in the content of interstitial fluid in the tissue adjacent to the lateral ventricles (transependymal flow), readily detected by MRI (see Fig. 30-2). Myelinated fibers and axons are injured, but not to the extent that one might expect from the degree of compression; minor degrees of astrocytic gliosis and loss of oligodendrocytes in the affected tissue are present to a decreasing extent away from the ventricles and represent a chronic hydrocephalic atrophy of the brain. The ventricles are characteristically denuded of ependyma, and the choroid plexuses are flattened and fibrotic. The lumens of cerebral capillaries in biopsy preparations are said to be narrowed—a finding that is difficult to evaluate.

NORMAL-PRESSURE HYDROCEPHALUS

In meningeal and ependymal diseases, hydrocephalus may develop and reach a stable state. It is then said to be "compensated" in the sense that formation of CSF equilibrates with absorption. Once equilibrium is attained, the ICP gradually falls, though it still maintains a gradient from ventricle to basal cistern to cerebral subarachnoid space. A stage is reached where the CSF pressure reaches a high normal level of 150 to 200 mm H_2O, but the patient nonetheless eventually manifests the cerebral effects of the hydrocephalic state. The name given to this condition by Adams, Fisher, and Hakim was *normal-pressure hydrocephalus* (NPH).

A *triad of clinical findings* is characteristic of NPH: a slowly progressive gait disorder is usually the earliest feature, followed by impairment of mental function and later, sphincteric incontinence. The reader should be alerted to the fact that the fully developed triad is not usually present in the early stages of the process. Grasp reflexes in the feet and falling attacks may also occur, but there are no Babinski signs. Headaches are infrequently a complaint, and there is no papilledema.

The *gait disturbance* that accompanies NPH may be of several different types, as discussed in Chap. 7. These are difficult to classify and only vaguely simulate the patterns observed in Parkinson disease or cerebellar ataxia, but certain features predominate. Most often, there is unsteadiness and impairment of balance and shortening of the step length, with the greatest difficulty being encountered on stairs and curbs (Fisher). Weakness and tiredness of the legs are frequent complaints, although examination discloses no paresis or ataxia. An impression of Parkinson disease may be conveyed, with short steps and slightly stooped, forward-leaning posture, but there is typically no shuffling early on, nor is there festination, rigidity, slowness of alternating movement, or tremor. Some patients present with unexplained falls, often helplessly backward, but on casual inspection the gait may betray little abnormality except a minimal reduction in step length and overall slowness. When the condition remains untreated, the steps become shorter, with more frequent shuffling and falls; eventually standing and sitting and even turning over in bed become impossible. Fisher referred to this advanced state as "hydrocephalic astasia–abasia."

The mental changes in the cases we have encountered have been, broadly speaking, "frontal" in character and embodied mainly apathy, dullness in thinking and actions, and slight inattention. Memory trouble is eventually a component of the overall problem and has been predominant in some cases, for which reason the diagnosis of Alzheimer disease is sometimes considered before the discovery of hydrocephalus, but as a rule, the gait derangement of NPH is fairly obvious by the time memory function is substantially impaired. There is usually a degree of affective indifference, but the patient reports little in the way of emotionality. Patients who display gait difficulty with prominent and progressive verbal, graphical, and calculation difficulties are more likely to have a degenerative or cerebrovascular disease. In those cases, the difficulty with walking and stability is ostensibly a result of frontal lobe disease, either degenerative or infarctive, as discussed in Chap. 7. Unfortunately, beyond the above-noted defects that are elicitable by routine testing, we have not found neuropsychologic tests of great value in the diagnosis of NPH.

Urinary symptoms appear relatively later in the illness. Initially, they consist of urinary urgency and frequency. Later, the urgency is associated with incontinence, and ultimately there is "frontal lobe incontinence," in which the patient is indifferent to his lapses of continence, and bowel control becomes similarly disordered.

The cause of the syndrome of NPH in most cases cannot be established and on weak grounds, an asymptomatic fibrosing meningitis is presumed to have been present. An uncertain proportion of cases can be traced to congenital aqueductal stenosis that has allowed normal brain function into adulthood and, for unknown reasons, decompensates; a few of our patients have become symptomatic after mild head trauma. This is probably the most common imputed cause of the syndrome but again, on uncertain grounds. An identical syndrome may follow subarachnoid hemorrhage from ruptured aneurysm, resolved acute meningitis or a chronic meningitis (tubercular, fungal, syphilitic, or other), Paget disease of the base of the skull, mucopolysaccharidosis of the meninges, and achondroplasia.

That the mechanical effect of ventricular enlargement on the adjacent brain is responsible for the syndrome is supported by Fisher's observations that a reduction in ventricular size caused by extrinsic compression from subdural collections has been associated with clinical improvement. One presumes that the main clinical features are due to dysfunction of the frontal lobes and their connections with the striatum, from mechanical pressure or distortion but this is conjecture.

Diagnosis of NPH

Verification of the diagnosis of NPH, and the selection of patients for ventriculoatrial or ventriculoperitoneal shunt has presented difficulties. The CT scan, as shown in Fig. 30-3, displays enlarged ventricles without convolutional atrophy. This disproportionate enlargement of the ventricular system in comparison to the degree

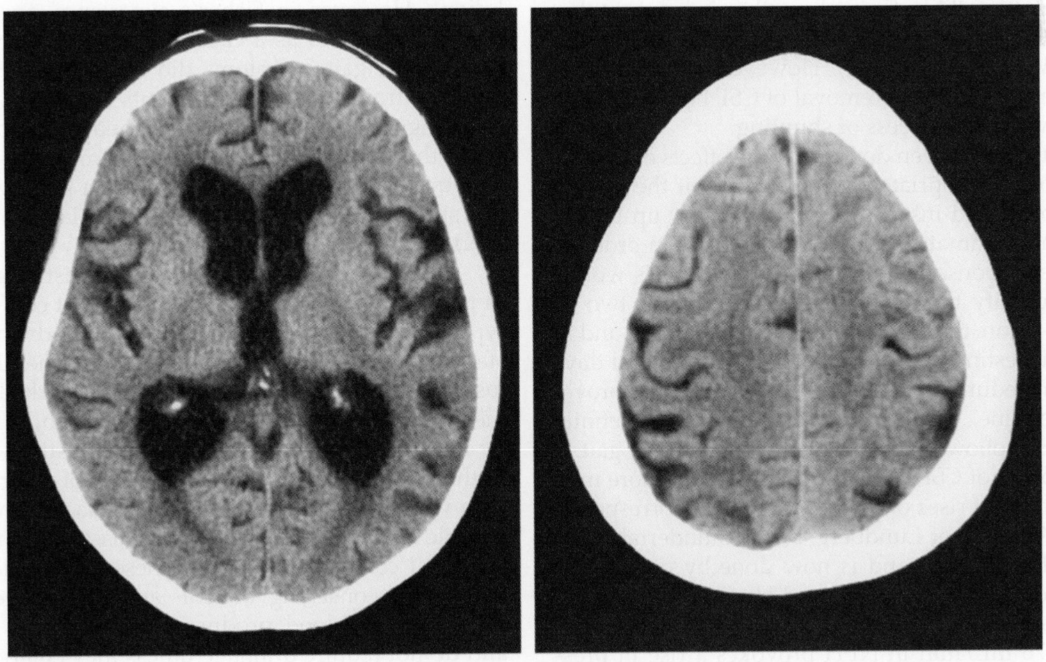

Figure 30-3. CT of a patient with normal-pressure hydrocephalus. There is enlargement of all the ventricles, particularly of the frontal horns of the lateral ventricles (*left*), which is roughly disproportionate to the cortical atrophy (*right*). The frontal horn span is over 40 mm. Various formulas have been devised to quantitate the imaging features, but they are difficult to apply.

of cortical atrophy is judged by the CT and MRI appearance, but there is no broadly agreed upon method for its determination. Various unwieldy formulas have been designed to assess this ratio. As a group, patients who have a sustained response to drainage of CSF by shunting, as described below, have had the first two elements of the clinical triad (fewer than half of our successfully treated patients have reached the point of incontinence) and their lateral ventricular span at the level of the anterior horns has been in excess of approximately 40 mm (a true dimension calculated from CT or MRI scans). MRI may show some degree of transependymal egress of water surrounding the ventricles, but this is not usually the case, and this sign is sometimes difficult to differentiate from the periventricular white matter change that is ubiquitous in the elderly. There may be an indication of inadequate pulsatile flow of CSF through the aqueduct as appreciated on T-2-weighted MRI.

A lumbar puncture is often performed for diagnostic purposes and the pressure measured carefully but here too, there is no uniformly agreed upon approach. In most cases of NPH, the CSF pressure is above 150 mm H_2O with the patient fully relaxed, but the disorder has occurred, at least as judged by improvement with shunting, with lower pressures, in a few instances as low as 120 mm H_2O. Drainage of large amounts of CSF (20 to 30 mL or more) by lumbar puncture often results in clinical improvement in stance and gait for a few days, usually with a delay of hours or a day so the patient and family must be depended upon to report these changes and these reports are prone to excessive optimism. Objective improvement in gait after spinal drainage, measured by reduced time to walk a predetermined distance, is one way to select patients for shunt operations when the clinical picture is not entirely clear, but the even this test is not infallible. Several small series suggest that a negative test does not preclude benefit from shunting (see, e.g., Walchenbach et al). However, in these same series, improvement after removal of CSF has had a high predictive value for success of shunting.

When there has been doubt as to the effects of lumbar puncture, one appropriate course is to admit the patient to the hospital, and insert a lumbar drain for up to 3 d, removing approximately 50 mL of CSF daily in order to observe the response in gait and mentation. It is worthwhile to quantify the speed and facility of gait two or three times before the lumbar puncture or drainage and to perform this testing at periodic intervals for several days after the procedure in order to be certain that improvement is genuine. Even more persuasive is a definite improvement followed days later by worsening of gait.

Monitoring of CSF pressure over a day or more may show intermittent rises of pressure, possibly corresponding to the A waves of Lundberg, but this undertaking is not generally practical and is now done by only a few centers. According to Katzman and Hussey, the infusion of normal saline into the lumbar subarachnoid space at a rate of 0.76 mL/min in NPH provokes a rise in pressure to greater than 300 mm H_2O that is not observed in normal individuals. Theoretically, this test or any of its derivatives, such as the one proposed by Børgesen and Gjerris, should reflect the adequacy of CSF absorption, but they too, have yielded unpredictable results. Radionuclide cisternography had been used in the past to demonstrate persistence of CSF labeling in the ventricles, but it is no longer considered a compelling test for NPH.

Treatment of NPH in Adults

The development of ventricular shunt tubing with one-way valves opened the way to successful treatment of hydrocephalus. CSF is diverted directly into the peritoneal cavity (ventriculoperitoneal shunt), of less often, a ventriculatrial or ventriculopleural shunt is used. The valve can be selected for a desired fixed opening pressure, or a variable valve can be inserted and adjustments can be made by an external magnetic device. Gratifying success can be obtained, often a complete or nearly complete restoration of mental function and gait after several weeks or months, by the placement of a shunt.

The most consistent improvement has been attained in the minority of patients in whom a cause could be established (subarachnoid hemorrhage, chronic meningitis, or tumor of the third ventricle). As already noted, other predictors of success are considerable enlargement of the ventricles in comparison to the degree of cortical atrophy, CSF pressures above 150 mm H_2O, and improvement after spinal puncture, but none of these is entirely dependable.

Deviations from the characteristic syndrome such as the occurrence of dementia without gait disorder or the presence of apraxias, aphasias, and other focal cerebral signs are associated with poorer outcomes after shunting. Fisher, on analyzing successfully shunted cases, noted that almost without exception gait disturbance was an early and prominent symptom. Uncertainties of diagnosis increase with advancing age owing to the frequent association of degenerative dementia and vascular lesions. However, in Fisher's experience, age alone did not exclude NPH as a cause of gait disorder, and long duration of gait symptoms did not preclude a salutary outcome from shunting. In patients who are averse to the shunting procedure or who have medical conditions that make the surgery inadvisable, it is sometimes possible to produce a reasonable improvement in gait by repeating the spinal puncture and drainage of large amounts of fluid every few weeks or months.

The potential failure of shunting must be anticipated in patients whose clinical features do not conform to the typical syndrome or whose disease has advanced to the stage of long-standing incontinence or dementia. In some instances, a lack of improvement, or marked improvement followed by subacute deterioration, is explained by inadequate decompression, which justifies a revision of the shunt or downward adjustment of a variable pressure valve. Overdrainage causes headaches that may be chronic or orthostatic and may be associated with small subdural collections of fluid. These fluid collections, or hygromas, consisting of CSF and proteinaceous fluid derived from blood products, are generally innocuous and do not require drainage unless they enlarge or cause focal neurologic symptoms or, rarely, seizures.

Although shunting is relatively simple as a surgical procedure, it is associated with complications, the main ones being a postoperative subdural hematoma (the bridging dural veins stretch and rupture but the procedure has been performed safely in patients who must take anticoagulants after shunting); infection of the valve and catheter, sometimes with ventriculitis and occasionally bacteremia; occlusion of the tip of the catheter in the ventricle; and, particularly in infants and children, the "slit ventricle syndrome" (see below). Orthostatic headaches can be overcome by raising the opening pressure of the shunt valve. Misplacement of the catheter may rarely transect tracts in the deep hemispheral white matter and cause serious neurologic deficits, mainly hemiplegia. It is our impression that this occurs more often when the catheter is inserted from the posterior rather than through the frontal or parietal regions. The incidence of catheter blockage is reduced by placing it in the anterior horn of the ventricle (usually the right side is used), where there is no choroid plexus. Meticulous aseptic technique, and the preoperative and postoperative administration of antibiotics have apparently reduced the incidence of shunt infections. Most shunts in adults are brought to termination in the peritoneum (ventriculoperitoneal shunt). Perforation of the stomach or bowel is possible. Rare complications of ventriculoatrial shunting are pulmonary hypertension and pulmonary embolism and nephritis, which are caused by low-level infection of the shunt tube with *Staphylococcus*.

Puncture of the floor of the third ventricle by endoscopic techniques ("third ventriculostomy") has been explored as an alternative to shunting, especially in children with congenital aqueductal stenosis. Cinalli and colleagues have suggested, and we concur based on experience with a limited number of our own adult patients, that third ventriculostomy is sometimes an effective treatment of shunt failure.

Once the CSF is shunted, the ventricles diminish in size within a week or two, even when the hydrocephalus has been present for a year or more. This indicates that hydrocephalic compression of the cerebrum is at least partly reversible. Indeed, in Black's series, the ventricles failed to return to normal in only 1 of his 11 shunted patients, and in that patient, there was no clinical improvement. Clinical improvement occurs within a few weeks, the gait disturbance being slower to reverse than the mental disorder. Symptoms of cerebral atrophy because of Alzheimer disease and related conditions are not altered by shunting, but this approach to the treatment of degenerative dementia has been periodically, and unadvisedly, resurrected, as discussed by Silverberg and associates.

Treatment of Infantile and Childhood Hydrocephalus

Here one encounters more difficulties than in the treatment of the adult disorder. The ventricular catheter may wander or become obstructed and require revision. Peritoneal pseudocysts may form (most shunts in children are ventriculoperitoneal). Another unexpected complication has been collapse of the ventricles, the so-called "slit ventricle" syndrome (the appearance of the ventricles on imaging studies is slit-like). This occurs more frequently in young children, although we have observed it in adults. These patients develop an intracranial low-pressure syndrome with severe generalized headaches, often with nausea and vomiting, whenever they sit up or stand. Some children become ataxic, irritable, or obtunded, or may vomit repeatedly. The CSF pressure is extremely low and the volume of CSF much reduced. In babies, the cranium may fail to grow even though the brain is of normal size. In most shunted patients with slit ventricle syndrome, the ICP in the upright position is diminished to 30 mm H_2O. To correct the condition, one would imagine that replacing the shunt valve with another that opens under a higher pressure or raising the opening pressure of an adjustable valve would suffice. Indeed, this may be successful. But once the condition is established, the most effective measure has been the placement of an antisiphon device, which prevents valve flow when the patient stands. (See further on for a discussion of intracranial hypotension in adults.)

Whether to shunt all hydrocephalic infants soon after birth is a controversial issue. In several series of cases that have been treated in this way, the number surviving with normal mental function has been small (see review of Leech and Brumback). The report of Dennis and associates is representative. They examined 78 shunted hydrocephalic children and found that 56 (72 percent) had full-scale IQs between 70 and 100; in 22 patients, the IQ was between 100 and 115; in 3 patients, it was below 70, and in 3 others, it was above 115. Mental functions improved unevenly and performance scores lagged behind verbal ones at all levels.

The use of the carbonic anhydrase inhibitor acetazolamide or other diuretics to inhibit CSF formation in children with hydrocephalus has not been successful in the hands of our colleagues, but several authors believe that by giving 250 to 500 mg of acetazolamide orally daily, shunting can be avoided in both adult normal-pressure, and infantile hydrocephalus (Aimard et al; Shinnar et al).

Parkinsonism and Midbrain Syndromes With Hydrocephalus and Shunting

Usually in the context of adult hydrocephalus due to aqueductal stenosis, a rare but distinct parkinsonian syndrome occurs that may be responsive to levodopa (Zeidler). It is particularly prone to occur if there is shunted hydrocephalus and has also been a craniotomy without replacement of the bone. The syndrome usually indicates failure of the shunt. MRI sometimes shows periaqueductal and dorsal midbrain edema, including in the region of the substantia nigra (Fig. 30-4); the mechanism of these changes is not clear. Positron emission tomography performed with ^{18F}DOPA has given evidence of reduced uptake in the caudate and putamen, suggesting a functional failure of the nigrostriatal dopamine system (Racette). Shunt malfunction in children also may be heralded by upward gaze palsy ("setting-sun sign") or even a dorsal midbrain (Parinaud) syndrome, including abnormal papillary reaction, upper lid retraction, paralysis of convergence, skew deviation, and convergence–retraction nystagmus. Shunting or shunt revision usually leads to reversal of both syndromes, but there may be a delay of days or weeks, and it is often difficult to find the ideal pressure setting for the valve.

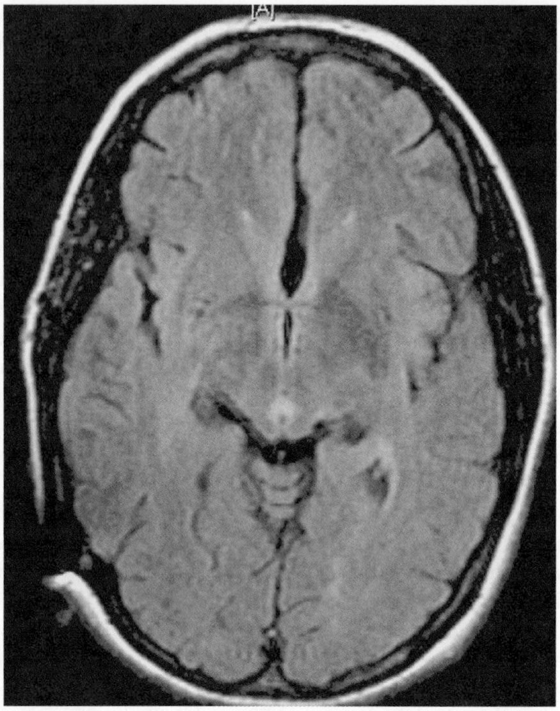

Figure 30-4. Fluid-attenuated inversion recovery (FLAIR) MRI sequence in a woman with hydrocephalus, shunt failure, and L-dopa-responsive parkinsonism. There is signal change in the dorsal midbrain and periaqueductal region.

INCREASED INTRACRANIAL PRESSURE DUE TO CEREBRAL VENOUS OBSTRUCTION

Occlusion of the major dural venous sinuses (superior longitudinal and lateral) results in increased ICP. This is not surprising in view of the direct effect of venous obstruction on CSF pressure. One such form, caused by lateral sinus thrombosis, was referred to by Symonds as "otitic hydrocephalus," a name that he later conceded was inaccurate insofar as the ventricles are not enlarged in this circumstance. Venous congestion that complicates heart failure and superior mediastinal obstruction also raise the CSF pressure, again without enlargement of the ventricles. This may happen as well with large, high-flow arteriovenous malformations of the brain. The effects of cerebral venous occlusion are considered further in the discussion of pseudotumor cerebri (below) and in Chap. 34 in the context of thrombosis of the cerebral venous sinuses. The role of compression of the large venous channels in cases of raised ICP from a mass has not been fully explored, but it may explain some of the intractable aspects of these cases.

PSEUDOTUMOR CEREBRI

This term was coined by Nonne in 1914 and has remained a useful means of designating a syndrome of headache, papilledema (unilateral or bilateral), minimal or absent focal neurologic signs, and normal CSF composition, all occurring in the absence of enlarged ventricles, or an intracranial mass on CT scanning, or MRI. Being a syndrome and not a disease, pseudotumor cerebri has a number of causes or pathogenetic associations. However, the most common form of the syndrome has no firmly established cause, i.e., it is idiopathic, and is generally referred to as *idiopathic intracranial hypertension*.

This syndrome was first described in 1897 by Quincke, who called it "serous meningitis." It is particularly frequent in overweight adolescent girls and young women, attaining an incidence of 19 to 21 per 100,000 in this group, as compared with 1 to 2 per 100,000 in the general population (Radhakrishnan et al). The features of increased ICP develop over a period of weeks or months. Relatively unremitting but fluctuating headache, described as dull or a feeling of pressure, is the cardinal symptom; it can be mainly occipital, generalized, or somewhat asymmetrical. Other, less-frequent complaints are blurred vision, a vague dizziness, minimal horizontal diplopia, transient visual obscurations that often coincide with the peak intensity of the headache, shoulder and neck pains, or a trifling numbness of the face on one side. Rarely, the presenting feature may be a nasal CSF leak, as pointed out by Clarke and colleagues. Self-audible bruits have been reported by some patients; this has been attributed to turbulence created by differences in pressure between the cranial and jugular veins.

The patient is then discovered to have flagrant papilledema (see Figs. 13-9 and 13-10), immediately raising the specter of a brain tumor. Rarely, papilledema is only minimally developed or absent or, conversely, papilledema alone, without headache, is the only manifestation of the disease. The risk of visual loss, and the severity of headache make the formerly used term *benign intracranial hypertension* less appropriate.

The CSF pressure is found to be elevated by lumbar puncture, usually in the range of 250 to 450 mm H_2O, but it is not clear whether the brain itself is swollen or, as is more likely, the increased pressure is the result of a change in the pressure within the CSF and venous compartments. When the CSF pressure is monitored for many hours, there are fluctuations taking the form of irregularly occurring plateau waves of increased pressure lasting 20 to 30 min, and then falling abruptly near to normal (Johnston and Paterson).

Aside from papilledema, there is remarkably little to be found on neurologic examination, perhaps slight unilateral or bilateral abducens palsy, fine nystagmus on far lateral gaze, or minor sensory change on the face or trunk. Visual field testing usually shows minor peripheral constriction with enlargement of the blind spots. As the process continues, more severe constriction of the fields, with greater nasal or inferior nasal loss, is found, often inevident to the patient. These issues are elaborated below. Enlargement of the blind spot is the result of displacement of the retina from the edges of the swollen disc. Central acuity is spared initially and the patient, in advanced cases, is left with an island of preserved central vision. These patients are at particular risk of visual loss. A study of 66 men with pseudotumor (9 percent of a larger cohort) by Bruce and colleagues suggested that there is a higher risk of vision loss than in women. Profound disc edema, significant early visual loss and perhaps being of African-American descent are other risks for visual loss.

Exceptionally, particularly in children, an otherwise typical Bell's palsy may occur (Chutorian et al). Mentation and alertness are preserved, and the patient seems surprisingly well aside from the headaches, which infrequently become severe enough to limit daily activity.

Examinations by CT and MRI show the ventricles to be normal in size or small. The sella may be enlarged and filled with CSF ("empty sella," Chap. 31), the posterior globes may be compressed and the perioptic subarachnoid spaces, expanded. Variable attenuation of the transverse sinuses has also been pointed out (see Friedman and colleagues). These are helpful but not indispensible features of the syndrome. There is no MRI evidence of change in the density of the brain, but edema may be seen in the optic nerves.

As remarked above, most affected patients are overweight young women of short stature, often with menstrual irregularities, but the condition also occurs in children or adolescents, in whom there is no clear sex predominance, and in men (Digre and Corbett). We have had experience with several familial instances, e.g., affecting mother and daughter. In obese women without the pseudotumor syndrome, CSF pressure usually does not differ from that of normal individuals (Corbett and Mehta).

Several endocrine and menstrual abnormalities (particularly amenorrhea), as well as the use of oral contraceptives, have been postulated as causative factors, but none has been substantiated. Cases have been reported during pregnancy, both those who have symptoms for the first time during pregnancy and a larger group with ongoing pseudotumor who become pregnant. Despite the theoretical appeal of relating the endocrine and other changes of pregnancy to the increased ICP, no suitable connection has been found, and there is no evidence that premature delivery or termination of the pregnancy ameliorates the pseudotumor. Nonetheless, our obstetric colleagues have often recommended delivery when safe for the fetus if the mother's vision is threatened. Most of the standard medical treatments detailed below have been used with some benefit during pregnancy, as in the series reported by Huna-Baron and Kupersmith.

Pathophysiology

The mechanism of increased CSF pressure in the idiopathic form of the disorder has remained elusive, but some recent experience suggests that, in at least some cases, there is a functional obstruction to outflow in the venous sinuses. Karahalios and colleagues and others have found the cerebral venous pressure to be consistently elevated in pseudotumor cerebri; in half of their patients, there was a venous outflow obstruction demonstrated by venography, often with a pressure gradient across the site. These authors have proposed that venous hypertension increases the resistance to CSF absorption and is the proximate mechanism underlying pseudotumor. Similarly, Farb and colleagues, using sophisticated MRI venography, found venous stenosis in 27 of 29 patients with pseudotumor (and in 4 of 59 control subjects). In both studies and in others like them, the nature of the obstruction was not clear, but the fact that in some series, it was bilateral and focal suggests that the stenosis was not simply the passive result of raised ICP. This issue is not yet resolved, as noted below.

A related finding in some cases, pointed out to us some time ago by Fishman, is one of partial obstruction of the lateral sinuses by enlarged pacchionian granulations (seen during the venous phase of conventional angiography). It is here that the evidence has been most provocative. Intervention by stenting of a venous sinus at the sites of apparent obstruction has resulted in clinical improvement, and a reduction in CSF pressure. For example, 5 of 12 patients treated by Higgins and colleagues became asymptomatic, but this was a population selected by the demonstration of a focal pressure gradient in the lateral sinus during venography. Karahalios and colleagues had similar success in several patients. What is not clear is how prevalent these partial venous obstructions are and what precisely is their nature (if not simply enlarged granulations). In some series, the abnormality has been found in 10 to 25 percent of patients who lack any features of pseudotumor (Leach et al). We have seen an obese patient of short stature who presented with typical pseudotumor cerebri, but who was found to have, in addition, anticardiolipin antibodies that resulted in thrombosis of the right transverse sinus; lysis of the clot led to resolution of the pseudotumor syndrome.

In an attempt to settle the role of the venous stenosis, King and colleagues measured intracranial venous pressure while withdrawing spinal fluid from the cervical subarachnoid space in patients with idiopathic pseudotumor cerebri. Their observation that the venous pressure drops immediately upon the reduction in CSF pressure supports the notion that the increased venous pressure is secondary (furthermore, they describe patients with pseudotumor and normal venous pressures in the sagittal and transverse sinuses). The unsatisfactory nature of all the currently offered theories of causation of pseudotumor cerebri are reviewed by Walker, but at the moment our reading of the literature suggests that venous stenosis from granulations or from some as yet undefined functional change, does account for a proportion of what had previously been considered to be idiopathic cases. How the venous changes relate to obesity and sex is also unclear. Perhaps some individuals have a congenital configuration of the venous sinuses that is exaggerated with obesity and elevated systemic venous pressures.

Some additional comments about the physiologic changes in CSF flow and pressure in relation to alternative mechanisms of pseudotumor may be informative. Using the method of constant infusion manometrics, Mann and coworkers demonstrated an increased resistance to CSF outflow, in their view, caused by an impaired absorptive function of the arachnoid villi. Other authors have attributed intracranial venous hypertension to raised intraabdominal and cardiac filling pressures, the mechanical result of obesity (Sugerman et al, 1995). On inconclusive evidence, benign intracranial hypertension was in the past attributed to an increase in brain volume secondary to an excess of extracellular fluid or blood volume within the cranium (Sahs and Joynt, Raichle et al). An interesting related finding has been an elevated level of vasopressin in the CSF but not in the blood (Seckl and Lightman). In the goat, this peptide causes a rise in ICP and a reduction in CSF absorption, raising the possibility that the pseudotumor state is caused by an aberration of the transit of water in the cerebrum. Finally, Jacobson and colleagues have made the observation that serum vitamin A levels (in the form of retinol) are 50 percent higher than expected, in patients with pseudotumor—a difference that is not explained by obesity. Because the levels were considerably lower than in cases of hypervitaminosis A with symptomatic forms pseudotumor (see below), the meaning of these findings is uncertain.

Symptomatic Causes of Pseudotumor Cerebri (See Table 30-1)

The main considerations in cases of generalized elevation of ICP and papilledema in the absence of an intracranial mass are, foremost, covert occlusion of the dural venous sinuses and then, a list of less-common conditions, including gliomatosis cerebri, occult arteriovenous malformation, and carcinomatous, infectious, or granulomatous meningitis. Although occlusion of the dural venous sinuses and their large draining veins is sometimes equated with pseudotumor, these cases are not, of course, idiopathic. When papilledema occurs in the context of a persistent headache, particularly if the cranial pain is centered near the vertex or medial parietal areas or if there are seizures, venous occlusion is likely. Venous sinus thrombosis can be detected in most instances by careful attention to the appearance of the superior sagittal and transverse sinuses on the T1-weighted MRI or on the contrast-enhanced CT scan, as discussed in Chap. 34 under "Thrombosis of Cerebral Veins and Venous Sinuses." Isolated cortical vein thrombosis on the cerebral convexity does not cause pseudotumor (but does induce seizures).

A large cerebral arteriovenous malformation (AVM), by causing an increase both of venous pressure and cerebral blood volume, can give rise to a pseudotumor syndrome. In a few of our cases, these changes in the physiology of the cerebral circulation were made evident by the appearance of early venous flow on the angiogram or by thrombosis of the superior sagittal sinus.

Several systemic diseases that are associated with raised CSF protein concentration have given rise to a pseudotumor syndrome, including the Guillain-Barré syndrome, systemic lupus, and spinal tumors, particularly oligodendroglioma. Elevated spinal fluid pressure has been attributed to a blockage of CSF absorption by the proteinaceous fluid in Guillain-Barré syndrome, but this mechanism has never been validated and fails to explain those few instances in which pseudotumor syndromes has been associated with a near-normal protein content of the CSF. This explanation is even less compelling if one recalls that the protein concentration of the fluid in the cerebral spaces is considerably lower than in the spinal ones. Also, as we have pointed out, when calculated correctly, neither the resistance to CSF absorption nor the colloid osmotic effect attributable to an increased protein content in the spinal fluid is adequate to explain the pressure elevation (Ropper and Marmarou). The mechanism of this type of pseudotumor syndrome is presently unknown.

In addition to mechanical factors, a number of toxic and metabolic disturbances may give rise to a pseudotumor syndrome. In children, as chronic corticosteroid therapy is withdrawn, there may be a period of headache, papilledema, and elevated ICP with little or no enlargement of the lateral ventricles. Lead toxicity in children may be marked by brain swelling and papilledema. Excessive doses of tetracycline (particularly outdated medication) and vitamin A (particularly in the form of isotretinoin, an oral vitamin A derivative used in the treatment of severe acne) also have been shown to cause intracranial hypertension in children and adolescents. Ingestion of large quantities of bear liver by hunters is another curious source of intoxication with vitamin A underlying pseudotumor. Isolated instances of hypo- or hyperadrenalism, myxedema, and hypoparathyroidism have been associated with increased CSF pressure and papilledema, and occasionally the administration of estrogens, phenothiazines, lithium, the antiarrhythmic drug amiodarone, and quinolone antibiotics has the same effect, for reasons not known.

Table 30-1

CAUSES AND ASSOCIATIONS OF PSEUDOTUMOR CEREBRI

I. Idiopathic intracranial hypertension
II. Cerebral venous hypertension (diagnosis by imaging of cerebral vasculature)
   A. Occlusion of superior sagittal or transverse venous sinus:
      1. Hypercoagulable states (cancer, birth control pills, dehydration, antiphospholipid antibody)
      2. Traumatic
      3. Postsurgical
      4. Infectious (mainly of transverse venous sinus due to mastoiditis)
   B. Increased blood volume due to high-flow arteriovenous malformation, dural fistulas, and other vascular anomalies
III. Meningeal diseases (diagnosis by examination of CSF)
   A. Carcinomatous and lymphomatous meningitis
   B. Chronic infectious and granulomatous meningitis (fungal, tuberculous, spirochetal, sarcoidosis)
IV. Gliomatosis cerebri
V. Toxic
   A. Hypervitaminosis A (especially isotretinoin, used for the treatment of acne)
   B. Lead intoxication
   C. Tetracycline, minocylcine, doxycycline
   D. Infrequent idiosyncratic effect of various drugs (amiodarone, quinolone and sulfa antibiotics, estrogen, phenothiazines, lithium)
VI. Metabolic disturbances
   A. Administration or withdrawal of corticosteroids
   B. Hyper- and hypoadrenalism
   C. Myxedema
   D. Hypoparathyroidism
VII. Greatly elevated protein concentration in the CSF
   A. Guillain-Barré syndrome
   B. Spinal oligodendroglioma
   C. Systemic lupus erythematosus

The first step in differential diagnosis is to exclude an underlying tumor or the nontumorous causes of raised ICP, mainly dural venous occlusion, and meningeal inflammation. This can be accomplished by CT and MRI, although it should be borne in mind that certain chronic meningeal reactions (e.g., those caused by sarcoidosis or to tuberculous or carcinomatous meningitis), which give rise to headache and papilledema, may sometimes elude detection by these imaging procedures. In these cases, however, lumbar puncture will disclose the diagnosis. It should be emphasized that *the diagnosis of idiopathic pseudotumor cerebri should not be accepted when the CSF content is abnormal.*

Visual Loss in Pseudotumor

Careful evaluations of the visual fields and of acuity is required soon after the diagnosis of idiopathic pseudotumor is established. Repeated examination of visual function, preferably in collaboration with an ophthalmologist, is essential in detecting early and potentially reversible visual loss. At the same time, it must be acknowledged that measurements of visual acuity (and of confrontation fields) are relatively insensitive means of detecting early visual loss and that abnormalities in these tests indicate that damage to the optic nerve head has already occurred. Quantitative perimetry, using the kinetic Goldmann technique, has been more informative than other methods. The neurologist probably advised to refer the patient for perimetry as an adjunctive test. Fundus photographs are also a reasonable means of assessing the course of papilledema. A reduction in previously normal acuity to less than 20/20 corrected, enlargement of the blind spot, or the appearance of sector field defects, usually inferonasal, are indications for prompt treatment of raised ICP.

If intracranial hypertension and papilledema are left untreated or fail to respond to the measures outlined below, there is danger of permanent visual loss from compressive damage to the optic nerve fibers and compression of the central retinal veins. Corbett and associates, who described a group of 57 patients followed for 5 to 41 years, found severe visual impairment in 14, and Wall and George, using refined perimetric methods, reported an even higher incidence of visual loss. Moreover, children with pseudotumor share the same visual risks as adults (Lessell and Rosman). Sometimes, vision is lost abruptly, either without warning or following one or more episodes of monocular or binocular visual obscurations.

Treatment

Most patients with idiopathic intracranial hypertension will be found initially to have no, or minor visual changes aside from the papilledema; the headache and lumbar puncture pressure then guide treatment. Besides symptomatic relief of headaches, the progression of visual loss is the main concern. At least one-fourth of patients have recovered within 6 months after treatment by repeated lumbar punctures and drainage of sufficient CSF to maintain the pressure at normal or near-normal levels (less than 200 mm H_2O). The lumbar punctures have been performed daily or on alternate days at first, and then at longer intervals, according to the level of pressure. While cumbersome and sometimes impractical, evidently, this is sometimes sufficient to restore the balance between CSF formation and absorption for at least several months. At the same time, weight loss has been encouraged and the best results have been reported when weight reduction was successful (see further on regarding weight loss).

Acetazolamide and Osmotic Agents This approach has been considered the first step in treatment for patients who are not losing visual acuity rapidly. Large doses of acetazolamide in the range of 1 to 5 g/d, are required and the expected side effects of paresthesias and nauseas may not be tolerated. Sustained use of the drug has a risk of kidney stones. Oral hyperosmotic agents—such as glycerol (15 to 60 mg four to six times daily), or furosemide 20 to 80 mg bid—to reduce CSF formation all have their advocates, but they generally have only a short-term impact on vision and headaches.

Weight Reduction This is always advised if the patient is markedly overweight but is difficult to accomplish. In two pathologically obese patients, we have resorted to bariatric surgical approaches, which had a beneficial effect on the pseudotumor but left the patient for a time with the gastrointestinal disturbances that commonly complicate these procedures. Sugerman and associates (1999) studied 24 obese women wit pseudotumor who had operations and found the results to be satisfactory over several years. Two of our patients developed a sensory polyneuropathy after surgery. The use of bariatric procedures is currently undergoing reevaluation for obesity in general, but in the circumstances of pseudotumor with visual loss, it is a reasonable alternative. The effect of weight loss in less overweight individuals is uncertain.

Lumbar–Peritoneal Shunting In patients whose headaches are unresponsive to the usual therapeutic measures—mainly acetazolamide and weight reduction—a treatment method that may have considerable temporary success is a lumbar–peritoneal shunt. Only a few of our patients have undergone this surgical procedure. It has been relatively safe and effective, but because of a tendency for the shunt to become obstructed or to be dislodged in obese patients, sometimes causing back or sciatic pain, the procedure has less appeal than in the past. Burgett et al, who treated 30 patients in this manner, reported success in reducing headache in almost all and in improving vision in 70 percent. Despite its shortcomings, this procedure may be preferable to the optic nerve fenestration described below. We have not had to resort to cranial subtemporal decompression, a procedure that was formerly used when vision was threatened.

Corticosteroids Most authorities eschew the use of corticosteroids and had objected strenuously to their inclusion as a treatment for pseudotumor in previous editions of this book. Nonetheless, with the administration of prednisone (40 to 60 mg/d) we have occasionally observed a gradual recession of papilledema and a lowering of CSF pressure, but such responses were not consistent or sustained and it has been difficult to decide whether this represented the effect of treatment or the natural course of the disease. Greer, who has reported on 110 patients, 11 of whom were treated with these agents, decided that they were of no value. Moreover, in patients whose papilledema seems to recede under the influence of corticosteroids, there is always a danger that it will recur when the drug is tapered. Considering the potential for undesirable side effects of corticosteroids, we have used them very sparingly and only for brief periods while preparing the patient for more definitive treatment.

Fenestration of the Optic Nerve Sheath For patients who are losing vision, unilateral fenestration of the optic nerve sheath is a procedure favored by some ophthalmologists. According to Corbett and colleagues, this procedure—which consists of partial unroofing of the orbit and the creation of an intraorbital window opening in the dural–arachnoid sheaths surrounding the optic nerve—effectively preserved or restored vision in 80 to 90 percent of patients. Even when the procedure is performed on only one side, its effect on vision is often bilateral and about two-thirds of patients have some relief of headache as well, although this has been transient in most of our patients.

However, the operation carries a moderately high risk of orbital vascular obstruction and unilateral visual loss, as happened in two of our patients. The causes of visual loss after this operation by various reports have included central retinal artery or vein occlusion, choroidal infarction, optic nerve trauma, hemorrhage into the nerve sheath, and infection. Over the past decades, enthusiasm for the procedure had diminished after publication of several series in which there was visual loss in 2 to 11 percent of patients. Some of these data come from studies of sheath fenestration for ischemic optic neuropathy, a condition not comparable to the disc swelling of pseudotumor. Follow-up studies have indicated that the reduction in ICP was limited to 1 year or less. As a result of recent reexamination of the complications of this procedure, there is renewed interest for the procedure over lumbar peritoneal shunting.

Relief of Venous Obstruction In a number of patients, the CSF pressure remains elevated and the papilledema becomes chronic despite one of the above-described treatments. It is the management of this group that is the most difficult and controversial. A careful search should then be made for anatomic and hematologic causes that might underlie cerebral venous dural sinus disease. Sometimes it is useful to treat venous occlusion using interventional vascular techniques. In cases of venous thrombosis antiphospholipid antibody syndrome, sickle cell disease, hormonally induced clotting, and related disorders, medical measures may be tried first, but intravascular thrombolysis remains an option.

The more complex decision to apply stenting to the partial occlusion of the transverse sinus by generous pacchionian granulations should probably be guided by the same principles, i.e., failure of medical treatment to adequately control CSF pressure, or relive the threat to vision. In a series of 10 patients with intractably raised CSF pressure and morphologic obstruction in the venous sinuses, Donnet and colleagues were able to provide complete relief by stenting in 6 patients and partial relief in 2 patients, with follow-up ranging from 6 to 36 months. In a summary of published cases and series of patients with pseudotumor cerebri treated by endovascular stenting of venous sinus stenosis, Aroc and colleagues concluded that approximately 80 percent were relieved of their main symptoms, and a similar proportion showed resolution, or improvement in papilledema. This is a selected group of patients.

In summary, the clinician is left with only incomplete guidance as to the course of treatment of pseudotumor cerebri. In cases with no visual impairment and with moderate headaches, we have favored aggressive weight reduction, acetazolamide, and repeated lumbar punctures. For more severe cases, we perform careful vascular imaging and correction of venous sinus occlusions as noted above. Failing this, we have advised lumbar drainage to the peritoneum. If vision is imminently threatened, optic sheath fenestration is probably the best course.

We have been impressed with the persistence of a complex migraine- or tension-like headache in some patients whose CSF pressure has been adequately reduced by repeated lumbar punctures, shunting, or optic nerve fenestration. After it has been confirmed that the pressure is not elevated, these headaches may be treated in a manner similar to the usual types of chronic headaches, as outlined in Chap. 10, especially with topiramate, which has the potential benefit of facilitating weight reduction. A recent review of the subject of surgical treatment, extensively referenced, has been given by Brazis. He was unable to conclude that any one approach was superior.

PNEUMOCEPHALUS AND PNEUMOCRANIUM

These disorders, in which air enters the ventricular system or the subarachnoid spaces, are discussed in relation to cranial injury, and the postoperative state (see Chap. 35). In the case of pneumocranium, the collection of air may act as a mass that compresses adjacent brain tissue, and requires relief by aspiration.

INTRACRANIAL HYPOTENSION (See also "Low-Pressure and Spinal Puncture Headache" in Chap. 10)

After lumbar puncture, this syndrome phenomenon is usually attributable to a lowering of ICP by leakage of CSF through the needle track into the paravertebral muscles. The headache may last for days or, rarely, weeks. Most characteristic is the relation of the cranial pain to upright posture, and its relief within moments after assuming the recumbent position. Actually, the syndrome includes more than headache. There may be pain at the base of the skull posteriorly and in the back of the neck and upper thoracic spine, mild stiffness of the neck and shoulders, and nausea and vomiting. At times, the signs of meningeal irritation are so prominent as to raise the question of postlumbar puncture meningitis, although lack of fever usually excludes this possibility. In addition to a low or unmeasurable CSF pressure if another spinal tap is performed (the CSF pressure is found to be in the range of 0 to 60 mm H_2O), there are occasionally a few to a dozen white cells in the CSF, which may further raise concern of meningitis. In the infant or young child, stiffness of the neck may be accompanied by irritability, unwillingness to move, and refusal of food. If the headache is protracted, recumbency still reduces it, but a feeling of dull pressure may remain, which the patient continues to report as pain. Many patients also report that shaking the head produces a cephalic pain. Occasionally, there will be unilateral or bilateral sixth nerve palsy or a self-audible bruit from turbulence in the intracranial venous system. Hearing loss is a far less common complication (see Chap. 2). A rare syndrome that has been attributed to sagging of the frontal lobes in low CSF pressure situations has been described by Wicklund and coworkers. Patients are apathetic and disinhibited and have prominent daytime somnolence.

It has been recognized that low CSF pressure is associated on the MRI with variable dural enhancement by gadolinium (Fig. 30-5) and, when the syndrome is protracted and severe, there may be small subdural effusions

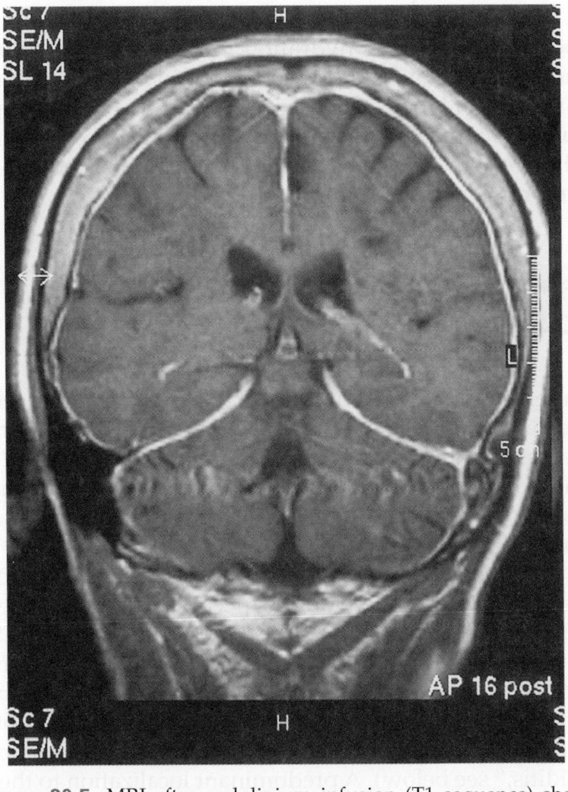

Figure 30-5. MRI after gadolinium infusion (T1 sequence) showing the widespread dural enhancement that is typical of low CSF pressure after lumbar puncture, spontaneous CSF leakage, or shunt overdrainage. Similar changes may be found in the spinal dura.

(see below). In older patients taking warfarin, a subdural hematoma may be found.

The use of a 22- to 24-gauge needle and the performance of a single clean (atraumatic) tap seemingly reduce the likelihood of a postlumbar puncture headache, as discussed in Chap. 2. A period of enforced recumbency, although widely practiced as a means of preventing headache, probably does not lessen its incidence (Carbaat and van Crevel). The ingestion of large volumes of fluids, the infusion of 1,000 to 2,000 mL of 5 percent glucose, and various forms of caffeine (see further on) are usually recommended, but are of uncertain benefit.

The most dependable treatment is a "blood patch" (spinal epidural injection of approximately 20 mL of the patient's own blood). At least 75 percent of patients are thus relieved of the headache according to Safa-Tisseront and colleagues; they report that after a second injection, improvement occurs in 97 percent. Many patients have transient back or radicular pain (sciatica) following the blood patch. Curiously, the headache is often relieved almost immediately, even if the blood is injected at some distance from the original puncture (although the procedure is usually done at the same level as the previous spinal tap). Moreover, the volume of blood injected, usually about 20 mL, is not related to the chances of success. The mechanism of this rapid improvement, therefore, may not simply be the plugging of a dural leak. A number of patients fail to benefit or have only transient effects; it is then unclear whether repeating the procedure is helpful. The administration of caffeine–ergotamine preparations or intravenous caffeine may also have a salutary, although temporary, effect on the orthostatic headache. The addition of analgesic medication is required if the patient must get up to care for himself or to travel. In protracted cases, patience is called for, as most headaches will resolve in 2 weeks or less.

As to mechanism, the pain is presumed to be from tugging on cerebral veins or assuming the upright position. Panullo and colleagues also showed that there is a downward displacement of the upper brainstem and posterior fossa contents when the patient assumes the upright position; but, as pointed out in Chap. 17, only rarely are there associated signs of brain herniation, the exceptions being some of the unusual cases discussed below. Miyazawa and colleagues have proposed that hypovolemia of the CSF, rather than lowered pressure, is the cause of downward displacement of the brain and dilatation of cerebral and spinal epidural veins. They propose that the buoyancy provided by the spinal fluid is lost in these cases.

The same problem of low pressure as that which follows lumbar puncture can occur after straining, a nonhurtful fall, or for no known reason. The cardinal feature is orthostatic headache and only rarely are there other neurologic complaints, such as diplopia from sixth-nerve palsy or a self-audible bruit. In these cases, the CSF pressure is low (60 mm H_2O or less) or not measurable; the fluid may contain a few mononuclear cells but is most often normal. A few cases have presented with stupor as a result of downward transtentorial displacement of the diencephalic region (Pleasure et al) or an upper cervical myelopathy caused by downward deformation and displacement of the spinal cord (Miyazaki et al).

Some surveys suggest that patients with structural disorders of connective tissue are at greater risk for spontaneous CSF leaks than others. The Marfan and Ehlers-Danlos syndrome as well as autosomal dominant polycystic kidney disease are risk factors as summarized by Schievink.

In many such patients with ostensibly idiopathic low CSF pressure syndromes, there has been a tear in the delicate arachnoid surrounding a nerve root, with continuous leakage of CSF. The site of the leak is difficult to ascertain except when it occurs into the paranasal sinuses (causing CSF rhinorrhea). In a series of 11 patients with spontaneous intracranial hypotension, a putative leak was found by radionuclide cisternography or CT myelography (the preferred procedure) in the cervical region or at the cervicothoracic junction in 5 patients, in the thoracic region in 5, and the lumbar region in 1 (Schievink et al). In the patients who underwent surgical repair, a leaking meningeal diverticulum (Tarlov cyst) was found and could be ligated. This seems to be the most common structural cause. A blood patch, as described above, may be useful and should be attempted before resorting to surgical repair of the cyst. Recumbency for a few days thereafter permits the pressure to build up, and there has been no recurrence in all but a few of the cases that we have encountered. Others, however, have reported repeated episodes of orthostatic headache. Rarely, a case of intracranial hypotension becomes chronic; the headache is then no longer responsive to recumbency. Mokri and colleagues (1998) have also made the point that orthostatic headache and diffuse pachymeningeal enhancement on MRI may occur in the presence of normal CSF pressures.

One of the most remarkable syndromes associated with low CSF pressure is that following spinal surgery that utilizes suction drainage of the lumbar wound. The patient may fail to awaken from anesthesia or show signs such as pupillary asymmetry or a seizure. Imaging studies show features usually associated with global brain hypoxia-ischemia including signal changes in the basal ganglia, thalamus, and deep cerebellar nuclei. This syndrome apparently occurs if there has been a dural spinal leak and a high volume of CSF drainage by the suction device (Parpaley et al). The mechanism is not clear, but cerebral venous congestion has been implicated.

As noted, a helpful diagnostic sign of low CSF pressure is prominent dural enhancement with gadolinium on the MRI (see Fig. 30-5), a phenomenon attributed by Fishman and Dillon to dural venous dilatation; this finding may extend to the pachymeninges of the posterior fossa and the cervical spine. According to Mokri and colleagues (1995), biopsy of the dura and underlying meninges in these cases shows fibroblastic proliferation and neovascularity with an amorphous subdural fluid that is hard to interpret. There may be additional subdural effusions and mass effect, either on the cerebral convexities, temporal lobes, optic chiasm, or cerebellar tonsils. Using ultrasonography, Chen and colleagues have described an enlarged superior ophthalmic vein and increased blood flow velocity in this vessel, both of which normalized after successful treatment. The pituitary gland is usually hyperemic as well.

In the most severe cases of low-CSF pressure syndrome, downward sagging of the entire cerebrum with stupor, as described in Chap. 17, or stretching of the vein of Galen and consequent impairment of venous drainage may cause life-threatening swelling of diencephalic and mesencephalic structures (see Savoiardo et al and Schievink).

The use of a one-way shunt valve in hydrocephalus may be complicated by a syndrome of low CSF pressure. Reference has already been made to this syndrome, and to the slit ventricles in children who have been treated for hydrocephalus, and to midbrain syndromes from brain displacement (see Fig. 30-4). Usually the valve setting is too low, and readjustment to maintain a higher pressure is corrective.

Also appropriate to mention here are CSF leaks that occur after cranial, nasal, or spinal surgery. These are suspected in the postoperative period, although the precise origin of the leak may be difficult to determine, but they give rise to some of the most intractable low-pressure syndromes and must be investigated by radiologic and nuclide studies. In our experience, several such leaks have been intermittent, adding to the difficulty in diagnosis.

The treatment of spontaneous intracranial hypotension is similar to that mentioned earlier under the treatment of postlumbar puncture headache. Kantor and Silberstein pointed out that some patients who fail to respond to conservative management with bed rest, abdominal binders, hydration, caffeine, theophylline, and corticosteroids, and who have also failed with lumbar epidural blood patch, will respond to a cervical epidural blood patch. This should be administered by those who are skilled in their use and are aware of the risk of compression of the spinal cord.

SPECIAL MENINGEAL AND EPENDYMAL DISORDERS

The effects of bacterial invasion of the pia-arachnoid, cerebrospinal subarachnoid space, ventricles, and ependyma are described in Chap. 32 and summarized in Table 32-1. The point being made here is that these structures may also be involved in a number of noninfective processes, some of obscure origin.

Because the ventricular and subarachnoid spaces are in continuity, one would expect that a noxious agent entering any one part would extend throughout the CSF pathway. Such is not always the case. The lower spinal roots or spinal cord alone may be implicated in "spinal arachnoiditis." A similar process may affect the optic nerves and chiasm exclusively ("opticochiasmatic arachnoiditis," see below). A predominant localization to these basal or cervical structures may be apparent even in cases of diffuse cerebrospinal meningeal reactions, perhaps because of an uneven concentration of the noxious agent. The mechanisms by which these meningeal reactions affect parenchymal structures (brain, cord, and nerve roots) are not fully understood. The most obvious sequela is an obstruction to the flow of CSF in hydrocephalus; here, simple fibrotic narrowing of the CSF circulatory pathway is causative. Progressive constriction of nerve roots and spinal cord, literally a strangulation of these structures, is another plausible mechanism, but it is difficult to separate vascular factors from mechanical ones. Because any toxic agent introduced into the subarachnoid space has free access via Virchow-Robin spaces and thereby to the superficial parts of the brain and spinal cord, direct parenchymal injury may follow. Perivascular reactions of subpial vessels, as in infectious processes, would be a plausible mechanism of injury to optic nerves and spinal cord, where long stretches of myelinated fibers abut the pia.

Regional Arachnoiditis

Arachnoiditis limited to the lumbosacral roots has followed ruptured discs, myelograms, and spinal surgery. Usually, there is sciatica and chronic pain in the back and lower extremities, but sensorimotor and reflex changes in the legs are variable. The MRI shows irregularly enhancing roots and arachnoidal thickening; myelography discloses loculated pockets of imaging media. This condition is discussed further in Chap. 11.

Another form of spinal arachnoiditis, in which both the spinal cord and roots are entrapped in thickened pia-arachnoid, sometimes with arachnoid-dural adhesions, is a rare but well-known and often idiopathic entity. An account of this condition is included with the spinal cord diseases (see Chap. 44). The etiologic factors have been singularly elusive, although in the past it followed the instillation of iophendylate (Pantopaque) for myelography and corticosteroids (for pain or multiple sclerosis) and other irritative agents, particularly chemically contaminated spinal anesthetics. Our colleagues saw more than 40 cases of the latter type, now rare, dating from the time when vials of anesthetic were stored in detergent sterilizing solutions. Instillation of the anesthetic agent was followed immediately by back pain and a rapidly progressive lumbosacral root syndrome (areflexic paralysis, anesthesia of the legs, and paralysis of sphincters). Several cases have, in our recent experience, followed prolonged spinal anesthesia with the patient in a decubitus position, usually for orthopedic procedures, but the resulting myelopathy or cauda equina radiculopathy was difficult to separate from a direct toxic effect of the anesthetic. The CSF protein rises rapidly in cases that were precipitated by injection of substances into the subarachnoid space, but pleocytosis is minimal. In other instances, protracted back pain lasting days to weeks is the only effect in the post anesthetic period but is followed, after months or years, by a progressive myelopathy. This takes the form of some combination of spinal arachnoiditis with ataxic paraparesis and sensory disturbance, hydrocephalus, or opticochiasmatic arachnoiditis. The point to be made is that there is always some risk attached to the subarachnoid instillation of any foreign agent.

Opticochiasmatic Arachnoiditis

This condition was well known to neurologists during the period when neurosyphilis was a common disease. It occurs after years of chronic syphilitic meningitis, sometimes in conjunction with tabes dorsalis or meningomyelitis. However, there were always nonsyphilitic cases, the cause of which was never determined. A constriction of visual fields, usually bilateral and asymmetrical (rarely scotomas), developed insidiously and progressed. Pathologically, the optic nerves were found to be enmeshed in thickened, opaque pia-arachnoid. The optic nerves are atrophic in appearance. Idiopathic cases are likely to be confused with multiple sclerosis.

Pachymeningitis

This term refers to a chronic, inflammatory thickening of the dura. The term is somewhat confusing insofar as the pia and arachnoid may be equally involved in the inflammatory thickening and all three membranes are bound together by dense fibrous adhesions. This type of meningeal reaction, which is now uncommon, was first described by Charcot and Joffroy. It occurred mainly in the cervical region (hence the name *pachymeningitis cervicalis hypertrophica*) and was attributed to syphilis. Indeed, in some instances there was a gummatous thickening of the dura. Involvement of cervical roots and compression of the spinal cord gave rise to variable degrees of paraparesis in association with root pain, paresthesia, sensory loss, and amyotrophy of the upper limbs. In the modern era, rheumatoid arthritis (Fig. 30-6), sarcoidosis, and

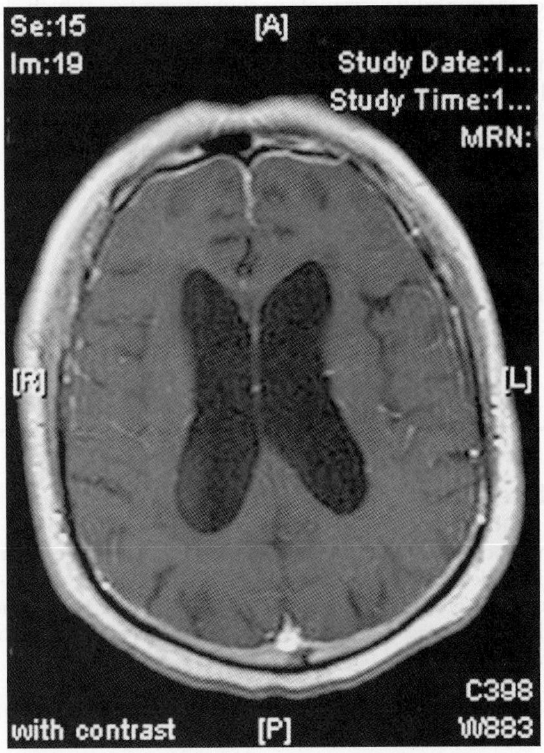

Figure 30-6. MRI with gadolinium infusion showing diffuse rheumatoid pachymeningitis in an older man with minimal systemic disease. He had severe headaches, hydrocephalus, and mental dullness.

chronic local infection (fungal, tuberculous) have been the main causes, but many cases remain unexplained. Idiopathic hypertrophic pachymeningitis continue to be reported; a summary of published cases and two personally studied ones is given by Dumont and colleagues and by Jimenez-Caballero and coworkers.

A condition associated with plasma cells proliferation that contain IgG-4 receptors has been reported to involve the pachymeninges. The process has a similar appearance to rheumatoid granulomatous infiltration and it is responsive to corticosteroids. In addition to evident thickening and gadolinium enhancement of the dura on imaging studies, the characteristic features are an elevation of the IgG fraction in the serum and in CSF and infiltration of meningeal tissue by uniform plasma cells that exhibit IgG-4 markers (Plasma cells are not prominent in the CSF in this condition; they are found in other states such as Listeria meningitis and neurosyphilis.). This process has been known to occur in other organs such as the salivary glands, lung and kidney; it tends to occur in men in their fifth or sixth decade according to the case series of pathologic samples reported by Lindstrom and colleagues.

The subdural space and dura can be involved by extension of a pathologic process from the arachnoid, especially in infants and children, in whom subdural hygromas regularly follow meningitis. The fibrous connective tissue of which the dura is composed may also undergo pronounced thickening in the course of a mucopolysaccharidosis, especially in cases where fibroblasts are implicated. The basal pia-arachnoid may be involved, leading to obstructive hydrocephalus. Older medical writings often made reference to syphilitic cranial pachymeningitis, which later proved to be the thickened membranes of subdural hematomas. The neovascular response and fibrosis of the dura and meninges that result from low CSF pressures and give the same appearance as pachymeningitis on enhanced CT scans and MRI were discussed earlier in the chapter.

Superficial Siderosis of the Meninges

Superficial siderosis is clearly the consequence of repeated contamination of the meninges by blood (McDougal and Adams; Fishman). An oozing vascular malformation or tumor has been the usual cause in our experience, although there have been instances in which the source of the blood could not be found; in these a past history of head trauma is common. The red blood corpuscles are phagocytosed, with the formation of hemosiderin, and gradually both iron pigment and ferritin are released into the CSF. As a result, the surface of the cerebellum, spinal cord, hippocampi, and olfactory bulbs are stained orange-brown. Iron pigments and ferritin, which are toxic, gradually diffuse through the pia into superficial parts of the cerebellum, eighth cranial nerve, and spinal cord, destroying nerve cells and exciting a glial reaction. In microscopic sections stained for iron, the histiocyte–microglial cells contain iron and ferritin, and particles of iron can be seen studding nerve and glial cells for a distance of several millimeters beneath the pia.

The clinical syndrome of siderosis of the meninges consists essentially of a progressive ataxia and nerve deafness; sometimes a spastic paraparesis is added and, rarely, mental impairment, probably from hydrocephalus. The hemosiderin and iron-stained meninges are readily visualized by MRI, as iron is strongly paramagnetic. All the iron-impregnated tissues are hypointense in T2-weighted images. Koeppen and associates attributed the vulnerability of the acoustic nerves to their extended meningeal exposure before acquiring a fibroblastic perineurium and epineurium. There is no treatment other than finding the source of the meningeal blood and preventing further hemorrhage and treating hydrocephalus if it is present. Kumar has provided a useful review of the problem of superficial siderosis. Curiously, the systemic disease hemochromatosis, does not affect the brain or meninges.

Oculoleptomeningeal Amyloidosis

Transthyretin amyloidosis can present as an infiltration of the leptomeninges by amyloidosis. The clinical syndrome includes dementia, seizures, stroke-like episodes, subarachnoid hemorrhage, ataxia, myelopathy, deafness, radiculopathy, and ocular amyloidosis, usually affecting the vitreous. The leptomeninges enhance with gadolinium on MRI; the CSF has elevated protein but is otherwise nondescript. There is no proven therapy, but liver transplantation could theoretically be effective.

References

Adams RD, Fisher CM, Hakim S, et al: Symptomatic occult hydrocephalus with "normal" cerebrospinal fluid pressure: A treatable syndrome. *N Engl J Med* 273:117, 1965.

Aimard G, Vighetto A, Gabet JY, et al: Acetazolamide: An alternative to shunting in normal pressure hydrocephalus? Preliminary results. *Rev Neurol* 146:437, 1990.

Ames A, Sakanoue M, Endo S: Na, K, Ca, Mg and Cl concentrations in choroid plexus fluid and cisternal fluid compared with plasma ultrafiltrate. *J Neurophysiol* 27:672, 1964.

Arac A, Lee M, Steinberg GK, et al: Efficacy of endovascular stenting in dural venous sinus stenosis for the treatment of idiopathic intracranial hypotension. *Neurosurg Focus* 27:1, 2009.

Black PM: Idiopathic normal pressure hydrocephalus: Results of shunting in 62 patients. *J Neurosurg* 53:371, 1980.

Blevins G, Macauley R, Harder A. et al. Oculoleptomeningeal amyloidosis in a large kindred with a new transthyretin variant Tyr69His. *Neurology* 60:1625, 2003.

Børgesen SE, Gjerris F: The predictive value of conductance to outflow of CSF in normal pressure hydrocephalus. *Brain* 105:65, 1982.

Brazis PW: Clinical review: the surgical treatment of idiopathic pseudotumor cerebri. *Cephalalgia* 28:1361, 2008.

Bruce BB, Kedar S, Van Stavern GP, et al: Idiopathic intracranial hypertension in men. *Neurology* 72:304, 2009.

Burgett RA, Purvin VA, Kawasaki A: Lumboperitoneal shunting for pseudotumor cerebri. *Neurology* 49:734, 1997.

Carbaat P, Van Crevel H: Lumbar puncture headache: Controlled study on the preventive effect of 24 hours' bed rest. *Lancet* 2:1133, 1981.

Chen CC, Luo CL, Wang SJ, et al: Colour Doppler imaging for diagnosis of intracranial hypotension. *Lancet* 354:826, 1999.

Chesnut, RM, Temkin, N, Carney, N, et al: A Trial of Intracranial-Pressure Monitoring in Traumatic Brain Injury. *N Engl J Med* 367;2471, 2012.

Chutorian AM, Gold AP, Braun CW: Benign intracranial hypertension and Bell's palsy. *N Engl J Med* 296:1214, 1977.

Cinalli G, Sainte-Rose C, Simon I, et al: Sylvian aqueduct syndrome and global rostral midbrain dysfunction associated with shunt malfunction. *J Neurosurg* 90:227, 1999.

Clarke D, Bullock P, Hui T, Firth J: Benign intracranial hypertension: A cause of CSF rhinorrhea. *J Neurol Neurosurg Psychiatry* 57:847, 1994.

Corbett JJ: Problems in the diagnosis and treatment of pseudotumor cerebri. *Can J Neurol Sci* 10:221, 1983.

Corbett JJ, Mehta MP: Cerebrospinal fluid pressure in normal obese subjects and patients with pseudotumor cerebri. *Neurology* 33:1386, 1983.

Corbett JJ, Nerad JA, Tse DT, Anderson RL: Results of optic nerve sheath fenestration for pseudotumor cerebri. *Arch Ophthalmol* 106:1391, 1988.

Corbett JJ, Thompson HS: The rational management of idiopathic intracranial hypertension. *Arch Neurol* 46:1049, 1989.

Cutler RWP, Spertell RB: Cerebrospinal fluid: A selective review. *Ann Neurol* 11:1, 1982.

Dandy WE: Experimental hydrocephalus. *Ann Surg* 70:129, 1919.

Dandy WE, Blackfan KD: Internal hydrocephalus: An experimental, clinical, and pathological study. *Am J Dis Child* 8:406, 1914.

Davson H, Welch K, Segal MB: *Physiology and Pathophysiology of the Cerebrospinal Fluid*. New York, Churchill Livingstone, 1987.

Dennis M, Fritz CR, Netley CT, et al: The intelligence of hydrocephalic children. *Arch Neurol* 38:607, 1981.

Digre KB, Corbett JJ: Pseudotumor cerebri in men. *Arch Neurol* 45:866, 1988.

Donnet A, Metellus P, Levrier O, et al: Endovascular treatment of idiopathic intracranial hypertension. *Neurology* 70:641, 2008.

Dumont AS, Clark AW, Sevick RJ, Miles T: Idiopathic hypertrophic pachymeningitis: A report of two cases and review of the literature. *Can J Neurol Sci* 27:383, 2000.

Farb RI, Vanek I, Scott JN, et al: Idiopathic intracranial hypertension. The prevalence and morphology of sinovenous stenosis. *Neurology* 60:1418, 2003.

Fisher CM: Hydrocephalus as a cause of disturbances of gait in the elderly. *Neurology* 32:1358, 1982.

Fisher CM: Reversal of normal pressure hydrocephalus symptoms by subdural hematoma. *Can J Neurol Sci* 29:171, 2002.

Fishman RA: *Cerebrospinal Fluid in Diseases of the Nervous System*, 2nd ed. Philadelphia, Saunders, 1992.

Fishman RA: Superficial siderosis. *Ann Neurol* 34:635, 1993.

Fishman RA: The pathophysiology of pseudotumor cerebri: An unsolved puzzle (editorial). *Arch Neurol* 41:257, 1984.

Fishman RA, Dillon WP: Dural enhancement and cerebral displacement secondary to intracranial hypotension. *Neurology* 43:609, 1993.

Foley J: Benign forms of intracranial hypertension—"toxic" and "otitic" hydrocephalus. *Brain* 78:1, 1955.

Friedman DI, Liu GT, Digre KB: Revised diagnostic criteria for the pseudotumor cerebri syndrome in adults. *Neurology* 81:1159, 2013.

Gilles FH, Davidson RI: Communicating hydrocephalus associated with deficient dysplastic parasagittal arachnoid granulations. *J Neurosurg* 35:421, 1971.

Greer M: Benign intracranial hypertension, in Vinken PJ, Bruyn GW (eds): *Handbook of Clinical Neurology*. Vol 16. Amsterdam, North-Holland, 1974, pp 150–166.

Hakim S, Adams RD: The special clinical problem of symptomatic hydrocephalus with normal cerebrospinal fluid pressure. *J Neurol Sci* 2:307, 1965.

Higgins JNP, Cousings C, Owler BK, et al: Idiopathic intracranial hypertension: 12 cases treated by venous sinus stenting. *J Neurol Neurosurg Psychiatry* 74:1662, 2003.

Huh JW, Boswinkel J, Ruppe MD, et al: Reference range for cerebrospinal fluid opening pressure in children. *N Engl J Med* 363:891,2010.

Huna-Baron R, Kupersmith MJ: Idiopathic intracranial hypertension in pregnancy. *J Neurol* 249:1078, 2002.

Hussey F, Schanzer B, Katzman R: A simple constant-infusion manometric test for measurement of CSF absorption: II. Clinical studies. *Neurology* 20:665, 1970.

Jacobson DM, Berg R, Wall M, et al: Serum vitamin A concentration is elevated in idiopathic intracranial hypertension. *Neurology* 53:1114, 1999.

Jimenez-Caballero PE, Deamontopoulos Fernandez J, Camacho-Castaneda I: Hypertrophic cranial and spinal pachymeningitis: A description of four cases and a review of the literature. *Rev Neurol* 43:470, 2006.

Johnson RT, Johnson DP, Edmonds CS: Virus-induced hydrocephalus: Development of aqueductal stenosis in hamsters after mumps infection. *Science* 157:1066, 1967.

Johnston I, Paterson A: Benign intracranial hypertension. *Brain* 97:289, 301, 1974.

Kantor D, Silberstein SD: Cervical epidural blood patch for low CSF pressure headaches. *Neurology* 65:1138, 2005.

Karahalios DG, Rekate HL, Khayata MH, Apostolides PJ: Elevated intracranial venous pressure as a universal mechanism in pseudotumor cerebri of varying etiologies. *Neurology* 46:198, 1996.

Katzman R, Hussey F: A simple constant-infusion manometric test for measurement of CSF absorption: I. Rationale and method. *Neurology* 20:534, 1970.

King JO, Mitchell PJ, Thomson KR, Tress BM: Manometry combined with cervical puncture in idiopathic intracranial hypertension. *Neurology* 58:26, 2002.

Koeppen AH, Dickson AC, Chu RC, Thach RE: The pathogenesis of superficial siderosis of the nervous system. *Ann Neurol* 34:646, 1993.

Kumar N: Superficial siderosis: Associations and therapeutic implications. *Arch Neurol* 64:491, 2007.

Leach IL, Jones BV, Tomsick TA, et al: Normal appearance of arachnoid granulations on contrast enhanced CT and MRI of the brain: Differentiation from dural sinus disease. *AJNR Am J Neuroradiol* 17:1523, 1996.

Leech RW, Brumback RA: *Hydrocephalus: Current Clinical Concepts*. St. Louis, MO, Mosby–Year Book, 1990, pp 86–90.

Lessell S, Rosman P: Permanent visual impairment in childhood pseudotumor cerebri. *Arch Neurol* 43:801, 1986.

Lindstrom KM, Cousar JB, Lopes MB: IgG4-related meningeal disease: Clinico-pathologic features and proposal for diagnostic criteria. *Acta Neuropathol* 120:765, 2010.

Lundberg N: Continuous recording and control of ventricular fluid pressure in neurosurgical practice. *Acta Psychiatr Scand* 36(Suppl 149):1, 1960.

Mann JD, Johnson RN, Butler AB, Bass NH: Impairment of cerebrospinal fluid circulatory dynamics in pseudotumor cerebri and response to steroid treatment. *Neurology* 29:550, 1979.

McDougal WB, Adams RD: The neurological changes in hemochromatosis. *Trans Am Neuropathol Soc* 9:117, 1950.

Meese W, Kluge W, Grumme T, Hopfenmuller W: CT evaluation of the CSF spaces in healthy persons. *Neuroradiology* 19:131, 1980.

Merritt HH, Fremont-Smith F: *The Cerebrospinal Fluid*. Philadelphia, Saunders, 1937.

Mestrezat W: *Le liquide cephalo-rachidien normal et pathologique*. Paris, Maloine, 1912.

Miyazaki T, Chiba A, Nishina H, et al: Upper cervical myelopathy associated with low CSF pressure: A complication of ventriculoperitoneal shunt. *Neurology* 50:1864, 1998.

Miyazawa K, Shiga Y, Hasegawa T, et al: CSF hypovolemia vs intracranial hypotension in "spontaneous intracranial hypotension syndrome." *Neurology* 60:941, 2003.

Mokri B, Hunter SF, Atkinson JL, Piepgras DG: Orthostatic headaches caused by CSF leak but with normal CSF pressures. *Neurology* 51:786, 1998.

Mokri B, Parisi JE, Scheithauer BW, et al: Meningeal biopsy in intracranial hypotension: Meningeal enhancement on MRI. *Neurology* 45:1801, 1995.

Panullo SC, Reich JB, Krol G, et al: MRI changes in intracranial hypotension. *Neurology* 43:919, 1993.

Pappenheimer JR, Heisey SR, Jordan EF, Downer J: Perfusion of the cerebral ventricular system in unanesthetized goats. *Am J Physiol* 203:763, 1962.

Parpaley Y, Urbach H, Kovacs A, et al: Pseudohypoxic brain swelling (postoperative intracranial hypotension-associated venous congestion) after spinal surgery: Report of 2 cases. *Neurosurgery* 68:E277, 2011.

Pleasure SJH, Abosch A, Friedman, et al: Spontaneous intracranial hypotension resulting in stupor caused by diencephalic compression. *Neurology* 50:1854, 1998.

Quincke H: Die Lumbarpunktion des Hydrocephalus. *Klin Wochenschr* 28:929, 965, 1891.

Racette BA, Esper GJ, Antenor J, et al: Pathophysiology of parkinsonism due to hydrocephalus. *J Neurol Neurosurg Psychiatry* 75:1617, 2004.

Radhakrishnan K, Ahlskog JE, Garrity JA, Kurland LT: Idiopathic intracranial hypertension. *Mayo Clin Proc* 69:169, 1994.

Raichle ME, Grubb RL, Phelps ME, et al: Cerebral hemodynamics and metabolism in pseudotumor cerebri. *Ann Neurol* 4:104, 1978.

Ropper AH (ed): *Neurological and Neurosurgical Intensive Care*, 4th ed. Baltimore, MD, Lippincott Williams & Wilkins, 2004.

Ropper AH, Marmarou A: Mechanism of pseudotumor in Guillain-Barré syndrome. *Arch Neurol* 41:259, 1984.

Rosman NP, Shands KN: Hydrocephalus caused by increased intracranial venous pressure: A clinicopathological study. *Ann Neurol* 3:445, 1978.

Rosner MJ, Becker DP: Origin and evolution of plateau waves. *J Neurosurg* 60:312, 1984.

Russell DS: *Observations on the Pathology of Hydrocephalus*. London, His Majesty's Stationery Office, 1949.

Safa-Tisseront V, Thromann F, Malassine P, et al: Effectiveness of epidural blood patch in the management of postdural puncture headache. *Anesthesiology* 95:2, 2001.

Sahs A, Joynt RJ: Brain swelling of unknown cause. *Neurology* 6:791, 1956.

Samuels MA, Gonzolez RG, Yim AY, Stemmer-Rachaminov A: Cabot Case 34–2007: A 77-year-old man with ear pain, difficulty speaking, and altered mental status. *N Engl J Med* 357:1957, 2007.

Savoiardo M, Minati L, Farina L, et al: Spontaneous intracranial hypotension with deep brain swelling. *Brain* 130:1884, 2007.

Schievink WI: Spontaneous spinal cerebrospinal fluid leaks and intracranial hypotension. *JAMA* 295:2286, 2006.

Schievink WI, Meyer FB, Atkinson JL, Mokri B: Spontaneous spinal cerebrospinal fluid leaks and intracranial hypotension. *J Neurosurg* 84:598, 1996.

Seckl J, Lightman S: Cerebrospinal fluid neurohypophysial peptides in benign intracranial hypertension. *J Neurol Neurosurg Psychiatry* 51:1538, 1988.

Shinnar S, Gammon K, Bergman EW Jr, et al: Management of hydrocephalus in infancy: Use of acetazolamide and furosemide to avoid cerebrospinal fluid shunts. *J Pediatr* 107:31, 1985.

Silverberg GD, Levinthal E, Sullivan EV, et al: Assessment of low-flow CSF drainage as a treatment for AD: Results of a randomized pilot study. *Neurology* 59:1139, 2002.

Sugerman HJ, Demaria EJ, Sismanins A: Gastric surgery for pseudotumor cerebri associated with obesity. *Ann Surg* 229:634, 1999.

Sugerman HJ, Felton WL, Salvant JB, et al: Effects of surgically induced weight loss on idiopathic intracranial hypertension in morbid obesity. *Neurology* 45:1655, 1995.

Symonds CP: Otitic hydrocephalus. *Brain* 54:55, 1931.

Tripathi BS, Tripathi RC: Vacuolar transcellular channels as a drainage pathway for CSF. *J Physiol* 239:195, 1974.

Van Crevel H: Papilledema, CSF pressure, and CSF flow in cerebral tumours. *J Neurol Neurosurg Psychiatry* 42:493, 1979.

Walchenbach R, Geiger E, Thomeer RJ, et al: The value of temporary external lumbar CSF drainage in predicting the outcome of shunting on normal pressure hydrocephalus. *J Neurol Neurosurg Psychiatry* 72:503, 2002.

Walker RWH: Idiopathic intracranial hypertension: Any light on the mechanism of raised pressure? *J Neurol Neurosurg Psychiatry* 71:1, 2001.

Wall M, George D: Visual loss in pseudotumor cerebri. *Arch Neurol* 44:170, 1987.

Weed LH: Certain anatomical and physiological aspects of the meninges and cerebrospinal fluid. *Brain* 58:383, 1935.

Zeidler M, Dorman PJ, Furguson IT, Bateman DE: Parkinsonism associated with obstructive hydrocephalus due to idiopathic aqueductal stenosis. *J Neurol Neurosurg Psychiatry* 64:657, 1998.

31

Intracranial Neoplasms and Paraneoplastic Disorders

Tumors of the central nervous system (CNS) constitute a bleak but vitally important chapter of neurologic medicine. Their importance derives from their great variety; the numerous neurologic symptoms caused by their size, location, and invasive qualities; the destruction and displacement of tissues in which they are situated; the elevation of intracranial pressure they cause; and, most of all, their lethality. Slowly, this dismal state of affairs is changing as a result of advances in anesthesiology, stereotactic and microneurosurgical techniques, focused radiation therapy, and the use of new chemotherapeutic agents.

For clinicians, the several generalizations should be a matter of general knowledge about brain tumors. *First*, many types of tumor, both primary and secondary, occur in the cranial cavity and spinal canal but certain ones are much more frequent than others and are prone to occur in particular age groups. Secondary metastatic deposits are more common than primary brain tumors in adults and the opposite is true in children. Furthermore, certain cancers (breast, lung, melanoma, renal cell cancer) display a tendency to metastasize to nervous tissue and many others do not do so. *Second*, some primary intracranial and spinal tumors, such as craniopharyngioma, meningioma, and schwannoma, have a disposition to grow in particular parts of the cranial cavity, thereby producing characteristic neurologic syndromes. *Third,* the presence of a state of immunosuppression such as AIDS or cancer chemotherapy, special inherited disorders such as neurofibromatosis, and exposure to radiation each predispose to the development of tumors of the nervous system. *Fourth,* the growth rates and invasiveness of tumors vary; some, like glioblastoma, are highly malignant, invasive, and rapidly progressive and others, like meningioma, are most often benign, slowly progressive, and compressive. These different qualities have substantial clinical implications, frequently providing the explanation of slowly or rapidly evolving clinical states as well as potential surgical cure and prognosis.

Finally, a special class of disorders result from the production of autoantibodies that are elaborated by systemic, nonneural, tumors and target cerebral and spinal neurons. These remote effects, referred to as *paraneoplastic*, often constitute the initial or only clinical manifestation of the underlying neoplasm.

A comprehensive reference on brain tumors is the text edited by Kaye and Laws.

Incidence of CNS Tumors and Their Types

Currently, in each year there are an estimated 600,000 deaths from cancer in the United States. Of these, the number of patients who died of primary tumors of the brain seems comparatively small (approximately 20,000, half of them malignant gliomas), but in roughly another 130,000 patients the brain is affected at the time of death by metastases. Thus, in approximately 25 percent of all the patients with cancer, the brain or its coverings are involved by neoplasm at some time in the course of the illness. Among causes of death from intracranial disease in adults, tumor is exceeded in frequency only by stroke, whereas in children primary brain tumors constitute the most common solid tumor and represent 22 percent of all childhood neoplasms, second in frequency only to leukemia. Viewed from another perspective, in the United States, the yearly incidence of all tumors that involve the brain is 46 per 100,000, and of primary brain tumors, 15 per 100,000.

It is difficult to obtain accurate statistics as to the types of intracranial tumors, for most of them have been obtained from university hospitals with specialized cancer and neurosurgical centers. From the figures of Posner and Chernik, one can infer that secondary tumors of the brain greatly outnumber primary ones; yet in the large series reported in the past (those of Cushing [1932], Olivecrona, Zülch, and Zimmerman), only 4 to 8 percent were of this type. In the autopsy statistics of municipal hospitals, where one would expect a more natural selection of cases, the figures for metastatic tumors vary widely, from 20 to 42 percent (Rubinstein, 1972). Even these estimates probably underestimate the incidence, particularly of metastatic disease. With these qualifications, the figures in Table 31-1 may be taken as representative.

Most primary brain tumors are of presumed glia cell origin—i.e., gliomas—a category that includes astrocytomas (which occur in several grades of malignancy), oligodendrogliomas, ependymomas (which may have characteristics of both glia and of epithelium), and a number of rarer types. Other brain tumors arise from ectodermal structures related to the brain (meningioma), from lymphocytes (CNS lymphoma), or from precursor neuronal elements (neuroblastoma, medulloblastoma),

Table 31-1

TYPES OF INTRACRANIAL TUMORS IN THE COMBINED SERIES OF ZÜLCH, CUSHING, AND OLIVECRONA, EXPRESSED IN PERCENTAGE OF TOTAL (APPROXIMATELY 15,000 CASES)

TUMOR	PERCENT OF TOTAL
Gliomas[a]	
Glioblastoma multiforme	20
Astrocytoma	10
Ependymoma	6
Medulloblastoma	4
Oligodendroglioma	5
Meningioma	15
Pituitary adenoma	7
Neurinoma (schwannoma)	7
Metastatic carcinoma	6
Craniopharyngioma, dermoid, epidermoid, teratoma	4
Angiomas	4
Sarcomas	4
Unclassified (mostly gliomas)	5
Miscellaneous (pinealoma, chordoma, granuloma, lymphoma)[b]	3
Total	100

[a]In *children*, the proportions differ: astrocytoma, 48 percent; medulloblastoma, 44 percent; ependymoma, 8 percent. Seventy percent of gliomas in children are infratentorial; in adults, 70 percent are supratentorial. Craniophrayngioma also occurs mainly in younger age groups.
[b]The incidence of lymphoma was negligible when these series were collected, but it has increased markedly since then (see text).

Table 31-2

AGE-SPECIFIC FREQUENCY OF TUMOR TYPES WITH AGE

TUMOR	CHILDHOOD, PERCENT	ADULT, PERCENT	OLDER ADULT, PERCENT
Neuroepithelial tumors (glial origin)	78.1	44.6	41.9
Pilocytic astrocytoma	19.8	0.7	0
Glioblastoma	3.8	23.2	29.3
Malignant glioma	8.9	1.5	3.1
Diffuse astrocytoma	1.5	0.8	0.6
Anaplastic astrocytoma	2.5	4.4	2.7
Other astrocytoma	9.2	4.1	3.8
Oligodendroglioma	2.3	3.4	0.7
Anaplastic oligodendroglioma	0.8	1.5	0.4
Ependymomas	6.4	0.5	0.4
Mixed glioma	0.8	1.1	0.2
Embryonal/primitive/medulloblastoma	16.0	0.5	0
Meningeal tumors	4.3	29.9	39.6
Meningioma	3.1	28.4	39.1
Hemangioblastoma	0.8	1.2	0.4
Lymphoma	0.5	2.4	2.7
Sellar tumors	6.4	8.7	3.9
Pituitary adenoma	0.8	8.0	3.8
Craniopharyngioma	3.6	0.6	0
Cranial and spinal nerve tumors	2.0	11.3	3.4
Germ cell tumors	4.3	0	0
Local extension from regional tumors	0.5	0.2	0
Unclassified	3.8	2.8	8.5
Total	100.0	100.0	100.0

Source: Adapted from the Central Brain Tumor Registry for the United States, 1995–1999; http://www.cbtrus.org.

germ cells (germinoma, craniopharyngioma, teratoma), or endocrine elements (pituitary adenoma). Table 31-2 provides a detailed tabulation compiled by the Central Brain Tumor Registry. Notable in all series, and emphasized in this table, is the higher frequency of certain tumors during childhood.

The main change since the first edition of this book in 1977 is the increase in incidence of primary CNS lymphomas. At that time, the incidence of this tumor, formerly called reticulum cell sarcoma, was negligible. In the last 25 years, the number in our hospitals has more than tripled; in specialized centers such as the Memorial Sloan-Kettering Cancer Center, the increase has been even more dramatic (DeAngelis). It now represents over 3 percent of all brain tumors. This increase is only partly attributable to the rise in number of immunosuppressed individuals, particularly of those with AIDS, as the tumor appears to be increasing in incidence even in those with normal immune function.

Classification and Grading of Nervous System Tumors

Classifications and grading systems of intracranial tumors abound and are often confusing to the general neurologist. Most classifications have been based on the presumed cell of origin of the neoplasm, while grading systems are meant to be an estimate of the rate of growth and clinical behavior, but the two are often concordant. The most recent World Health Organization (WHO) classification (the fourth revision, 2007) represents the current view of tumor specialists but the entire list is unwieldy for most clinicians. Table 31-3 shows the main items and a discussion of this system can be found in the article by Louis and colleagues (2007). In the past, the numerical grading system of Daumas-Duport and coworkers (also known as the St. Anne–Mayo system) and the three-tiered system of Ringertz (which correlates most closely with clinical survival) were widely used

Table 31-3

MAIN CATEGORIES OF THE WHO BRAIN TUMOR CLASSIFICATION

I. Astrocytic tumors
   A. Noninvasive: Pilocytic and subependymal giant cell astrocytomas and pleomorphic xanthoastrocytoma (grade I)
   B. Diffuse astrocytoma (grade II)
   C. Anaplastic astrocytoma (grade III)
   D. Glioblastoma multiforme (grade IV)
II. Oligodendroglial tumors
   A. Oligodendroglioma (grade II)
   B. Anaplastic (malignant) oligodendroglioma (grade III)
III. Ependymal cell tumors
   A. Ependymoma (grade II)
   B. Anaplastic ependymoma (grade III)
   C. Myxopapillary ependymoma
   D. Subependymoma (grade I)
IV. Mixed gliomas
   A. Mixed oligoastrocytoma (grade II)
   B. Anaplastic (malignant) oligoastrocytoma (grade III)
   C. Others (e.g., ependymoastrocytoma)
V. Neuroepithelial tumors of uncertain origin
   A. Polar spongioblastoma (grade IV)
   B. Astroblastoma (grade IV)
VI. Tumors of the choroid plexus
VII. Neuronal and mixed neuronal-glial tumors
   A. Gangliocytoma
   B. Dysplastic gangliocytoma of cerebellum (Lhermitte-Duclos)
   C. Ganglioma
   D. Anaplastic (malignant) ganglioglioma
   E. Desmoplastic infantile ganglioglioma
   F. Central neurocytoma
   G. Olfactory neuroblastoma (esthesioneuroblastoma)
VIII. Pineal parenchyma tumors
   A. Pineocytoma
   B. Pineoblastoma
   C. Mixed pineocytoma/pineoblastoma
IX. Tumors with neuroblastic or glioblastic elements (embryonal tumors)
   A. Primitive neuroectodermal tumors with multipotent differentiation
      1. Medulloblastoma
      2. Cerebral primitive neuroectodermal tumor
   B. Neuroblastoma
   C. Retinoblastoma
   D. Ependymoblastoma

Other CNS Neoplasms

I. Tumors of the sellar region
   A. Pituitary adenoma
   B. Pituitary carcinoma
   C. Craniopharyngioma
II. Hematopoietic tumors
   A. Primary malignant lymphomas
   B. Plasmacytoma
   C. Granulocytic sarcoma
III. Germ cell tumors
   A. Germinoma
   B. Embryonal carcinoma
   C. Yolk sac tumor (endodermal sinus tumor)
   D. Choriocarcinoma
   E. Teratoma
   F. Mixed germ cell tumors
IV. Tumors of the meninges
   A. Meningioma
   B. Atypical meningioma
   C. Anaplastic (malignant) meningioma
V. Nonmeningothelial tumors of the meninges
   A. Benign mesenchymal including lipoma
   B. Malignant mesenchymal including hemangiopericytoma
   C. Primary melanocytic lesions
   D. Hemopoietic neoplasms—malignant lymphoma
   E. Tumors of uncertain histogenesis
      1. Hemangioblastoma (capillary hemangioblastoma)
VI. Tumors of cranial and spinal nerves
   A. Schwannoma (neurinoma, neurilemoma)
   B. Neurofibroma
   C. Malignant peripheral nerve sheath tumor (malignant schwannoma)
VII. Local extensions from regional tumors
   A. Paraganglioma (chemodectoma)
   B. Chordoma
   C. Chondroma
   D. Chondrosarcoma
   E. Carcinoma
VIII. Metastatic tumors
IX. Cysts and tumor-like lesions
   A. Rathke cleft cyst
   B. Epidermoid
   C. Dermoid
   D. Colloid cyst of the third ventricle
   E. Hypothalamic neuronal hamartoma

(Continued)

Table 31-3

MAIN CATEGORIES OF THE WHO BRAIN TUMOR CLASSIFICATION (*CONTINUED*)

GRADE	I	II	III	IV
Astrocytic tumors				
Subependymal giant cell astrocytoma	•			
Pilocytic astrocytoma	•			
Pilomyxoid astrocytoma		•		
Diffuse astrocytoma		•		
Pleomorphic xanthoastrocytoma		•		
Anaplastic astrocytoma			•	
Glioblastoma				•
Giant cell glioblastoma				•
Gliosarcoma				•
Oligodendroglial tumors				
Oligodendroglioma		•		
Anaplastic oligodendroglioma			•	
Oligoastrocytic tumors				
Oligoastrocytoma		•		
Anaplastic oligoastrocytoma			•	
Ependymal tumors				
Subependymoma	•			
Myxopapillary ependymoma	•			
Ependymoma		•		
Anaplastic ependymoma			•	
Choroid plexus tumors				
Choroid plexus papilloma	•			
Atypical choroid plexus papilloma		•		
Choroid plexus carcinoma			•	
Other neuroepithelial tumors				
Angiocentric glioma	•			
Choroid glioma of the third ventricle		•		
Neuronal and mixed neuronalglial tumors				
Gangliocytoma	•			
Ganglioglioma	•			
Anaplastic ganglioglioma			•	
Desmoplastic infantile astrocytoma and ganglioglioma	•			
Dysembryoplastic neuroepithelial tumor	•			
Central neurocytoma		•		
Extraventricular neurocytoma		•		
Cerebellar liponeurocytoma		•		
Paraganglioma of the spinal cord	•			
Papillary glioneuronal tumor	•			
Rosette-forming glioneuronal tumor of the fourth ventricle	•			
Pineal tumors				
Pineocytoma	•			
Pineal parenchymal tumor of intermediate differentiation		•	•	
Pineoblastoma				•
Papillary tumor of the pineal region		•	•	

Table 31-3

MAIN CATEGORIES OF THE WHO BRAIN TUMOR CLASSIFICATION

GRADE	I	II	III	IV
Embryonal tumors				
Medulloblastoma				•
CNS primitive neuroectodermal tumor (PNET)				•
Atypical teratoid/rhabdoid tumor				•
Tumors of the cranial and paraspinal nerves				
Schwannoma	•			
Neurofibroma	•			
Perineurioma	•	•	•	
Malignant peripheral nerve sheath tumor (MPNST)		•	•	•
Meningeal tumors				
Meningioma	•			
Atypical meningioma		•		
Anaplastic/malignant meningioma			•	
Hemangiopericytoma		•		
Anaplastic hemangiopericytoma			•	
Hemangioblastoma	•			
Tumors of the sellar region				
Craniopharyngioma	•			
Granular cell tumor of the neurohypophysis	•			
Pituicytoma	•			
Spindle cell oncocytoma of the adenohypophysis	•			

and are cited in the literature. The various classification systems notwithstanding, it is clear that there are practical and prognostic consequences to subclassifying tumors by additional molecular methods that are predictive of outcome and of treatment response (see further on).

The *astrocytic tumors*, the most common forms of glioma, have been subdivided into diffuse well-differentiated astrocytoma (grade II), anaplastic astrocytoma (grade III), and glioblastoma (glioblastoma multiforme, or "GBM," grade IV). These grades represent a spectrum in terms of growth potential (degree of nuclear atypia, cellularity, mitoses, and vascular proliferation) and prognosis. The glioblastomas are largely defined by the features of necrosis and anaplasia of nonneural elements such as vascular proliferation and are set apart from anaplastic astrocytomas on the basis not only of their histology but also by a later age of onset than astrocytoma and a more rapid course. The grade I classification for astrocytomas is reserved for the relatively benign group that includes pilocytic astrocytomas (well-differentiated tumors mostly of children and young adults); the pleomorphic xanthoastrocytoma (with lipid-filled cells), and the subependymal giant cell astrocytoma (associated with tuberous sclerosis). They have been set apart because of their different growth patterns, pathologic features, and better prognosis.

The *ependymomas* are subdivided into cellular, myxopapillary, clear cell, and mixed types; the anaplastic ependymoma and the subependymoma are given separate status. The pathologic criteria of malignant astrocytoma do not apply to *oligodendroglioma*, for reasons elaborated further on. They are subdivided into tumors of pure oligodendroglial composition and those with mixed astrocytes and oligodendroglia.

Meningiomas are classified on the basis of their cytoarchitecture and genetic origin into 4 categories: (1) the common meningothelial or syncytial type, (2) the fibroblastic and (3) angioblastic variants, and (4) the malignant type. Tumors of the pineal gland, which were not included in earlier classifications, comprise germ cell tumors, the rare pineocytomas, and pineoblastomas. The *medulloblastoma* has been reclassified with other tumors of presumed neuroectodermal origin, namely neuroblastoma, retinoblastoma, neuroepithelioma, and ependymoblastoma. Tumors derived from the choroid plexus are divided into two classes, both rare: papillomas and carcinomas.

Given separate status also are the intracranial midline germ cell tumors, such as germinoma, teratoma, choriocarcinoma, and endodermal sinus carcinoma. A miscellaneous group comprises CNS lymphoma, hemangioblastoma, chordoma, hemangiopericytoma, spongioblastoma, and ganglioneuroma.

Tumors of cranial and peripheral nerves differentiate into three main types: schwannomas, neurofibromas, and neurofibrosarcomas. Most are sporadic but the neurofibromas assume special importance in neurofibromatosis.

Biology of Nervous System Tumors

In considering this subject, one of the first problems is with the definition of neoplasia. It is well known that a number of lesions may simulate brain tumors in their clinical manifestations and histologic appearance but are really hamartomas and not true tumors. A hamartoma is a "tumor-like formation that has its basis in maldevelopment" (Russell) and undergoes little change during the life of the host. The difficulty one encounters in distinguishing it from a true neoplasm, whose constituent cells multiply without restraint, is well illustrated by tuberous sclerosis and von Recklinghausen neurofibromatosis, where hamartomas and neoplasms are both found. Similarly, in a number of mass lesions—such as certain cerebellar astrocytomas, bipolar astrocytomas of the pons and optic nerves, von Hippel-Lindau cerebellar cysts, and pineal teratomas—a clear distinction between neoplasms and hamartomas is often not possible.

Many studies of the *pathogenesis of brain tumors* have gradually shed light on their origin. Johannes Müller (1838), in his atlas *Structure and Function of Neoplasms*, first enunciated the appealing idea that tumors might originate in embryonic cells left in the brain during development. This idea was elaborated upon by Cohnheim (1878), who postulated that the source of tumors was an anomaly of the embryonic anlage. Ribbert, in 1904, extended this hypothesis by postulating that the potential for differentiation of these stem cells would favor blastomatous growth.

For many years, thinking about the pathogenesis of primary CNS tumors was dominated by the *histogenetic theory* of Bailey and Cushing, which was based on the assumed embryology of nerve and glia cells. Although it is not a popular notion today, Bailey and Cushing attached the suffix *blastoma* to indicate all tumors composed of primitive-looking cells, such as glioblastoma and medulloblastoma. One prominent theory was that most tumors arise from neoplastic transformation of mature adult cells (*dedifferentiation*). A normal astrocyte, oligodendrocyte, microgliocyte, or ependymocyte is transformed into a neoplastic cell and, as it multiplies, the daughter cells become variably anaplastic, more so as the degree of malignancy increases. (*Anaplasia* refers to the more primitive undifferentiated state of the constituent cells.)

In fact, the cells of origin of the major types of brain tumors have not been unequivocally identified or, in many cases, they appear to arise from pluripotential stem cells that reside in the brain, a concept not known in Bailey's time. If this is indeed the case, it may be that the apparent dedifferentiation of tumor cells is an artifact of their histologic appearance and not a fundamental property.

The factor of age plays a central role in the biology of brain tumors. Medulloblastomas, polar spongioblastomas, optic nerve gliomas, and pinealomas occur mainly before the age of 20 years, and meningiomas and glioblastomas are most frequent in the sixth decade of life. A number of mutations, only some inherited, also figure greatly in the genesis of certain tumors, particularly retinoblastomas, neurofibromas, and hemangioblastomas. The gliomas associated with neurofibromatosis and tuberous sclerosis and the cerebellar hemangioblastomas of von Hippel-Lindau are the best examples of a genetic determinant. The rare familial disorders of multiple endocrine neoplasia and multiple hamartomas are associated with an increased incidence of anterior pituitary tumors and meningiomas, respectively. Glioblastomas and cerebral astrocytomas have also been reported occasionally in more than one member of a family but the study of such families has not disclosed the operation of an identifiable genetic factor.

Although there is only indirect evidence for an association between viruses and certain primary tumors of the nervous system, epidemiologic and experimental data—drawn from studies of the human papillomavirus and the hepatitis B, Epstein-Barr, and human T-lymphotropic viruses—indicate that they may be involved or act as risk factors in certain human cancers. The genes of Epstein-Barr virus (EBV), for example, are incorporated into the DNA of many cerebral lymphomas. In transgenic mice, certain viruses are capable of inducing olfactory neuroblastomas and neurofibromas. Each of these viruses possesses a small number of genes that are incorporated in a cellular component of the nervous system (usually a dividing cell such as an astrocyte, oligodendrocyte, ependymocyte, endothelial cell, or lymphocyte). The virus is believed to act to force the cell from its normal activity into an unrestrained replicative cycle. Because of this capacity to transform the cellular genome, the virus product is called an *oncogene*; such oncogenes are capable of immortalizing, so to speak, the stimulated cell to form a tumor. Oncogenes are also found in normal cells and may contain mutations or are capable of being activated by cellular and environmental (epigenetic) events as noted later.

Molecular and Genetic Features of Brain Tumors The above concepts have been expanded greatly by the identification of certain genetic aberrations that arise in tumor cells of the nervous system. What has emerged from these studies is the view that the biogenesis and progression of brain tumors are a consequence of defects in the control of the cell cycle. Some molecular defects predispose to tumor genesis; others underlie subsequent progression and accelerated malignant transformation and yet others may confer sensitivity or resistance to chemotherapeutic agents. This model presupposes the acquisition of multiple genetic defects over time since, with the exception of special inherited conditions such as neurofibromatosis, ataxia telangectasia, and a few others, these are not germ line mutations but are acquired as somatic events in the course of tumor evolution.

In cases that have an inherited and transmissible germ line defect there may be additional events that also cause somatic genetic mutations. Typically, inherited mutations affect only one of two copies of a tumor suppressor gene that, by itself, does not cause cancer. However, if the second copy of the gene acquires a mutation (e.g., from a chemical toxin or irradiation) the tumor suppression function of the gene is lost and neoplastic transformation of the cell becomes likely. These ideas are consistent with the observation that many of the gene defects that predispose to cancer are dominantly inherited. More recently, single nucleotide polymorphisms have been identified that in combination predispose to certain childhood tumors such as neuroblastoma, or to the more aggressive forms of various tumors.

The above model is illustrated by consideration of the astrocytoma. Among the first detectable changes are mutations acquired in the act of neoplastic cell division that inactivate the tumor suppressor gene *p53* on chromosome 17p; over 50 percent of astrocytomas have deletions within this gene. Other early changes include overexpression of genes that control growth factors or their receptors as noted below. After the tumor develops, progression to a more malignant grade of astrocytoma or to a glioblastoma may be triggered by defects in the *p16*-retinoblastoma gene signaling pathway, loss of chromosome 10 (seen in approximately 90 percent of high-grade gliomas), or overexpression of the epidermal growth factor gene. In fact, it is striking that analysis of the patterns of these defects in some tumors correlates with the staging and aggressive characteristics of these tumors. The events that lead to their accumulation are not clear, as noted below. Also, mutations in the genes that code for isocitrate dehydrogenase(IDH1 and 2) are common in gliomas and oligodendrogliomas and their presence relates to less tumor progression.

Knowledge of the molecular signatures of certain tumors may have considerable clinical value. For example, oligodendrogliomas that have combined deletions in chromosomes 1p and 19q respond well to chemotherapy and this property increases survival (Reifenberger and Louis; Louis et al, 2002). The childhood tumors of neuroectodermal origin would seem to be particularly attractive as models to explore genetic alterations and indeed, various changes such as the amplification of the *MYCN* oncogene has been associated with an aggressive clinical course and poor outcome in neuroblastoma and medulloblastoma.

Much of the modern genetic understanding of brain tumors is derived from the technical gene microarrays. The patterns of these multiple gene analyses are able to distinguish some types of medulloblastomas from the similar-appearing, primitive neuroectodermal tumors; the medulloblastomas express classes of genes that are characteristic of cerebellar granule cells, suggesting they arise from these cells. Also, gene expression signatures confer useful prognostic information in a more general way than noted above for oligodendroglioma. For example, medulloblastomas that express genes indicative of cerebellar differentiation are associated with longer survival than those expressing genes related to cell division (Pomeroy et al).

As alluded to earlier, in approximately 50 percent of gliomas there is an overexpression or a mutant form of epidermal growth factor receptor (EGFR) and of platelet-derived transforming growth factor receptor (PDGFR), suggesting a role for these in the progression of certain tumor types. Other trophic factors are overexpressed in yet other brain neoplasms and perhaps contribute to their morphology and growth pattern; for example, vascular endothelial growth factor (VEGF) is found in extremely high concentrations in meningiomas, which are highly vascular by nature. These findings, taken together, suggest an autocrine stimulation of growth by these factors and an interaction with some of the aforementioned gene defects. However, having emphasized molecular and chromosomal changes, it is not yet clear that any of them is truly causative or if they simply reflect an aberrant genetic process that accompanies the evolution of tumor growth and progression.

Finally, epigenetic events related to the attachment of histones to various tumor genes alter transcription in ways that may be relevant to growth and treatment effects. The best studied of these is the methylation status of the promoter of MGMT, a methyltransferase that alters sensitivity of the glioma to chemotherapy (see further on).

On the basis of this molecular information, views of the pathogenesis of neoplasia are being cast along new lines. Some of the specifics of these new data are presented in the following discussions of particular tumor types. A more extensive review can be found in the article by Osborne and colleagues, and the text by Kaye and Laws.

Pathophysiology of Brain Tumors

The production of symptoms by tumor growth is governed by certain principles of mechanics and physiology, some of which were discussed in Chaps. 17 and 30. There it was pointed out that the cranial cavity has a restricted volume, and the three elements contained therein—the brain (about 1,200 to 1,400 mL), cerebrospinal fluid (CSF; 70 to 140 mL), and blood (150 mL)—are relatively but not entirely incompressible, particularly the brain substance, and each is subject to displacement by a localized mass lesion. According to the Monro-Kellie doctrine, the total bulk of the three elements is at all times constant, and any increase in the volume of one of them must be at the expense of the others, as discussed in Chap. 30. A tumor growing in one part of the brain therefore compresses the surrounding brain tissue and displaces CSF and blood; once the limit of this accommodation is reached, the intracranial pressure (ICP) rises. The elevation of ICP and perioptic pressure impairs axonal transport in the optic nerve and the venous drainage from the optic nerve head and retina, manifesting in papilledema.

Only some brain tumors cause papilledema and many others—often quite as large—do not. Thus one may question whether the Monro-Kellie doctrine and its simple implied relationships of intracranial volume and CSF pressure fully account for the development of raised ICP and papilledema with brain tumors. This discrepancy is in part because in a slow process, such as tumor growth, brain tissue is to some degree compressible, as one might suspect from the large indentations of brain produced by massive meningiomas.

The slow growth of most tumors permits accommodation of the brain to changes in cerebral blood flow and ICP. Only in the advanced stages of tumor growth do the compensatory mechanisms fail and CSF pressure and ICP rise, with consequences described in Chap. 30. Once pressure is raised in a particular compartment of the cranium, the tumor begins to displace tissue at first locally and at a distance from the tumor, resulting in a number of *false localizing* signs, including coma, described in Chap. 17. Indeed, the transtentorial herniations, the paradoxical corticospinal signs of Kernohan and Woltman, sixth- and third-nerve palsies, occipital lobe infarcts, midbrain hemorrhages, and secondary hydrocephalus were all originally described in tumor cases (see further on, under "Brain Displacements and Herniations").

Brain Edema

Brain edema is such a prominent feature of cerebral neoplasm that this is a suitable place to summarize what is known about it. With tumor growth, the venules in the cerebral tissue adjacent to the tumor are compressed, with resulting elevation of capillary pressure, particularly in the cerebral white matter where edema is most prominent.

It has been recognized that conditions leading to peripheral edema, such as hypoalbuminemia and increased systemic venous pressure, do not have a similar effect on the brain. By contrast, lesions that alter the blood–brain barrier cause rapid swelling of brain tissue. Klatzo specified two categories of edema: *vasogenic* and *cytotoxic*. Fishman added a third, which he called *interstitial* edema. An example of the latter is the edema that occurs with obstructive hydrocephalus, especially when the ependymal lining is disrupted and CSF seeps into the periventricular tissues in the spaces between cells and myelin. Most neuropathologists use the term *interstitial* to refer to any increase in the extravascular intercellular compartment of the brain; this would include both vasogenic and interstitial edema.

Vasogenic edema is the type seen in the vicinity of tumor growths and other localized processes as well as in more diffuse injury to the blood vessels (e.g., lead encephalopathy, malignant hypertension). It is practically limited to the white matter and is evidenced by decreased attenuation on CT and by hyperintensity on T2-weighted MRI and elevated diffusivity (reduced anisotropy) on diffusion-weighted MRI. Presumably, there is increased permeability of the capillary endothelial cells so that plasma proteins exude into the extracellular spaces (Fig. 31-1A). This heightened permeability has been attributed to a defect in the tight endothelial cell junctions, but current evidence indicates that active vesicular transport of water across the endothelial cells is a more important factor.

Microvascular transudative factors, such as proteases released by tumor cells, also contribute to vasogenic edema by loosening the blood–brain barrier and allowing passage of blood proteins. The small protein fragments that are generated by this protease activity may exert osmotic effects as they spread through the white matter of the brain. This is the postulated basis of the regional swelling, or *localized cerebral edema* that surrounds the tumor. Experimentally, the increase in permeability has been shown to vary inversely with the molecular weight of various markers; e.g., inulin (molecular weight: 5,000) enters the intercellular space more readily than albumin (molecular weight: 70,000).

The vulnerability of white matter to vasogenic edema is not well understood; probably its loose structural organization offers less resistance to fluid under

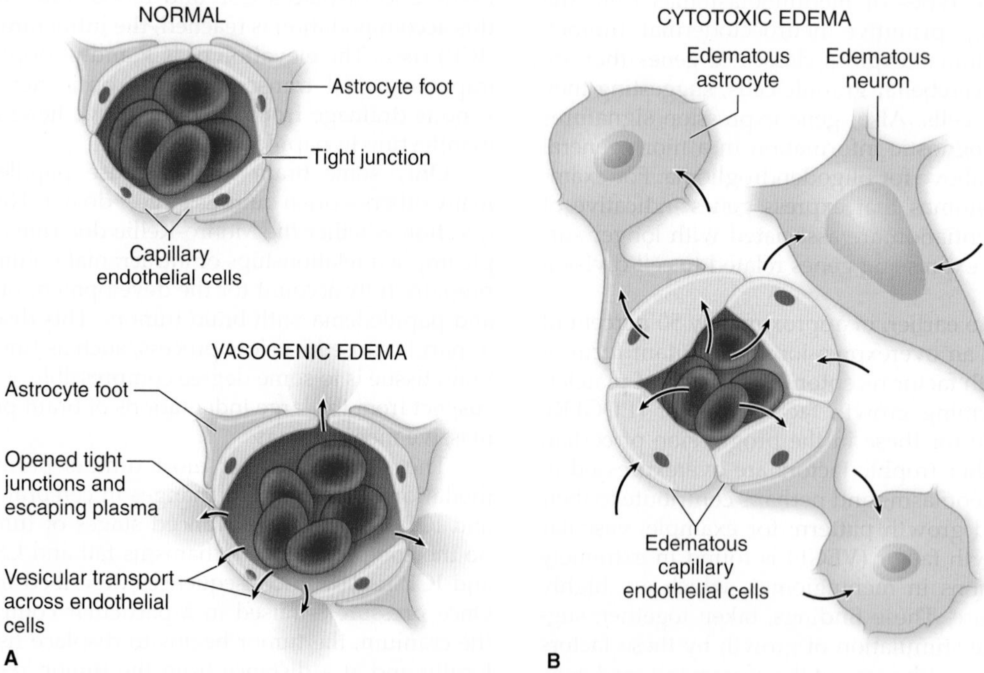

Figure 31-1. *A.* Schematic representation of the astrocytes and endothelial cells of the capillary wall in the normal state (*above*) and in vasogenic edema (*below*). Heightened permeability in vasogenic edema is partly the result of a defect in tight endothelial junctions, but mainly a result of active vesicular transport across endothelial cells. *B.* Cellular (cytotoxic) edema, showing swelling of the endothelial, glial, and neuronal cells at the expense of the extracellular fluid space of the brain. (Reproduced by permission from Fishman.)

pressure than the gray matter. There may also be special morphologic characteristics of white matter capillaries. The accumulation of plasma filtrate, with its high protein content, in the extracellular spaces and between the layers of myelin sheaths would be expected to alter the ionic balance of nerve fibers, impairing their function but this has never been demonstrated satisfactorily.

By contrast, in *cytotoxic edema*, all the cellular elements (neurons, glia, and endothelial cells) swell with fluid and there is a corresponding reduction in the extracellular fluid space. Because a shift of water occurs from the extracellular to the intracellular compartment, there is relatively little mass effect, the opposite of what occurs with the vascular leak of vasogenic edema. This cellular edema occurs typically with hypoxic–ischemic injury but it may also complicate acute hypoosmolality of the plasma, acute hepatic encephalopathy, inappropriate secretion of antidiuretic hormone, and the osmotic disequilibrium syndrome of hemodialysis (see discussion of hyponatremia and "dialysis disequilibrium syndrome" in Chap. 40). The effect of oxygen deprivation is the cause of failure of the adenosine triphosphate (ATP)-dependent sodium pump within cells; sodium accumulates in the cells, and water follows (Fig. 31-1B). The term *cellular edema* may be preferable to *cytotoxic edema* because it emphasizes intracellular ionic movement and not the implication of a toxic factor.

Like vasogenic edema, cytotoxic edema results in decreased attenuation in CT and hyperintensity on T2-weighted MRI. However, it is coupled with reduced diffusivity (increased anisotropy) rather than elevated diffusivity on diffusion-weighted MRI. In the case of cerebral infarction, an initial phase of cytotoxic edema precedes the onset of vasogenic edema, manifest as early reduced diffusivity followed by later elevated diffusivity on diffusion-weighted MRI.

Interstitial (hydrocephalic) edema, as defined by Fishman, is a recognizable condition but is probably of less clinical significance than cytotoxic or cellular edema. In tension hydrocephalus, the edema can extend for up to 2 to 3 mm from the ventricular wall. However, MRI suggests that the periventricular edema is more extensive than what is observed pathologically. There are also experimental data to show that a transependymal or periventricular route is utilized for absorption of CSF in hydrocephalus (Rosenberg et al).

Treatment of Brain Edema and Raised ICP

(See "Management of Raised Intracranial Pressure" in Chap. 35)

The treatment of brain edema and elevated ICP is governed by the underlying disease (excision of a tumor, treatment of intracranial infection, placement of a shunt, etc.). Here we consider the therapeutic measures that can be directed against the edema itself and the raised ICP as they apply to brain tumor.

The use of high-potency glucocorticosteroids has a beneficial effect on the vasogenic edema associated with tumors, both primary and metastatic, sometimes beginning within hours. Probably these steroids act directly on the endothelial cells, reducing their permeability. Steroids also shrink normal brain tissue, thus reducing overall intracranial pressure. Drugs such as dexamethasone also reduce the vasogenic edema associated with brain abscess and head injury, but their usefulness in these cases and in large cerebral infarctions, contusions, and hemorrhage is less clear; in fact, most attempts to demonstrate benefit in all conditions but brain tumors have proven negative. The swelling surrounding necrotic tissue is reduced; however, there is no evidence that cytotoxic or cellular edema responds to administration of glucocorticoids.

For patients with brain tumor, it is common practice initially to use doses of dexamethasone of approximately 4 mg q6h, or the equivalent dose of methylprednisolone. Although a few patients require a rigid schedule, a dose with meals and at bedtime usually suffices to suppress headache and focal tumor signs. In patients with large tumors and marked secondary edema, further benefit is sometimes achieved by the administration of extremely high doses of dexamethasone, to a total of 100 mg/d or more for a brief time. An initial dose may be given intravenously. Always to be kept in mind are the potentially serious side effects of sustained steroid administration, even at standard dose levels. Rare complications, such as aseptic necrosis of the hip, are sometimes idiosyncratic; consequently, the schedule should be organized around the desired clinical effect. It is also recognized that these drugs interfere with the metabolism of certain anticonvulsants commonly used in brain tumor patients.

In patients who have brain edema and who require intravenous fluids, one avoids solutions containing water ("free water") not matched by equivalent amounts of sodium. Normal saline (314 mOsm/L) is preferable, and lactated Ringer solution (osmolarity 289 mOsm/L) is acceptable, but dextrose solutions alone, in any concentration (except D5/NS), are avoided because of their hypoosmolar concentration.

The parenteral administration of hypertonic solutions, to which the brain is only partially permeable (mannitol, hypertonic saline, urea, glycerol), by shifting water from brain to plasma, is an effective means of rapidly reducing brain volume and lowering ICP as discussed more extensively in Chap. 35 in relation to trauma as we have summarized elsewhere in a review (Ropper). These agents are useful in urgent circumstances but have a diminishing effect over days. Edema, however, is actually little affected by shrinkage of the remaining normal brain provides most of the internal decompression.

Mannitol is the most widely used osmotic agent; a 25 percent solution is administered parenterally in a dose of 0.5 to 1.0 g/kg body weight over a period of 2 to 10 min. Hypertonic saline solutions (3, 7, or 23 percent) are equally effective. Repeated use on a regular schedule can lead to a reduction in headache and stabilization of some of the deleterious effects of a tumor. Diuretic drugs, notably acetazolamide and furosemide, may be helpful in special instances (interstitial edema, pseudotumor cerebri) by virtue of creating a hyperosmolar state and by reducing the formation of CSF. However, their effects are usually mild and transient.

Highly permeable solutes such as glucose do little to reduce brain volume, as they do not create an osmolar gradient that shifts water from the brain to the vasculature.

Furthermore, with repeated administration of hyperosmolar solutions such as mannitol or with diuretics, the brain gradually increases its osmolality—the result of added intracellular solute; thus these agents are not suitable for long-term use. The notion that hyperosmolar agents might exaggerate tissue shifts by shrinking normal brain tissue has not been substantiated. The net effect of hyperosmolar therapy is reflected roughly by the degree of hyperosmolarity and hypernatremia that is attained.

Controlled hyperventilation is another method of rapidly reducing brain volume by producing respiratory alkalosis and cerebral vasoconstriction; it is used mainly in cases of brain trauma with high ICP (see Chap. 35), during intracranial surgery, and in the management of patients who have become acutely comatose from the mass effect of a tumor, but its effect is brief.

Brain Displacements and Herniations

(See also Chap. 17)

An understanding of the effects of elevated intracranial pressure, localized vasogenic edema, and displacements of tissue and herniations are absolutely essential to understanding the clinical behavior of intracranial tumors and mass lesions of any type. Often the symptoms of intracranial tumors are related more to these effects than to invasion or destruction of neurologic structures by the tumor. The several "false localizing" signs (coma, unilateral or bilateral abducens palsy, pupillary changes, ipsilateral or bilateral corticospinal tract signs, etc.) are also attributable to these mechanical changes and tissue displacements. The main aspects of this problem, particularly the coma-producing mechanisms, were considered in Chap. 17. The pressure from a mass within any one dural compartment causes shifts or herniations of brain tissue to an adjacent compartment where the pressure is lower. The three well-known herniations are *subfalcial*, *transtentorial*, and *cerebellar–foramen magnum* (see Fig. 17-1), and there are several less familiar ones (*upward cerebellar-tentorial*, *diencephalic–sella turcica*, and *orbital frontal–middle cranial fossa [transalar]*). Herniation of swollen brain through an acquired defect in the calvarium, in relation to craniocerebral trauma or surgical craniotomy, is yet another (transcalvarial) type.

Subfalcial herniation, in which the cingulate gyrus is pushed under the falx, occurs frequently, but little is known of its clinical manifestations except that there may be occlusion of an anterior cerebral artery and resultant frontal lobe infarction. The *cerebellar–foramen magnum herniation* or *pressure cone* described by Cushing in 1917 consists of downward displacement of the inferomedial parts of the cerebellar hemispheres (mainly the ventral paraflocculi or tonsillae) through the foramen magnum, dorsolateral to the cervical cord. The clinical manifestations are less well delineated than those of the temporal lobe–tentorial herniation. Cushing considered the typical signs of cerebellar herniation to be episodic tonic extension and arching of the neck and back and extension and internal rotation of the limbs, with respiratory disturbances, cardiac irregularity (bradycardia or tachycardia), and loss of consciousness.

Other signs with subacutely evolving masses in the posterior fossa include pain in the neck, stiff neck, head tilt, and paresthesias in the shoulders, dysphagia, and loss of tendon reflexes in the arms. Head tilt, stiff neck, arching of the neck, and paresthesias over the shoulders are attributable to the herniation of the cerebellar tonsils into the foramen magnum, and tonic extensor spasms of the limbs and body (so-called cerebellar fits) and coma are caused by the compressive effects of the cerebellar mass on medullary structures or of hydrocephalus on upper brainstem structures. In any case, *respiratory arrest* is the feared and often fatal effect of medullary compression by a "cerebellar pressure cone." It may occur suddenly, without the aforementioned additional signs. With cerebellar mass lesions there may also be *upward herniation* of the cerebellum through the incisura of the tentorium. The clinical effects have not been clearly determined, but Cuneo and colleagues have attributed decerebrate posturing and pupillary changes—initially both pupils are miotic but still reactive, progressing to anisocoria and enlargement—to this type of brain displacement.

CLINICAL AND PATHOLOGIC CHARACTERISTICS OF BRAIN TUMORS

It should be stated at the outset that tumors of the brain often exist with hardly any symptoms. A slight bewilderment, slowness in comprehension, or loss of capacity for sustained mental activity may be the only deviations from normal, and signs of focal cerebral disease are wholly lacking. In some patients, on the other hand, there is early indication of cerebral disease in the form of a progressive hemiparesis, a seizure occurring in a previously well person, or some other dramatic symptom. In a third group, the existence of a brain tumor can be assumed because of the presence of increased intracranial pressure with or without localizing signs of the tumor. In yet another group, the symptoms are so definite as to make it likely that not only is there an intracranial neoplasm but that it is of a certain type and is located in a particular region. These localized growths create certain syndromes seldom caused by any other disease.

In the further exposition of this subject, intracranial tumors are considered in relation to these common modes of clinical presentation:

1. Patients who present with focal cerebral signs and general impairment of cerebral function, headaches, or seizures
2. Patients who present with evidence of increased intracranial pressure
3. Patients who present with specific intracranial tumor syndromes

Patients Presenting with General Impairment of Cerebral Function, Headaches, and Seizures

Altered mental function, headache, dizziness, and seizures are the usual manifestations in this group of patients. Until the advent of modern imaging procedures, these were the patients who presented the greatest difficulty in diagnosis and about whom decisions were often made with a great degree of uncertainty. Their initial symptoms are vague, and not until some time has elapsed will signs of focal brain disease appear; when they do, they are not always of accurate localizing value.

Changes in Mental Function

A lack of persistent application to everyday tasks, undue irritability, emotional lability, mental inertia, faulty insight, forgetfulness, reduced range of mental activity (judged by inquiring about the patient's introspections and manifested in his conversation), indifference to common social practices, lack of initiative and spontaneity—all of which may be misattributed to anxiety or depression—make up the cognitive and behavioral abnormalities seen in this clinical circumstance. Inordinate drowsiness or apathy may be prominent. We have sought a convenient term for this complex of symptoms, which is perhaps the most common type of mental disturbance encountered with neurologic disease, but none seems entirely appropriate. There is both a reduction in the amount of thought and action and a slowing of reaction time. MacCabe referred to this condition as "mental asthenia," which has the merit of distinguishing it from depression.

Much of this change in behavior is accepted by the patient with forbearance; if any complaint is made, it is of being weak, tired, or dizzy (nonvertiginous). Within a few weeks or months, these symptoms become more prominent. When the patient is questioned, a long pause precedes each reply (abulia); at times the patient may not respond at all. Or, at the moment the examiner decides that the patient has not heard the question and prepares to repeat it, an appropriate answer is given, usually in few words. Moreover, the responses are often more intelligent than one would expect, considering the patient's torpid mental state. Many of these features will be recognized as components of a frontal lobe syndrome, but the tumor is often situated elsewhere, or is diffusely infiltrative. There are, in addition, patients who are overtly confused or demented. If the condition remains untreated, dullness and somnolence increase gradually and, finally, as increased intracranial pressure supervenes, the patient progresses to stupor or coma.

Headaches (See also "Headaches of Brain Tumor" in Chap. 10)

These are an early symptom in fewer than 25 percent of patients with brain tumor and are variable in nature. In some, the pain is slight, dull, and episodic; in others, it is severe and either dull or sharp but also intermittent. If there are any characteristic features of the headache, they would be its nocturnal occurrence or presence on first awakening and perhaps its deep, nonpulsatile quality. However, these are not specific attributes, as migraine and hypertensive vascular headaches may also begin in the early morning hours or upon awakening. But if vomiting occurs at the peak of the head pain, tumor is more likely, as noted later. Occipitonuchal headache with vomiting is indicative of a tumor in or near the cerebellum and foramen magnum and is one typical presentation in children.

Patients with brain tumors do not always complain of head pain even when it is present, but they may betray its existence by placing their hands to their heads and looking distressed. When headache appears in the course of the psychomotor asthenia syndrome, it serves to clarify the diagnosis, but not nearly as much as does the occurrence of a seizure.

The mechanism of the headache is not fully understood and there may be more than one pathophysiology. In the majority of instances, the CSF pressure is normal during the first weeks when the headache is present, and one can attribute it only to local swelling of tissues and to distortion of blood vessels in the dura overlying the tumor. Later, the headache may be related to increases in intracranial pressure, thus the early morning occurrence after recumbency and vomiting, as discussed in Chap. 10. Tumors above the tentorium cause headache on the side of the tumor and in its vicinity, in the orbitofrontal, temporal, or parietal region; tumors in the posterior fossa usually cause ipsilateral retroauricular or occipital headache. With elevated intracranial pressure, bifrontal or bioccipital headache is the rule regardless of the location of the tumor.

Vomiting and Dizziness

Vomiting appears in a relatively small number of patients with a tumor syndrome and usually accompanies the headache when the latter is severe. It is more frequent with tumors of the posterior fossa. The most persistent vomiting (lasting several weeks) that we have observed has been in patients with low brainstem gliomas, fourth ventricular ependymomas, and subtentorial meningiomas. Some patients may vomit unexpectedly and forcibly without preceding nausea ("projectile vomiting"), a sign that is fairly specific to tumor in children, but others suffer nausea and severe discomfort. Usually the vomiting is not related to the ingestion of food, and, often, it occurs before breakfast.

No less frequent is the complaint of *dizziness*. As a rule it is not described with accuracy and consists of an unnatural sensation in the head, coupled with feelings of strangeness and insecurity when the position of the head is altered. Positional vertigo can be a symptom of a tumor in the posterior fossa affecting vestibular structures, but has many other more common and benign causes (see Chap. 15).

Seizures

The occurrence of focal or generalized seizures is the other major manifestation of brain tumor besides slowing of mental functions and signs of focal brain damage. Convulsions have been observed in 20 to 50 percent of all patients with cerebral tumors. *A first seizure during adulthood is always suggestive of brain tumor and, in the authors' experience, has been the most common initial manifestation of primary and metastatic neoplasm.* The localizing significance of seizure patterns was discussed in Chap. 16. Seizures caused by brain tumor most often have a focal onset and may secondarily generalize. There may be one seizure or many, and they may follow the other symptoms or precede them by weeks or months or—exceptionally, in patients with low-grade astrocytoma, oligodendroglioma, or meningioma—by several years. Status epilepticus as an early event from brain tumor is rare but has occurred in a few of our patients. As a rule, the seizures respond to standard antiepileptic medications and may improve after surgery for tumor resection.

Patients Presenting with Regional or Localizing Symptoms and Signs (Glioblastoma Multiforme, Astrocytoma, Oligodendroglioma, Ependymoma, Metastatic Carcinoma, Meningioma, and Primary Lymphoma

Sooner or later, focal cerebral signs will be discovered in most patients with brain tumors. Most often the focal signs are at first slight and subtle, but some patients present with such signs. In the modern era of ubiquitous imaging for all manner of cerebral complaints, CT or MRI often will have disclosed the presence of a tumor before either focal cerebral signs or the signs of increased intracranial pressure have become evident.

The cerebral tumors that are most likely to produce the syndromes of asthenia, headache, seizures, or focal signs are the ones listed above in the heading. The clinical aspects of these diseases, which happen to be the most common brain tumors in adults, are discussed in the sections below.

Glioblastoma Multiforme and Anaplastic Astrocytoma

These high-grade gliomas account for approximately 20 percent of all intracranial tumors and for more than 80 percent of gliomas of the cerebral hemispheres in adults. Although predominantly cerebral in location, they may also arise in the brainstem, cerebellum, or spinal cord. The peak incidence is in middle adult life (mean age for the occurrence of glioblastoma is approximately 60 years, and 46 years for anaplastic astrocytoma), but no age group is exempt. The incidence is higher in men (ratio of approximately 1.6:1). Almost all of the high-grade gliomas occur sporadically, without a familial predilection.

The glioblastoma, known since the time of Virchow, was definitively recognized as a glioma by Bailey and Cushing and given a place in their histogenetic classification. They are now listed as grade IV glial tumors in the WHO classification. Most arise in the deep white matter as a heterogenous mass and quickly infiltrate the brain extensively, sometimes attaining enormous size before attracting medical attention.

The tumor may extend to the meningeal surface or the ventricular wall, which probably accounts for the increase in CSF protein (more than 100 mg/dL in many cases), as well as for an occasional pleocytosis of 10 to 100 cells or more, mostly lymphocytes. The CSF is usually normal, however. Malignant cells, carried in the CSF, rarely may form distant foci on spinal roots or cause a widespread meningeal gliomatosis. Extraneural metastases, involving bone and lymph nodes, are very rare; usually they occur only after a craniotomy has been performed. Approximately 50 percent of glioblastomas occupy more than one lobe of a hemisphere; between 3 and 6 percent show multicentric foci of growth and thereby simulate metastatic cancer. A legitimate question is whether these tumors can have a multicentric origin or spread via CSF pathways. We have the impression that the first configuration does exist.

The tumor has a variegated appearance, being a mottled gray, red, orange, or brown, depending on the degree of necrosis and presence of hemorrhage, recent or old. The imaging appearance is usually that of an inhomogeneous mass, often with a center that is hypointense and nonenhancing. An irregular rim of enhancement surrounds the core lesion, and is surrounded by nonenhancing edematous brain tissue, consisting of a combination of infiltrating tumor cells and vasogenic edema (Fig. 31-2). It is not uncommon to see small nodular enhancing lesions adjacent to, but distinct from, the primary lesion. Part of one lateral ventricle is often distorted, and both lateral and third ventricles may be displaced.

The characteristic histologic findings of glioblastoma are hypercellularity with pleomorphism of cells and nuclear atypia; identifiable astrocytes with fibrils in combination with primitive forms in many cases; tumor giant cells and cells in mitosis; hyperplasia of endothelial cells of small vessels; and necrosis, hemorrhage, and thrombosis of vessels. This variegated appearance distinguishes glioblastoma from the anaplastic astrocytomas, which show frequent mitoses and atypical cytogenic features but no grossly necrotic or hemorrhagic areas. It is the necrotic and sometimes cystic areas that appear hypointense on imaging studies. An MRI study by Ulmer and colleagues showed that 70 percent of patients show evidence of a small region of infarction immediately surrounding the tumor in the postoperative period;

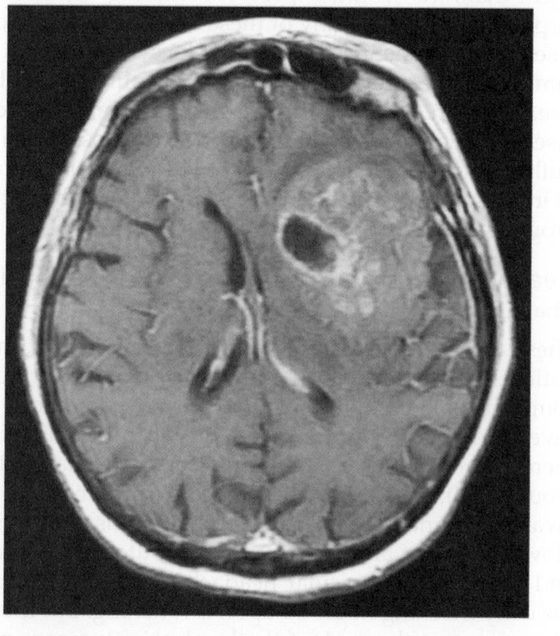

Figure 31-2. Glioblastoma multiforme. Contrast-enhanced T1-weighted MRI illustrates a large irregularly enhancing tumor with internal necrosis deep within the left cerebral hemisphere.

most of the affected areas also demonstrate these cystic encephalomalacic areas. The vasculature and fibroblasts can undergo a sarcomatous transformation giving the tumor a mixed appearance that is termed *gliosarcoma*.

Originally, glioblastoma was thought to be derived from and composed of primitive embryonal cells, or, in the late decades of the twentieth century, to arise through anaplasia of maturing astrocytes. However, these views have been called into question because models of malignant transformation of neural stem cells or of glial progenitor cells explain many of the characteristics and behavior of gliomas. The location, cellular and genetic heterogeneity, and manner of growth and spread of these tumors are consistent with an origin in a primitive cell. Sanai and colleagues have summarized the case for stem cell origin, but this notion is not universally accepted and potential deficiencies in this theory are noted by Reid and coworkers. The genetic or epigenetic events that putatively lead to a malignant evolution of these progenitor cells are not known. Ironically, this is a reversion to the idea of the early last century that posited an embryonal origin of glioma.

The histologic grade may vary from site to site within a tumor and it is common for sites of low-grade astrocytoma and glioblastoma to coexist; in some high-grade tumors there are even sites of well-differentiated astrocytoma. This relates to a problem that arises in interpreting single small biopsy samples taken for diagnosis. It is a fair statement that the most aggressive component (e.g., glioblast elements) determines the tumor's behavior.

To some extent, this behavior is also related to the genetic changes described earlier under "Molecular and Genetic Features of Brain Tumors." Amplification of the *EGFR* gene is characteristic in older patients with tumors that begin entirely as glioblastomas, whereas acquired mutations of the *p53* gene tend to occur in younger individuals whose tumors progress from an astrocytoma to a glioblastoma. More recently, the progression of astrocytomas and oligodendrogliomas to more malignant forms has been related to the enzyme isocitrate dehydrogenase, encoded by the genes *IDH1* and *IDH2*. Patients with mutations in these genes had better outcomes and slower tumor progression as presented by Yan and colleagues. The change in EGFR, a receptor tyrosine kinase that is implicated in the growth of a number of solid tumors, and other acquired mutations and epigenetic alterations, such as in the MGMT promoter gene discussed further on, are proving to be predictors of responsiveness to chemotherapeutic agents and of prognosis, as noted later in the chapter. Other tumors display underexpression of the tumor suppressor gene *PTEN*. It is likely that genetic analyses of tumor material from individual patients will become an increasingly important part of therapeutic decisions.

The natural history of untreated glioblastoma is well characterized. Fewer than 20 percent of patients survive for 1 year after the onset of symptoms and only about 10 percent live beyond 2 years (Shapiro). Age is an important prognostic factor; fewer than 10 percent of patients older than age 60 years survive for 18 months, in comparison to two-thirds of patients younger than age 40 years. Survival with anaplastic astrocytoma is somewhat better, typically 3 to 5 years. Cerebral edema and increased intracranial pressure are usually the causes of death. Survival rates with treatment are discussed below.

The diagnosis must be confirmed by a stereotactic biopsy or by a craniotomy that aims to remove as much tumor as is feasible at the same time.

Treatment At operation, usually only part of the tumor can be removed; its multicentricity and diffusely infiltrative character defy the scalpel. Partial resection of the tumor ("debulking"), however, seems to prolong survival as noted below. Neurosurgeons have developed a number of cortical electrophysiologic mapping and imaging techniques to facilitate maximal resection without injuring adjacent brain tissue.

Except for palliation, little can be done to alter the course of glioblastoma. For a brief period, corticosteroids, usually dexamethasone in doses of 4 to 10 mg q6–12h, are helpful if there are symptoms of mass effect, such as headache or drowsiness; local signs and surrounding edema tend to improve as well. Antiepileptic medications are not required unless there have been seizures. Although some neurologists and neurosurgeons still administer them in order to preempt a convulsion, several series have found antiepileptic medications to be unnecessary for this purpose. Serious skin reactions (erythema multiforme and Stevens-Johnson syndrome) may occur in patients receiving phenytoin at the same time as cranial radiation (Delattre et al). A maximally feasible resection, the debulking described above, is combined with radiation and chemotherapy. Cranial irradiation to a total dose of 6,000 cGy increases survival by 5 months on average (see below). This is true even in the elderly who have had only a biopsy without resection according to a trial conducted by Keime-Guibert and colleagues.

It had been considered for several decades that the addition of chemotherapeutic nitrosourea agents such as carmustine (BCNU) or lomustine (CCNU) increase survival slightly. Cisplatin and carboplatin have provided similar small marginal improvements in survival beyond that obtained by debulking and radiation therapy. Several randomized trials, however, have failed to show substantial benefit of chemotherapy but the Glioma Meta-analysis Trialists (GMT) Group had concluded in 2002 that there was a clear but quite small benefit of chemotherapy.

The methylating agent temozolomide, given in the form of an orally administered prodrug, has lower toxicity and has been shown in several trials to produce slightly superior results to the aforementioned agents. In a large trial conducted by Stupp and colleagues, the median survival was 14.6 months with radiation and temozolomide, compared to 12.1 months with radiation alone, but 2-year survival was more than doubled from 10 to 27 percent. The drug is administered daily (75 mg/m^2) concurrently with radiotherapy and, after a hiatus of 4 weeks, given for 5 d every 28 d for 6 cycles. Its main complications are thrombocytopenia or leukopenia in 5 to 10 percent of patients, and rare cases of *Pneumocystis carinii* pneumonia. Furthermore, high levels of a methyltransferase protein (MGMT) in some glioblastomas lead to resistance to chemotherapy. Hegi and colleagues found a relationship between the epigenetic silencing of the promoter of this gene ("methylation status") and the response to temozolomide. In fact, almost all the marginal benefit of the drug in their study could be attributed to improved survival in this group who displayed a methylated gene. However, there is still activity of temozolomide in nonmethylated tumors and is used in almost all cases. Additionally, there may be an interaction between MGMT methylation and mutations in other genes such as *IDH1* (Wick et al).

Tyrosine kinase inhibitors (erlotinib, gefitinib) have been developed in response to the upregulation of EGFR mentioned earlier. In a preliminary but provocative study, Mellinghoff and coworkers found that a deletion mutation of the gene for this protein and expression of the tumor suppression protein PTEN predicted responsiveness of recurrent gliomas to treatment with EGFR kinase inhibitors. This represents one example in a growing field of prediction of treatment response in relation to tumor genetics.

Brachytherapy (implantation of iodine-125 or iridium-193 beads or needles) and high-dose focused radiation (stereotactic radiosurgery) have so far not significantly altered survival times but continue to be studied.

The treatment of recurrent glioblastoma or anaplastic astrocytoma after surgery and radiation, almost inevitable occurrences, is controversial and must be guided by the location and pattern of tumor growth and the patient's age and relative state of health. Almost all glioblastomas recur within 2 cm of their original site and 10 percent develop additional lesions at distant locations. Reoperation is sometimes undertaken for local recurrences. The most aggressive approach—a second surgery and chemotherapy—can prove effective and has been generally used in patients younger than age 40 years whose original operation was many months earlier. If the PCV regimen discussed earlier has not already been used, some neurooncologists resort to that combination or the newer and better-tolerated alkylating agent temozolomide (which may be used if the PCV regimen was administered previously). These chemotherapeutic drugs may prolong the symptom-free interval but have little effect on survival. A promising approach for recurrent malignant gliomas is the use of drugs that target the tumor's vasculature. Antiangiogenic agents such as bevacizumab, a VEGF inhibitor, sometimes given in combination with chemotherapy, may delay progression and greatly reduce cerebral edema, therefore diminishing the requirement for corticosteroids, but also do not prolong survival. A recent but preliminary provocative observation from retrospective series has been that patients with glioblastoma receiving valganciclovir, ostensibly for concurrent CMV infections, had better survival than those who did not receive the drug (Söderberg-Nauclér and colleagues).

With aggressive surgical removal and radiotherapy, as described above, median survival for patients with glioblastoma is 12 months, compared to 7 to 9 months without such treatment.

Low- and Intermediate-Grade Astrocytoma

The lower-grade astrocytomas (grade II in the WHO classification), which constitute between 25 and 30 percent of cerebral gliomas, may occur anywhere in the brain or spinal cord. The median survival in cases of anaplastic astrocytoma is considerably longer than for glioblastoma, 2 to 5 years, often longer. Favored sites of occurrence are the cerebrum, cerebellum, hypothalamus, optic nerve and chiasm, and pons. In general, the location of the tumor appears to be influenced by the age of the patient. Astrocytomas of the cerebral hemispheres arise mainly in adults in their third and fourth decades or earlier; astrocytomas in other parts of the nervous system, particularly the posterior fossa and optic nerves, are more frequent in children and adolescents. These tumors are classified further according to their histologic characteristics: protoplasmic or fibrillary; gemistocytic (enlarged cells distended with hyaline and eosinophilic material); pilocytic (elongated, bipolar cells); and mixed astrocytoma-oligodendroglioma types. The most common type is composed of well-differentiated fibrillary astrocytes. The tumor cells contain glial fibrillary acidic protein (GFAP), which is a useful diagnostic marker in biopsy specimens. Some cerebral astrocytomas present as mixed astrocytomas and glioblastomas. The most common low-grade fibrillary type (grade II) is distinguished from the more benign WHO grade I pilocytic tumor and the rare pleomorphic xanthoastrocytoma. These distinctions correlate to a degree with the biologic behavior of the astrocytomas and therefore have prognostic importance.

Cerebral astrocytoma is a slowly growing tumor of infiltrative character with a tendency in some cases to form large cavities or pseudocysts. Other tumors of this category are noncavitating and appear grayish white, firm, and relatively avascular, almost indistinguishable from normal white matter, with which they merge imperceptibly. Fine granules of calcium may be deposited in parts of the tumor, but calcium in a slow-growing intracerebral tumor is more characteristic of an oligodendroglioma. The CSF is acellular; the only abnormalities in some cases are the increased pressure and protein content. The tumor may distort the lateral and third ventricles and displace adjacent cerebral vessels (Fig. 31-3). It may not be possible on clinical or imaging grounds to distinguish low-grade gliomas from a number of rare tumors in childhood such as the dysembryoplastic neuroepithelioma (DNET) discussed further on.

In about two-thirds of patients with astrocytoma, the first symptom is a focal or generalized seizure, and between 60 and 75 percent of patients have recurrent seizures in the course of their illness. Other subtle cerebral symptoms follow after months, sometimes after years. Headaches and signs of increased intracranial pressure are relatively late occurrences.

MRI may be helpful in distinguishing the more frequent fibrillary type of tumor under discussion from pilocytic astrocytomas. Pilocytic types are sharply demarcated, with smooth borders and little edema. On T1-weighted MRI, they are isointense or hypointense; on T2 sequences, hyperintense, and there tends to be marked enhancement of the nodular solid portion of the tumor after gadolinium infusion. Cyst formation and small amounts of calcification are common, especially in cerebellar tumors. The fibrillary tumors have a less-stereotyped appearance, generally taking the form of a more homogenous T1 hypointense and T2 hyperintense infiltrating mass with less well-defined borders and little or no contrast enhancement.

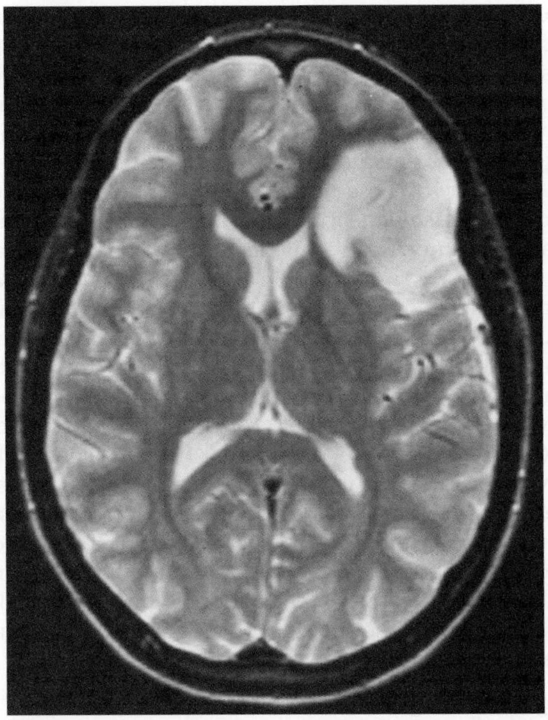

Figure 31-3. Astrocytoma of the left frontal lobe; the T2-weighted MRI shows an infiltrating tumor with minimal mass effect and mild edema. The degree of contrast enhancement is variable but most often less than glioblastoma.

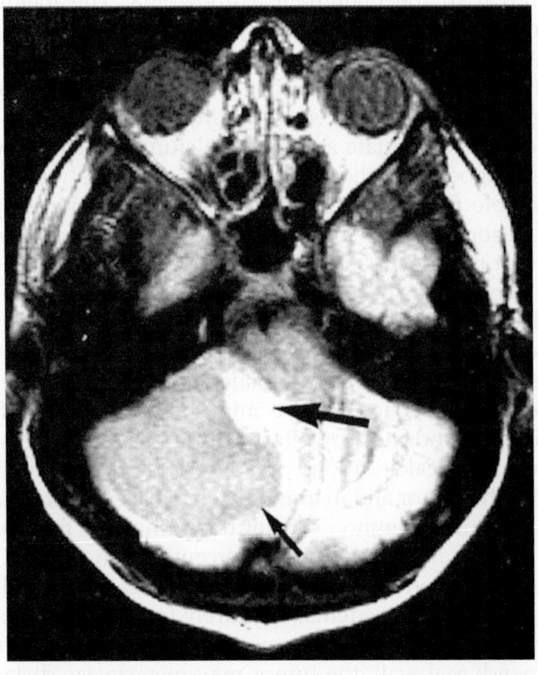

Figure 31-4. Cystic astrocytoma of the right cerebellum. MRI demonstrates the large cystic component of the tumor (*smaller arrow*) which appears hypointense compared to the solid tissue component (*larger arrow*). (Reproduced by permission from Bisese JH: *Cranial MRI*. New York, McGraw-Hill, 1991.)

In children, astrocytic tumors usually arise in the cerebellum (Fig. 31-4) and declare themselves by some combination of gait unsteadiness, unilateral ataxia, and increased intracranial pressure (headaches, vomiting).

Treatment One of the more interesting developments in the treatment of low-grade tumors has been the comparison made by Jakola and colleagues between the practices in two Norwegian centers, one which practiced an aggressive approach of removing accessible tumors when they are discovered, and another, of observing the patient by sequential imaging to determine if the tumor has transformed into a more aggressive mode. While a small, and not a randomized trial, surgical excision resulted in longer survival.

Excision of part of a cerebral astrocytoma can improve survival in a good functional state for many years. The cystic astrocytoma of the cerebellum is relatively benign in its overall behavior. In such cases, resection of the tumor nodule is of singular importance in delaying or preventing a recurrence. In recent series, the rate of survival 5 years after successful surgery has been greater than 90 percent (Pencalet et al). The outcome is less assured when the tumor also involves the brainstem and cannot be safely resected.

The natural history of the low-grade gliomas is to grow slowly and eventually undergo malignant transformation. The duration of progression before this transformation occurs and the latency to recurrence with modern treatment may extend for many years. A survey of the outcome of these low-grade supratentorial tumors showed that 10-year survival after operation was from 11 to 40 percent provided that 5,300 cGy was given postoperatively (Shaw et al). This, of course, is quite in contrast to the figures for glioblastoma.

In younger patients, particularly if the neurologic examination is normal or nearly so, radiation can be delayed and the course of the tumor evaluated by serial imaging. A number of studies have come to the conclusion that delaying radiation in younger patients may avoid the consequences of dementia and hypopituitarism (Peterson and DeAngelis), but others have suggested that the tumor itself and antiepileptic drugs cause more difficulty than high-dose radiation. An extensive randomized trial of early radiotherapy in adults demonstrated that median progression-free survival was extended to 5.3 years by early treatment in comparison to 3.4 years for observation only and radiation treatment that was initiated when signs of progression occurred, but that overall survival was unaffected, averaging just over 7 years in both groups (van den Bent et al).

Lacking any clear benefit on survival, it seems to us that radiation may be withheld initially. An increase in seizures or worsening neurologic signs then presses one to turn to radiation or further surgery. Repeated operations prolong life in some patients. Although chemotherapy has as yet no established place in the treatment of low-grade pure astrocytomas, tumors with an oligodendroglial component respond well to combination chemotherapy used for the treatment of anaplastic oligodendroglioma, as described later.

The special features of astrocytomas of the pons, hypothalamus, optic nerves, and chiasm, which produce highly characteristic clinical syndromes and do not behave like a cerebral mass, are discussed further on in this chapter.

Gliomatosis Cerebri

In this variant of high-grade glioma there is a diffuse infiltration of neoplastic glial cells, involving much of one or both cerebral hemispheres with sparing of neuronal elements but without a discrete tumor mass. Whether this type of "gliomatosis" represents neoplastic transformation of multicentric origin or direct spread from one or more small neoplastic foci is not known. For these and other reasons, the tumor is impossible to classify (or to grade) using the conventional brain tumor schemes, though the genetic and molecular alterations found in high-grade gliomas, as described earlier, are seen in some cases of gliomatosis cerebri as well.

Many small series of gliomatosis cerebri have been reported since Nevin introduced the term in 1938, but no truly distinctive clinical picture has emerged (Dunn and Kernohan). Impairment of intellect, headache, seizures, and papilledema are the major manifestations and do not set these cases apart on a clinical basis from the malignant astrocytoma, in which the tumor may also be more widespread than the macroscopic picture suggests. If there is a syndrome that can be associated early on with gliomatosis, in our experience it has been a nondescript frontal lobe behavioral syndrome sometimes mistaken for depression or a subacute dementia, or pseudobulbar palsy may be the first manifestation. The prognosis is variable but generally poor, measured in months to a few years from the time of diagnosis.

CT and MRI reveal small ventricles and one or more large confluent areas of signal change (Fig. 31-5). Imaging studies characteristically show the tumor crossing and thickening the corpus callosum. Contrast enhancement is scant, differentiating the tumor from cerebral lymphoma, which otherwise may have a similar appearance. As the tumor advances, enhancing nodules may appear, suggesting the emergence of foci of high-grade glioma.

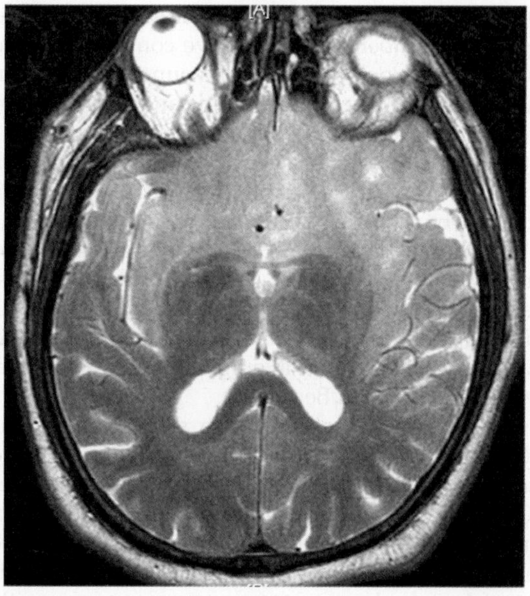

Figure 31-5. Gliomatosis cerebri invading both hemispheres. T2-weighted MRI shows a large confluent area of involvement in the frontal lobes with effacement of overlying cortical sulci. There was slight enhancement along the margins of the lesions after gadolinium infusion. The patient was mentally slow but had no other neurologic signs.

Treatment These tumors are too infrequent for categorical assessments of therapy, but the overall response to all antitumor treatments has been disappointing and the prognosis, as mentioned, is poor, survival usually being measured in months. Corticosteroids have little clinical effect, probably because of a paucity of vasogenic edema. Most trials suggest a benefit to radiation treatment, but the absolute prolongation of life has been only several weeks (Leibel et al). The addition of chemotherapy may confer a marginal further benefit when survival at 1 year is considered. Small series of patients treated with temozolomide suggest it may be a promising agent for this tumor but it will be difficult to conduct a randomized trial given its rarity. When a large region is infiltrated, particularly in the temporal lobe, surgical debulking may prolong life, but otherwise surgery is futile except to obtain a diagnosis.

Oligodendroglioma

This tumor was first identified by Bailey and Cushing in 1926 and described more fully by Bailey and Bucy in 1929. It is derived from oligodendrocytes or their precursor cells and may occur at any age, most often in the third and fourth decades, with an earlier peak at 6 to 12 years. It is relatively infrequent, constituting approximately 5 to 7 percent of all intracranial gliomas. From the time of its original descriptions, it was recognized as being more benign than the malignant astrocytoma. The incidence in men is twice that in women. In some cases the tumor may be recognized at surgery by its pink-gray color and multilobular form, its relative avascularity and firmness (slightly tougher than surrounding brain), and its tendency to encapsulate and form calcium and small cysts. Most oligodendrogliomas, however, are grossly indistinguishable from other gliomas, and a proportion—up to half in some series—are mixed *oligoastrocytomas*, suggesting that the precursor cell is pluripotential.

The neoplastic oligodendrocyte has a small round nucleus and a halo of unstained cytoplasm ("fried egg" appearance). The cell processes are few and stubby, visualized only with silver carbonate stains. Some of the oligodendrocytes have intense immunoreactivity to GFAP, similar to normal myelin-forming oligodendrocytes. Microscopic calcifications are observed frequently, both within the tumor and in immediately adjacent brain tissue.

The most common sites of this tumor are the frontal and temporal lobes (40 to 70 percent), often deep in the white matter, with one or more streaks of calcium but little or no surrounding edema. It is rarely found in other parts of the nervous system. By extending to the pial surface or ependymal wall, the tumor may metastasize distantly in ventricular and subarachnoid spaces, accounting for 11 percent of the series of gliomas with meningeal dissemination reported by Polmeteer and Kernohan (less frequent than medulloblastoma and glioblastoma; see also

Yung et al). The tumor does not lend itself easily to any of the grading scales, but a distinction is made between low grade (grade II) and a malignant type with degeneration, evidenced by greater cellularity and by numerous and abnormal mitoses; necrosis may occur in small regions of the tumor in about one-third of cases. In the oligoastrocytomas, either cell type may be anaplastic.

The typical oligodendroglioma grows slowly. As with astrocytomas, the first symptom in more than half of patients is a focal or generalized seizure; seizures often persist for many years before other symptoms develop. Approximately 15 percent of patients have early symptoms and signs of increased intracranial pressure; an even smaller number have focal cerebral signs (hemiparesis). Much less frequent are unilateral extrapyramidal rigidity, cerebellar ataxia, Parinaud syndrome, intratumoral hemorrhage, and meningeal oligodendrogliosis (cranial–spinal nerve palsies, hydrocephalus, lymphocytes, and tumor cells in CSF).

The appearance on imaging studies is variable, but the most typical is a hypodense (on CT) or T2 hyperintense (on MRI) heterogenous mass near the cortical surface with relatively well-defined borders (Fig. 31-6). Intratumoral calcification can be seen in more than half the cases and is a helpful diagnostic sign, but in the context of seizures, this finding also raises the possibility of an arteriovenous malformation or a low-grade astrocytoma. Approximately half of oligodendrogliomas demonstrate some contrast enhancement, and leptomeningeal enhancement adjacent to the tumor can be seen but is rare.

In recent years, a remarkable degree of progress has been made in understanding the genetic aberrations that

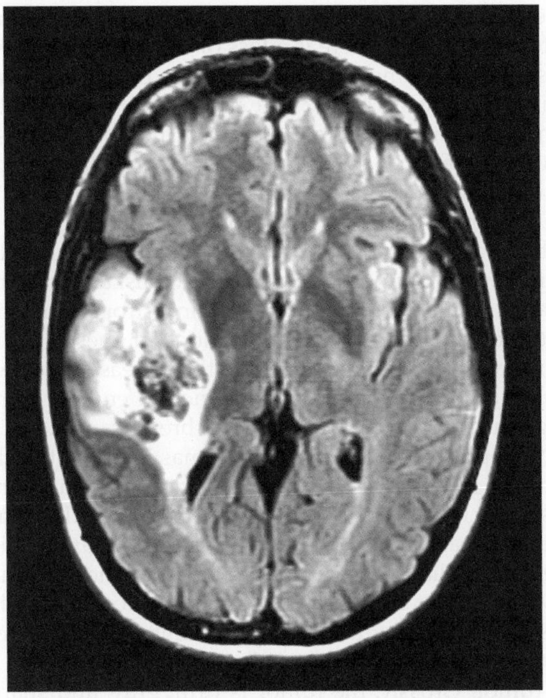

Figure 31-6. A partially cystic oligodendroglioma of the right frontotemporal region. There was no abnormal contrast enhancement.

occur as acquired somatic mutation within these tumors and the relationship of these changes to the prognosis and response to therapy. Specifically, loss of certain alleles on chromosome 1p has been predictive of a high degree of responsiveness to the below-described PCV chemotherapy regimen, and a similar loss on chromosome 19q has been associated with longer survival.

Treatment Surgical excision followed by radiation therapy has been the conventional treatment for oligodendroglioma. However, because of uncertainty as to the histologic classification of many of the reported cases, it is not clear whether radiation therapy is attended by longer survival. Well-differentiated oligodendrogliomas should probably not receive radiation if seizures are well controlled and there are no neurologic deficits. As mentioned earlier, in the discovery by Cairncross and MacDonald of considerable importance is that many oligodendrogliomas, especially anaplastic ones, respond impressively to chemotherapeutic agents. This has been studied with the PCV regimen (procarbazine, cyclophosphamide, and vincristine) given in approximately 6 cycles, but also applies to the better-tolerated temozolomide, which has become the preferred treatment.

The identification by Cairncross and others of genetic markers has been of great interest. For example, of 50 patients who had loss of regions on 1p, median survival was over 10 years. These findings have been variably adopted into general clinical practice and it is likely that refinements in this approach will be forthcoming (see Louis et al [2007] and Reifenberger and Louis for discussion). Mutations in IDH1 also appear to confer survival benefit. Mixed oligodendrogliomas and astrocytomas should generally be treated like astrocytomas, but temozolomide probably suffice to treat both components. An adequate direct comparison between temozolomide and PCV is awaited.

Ependymoma (See also "Ependymoma and Papilloma of the Fourth Ventricle" further on)

This tumor proves to be more complex and variable than other gliomas. Correctly diagnosed by Virchow as early as 1863, its origin from ependymal cells was first suggested by Mallory, who found the typical blepharoplasts (small, darkly staining cytoplasmic dots that are the basal bodies of the cilia as seen by electron microscopy). Two types were recognized by Bailey and Cushing: one was the ependymoma, and the other, with more malignant and invasive properties, the ependymoblastoma, now recognized as an anaplastic ependymoma. Approximately 6 percent of all intracranial gliomas are ependymomas, the percentage being slightly higher in children (8 percent). Approximately 40 percent of the infratentorial ependymomas occur in the first decade of life, a few as early as the first year. The supratentorial ones are more evenly distributed among all age groups, but in general the age incidence is lower than that of other malignant gliomas.

There is also a myxopapillomatous type of ependymoma, localized exclusively in the filum terminale of the spinal cord as discussed further on in the chapter. The latter gives rise to a special syndrome that variably combines symptoms and signs of the conus medullaris and the cauda equina such as sciatica or femoral pain, bladder difficulty, saddle anesthesia, and spastic leg weakness.

Ependymomas are derived from ependymal cells, i.e., the cells lining the ventricles of the brain and the central canal of the spinal cord; this is the most common glioma of the spinal cord. These cells have both glial and epithelial characteristics. As one might expect, the tumors grow either into the ventricle or adjacent brain tissue. The most common cerebral site is the fourth ventricle; less often they occur in the lateral or third ventricles. Grossly, those in the fourth ventricle are grayish pink, firm, cauliflower-like growths; those in the cerebrum, arising from the wall of the lateral ventricle, may be large (several centimeters in diameter), reddish gray, and softer and more clearly demarcated from adjacent tissue than astrocytomas, but they are not encapsulated. The tumor cells tend to form rosettes with central lumens or, more often, circular arrangements around blood vessels (pseudorosettes). Some ependymomas, called epithelial, are densely cellular; others form papillae. Some of the well-differentiated fourth ventricular tumors are probably derived from subependymal astrocytes (see later in this chapter and also Fig. 31-12).

Anaplastic ependymomas are identified by their high mitotic activity and endothelial proliferation, nuclear atypia, and necrosis. However, correlations between histopathologic features and clinical outcomes have not been well defined.

The *symptomatology* depends on the location of the neoplasm. The clinical manifestations of fourth ventricular tumors are described further on in this chapter; the point to be made here is the frequent occurrence of hydrocephalus and signs of raised intracranial pressure (manifest in children by lethargy, nausea, vomiting, and papilledema). Cerebral ependymomas otherwise resemble the other gliomas in their clinical expression in that seizures occur in approximately one-third of the cases.

The imaging characteristics are rather different from those of other tumors. With CT one observes a well-demarcated heterogeneous hyperdense mass with fairly uniform contrast enhancement. Calcification and some degree of cystic change are common in supratentorial tumors, but less so in infratentorial ones. There are mixed signal characteristics on MRI, generally hypointense on T1 sequences and hyperintense on T2. *An intraventricular location supports the diagnosis of ependymoma*, but meningioma and a number of other tumors may be found in this location. In keeping with the variability of anaplasia, the interval between the first symptom and the diagnosis ranges from 4 weeks in the most malignant types, to 7 to 8 years.

Treatment and Outcome In a follow-up study of 101 cases in Norway, where ependymomas made up 1.2 percent of all primary intracranial tumors (and 32 percent of intraspinal tumors), the postoperative survival was poor. Within a year, 47 percent of the patients had died, although 13 percent were alive after 10 years. Doubtless the prognosis depends on the degree of anaplasia (Mørk and Løken), the location of the tumor, and whether it is operable but the lack of certainty of these dicta have been alluded to earlier. Surgical removal is supplemented by radiation therapy, particularly to address the high rate of seeding of the ventricles and spinal axis. In the treatment of anaplastic ependymomas, antineoplastic drugs are often used in combination with radiation therapy.

Meningioma (See also "Meningioma of the Sphenoid Ridge" further on)

This is a tumor, first illustrated by Matthew Bailie in his *Morbid Anatomy* (1787) and first identified properly by Bright, in 1831, originating from the dura mater or arachnoid. It was analyzed from every point of view by Harvey Cushing and was the subject of one of his most important monographs (Cushing, 1962).

Meningiomas represent approximately 15 percent of all primary intracranial tumors; they are more common in women than in men (2:1) and have their highest incidence in the sixth and seventh decades of life. Some are familial. There is evidence that persons who have undergone radiation therapy to the scalp or cranium are vulnerable to the development of meningiomas and that the tumors appear at an earlier age in such individuals (Rubinstein et al). Radiofrequency energy exposure from portable cellular devices has failed to be linked to elevated incidence of meningiomas (or gliomas), however due to some inconclusive data, and mainly social pressure, the International Agency for Research on Cancer has classified radiofrequency electromagnetic fields as "possibly carcinogenic." There are also a number of reports of a meningioma developing at the site of previous trauma, such as a cranial fracture line, but the association is uncertain.

The most frequent acquired genetic defects of meningiomas are truncating (inactivating) mutations in the neurofibromatosis 2 gene (merlin) on chromosome 22q. These are present in the great majority of certain meningiomas (e.g., fibroblastic and transitional types), but not others. Merlin deletions probably also play a role in those instances in which there is a loss of the long arm of chromosome 22. In meningiomas of both the sporadic and neurofibromatosis type 2 (NF2)–associated types, other somatic genetic defects are found, including deletions on chromosomes 1p, 6q, 9p, 10q, 14q, and 18q. Meningiomas also elaborate a variety of soluble proteins, some of which (VEGF) are angiogenic and probably relate to both the highly vascularized nature of these tumors and their prominent surrounding edema (see Lamszus for further details). Some meningiomas contain estrogen and progesterone receptors. The implications of these findings are not yet clear, but may relate to the increased incidence of the tumor in women, its tendency to enlarge during pregnancy, and an association with breast cancer.

The precise origin of meningiomas is still not settled. According to Rubinstein, they may arise from dural fibroblasts, but it was the opinion of our colleague R.D. Adams that, they are more clearly derived from arachnoidal (meningothelial) cells, in particular from those forming the arachnoid villi. Because the clusters of arachnoidal cells penetrate the dura in largest number in the vicinity of venous sinuses, these are the sites of predilection for the tumor. Grossly, the tumor is firm, gray, and sharply circumscribed, taking the shape of the space in which it grows; thus, some tumors are flat and plaque-like, others round and lobulated. They may indent the brain and acquire a pia-arachnoid covering as part of their capsule, but they are clearly demarcated from the brain tissue (extraaxial) except in the unusual circumstance of a malignant invasive meningioma. Infrequently, they arise from arachnoidal cells within the choroid plexus, forming an intraventricular meningioma.

The cells of meningiomas are relatively uniform, with round or elongated nuclei, visible cytoplasmic membrane, and a characteristic tendency to encircle one another, forming whorls and *psammoma bodies* (laminated calcific concretions). A notable electron microscopic characteristic is the formation of very complex interdigitations between cells and the presence of desmosomes (Kepes). Cushing and Eisenhardt and, more recently, the World Health Organization (Lopes et al) have divided meningiomas into many subtypes depending on their mesenchymal variations, the character of the stroma, and their relative vascularity, but the value of such classifications is debatable. Currently neuropathologists recognize a meningothelial (syncytial) form as being the most common. It is readily distinguished from other similar but nonmeningothelial tumors such as hemangiopericytomas, fibroblastomas, and chondrosarcomas.

Meningiomas occur at sites of dural folds, most commonly the frontoparietal parasagittal convexities, falx, tentorium cerebelli, sphenoid wings, olfactory groove, and tuberculum sellae. Ninety percent of meningiomas are supratentorial, and the majority of infratentorial meningiomas occur at the cerebellopontine angle. Some meningiomas—such as those of the olfactory groove, sphenoid wing, and tuberculum sellae—express themselves by highly distinctive syndromes that are almost diagnostic; these are described further on in this chapter. Rarely, the tumors are multiple. Inasmuch as the meningioma extends from the dural surface, it commonly incites hyperostosis of adjacent bone and can, in more malignant cases, invade and erode the cranial bones or excite an osteoblastic reaction, giving rise to an exostosis on the external surface of the skull. Most of the following remarks apply to meningiomas of the parasagittal, sylvian, and other surface areas of the cerebrum.

Small meningiomas, less than 2.0 cm in diameter, are often found at autopsy in middle-aged and elderly persons without having caused symptoms. Only when they exceed a certain size and indent the brain or cause a seizure do they alter function. The size that must be reached before symptoms appear varies with the size of the space in which the tumor grows and the surrounding anatomic arrangements. Focal seizures are an early sign of meningiomas that overlie the cerebrum. The parasagittal frontoparietal meningioma may cause a slowly progressive spastic weakness or numbness of one leg and later of both legs, and incontinence in the late stages. The larger sylvian tumors are manifest by a variety of motor, sensory, and aphasic disturbances in accord with their location, and by seizures.

Before brain imaging became widely available, a meningioma often gave rise to neurologic signs for many years before the diagnosis was established, attesting to its slow rate of growth. Even now some tumors reach enormous size, to the point of causing papilledema, before the patient comes to medical attention. Many are detected on CT in individuals with unrelated neurologic diseases. The diagnosis of meningioma is greatly facilitated by their ready visualization with contrast-enhanced CT and MRI (Figs. 31-7 and 31-8), which reveal their tendency to calcify as well as their prominent vascularity. These changes are reflected by homogeneous contrast enhancement and by "tumor blush" on angiography. Typically the tumor takes the form of a smoothly contoured mass sometimes lobulated, with one edge abutting the inner surface of the skull, along the dura. On CT performed without contrast they are isointense or slightly hyperintense; calcification

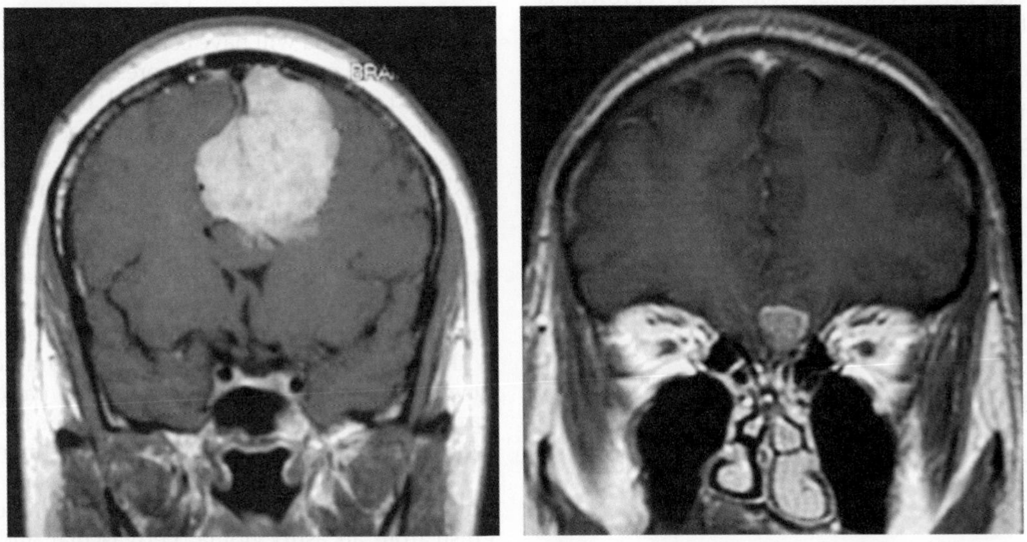

A B

Figure 31-7. *A*. Parafalcine meningioma; coronal image, MRI with gadolinium. Note the rightward displacement of an anterior cerebral artery (hypointense flow void) trapped between the right lateral margin of the mass and the right medial frontal lobe. *B*. Small and asymptomatic left olfactory groove meningioma, MRI with gadolinium.

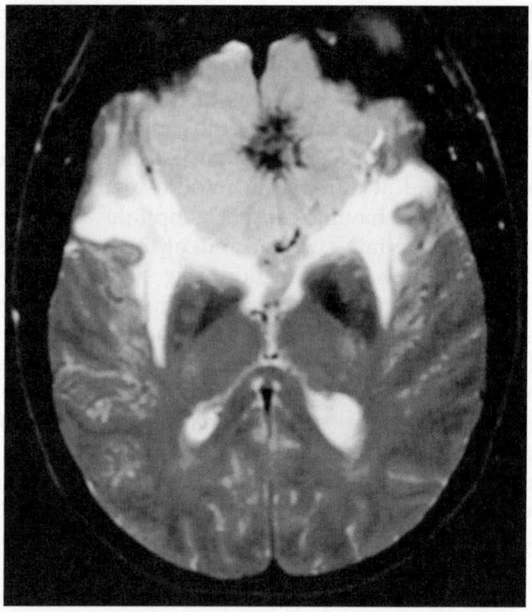

Figure 31-8. Gadolinium-enhanced MRI of meningioma. Large subfrontal extraaxial mass with central calcification and surrounding vasogenic edema. Homogeneous avid enhancement is characteristic of the tumor.

at the outer surface or heterogeneously throughout the mass is common. The amount of edema surrounding the tumor is highly variable and may relate to the extent of local brain symptoms. The CSF protein is usually elevated.

Treatment Surgical excision should afford long-term or permanent cure in most symptomatic and accessible tumors. Recurrence is likely if removal is incomplete, as is often the case, but for some the growth rate is so slow that there may be a latency of many years or decades. A few tumors show malignant qualities; i.e., a high mitotic index, nuclear atypia, marked nuclear and cellular pleomorphism, and invasiveness of brain. Their regrowth is then rapid if they are not completely excised. Tumors that lie beneath the hypothalamus, along the medial part of the sphenoid bone and parasellar region, or anterior to the brainstem are the most difficult to remove surgically. By invading adjacent bone, they may become impossible to remove totally. Carefully planned radiation therapy, including various forms of stereotactic treatment, is beneficial in cases that are inoperable and when the tumor is incompletely removed or shows malignant characteristics.

Smaller tumors at the base of the skull can be obliterated or reduced in size by focused radiation, probably with comparable or less risk than posed by surgery (see discussion by Chang and Alder). Conventional chemotherapy and hormonal therapy are probably ineffective, but the latter has been a subject of interest. Investigations are being undertaken with antiangiogenic antibodies for recurrent tumors.

Primary Central Nervous System Lymphoma

This tumor has assumed increasing significance in the last few decades because of its increased incidence in patients with AIDS and other immunosuppressed states. There is a preponderance of men, with the peak incidence in the fifth through seventh decades of life, or in the third and fourth decades in patients with AIDS.

For many years, the cell of origin of this tumor was attributed to the reticulum cell, a histiocytic component of the germinal center of lymph nodes that produces the reticulum stroma of the nodes, and the tumor was termed "reticulum cell sarcoma." The meningeal histiocyte and microgliacytes are the equivalent cells in the brain to the reticulum cell and considered then the origin of the tumor. Later, it was recognized that the malignant cells were lymphocytes and lymphoblasts, leading to its reclassification as a lymphoma (diffuse large cell type). It has been appreciated, on the basis of immunocytochemical studies, that the tumor cells are B lymphocytes. There is a fine reticulum reaction between the reticulum cells derived from fibroblasts and microglia or histiocytes. The disproportionate emphasis on this reticular stroma was in part the result of staining methods that brought it into relief with the lymphocytes. The B lymphocyte or lymphoblast is the tumor cell, whereas the fine reticulum and "microgliacytes" are secondary interstitial reactions.

In contrast, T-cell lymphomas of the nervous system are rare but do occur in both immunocompetent and immunosuppressed patients. Because the brain is devoid of lymphatic tissue, it is uncertain how this tumor arises; one theory holds that it represents a systemic lymphoma with a particular propensity to metastasize to the nervous system. This seems unlikely to the authors; systemic lymphomas of the usual kind rarely metastasize, as discussed further on, under "Involvement of the Nervous System in Systemic Lymphoma."

Primary CNS lymphoma may arise in any part of the cerebrum, cerebellum, or brainstem, with 60 percent being in the cerebral hemispheres; they may be solitary or multifocal. A periventricular localization is common. Vitreous, uveal, and retinal (ocular) involvement occurs in 10 to 20 percent of cases; here vitreous biopsy may be diagnostic, but it is not often performed. (Two-thirds of patients with ocular lymphoma will have cerebral involvement within a year.) Lai and colleagues have presented evidence that, in advanced cases that were autopsied, microscopic deposits of tumor found their way to many regions of the brain and not solely in areas indicated by nodular enhancement on MRI. Whether this indicates a widespread or multifocal origin of brain lymphoma is not clear.

The pia and arachnoid may be infiltrated, and a purely meningeal form of B-cell lymphoma that involves peripheral and cranial nerves is also known. Most such cases of what has been termed *neurolymphomatosis* present with painful, predominantly motor polyradiculopathies. One such patient of ours had a flaccid paraparesis and back and sciatic pain; MRI showed tumor infiltrating the cauda equina nerve roots and contiguous meninges.

The tumor forms a pinkish gray, soft, ill-defined, infiltrative mass in the brain, difficult at times to distinguish from an astrocytoma. Perivascular and meningeal spread results in shedding of cells into the CSF, accounting perhaps for the multifocal appearance of the tumor in many cases. The neoplasm is highly cellular and grows around and into blood vessels ("angiocentric" pattern) but elicits no tendency to necrosis. The nuclei are oval or bean-shaped with scant cytoplasm, and mitotic figures are numerous. B-cell markers applied to fixed tissue define the lymphoblastic cell population as monoclonal and identify the tumor cell type. The stainability of reticulum and microglial cells also serves to distinguish this tumor microscopically. There is no tumor tissue outside the brain.

Several of our cases of meningeal and cranial nerve lymphoma with similar histologic characteristics to primary CNS lymphoma were complications of chronic lymphatic leukemia, a type of so-called Richter transformation.

Primary lymphoma involving the cerebral hemispheres initially pursues a clinical course somewhat similar to that of the gliomas but with a vastly different response to treatment. Behavioral and personality changes, confusion, dizziness, and focal cerebral signs predominate over headache and other signs of increased intracranial pressure as presenting manifestations. Seizures may occur but are less common, in our experience, than they are as the introductory feature of gliomas. Most cases occur in adult life, but some have been observed in children, in whom the tumor may simulate the cerebellar symptomatology of medulloblastoma.

The finding on CT and MRI of one or several dense (hypercellular), homogeneous, enhancing, infiltrating, nonnecrotic, nonhemorrhagic, periventricular masses is characteristic (Fig. 31-9). However, rim enhancement also occurs, and any part of the brain may be involved. The radiologic appearance in the immunosuppressed patient is less predictable and may be difficult to distinguish from that of toxoplasmosis or another process with which lymphoma may coexist.

In some cases, a multitude of deep cerebral white matter lesions, some radially oriented and thereby simulating multiple sclerosis, are seen. Tumor enhancement with contrast agents tends to be more prominent and homogeneous than with the acute lesions of multiple sclerosis. A similar multinodular appearance occurs with intravascular lymphoma discussed in a later section.

Characteristic of primary CNS lymphoma is the disappearance on imaging of the lesions or complete but transient resolution of contrast enhancement in response to corticosteroids. Lymphocytic and mononuclear pleocytosis of CSF is more frequent than with gliomas and metastatic tumors. The immunohistochemical demonstration in CSF of monoclonal lymphocytes or an elevated beta microglobulin points to leptomeningeal spread of the tumor (Li et al), but frequently the diagnosis is not possible from CSF cytologic examination.

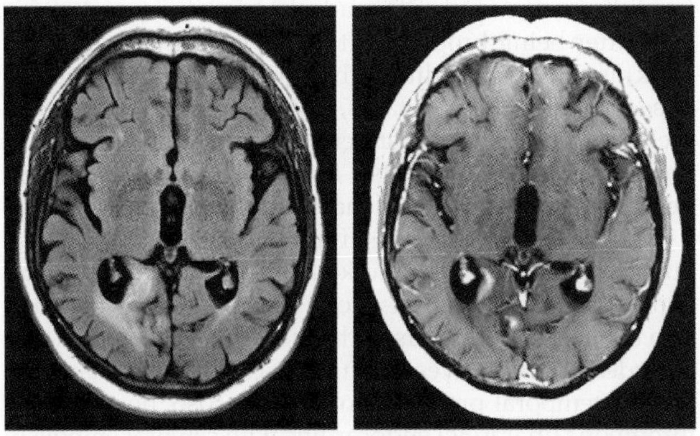

Figure 31-9. Cerebral lymphoma. *Left*: Axial T2-FLAIR MRI showing hyperintensity in the right periatrial white matter, without mass effect. *Right*: Contrast-enhanced MRI reveals two foci of nodular enhancement.

Patients with AIDS and less-common immunodeficiency states, such as the Wiskott-Aldrich syndrome and ataxia-telangiectasia, and those who are receiving immunosuppressive drugs for long periods, as for example, in renal transplantation, are particularly liable to develop this type of lymphoma. Many of the tumors in immunosuppressed patients contain the EBV genome, suggesting a pathogenetic role for the virus (Bashir et al); however, the EBV genome has also been found in the tumors of a few immunocompetent patients (Hochberg and Miller). Sometimes this tumor appears as a complication of an obscure medical condition such as salivary and lacrimal gland enlargement (Mikulicz syndrome) or Sjögren syndrome.

Stereotactic needle biopsy is the preferred method of establishing the histologic diagnosis in sporadic cases. In immunosuppressed patients, the differential diagnosis of a solitary brain nodule that is suspected to be lymphoma is aided by the response, or lack thereof, to treatment for toxoplasmosis, the main alternative diagnosis (see "Toxoplasmosis" in Chap. 32). Reduction in the size of the lesion with antimicrobial drugs makes biopsy unnecessary.

Treatment Because the tumors are deep and often multicentric, surgical resection is ineffective except in rare instances. Treatment with cranial irradiation and corticosteroids often produces a partial or, transiently, a complete response, but the tumor recurs in greater than 90 percent of patients. Until recently, the median survival of patients treated in this way has been 10 to 18 months and less in those with AIDS and in individuals who are otherwise immunocompromised. In immunocompetent patients, the addition of intrathecal methotrexate and intravenous cytosine arabinoside has increased median survival to more than 3 years (DeAngelis), and apparent cure is not unknown. However, this combined treatment is associated with a high risk of a leukoencephalopathy (see further on and Fig. 31-25) and causes considerable systemic side effects.

Glass and colleagues (1994) recommended a treatment regimen consisting of several cycles of intravenous methotrexate (3.5 g/m^2) and citrovorum, administered at 2- to 3-week intervals and at times continued indefinitely if the treatment is tolerated. More recently, methotrexate plus either cytarabine or a combination of rituximab and temozolomide has been favored. Cranial irradiation is not typically part of the initial treatment. Ocular lymphoma is eradicated only by radiation therapy. Corticosteroids are added at any point to control neurologic symptoms. The median survival time with this approach in the non-AIDS patient is in the range of 3.5 years with intravenous methotrexate alone and 4 years or more if radiation is given subsequently. Some patients are alive at 10 years.

Intracranial Metastatic Carcinoma

These are far more common than are primary brain tumors. Among secondary intracranial tumors, only metastatic carcinoma occurs with high frequency. Occasionally one encounters a rhabdomyosarcoma, Ewing tumor, carcinoid, and others that have metastasized, but these have such low incidence that cerebral metastases seldom become a matter of diagnostic concern. The interesting pathobiology of metastatic carcinoma—the complex biologic mechanisms that govern the detachment of tumor cells from the primary growth, their transport to distant tissues, and their implantation on the capillary endothelium of the particular organ in which they will eventually grow is of research interest. Suffice it to say that tumor cell adhesion molecules, the vasculature, and a number of other cellular events participate in the implantation of what is essentially a neoplastic embolus.

Autopsy studies disclose intracranial metastases in approximately 25 percent of patients who die of cancer (Posner, 1978). Approximately 80 percent are in the cerebral hemispheres and 20 percent in posterior fossa structures, corresponding roughly to the relative size and weights of these portions of the brain and their blood flow. Cancers of the pelvis and colon are exceptional in this respect, having a somewhat higher tendency than this to spread to the posterior fossa. Intracranial metastases assume three main patterns—those to the skull and dura, those to the brain itself, and those spreading diffusely through the craniospinal meninges (meningeal carcinomatosis). As common as intracranial metastases are, metastases to the vertebral column, which eventually cause compression of the spinal cord and nerve roots. This separate problem is discussed in Chap. 44. Metastatic deposits in the spinal cord itself are infrequent but are seen from time to time; they are more common, however, than another cancer-associated spinal cord lesion, paraneoplastic necrotic myelopathy (see further on).

Metastases to the skull and dura occur with any tumor that metastasizes to bone, but they are particularly common with carcinoma of the breast and prostate and in the special case of multiple myeloma. Secondary deposits usually occur without metastases to the brain itself and reach the skull either via the systemic circulation (as in carcinoma of the breast) or via the Batson vertebral venous plexus—a valveless system of veins that runs the length of the vertebral column from the pelvic veins to the large venous sinuses of the skull, bypassing the systemic circulation (the route presumably taken by carcinoma of the prostate). Metastatic tumors of the convexity of the skull are usually asymptomatic but those at the base may implicate the cranial nerve roots or the pituitary gland. Bony metastases are readily recognized on radionuclide bone and CT scans and most are evident in plain films. Occasionally, a carcinoma metastasizes to the subdural surface dura and compresses the brain, comparable to a subdural hematoma. Many metastases in the skull and dura, perhaps most, are asymptomatic.

Apart from the above, most carcinomas reach the brain by hematogenous spread. Almost one-third of metastases to the brain originate in the lung and half this number in the breast; melanoma is the third most frequent source in most series, and the gastrointestinal tract (particularly the colon and rectum) and kidney are the next most common, in part reflecting the prevalence of each of these tumors but also because of a tropism for the nervous system, as noted below. Carcinomas of the gallbladder, liver, thyroid, testicle, uterus, ovary, pancreas, etc., account for the remainder. Tumors originating in the prostate, esophagus, oropharynx, and skin (except for melanoma) only rarely metastasize to the substance of the brain. From a different perspective, certain neoplasms are particularly prone to metastasize to the brain—75 percent of melanomas do so, 55 percent of testicular tumors, and 35 percent of bronchial carcinomas, of which 40 percent are small cell tumors according to Posner and Chernik. They describe a solitary metastasis in 47 percent of cases, a somewhat higher figure than that observed in our practice and reported by others (see Henson and Urich). The metastatic tumors most likely to be single come from kidney, breast, thyroid, and adenocarcinoma of the lung. Small cell carcinomas and melanomas more often tend to be multiple, but exceptions abound.

Generally, the cerebral metastasis forms a circumscribed mass, usually solid but sometimes in the form of a ring (i.e., cystic), that excites little glial reaction but much regional vasogenic edema. Edema alone is often evident on imaging studies until the administration of contrast exposes small tumor nodules (Fig. 31-10).

Metastases from melanoma and chorioepithelioma are often hemorrhagic, but some from the lung, thyroid, and kidney exhibit this characteristic as well. In a number of these cases, one-quarter in some series, the first manifestation of the metastasis is an intratumoral hemorrhage. The relative frequency of lung cancer makes it the most common metastatic tumor to bleed, even though only a small proportion does so.

The usual clinical picture of *metastatic carcinoma of the brain* is much like that of glioma. Seizures, headache, focal weakness, mental and behavioral abnormalities, ataxia, aphasia, and signs of increased intracranial pressure—all inexorably progressive over a few weeks or months—are the common clinical manifestations. In addition, a number of unusual syndromes may occur. One that presents particular difficulty in diagnosis is a diffuse cerebral disturbance with headache, nervousness, depressed mood, trembling, confusion, and forgetfulness, resembling a relatively rapid dementia from degenerative disease. *Cerebellar metastasis*, with headache, dizziness, and ataxia (the latter being brought out only by having the patient walk) is another condition that may be difficult to diagnose. Brainstem metastases, most often originating in the lung, are rare but distinctive, giving rise to diplopia, imbalance, and facial palsy, as in the characteristic case described by Weiss and Richardson.

The onset of symptoms from brain metastases is infrequently abrupt or even "stroke-like" rather than insidious. Some cases of sudden onset can be explained by bleeding into the tumor and others perhaps by tumor embolism that occludes a cerebral vessel. In most cases, the explanation for this temporal profile is not known. Also, non-bacterial thrombotic (marantic) endocarditis with cerebral embolism must be suspected when a stroke-like event occurs in a cancer patient. It is not unusual for one or other of these neurologic manifestations to precede the discovery of a pancreatic, bowel, gastric, breast, or lung carcinoma.

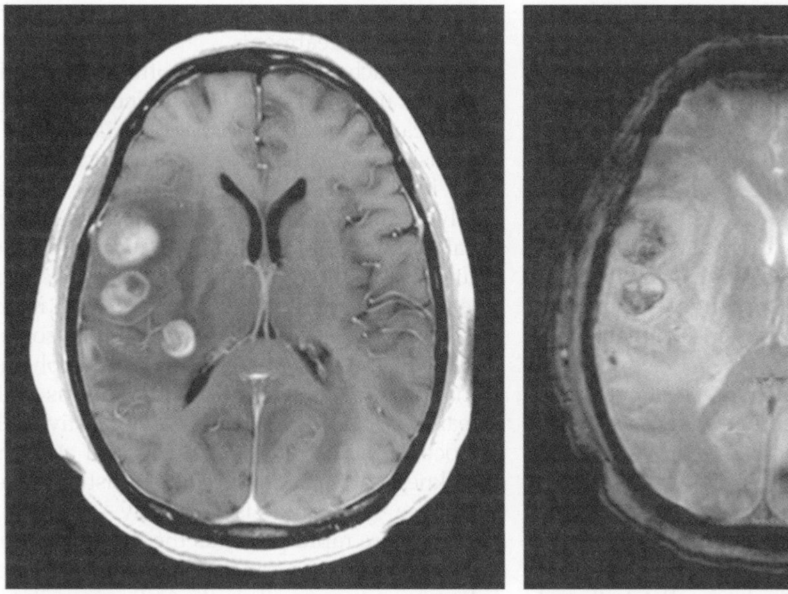

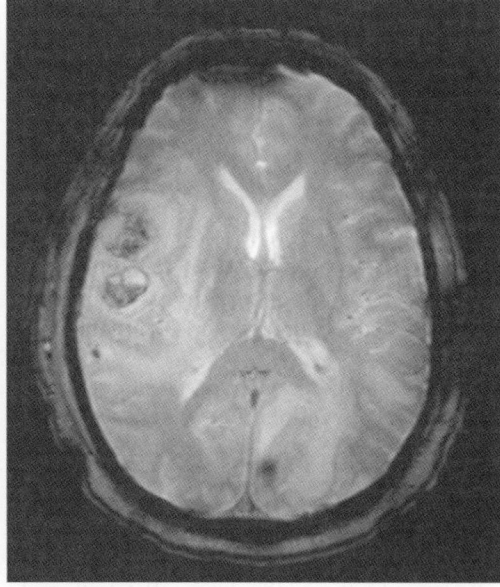

Figure 31-10. Contrast-enhanced MRI (*left*) showing multiple metastases from renal cell carcinoma. Note the extensive hypointense edema surrounding each lesion. The right image is a gradient echo MRI in which blood products appear hypointense. This sequence can aid in detection of small or nonenhancing hemorrhagic metastases, such as the lesion in the left occipital lobe.

When any of the several clinical syndromes caused by metastatic tumor is fully developed, diagnosis is relatively easy. If only headache and vomiting are present, a common problem is to attribute them to migraine or tension headache. One should invoke such explanations only if the patient has the standard symptoms of one of these conditions. CT, with and without contrast, will detect practically all sizable (1 cm) metastases though MRI is more sensitive especially for cerebellar and subcentimeter lesions, and will expose associated leptomeningeal disease. *Multiple nodular deposits of tumor in the brain on imaging studies most clearly distinguish metastatic cancer from other tumors* but this pattern may also occur with brain abscesses, brain lymphoma, and glioblastoma.

Solitary metastatic disease must be distinguished from a primary tumor of the brain and from infective abscess. Multiple brain metastases must not be confused with the neurologic syndromes that sometimes accompany carcinoma but are not caused by the invasion or compression of the nervous system by tumor. The latter, referred to as *paraneoplastic disorders*, include sensory neuronopathies and the Lambert-Eaton myasthenic syndrome (usually with carcinoma of the lung), cerebellar degeneration (ovarian and other carcinomas and Hodgkin disease), necrotizing myelopathy (rare), limbic encephalitis, and the opsoclonus–myoclonus syndrome. These paraneoplastic syndromes are discussed further on, under "Remote Effects of Neoplasia on the Nervous System (Paraneoplastic Disorders)."

In addition to the aforementioned conditions, there are many patients with cancer who exhibit symptoms of an altered mental state without evidence of metastases or a recognizable paraneoplastic disorder. These symptoms usually have their basis in systemic metabolic disturbances (hypercalcemia in particular), drugs, and psychologic reactions, some of which have yet to be clearly delineated. Problems of this type were noted in a high percentage of cancer patients seen in consultation at the Memorial Sloan-Kettering Cancer Center (Clouston et al) and are seen almost daily on the wards of our hospital. Once chemotherapy or brain radiation has been administered, the secondary effects of these treatments further cloud the picture.

Treatment The treatment of secondary (metastatic) tumors of the nervous system is undergoing a change. Current programs utilize various combinations of corticosteroids, brain irradiation, surgical intervention, and chemotherapy. Corticosteroids produce prompt improvement, probably on the basis of a reduction in the edema surrounding the lesion(s), but sustained use is restricted by side effects and eventual loss of efficacy. Most patients also temporarily benefit from the use of whole-brain irradiation, usually administered over a 2-week period, in 10 doses of 300 cGy each. High-dose focused radiotherapy is a suitable alternative for single or several cerebral metastases.

One randomized trial comparing stereotactic radiotherapy alone, or combined with whole-brain radiation for 1 to 4 metastases, found no difference in survival but there was a reduction in the frequency of recurrence at other sites in the brain when whole-brain treatment was added (Aoyama et al). Several other studies have suggested that control of local symptoms related to a metastasis is better with focused radiotherapy. However, with the exception of a single lesion from small cell lung cancer, there does not seem to be an advantage to either approach. If focused treatment has been used, whole-brain radiation can still be instituted at the time of a recurrence. Whether there is evidence to justify the routine implementation of this approach is not clear, especially as overall measures of the quality of life are not generally improved. An arbitrary limit of stereotactic treatment of four metastases arose as the field evolved but it appears that the results are similar with even greater numbers.

The issue of prophylactic radiation of the entire cranium in the case of certain tumors is more controversial. The best current information is from a trial by Slotman and colleagues and an older one by Aupérin and coworkers in patients with chemotherapy-responsive small cell lung cancer. Prophylactic radiation prolonged survival by 1.5 months and reduced the later emergence of metastasis to the brain.

In patients with a single parenchymatous metastasis (shown to be solitary by gadolinium-enhanced MRI), surgical extirpation may be undertaken provided that growth of the primary tumor and its systemic metastases is under good control and the metastasis is accessible to the surgeon and not located in a strategic motor or language area of the brain; usually excision is followed by radiation therapy to the entire brain. Patchell and coworkers have shown that survival and the interval between treatment and recurrence are longer and that the quality of life is better in patients treated in this way than in comparable patients treated with whole-brain radiation alone. Single or dual metastases from renal cell cancer, melanoma, and adenocarcinoma of the gastrointestinal tract lend themselves best to surgical removal, sometimes repeatedly.

There is increasing evidence that some metastatic brain tumors are sensitive to chemotherapeutic agents, especially if the primary tumor is similarly responsive. Intrathecal and intraventricular chemotherapy are not thought to be of value in the treatment of parenchymal metastases. Immunotherapy has not yet been widely employed.

Prophylactic antiepileptic drugs are generally not employed as they do not appear to prevent a first seizure, as mentioned earlier. Several studies, some well controlled, corroborate this as discussed in Chap. 16.

Despite all of these measures, survival is only slightly prolonged by treatment. The average period of survival in cases of brain metastases, even with therapy, is about 6 months, but it varies widely and is dominated by the extent of other systemic metastases. Between 15 and 30 percent of patients live for a year and 5 to 10 percent for 2 years; with certain radiosensitive tumors (lymphoma, testicular carcinoma, choriocarcinoma, some breast cancers), however, survival can be much longer. Patients with bone metastases tend to live longer than those with brain and meningeal metastases.

Carcinomatous Meningitis

Widespread dissemination of tumor cells throughout the meninges and ventricles, a special form of metastatic cancer, is the pattern in approximately 5 percent of cases of adenocarcinoma of breast, lung, and gastrointestinal tract, melanoma, childhood leukemia, and systemic lymphoma. This is among the most deceptive of neurologic diagnoses. With certain carcinomas, notably gastric, it may be the first manifestation of a neoplastic illness, although more often the primary tumor has been present and is under treatment.

Headache and backache, often with sciatica, are common but not invariable. Polyradiculopathies (particularly of the cauda equina), multiple cranial nerve palsies, and a confusional state have been the principal manifestations, and many cases are restricted to one of these features. Only a small number have an uncomplicated meningeal syndrome of headache, nausea, and meningismus, but these features develop within weeks in many cases. Delirium, stupor, and coma follow. Focal neurologic signs and seizures may be associated, and somewhat fewer than half the patients develop hydrocephalus. The combination of a cranial neuropathy, such as unilateral facial weakness, hearing loss (always suggestive of lymphoma), or ocular motor palsy, with bilateral asymmetrical limb weakness is particularly characteristic. The evolution in all these syndromes is generally subacute over weeks with a more rapid phase as the illness progresses.

The diagnosis can be established in most cases by identifying tumor cells in the CSF using cytology and flow cytometry techniques. More than one examination, using generous quantities of CSF, may be needed. Increased pressure in the subarachnoid space, elevation of CSF protein and low glucose levels, and lymphocytic pleocytosis (up to 100 cells but typically much fewer) are other common findings. Nevertheless, in a few patients, the CSF remains persistently normal. Measurement of certain biochemical markers of cancer in the CSF—such as lactate dehydrogenase, β-glucuronidase, β_2-microglobulin, and carcinoembryonic antigen (CEA)—offers another means of making the diagnosis and following the response to therapy. These markers are most likely to be abnormal in hematologic malignancies but may also be altered in some cases of intracranial infection and parenchymal metastases (Kaplan et al). In a few of the cases of meningeal carcinomatosis, there are also parenchymal brain metastases.

Also known is a rare primary malignant melanoma of the meninges that acts in a similar way to carcinomatous meningitis but has the striking feature of bloody CSF (1,000 to 10,000 red blood cells per mm^3). The origin of the neoplasm is from native melanotic cells in the meninges. The prognosis is as bleak as it is for metastatic carcinomatous meningitis as discussed by Liubinas et al.

Treatment and Outcome of Carcinomatous Meningitis This consists of radiation therapy to the symptomatic areas (cranium, posterior fossa, or spine) followed in selected cases by the intraventricular administration of methotrexate, but these measures rarely stabilize neurologic symptoms for more than a few weeks. The methotrexate is administered into the lateral ventricle via an Ommaya reservoir (12 mg diluted in preservative-free saline) or into the lumbar subarachnoid space through a lumbar puncture needle (12 to 15 mg). Several regimens have been devised, including daily instillation for 3 to 4 days followed by radiation, or methotrexate doses on days 1, 4, 8, 11, and 15. Involvement of the cranial nerves or an encephalopathy caused by widespread infiltration of the cranial meninges has been treated with whole-brain radiation, 3,000 cGy, given in fractions of 300 cGy per day for 10 days. Spinal root infiltration responds to spinal radiation, and regional treatments are helpful temporarily for local seeding of the lumbar roots.

The median duration of survival after diagnosis of meningeal carcinomatosis was 6 months in the large series reported by Wasserstrom and colleagues, but only 43 days in the series of Sorenson and coworkers. An encephalopathy caused by widespread tumor infiltration is a highly concerning and usually preterminal sign. The leukoencephalopathy that follows the combined use of intrathecal methotrexate and radiation therapy is described later. The best response to treatment occurs in patients with lymphoma and breast and small cell lung cancers; cases of meningeal infiltration by other lung cancers, melanoma, and adenocarcinoma do most poorly.

Involvement of the Nervous System in Leukemia

Almost one-third of all leukemic patients have evidence of diffuse infiltration of the leptomeninges and cranial and spinal nerve roots at autopsy (Barcos et al). The incidence is greater in acute than in chronic leukemia and greater in lymphocytic than in myelocytic leukemia; it is also far more frequent in children than in adults. The highest incidence is in children with acute lymphocytic (lymphoblastic) leukemia who relapse after treatment with combination chemotherapy (60 to 70 percent at time of death). The clinical and CSF picture of meningeal leukemia is much the same as that of meningeal carcinomatosis discussed earlier, with the qualification that leukemic cells are more likely to be found by cytologic examination of the spinal fluid. The treatment of the two disorders is also similar.

The studies of Price and Johnson demonstrated that CNS leukemia is primarily a pial disease. The earliest evidence of leukemia is detected in the walls of pial veins, with or without cells lying freely in the CSF. The leukemic infiltrate in our pathologic material has extended to the deep perivascular spaces, where the pial-glial membrane often confines it; at this stage the CSF consistently contains leukemic cells. Depending on the severity of meningeal involvement, transgression of the pial-glial membrane eventually occurs, with varying degrees of superficial parenchymal infiltration by collections of leukemic cells. Hemorrhages of varying sizes are another common complication and are sometimes lethal. Chloroma, a solid green-colored mass of myelogenous leukemic cells, may infiltrate the dura or, less often, the brain, but it is distinctly uncommon.

Cranial radiation, combined with methotrexate given intrathecally or intravenously, has been effective in the prevention and treatment of meningeal involvement in childhood leukemia. However, in a significant number of patients this combination gives rise to a distinctive *necrotizing leukoencephalopathy* within several days to months after the last administration of methotrexate and several months after completion of radiotherapy (Robain et al). The leukoencephalopathy occurs most frequently and is most severe when all three modalities of treatment, i.e., cranial irradiation and intrathecal and intravenous methotrexate, are used. The initial symptoms—consisting of apathy, drowsiness, depression of consciousness, and behavioral disorders—evolve over a few weeks to include cerebellar ataxia, spasticity, pseudobulbar palsy, extrapyramidal motor abnormalities, and akinetic mutism. Large hypodense areas of varying size appear on CT but—unlike the case with tumor metastases—there is no contrast enhancement. On MRI these lesions appear T2 hyperintense, but compared with pure radiation necrosis (see further on), they have poorly demarcated borders and like on CT, do not enhance. In some patients the condition stabilizes or improves, with corresponding radiographic resolution of the lesions. More often the patient is left with severe persistent sequelae; in most, death occurs within several weeks or months of onset but a few survive for years. Radiation injury seems to be the most important factor, coupled with the age of the patient (most are younger than 5 years old). In an attempt to reduce the cognitive sequela of cranial radiation in children with leukemia, Pui and coworkers conducted a study and found that it could be safely omitted if all other aspects of therapy have been optimized.

Involvement of the Nervous System in Systemic Lymphoma

Extradural compression of the spinal cord or cauda equina is the most common neurologic complication of all types of lymphoma, the result of extension from vertebrae or paravertebral lymph nodes. Treatment is with radiation to the affected portion of the neuraxis or, if a tissue diagnosis is lacking, surgical decompression. Systemic lymphoma rarely metastasizes to the brain. In a review of more than 100 autopsies at the Mallory Institute of Pathology, our colleague R.D. Adams observed only a half-dozen instances where patients with lymphomas had deposits of tumor cells in the brain and in none of these cases were they from multiple myeloma (Sparling et al). In the series of Levitt and associates, comprising 592 patients with non-Hodgkin lymphoma, there were only 8 with intracerebral metastases.

Much more common is meningeal dissemination of non-Hodgkin lymphoma (the earlier mentioned *neurolymphomatosis*), the clinical and CSF pictures being similar to those of meningeal leukemia and carcinomatosis described earlier. In the rare cases of meningeal involvement with Hodgkin lymphoma, there may be an eosinophilic pleocytosis. Leptomeningeal dissemination occurs almost exclusively in high-grade lymphomas with diffuse (rather than nodular) changes in the lymph nodes. Cranial nerve palsies are common, with a predilection for the eighth nerve; the cauda equina is involved eventually in most cases. The optimal treatment has not yet been ascertained. Radiotherapy and systemic and intraventricular chemotherapy have all met with some degree of success in small series.

Intravascular Lymphoma and Related Disorders (Malignant Angioendotheliomatosis, Angiotropic or Angioblastic Lymphoma, Lymphomatoid Granulomatosis, Castleman Disease)

These conditions are presented here with other forms of lymphoma, although their clinical behavior is as much in keeping with a vasculitic or prelymphomatous process. Although considered rare, we encounter several new cases yearly in our service. The nomenclature is confusing and the original term, *lymphomatoid granulomatosis* (also known as Castleman disease), is not equivalent to the more recently elucidated process of intravascular lymphoma; it is more accurate to consider the former a prelymphomatous process. As described by Liebow and colleagues, lymphomatoid granulomatosis is a systemic disease with prominent nodular pulmonary lesions, dermal, and lymph node changes and, in approximately 30 percent of cases, involvement of the CNS. In a small proportion, the changes are confined to the nervous system. According to Katzenstein and associates, a systemic malignant lymphoma develops in 12 percent of such patients, but others have noted this transformation in a considerably higher number. The genomic sequences of EBV, HHV-6, or HHV-8 have been found in most of these lesions.

The *angioblastic or intravascular lymphoma*, on the other hand, is regarded as a multifocal neoplasm of large anaplastic monoclonal lymphocytes that infiltrate the walls of blood vessels and surrounding areas (Sheibani et al) or grow intravascularly and cause occlusion of small and moderate-sized vessels, hence the several alternative designations for the same process. The disease can be distinguished from primary CNS lymphoma, which is also typically "angiocentric," meaning centered around vessels, but does not selectively invade and occlude vascular structures. In the brain and spinal cord there are lesions of various sizes that represent the combined effects of occlusion of small vessels and concentric infiltration of the adjacent tissue by neoplastic cells. In half of the cases, meningeal vessels are involved and in a few, the peripheral nerves, or more particularly the endoneurial vessels within spinal roots, have been involved by the neoplasm, and we have seen two cases with a flaccid paraplegia on this basis.

Although the lymphoid origin of the intravascular anaplastic cells is clear, not all are T cells as was at one time believed; an equal number are B cells. As in some cases of primary CNS lymphoma, portions of the genome of EBV have been isolated from the malignant B cells in a few cases. It has been proposed that the disorder in some cases represents an EBV-induced proliferation of B cells with a prominent inflammatory T-cell reaction (Guinee et al).

Because of the inconsistent location and size of the nervous system lesions there is no uniform syndrome, but intravascular lymphoma should be suspected in patients with a subacute encephalopathy and indications of focal brain and spinal cord or nerve root lesions. Headache is a prominent early component in some cases. One of our patients had intermittent seizures 3 months before confusion and progressive encephalopathy. The variety of clinical presentations is emphasized in the reviews of cases by Beristain and Azzarelli and the article by Glass and associates (1993). All had focal cerebral signs, 7 had dementia, 5 had seizures, and 2 had myelopathy. Some of our own patients, as mentioned above, have also had a flaccid paraplegia as a result of infiltration of the cauda roots; this peripheral involvement has been commented on by other authors. Only a few patients will have nodular or multiple infiltrative pulmonary lesions, skin lesions, or adenopathy; almost all of our cases were restricted to the brain and spinal cord, but other reports suggest systemic disease in a high proportion, including infiltration of the adrenal glands.

MRI shows multiple nodular or variegated abnormalities on T2-weighted images throughout the white matter of the brain; most lesions are enhanced by gadolinium, and some demonstrate restricted diffusion resulting from microvascular occlusion and infarction. In one of the cases we studied there were numerous hemorrhagic lesions. Definitive diagnosis is possible only through a biopsy of radiographically involved lung or nervous tissue that includes tissue with numerous intrinsic blood vessels. A helpful diagnostic feature may be the presence of antibodies to nuclear cytoplasmic antigens (c-ANCA), in some cases, as they are in a number of other vasculitic and granulomatous processes. A small number of our patients have also had adrenal or renal enlargement, as mentioned earlier, presumably because of infiltration of the vessels of these organs by the neoplasm. The spinal fluid has a variable lymphocytic pleocytosis and protein elevation, but malignant cells are not found. The sedimentation rate and serum lactate dehydrogenase (LDH) are said to be elevated in most patients, but this has not been consistently so in our experience.

Similar to demyelinating and lymphomatous lesions, these abnormalities may recede temporarily in response to treatment with corticosteroids and there is corresponding clinical improvement. The course tends to be fluctuating over months, although one of our patients died within weeks despite treatment. In a few cases, whole-brain irradiation has been successful in prolonging survival, but the outlook in most instances is poor.

An uncertain number of these patients have AIDS, although we have not encountered this combination. The illness must be distinguished from multiple sclerosis, primary CNS lymphoma, gliomatosis cerebri, and a process that simulates it closely, sarcoidosis (which produces brain and lung lesions) as well as from the cerebral vasculitides and Behçet disease, but intravascular lymphoma is more rapidly progressive than most of these conditions.

Sarcomas of the Brain

These are malignant tumors composed of cells derived from connective tissue elements (fibroblasts, rhabdomyocytes, lipocytes, osteoblasts, smooth muscle cells). They take their names from their histogenetic derivation—namely, fibrosarcoma, rhabdomyosarcoma, osteogenic sarcoma, and chondrosarcoma—and sometimes from the tissue of which the cells are a part, such as adventitial sarcomas and hemangiopericytoma.

All these tumors are rare. They constitute from 1 to 3 percent of intracranial tumors, depending on how wide a range of neoplasms one chooses to include in this group (see below). Occasionally one or more cerebral deposits of these types of tumors will occur as a metastasis from a sarcoma in another organ. Almost all others are primary in the cranial cavity and exhibit as one of their unique properties a tendency to metastasize to nonneural tissues—a decidedly rare occurrence with primary glial tumors. It is a disturbing fact that a few sarcomas have developed 5 to

10 years after cranial irradiation or, in one instance among 3,000 patients of which we are aware, after proton beam irradiation of the brain. Fibrosarcomas have occurred after radiation of pituitary adenomas and osteogenic sarcoma after other types of radiation, all localized to bone or meninges. Our experience with hemangiopericytoma has included to two intracranial lesions that simulated meningiomas and two others that arose in the high cervical spinal cord and caused subacute quadriparesis initially misdiagnosed as a polyneuropathy.

A number of other cerebral tumors, described in the literature as sarcomas, are probably tumors of other types. The rapidly growing, highly malignant "monstrocellular sarcoma" of Zülch or "giant cell fibrosarcoma" of Kernohan and Uihlein, so named for their multinucleated giant cells, were reinterpreted by Rubinstein (1972) as a form of giant cell glioblastoma or mixed glioblastoma and fibrosarcoma. The "hemangiopericytoma of the leptomeninges," also classified by Kernohan and Uihlein as a form of cerebral sarcoma, is considered by Rubinstein (1972) to be a variant of the angioblastic meningioma.

Patients who Present Primarily with Signs of Increased Intracranial Pressure (Medulloblastoma, Ependymoma of the Fourth Ventricle, Hemangioblastoma of the Cerebellum, Pinealoma, Colloid Cyst of the Third Ventricle and Rarer Related Tumors)

Upon first presentation, a number of patients show the characteristic symptoms and signs of increased intracranial pressure: periodic bifrontal and bioccipital headaches that awaken the patient during the night or are present upon awakening, projectile vomiting, mental torpor, unsteady gait, sphincteric incontinence, and papilledema. Most of these symptoms and the increased ICP are the result of hydrocephalus.

The diagnostic problem is resolved by CT or MRI, which should be obtained in all patients with symptoms of increased intracranial pressure with or without focal signs. In addition to the tumors listed in the heading above, other tumors that may present in this way are central neurocytoma, craniopharyngioma, and a high spinal cord tumor. In addition, with some of the gliomas discussed in the preceding section, increased intracranial pressure may occasionally precede the first focal cerebral signs.

Medulloblastoma, Neuroblastoma, and Retinoblastoma

Medulloblastoma Medulloblastoma is an invasive and rapidly growing tumor, mainly of childhood, that arises in the posterior part of the cerebellar vermis and neuroepithelial roof of the fourth ventricle in children. It accounts for 20 percent of childhood brain tumors. Rarely, it presents elsewhere in the cerebellum or other parts of the brain in adults (Peterson and Walker).

The origin of this tumor remained in doubt for a long time and is still not entirely settled, but some recent insights are notable. Bailey and Cushing introduced the name *medulloblastoma,* although medulloblasts have never been identified in the fetal or adult human brain; nevertheless the term has been retained for no reason other than its familiarity. The current view of the tumor is that it originates from pluripotential stem cells (that can differentiate into neuronal or glial elements) that have been prevented from maturing to their normal growth-arrested state. For this reason, newer classifications include it among the primitive neuroectodermal tumors (PNETs).

The tumor may differentiate uni- or pluripotentially, varying from case to case, and accounting for the recognized histologic variants, ranging from the undifferentiated medulloblastoma to medulloblastoma with glial, neuronal, or even myoblastic components. Rosette formation, highly characteristic of the below-described neuroblastoma is seen in half of medulloblastomas. Certain molecular genetic similarities relate the medulloblastoma to retinoblastomas and pineal cell tumors, and, rarely, to autosomal dominant diseases such as nevoid basal cell carcinoma. Chromosomal studies of medulloblastomas reveal a deletion on the distal part of chromosome 17 distal to the *p53* region. Schmidek has proposed that this accounts for the neoplastic transformation of cerebellar stem cells at various stages of their differentiation into tumor cells. It is also notable that medulloblastomas are encountered in Gorlin syndrome, caused by mutations in the gene encoding "patched," the receptor for sonic hedgehog ligand, and in Turcot syndrome, as a consequence of mutations in DNA repair genes (Louis et al). Gene expression profiling has given preliminary evidence that amplification or overexpression of the transcription factor MYCN (N-MYC) is associated with a poorer prognosis (as it is in neuroblastoma). Aberrations in the copy number of chromosomes 6q and 17q also appear to have predictive value for the behavior of the tumor. Maris has reviewed the complex genetic aspects of the tumor and has introduced the possibility that a combination of common variants may be a risk factor for its development. Another line of research has implicated the JC virus, the same agent that causes progressive multifocal leukoencephalopathy (Chap. 33). Genomic sequences from this virus have been found in 72 percent of tumors in some series (Khalili et al), and an experimental transgenic model in which the JC protein is expressed is characterized by a cerebellar tumor that resembles the medulloblastoma.

The majority of the patients are children 4 to 8 years of age, and males outnumber females 3:2 or 3:1 in most reported series. As a rule, symptoms have been present for 1 to 5 months before the diagnosis is made. The clinical picture is fairly distinctive and derives from secondary hydrocephalus and raised intracranial pressure as a result of blockage of the fourth ventricle. Typically, the child becomes listless, vomits repeatedly, and has a morning headache. The first diagnosis that suggests itself may be gastrointestinal disease or abdominal migraine. Soon, however, a stumbling gait, frequent falls, and diplopia as well as strabismus lead to a neurologic examination and the discovery of papilledema or sixth nerve palsies. However, when the tumor is located in the lateral cerebellum or in the cerebrum, as it usually is in adults, signs of raised intracranial pressure may be delayed. Dizziness (positional) and nystagmus are then frequent. A small proportion of children have a slight sensory loss on one side of the face and a mild facial weakness. Head tilt, the occiput being tilted back and away from the side of the tumor, indicates a developing cerebellar-foraminal herniation. Rarely, signs of spinal root and subarachnoid metastases precede cerebellar signs.

Extraneural metastases (cervical lymph nodes, lung, liver, and particularly bone) may occur, but usually only after craniotomy, which may allow tumor cells to reach scalp lymphatics. In rare instances the tumor cells may be spontaneously blood-borne and become metastatic to lung or liver. Decerebrate attacks ("cerebellar fits") appear in the late stages of the disease.

The radiologic appearance is also distinctive: high signal intensity on both T1- and T2-weighted MRIs, heterogeneous enhancement, and, of course, the typical location adjacent to and extending into the fourth ventricle. The tumor frequently fills the fourth ventricle and infiltrates its floor (Fig. 31-11). Seeding of the tumor may occur on the ependymal and meningeal surfaces of the cisterna magna and around the spinal cord. The tumor is solid, gray-pink in color, and fairly well demarcated from the adjacent brain tissue. It is very cellular, and the cells are small and closely packed with hyperchromatic nuclei, little cytoplasm, many mitoses, and a tendency to form clusters and pseudorosettes. The interstitial tissue is sparse.

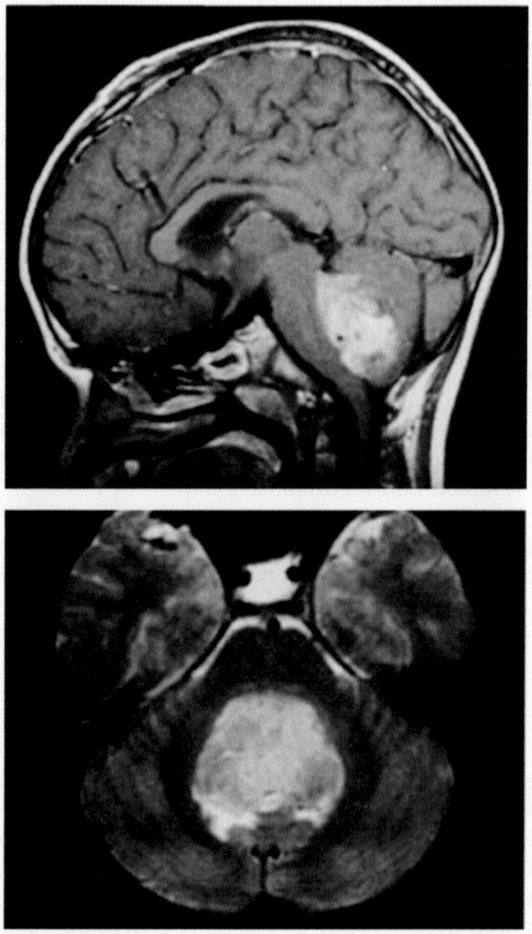

Figure 31-11. Medulloblastoma. MRI in the sagittal (*above*) and axial (*below*) planes, illustrating involvement of the cerebellar vermis and neoplastic obliteration of the fourth ventricle.

Treatment Maximal resection of the tumor is recommended. The addition of chemotherapy and radiotherapy of the entire neuraxis improves the rate and length of disease-free survival even for those children with the most extensive tumors at the time of diagnosis (Packer). The combination of surgery, radiation of the entire neuraxis, and chemotherapy permits a 5-year survival in more than 80 percent of cases.

Fear of radiation-induced cognitive deficits in the young children most often affected by this tumor has led to exploration of postoperative chemotherapy without radiation. Rutkowski and colleagues have reported some promising results, especially in those who had gross total tumor resection, but a large number nonetheless acquired a leukoencephalopathy that was said to be asymptomatic. The presence of desmoplastic features (i.e., connective tissue formations) is associated with a better prognosis independent of the type or treatment. Children who have residual tumor, and more so those with metastases, have a much poorer prognosis. Any of the features of brainstem invasion, spinal subarachnoid metastases, incomplete removal, and very early age of onset (younger than 3 years) greatly reduce the period of survival. Acquired genetic alterations in the tumor cells that have prognostic influence have been summarized earlier. A novel inhibitor of the abnormal hedgehog pathway in medulloblastoma cells had a marked effect in one adult patient (Rudin et al).

Neuroblastoma This, the most common solid tumor of childhood, is a different entity from medulloblastoma but of nearly identical histologic appearance, arising in the adrenal medulla and sometimes metastasizing widely. Usually it remains extradural even if it invades the cranial and spinal cavities. The main neurologic interest is a syndrome of *polymyoclonus with opsoclonus and ataxia* that occurs as a paraneoplastic complication as discussed further on. A rare form of neuroblastic medulloblastoma in adults tends to be more benign (Rubinstein, 1985).

In keeping with the genetic determinants of prognosis in this broad class of tumors, a loss of heterozygosity of certain sites on chromosomes 1 and 11 has been associated with somewhat poorer outcomes by Attiyeh and colleagues. MYCN amplification or overexpression is a poor prognostic factor, as it is in medulloblastoma. Various acquired chromosomal deletions and gains may also have predictive importance. More provocative are findings that suggest the emergence of an aggressive tumor based on polymorphisms in chromosome 6p. Maris has provided a review of the interesting genetic aspects of the tumor.

Several staging systems have evolved for neuroblastoma and The Children's Oncology Group has produced a risk-based system that includes the status of chromosomal changes (17q, 1p, 11q), but these approaches are under frequent revision.

Treatment is predicated on clinical staging, with the lowest risk category allowing observation because some lesions regress spontaneously. Those patients who are at intermediate risk are treated with chemotherapy and high-risk children have surgical resection and receive intensive chemotherapy, radiation, and in selected cases, hematopoietic stem cell transplantation. The two better-risk strata have survival rates exceeding 90 percent, but the highest risk group has a 30 percent survival rate.

Retinoblastoma Another closely related tumor is *retinoblastoma*. This proves to be one of the most frequent extracranial malignant tumors of infancy and childhood. Eighty percent develop before the fifth year of life. It is a small cell tumor with neurofibrils and, like neuroblastoma, has a tendency to form rosettes. The tumor develops within the eye and the blindness that it induces may be overlooked in an infant or small child. It is easily seen ophthalmoscopically, because it arises from cells of the developing retina. An abnormal protein encoded by a growth-suppressor or antioncogenic gene (Rb), mentioned earlier in relation to the genetics of brain tumors, has been identified. It is postulated that an inherited mutation affects one allele of the normal gene, and only if this is accompanied by a mutation that eliminates the function of the second allele will the tumor develop. Early recognition and radiation or surgery effect cure.

Ependymoma and Papilloma of the Fourth Ventricle

Ependymomas, as pointed out earlier in this chapter, arise from the lining cells in the walls of the ventricles. Approximately 70 percent of them originate in the fourth ventricle, according to Fokes and Earle (Fig. 31-12). Postmortem, some of these tumors, if small, are found protruding into the fourth ventricle, never having produced local symptoms. Whereas the supratentorial ependymoma occurs at all ages, fourth ventricular ependymomas appear mostly in childhood. In the large series of Fokes and Earle (83 cases), 33 developed in the first decade of life, 6 in the second decade, and 44 after the age of 20 years. Males have been affected almost twice as often as females.

Cerebral ependymomas usually arise from the floor of the fourth ventricle and extend through the foramina of Luschka and Magendie. They may later invade the medulla. These tumors produce a clinical syndrome much like that of the medulloblastoma except for their more protracted course and lack of early cerebellar signs. The histologic features of this tumor were described earlier in this chapter. The degree of anaplastic change varies and has prognostic significance. The most anaplastic form is the *ependymoblastoma*, a highly aggressive tumor that falls within the spectrum of primitive neuroectodermal tumors (see later).

Symptoms may be present for 1 or 2 years before diagnosis and operation. About two-thirds of the patients come to notice because of increased intracranial pressure; in the remainder, vomiting, difficulty in swallowing, paresthesia of the extremities, abdominal pain, vertigo, and neck flexion or head tilt are prominent manifestations. Some patients with impending cerebellar–tonsillar herniation are disinclined to sit and have vertical downbeating nystagmus. Surgical removal offers the only hope of survival. The addition of radiation therapy and sometimes ventriculoperitoneal shunting of CSF may prolong life. Myxopapillary ependymomas of the spinal cord and filum are discussed with the spinal cord tumors.

Papillomas of the choroid plexus are about one-fifth as frequent as ependymomas. They arise mainly in the lateral and fourth ventricles, occasionally in the third. Two authoritative studies (Laurence et al; Matson and Crofton) give the ratios of lateral/third/fourth ventricular locations as 50:10:40. The tumor, which takes the form of a giant choroid plexus, has as its cellular element the cuboidal epithelium of the plexus, which is closely related embryologically to the ependyma. An oncogene

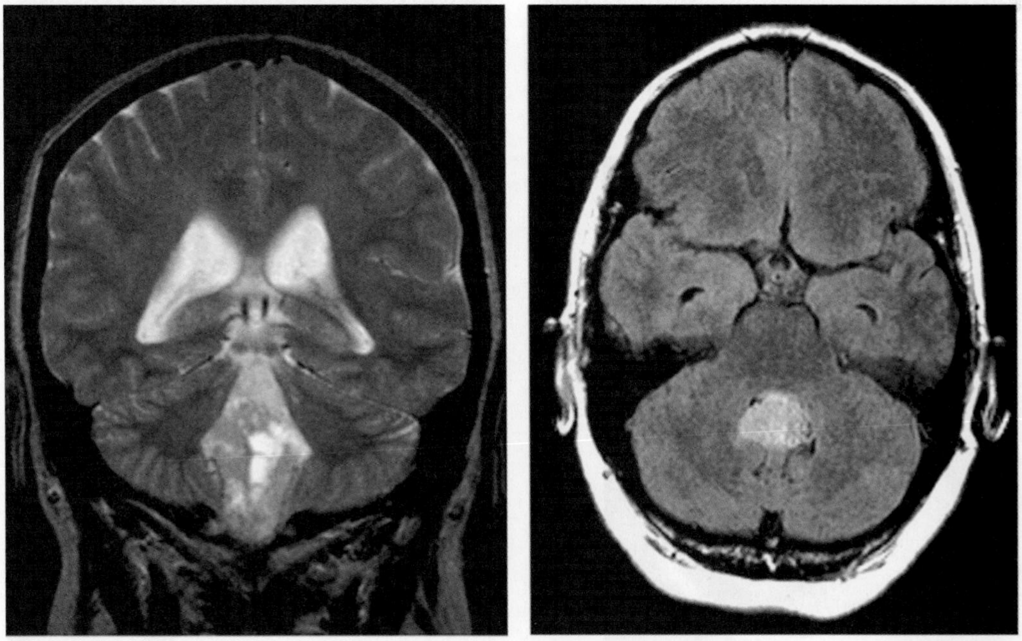

A B

Figure 31-12. Ependymoma of the fourth ventricle. *A*. Coronal T2 MRI shows an ependymoma growing out of the fourth ventricle. *B*. Axial T2 FLAIR MRI shows that the mass completely obliterates the fourth ventricle.

T (tumor) antigen of the SV40 virus is possibly involved in tumor induction (see Schmidek). Essentially, these are tumors of childhood. Fully 50 percent cause symptoms in the first year of life and 75 percent in the first decade. In the younger patient, hydrocephalus is usually the presenting syndrome, sometimes aggravated acutely by hemorrhage; there may be papilledema, an unusual finding in a hydrocephalic infant with enlarging head. Headaches, lethargy, stupor, spastic weakness of the legs, unsteadiness of gait, and diplopia are more frequent in the older child. Tumors that arise from the choroid plexus and project into the lateral recess of the fourth ventricle may present with a syndrome of the cerebellopontine angle (see further on). One consequence of the tumor (rather uncertain or inconsistent) may be increased CSF formation, which contributes to the hydrocephalus. Some of the tumors acquire more malignant attributes (mitoses, atypia of nuclei) and invade surrounding brain. They have the appearance of a carcinoma and may be mistaken for an epithelial metastasis from an extracranial site.

Treatment by surgical excision is usually curative, but palliative ventricular shunting may be needed first if the patient's condition does not permit surgery. The prognosis of the rare choroid plexus carcinomas is poor.

Primitive Neuroectodermal Tumor

This term was introduced by Hart and Earle in 1973 to describe tumors that have the histologic features of medulloblastoma but occur supratentorially. Various poorly differentiated or embryonal tumors of infancy and childhood were in the past included in this group: medulloblastoma, neuroblastoma, retinoblastoma, ependymoblastoma, and pineoblastoma (described further on). Subsequent authors have broadened the category of PNETs to include all CNS neoplasms of neuroectodermal origin. With the advent of immunohistochemical techniques, many of these poorly differentiated neoplasms of infancy came to be recognized as small cell gliomas (Friede et al); others, after ultrastructural study, could be classified as other types of primitive neoplasms. To some pathologists, the term *primitive neuroectodermal tumors* has appeal but has added little to our understanding of their undifferentiated embryonal origin. In practical terms, the prognosis and treatment of all these tumors are much the same, regardless of what they are called (see Duffner et al). Certain patterns of gene expression are used to distinguish this group of tumors from histologically similar medulloblastomas.

Hemangioblastoma of the Cerebellum

This tumor is referred to most often in connection with von Hippel-Lindau disease. Dizziness, ataxia of gait or of the limbs on one side, symptoms and signs of increased ICP from compression of the fourth ventricle, and in some instances an associated retinal angioma or hepatic and pancreatic cysts (disclosed by CT or MRI) constitute the syndrome. There is a tendency later for the development of malignant renal or adrenal tumors. Many patients have polycythemia as a result of elaboration of an erythropoietic factor by the tumor.

The age of onset is usually between 15 and 50 years. Blacks, whites, and Asians are equally affected. Dominant inheritance of von Hippel-Lindau disease is well known. Seizinger and coworkers, in cases associated with renal cell carcinoma and pheochromocytoma, localized a defect in a tumor suppressor gene (termed *VHL*; see Chap. 38).

The diagnosis can be deduced from the appearance on CT or MRI of a cerebellar cyst containing an enhancing nodular lesion on its wall. Often the associated retinal hemangioma will be disclosed by the same imaging procedure. The angiographic picture is also characteristic: a cluster of small vessels forming a mass 1.0 to 2.0 cm in diameter (Fig. 31-13). Craniotomy with opening of the cerebellar cyst and excision of the mural hemangioblastomatous nodule is usually curative, but there is a high rate of recurrence if the entire tumor, including the nodule, is not completely removed. In the series of Boughey and colleagues, the lesion was successfully excised in 80 percent

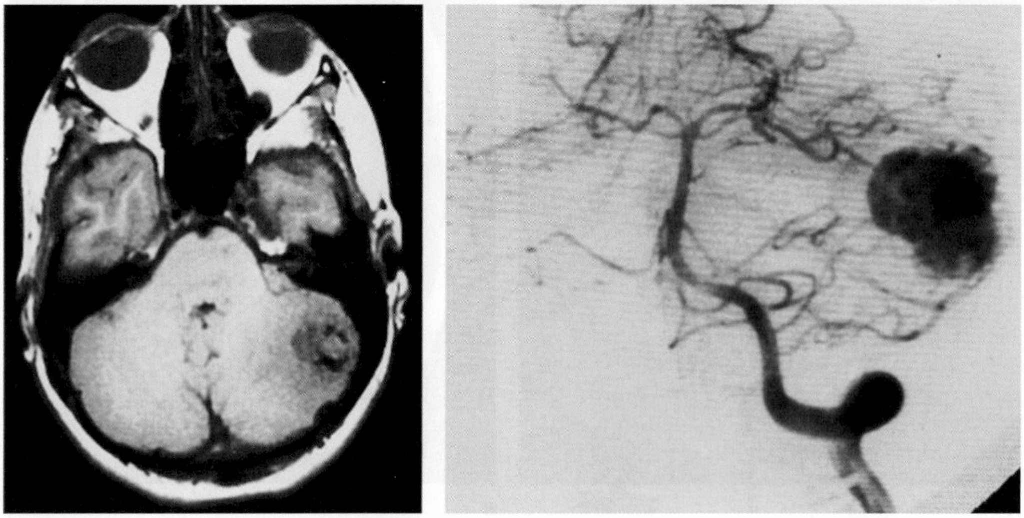

Figure 31-13. Hemangioblastoma. Contrast-enhanced MRI in the axial plane (*left*) shows the vascular tumor in the left cerebellar hemisphere. Selective left vertebral angiogram (*right*) defines a hypervascular nodule with dilated draining veins.

of patients; 15 percent of patients, who had only partial resection of an isolated cerebellar lesion, developed recurrent tumors. More recently, several groups have used endovascular embolization of the vascular nodule prior to surgery, but it is not clear if this reduces the incidence of recurrence. Treatment with focused radiation is also being undertaken, particularly for multifocal or surgically inaccessible lesions, and several modern case series using either stereotactic radiosurgery, or external or proton beam radiation indicate results that may be comparable to conventional treatment.

Hemangioblastomas of the spinal cord are frequently associated with a syringomyelic lesion (greater than 70 percent of cases); such lesions may be multiple and are located mainly in the posterior columns. A retinal hemangioblastoma may be the initial finding and leads to blindness if not treated by laser. New lesions continue to be formed over a period of years while the patient is under observation. The children of a parent with a hemangioblastoma of the cerebellum should be examined regularly for an ocular lesion and renal cell carcinoma.

Pineal Tumors

There has been much uncertainty as to the proper classification of pineal tumors. Originally they were all thought to be composed of pineal cells; hence they were classified as true *pinealomas*, a term suggested by Krabbe. Globus and Silbert believed that these originated from embryonic pineal cells but Russell later pointed out that some tumors in the pineal region are really atypical teratomas resembling the seminoma of the testicle. Four types of pineal tumors are now recognized: *germinoma*, nongerminatous germ cell tumors, *pinealoma* (pineocytoma, atypical pineocytoma, and pineoblastoma), and a *glioma* originating in astroglial cells of the pineal body. Some would include teratomas in this group.

The germinoma is a firm, discrete mass that usually reaches 3 to 4 cm in greatest diameter. It compresses the superior colliculi and sometimes the superior surface of the cerebellum and narrows the aqueduct of Sylvius. Often it extends anteriorly into the third ventricle and may then compress the hypothalamus. A germinoma may also arise in the *suprasellar area*. Microscopically, these tumors are composed of large, spherical epithelial cells separated by a network of reticular connective tissue and containing many lymphocytes.

Of the four groups of pineal tumors, approximately 50 percent are germinomas. Pinealomas, pineoblastomas, and gliomas are infrequent. Children, adolescents, and young adults—males more than females—are affected. Only rarely does one see a patient with a pineal tumor that has developed after the thirtieth year of life.

The *pineocytoma, atypical pineocytoma,* and *pineoblastoma* reproduce the normal structure of the pineal gland. These tumors enlarge the gland, are locally invasive, and may extend into the third ventricle and seed along the neuraxis. Cytologically, the pineocytoma is a moderately cellular tumor with none of the histologic attributes of anaplasia. The tumor cells tend to form circular arrangements, so-called pineocytomatous rosettes. Pinealocytes may be impregnated by silver carbonate methods, and some contain the retinal S antigen of photoreceptor cells. Pineoblastomas are highly cellular and composed of small, undifferentiated cells bearing some resemblance to medulloblasts. The *teratoma* and *dermoid* and epidermoid cysts of the pineal body have no special features—some are quite benign. The gliomas have the usual morphologic characteristics of an astrocytoma of varying degrees of malignancy. In some cases, the clinical syndrome of the several types of pineal tumors consists solely of symptoms and signs of increased intracranial pressure. Beyond this, the most characteristic localizing signs are an inability to look upward and slightly dilated pupils that react on accommodation but not to light (Parinaud syndrome). Sometimes ataxia of the limbs, choreic movements, or spastic weakness appears in the later stages of the illness. It is uncertain whether the ocular and motor signs are caused by neoplastic compression of the brachia conjunctivae and other tegmental structures of the upper midbrain or to hydrocephalus (dilatation of the posterior part of the third ventricle). Probably both mechanisms are operative. Precocious puberty occurs in males who harbor a germinoma. Although the pineal gland is the source of melatonin, sleep is not affected to an important degree in patients with these tumors, as discussed in "The Pineal Gland and Melatonin" in Chap. 27. Measurement of CSF or serum melatonin is useful mainly in the detection of tumor recurrence after surgical extirpation. In patients with a germ cell tumor, the CSF or serum may show elevations of β-human choriogonadotropin or alpha-fetoprotein. The diagnosis is made by neuroimaging (Fig. 31-14). The CSF may contain tumor cells and lymphocytes but may also be entirely normal.

Treatment These lesions were formerly judged to be inoperable. However, the use of the operating microscope now makes it possible to excise them by a supracerebellar or transtentorial approach. Operation for purposes of excision and histologic diagnosis is advised because each type of pineal tumor must be managed differently. Moreover, one may occasionally find an arachnoidal cyst that needs only excision. The germ cell tumors should be removed insofar as possible and the ventricular region radiated for germinomas, and the whole neuraxis is treated in the case of nongerminomatous lesions. The use of chemotherapy in addition to or instead of cranial irradiation is still being evaluated. Several of our patients have survived more than 5 years after the removal of a pineal glioma.

Neuroepithelial Tumors (DNET), Germinomas, Gangliocytomas, Mixed Neuronal-Glial Tumors, and Lhermitte-Duclos Disease

Malignant germ cell tumors occurring in locations other than the pineal body are usually found in the suprasellar space and rarely in the roof of the third. Germinoma is the most common of this rare group of neoplasms, which also includes choriocarcinoma, embryonal cell carcinoma, endodermal sinus tumors, and malignant teratomas. Certain biochemical markers of these tumors are of interest and of clinical utility, because they may be detected in samples of the blood and CSF. The beta subunit of human chorionic gonadotropin (hCG) is elaborated by choriocarcinoma and alpha-fetoprotein, and by endodermal sinus tumors and

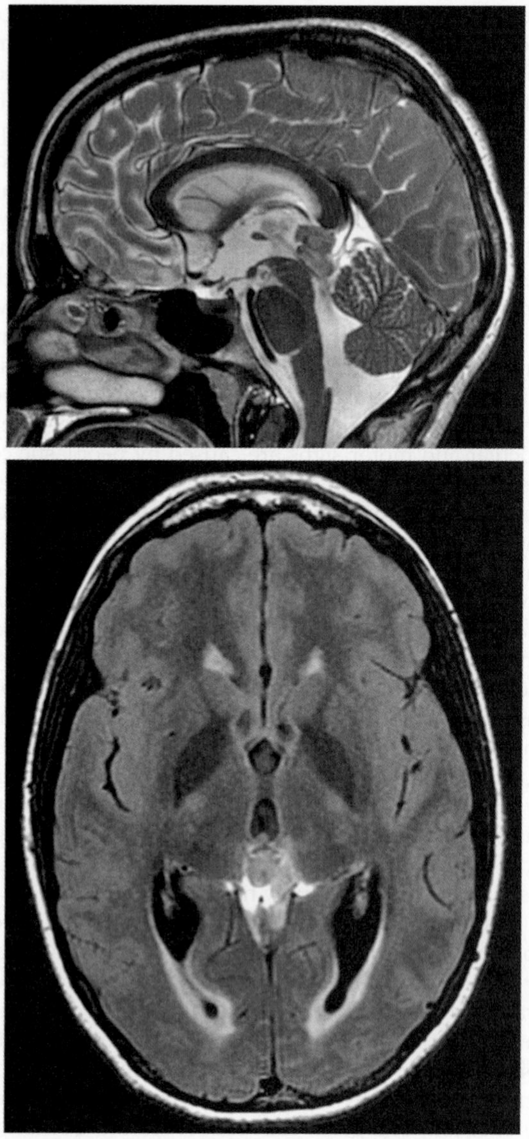

Figure 31-14. Pineal tumor. T2-weighted MRI in the sagittal plane (*above*) demonstrates a tumor that compresses the tectum and the cerebral aqueduct. Axial T2 FLAIR MRI (*below*) shows the tumor and evidence of hydrocephalus and transependymal flow of CSF from the lateral ventricles, resulting from aqueductal compression.

immature teratomas. Typical germinomas have shown little elevation of either. Most often these markers indicate the presence of complex mixed germ cell tumors.

Gangliogliomas and mixed neuronal–glial tumors are special tumor types, more frequent in the young and of variable but usually low-grade malignancy. They are composed both of differentiated glial cells, usually astrocytes, and of neurons in various degrees of differentiation. The latter, which may resemble glial cells, can be identified by Nissl stains, silver stains, and immunochemical reactions for cytoskeletal proteins. Inflammation is common in the parenchyma and adjacent to these tumors; this has led to the erroneous diagnosis of a nonneoplastic inflammatory condition if only limited biopsy samples are taken.

Some of these developmental tumors are difficult to separate from hamartomas or from the tubers of tuberous sclerosis. In the case of hamartomas, it may be difficult to determine if the tumor or the associated developmental abnormality is the cause of seizures. Some of these tumors take the form of large, slowly growing cystic lesions.

The best characterized, albeit rare, type in this group is the *gangliocytoma*, a tumor that occurs in the adrenal gland, retroperitoneal and thoracic sympathetic chain, internal auditory canal, and in the spinal cord. One form is the dysplastic gangliocytoma of the cerebellum (Lhermitte-Duclos disease). This is a slowly evolving lesion that forms a mass in the cerebellum; it is composed of granule, Purkinje, and glia cells. Reproduced therein, in a disorganized fashion, is the architecture of the cerebellum with no clear plane from normally structured cerebellar tissue. The importance of distinguishing this disease from other cerebellar tumors is its lack of growth potential and favorable prognosis. It should, however, be excised if symptomatic. The appearance on imaging is highly characteristic; a cerebellar hemisphere is occupied with an indistinct mass of "tiger stripe" appearance as a result of alternating layers of dysmorphic cerebellar cells (Fig. 31-15). Interest in this entity derives from its association with a germ line mutation in the *PTEN* gene that relates the disease to other gangliocytomas and to Cowden syndrome of multiple skin hamartomas and cancers of the gynecologic, breast, and thyroid glands (and which may include Lhermitte-Duclos as a component). Mice with the *PTEN* gene knocked-out have abnormal synaptic structure and dysplasia of the cerebellar granule cells.

Other forms of gangliogliomas include the *desmoplastic infantile ganglioglioma*, some of the *xanthoastrocytomas*, and the *dysembryoplastic neuroepithelioma tumor* (DNET).

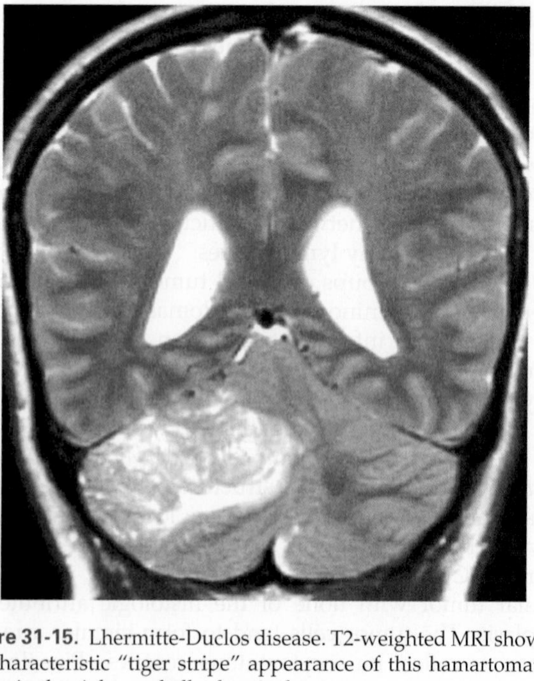

Figure 31-15. Lhermitte-Duclos disease. T2-weighted MRI showing the characteristic "tiger stripe" appearance of this hamartomatous tumor in the right cerebellar hemisphere.

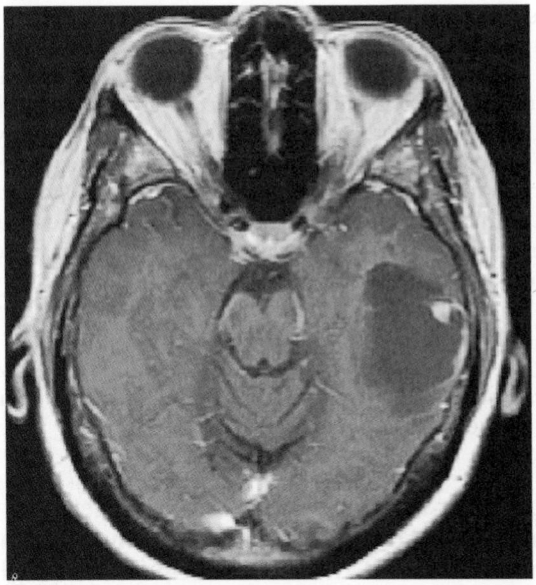

Figure 31-16. Contrast-enhanced MRI of a cystic and nodular dysembryoplastic neuroepithelial tumor (DNET) of the left temporal lobe in an adult who had a single seizure. The nodule had an inflammatory component and the seizures ceased with resection.

This last of these tumors, DNET, is worthy of comment as it often causes seizures that may be difficult to control in children. We have encountered them mostly in young adults after a single seizure or as an incidental finding on MRI. Although the tumors may be located in any part of the brain, there is a proclivity for the superficial (juxtacortical or intracortical) lateral or medial temporal lobe. The radiologic appearance is usually of a nodule or small cyst, or more specific to this entity, a cluster of several adjacent small cystic lesions, generally not enhancing and hyperintense on T2-weighted MRI (Fig. 31-16). The lesion is very slow growing and, if appropriately situated, may remodel the bone of the orbital roof or calvarium. The tumors originate from dysplastic cells in the germinal matrix that become arrested during migration toward the cortex; they are often associated with an adjacent region of cortical heterotopia. The histologic appearance varies but has as its main element a collection of neuroepithelial cells and clusters of oligodendrocytes with multinodular architecture that create mucinous cysts in some cases. When the lesion is single and has a nonspecific radiologic appearance, a biopsy or resection is required to differentiate it from a low-grade glioma or oligodendroglioma. Biopsy alone may be misleading in showing only the adjacent inflammation, at times prominent enough to appear almost granulomatous. Resection is curative and often eliminates the seizures but it is not clear what the best course of action is for asymptomatic lesions.

Another tumor that may be considered in this group is the subependymal giant cell astrocytoma that is found in up to 20 percent of patients with tuberous sclerosis. These are very slowly growing tumors that arise mostly near the foramen of Munro. Repeated resection is sometimes required to treat hydrocephalus. Krueger and colleagues have reported that everolimus, an inhibitor of the mTOR complex, which is disrupted in this phakomatosis, reduces the size of the tumor and ameliorates seizures. The remaining tumors mentioned earlier are rare and affect children mostly; therefore, they are not discussed further here. Good descriptions are to be found in the monographs of Russell, of Rubinstein (1972), of Levine (both articles from 1993), and of Schmidek, and in the article by Zentner and coworkers.

Colloid (Paraphysial) Cyst and Other Tumors of the Third Ventricle

The most important of these is the colloid tumor, which is derived from ependymal cells of a vestigial third ventricular structure known as the *paraphysis*. The cysts formed

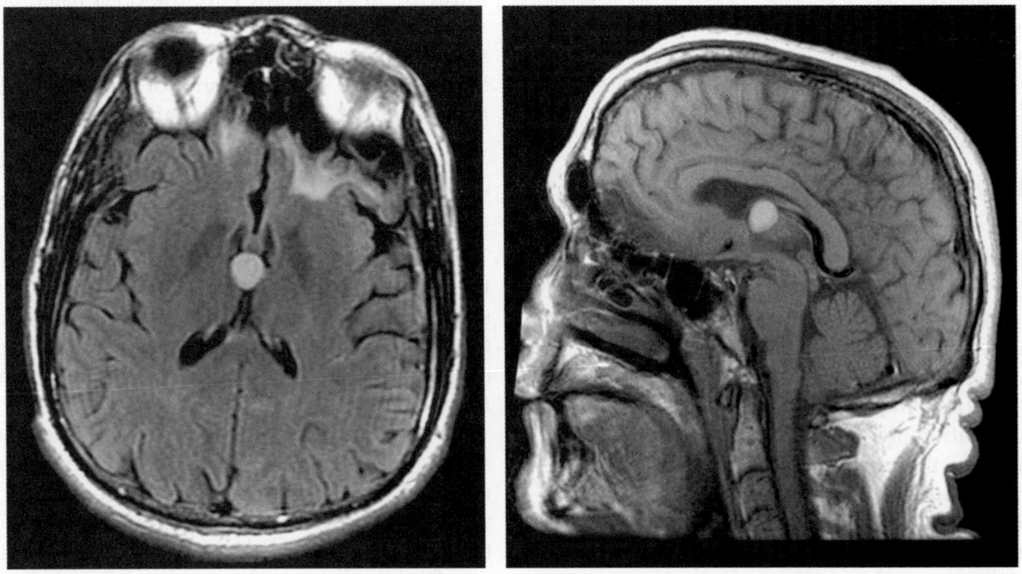

Figure 31-17. Colloid cyst of the third ventricle. MRI in the axial and sagittal planes. Hydrocephalus due to obstruction at the foramen of Monro can occur, but is not apparent here.

in this structure are always situated in the anterior portion of the third ventricle between the interventricular foramina and are attached to the roof of the ventricle (Fig. 31-17). They vary from 1 to 4 cm in diameter, are oval or round with a smooth external surface, and are filled with a gelatinous material containing a variety of mucopolysaccharides. The wall is composed of a layer of epithelial cells, some ciliated, surrounded by a capsule of fibrous connective tissue. Although congenital, the cysts practically never declare themselves clinically until adult life, when they block CSF outflow through the foramen of Monro and produce an obstructive hydrocephalus.

Suspicion of this tumor is occasioned by intermittent, severe bifrontal–bioccipital headaches, sometimes modified by posture ("ball valve" obstruction) or with crises of headache and obtundation, incontinence, unsteadiness of gait, bilateral paresthesias, dim vision, and weakness of the legs, with sudden falls but no loss of consciousness ("drop attacks"). Stooping may result in an increase or onset of headache and loss of balance. However, this intermittent obstructive syndrome has been infrequent in our experience. More often the patient has no headache and presents with the symptoms comparable to those of normal-pressure hydrocephalus or, as frequently, the tumor is found incidentally on CT or MRI. On CT and MRI, the lesion density depends on the hydration state of the mucopolysaccharides. These lesions do not restrict diffusion or enhance with contrast. Subtle behavioral changes are common and a few patients, as emphasized by Lobosky and colleagues, experience mild confusion and changes in personality that may reach the extreme of psychotic behavior. In our experience, chronic headache or gait difficulty is usually present by that time.

The treatment for many years has been surgical excision, which always carries some risk, but satisfactory results have also been obtained by ventriculoperitoneal shunting of the CSF, leaving the benign growth untouched. Decompression of the cyst by aspiration under stereotactic control has also become an increasingly popular procedure.

Other tumors found in the third ventricle and giving rise mainly to obstructive symptoms are craniopharyngiomas (see later), papillomas of the choroid plexus, and ependymomas (discussed earlier).

Arachnoid Cyst

This CSF-filled lesion, which is probably congenital, presents clinically at all ages but may become evident only in adult life, when it gives rise to symptoms of increased intracranial pressure and sometimes to focal cerebral or cerebellar signs, simulating intracranial neoplasm. Seizures may occur but are not characteristic. In infants and young children, macrocrania and extensive unilateral transillumination are characteristic features. Usually these cysts overlie the sylvian fissure or temporal pole; occasionally they are interhemispheric under the frontal lobes or lie in the pineal region or under the cerebellum. They may attain a large size, to the point of enlarging the middle cranial fossa and remodeling and elevating the lesser wing of the sphenoid, but they do not communicate with the ventricles. Rarely, one of these cysts may cover the entire surface of both cerebral hemispheres and create a so-called external hydrocephalus.

The cysts are readily recognized (often accidentally) on unenhanced CT or MRI, showing a circumscribed tissue defect filled with fluid that has the density of CSF (Gandy and Heier). If these cysts are completely asymptomatic, they should be left alone; if symptomatic, additional MRI studies are indicated, so as not to overlook a chronic subdural hematoma, which is often associated and may not be visualized on the unenhanced CT. Suprasellar arachnoid cysts are discussed further on, under "Empty Sella Syndrome."

The treatment of enlarging and symptomatic cysts is marsupialization or, less preferably, by shunting from the cyst to the subarachnoid space.

Skull Base and Other Regional Intracranial Tumor Syndromes (Vestibular Schwannoma, Other Tumors of the Cerebellopontine Angle, Craniopharyngioma, Pituitary, Meningioma of the Sphenoid Ridge and Olfactory Groove, Glioma of the Optic Nerve, Pontine Glioma, Chordoma Chondrosarcoma, Glomus Jugulare and Carotid Body Tumors, Nasopharyngeal Carcinoma)

In this group of tumors, symptoms and signs of general cerebral impairment and increased pressure occur late or not at all. Instead, special syndromes referable to particular intracranial loci arise and progress slowly. One arrives at the correct diagnosis by localizing the lesion accurately from the neurologic findings and by reasoning that the etiology must be neoplastic because of an afebrile and steadily progressive nature. Investigation by CT, MRI, and other special studies will usually confirm the clinical impression.

The tumors that most often produce these unique intracranial syndromes are the ones listed above as well as a number of other erosive tumors at the base of the skull. The aforementioned medulloblastoma, hemangioblastoma, and ependymoma of the fourth ventricle may have a similar regional clinical signature.

Vestibular Schwannoma (Acoustic Neuroma)

This tumor was first described as a pathologic entity by Sandifort in 1777, diagnosed clinically by Oppenheim in 1890, and recognized as a surgically treatable disease in the early 1900s. Cushing's monograph (1917) was a milestone, and the papers of House and Hitselberger and of Ojemann and colleagues provide valuable descriptions of diagnostic tests and surgical treatment in the era before modern imaging.

Approximately 3,000 new cases of acoustic neuroma are diagnosed each year in the United States (incidence rate of 1 per 100,000 per year). The tumor occurs occasionally as part of von Recklinghausen neurofibromatosis, in which case it takes one of two forms. In classic von Recklinghausen disease (peripheral or type 1 neurofibromatosis), a schwannoma may sporadically involve the eighth nerve, usually in adult life, but it may involve

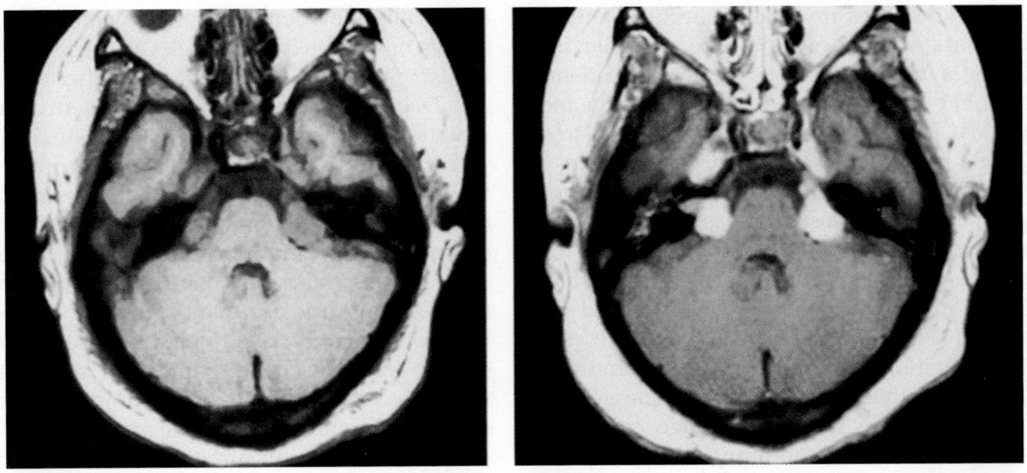

Figure 31-18. Bilateral vestibular schwannomas in neurofibromatosis type 2. T1-weighted MRI in the axial plane before (*left*) and after (*right*) contrast administration.

any other cranial (particularly trigeminal) or spinal nerve root. Rarely, if ever, do *bilateral acoustic neuromas* occur in this form of the disease. However, bilateral acoustic neuromas are the hallmark of the genetically distinct neurofibromatosis type 2 (NF2), in which they practically always occur before the age of 21 and show a strong (autosomal dominant) heredity (Fig. 31-18). Schwannomas are distinguished from neurofibromas (composed of both Schwann cells and fibroblasts) found in peripheral nerves of type 1 von Recklinghausen disease. A small percentage of neurofibromas become malignant, a phenomenon that is highly unusual in schwannomas.

In this context, a rare form of familial schwannomatosis should be mentioned, characterized by multiple schwannomas without vestibular tumors, which maps genetically to chromosome 22 but is distinct from NF2. The primary gene defect in this familial schwannomatosis has not been defined (MacCollin et al), although mutations in the *SMARCB1* gene on chromosome 22 locus have been identified in some patients.

The typical vestibular schwannoma in adults presents as a solitary tumor. Being a schwannoma, it originates in nerve. The examination of small tumors reveals that they practically always arise from the vestibular rather than the cochlear division of the eighth nerve, just within the internal auditory canal (Fig. 31-19). As the eighth nerve schwannoma grows, it extends into the posterior fossa to occupy the angle between the cerebellum and pons (cerebellopontine angle). In this lateral position, it is so situated as to compress the seventh, fifth, and less often the ninth and tenth cranial nerves, which are implicated in various combinations. Later it displaces and compresses the pons and lateral medulla and obstructs the CSF circulation; very rarely, it is a source of subarachnoid hemorrhage.

Certain biologic and clinical data assume clinical importance. The highest incidence is in the fifth and sixth

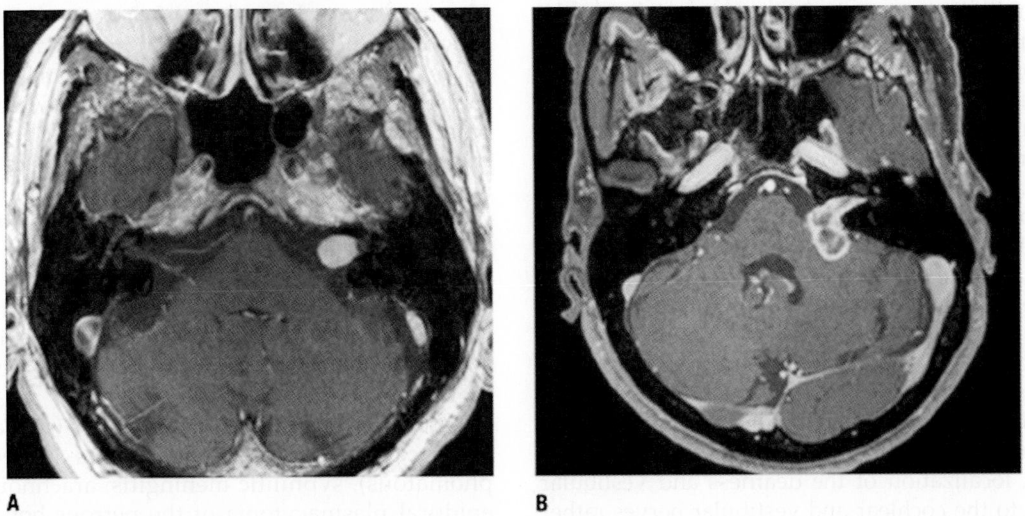

Figure 31-19. *A.* MRI of a small vestibular schwannoma emanating from the left porus acusticus, showing typical homogenous gadolinium enhancement. *B.* A larger atypical vestibular schwannoma with rim enhancement, causing compression of the left middle cerebellar peduncle.

decades of life, and the sexes are equally affected. Familial occurrence is a mark, usually, of von Recklinghausen disease. The earliest symptom reported by the 46 patients in the decades-old but instructive series of Ojemann and coworkers was loss of hearing (33 of 46 patients); headache (4 patients); disturbed sense of balance (3 patients); unsteadiness of gait (3 patients); and facial pain, tinnitus, and facial weakness, each in a single case. Some patients sought medical advice soon after the appearance of the initial symptom, some later, after other symptoms had occurred. One-third of the patients were troubled by vertigo associated with nausea, vomiting, and pressure in the ear. The vertiginous symptoms differed from those of Ménière disease in that discrete attacks separated by periods of normalcy were rare. The vertigo coincided more or less with hearing loss and tinnitus (most often a unilateral high-pitched ringing, sometimes a machinery-like roaring or hissing sound, like that of a steam kettle). Some of our patients ignored their deafness for many months or years; often the first indication of the tumor in such patients is a shift to the unaccustomed ear (usually right to left) in the use of the telephone. Others neglected these symptoms to a point where they presented with impaired mentation, imbalance, and sphincteric incontinence because of brainstem compression and secondary hydrocephalus.

The neurologic findings at the time of examination in the series mentioned above were as follows: eighth nerve involvement (auditory and vestibular; 45 of 46 patients), facial weakness including disturbance of taste (26 patients), sensory loss over the face (26 patients), gait abnormality (19 patients), and unilateral ataxia of the limbs (9 patients). Inequality of reflexes and eleventh- and twelfth-nerve palsies were present in only a few patients. Signs of increased intracranial pressure appear late and have been present in fewer than 25 percent of our patients. These findings are comparable to those reported by House and Hitselberger and by Harner and Laws. With the shift in recent years to fairly routine investigation of unilateral hearing loss by cerebral imaging, it is common to find these tumors at a far earlier stage, if as an incidental finding on cerebral imaging, well before the tumor becomes symptomatic.

The contrast-enhanced CT will detect practically all vestibular schwannomas that are larger than 2.0 cm in diameter and project further than 1.5 cm into the cerebellopontine angle. Much smaller intracanalicular tumors (i.e., restricted to within the internal acoustic canal) can be detected reliably by MRI with gadolinium (see Fig. 31-19). Specialized thin-slice MRI sequences such as steady-state free precession can accurately define anatomic relationships between the tumor and adjacent cranial nerves and vessels with high resolution.

Audiologic and vestibular evaluation includes the various tests described in Chap. 15, the brainstem auditory evoked response probably being the most sensitive to the presence of acoustic schwannoma. In combination, they permit localization of the deafness and vestibular disturbance to the cochlear and vestibular nerves rather than to their end organs. The CSF protein is raised in two-thirds of the patients (greater than 100 mg/dL in one-third); a clinically inevident acoustic schwannoma is one of the causes of an unexpectedly elevated CSF protein when a lumbar puncture is performed for other reasons.

Treatment The preferred treatment in most symptomatic cases has been surgical excision. Neurosurgeons who have had a lot of experience with these tumors favor a microsurgical suboccipital transmeatal approach (Martuza and Ojemann). The facial nerve can usually be preserved by intraoperative monitoring of brainstem auditory responses and facial nerve electromyography (EMG); in experienced hands, hearing can be preserved in approximately one-third of patients with tumors smaller than 2.5 cm in diameter. If no attempt is to be made to save hearing, small tumors can be removed safely by the translabyrinthine approach.

An alternative to surgery is focused radiation, which controls the growth of many of the smaller tumors. In a large series of patients treated with radiosurgery, facial motor and sensory functions were preserved in 75 percent of cases and, after 28 months of observation, no new neurologic deficits were detected (Kondziolka et al). This approach is favored in older patients with few symptoms but is being adopted increasingly for others. The rates of hearing loss and facial numbness and weakness are comparable or lower than with surgery, but the follow-up period in most series is less than 5 years (Flickinger et al). Focused radiation with the gamma Knife or proton beam also appears to be preferable to surgery in cases of recurrent tumor. The antiangiogenic agent, bevacizumab, in preliminary reports has reduced the size of these tumors in patients with NF2 (Plotkin et al).

There is no consensus on the management of an incidentally identified tumors but it is reasonable to follow these with audiograms and serial imaging. Some sources suggest that half of lesion smaller than 2 cm in diameter will not progress, or do so slowly enough that hearing and balance are not impaired. However, lesions larger than this size are associated with more surgical complications and make sparing of hearing less likely.

Other Tumors of the Cerebellopontine Angle

Neurinoma or schwannoma of the trigeminal (gasserian) ganglion or neighboring cranial nerves and *meningioma of the cerebellopontine angle* may, in some instances, be indistinguishable from a vestibular schwannoma. Fifth cranial nerve tumors should always be considered if deafness, tinnitus, and lack of response to caloric stimulation ("dead labyrinth") are not the initial symptoms of a cerebellopontine angle syndrome. A true *cholesteatoma (epidermoid cyst)* is a relatively rare tumor that is most often located in the cerebellopontine angle where it may simulate an acoustic neuroma but usually causes more severe facial weakness. Spillage of the contents of the cyst may produce intense chemical meningitis. Other disorders that enter into the differential diagnosis are glomus jugulare tumor (see later), metastatic cancer, neoplastic meningitis (especially lymphomatous), syphilitic meningitis, arachnoid cyst, and epidural plasmacytoma of the petrous bone. All these disorders may produce a cerebellopontine angle syndrome consisting of imbalance and unilateral hearing loss, but they are more likely to cause multiple lower cranial neuropathies and their temporal course differs from that of vestibular schwannoma. Occasionally, a tumor that originates in the pons or in the fourth ventricle (ependymoma, astrocytoma, papilloma, medulloblastoma) or a nasopharyngeal carcinoma may present as a cerebellopontine angle syndrome.

Craniopharyngioma (Suprasellar Epidermoid Cyst, Rathke Pouch or Hypophyseal Duct Tumor, Adamantinoma)

This is a histologically benign epithelioid tumor, generally assumed to originate from cell rests (remnants of the Rathke pouch [or adenohypophyseal diverticulum]) at the junction of the infundibular stem and pituitary gland. By the time the tumor has attained a diameter of 3 to 4 cm, it is almost always cystic and partly calcified. Usually it lies above the sella turcica, compressing and elevating the optic chiasm and extending up into the third ventricle. Less often it is subdiaphragmatic, i.e., within the sella, where it compresses the pituitary body and erodes one part of the wall of the sella or a clinoid process; seldom it balloons the sella like a pituitary adenoma. Large tumors may obstruct the flow of CSF.

The tumor is oval, round, or lobulated and has a smooth surface. The wall of the cyst and the solid parts of the tumor consist of cords and whorls of epithelial cells (often with intercellular bridges and keratohyalin) separated by a loose network of stellate cells. If there are bridges between tumor cells, which have an epithelial origin, the tumor is classed as an *adamantinoma*. The cyst contains dark albuminous fluid, cholesterol crystals, and calcium deposits; the calcium can be seen in plain films or CT of the suprasellar region in 70 to 80 percent of cases. The sella beneath the tumor tends to be flattened and enlarged. The majority of the patients are children, but the tumor is not infrequent in adults, and we have encountered patients up to 60 years of age.

The presenting syndrome may be one of increased intracranial pressure, but more often it takes the form of a combined pituitary-hypothalamic-chiasmal derangement. The symptoms are often subtle and long standing. In children, visual loss and diabetes insipidus are the most frequent findings, followed in a few cases by adiposity, delayed physical and mental development, headaches, and vomiting. The visual disorder takes the form of dim vision, chiasmal field defects, optic atrophy, or papilledema, as emphasized long ago by Kennedy and Smith. In adults, waning libido, amenorrhea, slight spastic weakness of one or both legs, headache without papilledema, failing vision, and mental dullness and confusion are the usual manifestations. One of the most remarkable cases in our experience was a middle-aged nurse who became distractible and ineffective at work and was thought for many months to be simply depressed. Often it is observed that drowsiness, ocular palsies, diabetes insipidus, and disturbance of temperature regulation (indicating hypothalamic involvement) occur later. Spontaneous rupture of the cystic lesion can incite severe aseptic meningitis, at times with depressed glucose in the CSF, a syndrome similar to that caused by rupture of the earlier described cholesteatoma.

In the *differential diagnosis* of the several craniopharyngioma syndromes, a careful clinical analysis is often more informative than laboratory procedures. Among the latter, MRI is likely to give the most useful information. Often, because of the cholesterol content, the tumor gives an increased signal on T1-weighted images. Usually, the cyst itself is isointense, like CSF, but occasionally it may give a decreased T2 signal.

Treatment Modern microsurgical techniques, reinforced by corticosteroid therapy before and after surgery and careful control of temperature and water balance postoperatively, permit successful excision of all or part of the tumor in the majority of cases. Although smaller tumors can be removed by a transsphenoidal approach, attempts at total removal require craniotomy and remain a challenge because of frequent adherence of the mass to surrounding structures (Fahlsbusch et al), as well as the potential for postoperative chemical meningitis from cyst contents. Partial removal practically ensures recurrence of the tumor, usually within 3 years, and the surgical risks of reoperation are considerable (10 percent mortality in large series). In 21 of our 35 patients, only partial removal was possible; of these, 8 died, most in the first postoperative year. Stereotactic aspiration is sometimes a useful palliative procedure, as are focused radiation therapy and ventricular shunting in patients with solid, nonresectable tumors. Endocrine replacement is necessary for an indefinite time. We have several times seen a syndrome of prolonged but reversible delirium after tumor resection.

Glomus Jugulare Tumor

This tumor is relatively rare but of interest to neurologists nonetheless. It is a purplish red, highly vascular tumor composed of large epithelioid cells, arranged in an alveolar pattern and possessing an abundant capillary network. The tumor is thought to be derived from minute clusters of nonchromaffin paraganglioma cells (glomus bodies) found mainly in the adventitia of the dome of the jugular bulb (*glomus jugulare*) immediately below the floor of the middle ear, as well as in multiple other sites in and around the temporal bone. These clusters of cells are part of the chemoreceptor system that also includes the carotid, vagal, ciliary, and aortic bodies.

The fully developed syndrome consists of partial deafness, facial palsy, dysphagia, and unilateral atrophy of the tongue combined with a vascular polyp in the external auditory meatus and a palpable mass below and anterior to the mastoid eminence, occasionally with a bruit that may be audible to the patient ("self-audible bruit"). Other neurologic manifestations are phrenic nerve palsy, numbness of the face, a Horner syndrome, cerebellar ataxia, and temporal lobe epilepsy. As with vestibular schwannoma, the availability of MRI has led to the earlier discovery of these tumors.

The jugular foramen is eroded and CSF protein may be elevated. Women are affected more than men, and the peak incidence is during middle adult life. The tumor grows slowly over a period of many years, sometimes 10 to 20 or more. Treatment in the past has consisted of radical mastoidectomy and removal of as much tumor as possible, followed by radiation. The combined intracranial and extracranial two-stage operation has resulted in the cure of many cases (Gardner et al). Embolization prior to resection is now also employed. A detailed account of this tumor can be found in the article by Kramer.

Carotid Body Tumor (Paraganglioma)

This is a generally benign but potentially malignant tumor originating in a small aggregate of paraganglioma cells of neuroectodermal type. The normal carotid body is small (4 mm in greatest diameter and 10 mg in weight) and is located at the bifurcation of the common carotid artery. The cells are of uniform size, have an abundant cytoplasm, are rich in substance P, and are sensitive to changes in Po_2, Pco_2, and pH (i.e., they are chemoreceptors, not to be confused with baroreceptors). The tumors that arise from these cells are identical in appearance to tumors of other chemoreceptor organs such as the glomus jugulare neoplasm described in the preceding section (paragangliomas). Interestingly, they are many times more frequent in individuals living at high altitudes.

The usual presentation is of a painless mass at the side of the neck below the angle of the jaw; thus it must be differentiated from the branchial cleft cyst, mixed tumor of the salivary gland, and carcinomas and aneurysms in this region. As the tumor grows (at an estimated rate of 2.0 cm in diameter every 5 years) it may implicate the sympathetic, glossopharyngeal, vagus, spinal accessory, and hypoglossal nerves (syndrome of the retroparotid space; see Chap. 47). Hearing loss, tinnitus, and vertigo are present in some cases. Tumors of the carotid body have been a source of transient ischemic attacks in 5 to 15 percent of the 600 or more reported cases. One of the most interesting presentations has been with sleep apnea, particularly with bilateral tumors (see later); respiratory depression as well as lability of blood pressure are common postoperative problems. Malignant transformation occurs in 5 percent of cases.

A similar *paraganglioma of the vagus nerve* has been reported; it occurs typically in the jugular or nodose ganglion but may arise anywhere along the course of the nerve. These tumors may also undergo malignant transformation in about 5 percent of cases, metastasize, or invade the base of the skull.

Carotid body tumor has been seen in combination with von Recklinghausen neurofibromatosis type 1 (NF1) and in von Hippel-Lindau disease. Familial cases are known, especially with bilateral carotid body tumors (about 5 percent of these tumors are bilateral). The treatment is surgical excision with or without prior intravascular embolization; radiation therapy has not been advised.

Pituitary Adenoma (See also "Pituitary Insufficiency" in Chap. 27)

Tumors arising in the anterior pituitary are of considerable interest to neurologists because they often cause visual and other symptoms related to involvement of structures bordering upon the sella turcica, before an endocrine disorder becomes apparent. Pituitary tumors are age-linked; they become increasingly numerous with each decade. By the eightieth year, small adenomas are found in more than 20 percent of pituitary glands. In some cases, an apparent stimulus to adenoma formation is endocrine end-organ failure, as occurs, for example, with ovarian atrophy that induces a basophilic adenoma. Only a small proportion (6 to 8 percent) enlarge the sella, i.e., most are "microadenomas," as discussed below.

On the basis of conventional hematoxylin-eosin-staining methods, cells of the normal pituitary gland were for many years classified as chromophobe, acidophil, and basophil, these types being present in a ratio of 5:4:1. Adenomas of the pituitary are most often composed of chromophobe cells (4 to 20 times as common as acidophil cell adenomas); the incidence of basophil cell adenomas is uncertain. Histologic study is now based on immunoperoxidase-staining techniques that define the nature of the hormones within the pituitary cells—both of the normal gland and of pituitary adenomas. These methods have shown that either a chromophobe or an acidophil cell may produce prolactin, growth hormone (GH), and thyroid-stimulating hormone (TSH), whereas the basophil cells produce adrenocorticotropic hormone (ACTH), β-lipotropin, luteinizing hormone (LH), and follicle-stimulating hormone (FSH).

The development of sensitive methods for the measurement of pituitary hormones in the serum has made possible the detection of adenomas at an early stage of their development and the designation of several types of pituitary adenomas on the basis of the endocrine disturbance. Hormonal tests for the detection of pituitary adenomas, preferably carried out in an endocrine clinic, are listed in Table 31-4. Between 60

Table 31-4

HORMONAL TESTS FOR DETECTION OF PITUITARY ADENOMAS

HORMONE	TEST
Prolactin	Serum prolactin level, chlorpromazine- or TRH-provocative tests, L-dopa suppression
Somatotropin (GH)	Serum GH level, glucagon, L-dopa, glucose-GH suppression, somatomicid C
Adrenocorticotropin	Serum cortisol, urinary steroids, metyrapone test, dexamethasone suppression
Gonadotropin	Serum FSH, LH, estradiol, testosterone, GnRH stimulation
Thyrotropin	TSH, T_4, TRH
Vasopressin	Urine and serum osmolality after water restriction for deficiency of hormone; without water restriction for excess of hormone

FSH, follicle-stimulating hormone; GH, growth hormone; GnRH, gonadotropin-releasing hormone; LH, luteinizing hormone; T_4, thyroxine; TRH, thyrotropin-releasing hormone; TSH, thyroid-stimulating hormone.

and 70 percent of tumors in both men and women are prolactin secreting. About 10 to 15 percent secrete growth hormone, and a smaller number secrete ACTH. Tumors that secrete gonadotropins and TSH are quite rare. These tumors may be monohormonal or plurihormonal and approximately one-third are composed of nonfunctional (null) cells.

Pituitary tumors usually arise as discrete nodules in the anterior part of the gland (adenohypophysis). They are reddish gray, soft (almost gelatinous), and often partly cystic, with a rim of calcium in some instances. The adenomatous cells are arranged diffusely or in various patterns, with little stroma and few blood vessels; less frequently the architecture is sinusoidal or papillary in type. Variability of nuclear structure, hyperchromatism, cellular pleomorphism, and mitotic figures are interpreted as signs of malignancy, which is exceedingly rare. Tumors less than 1 cm in diameter are referred to as *microadenomas* and are at first confined to the sella. As the tumor grows, it first compresses the pituitary gland; then, as it extends upward and out of the sella, it compresses the optic chiasm; later, with continued growth, it may extend into the cavernous sinus, third ventricle, temporal lobes, or posterior fossa. Recognition of an adenoma when it is still confined to the sella is of considerable practical importance, since total removal of the tumor by transsphenoidal excision or some form of stereotactic radiosurgery is possible at this stage with prevention of further damage to normal glandular structure and the optic chiasm. Penetration of the diaphragm sellae by the tumor and invasion of the surrounding structures make treatment more difficult.

Pituitary adenomas come to medical attention because of endocrine or visual abnormalities. Headaches are reported by nearly half of patients with macroadenomas but are not clearly part of the syndrome. The visual disorder usually proves to be a *complete or partial bitemporal hemianopia*, which has developed gradually and may not be evident to the patient (see the description of the chiasmatic syndromes in "Neurologic Causes of Reduced Vision" in Chap. 13). Early on, the upper parts of the visual fields may be affected predominantly, since those fibers run along the inferior optic nerve and chiasm. A small number of patients will be almost blind in one eye and have a temporal hemianopia in the other. Bitemporal central hemianopic scotomata are a less-frequent finding. A postfixed (situated relatively posteriorly) chiasm may be compressed in such a way that there is an interruption of some of the nasal retinal fibers, which, as they decussate, project into the base of the opposite optic nerve (Wilbrand knee); the controversy regarding the validity of this projection in humans is mentioned in Chap. 13. This results in a central scotoma on one or both sides (junctional syndrome) in addition to the classic temporal field defect (see Fig. 13-2).

If the visual disorder is longstanding, the optic nerve heads are atrophic. In 5 to 10 percent of cases, the pituitary adenoma extends into the cavernous sinus, causing some combination of ocular motor palsies as well as potential compression of the cavernous segment of the internal carotid artery. Other neurologic abnormalities, rare to be sure, are seizures from indentation of the medial temporal lobe, CSF rhinorrhea from erosion of the sella, and diabetes insipidus, hypothermia, and somnolence from hypothalamic compression.

With regard to differential diagnosis, *bitemporal hemianopia with a normal-size sella* indicates that the causative lesion is probably a saccular aneurysm of the circle of Willis or a meningioma of the tuberculum sellae; multiple sclerosis may simulate this pattern and eventration of a greatly hydrocephalic third ventricle is an uncertain cause (see Chap. 13). The idiopathic syndrome of an "empty sella" also can cause bitemporal hemianopia and is discussed further on.

The major endocrine syndromes associated with pituitary adenomas are described briefly in the following pages. Their functional classification can be found in the monograph edited by Kovacs and Asa. A detailed discussion of the diagnosis and management of hormone-secreting pituitary adenomas is given in the reviews of Klibanski and Zervas and of Pappas and colleagues; recommended also is an article that details the neurologic features of pituitary tumors by Anderson and colleagues. Worthy of emphasis is the catastrophic syndrome of pituitary apoplexy discussed further on.

Amenorrhea-Galactorrhea Syndrome As a rule, this syndrome becomes manifest during the childbearing years. The history usually discloses that menarche had occurred at the appropriate age; primary amenorrhea is rare. A common history is that the patient took birth control pills, only to find, when she stopped, that the menstrual cycle did not reestablish itself. On examination, there may be no abnormalities other than galactorrhea. Serum prolactin concentrations are increased (usually in excess of 100 ng/mL). In general, the longer the duration of amenorrhea and the higher the serum prolactin level, the larger the tumor (prolactinoma). The elevated prolactin levels distinguish this disorder from idiopathic galactorrhea, in which the serum prolactin concentration is normal.

Males with prolactin-secreting tumors rarely have galactorrhea and usually present with a larger tumor and complaints such as headache, impotence, and visual abnormalities. In normal persons, the serum prolactin rises markedly in response to the administration of chlorpromazine or thyrotropin-releasing hormone (TRH); patients with a prolactin-secreting tumor fail to show such a response. With large tumors that compress normal pituitary tissue, thyroid and adrenal function will also be impaired. It should be emphasized that large, nonfunctioning pituitary adenomas also cause modest hyperprolactinemia by distorting the pituitary stalk and reducing dopamine delivery to prolactin-producing cells.

Acromegaly This disorder consists of acral growth and prognathism in combination with visceromegaly, headache, and several endocrine disorders (hypermetabolism, diabetes mellitus). The highly characteristic facial and bodily appearance, well known to all physicians, is caused by an overproduction of GH after puberty; prior to puberty, an oversecretion of GH leads to gigantism. In a small number of acromegalic patients, there is an excess secretion of both GH and prolactin, derived apparently from two distinct populations of tumor cells. The diagnosis of this disorder, which is often long delayed, is made on the basis of the characteristic clinical changes, the finding of elevated serum GH values (0.10 ng/mL), and the failure of the serum GH concentration to rise in response to the administration of glucose or TRH. The new growth hormone-receptor antagonist pegvisomant was introduced to reduce many of the manifestations of acromegaly (see the review by Melmed).

Cushing Disease Described in 1932 by Cushing, this condition is only about one-fourth as frequent as acromegaly. A distinction is made between *Cushing disease* and *Cushing syndrome*, as indicated in Chap. 27. The former term is reserved for cases that are caused by the excessive secretion of pituitary ACTH, which, in turn, causes adrenal hyperplasia; the usual basis is a pituitary adenoma. *Cushing syndrome* refers to the effects of cortisol excess from any one of several sources—excessive administration of steroids (the most common cause), adenoma of the adrenal cortex, ACTH-producing bronchial carcinoma, and, very rarely, other carcinomas that produce ACTH. The clinical effects are the same in all of these disorders and include truncal obesity, hypertension, proximal muscle weakness, amenorrhea, hirsutism, abdominal striae, hyperglycemia, osteoporosis, and in some cases a characteristic mental disorder (see "Cushing Disease and Corticosteroid Psychoses" in Chap. 53).

Although Cushing originally referred to the disease as pituitary basophilism and attributed it to a basophil adenoma, the pathologic change may consist only of hyperplasia of basophilic cells or of a nonbasophilic microadenoma. Seldom is the sella turcica enlarged: Consequently, visual symptoms or signs as a result of involvement of the optic chiasm or nerves and extension to the cavernous sinus are rare. The diagnosis of Cushing disease is made by demonstrating increased concentration of plasma and urinary cortisol; these levels are not suppressed by the administration of relatively small doses of dexamethasone (0.5 mg qid), but they are suppressed by high doses (8 mg daily). A low level of ACTH and a high level of cortisol in the blood, increased free cortisol in the urine, and nonsuppression of adrenal function after administration of high doses of dexamethasone are evidence of an adrenal source of the Cushing syndrome—usually a tumor and less often a micronodular hyperplasia of the adrenal gland.

Diagnosis of Pituitary Adenoma This is virtually certain when a chiasmal syndrome is combined with an endocrine syndrome of either hypopituitary or hyperpituitary type. Laboratory data that are confirmatory of an endocrine disorder, as described above, and sometimes a ballooned sella turcica on plain films of the skull are occasionally found. Patients who are suspected of having a pituitary adenoma should be examined by MRI with gadolinium; this procedure will visualize pituitary adenomas as small as 3 mm in diameter and show the relationship of the tumor to the optic chiasm (Fig. 31-20). This also provides the means of following the tumor's response to therapy. It should be kept in mind that pituitary tissue normally enhances on CT and MRI, revealing small tumors as relatively hypoenhancing nodules.

Tumors and lesions other than pituitary adenomas may sometimes expand the sella. Enlargement may be the result of an intrasellar craniopharyngioma, meningioma, carotid aneurysm, or cyst of the pituitary gland. Intrasellar epithelium-lined cysts are rare lesions. They originate from the apex of the Rathke pouch, which may persist as a cleft between the anterior and posterior lobes of the hypophysis. Rarer still are intrasellar cysts that have no epithelial lining and contain thick, dark brown fluid, the product of intermittent hemorrhages. Both types of intrasellar cysts may compress the pituitary gland and mimic the endocrine-suppressive effects of pituitary adenomas. Neoplasms originating in the nasopharynx or sinuses may invade the sella and pituitary gland, and sarcoid lesions at the base of the brain may do the same. Also, the pituitary gland and the infundibulum

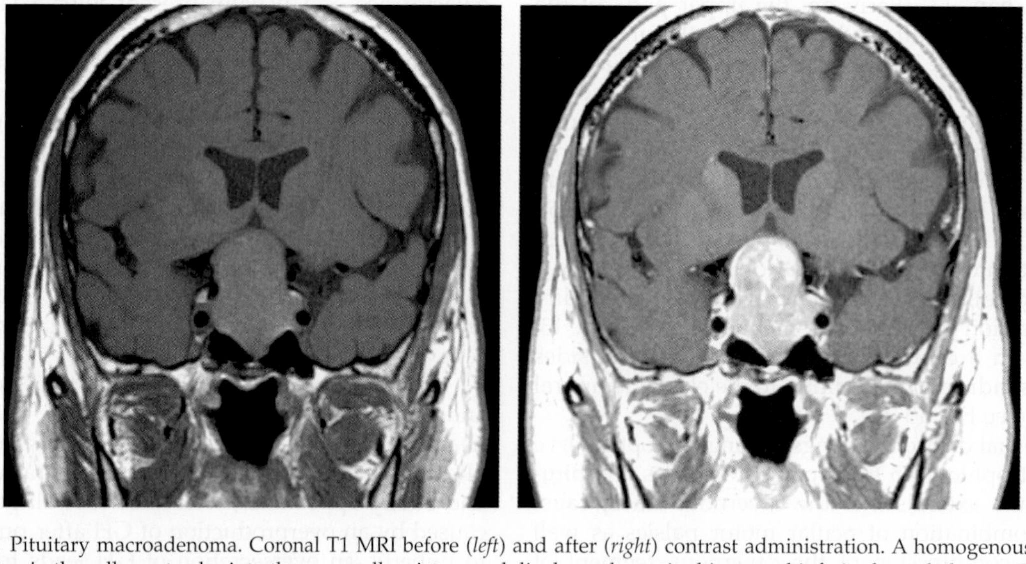

Figure 31-20. Pituitary macroadenoma. Coronal T1 MRI before (*left*) and after (*right*) contrast administration. A homogenously enhancing mass originating in the sella protrudes into the suprasellar cistern and displaces the optic chiasm and inferior hypothalamus. The lesion also extends into the left greater than right cavernous sinuses.

(and the chiasm) may be the site of metastases, most of them from the lung and breast (Morita et al); they give rise to diabetes insipidus, pituitary insufficiency, or orbital pain, and rarely may be the first indication of a systemic tumor.

Empty Sella Syndrome More common than the aforementioned conditions is a *nontumorous enlargement of the sella* ("empty sella"). This results from a defect in the dural diaphragm, which may occur without obvious cause or with states of raised intracranial pressure, such as pseudotumor cerebri (see Chap. 30) or hydrocephalus, or may follow surgical excision of a pituitary adenoma or meningioma of the tuberculum sellae or pituitary apoplexy (see later). The arachnoid covering the diaphragm sellae will bulge downward through the dural defect, and the sella then enlarges gradually, presumably because of the pressure and pulsations of the CSF acting on its walls. In the process, the pituitary gland becomes flattened, sometimes to an extreme degree; however, the functions of the gland are usually unimpaired. Flattening of the pituitary gland precedes bony expansion of the sella in many cases. Erosion or dishiscence of the sellar floor does not occur and the appearance of these changes implicates another type of lesion. Downward herniation of the optic chiasm occurs occasionally and may cause visual disturbances simulating those of a pituitary adenoma (Kaufman et al). As mentioned earlier, a bitemporal hemianopia with a normal-sized sella is usually caused by a primary suprasellar lesion (saccular aneurysm of the distal carotid artery, meningioma, or craniopharyngioma).

Treatment This varies with the type and size of the pituitary tumor, the status of the endocrine and visual systems, and the age and childbearing plans of the patient. The administration of the dopamine agonist *bromocriptine* (which inhibits prolactin) in a beginning dosage of 0.5 to 1.25 mg daily (taken with food) may be the only therapy needed for small or even large prolactinomas, and is a useful adjunct in the treatment of the amenorrhea–galactorrhea syndrome. The dose should be slowly increased by 2.5 mg or less every several days until a therapeutic response is obtained. Under the influence of bromocriptine, the tumor decreases in size within days, the prolactin level falls, and the visual field defect improves.

Some cases of acromegaly also respond to the administration of bromocriptine but even better to *octreotide*, an analogue of somatostatin. The initial dose of octreotide is 200 mg/d, increased in divided doses to 1,600 mg by increments of 200 mg weekly. In Lamberts' series of acromegaly patients, the growth hormone levels returned to normal and tumor size was reduced in 12 of 15 cases. Treatment with bromocriptine and octreotide must be continuous to prevent relapse. Newer slow-release somatostatin analogues and long-acting dopamine agonists such as cabergoline have been developed for use in patients who do not respond to the conventional agents (Colao and Lombardi).

If the patient is intolerant of medication (or, in the case of acromegaly, to octreotide and newer drugs), the treatment is surgical, using a transsphenoidal microsurgical approach, with an attempt at total removal of the tumor and preservation of normal pituitary function. Unfortunately, approximately 15 percent of GH-secreting tumors and prolactinomas will recur at 1 year. For this reason, incomplete removal or recurrence of the tumor (or tumors that are unresponsive to hormonal therapy) should be followed by radiation therapy.

Alternative primary treatment for intrasellar tumors is forms of stereotactic radiosurgery, *provided that vision is not being threatened and there is no other urgent need for surgery.* These forms of radiation can be focused precisely on the tumor and will destroy it. Kjellberg and colleagues and Chapman, using proton beam radiation, in the past treated more than 1,100 pituitary adenomas without a fatality and with few complications (Kliman et al). A single brief exposure was all that was necessary. An endocrine deficit will follow in most instances and must be corrected by hormone replacement therapy. Several equivalent methods (gamma Knife, Cyberknife) are more accessible and have become widely used. The advantage of these radiotherapeutic methods is that tumor recurrence is rare. A disadvantage is that the radiation effect is obtained only after several months. Estrada and colleagues have also reported that external beam-radiation therapy may be employed after unsuccessful transsphenoidal surgery for Cushing disease. After approximately 3.5 years following radiation, 83 percent of their patients showed no signs of tumor growth. There are a few reports, however, of a decline in memory ability after radiation treatment of all types.

Large extrasellar extensions of a pituitary growth must be removed by craniotomy, usually with a transfrontal approach, followed by radiation therapy. Visual field defects often remain, but some improvement in vision can be anticipated.

Pituitary Apoplexy This syndrome, described originally by Brougham, Heusner, and Adams, occurs as a result of infarction of an adenoma that has outgrown its blood supply. It is characterized by the acute onset of severe headache that may be retro-orbital, frontal, bitemporal, or generalized ophthalmoplegia; bilateral visual loss; and in severe cases, drowsiness or coma, with either subarachnoid hemorrhage or pleocytosis and elevated protein in the CSF. The CT or MRI shows infarction of tumor, often with hemorrhage in and above an enlarged sella. Pituitary apoplexy may threaten life unless the acute addisonian state is treated by hydrocortisone. Blindness is the other dreaded complication. If there is no improvement after 24 to 48 h, or if vision is markedly affected, transsphenoidal decompression of the sella is indicated. Factors that may precipitate the necrosis or hemorrhage of a pituitary tumor are anticoagulation, pituitary function testing, radiation, bromocriptine treatment, and head trauma; most cases, however, occur spontaneously. Some pituitary adenomas have been cured by this accident.

Ischemic necrosis of the pituitary, without the presence of a tumor followed by hypopituitarism, occurs under a variety of circumstances, the most common being in the partum or postpartum period (Sheehan syndrome).

Meningioma of the Sphenoid Ridge

This tumor, mentioned earlier in the chapter, is situated over the lesser wing of the sphenoid bone. As it grows, it may expand medially to involve structures in the wall of the cavernous sinus, anteriorly into the orbit, or laterally into the temporal bone. Fully 75 percent of such tumors occur in women, and the average age at onset is 50 years. Most prominent among the symptoms are a slowly developing unilateral exophthalmos, slight bulging of the bone in the temporal region, and radiologic evidence of thickening or erosion of the lesser wing of the sphenoid bone. Variants of the clinical syndrome include anosmia; oculomotor palsies; painful ophthalmoplegia (sphenoidal fissure and Tolosa-Hunt syndromes; see Table 47-2); blindness and optic atrophy in one eye, sometimes with papilledema of the other eye (Foster Kennedy syndrome); mental changes; seizures ("uncinate fits"); and increased intracranial pressure. Rarely, a skull bruit can be heard over a highly vascular tumor. Sarcomas arising from skull bones, metastatic carcinoma, orbitoethmoidal osteoma, benign giant cell bone cyst, tumors of the optic nerve, and angiomas of the orbit must be considered in the differential diagnosis. Neuroimaging with contrast provides the definitive diagnosis. The tumor is resectable without further injury to the optic nerve if the bone has not been invaded.

Meningioma of the Olfactory Groove

This tumor originates in arachnoidal cells along the cribriform plate. The diagnosis depends on the finding of ipsilateral or bilateral anosmia or ipsilateral or bilateral blindness—often with optic atrophy and mental changes. The tumors may reach enormous size before coming to the attention of the physician but as many are small and found incidentally with cerebral imaging (see Fig. 31-7B). If the anosmia is unilateral, it is rarely if ever reported by the patient. The unilateral visual disturbance may consist of a slowly developing central scotoma. Abulia, confusion, forgetfulness, and inappropriate jocularity (*witzelsucht*) are the usual psychic disturbances from compression of the inferior frontal lobes (see Chap. 22). The patient may be indifferent to or joke about his blindness. Usually there are radiographic changes along the cribriform plate. MRI with gadolinium is diagnostic. Except for the largest and most invasive tumors, surgical removal is possible.

Meningioma of the Tuberculum Sella

Cushing was the first to delineate the syndrome caused by this tumor. All of his 23 patients were female. The presenting symptoms were visual failure—a slowly advancing bitemporal hemianopia with a sella of normal size. Often the field defects are asymmetrical, indicating a combined chiasmal–optic nerve involvement. Usually there are no hypothalamic or pituitary deficits. If the tumor is not too large, complete excision is possible. If removal is incomplete or the tumor recurs or undergoes malignant changes, radiation therapy of one type or another is indicated. The outlook is then guarded; several of our patients succumbed within a few years.

Glioma of the Brainstem

Astrocytomas of the brainstem are relatively slow-growing tumors that infiltrate tracts and nuclei. They produce a variable clinical picture depending on their location in the medulla, pons, or midbrain. Most often, this tumor begins in childhood (peak age of onset is 7 years), and 80 percent appear before the twenty-first year. Symptoms have usually been present for 3 to 5 months before coming to medical notice. In most patients the initial manifestation is a palsy of one or more cranial nerves, usually the sixth and seventh on one side, followed by long tract signs—hemiparesis, unilateral ataxia, ataxia of gait, paraparesis, and hemisensory and gaze disorders in addition to pseudobulbar dysarthria and palsy. In the remaining patients the symptoms occur in the reverse order—i.e., long tract signs precede the cranial nerve abnormalities. Patients in the latter group survive longer than those whose illness begins with cranial nerve palsies. Headache, vomiting, and papilledema may occur, usually late in the illness. The course is slowly progressive over several years unless some part of the tumor becomes more malignant (anaplastic astrocytoma or glioblastoma multiforme) or, as rarely happens, spreads to the meninges (meningeal gliomatosis), in which instance the illness may terminate fatally within months.

The main problem in diagnosis is to differentiate this disease from a pontine form of multiple sclerosis, a vascular malformation of the pons (usually a cavernous hemangioma), or brainstem encephalitis, and to distinguish the focal from the diffuse type of glioma (see below). The most helpful procedure in diagnosis and prognosis is contrast-enhanced MRI (Fig. 31-21).

A study of 87 patients by Barkovich and coworkers emphasized the importance of distinguishing between diffusely infiltrating and focal nodular tumors. In the more common diffuse type, there is mass effect with hypointense signal on T1-weighted MRI and heterogeneously increased T2 signal, which reflects edema and tumor infiltration. These diffusely infiltrating tumors, usually showing an asymmetrical enlargement of the pons, have a poorer prognosis than the focal or nodular tumors, which tend to occur in the dorsal brainstem and

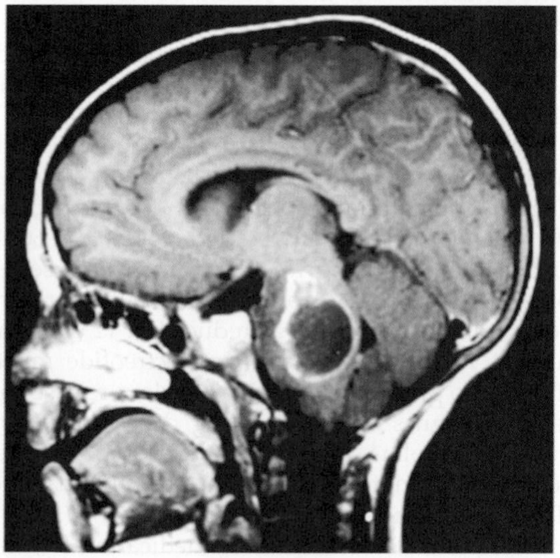

Figure 31-21. Pontine glioma. Contrast-enhanced T1 MRI demonstrates a mass with prominent irregular peripheral gadolinium enhancement. The patient was a 3-year-old male with progressive cranial nerve and long tract deficits.

often protrude in an exophytic manner. In a few instances of diffuse brainstem glioma, surgical exploration is necessary to establish the diagnosis (inspection and possibly biopsy). However, the histologic characteristics of a minute biopsy specimen of the tumor are not particularly helpful in determining prognosis or treatment and the general practice is to avoid surgery unless the tumor exhibits unusual clinical behavior or does not conform to the typical MRI appearance of the diffuse type.

Treatment The treatment of the diffuse infiltrative type is radiation, and if increased intracranial pressure develops as a result of hydrocephalus, ventricular shunting of CSF becomes necessary. Adjuvant chemotherapy has not been helpful. A series of 16 patients treated by Pollack and colleagues emphasizes that the focal and exophytic brainstem tumors are almost all low-grade astrocytomas; these tumors, in contrast to the more diffuse type, usually respond well to partial resection and permit long-term survival because they recur only slowly and do not undergo malignant transformation. Gangliocytomas or mixed astrogangliocytomas are rare imitators of nodular glioma in the brainstem. The rarer cystic glioma of the brainstem (see Fig. 31-19), a pilocytic tumor like its counterpart in the cerebellum, is treated by resection of the mural nodule and, as mentioned earlier, has an excellent prognosis. Landolfi and colleagues emphasized the longer survival in adults with pontine glioma (median 54 months) as compared to children. Most of the patients with pontine tumors with which we are familiar proved to have malignant gliomas.

Glioma of the Optic Nerves and Chiasm

This tumor, like the brainstem glioma, occurs most frequently during childhood and adolescence. In 85 percent of cases, it appears before the age of 15 years (average 3.5 years), and it is twice as frequent in girls as in boys (Cogan). The initial symptoms are dimness of vision with constricted fields, followed by bilateral field defects of homonymous, heteronymous, and sometimes bitemporal type and progressing to blindness and optic atrophy with or without papilledema. Ocular proptosis from the orbital mass is the other main feature. Hypothalamic signs (adiposity, polyuria, somnolence, and genital atrophy) occur occasionally as a result of proximal tumor extension. CT, MRI, and ultrasonography will usually reveal the tumor, and radiographs will show an enlargement of the optic foramen (greater than 7.0 mm). This finding and the lack of ballooning of the sella or of suprasellar calcification will exclude pituitary adenoma, craniopharyngioma, Hand-Schüller-Christian disease, and sarcoidosis. In adolescents and young adults, the medial sphenoid, olfactory groove, and intraorbital meningiomas (optic nerve sheath meningioma) are other tumors that cause monocular blindness and proptosis. If the entire tumor is prechiasmatic (the less-common configuration), surgical extirpation can be curative. For tumors that have infiltrated the chiasm or are causing regional symptoms and hydrocephalus, partial excision followed by radiation is all that can be offered. Both gliomas and nontumorous gliotic (hamartomatous) lesions of the optic nerves may occur in von Recklinghausen disease; the latter are sometimes impossible to distinguish from optic nerve gliomas and should be followed closely.

Chordoma

This is a soft, jelly-like, gray-pink growth that arises from remnants of the primitive notochord. It is located most often within the clivus (from dorsum sellae to foramen magnum) and in the sacrococcygeal region. It affects males more than females, usually in early or middle adult years and is one of the rare causes of syndromes involving multiple cranial nerves or the cauda equina. Approximately 40 percent of chordomas occur at each of these two ends of the neuraxis; the rest are found at any point in the vertebral bodies in between. The tumor is made up of cords or masses of large cells with granules of glycogen in their cytoplasm and often with multiple nuclei and intracellular mucoid material. Chordomas are locally invasive, especially of surrounding bone, but they do not metastasize.

The cranial neurologic syndrome caused by this tumor is remarkable in that all or any combination of cranial nerves from the second to twelfth on one or both sides may be involved. Associated signs in the series of Kendall and Lee were facial pain, conductive deafness, and cerebellar ataxia, the result of pontomedullary and cerebellar compression. A characteristic feature is neck pain radiating to the vertex of the skull on neck flexion. The tumors at the base of the skull may destroy the clivus and bulge into the nasopharynx, causing nasal obstruction and discharge and sometimes dysphagia. Extension to the cervical epidural space may result in cord compression. Thus, chordoma is one of the lesions that may present both as an intracranial and extracranial mass, the others being meningioma, neurofibroma, glomus jugulare tumor, and carcinoma of the sinuses or pharynx. CT of the skull base is useful for defining the bony margins of the tumor, and MRI can identify involved and adjacent neural and vascular structures. Midline (Wegener) granulomas, histiocytosis, Erdheim-Chester disease, and sarcoidosis also figure in the differential diagnosis. Chondrosarcoma of the clivus produces a similar syndrome.

Treatment of the chordoma is surgical excision and radiation (focused radiation). This form of treatment has effected a 5-year survival without recurrence in approximately 80 percent of patients.

Nasopharyngeal Growths That Erode the Base of the Skull (Nasopharyngeal Transitional Cell Carcinoma, Schmincke Tumor)

These are seen regularly in a general hospital; they arise from the mucous membrane of the paranasal sinuses or the nasopharynx near the eustachian tube, i.e., the fossa of Rosenmüller. In addition to symptoms of nasopharyngeal or sinus disease, which may not be prominent, facial pain and numbness, abducens, and other cranial nerve palsies may occur. Diagnosis depends on inspection and biopsy of a nasopharyngeal mass or an involved cervical lymph node and radiologic evidence of erosion of the base of the skull. Bone scans and CT are helpful in diagnosis (see Fig. 47-5). The treatment is surgical resection and radiation but chemotherapy is increasingly being included. Carcinoma of the ethmoid or sphenoid sinuses and postradiation neuropathy, coming on years after the treatment of a nasopharyngeal tumor, may produce similar clinical pictures and are difficult to differentiate. The syndromes resulting from nasopharyngeal tumors are discussed in Chap. 47, under "Diseases of the Cranial Nerves."

Other Tumors of the Base of the Skull

In addition to meningioma, nasopharyngeal tumors, and the other tumors enumerated earlier, there are a large variety of tumors, rare to be sure, that derive from tissues at the base of the skull and paranasal sinuses, ears, and other structures and give rise to distinctive syndromes. Included in this category are osteomas, chondromas, ossifying fibromas, giant cell tumors of bone, lipomas, epidermoids, teratomas, mixed tumors of the parotid gland, and hemangiomas and cylindromas (adenoid cystic carcinomas of salivary gland origin) of the sinuses and orbit; sarcoid granulomas may produce the same effect. Most of these tumors are benign, but some have a potential for malignant change. To the group must be added the *esthesioneuroblastoma* (of the nasal cavity) with anterior fossa extension and, perhaps most common of all of these, the *systemic malignant tumors that metastasize to basal skull bones* (prostate, lung, and breast being the most common sources), or involve them as part of a multicentric neoplastic process, e.g., primary lymphoma, multiple myeloma, plasmacytoma, and lymphocytic leukemia.

Suprasellar arachnoid cysts also occur in this region. CSF flows upward from the interpeduncular cistern but is trapped above the sella by thickened arachnoid (membrane of Liliequist). As the CSF accumulates, it forms a cyst that invaginates the third ventricle; the dome of the cyst may intermittently block the foramina of Monro and cause hydrocephalus (see Fox and Al-Mefty). Children with this condition exhibit a curious to-and-fro bobbing and nodding of the head, like a doll with a weighted head resting on a coiled spring. This has been referred to as the "bobble-head doll syndrome" by Benton and colleagues; it can be cured by emptying the cyst. Seesaw and other pendular and jerk types of nystagmus may also result from these suprasellar lesions.

Tables 31-5 and 47-1, adapted from Bingas' large neurosurgical service in Berlin, summarizes the facts about the focal syndromes of the skull base; his authoritative article and the more recent one by Morita and Piepgras, both in the *Handbook of Clinical Neurology*, are recommended references.

Modern imaging techniques now serve to clarify many of the diagnostic problems posed by these tumors. MRI is particularly helpful in delineating structures at the base of the brain and in the upper cervical region. CT is also capable of determining the absorptive values of the tumor itself and the sites of bone erosion. When the lesion is analyzed in this way, an etiologic diagnosis often becomes possible. For example, the absorptive value of lipomatous tissue is different from that of brain tissue, glioma, blood, and calcium. Bone scans (technetium and gallium) display active destructive lesions with remarkable fidelity, but in some cases, even when the tumor is seen with various studies, it may be difficult to obtain a satisfactory biopsy.

Tumors of the Foramen Magnum

Tumors in the region of the foramen magnum are of particular importance because of the need to differentiate them from diseases such as multiple sclerosis, Chiari malformation, syringomyelia, and bony abnormalities of the craniocervical junction. Failure to recognize these tumors is a consequential matter because the majority are benign and extramedullary, i.e., potentially resectable and curable. If unrecognized, they terminate fatally by causing medullary and high spinal cord compression.

Although these tumors are not common (approximately 1 percent of all intracranial and intraspinal tumors) sizable series have been collected by several clinicians (see Meyer et al for a complete bibliography). In all series, meningiomas, schwannomas, neurofibromas, and dermoid cysts are the most common types; others, all rare, are teratomas, dermoids, granulomas, cavernous hemangiomas, hemangioblastomas, hemangiopericytomas, lipomas, and epidural carcinomas.

Pain in the suboccipital or posterior cervical region, mostly on the side of the tumor, is usually the first and by far the most prominent complaint. In some instances the pain may extend into the shoulder and even the arm. The latter distribution is more frequent with tumors arising in the spinal canal and extending intracranially than the reverse. For uncertain reasons, the pain may radiate down the back, even to the lower spine. Both spine and root pain can be recognized, the latter because of involvement of either the C2 or C3 root or both.

One pattern is weakness of a shoulder and arm progressing to the ipsilateral leg and then to the opposite leg and arm ("around-the-clock" paralysis) as discussed in Chap. 3. Another configuration is triplegia that is a characteristic but not invariable sequence of events, caused by the encroachment of tumor upon the decussating corticospinal tracts at the foramen magnum. Occasionally, both upper limbs are involved alone; surprisingly, there may be atrophic weakness of the hand or forearm or even intercostal muscles with diminished tendon reflexes well below the level of the tumor, an observation made originally by Oppenheim. Involvement of sensory tracts also occurs; more often it is posterior column sensibility that is impaired on one or both sides, with patterns of progression similar to those of the motor paralysis. Sensation of intense cold in the neck and shoulders has been another unexpected complaint, and also "bands" of hyperesthesia around the neck and back of the head. Segmental bibrachial sensory loss has been demonstrated in a few of the cases and a Lhermitte sign (really a symptom) of electric-like sensations down the spine and limbs upon flexing the neck has been reported frequently. The cranial nerve signs most frequently conjoined and indicative of intracranial extension of a foramen magnum tumor are dysphagia, dysphonia, dysarthria, and drooping shoulder (because of vagal, hypoglossal, and spinal accessory involvement); included less often are nystagmus and episodic diplopia, sensory loss over the face and unilateral or bilateral facial weakness, and a Horner syndrome.

Table 31-5

CLINICAL SYNDROMES CAUSED BY TUMORS AT THE BASE OF THE SKULL

SITE OF LESION	EPONYM	CLINICAL SYMPTOMS	ETIOLOGY[a]
Anterior part of the base of the skull		Olfactory disturbances (uni- or bilateral anosmia), possibly psychiatric disturbances, seizures.	Tumors that invade the anterior part of the base of the skull from the frontal sinus, nasal cavity, or the ethmoid bone, osteomas. Meningiomas of the olfactory groove.
Superior orbital fissure	Rochon-Duvigneau; syndrome of the pterygopalatine fossa (Behr) and the base of the orbit (DeJean) commencing with a lesion of the maxillary and pterygoid rami and evolving into the superior orbital fissure syndrome.	Lesions of the third, fourth, sixth, and first divisions of the fifth nerves with ophthalmoplegia, pain, and sensory disturbances in the area of V_1; often exophthalmos, some vegetative disturbances.	Tumors: meningiomas, osteomas, dermoid cysts, giant-cell tumors, tumors of the orbit, nasopharyngeal tumors; more rarely, optic nerve gliomas; eosinophilic granulomas, angiomas, local or neighboring infections, trauma.
Apex of the orbit	Jacod-Rollet (often combined with the syndrome of the superior orbital fissure); infraclinoid syndrome of Dandy.	Visual disturbances, central scotoma, papilledema, optic nerve atrophy; occasional exophthalmos, chemosis.	Optic nerve glioma, infraclinoid aneurysm of the internal carotid artery, trauma, orbital tumors, Paget disease.
Cavernous sinus	Foix-Jefferson; syndrome of the sphenopetrosal fissure (Bonnet and Bonnet) corresponding in part to the cavernous sinus syndrome of Raeder.	Ophthalmoplegia caused by lesions of the third, fourth, sixth, and often fifth nerves; exophthalmos; vegetative disturbances. Jefferson distinguished three syndromes: (1) the anterior-superior, corresponding to the superior orbital fissure syndrome; (2) the middle, causing ophthalmoplegia and lesions of V_1 and V_2; (3) the caudal, in addition affecting the whole trigeminal nerve.	Tumors of the sellar and parasellar area, infraclinoid aneurysms of the internal carotid artery, nasopharyngeal tumors, fistulas of the sinus cavernosus and the carotid artery (traumatic), tumors of the middle cranial fossa, e.g., chondromas, meningiomas, and neurinomas.
Apex of the petrous temporal bone	Gradenigo-Lannois	Lesions of the fifth and sixth nerves with neuralgia, sensory, and motor disturbances, diplopia.	Inflammatory processes (otitis), tumors such as cholesteatomas, chondromas, meningiomas, neurinomas of the gasserian ganglion and trigeminal root, primary and secondary sarcomas at the base of the skull.
Sphenoid and petrosal bones (petrosphenoidal syndrome)	Jacod	Ophthalmoplegia caused by loss of function of the third, fourth, and sixth nerves; amaurosis; trigeminal neuralgia possibly with sensory signs.	Tumors of the sphenoid and petrosal bones and middle cranial fossa, nasopharyngeal tumors, metastases.
Jugular foramen	Vernet	Lesions of ninth, tenth, and eleventh nerves with disturbance of deglutition; curtain phenomenon; sensory disturbances of the tongue, soft palate, pharynx, and larynx; hoarseness; weakness of the sternocleidomastoid and trapezius.	Tumors of the glomus jugulare; neurinomas of eighth, ninth, tenth, and eleventh nerves; chondromas, cholesteatomas, meningiomas, nasopharyngeal and ear tumors; infections, angiomas, rarely trauma.
Anterior occipital condyles	Collet-Sicard (Vernet-Sargnon)	Loss of twelfth nerve function (loss of normal tongue mobility) in addition to the symptoms of the jugular foramen.	Tumors of the base of the skull, ear, parotid; leukemic infiltrates; aneurysms, angiomas, and inflammations.
Retroparotid space (retropharyngeal syndrome)	Villaret	Lesions of the lower group of nerves (Collet-Sicard) and Bernard-Horner syndrome with ptosis and miosis.	Tumors of the retroparotid space (carcinomas, sarcomas), trauma, inflammations.
Half of the base of the skull	Garcin (Guillain-Alajouanine-Garcin); also described by Hartmann in 1904.	Loss of function of all twelve cranial nerves of one side; in many cases, isolated cranial nerves spared; rarely signs of raised intracranial pressure or pyramidal tract symptoms.	Nasopharyngeal tumors, primary tumors at the base of the skull, leukemic infiltrates of basal meninges, trauma, metastases.

(Continued)

Table 31-5

CLINICAL SYNDROMES CAUSED BY TUMORS AT THE BASE OF THE SKULL (*CONTINUED*)

SITE OF LESION	EPONYM	CLINICAL SYMPTOMS	ETIOLOGY[a]
Cerebellopontine angle		Loss of function of eighth nerve (hearing loss, vertigo, nystagmus); cerebellar disturbances; lesions of the fifth, seventh, and possibly ninth and tenth cranial nerves. Signs of raised intracranial pressure, brainstem symptoms.	Acoustic neuromas (raised protein in CSF), meningiomas, cholesteatomas, metastases, cerebellar tumors, neurinomas of the caudal group of nerves and the trigeminal nerve, vascular processes such as angiomas, basilar aneurysms.

[a]Metastatic deposits may produce any of these syndromes.
Source: Adapted from Bingas. (See also Tables 47-1 and 47-2.)

The clinical course of such lesions often extends for years, with deceptive and unexplained fluctuations. The important diagnostic procedure is contrast-enhanced MRI (Fig. 31-22). With *dermoid cysts* of the upper cervical region, as in the case reported by Adams and Wegner, complete and prolonged remissions from quadriparesis may occur.

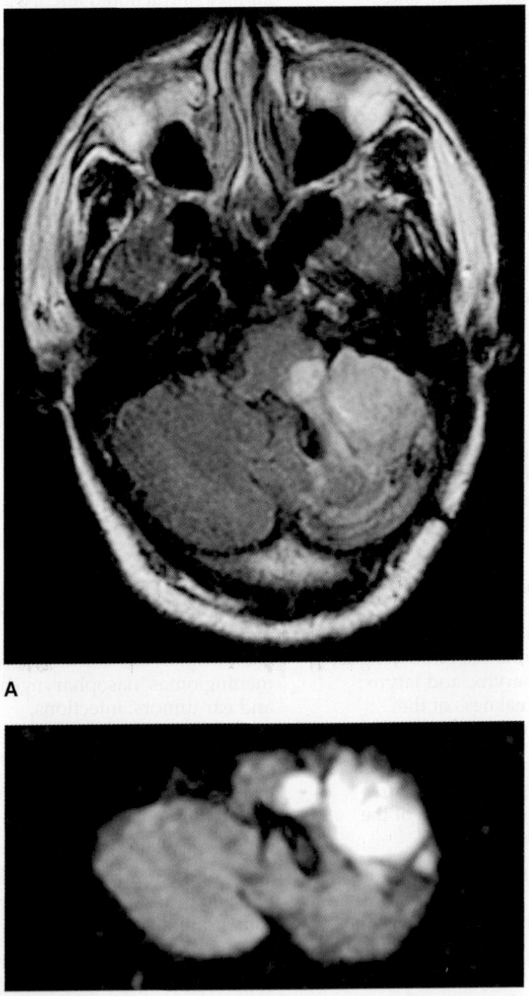

A

B

Figure 31-22. MRI demonstrating an epidermoid cyst in the left cerebellopontine angle just above the foramen magnum. The cyst is heterogenous and hyperintense on T2-weighted MRI (*A*) and demonstrates reduced diffusivity (*B*), a characteristic feature.

Tumors of the foramen magnum, as mentioned, should be differentiated from spinal or brainstem-cerebellar multiple sclerosis, Chiari malformation with syrinx, and bony compression. Persistent occipital neuralgia with a foramen magnum syndrome is particularly suggestive of a tumor at that site. The early occipitonuchal pain must be differentiated from mundane crucial osteoarthritis. Treatment is surgical excision (Hakuba et al) followed by focused radiation if the resection is incomplete and the tumor is known to be radiosensitive.

REMOTE EFFECTS OF NEOPLASIA ON THE NERVOUS SYSTEM (PARANEOPLASTIC DISORDERS) (TABLE 31-6)

In the past 50 years a group of neurologic disorders has been delineated that occur in patients with systemic neoplasia even though the nervous system is not the site of metastases or direct invasion or compression by the tumor. These so-called paraneoplastic disorders are not specific or confined to cancer, but the conditions are linked far more frequently than could be accounted for by chance. They assume special importance because in many cases the neurologic syndrome becomes apparent before the underlying tumor is found. The great variety of clinical presentations of paraneoplastic encephalitis disease can be appreciated from early series reported by Graus and colleagues of 200 patients: sensory neuropathy, 54 percent; cerebellar ataxia, 10 percent; limbic encephalitis, 9 percent; and others, including multiple sites, in 11 percent. Some of the paraneoplastic disorders that involve nerve and muscle—namely, polyneuropathy, polymyositis, and the myasthenic-myopathic syndrome of Lambert-Eaton—are described in later chapters on these subjects. Here we present the paraneoplastic processes that involve the spinal cord, cerebellum, brainstem, and cerebral hemispheres.

Comprehensive accounts of the paraneoplastic disorders may be found in the writings of Posner (1995), Darnell and Posner, and Dalmau and Rosenfeld. Some are associated with immunoglobulin G (IgG) autoantibodies (see Table 31-5), but it should be remarked that although certain antibodies are associated with specific syndromes, they are not invariably linked to particular cancers and vice versa. Furthermore, the same

Table 31-6

THE MAIN PARANEOPLASTIC DISORDERS AND THEIR ASSOCIATED AUTOANTIBODIES[a]

NEUROLOGIC DISORDER	CLINICAL FEATURES	PREDOMINANT AUTOANTIBODY	TUMOR
Cerebellar degeneration	Ataxia, subacute	Anti-Yo (anti-Purkinje cell)	Ovary, fallopian tube, lung, Hodgkin disease (anti-Tr)
Encephalomyelitis including limbic and brainstem encephalitis	Subacute confusion, brainstem signs, myelitis	Anti-Hu (ANNA 1) Anti-Ma, Anti-CRMP-5, Anti-Caspr2	Small cell lung, neuroblastoma, prostate, breast, Hodgkin, testicular (Ma)
	Psychosis, seizures, hypersympathetic state	Anti-NMDA, Anti-mGluR5	Ovarian (and other site) teratoma
Opsoclonus–myoclonus–ataxia	Ocular movement disorder, gait ataxia	Anti-Ri (ANNA 2)	Breast, fallopian tube, small cell lung
Retinal degeneration	Scotomas, blindness, disc swelling	Antirecoverin (Anti-CAR)	Small cell lung, thymoma, renal cell, melanoma
Subacute sensory neuropathy and neuronopathy	Distal or proximal sensory loss	Anti-Hu (ANNA-1)	Small cell lung, Hodgkin, other lymphomas
Lambert-Eaton myasthenic syndrome	Proximal fatiguing weakness, autonomic symptoms (dry mouth)	Anti-voltage-gated (VGCG) calcium channel	Small cell lung, Hodgkin, other lymphomas
Stiff person syndrome and neuromyotonia	Muscle spasms and rigidity	Antiamphiphysin, Anti-Caspr2, Anti-GAD	Breast, lung
Chorea	Bilateral choreoathetosis	Anti-Hu, Anti-CRMP-5	Lung, Hodgkin, others
Optic neuropathy	Blindness	Anti-CRMP-5	Lung

[a]In many cases, a particular autoantibody is associated with a specific tumor type rather than with the clinical syndrome (e.g., small cell lung cancer and polyneuropathy with ANNA 1, breast cancer with anti-Purkinje cell antibody, testicular tumors with anti-Ma). Clinical syndromes similar to each of these may occur with non–small cell lung cancer and lymphoma, most often in the absence of detectable antibodies.

syndromes and antibodies occur sometimes without an evident tumor. This was emphasized in the survey by Pittock and colleagues at the Mayo Clinic, who found that one-third of sera from patients with paraneoplastic neurologic disorders had more than one antibody. They have suggested that this reflects the numerous immunogenic onconeural proteins that are expressed by tumors. Consequently, the relationships between particular antibodies and a clinical syndromes listed in Table 31-6 should be taken as approximate, or nonexclusive. Nonetheless, certain syndromes seem to occur disproportionately often with particular antibodies. Small cell cancer of the lung, adenocarcinoma of the breast and ovary, and Hodgkin disease are the tumors most often associated with these disorders, but the paraneoplastic neurologic syndromes occur in only a very small proportion of patients with these tumors.

The mechanisms by which carcinomas produce their remote effects are incompletely understood. Perhaps the most plausible theory, as intimated above, is that they have an autoimmune basis. According to this theory, antigenic molecules are shared by certain tumors and central or peripheral neurons. The immune response is then directed to the shared antigen in both the tumor and the nervous system. The evidence for such an autoimmune mechanism is most clearly exemplified by the Lambert-Eaton syndrome, in which an antibody derived from a tumor binds to voltage-gated calcium channels at neuromuscular junctions (see Chap. 49).

Furthermore, in some types of paraneoplastic disorders, there is provocative evidence that the inciting tumor has antigen on its surface and self-binding of the antibody may inhibit tumor growth. This may account for the difficulty in detecting diminutive small cell lung cancers that underlie some of the paraneoplastic syndromes. It should be noted, however, that there is no evidence that suppressing or removing the antibody leads to growth of the tumor.

Encephalomyelitis Associated with Carcinoma and "Limbic Encephalitis"

The occurrence of regional and bilateral encephalomyelitic changes in association with carcinoma has been described by several authors (Corsellis et al; Henson and Urich; Posner, 1995). In most of the reported cases, the encephalitic process has been associated with carcinoma of the bronchus, usually of the small cell type, but all types of neoplasms, including Hodgkin disease, have been implicated. Histologically, this group of paraneoplastic disorders is characterized by extensive loss of neurons, accompanied by microglial proliferation, small patches of necrosis, and marked perivascular cuffing by lymphocytes and monocytes. Foci of lymphocytic infiltration have been observed in the leptomeninges as well. These pathologic changes may involve the brain and spinal cord diffusely, but more often they predominate in a particular part of the nervous system, notably in the medial temporal lobes and adjacent nuclei ("limbic encephalitis," Fig. 31-23), the brainstem, the cerebellum (see earlier), or the gray matter of the spinal cord. The symptoms will, of course, depend on the location and severity of the inflammatory changes and may overlap. Most cases are subacute, meaning specifically a progression over a few weeks or months, but often the main symptoms in mild form become apparent in a matter of days. Rare instances of remission have been reported.

The most distinctive features of *paraneoplastic limbic encephalitis* consists of a confusional–agitated state, memory defect (Korsakoff syndrome), seizures, sometimes focal, hallucinations, and dementia—singly or in various combinations and evolving subacutely (Gultekin et al); an amnestic component is almost universal and the central feature in most cases.

Vertigo, nystagmus, ataxia, nausea and vomiting, and a variety of ocular and gaze palsies reflect a different process of *paraneoplastic brainstem encephalitis*. As indicated above, these symptoms may be joined with cerebellar ataxia, and another group has an additional sensory neuropathy. We have seen instances of this condition involving only the midbrain and others involving only the medulla, the latter with unusual breathing patterns including gasping, inspiratory breathholding, and vocal–respiratory incoordination, and yet others with chorea and additional basal ganglionic features. Pathologic studies have partially clarified this form of paraneoplastic disorder. In some cases, few changes were demonstrable in the brain, even though there had been a prominent dementia during life. Contrariwise, widespread inflammatory changes may be found without clinical abnormalities having been recorded during life.

In most of these cases, MRI shows abnormal T2 hyperintensity and edema in affected regions; in severe cases, zones of focal necrosis may be seen. Odd seizures, including epilepsia partialis continua, have been observed with this disorder, but they must be uncommon. Sensory symptoms may be related to neuronal loss in the posterior horns, traced to the commonly associated loss of neurons in the dorsal root ganglia (sensory neuronopathy and sensory neuropathy) as mentioned earlier and discussed further on.

Most patients with small cell lung cancer and any of the types of paraneoplastic encephalomyelitis have been found to harbor circulating polyclonal IgG antibodies (*anti-Hu*, or *antineuronal antibody type 1*) that bind to the nuclei of neurons in many regions of the brain and spinal cord, dorsal root ganglion cells, and peripheral autonomic neurons. The antibodies are reactive with certain nuclear RNA-binding proteins. Cancers of the prostate and breast and neuroblastoma may rarely produce a similar antibody. The antibody titer is higher in the CSF than in the serum (as it is for anti-Yo with cerebellar degeneration), indicating production of antibody within the nervous system. Low titers of anti-Hu are found in approximately 15 percent of patients with small cell cancer who are neurologically normal, probably because these tumors have expressed only low levels of antigens that are recognized by anti-Hu. Antibodies to voltage-gated potassium channels (VGKC) have been identified in patients with limbic encephalitis without, or less often with, cancer (Vincent et al). A number of these cases respond to plasma exchange. The anti-VGKC disorders tend to be slower in evolution and less severe than the typical paraneoplastic neurologic syndromes.

Treatment Despite a few reports of improvement with plasma exchange or intravenous gamma globulin, the results of treatment have been disappointing. However, those few patients who did improve had treatment from the onset of symptoms, and this is possibly a way of limiting the neuronal loss.

Anti-NMDA Encephalitis

A special form of paraneoplastic encephalitis presents itself as an acute or subacute psychiatric syndrome consisting of some combination of hallucinations, panic, delusions, and incoherence, coupled with seizures, memory disturbance and hypoventilation has been described by Vitaliani and colleagues in four women with ovarian teratoma. Many patients have a non-descript prodrome of malaise, fatigue, headache excessive sleepiness, or low fever. Dalmau and coworkers (2007) demonstrated that this syndrome is associated with antibodies against a component of the NMDA receptor. The teratoma in one of their patients was located in the mediastinum instead of the ovary and rare cases have occurred with small cell lung cancer, including in men. Dalmau's series of 100 patients (2008) is instructive in that they were very predominantly women in their twenties with presentations or psychiatric or memory deterioration but a large number had dyskinesias, seizures, or hypoventilation. Almost all had several or dozens of white blood cells in the CSF, a majority had oligoclonal bands and the MRI showed abnormal T2 hyperintensity in the medial temporal lobes, similar to those of the anti-Hu type of limbic encephalitis.

We have been impressed with the autonomic overactivity in the patients under our care with this syndrome. Episodes of hypertension, tachycardia and diaphoresis can be pronounced, as is excessive salivation, pupillary dilation, and other signs of sympathetic dysfunction, individually or concurrently.

Dalmau and colleagues have identified the target of the antibody as the subunit of the NMDA receptor, NR1. There is a reasonable degree of certainty that the antibody is pathogenic.

Another peculiar syndrome associated with prostate cancer, which we have encountered once, was described by Baloh and colleagues prior to the discovery of most of the currently known paraneoplastic antibodies. These patients display brainstem signs, particularly loss of horizontal gaze, and facial and pharyngeal spasms or abdominal myoclonus. Whether this process will be subsumed under one or another of the known antibody syndromes is not known but it is notable because prostate cancer otherwise rarely gives rise to paraneoplastic disease.

Treatment A premium is attached to early identification of this disorder and rapid removal of the ovary containing the teratoma or resection of another inciting tumor. Vaginal ultrasound may be necessary for the demonstration of the ovarian lesion but a more extensive examination such as CT or PET is needed for the detection of other tumors. Improvement after tumor removal is associated with subsidence of the antibody titer over many weeks and a good outcome occurs in a majority of cases. Decisions regarding oophorectomy are difficult in view of reducing fertility in young women.

It has become apparent that a fair proportion of cases with circulating anti-NMDA antibody do not have a tumor that is detectable and immune treatments such as intravenous gamma globulin may then be used. It is reasonable to start these same immune treatments while awaiting surgery in cases that are highly symptomatic.

Paraneoplastic Sensory Neuronopathy

(See also Chap. 46)

This is a distinctive syndrome that is associated in most cases with the anti-Hu antibody. It should be emphasized that a nondescript, mainly sensory neuropathy is a more common accompaniment of systemic cancer, and it may or may not be associated with the anti-Hu antibody. As discussed further in Chap. 46, a sensory polyneuropathy from chemotherapeutic agents, notably the platinum-based ones and vincristine, also needs to be distinguished from the anti-Hu neuropathy syndrome.

The sensory neuronopathy and neuropathy were first described by Denny-Brown in 1948 and are notable because they served to introduce the modern-day concept of paraneoplastic neurologic disease. The initial symptoms in both processes are numbness or paresthesia, sometimes painful, in a limb or in both feet. There may be lancinating pains at the onset. Over a period of days in some cases, but more typically over weeks, the initially focal symptoms become bilateral and may spread to all limbs and their proximal portions and then to the trunk. It is this widespread and proximal distribution and the involvement of the face, scalp, and often the oral and genital mucosa that mark the process as a sensory ganglionitis and radiculitis and when subacute are highly suggestive of a paraneoplastic process.

As the illness progresses, all forms of sensation are greatly reduced, resulting in *disabling ataxia* and pseudoathetoid movements of the outstretched hands. The reflexes are lost, but not always at the outset, and strength is relatively preserved. *Autonomic dysfunction*—including constipation or ileus, sicca syndrome, pupillary areflexia, and orthostatic hypotension—is sometimes associated. Also, a virtually pure form of peripheral autonomic failure has been recorded as a paraneoplastic phenomenon (*paraneoplastic dysautonomia*). One of our patients with sensory neuronopathy had gastric atony with fatal aspiration after vomiting and another died of unexpected cardiac arrhythmia. Very early in the illness, the electrophysiologic studies may be normal, but this soon gives way to a loss of all sensory potentials, sometimes with indications of a mild motor neuropathy.

The spinal fluid usually contains an elevated protein and a few lymphocytes. As with paraneoplastic encephalomyelitis, most of the cases associated with small cell lung cancer demonstrate the anti-Hu antibody. As mentioned, neuropathy and encephalomyelitis often occur together. The sensory neuronopathy–ganglionopathy that is related to Sjögren disease and an idiopathic variety do not have this antibody, making its presence a reliable marker for lung cancer in patients with sensory neuronopathy. The polyneuropathy is refractory to almost all forms of treatment, or there is a transient benefit, and most patients die within months of onset, but there have been reports of brief remissions with plasma exchange and intravenous gamma globulin applied early in the illness. Resection of the lung tumor may halt progression of the neurologic illness.

Paraneoplastic Cerebellar Degeneration

For many years, this disorder was considered to be quite uncommon, but it is perhaps the most characteristic of the paraneoplastic syndromes. In reviewing this subject in 1970, Adams and Victor were able to find only 41 pathologically verified cases; in a subsequent review (Henson and Urich), only a few more cases were added. The actual incidence is much higher than these figures would indicate. At the Cleveland Metropolitan General Hospital, in a series of 1,700 consecutive autopsies in adults, there were 5 instances of cerebellar degeneration associated with neoplasm. In the experience of Henson and Urich, about half of all patients with nonfamilial, late-onset cerebellar degeneration proved sooner or later to be harboring a neoplasm. Large series of cases have been reported from the Mayo Clinic and the Memorial Sloan-Kettering Cancer Center (Hammock et al and N.E. Anderson et al, respectively). We see several such cases yearly, but have also encountered numerous instances of an identical syndrome with no cancer evident and no antibodies that are probably a result of diverse causes summarized in Chap. 5 and Table 5-1.

In approximately one-third of the cases, the underlying neoplasm has been in the lung (most often a small cell carcinoma)—a figure reflecting the high incidence of this tumor. However, the association of ovarian carcinoma and lymphoma, particularly Hodgkin disease, accounting for approximately 25 and 15 percent, respectively, is considerably higher than would be expected on the basis of the frequency of these malignancies. Carcinomas of the breast, bowel, uterus, and other viscera have accounted for most of the remaining cases (Posner, 1995).

The cerebellar symptoms have a subacute onset and steady progression over a period of weeks to months; in more than half the cases, the cerebellar signs are recognized before those of the associated neoplasm. Symmetrical ataxia of gait and limbs—affecting arms and legs more or less equally—dysarthria, and nystagmus are the usual manifestations; some have vertigo. Striking in fully developed cases has been the severity of the ataxia, matched by few other diseases. Occasionally, myoclonus and opsoclonus or a fast-frequency myoclonic tremor may be associated ("dancing eyes–dancing feet," as noted later). In addition, there are quite often symptoms and signs not strictly cerebellar in nature, notably diplopia, vertigo, Babinski signs (common in our cases), sensorineural hearing loss, disorders of ocular motility, and alteration of affect and mentation—findings that serve to distinguish paraneoplastic from alcoholic and other varieties of cerebellar degeneration. Lambert-Eaton syndrome is known to occur with cerebellar degeneration as paraneoplastic illnesses. These are well emphasized in the series of 47 patients collected by Anderson and colleagues and the 55 cases by Peterson et al, who tabulated these noncerebellar neurologic features.

The CSF may show a mild pleocytosis (up to 50 cells/mm^3 in a few of our patients) and increased protein, or it may be entirely normal. Early in the course of the disease, CT and MRI show no abnormality, but after a few months, atrophy of the brainstem and cerebellum may appear. In a few cases, T2-weighted MRI discloses increased signal of the cerebellar white matter (Hammock et al), but this has not been uniform in our experience, and furthermore does not correlate well to the degree of Purkinje cell loss (Fig. 31-23).

Pathologically, there are diffuse degenerative changes of the cerebellar cortex and deep cerebellar nuclei. Purkinje cells are affected prominently and all parts of the cerebellar cortex are involved. Degenerative changes in the spinal cord, involving the posterior columns and spinocerebellar tracts, have been found rarely. The cerebellar neuronal degeneration is frequently associated with perivascular and meningeal clusters of inflammatory cells. Henson and Urich regard the inflammatory changes as an independent process, part of a subacute paraneoplastic encephalomyelitis (see below). This view is supported by the finding that the specific antibodies linked to cerebellar degeneration differ from those found in paraneoplastic inflammatory lesions in other parts of the nervous system.

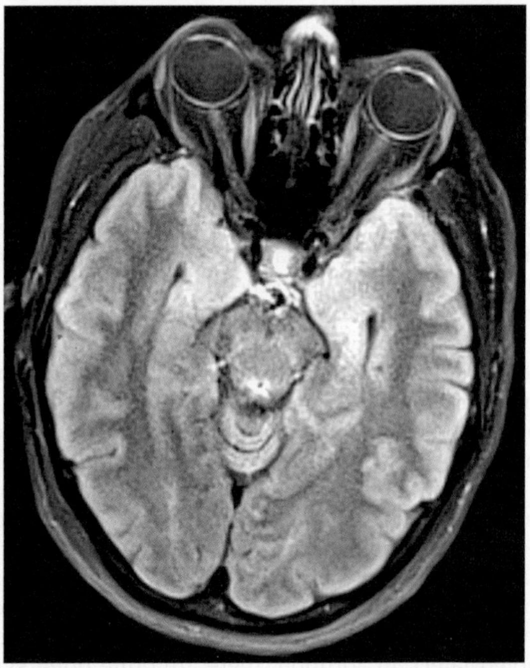

Figure 31-23. Axial T2 FLAIR MRI from a woman with anti-voltage-gated potassium channel (VGKC) paraneoplastic limbic encephalitis associated with thyroid cancer. The hippocampus and amygdala appear abnormally T2 hyperintense.

Anti-Purkinje cell antibodies (termed "anti-Yo") can be found in the sera of about half of patients with paraneoplastic cerebellar degeneration and in the large majority of those related to carcinoma of the breast or female genital tract, linking the clinical syndrome and this antibody closely. Antibodies against a nuclear antigen, termed anti-Hu, may also be present; they are more closely linked to the paraneoplastic encephalomyelitis discussed further on. (Hu and Yo are taken from the names of patients in whom the antibody was first found.) In the Mayo Clinic series of 32 patients with paraneoplastic cerebellar degeneration, 16 had such antibodies; all were women and most of them had breast or ovarian cancers. Anderson and colleagues report a similar proportion but point out that several anti-Purkinje antibodies besides the highly characteristic one may be found by special techniques. Death occurred in 4 to 18 months. In an equal number of cases without antibodies, half are men with lung cancer, some of whom display the anti-Hu antibody. This leaves a proportion who have no circulating antibody but who are nonetheless found to have a concealed tumor that must be sought by other ancillary tests including positron emission tomography (PET) of the entire body. In another small group, it must be conceded that no underlying tumor can be found despite extensive examinations and even at autopsy. The death rate in these cases has varied widely from 6 months to several years and depends on the behavior of the underlying tumor.

Whether the anti-Yo antibodies are merely markers of an underlying tumor or the agents of destruction of the Purkinje cells is not clear. They bind to a C-myc protein that initiates a degeneration of Purkinje cells. Regardless of the pathogenic significance of the antibodies, their presence in a patient with the typical neurologic disorder has considerable diagnostic significance. As mentioned above, they usually indicate that there is an underlying breast or ovarian cancer, which may be asymptomatic and small enough to be resected successfully. Other antibodies besides anti-Yo and anti-Hu are found on occasion, such as those against a glutamate receptor in patients with Hodgkin disease (Smitt et al). The differential diagnosis of subacute cerebellar ataxia is broad, as indicated in Table 5-1. The main considerations are a variant of Creutzfeldt-Jakob disease, postinfectious cerebellitis, and various intoxications.

Treatment Reports of aggressive plasma exchange or intravenous immunoglobulin treatment early in the course suggest some benefit, but it should not be assumed that this approach will succeed in most patients, and our own experience has been discouraging in this regard. There are also on record several cases in which there was a partial or complete remission of symptoms after removal of the primary tumor (Paone and Jeyasingham). Furthermore, in some cases associated with Hodgkin disease, there has been spontaneous improvement of the cerebellar symptoms.

Opsoclonus–Myoclonus–Ataxia Syndrome

In children, this syndrome is usually a manifestation of neuroblastoma, but it is more common and occurs in adults in relation to breast cancer and small cell lung cancer. The unique feature of the neuroblastoma is a response of this syndrome to corticosteroids and ACTH in most children and in some adults, and resolution of the neurologic signs when the neuroblastoma is removed. A subgroup of breast cancers produce an antineuronal antibody directed against a different RNA-binding antigen from the anti-Hu antibody; thus it has been termed "anti-Ri" (*antineuronal antibody type* 2). This antibody is not found in the opsoclonus–ataxic syndrome of neuroblastoma and is present only rarely with small cell lung cancer. There have also been a limited number of positive serologic tests in children with opsoclonus, apparently without an underlying tumor. A few such patients have had a mild pleocytosis in the CSF; the MRI is usually normal. More complex syndromes have been reported with the anti-Ri antibody, manifest by rigidity and intense stimulus-sensitive myoclonus in addition to the core features of opsoclonus and ataxia.

The neuropathologic findings have not been distinctive; mild cell loss has been described in the Purkinje cell layer, inferior olives, and brainstem, with mild inflammatory changes (Luque et al).

Besides breast cancer, we have observed the opsoclonus–myoclonus syndrome in a middle-aged woman with bronchial carcinoma and in a man with gastric carcinoma. Similar cases occur with both cerebellar ataxia and an irregular tremor, which we have interpreted as myoclonic in character. These patients were found to have marked degeneration of the dentate nuclei. The prognosis in this syndrome is somewhat better than that for the other paraneoplastic diseases, but besides a trial of ACTH, there is little that can be done but search for the tumor and resect it if possible.

Carcinomatous Myelopathy and Motor Neuronopathy

In addition to subacute degeneration of spinal cord tracts that may be associated with paraneoplastic cerebellar degeneration (see earlier), there has been described a rapidly progressive form of more widespread degeneration of the spinal cord (Mancall and Rosales). The myelopathy is characterized by a rapidly ascending sensorimotor deficit that terminates fatally in a matter of weeks. There is a roughly symmetrical necrosis of both the gray and white matter of most of the cord. This necrotizing *myelopathy* is distinctly rare, being far less common than compression of the spinal cord from cancer and even less frequent than intramedullary spinal cord metastases. Flanagan and colleagues have summarized a large series of their cases and described a variety of presentations including longitudinally extensive involvement on imaging studies that simulate the pattern seen with anti-aquaproin antibodies of Devic disease as described in Chaps. 36 and 44. It can therefore be said that there is a paraneoplastic type of neuromyelitis optica. Most of their cases had a CSF pleocytosis, half had oligoclonal bands, and one of the known paraneoplastic autoantibodies was found the majority.

Better defined is *subacute motor neuronopathy* that occurs as a remote effect of bronchogenic carcinoma, Hodgkin disease, and other lymphomas as mentioned earlier in the discussion of encephalomyelitis (Schold et al). Some cases take the form of a relatively benign, purely motor weakness of the limbs, the course and severity of which are independent of the underlying neoplasm. Other cases are severe and progressive, causing respiratory failure and death, thus simulating amyotrophic lateral sclerosis (ALS); some of these will have the anti-Hu antibody (Verma et al; Forsyth et al). The basic neuropathologic change is a depletion of anterior horn cells; also seen are inflammatory changes and neuronophagia as in chronic poliomyelitis. The few autopsied cases have shown gliosis of the posterior columns, pointing to an asymptomatic affection of the primary sensory neuron, as well as a reduction in the number of Purkinje cells.

Forsyth and colleagues subdivided their cases of *paraneoplastic motor neuron syndromes* into three groups: (1) rapidly progressive amyotrophy and fasciculations with or without brisk reflexes—all of their 3 patients displayed anti-Hu antibodies, 2 with small cell lung cancer and 1 with prostate cancer; (2) a predominantly corticospinal syndrome that affected the oropharyngeal or limb musculature, without definite evidence of denervation, thus resembling primary lateral sclerosis—all were breast cancer patients and none showed antineuronal antibodies; and (3) a syndrome indistinguishable from ALS in 6 patients with breast or small cell lung cancer, Hodgkin disease, or ovarian cancer, none of whom had antineuronal antibodies. In the latter two groups one cannot be certain that the condition was not a chance occurrence of the idiopathic variety of motor neuron disease. Nevertheless, this is such a rare cause of motor neuron disease that an evaluation for tumor is not required in the typical case of ALS.

A rare paraneoplastic syndrome of spinal myoclonus with tonic spasms can occur and is assumed to be from inflammation of the spinal cord gray matter as discussed in Chaps. 6 and 44.

Other Paraneoplastic Disorders

Several more recently discovered antibodies, such as CRMP-5 (collapsin-responsive mediator protein) and anti-Ma1 and -Ma2, have been detected in cases of brainstem encephalitis including with ophthalmoplegia but there have been associations with limbic and diencephalic syndromes as well and a hypokinetic parkinsonian appearance (Dalmau et al 2004). The anti-Ma antibodies cross-react with testicular antigens and a search for a testicular tumor is undertaken (Voltz et al). Although rare, the clinical syndromes associated with the anti-Ma antibody and testicular tumors are diverse: limbic, brainstem, or hypothalamic inflammation and an ataxic–opsoclonic syndrome that is more typical of anti-Ri antibody (see earlier).

The antibody to CRMP-5 is reported in some series to be second in frequency only to anti-Hu. Lung carcinoma has been the most common source in the series of Yu and colleagues, with thymoma, renal cell, and other neoplasms accounting for a few of the cases. The clinical features have been as diverse as for anti-Hu, including seizures, dementia, confusion, depression, as well as a variety of peripheral and cranial neuropathies and, surprisingly, the Lambert-Eaton syndrome.

An illness similar to the one caused by anti-NMDA antibodies, under the name of Ophelia syndrome, has been reported as a paraneoplastic syndrome that is due to antibodies directed against the metabotropic glutamate receptor, mGluR5 (see Lancaster et al).

Paraneoplastic Optic Neuropathy

An optic neuropathy is probably the most specific associated syndrome with the CRMP-5 antibody, as described by Cross and colleagues. There is subacute visual loss, disc swelling, and a cellular reaction in the vitreous. Most patients have features of another paraneoplastic syndrome. Several authors have remarked on the occurrence of chorea as a presenting symptom along with basal ganglionic changes on MRI. It is difficult for us to make sense of the clinical features aside from the optic neuropathy (really an optic neuritis), but they seem comparable to the perivenous inflammatory encephalitis and neuritis of the anti-Hu syndromes. Presumably this antibody accounts for some of the odd subacutely progressive syndromes previously thought to be antibody-negative; testing for this antibody might be included when an unusual paraneoplastic syndrome is suspected. The heterogeneity of antibody response to these expressed proteins may account for different clinical manifestations of the immune process but there is no certain evidence yet of their pathogenetic role.

Paraneoplastic Retinopathy

In recent years, there have been reports of retinopathy as a paraneoplastic syndrome that is distinct from the above-described optic neuropathy. Small cell carcinoma of the lung has been the most common underlying malignancy. In about half of the reported cases, retinal symptoms preceded the discovery of the tumor by several months. The lesion is in the photoreceptor cells, and antiretinal antibodies (directed against a calcium-binding protein, recoverin) have been identified in the serum. Photosensitivity, ring scotomas, and attenuation of the retinal arterioles are the main clinical features; Jacobson and coworkers suggested that they constitute a diagnostic triad.

Paraneoplastic Stiff Man Syndrome and Related Neuromuscular Disorders (See Chap. 48)

Occasionally this disorder (stiff man syndrome) occurs as a paraneoplastic disease. Lesser degrees of unexplained mild rigidity are seen from time to time, perhaps as a consequence of loss of spinal cord interneurons. In what might be called "stiff woman syndrome," Folli and associates described 3 female patients with breast cancer who developed a state of generalized motor hyperexcitability and rigidity. These patients generally have no antibodies to glutamic acid decarboxylase (GAD), as in the sporadic cases of "stiff man syndrome"; probably there are antibodies to other synaptic proteins.

The "chorée fibrillaire" of Morvan is an extraordinary disorder of continuous muscle fiber activity, insomnia, and hallucinosis that may be caused by a paraneoplastic antibody to voltage-gated potassium channels, as discussed in Chap. 48 and 50s. This same antibody, as well as acetylcholine receptor antibodies, has been associated with neuromyotonia of *Isaac syndrome*, seen in cases of lung cancer, lymphoma, and thymoma.

The Lambert-Eaton syndrome is perhaps the most common paraneoplastic neurologic syndrome; it is associated with antibodies directed against calcium channels, as mentioned earlier. This disorder, which may occur concurrently with other paraneoplastic syndromes such as cerebellar ataxia, is discussed in Chap. 53. Basal ganglia syndromes, chorea in particular, are associated with the anti-Hu and CRMP-5 antibodies as already noted. A myoclonus syndrome without ataxia or opsoclonus is reported from time to time in the literature and probably is a derivative of one of the better-characterized antibody diseases.

Radiation Injury of the Brain

Injury to the CNS from radiation is appropriately discussed here, since it occurs mainly in relation to therapy of brain tumors. Three syndromes of radiation damage have been delineated: acute, early delayed, and late delayed, although these syndromes often blend into one another. The acute reaction may begin during the latter part of a series of fractionated treatments or soon thereafter. There may be a seizure, a transitory worsening of the tumor symptoms, or signs of increased intracranial pressure. Although the condition has been attributed to brain edema, this is not always visible on MRI and its basis is unknown. The symptoms subside in days to weeks. Corticosteroids are usually administered, but with the exception of cases with demonstrable edema, their effect is uncertain. A novel syndrome of migraine-like headache and focal neurologic deficits, developing many years after cranial radiation, has also been described and is referred to below.

The early radiation syndrome has been more troublesome in our experience that has the very acute form. As with the acute syndrome, focal tumor symptoms may increase, and as seen on MRI (Fig. 31-25), the tumor mass enlarges, raising the possibility of further tumor growth, but again the symptoms usually reflect extensive demyelination, loss of oligodendrocytes beyond the confines of the tumor, and varying degrees of tissue necrosis. Possibly the administration of dexamethasone or a similar corticosteroid hastens resolution of this condition.

The late-delayed process is the most serious of radiation complications. Here one finds—in structures adjacent to a cerebral neoplasm, the pituitary gland, or other structures of the head and neck—necrosis of the white matter of the brain and, occasionally, of the brainstem. In some areas, the tissue undergoes softening and liquefaction, with cavitation. With lesser degrees of injury, the process is predominantly a demyelinating one, with partial preservation of axons. Later reactions are thought to be caused by diffuse vascular changes as a result of radiation energy. Endothelial cells frequently multiply and, because ionization injures dividing cells, the vessels are most vulnerable. The result is hyaline thickening of vessels with fibrinoid necrosis and widespread microthrombosis. There is a lesser degree of damage to glial cells. Neurons are relatively resistant though they can be secondarily affected by loss of glial support as well as reduced tissue perfusion.

The symptoms of delayed injury, coming on 3 months to many years after radiation therapy, are either those of a subacutely evolving mass, difficult to separate from those of tumor growth, or of a subacute dementia. The clinical pattern varies with the site of the lesion: focal or generalized seizures, impairment of mental function, and, sometimes, increased ICP. Whole-brain radiation for metastatic tumor or acute lymphoblastic leukemia can lead to multifocal zones of necrosis and holohemispheric spongiform changes in the white matter, with diffuse cerebral atrophy and enlarged ventricles. Progressive dementia, ataxia, and urinary incontinence are the main clinical features of this state (DeAngelis et al). In its mildest form there are no radiographic changes aside from the tumor, but the patient becomes mentally dull, slightly disinhibited, and often sleepy for large parts of the day. Panhypopituitarism is another complication of whole-brain radiotherapy, particularly in children, who may also suffer growth retardation. Radiation necrosis of the spinal cord is described in Chap. 44.

In the production of radiation necrosis, the total and fractional doses of radiation and the time over which treatment is administered are obviously important factors, but the exact amounts that produce such damage cannot be stated. Accepted levels of large-field radiation are tolerated in amounts approaching 6,000 cGy, provided it is given in small daily doses (200 to 300 cGy) 5 days per week over a period of 6 weeks. Other factors, still undefined, must play a part, as similar courses of radiation treatment may damage one patient and leave another unaffected. The severe necrotizing encephalopathy that has followed the combined use of methotrexate (intrathecally but also intravenously) was discussed earlier, under "Involvement of the Nervous System in Leukemia," the condition in which it was first described and formerly was most prevalent.

CT and MRI show a contrast-enhancing lesion, and by angiography there is an avascular mass. Small calcifications may appear many years after the radiation. MRI is somewhat more sensitive in distinguishing radiation necrosis from tumor and peritumor products, but PET is the most reliable way of differentiating the two, perhaps obviating the need for biopsy (Glantz et al, 1991). Single-photon emission tomography (SPECT) can be useful for this purpose as well (Carvalho et al). CT or MRI perfusion imaging can also be used to differentiate radiation necrosis from tumor progression; cerebral blood volume is reduced in the former and most often elevated in the latter.

Treatment has consisted of the administration of corticosteroids, which may cause regression of symptoms and of edema surrounding the lesion. Very high doses may be necessary, 40 mg or more of dexamethasone (or its equivalent) daily. Rarely, surgical resection of a necrotic mass has been attempted, with uncertain results.

A difficult to classify migraine-like syndrome following cranial irradiation has been described by Partap and colleagues and by Pruitt and coworkers. This syndrome has been given the acronym *SMART*, for stroke-like migraine attacks after radiation therapy. The typical case is of a young adult who, years or decades after receiving radiation as a child for an intracranial neoplasm, develops episodes of severe headache and simultaneous symptoms such as aphasia, hemiparesis, or hemianopia, sometimes lasting days. There may be an independent headache suggestive of migraine. The CSF protein is often elevated. In some cases there is diffuse gyriform enhancement over a large region of cortex spanning several arterial territories, and focal narrowing of intracranial vessels or capillary telangiectasias can be seen as well, both interpreted by the above authors as radiation-induced change. Corticosteroids seemed helpful in some cases.

It is also known that tumors, usually sarcomas, can be induced by radiation, as mentioned earlier (Cavin et al). While well documented, this occurs rarely and only after an interval of many years. We have also seen two cases of fibrosarcoma of the brachial plexus region in the radiation field for breast tumors (Gorson et al). These lesions appeared more than 10 years after the initial treatment, and many cases of even longer latency are on record.

Tumors of the spinal cord and peripheral nerves are discussed in Chaps. 44 and 46, respectively. The various neurologic effects of chemotherapy for systemic tumors, especially polyneuropathy, are discussed in Chaps. 43 and 46. The interesting problem of the effects on the nervous system of graft-versus-host disease are taken up in Chap. 36 with other inflammatory conditions (Figs. 31-24 and 31-25).

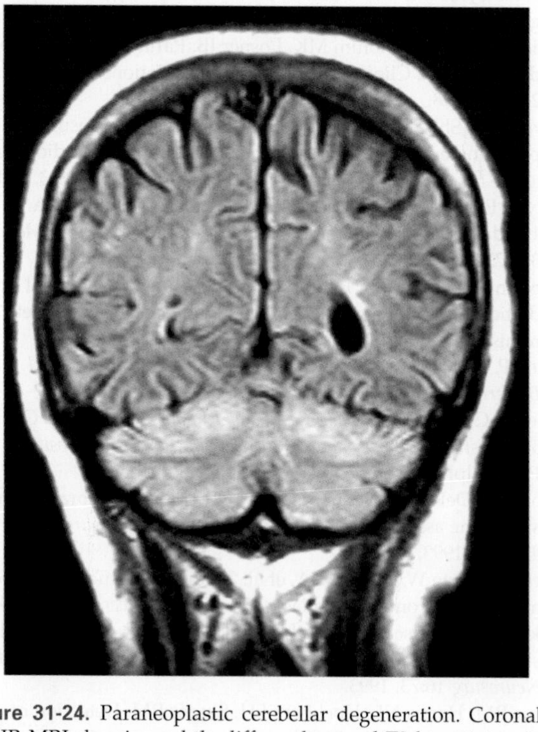

Figure 31-24. Paraneoplastic cerebellar degeneration. Coronal T2 FLAIR MRI showing subtle diffuse abnormal T2 hyperintensity of the cerebellar cortex.

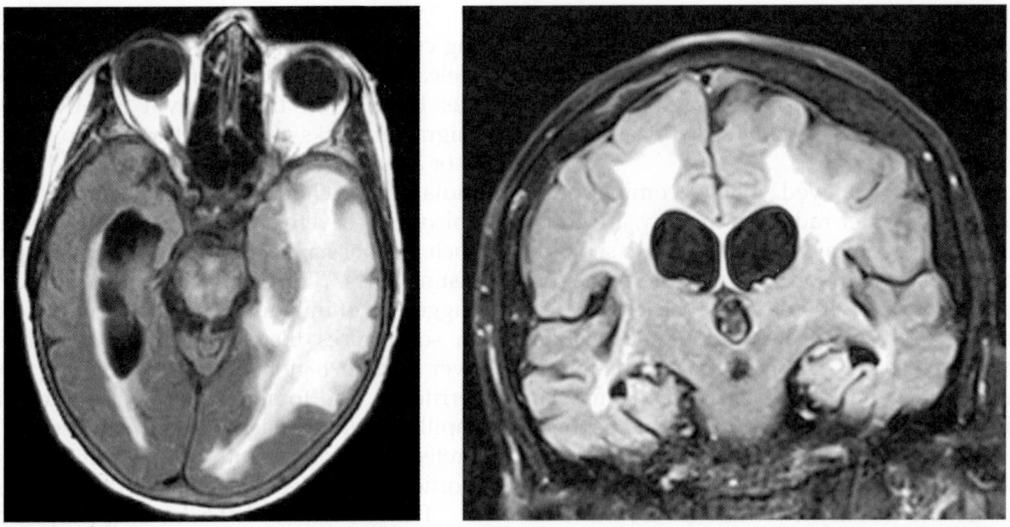

Figure 31-25. Radiation leukoencephalopathy. A patient who underwent proton beam radiation therapy for carcinoma of the mastoid area presented several years later with a seizure and was found to have extensive abnormal T2 hyperintensity in the adjacent left hemisphere (*left*), consistent with radiation necrosis. Another patient with lung cancer who was treated with prophylactic whole-brain radiation, presented several years later with gait difficulties and cognitive decline and was found to have extensive symmetric leukoencephalopathy with ex vacuo ventricular dilation.

References

Adams RD, Wegner W: Congenital cyst of the spinal meninges as cause of intermittent compression of the spinal cord. *Arch Neurol Psychiatry* 58:57, 1947.

Allen JC: Controversies in the management of intracranial germ cell tumors. *Neurol Clin* 9:441, 1991.

Anderson JR, Antoun N, Burnet N, et al: Neurology of the pituitary gland. *J Neurol Neurosurg Psychiatry* 66:703, 1999.

Anderson NE, Rosenblum MK, Posner JB: Paraneoplastic cerebellar degeneration: Clinical-immunologic correlations. *Ann Neurol* 24:559, 1998.

Aoyama H, Shirato H, Tago M, et al: Stereotactic radiosurgery plus whole-brain radiation therapy vs stereotactic radiosurgery alone for treatment of brain metastases. *JAMA* 295:2683, 2006.

Attiyeh EF, London WB, Mossé YP, et al: Chromosome 1p and 11q deletions and outcome in neuroblastoma. *N Engl J Med* 353:2243, 2005.

Aupérin A, Arrigada R, Pignon JP, et al: Prophylactic cranial irradiation for patients with small-cell lung cancer in complete remission. *N Engl J Med* 341:476, 1999.

Bailey P, Bucy PC: Oligodendrogliomas of the brain. *J Pathol Bacteriol* 32:735, 1929.

Bailey P, Cushing H: *A Classification of Tumors of the Glioma Group on a Histogenetic Basis with a Correlated Study of Prognosis*. Philadelphia, Lippincott, 1926.

Baloh RW, DeRossett SE, Cloughessy TF, et al: Novel brainstem syndrome associated with prostate carcinoma. *Neurology* 43:2591, 1993.

Barcos M, Lane W, Gomez GA, et al: An autopsy study of 1,206 acute and chronic leukemias (1958–1982). *Cancer* 60:827, 1987.

Barkovich AJ, Krischer J, Kun LE, et al: Brainstem gliomas: A classification system based on magnetic resonance imaging. *Pediatr Neurosurg* 16:73, 1993.

Bashir RM, Harris NL, Hochberg FH, Singer RM: Detection of Epstein-Barr virus in CNS lymphomas by in situ hybridization. *Neurology* 39:813, 1989.

Benton JW, Nellhaus G, Huttenlocher PR, et al: The bobble-head doll syndrome. *Neurology* 16:725, 1966.

Beristain X, Azzarelli B: The neurological masquerade of intravascular lymphomatosis. *Arch Neurol* 59:439, 2002.

Bigner DD, McLendon RE, Bruner JM (eds): *Russell and Rubinstein's Pathology of Tumors of the Nervous System*, 6th ed. London, Arnold, 1998.

Bingas B: Tumors of the base of the skull, in Vinken PJ, Bruyn GW (eds): *Handbook of Clinical Neurology*. Vol 17. Amsterdam, North-Holland, 1974, pp 136–233.

Boughey AM, Fletcher NA, Harding AE: Central nervous system hemangioblastoma: A clinical and genetic study of 52 cases. *J Neurol Neurosurg Psychiatry* 53:644, 1990.

Brougham M, Heusner AP, Adams RD: Acute degenerative changes in adenomas of the pituitary body—with special reference to pituitary apoplexy. *J Neurosurg* 7:421, 1950.

Cairncross JG, MacDonald DR: Chemotherapy for oligodendroglioma: Progress report. *Arch Neurol* 48:225, 1991.

Carvalho PA, Schwartz RB, Alexander E, et al: Detection of recurrent gliomas with quantitative thallium-201/technetium-99m HMPAO single-photon emission computerized tomography. *J Neurosurg* 77:565, 1992.

Cavin LW, Dalrymple GV, McGuire EL, et al: CNS tumor induction by radiotherapy: A report of four new cases and estimate of dose required. *Int J Radiat Oncol Biol Phys* 18:399, 1990.

Chang SD, Alder JR: Treatment of cranial base meningiomas with linear accelerator radiosurgery. *Neurosurgery* 41:1019, 1997.

Clouston PD, DeAngelis LM, Posner JB: The spectrum of neurological disease in patients with systemic cancer. *Ann Neurol* 31:268, 1992.

Cogan DG: Tumors of the optic nerve, in Vinken PJ, Bruyn GW (eds): *Handbook of Clinical Neurology*. Vol 17. Amsterdam, North-Holland, 1974, pp 350–374.

Colao A, Lombardi G: Growth-hormone and prolactin excess. *Lancet* 352:1455, 1998.

Corsellis JAN, Goldberg GJ, Norton AR: Limbic encephalitis and its association with carcinoma. *Brain* 91:481, 1968.

Cross SA, Salomano DR, Parisi JE, et al: Paraneoplastic autoimmune optic neuritis with retinitis defined by CRMP-5-IgG. *Ann Neurol* 54:38, 2003.

Cuneo RA, Caronna JJ, Pitts L, et al: Upward transtentorial herniation. Seven cases and literature review. *Ann Neurol* 36:618, 1979.

Cushing H: *Intracranial Tumors: Notes upon a Series of 2000 Verified Cases with Surgical-Mortality Percentages Pertaining Thereto*. Springfield, IL, Charles C Thomas, 1932.

Cushing H: Some experimental and clinical observations concerning states of increased intracranial tension. *Am J Med Sci* 124:375, 1902.

Cushing H: *The Pituitary Body and Its Diseases*. Philadelphia, Lippincott, 1912.

Cushing H: *Tumors of the Nervus Acousticus and Syndrome of the Cerebellopontine Angle*. Philadelphia, Saunders, 1917.

Cushing H, Eisenhardt L: *Meningiomas*. New York, Hafner, 1962.

Dalmau J, Gleichman AJ, Hughes EG, et al: Anti-NMDA-receptor encephalitis: Case series and analysis of the effects of antibodies. *Lancet Neurology* 7:1091, 2008.

Dalmau J, Graus F, Villarejo A, et al: Clinical analysis of anti-Ma1 associated encephalitis. *Brain* 127:1831, 2004.

Dalmau J, Rosenfeld MR: Paraneoplastic syndromes of the CNS. *Lancet Neurol* 7: 327, 2008.

Dalmau J, Tüzün E, Wu H, et al: Paraneoplastic anti-*N*-methyl-D-aspartate receptor encephalitis associated with ovarian teratoma. *Ann Neurol* 61:25, 2007.

Darnell RB, Posner JB: Paraneoplastic syndromes involving the nervous system. *N Engl J Med* 349:1543, 2003.

Daumas-Duport C, Scheithauer B, O'Fallon J, Kelly P: Grading of astrocytomas: A simple and reproducible method. *Cancer* 62:2152, 1988.

DeAngelis LM: Current management of primary central nervous system lymphoma. *Oncology* 9:63, 1995.

DeAngelis LM, Delattre J-Y, Posner JB: Radiation-induced dementia in patients cured of brain metastases. *Neurology* 39:789, 1989.

Delattre J-Y, Safai B, Posner JB: Erythema multiforme and Stevens Johnson syndrome in patients receiving cranial irradiation and phenytoin. *Neurology* 38:194, 1988.

Duffner PK, Cohen ME: Primitive neuroectodermal tumors, in Vecht CJ, Vinken PJ, Bruyn GW (eds): *Handbook of Clinical Neurology*. Vol 28. Amsterdam, Elsevier, 1997, pp 221–227.

Duffner PK, Cohen ME, Myers MH, Heise HW: Survival of children with brain tumors: SEER program, 1973–1980. *Neurology* 36:597, 1986.

Dunn J, Kernohan JW: Gliomatosis cerebri. *AMA Arch Pathol* 64:82, 1957.

Estrada J, Boronat M, Mielgo M, et al: The long-term outcome of pituitary irradiation after unsuccessful transsphenoidal surgery in Cushing's disease. *N Engl J Med* 336:172, 1997.

Fahlbusch R, Honegger J, Paulis W, et al: Surgical treatment of craniopharyngiomas: Experience with 168 patients. *J Neurosurg* 90:237, 1999.

Feigenbaum L, Ueda H, Jay G: Viral etiology of neurological malignancies in transgenic mice, in Levine AJ, Schmidek HH (eds): *Molecular Genetics of Nervous System Tumors*. New York, Wiley-Liss, 1993, pp 153–161.

Fishman RA: *Cerebrospinal Fluid in Diseases of the Nervous System*, 2nd ed. Philadelphia, Saunders, 1992.

Flanagan EP, McKeon A, Lennon VA, et al: Paraneoplastic isolated myelopathy. Clinical course and neuroimaging. *Neurology* 76:2089, 2011.

Flickinger JC, Kondziolka D, Niranjan A, et al: Results of acoustic neuroma radiosurgery: An analysis of 5 years' experience using current methods. *Neurosurgery* 94:1, 2001.

Fokes EC Jr, Earle KM: Ependymomas: Clinical and pathological aspects. *J Neurosurg* 30:585, 1969.

Folli F, Solimena M, Cofiell R, et al: Autoantibodies to a 128-kD synaptic protein in three women with the stiff-man syndrome and breast cancer. *N Engl J Med* 328:546, 1993.

Forsyth PA, Dalmau J, Graus F, et al: Motor neuron syndromes in cancer patients. *Ann Neurol* 41:722, 1997.

Fox JL, Al-Mefty O: Suprasellar arachnoid cysts: An extension of the membrane of Liliequist. *Neurosurgery* 7:615, 1980.

Friede RL, Janzer RC, Roessmann U: Infantile small-cell gliomas. *Acta Neuropathol* 57:103, 1982.

Gandy SE, Heier LA: Clinical and magnetic resonance features of primary intracranial arachnoid cysts. *Ann Neurol* 21:342, 1987.

Gardner G, Cocke EW Jr, Robertson JT, et al: Combined approach surgery for removal of glomus jugulare tumors. *Laryngoscope* 87:665, 1977.

Glantz MJ, Cole BF, Friedberg MH, et al: A randomized, blinded, placebo-controlled trial of divalproex sodium in adults with newly discovered brain tumors. *Neurology* 46:985, 1996.

Glantz MJ, Hoffman JM, Coleman RE, et al: Identification of early recurrence of primary central nervous system tumors by [18F] fluorodeoxyglucose positron emission tomography. *Ann Neurol* 29:347, 1991.

Glass J, Gruber ML, Cher L, Hochberg FH: Preirradiation methotrexate chemotherapy of primary central nervous system lymphoma: Long-term outcome. *J Neurosurg* 81:188, 1994.

Glass J, Hochberg FH, Tultar DC: Intravascular lymphomatosis. A systemic disease with neurologic manifestations. *Cancer* 71:3156, 1993.

Glioma Meta-analysis Trialists (GMT) Group: Chemotherapy in adult high-grade glioma: A systematic review and meta-analysis of individual patient data from 12 randomised trials. *Lancet* 359:1015, 2002.

Globus JH, Silbert S: Pinealomas. *Arch Neurol Psychiatry* 25:937, 1931.

Gorson KC, Musaphir S, Lathi ES, Wolfe G: Radiation-induced malignant fibrous histiocytoma of the brachial plexus. *J Neurooncol* 26:73, 1995.

Graus F, Keime-Guibert F, Rene R, et al: Anti-Hu-associated paraneoplastic encephalomyelitis: Analysis of 200 patients. *Brain* 124:1138, 2001.

Guinee D Jr, Jaffe E, Kingma D, et al: Pulmonary lymphomatoid granulomatosis. *Am J Surg Pathol* 18:753, 1994.

Gultekin SH, Rosenfeld MR, Voltz R, et al: Paraneoplastic limbic encephalitis: Neurologic symptoms, immunological findings and tumor association in 50 patients. *Brain* 123:1481, 2000.

Hakuba A, Hashi K, Fujitani K, et al: Jugular foramen neurinomas. *Surg Neurol* 11:83, 1979.

Hammack JE, Kimmel DW, O'Neill BP, et al: Paraneoplastic cerebellar degeneration: A clinical comparison of patients with and without Purkinje cell antibodies. *Mayo Clin Proc* 65:1423, 1990.

Harner SG, Laws ER: Clinical findings in patients with acoustic neurinoma. *Mayo Clin Proc* 58:721, 1983.

Hart MN, Earle KM: Primitive neuroectodermal tumors of children. *Cancer* 32:890, 1973.

Hegi ME, Diserens A, Gorlia T, et al: MGMT gene silencing and benefit from temozolomide in glioblastoma. *N Engl J Med* 352:997, 2005.

Henson RA, Urich H: *Cancer and the Nervous System*. Oxford, England, Blackwell, 1982.

Hochberg FH, Miller DC: Primary central nervous system lymphoma. *J Neurosurg* 68:835, 1988.

House WF, Hitselberger WE: Acoustic tumors, in Vinken PJ, Bruyn GW (eds): *Handbook of Clinical Neurology*. Vol 17. Amsterdam, North-Holland, 1974, pp 666–692.

Jacobson DM, Thirkill CE, Tipping SJ: A clinical triad to diagnose paraneoplastic retinopathy. *Ann Neurol* 28:162, 1990.

Jakola AS, Myrmel KS, Kloster R, et al: Comparison of a strategy favoring early surgical resection vs a strategy favoring watchful waiting in low-grade glioma. *JAMA* 308:1881, 2011.

Jefferson G: The tentorial pressure cone. *Arch Neurol Psychiatry* 40:837, 1938.

Kaplan JG, DeSouza TG, Farkash A, et al: Leptomeningeal metastases: Comparison of clinical features and laboratory data of solid tumors, lymphoma, and leukemias. *J Neurooncol* 9:225, 1990.

Katzenstein AA, Carrington CB, Liebow AA: Lymphomatoid granulomatosis. A clinicopathologic study of 12 cases. *Cancer* 43:360, 1979.

Kaufman B, Tomsak RL, Kaufman BA, et al: Herniation of the suprasellar visual system and third ventricle into empty sellae: Morphologic and clinical considerations. *AJR Am J Roentgenol* 152:597, 1989.

Kaye AH, Laws ER: *Brain Tumors. An Encyclopedic Approach*, 2nd ed. London, Churchill Livingstone, 2001.

Keime-Guibert F, Chinot O, Taillandier L, et al: Radiotherapy for glioblastoma in the elderly. *N Engl J Med* 356:1527, 2007.

Kendall BE, Lee BCP: Cranial chordomas. *Br J Radiol* 50:687, 1977.

Kennedy HB, Smith RJ: Eye signs in craniopharyngioma. *Br J Ophthalmol* 59:689, 1975.

Kepes JJ: *Meningiomas: Biology, Pathology, and Differential Diagnosis*. New York, Masson, 1982.

Kernohan JW, Sayre GP: Tumors of the central nervous system: Fasc 35, in *Atlas of Tumor Pathology*. Washington, DC, Armed Forces Institute of Pathology, 1952.

Kernohan JW, Uihlein A: *Sarcomas of the Brain*. Springfield, IL, Charles C Thomas, 1962.

Kernohan JW, Woltman HW: Incisura of the crus due to contralateral brain tumor. *Arch Neurol Psychiatry* 21:274, 1929.

Khalili K, Krynska B, Del Valle L, et al: Medulloblastomas and the human neurotropic polyomavirus JC virus. *Lancet* 353:1152, 1999.

Klatzo I: Neuropathological aspects of brain edema. *J Neuropathol Exp Neurol* 26:1, 1967.

Klibanski A, Zervas NT: Diagnosis and management of hormone-secreting pituitary adenomas. *N Engl J Med* 324:822, 1991.

Kliman B, Kjellberg RN, Swisher B, Butler W: Proton beam therapy of acromegaly: A 20-year experience, in Black PM (ed): *Secretory Tumors of the Pituitary Gland*. New York, Raven Press, 1984, pp 191–211.

Kondziolka D, Lunsford D, McLaughlin MR, Flickinger JC: Long-term outcomes after radiosurgery for acoustic neuroma. *N Engl J Med* 339:1426, 1998.

Kovacs K, Asa SL: *Functional Endocrine Pathology*. Boston, Blackwell Scientific, 1991.

Kramer W: Glomus jugulare tumors, in Vinken PJ, Bruyn GW (eds): *Handbook of Clinical Neurology*. Vol 18. Amsterdam, North-Holland, 1975, pp 435–455.

Kruger DA, Case MM, Holland K, et al: Everolimus for subependymal giant-cell astrocytomas, *N Engl J Med* 363:1801, 2010.

Lai R, Rosenblum MK, DeAngelis LM: Primary CNS lymphoma. A whole brain disease? *Neurology* 59:1557, 2002.

Lamberts SWJ: The role of somatostatin in the regulation of anterior pituitary hormone secretion and the use of its analogs in the treatment of human pituitary tumors. *Endocr Rev* 9:417, 1988.

Lamszus K: Meningoma pathology, genetics, and biology. *J Neuropathol Exp Neurol* 63:275, 2004.

Lancaster E, Martinez-Hernandez E, Titulaer MJ, et al: Antibodies to metabotropic glutamate receptors in the Ophelia syndrome. *Neurology* 77:1698, 2011.

Landolfi JC, Thaler HT, DeAngelis LM: Adult brainstem gliomas. *Neurology* 51:1136, 1998.

Laurence KM, Hoare RD, Till K: The diagnosis of choroid plexus papilloma of the lateral ventricle. *Brain* 84:628, 1961.

Leibel SA, Scott CB, Loeffler JS: Contemporary approaches to the treatment of malignant gliomas with radiation therapy. *Semin Oncol* 21:198, 1994.

Levin VA, Edwards MS, Wright DC, et al: Modified procarbazine, CCNU, and vincristine (PCV 3) combination chemotherapy in the treatment of malignant brain tumors. *Cancer Treat Rep* 64:237, 1980.

Levine AJ: Tumor suppressor genes, in Levine AJ, Schmidek HH (eds): *Molecular Genetics of Nervous System Tumors*. New York, Wiley-Liss, 1993, pp 137–143.

Levine AJ: The oncogenes of the DNA tumor viruses, in Levine AJ, Schmidek HH (eds): *Molecular Genetics of Nervous System Tumors*. New York, Wiley-Liss, 1993, pp 145–151.

Levitt LJ, Dawson DM, Rosenthal DS, Moloney WC: CNS involvement in the non-Hodgkin's lymphomas. *Cancer* 45:545, 1980.

Li C-Y, Witzig TE, Phyliky RL, et al: Diagnosis of B-cell non-Hodgkin's lymphoma of the central nervous system by immunocytochemical analysis of cerebrospinal fluid lymphocytes. *Cancer* 57:737, 1986.

Liebow AA, Carrington CR, Friedman PJ: Lymphomatoid granulomatosis. *Hum Pathol* 3:457, 1972.

Liubinas SV, Maartens N, Drummond KJ: Primary melanocytic neoplasms of the central nervous system. *J Clin Neurosci* 17:1227, 2010.

Lobosky JM, Vangilder JC, Damasio AR: Behavioural manifestations of third ventricular colloid cysts. *J Neurol Neurosurg Psychiatry* 47:1075, 1984.

Lopes MBS, Vandenberg SR, Scheithauer BW: The World Health Organization classification of nervous system tumors in experimental neurooncology, in Levine AJ, Schmidek HH (eds): *Molecular Genetics of Nervous System Tumors*. New York, Wiley-Liss, 1993, pp 1–36.

Louis DN, Ohgakin, Wiestler DD, et al: The 2007 WHO classification of tumors of the central nervous system. *Acta Neuropathol* 114:97, 2007.

Louis DN, Pomeroy SL, Cairncross JG: Focus on central nervous system neoplasia. *Cancer Cell* 1:125, 2002.

Ludwig CL, Smith MT, Godfrey AD, Armbrustmacher VW: A clinicopathological study of 323 patients with oligodendrogliomas. *Ann Neurol* 19:15, 1986.

Luque FA, Furneaux HM, Ferziger R, et al: Anti-Ri: An antibody associated with paraneoplastic opsoclonus and breast cancer. *Ann Neurol* 29:241, 1991.

MacCabe JJ: Glioblastoma, in Vinken PJ, Bruyn GW (eds): *Handbook of Clinical Neurology*. Vol 18. Amsterdam, North-Holland, 1975, pp 49–71.

MacCollin M, Willett C, Heinrich B, et al: Familial schwannomatosis: Exclusion of the NF-2 locus as the germline event. *Neurology* 60:1968, 2003.

Mancall EL, Rosales RK: Necrotizing myelopathy associated with visceral carcinoma. *Brain* 87:639, 1964.

Martuza RL, Ojemann RG: Bilateral acoustic neuromas: Clinical aspects, pathogenesis and treatment. *Neurosurgery* 10:1, 1982.

Matson DD, Crofton FDL: Papilloma of choroid plexus in childhood. *J Neurosurg* 17:1002, 1960.

Maris JM: Recent advances in neuroblastoma. *N Engl J Med* 302:2202, 2010.

Melmed S: Acromegaly. *N Engl J Med* 355:2558, 2006.

Mellinghoff IK, Wang WY, Vivanco I, et al. Molecular determinants of the response of glioblastomas to EGFR kinase inhibitors. *N Engl J Med* 353:2012, 2005.

Meyer A: Herniation of the brain. *Arch Neurol Psychiatry* 4:387, 1920.

Meyer FB, Ebersold MJ, Reese DF: Benign tumors of the foramen magnum. *J Neurosurg* 61:136, 1984.

Morita A, Meyer FB, Laws ER: Symptomatic pituitary metastases. *J Neurosurg* 89:69, 1998.

Morita A, Piepgras DG: Tumors of the base of the skull, in Vinken PJ, Bruyn GW, Vecht C (eds): *Handbook of Clinical Neurology*. Vol 68. Amsterdam, Elsevier 1997, pp 465–496.

Mørk SJ, Løken AC: Ependymoma—a follow-up study of 101 cases. *Cancer* 40:907, 1977.

Nevin S: Gliomatosis cerebri. *Brain* 61:170, 1938.

Ojemann RG, Montgomery W, Weiss L: Evaluation and surgical treatment of acoustic neuroma. *N Engl J Med* 287:895, 1972.

Olivecrona H: The surgical treatment of intracranial tumors, in Olivecrona H, Tonnis W (eds): *Handbuch der Neurochirurgie*. Vol IV. Berlin, Springer-Verlag, 1967, pp 1–300.

O'Neill BP, Buckner JC, Coffey RJ, et al: Brain metastatic lesions. *Mayo Clin Proc* 69:1062, 1994.

Osborne RH, Houlsen MP, Tijssen CC, et al: The genetic epidemiology of glioma. *Neurology* 57:1751, 2001.

Packer RJ: Chemotherapy for medulloblastoma/primitive neuroectodermal tumors of the posterior fossa. *Ann Neurol* 28:823, 1990.

Paone JF, Jeyasingham K: Remission of cerebellar dysfunction after pneumonectomy for bronchogenic carcinoma. *N Engl J Med* 302:156, 1980.

Pappas CTE, White WL, Baldree ME: Pituitary tumors: Anatomy, microsurgery, and management. *Barrow Neurol Inst Q* 6:2, 1990.

Partap S, Walker M, Longstreth WT, Spence AM: Prolonged but reversible migraine-like episodes long after cranial irradiation. *Neurology* 66:1105, 2006.

Patchell RA, Tibbs PA, Walsh JW, et al: A randomized trial of surgery in the treatment of single metastases to the brain. *N Engl J Med* 322:494, 1990.

Pencalet P, Maixner W, Sainte-Rose C, et al: Benign cerebellar astrocytoma in children. *J Neurosurg* 90:265, 1999.

Peterson K, DeAngelis LM: Weighing the benefits and risks of radiation therapy for low-grade glioma. *Neurology* 56:1225, 2001.

Peterson K, Rosenblum MK, Katanider H, Posner JB: Paraneoplastic cerebellar degeneration: I. A clinical analysis of anti-Yo antibody-positive patients. *Neurology* 42:1931, 1992.

Peterson K, Walker RW: Medulloblastoma/primitive neuroectodermal tumor in 45 adults. *Neurology* 45:440, 1995.

Pittock SJ, Kryzer TJ, Lennon VA: Paraneoplastic antibodies coexist and predict cancer, not neurological syndrome. *Ann Neurol* 56:715, 2004.

Plotkin SR, Stermer-Rachaminov AO, Barker FG, et al: Hearing improvement after bevicizumab in patients with neurofibromatosis type 2. *N Engl J Med* 361:358, 2009.

Pollack IF, Hoffman HJ, Humphreys RP, et al: The long-term outcome after surgical resection of dorsally exophytic brain-stem gliomas. *J Neurosurg* 78:859, 1993.

Pollock BE, Huston J: Natural history of asymptomatic colloid cysts of the third ventricle. *J Neurosurg* 91:364, 1999.

Polmeteer FE, Kernohan JW: Meningeal gliomatosis. *Arch Neurol Psychiatry* 57:593, 1947.

Pomeroy SL, Tamayo P, Gassenbeek M, et al: Prediction of central nervous system embryonal tumour outcome based on gene expression. *Nature* 415:436, 2002.

Posner J, Chernik NL: Intracranial metastases from systemic cancer. *Adv Neurol* 19:575, 1978.

Posner JB: Primary lymphoma of the CNS. *Neurol Alert* 5:21, 1987.

Posner JB, Saper CF, Schiff ND, Plum F: *Plum and Posner's Diagnosis of Stupor and Coma*. New York, Oxford University Press, 2007.

Price RA, Johnson WW: The central nervous system in childhood leukemia: I. The arachnoid. *Cancer* 31:520, 1973.

Pruitt A, Dalmau J, Detre J, et al: Episodic neurologic dysfunction with migraine and reversible imaging findings after radiation. *Neurology* 67:676, 2006.

Pui CH, Campano D, Pei D, et al: Treating childhood acute lymphoblastic leukemia without cranial irradiation. *N Engl J Med* 360:2730, 2009.

Reid T, Hedegus B, Wechsler-Reya R, Gutman DH: The neurobiology of neurooncology. *Ann Neurol* 60:3, 2006.

Reifenberger G, Louis DN: Oligodendroglioma: Toward molecular definitions in diagnostic neuro-oncology. *J Neuropathol Exp Neurol* 62:111, 2003.

Ribbert H: *Geschwulstlehre*. Bonn, Verlag Cohen, 1904.

Ringertz N: Grading system of gliomas. *Acta Pathol Microbiol Scand* 27:51, 1950.

Robain O, Dulac O, Dommergues JP, et al: Necrotising leukoencephalopathy complicating treatment of childhood leukaemia. *J Neurol Neurosurg Psychiatry* 47:65, 1984.

Ropper AH: Hyperosmolar therapy for raised intracranial pressure. *N Engl J Med* 367:746, 2012.

Rosenberg GA, Saland L, Kyner WT: Pathophysiology of periventricular tissue changes with raised CSF pressure in cats. *J Neurosurg* 59:606, 1983.

Rubinstein AB, Shalit MN, Cohen ML, et al: Radiation-induced cerebral meningioma: A recognizable entity. *J Neurosurg* 61:966, 1984.

Rubinstein LJ: Embryonal central neuroepithelial tumors and their differentiating potential. *J Neurosurg* 62:795, 1985.

Rubinstein LJ: Tumors of the central nervous system: Fasc 6, 2nd series, in *Atlas of Tumor Pathology*. Washington, DC, Armed Forces Institute of Pathology, 1972.

Rudin CM, Hann CL, Laterra J, et al: Treatment of medulloblastoma with hedgehog inhibitor GDC-0449. *N Engl J Med* 361:1173, 2009.

Russell DS: Cellular changes and patterns of neoplasia, in Haymaker W, Adams RD (eds): *Histology and Histopathology of the Nervous System*. Springfield, IL, Charles C Thomas, 1982, pp 1493–1515.

Rutkowski S, Bode U, Deinlein F, et al: Treatment of early childhood medulloblastoma by postoperative chemotherapy alone. *N Engl J Med* 352:978, 2005.

Sanai N, Alvarez-Buylla A, Berger MS: Neural stem cells and the origin of gliomas. *N Engl J Med* 353:811, 2005.

Schmidek HH: Some current concepts regarding medulloblastomas, in Levine AJ, Schmidek HH (eds): *Molecular Genetics of Nervous System Tumors*. New York, Wiley-Liss, 1993, pp 283–286.

Schold SC, Cho E-S, Somasundaram M, Posner JB: Subacute motor neuronopathy: A remote effect of lymphoma. *Ann Neurol* 5:271, 1979.

Seizinger BR, Roulean GA, Ozelius LJ, et al: Von Hippel–Lindau disease maps to the region of chromosome 3 associated with renal carcinoma. *Nature* 332:268, 1988.

Shapiro WR: Therapy of adult malignant brain tumors: What have the clinical trials taught us? *Semin Oncol* 13:38, 1986.

Shaw EG, Daumas-Duport C, Scheithauer BS, et al: Radiation therapy in the management of low-grade supratentorial astrocytomas. *J Neurosurg* 70:853, 1989.

Sheibani K, Battifora H, Winberg CD, et al: Further evidence that "malignant angioendotheliomatosis" is an angiotropic large-cell lymphoma. *N Engl J Med* 314:943, 1986.

Slotman B, Faivre-Finn C, Kramer G, et al: Prophylactic cranial irradiation in extensive small-cell lung cancer. *N Engl J Med* 357:664, 2007.

Smitt PS, Kinoshita A, Leeuw B, et al: Paraneoplastic cerebellar ataxia due to autoantibodies against a glutamate receptor. *N Engl J Med* 342:21, 2000.

Söderberg-Nauclér C, Rahbar A, Stragliotto G: Survival in patients with glioblastoma receiving valgangciclovir. *N Engl J Med* 369:985, 2013.

Sorenson SC, Eagan RT, Scott M: Meningeal carcinomatosis in patients with primary breast or lung cancer. *Mayo Clin Proc* 59:91, 1984.

Sparling HJ, Adams RD, Parker F: Involvement of the nervous system by malignant lymphoma. *Medicine* 26:285, 1947.

Stupp R, Mason W, van den Bent M, et al: Radiotherapy plus concomitant and adjuvant temozolomide for glioblastoma. *N Engl J Med* 352:987, 2005.

Tomlinson BE, Perry RH, Stewart-Wynne EG: Influence of site of origin of lung carcinomas on clinical presentation and central nervous system metastases. *J Neurol Neurosurg Psychiatry* 42:82, 1979.

Ulmer S, Braga TA, Barker FG, et al: Clinical and radiographic features of peritumoral infarction following resection of glioblastoma. *Neurology* 67:1688, 2006.

van den Bent MJ, Afra D, de Witte O, et al: Long-term efficacy of early versus delayed radiotherapy for low-grade astrocytoma and oligodendroglioma in adults: the EORTC 22845 randomised trial. *Lancet* 366:985, 2005.

Verma A, Berger JR, Snodgrass S, Petito C: Motor neuron disease: A paraneoplastic process associated with anti-Hu antibody and small-cell lung carcinoma. *Ann Neurol* 40:112, 1996.

Vincent A, Buckley C, Schott JM, et al: Potassium channel antibody-associated encephalopathy: A potentially immunotherapy-responsive form of limbic encephalitis. *Brain* 127:701, 2004.

Vitaliani R, Mason W, Ances B, et al: Paraneoplastic encephalitis, psychiatric symptoms, and hypoventilation in ovarian teratoma. *Ann Neurol* 58:594, 2005.

Voltz R, Gultekin SH, Rosenfeld MR, et al: A serologic marker of paraneoplastic limbic and brain-stem encephalitis in patients with testicular cancer. *N Engl J Med* 340:1788, 1999.

Waga S, Morikawa A, Sakakura M: Craniopharyngioma with midbrain involvement. *Arch Neurol* 36:319, 1979.

Wasserstrom WR, Glass JP, Posner JB: Diagnosis and treatment of leptomeningeal metastases from solid tumors: Experience with 90 patients. *Cancer* 49:759, 1982.

Weiss HD, Richardson EP: Solitary brainstem metastasis. *Neurology* 28:562, 1978.

Wick W, Meisner C, Hentschl B, et al: Prognostic or predictive value of MGMT promoter methylation in gliomas depends on IDH1 mutation. *Neurology* 81:1515, 2013.

Yan H, Parsons DW, Jin, GJ, et al: IDH1 and IDH2 mutations in gliomas. *N Engl J Med* 360:765, 2009.

Yu Z, Kryzer TJ, Griesmann GE, et al: CRMP-5 neuronal antibody: Marker of lung cancer and thymoma-related autoimmunity. *Ann Neurol* 49:164, 2001.

Yung WA, Horten BC, Shapiro WR: Meningeal gliomatosis: A review of 12 cases. *Ann Neurol* 8:605, 1980.

Zentner J, Wolf HK, Ostertun B, et al: Gangliogliomas: Clinical, radiological, and histopathological findings in 51 patients. *J Neurol Neurosurg Psychiatry* 57:1497, 1994.

Zimmerman HM: Brain tumors: Their incidence and classification in man and their experimental production. *Ann N Y Acad Sci* 159:337, 1969.

Zülch KJ: *Brain Tumors, Their Biology and Pathology*, 3rd ed. New York, Springer-Verlag, 1986.

32

Infections of the Nervous System (Bacterial, Fungal, Spirochetal, Parasitic) and Sarcoidosis

This chapter is concerned mainly with bacterial infections of the central nervous system (CNS), particularly bacterial meningitis, septic thrombophlebitis, brain abscess, epidural abscess, and subdural empyema. The granulomatous infections of the CNS, notably tuberculosis, syphilis and other spirochetal infections, and certain fungal infections are also discussed in some detail. In addition, consideration is given to sarcoidosis, a granulomatous disease of uncertain etiology, and to the CNS infections and infestations caused by certain rickettsias, protozoa, worms, and ticks.

A number of other important infectious diseases of the nervous system are discussed elsewhere in this book. Viral infections, because of their frequency and importance, are allotted a chapter of their own (see Chap. 33). Diseases caused by bacterial exotoxins—diphtheria, tetanus, botulism—are considered with other toxins that affect the nervous system (see Chap. 43). Leprosy, which is essentially a disease of the peripheral nerves, is described in Chap. 46, and trichinosis, mainly a disease of muscle, in Chap. 48.

BACTERIAL INFECTIONS OF THE CENTRAL NERVOUS SYSTEM

These infections reach the intracranial structures by one of two pathways, either by hematogenous spread (emboli of bacteria or infected thrombi) or by extension from cranial structures adjacent to the brain (ears, paranasal sinuses, osteomyelitic foci in the skull, penetrating cranial or congenital sinus tracts). In a number of cases, infection is iatrogenic, being introduced in the course of cerebral or spinal surgery, the placement of a ventriculoperitoneal shunt or, rarely, by a lumbar puncture needle. Increasingly, craniospinal infections are nosocomial, i.e., acquired in-hospital; in urban hospitals, nosocomial meningitis is now as frequent as the non–hospital-acquired variety (Durand et al).

Surprisingly little is known about the mechanisms of hematogenous spread and animal experiments involving the injection of virulent bacteria into the bloodstream have yielded somewhat contradictory results. In most instances of bacteremia or septicemia, the nervous system seems not to be infected; yet sometimes a bacteremia caused by pneumonia or endocarditis is the only apparent predecessor to meningitis. With respect to the formation of brain abscess, cerebral tissue has a notable resistance to infection. Direct injection of virulent bacteria into the brain of an animal seldom results in abscess formation. In fact, this condition has been produced consistently only by injecting culture medium along with the bacteria or by causing necrosis of the tissue at the time bacteria are inoculated. In humans, infarction of brain tissue because of arterial occlusion (thrombosis or embolism) or venous occlusion (thrombophlebitis) appears to be a common and perhaps necessary antecedent by way of causing of a necrotic nidus.

The mechanism of meningitis and brain abscess from infection of the middle ear and paranasal sinuses is easier to understand. The cranial epidural and subdural spaces are practically never the sites of blood-borne infections, in contrast to the spinal epidural space, where such infections are either hemtogenous spread but can be from contiguous osteomyelitis. Furthermore, the cranial bones and the dura mater (which essentially constitutes the inner periosteum of the skull) protect the cranial cavity against the ingress of bacteria. This protective mechanism may fail if suppuration occurs in the middle ear, mastoid cells, or frontal, ethmoid, and sphenoid sinuses. Two pathways from these sources have been demonstrated: (1) infected thrombi may form in diploic veins and spread along these vessels into the dural sinuses (into which the diploic veins flow), and from there, in retrograde fashion, along the meningeal veins into the brain, and (2) an osteomyelitic focus may erode the inner table of bone and invade of the dura, subdural space, pia-arachnoid, and even brain. Each of these pathways has been observed by the authors in some fatal cases of epidural abscess, subdural empyema, meningitis, cranial venous sinusitis and meningeal thrombophlebitis, and brain abscess. However, in many cases coming to autopsy, the pathway of infection cannot be determined.

With a hematogenous infection in the course of a bacteremia, usually a single type of virulent bacterium gains entry to the cranial cavity. In the adult the most common pathogenic organisms are pneumococcus (*Streptococcus pneumoniae*), meningococcus (*Neisseria meningitidis*), *Haemophilus influenzae* in unvaccinated children, *Listeria monocytogenes*, and staphylococcus; in the neonate, *Escherichia coli* and group B streptococcus; in the infant and unvaccinated child, *H. influenzae*. By contrast, when septic material embolizes from infected lungs, pulmonary arteriovenous fistulas, or congenital heart lesions, or extends directly from ears or sinuses, more than one type of bacterial flora common to these sources may be transmitted. Such "mixed infections" pose difficult problems in therapy. Occasionally in these latter conditions, the demonstration of the causative organisms may be unsuccessful, even from the pus of an abscess (mainly because of inadequate culturing techniques for anaerobic organisms and the prior use of antibiotics). Infections that follow neurosurgery or the insertion of a cranial appliance are usually staphylococcal; a small number are a result of mixed flora, including anaerobic ones, or one of the enteric organisms. In determining the most likely invading organism, the age of the patient, the clinical setting of the infection (community-acquired, postsurgical, or nosocomial), the immune status of the patient, and evidence of systemic and local cranial disease all must be taken into account.

ACUTE BACTERIAL MENINGITIS (LEPTOMENINGITIS)

The Biology of Bacterial Meningitis

The immediate effect of bacteria or other microorganisms in the subarachnoid space is to cause an inflammatory reaction in the pia and arachnoid as well as in the cerebrospinal fluid (CSF). Because the subarachnoid space is continuous around the brain, spinal cord, and optic nerves, an infective agent gaining entry to any one part of the space allows it to spread rapidly to all of it, even its most remote recesses; in other words, meningitis is always cerebrospinal. Infection also reaches the ventricles, either directly from the choroid plexuses or by reflux through the foramina of Magendie and Luschka.

The first reaction to bacteria or their toxins is hyperemia of the meningeal venules and capillaries and an increased permeability of these vessels, followed shortly by exudation of protein and the migration of neutrophils into the pia and subarachnoid space. The subarachnoid exudate increases rapidly, particularly over the base of the brain; it extends into the sheaths of cranial and spinal nerves and, for a very short distance, into the perivascular spaces of the cortex. During the first few days, mature and immature neutrophils, many of them containing phagocytosed bacteria, are the predominant cells. Within a few days, lymphocytes and histiocytes increase gradually in numbers. During this time, there is exudation of fibrinogen, which is converted to fibrin after a few days. In the latter part of the second week, plasma cells appear and subsequently increase in number. At about the same time the cellular exudate becomes organized into two layers—an outer one, just beneath the arachnoid membrane, made up of neutrophils and fibrin, and an inner one, next to the pia, composed largely of lymphocytes, plasma cells, and mononuclear cells or macrophages. Although fibroblasts of the meninges begin to proliferate early, they are not conspicuous until later, when they take part in the organization of the exudate, resulting in fibrosis of the arachnoid and loculation of pockets of exudate.

During the process of resolution, the inflammatory cells disappear in almost the reverse order as they had appeared. Neutrophils begin to disintegrate by the fourth to fifth day, and soon thereafter, with treatment, no new ones appear. Lymphocytes, plasma cells, and macrophages disappear more slowly, and a few lymphocytes and mononuclear cells may remain in small numbers for several months. The completeness of resolution depends on the stage at which the infection is arrested. If it is controlled in the very early stages, there may not be any residual change in the arachnoid; following an infection of several weeks' duration, there is a permanent fibrous overgrowth of the meninges, resulting in a thickened, cloudy, or opaque arachnoid and often in adhesions between the pia and arachnoid and even between the arachnoid and dura.

From the earliest stages of meningitis, changes are also found in the small and medium-sized subarachnoid arteries. The endothelial cells swell, multiply, and crowd into the lumen. This reaction appears within 48 to 72 h and increases in the days that follow. The adventitial connective tissue sheath becomes infiltrated by neutrophils. Foci of necrosis of the arterial wall sometimes occur. Neutrophils and lymphocytes migrate from the adventitia to the subintimal region, often forming a conspicuous layer. Later there is subintimal fibrosis. This is a striking feature of nearly all types of subacute and chronic infections of the meninges but most notably of tuberculous and syphilitic meningitis (Heubner arteritis). In the veins, swelling of the endothelial cells and infiltration of the adventitia also occur. Subintimal layering, as occurs in arterioles, is not observed, but there may be a diffuse infiltration of the entire wall of the vessel. It is in veins so affected that focal necrosis of the vessel wall and mural thrombi are most often found. Cortical thrombophlebitis of the larger veins does not usually develop before the end of the second week of the infection.

The unusual prominence of the vascular changes may be related to their anatomic peculiarities. The adventitia of the subarachnoid vessels, both of arterioles and venules, is actually formed by an investment of the arachnoid membrane, which is invariably involved by the infectious process. Thus, in a sense, the outer vessel wall is affected from the beginning by the inflammatory process—an infectious vasculitis. The much more frequent occurrence of thrombosis in veins than in arteries is probably accounted for by the thinner walls and the slower current of blood flow in the former.

Although the spinal and cranial nerves are surrounded by purulent exudate from the beginning of the infection, the perineurial sheaths become infiltrated by inflammatory cells only after several days. Exceptionally, there is infiltration of the endoneurium and degeneration of myelinated fibers, leading to the appearance of fatty macrophages and proliferation of Schwann cells and fibroblasts. More often, there is little or no damage to nerve fibers. Occasionally cellular infiltrations may be found in the optic nerves or olfactory bulbs.

The arachnoid membrane tends to serve as an effective barrier to the spread of infection into the adjacent subdural compartment, but some secondary reaction in this space may occur nevertheless (subdural effusion). This happens far more often in infants than in adults; according to Snedeker and coworkers, approximately 40 percent of infants with meningitis younger than 18 months of age develop subdural effusions. As a rule, there is no subdural pus, only a sterile yellowish exudate. In an even higher percentage of cases, small amounts of fibrinous exudate are found in microscopic sections that include the spinal dura.

In the early stages of meningitis, very little change in the substance of the brain can be detected. Neutrophils appear in the Virchow-Robin perivascular spaces but enter the brain only if there is necrosis. After several days, microglia and astrocytes increase in number, at first in the outer zone and later in all layers of the cortex. The associated nerve cell changes may be very slight. Obviously some disorder of the cortical neurons must take place from the beginning of the infection to account for the stupor, coma, and convulsions that are sometimes observed, but several days must elapse before any change can be demonstrated microscopically. It is uncertain whether these cortical changes are a result of the diffusion of toxins from the meninges, of a circulatory disturbance, or of some other factor, such as increased intracranial pressure or cortical venous thrombosis. The aforementioned changes are not because of invasion of brain substance by bacteria and should therefore be regarded as a noninfectious encephalopathy. When macrophages are exposed to endotoxins, they synthesize and release cytokines, among which are interleukin-1 and tumor necrosis factor. These cytokines are believed to stimulate and modulate the local immune response but may also affect neurons.

There is also little change initially in the ependyma and the subependymal tissues; but in later stages of meningitis, conspicuous changes are invariably found. The most prominent finding is infiltration of the subependymal perivascular spaces and often of the adjacent brain tissue with neutrophilic leukocytes and later with lymphocytes and plasma cells. Microglia and astrocytes proliferate, the latter sometimes overgrowing and burying remnants of the ependymal lining. The bacteria may pass through the ependymal lining and set up this inflammatory reaction in part because this sequence of events is favored by a developing hydrocephalus, which stretches and breaks the ependymal lining. Collections of subependymal astrocytes then begin to protrude into the ventricle, giving rise to a granular ependymitis, which, if prominent, may narrow and obstruct the aqueduct of Sylvius. As any meningitis becomes more chronic, the pia-arachnoid exudate tends to accumulate around the base of the brain (basilar meningitis), obstructing the flow of CSF and giving rise to *hydrocephalus*. In a survey of community-acquired bacterial meningitis, hydrocephalus occurred in only 5 percent, but it was associated with poor outcome (Kasanmoentalib et al).

The reader may question this digression into matters that are more pathologic than clinical, but knowledge of the morphologic features of meningitis enables one to understand the clinical state and its sequelae. The meningeal and ependymal reactions to bacterial infection and the clinical correlates of these reactions are summarized in Table 32-1.

Table 32-1

PATHOLOGIC-CLINICAL CORRELATIONS IN ACUTE, SUBACUTE, AND CHRONIC MENINGEAL REACTIONS

I. In acute meningeal inflammation:
   A. *Pure pia-arachnoiditis:* headache, stiff neck, Kernig and Brudzinski signs.
   B. *Subpial encephalopathy:* confusion, stupor, coma, and convulsions. Cerebral infarction because of cortical vein thrombosis may underlie these symptoms in some cases.
   C. *Inflammatory or vascular involvement of cranial nerve roots:* ocular palsies, facial weakness, and deafness are the main signs. Deafness may also be caused by middle ear infection, by extension of meningeal infection to the inner ear, or by toxic effects of antimicrobial agents.
   D. *Thrombosis of meningeal veins:* focal seizures, focal cerebral defects such as hemiparesis, aphasia (rarely prominent), most often after the first week.
   E. *Ependymitis, choroidal plexitis:* it is doubtful if there are any recognizable clinical effects.
   F. *Cerebellar or cerebral hemisphere herniation:* caused by swelling causing upper cervical cord compression with quadriplegia or signs of midbrain–third-nerve compression.

II. In subacute and chronic forms of meningitis:
   A. *Hydrocephalus:* at first caused by purulent exudate around the base of the brain, later by meningeal fibrosis, and rarely by aqueductal stenosis.
   B. *Subdural effusion:* impaired alertness in a child, refusal to eat, vomiting, immobility, bulging fontanels, and persistence of fever despite clearing of CSF.
   C. *Venous or arterial infarction:* unilateral or bilateral hemiplegia, decorticate or decerebrate rigidity, cortical blindness, stupor or coma with or without seizures. Deep infarcts may occur from an infectious vasculitis at the base of the brain.

III. Late effects or sequelae:
   A. *Meningeal fibrosis around optic nerves or around spinal cord and roots:* blindness and optic atrophy, spastic paraparesis with sensory loss in the lower segments of the body (opticochiasmatic arachnoiditis and meningomyelitis, respectively).
   B. *Chronic meningoencephalitis with hydrocephalus:* dementia, stupor or coma, and paralysis (e.g., general paralysis of the insane). If lumbosacral posterior roots are chronically damaged, a tabetic syndrome results. Deep infarcts.
   C. *Persistent hydrocephalus in the child:* blindness, arrest of mental activity, bilateral spastic hemiplegia.

Types of Bacterial Meningitis

Almost any bacterium gaining entrance to the body may produce meningitis but by far the most common are *H. influenzae, N. meningitidis,* and *S. pneumoniae,* which account for approximately 75 percent of sporadic cases. Infection with *L. monocytogenes* is now the fourth most common type of nonsurgical bacterial meningitis in adults. The following are less frequent causes: *Staphylococcus aureus* and group A (*Streptococcus pyogenes*) and group D streptococci, usually in association with brain abscess, epidural abscess, head trauma, neurosurgical procedures, or cranial thrombophlebitis; *E. coli* and group B streptococci in newborns; *Pseudomonas* and the Enterobacteriaceae, such as *Klebsiella, Proteus,* which are usually a consequence of lumbar puncture, spinal anesthesia, or shunting procedures to relieve hydrocephalus. Less-common meningeal pathogens include *Salmonella, Shigella, Clostridium, Neisseria gonorrhoeae,* and *Acinetobacter calcoaceticus.* In endemic areas, *mycobacterial infections* (to be considered further on) are as frequent as those caused by other bacterial organisms. They now assume greater importance in developed countries as the number of immunosuppressed persons increases.

Epidemiology

Pneumococcal, influenzal (*H. influenzae*), and meningococcal forms of meningitis have a worldwide distribution, occurring mainly during the winter and early spring and, in the case of the first two, also in the fall, and predominating slightly in males. Each has a relatively constant incidence, although epidemics of meningococcal meningitis seem to occur roughly in 10-year cycles. Drug-resistant strains appear with varying frequency, and such information, gleaned from surveillance reports issued by the Centers for Disease Control and Prevention and from reports of local health agencies and hospital infection surveillance, are of great practical importance.

H. influenzae meningitis, formerly encountered mainly in infants and young children, has been nearly eliminated in this age group as a result of vaccination programs in developed countries. It continues to be common in less-developed nations and is now occurring with increasing frequency in adults. *Meningococcal meningitis* occurs most often in children and adolescents but is also encountered throughout much of adult life, with a sharp decline in incidence after the age of 50 years. *Pneumococcal meningitis* predominates in the very young and in older adults. Perhaps the greatest change in the epidemiology of bacterial meningitis, aside from the one related to *H. influenzae* vaccination, has been the increasing incidence of nosocomial infections, accounting for 40 percent of cases in large urban hospitals (Durand et al); staphylococcus and gram-negative bacilli account for a large proportion of these. Noteworthy is the report of Schuchat and colleagues, who found that in 1995, some 5 years after the introduction of the conjugate *H. influenzae* vaccine, the incidence of bacterial meningitis in the United States had been halved. The yearly incidence rate (per 100,000 population) of the responsible pathogens is approximately as follows: *S. pneumoniae,* 1.1; *N. meningitidis,* 0.6; group B streptococcus (newborns), 0.3; *L. monocytogenes,* 0.2; and *H. influenzae,* 0.2. In an informative epidemiologic survey of bacterial meningitis in the United States from 1998 to 2007, Thigpen and colleagues found the relative order of the frequency of various organisms to be much the same and again emphasized the decrease in incidence of the disease due mainly to the *H. influenza* vaccination program. They estimated the recent overall incidence to be 4,100 cases annually, resulting in 500 deaths. Their article is recommended for its detailed analysis of age, race, and underlying medical condition.

Pathogenesis

The most common meningeal pathogens are all normal inhabitants of the nasopharynx in a significant part of the population and depend on antiphagocytic capsular or surface antigens for survival in the tissues of the infected host. To a large extent they express their pathogenicity by extracellular proliferation. It is evident from the frequency with which the carrier state is detected that nasal colonization is not a sufficient explanation of infection of the meninges. Factors that predispose the colonized patient to invasion of the bloodstream, which is the usual route by which these bacteria reach the meninges, are obscure but include antecedent viral infections of the upper respiratory passages or, in the case of *S. pneumoniae,* infections of the lung. Once bloodborne, it is evident that pneumococci, *H. influenzae,* and meningococci possess a predilection for the meninges, although the precise factors that determine this tropism are not known. Whether the organisms enter the CSF via the choroid plexus or meningeal vessels is also unknown. It has been variously postulated that the entry of bacteria into the subarachnoid space is facilitated by disruption of the blood–CSF barrier by trauma, circulating endotoxins, or an initial viral infection of the meninges. These organisms, being commensal in most persons, create immunity, but bacteria may nonetheless penetrate the mucosa. Certain features of the organisms enhance their ability to cause infection; this is particularly true of the meningococcus (Rosenstein et al).

Avenues other than the bloodstream by which bacteria can gain access to the meninges include congenital neuroectodermal defects; craniotomy sites; diseases of the middle ear and paranasal sinuses, particularly perilymphatic fistulas; skull fractures; and, in cases of recurrent infection, dural tears from remote minor or major trauma. Occasionally, a brain abscess may rupture into the subarachnoid space or ventricles, thus infecting the meninges. The isolation of anaerobic streptococci, *Bacteroides, Actinomyces,* or a mixture of microorganisms from the CSF should suggest the possibility of a brain abscess with an associated meningitis.

Clinical Features

Adults and Children

The early clinical effects of acute bacterial meningitis are fever, headache, usually severe, and stiffness of the neck (resistance to passive movement on forward bending), and less often initially, generalized convulsions and a disorder of consciousness (i.e., confusion, drowsiness, stupor, and coma). Flexion at the hip and knee in response to forward flexion of the neck (Brudzinski sign) and inability to completely extend the legs with the hips flexed (Kernig sign) have the same significance as stiff neck but are less-consistently elicitable. Basically, all of these signs are part of a flexor protective reflex (one of the "nocifensive" responses in Fulton's terms). Stiffness of the neck that is part of paratonic or extrapyramidal rigidity should not be mistaken for that of meningeal irritation. The former is more or less equal in all directions of movement, in distinction to that of meningitis, which is present only or predominantly on forward flexion. Whether it is stiffness in the initial few degrees of flexion of the neck or in the subsequent part of the movement that is more specific for meningitis has been debated; our experience has been that the latter is more sensitive but also proves to be mistaken for other disorders; thus the first may be more specific for meningitis.

Diagnosis of meningitis may be difficult when the initial manifestations consist only of fever and headache, when stiffness of the neck has not yet developed, or when there is only pain in the neck or abdomen or a febrile confusional state or delirium. Also, stiffness of the neck may not be apparent in the deeply stuporous or comatose patient or in the infant or the elderly, as indicated further on.

The symptoms comprised by the meningitic syndrome are common to the three main types of bacterial meningitis, but certain clinical features and the setting in which each of them occurs correlate more closely with one type than another.

Meningococcal meningitis should be suspected when the evolution is extremely rapid (delirium and stupor may supervene in a matter of hours), when the onset is attended by a petechial or purpuric rash or by large ecchymoses and lividity of the skin of the lower parts of the body, when there is circulatory shock, and especially during local outbreaks of meningitis. Because a petechial rash accompanies approximately 50 percent of meningococcal infections, its presence dictates immediate institution of antibiotic therapy, even though a similar rash may be observed with certain viral (echovirus serotype 9 and some other enteroviruses), as well as *S. aureus* infections, and, rarely, with other bacterial meningitides.

Pneumococcal meningitis is often preceded by an infection in the lungs, ears, sinuses, or heart valves. In addition, a pneumococcal etiology should be suspected in alcoholics, in splenectomized patients, in the very elderly, and in those with recurrent bacterial meningitis, dermal sinus tracts, sickle cell anemia ("autosplenectomized"), and basilar skull fracture. On the other hand, *H. influenzae* meningitis usually follows upper respiratory and ear infections in the uninocualted child.

Other specific bacterial etiologies are suggested by particular clinical settings. Meningitis in the presence furunculosis or following a neurosurgical procedure directs attention to the possibility of a coagulase-positive staphylococcal infection. Ventricular shunts or drains inserted for the relief of hydrocephalus are particularly prone to infection with coagulase-negative staphylococci and *Proprionobacerium acnes* and *diphteroids*. HIV infection, myeloproliferative or lymphoproliferative disorders, defects in cranial bones (tumor, osteomyelitis), collagen diseases, metastatic cancer, and therapy with immunosuppressive agents are clinical conditions that favor invasion by such pathogens as Enterobacteriaceae, *L. monocytogenes*, *A. calcoaceticus*, *Pseudomonas*, and occasionally by parasites.

Focal cerebral signs in the early stages of the disease, although seldom prominent, are most frequent in pneumococcal and *H. influenzae* meningitides. Some of the transitory focal cerebral signs may represent postictal phenomena (Todd paralysis); others may be related to an unusually intense focal meningitis, for example, purulent material collected in one sylvian fissure. Seizures are encountered most often with *H. influenzae* meningitis. Although seizures are most common in infants and children, it is difficult to judge the significance, because young children may convulse with fever of any cause. Persistent focal cerebral lesions or intractable seizures usually develop in the second week of the meningeal infection and are caused by an infectious vasculitis, as described earlier, usually with occlusion of surface cerebral veins and consequent infarction of cerebral tissue. Cranial nerve abnormalities are particularly frequent with pneumococcal meningitis, the result of invasion of the nerve by purulent exudate and possibly ischemic damage as the nerve traverses the subarachnoid space.

Infants and Newborns

Acute bacterial meningitis during the first month of life is said to be more frequent than in any subsequent 30-day period of life. It poses a number of special problems. Infants, of course, cannot complain of headache, stiff neck may be absent, and one has only the nonspecific signs of a systemic illness: fever, irritability, drowsiness, vomiting, convulsions, and a bulging fontanel to suggest the presence of meningeal infection. Signs of meningeal irritation do occur, but only late in the course of the illness. A high index of suspicion and liberal use of the lumbar puncture needle are the keys to early diagnosis. Lumbar puncture is ideally performed before any antibiotics are administered for other neonatal infections. An antibiotic regimen sufficient to control a septicemia may allow a meningeal infection to smolder and to flare up after antibiotic therapy for the systemic infection has been discontinued.

A number of other facts about the natural history of neonatal meningitis are noteworthy. It is more common in males than in females, in a ratio of about 3:1. Obstetric abnormalities in the third trimester (premature birth, prolonged labor, premature rupture of fetal membranes) occur frequently in mothers of infants who develop meningitis in the first weeks of life. The most significant factor in the pathogenesis of the meningitis is maternal infection (usually a urinary tract infection or puerperal fever of unknown cause). The infection in both mother and infant is most often caused by gram-negative enterobacteria, particularly *E. coli*, and group B streptococci, and less often to *Pseudomonas*, *Listeria*, *S. aureus* or *epidermidis* (formerly *albus*), and group A streptococci. Analysis of postmortem material indicates that in most cases infection occurs at or near the time of birth, although clinical signs of meningitis may not become evident until several days or a week later.

In infants with meningitis, one should be prepared to find a unilateral or bilateral sympathetic *subdural effusion* regardless of bacterial type. Young age, rapid evolution of the illness, low polymorphonuclear cell count, and markedly elevated protein in the CSF correlate to some extent with the formation of effusions, according to Snedeker and coworkers. Also, these attributes greatly increase the likelihood of the meningitis being associated with neurologic signs. Transillumination of the skull is the simplest method of demonstrating the presence of an effusion, but CT and MRI are the definitive diagnostic tests. When aspirated, most of the effusions prove to be sterile. If recovery is delayed and neurologic signs persist, a succession of aspirations is required. Children in whom meningitis is complicated by subdural effusions are no more likely, according to authorative sources, to have residual neurologic signs and seizures than are those without effusions.

Spinal Fluid Examination

As already indicated, *the lumbar puncture is an indispensable part of the examination of patients with the symptoms and signs of meningitis or of any patient in whom this diagnosis is suspected.* Bacteremia is not a contraindication to lumbar puncture. The dilemma concerning the risk of promoting transtentorial or cerebellar herniation by lumbar puncture, even without a cerebral mass, as indicated in Chaps. 2 and 17, has been settled in favor of performing the tap if there is a reasonable suspicion of meningitis. The highest estimates of risk come from studies such as those of Rennick, who reported a 4 percent incidence of clinical worsening among 445 children undergoing lumbar puncture for the diagnosis of acute meningitis; most other series give a lower number. It must be pointed out that a cerebellar pressure cone (tonsillar herniation) may occur in fulminant meningitis independent of lumbar puncture; therefore the risk of the procedure is probably even less than usually stated.

If there is clinical evidence of a focal lesion with increased intracranial pressure, then CT or MRI scanning of the head, looking for a mass lesion, is a prudent first step, but *in most cases this is not necessary and should not delay the administration of antibiotics.* In an attempt to determine the utility of the CT scan performed prior to a lumbar puncture, Hasbun and colleagues were able to identify several clinical characteristics that were likely to be associated with an abnormality on the scan in patients with suspected meningitis; these included a recent seizure, coma or confusion, gaze palsy, and others. The more salient finding from this study in our opinion was that only 2 percent of 235 patients had a focal mass lesion that was judged a risk for lumbar puncture; many others had CT findings of interest, including some with diffuse mass effect. This study does not entirely clarify the issue of the safety of lumbar puncture but it emphasizes that patients who lack major neurologic findings are unlikely to have findings on the scan that will preclude lumbar puncture.

Only a sizable brain abscess or substantial brain swelling entirely interdicts a lumbar puncture in suspected bacterial meningitis. Furthermore, the fact that death results from cerebral herniation in many fatal cases of bacterial meningitis does not, of course, mean that lumbar puncture precipitated the demise. When there are signs of impending herniation or indications of a dangerous configuration on cerebral images, one may wish to draw blood cultures and and institute empiric treatment rather than take the small risk of precipitation herniation with a lumbar puncture. Any coagulopathy that is deemed a risk for hemorrhagic complication of lumbar puncture should be rapidly reversed if possible.

The spinal fluid *pressure* is so consistently elevated (above 180 mm H_2O) that a normal pressure on the initial lumbar puncture in a patient with suspected bacterial meningitis suggests another diagnosis or raises the possibility that the needle is partially occluded or the spinal subarachnoid space is blocked. Pressures over approximately 350 mm H_2O suggest the presence of brain swelling and the potential for cerebellar herniation. Many neurologists favor the administration of intravenous mannitol if the pressure is this high, but this practice does not provide assurance that herniation will be avoided.

A *pleocytosis* in the spinal fluid is diagnostic. The number of leukocytes ranges from 250 to 100,000/mm^3, but the usual number is from 1,000 to 10,000. Occasionally, in pneumococcal and influenzal meningitis, the CSF may contain a large number of bacteria but few, if any, neutrophils for the first few hours. Cell counts of more than 50,000/mm^3 raise the possibility of a brain abscess having ruptured into a ventricle. Neutrophils predominate (85 to 95 percent of the total), but an increasing proportion of mononuclear cells is found as the infection continues for days, and especially in partially treated meningitis. In the early stages, careful cytologic examination may disclose that some of the mononuclear cells are myelocytes or young neutrophils. Later, as treatment takes effect, the proportions of lymphocytes, plasma cells, and histiocytes steadily increase.

Substantial hemorrhage or substantial numbers of red cells in the CSF are uncommon in meningitis, the exceptions being anthrax meningitis (see Lanska) as well as certain rare viral infections (Hantavirus, dengue fever, Ebola virus, etc.) and some cases of amebic meningoencephalitis.

The *protein* content is higher than 45 mg/dL in more than 90 percent of the cases; in most cases, it falls in the range of 100 to 500 mg/dL. The *glucose* content is diminished, usually to a concentration below 40 mg/dL, or less than 40 percent of the blood glucose concentration (measured concomitantly or within the previous hour), provided that the latter is less than 250 mg/dL. However, in atypical or *culture-negative cases*, other conditions associated with a reduced CSF glucose should be considered. These include hypoglycemia from any cause; sarcoidosis of the CNS; fungal or tuberculous meningitis; and some cases of subarachnoid hemorrhage, meningeal carcinomatosis, chemically induced inflammation from craniopharyngioma or teratoma, and meningeal gliomatosis. The factors that alter CSF glucose concentration, especially at the extremes of blood glucose, are discussed in Chap. 2.

A special problem pertains to identifying patients with a meningitic syndrome and CSF pleocytosis who do not, in fact, have bacterial meningitis but likely have a viral or other cause for their syndrome. This is driven by a desire to avoid exposure to high-potency intravenous antibiotics that are expensive and potentially dangerous. To address this problem, Nigrovic and colleagues have developed a clinical prediction rule that classifies patients at very low risk for bacterial meningitis if they lack all of the following criteria: positive CSF Gram stain, CSF absolute neutrophil count of at least 1,000 cells/mL, CSF protein of at least 80 mg/dL, peripheral absolute neutrophil count of at least 10,000 cells/mL, and a history of a seizure at or after the time of presentation. This rule was validated in a multicenter retrospective cohort study that encompassed 3,295 patients. Of those who were categorized at very low risk, only 2 had bacterial meningitis. Whether this low rate justifies withholding antibiotics is, of course, a clinical judgement made at the bedside.

The *Gram stain of the spinal fluid* sediment permits identification of the causative agent in most cases of bacterial meningitis; pneumococci and *H. influenzae* are identified more readily than meningococci. Small numbers of gram-negative diplococci in leukocytes may be indistinguishable from fragmented nuclear material, which may also be gram-negative and of the same shape as bacteria. In such cases, a thin film of uncentrifuged CSF may lend itself more readily to morphologic interpretation than a smear of the sediment. The most common error in reading Gram-stained smears of CSF is the misinterpretation of precipitated dye or debris as gram-positive cocci or the confusion of pneumococci with *H. influenzae*. The latter organism may stain heavily at the poles, so that they resemble gram-positive diplococci, and older or rapidly growing pneumococci often lose their capacity to take a gram-positive stain.

Cultures of the spinal fluid, which prove to be positive in 70 to 90 percent of cases of bacterial meningitis, are best obtained by collecting the fluid in a sterile tube and immediately inoculating plates of blood, chocolate, and MacConkey agar; tubes of thioglycolate (for anaerobes); and at least one other broth. The advantage of using broth media is that large amounts of CSF can be cultured. The importance of obtaining blood cultures is mentioned below.

The problem of identifying causative organisms that cannot be cultured, particularly in patients who have received antibiotics, may be overcome by the application of special laboratory techniques. One of these is counterimmunoelectrophoresis (CIE), a sensitive test that permits the detection of bacterial antigens in the CSF in a matter of 30 to 60 min. It is particularly useful in patients with partially treated meningitis, in whom the CSF still contains bacterial antigens but no organisms on a smear or grown in culture.

Several more recently developed serologic methods, radioimmunoassay (RIA) and latex-particle agglutination (LPA), as well as an enzyme-linked immunosorbent assay (ELISA), may be even more sensitive than CIE. An argument has been made that these procedures are not cost-effective, as—in virtually all instances in which the bacterial antigen can be detected—Gram stain also shows the organism. Our sense is that the more expensive tests are of some assistance if Gram stain is difficult to interpret and one or more doses of antibiotics render the cultures negative. Gene amplification by the polymerase chain reaction (PCR) is the most recently developed and most sensitive technique. As it has become more widely available in clinical laboratories, rapid diagnosis has been facilitated (Desforges; Naber), but the use of carefully Gram-stained preparations still needs to be encouraged.

It is of interest that chloride concentrations in the CSF are usually found to be low, possibly reflecting dehydration and low serum chloride levels. In contrast, CSF lactate dehydrogenase (LDH), although also infrequently measured, can be of diagnostic and prognostic value. A rise in total LDH activity is consistently observed in patients with bacterial meningitis; most of this is because of fractions 4 and 5, which are derived from granulocytes. Fractions 1 and 2 of LDH, which are presumably derived from brain tissue, are only slightly elevated in bacterial meningitis but rise sharply in patients who develop neurologic sequelae or later die. Various enzymes in the CSF, derived from leukocytes, meningeal cells, or plasma, may also be increased in meningitis, but the clinical significance of this observation is unknown. Levels of lactic acid in the CSF (determined by either gas chromatography or enzymatic analysis) are also elevated in both bacterial and fungal meningitides (greater than 35 mg/dL) and may be helpful in distinguishing these disorders from viral meningitides, in which lactic acid levels remain normal; however, these ancillary tests are infrequently performed.

Other Laboratory Findings

In addition to CSF cultures, *blood cultures* should be obtained if possible because they are positive in 40 to 60 percent of patients with *H. influenzae*, meningococcal, and pneumococcal meningitis, and may provide the only definite clue as to the causative agent. Routine cultures of the oropharynx are as often misleading as helpful, because pneumococci, *H. influenzae*, and meningococci are common in the throats of healthy persons. In contrast, *cultures of the nasopharynx* may aid in diagnosis, although often not in a timely way; the finding of encapsulated *H. influenzae* or groupable meningococci may provide the clue to the etiology of the meningeal infection. Conversely, the absence of such a finding prior to antibiotic treatment makes an *H. influenzae* and meningococcal etiology unlikely. The leukocyte count in the blood is generally elevated, and immature forms are usually present. Meningitis may be complicated after several days by severe hyponatremia, the result of inappropriate secretion of antidiuretic hormone (ADH).

Imaging Studies

In patients with bacterial meningitis, chest films are essential because they may disclose an area of pneumonia or abscess. Sinus and skull films may provide clues to the presence of cranial osteomyelitis, paranasal sinusitis, mastoiditis, or cranial osteomyelitis, but these structures are better visualized on CT scans, which have supplanted conventional films in most cases. The CT scan is particularly useful in detecting lesions that erode the skull or spine and provide a route for bacterial invasion, such as tumors or sinus wall defects, as well as in demonstrating a brain abscess or subdural empyema. MRI with gadolinium enhancement may display the meningeal exudate and cortical reaction, and both types of imaging, with appropriate techniques, will demonstrate venous occlusions and adjacent infarctions. The issues pertaining to an abscess and to brain swelling in meningitis have already been noted and are disucussed further on as well.

Recurrent Bacterial Meningitis

This is observed most frequently in patients who have had some type of shunting procedure for the treatment of hydrocephalus or who have an incompletely closed dural opening after cranial or spinal surgery. When the origin of the recurrence is inapparent, one should suspect a congenital neuroectodermal sinus or a fistulous connection between the nasal sinuses and the subarachnoid space. The fistula in these latter cases is more often traumatic than congenital in origin (e.g., a previous basilar skull fracture), although the interval between injury and the initial bout of meningitis may be several years. The site of trauma is in the frontal or ethmoid sinuses or the cribriform plate, and *S. pneumoniae* is the usual pathogen. Often it reflects the predominance of such strains in nasal carriers. These cases usually have a good prognosis; mortality is much lower than in ordinary cases of pneumococcal meningitis.

CSF rhinorrhea is present in most cases of posttraumatic meningitis, but it may be transient and difficult to find. Suspicion of its presence is raised by the recent onset of anosmia or by the occurrence of a watery nasal discharge that is salty to the taste and increases in volume when the head is dependent. One way of confirming the presence of a CSF leak is to measure the glucose concentration of nasal secretions; ordinarily they contain little glucose, but in CSF rhinorrhea the amount of glucose approximates that obtained by lumbar puncture (two-thirds of the serum value). A "dipstick" used for urine testing is sometimes adequate but these are regrettably decresingly available on general hospital wards. Another bedside test for CSF rhinorrhea or otorrhea is to estimate the amount of protein in the fluid. A high protein, sufficient to make a handkerchief stiff on drying, suggests it is of nasal mucosal origin. If the fluid fails to cause a handkerchief to stiffen on drying, a spinal fluid leak is suspected. The most specific and sensitive test for CSF otorrhea and rhinorrhea is the finding of beta$_2$-transferrin (tau), not found in fluids other than CSF.

The site of a CSF leak can sometimes be demonstrated by injecting a dye, radioactive albumin, or water-soluble contrast material into the spinal subarachnoid space and detecting its appearance in nasal secretions or its site of exit by CT scanning. This testing is best performed after the acute infection has subsided. Persistence of CSF rhinorrhea or a spinal CSF leak usually requires surgical repair.

Differential Diagnosis

The diagnosis of bacterial meningitis is usually not difficult in an immunocompetent individual. *Febrile patients with lethargy, headache, stiff neck, or confusion of sudden onset—even those with low-grade fever—should generally undergo lumbar puncture* if no alternative explanation for the state is evident. It is particularly important to recall the possibility of meningitis in drowsy, febrile, and septic patients in an intensive care unit when no obvious source of fever is apparent. Overwhelming sepsis itself, or the multiorgan failure that it engenders, may cause an encephalopathy; but if there is meningitis, it is imperative, in deciding on the choice of antibiotics, to identify it early. The same can be said for the confused alcoholic patient. Too often, the symptoms are ascribed to alcohol intoxication or withdrawal, or to hepatic encephalopathy, until examination of the CSF reveals meningitis. Although this approach undoubtedly results in many negative spinal fluid examinations, it is preferable to the consequence of overlooking bacterial meningitis. Viral meningitis (which is far more common than bacterial meningitis), subarachnoid hemorrhage, chemical meningitis (following lumbar puncture, spinal anesthesia, or myelography), and tuberculous, leptospiral, sarcoid, and fungal meningoencephalitis, and allergic-immune reactions enter into the differential diagnosis as well, as discussed in later sections.

A number of nonbacterial meningitides must be considered in the differential diagnosis when the meningitis recurs repeatedly and all cultures are negative. Included in this group are Epstein-Barr virus (EBV) infections; Behçet disease, which is characterized by recurrent oropharyngeal mucosal ulceration, uveitis, orchitis, and meningitis; Mollaret meningitis, which consists of recurrent episodes of fever and headache in addition to signs of meningeal irritation (in many cases caused by herpes simplex, as discussed in Chap. 33); and the Vogt-Koyanagi-Harada syndrome, in which recurrent meningitis is associated with iridocyclitis and depigmentation of the hair and skin (poliosis and vitiligo). The CSF in these recurrent types may contain large numbers of lymphocytes or polymorphonuclear leukocytes but no bacteria, and the glucose content is not reduced (see discussion of Chronic and Recurrent Meningitis Chap. 33). These recurrent syndromes rarely present in the fulminant manner of acute bacterial meningitis but sometimes they do, and the CSF formulas can be similar, including a reduction in glucose concentration. Rarely, a fulminant case of cerebral angiitis or intravascular lymphoma will present with headache, fever, and confusion in conjunction with a meningeal inflammatory reaction.

The other intracranial purulent diseases and their differentiation from bacterial meningitis are considered further on in this chapter.

Treatment

Bacterial meningitis is a medical emergency. The first therapeutic measures are directed to sustaining blood pressure and treating septic shock (volume replacement, pressor therapy). A premium is then placed on choosing an antibiotic that is known both to be bactericidal for the suspected organism and is able to enter the CSF in effective amounts. *Treatment should begin while awaiting the results of diagnostic tests* and may be altered later in accordance with the laboratory findings. Whereas penicillin formerly sufficed to treat almost all meningitides acquired outside the hospital, the initial choice of antibiotic has become increasingly complicated as resistant strains of meningitic bacteria have emerged. The selection of drugs to treat nosocomial infections also presents special difficulties.

In recent years, many reports have documented an increasing incidence of pneumococcal isolates that have a relatively high resistance to penicillin, reaching 50 percent in some European countries. Current estimates are that, in some areas of the United States, 15 percent of these isolates are penicillin-resistant to some degree (most have a relatively low level of resistance). In the 1970s, *H. influenzae* type B strains producing beta-lactamase, which are resistant to ampicillin and penicillin, were recognized. Currently, 30 percent of *H. influenzae* isolates produce the beta-lactamase enzyme, but almost all remain sensitive to third-generation cephalosporins (e.g., cefotaxime, ceftizoxime, ceftriaxone).

Recommendations for the institution of empiric treatment of meningitis have been reviewed by van de Beek and colleagues (2006) and by Tunkel and colleagues, often updated, and are summarized in modified form in Table 32-2. The choice of agents varies every few years based on epidemiology and geographic region, but these ones given here are a good approximation to current practice in developed countries.

Table 32-2

EMPIRIC THERAPY OF BACTERIAL MENINGITIS

AGE OF PATIENT	ANTIMICROBIAL THERAPY[a]
0–4 wk	Cefotaxime plus ampicillin
4–12 wk	Third-generation cephalosporin plus ampicillin (plus dexamethasone)
3 mo–18 y	Third-generation cephalosporin plus vancomycin (± ampicillin)
18–50 y	Third-generation cephalosporin plus vancomycin (± ampicillin)
>50 y	Third-generation cephalosporin plus vancomycin plus ampicillin
Immunocompromised state	Vancomycin plus ampicillin and ceftazidime
Basilar skull fracture	Third-generation cephalosporin plus vancomycin
Head trauma; neurosurgery	Vancomycin plus ceftazidime
CSF shunt	Vancomycin plus ceftazidime

[a]For all ages from 3 months onward, an alternative treatment is meropenem plus vancomycin (does not provide coverage for *Listeria*). For severe penicillin allergy, consider vancomycin and chloramphenicol (for meningococcus) and trimethoprim-sulfamethoxazole (for *Listeria*). A high failure rate has been reported with chloramphenicol in patients with drug-resistant pneumococcus.

In children and adults, third-generation cephalosporins such as ceftriaxone, combined with vancomycin is probably the best initial therapy for the three major types of community-acquired meningitides. In areas with low numbers of high-level penicillin-resistant pneumococci, it is possible to avoid adding vancomycin or rifampin. Ampicillin should be added to the regimen in cases of suspected *Listeria* meningitis, particularly in an immunocompromised patient. Intravenous drug abusers have high rates of meningitis due to *S. Aureus* and should receive cefepime or ceftazidime with vancomycin. When serious allergy to penicillin and cephalosporins precludes their use, chloramphenicol may be a suitable alternative in some regions, but not for *Listeria*.

Isolation from the blood or CSF of a resistant organism requires the use of ceftriaxone with the addition of vancomycin and rifampin. *N. meningitides*, at least in the United States, remains highly susceptible to penicillin and ampicillin. Regional variations and ongoing antibiotic-induced changes in the infecting microorganisms underscore the need for constant awareness of drug resistance in the physician's local area, especially in the case of pneumococcal infections. Throughout the course of treatment, it is necessary to have access to a laboratory that can carry out rapid and detailed drug-resistance testing.

Nosocomial Meningitis In cases of meningitis caused by coagulase-positive *S. aureus*, including those that occur after neurosurgery or major head injury, administration of vancomycin plus a third-generation cephalosporin (e.g., cefepime, ceftazadime, or meropenem) is a reasonable first approach. If *Pseudomonas* is considered possible, such as after neurosurgery, an antipseudomonal cephalosporin such as ceftazidime or cefapime should be added. Once the sensitivity of the organism has been determined, therapy may have to be altered or may be simplified by using vancomycin or nafcillin alone. These approaches have been reviewd by van de Beek and colleagues (2010). They note that the CSF cell count may be low in cases of ventricular catheter-associated meningitis. They also provide recommendations on the use of prophylactic antibiotics after a basilar skull fracture, a controversial problem that is reviewed in Chap. 35.

Table 32-3 lists the approximate dosages of the most used antibiotics, and Table 32-4 gives reasonable choices of antibiotic for the treatment of specific bacterial isolates.

Duration of Therapy Most cases of bacterial meningitis should be treated for a period of 10 to 14 days except when there is a persistent parameningeal focus of infection (otitic or sinus origin), in which cases longer treatment may be needed. Antibiotics should be administered in full doses parenterally (preferably intravenously) throughout the period of treatment. Treatment failures with certain drugs, notably ampicillin, may be attributable to oral or intramuscular administration, resulting in inadequate concentrations in the CSF. Repeated lumbar punctures are not necessary to assess the effects of therapy as long as there is progressive clinical improvement. The CSF glucose may remain low for many days after other signs of infection have subsided and should occasion concern only if bacteria are present in the fluid and the patient remains febrile and ill.

Table 32-3

RECOMMENDED DOSAGES OF ANTIMICROBIAL AGENTS FOR BACTERIAL MENINGITIS IN ADULTS WITH NORMAL RENAL AND HEPATIC FUNCTION[a]

ANTIMICROBIAL AGENT	TOTAL DAILY DOSE	DOSING INTERVAL, HOURS
Amikacin[b]	15 mg/kg	8
Ampicillin	12 g	4
Cefepime	4–6 g	8–12
Cefotaxime	12 g	4–6
Ceftazidime	6 g	8
Ceftriaxone	4 g	12–24
Chloramphenicol[c]	6 g	6
Ciprofloxacin	800–1, 200 mg	12
Gentamicin[b]	5 mg/kg	8
Linezolid	1,200 mg	12
Meropenem[d]	3–6 g	8
Nafcillin	9–12 g	4
Oxacillin	9–12 g	4
Penicillin G	24 million units	4
Quinupristin-dalfopristin	22.5 mg/kg	8
Rifampin[e]	600 mg	24
Tobramycin[b]	5 mg/kg	8
Trimethoprim-sulfamethoxazole[f]	20 mg/kg	6–12
Vancomycin[b,g]	2–4 g	6–12

[a]Unless indicated, therapy is administered intravenously.
[b]Aminoglycosides are not used as sole treatment for meningitis. Peak and trough serum concentrations should be monitored.
[c]Higher dose recommended for pneumococcal meningitis.
[d]Risk of seizures with meropenem.
[e]Oral administration.
[f]Dosage based on trimethoprim component.
[g]CSF concentrations may have to be monitored in severely ill patients.
Newer drugs are available for methicillin-resistant staphyloccocal infections but are not well studied for staphylococcal meningitis: linezolid, quinupristin-dalfopristin, and daptomycin.

Persistence of fever or the late appearance of drowsiness, hemiparesis, or seizures should raise the suspicion of subdural effusion, mastoiditis, venous sinus thrombosis, cortical vein or jugular phlebitis, or brain abscess; all require that therapy be continued for a longer period. Bacteriologic relapse after treatment is discontinued requires reinstitution of therapy and exploration for a persistent parameningeal focus of infection, such as in the spinal column.

Corticosteroids Controlled studies several decades ago were unable to demonstrate beneficial effects of corticosteroids in the treatment of bacterial meningitis. More recent studies have given another perspective of the therapeutic value of dexamethasone in children and adults with meningitis. In children, although mortality was not affected in the main study conducted by Lebel and colleagues, fever subsided more rapidly and the incidence of sensorineural deafness and other neurologic sequelae was reduced, particularly in those children with *H. influenzae* meningitis. On these grounds, it has been recommended that the treatment of childhood meningitis include dexamethasone in high doses (0.15 mg/kg qid for 4 days), instituted as soon as possible.

Despite similarly conflicting results from earlier studies of corticosteroids in adults, the trial by deGans and van de Beck has demonstrated a reduction in mortality and improved overall outcome if dexamethasone 10 mg is given just before the first dose of antibiotics and then repeated q6h for 4 days. The improvement was largely in patients who were infected with pneumococcus. Seizures and coma were reduced in incidence as a result of the administration of corticosteroids, but neurologic sequelae, such as hearing loss, were not affected. Based on a number of smaller studies, some authorities in the field of bacterial meningitis have endorsed the administration of dexamethasone in the doses mentioned above, but only if they can be started before antibiotics, and only in those with presumed pneumococcal infection (see Tunkel and Scheld). They also advise against the use of the drug if there is septic shock. In developing countries, especially those with high rates of AIDS, the benefits of adjuvant dexamethasone have not been clear. Improved survival was limited to those who ultimately had bacteria isolated from the CSF, in contrast to those with suspected meningitis but negative cultures.

Nonetheless, the incidence of deafness was reduced (Nguyen et al; Scarborough et al). The use of corticosteroids is therefore suggested in cases with overwhelming infection at any age (very high CSF pressure or signs of herniation, high CSF bacterial count with minimal pleocytosis, and signs of acute adrenal insufficiency, i.e., the Waterhouse-Friderichsen syndrome). It is not always possible to determine with certainty at the first presentation those cases that will be culture positive but one is referred back to the prediction "rules" validated by Nigrovic and colleagues.

Other Forms of Therapy There is no evidence that repeated drainage of CSF is therapeutically effective. In fact, increased CSF pressure in the acute phase of bacterial meningitis is largely a consequence of cerebral edema, in which case the lumbar puncture may predispose to cerebellar herniation. As already mentioned, a second lumbar puncture to gauge the effectiveness of treatment is generally not necessary, but it may be of value if the patient is worsening without explanation. Mannitol and urea have been employed with apparent success in some cases of severe brain swelling with unusually high initial CSF pressures (400 mm H_2O). Acting as osmotic diuretics, these agents enter cerebral tissue slowly, and their net effect is to decrease brain water. However, neither mannitol nor urea has been studied in controlled fashion in the management of meningitis. An adequate but not excessive amount of intravenous normal saline (and avoiding fluids with free water) should be given. Particular care should be taken with children to avoid hyponatremia and water intoxication—potential causes of brain swelling.

Antiepileptic drugs need not be administered routinely but should be given if a seizure has occurred or there is evidence of cortical vein thrombosis.

Prophylaxis Household contacts of patients with meningococcal meningitis should be protected with antibiotic treatment. The risk of secondary cases is small for adolescents and adults, but ranges from 2 to 4 percent for those younger than 5 years of age and is probably higher

Table 32-4

SPECIFIC ANTIMICROBIAL THERAPY FOR ACUTE MENINGITIS

MICROORGANISM	STANDARD THERAPY	ALTERNATIVE THERAPIES
Haemophilus influenzae		
Beta-lactamase–negative	Ampicillin	Third-generation cephalosporin[a]; chloramphenicol
Beta-lactamase–positive	Third-generation cephalosporin[a]	Chloramphenicol; cefepime
Neisseria meningitidis	Penicillin G or third-generation cephalosporin[a]	Chloramphenicol
Streptococcus pneumoniae		
Penicillin MIC <0.1 μg/mL (sensitive)	Penicillin G or ampicillin	Third-generation cephalosporin[a]; chloramphenicol; vancomycin plus rifampin
Penicillin MIC 0.1–1.0 μg/mL (intermediate sensitivity)	Third-generation cephalosporin[a]	Vancomycin; meropenem
Penicillin MIC ≥2.0 μg/mL (highly resistant)	Vancomycin plus third-generation cephalosporin	Meropenem
Enterobacteriaceae	Third-generation cephalosporin[a]	Meropenem; fluoroquinolone; trimethoprim-sulfamethoxazole, or cefepime
Pseudomonas aeruginosa	Ceftazidime or cefepime[b]	Meropenem; fluoroquinolone[b]; piperacillin
Listeria monocytogenes	Ampicillin or penicillin G[b]	Trimethoprim-sulfamethoxazole
Streptococcus agalactiae	Ampicillin or penicillin G[b]	Third-generation cephalosporin[a]; Vancomycin
Staphylococcus aureus		
Methicillin-sensitive	Nafcillin or oxacillin plus third-generation cephalosporin	Vancomycin
Methicillin-resistant[d]	Vancomycin[c] plus third-generation cephalosporin	Linezolid, quinupristin-dalfopristin, tigecycline
Staphylococcus epidermidis	Vancomycin[c]	Linezolid, tigecycline

MIC, minimal inhibitory concentration.
[a]Cefotaxime or ceftriaxone.
[b]Addition of an aminoglycoside should be considered.
[c]Addition of rifampin should be considered.
[d]Linezolid, quinupristin-dalfopristin, and daptomycin are newer alternatives for methicillin-resistant *Staphylococcus*, but few cases have been studied.

in the elderly. A single dose of ciprofloxacin is effective. An alternative is a daily oral dose of rifampin—600 mg q12h in adults and 10 mg/kg q12h in children—for 2 days. If 2 weeks or more have elapsed since the index case was found, no prophylaxis is needed.

As mentioned, immunization against *H. influenzae* is steadily reducing the incidence of meningitis from this organism. Also, many institutions housing young adults, such as colleges and the military, have instituted programs of immunization against *N. meningitidis*.

Prognosis and Sequelae of Meningitis

Untreated, bacterial meningitis is usually fatal. The overall mortality rate of uncomplicated but treated *H. influenzae* and meningococcal meningitis has remained at approximately 5 percent for many years; in pneumococcal meningitis, the rate is considerably higher (approximately 15 percent), perhaps related to the older and sicker population that is affected. Fulminant meningococcemia, with or without meningitis, also has a high mortality rate because of the shock associated with adrenocortical hemorrhages (Waterhouse-Friderichsen syndrome). A disproportionate number of deaths from meningitis occur in infants and in the aged. The mortality rate is highest in neonates, from 40 to 75 percent in several reported series, and at least half of those who recover show serious neurologic sequelae. In adults, the presence of bacteremia, coma, seizures, and a variety of concomitant diseases—including alcoholism, diabetes mellitus, multiple myeloma, and head trauma—all worsen the prognosis. The triad of pneumococcal meningitis, pneumonia, and endocarditis (Osler triad) has a particularly high fatality rate.

Suprisingly often, it is impossible to explain the death of a patient with meningitis or at least to trace it to a single specific mechanism. The effects of overwhelming infection, with bacteremia and hypotension, or brain swelling and cerebellar herniation, are clearly implicated in some patients during the initial 48 h. These events may occur in bacterial meningitis of any etiology; however, they are far more frequent in meningococcal and pneumococcal infection. Some of the deaths occurring later in the course of the illness are attributable to respiratory failure, often consequent to aspiration pneumonia.

It has been stated that relatively few adult patients who recover from meningococcal meningitis show residual neurologic defects, whereas such defects are encountered in at least 25 percent of children with *H. influenzae* meningitis and up to 30 percent of child and adult patients with pneumococcal meningitis. Kastenbauer and Pfister, reporting on adults with pneumococcal meningitis, have emphasized that the mortality remains quite high and that cerebral venous or arterial thrombosis occurred in almost a third of cases, as discussed further on. They also had two patients with an associated myelitis. We have seen several instances of upper cervical cord and lower medullary infarction in bacterial meningitis; quadriparesis and respiratory failure were the result of compression from descent of the cerebellar tonsils (Ropper and Kanis). As already discussed, the role of lumbar puncture in promoting this complication of cerebellar herniation has not been clarified.

Among infants who survive *H. influenzae* meningitis, Ferry and coworkers, in a prospective study of 50 cases, found that about half were normal, whereas 9 percent had behavioral problems and about 30 percent had neurologic deficits (seizures or impairment of hearing, language, mentation, and motor function). In a report of a series of 185 children recovering from bacterial meningitis, Pomeroy and associates found that 69 were not normal neurologically at the end of a month; however, at the end of a year, only 18 were left with a hearing deficit, 13 with late afebrile seizures, and 8 with multiple deficits. The presence of a persistent neurologic deficit was the only independent predictor of later seizures. Dodge and colleagues in past decades found that 31 percent of children with pneumococcal meningitis were left with persistent sensorineural hearing loss; for meningococcal and *H. influenzae* meningitis, the figures were 10.5 and 6 percent, respectively. These events are seemingly less frequent now, specifically in developed countries, but still reflect the seriousness of these sequealae in less advantaged regions of the world.

Cranial nerve palsies other than deafness, if they occur, tend to disappear after a few weeks or months. Deafness in these infections is a result of suppurative cochlear destruction or, less often now, of the ototoxic effects of aminoglycoside antibiotics. Bacteria reach the cochlea mainly via the cochlear aqueduct, which connects the subarachnoid space to the scala tympani. This occurs quite early in the course of infection, hearing loss being evident within a day of onset of the meningitis; in about half or most of such cases, the acute deafness resolves. Hydrocephalus is an infrequent complication that may become manifest months after treatment and then requires shunting if gait or mentation is affected. It may be difficult to determine on clinical grounds whether a residual state of imbalance is the result of hydrocephalus or of eighth nerve damage. The acute complications of bacterial meningitis, the intermediate and late neurologic sequelae, and the pathologic basis of these effects are summarized in Table 32-1.

ENCEPHALITIS DUE TO BACTERIAL INFECTIONS

Quite apart from acute and subacute bacterial endocarditis, which may give rise to cerebral embolism and characteristic inflammatory reactions in the brain (see further on), there are several systemic bacterial infections that are complicated by a special type of encephalitis or meningoencephalitis. Three common ones are *Mycoplasma pneumoniae* infections, *L. monocytogenes meningoencephalitis*, and *Legionnaire disease*. Probably Lyme borreliosis should be included in this category but it is more chronic and is described further on in this chapter with the spirochetal infections. The rickettsial encephalitides (particularly Q fever), which mimic bacterial meningoencephalitis, are also addressed later in the chapter. Catscratch disease is another rare cause of bacterial meningoencephalitis. Meningoencephalitis caused by brucellosis occurs very rarely in the United States. Whipple disease, discussed later, which appears to be a focal invasion of the brain by an unusual intracellular bacterium, is an oddity but also belongs in this category.

Mycoplasma pneumoniae

This organism, which causes 10 to 20 percent of all pneumonias, is associated with a number of neurologic syndromes. Guillain-Barré polyneuritis, cranial neuritis, acute myositis, aseptic meningitis, transverse myelitis, global encephalitis, seizures, cerebellitis, acute disseminated (postinfectious) encephalomyelitis, and acute hemorrhagic leukoencephalitis (Hurst disease) have all been reported in association with mycoplasmal pneumonias or with serologic evidence of a recent infection (Westenfelder et al; Fisher et al; Rothstein and Kenny). We have observed several patients with striking cerebral, cerebellar, brainstem, or spinal syndromes incurred during or soon after a mycoplasmal pneumonia or tracheobronchitis. In addition to the cerebellitis, which is clinically similar to the illness that follows varicella, unusual encephalitic syndromes of choreoathetosis, seizures, delirium, hemiparesis, and acute brain swelling (Reye syndrome) have each been reported in a few cases. The incidence of these complications has been estimated as 1 in 1,000 mycoplasmal infections, but it may approach 5 percent when more careful surveillance is carried out during epidemics. A severe prodromal headache has occurred in most of our cases. At the time of onset of the neurologic symptoms, there may be scant signs of pneumonia, and in some patients, only an upper respiratory syndrome occurs.

The mechanism of cerebral damage that complicates mycoplasmal infections has not been established, but recent evidence suggests that the organism is present in the CNS during the acute illness. To our knowledge, the organism has been cultured from the brain in only one fatal case, but PCR techniques have detected fragments of mycoplasmal DNA in the spinal fluid from several patients (Narita et al). In other instances, the nature of the neurologic complications and their temporal relationship to the mycoplasmal infection clearly suggest that secondary autoimmune factors are operative, i.e., that these are instances of postinfectious encephalomyelitis (a type of acute disseminated encephalomyelitis described in Chap. 36). This is almost certainly the mechanism of postmycoplasmal Guillain-Barrè syndrome. Most of the patients with the infectious variety have recovered with few or no sequelae, but rare fatalities are reported.

The CSF usually contains small numbers of lymphocytes and other mononuclear cells and an increased protein content. The diagnosis can be established by culture of the organism from the respiratory tract (which is difficult), by rising serum titers of complement-fixing immunoglobulin IgG and IgM antibodies and cold agglutinin antibodies in the blood and CSF, or by DNA detection techniques from the CSF.

Treatment Macrolide antibiotics such as azithromicin and clarithromicin but also erythromycin and tetracycline derivatives reduce morbidity, mainly by eradicating the pulmonary infection, but the effects of antibiotics on the nervous system complications are not known.

Listeria monocytogenes

Meningoencephalitis from this organism is most likely to occur in immunosuppressed and debilitated individuals and is a well-known and occasionally fatal cause of meningitis in the newborn. Meningitis is the usual neurologic manifestation, but there are numerous recorded instances of isolated focal bacterial infectious encephalitis, rarely with a normal CSF, most cases showing a pleocytosis that may be initially polymorphonuclear. Between 1929, when the organism was discovered, and 1962, when Gray and Killinger collected all the reported cases, it was noted that 35 percent of patients had either meningitis or meningoencephalitis as the primary manifestation.

The infection may take the form of a brainstem encephalitis, or "rhombencephalitis," specifically with several days of headache, fever, nausea, and vomiting followed by asymmetrical cranial-nerve palsies, signs of cerebellar dysfunction, hemiparesis, quadriparesis, or sensory loss. Respiratory failure has been reported. Of 62 cases of *Listeria* brainstem encephalitis reported by Armstrong and Fung, 8 percent were in immunosuppressed patients, meningeal signs were present in only half the patients, and the spinal fluid often showed misleadingly mild abnormalities. CSF cultures yielded *Listeria* in only 40 percent of cases (blood cultures were even more often normal). Consistent with our experience, the early CT scan was often normal; MRI, however, has revealed abnormal signals in the parenchyma of the brainstem.

The monocytosis, which gives the organism its name, refers to the reaction in the peripheral blood in rabbits but these cells have not been prominent in the blood or CSF of patients. One patient described by Lechtenberg and coworkers had a proven brain abscess; other patients have had multiple small abscesses (Uldry et al) but it is not clear if this is a uniform feature of the illness that explains the rhombencephalitis. Judging from the clinical signs in some cases, the infection appears to affect both the brainstem parenchyma and the extraaxial portion of the lower cranial nerves.

Treatment The treatment is ampicillin (2 g intravenously q4h) in combination with gentamicin (5 mg/kg intravenously in 3 divided doses daily). If the condition of the host is compromised, the outcome is often fatal, but most of our patients without serious medical disease have made a full and prompt recovery with treatment.

Melioidosis

In India and Southeast Asia, particularly Cambodia and Thailand, a brainstem, cerebellar, and meningitic illness, similar to that caused by *Listeria,* results instead from melioidosis (*Burkholderia pseudomallei*). It should be suspected in returning travelers from that region but the disease is, of course, well known to physicians in areas endemic for the organism. Diabetics are particularly prone to this infection. The CSF shows one to several dozen white blood cells and raised protein but glucose may be normal. There is usually an associated pulmonary infection but this may be minor and the degree of temperature elevation varies. The diagnosis can be made by the culture of the organism from any body site, CSF, pharynx, blood, urine or sputum, as it is not a normal commensal bacterium but both blood agar and special Ashdown's medium containg gentamicin are required. There is a commercial serologic test but there are high background rates of positivity in endemic regions.

Treatment This is in two phases, an intesive eradication component with high intravenous doses of ceftazidime (or several equivalent regimens) for 10 to 14 days, followed by an eradication phase that is necessary to prevent relapse, using co-trimoxazole alone or accompanied by doxycycline.

Legionella

This potentially fatal respiratory disease caused by the gram-negative bacillus *Legionella pneumophila,* first came to medical notice in July 1976, when a large number of members of the American Legion fell ill at their annual convention in Philadelphia. The fatality rate was high. In addition to the obvious pulmonary infection, manifestations referable to the CNS and other organs were observed regularly. Lees and Tyrrell described patients with severe and diffuse cerebral involvement, and Baker and associates and Shetty and colleagues described others with cerebellar and brainstem syndromes. The clinical details have varied. One constellation consisted of headache, obtundation, acute confusion or delirium with high fever, and evidence of pulmonary distress; another took the form of tremor, nystagmus, cerebellar ataxia, extraocular muscle and gaze palsies, and dysarthria.

Other neurologic abnormalities have been observed, such as inappropriate ADH secretion, or a syndrome of more diffuse encephalomyelitis or transverse myelitis, similar to that observed with *Mycoplasma* infections. The CSF is usually normal and CT scans of the brain are negative, a circumstance that makes diagnosis difficult. The neuropathologic abnormalities have not been studied. Suspicion of the disease, based on exposure or on the presence of an atypical pneumonia, should prompt urine antigen and culture of blood and CSF. Serologic tests are available but require paired sera and have little impact on clinical decision making. In most patients the signs of CNS disorder resolve rapidly and completely, although residual impairment of memory and a cerebellar ataxia have been recorded. To date, the *Legionella* bacillus has not been isolated from the brain or spinal fluid.

Treatment Treatment in adults has consisted of one of levofloxacin, moxifloxacin, or azithromycin; rifampin is sometimes used. In the past, erythromycin, 0.5 to 1.0 g was used intravenously q6h for a 7 to 10 days.

Catscratch Fever (*Bartonella henselae*)

Reports of over 100 cases of encephalitis from *catscratch disease* have appeared in the medical literature and several have occurred on our services over the years, for which reason we do not consider it rare. The causative organism is a gram-negative bacillus now called *Bartonella henselae* (formerly *Rochalimaea henselae*). The illness begins as unilateral axillary or cervical adenopathy occurring after a seemingly innocuous scratch (rarely a bite) from an infected cat. The cases with which we are familiar began with an encephalopathy and high fever (higher temperature than with most of the other organisms that are capable of causing a bacterial encephalitis), followed by seizures or status epilepticus. The organism has also been implicated in causing a focal cerebral vasculitis in AIDS patients as well as neuroretinitis in both immunocompromised and immunocompetent patients. Demonstration of elevated complement-fixing titers and detection of the organism by PCR or by silver staining from an excised lymph node are diagnostic. A single high antibody titer is probably inadequate for this purpose.

Treatment First-line treatment is with azithromycin or doxycycline, sometimes with rifampin in recalcitrant cases. Erythromycin is used less frequently. Most patients recover completely, but one of our patients and a few reported by others have died.

Anthrax

This rare form of meningoencephalitis is included here because of the current interest in *Bacillus anthracis* as a bioweapon. Lanska was able to collect from the literature 70 patients with meningeal infection, most of whom were encephalopathic. He has estimated that fewer than 5 percent of infected individuals will acquire a meningoencephalitis; in a 2001 U.S. outbreak, only 1 of 11 cases with anthrax pneumonitis developed this complication. Reflecting the main site of natural infection, the majority of cases originated in cutaneous anthrax. In addition to a typically fulminating course after a prodrome of one or several days, the exceptional feature was a hemorrhagic and inflammatory spinal fluid formula. Subarachnoid hemorrhage was prominent in autopsy material, presumably reflecting necrosis of the vessel walls as a toxic effect of *B. anthracis*.

Treatment Although natural isolates are sensitive to penicillin, bioengineered strains are resistant; therefore, combined treatment with ciprofloxacin with clindamycin, rifampin, or meropenem has been recommended initially. The benefit of specific antitoxin is uncertain once meningoencephalitis has occurred.

Recently, very similar overwhelming cases with meningitis and subarachnoid hemorrhage caused by *Bacillus cereus* have appeared in immunosuppressed patients.

Brucellosis

This worldwide disease of domesticated livestock is frequently transmitted to humans in areas where the infection is enzootic. In the United States, it is distinctly rare, with 200 cases or less being reported annually since 1980, some in abattoir workers. During the 1950s it was a fashionable explanation for chronic fatigue. In the Middle East, infection with *Brucella* is still frequent, attributable to the ingestion of raw milk. In Saudi Arabia, for example, al Deeb and coworkers reported on a series of 400 cases of brucellosis, of which 13 presented with brain involvement (acute meningoencephalitis, papilledema and increased intracranial pressure, and meningovascular manifestations). The CSF showed a lymphocytic pleocytosis and increased protein content. Blood and CSF antibody titers to the organism were greater than 1:640 and 1:128, respectively.

Treatment Prolonged treatment with doxycycline with streptomycin or gentamicin; an alternative is doxycycline plus rifampin to suppress the infection.

Whipple Disease

This is a rare but often-discussed disorder, predominantly of middle-aged men. Weight loss, fever, anemia, steatorrhea, abdominal pain and distention, arthralgia, lymphadenopathy, and hyperpigmentation are the usual systemic manifestations. Less often, infection is associated with a number of neurologic syndromes. It is caused by a gram-positive bacillus, *Tropheryma whipplei*, which resides predominantly in the gut. Biopsy of the jejunal mucosa, which discloses macrophages filled with the periodic acid-Schiff (PAS)-positive organisms, is diagnostic. PAS-positive histiocytes have also been identified in the CSF, as well as in periventricular regions, in the hypothalamic and tuberal nuclei, and diffusely scattered in the brain.

The neurologic manifestations most often take the form of a slowly progressive memory loss or dementia of subacute or early chronic evolution. Supranuclear ophthalmoplegia, ataxia, seizures, myoclonus, nystagmus, and a highly characteristic oculomasticatory movement described as myorhythmia (which looks to us like rhythmic myoclonus) have been noted less often than the dementing syndrome. The rhythmic myoclonus or spasm occurs in synchronous bursts involving several adjacent regions, mainly the eyes, jaw, and face. This movement disorder is fairly specific but insensitive for Whipple disease, occurring in only approximately 10 percent of patients. As pointed out by Matthews and colleagues, cerebellar ataxia, although obviously much less specific for Whipple disease of the brain, is more frequent, occurring in about half the documented cases. Almost always, the myorhythmias are accompanied by a supranuclear vertical gaze paresis that sometimes affects horizontal eye movements as well. Presumably, the neurologic complications are the result of infiltration of the brain by the organism, but this has not been satisfactorily established.

Approximately half of the patients have a mild pleocytosis and some of these have PAS-positive material in the CSF. A variety of brain imaging abnormalities have been recorded, none characteristic, but either enhancing focal lesions or a normal scan may be found. The diagnosis is made mainly from PAS staining of an intestinal (jejunal) biopsy, as already mentioned, supplemented by PCR testing of the bowel tissue or biopsy material from brain or lymph node. In cases of subacute progressive limb and gait ataxia occurring in middle-aged or older men in whom no cause is uncovered by less-invasive means, it is justifiable to perform these tests (see Chap. 5). Rarely, the neurologic symptoms may occur in the absence of gastrointestinal disease (Adams et al, 1987). In the review of 84 cases of cerebral Whipple disease by Louis and colleagues, 71 percent had cognitive changes, half with psychiatric features; 31 percent had myoclonus; 18 percent had ataxia; and 20 percent had the oculomasticatory and skeletal myorhythmias (Schwartz et al).

Treatment A course of induction by penicillin or ceftriaxone for 2 weeks followed by trimethoprim-sulfamethoxazole or doxycycline continued for 1 year are the currently recommended regimens. An alternative approach is 2 weeks of ceftriaxone followed by treatment with trimethoprim-sulfamethoxazole or a tetracycline for a year. Antibiotic-resistant cases and instances of relapse after antibiotic treatment are known. The review by Anderson may be consulted for details.

"Acute Toxic Encephalopathy"

We are uncertain of its status but have been shown putative cases of this disorder described by Lyon and colleagues as "acute encephalopathy of obscure origin in children," a febrile and sometimes fatal illness that could not be ascribed to direct infection of the nervous system. During the height of a systemic bacterial or sometimes viral infection, the child sinks into coma, seizures are infrequent, the neck is supple, and the spinal fluid shows no changes or only a few cells. This is undoubtedly an illness of diverse causes, common among them being fluid overload and electrolyte imbalance, Reye syndrome (see Chap. 30) and, possibly most commonly, the immune condition of postinfectious encephalitis (see Chap. 36). Nonetheless, cases continue to be reported, such as those of Thi and colleagues, which can only be classified as a noninfectious bacterial encephalopathy or encephalitis. A relationship to the "septic encephalopathy" of adults, which has been emphasized by the group from London, Ontario, is possible but unproved. The term *acute toxic encephalopathy* still has some utility in cases of obscure cause, but a careful search for better-characterized causes of febrile coma must be undertaken. The acute necrotizing encephalopathy that has been reported, particularly in Asian children after influenza, belongs to this category and consists of a number of diseases as discussed by Mizuguchi and coworkers.

SUBDURAL EMPYEMA

Subdural empyema is an intracranial (rarely intraspinal) purulent process between the inner surface of the dura and the outer surface of the arachnoid that occurs mainly in children. The term *subdural abscess*, among others, had been applied to this condition but the proper name is *empyema*, indicating suppuration in a preformed space. Thrombosis of the underlying cortical veins and dural sinuses is a common accompaniment. Contrary to prevailing opinion, subdural empyema is not a rarity (although it is only about one-fifth as frequent as cerebral abscess) and is increasingly the result of surgical procedures on the sinuses and cranium.

The infection usually originates in the frontal or ethmoid or, less often, the sphenoid sinuses and in the middle ear and mastoid cells. As with bacterial meningitis, in the last decade there have been an increasing number of cases that follow surgery of the sinuses and other cranial structures. In infants and children, and infrequently in adults, there may be a spread from a leptomeningitis. Infection gains entry to the subdural space by direct extension through bone and dura or by spread from septic thrombosis of the venous sinuses, particularly the superior longitudinal sinus. Rarely, the subdural infection is metastatic from infected lungs; hardly ever is it secondary to bacteremia or septicemia. Occasionally it extends from a brain abscess.

It is of interest that cases of sinus origin have predominated in adolescent and young adult men (Kaufman et al), a distinction for which there is no explanation. In such cases, streptococci (nonhemolytic and *viridans*) are the most common organisms, followed by facultative anaerobic streptococci (often *Streptococcus milleri*) or *Bacteroides*. Less often *S. aureus*, *E. coli*, *Proteus*, and *Pseudomonas* are causative. In about half the cases unrelated to surgery, no organisms can be cultured or seen on Gram stain.

Pathology

A collection of subdural pus ranging from a few milliliters to 100 to 200 mL lies over the cerebral hemisphere. Pus may spread into the interhemispheric fissure or be confined there; occasionally it is found in the posterior fossa, covering the cerebellum. The arachnoid, when cleared of exudate, is cloudy, and thrombosis of meningeal veins may be seen. The underlying cerebral hemisphere is compressed, and in fatal cases there is often an ipsilateral temporal lobe herniation. Microscopic examination discloses various degrees of organization of the exudate on the inner surface of the dura and infiltration of the underlying arachnoid with small numbers of neutrophilic leukocytes, lymphocytes, and mononuclear cells. Thrombi in cerebral veins seem to begin on the sides of the veins nearest the subdural exudate. The superficial layers of the cerebral cortex undergo ischemic necrosis, which probably accounts for focal seizures and other signs of disordered cerebral function (Kubik and Adams).

Symptomatology and Laboratory Findings

Usually the history includes reference to chronic sinusitis or mastoiditis with a recent flare-up causing local pain and increase in purulent nasal or aural discharge. In sinus cases, the pain is over the brow or between the eyes; it is associated with tenderness on pressure over these parts and sometimes with orbital swelling. General malaise, fever, and headache—at first localized, then severe and generalized and associated with vomiting are the first indications of intracranial spread. They are followed in a few days by drowsiness and increasing stupor, rapidly progressing to coma. At about the same time, focal neurologic signs appear, the most important of which are unilateral motor seizures, hemiplegia, hemianesthesia, aphasia, and paralysis of lateral conjugate gaze. Fever and leukocytosis are always present and the neck is stiff. Cases that follow surgery may be more indolent.

The usual CSF findings are an increased pressure, pleocytosis in the range of 50 to 1,000/mm^3, a predominance of polymorphonuclear cells, elevated protein content (75 to 300 mg/dL), and normal glucose values. The spinal fluid is often sterile, but on occasion an organism is cultured. If the patient is stuporous or comatose, there is a risk associated with performing a lumbar puncture, and one should proceed first with imaging procedures.

By CT scanning one can see the ear or sinus lesions or bone erosion. The meninges around the empyema enhance and the collection of pus can be visualized more dependably with MRI. Empyema that follows meningitis in children tends to localize on the undersurface of the temporal lobe and may require coronal views to be well visualized.

Several conditions must be distinguished clinically from subdural empyema: a treated subacute bacterial meningitis, cerebral thrombophlebitis, brain abscess (see further on), herpes simplex encephalitis (see Chap. 33), acute disseminated encephalomyelitis and necrotizing hemorrhagic leukoencephalitis (see Chap. 36), and septic embolism because of bacterial endocarditis (see further on in this chapter).

Treatment

Most subdural empyemas, by the time they are recognized clinically, require drainage through multiple burr holes, or through a craniotomy in cases with an interhemispheric, subtemporal, or posterior fossa location. The surgical procedure should be coupled with appropriate antibiotic therapy, generally a third-generation cephalosporin and metronidazole. Bacteriologic findings or an unusual presumed source may dictate a change to different drugs, particularly to later-generation cephalosporins. Without such massive antimicrobial therapy and surgery, some patients will die, usually within 7 to 14 days. On the other hand, patients who are treated promptly may make a surprisingly good recovery, including full or partial resolution of their focal neurologic deficits.

As with certain small brain abscesses, small subdural collections of pus that are recognized by CT scanning or MRI before stupor and coma have supervened may respond to treatment with large doses of antibiotics alone. The resolution (or lack thereof) of the empyema can be readily followed by repeated imaging of the brain (Leys et al).

CRANIAL EPIDURAL ABSCESS

This condition is usually associated with osteomyelitis in a cranial bone and originates from an infection in the ear or paranasal sinuses, or it is from a surgical procedure, particularly if the frontal sinus or mastoid had been opened or a foreign device inserted. Rarely, the infection is metastatic or spreads outward from a dural sinus thrombophlebitis. Pus and granulation tissue accumulate on the outer surface of the dura, separating it from the cranial bone. The symptoms are those of a local inflammatory process: frontal or auricular pain, purulent discharge from sinuses or ear, and fever and local tenderness. Sometimes the neck is slightly stiff. Localizing neurologic signs are usually absent. Rarely, a focal seizure may occur, or the fifth and sixth cranial nerves may be involved with infections of the petrous part of the temporal bone. The CSF is usually clear and under normal pressure but may contain a few lymphocytes and neutrophils (20 to 100 per milliliter; fewer than in subdural empyema) and a slightly increased amount of protein. Treatment consists of antibiotics, usually vancomycin alone or with a cephalosporin, aimed at the appropriate pathogen(s)—often *S. aureus*. Later, the diseased bone in the frontal sinus or the mastoid, from which the extradural infection had arisen, may have to be removed. Results of treatment are usually good.

Spinal Epidural and Subdural Abscesses
(See Chap. 44)

These types of abscesses possess unique clinical features and constitute important neurologic and neurosurgical emergencies. They are discussed in Chap. 44 with other diseases of the spinal column and spinal cord.

INTRACRANIAL SEPTIC THROMBOPHLEBITIS (SEE ALSO CHAP. 34)

The dural sinuses drain blood from all of the brain into the jugular veins. The largest and most important of these, and the ones usually involved by infection, are the lateral (transverse), cavernous, petrous, and, less frequently, the longitudinal (sagittal) sinuses. A complex system of lesser sinuses and cerebral veins connects these large sinuses to one another as well as to the diploic and meningeal veins and veins of the face and scalp. The basilar venous sinuses are contiguous to several of the paranasal sinuses and mastoid cells.

Usually there is evidence that septic thrombophlebitis of the large dural sinuses has extended from an infection of the middle ear and mastoid cells, the paranasal sinuses, or skin around the upper lip, nose, and eyes. Other forms of intracranial infection frequently complicate these cases, including meningitis, epidural abscess, subdural empyema, and brain abscess. Occasionally, infection may be introduced by direct trauma to large veins or dural sinuses. A variety of organisms, including all the ones that ordinarily inhabit the paranasal sinuses and skin of the nose and face, may give rise to intracranial thrombophlebitis. Streptococci and staphylococci are the ones most often incriminated. With the exception of fever and poorer outcome, the syndromes associated with septic phlebitis discussed below are similar to those produced by bland thrombosis of the veins, as discussed in Chap. 34, on cerebrovascular diseases.

Septic Lateral (Transverse) Sinus Thrombophlebitis

In lateral (transverse) sinus thrombophlebitis, which usually follows chronic infection of the middle ear, mastoid, or petrous bone, earache and mastoid tenderness are succeeded, after a period of a few days to weeks by generalized headache and in some instances, papilledema. If the thrombophlebitis remains confined to the transverse sinus, there are no other neurologic signs. Spread to the jugular bulb may give rise to the syndrome of the jugular foramen (see Table 47-1) and involvement of the torcula, leading to increased intracranial pressure. One lateral sinus, usually the right, is normally larger than the other, which may account for greatly elevated pressure when it is occluded. However, contiguous involvement of the superior sagittal sinus and cortical veins emanating from it causes seizures and focal cerebral signs (see below). Fever, as in all forms of septic intracranial thrombophlebitis tends to be present but intermittent, and other signs of the septic state may be prominent. The CSF has increased pressure but the formula is usually normal but may show a small number of cells and a modest elevation of protein content. The term "otitic hydrocephalus" was introduced for this condition by Sir Charles Symonds, giving the erroneous impression that hydrocephalus was the cause of raised intracranial pressure. It is mentioned here because his clinical description, as for many other conditions, remains an outstanding source.

Imaging by MR and CT with contrast infusion has supplanted cerebral venography, arteriography, and the various older tests involving compression of the jugular veins in the diagnosis of venous sinus thrombosis. MRI sequences that are appropriate to the slow blood flow in the cerebral venous system must be selected and imaging planes carefully chosen to pass through the venous sinuses. CT and MRI are also able to detect abscess and hydrocephalus.

Prolonged administration of high doses of antibiotics is the mainstay of treatment. Anticoagulation, shown to be beneficial in aseptic venous occlusion, is still of uncertain value, but it is usually administered as well (see Chap. 34).

Septic Cavernous Sinus Thrombophlebitis

This condition is usually secondary to infections of the ethmoid, sphenoid, or maxillary sinuses or the skin around the eyes and nose, sometimes originating in a seemingly innocuous lesion. Occasionally, no antecedent infection can be recognized. In addition to headache, high fluctuating fever, and signs of systemic toxicity, there are characteristic local effects. Obstruction of the ophthalmic veins leads to chemosis, proptosis, and edema of the ipsilateral eyelids, forehead, and nose. The retinal veins become engorged, which may be followed by retinal hemorrhages and papilledema. More often, however, vision in the affected eye is lost by a yet undefined type of optic neuropathy as noted below, without visible alterations in the fundus. Involvement of the third, fourth, sixth, and ophthalmic division of the fifth cranial nerves, which lie in the lateral wall of the cavernous sinus (see Chap 34), leads to ptosis, varying degrees of ocular palsy, pain around the eye, and sensory loss over the forehead. Within a few days, spread through the circular sinus to the opposite cavernous sinus results in bilateral symptoms. The posterior part of the cavernous sinus may become infected via the superior and inferior petrosal veins without the occurrence of orbital edema or ophthalmoplegia but usually with abducens and facial paralysis. The CSF is usually normal unless there is an associated meningitis or subdural empyema.

The only effective therapy in the fulminant variety, associated with thrombosis of the anterior portion of the sinus, is the administration of high doses of antibiotics aimed at coagulase-positive staphylococci, and probably gram-negative pathogens and at anaerobes if there has been sinusitis. As with septic lateral sinus phlebitis, anticoagulants have been used, but their value has not been proved. In our cases, the cranial-nerve palsies have resolved to a large extent, but visual loss, if it occurs, tends to remain, with findings suggestive of infarction of the retroorbital part of the optic nerve; the mechanism of this complication is not clear. Cavernous sinus thrombosis must be differentiated from mucormycosis infection of the sinuses and from orbital cellulitis, which usually occur in patients with uncontrolled diabetes, and from other fungus infections (notably *Aspergillus*), carcinomatous invasion of the sphenoid bone, Wegener granulomatosis, and sphenoid wing meningioma.

Septic Thrombosis of the Superior Sagittal Sinus

Now less common than at a time when uncontrolled ear and sinus infections were common, this may be asymptomatic but more often there is a clinical syndrome of fever, headache, unilateral convulsions, and motor weakness, first on one side of the body, then on the other, as a result of extension of the thrombophlebitis into the superior cerebral veins. Papilledema and increased intracranial pressure almost always accompany these signs. Severe generalized and vertex headache is a typical but not invariable complaint. Because of the localization of function in the cortex that is drained by the sinus, the weakness may take the form of a crural (lower limb) monoplegia or, less often, of paraplegia. A corticosensory loss may occur in the same distribution. Homonymous hemianopia or quadrantanopia, aphasia, paralysis of conjugate gaze, and urinary incontinence (in bilateral cases) have also been observed.

As in the case of aseptic thrombosis, loss of the flow void in the superior sagittal sinus in the MRI is diagnostic, and the clot may be visualized if the correct imaging sequences are used. A similar change can be seen on axial images of the contrast-enhanced CT scan by altering the viewing windows so as to show the clot within the posterior portion of the sagittal sinus. The CT scan performed early in the illness without contrast infusion usually shows the high-density clot within cortical veins as well, but only if carefully studied by altering the viewing window at the machine's console.

Treatment consists of high doses of antibiotics and temporization until the thrombus recanalizes. Although not of proven benefit (as it is in bland cerebral vein thrombosis), we have used heparin in these circumstances unless there are very large biparietal hemorrhagic infarctions. Because of the highly epileptogenic nature of the attendant venous infarction, we have also administered antiepileptic drugs prophylactically, but there is no clinical study to guide the clinician in this regard. Recovery from paralysis may be complete, or the patient may be left with seizures and varying degrees of spasticity in the lower limbs.

It should be reiterated that all types of thrombophlebitis, especially those related to infections of the ear and paranasal sinuses, may be simultaneously associated with other forms of intracranial purulent infection, namely bacterial meningitis, subdural empyema, or brain abscess. Therapy in these complicated forms of infection must be individualized. As a rule, the best plan is to institute antibiotic treatment of the intracranial disease and to decide, after it has been brought under control, whether surgery on the offending ear or sinus is necessary. To operate on the primary focus before medical treatment has taken hold is to court disaster. In cases complicated by bacterial meningitis, treatment of the latter usually takes precedence over the surgical treatment of complications, such as brain abscess and subdural empyema.

Aseptic thrombosis of intracranial venous sinuses and cerebral veins is discussed in Chap. 34 on cerebrovascular disease; aspects related to intracranial pressure are discussed in Chap. 30, on CSF circulation.

BRAIN ABSCESS

With the exception of a small proportion of cases (approximately 10 percent) in which infection is introduced from the outside (compound fractures of the skull, intracranial operation, bullet wounds), brain abscess is always secondary to bacteremia and a bacterial focus elsewhere in the body. Purulent pulmonary infections (abscess, bronchiectasis) and bacterial endocarditis account for the largest number of brain abscesses in the modern era. A decreasing proportion of brain abscesses in the current era is related to disease of the paranasal sinuses, middle ear, and mastoid cells. Of those originating in the ear, about one-third lie in the anterolateral part of the cerebellar hemisphere; the remainder occurs in the middle and inferior parts of the temporal lobe. The sinuses most frequently implicated are the frontal and sphenoid, and the abscesses derived from them are in the frontal and temporal lobes, respectively.

Pathogenesis

Otogenic and rhinogenic abscesses reach the nervous system by direct extension, in which the bone of the middle ear or nasal sinuses becomes the seat of an osteomyelitis, with penetration of the dura and leptomeninges, infection may spread along the major intracranial veins. Thrombophlebitis of the pial veins and dural sinuses, by infarcting brain tissue, renders the latter more vulnerable to invasion by infectious material. The close anatomic relationship of the lateral (transverse) sinus to the cerebellum explains the frequency with which this portion of the brain is infected via the venous route. The spread along venous channels also explains how an abscess may sometimes form at a considerable distance from the primary focus in the middle ear or paranasal sinuses.

As mentioned, the majority of brain abscesses is metastatic, i.e., hematogenous. These are traceable to bacterial endocarditis or to a primary septic focus in the lungs or pleura, as indicated earlier. Other metastatic abscesses are related to a congenital cardiac defect or pulmonary arteriovenous malformation that permits infected emboli to bypass the pulmonary circulation and reach the brain. Occasional cases are associated with infected pelvic organs, skin, tonsils, abscessed teeth, and osteomyelitis of noncranial bones. In approximately 20 percent of cases, the source cannot be ascertained.

Metastatic abscesses from hematogenous spread are usually situated in the distal territory of the middle cerebral arteries (Fig. 32-1), and they sometimes multiply, in contrast to otogenic and rhinogenic abscesses. Also, almost all deep cerebral abscesses have a systemic source. It should also be noted that the clinical and radiologic features of a solitary abscess mimic those of a brain tumor. Small and miliary abscesses may progress to large ones.

A careful distinction had in the past been made between the neuropathologic effects of endocarditis caused by different organisms. What had been divided into acute bacterial endocarditis (ABE) and subacute bacterial endocarditis (SBE) are now instead characterized by the virulence of the causative organism. For example, endocarditis from the implantation in the brain of streptococci of low virulence (alpha and gamma streptococci) or similar organisms on valves previously damaged by rheumatic fever seldom gives rise to a brain abscess. In contrast, organisms such as *S. aureus* and gram-negative bacteria have a propensity to cause abscesses. The cerebral lesions in all forms of endocarditis are a result of embolic occlusion of vessels by fragments of vegetations and bacteria, which cause infarction of brain tissue and a restricted inflammatory response around the involved blood vessels and the overlying meninges (cerebritis). It is the subsequent evolution of the process that is dependent on the inherent tendency of the organism to be invasive. Therefore, the former distinction between acute and subacute bacterial endocarditis has become less useful. The cerebral symptoms of a stroke may be the first clinical manifestations of the disease. Over time, sometimes within days but usually longer, the inflamed artery may form an aneurysm (mycotic aneurysm) that later gives rise to parenchymal or subarachnoid hemorrhage (see Chap. 34). Bacterial meningitis rarely develops with abscess and most often the CSF is sterile but there are exceptions.

Rapidly evolving cerebral signs in patients with acute endocarditis are nearly always caused by septic embolic infarction or hemorrhage. Anticoagulation has not been shown to reduce the incidence of embolization from endocarditis; the risk of inducing hemorrhage is uncertain but may have been overestimated in the past. In patients with endocarditis on a prosthetic heart valve, anticoagulation may be continued, but this treatment is suspended if there is a hemorrhagic brain infarction.

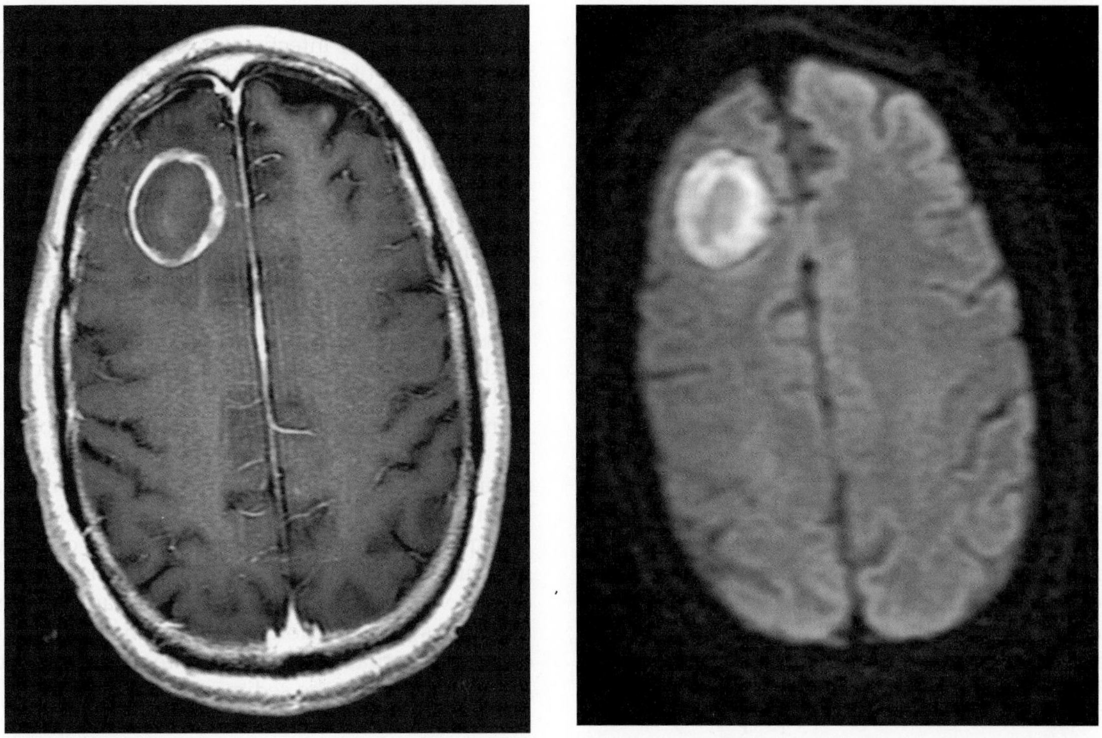

Figure 32-1. MRI showing a right frontal brain abscesses associated with bacterial endocarditis (*S. aureus*) in a 55-year-old man. There is characteristic rim enhancement with gadolinium (*left panel*) and restricted diffusion within the abscess (*right panel*).

Existing anticoagulation need not be reversed unless a cerebral hemorrhage evolves.

It is estimated that 5 percent of cases of *congenital heart disease* are complicated by brain abscess (Cohen; Newton). Viewed from another perspective, in children, more than 60 percent of cerebral abscesses are associated with congenital heart disease. The abscess is usually solitary; this fact, coupled with the potentially correctable underlying cardiac abnormality, makes the recognition of brain abscess in congenital heart disease a matter of considerable practical importance. For some unknown reason, brain abscess associated with congenital heart disease is rarely seen before the third year of life. The tetralogy of Fallot is by far the most common anomaly implicated, but the abscesses may occur with any right-to-left intracardiac or pulmonary shunt that allows venous blood returning to the heart to enter the systemic circulation without first passing through the lungs. Pulmonary emboli, by increasing the back pressure in the right heart, may open (make patent) an occult foramen ovale. A pulmonary arteriovenous malformation has a similar effect. Nearly half of the reported cases of pulmonary arteriovenous fistulas have *Osler-Rendu-Weber telangiectasia.* When the filtering effect of the lungs is thus circumvented, pyogenic bacteria or infected emboli from a variety of sources may gain access to the brain, where, aided by the effects of venous stasis and perhaps of infarction, an abscess is established.

Etiology

The most common organisms causing bacterial cerebral abscess are virulent streptococci, many of which are anaerobic or microaerophilic. These organisms are often found in combination with other anaerobes, notably *Bacteroides, Fusibacterium,* and *Prevotella and less often, Propionibacterium* (diphtheroids), and may be combined with *Hemophilus species,* Enterobacteriaceae, such as *E. coli* and *Proteus.* Staphylococci also commonly cause brain abscess, but pneumococci, meningococci, and *H. influenzae* rarely do. In addition, the gram-positive higher bacteria *Actinomyces* and *Nocardia* and certain fungi discussed later, notably *Candida, Mucor,* and *Aspergillus,* are isolated in some cases.

The type of organism tends to vary with the source of the abscess; staphylococcal abscesses are usually a consequence of accidental or surgical trauma, sometimes of endocarditis, especially in drug addicts who inject themselves; enteric organisms are almost always associated with otitic infections; and anaerobic streptococci are commonly metastatic from the lung and paranasal sinuses. Predisposing to nocardial brain abscess is pulmonary nocardial infection, often in immunosuppressed patients; this diagnosis is doubtful without a pneumonic infiltrate. Thus knowledge of the antecedent history enables one to institute appropriate therapy while awaiting the results of bacterial and fungal cultures. In immunosuppressed patients, brain abscess is usually from a nonbacterial organism; fungi and parasites (toxoplasmosis) prevail.

Pathology

Localized inflammatory exudate, septic thrombosis of vessels, and aggregates of degenerating leukocytes represent the early reaction to bacterial invasion of the brain. Surrounding the necrotic tissue are macrophages, astroglia, microglia, and many small veins, some of which show endothelial hyperplasia, contain fibrin, and are cuffed with polymorphonuclear leukocytes. There is interstitial edema in the surrounding white matter. At this stage, which is rarely observed postmortem, the lesion is poorly circumscribed and tends to enlarge by a coalescence of inflammatory foci. The term *cerebritis* is loosely applied to this local suppurative encephalitis or immature abscess.

Within several days, the intensity of the reaction begins to subside and the infection tends to become delimited. The center of the abscess takes on the character of pus; at the periphery, fibroblasts proliferate from the adventitia of newly formed blood vessels and form granulation tissue, which is readily identified pathologically within 2 weeks of the onset of the infection but it is evident earlier as restriction of diffusion on MRI. As the abscess becomes more chronic, the granulation tissue is replaced by collagenous connective tissue. It has also been noted, both in experimental animals and in humans, that the capsule of the abscess is not of uniform thickness, frequently being thinner on its medial (paraventricular) aspect. These factors account for the propensity of cerebral abscesses to spread deeply into the white matter and to produce daughter abscesses or a chain of abscesses and extensive surrounding cerebral edema. In some instances, the process culminates in a catastrophic rupture into the ventricles.

Clinical Manifestations

Headache is probably the most frequent initial symptom of intracranial abscess but this varies and a considerable number of cases are revealed incidentally. Other early symptoms, roughly in order of their frequency are drowsiness and confusion; focal or generalized seizures; and focal motor, sensory, or speech disorders. Fever and leukocytosis are not consistently present, depending on the phase of the development of the abscess at the time of presentation (see below). In patients who harbor chronic ear, sinus, or pulmonary infections, a recent activation of the infection frequently precedes the onset of cerebral symptoms. In patients without an obvious focus of infection, headache or other cerebral symptoms may appear abruptly on a background of mild general ill health or congenital heart disease. In some patients, bacterial invasion of the brain may be asymptomatic or may be attended only by a transitory focal neurologic disorder, as might happen when a septic embolus briefly lodges in a brain artery. Sometimes stiff neck accompanies generalized headache, suggesting the diagnosis of meningitis (especially a partially treated one).

Localizing neurologic signs become evident sooner or later, but, like papilledema, they occur relatively late in the course of the illness. The nature of the focal neurologic defect will, of course, depend on the location of the abscess as fully explicated in Chap. 22. In *cerebellar abscess*, the headache is generally postauricular or occipital; the signs are those expected for disease of this part of the brain.

The treacherous aspect of brain abscess is that the signs of systemic infection may be entirely absent. The invasive stage of cerebral infection may be so inconspicuous, and the course so indolent, that the entire clinical picture may not differ from that of malignant brain tumor. Although slight *fever* is characteristic of the early invasive phase of cerebral abscess, the temperature may return to normal as the abscess becomes encapsulated; the same is true of leukocytosis. The sedimentation rate is usually elevated. Although lumbar puncture is not recommended, in the early stages of abscess formation the CSF pressure is moderately increased; and there is a mild to moderate pleocytosis with 10 to 80 percent neutrophils; and the protein content is modestly elevated, rarely more than 100 mg/dL. Glucose values are not lowered, and the CSF is sterile unless there is concomitant bacterial meningitis. As already mentioned, the combination of brain abscess and acute bacterial meningitis occurs only infrequently. In some patients, abscess is combined with subdural empyema; in these instances the clinical picture can be very complicated, although headache, fever, and focal signs again predominate. In a small number of cases, especially partially treated ones, there are no spinal fluid abnormalities and the sedimentation rate may be normal.

It is apparent from this overview that the clinical picture of brain abscess is far from stereotyped. Whereas headache is the most prominent feature in most patients, seizures or certain focal signs may predominate in others, and a considerable number of patients will present with only signs of increased intracranial pressure. In some instances the symptoms evolve swiftly over a week, new ones being added day by day. In such cases the abscess may become apparent only when cerebral imaging performed for the evaluation of headache or other symptoms discloses a ring-enhancing mass. Even then, the radiologic distinction between tumor and abscess is not straightforward, depending often on the presence of a uniform, enhancing capsule that is typical of a mature abscess (see below). An impressive feature of cerebral abscess is the unpredictability with which the symptoms may evolve, particularly in children. Thus, a patient whose clinical condition seems to have stabilized may, in a matter of hours or a day or two, advance to an irreversible state of coma. Often this is caused by rupture of the abscess into the subarachnoid or ventricular CSF.

Diagnosis

CT and MRI are the most important diagnostic tools. In the CT scan, the capsule of the abscess enhances and the center of the abscess and surrounding edematous white matter are hypodense. With MRI, in T1-weighted images, the capsule enhances and the interior of the abscess is hypointense and shows restricted diffusion; in T2-weighted images, the surrounding edema is apparent and the capsule is hypointense and there is variable diffusion restriction within the lesion (Fig. 32-1, right). The abscess capsule tends to be thinner on the side directed to the lateral ventricle. Cerebritis appears as dot-sized areas of decreased density that enhance with gadolinium. Practically all abscesses larger than 1 cm produce positive scans. There is almost no likelihood of cerebral abscess if enhanced CT and MRI studies are negative. Blood cultures, sedimentation rate, and chest radiography are indispensable in the complete diagnosis of brain abscess, although it must be acknowledged that blood cultures are likely to be unrevealing except in cases of acute endocarditis.

If there is no apparent source of infection and there are only signs and symptoms of a mass lesion, the differential diagnosis includes tuberculous or fungal abscess, glioma, metastatic carcinoma, toxoplasmosis, subdural hematoma, subacute infarction of the basal ganglia or thalamus, and resolving cerebral hemorrhage or infarction. Sometimes only surgical exploration will settle the issue, but one must be cautious in interpreting the stereotactic biopsy if only inflammatory and gliotic tissue is obtained, as these changes may appear in the neighborhood of either abscess or tumor.

Treatment

During the stage of cerebritis and early abscess formation, which is essentially an acute focal encephalitis, intracranial operation accomplishes little and probably adds only further injury and swelling of brain tissue and possibly dissemination of the infection. Some cases can be cured at this stage by the adequate administration of high-dose antibiotics. Even before bacteriologic examination of the intracerebral mass, certain antibiotics can be given, with the choice based on the predisposing condition (vancomycin, a second- or third-generation cephalosporin such as ceftriaxone, and either meropenem or metronidazole). If a penicillin- or oxacillin-sensitive organism is suspected or isolated, those agents are superior to vancomycin. These drugs are given intravenously in divided daily doses. Metronidazole is so well absorbed from the gastrointestinal tract that it can be administered orally, 500 mg q6h.

This choice of antimicrobial agents is based on the fact that anaerobic streptococci and *Bacteroides* are often among the causative organisms. Evidence of staphylococcal infection can be presumed if there has been recent neurosurgery or head trauma or a demonstrable bacterial endocarditis with this organism. Abscesses caused by bacteria of oral origin do not respond well to any of these regimens because of the frequency of gram-negative organisms; penicillin and metronidazole are usually adequate for odontogenic infections but a third- or fourth-generation cephalosporin, such as cefotaxime, 2 g q4h intravenously, is often used. In all cases, several weeks of treatment are advised.

The initial elevation of intracranial pressure and threatening temporal lobe or cerebellar herniation can be managed by the use of intravenous mannitol (or hypertonic saline) and dexamethasone, 6 to 12 mg q6h. If improvement does not begin promptly, it becomes necessary to aspirate the abscess stereotactically or remove it by an open procedure that also allows precise etiologic diagnosis (Gram stain and culture). The decision regarding aspiration or open removal of the abscess is governed by its location and the course of clinical signs and by the degree of mass effect and surrounding edema as visualized by repeated scans.

Only if the abscess is solitary, superficial, and well encapsulated or associated with a foreign body should total excision be attempted; if the abscess is deep, aspiration performed stereotactically and repeated if necessary is currently the method of choice. If the location of the abscess is such that it causes obstructive hydrocephalus, for example, in the thalamus adjacent to the third ventricle or in the cerebellum, it is advisable to remove or aspirate the mass and to drain the ventricles externally for a limited time. While it has been our practice to recommend either complete excision for posterior fossa and fungal abscesses or aspiration if they are deep, there is still a lack of unanimity as to the optimal surgical approach. Some neurosurgeons instill antibiotics into the abscess cavity following aspiration, but the efficacy of this treatment is difficult to judge.

The least satisfactory results are obtained if the patient is comatose before treatment is started; more than 50 percent of such patients in the past have died. If treatment is begun while the patient is alert, the mortality is in the range of 5 to 10 percent, and even multiple metastatic abscesses may respond. Approximately 30 percent of surviving patients are left with neurologic residua. Of these, focal epilepsy is the most troublesome. Following successful treatment of a cerebral abscess in a patient with congenital heart disease, correction of the cardiac anomaly is indicated to prevent recurrence. One may even consider closing a patent foramen ovale using interventional or open surgical methods if no other explanation for the abscess is apparent.

SUBACUTE AND CHRONIC FORMS OF MENINGITIS

There are many infectious processes that induce an inflammation of the leptomeninges of lesser intensity and more chronicity than the acute forms described earlier. Included are some bacterial and most fungal infections, tuberculosis, syphilis, Lyme disease, HIV infection, and presumed noninfectious causes, such as lymphoma, sarcoidosis, Wegener granulomatosis, and others. As pointed out by Ellner and Bennett many decades ago, the clinical syndrome of chronic meningitis comprises confusion or cognitive decline, seizures, an absence of lateralizing and focal cerebral signs, with or without headache, and mild stiffness of the neck. In most cases there is little or no fever or other manifestation of infection. The CSF will often not divulge the causative agent, as the organisms are usually by nature more difficult to detect and culture. The main identifiable forms of subacute and chronic meningitis are described below. Chapter 33 addresses the approach to the complicated problem of chronic nonbacterial meningitis (aseptic meningitis) in which no cause can be found, and should be referred to along with this section.

Tuberculous Meningitis

In the United States and in most western countries, the incidence of tuberculous meningitis, which parallels the frequency of systemic tuberculosis, has, until recently, decreased steadily and markedly since World War II. Since 1985, however, there has been a moderate increase in the incidence of systemic tuberculosis (and tuberculous meningitis) in the United States—a 16 percent annual increase compared to an average annual decline of 6 percent during the preceding 30 years (Snider and Roper). This trend has recently been reversed in the United States because HIV is under better control. In fact, tuberculosis may be the first clinical manifestation of HIV infection (Barnes et al); among patients with full-blown AIDS, the incidence of tuberculosis is almost 500 times the incidence in the general population (Pitchenik et al). In developing countries, particularly in sub-Saharan Africa, recent estimates of the incidence of tuberculosis suggest that it is 25 times more frequent than in the United States, again largely because of the prevalence of HIV infection.

Pathogenesis

Tuberculous meningitis is usually caused by the acid-fast organism *Mycobacterium tuberculosis* and exceptionally by *Mycobacterium bovis, Mycobacterium avian, Mycobacterium kansasii,* and *Mycobacterium fortuitum* (the last of these after neurosurgical procedures and cranial trauma). The emergence of AIDS has led to a marked increase in cases caused by both the main organism and also by the two atypical mycobacteria. In a monograph as informative today as it was 70 years ago, Rich described two stages in the pathogenesis of tuberculous meningitis: first a bacterial seeding of the meninges and subpial regions of the brain with the formation of tubercles, followed by the rupture of one or more of the tubercles and the discharge of bacteria into the subarachnoid space. Whether the meningitis always originates in this way is unlikely. It can be said, however, that the meningitis may occur as a terminal event in cases of miliary tuberculosis or as part of generalized tuberculosis with only a single focus (tuberculoma) in the brain.

Pathologic Findings

Small, discrete white tubercles are scattered over the base of the cerebral hemispheres and to a lesser degree on the convexities. The brunt of the pathologic process falls on the basal meninges, where a thick, gelatinous exudate accumulates, obliterating the pontine and interpeduncular cisterns and extending to the meninges around the medulla, the floor of the third ventricle and subthalamic region, the optic chiasm, and the undersurfaces of the temporal lobes. There may be multiple small abscesses (Fig. 32-2) or a more uniform exudate in the leptomeninges. By comparison, the convexities are little involved, possibly because the associated hydrocephalus obliterates the cerebral subarachnoid space. Microscopically, the meningeal tubercles are like those in other parts of the body, consisting of a central zone of caseation surrounded by epithelioid cells and some giant cells, lymphocytes, plasma cells, and connective tissue. The exudate is composed of fibrin, lymphocytes, plasma cells, other mononuclear cells, and some polymorphonuclear leukocytes. The ependyma and choroid plexus are studded with minute glistening tubercles. The exudate also surrounds the spinal cord. Unlike the typical bacterial meningitides, the disease process is not confined to the subarachnoid space but frequently penetrates the pia and ependyma and invades the underlying brain, so that the process is truly a *meningoencephalitis*.

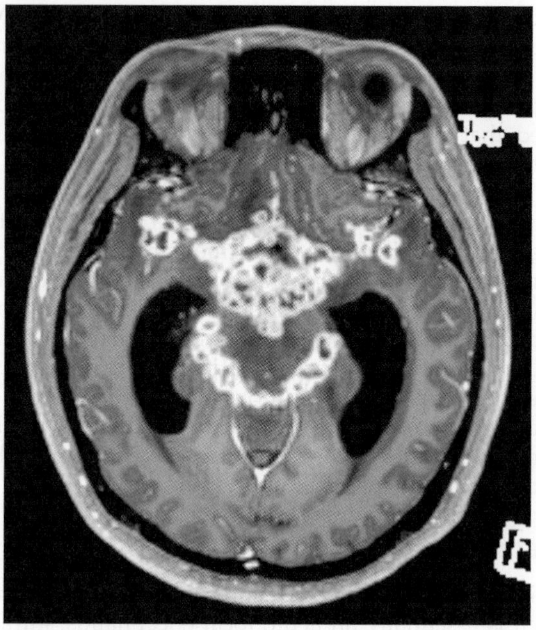

Figure 32-2. MRI in tuberculous meningitis showing gadolinium enhancement of the basal meninges, reflecting microabscesses and intense inflammation, accompanied by hydrocephalus and cranial nerve palsies.

Other pathologic changes depend on the chronicity of the disease process and recapitulate the changes that occur in the subacute and chronic stages of the other bacterial meningitides (see Table 32-1). Cranial nerves are often involved by the inflammatory exudate as they traverse the subarachnoid space, indeed, far more often than with typical bacterial meningitis. Arteries may become inflamed and occluded, with infarction of brain. Blockage of the basal cisterns frequently results in a meningeal, obstructive hydrocephalus. Marked ependymitis with blocking of the CSF in the aqueduct or fourth ventricle is a less-common cause. The exudate occasionally predominates around the spinal cord, leading to multiple spinal radiculopathies and compression of the cord.

Clinical Features

Tuberculous meningitis occurs in persons of all ages. Formerly, it was more frequent in young children, but now it is more frequent in adults, at least in the United States. The early manifestations are usually low-grade fever, malaise, headache (more than 50 percent of cases), lethargy, confusion, and stiff neck (75 percent of cases), with Kernig and Brudzinski signs. Characteristically, these symptoms evolve much less rapidly in tuberculous than in bacterial meningitis, usually over a period of a week or two, sometimes longer. In young children and infants, apathy, hyperirritability, vomiting, and seizures are the usual symptoms; however, stiff neck may not be prominent or may be absent altogether.

Because of the inherent chronicity of the disease, signs of cranial nerve involvement (usually ocular palsies, less-often facial palsies or deafness) and papilledema may be present at the time that the infection is recognized (20 percent of cases). Occasionally, the disease may present with the rapid onset of a focal neurologic deficit because of hemorrhagic infarction, with signs of raised intracranial pressure or with symptoms referable to the spinal cord and nerve roots. Hypothermia and hyponatremia have been additional features in several of our cases at the time of discovery of the meningitis.

In approximately two-thirds of patients with tuberculous meningitis there is evidence of active tuberculosis elsewhere, usually in the lungs and occasionally in the small bowel, bone, kidney, or ear. In some patients, however, only inactive pulmonary lesions are found, and in others there is no evidence of tuberculosis outside of the nervous system. As mentioned, among our adult patients, tuberculous meningitis is now seen largely in those with AIDS, but also in alcoholics, and in people who have emigrated from Asia, Africa, and India, and certain locations in the former Soviet Union. Except for the emergence of drug-resistant organisms, the HIV infection does not appear to much change the clinical manifestations or the outcome of tuberculous meningitis. However, others disagree with this statement, pointing out that the course of the bacterial infection is accelerated in AIDS patients, with more frequent involvement of organs other than the lungs. Whether or not HIV infection alters the natural history of tuberculous meningitis, treatment of the HIV infection is of paramount importance and should be started within 2 weeks of the onset of antituberculous therapy.

If tuberculous meningitis is untreated, its course is characterized by confusion and progressively deepening stupor and coma, coupled with cranial-nerve palsies, pupillary abnormalities, focal neurologic deficits, raised intracranial pressure, and decerebrate postures; invariably, untreated, a fatal outcome then follows within 4 to 8 weeks of the onset.

Laboratory Studies

The most important diagnostic test is lumbar puncture, which preferably should be performed before the administration of antibiotics. The CSF is usually under increased pressure and contains between 50 and 500 white cells per cubic millimeter, rarely more. Early in the disease there may be a more-or-less-equal number of polymorphonuclear leukocytes and lymphocytes, but after several days lymphocytes predominate in the majority of cases. In some cases, however, *M. tuberculosis* causes a *persistent polymorphonuclear pleocytosis*, the other usual causes of this CSF formula being *Nocardia*, *Aspergillus*, and *Actinomyces* (Peacock). The protein content of the CSF is always elevated, between 100 and 200 mg/dL in most cases, but much higher if the flow of CSF is blocked around the spinal cord. Glucose is reduced to levels below 40 mg/dL, but rarely to the very low values observed in pyogenic meningitis; the glucose falls slowly and a reduction may become manifest only several days after the patient has been admitted to the hospital. The serum sodium and chloride and CSF chloride are often reduced, in most instances because of inappropriate ADH secretion or an addisonian state due to tuberculosis of the adrenals.

Most children with tuberculous meningitis have positive tuberculin skin tests (85 percent) but the rate is far lower in adults with or without AIDS: 40 to 60 percent in most series.

The previously conventional methods of demonstrating tubercle bacilli in the spinal fluid are inconsistent and often too slow for immediate therapeutic decisions. Success with the traditional identification of tubercle bacilli in smears of CSF sediment stained by the Ziehl-Neelsen method is a function not only of their number but also of the persistence with which they are sought. There are effective means of culturing the tubercle bacilli; because their quantity is usually small, however, attention must be paid to proper technique. The amount of CSF submitted to the laboratory is critical; the more that is cultured, the greater the chances of recovering the organism. Unless one of the newer techniques is used, growth in culture media is not seen for 3 to 4 weeks.

More widely used test now is polymerase chain reaction amplification from the CSF, which rapidly permits the detection of small amounts of tubercle bacilli. The sensitivity of this test is stated to be close to 80 percent but there is a 10 percent false-positive rate. There is also a rapid culture technique that allows identification of the organisms in less than 1 week. However, even these new diagnostic methods may give uncertain results or take several days to demonstrate the organism and they cannot be counted on to exclude the diagnosis. For these reasons, if a presumptive diagnosis of tuberculous meningitis has been made and cryptococcosis and other fungal infections and meningeal neoplasia have been reasonably excluded, treatment can be instituted without waiting for the results of bacteriologic study.

Other diagnostic procedures (CT, MRI) are necessary in patients who present with or develop raised intracranial pressure, hydrocephalus, or focal neurologic deficits. One or more tuberculomas may also be visualized (Fig. 32-2 and 32-3) or there may be deep cerebral infarction from occlusion of vessels of the circle of Willis or one of its primary branches. MR or CT angiography may demonstrate vascular occlusive disease from granulomatous infiltration of the walls of arteries.

Other Forms of Central Nervous System Tuberculosis

Tuberculous Serous Meningitis

This condition, which is essentially a self-limited meningitis, is observed with some frequency in countries where tuberculosis is prevalent. The CSF shows a modest pleocytosis in some, but not all, cases, a normal or elevated protein content, and normal glucose levels. Headache, lethargy, and confusion are present in some cases and there are mild meningeal signs. Lincoln, who was the first to call attention to this syndrome, believed it to be a meningeal reaction to an adjacent tuberculous focus that did not progress to frank meningitis but this form of meningitis is not always self-limited.

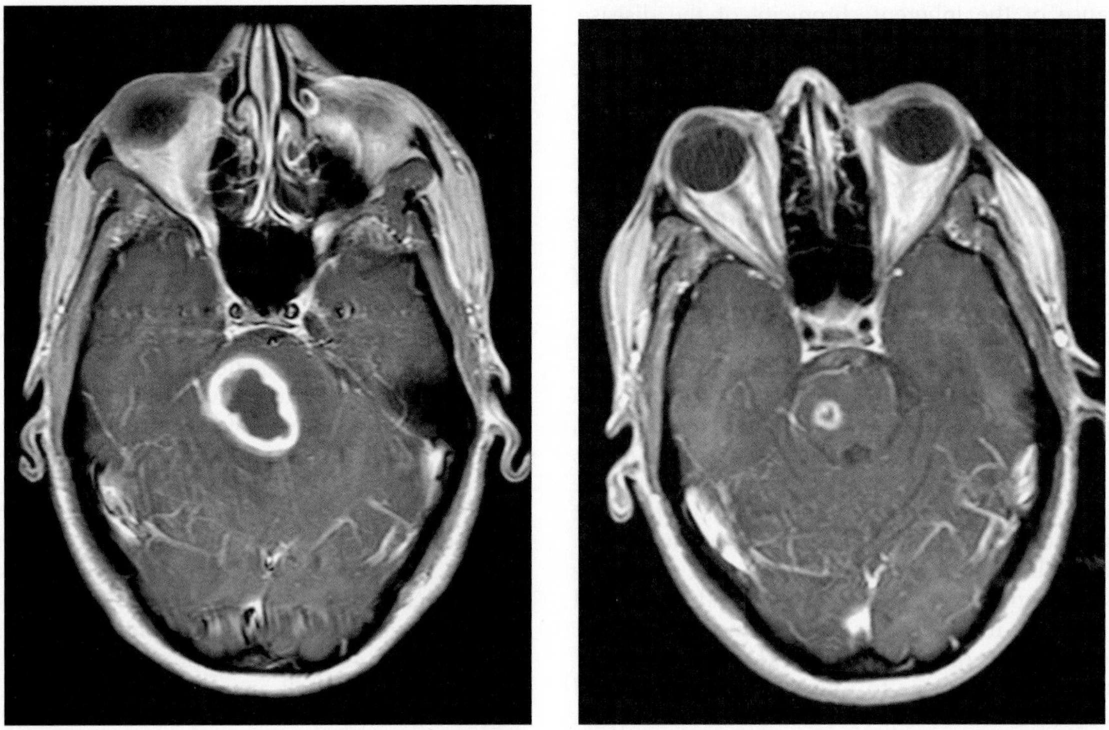

Figure 32-3. A tuberculoma of the pons on a gadolinium-enhanced MRI (*left panel*). There is a thick, uniform enhancing rim. The mass behaved clinically like a malignant brain tumor. The right panel shows the same lesion after antituberculous treatment.

Tuberculoma

These are tumor-like masses of tuberculous granulation tissue, most often multiple but also occurring singly, that form in the parenchyma of the brain and range from 2 to 12 mm in diameter (Fig. 32-3). The larger ones may produce symptoms of a space-occupying lesion and periventricular ones may cause obstructive hydrocephalus, but many are unaccompanied by symptoms of focal cerebral disease. In the United States, tuberculomas are rare; in developing countries, however, they constitute from 5 to 30 percent of all intracranial mass lesions. In some tropical countries, cerebellar tuberculomas are the most frequent intracranial tumors in children. Because of their proximity to the meninges, the CSF often contains a small number of lymphocytes and increased protein (serous meningitis), but the glucose level is not reduced. True tuberculous abscesses of the brain are rare except in AIDS patients. In two of our patients who presented with a brainstem tuberculoma, there was a serous meningitis that progressed to a fatal generalized tuberculous meningitis.

Myeloradiculitis

The spinal cord may be affected in a number of ways in the course of tuberculous infection. In addition to compressing spinal roots and cord, causing spinal block, the inflammatory meningeal exudate may invade the underlying parenchyma, producing signs of posterior and lateral column and spinal root disease. Spinal cord symptoms may also accompany tuberculous osteomyelitis of the spine with compression of the cord by an epidural abscess, a mass of granulation tissue (Pott disease, "Pott paraplegia"), or, less frequently, by the mechanical effects of angulation of the vertebral column. Pott disease, a tuberculous osteomyelitis of the spine that leads to compression of vertebral bodies and a highly characteristic kyphotic deformity at the thoracic or upper lumbar level, is discussed in Chap. 44.

Treatment of Central Nervous System Tuberculous Infections

The treatment of tuberculous meningitis consists of the administration of a combination of four drugs—isoniazid (INH), rifampin (RMP), ethambutol (EMB), and/or pyrazinamide (PZA) for the first 2 months. Some regimens omit the last drug but recent recommendations from various U.S. societies prefer the four-drug combination. An alternative regimen is INH, PZA, high-dose RMP, and moxifloxacin. All of these drugs have the capacity to penetrate the blood–brain barrier, with INH and PZA ranks higher than the others in this respect. Resistant strains of tuberculous organisms are emerging, requiring the use of second-line drugs. It has been pointed out that individuals from certain countries (e.g., Vietnam, Haiti, Philippines, former Soviet Union) have high rates of INH, and sometimes EMB-resistant organisms. In these cases of multidrug resistance, ethionamide (ETA) must be added as a fifth drug. Antibiotics must be given for a prolonged period, 9 to 12 months if first-line treatment has been given (although it may not be necessary to give all 3 or 4 drugs for the entire period).

INH is the single most effective drug. It can be given in a single daily dose of 5 mg/kg in adults and 10 mg/kg in children. Its most important adverse effects are neuropathy (see Chap. 40) and hepatitis, particularly in alcoholics. Neuropathy can be prevented by the administration of 50 mg pyridoxine daily. In patients who develop the symptoms of hepatitis or who have abnormal liver function tests, INH should be discontinued. The usual dose of RMP is 10 mg/kg daily for adults, 15 mg/kg for children. Ethambutol is given in a single daily dose of 15 mg/kg. The dosage of ETA is 15 to 25 mg/kg daily for adults; because of its tendency to produce gastric irritation, it is given in divided doses, after meals. The latter two drugs (EMB and ETA) may cause optic neuropathy, so that patients taking them should have regular examinations of visual acuity and red-green color discrimination. Pyrazinamide is given once daily in doses of 20 to 35 mg/kg. Rash, gastrointestinal disturbances, and hepatitis are the main adverse effects. Except for INH, all these drugs can be given only orally or by stomach tube. INH and rifampin may be given parenterally.

Corticosteroids may be used in patients whose lives are threatened by the effects of subarachnoid block or raised intracranial pressure but only in conjunction with antituberculous drugs. A randomized study conducted in Vietnam, including patients with and without AIDS, showed that the addition of intravenous dexamethasone (0.4 mg/kg daily for a week and then tapering doses for 3 to 6 weeks) reduced mortality from 41 percent to 32 percent but had no effect on residual disability (Thwaites et al).

Intracranial tuberculoma calls for a similar course of antibiotics, as outlined above. Under the influence of these drugs, the tuberculoma(s) may decrease in size and small ones ultimately disappear or calcify, as judged by the CT scan; if they do not, and especially if there is "mass effect," excision may be necessary. Patients with spinal osteomyelitis or localized granulomas with instability or spinal cord compression (Pott paraplegia) should be explored surgically after an initial course of chemotherapy, and an attempt should be made to excise the tuberculous focus. We have, however, dealt successfully with tuberculous osteomyelitis of the cervical spine (without significant abscess or cord compression) by immobilizing our patient in a hard collar and administering triple-drug therapy (at the suggestion of the patient's father, who was a physician in India), once it was established that the spinal column was stable, the collar could be removed. Thus, flexion–extension x-rays can be valuable if they can be obtained safely.

The overall mortality of patients with CNS tuberculosis is still significant (approximately 10 percent), infants and the elderly being at greatest risk. Among HIV-infected patients, the mortality from tuberculous meningitis is considerably higher (21 percent in the series of Berenguer et al)—the result of delays in diagnosis and, more importantly, of resistance to antituberculous drugs in some patients (Snider and Roper). Most resistant tuberculosis in developed countries is a result of intermittent, ineffective therapy. Therefore, directly observed therapy for at least 2 months–"short course" (DOTS) has become routine for patients in many areas. (See also "Tuberculous Myelitis" in Chap. 44.) Early diagnosis, as one might expect, enhances the chances of survival. In patients who are treated late in the disease, when coma has supervened, the mortality rate is nearly 50 percent. Between 20 and 30 percent of survivors manifest a variety of residual neurologic sequelae, the most important of which are diminished intellectual function, psychiatric disturbances, recurrent seizures, visual and oculomotor disorders, deafness, and hemiparesis. A detailed account of these has been given by Wasz-Hockert and Donner.

Sarcoidosis

The infectious etiology of sarcoidosis has never been established but the disease may suitably be considered at this point because of its close resemblance pathologically and clinically to tuberculosis and other granulomatous infections. Indeed, one still credible theory of causation considers sarcoidosis to be a modified form or product of the tubercle bacillus. This has not been proved, and the same can be said for various other infectious and noninfectious etiologies that from time to time have been proposed as the underlying cause. Current opinion favors the idea that sarcoidosis represents an exaggerated cellular immune response to a limited class of antigens or autoantigens (Baughman and Lower).

The essential lesion in sarcoidosis consists of focal collections of epithelioid cells surrounded by a rim of lymphocytes; frequently there are giant cells, but caseation is lacking. The sarcoid, noncaseating granuloma may be found in all organs and tissues, including the nerve roots, peripheral, and central nervous systems, but the most frequently involved are the mediastinal and peripheral lymph nodes, lungs, liver, skin, phalangeal bones, eyes, and parotid glands.

According to Iannuzzi and colleagues, sarcoidosis is accompanied by nervous system involvement (neurosarcoidosis) in approximately 25 percent of postmortem cases. This number overestimates the frequency of neurosarcoidosis because only a small percentage of all patients with sarcoidosis come to autopsy and among these, neurologic involvement is prevalent. Approximately 5 percent of patients with sarcoidosis prove to have nervous system involvement clinically. *Primary neurosarcoidosis*, by which is meant sarcoidosis isolated only to the nervous system, is even less common. If one excludes facial palsy, primary neurosarcoidosis is rare. Several other syndromes are caused by localized sarcoid involvement of the meninges, brain, and spinal cord (Table 32-5). In Scadding's series of 275 patients, only 3 developed CNS lesions; in other large series, the incidence of CNS involvement was greater but, as mentioned, most are in the range of 5 to 10 percent (of 285 studied by Chen and McLeod; and 33 of 649 studied by Stern et al). Delaney, in his review of the literature, found the neurologic involvement in sarcoidosis to be equally divided between the peripheral and central nervous systems.

Sarcoidosis in the nervous system may take one of several forms (see Table 32-5). As indicated in

Table 32-5

THE MAIN NERVOUS SYSTEM MANIFESTATIONS OF SARCOIDOSIS

Cranial neuropathy (see Chap. 47)
Facial palsy, unilateral, bilateral, or sequential[a]
Visual loss
Optic neuropathy
Uveitis
Retinal vasculopathy
Hearing loss, vertigo
Facial sensory loss or pain
Spinal cord and roots (see Chap. 44)
Polyradiculopathy
Granulomatous meningomyelitis, subacute or chronic
Cauda equina syndrome
Peripheral nervous system (see Chap. 46)
Lumbar or brachial plexopathy
Sensory-predominant polyneuropathy
Mononeuropathy and mononeuropathy multiplex
Brain lesions
Nodular masses
Perivascular infiltration
Basal granulomas with diabetes insipidus
Subacute meningitis and pachymeningitis

[a]Facial palsies account for the majority of neurosarcoidosis.

Chaps. 13, 46, and 47, isolated sarcoid granulomas may involve peripheral or cranial nerves, giving rise to a subacute or chronic polyradiculopathy, neuropathy, or plexopathy of asymmetrical type (Jefferson). Polyneuropathy may occur, but is infrequent; Zuniga and colleagues summarized our experience with this process. Of the cranial nerves, the facial is the most frequently involved, either as part of the uveoparotid syndrome (Heerfordt syndrome) or independently. The facial palsy may be unilateral or bilateral; if the latter, the nerves may be affected simultaneously or in succession. Blindness is a rare complication that follows basal infiltration that encompasses the optic nerves as noted later (Fig. 32-4). Other causes of visual disturbance include uveitis and optic neuropathy.

There is also a well-described myopathy associated with sarcoidosis; it is discussed below, and also considered in Chap. 49. The neuropathy of sarcoidosis is discussed further in Chap. 46.

In the CNS, sarcoidosis takes the form of a granulomatous infiltration of the meninges and underlying parenchyma, most frequent at the base of the brain (see Fig. 32-4). The process is subacute or chronic in nature, mimicking other granulomatous lesions and neoplasms. One particular syndrome that has been associated with sarcoidosis consists of a circumscribed lesion of the stalk of the pituitary gland, optic chiasm, and hypothalamus, it causes visual disturbances, polydipsia, polyuria, or somnolence. Hydrocephalus, seizures, cranial-nerve palsies, and corticospinal and cerebellar signs are other occasional manifestations.

Rarely, sarcoid can be a cause of a chronic recurrent or persistent meningitis, or severe, steroid-responsive headache. Granulomas may present as a mass or as one or more focal infiltrating cortical and subcortical lesions that tend to follow the course of superficial cortical veins. Focal

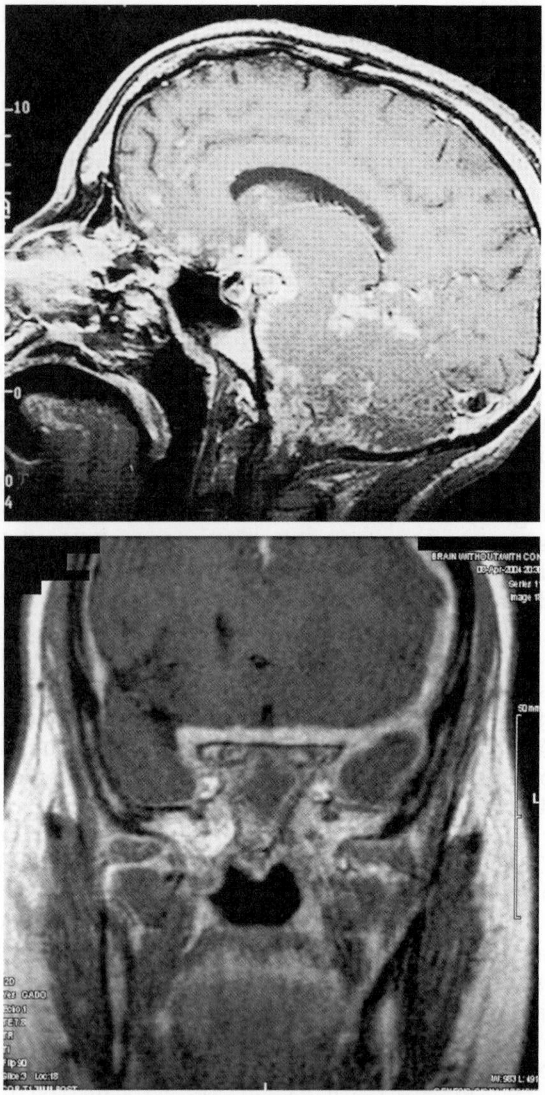

Figure 32-4. Cerebral sarcoid. Gadolinium-enhanced MRI of the brain. *Top panel:* Sarcoid lesions coat the base of the brain and cerebellum and surround the pituitary stalk. The patient had pulmonary sarcoid, marked abulia, and panhypopituitarism. *Bottom panel:* Sarcoid infiltration of the basal pachymeninges and both optic nerves causing blindness. Visual acuity returned almost to normal after 2 weeks of corticosteroid administration.

cerebral signs, including seizures, presumably caused by deposits of sarcoid in the brain, are observed but are uncommon. Among the odd focal syndromes reported are an amnestic or dementing condition from infiltration of the medial temporal lobes and psychotic and related behavioral aberrations. In addition to this leptomeningitis, there is an infiltration of the dura, a pachymeningitis.

The spinal meninges and spinal cord may be infiltrated, usually independently of brain involvement, imparting a picture of chronic adhesive arachnoiditis or an inflammatory myelopathy. There is more prominent focal contrast enhancement and T2 signal abnormality on MRI than is usual for a demyelinating disease. It is one of the causes of a "longitudinally extensive myelopathy" (see Chap. 36). Characteristic of the spinal lesion is enhancement on the surface of the cord and a degree of expansion at the level of the myelitic lesion (see "Sarcoid Myelitis" in Chap. 44). We have had experience with several such cases in which the only evidence of sarcoid was a lesion in the thoracic cord. Biopsy of the spinal cord lesion, a risky procedure, was necessary for diagnosis in some of these cases.

Diagnosis

A slight lymphocytic pleocytosis (10 to 200 cells/mm^3) and a moderate increase in protein content (generally without oligoclonal bands), consistent with meningeal involvement are the usual CSF findings but many cases show no change. The glucose content is normal or slightly reduced. The spinal form may be associated with CSF block and a resultant greatly raised protein content.

The *diagnosis* of neurosarcoidosis is made on the basis of the clinical features together with clinical and biopsy evidence of sarcoid granulomas in other tissues (lymph nodes, lungs, bones, uvea, skin, and muscle). The history or presence of erythema nodosum or iritis further raises suspicion of this process. If a conventional chest radiograph does not disclose the characteristic bilateral hilar adenopathy of sarcoidosis, a thoracic CT scan may be obtained. In patients in whom the clinical suspicion remains high, positron emission tomography (PET) scanning may be useful to identify inflamed lymph nodes that are amenable to biopsy. If PET scanning is not available, radionuclide scanning with gallium-67 also shows uptake in the chest, spleen, and salivary or lacrimal glands in almost half of patients and can be a useful ancillary test.

The contrast-enhanced CT or MRI are useful means of detecting meningeal involvement and MRI may disclose periventricular and white matter lesions, although the latter pattern is usually not at all specific. Nodular or streak-like perivenular enhancement may be found on the contrast-enhanced MRI, as described by Sherman and Stern and by Christoforidis and colleagues. The intensity of enhancement may be reduced after the administration of corticosteroids.

Of historical interest is the Kveim-Siltzbach skin reaction, a granuloma in response to homogenate of spleen or lymph node from patients with known sarcoidosis. Most patients are allergic to multiple antigens including purified protein derivative (for tuberculosis) and *Candida* antigen, injected intradermally. Mild anemia, lymphocytopenia (occasional eosinophilia), slightly elevated sedimentation rate, hypercalcemia, and hyperglobulinemia are common findings in active disease. Serum levels of angiotensin-converting enzyme (ACE) are increased in two-thirds of patients with active pulmonary sarcoid but only one-fifth of those with chronic disease. Therefore it may not be helpful in instances of neurosarcoidosis. There is scant evidence that the concentration of ACE in the spinal fluid is helpful in the diagnosis of CNS sarcoidosis.

The differential diagnosis of neurosarcoidosis is broad and includes multiple sclerosis as well as entities such as Sjögren syndrome, systemic lupus, lymphoma, lymphomatoid granulomatosis, cryptococcosis and other fungal infections that cause abscesses and chronic meningitis, syphilis, Wegener granulomatosis, Whipple disease, and, of course, tuberculosis.

Treatment

Administration of corticosteroids is the main therapy for neurosarcoidosis, but it has not been subjected to an adequate trial. Other immunosuppressive drugs are effective; methotrexate, cyclophosphamide, and the anti-TNF agents (infliximab, etanercept, and adalimumab). Radiation of focal lesions had in the past found favor but is now infrequently used.

The major problem is in knowing when to treat the patient, because neurosarcoid may remit spontaneously in about half the cases. The recent onset of neurologic symptoms, indicating an active phase of the disease, or a disabling syndrome such as myelopathy, is the most certain indication for steroid therapy. One approach is to use prednisone in daily doses of 40 mg, given for 2 weeks, followed by 2-week periods in which the dose is reduced by 5 mg, until a maintenance dose of 15 to 10 mg is reached. Therapy should be continued for at least several months and in many cases is required for several years. If patients become resistant or intolerant to corticosteroids, most often one of the anti-TNF drugs is added.

Neurosyphilis

The incidence of neurosyphilis, like that of CNS tuberculosis, declined dramatically in the decades following World War II, with the advent of penicillin. In the United States, for instance, the rate of first admissions to mental hospitals because of neurosyphilis fell from 4.3 per 100,000 population (in 1946) to 0.4 per 100,000 (in 1960). However, in more recent years, the number of reported cases of early syphilis has increased, both in nonimmunocompromised individuals and particularly in HIV-infected ones. Notable also is the shift in clinical presentation of neurosyphilis from parenchymal damage, now quite rare, to one of chronic meningovascular disease, particularly in patients with AIDS. Congenital syphilis represents a special problem, which is discussed with developmental diseases in Chap. 37.

Etiology and Pathogenesis

Syphilis is caused by *Treponema pallidum*, a slender, spiral, motile organism. In this chapter, only the basic facts regarding the neurosyphilitic infection are enumerated. Figure 32-5 summarizes the neurosyphilitic diseases.

The treponeme usually invades the CNS within 3 to 18 months of inoculation with the organism. If the nervous system is not involved by the end of the second year, as shown by completely negative CSF, there is only one chance in 20 that the patient will develop neurosyphilis as a result of the original infection; if the CSF is negative at the end of 5 years, the likelihood of developing neurosyphilis falls to 1 percent. *The initial event in the neurosyphilitic infection is meningitis, which occurs in approximately 25 percent of all cases of syphilis.* Usually the meningitis is asymptomatic and can be discovered only by lumbar puncture. Exceptionally, it is more intense and causes cranial-nerve palsies, seizures, stroke, and symptoms of increased intracranial pressure. In the current era, clinicians understandably neglect to consider

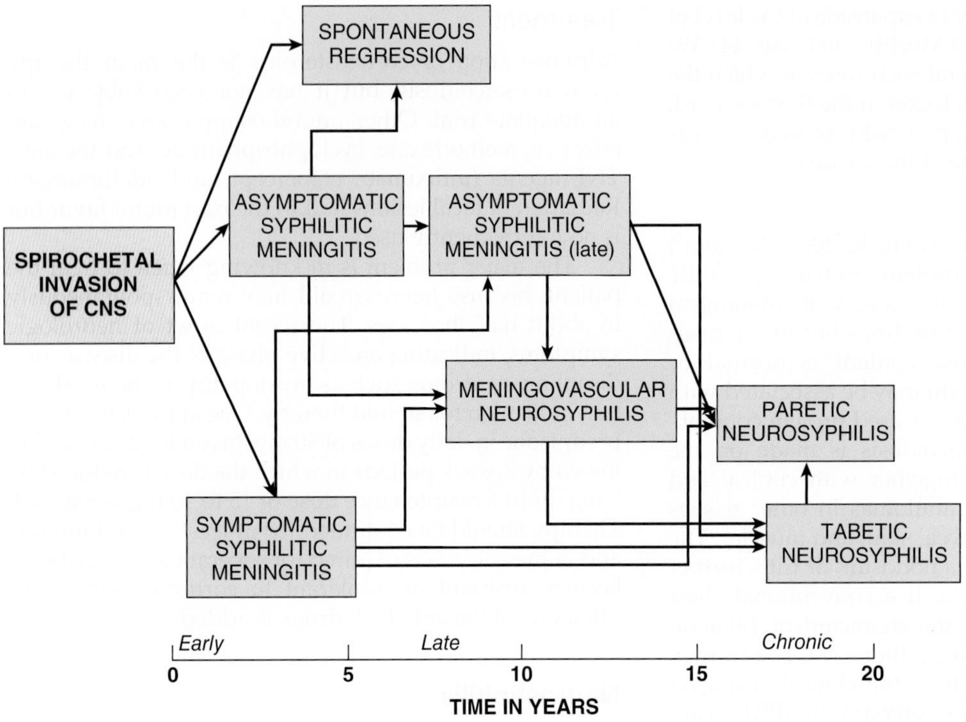

Figure 32-5. Diagram of the evolution of neurosyphilis.

the possibility of neurosyphilis with these syndromes. The meningitis may persist in an asymptomatic state and, ultimately, after a period of years, may lead to parenchymal damage. In some cases, however, there is a natural subsidence of the meningitis.

All forms of neurosyphilis begin as meningitis and meningeal inflammation are the invariable accompaniment of all forms of neurosyphilis. The early clinical syndromes are aseptic meningitis and meningovascular syphilis; the late (secondary) ones are vascular syphilis (1 to 12 years), followed even later by tertiary syphilis, general paresis, tabes dorsalis, optic atrophy, or subacute myelitis. In each case this pathologic sequence results from chronic syphilitic meningitis. The intermediate mechanisms, whereby transformation occurs from persistent asymptomatic syphilitic meningitis or relapsing meningitis, to the late forms of parenchymal neurosyphilis are unknown.

From a clinical point of view, asymptomatic neurosyphilis is perhaps the most important form because, if discovered and adequately treated, the symptomatic varieties would be prevented in most instances. Because asymptomatic neurosyphilis can be recognized only by the changes in the CSF, it is advisable that all patients with syphilis should have a spinal fluid examination.

Clinical syndromes such as syphilitic meningitis, meningovascular syphilis, general paresis, tabes dorsalis, optic atrophy, and meningomyelitis *seldom exist in pure form*. Because all of them appear to have a common origin in meningitis, there is usually a combination of two or more syndromes with one predominating, e.g., meningitis and vascular syphilis, tabes and paresis. Even though the patient's symptoms may have been referable to only one part of the nervous system, postmortem examination usually discloses diffuse changes, in both brain and spinal cord, which were of insufficient severity to be detected clinically.

The clinical syndromes and pathologic reactions of *congenital syphilis* are similar to those of the late-acquired forms, differing only in the age at which they occur. All the aforementioned biologic events are equally applicable to congenital and childhood neurosyphilis.

The CSF has been a sensitive indicator of the presence of active neurosyphilitic infection. The CSF abnormalities consist of (1) a pleocytosis of up to 100 cells/mm^3, sometimes higher, mostly lymphocytes and a few plasma cells and other mononuclear cells (the counts may be lower in patients with AIDS and those with leukopenia); (2) elevation of the total protein, from 40 to 200 mg/dL; (3) an increase in gamma globulin (IgG), usually with oligoclonal banding; and (4) positive serologic tests. Elevated gamma globulin in the CSF is produced intrathecally and has been shown to be adsorbed to *T. pallidum* (Vartdal et al). Hence the gamma globulin represents a specific antibody response to this organism and is recognized as the presence of oligoclonal banding of CSF protein. The glucose content is usually normal. In congenital (but not adult) neurosyphilis, the earliest changes in the CSF, consisting of pleocytosis and an elevation of protein, may occur in the first few weeks of the infection, before the serologic tests become positive. Later, the CSF changes may vary. With either spontaneous or therapeutic remission of the disease, the cells disappear first; next the total protein returns to normal; then the gamma globulin concentration is reduced. The positive serologic tests are the last to revert to normal. Some caution is advisable in interpreting the CSF results in patients with concurrent

AIDS. On the one hand, an aseptic reaction may be the result of HIV alone; on the other hand, those with profound leukopenia or T-cell deficiencies may show little or no cellular reaction in the CSF.

Frequently, the CSF serology remains positive, despite repeated courses of therapy and the subsidence of all signs of inflammatory activity. When this occurs, it may be safely concluded that the syphilitic inflammation in the nervous system is burned out and that further progression of the disease probably will not occur. If treatment restores the CSF to normal, particularly the cell count and protein, arrest of the clinical symptoms almost always occurs. A return of cells and elevation of protein precedes or accompanies clinical relapse.

Serologic Diagnosis of Syphilis This depends on the demonstration of one of two types of antibodies: nonspecific or nontreponemal (reagin) antibodies and specific treponemal antibodies. The common tests for reagin are the Kolmer, which uses a complement fixation technique, and the Venereal Disease Research Laboratory (VDRL) slide test, which uses a flocculation technique. These reagin tests, *if positive in the CSF*, are virtually diagnostic of neurosyphilis. Serum reactivity alone demonstrates exposure to the organism in the past, but does not imply the presence of neurosyphilis. However, serum reagin tests are negative in a significant proportion of patients with late syphilis and in those with neurosyphilis in particular (*seronegative syphilis*). In such patients (and in patients with suspected false-positive test in the serum) it is essential to employ tests for antibodies that are directed specifically against treponemal antigens. The latter are positive in the serum of practically every instance of neurosyphilis. The fluorescent treponemal antibody absorption (FTA-ABS) test is more than adequate for the majority of clinical situations. The *T. pallidum* immobilization (TPI) test is the most reliable, but it is expensive, difficult to perform, and available in only a few laboratories.

Principal Types of Neurosyphilis

Asymptomatic Neurosyphilis

In this condition, there are no symptoms or physical signs except, in rare cases, abnormal pupils, which are light-unreactive but constrict as part of the near response (accommodate with convergence) (Argyll Robertson pupils, Chap. 14). The diagnosis is based entirely on the CSF findings, which vary, as mentioned above.

Meningeal Syphilis

Symptoms of meningeal involvement may occur at any time after infection but typically does so within the first 2 years. The most common symptoms are headache, stiff neck, cranial-nerve palsies, convulsions, and mental confusion. Occasionally, headache, papilledema, nausea, and vomiting—as a result of the presence of increased intracranial pressure—are added to the clinical picture. The patient is afebrile, unlike the case in tuberculous meningitis. The CSF always has a lymphocytic reaction, more so than in asymptomatic syphilitic meningitis. Obviously the meningitis is more intense in the symptomatic type and may be associated with hydrocephalus. With adequate treatment, the prognosis is good. The symptoms usually disappear within days to weeks, but if the CSF remains abnormal, it is likely that some other form of neurosyphilis will subsequently develop if treatment is not continued.

Meningovascular Syphilis

As indicated earlier, this clinical syndrome is now probably the most common form of neurosyphilis. Whereas in the past, strokes from syphilitic meningitis accounted for only 10 percent of neurosyphilitic syndromes, their frequency is now estimated to be 35 percent. The most common time of occurrence of meningovascular syphilis is 6 to 7 years after the original infection, but it may be as early as 9 months or as late as 10 to 12 years. It is therefore the main manifestation of what has been termed "secondary syphilis."

The CSF almost always shows some abnormality, usually an increase in cells, protein content, and gamma globulin, as well as a positive serologic test.

The pathologic changes in this disorder consist not only of meningeal infiltrates but also of inflammation and fibrosis of small arteries (*Heubner arteritis*), which lead to narrowing and, finally, occlusion. Most of the infarctions occur in the distal territories of medium- and small-caliber lenticulostriate branches that arise from the stems of the middle and anterior cerebral arteries. Most characteristic perhaps is an internal capsular lesion, extending to the adjacent basal ganglia. The presence of multiple small but not contiguous lesions adjacent to the lateral ventricles is another common pattern. Small, asymptomatic lesions are often seen in the caudate and lenticular nuclei. Several of our patients have had transient prodromal neurologic symptoms.

The neurologic signs that remain after 6 months will usually be permanent but adequate treatment will prevent further vascular episodes. If repeated strokes occur despite adequate therapy, one should consider the possibility of nonsyphilitic vascular disease of the brain.

Paretic Neurosyphilis (General Paresis, Dementia Paralytica)

The general setting of this form of cerebral syphilis is long-standing meningitis hence, with tabes, it is a form of "tertiary syphilis." As remarked above, some 15 to 20 years usually separate the onset of general paresis from the original infection. The history of the disease is entwined with many of the major historical events in neuropsychiatry. Haslam in 1798 and Esquirol at about the same time first delineated the clinical state. Bayle in 1822 commented on the arachnoiditis and meningitis, and Calmeil, on the encephalitic lesion. Nissl and Alzheimer added details to the pathologic descriptions. The syphilitic nature of the disease was suspected by Lasegue and others long before Schaudinn's discovery of the spirochete; it was finally confirmed by Noguchi in 1913. Kraepelin's monograph *General Paresis* (1913) is one of the classic reviews (see Merritt et al for these and other historical references).

Once a major cause of various forms of mental illness, accounting for some 4 to 10 percent of admissions to asylums (hence the term "general paresis of the insane," or GPI), general paresis is now a rarity. Because syphilis is acquired mainly in late adolescence and early adult life, the middle years (35 to 50) are the usual time of onset of the paretic symptoms. There have not been many cases of this process in patients with AIDS; possibly the immunodeficiency has altered the biologic reaction to the organism.

The clinical picture in its fully developed form includes progressive dementia, dysarthria, myoclonic jerks, action tremor, seizures, hyperreflexia, Babinski signs, and Argyll Robertson pupils. However, greater importance attaches to diagnosis at an earlier stage, when few of these manifestations are conspicuous. The insidious onset of memory defect, impairment of reasoning, and reduction in critical faculties—along with minor oddities of deportment and conduct, irritability, and lack of interest in personal appearance—are not too different from the general syndrome of dementia outlined in Chap. 21, especially of the frontotemporal variety. One can appreciate how elusive the disease may be at any one point in its early evolution. Indeed, with the currently low index of suspicion of the disease, diagnosis at this predemented stage is more often accidental than deliberate.

Although former writings have stressed the development of delusional systems, most dramatically in the direction of mania, such symptoms are exceptional in the early or preparalytic phase. More usual has been a simple dementia with reduction of intellectual capacities, forgetfulness, disorders of speaking and writing, and vague concerns about health. In a few patients the first hint of a syphilitic encephalitis, as mentioned earlier, may be facial quivering; tremulousness of the hands; indistinct, hurried speech; myoclonus; and seizures—reminiscent of delirium or acute viral encephalitis. As the deterioration continues into the paralytic stage, intellectual function progressively declines, and aphasias, agnosias, and apraxias intrude themselves.

Physical dissolution progresses concomitantly—impaired station and gait, debility, unsteadiness, dysarthria, and tremor of the tongue and hands. All these disabilities lead eventually to a bedridden state; hence the term *paretic*. Other symptoms are hemiplegia, hemianopia, aphasia, cranial-nerve palsies, and seizures with prominent focal signs of unilateral frontal or temporal lobe disease—a syndrome known pathologically as Lissauer cerebral sclerosis.

Agitated, delirious, depressive, and schizoid psychoses are special psychiatric syndromes that can be differentiated from general paresis by the lack of mental decline, neurologic signs, and CSF findings. The neuropsychiatric features of this disease create a picture unlike that of most degenerative diseases—with the notable exception of the category of frontotemporal dementias discussed in Chap. 39. It is well to remember that many of our ideas about the brain and the mind were shaped historically by this disease.

Pathologic Changes This consists of meningeal thickening, brain atrophy, ventricular enlargement, and granular ependymitis. Microscopically, the perivascular spaces are filled with lymphocytes, plasma cells, and mononuclear cells; nerve cells have disappeared; there are numerous rod-shaped microgliacytes and plump astrocytes in parts of the cortex devastated by neuronal loss; iron is deposited in mononuclear cells; and, with special stains, spirochetes are visible in the cortex. The changes are most pronounced in the frontal and temporal lobes. The ependymal surfaces of the ventricles are studded with granular elevations protruding between ependymal cells (granular ependymitis). Meningeal fibrosis with obstructive hydrocephalus is present in many cases.

Treatment The prognosis in early treated cases with antibiotics has in the past been fairly good; 35 to 40 percent of patients made some occupational readjustment; in another 40 to 50 percent, the disease was arrested but left the patient dependent. Without treatment as discussed below there is progressive mental decline, and death occurs within 3 to 4 years.

Tabetic Neurosyphilis (Tabes Dorsalis)

This type of neurosyphilis, described by Duchenne in his classic monograph *L'ataxie locomotrice progressive* (1858), usually develops 15 to 20 years after the onset of the infection. The major symptoms are lightning pains, ataxia, and urinary incontinence; the chief signs are absent tendon reflexes at knee and ankle, impaired vibratory and position sense in feet and legs, and a Romberg sign. The ataxia is purely a result of the sensory defect. Power, by contrast, is fully retained in most cases. The pupils are abnormal in more than 90 percent of cases, usually Argyll Robertson in type, and the majority of patients show ptosis or some degree of ophthalmoplegia. Optic atrophy is frequent. The lancinating or lightning pains (present in more than 90 percent of cases) are, as their name implies, sharp, stabbing, and brief, like a flash of lightning. They are more frequent in the legs than elsewhere but roam over the body from face to feet, sometimes playing persistently on one spot "like the repeated twanging of a fiddle string," as Wilson remarked. They may come in bouts lasting several hours or days. "Pins and needles" feelings, coldness, numbness, tingling, and other paresthesias are also present and are associated invariably with impairment of tactile, pain, and thermal sensation. The bladder is insensitive and hypotonic, resulting in unpredictable overflow incontinence. Constipation and megacolon as well as impotence are other expressions of dysfunction of the sacral roots and ganglia.

In the established phase of the disease, now seldom seen, ataxia is the most prominent feature. The patient totters and staggers while standing and walking. In mild form it is best seen as the patient walks between obstacles or along a straight line, turns suddenly, or halts. To correct the instability, the patient places his feet and legs wide apart, flexes his body slightly, and repeatedly contracts the extensor muscles of his feet as he sways (*la danse des tendons*). In moving forward, the patient flings his stiffened leg abruptly, and the foot strikes the floor with a resounding thump in a manner quite unlike that seen in the ataxia of cerebellar disease. The patient clatters along in this way with eyes glued to the floor. If his vision is blocked, he is rendered helpless. When the ataxia is severe, walking becomes impossible despite relatively normal strength of the leg muscles. A Romberg sign is grossly manifest.

Trophic lesions, perforating ulcers of the feet, and Charcot joints are characteristic complications of the tabetic state.

The deformity of deafferented *Charcot joints* occurs in less than 10 percent of tabetics (the most common cause nowadays is diabetic neuropathy, which is also a cause of lancinating pains). Most often the hips, knees, and ankles are affected, but occasionally also the lumbar spine or upper limbs are affected. The process generally begins as an osteoarthritis, which, with repeated injury to the insensitive joint, progresses to destruction of the articular surfaces. Osseous architecture disintegrates, with fractures, dislocations, and subluxations, only some of which occasion discomfort. The arthropathy has been observed to occur as frequently in the burned-out as in the active phase of tabes; hence it is only indirectly related to the syphilitic process. Although the basic abnormality appears to be repeated injury to an anesthetic joint, the process need not be painless. Presumably a deep and incomplete hypalgesia and loss of autonomic function are enough to interfere with protective mechanisms. The Charcot joint is addressed further in Chap. 46 in the context of sensory polyneuropathies. Visceral crises represent another interesting manifestation of this disease, now rarely seen. The gastric ones are the best known. The patient is seized abruptly with epigastric pain that spreads around the body or up over the chest. There may be a sense of thoracic constriction as well as nausea and vomiting—the latter repeated until nothing but blood-tinged mucus and bile are raised. The symptoms may last for several days; a barium swallow sometimes demonstrates pylorospasm. The attack subsides as quickly as it came, leaving the patient exhausted, with a soreness of the epigastric skin. Intestinal crises with colic and diarrhea, pharyngeal and laryngeal crises with gulping movements and dyspneic attacks, rectal crises with painful tenesmus, and genitourinary crises with strangury and dysuria are all less frequent but well-documented types.

In most cases now seen, the CSF is normal when the patient is first examined (so-called burned-out tabes). It is abnormal less often than in general paresis.

Pathology *Pathologic study* reveals a striking thinness and grayness of the posterior roots, principally lumbosacral, and thinning of the spinal cord mainly as a result of the degeneration of the posterior columns. Only a slight outfall of neurons is observed in the dorsal root ganglia; the peripheral nerves are essentially normal. For many years there was an argument as to whether the spirochete first attacked the posterior columns of the spinal cord, the posterior root as it pierced the pia, the more distal part of the radicular nerve where it acquires its arachnoid and dural sheaths, or the dorsal root ganglion cell. The observations of our colleagues of rare active cases have shown the inflammation to be all along the posterior root; the slight dorsal ganglion cell loss and posterior column degeneration were found to be secondary.

The hypotonia, areflexia, and ataxia relate to destruction of proprioceptive fibers in the sensory roots. The hypotonia and insensitivity of the bladder are caused by deafferentation at the S2 and S3 levels; the same is true of the impotence and obstipation. Lightning pains and visceral crises cannot be fully explained but are probably attributable to incomplete posterior root lesions at different levels. Analgesia and joint insensitivity relate to the partial loss of A and C fibers in the roots.

Treatment If the CSF is positive, the patient should be treated with penicillin, as described below. If, however, there is no pleocytosis, the CSF protein content is normal, and there is no evidence of cardiovascular or other types of syphilis, antisyphilitic treatment is not necessary. We are uncertain of the proper course of treatment in patients with tabes who have survived many decades with HIV. Residual symptoms in the form of lightning pains, gastric crises, Charcot joints, or urinary incontinence frequently continue long after all signs of active neurosyphilitic infection have disappeared. These should be treated symptomatically rather than by antisyphilitic drugs.

Syphilitic Optic Atrophy

This takes the form of progressive blindness beginning in one eye and then involving the other. The usual finding is a constriction of the visual fields, but scotomata may occur in rare cases. The optic discs are gray-white. Other forms of neurosyphilis, particularly tabes dorsalis, not infrequently coexist. The CSF is almost invariably abnormal, although the degree of abnormality may be slight in some cases. The prognosis is poor if vision in both eyes is greatly reduced. If only one eye is badly affected, sight in the other eye can usually be saved. In exceptional cases, visual impairment may progress, even after the CSF becomes negative. The pathologic changes consist of perioptic meningitis, with subpial gliosis and fibrosis replacing degenerated optic nerve fibers. Exceptionally there are vascular lesions with infarction of central parts of the nerve.

Spinal Syphilis

There are several types of spinal syphilis other than tabes. Two of them, *syphilitic meningomyelitis* (formerly called Erb spastic paraplegia because of the predominance of bilateral corticospinal tract signs) and *spinal meningovascular syphilis*, are observed from time to time, although less often than tabes. Spinal meningovascular syphilis may occasionally take the form of an anterior spinal artery syndrome. In meningomyelitis, there is subpial loss of myelinated fibers and gliosis as a direct result of the chronic fibrosing meningitis. Gumma of the spinal meninges and cord seldom is found. It was not present in a single case in Merritt and Adams' study of spinal syphilis. Progressive muscular atrophy (syphilitic amyotrophy) is a very rare disease of questionable syphilitic etiology; most cases are degenerative (see Chap. 39). Also rare is syphilitic hypertrophic pachymeningitis or arachnoiditis, which allegedly gives rise to radicular pain, amyotrophy of the hands, and signs of long tract involvement in the legs (*syphilitic amyotrophy with spastic-ataxic paraparesis*). In all these syndromes there is an abnormal CSF, unless, of course, the neurosyphilitic infection is burned out (see Chap. 44).

The prognosis in spinal neurosyphilis is uncertain. There is improvement or at least an arrest of the disease process in most instances, although a few patients may progress slightly after treatment is begun. A steady advance of the disease in the face of a negative CSF usually means that there has been a secondary constrictive myelopathy or that the original diagnosis was incorrect and the patient suffers from some other disease, e.g., a spinal form of multiple sclerosis as a degenerative disease.

Syphilitic Nerve Deafness and Vestibulopathy

This may occur in either early or late syphilitic meningitis and may be combined with other syphilitic syndromes. Because this may produce a treatable vestibular syndrome of vertigo, with or without hearing loss, syphilis serology should be tested in patients with cryptic vestibular dysfunction. Some of the characteristics of vestibular neurosyphilis are identical to those of Ménière disease, including episodic loss of function (Baloh and Honrubia). Curiously, there is seldom a history of clear primary syphilitic infection. The pathology, mainly endarteritis in the cochlea and labyrinths, is identical to the more common congenital syphilitic deafness, which is described in Chap. 37.

Treatment of Neurosyphilis

The treatment of all of these forms of neurosyphilis consists of the administration of penicillin G, given intravenously in a dosage of 18 to 24 million units daily (3 to 4 million units q4h) for 10 to 14 days. The CDC recommends procaine penicillin and probenecid and ceftriaxone as an alternative. Penicillin is so much preferred that even these patients are ideally desensitized to the drug. The Jarisch-Herxheimer reaction, which occurs after the first dose of penicillin and is a matter of concern in the treatment of primary syphilis, is of little consequence in neurosyphilis; it usually consists of no more than a mild temperature elevation and leukocytosis.

The effects of treatment on certain symptoms of neurosyphilis, especially of tabetic neurosyphilis, are unpredictable and often little influenced by treatment with penicillin; they require symptomatic measures. Lightning pains may respond to gabapentin or carbamazepine. Analgesics may be helpful, but opiates should generally be avoided. Neuropathic (Charcot) joints require bracing or fusion. Atropine and phenothiazine derivatives are said to be useful in the treatment of visceral crises.

In all forms of neurosyphilis, the patient should be reexamined every 3 to 6 months after treatment and the CSF should be retested after a 6-month interval. If after 6 months the patient is free of symptoms and the CSF abnormalities have been reversed (disappearance of cells as well as reduction in protein, gamma globulin, and serology titers), no further treatment is indicated. Followup should include clinical examinations at approximately 12 months and another lumbar puncture. If a pleocytosis remains, these procedures should be repeated every 6 months. In the opinion of most experts, a persistent weakly positive serologic (VDRL) test after the cells and protein levels have returned to normal does not constitute an indication for additional treatment. Such a CSF formula ensures that the disease is quiescent or arrested. Others are not convinced of the reliability of this concept and prefer to give more penicillin. If at the end of 6 months there are still an increased number of cells and an elevated protein in the fluid, another full course of penicillin should be given. Clinical relapse is almost invariably attended by recurrence of cells and increase in protein levels. Rapid clinical progression in the face of a negative CSF suggests the presence of a nonsyphilitic disease of the brain or cord.

Lyme Disease (Erythema Chronicum Migrans; Borreliosis)

Until comparatively recently, the nonvenereal spirochetes were of little interest to neurologists of the Western world. Yaws, pinta, and endemic syphilis rarely, if ever, affected the nervous system. Leptospirosis was essentially an acute liver disease with only one variant causing nonicteric lymphocytic meningitis; tick- and louse-borne relapsing fevers were medical curiosities that did not involve neurologists. However, in the late 1970s, a multisystem disease with prominent neurologic features was recognized in the eastern United States (it had been known in Northern Europe). It was named after the town of Lyme, Connecticut, where a cluster of cases was first recognized in 1975. An early skin manifestation of the disease had previously been described in Western Europe and referred to as *erythema chronicum migrans*. In 1982, Burgdorfer and colleagues identified the causative spirochetal agent, *Borrelia burgdorferi*. Later manifestations of the disease—taking the form of acute radicular pain followed by chronic lymphocytic meningitis and frequently accompanied by peripheral and cranial neuropathies—had long been known in Europe as the Bannwarth or Garin-Bujadoux syndrome. The identity of these diseases has been established, as well as their close relationship to relapsing fever—a disease that is also caused by spirochetes of the genus *Borrelia* and transmitted by ticks. The entire group is now classed as the borrelioses but there are notable clinical and serologic differences between the American and European varieties of the disease.

In humans, all these spirochetoses, if untreated, induce a subacute or chronic illness that evolves in ill-defined stages, with early spirochetemia, vascular damage in many organs, and a high level of neurotropism. As in syphilis, the nervous system is invaded early in the form of asymptomatic meningitis. Later, neurologic abnormalities appear, but only in small a proportion of such cases. The early neurologic complications are mainly derivations of meningitis. Unlike syphilis, peripheral and cranial nerves are often damaged (see further on and Chap. 46). Immune factors may be important in the later phases of the disease and in the development of the neurologic syndromes.

Lyme disease is less acute than leptospirosis (Weil disease) and less chronic than syphilis. It successively involves the skin, nervous system, heart, and articular structures over a period of a year or longer although one aspect or another may predominate. The responsible organism, as stated earlier, is the spirochete *B. burgdorferi* and the vector in the United States is the common ixodid tick. The precise roles of the infecting spirochete, the antibodies it induces, and other features of the human host response in the production of clinical symptoms and signs are not fully understood, but the development of an animal model by Pachner and colleagues suggests that there may be a chronic form of *Borrelia* infection.

Lyme borreliosis has a worldwide distribution but the typical neurologic manifestations differ slightly in Europe and America, as emphasized in the review by Garcia-Monico and Benach (as does the serologic testing). In the United States, where approximately 15,000 cases are reported annually, the disease is found mainly in the Northeast and the North Central states. Most infections are acquired from May to July. In 60 to 80 percent of cases, a skin lesion (erythema chronicum migrans, or erythema migrans) at the site of a tick bite is the initial manifestation, occurring within 30 days of exposure. It is a solitary, enlarging, ring-like erythematous lesion that may be surrounded by annular satellite lesions. Usually fatigue and influenza-like symptoms (myalgia, arthralgia, and headache) are associated, and these seem to be more prominent in the North American (*B. burgdoferii*) than the European form of the illness (*Borrelia afzelii and Borrelia garinii*)—possibly attributable to a more virulent species of spirochete (Nadelman and Wormser). This assumes importance in patients who may have acquired the illness in another part of the world in whom the correct diagnosis may be missed if the specific antibody for the regional organism is not sought. The European variant has a propensity to cause the painful lymphocytic meningoradiculitis, Bannwarth syndrome, as summarized in the review by Pachner and Steiner.

Weeks to months later, neurologic or cardiac symptoms appear in 15 and 8 percent of the cases, respectively. Still later, if the patient remains untreated, arthritis or, more precisely, synovitis develops in approximately 60 percent of the cases. Death from this disease does not occur; consequently, little is known of the pathology. A long period of disability is to be expected if the disease is not recognized and treated.

Diagnosis is not difficult during the summer season in regions where the disease is endemic and when all the clinical manifestations are present. But in some cases, a skin lesion is not observed or may have been forgotten, or there may have been only a few or no secondary lesions and the patient is first seen in the neurologic phase of the illness. Then clinical diagnosis may be difficult.

Neurologic Manifestations

The usual pattern of neurologic involvement is one of aseptic meningitis or a fluctuating meningoencephalitis with cranial or peripheral neuritis, lasting for months (Reik). By the time the neurologic disturbances appear, the systemic symptoms and skin lesions may have long since receded, usually by many weeks or months. A cardiac disorder, which may accompany or occur independently of the neurologic changes, takes the form of myocarditis, a pericarditis, or an atrioventricular block.

The initial nervous system symptoms are rather nonspecific. They consist of headache, mild stiff neck, nausea and vomiting, malaise, and chronic fatigue, fluctuating over a period of weeks to months. Mild meningism without pleocytosis has been seen early in the syndrome and it may be worth repeating the studies in highly suspicious cases. These symptoms relate to the meningitis. There is a CSF lymphocytosis with cell counts from 50 to 3,000/mL and protein levels from 75 to 400 mg/dL, but both values are typically in the lower part of the range. Polymorphonuclear cells may be prominent in the early part of the illness. Usually the glucose content is normal. Somnolence, irritability, faulty memory, depressed mood, and behavioral changes have been interpreted as marks of encephalitis but are difficult to separate from the effects of meningitis. Seizures, choreic movements, cerebellar ataxia, and dementia have been reported but are infrequent. A myelitic syndrome, causing quadriparesis, is also documented as another rare manifestation.

In about half the cases, cranial neuropathies become manifest within weeks of onset of the meningitic illness. The most frequent is a unilateral or bilateral facial palsy but involvement of other cranial nerves, including the abducens and optic nerve has been observed, usually in association with meningitis. One-third to one-half of the patients with meningitis have multiple radicular or peripheral nerve lesions in various combinations. These are described in Chap. 46. In addition to facial palsies, a severe and painful meningoradiculitis of the cauda equina (Bannwarth syndrome) is particularly characteristic and seems to be more common in Europe than in the United States (there are other causes of this syndrome, including herpesvirus and cytomegalovirus). There is also an infrequent occurrence of Guillain-Barré syndrome following Lyme infection, again apparently more common in Europe, but there is no reason to believe that the illness then differs from other cases of the acute inflammatory demyelinating polyneuropathy that follows numerous other infections.

Because of the paucity of autopsy material, knowledge of the nature of Lyme encephalitis is still imprecise. Such pathologic material as is available has shown a perivascular lymphocytic inflammatory process of the leptomeninges and the presence of subcortical and periventricular demyelinative lesions, like those of multiple sclerosis. Oksi and colleagues have recovered *B. burgdorferi* DNA from the involved areas, suggesting that the encephalitis is caused by direct invasion by the spirochete.

In the peripheral nerves (see Chap. 46) there are scattered lymphocytic infiltrates, without vasculitis. It seems likely to us that the organism will eventually be found in nervous tissue as the cause of disease, as there is active antibody production reflected in the CSF.

A problematic aspect of Lyme disease relates to the development in some patients of a mild chronic encephalopathy coupled with fatigue. That such a disorder may occur after a well-documented attack of Lyme disease is undoubted. However, in the absence of a history of the characteristic rash, arthritis, or aseptic meningitis, the attribution to Lyme disease of fatigue alone or various other vague mental symptoms, such as difficulty in concentration, is almost always erroneous, even if there is serologic evidence of exposure to the spirochete. It would be an understatement that a large number of patients are persuaded that various symptoms are the result of Lyme infection and seek and receive unnecessary treatment.

Laboratory Diagnosis

In acute and subacute cases that involve the spinal or cranial nerve roots or spinal cord, the CSF routinely shows a pleocytosis (20 to 250 lymphocytes/mm^3) with moderately elevated protein; the glucose concentration is usually normal but may be slightly depressed. The majority of cases with facial palsy alone are associated with this CSF formula, but there are exceptions.

Serologic tests are of great value but must be interpreted with caution if there has not been an inciting clinical syndrome of erythema migrans or arthritis or a well-documented tick bite. The most valuable initial screening is performed by the ELISA; if both acute and convalescent sera are tested, approximately 90 percent of patients have a positive IgM response. After the first few weeks, most patients have elevated IgG antibody responses to the spirochete (Berardi et al); a positive test of this nature may simply reflect prior exposure. The ratio of IgG intrathecal anti-*Borrelia* antibody to that of the serum is greater than 2 in cases of neuroborreliosis; this elevated ratio is a necessary criterion for the diagnosis in Europe. However, Blanc and colleagues studied a sample of 123 consecutive patients with clinical signs of neurologic involvement and found the sensitivity of the index was only 75 percent and the specificity was 97 percent. These authors have proposed more pragmatic diagnostic, but somewhat contrived, criteria for neuroborreliosis, consisting of the presence of 4 of the following 5 items: no past history of neuroborreliosis, active CSF ELISA serology, anti-*Borrelia* antibody index greater than 2, favorable outcome after specific antibiotic treatment, and no alternative diagnosis. False-positive tests do occur in some of the conditions that react to syphilitic reagin; *B. burgdorferi*–specific antibodies can also be demonstrated in the CSF (these are also reflected by the presence of oligoclonal bands).

Positive ELISA testing should be pursued further with Western blot or immunoblot analysis or other more specific serologies in clinically uncertain cases. Although these latter tests are difficult to carry out and have not been entirely standardized, the presence of both IgG and IgM antibodies is strongly supportive of a recent infection, whereas the IgG is useful in later cases. These laboratory diagnostic issues are discussed and put in perspective by Golightly. If the European variety of borreliosis is suspected, different serologic tests are required but the general principles of diagnosis are the same as for cases in the United States and elsewhere.

In only approximately 30 percent of cases, the organism can be detected in the spinal fluid using PCR techniques, usually early in the neurologic illness.

In the chronic phase of the disease, CT and MRI in cases of encephalopathy may display multifocal and periventricular cerebral lesions but these are by no means indicative alone of Lyme disease, as they also appear in numerous other conditions.

Treatment

The recommended treatment in the first stage of the disease, mainly referring to the initial rash and the subsequent presence of facial or other cranial nerve palsies alone, is oral or doxycycline (100 mg bid) for 14 days. Alternate therapies include amoxicillin 500 mg tid, used sometimes in children, or cefuroxime axetil 500 mg bid. CNS cardiac and arthritic disease can thereby be prevented in almost all cases. It follows that one is justified in being suspect of cases of "late Lyme" that have undergone adequate early treatment. Once the meninges and central or peripheral nervous system are implicated probably most effective is ceftriaxone, 2 g daily, usually given intravenously for a similar period.

Tetracycline, 500 mg qid for 30 days, is recommended by Reik for patients who are allergic to these intravenous drugs. Other alternative drugs are cefotaxime 2 g IV q8h and penicillin G 18 to 20 million units per day in divided doses q4h. For late abnormalities, no treatment has proved to be effective. However, most of the symptoms tend to regress regardless of the type of treatment given.

According to Kaiser, more than 90 percent of subacute neuropathies and facial palsies resolve by 1 year after treatment, but a smaller proportion of spastic and ataxic myelopathy cases are improved. In other studies, up to a fifth of children with facial palsies have residual weakness.

Leptospirosis

This systemic spirochetal infection, caused by *Leptospira interrogans*, is characterized primarily by hepatitis but may include aseptic meningitis during the second part of a biphasic illness. Initially there is high fever, tender muscles, chest and abdominal pain, and cough. An extreme form (Weil disease) comprises hepatic and renal failure. Prominent conjunctival suffusion and photophobia are typical of leptospirosis and should draw attention to the diagnosis. The CSF during the meningitic stage contains approximately 100 lymphocytes/mm^3, but cell counts in excess of 10,000 have been reported and the protein concentration may reach high levels. Subarachnoid and intracerebral bleeding, probably from inflamed blood vessels, is known to occur. The diagnosis is made by serologic methods (ELISA, indirect hemoglutination assay, followed by specific agglutination tests and culture).

Treatment Antibiotic treatment seems to be effective only if implemented during the initial febrile phase. Penicillin, doxycycline, or ceftriaxone have been used. The meningitis is usually self-limited.

FUNGAL INFECTIONS OF THE NERVOUS SYSTEM

Described in the following pages are a number of infectious diseases, much less common than bacterial ones, in which a systemic fungal infection secondarily involves the CNS. For the neurologist, the diagnosis rests on two lines of clinical information: evidence of infection in the lungs, skin, or other organs and the appearance of a subacute meningeal or multifocal encephalitic disorder. Although a large number of fungal diseases may involve the nervous system, only a few do so with regularity. Of 57 cases assembled by Walsh and coworkers, there were 27 of candidiasis, 16 of aspergillosis, and 14 of cryptococcosis. Among the opportunistic mycoses (see below), the majority is accounted for by species of *Aspergillus* and *Candida*. Mucormycosis and coccidioidomycosis are less frequent, and blastomycosis and actinomycosis (*Nocardia*) occur in isolated instances. However, of all of these infections, cryptococcal meningitis, which can occur in immunocompetent patients, is being seen more frequently as a result of its association with AIDS. Infections related to impairment of the body's protective mechanisms are referred to as *opportunistic* and include not only fungal infections but also those caused by certain bacteria (*Pseudomonas* and other gram-negative organisms, *L. monocytogenes*), protozoa (*Toxoplasma*), and viruses (cytomegalovirus, herpes simplex, and varicella zoster). It follows that these types of infections should be considered in the aforementioned clinical situations.

General Features

Fungal infections of the CNS may arise without obvious predisposing cause, but they typically complicate some other disease process that suppresses immune function such as AIDS, cancer chemotherapy, organ transplantation, severe burns, leukemia, lymphoma or other malignancy, diabetes, collagen vascular disease, or prolonged corticosteroid therapy. The factors operative in these clinical situations are the interference with the body's normal flora and impaired T-cell and humoral responses. Thus fungal infections tend to occur in patients with leukopenia, inadequate T-lymphocyte function, or insufficient antibodies.

Fungal meningitis develops insidiously, as a rule, over a period of several days or weeks, similar to tuberculous meningitis; the symptoms and signs are also much the same as with tuberculous infection. Involvement of several cranial nerves, arteritis with thrombosis and infarction of brain, multiple cortical and subcortical microabscesses, and hydrocephalus frequently complicate the course of fungal meningitis, just as they do in all chronic meningitides. Sometimes the patient is afebrile or has only intermittent fever.

The spinal fluid changes in fungal meningitis are like those of tuberculous meningitis. Pressure is elevated to a varying extent, pleocytosis is moderate and lymphocytes predominate. Exceptionally, in acute cases, a pleocytosis above 1,000/mm^3 and a predominant polymorphonuclear response are observed (also seen with the bacterial infections, nocardia, and actinomycosis). On the other hand, in patients with AIDS or with pronounced leukopenia for other reasons, the pleocytosis may be minimal or even absent. Glucose is subnormal and protein is elevated, sometimes to very high levels.

The specific diagnosis is made from smears of the CSF sediment, from cultures and by demonstrating antigens of the organism by immunodiffusion, latex particle agglutination, or comparable antigen recognition tests. The CSF examination should also include a search for tubercle bacilli and abnormal white cells because of the not infrequent concurrence of fungal infection and tuberculosis, leukemia, or lymphoma.

Some of the special features of the more common fungal infections are indicated later.

Cryptococcosis (Torulosis, European Blastomycosis)

Cryptococcosis (formerly called *torulosis*) is one of the more frequent fungal infections of the CNS and it occurs in both normal and immunocompromised hosts. The causative organism is usually *Cryptococcus neoformans* but *Cryptococcus gattii* has also been implicated. Cryptococcus is a common soil fungus found in the roosting sites of birds, especially pigeons. Usually the respiratory tract is the portal of entry, less often the skin and mucous membranes. The pathologic changes are those of granulomatous meningitis; in addition, there may be small granulomas and cysts within the cerebral cortex, and sometimes larger granulomas and cystic nodules deep in the brain (cryptococcomas). The cortical cysts contain a gelatinous material and large numbers of organisms; the solid granulomatous nodules are composed of fibroblasts, giant cells, aggregates of organisms, and areas of necrosis.

Cryptococcal meningitis has an indistinct clinical syndrome. Most cases evolve subacutely, like other fungal infections and tuberculosis. In most cases, headaches, fever, and stiff neck are lacking altogether, and the patient presents with symptoms of gradually increasing intracranial pressure because of hydrocephalus (papilledema is present in half such patients) or with a confusional state, dementia, cerebellar ataxia, or spastic paraparesis, usually without other focal neurologic deficit. A few cases have had an explosive onset, rendering the patient quite ill in a day. Large series of affected patients indicate that 20 to 40 percent of patients have no fever when first examined (the figure applies to patients without AIDS). Cranial-nerve palsies are infrequent. Rarely, a granulomatous lesion forms in one part of the brain, and the only clue to the etiology of the cerebral mass is a lung lesion and an abnormality of the CSF.

Meningovascular lesions, presenting as small deep strokes in an identical manner to meningovascular syphilis, may be superimposed on the clinical picture. A pure motor hemiplegia, like that caused by a hypertensive lacune, has been the most common type of stroke in our experience.

The course of the disease is quite variable. It may be fatal within a few weeks if untreated. More often, it is steadily progressive over a period of several weeks or months; in a few patients, it may be remarkably indolent, lasting for years, during which there may be periods of clinical improvement and normalization of the CSF. Lymphoma, Hodgkin disease, leukemia, carcinoma, tuberculosis, and other debilitating diseases that alter the immune responses are predisposing factors in as many as half the patients. As already emphasized, patients with AIDS are particularly vulnerable to cryptococcal infection; estimates are that 6 to 12 percent of AIDS patients are subject to meningoencephalitis with the organism but this seems higher than we have observed.

The spinal fluid shows a variable lymphocytic pleocytosis, usually less than 50 cells/mm^3, but there may be few or no cells in a patient with AIDS (two-thirds have 5 or fewer cells/mm^3). The initial CSF formula may display polymorphonuclear cells but it rapidly changes to a lymphocytic predominance. The glucose is reduced in three-fourths of cases (again, it may be normal in AIDS patients) and the protein may reach high levels.

Specific diagnosis in developed regions depends on finding *C. neoformans* antigens in the CSF. The organism may be seen as spherical cells, 5 to 15 μm in diameter, which retain Gram stain and are surrounded by a thick, refractile capsule. India ink preparations are distinctive and diagnostic in experienced hands (debris and talc particles from the gloves used in lumbar puncture may be mistaken for the organism) but the rate of positive tests under the best circumstance is 75 percent. The carbon particles of the dye fail to penetrate the capsule, leaving a wide halo around the doubly refractile wall of the organism. Large volumes of CSF (20 to 40 mL) may be needed to find the organism, but in others they are prolific. The search for these organisms is particularly important in AIDS patients, in whom the CSF values for cells, glucose, and proteins may be entirely normal but difficulties interpreting the India ink preparation have led to its being used less often. A latex agglutination test for the cryptococcal polysaccharide antigen in the CSF is now widely available and gives rapid results. The latter test, if negative, excludes cryptococcal meningitis with approximately 90 percent reliability in AIDS patients and slightly less in others (Chuck and Sande). In most cases the organisms grow readily in Sabouraud glucose agar at room temperature and at 37°C (98.6°F), but these results may not appear for days. Newer enzyme-linked immunoadsorption tests are being evaluated.

The principal diseases to be considered in diagnosis are tuberculous meningitis; granulomatous cerebral vasculitis (normal glucose values in CSF); unidentifiable forms of viral meningoencephalitis (normal CSF glucose values); sarcoidosis; and lymphomatosis or carcinomatosis of meninges (neoplastic cells in CSF).

Treatment In patients without AIDS, this consists of intravenous administration of amphotericin B, given in a dose of 0.7 to 1.0 mg/kg/d. Intrathecal administration of the drug in addition to the intravenous route appears not to be essential. Administration of the drug should be discontinued if the blood urea nitrogen reaches 40 mg/dL and resumed when it descends to normal levels. Renal tubular acidosis also frequently complicates amphotericin B therapy. The addition of flucytosine (100 mg/kg/d) to amphotericin B results in fewer failures or relapses, more rapid sterilization of the CSF, and less nephrotoxicity than the use of amphotericin B alone because it permits the reduction of the amphotericin dose to 0.3 to 0.5 mg/kg/d. Both medications are usually continued for at least 6 weeks—longer if CSF cultures remain positive.

However, this regimen, which has a success rate of 75 to 85 percent in immunocompetent patients, has proven to be much less effective in patients with AIDS. The recommended treatment in these circumstances is amphotericin supplemented by flucytosine for 2 weeks. Subsequently, fluconazole, an oral triazole antifungal agent, is given (or less preferably, oral itraconazole), for up to 1 year or indefinitely to prevent relapse (Saag et al; Powderly et al). The optimum use of these drugs has not been settled, and some trials have yielded ambiguous results in both AIDS and other patients. A current perspective on treatment can be obtained in the reference of Tunkel and Scheld and details of a randomized trial in AIDS comparing amphotericin as above to a regimen of additional flucytosine is given by Day and colleagues. They showed no advantage to an initial regimen of both drugs over amphotericin alone.

Mortality from cryptococcal meningoencephalitis, even in the absence of AIDS or other disease, is high.

Candidiasis (Moniliasis)

Candidiasis is probably the most frequent opportunistic fungus infection. The notable antecedents of *Candida* sepsis are severe burns and the use of total parenteral nutrition, especially in children. Urine, blood, skin, and particularly the heart (myocardium and valves) and lungs (alveolar proteinosis) are the usual sites of primary infection. No special features distinguish this fungal infection from others; meningitis, meningoencephalitis, and cerebral abscess, usually multiple and small, are the main modes of clinical presentation. Generally, the CSF contains several hundred (up to 2,000) cells/mm^3. Yeast can be seen on direct microscopy in half the cases. Even with treatment (intravenous amphotericin B), the prognosis is extremely grave.

Aspergillosis

In most instances, this infection has presented as a chronic sinusitis (particularly sphenoidal), with osteomyelitis at the base of the skull or as a complication of otitis and mastoiditis. Cranial nerves adjacent to the infected bone or sinus may be involved. We have also observed brain abscesses and cranial and spinal dural granulomas. In one of our patients, the *Aspergillus* organisms had formed a granulomatous mass that compressed the cervical spinal cord. Aspergillosis does not present as meningitis but hyphal invasion of cerebral vessels may occur, with thrombosis, necrosis, and hemorrhage; i.e., it is an infectious vasculitis. In some cases, the infection is acquired in the hospital, and in most it is preceded by a pulmonary infection that is unresponsive to antibiotics. Diagnosis can often be made by finding the organism in a biopsy specimen or by culturing it directly from a lesion. Also, specific antibodies and galactomannan are detectable in the blood.

Treatment Liposoma amphotericin in combination with voriconazole, and echinocandins in some cases, is the recommended treatment, but this regimen is not as effective for aspergillosis as it is for cryptococcal disease. The addition of itraconazole, 200 mg bid, in less-immunocompromised patients is recommended. If amphotericin B is given after surgical removal of the infected material, some patients recover.

Mucormycosis (Zygomycosis, Phycomycosis)

This is a malignant infection of cerebral vessels with one of the Mucorales. It occurs as a rare complication in patients with diabetes, especially during diabetic acidosis, in drug addicts, and in those with leukemia and lymphoma, particularly those treated with corticosteroids and cytotoxic agents.

The cerebral infection begins in the nasal turbinates and paranasal sinuses and spreads from there along infected vessels to the retroorbital tissues (where it results in proptosis, ophthalmoplegia, and edema of the lids and retina) and then to the adjacent brain, causing hemorrhagic infarction. Numerous hyphae are present within the thrombi and vessel wall, often invading the surrounding parenchyma. The cerebral form of mucormycosis is usually fatal in short order. Rapid correction of hyperglycemia and acidosis and treatment with liposomal amphotericin or posaconazole have resulted in recovery in some patients. The differential diagnosis is typically from septic cavernous sinus thrombosis in a diabetic.

Coccidioidomycosis, Histoplasmosis, Blastomycosis, and Actinomycosis

Coccidioidomycosis is a common infection in the southwestern United States. It usually causes only a benign, influenza-like illness with pulmonary infiltrates that mimic those of nonbacterial pneumonia, but in a few individuals (0.05 to 0.2 percent), the disease takes a disseminated form, of which meningitis may be a part. The pathologic reactions in the meninges and CSF and the clinical features are very much like those of tuberculous meningitis. *Coccidioides immitis* is recovered with difficulty from the CSF but readily from the lungs, lymph nodes, and ulcerating skin lesions. Diagnosis is made from CSF serology.

Treatment consists of the intravenous administration of amphotericin B coupled with implantation of an Ommaya reservoir into the lateral ventricle, permitting injection of the drug for a period of years. Instillation of the drug by repeated lumbar punctures is an alternative, albeit cumbersome, procedure. Even with the most assiduous programs of treatment, only about half the patients with meningeal infections survive.

A similar type of meningitis may occasionally complicate *histoplasmosis, blastomycosis,* and the anaerobic bacterium *actinomycosis*. These chronic meningitides possess no specific features except that actinomycosis, like some cases of tuberculosis and nocardiosis, may cause a *persistent polymorphonuclear pleocytosis* (see "Chronic Persistent and Recurrent Meningitis" in Chap. 33). The CSF yields an organism in a minority of patients, so that diagnosis depends on culture from extraneural sites, biopsy of brain abscesses if present, as well as knowledge of the epidemiology of these fungi. Patients with chronic meningitis in whom no cause can be discovered should also have their CSF tested for antibodies to *Sporothrix schenckii*, an uncommon fungus that is difficult to culture. Several even rarer fungi that must be considered in the diagnosis of chronic meningitis are discussed in the article by Swartz.

Treatment The current preferred treatment is fluconazole and amphotericin B and supplemental antifungal agents are used in the others. Intrathecal via a reservoir amphotericin is administered in patients who relapse.

INFECTIONS CAUSED BY RICKETTSIAS, PROTOZOA, AND WORMS

Rickettsial Diseases

Rickettsias are obligate intracellular parasites that appear microscopically as pleomorphic coccobacilli. The major ones are maintained in nature by a cycle involving an animal reservoir, an insect vector (lice, fleas, mites, and ticks), and humans. Epidemic typhus is an exception, involving only lice and human beings, and Q fever is probably contracted by inhalation. At the time of World War I, the rickettsial diseases, typhus in particular, were remarkably prevalent and of the utmost gravity. In Eastern Europe, between 1915 and 1922, there were an estimated 30 million cases of typhus with 3 million deaths. Now, the rickettsial diseases are of minor importance, the result of insect control by dichlorodiphenyltrichloroethane (DDT) and other chemicals and the therapeutic effectiveness of broad-spectrum antibiotics. In the United States these diseases are quite rare, but they assume significance because, in some types, up to one-third of patients have neurologic manifestations. About 200 cases of Rocky Mountain spotted fever (the most common rickettsial disease) occur each year in the United States, with a mortality of 5 percent or less. Neurologic manifestations occur in a small portion, and neurologists may not encounter a single instance in a lifetime of practice. For this reason, the rickettsial diseases are simply tabulated here.

The following are the major rickettsial diseases:

1. *Epidemic typhus*, small pockets of which are present in many undeveloped parts of the world. It is transmitted from lice to humans and from person to person.
2. *Murine (endemic) typhus*, which is present in the same areas as Rocky Mountain spotted fever (see below). It is transmitted by fleas from rats to humans.
3. *Scrub typhus* or *tsutsugamushi fever*, which is confined to eastern and southeastern Asia. It is transmitted by mites from infected rodents or humans.
4. *Rocky Mountain spotted fever*, first described in Montana, is most common in Long Island, Tennessee, Virginia, North Carolina, and Maryland. It is transmitted by special varieties of ticks.
5. *Q fever*, which has a worldwide distribution (except for the Scandinavian countries, New Zealand, and the tropics). It is transmitted in nature by ticks but also by inhalation of dust and handling of materials infected by the causative organism, *Coxiella burnetii*.

With the exception of Q fever, the clinical manifestations and pathologic effects of the rickettsial diseases are much the same, varying only in severity. Typhus may be taken as the prototype. The incubation period varies from 3 to 18 days. The onset is usually abrupt, with fever rising to extreme levels over several days; headache, often severe; and prostration. A macular rash, which resembles that of measles and involves the trunk and limbs, appears on the fourth or fifth febrile day. An important diagnostic sign in scrub typhus is the necrotic ulcer and eschar at the site of attachment of the infected mite. Delirium—followed by progressive stupor and coma, sustained fever, and occasionally focal neurologic signs and optic neuritis—characterizes the untreated cases. Stiffness of the neck is noted only rarely, and the CSF may be entirely normal or show only a modest lymphocytic pleocytosis.

In fatal cases, the rickettsial lesions are scattered diffusely throughout the brain, affecting gray and white matter alike. The changes consist of swelling and proliferation of endothelial cells of small vessels and a microglial reaction, with the formation of so-called typhus nodules.

Q fever, unlike the other rickettsioses, is not associated with an exanthem. In the few cases with which we are familiar, the main symptoms were those of a low-grade meningitis. Rare instances of encephalitis, cerebellitis, and myelitis are also reported, possibly as postinfectious complications. There is usually a tracheobronchitis or atypical pneumonia (one in which no organism can be cultured from the sputum) and a severe prodromal headache. In these respects, the pulmonary and neurologic illnesses resemble that of the other main cause of "atypical pneumonia," *M. pneumoniae*. The Q fever agent (*Coxiella*) should be suspected if there are concomitant respiratory and meningoencephalitic illnesses and there has been exposure to parturient animals, to livestock (including abattoir workers, who are also exposed to *Brucella* and anthrax), or to wild deer or rabbits. The diagnosis can be made by the finding of a severalfold increase in specific immunofixation antibodies. Patients who survive the illness usually recover completely; a few are left with residual neurologic signs.

Treatment

This consists of the administration of doxycycline or chloramphenicol, which are highly effective in all rickettsial diseases. If these drugs are given early, coincident with the appearance of the rash, symptoms abate dramatically and little further therapy is required. Cases recognized late in the course of the disease require considerable supportive care, including the administration of corticosteroids, maintenance of blood volume to overcome the effects of the septic-toxic reaction, and hypoproteinemia.

Protozoal Diseases

Toxoplasmosis

This disease is caused by *Toxoplasma gondii*, a tiny (2- to 5-μm), obligate, intracellular parasite that is readily recognized in Wright- or Giemsa-stained preparations. It has assumed greater importance in recent decades because of the frequency with which it involves the brain in patients with AIDS. Infection in humans is either congenital or acquired postnatally. Congenital infection is the result of parasitemia in the mother who happens to be pregnant at the time of her initial (asymptomatic) *Toxoplasma* infection. (Treated mothers can be assured, therefore, that there is little carryover risk of producing a second infected infant.) Several modes of transmission of the late-acquired form have been described—eating raw beef, handling uncooked mutton (in Western Europe), and, most often, contact with cat feces, the cat being the natural host of *Toxoplasma*. Most infections in AIDS patients occur in the absence of an obvious source.

The *congenital infection* has attracted attention because of its severe destructive effects on the neonatal brain, as discussed in Chap. 38. Signs of active infection—fever, rash, seizures, hepatosplenomegaly—may be present at birth. More often, chorioretinitis, hydrocephalus or microcephaly, cerebral calcifications, and psychomotor retardation are the major manifestations. These may become evident soon after birth or, more often, the infection is asymptomatic and becomes manifest only several months or years later with choriretinitis. Most infants succumb; others survive with varying degrees of the aforementioned abnormalities.

Serologic surveys indicate that the *exposure to toxoplasmosis* in adults is widespread (approximately 40 percent of American city dwellers have specific antibodies); cases of clinically evident active infection, however, are rare. It is of interest that in 1975 the medical literature contained only 45 well-documented cases of acquired adult toxoplasmosis (Townsend et al); moreover, in half of them there was an underlying systemic disease (malignant neoplasms, renal transplants, collagen vascular disease) that had been treated intensively with immunosuppressive agents. Now, innumerable cases of acquired toxoplasmosis are being seen because it is the most common cause of focal cerebral lesions in patients with AIDS (see Chap. 33). Frequently, the symptoms and signs of infection with *Toxoplasma* are assigned to the primary disease with which toxoplasmosis is associated, and an opportunity for effective therapy is missed.

Most cases in adults are reactivations of the congenital infection. The clinical picture in patients without AIDS varies. Most often it is a subclinical process or manifested by a painless lymphadenopathy, a mononucleosis-like syndrome, or acute chorioretinitis. There is a rare fulminant, widely disseminated infection with a rickettsia-like rash, encephalitis, myocarditis, and polymyositis. Or the neurologic signs may consist only of myoclonus and asterixis, suggesting a metabolic encephalopathy. Often, there are signs of a meningoencephalitis, i.e., seizures, mental confusion, meningeal irritation, coma, and a lymphocytic pleocytosis and increased CSF protein. The brain in such cases shows one or more foci of inflammatory necrosis, essentially an abscess, (Fig. 32-6), with free and encysted *T. gondii* organisms scattered throughout the white and gray matter. Rarely, large areas of necrosis manifest themselves as one or more mass lesions. Sometimes, a nodular lesion is detected on MR or CT imaging that is performed for other reasons.

A presumptive diagnosis can be made on the basis of a rising antibody titer or a positive IgM indirect fluorescent antibody or other serologic test. The diagnosis may be confirmed by the infrequent finding of organisms in CSF sediment and in biopsy specimens of muscle or lymph node. Patients with AIDS and those who are otherwise immunocompromised, however, usually do not display an antibody response or an elevation of titers (those with lymphoma do have positive serologic tests). Excepting AIDS cases, a clinical syndrome and radiologic

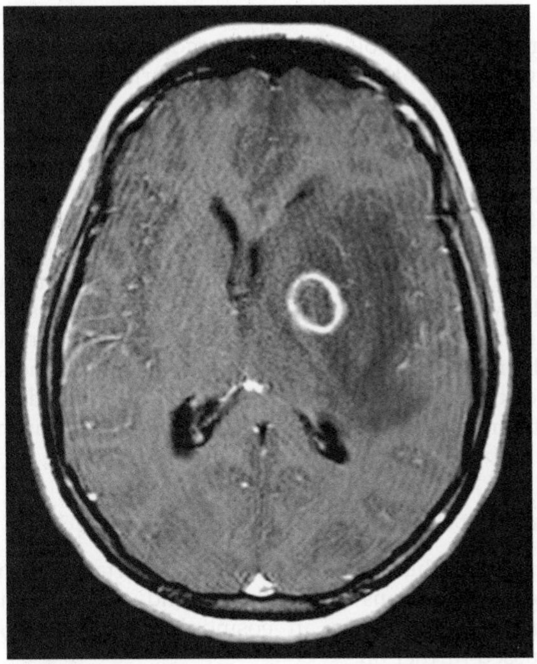

Figure 32-6. MRI showing a rim-enhancing *Toxoplasma* abscess in the deep left cerebral hemishepere in an AIDS patient. There is mass effect and surrounding edema, features which are variable in other similar cases.

features that are consistent with toxoplasmosis and a greatly elevated IgG titer are thought to be diagnostic. In the setting of AIDS, patients with multiple nodular or ring-enhancing brain lesions are treated initially with antibiotics for toxoplasmosis, and further evaluation (mainly for cerebral lymphoma) is undertaken only if there is no response, as discussed in Chap. 33.

Treatment Patients with a presumptive diagnosis are treated with oral sulfadiazine (4 g initially, then 4 to 6 g daily) and pyrimethamine (200 mg initially, then 50 to 100 mg daily). Leucovorin, 15 to 20 mg daily, should be given to counteract the antifolate action of pyrimethamine. Treatment must be continued for at least 6 weeks. In patients with AIDS, treatment at lower doses is continued until the CD4 count exceeds 200 to 250 for 6 months or more; otherwise treatment must be lifelong so as to prevent relapses.

Amebic Meningoencephalitis

This disease is caused by free-living flagellate amoebae, usually of the genus *Naegleria* and less frequently of the genera *Acanthamoeba* and *Balamuthia*. *Naegleria* is acquired by swimming in ponds or lakes where there is warm fresh water. One outbreak in Czechoslovakia followed swimming in a chlorinated indoor swimming pool. Most of the cases in the United States have occurred in the Southeastern states. It is a rare but lethal illness with several dozen instances in the last decade in the United States.

The onset of the illness caused by *Naegleria* is usually abrupt, with severe headache, fever, nausea and vomiting, and stiff neck. The course is inexorably progressive—with seizures, increasing stupor and coma, and focal neurologic signs—and the outcome is practically always fatal, usually within a week of onset. The reaction in the CSF is like that in acute bacterial meningitis: increased pressure, a large number of polymorphonuclear leukocytes (not eosinophils, as in the parasitic infestations discussed further on), and increased protein and decreased glucose content. The diagnosis is supported by a history of swimming in fresh warm water, particularly of swimming underwater for sustained periods, and on finding viable trophozoites in a wet preparation of unspun spinal fluid. Gram stain and ordinary cultures do not reveal the organism.

Autopsy discloses purulent meningitis and numerous quasigranulomatous microabscesses in the underlying cortex.

Subacute and chronic granulomatous meningoencephalitis from ameba is a rare disease in humans. Isolated instances have been reported in debilitated and immunosuppressed patients (Gonzalez et al). The organism may be difficult to culture from the CSF; most diagnoses are made from biopsy. A fatal case of ours, in a leukopenic patient who had been receiving granulocyte-stimulating factor, ran a subacute course over 1 month with headache, mild fever, stupor, and unmeasurably low CSF glucose toward the end of life (Katz et al). Initially, there were scattered, round, enhancing lesions on the MRI that disappeared with corticosteroids, much like lymphoma; later, there were more irregular confluent white matter lesions. A brain biopsy revealed amoebae that could have been easily mistaken for macrophages or cellular debris; the organism proved to be *Balamuthia*.

Treatment with the usual antiprotozoal agents is largely ineffective. Because of the in vitro sensitivity of *Naegleria* to amphotericin B, this drug should be used by the same schedule as for cryptococcal meningitis. With such a regimen in combination with rifampin, recovery is rarely possible.

Malaria

A number of other protozoal diseases are of great importance in tropical regions. One is *cerebral malaria*, which complicates approximately 2 percent of cases of *falciparum malaria*. This is a rapidly fatal disease characterized by headache, seizures, and coma, with diffuse cerebral edema and only very rarely by focal features such as hemiplegia, aphasia, hemianopia, or cerebellar ataxia. Bruxism and hiccoughs have been commented on as common features in case reports. Cerebral capillaries and venules are packed with parasitized erythrocytes and the brain is dotted with small foci of necrosis surrounded by glia (Dürck nodes). A retinopathy consisting of macular whitening, orange or white discoloration of retinal vessels, and intraretinal blot-type hemorrhages, has been suggested as a dependable sign of severe malaria as summarized by Beare and colleagues.

These findings have been the basis of several hypotheses (one of which attributes the cerebral symptoms to mechanical obstruction of the vessels), but none is entirely satisfactory. Also, it seems unlikely that a disorder of immune mechanisms is directly involved in the pathogenesis (see the reviews by Newton et al and by Turner for a discussion of current hypotheses).

Usually the neurologic symptoms appear in the second or third week of the infection, but they may be the initial manifestation. Children in hyperendemic regions are the ones most susceptible to cerebral malaria. Among adults in nonenedmic areas, only pregnant women and nonimmune individuals who discontinue prophylactic medication are liable to CNS involvement (Toro and Roman). Useful laboratory findings are anemia and parasitized red blood cells. The CSF may be under increased pressure and sometimes contains a few white blood cells, and the glucose content is normal. With *Plasmodium vivax* infections, there may be drowsiness, confusion, and seizures without invasion of the brain by the parasite.

Treatment Quinine and artesunate, and related drugs are curative if the cerebral symptoms are not pronounced, but once coma and convulsions supervene, 20 to 30 percent of patients do not survive. Newer drugs such as mefloquine, artemether with lumefantrine, and atovaquone are increasingly used. It had been stated that the administration of large doses of dexamethasone, given as soon as cerebral symptoms appear, may be lifesaving, but most studies, including those of our colleagues, demonstrate that corticosteroids are ineffective. Blood or exchange transfusions may confer a modest benefit on survival in severe cases.

Trypanosomiasis

This is a common disease in equatorial Africa and in Central and South America. The African type ("sleeping sickness") is caused by *Trypanosoma brucei, rhodesiense, and gambiense* and is transmitted by several species of the tsetse fly. Most cases in the United States have been due to the second type in travelers returning from safari. There was an alarming increase in this disease in sub-Saharan Africa during past decades but now, fewer than several thousand cases have been reported because of active control interventions. The infection begins with a chancre at the site of inoculation and localized lymphadenopathy. Posterior cervical adenopathy is highly characteristic of CNS infection (Winterbottom sign); another sign of neurologic interest is pronounced pain at sites of minor injury (called Kerandel hyperesthesia). Later, episodes of parasitemia occur, and at some time during this stage of dissemination, usually in the second year of the infection, the trypanosomes give rise to a diffuse meningoencephalitis. The latter expresses itself clinically as a chronic progressive neurologic syndrome consisting of a reversal or disruption of circadian sleep rhythm, vacant facial expression, and in some, ptosis and ophthalmoplegia, dysarthria, and then muteness, seizures, progressive apathy, stupor, and coma.

The South American variety of trypanosomiasis (Chagas disease) is caused by *Trypanosoma cruzi* and is transmitted from infected animals to humans by the bite of reduviid bugs. There have been rare cases from blood transfusion and organ transplantation. The sequence of local lymphadenopathy, hematogenous dissemination, and chronic meningoencephalitis is like that of African trypanosomiasis. Serologic tests are available to confirm the diagnosis.

Treatment Treatment is with pentavalent arsenicals, mainly melarsoprol, which are more effective in the African than in the South American form of the disease but is highly toxic. An encephalopathy occurs in 10 percent of cases during the institution of treatment; half of these are fatal. As pointed out by Braakman and colleagues, the arsenical encephalopathy is characterized by multiple white matter lesions, sometimes with hemorrhage, and is often quite severe, lethal in between 50 and 75 percent of cases. Newer drugs or combinations, particularly eflornithine with nifurtimox are being used for the gambiense disease. Unusually high rates of relapse are being reported after treatment. A review of the subject of trypanosomiasis has been given by Kennedy. The treatment of Chagas disease has been with nifurtimox and benznidazole.

Diseases Caused by Nematodes (Table 32-6)

Of these, trichinosis is of greatest importance to neurologists. Infections with other roundworms, such as *Angiostrongylus*, cause an eosinophilic meningitis, as discussed further on.

Trichinellosis, Trichinosis (See also Chap. 49)

This disease is caused by the intestinal nematode *Trichinella spiralis*. Infection in humans results from the ingestion of uncooked or undercooked pork (occasionally bear meat) containing the encysted larvae of *T. spiralis*. The larvae are liberated from their cysts by the gastric juices and develop into adult male and female worms in the duodenum and jejunum. After fertilization, the female burrows into the intestinal mucosa, where she deposits several successive batches of larvae. These make their way—via the lymphatics, regional lymph nodes, thoracic duct, and bloodstream—into all parts of the body. The new larvae penetrate all tissues but survive only in striated muscle, where they become encysted and eventually calcify. Animals are infected in the same way as humans, and the cycle can be repeated only if a new host ingests the encysted larvae. Gould has written an authoritative review of this subject.

The early symptoms of the disease, beginning a day or two after the ingestion of pork, are those of a mild gastroenteritis. Later symptoms coincide with invasion of muscle by larvae. The latter begins about the end of the first week and may last for 4 to 6 weeks. Low-grade fever, pain and tenderness of muscles, edema of the conjunctivae and particularly of the eyelids, and fatigue are the usual manifestations. The myopathic aspects of *Trichinella* infestation are considered fully in Chap. 49.

Particularly heavy infection may be associated with a CNS disorder from larval migration through the nervous system without encystation. Headache, stiff neck, and a mild confusional state are the usual symptoms. Delirium, coma, hemiplegia, and aphasia have also been observed on occasion. The spinal fluid is usually normal but may contain a moderate number of lymphocytes and, rarely, parasites.

An eosinophilic leukocytosis usually appears when the muscles are invaded. Serologic (precipitin) tests

Table 32-6

PARASITIC CAUSES OF CENTRAL NERVOUS SYSTEM LESIONS

DISEASE (ORGANISM)	CLINICAL FEATURES	RADIOGRAPHIC FEATURES
Cestodes (tapeworms)		
Cysticercosis (*Taenia solium*) and coenuriasis (*Taenia multiceps*)	Seizures with mature lesions, hydrocephalus, ventricular and multiple subarachnoid implantation	Cyst with scolex; late calcification
Sparganosis (*Spirometra*)	Subcutaneous nodule, seizures	Migrating granuloma or mass
Hydatid disease (*Echinococcus*)	Focal cerebral findings, raised intracranial pressure	Large fluid-filled cyst, solid "chitinoma"
Nematodes (roundworms)		
Trichinosis	Skin lesions, severe myositis, brain lesions, eosinophilia, meningitis, encephalitis (rare)	Granuloma
Angiostrongyloidiasis (*Angiostrongylus cantonensis*)	Meningoencephalitis, eosinophilia	Granuloma, nodule, migrating track
Gnathostomiasis (*Gnathostoma spinigerum*)	Eosinophilic meningoencephalitis	
Baylisascariasis (*Baylisascarus procyonis*)	Eosinophilic meningoencephalitis (from racoon bites)	
Strongyloidiasis (*Strongyloides stercoralis*)	Encephalitis, myelitis, seizures	Irregular nodular enhancing lesions, may change position
Visceral larva migrans (*Toxocara canis, T. cati*)	Eosinophilic meningoencephalitis	
Trematodes (flukes)		
Schistosomiasis (*Schistosoma japonicum, S. mansoni, S. haematobium*)	Myelopathy, seizures, tumor symptoms, swimmer's itch	Single granuloma, may be large
Paragonimiasis	Seizures, meningoencephalitis, pulmonary lesions	Single granuloma
Other tropical and parasitic infections		
Toxoplasmosis (*T. gondii*)	Seizures, focal cerebral findings	Single or multiple enhancing lesions
Amebiasis	Colitis, liver abscess, rare brain abscess	Abscess or encephalopathy
Entamoeba histolytica, N. fowleri, B. mandrallis	Primary amebic meningoencephalitis, seizures (after swimming)	Multiple small abscess lesions
	Granulomatous encephalitis	
Tuberculoma (*M. tuberculosis* and atypical forms)	Seizure	Granuloma

become positive early in the third week. The heart is often involved, manifested by tachycardia and electrocardiographic changes; sterile brain embolism may follow the myocarditis. These findings may aid in the diagnosis, which can be confirmed by finding the larvae in a muscle biopsy, using the technique of low-power scan of wet tissue pressed between two glass slides.

Trichinosis is seldom fatal. Most patients recover completely, although myalgia may persist for several months. Once recurrent seizures and focal neurologic deficits appear, they may persist indefinitely. The latter are based on the rare occurrence of trichina encephalitis (the filiform larvae may be seen in cerebral capillaries and in cerebral parenchyma) and emboli from mural thrombi arising in infected heart muscle.

Treatment (See also Chap. 49.) In the *treatment of severe trichinosis*, albendazole, an antihelminthic agent, and corticosteroids are of value. This drug prevents larval reproduction and is therefore useful in patients known to have ingested trichinous meat. It also interferes with the metabolism of muscle-dwelling larvae. Fever, myalgia, and eosinophilia respond well to the antiinflammatory and immunosuppressant effects of prednisone (40 to 60 mg daily), and a salutary effect has been noted on the cardiac and neurologic complications as well.

Other nematodes, mainly toxocara (the cause of visceral larva migrans), strongyloides, and angiostrongyloides may rarely migrate to the brain, but each is characterized by a systemic illness, which is far more common than the neurologic one. Parasitic meningitis is discussed later.

Diseases Caused by Cestodes

Cysticercosis (See Table 32-6)

This is the larval or intermediate stage of infection with the pork tapeworm *Taenia solium*. In Central and South America and in parts of Africa and India, cysticercosis is a leading cause of epilepsy and other neurologic disturbances. Because of a considerable emigration from these endemic areas, patients with cysticercosis are now being seen with some regularity in countries where the disease had previously been unknown. Usually the diagnosis is suggested by CT or MRI of the brain but can also be made by the presence of multiple calcified lesions in the thigh, leg, and shoulder muscles and in the cerebrum.

The cerebral manifestations of cysticercosis are diverse, related to the encystment and subsequent calcification of the larvae in the cerebral parenchyma, subarachnoid space, and ventricles (Fig. 32-7). The lesions are most

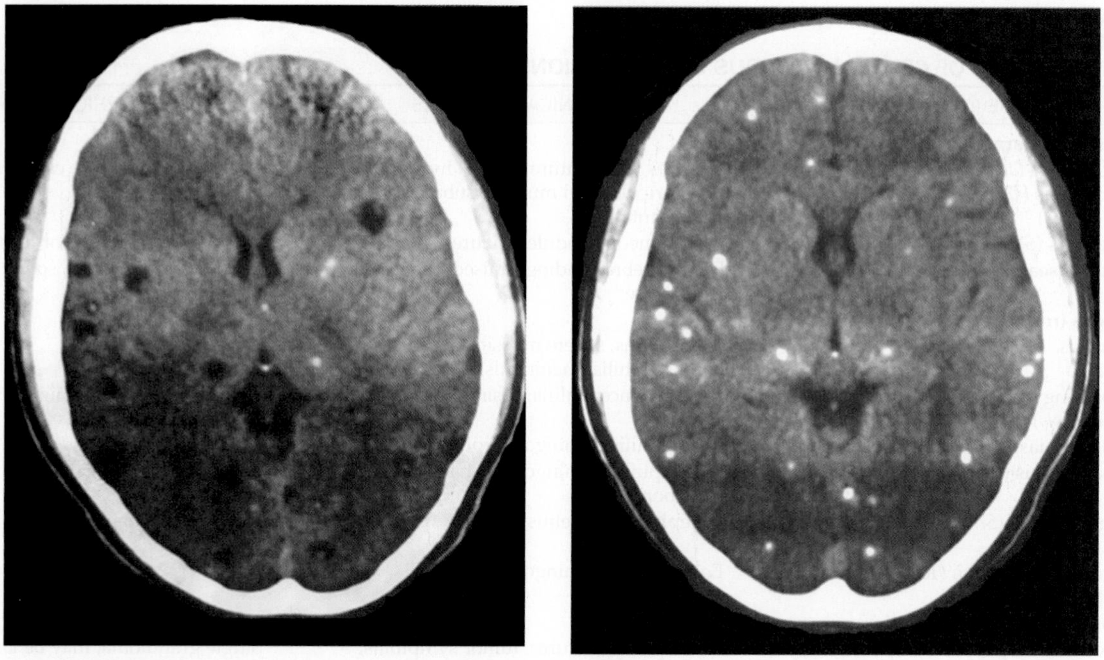

Figure 32-7. Cysticercosis on CT without contrast. Multiple vesicular lesions, some with visible scolices and without mass effect (*left panel*) that became calcified 2 years later (*right panel*).

often multiple but may be solitary; in the United States and nonendemic countries, single cysts are more common. Before the cyst degenerates and eventually calcifies, CT scanning and MRI may actually visualize the scolex. Most often the neurologic disease presents with seizures, although many patients are entirely asymptomatic, the cysts being discovered radiologically. It is only when the cyst degenerates, many months or years after the initial infestation that an inflammatory and granulomatous reaction is elicited and focal symptoms arise.

In some patients, a large subarachnoid or intraventricular cyst may obstruct the flow of CSF, in which case the surgical removal of the cyst or a shunt procedure becomes necessary. Proano and colleagues, however, have reported on a series of such cases with cysts larger than 5 cm in diameter, which they have treated medically. In a more malignant form of the disease, the cysticerci are located in the basilar subarachnoid space, where they induce an intense inflammatory reaction leading to hydrocephalus, vasculitis, and stroke as well as cranial nerve palsies. This so-called racemose form of the illness is little altered by the use of praziquantel or any other form of therapy (Estanol et al) but responds less well than the cystic form.

Treatment For a comprehensive treatment of the subject of neurocysticercosis the reader is referred to the review by Nash and colleagues. The following is a summary of current treatment principles. The therapy of this disorder has been greatly improved in recent years by the use of CT and MRI and the administration of albendazole or praziquantel, an antihelminthic agent that is also active against all species of schistosomes. Albendazole is given as 5 mg/kg tid for 15 to 30 days. Initially, treatment may seem to exacerbate neurologic symptoms, with an increase in cells and protein in the CSF, but then the patient improves and may become asymptomatic, with a striking decrease in the size and number of cysts on CT scanning. Corticosteroids are usually used at the onset of antihelminthic treatment and particularly if a large single lesion is causing symptoms by its mass effect.

Other Cestode Infections

Infection with *Echinococcus* occasionally affects the brain. The usual sources of infection are water and vegetables contaminated by canine feces. After they are ingested, the ova hatch and the freed embryos migrate, primarily to lung and liver, but sometimes to brain (approximately 2 percent of cases), where a large solitary (hydatid) cyst may be formed. The typical lesion is a large fluid-filled cyst with the parasite visible by imaging procedures, but a solid nodular brain lesion, a "chitinoma," is also known to occur. We have also observed a compressive spinal cord lesion. Treatment with the albendazole or mebendazole is recommended when surgery is not feasible.

Cerebral coenuriasis (*coenurus cerebralis*) is an uncommon infestation by larvae of the tapeworm *Taenia multiceps*. It occurs mainly in sheep-raising areas where there are many dogs, the latter being the definitive hosts. The larvae form grape-like cysts, most often in the posterior fossa, which obstruct the spinal fluid pathways and cause signs of increased intracranial pressure. Surgical removal is possible.

Another cestode, *Spirometra mansoni*, may migrate within the brain, leaving a visible track as it moves. Subcutaneous nodules are the most common lesions. This parasite is found predominantly in the Far East.

The nervous system may also be invaded directly by certain worms (*Ascaris*, *filaria*) and flukes (*Schistosoma*, *Paragonimus*). These diseases are virtually nonexistent in the United States except among those who have recently returned from endemic areas. Schistosomiasis, however, is of such great importance and often invades the nervous system in such characteristic ways that it is considered below in detail.

Diseases Caused by Trematodes

Schistosomiasis (See Table 32-6)

The ova of *trematodes* seldom involve the nervous system, but when they do, the infecting organism is usually *Schistosoma japonicum* and, less often, *Schistosoma haematobium* or *Schistosoma mansoni*. It is said that *S. japonicum* has a tendency to localize in the cerebral hemispheres and *S. mansoni* in the spinal cord, but there have been many exceptions. The cerebral lesions form in relation to direct parasitic deposition of eggs in blood vessels and take the form of mixed necrotizing and ischemic parenchymal foci that are infiltrated by eosinophils and giant cells (Fig. 32-8) (Scrimgeour and Gajdusek). The lesions do not calcify.

Schistosomiasis is widespread in tropical regions; 80 percent of cases are in sub-Saharan Africa. North American neurologists have little contact with it except in travelers who have bathed in lakes or rivers where the snail hosts of the parasite are plentiful. The initial manifestation may be a local skin irritation at the site of entry of the parasite (swimmer's itch), or a large serpiginous urticarial rash on the trunk, Katayama fever, particularly likely to occur in prior exposure, but the patient frequently does not offer this information unless sought. A small proportion of patients develop neurologic symptoms several months after exposure.

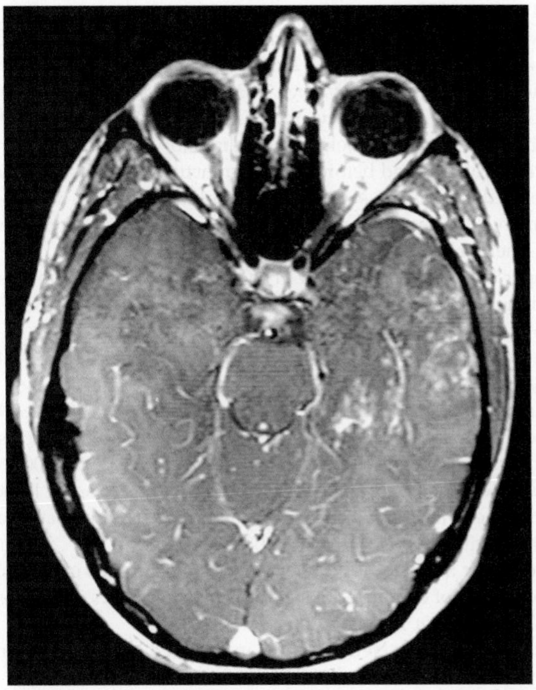

Figure 32-8. MRI of schistosomiasis (*S. mansoni*) with gadolinium enhancement of patchy lesions in the left temporal lobe in a traveler returning from Ghana.

Headaches, convulsions (either focal or generalized), and other cerebral signs appear; with lesions of larger size, papilledema may develop, simulating a brain tumor. It has been hypothesized that travelers are more prone to develop symptomatic nervous system disease because of an intense inflammatory reaction surrounding the deposited eggs.

Some types of *Schistosoma* infections (also called *Bilharzia*), mainly *mansoni*, tend to localize in the spinal cord, causing an acute or subacute myelitis that is concentrated in the conus medullaris. The clinical picture is of a subacutely developing transverse cord lesion. There is often preceding leg or radicular pain and bladder control is affected prominently. We have observed a few cases in students returning from Africa; their lesions were in the conus. Unless treated immediately, there may be permanent paralysis of the legs and bladder from inflammatory and microvascular destruction of the lower cord.

Eosinophilia is common in symptomatic individuals and there is a serologic test but it often becomes negative soon after the initial infection. Examination of the CSF in the myelitic form discloses a pleocytosis, sometimes with an increase in eosinophils (more than half of patients), increased protein content, and increased pressure. Diagnosis is made by the finding of eggs in stool or urine. Serology is probably more sensitive. The other major trematode, *Paragonimus*, has been known to invade the brain in up to one-quarter of cases, where it creates a solitary granulomatous nodule comparable to that seen in schistosomiasis.

Treatment This consists of praziquantel orally in a dosage of 20 mg/kg tid. In one series, 8 of 9 patients with epilepsy caused by cerebral schistosomiasis became seizure-free after treatment with praziquantel. Surgical excision of spinal granulomatous tumors is sometimes indicated, but the results are unpredictable. Corticosteroids are often given concurrently.

Eosinophilic Meningoencephalitis and Meningitis Caused by Parasites

An eosinophilic meningoencephalitis, often with cranial nerve and painful polyradicular findings, has been reported with *Angiostrongylus cantonensis*, *Gnathostoma*, *Paragonimus*, and *Toxocara canis* and *cati* infections. In *Angiostrongylus* infections, snails, freshwater prawns, and unwashed lettuce carry the nematode. The resulting illness may last for weeks to months, with pain, paresthesias, sensorimotor abnormalities, and a confusional state as the main manifestations. Cook has reviewed these and other protozoan and helminthic infections of the CNS. An interesting outbreak in a group of medical students who returned to the United States from Jamaica has been described by Slom and colleagues; they highlighted paresthesias and dysesthesias but noted eosinophilia in the blood or CSF in only half of their patients. Meningeal Hodgkin disease, other lymphomas, and cholesterol emboli also occasionally incite eosinophilic meningitis.

More detailed descriptions of parasitic diseases of the nervous system can be found in the monographs of Bia and of Gutierrez.

References

Adams M, Rhyner PA, Day J, et al: Whipple's disease confined to the central nervous system. *Ann Neurol* 21:104, 1987.

Adams RD, Kubik CS, Bonner FJ: The clinical and pathological aspects of influenzal meningitis. *Arch Pediatr* 65:354, 1948.

Al Deeb SM, Yaqub BA, Sharif HS, Phadke JG: Neurobrucellosis: Clinical characteristics, diagnosis, and outcome. *Neurology* 39:498, 1989.

Anderson M: Neurology of Whipple's disease. *J Neurol Neurosurg Psychiatry* 68:1, 2000.

Armstrong RW, Fung PC: Brainstem encephalitis (rhombencephalitis) due to *Listeria monocytogenes*: Case report and review. *Clin Infect Dis* 16:689, 1993.

Baker P, Price T, Allen CD: Brainstem and cerebellar dysfunction with legionnaires' disease. *J Neurol Neurosurg Psychiatry* 44:1054, 1981.

Baloh RW, Honrubia V: *Clinical Neurophysiology of the Vestibular System*. Oxford, Oxford University Press, 2001, pp 232–234.

Bannwarth A: Chronische lymphocytare Meningitis, entzundliche Polyneuritis und "Rheumatismus." *Arch Psychiatr Nervenkr* 113:284, 1941.

Barnes PF, Bloch AB, Davidson PT, Snider DE Jr: Tuberculosis in patients with human immunodeficiency virus infection. *N Engl J Med* 324:1644, 1991.

Baughman RP, Lower EE: Sarcoidosis, in Fauci AS, Braunwald E, Kasper DL, et al (eds): *Harrison's Principles of Internal Medicine*, 17th ed. New York, McGraw-Hill, 2008, pp 2135–2141.

Beare NAV, Taylor TE, Harding SP, et al: Malarial retinopathy: A newly established diagnostic sign in malaria. *Am J Trop Med Hyg* 75:790, 2006.

Berardi VE, Weeks KE, Steere AC: Serodiagnosis of early Lyme disease: Evaluation of IgM and IgG antibody responses by antibody capture enzyme immunoassay. *J Infect Dis* 158:754, 1988.

Berenguer J, Moreno S, Laguna F, et al: Tuberculous meningitis in patients infected with the human immunodeficiency virus. *N Engl J Med* 326:668, 1992.

Berman PH, Banker BQ: Neonatal meningitis: A clinical and pathological study of 29 cases. *Pediatrics* 38:6, 1966.

Bhandari YS, Sarkari NBS: Subdural empyema: A review of 37 cases. *J Neurosurg* 32:35, 1970.

Bia F (ed): Parasitic diseases of the nervous system. *Semin Neurol* 13(2):1, 1993.

Blanc F, Jaulhac B, Fleury M, et al. Relevance of the antibody index to diagnose Lyme neuroborreliosis among seropositive patients. *Neurology* 69:953, 2007.

Braakman HM, van de Molengraft FJJ, Hubert WW, et al: Lethal African trypanosomiasis in a traveler: MRI and neuropathology. *Neurology* 66:1094, 2006.

Brisson-Noël A, Aznar C, Chureau C, et al: Diagnosis of tuberculosis by DNA amplification in clinical practice. *Lancet* 338:364, 1991.

Burgdorfer W, Barbour AG, Hayes SF, et al: Lyme disease CA tick-borne spirochetosis. *Science* 216:1317, 1982.

Chen RC, McLeod JG: Neurological complications of sarcoidosis. *Clin Exp Neurol* 26:99, 1989.

Christoforidis GA, Spickler EM, Recio MV, Mehta BM: MR of CNS sarcoidosis: Correlation of imaging features to clinical symptoms and response to treatment. *AJNR Am J Neuroradiol* 20:655, 1999.

Chuck SL, Sande MA: Infection with *Cryptococcus neoformans* in the acquired immunodeficiency syndrome. *N Engl J Med* 321:794, 1989.

Cohen MM: The central nervous system in congenital heart disease. *Neurology* 10:452, 1960.

Cook GC: Protozoan and helminthic infections, in Lambert HP (ed): *Infections of the Central Nervous System*. Philadelphia, Decker, 1991, pp 264–282.

Day JN, Chau TTH, Wolbers M, et al: Combination antifungal therapy for cryptococcal meningitis. *N Engl J Med* 368:1291, 2013.

deGans J, van de Beck D, et al: Dexamethasone in adults with bacterial meningitis. *N Engl J Med* 347:1549, 2002.

Delaney P: Neurologic manifestations in sarcoidosis: Review of the literature, with a report of 23 cases. *Ann Intern Med* 87:336, 1977.

Dismukes WE: Cryptococcal meningitis in patients with AIDS. *J Infect Dis* 157:624, 1988.

Dodge PR, Davis H, Feigin RD, et al: Prospective evaluation of hearing impairment as a sequela of acute bacterial meningitis. *N Engl J Med* 311:869, 1984.

Durand ML, Calderwood SB, Weber DJ, et al: Acute bacterial meningitis: A review of 493 episodes. *N Engl J Med* 328:21, 1993.

Ellner JJ, Bennett JE: Chronic meningitis. *Medicine (Baltimore)* 55:341, 1976.

Estanol B, Corona T, Abad P: A prognostic classification of cerebral cysticercosis: Therapeutic implications. *J Neurol Neurosurg Psychiatry* 49:1131, 1986.

Ferry PC, Culbertson JL, Cooper JA, et al: Sequelae of *Haemophilus influenzae* meningitis: Preliminary report of a long-term follow-up study, in Sell SH, Wright PF (eds): *Haemophilus Influenzae—Epidemiology, Immunology and Prevention of Disease*. New York, Elsevier, 1982, sec 3, pp 111–116.

Fisher RS, Clark AW, Wolinsky JS, et al: Postinfectious leukoencephalitis complicating *Mycoplasma pneumoniae* infection. *Arch Neurol* 40:109, 1983.

Garcia-Monico JC, Benach JL: Lyme neuroborreliosis. *Ann Neurol* 37:691, 1995.

Golightly MG: Lyme borreliosis: Laboratory considerations. *Semin Neurol* 17:11, 1997.

Gonzalez MM, Gould E, Dickinson G, et al: Acquired immunodeficiency syndrome associated with *Acanthamoeba* infection and other opportunistic organisms. *Arch Pathol Lab Med* 110:749, 1986.

Gould SE: *Trichinosis in Man and Animals*. Springfield, IL, Charles C Thomas, 1970.

Gray ML, Killinger AH: *Listeria monocytogenes* and *Listeria* infections. *Bacteriol Rev* 30:309, 1966.

Gutierrez Y: *Diagnostic Pathology of Parasitic Infections with Clinical Correlations*, 2nd ed. New York, Oxford University Press, 2000.

Hasbun R, Abrahams J, Jekel J, Quagliarello VJ: Computed tomography of the head before lumbar puncture in adults with suspected meningitis. *N Engl J Med* 345:1727, 2001.

Hinman AR: Tuberculous meningitis at Cleveland Metropolitan General Hospital. *Am Rev Respir Dis* 94:465, 1966.

Hooper DC, Pruitt AA, Rubin RH: Central nervous system infections in the chronically immunosuppressed. *Medicine (Baltimore)* 61:166, 1982.

Iannuzzi MC, Rybicki BA, Teirstein AS: Sarcoidosis. *N Engl J Med* 357:2153, 2007.

Jefferson M: Sarcoidosis of the nervous system. *Brain* 80:540, 1957.

Kaiser R: Clinical courses of acute and chronic neuroborreliosis following treatment with ceftriaxone. *Nervenarzt* 75:553, 2004.

Kasanmoentalib ES, Brouwer MC, vander Ende A, von de Beek D: Hydrocephalus in adults with community-acquired bacterial meningitis. *Neurology* 75:918, 2010.

Kastenbauer S, Pfister HW: Pneumococcal meningitis in adults. Spectrum of complications and prognostic factors in a series of 87 cases. *Brain* 126:1015, 2003.

Katz DA, Berger JR: Neurosyphilis in acquired immunodeficiency syndrome. *Arch Neurol* 46:895, 1989.

Katz JD, Ropper AH, Adelman L, et al: A case of *Balamuthia mandrillaris* meningoencephalitis. *Arch Neurol* 57:1210, 2000.

Kaufman DM, Litman N, Miller MH: Sinusitis-induced subdural empyema. *Neurology* 33:123, 1983.

Kennedy PGE: The continuing problem of human African Trypanosomiasis (sleeping sickness). *Ann Neurol* 64:116, 2008.

Kubik CS, Adams RD: Subdural empyema. *Brain* 66:18, 1943.

Lambert HP (ed): *Infections of the Central Nervous System*. Philadelphia, Decker, 1991.

Lanska DJ: Anthrax meningoencephalitis. *Neurology* 59:327, 2002.

Lebel MH, Freij BJ, Syrogiannopoulos GA, et al: Dexamethasone therapy for bacterial meningitis. Results of two double-blind trials. *N Engl J Med* 319:964, 1988.

Lechtenberg R, Sterra MF, Pringle GF, et al: *Listeria monocytogenes*: Brain abscess or meningoencephalitis? *Neurology* 29:86, 1979.

Lees AW, Tyrrell WF: Severe cerebral disturbance in legionnaires' disease. *Lancet* 2:1331, 1978.

Lewis JL, Rabinovich S: The wide spectrum of cryptococcal infection. *Am J Med* 53:315, 1972.

Leys D, Destee A, Petit H, Warot P: Management of subdural intracranial empyemas should not always require surgery. *J Neurol Neurosurg Psychiatry* 49:635, 1986.

Lincoln EM: Tuberculous meningitis in children. Serous meningitis. *Annu Rev Tuberculosis* 56:95, 1947.

Louis ED, Lynch T, Kaufmann P, et al: Diagnostic guidelines in central nervous system Whipple's disease. *Ann Neurol* 40:561, 1996.

Lyon G, Dodge PR, Adams RD: The acute encephalopathies of obscure origin in children. *Brain* 84:680, 1961.

Matthews BR, Jones LK, Saad DA, et al: Cerebellar ataxia and central nervous system Whipple disease. *Arch Neurol* 62:618, 2005.

Merritt HH, Adams RD, Solomon H: *Neurosyphilis*. New York, Oxford University Press, 1946.

Mizuguchi M, Yamanouchi H, Ichiyama T, et al: Acute encephalopathy associated with influenza and other viral infections. *Acta Neurol Scand* 115:45, 2007.

Naber SP: Molecular pathology—diagnosis of infectious disease. *N Engl J Med* 331:1212, 1994.

Nadelman RB, Wormser GP: Lyme borreliosis. *Lancet* 352:557, 1998.

Narita M, Matsuzono Y, Togashi T, et al: DNA diagnosis of central venous system infection by *Mycoplasma pneumoniae. Pediatrics* 90:250, 1992.

Nash TE, Singh G, White AC, et al: Treatment of neurocysticercosis: current status and future research needs. *Neurology* 67:1120, 2006.

Newton CRJ, Hien TT, White N: Cerebral malaria. *J Neurol Neurosurg Psychiatry* 69:433, 2000.

Newton EM: Hematogenous brain abscess in cyanotic congenital heart disease. *Q J Med* 25:201, 1956.

Nguyen TH, Tran TH, Thwaites G, et al: Dexamethasone in Vietnamese adolescents and adults with bacterial meningitis. *N Engl J Med* 357:2431, 2007.

Nigrovic LE, Kuppermann N, Macias CG, et al: Clinical prediction rule for identifying children with cerebrospinal fluid pleocytosis at very low risk of bacterial meningitis. *JAMA* 297:52, 2007.

Oksi J, Kalimo H, Marttila RJ, et al: Inflammatory brain changes in Lyme borreliosis. *Brain* 119:2143, 1996.

Pachner AR, Delaney E, O'Neill T: Neuroborreliosis in the nonhuman primate: *Borrelia burgdorferi* persists in the central nervous system. *Ann Neurol* 38:667, 1995.

Peacock JE: Persistent neutrophilic meningitis. *Infect Dis Clin North Am* 4:747, 1990.

Pitchenik AE, Fertel D, Bloch AB: Mycobacterial disease: Epidemiology, diagnosis, treatment, and prevention. *Clin Chest Med* 9:425, 1988.

Poachner AR, Steiner I: Lyme neuroborreliosis: Infection, immunity, and inflammation. *Lancet Neurol* 6:544, 2007.

Pomeroy SL, Holmes SJ, Dodge PR, Feigin RD: Seizures and other neurologic sequelae of bacterial meningitis in children. *N Engl J Med* 323:1651, 1990.

Powderly WG, Saag MS, Cloud GA, et al: A controlled trial of fluconazole or amphotericin B to prevent relapse of cryptococcal meningitis in patients with the acquired immunodeficiency syndrome. *N Engl J Med* 326:793, 1992.

Proano JV, Madrazo I, Avelar F, et al: Medical treatment for neurocysticercosis characterized by giant subarachnoid cysts. *N Engl J Med* 345:879, 2001.

Quagliarello VJ, Scheld WM: Treatment of bacterial meningitis. *N Engl J Med* 336:708, 1997.

Reik L: Spirochetal infections of the nervous system, in Kennedy PGE, Johnson RT (eds): *Infections of the Nervous System*. Oxford, Butterworth, 1987, pp 43–75.

Rennick G: Cerebral herniation during bacterial meningitis in children. *BMJ* 306:953, 1993.

Rich AR: *The Pathogenesis of Tuberculosis*, 2nd ed. Oxford, England, Blackwell, 1951.

Ropper AH, Kanis KB: Flaccid quadriplegia from tonsillar herniation in pneumococcal meningitis. *J Clin Neurosci* 7:330, 2000.

Rosenstein NE, Perkins BA, Stephens DS, et al: Meningococcal disease. *N Engl J Med* 344:1378, 2001.

Rothstein TL, Kenny GE: Cranial neuropathy, myeloradiculopathy, and myositis: Complications of *Mycoplasma pneumoniae* infection. *Arch Neurol* 36:476, 1979.

Saag MS, Powderly WG, Cloud GA, et al: Comparison of amphotericin B with fluconazole in the treatment of acute AIDS-associated cryptococcal meningitis. *N Engl J Med* 326:83, 1992.

Scadding JG: *Sarcoidosis*. London, Eyre and Spottiswoode, 1967.

Scarborough M, Gorodon SB, Whitty CJ, et al: Corticosteroids for bacterial meningitis in adults in sub-Saharan Africa. *N Engl J Med* 357:2441, 2007.

Schuchat A, Robinson K, Wenger JD, et al: Bacterial meningitis in the United States. *N Engl J Med* 337:970, 1997.

Schwartz MA, Selhorst JB, Ochs AL, et al: Oculomasticatory myorhythmia: A unique movement disorder occurring in Whipple disease. *Ann Neurol* 20:677, 1986.

Scrimgeour EM, Gajdusek DC: Involvement of the central nervous system in *Schistosoma mansoni* and *S. haematobium* infection. *Brain* 108:1023, 1985.

Seidel JS, Harmatz P, Visvesvara GS, et al: Successful treatment of primary amebic meningoencephalitis. *N Engl J Med* 306:346, 1982.

Sherman JL, Stern BJ: Sarcoidosis of the CNS: Comparison of unenhanced and enhanced MR images. *AJNR Am J Neuroradiol* 11:915, 1990.

Shetty KR, Cilvo CL, Starr BD, Harter DH: Legionnaires' disease with profound cerebellar involvement. *Arch Neurol* 37:379, 1980.

Siltzbach LE, James DG, Neville E, et al: Course and prognosis of sarcoidosis around the world. *Am J Med* 57:847, 1974.

Slom TJ, Cortese MM, Gerber SJ, et al: An outbreak of eosinophilic meningitis caused by *Angiostrongylus cantonensis* in travelers returning from the Caribbean. *N Engl J Med* 346:688, 2002.

Snedeker JD, Kaplan SL, Dodge PR, et al: Subdural effusion and its relationship with neurologic sequelae of bacterial meningitis in infancy: A prospective study. *Pediatrics* 86:163, 1990.

Snider DE, Roper WL: The new tuberculosis. *N Engl J Med* 326:703, 1992.

Sotelo J, Escobedo F, Rodriguez-Carbajal J, et al: Therapy of parenchymal brain cysticercosis with praziquantel. *N Engl J Med* 310:1001, 1984.

Stern BJ, Krumholz A, John SC, et al: Sarcoidosis and its neurological manifestations. *Arch Neurol* 42:909, 1985.

Swartz MN: "Chronic meningitis"—many causes to consider. *N Engl J Med* 317:957, 1987.

Swartz MN, Dodge PR: Bacterial meningitis: A review of selected aspects. *N Engl J Med* 272:725, 779, 842, 898, 1965.

Symonds, C: Hydrocephalic and focal cerebral symptoms in relation to thrombophlebitis of the dural sinuses and cerebral veins. *Brain* 60:531, 1937.

Thi VA, Nordmann P, Landrieu P: Encéphalopathie associée aux infections bactériennes sévères de l'enfant: ("encéphalite presuppurative" ou "syndrome toxi-infectieux"). *Rev Neurol* 158:709, 2002.

Thigpen MC, Whitney CG, Messonnier et al: Bacterial meningitis in the United States, 1998-2007. *N Engl J Med* 364:2016, 2011.

Thompson RA: Clinical features of central nervous system fungus infection, in Thompson RA, Green JR (eds): *Advances in Neurology*. Vol 6. New York, Raven Press, 1974, pp 93–100.

Thwaites GE, Bang ND, Dung NH, et al: Dexamethasone for the treatment of tuberculous meningitis in adolescents and adults. *N Engl J Med* 351:1741, 2004.

Tompkins LS: The use of molecular methods in infectious diseases. *N Engl J Med* 327:1290, 1992.

Toro G, Roman G: Cerebral malaria. *Arch Neurol* 35:271, 1978.

Townsend JJ, Wolinsky JS, Baringer JR, Johnson PC: Acquired toxoplasmosis. *Arch Neurol* 32:335, 1975.

Tunkel AR, Hartman BJ, Kaplan SL, et al: Practice guidelines of the management of bacterial meningitis. *Clin Infect Dis* 39:1267, 2004.

Tunkel AR, Scheld WM: Corticosteroids for everyone with meningitis? *N Engl J Med* 347:1613, 2002.

Turner G: Cerebral malaria. *Brain Pathol* 7:569, 1997.

Tyler KL, Martin JB: *Infectious Diseases of the Nervous System*. Philadelphia, Davis, 1993.

Uldry PA, Kuntzer T, Bogousslavsky J, et al: Early symptoms and outcome of *Listeria monocytogenes* rhombencephalitis: 14 adult cases. *J Neurol* 240:235, 1993.

van de Beek D, de Gans J, Tunkel AR, Wijdicks EFM: Community-acquired bacterial meningitis in adults. *N Engl J Med* 354:44, 2006.

van de Beek D, Drake JM, Tunkel AR: Nosocmial bacertial meningitis. *N Engl J Med* 362:146, 2010.

Vartdal F, Vandvik B, Michaelsen TE, et al: Neurosyphilis: Intrathecal synthesis of oligoclonal antibodies to *Treponema pallidum*. *Ann Neurol* 11:35, 1982.

Walsh TJ, Hier DB, Caplan LR: Fungal infections of the central nervous system: Comparative analysis of risk factors and clinical signs in 57 patients. *Neurology* 35:1654, 1985.

Wasz-Hockert O, Donner M: Results of the treatment of 191 children with tuberculous meningitis. *Acta Paediatr* 51(Suppl 141):7, 1962.

Watt G, Adapon B, Long GW, et al: Praziquantel in treatment of cerebral schistosomiasis. *Lancet* 2:529, 1986.

Westenfelder GO, Akey DT, Corwin SJ, Vick NA: Acute transverse myelitis due to *Mycoplasma pneumoniae* infection. *Arch Neurol* 38:317, 1981.

Zuniga G, Ropper AH, Frank J: Sarcoid peripheral neuropathy. *Neurology* 41:1558, 1991.

33

Viral Infections of the Nervous System, Chronic Meningitis, and Prion Diseases

A number of viruses share the unique tendency to primarily affect the human nervous system. Included in this group are the human immunodeficiency viruses (HIV-1 and HIV-2), herpes simplex viruses (HSV-1 and HSV-2), herpes zoster or varicella zoster virus (VZV), Epstein-Barr virus (EBV), cytomegalovirus (CMV), poliovirus, rabies, and several seasonal arthropod-borne viruses (Flaviviruses). Some of these are neurotropic, exhibiting an affinity for certain types of neurons: for example, poliomyelitis viruses and motor neurons, VZV and peripheral sensory neurons, and rabies virus and brainstem neurons. Yet others attack nonneuronal supporting glial cells; JC virus causing progressive multifocal leukoencephalopathy is the prime example. For many of the rest, the affinity is less selective in that all elements of the nervous system are involved. Herpes simplex, for example, may devastate the medial parts of the temporal lobes, destroying neurons, glia cells, myelinated nerve fibers, and blood vessels; and HIV may induce multiple foci of tissue necrosis throughout the cerebrum. These relationships and many others, which are the subject of this chapter, are of wide interest in medicine. In some conditions, the systemic effects of the viral infection are negligible; it is the neurologic disorder that brings them to medical attention.

Pathways of Infection

Viruses gain entrance to the body by one of several ways. Mumps, measles, and VZV enter via the respiratory passages. Polioviruses and other enteroviruses enter by the oral–intestinal route, and HSV enters mainly via the oral or genital mucosal route. Other viruses are acquired by inoculation, as a result of the bites of animals (e.g., rabies), ticks, mites, or mosquitoes (arthropod-borne or arbovirus infections). The fetus may be infected transplacentally by rubella virus, CMV, and HIV. In all these cases, viremia is an intermediate step to seeding the brain or CSF.

Another pathway of infection is along peripheral nerves; centripetal movement of virus is accomplished by the retrograde axoplasmic transport system. HSV, VZV, and rabies virus utilize this peripheral nerve pathway, which explains why the initial symptoms of rabies occur locally, at a segmental level corresponding to the animal bite. It has been shown experimentally that HSV may spread to the CNS by involving olfactory neurons in the nasal mucosa; the central processes of these cells pass through openings in the cribriform plate and synapse with cells in the olfactory bulb (CNS). Another potential pathway is the trigeminal nerve and gasserian ganglion, however, the role of these pathways in human infection is not certain. Of the different routes of infection, the hematogenous one is by far the most important for the majority of viruses.

Additionally, VZV resides in the sensory ganglia and becomes reactivated later in life, causing shingles decades after the primary infection that produces chicken pox. The JC virus also is latent in tissues, possibly the kidney and bone marrow, only to reemerge under conditions of immunosuppression, to infect the brain.

Mechanisms of Viral Infections

Viruses, once they invade the nervous system, have numerous clinical and pathologic effects. One reason for this diversity is that different cell populations within the CNS vary in their susceptibility to infection with different viruses. To be susceptible to a viral infection, the host cell must have on its cytoplasmic membrane specific receptor sites to which the virus attaches. Thus, some infections are confined to meningeal cells, enteroviruses being the most common, in which case the clinical manifestations are those of aseptic meningitis. Other viruses involve particular classes of neurons of the brain or spinal cord, giving rise to the more serious disorders such as encephalitis and poliomyelitis. The virus or its nucleocapsid must be capable of penetrating the cell, mainly by the process of endocytosis, and of releasing its protective nucleoprotein coating. For viral reproduction to occur, the cell must have the metabolic capacity to transcribe and translate virus-coated proteins, to replicate viral nucleic acid, and, under the direction of the virus's genome, to assemble virions. Certain agents depend on cell-surface receptors to ingress into the cell; these relationships have potential therapeutic interest as, for example, the use of serotonin receptor for entry of the JC virus into oligodendrocytes.

The pathologic effects of viruses on susceptible cells vary greatly. In acute encephalitis, neurons are invaded directly by virus and the cells undergo lysis. There is a corresponding glial and inflammatory reaction. Neuronophagia (phagocytosis of affected neurons and their degenerative products by microglia) is a mark of this phenomenon. In progressive multifocal leukoencephalopathy (PML), there is a selective lysis of oligodendrocytes, resulting in foci of demyelination. In certain congenital infections, e.g., measles and rubella, the virus persists in nervous tissue for months or years. In still other circumstances, a viral infection may exist in the nervous system for a long period before exciting an inflammatory reaction (e.g., subacute sclerosing panencephalitis, SSPE); in these cases the disease may be so indolent as to simulate a degenerative disease.

Differentiating cells of the fetal brain have particular vulnerabilities, and viral incorporation may give rise to malformations and to hydrocephalus; an example is mumps virus with ependymal destruction and aqueductal stenosis.

In experimental animals cerebral neoplasms can be induced when certain viral genomes are incorporated into the DNA of the host cell. There is suggestive evidence of such a mechanism relating to EBV in B-cell lymphoma of the brain. The prions have yet other means of affecting cells that do not conform to the traditional concepts of infection and are discussed in a later section of this chapter.

CLINICAL SYNDROMES

A large number of viruses are able to affect the nervous system. Among the enteroviruses alone, nearly 70 distinct serologic types are associated with CNS disease, and additional types from this family of viruses and others are still being discovered. There is no need, however, to consider them individually, as there are only a limited number of ways in which they express themselves clinically: (1) acute aseptic ("lymphocytic") meningitis; (2) a less-common recurrent meningitis; (3) acute encephalitis and meningoencephalitis; (4) ganglionitis (herpes zoster); (5) chronic invasion of nervous tissue by retroviruses, i.e., HIV and tropical spastic paraparesis (TSP); (6) acute anterior poliomyelitis; (7) chronic viral infections including the agent causing PML and subacute sclerosing panencephalitis (SSPE) and (8) the prion agents that are discussed later in the chapter.

ACUTE ASEPTIC MENINGITIS

The term *aseptic meningitis* was first introduced to designate what was thought to be a specific disease—"aseptic" because bacterial cultures were negative. The term is now applied to a symptom complex that is produced by any one of a number of infective agents, the majority of which are viral but a few of which are bacterial (mycoplasma, Q fever, other rickettsial infections). Because aseptic meningitis is rarely fatal, the precise pathologic changes are uncertain but are presumably limited to the meninges. Conceivably, there may be some minor changes in the underlying brain itself, but these are of insufficient severity to cause neurologic symptoms and signs or to show changes on imaging studies.

In outline, the clinical syndrome of aseptic meningitis consists of fever, headache, signs of meningeal irritation, and a predominantly lymphocytic pleocytosis in the spinal fluid with normal glucose. Usually the onset is acute and the temperature is elevated, from 38 to 40°C (100.4 to 104°F). Headache that is more severe than that associated with other febrile states is the most frequent symptom. A variable but usually mild degree of lethargy, irritability, and drowsiness may occur. Photophobia and pain on movement of the eyes are common additional complaints. Stiffness of the neck and spine on forward bending attests to the presence of meningeal irritation (meningismus), but at first it may be so slight as to pass unnoticed. Here the Kernig and Brudzinski signs help little, for they are often absent in the presence of manifest viral meningitis. When there are accompanying neurologic signs, they too tend to be mild or fleeting: paresthesia in an extremity, or wavering Babinski signs.

Systemic symptoms and signs aside from fever are infrequent and depend mainly on the more mundane effects of the invading virus; these include sore throat, nausea and vomiting, vague weakness, pain in the back and neck, conjunctivitis, cough, diarrhea, vomiting, rash, petechia, hepatitis, adenopathy, or splenomegaly. The childhood exanthems associated with meningitis and encephalitis (varicella, rubella, mumps) produce well-known eruptions and other characteristic signs. An erythematous papulomacular, nonpruritic rash, confined to the head and neck or generalized, may also be a prominent feature, particularly in children, of certain echoviruses and Coxsackie viruses. An enanthem (herpangina), taking the form of a vesiculoulcerative eruption of the buccal mucosa, may also occur with these viral infections.

In milder cases, in the first hours or day of the illness, there may be no abnormalities of the spinal fluid, and the patient may erroneously be thought to have migraine or a headache induced by a systemic infectious illness. Microorganisms cannot be demonstrated by conventional smear or culture. As a rule, the glucose content of the CSF is normal; but infrequently, mild depression of the CSF glucose (never below 25 mg/dL) occurs with the meningitis caused by mumps, HSV-2, lymphocytic choriomeningitis, or VZV.

Causes of Acute Aseptic Meningitis

Aseptic meningitis is a common occurrence, with an annual incidence of approximately 20 cases per 100,000 population (Beghi et al; Ponka and Pettersson). Most are caused by viral infections. Of these, the most common are from enterovirus—mainly echovirus and Coxsackie virus. These make up 80 percent of cases in which a specific viral cause can be established. HSV-2 is perhaps next in frequency in adults, followed by varicella, HIV, mumps in children, lymphocytic choriomeningitis (LCM), HSV-1, and adenovirus infections. The next most frequent group comprise EBV (infectious mononucleosis), CMV, leptospira, HSV-1, and the bacterium *Mycoplasma pneumoniae* (see Chap. 32), and in some parts of the world, tick-borne encephalitis virus and *Borrelia*, including the Lyme agent (Kupila et al), or during local outbreaks anywhere, arboviruses. Influenza virus, adenoviruses, and numerous sporadic and otherwise innocuous agents are at times isolated from the spinal fluid in cases of aseptic meningitis. The California and West Nile viruses, which are arthropod-borne viruses ("arboviruses" in the family of Flaviviruses) are responsible for a small number of cases; they usually cause an encephalitis or meningoencephalitis in brief regional outbreaks as discussed further on.

It is also recognized that infection with HIV may present as acute, self-limited aseptic meningitis with an infectious mononucleosis-like clinical picture. While HIV has been obtained from the CSF in the acute phase of the illness, seroconversion occurs only later, during convalescence from the meningitis (see further on). HSV-1 has been isolated from the CSF of patients with recurrent bouts of benign aseptic meningitis (so-called Mollaret meningitis), but this finding has not been consistent (Steel et al). As discussed in Chap. 47, it is now believed that this virus also underlies many if not most cases of what has been traditionally considered idiopathic Bell's palsy.

Two other aspects of the virology of aseptic meningitis should be noted: first, in most published series of cases from virus isolation centers, a specific cause cannot be established in one-third or more of cases of presumed viral origin; second, most agents capable of producing aseptic meningitis also sometimes cause encephalitis.

Differential Diagnosis of the Cause of Viral Meningitis

Clinical distinctions between the many viral causes of aseptic meningitis cannot be made with high reliability, but useful clues can be obtained by attention to certain details of the clinical history and physical examination. Inquiry should be made regarding recent respiratory or gastrointestinal symptoms, immunizations, past history of infectious disease, family outbreaks, insect bites, contact with animals, and areas of recent travel. The presence of a local epidemic, the season during which the illness occurs, and the geographic location, are other helpful data.

Because the common enteroviruses, including polio, grow in the intestinal tract and are spread mainly by the fecal–oral route, family outbreaks are usual and the infections are most common among children. A number of echovirus and Coxsackie virus (particularly group A) infections are associated with exanthemata and may be associated with the grayish vesicular lesions of oral herpangina. Pleurodynia, brachial neuritis, pericarditis, and orchitis are characteristic of some cases of group B Coxsackie virus infections and there are certainly other causes. Pain in the back and neck and in the muscles should suggest poliomyelitis or dengue. Lower motor neuron weakness may also occur with echo, West Nile, and Coxsackie virus infections, but it is usually mild and transient in nature. The peak incidence of enteroviral infections is in August and September.

Mumps meningitis occurs sporadically throughout the year, but the highest incidence is in late winter and spring. Males are affected three times more frequently than females. Other manifestations of mumps infection—parotitis, orchitis, mastitis, oophoritis, and pancreatitis—may be, but most often are not, present. It should be noted that orchitis is not specific for mumps but occurs occasionally with group B Coxsackie virus infections, infectious mononucleosis, and lymphocytic choriomeningitis. A definite past history of mumps aids in excluding the disease as an attack confers lifelong immunity.

The natural host of the *LCM virus* is the common house mouse, *Mus musculus*. Humans acquire the infection by contact with infected hamsters or with dust contaminated by mouse excreta. Laboratory workers who handle rodents may be exposed to LCM. The meningitis may be preceded by respiratory symptoms, sometimes with pulmonary infiltrates. The infection is particularly common in late fall and winter, presumably because mice enter dwellings at that time.

Parvovirus causes fifth disease in young children, characterized by high fever and markedly flushed cheeks but not associated with neurologic symptoms beyond irritability and sometimes, febrile seizures. However, when contracted from the child by an adult, various neurologic manifestations such as brachial neuritis can occur. There have also been reports of encephalitis and meningitis with the B-19 strain, particularly in children and sometimes in individuals with altered immunity. By a difficult to understand complication, some patients have had strokes as discussed in the review by Douvoyiannis and colleagues.

HSV and HIV meningitis may be associated with a cauda equina neuritis. In the case of HSV, there is often a preceding genital infection with the virus (see Chap. 46). The presence of sore throat, generalized lymphadenopathy, transient rash, and mild icterus is suggestive of *infectious mononucleosis caused by EBV* or, at times, *CMV infection*. Icterus is a prominent manifestation of viral hepatitis and some serotypes of leptospirosis and, at times, of Q fever. Among the bacterial and spirochetal cause of an aseptic meningitis syndrome, *leptospirosis, M. pneumoniae,* and *Lyme borreliosis* are notable as discussed in the previous chapter.

Certain forms of encephalitis occur particularly in individual who are immunosuppressed from HIV, chemotherapy for neoplasm, organ transplantation, or hematologic and lymphoid malignancy. The manifestation is usually encephalitis but aseptic meningitis is known to occur. The main causative organisms in this group are HHV-6, CMV, and VZV.

Laboratory findings suggest certain organisms as the cause of aseptic meningitis. Most cases of infectious mononucleosis can be identified by the blood smear and specific serologic tests (heterophil or others). LCM should be suspected if there is an intense lymphocytic pleocytosis. Counts above 1,000 cells/mm^3 in the spinal fluid, particularly if the cells are all lymphocytes, are most often due to LCM but may occur occasionally with mumps or echovirus 9. In the last of these agents, neutrophils may predominate in the CSF for a week or longer. Slightly depressed glucose in the spinal fluid is consistent with mumps meningitis and with the viruses mentioned earlier, but it is more often indicative of bacterial or fungal infection.

Liver function tests are abnormal in many patients with EBV infection and leptospiral infections; the hepatitis viruses are not known to produce meningitis. In the majority of patients with *M. pneumoniae* infections, cold agglutinins appear in the serum toward the end of the first week of the illness.

Panels of serologic tests for the main viruses that cause aseptic meningitis are available; most use complement fixation or enzyme-linked immunosorbent assay (ELISA) techniques; an infection is demonstrated by a fourfold increase in titer from acute to convalescent serum drawn at least 10 days apart, but these, of course, do no more than confirm the diagnosis after the illness has mostly passed. In some instances, elevation of specific IgM antibody directed at an infectious agent is useful. Serologic reactions of CSF for syphilis should be interpreted with caution, because inflammation of many types, including infectious mononucleosis, can produce a false-positive reaction. In the last few years, the polymerase chain reaction (PCR) has been applied to the diagnosis of viral infections of the nervous system, among them being CMV and HSV. The test is most sensitive during the active stage of viral replication, in contrast to serologic tests, which are more accurate later in the course of the infection. There are numerous false-negative and fewer false-positive PCR tests for CMV, but they are nonetheless useful in some circumstances, such as the early diagnosis of fulminant CMV infection in AIDS patients (see later in this chapter). For the most part, neither serologic nor PCR testing is required in clinical practice.

Nonviral Causes of Aseptic, Chronic, and Recurrent Meningitis

In addition to the aforementioned bacterial infections that can cause meningitis, several other categories of disease may cause a sterile, predominantly lymphocytic or mononuclear reaction in the leptomeninges: (1) foci of bacterial infection lying adjacent to the meninges, such as spinal or cranial epidural abscess (parameningeal infection); (2) partially treated bacterial meningitis; (3) meningeal infections in which the organism is difficult or impossible to isolate—fungal and tuberculous meningitis are at times in this category and parasitic infections are in this group; (4) neoplastic invasion of the leptomeninges (lymphomatous and carcinomatous meningitis); (5) granulomatous, vasculitic, or other inflammatory diseases such as sarcoidosis, Behçet disease, and granulomatous angiitis; and (6) acute or chronic recurrent inflammatory meningitides as a result of chemical irritation, drug-induced allergic reactions, including an aseptic *chemical meningitis* incited by rupture of a craniopharyngioma or other cystic structure containing proteinaceous fluid. These are described further on under "Chronic Persistent and Recurrent Meningitis." (7) Rarely, children with scarlet fever or streptococcal pharyngitis develop meningeal signs and slight pleocytosis, the result of a sterile serous inflammation that does not involve invasion of the meninges by organisms. The same occurs in bacterial endocarditis.

An idiosyncratic, presumably immunologic meningitis may result from the use of nonsteroidal antiinflammatory drugs, intravenous immune globulin (due probably to a carrier chemical in the solution), and, rarely, from other drugs, including certain antibiotics. Individuals with systemic lupus erythematosus have an increased risk of aseptic meningitic reactions to antiinflammatory medications.

In respect to the first two categories, parameningeal and partially treated bacterial infections, smoldering paranasal sinusitis or mastoiditis may produce a CSF picture of aseptic meningitis because of epidural or subdural extension into the intracranial compartments; it is infrequent that the entire syndrome of meningitis is present. Uncomplicated sinusitis alone does not cause a meningeal reaction.

Antibiotic therapy given for a systemic or pulmonary infection may suppress a bacterial meningitis to the point where mononuclear cells predominate, glucose is near normal, and organisms cannot be cultured from the CSF although they may still be evident by Gram stain. Careful attention to the history of recent antimicrobial therapy permits recognition of these cases.

Syphilis, cryptococcosis, and tuberculosis are the important members of the third group that cause aseptic meningitis and in which the organism may be difficult to culture, as detailed in Chap. 32. Tuberculous meningitis, in its initial stages, may masquerade as innocent aseptic meningitis and the diagnosis may be delayed. Similarly, the diagnosis of cryptococcosis, other fungal infection, or nocardiosis is occasionally missed because the organisms may be present in such low numbers as to be overlooked in smears, especially in AIDS patients. Brucellosis (Mediterranean fever, Malta fever) is a rare disease that may present as an acute meningitis or meningoencephalitis, with the CSF findings of aseptic meningitis. The diagnosis depends on the detection of high serum antibody titers and *Brucella*-specific immunoglobulins, using the ELISA or serum agglutination testing.

In the neoplastic group, leukemias and lymphomas are the most common sources of meningeal infiltrations. In children, leukemic "meningitis" with cells (lymphoblasts or myeloblasts) in the CSF numbering in the thousands may occur. In leptomeningeal metastases (carcinomatous meningitis), neoplastic cells extend throughout the leptomeninges and involve cranial and spinal nerve roots, producing a picture of meningoradiculitis with normal or low CSF glucose values. Lymphocytic meningitis that is accompanied by cranial-nerve palsies may prove to be tuberculous if the patient is febrile and the CSF glucose is low (or even without these signs in an endemic area); it is likely to be neoplastic if the patient is afebrile and the CSF glucose is normal or mildly decreased. Concentrated cytologic preparations usually permit identification of the tumor cells. Chapter 31 discusses neoplastic meningitis in detail.

Occlusion of many small cerebral blood vessels by cholesterol emboli may also excite a reaction in meningeal vessels and a pleocytosis that includes eosinophils.

CHRONIC PERSISTENT AND RECURRENT MENINGITIS (Table 33-1)

Chronic and recurrent meningitides always pose diagnostic problems. Such patients may have a low-grade fever, headache of varying severity, stiff neck, and a

Table 33-1

CAUSES OF CHRONIC AND RECURRENT ASEPTIC MENINGITIS

Infectious	
	Tuberculosis and atypical mycobacterial
	Fungal (cryptococcal, coccidial, histoplasmal, blastomyces, etc.)
	Nocardia
	HIV
	Herpes type 2 (recurrent Mollaret meningitis)
	Lyme disease
	Syphilis
	Brucellosis
	Epidural abscess or hematoma
	Incompletely treated bacterial meningitis
Granulomatous and vasculitic	
	Sarcoidosis
	Wegener granulomatosis
	Behçet disease
	Vasculitis
	IgG-4 pachymeningitis
Neoplastic	
	Carcinomatous
	Lymphomatous
	Leukemic
Allergic	
	Nonsteriodal antiinflammatory drugs
	IVIg
	Antibiotics
	Other medications
Chemical	
	Leakage from epidermoid tumor, dermoid cyst, craniopharyngioma, or teratoma
	Instillation of irritative substances by lumbar puncture, spinal anesthesia, or surgery
Idiopathic	
	Vogt-Kayanagi-Harada disease
	No cause determined in one-third of cases

predominantly mononuclear pleocytosis, sometimes with slightly raised CSF pressure. There may be limited focal neurologic signs such a slight pronator drift or Babinski sign. A viral or some other type of infective inflammation is always suspected, but a search by culture methods and serology usually yields negative results. Herpesvirus has been demonstrated to be the cause of a few cases, as in the recurrent Mollaret type of meningitis noted later. The process often improves without identification of the cause over a period of months or a year or more; in other cases, the cause is eventually found. Only a few end fatally.

In a group of such patients studied at the Mayo Clinic, 33 of 39 underwent a natural resolution and 2 died; 14 were still symptomatic at the time of the report (Smith and Aksamit). In another series from New Zealand of 83 patients, Anderson and colleagues ultimately found tuberculosis to be the most common identifiable cause, a smaller number being accounted for by neoplastic and cryptococcal meningitis; in fully one-third of the patients, no cause could be established. Charleston and colleagues reported a subgroup of these patients who were responsive to steroids; in only 7 of 17 patients could medication eventually be withdrawn without recurrence; 4 required treatment indefinitely; and the remaining 6 died after many months or years. The outcome and response to steroids in our patients have been much the same. These series excluded chemical or irritative meningitis, which should be considered if there had been spinal surgery or infusion of even apparently innocuous substances into the spinal space.

The special problem of *chronic neutrophilic meningitis* has been mentioned in the preceding chapter in relation to *Nocardia, Aspergillus, Actinomyces,* or certain *Mycobacterium* species; other causes include coccidioidomycosis, histoplasmosis, and blastomycosis, (see Peacock, cited in Chap. 32).

A reasonable approach in patients with chronic meningitis is to repeat the lumbar puncture several times to obtain all cultures including for fungi and cytology of CSF, using markers to detect uniform populations of B and T lymphocytes and tumor cells, biochemical tests that are sensitive to neoplastic meningitis (such as β_2-microglobulin, lactate dehydrogenase [LDH]), and PCR amplification of herpesviruses, serologic tests mainly for HIV, syphilis, coccidioidomycosis, *Brucella*, and Lyme disease. MRI of the brain and spinal cord with gadolinium should also be performed to detect parameningeal collections. If hydrocephalus develops, it should be managed along the lines described in Chap. 30.

A trial of antiviral agents and broad-spectrum antibiotics may be justified, although we have had limited success with them in our last several patients. We resort to a biopsy of the meninges over the frontal convexity or at a site that demonstrates infiltration or marked enhancement if the diagnosis has not been clarified in 6 to 12 months or if febrile meningitis persists for more than several weeks, but examination of this tissue has also proved to be of limited value. In Anderson's (1995) series, mentioned earlier, biopsy yielded a diagnosis in 5 of 25 patients. Finally, if bacterial infection has been reasonably excluded, corticosteroids are administered for several weeks and then tapered while observing the patient and resampling the CSF.

The CSF formula in a number of other *chronic or acutely recurring meningitides* corresponds to that of aseptic meningitis. These include (1) the Vogt-Koyanagi-Harada syndrome, which is characterized by combinations of iridocyclitis, depigmentation of a thick swath of hair (poliosis circumscripta) and of the skin, vitiligo, around the eyes, loss of eyelashes, dysacusis, and deafness (the pathologic basis of the syndrome is not known); and (2) Mollaret recurrent meningitis, many instances of which have been associated with HSV-1 (Steel) and others (perhaps most) with HSV-2 infection (Cohen et al). The syndrome is characterized by episodes of acute meningitis with severe headache and sometimes low-grade fever, lasting for about 2 weeks, and recurring over a period of several months or years. In a few patients of ours, in whom no virus could be identified in the CSF, antiviral therapy met with some success, although corticosteroids seemed to reduce the severity of acute episodes. A proportion of these cases follow bouts of genital herpes and individual cases have been reported with EBV, herpes-6 in children, and other viruses. A special syndrome that has been associated with HSV-2 is that of aseptic meningitis and bladder failure and vaginal or vulvar pain after a bout of genital herpes (Elsberg syndrome as reviewed by Ellie and colleagues); (3) In some patients, the recurrent attacks are associated with encephalopathy and headache; this is probably identical to the illness called "pseudomigraine with temporary neurological symptoms" by Gomez-Aranda and described earlier by Bartleson. The entity, also known as HaNDL syndrome ("headache neurologic deficit and lymphocytic pleocytosis") is allied more closely with the headache syndromes as discussed and cited in Chap. 10. (4) Allergic or hypersensitivity meningitis, in the past occurring in the course of serum sickness and now more commonly of autoimmune diseases such as lupus erythematosus, and in relation to certain medications such as nonsteroidal antiinflammatory drugs and intravenously administered immunoglobulin. (5) Behçet disease, which is an important acute, recurrent inflammatory CNS disease, particularly in individuals of Middle Eastern origin. It is essentially a diffuse inflammatory disease of small blood vessels that has several other characteristic features such as oral and genital ulcers and is more appropriately considered with the vasculitides in Chap. 34.

In summary, the temporal history of the illness, associated clinical findings, and laboratory tests usually provide clues to the diagnosis of nonviral and chronic forms of aseptic meningitis. It is useful to keep in mind the possibility of neoplasia, HIV, tuberculosis, cryptococcosis, sarcoidosis, syphilis, borreliosis, parameningeal collection, and inadequately treated bacterial meningitis—each of which presents an urgent diagnostic problem.

ACUTE ENCEPHALITIS

From the foregoing discussion it is evident that the separation of the clinical syndromes of aseptic meningitis and encephalitis is not always clear. In some patients with aseptic meningitis, mild drowsiness or confusion may be present, suggesting cerebral involvement. Conversely, in some patients with encephalitis, the cerebral symptoms may be mild and meningeal symptoms and CSF abnormalities predominate. The common practice is to assume that viral meningitis causes only fever, headache, stiff neck, and photophobia; if any other CNS symptoms are added, the condition is generally called meningoencephalitis. As has been emphasized, the same spectrum of viruses gives rise to both meningitis and encephalitis. It is our impression that many cases of enteroviral and practically all cases of mumps and LCM encephalopathy are little more than examples of intense meningitis in which the subpial surface of the brain is inflamed. Rarely have they caused demonstrable postmortem cerebral lesions, and surviving patients have no residual neurologic signs. Conversely, several agents, notably the arboviruses, may cause encephalitic lesions with only mild meningeal symptoms.

The core of the *encephalitis syndrome* consists of an acute febrile illness with evidence of various combinations of seizures, delirium, confusion, stupor or coma; aphasia, hemiparesis with asymmetry of tendon reflexes and Babinski signs, involuntary movements, ataxia, and myoclonic jerks; and nystagmus, ocular palsies, and facial weakness. The meningitic component may be intense, have mild manifestations such as headache, or be entirely inapparent. The spinal fluid invariably shows a cellular reaction and the protein is slightly elevated. Imaging studies of the brain are most often normal but may show diffuse edema or enhancement of the cortex and, in certain infections, subcortical and deep nuclear involvement as well as, in the special case of HSV encephalitis, selective damage of the inferomedial temporal and frontal lobes.

Differentiation of Viral from Postinfectious Encephalitis (See also Chap. 36) The acute encephalitis syndrome described above may take two forms: the more common direct invasion of brain and meninges (true viral encephalitis) and a postinfectious encephalomyelitis that is presumably based on an autoimmune reaction to the systemic viral infection but in which virus is not present in neural tissue. The distinction between postinfectious encephalomyelitis and infectious encephalitis may be difficult, especially in younger patients who have a proclivity to develop the postinfectious variety with fever. The latter, termed acute disseminated encephalomyelitis (ADEM), occurs after a latency of several days, as the infectious illness is subsiding. It is expressed by a low-grade fever and cerebral symptoms such as confusion, seizures, coma, or ataxia. The spinal fluid shows slight inflammation and elevation of protein—sometimes a more intense reaction, and there are usually characteristic confluent, scattered, bilateral lesions in the white matter in imaging studies, findings that differ from those of viral encephalitis. When there is no coexistent epidemic of encephalitis to suggest the diagnosis, or the preceding systemic illness is absent or obscure, a differentiation between the two may not be possible on clinical grounds alone. The fever is generally higher in the infectious type but even this difference does not always hold in young children with ADEM. The encephalitis that follows certain childhood exanthems (postexanthematous) and vaccinations at any age (postvaccinal) are essentially forms of ADEM.

Because ADEM is predominantly an inflammatory and demyelinative process, we mention it here but discuss its clinical features and imaging more fully in Chap. 36, with the other demyelinating diseases such as multiple sclerosis, with which it shares some features. We also place in special categories further on the now rare Reye syndrome of postinfectious acute encephalopathy with hepatic failure that follows influenza, and other viral infections and postinfectious cerebellitis.

Etiology

Whereas numerous viral, bacterial, fungal, and parasitic agents are cited as causes of the encephalitis syndrome, only the viral ones are considered here, for they are the most common and it is to these that one usually refers when the term *encephalitis* is used. The nonviral forms (mycoplasmal, rickettsial, Lyme, etc.) are considered in Chap. 32, under "Encephalitis Caused by Bacterial Infections," and should be reviewed with this section.

According to the Centers for Disease Control and Prevention, approximately 20,000 cases of acute viral encephalitis are reported annually in the United States. Death occurs in 5 to 20 percent of these patients and residual signs, such as mental deterioration, amnesic defect, personality change, recurrent seizures, and hemiparesis, are seen in approximately another 20 percent. However, these overall figures fail to reflect the widely varying incidence of mortality and residual neurologic abnormalities that follow infections by different viruses. In herpes simplex encephalitis, for example, approximately 50 percent of patients die or are left with some impairment, and in eastern equine encephalitis, the figures are even higher. On the other hand, death and serious neurologic sequelae have been observed in only 5 to 15 percent of those with western equine and West Nile infections and in even fewer patients with Venezuelan, St. Louis, and La Crosse encephalitides.

The types of viral encephalitis that occur with sufficient frequency to be of clinical importance are relatively few. HSV is by far the most common sporadic cause of encephalitis and has no seasonal or geographic predilections. Its age distribution is slightly skewed and biphasic, affecting persons mainly between ages 5 and 30 years and those older than age 50 years. Many other viruses, exemplified by the arboviral encephalitides, have a characteristic geographic and seasonal incidence. The most important of these is the Japanese encephalitis serogroup (Flaviviruses), of which the now common West Nile virus is a member. In recent outbreaks in the United States, the West Nile virus has been more frequent than any of the other arboviruses and has had a wide geographic distribution (Solomon). In the United States, eastern equine encephalitis, as the name implies, is observed mainly in the eastern states and on both the Atlantic and Gulf coasts. Western equine encephalitis is fairly uniformly distributed west of the Mississippi. St. Louis encephalitis, another arthropod-borne late-summer encephalitis, occurs nationwide but especially along the Mississippi River in the South; outbreaks occur in August through October, slightly later than is customary for the other arboviruses. Venezuelan equine encephalitis is common in South and Central America; in the United States it is practically confined to Florida and the southwestern states. California virus encephalitis predominates in the northern Midwest and northeastern states. After West Nile, the La Crosse variety is perhaps the most frequent identifiable arbovirus encephalitis in the United States.

Rabies infections occur worldwide, but in the United States they are seen mostly in the Midwest and along the West Coast. Japanese B encephalitis (the most common encephalitis outside of North America), Russian spring-summer encephalitis, Murray Valley encephalitis (Australian X disease), and several less common viral encephalitides are infrequent in the United States or, as in the case of West Nile fever, have appeared only recently. With the ease and rapidity of travel, many of these will undoubtedly increase in number in North America and parts of Europe where they have not been seen hitherto.

Infectious mononucleosis, which is a primary infection with EBV, is complicated by meningitis, encephalitis, facial palsy, or polyneuritis of the Guillain-Barré type in a small proportion of cases. Each of these neurologic complications can occur in the absence of the characteristic fever, pharyngitis, and lymphadenopathy of infectious mononucleosis. The same is true of *M. pneumoniae*. In these two diseases there is still uncertainty as to whether they are true infectious encephalitides or postinfectious complications, as discussed in Chap. 32. Evidence from PCR testing of spinal fluid is consistent with a direct infection in some cases. Varicella zoster and CMV are other herpes-type viruses that may cause encephalitis. They are discussed in relation to the particular clinical settings in which they occur. Definite cases of "epidemic encephalitis" (encephalitis lethargica) have not been observed in acute form since 1930, although an occasional surviving patient with a residual parkinsonian syndrome is still seen in neurology clinics. However, various movement disorders, including parkinsonism, are being seen as a residua of encephalitis from the Flaviviruses. The latency from infection to these complications is brief, or may be present from the outset, quite unlike encephalitis lethargica. There may also be a postinfectious-immune variety of this midbrain encephalitis.

More recently, a sometimes overwhelming encephalitis has been recognized as a rare manifestation of influenza infection, particularly the H1N1 strain that has infected mainly children in Southeast Asian countries, but also other serotypes of influenza including mundane influenza viruses that cause yearly outbreaks. The disorder has been called an "encephalopathy" in research publications but convulsions, delirium, and coma suggest that the neurologic aspects are from encephalitis.

The relative frequency of the various viral infections of the nervous system can be appreciated from several studies. An early series from the Walter Reed Army Institute comprising 1,282 patients is particularly noteworthy in that a positive laboratory diagnosis was achieved in more than 60 percent of cases (Buescher et al)—a higher rate than in almost any subsequent study of comparable size. Aside from the poliovirus (some of the data were gathered before 1959) the common infective agents in cases of both aseptic meningitis and encephalitis were group B Coxsackie virus, echovirus, mumps virus, lymphocytic choriomeningitis virus, arboviruses, HSV, and *Leptospira*, in that order. In a later prospective virologic study of all children examined at the Mayo Clinic during the years 1974 to 1976, a diagnosis of aseptic meningitis, meningoencephalitis, or encephalitis was entertained in 42 cases and an infectious agent was identified in 30 of them (Donat et al). The California virus was isolated in 19 cases and one of the enteroviruses (echovirus types 19, 16, 21, or Coxsackie virus) in 8 cases; mumps, rubeola, HSV, adenovirus 3, and *M. pneumoniae* were detected in individual cases (several patients had evidence of combined infections). As mentioned, recent outbreaks of *West Nile virus*, close to 3,000 cases yearly in the United States, make it of more current import than some of the viral infections listed here. The related Japanese encephalitis virus is even more ubiquitous on a worldwide basis, causing 10,000 deaths in Asia each year.

In a more contemporary and impressively large series of viral infections of the nervous system from the United Kingdom involving more than 2,000 patients, viral identification in the CSF was attempted by means of PCR with positive results in only 7 percent, half of which were various enteroviruses (Jeffery et al). The other organisms commonly identified were HSV-1, followed by VZV, EBV, and other herpesviruses. In patients with AIDS, however, the relative frequencies of the organisms that cause meningoencephalitis are quite different and include special clinical presentations; this applies particularly to CMV infection of the nervous system, as discussed further on, under "Opportunistic Infections and Neoplasms of the CNS in AIDS." Our personal experience has been heavily biased toward HSV encephalitis, seasonal outbreaks of eastern equine or West Nile encephalitis, and AIDS-related cases.

Arboviral Encephalitis

The common arthropod-borne viruses (arboviruses) that cause encephalitis in the United States and their geographic range have been mentioned earlier. Most of the agents are in the category of Flaviviruses. There are alternating cycles of viral infection in mosquitoes and vertebrate hosts; the mosquito becomes infected by taking a blood meal from a viremic host (horse or bird) and injects virus into the host, including humans. The seasonal incidence of these infections is practically limited to the summer and early fall, when mosquitoes are biting. In the equine encephalitides, regional deaths in horses usually precede human epidemics. For St. Louis encephalitis, the urban bird or animal or possibly the human becomes the intermediate host. West Nile outbreaks are preceded by illness in common birds such as crows and jays. St. Louis, California, and La Crosse agents are endemic in the United States because of the cycle of infection in small rodents. Powassan virus from the deer tick has been added to the list of causes of Flavivirus encephalitis in North America as in the report by Tavakoli and coworkers.

The clinical manifestations of the arbovirus infections are almost indistinguishable from one another, although they do vary with the age of the patient. The incubation period after mosquito or tick bite transmission is 5 to 15 days. There may be a brief prodromal fever with arthralgia or rash (e.g., West Nile fever). In infants, there may be only an abrupt onset of fever and convulsions, whereas in older children and adults the onset is usually less abrupt, with complaints of headache, listlessness, nausea or vomiting, drowsiness, and fever for several days before medical attention is sought; convulsions, confusion, stupor, and varying degrees of stiff neck then become prominent. Photophobia, diffuse myalgia, and tremor (of either action or intention type) may be observed. Asymmetry of tendon reflexes, hemiparesis, extensor plantar signs, myoclonus, chorea, and sucking and grasping reflexes may also occur. McJunkin and colleagues described the clinical features of 127 patients with La Crosse infection seen at their medical center over a decade, and their descriptions are representative of other arboviral infections. In addition to the typical features of viral encephalitis they emphasize aspects that occur in a proportion of patients: hyponatremia, raised intracranial pressure with cerebral swelling, and, most notable to us, signal changes in the MRI that simulate herpes encephalitis.

A special syndrome of febrile, flaccid, paralytic poliomyelitis resulting from West Nile virus infection is now also well known. It evolves over several days and in a few cases is accompanied by facial paralysis (Jeha et al). A few cases have had an early extrapyramidal syndrome; any of these features may occur with the other Flaviviruses.

The fever and neurologic signs of arboviral encephalitis subside after 4 to 14 days unless death supervenes or destructive CNS changes have occurred. No antiviral agents are known to be effective; one must rely entirely on supportive measures. On occasion, brain swelling reaches a degree that requires specific therapy, as outlined in "Management of the Acutely Comatose Patient and Management of Raised Intracranial Pressure" in Chap. 17.

Of the arbovirus infections in the United States, eastern equine encephalitis (EEE) is among the most serious, as a large proportion of those infected develop encephalitis; approximately one-third die and a similar number, more often children, are left with disabling abnormalities—mental retardation, emotional disorders, recurrent seizures, blindness, deafness, hemiplegia, extrapyramidal motor abnormalities, and speech disorders. While only a small proportion of those exposed become infected, the poliomyelitis and parkinsonian syndromes of the Flaviviruses may be permanent residua as mentioned earlier (Solomon). On the other extreme, La Crosse encephalitis, which affects mostly children, has an almost uniformly benign outcome. The rate of progression from a nondescript febrile viral syndrome to encephalitis is similarly low in the arbovirus infections and mortality rate varies from 2 to 12 percent in different outbreaks.

Diagnosis The CSF findings are much the same as in aseptic meningitis (lymphocytic pleocytosis, mild protein elevation, normal glucose values). Recovery of virus from blood or CSF is usually not possible and PCR testing is routinely only applied during local epidemics. However, antiviral immunoglobulin (Ig) M antibody is present in the serum and CSF within the first days of symptomatic disease and can be detected and quantified by means of ELISA, making it preferable to other testing for specific diagnosis. Some patients have not developed antibodies by the time of admission to the hospital and the test may have to be repeated in several days. The MRI may be normal or show signal changes and edema in the cortex, basal ganglia, or thalamus (the latter is described particularly in the Japanese B virus group, West Nile, EEE, and rabies).

Pathology Perivascular cuffing by lymphocytes and other mononuclear leukocytes and plasma cells, as well as a patchy infiltration of the meninges with similar cells, are the usual histopathologic hallmarks of viral encephalitis. There is widespread degeneration of single nerve cells, with neuronophagia as well as scattered foci of inflammatory necrosis involving both the gray and white matter. The brainstem is relatively spared. In some cases of eastern equine encephalitis, the destructive lesions may be massive, involving the major part of a lobe or hemisphere and are readily displayed by MRI, but in the other arbovirus infections the foci are microscopic in size (Deresiewicz et al). West Nile virus may produce a regional pattern of neuronal damage that affects the anterior horn cells of the spinal cord, a poliomyelitis, as mentioned earlier. Pathologic descriptions of this process have been provided by our colleagues and by others (see Asnis et al).

Herpes Simplex Encephalitis

Of the common viral encephalitides, this is perhaps the gravest and is by far the most common. About 2,000 cases occur yearly in the United States, accounting for approximately 10 percent of all cases of encephalitis. Between 30 and 70 percent are fatal, and the majority of patients who survive are left with serious neurologic abnormalities. HSV encephalitis occurs sporadically throughout the year and in patients of all ages and in all parts of the world. It is almost always caused by HSV-1, which is also the cause of the common herpetic lesions of the oral mucosa; only rarely, however, are the oral and encephalitic lesions concurrent. The type 2 herpesvirus may also cause acute generalized encephalitis, usually in the neonate and in relation to genital herpetic infection in the mother. Type 2 infection in the adult more typically causes an aseptic meningitis and sometimes a polyradiculitis or myelitis, again in association with a recent genital herpes infection. Exceptionally, the localized adult type of encephalitis is caused by the type 2 virus and the diffuse neonatal encephalitis by type 1.

Clinical Features

The symptoms, which evolve over several days, are in most cases like those of any other acute encephalitis—namely, fever, headache, seizures, confusion, stupor, and coma. In some patients these manifestations are preceded by symptoms and findings that betray the predilection of this disease for the inferomedial or lateral portions of the frontal and temporal lobes and the insula. The symptoms and findings include olfactory or gustatory hallucinations, anosmia, temporal lobe seizures, personality change, bizarre or psychotic behavior or delirium, aphasia, and hemiparesis. Although several seizures at the onset of illness are not an uncommon presentation, status epilepticus is rare. Disturbed memory function can often be recognized, but usually this becomes evident only later in the convalescent stage as the patient awakens from stupor or coma. Hemorrhagic swelling and herniation of one or both temporal lobes through the tentorial opening may occur, leading to coma during the first few days of the illness, a very poor prognostic sign.

The CSF is typically under increased pressure and almost invariably shows a pleocytosis (range 10 to 200 cells/mm^3; infrequently greater than 500 cells/mm^3). The cells are mostly lymphocytes, but there may be a significant number of neutrophils early on. In a few cases, 3 to 5 percent in some large series, the spinal fluid was normal in the first days of the illness, only to become abnormal when reexamined. The hemorrhagic nature of brain tissue destruction with this infection may be reflected in the spinal fluid. In fact, in only a minority of cases, red cells, sometimes numbering in the thousands but usually far fewer, and xanthochromia are found. The protein content is increased in most cases. Rarely, the CSF glucose levels may be reduced to slightly less than 40 mg/dL, creating confusion with tuberculous and fungal meningitides. The cerebral imaging appearance, giving highly characteristic features, is discussed later in the section on "Diagnosis."

Pathology

The lesions take the form of an intense hemorrhagic necrosis of the inferior and medial temporal lobes and the mediorbital parts of the frontal lobes. The region of necrosis may extend upward along the cingulate gyri and sometimes to the insula or the lateral parts of the temporal lobes or caudally into the midbrain but always contiguous with areas of mediotemporal lobe necrosis. The temporal lobe lesions are usually bilateral but not symmetrical. This distribution of lesions is so characteristic that the diagnosis can be made by gross inspection or by their location and appearance on imaging studies. Cases described in past years as "acute necrotizing encephalitis" and "inclusion body encephalitis" were likely to have been instances of HSV encephalitis. In the acute stages, intranuclear eosinophilic inclusions are found in neurons and glia cells, in addition to the usual microscopic abnormalities of acute encephalitis and hemorrhagic necrosis. Specific intracellular staining with antibody to various portions of the virus is perhaps the most definitive demonstration of the disease.

The characteristic localization of the lesions in this disease has been putatively explained by the virus' route of entry into the CNS. Two such routes have been suggested (Davis and Johnson). The virus may, for example, be latent in the trigeminal ganglia and, with reactivation, infect the nose and then the olfactory tract. Alternatively, with reactivation in the trigeminal ganglia, the infection may spread along nerve fibers that innervate the leptomeninges of the anterior and middle fossae. The lack of lesions in the olfactory bulbs in as many as 40 percent of fatal cases (Esiri) is a point in favor of the second pathway.

Diagnosis

Acute herpes simplex encephalitis must be distinguished from other types of viral encephalitis, from acute hemorrhagic leukoencephalitis, and from paraneoplastic and other forms of limbic encephalitis, tumor, cerebral abscess, cerebral venous thrombosis, and septic embolism (see Chap. 32). When aphasia is the initial manifestation of the illness, it may be mistaken for a stroke. The CSF findings have been mentioned and are typical of a meningoencephalitis. Spinal fluid that contains a large number of red cells may be attributed to a ruptured saccular aneurysm. The electroencephalographic (EEG) changes, consisting of lateralized periodic high-voltage sharp waves in the temporal regions and slow-wave complexes at regular 2 to 3/s intervals, are highly suggestive in the appropriate clinical context, though they are not

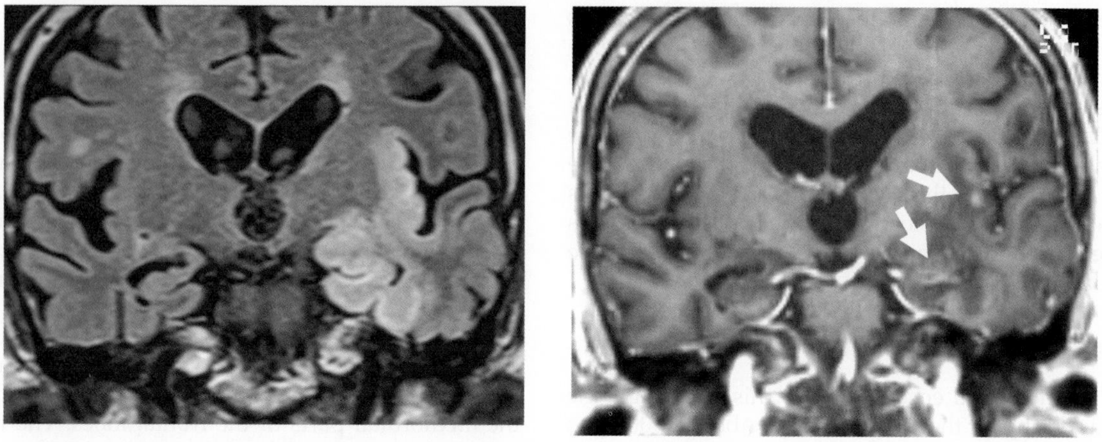

Figure 33-1. Herpes simplex encephalitis. *Left panel*: T2-FLAIR coronal MRI, taken during the acute stage of the illness. There is increased signal in the inferior and medial temporal lobe and the insular cortex of the left hemisphere. *Right panel*: T1-weighted image after gadolinium infusion showing enhancement of the left insular and medical temporal cortices (arrows).

specific for the disease and their sensitivity has not been established with certainty.

CT shows hypodensity of the affected temporal lobe areas in perhaps two-thirds of cases and MRI shows signal changes in almost all (increased signal in T2-weighted images; Fig. 33-1). T1-weighted images demonstrate areas of low signal intensity with surrounding edema and sometimes with scattered areas of hemorrhage occupying the inferior parts of the frontal and temporal lobes. The lesions almost always enhance to some degree with contrast infusion or with gadolinium, indicating cortical and pial abnormalities of the blood–brain barrier. It should be noted that these destructive lesions, and certainly their degree, are almost unique among the viral encephalitides, being seen only occasionally in other viral infections of the brain.

A rising titer of neutralizing antibodies can be demonstrated from the acute to the convalescent stage, but this is not of diagnostic help in the acutely ill patient and may not be significant in patients with recurrent herpes infections of the oral mucosa. Tests for the detection of HSV antigen in the CSF by the application of PCR have been developed and are useful in diagnosis while the virus is replicating in the first few days of the illness (Rowley et al). A refinement in this technique (a nested PCR assay described by Aurelius and coworkers) reportedly has a sensitivity of 95 percent and gives very few false-positive tests in the first 3 weeks of illness. In the experience of Lakeman and colleagues, the test was 98 percent positive in cases proven by cultures of brain biopsy material and gave 6 percent false positives. Antiviral treatment did not appear to affect the results. False-negative tests are most likely to occur in the first 48 h of febrile infection. When the clinical features are consistent with the disease and the PCR test is negative, it is advisable to repeat it in several days, perhaps in another laboratory and to obtain PCR testing for HSV-2 as well.

The only alternative way to establish the diagnosis of acute HSV encephalitis is by fluorescent antibody study and by viral culture of cerebral tissue obtained from brain biopsy. The approach to biopsy as a diagnostic test is now infrequently employed with the availability of the PCR test. We have now found it necessary to perform biopsy in only a very few cases, preferring to treat the patient with antiviral agents based on compatible clinical, radiologic, and CSF findings while awaiting serologic and PCR test results.

Treatment

Until the late 1970s, there was no specific treatment for HSV encephalitis. A collaborative study sponsored by the National Institutes of Health and also a Swedish trial indicated that the antiviral agent acyclovir significantly reduces both mortality and morbidity from the disease (Whitley et al; Sköldenberg et al). For this reason, it has become general practice to initiate treatment while confirmatory testing is being carried out. Acyclovir is given intravenously in a dosage of 30 mg/kg/d and continued for 10 to 14 days in order to prevent relapse. Acyclovir carries limited risk and can be discontinued if further clinical or laboratory features point to another diagnosis. The main problems that arise from the drug are local irritation of the veins used for infusion, mild elevation of hepatic enzymes, or transient impairment of renal function. Nausea, vomiting, tremor, or an encephalopathy that is difficult to distinguish from the encephalitis itself occurs in a very few patients.

The matter of *relapse after treatment* with acyclovir has been recognized, particularly in children. Several potential mechanisms have been suggested by Tiége and colleagues, including an immune-mediated inflammatory response, but treatment with too low a dose or for too brief a period is undoubtedly the main cause of the rare relapses that occur in adults. In children, a second course of acyclovir is usually successful.

When a large volume of brain tissue is involved, the hemorrhagic necrosis and surrounding edema act as an enlarging mass that requires separate attention. Coma and pupillary changes should not be attributed to the mass effect unless compression of the upper brainstem is evident on brain imaging, as the infection is capable of spreading to the mesencephalon from the contiguous deep temporal lobe, thereby causing coma by a direct destructive effect. All measures used in the management of brain edema from mass lesions are applicable here, but there are insufficient data by which to judge their effectiveness. The concern that corticosteroids may aggravate the infection has not been borne out by clinical experience, but a detrimental effect cannot be discounted and their value is uncertain. Our experience (reported by Barnett et al) and that of Schwab and colleagues have been that the presence of raised intracranial pressure early in the illness presages a poor outcome. Seizures are usually brought under control by high doses of conventional antiepileptic drugs. The use of these medications prophylactically for seizures has not been resolved.

Prognosis The outcome of this disease, both mortality and morbidity, is governed to a large extent by the patient's age and state of consciousness, particularly at the time of institution of acyclovir therapy. If the patient is unconscious (except immediately after a convulsion), the outcome is usually poor. However, if treatment is begun within 4 days of onset of the illness in an awake patient, survival is greater than 90 percent (Whitley, 1990). Evaluation of patients 2 years after treatment showed 38 percent to be normal or nearly normal, whereas 53 percent were dead or severely impaired. The neurologic sequelae are often of the most serious type, consisting of a Korsakoff amnesic defect or a global dementia, seizures, and aphasia as described by Drachman and Adams in the era before treatment became available. If there were seizures during the acute illness, it is advisable to continue antiepileptic medications for a year or more and then judge the risk of discontinuing them on the basis of further seizures, the EEG, and the patient's exposure to situations that pose a danger, such as driving. With the exception of the rare relapsing cases mentioned earlier, the infection does not recur.

HHV-6 Encephalitis in Stem Cell Transplant

This agent, the cause of roseola (exanthema subitum), has had a controversial role in a number of acute febrile neurologic illnesses, including febrile seizures in infants and young children, subsequent temporal lobe epilepsy, cranial-nerve palsies, and other conditions. However, it is fairly firmly established as the cause of a medial temporal lobe (limbic) encephalitis in adult patients following allogenic hematopoietic stem cell bone marrow transplantation, as summarized by Seeley and colleagues. All of their patients also developed a graft-versus-host reaction. The clinical and imaging features closely resemble the paraneoplastic and anti–voltage-gated potassium channel limbic encephalitis that is discussed in Chap. 31. The prognosis is far better than in herpetic encephalitis. It is mentioned here that mundane adenoviruses can also produce a severe medial temporal lobe encephalitis in bone marrow transplant cases, in one of our patients associated with gray matter damage in the spinal cord.

The other viral agents that appear as causes of encephalitis with some regularity in stem-cell and organ transplant patients include parvovirus, CMV, EBV, adenovirus, HSV, and varicella zoster virus. Quite often, these infections are but one component of multiorgan viral infection. Some of these agents also cause manifestations of infection in peripheral and cranial nerves.

Rabies

This disease also stands apart from other acute viral infections by virtue of the latent period that follows inoculation with the virus and its stunningly distinctive clinical and pathologic features. Human examples of this disease are rare in the United States; between 1980 and 1997, only 34 instances were known to have occurred and since 1960, there have not been more than 5 or so cases in any 1 year. In some areas (Australia, Hawaii, Great Britain, and the Scandinavian peninsula), no indigenous cases have ever been reported. In contrast, in India there is a high incidence. The importance of this disease derives from the fact that it is almost invariably fatal once the characteristic clinical features appear, making survival of the infected individual dependent on the institution of specific therapeutic measures before the infection becomes clinically evident. Furthermore, each year 20,000 to 30,000 individuals are treated with rabies vaccine, having been bitten by animals that possibly were rabid, and although the incidence of complications with the newer rabies vaccination is much lower than before, a few serious reactions continue to be encountered (see further on and also Chap. 36).

Etiology

Practically all cases of rabies are the result of transdermal viral inoculation by an animal bite. In developing countries, where rabies is relatively common, the most frequent source is the rabid dog. In Western Europe and the United States, the most common rabid species are raccoons, skunks, foxes, and bats among wild animals and dogs and cats among domestic ones. Because rabid animals commonly bite without provocation, the nature of the attack should be determined. Also, the prevalence of animal rabies virus varies widely in the United States, and local presence of the disease is useful in assessing risk. Rare cases have been caused by inhalation of the virus shed by bats; a history of spelunking suggests this mode of acquiring the infection. In a few cases the source of the infection may not be identifiable. The epidemiology and public health aspects of rabies have been reviewed by Fishbein and Robinson.

Clinical Features

The incubation period is usually 20 to 60 days but may be as short as 14 days, especially in cases involving multiple deep bites around the face and neck. Tingling or numbness at the site of the bite, even after the wound has healed, is characteristic. This is thought to reflect an inflammatory response that is incited when the virus reaches the sensory ganglion.

The main neurologic symptoms, following a 2- to 4-day prodromal period of fever, headache, and malaise consist of apprehension, dysarthria, and psychomotor overactivity, followed by dysphagia (hence salivation and "frothing at the mouth"), spasms of throat muscles induced by attempts to swallow water or in rare cases by the mere sight of water ("hydrophobia"), dysarthria, numbness of the face, diplopia, and spasms of facial muscles. These features indicate the involvement of the tegmental medullary nuclei. Generalized seizures, confusional psychosis, and a state of agitation may follow. A less common paralytic form ("dumb" rabies of older writings, in distinction to the above described "rabid" form) as a result of spinal cord infection may accompany or replace the state of excitement. The paralytic form is most likely to follow bat bites or, in the past, the administration of rabies vaccination. Coma gradually follows the acute encephalitic symptoms and, with rare exceptions as noted below, death ensues within 4 to 10 days, or longer in the paralytic form.

Pathologic Features

The disease is distinguished by the presence of cytoplasmic eosinophilic inclusions, the Negri bodies. They are most prominent in pyramidal cells of the hippocampus and Purkinje cells but have been seen in nerve cells throughout the brain and spinal cord. In addition there is widespread perivascular cuffing and meningeal infiltration with lymphocytes and mononuclear cells and small foci of inflammatory necrosis, such as those seen in other viral infections. The inflammatory reaction is most intense in the brainstem. The focal collections of microglia in this disease are referred to as *Babes nodules* (named for Victor Babes, a Romanian microbiologist).

Treatment

Bites and scratches from a potentially rabid animal should be thoroughly washed with soap and water and, after all soap has been removed, cleansed with benzyl ammonium chloride (Zephiran), which has been shown to inactivate the virus. Wounds that have broken the skin also require tetanus prophylaxis.

After a bite by a seemingly healthy animal, surveillance of the animal for a 10-day period is necessary. Should signs of illness appear in the animal, it should be killed and the brain sent, under refrigeration, to a government-designated laboratory for appropriate diagnostic tests. Wild animals, if captured, should be killed and the brain examined in the same way.

If the animal is found by fluorescent antibody or other tests to be rabid, or if the patient was bitten by a wild animal that escaped, *postexposure prophylaxis* should be given. Human rabies immune globulin (HRIG) is injected in a dose of 20 U/kg of body weight (one-half infiltrated around the wound and one-half intramuscularly). This provides passive immunization for 10 to 20 days, allowing time for active immunization. Duck embryo vaccine (DEV) was previously used for this purpose and greatly reduced the danger of serious allergic encephalomyelitis from about 1 in 1,000 cases (with the formerly used equine vaccine) to 1 in 25,000 cases; it is still used in many parts of the world. The more recently developed rabies vaccine grown on a human diploid cell line (human diploid cell vaccine [HDCV]) has reduced the doses needed to just 5 (from the 23 needed with DEV); these are given as 1-mL injections on the day of exposure and then on days 3, 7, 14, and 28 after the first dose. The HDCV vaccine has increased the rate of antibody response and reduced even further the allergic reactions by practically eliminating foreign protein. A thorough trial of the new antiviral agents in patients already symptomatic has not been undertaken. Persons at risk for rabies, such as animal handlers and laboratory workers, should receive preexposure vaccination with HDCV. A preventative DNA rabies vaccine has been genetically engineered and is being tested for use in animal handlers and others at high risk.

With modern intensive-care techniques, there have been a number of survivors of the encephalitic illness, all of whom had received postexposure immunization. In addition to mechanical respiratory support, several secondary abnormalities must be addressed, including raised intracranial pressure, excessive release of antidiuretic hormone, diabetes insipidus, and extremes of autonomic dysfunction, especially hyper- and hypotension. Willoughby and colleagues were successful in treating a 15-year-old girl who had not received vaccine by using an empirical approach of induced coma with ketamine and midazolam supplemented by ribavirin and amantadine. The goal was to support the patient while her antibody response matured. At least two other cases treated in a similar manner, reported anecdotally, did not survive.

Acute Cerebellitis (Acute Ataxia of Childhood)

A comment is made here concerning a dramatic syndrome of acute ataxia that occurs in the context of an infectious illness, mainly in children. The syndrome was originally described by Westphal in 1872 following smallpox and typhoid fever in adults, but Batten is credited with drawing attention to the more common ataxic illness that occurs after common childhood infections such as measles, pertussis, and scarlet fever. Currently, acute ataxia of childhood is most often associated with chickenpox (about one-quarter of 73 consecutive cases reported by Connolly et al), but it can occur during or after any of the childhood exanthems, as well as in association with infections caused by enteroviruses (mainly Coxsackie virus), EBV, *Mycoplasma*, CMV, Q fever, vaccinia, a number of vaccinations, rarely following HSV, and also after nondescript respiratory infections (see Weiss and Guberman). The condition, as mentioned, is far less frequent in adults, but we encounter a case every few years in adolescents and individuals in their twenties; besides a case of varicella that we observed in a 25-year-old, the most common preceding organisms in these individuals have been EBV and *Mycoplasma*.

This illness, which is essentially a "meningocerebellitis," appears relatively abruptly, over a day or so, and consists of limb and gait ataxia and often, but not uniformly, dysarthria and nystagmus. Additional signs include increased limb tone, Babinski signs, or confusion. The fever of the original infection may have abated, or it may persist through the early stages of the ataxic illness. As a rule, there is a mild pleocytosis; the CSF protein is elevated or may be normal. The MRI is normal in the majority of cases but some show enhancement with gadolinium of the cerebellar cortical ribbon. Most patients make a slow recovery, but permanent residua are known to follow. Because the benign nature of the illness has precluded extensive pathologic study, there is uncertainty regarding the infectious or postinfectious nature of these ataxic illnesses. Some cases have shown an inflammatory pathology most suggestive of a postinfectious process (see Chap. 36), but the finding of fragments of VZV and *Mycoplasma* genomes in the spinal fluid by means of DNA amplification techniques favors a primary infectious encephalitis, at least in some instances.

SYNDROMES OF HERPES ZOSTER

Herpes zoster ("shingles," "zona") is a common viral infection of the nervous system occurring at an overall rate of 3 to 5 cases per 1,000 persons per year, with higher rates in the elderly. Shingles is distinctly rare in childhood. It is characterized clinically by radicular pain, a vesicular cutaneous eruption, and, less often, by segmental sensory and delayed motor loss. The pathologic changes consist of an acute inflammatory reaction in isolated spinal or cranial sensory ganglia and lesser degrees of reaction in the posterior and anterior roots, the posterior gray matter of the spinal cord, and the adjacent leptomeninges.

The neurologic implications of the segmental distribution of the rash were recognized by Richard Bright as long ago as 1831. Inflammatory changes in the corresponding ganglia and related portions of the spinal nerves were first described by von Barensprung in 1862. The concept that varicella and zoster are caused by the same agent was introduced by von Bokay in 1909 and was subsequently established by Weller and his associates (1958). The common agent is varicella or VZV, a DNA virus that is similar in structure to the virus of herpes simplex. These and other historical features of herpes zoster were reviewed by Denny-Brown, Adams, and Fitzgerald and by Weller, Witton, and Bell.

Pathology and Pathogenesis

The pathologic changes in VZV infection consist of one or more of the following: (1) an inflammatory reaction in several unilateral adjacent sensory ganglia of the spinal or cranial nerves, frequently of such intensity as to cause necrosis of all or part of the ganglion, with or without hemorrhage; (2) an inflammatory reaction in the spinal roots and peripheral nerve contiguous with the involved ganglia; (3) a less-common poliomyelitis that closely resembles acute anterior poliomyelitis but is readily distinguished by its unilaterality, segmental localization, and greater involvement of the dorsal horn, root, and ganglion, sometimes with necrosis; and (4) a relatively mild leptomeningitis, largely limited to the involved spinal or cranial segments and nerve roots. These pathologic changes are the substrate of the neuralgic pains, the pleocytosis, and the local palsies that may attend and follow the VZV infection. There may also be a delayed cerebral vasculitis (see further on).

As to *pathogenesis*, herpes zoster represents a spontaneous reactivation of VZV infection, which becomes latent in the neurons of sensory ganglia following a primary infection with chickenpox (Hope-Simpson). This mechanism is consistent with the differences in the clinical manifestations of chickenpox and herpes zoster, even though the same virus causes both. Chickenpox is highly contagious by respiratory aerosol, has a well-marked seasonal incidence (winter and spring), and tends to occur in epidemics. Zoster, on the other hand, is not communicable (except to a person who has not had chickenpox), occurs sporadically throughout the year, and shows no increase in incidence during epidemics of chickenpox. In patients with zoster, there is practically always a past history of chickenpox. Such a history may be lacking in rare instances of herpes zoster in infants, but in these cases there has usually been prenatal maternal contact with VZV.

VZV DNA is localized primarily in trigeminal and thoracic ganglion cells, corresponding to the dermatomes in which chickenpox lesions are maximal and that are most commonly involved by VZV (Mahalingam et al). The supposition is that the virus makes its way from the cutaneous vesicles of chickenpox along the sensory nerves to the ganglion, where it remains latent until activated, at which time it progresses down the axon to the skin. Multiplication of the virus in epidermal cells causes swelling, vacuolization, and lysis of cell boundaries, leading to the formation of vesicles and so-called Lipschütz inclusion bodies. Alternatively, the ganglia could be infected during the viremia of chickenpox, but then one would have to explain why only one or a few sensory ganglia become infected. Reactivation of virus is attributed to waning immunity, which would explain the increasing incidence of zoster with aging and with lymphomas, administration of immunosuppressive drugs, AIDS, and after radiation therapy.

The subject of pathogenesis of herpes zoster has been reviewed by Gilden and colleagues (2000) and in the monograph by Rentier, who describes the molecular and immune investigations pertaining to VZV.

Clinical Features

As indicated above, the incidence of herpes zoster rises with age. Hope-Simpson has estimated that if a cohort of 1,000 people lived to 85 years of age, half would have had one attack of zoster and 10 would have had two attacks. The notion that one attack of zoster provides lifelong immunity is incorrect, although recurrent attacks are rare and most localized repeated herpetic eruptions are caused by HSV. The sexes are equally affected, as is each side of the body. Herpes zoster occurs in up to 10 percent of patients with lymphoma and 25 percent of patients with Hodgkin disease—particularly in those who have undergone splenectomy or received radiotherapy. Conversely, approximately 5 percent of patients who present with herpes zoster are found to have a concurrent malignancy (about twice the number that would be expected), and the proportion appears to be even higher if more than two adjacent dermatomes are involved.

The vesicular eruption is usually preceded for several days by itching, tingling, or burning sensations in the involved dermatome, and sometimes by malaise and fever. Or there is severe localized or radicular pain that may be mistaken for pleurisy, appendicitis, cholecystitis, muscle strain, or, quite often, ruptured intervertebral disc, until the diagnosis is clarified by the appearance of vesicles (nearly always within 72 to 96 h).

The rash consists of clusters of tense clear vesicles on an erythematous base, which become cloudy after a few days (as a result of accumulation of inflammatory cells), and dry, crusted, and scaly after 5 to 10 days. In a small number of patients, the vesicles are confluent and hemorrhagic, and healing is delayed for several weeks. In most cases, pain and dysesthesia last for 1 to 4 weeks; but in the others (7 to 33 percent in different series) the pain persists for months or, in different forms, for years, and presents a difficult problem in management. Impairment of superficial sensation in the affected dermatome(s) is common, and segmental weakness and atrophy are added in approximately 5 percent of patients. In the majority of patients the rash and sensorimotor signs are limited to the territory of a single dermatome, but in some, particularly those with cranial or limb involvement, two or more contiguous dermatomes are involved.

Rarely (and usually in association with malignancy) the rash is generalized, like that of chickenpox, or it is altogether absent (*zoster sine herpete*) in which case, the pain is often attributed to another more mundane process such as sciatica.

In more than half of the cases, the CSF shows a mild increase in cells, mainly lymphocytes, and a modest increase in protein content (although lumbar puncture is not performed to establish the diagnosis). The herpetic nature of the eruption can be confirmed by direct immunofluorescence of a biopsied skin lesion, using antibody to VZV, or inferred by finding multinucleated giant cells in scrapings from the base of an early vesicle (Tzanck smear). The spinal fluid also contains antibodies to the virus or evidence of the organism by PCR testing in 35 percent of cases according to a prospective study by Haanpää and colleagues.

Virtually any dermatome may be involved in zoster, but some regions are far more frequent than others. The thoracic dermatomes, particularly T5 to T10, are the most common sites, accounting for more than two-thirds of all cases, followed by the craniocervical regions. In the latter cases the disease tends to be more severe, with greater pain, more frequent meningeal signs, and involvement of the mucous membranes. Another rare complication of zoster, taking the form of a subacute amyotrophy (*zoster paresis*) of a portion of a limb or trunk, is probably linked to a restricted form of VZV myelitis.

There are two rather characteristic cranial herpetic syndromes—ophthalmic herpes and geniculate herpes. In *ophthalmic herpes*, which accounts for 10 to 15 percent of all cases of zoster, the pain and rash are in the distribution of the first division of the trigeminal nerve, and the pathologic changes are centered in the gasserian ganglion. The main hazard in this form of the disease is herpetic involvement of the cornea and conjunctiva, resulting in corneal anesthesia and residual scarring. Palsies of extraocular muscles, ptosis, and mydriasis are frequently associated, indicating that the third, fourth, and sixth cranial nerves are affected in addition to the gasserian ganglion. The less common but also characteristic cranial nerve syndrome consists of a facial palsy in combination with a herpetic eruption of the external auditory meatus, sometimes with tinnitus, vertigo, and deafness. Ramsay Hunt (whose name has been attached to the syndrome) attributed this illness to herpes of the geniculate ganglion. Denny-Brown, Adams, and Fitzgerald found the geniculate ganglion to be only slightly affected in a man who died 64 days after the onset of a so-called *Ramsay Hunt syndrome* (during which time the patient had recovered from the facial palsy); there was, however, inflammation of the facial nerve.

Herpes zoster of the palate, pharynx, neck, and retroauricular region (*herpes occipitocollaris*) depends on herpetic infection of the upper cervical roots and the ganglia of the vagus and glossopharyngeal nerves. Herpes zoster in this distribution may also be associated with the Ramsay Hunt syndrome. The relative frequency of distribution of zoster in these truncal dermatomes and a proclivity for facial eruption, suggests to us that herpetic neurologic syndromes are more likely to occur if the distance of the ganglia from the skin is short.

Encephalitis and *cerebral angiitis* (see below) are rare but well-described complications of cervicocranial zoster, as discussed below, and a restricted but destructive myelitis is a similarly rare but often quite serious complication of thoracic zoster. Devinsky and colleagues reported their findings in 13 patients with zoster myelitis (all of them immunocompromised) and reviewed the literature on this subject. The signs of spinal cord involvement appeared 5 to 21 days after the rash and then progressed for a similar period of time. Asymmetrical paraparesis and sensory loss, sphincteric disturbances, and, less often, a Brown-Séquard syndrome were the usual clinical manifestations. The CSF findings were more abnormal than in uncomplicated zoster (pleocytosis and raised protein) but otherwise similar. The pathologic changes, which take the form of a necrotizing inflammatory myelopathy and vasculitis, involve not just the dorsal horn but also the contiguous white matter, predominantly on the same side and at the same segment(s) as the affected dorsal roots, ganglia, and posterior horns. Early therapeutic intervention with acyclovir appeared to be beneficial. Our experience with the problem includes an elderly man who was not immunosuppressed; he remained with an almost complete transverse myelopathy.

Many of the writings on *zoster encephalitis* give the impression of a severe illness that occurs temporally remote from the attack of shingles in an immunosuppressed patient. Indeed, such instances have been reported in patients with AIDS and may be concurrent with the small vessel vasculitis described below. However, our experience is more in keeping with that of Jemsek and colleagues and of Peterslund, who described a less severe form of encephalitis in patients with normal immune systems. Our several patients with this process, all elderly women, developed self-limited encephalitis during the latter stages of an attack of shingles. They were confused and drowsy, with low-grade fever but little meningismus, and a few had seizures. Recovery was complete and the MRI was normal, in distinction to the vasculitic syndromes. In some reported cases, VZV has been isolated from the CSF and specific antibody to VZV membrane antigen (VAMA) has been found in the CSF and serum, although it is hardly needed for purposes of diagnosis. (The differential diagnosis in these elderly patients also includes a drowsy confusional state induced by narcotics given for the control of pain.) *Varicella cerebellitis*, a post- or parainfectious condition, was discussed earlier in the chapter.

Zoster Angiitis

A *cerebral angiitis* that occasionally complicates VZV infection is histologically similar to granulomatous angiitis and to Wegener granulomatosis. Typically, 2 to 10 weeks after the onset specifically of ophthalmic zoster, the patient develops an acute hemiparesis, hemianesthesia, aphasia, or other focal neurologic or retinal deficits associated with a mononuclear pleocytosis in the spinal fluid and elevated IgG indices in the CSF. Nagel and colleagues have found that specific antibodies in the CSF to the virus were more sensitive for the diagnosis of this condition than was detection of viral DNA. CT or MRI scans demonstrate small, deep infarcts in the hemisphere ipsilateral to the outbreak of shingles on the face. Angiograms show narrowing or occlusion of the internal carotid artery adjacent to the ganglia; but in some cases, vasculitis is more diffuse, even involving the contralateral hemisphere.

Whether the angiitis results from direct spread of the viral infection via neighboring nerves as postulated by Linnemann and Alvira, or represents an allergic reaction during convalescence from zoster, has not been settled. VZV-like particles have been found in the vessel walls, suggesting a direct infection and viral DNA has been extracted in a few cases from affected vessels. Because the exact pathogenetic mechanism is uncertain, treatment with both intravenous acyclovir and corticosteroids may be justified. There are occasional instances of a cerebral vasculitis following dermatomal zoster on the trunk.

An entirely different type of delayed *vasculitis that affects small vessels*, with which we have had limited experience, is being reported in patients with AIDS and other forms of immunosuppression. In this condition, weeks or months after one or more attacks of zoster, a subacute encephalitis ensues, including fever and focal signs. Some cases apparently arise without a rash, but viral DNA and antibodies to VZV are found in the CSF. The MRI shows multiple cortical and white matter lesions, the latter being smaller and less confluent than in progressive multifocal leukoencephalopathy. There is usually a mild pleocytosis. Almost all cases have ended fatally. The vasculitic and other neurologic complications of zoster have been reviewed by Gilden and colleagues (2002). Nagel and coworkers from Gilden's laboratory have also found cases in which the temporal arteries contain VZV particles and they have suggested that the vascular changes caused by the virus may simulate temporal arteritis.

Finally, as mentioned earlier, a facial palsy or pain in the distribution of a trigeminal or segmental nerve (usually lumbar or intercostal) as a result of herpetic ganglionitis, may occur rarely without involvement of the skin (*zoster sine herpete*); lumbar disc herniation may be suspected. In a few such cases, an antibody response to VZV has been found (Mayo and Booss), and Dueland and associates have described an immunocompromised patient who developed a pathologically and virologically proved zoster infection in the absence of skin lesions. Similarly, Gilden and colleagues (2002) recovered VZV DNA from two otherwise healthy immunocompetent men who had experienced chronic radicular pain without a zoster rash. But practically no instances of Bell's palsy, tic douloureux, and intercostal neuralgia are associated with serologic evidence of activation of VZV (Bell's palsy has instead been associated with HSV, as indicated in Chap. 47).

Treatment

An important inception for shingles has been a live, attenuated vaccine that can be administered to adults over age 60. It has been shown to reduce the emergence of shingles and to decrease the incidence of postherpetic complications by two-thirds (Oxman et al).

During the acute stage of shingles, analgesics and drying and soothing lotions, such as calamine, help to blunt the pain. Nerve root blocks may provide temporary relief but are not often used. After the lesions have dried, the repeated application of capsaicin ointment (derived from hot peppers) may relieve the pain in some cases by inducing a cutaneous anesthesia. When applied too soon after the acute stage, however, capsaicin is highly irritating and should be used cautiously.

Acyclovir shortens the duration of acute pain and speeds the healing of vesicles, provided that treatment is begun within approximately 48 h (some authorities say 72 h) of the appearance of the rash (McKendrick et al, 1986). Several studies have suggested that the duration of postherpetic neuralgia is reduced by treatment during the acute phase with famciclovir or valacyclovir, but the incidence of this complication is not markedly affected. Famciclovir (500 mg tid for 7 d) or the better absorbed valacyclovir (2 g orally qid) are possibly better alternatives than the previously favored acyclovir (see below on the subject of postherpetic neuralgia). Other studies have shown favorable results in preventing postherpetic pain by starting a tricyclic antidepressant during the acute phase.

All patients with ophthalmic zoster should receive acyclovir or valacyclovir orally; in addition, acyclovir applied topically to the eye, in either a 0.1 percent solution every hour or a 0.5 percent ointment 4 or 5 times a day, is recommended by some ophthalmologists. Patients who are immunocompromised or have disseminated zoster (lesions in more than 3 dermatomes) should generally receive intravenous acyclovir for 10 days. There is now available (from state health agencies) a VZV immune globulin (VZIG) that may protect against dissemination in immunosuppressed patients but is not indicated for established disease. Although it may reduce the incidence of postherpetic neuralgia (Hugler et al), this is not its main purpose and it does not appear to prevent or ameliorate CNS complications.

Postherpetic Neuralgia

(See also Chaps. 8 and 10)

This severely painful syndrome follows shingles in 5 to 10 percent of patients but occurs almost three times more often among individuals older than age 60 years. The possible effect of acute treatment on the severity of postherpetic neuralgia is mentioned above but potential prevention with the vaccine is even more appealing.

The management of *postherpetic pain* and dysesthesia can be a trying matter for both the patient and the physician. It is likely that incomplete interruption of nerve impulses results in a hyperpathic state in which every stimulus excites pain. In a number of controlled studies, amitriptyline proved to be an effective therapeutic measure. Initially, it is given in doses of approximately 50 mg at bedtime; if needed, the dosage can be increased gradually to 125 mg daily. The addition of carbamazepine, gabapentin, pregabalin, or valproate may further moderate the pain, particularly if it is of lancinating type.

Capsaicin ointment can be applied to painful skin, as noted above. A salve of two aspirin tablets, crushed and mixed with cold cream or chloroform (15 mL) and spread on the painful skin, was reported to be successful in relieving the pain for several hours (King). The effect of nerve root blocks is inconsistent, but this procedure may afford temporary relief. In one randomized trial, the preemptive use of epidural steroids at the onset of the rash had minimal effects (van Wijck et al). It should be emphasized that postherpetic neuralgia eventually subsides even in the most severe and persistent cases but the short-term use of narcotics is appropriate when the pain is severe. Until the pain subsides, the physician must exercise skill and patience and avoid the temptation of subjecting the patient to one of the many surgical measures that have been advocated for this disorder (see Chap. 9 for further discussion of pain management). Some patients with the most persistent complaints, beyond a year, have symptoms of a depressive state and will be helped by antidepressive medications.

NEUROLOGIC DISEASES INDUCED BY RETROVIRUSES INCLUDING HIV AND SECONDARY OPPORTUNISTIC INFECTIONS

Retroviruses are a large group of RNA viruses, so called because they contain the enzyme reverse transcriptase, which permits the reverse flow of genetic information from RNA to DNA. Two families of retroviruses are known to infect humans: (1) the *lentiviruses*, the most important of which is the HIV, the cause of AIDS, and (2) the *oncornaviruses*, which include the human T-cell lymphotropic viruses (HTLV-I), the agents that induce chronic T-cell leukemias and lymphomas (HTLV-II) and tropical spastic paraparesis (HTLV-I). A comprehensive account of the neurobiology, pathology, and clinical features of these infections can be found in the appropriate sections of *Harrison's Principles of Internal Medicine* and authoritative information regarding treatment is given in the text by Rubin and Young.

The Acquired Immunodeficiency Syndrome

In 1981, physicians became aware of the frequent occurrence of otherwise rare opportunistic infections and neoplasms—notably *Pneumocystis carinii* pneumonia and Kaposi sarcoma—in otherwise healthy young homosexual men. The study of these patients led to the recognition of a new viral disease, AIDS.

HIV infection is characterized by an acquired and usually profound depression of cell-mediated immunity as manifest by cutaneous anergy, lymphopenia, reversal of the T-helper–to–T-suppressor cell ratio—more accurately, CD4+/CD8+ lymphocytes, as a result of reduction in CD4+ cells—and depressed in vitro lymphoproliferative response to various antigens and mitogens. It is this failure of immune function that explains the development of a wide range of opportunistic infections and unusual neoplasms. Virtually all organ systems are vulnerable, including all parts of the CNS, the peripheral nerves and roots, and muscle. Moreover, the nervous system is susceptible to a number of unusual syndromes that are the direct result of the AIDS virus infection.

Epidemiology

In a span of 25 years, HIV infection and AIDS have attained pandemic proportions. At the time of this writing it was estimated by the World Health Organization (WHO) that approximately 34 million persons are infected worldwide and that approximately 1 million adults in the United States are seropositive for the virus with 50,000 new cases yearly. The CDC furthermore estimates that 18 percent of infections have not been diagnosed. Though the incidence is decreasing, particularly startling are the statistics from sub-Saharan Africa and Southeast Asia, where the WHO estimated that approximately 25,000,000 adults—or almost 9 percent of the adult population—were infected. In some areas of East Africa, 30 percent of adults are infected with the virus.

In the United States, AIDS affects mainly homosexual and bisexual males (two-thirds of all cases) and male and female drug users (almost one-third of cases). Somewhat less than 2 percent of patients who are at risk are hemophiliacs and others who receive infected blood or blood products, and the disease has occurred in infants born of mothers with AIDS. Moreover, the virus may be transmitted by asymptomatic and still immunologically competent mothers to their offspring. Spread of the disease by heterosexual contact accounts for approximately 5 percent of cases, but this number is gradually increasing, partly through the activities of intravenous drug users. By contrast, an estimated 80 percent of African AIDS patients acquire their disease through heterosexual contact.

The related but less common entity of HIV-2 infection causes a generally less severe illness than HIV-1 but may include almost any of the features described below, including dementia. The virus is currently most prolific in Brazil, Cape Verde, and West African countries. The diagnosis is made complicated by the usual findings of a positive ELISA test but a negative or indeterminate Western blot results when conventional methods are used. A specific Western blot is available for HIV-2.

Clinical Features

Infection with HIV produces a spectrum of disorders, ranging from *clinically inevident seroconversion* to widespread lymphadenopathy and other systemic manifestations such as diarrhea, malaise, and weight loss, which comprises the direct effects of the virus on all organ systems as well as the complicating effects of a multiplicity of secondary parasitic, fungal, viral, and bacterial infections and a number of neoplasms, all of which require cell-mediated immunity for containment. Until the recent advent of multiple antiviral drug therapy, once the manifestations of AIDS had become established, half of patients died by 1 year and most by 3 years. Neurologic abnormalities had been found in about one-third of untreated patients with AIDS, but at autopsy the nervous system is affected in nearly all of them. Table 33-2 lists the main infections and neoplastic lesions of the nervous system that complicate AIDS.

It has already been mentioned that HIV infection may present as an acute *asymptomatic meningitis* with a mild lymphocytic pleocytosis and modest elevation of CSF protein. The acute illness may also take the form of a *meningoencephalitis* or even a *myelopathy* or *neuropathy* (see further on). Most patients recover from the initial acute neurologic illnesses; the relationship to AIDS may pass unrecognized, as these illnesses are quite nonspecific clinically and may precede or coincide with seroconversion. Once seroconversion has occurred, the patient becomes vulnerable to all the late complications of HIV infection. In adults, the interval between infection and the development of AIDS ranges from several months to 15 years or even longer; the mean latency is 8 to 10 years and 1 year or less in infants.

HIV-2 may display special features of a subacute confusional-dementing illness with deep white matter and basal ganglionic damage.

Table 33-2

NEUROLOGIC COMPLICATIONS OF HIV-AIDS

Brain
- *Encephalitis*
  - HIV encephalitis
  - Cytomegalovirus encephalitis
  - Varicella zoster virus encephalitis
  - Herpes simplex virus encephalitis
- *Focal lesion*
  - Cerebral toxoplasmosis
  - Brain lymphoma
  - Progressive multifocal leukoencephalopathy
  - Cryptococcoma
  - Bacterial brain abscess
  - Tuberculoma
- *Cerebrovascular disorders*—nonbacterial endocarditis, cerebral hemorrhages associated with thrombocytopenia, and vasculitis
- *HIV dementia*

Spinal cord
- Vacuolar myelopathy
- Herpes simplex or zoster myelitis

Meningitis
- Acute and chronic lymphocytic meningitis
- Cryptococcal and other fungal types
- Tuberculous
- Syphilitic
- Herpes zoster

Peripheral nerve and root
- Distal sensory polyneuropathy
- Herpes zoster
- Cytomegalovirus lumbar polyradiculopathy
- Acute and chronic inflammatory polyneuritis
- Mononeuritis multiplex
- Sensorimotor demyelinating polyneuropathy
- Diffuse infiltrative lymphocytic syndrome (DILS)
- Leprosy

Muscle
- Polymyositis and other myopathies (including drug induced)

HIV-Associated Neurocognitive Disorders (AIDS Dementia Complex)

In the later stages of HIV infection, the most common neurologic complication is a subacute or chronic HIV encephalitis presenting as a form of dementia; formerly it was called AIDS encephalopathy or encephalitis, but it is now generally referred to as AIDS dementia complex (ADC; Navia, Jordan, and Price). It has been estimated that only 3 percent of AIDS cases present in this manner, but the frequency is far higher, close to two-thirds, after the constitutional symptoms and opportunistic infections of AIDS have become established. In children with AIDS, dementia is more common than all opportunistic infections, more than 60 percent of children eventually being affected.

The disorder in adults takes the form of a slowly or subacutely progressive dementia (loss of retentive memory, inattentiveness, language disorder, and apathy) accompanied variably by abnormalities of motor function. Patients complain of being unable to follow conversations, taking longer to complete daily tasks, and becoming forgetful. Incoordination of the limbs, ataxia of gait, and impairment of smooth pursuit and saccadic eye movements may be early accompaniments of the dementia. Heightened tendon reflexes, Babinski signs, grasp and suck reflexes, weakness of the legs progressing to paraplegia, bladder and bowel incontinence reflecting spinal cord or cerebral involvement, and abulia or mutism are prominent in the later stages of the disease. In the untreated case, the dementia evolves, over a period of weeks or months; survival after the onset of dementia is generally 3 to 6 months but may be considerably longer if treatment is instituted. Treatment with antiretroviral drugs can result in cognitive improvement. There is an interest in rare cases of poor penetration of antiretroviral drugs into the central nervous system, allowing for viral replication and reemergence despite elimination of HIV from the peripheral blood.

Tests of psychomotor speed seem to be most sensitive in the early stages of dementia (e.g., trail making, pegboard, and symbol-digit testing). Epstein and colleagues have described a similar disorder in children, who develop a progressive encephalopathy as the primary manifestation of AIDS. The disease in children is characterized by an impairment of cognitive functions

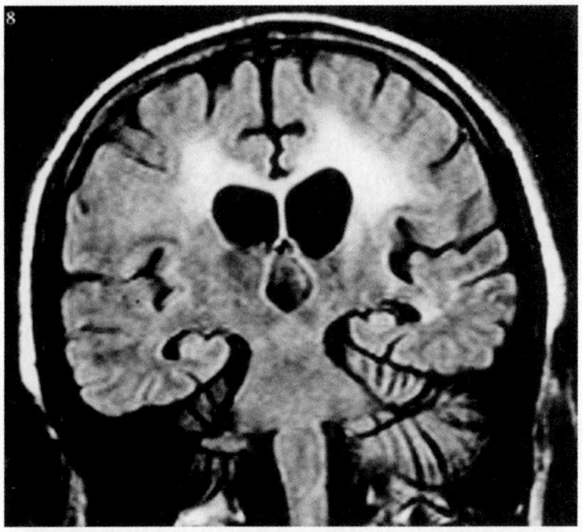

Figure 33-2. MRI of HIV leukoencephalopathy. There are large areas of white matter change that underlie one form of AIDS dementia; cortical atrophy and ventricular enlargement are evident.

and spastic weakness and secondarily by impairment of brain growth.

The CSF (including those lacking other manifestations of AIDS) may be normal or show only a slight elevation of protein content and, less frequently, a mild lymphocytosis. HIV can be isolated from the CSF. In the CT scan there is widening of the sulci and enlargement of the ventricles; MRI may show patchy but confluent or diffuse white matter changes with ill-defined margins (Fig. 33-2). These findings are useful in diagnosis, although CMV infection of the brain in AIDS produces a similar MRI appearance, as described further on.

The pathologic basis of the dementia appears to be a diffuse and multifocal rarefaction of the cerebral white matter accompanied by scanty perivascular infiltrates of lymphocytes and clusters of a few foamy macrophages, microglial nodules, and multinucleated giant cells (Navia, Chos, Petito et al). Evidence of CMV infection may be added, but accumulating virologic evidence indicates that the AIDS dementia complex is a result of direct infection with HIV. Which of these changes corresponds most closely to the presence and severity of dementia has not been settled. The pathologic changes in AIDS dementia are actually not as uniform as portrayed here. In one group of patients, there is a diffuse pallor of the cerebral white matter, most obvious with myelin stains, accompanied by reactive astrocytes and macrophages; the myelin pallor seems to reflect a breakdown of the blood–brain barrier.

In another form of this process, referred to as "diffuse poliodystrophy," there is widespread astrocytosis and microglial activation in the cerebral cortex, with little recognizable neuronal loss. In yet other patients, small or large perivascular foci of demyelination, like those of postinfectious encephalomyelitis, are observed; the nature of this diffuse white matter lesion is not understood. These forms of pathologic change may occur singly or together and all correlate poorly with the severity of the dementia. Progressive multifocal leukoencephalopathy also occurs in patients with AIDS and is simulated by the primary white matter encephalopathy.

HIV Myelopathy, Peripheral Neuropathy, and Myopathy

A *myelopathy*, taking the form of a vacuolar degeneration that bears a marked pathologic resemblance to subacute combined degeneration because of vitamin B_{12} deficiency, is sometimes associated with the AIDS dementia complex; or the myelopathy may occur in isolation, as the leading manifestation of the disease (Petito et al). This disorder of the spinal cord is discussed further in Chap 47.

AIDS may also be complicated by several forms of *peripheral neuropathy*, as discussed in Chap 46. A distal, symmetrical, axonal polyneuropathy, predominantly sensory and dysesthetic in type has been the most common neuropathic pattern. The HIV virus has been isolated from the peripheral nerves and ganglia. In fact, this stands as the first proven viral polyneuritis in humans (zoster being more a ganglionopathy). In other patients, a painful *mononeuropathy multiplex* occurs, seemingly related to a focal vasculitis, or there may be a subacute inflammatory cauda equina syndrome (a *polyradiculitis*) that is usually caused by an accompanying *CMV* infection (Eidelberg et al). Cornblath and colleagues have documented the occurrence of an *inflammatory demyelinating peripheral neuropathy*, of both the acute (Guillain-Barré) and chronic types, in otherwise asymptomatic patients with HIV infection. Most of these patients had a mild pleocytosis in addition to an elevated CSF protein content. Most patients with inflammatory demyelinating neuropathy have recovered—either spontaneously or in response to plasma exchange—suggesting an immunopathogenesis similar to that of the Guillain-Barré syndrome. Cornblath and associates suggest that all patients with inflammatory demyelinating polyneuropathies should now be tested for the presence of HIV infection. *Facial palsy* is being reported with increasing frequency as a feature of AIDS; its relationship to the generalized polyneuritis of AIDS is uncertain.

In a rare peripheral neuropathy of AIDS termed *diffuse infiltrative lymphocytosis syndrome* (DILS), a variety of clinical syndromes have been described including all patterns of the usual AIDS polyneuropathies. Some instances of polyneuropathy in AIDS patients are probably caused by the nutritional depletion that characterizes advanced stages of the disease and to the effects of therapeutic agents. These AIDS-related neuropathies are discussed in Chap. 46 and are summarized by Wulff and Simpson.

A primary *myopathy*, taking the form of an inflammatory polymyositis, has been described in HIV patients at any stage of the disease (Simpson and Bender). In some of these cases, the myopathy has improved with corticosteroid therapy. The original anti-AIDS drug, zidovudine (AZT), has caused a myopathy, probably because of its effect on mitochondria, but some investigators have attributed almost all such cases to be attributable to the

AIDS virus itself (see "HIV and HTLV-I Myositis" in Chap. 49). It is apparent that this remains an area of some controversy.

Opportunistic Infections and Neoplasms of the CNS in AIDS

In addition to the direct neurologic effects of HIV infection, a variety of opportunistic disorders, both focal and generalized, occur in such patients as outlined in Table 33-2. Interestingly, there appears to be a predilection for certain ones—toxoplasmosis, CMV infection, primary B-cell lymphoma, cryptococcosis, and progressive multifocal leukoencephalopathy, in approximately this order of frequency (Johnson). The focal encephalitis and vasculitis of VZV infection, considered earlier in this chapter, and unusual types of tuberculosis and syphilis are other common opportunistic infections of AIDS. Usually *P. carinii* infection and Kaposi sarcoma do not spread to the nervous system. In almost of these categories, the infectious process is accelerated or intensified by the presence of the HIV infection.

Toxoplasmosis Of the focal infectious complications, cerebral toxoplasmosis is the most frequent (and treatable; see Chap 32). In the autopsy series of AIDS reported by Navia, Petito, Gold, and colleagues, areas of inflammatory necrosis caused by *Toxoplasma* were found in approximately 13 percent (see Fig. 32-6). Lumbar puncture, contrast-enhanced CT scanning, and MRI are useful in diagnosis. The spinal fluid usually shows an elevation of protein in the range of 50 to 200 mg/dL, and one-third of patients have a lymphocytic pleocytosis. Because the disease usually represents reactivation of a prior *Toxoplasma* infection, it is important to identify *Toxoplasma*-seropositive patients early in the course of AIDS and to treat them with oral pyrimethamine (100 mg initially and then 25 mg daily) and a sulfonamide (4 to 6 g daily in four divided doses). Curiously, the toxoplasmosis, so common in the brains of AIDS patients, is not a frequent cause of one of its more typical manifestation, myositis. The main clinical problem in reference to toxoplasmosis in AIDS is its differentiation from cerebral lymphoma as discussed below and in Chap. 31.

In a series from Johns Hopkins (see Johnson, 1998), approximately 11 percent of AIDS patients developed a *primary CNS lymphoma*, which may, in some cases, be difficult to distinguish from toxoplasmosis clinically and radiologically. If the cytologic study of the CSF is negative and there has been no response to antibiotics (see below), stereotaxic brain biopsy may be necessary for diagnosis. The prognosis in such patients is considerably less favorable than in non-AIDS patients; the response to radiation therapy, methotrexate, and corticosteroids is short-lived, and survival is usually measured in months.

In the face of enhancing focal brain lesions in AIDS, the current approach is to initially assume the presence of toxoplasmosis, which is treatable. Antibody tests for toxoplasmosis should be obtained; the absence of IgG antibodies mandates that treatment be changed in order to address the problem of brain lymphoma. Also, if antitoxoplasmal therapy with pyrimethamine and sulfadiazine fails to reduce the size of the lesions within several weeks, another cause should be sought, again mainly lymphoma. In those patients who cannot tolerate the frequent side effects of pyrimethamine or sulfonamides (rash or thrombocytopenia), clindamycin may be of value. Recently, it has been suggested that positron emission tomography (PET) and other metabolic imaging techniques can identify lymphoma as the cause of a mass lesion in the HIV patient. The less frequent possibilities of tuberculous or bacterial brain abscess should be kept in mind if none of these avenues allow a confident diagnosis.

Cytomegalovirus Among the nonfocal neurologic complications of AIDS, the most common are CMV and *cryptococcal* infections. At autopsy, about one-third of AIDS patients are found to be infected with CMV. However, the contribution of this infection to the total clinical picture is often uncertain. Despite this ambiguity, certain features have emerged as typical of CMV encephalitis in the AIDS patient. According to Holland and colleagues, late in the course of AIDS and usually concurrent with CMV retinitis, the encephalopathy evolves over 3 to 4 weeks. Its clinical features include an acute confusional state or delirium combined in a small proportion of cases with cranial nerve signs including ophthalmoparesis, nystagmus, ptosis, facial nerve palsy, or deafness. In one of our patients, there were progressive oculomotor palsies that began with light-fixed pupils.

Pathologic specimens and MRI show the process to be concentrated in the ventricular borders, especially evident as T2 signal hyperintensity in these regions. The lesions may extend more diffusely through the adjacent white matter and be accompanied by meningeal enhancement by gadolinium in a few cases. Extensive destructive lesions have also been reported; this has been true in two of our own cases. Such lesions may be associated with hemorrhagic changes in the CSF in addition to showing an inflammatory response. CMV may also produce a painful lumbosacral polyradiculitis in AIDS (Chap. 44).

The diagnosis of CMV infection during life is often difficult. Cultures of the CSF are usually negative and IgG antibody titers are nonspecifically elevated. Newer PCR methods prove useful here. Where the diagnosis is strongly suspected, treatment with the antiviral agents ganciclovir and foscarnet has been recommended, but, as pointed out by Kalayjian and colleagues, the CMV disease may develop and progress while patients are taking these medications as maintenance therapy.

Cryptococcal Infection *Meningitis* with this fungus and less often, *solitary cryptococcoma* are the most frequent fungal complications of HIV infection. Flagrant symptoms of meningitis or meningoencephalitis may be lacking and the CSF may show little abnormality with respect to cells, protein, and glucose. For these reasons, evidence of cryptococcal infection of the spinal fluid should be actively sought with antigen testing, and fungal cultures. India ink preparations are still valuable and rapid but are not currently performed consistently and well enough in many hospitals to be entirely dependable. Treatment is along the lines outlined in Chap. 32.

Varicella Zoster Cerebral infections with this virus are less common complications of AIDS, but when they do occur, they tend to be severe. They take the form of multifocal lesions of the cerebral white matter, somewhat like those of progressive multifocal leukoencephalopathy, a cerebral vasculitis with hemiplegia (usually in association with ophthalmic zoster), or, rarely, a myelitis. Encephalitis caused by HSV-1 and HSV-2 has also been identified in the brains of AIDS patients, but the clinical correlates are unclear. Shingles involving several contiguous dermatomes is known to occur in AIDS with CD4 counts below 500, as in other immunosuppressed conditions.

Tuberculosis Two particular types of mycobacterial infection tend to complicate AIDS—*Mycobacterium tuberculosis* and *Mycobacterium avium-intracellulare*. Tuberculosis predominates among drug abusers and HIV patients in developing countries, and a higher-than-usual proportion of these immunosuppressed individuals develop tuberculous meningitis. Diagnosis and treatment are along the same lines as in non-AIDS patients.

Neurosyphilis *Syphilitic meningitis* and *meningovascular syphilis* appear to have an increased incidence in AIDS patients. Cell counts in the CSF are unreliable as signs of activity; diagnosis depends entirely upon serologic tests. It is possible that AIDS causes false-positive tests for syphilis. It appears that the presence of HIV infection accelerates the transition of syphilis to later stages, including infection of the nervous system. Indeed, a category of quaternary syphilis has emerged that consists of an aggressive and rapidly progressive necrotizing process that causes strokes and dementia as a result of involvement of brain parenchyma and vessels. The incidence of relapse of syphilis and resistance to conventional doses of antisyphilitic medication are probably increased with HIV coinfection. It is unclear, however, if the tertiary forms of syphilis, general paresis and tabes dorsalis, are increased in incidence because of AIDS; they may require the chronicity of meningovascular syphilis to evolve. Readers are referred to the review by Marra.

Other rare organisms, such as *Bartonella henselae*, the cause of cat scratch fever, are found rarely in AIDS patients and have been implicated in an encephalitis. Progressive multifocal leukoencephalopathy, a viral disease now closely linked with the immunosuppressed state of AIDS and seen in high numbers, is discussed further on in this chapter.

Treatment

The treatment of HIV infection/AIDS, as is true for any chronic, life-threatening disease, is difficult. Treatment with several antiretroviral drugs is required not just for control of the neurologic manifestations of retroviral infection but also to control secondary infections. Recommendations regarding drug therapy for HIV infection change rapidly (Rubin and Young) and the reader is referred to any of the modern sources for the details of treatment, including *Harrison's Principles of Internal Medicine*. It is believed that these approaches will prolong survival but it might be expected also to increase the prevalence of neurologic complications of AIDS, each of which needs to be treated as it is recognized. A special result of HIV antiretroviral treatment may induce an intense inflammatory response to a coexistent infection. This complication, immune reconstitution inflammatory syndrome, or *IRIS*, is perhaps most pertinent to progressive multifocal leukoencephalopathy discussed later.

Tropical Spastic Paraparesis, HTLV-I Infection

This is an endemic neurologic disorder in many tropical and subtropical countries. Its cause was overlooked until 1985, when Gessain and coworkers found IgG antibodies to HTLV-I in the sera of 68 percent of tropical spastic paraparesis (TSP) patients in Martinique. The same antibodies were then identified in the CSF of Jamaican and Colombian patients with TSP, and in patients with a similar neurologic disorder in the temperate zones of southern Japan. The latter disorder was originally called HTLV-I–associated myelopathy (HAM), but it is now considered to be identical to HTLV-I–positive TSP (Roman and Osame). It is a curious feature of this disorder that only a small proportion of HTLV-I–infected persons (estimated at 2 percent) develop a myelopathy. Sporadic instances have now been reported from many parts of the Western world. The virus is transmitted in one of several ways—from mother to child, across the placenta or in breast milk; by intravenous drug use or blood transfusions; or by sexual contact. The age of onset is in mid adult life, and it is more common in females than in males, in a ratio of 3:1.

The clinical and pathologic features of the disease are described in Chap. 44 and in several recommended reviews (Rodgers-Johnson et al); the differentiation from the progressive spinal form of multiple sclerosis and with subacute combined degeneration, with which it is most likely to be confused, is discussed further on under "Differential Diagnosis." There are also clinical and pathologic differences from the myelopathy caused directly by HIV infection. No form of treatment has proved effective in reversing this disorder, although there are anecdotal reports that the intravenous administration of immune globulin may halt its progress.

The retrovirus HTLV-II is less common than HTLV-I but the two are virologically very similar. There is a high rate of infection with HTLV-II among drug users who are coinfected with HIV. A few cases of myelopathy have been reported in HTLV-II–infected patients, similar in all respects to HTLV-I–associated myelopathy (Lehky et al).

VIRAL INFECTIONS OF THE DEVELOPING NERVOUS SYSTEM (See Chap. 38)

Viral infections of the fetus, notably rubella, CMV, HIV, herpes zoster, Epstein-Barr, and HSV infection of the newborn are important causes of CNS abnormalities. This subject is covered in detail in "Intrauterine and Neonatal Infections" in Chap. 38.

ACUTE ANTERIOR POLIOMYELITIS

In the past, this syndrome was almost invariably the result of infection by one of the three types of poliovirus. However, illnesses that clinically resemble poliovirus infections can be caused by other enteroviruses such as the Coxsackie groups A and B and Japanese encephalitis, as well as by West Nile virus. Epidemics of hemorrhagic conjunctivitis (caused by enterovirus 70 and formerly common in Asia and Africa) can also be associated with a lower motor neuron paralysis resembling poliomyelitis (Wadia et al). In countries with successful poliomyelitis vaccination programs, these other viruses are now the most common causes of the anterior poliomyelitis syndrome. In some cases, the illnesses induced by these viruses are benign and the associated paralysis is insignificant. West Nile virus is an exception that has been associated with a severe and persistent asymmetrical flaccid poliomyelitis.

The important (paralytic) disease in this category nonetheless remains poliomyelitis. Although no longer a scourge in areas where vaccination is routine, its lethal and crippling effects are still fresh in the memory of physicians who practiced in the 1950s. In the summer of 1955, when New England experienced its last epidemic, 3,950 cases of acute poliomyelitis were reported in Massachusetts alone, and 2,771 were paralytic. The details of this epidemic described by Pope and colleagues are worth reviewing by any student of the disease. Polio has essentially from the Americas, the only cases currently being imported ones. Live polio vaccine, which had been the source of approximately 150 cases in previous decades, is no longer used in the United States.

Of course, because it is highly communicable, acute poliomyelitis still occurs in regions of the world where large-scale and recurrent vaccination is not practiced. In a recent year, there were fewer than 2,000 cases in the world but there are periodic small outbreaks. For these reasons and also because it stands as a prototype of a neurotropic viral infection, the main features of the disease should be known to neurologists.

The paralytic residua of previous epidemics can still be seen. In these cases, a delayed progression of muscle weakness may appear many years after the acute paralytic illness—a condition termed postpolio syndrome (see discussion of amyotrophic lateral sclerosis [ALS] in Chap. 39).

Etiology

The poliomyelitis agent is a small RNA virus that is a member of the enterovirus group of the picornavirus family. Three antigenically distinct types have been defined and infection with one does not protect against the others. Poliomyelitis is a highly communicable disease. The main reservoir of infection is the human intestinal tract (humans are the only known natural hosts), and the main route of infection is fecal-oral, i.e., hand to mouth, as with other enteric pathogens. The virus multiplies in the pharynx and intestinal tract. During the incubation period, which is from 1 to 3 weeks, the virus can be recovered from both of these sites. In only a small fraction of infected patients is the nervous system invaded. Between 95 and 99 percent of infected patients are asymptomatic or experience only a nonspecific febrile illness. It is the latter type of patient—the carrier with inapparent infection—who is most important in the spread of the virus from one person to another.

Clinical Manifestations

In the *inapparent infections, and those in which* there are only mild systemic symptoms with pharyngitis or gastroenteritis had been called *abortive poliomyelitis*. The mild symptoms correspond to the period of viremia and dissemination of the virus; they give rise in most cases to an effective immune response—a feature that accounts for the failure to cause meningitis or poliomyelitis. In the relatively small proportion of patients in whom the nervous system is invaded, the illness still has a wide range of severity from mild aseptic meningitis (*nonparalytic* or preparalytic poliomyelitis) to the most severe forms of paralytic poliomyelitis.

Nonparalytic Poliomyelitis The prodromal symptoms consist of listlessness, generalized, nonthrobbing headache, fever of 38 to 40°C (100.4 to 104°F), stiffness and aching in the muscles, sore throat in the absence of upper respiratory infection, anorexia, nausea, and vomiting. These symptoms may subside to a varying extent, to be followed after 3 to 4 days by recrudescence of headache and fever and by symptoms of nervous system involvement; more often the second phase of the illness blends with the first. Tenderness and pain in the muscles, tightness of the hamstrings (spasm), and pain in the neck and back become increasingly prominent. Other early manifestations of nervous system involvement include irritability, restlessness, and emotional instability; these are frequently a prelude to paralysis. Added to these symptoms are stiffness of the neck on forward flexion and the characteristic CSF findings of aseptic meningitis. This may constitute the entire illness; alternatively, paralysis may follow the preparalytic symptoms.

Paralytic Poliomyelitis Weakness becomes manifest while the fever is at its height, or, just as frequently, as the temperature falls and the general clinical picture seems to be improving. Muscle weakness may develop rapidly, attaining its maximum severity in 48 h or even less; or it may develop more slowly or in stuttering fashion over a week, rarely even longer. As a general rule, there is no progression of weakness after the temperature has been normal for 48 h. The distribution of spinal paralysis is quite variable; rarely there may be an acute symmetrical paralysis of the muscles of the trunk and limbs as occurs in the Guillain-Barré syndrome. Excessive physical activity and local injections during the period of asymptomatic infection were thought to favor the development of paralysis of the exercised or injected limbs.

Coarse fasciculations are seen as the muscles weaken; they are transient as a rule, but occasionally they persist. Tendon reflexes are diminished and lost as the weakness evolves and paralyzed muscles become flaccid. Patients frequently complain of paresthesias in the affected limbs but objective sensory loss is seldom demonstrable.

Retention of urine is a common occurrence during the early phase in adult patients, rarely persisting. Atrophy of muscle can be detected within 3 weeks of onset of paralysis, is maximal at 12 to 15 weeks, and is permanent.

Bulbar paralysis is more common in young adults, but usually such patients have spinal involvement as well. The most frequently involved cranial muscles are those of deglutition, reflecting involvement of the nucleus ambiguus. The other great hazards of medullary disease are disturbances of respiration and vasomotor control—hiccough, shallowness and progressive slowing of respiration, cyanosis, restlessness and anxiety from air hunger, hypertension, and, ultimately, hypotension and shock. When these disturbances are added to paralysis of diaphragmatic and intercostal musculature, the patient's survival is threatened and the institution of respiratory assistance and intensive care becomes urgent.

Pathologic Changes and Clinicopathologic Correlations

In fatal infections, lesions are found in the precentral (motor) gyrus of the brain (usually of insufficient severity to cause symptoms), brainstem, and spinal cord. The brunt of the disease in these cases is borne by the hypothalamus, thalamus, motor nuclei of the brainstem and surrounding reticular formation, vestibular nuclei and roof nuclei of the cerebellum, and mainly the neurons of the anterior and intermediate gray matter of the spinal cord. In these areas, nerve cells are destroyed and phagocytosed by microgliacytes (neuronophagia). A local leukocytic reaction is present for only a few days, but mononuclear cells persist as perivascular accumulations for many months. Inclusion bodies are not seen. The earliest histopathologic changes in the anterior horns of the cord are central chromatolysis of the nerve cells, along with an inflammatory reaction. These changes correlate with a multiplication of virus in the CNS and, in the infected monkey, precede the onset of paralysis by one or several days.

In Bodian's experimental material, the infected motor neurons continued to function until a stage of severe chromatolysis was reached. Moreover, if damage to the cell had attained only the stage of central chromatolysis, complete morphologic recovery could be expected—a process that took a month or longer. After this time, the degrees of paralysis and atrophy were closely correlated with the number of motor nerve cells that had been destroyed; where limbs remain atrophic and paralyzed, less than 10 percent of neurons survived in corresponding cord segments. Lesions in the motor nuclei of the brainstem are associated with paralysis in corresponding muscles. Disturbances of swallowing, respiration, and vasomotor control are related to neuronal lesions in the medullary reticular formation, centered in the region of the nucleus ambiguus, as mentioned earlier.

Atrophic, areflexic paralysis of muscles of the trunk and limbs relates, of course, to destruction of neurons in the anterior and intermediate horns of the corresponding segments of the spinal cord gray matter. The affected regions can be quite focal or scattered, giving rise, for instance, to permanent paralysis of only one limb. Stiffness and pain in the neck and back, attributed to "meningeal irritation," are probably related to the mild inflammatory exudate in the meninges and to the generally mild lesions in the dorsal root ganglia and dorsal horns. These lesions also account for the muscle pain and paresthesia in parts that later become paralyzed. Abnormalities of autonomic function are attributable to lesions of autonomic pathways in the reticular substance of the brainstem and in the lateral horn cells in the spinal cord.

It is of interest that poliovirus has been readily isolated from CNS tissue of fatal cases but can rarely be recovered from the CSF during clinical disease. This is in contrast to the closely related Coxsackie and echo picornaviruses, which have been isolated frequently from the CSF during the neurologic illness.

Treatment

Patients in whom acute poliomyelitis is suspected require careful observation of swallowing function, vital capacity, heart rate, and blood pressure in anticipation of respiratory and circulatory complications. With paralysis of limb muscles, footboards, hand and arm splints, and knee and trochanter rolls prevent foot-drop and other deformities. Frequent passive movement prevents contractures, ankylosis, and pressure sores.

Respiratory failure as a result of paralysis of the intercostal and diaphragmatic muscles or of depression of the respiratory centers in the brainstem calls for the use of a positive-pressure respirator and in most patients, for a tracheostomy as well. It was during the epidemics of the mid-twentieth century that the use of Drinker's "iron lung" attained widespread use. The management of the pulmonary and circulatory complications does not differ from their management in diseases such as myasthenia gravis and Guillain-Barré syndrome and is best carried out in special respiratory or neurologic intensive care units.

The authors know of no systematic study of the potency of antiviral agents in this disease.

Prevention

Prevention, of course, has proved to be one of the outstanding accomplishments of modern medicine. The cultivation of poliovirus in cultures of human embryonic tissues and monkey kidney cells—the achievement of Enders and associates—made possible the development of effective vaccines. The first of these was the injectable Salk vaccine, containing formalin-inactivated virulent strains of the three viral serotypes. This was followed by the Sabin vaccine, which consists of attenuated live virus, administered orally in two doses 8 weeks apart; boosters are required at 1 year of age and again before starting school. Since 1965, the reported annual incidence rate of poliomyelitis in the United States has been less than 0.01 per 100,000 (compared to a rate of 24 cases per 100,000 during the years 1951 to 1955). Very rarely in the past, poliomyelitis followed vaccination with the attenuated live virus (0.02 to 0.04 cases per 1 million doses). The virus is not used in the United States and polio is essentially eradicated in the Americas. The only obstacle to eradication of the disease elsewhere is inadequate utilization of the vaccine. Conceivably, with an increasing lack of immunity in underdeveloped nations (so-called herd immunity), outbreaks of poliomyelitis could occur once again.

Prognosis

Mortality from acute paralytic poliomyelitis is between 5 and 10 percent—higher in the elderly and very young. If the patient survives the acute stage, paralysis of respiration and deglutition usually recovers completely; in only a small fraction of such patients is chronic respiratory care necessary. Many patients also recover completely from early muscular weakness, and even the most severely paralyzed often improve to some extent. The return of muscle strength occurs mainly in the first 3 to 4 months and is probably the result of morphologic restitution of partially damaged nerve cells. Branching of axons of intact motor cells with collateral reinnervation of muscle fibers of denervated motor units may also play a part. Slow recovery of slight degree may then continue for a year or more. The postpolio syndrome is discussed in "Differential Diagnosis of ALS" in Chap. 39 and in Chap. 48.

Nonpoliovirus Poliomyelitis

As indicated earlier, a number of RNA viruses that normally cause mundane upper respiratory or enteric infections are now the main causes of a sporadic poliomyelitic syndrome. Fifty-two such cases were recorded by the Centers for Disease Control over a 4-year period. Most of them were caused by one of the echoviruses and a smaller number to Coxsackie enteroviruses, particularly strains 70 and 71. The former illness leaves little residual paralysis, but the Coxsackie viruses, which have been studied in several outbreaks in the United States, Bulgaria, and Hungary, have had more variable effects. Enterovirus 70 causes acute hemorrhagic conjunctivitis in limited epidemics and is followed by a poliomyelitis in 1 of every 10,000 cases. European outbreaks of enterovirus 71, known in the United States as a cause of hand-foot-and-mouth disease and of aseptic meningitis, have resulted in poliovirus-type paralysis, including a few fatal bulbar cases (Chumakov et al). In a recent outbreak of enterovirus 71 in Taiwan, Huang and associates described brainstem encephalitis with myoclonus and cranial nerve involvement in a high proportion of the patients. The tendency of West Nile virus to cause a poliomyelitis has already been mentioned.

Our own experience with this form of poliomyelitis has consisted of several patients who were referred over the years for paralyzing illnesses initially thought to be Guillain-Barré syndrome (Gorson and Ropper). In each case, the illness began with fever and aseptic meningitis (50 to 150 lymphocytes/mm^3 in the CSF), followed by backache and widespread, relatively symmetrical paralysis, including the oropharyngeal muscles in two cases and asymmetrical weakness limited to the arms in two patients. There were no sensory changes. One patient had a mild concurrent encephalitic illness and died months later. The evolving electromyographic changes indicated that the paralysis was caused by a loss of anterior horn cells rather than by a motor neuropathy or a purely motor radiculopathy, but this distinction was not always certain. MRI was remarkable in showing distinct changes in the gray matter of the cord, mainly ventrally (Fig. 33-3). No virus could be isolated from the CSF and serologic tests in our patients failed to implicate any of the usual encephalitic RNA viruses, including poliovirus. The patients had been immunized against the poliomyelitis viruses.

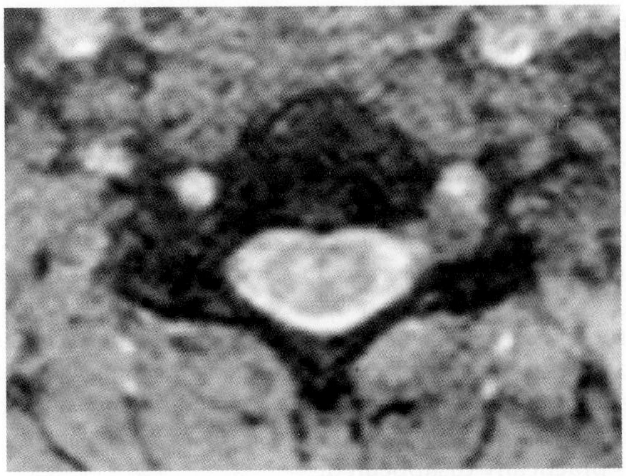

Figure 33-3. MRI of the cervical cord in a patient with nonpoliovirus poliomyelitis and an asymmetrical, flaccid, bibrachial paralysis. There is T2 signal change in the anterior regions of the gray matter.

SUBACUTE AND CHRONIC VIRAL INFECTIONS

The concept that viral infections may lead to chronic disease, especially of the nervous system, had been entertained since the 1920s, but only many decades later was it firmly established. Indirect and direct evidence supported this view: (1) the demonstration of a slowly progressive noninflammatory degeneration of nigral neurons long after an attack of encephalitis lethargica; (2) the finding of inclusion bodies in cases of subacute and chronic sclerosing encephalitis; (3) the discovery of chronic neurologic disease in sheep caused by a conventional RNA virus (visna)—it was in relation to this disease in sheep that Sigurdsson first used the term *slow virus infection* to describe long incubation periods during which the animals appeared well; and (4) the demonstration by electron microscopy of viral particles in the lesions of progressive multifocal leukoencephalopathy and, later, isolation of virus from the lesions. The suggestion that the late onset of progressive weakness after poliomyelitis ("postpolio syndrome") might represent a slow infection has never been verified. Claims have also been made numerous times over the years for a viral causation of multiple sclerosis, amyotrophic lateral sclerosis, and other degenerative diseases, but the evidence in all instances has been questionable.

The established human slow infections of the nervous system caused by conventional viruses include subacute sclerosing panencephalitis (measles virus), progressive rubella panencephalitis, and progressive multifocal leukoencephalopathy (JC virus). These diseases, except for PML, are decidedly rare. They are caused by conventional viruses and are not to be confused with a group of subacute and chronic neurologic diseases that are instead the result of *prions*, entirely distinct unconventional transmissible agents. These are accorded a separate section later in this chapter.

Subacute Sclerosing Panencephalitis

This disease was first described by Dawson in 1934 under the name "inclusion body encephalitis" and extensively studied by Van Bogaert, who renamed it *subacute sclerosing panencephalitis*. It is now recognized to be the result of chronic measles virus infection. Never a common disease, the condition occurred until recently at a rate of about 1 case per 1 million children per year and now, with the introduction and widespread use of measles vaccine, it has practically disappeared.

Children and adolescents were affected for the most part, the disease rarely appearing beyond the age of 10 years. Typically there is a history of primary measles infection at a very early age, often before 2 years, followed by a 6- to 8-year asymptomatic period. The illness evolved in several stages. Initially there was a decline in proficiency at school, temper outbursts and other changes in personality, difficulty with language, and loss of interest in usual activities. These soon give way to a severe and progressive intellectual deterioration in association with focal or generalized seizures, widespread myoclonus, ataxia, and sometimes visual disturbances caused by progressive chorioretinitis. As the disease advances, rigidity, hyperactive reflexes, Babinski signs, progressive unresponsiveness, and signs of autonomic dysfunction appear. In the final stage, the child lies insensate, virtually "decorticated."

The course is usually steadily progressive, death occurring within 1 to 3 years. A series of 39 such adult cases from India with mean age of 21 years was reported by Prashanth and coworkers, the oldest patient a 43-year old. The main features were similar in most ways to childhood cases, except that several had visual disturbances and two had extrapyramidal features, raising the possibility of prion disease. Myoclonus was present early in the illness in 26 and developed later in all cases; the movements were described as "slow," a characteristic alluded to in other series. In two cases that occurred in pregnant women, blurred vision and weakness of limbs was followed by akinetic mutism, without a trace of myoclonus or cerebellar ataxia. Nevertheless, the progressive ataxic-myoclonic chronic dementia in a child is so typical that bedside diagnosis was usually possible.

The EEG shows a characteristic abnormality consisting of periodic (every 5 to 8 s) bursts of 2 to 3/s high-voltage waves, followed by a relatively flat pattern. The CSF contains few or no cells, but the protein content is increased, particularly the gamma globulin fraction, and agarose gel electrophoresis discloses oligoclonal bands of IgG. These proteins have been shown to represent measles-virus-specific antibody (Mehta et al). MRI changes begin in the subcortical white matter and spread to the periventricular region (Anlar et al).

Histologically, the lesions involve the cerebral cortex and white matter of both hemispheres and the brainstem. The cerebellum is usually spared. Destruction of nerve cells, neuronophagia, and perivenous cuffing by lymphocytes and mononuclear cells indicate the viral nature of the infection. In the white matter there is degeneration of medullated fibers (both myelin and axons), accompanied by perivascular cuffing with mononuclear cells and fibrous gliosis (hence the term *sclerosing encephalitis*). Eosinophilic inclusions, the histopathologic hallmark of the disease, are found in the cytoplasm and nuclei of neurons and glia cells. Virions, thought to be measles nucleocapsids, have been observed in the inclusion-bearing cells examined electron microscopically.

How a ubiquitous and transient viral infection in a seemingly normal young child allows the development, many years later, of a rare encephalitis is a matter of speculation. Sever believes that there is a delay in the development of immune responses during the initial infection and a later inadequate immune response that is incapable of clearing the suppressed infection.

The differential diagnosis of SSPE includes the childhood and adolescent dementing diseases such as lipid storage diseases (see Chap. 37), prion disease (Creutzfeldt-Jakob), and Schilder-type demyelinative disease (see Chap. 36). In presumptive clinical cases of SSPE, the findings of periodic complexes in the EEG, elevated gamma globulin and oligoclonal bands in the CSF, and elevated measles antibody titers in the serum and CSF are sufficient to make the diagnosis.

No effective treatment is available. The administration of amantadine and inosine pranobex (formerly inosiplex) was found by some investigators to lead to improvement and prolonged survival, but these effects have not been corroborated.

Subacute Measles Encephalitis with Immunosuppression

Whereas SSPE occurs in children who were previously normal, another rare type of measles encephalitis has been described that affects both children and adults with defective cell-mediated immune responses (Wolinsky et al). In this type, measles or exposure to measles precedes the encephalitis by 1 to 6 months. Seizures (often epilepsia partialis continua), focal neurologic signs, stupor, and coma are the main features of the neurologic illness and lead to death within a few days to a few weeks. The CSF may be normal, and levels of measles antibodies do not increase. Aicardi and colleagues have isolated measles virus from the brain of such a patient. The lesions are similar to those of SSPE (eosinophilic inclusions in neurons and glia, with varying degrees of necrosis) except that inflammatory changes are lacking. In a sense, this subacute measles encephalitis is an opportunistic infection of the brain in an immunodeficient patient. The relatively short interval between exposure and onset of neurologic disease, the rapid course, and lack of antibodies distinguish this form of subacute measles encephalitis from both SSPE and postmeasles (postinfectious) encephalomyelitis (see Chap. 36).

Progressive Rubella Panencephalitis

The deficits associated with congenital rubella infection of the brain are nonprogressive at least after the second or third year of life. There are, however, descriptions of children with the congenital rubella syndrome in whom a progressive neurologic deterioration occurred after a stable period of 8 to 19 years (Townsend et al; Weil et al). In 1978, Wolinsky described 10 instances, a few of them apparently related to acquired rather than to congenital rubella. Since then, this late-appearing progressive syndrome seems to have disappeared, no definite new cases having been reported in the past 30 years but it nonetheless remains of biological interest.

The clinical syndrome was quite uniform. On a background of the features of congenital rubella, a decade later there occurred a deterioration in behavior and school performance, often associated with seizures, and, soon thereafter, a progressive impairment of mental function (dementia). Clumsiness of gait was an early symptom, followed by a frank ataxia of gait and then of the limbs. Spasticity and other corticospinal tract signs, dysarthria, and dysphagia ensue.

Progressive Multifocal Leukoencephalopathy

This disorder, first observed clinically by Adams and colleagues in 1952, was described morphologically in 1958 by Åstrom and coworkers, and then with a larger body of material by Richardson in 1961. It is characterized by widespread demyelinating lesions, mainly of the cerebral hemispheres but sometimes of the brainstem and cerebellum, and, rarely, of the spinal cord. The lesions vary greatly in size and severity—from microscopic foci of demyelination to massive multifocal zones of destruction of both myelin and axons involving large parts of a cerebral or cerebellar hemisphere. The abnormalities of the glia cells are distinctive. Many of the reactive astrocytes in the lesions are gigantic and contain deformed and bizarre-shaped nuclei and mitotic figures, changes that are seen otherwise only in malignant glial tumors. Also, at the periphery of the lesions, the nuclei of oligodendrocytes are greatly enlarged and contain abnormal inclusions. Many of these cells are destroyed, accounting for the demyelination. Vascular changes are lacking, and inflammatory changes are present but usually insignificant, except in a small number of interesting cases in which immune reconstitution by retroviral drugs for AIDS allows the emergence of intense inflammation.

Clinical Features

An uncommon disease of late adult life, PML usually develops in a patient with a neoplasm or chronic immunodeficiency state. The large majority of cases are now observed in patients with AIDS in whom the incidence of PML approaches 5 percent. Viewed from another perspective, more than 75 percent of cases of PML in the current era are associated with HIV. Indeed, the incidence is so much higher than in any other form of immunosuppression that an interaction between HIV and the causative virus of PML has been suggested. Other important associations are with chronic neoplastic disease (mainly chronic lymphocytic leukemia, Hodgkin disease, lymphosarcoma, and myeloproliferative disease) and less often, with nonneoplastic granulomatosis, such as tuberculosis or sarcoidosis. A number of cases occur in patients receiving immunosuppressive drugs for renal transplantation, multiple sclerosis (see Chap. 36), or for other reasons.

Personality changes and intellectual impairment may introduce the neurologic syndrome, which then evolves over a period of several days to weeks. Any one or some combination of hemiparesis progressing to quadriparesis, visual field defects, cortical blindness, aphasia, ataxia, dysarthria, dementia, confusional states, and coma are manifestations. Some of the cases under our observation had a predominantly cerebellar syndrome. Seizures are infrequent, occurring in only about 10 percent of cases. In most cases, death occurs in 3 to 6 months from the onset of neurologic symptoms and even more rapidly in patients with AIDS unless aggressive antiretroviral treatment is undertaken. The CSF is usually normal. CT and MRI localize the nonenhancing demyelinating lesions with clarity (Fig. 33-4) but the variability in size, location, and multiplicity make the diagnosis more dependent on viral DNA isolation from CSF and on the context of immunosuppression.

Pathogenesis

Waksman's original suggestion (quoted by Richardson) that PML could be caused by viral infection of the CNS in patients with impaired immunologic responses proved to be correct. ZuRhein and Chou, in an electron microscopic study of cerebral lesions from a patient with PML later demonstrated crystalline arrays of particles resembling papovaviruses in the inclusion-bearing oligodendrocytes. Since then a human polyomavirus, designated "JC virus" or JCV (initials of the patient from whom the virus was originally isolated), has definitively been shown to be the causative agent. JCV is ubiquitous, as judged by the presence of antibodies to the virus in approximately 70 percent of the normal adult population. It is thought to be dormant in the kidney or bone marrow until an immunosuppressed state permits its active replication. The virus has been isolated from the urine, blood lymphocytes, bone marrow, and kidney, but there is no clinical evidence of damage to extraneural structures.

Treatment

The disease is generally believed to be untreatable in the non-AIDS patient. Anecdotal reports of the efficacy of various medications such as cytosine arabinoside, cidofovir, mirtazapine, interferon, and topotecan, either have not been tested in, or have failed to be sustained in larger trials. In AIDS patients, aggressive treatment using antiretroviral drug combinations, including protease inhibitors, greatly slows the progression of PML and has led to remission in almost half of cases for a year, as in the large series reported by Antinori and colleagues. Several retrospective series found that a CD4 count below 100 cells/μL is a poor prognostic sign for recovery from PML. A review of these issues, particularly relating to AIDS and PML, is in the report by Mangi and Miller.

A special comment should be made regarding the transient but sometimes severe clinical worsening of PML that may occur during the initial treatment of HIV

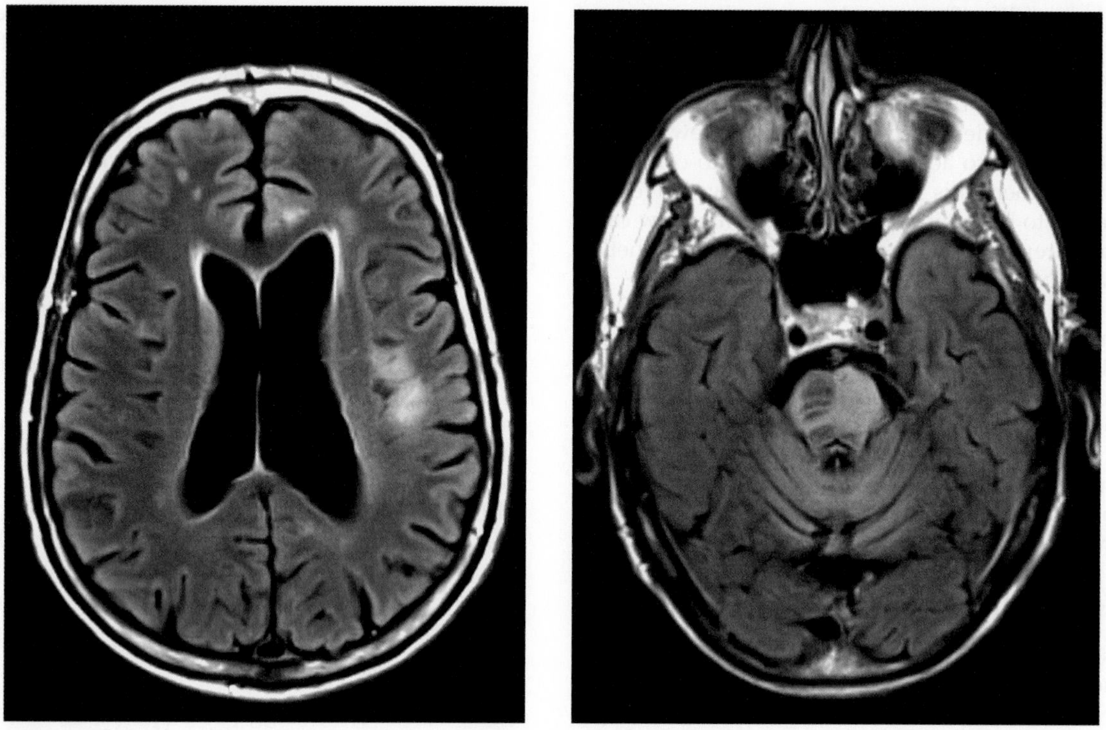

Figure 33-4. Progressive multifocal leukoencephalopathy (PML). MRI, T2-FLAIR, demonstrates multiple subcortical white matter lesions in both hemispheres (*left panel*) and in the left pons (*right panel*) in a 31-year-old male with AIDS. The lesions did not enhance.

infection with antiretroviral drugs. This syndrome has been attributed to the emergence of acute inflammation surrounding the demyelinating lesions as a result of reconstitution of the immune system (immune reconstitution syndrome or *IRIS* that has been mentioned in the section on the treatment of HIV). In support of this mechanism, there is a parallel blossoming of the lesions with gadolinium enhancement on MRI. Treatment with corticosteroids has been suggested and is said to allow survival and temporary remission of PML, although we have seen at least one dramatic exception. Judicious use of corticosteroids is implemented to mute this reaction.

Encephalitis Lethargica (von Economo Disease, Sleeping Sickness)

Although examples of a somnolent-ophthalmoplegic encephalitis dot the early medical literature (e.g., nona, fébre lethargica, Schlafkrankheit), it was in the wake of the influenza pandemic of World War I that this disease appeared prominently and continued to reappear for about 10 years. The viral agent was never identified, but the clinical and pathologic features were typical of viral infection. Nonetheless recent testing of archived brain material has failed to reveal influenzal RNA, so that encephalitis lethargica may be considered a putative viral disease. An alternative view of an immune pathogenesis is presented below.

The importance of encephalitis lethargica relates to its unique clinical syndromes and sequelae and to its place as the first recognized "slow virus infection" (ironically, without identification of the agent) of the nervous system in humans. The unique symptoms were ophthalmoplegia and pronounced somnolence, from which the disease took its name. Some patients were overly active, and a third group manifested a disorder of movement in the form of bradykinesia, catalepsy, mutism, chorea, or myoclonus. Lymphocytic pleocytosis was found in the spinal fluid of half the patients, together with variable elevation of the CSF protein content. More than 20 percent of the victims died within a few weeks, and many survivors were left with varying degrees of impairment of mental function. However, the most extraordinary feature was the appearance of a parkinsonian syndrome, after an interval of weeks or months (occasionally years), in a high proportion of survivors. Myoclonus, dystonia, oculogyric crises (Chap. 14) and other muscle spasms, bulimia, obesity, reversal of the sleep pattern, and, in children, a change in personality with compulsive behavior ("organic driveness") were other distressing sequelae. This is not the only form of encephalitis known to cause a delayed extrapyramidal syndrome of this type (a similar though not identical syndrome with a much shorter latency may follow Japanese B encephalitis and other arboviral encephalitis).

The pathology was typical of a viral infection, localized principally to the midbrain, subthalamus, and hypothalamus. In the patients who died years later with Parkinson syndrome, the main findings were depigmentation of the substantia nigra and locus ceruleus because of nerve cell destruction. Neurofibrillary changes in the surviving nerve cells of the substantia nigra and the oculomotor and adjacent nuclei were also described, indistinguishable from those of progressive supranuclear palsy. Lewy bodies were not seen, in contrast to idiopathic Parkinson disease, where they are consistently present. Only a few new cases of postencephalitic type have been seen in the United States and western Europe since 1930. Sporadic cases, such as the four reported by Howard and Lees, may be examples of this disease, but there is no way of proving their identity.

More often currently, a postinfectious extrapyramidal syndrome is putatively the result of circulating autoantibodies. While not necessarily viral in origin, this is an appropriate place to summarize the recent findings of Dale and colleagues, who have studied the problem carefully and presented 20 cases that were remarkably similar to the ones described by von Economo. Half of their patients had a preceding pharyngitis that was followed by somnolence or pathologic insomnia, parkinsonism, dyskinesias, and psychiatric symptoms. Many had oligoclonal bands in the cerebrospinal fluid and some had changes on MRI in the basal ganglia. Their singular finding was that 95 percent had serum autoantibodies against basal ganglia neural antigens (two-thirds also had antibodies to anti–streptolysin O). Pathologic examination in one case showed perivascular inflammation. Thus, the long-held notion that this form of encephalitis was, and is, a viral illness might be challenged. Dale and colleagues comment that von Economo and his contemporaries in fact doubted that there was a connection to influenza.

Other Forms of Subacute Encephalitis

A number of uncommon conditions not covered above are characterized by regional inflammation in the cerebrum. Among these, *Rasmussen encephalitis,* which causes intractable focal seizures and progressive hemiparesis (see Chap. 16), has been tentatively connected to infections by CMV and HSV-I in various studies that used PCR techniques but the presence of autoantibodies to glutamate receptors suggest this is an immune process. However, a specific immune reaction consisting of antibodies to glutamate receptors has been implicated more consistently and immunosuppressive treatments may be effective. It is not clear whether this process can be classed with the infectious encephalitides; it is discussed in detail with other epileptic diseases in Chap. 16. Similarly, the restricted inflammatory conditions called *limbic encephalitis* and "brainstem encephalitis"—most often a distant effect of lung cancer—have some characteristics of a subacute viral encephalitis, but no agent has been consistently isolated and they are also best considered immunologic reactions. They are included in the discussion of paraneoplastic illnesses in Chap 31.

PRION DISEASES

This category of infections includes a quartet of human diseases—Creutzfeldt-Jakob disease (and a variant that infects cows and may be rarely transmitted to humans), the Gerstmann-Sträussler-Scheinker syndrome, kuru, and fatal familial insomnia.

Although this group of diseases has been included for discussion in the chapter on viruses that affect the nervous system, it has been evident for some time that the cause of these diseases is neither a virus nor a viroid (nucleic acid alone, without a capsid structure). The transmissible, or "infectious" nature of prions was discovered by Gadjusek and Gibbs in the Fore tribes of New Guinea, who practiced ritual cannibalism and ate the brains of the deceased. The resulting disease, kuru, is described further on but the important point is that the aforementioned workers were able to transmit the disease to chimpanzees after a long latent period of years. Prusiner is credited with doggedly pursuing this problem, for which he was awarded the Nobel Prize. He (1993, 1994, 2001) has presented evidence that the transmissible pathogen is a proteinaceous infectious particle that is devoid of nucleic acid, resists the action of enzymes that destroy RNA and DNA, fails to produce an immune response, and electron microscopically does not have the structure of a virus. To distinguish this pathogen from viruses and viroids, Prusiner introduced the term *prion*.

The very same prion protein (PrP) is normally encoded by a gene on the short arm of chromosome 20 in humans. The discovery of mutations in the PrP genes of patients with familial Creutzfeldt-Jakob disease and Gerstmann-Sträussler-Scheinker syndrome (described below) attests to the fact that prion diseases may be both genetic and infectious. This is another way in which prions are unique among all pathogens. It is now possible to detect inherited types of prion diseases during life, using DNA extracted from leukocytes. How prions arise in sporadic forms of spongiform encephalopathy is not fully understood. The conversion of the normal cellular protein to the infectious form involves a conformational change in the protein structure as described in Prusiner's review in 2001. Remarkably, as discussed below, the current theory holds that an abnormally folded prion protein can act as a template for the conversion of normal PrP to PrPsc (the latter denoting the scrapie prion; see further on). A description of the human prion diseases is given here, the most important by far being Creutzfeldt-Jakob disease.

Creutzfeldt-Jakob Disease (Subacute Spongiform Encephalopathy)

These terms refer to a distinctive cerebral disease in which a rapidly or subacutely progressive and profound dementia is associated with diffuse myoclonic jerks and a variety of other neurologic abnormalities, mainly visual or cerebellar. The major neuropathologic changes are found in the cerebral and cerebellar cortices, and the outstanding features are widespread neuronal loss and gliosis accompanied by a striking vacuolation or spongy state of the affected regions—hence the designation *subacute spongiform encephalopathy (SSE)*. Less severe changes in a patchy distribution are found in cases with a briefer clinical course.

The widely used term Creutzfeldt-Jakob disease (CJD) may be an inappropriate eponym as it is most unlikely that the patient described by Creutzfeldt and at least three of the five patients described by Jakob did not have the same disease that we now recognize as subacute spongiform encephalopathy. However, decades of use make it virtually impossible to displace.

One of the more interesting aspects of the development of the prion concept has been the hypothesis that many conditions, most in the category of degenerative neurologic disease and characterized by the accumulation of specific proteins such as amyloid, tau, synuclein, and ubiquitin may have a similar mechanism in sequential, contiguous conformational change in protein aggregation.

Epidemiology and Pathogenesis

The disease appears in all parts of the world and in all seasons, with an annual incidence of 1 to 2 cases per million of population. The incidence is higher in Israelis of Libyan origin, in immigrants to France from North Africa, and perhaps in Slovakia. The incidence of spongiform encephalopathy is somewhat higher in urban than in rural areas, but a consistent temporal or spatial clustering of cases has not been observed, at least in the United States. A small proportion of all series is familial—varying from 5 percent reported by Cathala and associates to 15 percent of 1,435 cases analyzed by Masters and coworkers (1979). The occurrence of familial cases that are not in the same household probably indicates a genetic susceptibility to infection, although the possibility of common early exposure to the transmissible agent cannot be excluded. A small number of conjugal cases have also been reported. The only clearly demonstrated mechanism of spread of the usual type of CJD is iatrogenic, having occurred in a few cases after transplantation of corneas or dural grafts from infected individuals, after implantation of infected electroencephalographic depth electrodes, and after the injection of human growth hormone or gonadotropins that had been prepared from pooled cadaveric sources. At least one neurosurgeon is known to have acquired the disease. Of some interest is the finding by Zanusso and colleagues of the infectious prion protein in the nasal mucosa of all nine patients studied with the sporadic disease. This suggests a route for entry into the nervous system of the aberrant prion and also a potential diagnostic test. As noted further on, the tonsils of patients affected with variant CJD may also show immunostaining for prions.

Attention has been drawn to an outbreak of prion disease among cows in the British Isles ("mad cow disease," bovine spongiform encephalopathy, BSE). Cows elsewhere have sporadically been found to be infected. The mini-epidemic began in 1986, with putative transmission of the disease to some 24 humans. These patients were younger (average age of onset 27 years) than those with typical CJD (average age of onset 65 years) and manifested psychiatric and sensory symptoms as the first sign of illness; they did not exhibit the usual EEG findings even as the illness advanced to its later stages (Will et al). This has been called "new variant Creutzfeldt-Jakob disease (vCJD)." One reason for including a lengthy explanation of this illness is the potential for cases to appear in future years. It was shown that the prion strain in affected patients is identical to the one from affected cattle and different from the prion agent that causes sporadic CJD. The mode of transmission, presumed to be the ingestion of infected meat, is reminiscent of the propagation of kuru in New Guinea by ceremonial ingestion of brain tissue from infected individuals that opened the era of understanding of prion disease.

Prion (spongiform) encephalopathy or all types has now been firmly associated with the conversion of a normal cellular protein, PrPc to an abnormal isoform, PrPsc. The transformation involves a change in the physical conformation of the protein in which its helical proportion diminishes and the proportion of the β pleated sheet increases (see reviews by Prusiner). The current understanding is that the "infectivity" of prions and their propagation in brain tissue result from the susceptibility of the native PrP to alter its shape as a result of physical exposure to the abnormal protein, a so-called conformational disease. Conformationally altered prions have a tendency to aggregate, and this may be the mode of cellular destruction that leads to neuronal disease. In contrast, familial cases of prion disease are thought to be the result of one of several gene aberrations residing in the region that code for PrPc.

As the isoforms of the prions that causes the sporadic disease have been characterized, clinical patterns have emerged as more or less typical of certain protein configurations and their underlying genotypes. Several competing classification systems have been devised that are based on both the presence of methionine (M) or valine (V) at codon 129 of the prion protein and on which of two physicochemical properties it displays (termed types 1 or 2; see Parchi et al). The most common variant in most studies has been MM and the least common, VV, and type 1 is more frequent than type 2 (hence MM1 is the most common type overall, present in approximately two-thirds of sporadic cases). However, classification is complicated by the fact that some brain samples show more than one type of protein. Although several studies conflict on these points, a typical EEG pattern was most common in type 1 cases with at least one methionine, whereas MV2 cases were most likely to have MRI changes (see further on). Some studies have suggested that the MV2 subtype, comprising a small proportion of cases, was likely to present with ataxia, psychiatric changes, a lack of positive sharp waves on EEG, and a prolonged duration of disease, but none of the distinctions has been even close to absolute. There has also been controversy regarding the relationship of the genotype to the sensitivity of diagnostic tests discussed below. Details of these putative associations can be found in an extensive international study of 2,541 pathologically confirmed cases of CJD reported by Collins and colleagues.

Clinical Features

Prion encephalopathy is in most cases a spontaneously occurring disease of late middle age, although it occurs in young adults. The sexes are affected equally. In the large series of pathologically verified cases reported by Brown and coworkers, prodromal symptoms—consisting of fatigue, depression, weight loss, and disorders of sleep and appetite lasting for several weeks—were observed in about one-third of the patients.

The early stages of the neurologic disease are characterized by a great variety of clinical manifestations, but the most frequent are changes in behavior, emotional response, and intellectual function, often followed by ataxia and abnormalities of vision, such as distortions of the shape and alignment of objects or impairment of visual acuity. Typically, the early phase of the disease is dominated by symptoms of confusion, with hallucinations, delusions, and agitation. In other instances, cerebellar ataxia (Brownell-Oppenheimer variant) or visual disturbances (Heidenhain variant) precede the mental changes and may be the most prominent features for several months. Headache, vertigo, and sensory symptoms are complaints in some patients but become quickly obscured by dementia and muteness.

As a rule, the disease progresses rapidly, so that obvious deterioration is seen from week to week and even day to day. Sooner or later, in almost all cases, myoclonic contractions of various muscle groups appear, perhaps unilaterally at first but later becoming generalized. Or, infrequently, the myoclonus may not appear for weeks or months after the initial mental changes. In a few patients, a startle response, that is elicitable for a brief period of time, is the only manifestation of myoclonus. In general, the myoclonic jerks are evocable by sudden sensory stimuli of all sorts, a startle response (to noise, bright light, touch) but they occur spontaneously as well. Twitches of individual fingers are typical but it should be emphasized that well-formed seizures are not a component of the illness. These changes gradually give way to a mute state, stupor, and coma, but the myoclonic contractions may continue to the end. Signs of degeneration of the pyramidal tracts or anterior horn cells, palsies of convergence and upgaze, and extrapyramidal signs occur in a small number of patients as the disease advances.

The clinical diagnosis during life rests mostly on the recognition of one of the clusters of typical clinical features, particularly the special rate of rapid progression of dementia—much more quickly than that of common degenerative diseases—coupled with stimulus-sensitive myoclonus and the characteristic MRI and EEG changes that occur in most patients (see below).

The disease is invariably fatal, usually in a few months and almost always less than a year from the onset. In approximately 10 percent of patients, the illness begins with almost stroke-like suddenness and runs its course rapidly, in a matter of a few weeks. At the other extreme, a small number of patients have reportedly survived for 2 to 10 years, but these reports should be accepted with caution; in some of them, the illness appears to have been superimposed on Alzheimer or Parkinson disease or some other chronic condition that predated the prion illness.

Laboratory Diagnosis

The routine CSF and other laboratory tests are normal—useful findings in that they exclude a number of chronic inflammatory causes of dementia such as neurosyphilis. In most patients, the EEG pattern is distinctive, changing over the course of the disease from one of diffuse and nonspecific slowing to one of stereotyped high-voltage slow- (1- to 2-Hz) and sharp-wave complexes on an increasingly slow and low-voltage background (see Fig. 2-5G). The high-voltage sharp waves, which give the appearance of periodicity (they have been called pseudo-periodic), are synchronous with the myoclonus, but may persist in its absence.

MRI of the brain has now been appreciated to show hyperintensity of the lenticular nuclei on T2-weighted and diffusion-weighted images in the basal ganglia and cortex when the disease is fully established (Fig. 33-5). Long contiguous segments of the cortex, as well as various parts of the basal ganglia, show these alterations in a pattern that is characteristic and mistakable only perhaps for the appearance of diffuse cerebral anoxia. According to Shiga and colleagues, these changes occur in 90 percent of cases (cortex more often than caudate or lenticular nuclei and sometimes both), making them potentially the most sensitive test for the disease but the proportion has been lower in our patients. Complicating the interpretation of the MRI findings in this disease have been reports from Japan of extensive white matter lesions in several autopsy-proven cases (Matsusue et al).

There are helpful confirmatory diagnostic tests but they are not always necessary. Hsich and colleagues described a now widely used test of CSF—the finding by immunoassay of peptide fragments of normal brain proteins, termed "14-3-3." This test is particularly useful in separating CJD from other chronic noninflammatory dementing diseases but it has been sometimes disappointing on our wards, giving both false-positive and false-negative results. Several studies have given conflicting information on the sensitivity of the 14-3-3 test in relation to the various forms of prions and differing clinical presentations, but all seem to converge on the fact that repeated testing, up to three times is more likely to give positive results. A summary publication has indicated an overall sensitivity from pooled reports of 92 percent and specificity of 80 percent (report of the Guidelines Development Committee of the American Academy of Neurology). Also, enolase and neopterin concentrations in CSF are elevated in most cases, but the release of these substances is found with other types of brain lesions, particularly infarction. A number of other tests are emerging from specialized laboratories that are able to detect the specific abnormal PrPsc isoform of the prion protein in the spinal fluid. Prusiner's laboratory has been able to detect eight prion strains but it is not yet clear if this scientific advance can be put to clinical use.

Tonsillar material from patients with new variant Creutzfeldt-Jakob disease ("mad cow disease") stains

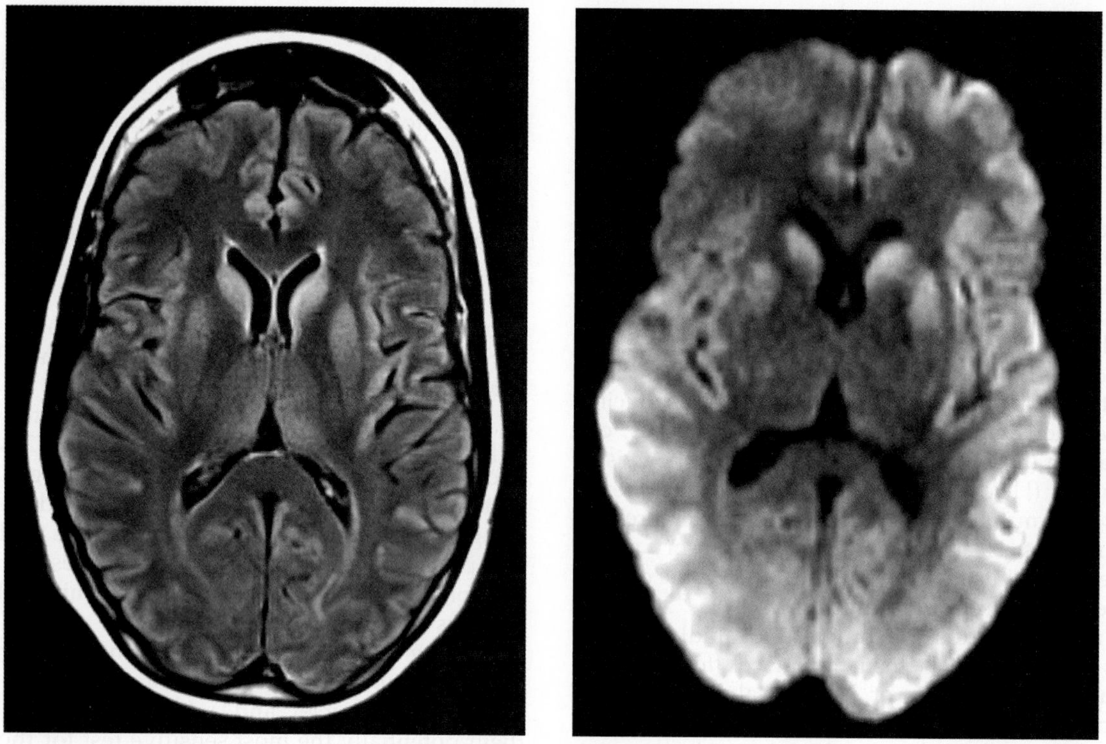

Figure 33-5. MRI showing T2 signal changes in the striatum in a patient with sporadic CJD (*left*) of 1 month's duration. DWI sequence showing restriction of diffusion in contiguous bands of cortex and in the striatum (*right*) in the same case.

with antibodies against abnormal prion protein, but this technique does not appear to be applicable to the early diagnosis of the sporadic disease (Hill). Whether the earlier-mentioned finding of infectious prion material in the nasal mucosa in the sporadic form will prove to have practical value in diagnosis is yet to be determined.

The National Prion Disease Pathology Surveillance Center, which was established at Case Western Reserve University, is available to assist clinicians by performing, free of charge, a variety of specific diagnostic tests (accessible through *http://www.cjdsurveillance.com*).

Pathology The disease affects principally the cerebral and cerebellar cortices, generally in a diffuse fashion, although in some cases the occipitoparietal regions are almost exclusively involved, as in those described by Heidenhain. In others, such as the cases of Brownell and Oppenheimer alluded to earlier, the cerebellum has been most extensively affected, with early and prominent ataxia. The degeneration and disappearance of nerve cells are associated with extensive astroglial proliferation; ultrastructural studies have shown that the microscopic vacuoles, which give the tissue its typically spongy appearance, are located within the cytoplasmic processes of glia cells and dendrites of nerve cells. The loss in particular of certain inhibitory neurons in the thalamic reticular nuclei seems to correspond to the presence of myoclonus and positive sharp waves in the EEG according to Tschampa and colleagues. Despite the fact that the disease is caused by a transmissible agent, the lesions show no evidence of an inflammatory reaction and no viral particles are seen.

Differential Diagnosis The diagnosis of most cases presents no difficulty if the rapidity of progression and the myoclonus are recognized. Not infrequently, however, we have been surprised by a "typical" case that proves to be some other disease. Lithium intoxication, Hashimoto encephalopathy (as emphasized by Seipelt and colleagues who found a number of these cases in an epidemiologic survey of SSE; Chap. 40), Whipple disease (see Chap. 32), intravascular lymphoma, and carcinomatous meningitis—all of them characterized by myoclonus and dementia—may mimic CJD in the early weeks of illness. Contrariwise, the early mental changes of SSE may be misinterpreted as an atypical or unusually intense emotional reaction, as one of the major psychoses, as an unusual form of Alzheimer disease with myoclonus, corticobasal degeneration (see Chap. 39), or as Lewy-body disease. Despite the designation of CJD as a progressive dementia, the similarities to even rapidly developing Alzheimer disease are superficial. Also, diagnosis may be difficult in patients who present with dizziness, gait disturbance, diplopia, or visual disturbances until the rapidly evolving clinical picture clarifies the issue. Subacute sclerosing panencephalitis (see earlier in this chapter) in its fully developed form may resemble CJD, but the former is chiefly a disease of children or young adults, and the CSF shows elevation of gamma globulin (IgG), whereas the latter is essentially a disease of middle age and the presenile period and the CSF is normal. Limbic-brainstem-cerebellar encephalitis in patients with an occult tumor and AIDS dementia (discussed earlier) also figure in the differential diagnosis. Cerebral lipidosis in children or young adults can result in a similar combination of myoclonus and dementia, but the clinical course in such cases is extremely chronic and there are retinal changes that do not occur in spongiform encephalopathy. Well-formed convulsions should direct attention to another diagnosis.

Management No specific treatment is known. Antiviral agents have been ineffective. In view of the transmissibility of the disease from humans to primates and iatrogenically from person to person with infected materials, certain precautions should be taken in the medical care and handling of materials from affected patients. Special isolation rooms are unnecessary, and the families of affected patients and nursing staff can be reassured that casual contact poses no risk. Needle punctures and cuts are not thought to pose a risk, but some uncertainty remains. The transmissible agent is resistant to boiling, treatment with formalin and alcohol, and ultraviolet radiation but can be inactivated by autoclaving at 132°C (269.6°F) at 15 lb/in^2 for 1 h or by immersion for 1 h in 5 percent sodium hypochlorite (bleach). Workers exposed to infected materials (butchers, abattoir workers, healthcare workers) should wash thoroughly with ordinary soap. Needles, glassware, needle electrodes, and other instruments should be handled with great care and immersed in appropriate disinfectants and autoclaved or incinerated. The performance of a brain biopsy or autopsy requires that a set of special precautions be followed, as outlined by Brown but this surgical procedure is not necessary as more diagnostic tools have become available. Obviously such patients or any others known to have been demented should not be donors of organs or corneas for transplantation or blood for transfusion.

Gerstmann-Sträussler-Scheinker Syndrome

This is a rare, strongly familial disease inherited as an autosomal dominant trait. It begins insidiously in midlife and runs a chronic course (mean duration 5 years). The main characteristics are progressive cerebellar ataxia, corticospinal tract signs, dysarthria, and nystagmus. Dementia is often associated but is relatively mild.

Dysesthesias and proximal weakness of the legs have been emphasized as an early feature by Arata and colleagues. Their report may be consulted for details of 11 well-studied cases. The MRI is usually normal; with progression, generalized atrophy is found.

There are characteristic spongiform changes in brain tissue, as in CJD. Brain tissue from patients with this disease, when inoculated into chimpanzees, has produced a spongiform encephalopathy (Masters et al, 1981). Molecular genetic studies of affected family members demonstrate a mutation of the prion protein gene. This syndrome should be considered as a small familial subset of SSE, of slowly progressive type.

Fatal Insomnia (Familial and Sporadic)

This is another rare and usually familial disease in the spongiform encephalopathy group. It is characterized by intractable insomnia, sympathetic overactivity, and dementia, leading to death in 7 to 15 months (see also Chap. 16). The pathologic changes, consisting of neuronal loss and gliosis, are found mainly in the medial thalamic nuclei. Studies of a few families have shown a mutation of the prion protein gene and brain material was found to contain a protease-resistant form of the gene that is characterized by a mutation in the prion gene at codon 178 in conjunction with the presence of methionine at codon 129 on chromosome 20, the latter being a feature of sporadic CJD. Transmission of the disease by inoculation of infected brain material has not been accomplished (Medori et al). There is also a rare sporadic form of this disease and the configuration of the prion alteration is different from the familial variety.

Kuru

This disease occurs exclusively among the Fore linguistic group of natives of the New Guinea highlands and is included here because of its historical interest as the first slow infection caused by an unconventional transmissible agent to be documented in human beings. Clinically the disease takes the form of an afebrile, progressive cerebellar ataxia, with abnormalities of extraocular movements, weakness progressing to immobility, incontinence in the late stages, and death within 3 to 6 months of onset. In some ways it is similar to the ataxic (Brownell-Oppenheimer) variant of CJD. The remarkable epidemiologic and pathologic similarities between kuru and scrapie in sheep were pointed out in 1959 by Hadlow, who suggested that it might be possible to transmit kuru to subhuman primates. This was accomplished in 1966 by Gajdusek and coworkers; inoculation of chimpanzees with brain material from affected humans produced a kuru-like syndrome in chimpanzees after a latency of 18 to 36 months. Since then the disease has been transmitted from one chimpanzee to another and to other primates by using both neural and nonneural tissues. The pioneering work in this field led to the awarding of a Nobel Prize to these workers and the same prize was awarded to Prusiner 23 years later, representing a landmark in which the Nobel was awarded twice for work regarding the same disease. Histologically there is a noninflammatory loss of neurons and spongiform change throughout the brain, but predominantly in the cerebellar cortex, with astroglial proliferation and periodic acid-Schiff–positive stellate plaques of amyloid-like material ("kuru plaques"). The transmissible agent has not been visualized, however.

Kuru has gradually disappeared because of the cessation of ritual cannibalism by which the disease had been transmitted. In this ritual, infected brain tissue was ingested and rubbed over the body of the victim's kin (women and young children of either sex), permitting absorption of the infective agent through conjunctivae, mucous membranes, and abrasions in the skin.

References

Adams H, Miller D: Herpes simplex encephalitis: A clinical and pathological analysis of twenty-two cases. *Postgrad Med J* 49:393, 1973.

Aicardi J, Gouthieres F, Arsenio-Nunes HL, Lebon P: Acute measles encephalitis in children with immunosuppression. *Pediatrics* 55:232, 1977.

Anderson NE, Willoughby EW: Chronic meningitis without predisposing illness—a review of 83 cases. *Q J Med* 63:283, 1987.

Anderson NE, Willoughby EW, Synek BK: Leptomeningeal and brain biopsy in chronic meningitis. *Aust N Z J Med* 26:703, 1995.

Anlar B, Saatçi I, Köse, et al: MRI finding in subacute sclerosing panencephalitis. *Neurology* 47:1278, 1996.

Antinori A, Cingolani A, Lorenzini P, et al: Clinical epidemiology and survival of progressive multifocal leukoencephalopathy in the era of highly active antiretroviral therapy: data from the Italian Registry Investigative Neuro AIDS (IRINA). *J Neurovirol* 9(Suppl 1):47, 2003.

Arata H, Takashima H, Hirano R, et al: Early clinical signs and imaging findings in Gerstmann-Sträussler-Scheinker syndrome (Pro102Leu). *Neurology* 66:1672, 2006.

Asnis DS, Conetta R, Teixeira AA, et al: The West Nile virus outbreak of 1999 in New York: The Flushing Hospital experience. *Clin Infect Dis* 30:413, 2000.

Åstrom KE, Mancall EL, Richardson EP Jr: Progressive multifocal leukoencephalopathy. *Brain* 81:93, 1958.

Aurelius E, Johansson B, Sköldenberg B, et al: Rapid diagnosis of herpes simplex encephalitis by nested polymerase chain reaction assay of cerebrospinal fluid. *Lancet* 337:189, 1991.

Barnett GH, Ropper AH, Romeo J: Intracranial pressure and outcome in adult encephalitis. *J Neurosurg* 68:585, 1988.

Bartleson JD, Swanson JW, Whisnant JP: A migrainous syndrome with cerebrospinal fluid pleocytosis. *Neurology* 31:1257, 1981.

Beghi E, Nicolosi A, Kurland LT, et al: Encephalitis and aseptic meningitis, Olmstead County, Minnesota, 1950–1981: Epidemiology. *Ann Neurol* 16:283, 1984.

Bell JE: The neuropathology of adult HIV infection. *Rev Neurol* 154:816, 1998.

Bodian D: Histopathologic basis of clinical findings in poliomyelitis. *Am J Med* 6:563, 1949.

Brown P: Guidelines for high risk autopsy cases: Special precautions for Creutzfeldt-Jakob disease, in *Autopsy Performance and Reporting*. Northfield, IL, College of American Pathologists, 1990, pp 67–74.

Brown P, Cathala F, Castaigne P, et al: Creutzfeldt-Jakob disease: Clinical analysis of a consecutive series of 230 neuropathologically verified cases. *Ann Neurol* 20:597, 1986.

Brownell B, Oppenheimer DR: An ataxic form of subacute presenile polioencephalopathy (Creutzfeldt-Jakob disease). *J Neurol Neurosurg Psychiatry* 20:350, 1965.

Buescher EL, Artenstein MS, Olson LC: Central nervous system infections of viral etiology: The changing pattern, in Zimmerman HM (ed): *Infections of the Nervous System*. Baltimore, Williams & Wilkins, 1968, pp 147–163.

Cathala F, Brown P, Chatelain J, et al: Maladie de Creutzfeldt-Jacob en France: Intérêt des formes familiales. *Presse Med* 15:379, 1986.

Charleston AJ, Anderson NE, Willoughby EW: Idiopathic steroid responsive chronic lymphocytic meningitis: Clinical features and long term outcome in 17 patients. *Aust N Z J Med* 28:784, 1998.

Chesebro B: BSE and prions: Uncertainties about the agent. *Science* 279:42, 1998.

Chumakov M, Voroshilova M, Shindarov L, et al: Enterovirus 71 isolated from cases of epidemic poliomyelitis-like disease in Bulgaria. *Arch Virol* 60:329, 1979.

Cohen BA, Rowley AH, Long CM: Herpes simplex type 2 in a patient with Mollaret's meningitis: Demonstration by polymerase chain reaction. *Ann Neurol* 35:112, 1994.

Collins SJ, Sanchez-Juan P, Masters CL, et al: Determinants of diagnostic investigation sensitivities across the clinical spectrum of sporadic Creutzfeldt-Jakob disease. *Brain* 239:2278, 2006.

Connolly AM, Dodson WE, Prensky AL, Rust RS: Cause and outcome of acute cerebellar ataxia. *Ann Neurol* 35:673, 1994.

Cornblath DR, McArthur JC, Kennedy PGE, et al: Inflammatory demyelinating peripheral neuropathies associated with human T-cell lymphotropic virus type III infection. *Ann Neurol* 21:32, 1987.

Dale RC, Church AJ, Surtees RA, et al: Encephalitis lethargica syndrome: 20 new cases and evidence of basal ganglia autoimmunity. *Brain* 127:21, 2004.

Davis LE, Johnson RT: An explanation for the localization of herpes simplex encephalitis. *Ann Neurol* 5:2, 1979.

Dawson JR: Cellular inclusions in cerebral lesions of epidemic encephalitis. *Arch Neurol Psychiatry* 31:685, 1934.

Denny-Brown D, Adams RD, Fitzgerald PJ: Pathologic features of herpes zoster: A note on "geniculate herpes." *Arch Neurol Psychiatry* 51:216, 1944.

Deresiewicz RL, Thaler SJ, Hsu L, et al: Clinical and neuroradiologic manifestations of eastern equine encephalitis. *N Engl J Med* 336:1867, 1997.

Devinsky O, Cho E-S, Petito CK, Price RW: Herpes zoster myelitis. *Brain* 114:1181, 1991.

Donat JF, Rhodes KH, Groover RV, et al: Etiology and outcome in 42 children with acute nonbacterial encephalitis. *Mayo Clin Proc* 55:156, 1980.

Douvoyiannis M, Litman, Goldman, DL: Neurologic manifestations associated with parvovirus B-19 infection. *CID* 48:1713, 2009.

Drachman DA, Adams RD: Herpes simplex and acute inclusion-body encephalitis. *Arch Neurol* 7:45, 1962.

Dueland AN, Devlin M, Martin JR, et al: Fatal varicella-zoster virus meningoradiculitis without skin involvement. *Ann Neurol* 29:569, 1991.

Eidelberg D, Sotrel A, Vogel H, et al: Progressive polyradiculopathy in acquired immune deficiency syndrome. *Neurology* 36:912, 1986.

Ellie E, Rozenberg F, Dousset V, Beylot-Barry M. Herpes simplex virus type 2 ascending myeloradiculitis: MRI findings and rapid diagnosis by the polymerase chain method. *J Neurol Neurosurg Psychiatry* 57: 869,1994.

Enders JF, Weller TH, Robbins FC: Cultivation of Lansing strain of poliomyelitis virus in cultures of various human embryonic tissues. *Science* 109:85, 1949.

Epstein LG, Sharer LR, Choe S, et al: HTLV-III/LAV-like retrovirus particles in the brains of patients with AIDS encephalopathy. *AIDS Res* 1:447, 1985.

Esiri MM: Herpes simplex encephalitis: An immunohistological study of the distribution of viral antigen within the brain. *J Neurol Sci* 54:209, 1982.

Fauci AS, Lane HC: Human immunodeficiency virus (HIV) disease: AIDS and related disorders, in Fauci A, Braunwald E, Kasper D, et al (eds): *Harrison's Principles of Internal Medicine*, 17th ed. New York, McGraw-Hill, 2008, pp 1137–1204.

Fishbein DB, Robinson LE: Rabies. *N Engl J Med* 329:1632, 1993.

Gajdusek DC, Gibbs CJ Jr, Alpers M: Experimental transmission of a kuru-like syndrome to chimpanzees. *Nature* 209:794, 1966.

Gallo RC, Salahuddin SZ, Popovic M, et al: Frequent detection and isolation of cytopathic retroviruses (HTLV-III) from patients with AIDS and at risk for AIDS. *Science* 224:500, 1984.

Gessain A, Barin F, Vernant JC, et al: Antibodies to human T-lymphotropic virus type-I in patients with tropical spastic paraparesis. *Lancet* 2:407, 1985.

Gibbs CJ Jr, Gajdusek DC, Asher DM, Alpers MP: Creutzfeldt-Jakob disease (spongiform encephalopathy): Transmission to the chimpanzee. *Science* 161:388, 1968.

Gibbs CJ, Joy A, Heffner R, et al: Clinical and pathological features and laboratory confirmation of Creutzfeldt-Jakob disease in a recipient of pituitary derived growth hormone. *N Engl J Med* 313:734, 1985.

Gilden DH, Beinlich BR, Rubinstein EM, et al: Varicella-zoster virus myelitis: An expanding spectrum. *Neurology* 44:1818, 1994.

Gilden DH, Klein Schmidt-DeMasters BK, Laggard JS, et al: Neurologic complications of the reactivation of varicella-zoster virus. *N Engl J Med* 342:635, 2000.

Gilden DH, Lipton HL, Wolf JS, et al: Two patients with unusual forms of varicella-zoster virus vasculopathy. *N Engl J Med* 347:1500, 2002.

Gilden DH, Wright RR, Schneck SA, et al: Zoster sine herpete, a clinical variant. *Ann Neurol* 35:530, 1994.

Gomez-Aranda F, Cañadillas F, Martí-Massó JF, et al: Pseudomigraine with temporary neurological symptoms and lymphocytic pleocytosis: A report of 50 cases. *Brain* 120:1105, 1997.

Gorson KC, Ropper AH: Nonpoliovirus poliomyelitis simulating Guillain-Barré syndrome. *Arch Neurol* 58:1460, 2001.

Haanpää M, Dastidar P, Weinberg A, et al: CSF and MRI findings in patients with acute herpes zoster. *Neurology* 51:1405, 1998.

Hadlow WJ: Scrapie and kuru. *Lancet* 2:289, 1959.

Heidenhain A: Klinische und anatomische Untersuchungen uber eine eigenartige organische Erkrankung des Zentralnervensystems im Praesenium. *Z Gesamte Neurol Psychiatry* 118:49, 1929.

Henson RA, Urich H: *Cancer and the Nervous System*. Oxford, Blackwell Scientific, 1982, pp 319–322.

Hill AF, Butterworth J, Joiner S, et al: Investigation of variant Creutzfeldt-Jakob disease and other human prion diseases with tonsil biopsy samples. *Lancet* 353:183, 1999.

Hilt DC, Buchholz D, Krumholz A, et al: Herpes zoster ophthalmicus and delayed contralateral hemiparesis caused by cerebral angiitis: Diagnosis and management approaches. *Ann Neurol* 14:543, 1983.

Holland NR, Power C, Mathews VP, et al: Cytomegalovirus encephalitis in acquired immunodeficiency syndrome (AIDS). *Neurology* 44:507, 1994.

Hope-Simpson RE: The nature of herpes zoster: A long-term study and a new hypothesis. *Proc R Soc Med* 58:9, 1965.

Howard RS, Lees AJ: Encephalitis lethargica: A report of four cases. *Brain* 110:19, 1987.

Hsich G, Kenney K, Gibbs CJ, et al: The 14-3-3 brain protein in cerebrospinal fluid as a marker for transmissible spongiform encephalopathies. *N Engl J Med* 335:924, 1996.

Huang CC, Liu CC, Chang YC, et al: Neurologic complications in children with enterovirus 71 infection. *N Engl J Med* 341:936, 1999.

Hugler P, Siebrecht P, Hoffman K, et al: Prevention of postherpetic neuralgia with use of varicella-zoster hyperimmune globulin. *Eur J Pain* 6:435, 2002.

Jeffery KJ, Read SJ, Petro TE, et al: Diagnosis of viral infections of the central nervous system: Clinical interpretation of PCR results. *Lancet* 349:313, 1997.

Jeha LE, Sila CA, Lederman RJ, et al: West Nile virus infection. A new acute paralytic illness. *Neurology* 61:55, 2003.

Jemsek J, Greenberg SB, Taber L, et al: Herpes zoster associated encephalitis: Clinicopathologic report of 12 cases and review of the literature. *Medicine (Baltimore)* 62:81, 1983.

Johnson RT: Arboviral encephalitis, in Warren KS, Mahmoud AAF (eds): *Tropical and Geographical Medicine*. New York, McGraw-Hill, 1990, pp 691–699.

Johnson RT: Selective vulnerability of neural cells to viral infections. *Brain* 103:447, 1980.

Johnson RT: *Viral Infections of the Nervous System*, 2nd ed. Philadelphia, Lippincott-Raven, 1998.

Kalayjian RC, Coehn ML, Bonomo RA, et al: Cytomegalovirus ventriculoencephalitis in AIDS: A syndrome with distinct clinical and pathological features. *Medicine (Baltimore)* 72:67, 1993.

King RB: Concerning the management of pain associated with herpes zoster and of post-herpetic neuralgia. *Pain* 33:73, 1988.

Kupila L, Vuorinen T, Vanjonpää R, et al: Etiology of aseptic meningitis and encephalitis in adult population. *Neurology* 66:75, 2006.

Lakeman FD, Whitley RJ: Diagnosis of herpes simplex encephalitis: Application of polymerase chain reaction to cerebrospinal fluid from brain-biopsied patients and correlation with disease. *J Infect Dis* 171:857, 1995.

Lehky TJ, Flerlage N, Katz D, et al: Human T-cell lymphotropic virus type II-associated myelopathy: Clinical and immunologic profiles. *Ann Neurol* 40: 714, 1996.

Linnemann CC Jr, Alvira MM: Pathogenesis of varicella-zoster angiitis in the CNS. *Arch Neurol* 37:239, 1980.

Mahalingam R, Wellis M, Wolf W, et al: Latent varicella-zoster viral DNA in human trigeminal and thoracic ganglia. *N Engl J Med* 323:627, 1990.

Mangi H, Miller RC: Progressive multifocal leukoencephalopathy: Progress in the AIDS era. *J Neurol Neurosurg Psychiatry* 69:569, 2000.

Masters CL, Gajdusek DC, Gibbs CJ Jr: Creutzfeldt-Jakob disease virus isolations from the Gerstmann-Sträussler syndrome. *Brain* 104:559, 1981.

Masters CL, Harris JO, Gajdusek C, et al: Creutzfeldt-Jakob disease: Patterns of worldwide occurrence and the significance of familial and sporadic clustering. *Ann Neurol* 5:177, 1979.

Matsusue E, Kinoshita T, Sugihara S, et al: White matter lesions in panencephalopathic type of Creutzfeldt-Jakob disease: MR imaging and pathologic correlation. *AJNR Am J Neuroradiol* 25:910, 2004.

Marra CM: Update on neurosyphilis. *Curr Infect Dis Rep.* 11:127-34. 2009.

Mayo DR, Booss J: Varicella zoster-associated neurologic disease without skin lesions. *Arch Neurol* 46:313, 1989.

McJunkin JE, De los Reyes E, Irazuzta JE, et al: La Crosse encephalitis in children. *N Engl J Med* 344:801, 2001.

McKendrick MW, McGill JI, White JE, Wood MJ: Oral acyclovir in acute herpes zoster. *Br Med J* 293:1529, 1986.

McKendrick MW, McGill JI, Wood MJ: Lack of effect of acyclovir on postherpetic neuralgia. *BMJ* 298:431, 1989.

Medori R, Tritschler HJ, LeBlanc A, et al: Fatal familial insomnia: A prion disease with a mutation at codon 178 of the prion protein gene. *N Engl J Med* 326:444, 1992.

Mehta PD, Patrick BA, Thormar H: Identification of virus-specific oligoclonal bands in subacute sclerosing panencephalitis by immunofixation after isoelectric focusing and peroxidase staining. *J Clin Microbiol* 16:985, 1982.

Murakami S, Mizobuchi M, Nakashiro Y, et al: Bell's palsy and herpes simplex virus: Identification of viral DNA in endoneural fluid and muscle. *Ann Intern Med* 124:27, 1996.

Nagel MA, Bennett JL, Khmeleva N, et al: Multifocal VZV vasculopathy with temporal artery infection mimics giant cell arteritis. *Neurology* 80:2017, 2013.

Nagel MA, Forghani B, Mahalingam R, et al: The value of detecting anti-VZV IgG antibody in CSF to diagnose V2V vasculopathy. *Neurology* 68:1069, 2007.

Navia BA, Chos E-S, Petito CK, et al: The AIDS dementia complex: II. Neuropathology. *Ann Neurol* 19:525, 1986.

Navia BA, Jordan BD, Price RW: The AIDS dementia complex: I. Clinical features. *Ann Neurol* 19:517, 1986.

Navia BA, Petito CK, Gold JWM, et al: Cerebral toxoplasmosis complicating the acquired immune deficiency syndrome: Clinical and neuropathological findings in 27 patients. *Ann Neurol* 19:224, 1986.

Navia BA, Price RW: The acquired immunodeficiency syndrome dementia complex as the presenting or sole manifestation of human immunodeficiency virus infection. *Arch Neurol* 44:65, 1987.

Oxman MN, Levin MJ, Johnson GR, et al: A vaccine to prevent herpes zoster and postherpetic neuralgia in older adults. *N Engl J Med* 352:2271, 2005.

Padgett BL, Walker DL, ZuRhein GM, Eckroade RJ: Cultivation of papova-like virus from human brain with progressive multifocal leukoencephalopathy. *Lancet* 1:1257, 1971.

Parchi P, Giese A, Capellari S, et al: Classification of sporadic Creutzfeldt-Jakob disease based on molecular and phenotypic analysis of 300 subjects. *Ann Neurol* 46:224, 1999.

Peterslund NA: Herpes zoster associated encephalitis: Clinical findings and acyclovir treatment. *Scand J Infect Dis* 20:583, 1988.

Petito CK, Navia BA, Cho E-S, et al: Vacuolar myelopathy pathologically resembling subacute combined degeneration in patients with acquired immunodeficiency syndrome (AIDS). *N Engl J Med* 312:874, 1985.

Ponka A, Pettersson T: The incidence and aetiology of central nervous system infections in Helsinki in 1980. *Acta Neurol Scand* 66:529, 1982.

Pope AS, Feemster RF, Rosengard DE, et al: Evaluation of poliomyelitis vaccination in Massachusetts. *N Engl J Med* 254:110, 1956.

Prashanth LK, Taly AB, Ravi V, et al: Adult onset subacute sclerosing panencephalitis: Clinical profile of 39 patients from a tertiary care centre. *J Neurol Neurosurg Psychiatry* 77:630, 2006.

Price RW: Neurological complications of HIV infection. *Lancet* 348:445, 1996.

Prusiner SB: Genetic and infectious prion disease. *Arch Neurol* 50:1129, 1993.

Prusiner SB: Prion diseases and the BSE crisis. *Science* 278:245, 1997.

Prusiner SB: Shattuck Lecture—neurodegenerative diseases and prions. *N Engl J Med* 344:1516, 2001.

Prusiner SB, Hsiao KK: Human prion disease. *Ann Neurol* 35:385, 1994.

Rentier B: Second International Conference on the varicella-zoster virus. *Neurology* 45(Suppl 8):S18, 1995.

Report of the Guidelines Development Committee of the American Academy of Neurology: Evidence-based guideline: Diagnostic accuracy of CSF 14-3-3 protein in sporadic Creutzfeldt-Jakob disease. *Neurology* 79:1499, 2012.

Richardson EP Jr: Progressive multifocal leukoencephalopathy. *N Engl J Med* 265:815, 1961.

Rodgers-Johnson PE: Tropical spastic paraparesis HTLV-1 associated myelopathy: Etiology and clinical spectrum. *Mol Neurobiol* 8:175, 1994.

Roman GC, Osame M: Identity of HTLV-I associated tropical spastic paraparesis and HTLV-I associated myelopathy. *Lancet* 1:651, 1988.

Rosenblum ML, Levy RM, Bredesen DE (eds): *AIDS and the Nervous System*. New York, Raven Press, 1988.

Rowley AH, Whitley RJ, Lakeman FD, Wolinsky SM: Rapid detection of herpes-simplex-virus DNA in cerebrospinal fluid of patients with herpes simplex encephalitis. *Lancet* 335:440, 1990.

Rubin RH, Young LS: *Clinical Approach to Infection in the Compromised Host*, 4th ed. New York, Kluwer Academic, 2002.

Schwab S, Jünger E, Spranger M, et al: Craniectomy: An aggressive treatment approach in severe encephalitis. *Neurology* 48:413, 1997.

Seeley WW, Marty FM, Holmes TM, et al: Post-transplant acute limbic encephalitis. Clinical features and relationship to HHV-6. *Neurology* 69:156, 2007.

Seipelt M, Zerr I, Nau R, et al: Hashimoto's encephalitis as a differential diagnosis of Creutzfeldt-Jakob disease. *J Neurol Neurosurg Psychiatry* 66:172, 1999.

Selby G, Walker GL: Cerebral arteritis in cat-scratch fever. *Neurology* 29:1413, 1979.

Sever JL: Persistent measles infection in the central nervous system. *Rev Infect Dis* 5:467, 1983.

Shiga Y, Miyazawa K, Sato S, et al: Diffusion-weighted MRI abnormalities as an early diagnostic marker for Creutzfeldt-Jakob disease. *Neurology* 63:443, 2004.

Sigurdsson B: Rida: A chronic encephalitis of sheep, with general remarks on infections which develop slowly and some of their special characteristics. *Br Vet J* 110:341, 1954.

Simpson DM, Bender AN: HTLV-III associated myopathy (abstr). *Neurology* 37(Suppl):319, 1987.

Sköldenberg B, Forsgren M, Alestig K, et al: Acyclovir versus vidarabine in herpes simplex encephalitis: Randomised multicentre study in consecutive Swedish patients. *Lancet* 2:707, 1984.

Smith JE, Aksamit AJ: Outcome of chronic idiopathic meningitis. *Mayo Clin Proc* 69:548, 1994.

Solomon J, Dung NM, Kneen R, et al: Japanese encephalitis. *J Neurol Neurosurg Psychiatry* 68:405, 2000.

Solomon T: Flavivirus encephalitis. *N Engl J Med* 351:370, 2004.

Steel JG, Dix RD, Baringer JR: Isolation of herpes simplex virus type I in recurrent Mollaret meningitis. *Ann Neurol* 11:17, 1982.

Tavakoli NP, Wang HW, Dupuis M, et al: Fatal case of deer tick encephalitis. *N Engl J Med* 360:2099, 2009.

Tiége XD, Rozenberg F, Des Portes V, et al: Herpes simplex encephalitis relapses in children. Differentiation of two neurologic entities. *Neurology* 61:241, 2003.

Towsend JJ, Baringer JR, Wolinsky JS, et al: Progressive rubella panencephalitis: Late onset after congenital rubella. *N Engl J Med* 292:990, 1975.

Tschampa HJ, Herms JW, Scholz-Schaffer WJ, et al: Clinical findings in sporadic Creutzfeldt-Jacob disease correlate with thalamic pathology. *Brain* 125:2558, 2002.

Twyman RE, Gahring LC, Spiess J, Rogers SW: Glutamate receptor antibodies activate a subset of receptors and reveal agonist binding sites. *Neuron* 14:755, 1995.

van Wijck AJM, Opstelten W, Moons KG, et al: The PINE study of epidural steroids and local anesthetics to prevent postherpetic neuralgia. *Lancet* 367:219, 2006.

von Economo C: *Encephalitis Lethargica*. New York, Oxford University Press, 1931.

Wadia NH, Katrak SM, Misra VP, et al: Polio-like motor paralysis associated with acute hemorrhagic conjunctivitis in an outbreak in 1981 in Bombay, India: Clinical and serologic studies. *J Infect Dis* 147:660, 1983.

Weil ML, Itabashi HH, Cremer NE, et al: Chronic progressive panencephalitis due to rubella virus simulating subacute sclerosing panencephalitis. *N Engl J Med* 292:994, 1975.

Weiss S, Guberman A: Acute cerebellar ataxia in infectious disease, in Vinken PJ, Bruyn GW (eds): *Handbook of Clinical Neurology*. Vol 34. Amsterdam, North-Holland, 1978, pp 619–639.

Weller TH, Witton HM, Bell EJ: Etiologic agents of varicella and herpes zoster. *J Exp Med* 108:843, 1958.

Whitley RJ: The frustrations of treating herpes simplex virus infections of the central nervous system. *JAMA* 259:1067, 1988.

Whitley RJ: Viral encephalitis. *N Engl J Med* 323:242, 1990.

Whitley RJ, Alford CA, Hirsch MS, et al: Vidarabine versus acyclovir therapy in herpes simplex encephalitis. *N Engl J Med* 314:144, 1986.

Will RG, Zerdler M, Stewart GE, et al: Diagnosis of new variant Creutzfeldt-Jakob disease. *Ann Neurol* 47:575, 2000.

Willoughby RE, Tieves KS, Hoffman GH, et al: Survival after treatment of rabies with induction of coma. *N Engl J Med* 352:2508, 2005.

Wolinsky JS: Progressive rubella panencephalitis, in Vinken PJ, Bruyn GW (eds): *Handbook of Clinical Neurology*. Vol 34. Amsterdam, North-Holland, 1978, pp 331–342.

Wolinsky JS, Swoveland P, Johnson KP, Baringer JR: Subacute measles encephalitis complicating Hodgkin's disease in an adult. *Ann Neurol* 1:452, 1977.

Wulff EA, Simpson DM: Neuromuscular complications of the human immunodeficiency virus type 1 infection. *Semin Neurol* 19:157, 1999.

Zanusso G, Ferrari S, Cardone F, et al: Detection of pathologic prion protein in the olfactory epithelium in sporadic Creutzfeldt-Jakob disease. *N Engl J Med* 348:711, 2003.

Zeidler M, Stewart GE, Barraclough CR, et al: New variant Creutzfeldt-Jakob disease: Neurological features and diagnostic tests. *Lancet* 350:903, 1997.

Zerr I, Bodemer M, Otto M, et al: Diagnosis of Creutzfeldt-Jakob disease by two-dimensional gel electrophoresis of cerebrospinal fluid. *Lancet* 348:846, 1996.

ZuRein GM, Chou SM: Particles resembling papova-viruses in human cerebral demyelinative disease. *Science* 148:1477, 1965.

34

Cerebrovascular Diseases

Among all the neurologic diseases of adult life, stroke ranks first in frequency and importance. The common mode of expression of *stroke* is a relatively sudden occurrence of a focal neurologic deficit. Strokes are broadly categorized as ischemic or hemorrhagic. *Ischemic stroke* is due to occlusion of a cerebral blood vessel and causes cerebral infarction. The resultant neurologic syndrome corresponds to a portion of the brain that is supplied by one or more cerebral vessels. Knowledge of the stroke syndromes, the signs and symptoms that correspond to the region of brain that is supplied by each vessel, allows a degree of precision in determining the particular vessel that is occluded and from the temporal evolution of the syndrome, the underlying cause of vascular occlusion can be deduced.

Ischemic strokes are classified by the underlying cause of the vascular occlusion. One of three main processes is usually operative: (i) atherosclerosis with superimposed thrombosis affecting large cerebral or extracerebral blood vessels, (ii) cerebral embolism, and (iii) occlusion of small cerebral vessels within the parenchyma of the brain. There are many other pathologic processes that lead to ischemic brain damage, not all associated with occlusion of cerebral vessels, including arterial dissection, inflammatory conditions such as vasculitis, thrombosis of cerebral veins and dural sinuses, in situ thrombosis of large or small cerebral vessels due to hypercoagulable conditions, vasospasm from any of several mechanisms, unusual types of embolic materials such as fat, tumor, cholesterol, and several unique diseases that involve the cerebral vasculature (see further on). Closely allied with ischemic strokes is the transient ischemic attack (TIA), a temporary neurologic deficit caused by a cerebrovascular disease that leaves no clinical or imaging trace. The causes of stroke are so numerous that the listing given in Table 34-1 offers only a guide to the remainder of this chapter. As helpful is knowledge of the major causes of stroke by each epoch of age, particularly in childhood and young adults, a subject taken up in a later section and summarized in Table 34-2.

The second broad category consists of *hemorrhage, which* occurs either within the substance of the brain, intracerebral hemorrhage, or contained within the subarachnoid spaces and ventricular system, subarachnoid hemorrhage. The causes of the first category are numerous and include chronic hypertension, coagulopathies that arise endogenously or as a result of anticoagulant medications, vascular malformations of the brain, cranial trauma, and hemorrhage that occurs within the area of an ischemic stroke. Subarachnoid hemorrhage has fewer fundamental causes, the most common being the rupture of a developmental aneurysm arising from the vessels of the circle of Willis, but also includes cerebral trauma and arteriovenous malformations, and rarer processes.

THE CLINICAL STROKE SYNDROME

There are all gradations of severity, but in all forms of stroke the essential feature is abruptness with which the neurologic deficit develops—usually a matter of seconds that stamps the disorder as vascular. In its most severe form, the patient with a stroke becomes hemiplegic or even comatose—an event so dramatic that it had in the past been given vivid designations: *apoplexy, cerebrovascular accident (CVA)*, or shock (colloquial). However, *stroke* is the preferred term.

In its mildest form, a stroke may consist of a trivial and transient neurologic disorder insufficient for the patient even to seek medical attention. Most embolic strokes occur suddenly and the deficit reaches its peak almost at once. Thrombotic strokes tend to evolve somewhat more slowly over a period of minutes or hours and occasionally days; in the latter case, the stroke usually progresses in a saltatory fashion, i.e., in a series of steps rather than smoothly. In cerebral hemorrhage, also abrupt in onset, the deficit may be virtually static or steadily progressive over a period of minutes or hours, while subarachnoid hemorrhage is almost instantaneous. It follows that gradual downhill course over a period of several days or weeks will usually be traced to a nonvascular disease. There are, however, many exceptions, such as the additive effects of multiple vascular occlusions and the progression that is caused by secondary brain edema surrounding large infarctions and cerebral hemorrhages. At the other extreme is rapid regression of a focal stroke syndrome that reverses itself entirely and dramatically over a period of minutes or up to an hour; this defines the TIA.

The second essential feature of stroke is its focal signature. The neurologic deficit reflects both the location

Table 34-1

CAUSES OF ISCHEMIC AND HEMORRHAGIC STROKE

1. Atherosclerotic thrombosis
2. Transient ischemic attacks
3. Embolism
4. Hypertensive hemorrhage
5. Ruptured or unruptured saccular aneurysm or arteriovenous malformation
6. Arteritis
   a. Meningovascular syphilis, arteritis secondary to pyogenic and tuberculous meningitis, rare infective types (typhus, schistosomiasis, malaria, mucormycosis, etc.)
   b. Autoimmune vasculopathies (polyarteritis nodosa, lupus erythematosus), necrotizing arteritis. Wegener arteritis, temporal arteritis, Takayasu disease, granulomatous or giant cell arteritis of the aorta, and giant cell granulomatous angiitis of cerebral arteries
7. Cerebral thrombophlebitis: secondary to infection of ear, paranasal sinus, face, etc.; with meningitis and subdural empyema; debilitating states, postpartum, postoperative, cardiac failure, hematologic disease (polycythemia, sickle cell disease), and of undetermined cause
8. Hematologic disorders: anticoagulants and thrombolytics, clotting factor disorders, polycythemia, sickle cell disease, thrombotic thrombocytopenic purpura, thrombocytosis, intravascular lymphoma, etc.
9. Trauma and dissection of carotid and basilar arteries
10. Amyloid angiopathy
11. Dissecting aortic aneurysm
12. Complications of arteriography
13. Complex migraine with persistent deficit
14. With tentorial, foramen magnum, and subfalcial herniations
15. Miscellaneous types: fibromuscular dysplasia, with local dissection of carotid, middle cerebral, or vertebrobasilar artery, x-irradiation, unexplained middle cerebral infarction in closed head injury, pressure of unruptured saccular aneurysm, complication of oral contraceptives, moyamoya disease
16. Genetic causes in children and young adults and others

and the size of the infarct or hemorrhage. Hemiplegia stands as the most typical sign of cerebrovascular diseases, whether in the cerebral hemisphere or brainstem, but there are many other manifestations, occurring in recognizable combinations. These include paralysis, numbness, and sensory deficits of many types on one side of the body, aphasia, visual field defects, diplopia, dizziness, dysarthria, and so forth. The neurovascular syndromes enable the physician to localize the lesion—sometimes so precisely that even the affected arterial branch can be specified—and to indicate whether the lesion is an infarct or a hemorrhage. These syndromes are described in the sections that follow. This group of diseases has also provided the most instructive approach to localization in neurology. As our colleague C.M. Fisher aptly remarked, neurology is learned "stroke by stroke." Also, the focal ischemic lesion has divulged some of our most important ideas about the function of the human brain.

The analysis of a stroke involves several steps. First, the clinician must determine whether the event is a stroke rather than some other process that may have a similar sudden onset, such as migraine, seizure, or syncope. Second, if the event is considered likely to be a stroke or TIA, then the pathophysiology must be ascertained (e.g., cerebral embolism from the heart or a proximal artery, large vessel atherothrombotic occlusion, venous occlusive disease). Third, acute treatment (e.g., tissue plasminogen activator) is initiated, if appropriate. Fourth, a plan for the prevention of future strokes is undertaken.

Table 34-2

CEREBROVASCULAR DISEASES CHARACTERISTIC OF EACH AGE PERIOD

1. Prenatal circulatory diseases leading to
   a. Porencephaly
   b. Hydranencephaly
   c. Hypoxic-ischemic damage
   d. Unilateral cerebral infarction
2. Perinatal and postnatal circulatory disorders resulting in
   a. Cardiorespiratory failure and generalized ischemia—*état marbre*
   b. Periventricular infarcts
   c. Matrix hemorrhages and ischemic foci in premature infants
   d. Hemorrhagic disease of the newborn
3. Infancy and childhood: vascular diseases associated with
   a. Ischemic infarction
   b. Congenital heart disease and paradoxical embolism
   c. Moyamoya disease
   d. Bacterial endocarditis, rheumatic fever, lupus erythematosus
   e. Sickle cell anemia
   f. Mitochondrial disorders (MELAS)
   g. Homocystinuria and Fabry angiokeratosis
4. Adolescence and early adult life: vascular occlusion or hemorrhage with
   a. Pregnancy and puerperium
   b. Estrogen-related stroke
   c. Migraine
   d. Vascular malformations
   e. Premature atherosclerosis
   f. Arteritis
   g. Valvular heart disease
   h. Sickle cell anemia
   i. Antiphospholipid arteriopathy, plasma C-protein deficiency, and other coagulopathies
   j. Moyamoya, Takayasu diseases
   k. Arterial dissections
   l. Amyloid angiopathy
5. Middle age
   a. Atherosclerotic thrombosis and embolism
   b. Cardiogenic embolism
   c. Primary (hypertensive) cerebral hemorrhage
   d. Ruptured saccular aneurysm
   e. Arterial dissection
   f. Fibromuscular dysplasia
6. Late adult life
   a. Atherosclerotic thrombotic occlusive disease
   b. Embolic disease
   c. Lacunar stroke
   d. Brain hemorrhage (multiple causes)
   e. Multiinfarct dementia
   f. Binswanger disease

MELAS, mitochondrial encephalomyopathy, lactic acidosis, and stroke.
Source: Reproduced by permission from Salam-Adams and Adams.

In the last decades, extraordinary imaging technology has been introduced that allow the physician to make physiologic distinctions among normal, ischemic, and infarcted brain tissue. This approach to stroke will likely guide the next generation of treatments and has already had a pronounced impact on the direction of research in the field. Salvageable brain tissue in the acute phase of stroke can be delineated by these methods. To identify such ischemic but not yet infarcted tissue is a major goal of modern acute stroke medicine. In particular, diffusion-weighted magnetic resonance imaging has already altered the understanding and management of stroke patients.

The introduction of effective treatments for acute stroke has led to greater dependence on these sophisticated imaging techniques, but the authors believe it remains essential for the neurologist to understand the details of the cerebral vascular anatomy and the corresponding stroke syndromes for several reasons. Imaging techniques, though increasingly accurate, are not perfect. In cases in which the imaging does not reveal a stroke, the clinician remains dependent on careful history and neurologic examination. Furthermore, in many parts of the world, imaging techniques are unavailable at the pace necessary to initiate acute treatment. Finally, understanding the detailed anatomy helps the neurologist understand how the nervous system functions, lessons which are applicable to many other categories of illness other than stroke.

Despite these valuable imaging and therapeutic advances in stroke neurology, three points should be made. First, all physicians have a role to play in the prevention of stroke by encouraging the reduction of risk factors, such as hypertension, smoking, and hyperlipidemia and the identification of signs of potential impending stroke, such as transient ischemic attacks, atrial fibrillation, and carotid artery stenosis. Second, careful clinical evaluation integrated with the newer testing methods still provides the most powerful approach to this category of disease. Finally, there has been a departure from the methodical clinicopathologic studies that have been the foundation of our understanding of cerebrovascular disease. Increasingly, randomized trials involving several hundred and even thousands of patients and conducted simultaneously in dozens of institutions have come to dominate investigative activity in this field. These multicenter trials have yielded highly valuable information about the treatment of a variety of cerebrovascular disorders, both symptomatic and asymptomatic. However, this approach suffers from a number of inherent limitations, the most important of which is that the homogenized data derived from an aggregate of patients is difficult to apply to a specific case at hand or the data is not available to resolve each patient's particular problem. Most large studies show only modest or marginal differences between treated and control groups and correspondingly give guidance in large populations. These multicenter studies will be critically appraised at appropriate points in the ensuing discussion.

Differentiation of Stroke from Other Neurologic Illnesses

The diagnosis of a vascular lesion therefore rests essentially on recognition of the stroke syndrome; without evidence of this, the diagnosis must always be in doubt. The three criteria by which the stroke is identified should be reemphasized: (1) the temporal profile of the clinical syndrome, (2) evidence of focal brain disease, and (3) the clinical setting. Definition of the temporal profile requires a clear history of the premonitory phenomena, the mode of onset, and the evolution of the neurologic disturbance in relation to the patient's medical status. Here, an inadequate history is the most frequent cause of diagnostic error. If these data are lacking, the stroke profile may still be determined by extending the period of observation for a few days or weeks, thus invoking the clinical rule that the physician's best diagnostic tool is a second and third examination. The first distinction is to separate ischemic from hemorrhagic stroke; features that are characteristic of the latter such as headache and vomiting at the onset, rapid progression to coma, and sever hypertension are emphasized in the later section on cerebral hemorrhage. Often, however, the distinction is not so clear because sudden onset of a focal neurologic problem is the core syndrome of both processes.

There are few categories of neurologic disease whose temporal profile mimics that of the cerebrovascular disorders. Migraine may do so, but the history usually provides the diagnosis. A seizure may be followed by a prolonged focal deficit (Todd paralysis) but is rarely the initial event in a stroke; the setting in which these symptoms occur and their subsequent course clarify the clinical situation. Tumor, infection, inflammation, degeneration, and nutritional deficiency are unlikely to manifest themselves precipitously, although rarely a primary or metastatic brain tumor produces a focal deficit of abrupt onset (see later). Trauma, of course, occurs abruptly but usually offers no problem in diagnosis. In multiple sclerosis and other demyelinative diseases, there may be an abrupt onset or exacerbation of symptoms, but for the most part they occur in a different age group and clinical setting. Conversely, a stroke-like onset of cerebral symptoms in a young adult should always raise a suspicion of demyelinative disease. A stroke developing over a period of several days usually progresses in a stepwise fashion, increments of deficit being added abruptly from time to time. A slow, gradual, downhill course over a period of 2 weeks or more indicates that the lesion is probably not vascular but rather neoplastic, demyelinative, infectious (abscess) or granulomatous, or a subdural hematoma.

In regard to the *focal neurologic deficits* of cerebrovascular disease, many of the nonvascular diseases may produce symptoms that are much the same, and the diagnosis cannot rest solely on this aspect of the clinical picture. Nonetheless, specific patterns of neurologic signs are so highly characteristic of vascular occlusion—e.g., the lateral medullary syndrome—that they mark the disease as a stroke. Conversely, certain disturbances are hardly ever attributable to ischemic stroke—e.g., diabetes insipidus, fever, bitemporal hemianopia, parkinsonism, generalized myoclonus, repeated falls, and isolated cranial-nerve palsies—and their presence may be of help in excluding vascular disease. Finally, the diagnosis of cerebrovascular disease should always be made on positive data, not by exclusion.

A few conditions are so often confused with cerebrovascular diseases that they merit further comment. Miscellaneous conditions occasionally taken to be a stroke are migraine; Bell's palsy; Stokes-Adams syncopal attacks; a severe attack of labyrinthine vertigo; diabetic ophthalmoplegia; acute ulnar, radial, or peroneal palsy; embolism to a limb; and temporal arteritis associated with blindness all of which are discussed in later parts of this chapter.

A brain tumor, especially a rapidly growing glioblastoma or lymphoma, may produce a severe hemiplegia rapidly. Also, the neurologic deficit caused by cancer metastatic to the cerebrum may evolve rapidly, almost at a stroke-like pace. Moreover, in rare cases of brain tumor, a hemiplegia may be preceded by transitory episodes of neurologic deficit, indistinguishable from TIAs. The presence of the tumor and its effects on the cerebrum may make it difficult for the patient to articulate a clear history. A lack of detailed history may also be responsible for the opposite diagnostic error, i.e., mistaking a relatively slowly evolving stroke (usually caused by internal carotid artery or basilar occlusion) for a tumor. CT and MRI usually settle the problem. A brain abscess or inflammatory necrotic lesion—e.g., herpes encephalitis or toxoplasmosis—may also develop rapidly.

Contrariwise, certain manifestations of stroke may be incorrectly interpreted as evidence of some other neurologic disorder. *Headache*, at times severe, often occurs as a prodrome of a thrombotic stroke or subarachnoid hemorrhage; unless this is appreciated, a diagnosis of migraine may be made. *Dizzy spells, vertigo, vomiting, or brief intermittent lapses of equilibrium* as a result of vascular disease of the brainstem may be ascribed to vestibular neuritis, Ménière disease, Stokes-Adams syncope, or gastroenteritis. A detailed account of the attack will usually avert this error. A strikingly focal monoplegia of cerebral origin, causing only weakness of the hand or arm or foot-drop, is not infrequently misdiagnosed as a peripheral neuropathy or plexopathy.

Epidemiology of Cerebrovascular Diseases

Stroke, after heart disease and cancer, is the third most common cause of death in the United States. Every year there are in the United States approximately 700,000 cases of stroke—roughly 600,000 ischemic lesions and 100,000 hemorrhages, intracerebral or subarachnoid—with 175,000 fatalities from these causes combined. Since 1950, coincident with the introduction of effective treatment for hypertension, there has been a substantial reduction in the frequency of stroke. Both sexes have shared in the reduced incidence. During this period, the incidence of coronary artery disease and uncontrolled hypertension also fell significantly. By contrast, there has been no change in the frequency of aneurysmal rupture. In the last two decades, according to the American Heart Association, the mortality rate from stroke has declined by 12 percent, but the total number of strokes may again be rising. Stroke assumes importance both because of its high rate of mortality and the residual disability that it causes.

The burden of stroke has far wider implications when viewed from an international perspective. Cerebrovascular disease is estimated to account for 7.8 million deaths yearly throughout the world and represents about 13 percent of all causes of death. In developed countries, stroke mortality is only surpassed by cardiac ischemic diseases and close to equivalent to the cancers collectively (mainly lung cancer) in the most recent Global Burden of Disease study undertaken in 2004. Stroke remains among the five leading causes of death across every income group in most countries in the last comprehensive review by the World Health Organization in 2004. They cause significant physical, emotional, and cognitive disabilities among survivors, accounting for 3.6 percent of the total disability-adjusted life years (DALYs) and thus placing stroke within the 10 leading causes of disability irrespective of the development status of countries (see http://www.who.int/healthinfo/global_burden_disease/GBD_report_2004update_part2.pdf).

Risk Factors for Stroke

This is an area of major public health importance in that several modifiable factors are known to increase the liability to stroke. The most important of these are hypertension, atrial fibrillation, diabetes mellitus, cigarette smoking, and hyperlipidemia. Others, such as systemic diseases associated with a hypercoagulable state and the use of contraceptives, also contribute, but only in special circumstances. Hypertension is also the most readily recognized factor in the genesis of primary intracerebral hemorrhage. It appears that the stroke-producing potential of hypertension is as much the product of heightened systolic pressure, as of diastolic pressure (Rabkin et al). The cooperative studies of the Veterans Administration (see Freis et al) and the report by Collins and associates (collating 14 randomized trials of antihypertensive drugs) convincingly demonstrated that the long-term control of hypertension decreased the incidence of both ischemic infarction and intracerebral hemorrhage. It has been found that simple measures such as the use of hydrochlorothiazide for blood pressure control may be, overall, the most effective. The presence of congestive heart failure and coronary atherosclerosis also increases the probability of stroke. As for embolic strokes, the most important risk factors are structural cardiac disease and arrhythmias, mostly atrial fibrillation, which increases the incidence of stroke about 6-fold, and by 18-fold if, as was common in the past, there is also rheumatic valvular disease.

Diabetes hastens the atherosclerotic process in both large and small arteries. Weinberger and colleagues and Roehmholdt and coworkers found diabetic patients to be twice as liable to stroke as age-matched nondiabetic groups. The importance of long-duration cigarette smoking in the development of carotid atherosclerosis has long been known and was quantitated by Ingall and colleagues. The interactions between diabetes and hypertension on the one hand, and intracerebral hemorrhage and atherothrombotic infarction on the other, as well as the association of cardiac disease and cerebral embolism, are considered further on in this chapter in relation to each of these categories of cerebrovascular disease. Numerous clinical trials have also shown a marked reduction in stroke incidence with the use of cholesterol-lowering drugs. As in the case of coronary artery disease, the level of low-density lipoprotein (LDL) cholesterol has the most impact on the incidence of stroke but elevated triglycerides may also confer risk. Subsidiary factors, such as low potassium intake and reduced serum levels of potassium, are associated with an increased stroke rate in several studies, including one in which we participated, but the mechanism of this effect is obscure (Green et al); a detrimental effect on blood pressure is possible. Public health measures designed to detect and reduce the aforementioned risk factors offer the most intelligent long-range approach to the prevention of cerebrovascular disease.

Finally, in keeping with the emerging field of genetic risk factors in human disease, several genetic loci have been found that putatively impart a risk of stroke in various populations. The largest of these, reported by Ikram and associates, has implicated a polymorphism on chromosome 12, encompassing several genes that have putative connections to vascular disease. However, other groups, such the International Stroke Genetics Consortium, were unable to confirm this. It seems likely that more refined definitions of stroke subtypes and careful genotyping of circumscribed populations will be necessary if genetic risk factors for stroke are to be be found that are not simply markers for vasculopathy, inducing diseases such as diabetes, hyperlipidemia, and hypertension.

The Major Causes of Cerebral Vascular Occlusion and Ischemic Stroke

Two causes of ischemic stroke stand out: atherosclerotic–thrombotic disease of the cerebral or extracerebral vessels, and cerebral embolism. An understanding of the biology of these two processes is essential for the analysis of the clinical, laboratory, and imaging features of stroke and its treatment. All other causes of vascular occlusion taken together, account for far fewer strokes. These are also important and they are accorded their own sections later in the chapter.

Atherothrombosis

The evolution of clinical phenomena in cerebral thrombosis, both of large intracranial (basilar, carotid) or extracranial (carotid, vertebral) and small vessels (lacunes), is more variable than that of embolism and hemorrhage. In approximately half of patients the stroke is preceded by minor signs or one or more transient attacks of focal neurologic dysfunction, TIAs, discussed further on. These transient *prodromal episodes* may herald the oncoming vascular event caused by atherothrombotic stroke. Occasionally embolism is preceded by a transient neurologic disorder but TIAs are generally considered as more closely aligned with atherothrombotic stroke.

The thrombotic stroke syndrome develops in one of several ways. There may be a single episode, but typically the whole stroke evolves over a few minutes or hours or less. Characteristic is a "stuttering" or intermittent progression of neurologic deficits extending over several hours or a day or longer. This is a starkly different profile from the abrupt onset of stroke that characterizes the embolic mechanism discussed further on. In thrombosis, a partial stroke may occur and even recede temporarily for several hours, after which there is rapid progression to the completed deficit—or several fleeting episodes may be followed by a longer one and, hours or a day or two later, by a major stroke. Several parts of the body may be affected at once or only one part, such as a limb or one side of the face, the other parts becoming involved serially in step-like fashion until the stroke is fully developed. Sometimes the deficit is episodic; spells of weakness or involuntary movement of a hand or arm or dimness of vision, lasting 5 to 10 min, occur spontaneously or are brought on by standing or walking. Each of the partial attacks may reproduce the profile of the stroke in miniature. In other words, the principle of intermittency seems to characterize the thrombotic process from beginning to end.

Also characteristic of atherothrombotic events in many, but not all cases, is the occurrence of the stroke during sleep; the patient awakens paralyzed, either during the night or in the morning. Unaware of any difficulty, he may arise and fall helplessly to the floor with the first step. This is the story given by half of our patients with thrombotic strokes, as well as by a smaller number with embolic strokes.

Most deceptive are the few instances, in which the neurologic disorder evolves very gradually, over several days or longer ("slow stroke"). One's first impulse is to make a diagnosis of brain tumor, abscess, or subdural hematoma. This error can usually be avoided by a careful analysis of the course of the illness, which will disclose an uneven, saltatory progression. There are also cases—and these are usually instances of pure motor hemiplegia—in which the evolution of a thrombotic stroke is evenly progressive over a period of days. It is likely also that the abrupt development of a thrombus on an atherosclerotic plaque in a distal cerebral vessel (beyond the circle of Willis) can also cause a fairly sudden or at least rapid evolution of stroke, but this is not characteristic.

Atheromatous plaques preferentially form at branching points and curves of the cerebral arteries. *The most frequent sites are* (1) in the *internal carotid artery* at its origin from the common carotid; (2) in the *cervical part of the vertebral arteries and at their junction to form the basilar artery*; (3) in the *stem or at the main bifurcation of the middle cerebral arteries*; (4) in the proximal *posterior cerebral arteries* as they wind around the midbrain; and (5) in the proximal *anterior cerebral arteries* as they pass anteriorly and curve over the corpus callosum. The last two sites are far less frequent than the first three. It is infrequent for the cerebral arteries to develop significant plaques beyond their first major branching after the circle of Willis. Also, it is unusual for the cerebellar and ophthalmic arteries to show atheromatous involvement. The common carotid and vertebral arteries at their origins from the aorta are additional frequent sites of atheromatous deposits, but because of abundant collateral arterial pathways, occlusions at these sites are less commonly associated with cerebral ischemia as discussed further on.

Atherothrombosis may cause cerebral infarction in several ways. The most obvious is that an occlusive plaque or a thrombus formed on a plaque occupies the lumen of a major intracerebral vessel, such as the middle cerebral artery, and stops flow to the areas of the brain supplied by the vessel. A variation of this mechanism is one of occlusion by atherosclerosis of a more proximal vessel, such as the distal carotid artery. This leads to infarction in the territory between major branches of the internal carotid circulation that are most susceptible to reduced blood flow—termed "watershed infarction." Or, an atherothrombotic lesion in a proximal vessel may serve as the nidus for the formation of an embolus that manifests itself as a stroke in one of the territories of that vessel—called "artery-to-artery" embolism. The essential issue here is that it is almost always severe stenosis of a proximal internal carotid artery that produces either ischemic or embolic stroke; milder degrees are usually not implicated. A separate mechanism pertains when an atherosclerotic plaque in a large vessel of the circle of Willis occludes the orifices of small penetrating vessels, most often the lenticulostriate branches of the middle cerebral artery or the thalamostriate vessels of the posterior cerebral artery, and cause small, or more confluent, strokes deep in the brain.

Whether plaque rupture plays a role in vessel occlusion or thrombus formation, as it does in the coronary artery, is not clear. In the carotid artery, Hosseini and coworkers found evidence of intraplaque hemorrhage using special MRI techniques and found these changes to be predictive of stroke in the distal distribution of the artery. Previous work by Fisher and Ojemann, cited in the references, involving the serial sectioning of carotid plaques removed at surgery, suggested otherwise. It is clear that the more severe the focal atheromata, the more likely a thrombotic complication will occur. Whether the complexity of a carotid artery plaque with ulcerations is an important component of stroke risk, for example, by originating small emboli, is not entirely settled. Again, it is the high degree of stenosis, usually above 90 percent of the original lumen compromised, or a residual lumen of less than approximately 2 mm, of the carotid artery that is most likely to be associated with strokes in the distal territory of the vessel.

Atheromatous lesions may regress to some extent under the influence of diet and lipid-lowering drugs. Hennerici and colleagues followed a series of patients with carotid stenosis for a period of 18 months and observed spontaneous regression in nearly 20 percent of the lesions. In the large majority of cases, however, atherosclerosis is a progressive disease.

The hemostatic elements, both clotting factors and platelets, which produce a thrombus within a vessel are complex and have been the object of intense study (see Furie and Furie for a discussion of this field). However, just as in the case of coronary artery disease, it is often the development and enlargement of the thrombus that acts as the final element in cerebral vascular occlusion and an ischemic stroke. It seems plausible, although not adequately studied, that the temporal profile of atherothrombotic stroke reflects this accretion of clot in a vessel. These biologic mechanisms have bearing on the treatment and prevention of stroke.

Cerebral Embolism

This is the most common cause of ischemic strokes and of all the types of stroke, cerebral embolism develops most rapidly, "like a bolt out of the blue." As a rule, the full-blown picture evolves within seconds, exemplifying most perfectly the idealized temporal profile of a stroke. Although the abruptness with which the stroke develops and the lack of prodromal symptoms point strongly to embolism, the diagnosis is based on the total clinical circumstances. Embolism always merits careful consideration in young persons, in whom atherosclerosis is less common. Only occasionally does the problem unfold more gradually, over many hours, with some fluctuation of symptoms. Possibly, in these cases the embolus initiates a propagating thrombotic process in the occluded vessel.

In most cases, the embolic material consists of a fragment that has broken away from a thrombus within the heart ("cardioembolic"). Somewhat less frequently, the source is intraarterial from the distal end of a thrombus within the lumen of an occluded or severely stenotic carotid or vertebral artery, or a clot that originates in the systemic venous system and passes through an aperture in the heart walls, or the origin of an embolus may be from large atheromatous plaques in the aorta. Thrombotic or infected material (endocarditis) that adheres to the aortic or mitral heart valves and breaks free are also well-appreciated sources of embolism, as are clots originating on prosthetic heart valves. Embolism caused by fat, tumor cells (atrial myxoma), fibrocartilage, amniotic fluid, or air enters into the differential diagnosis of stroke only in special circumstances.

The embolus usually becomes arrested at a bifurcation or other site of natural narrowing of the lumen of an intracranial vessel. The resultant infarction is pale, hemorrhagic, or mixed; hemorrhagic infarction nearly always indicates embolism (although venous occlusion can do the same). Any region of the brain may be affected, the territories of the middle cerebral artery, particularly the superior division, being most frequently involved. The two cerebral hemispheres are approximately equally affected. Large embolic clots can block large vessels (e.g., the carotid arteries in the neck or at their termination intracranially), while tiny fragments may reach vessels as small as 0.2 mm in diameter, usually with inconsequential effects. The embolic material may remain arrested and plug the lumen solidly, but more often it breaks into fragments that enter smaller vessels so that even careful pathologic examination fails to reveal their final location. In this instance, the clinical effects may abate. Because of the rapidity with which embolic occlusion develops, useful collateral influx does not become established. Thus, sparing of the brain territory distal to the site of occlusion is usually not as evident as in thrombosis that develops more slowly.

According to the Framingham Heart Study, patients with chronic atrial fibrillation are approximately six times more liable to stroke than an age-matched population with normal cardiac rhythm (Wolf et al, 1983) and the risk is considerably higher if there is also rheumatic valvular disease, now far less prevalent than in the past. Furthermore, the risk for stroke conferred by the presence of atrial fibrillation varies with age, being 1 percent per year in persons younger than age 65 years, and as high as 8 percent per year in those older than age 75 years with additional risk factors. These levels of risk are of prime importance in determining the potential benefit of chronic anticoagulation, as discussed later. Embolism may also occur in cases of paroxysmal atrial fibrillation or flutter and various studies have suggested that the risk of stroke is even greater than for the chronic arrhythmia. Even more vexing, intermittent and asymptomatic atrial fibrillation is difficult to detect except with long periods of rhythm monitoring. For example, in a study of patients with implanted pacemakers or defibrillators but not known to have atrial fibrillation by Healy and colleagues, a substantial number of atrial arrhythmias were uncovered and raised the risk of stroke fivefold. In related studies by Gladstone and coworkers and by Gaillard and colleagues, suggest that recording heart rhythm for longer periods with a loop monitor increases the rate of detection of episodic atrial fibrillation to approximately 15 percent, from approximately 3 percent with conventional Holter monitoring. Whether such long-term monitoring should be adopted in routine practice is not yet certain, but it is being increasingly added in the evaluation of "cryptogenic" stroke.

Several scoring systems have been developed to gauge the future likelihood of stroke from atrial fibrillation. The CHADS$_2$ and related systems are shorthand methods to quantitate the risk factors that modulate risk for stroke in a patient with atrial fibrillation. A refinement of this system, CHA$_2$DA$_2$-VASc is purported to improve these predictions but the confidence intervals around the point estimates of predictive values in both scales are considerable and clinical judgment must be exercised in their use. This is reflected in part by the observation that the second score does not confer increased risk of stroke in a continuous fashion with each increase in score. The scores, subject to replacement by future ones, are given in Table 34-3. Furthermore, the goal of most of these systems is to make choices regarding warfarin or similar anticoagulation for the prevention of embolic stroke from the arrhythmia as discussed later in the chapter, or as pertinently to identify patients who have such a low risk of stroke that the risks of anticoagulation may not be justified. Epidemiologic and clinical aspects of the protective effects of anticoagulation have their own imprecisions.

Table 34-3

SCORING SYSTEMS TO PREDICT THE RISK OF STROKE IN PATIENTS WITH ATRIAL FIBRILLATION (CHADS$_2$ AND CHA$_2$DS$_2$-VASC)

CHADS$_2$	POINTS ASSIGNED FOR EACH ITEM	PREDICTED YEARLY STROKE RISK BY TOTAL SCORE
Congestive heart failure	1	0.... 1.9%
Hypertension	1	1..... 2.8%
Stroke, TIA in past	2	2..... 4.0%
Vascular disease	1	3... 5.9%
Diabetes	1	4... 8.5%
Female	1	5.. 12.5%
Age		
<65 years	0	4..... 8.5%
65–74 years	1	5....12.5%
>75 years	2	6....18.2%
CHA$_2$DS$_2$-VASC	**POINTS ASSIGNED FOR EACH ITEM**	**0.... 0%**
Heart failure or ejection fraction <35%	1	1...... 1.3%
Hypertension	1	2...... 2.2%
Age <65 years	0	3...... 3.2%
66–74 years	1	
>75 years	2	
Previous stroke or TIA	2	4...... 4.0%
Diabetes	1	5.......6.7%
Coronary or peripheral vascular disease	1	6...... 9.8%
Female	1	7..... 6.9%
		8..... 6.7%
		9..... 15.5%

Mural thrombus deposited on the damaged endocardium overlying a myocardial infarct in the left ventricle, particularly if there is an aneurysmal sac, is an important source of cerebral emboli, as is a thrombus associated with severe mitral stenosis without atrial fibrillation, now a far less common circumstance than when rheumatic fever was prevalent. Emboli may occur in the first few weeks after an acute myocardial infarction but Loh and colleagues found that a lesser degree of risk persists for up to 5 years. Cardiac catheterization or surgery, especially valvuloplasty, may disseminate fragments from a thrombus or a calcified valve. Mitral and aortic valve prostheses are, as mentioned, additional important sources of embolism.

Another source of embolism is the carotid or vertebral artery, where clot forming on an ulcerated atheromatous plaque may be detached and carried to an intracranial branch (artery-to-artery embolism). A similar phenomenon occurs with arterial dissections, discussed in a later section, "Less Common Causes of Ischemic Cerebrovascular Disease," and sometimes with fibromuscular disease of the carotid or vertebral arteries.

Atheromatous plaques in the ascending aorta have been recognized to be a more frequent source of embolism than had been previously appreciated. Amarenco and colleagues reported that as many as 38 percent of a group of patients with no discernible cause for embolic stroke had echogenic atherosclerotic plaques in the aortic arch that were greater than 4 mm in thickness, a size found to be associated on a statistical basis with strokes. Disseminated cholesterol emboli from the aorta are known to occur in the cerebral circulation and may be dispersed to other organs as well; rarely, this is sufficiently severe to cause an encephalopathy and pleocytosis in the spinal fluid.

Also of interest are the symptoms caused by an embolus as it traverses a large vessel. This *migrating* or *traveling embolus syndrome* is most evident in cases of posterior cerebral artery occlusion, either from a cardiogenic source or from a thrombus in the proximal vertebral artery ("artery-to-artery" embolism; see Koroshetz and Ropper). Minutes or more before the hemianopia develops, the patient reports fleeting dizziness or vertigo, diplopia, or dysarthria, the result of transient occlusion of the origins of penetrating vessels as the clot material traverses the basilar artery. Small residual areas of infarction within the brainstem or cerebellum can be seen on MRI or found at autopsy, and some of the signs of brainstem infarction may persist. The basilar artery is singularly susceptible to this syndrome because the vertebral arteries are smaller in caliber than the basilar, allowing a clot to slowly traverse the larger vessel; furthermore, a clot in the basilar artery is prone to occlude the small orifices of arteries that supply blood to the brainstem.

Paradoxical embolism occurs when an abnormal communication exists between the right and left sides of the heart (particularly a patent foramen ovale [PFO]) or the alternative route of connection via a pulmonary arteriovenous fistula. Embolic material arising in the veins of the lower extremities or pelvis or elsewhere in the systemic venous circulation bypasses the pulmonary circulation and reaches the cerebral vessels. Pulmonary hypertension (often from previous pulmonary embolism) favors the occurrence of paradoxic embolism, but these strokes occur even in the absence of pulmonary hypertension. Several studies indicate that the presence of a small atrial septal aneurysm adjacent to the patient foramen increases the likelihood of stroke. In the series reported by Mas and colleagues (2001), patients ages 18 to 55 years who had a stroke were followed for 4 years; the risk of second stroke was 2 percent in those with a PFO alone and 15 percent among those with both a PFO and an atrial septal aneurysm (curiously, the risk among those with neither congenital abnormality was 4 percent—higher than for those with a PFO alone). This mechanism comes into play mainly in considering the causes of stroke in the younger patient, but Handke and colleagues published a series in which there was a slightly increased risk of stroke in patients who were older than age 55 and had PFO. It must be emphasized, however, that about one-third of patients in all age groups will be found to have a PFO, and anticoagulation or repair of these lesions in older patients with embolic stroke has not been shown to be beneficial (see further on for discussion of treatment of PFO). Subendocardial fibroelastosis, idiopathic myocardial hypertrophy, cardiac myxomas, and myocardial lesions of trichinosis are additional rare causes of embolism from a cardiac source. The vegetations of infective and noninfective (marantic) endocarditis give rise to several different lesions in the brain as described in Chap. 32.

Mitral valve prolapse, in the past considered a common source of emboli, especially in young patients, is no longer currently thought to be an important origin. The initial impetus for considering this abnormality as a source of embolus came from the study of Barnett and colleagues (1980) of a group of 60 patients who had TIAs or small strokes and were younger than 45 years of age; mitral prolapse was detected (by echocardiography and a characteristic midsystolic click) in 24 patients, but in only 5 of 60 age-matched controls. However, several subsequent large studies (Sandok and Giuliani; Jones et al) found that only a very small proportion of strokes in young patients could be attributed to prolapse; even then, the connection was inferred by the exclusion of other causes of stroke. Indeed, in a study using stringent criteria for the echocardiographic diagnosis of prolapse, Gilon and colleagues were unable to establish a relation to stroke. Usually, when valvular prolapse is associated with stroke, it is usually severe with ballooning of the valve and a propensity to accumulate clot behind the valve. Of interest, Rice and colleagues described a family with premature stroke in association with valve prolapse and a similar relationship has been reported in twins; the same may occur in Ehlers-Danlos disease.

The *pulmonary veins* are a potential, if infrequent, source of cerebral emboli, as reflected by the occurrence of cerebral abscesses in association with pulmonary infectious disease (and by the high incidence of cerebral deposits secondary to pulmonary carcinoma). In Osler-Weber-Rendu disease, pulmonary shunts serve as a conduit for emboli. A rare type of embolism follows thyroidectomy, where thrombosis in the stump of the superior thyroid artery extends proximally until a section of the clot, protruding into the lumen of the carotid artery, is carried into the cerebral circulation.

During *cerebral arteriography*, emboli may arise from the tip of the catheter, or manipulation of the catheter may dislodge atheromatous material from the aorta or carotid or vertebral arteries and account for some of the strokes during this procedure. Monitoring of the cerebral arteries by transcranial Doppler insonation has suggested that small emboli frequently arise during angiographic procedures. For example, a study by Bendszus and colleagues found that 23 of 100 consecutive patients had new cortical lesions shown on diffusion-weighted MRI just after cerebral arteriography. However, none of these patients was symptomatic, and with good technique, emboli from vascular catheters are infrequent.

Cerebral embolism of special type must always have occurred when secondary metastatic tumor is deposited in the brain but a mass of tumor cells is seldom large enough to occlude a cerebral artery and produce the picture of a stroke. Nevertheless, tumor embolism with stroke is known from cardiac myxoma and fibroelastoma, and occasionally with other tumors, even systemic ones; in some of these cases it is a thrombus in the primary lesion that offers a source of embolism. This syndrome must be distinguished from embolism caused by nonbacterial endocarditis that complicates malignant neoplasms (nonbacterial thrombotic endocarditis is discussed further on). This special source of cerebral embolism is a component of a hypercoagulable state that especially accompanies adenocarcinoma and cachexia.

Diffuse cerebral *fat embolism* is related to severe bone trauma. As a rule, the emboli are minute and widely dispersed, giving rise first to pulmonary symptoms and then to multiple dermal (anterior axillary fold and elsewhere) and cerebral petechial hemorrhages. Accordingly, the clinical picture is more of an encephalopathy and not strictly focal as it is in a stroke, although in some instances there may be focal features. Cerebral *air embolism* is a rare complication of abortion, scuba diving, or cranial, cervical, or thoracic operations involving large venous structures or venous catheter insertion; it was formerly encountered as a complication of pneumothorax therapy. Clinically, cerebral air embolism may be difficult to separate from the deficits following hypotension or hypoxia with which it frequently coexists. Hyperbaric treatment may be effective if instituted early.

Despite the large number of established sources of emboli, the point of origin cannot be determined in 20 to 30 percent or more of presumed embolic strokes. In such cases, emboli likely have originated from thrombi in the cardiac chambers but have left behind no residual clot and may be undetectable even by sophisticated methods, such as transesophageal echocardiography and newer MR techniques. Other cases may be a result of atheromatous material arising from the aorta or paradoxical embolism. If extensive evaluation fails to disclose the origin, the odds still favor a source in the left heart. Often, the diagnosis of cerebral embolism is made at autopsy without finding a source. In these cases, one presumes that the search for a thrombotic nidus may not have been sufficiently thorough and small thrombi in the atrial appendage, endocardium (between the papillary muscles of the heart), the aorta and its branches, or pulmonary veins may have been overlooked. Nevertheless, the source of embolic material is not revealed in a number of cases.

Transient Ischemic Attacks (TIAs)

When brief ischemic attacks precede a stroke but disappear entirely, leaving no clinical or imaging trace of cerebral infarction, they almost always stamp the underlying process as atherothrombotic involving a large or small blood vessel. Transient ischemic attacks can reflect the involvement of virtually any cerebral artery: common or internal carotid; middle, posterior, or anterior cerebral; ophthalmic; vertebral, basilar, or cerebellar; or a penetrating branch to the internal capsule, thalamus, or brainstem (lacunar TIAs). Thus, they may present themselves as transient spells of hemiparesis, aphasia, numbness or tingling on one side of the body, dysarthria, diplopia, ataxia, obscuration of a visual field, or combinations thereof that replicate the stroke syndromes. TIAs may precede, accompany, or infrequently follow the development of a stroke, or they can occur by themselves without leading to a stroke—a fact that makes any form of therapy difficult to evaluate. Transient ischemic episodes must be distinguished from other brief neurologic attacks that are from seizures, migraine and its variants, transient global amnesia, syncope, vertigo from labyrinthine disease, and psychogenic episodes as emphasized further on. The differentiation of TIAs from other similar transient spells is not always straightforward and occupies considerable attention from neurologists; the implications of these distinctions have serious implications with regard to evaluation and treatment.

Although there is little doubt that TIAs are caused by transient focal ischemia, their mechanism is not fully understood. Current opinion holds that TIAs are brief, reversible episodes of focal ischemic brain disturbance without evidence of cerebral infarction. The consensus had in the past been that their duration should be less than 24 h, an idea introduced 40 years ago by a committee assigned to study the problem. It is more useful clinically to separate attacks that last only a few minutes (up to 1 h) and leave no permanent signs, from those of longer duration, which are almost invariably a result of embolism that shows evidence of infarction on imaging studies and therefore carry an entirely different connotation than briefer TIAs. Whether to redefine TIAs by the presence or absence of imaging abnormalities after a transient focal neurologic episode may be semantic because, in either case, embolus or atherosclerosis may be responsible for the following stroke and the evaluation for the source of the difficulty is essentially the same in both circumstances.

In the clinical analysis of TIAs, it is also useful to separate a single transient episode from repeated ones that are all of uniform type. The latter are more a warning of impending vascular occlusion, particularly of the internal carotid artery, whereas the former, especially when prolonged, are again often caused by an embolus that leaves no lasting clinical effect. Prolonged, fluctuating TIAs are the most ominous. Approximately 20 percent of infarcts that follow TIAs occur within a month after the first attack, and approximately 50 percent within a year (Whisnant et al). In an attempt to provide a predictive tool, various scales have been devised, among them the "ABCD" system devised by Rothwell and colleagues (2005) and derivatives of this scale. Blood pressure, unilateral weakness, speech disturbance, and the duration of symptoms (all less than 1 h) are added to produce a predictive score for stroke within 1 week. Studies subsequent to the original one have given variable sensitivities, for which reason this interesting approach must be considered in clinical context. In the original study, unilateral weakness and duration lasting over an hour were most predictive of stroke. The problem of determining the cause of a prolonged TIA has been alluded to—many of these cases are a result of emboli.

In a prospective study of a large group of patients with TIAs caused by atherosclerotic vascular disease, the 5-year cumulative rate of fatal or nonfatal cerebral infarction was 23 percent (Heyman et al). Interestingly, the rate of myocardial infarction in this group of patients, particularly in those with carotid lesions, was almost as high (21 percent), and in other series it has exceeded the risk of stroke. Thus the occurrence of carotid TIAs is a predictor not only of cerebral infarction but also of myocardial infarction. About two-thirds of all patients with TIAs are men with hypertension, reflecting the higher incidence of atherosclerosis in this group. Occasionally, in younger adults, TIAs may occur as relatively benign phenomena, without recognizable features of atherosclerosis or risk factors for it. Migraine is suspected in such patients (see further on); other such instances are a result of special hematologic disorders such as the antiphospholipid antibody discussed later in the chapter.

It should also be pointed out that blood diseases that cause excessive viscosity or sludging of blood (polycythemia vera, sickle cell disease, thrombocytosis, leukemia, and hyperglobulinemic states) may also cause TIAs prior to a stroke.

Transient Monocular Blindness

In the transient ischemic attack of the eye, *transient monocular blindness* (also called *amaurosis fugax* or *TMB*) is the usual symptom. Most of the visual episodes evolve swiftly, over 5 to 30 s, and are described as a horizontal shade falling (or rising) smoothly over the visual field until the eye is completely but painlessly blind. The attack clears slowly and uniformly. Sometimes the attack takes the form of a wedge of visual loss, sudden generalized blurring, or, a gray or bright light obscuring vision. Transient attacks of monocular blindness are usually more stereotyped with repeated episodes than are hemispheric attacks. TIAs consisting of a homonymous hemianopia should suggest a stenosis of the posterior cerebral artery but it is often difficult for the patient to make the distinction from monocular blindness.

The implications of amaurosis fugax have been evaluated by several investigators and found not to be quite as ominous as those of hemispheral TIAs, particularly in younger patients. Poole and Ross Russell observed a group of 110 patients for periods of 6 to 19 years following an episode of amaurosis fugax (exclusive of the type caused by cholesterol emboli). At the end of 6 years, the mortality rate (mainly because of heart disease) was 21 percent, but the incidence of stroke was 13 percent (compared to expected figures of 15 and 3, respectively, percent in an age-matched population). Of the patients who were alive at the end of the observation period, 43 percent had had no further attacks of amaurosis fugax following the initial episode. Noteworthy also was the finding that among patients with normal carotid arteriograms, only 1 of 35 had had a stroke during the followup period, whereas stroke had occurred in 8 of 21 patients in whom the internal carotid artery was occluded or stenotic. As pointed out by Benavente and colleagues, the risk of stroke over the 3 years following an attack is as low as 2 percent if there are no other issues such as diabetes, but it may be as high as 24 percent in older patients with risk factors for atherosclerosis. Tippin and coworkers reviewed the records of 83 patients with onset of amaurosis fugax before the age of 45 years and found evidence of stroke in none; moreover, 42 of these patients were examined after a mean period of 5.8 years during which no stroke had occurred. It is evident that in this younger group a mechanism other than atherosclerosis was operative, such as migraine or an antiphospholipid antibody (discussed further on).

It is perhaps not surprising that the risk of stroke after transient monocular blindness is lower than for cerebral TIAs from carotid atherosclerotic disease. The size of particulate material that occludes the ophthalmic and its branches' vessels is so small that a similar event in the cerebral hemispheres would be less likely to produce symptoms. Furthermore, ischemia of the retina produces symptoms that are hard for the patient to ignore. While there are other underlying causes of TMB, these notions taken together could explain a large part of the difference in risk between conventional TIA and TMB.

Lacunar Transient Ischemic Attacks

It has been recognized that strokes caused by occlusion of small penetrating vessels of the brain have a propensity to be intermittent ("stuttering") at their onset and occasionally to allow virtually complete restitution of function between discrete episodes. Whether this constitutes a "lacunar TIA" has been debated, but it seems to us that the more important problem is our inability to distinguish a transitory occlusion of a small vessel from that of a larger vessel. Donnan and colleagues (1993) speak of a "capsular warning syndrome," which we have seen a number of times, consisting of escalating episodes of weakness in the face, arm, and leg and culminating in a capsular lacunar stroke. We conclude that lacunar symptoms at their onset may stutter or remit for hours or days, and there is no doubt that one or many of them may precede a lacunar stroke. Nevertheless, the basic pattern of a small deep stroke remains identifiable in mild form; partial syndromes that simulate cortical TIA are less common. Lacunar stroke is discussed extensively further on.

Mechanism of Transient Ischemic Attacks

The question here, so far not satisfactorily answered, is whether reduced blood flow or embolic particles are responsible for TIAs. Whatever the cause of the attacks, they are in most cases intimately related to vascular stenosis and, usually, to ulceration as a result of atherosclerosis and thrombus formation. Embolization of fibrin-platelet material from atherosclerotic sites indeed may be the cause of attacks in some cases, but it is difficult to understand how attacks of identical pattern could be caused by successive emboli from a distance that enter the same arterial branch each time. Moreover, one would expect the involved cerebral tissue to be at least partially damaged by embolism, leaving some residual signs. When a single transient episode has occurred, particularly if prolonged, the factor of recurrence does not enter into the diagnosis, and cerebral embolism must, of course, then be considered. In some cases of documented embolism, the neurologic state fluctuates from normal to abnormal repeatedly for as long as 36 h, giving the appearance of TIAs ("accelerated TIAs"); in others, a deficit of several hours' duration occurs, fulfilling the traditional (now largely discarded) criterion for TIAs. As already noted, the same sequence of events can precede lacunar infarction and seem far more likely to be the result of locally reduced blood flow than to recurrent emboli. *Restated, a single transitory episode, especially if it lasts longer than 1 h, and multiple episodes of different pattern, suggest embolism and must be distinguished from brief (2- to 10-min) recurrent attacks of the same clinical pattern, which suggest TIAs from atherosclerosis and thrombosis in a large vessel.*

Ophthalmoscopic observations of the retinal vessels made during episodes of transient monocular blindness may infrequently show either an arrest of blood flow in the retinal arteries and breaking up of the venous columns to form a "boxcar" pattern or scattered bits of white material temporarily blocking the retinal arteries. These observations indicate that in some cases of ischemic attacks involving the retinal vessels, a temporary, complete, or relatively complete cessation of blood flow occurs locally. Whether this is a result of platelet or fibrin emboli or of platelet aggregation in situ because of decreased perfusion pressure remains unsettled.

On the other hand, exercise and postural TIAs, when they do occur, are particularly suggestive of stenosis of aortic branches, as occurs in Takayasu disease (see further on) and in dissection of the aortic arch and, occasionally, in a fixed atherosclerotic carotid stenosis. TIAs induced by hyperventilation are said to be characteristic of moyamoya disease, a progressive stenosis of intracranial vessels discussed in a later section.

In states of anemia, polycythemia, thrombocythemia, extreme hyperlipidemia, hyperviscosity from macroglobulinemia, sickle cell anemia, and extreme hyper- or hypoglycemia, there may be transient neurologic deficits related to rheologic or other changes in blood, as already mentioned. In some of these cases, the metabolic or rheologic change appears to have brought out symptoms of stenosis in a large or small vessel, but just as often the vasculature is normal. Patients with antiphospholipid antibodies may have TIAs, the mechanism of which is undefined.

In some instances the TIAs begin after the artery has already been occluded by thrombus. As shown by Barnett, emboli may arise from the distal end of the thrombus or enter the upper part of the occluded vessel through a collateral artery. However, almost one-fifth of "carotid TIAs" in the series of Pessin and colleagues (1977), and a somewhat larger proportion of cases reported by Ueda and coworkers, had neither stenosis nor ulceration of the carotid arteries. In most of the cases with normal carotid arteries, the ischemic attacks exceeded 1 h in duration, suggesting embolism from the heart or great vessels including the aortic arch; but there were also a small number of brief ischemic attacks that were unexplained even after arteriography.

In general, hemodynamic changes in the retinal or cerebral circulation make their appearance when the lumen of the internal carotid artery is reduced to 2.0 mm or less (normal diameter, 7.0 mm; range, 5 to 10 mm, lower part of this range in women). This corresponds to a reduction in cross-sectional area of the vessel of more than 95 percent. The exact degree of stenosis that may cause TIAs and the risk of stroke with mild and moderate degrees of stenosis are controversial and are addressed further on.

Differential Diagnosis of TIA

Transient focal neurologic symptoms are ubiquitous in neurologic practice. They may be a result of seizures, migraine, syncope, or other conditions such as transient global amnesia (see Chap. 21), and they occur occasionally in patients with multiple sclerosis. The clinical setting in which they occur assists in making clear the nature of the attack. Furthermore, transient and reversible episodes of focal cerebral symptoms, indistinguishable from TIAs, are known to occur in patients with meningioma, glioblastoma, metastatic brain tumors situated in or near the cortex, and even with subdural hematoma. Although infrequent, these attacks are important mainly because the use of anticoagulants is relatively contraindicated in some of these circumstances. We have seen these episodes mainly with meningiomas and subdural hematomas; they have consisted of transient aphasia or speech arrest lasting from 2 min to several hours, but sensory symptoms with or without spread over the body, arm weakness, and hemiparesis have also been reported. Some remarkable cases of meningioma have involved repeated transient attacks for decades. Seizures are always suspected in these cases but are rarely proved. It has been speculated that a local vascular disturbance of some kind is operative, but the mechanism is not understood. As far as we can determine, mass lesions have not caused episodes that simulate posterior circulation TIAs.

The issue of the uncertainty regarding vertigo alone as a manifestation of a TIA referable to the basilar or vertebral artery was addressed in Chap. 15. There are occasional cases in which multiple brief episodes of vertigo, lasting perhaps a minute or less and fluctuating in intensity, may be interspersed with additional signs of brainstem ischemia. Careful questioning of the patient usually settles the question but imaging may be necessary in cases where uncertainty remains. Even then, more instances of vertigo than are justified are attributed to atherosclerotic disease in the posterior vessels. In some patients, the complaint of "dizziness" will prove, however infrequently, to be part of a carotid TIA; hence this symptom, in our experience and that of Ueda and associates, is not a totally reliable indicator of the vascular territory involved. According to Ross Russell, so-called drop attacks (see Chap. 7) have been recorded in 10 to 15 percent of patients with vertebrobasilar insufficiency but we have never observed such attacks as a recurrent ischemic phenomenon or a manifestation of other forms of cerebrovascular disease and the syndrome has usually been due to syncope, seizure, or has been of obscure origin.

Pathophysiology of Ischemic Infarction

Cerebral infarction basically comprises two pathophysiologic processes: one, a loss of the supply of oxygen and glucose secondary to vascular occlusion, and the other, an array of changes in cellular metabolism consequent to the collapse of energy-producing processes, ultimately with disintegration of cell structures and their membranes, a process subsumed under the term necrosis. Of potential therapeutic importance are the observations that some of the cellular processes leading to neuronal death are not irrevocable and may be reversed by early intervention, either through restoration of blood flow, by prevention of the influx of calcium into cells, or by interdicting intermediary processes involved in cell death.

At the center of an ischemic stroke is a zone of infarction. The necrotic tissue swells rapidly, mainly because of excessive intracellular water content (cytotoxic edema). Because anoxia also causes necrosis and swelling of cerebral tissue, oxygen lack must be a factor common to both infarction and anoxic encephalopathy. The effects of ischemia, whether functional and reversible or structural and irreversible, depend on its degree and duration. The margins of the infarct are hyperemic, being supplied by meningeal collaterals, and here there is only minimal or no parenchymal damage.

Implicit in discussions of ischemic stroke and its treatment is the existence of a "penumbra" zone that is marginally perfused and contains at-risk but viable neurons. Presumably this zone exists at the margins of an infarction, which at its core has irrevocably damaged tissue that is destined to become necrotic. Using various methods, such a penumbra can be demonstrated in association with some infarctions but not all, and the degree of reversible tissue damage is difficult to determine. The neurons in the penumbra are considered to be physiologically "stunned" by moderate ischemia and subject to salvage if blood flow is restored in a certain period of time. Olsen and colleagues demonstrated hypoperfused penumbral zones but, interestingly, found that regions just adjacent to them are hyperperfused. These concepts find a parallel in attempts to demonstrate by imaging matching of perfusion and infarction (detected by diffusion-weighted images on MRI) in patterns with acute stroke as discussed in the section on treatment. Elevating the systemic blood pressure or improving the rheologic flow properties of blood in small vessels by hemodilution improves flow in the penumbra; however, attempts to use these techniques in clinical work have met with mixed success.

Vascular Factors

The effects of a focal arterial occlusion on brain tissue vary depending on the location of the occlusion and on available collateral and anastomotic channels. In occlusion of the internal carotid artery in the neck, there may be anastomotic flow through the anterior and posterior communicating arteries of the circle of Willis from the external carotid artery through the ophthalmic artery or via other smaller external-internal connections (Fig. 34-1). With blockage of the vertebral artery, the anastomotic flow may be via the deep cervical, thyrocervical, or occipital arteries or retrograde from the other vertebral artery and again through the posterior communicating arteries. If the occlusion is in the stem portion of one of the cerebral arteries, i.e., distal to the circle of Willis, a series of meningeal interarterial anastomoses may carry sufficient blood into the compromised territory to lessen ischemic damage (Fig. 34-2). There is also a capillary anastomotic system between adjacent arterial branches, and although it may reduce the size of an ischemic territory, it is usually not adequate to prevent infarction. Thus, in the event of occlusion of a major arterial trunk, the extent of infarction ranges from none at all to the entire vascular territory of that vessel. Between these two extremes are all degrees of variation in the extent of infarction and its degree of completeness.

The phenomenon of cerebrovascular *autoregulation* is appropriately introduced here. Over a range of mean blood pressures of approximately 50 to 150 mm Hg, the small pial vessels are able to dilate and to constrict in order to maintain cerebral blood flow (CBF) in a relatively narrow range. This accommodation eventually fails at the extremes of blood pressure, after which CBF follows systemic pressure passively, either falling precipitously or rising to levels that damage the walls of small vessels. The conditions in which the limits of autoregulation are exceeded are at the extremes of hypertensive encephalopathy at one end and circulatory failure at the other, both of which are discussed in later sections of the chapter.

If brain tissue is observed in experimental circumstances at the time of arterial occlusion, the venous blood is first seen to darken, owing to an increase in deoxygenated hemoglobin. The viscosity of the blood and resistance to flow both increase, and there is sludging of formed blood elements within vessels. The tissue becomes pale. Arteries and arterioles become narrowed. Upon reestablishing flow in the occluded artery, the sequence is reversed and there may be a slight hyperemia.

Metabolic and Physiologic Factors

Many of these factors relating to cerebral blood flow have been studied by Heiss and by Siesjo and others and are reviewed in detail by Hossman. They have determined the critical threshold of CBF, measured by xenon clearance, below which functional impairment occurs. In several animal species, including macaque monkeys and gerbils, the critical level was 23 mL/100 g/min (normal is 55); if, after a short period of time, CBF is restored to higher levels, the impairment of function can be reversed. Reduction of CBF below 10 to 12 mL/100 g/min causes infarction, almost regardless of its duration. The critical level of hypoperfusion that abolishes function and leads to tissue damage is therefore a CBF between 12 and 23 mL/100 g/min. At these levels of blood flow the electroencephalogram (EEG) is slowed, and below this level it becomes isoelectric. In the region of marginal perfusion, the K level increases (as a result of efflux from injured depolarized cells) and adenosine triphosphate (ATP) and creatine phosphate are depleted. These biochemical abnormalities are reversible if the circulation is quickly restored to normal. Disturbance of calcium ion homeostasis and accumulation of free fatty acids interfere with full recovery of cells. A CBF of 6 to 8 mL/100 g/min causes marked ATP depletion, increase in extracellular K, increase in intracellular Ca, and cellular acidosis, invariably leading to histologic signs of necrosis. These changes do not become apparent for several hours. Free fatty acids (appearing as phospholipases) are activated and destroy the phospholipids of neuronal membranes. Prostaglandins, leukotrienes, and free radicals accumulate, and intracellular proteins and enzymes are denatured. Cells then swell, a process called *cellular*, or *cytotoxic, edema* (see "Brain Edema" in Chap. 31). Similar abnormalities affect mitochondria even before other cellular changes are evident.

Regarding anoxic damage of the brain, Ames and Nesbett, in a series of articles, studied the rabbit retina

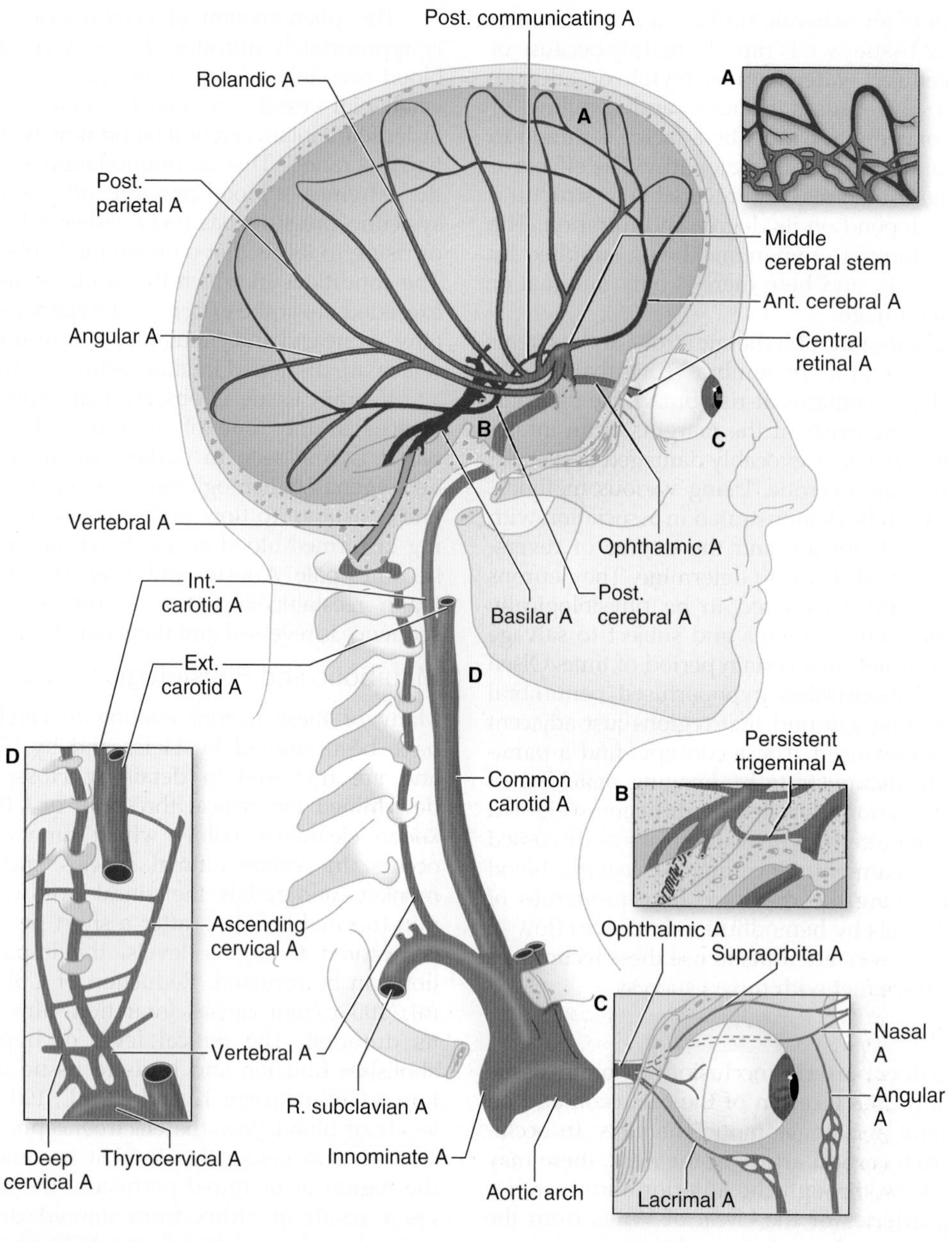

Figure 34-1. Arrangement of the major arteries on the right side carrying blood from the heart to the brain. Also shown are collateral vessels that may modify the effects of cerebral ischemia. For example, the posterior communicating artery connects the internal carotid and the posterior cerebral arteries and may provide anastomosis between the carotid and basilar systems. Over the convexity, the subarachnoid interarterial anastomoses linking the middle, anterior, and posterior cerebral arteries are shown, with inset *A* illustrating that these anastomoses are a continuous network of tiny arteries forming a border zone between the major cerebral arterial territories. Occasionally a persistent trigeminal artery connects the internal carotid and basilar arteries proximal to the circle of Willis, as shown in inset *B*. Anastomoses between the internal and external carotid arteries via the orbit are illustrated in inset *C*. Wholly extracranial anastomoses from muscular branches of the cervical arteries to vertebral and external carotid arteries are indicated in inset *D*.

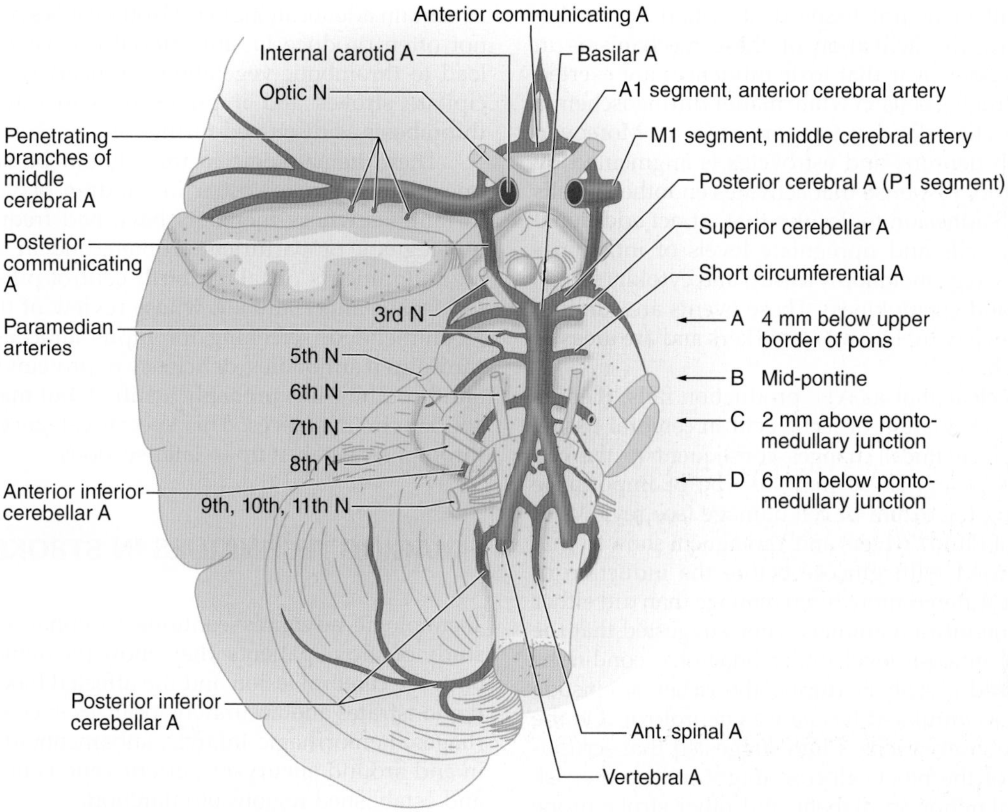

Figure 34-2. Diagram of the base of the brain showing the principal vessels of the vertebrobasilar system (the circle of Willis and its main branches). The term *M1* is used to refer to the initial (stem) segment of the middle cerebral artery; *A1* to the initial segment of the anterior cerebral artery proximal to the anterior communicating artery; *A2* to the postcommunal segment of the anterior cerebral artery; and *P1* and *P2* to the corresponding pre- and post-communicating segments of the posterior cerebral artery. The letters and arrows on the right indicate the levels of the four cross-sections following: *A* = Fig. 34-15; *B* = Fig. 34-14; *C* = Fig. 34-13; *D* = Fig. 34-12. Although vascular syndromes of the pons and medulla have been designated by sharply outlined shaded areas, one must appreciate that because satisfactory clinicopathologic studies are scarce, the diagrams do not always represent established fact. The frequency with which infarcts fail to produce a well-recognized syndrome and the special tendency for syndromes to merge with one another must be emphasized.

in an immersion chamber in which O_2 and various substrates could be altered directly rather than through the vasculature. They found that cells could withstand complete absence of O_2 for 20 min. After 30 min of anoxia, there was irreversible damage, reflected by an inability of the tissue to utilize glucose and to synthesize protein. Hypoglycemia further reduced the tolerance to hypoxia, whereas the tolerance could be prolonged by reducing the energy requirements of cells (increasing magnesium in the medium). Ames and colleagues (1968) postulated that the long period of tolerance of retinal neurons to complete anoxia in vitro, in comparison to that in vivo, is related to what he called the no-reflow phenomenon (swelling of capillary endothelial cells, which prevents the restoration of circulation), as mentioned earlier. Body temperature is yet another important factor in determining the extent of infarction. A reduction of even 2 to 3°C (3.6 to 5.4°F) reduces the metabolic requirements of neurons and increases their tolerance to hypoxia by 25 to 30 percent.

One area of interest has focused on the role of excitatory neurotransmitters in stroke, particularly glutamate and aspartate, which are formed from glycolytic intermediates of the Krebs cycle. These neurotransmitters, released by ischemic cells, excite neurons and produce an intracellular influx of Na and Ca. These changes are in part responsible for irreversible cell injury, but this must be an oversimplification. Some current attempts at therapy, for example, are directed at limiting the extent of infarction by blocking the glutamate receptor, particularly the NMDA (*N*-methyl-D-aspartate) channel—one of several calcium channels that open under conditions of ischemia and set in motion a cascade of cellular events eventuating in neuronal death (*apoptosis*). However, even complete blockade of the NMDA channels has not prevented cellular death, presumably because dysfunction of several other types of calcium channels continues and allows calcium entry to cells. Additional biochemical events must be induced by ischemia, including the production of free radicals, which leads to peroxidation and disruption of the outer cell and mitochondrial membranes. Clearly, the cascade of intracellular events that lead to neuronal death is likely to be more complex than is currently envisioned.

The extent of neural tissue dysfunction is not dictated solely by the activation of these mechanisms in neurons. It is now clear that toxic influences are exerted on oligodendroglial cells in white matter during ischemia and on astrocytic cells that support neurons. Moreover, injury to both neurons and astroyctes is augmented by an inflammatory response that activates endothelial cells to express cell adhesion molecules that attract additional inflammatory cells and upregulate levels of inflammatory proteases (e.g., metalloproteases) and cytokines (e.g., interleukins and chemokines). These events are summarized in the review by Lo and coworkers and are areas of active research.

It is also clear that as ATP production fails, there is significant accumulation of lactic acid in cerebral tissue, and all the biochemical changes consequent to the cellular acidosis occur. These may also be of importance in determining the extent of cell damage (see reviews of Raichle and of Plum). Myers and Yamaguchi showed that monkeys infused with glucose before the induction of cardiac arrest suffered more brain damage than did either fasted or saline-infused animals. They suggested that the high cerebral glucose level under anaerobic conditions led to increased glycolysis during the ischemic episode and that the accumulated lactate was neurotoxic. On the basis of such observations, Plum suggested that scrupulous control of the blood glucose might reduce the risk of cerebral infarction in diabetic and other stroke-prone patients, and during conditions of potential hyperglycemia. Clinical implementation of this idea is difficult and its advantages remain to be established. Nonetheless, these multiple molecular pathways for neuronal damage provide opportune points for therapeutic intervention.

Hematologic Factors

Involved in the process of thrombosis are changes in a number of natural anticoagulant factors such as heparin cofactor 2, antithrombin III, protein C, and protein S. Some of these are extrinsic to the blood vessels and hence may result in thrombosis in one or in multiple sites even without prior vascular injury. These are discussed by Furie and Furie. Protein C is a vitamin K-dependent protease that, in combination with its cofactors protein S and antithrombin III, inhibits coagulation. A deficiency of any of these factors may predispose to in situ thrombosis within either the arterial or venous systems and is a cause of otherwise unexplained strokes in young persons. For example, protein C deficiency (heterozygous in one of every 16,000 individuals) is a cause of thrombosis of both veins and arteries; a resistance to activated protein C has also been described (causing venous thrombosis almost exclusively). Antiphospholipid antibody is yet another cause of vascular occlusion that is not incited by damage to the vessel wall (see later in chapter). The metabolic disturbances in a number of metabolic diseases such as Fabry disease also favor cerebrovascular clotting. Persons with inflammatory bowel diseases (ulcerative colitis, Crohn disease) are known to be prone to thrombotic strokes. Whether inflammation elsewhere in the body predisposes to cerebral vascular occlusions is an open question. Curiously, the hypercoagulable state induced by certain adenocarcinomas (Trousseau's syndrome) does not often produce in situ arterial occlusion but it does lead to thrombotic vegetations on heart valves that precipitate strokes and it predisposes to cerebral venous thrombosis as discussed further on.

These hematologic factors should be sought when unexplained strokes occur in children or young adults, in families whose members have had frequent strokes, in pregnant or parturient women, and in women who are migraineurs or taking birth control pills. According to Markus and Hambley, whose review of this subject is recommended, screening for lupus anticoagulant, anticardiolipin antibodies, deficiency of proteins C and S, and antithrombin III is probably justified, but mainly in these special circumstances. This special category of vascular thrombosis is taken up in later sections.

IMAGING TECHNIQUES IN STROKE

Technologic advances continue to enhance the clinical study of stroke patients; they allow the demonstration of both the cerebral lesion and the affected blood vessel. CT demonstrates and accurately localizes even small hemorrhages, hemorrhagic infarcts, subarachnoid blood, clots in and around aneurysms, arteriovenous malformations, and established regions of infarction.

Magnetic resonance imaging is able to reveal flow voids in vessels, hemosiderin and iron pigment, and the alterations resulting from ischemic necrosis and gliosis. MRI is particularly advantageous in demonstrating small lacunar lesions deep in the hemispheres and abnormalities in the brainstem (a region obscured by adjacent bone in CT). However, the main advance has been the introduction of diffusion-weighted magnetic resonance techniques, which allow the detection of an infarctive lesion within minutes of the stroke, i.e., considerably earlier than CT and other MRI sequences (Fig. 34-3). The various MRI imaging sequences used in the diagnosis and dating of stroke are discussed below and in Chap. 2 and in Table 34-4.

Arteriography, enhanced by digital processing of images, accurately demonstrates stenoses and occlusions of the intracranial and extracranial vessels as well as aneurysms, vascular malformations, and other blood vessel diseases such as arteritis and vasospasm. To a large extent, conventional contrast angiography has been supplanted by magnetic resonance angiography (MRA), venography (MRV), and CT angiography for the visualization of large intracranial arteries and veins (see Fig. 2-2*J* and *K*). These techniques have the advantage of relative safety (injection of contrast media is required for CT angiography) but do not give refined images of the smaller blood vessels. MRA depicts the "time of flight" of blood through vessels and is not as accurate as CT angiography in measuring the degree and morphology of changes within a cerebral or intracranial vessel. Vascular imaging by MRI has the advantage that areas of restricted diffusion can be detected during the same imaging session, while the CT technique, in addition to better resolution of vascular

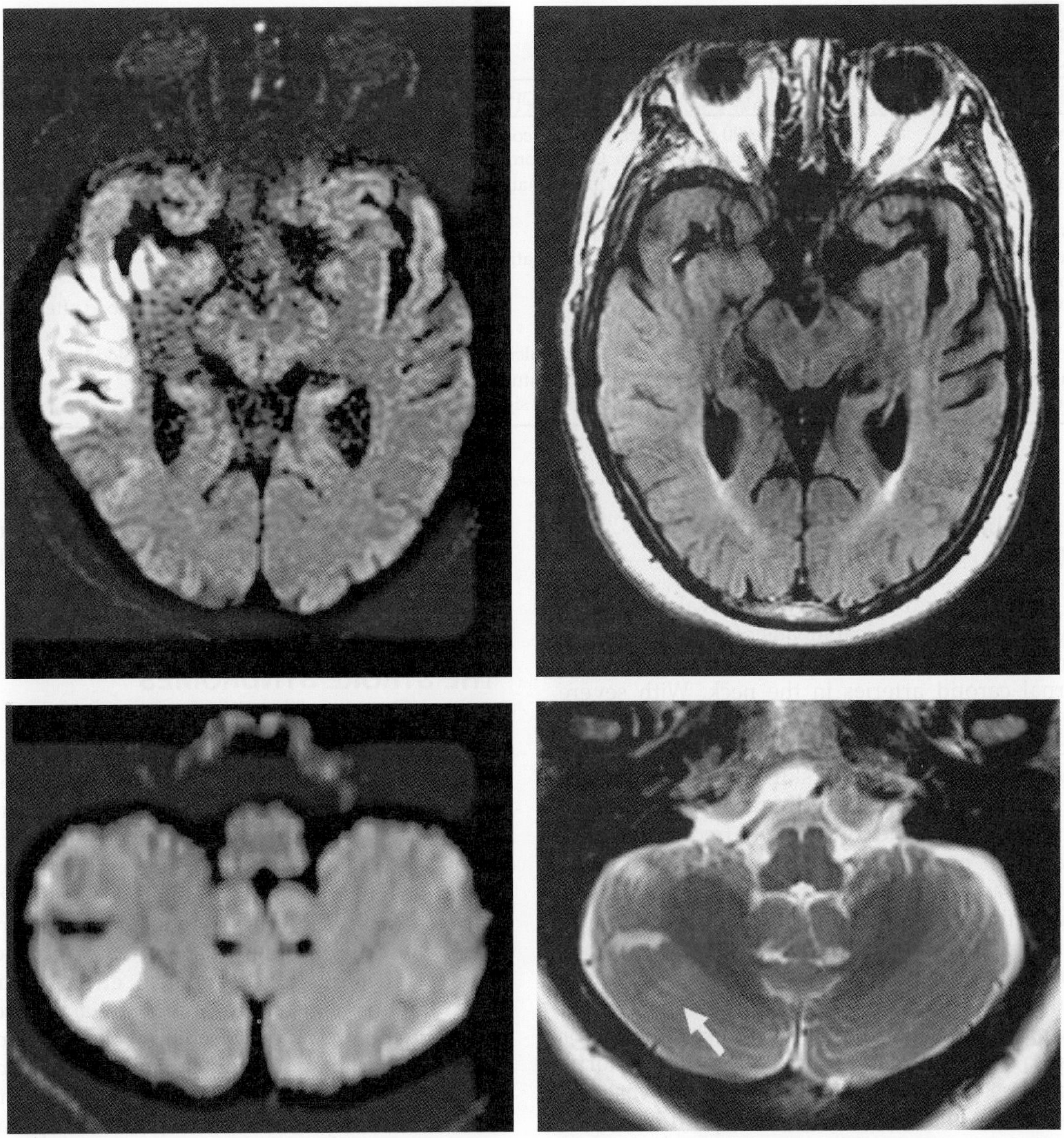

Figure 34-3. MRI showing acute infarctions. The upper images show a right middle cerebral artery infarction that appears bright on diffusion-weighted imaging (DWI) (*upper left*). There is subtle hyperintensity representing early vasogenic edema on T2-FLAIR sequence (*upper right*). The lower images show an acute cerebellar infarction in the territory of the posterior inferior cerebellar artery (PICA) that is bright on DWI (*lower left*) and faintly bright on T2-FLAIR (*arrow, lower right*). There is also a previous infarction just anterior to the acute cerebellar stroke that is dark on DWI and bright on T2 due to gliosis.

lumens, is preferable in circumstances requiring the demonstration of soft tissues and bone adjacent to blood vessels, thereby providing the surgeon with important anatomic information (see Chap. 2).

Other procedures for the investigation of cerebrovascular disease include Doppler ultrasound flow studies, which demonstrate atheromatous plaques and stenoses of large vessels, particularly of the carotid but also of the vertebrobasilar arteries. The transcranial Doppler technique has reached a degree of precision whereby occlusion or spasm of the main vessels of the circle of Willis can be detected and roughly quantitated. Various methods of measuring regional blood flow with positron emission tomography (PET) and radionuclide imaging find use in special instances discussed in appropriate sections of the chapter.

The EEG and lumbar puncture have lost favor in stroke diagnosis but the former is possibly underused as a readily available means of detecting cortical infarction in the wake of ischemia of a region of one hemisphere. It allows a distinction to be made between occlusion of a small and a large vessel, because focal EEG abnormalities are sparse or absent with a deep lacunar stroke. The technique finds more use in distinguishing between transient alterations in nervous function that are a result of seizures and episodes caused by focal ischemia.

Table 34-4

MRI SEQUENCES IN THE DIAGNOSIS OF STROKE

SEQUENCE	TE	TR	GOOD FOR	BRIGHT	DARK
T1-weighted	<50	<1,000	Subacute blood, contusions, CSF disorders	CSF, bone, edema, deoxyhemoglobin mineralization	
T2-weighted	>80	>2,000	Infarcts, inflammation, tumors	CSF, liquids, edema	Solids, calcium
Proton (spin) density	<50	>2,000		"Most pathology"	Fat, water, acute blood
Fluid-attenuated inversion recovery (FLAIR)	>80	>10,000	Edema, inflammation	Edema, inflammation, gliosis	CSF; otherwise like T2
Diffusion-weighted image (DWI)			Acute infarcts		Blood after several days
Susceptibility sequence			Hemorrhages, calcification		Blood
Short tau inversion recovery (STIR)			Spine and orbit studies (eliminates fat signals)		

Neurovascular Examination and Carotid Artery Bruit

Whereas most cerebral arteries can be evaluated only indirectly, more direct clinical means of physical examination are available for the evaluation of the common and internal carotid arteries in the neck. With severe atherosclerotic stenosis at the level of the carotid sinus auscultation discloses a *bruit*, best heard with the bell of the stethoscope held against the skin just tightly enough to create a seal (excessive pressure creates a diaphragm of the skin and filters the low-pitched frequencies that are typical of the bruit of carotid stenosis). Occasionally, a bruit at the angle of the jaw is caused by stenosis at the origin of the external carotid artery or is a radiated murmur from the aortic valve and can then be misleading. If the bruit is loudest at the angle of the jaw, the stenosis usually lies at the proximal internal carotid; if heard lower in the neck, it is in the common carotid or subclavian artery and may be radiated from the aortic valve. Rarely, stenosis in vertebral arteries or vascular malformations at the base of the brain produce bruits that are heard posteriorly in the neck.

The presence of a bruit in the neck is an indication of cerebrovascular disease but its detection is not highly correlated with the presence of severely stenotic lesions as assessed by ultrasonography or angiography. In the past, the physician was almost completely dependent on the details of the nature of the bruit but these details are now of limited interest. An additional though infrequent sign of carotid occlusion is the presence of a bruit over the opposite carotid artery, heard by placing the bell of the stethoscope over the eyeball (ocular bruit). As pointed out by Pessin and colleagues (1983), this murmur is often caused by augmented circulation through the patent vessel but there have been as many instances in our experience when a bruit over the eye instead reflects a stenosis in the intracranial portion of the carotid artery on that side. These and other tests for assessing carotid flow have been supplanted by ultrasound insonation and imaging of the carotid artery, but retinal examination remains valuable in that it may demonstrate *emboli* within retinal arteries, either shiny white or reddish in appearance; this is another important sign of carotid disease (crystalline cholesterol, termed Hollenhorst plague, is sloughed from an atheromatous ulcer).

THE STROKE SYNDROMES

The clinical picture that results from an occlusion of any one artery differs in minor ways from one patient to another, but there is sufficient uniformity to justify the assignment of a typical syndrome to each of the major cerebral arteries and their branches and their identification by careful examination of highly specific neurovascular syndromes is one of the cardinal skills of the clinical neurologist. The following descriptions apply particularly to the clinical effects of ischemia and infarction caused by embolism and thrombosis. The distinction between vascular occlusion from a local atherosclerotic plaque with superimposed thrombosis and an embolic occlusion is made largely on the basis of factors already enumerated: (1) the temporal profile of the stroke syndrome, an immediate stroke favoring embolus, and a slowly evolving or "stuttering" onset or emergence form sleep with a stroke favoring atherosclerosis, and (2) associated medical risk factors such as atrial fibrillation (strongly favoring embolus) or diabetes, hypertension, hyperlipidemia and smoking, together favoring atherosclerosis of the small penetrating, or large trunk vessels. Although hemorrhage within a specific vascular territory may give rise to many of the same effects, the total clinical picture is different because it usually involves regions supplied by more than one artery and, by its deep extension and pressure effects, causes secondary features of headache, vomiting, and hypertension, as well as a series of falsely localizing signs, as described in Chaps. 17 and 31.

Carotid Artery Syndromes

The carotid system consists of three major arteries: the common carotid, internal carotid, and external carotid. As indicated in Fig. 34-1, the right common carotid artery arises at the level of the sternoclavicular notch from the innominate (brachiocephalic) artery, and the left common carotid comes directly from the aortic arch. The common carotid arteries ascend in the neck to the C4 level, just below the angle of the jaw, where each divides into external and internal branches (sometimes the bifurcation is slightly above or below this point). This part of the extracerebral circulation is essential to an understanding of stroke. The carotid vessels are subject to atherosclerotic narrowing, atherothrombotic occlusion, arterial dissection and rarely, other processes such as various forms of vasculitis.

Occlusion of the common carotid artery accounts for less than 1 percent of cases of carotid artery syndrome, the remainder being because of disease of the internal carotid artery itself. Nevertheless, the common carotid can be occluded by an atheromatous plaque at its origin in the thorax, more often on the left side. Atherosclerotic stenosis or occlusion of the midportion of the common carotid may also occur years after radiation therapy for laryngeal, thyroid, or other head and neck cancer. If the bifurcation is patent, few if any symptoms may result because retrograde flow from the external carotid maintains internal carotid flow and perfusion of the brain.

The remainder of this discussion is concerned with disease of the *internal carotid artery*. The territory supplied by this vessel and its main branches is shown in Figs. 34-1, 34-4 and 34-5.

The territory affected by diminished blood flow in the brain in cases of carotid occlusion is highly dependent on the configuration of the circle of Willis. For example, when the anterior communicating artery is very small, the ipsilateral anterior cerebral territory is affected as well. In extreme instances where the circle of Willis provides no communication to the side of an occluded carotid artery, thus isolating the hemisphere from other blood flow, massive infarction involving the anterior two-thirds or all of the cerebral hemisphere results. If the two anterior cerebral arteries arise from a common stem on one side, infarction may occur in the territories of both vessels. The territory supplied by the posterior cerebral artery will also be included if this vessel is supplied by the internal carotid rather than the basilar artery (a configuration that reflects a residual fetal origin of the posterior cerebral artery). The clinical manifestations of atherosclerotic thrombotic disease of this artery are among the most variable of any cerebrovascular syndrome because the internal carotid is not an end vessel. In most individuals it is in continuity with the vessels of the circle of Willis and those of the orbit, and no part of the brain is completely dependent on it. Therefore occlusion, which occurs most frequently in the first part of the internal carotid artery immediately beyond the carotid bifurcation, may be silent (30 to 40 percent of cases).

If one internal carotid artery had been occluded at an earlier time, occlusion of the other may cause bilateral cerebral infarction. The clinical effects in such cases may

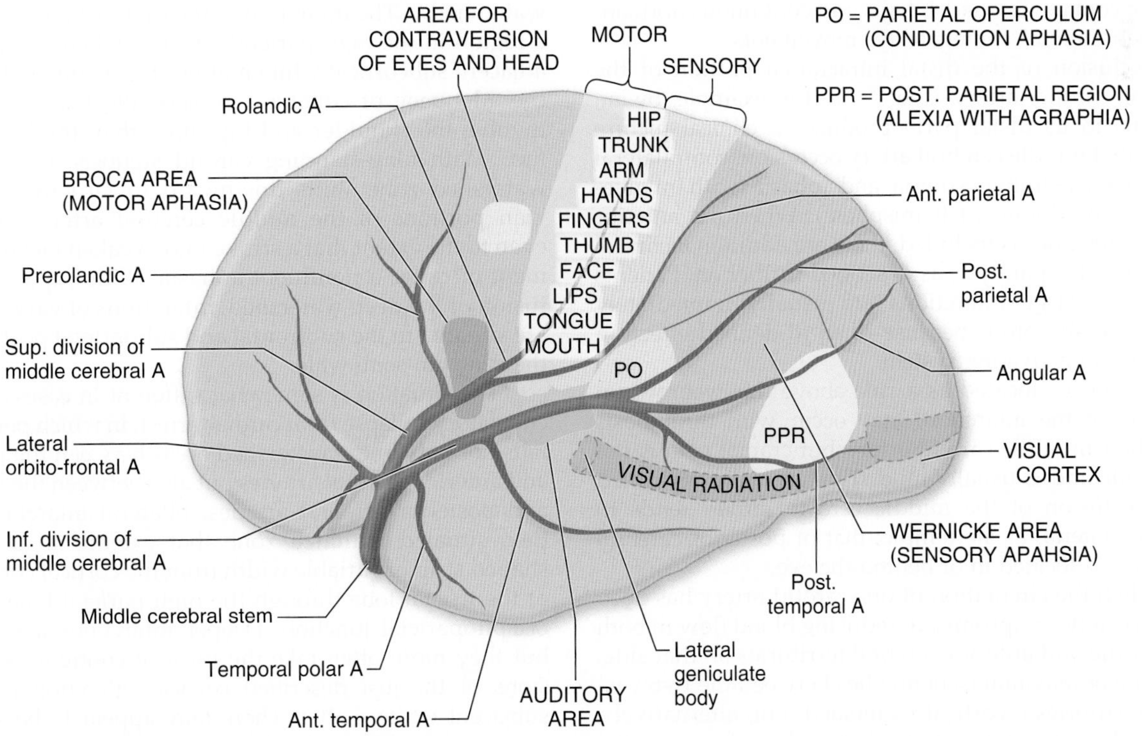

Figure 34-4. Diagram of the left cerebral hemisphere, lateral aspect, showing the courses of the middle cerebral artery and its branches and the principal regions of cerebral localization. Below is a list of the clinical manifestations of infarction in the territory of this artery and the corresponding regions of cerebral damage.

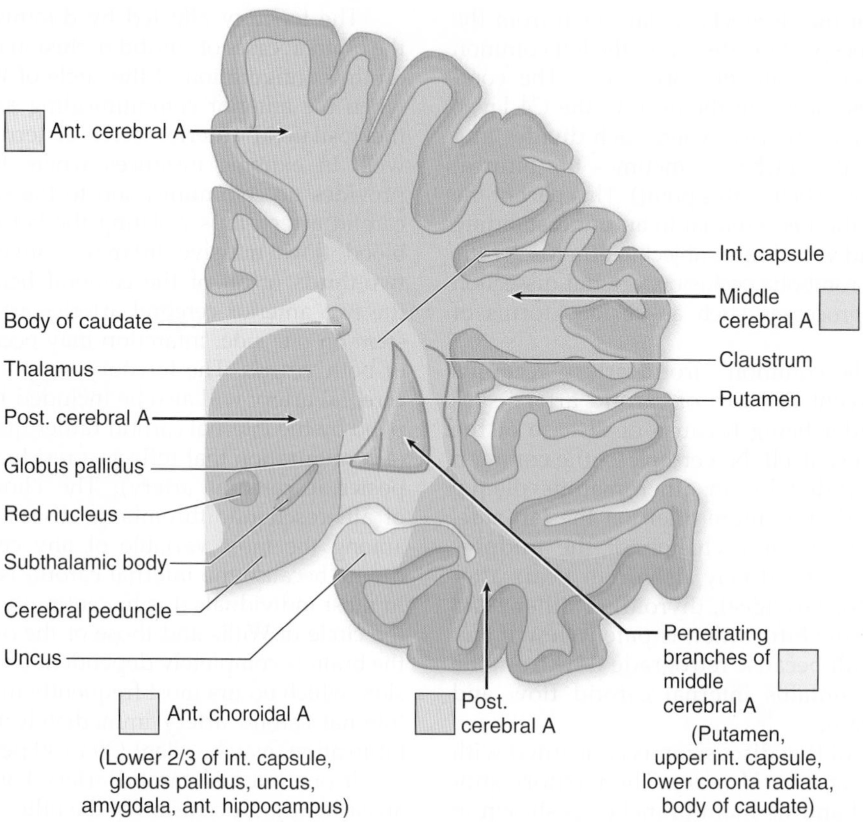

Figure 34-5. Diagram of one cerebral hemisphere, coronal section, showing the regions of blood supply of the major cerebral vessels.

include coma with quadriplegia and continuous horizontal "metronomic" conjugate eye movements.

Occlusion of the distal intracranial portion of the internal carotid artery (the "T")—for example by an embolus to its distal part—produces a clinical picture like that of middle cerebral artery occlusion: contralateral hemiplegia, hemihypesthesia, and aphasia (with involvement of the dominant hemisphere). When the anterior cerebral territory is included, there are additional clinical features of leg paralysis as described further on. Patients with such large infarctions are usually immediately drowsy or stuporous because of an ill-defined effect on the reticular activating system.

Headache, located as a rule above the eyebrow, on the side of the infarction, may occur with thrombosis or embolism of the carotid artery, but cranial pain is not invariable and is usually mild. The headache associated with occlusion of the middle cerebral artery tends to be more lateral, at the temple; that of posterior cerebral occlusion is located in or behind the eye.

When the circulation of one carotid artery has been incompletely compromised, reducing blood flow in both the middle and anterior cerebral territories on that side, the zone of maximal ischemia lies between the two vascular territories ("cortical watershed") or, alternatively, in the deep portions of the hemisphere between the territories of the lenticulostriate branches and the penetrating vessels from the convexity ("internal" or "deep watershed"). The infarction in the first instance occupies a region in the high parietal and frontal cortex and the adjacent subcortical white matter. Its size depends upon the adequacy of collateral vessels. Weakness tends to involve the shoulder and hip more than the hand and face. With long-standing carotid stenosis, the cortical watershed zone shifts downward toward the perisylvian portions of the middle cerebral artery territory, even to the extent that a stroke may weaken facial movement or cause a nonfluent aphasia. With impaired perfusion of the deep watershed, infarctions of varying size are situated in the subfrontal and subparietal portions of the centrum semiovale.

The situation is somewhat different in cases of total circulatory collapse from cardiac arrest, in which perfusion fails not only in the watershed areas between the middle and anterior cerebral arteries but also between the middle and posterior cerebral arteries. Bilateral infarctions are then situated within a zone that extends in a sickle-shaped strip of variable width from the cortical convexity of the frontal lobe through the high parietal lobe, to the occipitoparietal junction. Deeper infarctions also occur, but they more often take the form of contiguous extensions of the just described cortical infarction into the subjacent white matter. There may appear to be several separate infarctions after hypoperfusion states, but these often turn out to be radiographically visible portions of a larger border-zone lesion.

The internal carotid artery also nourishes the optic nerve and retina. For this reason, *transient monocular blindness* occurs prior to the onset of stroke in 10 to 25 percent of cases of symptomatic carotid occlusion. Yet central retinal artery ischemia is a relatively rare manifestation of carotid artery occlusion, presumably because of efficient collateral supply in the globe.

Signs of carotid occlusion include transient monocular blindness or visual loss or dimness of vision with exercise, after exposure to bright light, or on assuming an upright position; retinal atrophy and pigmentation; atrophy of the iris; peripapillary arteriovenous anastomoses in the retinae; and claudication of jaw muscles. However, the cardinal clinical signs of stenoses, ulcerations, and dissections of the internal carotid artery are TIAs. It is a subject of debate whether these are the result of fibrin platelet emboli or a reduction in blood flow. TIAs were discussed earlier, but here it can be stated again that they represent an important risk factor for stroke.

Middle Cerebral Artery Stroke Syndromes

The middle cerebral artery (MCA) has superficial and deep hemispheral branches that together supply the largest portion of the cerebral hemisphere. Through its *cortical branches*, it supplies the lateral (convexity) part of the cerebral hemisphere (see Fig. 34-4) encompassing (1) the cortex and white matter of the lateral and inferior parts of the frontal lobe—including motor areas 4 and 6, contraversive centers for lateral gaze and the motor speech area of Broca (dominant hemisphere); (2) the cortex and white matter of the parietal lobe, including the primary and secondary sensory cortices and the angular and supramarginal gyri; and (3) the superior parts of the temporal lobe and insula, including the receptive language area of Wernicke. The deep *penetrating* or *lenticulostriate branches* of the MCA supply the putamen, a large part of the head and body of the caudate nucleus (shared with the Heubner artery, see further on), the outer globus pallidus, the posterior limb of the internal capsule, and the corona radiata (see Fig. 34-5).

MCA Stem (M1) Occlusion Syndrome

The MCA may be occluded in its longitudinal portion, or the stem, that is proximal to its bifurcation (the term *M1* is used by radiologists to denote this portion of the vessel). An occlusion at this site blocks the flow in the small deep penetrating vessels as well as in superficial cortical branches. An occlusion at the distal end of the stem blocks only the orifices of the divisions of the artery in the sylvian sulcus but leaves unaffected the deep penetrating vessels. The picture of *total occlusion of the stem is one of contralateral hemiplegia (involving the face, arm, and leg as a result of infarction of the posterior limb of the internal capsule), hemianesthesia, and homonymous hemianopia* (because of infarction of the lateral geniculate body), with *deviation of the head and eyes toward the side of the lesion*. In addition, there is a variable but usually *global aphasia with left hemispheric lesions and anosognosia and amorphosynthesis with right-sided lesions* (see Chap. 22). In the beginning, the patient may be drowsy or stuporous because of an ill-defined effect of widespread paralysis of neurologic function. Once fully established, the motor, sensory, and language deficits remain static or improve little as months and years pass. If the patient is globally aphasic for many months, he seldom ever again communicates effectively (see Chap. 23 for a discussion of the aphasic disorders). If there are adequate collateral vessels over the surface of the hemisphere, only those components of the stroke referable to the deep structures are evident (mainly hemiplegia encompassing the contralateral limbs and face) as discussed below, the cortical elements of aphasia, agnosia, and apraxia then being absent or mild.

Occlusion of the stem of the MCA is usually caused by embolus and less often by a thrombus superimposed on an atherosclerotic plaque. Studies over the years have affirmed that most carotid occlusions are thrombotic, whereas most middle cerebral occlusions are embolic (Fisher, 1975; Caplan, 1989). The emboli may lodge in the stem or, more often, drift into the cortical branches as described below; not more than 1 in 20 will enter deep penetrating branches that originate in the stem. In the less-common circumstance, the MCA may become stenotic from atherosclerosis. The stroke is then the result of occlusion of the vessel by a superimposed thrombus. In several series of such cases, the stroke was preceded by TIAs, producing a picture resembling that of carotid stenosis (see Caplan, 1989). Transient monocular blindness does not occur in this situation because the occlusion is distal to the ophthalmic artery. In epidemiologic studies, certain populations such as Asians are disproportionally affected by this form of intracranial atherosclerosis, as are diabetics.

Striatocapsular Infarction A number of interesting syndromes occur with deep lesions in the territory of the penetrating, lenticulostriate, vessels of the MCA (see Figs. 34-5 and 34-7). Most, as mentioned, are attributable to emboli that lodge in the stem of the main vessel, although imaging studies may show a patent vessel and others are undoubtedly atherothrombotic. There have been few adequate pathologic studies. Although the infarction is centered in the deep white matter, most of the syndromes are fragments of the cortical–subcortical stroke patterns described further on. The most common type in our experience has been a *large striatocapsular infarction*, similar to that described by Weiller and colleagues. All of their patients had a degree of hemiparesis and one-fifth had aphasia or hemineglect. Aphasia, when it occurred, tended to be a limited form of the Broca type and in our experience, has been short-lived. With smaller deep strokes we have most often encountered incomplete motor syndromes affecting only the arm and hand, without language disturbance or neglect; these are difficult to differentiate from small embolic cortical strokes. The lesions in the corona radiata are larger than typical lacunar infarctions (see further on) but probably have a similar pathophysiology.

Homonymous hemianopia may occur with posterior capsular lesions, probably as a result of damage to the region of the lateral geniculate nucleus, but it is infrequent and must be distinguished from visual hemineglect of contralateral space. Bilateral cerebral infarctions involving mainly the insular–perisylvian (anterior opercular) regions manifest themselves by a diplegia of the face, tongue, and masseters that results in anarthria without aphasia (see Mao et al).

MCA Branch Syndromes

Superior Division An embolus entering the middle cerebral artery most often lodges in one of its two main branches, the superior division (supplying the rolandic and prerolandic areas) or the inferior division (supplying the lateral temporal and inferior parietal lobes). Atherothrombotic occlusion of this vessel is infrequent. Major infarction in the territory of the *superior division* causes a *dense sensorimotor deficit in the contralateral face, arm, but, to a lesser extent the leg, as well as ipsilateral deviation of the head and eyes*; i.e., it differs from the MCA stem occlusion syndrome in that the leg and foot are partly spared and less involved with weakness than the arm and face ("brachiofacial," or chierobrachial "paralysis"); there is no impairment of alertness. If the occlusion is long-lasting (not merely transient ischemia with disintegration of the embolus) there will be slow improvement; after a few months, the patient is able to walk with a spastic leg, while the motor deficits of the arm and face remain. The sensory deficit may be profound, resembling that of a thalamic infarct (as described in Chaps. 8 and 9) but more often it is less severe than the motor deficit, taking the form of stereoanesthesia, agraphesthesia, impaired position sense, tactile localization, and two-point discrimination, as well as variable changes in touch, pain, and temperature sense (see Chap. 22). With *left-sided lesions there is initially a global aphasia, which changes to a predominantly nonfluent (Broca's) aphasia*, with the emergence of an effortful, hesitant, grammatically simplified, and dysmelodic speech (see Chap. 23); or quite often there is *Broca's aphasia from the outset*.

Embolic occlusion limited to one of the *distal branches of the superior division*, perhaps the most common stroke seen in clinical practice, produces a more circumscribed infarct that further fractionates the above-described syndrome. With occlusion of the ascending frontal branch, the motor deficit is limited to the face and arm with little or no weakness of the leg, and the latter, if weakened at all, soon improves; with left-sided lesions, there is dysfluent and agrammatic speech and normal comprehension (Broca's aphasia). Embolic occlusion of the left rolandic branch alone results in sensorimotor paresis with severe dysarthria but little evidence of aphasia. A cortical–subcortical branch occlusion may give rise solely to a brachial monoplegia or hand weakness that simulates a problem in the peripheral nervous system. Embolic occlusion of ascending parietal and other posterior branches of the superior division may cause no sensorimotor deficit but only a conduction aphasia (see Chap. 23) and ideomotor apraxia. There are many other limited stroke syndromes or combinations of the aforementioned deficits relating to small regions of damage in the frontal, parietal, or temporal lobes. Among these are the Gerstmann syndrome and various forms of agnosia (in some patients, these may be in the territory of the inferior division of the MCA discussed below). Most of these are discussed in Chap. 22, which details the result of lesions in particular parts of the cerebrum. Improvement can be expected within a few weeks to months but some remnant of the original problem usually remains in place. As indicated earlier, the distal territory of the middle cerebral artery may also be rendered ischemic by failure of the systemic circulation, especially if the carotid artery is stenotic; this situation may simulate embolic branch occlusions.

Inferior Division Occlusion of the *inferior division* of the MCA is slightly less frequent than occlusion of the superior one, but again is nearly always the result of embolism. The usual result in left-sided lesions is a *Wernicke's aphasia*, which generally remains static for days or weeks after which some improvement can be expected. In less-extensive infarcts that are the result of selective distal branch occlusions (superior parietal, angular, or posterior temporal), the deficit in comprehension of spoken and written language may be especially severe. Again, after a few months, the deficits usually improve, often to the point where they are evident only in self-generated efforts to read and copy visually presented words or phrases. With either right- or left-hemispheric lesions, there is usually a *superior quadrantanopia or homonymous hemianopia* and, *with right-sided ones, a left visual neglect* and other signs of amorphosynthesis. Rarely, an agitated confusional state, presumably from nondominant temporal lobe damage, may be a prominent feature of dominant hemispheral lesions and sometimes of nondominant ones. Some of the syndromes applicable to the angular gyrus and the supramarginal gyrus may occur in strokes within this division, depending on the distributions of the vessels in an individual.

Anterior Cerebral Artery Stroke Syndromes

This artery, through its cortical branches, supplies the anterior three-quarters of the medial surface of the frontal lobe, including its medial-orbital surface, the frontal pole, a strip of the lateral surface of the cerebral hemisphere along its superior border, and the anterior four-fifths of the corpus callosum. Deep branches, arising near the circle of Willis (proximal and distal to the anterior communicating artery) supply the anterior limb of the internal capsule, the inferior part of the head of the caudate nucleus, and the anterior part of the globus pallidus (see Figs. 34-5, 34-6, and 34-7). The largest of these deep branches is the artery of Heubner ("recurrent artery of Heubner"). This artery, which may, in fact, be up to four small vessels, shares its territory of supply with anteriorly placed lenticulostriate arteries that emanate from the middle cerebral artery. Strokes in this territory cause infarction of the head of the caudate. Most strokes are of the embolic variety, far less often atherosclerotic, and occasionally due to other processes such as vasospasm or vasculitis.

The clinical picture of anterior cerebral artery stroke will depend on the location and size of the infarct, which, in turn, relates to the site of the occlusion (proximal or

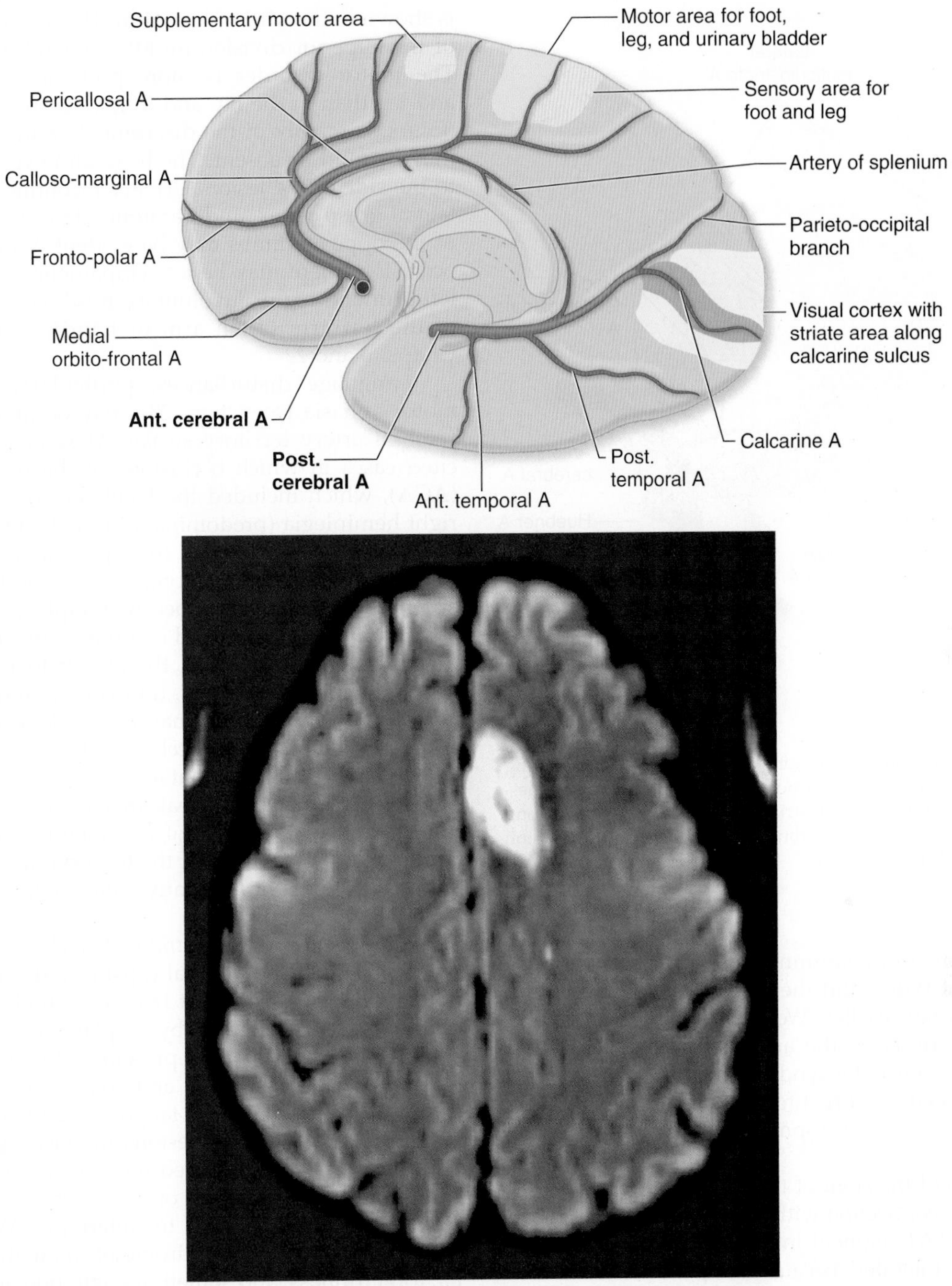

Figure 34-6. *A*. Diagram of the right cerebral hemisphere, medial aspect, showing the branches and distribution of the *anterior cerebral artery* and the principal regions of cerebral localization. Below is a list of the clinical manifestations of infarction in the territory of this artery and the corresponding regions of cerebral damage. Also shown is the course of the main branch of the *posterior cerebral artery* on the medial side of the hemisphere. *Note*: Hemianopia does not occur; transcortical aphasia occurs rarely (isolation of the language areas) (see Chap. 23). *B*. Axial diffusion-weighted MRI showing an acute ischemic infarction in the anterior cerebral artery territory.

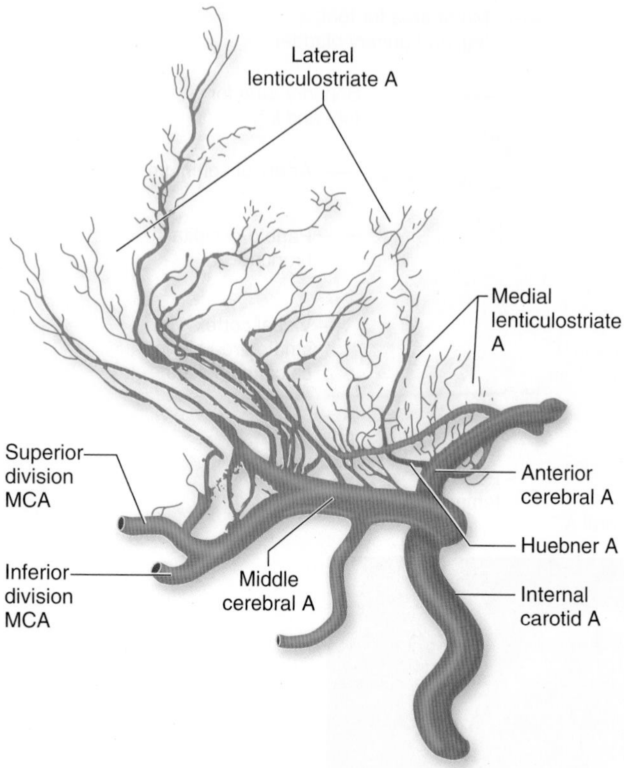

Figure 34-7. Corrosion preparations with plastics demonstrating penetrating branches of the anterior and middle cerebral arteries. The medial and lateral lenticulostriate arterioles are labeled, along with the recurrent artery of Heubner. (Reproduced by permission from Krayenbühl and Yasargil.)

distal to the anterior communicating artery), the pattern of the circle of Willis, and the other ischemia-modifying factors mentioned earlier. Well-studied cases of infarction in the territory of the anterior cerebral artery are not numerous; hence the syndromes have not been completely elucidated (see Brust for a review of the literature and a description of developmental abnormalities of the artery).

Occlusion of the stem of the anterior cerebral artery, proximal to its connection with the anterior communicating artery (the A1 segment in neuroradiologic parlance) is usually well tolerated, because adequate collateral flow is provided by the anterior or cerebral artery of the opposite side. Maximal disturbance occurs when both arteries arise from one anterior cerebral stem, in which case there is infarction of the anterior and medial parts of both cerebral hemispheres resulting in paraplegia, incontinence, abulia and nonfluent aphasic symptoms, and frontal lobe personality changes (see Chap. 22). Occlusion of the anterior cerebral arteries is usually embolic, but atherothrombotic lesions are known and instances because of surgical occlusion by an aneurysm clip are well described.

Complete infarction as a result of *occlusion of one anterior cerebral artery distal to the anterior communicating artery (A2 segment) results in a sensorimotor deficit of the opposite foot and leg and, to a lesser degree, of the shoulder and arm, with sparing of the hand and face* (the distribution of which is shown in the MRI of Fig. 34-6). This is the complement of the superior division middle cerebral artery pattern. The motor disorder is more pronounced in the foot and leg than in the hip and thigh. Sensory loss, when it occurs, is mainly of the discriminative modalities but it may be mild or absent. The head and eyes may deviate to the side of the lesion. Urinary incontinence, a contralateral grasp reflex, and paratonic rigidity (gegenhalten) of the opposite limbs may be evident. With a left-sided occlusion, there may be a "sympathetic apraxia" of the left arm and leg or involuntary misdirected movements of the left arm (alien arm or hand), as described in Chaps. 3 and 22.

Language disturbances, particularly transcortical motor aphasia (see Chap. 23), may occur with anterior cerebral artery territory stroke. Alexander and Schmitt cited cases in which occlusions of the proximal artery (ACA), which included the Heubner artery, resulted in right hemiplegia (predominant in the leg) with grasping and groping responses of the right hand and buccofacial apraxia that were accompanied by a diminution or absence of spontaneous speech, agraphia, and a limited ability to name objects and compose word lists but with a striking preservation of the ability to repeat spoken and written sentences (i.e., transcortical motor aphasia). *Disorders of behavior* that may be overlooked in cases of anterior cerebral artery occlusion; they are abulia, or a slowness and lack of spontaneity in all reactions, muteness or a tendency to speak in whispers, and distractibility. Branch occlusions of the anterior cerebral artery produce only fragments of the total syndrome, usually a spastic weakness or associative sensory loss in the opposite foot and leg.

With occlusion of *penetrating branches of the ACA,* the anterior limb of the internal capsule and caudate is usually involved. In a series of 18 cases of unilateral caudate region infarcts collected by Caplan and associates, a transient hemiparesis was present in 13. Dysarthria and either abulia or agitation and hyperactivity were also common. Stuttering and language difficulty occurred with two of the left-sided lesions and visuospatial neglect with three of the right-sided ones. To what extent these symptoms were the result of a disturbance of neighboring structures is difficult to determine. With bilateral caudate infarctions, a syndrome of inattentiveness, abulia, forgetfulness, and sometimes agitation and psychosis was observed. Transitory choreoathetosis and other dyskinesias (we have seen two cases of ballismus) have also been attributed to ischemia of the caudate and anterior basal ganglia, occurring sometimes under conditions of prolonged standing and exercise (Caplan and Sergay; Margolin and Marsden).

Anterior Choroidal Artery Stroke Syndrome

This is a long, narrow artery that springs from the internal carotid, just above the origin of the posterior communicating artery. It supplies the internal segment of the globus pallidus and posterior limb of the internal capsule and several contiguous structures including (in most patients) the optic tract (see Fig. 34-5). It then penetrates the temporal horn of the lateral ventricle, where it supplies the choroid plexus and anastomoses with the posterior choroidal artery. This being a small caliber branch, most strokes in this territory are due to in situ atherosclerosis of the type that occurs in diabetics but occlusion of the orifice of the vessel by an embolus is possible and it is a known complication of clipping of an aneurysm at the upper reaches of the carotid artery.

Only a few complete clinicopathologic studies have been made of the distinctive syndrome caused by occlusion of this artery. It was found by Foix and colleagues to consist of *contralateral hemiplegia, hemihypesthesia,* and *homonymous sectorial hemianopia* (not reaching the vertical meridian of the visual fields) as a result of involvement of the posterior limb of the internal capsule and white matter posterolateral to it, through which the geniculocalcarine tract passes, and the lateral geniculate nucleus. This combination of extensive unilateral motor, sensory, and visual impairment in an individual with well-preserved language and cognition distinguishes this stroke syndrome from the more common ones involving the major cerebral arteries. Decroix and colleagues reported 16 cases (identified by CT) in which the lesion appeared to lie in the vascular territory of this artery. In most of their cases, the clinical syndrome fell short of what was expected on anatomic grounds or had additional features.

With right-sided lesions, there may be a left spatial neglect and constructional apraxia; slight disorders of speech and language may accompany left-sided lesions. Hupperts and colleagues have discussed the controversy regarding the effects of occlusion of the artery and in particular the variability of its supply to the posterior paraventricular area of the corona radiata and adjacent regions. They concluded, also from a survey of CT images, that there was no uniform syndrome attributable to occlusion of the vessel and that in most cases its territory of supply was overlapped by small surrounding vessels. It may be remembered that for a time, in order to abolish the tremor and rigidity of unilateral Parkinson disease, the anterior choroidal artery was being surgically ligated without these other effects having been produced.

Posterior Cerebral Artery Stroke Syndromes

In approximately 70 percent of individuals, both posterior cerebral arteries are formed by the bifurcation of the basilar artery and thin posterior communicating arteries join this system to the internal carotid arteries. In 20 to 25 percent, one posterior cerebral artery arises from the basilar in the usual way, but the other arises from the internal carotid, a persistent fetal pattern of circulation; fewer than 5 percent have the unusual configuration in which both arise from the corresponding carotid arteries. Most strokes in this territory are embolic in origin but some individuals are predisposed to atherosclerosis in the proximal posterior cerebral artery. There is also the possibility of ischemia in this territory from occlusion of more proximal vessels, particularly the basilar artery, or infraction in the distal territory of the vessel as a result of global failure of cerebral perfusion, as in severe hypotension.

The configuration and branches of the *proximal segment of the posterior cerebral artery* (P1 segment) are illustrated in Figs. 34-6, 34-8, and 34-9. The *interpeduncular branches,* which arise just above the basilar bifurcation, supply the red nuclei, the substantia nigra bilaterally, medial parts of the cerebral peduncles, oculomotor and trochlear nuclei and nerves, reticular substance of the upper brainstem, decussation of the superior cerebellar peduncles, medial longitudinal fasciculi, and medial lemnisci. The P1 portion of the posterior cerebral artery, giving rise to the interpeduncular branches (that portion between the bifurcation of the basilar artery and the ostium of the posterior communicating artery), is also referred to as the *mesencephalic artery* or the *basilar communicating artery*. As pointed out by Percheron (whose name is often applied to the largest of these vessels), the arterial configuration of the paramedian mesencephalic arteries varies considerably: in some cases, two small vessels arise symmetrically, one from each side; in others, a single artery arises from one posterior cerebral stem (proximal P1), which then bifurcates. In the latter case, one posterior cerebral stem supplies the medial thalamic territories on both sides, and an occlusion of this artery or one common paramedian trunk produces a bilateral butterfly-shaped lesion in the medial parts of the diencephalon. These are elaborated and illustrated by Castaigne et al.

The *thalamoperforate branches* (also called *paramedian thalamic arteries*) arise slightly more distally from the stem, nearer the junction of the posterior cerebral and posterior communicating arteries (P2 segment of the artery) and supply the inferior, medial, and anterior parts of the thalamus. The *thalamogeniculate* branches arise still more distally, opposite the lateral geniculate body, and supply the geniculate body and the central and posterior parts of the thalamus. Medial branches emerging from the posterior cerebral artery as it encircles the midbrain, supply the lateral part of the cerebral peduncle, lateral tegmentum and corpora quadrigemina, and pineal gland. Posterior choroidal branches run to the posterosuperior thalamus, choroid plexus, posterior parts of the hippocampus, and psalterium (decussation of deep white matter fornices).

Most importantly, the terminal or *cortical branches of the posterior cerebral artery* supply the inferomedial part of the temporal lobe and the medial occipital lobe, including the lingula, cuneus, precuneus, and visual Brodmann areas 17, 18, and 19 (see Figs. 34-6, 34-8, and 34-9).

Occlusion of the posterior cerebral artery produces a greater variety of clinical effects than occlusion of any other artery because both the upper brainstem, which is replete with important structures, and the inferomedial parts of the temporal and occipital lobes lie within its supply. The site of the occlusion and the arrangement of the circle of Willis will, in large measure, determine the location and extent of the resulting infarct. For example, occlusion proximal to the posterior communicating artery may be asymptomatic or have only transitory effects if the collateral flow is adequate from the opposite posterior cerebral vessel (see Fig. 34-8; see also Fig. 34-9). Even distal to the posterior communicating artery, an occlusion may cause relatively little damage if the collateral flow

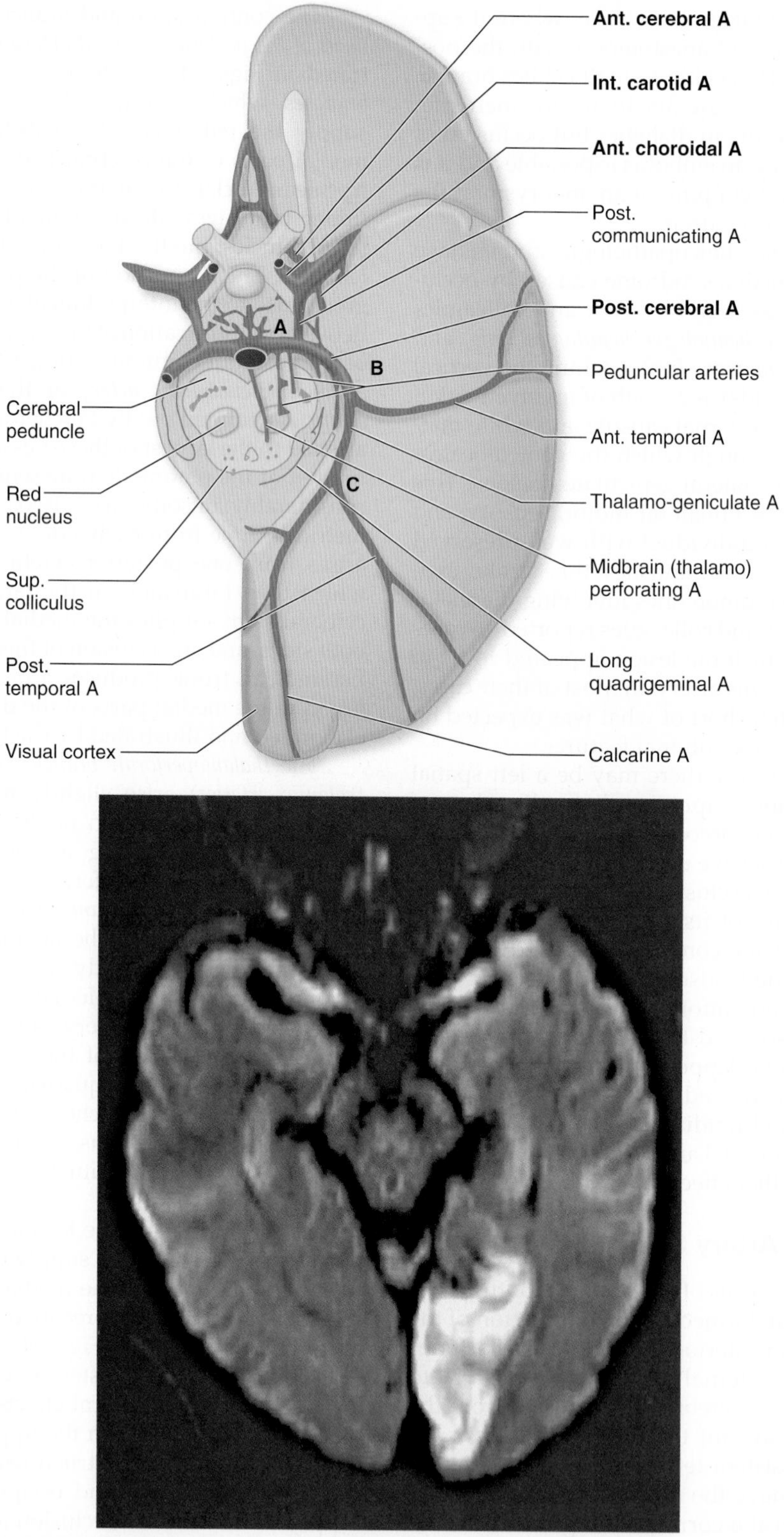

Figure 34-8. *A.* Inferior aspect of the left hemisphere showing the branches and distribution of the posterior cerebral artery and the principal anatomic structures supplied. The vessel is considered from the perspective of its proximal and distal territories. Listed below are the clinical manifestations produced by infarction in these territories and the corresponding regions of damage. Tremor in repose has been omitted because of the uncertainty of its occurrence in the posterior cerebral artery syndrome. Peduncular hallucinosis may occur in thalamic-subthalamic ischemic lesions, but the exact location of the lesion is unknown. *B.* Axial diffusion-weighted MRI showing an acute ischemic infarction in the posterior cerebral artery territory.

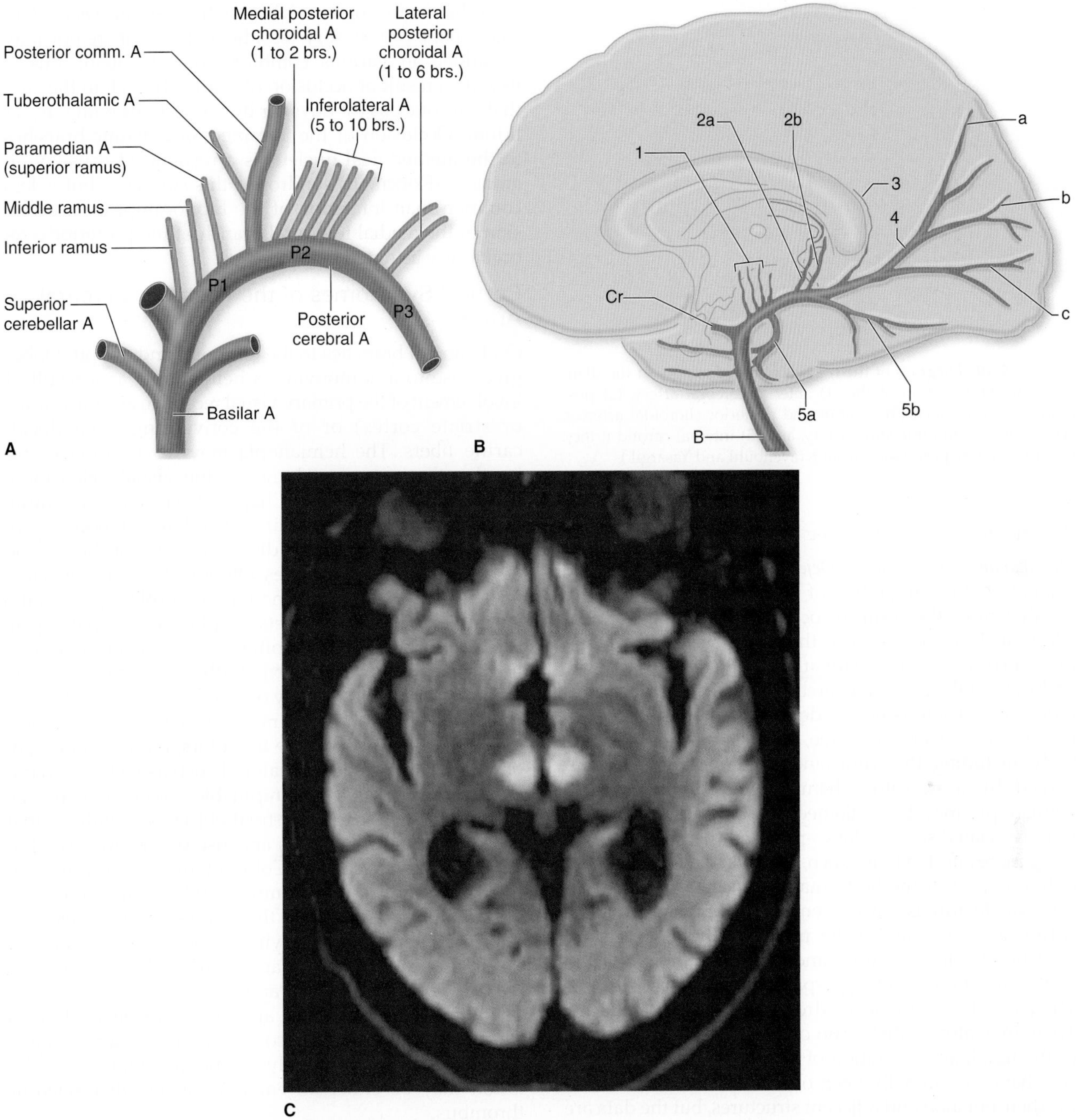

Figure 34-9. The posterior cerebral and basilar arteries. *A*. The terminus of the basilar artery and branches originating from the P1 through P3 segments. (Reproduced by permission from *Stroke* 34:2264, 2003.) *B*. Lateral view of the brain showing the branches of the posterior cerebral artery. (Reproduced by permission from Krayenbühl and Yasargil.) *C*. Axial diffusion-weighted MRI showing an acute ischemic infarction due to occlusion of an artery of Percheron, an anatomic variant, in which an azygos paramedian artery supplies both sides of the posterior-medial thalamus.

through border-zone collaterals from anterior and middle cerebral arteries is sufficient.

In the series of posterior cerebral artery strokes studied by Milandre and coworkers, the causes were, in general, similar to those of strokes in other vascular territories except that there was a higher incidence of atherosclerotic occlusion (35 patients) in contrast to cardioembolic types (15 patients). Two of their stroke cases were attributed to migraine. Our experience has differed in that the proportion of presumed embolic occlusions has been far greater than that of other causes.

For convenience of exposition, it is helpful to divide the posterior cerebral artery syndromes into three groups: (1) proximal (involving interpeduncular, thalamic perforant, and thalamogeniculate branches), (2) cortical (inferior temporal and medial occipital), and (3) bilateral.

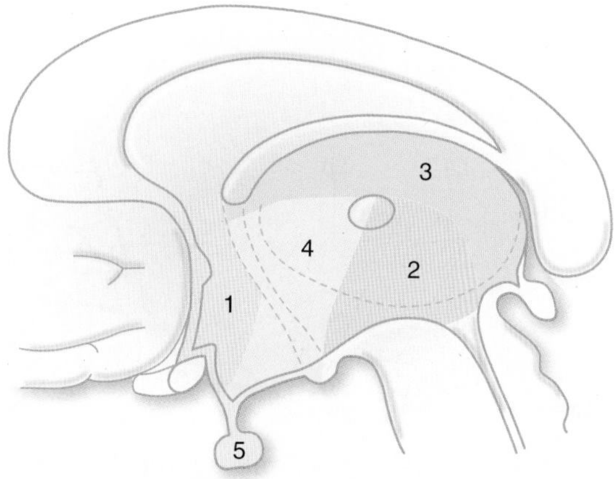

Figure 34-10. Diagram of the regions of blood supply of the diencephalon. Distribution of the (1) anterior cerebral artery, (2) posterior cerebral artery, (3) anterior and posterior choroidal arteries, (4) posterior communicating artery, and (5) internal carotid artery. (Reproduced by permission from Krayenbühl and Yasargil.)

Proximal Syndromes (See Figs. 34-9 and 34-10)

The thalamic syndrome of Dejerine and Roussy (see also Chap. 8) follows infarction of the sensory relay nuclei in the thalamus, the result of occlusion of thalamogeniculate branches. Occlusion of the small vessels supplying these territories from in situ atherothrombosis or embolic occlusion of the posterior cerebral artery is the most common cause. There is both a deep and cutaneous sensory loss, usually severe in degree, of the opposite side of the body, including the trunk and face, sometimes accompanied by a transitory hemiparesis. A homonymous hemianopia may be conjoined. In some instances there is a dissociated sensory loss—pain and thermal sensation being more affected than touch, vibration, and position—or only one part of the body may be anesthetic. The characteristic feature is always sensory loss that includes the entire hemibody up to the midline. After an interval, sensation begins to return, and the patient may develop pain, paresthesia, and hyperpathia in the affected parts. The painful paresthetic syndrome may persist for years. There may also be distortion of taste, athetotic posturing of the hand, and alteration of mood. Mania and depression have occasionally been observed with infarction of the diencephalon and adjacent structures, but the data are usually incomplete.

Central midbrain and subthalamic syndromes are a result of occlusion of the interpeduncular branches of the posterior cerebral artery. The clinical syndromes include palsies of vertical gaze, stupor, or coma. Syndromes of the *paramedian arteries*, including the proximal posterior cerebral artery, have as their main feature a third-nerve palsy combined with contralateral hemiplegia (*Weber syndrome*), contralateral ataxic tremor (*Claude syndrome*), or homolateral ataxia, hemiplegia with contralateral third-nerve palsy (*Benedikt syndrome*), as summarized in Table 34-5.

Anteromedial-inferior thalamic syndromes follow occlusion of the thalamoperforant branches. Here the most common effect is an extrapyramidal movement disorder (hemiballismus or hemichoreoathetosis or less often, asterixis). Deep sensory loss, hemiataxia, or tremor may be added in various combinations. Hemiballismus is usually a result of occlusion of a small branch to the subthalamic nucleus (of Luys) or its connections with the pallidum. Occlusion of the paramedian thalamic branches to the mediodorsal nucleus is a recognized cause of an amnesic (Korsakoff) syndrome; this simulates but is less common than infarction of the hippocampi from occlusion of the medial temporal branch of the posterior cerebral artery as noted below.

Cortical Syndromes of the Posterior Cerebral Artery

Occlusion of branches to the temporal and occipital lobes gives rise to a homonymous hemianopia as a result of involvement of the primary visual receptive areas (calcarine or striate cortex) or of the converging geniculocalcarine fibers. The hemianopia may be incomplete and involve the upper quadrants of the visual fields more than the lower ones (see Chap. 13). Macular, or central, vision is often spared because of collateral blood supply of the occipital pole from distal branches of the middle (or anterior) cerebral arteries. Other features seen in a few instances are visual hallucinations in the blind parts of the visual fields (Cogan) or metamorphopsia and palinopsia (Brust and Behrens). Occipital infarcts of the dominant hemisphere may cause alexia without agraphia, anomia (amnesic aphasia), a variety of visual agnosias, and rarely some degree of impaired memory. The anomias, when they occur, are most severe for colors, but the naming of other visually presented material such as pictures, mathematical symbols, and manipulable objects may also be impaired. The patient may treat objects as familiar—that is, describe their functions and use them correctly—but be unable to name them. Color anomia (a form of "central achromatopsia") and amnesic aphasia are more often present in this syndrome than is alexia. The defect in retentive memory is of varying severity and may or may not improve with the passage of time. These syndromes are described in Chaps. 22 and 23.

A complete proximal arterial occlusion leads to a syndrome that combines cortical and anterior-proximal syndromes in part or totally. As mentioned, the vascular lesion may be either an embolus or an atherosclerotic thrombus.

Bilateral Posterior Cerebral Artery Stroke Syndromes

These occur as a result of successive infarctions or from a single embolic or thrombotic occlusion of the upper basilar artery, especially if the posterior communicating arteries are unusually small or absent, or from global failure of circulation.

Bilateral lesions of the occipital lobes, if extensive, cause "cortical blindness" that is essentially bilateral homonymous hemianopia, sometimes accompanied by unformed visual hallucinations. The pupillary reflexes are preserved and the optic discs appear normal. Sometimes the patient is unaware of being blind and denies the problem even when it is pointed out to him (Anton syndrome).

Table 34-5

INTRAMEDULLARY BRAINSTEM SYNDROMES[a]

EPONYM[b]	SITE	CRANIAL NERVES INVOLVED	TRACTS INVOLVED	SIGNS	USUAL CAUSE
Weber syndrome	Base of midbrain	III	Corticospinal tract	Oculomotor palsy with crossed hemiplegia	Vascular occlusion, tumor, aneurysm
Claude syndrome	Tegmentum of midbrain	III	Red nucleus, superior cerebellar peduncles after decussation	Oculomotor palsy with contralateral cerebellar ataxia and tremor	Vascular occlusion, tumor, aneurysm
Benedikt syndrome	Tegmentum of midbrain	III	Red nucleus, corticospinal tract, and superior cerebellar peduncles after decussation	Oculomotor palsy with contralateral cerebellar ataxia, tremor, and corticospinal signs, may have choreoathetosis	Infarct, hemorrhage, tuberculoma, tumor
Nothnagel syndrome	Tectum of midbrain	Unilateral or bilateral III	Superior cerebellar peduncles	Ocular palsies (IV), paralysis of gaze, nystagmus, and ataxia	Tumor
Parinaud syndrome	Dorsal midbrain		Supranuclear mechanism for upward gaze and other structures in periaqueductal gray matter	Paralysis of upward gaze and accommodation; fixed pupils	Pinealoma and other lesions of dorsal midbrain, hydrocephalus
Millard-Gubler syndrome and Raymond-Foville syndrome	Base of pons	VII and often VI	Corticospinal tract	Facial and abducens palsy and contralateral hemiplegia; sometimes gaze palsy to side of lesion	Infarct or tumor
Avellis syndrome	Tegmentum of medulla	X	Spinothalamic tract; sometimes descending pupillary fibers, with Bernard-Horner syndrome	Paralysis of soft palate and vocal cord and contralateral hemianesthesia	Infarct or tumor
Jackson syndrome	Tegmentum of medulla	X, XII	Corticospinal tract	Avellis syndrome plus ipsilateral tongue paralysis	Infarct or tumor
Wallenberg syndrome	Lateral tegmentum of medulla	Spinal V, IX, X, XI	Lateral spinothalamic tract Descending pupillodilator fibers Spinocerebellar and olivocerebellar tracts	Ipsilateral V, IX, X, XI palsy, Horner syndrome, and cerebellar ataxia; contralateral loss of pain and temperature sense	Occlusion of vertebral or posterior–inferior cerebellar artery

[a]See also Table 47-1, which lists the brainstem syndromes due to extramedullary lesions.
[b]See Wolf JK: *The Classical Brainstem Syndromes.* Springfield, IL, Charles C Thomas, 1971, for translations of original reports.

More frequently, the lesions are incomplete, and a sector of the vision, usually on one side, remains intact. When the visual remnant is small, vision may seemingly fluctuate from moment to moment as the patient attempts to capture the image in the island of intact vision, in which case hysteria may be incorrectly inferred. In bilateral lesions confined to the occipital poles, there may be a loss of central vision only (homonymous central scotomas). With more anteriorly placed lesions of the occipital pole, there may be homonymous paracentral scotomas, or the occipital poles may be spared, leaving the patient with only central vision. Horizontal or altitudinal field defects are usually a result of similar restricted lesions affecting the upper or lower banks of the calcarine sulci. The Balint syndrome (see Chap. 22) is an effect of bilateral occipito-parietal border-zone lesions.

With bilateral lesions that involve the inferomedial portions of the temporal lobes, including the hippocampi and their associated structures, the impairment of memory may be severe, causing the Korsakoff amnesic state. In several of our patients, a solely left-sided infarction of the inferomedial temporal lobe impaired retentive memory. Bilateral mesiotemporal-occipital lesions also cause a lack of recognition of faces (prosopagnosia). These and other effects of temporal and occipital lesions are discussed in Chaps. 13 and 22.

Vertebral Artery Stroke Syndromes

The vertebral arteries are the chief arteries of the medulla; each supplies the lower three-fourths of the pyramid, the medial lemniscus, all or nearly all of the retroolivary (lateral medullary) region, the restiform body, and the posteroinferior part of the cerebellar hemisphere through the posterior inferior cerebellar arteries (Fig. 34-11). The relative sizes of the vertebral arteries vary considerably, and in approximately 10 percent of cases, one vessel is so small that the other is essentially the only artery of supply to the brainstem. In the latter cases, if there is no collateral flow from the carotid system via the circle of Willis,

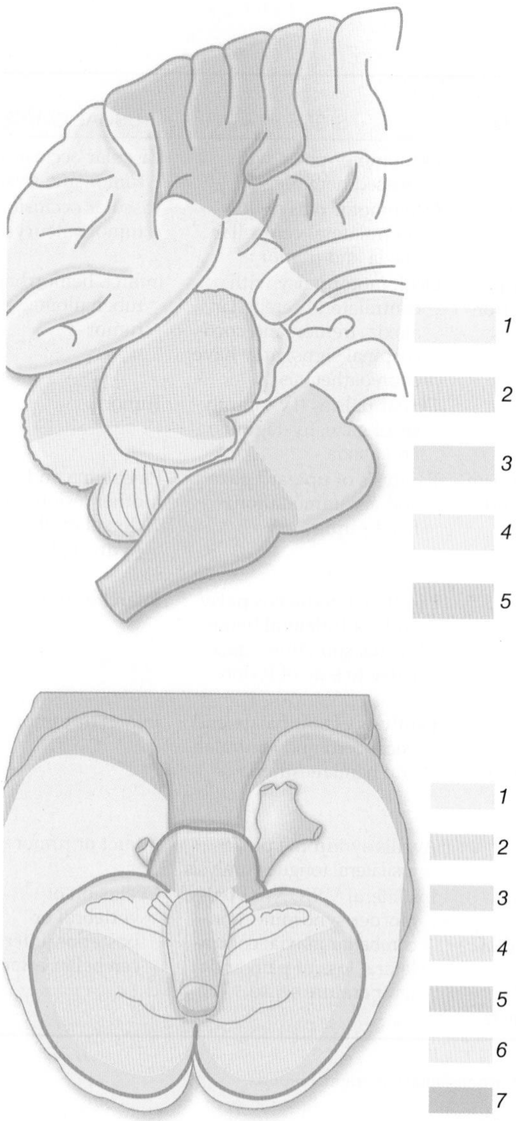

Figure 34-11. Regions supplied by the posterior segment of the circle of Willis, lateral view (*A*) and basal view (*B*). *A*. (1) Posterior cerebral artery; (2) superior cerebellar artery; (3) basilar artery and superior cerebellar artery; (4) posterior inferior cerebellar artery; (5) vertebral artery (posterior inferior cerebellar artery, anterior spinal artery, posterior spinal artery). *B*. (1) Posterior cerebral artery; (2) superior cerebellar artery; (3) paramedian branches of the basilar artery and spinal artery; (4) posterior inferior cerebellar artery; (5) vertebral artery; (6) anterior inferior cerebellar artery; (7) dorsal spinal artery. (Reproduced by permission from Krayenbühl and Yasargil.)

occlusion of the one functional vertebral artery is equivalent to occlusion of the basilar artery (see below). The posteroinferior cerebellar artery (PICA) is usually a branch of the vertebral artery but can have a common origin and form a loop with the anteroinferior cerebellar artery (AICA) from the basilar artery. It is necessary to keep these anatomic variations in mind in considering the effects of vertebral artery occlusion.

The vertebral arteries are most often occluded by atherothrombosis in their intracranial portion. Because the vertebral arteries have a long extracranial course and pass through the transverse processes of C6 to C1 vertebrae before entering the cranial cavity, one might expect them to be subject to trauma, spondylotic compression, and a variety of other vertebral diseases. With the exception of arterial dissection, in our experience the other causes of vascular occlusion happen only infrequently. We rarely see convincing examples of spondylotic occlusion but several such cases have been reported. Extreme extension of the neck, as experienced by women who are having their hair washed in beauty salons, or during yoga positions, may give rise to transient symptoms in the territory of the vertebral artery.

Dissection of the vertebral artery by contrast is well described; it declares itself by cervicooccipital pain and deficits of brainstem function. One's attention is drawn to the diagnosis of vertebral dissection where there have been vigorous and protracted bouts of coughing or trauma to the neck or head. Dissection of the extracranial vessels is discussed in more detail further on. Examples of posterior circulation stroke in children have been reported in association with odontoid hypoplasia and other atlantoaxial dislocations, causing the vertebral arteries to be stretched or kinked in their course through the transverse processes of C1-C2 (Phillips et al).

The results of vertebral artery occlusion are quite variable. If the occlusion of the vertebral artery is so situated as to block the posterior inferior cerebellar artery supplying the lateral medulla and inferior cerebellum (PICA), a characteristic syndrome results with vertigo being a prominent symptom (see "Lateral Medullary Syndrome" described below). If the subclavian artery is blocked proximal to the origin of the left vertebral artery, exercise of the arm on that side may draw blood from the right vertebral and basilar arteries, retrograde down the left vertebral and into the distal left subclavian artery—sometimes resulting in the symptoms of basilar insufficiency. This phenomenon, described in 1961 by Reivich and colleagues, was referred to by Fisher (1961) as the *subclavian steal*. Its most notable features are vertigo and other brainstem signs coupled with transient weakness on exercise of the left arm. There may also be headache and claudication or pain of the arm. In an unusual configuration in which one vertebral artery is occluded just proximal to the origin of its PICA branch, and the opposite vertebral artery is open and sufficient in size, there may be no symptoms because the PICA is still filled by retrograde flow through its vertebral artery.

Less often, occlusion of the vertebral artery or one of its medial branches produces an infarct that involves the medullary pyramid, the medial lemniscus, and the emergent hypoglossal fibers; the resultant syndrome consists of a contralateral paralysis of arm and leg (with sparing of the face), contralateral loss of position and vibration sense, and ipsilateral paralysis and later atrophy of the tongue. This is the *medial medullary syndrome* (Fig. 34-12). A more limited lesion, from occlusion of one spinal artery arising from the vertebral artery, gives rise to a contralateral hemiplegia (rarely a quadriplegia) that spares the face. When the vertebral branch to the anterior spinal artery is blocked, flow from the other (corresponding)

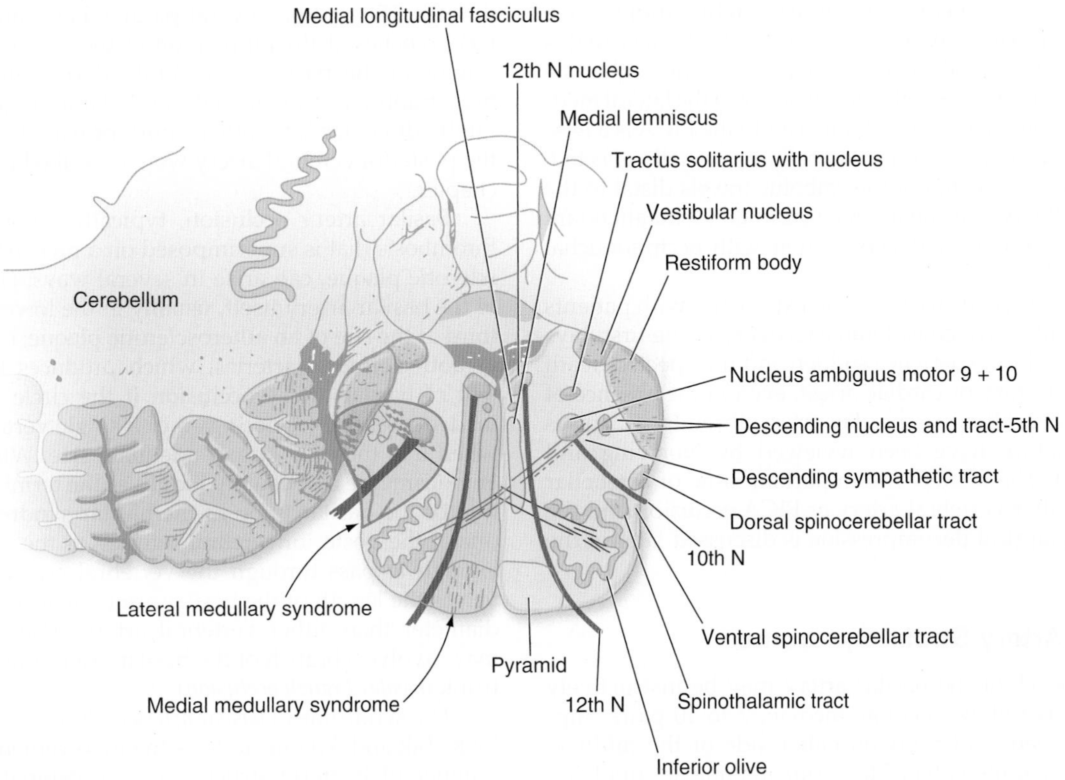

Figure 34-12. Transverse section through the upper medulla, reflecting regions supplied by the vertebral arteries and their branches.

branch is usually sufficient to prevent infarction of the cervical cord, but we and others have described solely pyramidal infarction with hemiplegia or quadriplegia that spares the face (Ropper et al). Occlusion of a vertebral artery low in the neck is usually compensated by anastomotic flow to the upper part of the artery via the thyrocervical, deep cervical, and occipital arteries or by reflux from the circle of Willis.

Lateral Medullary Syndrome

Known also as the *Wallenberg syndrome* (who described a case in 1895), this common stroke is produced by infarction of a wedge of lateral medulla lying posterior to the inferior olivary nucleus (see Fig. 34-12). The complete syndrome, as outlined by Fisher and colleagues (1961), comprises (a) symptoms derived from the vestibular nuclei (vertigo, nystagmus, oscillopsia, vomiting); (b) spinothalamic tract (contralateral or, less often, ipsilateral impairment of pain and thermal sense over half the body); (c) descending sympathetic tract (ipsilateral Horner syndrome—miosis, ptosis, decreased sweating); (d) issuing fibers of the ninth and tenth nerves (hoarseness, dysphagia, hiccough, ipsilateral paralysis of the palate and vocal cord, diminished gag reflex); (e) utricular nucleus (vertical diplopia and illusion of tilting of vision and rotation of the vertical meridian, rarely so severe as to produce upside down vision); (f) olivocerebellar, spinocerebellar fibers, restiform body and inferior cerebellum (*ipsilateral* ataxia of limbs, falling or toppling to the ipsilateral side, and the sensation of lateropulsion); (g) descending tract and nucleus of the fifth nerve (pain, burning, and impaired sensation over ipsilateral half of the face); (h) nucleus and tractus solitarius (loss of taste); and rarely, (i) cuneate and gracile nuclei (numbness of *ipsilateral* limbs). Fragmentary syndromes are more frequent, especially at the onset of the stroke. These subsyndromes may consist of vertigo and ptosis, toppling and vertical diplopia, hoarseness and disequilibrium, or other combinations short of the entire syndrome. While vertigo is the most frequent feature alone, it is not usually an indication of lateral medullary infarction. The smallest infarction we have studied gave rise only to symptoms of lateropulsion and mild ipsilateral limb ataxia.

The eye signs of lateral medullary infarction are also varied and quite interesting. There is often a fragment of an internuclear ophthalmoplegia or a skew deviation (the globe on the affected side usually being higher). Direction- changing nystagmus (with different head positions) is a useful feature that suggests labyrinthine disease from brainstem forms of nystagmus, but infarction of the vestibular nucleus as part of the lateral medullary syndrome may also produce this sign (see Chap. 15).

The entire lateral medullary syndrome, one of the most striking in neurology, is almost always caused by infarction, with only a small number of cases being the result of hemorrhage, demyelination, or tumor. Although it has traditionally been attributed to occlusion in the course of the PICA, as mentioned earlier, careful studies have shown that in 8 of 10 cases it is the vertebral artery that is occluded by atherothrombosis; in the remainder, either the posterior inferior cerebellar artery or one of the lateral medullary arteries is occluded. Embolism to the PICA is a less-frequent cause. The inferior cerebellum is usually affected, sometimes in isolation if the embolus travels distal to the origin of PICA, causing a cerebellar infarct with attendant vomiting, vertigo, and ataxia often with occipitonuchal headache.

In recent years, we have had experience with patients who initially have considerable recovery in the first days and weeks, but experience sudden and unexpected death from respiratory or cardiac arrest, even in the absence of cerebellar swelling or basilar artery thrombosis. Cases of this nature have been reviewed by Norrving and Cronqvist. The related and important issue of cerebellar swelling after vertebral artery or PICA occlusion and the need for surgical decompression is discussed later in the chapter.

Basilar Artery Stroke Syndromes

The branches of the basilar artery may be instructively grouped as follows: (1) paramedian, 7 to 10 pairs, supplying a wedge of pons on either side of the midline; (2) short circumferential, 5 to 7 pairs in number, supplying the lateral two-thirds of the pons and the middle and superior cerebellar peduncles; (3) long circumferential, 2 on each side (the superior and anterior inferior cerebellar arteries), which run laterally around the pons to reach the cerebellar hemispheres (see Figs. 34-11 and 34-13 through 15); and (4) several paramedian (interpeduncular) branches at the bifurcation of the basilar artery and origins of the posterior cerebral arteries supplying the high midbrain and medial subthalamic regions. These interpeduncular and other short proximal branches of the posterior cerebral artery were described earlier in the chapter.

Basilar artery occlusion, typically because of local thrombosis that is superimposed on a preexisting atherosclerotic plaque, can arise in several ways: (1) occlusion of the basilar artery itself, usually in the lower or middle third at the site of an atherosclerotic plaque; (2) occlusion of both vertebral arteries, which produces the equivalent of basilar artery occlusion if the circle of Willis is inadequate; and (3) occlusion of a single vertebral artery when it is the only one of adequate size. When there is embolism, the clot usually lodges at the terminal bifurcation of the basilar ("top-of-the-basilar syndrome") or in one of the posterior cerebral arteries, as the clot, if small enough to pass through the vertebral artery, easily traverses the length of the basilar artery, which is of greater diameter than either vertebral artery. Also, thrombosis may involve a branch of the basilar artery rather than the trunk (*basilar branch occlusion*).

The syndrome of *basilar artery occlusion*, as delineated by Kubik and Adams, reflects the involvement of a large number of bilateral structures: corticospinal and corticobulbar tracts; cerebellum, middle and superior cerebellar peduncles; medial and lateral lemnisci; spinothalamic tracts; medial longitudinal fasciculi; pontine nuclei; vestibular and cochlear nuclei; descending hypothalamospinal sympathetic fibers; and the third through eighth

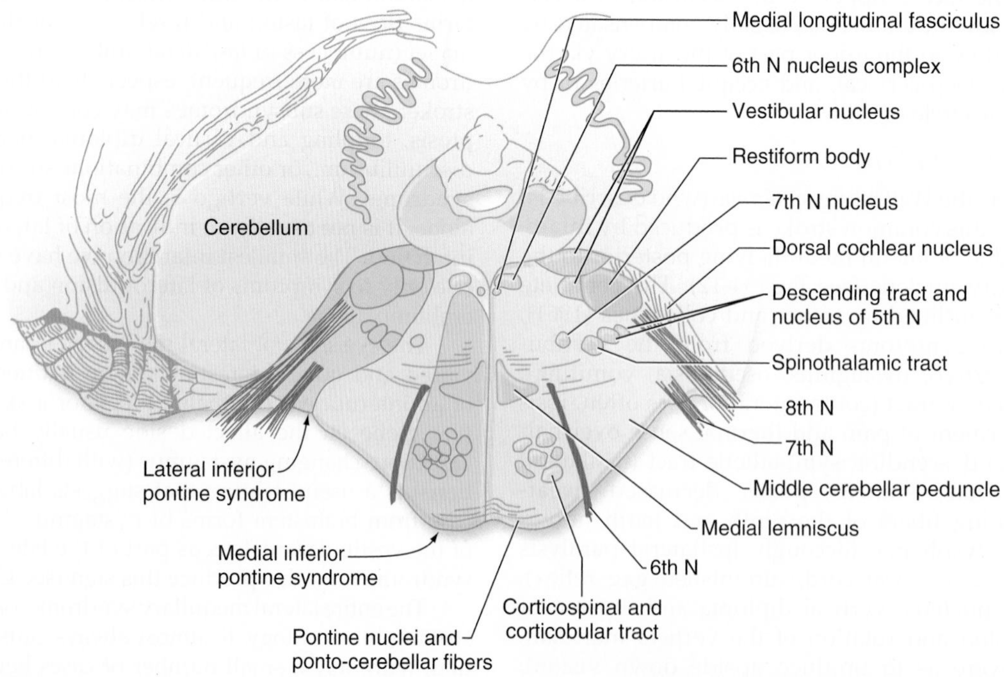

Figure 34-13. Transverse section through the lower pons, reflecting the regions supplied by the lower basilar artery including its anterior inferior cerebellar artery branch.

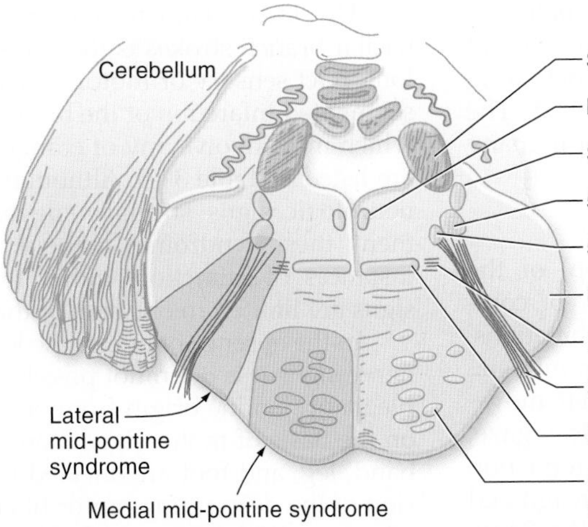

Figure 34-14. Transverse section through the midpons in the regions supplied by the mid-basilar artery and its short circumferential and paramedian branches.

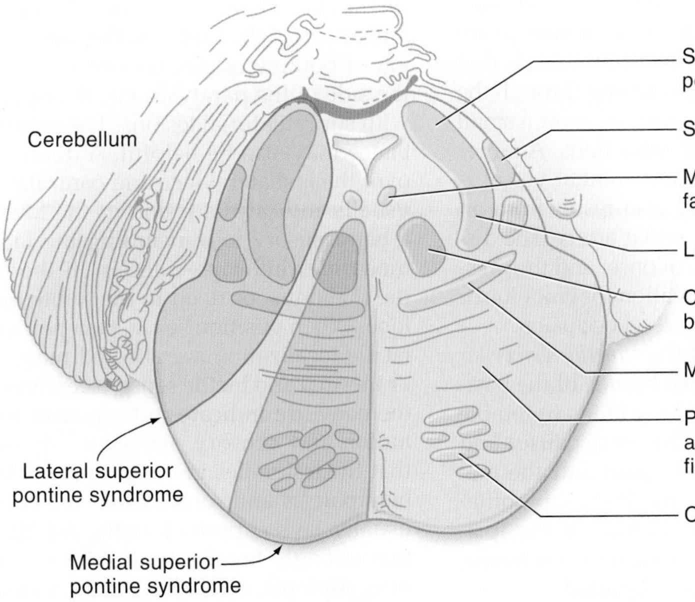

Figure 34-15. Transverse section through the upper pons and the regions supplied by the upper basilar artery and its superior cerebellar artery branch.

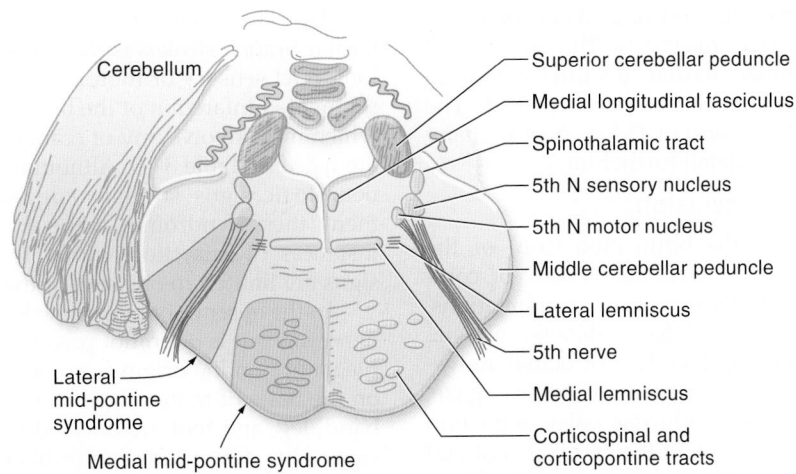

cranial nerves (the nuclei and their segments within the brainstem). Thus the *complete syndrome* comprises bilateral long tract signs (sensory and motor) with variable cerebellar, cranial nerve, and other segmental abnormalities of the brainstem.

Another important syndrome, the result of occlusion of the distal end of the basilar artery, consists of coma from infarction of the high midbrain reticular activating system. This "top of the basilar" artery occlusion is most often embolic and characterized by transient loss of consciousness, oculomotor disturbances (roving eye movements or eyes looking downward and inward with inability to reflexly elicit upward movements), hemianopia, bilateral ptosis, and pupillary enlargement with preserved reaction to light. Spontaneous recanalization of the vessel is frequent, but occurs in a delayed fashion, after the infarct has been established. MRI demonstrates a characteristic pattern of central midbrain, bilateral posterior thalamic, and, more variably, uni- or bilateral posterior territory infarction as discussed below.

Yet another configuration, the result of occlusion of the midbasilar artery, gives rise to the locked-in syndrome, in which the patient is mute and quadriplegic but conscious, reflecting interruption of descending motor pathways in the base of the pons but sparing of the reticular activating system ("locked-in" syndrome; see Chap. 17). Horizontal eye movements are obliterated but vertical ones and some ability to elevate the eyelids are spared. The pupils become extremely small but retain some reaction to light. Midbasilar disease may also cause coma if the posterior communicating arteries are inadequate to perfuse the distal basilar artery territory.

In the presence of the full syndrome, it is usually not difficult to make the correct diagnosis. The aim should be, however, to recognize basilar insufficiency long before the stage of total deficit has been reached. The early manifestations (in the form of TIAs) occur in many combinations, described in detail further on.

Basilar Artery Branch Occlusion

Occlusion of branches at the bifurcation (top) of the basilar artery results in a remarkable number of complex syndromes that include, in various combinations, somnolence or coma, memory defects, akinetic mutism, visual hallucinations, ptosis, disorders of ocular movement (convergence spasm, paralysis of vertical gaze, retraction nystagmus, pseudoabducens palsy, retraction of upper eyelids, skew deviation of the eyes), an agitated confusional state, and visual field defects (see Fig. 34-9). These have been summarized by Petit and coworkers and Castaigne and associates and categorized as paramedian thalamic, subthalamic, and midbrain syndromes, and by Caplan as parts of the "top of the basilar" syndrome. Limited, small infarctions on one side of the brainstem are usually due to occlusion of small penetrating vessels that originate in the basilar artery. Emboli coursing through the basilar artery can also occlude the mouths of several small penetrating vessels and cause larger infractions. A larger infarction in the territory of one circumferential vessel is usually due to an embolus but may also result from an atherosclerotic plaque in the parent basilar artery. The distinction is often made by the rapidity of onset and the presence of risk factors such as atrial fibrillation for embolus or diabetes and hypertension for small vessel occlusion.

The main signs of occlusion of the *superior cerebellar artery*, the most rostral circumferential branch of the basilar, are ipsilateral cerebellar ataxia of the limbs (referable to middle and superior cerebellar peduncles); nausea and vomiting; slurred speech; and loss of pain and thermal sensation over the opposite side of the body (spinothalamic tract). Partial deafness, static tremor of the ipsilateral upper extremity, an ipsilateral Horner syndrome, and palatal myoclonus have also been reported.

With occlusion of the *anterior inferior cerebellar artery* (AICA), the extent of the infarct is extremely variable, as the size of this artery and the territory it supplies vary inversely with the size and territory of supply of the PICA. The principal findings are vertigo, vomiting, nystagmus, tinnitus, and sometimes unilateral deafness; facial weakness; ipsilateral cerebellar ataxia (inferior or middle cerebellar peduncle); an ipsilateral Horner syndrome and paresis of conjugate lateral gaze; and contralateral loss of pain and temperature sense of the arm, trunk, and leg (lateral spinothalamic tract) as shown in Fig. 34-14. The tinnitus, if present at all, may be overwhelming, called "screaming" by some of our patients. If the occlusion is close to the origin of the artery, the corticospinal fibers may also be involved, producing a hemiplegia; if distal, there may be cochlear and labyrinthine infarction. Cerebellar swelling did not occur with AICA territory infarction in the 20 collected by Amarenco and Hauw but it has been a more common occurrence in our material.

The most characteristic manifestation of all these basilar branch strokes is the "crossed" cranial nerve and long tract sensory or motor deficit reflecting a unilateral segmented infarction of the brainstem. These syndromes, which may involve any of cranial nerves III through XII, are listed in Table 34-5. Although the finding of bilateral neurologic signs strongly suggests brainstem involvement, these syndromes make it apparent that in many instances of infarction within the basilar territory, the signs are limited to one side of the body.

In the absence of one of the localizing crossed cranial nerve signs it is often not possible to distinguish a hemiplegia of pontine origin from one of deep cerebral origin on the basis of motor signs alone. In both, the face, arm, hand, leg, and foot are affected because of the compression of the descending motor fibers into a small segmental region. With brainstem lesions as with cerebral ones, a flaccid paralysis gives way to spasticity after a few days or weeks, and there is no satisfactory explanation for the occurrence in some cases of spasticity from the onset of the stroke. There is also often a combined hemiparesis and ataxia of the limbs on the same side. With a hemiplegia of pontine origin, however, the eyes may deviate to the side of the paralysis, i.e., the opposite of what occurs with supratentorial lesions. The pattern of sensory disturbance may also be helpful. A dissociated sensory deficit over the ipsilateral face and contralateral half of the body usually indicates a lesion in the lower brainstem, while a hemisensory loss including the face and involving all modalities indicates a lesion in the upper brainstem, in the thalamus, or deep in the white matter of the parietal lobe. When position sense, two-point discrimination, and tactile localization are affected relatively more than pain or thermal and tactile sense, a cerebral lesion is suggested; the converse indicates a brainstem localization. Bilateral motor and sensory signs are almost certain evidence that the lesion lies in the brainstem. When hemiplegia or hemiparesis and sensory loss are coextensive, the lesion usually lays supratentorially. Additional manifestations that strongly favor a brainstem site are rotational dizziness, diplopia, cerebellar ataxia, a Horner syndrome, and deafness. The numerous brainstem syndromes illustrate the important point that the cerebellar pathways, spinothalamic tract, trigeminal nucleus, and sympathetic fibers can be involved at different rostral-caudal levels so that "neighboring" phenomena are required to identify the exact site of the infarction.

A myriad of proper names have been applied to the brainstem syndromes, as noted in Tables 34-5 and 47-1. Many of them were originally described in relation to tumors, trauma, and other nonvascular diseases. The diagnosis of vascular disorders in this region of the brain is not greatly facilitated by knowledge of these eponymic syndromes; it is much more profitable to be closely familiar with the anatomy of the brainstem. To recapitulate, the principal syndromes to be recognized are the full basilar, vertebral–PICA, posteroinferior cerebellar, anteroinferior cerebellar, superior cerebellar, pontomedullary, and medial medullary. Figures 34-12 through 34-15, supplied by C.M. Fisher and used in all previous editions of this book, present both medial and lateral syndromes at several levels of the medulla and pons. Other syndromes can usually be identified as fragments or combinations of the major ones.

Lacunar Stroke

As one might surmise, small penetrating branches of the cerebral arteries may become occluded, and the resulting infarcts may be so small or so situated as to cause no symptoms whatsoever. As the softened tissue is removed by macrophages, a small cavity, or lacune, remains. Early in the twentieth century, Pierre Marie referred to the condition as *état lacunaire* (the lesions were first described by Durant-Fardel in 1843). He distinguished these lesions from a fine loosening of tissue around thickened small vessels that enter the anterior and posterior perforated spaces, a change to which he gave the name *état criblé* (cribriform change). Pathologists have not always agreed on these distinctions, but we have adhered to the view of Fisher and Adams that lacunes are usually caused by occlusion of small arteries, 50 to 200 microns in diameter, and the cribriform state, to mere thickening of vessels and fraying of the surrounding tissue—i.e., dilated perivascular spaces (Virchow-Robin spaces) that do not have a corresponding neurologic disease.

In almost all clinical and pathologic material, there has been a strong relationship between the lacunar state and chronic hypertension, but also diabetes and hyperlipidemia. Sacco and colleagues (1991), in a population-based study in Rochester, Minnesota, found that 81 percent of patients with lacunar infarctions were also hypertensive. There appear to be three mechanisms for lacunar infarction but variants of atherothrombosis are foremost. The first, and the one most characteristically tied to lacunes, is a local type of fibrohyalinoid arteriolar sclerosis that involves the orifice or proximal part of a small penetrating blood vessel (lipohyalinosis as described below). The second is atherosclerosis of a large trunk vessel that occludes the origin of these same small vessels. This is prone to involve several adjacent vessels and cause, at times, larger lacunes or the atherosclerosis extends from a trunk vessel into a smaller one. Third is the entry of small embolic material into one of the vessels. The relative frequency of these three pathologies is not known, but the first seems to be most common and occurs without pathologic change in the trunk vessel of the circle of Willis whereas the embolic type is least frequent. When Fisher (1975) examined a series of such lesions in serial sections, from a basal parent artery up to and through the lacune, he was able to confirm a lipohyalin degeneration of the vessel wall and occlusion in the initial course of small vessels in most cases. In some, lipohyalinotic changes had resulted in false aneurysm formation, resembling the Charcot-Bouchard aneurysms, another hypertension-related change that underlies brain hemorrhage (see further on). In a series of 1,042 consecutive adults whose brains were examined postmortem, Fisher (1965b) observed one or more lacunes in 11 percent. He found 4 to 6 and sometimes up to 10 to 15 lacunes in any given brain specimen. In recent years, better treatment of hypertension has greatly reduced this number and the overall frequency of lacunar infarction, at least as judged by MRI.

Lacunes are situated, in descending order of frequency, in the putamen and caudate nuclei, thalamus, basis pontis, internal capsule, and deep in the central hemispheral white matter. The cavities range from 3 to 15 mm in diameter, and whether they cause symptoms depends entirely on their location.

Lacunar strokes tend to evolve quickly but not typically as suddenly as an embolus, for example. These clinical aspects are discussed extensively in the earlier section "Lacunar TIA." In broad terms, the essential feature of these deep strokes is the uniform and striking absence of cortical deficits; that is, seizures, aphasia or amnesia (except in limited circumstances of small thalamic infarction), agnosia, apraxia, dysgraphia, alexia, and, a large number of similar cognitive changes that only begin to appear when there are multiple deep strokes and a dementia of the type discussed in Chap. 21. Furthermore, because of the small size of the strokes, certain clinical syndromes that might be expected to result from deep lesions, such as hemianopia, also do not occur. Fisher, in several papers, has delineated the most frequent symptomatic forms of lacunar stroke:

1. Pure motor hemiplegia
2. Pure sensory stroke
3. Clumsy hand–dysarthria
4. Ipsilateral hemiparesis–ataxia

A lacune in the territory of a lenticulostriate artery, i.e., in the internal capsule or adjacent corona radiata, usually causes a highly characteristic syndrome of *pure motor hemiplegia* involving the opposite face, arm, hand, leg, and foot in approximately equal measure. A lacune situated in the ventral pons causes an identical syndrome (Fig. 34-16). In both cases, the lacunar syndrome is identified as much by its signature deficits as by those features that are absent; aphasia, apraxia, agnosia, and visual field defect. Symptoms may be abrupt in onset or evolve over several hours, but in some instances the neurologic deficit evolves stepwise and relatively slowly, over as long a period as 2 to 3 days. Our experience has tended toward the shorter time frame, with most patients reporting that the full deficit is present not instantaneously but within minutes. Recovery, which may begin within hours, days, or weeks, is sometimes nearly complete even in the face of a severe initial stroke. However, many patients are left with some degree of clumsiness or slowness of movement of the affected side.

The motor disorder may take the form of a hemiparesis of the face and arm or arm and leg, or predominantly arm and proximal leg weakness; these fragmented patterns are indicative of a lesion located higher than the internal capsule, in the centrum semiovale. In these cases the stroke simulates an embolic stroke affecting the cortex.

A lacune of the lateral thalamus or (less often of the deep parietal white matter) is the cause of hemisensory defect involving the limbs, face, and trunk extending to the midline with no motor or language difficulty, a *pure sensory stroke*. Partial sensory syndromes involving only parts of the hemibody are less frequent than in motor lacunar strokes. The incidence, course, and outcome are much the same as in a pure hemiplegia.

As mentioned, in the ventral pons, the lacunar syndrome may be one of pure motor hemiplegia, mimicking that of internal capsular infarction except at times for relative sparing of the face and the presence of an ipsilateral paresis of conjugate gaze in some cases; or there is another highly characteristic lacunar syndrome of a combination of *dysarthria and clumsiness* of one hand. This "clumsy hand–dysarthria" stroke is usually located in the paramedian midpons on the side opposite the clumsy limb but a lacune in the posterior portion of the internal capsule on the side opposite the affected limb. Occasionally a lacunar infarction of the pons, midbrain, internal capsule, or parietal white matter gives rise to a *hemiparesis with ataxia* on the same side as the weakness (Fisher, 1965a; Sage and Lepore). Some of the brainstem syndromes may blend with basilar branch syndromes.

There are many other, less frequent, lacunar configurations but they can be identified by their similarity to one of the archetypal syndromes; they tend to affect one limited system or are fragments of a typical syndrome. Indeed, Fisher (1982) described 20 such variant types and several "miscellaneous" patterns. Some of these are difficult to accept, such as pure motor hemiparesis with confusion and loss of memory, but we have encountered many of the others, admittedly infrequently, including pure dysarthria, hemiballismus, virtual locked-in syndrome from bilateral lacunes in the base of the pons, and pure motor hemiplegia with sixth nerve palsy.

Some strokes that carry the term "lacune" are simply the result of larger deep cerebral infarctions along the lines of the striatocapsular stroke discussed earlier. In order to retain its clinical utility, the term lacune is probably best applied to small deep lesions that are the result of occlusion of a correspondingly small vessel and not to those strokes that result from occlusion of the orifices of several adjacent small vessels and are typically from larger atheromas in a parent vessel.

Multiple lacunar infarcts involving the corticospinal and corticobulbar tracts are a common cause of pseudobulbar palsy in clinical practice (trailed in frequency by amyotrophic lateral sclerosis and infiltrating tumors). Undoubtedly, an accumulation of lacunes deep in both hemispheres can give rise to gait disorders and also to mental dulling sometimes referred to as multiinfarct dementia (see further on and Chap. 21). The main differential diagnostic considerations are normal-pressure hydrocephalus (see Chap. 31) and the common degenerative brain conditions that affect the frontal lobes and basal ganglia (see Chap. 39).

Finally, it should be emphasized that what appears initially to be a lacunar syndrome may be the initial component or warning sign of a large deep territory infarction in the middle, posterior cerebral, or basilar arteries.

As mentioned earlier, MRI is more reliable than CT in demonstrating the lacunes. Initially, lacunes are seen on the MRI as deep oval or linear areas of T2, fluid-attenuated inversion recovery (FLAIR), and, especially, diffusion-weighted signal abnormality; later they become cavitated. Representative lacunar infarctions are shown in Fig. 34-16.The EEG, while little used for this purpose nowadays, may be helpful in a negative sense; in the case of lacunes in the pons or the internal capsule, there is a notable discrepancy between the unilateral paralysis or sensory loss and the negligible electrical changes over

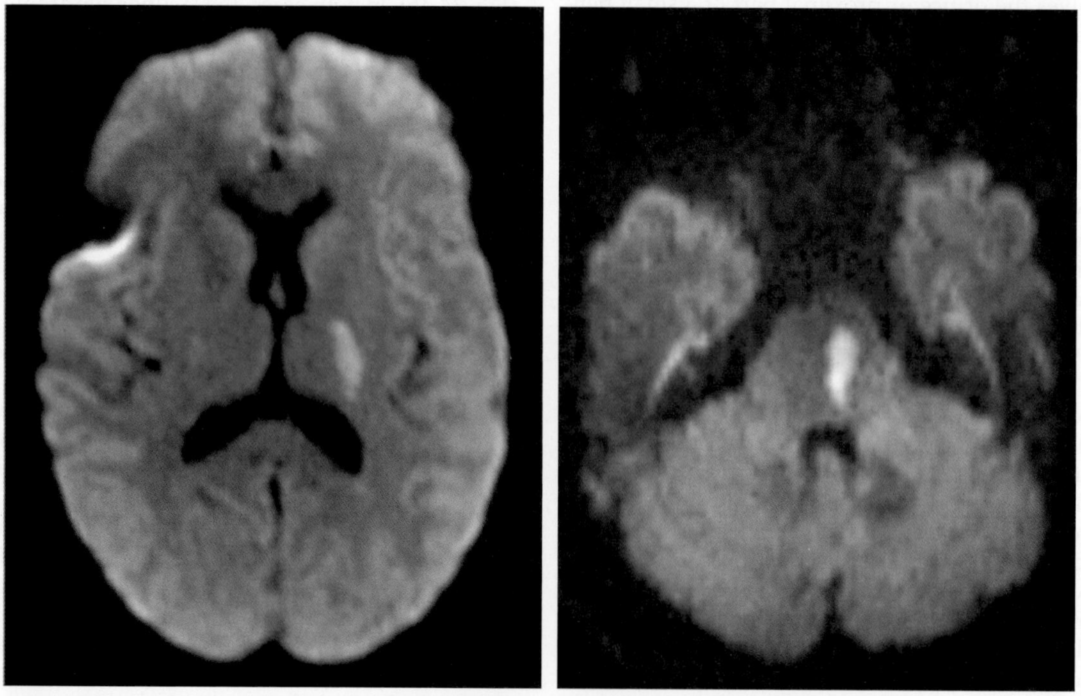

Figure 34-16. Axial diffusion-weighted MRI of acute lacunar infarctions. *A*. Left capsular infarction causing a right pure motor hemiplegia. *B*. Left pontine infarction causing a clumsy hand–dysarthria syndrome.

the affected hemisphere and, even with lacunes of the cerebrum, any EEG changes are disproportionately mild in comparison to the deficit.

TREATMENT OF ISCHEMIC STROKE

The main objective in these forms of ischemic cerebrovascular disease is the amelioration of the existing deficit and the prevention of future stroke. It is now a major goal of general medicine to reduce the incidence of stroke in the general population by the control of modifiable risk factors ("primary prevention"). In addition to reduction of known risk factors such as hypertension, smoking, and glucose control in diabetics, the widespread use of cholesterol-lowering statin medications has been shown in some studies to reduce the primary incidence of and recurrence of stroke. The treatment of stroke may be divided into three parts: management in the acute phase by measures to restore the circulation and arrest the pathologic process, physical therapy and rehabilitation, and measures to prevent further strokes and progression of vascular disease.

Management in the Acute Phase

The relative advantages of placing the seriously ill acute stroke patient in a special "stroke" unit have been the subject of much study. The outcome in these patients in terms of morbidity and mortality is improved, although the differences have been small and difficult to document. However, this organizational plan has not been widely implemented and instead protocols for rapid evaluation of stroke and the emergence of a specialty of stroke neurology have proliferated instead. If nothing else, this is the result of a general recognition that stroke, like myocardial infarction, requires special expertise and focus. Protocols to prevent excessive hypertension after thrombolytic treatment are best instituted in units that have staffing patterns that create familiarity with these and other protocols. As already emphasized, the prevention of aspiration and pneumonia is paramount by identifying those patients at risk. The patients at risk also benefit from systematic application of protocols. Also deserving attention is the prevention of venous thrombosis in the legs, pulmonary embolism, and coronary syndromes. Some units find it advisable to keep patients supine for the first hours or day after an ischemic stroke, mainly to prevent hypotension and cerebral hypoperfusion; this approach has not been studied systematically. When sitting and walking begin, special attention should be given to the maintenance of normal blood pressure.

Several studies have confirmed the high prevalence of new or enhanced levels of hypertension immediately following an ischemic stroke and its tendency to decline over subsequent days even without medications. The treatment of previously unappreciated hypertension is preferably deferred until the neurologic deficit has stabilized. As suggested by Britton and colleagues, it is prudent to avoid antihypertensive drugs in the first few days unless there is active myocardial ischemia or the blood pressure is high enough to pose a risk to other organs, particularly the kidneys, or there is a special risk of cerebral hemorrhage as a result of the use of thrombolytic drugs.

Measures to Restore the Circulation and Arrest the Pathologic Process

Efforts are directed at establishing a diagnosis of thrombotic stroke at the earliest possible stage and circumventing the full deficit by all means available without risking the safety of the patient. Even when the symptoms and signs have become static, some of the affected tissue may not be irreversibly damaged and will survive if perfusion can be reestablished (the penumbra). If the patient is under care within 4.5 h of onset of the first symptom and this time can be established with confidence, thrombolytic therapy with tissue plasminogen activator (tPA) is usually indicated. The contraindications and implementation of thrombolytic therapy is given in detail in the next section.

Intravenous Thrombolytic Agents

Tissue plasminogen activators (recombinant tPA) convert plasminogen to plasmin. These drugs are effective in the treatment of coronary artery occlusion (but are associated with a 1 percent risk of cerebral hemorrhage) and have a reasonably clear role in the treatment of acute ischemic stroke. As an alternative to the usual form of tPA, alteplase and tenecteplase are genetically engineered mutant form of plasminogen activators. In the following discussion, we use "tPA" to represent all of the tissue plasminogen activators.

The benchmark study organized by the National Institute of Neurological and Communicative Disorders and Stroke (see the NINCDS and Stroke rtPA Stroke Study Group in the references) has provided evidence of benefit later from *intravenous tPA* when patients were examined months later. Treatment within 3 h of the onset of symptoms led to a 30 percent increase in the number of patients who remained with little or no neurologic deficit when reexamined 3 months after the stroke; this benefit persisted when assessed 1 year later in the study by Kwiatkowski and associates. It is not easy to comprehend why the benefits extended to all types of ischemic strokes, including those caused by occlusion of small vessels (lacunes) and why improvement was not apparent in the days immediately following treatment, only at later times.

The tPA in the NIH study was administered in a dose of 0.9 mg/kg, 10 percent of which was given as an initial bolus, followed by an infusion of the remainder over 1 h. This has been adopted as a conventional approach in practice. A dose of 90 mg was not exceeded, this being lower than the dose used for myocardial infarction. The relative improvement in neurologic state came at the expense of a 6 percent risk of symptomatic cerebral hemorrhage, i.e., a far lower rate than in most previous studies but twice the expected rate without thrombolysis (some of the hemorrhages were into the area of infarction and did not cause symptomatic worsening). Patients were excluded from the study if they had massive infarctions (encompassing more than two-thirds of the territory of the middle cerebral artery), had high scores on a clinical stroke scale that was devised for the National Institutes of Health (NIH) study (available at: http://www.ninds.nih.gov/doctors/NIH_Stroke_Scale.pdf and from other sources) had uncontrolled hypertension, were more than 80 years of age, or had recently received anticoagulants (except aspirin). Further analysis of the NINCDS trial revealed that patients who were treated earliest within the 3-h time frame had more benefit than those treated later; indeed, the administration of tPA in the time period between 2.5 and 3 h after the stroke was of less value.

Attempts to establish that patients with a longer duration of ischemic symptoms benefit from tPA have varied in success but have favored an effect up to 4.5 h as noted below. In particular, a subgroup of patients with carotid–middle cerebral artery strokes of moderate severity did appear to benefit. In some patients with basilar artery occlusion and coma of brief duration and those without extensive thrombosis, prompt tPA treatment also resulted in an overall improvement in neurologic function, but there were numerous exceptions. Following from these findings, a randomized trial of over 800 patients receiving tPA between 3 and 4.5 h after the onset of symptoms demonstrated that 10 percent more achieved a good outcome if given the drug than placebo and, although more had cerebral hemorrhages, the overall mortality was the same in the treated and untreated groups (Hacke et al, 2008). This study has altered practice to extend the acceptable interval for drug administration to 4.5 h if proper care is taken to select low-risk patients and prevent excessive blood pressure after tPA is given. A summary of the sequence of clinical trials that have led to the current recommendations for the use of tPA in acute stroke has been reviewed by Wechsler. Taken from a summary by the American Heart Association are the generally agreed upon inclusion and exclusion criteria for the use of intravenous tPA in Table 34-6. Intracranial and systemic bleeding is, of course, the great concern but a minor but interesting point is that some patients, who had been receiving angiotensin-converting enzyme inhibitors for the treatment of hypertension, seem to display angioneurotic edema as a side effect of tPA.

Generally excluded are those in whom the deficit is either very small (e.g., hand affected only, dysarthria alone, minor aphasia) or, more importantly, is so large as to implicate almost the entire territory of the middle cerebral artery. Many centers have expanded their practices beyond the confines of the NIH study, treating patients older than age 80 years and some with large strokes. Attempts are currently being made to identify patients in whom there is a mismatch between regional cerebral perfusion and preservation of brain tissue (typically shown by the absence of restricted water diffusion on MRI), but several studies so far have failed to demonstrate that selection of patients on this basis improves clinical outcome. Also ambiguous is the treatment of patients with acute stroke in whom the referable cerebral vessels are entirely patent.

An apparently effective ancillary technique has been to supplement intravenously administered tPA with 2 h of continuously applied transcranial ultrasound aimed at the occluded vessel. According to Alexandrov and colleagues, complete recanalization of the middle cerebral artery or clinical recovery occurred within 2 h but the outcome at 3 months did not differ from those who did not receive ultrasound in part because other similar trials were terminated prematurely as a result of high rates of cerebral hemorrhage. The technique has not been adopted into general clinical work. At least one small trial has shown alteplase to be slightly superior to tPA in restoring vascular patency if certain technical features of maintained cerebral perfusion were used to select patients (see Parsons and coworkers).

Although a valid approach to acute stroke, the use of acute thrombolytic therapy depends on the early identification of an as yet limited group of patients who arrive under care well before the 4.5 h from the onset; therefore this therapy is applicable to only a proportion of patients who present to the emergency department soon after the first symptoms (approximately 10 percent in most surveys) or those who have strokes while under observation in the hospital. It is noteworthy that attempts to

Table 34-6

CRITERIA FOR THE USE OF INTRAVENOUS TPA IN ACUTE ISCHEMIC STROKE[a]

Inclusion criteria

- Acute ischemic stroke with measurable neurologic deficit
- Onset of symptoms less than 3 h before institution of treatment (all preliminary diagnostic tests must be completed)
- Onset of symptoms between 3 and 4.5 h and patient younger than 80 years, and with NIH stroke score below 25, nondiabetic, and having received no recent anticoagulant medication, regardless of INR[b]
- Age over 18 years

Exclusion criteria

- Cerebral imaging showing intracerebral hemorrhage
- Cerebral imaging demonstrating large infarction, >1/3 territory of a cerebral hemisphere (CT hypodensity or diffusion restriction on MRI)
- Head trauma within 3 months prior to stroke
- History of intracranial hemorrhage
- Elevated blood pressure; systolic >185 mm Hg or diastolic >110 mm Hg that has not responded to medications
- Active bleeding or arterial puncture at noncompressible site
- Hematologic alternations including
  - Platelet count <100,000/mm^3
  - Heparin administered within 48 h resulting in a PTT above normal range
  - Current use of anticoagulation with INR >1.7 or prothrombin time >15 s
- Blood glucose <50 mg/dL (2.7 mmol/L)

Relative contraindications

- Minor or resolving stroke
- Seizure at onset
- Major surgery or trauma within 14 days
- Gastrointestinal or urinary bleeding within 21 days
- Myocardial infarction within 3 months

[a]Adapted from 2010 American Heart Association Guidelines.
[b]Additional restrictions for the time period 3 to 4.5 h are taken from the European Cooperative Acute Stroke Study III (ECASS III); see Hacke, 2008.

reproduce the beneficial effects of tPA in a community setting have demonstrated deviations from treatment guidelines and an excess number of hemorrhages (Katzan et al). Nonetheless, acute intravenous thrombolysis that is managed by experienced individuals using validated protocols is an appropriate treatment for acute ischemic stroke. Public health education should increase the numbers of stroke patients who seek early attention and thus raise the proportion who are eligible for tPA treatment.

Intraarterial Thrombolysis

Thrombolytic substances injected intraarterially, or mechanical lysis for disruption or removal of an intravascular clot, can in some instances restore blood flow of the middle cerebral and basilar arteries. There is a high incidence of reocclusion of the treated vessel unless anticoagulants and stenting are also used. The most recent approaches involve one of a number of devices that retrieve clots from the intravascular lumen. Although early studies suggested that the results of intravascular clot lysis or removal were somewhat better than for intravenous or intraarterial thrombolysis, when more rigid criteria and trial design were applied, no such benefit has been shown.

In particular, three studies with different approaches to comparing these methods showed no clinical benefit for intraarterial means of restoring vascular patency in comparison to intravenous tPA (Broderick et al, and also Ciccone et al); and interventional methods were not superior when patients were selected on the basis of imaging patterns that demonstrated an area of ischemic tissue that was not yet infarcted (Kidwell and coworkers). Arguments notwithstanding that better mechanical devices will lead to improved outcomes, the results of systematic studies so far make it difficult to endorse intraarterial methods to revascularize cerebral vessels after acute stroke outside the confines of a clinical trial. The question of reversing the neurologic deficit from basilar artery thrombosis without cerebellar infarctions is nonetheless being studied.

Acute Surgical Revascularization

This refers to the opening of the carotid artery or an area of intracranial atherosclerosis immediately after a stroke with the intention of improving the clinical outcome; the issue of endarterectomy for the prevention of future strokes is another matter and is taken up in a later section. In past decades, there had been limited experience with immediate surgical removal of a clot from the carotid artery or the performance of a bypass to restore function. Ojemann and colleagues (1995) operated on 55 such patients as an emergency procedure; 26 of these had stenotic vessels and 29 acutely thrombosed vessels. Of the latter, circulation was restored in 21, with an excellent or good clinical result in 16. In 26 patients with stenotic carotid arteries, an excellent or good result was obtained in 19. Usually several hours will have elapsed before the diagnosis is established. If the interval is longer than 12 h, opening the occluded vessel is usually of little value and may present additional dangers. In any case, this approach has been largely supplanted by the above-described endovascular techniques. Reoperation because the vessel has closed or caused an embolus immediately after carotid endarterectomy is a special circumstance in which rapid removal of a clot or repair of an intimal tear is performed more or less routinely and is also mentioned in a later section. This subject is reviewed again further on.

The separate issue of the endovascular treatment of intracranial atherosclerosis is considered here for convenience. The risks of manipulating intracranial vessels are obvious, particularly those of the circle of Willis with no surrounding tissue because they are located within the subarachnoid space. In an attempt to determine if a stent and angioplasty would improve outcome in patients who had TIAs or minor strokes as a result of an intracranial stenosis, Chimowitz and colleagues (2011) reported that their trial was stopped early because of poor outcomes of the group who were treated by stent in comparison to medical management. The treatment of symptomatic intracranial atherosclerosis therefore remains problematic and is delegated to the antiplatelet drugs and lipid-lowering agents discussed further on.

Anticoagulation

Several considerations weigh in any discussion of the institution and choice of antiplatelet or anticoagulant treatment (meant here to denote the agents that alter the clotting cascade) for stroke. First is the distinction between anticoagulation to prevent the progression of an acute stroke and the prophylactic use of anticoagulation for the prevention of future strokes. The pivotal issue in prevention of further strokes is whether the stroke or TIA is atherothrombotic or cardioembolic. As discussed further on, several studies point conclusively to a role for anticoagulation in stroke due to certain cardioembolic sources, particularly atrial fibrillation, while the indications in atherothrombotic disease are less certain.

Heparin Treatment during an Acute Evolving Stroke Although not intuitive, if one holds the concept that a thrombus must form on an atherosclerotic plaque in order to cause stroke, it is apparent that anticoagulants have little effect at preventing the recurrence or progression of a thrombotic stroke and are certainly no more effective than agents that interfere with platelet aggregation. The two situations in which the immediate administration of heparin or an equivalent agent such as enoxaparin have drawn the most support from clinical practice are in basilar artery thrombosis with fluctuating deficits and in impending carotid artery occlusion from thrombosis or dissection. In these situations, the administration of heparin may be initiated while the nature of the illness is being clarified; the drug is then discontinued if contraindicated by new findings. Satisfactory clinical studies in support of this approach of acute anticoagulation have not been carried out and most authoritative writers find no evidence for the use of heparin in these situations (see, for example, Report of the Joint Stroke Guideline Development Committee authored by Coull et al). One fact seems fairly clear—that the administration of anticoagulants is not of great value once the stroke is fully developed.

Swanson has reviewed several trials evaluating heparin (including the International Stroke Trial and the TOAST study) and suggested that there was no net benefit from heparin in acute stroke because of an excess of cerebral hemorrhages. However, in these series there was a low incidence, estimated as 2 percent, of recurrent stroke in the first weeks after a cerebral infarction in the untreated groups. An early recurrent stroke rate this low almost precludes demonstrating a benefit from the use of heparin or heparinoid drugs. The issue of administering heparin in cases of recent cardioembolic cerebral infarction, particularly as a "bridge," while waiting for the effects of warfarin to be established is addressed further on.

In the event heparin is used, and assuming tPA has not been used in the preceding 24 h, heparin may be given intravenously, beginning with a bolus of 100 U/kg followed by a continuous drip (1,000 U/h) and adjusted according to the partial thromboplastin time (PTT). Bleeding into any organ may occur when the PTT is greater than 3 times the pretreatment level. When the PTT exceeds 100 s, it is preferable to discontinue the infusion, check the blood clotting values, and then reinstitute the infusion at a lower rate based on the test results (rather than simply lower the infusion rate). In circumstances of fluctuating basilar artery ischemia, it is our practice to permit higher values of PTT.

The use of low-molecular-weight heparin (enoxaparin or nadroparin) given subcutaneously within the first 48 h of the onset of symptoms have uncertain benefit. In a limited trial, there was no increase in the frequency of hemorrhagic transformation of the ischemic region when compared to placebo treatment (Kay et al). Because the outcome measures in this study were coarse (death or dependence 6 months after stroke), further investigations of this approach need to be carried out. We can only infer that the use of low-molecular-weight heparin (approximately 4,000 U subcutaneously, tid) appears to be safe but there is no compelling evidence supporting their use in acute ischemic stroke.

Warfarin for the Prevention of Recurrent Strokes from Atrial Fibrillation (see Table 34-3) The most convincing evidence favoring the efficacy of anticoagulants in the prevention of embolism comes from the Boston Area Anticoagulant Trial for Atrial Fibrillation. A group of patients at risk for stroke from chronic atrial fibrillation was randomized to be maintained for 2 years on warfarin (INR of 1.5 to 2) or no anticoagulation; there were 212 anticoagulated patients and 208 controls. Recurrent strokes were reduced by 86 percent in the warfarin group and the death rate was lower. One fatal hemorrhage occurred in each group; minor hemorrhages occurred in 38 of the warfarin-treated group and in 21 of the control group. In a similar study from Copenhagen, the incidence of stroke in a group receiving warfarin was calculated to be 2 percent per year in comparison to 5.5 percent per year in an untreated group. Several subsequent trials have attested to the efficacy of warfarin in the prevention of stroke in patients with nonrheumatic atrial fibrillation (see Singer). Subsequent studies suggest that an INR between 2 and 3 confers better protection than levels below 2. It should be pointed out, however, that patients younger than 65 years of age in these trials did not clearly benefit from long-term prophylactic anticoagulation unless there were additional cerebrovascular risk factors such as diabetes, hypertension, congestive heart failure, or cardiac valvular disease. Those younger than 65 years old and without such additional features (*lone fibrillators*), constituting about one-third of adults with atrial fibrillation, have a low risk of stroke. These observations are incorporated into the CHADS scores summarized in Table 34-3. Aspirin does not appear to afford the same degree of protective benefit as does anticoagulation, but some studies suggest a slightly better outcome than with no treatment; it has been used in the younger group of patients and in those unable to take warfarin.

Intracranial hemorrhage must be excluded by CT or MRI. A determination of prothrombin and partial thromboplastin activity is needed before therapy is started, but if this is not feasible, the initial doses of anticoagulant drugs can usually be given safely if there is no clinical evidence of bleeding anywhere in the body and there has been no recent surgery. Warfarin therapy, beginning with a dose of 5 to 10 mg daily, is relatively safe provided that the international normalized ratio (INR) is brought to 2 to 3 (formerly measured as a prothrombin time between 16 and 19 s) and the level is determined regularly (an approximate plan is once a day for the first 5 days, then 2 or 3 times a week for 1 to 2 weeks, and finally once every several weeks). Because there is no reliable evidence that complications are more frequent in the presence of mild to moderate hypertension if the INR is not allowed to exceed 2 to 3 times normal, we have not withheld anticoagulant therapy in these patients. However, when the blood pressure is greater than 220/120 mm Hg, an attempt is made to lower it gradually at the same time. Numerous drugs may alter the anticoagulant effects of the coumarins or add to the risk of bleeding—aspirin, cholestyramine, alcohol, carbamazepine, cephalosporin and quinolone antibiotics, sulfa drugs, and high-dosage penicillin being the most important ones. Hemorrhagic skin necrosis is a rare but dangerous complication. It is the result of a paradoxical microthrombosis of skin vessels and is liable to occur in patients with unsuspected deficiencies of endogenous clotting proteins (S and C). Although the disseminated form of skin necrosis occurs within days of initiating warfarin therapy, we have seen one patient with a form of this lesion following local skin injury after months on treatment.

For patients with atrial fibrillation of recent onset, an attempt should be made to restore normal sinus rhythm by the use of electrical cardioversion or a trial of antiarrhythmic drugs. If these fail, prophylactic anticoagulant therapy is recommended. Before attempting cardioversion of more long-standing atrial fibrillation anticoagulation for several days or longer is advisable to reduce emboli.

As noted below, opinions vary about the use and precise timing of instituting anticoagulation with warfarin after an embolic stroke, in part because the risk of recurrent stroke in the first days and weeks is low. In the past, there had been a theoretical risk of transient hypercoagulability when starting warfarin (on the basis of upregulation of protein S); this, and a desire to institute anticoagulation rapidly, led to a strategy of "bridging" with heparin or a low-molecular-weight heparin while awaiting the effects of warfarin to be evident. This risk has seemingly not had clinical significance. Therefore, on the basis of the aforementioned trials of acute anticoagulation that showed only a 1 to 2 percent frequency of early recurrent stroke, most clinicians have eschewed the "bridging" approach. The view that opposes heparin or a similar anticoagulant is based also on a retrospective study by Hallevi and colleagues, supported by a meta-analysis reported by Whiteley and coworkers, that found higher rates of symptomatic and serious bleeding in the brain or systemically with the bridging strategy.

In patients with very large cerebral infarcts that have a component of deep (basal ganglionic) tissue damage, especially in those patients who are also hypertensive, there may be a risk of anticoagulant-related hemorrhage into the acute infarct—"hemorrhagic conversion" (Shields et al). With the exception of urgent circumstances such as a mechanical heart valve that requires continuous anticoagulation, current practice has been to delay instituting warfarin when the stroke is large, a definition that is admittedly difficult to quantify—perhaps greater than half or a third of the territory of the middle cerebral artery supply. In these patients, anticoagulation therapy perhaps should be delayed for several weeks but even this is uncertain.

A frequent clinical problem arises in an elderly patient with atrial fibrillation who is at risk of falling from any of a number of causes including the stroke itself. In a review of selected administrative database records, Gage and colleagues concluded that the overall risk of inducing cerebral hemorrhage in older patients with atrial fibrillation treated with warfarin was lower than the risk of recurrent stroke. In those patients who had hemorrhages while receiving warfarin, they were, however, more likely to be fatal. Of course, decisions about anticoagulation must be tailored to the conditions of the individual patient. Alternatives to warfarin in patients with atrial fibrillation have been explored, such as the thrombin inhibitor ximelagatran, which has the advantage of not requiring monitoring by blood tests (see the Stroke Prevention Using an Oral Thrombin Inhibitor in Atrial Fibrillation [SPORTIF] trial).

Anticoagulant therapy may also be desirable for at least several weeks in patients with acute myocardial infarction, especially if the left side of the heart is involved. No guidelines have been established in these circumstances; the new common use of one or more platelet aggregation inhibitor drugs after myocardial infarction may preclude the concurrent use of warfarin. In cerebral embolism associated with bacterial endocarditis, anticoagulant therapy should be used cautiously because of the danger of intracranial bleeding, and one proceeds instead with antibiotics. Generally, we have not anticoagulated these patients.

Warfarin for the Prevention of Further Strokes in the Weeks and Months after a First Stroke Not due to Atrial Fibrillation Despite its established benefit in preventing embolic strokes from atrial fibrillation, whether warfarin is effective in preventing strokes in patients with TIAs or recent stroke that are not due to atrial fibrillation is a question that has never been answered satisfactorily. Decisions regarding this matter depend not only on the putative ability of warfarin to prevent stroke but on an assessment of the relative risk of causing cerebral or systemic hemorrhage. The problem that continues to plague all attempts to use long-term anticoagulants, as already noted in the discussion regarding heparin in the acute situation, is the risk of hemorrhage estimated by Whisnant and colleagues to be 5 percent overall and considerably higher in elderly patients who have been treated for more than 1 year.

There had been a notion that warfarin is of some value in the first 2 to 4 months following the onset of an ischemic stroke due to *atherosclerotic* disease. However, the results of controlled studies have indicated that there is no reason to favor warfarin in comparison to aspirin in cases of atherothrombotic stroke. This was amply shown in the Warfarin-Aspirin Recurrent Stroke Study (WARSS; not including cardioembolic stroke) reported by Mohr and colleagues (2001); over 2 years the recurrent stroke rate was about 16 percent in both groups, and, surprisingly, the rate of cerebral hemorrhage was similar (near 2 percent). Similarly, for the special case of TIA or stroke that is shown to be because of intracranial atherosclerosis, Chimowitz and colleagues in the Warfarin-Aspirin Symptomatic Intracranial Disease (WASID) trial have suggested that warfarin provided no benefit over aspirin in preventing subsequent cerebrovascular events but warfarin had more risk as commented below. The WASID trial exposed not so much the deficiency of warfarin in prevention of stroke as much as the difficulties in its use, as pointed out by Koroshetz.

In contrast to the situation with atherothrombotic disease, warfarin is still used by some clinicians for prevention of a second stroke in *cardioembolic* disease. This applies more specifically to instances of a demonstrated source for the embolus in the cardiac chambers, valves, or through a patent foramen ovale as well as atrial fibrillation discussed earlier. The larger number of "*cryptogenic strokes*," many of which may nevertheless be cardioembolic, cannot be confidently treated with warfarin. Of course, the extent of the evaluation to establish that an embolic stroke may have its origin in the heart, determines the likelihood of delineating a stroke as cryptogenic. In particular, several studies have shown that prolonged heart rhythm monitoring (event monitors) for up to 30 days moderately increases the rate of detection of atrial fibrilation. This creates a conundrum for the clinician confronted with a patient with an otherwise unexplained embolic stroke. There is therefore some latitude in deciding on treatment to prevent stroke in the subsequent months: none, aspirin (see below), or warfarin, as older studies had suggested. The issue of delaying anticoagulation after a large ischemic stroke was discussed in the preceding section.

The justification for, and excess risk of hemorrhage, when combining an antiplatelet agent with warfarin, has not been quantified. There seems to be relatively small risk if low-dose (81 mg) aspirin is included in a regimen of warfarin for atrial fibrillation. Beyond this statement, little can be said with authority but our personal experience, certainly tainted by the weaknesses engendered by the availability heuristic, is that subdural hematomas abound in elderly patients, with or without falls, who are on one or more agents. Even the relatively rapid reversal of anticoagulation with vitamin K and one of the clotting factor preparations or fresh plasma do little more than allow for safer surgery to remove intracerebral clots. Certain conditions such as chronic renal failure may confer a greater risk of cerebral hemorrhage with either drug, but the stroke risk from atrial fibrillation is also increased in comparison to patients with normal renal function as described in the epidemiologic study by Olesen and colleagues.

The introduction of factor Xa inhibitors has offered an alternative to the vitamin K antagonist, warfarin, for reducing strokes in patients with atrial fibrillation. In one study by Granger and coworkers that introduced apixaban for this purpose, there were slightly fewer strokes and fewer cerebral hemorrhages than with warfarin when the intended goal with warfarin was to keep the INR between 2 and 3. Dabigatran and rivaroxaban confer similar reductions in stroke to apixaban and warfarin (c.f., Patel et al). These drugs have the advantage over warfarin of not requiring regular blood tests for the measurement of the INR and of having fewer drug interactions. However, although they have short half-lives compared to warfarin, they are still present for many hours after discontinuation and anticoagulation is not easily reversible should there be systemic or cerebral bleeding.

Any type of serious bleeding with warfarin, even if not a result of overdosage, justifies immediate administration of fresh-frozen plasma and large doses of vitamin K. An INR above 5 in a patient who must remain anticoagulated—for example, one with a prosthetic heart valve—may be corrected with small doses of vitamin K (0.5 to 2 mg), preferably given intravenously.

Thus, it would appear that with long-term administration of warfarin, except in certain circumstances—such as a severely stenotic cerebral vessel, atrial fibrillation, prosthetic heart valve, and certain blood disorders—the risk of hemorrhage outweighs the benefit from prevention of stroke.

Antiplatelet Drugs

Aspirin has proved to be the most consistently useful drug in the prevention of thrombotic and possibly, embolic strokes. One currently favored approach, based in part on the above-mentioned WARSS trial, is to simply administer aspirin in all cases of acute stroke (except perhaps if tPA has been used). This approach is further endorsed by the WASID trial comparing aspirin (1,300 mg/d) to warfarin for treatment of intracranial arterial stenosis on the basis that warfarin was no better at preventing strokes while aspirin was associated with fewer gastrointestinal hemorrhages and a lower overall death rate. Confirmation of this approach was given by the IST and CAST trials that established a modest reduction in mortality and stroke recurrence if aspirin was given within 48 h of stroke.

The acetyl moiety of aspirin combines with the platelet membrane and inhibits platelet cyclooxygenase, thus preventing the production of thromboxane A_2, a vasoconstricting prostaglandin, and also prostacyclin, a vasodilating prostaglandin. In patients who cannot tolerate aspirin, the platelet aggregate inhibitor clopidogrel or a similar drug (such as *ticlopidine* or *dipyridamole*) can be substituted (see below).

A number of controlled studies have attested to the therapeutic value of aspirin and ticlopidine, clopidogrel, or dipyridamole in stroke prevention (not acute treatment as discussed above), but it is important not to exaggerate the magnitude of their effects. With few exceptions, it can be concluded that aspirin is beneficial in preventing stroke; whether low doses (50 to 100 mg) and high doses (1,000 to 1,500 mg) provide equivalent protection is still uncertain.

From a review of several studies, it appears that both dosages are effective and that the addition of dipyridamole further reduces the risk of stroke by a small amount. Ticlopidine and clopidogrel are considered, on the basis of clinical trials, to be equivalent to or marginally more effective than aspirin for the prevention of stroke but they are more expensive. Furthermore, both drugs are potentially toxic; ticlopidine may produce neutropenia and clopidogrel may cause thrombotic thrombocytopenic purpura. Dipyridamole in high doses has not been as well tolerated by many of our patients because of dizziness induced by peripheral vasodilatation.

The combined use of these antiplatelet drugs with aspirin has generally been slightly superior to aspirin alone in secondary stroke prevention, but with an increased risk of cerebral hemorrhage in some studies. In most large trials, the incremental benefits of adding one of these drugs to aspirin has been of the order of 1 to 3 percent (see the ESPRIT study and Bhatt et al and Sacco et al, a trial that failed to show benefit for the addition of extended release of dipyridamole to aspirin). A recent study with over 5,000 patients from China, the CHANCE trial reported by Wang and coworkers, did demonstrate a reduction in stroke recurrence during the first 90 days after the first minor stroke or TIA by adding clopidogrel to aspirin, either 75 mg or 300 mg, and no increase in cerebral hemorrhages. All that can be said at the moment is that the use of dual antiplatelet function agents may confer slight benefit over aspirin alone after a stroke but we remain wary of the potential risks.

In trials comparing aspirin to anticoagulation for stroke prevention in atrial fibrillation, anticoagulation has still been superior (see ACTIVE Writing Group). These studies notwithstanding, the therapeutic effectiveness of aspirin is still rather slight and the addition of clopidogrel to aspirin in patients who were not deemed suitable for warfarin reduces strokes over several years of observation but increases the risk of major bleeding so that the combination cannot be endorsed (ACTIVE Investigators). Moreover, in each of the trials, a significant number of subsequent ischemic strokes occurred in patients while they were receiving aspirin.

The best course of treatment for patients who have lacunar or atherothrombotic strokes while already receiving antiplatelet medications is not clear. Switching to warfarin from antiplatelet agents is sensible in some circumstances but should be done with caution. Control of blood pressure and the administration of a lipid-lowering drug are advisable, even if lipid levels are normal. In the most comprehensive study of statins to date, the institution of high doses of drug reduced the incidence of subsequent stroke after a TIA or first stroke by 2 percent over 5 years (see Stroke Prevention by Aggressive Reduction in Cholesterol Investigators [SPARCL trial]). This was at the expense of a slight increase in the other large studies that have not shown this effect with lower doses of statin drugs. Whether this is adequate to adapt into routine practice is unclear to us.

Other Forms of Medical Treatment

In the past, treatment by hemodilution was popularized by the studies of Wood and Fleischer, who showed a high incidence of short-term improvement when the hematocrit was reduced to approximately 33 percent. That lowering blood viscosity improves regional blood flow in the heart had been known for some time, and a similar effect on the brain has been demonstrated by CBF studies. Earlier observations had shown a reduction in the overall neurologic deficit, but almost all larger randomized trials—which included patients in many settings who were treated at various times up to 48 h after stroke—failed to confirm any such benefit, and the use of this treatment has been virtually abandoned. While this treatment cannot be recommended as a routine approach, it may have some merit in selected situations, such as fluctuating stroke. Therapies aimed at improving blood flow by enhancing cardiac output (aminophylline, pressor agents), by improving the microcirculation (mannitol, glycerol, dextran), or by use of a large number of vasodilating drugs (see below) have failed to show consistent benefits, but several are still under study. Normobaric and hyperbaric oxygen may reduce ischemic deficits temporarily but have no sustained effect. Induced hypothermia limits the size of ischemic stroke, but it is technically difficult to administer and often has serious side effects.

Calcium channel blockers of the types administered for cardiac disease have also been found to increase CBF and to reduce lactic acidosis in stroke patients. However, several multicenter clinical trials that compared calcium channel blockers with placebo did not establish a difference in outcome in the two groups. There has also been interest, as noted earlier in this chapter, in drugs that inhibit excitatory amino acid transmitters and free-radical scavengers such as dimethyl sulfoxide (DMSO) and growth factors, but so far none of these has been successfully applied to humans.

Despite some experimental evidence that certain vasodilators, such as CO_2 and papaverine, increase CBF, none has proved beneficial in carefully studied human stroke cases at the stage of TIAs, thrombosis in evolution, or established stroke. Vasodilators may actually be harmful, at least on theoretical grounds, because by lowering the systemic blood pressure or dilating vessels in normal brain tissue (the autoregulatory mechanisms are lost in vessels within the infarct); they may reduce the intracranial anastomotic flow. Moreover, the vessels in the margin of the infarct (border zone) are already maximally dilated. New discoveries regarding the role of nitric oxide in vascular control will probably give rise to new pharmacologic agents that will require evaluation. The metabolic stresses of ischemia and the production of destructive oxygen-free radicals were referred to earlier. Among the numerous "brain-sparing" agents that have been tried in an attempt to reduce the size of infarction, certain ones have had erratic results in large randomized trials. Two recent trials, for example, gave initially promising results and later proved ineffective (Shuaib et al). These agents were of interest because they can be administered up to several hours after the stroke (continuing for 72 h). So far, the results of neuroprotective agents in stroke have been discouraging.

Closure of Patent Foramen Ovale (PFO)

The role of the patent foramen ovale as a cause of stroke that is otherwise cryptogenic, has been a matter of contention for three decades. Certainly in some instances, such as a young individual who has demonstrable clots in the venous system of the legs or pelvis or who has had a recent pulmonary embolism, this mechanism becomes an appealing explanation. As mentioned earlier in the chapter, several epidemiologic and other studies have demonstrated a statistical association between strokes in the presence of a PFO. In other studies of older patients, however, the presence of a patent foramen did not increase the risk of stroke or TIA. It has also been a matter of some contention whether the size of the cardiac defect or the presence of an associated atrial septal aneurysm raise the risk of stroke. Even in younger patients, simply the discovery of a PFO with the use of echocardiography and injection of agitated saline or similar method that highlights the potential for movement of material from the right into the left atrium is not nearly proof of a causative mechanism. Our practice has been to perform noninvasive studies in younger patients with a PFO in order to determine if there are clots present, and in younger women, to consider imaging procedures of the pelvic veins.

Even if a putative relationship between cryptogenic stroke and PFO were established, it has been difficult to demonstrate that closing the defect provides protection against further strokes. Moreover, the value of anticoagulation, either alone or in comparison to closure of the PFO, has been uncertain. Two studies, one by Furlan and associates and the other by Meier and coworkers, have shown that closure of a PFO in a patient had a stroke, does not provide benefit, at least for 2 to 4 years after the procedure. It is instructive from both of these studies that the rate of recurrent stroke was close to 1 to 2 percent per year in both the groups who had a procedure to close the defect and those who were treated with either warfarin or aspirin. Although neither trial was designed to settle the question of which form of medical treatment was superior, at least over the short duration of these studies, the results were similar. At this time, closure of the PFO is recommended only as a component of a clinical trial and the clinician is left with limited direction regarding the need for, and type of, anticoagulation. There may be instances in which repeated strokes, coupled with known thrombi in lower extremity or pelvic veins, coupled with a sizable PFO might justify the procedure.

Treatment of Infarctive Brain Swelling and Raised Intracranial Pressure (See also Chap. 35)

In the first few days following massive cerebral infarction, brain edema of the necrotic tissue may threaten life. Most often this occurs with a complete infarction in the territory of the middle cerebral artery, i.e., encompassing the deep and distal vascular territory. Some degree of mass effect may be evident on a CT in the first 24 h. Additional infarction in the territory of the anterior cerebral artery (total carotid occlusion) worsens the situation. Clinical deterioration occurs usually on the third to fifth days, sometimes later, but may rarely evolve as quickly as several hours after the onset (Fig. 34-17). The clinical indicators of worsening—drowsiness, a fixed (but not necessarily enlarged) pupil, a Babinski sign on the side of the infarction (on the preserved side of the body), and changes in breathing pattern, as well as characteristic imaging signs—are all a result of secondary tissue shifts, as described in Chaps. 17 and 30 and are detailed in the studies of Hacke and colleagues (1996), and Ropper and Shafran. Frank has shown that clinical deterioration is not always associated with an initial elevation of intracranial pressure (ICP). It is not clear if it is advisable, in selected cases, to measure the ICP directly before embarking on an aggressive medical regimen to lower the pressure.

Intravenous mannitol in doses of 1 g/kg, then 50 g every 2 or 3 h, may forestall further deterioration, but most of these patients, once comatose, are likely to die unless drastic measures are taken. In such instances, controlled hyperventilation may be useful as a temporizing maneuver. Corticosteroids are probably of little value; several trials have failed to demonstrate their efficacy.

In the past several years there has been interest in *hemicraniectomy* as a means of reducing the mass effect and intracranial pressure in these extreme circumstances. One favored approach has been to perform hemicraniectomy fairly early in the course of brain swelling, in the first 2 or 3 days, when the patient is drowsy but before coma supervenes. A pooled analysis of three randomized trials based on this premise has been given by Vahedi and colleagues. Excluding patients older than age 60 years, a total of 93 patients who were not fully alert could be analyzed. A large advantage in survival was found favoring the group operated within 48 h. There has been controversy regarding the functional status of survivors and this involves the matter of the desirability of patients remaining with modified Rankin scale scores of 4, meaning they are dependent on others for their personal care. A more carefully controlled trial conducted in patients over age 60 has confirmed a beneficial effect of hemicraniectomy in preventing death from brain swelling after stroke. However, not surprisingly, the proportion of survivors with good functional outcomes in this older group was not as high as for younger patients.

Our recent practice has been to wait for signs of deterioration, generally leading to operation on fewer than half of patients with large MCA territory strokes and, generally having operations from the third through fifth days. The family must understand the risks involved and the likelihood that the stroke deficits will persist so that approximately a third of surviving patients will be dependent for care. Hemicraniectomy combined with an overlying duraplasty is then undertaken if the patient is progressing from a stuporous state to coma and imaging studies show increasing mass effect. Whether anterior temporal lobectomy is of added benefit is not known, but it is now infrequently included. The value of surgical decompression has not been limited to patients with right-hemispheric strokes; those with initially limited

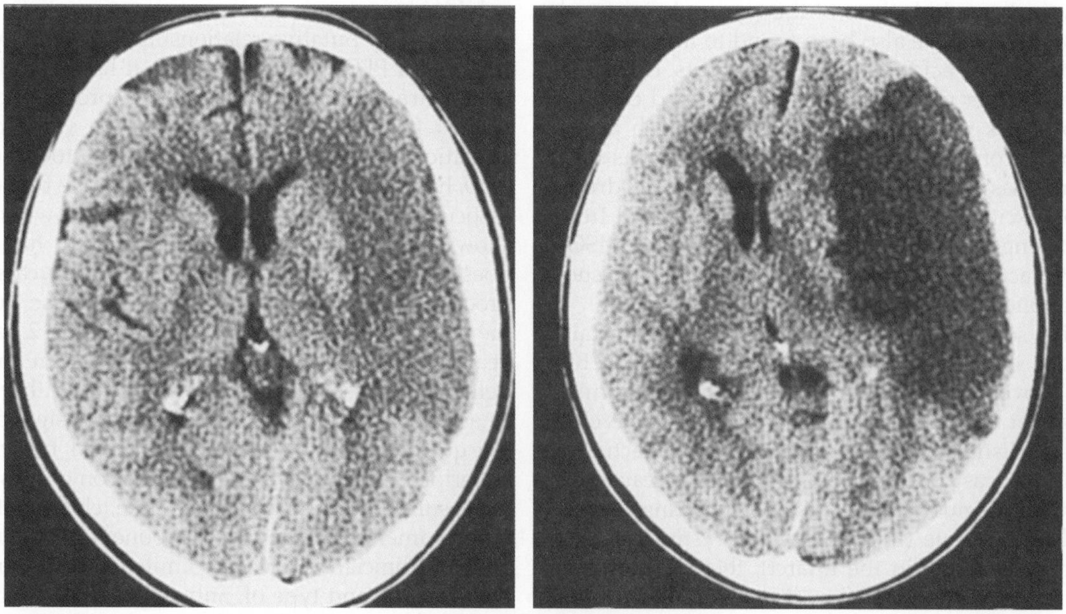

Figure 34-17. Large ischemic infarction of the left cerebral hemisphere mainly in the distribution of the superior division of the middle cerebral artery. CT at 24 h (*left*) and 72 h (*right*) following the onset of stroke symptoms. The second scan (*right*) demonstrates marked swelling of the infarcted tissue and rightward displacement of central structures.

degrees of aphasia may also be appropriate candidates. After a protracted period of coma with bilaterally enlarged pupils or with evidence that the midbrain has been irrevocably damaged, the procedure may be futile.

In the special case of large *cerebellar infarctions*, usually from occlusion of a vertebral artery, swelling may compress the lower brainstem within hours or days. This complication carries the risk of sudden respiratory arrest. Cerebellar swelling may occur with or without an associated lateral medullary stroke and the situation is comparable to medullary compression caused by cerebellar hemorrhage. Hydrocephalus usually develops as a prelude to deterioration and is manifest as drowsiness and stupor, increased tone in the legs, and Babinski signs; other sentinel signs of compression of the brainstem are gaze paresis, sixth nerve palsy, or hemiparesis ipsilateral to the ataxia (Kanis and Ropper). It is at times difficult to differentiate the effects of increasing hydrocephalus from those of brainstem infarction from thrombus propagation in the basilar artery (Lehrich et al). Surgical decompression of the infarcted and swollen tissue should be undertaken almost as soon as cerebellar edema becomes clinically apparent by the emergence of hydrocephalus or brainstem signs, as further swelling can be anticipated. A brief period of observation before committing to surgery is not unreasonable if the fourth ventricle and peribrainstem cisterns are open and the patient is awake. Mannitol may be used to prepare the patient for surgery or if a period of observation is anticipated but its value is not clear. As in the case of cerebellar hemorrhage, ventricular drainage alone is usually inadequate and, in any case, is unnecessary if the pressure is relieved by hemicraniectomy and resection of infarcted tissue.

Carotid Artery Stenosis

Comments have already been made concerning the opening of an occluded carotid artery soon after a stroke. Here we discuss the patient who has had TIAs or who has passed the acute period of stroke, when surgery is considered to be safer. The region that most often lends itself to such therapy is the carotid sinus (the bulbous expansion of the internal carotid artery just above its origin from the common carotid). Other sites suitable for surgical management include the common carotid, innominate, and subclavian arteries. Operation on the vertebral artery at its origin has proved successful only in exceptional circumstances. In recent years, balloon angioplasty and stenting of the carotid artery have become increasingly popular as an alternative to surgery (see below).

Surgery and angioplasty, in our opinion, are as yet applicable mainly to the group of patients with *symptomatic* carotid artery stenosis (the asymptomatic ones are discussed below) who have substantial extracranial stenosis but not complete occlusion, and, in special instances, in those with nonstenotic ulcerated plaques. Those with stenosis constitute less than 20 percent of all patients with TIAs (Marshall); but from the perspective of surgical therapy, the term *symptomatic* encompasses both TIAs and large or small strokes ipsilateral to the stenosis, some of which may be evident only with cerebral imaging. There is evidence that well-executed surgery in appropriately chosen cases arrests the TIAs and diminishes the risk of future strokes. These views received strong affirmation from two often-cited randomized studies—the North American Symptomatic Carotid Endarterectomy Trial (NASCET) and the European Carotid Surgery Trial (ECST). The conclusion reached in each of these studies was that carotid endarterectomy for symptomatic lesions causing degrees of stenosis greater than 70 to 80 percent in diameter reduces the incidence of ipsilateral hemispheral strokes and shows greater benefit with increasing degrees of stenosis. These two trials differed in the method of estimating the degree of stenosis, but when adjustments are made, the results are comparable (Donnan et al, 1998). Further analysis of the North American trial by Gasecki and colleagues indicated that the risk of cerebral infarction on the side of the symptomatic stenosis is increased if there is a contralateral carotid stenosis but that operated patients (on the side of symptomatic stenosis) still had fewer strokes than those treated with medication alone. In those with bilateral carotid disease, the risk of stroke after 2 years was 69 percent, and if operated, 22 percent.

As to the timing of endarterectomy, opinions have diverged but a metaanalysis reported by Rothwell and colleagues (2004) has suggested that the maximum benefit is accrued if surgery is performed within 2 weeks of a TIA or minor stroke.

In the final analysis, the relative benefits of surgery or medical treatment (anticoagulation or aspirin) depend mainly on the actual surgical risk—i.e., on the record of an individual surgeon. If there is an established operative complication rate of less than 3 percent, then surgery can be recommended in symptomatic patients with carotid stenosis greater than 70 percent. This benefit extends to elderly patients and, indeed, it has been shown on a statistical basis to be most evident in patients older than age 75 (see the post hoc analysis of NASCET data by Alamowitch et al).

Before operation or angioplasty, the existence of the carotid lesion and its extent must be determined. Conventional arteriography, the procedure that yields the best images and most accurate measurements of the residual lumen, carries a small risk of worsening the stroke or producing new focal signs though this notion has never been documented systematically. CTA and MRA have emerged as a surrogate that well demonstrates the carotid bulb and carries only the risk of renal damage from dye infusion (Fig. 34-18). Severe stenosis is also indirectly reflected in angiography by the filling of the distal branches of the external carotid artery before the branches of the middle cerebral artery are opacified—a reversal of the usual filling pattern. Increasingly, the diagnosis of carotid stenosis is being initially made by less invasive methods, but with ultrasonography and magnetic resonance arteriography there is some difficulty in quantifying severe stenosis and in separating it from complete carotid artery occlusion. If the patient is in good medical condition, has normal vessels on the contralateral side, and has normal cardiac function (no heart failure, uncontrolled angina, or recent infarction), symptomatic lesions with greater than 70 percent stenosis, roughly corresponding to a residual luminal diameter

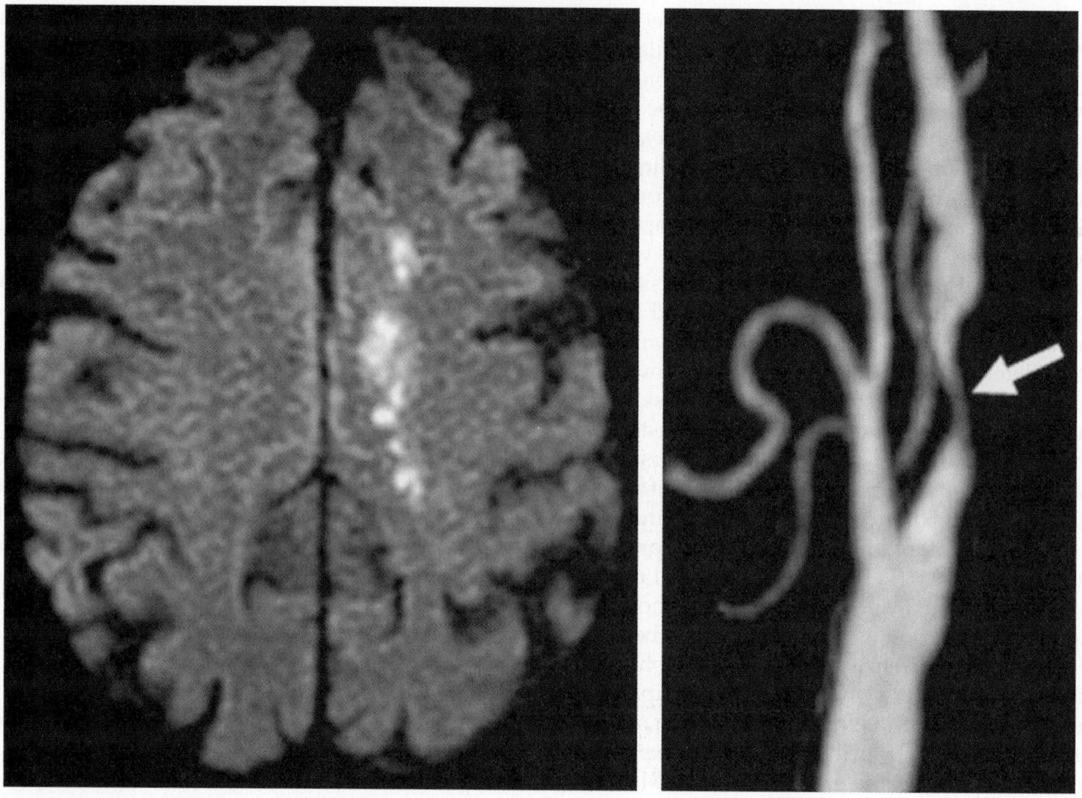

A B

Figure 34-18. *A.* Axial diffusion-weighted MRI showing multifocal acute infarctions in the left ACA-MCA arterial border zone. *B.* Magnetic resonance angiography displays severe stenosis of the left internal carotid artery (*arrow*), just above the common carotid artery bifurcation.

of less than 2 mm, can usually be dealt with safely by endarterectomy.

Carotid angioplasty and stenting were mentioned earlier. The role of this approach in clinical practice in comparison to endarterectomy has been recently clarified. Stenting offers an alternative for the patient who is too ill to undergo surgery. Direct comparisons have been made in several organized studies. In one early trial reported by the CAVATAS investigators (Carotid and Vertebral Artery Transluminal Angioplasty Study), the incidence of minor (nonstroke) complications was lower in patients who had angioplasty and stenting. Also, a higher proportion of patients undergoing angioplasty had restenosis. Otherwise, the recurrent stroke rates were similar, 10 percent for both groups. A useful comparison between angioplasty and surgical endarterectomy has been made in the trial reported by Mas and associates (2006) and in the "SPACE" trial. While the first of these favored a surgical approach for severe symptomatic stenosis, the second gave equivalent results of approximately 6 percent combined stroke and death rates with either procedure.

Endarterectomy, in a small number of cases may be followed by a *new hemiplegia or aphasia that becomes evident in the hours after the procedure*, usually by the time the patient arrives in the recovery room. In these cases, surgeons prefer to return the patient to the operating room and open the artery, as discussed earlier on. An intimal flap at the distal end of the endarterectomy and varying amounts of fresh clot proximal to it are usually encountered; but after removal and repair of the vessel, the effects of the stroke, if one has occurred, are not usually improved. The postoperative care of carotid endarterectomy focuses on reversing reflex hypotension that is induced by exposing the carotid wall to high perfusion pressure. This phenomenon can be reduced by infiltrating the carotid sinus with anesthetic prior to the operation. An uncommon but rather striking *hyperperfusion syndrome* develops several days to a week after carotid endarterectomy. The features are headache, focal deficits, seizures, brain edema, or cerebral hemorrhage. These are thought to reflect autoregulatory failure of the cerebral vasculature in the face of abrupt restoration of normal blood pressure and perfusion. After a long period of autoregulatory compensation for a stenotic carotid artery, then a normal cerebral perfusion pressure may result in endothelial incompetence with leakage of water across the blood–brain barrier. Unilateral severe headache is the most common symptom and may be the only manifestation. On occasion, cerebral edema is so massive as to lead to death (Breen et al). Treatment is by control of hypertension; it is unclear whether antiepileptic medications are required if there has been a seizure as a component of the syndrome. We mention here that an identical syndrome of focal cerebral deficits and brain edema, perhaps with the exception of seizures, has been seen, rarely and with no explanation, in migraineurs, including two patients under our care.

For intracranial internal carotid occlusion that extends into the siphon and distally, a transcranial (superficial temporal–middle cerebral) anastomosis had been employed in the past. Although this operation is technically feasible, its therapeutic value has been questioned by the multicenter study of Barnett and collaborators (1985), who found that it did not produce a reduction in TIAs, strokes, or deaths. That study was criticized for having a skewed patient selection and several smaller and uncontrolled trials have suggested that the procedure may benefit some patients. There may be particular circumstances that justify its use; for example, when there are ongoing TIAs in relation to upright posture or with episodes of mild hypotension. Bypass procedures and their derivatives such as temporal-pial synangiosis may be useful in reestablishing flow to a hemisphere when there has been progressive intracranial carotid stenosis. Testament to the success of the bypass procedure is the regression of symptoms and of the network of collateral vessels in moyamoya disease (see further on).

Asymptomatic Carotid Stenosis

Finally, there is the problem of the asymptomatic bruit over a carotid artery or incidentally discovered carotid artery stenosis. A bruit generally corresponds to the reduction in luminal diameter of the artery to 2 mm or less and, while found in a large proportion of patients with severe stenosis, it is not specific and is heard in up to 10 percent of older patients who have little or no stenosis. The population studies by Heyman and associates over 30 years ago shed some light on this. They found, not surprisingly, that cervical bruits in men constituted a risk for death from ischemic heart disease, and that the presence of asymptomatic bruits in men (but not in women) carried a slightly increased risk of stroke. Notably, the subsequent stroke often did not usually coincide in its angioanatomic locus and laterality with the cervical bruit so that asymptomatic stenosis is in the short term a general marker for atherosclerosis more so than for a proximate stroke. Other investigators have reported similar findings. On the other hand, Wiebers and colleagues (1990) found that patients with asymptomatic carotid bruits who were followed for 5 years were approximately three times more likely to have ischemic strokes than an age- and sex-matched population sample without carotid bruits.

The appropriate step when a carotid bruit is found during a routine examination is probably to obtain ultrasonography in order to quantify the presence of and degree of stenosis and to make subsequent decisions cautiously based on the studies discussed below. We usually also obtain imaging of the brain to determine if there has been a stroke on the side of the carotid disease—this aids in decisions regarding therapy. A note is made here regarding the *self-audible bruit*, which occasionally indicates carotid stenosis, dissection, or fibromuscular dysplasia, but is usually of less consequence and in some instances is associated with an enlarged and superiorly located jugular bulb—a benign anatomic variant that can be discerned on CT (Adler and Ropper).

Many attempts have been made to clarify the role of surgically correcting asymptomatic carotid stenosis by means of endarterectomy. The Asymptomatic Carotid Atherosclerotic Study (ACAS), as reported by its Executive Committee, found that the frequency of strokes could be reduced from 11 percent to 5 percent over 5 years by removing the plaque if there was a stenosis greater than 60 percent (in diameter). These conclusions have been tempered by a reanalysis of the ACAS data, in which almost half of the strokes were of lacunar or cardioembolic (Inzitari et al). Data from a European trial, encompassing 3,120 patients (MRC Asymptomatic Carotid Surgery Trial [ACST] Collaborative Group), have indicated that asymptomatic carotid stenosis of more than 70 percent carries a 2 percent annual risk of stroke over a 5-year period and that the risk is reduced to 1 percent with endarterectomy. It was concluded that endarterectomy may be justified for asymptomatic carotid stenosis of this degree in men (not so in women) but that an audited surgical risk below 3 percent was required to obtain favorable results (just as for symptomatic carotid stenosis). However, all of these trials were conducted before the ubiquitous use of statin drugs, which seemingly stabilize carotid plaques. Several trials comparing endarterectomy to stenting, some of which were commented on earlier, included asymptomatic patients but there were too few on which to base conclusions.

From these and other trials it can be inferred that endarterectomy does not reduce the incidence of strokes in patients who have asymptomatic carotid stenosis with luminal narrowing that is less than 60 to 70 percent of normal diameter. For those with greater degrees of stenosis, the benefits are slight and apply predominantly to men. It is not clear if the presence of an ulcerated plaque or heavy calcification alters this view but it probably does not. These comments also apply to patients with asymptomatic carotid stenosis who are about to undergo major surgery such as cardiac bypass grafting, but adequate studies in this circumstance have not been performed. As already noted, any advice should be tempered by the surgical risk in a particular institution. Our usual practice with asymptomatic cases has been to reevaluate the lumen of the internal carotid artery (using ultrasonography) at 6- to 12-month intervals. If the stenosis is advancing and becomes narrowed to about 2 mm or less, or if there is an event that could be construed as a TIA referable to the stenotic side, then surgery is considered. In the case of an asymptomatic but progressive stenosis, statin agents, accompanied by smoking cessation, aspirin therapy, and glucose control where applicable, are a reasonable alternative approach.

These comments reflect the guidelines for carotid endarterectomy set forth by the American Heart Association as reported by Moore and colleagues (1995) but there must be a careful evaluation of the circumstances in each patient and a recognition that residual lumen diameters and percent stenoses are measured in different ways by varying techniques, both in the above-described studies and in clinical practice.

Course and Prognosis of Ischemic Stroke

It is a fair statement that no rules have yet been formulated that allow prediction of the early or late course of stroke. A mild paralysis may become a disastrous hemiplegia or the patient's condition may worsen only temporarily. In cases of basilar artery occlusion, dizziness and dysphagia may progress in a few days to total paralysis and deep coma. Or, in both cases, the deficit may completely resolve. Anticoagulation and thrombolytic therapy may alter the course as discussed further on, but cerebral thrombosis is so often progressive that a cautious attitude on the part of the physician in what first appears to be a mild stroke is usually justified, at least for the first day.

During the period 1970–1974 in Rochester, Minnesota, 94 percent of patients with ischemic strokes survived for 5 days and 84 percent for 1 month (Garraway et al, 1983a and b). The *survival rate* was 54 percent at 3 years and 40 percent at 7 years. These were significantly greater than had been the case during the period 1965–1969. These figures, which were gathered retrospectively, are comparable to more recent ones reported by Bamford and colleagues from patients who had strokes in the 1980s. The mortality rate following cerebral infarcts (no separation being made between thrombotic and embolic types) at the end of 1 month was 19 percent and at the end of 1 year, 23 percent. Of the survivors, 65 percent were capable of an independent existence. In every series, among long-term survivors, heart disease is a more frequent cause of death than additional strokes. It has been repeatedly pointed out that pneumonia as a result of faulty swallowing is a major determinant of survival; further discussion regarding aspiration problems following stroke are found in later sections of the chapter.

Several other circumstances influence the *early prognosis* in cerebral infarction. In the case of very large infarcts in the middle cerebral artery territory, swelling of the infarcted tissue may occur, followed by displacement of central structures, transtentorial herniation, and death of the patient after several days. This can at times be anticipated by the sheer volume of the infarct and is usually evident on the CT or MRI scan within a day of the stroke. Smaller infarcts of the inferior surface of the cerebellum may also cause a fatal herniation into the foramen magnum. Milder degrees of swelling and increased intracranial pressure in both of the above-cited cases may progress slightly for 2 to 3 days but do not prove fatal. (See earlier under "Treatment of Infarctive Brain Swelling and Raised Intracranial Pressure.")

In extensive brainstem infarction associated with deep coma caused by basilar artery occlusion, the early mortality rate approaches 40 percent. In any type of stroke, if coma or stupor is present from the beginning, survival is largely determined by success in keeping the airway clear, controlling brain swelling, preventing aspiration pneumonia, and maintaining fluid and electrolyte balance, as described further on. With smaller thrombotic infarcts, the mortality is 3 to 6 percent, much of it from myocardial infarction and aspiration pneumonia.

As for the *eventual prognosis* of the neurologic deficits, some improvement is the rule if the patient survives. The patient with a lacunar infarct usually fares well but may take months to improve to the maximum extent. With other small infarcts, recovery may start within a day or two, and restoration may be complete or nearly complete within a week. In cases of severe deficit, there may be little significant recovery; after months of assiduous efforts at rehabilitation, the patient may remain bereft of speech and understanding, with the upper extremity still useless and the lower extremity serving only as an uncertain prop during attempts to walk. Between these two extremes there is every gradation of recovery. Measurement of central motor conduction by magnetic stimulation has been predictive of recovery but is not widely used for clinical work. If clinical recovery does not begin in 1 or 2 weeks, the outlook is poor for both motor and language functions. Constructional apraxia, uninhibited anger (with left and rarely with right temporal lesions), nonsensical logorrhea and placidity, unawareness of the paralysis and neglect (with nondominant parietal lesions), and confusion and delirium (with nondominant temporal lesions) all tend to diminish and may disappear within a few weeks. A hemianopia that has not cleared in a few weeks will usually be permanent, although reading and color discrimination may continue to improve. In lateral medullary infarction, difficulty in swallowing may be protracted, lasting 4 to 8 weeks or longer, yet relatively normal function is finally restored in nearly every instance. Aphasia, dysarthria, cerebellar ataxia, and walking may improve for a year or longer, but for all practical purposes it may be said that whatever motor and language deficits remain after 5 to 6 months will be permanent.

Characteristically, the paralyzed muscles are flaccid in the first days or weeks following a stroke; the tendon reflexes are usually unchanged but may be slightly increased or decreased. Gradually spasticity develops, and the tendon reflexes become brisker. The arm tends to assume a flexed adducted posture and the leg an extended one. Function is rarely if ever restored after the slow evolution of spasticity; however, the use of botulinum toxin may help considerably in relieving the spasticity. Conversely, the early development of spasticity in the arm or the early appearance of a grasp reflex may presage a favorable outcome. In some patients with extensive temporoparietal lesions, the hemiplegia remains flaccid; the arm dangles and the slack leg must be braced to stand. The physiologic explanation of this remains obscure. If the internal capsule is not interrupted completely in a stroke that involves the lenticular nucleus or thalamus, the paralysis may give way to hemichoreoathetosis, hemitremor, or hemiataxia, depending on the particular anatomy of the lesion. Bowel and bladder control usually returns; sphincteric disorders persist in only a few cases. Physical therapy should be initiated early in order to prevent pseudocontracture of muscles and capsulitis at the shoulder, elbow, wrist, knuckles, knee, and ankle. These are frequent complications and often a source of pain and added disability, particularly of the shoulder. Occasionally, atrophy of bone and pain in the hand may accompany the shoulder pain (shoulder–hand syndrome). An annoying dizziness and unsteadiness often persists after damage to the vestibular system in brainstem infarcts.

Seizures are a relatively uncommon sequel of thrombotic strokes in comparison to embolic cortical infarcts, which are followed by seizures in up to 10 percent of patients. Most often in our experience, the EEG in these cases had never normalized and showed sharp activity over the region of the infarct even many months after the stroke (see further on for advice on the treatment of seizures after stroke).

Many patients complain of fatigability and are depressed, possibly more so after strokes that involve the left frontal lobe (Starkstein et al); other studies implicate an infarct on either side of the brain. The explanation of these symptoms is uncertain; some are certainly expressions of a reactive depression. Several small series have suggested that prophylactic treatment with antidepressants reduce the incidence of depression as described in the review by Chen and colleagues, but the routine administration of these medications has not found its way into general practice. Only a few patients develop serious behavior problems or are psychotic after a stroke, but paranoid trends, confusion, stubbornness, and peevishness may appear, or an apathetic state ensues. Large lesions affect concentration as well as synthetic and executive mental functions in rough proportion to their size; these mental changes are independent of any disturbances in language function.

When multiple infarcts occur over a period of months or years, special types of dementia and gait failure may develop. In some, the major lesions involve the white matter and spare, relatively, the cortex and basal ganglia; the lesions may be lacunar or larger infarctions. This disorder, referred to as arteriosclerosis dementia and *Binswanger subcortical leukoencephalopathy*, probably represents the accumulation of multiple white matter infarcts and lacunes (see further on and the papers by Mohr and Mast and by Babikian and Ropper). The white matter that is destroyed tends to lie in the border zones between the penetrating cortical and basal ganglionic arteries. Large patches of subcortical myelin loss and gliosis, in combination with small cortical and subcortical infarcts, are evident with brain imaging. This process and the histologically similar but biologically unique inherited condition of white matter termed *CADASIL (cerebral autosomal dominant arteriopathy with subcortical infarct and leukoencephalopathy)* are discussed further on.

Physical Therapy and Rehabilitation

In all but the most seriously ill patients, beginning within a few days of the stroke the paralyzed limbs ideally should be carried through a full range of passive movement several times a day. The purpose is to avoid contracture (and capsulitis), especially at the shoulder, elbow, hip, and ankle. Soreness and aching in the paralyzed limbs should not be allowed to interfere with exercises to the extent possible. Patients should be moved from bed to chair as soon as the stroke is completed and blood pressure is stable. Prophylaxis for deep venous thrombosis with compression boots or anticoagulation is appropriate if the patient cannot be mobilized. An assessment for swallowing difficulty should be made early during recovery and dietary adjustments on the insertion of a nasogastric tube made if there is a risk of aspiration. Nearly all hemiplegic patients regain the ability to walk to some extent, usually within a 3- to 6-month period, and this should be a primary aim in rehabilitation. The presence of deep sensory loss or anosognosia in addition to hemiplegia, are the main limiting factors. A short or long leg brace is often required. By teaching patients with cerebellar ataxia new strategies, balance and gait disorders can be made less disabling. As motor function improves and if mentality is preserved, instruction in the activities of daily living and the use of various special devices can help the patient become at least partly independent at home. Whatever little research is available on the effectiveness of stroke rehabilitation suggests that a greater intensity of physical therapy does indeed achieve better scores on some measures of walking ability and dexterity. In a randomized trial, Kwakkel and colleagues achieved these results by applying an additional 30 min per day beyond conventional physical therapy of focused treatments to the leg or arm, 5 days per week, for 20 weeks. Other studies have demonstrated clearly the undesirable effects of immobilizing a limb in a splint after a stroke.

Experimental work in monkeys and limited data from patients suggest that improvement can be obtained by restraining the normal limb and forcing use of the sound limb. In a randomized trial, Wolf and colleagues (2006) were able to demonstrate a benefit from this form of *"constraint therapy"* by forcing the patient to wear a mitt on the good hand while engaging in persistent exercises with the hemiplegic limb for more than 90 percent of their waking time through 2 weeks. This may reflect functional expansion of the cortical motor representation into adjacent undamaged cortical areas, indicating the potential for some degree of reorganization that corresponds to clinical recovery. A related approach, *"mirror therapy"* confronts the patient with a mirror that creates an illusion of moving the paretic side when the good side is activated. The Cochrane metaanalysis of 14 such studies indicates a modest benefit in motor recovery and a more prominent benefit for relief of pain and quality of life improvement (Thieme and colleagues).

The neural substrates of improvement after stroke are just beginning to be studied. Considerable clinical experience and physiologic data such as those reported by Luft and colleagues have demonstrated that the injured brain has some degree of plasticity; remodeling of brain tissue and reorganization of neural function may occur with training even months after large strokes.

Speech and language therapy is particularly valuable in identifying the risk of aspiration as noted above. Specific therapy should be given in appropriate cases and certainly improves the morale of the patient and family. Further comments on the value of such treatments can be found in Chap. 23.

Secondary Preventive Measures

Because the primary objective in the treatment of atherothrombotic disease is prevention, efforts to control the risk factors must continue after stroke. The carotid vessels, being readily accessible, may be examined for the presence of a bruit; the latter often indicates a stenosis, although not all stenoses cause a bruit and many bruits heard are transmitted sounds from a stenotic aortic valve.

Ultrasonography, CT, or MRA examination of the cervical and intracranial vessels is justified in almost all patients with TIAs and ischemic stroke. The management of patients with asymptomatic carotid bruits has been considered above.

For patients who have had a stroke from atherothrombotic disease, preventive measures include the following: (1) aspirin, which reduces the risk of second stroke slightly, but its effect, as already noted, is modest (see earlier under "Antiplatelet Drugs"); (2) administration of any required antihypertensive agents but with caution in the first days after ischemic stroke; (3) administration of cholesterol-lowering drugs as commented below; (4) smoking cessation; and (5) during future general surgical procedures, maintenance of systemic blood pressure and oxygenation, especially in elderly patients. Regarding the appropriate dose of aspirin, a consensus has been that 50 to 100 mg is adequate as a preventative measure (typically 81 mg in the United States) and that higher doses do not offer additional benefit. Many patients are taking the higher dose levels for peripheral or coronary artery disease.

The issue of "aspirin resistance" has not been resolved but it can be stated that no laboratory test has been devised to accurately predict the clinical effects of aspirin dose. "Aspirin failure" on the other hand, refers to continued TIAs or strokes while on low doses of the medication. It has not been established that changing to a higher dose level is the correct course of action; many clinicians do so and others instead add a second antiplatelet agent or switch to another drug.

There may be additional but modest value in administering high doses of statin drugs even in patients with normal cholesterol levels who have had an atherothrombotic stroke. A large study mentioned earlier, the Stroke Prevention by Aggressive Reduction in Cholesterol Levels (SPARCL) trial, has shown that secondary stroke prevention is possible in patients with TIA or stroke in the prior 6 months with the use of high-dose atorvastatin (80 mg) but the magnitude of benefit was small (approximately 3 percent). The trial included mainly patients whose LDL cholesterol levels were modestly elevated. The clinician should be mindful of the risk of a statin-induced myopathy, and it is not known if lower doses of medication have the same preventative effect. Consistent with some other trials using statins, there was a slight increase in the number of hemorrhages in the treated group compared to the placebo group. The higher rate of cerebral hemorrhage in this study, however, contrast with at least one other large secondary prevention trial (the Heart Protection Collaborative Study) that used simvastatin at lower doses.

GENERALIZED BRAIN ISCHEMIA AND HYPOXIA (See also Chap. 40)

This constitutes a special type of infarction that follows cardiac arrest and other forms of prolonged hypotension or hypoxia. The most typical configuration, seen with imaging, is of widespread cortical infarction affecting also the deep nuclei, i.e., the most metabolically active regions of the cerebral hemispheres. In the case of reduced blood flow to the cerebral hemispheres, there is a tendency for regional infarctions to occur in the areas of lowest blood flow that lie between the major surface arteries, referred to metaphorically as a watershed infarction. An important distinction is drawn between the concept of end-arterial distribution, the site of distal embolization, and the area of lowest flow between two or more end territories, which is compromised in any form of globally returned blood flow. In extreme cases of hypotension, there is global infarction of the brain accompanied by the clinical syndrome of brain death.

Pure hypoxia-anoxia without hypotension produces another type of damage in areas susceptible to reduced oxygen delivery, mainly affecting the hippocampi; a Korsakoff syndrome results. Most often, ischemic and hypoxic states coexist and produce complex patterns of cerebral damage. This topic is discussed fully in Chap. 40. The special problem of cerebral ischemia during cardiac surgery with the use of a bypass pump is discussed further on in the section "Stroke With Cardiac Surgery."

LESS-COMMON CAUSES OF ISCHEMIC CEREBROVASCULAR DISEASE

Fibromuscular Dysplasia

This is a segmental, nonatheromatous, noninflammatory arterial disease of unknown etiology, almost exclusively in women. It is uncommon (0.5 percent of 61,000 arteriograms in the series of So et al) but is being reported with increasing frequency because of improved arteriographic techniques. In our experience, it has often been an incidental finding in asymptomatic individuals undergoing vascular imaging for other reasons. Approximately 10 percent of cases have been reported to be familial.

First described in the renal artery by Leadbetter and Burkland in 1938, fibromuscular dysplasia is now known to affect other vessels including cervicocerebral ones. The internal carotid artery is involved most frequently, followed by the vertebral and cerebral arteries. The radiologic picture is of a series of transverse constrictions, giving the appearance of an irregular string of beads or a tubular narrowing; it is observed bilaterally in 75 percent of cases. Usually only the extracranial part of the artery is involved. A single transverse web that occupies a portion of the carotid lumen is probably a variant of the fibromuscular condition or could conceivably represent an entirely different static congenital process. In the series of Houser and colleagues, 42 of 44 patients were women and 75 percent were older than 50 years of age. All of the patients reported by So and coworkers were women, ranging in age from 41 to 70 years. Cerebral ischemia may be associated with the process but the rate of this complication has not been established; our impression is that it is low. In the study by Corrin and colleagues, among 79 untreated asymptomatic patients followed for an average of 5 years, 3 had a cerebral infarct 4 to 18 years after the initial diagnosis. Also, between 7 and 20 percent of affected individuals are found to have intracranial saccular aneurysms (rarely a giant aneurysm), which may be sources of subarachnoid hemorrhage, and up to 12 percent develop arterial dissections, as described below.

The narrowed arterial segments show degeneration of elastic tissue and irregular arrays of fibrous and smooth muscle tissue in a mucous ground substance. Interspersed dilatations are a result of atrophy of the coat of the vessel wall. There is atherosclerosis in some and small degrees of arterial dissection in others. Usually vascular occlusion is not present, though there may be marked stenosis. Schievink and colleagues have summarized the pathology of this disease. In some instances the mechanism of the cerebral ischemic lesion is unexplained, but is presumed to be from thrombi in the pouches or in relation to intraluminal septa.

The disease is not amenable to endarterectomy. So and colleagues have recommended excision of the affected segments of the carotid artery if ischemic neurologic symptoms are related to them, and conservative therapy if the fibromuscular dysplasia is an incidental and asymptomatic arteriographic finding. It is now possible to dilate the affected vessel by means of endovascular techniques and several case reports have suggested that benefit is achieved at lower risk than with surgical excision. Intracranial saccular aneurysms, which may accompany this disease as noted above, should be sought by arteriography, CT, or MRA and obliterated if their size warrants. It is not known if anticoagulation or antiplatelet therapy confers protection from stroke.

Dissection of the Cervical and Intracranial Arteries

Internal Carotid Artery Dissection

It has long been appreciated that the process formerly known as Erdheim's medionecrosis aortica cystica, the main cause of aortic dissection, may independently involve or extend into the common carotid arteries, occluding them and causing massive infarction of the cerebral hemispheres. Examples of such occurrences were cited by Weisman and Adams in 1944 in their study of the neurology of dissecting aneurysms of the aorta, and Chase and colleagues gave the clinicopathologic details of 16 cases they studied. The principal neurologic features in both series were syncope, hemiparesis, or coma. The frequency of cerebral stroke with aortic dissection has varied from 10 to 50 percent and that of spinal stroke has been approximately 10 percent (see Chap. 44).

In more recent years, attention has been drawn to the occurrence of both spontaneous and traumatic dissection of the internal carotid artery, not necessarily associated intrinsic disease of the vessel walls, as an important cause of nonatherosclerotic stroke in young adults. Many large series of such cases have been reported in separate studies by Ojemann and colleagues (1972) and by Mokri and coworkers (1986). Although the disease is overrepresented in women, it occurs frequently in men, typically in their late thirties or early forties for either sex. It is a spontaneous event or arises in relation to a whiplash injury, bouts of violent coughing, or direct trauma to the head or neck, which need not be severe—e.g., being struck in the neck by a golf or tennis ball. We have encountered cases that occurred during pregnancy and immediately after delivery. Indeed, it is questionable if most cervical arterial dissections are truly "spontaneous," as many can be connected to some strenuous event but a relation to trauma is often only presumed. Three of our patients over the years had a carotid dissection that was manifest as a hemiplegia days after blunt head injury.

A small number of patients have fibromuscular disease as discussed above. The Ehlers-Danlos and Marfan syndromes, osteogenesis imperfecta, Loeys-Dietz syndrome (transforming growth factor [TGF]-β receptor mutation), and alpha$_1$-antitrypsin deficiency are also associated with an increased risk of vascular dissection. One of these conditions should be suspected if multiple extracranial vessels are involved in spontaneous dissections or if there is joint and skin laxity or widespread vascular tortuosity (neck and thoracic trauma or aortic arch dissection are more common causes of multiple extracranial dissections).

A few patients with carotid dissection have had preceding unilateral cranial or facial pain lasting days, followed by stroke in the territory of the internal carotid artery. The pain is aching, may fluctuate in severity, and is centered most often in and around the eye; less often, it is in the frontal or temporal regions, angle of the mandible, or high anterior neck over the carotid artery. Rapid and marked relief of the pain after the administration of corticosteroids in a young person may be a helpful diagnostic feature (see below). Neck pain over a site of dissection is usually present as well; however, it may be absent, particularly if the dissection originates near the base of the skull.

The ischemic manifestations consist of transient attacks in the territory of the internal carotid, followed frequently by the signs of hemispheral stroke, which may be abrupt or evolve smoothly over a period of minutes to hours or over several days in a fluctuating or stepwise fashion. A unilateral Horner syndrome is often present. A cervical bruit, sometimes audible to the patient, amaurosis fugax, faintness and syncope, and facial numbness are less common symptoms. Most of the patients described by Mokri and colleagues (1986) had one of two distinct syndromes: (1) unilateral headache associated with an ipsilateral Horner syndrome, essentially the Raeder syndrome, or (2) unilateral headache and delayed focal cerebral ischemic symptoms. One lesson is that a *painful Horner syndrome* is usually due to an underlying structural lesion. Some patients have evidence of involvement of one or more of the vagi, spinal accessory, or hypoglossal nerve on the side of a carotid dissection; these nerves lie in close proximity to the carotid artery and are nourished by small branches from it.

In most cases, dissection of the internal carotid artery can be detected by ultrasonography and confirmed by MRI and CTA, which show a double lumen (Fig. 34-19) within the vessel on axial MRI sections. Arteriography by any of these methods, including by conventional

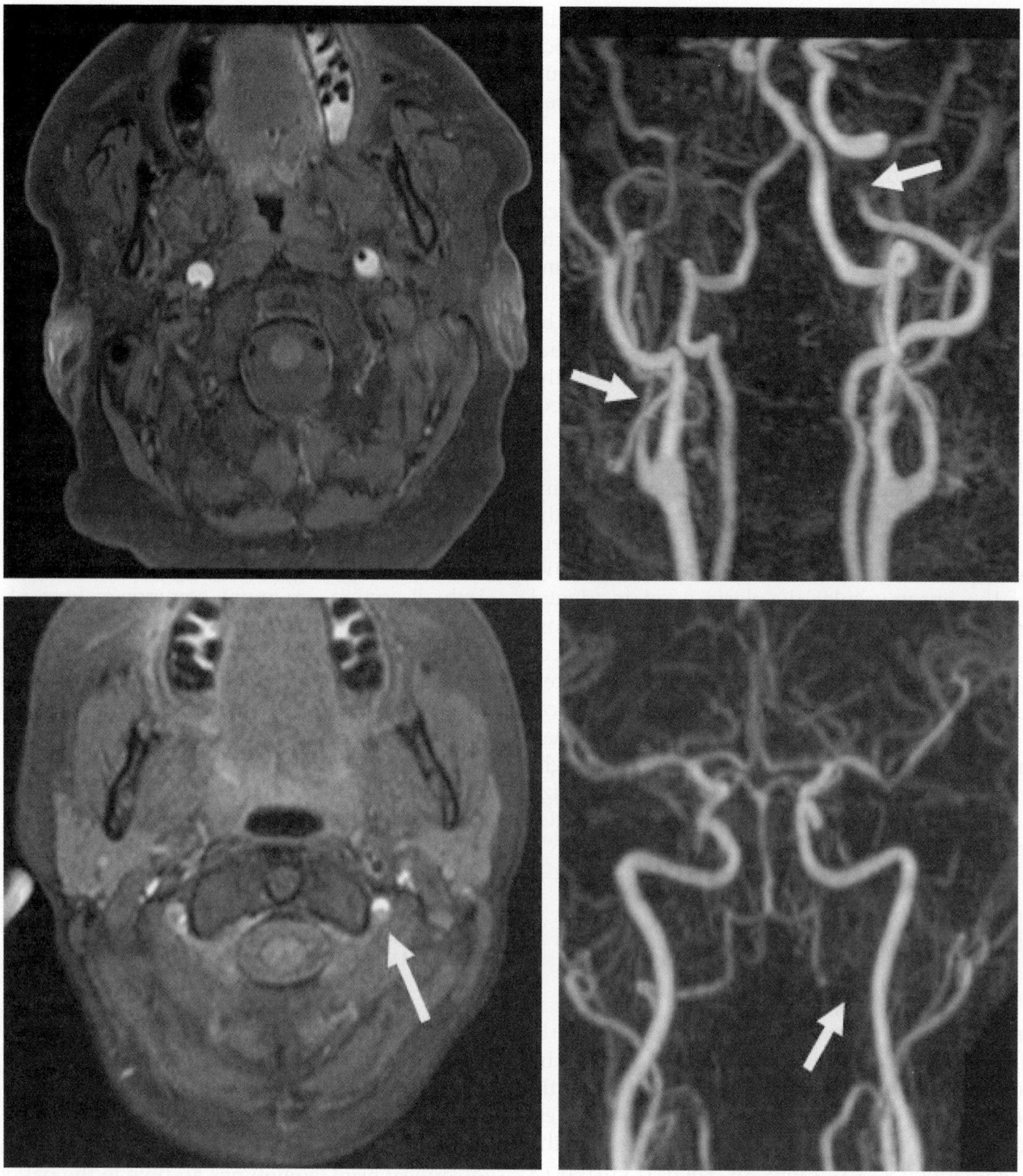

Figure 34-19. Cervical artery dissections. T1 MRI with fat saturation *(left)* and magnetic resonance angiography *(right)*. The upper images show bilateral internal carotid artery dissections *(arrows)*. The lower images show a left vertebral artery dissection *(arrows)*. The T1 hyperintensity that is shown in the left upper and lower images is due to thrombus within the false lumen of the vessel.

angiography usually reveals an elongated, but variable length, irregular narrow column of dye, usually beginning 1.5 to 3 cm above the carotid bifurcation and extending to the base of the skull, a picture that Fisher has called the *string sign*. There may be a characteristic tapered occlusion or an outpouching at the upper end of the string. It is the site and the shape of the occlusion that are helpful in identifying dissection. Less often the dissection is confined to the midcervical region, and occasionally it extends into the middle cerebral artery or involves the opposite carotid artery or the vertebral and basilar arteries.

The pathogenesis of spontaneous carotid dissection is at present uncertain. In most reported cases, cystic medial necrosis has not been found on microscopic examination of the involved artery. In some, there has been disorganization of the media and internal elastic lamina, but the specificity of these changes is in doubt, as Ojemann and colleagues (1972) noted similar changes in some of their control cases. In a small proportion of cases there are the changes of fibromuscular dysplasia, as noted earlier. Several groups have found structural collagen abnormalities in the skin biopsies of patients with dissection. A more thorough study of these vessels is needed.

Vertebral Artery Dissection

Dissection of these arteries may originate in the neck and extend into the intracranial portion of the vessel or remain isolated to either of these segments as noted below. In both instances there is a tendency to form pseudoaneurysms, mostly with the intracranial type, and in the latter there is a risk of rupture through the adventitia leading to a subarachnoid hemorrhage. Rapid and extreme rotational movement of the neck is the most common identifiable cause of vertebral artery dissection, as in turning the head to back up a car or with chiropractic manipulation. Extending the neck to have one's hair washed, swinging a golf club, and direct neck trauma have also been precipitants. Forceful coughing may also cause dissection, as it may in the carotid vessels. There is no clear female predominance (as there may be in carotid dissection) but the previously cited intrinsic weaknesses of the vascular wall from Ehlers-Danlos disease and fibromuscular dysplasia are risk factors.

The dissection most commonly originates in the C1-C2 segment of the vessel, where it is mobile but tethered as it leaves the transverse foramen of the axis and turns sharply to enter the cranium. The symptoms, mainly vertigo, are fragments of the lateral medullary syndrome, often with additional features referable to the pons or midbrain, particularly diplopia and dysarthria. The clinical manifestations in our experience have fluctuated over minutes and hours, quite unlike the usual vertebrobasilar TIA.

Less-common strokes include artery-to-artery embolism to the posterior cerebral territory or, a syndrome that has come to our attention several times in the past few years, a centrally placed infarction of the cervical spinal cord with bibrachial weakness, presumably from occlusion of the anterior spinal arteries. Another interesting but rare association with dissection has been the reversible cerebral vasoconstriction syndrome. Mawet and colleagues reported on 20 cases they extracted from their experience but could not determine which process occurred first and could only speculate as to the relationship. Dissection of the vertebral artery was a more common association with "RCVS" than was carotid artery dissection.

The diagnosis of vertebral dissection should be suspected if persistent occipitonuchal pain and vertigo or related medullary symptoms arise following one of the known precipitants—such as chiropractic manipulation of the neck, head trauma, or Valsalva straining or coughing activities—but it may otherwise escape detection until the full-blown medullary or cerebellar stroke is established. The stroke may follow the inciting event by several days or weeks or even longer, obscuring the relationship. Axial MRI images, particularly the T1-weighted sequences, show a double lumen in the dissected vessel, as described for carotid artery dissection earlier, and skillful ultrasound investigation documents the same. Some patients will be found to have evidence of spontaneous or traumatic dissection of multiple extracranial vessels; this also occurs as a consequence of dissection of the aortic arch from chest trauma.

No generally agreed upon method has been devised to detect the infrequent instance of subarachnoid hemorrhage from dissection. Lumbar puncture is not routinely performed. CT is probably adequate for this purpose but it must be acknowledged that it, too, is not often obtained, except in cases of strong suspicion that the dissection has extended into the subarachnoid space, as evidenced by lower cranial-nerve palsies.

Once a stroke has occurred, even though embolic in most cases, prompt reopening of the artery can at times prove beneficial; this is currently performed by endovascular techniques. Most neurologists take the approach that warfarin, if used, may be discontinued after several months or a year, when angiography or MRA shows the lumen of the carotid artery to be patent, or at least reduced to no more than 50 percent of the normal diameter, and smooth walled. Despite numerous publications demonstrating the ability of skilled operators to reopen a dissection by endovascular methods, acute intervention has not been studied in a way that allows a judgment regarding its value. Of both therapeutic and diagnostic value is the relief of pain afforded by corticosteroids in cervical and intracranial dissections, as mentioned earlier. Pseudoaneurysms in the cervical portions of the vessels generally do not require specific treatment; the series of 38 cases collected by Benninger and colleagues is instructive in that none of the aneurysms ruptured during several years of followup and one had a delayed ischemic strokes.

The study by Mokri and colleagues (1988) reported a complete or excellent recovery in 85 percent of patients with the angiographic signs of cervical artery dissection; mainly, these were patients who had fluctuating ischemic symptoms but without stroke. The outcome in cases complicated by stroke is far less benign. Approximately 25 percent of such patients succumb and most others remain seriously impaired. If early recanalization of the occluded artery is observed (as determined by ultrasonography), there may also be good functional recovery. Local pseudoaneurysms form in a small proportion of patients and generally do not require surgical repair; they also do not preclude cautious anticoagulation. Subarachnoid hemorrhage from transmural rupture is mostly a complication of vertebral artery dissection discussed below.

Intracranial Arterial Dissection

Dissections of intracranial arteries are less common than extracranial ones and they present in several unusual ways. A number of times we have misinterpreted the arteriographic appearance of a short segment of narrowing of the basilar or proximal middle cerebral arteries, assuming these changes to represent embolism or arteritis when in fact they proved to be dissections of the vessel wall. In the case of purely intracranial dissection of the middle cerebral or basilar arteries, there is usually no preceding trauma, but a few patients have had minor head injuries, extreme coughing, or other recently Valsalva-producing events (e.g., after childbirth)—or they had used cocaine. The typical picture is of fluctuating symptoms referable to the affected circulation and severe cranial pain on the side of the occlusion—retroorbital in the case of middle cerebral dissection, occipital in the case of basilar dissection, occipital combined with supraorbital in the case of vertebral dissection (see above). A few patients have had sudden strokes that suggested embolic infarction, and a small number present with subarachnoid hemorrhage.

Treatment of Cervical Artery Dissection

As an overall comment pertaining to dissection, treatment is primarily with anticoagulation for several weeks or months and followed up with some form of arteriography. The choice between aspirin and warfarin has not been clarified as the rate of stroke is low, in the range of 5 percent or less, and remains so with either agent (Georgiadis and colleagues); however, there have not been adequately controlled trials to determine if this is true for large groups of patients. If the dissection has produced complete occlusion of the vessel, the role of anticoagulation is less clear. Endovascular revascularization has been attempted with mixed results, the main problem being catastrophic and sometimes fatal vessel rupture during angioplasty. An issue pertaining to treatment is in establishing the presence of dissection into the subarachnoid space of the intracranial compartment. For carotid dissection, such extensions would seem to present a risk of subarachnoid hemorrhage if the lesion reaches beyond the cavernous sinus. Within the sinus, any bleeding would create a cavernous-carotid fistula, which is not usually fatal. In vertebral dissection, this question arises when the false lumen extends into the foramen magnum, beyond the dural entry of the vessel.

Although there are no data to determine the proper approach to anticoagulation in these circumstances that entail a risk of a subarachnoid hemorrhage, in general we do use heparin and warfarin for a brief period because of the greater concern for embolus, unless there is existing subarachnoid blood on a CT scan or if there is a pseudoaneurysm within the intracranial portion of the dissection (see Metso et al). Some stroke specialists have suggested that a lumbar puncture be performed before initiating anticoagulation but this has not been our practice.

Moyamoya Disease

Moyamoya is a Japanese word for a "haze," "puff of smoke"; it has been used to refer to an *extensive basal cerebral rete mirabile*—a network of small anastomotic vessels at the base of the brain around and distal to the circle of Willis, seen in carotid arteriograms, associated with segmental stenosis or occlusion of the terminal intracranial parts of both internal carotid arteries (Fig. 34-20). This form of cerebrovascular disease is predominant in,

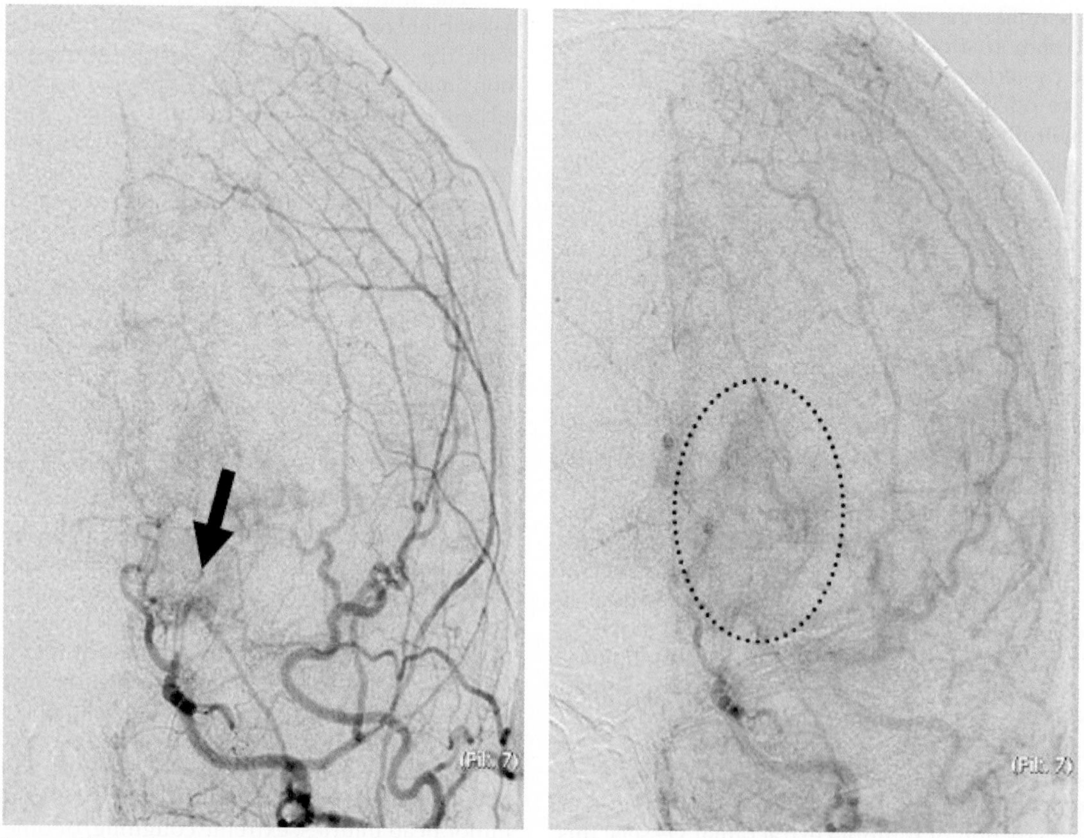

Figure 34-20. Moyamoya disease. Digital subtraction angiography in the coronal plane of the left common carotid artery. On the left image, there is occlusion of the left internal carotid artery near its terminus, and evidence of abnormal vascular proliferation involving the lenticulostriate vessels (*arrow*). The external carotid artery branches fill normally. The right image shows the same contrast injection during the early capillary phase; the characteristic "puff of smoke" is encircled.

but not limited to the Japanese. The authors have periodically observed such patients, as have others, in the United States, Western Europe, and Australia. Certain hemoglobinopathies, particularly sickle cell anemia, may cause a vasoocculsive condition equivalent to moyamoya disease, possibly because of sickling of red blood cells in the vasa vasorum of the supraclinoid carotid artery. An association between moyamoya, Down syndrome, and certain human leukocyte antigen (HLA) types favors a hereditary basis (Kitahara et al). A familial component has long been suspected but can be established in only 10 percent of cases, possibly in an autosomal dominant pattern with incomplete penetrance due to a site on chromosome 17q that has been implicated as one possible locus. Also, a rare condition in either Asians or Europeans of atherosclerotic occlusion of the distal intracranial carotid arteries can cause deep collateral vessels to enlarge and simulate moyamoya. In this way, moyamoya can be considered either a radiologic pattern or a disease process.

Nishimoto and Takeuchi reported on 111 cases that were selected on the basis of the two main radiologic criteria. The condition was observed mainly in infants, children, and adolescents (more than half the patients were younger than 10 years of age, and only 4 were older than age 40 years). All of their patients were Japanese, in whom the disease seems disproportionately prevalent; both males and females were affected, and 8 were siblings. The symptom that led to medical examination was usually a sudden weakness of an arm, leg, or both on one side. The symptoms tended to clear rapidly but recurred in some instances. Headache, convulsions, impaired mental clarity, visual disturbance, and nystagmus were less frequent. In older patients, subarachnoid hemorrhage was the most common initial manifestation. Other symptoms and signs were speech disturbance, sensory impairment, involuntary movements, and unsteady gait. Characteristics noted in other series have included prolonged TIAs (this accords with our experience), characteristically induced by hyperventilation or hyperthermia, parenchymal rather than subarachnoid hemorrhages (most situated in the basal ganglia or thalamus), and an unusual "rebuildup" EEG phenomenon in which high-voltage slow waves reappear 5 min after the end of hyperventilation.

Postmortem examinations of cases of moyamoya have yielded a reasonably clear picture of the intracranial distal carotid lesion. The adventitia, media, and internal elastic laminae of the stenotic or occluded arteries were normal, but the intima was greatly thickened by fibrous tissue. No inflammatory cells or atheromata were seen. In a few cases, hypoplasia of the vessel with absent muscularis has been described. The profuse rete mirabile consists of a fine network of vessels over the basal surface of the brain (in the pia-arachnoid), which, according to Yamashita and coworkers, reveals microaneurysm formation because of weakness of the internal elastic lamina and thinness of the vessel wall. The latter lesion is the source of subarachnoid hemorrhage. Thus one part of the symptomatology is traced to the distal carotid stenosis and another to the rupture of the vascular network. Opinion is divided as to whether the basal rete mirabile represents a congenital vascular malformation (i.e., a persistence of the embryonal network) or a rich collateral vascularization secondary to a congenital hypoplasia, acquired stenosis, or occlusion of the internal carotid arteries early in life.

Treatment The treatment of moyamoya is far from satisfactory. Certain surgical measures have been employed, including transplantation of a vascular muscle flap, omentum, or pedicle containing the superficial temporal artery to the pial surface of the frontal lobe temporal pial synangiosis with the idea of creating neovascularization of the cortical convexity. These measures have reportedly reduced the number of ischemic attacks, but whether they alter the natural history of the illness cannot be stated. Anticoagulation is considered risky in view of the possibility of cerebral hemorrhage, but there have not been systematic studies. The reader is referred to a contemporary review of the clinical features and surgical treatments by Scott and Smith.

Binswanger Disease

This entity was mentioned briefly in the discussion of the course and prognosis of atherothrombotic infarction and as a cause of dementia in Chaps. 21 and 39. The term has come to denote a widespread degeneration of cerebral white matter having a vascular causation and observed in the context of hypertension, atherosclerosis of the small blood vessels, and multiple strokes. Hemiparesis, dysarthria, TIAs, and typical lacunar or cortical strokes are admixed in many cases. The process has been associated with a particular radiologic appearance that reflects confluent areas of white matter signal change. The term *leukoaraiosis* describes the imaging appearance of hypointense periventricular tissues, presumably damaged by chronic ischemia. It is likely that leukoaraiosis exist in a continuum with Binswanger disease and many elderly individuals who have these changes show cognitive impairment as discussed below. Whether multiple discrete lacunes in the deep white matter constitute Binswanger disease may be a semantic issue, but we adhere to the notion that the former is characterized by a more widespread ischemic and gliotic change in the deep white matter.

Dementia, a pseudobulbar state, and a gait disorder, alone or in combination, are the main features of Binswanger cases. They have been attributed to the cumulative effects of the ischemic changes producing a white matter degeneration. It is likely that the pathologic basis of such a clinical entity is arteriolar sclerosis but surprisingly, as pointed out in Fisher's review, the lumens are open. Yet another problem is to distinguish such a state from deficits produced by the cumulative effect of numerous larger lacunes, which have for a century been known to cause the aforementioned syndromes of dementia, gait disturbance, and a pseudobulbar syndrome. From time to time, imaging studies of the brain disclose large regions of white matter change or the occurrence of multiple infarctions in the absence of hypertension, and it is not clear how such cases should be classified. Some prove to be areas of demyelination or metabolic dysmyelination;

others are mitochondrial disorders, and perhaps some are related to the familial CADASIL syndrome or Susac syndrome discussed below. Fabry disease also enters into the differential diagnosis of multiple small infarctions in the cerebrum that may coalesce into areas of white matter damage. Readers may consult the reviews on the subject by Babikian and Ropper, by Caplan (1995), and the mentioned review by CM Fisher.

Familial Subcortical Infarction (CADASIL and CARASIL)

A process with an imaging appearance of large confluent cerebral white matter changes, somewhat similar to Binswanger leukoencephalopathy, has been identified as an autosomal dominant familial trait linked in several families to a missense mutation on chromosome 19. In the past, it had been described under a number of names, including *hereditary multiinfarct dementia*. The acronym *CADASIL* (cerebral autosomal dominant arteriopathy with subcortical infarcts and leukoencephalopathy) is now applied. In these patients recurrent small strokes beginning in early adulthood culminate in a subcortical dementia (see Chap. 21). Migraine headaches, often with neurologic accompaniments, may precede the strokes by several years, as may numerous and varied TIAs that are attributed, probably incorrectly, to the migraine. On the other hand, some individuals display few clinical changes while yet others are demented or have strokes that simulate lacunes. We are unable to comment on the encephalopathy and coma accompanied by fever described by Schon and colleagues that has been attributed to this condition.

The familial nature of the process may not be appreciated because genetic penetrance is not complete until after 60 years of age. On MRI, clinically unaffected family members may show substantial changes in the white matter well before strokes or dementia arises (Fig. 34-21). A syndrome of early alopecia and lumbar spondylosis with the white matter changes typical of CADASIL has been identified as a recessively inherited disease (cerebral autosomal recessive arteriopathy with subcortical infarcts and leukoencephalopathy [CARASIL]) and is discussed separately below.

The MRI and CT appearance is of multiple confluent white matter lesions of various sizes, many quite small and concentrated around the basal ganglia and periventricular areas. Lesions anterior to the temporal horns of the lateral ventricles are particularly characteristic of the entity. When the affected regions are asymmetrical and periventricular, they are difficult to distinguish from the lesions of multiple sclerosis. In the autopsy cases studied by Jung and colleagues, numerous partially cavitated infarctions were found in the white matter and basal ganglia. Small vessels in the regions of these infarctions, 100- to 200-mm diameters, contained basophilic granular deposits in the media with degeneration of smooth muscle fibers. Attribution of the white matter lesions to these vascular changes presents the same problems as in Binswanger disease, particularly in view of patency of most of the many small vessels in the examined material. Nevertheless, CADASIL is probably the main cause of sporadic instances of what otherwise

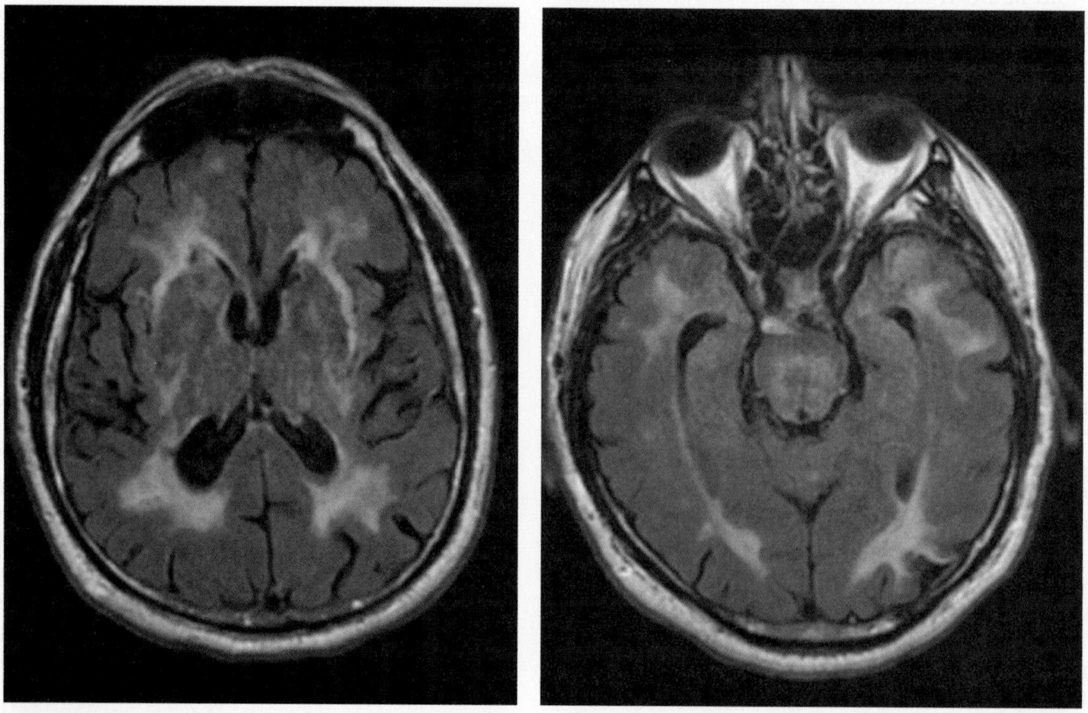

Figure 34-21. Axial T2-FLAIR MRI of cerebral autosomal dominant arteriopathy with subcortical infarcts and leukoencephalopathy (CADASIL). There is confluent symmetric abnormal hyperintensity within the periventricular white matter and internal and external capsules (*left*) and characteristically, also in the anterior temporal lobes (*right*).

passes for Binswanger disease; the anterior temporal changes, however, are typical of the former. Also, migraine headaches are not a component of Binswanger disease.

The responsible mutation is a missense change on chromosome 19 of the *NOTCH 3* gene, in the same locus as the gene for familial hemiplegic migraine, and has been characterized by Joutel and colleagues; this provides a diagnostic test that can be performed on the blood or skin. The gene may now be sequenced in commercial laboratories. The diagnosis can also be confirmed by finding eosinophilic inclusions in the arterioles of a skin biopsy (osmophilic with electron microscopy).

An entirely different vasculopathy with widespread white matter signal change has been reported in Japan. Migraine is not a component of the syndrome, and the *NOTCH* gene, implicated in CADASIL, is normal. Inheritance is as a recessive trait (hence, CARASIL) from a mutation in the *HTAR1* gene (see Hara et al). The result is fragmentation and duplication of the internal elastic lamina of cerebral vessels with narrowing of their lumens. As intriguing from this mutation is an associated osteoid growth that causes severe lumbar stenosis and alopecia.

An interesting mutation of the *COL4A*1 gene for type 4 collagen leads to familial small vessel disease and intracerebral hemorrhage in mice and humans (Gould et al). More often, as in the cases described by Verreault and colleagues, there are numerous white matter infarctions that are not explained by hypertension and similar lesions may be found in family members by MRI.

Under the terms HERNS (hereditary endotheliopathy, retinopathy, nephropathy, and strokes) and CRV (cerebroretinal vasculopathy), rare dominantly inherited conditions have been described that cause subcortical white matter degeneration, presumably on a microvascular occlusive basis. Ocular symptoms and retinopathy are the main features and the neurologic aspects. Awareness of these vascular forms of white matter degenerations adds to the list of inherited leukoencephalopathies discussed in Chap. 38 and the action of the implicated genes reveals novel mechanisms of damage to small cerebral vessels.

Strokes in Children and Young Adults

As indicated in Table 34-2 in an earlier section, ischemic necrosis of cerebral tissue can occur in utero. The resulting stroke is usually referred to as *congenital hemiplegia* but there are heterogeneous causes and in most instances, the underlying vascular disease cannot be discerned. The adjacent ventricular region tends to expand into the stroke cavity and may cause a porencephalic cyst.

Acute hemiplegia in infants and children is a rare but well-recognized phenomenon. In a series of 555 consecutive postmortem examinations at the Children's Medical Center in Boston (now Boston Children's Hospital), there were 48 cases (8.7 percent) of occlusive vascular disease of the brain (Banker). The occlusions, studied neuropathologically, were both embolic (mainly associated with congenital heart disease) and thrombotic, and the latter were actually more common in veins than in arteries.

Similarly, stroke is not an uncommon event in young adults (ages 15 to 45 years), accounting for an estimated 3 percent of cerebral infarctions in typical series. In terms of causation, this group is also remarkably heterogeneous. Among 144 such patients, more than 40 possible etiologies were identified by H.P. Adams and colleagues. Nevertheless, most of the strokes could be accounted for by three categories, more or less equal in size: (1) atherosclerotic thrombotic infarction (usually with a recognized risk factor); (2) cardiogenic embolism (particularly in the past association with rheumatic heart disease, infective and noninfective endocarditis, paradoxic embolism through patent foramen ovale and other cardiac defects, and prosthetic heart valves); and (3) one of several nonatherosclerotic vasculopathies (arterial trauma, dissection of the carotid artery, moyamoya, lupus erythematosus, drug-induced vasculitis). Hematologically related disorders—use of oral contraceptives (discussed further on), the postpartum state, and other hypercoagulable states—were the probable causes in 15 percent patients. The presence of antiphospholipid or anticardiolipin antibodies (lupus anticoagulant) explains some of these cases and is discussed further in the section on "Stroke as a Complication of Hematologic Disease"; the majority of these patients are women in their thirties without manifest systemic lupus erythematosus.

Despite the attention they have received recently as a cause of strokes in the juvenile and young adult period, the frequency of inherited deficiencies of naturally occurring anticoagulant factors as a cause of stroke is low. Table 34-7 summarizes the main inherited prothrombotic clotting defects. They predispose primarily to cerebral venous thrombosis. Most arise from partial protein deficiencies as a result of heterozygous mutations in the genes encoding proteins in the clotting cascade (antithrombin III, proteins S and C) and from those that disturb clotting balance (resistance to activated protein C, or factor V Leiden mutation, and prothrombin mutations as well as excess factor VIII) (see discussion by Brown and Bevan). When homozygous, these mutations may be associated with devastating neonatal hemorrhagic conditions. In some series that report cases of strokes in youth, such as the one reported by Becker and colleagues, up to half of stroke cases had one of these disorders, the most common being the factor V Leiden mutation, but others have found this mutation to be much less frequent, which is more consonant with our experience. Nevertheless, in children with unexplained stroke, particularly venous ones or if there is a family history of stroke in early life, and especially if there has been a previous thrombosis or if the strokes are recurrent, it is advisable to carry out an extensive hematologic investigation, including testing for antiphospholipid antibody (an acquired defect), as described in the later section on "Antiphospholipid Antibody (Hughes) Syndrome." Establishing a diagnosis of a prothrombotic clotting gene variant has further significance because strokes are prone to occur in the setting of additional risks, such as the use of oral contraceptives and smoking. In adults, the evaluation for inherited clotting defects is less fruitful. Furthermore, it should be kept in mind that the levels of proteins C and S and of antithrombin are temporarily depressed after stroke, so that any detected abnormalities must be confirmed months later and in the absence of anticoagulation.

Table 34-7

STROKE ASSOCIATED WITH GENETIC DISORDERS

	GENE	INHERITANCE	STRUCTURES AFFECTED	GENERAL POPULATION (%)	WITH CEREBRAL THROMBOSIS (%)
Causes of arterial or venous infarction					
Activated protein C resistance	Leiden factor V mutation	AR	v	2–15	5–20
Prothrombin 20210	Prothrombin	AR	v	0.1	1–5
Protein C deficiency	Protein C gene	AR	v	0.2–0.4	3–6
Protein S deficiency	Protein S gene	AR	v	0.03–0.13	1–5
Increased factor VIII	von Willebrand factor deficiency	AR	v	10	25
Antithrombin III deficiency	Antithrombin III	AR	v	Rare	3–8
Plasminogen deficiency	Plasminogen activator-1	AR	v		
Lipoprotein (a)	Apolipoprotein (a)	AR	v		
Marfan syndrome	Fibrillin 1		v, h, ao	0.03	
Fabry disease	Alpha-galactosidase	AR	v		
Sickle cell syndrome	Globin genes		v, a		
Heparin cofactor II	Heparin cofactor II	AR	v	Rare	? 5
Platelet collagen receptor	Platelet collagen receptor	AR	v		
Factor XII	Factor XII	AR	v		
Phosphodiesterase 4D	Phosphodiesterase 4D	Complex	a		
CADASIL	Notch 3	AD	a		
CARASIL	HTAR1	AR	a		
Hyperhomocysteinemia	Methylene tetrahydrofolate reductase	AR	a	Rare	20 in young
Homocysteinemia	Cystathionine beta-synthase	AR	a		
Homocysteinemia	Homocysteine methyl transferase	AR	a		
Ehlers Danlos disease	Collagen type III, numerous mutations	Mainly AD	a		
MELAS (mitochondrial)	mtDNA	Maternal			
Causes of cerebral hemorrhage associated with congenital diseases					
von Hippel-Lindau (see Chap. 31)	pVHL	AD	hemorrhage		
Cavernous malformations	Cerebral cavernous malformations (CCM1)	AD	"		
Cerebral amyloidosis	Apolipoprotein E_4	Complex	"		
Cerebral hemorrhage with amyloidosis			"		
Dutch type	Amyloid precursor protein	AD	"		
Icelandic type	Cystatin C	AD	"		
Hereditary hemorrhagic telangiectasia	Endoglin	AD	"		
Hereditary hemorrhagic telangiectasia	Activin receptor-like kinase (ALK-1)	AD	"		
Polycystic kidney disease	Polycystin 1, 2	AD	"		

a, arterial; AD, autosomal dominant; ao, aorta; AR, autosomal recessive; h, heart; v, venous.

Persistent cerebral ischemia and infarction may occasionally complicate migraine in young persons as discussed in Chap. 10. Wolf and colleagues identified a prolonged aura in young women with an established history of migraine as a risk for strokes, most of which occurred in the posterior circulation. The combination of migraine and oral contraception is particularly hazardous, as detailed below. Despite the common occurrence of mitral valve prolapse in young adults, it is probably only rarely a cause of stroke (see previous comments). Stroke because of either arterial or venous occlusion occurs occasionally in association with inflammatory bowel disease in young persons. Evidence points to a hypercoagulable state during exacerbations of the enteritis but a precise defect in coagulation has not been identified. Meningovascular syphilis and fungal and tuberculous meningitis and other forms of chronic basal meningitis are also considerations in this age group; the strokes are usually of the lacunar type, resulting from inflammatory occlusion of small basal vessels.

Sickle cell anemia is a rare but important cause of stroke in children of African ancestry; acute hemiplegia is the most common manifestation but all types of focal cerebral disorders have been observed. The pathologic findings are those of infarction, large and small; their basis is assumed to be vascular obstruction associated with the sickling process. The association of sickle cell anemia with the moyamoya syndrome was mentioned earlier and surveillance for the development of supraclinoid stenosis may be undertaken by transcranial Doppler. Exchange transfusions have prevented or retarded the formation of moyamoya and the report by RJ Adams and colleagues indicates that the procedure may reduce the risk of stroke if the arteriopathy is detected. Intracranial bleeding (subdural, subarachnoid, and intracerebral) and cerebral venous thrombosis may also complicate sickle cell anemia, and—probably because of autosplenectomy—there is an increased incidence of pneumococcal meningitis. Treatment of the cerebral circulatory disorder, based presumably on sludging of red blood cells, is with intravenous hydration and transfusion. Cerebral venous sinus thrombosis in young children and neonates from various causes represents a special problem, difficult to diagnose, and with a poor prognosis (see deVeber et al).

Certain hereditary metabolic diseases (*homocystinuria* and *Fabry angiokeratosis*) and the mitochondrial disorder *MELAS* (mitochondrial encephalomyopathy, lactic acidosis, and stroke-like episodes) may give rise to strokes in children or young adults; investigation of these causes is undertaken if the aforementioned clotting disorders have been excluded or if there is a family history. Figure 34-22 demonstrates an example of stroke related to MELAS.

Overall, in children and young adults with ischemic stroke, the main diagnoses to be considered are carotid and vertebral dissection, drug abuse (mainly cocaine), thrombosis induced by contraceptive estrogens (see below), antiphospholipid antibody syndrome, and cardiac disease including patent foramen ovale (PFO). Migraine might be added to this list, but it is a diagnosis by exclusion in these circumstances and CADASIL, albeit rare, should also be considered if migraine headaches and TIAs precede a stroke. Inherited prothrombotic states—such as those caused by the various clotting factor deficiencies discussed above, Fabry disease, moyamoya, and Takayasu arteritis—arise in the younger age group and require exploration if clinical circumstances suggest one of these processes on the basis of unusual TIAs (orthostatic, hyperventilation, or fever induced), Down syndrome, or strong family history of strokes in youth.

Oral Contraceptives, Estrogen, and Cerebral Infarction

The early studies of Longstreth and Swanson and of Vessey and associates indicated that women who take oral contraceptives in the childbearing years—particularly if they are older than 35 years of age and also smoke, are hypertensive, or have migraine—are at increased risk of cerebral infarction. Stroke in these cases is usually a result of arterial occlusion, occurring in both the carotid–middle cerebral and vertebrobasilar territories and sometimes to occlusion of cerebral veins. In most of the reported fatal cases, the thrombosed vessel has been free of atheroma or other disease. The vascular lesion underlying cerebral thrombosis in women taking oral contraceptives was studied by Irey and colleagues. It consists of nodular intimal hyperplasia of eccentric distribution with increased acid mucopolysaccharides and replication of the internal elastic lamina. Similar changes have been found in pregnancy and in humans and animals receiving exogenous steroids, including estrogens. These observations, coupled with evidence that estrogen alters the coagulability of the blood, suggest that a state of hypercoagulability is the important factor in the genesis of contraceptive-associated infarction.

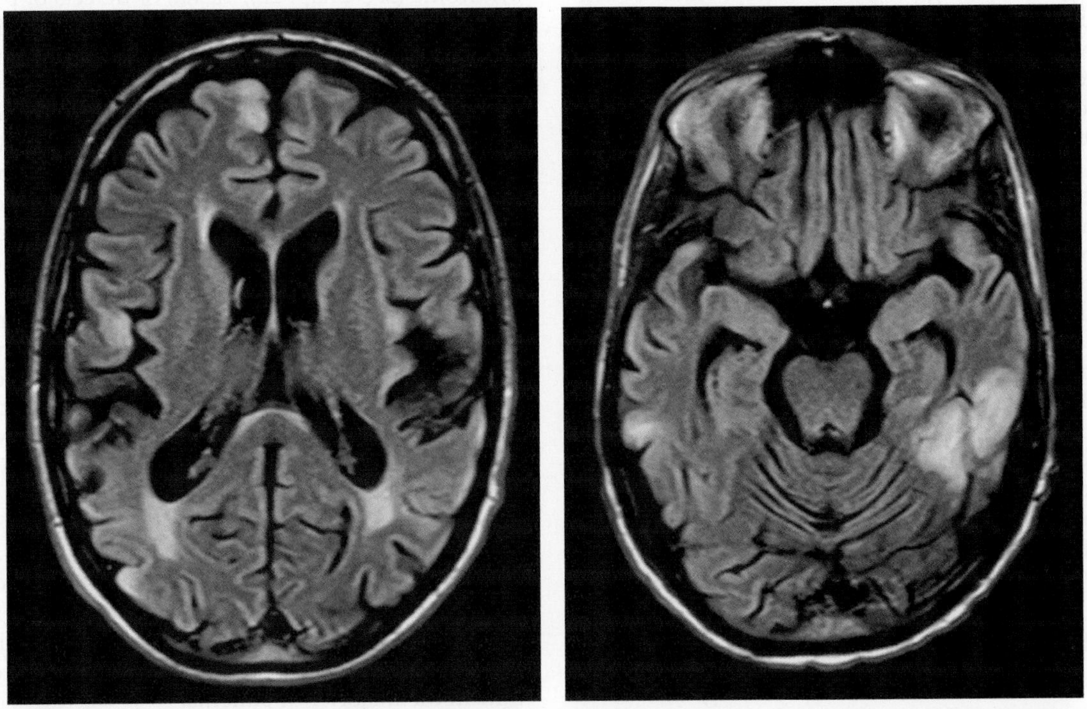

Figure 34-22. Two axial T2-FLAIR images of mitochondrial encephalomyopathy with lactic acidosis and stroke-like episodes (MELAS). Multifocal asymmetric areas of cortical and subcortical T2 hyperintensity are seen.

Mainly at increased risk of stroke are women taking high-dose (0.50-mg) estrogen pills; in recent years, lowering the estrogen content has substantially reduced, but not eliminated, this risk. The use of progestin-only pills or of subcutaneously implanted capsules of progestin has not been associated with stroke as far as can be currently determined (Petitti et al). The epidemiologic study reported by Lidegaard and colleagues puts the risk of hormonal contraception in perspective; in a large cohort of Danes, the risks of thrombotic strokes and myocardial infarction over 15 years was very low with estradiol-containing compounds but it increased with age and with the dose of estradiol. It has also become apparent that mutations of the prothrombin gene are more frequent in patients who have cerebral venous thrombosis while on oral contraceptive pills than they are in the general population. Martinelli and associates propose that these genetic abnormalities account for 35 percent of idiopathic cases of cerebral vein thrombosis; and they have contended that contraceptives increase this risk 20-fold.

Stroke in Pregnancy and the Postpartum Period

In addition to the eclamptic-hypertensive state, there is an increased incidence of cerebrovascular events during pregnancy and the postpartum period. The risk of both cerebral infarction and intracerebral hemorrhage appears to be mainly in the 6-week period after delivery rather than during the pregnancy itself (Kittner et al). Fisher (1971) reviewed the literature and analyzed 12 postpartum, 9 puerperal, and 14 contraceptive cases, as well as 9 patients receiving estrogen therapy; arterial thrombosis was demonstrated in half of these cases. Most of the focal vascular lesions during pregnancy were a result of arterial occlusion in the second and third trimesters and in the first week after delivery. Venous occlusion tended to occur 1 to 4 weeks postpartum. In Rochester, New York, the incidence rate of stroke during pregnancy was 6.2 per 100,000, but it doubled with each advance in age from 25 to 29, 30 to 39, and 40 to 49 years. Included in most past series are cases with cardiac disease, particularly valve-related embolism. It is perhaps surprising that subarachnoid hemorrhage is not more frequent during the Valsalva activity of childbirth. Carotid artery dissection may also be encountered late in pregnancy or soon after delivery.

The occurrence of paradoxical embolus is always a consideration in pregnancy because of a tendency to form clots in the pelvic and leg veins, coupled with increased right heart pressures. Amniotic fluid embolus may rarely cause stroke in this manner and should be suspected in multiparous women who have had uterine tears; there are almost invariably signs of acute pulmonary disease from simultaneous occlusion of lung vessels. A rare peripartum cardiomyopathy is yet another source of embolic stroke.

Stroke With Cardiac Surgery

Incident to cardiac arrest and bypass surgery, there is risk of both generalized and focal ischemia of the brain. Improved operative techniques have lessened the frequency of these complications but they are still distressingly frequent. Fortunately, most are transient. Atherosclerotic plaques may be dislodged during cross-clamping of the proximal aorta and are an important source of cerebral emboli. In the last decade, the incidence of stroke related to cardiac surgery has dropped to between 2 and 3 percent in large series numbering thousands of patients (Libman et al; Ahlgren and Arén). Advanced age, congestive heart failure, and more complex surgeries have been listed as risk factors for stroke from various reports.

Representative is a retrospective study by Dashe and colleagues, in which 2 percent had strokes; most minor, but the risk was greatly increased on the side of a carotid stenosis. Curiously, almost one-fifth of postoperative strokes in some series have been of lacunar type. In one prospective study of 2,108 patients who underwent coronary operations in several institutions, 3 percent had strokes or TIAs; the adverse effects mostly occurred in older patients and were transient (Roach et al). Mohr and coworkers (1978) examined 100 consecutive cases pre- and postoperatively and observed two types of stroke-like complications—one occurring immediately after the operation and the other after an interval of days or weeks. The immediate neurologic disorder consisted of a delay in awakening from the anesthesia; subsequently there was slowness in thinking, disorientation, agitation, combativeness, visual hallucinations, and poor registration and recall of what was happening. These symptoms, in the form of a confusional state sometimes verging on delirium or acute psychosis, usually cleared within 5 to 7 days, although some patients were not entirely normal mentally some weeks later. As the confusion cleared, about half of the patients were found to have small visual field defects, dyscalculia, Balint syndrome (see Chap. 22), alexia, or defects of perception suggestive of lesions in the parietooccipital regions. The immediate effects were attributed to hypotension and various types of embolisms (atherosclerotic, air, silicon, fat, platelets). The delayed effects were more clearly embolic and were especially frequent in patients having prosthetic valve replacements or other valve repairs.

In addition to overt and covert strokes detected only by imaging, a degree of cognitive decline and depression is to be expected in a proportion of patients undergoing coronary artery bypass grafting. The frequency of these changes is reported to be between 40 and 70 percent (see Chap. 20). It is our impression that many of these neurologic complications, both small strokes and cognitive abnormalities, pass unnoticed in many cardiac surgical units. This was emphasized in the study by McKhann and colleagues, who tested several neuropsychologic functions and found that only 12 percent of patients escaped some type of early cognitive problem. However, his group and others, for example, Mülges and colleagues, have shown that only a small proportion (13 percent in the latter series) retained permanent effects 5 years after operation. Others have reported higher rates, but it is clear that the cognitive problems improve over time in the majority of patients.

The use of Doppler insonation of the middle cerebral arteries is being studied to detect transient signals called

HITs (high-intensity transients) as a manifestation of small emboli during surgery but, as for the transients frequently noted during cerebral arteriography, the clinical importance of these emboli is not known. In an attempt to avoid neurologic complication related to extracorporeal circulation, off-pump coronary artery bypass has been popularized in many centers. Unfortunately, most studies have found no fewer cognitive complications as compared to conventional coronary artery bypass surgery (e.g., see Shroyer et al). This is contrary to the notion that the extracorporeal apparatus is the cause of the problem. The issue of the neurologic complications of cardiac surgery may be summarized by noting that strokes originating from the aorta are the main cause of cognitive failure. The clinical syndromes seem to fall on a continuum; a few strokes (less than 3 percent) are recognizable as obvious deficits (e.g., hemiplegia), instead, many have multiple small emboli that are evident with imaging and these are manifest as an acute encephalopathy. When the burden of emboli is lower, no deficit is recognized in the acute period. It is likely that in patients with premorbid presymptomatic Alzheimer disease, confusion and dementia are made manifest by the stress of cardiac surgery and the surgery is then blamed for the emergence of an ostensibly new problem (see Samuels).

The other special stroke problems relating to prosthetic heart valves—mainly infective endocarditis causing embolic strokes and anticoagulant-related cerebral hemorrhage—are described in later sections of this chapter.

Table 34-8

CAUSES OF CEREBRAL HEMORRHAGE (INCLUDING INTRACEREBRAL, SUBARACHNOID, AND VENTRICULAR)

1. Primary (hypertensive) intracerebral hemorrhage
2. Ruptured saccular aneurysm
3. Ruptured arteriovenous malformation; less often, venous and dural vascular malformations
4. Cavernous angioma
5. Trauma including posttraumatic delayed apoplexy
6. Hemorrhagic disorders: leukemia, aplastic anemia, thrombocytopenic purpura, liver disease, complication of anticoagulant or thrombolytic therapy, hypofibrinogenemia, hemophilia, etc.
7. Hemorrhage into primary and secondary brain tumors
8. Septic embolism, mycotic aneurysm
9. With hemorrhagic infarction, arterial or venous
10. With inflammatory and infectious disease of the arteries and veins
11. With cerebrovascular amyloidosis
12. Pituitary apoplexy
13. Postcraniotomy or brain biopsy
14. Primary intraventricular hemorrhage
15. Miscellaneous rare types: vasopressor drugs, cocaine, moyamoya, herpes simplex encephalitis, meningeal melanomatosis, acute necrotizing hemorrhagic encephalitis (Hurst disease), tularemia, anthrax, etc.

INTRACEREBRAL HEMORRHAGE

This is the third most frequent cause of stroke, following cerebral embolism and thrombotic disease. Although more than a dozen causes of nontraumatic intracranial hemorrhage are listed in Table 34-8, hypertensive primary ("spontaneous") intracerebral hemorrhage, ruptured saccular aneurysm and vascular malformation, and hemorrhage associated with the use of anticoagulants or thrombolytic agents account for the majority. Cerebrovascular amyloidosis and acquired or congenital bleeding disorders account for a smaller number. The small brainstem hemorrhages secondary to temporal lobe herniation and brainstem compression (Duret hemorrhages), hypertensive encephalopathy, and brain purpura might be included in this group, but they do not simulate a stroke.

Primary Intracerebral Hemorrhage

This is the often devastating "spontaneous" brain hemorrhage. It is predominantly a result of chronic hypertension and degenerative changes in cerebral arteries. In recent decades, with increased awareness of the need to control blood pressure, the proportion of hemorrhages attributable to causes other than hypertension, mainly anticoagulation, has greatly increased so that more than half such hemorrhages on our services now occur in normotensive individuals, and the hemorrhages more often arise in locations that are not typical for hypertension. Nevertheless, the hypertensive cerebral hemorrhage serves as a model for understanding and managing other cerebral hemorrhages.

In approximate order of frequency, the most common sites of a cerebral hemorrhage are (1) the putamen and adjacent internal capsule (50 percent); (2) the central white matter of the temporal, parietal, or frontal lobes (lobar hemorrhages, not strictly associated with hypertension); (3) the thalamus; (4) one or the other cerebellar hemisphere; and (5) the pons. The vessel that ruptures, giving rise to the hemorrhage, is usually a small penetrating artery that originates from a larger trunk. Approximately 2 percent of primary hemorrhages are multiple. Multiple, nearly simultaneous intracerebral hemorrhages raise the possibility of amyloid angiopathy or a bleeding diathesis (see further on) but may occur when one conventional hypertensive intracerebral hemorrhage causes hypertension, which in turn leads to one or more additional hemorrhages.

The extravasation of blood into the substance of the brain forms a roughly circular or oval mass that disrupts the tissue and can grow in volume if the bleeding continues. Adjacent brain tissue is distorted and compressed. If the hemorrhage is large, midline structures are displaced to the opposite side of the cranium and the reticular activating and respiratory centers are compromised, leading to coma and death in the manner described in Chap. 17. It has been long known that both the size and the location of the clot determine the degree of secondary brainstem compression and this was confirmed by Andrew and associates. Rupture or seepage of blood into the ventricular system or rarely to the surface subarachnoid space may occur, and the CSF becomes bloody in these cases.

In the first hours and days following the hemorrhage, varying degrees of edema evolve around the clot and add to the mass effect. Hydrocephalus may occur as a result of bleeding into the ventricular system or from compression of the third ventricle.

The extravasated blood undergoes a predictable series of changes. At first fluid, the collection becomes a clot within hours. Before the clot forms, red cells settle in the dependent part of the hematoma and form a meniscus with the plasma above; this is particularly prone to occur in cases of anticoagulant-induced hemorrhage. The resultant fluid–fluid level can be observed on CT and MRI ("hematocrit effect"). Hematomas, when examined in autopsy material, contain only masses of red blood cells and proteins; rarely one sees a few remnants of destroyed brain tissue. The hematoma is often surrounded by petechial hemorrhages from torn arterioles and venules. Within a few days, hemoglobin products, mainly hemosiderin and hematoidin, begin to appear. The hemosiderin forms within histiocytes that have phagocytized red blood cells (RBCs) and takes the form of ferritin granules that stain positively for iron. As oxyhemoglobin is liberated from the RBCs and becomes deoxygenated, methemoglobin appears. This begins within a few days and imparts a brownish hue to the periphery of the clot. Phagocytosis of red cells begins within 24 h, and hemosiderin is first observed around the margins of the clot in 5 to 6 days. The clot changes color gradually over a few weeks from dark red to pale red, and the border of golden-brown hemosiderin widens. The edema disappears over many days or weeks. In 2 to 3 months, larger clots are filled with a chrome-colored thick fluid, which is slowly absorbed, leaving a smooth-walled cavity or a yellow-brown scar. The iron pigment (hematin) becomes dispersed and studs adjacent astrocytes and neurons and may persist well beyond the border of the hemorrhage for years.

Imaging techniques demonstrate a predictable sequence of changes as shown in Fig. 34-23. On CT, fresh blood is visualized as a white mass as soon as it is shed. The "spot sign," the appearance of contrast within the hemorrhage during CT angiography, is associated with a high rate of hematoma expansion. The mass effect and the surrounding extruded serum and edema are hypodense on CT. After 2 to 3 weeks, the surrounding edema begins to recede and the density of the hematoma decreases, first at the periphery. Gradually the clot becomes isodense with brain. There may be a ring of enhancement from the hemosiderin-filled macrophages and the reacting cells that form a capsule for the hemorrhage. At one point several weeks after the bleed, the appearance may transiently simulate a tumor or abscess. By MRI, either in conventional T1- or T2-weighted images, the hemorrhage is not easily visible in the 2 or 3 days after bleeding, as oxyhemoglobin is diamagnetic or, at most, is slightly hypointense, so that only the mass effect is evident. MR gradient echo or equivalent sequences that display areas of magnetic susceptibility show hemorrhages earlier and detect remnants of deposited hemosiderin even years afterward.

After several days the surrounding edema is hyperintense in T2-weighted images. As deoxyhemoglobin and methemoglobin form, the hematoma signal becomes bright on T1-weighted images and dark on T2. The hematoma is then subacute and the dark signal gradually brightens. When methemoglobin disappears and only hemosiderin remains, the entire remaining mass is hypodense on T2-weighted images, as are the surrounding deposits of iron. The sizes of cerebral hemorrhages vary widely. *Massive* refers to hemorrhages several centimeters in diameter, usually larger than 50 mL; *small* applies to those 1 to 2 cm in diameter and less than 20 mL in volume. The volume and location relate to outcome and the nature of the initial neurologic deficit.

Pathogenesis

The hypertensive vascular lesion that leads to arteriolar rupture in most cases appears to arise from an arterial wall altered by the effects of hypertension, i.e., the change referred to in a preceding section as segmental lipohyalinosis and the false aneurysm (microaneurysm) named for Charcot and Bouchard. Ross Russell's work affirmed the relationship of these microaneurysms to hypertension and hypertensive hemorrhage and their frequent localization on penetrating small arteries and arterioles of the basal ganglia, thalamus, pons, and subcortical white matter. However, in the few hemorrhages examined in serial sections by our colleague C.M. Fisher, the bleeding could not be traced to Charcot-Bouchard aneurysms. Takebayashi and coworkers, in an electron microscopic study, found breaks in the elastic lamina at multiple sites, almost always at bifurcations of the small vessels. Possibly these represented points of secondary rupture from tearing of small vessels by the expanding hematoma. Amyloid impregnation of vessel walls represents a different mechanism for vessel rupture, as discussed further on.

Clinical Syndrome

Of all the cerebrovascular diseases, brain hemorrhage is the most dramatic and from ancient times has been given its own name, "apoplexy." The prototype was an obese, plethoric, hypertensive male who falls senseless to the ground—impervious to shouts, shaking, and pinching—breathes stertorously, and dies in a few hours. A massive blood clot escapes from the brain as it is removed postmortem. With smaller hemorrhages, the clinical picture conforms more closely to the usual temporal profile of a stroke, i.e., an abrupt onset of symptoms that evolve gradually and steadily over minutes or hours, depending on the speed and expansion of bleeding.

Several general features of intracerebral hemorrhage should be emphasized. *Acute reactive hypertension*, far exceeding the patient's chronic hypertensive level, is a feature that, in the context of a stroke, suggests hemorrhage; it is seen particularly with moderate and large clots situated in deep regions. *Vomiting* at the onset of intracerebral hemorrhage occurs much more frequently than with infarction and likewise suggests bleeding as the cause of an acute hemiparesis. Severe headache is generally considered to be an accompaniment of intracerebral hemorrhage and in many cases it is, but in almost half of cases it has been absent or mild. *Nuchal rigidity* is infrequent. If there is stiffness of the neck, it characteristically

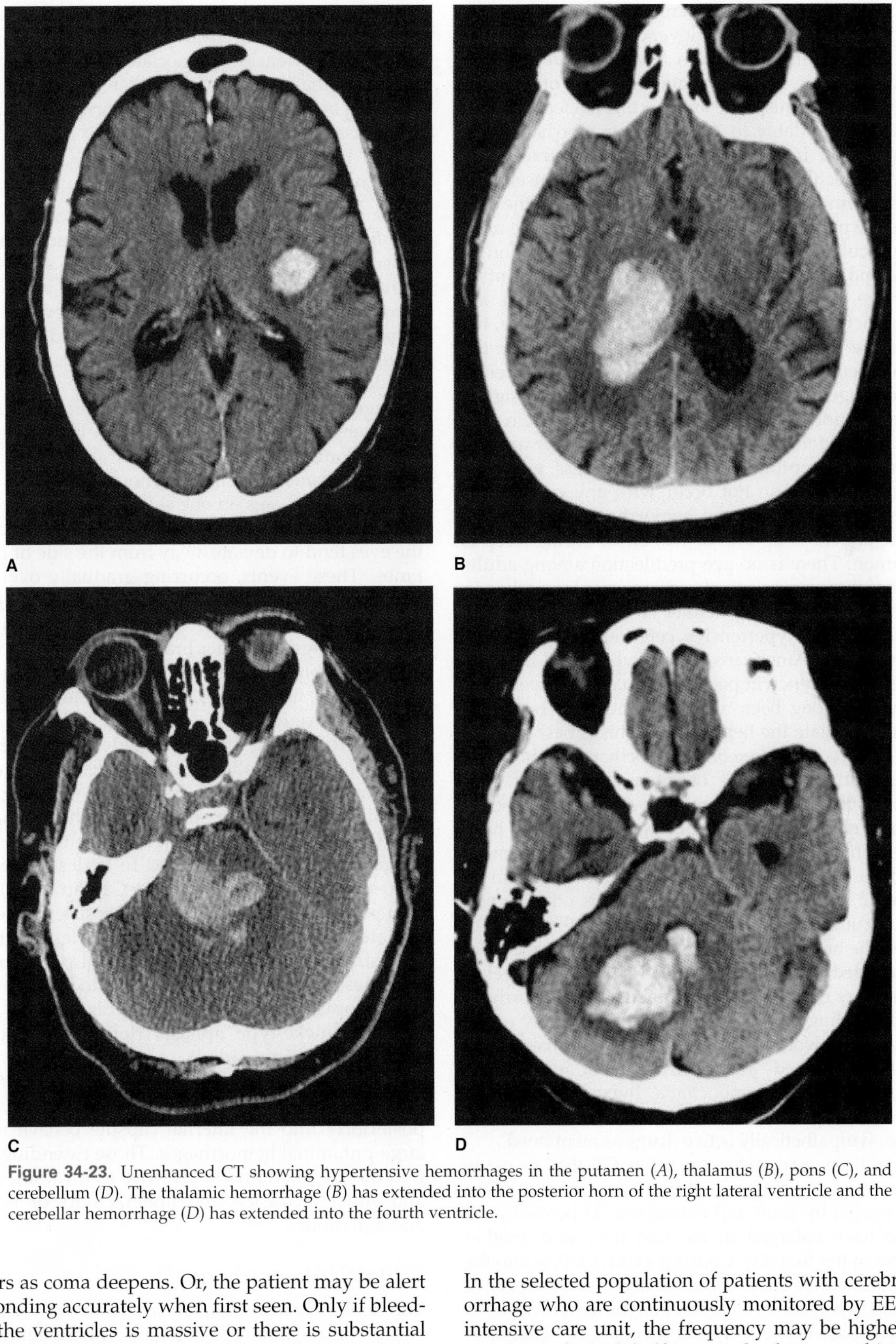

Figure 34-23. Unenhanced CT showing hypertensive hemorrhages in the putamen (*A*), thalamus (*B*), pons (*C*), and cerebellum (*D*). The thalamic hemorrhage (*B*) has extended into the posterior horn of the right lateral ventricle and the cerebellar hemorrhage (*D*) has extended into the fourth ventricle.

disappears as coma deepens. Or, the patient may be alert and responding accurately when first seen. Only if bleeding into the ventricles is massive or there is substantial distortion of the midbrain, does coma result.

Seizures, usually focal, occur in the first few days in only 10 percent of cases of supratentorial hemorrhage, rarely at the time of the ictus and more commonly as a delayed event, months or years after the hemorrhage. In the selected population of patients with cerebral hemorrhage who are continuously monitored by EEG in an intensive care unit, the frequency may be higher, up to one-third of which half are purely electrographic, according to Claassen and associates. This finding is interesting but does not seem to justify routine EEG monitoring.

The fundi often show hypertensive changes in the arterioles. Infrequently, fresh preretinal (subhyaloid) hemorrhages occur; the latter are much more common with ruptured aneurysm, arteriovenous malformation, or severe cranial trauma. Therefore, *headache, acute hypertension,* and *vomiting* with hemiplegia in the case of bleeding into the cerebral hemisphere are the cardinal features and serve most dependably to distinguish hemorrhage from ischemic stroke. In the localization of an intracerebral hemorrhage, ocular signs may be particularly useful. In putaminal hemorrhage, the eyes are deviated to the side opposite the paralysis; in thalamic hemorrhage, the most common ocular abnormality is downward deviation of the eyes and the pupils may be unreactive; in pontine hemorrhage, the eyeballs are fixed and the pupils are tiny but reactive; and in large cerebellar hemorrhage, the eyes may be deviated laterally to the side opposite the lesion and ocular bobbing may occur (as often in cerebellar hemorrhage in awake patients there are no eye signs).

Small hemorrhages in some regions of the brain may escape clinical detection. Usually there are no warnings or prodromal symptoms; headache, dizziness, epistaxis, or other symptoms do not occur with any consistency. In the majority of cases, the hemorrhage has its onset while the patient is up and active; onset during sleep is not common. There is no age predilection among adults except that the average age of occurrence is lower than in thrombotic infarction and neither sex is more disposed. The incidence of hypertensive cerebral hemorrhage is higher in African Americans than in whites and it occurs with higher frequency in people of Japanese descent.

There has long been a notion that acute hypertension can precipitate the hemorrhage. This is based on the known occurrence of cerebral hemorrhage at moments of extreme fright or anger or intense excitement, presumably as the blood pressure rises abruptly beyond its chronically elevated level. Similarly, hemorrhages have been described in relation to taking sympathomimetic medications such as phenylpropanolamine (Kernan et al), ephedra, or cocaine, and to numerous other hypertensive circumstances. However, in fully 90 percent of instances, the hemorrhage occurs when the patient is calm and unstressed, according to Caplan (1993). The level of blood pressure rises early in the course of the hemorrhage but the preceding chronic hypertension is usually of the "essential" type. Nonetheless, causes of hypertension must always be considered—renal disease, renal artery stenosis, eclampsia, pheochromocytoma, hyperaldosteronism, adrenocorticotropic hormone or corticosteroid excess and, of course, sympathetically active drugs as mentioned.

It has been recognized by serial CT that in many instances, there is enlargement of the hematoma. In the series reported by Brott and colleagues, 25 percent were found to have enlarged in the first hour and another 12 percent in the first day. Contrast extravasation into the adjacent brain after CTA was associated in a retrospective study with expansion of a hematoma, the aforementioned "spot sign" (Goldstein et al), but there are no other clear predictive factors of expansion of the clot. Blood in cerebral tissue is absorbed slowly over months during which time symptoms and signs recede. Hence the neurologic deficit is never transitory in intracerebral hemorrhage, as it so often is in TIA or embolism.

The main types and locations of cerebral hemorrhage are described below and shown in Fig. 34-23. Chronic hypertension is associated with bleeding into the putamen, thalamus, pons, and cerebellum. Intracerebral bleeding at other sites, "lobar hemorrhages," has numerous causes.

Putaminal Hemorrhage

The most common syndrome is the one caused by *putaminal hemorrhage* with extension to the adjacent internal capsule (see Fig. 34-23*A*). Neurologic symptoms and signs vary slightly with the precise site and size of the extravasation, but hemiplegia from interruption of the capsule is a consistent feature of medium-sized and large clots. Vomiting occurs in about half the patients. Headache is frequent but not invariable. With large hemorrhages, patients lapse almost immediately into a stupor with hemiplegia and their condition visibly deteriorates as the hours pass. As often, there is headache or some other abnormal cephalic sensation. Within a few minutes or less the face sags on one side, speech becomes slurred or aphasic, the arm and leg weaken and are flaccid, and the eyes tend to deviate away from the side of the paretic limbs. These events, occurring gradually over a period of several minutes or more, are strongly suggestive of intracerebral bleeding. More advanced stages are characterized by signs of upper brainstem compression (coma); bilateral Babinski signs; irregular or intermittent respiration; dilated, fixed pupils, first on the side of the clot; and decerebrate rigidity.

Neuroimaging has disclosed the frequent occurrence of many smaller putaminal hemorrhages, which in former years would have been misdiagnosed as embolic or thrombotic strokes. With hemorrhages confined to the anterior segment of the putamen, the hemiplegia and hyperreflexia tend to be less severe and to clear more rapidly according to Caplan (1993). There is also prominent abulia, motor impersistence, temporary unilateral neglect, and with left-sided lesions, nonfluent aphasia, and dysgraphia. With small posterior lesions, weakness is also mild and is attended by sensory loss, hemianopia, impaired visual pursuit to the opposite side, Wernicke-type aphasia (left-sided lesions), and anosognosia (right-sided).

The effects of relatively pure *caudate hematoma* have been difficult to define. Those extending laterally and posteriorly into the internal capsule behave much like large putaminal hemorrhages. Those extending medially into the lateral ventricle give rise to drowsiness, stupor, and either confusion and underactivity or restlessness and agitation.

Thalamic Hemorrhage

The central feature here is severe sensory loss on the entire contralateral body. If large or moderate in size, thalamic hemorrhage also produces a hemiplegia or hemiparesis by compression or destruction of the adjacent internal capsule (see Fig. 34-23*B*). The sensory deficit involves all of the opposite side including the trunk and may exceed the motor weakness. A fluent aphasia or anemia may be present with lesions of the dominant side and contralateral neglect, with lesions of the nondominant side. A homonymous field defect, if present, usually clears in a few days.

Thalamic hemorrhage, by virtue of its extension into the subthalamus and high midbrain, may also cause a series of ocular disturbances—pseudoabducens palsies with one or both eyes turned asymmetrically inward and slightly downward, palsies of vertical and lateral gaze, forced deviation of the eyes downward, inequality of pupils with absence of light reaction, skew deviation with the eye ipsilateral to the hemorrhage assuming a higher position than the contralateral eye, ipsilateral ptosis and miosis (Horner syndrome), absence of convergence, retraction nystagmus, and tucking in (retraction) of the upper eyelids. Extension of the neck may be observed. Compression of the adjacent third ventricle leads to enlargement of the lateral ventricles that may require temporary drainage. Small and moderate-sized hemorrhages that rupture into the third ventricle have been associated with fewer neurologic deficits and better outcomes, but early hydrocephalus is common.

Pontine Hemorrhage

Hemorrhage into the pons is almost invariably associated with deep coma within a few minutes; the remainder of the clinical picture is dominated by total paralysis with bilateral Babinski signs, decerebrate rigidity, and small (1-mm) pupils that react to light. Lateral eye movements, evoked by head turning or caloric testing, are impaired or absent. Death usually occurs within a few hours, but there are exceptions in which consciousness is retained and the clinical manifestations indicate a smaller lesion in the tegmentum of the pons (disturbances of lateral ocular movements, crossed sensory or motor disturbances, small pupils, and cranial-nerve palsies) in addition to signs of bilateral corticospinal tract involvement. A number of our patients with limited tegmental hemorrhages and blood in the CSF have survived with good functional recovery. In a series of 60 patients with pontine hemorrhage reviewed by Nakajima, 19 survived (8 of whom had remained alert). Similarly, Wijdicks and St. Louis reported that 21 percent made a good recovery—mostly those who were awake on admission. Figure 34-23C depicts a typical pontine hemorrhage.

Cerebellar Hemorrhage

This usually develops over a period of 1 or more hours, and loss of consciousness at the onset is unusual. Repeated vomiting is a prominent feature, with occipital headache, vertigo, and inability to sit, stand, or walk. Often these are the only abnormalities, making it imperative to have the patient attempt to ambulate; otherwise the examination may erroneously seem to be normal. In the early phase of the illness other clinical signs of cerebellar disease are usually minimal or lacking; only a minority of cases show nystagmus or cerebellar ataxia of the limbs, although these signs must always be sought. A mild ipsilateral facial weakness, diminished corneal reflex, paresis of conjugate lateral gaze to the side of the hemorrhage, or an ipsilateral sixth-nerve weakness occur with larger hemorrhages that compress the pons or extend into the cerebellar peduncle. Dysarthria and dysphagia may be prominent in some cases but usually are absent. Other infrequent ocular signs include blepharospasm, involuntary closure of one eye, skew deviation, "ocular bobbing," and small, often unequal pupils that continue to react until very late in the illness. Contralateral hemiplegia and ipsilateral facial weakness occur if there is marked displacement and compression of the medulla against the clivus.

Occasionally at the onset there is a spastic paraparesis or a quadriparesis with preservation of consciousness. The plantar reflexes are flexor in the early stages but extensor later. When these signs occur, hydrocephalus is usually found and may require drainage. In the series collected by St. Louis and colleagues, patients with vermian clots and hydrocephalus were at the highest risk for rapid deterioration. As the hours pass, and occasionally with unanticipated suddenness, the patient becomes stuporous and then comatose or suddenly apneic as a result of brainstem compression, at which point reversal of the syndrome, even by surgical therapy, is seldom successful. As discussed further on, cerebellar hemorrhage is the most amenable to surgical evacuation with good results. A typical case is shown with imaging in Fig. 34-23*D*.

Lobar Hemorrhage

Bleeding in areas other than those listed above, specifically in the subcortical white matter of one of the lobes of the cerebral hemisphere, is not associated strictly with hypertension. Any number of other causes are usually responsible, the main ones being anticoagulation or thrombolytic therapy, acquired coagulopathies, cranial trauma, arteriovenous malformation (discussed further on), trauma, and, in the elderly, amyloidosis of the cerebral vessels. The role of antiplatelet agents in precipitating intracerebral hemorrhage has been a matter of contention with numerous surveys and studies giving divergent results regarding larger, expanding or more clinically destructive hematomas.

Most lobar hemorrhages are spherical or ovoid, but a few follow the contour of the subcortical white matter tracts and take the form of a slit (subcortical slit hemorrhage). It is our impression that many of these are the result of a bleeding diathesis, such as thrombocytopenia.

In a consecutive series of 26 cases of lobar hemorrhage, we found 11 to lie within the occipital lobe, causing pain around the ipsilateral eye and a dense homonymous hemianopia; 7 in the temporal lobe that produced pain in or anterior to the ear, partial hemianopia, and fluent aphasia; 4 in the frontal lobe, with frontal headache and contralateral hemiplegia, mainly of the arm; and 3 in the parietal lobe that presented with anterior temporal headache and hemisensory deficit contralaterally (Ropper and Davis). The smaller hematomas simulate an embolic stroke in the same territory. The occurrence of a progressively worsening headache, vomiting, or drowsiness in conjunction with any one of these syndromes is virtually diagnostic, and, of course, the presence of a lobar hemorrhage is readily corroborated by an unenhanced CT. Of our 26 patients, 14 had normal blood pressure, and in several of the fatal cases there was amyloidosis of the affected vessels; 2 patients were receiving anticoagulants,

2 had an arteriovenous malformation, and 1 had a metastatic tumor. Similarly, in the series of 22 patients with lobar clots reported by Kase and colleagues, 55 percent were normotensive; metastatic tumors, arteriovenous malformations, and blood dyscrasias were found in 14, 9, and 5 percent of the patients, respectively. The role of amyloid angiopathy in lobar hemorrhage in the elderly patient is discussed further on.

Laboratory Findings

For the rapid diagnosis of intracerebral hemorrhage, the CT occupies the foremost position (see Fig. 34-23). It is reliable in the detection of hemorrhages that are less than 1.0 cm in diameter. Very small pontine hemorrhages may be overlooked because of the artifact produced by adjacent bone. The spot sign on CT angiography has been mentioned above in relation to hematoma expansion. At the same time, coexisting hydrocephalus, tumor, cerebral swelling, and displacement of the intracranial contents are readily appreciated. MRI is particularly useful for demonstrating brainstem hemorrhages and residual hemorrhages, which remain visible long after they are no longer detectable on the CT (after 4 to 5 weeks). Hemosiderin and iron pigment have characteristic appearances, as described earlier and in Chap. 2.

In general, lumbar puncture is ill advised, for it may precipitate or aggravate an impending shift of central structures and herniation. The white cell count in the peripheral blood may rise transiently to 15,000/mm^3, a higher figure than in thrombosis, but it is most often normal. The sedimentation rate may be mildly elevated in some patients. Determination of the INR, partial thromboplastin time, and platelet count is advisable.

Course and Prognosis

The immediate prognosis for large and medium-sized cerebral clots is grave; some 30 to 35 percent of patients die in 1 to 30 days. In these cases, either the hemorrhage has extended into the ventricular system or intracranial pressure becomes elevated to levels that preclude normal perfusion of the brain. Or the hemorrhage seeps into vital centers such as the hypothalamus or midbrain. A formula that predicts outcome of hemorrhage based on clot size was devised by Broderick and coworkers (1993); it is mainly applicable to putaminal and thalamic clots. A volume of 30 mL or less, calculated by various methods from the CT predicted a generally favorable outcome; only 1 of their 71 patients with clots larger than 30 mL had regained independent function by 1 month. By contrast, in patients with clots of 60 mL or larger and an initial Glasgow Coma Scale score of 8 or less, the mortality was 90 percent (this scale is detailed in Table 35-1). As remarked earlier, it is the location of the hematoma, not simply its size that determines the clinical effects. A clot 60 mL in volume is almost uniformly fatal if situated in the basal ganglia but may allow reasonably good outcome if located in the frontal or occipital lobe. From the studies of Diringer and colleagues (1998), hydrocephalus is also an important predictor of poor outcome, and this accords with our experience. Prompt drainage of the ventricles can markedly improve the clinical state.

Several other scoring systems that predict prognosis fairly well have been devised and validated as predictive of outcome. The two in main use, shown in Table 34-9, are "FUNC" produced by Rost and coworkers, which incorporates the patient's age, size and location of hematoma, the presence of preexisting cognitive impairment, and Glasgow Coma score (see Chap. 17); and the "ICH score" devised by Hemphill and colleagues that uses GCS, volume, presence of intraventricular hemorrhage, the location—supra- or infratentorial, and age above or below 80 years. The value of these scores may be in advising families regarding the appropriate intensity of medical care but it must be realized that these point estimates of outcomes based on numerical scores have wide confidence intervals. Indeed, of all the cerebrovascular diseases, cerebral hemorrhage may give the most discouraging clinical

Table 34-9

SCORING SYSTEMS FOR PREDICTION OF OUTCOME IN INTRACEREBRAL HEMORRHAGE (ICH AND FUNC SCORES)

ICH Score

GLASGOW COMA SCORE	POINTS ASSIGNED	MORTALITY POINT ESTIMATE PREDICTION	
3–4	2	5+	100%
5–12	1	4	97%
13–15	0	3	72%
ICH volume (mL)		2	26%
≥30	1	1	13%
<30	0	0	0%
Age			
≥80	1		
<80	0		
Infratentorial location	1		
Intraventricular hemorrhage	1		

FUNC Score

GLASGOW COMA SCORE		FUNCTIONAL INDEPENDENCE AT 90 DAYS POINT ESTIMATE	
≥9	2	0–4	0%
<9	0	5–7	13%
ICH volume (mL)		8	42%
<30	4	9–10	66%
30–60	2	11	82%
≥60	0		
Age			
<70	2		
70–79	1		
≥80	0		
ICH location			
Lobar	2		
Deep	1		
Infratentorial	0		
Pre-ICH cognitive impairment			
No	1		
Yes	0		

ICH score adapted from Hemphill and colleagues; FUNC adopted from Rost et al.

picture initially and yet have a reasonable clinical outcome and such scores must be tempered by clinical experience.

In patients who survive, there can be a surprising degree of restoration of function, because, in contrast to infarction, the hemorrhage has to some extent pushed brain tissue aside rather than destroyed it. Function returns very slowly, however, because extravasated blood takes time to be removed from the tissues. Healed scars impinging on the cortex are liable to be epileptogenic; the frequency of seizures after each type of hemorrhage has not been established, but it is lower than for ischemic strokes. There is no need to administer anticonvulsive medication unless a seizure has occurred.

The poor prognosis of all but the smallest pontine hemorrhages has already been mentioned. Cerebellar hemorrhages present special problems that are discussed below.

Treatment

The management of patients with large intracerebral hemorrhages and coma includes the maintenance of adequate ventilation, selective acute use of controlled hyperventilation to a Pco_2 of 25 to 30 mm Hg, monitoring of intracranial pressure in some cases and its control by the use of tissue-dehydrating agents such as mannitol (osmolality kept at 295 to 305 mOsm/L and Na at 145 to 150 mEq), and limiting intravenous infusions to normal saline. Qureshi's group offered data suggesting that aggressive measures to reduce intracranial pressure may be lifesaving and result in good outcome even in patients who have signs of transtentorial herniation. In our experience, this type of recovery is exceptional, but medical treatment of raised intracranial pressure may be justified in patients whose medical condition allows it.

As mentioned, virtually all patients with intracerebral hemorrhage are hypertensive immediately after the stroke because of a generalized sympathoadrenal response. The natural trend is for the blood pressure to diminish over several days; therefore active treatment in the acute stages has been a matter of controversy. Rapid reduction of moderately elevated blood pressure (between 140 and 160 mm Hg systolic), in the hope of reducing further bleeding, is not recommended, because it risks compromising cerebral perfusion in cases of raised intracranial pressure. On the other hand, sustained mean blood pressures of greater than 110 mm Hg (generally above 160 mm Hg systolic) may exaggerate cerebral edema and perhaps enhance the risk extension of the clot. It is at approximately this level of acute hypertension that the use of beta-blocking drugs (esmolol, labetalol) or angiotensin-converting enzyme (ACE) inhibitors is recommended. The major calcium channel-blocking drugs are used less often for this purpose because of reports of adverse effects on intracranial pressure, although this information derives mainly from patients with brain tumors. Hayashi and associates have shown that although blood pressure is lowered with nifedipine after cerebral hemorrhage, intracranial pressure is raised, resulting in an unfavorable net reduction in cerebral perfusion pressure. Nevertheless, we have used all classes of medication in patients with small- and medium-sized clots without adverse effects. Diuretics are helpful in combination with any of the antihypertensive medications. More rapidly acting and titratable agents such as nitroprusside may be used in extreme situations, recognizing that they may further raise intracranial pressure.

Although it would appear intuitively that *evacuation of a hematoma might be beneficial,* surgical results have not been superior to those with medical measures alone (Waga and Yamamoto; Batjer et al; Juvela et al; Rabinstein et al). A large, multicenter, randomized study involving 1,033 patients with supratentorial hemorrhage, under the auspices of the Surgical Trial in Intracerebral Haemorrhage (STICH) study reported by Mendelow and colleagues, has failed to show a benefit from early surgery on survival or neurologic functioning at 6 months. This negative result extended to almost all levels of neurologic deficit and all age groups. In a post hoc analysis, clots that were small and close to the surface of the brain may have benefited from evacuation. As a result, a direct surgical approach has been used less frequently than in the past, but we acknowledge that in a few instances with ongoing deterioration in young patients with hematomas that were easily accessible from the cortical surface, we have asked our neurosurgical colleagues to undertake evacuation of the clot.

Mayer and coworkers studied the promising approach of administering clotting factor VII within 4 h of hemorrhage. In a preliminary study, survival was improved and there was a reduction in enlargement of the hematoma, but their subsequent series has failed to confirm the benefit on survival so that infusion of factor VII is not currently part of routine practice.

If acute hydrocephalus has resulted from a centrally placed hemorrhage or rupture into the ventricular system, a drain is needed. It has been appreciated for some time that intraventricular extension of cerebral hemorrhage generally denotes a poor outcome. An exception may be small thalamic hemorrhages. There was an ongoing study of the reduction of intraventricular hemorrhage size by the use of infused tissue plasminogen activator through a ventricular catheter. Preliminary results suggest that this approach may reduce mortality, and similar practices have been adopted for some time on many neurosurgical services.

Once the patient with a supratentorial hemorrhage becomes deeply comatose with dilated fixed pupils, the chance of recovery is negligible. Even in retrospective studies in which clinical worsening was the reason for surgery, such as the one by Rabinstein and colleagues, only 25 percent of patients attained a state of functional independence and all of their patients who lost their brainstem reflexes and had extensor posturing died despite surgery; there have been a few exceptions to this observation.

In comatose patients with large hemorrhages, the placement of a device for monitoring of intracranial pressure enables the clinician to use medical measures with greater precision, as outlined in Chap. 17, but there is no evidence that outcome is significantly improved (Ropper and King). Whether hemicraniectomy is of value, as it is with large hemispheral strokes, is not known but it seems unlikely.

The issue often arises of the appropriate timing of restarting anticoagulation in patients whose hemorrhage occurred on warfarin. In some instances, such as a prosthetic heart valve requires warfarin, medication is often reintroduced after a week or two. However, for the more common indication of this drug, namely atrial fibrillation, there have been diverging suggestions from different surveys. In an often-cited study by Majeed and colleagues, a retrospective review of almost 3,000 patients over 6 years suggested that the risk of creating another hemorrhage by restarting warfarin earlier than 10 to 30 weeks after the initial stroke was quite high.

Surgical Evacuation of Cerebellar Hematoma In contrast, the *surgical evacuation of cerebellar hematomas* is a generally accepted treatment and is a more urgent matter because of the proximity of the mass to the brainstem and the risk of abrupt progression to coma and respiratory failure. Also, hydrocephalus from compression of the fourth ventricle more often complicates the clinical picture and further raises intracranial pressure (St. Louis et al). As a rule, a cerebellar hematoma less than 2 cm in diameter leaves most patients awake and infrequently leads to deterioration, therefore generally not requiring surgery. Hematomas that are 4 cm or more in largest diameter, especially if located in the vermis, pose the greatest risk, and some surgeons have recommended evacuation of lesions of this size no matter what the clinical status of the patient. In determining the need for surgical evacuation, we have been guided by the patient's state of consciousness, the mass effect caused by the clot as visualized on CT (particularly the degree of compression of the quadrigeminal cistern, as pointed out by Taneda and colleagues), and the presence or absence of hydrocephalus. Assessment may require daily or even more frequent CT. The patient who is stuporous or displays arrhythmic breathing is best intubated and brought to the operating room within hours or sooner. Once coma and pupillary changes supervene, few patients survive, even with surgery; however, rapid medical intervention with mannitol and hyperventilation, followed by surgical evacuation of the clot and drainage of the ventricles within hours of the onset of coma has been successful in a few cases. Patients who are drowsy and those with hematomas of 2 to 4 cm in diameter in the cerebellar hemisphere pose the greatest difficulty in determining if, and when, surgery is advisable. If the level of consciousness is fluctuating or if there is obliteration of the perimesencephalic cisterns, particularly if coupled with hydrocephalus, we believe that the risk of surgery is less than that of a sudden deterioration. In only a very limited number of patients have we found it practical to perform only drainage of the enlarged ventricles, although some groups still favor this procedure and eschew a posterior fossa operation. Evacuation of the clot in our experience has been more important than reduction of the hydrocephalus.

SPONTANEOUS SUBARACHNOID HEMORRHAGE AND RUPTURED SACCULAR ANEURYSM

This is the fourth most frequent cerebrovascular disorder—following atherothrombosis, embolism, and primary intracerebral hemorrhage, but one that is often disastrous. Saccular aneurysms also have been called "berry" aneurysms. They take the form of small, thin-walled blisters protruding from arteries of the circle of Willis or its major branches. Their rupture causes a flooding of the subarachnoid space with blood under high pressure. As a rule, the aneurysms are located at vessel bifurcations and branchings (Fig. 34-24) and are generally presumed

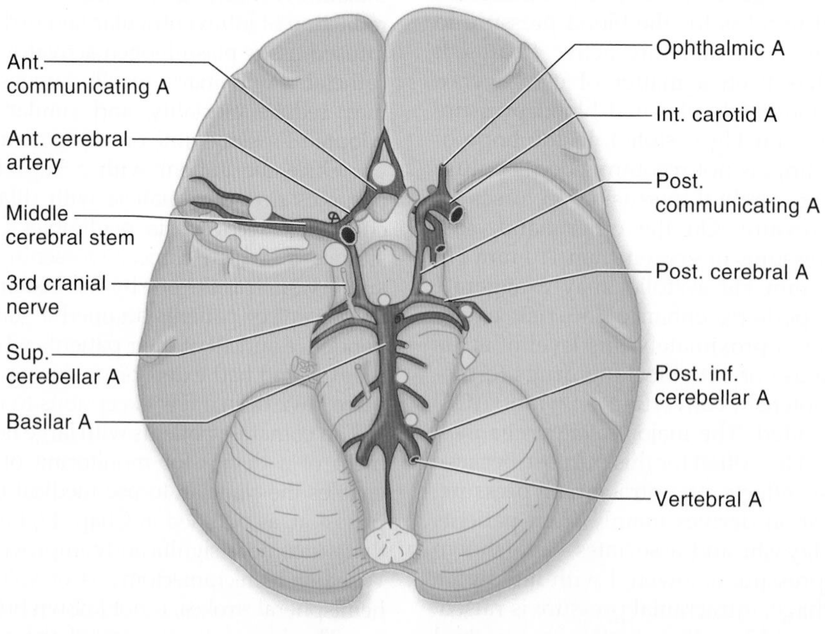

Figure 34-24. Diagram of the circle of Willis showing the principal sites of intracranial aneurysms. Approximately 90 percent of aneurysms arise from branches of the anterior half of the circle. The sizes of the aneurysms depicted correspond roughly to the frequency of occurrence at those sites.

to result from developmental defects in the media and elastica of the arteries. An alternate theory holds that the aneurysmal process is initiated by focal destruction of the internal elastic membrane, which is produced by hemodynamic forces at the apices of bifurcations (Ferguson). As a result of the local weakness in the vessel wall, the intima bulges outward, covered only by adventitia; the sac then gradually enlarges and may finally rupture. Cerebral aneurysms vary in size from 2 mm to 2 or 3 cm in diameter, averaging 7.5 mm (Wiebers et al, 1981 and 1987). Those that rupture usually have a diameter of 10 mm or more, but rupture also occurs, albeit less often, in those of smaller size. Aneurysms vary greatly in form. Some are round and connected to the parent artery by a narrow stalk; others are broad-based without a stalk; and still others take the form of narrow cylinders. The site of rupture is usually at the dome of the aneurysm, which may have one or more secondary sacculations. A review of the subject by Schievink gives further details of this extensively studied subject.

The incidence of unruptured aneurysms in routine autopsies is almost 2 percent—excluding minor vessel outpouchings of 3 mm or less. Moreover, aneurysms are multiple in 20 percent of patients. In the past, it was estimated that 400,000 Americans harbored unruptured aneurysms and that there were 26,000 aneurysmal subarachnoid hemorrhages per year (Sahs et al, 1981 and 1984). Rupture of saccular aneurysms in childhood is rare, and they are seldom found at routine postmortem examination in this age group; beyond childhood, they gradually increase in frequency to reach their peak incidence between ages 35 and 65 years. Therefore aneurysms cannot be regarded as fully formed congenital anomalies; rather, they appear to develop over the years on the basis of either a developmental or acquired arterial defect. There is an increased incidence of congenital polycystic kidneys, fibromuscular dysplasia of the extracranial arteries, moyamoya, arteriovenous malformations of the brain, and coarctation of the aorta among persons with saccular aneurysms and vice versa. An accompanying saccular aneurysm occurs in approximately 5 percent of cases of cerebral arteriovenous malformation, usually on the main feeding artery of the malformation.

Numerous reports have documented a familial occurrence of saccular aneurysms, lending support to the idea that genetic factors play a role in their development. The number of first-degree relatives found to harbor an unsuspected aneurysm has been approximately 4 percent in most series. This low rate, the finding that half of the discovered aneurysms are small, and the complications of surgery make routine screening of siblings, children, and parents of patients with ruptured aneurysms impractical, according to the Magnetic Resonance Angiography in Relatives of Patients with Subarachnoid Hemorrhage Study Group. However, because aneurysms of the familial variety tend to be larger at the time of rupture and more numerous than in patients who have sporadic ones, there are exceptions to this statement (Ruigrok et al), and there is little question that, in practice, the close relatives of patients with ruptured aneurysms ask for, and are accommodated, screening for aneurysms. From a survey in Scotland, the lifetime risk of hemorrhage was only 4.7 percent for a first-degree relative and 1.9 percent for a second-degree relative (Teasdale et al). From several series, it is apparent that the risk is highest for individuals with two or more first-degree relatives and negligible for one second-degree relative.

Although hypertension is more frequently present than in the general population, aneurysms most often occur in persons with normal blood pressure. Pregnancy does not appear to be associated with an increased incidence of aneurysmal rupture, although there is always concern about the possibility of inducing bleeding during the straining of natural delivery. Atherosclerosis, although present in the walls of some saccular aneurysms, probably plays no part in their formation or enlargement.

Approximately 90 to 95 percent of saccular aneurysms lie on the anterior part of the circle of Willis (see Fig. 34-24). The four most common sites are (1) the proximal portions of the anterior communicating artery, (2) at the origin of the posterior communicating artery from the stem of the internal carotid, (3) at the first major bifurcation of the middle cerebral artery, and (4) at the bifurcation of the internal carotid into middle and anterior cerebral arteries. Other sites include the internal carotid artery in the cavernous sinus, at the origin of the ophthalmic artery, the junction of the posterior communicating and posterior cerebral arteries, the bifurcation of the basilar artery, and the origins of the cerebellar arteries. Aneurysms of the carotid artery that rupture in the cavernous sinus give rise to an arteriovenous fistula (see further on).

There are several types of aneurysms other than saccular, e.g., mycotic, fusiform, diffuse, and globular. The mycotic aneurysm is caused by a septic embolus that weakens the wall of the vessel in which it lodges, almost always at a site in a distal cerebral vessel, well beyond the circle of Willis. These lesions are discussed separately in a later section of this chapter. The others are named for their predominant morphologic characteristics and consist of enlargement or dilatation of the entire circumference of the involved vessels, usually the internal carotid, vertebral, or basilar arteries. Fusiform deformities are also referred to as arteriosclerotic aneurysms, as they frequently show atheromatous deposition in their walls, but it is likely that they are at least partly developmental in nature. Some are very large (so-called giant aneurysms) and press on neighboring structures or become occluded by thrombus, but they rupture only infrequently (as discussed further on).

Clinical Syndrome

With rupture of the aneurysm, blood under high pressure is forced into the subarachnoid space and the resulting clinical events assume one of three patterns: (1) the patient is stricken with an excruciating generalized headache and vomiting and falls unconscious almost immediately; (2) severe generalized headache develops in the same instantaneous manner but the patient remains relatively lucid with varying degrees of stiff neck—the most common syndrome; (3) rarely, consciousness is lost so quickly that there is no preceding complaint. If the hemorrhage is massive, death may ensue in a matter of minutes or hours, so that ruptured aneurysm must be considered in the differential diagnosis of sudden death. A considerable proportion of such patients probably never reach a hospital. Decerebrate rigidity and brief clonic jerking of the limbs may occur at the onset of the hemorrhage, always in association with unconsciousness. Persistent deep coma is accompanied by irregular respirations, attacks of extensor rigidity, and finally respiratory arrest and circulatory collapse. In these rapidly evolving cases, the subarachnoid blood has greatly increased the intracranial pressure to a level that approaches arterial pressure and caused a marked reduction in cerebral perfusion. In some instances, the hemorrhage has dissected intracerebrally and entered the brain or ventricular system.

Rupture of the aneurysm usually occurs while the patient is active rather than during sleep, and in a few instances during sexual intercourse, straining at stool, lifting heavy objects, or other sustained exertion (see "Headaches Related to Sexual Activity" in Chap. 10). A momentary Valsalva maneuver, as in coughing or sneezing, has generally not caused aneurysmal rupture (it may cause arterial dissection). In patients who survive the initial rupture, the most feared complication is rerupture, an event that may occur at any time from minutes up to 2 or 3 weeks.

In less-severe cases, consciousness, if lost, may be regained within minutes or hours, but a residuum of drowsiness, confusion, and amnesia accompanied by severe headache and stiff neck persists for at least several days. Because the hemorrhage in most cases is confined to the subarachnoid space, there are few if any focal neurologic signs. That is to say, hemiparesis, hemianopia, and aphasia are absent. On occasion, a jet of blood emanating from an aneurysm ruptures into the adjacent brain or insular cistern and produces a hemiparesis or other focal syndrome. This may be more common when the aneurysm has bled in the past, after which it adheres to the brain, thus predisposing to intracerebral hemorrhage at the time of subsequent rupture. There is, however, a transient focal acute syndrome that occasionally occurs in the territory of the aneurysm-bearing artery. The pathogenesis of such manifestations is not fully understood, but a transitory fall in pressure in the circulation distal to the aneurysm or some form of acute transient vasospasm has been postulated. An entirely separate problem of delayed vasospasm is responsible for focal signs that emerge after several days as discussed below. Transient deficits when they do occur constitute reliable indicators of the site of the ruptured aneurysm (see below).

Convulsive seizures, usually brief and generalized, occur in 10 to 25 percent of cases according to Hart and associates (but far less often in our experience) in relation to acute bleeding or rebleeding. These early seizures do not correlate with the location of the aneurysm and do not appear to alter the prognosis.

Prior to rupture, saccular aneurysms are usually asymptomatic. Exceptionally, if large enough to compress pain-sensitive structures, they may cause localized cranial pain. With a cavernous or anterolaterally situated aneurysm on the first part of the middle cerebral artery, the pain may be projected to the orbit. An aneurysm on the posteroinferior or anteroinferior cerebellar artery may cause unilateral occipital or cervical pain. The presence of a partial oculomotor palsy with dilated pupil may be indicative of an aneurysm of the posterior communicating–internal carotid junction or at the posterior communicating–posterior cerebral junction. Occasionally, large aneurysms just anterior to the cavernous sinus compress the optic nerves or chiasm, third nerve, hypothalamus, or pituitary gland. A monocular visual field defect may also develop with a supraclinoid aneurysm near the anterior and middle cerebral bifurcation or the ophthalmic–carotid bifurcation. In the cavernous sinus, they may compress the third, fourth, or sixth nerve, or the ophthalmic division of the fifth nerve.

Whether a small leak of blood from an aneurysm may serve as a warning sign of a subsequent more catastrophic rupture ("warning leak") has been disputed. An entity known as "sentinel headache" has been used in an imprecise way to refer to both a headache that precedes subarachnoid hemorrhage and to a small leakage prior to a major rupture. The former in our view has little validity, as headaches are so ubiquitous that many, even severe ones, are coincidental in relation to subarachnoid hemorrhage. The frequency of true warming leaks is unknown but is not likely to be high. We have seen several cases where an acute and severe exertional or spontaneous headache was found to be associated with a small subarachnoid hemorrhage that was discovered by lumbar puncture; more often the headache is unrelated to hemorrhage and is attributable to migraine. This type of "thunderclap headache," may be a variant of migraine, or less often, cerebral venous thrombosis, diffuse vasospasm (the Call-Fleming syndrome), or even less often, pituitary apoplexy, hypertensive encephalopathy, intracranial hypotension, and intracranial or extracranial arterial dissection. The details of the CSF examination assume great importance in the diagnosis of subarachnoid hemorrhage and the exclusion of the disorders mentioned above.

Laboratory Findings

A CT will detect blood locally or diffusely in the subarachnoid spaces or within the brain or ventricular system in more than 90 percent of cases and in practically all cases in which the hemorrhage has been severe enough to cause momentary or persistent loss of consciousness (Fig. 34-25). Therefore, this should be the initial investigative procedure. Because the blood may appear as a subtle shadow along the tentorium or in the sylvian or adjacent fissures, it is more easily appreciated in the noncontrast study. A large localized collection of subarachnoid blood or a hematoma in brain tissue or within the sylvian fissure indicates the adjacent location of the aneurysm and the likely region of subsequent vasospasm, as already noted. When two or more aneurysms are visualized, the CT can identify the one that had ruptured by the clot that surrounds it. Also, coexistent hydrocephalus will be demonstrable. If the CT documents subarachnoid blood with certainty, a spinal tap is not necessary. MRI can

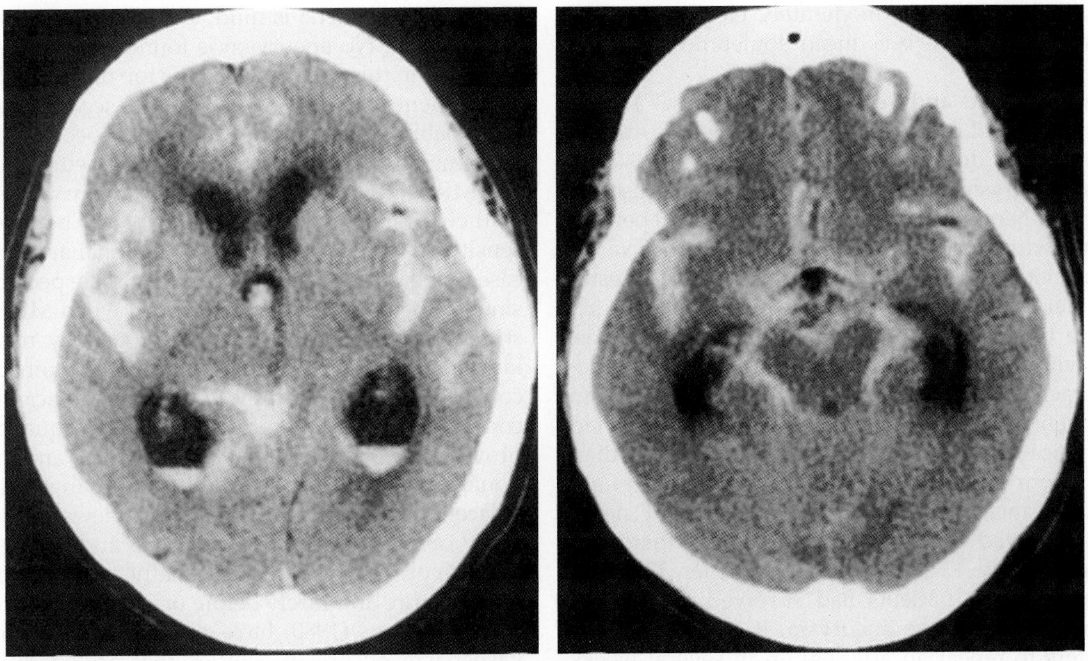

Figure 34-25. Subarachnoid hemorrhage as a result of rupture of a basilar artery aneurysm. *Left*: Axial CT at the level of the lateral ventricles showing widespread hyperdense blood in the subarachnoid spaces and layering within the ventricles with resultant hydrocephalus. There is a blood–CSF level in the posterior horns of the lateral ventricles, typical of recent bleeding. *Right*: At the level of the basal cisterns, blood can be seen surrounding the brainstem, in the anterior sylvian fissures, and the anterior interhemispheric fissure. The temporal horns of the lateral ventricles are enlarged, reflecting acute hydrocephalus.

also detect blood in the proton-density sequence; after a day has passed, this is also appreciated with the FLAIR technique.

In all other cases where subarachnoid hemorrhage is suspected but not apparent on imaging studies, a lumbar puncture should be undertaken. Usually the CSF becomes grossly bloody within 30 min or sooner of the hemorrhage, with RBC counts up to 1 million/mm^3 or even higher. Blood may not be easily apparent in a lumbar puncture minutes after the hemorrhage. With a relatively mild hemorrhage, there may be only a few thousand cells, a severe headache syndrome from subarachnoid hemorrhage is associated with at least several hundred cells. It is also probably not possible for an aneurysm to rupture entirely into brain tissue without some leakage of blood into the subarachnoid fluid. In other words, the diagnosis of ruptured saccular aneurysm is essentially excluded if blood is not present in the CSF, provided the spinal fluid is examined more than 30 min after the event. Xanthochromia is found after centrifugation if several hours or more have elapsed from the moment of the ictus. In a patient who reports a headache that was consistent with subarachnoid hemorrhage but that had occurred several days earlier, the CT may be normal and xanthochromia is the only diagnostic finding. To determine whether xanthochromia is present, fresh CSF must be centrifuged in a tube with a conical bottom and the supernatant compared to clear water in good light or examined by spectrophotometric techniques. It has been our experience that most hospital laboratories cannot be depended on to give accurate results for this test. Also helpful after several days is the MRI taken with the FLAIR sequence as mentioned, which will demonstrate blood (the proton-density sequence is more sensitive to blood in the first day).

The problem of a "traumatic tap" often clouds the early diagnosis, and several aids to detecting this misleading laboratory result are discussed in Chap. 2. Here it is reiterated that in addition to the absence of xanthochromia, the most important features indicating that blood has been spuriously introduced by entering small veins in the epidural space with the lumbar puncture needle are the clearing of blood as one continues to collect fluid and a marked reduction in the number of RBCs in serial tubes of spinal fluid. A normal opening pressure also suggests puncture of a local vessel rather than a ruptured aneurysm. The combination of subarachnoid hemorrhage and a traumatic tap generally requires that vascular imaging procedures be performed to resolve the issue. The CSF in the first days is under increased pressure, as high as 500 mm H_2O—but usually closer to 250 mm H_2O—an important finding in differentiating spontaneous subarachnoid hemorrhage from a traumatic tap. In both a traumatic puncture and early in subarachnoid hemorrhage, the proportion of WBCs to RBCs in the CSF is usually the same as in the circulating blood (approximately 1:700), but in some patients with genuine hemorrhage a brisk CSF leukocytosis appears within 48 h, sometimes reaching more than 1,000 cells/mm^3.

The protein is slightly or moderately elevated and in some instances glucose is reduced sometimes dramatically so.

Bilateral carotid and vertebral ("four-vessel") angiography is the most dependable means of demonstrating an aneurysm and does so in essentially all patients who harbor an aneurysm, but in addition to other causes of subarachnoid hemorrhage, approximately 5 to 10 percent of patients with aneurysmal rupture will not have an aneurysm evident. Some of these instances are a result of the obliteration of the lesion in the process of rupture. Others are because of somewhat more benign lesions. Patients with the typical clinical picture of spontaneous subarachnoid hemorrhage in whom an aneurysm or arteriovenous malformation cannot be demonstrated angiographically have a distinctly better prognosis than those in whom the lesion is visualized (Nishioka et al). For example, in a series of 323 angiographically negative cases followed for an average of 10 years, there was rebleeding in only 12 (Hawkins et al). After 22 years, 69 percent of these patients had survived. If the first study does not reveal an aneurysm, it is customary in most centers to repeat an arteriogram in several weeks because it has been observed that vascular spasm may have earlier obscured the aneurysm. Even when there is no vasospasm visualized, it is sometimes the case that a second study shows the lesion. It is advantageous to obtain images from several different angles in order to expose those views that may be obscured by adjacent overlying vessels. If the first study involves all cerebral vessels and uses several views of the basal circulation, it has been our experience that the second arteriogram is infrequently revealing, but we follow general practice and repeat it nonetheless.

Another clinical circumstance with a favorable outcome is a limited *perimesencephalic hemorrhage* as described by van Gijn and colleagues. The cisterns surrounding the midbrain and upper pons are symmetrically filled with blood, the headache is mild, and signs of vasospasm do not develop. No aneurysm is found at the expected site for blood in this region, i.e., at the top of the basilar artery. The patient usually does well and a second arteriogram is probably not required. It has been speculated that the bleeding has a venous rather than an aneurysmal source.

MRI detects most aneurysms of the basal vessels and of their first branches but may not yet be of sufficient sensitivity to replace CT or conventional angiography in cases where an aneurysm is strongly suspected but too small to be detected by MRA. Even when MRA demonstrates the aneurysm, the surgeon usually requires the kind of anatomic definition that can be obtained only by conventional angiography. CT technology scanning with contrast infusion has certainly begun to equal the detail provided by conventional angiography and has additional advantages of showing the lesion in relation to the adjacent brain and skull in multiple views (Fig. 34-26).

Vasospasm *Delayed hemiplegia* and other deficits because of focal vasospasm usually appear 3 to 10 days after rupture and rarely before or after this period. Fisher and coworkers (1980) have shown that the most severe vasospasm occurs in arteries that are surrounded by collections of clotted subarachnoid blood after 24 h. These same authors devised a widely used scale that rates the extent and location of remaining clot. The reduction in the caliber of blood vessels (vasospasm) appears to be a direct effect of some blood product on the adventitia of the adjacent artery. Areas of ischemic infarction in the territory of the vessel bearing the aneurysm, without thrombosis or other intraluminal changes in the vessel, is the usual finding in such cases. The mechanism is presumed to be purely a reduction in blood flow distal to the area of vasospasm but therefore influenced by systemic blood pressure and by collateral circulation in the cortex. The ischemic lesions are often multiple and had in the past occurred with great frequency, according to Hijdra and associates.

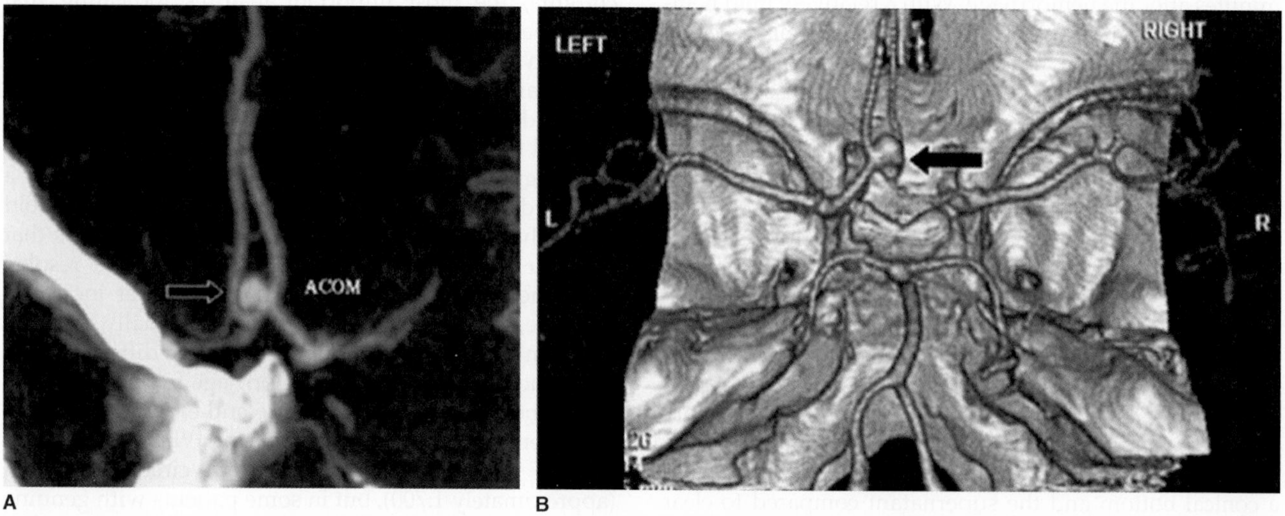

A B

Figure 34-26. Berry aneurysm of the anterior communicating artery. *Left*: CT angiogram showing the aneurysm (*arrow*) arising from the branch point of the anterior communicating artery and the A1 segment; *Right*: Reconstructed image from CT angiogram data showing the aneurysm (*arrow*) in relation to the adjacent bony and vascular structures.

After a few days, arteries in chronic spasm undergo a series of morphologic changes. The smooth muscle cells of the media become necrotic, and the adventitia is infiltrated with neutrophilic leukocytes, mast cells, and red blood corpuscles, some of which have migrated to a subendothelial position. The current notion is that these changes are caused by products of hemolyzed blood seeping inward from the pia-arachnoid into the muscularis of the artery.

The clinical features of delayed cerebral vasospasm depend on the affected blood vessel but typically include a fluctuating hemiparesis or aphasia and increasing confusion that must be distinguished from the effects of hydrocephalus (see below). In the past, an arteriogram was required to verify the diagnosis, although it is not often performed now because of the slight associated risk of worsening vascular spasm and the ease with which the condition can be recognized by its clinical presentation. Severe vasospasm is also visualized with MRA and CT techniques (Fig. 34-27). Transcranial Doppler ultrasonography measurements provide an indirect way of following, by observations of blood flow velocity, the caliber of the main vessels at the base of the brain but they are somewhat imprecise for this purpose. Almost all patients have a greatly increased velocity of blood flow in the affected vessel that can be detected by ultrasound in the days after hemorrhage. However, progressive elevation of flow velocity in any one vessel (especially if over 175 cm/s) suggests that focal vasospasm is occurring. There is a reasonable correlation between these findings and the radiographic appearance of vasospasm, but the clinical manifestations of ischemia depend on additional factors such as collateral blood supply and the cerebral perfusion pressure.

Hydrocephalus If a large amount of blood ruptures into the ventricular system or floods the basal subarachnoid space, it may find its way into the ventricles through the foramina of Luschka and Magendie. The patient then becomes confused or unconscious as a result of *acute hydrocephalus*. The clinical signs are reversed by draining the ventricles, either by external ventriculostomy or, in selected cases, by lumbar puncture, but the routine use of ventricular drainage after subarachnoid hemorrhage is not uniformly agreed upon.

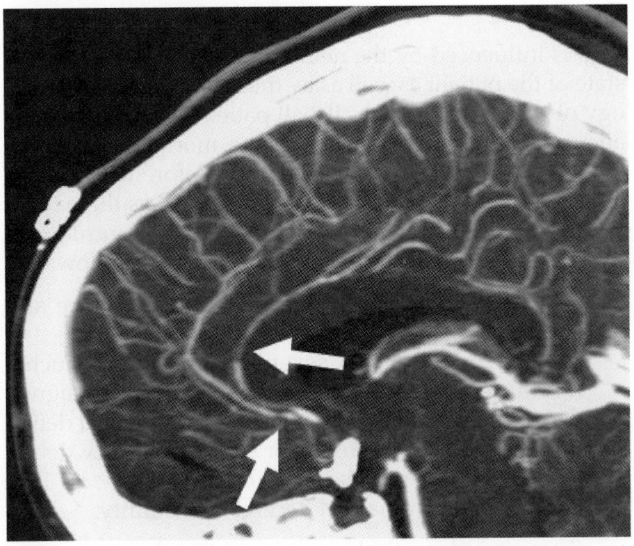

Figure 34-27. Vasospasm following subarachnoid hemorrhage due to rupture of an anterior communicating artery aneurysm. Sagittal CT angiography reveals multifocal narrowing of segments of the anterior cerebral artery (*arrows*).

Delayed and *subacute hydrocephalus* as a result of blockage of the CSF pathways by blood may appear after 2 to 4 weeks and is managed similarly. Many of these latter cases improve. There are further instances of long-delayed hydrocephalus that present as normal-pressure hydrocephalus (NPH) months or years after subarachnoid hemorrhage, as described in Chap. 30.

Anatomic–Clinical Correlations of Aneurysms

In most patients, the neurologic manifestations do not point to the exact site of the aneurysm, but it can often be inferred from the location of the main clot on CT. A collection of blood in the anterior interhemispheric fissure indicates rupture of an anterior communicating artery aneurysm; in the sylvian fissure, a middle cerebral artery aneurysm; in the anterior perimesencephalic cistern, a posterior communicating or distal basilar artery aneurysm. In other instances clinical signs provide clues to its localization, as follows: (1) third-nerve palsy (ptosis, diplopia, dilatation of pupil, and divergent strabismus), indicates an aneurysm at the junction of the posterior communicating artery and the internal carotid artery—the third nerve passes immediately lateral to this point or at the posterior cerebral-posterior communicating artery junction; (2) transient paresis of one or both of the lower limbs at the onset of the hemorrhage suggests an anterior communicating aneurysm that has interfered with the circulation in the anterior cerebral arteries; (3) hemiparesis or aphasia points to an aneurysm at the first major bifurcation of the middle cerebral artery; (4) unilateral blindness indicates an aneurysm lying anteromedially in the circle of Willis (usually at the origin of the ophthalmic artery or at the bifurcation of the internal carotid artery); (5) a state of retained consciousness with akinetic mutism or abulia favors a location on the anterior communicating artery; (6) the side on which the aneurysm lies may be indicated by a unilateral preponderance of headache or by unilateral preretinal (subhyaloid) hemorrhage (Terson syndrome), the occurrence of monocular pain, or, rarely, lateralization of an intracranial sound heard at the time of rupture of the aneurysm. Sixth-nerve palsy, unilateral or bilateral, is usually attributable to raised intracranial pressure and is less often of localizing value.

In summary, the clinical sequence of sudden severe headache, vomiting, collapse, relative preservation of consciousness with few or no lateralizing signs, and neck stiffness is diagnostic of subarachnoid hemorrhage caused by a ruptured saccular aneurysm.

Other clinical data may be of assistance in reaching a correct diagnosis. Levels of blood pressure of 200 mm Hg systolic are seen occasionally just after rupture, but usually the pressure is elevated only moderately and fluctuates with the degree of head pain. Nuchal rigidity is usually present but occasionally absent, and the main complaint of pain may be referable to the interscapular region or even the low back rather than to the head. Examination of the fundi frequently reveals smooth-surfaced, sharply outlined collections of blood that cover the retinal vessels—preretinal or subhyaloid hemorrhages (Terson syndrome); Roth spots are seen occasionally. Bilateral Babinski signs are found in the first few days following rupture if there is hydrocephalus. Fever up to 39°C (102.2°F) may be seen in the first week, but most patients are afebrile. Rarely, escaping blood enters the subdural space and produces a hematoma, evacuation of which may be lifesaving.

Systemic Changes Associated With Subarachnoid Hemorrhage

Acute subarachnoid hemorrhage is associated with several characteristic responses in the systemic circulation, water balance, and cardiac function. The ECG changes include symmetrically large peaked T waves ("cerebral T waves") and other alterations, suggesting subendocardial or myocardial ischemia. There may be a minor elevation of troponin and the myocardial band (MB) of creatine phosphokinase (CPK). In some patients, the cardiac dysfunction is severe enough to seriously reduce the ejection fraction and cause heart failure. There is a tendency to develop hyponatremia; this abnormality and its relationship to intravascular volume depletion play a key role in treatment, as discussed further on. Albuminuria and glycosuria may be present for a few days. Rarely, diabetes insipidus occurs in the acute stages, but water retention or a natriuresis is more frequent. There may be a leukocytosis of 15,000 to 18,000 cells/mm^3, but the sedimentation rate and C-reactive protein are usually normal, or any elevation is attributable to another cause.

Rebleeding and Prognosis

The outstanding characteristic of this condition, mentioned earlier, is the tendency for the hemorrhage to recur from the same site in more than one-third of patients, often catastrophically. This threat colors all prognostications and dominates modern treatment strategies. There does not appear to be a way of determining reliably which patients will bleed again. The cause of recurrent bleeding is not understood but is related to naturally occurring mechanisms of clot lysis at the site of initial rupture, usually at the dome of the aneurysm.

As regards prognosis of aneurysmal hemorrhage, McKissock and colleagues decades ago found that the patient's state of consciousness at the time of arteriography was the single best index of outcome, and this remains largely true today. Their data, representative of the status of aneurysm management in the 1950s and consonant with the natural history before the advent of modern surgical and intensive care techniques, indicated that of every 100 patients reaching a hospital and coming to arteriography, 17 were stuporous or comatose and 83 appeared to be recovering from the ictus. At the end of 6 months, 8 of every 100 patients had died of the original hemorrhage and 59 had a recurrence (with 40 deaths), making a total of 48 deaths and 52 survivors. In regard to recurrence of bleeding, it was found that of 50 patients seen on the first day of the illness, 5 rebled in the first week (all fatal), 8 in the second week (5 fatal), 6 in the third and fourth weeks (4 fatal), and 2 in the next 4 weeks (2 fatal), making a total of 21 recurrences (16 fatal) in 8 weeks.

The most comprehensive long-term analysis of the natural history of the disease, outdated but still instructive, is contained in the report of the Cooperative Study of Intracranial Aneurysms and Subarachnoid Hemorrhage (Sahs et al, 1984). The study was based on long-term observations of 568 patients who sustained an aneurysmal bleed between 1958 and 1965 and were managed only by a conservative medical program. A followup search in 1981 and 1982 disclosed that 378, or two-thirds of the patients, had died; 40 percent of the deaths had occurred within 6 months of the original hemorrhage. For the patients who survived the original hemorrhage for 6 months, the chances of survival during the next two decades were significantly worse than those of a matched normal population. Rebleeding occurred at a rate of 2.2 percent per year during the first decade and 0.86 percent per year during the second, and these were fatal in 78 percent of cases. Although these statistics reflect the outcome prior to the modern era of microsurgery and neurologic intensive care management, current figures are only modestly better. In a prospective clinical trial conducted by the International Cooperative Study in 1990 and based on observations of 3,521 patients (surgery performed in 83 percent), it was found at the 6-month evaluation that 26 percent had died and 58 percent had made a good recovery (Kassell et al). Vasospasm and rebleeding were the leading causes of morbidity and mortality in those who survived the initial hemorrhage.

In respect to rebleeding, all series indicate that the risk is greatest in the first day but extends for weeks. The observations of Aoyagi and Hayakawa are representative of other series; they found that rebleeding occurred within 2 weeks in 20 percent of patients, with a peak incidence in the 24 h after the initial episode. Surgical treatment is largely oriented toward reducing this complication.

Treatment

This is influenced by the neurologic and general medical state of the patient as well as by the location and morphology of the aneurysm. Ideally, all patients should have the aneurysmal sac obliterated, but the mortality is high if the patient is stuporous or comatose. Before deciding on a course of action, it has been useful to assess the patient with reference to the widely employed scale introduced by Botterell and refined by Hunt and Hess, as follows:

Grade I. Asymptomatic or with slight headache and stiff neck
Grade II. Moderate to severe headache and nuchal rigidity but no focal or lateralizing neurologic signs
Grade III. Drowsiness, confusion, and mild focal deficit
Grade IV. Persistent stupor or semicoma, early decerebrate rigidity and vegetative disturbances
Grade V. Deep coma and decerebrate rigidity

The general medical management in the acute stage includes the following, all or in part: bed rest, fluid administration to maintain above-normal circulating blood volume and central venous pressure; use of elastic stockings and stool softeners; administration of calcium channel blockers to reduce infarction from vasospasm (see below); additional beta-adrenergic blockers, intravenous nitroprusside, or other medication to reduce greatly elevated blood pressure and then maintain systolic blood pressure at 150 mm Hg or less; and pain-relieving medication for headache (this alone will often reduce the hypertension). The prevention of systemic venous thrombosis is critical; it usually is accomplished by the use of cyclically inflated whole-leg compression boots. The use of antiepileptic drugs is controversial; many neurosurgeons administer them early, with a view of preventing a seizure-induced risk of rebleeding. Several small studies suggest they may be detrimental and we have generally avoided them unless a seizure has occurred.

Calcium channel blockers are used to reduce the incidence of stroke from vasospasm. Nimodipine 60 mg administered orally every 4 h is currently favored. Although calcium channel blockers do not alter the incidence of angiographically demonstrated vasospasm, they have reduced the number of strokes in each of five randomized studies, beginning with the one conducted by Allen and colleagues. Several groups use angioplasty techniques to dilate vasospastic vessels and report symptomatic improvement, but there are as yet insufficient controlled data to judge the merits and safety of this procedure.

The most notable advances in this disease have been in the techniques for the early obliteration of aneurysms, particularly the operating microscope and endovascular approaches, and in the management of circulatory volume. In the majority of patients, intravascular volume is depleted in the days after subarachnoid hemorrhage. This, in turn, greatly increases the chances of ischemic infarction from vasospasm. In part, this volume contraction can be attributed to bed rest, but sodium loss, probably resulting from the release of atrial natriuretic factor (ANF), a potent oligopeptide stimulator of sodium loss in renal tubules, may also be a factor. Hyponatremia develops in the first week after hemorrhage, but it is unclear whether this also results from the natriuretic effects of ANF or is an effect of antidiuretic hormone, causing water retention. The work of Diringer and coworkers (1988) suggests that both mechanisms are operative but it is the volume depletion, not hyponatremia per se, that is of the greatest clinical consequence.

Both the risk of rerupture of the aneurysm and some of the secondary problems that arise because of blood in the subarachnoid space can be obviated by early obliteration of the aneurysm. Because of the changes in water balance and the risk of delayed stroke from vasospasm, there has been an emphasis on early volume expansion and sodium repletion by the intravenous infusion of crystalloids. As Solomon and Fink point out, this can be accomplished without fear of aneurysmal rupture if blood pressure is allowed to rise only minimally. Of course, fluid replacement and a modest elevation of blood pressure become completely safe if the aneurysm has been surgically occluded. Thus the current approach is to operate or eliminate the aneurysm by endovascular means early, within 24 h if possible, for patients in grades I and II, and then to increase intravascular volume and maintain normal or above-normal blood pressures. This precludes rebleeding, with its high mortality, and ameliorates the second cause of morbidity, stroke from vasospasm. The timing of surgery or endovascular treatment for grade III patients is still controversial but if their medical condition allows, they, too, probably benefit from the same early and aggressive approach. In grade IV patients, the outcome is generally dismal, no matter what course is taken, but we have usually counseled against early operation; some neurosurgeons disagree. The insertion of ventricular drains into both frontal horns has occasionally raised a patient with severe hydrocephalus to a better grade and facilitated early operation. In the hands of experienced anesthesiologists and cerebrovascular surgeons, the operative mortality, even in grades III and IV patients, has now been reduced to 2 to 3 percent. For a detailed account of the operative approach to each of the major classes of saccular aneurysm, the reader is referred to the monograph by Ojemann and colleagues (1995).

Several alternative therapeutic measures are in common use but are still being studied. Among these, endovascular obliteration of the lumen of the aneurysm holds the most promise. This has become the preferred approach for aneurysms that are surgically inaccessible—for example, those in the cavernous sinus—and for patients whose medical state precludes an operation. Among several trials that have compared surgery with endovascular placement of coils in the aneurysm, most have shown equivalence or a slight superiority of the latter. For example, the International Subarachnoid Aneurysm Trial Group randomly assigned more than 2,000 patients to surgery or coil deployment; the overall rate of death or dependence at 1 year was 24 percent in the endovascular group and 31 percent in the operated group, a difference that was sustained at 2 years of followup (Molyneux et al). Doubtless, further studies will continue to clarify the relative benefits of the treatment. It is self-evident that the skill of the surgeon and the quality of postoperative care are major determinants of outcome; perhaps the simplicity of endovascular treatment and the improvements in the training of interventional specialists will prove its advantage over time.

Because of the current approach of ablating the aneurysm early, the previously popular use of antifibrinolytic agents as a means of impeding lysis of the clot at the site of aneurysmal rupture has been generally abandoned. Repeated drainage of the CSF by lumbar puncture is also no longer practiced as a routine. One lumbar puncture is generally carried out for diagnostic purposes if the CT is inconclusive; thereafter, spinal fluid drainage is performed only for the relief of intractable headache or to detect recurrence of bleeding. As mentioned earlier, patients with stupor or coma who have massive hydrocephalus often benefit from decompression of the ventricular system. This is accomplished initially by external drainage and may require permanent shunting if the hydrocephalus returns. The common practice of draining milder degrees of hydrocephalus has not been proven to be helpful. Some risk may attend rapid removal of CSF by this method or lumbar puncture. The risk of infection of the external shunt tubing is high if it is left in place for much more than 3 days. Replacement with a new drainage tube, preferably at another site, reduces this risk.

Unruptured Intracranial Aneurysms

Quite often in clinical practice, cerebral angiography, MRI, MRA, or CT performed for an unrelated reason discloses the presence of an unruptured saccular aneurysm. Or, a second or third aneurysm is found during the angiogram to assess a ruptured one. There is now a reasonably sound body of information about the natural history of these lesions. Wiebers and colleagues (1987) observed 65 patients with one or more unruptured aneurysms for 5 years or longer after their detection. The only feature of significance relative to rupture was aneurysmal size. Of the 44 aneurysms smaller than 10 mm in diameter, none had ruptured, whereas 8 of 29 aneurysms 1 cm or larger eventually did so, with a fatal outcome in 7 cases. Two large studies have attempted to refine these statistical data. In the older Cooperative Study of Intracranial Aneurysms, none of the aneurysms less than 7-mm diameter "had further trouble." A more recent and sizable cooperative study that included 4,060 patients and gathered data prospectively for 5 years, conducted by the International Study of Unruptured Intracranial Aneurysms Investigators, found an extremely low rate of rupture, approximately 0.1 percent yearly, for aneurysms smaller than 7 mm in diameter, an annual risk of 0.5 percent for aneurysms between 7 and 10 mm, and a risk ranging from 0.6 to 3.5 percent for lesions between 13 and 24 mm (depending on location). The risk ranged up to 10 percent for aneurysms greater than 25-mm diameter. The yearly rates for rupture were higher in all categories if there had been prior bleeding from another site. The location of the lesion also had great bearing on the risk of rupture, as did increasing age; notably, vertebrobasilar and posterior cerebral aneurysms bled at a rate many times higher than the others. Such data aids in comparing the risk of surgery and endovascular treatment, which, for example, exceed the risk of bleeding within 5 years for small aneurysms located in the carotid circulation. In almost all other circumstances, there is overall benefit to obliterating the unruptured aneurysm.

A special problem pertains to clots within an aneurysm that cause transient ischemic attacks or small strokes in the vascular territory distal to the site. The frequency of this complication is not clear and it occurs at times without evident intraluminal clot on an angiogram.

Giant Cerebral Aneurysms

These are believed to be congenital anomalies even when there is considerable atherosclerosis in their walls. They may become enormous in size, by definition greater than 2.5 cm in diameter, but sometimes twice or more as large. Most are located on a carotid, basilar, anterior, or middle cerebral artery, but also are found on the vertebral artery (Fig. 34-28). They grow slowly by accretion of blood clot within their lumens or by the organization of surface blood clots from small leaks. At a certain point they may compress adjacent structures, e.g., those in the cavernous sinus, optic nerve, or lower cranial nerves. The giant fusiform aneurysm of the midbasilar artery, with signs of brainstem ischemia and lower cranial-nerve palsies, is a relatively common form. Clotting within the aneurysm may cause ischemic infarction in its territory of supply, as mentioned in the case of berry aneurysms. Giant aneurysms may also rupture and cause subarachnoid hemorrhage, but not nearly as often as saccular aneurysms. These clinical observations were confirmed by the International Study, referred to above.

Treatment of saccular aneurysms is surgical if the lesion is symptomatic and it is accessible; endovascular techniques have been employed if the lesion is in the vertebral or midbasilar artery. Obliteration of the lumen,

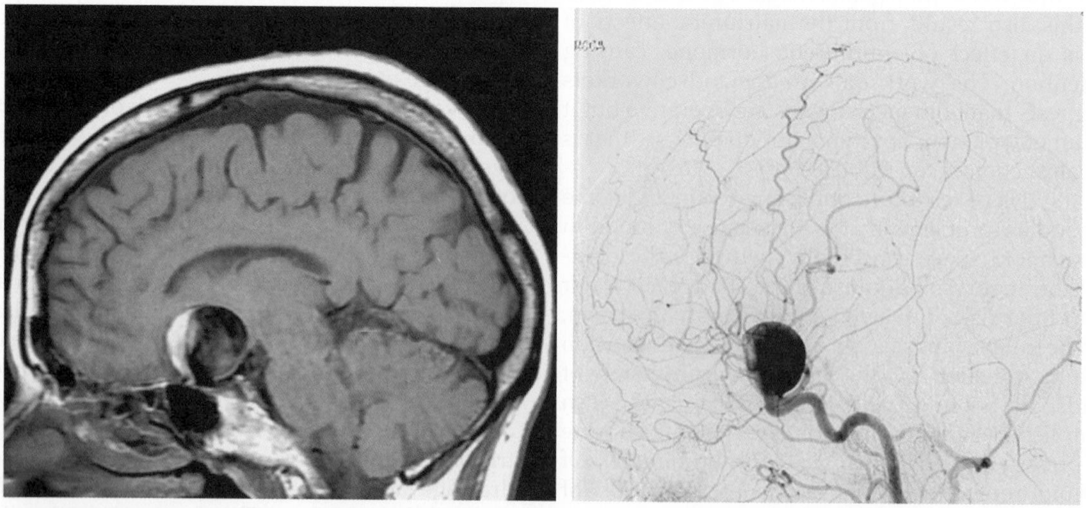

Figure 34-28. Giant aneurysm of the anterior cerebral artery. *Left:* T1-weighted MRI without gadolinium infusion. The white signal is thrombus within the anterior aspect of the aneurysm; there is some blood flow within the lesion evidenced by the darker signal. *Right:* Cerebral angiogram, left common carotid injection, lateral view, showing the residual flow in the posterior aspect of the aneurysm.

coupled with vascular bypass procedures, has been successful in the hands of cerebrovascular neurosurgeons, but the morbidity is high. Some giant aneurysms can be ligated at their necks, others by trapping or by the use of an intravascular detachable balloon. Drake summarized his surgical experience in the treatment of 174 such cases. Some fusiform aneurysms have been wrapped in muslin or similar material with mixed results. We have followed one such patient who had been operated on by T. Sundt more than 35 years ago. Recent attempts at stabilizing the expansion of the aneurysm by deploying an intravascular stent are under study.

Mycotic Aneurysm

The term *mycotic aneurysm* designates an aneurysm caused by a localized bacterial or fungal inflammation of an artery. (Osler introduced the misnomer *mycotic* aneurysm to describe an infectious process in the wall of a vessel.) With the introduction of antibiotics, mycotic aneurysms have become less frequent, but they are still being seen in patients with bacterial endocarditis and in intravenous drug abusers. Peripheral arteries are involved more often than intracranial ones; about two-thirds of the latter are associated with bacterial endocarditis caused by streptococcal infections. In recent years, the number of mycotic aneurysms caused by staphylococcal infections and acute endocarditis has increased. The usual pathogenic sequence is an embolic occlusion of a small artery, which may announce itself clinically by an ischemic stroke with white blood cells in the CSF. Later, or sometimes as the first manifestation, the weakened vessel wall ruptures and causes a subarachnoid or brain hemorrhage. An important point is that the aneurysm may appear within days of seeding of the vessel and rupture at any time, although the rates of rupture with subarachnoid hemorrhage are low.

The mycotic aneurysm may appear on only one artery or several arteries, and the hemorrhage, if it has happened, may recur. A consensus regarding the treatment of mycotic aneurysm has not been reached. The underlying endocarditis or bacteremia mandates appropriate antibiotic therapy and, in at least 30 percent of cases, healing of the aneurysm can be observed in successive arteriograms with this approach alone. Antibiotic or antifungal treatment is usually continued for at least 6 weeks. Some neurosurgeons favor excising an accessible aneurysm if it is solitary and the systemic infection is under control. Many mycotic aneurysms do not bleed, and in our view medical therapy takes precedence over surgical therapy.

Convexity Subarachnoid Hemorrhage

The finding of blood over a convexity of the cerebral hemisphere, usually discovered because of an evaluation for sudden headache, has become a common occurrence. The causes for this bleeding are numerous, the most obvious being cranial trauma but a diversity of processes may be responsible including cerebral amyloid angiopathy, reversible cerebral vasoconstriction syndrome, cortical vein thrombosis, the use of cocaine, cavernous angioma, dural arteriovenous fistula, and posterior reversible leukoencephalopathy. It is interesting to note that this list largely overlaps with the causes of "thunderclap headache," discussed earlier and in Chap. 10. Of course, in the appropriate clinical circumstances, ruptured aneurysm and mycotic aneurysm are still concerns. In a survey conducted by Kumar and associates, it was suggested that younger patients present with abrupt headache and older ones, with TIA-like symptoms and imaging findings that were consistent with cerebral amyloid angiopathy. Further notable is the later occurrence of meningeal hemosideriosis as a result of these lesions, particularly with amyloid angiopathy (see Linn and colleagues).

ARTERIOVENOUS MALFORMATIONS OF THE BRAIN

An arteriovenous malformation (AVM) consists of a tangle of dilated vessels that form an abnormal communication between the arterial and venous systems. These developmental abnormalities represent persistence of an embryonic pattern of blood vessels and not a neoplasm, but the constituent vessels may proliferate and enlarge with the passage of time. Venous malformations, consisting purely of distended veins deep in the white matter, are a separate entity; they may be the cause of seizures and headaches but seldom of hemorrhage. When a small hemorrhage occurs, it is usually the result of an associated malformation of the so-called cavernous type; these are small hamartomatous lesions of multiple juxtaposed endothelium-lined cavities without interposed neural tissue. These are discussed further on.

True vascular malformations vary in size from a small blemish a few millimeters in diameter lying in the cortex or white matter to a huge mass of tortuous channels constituting an atrioventricular (AV) shunt of sufficient magnitude to raise cardiac output. Hypertrophic dilated arterial feeders can be seen approaching the main lesion and to break up into a network of thin-walled blood vessels that connect directly with draining veins. The latter often form greatly dilated, pulsating channels, carrying away arterial blood. The tangled blood vessels interposed between arteries and veins are abnormally thin and do not have the structure of normal arteries or veins. AVMs occur in all parts of the cerebrum, brainstem, and cerebellum (and spinal cord), but the larger ones are more frequently found in the central part of a cerebral hemisphere, commonly forming a wedge-shaped lesion extending from the cortex to the ventricle. Some lie on the dural surface of the brain or spinal cord, but these more often turn out to be direct arteriovenous fistulas, as discussed further on.

When hemorrhage occurs from an AVM, blood may enter the subarachnoid space, producing a picture almost identical to that of a ruptured saccular aneurysm, but generally less severe. Because most AVMs lie within cerebral tissue, bleeding is more than likely to be intracerebral as well, or to be solely intracerebral, causing a hemiparesis, hemiplegia, and so forth, or even death.

AVMs are about one-tenth as common as saccular aneurysms and about equally frequent in males and females. The two lesions—AVM and saccular aneurysm (on the main feeding artery of the AVM)—are associated in approximately 5 percent of cases; the conjunction increases with the size of the AVM and the age of the patient (Miyasaka et al). AVMs rarely occur in more than one member of a family in the same generation or successive ones.

For a review of the embryologic theories of formation of AVMs, the reader is directed to the article by Fleetwood and Steinberg.

Clinical Features

Bleeding or seizures are the main modes of presentation. Most AVMs are clinically silent for a long time. Although the lesion is present from birth, onset of symptoms is most common between 10 and 30 years of age; occasionally it is delayed to age 50 or even beyond. In almost half of patients, the first clinical manifestation is a cerebral subarachnoid hemorrhage; in 30 percent, a seizure is the first and only manifestation; and in 20 percent, the only symptom is headache. Progressive hemiparesis or other focal neurologic deficit is present in approximately 10 percent of patients. The first hemorrhage may be fatal, but in more than 90 percent of cases the bleeding stops and the patient survives. Most often there are no symptoms before rupture. Chronic, recurrent headache may be a complaint; usually it is of a nondescript type but a classic migraine with or without neurologic accompaniment occurs in approximately 10 percent of patients—probably with greater frequency than it does in the general population. Most of the malformations associated with migraine-like headaches lie in the parietooccipital region of one cerebral hemisphere, and about two-thirds of such patients have a family history of migraine.

Huge AVMs may produce a slowly progressive neurologic deficit because of compression of neighboring structures by the enlarging mass of vessels and by shunting of blood through greatly dilated vascular channels. It has also been proposed that an "intracerebral steal" can result in hypoperfusion of the surrounding brain (Homan et al). When the vein of Galen is enlarged as a result of drainage from an adjacent AVM, hydrocephalus may result, particularly in children. With moderate size and large lesions, one or both carotid arteries frequently pulsate unusually forcefully in the neck. A systolic bruit heard over the carotid in the neck or over the mastoid process or the eyeballs in a young adult is suggestive of an AVM. However, such bruits have been heard in fewer than 25 percent of our patients. Exercise such as repeated squatting that increases the pulse pressure may bring out a bruit if none is present at rest. There is no relation of the existence of an AVM, or its rupture, to chronic hypertension (the same pertains to cerebral aneurysms).

Inspection of the eye grounds will rarely disclose a retinal vascular malformation that is coextensive with a similar lesion of the optic nerve and basal portions of the brain. Cutaneous, orbital, and nasopharyngeal AVMs may occasionally be found in relation to a cerebral lesion. Skull films rarely show crescentic linear calcifications in the larger malformations.

To summarize the size, location, and venous drainage characteristics of a cerebral AVM for surgical planning, Spetzler and Martin devised a widely used grading scale. The summed score gives guidance as to the difficulty in surgical removal and has a less certain relationship to the clinical behavior of the lesion. Lesions 1 to 3 mm are considered small, and give 1 point; 3 to 6 mm are medium sized and 2 points; over 6 mm are large and assigned 3 points; location in an eloquent site gives 1 point and venous drainage to the deep veins gives another point (the summed score is between 1 and 5). The use of this scale to plan treatment is discussed in the next section.

Features that have been related to risk of bleeding in some series have been a deep location of the AVM or deep venous drainage channels, and mostly, a previous hemorrhage summarized by Stapf and colleagues. The natural history of AVMs has been studied by Ondra and colleagues, who have presented data on a large and comprehensive series of untreated malformations in Finland over a 30-year period, and another similar series has been reported by Crawford and coworkers in Great Britain. The rate of rebleeding in most series has been 2 to 4 percent per year over decades but may be as high as 6 to 9 percent in the year after a first hemorrhage. In the latter study, comprising 343 patients, 217 were managed without surgery and observed for many years (mean: 10.4 years). Hemorrhage occurred in 42 percent and seizures in 18 percent. By 20 years after diagnosis, 29 percent had died and 27 percent of the survivors had a neurologic handicap. In a series of 1,000 patients referred mainly for proton-beam radiation of an AVM and studied by our colleague R.D. Adams, 464 had a hemorrhage as the first manifestation and 218 had a seizure (mainly with frontal and frontoparietal lesions). In those few AVMs that came to attention as a result of a progressive neurologic deficit, most were situated in the posterior fossa or axially in the cerebrum. The combination of a prolonged history of headaches, seizures, and a progressive deficit in Adams' series almost always indicated a large malformation. The matter of an increased risk of AVM rupture during pregnancy has been disputed. The weight of evidence suggests that the risk is not raised by pregnancy alone.

Fully 90 percent of AVMs are disclosed by CT if performed with contrast infusion, and an even larger number by MRI (Fig. 34-29). Magnetic-susceptibility MRI shows small areas of previous bleeding around AVMs. Arteriography is usually necessary to establish the diagnosis with certainty and will demonstrate AVMs larger than 5 mm in diameter; MRI may fail to reveal smaller lesions. Another value of arteriography, particularly if performed with rapid sequential and delayed images is to define all of the feeding arteries, the presence of an associated aneurysm and the channels of venous drainage, all of which inform the expectations of future bleeding and the most advisable methods of obliterating the lesion. The decision to obtain imaging to detect an AVM in cases of typical cerebral hemorrhage of the type discussed in earlier sections is based on factors such as young age (childhood and adolescence onset is particularly suggestive), a history of an unusual unilateral headache syndrome, a focal seizure disorder, the absence

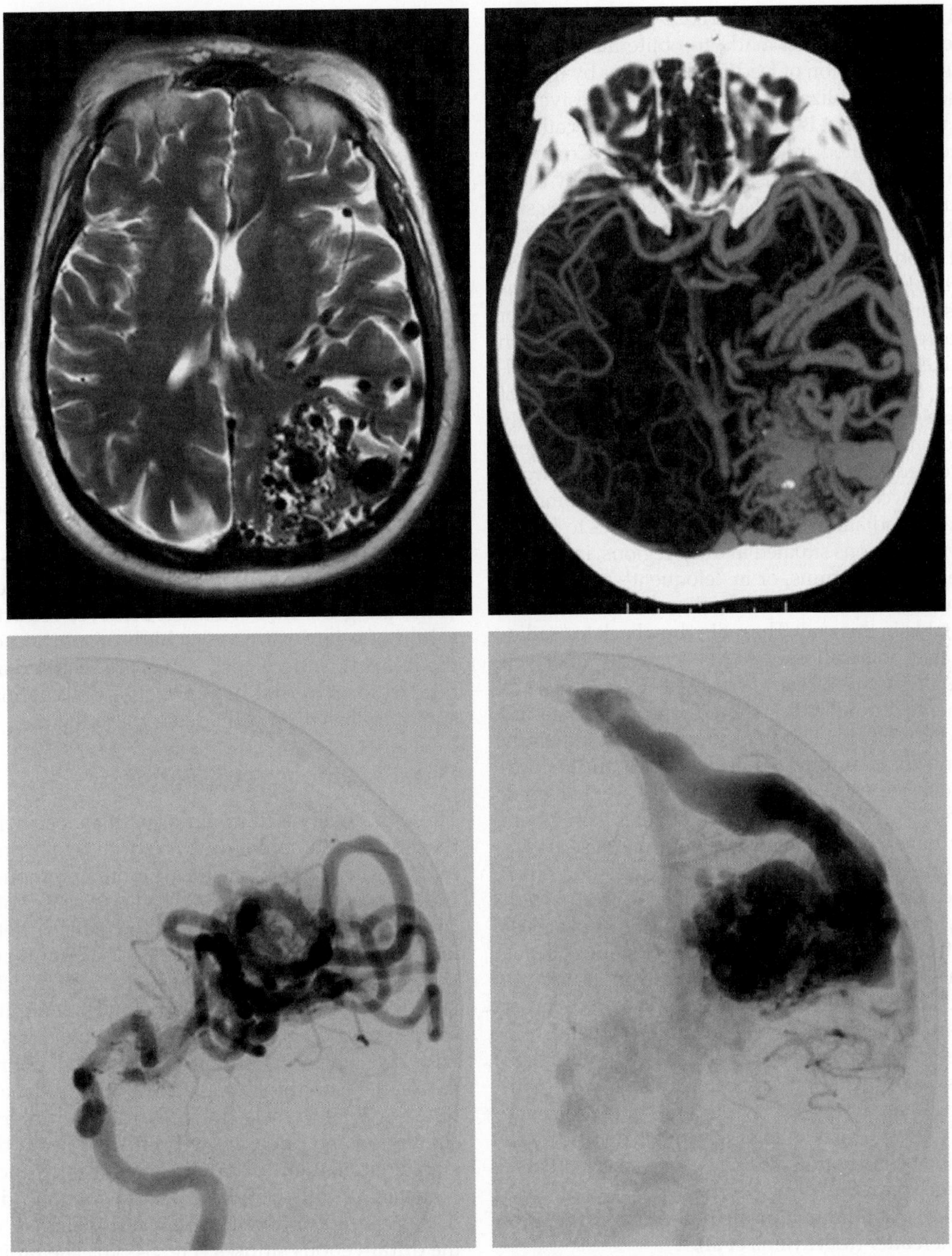

Figure 34-29. Left parietal arteriovenous malformation. *Upper left*: T2-weighted MRI shows a tangle of vessels interspersed throughout the parietal lobe. The largest of these vessels are dilated draining veins. *Upper right*: CT angiography demonstrates enhancement of the abnormal vessels throughout the left hemisphere. The AVM is fed primarily via branches of the left MCA. Cerebral angiography. Contrast injected into the left internal carotid artery reveals the feeding arteries (*lower left*) and abnormal early filling of dilated draining veins (*lower right*) due to blood bypassing the capillary bed.

of other apparent cause (e.g., coagulopathy, chronic hypertension, metastatic tumor), but most of all, recurrent bleeding in one location of the brain.

Treatment

The preferred approach in most centers is surgical excision. The Spetzler-Martin Scale gives guidance as to the surgical difficulty and risk. Grades IV and V are generally not resected; grade III lesions may be approached surgically but often with preceding interventional embolization of parts of the lesion. Some 20 to 40 percent of AVMs are amenable to block dissection, with an operative mortality rate of 2 to 5 percent and a morbidity of 5 to 10 percent (see Fleetwood and Steinberg for a summary of reported surgical results up to 2002). For inaccessible lesions, attempts have been made to obliterate the malformed vessels by ligation of feeding arteries or by the use of endovascular embolization with liquid adhesives or particulate material that is injected via a balloon catheter that has been navigated into a feeding vessel. Complete obliteration of large AVMs is usually not possible by these methods but they are highly effective in reducing the size of the AVM prior to surgery.

Several modes of radiosurgery are used to decrease the size of the lesion, albeit with a substantial delay. This approach is utilized most often with AVMs of 3 cm or smaller located in an area of the brain in which resection would be likely to produce a serious neurologic disability. Kjellberg and Chapman pioneered the treatment of AVMs using a single dose of subnecrotizing stereotactically directed proton radiation. The technique of radiosurgery has been adopted by others using photon radiation sources, such as a linear accelerator, gamma Knife, and other modes of focused x-ray radiation as accepted alternatives to operative treatment of lesions situated in deep regions, including the brainstem, the thalamus, or in "eloquent" areas of the cortex. Generally, malformations smaller than 3 cm diameter are treatable in this way. The main drawback to "radiosurgery" is that obliteration of AVMs occurs in a delayed manner, usually with a latency of at least 18 to 24 months after treatment, during which the patient is unprotected from rebleeding. The likelihood of successful radiotherapy treatment and the nature of the risks depend on the location and size of the AVM and the radiation dose delivered. After 2 years, 75 to 80 percent of AVMs smaller than 2.5 cm in diameter have been obliterated. Even for those AVMs that have not been totally eliminated, the radiation effect appears to confer some long-term protection from bleeding. Of the larger ones, a majority shrink or appear less dense. The rest show no change at this low-dose level, but even in this group, the morbidity and mortality are lower than in the untreated group. A proportion of larger AVMs that are initially obliterated will later recanalize, and many of these will subsequently bleed. Among more than 250 patients whose AVMs disappeared following proton-beam therapy, there has been no recurrence of hemorrhage for up to 10 years. The results of treatment with focused radiation have been about the same. In one study, the risk of hemorrhage was reduced by 54 percent between the time of radiation and obliteration of the malformation and by 88 percent thereafter (Maruyama et al).

Two types of complications of radiation occur at a combined rate of approximately 2 to 4 percent. The first is delayed radiation necrosis, which is predictable based on the radiation dose, and the second is venous congestion that occurs several weeks or months after treatment. The latter is indicative of the desired effect of thrombosis of the malformation. Both may cause local symptoms for weeks or months. Radiation necrosis may be reduced by the administration of corticosteroids but the vascular problem generally is not helped.

The treatment of AVMs by endovascular techniques is increasingly being used but is only recently being fully evaluated. Nearly every AVM has several feeding arteries, some not reachable by a catheter, and some part of the AVM may remain after treatment. In most series, 25 percent or more of AVMs, mostly of small and medium size, have been completely obliterated, with a mortality rate below 3 percent and morbidity of 5 to 7 percent, both of which compare favorably with surgical outcomes. These techniques are also particularly suited to lesions of a combined AVM and an aneurysm on the feeding vessel.

In the past several years, combined therapy that begins with endovascular reduction of the lesion and is followed by either surgery or radiation has been viewed favorably. Using this approach, more than 90 percent of lesions can be obliterated with a very low rebleeding rate over several years. It is clear that the plan for each patient must be individualized based on the size, location, nature of feeding vessels, the presence of other vascular lesions (aneurysm or additional AVM), and the age of the patient. Another strategy for otherwise untreatable grade IV and V lesions has been to stage radiosurgery in order to reduce parts of the lesions sequentially as described by Sirin and colleagues. Even then, there will be differences of opinion based on local resources and experience.

Finally, if the primary problem is recurrent seizure, eliminating the malformation achieves reduction or cessation of seizures in a very high proportion of cases. In the interval, antiepileptic drugs are required and may be needed for a period of years after obliteration. A recent summary has been provided by Friedlander.

Dural Arteriovenous Fistula

These curious vascular abnormalities, occurring in both the cranial and spinal dura, have different presentations at each site. The spinal form, more common in general experience, is discussed with other diseases of the spinal cord in Chap. 44. The cranial type is being detected with increasing frequency as refinements continue to be made in imaging of the cerebral vessels, but its incidence and pathogenesis are not fully known. The defining features are radiologic—a nidus of abnormal arteries and veins with arteriovenous shunting contained entirely within the leaflets of the dura. The lesion is usually fed by dural arterial vessels derived from the internal cranial circulation and often, more prolifically, from the external cranial circulation (external carotid artery and muscular branches of the vertebral artery). Venous drainage of these lesions is often complex and is largely directed to the dural venous sinuses (Fig. 34-30). The rapid transit of injected angiographic dye through dural fistulas accounts for the early opacification of the draining venous structures. In the case of high-flow connections, this may not be seen unless images are taken almost immediately after the injection. A number of potential feeding vessels must be individually opacified to demonstrate all the conduits into the lesion. On CT and MRI, the fistula is sometimes detected as a thickening or enhancement of a region of dura, generally close to a large dural venous sinus. In other cases, the dilated draining vessels may be seen only with the injection of dye or gadolinium. Probably, many are not detected by either of these techniques.

Several classification systems (Borden; Cognard) have been developed that are based on the nature and

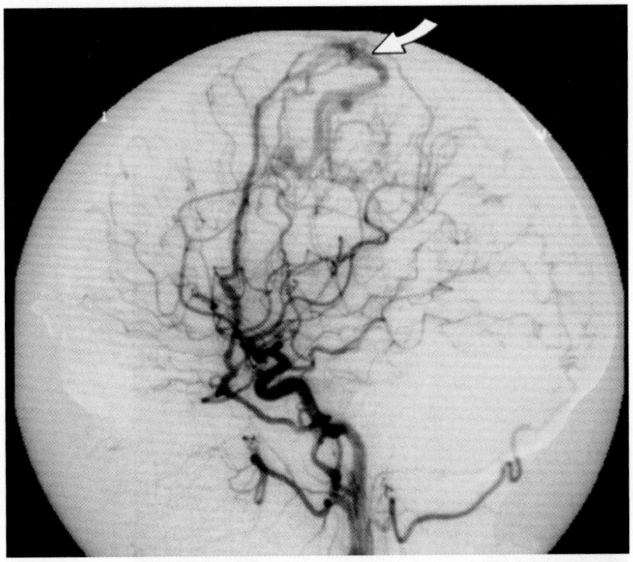

Figure 34-30. Cerebral angiogram of a cerebral dural arteriovenous malformation. The nidus is located at the cerebral convexity (*arrow*). There is rapid filing of the cerebral venous system after injection of contrast into one internal carotid artery.

direction of the drainage of the lesion. There are some associations between the nature of these drainage patters, as summarized by the classification systems, and clinical presentation.

The origin of these vascular lesions has not been settled—several mechanisms may be involved. Most evidence suggests that at least some of them, unlike conventional cerebral AVMs and aneurysms, are not developmental in origin. The best-defined examples of acquired fistulas are those that arise adjacent to a venous sinus thrombosis or in association with a vascular atresia, most often of the transverse sigmoid sinus or adjacent to the cavernous sinus. However, it is not always clear whether the abnormality of the venous sinus is the cause or the result of the dural fistula. In a number of cases, a dural fistula has appeared after a forceful head injury, often in a region remote from the site of impact. Another small group that is clearly developmental is associated with the Klippel-Trenaunay or Osler-Weber-Rendu syndromes, diseases in which a conjunction with AVMs is well known. (In the first of these, they may also be an associated enlargement of the affected limb.) Usually, these causes can be excluded by physical examination and an absence of family history and the largest group remains idiopathic.

A major obstacle to understanding of dural fistula is the varied ways in which this lesion presents itself clinically. Subdural hemorrhage is an infrequent but dramatic mode of presentation, sometimes creating a large and fatal clot; another syndrome is a cerebral–subarachnoid hemorrhage, although this occurs with not nearly the same frequency or severity as bleeding from brain AVMs. Indeed, the risk of bleeding from dural fistulas and the evolution of these lesions is far less precise than it is for cerebral AVMs. It appears that the dural lesions most at risk of bleeding are those located in the anterior cranial fossa and those at the tentorial incisura. Seizures are distinctly uncommon. Yet another special syndrome linked to dural AVMs, although it may occur also with high-flow cerebral malformations, is of headache, vomiting, and papilledema—namely, *pseudotumor cerebri* (see Chap. 30). Whether the increased intracranial pressure is the cause or the result of the fistula is unsettled, but relief of venous insufficiency may result in regression of fistulae. A cranial bruit, audible to either the examiner or patient, is infrequent with fistula but may be sought. In small children, the high-flow lesions may shunt so much blood as to cause congestive heart failure, similar to arteriovenous malformations of the vein of Galen.

Treatment is by surgical extirpation or endovascular embolization, at times a painstaking procedure because of the multitude of potential feeding vessels. Surgery seems preferable for the smaller lesions and embolization for larger and inaccessible ones. Slowed flow in a venous sinus that is draining a malformation risks venous thrombosis but the issue of anticoagulation in this circumstance remains uncertain.

Cavernous Malformations (Cavernoma)

Vascular malformations composed mainly of clusters of thin-walled veins without important arterial feeders and with little or no intervening nervous tissue make up a significant group, some 7 to 8 percent of AVMs. Conventional subdivisions of this group into cavernous, venous, and telangiectatic types have not proven useful. Most clinicians roughly designated them all as *cavernous*. Several attributes set them apart from other vascular malformations. Their tendency to bleed is probably no less than that of the more common AVMs, and far more often, the hemorrhages are small and clinically silent. The incidence of bleeding is uncertain but is estimated to be less than 1 percent per year per lesion but quite often they are multiple lesions so that the cumulative risk in any one patient is higher. Flemming and colleagues, in a survey of 292 patients followed for an average of almost 10 years, gave the rate as 0.3 percent annually for asymptomatic lesions and found that individuals who had a previous episode of bleeding or had more than one lesion were 2.5 times more likely to have another hemorrhage.

As mentioned, approximately 10 percent of these lesions are multiple and 5 percent are familial. In one family we followed, there were 29 affected members in three generations; the inheritance followed an autosomal dominant pattern. At the present, several genes have been identified as possibly causative in certain families. One interesting characteristic of this group, as pointed out by Labauge and colleagues, is the appearance over time of new lesions in one-third of patients. The followup of some of our patients has affirmed this.

The diagnosis is based on clinical manifestations and MRI, which discloses a cluster of vessels surrounded by a zone of hypodense ferritin in the T1-weighted images (Fig. 34-31), the product of previous small episodes of bleeding. An uncertain number is associated with adjacent deep venous anomaly visualized by imaging studies and these are discussed in a separate section below.

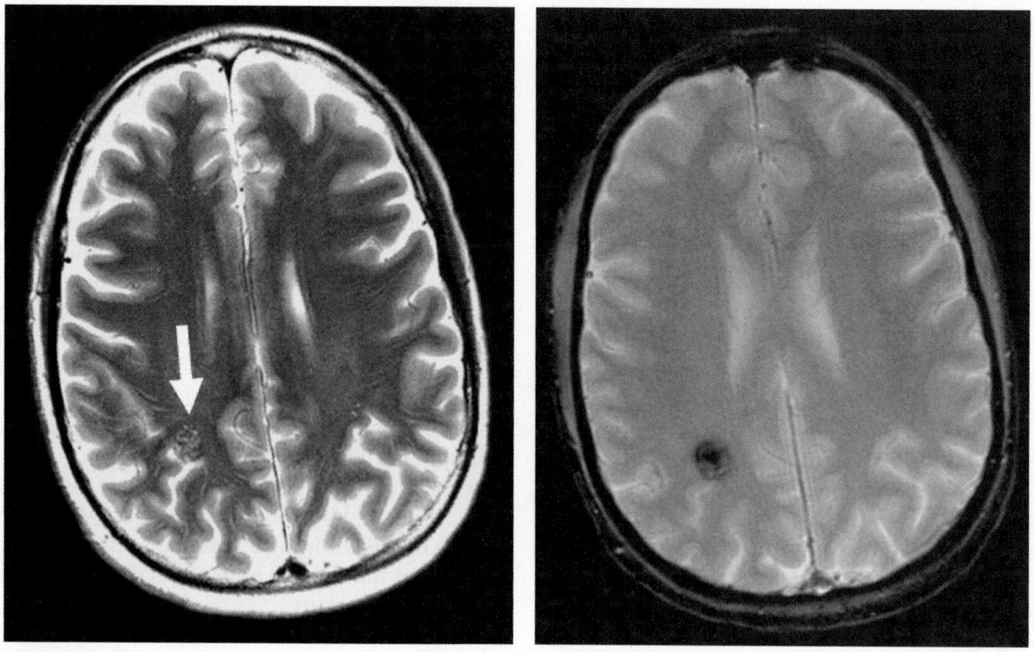

Figure 34-31. Cavernous malformation in the right parietal lobe. Axial T2 MRI (*left*) shows a round lesion which is heterogeneously hyperintense and hypointense. This appearance is due to vascular channels which are immediately adjacent to each other without interspersed normal brain tissue, containing blood products in different stages of degradation. An axial gradient echo MRI (*right*) shows that the lesion is hypointense, again due to blood products.

About one-half of all cavernous angiomas lie in the brainstem, and in the past (before the availability of MRI), many of them were misdiagnosed as multiple sclerosis because of the stepwise accumulation of neurologic deficits with each hemorrhage. A large series of cavernous malformations of the brainstem, most in the pons, has been described by Porter and colleagues. They describe a higher rate of bleeding than had been reported for similar malformations in the cerebral hemispheres, frequent adjacent venous anomalies, and good results from surgical ablation. They estimated the rate of bleeding to be 5 percent per year and the rate of rebleeding close to 30 percent per year.

Treatment Cavernous angiomas on the surface of the brain, within reach of the neurosurgeon, even those in the brainstem, can be plucked out like blackberries, with low morbidity and mortality. Kjellberg and colleagues treated 89 deeply situated cavernous angiomas with low-dose proton radiation, but our impression is that these vascular malformations, like hemangioblastomas, respond poorly to radiation and are not amenable to treatment by endovascular techniques.

Lesions that cause recurrent bleeding and are surgically accessible with little risk are often removed but incidentally discovered angiomas, even if they have caused a small hemorrhage, and those that are inaccessible may be left alone. Although this conservative approach is usually taken, there are not adequate data on the rate and risk of bleeding to determine the proper course of action.

Deep (Developmental) Venous Anomaly

This is perhaps the most common cerebral vascular malformation, estimated to occur in almost 3 percent of large autopsy series (attributed to Swar and McCormick). As with cavernous angiomas, these lesions are frequently detected as asymptomatic problems in brain imaging. The defining characteristics are of a caput medusa draining into a small collecting vein. The draining vein itself is often visualized most easily and fills with contrast concurrently with normal cerebral (Fig. 34-32). As mentioned

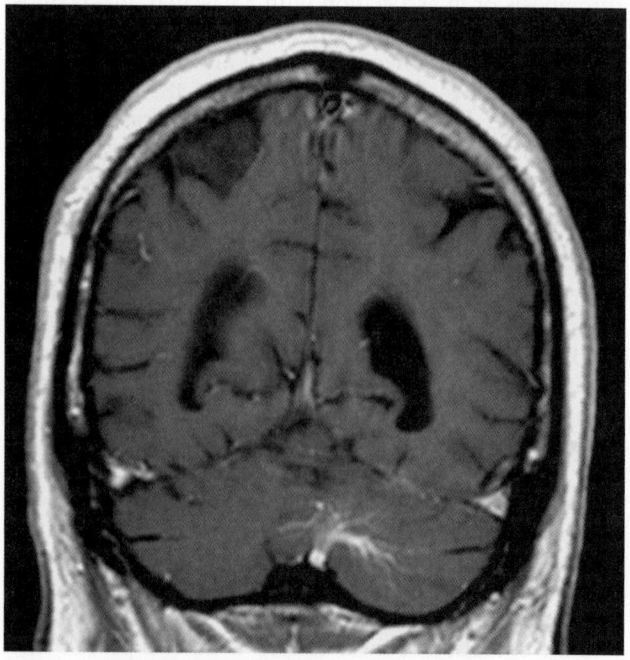

Figure 34-32. A developmental venous anomaly (DVA) and its collecting vein in the left cerebellum on a T1-weighted MRI with contrast.

above, perhaps up to 40 percent of cavernous malformations (probably fewer) have an associated deep venous anomaly. Although the risks of stroke in relation to one of these anomalies is low, certainly less than 1 percent per year, small hemorrhage or infarction surrounding a deep venous anomaly may result from acute thrombosis in a collecting vein. An extensive summary of the clinical and imaging features of venous anomalies is given by Ruiz and colleagues. They reviewed the interesting cases reported in the literature in which the anomaly has thrombosed, and discuss the possible pathophysiologic relationship between the vein and the development of a cavernous malformation.

The management of developmental venous anomalies has not been clarified although numerous forms of surgery, embolization, or focused radiation, have been used depending on the nature of an associated lesion such as cavernous malformation, and the occurrence of repeated bleeding. In general, incidentally discovered lesions are simply followed with imaging at reasonable intervals.

Other Causes of Intracranial Bleeding and Multiple Cerebral Hemorrhages

Next in frequency to hypertension, *anticoagulant therapy* is currently the most common cause of cerebral hemorrhage. The hemorrhages that develop, although sometimes situated in the sites of predilection of hypertensive hemorrhage, are more likely to occur elsewhere, mainly in the lobes of the brain. When the bleeding is precipitated by warfarin therapy, treatment with fresh-frozen plasma and vitamin K, sometimes prothrombin complex concentrate (PCC) and similar products, which contains clotting factors, is recommended. The use of *thrombolytic drugs* in the treatment of stroke or myocardial infarction is complicated by intracranial hemorrhage in 6 to 20 percent of cases, depending on the dose and timing of drug administration in relation to the onset of symptoms, as discussed in the section earlier on "Thrombolytic Agents." The newer antifactor X and direct thrombin-inhibiting anticoagulants are not as easily subject to reversal. When bleeding is associated with aspirin therapy or other agents that affect platelet function, fresh platelet infusion, often in massive amounts, may be used to control the hemorrhage, however, their effectiveness in management of cerebral hemorrhage has been questioned.

In the elderly, *amyloid angiopathy* appears to be a major cause of lobar bleeding, especially if hemorrhages appear in succession or are multiple. Several of our patients who later proved to have amyloid angiopathy had minor head injuries in the weeks before hemorrhage. In our own material, only severe impregnation of vessels with amyloid and fibrinoid change in the vessel wall were associated with hemorrhage (Vonsattel et al). Greenberg and colleagues found that apolipoprotein E4, the same marker that is overrepresented in Alzheimer disease, is associated with severe amyloid angiopathy and a risk of intracerebral hemorrhage, but others have found an association with the E2 allele. Contrary to previous pronouncements, there is probably no greater risk in evacuating these clots surgically than in the case of other cerebral hemorrhages, but most of them are of a size that allows conservative management and evidence is lacking that surgery improves outcome as discussed earlier.

Several *primary hematologic disorders* are also complicated by hemorrhage into the brain. The most frequent of these are leukemia, aplastic anemia, and thrombocytopenia of various causes. Often they give rise to multiple intracranial hemorrhages, some in the subdural and subarachnoid spaces. As a rule, this complication signals a fatal outcome. Other, less-common causes of intracerebral bleeding are advanced *liver disease*, uremia that is being treated with dialysis, and lymphoma. Usually several factors are operative in these hematologic cases: reduction in prothrombin or other clotting elements (fibrinogen, factor V), bone marrow suppression by antineoplastic drugs, and disseminated intravascular coagulation. Any part of the brain may be involved, and the hemorrhagic lesions are usually multiple. Frequently there is also evidence of abnormal bleeding elsewhere (skin, mucous membranes, kidney) by the time cerebral hemorrhage occurs. Plasma exchange, used in the treatment of myasthenia gravis and Guillain-Barré disease, lowers the serum fibrinogen to a marked degree, but we have not observed a single instance of intracerebral hemorrhage in more than 500 patients treated in this way.

Occasionally the origin of intracranial hemorrhage cannot be determined clinically or pathologically. In some postmortem cases, a careful microscopic search discloses a small arteriovenous malformation; this is the basis for suspecting that an overlooked lesion of this type may be the cause of cerebral hemorrhage in other cases. *Primary intraventricular hemorrhage*, a rare event in adults, can sometimes be traced to a vascular malformation or neoplasm of the choroid plexus or one of the choroidal arteries; more often, such a hemorrhage is the result of periventricular bleeding often from a medial thalamic hemorrhage, in which blood enters the ventricle without producing a large parenchymal clot.

Hemorrhage into primary and secondary brain tumors is not rare. When this is the first clinical manifestation of the neoplasm, diagnosis may be difficult. Choriocarcinoma, melanoma, renal cell and bronchogenic carcinoma, pituitary adenoma, thyroid cancer, glioblastoma multiforme, intravascular lymphoma, carcinoid, and medulloblastoma may present in this way, but bleeding is most characteristic of the first three types. Careful inquiry will usually disclose that neurologic symptoms compatible with intracranial tumor growth had preceded the onset of hemorrhage or the primary neoplasm had been revealed previously. Needless to say, a thorough search should be made in these circumstances for evidence of intracranial tumor or of secondary tumor deposits in other organs, particularly the lungs.

A number of disparate diseases may result in a multitude of simultaneous or at least temporally clustered cerebral hemorrhages. Among the most common causes are cerebrovascular amyloidosis (amyloid angiopathy) as mentioned earlier, those related to hematologic and clotting disease, particularly ones that progress rapidly, such as leukemia, but almost any coagulopathy, including those brought on by the administration of medications. The most overwhelming examples in our experience have occurred in the hours after injecting tPA for acute stroke. Serious cranial injury itself may produce a passel of scattered contusions, some of which have the appearance of ball hemorrhages, but most are recognized to be along force lines (see Chap. 35). Occlusion of cerebral veins, particularly of the superior sagittal sinus, causes several biparietal hemorrhages.

Multiple small hemorrhages, brain "microbleeds," are most commonly considered to be the result of vascular amyloid as discussed in the next section, but may also be associated with chronic hypertension according to Cordonnier and colleagues, but we have been unable to confirm this latter view from our own material. Often, these dozens of small areas of residual blood products or acute hemorrhages do not cause symptoms and are revealed on MRI that is performed for other reasons with gradient-echo and other susceptibility sequences (Fig. 34-33). Certainly, other forms of cerebrovascular disease are found disproportionately in these patients and several series suggest that they represent a risk for future bleeding or ischemic stroke, including lacunes. Multiple cavernous angiomas, the earlier-described amyloid angiopathy, CADASIL, bacterial endocarditis, moyamoya, and mutations that affect blood vessel integrity may also be implicated but the cause in any individual case often remains uncertain.

The pathologic entity called *brain purpura* (pericapillary encephalorrhagia), incorrectly referred to as "hemorrhagic encephalitis," consists of multiple petechial hemorrhages scattered throughout the white matter of the brain. The clinical picture is that of a diffuse encephalopathy, but diagnosis is essentially a pathologic one. Blood does not appear in the CSF, and the condition should not be confused with a stroke. The pathologic appearance is highly characteristic. The lesions in brain purpura are small, 0.1 to 2.0 mm in diameter, and are confined to the white matter, particularly the corpus callosum, centrum ovale, and middle cerebellar peduncles. Each lesion is situated around a small blood vessel, usually a capillary. In this para-adventitial area, both the myelin and axis cylinders are destroyed, and the lesion is usually though not always hemorrhagic. Fibrin exudation, perivascular and meningeal infiltrates of inflammatory cells, and widespread necrosis of tissue are not observed. In these respects, brain purpura differs fundamentally from acute necrotizing hemorrhagic leukoencephalitis. Usually the patient becomes stuporous and comatose without focal neurologic signs.

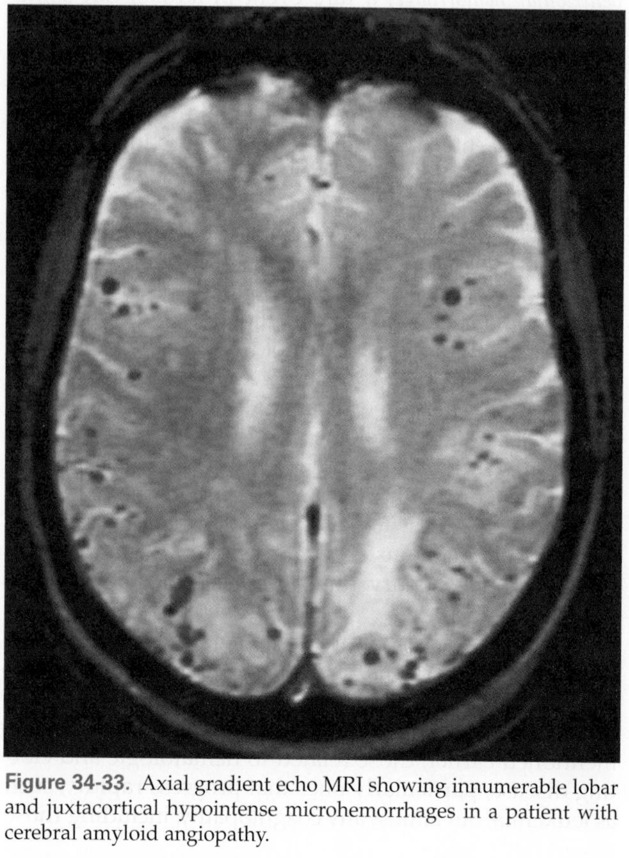

Figure 34-33. Axial gradient echo MRI showing innumerable lobar and juxtacortical hypointense microhemorrhages in a patient with cerebral amyloid angiopathy.

The etiology of brain purpura is quite obscure and there may be several causes. It may complicate viral pneumonia, uremia, promyelocytic leukemia, arsenical intoxication, and, rarely, metabolic encephalopathy and sepsis, or there may be no associated disease. Amyloid angiopathy and an uncharacterized cerebral small vessel disease also have caused this picture of a multiplicity of small hemorrhages. Primary or secondary thrombotic thrombocytopenic purpura (TTP) may be the final common pattern for this entity.

A degree of brain hemorrhage is to be expected in acute hemorrhagic leukoencephalitis (Hurst type), which represents an extreme form of acute disseminated encephalomyelitis (see Chap. 36), and in herpes encephalitis (see Chap. 33).The other rare types of hemorrhages, listed in Table 34-8, are self-explanatory.

Hemorrhages of *intraspinal* origin, all of them rare, may be the result of trauma, AVM (the usual cause of nontraumatic hematomyelia), dural AV fistula, anterior spinal artery aneurysms, or bleeding into tumors such as hemangioblastoma. Spinal subarachnoid hemorrhage from an AVM may simulate an intracranial subarachnoid hemorrhage, causing a stiff neck, headache, and even subhyaloid hemorrhages. Subarachnoid hemorrhage in which interscapular or neck pain predominates should raise the suspicion of an aneurysm of the anterior spinal artery or of a spinal AVM or cavernous angioma. Angiographic study of the radicular spinal vessels and the origins of the anterior spinal arteries from the vertebral arteries may disclose the source of bleeding. Extradural and subdural spinal extravasations may be *spontaneous* (sometimes in relation to rheumatoid arthritis) but are far more often a result of trauma, anticoagulants, or both. Extradural spinal hemorrhage causes the rapid evolution of paraplegia or quadriplegia; diagnosis must be prompt if function is to be salvaged by surgical drainage of the hematoma. These entities are discussed further in Chap. 44.

Cerebral Amyloid Angiopathy

This angiopathy consists of the deposition of amyloid in the media and adventitia of small vessels, predominantly in the meninges, cortex, and cortical penetrating vessels. The incidence at autopsy of vascular amyloid deposition in the brain is related to the age of the population studied; rates of 12 percent are cited in patients older than 85 years of age (the same changes are present in more than 25 percent of individuals with Alzheimer disease, but the nature of the amyloid [Aβ40 in the pure cerebrovascular form] is different in the two conditions). The result of this deposition is several large or numerous small hemorrhages at various ages, mainly deposited in the cerebral hemispheres. There is a propensity for hemorrhages in the posterior parts of the brain. A strong association has been found with the homozygous APOE ε4/ε4 genotype. As alluded to several times in earlier sections on cerebral hemorrhage, this is the main cause of otherwise unexplained single of multiple cerebral hemorrhage in older people. Telltale signs of multiple small and larger hemorrhages are often present in these cases; they are seen to advantage with gradient-echo sequences on the MRI. The location of these hemorrhages, subcortical, frequently posteriorly in the brain, and sometimes subpial, imparts a distinctive pattern that is characteristic of this disease. The biology of cerebrovascular amyloid is summarized by Viswanathan and Greenberg.

Some reports have emphasized multiple TIA-like syndromes, some with migrainous features such as spreading sensory symptoms; these are not consistently ischemic and may be associated with microhemorrhages, or white matter changes of uncertain nature. In some cases, there is a fairly rapid progression to dementia but that is more characteristic of the inflammatory type of cerebrovascular amyloid discussed just below.

Over the last few years, our colleague S.M. Greenberg has emphasized certain clinical features associated with a rare inflammatory type of cerebrovascular amyloidosis (see Kinnecom et al). The MRI appearance is of large subcortical patches of T2 signal change suggestive of cerebral edema. Included in the clinical picture are encephalopathy, seizures, and focal cerebral symptoms such as aphasia. The frequency of this interesting condition in the elderly is unclear. It is treated with a short course of high-dose corticosteroids.

There is a separate familial amyloidotic condition of diffuse white matter degeneration with dementia, associated in some families with calcification in the occipital lobes, and the aforementioned mutations in the *COL4A* gene cause a disruption of the small vessel wall that can cause small cerebral hemorrhages that are similar to those of cerebrovascular amyloid.

HYPERTENSIVE ENCEPHALOPATHY (POSTERIOR REVERSIBLE ENCEPHALOPATHY SYNDROME [PRES], REVERSIBLE POSTERIOR LEUKOENCEPHALOPATHY [RPLE])

Clinical Features

Hypertensive encephalopathy is the term applied to a relatively rapidly evolving syndrome of severe hypertension in association with headache, nausea and vomiting, visual disturbances, confusion, and—in advanced cases—stupor and coma. Multiple seizures may occur and may be more marked on one side of the body. In special circumstances, the absolute level of blood pressure seems less pertinent that is a rapid rise in pressure as occurs in eclampsia and with exposure to certain drugs. The neurologic syndrome is usually dominated by symptoms referable to the occipital and adjacent parietal region. There may be field deficits, hallucinations, Balint syndrome, and cortical blindness. An indistinguishable syndrome with similar imaging characteristics also occurs with the use of a variety of mainly cancer chemotherapeutic agents as discussed in Chap. 43 and Table 43-1.

Diffuse cerebral disturbance may be accompanied by focal or lateralizing neurologic signs, either transitory or lasting, which may suggest cerebral hemorrhage or infarction, i.e., the more common cerebrovascular complications of severe chronic hypertension. A clustering of multiple microinfarcts and petechial hemorrhages (the basic neuropathologic changes in hypertensive encephalopathy) in one region may occasionally result in a mild hemiparesis, aphasic disorder, or rapid failure or the above-noted distortion of vision. The last of these, as mentioned, is particularly characteristic of accelerated hypertension and has special features of signal changes in the occipital white matter; for which reason the terms reversible posterior leukoencephalopathy (RPLE) and posterior or reversible leukoencephalopathy syndrome (PRES) have been applied to this condition, as noted below and shown in Fig. 34-34.

In instances of typical accelerated hypertension, by the time the neurologic manifestations appear, the hypertension has usually reached the malignant stage, with diastolic pressures above 125 mm Hg, retinal hemorrhages, exudates, papilledema, and evidence of renal and cardiac disease. However, instances of encephalopathy at lower pressures are common, especially if the rise in pressure has been abrupt (see below). If the rate of elevation is high enough, the syndrome may be seen with blood pressure considered to be close to the normal range. Presumably, these circumstances have to do with a change in the permeability of cerebral vessels that is part of the process in special cases such as eclampsia and the hemolysis, elevated liver enzymes, low platelet count (HELLP) syndrome that are mentioned further on. The term *hypertensive encephalopathy* should probably be reserved for the above syndrome and should not be used to refer to chronic recurrent headaches, dizziness, epileptic seizures, TIAs, or strokes, which may occur in association with elevated blood pressure.

Encephalopathy may complicate extreme hypertension from any cause (chronic renal disease, renal artery stenosis, acute glomerulonephritis, acute toxemia, pheochromocytoma, Cushing syndrome), cocaine, or administration of drugs such as aminophylline or phenylephrine, but it occurs most often in patients with rapidly worsening "essential" hypertension.

In *eclampsia*, which from a neurologic perspective may be considered a special form of hypertensive encephalopathy, and in *acute renal disease*, particularly in children, encephalopathic symptoms may develop at blood pressure levels considerably lower than those of hypertensive encephalopathy of "essential" type. Eclamptic retinal and cerebral lesions are the same as those that complicate

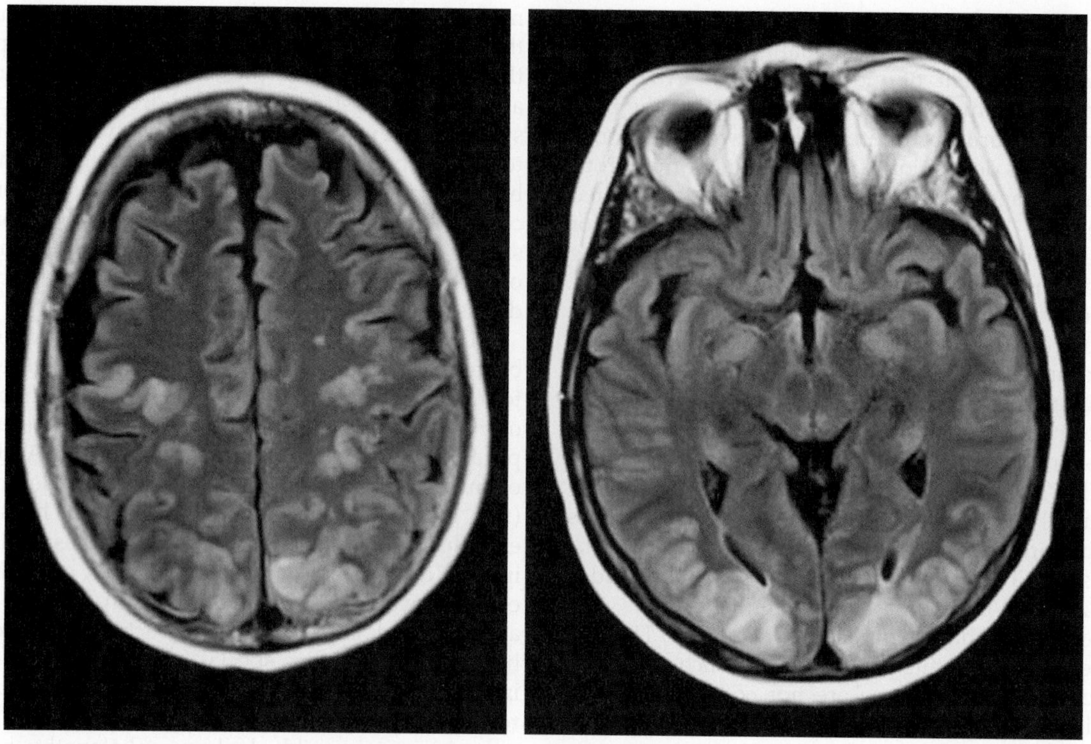

Figure 34-34. Hypertensive encephalopathy. Axial T2-FLAIR images showing fairly symmetric abnormal hyperintensity predominately in the parietooccipital lobes. The lesion affects the cortex and subcortical white matter and there is little mass effect. In severe cases, there may be hemorrhage and heterogeneous infarction in the cerebral cortex. The same imaging findings may occur in eclampsia (see also Chap. 43).

malignant nephrosclerosis; in both there is also failure of autoregulation of the cerebral arterioles. A discussion of eclamptic seizures can be found in the section on that subject in Chap. 16.

Imaging Features

Hypertensive encephalopathy is marked by changes already alluded to on CT and MRI. The findings are of large areas of white matter signal change of edema, but their tendency to normalize over several weeks is remarkable. As summarized by Hauser and coworkers, the main feature is a bilateral increase in T2 signal intensity in the white matter on MRI and a corresponding reduced density on CT, usually concentrated in the posterior part of the hemispheres (see Fig. 34-34). Thus the condition is one of the causes of reversible posterior leukoencephalopathy. These imaging characteristics are a result of an accumulation of fluid, but—unlike the edema in trauma, neoplasm, or stroke—there is little or no mass effect and the water does not tend to course along white matter tracts such as the corpus callosum. In addition, scattered cortical lesions may occur in a watershed vascular distribution and probably correspond to small infarctions. These same findings in the white matter and cortex occur in eclampsia and have been seen in cases of diffuse vasospasm caused by sympathomimetic and serotonergic drugs, discussed further on.

Hypertensive encephalopathy and eclampsia may cause subarachnoid hemorrhage. Most such cases are not caused by the rupture of an intracranial aneurysm and are not as overwhelming as in aneurysmal hemorrhage; indeed, the headache associated with PRES tends to be milder than with aneurysmal rupture and it may be absent. The bleeding, if it occurs, is mainly a feature that is appreciated on MRI examination, as described by Shah. The mechanism is obscure.

In many, but not all, cases, the CSF pressure and protein values are elevated; the latter to more than 100 mg/dL, but there is no cellular reaction.

Pathophysiology

Neuropathologic examination reveals a rather normal-looking brain, but in some cases cerebral swelling, hemorrhages of various sizes, or both will be found. In extreme instances, a cerebellar pressure cone reflects an increased volume of tissue and increased pressure in the posterior fossa; lumbar puncture appears to have only rarely precipitated fatalities. Microscopically there are widespread minute infarcts in the brain, the result of fibrinoid necrosis of the walls of arterioles and capillaries and occlusion of their lumens by fibrin thrombi (Chester et al). This is often associated with zones of cerebral edema. Similar vascular changes are found in other organs, particularly in the retinae and kidneys.

Volhard originally attributed the symptoms of hypertensive encephalopathy to vasospasm. This notion was reinforced by Byrom, who demonstrated, in rats, a segmental constriction and dilatation of cerebral and retinal arterioles in response to severe hypertension. However, the observations of Byrom and of others indicate that overdistention of the arterioles (which have lost their adaptive capacity), rather than excessive constriction, may be responsible for the necrosis of the vessel wall (see reviews of Auer and of Chester et al). The brain edema is the result of active exocytosis of water rather than simply a passive leak from vessels subjected to high pressures. In toxemia or eclampsia, rising levels of the antiangiogenic proteins endoglin, vascular endothelial growth factor, and placental growth factor had been postulated to play a role (Levine et al, 2006) but this has not been fully corroborated. The net result is of various forms of endothelial dysfunction, including presumably, in the brain. We have been impressed that the distribution of lesions on the MRI differs between eclamptic and older hypertensive patients, suggesting some difference in pathophysiology, or perhaps simply that chronic hypertension in the latter group predisposes to the occipital lesions. The forms of PRES that are induced by chemotherapeutic and other agents are more complex and are discussed in Chap. 43. A few eclamptic women will develop hemolysis, hepatic failure, and thrombocytopenia—HELLP syndrome—an illness that has similarities to TTP and the hemolytic uremic syndrome (HUS). The interplay between eclampsia and HELLP syndrome in relation to cerebral lesions is complex and not fully understood.

Treatment

In the past, when effective treatment was not available, the outcome was often fatal. Lowering of the blood pressure with antihypertensive drugs may reverse the picture in a day or two. The same can be accomplished by administering magnesium sulfate in the eclamptic woman. However, antihypertensive drugs must be used cautiously; a safe target is a pressure of 150/100 mm Hg or a 20 percent reduction in mean pressure. One may use intravenous sodium nitroprusside, 0.5 to 0.8 mg/kg/min; a calcium channel blocker such as nifedipine, 10 to 20 mg sublingually; or intravenous beta-adrenergic blockers (labetalol, 20 to 40 mg intravenously followed by an infusion at 2 mg/min, or esmolol are favored). Longer-acting antihypertensive agents, such as ACE inhibitors and calcium channel blockers, must follow these. If there is already evidence of brain edema and increased intracranial pressure, dexamethasone, 4 to 6 mg every 6 h, is sometimes added, but its effect, and the use of hyperosmolar therapy, have not been studied systematically; our clinical impression is that they have little effect.

DIFFUSE CEREBRAL VASOSPASM (REVERSIBLE CEREBRAL VASOCONSTRICTION SYNDROME [RCVS], CALL-FLEMING SYNDROME)

A widespread multifocal or diffuse reduction in the caliber of the cerebral vessels and their branches constitutes a special syndrome of several causes. Vasospasm is, of course, a well-known complication of subarachnoid hemorrhage as described earlier. But the process under discussion has different characteristics. Some degree of attenuation of large cerebral vessels is observed in hypertensive encephalopathy and eclampsia, but a more diffuse and sustained reduction in vascular caliber can result from various causes summarized in Table 34-10.

Table 34-10

CONDITIONS THAT HAVE BEEN ASSOCIATED WITH DIFFUSE OR WIDESPREAD CEREBRAL VASOSPASM
Idiopathic
Postpartum state
Eclampsia
Hypertensive encephalopathy
Massive subarachnoid hemorrhage
Ergot, sympathomimetic, and serotoninergic drugs including "triptans" and cocaine
"Thunderclap headache" (see Chap. 10)
Head trauma
Cervical arterial dissection, mainly vertebral
Acute porphyria
Hypercalcemia
Migraine?

This type of vasculopathy is produced by sympathomimetic drugs alone, such as ephedra in health food supplements, phenylpropanolamine, pseudoephedrine, methamphetamine, and cocaine, but there are few well-studied cases, as also discussed just below. In all cases, including those noted above, the treatment is cessation of the offending drugs; calcium channel blockers, corticosteroids, nitroglycerin, nitroprusside, and beta-adrenergic or papaverine infusions have been tried with uncertain effect. We have generally prescribed calcium channel-blocking drugs orally. Singhal and colleagues and others have brought to attention that serotonergic drugs may produce reversible multifocal vasospasm, severe headache, and stroke. One of their patients was using the antimigraine medicine sumatriptan; others were using serotonin reuptake inhibitor antidepressants and, in addition, had taken over-the-counter cold remedies that included pseudoephedrine and dextromethorphan; we are aware of other similar cases. These authors proposed that in these cases a "serotonin syndrome" had occurred, similar to what has been seen with overdoses of this class of antidepressants.

In addition, there is a less well-defined syndrome that is apparent on vascular imaging and affects few or many vessels distal to the circle of Willis (Fig. 34-35). Call and colleagues have described a striking idiopathic widespread segmental vasospasm of cerebral vessels that is characterized clinically by severe headache (often of the "thunderclap" variety, as described in Chap. 10) and fluctuating TIA-like episodes (termed Call-Fleming syndrome). The middle cerebral artery and its branches are mainly affected; the angiographic appearance may be mistaken for arteritis. The patients we have seen with this process, after several days or weeks of dramatically fluctuating focal neurologic symptoms and disabling headache, have recovered completely or nearly so, but several

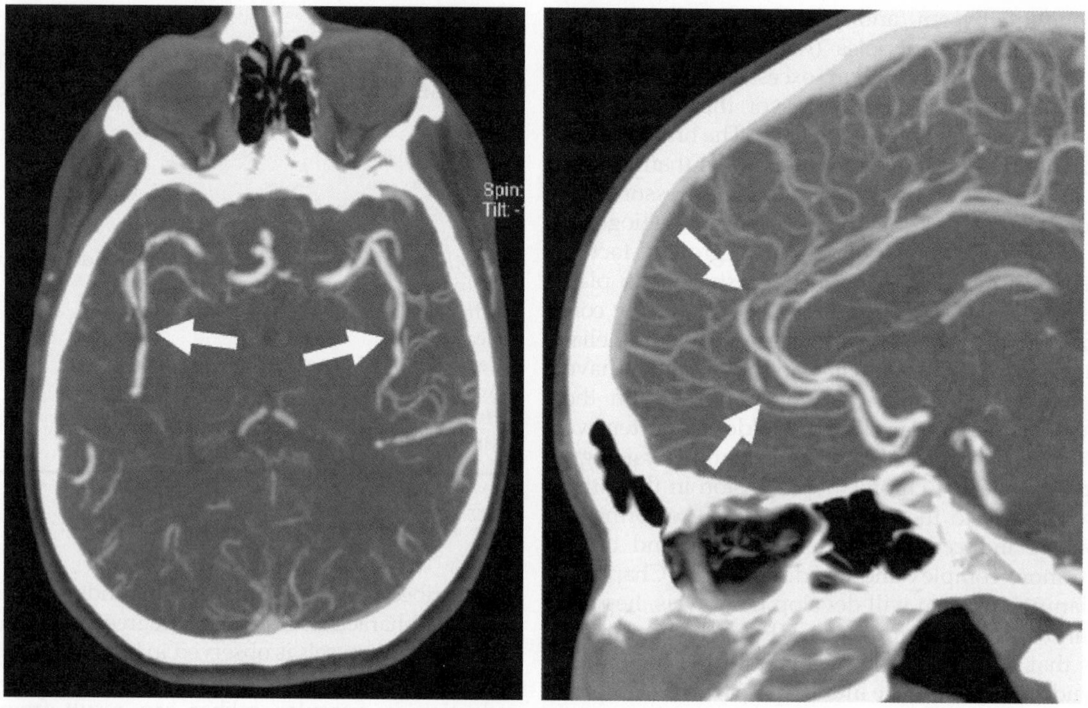

Figure 34-35. Reversible cerebral vasoconstriction syndrome. Axial (*left*) and sagittal (*right*) CT angiogram showing segmental narrowing of the middle and anterior cerebral artery branches (*arrows*).

have had small strokes. There may be an associated posterior leukoencephalopathy that is similar to the imaging appearance in hypertensive encephalopathy. Sometimes the headache is minimal and the attenuation of vessels is found in imaging performed for other reasons. The spinal fluid, except perhaps for elevated pressure, is normal.

The nature of this condition when there is no hyperadrenergic precipitant, trauma, or arterial dissection, is unknown. A relationship to hypertensive encephalopathy or to delayed postpartum eclampsia has been suggested because of the aforementioned white matter changes and the observation of widespread vasospasm in eclamptic women. Two of our patients have been in the postpartum period and other such patients with Call-Fleming have been described in the first 3 weeks after delivery. It is clear that, in addition to the idiopathic variety, several disorders cause this type of vasculopathy (see Table 34-10).

CEREBRAL VASCULITIS

Infectious Vasculitis

Inflammatory diseases of the blood vessels that are of infectious origin and their effects upon the nervous system are considered in detail in Chap. 32. There it was pointed out that meningovascular syphilis, tuberculous meningitis, fungal meningitis, and the subacute (untreated or partially treated) forms of bacterial meningitis may be accompanied by inflammatory changes in the walls of vessels that pass through the subarachnoid space and result in occlusion of the arteries or veins. For example, a small deep stroke is the first clinical sign of chronic basilar meningitis, but more often it develops well after the meningeal symptoms are established. The nature of the cerebral vasculitis that may rarely accompany AIDS is unclear. Independent of this possible mechanism, an increasing incidence of stroke in patients with AIDS has drawn considerable attention, for example, the epidemiologic survey by Ovbiagele and Nath has indicated a 60 percent increase in hospitalizations for stroke in HIV patients over a recent decade. However, the autopsy study carried out by Connor and coworkers emphasized that the causes of stroke were of the mundane types seen in others, and, while some nondescript vasculopathy was seen in small vessels, this was not related to vasculitis.

Typhus, schistosomiasis, mucormycosis, aspergillosis, malaria, and trichinosis are infrequent causes of inflammatory arterial disease, which, unlike the above-mentioned infections, are not secondary to meningeal infections. In *typhus and other rickettsial diseases*, capillary and arteriolar changes and perivascular inflammatory cells are found in the brain; presumably they are responsible for the seizures, acute psychoses, cerebellar syndromes, and coma characterizing the neurologic disorder in these diseases. The internal carotid artery may be secondarily occluded in diabetic patients as part of the orbital and cavernous sinus infections with *mucormycosis*. In *trichinosis*, the cause of the cerebral symptoms has not been clearly established. Parasites have been found in the brain; in one of our patients the cerebral lesions were produced by bland emboli arising in the heart and related to a severe myocarditis. In *cerebral malaria*, convulsions, coma, and, sometimes, focal symptoms appear to be due to the blockage of capillaries and precapillaries by masses of parasitized red blood corpuscles. Schistosomiasis may invade cerebral or spinal arteries. These diseases are discussed further in Chap. 32.

Noninfectious Inflammatory Diseases of Cranial Arteries

Included under this heading is a diverse group of arteritides that have little in common except their tendency to involve the cerebral vasculature. One group involves the larger caliber vessels and includes the *giant cell arteritides*—extracranial (temporal) arteritis; granulomatous arteritis of the brain; and aortic branch arteritis, one form of which is known as Takayasu disease.

A second group that affects the medium- and smaller-sized vessels includes polyarteritis nodosa, the Churg-Strauss type of arteritis, Wegener granulomatosis, systemic lupus erythematosus, Behçet disease, hypersensitivity angiitis, Kohlmeier-Degos disease, and the small vessel disorder of Susac syndrome. Immunologic studies show that in most of these processes there is an abnormal deposit of complement-fixing immune complex on the endothelium, leading to inflammation, vascular occlusion, or rupture with small hemorrhage. The initial inflammatory event is thought in some cases to be evoked by a virus, bacterium, or drug, but these are rarely proven in any one case. It is postulated by some immunologists that in the *granulomatous arteritides*, a different mechanism is operative—that an exogenous antigen induces antibodies that attach to the primary target (the vessel wall) as immune complexes, damage it, and attract lymphocytes and mononuclear cells. The giant cells form around remnants of the vessel wall. Wegener granulomatosis may fit this model. An acute necrotizing cerebral angiitis sometimes complicates ulcerative colitis and responds to treatment with prednisone and cyclophosphamide; it may also belong in this category. Mixed essential cryoglobulinemia, a vasculitic disorder that more often affects the peripheral than the central nervous system, may nonetheless produce an encephalopathy.

Temporal Arteritis (Giant Cell Arteritis, Cranial Arteritis) (See also Chap. 10)

In this disease, which is common among older persons, arteries of the external carotid system, particularly the temporal branches, are the sites of a subacute granulomatous inflammatory exudate consisting of lymphocytes and other mononuclear cells, neutrophilic leukocytes, and giant cells. The most severely affected parts of the artery usually become thrombosed. The sedimentation rate is characteristically elevated above 80 mm/h and sometimes exceeds 120 mm/h, but a small number of cases occur with values below 50 mm/h. The disease is included in this chapter because it uncommonly affects the extracranial internal and vertebral arteries and may result in stroke on the basis of ischemic occlusion or secondary embolus. However, significant inflammatory involvement of *intracranial arteries* from temporal arteritis is uncommon, perhaps because of a relative lack of elastic tissue.

Regional or bilateral headache or head pain is the chief complaint, and there may be severe pain, aching, and stiffness in the proximal muscles of the limbs associated with the markedly elevated sedimentation rate. Thus the clinical picture overlaps that of *polymyalgia rheumatica* as discussed in Chap. 10. Occlusion of branches of the ophthalmic artery (mainly those to the posterior ciliary artery and the choroidal circulation that supply the anterior optic nerve) results in blindness in one or both eyes, is the most feared complication, often unpredictably. This is one of the main forms of anterior ischemic optic neuropathy discussed in Chap. 13. In a few cases, blindness is preceded by transient visual loss, thereby simulating a TIA (transient monocular blindness). Other symptoms include jaw claudication due to ischemia of the masseter muscles. Occasionally the arteries of the oculomotor nerves are also involved, causing various ophthalmoplegias.

The administration of prednisone, 50 to 75 mg/d, provides striking relief of the headache and polymyalgic symptoms within days and sometimes within hours, and also prevents blindness. The medication must be given in very gradually diminishing doses for at least several months or longer, guided by the symptoms and the sedimentation rate. The latter begins to drop within days but seldom falls below 25 mm/h. These issues are discussed in greater detail in Chap. 10.

Intracranial Granulomatous Arteritis

Scattered examples of small- and medium-sized vessel giant cell arteritis of undetermined etiology in which only brain vessels are affected have come to medical attention over the years. The clinical aspects have taken diverse forms, sometimes presenting as low-grade, nonfebrile meningitis with sterile CSF followed by infarction of one or several parts of the cerebrum or cerebellum. In other cases it has evolved over a period of weeks, with strokes or an unusual dementia. Headaches (variable in our experience but sometimes severe), focal cerebral or cerebellar signs of gradual (occasionally stroke-like) evolution, confusion with memory loss, pleocytosis and elevated CSF protein, and papilledema as a result of increased intracranial pressure (in about half of reported cases but far fewer in our experience) constitute the most frequently encountered syndromes. The symptoms usually persist for several months. In contrast to temporal arteritis, the sedimentation rate is generally normal or only slightly elevated. An extensive early report given by Kolodny and colleagues still serves as a useful reference.

In about half the patients can the diagnosis be made by angiography, which demonstrates an irregular narrowing and in some cases blunt ending of several medium-sized cerebral arteries (Fig. 34-36). CT and MRI show multiple irregular white matter and cortical changes and small cortical lesions; sometimes these cannot be differentiated from a tumor or demyelinative or infectious process. If the white matter abnormalities become confluent, the radiologic appearance simulates Binswanger disease. The diagnosis is made most often by a brain biopsy, which includes a sample of the meninges with vessels, but even

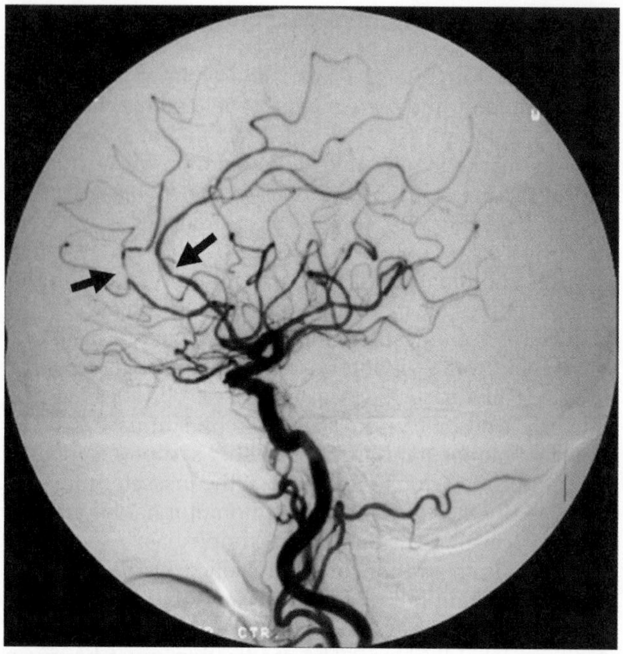

Figure 34-36. Granulomatous angiitis of the brain. Cerebral arteriogram from a common carotid artery injection, lateral projection, demonstrating numerous areas of irregular narrowing (*arrows*) and, in some areas, contiguous slight dilatation ("beading"), particularly in the anterior cerebral artery.

with tissue sampling, about half of suspected cases show the typical histopathologic changes. It is not unusual, however, for patients with normal angiograms to have the typical arteritic findings on biopsy. Tissue excised during an operation (or brain biopsy) for a suspected brain tumor, lymphoma, or white matter disease has revealed the characteristic vasculitis in some of our patients; in others, the diagnosis has been made only at autopsy, the findings coming as a distinct surprise.

The affected vessels are mainly in the 100- to 500-mm diameter arteries and arterioles and are surrounded and infiltrated by lymphocytes, plasma cells, and other mononuclear cells; giant cells are distributed in small numbers in the media, adventitia, or perivascular connective tissue. Infarction of brain tissue can be traced to widespread thrombosis in these vessels. The meninges are variably infiltrated with inflammatory cells. Sometimes only a part of the brain has been clinically affected—in one of our cases the cerebellum, in another, one frontal lobe and the opposite parietal lobe.

Among the most important considerations in this disease is the cerebral arteritis caused by varicella zoster virus of the ophthalmic division of the trigeminal nerve; it simulates in radiographic appearance granulomatous arteritis and giant cell arteritis. On occasion, intravascular lymphoma may present a similar picture and sympathomimetic agents, as mentioned earlier, cause a vasculopathy with segmental narrowing of cerebral vessels that has many similarities. The clinical and radiologic appearance of brain arteritis also raises the question of sarcoidosis, which is sometimes limited to the nervous system, of CADASIL, Antiphospholipid Antibody syndrome, or of the polyarteritis (allergic granulomatous angiitis) described by Churg and Strauss. Unlike some of these diseases, however, the lungs and other organs are spared; there is no systemic eosinophilia, increase in sedimentation rate or antineutrophil cytoplasmic antibodies (ANCA), or anemia.

Some patients with isolated angiitis of nervous system presenting as an aseptic meningitis and multiple cerebral infarcts have responded to corticosteroid and cyclophosphamide therapy (Moore, 1994), and we have used this combined approach from the time the diagnosis is established. The severity and configurations of the process are so variable that judging the effects of treatment is difficult, but our untreated patients have uniformly deteriorated or died without treatment.

Takayasu Disease ("Pulseless Disease")

This is a nonspecific chronic arteritis involving mainly the aorta and the large arteries arising from its arch. It is similar in some ways to giant cell arteritis except for its propensity to involve the proximal rather than the distal branches of the aorta. Most of the patients have been young Asian women, but there are now numerous reports of similar cases from the United States, Latin America, and Europe. The etiology has never been ascertained but an autoimmune mechanism is suspected.

Constitutional symptoms such as malaise, fever, anorexia, weight loss, and night sweats usually introduce the illness. The erythrocyte sedimentation rate is elevated in the early and active stages. Later there is evidence of occlusion of the brachiocephalic, subclavian, carotid, vertebral, and other arteries that may be asymptomatic or cause neurologic ischemic symptoms. The affected arteries no longer pulsate, hence the descriptive term *pulseless disease*. When renal arteries are involved, hypertension results, and there may be coronary occlusion, which may be fatal. Involvement of the pulmonary artery may lead to pulmonary hypertension. Coolness of the hands and weak radial pulses are common indicators of the disease and headaches are frequent. Blurring of vision, especially upon physical activity or fever, dizziness, and hemiparetic and hemisensory syndromes are the usual neurologic manifestations (Lupi-Herrera et al). The frequency of posturally induced neurologic symptoms has been emphasized, as well as the relative infrequency of major strokes despite multiple TIA-like spells. The inflamed vessels in the thorax are revealed by radionuclide scans using gallium. Pathologic studies disclose a periarteritis of the large vessels, often with giant cells and reparative fibrosis.

Many of the patients die in 3 to 5 years. According to Ishikawa and colleagues, the administration of corticosteroids in the acute inflammatory stage of the disease improves the prognosis. Reconstructive vascular surgery has helped some of the patients in the later stages of the disease.

Polyarteritis Nodosa and Churg-Strauss Angiitis of Cerebral Vessels

The inflammatory necrosis of arteries and arterioles throughout the body in this disease rarely affects the central (in contrast to frequent involvement of the peripheral) nervous system. The lungs are usually spared, which is the basis of distinguishing polyarteritis vasculitis from the Churg-Strauss granulomatous angiitis. It has been estimated that the brain is involved in fewer than 5 percent of cases of either of these processes and takes the form of one or more microinfarcts; macroscopic infarction is a rarity. The clinical manifestations vary and have included headache, confusion and fluctuating cognitive disorders, convulsions, hemiplegia, and brainstem signs. We have also observed one instance of acute spinal cord lesions. Brain hemorrhage is rare and usually occurs in a setting of extreme renal hypertension. Both of these diseases assume greater importance in the field of vasculitic neuropathy as discussed in Chap. 46.

Wegener Granulomatosis

This is a rare disease of unknown cause, affecting adults as a rule and favoring males slightly. A subacutely evolving vasculitis with necrotizing granulomas of the upper and lower respiratory tracts followed by necrotizing glomerulonephritis are its main features. Neurologic complications come later in one-third to one-half of cases and take two forms: (1) a peripheral neuropathy either in a pattern of polyneuropathy or, far more frequently, in a pattern of mononeuropathy multiplex (see discussion in Chap. 46), and (2) multiple cranial neuropathies as a result of direct extension of the nasal and sinus granulomas into adjacent upper cranial nerves and from adjacent to pharyngeal lesions to the lower cranial nerves (see Chap. 47). We have seen this disease produce the syndrome of episodic hemicrania, with periorbital ecchymosis. The basilar parts of the skull may be eroded, with spread of granuloma to the cranial cavity and more remote parts. A description is included here because cerebrovascular events, seizures, and cerebritis are less common but well-described neurologic complications. Spastic paraparesis, temporal arteritis, Horner syndrome, and papilledema have been observed but are rare (see Nishino et al). The orbits are involved in 20 percent of patients and lesions here simulate the clinical and radiologic appearance of orbital pseudotumor, cellulitis, or lymphoma. Pulmonary granulomas, usually asymptomatic but evident on a chest CT, are also common.

The vasculitis implicates both small arteries and veins. There is a fibrinoid necrosis of their walls and an infiltration by neutrophils and histiocytes. The sedimentation rate is elevated, as are the rheumatoid and antiglobulin factors. The presence in the blood of cytoplasmic antineutrophil cytoplasmic antibodies (cANCA) has been found to be relatively specific and sensitive for Wegener disease but it may also be present in intravascular lymphoma.

A degree of therapeutic success in this formerly fatal disease has been achieved by the use of cyclophosphamide, chlorambucil, rituximab, or azathioprine. Cyclophosphamide in oral doses of 1 to 2 mg/kg per day has ameliorated 90 to 95 percent of the cases. In acute cases, rapidly acting steroids—prednisone, 50 to 75 mg/d—is usually given in conjunction with the immunosuppressant drug(s).

Systemic Lupus Erythematosus

Involvement of the nervous system is an important aspect of this disease. In the pathologic and clinical series reported by Johnson and Richardson, the central nervous system (CNS) was affected in 75 percent of cases, but our recent experience has suggested a lower frequency of clinical manifestations, especially if minor neurologic aspects such as headache are excluded. Disturbances of mental function—including alteration of consciousness, seizures, and signs referable to cranial nerves—are the usual neurologic manifestations; most often they develop in the late stages of the disease, but they may occur early and may be mild and transient. Hemiparesis, paraparesis, aphasia, homonymous hemianopia, movement disorders (chorea), and derangements of hypothalamic function occur but have been infrequent in our experience. Larger infarcts are usually traceable to emboli from Libman-Sacks (a form of nonbacterial thrombotic) endocarditis.

In some instances the CNS manifestations resemble multiple sclerosis, especially when there is an optic neuritis or myelopathy. Two manifestations that should be noted are of "longitudinally extensive myelopathy" that simulates Devic disease, and of white matter changes in the cerebral hemispheres with varied clinical manifestations, ("Sjogren sclerosis," or "lupus sclerosis"). These are discussed in Chap. 36 with multiple sclerosis and diseases that simulate it. The presence of serum antinuclear antibodies is of help in the differentiation of lupus erythematosus but in itself does not establish the diagnosis. Antibodies to double-stranded DNA (anti-dsDNA) are a sensitive indicator of the disease. The CSF is normal or shows only a mild lymphocytic pleocytosis and slight increase in protein content, although in some patients—primarily those with peripheral neuropathy and myelopathy—the protein content may be greatly increased.

Some of the neurologic manifestations can be accounted for by widespread microinfarcts in the cerebral cortex and brainstem; these, in turn, are related to destructive and proliferative changes in arterioles and capillaries. The acute lesion is subtle; it is not a typical fibrinoid necrosis of the vessel wall, like that in hypertensive encephalopathy, and there is no cellular infiltration. Attachment of immune complexes to the endothelium is the postulated mechanism of vascular injury. Thus, the changes do not represent a vasculitis in the strict sense of the word. However, there is also an immune component to some of the white matter and cord lesions that do not require implicating a vasculopathy (see Chap. 36).

Other neurologic manifestations are related to hypertension, which frequently accompanies the disease and may precipitate cerebral hemorrhage; to endocarditis, which may give rise to cerebral embolism; to thrombotic thrombocytopenic purpura, which commonly complicates the terminal phase of the disease (Devinsky et al); and to treatment with corticosteroids, which may precipitate or accentuate muscle weakness, seizures, and psychosis. In other cases, steroids appear to improve these neurologic manifestations. A similar set of neurologic problems arises in relation to the antiphospholipid antibody syndrome, which may be a feature of lupus or arise independently (see "Antiphospholipid Antibody (Hughes) Syndrome"). It is not entirely clear to us what proportion of the cerebrovascular features of lupus might be explained on the basis of the coagulation disorder or Libman-Sacks endocarditis.

Arteritis Symptomatic of Underlying Systemic Disease and Sympathomimetic Drug Ingestion

Drug-induced vasculitis, typical of the ingestion of sympathomimetic compounds, is difficult to distinguish from a more common state of focal vasospasm that may also be induced by these same agents, as discussed earlier under "Diffuse and Focal Cerebral Vasospasm, Call-Fleming Syndrome, Postpartum Cerebral Vasculopathy." A true cerebral or spinal cord vasculitis can occur in association with systemic lymphoma, particularly with Hodgkin disease. The nature of this process is indeterminate but may be related to the deposition of circulating immune complexes in the walls of cerebral vessels.

The cerebrovascular problems resulting from cocaine use are quite varied. Seizures and death may occur as a result of a syndrome of delirium and extreme hyperthermia. More pertinent to this chapter are the strokes that arise during and just after cocaine use. Here, as emphasized by Levine and colleagues (1991), a clear distinction should be made between the complications of cocaine hydrochloride (the usual form of ingestible cocaine) and the alkaloid form, or "crack cocaine." The former, when injected intravenously more so than when used intranasally, is prone to cause cerebral hemorrhage as a result of acute hypertension, similar to the bleeding that may be precipitated by other sympathomimetic drugs such as amphetamine and phenylpropanolamine. Both subarachnoid and intracerebral hemorrhage may result. Or, the features of hypertensive encephalopathy are precipitated, including changes in the posterior white matter of the cerebral hemispheres that are so striking on imaging studies (PRES, as discussed earlier). The strokes with crack cocaine, however, are more often ischemic, typically involving the territory of a large vessel. Some ambiguity attends the vasculopathy induced by crack cocaine, cocaine hydrochloride, and the amphetamines, particularly the first of these. There are undoubted instances of a true cerebral inflammatory vasculitis, perhaps of a hypersensitivity type such as those reported with biopsy verification by Krendel and colleagues, by Merkel and associates, and by others. What is confusing about these cases is the normal angiographic appearance in many instances and large vessel occlusions in others, in contrast to the pathologic changes, which are concentrated in small cortical vessels. Many cases seem to be of an entirely different type, displaying long segments of vascular attenuation in the angiogram and no evidence of an inflammatory process in biopsy or autopsy material. The correct treatment, aside from lowering the blood pressure, is uncertain. A similar apparently vasospastic disorder is emerging from the use of *high-potency cannabinoids* (e.g., K-2, "spice"), including strokes.

Whether there is an increased incidence of arteriovenous malformation and cerebral aneurysm in patients who have cerebral hemorrhages after ingestion of cocaine, as suggested in several articles, is uncertain but this, in any case, suggests that sympathomimetic drugs can precipitate hemorrhage from an underlying developmental vascular lesion (Fessler et al).

Crack cocaine may also cause a choreiform disorder ("crack dancing"), not unlike that associated with antiphospholipid antibody but generalized rather than focal (see further on); usually there are small infarctions in the basal ganglia, but an immune mechanism has also been suggested.

Another entirely different type of small vessel arteritis occurs as a hypersensitivity phenomenon. Often it is associated with an allergic skin lesion (Stevens-Johnson vasculopathy or a leukocytoclastic vasculitis). The clinical picture does not resemble that of polyarteritis nodosa, but the central or peripheral nervous system is affected in rare instances. The response to corticosteroids is excellent.

The special case of intravascular lymphoma, which closely simulates a cerebral vasculitis, is discussed in Chap. 31.

Susac Syndrome

This is yet another poorly understood form of vasculitis, consisting of a microangiopathy affecting mainly the brain and retina. Psychiatric symptoms, headache, dementia, sensorineural deafness, vertigo, and impairments of vision are the clinical manifestations. Funduscopy (multiple retinal artery branch occlusions) and retinal angiography manifest evidence of the vasculopathy (Susac and colleagues, 1979). The MRI may show characteristic white matter lesions, particularly in the corpus callosum (see Susac and colleagues, 2003). Antibodies to endothelial cells have been identified by Magro and colleagues in many of the cases. The patients seem to respond to steroid therapy. Only biopsy material has been examined.

Behçet Disease

This disorder is suitably considered here because it is a chronic, recurrent vasculitis, involving small vessels, with prominent neurologic manifestations. It is most common in Turkey, where it was first described, in other Mediterranean countries, and in Japan, but it occurs throughout Europe and North America, affecting men more often than women. The disease was originally distinguished by the triad of relapsing iridocyclitis and recurrent oral and genital ulcers, but it is now recognized to be a systemic disease with a much wider range of symptoms, including erythema nodosum, thrombophlebitis, polyarthritis, ulcerative colitis, and a number of neurologic manifestations, some of them encephalitic or meningitic in nature. The most reliable diagnostic criteria, according to the International Study Group that assembled data on 914 cases from 12 medical centers in 7 countries, were recurrent aphthous or herpetiform oral ulceration, recurrent genital ulceration, anterior or posterior uveitis, cells in the vitreous or retinal vasculitis, and erythema nodosum or papulopustular lesions.

The nervous system is affected in approximately 30 percent of patients with Behçet disease (Chajek and Fainaru); the manifestations are recurrent meningoencephalitis, cranial nerve (particularly abducens) palsies, cerebellar ataxia, corticospinal tract signs, and venous occlusion disease. There may be episodes of diencephalic and brainstem dysfunction resembling minor strokes. A few postmortem examinations have related these small foci of necrosis to a vasculitis, including perivascular and meningeal infiltration of lymphocytes. There may also be cerebral venous thrombosis. The neurologic symptoms usually have an abrupt onset and are accompanied by a brisk spinal fluid pleocytosis (lymphocytes or neutrophils may predominate), along with elevated protein but normal glucose values (in one of our patients, 3,000 neutrophils per cubic millimeter were found at the onset of an acute meningitis). As a rule, neurologic symptoms clear completely in several weeks, but they have a tendency to recur, and some patients are left with persistent neurologic deficits. Rarely, the clinical picture is that of a progressive confusional state or dementia (see the reviews of Alema and of Lehner and Barnes for detailed accounts).

The cause of Behçet disease is unknown. A pathergy skin test—the formation of a sterile pustule at the site of a needle prick—is listed as an important diagnostic test by the International Study Group, but on the basis of admittedly limited U.S. experience, we and our colleagues have found it to be of questionable value. Administration of corticosteroids has been the usual treatment, on the assumption of an autoimmune etiology. Because the episodes of disease naturally subside and recur, evaluation of treatment is difficult.

THROMBOSIS OF CEREBRAL VEINS AND VENOUS SINUSES

Thrombosis of the cerebral venous sinuses, particularly of the superior sagittal or lateral sinus and the tributary cortical and deep veins, gives rise to a number of important neurologic syndromes. Cerebral vein thrombosis may develop in relation to infections of the adjacent ear and paranasal sinuses or to bacterial meningitis, as described in Chap. 32. More common is noninfectious venous occlusion resulting from one of the many hypercoagulable states discussed below.

Occlusion of cortical veins that are the tributaries of the dural sinuses takes the form of a venous infarctive stroke. It may be difficult to determine if the thrombus originated in the dural sinuses and propagates to the tributary cortical veins, or the reverse. The diagnosis is difficult except in certain clinical settings known to favor the occurrence of venous thrombosis, such as the taking of birth control pills or postpartum and postoperative states, which are often characterized by thrombocytosis and hyperfibrinogenemia. Hypercoagulable conditions also occur in cancer (particularly of the pancreas and colon and other adenocarcinomas), cyanotic congenital heart disease; cachexia in infants; sickle cell disease; antiphospholipid antibody syndrome, the aforementioned Behçet disease, factor V Leiden mutation, protein S or C deficiency, antithrombin III deficiency, resistance to activated protein C; primary or secondary polycythemia and thrombocythemia; and paroxysmal nocturnal hemoglobinuria.

The administration of drugs such as tamoxifen, bevacizumab, and erythropoietin, and even the hypercoagulable reaction to heparin that is associated with thrombocytopenia have all been cited as risks for cerebral venous thrombosis.

The study by Martinelli and colleagues, mentioned earlier in the chapter, attributed 35 percent of cases of cerebral vein thrombosis in the context of oral contraceptive use to a mutation in the factor V or in the prothrombin gene. Averback, who reported seven cases of venous thrombosis in young adults, has emphasized the diversity of the clinical causes. Two of his patients had carcinoma of the breast and one had ulcerative colitis. A few cases will follow head injury or remain unexplained.

A stroke in a patient suffering from any one of these systemic conditions should suggest venous thrombosis, although in some instances—e.g., postpartum strokes—arteries are occluded as often as veins. A slower evolution of the clinical stroke syndrome, the presence of multiple cerebral lesions not in arterial territories, and a convulsive and hemorrhagic character favor venous over arterial thrombosis.

The reasons for these clinical features and their variability as well as the differences from ischemic brain damage caused by arterial occlusion become apparent in the discussions below. Stam has undertaken a review of this subject.

Cortical Vein Thrombosis (Superficial Thrombosis of Cortical Veins)

Certain syndromes occur with sufficient regularity that they suggest thrombosis of a particular vein or sinus. The signature features of isolated *thrombosis of superficial cortical veins* are the presence of large superficial (cortex and subjacent white matter) hemorrhagic infarctions and a marked tendency to focal seizures. Hemiparesis, incomplete hemianopia, and aphasia, any of which may fluctuate over days, are also characteristic according to Jacobs and colleagues. These variable syndromes reflect the inconstant location of the main surface veins. Thrombosis of the vein of Labbé causes infarction of the underlying superior temporal lobe, and occlusion of the vein of Trolard implicates the parietal cortex. A concern is the propagation of the clot into the larger draining veins or dural sinuses.

Quite often, in our experience, the focal deficit worsens immediately after a focal seizure. The intracranial pressure is not elevated, as it is when the dural venous sinuses are occluded. The diagnosis is made by careful examination of the MRV or by the venous phase of the conventional angiogram. Cortical vein thrombosis should be suspected in the situation of multiple hemorrhagic infarctions in one hemisphere without a source of embolism or atherothrombosis.

Dural Sinus Thrombosis

Sagittal and Transverse (Lateral) Sinus Thrombosis In the case of *sagittal sinus thrombosis*, intracranial hypertension with headache, vomiting, and papilledema may constitute the entire syndrome; this is the main consideration in the differential diagnosis of pseudotumor cerebri (see Chaps. 13 and 30) or it may be conjoined with hemorrhagic infarction. Paraparesis, hemiparesis, fluctuating unilateral or bilateral sensory symptoms, or aphasia result only if the thrombosis propagates to surface veins. Focal or odd sensory or motor seizures occur on the same basis but are not as common as with cortical vein thrombosis.

The transverse sinuses are usually asymmetrical; slightly more than half of individuals have a dominant right vein and approximately a quarter are symmetrical. (The larger sinus corresponds to a smaller occipital lobe on that side—a *petalia*). Unilateral occlusion of the nondominant transverse sinus may not be symptomatic, whereas thrombosis of the dominant side generally gives the equivalent syndrome to blockage of the sagittal sinus. Increased intracranial pressure without ventricular dilatation occurs with thrombosis of the superior sagittal sinus, the main jugular vein, and the transverse sinus or the confluence of the sinuses.

The common imaging feature that results from occlusion of the superior sagittal sinus is of bilateral superficial paramedian parietal or frontal hemorrhagic infarctions or edematous venous congestion. In the case of CT with contrast infusion in axial images, a lack of dye opacification in the posterior sagittal sinus can be observed with careful adjustment of the viewing window ("empty delta sign"). The spinal fluid pressure is increased, and the fluid may be slightly sanguinous. Transverse sinus thrombosis causes hemorrhagic infarction of the temporal lobe convexity, usually with considerable vasogenic edema. The enhanced CT, arteriography (venous phase), and MRV (Fig. 34-37) facilitate diagnosis by directly visualizing the venous occlusion by showing an absence of opacification of a sinus or, at times, a clot within a vein. Once a venous thrombosis becomes established for several days or longer, the tributary surface veins take on a "corkscrew" appearance that is appreciated on the venous phase of an angiogram.

Cavernous Sinus Thrombosis As pointed out in Chaps. 13 and 14, in cases of *cavernous sinus thrombosis* there may be marked chemosis and proptosis, corresponding to a clot in the anterior portion of the sinus and there may be disordered function of cranial nerves III, IV, VI, and the ophthalmic division of V when the posterior portion is affected. If there is spread of the clot to the inferior petrosal sinus, palsies of cranial nerves VI, IX, X, and XI may result. Also involvement of the *superior petrosal sinus* may be accompanied by a fifth nerve palsy.

Thrombosis of the venous sinuses in neonates presents special problems in diagnosis. In the series reported by deVeber and colleagues, various perinatal complications, including systemic illness such as severe dehydration or infection were common precedents; the outcome was poor. In young children the risk factors differed, in that connective tissue and prothrombotic disorders and head and neck infections were more common.

Deep Cerebral Vein Thrombosis

Occlusion of the vein of Galen and of the internal cerebral veins is the least common and clinically most obscure of the venous syndromes.

From the few cases that have been studied, a picture of bithalamic infarction emerges, sometimes reversible, and consisting mainly of inattention, spatial neglect, and amnesia in the case reported by Benabdeljili and colleagues, and of akinetic mutism and apathy in the case of Gladstone and associates. The case series of van den Bergh and colleagues emphasizes the difficulty in diagnosis of partial syndromes of this nature. In most reports of this condition, it is the neuropsychologic aspects that are emphasized. Other cases have manifested coma and pupillary changes referable to the ischemic diencephalon and rostral midbrain. Perhaps most striking is the MRI, with a large bilobular region of signal change that encompasses the thalami. Much of the signal change probably represents reversible edema and venous congestion, because substantial clinical improvement may occur. Angiography is needed to confirm the diagnosis, most often a magnetic resonance venogram.

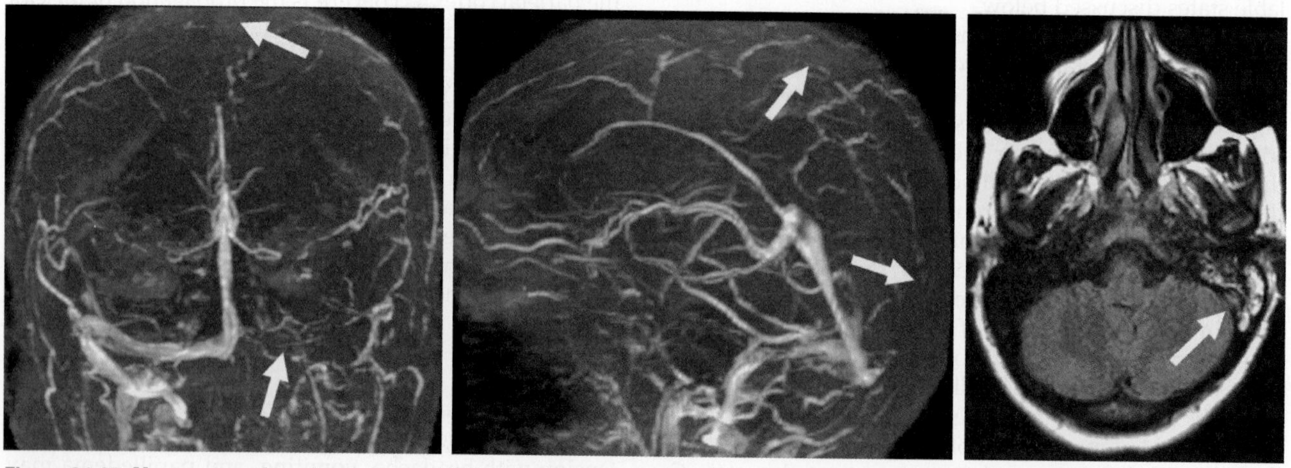

Figure 34-37. Venous sinus thrombosis. Coronal (*left*) and sagittal (*center*) magnetic resonance venogram demonstrating absence of flow in the superior sagittal and left transverse sinuses (*arrows*). Note that the straight sinus and right transverse sinuses remain patent. Axial T2-FLAIR MRI shows left otomastoiditis, which was the cause of the extensive thrombosis.

Treatment of Cerebral Venous Thrombosis

Anticoagulant therapy beginning with heparin or an equivalent for several days, followed by warfarin, and combined with antibiotics if the venous occlusion is infectious (it rarely is in recent times) has been lifesaving in some cases. Nonetheless, the overall mortality rate remains high, with large hemorrhagic venous infarctions found in 10 to 20 percent of cases. The clinical trial conducted by Einhaupl and colleagues generally settled the question of therapy in favor of aggressive anticoagulation, but this could not be confirmed by de Bruijn and coworkers, who found a minimal difference between patients who were treated with low-molecular-weight heparin followed by oral anticoagulation. Most treated patients do well, but it may take weeks for the headaches to remit. Coma and multiple cerebral hemorrhages, on the other hand, are usually fatal.

The local infusion of tPA has been used, but not subjected to the same randomized testing. Thrombolytic therapy by local venous or systemic infusion has been successful in small series of cases, such as the 5 patients treated with urokinase and heparin by DiRocco and colleagues. We have reserved thrombolysis for extreme cases of dural sinus thrombosis with stupor or coma and greatly raised CSF pressure.

STROKE DUE TO HYPERCOAGULABLE STATES

Nonbacterial Thrombotic (Marantic) Endocarditis

Sterile vegetations, referred to also as *nonbacterial thrombotic endocarditis*, consist of fibrin and platelets and are loosely attached to the mitral and aortic valves and contiguous endocardium. They are a common source of cerebral embolism (almost 10 percent of all instances of cerebral embolism according to Barron et al, but lower in the experience of other series). In past series, almost half the patients had vegetations associated with a malignant neoplasm; the remainder occurs in patients debilitated by other diseases (Biller et al). Recent experience suggests that the majority is related to systemic cancer.

The setting in which embolism from nonbacterial endocarditis occurs is distinctive. There may also be prototypic clinical features that permit differentiation from other forms of cerebral embolism. In particular, the strokes may be multiple, sequential over days or weeks, and generally small, imparting a picture of incomplete stroke syndromes with a superimposed encephalopathy. The sudden nature of the embolic deficits helps to distinguish this process from the usual forms of cerebral metastases.

The disease is essentially a manifestation of chronic disseminated intravascular coagulation (DIC) discussed below and therefore it is not surprising that similar laboratory changes are found, including an elevation in circulating fibrin split products, specifically D-dimer and indications of microangiopathic hemolysis in the blood smear. There is typically moderate thrombocytopenia. The echocardiogram is often obtained but it is insensitive.

The hazards of using anticoagulants in gravely ill patients with widespread malignant disease may outweigh the benefits from this treatment, but drugs that prevent platelet aggregation, while possibly helpful, have not been studied systematically for this condition. Quite often the embolic strokes continue despite treatment.

Stroke as a Complication of Hematologic Disease

The brain is involved in the course of many hematologic disorders, some of which have already been mentioned. A number of the better-characterized ones are discussed here.

Disseminated Intravascular Coagulation

This is perhaps the most common and most serious disorder of coagulation affecting the nervous system. The basic process depends on the release of thromboplastic substances from damaged tissue, resulting in the activation of the coagulation process and the formation of fibrin, in the course of which clotting factors and platelets are consumed. Virtually any mechanism that produces tissue damage can result in the release of tissue thromboplastins into the circulation. Thus, disseminated intravascular coagulation (DIC) complicates a wide variety of clinical conditions—overwhelming sepsis, massive trauma, cardiothoracic surgery, heat stroke, burns, incompatible blood transfusions and other immune complex disorders, diabetic ketoacidosis, leukemia, obstetric complications, cyanotic congenital heart disease, and shock from many causes.

The essential pathologic change in DIC is the occurrence of widespread fibrin thrombi in small vessels, resulting in numerous small infarctions of many organs, including the brain. Sometimes DIC is manifest by a hemorrhagic diathesis in which petechial hemorrhages are situated around small penetrating vessels. In some cases, cerebral hemorrhage is quite extensive, similar to a primary hypertensive hemorrhage. The main reason for the hemorrhage is the consumption of platelets and various clotting factors that occurs during fibrin formation; in addition, fibrin degradation products have anticoagulant properties of their own.

The diffuse nature of the neurologic damage may suggest a metabolic rather than a vascular disorder of the brain. In the absence of a clear metabolic, infective, or neoplastic cause of an encephalopathy, the onset of acute and fluctuating focal neurologic abnormalities or a generalized and sometimes terminal neurologic deterioration during the course of a severe illness should arouse suspicion of DIC, and coagulation factors and fibrin split products should be measured. Platelet counts are invariably depressed and there is evidence of consumption of fibrinogen and other clotting factors, indicated by prolonged prothrombin and partial thromboplastin times.

In the related illness abbreviated as HELLP mentioned earlier in the sections on hypertensive and eclamptic encephalopathy, women with eclampsia develop liver failure and thrombocytopenia; the contribution of this limited form of DIC to the eclamptic effects on the nervous system have not been established (see earlier discussion of eclampsia).

Antiphospholipid Antibody (Hughes) Syndrome

This condition, in which TIAs, or stroke, migraine, and thrombocytopenia in various combinations, occur in young adults, has already been discussed under "Strokes in Children and Young Adults." Phospholipids are a family of lipoproteins that influence clotting. Some of the phospholipids with which the antibodies react are shared with clotting factors, particularly prothrombin. Autoantibodies directed at the binding protein of phospholipids thereby induce blood clotting. The first of the antibodies to be described were *lupus anticoagulant* and *anticardiolipin*. Most classifications of the antiphospholipid syndrome also include antibodies to β_2-glycoprotein 1, a protein that may be necessary for the binding and procoagulant effect of anticardiolipin antibody. The formal criteria for the diagnosis of the syndrome require that an ischemic event be accompanied by the detection of autoantibodies on two occasions at least 6 weeks apart.

Testing for this disease consists of detection of IgM, IgG, and mixed antibodies to each of these three main phospholipids; there is a partial overlap in many patients, in which more than one antibody subclass is present against more than one lipoprotein—80 percent of patients with lupus anticoagulant have anticardiolipin antibody but fewer than 50 percent of those with anticardiolipin antibody have lupus anticoagulant. Antibodies to β_2-glycoprotein 1 are most specific for the disease. Nonetheless, the main laboratory feature of the illness is a prolonged partial thromboplastin time. The titer of anticardiolipin broadly correlates with the risk of thrombosis and the specificity for the syndrome is higher for IgG than for IgM autoantibodies. An increased incidence of migraine has long been discussed and also disputed. A review has been given by Levine.

These comments pertain mainly to a "primary" idiopathic autoimmune form of the disease but many cases occur secondarily to lupus erythematosus, Sjögren disease, neuroleptic drugs such as the phenothiazines, butyrophenones and others drugs, and to certain infections.

The most frequent neurologic abnormality is a TIA, often taking the form of amaurosis fugax (transient monocular blindness), with or without retinal arteriolar or venous occlusion (Digre et al). Stroke-like phenomena are more frequent in patients who also have migraine, hyperlipidemia, or antinuclear antibodies, and in those who smoke or take birth control pills. Almost one-third of the 48 patients reported by Levine and associates (1990) had thrombocytopenia and 23 percent had a false-positive Venereal Disease Research Laboratory (VDRL) test. The vascular lesions are mainly in the cerebral white matter and are infarcts, seen well with MRI. Angiography reveals occlusions of arteries at unusual sites (Brey et al). The mechanism of stroke is not entirely clear and may derive from emboli originating on mitral valve leaflets similar to nonbacterial thrombotic endocarditis; alternatively, and more likely in our view, there is a noninflammatory in situ thrombosis of medium-sized cerebral vessels, as suggested by the limited pathologic material studied by Briley and colleagues.

These circulating antibodies may also cause a syndrome of transient bilateral chorea or hemichorea; some patients have an additional slight hemiparesis or other subtle focal signs. Almost all of the affected patients we have seen have been women with thrombocytopenia, some of whom probably had systemic lupus, at least on the grounds of laboratory studies. A direct connection of the choreic syndrome to the antibodies comparable to what is proposed in Sydenham chorea may be valid, but at the moment is unproven. Some cases display microinfarctions in the basal ganglia, perhaps on the basis of valvular vegetations. The choreic syndrome may be precipitated in these patients by the introduction of estrogen-containing birth control pills and is improved, usually promptly, by corticosteroids or antiplatelet agents.

The *Sneddon syndrome* is an arteriopathy producing deep blue-red skin lesions of livedo reticularis and livedo racemosa in association with multiple ischemic strokes. Many, but not all, patients have high titers of antiphospholipid antibodies. Although the skin lesions show a noninflammatory vasculopathy with intimal thickening, the pathology of the occlusive disease has not been adequately studied. In a report of 17 such patients by Stockhammer and coworkers, 8 had strokes and MRI showed lesions in 16 patients. The age of patients with strokes was 30 to 35 years; hence this condition is considered in young adults with cerebrovascular disease. Many of the lesions on MRI were small, deep, and multiple. Although there is a tendency for strokes to recur, many of the patients have remained well for years after a single stroke. Skin biopsy aids in diagnosis.

There are instances in which the radiologic changes caused by recurrent small infarctions of antiphospholipid syndrome are difficult to distinguish from multiple sclerosis, as discussed in several parts of Chap. 36, on demyelinative diseases. Associations of the antiphospholipid syndrome with transverse myelitis (see Chap. 44), hearing loss, and a number of other processes have been suspected but not proven.

Treatment During the period in which the diagnosis is being established by repeating the antibody tests, or after just a single arterial ischemic stroke, consensus groups have stated that it is reasonable to treat these patients with antiplatelet or anticoagulant agents (see Lim and colleagues). Warfarin, the definitive therapy, alters the testing for antibodies and several guidelines recommend confirming the presence of antibodies after an interval of two weeks before starting treatment. However, warfarin has been used with greatest benefit and we have sometimes started this medication on suspicion of the syndrome. Khamashta and colleagues have found that the INR must be maintained close to 3 for effective prevention of stroke. According to the study conducted by Crowther and colleagues, an INR of 2 to 3 conferred the same degree of protection from thrombosis as did higher levels, but the number of thrombotic events was low in both groups and there was only 1 stroke in 114 patients over a period of about 3 years. Patients with severe thrombocytopenia and with other intrinsic coagulopathies should be treated with warfarin very cautiously. Although the INR is used as a gauge of the level of anticoagulation, it is also altered by the antibodies; no ideal method for monitoring the treatment has been devised. Aspirin, on uncertain grounds, is thought not to confer protection for stroke, but in only a few small series has its effect been analyzed. In "catastrophic" cases with repetitive strokes, intravenous immunoglobulin and plasma exchange have been used with some effect.

It is important to eliminate smoking and estrogen-containing compounds, as these greatly raise the risk of stroke in this syndrome. Aspirin and heparin are favored in women with recurrent fetal loss related to antiphospholipid antibody (Lockshin and Sammaritano).

Thrombotic Thrombocytopenic Purpura (TTP, Moschcowitz Syndrome) and Hemolytic Uremic Syndrome

These are serious diseases of the small blood vessels combined with microangiopathic hemolytic anemia characterized by widespread occlusions of arterioles and capillaries involving practically all organs of the body, including the brain. It was described by Adams and colleagues (1948) and named thrombocytic acroangiothrombosis. Fibrin components have been identified by immunofluorescent techniques; some investigators have demonstrated disseminated intravascular platelet aggregation rather than fibrin thrombi. Sporadic TTP is caused by an acquired circulating IgG inhibitor of the von Willebrand factor-cleaving protease (termed "a disintegrin and metalloproteinase with thrombospondin type 1 motif, member 13 [ADAMTS13]"). A rarer familial form (The Upshaw-Shulman syndrome) is caused by an inherited deficiency of ADAMTS13.

Clinically, the main features of this disease are fever, anemia, symptoms of renal and hepatic disease, and thrombocytopenia—the latter giving rise to the common hemorrhagic manifestations (petechiae and ecchymoses of the skin, retinal hemorrhages, hematuria, gastrointestinal bleeding, etc.). Neurologic symptoms are practically always present and are the initial manifestation of the disease in about half the cases. Confusion, delirium, seizures, and hemiparesis—sometimes remittent or fluctuating in nature—are the usual manifestations of the nervous system disorder and are readily explained by the widespread microscopic ischemic lesions in the brain. Garrett and colleagues have emphasized the presentation of nonconvulsive status epilepticus in TTP, and we have encountered two such cases. Gross infarction was not observed. In most patients who survive, recovery of the focal neurologic deficits can be expected unless there is an identifiable infarction on CT or MRI. The CSF is normal except for elevated protein in some cases. To our knowledge, a mononeuritis multiplex does not occur.

The diagnosis is made by finding a microangiopathic hemolytic anemia in the context of the characteristic clinical picture. An assay for ADAMTS13 activity is available using an enzyme-linked immunosorbent assay but the initiation of treatment usually cannot await confirmation of the diagnosis. There is an important overlap among TTP, HUS, toxemia of pregnancy, the hemolytic anemia with elevated liver function tests and platelet count (HELLP syndrome), hypertensive encephalopathy, and other causes of the posterior reversible leukoencephalopathy syndrome (PRES, see earlier discussion). In all of them, the central nervous system problem is mediated by endothelial dysfunction with breakdown of the blood–brain barrier. The recommended treatment for TTP is plasma exchange or plasma infusion. Further details can be found in *Harrison's Principles of Internal Medicine*.

Polycythemia Vera, Thrombocytosis, and Thrombocythemia

Polycythemia vera is a myeloproliferative disorder of unknown cause, characterized by a marked increase in RBC mass and in blood volume and often by an increase in WBCs and platelets. The condition must be distinguished from the many secondary or symptomatic forms of polycythemia (erythrocytosis), in which the platelets and white cells remain normal. The slightly increased incidence of thrombosis in primary polycythemia is attributed to the high blood viscosity, engorgement of vessels, and reduced rate of blood flow. The majority of patients with cerebrovascular manifestations have TIAs and small strokes, but we have seen one case of sagittal sinus thrombosis. With very high hematocrit, sludging of red cells may be seen in the retinal vessels. The cause of cerebral hemorrhage in this disease is less clear, although a number of abnormalities of platelet function and of coagulation have been described (see Davies-Jones et al).

Instances of platelet counts above 800,000/mm^3 are considered to be a form of myeloproliferative disease allied with polycythemia vera. In some patients there is an enlarged spleen, polycythemia, chronic myelogenous leukemia, or myelosclerosis. In several of our patients, no explanation of the thrombocytosis was found. They presented with recurrent cerebral and systemic thrombotic episodes, often of minor degree and transient. Cytapheresis, to reduce the platelets, and antiplatelet drugs (hydroxyurea anagrelide) to suppress megakaryocyte formation, are helpful in ameliorating the neurologic symptoms. In one of the cases we followed, several small lesions, presumably infarctions, were situated in the white matter and simulated multiple sclerosis. Another patient with essential thrombocytosis developed dramatic new migraine with aura when her platelet counts exceeded 1,000,000/mm^3.

A wide variety of bleeding disorders—such as *leukemia*, *aplastic anemia*, *thrombocytopenic purpura*, and *hemophilia*—may also give rise to cerebral hemorrhage. Many rare forms of bleeding disease may be complicated by hemorrhagic manifestations; these are reviewed by Davies-Jones and colleagues.

Sickle Cell Disease

This inherited disease is related to the presence of the abnormal hemoglobin S in the red corpuscles. Clinical abnormalities occur mainly in patients with sickle cell disease—i.e., with the homozygous state, and not in those with the sickle cell trait, which represents the heterozygous state. We have seen neurologic symptoms in patients with a heterozygous mixed hemoglobinopathy, such as sickle-thalassemia, sickle-S, and sickle-D, but all are less severe and less frequent than in sickle cell anemia. The disease, which is practically limited to persons of central African and certain Mediterranean origins, begins early in life and is characterized by "crises" of infection (particularly pneumococcal meningitis), pain in the limbs and abdomen, chronic leg ulcers, and infarctions of bones and visceral organs. Ischemic lesions of the brain, both large and small, are the most common neurologic complications, but cerebral, subarachnoid, and subdural hemorrhage may also occur, and the vascular occlusions may be either arterial or venous. Patients with sickle cell anemia may develop progressive stenosis of the supraclinoid intracranial carotid artery with consequent collateral formation, producing a syndrome akin to moyamoya disease described earlier in the chapter. These fragile collateral vessels may rupture causing intracranial hemorrhage.

Lee and colleagues demonstrated that exchange transfusions with monitoring of the velocities of flow in the middle cerebral artery by transcranial Doppler examination reduces the risk of this important neurologic complication. In the stroke prevention trial of sickle cell anemia, the risk of first stroke was reduced by 90 percent in 63 children who received periodic transfusions as compared to 67 children who received only supportive care.

SPECIAL CLINICAL PROBLEMS IN CEREBROVASCULAR DISEASE

Inevitably, most patients are seen first by clinicians who may not be expert in all the fine points of cerebrovascular disease. Situations arise in which critical decisions must be made regarding anticoagulation, further laboratory investigation, and the advice and prognosis to be given to the family. The following are some of the situations encountered by the authors that may be of value to students and residents and to nonspecialists in the field.

The Patient With a History of an Ischemic Attack or Small Stroke in the Past

The patient may be functioning normally when examined, but it has been ascertained by the history or radiologic procedures that a stroke or TIA occurred in the past. The problem is what measures should be taken to reduce the risk of further strokes. This is particularly problematic if a surgical procedure is planned. A brief focal TIA, several minutes or less in duration, or many stereotyped spells usually represent severe stenosis of the internal carotid artery on the side of the affected cerebral hemisphere. If the symptoms have occurred recently, these may be forerunners of complete occlusion. If the TIA was far in the past—more than several weeks previously—the immediate risks of occlusion are reduced. The initial approach is to establish the patency of the carotid arteries by ultrasonography or MRA. If there is a reduction in diameter of greater than 70 percent when compared with an adjacent normal segment of vessel, and probably if there is a severely ulcerated but not critically stenotic plaque, carotid surgery (or angioplasty with stenting) is advisable. If a single TIA lasted more than an hour or the neurologic examination discloses minor signs referable to the region of the hemisphere affected by the TIA, a search for a source of embolus is indicated. Appropriate diagnostic studies include ECG, a transesophageal echocardiogram, monitoring for cardiac arrhythmia, ultrasonography of the carotid arteries, and a CT or MRI if it has not already been performed. Control of elevated blood pressure and addressing high cholesterol levels are ancillary steps. The mistake is to ignore the potential significance of a prior small stroke or TIA.

The Patient With a Recent Stroke That May Not Be Complete

If hours have passed since the first symptoms of stroke but the syndrome is fluctuating or advancing, the basic problem is whether a thrombotic infarction (venous or arterial) will spread and involve more brain tissue; or if embolic, whether the ischemic tissue will become hemorrhagic or another embolus will occur; or if there is an arterial dissection, whether it will give rise to emboli. Therapies are controversial in most of these circumstances. In some centers, it is the practice to try to prevent propagation of a thrombus by administering heparin (or low-molecular-weight heparin) followed by warfarin, as discussed earlier. Some stroke deficits fluctuate with blood pressure, suggesting occlusion of the carotid or of another large vessel. Attention to adequate cerebral perfusion by omitting the patient's usual blood pressure medications, assuring adequate hydration and avoiding hemoconcentration, and potentially utilizing a head-down position may all assist in stabilizing the situation.

The Inevident or Misconstrued Syndromes of Cerebrovascular Disease

Although hemiplegia is the typical manifestation of stroke, cerebrovascular disease may manifest itself by signs that spare the motor pathways but have the same serious diagnostic and therapeutic implications. The following stroke syndromes tend to be overlooked.

Sometimes disregarded is a leaking aneurysm presenting as a sudden and intense generalized headache lasting hours or days and unlike any headache in the past. Examination may disclose no abnormality except for a slightly stiff neck and raised blood pressure. Failure to investigate such a case by imaging procedures and examination of the CSF may permit the occurrence of a later massive subarachnoid hemorrhage. Small cerebral hemorrhages, subdural hematomas, and brain tumors figure into the differential diagnosis, which is usually settled by a CT or MRI.

A second nonobvious stroke is one caused by occlusion of the posterior cerebral artery, usually embolic. This may not be recognized unless the visual fields are carefully tested at the bedside. The patient himself may not be aware of the difficulty or will complain only of blurring of vision or the need for new glasses. Accompanying deficits are inability to name colors or recognize manipulable objects or faces, difficulty in reading, etc. MRI or CT usually corroborates the clinical diagnosis, and therapy is directed against further emboli or extension of the thrombosis.

An inapparent stroke that may be mistaken for psychiatric disease is an attack of paraphasic speech from embolic occlusion of a branch of the left middle cerebral artery. The patient talks in nonsensical phrases, appears confused, and does not fully comprehend what is said to him. He may perform satisfactorily at a superficial level and offer socially appropriate greetings and gestures. Only scrutiny of language function and behavior will lead to the correct diagnosis. Infarction of the dominant or nondominant temporal lobe and rarely of the caudate may produce an agitated delirium with few focal findings. This may be mistaken for a toxic or withdrawal state.

Parietal infarctions on either side (usually nondominant hemisphere) are often missed because the patient is entirely unaware of the problem or the symptoms create only a subtle confusional state, drowsiness, or only subtle problems with calculation, dialing a phone, reaching accurately for objects, or loss of ability to write. Extinction of bilaterally presented visual or tactile stimuli gives a clue; marked asymmetry of the optokinetic nystagmus response is sometimes the only definite sign.

A cerebellar hemorrhage may at first be difficult to recognize as a stroke. An occipital headache and complaint of dizziness with vomiting may be interpreted as a labyrinthine disorder, gastroenteritis, or myocardial infarction. A slight ataxia of the limbs, inability to sit or stand, and mild gaze paresis may not have been properly tested or have been overlooked. The entire syndrome may be missed if the patient is not asked to get off the gurney and walk. Early intervention by surgery may be lifesaving; but once the syndrome has progressed to the point of coma with pupillary abnormalities with bilateral Babinski signs, surgery is usually less likely to result in a good outcome. Similarly, a lateral medullary infarction causing incessant vomiting and dizziness may be mistaken for gastroenteritis unless nystagmus and gait ataxia are appreciated.

The Comatose Stroke Patient

The most common causes of vascular coma are intracranial hemorrhage—usually deep in the hemisphere, less often in the cerebellum or brainstem, extensive subarachnoid hemorrhage, and basilar artery occlusion. After several days, brain edema surrounding a large infarction in the territory of the middle cerebral artery or adjacent to a hemorrhage may compress the midbrain and produce the same effect. Certain remedial surgical measures are still available in these circumstances: drainage of blood from the ventricles, shunting of the ventricles in cases of secondary hydrocephalus due to obstruction of the third ventricle or aqueduct, evacuation of a cerebral hemorrhage in cases of recent decline into stupor and coma, and hemicraniectomy in the case of massive stroke edema. Also, thrombolytic therapy and anticoagulants are sometimes successful in reversing the progression of basilar artery thrombosis that has caused coma by ischemia or infarction of the upper brainstem.

Seizures Following Stroke

With the exception of infarction caused by cerebral venous occlusion, convulsive seizures following stroke are not a great problem. As mentioned earlier and in other chapters of the book, seizures are quite infrequent as the initial manifestation of an ischemic stroke, and when they do occur in this fashion, an embolus is usually the causative mechanism. More often, they are delayed by months or years after the infarction or hemorrhage. In the data presented by Lamy and colleagues (who were studying stroke in young patients with patent foramen ovale), when seizures occurred not at the outset but within the first week after stroke, as they did in 2 to 4 percent of their cases, about half had another seizure, usually single, during the next several years. However, the same was true for those with a first seizure after 1 week. Perhaps not surprisingly, the rate of seizures is higher after hemorrhagic than ischemic strokes and for the latter category, larger cortical strokes were more likely to result in a seizure disorder. An overview of the low rate of seizures that occurred soon after a stroke can be appreciated from the report by Beghi and colleagues, about 6 percent.

No satisfactory study has been conducted to determine if these patients benefit from antiepileptic therapy to prevent the second or subsequent seizures. Following the practice of most other neurologists, we prescribe one of the main epilepsy medications only if there has been a seizure, and continue it for about 12 months. If the EEG shows focal sharp waves or other epileptic activity at that time, we continue the drug; if not, we may discontinue the medication. It is also clear that prophylactic anticonvulsant treatment of all stroke patients is not necessary.

Dementia With Cerebrovascular Disease

Dementia of the Alzheimer type is often ascribed, on insufficient and conceptually incorrect grounds, to the occurrence of multiple small strokes. If vascular lesions are responsible, evidence of an acute stroke episode or episodes and of focal neurologic deficits to account for at least part of the syndrome are evident. However, there is a process in which diffuse white matter changes on the basis of vascular disease lead to a less saltatory decline in cognitive function—vascular dementia. Complicating the understanding of this syndrome is the frequent coexistence, and possibly interdependence, of the lesions of both vascular and Alzheimer disease. There may be difficulty in determining to what extent each of them is responsible for the neurologic deficits. Several studies have shown an increased incidence or an acceleration of Alzheimer dementia if there are concurrent vascular lesions.

References

ACTIVE Investigators: Effect of clopidogrel added to aspirin in patients with atrial fibrillation. *N Engl J Med* 360:2006, 2009.

ACTIVE Writing Group, The: Clopidogrel plus aspirin versus oral anticoagulation for atrial fibrillation in the atrial fibrillation clopidogrel trial with Irbesartan for prevention of vascular events (ACTIVE W)—a randomized trial. *Lancet* 367:1903, 2006.

Adams HP Jr, Butler MJ, Biller J, Toffol GN: Nonhemorrhagic cerebral infarction in young adults. *Arch Neurol* 43:793, 1986.

Adams RD: Mechanisms of apoplexy as determined by clinical and pathological correlation. *J Neuropathol Exp Neurol* 13:1, 1954.

Adams RD, Cammermeyer J, Fitzgerald PJ: The neuropathological aspects of thrombotic acroangiothrombosis. *J Neurol Neurosurg Psychiatry* 11:1, 1948.

Adams RD, Torvik A, Fisher CM: Progressing stroke: Pathogenesis, in Siekert RG, Whisnant JP (eds): *Cerebral Vascular Diseases, Third Conference*. New York, Grune & Stratton, 1961, pp 133–150.

Adams RD, Vander Eecken HM: Vascular disease of the brain. *Annu Rev Med* 4:213, 1953.

Adams RJ, McKie VC, Hsu L, et al: Prevention of first stroke by transfusion in children with sickle cell anemia and abnormal results on transcranial ultrasonography. *N Engl J Med* 339:5, 1998.

Adler JR, Ropper AH: Self-audible venous bruits and high jugular bulb. *Arch Neurol* 43:257, 1986.

Ahlgren E, Arén C: Cerebral complications after coronary artery bypass surgery and heart valve surgery: Risk factors and onset of symptoms. *J Cardiothorac Vasc Anesth* 12:270, 1998.

Alamowitch S, Eliasziw M, Algra A, et al: Risk, causes, and prevention of ischaemic stroke in elderly patients with symptomatic internal-carotid-artery stenosis. *Lancet* 357:1154, 2001.

Alema G: Behçet's disease, in Vinken PJ, Bruyn GW (eds): *Handbook of Clinical Neurology: Infection of the Nervous System*. Vol. 34: Part II. Amsterdam, North-Holland, 1978, pp 475–512.

Alexander MP, Schmitt MA: The aphasia syndrome of stroke in the left anterior cerebral artery territory. *Arch Neurol* 37:97, 1980.

Alexandrov AV, Molina CA, Grotta JC, et al: Ultrasound-enhanced systemic thrombolysis for acute ischemic stroke. *N Engl J Med* 351:2170, 2004.

Allen GS, Ahn HS, Preziosi TJ, et al: Cerebral arterial vasospasm: A controlled trial of nimodipine in patients with subarachnoid hemorrhage. *N Engl J Med* 308:619, 1983.

Amarenco P, Cohen A, Tzourio C, et al: Atherosclerotic disease of the aortic arch and the risk of ischemic stroke. *N Engl J Med* 331:1474, 1994.

Amarenco P, Hauw J-J: Cerebellar infarction in the territory of the anterior and inferior cerebellar artery: A clinicopathological study of 20 cases. *Brain* 113:139, 1990.

Ames A, Nesbett FB: Pathophysiology of ischemic cell death: I. Time of onset of irreversible damage: Importance of the different components of the ischemic insult. *Stroke* 14:219, 1983.

Ames A, Nesbett FB: Pathophysiology of ischemic cell death: II. Changes in plasma membrane permeability and cell volume. *Stroke* 14:227, 1983.

Ames A, Nesbett FB: Pathophysiology of ischemic cell death: III. Role of extracellular factors. *Stroke* 14:233, 1983.

Ames A, Wright RL, Kowada M, et al: Cerebral ischemia: II. The noreflow phenomenon. *Am J Pathol* 52:437, 1968.

Andrew BT, Chiles BW, Olsen WL, et al: The effects of intracerebral hematoma location on the risk of brainstem compression and clinical outcome. *J Neurosurg* 69:518, 1988.

Aoyagi N, Hayakawa I: Analysis of 223 ruptured intracranial aneurysms with special reference to rerupture. *Surg Neurol* 21:445, 1984.

Asherson CR, Tikly FJ, Chamorro PL, et al: Chorea in the antiphospholipid syndrome. Clinical, radiologic, and immunologic characteristics of 50 patients from our clinics and the recent literature. *Medicine (Baltimore)* 76:203, 1997.

Auer LM: The pathogenesis of hypertensive encephalopathy. *Acta Neurochir Suppl* 27:1, 1978.

Averback P: Primary cerebral venous thrombosis in young adults: The diverse manifestations of an unrecognized disease. *Ann Neurol* 3:81, 1978.

Babikian V, Ropper AH: Binswanger's disease: A review. *Stroke* 18:2, 1987.

Bamford J, Sandercock P, Dennis M, et al: A prospective study of acute cerebrovascular disease in the community: The Oxfordshire Community Stroke Project. 1981–1986. *J Neurol Neurosurg Psychiatry* 51:1373, 1988; also 53:16, 1990.

Banker BQ: Cerebral vascular disease in infancy and childhood: I. Occlusive vascular disease. *J Neuropathol Exp Neurol* 20:127, 1961.

Barnett HJM: The EC/IC Bypass Study Group. Failure of extracranial-intracranial arterial bypass to reduce the risk of ischemic stroke: Results of an international randomized trial. *N Engl J Med* 313:1191, 1985.

Barnett HJM, Boughner GR, Cooper PF: Further evidence relating mitral-valve prolapse to cerebral ischemic events. *N Engl J Med* 302:139, 1980.

Barnett HJM, Mohr JP, Stein BM, Yatsu FM (eds): *Stroke: Pathophysiology, Diagnosis, and Management*, 3rd ed. New York, Churchill Livingstone, 1998.

Barron KD, Siqueira E, Hirano A: Cerebral embolism caused by non-bacterial thrombotic endocarditis. *Neurology* 10:391, 1960.

Batjer HH, Reisch JW, Allen BC, et al: Failure of surgery to improve outcome in hypertensive putaminal hemorrhage. *Arch Neurol* 47:1103, 1990.

Becker S, Heller CH, Gropp F, et al: Thrombophilic disorders in children with cerebral infarction. *Lancet* 352:1756, 1998.

Beghi E, D'Allessandro R, Beretta S, et al. Incidence and predictors of acute symptomatic seizures after stroke. *Neurology* 77:1785, 2011.

Benabdeljlil M, El Alaoui Faris M, Kissani N, et al: Troubles neuropsychologiques apres infarctus bi-thalamique par thrombose veineuse profonde. *Rev Neurol (Paris)* 157:62, 2001.

Benavente O, Eliasziw M, Streifler JY, et al: Prognosis after transient monocular blindness associated with carotid-artery stenosis. *N Engl J Med* 345:1084, 2001.

Bendszus M, Koltzenberg M, Burger R, et al: Silent embolism in diagnostic cerebral angiography and neurointerventional procedures: A prospective study. *Lancet* 354:1594, 1999.

Benninger DH, Gandjour J, Georgiadis D, et al: Benign long-term outcome of conservatively treated cervical aneurysms due to carotid dissection. *Neurology* 69:486, 2007.

Bhatt DL, Fox KA, Hacke W, et al: Clopidogrel and aspirin versus aspirin alone for the prevention of atherothrombotic events. *N Engl J Med* 354:1706, 2006.

Biller J, Challa VR, Toole JF, Howard VJ: Nonbacterial thrombotic endocarditis. *Arch Neurol* 39:95, 1982.

Boston Area Anticoagulation Trial for Atrial Fibrillation Investigators: The effect of low-dose warfarin in the risk of stroke in patients with nonrheumatic atrial fibrillation. *N Engl J Med* 323:1505, 1990.

Botterell EH, Lougheed WM, Scott JW, Vandewater SL: Hypothermia, and interruption of carotid or carotid and vertebral circulation, in the surgical management of intracranial aneurysms. *J Neurosurg* 13:1, 1956.

Breen JC, Caplan LR, DeWitt D, et al: Brain edema after carotid surgery. *Neurology* 46:175, 1996.

Brey RL, Hart RG, Sherman DG, Tegeler CH: Antiphospholipid antibodies and cerebral ischemia in young people. *Neurology* 40:1190, 1990.

Briley DP, Coull BM, Goodnight SH: Neurological disease associated with antiphospholipid antibodies. *Ann Neurol* 25:221, 1989.

Britton M, DeFaire U, Helmers C: Hazards of therapy for excessive hypertension in acute stroke. *Acta Med Scand* 207:352, 1980.

Broderick JP, Brott TG, Buldner JE, et al: Volume of intracerebral hemorrhage. A powerful and easy-to-use predictor of 30-day mortality. *Stroke* 24:987, 1993.

Broderick JP, Palesch YY, Demchuck AM, et al. Endovascular therapy after intravenous t-Pa versus t-Pa alone for stroke. *N Engl J Med* 368:368, 2013.

Broderick JP, Phillips SJ, Whisnant JP, et al: Incidence rates of stroke in the eighties: The end of the decline in stroke? *Stroke* 20:577, 1989.

Brott T, Broderick J, Kothari R, et al: Early hemorrhage growth in patients with intracerebral hemorrhage. *Stroke* 28:1, 1997.

Brown MM, Bevan D: Is inherited thrombophilia a risk factor for arterial stroke? *J Neurol Neurosurg Psychiatry* 65:617, 1998.

Brust JCM: Anterior cerebral artery disease, in Barnett HJM, Mohr JP, Stein BM, Yalsu FM (eds): *Stroke: Pathophysiology, Diagnosis, and Management*, 2nd ed. New York, Churchill Livingstone, 1992, pp 337–360.

Brust JCM, Behrens MM: "Release hallucinations" as the major symptom of posterior cerebral artery occlusion: A report of 2 cases. *Ann Neurol* 2:432, 1977.

Byrom FB: The pathogenesis of hypertensive encephalopathy. *Lancet* 2:201, 1954.

Call G, Fleming M, Sealfon S, et al: Reversible cerebral segmental vasoconstriction. *Stroke* 19:1159, 1988.

Caplan LR: Binswanger's disease—revisited. *Neurology* 45:626, 1995.

Caplan LR: Intracranial branch atheromatous disease: A neglected, understudied, and overused concept. *Neurology* 39:1246, 1989.

Caplan LR: *Stroke: A Clinical Approach*, 2nd ed. Boston, Butterworth-Heinemann, 1993.

Caplan LR: "Top of the basilar" syndrome. *Neurology* 30:72, 1980.

Caplan LR, Schmahmann JD, Kase CS, et al: Caudate infarcts. *Arch Neurol* 47:133, 1990.

Caplan LR, Sergay S: Positional cerebral ischemia. *J Neurol Neurosurg Psychiatry* 39:385, 1976.

Carlberg B, Asplund K, Haag E: Factors influencing admission blood pressure levels in patients with acute stroke. *Stroke* 22:527, 1991.

Carter BS, Ogilvy CS, Candia GJ, et al: One-year outcome after decompressive surgery for massive nondominant hemispheric infarction. *Neurosurgery* 40:1168, 1997.

Castaigne P, Lhermitte F, Buge A, et al: Paramedian thalamic and midbrain infarcts: Clinical and neuropathological study. *Ann Neurol* 10:127, 1981.

CAVATAS Investigators: Endovascular versus surgical treatment in patients with carotid stenosis in the carotid and vertebral artery transluminal angioplasty study (CAVATAS): A randomised trial. *Lancet* 357:1729, 2001.

Chajek T, Fainaru M: Behçet's disease: Report of 41 cases and a review of the literature. *Medicine (Baltimore)* 54:179, 1975.

Chase TN, Rosman NP, Price DL: The cerebral syndromes associated with dissecting aneurysms of the aorta. A clinicopathologic study. *Brain* 91:173, 1968.

Chen Y, Patel NC, Guo JJ, Zhan S: Antidepressant prophylaxis for poststroke depression: a meta-analysis. *Int Clin Psychopharmacol* 22:159, 2007.

Chester EM, Agamanolis DP, Banker BQ, Victor M: Hypertensive encephalopathy: A clinicopathologic study of 20 cases. *Neurology* 28:928, 1978.

Chimowitz MI, Lynn MJ, Derdyn CP, et al: For the SMPRISS Trial investigators. *N Engl J Med* 365:993, 2011.

Chimowitz MI, Lynn MJ, Howlett-Smith H, et al: Comparison of warfarin and aspirin for symptomatic intracranial arterial stenosis. *N Engl J Med* 352:1305, 2005.

Churg J, Strauss L: Allergic granulomatosis, allergic angiitis and periarteritis nodosa. *Am J Pathol* 27:277, 1951.

Ciccone A, Valvassori L, Nichelatti M, et al. Endovascular treatment for acute ischemic stroke. *N Engl J Med* 368:904, 2013.

Claassen J, Jetté N, Chum R, et al: Electrographic seizures and periodic discharges after intracerebral hemorrhage. *Neurology* 69:1356, 2007.

Cogan DG: Visual hallucinations as release phenomena. *Graefes Arch Clin Exp Ophthalmol* 188:139, 1973.

Collins R, Peto R, MacMahon S, et al: Blood pressure, stroke, and coronary heart disease. *Lancet* 335:827, 1990.

Connor MD, Lammie GA, Bell JE, et al: Cerebral infarction in adults AIDS patients. Observations from the Edinburgh HIV autopsy cohort. *Stroke* 31:2117, 2000.

Cordonnier C, Salman RA, Wardlaw J: Spontaneous brain microbleeds: Systematic review, subgroup analyses and standards for study design and reporting. *Brain* 130:198, 2007.

Corrin LS, Sandok BA, Houser W: Cerebral ischemic events in patients with carotid artery fibromuscular dysplasia. *Arch Neurol* 38:616, 1981.

Coull BM, Williams LS, Goldstein LD, et al: Anticoagulants and antiplatelet agents in acute ischemic stroke. *Neurology* 59:13, 2002.

Crawford PM, West CR, Chadwick DW, et al: Arteriovenous malformations of the brain: Natural history in unoperated patients. *J Neurol Neurosurg Psychiatry* 49:1, 1986.

Crowther MA, Ginsberg JS, Julian J, et al: A comparison of two intensities of warfarin for the prevention of recurrent thrombosis in patients with antiphospholipid antibody syndrome. *N Engl J Med* 349:1133, 2003.

Dashe JF, Pessin MS, Murphy RE, Payne DD: Carotid occlusive disease and stroke risk in coronary artery bypass graft surgery. *Neurology* 49:678, 1997.

Davies-Jones GAB, Preston FE, Timperley WR: *Neurological Complications in Clinical Haematology*. Oxford, England, Blackwell, 1980.

de Bruijn SF, Stam J: Randomized, placebo-controlled trial of anticoagulant treatment with low-molecular-weight heparin for cerebral sinus thrombosis. *Stroke* 30:484, 1999.

Decroix JP, Graveleau R, Masson M, Cambier J: Infarction in the territory of the anterior choroidal artery. *Brain* 109:1071, 1986.

Déjerine J: *Sémiologie d'affections du systéme nerveux*. Paris, Masson, 1914.

Delshaw JB, Broaddus WC, Kassell NF, et al: Treatment of right hemisphere cerebral infarction by hemicraniectomy. *Stroke* 21: 874, 1990.

deVeber G, Andrew M, Adams C, et al: Cerebral sinovenous thrombosis in children. *N Engl J Med* 345:417, 2001.

Devinsky O, Petito CK, Alonso DR: Clinical and neuropathological findings in systemic lupus erythematosus: The role of vasculitis, heart emboli, and thrombotic thrombocytopenic purpura. *Ann Neurol* 23:380, 1988.

Digre KB, Durcan FJ, Branch DW, et al: Amaurosis fugax associated with antiphospholipid antibodies. *Ann Neurol* 25:228, 1989.

Diringer MN, Edwards DF, Zazulia AR: Hydrocephalus: A previously unrecognized predictor of poor outcome from supratentorial intra-cerebral hemorrhage. *Stroke* 29:1352, 1998.

Diringer MN, Ladenson PW, Stern BJ, et al: Plasma atrial natriuretic factor and subarachnoid hemorrhage. *Stroke* 19:1119, 1988.

DiRocco C, Ianelli A, Leone G, et al: Heparin-urokinase treatment in aseptic dural sinus thrombosis. *Arch Neurol* 38:431, 1981.

Donnan GA, Davis SM, Chambers BR, Gates PC: Surgery for prevention of stroke. *Lancet* 351:1372, 1998.

Donnan GA, O'Malley HM, Quang L, et al: The capsular warning syndrome: Pathogenesis and clinical features. *Neurology* 43:957, 1993.

Drake CG: Giant fusiform intracranial aneurysms: Review of 120 patients treated surgically from 1965 to 1992. *J Neurosurg* 87:141, 1997.

Einhaupl KM, Villringer A, Meister W: Heparin treatment in sinus venous thrombosis. *Lancet* 358:597, 1991.

ESPRIT Study Group, The: Aspirin plus dipyridamole versus aspirin alone after cerebra ischemia of arterial origin (ESPRIT): Randomized controlled trial. *Lancet* 367:1665, 2006.

European Carotid Surgery Trialists' Collaborative Group: Risk of stroke in the distribution of an asymptomatic carotid artery. *Lancet* 345:209, 1995.

Executive Committee for the Asymptomatic Carotid Atherosclerosis Study: Endarterectomy for asymptomatic carotid artery stenosis. *JAMA* 273:1421, 1995.

Ferguson GG: Physical factors in the initiation, growth, and rupture of human intracranial saccular aneurysms. *J Neurosurg* 37:666, 1972.

Fessler RD, Esshaki CM, Stankewitz RC, et al: The neurovascular complications of cocaine. *Surg Neurol* 47:339, 1997.

Fisher CM: A lacunar stroke: The dysarthria-clumsy hand syndrome. *Neurology* 17:614, 1967.

Fisher CM: A new vascular syndrome: "The subclavian steal." *N Engl J Med* 265:912, 1961.

Fisher CM: Binswanger's encephalopathy: A review. *J Neurol* 236:65, 1989.

Fisher CM: Capsular infarct: The underlying vascular lesions. *Arch Neurol* 36:65, 1979.

Fisher CM: Cerebral ischemia—less familiar types. *Clin Neurosurg* 18:267, 1971.

Fisher CM: Cerebral thromboangiitis obliterans. *Medicine (Baltimore)* 36:169, 1957.

Fisher CM: Homolateral ataxia and crural paresis: A vascular syndrome. *J Neurol Neurosurg Psychiatry* 28:48, 1965a.

Fisher CM: Lacunar strokes and infarcts: A review. *Neurology* 32:871, 1982.

Fisher CM: Late-life migraine accompaniments as a cause of unexplained transient ischemic attacks. *Can J Neurol Sci* 7:9, 1980.

Fisher CM: Small deep cerebral infarcts. *Neurology* 15:774, 1965b.

Fisher CM: The anatomy and pathology of the cerebral vasculature, in Meyer JS (ed): *Modern Concepts of Cerebrovascular Disease*. New York, Spectrum, 1975, pp 1–41.

Fisher CM: The pathologic and clinical aspects of thalamic hemorrhage. *Trans Am Neurol Assoc* 84:56, 1959.

Fisher CM, Adams RD: Observations on brain embolism with special reference to hemorrhagic infarction, in Furlan AJ (ed): *The Heart and Stroke: Exploring Mutual Cerebrovascular and Cardiovascular Issues*. Berlin, Springer-Verlag, 1987, pp 17–36.

Fisher CM, Karnes WE, Kubik CS: Lateral medullary infarction—the pattern of vascular occlusion. *J Neuropathol Exp Neurol* 20:323, 1961.

Fisher CM, Kistler JP, Davis JM: Relation of cerebral vasospasm to subarachnoid hemorrhage visualized by CT scanning. *Neurosurgery* 6:1, 1980.

Fisher CM, Ojemann RG: A clinico-pathologic study of carotid endarterectomy plaques. *Rev Neurol* 142:573, 1986.

Fleetwood IG, Steinberg GK: Arteriovenous malformations. *Lancet* 359:863, 2002.

Flemming KD, Link MJ, Christainson TJH, Brown RD: Prospective hemorrhage risk of intracerebral cavernous malformation. *Neurology* 78:632, 2012.

Foix C, Chavaney JA, Levy M: Syndrome pseudothalamique d'origine parietale. *Rev Neurol* 35:68, 1927.

Ford CS, Frye JL, Toole JF, Lefkowitz D: Asymptomatic carotid bruit and stenosis. *Arch Neurol* 43:219, 1986.

Frank JI: Large hemispheric infarction, deterioration, and intracranial pressure. *Neurology* 45:1286, 1995.

Freis ED, Calabresi M, Castle CH, et al: Veterans Administration Cooperative Study Group on Antihypertensive Agents: Effects of treatment on morbidity in hypertension II: Results in patients with diastolic blood pressure averaging 90 through 114 mm Hg. *JAMA* 213:1143, 1970.

Friedlander RM: Arteriovenous malformations of the brain. *N Engl J Med* 356:2704, 2007.

Furie B, Furie BC: Mechanism of thrombus formation. *N Engl J Med* 359:938, 2009.

Furlan AJ, Reisman M, Massaro J, et al. Closure or medical therapy for cryptogenic stroke with patent foramen ovale. *N Engl J Med* 266:991, 2012.

Gage B, Birman-Deych E, Kerzner R, et al: Incidence of intracranial hemorrhage in patients with atrial fibrillation who are prone to fall. *Am J Med* 118:612, 2005.

Gaillard N, Deltour S, Vilotijevic B, et al. Detection of paroxysmal atrial fibrillation with transtelephonic EKG in TIA or stroke patients. *Neurology* 74:1666, 2010.

Garraway WM, Whisnant JP, Drury I: The changing pattern of survival following stroke. *Stroke* 14:699, 1983a.

Garraway WM, Whisnant JP, Drury I: The continuing decline in the incidence of stroke. *Mayo Clin Proc* 58:520, 1983b.

Garrett WT, Chang CW, Bleck TP: Altered mental status in thrombotic thrombocytopenic purpura is secondary to nonconvulsive status epilepticus. *Ann Neurol* 40:245, 1996.

Gasecki AP, Eliasziw M, Ferguson GG, et al: Long-term prognosis and effect of endarterectomy in patients with symptomatic severe carotid stenosis and contralateral carotid stenosis or occlusion: Results from NASCET. *J Neurosurg* 83:778, 1995.

Georgiadis D, Arnold M, von Buedingen HC, et al: Aspirin vs anticoagulation in carotid artery dissection: A study of 298 patients. *Neurology* 72:1810, 2009.

Gilon D, Buonanno FS, Joffe MM, et al: Lack of evidence of an association between mitral-valve prolapse and stroke in young patients. *N Engl J Med* 3:41, 1999.

Gladstone DJ, Silver FL, Willinsky RA, et al: Deep cerebral venous thrombosis: An illustrative case with reversible diencephalic dysfunction. *Can J Neurol Sci* 28:159, 2001.

Goldstein JN, Fazen LE, Snider R, et al: Contrast extravasation on CT angiography predicts hematoma expansion in intracerebral hemorrhage. *Neurology* 68:889, 2007.

Gould DB, Phalan C, van Mil S, et al: Role of COL4A1 in small vessel disease and hemorrhagic stroke. *N Engl J Med* 354:1489, 2006.

Granger CB, Alexander JH, McMurray JJV, et al: Apixaban versus warfarin in patients with atrial fibrillation. *N Engl J Med* 365:981, 2011.

Green DM, Ropper AH, Kronmal RA, et al: Serum potassium level and dietary potassium intake as risk factors for stroke. *Neurology* 59:314, 2002.

Greenberg SM, Rebeck GW, Vonsattel JP, et al: Apolipoprotein E e4 and cerebral hemorrhage associated with amyloid angiopathy. *Ann Neurol* 38:254, 1995.

Greenberg SM, Vonsattel JP, Stakes JW, et al: The clinical spectrum of cerebral amyloid angiopathy: Presentations without lobar hemorrhage. *Neurology* 43:2073, 1993.

Hacke W, Kaste M, Fieschi C, et al: Randomised double-blind placebo-controlled trial of thrombolytic therapy with intravenous alteplase in acute ischaemic stroke. *Lancet* 352:1245, 1998.

Hacke W, Markku K, Bluhmki E, et al: Thrombolysis with alteplase 3 to 4.5 hours for acute stroke. *N Engl J Med* 359:1317, 2008.

Hacke W, Schwab S, Horn M, et al: "Malignant" middle cerebral artery territory infarction: Clinical course and prognostic signs. *Arch Neurol* 53:309, 1996.

Hallevi H, Albright KC, Martin-Schild S, et al: Anticoagulation after cardioembolic stroke: To bridge or not to bridge? *Arch Neurol* 65:1169, 2008.

Hallevi H, Albright KC, Martin-Schild S, et al: The complications of cardioembolic stroke: Lessons from the VISTA database. *Cerebrovasc Dis* 26:38, 2008.

Handke M, Harloff A, Olschewski M, et al: Patent foramen ovale and cryptogenic stroke in older patients. *N Engl J Med* 357:2262, 2007.

Hara K, Shiga A, Fukutake T, et al: Association of HTRA1 mutations and familial ischemic cerebral small-vessel disease. *N Engl J Med* 360:1729, 2009.

Hart RG, Byer JA, Slaughter JR, et al: Occurrence and implications of seizures in subarachnoid hemorrhage due to ruptured intracranial aneurysms. *Neurosurgery* 8:417, 1981.

Hart RG, Coull BM, Hart D: Early recurrent embolism associated with nonvalvular atrial fibrillation: A retrospective study. *Stroke* 14:688, 1983.

Hauser RA, Lacey M, Knight R: Hypertensive encephalopathy: Magnetic resonance imaging demonstration of reversible cortical and white matter lesions. *Arch Neurol* 45:1078, 1988.

Hawkins TD, Sims C, Hanka R: Subarachnoid haemorrhage of unknown cause: A long-term follow-up. *J Neurol Neurosurg Psychiatry* 52:230, 1989.

Hayashi M, Kobayashi H, Kanano H, et al: Treatment of systemic hypertension and intracranial hypertension in cases of brain hemorrhage. *Stroke* 19:314, 1988.

Healy JS, Connolly SJ, Gold MR, et al. Subclinical atrial fibrillation and the risk of stroke. *N Engl J Med* 366:120, 2012.

Heart Protection Collaborative Study Group: Effects of cholesterol-lowering with simvastatin on stroke and other major vascular events in 20,536 people with cerebrovascular disease or other high-risk conditions. *Lancet* 363:757, 2004.

Heiss WD: Flow thresholds of functional and morphological damage of brain tissue. *Stroke* 14:329, 1983.

Hemphill JC 3rd, Bonovich DC, Besmertis L, et al: The ICH score: A simple, reliable grading scale for intracerebral hemorrhage. *Stroke* 32:891, 2001.

Hennerici M, Trockel U, Rautenberg W, et al: Spontaneous progression and regression of carotid atheroma. *Lancet* 1:1415, 1985.

Heyman A, Wilkinson WE, Hurwitz BJ, et al: Risk of ischemic heart disease in patients with TIA. *Neurology* 34:626, 1984.

Hijdra A, VanGijn, Stefanko S, et al: Delayed cerebral ischemia after aneurysmal subarachnoid hemorrhage: Clinicoanatomic correlations. *Neurology* 36:329, 1986.

Homan RW, Devous MD, Stokely EM, Bonte FJ: Quantification of intracerebral steal in patients with arteriovenous malformation. *Arch Neurol* 43:779, 1986.

Hosseini AA, Kandiyil N, MacSweeney STS, et al: Carotid plaque hemorrhage on magnetic resonance imaging strongly predicts recurrent ischemia and stroke. *Ann Neurol* 73:774, 2013.

Hossman K-A: Pathophysiology of cerebral infarction, in Vinken PJ, Bruyn GW, Klawans HL (eds): *Handbook of Clinical Neurology*. Vol 53. Vascular Diseases. Part I. Amsterdam, Elsevier, 1988, pp 27–46.

Houser OW, Baker HL Jr, Sandok BA, Holley KE: Fibromuscular dysplasia of the cephalic arterial system, in Vinken PJ, Bruyn GW (eds): *Handbook of Clinical Neurology*. Vol 11. Vascular Disease of the Nervous System. Part 1. Amsterdam, North-Holland, 1972, pp 366–385.

Hunt WE, Hess RM: Surgical risk as related to time of intervention in the repair of intracranial aneurysms. *J Neurosurg* 28:14, 1968.

Hupperts RMM, Lodder J, Meuts-van Raak EPM, et al: Infarcts in the anterior choroidal artery territory: Anatomical distribution, clinical syndromes, presumed pathogenesis, and early outcome. *Brain* 117:825, 1994.

Ikram MA, Seshadri S, Bis JC, et al: Genomewide association studies in stroke. *N Engl J Med* 360:1718, 2009.

Ingall TJ, Homer D, Baker HL Jr, et al: Predictors of intracranial carotid artery atherosclerosis: Duration of cigarette smoking and hypertension are more powerful than serum lipid levels. *Arch Neurol* 48:687, 1991.

International Stroke Genetics Consortium and Wellcome Trust Case-Control Consortium-2: Failure to validate association between 12p13 variants and ischemic stroke. *N Engl J Med* 362:1547, 2010.

International Study of Unruptured Intracranial Aneurysms Investigators: Unruptured intracranial aneurysms: Natural history, clinical outcome, and risks of surgical and endovascular treatment. *Lancet* 362:103, 2003.

Inzitari D, Eliasziw M, Gates P, et al: The causes and risks of stroke in patients with asymptomatic internal-carotid-artery stenosis. *N Engl J Med* 342:1693, 2000.

Irey NS, McAllister HA, Henry JM: Oral contraceptives and stroke in young women: A clinicopathologic correlation. *Neurology* 28:1216, 1978.

Ishikawa K, Uyama M, Asayama K: Occlusive thromboaortopathy (Takayasu's disease): Cervical arterial stenoses, retinal arterial pressure, retinal microaneurysms and prognosis. *Stroke* 14:730, 1983.

Jacobs K, Moulin T, Bogousslavsky J, et al: The stroke syndrome of cortical vein thrombosis. *Neurology* 47:376, 1996.

Johnson RT, Richardson EP: The neurological manifestations of systemic lupus erythematosus. *Medicine (Baltimore)* 47:337, 1968.

Jones HR, Naggar CZ, Seljan MP, Downing LL: Mitral valve prolapse and cerebral ischemic events: A comparison between a neurology population with stroke and a cardiology population with mitral valve prolapse observed for five years. *Stroke* 13:451, 1982.

Joutel A, Vahedi K, Corpechot C, et al: Strong clustering and stereotyped nature of Notch 3 mutations in CADASIL patients. *Lancet* 350:1511, 1997.

Jung HH, Bassetti C, Tourier-Lasserve E: Cerebral autosomal dominant arteriopathy with subcortical infarcts and leukoencephalopathy: A clinicopathologic and genetic study of a Swiss family. *J Neurol Neurosurg Psychiatry* 59:138, 1995.

Junque C, Pujol J, Vendrell P, et al: Leuko-araiosis on magnetic resonance imaging and speed of mental processing. *Arch Neurol* 47:151, 1990.

Juvela S, Helskanen O, Poranen A, et al: The treatment of spontaneous intracerebral hemorrhage. *J Neurosurg* 70:755, 1989.

Kanis K, Ropper AH: Homolateral hemiparesis as an early sign of cerebellar mass effect. *Neurology* 44:2194, 1994.

Karlsson B, Lindquist C, Steiner L: Prediction of obliteration after gamma knife surgery for cerebral arteriovenous malformations. *Neurosurgery* 40:425, 1997.

Kase CS, Caplan LR: *Intracerebral Hemorrhage*. Boston, Butterworth-Heinemann, 1994.

Kase CS, Williams JP, Wyatt DA, Mohr JP: Lobar intracerebral hematomas: Clinical and CT analysis of 22 cases. *Neurology* 32:1146, 1982.

Kassell NF, Torner JC, Haley EC Jr, et al: The International Cooperative Study on the Timing of Aneurysm Surgery: Part 1. Overall management results. *J Neurosurg* 73:18, 1990; Part 2: Surgical results. *J Neurosurg* 73:37, 1990.

Katzan IL, Furlan AJ, Lloyd LE, et al: Use of tissue-type plasminogen activator for acute ischemic stroke: The Cleveland area experience. *JAMA* 288:1151, 2000.

Kay R, Wong KS, Ling YL, et al: Low-molecular-weight heparin for the treatment of acute ischemic stroke. *N Engl J Med* 333:1588, 1995.

Kernan WN, Viscoli CM, Brass LM, et al: Phenylpropanolamine and the risk of hemorrhagic stroke. *N Engl J Med* 343:1826, 2000.

Khamashta MA, Cuadro MJ, Mujic F, et al: The management of thrombosis in the antiphospholipid syndrome. *N Engl J Med* 332: 993, 1995.

Kidwell CS, Jahan R, Gornbein J, et al. A trial of imaging selection and endovascular treatment for ischemic stroke. *N Engl J Med* 368:914, 2013.

Kinnecom C, Lev MH, Wendell L, et al: Course of cerebral amyloid angiopathy-related inflammation. *Neurology* 68:1411, 2007.

Kistler JP, Buonanno FS, Gress DR: Carotid endarterectomy—specific therapy based on pathophysiology. *N Engl J Med* 325:505, 1991.

Kitahara T, Okumura K, Semba A, et al: Genetic and immunologic analysis on Moyamoya. *J Neurol Neurosurg Psychiatry* 45:1048, 1982.

Kittner SJ, Stern BJ, Feeser BR, et al: Pregnancy and the risk of stroke. *N Engl J Med* 335:768, 1996.

Kizer JR, Devereux RB: Patent foramen ovale in young adults with unexplained stroke. *N Engl J Med* 353:2361, 2005.

Kjellberg RN, Hanamura T, Davis KR, et al: Bragg-peak proton-beam therapy for arteriovenous malformations of the brain. *N Engl J Med* 309:269, 1983.

Kolodny EH, Rebeiz JJ, Caviness VS, Richardson EP: Granulomatous angiits of the central nervous system. *Arch Neurol* 19:510, 1968.

Koroshetz WJ: Warfarin, aspirin, and intracranial vascular disease. *N Engl J Med* 31:1368, 2005.

Koroshetz WJ, Ropper AH: Artery to artery embolism causing stroke in the posterior circulation. *Neurology* 37:292, 1987.

Krayenbühl H, Yasargil MG: Radiological anatomy and topography of the cerebral arteries, in Vinken PJ, Bruyn GW (eds): *Handbook of Clinical Neurology*. Vol 11. Vascular Diseases of the Nervous System. Part 1. Amsterdam, North-Holland, 1972, pp 65–101.

Krendel DA, Ditter SM, Frankel MR, et al: Biopsy-proven cerebral vasculitis associated with cocaine abuse. *Neurology* 40:1092, 1990.

Kubik CS, Adams RD: Occlusion of the basilar artery—a clinical and pathological study. *Brain* 69:73, 1946.

Kwakkel G, Wagenaar RC, Twisk JW, et al: Intensity of leg and arm training after primary middle-cerebral-artery stroke: A randomised trial. *Lancet* 354:191, 1999.

Kwiatkowski TG, Libman RB, Frankel M, et al: Effects of tissue plasminogen activator for acute ischemic stroke at one year. *N Engl J Med* 340:1781, 1999.

Labauge P, Brunereau L, Laberge S, et al: Prospective follow-up of 33 asymptomatic patients with familial cerebral cavernous malformations. *Neurology* 57:1825, 2001.

Lamy C, Domingo V, Samah F, et al: Early and late seizures after cryptogenic ischemic stroke in young adults. *Neurology* 60:400, 2003.

Lee MT, Piomelli S, Granger S, et al: Stroke prevention trial in sickle cell anemia (STOP) extended follow-up and final results. *Blood* 108:847, 2006.

Lehner T, Barnes CG (eds): *Behçet's Syndrome: Clinical and Immunological Features*. New York, Academic Press, 1980.

Lehrich J, Winkler G, Ojemann R: Cerebellar infarction with brainstem compression: Diagnosis and surgical treatment. *Arch Neurol* 22:490, 1970.

Leung DY, Black IW, Cranney GB, et al: Selection of patients for transesophageal echocardiography after stroke and systemic embolic events. *Stroke* 26:1820, 1995.

Levine RJ, Lam C, Qian C, et al: Soluble endoglin and other circulating antiangiogenic factors in preeclampsia. *N Engl J Med* 355:992, 2006.

Levine SR, Brust JCM, Futrell N, et al: A comparative study of the cerebrovascular complications of cocaine: Alkaloidal versus hydrochloride—a review. *Neurology* 41:1173, 1991.

Levine SR, Deegan MJ, Futrell N, Welch KMA: Cerebrovascular and neurologic disease associated with antiphospholipid antibodies: 48 cases. *Neurology* 40:1181, 1990.

Libman RB, Wirkowski E, Neystat M, et al: Stroke associated with cardiac surgery: Determinants, timing, and stroke subtypes. *Arch Neurol* 54:83, 1997.

Lidegaard Ø, Løkkegaard E, Jensen A, et al. Thrombotic stroke and myocardial infarction with hormonal contraception. *N Engl J Med* 366:2257, 2012.

Lim W, Crowther MA, Eikelboom JW, et al: Management of antiphospholipid antibody syndrome: A systematic review. *JAMA* 295:1050, 2006.

Linn J, Halpin A, Demaerel P, et al: Prevalence of superficial siderosis in patients with cerebral amyloid angiopathy. *Neurology* 74:1346, 2010.

Lo EH, Dalkara T, Moskowitz MA: Mechanisms, challenges, and opportunities in stroke. *Nat Rev Neurosci* 4:399, 2003.

Lockshin MD, Sammaritano LR: Antiphospholipid antibodies and fetal loss. *N Engl J Med* 326:951, 1992.

Locksley HB: Natural history of subarachnoid hemorrhage, intracranial aneurysms and arteriovenous malformations—based on 6368 cases in the cooperative study. *J Neurosurg* 25:219, 1966.

Lodder J, Van der Lugt PJM: Evaluation of the risk of immediate anticoagulant treatment in patients with embolic stroke of cardiac origin. *Stroke* 14:42, 1983.

Loh E, Sutton M, Wun C, et al: Ventricular dysfunction and the risk of stroke after myocardial infarction. *N Engl J Med* 336:251, 1997.

Longstreth WT, Swanson PD: Oral contraceptives and stroke. *Stroke* 15:747, 1984.

Luft AR, McCombe-Waller S, Whitall J, et al: Repetitive bilateral arm training and motor cortex activation in chronic stroke: A randomized controlled trial. *JAMA* 292:1853, 2004.

Lupi-Herrera E, Sanchez-Torres G, Marcushamer J, et al: Takayasu's arteritis: Clinical study of 107 cases. *Am Heart J* 93:94, 1977.

MacMahon S, Peto R, Cutler J, et al: Blood pressure, stroke, and coronary heart disease: Part I. Prolonged differences in blood pressure: Prospective observational studies corrected for the regression dilution bias. *Lancet* 335:765, 1990.

Magnetic Resonance Angiography in Relatives of Patients With Subarachnoid Hemorrhage Study Group, The: Risks and benefits of screening for intracranial aneurysms in first-degree relatives of patients with sporadic subarachnoid hemorrhage. *N Engl J Med* 341:1344, 1999.

Magro CM, Poe JC, Lubow M, Susac JO: Susac syndrome: An organ-specific autoimmune endotheliopathy syndrome associated with anti-endothelial cell antibodies. *Am J Clin Pathol* 136:903, 2011.

Majeed A, Kim Y-K, Roberts RS, et al: Optimal timing of resumption of warfarin after intracranial hemorrhage. *Stroke* 41:2860, 2010.

Mao C-C, Coull BM, Golper LAC, Rau MT: Anterior operculum syndrome. *Neurology* 39:1169, 1989.

Margolin DI, Marsden CD: Episodic dyskinesias and transient cerebral ischemia. *Neurology* 32:1379, 1982.

Markus HS, Hambley H: Neurology and the blood: Haematological abnormalities in ischaemic stroke. *J Neurol Neurosurg Psychiatry* 64:150, 1998.

Marshall J: Angiography in the investigation of ischemic episodes in the territory of the internal carotid artery. *Lancet* 1:719, 1971.

Martinelli I, Sacchi E, Landi G, et al: High-risk of cerebral-vein thrombosis in carriers of a prothrombin gene mutation and in users of oral contraceptives. *N Engl J Med* 338:1793, 1998.

Maruyama K, Kawahara N, Shin M, et al: The risk of hemorrhage after radiosurgery for cerebral arteriovenous malformations. *N Engl J Med* 352:146, 2005.

Mas JL, Arquizan C, Lamy C, et al: Recurrent cerebrovascular events associated with patent foramen ovale, atrial septal aneurysm, or both. *N Engl J Med* 345:1740, 2001.

Mas JL, Chatellier G, Beyssen B, et al: Endarterectomy versus stenting in patients with symptomatic severe carotid stenosis. *N Engl J Med* 355:1660, 2006.

Mawet J, Boukobza M, Franc J, et al: Reversible cerebral vasoconstriction syndrome and cervical artery dissection in 20 patients. *Neurology* 81:821, 2013.

Mayer SA, Brun NC, Begtrup K, et al: Efficacy and safety of recombinant activated factor VII for acute intracerebral hemorrhage. *N Engl J Med* 358:2127, 2008.

McKhann GW, Goldsborough MA, Borowicz LM, et al: Cognitive outcome after coronary artery bypass: A one-year prospective study. *Ann Thorac Surg* 63:510, 1997.

McKissock W, Paine KW, Walsh LS: An analysis of the results of treatment of ruptured intracranial aneurysms: A report of 722 consecutive cases. *J Neurosurg* 17:762, 1960.

Meier B, Kalesan, B, Mattle HP, et al. Percutaneous closure of patent foramen ovale in cryptogenic embolism. *N Engl J Med* 368:1083, 2013.

Mendelow AD, Gregson BA, Fernandes HM, et al: Early surgery versus initial conservative treatment in patients with spontaneous supratentorial intracerebral hematomas in the International Surgical Trial in Intracerebral Haemorrhage (STICH); a randomized trial. *Lancet* 365:387, 2005.

Merkel PA, Koroshetz WJ, Irizarry MC, et al: Cocaine-associated cerebral vasculitis. *Semin Arthritis Rheum* 25:172, 1995.

Metso TM, Metso AJ, Helenius J, et al: Prognosis and safety of anticoagulation in intracranial artery dissections in adults. *Stroke* 38:1837, 2007.

Milandre L, Brosset C, Botti G, Khawl R: A study of 82 cerebral infarctions in the area of posterior cerebral arteries. *Rev Neurol* 150:133, 1994.

Miyasaka K, Wolpert SM, Prager RJ: The association of cerebral aneurysms, infundibula, and intracranial arteriovenous malformations. *Stroke* 13:196, 1982.

Mohr JP, Caplan LR, Melski JW, et al: The Harvard Cooperative Stroke Registry: A prospective registry of patients hospitalized with stroke. *Neurology* 28:754, 1978.

Mohr JP, Thompson JL, Lazar RM, et al: A comparison of warfarin and aspirin for the prevention of recurrent ischemic stroke. *N Engl J Med* 345:1444, 2001.

Mokri B, Houser W, Sandok BA, Piepgras DG: Spontaneous dissections of the vertebral arteries. *Neurology* 38:880, 1988.

Mokri B, Sundt TM Jr, Houser W, Piepgras DG: Spontaneous dissection of the cervical internal carotid artery. *Ann Neurol* 19:126, 1986.

Molyneux A, Kerr R, Stratton I, et al: International Subarachnoid Aneurysm Trial (ISAT) Collaborative Group: International Subarachnoid Aneurysm Trial of neurosurgical clipping versus endovascular coiling in 2143 patients with ruptured intracranial aneurysms: A randomised trial. *Lancet* 360:1267, 2002.

Moore PM: Diagnosis and management of isolated angiitis of the central nervous system. *Neurology* 39:167, 1989.

Moore PM (ed): Vasculitis. *Semin Neurol* 14:291, 1994.

Moore WS, Barnett HJ, Beebe HG, et al: Guidelines for carotid endarterectomy: A multidisciplinary consensus statement from the ad hoc committee, American Heart Association. *Stroke* 26:188, 1995.

MRC Asymptomatic Carotid Surgery Trial (ACST) Collaborative Group: Prevention of disabling and fatal strokes by successful carotid endarterectomy in patients without recent neurological symptoms: Randomized controlled trial. *Lancet* 363:1491, 2004.

Mülges W, Babin-Ebel J, Reents W, Toyka KV: Cognitive performance after coronary bypass grafting: A follow-up study. *Neurology* 59:741, 2002.

Multicenter Acute Stroke Trial—Europe Study Group: Thrombolytic therapy with streptokinase in acute stroke. *N Engl J Med* 335:145, 1996.

Multicentre Acute Stroke Trial—Italy (MAST-I) Group: Randomised controlled trial of streptokinase, aspirin, and combination of both in treatment of acute ischaemic stroke. *Lancet* 346:1509, 1995.

Myers RE, Yamaguchi S: Nervous system effects of cardiac arrest in monkeys. *Arch Neurol* 34:65, 1977.

Nakajima K: Clinicopathological study of pontine hemorrhage. *Stroke* 14:485, 1983.

National Institute of Neurological Disorders and Stroke rt-PA Stroke Study Group: Tissue plasminogen activator for acute ischemic stroke. *N Engl J Med* 333:1581, 1995.

Nelson J, Barron MM, Riggs JE, et al: Cerebral vasculitis and ulcerative colitis. *Neurology* 36:719, 1986.

Nicholls ES, Johansen HL: Implications of changing trends in cerebrovascular and ischemic heart disease mortality. *Stroke* 14:153, 1983.

Nishimoto A, Takeuchi S: Moyamoya disease, in Vinken PJ, Bruyn GW (eds): *Handbook of Clinical Neurology*. Vol 12. Vascular Diseases of the Nervous System. Part 2. Amsterdam, North-Holland, 1972, pp 352–383.

Nishino H, Rubino FA, DeRemee RA, et al: Neurological involvement in Wegener's granulomatosis: An analysis of 324 consecutive patients at the Mayo Clinic. *Ann Neurol* 33:4, 1993.

Nishioka H, Torner JC, Graf CJ, et al: Cooperative study of intracranial aneurysms and subarachnoid hemorrhage: A long-term prognostic study: II. Ruptured intracranial aneurysms managed conservatively. *Arch Neurol* 41:1142, 1984.

North American Symptomatic Carotid Endarterectomy Trial Collaborators: Beneficial effect of carotid endarterectomy in symptomatic patients with high-grade carotid stenosis. *N Engl J Med* 325:445, 1991.

Norrving B, Cronqvist S: Lateral medullary infarction: Prognosis in an unselected series. *Neurology* 41:244, 1991.

Nubiola AR, Masana L, Masdeu S, et al: High-density lipoprotein cholesterol in cerebrovascular disease. *Arch Neurol* 38:468, 1981.

Ojemann RG, Fisher CM, Rich JC: Spontaneous dissecting aneurysms of the internal carotid artery. *Stroke* 3:434, 1972.

Ojemann RG, Ogilvy CS, Crowell RM, Heros RC: *Surgical Management of Neurovascular Disease,* 3rd ed. Baltimore, Williams & Wilkins, 1995.

Olesen J, Lip GYH, Kamper A-L, et al: Stroke and bleeding in atrial fibrillation with chronic kidney disease. *N Engl J Med* 367:625, 2012.

Olsen TS, Larsen B, Herning M, et al: Blood flow and vascular reactivity in collaterally perfused brain tissue. *Stroke* 14:332, 1983.

Ondra SL, Troupp H, George ED, Schwab K: The natural history of symptomatic arteriovenous malformations of the brain: A 24-year follow-up assessment. *J Neurosurg* 73:387, 1990.

Ovbiagele B, Nath A. Increasing incidence of ischemic stroke on patients with HIV infection. *Neurology* 16:444, 2011.

Parsons M, Spratt N, Bivard A, et al: A randomized trial of tenecteplase versus alteplase for acute ischemic stroke. *N Engl J Med* 366:1099, 2012.

Patel MR, Mahaffey KW, Garg J, et al and the ROCKET AF Steering Committee for the ROCKET AF Investigators. Rivaroxaban versus warfarin in nonvalvular atrial fibrillation. *N Engl J Med* 365:883, 2011.

Percheron G: Les artéres du thalamus humain: II. Artéres et territoires thalamiques paramédians de l'artére basilaire communicante. *Rev Neurol* 132:309, 1976.

Pessin MS, Duncan GW, Mohr JP, Poskanzer DC: Clinical and angiographic features of carotid transient ischemic attacks. *N Engl J Med* 296:358, 1977.

Pessin MS, Hinton RC, Davis KR, et al: Mechanisms of acute carotid stroke. *Ann Neurol* 6:245, 1979.

Pessin MS, Panis W, Prager RJ, et al: Auscultation of cervical and ocular bruits in extracranial carotid occlusive disease: A clinical and angiographic study. *Stroke* 14:246, 1983.

Petit H, Rousseaux M, Clarisse J, Delafosse A: Troubles oculocephalomoteurs et infarctus thalamo-sous-thalamique bilateral. *Rev Neurol* 137:709, 1981.

Petitti DB, Sidney S, Bernstein A, et al: Stroke in users of low-dose oral contraceptives. *N Engl J Med* 335:8, 1996.

Phillips PC, Lorentsen KJ, Shropshire LC, Ahn HS: Congenital odontoid aplasia and posterior circulation stroke in childhood. *Ann Neurol* 23:410, 1988.

Plum F: What causes infarction in ischemic brain? The Robert Wartenberg lecture. *Neurology* 33:222, 1983.

Poole CMJ, Ross Russell RW: Mortality and stroke after amaurosis fugax. *J Neurol Neurosurg Psychiatry* 48:902, 1985.

Porter RW, Detwiler PW, Spetzler RF, et al: Cavernous malformations of the brainstem: Experience with 100 patients. *J Neurosurg* 90:50, 1999.

Qureshi AI, Geocadin RC, Suarez JI, Ulatowski JA: Long-term outcome after medical reversal of transtentorial herniation in patients with supratentorial mass lesions. *Crit Care Med* 28:1556, 2000.

Rabinstein AA, Atkinson JL, Wijdicks EFM: Emergency craniotomy in patients worsening due to expanded cerebral hematoma: To what purpose? *Neurology* 58:1367, 2002.

Rabkin SW, Mathewson FAL, Tate RB: Long-term changes in blood pressure and risk of cerebrovascular disease. *Stroke* 9:319, 1978.

Raichle ME: The pathophysiology of brain ischemia. *Ann Neurol* 13:2, 1983.

Rauh R, Fischereder M, Spengel FA: Transesophageal echocardiography in patients with focal cerebral ischemia of unknown cause. *Stroke* 27:691, 1996.

Reivich M, Holling HE, Roberts B, Toole JF: Reversal of blood flow through the vertebral artery and its effect on cerebral circulation. *N Engl J Med* 265:878, 1961.

Rice GPA, Boughner DR, Stiller C, Ebers GC: Familial stroke syndrome associated with mitral valve prolapse. *Ann Neurol* 7:130, 1980.

Richardson AE, Jane JA: Long-term prognosis in untreated cerebral aneurysms: I. Incidence of late hemorrhage in cerebral aneurysm: Ten-year evaluation of 364 patients. *Ann Neurol* 1:358, 1977.

Roach GW, Kanchuger M, Mangano CM, et al: Adverse cerebral outcomes after coronary bypass surgery. *N Engl J Med* 335:1857, 1996.

Roehmholdt ME, Palumbo PJ, Whisnant JP, Elveback LR: Transient ischemic attack and stroke in a community-based diabetic cohort. *Mayo Clin Proc* 58:56, 1983.

Ropper AH: Neurologic intensive care, in Vinken PJ, Bruyn GW, Klawans HL (eds): *Handbook of Clinical Neurology. Vascular Diseases*. Part III. Vol 55. Amsterdam, Elsevier, 1990, pp 203–232.

Ropper AH, Davis KR: Lobar cerebral hemorrhages: Acute clinical syndromes in 26 cases. *Ann Neurol* 8:141, 1980.

Ropper AH, Fisher CM, Kleinman GM: Pyramidal infarction in the medulla. A cause of pure motor hemiplegia sparing the face. *Neurology* 21:91, 1979.

Ropper AH, King RB: Intracranial pressure monitoring in comatose patients with cerebral hemorrhage. *Arch Neurol* 41:725, 1984.

Ropper AH, Shafran B: Brain edema after stroke: Clinical syndrome and intracranial pressure. *Arch Neurol* 41:26, 1984.

Ross Russell RW: *Vascular Disease of the Central Nervous System*, 2nd ed. Edinburgh, Churchill Livingstone, 1983, pp 206–207.

Rost NS, Smith EE, Chang Y, et al: Prediction of functional outcome in patients with primary intracerebral hemorrhage: The FUNC score. *Stroke* 39:2304, 2008.

Rothwell PM, Giles MF, Flossman E, et al: A simple score (ABCD) to identify individuals at high risk of stroke after transient ischemic attack. *Lancet* 366:29, 2005.

Rothwell PM, Eliszíw M, Gutnikov SA, et al: Endarterectomy for symptomatic carotid artery stenosis in relation to clinical subgroups and timing of surgery. *Lancet* 363:915, 2004.

Ruigrok TM, Rinkel GJ, Algra A, et al: Characteristics of intracranial aneurysms in patients with familial subarachnoid hemorrhage. *Neurology* 62:891, 2004.

Ruiz DSM, Yilmaz Y, Gailloud P: Cerebral developmental venous anomalies: Current concepts. *Ann Neurol* 66:271, 2009.

Sacco RL, Ellenberg JH, Mohr JP, et al: Infarcts of undetermined cause: The NINCDS stroke data bank. *Ann Neurol* 25:382, 1989.

Sacco RL, Diener HC, Yusuf S, et al: Aspirin and extended-release dipyridamole versus clopidogrel for recurrent stroke. *N Engl J Med* 359:1238, 2008.

Sacco SE, Whisnant JP, Broderick JP, et al: Epidemiological characteristics of lacunar infarcts in a population. *Stroke* 22:1236, 1991.

Sage JI, Lepore FE: Ataxic hemiparesis from lesions of the corona radiata. *Arch Neurol* 40:449, 1983.

Sahs AL, Nibbelin KDW, Torner JC (eds): *Aneurysmal Subarachnoid Hemorrhage*. Baltimore, Urban & Schwarzenberg, 1981.

Sahs AL, Nishioka H, Torner JC, et al: Cooperative study of intracranial aneurysms and subarachnoid hemorrhage: A long term prognostic study. *Arch Neurol* 41:1140, 1142, 1147, 1984.

Salam-Adams M, Adams RD: Cerebrovascular disease by age group, in Vinken PJ, Bruyn GW, Klawans HL (eds): *Handbook of Clinical Neurology*. Vol 53. Vascular Diseases. Part I. Amsterdam, Elsevier, 1988, pp 27–46.

Samuels MA: Can cognition survive heart surgery? *Circulation* 113:2784, 2006.

Sandok BA, Furlan AJ, Whisnant JP, Sundt TM Jr: Guidelines for the management of transient ischemic attacks. *Mayo Clin Proc* 53:665, 1978.

Sandok BA, Giuliani ER: Cerebral ischemic events in patients with mitral valve prolapse. *Stroke* 13:448, 1982.

Sarrel PM, Lindsay DC, Poole-Wilson PA, Collins P: Hypothesis: Inhibition of endothelium-derived relaxing factor by haemoglobin in the pathogenesis of pre-eclampsia. *Lancet* 336:1030, 1990.

Schievink WI: Intracranial aneurysms. *N Engl J Med* 336:28, 1997.

Schievink WI, Bjornsson J, Parisi JE, Prakash UB: Arterial fibromuscular dysplasia associated with severe alpha 1-antitrypsin (alpha 1-AT) deficiency. *Mayo Clin Proc* 69:1040, 1994.

Schmidt WA, Kraft HE, Vorpahl K, et al: Color duplex ultrasonography in the diagnosis of temporal arteritis. *N Engl J Med* 337:1336, 1997.

Schon F, Martin RJ, Prevett M, et al: "CADASIL coma": An underdiagnosed acute encephalopathy. *J Neurol Neurosurg Psychiatry* 74:249, 2003.

Schwab S, Steiner T, Aschoff A, et al: Early hemicraniectomy in patients with complete middle cerebral artery infarction. *Stroke* 29:1888, 1998.

Scott RM, Smith ER: Moyamoya disease and moyamoya syndrome. *N Engl J Med* 360:1226, 2009.

Shah AK: Non-aneurysmal primary subarachnoid hemorrhage in pregnancy-induced hypertension and eclampsia. *Neurology* 61:117, 2003.

Shields RW Jr, Laureno R, Lachman T, Victor M: Anticoagulant-related hemorrhage in acute cerebral embolism. *Stroke* 15:426, 1984.

Shroyer AL, Grover FL, Hattler B, et al: On-pump versus off-pump coronary bypass surgery. *N Engl J Med* 361:1827, 2009.

Shuaib A, Lees KR, Lyden P, et al: NXY-059 for the treatment of acute ischemic stroke. *N Engl J Med* 357:562, 2007.

Siesjo BK: Historical overview: Calcium, ischemia, and death of brain cells. *Ann N Y Acad Sci* 522:638, 1988.

Sigsbee B, Deck MDF, Posner JB: Nonmetastatic superior sagittal sinus thrombosis complicating systemic cancer. *Neurology* 29: 139, 1979.

Singer DE: Randomized trials of warfarin for atrial fibrillation. *N Engl J Med* 327:1451, 1992.

Singhal AB, Caviness VS, Begleiter AF, et al: Cerebral vasoconstriction and stroke after use of serotonergic drugs. *Neurology* 58:130, 2002.

Sirin S, Kondziolka D, Niranjan A, et al: Prospective staged volume reduction for large arteriovenous malformations: Indications and outcomes in otherwise untreatable patients. *Neurosurgery* 58:17, 2006.

Sneddon JB: Cerebrovascular lesions and livedo reticularis. *Br J Dermatol* 77:180, 1965.

So EL, Toole JF, Dalal P, Moody DM: Cephalic fibromuscular dysplasia in 32 patients: Clinical findings and radiologic features. *Arch Neurol* 38:619, 1981.

Solomon RA, Fink ME: Current strategies for the management of aneurysmal subarachnoid hemorrhage. *Arch Neurol* 44:769, 1987.

SPACE Collaborative Group, The: 30 day results form the SPACE trial of stent-protected angioplasty versus carotid endarterectomy in symptomatic patients: a randomized non-inferiority trial. *Lancet Neurol* 368:1239, 2006.

Spetzler RF, Martin NA: A proposed grading system for arteriovenous malformations. *J Neurosurg* 65:476, 1986.

SPORTIF Executive Steering Committee for the SPORTIF V Investigators: Ximelagatran vs warfarin for stroke prevention in patients with nonvalvular atrial fibrillation. *JAMA* 293:690, 2005.

Stam J: Thrombosis of the cerebral veins and sinuses. *N Engl J Med* 352:1791, 2005.

Stapf C, Mast H, Sciacca RR, et al: Predictors of hemorrhage in patients with untreated brain arteriovenous malformations. *Neurology* 66:1350, 2006.

Starkstein SE, Robinson RG, Price TR: Comparison of cortical and subcortical lesions in the production of post-stroke mood disorders. *Brain* 110:1045, 1987.

Stewart RM, Samson D, Diehl J, et al: Unruptured cerebral aneurysms presenting as recurrent transient neurologic deficits. *Neurology* 30:47, 1980.

St. Louis, Wijdicks EF, Li H: Predicting neurologic deterioration in patients with cerebellar haematomas. *Neurology* 51:1364, 1998.

Stockhammer G, Felber SR, Zelger B, et al: Sneddon's syndrome: Diagnosis by skin biopsy and MRI in 17 patients. *Stroke* 24:685, 1993.

Strand T, Asplund K, Eriksson S, et al: A randomized control trial of hemodilution therapy in acute ischemic stroke. *Stroke* 15:980, 1984.

Stroke Prevention by Aggressive Reduction in Cholesterol Levels (SPARCL) Investigators, The: High-dose atorvastatin after stroke or transient ischemic attack. *N Engl J Med* 355:549, 2006.

Susac JO, Hardman JM, Selhorst JB: Microangiopathy of the brain and retina. *Neurology* 29:313, 1979.

Susac JO, Murtagh R, Egan RA, et al: MRI findings in Susac's syndrome. *Neurology* 61:1783, 2003.

Swanson RA: Intravenous heparin for acute stroke: What can we learn from the megatrials? *Neurology* 52:1746, 1999.

Takayasu M: A case with peculiar changes of the central retinal vessels. *Acta Soc Ophthalmol Jpn* 12:554, 1908.

Takebayashi S, Sakata N, Kawamura A: Reevaluation of miliary aneurysm in hypertensive brain: Recanalization of small hemorrhage? *Stroke* 21(Suppl):1, 1990.

Taneda M, Hayakawa T, Mogami H: Primary cerebellar hemorrhage: Quadrigeminal cistern obliteration as a predictor of outcome. *J Neurosurg* 67:545, 1987.

Taomoto K, Asada M, Kamazawa Y, Matsumoto S: Usefulness of the measurement of plasma-thromboglobulin (b-TG) in cerebrovascular disease. *Stroke* 14:518, 1983.

Teasdale GM, Wardlaw JM, White PM, et al: The familial risk of subarachnoid hemorrhage. *Brain* 128:1677, 2005.

Thieme H, Mehrholz J, Pohl M, et al: Mirror therapy for improving motor function after stroke. *Cochrane Database Syst Rev* 14:3, 2012.

Tippin J, Corbett JJ, Kerber RE, et al: Amaurosis fugax and ocular infarction in adolescents and young adults. *Ann Neurol* 26:69, 1989.

Ueda K, Toole JF, McHenry LC: Carotid and vertebral transient ischemic attacks: Clinical and angiographic correlation. *Neurology* 29:1094, 1979.

Vahedi K, Hofmeijer J, Juettler E, et al: Early decompressive surgery in malignant infarction of the middle cerebral artery—a pooled analysis of three randomized controlled trials. *Lancet Neurol* 6:215, 2007.

van den Bergh WM, van der Schaaf I, van Gijn J: The spectrum of presentations of venous infarction caused by deep cerebral venous thrombosis. *Neurology* 65:192, 2005.

Vander Eecken HM, Adams RD: Anatomy and functional significance of meningeal arterial anastomoses of human brain. *J Neuropathol Exp Neurol* 12:132, 1953.

van Gijn J, Van Donegen KJ, Vermeulen M, et al: Perimesencephalic hemorrhage: A nonaneurysmal and benign form of subarachnoid hemorrhage. *Neurology* 35:493, 1985.

Vernooij MW, Ikram MA, Tanghe HL, et al: Incidental findings on brain MRI in the general population. *N Engl J Med* 357:1821, 2007.

Verreault S, Joutel A, Riant F, et al: A novel hereditary small vessel disease of the brain. *Ann Neurol* 59:353, 2006.

Vessey MP, Lawless M, Yeates D: Oral contraceptives and stroke: Findings in a large prospective study. *Br Med J* 289:530, 1984.

Viswanathan A, Greenberg SM: Cerebral amyloid angiopathy in the elderly. *Ann Neurol* 70:871, 2011.

Volhard F: Clinical aspects of Bright's disease, in Berglund H, et al (eds): *The Kidney in Health and Disease*. Philadelphia, Lea & Febiger, 1935, pp 665–688.

Vonsattel JP, Myers RH, Hedley-Whyte ET, et al: Cerebral amyloid angiopathy without and with cerebral hemorrhages: A comparative histological study. *Ann Neurol* 30:637, 1991.

Waga S, Yamamoto Y: Hypertensive putaminal hemorrhage—treatment and results: Is surgical treatment superior to conservative? *Stroke* 14:480, 1983.

Wang Y, Wang Y, Zhao X, et al for the CHANCE Investigators: Clopidogrel with aspirin in acute minor stroke or transient ischemic attack. *N Eng J Med* 369:11, 2013.

Wechsler LR: Intravenous thrombolytic therapy for acute stroke. *N Engl J Med* 364:22, 2011.

Weiller C, Ringelstein B, Reiche W, et al: The large striatocapsular infarct. A clinical and pathophysiological entity. *Arch Neurol* 47:1085, 1990.

Weinberger J, Biscarra V, Weisberg MK: Factors contributing to stroke in patients with atherosclerotic disease of the great vessels: The role of diabetes. *Stroke* 14:709, 1983.

Weisman AD, Adams RD: The neurological complications of dissecting aortic aneurysm. *Brain* 67:69, 1944.

Whisnant JP, Matsumoto N, Elveback LR: Transient cerebral ischemic attacks in a community: Rochester, Minnesota, 1955 through 1969. *Mayo Clin Proc* 48:194, 1973.

White HD, Simes JS, Anderson NE, et al: Pravastatin therapy and the risk of stroke. *N Engl J Med* 343:317, 2000.

Whiteley WN, Adams, HP, Bath MWP, et al: Targeted use of heparin, heparinoids, or low-molecular-weight heparin to improve outcome after acute ischaemic stroke: An individual patient data meta-analysis of randomised controlled trials. *Lancet Neurol* 12: 539, 2013.

Wiebers DO: Ischemic cerebrovascular complications of pregnancy. *Arch Neurol* 42:1106, 1985.

Wiebers DO, Whisnant JP, O'Fallon WM: The natural history of unruptured intracranial aneurysms. *N Engl J Med* 304:696, 1981.

Wiebers DO, Whisnant JP, Sandok BA, O'Fallon WM: Prospective comparison of a cohort with asymptomatic carotid bruit and a population-based cohort without carotid bruit. *Stroke* 21:984, 1990.

Wiebers DO, Whisnant JP, Sundt TM, O'Fallon WM: The significance of unruptured intracranial saccular aneurysms. *J Neurosurg* 66:23, 1987.

Wijdicks EF, St. Louis E: Clinical profiles predictive of outcome in pontine hemorrhage. *Neurology* 49:1342, 1997.

Wijdicks EFM, Ropper AH, Hunnicut EJ, et al: Atrial natriuretic factor and salt wasting after subarachnoid hemorrhage. *Stroke* 22:1519, 1991.

Wijdicks EFM, Vermeulen M, Hudra A, et al: Hyponatremia and cerebral infarction in patients with ruptured intracranial aneurysms: Is fluid restriction harmful? *Ann Neurol* 17:137, 1985.

Wolf ME, Szabo K, Griebe M, et al: Clinical and MRI characteristics of acute migrainous infarction. *Neurology* 76:1911, 2011.

Wolf PA, Kannel WB, McGee DL, et al: Duration of atrial fibrillation and imminence of stroke: The Framingham Study. *Stroke* 14:664, 1983.

Wolf SL, Winsten CJ, Miller JP, et al: Effect of constraint-induced movement therapy on upper extremity function 3 to 9 months after stroke. *JAMA* 296:2095, 2006.

Wood JH, Fleischer AS: Observations during hypervolemic hemodilution of patients with acute focal cerebral ischemia. *JAMA* 248:2999, 1982.

Yamashita M, Oka K, Tanaka K: Histopathology of the brain vascular network in moyamoya disease. *Stroke* 14:50, 1983.

Yanagihara P, Piepgras DG, Klass DW: Repetitive involuntary movement associated with episodic cerebral ischemia. *Ann Neurol* 18:244, 1985.

35

Craniocerebral Trauma

Among the vast array of neurologic diseases, cerebral trauma ranks high in order of frequency and gravity. In the United States, trauma is the leading cause of death in persons younger than 45 years of age and more than half of these deaths are a result of head injuries. According to the American Trauma Society, an estimated 500,000 Americans are admitted to hospitals yearly following cerebral trauma; of these, 75,000 to 90,000 die and even larger numbers, most of them young and otherwise healthy, are left permanently disabled.

The basic problem in craniocerebral trauma is at once both simple and complex: simple because there is usually no difficulty in determining causation, namely, a blow to the head, and complex because of a number of delayed effects that complicate the injury. As for the trauma itself, little can be done, for it is finished before the physician or others arrive on the scene. At most there can be an assessment of the full extent of the immediate cerebral injury, an evaluation of factors conducive to complications and further lesions, and the institution of measures to avoid such additional problems. Specifically, the neck can be stabilized and adequate perfusion and oxygenation can be secured. But of the disastrous intracranial phenomena that can be initiated by head injury, few offer possibilities of treatment. New techniques of cellular biology are exposing phenomena that are set in motion by traumatic injury of nerve cells and glia. Some of these changes may be reversible, but at the moment, such knowledge is limited.

It is a common misconception that craniocerebral injuries are matters that concern only the neurosurgeon and not the general physician or neurologist. Actually, 80 percent of head injuries are first seen by a physician in an emergency department, and fewer than 20 percent ever require neurosurgical intervention of any kind, and even this number is decreasing. The neurologist must be familiar with the clinical manifestations and the natural course of primary brain injury and its complications and have a sound grasp of the underlying physiologic mechanisms. Such knowledge must also relate to the interpretation of CT and MRI, both of which have greatly enhanced our ability to deal with traumatic brain injury. The present chapter reviews the salient facts concerning craniocerebral injuries and outlines a clinical approach that the authors have found useful over the years. Matters pertaining to spinal injuries, often coexistent with head trauma, are considered in Chap. 44.

DEFINITIONS AND MECHANISMS

The very language that one uses to discuss certain types of head injuries divulges a number of misconceptions inherited from previous generations of physicians. Certain terms have crept into the medical vocabulary and have been retained long after the ideas for which they stood have been refuted, attesting to the disadvantage of premature adoption of explanatory terms rather than descriptive ones. The word *concussion*, for example, implies a violent shaking or jarring of the brain and a resulting transient functional impairment. Yet despite numerous postulates of physical changes within nerve cells, axons, or myelin sheaths (vibration effects, formation of intracellular vacuoles) that putatively occurred with concussion, confirmation of their existence has proved difficult in humans and experimental animals.

In all attempts to analyze the mechanisms of *closed*, or *blunt* (*nonpenetrating*), head injury, one fact is preeminent: there must be the sudden application of a physical force of considerable magnitude to the head. Unless the head is struck, the brain suffers no injury except in the rare instances of violent flexion–extension (whiplash) of the neck and possibly in explosion-blast injury with a sudden extreme increase of atmospheric pressure. In military medical practice, blast injuries assume great importance and in theory, challenge many concepts of loss of consciousness in closed head injury; i.e., there is no contact with, or sudden acceleration or deceleration of the cranium. The mechanical factors of importance in brain injury are the differential mobility of the head on the neck, and of the brain within the cranium, the tethering of the upper brainstem that allows movement of the cerebral hemispheres around that vertex, and the striking of parts of the brain on dural septa and bony prominences. As to concussive injuries, it is useful to point out that concussions usually involve a physical force that imparts motion to the stationary head or more commonly, a hard surface that arrests the motion of a moving head, i.e., concussion does not occur if the head remains stationary.

This sudden deceleration or acceleration of the cranium is the mechanism of most civilian head injuries, and they are notable in two respects: they often induce at least a temporary loss of consciousness, and the brain may suffer gross damage even though the skull is not penetrated, i.e., contusion, laceration, hemorrhage, and swelling. A theory that brings coherence to all of these physical and gross neuropathologic changes and their relation to transient loss of consciousness (concussion) and prolonged coma has only been tentatively formulated.

In contrast to closed head injury, high-velocity missiles penetrate the skull and cranial cavity, or rarely, the skull may be compressed between two converging forces that crush the brain without causing significant displacement of the head or the brain. In these circumstances, the patient may suffer severe and even fatal injury without preceding loss of consciousness. Hemorrhage, destruction of brain tissue, and, if the patient survives for a time, meningitis or abscess are the principal pathologic changes created by injuries of these types. They offer little difficulty to our understanding. Figure 35-1 illustrates these various types of head injuries.

The relation of *skull fracture* to brain injury has been viewed in changing perspective throughout the history of this subject. In the first half of the last century, fractures dominated the thinking of the medical profession, and cerebral lesions were regarded as secondary. Later, it became clear that the skull, although rigid, is still flexible enough to yield to a blow that injures the brain without causing fracture. Therefore the presence of a fracture, although a rough measure of the force to which the brain has been exposed, is not an infallible index of the presence of cerebral injury (see further on in discussion of predictive features for imaging abnormalities with concussion). Even in immediately fatal head injuries, autopsy reveals an intact skull in 20 to 30 percent of cases. Of course, many patients suffer skull fractures without serious or prolonged disorder of cerebral function, partly because the energy of a blow is dissipated in the fracture. Indeed, this diffusion of the impact might be expected to reduce underlying brain damage.

Nevertheless, fractures cannot be dismissed without further comment for several reasons. Overall, brain injury is estimated to be 5 to 10 times more frequent with skull fractures than without them and perhaps 20 times more frequent with severe and multiple fractures. Fractures assume further importance in providing an explanation for cranial-nerve palsies, and in creating potential pathways for the ingress of bacteria and air or the egress of cerebrospinal fluid (CSF leak). In these respects, fractures through the base of the skull are of special significance, and are considered below.

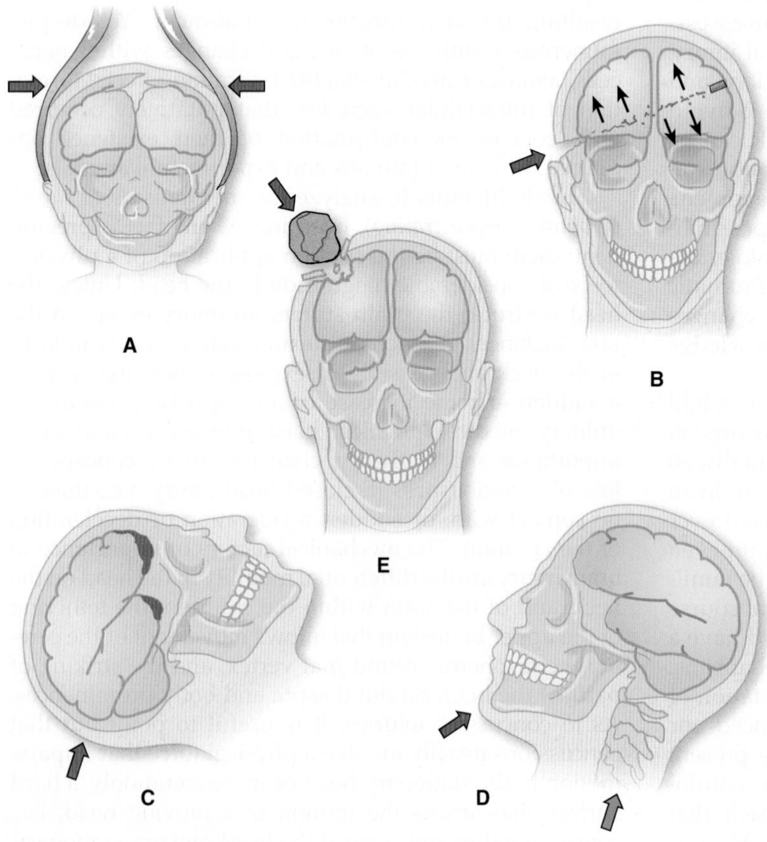

Figure 35-1. Mechanisms of craniocerebral injury. *A.* Cranium distorted by forceps (birth injury). *B.* Gunshot wound of the brain. *C.* Falls (also traffic accidents). *D.* Blows on the chin ("punch-drunk"). *E.* Injury to skull and brain by falling objects. (From Courville.)

Basal Skull Fractures and Cranial Nerve Injuries

Figure 35-2 illustrates the major sites and directions of basilar skull fractures. One can readily perceive the possibilities of injury to cranial nerves. Fractures of the base are difficult to detect in plain skull films and may be missed by other imaging techniques, but their presence should be suspected in the presence of any one of a number of characteristic clinical signs. Fracture of the petrous pyramid often deforms the external auditory canal or tears the tympanic membrane, with resultant leakage of CSF (otorrhea); or, blood may collect behind an intact tympanic membrane and discolor it. If the fracture extends more posteriorly, damaging the sigmoid sinus, the tissue behind the ear and over the mastoid process becomes boggy and discolored (Battle sign). Basal fracture of the anterior skull may also cause blood to leak into the periorbital tissues, imparting a characteristic "raccoon" or "panda bear" appearance. The presence of any of these signs calls for CT scanning of the skull base using bone window settings to detect a fracture.

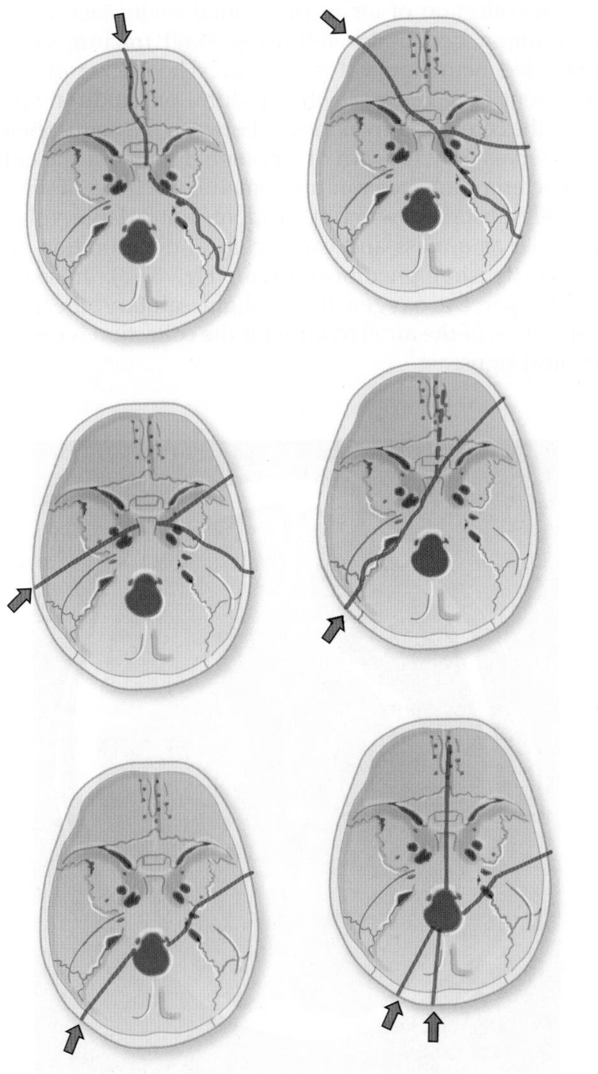

Figure 35-2. The course of fracture lines through the base of the skull. *Arrows* indicate point of application and direction of force. (From Courville.)

The existence of a basal fracture is also indicated by signs of cranial nerve damage. The olfactory, facial, and auditory nerves are the ones most liable to injury, but any one, including the twelfth, may be damaged. *Anosmia and an apparent loss of taste* (actually a loss of perception of aromatic flavors as the elementary modalities of taste are unimpaired) are frequent sequelae of head injury, especially with falls on the back of the head. In the majority of cases the anosmia is permanent. If unilateral, it will not be noticed by the patient. However, mechanism of these disturbances is thought to be a displacement of the brain and tearing of the olfactory nerve filaments in or near the cribriform plate, through which they course, rather than being attributable to a fracture. A fracture in or near the sella may tear the stalk of the pituitary gland with resulting *diabetes insipidus*. Rarely, such a fracture may cause bleeding from a preexisting pituitary adenoma and produce the syndrome of pituitary apoplexy (see Chap. 31). A fracture of the sphenoid bone may lacerate the optic nerve, with blindness from the beginning. The pupil is unreactive to a direct light stimulus but still reacts to a light stimulus to the opposite eye (consensual reflex). The optic disc becomes pale, i.e., atrophic, after an interval of several weeks. Partial injuries of the optic nerve result in scotomas and a troublesome blurring of vision.

Complete *oculomotor nerve injury* is characterized by ptosis and diplopia, a divergence of the globes with the affected eye resting in an abducted and slightly depressed position, loss of medial and most of the vertical movements of the eye, and a fixed, dilated pupil, as described in Chap. 13. The most common symptom is diplopia that is worse on looking down and compensatory tilting of the head indicating a *trochlear nerve* injury. In a series of 60 patients with head injury, Lepore confirmed that fourth-nerve palsy was the most common cause of diplopia, occurring unilaterally twice as often as bilaterally, followed in frequency by damage to one or both third nerves, then, least often, a unilateral or bilateral sixth-nerve palsy. Five of his patients had palsies that reflected damage to more than one nerve and seven had supranuclear disorders of convergence. The long, circumferential subarachnoid course of the fourth nerve is usually given as the explanation for its frequent injury, but this mechanism has never been validated. These optic and ocular motor nerve disorders must be distinguished from those caused by displacement of the globe or entrapment of an extraocular muscle as a result of direct injury to the orbit.

Injury to the *ophthalmic and maxillary divisions of the trigeminal nerve* may be the result of either a basal fracture across the middle cranial fossa or a direct extracranial injury to the branches of the nerves. Numbness and paresthesia of the skin supplied by the nerve branch or chronic neuralgia can be troublesome sequelae of these injuries.

The *facial nerve* may be involved in one of two ways. In the first type of injury, associated with transverse fractures through the petrous bone, there is an immediate facial palsy, probably caused by contusion or transection of the nerve. Surgical anastomosis has sometimes been successful in restoring function in this circumstance. The second, more common type, is associated with longitudinal fractures of the petrous bone, the facial palsy then often being delayed for several days, a sequence that may be misinterpreted as progression of the intracranial traumatic lesion. This latter type is usually transitory, and its mechanism is not known.

Injury to the *eighth cranial nerve* because of petrous fractures results in a loss of hearing or in postural vertigo and nystagmus coming on immediately after the trauma. Deafness as a result of nerve injury must be distinguished from the high-tone hearing loss due to *cochlear* injury and from deafness caused by bleeding into the middle ear and disruption of the ossicular chain (conduction deafness). Also, vertigo must be distinguished from the very common symptom of posttraumatic dizziness discussed in a later section. The rare condition of fracture through the hypoglossal canal causes weakness of one side of the tongue. It should be kept in mind that blows to the upper neck may also cause lower cranial-nerve palsies, either by direct injury to their peripheral extensions or as a result of *carotid artery dissection* in the cervical segment of the artery.

Carotid–Cavernous Fistula

A basal fracture through the sphenoid bone may lacerate the internal carotid artery or one of its intracavernous branches where it lies in the cavernous sinus. Within hours or a day or two, a disfiguring pulsating exophthalmos develops as arterial blood enters the sinus and distends the superior and inferior ophthalmic veins that empty into the sinus. The orbit feels tight and painful, and the eye may become partially or completely immobile because of pressure on the ocular nerves traversing the sinus (see Fig. 14-5). The sixth nerve is affected most often, and the third and fourth nerves less often. Also, there may be a loss of vision as a result of ischemia of the optic nerve and retina, although the mechanism has not been entirely clear; congestion of the retinal veins and glaucoma are potential factors in the visual failure. Some 5 to 10 percent of fistulas resolve spontaneously, but the remainder must be obliterated by interventional radiologic means (by a detachable balloon inserted into the carotid artery via a transfemoral catheter) or by a direct surgical repair of the fistula (see Stern).

Not all carotid–cavernous fistulas are traumatic. They may occasionally occur with rupture of an intracavernous saccular aneurysm or in Ehlers-Danlos disease, where the connective tissue is defective; or the cause may be unexplained. Occasionally, a dural-based arteriovenous fistula opens in the region of the cavernous sinus after an injury; most such cases are spontaneous and they cause less in the way of orbital swelling and congestion.

Pneumocephalus, Aerocele, and Rhinorrhea (Cerebrospinal Fluid Leak)

If the skin over a skull fracture is lacerated and the underlying meninges are torn, or if the fracture passes through the inner wall of a paranasal sinus, bacteria may enter the cranial cavity, with resulting meningitis or abscess formation. CSF that leaks into the sinus presents as a watery discharge from the nose (*CSF rhinorrhea*). The nasal discharge can be identified as CSF by testing it for glucose with diabetic test tape (mucus has no glucose) or by the presence of fluorescein or radionuclide-labeled dye that is injected into the lumbar subarachnoid space and then absorbed by pledgets placed in the nasal cavity. Mucus, when absorbed onto a handkerchief and allowed to dry, will leave the material stiff, whereas CSF, will not. A more elaborate test is to detect tau protein in the discharge; it is present only in CSF and not in mucus or blood. Most cases of acute CSF rhinorrhea heal by themselves. An indwelling lumbar drain for a few days may aid the process. If the condition is persistent or is complicated by an episode of meningitis, repair of the torn dura is indicated. The prophylactic use of antibiotics to prevent meningitis in cases of nasal CSF leak is controversial, but many neurosurgeons continue this practice, particularly in children.

A collection of air in the cranial cavity (aerocele) is a common occurrence following skull fracture or any extended neurosurgical procedure. The pocket of air is apparent by CT scan in the epidural or subdural space over the cerebral convexities or between the hemispheres, and serves only to warn of a potential route for the entry of bacteria into the cranium. Small collections of air are usually absorbed without incident, but a large volume may act as a mass and cause clinical deterioration after injury (tension pneumocranium; Fig. 35-3). Inhalation of 100 percent oxygen has a slight salutary effect, but aspiration of the air is required if the collection is causing clinical signs.

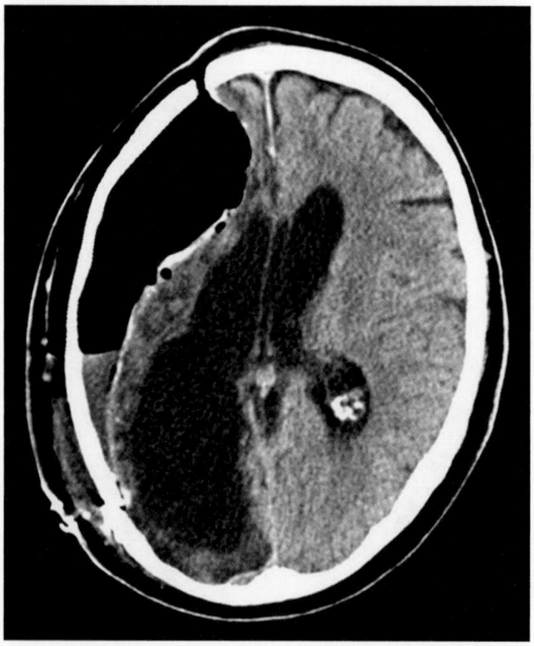

Figure 35-3. CT of postoperative tension pneumocranium (aerocele) that caused progressive drowsiness and required removal by aspiration. The air is apparent as a very-low-density collection that compresses the right frontal lobe.

Depressed skull fractures are of significance only if the underlying dura is lacerated or the brain is compressed by indentation of bone. They then are surgically elevated, preferably within the first 24 to 48 h.

Concussion

Much has been written about the mechanisms of concussion in closed head injury and its definition has undergone serial revision. In the past, a transient loss of consciousness and amnesia after a blow to the head had been considered necessary to qualify as concussion but lesser degrees of mild confusion, incoordination, or even symptoms such as headache and fatigue that follow mild head injury are now encompassed under the term. Whether all these problems derive from the same mechanism cannot be stated with confidence.

History of Concepts of Concussion The mechanism of concussive "cerebral paralysis" has been interpreted in various ways throughout medical history in light of the state of knowledge at a particular period of time. The favored hypotheses for the better part of a century were "vasoparalysis" (suggested by Fischer in 1870) or an arrest of circulation by an instantaneous rise in intracranial pressure (ICP) (proposed by Strohmeyer in 1864 and popularized by Trotter in 1932). Jefferson, in his essay on the nature of concussion (1944), convincingly refuted these vascular hypotheses. Later, Shatsky and coworkers, by the use of high-speed cineangiography, showed displacement of vessels but no arrest of circulation immediately after impact.

Beginning with the work of Denny-Brown and Russell in 1941, the physical factors involved in head and brain injuries were subjected to careful analysis. These investigators demonstrated that in monkey and cat the concussion resulted when the freely moving head was struck by a heavy mass. If the head was prevented from moving at the moment of impact, the same degree of force invariably failed to produce concussion. The importance of head motion was verified by Gennarelli and colleagues, who were able to induce concussion in primates by rapid acceleration of the freely moving head without impact, a condition that rarely occurs in humans.

Holbourn, a Cambridge physicist, from a study of gelatin models under conditions simulating head trauma, deduced that when the head is struck, movement of the partly tethered but suspended brain always lags (because of inertia), but inevitably the brain moves also, and when it does it must rotate in an arc because of attachment to the neck. Ommaya and Gennarelli (1974) proved the correctness of this assumption by photographing the brain through a transparent calvarium at the moment of impact. The brain was thus subjected to stresses set up by rotational forces mainly in the sagittal plane, centered at its point of tethering in the high midbrain. The torque at the level of the upper reticular formation would explain the immediate loss of consciousness, as described later. An extensive and scholarly review of the pathophysiology of concussion was done by Shaw (although we are uncertain of the validity of his view of a seizure-concussive mechanism).

Mechanism of Concussion The core features of loss of consciousness or confusion are notable for being immediate after trauma (not delayed even by seconds) and for being entirely reversible. This is the sense in which concussion was used to mean a *reversible traumatic paralysis of nervous function* and any physiologic explanation of the syndrome would have to incorporate this temporal sequence. However, the effects of concussion on brain function may last for a variable time (seconds, minutes, hours, or longer) and to set arbitrary limits on the duration of loss of consciousness, i.e., to consider a brief loss as indicative of concussion and a prolonged loss as indicative of contusion or other traumatic cerebral lesion, is unsound physiologically. As pointed out by Symonds, any such difference is quantitative, not qualitative. It is true that in the more prolonged states of stupor or coma, there is a far greater chance of finding hemorrhage and contusion, which undoubtedly contribute to the persistence of coma and the likelihood of irreversible change. Finally, the optimal condition for the production of concussion, demonstrated originally by Denny-Brown and Russell, is a sudden change in the momentum of the head; i.e., either movement is imparted to the stationary head by a blow or movement of the head is arrested by a hard, unyielding surface.

Rotational movements of the brain also provide a reasonable explanation for the occurrence of surface injuries in specific locations, i.e., where the swirling brain comes into contact with bony prominences on the inner surface of the skull (petrous and orbital ridges, sphenoid wings), and of injuries to the corpus callosum, which is flung against the falx. Not well explained by any of these mechanisms are concussions after *blast injuries*, a serious problem in military medicine. This syndrome possibly resurrects the notion that a shock wave travels through the brain and disrupts neural function throughout the cerebral hemispheres or in the reticular formation of the midbrain.

These views on the site and mechanism of concussion are not fully accepted but have been supported by a number of additional physiologic observations. Foltz and Schmidt, in 1956, suggested that the reticular formation of the upper brainstem was the anatomic site of concussive injury. They showed that in the concussed monkey, lemniscal sensory transmission through the brainstem was unaltered, but its effect in activating the reticular formation was blocked and that the electrical activity of the medial reticular formation was depressed for a longer time and more severely than that of the cerebral cortex.

What was further noteworthy in most of these cases, and in those reported by Jellinger and Seitelberger, was the presence of additional lesions in the region of the reticular activating system and small hemorrhagic softenings in the corpus callosum, superior cerebellar peduncles, and dorsolateral tegmentum of the midbrain. As discussed further on, Strich (1956) interpreted the extensive white matter lesions, both in the hemispheres and in the upper brainstem, to represent a degeneration of nerve fibers that had been stretched or torn by the shear stresses set up during rotational acceleration of the head, as had been postulated earlier by Holbourn. She suggested that if nerve fibers are stretched rather than torn, the lesions may be reversible and may play a part in the mechanism of concussion. Symonds elaborated on this view and saw in the shearing stresses, which are maximal at the point where the cerebral hemispheres rotate on the relatively fixed upper brainstem, the explanation of concussion.

Clinical Manifestations of Concussion

In its fullest form, the characteristic clinical signs of concussive brain injury are the immediate abolition of consciousness, suppression of supportive reflexes (falling to the ground if standing), transient arrest of respiration, a brief period of bradycardia, and fall in blood pressure following a momentary rise at the time of impact. Rarely, if these abnormalities are sufficiently intense, death may occur at the moment of impact, presumably from respiratory arrest. In its mildest form, there is no apparent loss of consciousness or collapse, only a brief period of stunned disorientation, staggering, and subsequent amnesia during which the individual appears outwardly normal. The vital signs usually return to normal and stabilize within a few seconds even if the patient remains unconscious.

Brief tonic extension of the limbs, clonic convulsive movements lasting up to approximately 20 s, and other peculiar movements may occur immediately after the loss of consciousness (see McCrory et al). These "concussive convulsions" are probably of little prognostic significance and have not been shown to confer an increased risk of later seizures. McCrory and colleagues noted an association between motor and convulsive movements and facial impact, and we have seen this feature several times in teenagers who collided while pursuing a ball.

In the period during which the patient is unconscious and for a few moments afterwards, the plantar reflexes are extensor. After a variable period of time, the patient begins to stir and opens his eyes. Corneal, pharyngeal, and cutaneous reflexes, originally depressed, return, and the limbs withdraw from painful stimuli. Gradually, contact is made with the environment and the patient begins to obey simple commands and respond slowly to questions. Memories are not formed during this period; the patient may even carry on a conversation, which he cannot later recall. Finally, there is ostensibly full neurologic recovery corresponding to the time when the patient can form consecutive memories of current experiences.

The time required for the patient to pass through these stages of recovery may be only a few seconds or minutes, several hours, or possibly a limited number of days; but again, between these extremes there seem to be only quantitative differences. To the observer, such patients are comatose only from the moment of injury until they open their eyes and begin to speak; however, for the patient, the period of unconsciousness in one limited perspective extends from a point before the injury occurred (*retrograde amnesia*) until the time when he is able to form consecutive memories at the end of the period of anterograde amnesia. The duration of the amnesic period, particularly of *anterograde amnesia*, is but one index of the severity of the concussive injury. Although momentary "stunning" without loss of consciousness represents the mildest degree of concussion, it is not known if it shares the same mechanism as overt loss of consciousness. The aftereffects of concussion in causing anxiety, sleep disturbance, mental fogginess and cognitive difficulty, and dizziness are common to both and are discussed further on.

Athletic Concussion

This is a topic of current interest and various guidelines regarding return to play have been published. A recent summary from the American Academy of Neurology can be consulted (authored by Giza and colleagues). The later-life development of dementia and other neurodegenerative conditions in professional athletes is discussed further on. Many useful observations have emerged from study of athletes after head injury. Foremost among these observations is that athletes who have had concussion are more likely than other players to have another concussion in the same playing season (Guskiewicz et al); whether this is a reflection of constitutional incoordination or the person's style of play, or another factor is not known. Second, most prospective studies show a decline in reaction time and in other neuropsychologic tests after concussion, which returns to baseline over several days or weeks. Third, there is an indication from several series of concussions in National Collegiate Athletic Association and National Football League players that the number of recollected concussions is proportional to the degree of impairment on neuropsychologic tests (McCrea et al). Similar results have been found in other pursuits such as jockeying (Wall et al), but there are few adequate prospective studies.

The appropriate duration of removal from play has been the subject of numerous and largely arbitrary systems. The basis of most rules has been an appropriate conservatism that requires the absence of cerebral symptoms both at rest and under physical stress testing such as running or repetitive squatting. The duration of loss of consciousness and of amnesia was formerly a major component of the decision about return to play. More current guidelines focus instead on slowness in answering questions, uncertainty about plays or game assignments, and clumsiness, with or without loss of consciousness or amnesia. All such players are removed from the game. After medical evaluation, which may include imaging and neuropsychologic testing, a program of physical and cognitive "rest" is followed by graduated physical and mental activity under observation and a return to a lower level if symptoms occur (McCrory et al). Specifically, light aerobic exercise is followed by sport-specific training and noncontact, then contact, drills.

Pathologic Changes Associated With Severe Head Injury

In contrast to concussion, in cases of traumatic brain injury that are fatal or very serious, the brain is usually bruised (contused), swollen, or lacerated, and there are hemorrhages, both meningeal and intracerebral, as well as hypoxic-ischemic lesions. A majority of patients who remain in a coma for more than 24 h after a head injury are found to have intracerebral hematomas and contusions. Of these lesions, the most frequent are contusions of the surface of the brain beneath the point of impact (*coup lesion*) and the sometimes more extensive lacerations and contusions on the side opposite the site of impact (*contrecoup lesion*), as shown in Fig. 35-4. Blows to the front of the head may produce mainly coup lesions, whereas blows to the back of the head may cause mainly contrecoup lesions. Blows to the side of the head produce either coup or contrecoup lesions, or both. Irrespective of the site of the impact, the common sites of cerebral contusions are in the frontal and temporal lobes, as illustrated in Figs. 35-4 and 35-5. The inertia of the malleable brain—which causes it to be flung against the side of the skull that is struck, to be pulled away from the contralateral side, and to be impelled against bony promontories within the cranial cavity, explains these coup–contrecoup patterns. Relative sparing of the occipital lobes in coup–contrecoup injury has been explained by the smooth inner surface of the occipital bones and subadjacent tentorium, as pointed out by Courville.

The contused cortex is diffusely swollen and hemorrhagic, most of the blood being found around parenchymal vessels. On CT scanning, the lesions appear as edematous regions of cortex and subcortical white matter admixed with areas of increased density representing leaked blood (Fig. 35-6). The bleeding points may coalesce and give the appearance of a unitary clot in the cortex and immediately adjacent white matter. The predilection of these lesions for the crowns of convolutions attests to their traumatic origin (being thrown against the overlying skull) and distinguishes them from cerebrovascular and other types of cerebral lesions. There may be ball hemorrhages within the hemispheres that are independent of contusions as discussed below. Not surprisingly, such deep areas of bleeding are common in patients receiving anticoagulant or antiplatelet medications.

Of equal importance are axonal lesions that occur at the time of impact or evolve soon afterwards. Strich (1961) described the neuropathologic findings in patients who died months after severe closed head injuries that had caused immediate and protracted coma. In all of her cases, in which there were no signs of skull fracture, raised intracranial pressure, or gross subarachnoid hemorrhage, she observed an uneven but diffuse degeneration of the cerebral white matter that has become the basis of all subsequent work on diffuse axonal shearing (*diffuse axonal injury, DAI*). In cases of shorter survival (up to 6 weeks), she observed ballooning and interruption of axis cylinders. These findings were subsequently confirmed and expanded by Nevin, by Adams and colleagues (1982), and by Gennarelli and coworkers, the last of these groups also working with monkeys.

The extension of Strich's concept, that postulates diffuse axonal injury throughout the cerebral white matter as the main cause of persistent unconsciousness, has been widely adopted. In relation to concussion, shearing

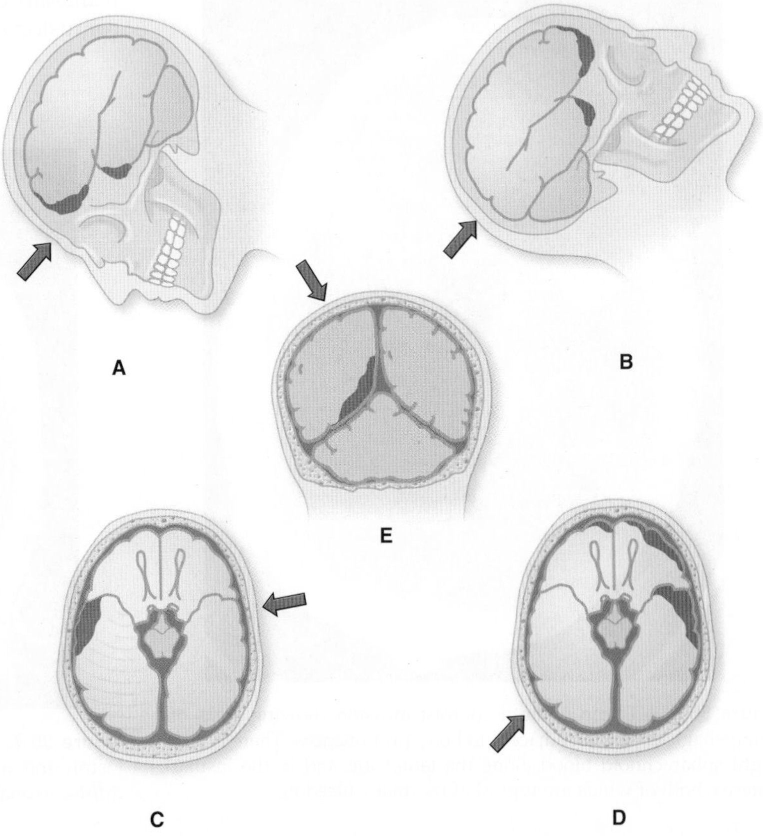

Figure 35-4. Mechanisms of cerebral contusion. *Arrows* indicate point of application and direction of force; *dark red areas* indicate location of contusion. *A*. Frontotemporal contusion consequent to frontal injury. *B*. Frontotemporal contusion following occipital injury. *C*. Contusion of temporal lobe because of contralateral injury. *D*. Frontotemporal contusion as a result of injury to opposite temporooccipital region. *E*. Diffuse mesial temporooccipital contusion caused by a blow on the vertex. (From Courville.)

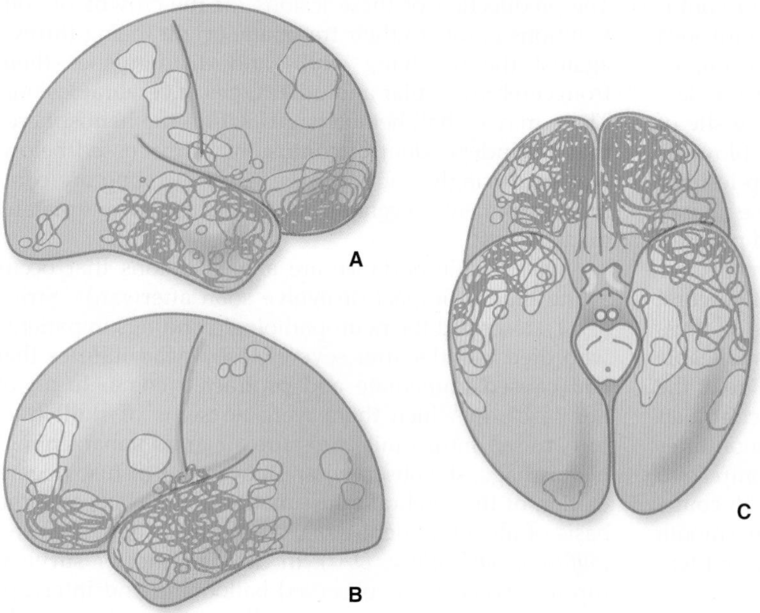

Figure 35-5. Distribution of contusions emphasizing the frontal and frontotemporal distribution in 40 consecutive autopsy cases collected by Courville. (From Courville.)

lesions are also seen in the midbrain and lower thalamus in severe injury, providing some evidence for this neuronal dysfunction in these regions as the cause of concussion.

In most cases of severe head injury, there is damage to the corpus callosum by impact with the falx; necrosis and hemorrhage are sometimes visible by CT and can be seen to spread bilaterally to adjacent white matter (Fig. 35-7). There may also be scattered hemorrhages in the white matter along lines of force from the point of impact to the contralateral side. The degeneration of white matter from diffuse axonal injury can be remarkably diffuse, with no apparent relationship to focal destructive lesions, although differentiating it from secondary wallerian change that originates in a surface or callosal contusion can be difficult. Investigations using MRI, such

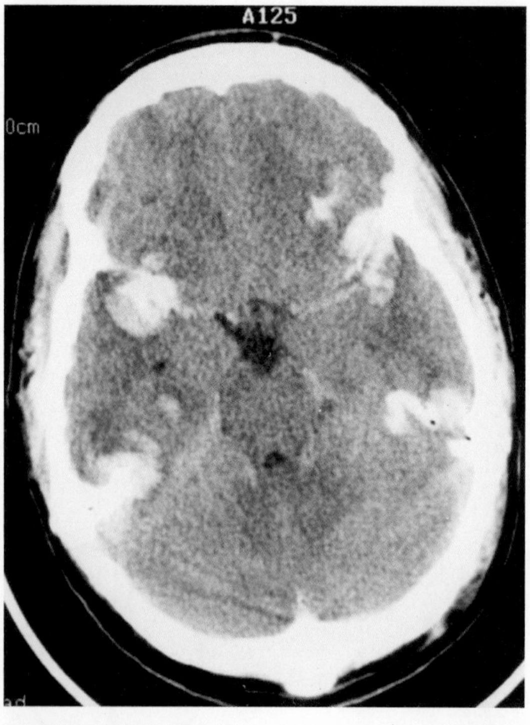

Figure 35-6. CT scan without contrast infusion showing areas of hemorrhagic contusion adjacent to bony prominences. There is also slight subarachnoid blood along the tentorium and in the insular cisterns, both of which are typical of traumatic bleeding.

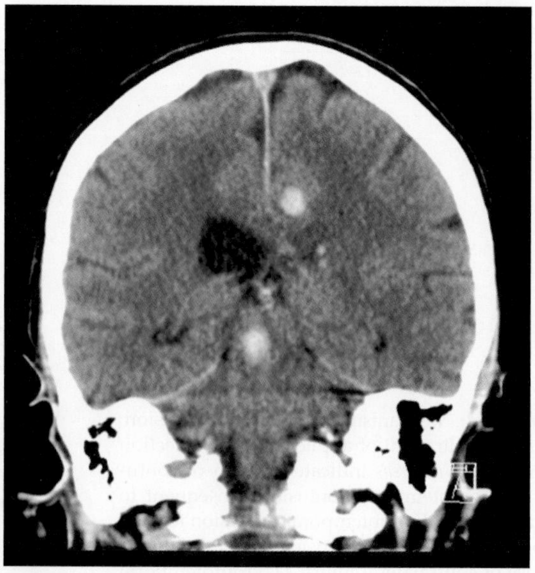

Figure 35-7. Coronal MRI showing small hemorrhages in the callosum and midbrain that are considered part of the spectrum of diffuse axonal shearing injuries.

as the series by Kampfl and colleagues, suggest that diffuse axonal injury may be the substrate of the persistent vegetative state. However, in most cases of severe cranial injury and protracted coma, there have been major sites of injury in the midbrain and subthalamus, i.e., in the zones subjected to the greatest torque, and these latter lesions may be the critical ones in persistent coma and vegetative state (Adams et al 2000, Ropper and Miller). This was true of the cases of persistent coma described by Jellinger and Seitelberger. Notable, again, was that these deep lesions coincided with the postulated locus of reversible concussive paralysis.

Primary brainstem hemorrhages due to torsion and tearing of tissue at the time of impact are distinguished from the secondary hemorrhages that are a result of the effects of downward displacement of the brainstem. Duret originally emphasized the medullary location of these secondary hemorrhages, but the term *Duret hemorrhage* has come to signify all brainstem hemorrhages when there is mass effect that distorts the brainstem.

In addition to contusions and extradural, subdural, subarachnoid, and intracerebral hemorrhages, closed head injury induces variable degrees of vasogenic edema that increases during the first 24 to 48 h and sometimes, small zones of infarction that have been attributed to vascular spasm caused by subarachnoid blood surrounding basal vessels. The frequency and importance of this type of secondary cerebral infarction have been debated. A retrospective imaging study by Marino and colleagues found that 17 of 89 patients had regions of stroke after moderate or severe head injury. Most were in the distribution of a major branch or penetrating cerebral vessel or in a watershed territory.

The presence of intracranial hypertension has also been associated with a higher incidence of infarction. Marmarou and colleagues demonstrated that *brain swelling* after head injury is essentially the result of edema and not of an increase in cerebral blood volume, as has long been postulated. In children, and in some cases in adults, the cerebral edema may be massive and lead to secondary brainstem compression.

Cerebral Fat Embolism

With fractures of large bones in cases of generalized trauma, with or without head injury, after 24 to 72 h there may be an acute onset of pulmonary symptoms (dyspnea and hyperpnea) followed by coma with or without focal signs or seizures. This sequence is a result of systemic fat embolism, first of the lungs and then of the brain. Cranial trauma is not required. In some cases the onset of pulmonary symptoms is associated with a petechial rash over the thorax, especially in the axillae and also in the conjunctivea and 1 in 3 cases is said to show fat globules in the urine. The specificity of the last of these findings has been questioned. Respiratory distress is the most important and often the only feature of the fat embolism syndrome, evident in the chest film as fluffy infiltrates in both lungs. In the brain, multiple small fat emboli cause widespread petechial hemorrhages and small infarctions, involving both white and gray matter and a few larger infarcts. Most patients with fat embolism recover spontaneously in 3 or 4 days, although a mortality rate of up to 10 percent is cited, usually related to underlying systemic and bony injuries. Treatment, aside from respiratory support, is supportive. Heparin, which had been used in the past, is not considered effective.

APPROACH TO THE PATIENT WITH HEAD INJURY

The physician first called on to examine a patient who has had a closed head injury will generally find one of three clinical conditions as indicated by the headings below, each of which is dealt with differently. It is usually possible to categorize the patient by assessing the mental and neurologic status when first seen and at intervals after the accident. The *Glasgow Coma Scale* is used as a rapid reference to accomplish this purpose (Table 35-1) but does not substitute for a fuller neurologic examination. The scale registers three aspects of neurologic function: eye opening, verbal response, and motor response to various stimuli. The scale uses a summed score with a maximum of 15; a score of 7 or less is considered to reflect severe trauma and a poor clinical state, 8 to 12, moderate injury,

Table 35-1

GLASGOW COMA SCALE (TOTAL SCORE IS USED FOR SERIAL ASSESSMENT AND PROGNOSIS)

EYES OPEN	
Never	1
To pain	2
To verbal stimuli	3
Spontaneously	4
BEST VERBAL RESPONSE	
No response	1
Incomprehensible sounds	2
Inappropriate words	3
Disoriented and converses	4
Oriented and converses	5
BEST MOTOR RESPONSE	
No response	1
Extension (decerebrate rigidity)	2
Flexion abnormal (decorticate rigidity)	3
Flexion withdrawal	4
Localizes pain	5
Obeys	6
Total	3–15

and higher scores, mild injury. The scores provided by this scale correspond roughly with the outcome of the head injury as discussed further on, but its main utility is in recording sequential changes in the patient's clinical state with an easily learned and reproducible tool.

Patients Who Are Conscious or Rapidly Regaining Consciousness (Concussion and Minor Head Injury)

This is the most frequently encountered clinical situation. Roughly, two degrees of disturbed function can be recognized within this category. In one, the patient was not unconscious at all but only stunned momentarily, "saw stars," or was briefly disoriented. This injury is insignificant when judged in terms of life or death and brain damage, although, as we point out further on, there is still the small possibility of a skull fracture or the later development of an epidural or subdural hematoma. Moreover, some patients are liable to a troublesome posttraumatic syndrome consisting of headache, giddiness, fatigability, insomnia, and nervousness that can appear soon after or within a few days of the injury. This problem is discussed in a later section. In the instance of consciousness that was temporarily abolished for a few seconds or minutes, recovery may already be complete, or the patient may be in one of the stages of partial recovery described earlier. Even though mentally clear, there is amnesia for events immediately preceding and following the injury. The latter produces a circumscribed confusional state that is usually confined to inattention and may be ongoing when the patient is first examined. It is characterized by a dazed appearance and repetitive questions from the patient about the circumstances that led to his being found.

In most such mild cases, a brief assessment for mental clarity, weakness, ocular abnormalities, and Babinski signs is appropriate, but there is little need of extensive neurologic consultation and hospitalization is not required, provided that a responsible family member is available to report any change in the clinical state. In only a small group of these patients, mainly in those who are slow in regaining consciousness or who have severe headache, vomiting, or a skull fracture, is there significant risk of intracerebral hemorrhage or other delayed complications.

Whether to obtain imaging of the head routinely in such patients is an unresolved problem. In our litigious society, the physician is inclined to obtain a CT scan. If there is no subarachnoid blood (a common finding) or intraparenchymal clot or contusion, and the patient is mentally clear there is little chance of developing an extradural hemorrhage. The presence of a fracture may increase these odds but most studies, such as the one by Lloyd and colleagues have found that the presence of a skull fracture in children proves to be a relatively poor indicator of intracranial injury. The exception is a fracture through the squamous bone and the groove of the middle meningeal artery, which represents a risk for arterial bleeding and epidural hemorrhage.

With the current focus on the cost-effective use of ancillary studies, criteria that justify obtaining a cranial CT following minor forms of head trauma have been developed. We have generally advised a CT in cases of head injury that was associated with prolonged loss of consciousness (more than 1 min), severe and persisting headache, nausea and vomiting, a confusional state, and any new, objective neurologic signs, but these are admittedly arbitrary criteria. The CT scan may be particularly important in elderly patients with minor head trauma, in whom the presence of an intracranial lesion (mainly subdural hematoma) may not be predicted by clinical signs. However, in children, it may be advisable to perform the scans more liberally. This is underscored by the results of a study of 215 children with minor head trauma conducted by Simon and colleagues: 34 children with no known loss of consciousness and a Glasgow Coma Scale score of 15 nonetheless displayed intracranial lesions, 3 of whom required surgery.

Several studies in adults have given broad guidance in choosing which patients to scan ("New Orleans Criteria" and "Canadian CT Head Rule"; Table 35-2). They include features that are sensitive but not specific for intracranial injury, such as age above 60 years, intoxication, more than 30 min of retrograde amnesia, suspected skull fracture, seizure, anticoagulation, and dangerous mechanism of injury, (see Smits et al and Stiell et al). These two validated schemes for assisting in the determination of need for CT scanning in the emergency department are included for the reader's reference but they should be viewed as broad guidelines with fairly

Table 35-2

THE NEW ORLEANS AND CANADIAN CLINICAL DECISION RULES FOR CT AFTER CONCUSSION

New Orleans Criteria[a]—Glasgow Coma Scale score of 15
Headache
Vomiting
Age >60 y
Drug or alcohol intoxication
Persistent anterograde amnesia (deficits in short-term memory)
Evidence of traumatic soft-tissue or bone injury above clavicles
Seizure
Canadian CT Head Rule[b]—Glasgow Coma Scale score of 13–15 for patients age 16 y and older
High risk of neurosurgical intervention
Glasgow Coma Scale score <15 within 2 h after surgery
Suspected open or depressed skull fracture
Any sign of basal skull fracture
Two or more episodes of vomiting
Age >54 y
Moderate risk of brain injury detected by CT
Retrograde amnesia for ≥30 min
Dangerous mechanism

[a]Adapted from Haydel et al.
[b]Adapted from Stiell et al.

high sensitivity for important lesions on the CT, but low specificity so that most CT scans done under these advisories can be expected to be normal. These issues are addressed in a review by Ropper and Gorson.

Minor and seemingly trivial head injuries may sometimes be followed by a number of puzzling and worrisome clinical phenomena, some insignificant, others serious and indicative of a pathologic process other than concussion. The latter are described below. When they occur, a neurologic or neurosurgical evaluation is indicated.

Drowsiness, Headache, and Confusion These symptoms occur most often in children, who, minutes or hours after a concussive head injury, seem not to be themselves. They lie down, are drowsy, complain of headache, and may vomit—symptoms that suggest the presence of an intracranial hemorrhage. Mild focal edema near the point of impact may be seen on MRI. There is usually no skull fracture but, as Nee and colleagues point out, vomiting is associated with an increase in the incidence of skull fracture and the New Orleans and Canadian CT rules found vomiting to be a factor associated with intracranial bleeding (Table 35-2). The symptoms subside after a few hours, attesting to the benign nature of the condition in most cases but some form of cerebral imaging is required.

Transient Paraplegia, Blindness, and Migrainous Phenomena With falls or blows on top of the head, both legs may become temporarily weak and numb, with wavering bilateral Babinski signs and sometimes with sphincteric incontinence. Impact over the occiput may cause temporary blindness. The symptoms disappear after a few hours. It seems possible that these transient symptoms represent a direct localized concussive effect, caused either by indentation of the skull or by impact on these parts of the brain against the inner table of the skull, but a vascular mechanism cannot be excluded. The blindness and paraplegia are usually followed by a throbbing, vascular type of headache. Transient migrainous visual phenomena, aphasia, or hemiparesis, followed by a headache, are observed sometimes after minimal concussion in athletes who participate in competitive contact sports. Possibly all of these phenomena are the result of an attack of migraine induced by a blow to the head. These focal syndromes can be perplexing for a few hours, especially if it is the first such attack of migraine in a child. Possibilities to be remembered, particularly in cases of acute quadriplegia, is traumatic cord compression or the rarer cartilaginous embolism of the cervical cord (see "Fibrocartilaginous Embolism" in Chap. 44). A concussion of the cervical portion of the spinal cord is another potential mechanism of transient paraplegia.

Episodes of transient global amnesia after minor head injury have been described by Haas and Ross, as mentioned in Chap. 21. The problem in interpreting these spells is their similarity to posttraumatic amnesia and the repetitive stereotyped questioning regarding orientation that is common to both processes. A duration of 2 to 24 h and the feature of repetitive querying were suggested by Haas and Ross as differentiating the two conditions but the separation on this basis is not compelling.

Delayed Hemiplegia The main causes of delayed hemiplegia are a late-evolving epidural or subdural hematoma and, in more severe injuries, an intracerebral hemorrhage. Most of these are associated with a diminution in the level of consciousness from the outset but there are exceptions.

Dissection of the internal carotid artery should always be considered in cases of delayed hemiplegia. The dissection may occur in the extracranial or the intracranial portion of the carotid artery and should be sought by vascular imaging study if the hemiparesis has no other explanation. In other instances, the hemiplegia has no clear explanation other than the blow to the head, perhaps related to the migraine phenomenon described earlier.

Serious Cerebral Damage Following a Lucid Interval

This group is smaller than the other two but is of importance because it includes a disproportionate number of patients who are in urgent need of surgical treatment. The initial loss of consciousness from concussion may have lasted only a few minutes or, exceptionally, there may have been no period of unresponsiveness at all, in which instance one might wrongly conclude that there was no concussion and little possibility of traumatic hemorrhage or other type of brain injury. Patients who display this sequence of events, in the past referred to vividly as "talk and die" by Marshall and associates (1983), have late deterioration because of the expansion of a subdural hematoma, worsening brain edema around a contusion, or the delayed appearance of an epidural clot. Among 34 such patients in the Traumatic Coma Data Bank who had this type of lucid interval, the majority showed substantial degrees of midline shift on the initial CT scan, reflecting the presence of early brain edema and contusion (Marshall et al, 1983). A somewhat related condition of delayed intracerebral hematoma (*spät apoplexie*), discussed further on, is a feature of a more severe initial head injury that usually produces coma from the onset. The problem of cerebral fat embolism, mentioned earlier, should be considered in these cases of delayed deterioration, especially if there is interposed respiratory failure.

Patients Who Remain Comatose from the Time of Head Injury

Here, the central problem, set forth by Symonds, is the relationship between concussion and contusion and other forms of persisting structural brain damage. Because consciousness is abolished at the moment of injury, one can hardly doubt the existence of concussion in such cases; but when hours pass without consciousness being regained, the second half of the usual definition of concussion—that the disruption of cerebral function be transitory—is not satisfied. Pathologic examination of such cases usually discloses evidence of increased intracranial pressure and of cerebral contusions, subarachnoid hemorrhage, zones of infarction, and scattered intracerebral hemorrhages both at the point of injury (coup) and on the opposite side (contrecoup), in the corpus callosum, and between these points, along the line of force of the impact. In some patients, the diffuse axonal type of injury is prominent or, as mentioned, there are separate but strategically placed ischemic and hemorrhagic lesions in the upper midbrain and lower thalamic region. Varying amounts of blood in the subarachnoid and subdural spaces are present. Displacement of the thalamus and midbrain may be present, with compression of the opposite cerebral peduncle against the free margin of the tentorium as well as secondary midbrain hemorrhages and zones of necrosis; in some cases, there is transtentorial herniation.

Severe head injury is often associated with an immediate arrest of respiration and sometimes with bradyarrhythmia and cardiac arrest. The immediate effects on the brain of these systemic changes may in themselves be sufficiently profound to cause coma. Intracranial pressure is almost always elevated and imaging of the brain shows various degrees of brain swelling, ventricular compression, and displacement of midline structure. Also, head injury often complicates alcohol and drug ingestion, so the possibility of a toxic or metabolic encephalopathy as the cause (or a contributing cause) of stupor must always be considered.

In all of these patients, following the initial period of stabilization, the matter of interest is the clinical and imaging assessment, with the purpose of uncovering a surgically remediable lesion, namely a subdural or epidural hematoma or a treatable intraparenchymal hematoma. In most cases, the discovery of such a mass lesion leads to surgical removal. But unless it is the only lesion, the procedure often proves to be insufficient and coma is likely to persist because of the associated cerebral damage. The recognition and management of these hematomas are described further on.

In the Traumatic Coma Data Bank, which included 1,030 gravely injured patients with Glasgow Coma Scale scores of 8 or less, 21 percent had subdural hematomas, 11 percent had intracerebral clots, and 5 percent had epidural hematomas. Notable, however, half the patients had no mass lesions on the CT scan. On this basis, these patients were thought to have diffuse axonal injury. However, in 50 consecutive autopsies of severely injured patients, summarized in an earlier era by Rowbotham, all but 2 showed macroscopic changes, suggesting the relative unreliability of CT analysis. The lesions in these cases consisted of surface contusions (48 percent), lacerations of the cerebral cortex (28 percent), subarachnoid hemorrhage (72 percent), subdural hematoma (15 percent), extradural hemorrhage (20 percent), and skull fractures (72 percent). As these figures indicate, several pathologic entities were found in the same patient.

There is that relatively small, distressing group of severely brain-injured patients in whom the vital signs become normal but who never regain full consciousness. As the weeks pass, the prospects become bleaker. Such a patient, especially if a child, may still emerge from coma after 6 to 12 weeks or longer and make a relatively good, although usually incomplete, recovery. Some of those who survive for long periods open their eyes and move their heads and eyes from side to side but betray no evidence of seeing or recognizing even the closest members of their families. They do not speak and are capable of only primitive postural or reflex withdrawal movements. Jennett and Plum referred to this as the "persistent vegetative state" (see Chap. 17 for a full discussion of this subject). Fourteen percent of the patients in the Traumatic Coma Data Bank remained in this state. Hemiplegia or quadriplegia with varying degrees of decerebrate or decorticate posturing are usually present. Life is terminated after several months or years by some medical complication but some of our patients have survived for decades. Our colleague R.D. Adams has examined the brains of 14 patients who remained in coma and in vegetative states from 1 to 14 years. All showed extensive zones of necrosis and hemorrhage in the upper brainstem. Among patients who survived and remained vegetative until death, Adams and colleagues (2000) found that 80 percent had thalamic damage and 71 percent had findings of diffuse axonal injury. Moreover, trauma of extracranial organs and tissues is frequent and obviously contributes to the fatal outcome. Recent functional studies have shown that a limited proportion of patients who are in a vegetative or minimally conscious state can be trained to purposefully engage parts of the cerebrum.

In generalizing about this category of head injury, the effects of contusion, hemorrhage, and brain swelling often become evident within 18 to 36 h after the injury and then may progress for several days. If a patient survives this period, his chances of dying from complications of these effects are greatly reduced. The mortality rate of those who reach the hospital in coma is approximately 20 percent, and most of the deaths occur in the first 12 to 24 h as a result of direct injury to the brain in combination with other nonneurologic injuries. Of those alive at 24 h, the overall mortality falls to 7 to 8 percent; after 48 h, only 1 to 2 percent of patients succumb. There is some evidence that transfer of such patients to an intensive care unit, where personnel experienced in the handling of head injury can monitor them, improves the chances for survival (see further on).

One modest advance in the medical treatment of traumatic unresponsiveness has come from a randomized trial by Giacino and colleagues. Amantadine accelerated slightly the emergence from the vegetative or minimally conscious state; it was given for 4 weeks between the fourth and twelfth weeks after injury, 100 mg twice per day and increasing to 200 mg twice per day. The effects were less evident by 6 weeks but this seems like a promising approach. In cases of longer standing, deep brain stimulation of thalamic nuclei has been explored intermittently in past decades and has had some notable successes.

SPECIFIC TRAUMATIC CRANIAL LESIONS (Table 35-3)

The following lesions are considered in all cases of serious initial injury. They each have characteristic clinical and imaging features but they may be admixed and the contribution of each to the clinical state must be assessed before deciding on a course of action.

Table 35-3

CLINICAL AND RADIOGRAPHIC CHARACTERISTICS OF THE MAIN TRAUMATIC BRAIN LESIONS

	EPIDURAL HEMATOMA	ACUTE SUBDURAL HEMATOMA	CHRONIC SUBDURAL HEMATOMA	CONTUSION/ PARENCHYMAL HEMORRHAGE	INTRAVENTRICULAR HEMATOMA	SUBARACHNOID HEMORRHAGE	SUBDURAL HYGROMA	DIFFUSE AXONAL INJURY
Causative factor	Laceration of middle cerebral artery or dural sinus	Tearing of bridging pial veins and arteries	Trauma (may be absent or minimal) Risk factors: coagulopathy and severe brain atrophy	Shearing of parenchymal vessels Risk factors: coagulopathy and amyloid vasculopathy	Shearing of parenchymal vessels; rule out vascular defects	Exclude underlying aneurysmal rupture	Arachnoid tear, following meningitis	Deceleration or rotational forces
Typical location	Lateral cerebral convexities	Lateral cerebral convexities	Lateral cerebral convexities, may be bilateral	Inferior frontal and temporal lobes	Lateral and third ventricles blood filled	Basilar cisterns	Lateral cerebral convexities	Deep white matter, corpus callosum, dorsolateral pons
Evolution	Hours	Many hours	Days to weeks	Expand over 12–48 h	Rapid	Minutes to hours	Days to weeks	From time of injury
Clinical profile	Typically, lucid interval then coma, but more variable; pupillary dilatation with contralateral then bilateral limb weakness; slowly evolving stupor then coma	Drowsiness, coma; pupillary dilatation with contralateral then bilateral limb weakness; progressive stupor then coma	Headache, progressive alteration in mental status ± focal neurologic signs	Stupor → coma, dilated pupil, progressive hemiplegia, spasticity	Progressive signs of hydrocephalus	Headache, meningismus, delayed manifestations, vasospasm	Mimics chronic subdural hematoma	Coma, posturing, normal intracranial pressure
Age at risk	Children, young adults	Any	Elderly	Any	Any	Any	Infants, children, adults	Any
Radiologic features	Acute bulging epidural clot bounded by cranial sutures; lenticular in shape	Acute blood rimming broad region of cerebral convexity	Hyper- or isodense, unilateral or bilateral	Multiple, confluent regions of edema intermixed with focal, acute blood	Focal, acute blood within ventricles; may layer with gravity	Acute blood lining cortex in subarachnoid space	Focal, CSF density, fluid collection	CT may be normal; MRI shows evolving small deep contusions
Surgical intervention	Urgent evacuation	Urgent evacuation if large enough to cause symptoms	Evacuation in some circumstances	Evacuate if large	Shunting	May cause secondary vasospasm or late hydrocephalus	Aspiration of fluid	None

Acute Epidural Hemorrhage

As a rule, epidural hematoma arises with a temporal or parietal fracture and laceration of the middle meningeal artery or vein. Less often, there is a tear in a dural venous sinus. The injury, even when it fractures the skull, may not have produced coma initially, or it may be part of a devastating craniocerebral injury. A typical example is that of a child who has fallen from a bicycle or swing or has suffered some other hard blow to the head and was unconscious only momentarily. A few hours later (exceptionally, with venous bleeding the interval may be several days or a week), headache of increasing severity develops, with vomiting, drowsiness, confusion, aphasia, seizures (which may be one-sided), hemiparesis with slightly increased tendon reflexes, and a Babinski sign. As coma develops, the hemiparesis may give way to bilateral spasticity of the limbs and Babinski signs. The heart rate is often slow (below 60 beats/min) and bounding, with a concomitant rise in systolic blood pressure (Cushing effect). The pupil may dilate on the side of the hematoma. Physicians need not be reminded that lumbar puncture is contraindicated in this setting, particularly now that CT and MRI are available. Death, which is almost invariable if an expanding clot is not removed surgically, comes at the end of a comatose period and is a result of respiratory arrest. The visualization of a fracture line across the groove of the middle meningeal artery and knowledge of which side of the head was struck (the clot is on that side) are of aid in diagnosis and lateralization of the lesion. However, meningeal vessels may occasionally be torn without fracture. The CT scan is definitive and reveals a lens-shaped clot with a smooth inner margin (Fig. 35-8).

Treatment of Epidural Hematoma The surgical procedure consists of placement of burr holes in an emergency situation or, preferably, a craniotomy, drainage of the hematoma, and identification and ligation of the bleeding vessel. The operative results are excellent except in cases with extended fractures and laceration of the dural venous sinuses, in which the epidural hematoma may be bilateral rather than unilateral. If coma, bilateral Babinski signs, spasticity, or decerebrate rigidity supervene before operation, it usually means that displacement of central structures and compression of the midbrain have already occurred; prognosis is then poor, but a few patients do well if surgery is not greatly delayed. Small epidural hemorrhages can be followed by serial CT scanning and will be seen to enlarge gradually for a week or two and then be absorbed. There is controversy about the benefit of removing these smaller clots in a patient who has no symptoms; with careful clinical and imaging surveillance, most can be left alone.

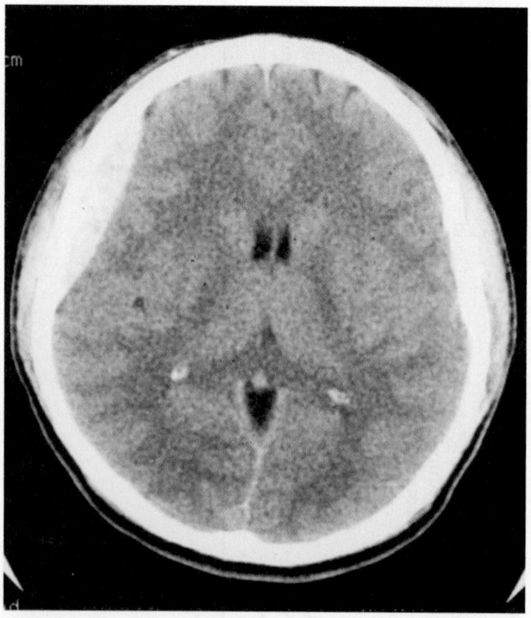

Figure 35-8. Acute epidural hematoma. Unenhanced CT scan showing a typical lens-shaped frontal epidural clot.

Acute and Chronic Subdural Hematomas

The problems created by acute and chronic subdural hematomas are so different that they must be considered separately. In *acute subdural hematoma*, which may be unilateral or bilateral, there may be a brief lucid interval between the blow to the head and the advent of coma. More often, the patient is comatose from the time of the injury and the coma deepens progressively. Acute subdural hematoma may be combined with epidural hemorrhage, cerebral contusion, or laceration. The clinical effects of these several lesions are difficult to distinguish and there are a few patients in whom it is impossible to state before operation whether the clot is epidural or subdural in location. Subdural clots more than a few millimeter in thickness can be accurately visualized by the CT scan in more than 90 percent of cases, but the window settings must be appropriate to avoid obscuring of the clot by adjacent bone (Fig. 35-9). A large acute clot causes a shift of midline structure as well as marked compression of one lateral ventricle; but if there are bilateral clots, there may be no shift and the ventricles may appear symmetrically compressed.

Rapidly evolving subdural hematomas are usually a result of tearing of bridging veins, and symptoms are caused by compression of the adjacent brain and of deep structures. Unlike epidural arterial hemorrhage, which is steadily progressive, the rising intracranial pressure usually arrests the venous bleeding.

Exceptionally, the subdural hematoma forms in the *posterior fossa* and gives rise to headache, vomiting, pupillary inequality, dysphagia, cranial-nerve palsies, and, rarely, stiff neck, and ataxia of the trunk and gait if the patient is well enough to be tested for these functions. Because of their apposition to bone or an axial orientation along the tentorial dura, posterior fossa clots are likely to be overlooked in CT scans.

In *chronic subdural hematoma*, the traumatic etiology is often less clear. The head injury, especially in elderly persons and in those taking anticoagulant drugs, may have been trivial and forgotten. A period of weeks then follows when headaches (not invariable), light-headedness, slowness in thinking, apathy and drowsiness, unsteady gait,

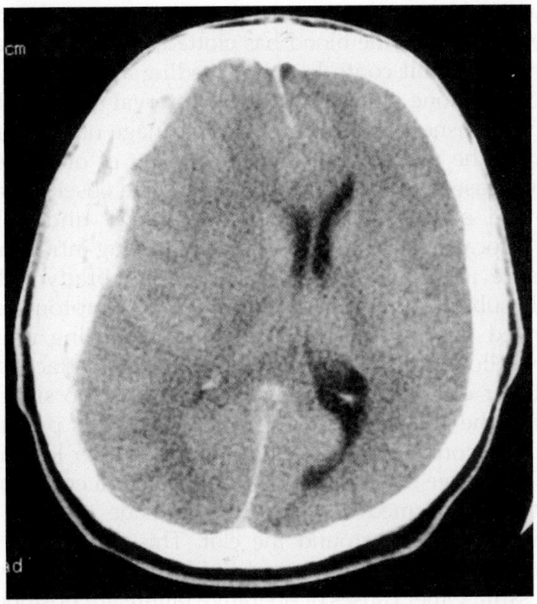

Figure 35-9. Acute subdural hematoma over the right convexity, with substantial mass effect (displacement) of brain tissue but little edema.

and occasionally a seizure are the main symptoms. The initial impression may be that the patient has a vascular lesion or brain tumor or is suffering from drug intoxication, a depressive illness, or Alzheimer disease. Gradual expansion of the hematoma by one of several mechanisms discussed further on is believed to cause the progression of symptoms. As with acute subdural hematoma, the disturbances of mentation and consciousness (drowsiness, inattentiveness, and confusion) are more prominent than focal or lateralizing signs, and they may fluctuate. Focal signs, when present, consist of mild hemiparesis and, rarely, an aphasic disturbance. Homonymous hemianopia is seldom observed, probably because the geniculocalcarine pathway is deep and not easily compressed; similarly, hemiplegia, i.e., complete paralysis of one arm and leg, is usually indicative of a lesion within the cerebral hemisphere rather than a compressive lesion on its surface. Hemiparesis from subdural hematoma may sometimes be ipsilateral to the clot, the result of compression of the contralateral cerebral peduncle against the free edge of the tentorium (Kernohan-Woltman sign; see "Pathoanatomy of Brain Displacement and Herniations" in Chap. 17). If the condition progresses, the patient becomes stuporous or comatose. But this course is often interrupted by striking fluctuations of awareness.

With both large acute and chronic hematomas, dilatation of the ipsilateral pupil is a fairly reliable indicator of the side of the hematoma, although this sign may be misleading, occurring on the opposite side in 10 percent of cases, according to Pevehouse and coworkers. Convulsions are seen occasionally, most often in alcoholics or in patients with cerebral contusions, but they cannot be regarded as a cardinal sign of subdural hematoma. Rare cases of internuclear ophthalmoplegia and of chorea have been reported but have not occurred in our material. Presumably they are a result of distortion of deep structures. Also, brief and self-limited disturbances of neurologic function simulating transient ischemic attacks (TIAs) may occur with chronic hematomas; their mechanism is uncertain, but they do not appear to represent seizures. In infants and children, enlargement of the head, vomiting, and convulsions are prominent manifestations of subdural hematoma.

CT scanning with contrast infusion and MRI are the most reliable diagnostic procedures. On CT scans, the acute clot is initially hyperdense but becomes slowly more isodense after a period of 1 or more weeks (Fig. 35-10). At that stage it may be difficult to detect except by the tissue shifts it causes. The fluid collection then becomes progressively hypodense (with respect to the cortex) over 2 to 6 weeks. The evolution of signal changes in the MRI is similar to the sequential imaging changes found with parenchymal hematomas. The acute clot is hypointense on T2-weighted images, reflecting the presence of deoxyhemoglobin. Over the subsequent weeks, all image sequences show it as hyperintense as a result of methemoglobin formation. Eventually the chronic clot again becomes hypointense on the T1-weighted images. With contrast infusion, both imaging procedures usually reveal the vascular and reactive border surrounding the clot. Usually, by the fourth week, sometimes later, the hematoma becomes very hypodense, giving rise to a chronic subdural hygroma that is indistinguishable from idiopathic ones that are presumably caused by a rent in the arachnoid that allows CSF to escape to the subdural compartment, as discussed further on.

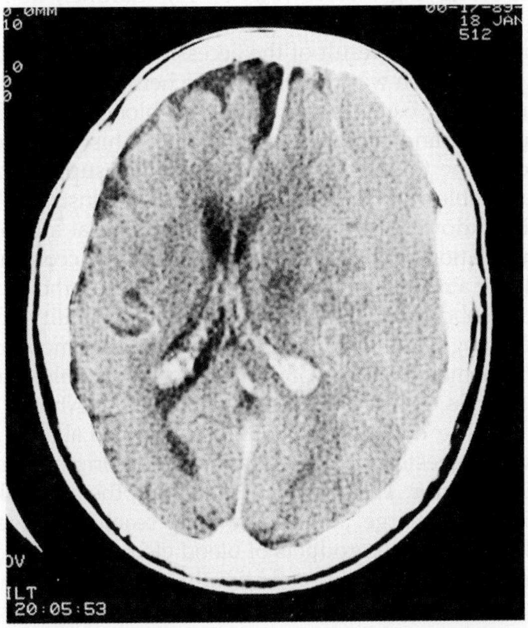

Figure 35-10. Subacute subdural hematoma on the left (*reader's right*). CT scans after administration of intravenous contrast material. The lesion is isodense to the adjacent brain tissue, but its margin can be appreciated with contrast enhancement. Note displacement of cerebral structures.

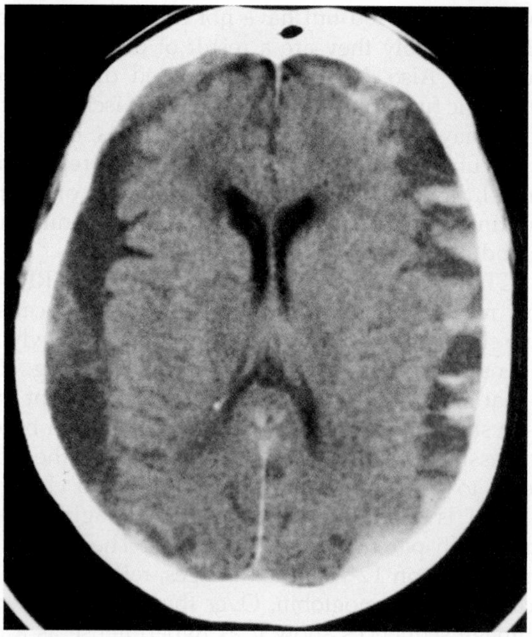

Figure 35-11. Chronic subdural hematomas over both cerebral hemispheres without shift of the ventricular system. Chronicity results in hypodense appearance of the clots. Some old blood can still be seen on the right side. The bilaterally balanced masses result in an absence of horizontal displacement, but they may compress the upper brainstem.

The chronic subdural hematoma becomes gradually encysted by fibrous membranes (pseudomembranes) that grow from the dura. Some hematomas, probably those in which the initial bleeding was slight (see below), resorb spontaneously. Others expand slowly and act as space-occupying masses (Fig. 35-11). Gardner, in 1932, first postulated that the gradual enlargement of the hematoma was a result of the accession of fluid, particularly CSF, which was drawn into the hemorrhagic cyst by its increasing osmotic tension as red blood cells (RBCs) hemolyzed and protein was liberated. This hypothesis, which came to be widely accepted, is not supported by the available data. Rabe and colleagues demonstrated that the breakdown of RBCs contributes little, if at all, to the accumulation of fluid in the subdural space. According to the latter authors, the most important factor in the expansion of subdural fluid is a pathologic permeability of the developing capillaries in the outer pseudomembrane of the hematoma. The CSF plays no discernible role in this process, contrary to the original view of Munro and Merritt. The experimental observations of Labadie and Glover suggested that the volume of the original clot is a critical factor: The larger its initial size, the more likely it will be to enlarge. An inflammatory reaction, triggered by the breakdown products of blood elements in the clot, appears to be an additional stimulus for growth as well as for neomembrane formation and its vascularization. In any event, as the hematoma enlarges, the compressive effects increase gradually.

Treatment of Subdural Hematoma In most cases of acute hematoma it is sufficient to place burr holes and evacuate the clot before coma has developed. Treatment of larger hematomas, particularly after several hours have passed and the blood has clotted, consists of craniotomy to permit control of the bleeding and removal of the clot. As one would expect, the interval between loss of consciousness and the surgical drainage of the clot is perhaps the most important determinant of outcome in serious cases. Thin, crescentic clots can be observed and followed over several weeks and surgery undertaken only if focal signs or indications of increasing intracranial pressure arise (headache, vomiting, and bradycardia). Small subdural hematomas causing no symptoms and followed by CT scans will self-absorb, leaving only a deep yellow, sometimes calcified membrane attached to the inner dural surface. If the acute clot is too small to explain the coma or other symptoms, there is probably extensive contusion of the cerebrum or another lesion.

To remove the more chronic hematomas a craniotomy must be performed and an attempt made to strip the membranes that surround the clot. This diminishes the likelihood of reaccumulation of fluid but it is not always successful. Other causes of operative failure are postoperative swelling of the compressed hemisphere or failure of the hemisphere to expand after removal of a large clot. The difficulty of managing these patients surgically should not be underestimated. Elderly patients may be slow to recover after removal of the chronic hematoma or may have a prolonged period of confusion. Postoperative expansion of the brain can be followed by serial CT scans and may take weeks. Small, asymptomatic chronic collections are usually left alone and followed serially by clinical and CT examination, first at several week and then longer intervals.

Although no longer a common practice, the administration of corticosteroids was an alternative to surgical removal of subacute and chronic subdural hematomas in patients with minor symptoms or with contraindications to surgery. This approach, reviewed by Bender and Christoff decades ago, has not been studied systematically but has been successful in a few of our patients (of course, they may have improved independent of the steroids).

Subdural Hygroma

This is a thinly encapsulated collection of clear or slightly xanthochromic fluid in the subdural space; such collections form after an injury, as well as after meningitis (in an infant or young child). As often, subdural hygromas appear without precipitant, presumably because of a ball-valve effect of an arachnoidal tear that allows cerebrospinal fluid to collect in the space between the arachnoid and the dura; brain atrophy is conducive to this process. Occasionally a hygroma originates from a tear in an arachnoidal cyst. It may be difficult to differentiate a long-standing subdural hematoma from hygroma, and some chronic subdural hematomas are probably the result of repeated small hemorrhages that arise from the membranes of hygromas. Shrinkage of the hydrocephalic brain after ventriculoperitoneal shunting is also conducive to the formation of a subdural hematoma or hygroma, in which case drowsiness, confusion, irritability, and low-grade fever are relieved when the subdural fluid is aspirated or drained. Intracranial hypotension is another cause of subdural hygromas. In adults, hygromas are usually asymptomatic and do not require treatment; they only are infrequently the cause of seizures.

Cerebral Contusion and Traumatic Intracerebral Hemorrhage

Severe closed head injury is almost universally accompanied by cortical contusions and surrounding edema. The mass effect of contusional swelling, if sufficiently large, becomes a major factor in the genesis of tissue shifts and raised intracranial pressure. The CT appearance of contusion was already described (see Figs. 35-4 and 35-5). In the first few hours after injury, the bleeding points in the contused area may appear small and innocuous. The main concern, however, is the tendency for a contused area to swell or to develop into a hematoma during the first several days after injury. This may give rise to delayed clinical deterioration, sometimes abrupt in onset and concurrent with the appearance of swelling of the damaged region on the CT scan. It has been claimed, on uncertain grounds, that the swelling in the region of an acute contusion is precipitated by excessive administration of intravenous fluids (fluid management is considered further on in this chapter). Craniotomy and decompression of the swollen brain may be of benefit in selected cases with elevated intracranial pressure but it has no effect on the focal neurologic deficit.

One or several intracerebral hemorrhages may be apparent immediately after head injury, or hemorrhage may be infrequently delayed in its development by several days (the earlier mentioned *spät apoplexie*). The bleeding is in the subcortical white matter of one lobe of the brain or in deeper structures such as the basal ganglia or thalamus. The injury had nearly always been severe; blood vessels as well as cortical tissue are torn.

The clinical picture of traumatic intracerebral hemorrhage is similar to that of hypertensive brain hemorrhage with deepening coma with hemiplegia, a dilating pupil, bilateral Babinski signs, and stertorous and irregular respirations. The additional mass may be manifest by an abrupt rise in blood pressure and in intracranial pressure.

Craniotomy with evacuation of an acute or delayed clot has given a successful result in some cases but the advisability of surgery is governed by several factors including the level of consciousness, the time from the initial injury, and the associated damage (contusions, subdural and epidural bleeding) shown by imaging studies. Application of intracranial pressure monitoring and of CT scans at intervals after the injury facilitates diagnosis. Boto and colleagues found that basal ganglia hemorrhages were prone to enlarge in the day or two after closed head injury and that those greater than 25 mL in volume were fatal in 9 of 10 cases.

It should be mentioned again that subarachnoid blood of some degree is very common after all degrees of head injury. A problem that sometimes arises in cases that display both contusions and subarachnoid blood is the possibility that a ruptured aneurysm was the initial event and that a resultant fall caused the contusions. In cases where the subarachnoid blood is concentrated around one of the major vessels of the circle of Willis, an angiogram is justified to exclude the latter possibility. Also in elderly patients, it has been difficult to determine whether a fall had been the cause or the result of a subarachnoid or an intracerebral hemorrhage. These subjects are addressed further in Chap. 34.

Acute Brain Swelling in Children

This condition is seen in the first hours after injury and may prove rapidly fatal. The CT scan shows enlargement of both hemispheres and compression of the basal cisterns and ventricles. There is usually no papilledema in the early stages, during which the child hyperventilates, vomits, and shows extensor posturing. The assumption has been that this represents a loss of regulation of cerebral blood flow and a massive increase in the blood volume of the brain. The administration of excessive water in intravenous fluids may contribute to the problem and should be avoided. Inappropriate secretion of antidiuretic hormone (ADH) also exaggerates the swelling in some children. We have not observed this complication in adults. Fear of massive brain swelling from a second impact after a concussion has been raised as a rationale for keeping youngsters from returning to athletic activity, but there is little evidence for the existence of this entity in adults as noted by McCrory and Berkovic.

"Shaken Baby" Syndrome

This form of craniocerebral trauma in infants is well known in large emergency practices and is now missed less frequently than in the past as practitioners have been sensitized to specifically consider it when an infant or child is injured. As the name implies, the inciting trauma is typically violent shaking of the body or head of an infant, resulting in rapid acceleration and deceleration of the cranium. The presence of this type of injury must often be inferred from the distribution and types of lesions on imaging studies or autopsy examination, but precision in examination is paramount because of its forensic and legal implications. The diagnosis is suspected from the combination of subdural hematomas and retinal hemorrhages, as summarized by Bonnier and colleagues. Sometimes there are occult skull fractures, but more often, there is little or no direct cranial trauma. Additional lesions may be evident on diffusion-weighted MRI, particularly in the white matter of the corpus callosum and the temporo-occipito-parietal region. This syndrome confers a high risk for slowing of cognitive development; in extreme cases there may be acquired microcephaly reflecting brain atrophy consequent to both contusions and infarctions. A low initial Glasgow Coma Scale score, severe retinal hemorrhages, and skull fractures are associated with poor outcomes. Old and recent fractures in other parts of the body should arouse suspicion of this syndrome.

Penetrating Wounds and Blast Injuries

Missiles and Fragments

The descriptions in the preceding pages apply to blunt, nonpenetrating injuries of the skull and their effects on the brain. In the past, the care of penetrating craniocerebral injuries was mainly the interest of the military surgeon, but—with the persistence of violent crime in society—such cases have also become commonplace on the emergency wards of general hospitals.

In civilian life, *missile injuries* are essentially caused by bullets fired from rifles or handguns at high velocities. Air is compressed in front of the bullet so that it has an explosive effect on entering tissue and causes damage for a considerable distance around the missile track. *Missile fragments*, or *shrapnel*, from exploding shells, mines, grenades, or bombs are the usual causes of penetrating cranial injuries in wartime. The cranial wounds that result from missiles and shrapnel have been classified by Purvis as tangential, with scalp lacerations, depressed skull fractures, and meningeal and cerebral lacerations; penetrating, with in-driven metal particles, hair, skin, and bone fragments; and through-and-through wounds.

In most penetrating injuries from high-velocity missiles, the object (such as a bullet) causes a high-temperature coagulative lesion that is sterile and does not require surgery if the projectile exits the skull. In these instances, the main considerations are the development of infection or CSF leaks or, in the long term, epilepsy or aneurysms in distal blood vessels. The latter are considered to be the result of disruption of the vessel wall by the local high-energy shock wave.

If the brain is penetrated at the lower levels of the brainstem, death is instantaneous because of respiratory and cardiac arrest. Even through-and-through wounds at higher levels, as a result of energy dissipated in the brain tissue, may damage vital centers sufficiently to cause death immediately or within a few minutes.

Once the initial complications are dealt with, the surgical problems, as outlined by Meirowsky, are reduced to three: prevention of infection by debridement accompanied by the administration of broad-spectrum antibiotics; control of increased intracranial pressure and shift of midline structures by removal of clots of blood and the administration of mannitol or other dehydrating agents, and the prevention of life-threatening systemic complications.

When first seen, the majority of patients with penetrating cerebral lesions are comatose. A small metal fragment may have penetrated the skull without causing concussion, but this is usually not true of high-velocity missiles. In a series of 132 patients analyzed by Frazier and Ingham, consciousness was lost initially in 120. The depth and duration of coma seemed to depend on the degree of cerebral necrosis, edema, and hemorrhage. In the series of the Traumatic Coma Data Bank, the mortality rate in 163 patients who were initially comatose from a cranial gunshot wound is 88 percent—more than twice the rate from severe blunt head injury. On emerging from coma, the patient passes through states of stupor, confusion, and amnesia, not unlike those following severe closed head injuries. Focal or focal and generalized seizures occur in the early phase of the injury in some 15 to 20 percent of cases.

Recovery may take many months. Frazier and Ingham commented on the "loss of memory, slow cerebration, indifference, mild depression, inability to concentrate, sense of fatigue, irritability, vasomotor, and cardiac instability, frequent seizures, headaches, and giddiness, all reminiscent of the residual symptoms from severe closed head injury with contusions." Every possible combination of focal cerebral symptoms may be caused by such lesions. The excellent older articles by Feiring and Davidoff, by Russell, and by Teuber are still very useful references on this subject.

Epilepsy is the most troublesome sequela and is described further on. Ascroft and also Caviness, in reviewing World War II cases, found that approximately half of all patients with bullet or shrapnel wounds that had penetrated the dura eventually developed seizures, most focal in nature; the figures reported by Caveness for Korean War veterans are about the same.

CSF rhinorrhea, discussed earlier and in Chap. 30, may occur as an acute manifestation of a penetrating injury that produces a fracture through the frontal, ethmoid, or sphenoid bones. Cairns listed these acute cases as a separate group in his classification of CSF rhinorrheas, the others being (1) a delayed form after craniocerebral injury, (2) a form that follows sinus and cranial surgery, and (3) a spontaneous variety. *Pneumoencephalocele (aerocele)*—i.e., air entering the cerebral subarachnoid space or ventricles spontaneously or as a result of sneezing or blowing the nose—is evidence of an opening from the paranasal sinus through the dura, as mentioned earlier in relation to skull fracture (see Fig. 35-3).

Blast Injuries

The shock wave of an explosive device such as bomb can propel objects into the cranium but there is also a direct form of organ damage from the dissipation of energy that occurs at the interfaces of tissues of different densities. This form of barotrauma invariably ruptures the tympanic membranes, a sign that is a marker of blast injury (Xydakis et al). Deafness, tinnitus, and vertigo are common accompaniments from cochlear concussion. The lung is next most often affected.

Loss of consciousness may occur but there is little understanding of the mechanism aside from the more conventional flinging of the skull from the pressure wave. As summarized in an editorial by one of the authors, the initial shock wave is followed by a supersonic blast wind and a reverse and prolonged front of underpressure. Tissues are damaged when energy is dissipated at the interface between air and liquid that presents a change in acoustic impedance. The subsequent blast wind is the source of separate injury, throwing people against fixed objects and dispersing projectiles that penetrate the body. Potential modes of conduction of the force of the blast to the cranial contents include the acceleration and deceleration of the head as a wave passes by, which essentially results in concussion; skull deformation which squeezes the brain; the indirect passage of the shock wave through the lungs; and the entry of the wave through the openings in the cranial vault, specifically, the acoustic and optic canals and the foramen magnum.

Acute gas embolism of the brain vessels has also been reported in the military medical literature. DePalma and colleagues have thoroughly reviewed blast injuries but the neurologic literature is quite deficient and does not settle whether the percussion wave can produce unconsciousness by direct "concussion" of brain tissue in the original meaning of the term.

SEQUELAE OF HEAD INJURY

Posttraumatic Epilepsy (See also Chap. 16)

Seizures are the most common delayed sequela of craniocerebral trauma, with an overall incidence of approximately 5 percent in patients with closed head injuries and 50 percent in those who had sustained a compound skull fracture and direct wounds of the brain. The basis is nearly always a contusion or laceration of the cortex. As one might expect, the risk of developing posttraumatic epilepsy is also related to the overall severity of the closed head injury. In a civilian cohort of 2,747 head-injured patients described by Annegers and colleagues (1980), the risk of seizures after severe head injury (defined by loss of consciousness or amnesia for more than 24 h, including subdural hematoma and brain contusion) was 7 percent within 1 year and 11.5 percent in 5 years. If the injury was only moderate (unconsciousness or amnesia for 30 min to 24 h or causing only a skull fracture), the risk fell to 0.7 and 1.6 percent, respectively. After mild injury (loss of consciousness or amnesia of less than 30 min), the incidence of seizures was not significantly greater than in the general population. In a subsequent study, Annegers and colleagues (1998) expanded the original cohort to include 4,541 children and adults with cerebral trauma. The results were much the same as those of the first study except that in patients with mild closed head injuries, there was only a slight excess risk of developing seizures—a risk that remained elevated only until the fifth year after injury. The likelihood of epilepsy is said to be greater in parietal and posterior frontal lesions, but it may arise from lesions in any area of the cerebral cortex. Also, the frequency of seizures is considerably higher after penetrating cranial injury, as cited earlier.

The interval between the head injury and the first seizure varies greatly. A small number of patients have convulsive movements within moments of the injury (*immediate epilepsy*). Usually this amounts to a brief tonic extension of the limbs, with slight shaking movements immediately after concussion, followed by awakening in a mild confusional state. Whether this represents a true epileptic phenomenon or, as appears more likely, is the result of arrest of cerebral blood flow or a transient brainstem dysfunction is unclear. Some 4 to 5 percent of hospitalized head-injured individuals are said to have one or more seizures within the first week of their injury (*early epilepsy*). The immediate seizures have a good prognosis and we tend not to treat them as if they represented epilepsy; on the other hand, late seizures are significantly more frequent in patients who had experienced epilepsy in the first week after injury (not including the convulsions of the immediate injury; Jennett). Seizures occurring minutes or hours after the injury in an otherwise fully awake patient have sometimes turned out to be factitious in our experience.

The term *posttraumatic epilepsy* usually refers to late epilepsy, i.e., to seizures that develop several weeks or months after closed head injury (1 to 3 months in most cases). Approximately 6 months after injury, half the patients who will develop epilepsy have had their first episode; by the end of 2 years, the figure rises to 80 percent (Walker). Data derived from a 15-year study of military personnel with severe (penetrating) brain wounds indicate that patients who escape seizures for 1 year after injury can be 75 percent certain of remaining seizure-free; patients without seizures for 2 years can be 90 percent certain; and for 3 years, 95 percent certain. For the less-severely injured (mainly closed head injuries), the corresponding times are 2 to 6 months, 12 to 17 months, and 21 to 25 months (Weiss et al). Despite this, there is no doubt that seizures in adulthood occur for which there is no other explanation than a small scarred cortical contusion that had been acquired decades before. The interval between head injury and development of seizures is said to be longer in children.

Posttraumatic seizures (both focal and generalized) tend to decrease in frequency as the years pass, and a significant number of patients (10 to 30 percent, according to Caviness) eventually stop having them. Status epilepticus is uncommon. Individuals who have early attacks (within a week of injury) are more likely to have a complete remission of their seizures than those whose attacks begin a year or so after injury. A low frequency of attacks is another favorable prognostic sign. Alcoholism is considered to have an adverse effect on this seizure state, but there are no systematic studies of this subject. Our colleague, M. Victor, observed some 25 patients with posttraumatic epilepsy in whom seizures had ceased altogether for several years, only to recur in relation to drinking. In these patients the seizures were precipitated by a weekend or even one evening of heavy drinking and occurred, as a rule, not when the patient was intoxicated but in the withdrawal period.

The nature of the epileptogenic lesion has been a cortical scar in most instances, but in some cases, particularly in alcoholics, it has been elusive. From the examination of old cortical contusions (*plaques jaunes*), one cannot, on morphologic grounds, determine whether a lesion had or had not been epileptogenic. Electrocorticograms of the brain in regions adjacent to old traumatic foci reveal a number of spontaneously electrically active zones adjacent to the scars.

Treatment and Prophylaxis The use of antiepileptic drugs to prevent a posttraumatic seizure and subsequent epilepsy after closed or penetrating cranial injury has its proponents and skeptics. In one study, patients receiving phenytoin developed fewer seizures at the end of the first year than a placebo group, but a year after medication was discontinued, the incidence was the same (and quite low) in the two groups. An extensive randomized study by Temkin and colleagues demonstrated that when administered within a day of injury and continuing for 2 years, phenytoin reduced the incidence of seizures in the first week, but not thereafter. Also, in a study of a large number of patients with penetrating head injuries, the prophylactic use of antiepileptic medications was ineffective in preventing early seizures (Rish and Caveness), and this is reflected in current guidelines (Chang and Lowenstein).

Usually, persistent seizures can be controlled by a single antiepileptic medication, and relatively few seizure disorders are recalcitrant to the point of requiring excision of the epileptic focus. In this small group, the surgical results vary according to the methods of patient selection and techniques of operation. Under the neurosurgical conditions of four decades ago, with careful selection of cases, Rasmussen (also Penfield and Jasper) was able to eradicate seizures in 50 to 75 percent of cases by excision of the focus; the results currently are somewhat better.

Autonomic Dysfunction ("Storm") Syndrome

A worrisome consequence of severe head injury, which is observed in some comatose patients and particularly in the vegetative state, is a syndrome of episodic vigorous extensor posturing, profuse diaphoresis, hypertension, and tachycardia lasting minutes to an hour. A slight fever may accompany the spells. Families and staff are greatly disturbed by the display, particularly when the patient's grimacing suggests suffering. These spells of excessive sympathetic activity and posturing may be precipitated by painful stimuli or by distention of a viscus, but often they arise spontaneously. The syndrome is often mistakenly identified as a seizure and in many texts is still referred to as "diencephalic epilepsy" but it is more likely the result of the removal of suppressive cortical influences on autonomic structures, allowing the hypothalamus to function independently of normal inhibitory mechanisms. A survey of 35 such patients by Baugley and colleagues identified diffuse axonal injury and a period of hypoxia as being the main associated injuries and this has been our experience as well.

Narcotics such as morphine and benzodiazepines have a slightly beneficial effect but bromocriptine, which may be used in combination with sedatives or with small doses of morphine, has been most effective according to Rossitch and Bullard.

Extrapyramidal and Cerebellar Disorders Following Trauma

The question of a causative relationship between cerebral trauma and the development of Parkinson disease has been a controversial issue for many years—usually with the conclusion that the condition does not exist and that any apparent relationship, particularly after a single brain injury, is coincidental. Some such patients probably had early symptoms of Parkinson disease brought to light by the head injury. There are, however, cases such as the one reported by Doder and colleagues, in which traumatic necrosis of the lenticular and caudate nuclei was followed after a period of 6 weeks by the onset of predominantly contralateral parkinsonian signs, including tremor, which progressed slowly and were unresponsive to L-dopa. There are also undoubted instances of parkinsonism following severe closed head injury and the vegetative state (Matsuda et al). An exception to these statements may be a parkinsonian syndrome in ex-boxers and in others who had frequent minor head injuries, as a manifestation of the "punch-drunk" syndrome. There remains the possibility that cranial trauma incites a series of cellular events that lead to the deposition of abnormal structural proteins such as synuclein (see below).

Cerebellar ataxia is another rare consequence of cranial trauma, often unexplained but also in cases complicated by cerebral anoxia (causing ataxia with myoclonus) or a by a hemorrhage strategically placed in the deep midbrain or cerebellum. When cerebellar ataxia is caused by the trauma itself, it is frequently unilateral and the result of injury to the superior cerebellar peduncle. We have experience with a severely ataxic patient who had only small lesions in the cerebellum after bilateral acute subdural hematomas from an assault with head trauma. An "apraxia" of gait may also reflect the presence of a communicating hydrocephalus (see below and Chap. 30).

Acute and Chronic Traumatic Encephalopathy

Acute Traumatic Encephalopathy In almost all patients with cerebral concussive injury, there remains a gap in memory (traumatic amnesia) spanning a variable period from before the accident to some point following it. This gap is permanent and is filled in only by what the patient is told. In addition, as stated in the introduction to this section, some degree of impairment of higher cortical function may persist for weeks (or be permanent) after moderate to severe head injuries, even after the patient has reached the stage of forming continuous memories. During the period of reduced mentation, the memory disorder is the most prominent feature; in that respect, the state resembles the alcoholic form of the Korsakoff amnesic state and has some resemblance to the state of transient global amnesia (see Chap. 21).

With more careful testing, other cognitive disorders are usually evident. Concussed patients, during the period of posttraumatic amnesia, rarely confabulate. Apart from disorientation in place and time, the head-injured patient also shows defects in attention, as well as showing distractibility, perseveration, and an inability to synthesize perceptual data. Judgment and executive function may be mildly impaired, rarely severely, during the amnestic epoch. A perseverative tendency interferes with both action and thought. Leininger and associates, for example, found that most of their 53 patients who suffered minor head injury in traffic accidents performed less well than controls on psychologic tests (category test, auditory verbal learning, copying of complex figures). The fact that those who were merely dazed did as poorly as those who were concussed and that litigation was involved in some cases would lead one to question these results. Perhaps most affected, and most evident to high-functional individuals, is a problem with overall planning and coherence that is attributable to a defect in frontal lobe executive functioning.

As a general rule, the lower the score on the Glasgow Coma Scale immediately after injury (see Table 35-1) and the longer the posttraumatic gap in the formation of new memories (anterograde amnesia), the more likely the patient is to suffer some permanent cognitive and personality changes. According to Jennett and Bond, patients with good recovery achieved their maximum degree of improvement within 6 months. Others have found that detailed and repeated psychologic testing over a prolonged period, even in patients with relatively minor cerebral injuries, discloses measurable improvement for as long as 12 to 18 months.

There are other mental and behavioral abnormalities of a more subtle type that remain as sequelae to serious cerebral injury. As the stage of posttraumatic dementia recedes, the patient may find it impossible to work or to adjust to his family situation. Such patients are often abnormally abrupt, argumentative, and suspicious. Unlike the postconcussion syndrome described above, in which there is a certain uniformity, these traits vary with the patient's age, past experience, and environmental stresses. Extremes of age have been particularly important in our experience. The most prominent behavioral abnormality in children, described by Bowman and colleagues, is a change in personality. They become impulsive, impatient, unable to sit still, or may become heedless of the consequences of their actions and lacking in appreciation of social norms—much like those who in the past had recovered from encephalitis lethargica. Some adolescents or young adults show the general lack of inhibition and impulsivity that one associates with frontal lobe disease. In the older person, it is the impairment of intellectual functions that assumes greater prominence. In most instances, these more serious behavioral changes can be traced to contusions in the frontal and temporal lobes. In cases without obvious structural brain damage, cognitive deficiency after trauma has been widely attributed to diffuse axonal injury. Attempts to validate this by modern techniques such as diffusion tensor imaging have met with some success, such as the series described by Kraus and colleagues.

The tendency is for many such symptoms to subside slowly although not always completely, even in those in whom an accident has provoked a frank outburst of psychosis (as may happen to a person who is bipolar or a paranoid schizophrenic). These forms of what had colorfully in the past been called "traumatic insanity" were analyzed for the first time by Adolf Meyer.

Chronic Traumatic Encephalopathy The cumulative effects of repeated or even single cerebral injuries, constitute a type of head injury that until recently was difficult to classify. The subject of a delayed neurodegenerative cerebral disease that follows mild traumatic brain injury after many years is best introduced by an exposition of the long-appreciated condition in boxers who had engaged in many bouts over a long period of time. This refers to the development, after many years in the ring, of dysarthric speech and a state of forgetfulness, slowness in thinking, and other signs of dementia. Movements are slow, stiff, and uncertain, especially those involving the legs, and there is a shuffling, wide-based gait. In other words, a parkinsonian and dementing syndrome emerges and sometimes a moderately disabling ataxia, but there is no mistaking these for idiopathic Parkinson or Alzheimer disease. The plantar reflexes may be extensor on one or both sides. The clinical syndrome was reanalyzed by Roberts and colleagues, who found it present to some degree in 37 of the 224 professional boxers they examined. More recent studies show that in about one-half of all professional boxers, both active and retired, the CT scan discloses ventricular dilatation and sulcal widening and a cavum septi pellucidi (why the latter, which is ostensibly a developmental anomaly, would be overrepresented in boxers is unclear). These anatomic abnormalities had been demonstrated many years before by pneumoencephalography and were found to be related to the number of bouts (Ross et al; Casson et al).

A pathologic study of this disorder specific to boxers was made by Corsellis and associates. They examined the brains of 15 retired boxers who had shown the punch-drunk syndrome and identified a group of cerebral changes that appeared to explain the clinical findings. Mild to moderate enlargement of the lateral ventricles and thinning of the corpus callosum were present in all cases. Also, as mentioned, practically all of them showed a greatly widened cavum septi pellucidi and fenestration of the septal leaves. Readily identified areas of glial scarring were situated on the inferior surface of the cerebellar cortex. In these areas, and well beyond them, Purkinje cells were lost and the granule cell layer was somewhat thinned. Surprisingly, cerebral cortical contusions were found in only a few cases. Notably absent also was evidence of previous hemorrhage. Of the 15 cases, 11 showed varying degrees of loss of pigmented cells of the substantia nigra and locus ceruleus, and many of the remaining cells showed Alzheimer neurofibrillary change but not Lewy bodies. Neurofibrillary changes were scattered diffusely through the cerebral cortex and brainstem but were most prominent in the mediotemporal gray matter. Noteworthy was the absence of discrete amyloid plaques in this material by the usual staining methods; however, all cases showed extensive immunoreactive deposits of beta-amyloid ("diffuse plaques").

However, these studies were performed before the advent of modern immunohistochemistry techniques. McKee and coworkers have drawn attention to the deposition of tau protein in autopsy material that has come to define chronic traumatic encephalopathy. They have found a fairly consistent neuropathologic pattern consisting mainly of perivascular hyperphosphorylated tau protein embedded in astrocytic or neurofibrillary tangles with a predilection for the depths of sulci of the frontal and temporal lobes but also in other areas of cortex, thalamus, and brainstem, and eventually appearing extensively in the medial temporal lobes. Among 85 subjects with repetitive mild traumatic brain injury they found these changes to varying degrees in 68. The majority had headaches, depression, impulsivity and aggression, to some extent independent of the severity of pathologic changes. As evident in others was poor cognitive performance in the spheres of executive function and memory. Only those with the most widespread and densest deposition of tau were overtly demented and many of those had gait difficulty. A few of these also had parkinsonian manifestations. A putative relationship to motor neuron disease has also been raised. This form of chronic encephalopathy and tau deposition has evinced great interest in relation to concussion sustained during athletics at all levels.

Posttraumatic Hydrocephalus

This is an uncommon complication, but one that is frequently imputed to severe head injury. It conforms to the category of normal pressure hydrocephalus, as discussed in Chap. 30. Intermittent headaches, vomiting, confusion, and drowsiness are the initial manifestations. Later on, mental dullness, apathy, and psychomotor retardation are seen; by this time the CSF pressure may have fallen to a normal level (normal-pressure hydrocephalus). Postmortem examinations in some cases have demonstrated an adhesive basilar arachnoiditis. Early subarachnoid hemorrhage may be involved in the mechanisms. The response to ventriculoperitoneal shunt may be dramatic. Zander and Foroglou have written informatively about this condition.

Postconcussion Syndrome

This troublesome and common problem has been mentioned earlier, as well as in Chap. 10 in relation to headache. When the syndrome is protracted, neurologists are vexed by the condition—a problem intensified by worried patients and family. It has some similarities to the *posttraumatic stress disorder*, and had in the past been termed *posttraumatic nervous instability syndrome* and *traumatic neurasthenia* by Sir Charles Symonds, among many other names. Headache, dizziness, poor endurance, and lack of mental clarity are the central symptoms.

The cranial pain is either generalized or localized to the part that had been struck and variously described as aching, throbbing, pounding, stabbing, pressing, or band-like; it is remarkable for its variability in an individual patient. The intensification of the headache and other symptoms by mental and physical effort, straining, stooping, and emotional excitement is characteristic; rest and quiet tend to relieve it. Headaches may present a major obstacle to convalescence.

Dizziness, another prominent symptom, is usually not a true vertigo but a giddiness or light-headedness. The patient may feel unsteady, dazed, weak, or faint. However, a certain number of patients describe symptoms that are at least consonant with labyrinthine disorder; objects in the environment move momentarily, and looking upward or to the side may cause a sense of imbalance. Labyrinthine tests may show hyporeactivity of one side of the vestibular apparatus but more often they disclose no abnormalities. McHugh found a high incidence of minor abnormalities by electronystagmography, both in concussed patients and in those suffering from whiplash injuries of the neck; but we find much of the data difficult to interpret. Exceptionally, vertigo is accompanied by diminished excitability of both the labyrinth and the cochlea (deafness), and one may assume the existence of direct injury to the eighth nerve or end organ. Intolerance of alcohol is reported by some patients.

These physical symptoms resolve in several weeks in the majority of patients. When the symptoms persist, the patient becomes intolerant of noise, emotional excitement, and crowds. Tenseness, restlessness, fragmentation of sleep, inability to concentrate, feelings of nervousness, fatigue, worry, apprehension, and an inability to tolerate the usual amount of alcohol complete the clinical picture. The resemblance of these symptoms to those of anxiety and depression and to other forms of "posttraumatic stress disorder" is apparent.

The postconcussion syndrome complicates all types of head injury, mild and severe. Once established, it may persist for months or even years, and it tends to resist all varieties of treatment. Any relationship to the earlier described CTE is uncertain. Strangely, this syndrome is almost unknown in children. Characteristic also is the augmentation of both the duration and intensity of this syndrome by problems with compensation and litigation, suggesting a psychologic factor. In countries where these matters are a less-prominent part of the social fabric, the occurrence of posttraumatic syndrome is far less frequent. Environmental stress assumes importance as well, for if too much is demanded of the patient soon after injury, irritability, insomnia, and anxiety are enhanced. In this connection, an interesting experiment was conducted by Mittenberg and colleagues (1992). A group of subjects with no personal experience or knowledge of head injury was asked to select from a list of those symptoms that they would expect after a concussive head injury. They chose a cluster of features virtually identical to that of the postconcussion syndrome. The high background rates of various components of the postconcussion syndrome make it appear to be more prevalent than it truly is. The prospective study by Meares and coworkers found that, when compared to a group of patients who had noncranial trauma, the rates of the features of the syndrome were the same and that the strongest predictor of its occurrence was a previous anxiety disorder. However, the symptoms undoubtedly occur in well-adjusted, high-functioning individuals and should not be dismissed as simply anxiety.

An approach to treating postconcussion symptoms is given below. It has also been reported that military personnel who experience head injuries of any degree have a higher incidence of posttraumatic stress disorder (PTSD) than those with other somatic injuries but again, the disorder is not easily predicated on psychologic factors. The same disorder can be detected in civilians after injury and it then blends clearly into the earlier-described postconcussion syndrome.

Hysterical symptoms that develop after head injury, both cognitive and somatic, appear to be more common than those following injury to other parts of the body. These symptoms are discussed in Chap. 51. They may be immediate or delayed and vary from amnesia to blindness, paralysis, stuttering, inability to stand, and even to catatonia.

TREATMENT OF HEAD INJURY

Patients With Concussion and Transient Symptoms

Patients with an uncomplicated concussive injury who have already regained consciousness by the time they are seen in a hospital and have a normal neurologic examination pose few difficulties in management. They should not be discharged until the appropriate examinations (CT scans, skull films, if necessary) have been obtained and the results prove to be negative. Also, the patient should not be released until the capacity for consecutive memories has been regained and arrangements have been made for observation by the family of signs of possible, although unlikely, delayed complications (subdural and epidural hemorrhage, intracerebral bleeding, and edema). A program instituted by Mittenberg and colleagues (2001) has shown that reassurance and explanation of the concussive injury and anticipated aftereffects reduce the incidence of postconcussive symptoms at 6 months. Most such patients become mentally clear, have mild or no headache, and are found to have a normal neurologic examination. They do not require hospitalization or special testing, but in the current litigious climate of the United States, some form of brain imaging is nonetheless often performed as discussed in an earlier section.

Acetaminophen may be prescribed for headache. Any increase in headache, vomiting, or difficulty arousing the patient should prompt a return to the emergency department. A written instruction sheet with symptoms to be expected and clear advice about returning for examination is very helpful.

Patients with persistent complaints of headache, dizziness, and nervousness, are the most difficult to manage. The main approach is to counsel patients while the symptoms resolve, coupled with a reduction in mental and physical effort that is commensurate with the patient's level of endurance. A program must be planned in accordance with the basic problem. If work or school work precipitate headaches, for example, plans should be made to have them curtailed. Half-time work may be suitable for some individuals but not for others. Similarly, some physical activity is to be encouraged but exertion that causes headaches or mental confusion to occur or worsen should be reduced. At the same time, a bedbound or homebound state is discouraged and the patient may walk, use the internet, watch television, or read up to the level of causing fatigue. Each of these activities is then increased at a gradual rate. In all instances, reassurance that these symptoms improve over weeks or more should be offered in order not to allow the individual to internalize the notions of chronic dementia after head injury that pervade the popular press. Some hard-driving patients return to work, only to find headache, confusion, and fatigue recur in a disabling way and must start the cycle of reduced effort over again.

If there is mainly an anxious depression, antidepressant medications—such as in a fluoxetine, paroxetine, or a tricyclic—may be useful, but their effects are often disappointing. Simple analgesics, such as acetaminophen or nonsteroidal antiinflammatory drugs, should be prescribed for the headache. Litigation should be settled as soon as possible. To delay settlement usually works to the disadvantage of the patient. Long periods of observation, repetition of a multitude of tests, and waiting only reinforce the patient's worries and fears and reduce the motivation to return to work. Neuropsychologic tests may be useful in the group with persistent cognitive difficulty, but the results should be interpreted with caution, as depression and poor motivation will degrade performance.

Patients With Severe Head Injury

If the physician arrives at the scene of an accident and finds an unconscious patient, a rapid examination should be made before the patient is moved. First it must be determined whether the patient is breathing and has a clear airway and obtainable pulse and blood pressure, and whether there is hemorrhage from a scalp laceration or injured viscera. Severe head injuries that arrest respiration are soon followed by cessation of cardiac function. Injuries of this magnitude are often fatal; if resuscitative measures do not restore and sustain cardiopulmonary function within 4 to 5 min, the brain is usually irreparably damaged. Bleeding from the scalp can usually be controlled by a pressure bandage unless an artery is divided; then a suture becomes necessary. Resuscitative measures (artificial respiration and cardiac compression) should be continued until they are taken over by ambulance personnel. Oxygen should then be administered.

The likelihood of a cervical fracture–dislocation, which may be associated with any severe head injury, is the reason for taking precautions in immobilizing the neck and in moving the patient. In the awake patient, neck pain calls attention to this complication. It should be recalled that even in the absence of a spinal fracture, the spinal cord may be threatened by the instability resulting from ligamentous injuries (posing the risk of subluxation). In the study of 292 patients with traumatic cervical injuries by Demetriades and colleagues, 31 (11 percent) showed subluxations without fracture and 11 (4 percent) had cord injuries with neither fracture nor subluxation. The combined use of standard cervical spine films and cervical CT scanning detected all cervical injuries. After severe head or neck injury, even without direct impact to the neck, it is advisable to obtain standard anteroposterior, lateral, and oblique neck films, with additional gentle flexion (20 degrees) and extension (30 degrees) views of the neck and a neck CT scan. If these are normal and there is little or no neck pain, the cervical collar is no longer required. If after these studies, or if they cannot be obtained, or if there is significant persistent pain or other neurologic findings induced by head movement, a cervical MRI is advisable. If there are signs of a myelopathy such as flaccid legs or incontinence, urgent MRI is advisable.

In the hospital, the first step is to clear the airway and ensure adequate ventilation by endotracheal intubation if necessary. A search for other injuries must be made, particularly of the abdomen, chest, spine, and long bones. Chestnut et al, in analyzing the data from the Traumatic Coma Data Bank, found that sustained early hypotension (systolic blood pressure <90 mm Hg) was associated with a doubling of mortality. If shock was present on admission to the emergency ward, the mortality was 65 percent. Although the hypotension that follows most injuries is a vasodepressor response and usually comes under control within approximately an hour without pressor drugs, a large, unimpeded intravenous line should be inserted. Persistent hypotension because of head injury alone is an uncommon occurrence and should always raise the suspicion of thoracic or abdominal internal bleeding, extensive fractures, or trauma to the cervical cord, or diabetes insipidus. Initially, the infused fluid should be normal saline, avoiding the administration of excessive "free water" because of its adverse effect on brain edema. Oxygen should continue to be administered until it can be shown that the arterial oxygen saturation is normal.

A rapid neurologic survey can then be made, with attention to the depth of coma, size of the pupils and their reaction to light, ocular movements, corneal reflexes, facial movements during grimace, swallowing, vocalization, gag reflexes, muscle tone and movements of the limbs, predominant postures, reactions to pinch, and reflexes. Bogginess of the temporal or postauricular area (Battle sign), bleeding from the nose or ear, and extensive conjunctival edema and hemorrhage are useful signs of an underlying basal skull fracture. However, it should be remembered that rupture of an eardrum or a blow to the nose may also cause bleeding from these parts. Fracture of the orbital bones may displace the eye, with resulting strabismus; fracture of the jaw results in malocclusion and discomfort on attempting to open the mouth. If urine is retained and the bladder is distended, a catheter should be inserted and kept there. Temperature, pulse, respiration, blood pressure, arterial oxygen saturation, and state of consciousness should be checked and charted every hour. The Glasgow Coma Scale, mentioned earlier, has provided a practical means by which the state of impaired consciousness can be evaluated at frequent intervals (see Table 35-1), but it should not be considered a substitute for a more complete neurologic examination.

CT and MRI scanning of the cranium have assumed central importance at this juncture. A sizable epidural, subdural, or intracerebral blood clot is an indication for immediate surgery. The presence of contusions, brain edema, and displacement of central structures calls for measures to monitor progression of these lesions and to control intracranial pressure. These measures are best carried out in a critical care unit.

Management of Raised Intracranial Pressure

There has been a presumption, not unreasonable, that high levels of intracranial pressure are deleterious after head injury, much as it is in other processes that involve an intracranial mass. At issue has been the precise pressure at which damage occurs, whether lowering ICP improves outcome, which treatments are best, and the role of monitoring in guiding treatment. Certainly there are many biologic processes in neurons and astrocytes that greatly influence outcome after traumatic brain injury, many set in motion at the time of impact and not referable to raised ICP. At times, these overwhelm the changes induced by intracranial pressure but they are not particularly remediable, producing an emphasis on reducing intracranial pressure as a means of preventing secondary brain damage. An approach to intracranial pressure treatment is given here and also addressed in Chap. 17 on coma and Chap. 31 on brain tumors.

ICP Monitoring In cases of moderate and severe head injury it has been the practice on most ICU services to insert one of several available devices that continuously record intracranial pressure (ICP). The rationale is ostensibly to gain control over a remediable cause of secondary brain damage, particularly if the patient's neurologic examination is reduced to a few sentinel signs such as pupillary enlargement or because sedating medications have obscured the examination. The ventricular catheter has been considered a "gold standard" of pressure measurements as it is directly coupled to the CSF compartment, which should best reflect the summated pressures within the cranium. It has the additional advantage of affording therapeutic drainage of CSF in order to reduce ICP. In comatose patients, monitoring of ICP could avoid excessive fluid administration, refine the amount of osmotic agent and hypertonic saline used to reduce pressure, and establishes the ideal level of hyperventilation. In these respects, monitoring can be helpful by guiding treatment and avoiding detrimental effects on ICP of treatments for head trauma.

However, there are few critical data to support the routine use of ICP monitoring. Certainly in the patient who is only drowsy or shows only minimal mass effect on CT, it is usually not necessary. Guidelines given by the American Association of Neurological Surgeons and allied groups have been that monitoring is appropriate if Glasgow Coma Scale is between 3 and 8 and there are abnormalities on CT scan, or if there is no abnormality on the CT but the patient has any two of age over 40, posturing, or has systolic blood pressure below 90 mm Hg. They set a desirable level of ICP of below 20 mm Hg and this has reinforced the role of ICP monitoring in head trauma management.

A reassessment of the effectiveness of ICP monitoring in a randomized trial reached the contrary conclusion that the information gained offers no advantage over clinical observation and imaging with CT scan. This trial was carried out by Chesnut and colleagues in developing countries and defined raised intracranial pressure at a level that has been criticized as too low (20 mm Hg). Nonetheless the study has demonstrated that the use of a clinical approach to management of raised ICP is as feasible as a program based on direct ICP measurement. This does not negate the desirability of keeping ICP controlled at some arbitrary level; it merely questions the need for direct monitoring as a guide to management.

As a practical matter, we use ICP monitoring in our unit to warn of impending deterioration from brain edema or hemorrhage if the patient cannot be effectively examined or shows poor responsiveness with evidence of mass effect on a CT scan. Although the risk of infection with a ventricular catheter is low, less than 3 percent, prolonged use may be complicated by bacterial meningitis. The catheter may be left in place for 3 to 5 days, or fewer if the clinical state and ICP are stable for 24 to 48 h. The current generation of ICP monitors employs fiberoptic strain gauges that can be inserted directly into the cerebral cortex without apparent damage.

General Measures The first step in lowering elevated ICP is to control the incidental factors that are known to raise pressure, such as hypoxia, hypercarbia, particularly hyperthermia, awkward head positions that compress the jugular veins, and high mean airway pressures from positive pressure ventilation (see the monograph by Ropper and colleagues [2004] and Chap. 30 for further details). The avoidance of hyponatremia and serum hypoosmolarity that would allow water to enter the brain and increase its volume is accomplished by infusing only isoosmolar or hyperosmolar solutions such as normal saline. Elevations in serum osmolality as a consequence of excessive concentrations of diffusible solutes such as glucose are not useful in reducing intracranial volume because they do not create gradient for water and solutes across the cerebral vasculature. Consequently, fluids such as 5 percent dextrose in water, 0.5 normal saline, and 5 percent dextrose in 0.5 normal saline are avoided; lactated Ringer solution is permissible; normal saline, with or without added dextrose, is ideal. In a post hoc study of a cohort of severely injured patients, resuscitation with albumin was found to have a detrimental effect compared to saline (SAFE Investigators).

Hyperosmolar Therapy The basis for this class of treatments is the creation of a gradient of water concentration from the brain to the blood that reduces brain volume. Mannitol, glycerol, and urea are effective in lowering ICP by producing serum hyperosmolarity initially and then causing a diuresis that sustains this state and secondarily causes hypernatremia and hypovolemia. Hyperosmolar saline, in contrast, raises serum sodium directly and expands intravascular volume.

The effects of mannitol have been of great interest to those who treat head trauma, but the ideal plan for its use has never been established. If intracranial pressure exceeds a predetermined level, for example 20 mm Hg as recommended by aforementioned guidelines for the treatment of traumatic brain injury, mannitol 20 percent, 0.25 to 1.0 g/kg is given every 3 to 6 h to maintain serum sodium above approximately 142 mEq/L and osmolarity of 290 to 315 mOsm/L. Even if ICP monitoring is not used, an attempt may be made to maintain this level of serum osmolality for the first days after injury if contusion and brain swelling are detected on the CT scan.

Mannitol in large amounts may cause renal failure, almost always reversible, though an uncertain mechanism perhaps having to do with renal blood flow. Limited evidence suggests that this complication occurs only with the use of more than 200 g of mannitol daily.

The relative merits of hypertonic saline and mannitol are frequently discussed and have been reviewed by one of us (Ropper, 2012). Several small series comparing the agents, referenced in the review, have shown too little difference to allow a choice between the two agents. Local experience and an overall assessment of the side effects of each typically dominate practice. Hypertonic saline (concentrations of 3 percent to 23 percent) has a comparable effect to mannitol in the treatment of raised ICP and has the advantage of avoiding severe dehydration because it increases osmolarity directly rather than through diuresis. The opposite also pertains, namely that patients with poor cardiac output may be subject to congestive heart failure with hypertonic saline in high volumes. Diuretics have been used to mitigate this effect. Either agent can produce a hyperglycemic, hyperosmolar state in diabetics, particularly in the elderly and in those receiving corticosteroids.

Hypertonic saline, 3 percent, can be used in boluses of 150 mL; a 7.5 percent solution, in 75 mL boluses; and 23 percent, in volumes of approximately 30 mL. All but the lowest concentration of saline require a central venous catheter to prevent sclerosis of veins. The same levels of sodium concentration as noted for mannitol are used as a reference to guide graduated increments of sodium administration, with serum sodium higher than about 156 mEq/L infrequently providing additional reductions in ICP.

Hypocarbia Hypocarbia, induced by hyperventilation, produces alkalosis of the CSF and cerebral vasoconstriction with a corresponding reduction in cerebral blood volume and ICP. It is effective for a limited period of time, as the pH of the spinal fluid equilibrates over hours by the elaboration of ammonium ions in the choroids plexus, allowing cerebral blood volume to return to its previous level. A single-step reduction in Pco_2 typically lowers ICP for approximately 20 to 40 min. Attempts to prolong the effect of hypocarbia and the alkalosis by the intravenous administration of ammonium buffers have met with mixed success.

It has been suggested that hyperventilation may be harmful to some head-injured patients because of a reduction in cerebral blood flow, but the risk, if any, appears to be minimal, at least in adults. In children, reductions in cerebral blood flow have been demonstrated by Skippen and colleagues at even modest levels of hypocarbia and three-quarters show slight brain ischemia when Pco_2 is below 25 mm Hg. For these reasons, hypocarbia is used in cases of head trauma mainly in acute circumstances and has been eschewed for chronic use. If the ICP continues to rise and brain swelling progresses despite these measures, the outlook for survival is poor. It should be mentioned that many patients, particularly children, hyperventilate spontaneously after head trauma.

Hypothermia Hypothermia and barbiturate anesthesia fairly consistently reduce ICP but relatively few patients respond to such measures for long and their clinical outcome is not improved. The main problem, aside from the difficulty maintaining lower body temperatures, is that rewarming induces substantial brain swelling and a return of ICP to prior levels or higher. A randomized controlled trial of cooling adult patients with severe closed head injury (Glasgow Coma Scale scores of 3 to 7) to 33°C (91.4°F) for 24 h appeared to hasten neurologic recovery and may have modestly improved outcome (Marion et al), but a larger and better-conducted study led by Clifton showed that attaining hypothermia of 33°C (91.4°F) within 8 h of injury failed to improve outcome and this approach cannot be endorsed except in special circumstances. The same lack of effect has been shown in studies with children (Hutchinson et al).

Although barbiturates lower ICP, they lower the blood pressure as well; hence they may diminish cerebral perfusion. However, an uncontrolled series by Marshall and coworkers (1979) claimed improved survival by using barbiturates even in cases where the ICP exceeded 40 mm Hg.

The more definitive randomized study by Eisenberg and associates showed no benefit from barbiturate-induced anesthesia in head-injured patients, and this class of drugs has been largely abandoned except for brief, acute control of ICP while other measures are being instituted.

Corticosteroids Several controlled studies have established that the administration of high-dose steroids does not improve the clinical outcome of severe head injury. Eclipsing smaller prior studies was the well-designed Clinical Randomization of an Antifibrinolytic in Significant Hemorrhage (CRASH) trial, conducted in more than 10,000 adults and controlled for varying degrees of injury as judged by the Glasgow Coma Scale and imaging features. The effect of the infusion of methylprednisolone 2 g, followed by 0.4 g/h for 48 h, favored survival in the untreated patients by a small but clear margin, leading to the current recommendation that steroids not be used routinely following head injury.

Blood Pressure Management The management of posttraumatic systemic hypertension represents a difficult problem. Within hours after head injury, the sympathoadrenal response and elevation of blood pressure recedes spontaneously in a matter of a few hours or days. Unless the blood pressure elevation is extreme (greater than 180/95 mm Hg), it can be disregarded in the early stages. In animal experiments, it has been found that severe hypertension leads to increased perfusion of the brain and an augmentation of the edema surrounding contusions and hemorrhages. As mentioned earlier, edema is the main element in the genesis of brain swelling and of raised ICP in most head-injured patients (Marmarou et al). This reflects a failure of autoregulatory vascular mechanisms, with resulting transudative edema in damaged areas of the brain. The control of high blood pressure must be balanced against the risk of reducing cerebral perfusion pressure and the observation that even a brief period of mild hypotension may provoke a cycle of cerebral vasodilatation, increased cerebral blood volume, and elevated ICP in the form of plateau waves (Rosner and Becker). Observations such as these emphasize the need for immediate correction of hypotension in severely head-injured patients.

Because most therapies for elevated ICP dehydrate the patient or reduce cardiac filling pressures, thereby leading to hypotension, a middle course of avoiding both severe hypertension and any degree of hypotension seems the best compromise. In lowering high levels of blood pressure, diuretics, beta-adrenergic blocking agents, or angiotensin-converting enzyme inhibitors are generally used, rather than agents that potentially dilate the cerebral vasculature (nitroglycerin and nitroprusside, hydralazine, and some of the calcium channel blockers may present this risk). Hypotension should be corrected by vasopressor agents such as phenylephrine or norepinephrine. The precise level of blood pressure that requires treatment must be judged in the context of the ICP and the presence of plateau waves, the goal being to maintain normal cerebral perfusion pressure of 60 to 80 mm Hg, as well as the patient's previous blood pressure level; evidence of organ failure from either hyper- or hypotension, such as cardiac or renal ischemia, must also be considered.

General Medical Measures

If coma persists for more than 48 h, a nasogastric tube should be passed and fluids and nutrition should be given by this route. A basilar skull fracture, especially if there is a CSF leak, may preclude this route and compel a directly situated gastric tube. Agents that reduce gastric acid production—or the equivalent, antacids by stomach tube to keep gastric acidity at a pH above 3.5—are of value in preventing gastric hemorrhage. The prophylactic use of antiepileptic drugs, as discussed earlier, under "Posttraumatic Epilepsy," recently has been favored, but there is no evidence that delayed epileptic seizures are reduced (see Chang and Lowenstein). Only if there has been a seizure are antiepileptics given.

Restlessness is controlled by diazepam, propofol, or a similar drug, but only if careful nursing fails to quiet the patient and provide sleep for a few hours at a time. Etomidate and dexmedetomidine may be preferable for reducing agitation because they are minimally sedating. Fever is counteracted by antipyretics such as acetaminophen and, if necessary, by a cooling blanket. The use of morphine or bromocriptine to quiet episodes of vigorous extensor posturing and accompanying adrenergic activity already has been mentioned.

Surgical Decompression

The need for surgical intervention during the acute posttraumatic period is decided by two factors: the clinical status of the patient and the findings on imaging. The presence of a subdural or epidural clot that is causing a shift of central brain structures calls for evacuation of the collection. The approach to these lesions has been discussed earlier. Should the elevated ICP not respond to this procedure or to the standard osmotic agents and other medical measures outlined earlier, or should the condition of the patient and vital signs then begin to deteriorate (heart rate rising, temperature rising or falling below normal, state of consciousness worsening, hemiplegia, plantar reflexes more clearly extensor), a renewed search must be undertaken for a late-occurring cerebral hemorrhage. Usually in these clinical circumstances, CT scanning will disclose a new or enlarged epidural, subdural, or intracerebral hematoma, or worsened cerebral edema. If death or severe disability is to be avoided, operation in these cases must be undertaken before the advanced signs of brainstem compression—decerebrate or decorticate posturing, hypertension, bradycardia—have appeared.

The use of *decompressive craniectomy* in patients with progressive and intractable traumatic brain swelling has been a subject of renewed interest, after having been practically abandoned several decades ago. Guerra and colleagues reported on 57 such patients, mostly young adults, who underwent wide frontotemporal craniectomy, unilateral in 31 and bilateral in 26. Of these, 58 percent attained surprisingly good states of rehabilitation. These authors were of the opinion that these results represented a significant improvement over the expected outcome in this particular group of patients. A similar open trial conducted by Aarabi and colleagues described

40 percent with good outcome. Similar results in children were reported by Polin and associates. The few cases with which we have been involved, mostly children operated late, have not been as encouraging.

However, these generally favorable results could not be validated in the randomized "DECRA" trial carried out by Cooper and colleagues. Decompression did indeed reduce ICP, as expected, when the intracranial contents are exposed to atmospheric pressure, but surgery did not improve outcome. The details of the operation and choice of ICP level that were chosen to trigger operation have been criticized, but this study remains the best information to date until further trials with different designs, some ongoing, clarify the issue of surgical decompression. Further trials of decompressive craniectomy after severe traumatic brain injury are being undertaken.

The treatment of the general medical diseases relating to protracted coma was outlined in Chap. 17. Each patient presents unique problems.

PROGNOSIS

As has been intimated, the outcome in severe injury is particularly discouraging, more so with increasing age. Some aspects of prognosis were mentioned earlier but the following general comments serve to frame the problem. In the survey of the large European Brain Injury Consortium, comprising 10,005 adult patients, the injury proved fatal in 31 percent; 3 percent were left in a persistent vegetative state, and 16 percent remained severely disabled neurologically (Murray et al). Data from the extensively analyzed Traumatic Coma Data Bank are comparable, as reported by Marshall and coworkers (1983). The signs of focal brain disease, whether because of closed head injuries or open and penetrating ones, tend always to ameliorate as the months pass. A hemiplegia is often reduced to a minimal hemiparesis or to ineptitude of voluntary motor function with exaggerated reflexes and an equivocal Babinski sign on that side, and aphasia is gradually transformed into a stuttering or hesitant paraphasia or dysnomia that is not disabling. Many of the signs of brainstem disease (cranial nerve dysfunction and ataxia) improve also, usually within the first 6 months after injury (Jennett and Bond) and often to a surprising extent. Most patients who had been in coma for many hours or days—i.e., those with severe brain injuries—are left with memory impairment and other cognitive defects and with personality changes. These may be the only lasting sequelae as detailed earlier. According to Jennett and Bond, these mental and personality changes are a greater handicap than focal neurologic ones as far as social adjustment is concerned. In open head wounds and penetrating brain injuries, Grafman and coworkers found that the magnitude of tissue loss and location of the lesion were the main factors affecting the outcome.

The prognosis of head injury is influenced by several other factors as mentioned. The *age of the patient* is the most important factor (Vollmer et al). Increasing age reduces the chances of survival and of good recovery. Older patients often remain disabled, especially when compensation is involved. Young and middle-aged patients do better, particularly if they are not entitled to compensation.

As a general statement, children recover more completely than adults. Russell pointed out long ago that the severity of the injury as measured by the duration of *traumatic amnesia* is a useful prognostic index. Of patients with a period of amnesia lasting less than 1 h, 95 percent were back at work within 2 months; if the amnesia lasted longer than 24 h, only 80 percent had returned to work within 6 months. However, approximately 60 percent of the patients in his large series still had symptoms at the end of 2 months, and 40 percent at the end of 18 months. Of the most severely injured (those comatose for several days), many remained permanently disabled. However, the degree of recovery was often better than one had expected; the motor impairment, aphasia, and dementia tended to lessen and sometimes cleared. Improvement could continue over a period of 3 or more years. Obviously, multiple-organ injury and, particularly, hypotension in the hours immediately after injury, have major effects, not just on survival, but in some studies, with neurocognitive and behavioral outcome.

The remarkable findings of voluntary activation of parts of the cerebral cortex in patients who are in a vegetative or minimally conscious state was mentioned earlier and in Chap. 17. These serve as a caution to the neurologist to assign the diagnostic labels of vegetative and minimally conscious state only after careful and preferably, repeated examinations and then to temper communication with the family and other physicians by an appropriate degree of uncertainty as to outcome. Nonetheless, most patients who are vegetative for 6 or more months after cranial trauma will not recover to a meaningfully independent life.

References

Aarabi B, Hesdorffer DC, Ahn ES, et al: Outcome following decompressive craniectomy for malignant swelling due to severe head injury. *J Neurosurg* 104:469, 2006.

Adams JH, Graham DI, Jennet B: The neuropathology of the vegetative state after an acute brain insult. *Brain* 123:1327, 2000.

Adams JH, Graham DI, Murray LS, Scott G: Diffuse axonal injury due to nonmissile head injury in humans: An analysis of 45 cases. *Ann Neurol* 12:557, 1982.

Annegers JF, Grabow JD, Groover RV, et al: Seizures after head trauma: A population study. *Neurology* 30:683, 1980.

Annegers JF, Hauser A, Coan SP, Rocca WA: A population-based study of seizures after traumatic brain injuries. *N Engl J Med* 338:20, 1998.

Ascroft RB: Traumatic epilepsy after gunshot wounds of the head. *Br Med J* 1:739, 1941.

Baugley IJ, Nicholls JL, Felmingham KL, et al: Dysautonomia after traumatic brain injury: A forgotten syndrome. *J Neurol Neurosurg Psychiatry* 67:39, 1999.

Bender MB, Christoff N: Nonsurgical treatment of subdural hematomas. *Arch Neurol* 31:73, 1974.

Bonnier C, Nassogne MC, Saint-Martin C, et al: Neuroimaging of intraparenchymal lesions predicts outcome in shaken baby syndrome. *Pediatrics* 112:808, 2003.

Boto GR, Lobato RD, Rivas JJ, et al: Basal ganglia hematomas in severely head injured patients: Clinicoradiological analysis of 37 cases. *J Neurosurg* 94:224, 2001.

Bowman KM, Blau A, Reich R: Psychiatric states following head injury in adults and children, in Feiring EH (ed): *Brock's Injuries of the Brain and Spinal Cord and Their Coverings*, 5th ed. New York, Springer-Verlag, 1974, pp 570–613.

Cairns H: Injuries of frontal and ethmoid sinuses with special reference to CSF rhinorrhea and aerocele. *J Laryngol Otol* 52: 289, 1937.

Casson IR, Sham RAJ, Campbell EA, et al: Neurological and CT evaluation of knocked-out boxers. *J Neurol Neurosurg Psychiatry* 45:170, 1982.

Caveness WF: Onset and cessation of fits following craniocerebral trauma. *J Neurosurg* 20:570, 1963.

Caveness WF: Post-traumatic sequelae, in Caveness WF, Walker AE (eds): *Head Injury*. Philadelphia, Lippincott, 1966, pp 209–219.

Caviness VS Jr: Epilepsy and craniocerebral injury of warfare, in Caveness WF, Walker AE (eds): *Head Injury*. Philadelphia, Lippincott, 1966, pp 220–234.

Chang BS, Lowenstein DH: Practice parameter: Antiepileptic drug prophylaxis in severe traumatic brain injury. Report of the Quality Standards Subcommittee of the American Academy of Neurology. *Neurology* 60:10, 2003.

Chesnut RM, Marshall SB, Piek J, et al: Early and late systemic hypotension as a frequent and fundamental source of cerebral ischemia following severe brain injury in the Traumatic Coma Data Bank. *Acta Neurochir (Wien)* 59(Suppl):121, 1993.

Chesnut RM, Temkin N, Carney N, et al: A trial of intracranial-pressure monitoring in traumatic brain injury. *N Engl J Med* 367:2471, 2012.

Clifton GL, Miller ER, Choi SC, et al: Lack of effect of induction of hypothermia after acute brain injury. *N Engl J Med* 344:556, 2001.

Copper DJ, Rosenfeld JD, Murray L, et al: Decompressive craniectomy in diffuse traumatic brain injury. *N Engl J Med* 364:1493, 2011.

Corsellis JAN, Bruton CJ, Freeman-Browne D: The aftermath of boxing. *Psychol Med* 3:270, 1973.

Courville CB: *Pathology of the Central Nervous System*: Part 4. Mountain View, CA, Pacific, 1937.

CRASH Trial Collaborators: Effect of intravenous corticosteroids on death within 14 days in 10008 adults with clinically significant head injury (MRC CRASH trial: randomized placebo-controlled trial). *Lancet* 364:1321, 2004.

Demetriades D, Charalambides K, Chahwan S, et al: Non-skeletal cervical spine injuries: Epidemiology and diagnostic pitfalls. *J Trauma* 48:724, 2000.

Denny-Brown D: Delayed collapse after head injury. *Lancet* 1:371, 1941.

Denny-Brown D, Russell WR: Experimental cerebral concussion. *Brain* 64:93, 1941.

DePalma RG, Burris DC, Champion HR, et al: Blast injuries. *N Engl J Med* 352:1335, 2005.

Doder M, Jahanshahi M, Turjanski N, et al: Parkinson's syndrome after closed head injury: A single case report. *J Neurol Neurosurg Psychiatry* 66:380, 1999.

Eisenberg HM, Frankowski HF, Conant LP, et al: High dose barbiturate control of elevated intracranial pressure in patients with severe head injury. *J Neurosurg* 69:15, 1988.

Feiring EH, Davidoff LM: Gunshot wounds of the brain and their complications, in Feiring EH (ed): *Brock's Injuries of the Brain and Spinal Cord and Their Coverings*, 5th ed. New York, Springer-Verlag, 1974, pp 283–335.

Foltz EL, Schmidt RP: The role of reticular formation in the coma of head injury. *J Neurosurg* 13:145, 1956.

Frazier CH, Ingham SD: A review of the effects of gunshot wounds of the head based on the observation of 200 cases at US Army General Hospital, No 11, Cape May, NJ. *Trans Am Neurol Assoc* 45:59, 1919.

Gennarelli TA, Thibault LE, Adams JH, et al: Diffuse axonal injury and traumatic coma in the primate. *Ann Neurol* 12:564, 1982.

Giacino JT, Whyte J, Bagiella E, et al: Placebo-controlled trial of amantadine for severe traumatic brain injury. *N Engl J Med* 366:819, 2012.

Giza CC, Kutcher JS, Ashwal S, et al: Summary of evidence-based guideline update: Evaluation and management of concussion in sports. Report of the Guideline Development Subcommittee of the American Academy of Neurology: Summary of evidence-based guideline update: Evaluation and management of concussion in sports. *Neurology* 80:2250, 2013.

Grafman J, Jonas BS, Martin A, et al: Intellectual function following penetrating head injury in Vietnam veterans. *Brain* 111:169, 1988.

Graham DI, Adams JH, Doyle D: Ischemic brain damage in fatal non-missile injuries. *J Neurol Sci* 39:213, 1978.

Guerra WK, Gaab MR, Dietz H, et al: Surgical decompression for traumatic brain swelling: Indications and results. *J Neurosurg* 90:187, 1999.

Guskiewicz KM, McCrea M, Marshall SW, et al: Cumulative effects associated with recurrent concussion in collegiate football players. *JAMA* 290:2549, 2003.

Haas DC, Ross GS: Transient global amnesia triggered by mild head trauma. *Brain* 109:251, 1986.

Haydel MJ, Preston CA, Mills TJ, et al: Indications for computed tomography in patients with minor head injury. *N Engl J Med* 343:100, 2000.

Hoge CW, McGurk D, Thomas JL, et al: Mild traumatic brain injury in U.S. soldiers returning from Iraq. *N Engl J Med* 358:453, 2008.

Holbourn AHS: Mechanics of head injury. *Lancet* 2:438, 1943.

Hutchinson JS, Ward RE, Lacroix J, et al: Hypothermia therapy after traumatic brain injury in children. *N Engl J Med* 358:2447, 2008.

Jefferson G: The nature of concussion. *Br Med J* 1:1, 1944.

Jellinger K, Seitelberger F: Protracted post-traumatic encephalopathy: Pathology, pathogenesis and clinical implications. *J Neurol Sci* 10:51, 1970.

Jennett B: *Epilepsy after Non-missile Head Injuries*, 2nd ed. London, Heinemann, 1975.

Jennett B, Bond M: Assessment of outcome after severe brain damage. *Lancet* 1:480, 1975.

Jennett B, Teasdale G: *Management of Head Injuries: Contemporary Neurology*, no 20. Philadelphia, Davis, 1981.

Kampfl A, Franz G, Aichner F, et al: The persistent vegetative state after closed head injury: Clinical and magnetic resonance imaging findings in 42 patients. *J Neurosurg* 88:809, 1998.

Kraus MF, Susmaras T, Caughlin BP, et al: White matter integrity and cognition in chronic traumatic brain injury. *Brain* 130:2508, 2007.

Labadie EL, Glover D: Physiopathogenesis of subdural hematomas. *J Neurosurg* 45:382, 393, 1976.

Leininger BE, Gramling SE, Farrell AD, et al: Neuropsychological deficits in symptomatic minor head injury patients after concussion and mild concussion. *J Neurol Neurosurg Psychiatry* 53:293, 1990.

Lepore FE: Disorders of ocular motility following head trauma. *Arch Neurol* 52:924, 1995.

Lloyd DA, Carty H, Patterson M, et al: Predictive value of skull radiography for intracranial injury in children with blunt head injury. *Lancet* 349:821, 1997.

Marino R, Gasparotti R, Pinelli L, et al: Posttraumatic cerebral infarction in patients with moderate or severe head trauma. *Neurology* 67:1165, 2006.

Marion DW, Penrod LE, Kelsey SF, et al: Treatment of traumatic brain injury with moderate hypothermia. *N Engl J Med* 336:540, 1997.

Marmarou A, Fatouros PP, Barzo P, et al: Contribution of edema and cerebral blood volume to traumatic brain swelling in head-injured patients. *J Neurosurg* 93:183, 2000.

Marshall LF, Smith RW, Shapiro HM: The outcome with aggressive treatment in severe head injury: Part II. Acute and chronic barbiturate administration in the management of head injury. *J Neurosurg* 50:26, 1979.

Marshall LF, Toole BM, Bowers SA: The National Traumatic Coma Data Bank: Part 2. Patients who talk and deteriorate: Implications for treatment. *J Neurosurg* 59:285, 1983.

Matsuda W, Matsumara A, Komatsu Y, et al: Awakenings from persistent vegetative state: Report of three cases with parkinsonism and brain stem lesions on MRI. *J Neurol Neurosurg Psychiatry* 74:1571, 2003.

McCrea M, Guskiewicz KM, Marshall SW, et al: Acute effects and recovery time following concussion in collegiate football players. The NCAA concussion study. *JAMA* 290:2556, 2003.

McCrory P, Meeuwisse W, Johnston K, et al: Consensus statement on concussion in sport. 3rd international conference on concussion in sport held in Zurich, November 2008. *Clin J Sport Med* 19:185, 2009.

McCrory PR, Berkovic SF: Second impact syndrome. *Neurology* 50:677, 1998.

McCrory PR, Berkovic SF: Video analysis of acute motor and convulsive movements in sport-related concussion. *Neurology* 54:1488, 2000.

McHugh HE: Auditory and vestibular disorders in head injury, in Caveness WF, Walker AE (eds): *Head Injury*. Philadelphia, Lippincott, 1966, pp 97–105.

McKee AC, Stein TD, Nowinski CJ, et al: The spectrum of disease in chronic traumatic encephalopathy. *Brain* 136:43, 2013.

Meares S, Shores EA, Taylor AJ, et al: Mild traumatic injury does not predict acute postconcussion syndrome. *J Neurol Neurosurg Psychiatry* 79:300, 2008.

Meirowsky AM: Penetrating craniocerebral trauma, in Caveness WF, Walker AE (eds): *Head Injury*. Philadelphia, Lippincott, 1966, pp 195–202.

Meyer A: The anatomical facts and clinical varieties of traumatic insanity. *Am J Insanity* 60:373, 1904.

Mittenberg W, Canyock EM, Condit D, Pottor C: Treatment of post-concussion syndrome following mild head injury. *J Clin Exp Neuropsychol* 23:829, 2001.

Mittenberg W, DiGiulio DV, Perrin S, Bass AE: Symptoms following mild head injury: Expectations as aetiology. *J Neurol Neurosurg Psychiatry* 55:200, 1992.

Munro D, Merritt HH: Surgical pathology of subdural hematoma based on a study of 105 cases. *Arch Neurol Psychiatry* 35:64, 1936.

Murray GD, Teasdale GM, Braakman, et al: The European Brain Injury Consortium survey of head injuries. *Acta Neurochir (Wien)* 141:223, 1999.

Nee PA, Hadfield JM, Yates DW, Faragher EB: Significance of vomiting after head injury. *J Neurol Neurosurg Psychiatry* 66:470, 1999.

Nevin NC: Neuropathological changes in the white matter following head injury. *J Neuropathol Exp Neurol* 26:77, 1967.

Ommaya AK, Gennarelli TA: Cerebral concussion and traumatic unconsciousness: Correlations and experimental and clinical observations on blunt head injuries. *Brain* 97:633, 1974.

Ommaya AK, Grubb RL, Naumann RA: Coup and contre-coup injury: Observations on the mechanics of visible brain injuries in the rhesus monkey. *J Neurosurg* 35:503, 1971.

Penfield W, Jasper HH: *Epilepsy and Functional Anatomy of the Human Brain*. Boston, Little, Brown, 1954.

Pevehouse BC, Blom WH, McKissock KW: Ophthalmologic aspects of diagnosis and localization of subdural hematoma. *Neurology* 10:1037, 1960.

Polin RS, Shaffrey ME, Bogaev CA, et al: Decompressive bifrontal craniectomy in the treatment of severe refractory posttraumatic cerebral edema. *Neurosurgery* 41:84, 1997.

Purvis JT: Craniocerebral injuries due to missiles and fragments, in Caveness WF, Walker AE (eds): *Head Injury*. Philadelphia, Lippincott, 1966, pp 133–141.

Rasmussen T: Surgical therapy of post-traumatic epilepsy, in Walker AE, Caveness WF, Critchley M (eds): *Late Effects of Head Injury*. Springfield, IL, Charles C Thomas, 1969, pp 277–305.

Rish BL, Caveness WR: Relation of prophylactic medication to the occurrence of early seizures following craniocerebral trauma. *J Neurosurg* 38:155, 1973.

Roberts AJ: *Brain Damage in Boxers: A Study of Prevalence of Traumatic Encephalopathy Among Ex-professional Boxers*. London, Pitman, 1969.

Roberts GW, Allsop D, Bruton C: The occult aftermath of boxing. *J Neurol Neurosurg Psychiatry* 53:373, 1990.

Ropper AH: Brain injuries from blasts. *N Engl J Med* 364:2156, 2011.

Ropper AH: Hyperosmolar therapy for raised intracranial pressure. *N Engl J Med* 367:746, 2012.

Ropper AH, Gorson KC: Concussion. *N Engl J Med* 356:166, 2007.

Ropper AH, Gress DR, Diringer MN, et al (eds): *Neurological and Neurosurgical Intensive Care*, 4th ed. Baltimore, MD, Lippincott Williams & Wilkins, 2004.

Ropper AH, Miller D: Acute traumatic midbrain hemorrhage. *Ann Neurol* 18:80, 1985.

Rosner MJ, Becker DP: Origin and evolution of plateau waves. *J Neurosurg* 60:312, 1984.

Ross RJ, Cole M, Thompson JS, Kim KH: Boxers—computed tomography, EEG, and neurological evaluation. *JAMA* 249:211, 1983.

Rossitch E, Bullard DE: The autonomic dysfunction syndrome: Aetiology and treatment. *Br J Neurosurg* 2:471, 1988.

Rowbotham GF (ed): *Acute Injuries of the Head*, 4th ed. Baltimore, MD, Williams & Wilkins, 1964.

Russell WR: *The Traumatic Amnesias*. London, Oxford, 1971.

SAFE Investigators: Saline or albumin for fluid resuscitation in patients with traumatic brain injury. *N Engl J Med* 357:874, 2000.

Shatsky SA, Evans DE, Miller F, Martins AN: High speed angiography of experimental head injury. *J Neurosurg* 41:523, 1974.

Shaw NA: The neurophysiology of concussion. *Prog Neurobiol* 67:281, 2002.

Simon B, Letourneau P, Vitorino E, et al. Pediatric head trauma: Indications for computed tomographic scanning revisited. *J Trauma* 51:231, 2001.

Skippen P, Seear M, Poskitt K, et al: Effect of hyperventilation on regional cerebral blood flow in head-injured children. *Crit Care Med* 25:1402, 1997.

Smits M, Dippel DW, de Haan GG, et al. External validation of the Canadian CT head rule and the New Orleans Criteria for CT scanning in patients with minor head injury. *JAMA* 294:1519, 2005.

Snoek JW, Minderhoud JM, Wilmink JT: Delayed deterioration following mild head injury in children. *Brain* 107:15, 1984.

Stern WE: Carotid-cavernous fistula, in Vinken PJ, Bruyn GW (eds): *Handbook of Clinical Neurology*. Vol 24. Amsterdam, North-Holland, 1975, pp 399–440.

Stiell IG, Clement C, Rowe BH, et al. Comparison of the Canadian CT Head Rule and the New Orleans Criteria in patients with minor head injury. *JAMA* 294:1511, 2005.

Strich SJ: Diffuse degeneration of the cerebral white matter in severe dementia following head injury. *J Neurol Neurosurg Psychiatry* 19:163, 1956.

Strich SJ: The pathology of severe head injury. *Lancet* 2:443, 1961.

Symonds CP: Concussion and contusion of the brain and their sequelae, in Feiring EH (ed): *Brock's Injuries of the Brain and Spinal Cord and Their Coverings*, 5th ed. New York, Springer-Verlag, 1974, pp 100–161.

Temkin NR, Dikman SS, Wilensky AJ et al: A randomized double-blind study of phenytoin for the prevention of seizures. *N Engl J Med* 323:497, 1990.

Teuber H-L: Effects of brain wounds implicating right or left hemisphere in man, in Mountcastle VB (ed): *Interhemispheric Relations and Cerebral Dominance*. Baltimore, MD, Johns Hopkins University Press, 1962, pp 131–157.

Trotter W: Certain minor injuries of the brain. *Lancet* 1:935, 1924.

Vollmer DG, Torner JC, Jane JA, et al: Age and outcome following traumatic coma: Why do older patients fare worse? *J Neurosurg* 75(Suppl):S37, 1991.

Walker AE: Post-traumatic epilepsy, in Rowbotham GF (ed): *Acute Injuries of the Head*, 4th ed. Baltimore, MD, Williams & Wilkins, 1964, pp 486–509.

Wall SE, Williams WH, Cartwright-Hatton S, et al: Neuropsychological dysfunction following repeat concussions in jockeys. *J Neurol Neurosurg Psychiatry* 77:518, 2006.

Weir B: The osmolality of subdural hematoma fluid. *J Neurosurg* 34:528, 1971.

Weiss GH, Salazar AM, Vance SC, et al: Predicting posttraumatic epilepsy in penetrating head injury. *Arch Neurol* 43:771, 1986.

Xydakis MS, Bebarta VS, Harrison CD, et al: Tympanic membrane perforation as a marker of concussive injury in Iraq. *N Engl J Med* 357:830, 2007.

Zander E, Foroglou G: Post-traumatic hydrocephalus, in Vinken PJ, Bruyn GW (eds): *Handbook of Clinical Neurology*. Vol 24. Amsterdam, North-Holland, 1976, pp 231–253.

36

Multiple Sclerosis and Other Inflammatory Demyelinating Diseases

It has long been the practice to set apart a group of diseases of the brain and spinal cord in which destruction of myelin, termed *demyelination*, is a prominent feature. To define these diseases precisely is difficult, for the simple reason that there is probably no disease in which myelin destruction is the exclusive pathologic change. The idea of a demyelinating disease is an abstraction that serves primarily to focus attention on one of the more striking and distinctive features of one group of pathologic processes. Another unifying feature of most of these processes is the participation of an inflammatory reaction in proximity to demyelination. The most common and important inflammatory demyelinating disease is multiple sclerosis (MS).

The generally accepted pathologic criteria of a demyelinating disease are (1) destruction of the myelin sheaths of nerve fibers with *relative* sparing of the other elements of nervous tissue, i.e., of axons, nerve cells, and supporting structures, which are less affected; (2) infiltration of inflammatory cells, particularly in a perivenous distribution; (3) lesions that are primarily in white matter, either in multiple small disseminated foci or in larger foci spreading from one or more centers. In most of the demyelinating diseases, it has been known since the early descriptions that there is some degree of neuronal and axonal degeneration, but it is the preferential effect on myelin that defines this group of disorder. In the language of neurology, therefore, the term *demyelination* has acquired a special meaning.

A broad classification of the inflammatory demyelinating diseases is given in Table 36-1. Like all classifications that are not based on etiology, this one has its limitations. For example, in some of the diseases here classified as demyelinating, notably, in necrotizing hemorrhagic leukoencephalitis and even in some cases of multiple sclerosis, the inflammatory process may be sufficiently intense so much so that there is destruction of all tissue in a region including vessels and axons.

In contrast, a number of diseases in which demyelination is a prominent feature are considered part of this category, as mentioned earlier. In some cases of anoxic encephalopathy, for example, the myelin sheaths of the radiating nerve fibers in the deep layers of the cerebral cortex or in ill-defined patches in the convolutional and central white matter are destroyed, while most of the axis cylinders are spared. A relatively selective degeneration of myelin may also occur in some small ischemic foci as a result of vascular occlusion or in larger confluent areas, as is the case in Binswanger disease (see Chap. 34). In subacute combined degeneration (SCD) of the spinal cord associated with pernicious anemia and in tropical spastic paraparesis (TSP), a demyelinating spinal cord disease, myelin may be affected earlier and to a greater extent than axons. The same is true of progressive multifocal leukoencephalopathy (PML), osmotic demyelination (also known as central pontine myelinolysis), and Marchiafava-Bignami disease. Some of these disorders and several others are not classified as demyelinating because the effects of the process are not primarily on myelin; furthermore, they are not based on an inflammatory component. In addition, for reasons that will become clear in subsequent discussion, the chronic progressive leukodystrophies of childhood and adolescence (e.g., globoid body, metachromatic, and adrenal leukodystrophies), although clearly diseases of myelin, are set apart and called *dysmyelinating* because of their unique genetic and morphologic features, and are discussed in Chap. 37. Occupying an uncertain place in this nosology are demyelinating lesions associated with connective tissue diseases or with autoantibodies directed against DNA or phospholipids. The central nervous system (CNS) lesions may be multiple and cannot easily be distinguished by imaging features from multiple sclerosis. But, as noted further on, their nature is uncertain, while some are clearly caused by a vasculopathy.

MULTIPLE SCLEROSIS

History Multiple sclerosis, called MS by most physicians, was referred to by the British as *disseminated sclerosis* and by the French as *sclérose en plaques*. The broad nature of disseminated lesions was known to pathologists in the early nineteenth century particularly as described by Carswell, Cruveilhier and later, Frerichs, but J.M Charcot at the Salpêtrière later in the century is justly credited with the first serious study of the clinical and pathologic aspects of the disease. He collected 34 cases and set a foundation for understanding the disease. With neurosyphilis, multiple sclerosis formed much of

Table 36-1

CLASSIFICATION OF THE INFLAMMATORY DEMYELINATIVE DISEASES

I. Multiple sclerosis
  A. Relapsing-remitting form
  B. Secondary progressive form
  C. Primary progressive form
  D. Acute multiple sclerosis (Marburg disease and tumefactive multiple sclerosis)
  E. Diffuse cerebral sclerosis (Schilder disease and concentric sclerosis of Balo)
II. Neuromyelitis optica (Devic disease, NMO) and progressive necrotic myelopathy
III. Acute disseminated encephalomyelitis (ADEM) and acute hemorrhagic encephalitis (Weston Hurst disease)
IV. Demyelination in association with autoimmune disease (SLE, Sjögren disease, and related conditions)
V. Sarcoid-related demyelination
VI. Graft-versus-host disease

the basis of early clinicopathologic correlation and the clinical method in neurology. It is therefore among the most venerable of neurologic diseases and one of the most important by virtue of its frequency, chronicity, and tendency to affect young adults. Cruveilhier (circa 1835), in his original description of the disease, attributed it to suppression of sweat, and since that time there has been endless speculation about the etiology. While many of the early theories are anachronistic in the light of present-day concepts, others are still of interest. There is little point in enumerating them here. The historical aspects can be found in the corresponding chapter of the text by Compston and colleagues.

Introductory Remarks Multiple sclerosis is a chronic condition characterized clinically by episodes of focal disorders of the optic nerves, spinal cord, and brain, which remit to a varying extent and recur over a period of many years and are usually progressive. The neurologic manifestations are protean, being determined by the varied location and extent of the demyelinating foci. Nevertheless, the lesions have a predilection for certain parts of the CNS, resulting in complexes of symptoms and signs and imaging appearances that can often be recognized as distinctive of MS as discussed in detail further on.

Typical features include weakness, paraparesis, paresthesias, loss of sight, diplopia, nystagmus, dysarthria, tremor, ataxia, impairment of deep sensation, and bladder dysfunction. The diagnosis may be uncertain at the onset and in the early years of the disease, when symptoms and signs point to a lesion in only one locus of the nervous system. Later, as the disease recurs and disseminates throughout the central nervous system, the diagnosis becomes quite certain. There may be a long period of latency (1 to 10 years or longer) between a minor initial symptom, which may not even come to medical attention, and the subsequent development of more characteristic symptoms. In most cases, there is initially a *relapsing-remitting* pattern, i.e., the signs and symptoms improve partially or completely, followed after a variable interval by the recurrence of the same abnormalities or the appearance of new ones in other parts of the nervous system. However, in fewer than half of patients, the disease takes the form a steadily progressive course, especially in patients older than 40 years of age at the time of onset (*primary progressive MS*). Or, as happens more often, an initially relapsing profile later becomes steadily progressive (*secondary progressive MS*).

A rule that had in the past guided clinicians is that the diagnosis of MS was not secure unless there was a history of remission and relapse and evidence on examination of more than one discrete lesion of the CNS. The advent of MRI and its capacity to identify clinically inevident lesions has replaced the exclusive dependence on clinical criteria for the diagnosis.

Pathologic Findings

Before being sectioned, the brain and spinal cord generally show no evidence of disease, but the surface of the spinal cord may appear and feel uneven. Sectioning of the brain and cord discloses numerous scattered patches where the tissue is slightly depressed below the cut surface and stands out from the surrounding white matter by virtue of its pink-gray color (a result of loss of myelin). The lesions may vary in diameter from less than a millimeter to several centimeters; they principally affect the white matter of the brain and spinal cord, and do not extend beyond the root entry zones of the cranial and spinal nerves. It is because of their sharp delineation that they were called *plaques* by French pathologists.

The topography of the lesions is noteworthy. A periventricular localization is characteristic, but only where subependymal veins line the ventricles (mainly adjacent to the bodies and atria of the lateral ventricles). Other favored structures are the optic nerves and chiasm (but rarely the optic tracts) and the spinal cord, where pial veins lie next to or within the white matter. The lesions are distributed randomly throughout the brainstem, spinal cord, and cerebellar peduncles without reference to particular systems of fibers, but always confined predominantly to the white matter. In the cerebral cortex and central nuclear and spinal structures, the acute lesions destroy myelin sheaths but leave the nerve cells mostly intact. Severe and more chronic lesions, however, may destroy axons and neurons in the affected region, but the dominant lesion is still demyelinating.

The histologic appearance of the lesion depends on its age. Relatively recent lesions show a partial or complete destruction and loss of myelin throughout a zone formed by the confluence of many small, predominantly perivenous foci; the axons in the same region are relatively spared or less affected. There is a variable but usually slight degeneration of oligodendroglia, a variable astrocytic reaction, and perivascular and para-adventitial infiltration with mononuclear cells and lymphocytes as discussed in detail further on. Later, large numbers of microglial phagocytes (macrophages) infiltrate the lesions and astrocytes in and around the lesions increase in number and size. Long-standing lesions, on the other hand, are composed of thickly matted, relatively acellular glial tissue, with only occasional perivascular lymphocytes and macrophages; in such lesions, a few intact axons may still be found. In old lesions with interruption of axons, there may be descending and ascending wallerian degeneration of long fiber tracts in the spinal cord. Partial remyelination is believed to take place on undamaged axons and to account for incompletely demyelinated "shadow patches" (Prineas and Connell). A few of the most severe older lesions will have undergone cavitation, indicating that the disease process has affected not only myelin and axons but also supporting tissues and blood vessels. All gradations of histopathologic change between these two extremes may be found in lesions of diverse size, shape, and age, consistent with the extended clinical course.

The relatively ineffective remyelination of the MS plaque leaves in its wake denuded axons that are thinly myelinated, creating the just mentioned shadow plaques. Histologic evidence suggests that some of the oligodendrocytes are destroyed in areas of active demyelination but also that the remaining ones have little ability to proliferate. Instead, there is an influx of oligodendroglial precursor cells, which mature into oligodendrocytes and provide the remaining axons with new myelin. Probably the astrocytic hyperplasia in regions of damage and the persistent inflammatory response account for some of the inadequacy of the reparative process (see Prineas et al).

An insight into the complexity of the immunopathologic process can be appreciated in the analyses by Lucchinetti and colleagues (2000) of autopsy and brain biopsy specimens from patients with MS. They separated the lesions into four histologic subgroups: inflammatory lesions made up of T cells and macrophages alone (pattern I); an autoantibody lesion mediated by immunoglobulin and complement (pattern II); those characterized by apoptosis of oligodendrocytes and absence of immunoglobulin, complement, and with partial remyelination (pattern III); and those showing only oligodendrocyte dystrophy and no remyelination (pattern IV). Two features are of interest here. First, each case demonstrated only one pattern of pathology, suggesting that perhaps different pathophysiologic processes operated in each patient. Moreover, the last two histopathologic types were considered to represent a primary oligodendroglial cell degeneration. Some confirmation of a primary process in oligodendrocytes is the material from newly symptomatic lesions reported by Barnett and Prineas, in which there was loss of these cells. In addition, early lesions have been found to contain areas of demyelination within the cerebral cortex and these are often in contiguity with meningeal inflammatory infiltrates, or lymphoid follicles (Lucchinetti et al 2011, Howell et al).

The overall implication is that the pathologic characteristics of the chronic progressive type of MS may differ from those of the typical relapsing type (see further on). Most data suggest that antibody and complement-mediated myelin phagocytosis are the dominant mechanism of demyelination in MS. At the moment, we continue to conceptualize MS as mainly an inflammatory-immune process that targets central myelin along the lines of the observations of Adams and Kubik in their earlier studies, who were aware of the axonal and cortical changes in pathologic material they collected in the 1940s.

Etiology and Epidemiology

The incidence of MS is two or three times higher in women than in men but the basis of this fact is unclear, the best current explanation being that women are generally more susceptible to immune and inflammatory conditions. The incidence in children is very low; only 0.3 to 0.4 percent of all cases appear during the first decade. In an analysis of a small number of childhood-onset cases, Hauser and colleagues (1982) found no phenotypic differences between childhood and adult cases, but Renoux and colleagues analyzed a cohort of 394 patients who had MS with an onset at 16 years or younger and found that these patients took longer to reach states of irreversible disability, but did so at a younger age than patients with adult-onset MS. Beyond childhood, the risk of first developing symptoms of the disease rises steeply with age, reaching a peak at about 30 years, remaining high in the fourth decade, then falling off sharply and becoming low in the sixth decade. On this basis it has been pointed out that MS has a unimodal age-specific onset curve, similar to that of infectious and connective tissue diseases.

In a smaller number, the disease appears to develop in late adult life (late fifties and sixties). In such patients, early symptoms may have been forgotten or may never have declared themselves clinically (we have several times found the typical lesions of MS in aged autopsied individuals who had no history of neurologic illness). Gilbert and Sadler report five such cases and from their pathologic findings suggest that the true incidence of MS may be three times higher than the stated figures.

Although the cause of MS remains undetermined, a number of epidemiologic facts have been established and will eventually have to be incorporated in any hypothesis. The disease has a prevalence of less than 1 per 100,000 in equatorial areas; 6 to 14 per 100,000 in the southern United States and southern Europe; and 30 to 80 per 100,000 in Canada, northern Europe, and the northern United States. Mayr and colleagues reported an incidence of 8 and a prevalence of 177 cases per 100,000 in Olmstead County, Minnesota; this prevalence has been stable for approximately 30 years. A less-well-defined gradient exists in the southern hemisphere. Kurland's studies indicated that there is a threefold increase in prevalence and a fivefold gradient in mortality rate between New Orleans (30 degrees north latitude) and Boston (42 degrees north) and Winnipeg (50 degrees north). In Japan, there is a similar although less distinct latitudinal gradient (the prevalence of MS there is much lower than in corresponding latitudes of North America and northern Europe).

The increasing risk of developing MS with higher and lower latitude has been confirmed by many epidemiologists following the work of Kurtzke (1975). In the United States, African Americans are at lower risk than whites at all latitudes, but both races show the same south-to-north gradient in risk, findings that invoked an environmental factor regardless of genetic predisposition. Supporting this view are the descriptions, by Kurtzke and Hyllested, of an "epidemic" of MS in the Faroe Islands of the North Atlantic. They found a much-higher-than-expected incidence of the disease, occurring as three separate outbreaks of decreasing extent between the years 1943 and 1973. (It should be pointed out that the largest outbreak consisted of only 21 cases.) It was their contention, confirmed by Poskanzer and colleagues, that the disease was the result of an unidentified infection introduced by British troops who occupied the islands in large numbers in the years immediately preceding the outbreak. Kurtzke and colleagues (1982) described a similar postwar epidemic in Iceland. The cause of these geographic distributions has been reinterpreted in terms of migration and population genetics rather than a number of other imputed causes, but they remain interesting (see Compston and Confavreaux for a complete discussion).

The role of Vitamin D and of sun exposure has become an area of related epidemiologic research. Some data suggest that the risk of MS is in part a result of a lack of exposure to these two related environmental features (Munger et al and van der Mei et al). Whether this partly explains the latitudinally graded risk is unclear. An observed seasonal fluctuation in the activity of established MS lesions may have a similar basis.

Several studies indicate that persons who migrate from a high-risk to a low-risk zone carry with them at least part of the risk of their country of origin and genetic makeup, even though the disease may not become apparent until 20 years after migration. Such a pattern has been demonstrated in both South Africa and Israel. Dean determined that the prevalence of MS in native-born white South Africans was 3 to 11 per 100,000, whereas the rate in immigrants from northern Europe was approximately 50 per 100,000, only slightly less than among the nonimmigrating natives of those countries. The data of Dean and Kurtzke indicate further that in persons who had immigrated before the age of 15, the risk was similar to that of native-born South Africans; whereas in persons who had immigrated after that age, the risk was similar to that of their birthplace. Alter and colleagues found that in the descendants of European immigrants born in Israel, the risk of MS was low, similar to that of other native-born Israelis, whereas among recent immigrants the incidence in each national group approached that of the land of birth. Again, the critical age of immigration appeared to be about 15 years. These older epidemiologic studies and others have suggested that MS is associated with particular localities rather than with a particular ethnic group in those localities, and implicate environmental factors but not to the exclusion of genetic susceptibility. However, more current studies suggest the opposite; that genetic factors in a population predominate.

A familial aggregation of MS is now well established. Approximately 15 percent of MS patients have an affected relative, with the highest risk of concurrence being observed in the patient's siblings (Ebers, 1983). In a large population-based study carried out in British Columbia by Sadovnick and colleagues (1988), it was found that almost 20 percent of index cases had an affected relative, again with the highest risk in siblings. In a subsequent study, Sadovnick and colleagues (1996) sought to determine the degree of heritability of MS by comparing the risk of disease in the half-sibs (one biologic parent in common) of affected individuals with the risk in full sibs; the risk for full sibs was two to three times greater than for half-sibs and they interpreted these results as clearly genetic in basis.

The case for heritability is further supported by studies of twins in whom one of each pair is known to have MS. In the most extensive of these studies (Ebers et al), the diagnosis was verified in 12 of 35 pairs of monozygotic twins (34 percent) and in only 2 of 49 pairs of dizygotic twins (4 percent). Furthermore, in two additional sets of monozygotic twins who were clinically normal, lesions were detected by MRI. The concordance rate in dizygotic pairs is similar to that in nontwin siblings. Despite these provocative findings, no consistent pattern of mendelian inheritance has emerged. Of course, one must not assume that all diseases with an increased familial incidence are hereditary in that instances of the same condition in several members of a family may simply reflect an exposure to a common environmental agent. Paralytic poliomyelitis, for example, was about eight times more common in immediate family members than in the population at large.

Further evidence of a genetic factor in the causation of MS is the finding that certain histocompatibility locus antigens (HLAs) are more frequent in patients with MS than in control subjects. The strongest association is with the DR locus on chromosome 6. Other HLA haplotypes that are overrepresented in MS (HLA-DR2 and, to a lesser extent, -DR3, -B7, and -A3) are thought to be markers for an MS "susceptibility gene"—possibly an immune response gene. The presence of one of these markers increases the risk that an individual will develop MS by a factor of 3 to 5. These antigens may indeed prove to be related to the frequency of the disease, but their presence is not invariable and their exact role is far from clear. A genome-wide association study identified several alleles, interleukin (IL)-2Rα, and IL7Rα in addition to the previously established HLA loci, as heritable risk factors for MS (International Multiple Sclerosis Genetics Consortium). These findings, although they apply to a small number of individuals, support the concept that dysregulation of the immune response is a factor in the risk for developing MS.

The low conjugal incidence of MS, on the other hand, indicates that any common exposure to an inciting infection or environmental agent must occur early in life. To test this hypothesis, Schapira and coworkers determined the periods of common exposure (common habitation periods) in members of families with two or more cases. From this they calculated the mean common exposure to have happened before 14 years of age, with a latency of about 21 years—figures that are in general agreement with those derived from the migration studies quoted above.

Several studies from northern Europe and Canada suggest that the likelihood of developing MS is somewhat greater among rural than among urban dwellers; studies of American army personnel indicate the opposite (Beebe et al). A number of surveys in Great Britain intimate that the disease is more frequent in the higher socioeconomic groups than in the lower ones. Yet in the United States, no clear relationship has been established to the poverty or social deprivations that are part of a low socioeconomic status. Numerous other environmental factors (surgical operations, trauma, anesthesia, exposure to household pets [small dogs], cobalamin deficiency or resistance, mercury in silver amalgam fillings in teeth), and Lyme disease have been proposed but are unsupported by firm evidence and probably are mostly spurious associations.

Pathogenesis

These epidemiologic data point to both a genetic susceptibility and some environmental factor that is encountered in childhood that, after years of latency, evokes the disease. Over the years, data favoring an infection, most often viral as the triggering factor, have had periods of support (see above). A body of indirect evidence has been marshaled in support of this idea, based largely on alterations in humoral and cell-mediated immunity to viral agents. To this day, however, no virus (including all known members of the human retrovirus family) has been seen in, or isolated from, the tissues of patients with MS despite innumerable attempts to do so. Moreover, no satisfactory viral model of MS has been produced experimentally. The bacterial agents *Chlamydia pneumoniae* and *Borrelia burgdorferi* (the agent of Lyme disease) and herpesvirus type 6 have been similarly implicated by the finding of their genomic material in MS plaques, but the evidence for their direct participation in the disease is, at the moment, not compelling.

If, indeed, some obscure infection is the initial event in the genesis of MS, then a secondary factor must be operative in later life to reactivate the disease and cause exacerbations. One view is that this secondary mechanism is an autoimmune reaction attacking some component of myelin and, in its most intense form, destroying all tissue elements, including axons. Several lines of argument have been advanced in support of this view. One is inclined to draw an analogy between the lesions of MS and those of acute disseminated encephalomyelitis, which is almost certainly an autoimmune disease of delayed hypersensitivity type (see further on). Also in support of this possibility is the finding of antibodies to specific myelin proteins—for example, myelin basic protein (MBP)—in both the serum and cerebrospinal fluid (CSF) of MS patients, and these antibodies, along with T cells that are reactive to MBP and to other myelin proteolipids, increase with disease activity; moreover, MBP cross-reacts to some extent with measles virus antibodies. The arguments that a chronic viral infection reactivates and perpetuates the disease are, however, less convincing than those proposing a role for viruses in the initiation of the process in susceptible individuals.

The relative roles of humoral and cellular factors in the production of MS plaques are not fully understood. The deposition of immunoglobulin in the plaques of patients with acute and relapsing–remitting disease, but not in the plaques of those with progressive MS, was alluded to earlier. That the humoral immune system is involved is evident from the presence in the CSF of most patients of oligoclonal immune protein antibodies, which are produced by B lymphocytes within the CNS. Sera from patients with MS (and some normal controls), when added to cultures of nervous system tissue from newborn mice in the presence of complement, can damage myelin, inhibit remyelination, and block axonal conduction. Antibodies to oligodendrocytes are present in the serum of up to 90 percent of patients in some studies, but far less frequently in others.

Autoantibodies have been found inconsistently that are directed against myelin oligodendrocyte glycoprotein (MOG) and MBP. It has also been demonstrated that subsets of T cells (CD41 Th2 cells) are activated by MBP and MOG to activate B cells, the production of oligoclonal bands and membrane attack complexes, and the release of cytokines (tumor necrosis factor-alpha [TNF-α], interleukins, interferon-gamma [IFN-γ]). The inflammatory process erodes the blood–brain barrier and ultimately destroys both oligodendroglia and axons. The eventual functional outcome reflects both the activity of this inflammatory cascade and the degree of axonal damage. In other cases, there may be a compromise of oligodendroglial function and axonal degeneration in the absence of prominent inflammation. Many times, one or another putative antigenic target has been found by immunologic techniques in one laboratory, only to fail to be replicated by another group. None of these provide a unifying etiology for the disease but the humoral aspects may provide insights particularly into the pauci-inflammatory type of oligodendrocyte degeneration that characterizes some lesions, as discussed in the section on pathology.

Nevertheless, most immunologists currently subscribe to the notion that MS is mediated by a T-cell sensitization to some component of myelin. This idea is supported by numerous lines of evidence, including the observation that T cells initiate the lesions of experimental allergic encephalomyelitis (EAE), which is assumed to be an approximate animal model of MS, as suggested originally by Waksman and Adams. It has been difficult, however, to produce a relapsing experimental form of the illness that would simulate MS. Although the entry of autoreactive T cells into the CNS results in a perivascular inflammatory reaction, its relationship to MS is unclear. Conceivably, intense T-cell stimulation is in itself sufficient to induce demyelination but it is also possible that the primary target of the immune reaction is the myelin sheath or some component thereof and that the T-cell infiltration is a reaction to demyelination. Most investigators believe that an additional insult is required, as illustrated by the EAE animal model, in which myelin alone is not a sufficient factor but always requires an adjuvant immune stimulus. EAE is clearly an imperfect model; it is not a naturally occurring disease but one in which a demyelination of the CNS is induced in susceptible animals in a single episode by autologous myelin antigens. The inducing antigen in EAE is known, whereas the putative antigens in MS are not.

Also incorporated into most theories of the immune pathogenesis is an alteration of the blood–brain barrier, represented by adhesion of lymphocytes to endothelial cells in the nervous system. Whether this is an active interaction or a passive event triggered by antigenic attraction is not clear; nonetheless, these cell–vascular interactions have been incorporated into pathogenic theories and are the basis of newer treatments for MS. Always in the background is the element of genetic susceptibility, presumably making certain individuals prone to these immunologic events as noted in the earlier sections.

The foregoing data notwithstanding, the immune mechanisms in MS are not fully specified and the autoimmune hypothesis is not beyond challenge. It is noteworthy that the prevalence of other diseases of presumed autoimmune origin in some series is no higher in MS patients than in the general population (De Keyser). However, various epidemiologic studies differ on this point and some have found an increase in autoimmune diseases in affected patients and in their families.

Physiologic Effects of Demyelination

The main physiologic effect of demyelination is to impede saltatory electrical conduction of nerve impulses from one node of Ranvier, where sodium channels are concentrated, to the next node. The resulting failure of electrical transmission is thought to underlie most of the abnormalities of function resulting from demyelinating diseases of both the central and peripheral nerves. As an example, the delay in electrical conduction in the optic nerve (found by using pattern-shifting visual stimuli in MS patients) raises a number of points about the pathophysiology of demyelination. When the demyelinating process is acute and reversible within a few days, the block in nerve fiber conduction is obviously physiologic rather than pathologic; in such a brief period, recovery is unlikely to have been a result of remyelination; recovery is probably a result of subsidence of the edema and acute inflammatory changes in and around the lesion. Remyelination probably does occur, but it is a slower process and partial at best, and its functional effects in the CNS are possibly expressed as a slowing of nerve conduction, which, if present in an eye with normal vision, may account for the reduction in flicker fusion and in the perception of multiple visual stimuli (Halliday and McDonald). It also explains one of the typical symptoms of optic neuritis—reduction in the intensity (desaturation) of the color red. It is clear, however, that many of the plaques in the cerebral hemispheres that are visualized on MRI are unaccompanied by corresponding symptoms. Either there has been complete remyelination in these plaques, sufficient to support clinical functioning, or, in the acute stage, the plaque may represent edema rather than demyelination.

Another typical feature of MS is the temporary induction, by heat or exercise, of symptoms such as unilateral visual blurring (the Uhthoff phenomenon) or tingling and weakness of a limb (the basis of the hot-tub test used in previous years). This has been shown experimentally to represent an extreme sensitivity of conduction in demyelinated nerve fibers to an elevation in temperature. A rise of only 0.5°C (0.9°F) can block electrical transmission in thinly myelinated or demyelinated fibers. Likewise, hyperventilation slows conduction of the visual evoked response, an effect that is rarely perceived by the patient. The remarkable sensitivity of demyelinated and remyelinated regions to subtle metabolic and environmental changes provides an explanation for the rapid onset of symptoms in some patients and the apparent fluctuations of MS that show no laboratory evidence of active inflammatory changes in the CNS. Smoking, fatigue, hyperventilation, and a rise in environmental temperature are all capable of briefly worsening neurologic functioning and are easily confused with relapses of disease.

Clinical Manifestations

Early Symptoms and Signs

Weakness or numbness, sometimes both, in one or more limbs is the initial symptom in about half the patients. Symptoms of tingling of the extremities and tight bandlike sensations around the trunk or limbs are commonly associated and are probably the result of involvement of the posterior columns of the spinal cord. The symptoms generally appear over hours or days, at times being so trifling that they are ignored, and less often, coming on so acutely and prominently as to bring the patient urgently to the doctor. The resulting clinical syndromes vary from a mere dragging or poor control of one or both legs to a spastic or ataxic paraparesis. The tendon reflexes are retained and later become hyperactive with extensor plantar reflexes; varying degrees of deep and superficial sensory loss may be associated. It is a useful adage that *the patient with MS presents with symptoms in one leg but with signs in both*; the patient will complain of weakness, incoordination, or numbness and tingling in one lower limb and prove to have bilateral Babinski signs and other evidence of bilateral corticospinal and posterior column disease.

There are, in addition, several syndromes that are typical of multiple sclerosis and may be the initial manifestations. These common modes of onset are: (1) optic neuritis, (2) transverse myelitis, (3) cerebellar ataxia, and (4) brainstem syndromes (vertigo, facial pain or numbness, dysarthria, diplopia). When these are unaccompanied by other features of MS, they are termed "clinically isolated syndrome" (CIS) but they are often aspects of the established disease as well. In the initial phases of the illness, they may pose diagnostic questions, as they also certainly occur with numerous diseases other than MS.

Flexion of the neck may induce a tingling, electric-like feeling down the shoulders and back and, less commonly, down the anterior thighs. This phenomenon is known as the *Lhermitte sign*, although it is more a symptom than a sign and was originally described by Babinski in a case of cervical cord trauma. Lhermitte's contribution was to draw attention to the frequent occurrence of this phenomenon in MS. It is probably attributable to an increased sensitivity of demyelinated axons to the stretch or pressure on the spinal cord induced by neck flexion, but it occurs in other conditions such as cervical spondylosis.

McAlpine and coworkers (1972) analyzed the mode of onset in 219 patients and found that in 20 percent the neurologic symptoms were fully developed in a matter of minutes, and, in a similar number, in a matter of hours. In approximately 30 percent the symptoms evolved more slowly, over a period of a day or several days, and in another 20 percent more slowly still, over several weeks to months. In the remaining 10 percent the symptoms had an insidious onset and slow, steady, or intermittent progression over months and years. The typical relapsing–remitting pattern of disease is more likely to appear in patients who are younger than 40 years of age. Certain paroxysmal symptoms and signs may occur in the established phase of the disease and discussed further on. The inflammatory process of MS affects no organ system other than the CNS.

Optic Neuritis (Retrobulbar Neuritis; Papillitis)

(See "Optic Neuritis" in Chap. 13)

In approximately 25 percent of all MS patients (and possibly in a larger proportion of children), the initial manifestation is an episode of *optic neuritis*. It will be recalled that the optic nerve is in fact a tract of the brain, and involvement of the optic nerves is therefore consistent with the rule that lesions of MS are confined to the CNS. Characteristically, over a period of several days, there is partial or total loss of vision in one eye. Many patients, for a day or two before the visual loss, experience pain within the orbit, worsened by eye movement or palpation of the globe. Rarely, the visual loss is steadily progressive for several weeks, mimicking a compressive lesion or intrinsic tumor of the optic nerve (Ormerod and McDonald). Usually a scotoma involving the macular area and blind spot (cecocentral) can be demonstrated, but a wide variety of other field defects may occur, rarely even hemianopic involvement (sometimes homonymous). In some patients, both optic nerves are involved, either simultaneously or, more commonly, within a few days or weeks of one another, and at least one in eight patients will have repeated attacks.

Serial examinations may disclose evidence of swelling or edema of the optic nerve head (papillitis) in about a tenth of the patients. The occurrence of papillitis depends on the proximity of the demyelinating lesion to the nerve head. As emphasized in Chap. 13, papillitis can be distinguished from the papilledema of increased intracranial pressure by the severe and acute visual loss that accompanies only the former. More often, the optic nerve head appears normal or nearly so; this represents *retrobulbar neuritis*. Subtle manifestations of optic nerve affection, such as an afferent pupillary defect, atrophy of retinal nerve fibers, or sheathing of retinal veins and abnormalities of the visual evoked response (Chap. 2), should be sought in patients who have no visual complaints but are suspected of having MS. In cases of substantial visual loss, there is a diminished pupillary response to light (afferent pupillary paralysis) and instability of the direct pupillary response but the pupil is not dilated in ambient light. If the optic neuritis is unilateral, the consensual light reflex from the normal eye is retained. (Demyelination of the third nerve in its brainstem course, however, may be associated with a fixed enlargement of the pupil.) Visual evoked potentials and optical coherence tomography (OCT) may be useful in detecting optic neuritis, as discussed in a later section and in Chap. 2.

As noted in Chap. 13, about half of patients with optic neuritis recover completely, and most of the remaining ones improve significantly, even those who present initially with profound visual loss and, later, pallor of the optic disc (Slamovitis et al). Any pain in the globe is short-lived and persistent pain should prompt an evaluation for local disease. In a cohort of 397 patients enrolled in the Optic Neuritis Treatment Trial and examined 5 years after the initial attack of optic neuritis, visual acuity had returned to 20/25 or better in 87 percent of patients and to 20/40 or better in 94 percent—even if there had been a recurrence of optic neuritis during the 5-year period. Moreover, the mode of treatment did not appear to influence the outcome. Dyschromatopsia, generally taking the form of a perceived desaturation of colors, frequently persists as does the Pulfrich effect, wherein an object such as a pendulum that is swinging perpendicular to the patient's line of sight, appears to moving in a three-dimensional, circular motion.

When improvement occurs, it usually begins within 2 weeks of onset, as is true of most acute manifestations of MS, perhaps sooner with corticosteroid treatment. Once improvement in neurologic function begins, it may continue for several months.

More than one-half of adult patients who present with optic neuritis will eventually develop other signs of MS. The prospective investigation of Rizzo and Lessell showed that MS developed in 74 percent of women and 34 percent of men by the fifteenth year after onset of visual loss; similar results were reported by the Optic Neuritis Study Group (Beck et al, 2003). The risk is much lower if the initial attack of optic neuritis occurs in childhood (26 percent developed after 40 years of followup [Lucchinetti et al 1997]); this suggests that some instances of the childhood disease may be of a different type, perhaps viral or postinfectious. The longer the period of observation and the greater the care given to detection of mild cases, the greater the proportion of patients who are found to develop signs of MS; however, most do so within 5 years of the original attack (Ebers, 1985; Hely et al). In fact, in many patients with clinically isolated optic neuritis, MRI has disclosed lesions of the cerebral white matter—suggesting that dissemination, albeit asymptomatic, had already occurred and thereby establishing the diagnosis of MS (Jacobs et al, 1986; Ormerod et al). The Optic Neuritis

Study Group has made the point, well known to neurologists, that the *recurrence* of optic neuritis greatly increases the chances of developing MS. Of practical value is the observation, in the study by Beck and colleagues (2003), that the risk of relapsing-remitting MS is also considerably lower (22 percent at 10 years) if the cranial MRI fails to reveal demyelinating lesions.

It is unclear whether optic neuritis that occurs alone and is not followed by other evidence of demyelinating disease is simply a restricted form of MS or a manifestation of some other disease process, such as postinfectious encephalomyelitis. By far the most common pathologic basis for optic neuropathy is demyelinating disease, although it is known that a vascular lesion or compression of an optic nerve by a tumor or mucocele may cause a central or cecocentral scotoma that is indistinguishable from the defect of optic neuritis. Also, there may be a special form of chronic relapsing optic neuritis that is the result of an undefined granulomatous process such as sarcoid, as suggested by Kidd and colleagues. Uveitis and sheathing of the retinal veins are other ophthalmic disorders that occur with higher than expected incidence in patients with MS. The retinal vascular sheathing is caused by T-cell infiltration, identical to that in typical plaques, but this is an unusual finding, because the retina usually contains no myelinated fibers (Lightman et al). Optic neuritis is, of course, a common feature in neuromyelitis optica (Devic disease), discussed in a later section.

The treatment of optic neuritis is discussed further on.

Acute Myelitis (Transverse Myelitis)

(See Chap. 44)

This is the common designation for an acutely evolving inflammatory–demyelinating lesion of the spinal cord, which proves in many, but not all, instances to be an expression of MS. In this sense, the myelitic lesion is analogous to that of optic neuritis. The term *transverse* in relation to the myelitis is somewhat imprecise, implying that all of the elements in the cord are involved in the transverse plane, usually over a short vertical extent. Instead, in MS, the spinal cord signs are asymmetrical and incomplete and involve only a part of the long ascending and descending tracts, i.e., paraplegia and complete sensory loss are unusual.

Clinically, the illness is characterized by a rapidly evolving (several hours or days) symmetrical or asymmetrical paraparesis or paraplegia, ascending paresthesia, loss of deep sensibility in the feet, a sensory level on the trunk, sphincteric dysfunction, and bilateral Babinski signs. The CSF shows a modest number of lymphocytes and increase in total protein but both may be normal early in the illness. As many as one-third of patients report an infectious illness in the weeks preceding the onset of neurologic symptoms, in which case a monophasic postinfectious demyelinating disease rather than MS is the likely cause of the myelitis. The MRI usually shows indications of focal demyelination in the spinal cord at the appropriate level and there may be enhancement with gadolinium infusion, but neither of these findings is invariable. The lesions, as shown in Fig. 36-1 (*lower right panel*), are almost indistinguishable from those of postinfectious myelitis. In those instances associated with existing MS, even if not previously symptomatic, MRI of the cerebral hemispheres will show lesions consistent with demyelination; the absence of such lesions, however, does not ensure that the myelitic illness is monophasic and will not evolve to MS. Some cases progress to a necrotic myelopathy, with or without optic neuropathy, that is an expression of neuromyelitis optica, as discussed in a later section.

Fewer than half the patients have evidence of an asymptomatic demyelinating lesion elsewhere in the nervous system or develop clinical evidence of dissemination within 5 years of the initial attack of acute myelitis (Ropper and Poskanzer). Not entirely in accord with our experience is the analysis of subgroups in a trial of interferon therapy conducted by Beck and colleagues (2002), in which the cumulative probability of developing MS after 2 years was similar after either optic neuritis or transverse myelitis. Our sense has been that acute transverse myelitis is somewhat less often an initial expression of MS than is optic neuritis.

A special problem is presented by patients with *recurrent myelitis* at one level of the spinal cord but in whom no other signs of demyelinating disease can be found by careful clinical examination or MRI. Some of them may even have oligoclonal bands in the CSF, which are commonly associated with MS (see further on). Enough cases of this limited nature have come to our attention to permit the conclusion that there is a recurrent form of spinal cord MS in which cerebral dissemination is infrequent (Tippett et al). Isolated recurrent myelitis or myelopathy occurs also with lupus erythematosus, sarcoidosis, Sjögren syndrome, mixed connective tissue disease, and the antiphospholipid antibody syndrome or in the presence of other autoantibodies, as well as with dural and cord vascular fistulas and arteriovenous malformations. An analogous situation pertains in respect to some instances of optic neuritis—repeated attacks that remain confined to the optic nerve.

Other aspects of transverse myelitis are discussed in Chap. 44, and later in this chapter.

Other Clinical Features of Acute Attacks

Like the modes of onset cited above, other early manifestations of MS are unsteadiness in walking, brainstem symptoms (diplopia, vertigo, vomiting), paresthesias or numbness of an entire arm or leg, facial pain often simulating tic douloureux, and disorders of micturition. Vertigo of central type is also a frequent initial sign of MS, but it more often appears in established cases. Discrete manifestations such as hemiplegia, pain syndromes, facial paralysis, deafness, or seizures occur in an only small proportion of cases. Most often the disease presents with more than one of the aforementioned symptoms almost simultaneously or in rapid succession. Another relatively isolated syndrome, occurring mainly in older women, is a slowly progressive cervical myelopathy with weakness and ataxia. This is particularly difficult to differentiate from cervical spondylosis.

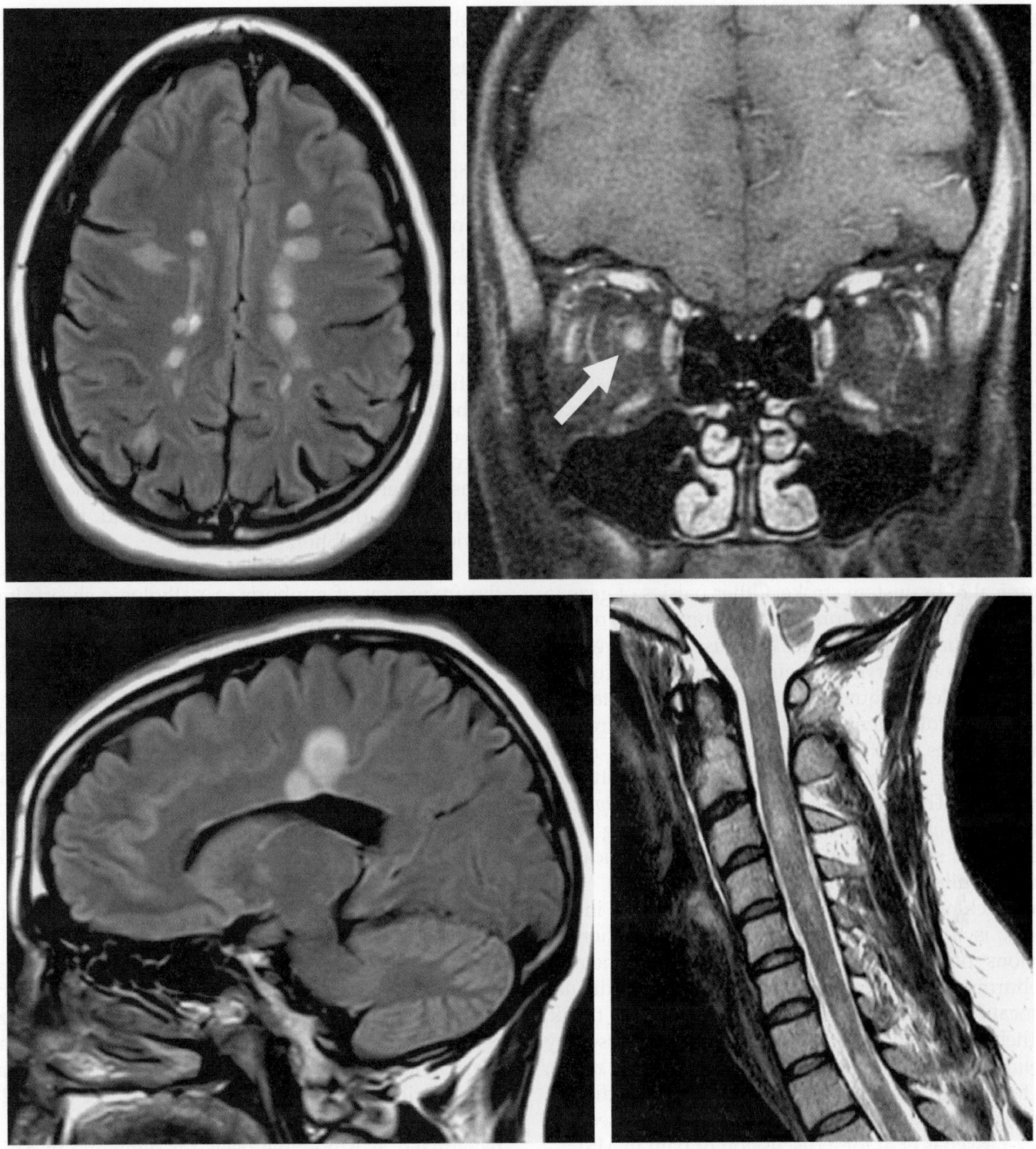

Figure 36-1. MRI in multiple sclerosis. *Upper left,* axial T2-FLAIR image showing multiple discrete periventricular hyperintense plaques, as well as two subcortical plaques in the right frontal and parietal lobes. *Upper right,* coronal T1-post gadolinium image showing abnormal enhancement of the right optic nerve in a case of acute optic neuritis (arrow). *Lower left,* sagittal T2-FLAIR image showing two hyperintense plaques emanating radially from the body of the corpus callosum ("Dawson fingers"). *Lower right,* sagittal T2 MRI showing multiple discrete hyperintense plaques within the cervical spinal cord. The lesion at C3 is acute with accompanying expansion of the cord. The lesion at the T1 level of the cord is chronic and shows cord atrophy.

Not infrequently a prominent feature of the disease is *nystagmus and ataxia,* with or without weakness and spasticity of the limbs, a syndrome that reflects involvement of the cerebellar and corticospinal tracts. Ataxia of cerebellar type can be recognized by scanning speech, rhythmic instability of the head and trunk, intention tremor of the arms and legs, and incoordination of voluntary movements and gait, as described in Chap. 5. The combination of nystagmus, scanning speech, and intention tremor is known as the *Charcot triad.* While this group of symptoms is often seen in the advanced stages of the disease, most neurologists would agree that it is not a common mode of presentation. The most severe forms of cerebellar ataxia, in which the slightest attempt to move the trunk or limbs precipitate a violent and uncontrollable ataxic tremor, are observed among patients with long-standing MS. The responsible lesion probably lies in the tegmentum of the midbrain and involves the dentatorubrothalamic tracts and adjacent structures. Cerebellar ataxia may be combined with sensory ataxia, owing to involvement of the posterior columns of the spinal cord or medial lemnisci of the brainstem. In most cases of this type, the signs of spinal cord involvement ultimately predominate; in others, the cerebellar signs are more prominent.

Diplopia is another common presenting complaint. It is most often a result of involvement of the medial longitudinal fasciculi, producing an internuclear *ophthalmoplegia* (see Chap. 14). The signs are characterized by paresis of the medial rectus on attempted lateral gaze, with a coarse nystagmus in the abducting eye; in MS, this abnormality is usually bilateral (unlike small pontine infarcts, which cause a unilateral internuclear ophthalmoplegia [INO]). As a corollary, *the presence of bilateral internuclear ophthalmoplegia in a young adult is virtually diagnostic of MS*. Occasionally, internuclear ophthalmoplegia in one direction is combined with a horizontal gaze paresis in the other, although this "one-and-a-half syndrome" is more typical of brainstem stroke. Other palsies of gaze (a result of interruption of supranuclear connections) or palsies of individual ocular muscles (because of involvement of the ocular motor nerves in their intramedullary course) also occur, but less frequently. Additional manifestations of brainstem involvement include myokymia or paralysis of facial muscles, deafness, tinnitus, vertigo—as noted above, vomiting (vestibular connections), and, rarely, stupor and coma. The occurrence of *transient facial hypesthesia or anesthesia or of trigeminal neuralgia* in a young adult should always suggest the diagnosis of MS implicating the intramedullary fibers of the fifth cranial nerve.

Dull, aching, but otherwise nondescript *pain* in the low back is a common complaint, but its relation to the lesions of MS is uncertain. Infrequently, there is sharp, burning, poorly localized, or lancinating radicular pain, localized to a limb or discrete part of the trunk. Nevertheless, these types of pains, presumably caused by demyelinating foci involving the dorsal root entry zones, have a few times been the presenting feature of the disease or have appeared at a later time in established cases (see Ramirez-Lassepas et al for a discussion of pain in MS).

Symptoms and Signs in the Established Disease

When the diagnosis of MS has become virtually certain, a number of clinical syndromes are observed to occur with regularity. Approximately one-half of the patients will manifest a clinical picture of *mixed* or *generalized type* with signs pointing to involvement of the optic nerves, brainstem, cerebellum, and spinal cord—specifically signs relating to the posterior columns and corticospinal tracts. Another 30 to 40 percent will exhibit only varying degrees of spastic ataxia and deep sensory changes in the extremities, i.e., essentially a *spinal form of the disease*. In either case, an asymmetrical spastic paraparesis with some degree of impaired joint position and vibration sense in the legs is probably the most common manifestation of progressive MS. A predominantly *cerebellar* or *brainstem–cerebellar form* occurs in approximately 5 percent of cases. Thus the mixed and spinal forms together have made up at least 80 percent of our clinical material.

It has become evident that some degree of cognitive impairment, and probably a progressive decline, is present in perhaps one-half of patients with long-standing MS. The process is characterized by reduced attention, diminished processing speed and executive skills, and memory decline, while language skills and other intellectual functions are preserved, features that have been subsumed under "subcortical dementia," as discussed in Chap. 21. Other mental disturbances, such as a loss of retentive memory, a global dementia, or a confusional–psychotic state, also occur in limited cases in the advanced stages of the disease, but we have found this degree of deterioration to be exceptional. The decline in cognitive functions correlates with quantifiable MRI measurements, particularly loss of white matter volume, thinning of the corpus callosum, and brain atrophy (reviewed by Bobholz and Rao).

Traditional teaching has probably overemphasized the frequency of euphoria, a pathologic cheerfulness or elation that seems inappropriate in the face of the obvious neurologic deficit. (Charcot spoke of this phenomenon as "stupid indifference" and Vulpian as "morbid optimism." It has often been referred to as "la belle indifférence.") Some patients do show this abnormality, usually in association with other signs of cerebral impairment. In some instances, it is manifestly a part of the syndrome of pseudobulbar palsy. A much larger number of patients, however, are depressed, irritable, and short-tempered, sometimes as a reaction to the disabling features of the disease but also apparently as a primary effect of the brain disease; the incidence of depression has been estimated to be as high as 25 to 40 percent in some series. Dalos and coworkers, in comparing MS patients with a group of traumatic paraplegics, found a significantly higher incidence of emotional disturbance in the former group, especially during periods of relapse. As mentioned above, the cognitive impairment is in keeping with what has been ascribed to "subcortical dementia" (see Chap. 21) but demyelination in the cortical layers is increasingly being recognized as a possible basis for dementia in MS. Loss of the volume of gray matter, for example, appears to be predictive of dementia as much as loss of central white matter. Either can give rise to global cerebral atrophy.

Symptoms of *bladder dysfunction*, including hesitancy, urgency, frequency, and incontinence, occur commonly with spinal cord involvement. Urinary retention, as a result of damage to sacral segments of the cord is less frequent (see Fig. 26-4). These symptoms are often associated with erectile dysfunction, a symptom that the patient may not report unless specifically questioned in this regard.

Paroxysmal attacks of neurologic deficit, lasting a few seconds or minutes and sometimes recurring many times daily, are relatively infrequent but well-recognized features of MS (see Mathews and also Osterman and Westerbey). Usually the attacks occur during the course of relapsing and remitting phase of the illness, rarely as an initial manifestation. These clinical phenomena are referable to any part of the CNS but tend to be stereotyped in an individual patient. The most common phenomena are dysarthria and ataxia, paroxysmal pain and dysesthesia in a limb, flashing lights, paroxysmal itching, or tonic "seizures", taking the form of flexion (dystonic) spasm of the hand, wrist, and elbow with extension of the lower limb. The paroxysmal symptoms, particularly the tonic spasms, may be triggered by sensory stimuli or can be elicited by hyperventilation. On a few occasions we have seen dystonic hand and arm spasms as the first symptoms; an acute plaque was detected in the opposite internal capsule. In advanced cases, the spasms may involve all four limbs and even a degree of opisthotonos. The cause of paroxysmal phenomena is uncertain. They have been attributed by Halliday and McDonald to ephaptic transmission ("cross-talk") between adjacent demyelinated axons within a lesion.

These transitory symptoms appear suddenly, may recur frequently for several days or weeks, sometimes longer, and then remit completely, i.e., they exhibit the temporal profile of a relapse or an exacerbation. It is sometimes difficult to determine whether they represent an exacerbation or a new lesion. Years ago, Thygessen pointed out, in an analysis of 105 exacerbations in 60 patients, that there were new symptoms in only 19 percent; in the remainder there was only a recurrence of old symptoms. Another problem is that the original lesion may have been asymptomatic. This is most obviously reflected in the many patients who are found to have impaired visual evoked responses but have never had symptomatic visual changes. Thus, new symptoms and signs may be manifestations of previously formed but asymptomatic plaques. However, the observations of Prineas and Connell indicate that symptoms and signs may progress without the appearance of new plaques. These and other factors need to be taken into consideration in evaluating the clinical course of the illness and the effects of a therapeutic program (see Poser, 1980). Carbamazepine is usually effective in controlling such spontaneous attacks, and acetazolamide blocks the painful tonic spasms that are elicited by hyperventilation.

Unusually severe *fatigue* is another peculiar symptom of MS; it is often transient and more likely to occur when there is fever or other evidence of disease activity but it can be a persistent complaint and a source of considerable distress. Depression may play a role in these recalcitrant cases, although the response to pharmacologic agents suggests that these two aspects of the disease are dissociable. Thus, antidepressants often do not improve fatigue, whereas drugs that alleviate fatigue, such as modafinil and amantadine, do not function as antidepressants.

A number of other interesting manifestations of MS have come to attention over the years and have given rise to difficulties in diagnosis. The occurrence of typical *tic douloureux* in young patients has already been mentioned; only their young age and the bilaterality of the pain in some of them raised the suspicion of MS, confirmed later by sensory loss in the face and other neurologic signs. It is notable, however, that facial palsy along the lines of Bell's palsy is almost never a sign of MS. Brachial, thoracic, or lumbosacral *pain* consisting mainly of thermal and algesic dysesthesias was a source of puzzlement in several of our patients until additional lesions developed. Other types of pain in MS have been addressed earlier.

In two of our cases, the relatively acute occurrence of a right hemiplegia and aphasia first raised the probability of a cerebrovascular lesion; in still others, a more slowly evolving hemiplegia had led to an initial diagnosis of a cerebral glioma. The dystonic and paroxysmal symptoms are mentioned earlier; they do not typically bring the diagnosis of MS to mind.

There may be a slightly increased incidence of seizures in patients with MS but the frequency of the problem varies greatly among studies. It should be emphasized that seizures are usually in relation to an obvious cerebral lesion and advanced disease of many years duration. Seizures at an early stage of illness are almost always attributable to previous head injury, idiopathic epilepsy, or withdrawal of sleep medication, but not to MS.

Several times we have seen coma during relapse of longstanding MS, and in each instance it continued to death. In one case it occurred in a 64-year-old woman who had had two previous episodes of nondisabling spinal MS at 30 and 44 years of age. A confusional state with drowsiness was the initial syndrome in another patient whom we saw later with a relapse involving the cerebellum and spinal cord. Another unusual syndrome is one of slow intellectual decline with slight cerebellar ataxia. The chronic progressive form of MS is addressed below.

Precipitating Factors for Acute Attacks

A variety of events occurring immediately before the initial symptoms or exacerbations of MS have been invoked as precipitating factors. The most common are infection, trauma, and pregnancy. However, in our view, none of these has been convincingly related to an increased risk of new attacks of MS, but there is little question that some febrile illnesses such as urinary infections can exaggerate the existing symptoms. The issue of truly precipitating a relapse as a result of a nondescript febrile illness is not resolved. Nonetheless, we have had experience with two patients who regularly had acute exacerbations of MS following each outbreak of labial genital herpes. The incidence of respiratory, urinary, or gastrointestinal viral infections that precede the onset or exacerbations of the disease varies greatly in different series, from 5 to 50 percent. The swine influenza vaccine, which was given to 45 million persons in the United States in late 1976, caused a slight increase in the incidence of Guillain-Barré disease but not of MS (Kurland et al), and more recent surveys of immunization programs, such as the one by Confavreux and colleagues (2001), have had similar results.

The possible role of trauma in precipitating MS is more difficult to assess. McAlpine and Compston found that the incidence of trauma within a 3-month period preceding the onset of MS was slightly greater than in a control group of hospital patients. Furthermore, there appeared to be a relationship between the site of the injury and the site of initial symptoms, particularly in patients who developed symptoms within a week of injury. We do not find this evidence convincing, particularly when given as an explanation for a large number of attacks. Other forms of trauma (including lumbar puncture and general surgical procedures) that occur after the onset of the neurologic disorder have not been shown to have an adverse effect on the course of the illness. Matthews, who has extensive personal experience with survivors of penetrating head wounds, did not find a single instance of MS among them. One of the most meaningful prospective studies of the relation of physical injury to MS is that of Sibley and colleagues, who followed 170 MS patients and 134 controls for an average of 5 years, during which they recorded all (1,407) instances of trauma and measured their effects on exacerbation rate and progression of the disease. With the possible exception of a case or two of electrical injury, there was no correlation between traumatic episodes and exacerbations. The current authoritative view on this subject is that the coincidence of trauma and new or exacerbated MS is incidental.

Certain other epidemiologic data have a bearing on this subject. There are, in the United States, 250,000 to 350,000 cases of physician-diagnosed MS (Anderson et al). Also, a study from the National Center for Health Statistics has determined that trauma sufficiently severe to be recalled at a periodic health examination occurs in one-third of the population of the United States (some 83 million persons) each year. Moreover, MS patients suffer physical injuries two or three times more often than normal persons (Sibley et al). In light of these data, it is perhaps not surprising that a traumatic event and an exacerbation should sometimes coincide, quite by chance.

Issues related to MS and pregnancy are addressed in a later section.

Variants of Multiple Sclerosis

Several variants of MS present special problems that are addressed in this and in later section.

Acute and Tumor-Like (Tumefactive) Multiple Sclerosis (Marburg Variant)

Rarely, MS takes a rapidly progressive and highly malignant form; Marburg's name has been attached to this variant. A combination of cerebral, brainstem, and spinal manifestations evolves over a few weeks, rendering the patient stuporous, comatose, or decerebrate with prominent cranial nerve and corticospinal abnormalities. Death may end the illness within a few weeks to months without any remission having occurred, or there may be partial recovery, as noted below. At autopsy the lesions are of macroscopic dimensions, in essence very large acute plaques of MS. The only difference from the usual form of MS is that many plaques are of the same age and the confluence of many perivenous zones of demyelination is more obvious. Two of our most striking examples of this rapidly fatal form were in a 6-year-old girl and a 16-year-old boy, both of whom died within 5 weeks of the onset of symptoms. Another was a 30-year-old man who lived 2 months. In none of them had there been a preceding exanthem or inoculation or any symptoms suggestive of demyelinating disease. Usually the CSF shows a cellular response but no oligoclonal bands. Some have made an astonishing recovery after several months, and a few have then remained well for 25 to 30 years. Others have relapsed, and the subsequent clinical course was typical of MS.

Among these cases are occurrences of large acute plaques with associated mass effect and enhancement that simulate a tumor on imaging (*tumefactive MS*, as described in the series by Kepes and shown in Fig. 36-2).

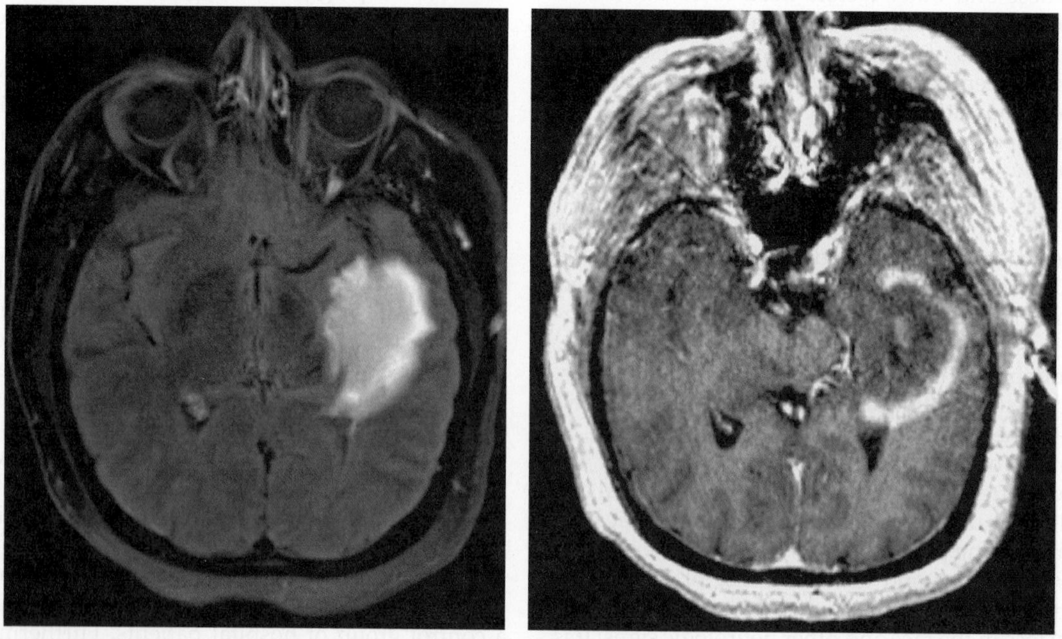

Figure 36-2. *Left* AxialT2 –FLAIR image of a tumefactive MS lesion in the left temporal lobe. *Right* T1-post gadolinium showing an "open ring" of abnormal contrast enhancement, a common imaging feature of acute demyelinating plaques that is less typical of tumors or abscesses.

The tumefactive lesion also occurs independently in cases of new or established disease that evolve in a manner that is more consistent with typical MS.

Balo and Schilder Diseases

The *concentric sclerosis of Balo* has as its distinguishing feature the occurrence of alternating bands of destruction and preservation of myelin in a series of concentric rings that represent alternating areas of myelin loss, and preservation. The configuration of lesions in this pattern suggests the centrifugal diffusion of some factor that is damaging to myelin. While usually a part of an acute illness, a similar pattern of lesions, although less extensive, is seen in occasional cases of chronic relapsing MS. Some studies have found a high incidence in the Philippines.

A related but confusing entity, which had been the subject of much discussion in the earlier part of the last century, is that of diffuse sclerosis, or Schilder disease. Exceptionally, the cerebrum is the site of diffuse and massive demyelination. Such cases are more frequent in childhood and adolescence than in adult life. Despite the undoubted occurrence of such cases, to call them "Schilder disease" is to refer to a clinical entity of ambiguous standing.

The term *diffuse sclerosis* was first used by Strümpell (1879) to describe the hard texture of the freshly removed brain of an alcoholic; later the term was applied to widespread cerebral gliosis of whatever cause. In 1912, Schilder described an instance of what he considered to be "diffuse sclerosis." The case was that of a 14-year-old girl with progressive mental deterioration and signs of increased intracranial pressure, terminating fatally after 19 weeks. Postmortem examination disclosed large, well-demarcated areas of demyelination in the white matter of both cerebral hemispheres, as well as a number of smaller demyelinating foci, resembling the common lesions of MS. Because of the similarities of the pathologic changes to those of MS (prominence of the inflammatory reaction and relative sparing of axons), Schilder called this disease *encephalitis periaxialis diffusa*, bringing it in line with *encephalitis periaxialis scleroticans*, a term that Marburg had used to describe a case of acute MS. Unfortunately, in subsequent publications, Schilder applied the same term to two other conditions of different types. One appears to have been a familial leukodystrophy (probably adrenoleukodystrophy) in a boy, and the other, quite unlike either of the first two cases, was suggestive of an infiltrative lymphoma. The last two reports seriously confused the subject, and for many years the terms *Schilder disease* and *diffuse sclerosis* were indiscriminately attached to quite different conditions.

If one sets aside the hereditary metabolic leukodystrophies and other childhood disorders of cerebral white matter, there remains a characteristic group of cases allied with multiple sclerosis that does, indeed, correspond to Schilder's original case description. They are most frequently encountered in children or young adults. As with the case reported by Ellison and Barron, the disease may follow the course of MS, either steady and unremitting or punctuated by a series of episodes of rapid worsening. The CSF may show changes similar to those in chronic relapsing MS. Death occurs in most patients within a few months or years, but some survive for a decade or longer. In the differential diagnosis, a diffuse cerebral neoplasm (gliomatosis or lymphoma), adrenoleukodystrophy, and progressive multifocal leukoencephalopathy (Chap. 33) are the main considerations. Histologically, the large single focus, as well as the smaller disseminated ones, shows the characteristic features of MS. These features were elaborated by Poser and colleagues in a subsequent (1986) review of this subject.

Multiple Sclerosis in Conjunction With Peripheral Neuropathy

From time to time there have been patients with MS who also have a polyneuropathy or mononeuropathy multiplex. This relationship always invites speculation and controversy especially as several autopsy cases have shown a coexistent demyelinating lesions in the central white matter and scattered in peripheral nerves but there are reasons for skepticism as vitamin deficiency polyneuropathy or multiple pressure palsies may be responsible. The rarity of the combination suggests a purely coincidental occurrence, perhaps with another underlying disease as an explanation (e.g., Lyme disease, AIDS). Another view, expressed by Thomas and colleagues and by Mendell et al, is that an autoimmune demyelination has been incited in both spinal cord and peripheral nerve, the latter taking the form of a chronic inflammatory polyradiculoneuropathy. Of course, radicular and neuropathic symptoms, motor and/or sensory, can result from the involvement of myelinated fibers in the root entry zone of the cord or fibers of exit in the ventral white matter. At the moment, we consider the two components to be most often different in origin.

Laboratory Findings in Typical Multiple Sclerosis

Cerebrospinal Fluid

In about one-third of all MS patients, particularly those with an acute onset or an exacerbation, there may be a slight to moderate mononuclear pleocytosis (usually in the range of 6 to 20 and in any case, less than 50 cells/mm^3). In rapidly progressive cases of neuromyelitis optica (see further on) and in certain instances of severe demyelinating disease of the brainstem, the total cell count may reach or exceed 100, and rarely in the hyper-acute cases 1,000, cells/mm^3 and in the last of these processes, the greater proportion of cells may be polymorphonuclear leukocytes. This pleocytosis may in fact be the only measure of activity of the disease.

It has been shown that the gamma globulin proteins in the CSF of patients with MS are synthesized in the CNS (Tourtellotte and Booe) and that they migrate in agarose electrophoresis as abnormal discrete populations, called *oligoclonal bands*. This is currently the most widely used CSF test for the confirmation of the diagnosis. Determination for oligoclonal IgG bands will show several bands in the CSF in more than 90 percent of cases of MS. A lower proportion of patients in Asian countries demonstrate bands. Such bands also appear in the CSF of patients with syphilis, Lyme, and subacute sclerosing panencephalitis, disorders that should not be difficult to distinguish from MS on clinical grounds. The demonstration of oligoclonal bands in the CSF and not in the blood is particularly helpful in confirming the diagnosis of MS, but they are not always found with the first attack or even in the later stages of the disease. The presence of bands in a first attack of MS is predictive of a chronic relapsing course, according to Moulin and coworkers and others. Oligoclonal bands are usually reported as being present if there is more than one band; the meaning of a single band is not clear, and we have treated this result as a negative test. As will be pointed out, the conditions of necrotic myelopathy and Devic disease generally lack oligoclonal bands.

Also, in approximately 40 percent of patients, the total protein content of the CSF is increased. The increase is slight, however, and a concentration of more than 100 mg/dL is so unusual that the possibility of another diagnosis should be entertained. Less used as a diagnostic test currently is measurement of IgG and the IgG index in the CSF. The latter refers to proportion of gamma globulin (mainly IgG) in reference to the total protein in CSF; a positive test is considered to be greater than 12 percent of the total protein. The same diseases mentioned above as being associated with oligoclonal bands can also increase the IgG index.

It has also been shown, by the use of a sensitive radio-immunoassay, that the CSF of many patients contains high concentrations of MBP during acute exacerbations of MS and that these levels are lower or normal in slowly progressive MS and normal during remissions of the disease. Other lesions that destroy myelin (e.g., infarction) can also increase the level of MBP in the spinal fluid. Thus the assay is not particularly useful as a diagnostic test and probably simply reflects the destruction of central myelin.

When cells, total protein, gamma globulin, and oligoclonal bands are all taken into account, some abnormality of the spinal fluid will be found in the great majority of patients with established MS. At present, the oligoclonal bands in the CSF is the most widely used of the CSF tests for MS, particularly when taken some interval after an acute exacerbation or during the chronic progressive phase of disease. The more complicated laboratory procedures, such as CSF measurements of globulin production or MBP provide little additional sensitivity.

Imaging

It is now widely appreciated that MRI is the most helpful ancillary examination in the diagnosis of MS, by virtue of its ability to reveal symptomatic and asymptomatic plaques in the cerebrum, brainstem, optic nerves, and spinal cord (Fig. 36-1). Most experience indicates that the incidence of lesions, if the cerebra and spinal cord are imaged, is greater than 90 percent in established cases of MS. It is remarkable that even when there are a multitude of cerebral lesions, they tend to be asymptomatic; by contrast, spinal cord lesions are almost always symptomatic.

Several MRI features are characteristic of the MS lesion. In general, MS plaques are hyperintense (white) on T2-weighted images and even more obvious on T2 fluid-attenuated inversion recovery (T2-FLAIR) images. The T2 sequence is particularly sensitive in detecting lesions in the brainstem, cerebellum, and spinal cord. Acute lesions tend to demonstrate tissue expansion due to edema that is evident as T1 hypointensity and T2 hyperintensity. Chronic lesions, in distinction, are usually contracted and hyperintense on T2 sequences. The presence of T1 hypointensity depends on the extent of remyelination of the lesion. If there is no or scant remyelination, the center of the chronic lesion gives the appearance of a "black hole." As assessed histologically with both autopsy and MRI studies, T1 hypointensity was inversely proportional to the degree of remyelination (Barkhof et al).

The individual cerebral lesions on MRI do not always ensure the diagnosis of MS, but the finding of multifocal, well-demarcated, oval or linear, radially oriented lesions adjacent to the ventricular surface usually denotes the typical relapsing-remitting form of MS. When viewed in sagittal images, they extend from the corpus callosum in a filiform pattern and have been termed "Dawson fingers." The radial orientation of these lesions corresponds to the course of venules embedded within the cerebral white matter. In addition to these periventricular lesions, subcortical and infratentorial lesions are frequently seen, most often in white matter tracts such as the cerebral and cerebellar peduncles and the medial longitudinal fasciculus. Lesions in MS do not conform to cerebral vascular territories and lack the wedge shape of typical embolic cerebral infarctions. Further assisting in distinguishing an MS lesion from an infarction, diffusivity in MS is variable.

Early in the evolution of an MS lesion, there is disruption of the blood–brain barrier, presumably as a consequence of inflammation. The MRI correlate of this inflammation is abnormal T1 hyperintensity (enhancement) following the administration of gadolinium. Gadolinium enhancement, may last for many weeks. One characteristic pattern is of a C-shaped partial or open ring of abnormal enhancement; which assists in differentiation a MS lesion from other lesions such as abscess and neoplasm. The open segment of the ring is most often medially situated. Many of these imaging characteristics are listed in Table 2-3 and displayed in Fig. 36-1.

In advanced cases of MS, the periventricular lesions may become confluent, usually at the poles of the ventricles. Infrequently, a large acute lesion may have a mass effect and a ring-like contrast-enhancing border, then resembling a glioblastoma or an infarct—the previously referred to "tumefactive" lesion (see Fig. 36-2).

As discussed below, in recent criteria for diagnosis, and in keeping with the traditional notion of MS as a disease that is "disseminated in time and space," the MRI is invaluable for demonstrating asymptomatic lesions. It is the discovery of these additional lesions in a patient with a single clinical episode that can establish the diagnosis of MS. Similarly, the unsuspected diagnosis of MS may be revealed on a single MRI by detecting one or more acute (enhancing) lesions with additional nonenhancing ones. Some of these asymptomatic lesions may be found in the spinal cord as discussed by Bot and colleagues. Furthermore, serial MRIs showing accumulating T2 hyperintense lesions over time are consistent with the diagnosis. As with other laboratory procedures, MRI changes assume maximal significance when they are consistent with the clinical findings.

Less evident than the focal lesions of MS is the progressive cerebral atrophy that accompanies most cases. This change probably reflects both the loss of glial cells and, importantly, wallerian degeneration and loss of axons triggered acutely by inflammation and more chronically by other neurodegenerative stimuli (Miller et al, 2002). Several studies document that slowly progressive brain atrophy, as gauged by volumetric MRI measurements of the cortical mantle, deep nuclei, and white matter, is a feature of MS. This is demonstrable both early and late in the disease and correlates particularly with cognitive disability.

The spinal lesions of MS occupy only a portion of the transverse surface of the cord, most commonly being situated in white matter tracts in a subpial location. The lesions infrequently extend longitudinally beyond three contiguous vertebral segments (Fig. 36-1), in contrast to those of neuromyelitis optica as discussed further on. As described above, acute lesions may cause focal expansion of the cord and enhance with contrast, while chronic lesions tend to produce atrophy.

It should be stressed that foci of periventricular T2 hyperintensity are observed with a variety of pathologic processes and even in normal persons, particularly older ones. Unlike the lesions of MS, these periventricular lesions are usually oriented parallel to the ventricular surfaces, are smoother in outline than the lesions of MS, and have been attributed to microvascular changes as discussed in Chapter 34. The same lack of specificity of cerebral lesions pertains to those in the spinal cord.

CT may also demonstrate cerebral lesions, sometimes unexpectedly, but with far less sensitivity than MRI. Two points worth noting about the CT are that acute plaques can appear as contrast-enhanced ring lesions, simulating abscess or tumor, and that some contrast-enhanced periventricular lesions become radiologically inevident after steroid treatment.

Evoked Potentials and Other Tests

When the clinical data point to only one lesion in the CNS, as often happens in the early stages of the disease or in the spinal form, a number of other sensitive physiologic and radiologic tests may establish the existence of additional asymptomatic lesions. These include visual, auditory, and somatosensory-evoked responses and the less standardized and infrequently tested perceptual delay on visual stimulation; electrooculography; altered blink reflexes; and a change in flicker fusion of visual images. Abnormalities of visual evoked responses have been found in approximately 70 percent of patients with the clinical features of definite MS and 60 percent of patients with probable or possible MS. The corresponding figures for somatosensory evoked responses have been 60 percent and 40 percent, and for brainstem auditory evoked responses (usually prolonged interwave latency or decreased amplitude of wave 5), approximately 40 percent and 20 percent, respectively (see Chap. 2). These tests had been used with greater frequency in the past and have been largely supplanted by MRI to detect dispersed demyelinating lesions.

Optical coherence tomography (OCT) is a technique for creating two- and three-dimensional images of the optic nerve and retina. By using near-infrared interferometry, it displays axonal loss and thinning of the retina that assists in the evaluation of optic neuritis and subsequent optic atrophy. It is used mainly to follow the course of optic neuritis.

Whether tests for serum antibodies against oligodendrocytes and myelin have the predictive value remains to be seen. Berger and colleagues published provocative findings in which 23 percent of patients who lacked such antibodies had further attacks after their first one, whereas 95 percent of those who had both antibodies suffered a relapse. Attempts to reproduce these findings by Kuhle and colleagues did not meet with success and there is no serum test for multiple sclerosis that has proven consistent, nor is there a predictive test for relapse. The importance of anti-aquaporin (NMO) antibodies in Devic disease will be discussed further on.

Diagnostic Criteria for Multiple Sclerosis

The clinician is well advised to make the diagnosis of MS on the firmest grounds possible and to withhold judgment unless the combination of clinical and laboratory features allows certainty. In the past, the passage of time was necessary to clarify the situation but presently, it is considered preferable to use MRI and other tests to attempt to establish the diagnosis at the time of the first symptoms. Certainly, the disease is likely when one of the usual syndromes, such as optic neuritis, bilateral brainstem symptoms, or transverse myelitis, occurs in a younger person. However, the time-honored—and still valid—criteria for diagnosis proposed by McAlpine and colleagues (1972), requiring several lesions that were "separated in time and space," have been broadened greatly by the ability to detect demyelinating lesions by nonclinical means. This approach, in essence, predicts the likelihood that a clinically isolated syndrome ("CIS") will disseminate over time and space and conform to the diagnosis of MS.

Polman and colleagues in 2011 have provided a diagnostic scheme based on previous consensus (2001, 2005 and 2010) that incorporates MRI changes into the criteria and further revisions have increased sensitivity (Table 36-2). These criteria are provided for the reader because they are often cited but they may prove unwieldy for routine clinical work. Our colleague Kurtzke apocryphally is said to have quipped "MS is what the experienced neurologist says it is." All such criteria are also relevant to predicting the course of illness, which is discussed below.

Table 36-2

DIAGNOSTIC CRITERIA FOR MS[a]

CLINICAL FEATURES	LABORATORY FEATURES
Two or more typical attacks of central nervous system demyelination with objective evidence on examination for both lesions (see text)	—
Two clinical attacks with objective evidence on examination for only one lesion	Lesions or T2 hyperintensity located in at least two of four typical locations (periventricular, juxtacortical, infratentorial, or spinal cord)
One attack with objective evidence on examination of two or more lesions	Dissemination over time: simultaneous enhancing and nonenhancing lesions in the above locations, or interval development of new T2 hyperintense lesions
One attack with objective evidence on examination for only one lesion (clinically isolated syndrome, CIS; see text)	Dissemination in space: lesions or T2 hyperintensity located in at least two of four typical locations (periventricular, juxtacortical, infratentorial, or spinal cord), and dissemination in time demonstrated by simultaneous enhancing and nonenhancing lesions in the above locations, or interval development of new T2 hyperintense lesions
Progressive, nonrelapsing, deficits suggestive of MS	One year of disease progression and dissemination in space as above and oligoclonal bands or elevated IgG index in the CSF

[a]Adapted from Polman 2011.

Clinical Course and Prognosis

The intermittency of the clinical manifestations—the disease advancing in a series of attacks, each permitting remission—is perhaps the most important clinical attribute of most cases of MS. Some patients will have a complete clinical remission after the initial attack, or, there may be a series of exacerbations, each with complete remission; rarely, such exacerbations may be severe enough to have caused quadriplegia and pseudobulbar palsy. The average relapse rate is 0.3 to 0.4 attacks per year according to the calculations of McAlpine and Compston, but the interval between the opening symptom and the first relapse is highly variable. It occurred within 1 year in 30 percent of McAlpine's cases and within 2 years in another 20 percent. A further 20 percent relapsed in 5 to 9 years, and another 10 percent in 10 to 30 years. Not only the length of this interval is remarkable, but also the fact that the basic pathologic process can remain potentially active for such a long time.

Weinshenker and colleagues (1989), on the basis of observations in 1,099 MS patients over a 12-year period, have identified a number of features of the early clinical course that were predictive, in a general way, of the outcome of the illness. Perhaps not surprisingly, they found that a high degree of disability, as measured by the Kurtzke Disability Status Scale, was reached earlier in patients with a higher number of attacks, a shorter first interattack interval, and a shorter time to reach a state of moderate disability. Kurtzke had earlier reported that the feature most predictive of long-term disability was the degree of disability at 5 years from the first symptom. Confavreux and colleagues (2000) analyzed a cohort of 1,844 patients with multiple sclerosis and found, somewhat surprisingly, that relapses did not significantly influence the progression of irreversible disability. Furthermore, large population studies (Pittock et al 2004; Tremlett et al) have shown that many patients develop only mild disability after long follow-up (so-called benign MS). Regardless of the age of onset, approximately 20 percent of patients do not become disabled, even after many decades of illness. These data should inform the use of the long-term disease-modifying therapies discussed in a later section but, as pointed out by Sayao and colleagues, reliable criteria for identifying patients who are destined to accumulate minimal or no disability are not available but are being sought.

After a number of years there is an increasing tendency for the patient to enter a phase of slow, steady, or fluctuating deterioration of neurologic function, attributable to the cumulative effect of increasing numbers of lesions (*secondary progressive MS* as described in the introductory section). However, in approximately 10 percent of cases, the clinical course lacks periodic relapses and is almost evenly progressive from the beginning (*primary progressive MS*; see Thompson et al). In these latter cases, the disease usually takes the form of a chronic asymmetrical spastic paraparesis and probably represents the most frequent type of difficult to diagnose as MS. In Thompson's review of primary progressive MS, there was little change over time in the MRI findings, a negligible response to therapy, and a poor outcome. The frequency with which acute MS blends into the progressive variety has already been emphasized. (See earlier comments regarding the pathologic distinctions between types of MS.)

Pregnancy is typically associated with clinical stability or even with improvement (as it is in a number of autoimmune diseases). The average relapse rate in established cases declines in each trimester, reaching a level less than one-third of the expected rate by the third trimester. However, there appears to be an increased risk of exacerbations, up to twofold, in the first few months postpartum (Birk and Rudick). An extensive study of 269 pregnancies by Confavreux and colleagues (1998) established a rate of relapse of 0.7 per woman per year before pregnancy and rates of 0.5 in the first, 0.6 in the second, and 0.2 in the third trimester, the rate then increasing substantially to 1.2 in the first 3 months postpartum.

The duration of the disease is exceedingly variable. A small number of patients die within several months or years of the onset, but the average duration of the illness is in excess of 30 years. A 60-year appraisal of the resident population of Rochester, Minnesota, disclosed that 74 percent of patients with MS survived 25 years, as compared with 86 percent of the general population. At the end of 25 years, one-third of the surviving patients were still working and two-thirds were still ambulatory (Percy et al). Other statistical analyses have given a less optimistic prognosis; these were reviewed by Matthews. Patients with mild and quiescent forms of the disease are, of course, less likely to be included in such surveys. Although exceptional, one of our patients relapsed and developed massive brainstem demyelination and coma after 30 years (confirmed by postmortem examination) and cases of an aggressive myelopathy that appears after years are well known.

No environmental, dietary, or activity-related changes are known to alter the course of the illness.

Differential Diagnosis

In the usual forms of MS—that is, in those with a relapsing and remitting course and evidence of disseminated lesions in the CNS—the diagnosis is rarely in doubt. Vascular malformations such as cavernous angiomas of the brainstem or spinal cord with multiple episodes of bleeding, brain lymphoma, lupus erythematosus, the antiphospholipid antibody syndrome, and Behçet disease all may simulate relapsing MS, and each has its own characteristic and diagnostic features. The list can be expanded by the inclusion of corticosteroid-responsive intravascular lymphoma and the other numerous causes of multiple, well-demarcated white matter abnormalities on MRI, such as embolic infarcts, progressive multifocal leukoencephalopathy, migraine-associated white matter lesions, Lyme disease, sarcoidosis, and tumors. Difficulties are most likely to arise when the standard clinical criteria for the diagnosis of MS are lacking, as occurs in the acute initial attack of the disease and in cases with an insidious onset and slow, steady progression. Other features that call for caution in diagnosis of MS are an absence of symptoms and signs of optic neuritis, the presence of widespread amyotrophy, entirely normal eye movements, a hemianopic field defect, pain as the predominant symptom, or a progressive nonremitting illness that begins in youth. Other points against MS are fever and nonneurologic features such as joint inflammation, skin rash, sicca syndrome, or evidence of peripheral neuropathy. The differentiation from Devic disease is discussed further on.

As has been stated, *the initial attack of MS* may mimic acute labyrinthine vertigo or tic douloureux (trigeminal neuralgia). Careful neurologic examination of such patients usually discloses other signs of a brainstem lesion; the CSF examination may be particularly helpful in these circumstances. Extensive brainstem demyelination of subacute evolution, involving tracts and cranial nerves sequentially, may be mistaken for a pontine glioma. With brainstem symptoms of acute onset, there may be difficulty in distinguishing an MS plaque from a small infarction because of a basilar branch occlusion. In several patients who we have observed, recurrent bleeding from cavernous vascular malformations and small brainstem arteriovenous malformations simulated MS clinically. Only with MRI, visualization of blood products surrounding the small vascular lesions may the diagnosis be clarified. Sequential MRIs and the course of the illness usually settle the matter.

Acute disseminated encephalomyelitis (ADEM; see further on) is an acute illness with widely scattered small demyelinating lesions but it is self-limited and monophasic. Furthermore, fever, stupor, and coma, which are characteristic of severe cases, rarely occur in MS. The encephalomyelitis may, however, progress for several weeks, making the distinction from MS difficult.

White Matter Lesions Associated With Systemic Autoimmune and Inflammatory Diseases

In systemic lupus erythematosus and less often in other autoimmune diseases (mixed connective tissue disease, Sjögren syndrome, scleroderma) there may be multiple lesions of the CNS white matter. These may parallel the activity of the underlying immune disease or the level of autoantibodies, particularly those against native DNA or phospholipids but myelitis or lesions in the cerebral hemispheres are known to occur before other organ systems are affected. Conversely, between 5 and 10 percent of MS patients have antinuclear or anti-double stranded DNA antibodies without signs of lupus, but the significance of this finding is not at all clear. In addition, as discussed in the introductory section relatives of patients with MS in some series have a higher than expected incidence of autoantibodies of various types, suggesting an as yet unproved connection between systemic autoimmune disease and MS.

On MRI, the lesions of lupus and of antiphospholipid antibody syndrome appear similar to plaques, and both the optic nerve (rarely) and the spinal cord may be involved, even repeatedly, in a succession of attacks resembling MS. The lesions may be small and single, multiple, or confluent in large regions (Akasbi). Nevertheless some of the lesions represent small zones of infarct necrosis rather than demyelination and are traceable to small-vessel occlusion. Others may be autoimmune and demyelinating and this group of processes that affect the cerebral white matter remains difficult to understand. In a few instances, inflammatory demyelination without vascular changes may be seen. It is best for the moment to consider these as special manifestations of lupus or related diseases that mimic MS. The neurologist should be cautious in initiating some of the treatments for MS, such as β-interferon, as they may worsen the systemic autoimmune illness.

Periarteritis nodosa or vasculitis confined to the nervous system may produce multifocal lesions simulating MS. The distinction may be particularly difficult in rare instances of the vasculitic process in which the neurologic manifestations take the form of a relapsing or steroid-responsive myelitis. In these cases, the CSF may contain 100 or more white blood cells/mm^3 and there may be no evidence of disease elsewhere in the nervous system. Occasionally, a young person with Lyme disease may have complaints of inordinate fatigue and vague neurologic symptoms coupled with hyperintense lesions on the T2-weighted cranial MRI. Close attention to the characteristic history (rash, arthritis, etc.) and serologic findings permit the distinction between MS and systemic diseases. The distinguishing features of Behçet disease are recurrent iridocyclitis and meningitis, mucous membrane ulcers of mouth and genitalia, and symptoms of articular, renal, lung, and multifocal cerebral disease. The chronic forms of brucellosis in the Mediterranean regions and Lyme borreliosis throughout North America and Europe may cause myelopathy or encephalopathy with multiple white matter lesions on imaging studies, but in each case the history and other features of the disease help to identify the infectious illness (see Chap. 32).

Spinal Multiple Sclerosis

The *purely spinal form of MS*, presenting as a progressive spastic paraparesis, hemiparesis, or, in several of our cases, spastic monoparesis of a leg with varying degrees of posterior column involvement, is a special source of diagnostic difficulty. A tendency to affect older women has already been mentioned. Such patients require careful evaluation for the presence of spinal cord compression from neoplasm or cervical spondylosis. Dural arteriovenous fistula is also a consideration as mentioned below. Radicular pain at some point in the illness is a frequent manifestation of these disorders and is much less frequent in MS. Pain in the neck, restricted mobility of the cervical spine, and severe muscle wasting as a result of spinal root involvement, as is sometimes seen in spondylosis, are almost unknown in MS. However, atrophy of the first dorsal interosseus muscles, a frequent finding in spondylosis, is also in MS. As a general rule, loss of abdominal reflexes, erectile dysfunction, and disturbances of bladder function occur early in the course of demyelinating myelopathy but late or not at all in cervical spondylosis. The CSF protein in cervical spondylosis is often elevated, but oligoclonal bands and elevated IgG are not found.

A special problem arises when imaging procedures reveal a regional swelling of the spinal cord suggestive of a tumor. In a patient with this finding and a subacute, saltatory myelopathy restricted to several adjacent levels (usually thoracic), a search for an arteriovenous malformation or fistula may be required. In several of our patients, this finding has led to an ill-advised attempt at spinal cord biopsy. Sarcoidosis affecting the cord presents similar problems; steroid-responsive granulomatous lesions of sarcoid that follow a venous pattern in the cerebrum may cause confusion with MS when viewed by MRI. A subpial pattern of enhancement with gadolinium is helpful in identifying sarcoid.

The problem of differentiating chronic spinal MS from tropical spastic paraparesis (human lymphotropic virus, myelitis of the HTLV-1 type) and progressive familial spastic paraplegia may also arise occasionally. Amyotrophic lateral sclerosis (ALS) and subacute combined degeneration (SCD) may be confused with MS, but ALS can be identified by the presence of muscle wasting, fasciculations, and the absence of sensory involvement, whereas SCD is characterized by symmetrical involvement of the posterior and then lateral columns of the spinal cord. Reports that vitamin B_{12} levels are marginally low in a proportion of MS patients have suggested an underlying disturbance of homocysteine metabolism but this has not been confirmed (Vrethem et al).

Platybasia and basilar impression of the skull should also be considered in the differential diagnosis, but patients with these conditions usually have a characteristic shortening of the neck; images of the base of the skull are diagnostic. Neurologic syndromes resulting from the Chiari malformation, syringomyelia, rheumatoid destruction of the upper cervical segments, and tumors of the foramen magnum, cerebellopontine angle, clivus, and other parts of the posterior fossa have been misdiagnosed clinically as MS. In each of these instances, a solitary, strategically placed lesion may give rise to a variety of neurologic symptoms and signs referable to the lower brainstem and cranial nerves, cerebellum, and upper cervical cord, giving the impression of dissemination of lesions. It is a dependable clinical dictum that a diagnosis of MS should be made with caution when all of the patient's symptoms and signs can be explained by a single lesion in one region of the neuraxis.

Occasionally, the chronic progressive form of MS may be confused with the hereditary ataxias, particularly the spinocerebellar types. The latter are generally distinguished by their familial incidence and other associated genetic traits; by their insidious onset and slow, steady progression; and by their relative symmetry and stereotyped clinical pattern. Intactness of abdominal reflexes and sphincter function and the presence of pes cavus, kyphoscoliosis, and cardiac disease are other features that favor the diagnosis of a heredodegenerative disorder (see Chap. 39).

Treatment of Multiple Sclerosis

As one might expect, numerous forms of treatment have been proposed over the years, and many were thought to be successful, no doubt because of the remitting nature of the disease. The many therapeutic trials of recent years, using mainly anti-inflammatory and immunosuppressive are summarized below. Typical relapsing-remitting MS that is associated with episodic inflammation is most responsive to immunomodulatory therapy; on the other hand, these measures may be ineffective for chronic progressive subtypes. Therefore, as discussed earlier, therapy should be guided by the nature of the disease in each individual and with consideration of the side effects and risks of each of the expanding group of available therapies. A current list of clinical trials is maintained by the National Multiple Sclerosis Society: http://www.nationalmssociety.org/research/clinical-trials/clinical-trials-in-ms/index.aspx

Although many writers on the subject indicate that virtually all patients with proven MS should be treated soon after the diagnosis is established, the long-term effects on the illness still remain to be clarified. From the numerous studies cited below, a concept has emerged that subclinical lesions may be of importance and that, over time, cognitive decline and neurologic deficits are more likely to occur if progression is not reduced by treatment. There are few circumstances where such treatment is mandated immediately, and we allow enough time for the patient to consider the alternatives and sometimes encourage serial examinations and MRI to determine the course of illness. With all of these treatments it should be acknowledged that there is no certain correlation between the number of relapses and the ultimate disability despite authoritative statements to the contrary (as expressed by Confavreux et al [2000]).

Corticosteroids Under the influence of corticosteroids, recovery from an acute attack, including an attack of optic neuritis, appears to be hastened. However, a substantial group of patients with acute exacerbations fails to respond; in others, benefit is not apparent for a month or longer after the course of treatment has been completed and therefore may reflect the natural course of disease. There is no evidence that steroids have a significant effect on the ultimate course of this disease or that they prevent recurrences. Accordingly, there is limited justification for steroid treatment over a period of many months or years except in those infrequent cases where withdrawal of the medication consistently leads to relapse (alternative diagnoses should be considered in this event). In a study of intravenous methylprednisolone administered at 1 g/d for 5 days per month over 5 years, there was a reduction in disability as well as in the degree of brain atrophy and total volume of hypodense lesions on T1-weighted MRI (Zivadinov et al).

As to the dosage of corticosteroids for an acute attack, it seems that initially a high dose is more effective but this has been disputed, as noted below. A randomized trial comparing oral and intravenous methylprednisolone in acute relapses of MS demonstrated no clear advantage of the intravenous regimen (Barnes et al), but many MS experts dispute this finding. The administration of adrenocorticotropic hormone (ACTH), which was popular during the 1970s, has been abandoned.

The intravenous administration of massive doses of methylprednisolone (a bolus of 500 to 1,000 mg daily for 3 to 5 days) followed by high oral doses of prednisone (beginning with 60 to 80 mg daily and tapering to a lower dosage over a 12- to 20-day period) is generally effective in aborting or shortening an acute or subacute exacerbation of MS or of optic neuritis. Whether the tapering oral course is necessary is unclear. When it is impractical to administer parenteral methylprednisolone, one may substitute oral methylprednisolone (48 mg in a single daily dose for 1 week, followed by 24 mg daily for 1 week, and finally 12 mg daily for 1 week) or the equivalent amount of prednisone (Barnes et al).

A brief period of corticosteroid administration generally produces few adverse effects but some patients complain of insomnia and a few will develop depressive or manic symptoms. Patients who, because of clinical relapse on withdrawal of the medication, require oral treatment for more than several weeks are subject to the effects of hypercortisolism, including the facial and truncal cosmetic changes of Cushing syndrome, hypertension, hyperglycemia and erratic diabetic control, osteoporosis, avascular necrosis of the head of the femur, and cataracts; less often, there may be gastrointestinal hemorrhage and activation of tuberculosis or pneumocystis. It must be acknowledged that the corticosteroid regimens and dosages in common use are derived from anecdotal experience (the Optic Neuritis Treatment Trial being an exception) and that certain patients appear, at least for a period of time, to respond better to one or another method of treatment.

As mentioned under "Acute Multiple Sclerosis," there may be a role for *plasma exchange* (see Weinshenker et al, 1999; Rodriguez et al) and perhaps immunoglobulin in fulminant cases, but these have not been tested rigorously. One limited trial has shown some benefit, in patients with relapsing–remitting disease, of monthly infusions of intravenous immunoglobulin (0.2 g/kg) for 2 years (Fazekas et al).

Treatment of Optic Neuritis (See Chap. 13) The Optic Neuritis Treatment Trial, reported by Beck and colleagues, cautioned against the use of oral prednisone in the treatment of acute optic neuritis (see also Lessell). In this study, it was found that the use of intravenous methylprednisolone followed by oral prednisone did, indeed, speed the recovery from visual loss, although at 6 months there was little difference between patients treated in this way and those treated with placebo. They reported that treatment with oral prednisone alone slightly increased the risk of new episodes of optic neuritis. In a subsequent randomized trial conducted by Sellebjerg and colleagues, it was found that methylprednisolone 500 mg orally for 5 days had a beneficial effect on visual function at 1 and 3 weeks. However, at 8 weeks, no effect could be shown (compared with the placebo-treated group), nor was there an effect on the subsequent relapse rate.

Interferon-Beta Interferon and glatiramer modestly alter the natural history relapsing-remitting MS. IFN-β-1b, a nonglycosylated bacterial cell product with an amino acid sequence identical to that of natural IFN-β, was the first of these agents to be tested (Arnason). Several trials have shown that the subcutaneous injection of this agent every second day for up to 5 years decreases the frequency and severity of relapses by almost one-third and also the number of new or enlarging lesions ("lesion burden") in serial MRIs. A large-scale trial (European Study Group, (PRISMS Study Group) has extended the observations with IFN-β-1b to patients with the secondarily progressive type of MS; progression of the disease was delayed for 9 to 12 months in a study period of 2 to 3 years. The treatment of relapsing–remitting MS with IFN-β-1a is probably equally effective but was tested in a once weekly intramuscular regimen, making direct comparisons to the -1b preparation difficult. The dose currently used is 30 mcg, or 6.6 million units.

One issue with the longer term administration of interferon is the development of antibodies to the drug. The rate of such antibody emergence increases with the frequency of use of interferon. After a period of years, 30 percent of patients demonstrate antibodies with daily administration, 18 percent with alternate-day use, and less than 5 percent with weekly use. More recent changes in the preparation of interferon have led to reported rates of only 2 percent with antibodies after 1 year of use. There is some evidence that the presence of these antidrug antibodies diminishes the effectiveness of interferon.

Overall, the side effects of these interferon agents are modest, consisting mainly of flu-like symptoms, sweating, and malaise beginning several hours after the injection and persisting for up to 14 h; they are reduced by pre- and post-treatment with nonsteroidal anti-inflammatory drugs and tend to abate with continued use of the agents. In severe cases, prednisone 10 mg taken an hour before, a few hours after, and again 6 to 8 hours after injection may be effective. Nevertheless, some patients cannot tolerate interferon. A few migraineurs complain of exacerbation of their headaches. There may also be a tendency to depression in susceptible patients treated with interferon, and in our experience, this information, when openly discussed with the patient, has sometimes influenced the decision regarding choice of treatment. A rare but notable problem is the induction of a "systemic capillary leak syndrome" in patients with a monoclonal gammopathy who receive interferon. With more than weekly use, there may be an increase in liver function enzymes.

The need to treat patients with optic neuritis alone with interferon has not been satisfactorily resolved. We have generally avoided this approach except in a few patients with repeated episodes involving both eyes at various times. Some guidance is given by the Controlled High Risk Subjects Avonex Multiple Sclerosis Prevention Study (CHAMPS), which examined the effect of interferon (weekly) in patients with a first episode of optic neuritis and at least two lesions on MRI that were compatible with MS. Over 3 years, there was a modest reduction in clinical progression or relapse from 37 percent to 28 percent; if further MRI lesions were used as evidence of clinical progression, the difference from placebo treatment was even greater. If nothing else, this points to the value of a cerebral MRI in patients who have their first optic attack.

Glatiramer Copolymer I (glatiramer acetate), which was synthesized to mimic the actions of myelin basic protein, a putative autoantigen in MS, is given daily in subcutaneous doses of 20 mg. Antibodies do not develop to glatiramer, and this has been emphasized as a relative advantage of the drug. The salutary effects of treatment are definite though limited. Patients receiving glatiramer acetate should be warned of a reaction consisting of flushing, chest tightness, dyspnea, palpitations, and severe anxiety. Injection site reactions occur with both classes of drugs but are rarely troublesome if the sites are rotated. Trials that combine interferon and glatiramer have not produced benefit over either agent alone (Lublin and colleagues).

Conventional Immunosuppressive Drugs A number of agents that modify immune reactivity have been tried with, until recently, limited success. Drugs such as azathioprine and cyclophosphamide, as well as total lymphoid irradiation and bone marrow transplantation, have been given to small groups of patients and seem to have improved the clinical course of some (Aimard et al; Hauser et al, 1983; Cook et al). However, the risks of prolonged use of immunosuppressive drugs, including a chance of neoplastic change and infection, will probably preclude their widespread use. The study by the British and Dutch Multiple Sclerosis Azathioprine Trial Group attributed no significant advantage to treatment with this drug.

For the chronic, progressive phase of the disease, an MS study group has reported a modest delay in the advance of the disease after a 2-year trial of prednisolone and cyclophosphamide. The group cautions, however, that the "burdensome and potentially serious toxicity must temper consideration of its use in this disease." At least one subsequent blinded, placebo-controlled study with cyclophosphamide has failed to show any benefit but many groups continue to use it for recalcitrant and severe acute cases. In one trial involving patients with chronic progressive MS, weekly low-dose oral methotrexate resulted in slight improvement difference and produced some reduction in the volume of cerebral lesions on the MRI compared with control cases (Goodkin et al, 1996). Because this regimen is well tolerated, it may still have some use in otherwise untreatable progressive cases. Among these more aggressive agents, mitoxantrone, a drug with broad immunosuppressant and cytotoxic activity, has attracted interest because one study has shown a slight beneficial effect on the progressive form of the disease (Hartung et al). Some have disputed the interpretation of these results; additionally, there is little effect on the number of MRI lesions. Mycophenolate and similar drugs have been tried with varying success.

These drugs, as a class, are being used less frequently, particularly as new oral agents become available.

Monoclonal Antibodies One novel approach to treatment has been the use of monoclonal antibodies to various components of the inflammatory response. Natalizumab is directed against alpha-integrin in order to block lymphocyte and monocyte adhesion to endothelial cells and their migration through the vessel wall. It has been used in rheumatoid arthritis and fistulizing Crohn disease. In a study that ran for 6 months, Miller and colleagues (2003) were able to demonstrate a reduction in the number of relapses and a slowing of the accumulation of MRI lesions. A double-blind, placebo-controlled study of 942 patients with relapsing–remitting MS (Polman et al; the AFFIRM study) showed a 68 percent reduction in relapses, an 80 percent reduction in new or enlarging T2 cerebral lesions and a 96 percent reduction in gadolinium-enhancing lesions on MRI after a year. This represents a twofold improvement in efficacy compared to what has been reported with interferon and glatiramer acetate. There was a 2 percent rate of anaphylactic reactions. Another study suggested that the use of interferon and natalizumab may give better results (Rudick et al, 2006; the SENTINEL study) but these two are no longer combined in practice.

The advantages of this drug are once monthly intravenous treatment and a virtual lack of acute side effects. However, the appearance of cases of progressive multifocal leukoencephalopathy (PML as discussed in Chap. 33) has led to a restriction on its use. As of the time just prior to this writing, there were over 300 cases of PML recorded in relation to the use natalizumab for MS. Programs are in place to facilitate the early detection of PML since recovery may be possible if the drug is stopped promptly and removed by plasma exchange. However, the methods to detect the infection and to predict which patients will become symptomatic are imperfect. It can be stated that the absence of both JC virus in the urine and of serum antibodies to JC virus makes it very unlikely that PML will occur but there still may be rare cases. In those who have anti-JC virus antibodies, the risk is dependent on the duration of use of natalizumab (particularly if over 24 months) and the prior or concurrent use of other immunosuppressive medications. With both of these factors present, the risk of PML is approximately 11 per 1000 patients (Bloomgren et al).

One remarkable observation has been that the use of plasma exchange to rapidly clear natalizumab has reversed PML and led to disappearance of JC virus from the cerebrospinal fluid. There may be an *immune reconstitution inflammatory syndrome* (IRIS) soon after the exchanges, which may be ameliorated by corticosteroids (Wenning et al; Lindå et al). Some patients have survived PML using this approach, 71 percent in one series reported by Vermersch and colleagues, in distinction to the almost uniform fatality in other circumstances.

Alemtuzumab is a monoclonal antibody that targets CD-52 antigen expressed on T and B lymphocytes, reduces the number of circulating B cells and, for a longer period, T cells. It is used in an annual cycle of intravenous administration for 5 consecutive days. A randomized trial conducted over 36 months comparing the drug to interferon-β-1a found it to be superior in preventing relapses and in the accumulation of disability (CAMMS223 Trial Investigators). A series of subsequent trials have confirmed its effectiveness in comparison to interferon (Cohen et al). The drug can produce idiopathic thrombocytopenic purpura and autoimmune thyroiditis that results in either hyper- or hypothyroidism. At the time of this writing, it is being used in Europe but has not yet been approved in the United States.

Rituximab, a B-cell-depleting monoclonal antibody that targets CD20 lymphocytes, has been tested in several trials and found to be effective in reducing relapses and the accumulation of MRI lesions in a trial of relapsing–remitting cases over 4 years, but long-term safety is still being established (Hauser et al, 2008). Numerous other drugs in this class have been explored for MS with varying but generally positive results. The limiting factors have been infection, later development of lymphoma, and a number of effects that are particular to each drug. A similar anti-CD20 drug, ocrelizumab, is effective in reducing new MRI lesions (Kappos 2011).

Oral Therapies Several novel oral agents have become available for the treatment of MS. Similar to the drugs described above, they each have particular idiosyncratic side effects, but it is patient preference in avoiding injections and infusions that is driving the development of this class.

One immunosuppressive drug that interferes with egress of lymphocytes from lymph nodes, fingolimod, has had a short-term effect on MRI lesion burden and relapse rate that is comparable or slightly superior to inject able agents in a randomized trial reported by Kappos and colleagues. The drug stands out because it is administered orally, once daily, and ostensibly has tolerable side effects. It causes a lymphopenia by restricting lymphocytes to the lymph nodes and causes adenopathy. Discontinuation of the drug is sometimes required because of extremes of bradycardia or atrioventricular block, macular edema, herpes infections and elevations in liver function tests, the last of these, in approximately 10 percent of patients.

Other oral drugs under study and in clinical use include: teriflunomide, laquinimod, cladribine, and dimethyl fumarate, not all of which have been accepted by various national drug approval agencies. The last of these has an interesting history and is perhaps notable because its mechanism of action in MS and psoriasis, the other main disease in which it is used, is not clear (Ropper 2012). Which of these orally administered drugs will be widely used remains to be determined.

General Measures Fatigue, a common complaint of MS patients, particularly in relation to acute attacks, responds to some extent to amantadine (100 mg morning and noon), modafinil (200 to 400 mg/d), or pemoline (20 to 75 mg each morning), methylphenidate, or dextroamphetamine. Confirmation of their benefit will be required before they come into general use. A number of agents exist that improve conduction through demyelinated central fibers and have been suggested as improving fatigue and gait (e.g., 4-aminopyridine).

Disorders of bladder function may raise serious problems in management. Where the major disorder is one of urinary retention, bethanechol chloride is helpful. In this situation, monitoring and reducing the residual urinary volume are important means of preventing infection; volumes up to 100 mL are generally well tolerated. Some patients with severe bladder dysfunction, particularly those with urinary retention, benefit from intermittent catheterization, which they can learn to do themselves and which lessens the constant risk of infection from an indwelling catheter. More often the problem is one of urinary urgency and frequency (spastic bladder), in which case the use of propantheline (Pro-Banthine) or oxybutynin (Ditropan) may serve to relax the detrusor muscle (Chap. 26). These drugs are best used intermittently. Severe constipation is best managed with properly spaced enemas. Often a program of bowel training can be successfully undertaken. Sexual dysfunction has been treated with sildenafil and similar drugs. When pain is a prominent symptom, its management follows the general principles of pain management outlined in Chap. 8. Carbamazepine or gabapentin are often helpful to reduce paroxysmal symptoms in MS.

In patients with severe spastic paralysis and painful flexor spasms of the legs, if local injection of botulinum toxin fails, oral and then intrathecal infusion of baclofen through an indwelling catheter and implanted pump, as in other spastic states, is sometimes of value. The selective injection of botulinum toxin into the most hypertonic muscles is an early resort. Patients with lesser degrees of spasticity have benefited from the oral administration of baclofen. An alternative to oral baclofen is tizanidine. Failing this measure, intrathecal baclofen infusion by pump may give relief for a prolonged period.

The severe and disabling tremor that is brought out by the slightest movement of the limbs, if unilateral, can be managed surgically by ventrolateral thalamotomy or implanted stimulator of the type used for the treatment of Parkinson disease. Most surgical series report that about two-thirds of patients achieve a satisfactory reduction in their intention tremor (Critchley and Richardson; Geny et al). In the experience of others, the results have not been quite this reliable. In the series of Hooper and Whittle, only 3 of 10 MS patients who underwent thalamotomy for a severe tremor had sustained improvement. Hallett and colleagues have reported that severe postural tremor of this type can be improved by the administration of isoniazid (300 mg daily, increased by weekly increments of 300 mg to a dose of 1,200 mg daily) in combination with 100 mg of pyridoxine daily. How isoniazid produces its beneficial effects is not known, and careful monitoring of liver tests is required. Variable success may also be achieved with carbamazepine or clonazepam. For the depression associated with the disease, there does not seem to be any superior antidepressant and donepezil has not been found to be helpful for cognitive problems.

There are no valid studies to substantiate claims that have been made for the value of synthetic polypeptides other than copolymer, for hyperbaric oxygen, low-fat and gluten-free diets, or linoleate supplementation of the diet. Necessary vaccinations are not prohibited in patients with MS.

The importance of an understanding and sympathetic physician in the care of patients with a chronic and potentially incapacitating neurologic disease that requires choices among many medications of this kind cannot be overemphasized. Enlisting the support of physical and occupational therapists, visiting nurses, and social workers can be equally important. From the beginning, when patients first inquire about the nature of their illness, they require advice about their daily routine, marriage, pregnancy, the use of drugs, inoculations, and so on. As indicated earlier, the term *MS* should not be introduced until the diagnosis is certain, and then it should be qualified by a balanced explanation of the symptoms, stressing always the optimistic aspects of the disease. Most patients desire an honest appraisal of their condition and prognosis; some consider the uncertainty of their prognosis worse than their actual disability.

Neuromyelitis Optica (Devic Disease, Necrotic Myelopathy) (See also Chap. 44)

This disease is characterized by a simultaneous or successive and usually severe involvement of optic nerves and spinal cord. The combination was remarked upon by Clifford Albutt in 1870, and Gault (1894), stimulated by his teacher Devic, devoted his thesis to the subject. Devic subsequently endeavored to crystallize medical thought about a condition that has come to be known as neuromyelitis optica. Its principal features are the acute to subacute onset of blindness in one or both eyes, preceded or followed within days or weeks by a severe transverse or ascending myelitis (Mandler et al, 1993). The singular modern insight in Devic disease has been the discovery by the group at the Mayo Clinic of a fairly specific circulating autoantibody to the aquaporin-4 water channel protein. After decades of debate, this has largely settled the controversy about Devic disease as an independent entity from MS.

In certain parts of the world, this form of aggressive and usually monophasic demyelinating disease is more common than is typical MS. The disease termed "Asian optic–spinal MS" almost certainly represents Devic disease and displays this antibody in the majority of cases. Most cases of neuromyelitis optica stand apart from MS by virtue of distinctive clinical and pathologic features, mainly, a failure to develop cerebral demyelinating lesions typical of MS even after years of illness; the absence of oligoclonal bands in the CSF; a tendency to CSF pleocytosis more so than in MS, and the necrotizing and cavitary nature of the spinal cord lesion, affecting white and gray matter alike with prominent thickening of vessels but with minimal inflammatory infiltrates. It is also quite unusual for MS to involve several contiguous longitudinal segments of the spinal cord, and this is a frequent finding in Devic disease (Fig. 36-3). It is not clear if events such as pregnancy that alter the course of MS have the same relationship to NMO (Bourre et al).

The spinal cord lesions in cases of neuromyelitis optica are often necrotizing, centrally located in the cord, and occupying several contiguous vertebral segments, leading eventually to cavitation. As would be expected, the clinical effects are more likely to be permanent than those of typical demyelination. A few affected patients have been children; in a number of instances, they have suffered only a single episode of neurologic illness. Despite the now clear distinction between Devic disease and MS, there remains a group of patients with the clinical syndrome of simultaneous or sequential optic neuritis and myelitis, who probably have the latter condition. The presence of the anti-aquaporin antibody (see below) and the MRI appearance of the cord lesion are able to differentiate most instances. In one memorable example, where hemiplegia and aphasia were followed within 2 weeks by a necrotizing myelitis from which there was no recovery, the patient later developed typical attacks of MS, including retrobulbar neuritis. Elsewhere in the brain and cord, the lesions were typically demyelinating.

Most compelling, the separation of Devic disease from MS is supported by evidence of a specific serum immunoglobulin (Ig) G antineural antibody directed against aquaporin-4, (*NMO antibody*) that binds complement. This has led to the conclusion that the Devic process is a humoral disease in contrast to the cellular mechanism that is proposed for MS (see Lucchinetti et al, 2002). Pittock and coworkers have explored the distribution of the antibody and found it to be located in astrocytic end feet adjacent to capillaries, pia, and Virchow-Robin spaces

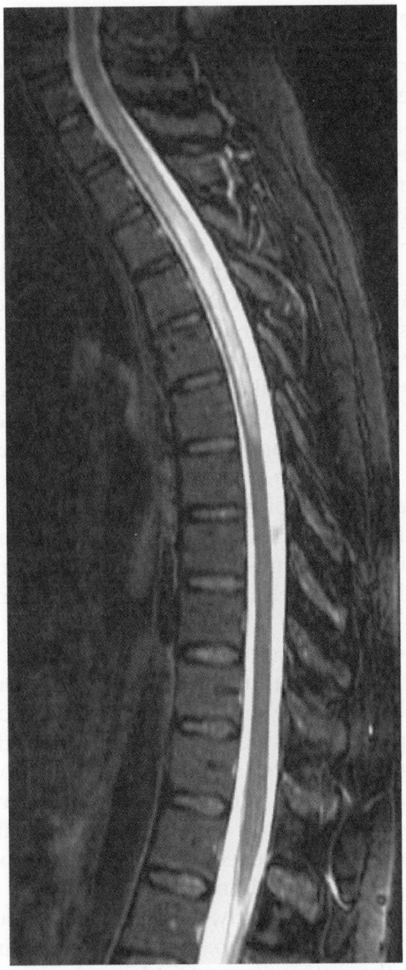

Figure 36-3. MRI of the spinal cord in neuromyelitis optica. Sagittal T2 image showing a hyperintense, longitudinally extensive, confluent cervico-thoracic lesion.

all in the periventricular region and surrounding the central canal of the spinal cord. This is concordant with the distribution of the lesions and many of the clinical characteristics such as the extensive myelitis but also unusual features such as *vomiting* and *hiccoughs*, which reflects damage in the area postrema.

Lennon and colleagues reported that the antibody is a marker for neuromyelitis optica in the majority of cases, and that it is virtually absent in MS. In the material of Wingerchuk and colleagues, the presence of the antibody was 76 percent sensitive and 94 percent specific. By using the additional criteria of the presence of two of the following, the sensitivity and specificity were 99 and 90 percent: longitudinally extensive myelopathy, positive antibodies and an initial MRI that is not characteristic for MS.

Occasionally, neuromyelitis optica occurs in the context of a connective tissue disease such as Sjögren syndrome or lupus, and many of these patients have this same circulating anti-aquaporin antibody. Pittock and colleagues (2008) give the frequency of these antibodies as approximately one-third in patients with systemic autoimmune disease and clinical features of Devic disease. It should also be noted that acute disseminated encephalomyelitis, discussed further on, may present as a neuromyelitis optica syndrome.

Differential Diagnosis There is in addition to the myelitis described earlier a progressive and sometimes saltatory *subacute necrotic myelopathy* without optic neuritis that shares all the features of Devic disease but not the optic neuropathy and, in our view, they probably represent the same entity (Katz and Ropper). The differential diagnosis is broader and includes vascular malformations of the cord or dura and infarction or neoplasm of the cord. Also, a rare isolated vasculitis of the cord may cause a necrotic myelopathy; it is associated with an active CSF pleocytosis (Ropper et al). The cord in the cases we have studied was swollen on MRI in the early stages, often with edema extending many segments above and below the area of primary disease, and later became atrophic, similar to what has been reported in Devic disease. Up to 50 cells are typical in the CSF and the protein is elevated but the spinal fluid may be normal during periods of clinical stability. Several, but not all, of these cases have had positive NMO IgG antibodies (see above), further supporting the notion that most of these aggressive, purely spinal cases are allied with Devic disease.

Treatment The treatment of neuromyelitis optica and of subacute necrotic myelopathy has been largely unsuccessful, most cases progressing despite aggressive therapy, including high-dose corticosteroids, plasma exchange, intravenous immunoglobulin, azathioprine, and cyclophosphamide. A study of several patients by Mandler and colleagues (1998) suggested that perhaps a combination of high-dose methylprednisolone and azathioprine led to clinical improvement; we cannot affirm this approach, but most other treatments have given poor results in our experience. Because a few individuals respond to them, it may be appropriate to try one or more of these therapies. A provocative approach that is being explored by Tradtrantip and colleagues is the use of blocking antibodies to the aquaporin antibody. A summary of treatment has been given by Collongues and de Seze.

ACUTE DISSEMINATED ENCEPHALOMYELITIS (ADEM); POSTINFECTIOUS, POSTEXANTHEM, POSTVACCINAL ENCEPHALOMYELITIS

Some of these terms, used originally to refer to the neurologic sequelae of infectious fevers, were introduced into medicine in the late nineteenth century but it was not until the late 1920s that Perdrau, Pette, Greenfield, and others identified a type of pathologic reaction common to a number of exanthems and vaccines. The current view of this entity is that it represents an acute inflammatory and demyelinating disease, distinguished pathologically by numerous foci of demyelination scattered throughout the brain and spinal cord. These lesions vary from 0.1 to several millimeters (when confluent) in diameter and invariably surround small and medium-sized veins. The axons and nerve cells remain more or less intact. Equally distinctive is the perivenular inflammatory reaction of lymphocytes and mononuclear cells. The adjacent regions of white matter are invaded by monocytes and microglia corresponding to the zones of demyelination. Multifocal meningeal infiltration is another invariable feature but is rarely severe. With the exception of this last feature, ADEM is indistinguishable on histopathologic grounds from acute MS. It is the postinfectious setting, temporal course, and certain special features of each that set them apart. Indeed, even the monophasic nature of ADEM and its clear separation from MS on clinical grounds has been questioned by Schwarz and colleagues, who found that 14 of 40 adults later developed clear signs of MS, usually within a year.

An acute encephalitic, myelitic, or encephalomyelitic process of this type is observed in a number of clinical settings and is more common in children. In our experience, the disease in children follows a febrile illness by days or infrequently up to 2 weeks; this is less often the case in adults. In the originally described form, it occurred within a few days of onset of the exanthem of measles, rubella, smallpox, or chickenpox. Prior to widespread immunization against measles, an epidemic in a large city might have resulted in 100,000 cases of measles and clinically evident neurologic complications in 1 in 800 to 1 in 2,000 cases. The mortality among patients with such complications ranged from 10 to 20 percent; about an equal number were left with persistent neurologic damage. The neurologic complications of measles alone provide sufficient justification for immunization against the disease. The incidence of encephalomyelitis was less following chickenpox and rubella, and much less following mumps (the latter never seen in our pathologic material). In the past, a similar illness was observed to follow vaccination against rabies and smallpox and, reportedly, after administration of tetanus antitoxin (rare), as discussed further on. Now, however, most cases, clinically and pathologically indistinguishable from these two categories of ADEM, appear to develop after seemingly banal respiratory infections and after documented infections with Epstein-Barr, cytomegalovirus, and *Mycoplasma pneumoniae* and even HIV (Narisco et al); occasionally there is no clearly defined preceding illness or inoculation. Many, if not most, instances of acute transverse myelitis may represent the same postinfectious process. The neurologic illness may coincide with the later stages of the manifestations of the infection, in which case the term *parainfectious* may be appropriate.

Irrespective of the clinical setting in which it occurs, disseminated encephalomyelitis in its severe form is of grave import because of the significant rate of neurologic defects in patients who survive. In children, recovery from the acute stage is sometimes followed by a permanent disorder of behavior, mental retardation, or epilepsy; paradoxically, most adults make good recoveries. The *cerebellitis* and acute ataxia that follow chickenpox and other infections are more benign, normally clearing over several months, and may represent a different process, as discussed further on.

Pathogenesis

The pathogenesis of disseminated encephalomyelitis is still unclear despite its obvious association with viral infections. In the postexanthem cases, a definite interval usually separates the onset of disseminated encephalomyelitis from the onset of the rash; also, the pathologic changes are quite different from those of viral infections and virus is rarely if ever recovered from the CSF or brains of patients with disseminated encephalomyelitis. For these reasons, it is believed that the disorder represents an immune-mediated complication of infection rather than a direct infection of the CNS, a process comparable to the Guillain-Barré syndrome. However, as discussed in Chap. 33, new molecular techniques have been able to detect fragments of DNA from varicella zoster virus, *Mycoplasma*, and other organisms in the CSF, so that the question of pathogenesis cannot be answered with finality. Nevertheless, Waksman and Adams found the pathologic changes in these two circumstances—postinfectious demyelination and direct viral infection of the CNS—to be quite different.

A laboratory model of the disease, EAE, has been produced by inoculating animals with a combination of sterile brain tissue and adjuvants. The experimental disease appears most commonly between the eighth and fifteenth days after sensitization (see below) and is characterized by the same perivenular demyelinating and inflammatory lesions that one observes in the human disease. Presumably the lesions are the result of a T-cell–mediated immune reaction to components of myelin or oligodendrocytes. Recently, evidence of antibody binding, complement activation, and eosinophilic infiltration has led to the notion that ADEM is a humoral disease, in contrast to the cellular mechanism that has been proposed for MS, but further confirmation of this notion is required (see Lucchinetti et al, 2000 and 2002).

The notion that EAE and disseminated encephalomyelitis have a similar pathogenesis has received support from the observations of R.T. Johnson and colleagues. They studied 19 patients with postinfectious encephalomyelitis complicating natural measles virus infections. Early myelin destruction was demonstrated by the presence of MBP in the CSF, and lymphocyte proliferative responses to MBP were found in 8 of 17 patients tested. Similar responses were observed in patients with encephalomyelitis after rabies vaccine and after varicella and rubella virus infections, suggesting a common immune-mediated pathogenesis. Moreover, the patients with postmeasles encephalomyelitis showed a lack of intrathecal synthesis of antibody against measles virus, indicating that the neurologic disease was not dependent on viral replication within the CNS.

Clinical Features

The encephalitic form is expressed more fully in children than in adults. As an acute infectious illness is resolving or after a latency of several days or longer, there is the abrupt onset, over hours or a day or two, of confusion, somnolence, and sometimes convulsions with headache, fever, and varying degrees of neck stiffness. Ataxia is common, but myoclonic movements and choreoathetosis are observed less frequently. In more severe cases, stupor, coma, and at times decerebrate rigidity may occur in rapid succession. In many cases, the disease is less severe and the patient suffers a transient encephalitic illness with headaches, confusion, and slight signs of meningeal irritation.

The latency between infection and the first neurologic symptoms that it is acceptable for this diagnosis is a matter of debate, but there are convincing cases (postexanthematous) in which the two phases of illness are separated by 3 or 4 weeks; several days is more typical, as noted below. Curiously, in the encephalitic form, new signs may continue to appear for up to 2 or 3 weeks from the onset. This is emphasized in the series of affected children collected by Hynson and colleagues. The imaging changes may also display delayed or continued evolution. These authors note that ataxia was the most common initial feature in their cases, which is not entirely in accordance with our experience.

In the myelitic form (*postinfectious myelitis, acute transverse myelitis*), there is partial or complete paraplegia or quadriplegia, diminution or loss of tendon reflexes, sensory impairment, and varying degrees of paralysis of bladder and bowel. A syndrome that simulates anterior spinal artery occlusion (spastic paraplegia and loss of pain sensation below a level on the trunk but tending to spare large-fiber sensibility) is not uncommon in our experience. Also, we have cared for a few patients with a limited sacral form of postinfectious myelitis. Midline back pain may be a prominent symptom at the onset.

In both the encephalitic and myelitic types, there may be slight fever, particularly in the more aggressive cases and in younger individuals, where we have seen temperatures reaching 39.4°C (103°F), but the peripheral white blood cell count is normal if the initiating infection has resolved. A few of our patients have had elevated sedimentation rates, but it is not possible to know whether this reflects the precipitating infection. Nonetheless, separating these two entities may be difficult, especially in children who have a greater tendency to develop fever and convulsions with ADEM. Either process may be associated with aseptic meningitis.

The CSF shows a slight increase in lymphocytes and protein content, but these are highly variable, with a few of our patients having only an increase in protein and no cells and others having up to several hundred cells. The MRI shows several bilateral confluent white matter lesions in both cerebral hemispheres early in the course of ADEM (Fig. 36-4); when these are large and numerous, the diagnosis is more certain. The lesions all appear to be of similar age, but we cannot account for several cases we have seen in which serial MRIs show new lesions accumulating over 2 or 3 weeks, as already noted. Moreover, as pointed out by Honkaniemi and colleagues, there may be a delay of several days between the clinical manifestations and the first appearance of changes in the MRI, a situation to which we can attest. Whether a single lesion on MRI can be considered compatible with ADEM is unclear.

In the case of postexanthem encephalomyelitis, the syndrome generally begins 2 to 4 days after the appearance of the rash. Usually the rash is fading and other symptoms are improving when the patient, typically a

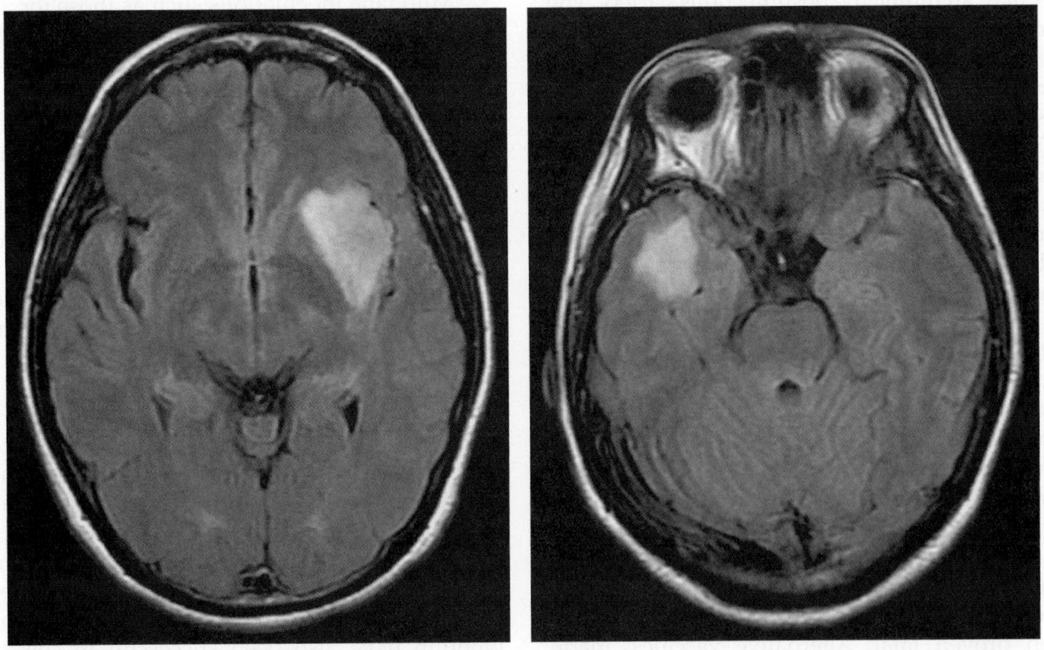

Figure 36-4. Acute (postinfectious) disseminated encephalomyelitis (ADEM). Axial T2-FLAIR images showing left inferior frontal (*left*) and right anterior temporal (*right*) edematous lesions.

child, suddenly develops a recrudescence of fever, convulsions, stupor, and sometimes coma. Less commonly, the patient may develop hemiplegia or a virtually pure cerebellar syndrome, as noted below (particularly after chickenpox), and occasionally a transverse myelitis, sphincteric disturbance, or other signs of spinal cord involvement. Choreoathetotic movements are seen infrequently. Likewise, optic neuritis is uncommon, but it does occur.

A variant of postinfectious encephalomyelitis that involves solely or predominantly the cerebellum deserves special comment. Typically, a mild ataxia with variable corticospinal or other signs appears within days of one of the childhood exanthems as well as after Epstein-Barr virus, *Mycoplasma*, *Legionella*, and cytomegalovirus infections, and after a number of vaccinations and nondescript respiratory infections. It is described in detail in Chap. 33 because it has a close relationship to certain viruses, particularly varicella, suggesting that some, if not most, cases are caused by an infectious meningoencephalitis. Others—for example, following mycoplasmal infection—occur after a long latency and show pathologic changes that are consistent with a postinfectious demyelination. Thus it is possible that there may be two types of acute cerebellitis, one para- or postinfectious and the other caused by a direct infection of the brain and meninges. The benign nature of the illness has precluded adequate pathologic examination; hence some of these statements are speculative.

Not all the neurologic complications of measles and other exanthems and acute viral infections are examples of postinfectious encephalomyelitis. As already noted, the illness is at times difficult to distinguish from viral meningoencephalitis. Infectious mononucleosis, herpes simplex, mycoplasmal infection, and other forms of encephalitis may all mimic the postinfectious variety. The Reye syndrome is usually not difficult to separate from postinfectious encephalomyelitis, even when it follows chickenpox or viral influenza, because of the normal CSF and high serum concentrations of liver enzymes and ammonia (see Chap. 33). In a child, the first attack of febrile seizures in the course of an exanthematous illness may raise the suspicion of encephalitis or postinfectious encephalomyelitis.

The MRI finding of large or multifocal areas of white matter damage can also be produced by intravascular lymphoma and progressive multifocal leukoencephalopathy (Chap. 31) and a rare leukoencephalopathy that follows inhaling heroin vapor (Chap. 43).

Postvaccinal ADEM Since late in the nineteenth century, it has been known that a severe form of encephalomyelitis may complicate the injection of rabies vaccine ("neuroparalytic accident"). Until quite recently, the rabies vaccine in common use consisted of killed virus that had been grown in rabbit brain tissue. Encephalomyelitis occurred in about 1 in 750 patients inoculated with this vaccine, and approximately 25 percent of cases with this complication proved fatal. Alternative vaccines, made from embryonated duck eggs (and later from human diploid cells) infected with fixed viruses, contain very little or no nerve tissue and are almost free of neurologic complications. In developing countries, where less-expensive brain-based vaccines are still in use, neuroparalytic accidents continue to occur. The observations of Hemachudha and colleagues indicate that the altered immune mechanism that is operative in the neuroparalytic accident is the same as that in postmeasles encephalomyelitis and experimental allergic encephalomyelitis.

There are numerous recorded instances in which the old rabies vaccine (with neural tissue) induced an attack of what subsequently appeared to be MS. Shiraki and Otani reported such examples from Japan. The evolution of symptoms was subacute, over a period of 2 to 4 weeks, and the demyelinating lesions were macroscopic—up to 1 to 2.0 cm in diameter—but composed of confluent perivenous lesions. The disease could be reproduced in dogs—persuasive evidence that one form of acute MS is a variant of ADEM. Encephalomyelitis following vaccination against smallpox has been known since 1860, having occurred about once in 4,000 vaccinations. That disease is now of historical interest only, insofar as smallpox has disappeared as a human illness.

The association of the neurologic disorder with vaccination usually leaves the diagnosis in little doubt, and the characteristic combination of encephalitic and myelitic features will help to distinguish the condition from meningitis, viral encephalitis, and poliomyelitis. Rarely, an atypical case may mimic any one of these disorders. On occasion, the disease may suggest involvement of nerve roots and peripheral nerves and resemble acute inflammatory polyneuritis (Guillain-Barré syndrome). In fact, the rabies vaccine produced in South America from suckling mouse brain causes this type of peripheral nerve disease more often than encephalomyelitis.

Mundane inoculations such as those for influenza or hepatitis must have a very small rate of ADEM, judging from surveillance studies; Ascherio and colleagues were unable to find any increase in cases among two large studies of nurses who received hepatitis B vaccine. The absence of a clear connection of MS to vaccination has already been mentioned.

The mortality rate of postvaccinal encephalomyelitis is high, between 30 and 50 percent. If recovery occurs, it may be surprisingly complete. However, a significant proportion of patients show residual neurologic signs, mainly in the form of seizures, intellectual impairment, or behavioral abnormalities.

Treatment

Corticosteroids given soon after the appearance of neurologic signs may modify the severity of experimental allergic encephalomyelitis; this provides the logic for their use in the human counterpart of this disease but controlled trials have not been carried out. We usually administer methylprednisolone in high doses intravenously for 3 to 5 days. Plasma exchange and intravenous immune globulin have also been successful in some fulminant cases (Kanter et al; Stricker et al) but only in a few we have observed.

Acute Necrotizing Hemorrhagic Encephalomyelitis (Acute Hemorrhagic Leukoencephalitis of Weston Hurst)

This, the most fulminant form of demyelinating disease, almost certainly the severe end of the spectrum of ADEM, affects mainly young adults and children. It is usually preceded by a respiratory infection of variable duration (1 to 14 days), sometimes caused by *M. pneumoniae* but more often following a mundane infection or of indeterminate cause. The neurologic symptoms appear abruptly, beginning with headache, fever, stiff neck, and confusion. These are followed in short order by signs of disease of one or both cerebral hemispheres and brainstem—focal seizures, hemiplegia or quadriplegia, pseudobulbar paralysis, and progressively deepening coma. Peripheral leukocytosis is usually present, sometimes reaching 30,000 cells/mm^3, and the sedimentation rate is elevated. The CSF is often under increased pressure; cells vary in number from a few lymphocytes to a polymorphonuclear pleocytosis of up to 3,000 cells/mm^3; red cells may be present in variable numbers; protein content is increased, but glucose values are normal. Diagnosis is greatly facilitated by CT scanning and MRI, which reveal bilateral but asymmetrical large, confluent, edematous lesions in the cerebral white matter with a myriad of punctate hemorrhages in gray and white matter (Fig. 36-5). The size of the lesions, their hemorrhagic character, and the extent of the surrounding edema distinguish them from the typical postinfectious ADEM. In many other ways they are similar, except for their severity. Many cases terminate fatally in 2 to 4 days, but in others, survival is longer. Patients with a similar clinical picture who are thought to have the same disease on the basis of brain biopsy examinations have recovered with almost no residual symptoms. In one of the fatal cases reported by Adams and colleagues, the illness evolved more slowly—over a period of 2 to 3 weeks—while another patient died with temporal lobe herniation within 12 h. A single recurrence of the disease after an interval of 2 years was observed in one of our patients.

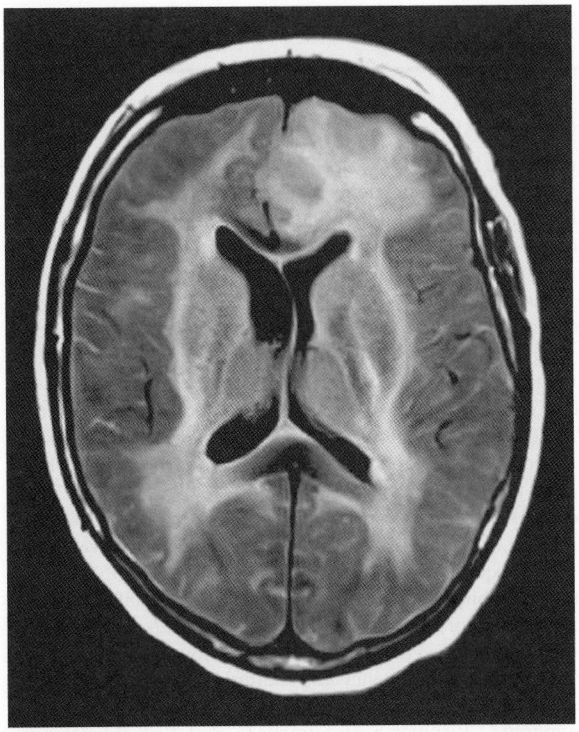

Figure 36-5. Acute necrotizing hemorrhagic leukoencephalitis. Axial T2-FLAIR MRI shows extensive abnormal hyperintensity throughout the hemispheric white matter as well as within the deep gray nuclei. Additional signal abnormality in the cortical sulci is due to subarachnoid hemorrhage.

Brain abscess, subdural empyema, focal embolic encephalomalacia, and acute encephalitis, especially as a result of type 1 herpes simplex virus, are the important considerations in the differential diagnosis.

The *pathologic findings* are distinctive. On sectioning of the brain, the white matter of one or both hemispheres is destroyed almost to the point of liquefaction. The involved tissue is pink or yellow-gray and flecked with multiple petechial hemorrhages. Similar changes are often found in the brainstem and cerebellar peduncles and probably in the spinal cord (one form of acute necrotizing myelitis and Devic disease). On histologic examination, one finds widespread necrosis of small blood vessels and brain tissue around the vessels, with intense cellular infiltration, multiple small hemorrhages, and an inflammatory reaction in the meninges of variable intensity. The pathologic picture resembles that of disseminated encephalomyelitis in its perivascular distribution, with the added features of a more widespread necrosis and a tendency of lesions to form large foci in the cerebral hemispheres. The vascular lesions result in a characteristic exudation of fibrin into the vessel wall and surrounding tissue. It is possible that certain patients who are showing an explosive myelitic illness are suffering from a necrotizing lesion of similar type, but pathologic evidence in support of this view has been difficult to obtain. Fibrin exudation in an acute fatal hemorrhagic myelitis was present in a case examined by Adams and colleagues. We also have experience with a case of this nature that evolved in steps over several months, resulting in death, with a cellular reaction in the spinal fluid on each of several lumbar punctures. There was partial steroid responsiveness.

The etiology of this condition remains obscure, but its resemblance to other demyelinating diseases should be emphasized. The similarities of the histologic changes to those of disseminated encephalomyelitis, noted above, suggest that the two diseases are related forms of the same fundamental process. In fact, cases combining both types of pathologic changes have been described (Fisher et al). It is noteworthy that, among the small number of patients who have recovered from what appeared to be a typical necrotizing hemorrhagic encephalitis, a few have gone on to develop typical MS.

Treatment of Hurst Disease

High-dose intravenous corticosteroids should be used in the treatment of acute necrotizing hemorrhagic encephalopathy; in several personally observed patients, we had the impression that corticosteroids produced a favorable result. The use of plasma exchange and intravenous immunoglobulin, as for acute disseminated encephalomyelitis, is being explored and has had success in single reported cases when instituted early.

Graft-Versus-Host Disease

This form of brain inflammation, pertinent to the special circumstance of bone marrow transplantation, is included here for lack of a better category with which to align it. Months or years after transplantation, subacute hemiparesis, seizures, behavioral changes, or ataxia arise and may be attributed to PML, a viral infection of the white matter (Chap. 33), or another viral process that is known to occur with circumstances of immunosuppression. The MRI shows white matter lesions that conform to an MS-like periventricular orientation or a more confluent leukoencephalopathy. A recent patient under our care demonstrated lesions in the splenium of the corpus callosum that extended into the adjacent centrum semiovale (Fig. 36-6). Several reports emphasize a mild vasculitis in the territory of the white matter lesions (Padovan et al). Almost all affected patients have concurrently displayed a tender eryhtemetous, macular rash that is typical of acute graft-versus-host disease. There are also rare, but well-characterized, neuromuscular complications of graft-versus-host disease.

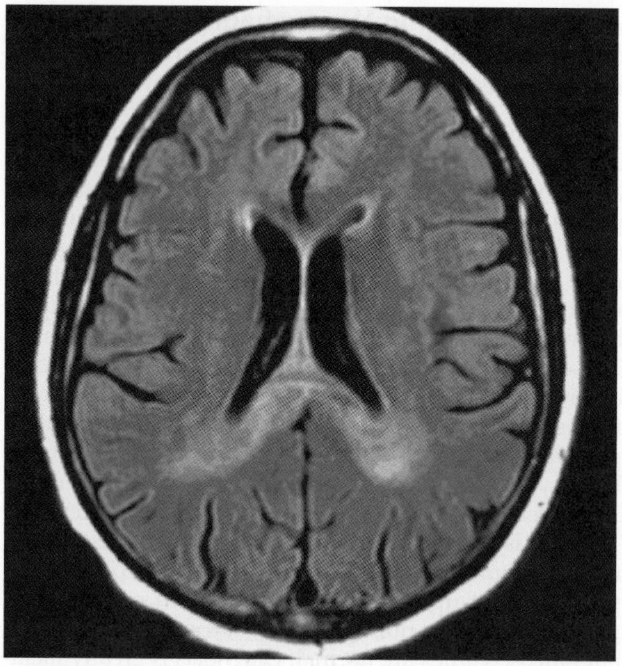

Figure 36-6. Abnormal T2 hyperintensity in the splenium of the corpus callosum in a patient with graft-versus-host disease 2 years following allogenic bone marrow transplantation.

References

Adams RD, Cammermeyer J, Denny-Brown D: Acute hemorrhagic encephalopathy. *J Neuropathol Exp Neurol* 8:1, 1949.

Adams RD, Kubik CS: The morbid anatomy of the demyelinating diseases. *Am J Med* 12:510, 1952.

Aimard G, Confavreux C, Ventre JJ, et al: Etude de 213 cas de sclerose en plaques traites par l'azathiaprine de 1967–1982. *Rev Neurol* 139:509, 1983.

Akasbi M, Berenguer A, Saiz A, et al: White matter abnormalities in primary Sjögren syndrome. *QJM* 105:433, 2012.

Allen IV, Miller JHD, Shillington RKA: Systemic lupus erythematosus clinically resembling multiple sclerosis and with unusual pathological ultrastructural features. *J Neurol Neurosurg Psychiatry* 42:392, 1979.

Alter M, Halpern L, Kurland LT, et al: Multiple sclerosis in Israel. *Arch Neurol* 7:253, 1962.

Anderson DW, Ellenberg JH, Leventhal CM, et al: Revised estimate of the prevalence of multiple sclerosis in the United States. *Ann Neurol* 31:333, 1992.

Arnason BGW: Interferon beta in multiple sclerosis. *Neurology* 43:641, 1993.

Ascherio A, Zhang SM, Hernan MA, et al: Hepatitis B vaccination and the risk of multiple sclerosis. *N Engl J Med* 344:327, 2001.

Barkhof F, Bruck W, De Groot CJ, et al: Remyelinated lesions in multiple sclerosis: Magnetic resonance image appearance. *Arch Neurol* 60:1073, 2003.

Barnes D, Hughes RAC, Morris RW, et al: Randomised trial of oral and intravenous methylprednisolone in acute relapses of multiple sclerosis. *Lancet* 349:902, 1997.

Barnett MH, Prineas JW: Relapsing and remitting multiple sclerosis. Pathology of the newly forming plaque. *Ann Neurol* 55:458, 2004.

Batten FE: Ataxia in childhood. *Brain* 28:484, 1905.

Beck RW, Chandler DL, Cole SR, et al: Interferon β-1a for early multiple sclerosis: CHAMPS trial subgroup analysis. *Ann Neurol* 51:481, 2002.

Beck RW, Cleary PA, Anderson MM Jr, et al: A randomized controlled trial of corticosteroids in the treatment of acute optic neuritis. *N Engl J Med* 326:581, 1992.

Beck RW, Trobe JD, Moke PS, et al: High- and low-risk profiles for the development of multiple sclerosis within 10 years after optic neuritis: Experience of the optic neuritis treatment trial. *Arch Ophthalmol* 121:944, 2003.

Beebe GW, Kurtzke JF, Kurland LT, et al: Studies on the natural history of multiple sclerosis: 3. Epidemiologic analyses of the Army experience in World War II. *Neurology* 17:1, 1967.

Berger T, Rubner P, Schautzer F, et al: Antimyelin antibodies as a predictor of clinically definite multiple sclerosis after a first demyelinating event. *N Engl J Med* 349:139, 2003.

Birk K, Rudick R: Pregnancy and multiple sclerosis. *Arch Neurol* 43:719, 1986.

Bloomgren G, Richman S, Hotermans C, et al. Risk of natalizumab-associated progressive multifocal leukoencephalopathy. *N Engl J Med* 366:1870, 2012.

Bobholz JA, Rao SM: Cognitive dysfunction in multiple sclerosis: A review of recent developments. *Curr Opin Neurol* 16:283, 2003.

Bornstein MB, Miller A, Slagle S, et al: A pilot trial of COP I in exacerbating-remitting multiple sclerosis. *N Engl J Med* 317:408, 1987.

Bot JC, Barkhof F, Polman CH, et al: Spinal cord abnormalities in recently diagnosed MS patients. Added value of spinal MRI examination. *Neurology* 62:226, 2004.

Bourre B, Marignier R, Zéphir H, et al: Neuromyelitis optica and pregnancy. *Neurology* 78:875, 2012.

British and Dutch Multiple Sclerosis Azathioprine Trial Group: Double masked trial of azathioprine in multiple sclerosis. *Lancet* ii:179, 1988.

CAMMS223 Trial Investigators et al: A randomized, rater-blinded, trial of alemtuzumab versus interferon beta-1a in early, relapsing remitting multiple sclerosis. *N Engl J Med* 359:1786, 2008.

CHAMPS Study Group: Interferon beta-1a for optic neuritis patients at high risk for multiple sclerosis. *Am J Ophthalmol* 132:463, 2001.

Cohen JA, Coles AJ, Arnold DL, et al: Alemtuzumab versus interferon beta 1a as first-line treatment for patients with relapsing-remitting multiple sclerosis: A randomised controlled phase 3 trial. *Lancet* 380:1819, 2012.

Collongues N, de Seze J: Current and future treatment approaches for neuromyelitis optica. *Ther Adv Neurol Disord* 4: 111, 2011.

Compston A, Confavreux C: The distribution of multiple sclerosis, in Compston A, Lassman H, McDonald I, et al (eds): *McAlpine's Multiple Sclerosis*, 4th ed. New York, Churchill Livingstone, 2006, pp 69–112.

Compston A, Lassmann H, McDonald I: The history of multiple sclerosis in Compston A, Lassman H, McDonald I, et al (eds): *McAlpine's Multiple Sclerosis*, 4th ed. New York, Churchill Livingstone, 2006, pp 3-68.

Confavreux C, Hutchinson M, Hours MM, et al: Rate of pregnancy related relapse in multiple sclerosis. *N Engl J Med* 339:285, 1998

Confavreux C, Suissa S, Saddier P, et al: Vaccinations and the risk of relapse in multiple sclerosis. *N Engl J Med* 344:319, 2001.

Confavreux C, Vukusie S, Moreau T, Adeleine P: Relapses and progression of disability in multiple sclerosis. *N Engl J Med* 343:1430, 2000.

Cook SD, Devereux C, Troiano R, et al: Effect of total lymphoid irradiation in chronic progressive multiple sclerosis. *Lancet* 1:1405, 1986.

Critchley GR, Richardson PL: Vim thalamotomy for the relief of the intention tremor of multiple sclerosis. *Br J Neurosurg* 12:559, 1998.

Dalos NP, Robins PV, Brooks BR, et al: Disease activity and emotional state in multiple sclerosis. *Ann Neurol* 13:573, 1983.

Dean G: The multiple sclerosis problem. *Sci Am* 233:40, 1970.

Dean G, Kurtzke JF: On the risk of multiple sclerosis according to age at immigration to South Africa. *Br Med J* 3:725, 1971.

DeJong RN: Multiple sclerosis: History, definition and general considerations, in Vinken PJ, Bruyn GW (eds): *Handbook of Clinical Neurology*. Vol 9. Amsterdam, North-Holland, 1970, pp 45–62.

De Keyser J: Autoimmunity in multiple sclerosis. *Neurology* 38:371, 1988.

Ebers GC: Genetic factors in multiple sclerosis. *Neurol Clin* 1:645, 1983.

Ebers GC: Optic neuritis and multiple sclerosis. *Arch Neurol* 42:702, 1985.

Ebers GC, Bulman DE, Sadovnick AD: A population-based study of multiple sclerosis in twins. *N Engl J Med* 315:1638, 1986.

Ellison PH, Barron KD: Clinical recovery from Schilder's disease. *Neurology* 29:244, 1979.

European Study Group: Interferon β-1b in secondary progressive MS. *Lancet* 352:1491, 1998.

Fazekas F, Deisenhammer F, Strasser-Fuchs S, et al: Randomised placebo-controlled trial of monthly intravenous immunoglobulin in relapsing-remitting multiple sclerosis. *Lancet* 349:589, 1997.

Fisher RS, Clark AW, Wolinsky JS, et al: Post-infectious leukoencephalitis complicating *Mycoplasma pneumoniae* infection. *Arch Neurol* 40:109, 1983.

Geny C, Ngeyen JP, Pollin B, et al: Improvement in severe postural cerebellar tremor in multiple sclerosis by thalamic stimulation. *Mov Disord* 11:489, 1996.

Gilbert JJ, Sadler M: Unsuspected multiple sclerosis. *Arch Neurol* 40:533, 1983.

Goodkin DE, Rudick RA, Medendorp V, et al: Low-dose oral methotrexate in chronic progressive multiple sclerosis. *Neurology* 47:1153, 1996.

Hallett M, Lindsey JW, Adelstein BD, Riley PO: Controlled trial of isoniazid therapy for severe postural cerebellar tremor in multiple sclerosis. *Neurology* 35:1314, 1985.

Halliday AM, McDonald WI: Pathophysiology of demyelinating disease. *Br Med Bull* 33:21, 1977.

Hartung HP, Gonsette R, Konig H, et al: Mitoxantrone in progressive multiple sclerosis: A placebo-controlled, double-blind randomised, multicentre trial. *Lancet* 360:2018, 2002.

Hauser SL, Bresnan MJ, Reinherz EL, Weiner HL: Childhood multiple sclerosis: Clinical features and demonstration of changes in T-cell subsets with disease activity. *Ann Neurol* 11:463, 1982.

Hauser SL, Dawson DM, Lehrich JR: Intensive immune suppression in progressive multiple sclerosis: A randomized three arm study of high-dose intravenous cyclophosphamide, plasma exchange and ACTH. *N Engl J Med* 308:173, 1983.

Hauser SA, Waubant E, Arnold DL, et al: B-cell depletion with rituximab in relapsing-remitting multiple sclerosis. *N Engl J Med* 358:676, 2008.

Hely MA, McManis PG, Doran TJ, et al: Acute optic neuritis: A prospective study of risk factors for multiple sclerosis. *J Neurol Neurosurg Psychiatry* 49:1125, 1986.

Hemachudha T, Griffin DE, Giffels JJ, et al: Myelin basic protein as an encephalitogen in encephalomyelitis and polyneuritis following rabies vaccination. *N Engl J Med* 316:369, 1987.

Honkaniemi J, Dastidar P, Kahara V, et al: Delayed MR imaging changes in acute disseminated encephalomyelitis. *AJNR Am J Neuroradiol* 22:1117, 2001.

Hooper J, Whittle IR: Long-term outcome after thalamotomy for movement disorders in multiple sclerosis. *Lancet* 352:1984, 1998.

Howell OW, Reeves CA, Nicholas R, et al. Meningeal inflammation is widespread and linked to cortical pathology in multiple sclerosis. *Brain* 134:2755, 2011.

Hughes RAC, Sharrack B: More immunotherapy for multiple sclerosis. *J Neurol Neurosurg Psychiatry* 61:239, 1996.

Hynson JL, Kornberg AJ, Coleman LT, et al: Clinical and neuroradiologic features of acute disseminated encephalomyelitis in children. *Neurology* 56:1308, 2001.

International Multiple Sclerosis Genetics Consortium: Risk alleles for multiple sclerosis identified by a genomewide study. *N Engl J Med* 357:851, 2007.

Jacobs L, Kinkel PR, Kinkel WR: Silent brain lesions in patients with isolated idiopathic optic neuritis. *Arch Neurol* 43:452, 1986.

Jacobs L, O'Malley JA, Freeman A, et al: Intrathecal interferon in the treatment of multiple sclerosis: Patient follow-up. *Arch Neurol* 42:841, 1985.

Johnson KP, Arrigo SC, Nelson BS, Ginsberg A: Agarose electrophoresis of cerebrospinal fluid in multiple sclerosis. *Neurology* 27:273, 1977.

Johnson KP, Likosky WH, Nelson BJ, Fine G: Comprehensive viral immunology of multiple sclerosis: I. Clinical, epidemiological, and CSF studies. *Arch Neurol* 37:537, 610, 616, 1980.

Johnson RT, Griffin DE, Hirsch RL, et al: Measles encephalomyelitis: Clinical and immunologic studies. *N Engl J Med* 310:137, 1984.

Kanter DS, Horensky D, Sperling RA, et al: Plasmapheresis in fulminant acute disseminated encephalomyelitis. *Neurology* 45:824, 1995.

Kappos L, Antel J, Comi G, et al: Oral fingolimod (FTY720) for relapsing multiple sclerosis. *N Engl J Med* 355:1124, 2006.

Kappos L, Li D, Calabresi PA, et al. Ocrelizumab in relapsing-remitting multiple sclerosis: A phase 2, randomised, placebo-controlled multicentre trial. *Lancet* 378: 1779, 2011.

Katz J, Ropper AH: Progressive necrotic myelopathy: Clinical course in 9 patients. *Arch Neurol* 57:355, 2000.

Kepes JJ: Large focal tumor-like demyelinating lesions of the brain: Intermediate entity between multiple sclerosis and acute disseminated encephalomyelitis: A study of 31 patients. *Ann Neurol* 33:18, 1993.

Kidd D, Burtan B, Plant GT, et al: Chronic relapsing inflammatory optic neuropathy. *Brain* 126:276, 2003.

Kuhle J, Pohl C, Mehling M, et al: Lack of association between antimyelin antibodies and progression to multiple sclerosis. *N Engl J Med* 356:371, 2007.

Kurland LT: The frequency and geographic distribution of multiple sclerosis as indicated by mortality statistics and morbidity surveys in the United States and Canada. *Am J Hyg* 55:457, 1952.

Kurland LT, Molgaard CA, Kurland EM, et al: Swine flu vaccine and multiple sclerosis. *JAMA* 251:2672, 1984.

Kurtzke JF: A reassessment of the distribution of multiple sclerosis. *Act Neurol Scand* 51:110, 1975.

Kurtzke JF: On the evaluation of disability in multiple sclerosis. *Neurology* 11:686, 1961.

Kurtzke JF: Optic neuritis or multiple sclerosis. *Arch Neurol* 42:704, 1985.

Kurtzke JF, Beebe GW, Nagler B, et al: Studies on the natural history of multiple sclerosis: Early prognostic features of the later course of the illness. *J Chronic Dis* 30:819, 1977.

Kurtzke JF, Beebe GW, Norman JE Jr: Epidemiology of multiple sclerosis in U.S. veterans: I. Race, sex, and geographic distribution. *Neurology* 29:1228, 1979.

Kurtzke JF, Gudmundsson KR, Bergmann S: Multiple sclerosis in Iceland: I. Evidence of a post-war epidemic. *Neurology* 32:143, 1982.

Kurtzke JF, Hyllested K: Multiple sclerosis in the Faroe Islands: II. Clinical update, transmission, and the nature of MS. *Neurology* 36:307, 1986.

Lennon VA, Wingerchuk DM, Kryzer TJ, et al: A serum autoantibody marker of neuromyelitis optica: Distinction from multiple sclerosis. *Lancet* 364:2106, 2004.

Lessell S: Corticosteroid treatment of acute optic neuritis. *N Engl J Med* 326:634, 1992.

Lightman S, McDonald WI, Bird AC, et al: Retinal venous sheathing in optic neuritis. *Brain* 110:405, 1987.

Lindå H, von Heijne A, Major EO, et al: Progressive multifocal leukoencephalopathy after natalizumab monotherapy. *N Engl J Med* 361:1081, 2009.

Lublin FD, Cofield SS, Cutter GR, et al: Randomized study combining interferon and glatiramer acetate in multiple sclerosis. *Ann Neurol* 73:327, 2013.

Lucchinetti CF, Brück W, Parisi J, et al: Heterogeneity of multiple sclerosis lesions: Implications for the pathogenesis of demyelination. *Ann Neurol* 47:707, 2000.

Lucchinetti CF, Kiers L, O'Duffy A, et al: Risk factors for developing multiple sclerosis after childhood optic neuritis. *Neurology* 49:1413, 1997.

Lucchinetti CF, Mandler RN, McGovern D, et al: A role for humoral mechanisms in the pathogenesis of Devic's neuromyelitis optica. *Brain* 125:1450, 2002.

Lucchinetti CF, Popescu BF, Bunyan RF, et al: Inflammatory cortical demyelination in early multiple sclerosis. *N Engl J Med* 365:2188, 2011.

Mandler RN, Ahmed W, Dencoff JE: Devic's neuromyelitis optica: A prospective study of seven patients treated with prednisone and azathioprine. *Neurology* 51:1219, 1998.

Mathews WB: Paroxysmal symptoms in multiple sclerosis. *J Neuro Neurosurg Psychiat* 38:617, 1975.

Mayr WT, Pittock SJ, McClelland RL, et al: Incidence and prevalence of multiple sclerosis in Olmsted County, Minnesota, 1985–2000. *Neurology* 61:1373, 2003.

McAlpine D, Compston MD: Some aspects of the natural history of disseminated sclerosis. *Q J Med* 21:135, 1952.

McAlpine D, Lumsden CE, Acheson ED: *Multiple Sclerosis: A Reappraisal*, 2nd ed. Edinburgh, UK, Churchill Livingstone, 1972.

McDonald WI: The mystery of the origin of multiple sclerosis. *J Neurol Neurosurg Psychiatry* 49:113, 1986.

McDonald WI, Compston A, Edan G, et al: Recommended diagnostic criteria for multiple sclerosis: guidelines from the International Panel on the diagnosis of multiple sclerosis. *Ann Neurol* 50:121, 2001.

McDonald WI, Halliday AM: Diagnosis and classification of multiple sclerosis. *Br Med Bull* 33:4, 1977.

Mendell JR, Kolkin S, Kissel JT, et al: Evidence for central nervous system demyelination in chronic inflammatory demyelinating polyradiculoneuropathy. *Neurology* 37:1291, 1987.

Miller DH, Barkhof F, Frank JA, et al: Measurement of atrophy in multiple sclerosis: Pathological basis, methodological aspects and clinical relevance. *Brain* 125:1676, 2002.

Miller DH, Khan OA, Sheremata WA, et al: A controlled trial of natalizumab for relapsing multiple sclerosis. *N Engl J Med* 348:15, 2003.

Moulin D, Paty DW, Ebers GC: The predictive value of CSF electrophoresis in "possible" multiple sclerosis. *Brain* 106:809, 1983.

Munger KL, Levin LI, Hollis BW, et al: Serum 25-hydroxyvitamin D levels and risk of multiple sclerosis. *JAMA* 296:2832, 2006.

Multiple Sclerosis Study Group, The: Efficacy and toxicity of cyclosporine in chronic progressive multiple sclerosis: A randomized, double-blinded, placebo-controlled clinical trial. *Ann Neurol* 27:591, 1990.

Narisco P, Galgani S, Del Grosso B, et al: Acute disseminated encephalomyelitis as manifestation of primary HIV infection. *Neurology* 57:1493, 2001.

National Center for Health Statistics, Collins JG: *Types of Injuries and Impairments Due to Injuries*. United States Vital Statistics. Series 10, no 159, DHHS, no (PHS) 871587. Washington, DC, U.S. Public Health Service, 1986.

Optic Neuritis Study Group: The five-year risk of MS after optic neuritis. *Neurology* 49:1404, 1997.

Ormerod IEC, McDonald WI, DuBoulay GH, et al: Disseminated lesions at presentation in patients with optic neuritis. *J Neurol Neurosurg Psychiatry* 49:124, 1986.

Osterman PO, Westerberg CE: Paroxysmal attacks in multiple sclerosis. *Brain* 98:189, 1975.

Padovan CS, Bise K, Hahn J, et al: Angiitis of the central nervous system after allogenic bone marrow transplantation? *Stroke* 30:1651, 1999.

Percy AK, Nobrega FT, Okazaki H: Multiple sclerosis in Rochester, Minnesota: A 60-year appraisal. *Arch Neurol* 25:105, 1971.

Pittock SJ, Lennon VA, de Seze J, et al: Neuromyelitis optica and non organ-specific autoimmunity. *Arch Neurol* 65:78, 2008.

Pittock SJ, Mayr WT, McClelland RL, et al: Disability profile of MS did not change over 10 years in a population-based prevalence cohort. *Neurology* 62:601, 2004.

Pittock SJ, Weinshenker BG, Lucchinetti CF, et al: Neuromyelitis optica brain lesions localized at sites of high aquaporin 4 expression. *Arch Neurol* 63:964, 2006.

Polman CH, O'Connor PW, Havardova E, et al: A randomized, placebo-controlled trial of natalizumab for relapsing multiple sclerosis. *N Engl J Med* 354:899, 2006.

Polman CH, Reingold SC, Banwell B, et al: Diagnostic criteria for multiple sclerosis: 2010 revisions to the McDonald criteria. *Ann Neurol* 69:292, 2011.

Poser CM: Exacerbations, activity and progression in multiple sclerosis. *Arch Neurol* 37:471, 1980.

Poser CM, Goutieres F, Carpentier M: Schilder's myelinoclastic diffuse sclerosis. *Pediatrics* 77:107, 1986.

Poser CM, Roman GC, Vernant J-C: Multiple sclerosis or HTLV-1 myelitis? *Neurology* 40:1020, 1990.

Poser CM, Van Bogaert L: Natural history and evolution of the concept of Schilder's diffuse sclerosis. *Acta Psychiatr Neurol Scand* 31:285, 1956.

Poskanzer DC, Schapira K, Miller H: Multiple sclerosis and poliomyelitis. *Lancet* 2:917, 1963.

Prineas JW, Barnard RO, Kwon EE, et al: Multiple sclerosis: Remyelination of nascent lesions. *Ann Neurol* 33:137, 1993.

Prineas JW, Connell F: The fine structure of chronically active multiple sclerosis plaques. *Neurology* 28:68, 1978.

PRISMS Study Group: Randomized double-blind placebo-controlled study of interferon β-1a in relapsing/remitting multiple sclerosis. *Lancet* 352:1498, 1998.

Ramirez-Lassepas M, Tullock JW, Quinones MR, Snyder BD: Acute radicular pain as a presenting symptom in multiple sclerosis. *Arch Neurol* 49:255, 1992.

Renoux C, Vukusic S, Mikaeloff Y, et al: Natural history of multiple sclerosis with childhood onset. *N Engl J Med* 356:2603, 2007.

Rizzo JF III, Lessell S: Risk of developing multiple sclerosis after uncomplicated optic neuritis: A long-term prospective study. *Neurology* 38:185, 1988.

Rodriguez M, Karnes WE, Bartelson JD, Pineda AA: Plasmapheresis in acute episodes of fulminant inflammatory demyelination. *Neurology* 43:1100, 1993.

Ropper AH: The "Poison Chair" Treatment for Multiple Sclerosis. *N Engl J Med* 367:1150, 2012.

Ropper AH, Ayata C, Adelman L: Vasculitis of the spinal cord. *Arch Neurol* 60:1791, 2003.

Ropper AH, Poskanzer DC: The prognosis of acute and subacute transverse myelitis based on early signs and symptoms. *Ann Neurol* 4:51, 1978.

Rudick RA, Stuart WH, Calabrese PA, et al: Natalizumab plus interferon beta-1a for relapsing multiple sclerosis. *N Engl J Med* 354:911, 2006.

Sadovnick AD, Baird PA, Ward RH: Multiple sclerosis: Updated risks for relatives. *Am J Med Genet* 29:533, 1988.

Sadovnick AD, Ebers GC, Dyment DA, et al: Evidence for a genetic basis for multiple sclerosis. *Lancet* 347:1728, 1996.

Sayao A-L, Devonshire V, Tremlett H. Longitudinal follow-up of "benign" multiple sclerosis at 20 years. *Neurology* 68:496, 2007.

Schapira K, Poskanzer DC, Miller H: Familial and conjugal multiple sclerosis. *Brain* 86:315, 1963.

Schiffer RB, Slater RJ: Neuropsychiatric features of multiple sclerosis: Recognition and management. *Semin Neurol* 5:127, 1985.

Schilder P: Zur Kenntniss der sogennanten diffusen Sklerose. *Z Gesamte Neurol Psychiatry* 10:1, 1912.

Schwarz S, Mohr A, Knauth M, et al: Acute disseminated encephalomyelitis. A follow-up study of 40 adult patients. *Neurology* 56:1313, 2001.

Sellebjerg F, Nielsen S, Frederikson JL, et al: A randomized controlled trial of oral high-dose methylprednisolone in acute optic neuritis. *Neurology* 52:1479, 1999.

Shiraki H, Otani S: Clinical and pathological features of rabies postvaccinal encephalomyelitis in man, in Kies MW, Alvord EC Jr (eds): *"Allergic" Encephalomyelitis*. Springfield, IL, Charles C Thomas, 1959, pp 58–129.

Sibley WA, Bamford CRF, Clark K, et al: A prospective study of physical trauma and multiple sclerosis. *J Neurol Neurosurg Psychiatry* 54:584, 1991.

Slamovitis S, Rosen CE, Cheng KP, et al: Visual recovery in patients with optic neuritis and visual loss to no light perception. *Am J Ophthalmol* 111:209, 1991.

Stricker RD, Miller RG, Kiprov DO: Role of plasmapheresis in acute disseminated (postinfectious) encephalomyelitis. *J Clin Apher* 7:173, 1992.

Thomas PK, Walker RWH, Rudge P, et al: Chronic demyelinating peripheral neuropathy associated with multifocal central nervous system demyelination. *Brain* 110:53, 1987.

Thompson AJ, Polman CH, Miller DH, et al: Primary progressive multiple sclerosis. *Brain* 120:1085, 1997.

Thygessen P: *The Course of Disseminated Sclerosis: A Close-Up of 105 Attacks*. Copenhagen, Rosenkilde and Bagger, 1953.

Tippett DS, Fishman PS, Panitch HS: Relapsing transverse myelitis. *Neurology* 41:703, 1991.

Tourtellotte WW, Booe IM: Multiple sclerosis: The blood-brain barrier and the measurement of de novo central nervous system IgG synthesis. *Neurology* 28(Suppl):76, 1978.

Tradtrantip L, Zhang H, Saadoun S, et al: Anti-aquaporin-4 monoclonal antibody blocker therapy for neuromyelitis optica. *Ann Neurol* 71:314, 2014.

Tremlett H, Paty D, Devonshire V. Disability progression in multiple sclerosis is slower than previously reported. *Neurology* 66:172, 2006.

van der Mei IA, Ponsonby AL, Dwyer T, et al: Vitamin D levels in people with multiple sclerosis and community controls in Tasmania, Australia. *J Neurol* 254:581, 2007.

Vermersch F, Kappos L, Gold R, et al: Clinical outcomes of natalizumab-associated progressive multifocal leukoencephalopathy. *Neurology* 76:1697, 2011.

Vrethem M, Mattsson E, Hebelka H, et al: Increased plasma homocysteine levels without signs of vitamin B_{12} deficiency in patients with multiple sclerosis assessed by blood and cerebrospinal fluid homocysteine and methylmalonic acid. *Mult Scler* 9:239, 2003.

Waksman BH, Adams RD: Studies of the effect of the Schwartzman reaction on the lesions of experimental allergic encephalomyelitis. *Am J Pathol* 33:131, 1957.

Weinshenker BG, O'Brien PC, Petterson TM, et al: A randomized trial of plasma exchange in acute central nervous system demyelinating inflammatory disease. *Ann Neurol* 46:878, 1999.

Weinshenker BG, Rice GP, Noseworthy JH, et al: The natural history of multiple sclerosis: A geographically based study: 2. Predictive value of the early clinical course. *Brain* 112:1419, 1989.

Wingerchuk DM, Lennon VA, Pittock SJ, et al: Revised diagnostic criteria for neuromyelitis optica. *Neurology* 66:1485, 2006.

Wenning W, Haghikia A, Laubenberger J, et al: Treatment of progressive multifocal leukoencephalopathy associated with natalizumab. *N Engl J Med* 361:1075, 2009.

Zivadinov R, Rudick RA, De Masi R, et al. Effects of IV methylprednisolone on brain atrophy in relapsing-remitting MS. *Neurology* 57:1239, 2001.

37

Inherited Metabolic Diseases of the Nervous System

Advances in biochemistry and molecular genetics have led to the discovery of such a large number of metabolic diseases of the nervous system that it taxes the mind just to remember their names. As the causes and mechanisms of the diseases included in this chapter are increasingly being expressed in terms of molecular genetics, it seems appropriate, by way of introduction, to consider briefly some basic facts pertaining to the genetics of neurologic disease. The reader is referred to the continuously updated database, *Online Mendelian Inheritance in Man* (*http://www.ncbi.nlm.nih.gov/omim*), to the four-volume text by Scriver and colleagues, which still serves as an excellent source, and to recent general reviews by Feero and colleagues, and on mitochondrial genetics, by Koopman and coauthors.

The brain is more frequently affected by a genetic abnormality than any other organ, probably because of the large number of genes implicated in its development (an estimated one-third of the human genome). Approximately one-third of all inherited diseases are neurologic in some respect; if one adds the inherited diseases affecting the musculature, skeleton, eye, and ear, the number rises to 80 to 90 percent. Approximately 7 percent of diseases in hospitalized children are estimated to be attributable to single-gene defects and 0.4 to 2.5 percent to a chromosomal abnormality. Another 22 to 31 percent have a disease putatively due to polymorphisms, most of which are yet to be specified. Mitochondrial inheritance of mutations is much less frequent but gives rise to several distinctive diseases.

Although only a minority of inherited diseases is identified as an enzymopathy, this group represents the most direct translation of mendelian disorders to primary defects in proteins. These constitute only one-third of the known recessive (autosomal and X-linked) disorders. Most enzymopathies become manifest in infancy and childhood; only a few appear as late as adolescence or adult life. Many damage the nervous system so severely that survival to adult years and reproduction are impossible, and some cause death in utero. As a group, these diseases—along with congenital anomalies (see Chap. 38), birth injuries, epilepsy, disharmonies of development, and learning disabilities (see Chap. 28)—make up the bulk of the clinical problems with which the pediatric neurologist must contend.

PATTERNS OF GENETIC ABERRATIONS AND INHERITANCE

The diseases grouped in this chapter, and many in the next, represent four particular categories of genetic abnormality: (1) monogenic disorders determined by a single mutation that follow a mendelian pattern of inheritance. These mutations can be of a single base pair (point mutation), an insertion or deletion of nucleotides, or structural rearrangements of a sequence of DNA, such as translocations or inversions; because the most important of these involve the coding (exonic) portion of DNA, they are likely to disrupt the structure and function of enzymes or cellular structural proteins. *Most of the diseases discussed in this chapter are of this variety*; (2) a type of monogenic mutation characterized by duplications or deletions of genes or parts of chromosomes, termed *copy number variations*; these account for some proportion the heritability of common diseases; (3) single nucleotide polymorphisms, which are variations from the most common, "wild type," sequence of a gene and are by convention present with a frequency of greater than 1 percent in the population; these play a role in the genesis of disease but do not obligatorily result in a somatic aberration or alternatively, they interact with exogenous environmental factors; and (4) mitochondrial gene mutations that are inherited in a nonmendelian, mainly maternally inherited pattern.

Autosomal and Sex-Linked Inheritance

Traditionally, the recognition of the broad categories of genetically determined diseases has rested on their pattern of occurrence in families, segregated according to mendelian inheritance into autosomal dominant, autosomal recessive, and sex-linked types. As mentioned, mutations of nuclear DNA account for the heritable autosomal and sex-linked diseases described in this chapter, and they are remarkably diverse in nature. Some are lethal and are therefore not transmitted to successive generations; others are less harmful and may conform to one of the classic mendelian patterns. The mutation may be large and result in duplication of a major part of a chromosome or even of the entire gene (diploidy or triploidy) or a deletion (haploidy). Other mutations are quite small, involving only a single base pair ("point mutation"). Between these two extremes are deletions or duplications that include a portion of a gene, an entire gene, or contiguous genes, as mentioned above.

The factors conducive to mutations are poorly understood. The parent's increasing age is important in relation to some mutations; the size, structure, and placement of the gene on the chromosome are important in others. A mutation of the DNA of a germ cell leaves unchanged the somatic phenotype of the individual in whom it occurs, but it may have a devastating effect on the descendants. Conversely, a DNA mutation of a somatic cell affecting only part of the cell population may change the individual harboring it but is not passed on to the descendants. Such an individual, with both normal cells and cells containing the mutant gene, is referred to as a *mosaic*. Mutations of somatic cells appear to be most pertinent to cancer and aging.

In the monogenic inheritance of all three mendelian patterns, the mutation usually causes an abnormality of a single protein. It may involve an enzyme, peptide hormone, immunoglobulin, collagen, membrane channel, or coagulation factor. Such abnormalities of single genes have been isolated in several hundred diseases, but less is known of their protein products. About one-quarter of these diseases are apparent soon after birth and more than 90 percent by puberty. More than half of them affect more than one organ. Of the 10 in every 1,000 live births with monogenic diseases, 7 are dominant, 2.5 are recessive, and the remainder are sex-linked.

Autosomal dominant mutations usually cause manifest disease in heterozygotes, but variations in the size of the gene abnormality can produce any one of several phenotypes. This poses a challenge to the current clinical and pathologic classifications of disease. Moreover, an identical clinical syndrome may be traced to a gene on two different chromosomes. Even more surprising, an estimated 28 percent of all gene loci have polymorphic rather than monomorphic effects—that is, the same mutation has several different phenotypic expressions. Another problem is that of differentiating dominant from recessive inheritance. In small families, in which only one descendant is afflicted and the parent is seemingly normal, one may mistakenly conclude that the inheritance is recessive. Other characteristics of mutational diseases are penetrance, a measure of the proportion of individuals with a given genotype who will show the phenotype, and expressivity, referring to the severity of disease in an affected individual. Variable degrees of penetrance and expressivity are characteristic features of dominant patterns of inheritance but not of recessive ones. There is also a general tendency for dominantly inherited disease to first appear long after birth.

Autosomal recessive forms of inherited metabolic diseases, in contrast to dominant ones, occur only in the homozygous state (both alleles are abnormal). They are usually characterized by an onset soon after birth. The basic abnormality in the recessively inherited diseases discussed in this chapter is more often an enzyme deficiency than an abnormality of some other protein.

In disorders of X-linked genes, in which the mutant gene affects mainly one sex, the female will suffer the same fate as the male if one X chromosome has been inactivated, as happens in most cells during embryonic development (the Lyon phenomenon). However, even if the abnormal X chromosome is not widely expressed, the female carrier may still exhibit minor abnormalities. In the latter case, sex-linked inheritance becomes difficult to distinguish from dominant inheritance. Also, sex linkage is deceptive when a disease is lethal to one sex. In contrast to autosomal recessive mutations, the abnormality has more often been one of a basic protein than an enzyme deficiency.

Multifactorial genetic diseases may also be familial. They may present as constitutional disorders with gene abnormalities located on several chromosomes (polygenic, or "complex genetics") or they may arise from single nucleotide polymorphisms or copy number variations. Here, the relative contributions of genetic and environmental influences are highly variable. The occurrence of many disorders that display high degrees of familial incidence, such as schizophrenia and Gilles de la Tourette syndrome, but do not strictly conform to classic genetic principles has been attributed to this type of complex genetics.

The Genetics of Mitochondrial Disease

An entirely different type of genetic transmission relating to the DNA that lies in the mitochondria has been elucidated. Mitochondria contain their own extrachromosomal DNA, distinct from nuclear DNA. Mitochondrial DNA ("the other human genome") is a double-stranded, circular molecule that encodes the protein subunits required mainly for translation of the proteins located on the mitochondrial inner membrane. Of the 37 mitochondrial genes, small in number by comparison with nuclear DNA, 13 partake in the cellular processes of oxidative phosphorylation and the production of adenosine triphosphate (ATP). A few genes in the cell's nucleus also code for a considerable number of oxidative enzymes of the mitochondria, but their inheritance follows a mendelian pattern; consequently, a mitochondrial disorder may fail to display maternal inheritance that is characteristic of mitochondrial mutations as described below.

Each mitochondrion contains up to 10 ringed DNA molecules, and each cell, of course, contains numerous mitochondria. In the cell, mitochondria with mutant genes may exist next to normal mitochondria (*heteroplasmy*), a state that permits an otherwise lethal mutation to persist (Johns). The presence of either completely normal or completely mutant mitochondrial DNA is termed *homoplasmy*. The essential feature of mitochondrial genes and the mutations to which they are subject is that they are inherited almost exclusively through *maternal* lineage. This is explained by the transmission of virtually all mitochondria from the ovum at the time of conception. Moreover, mitochondrial DNA does not recombine, thus permitting the accumulation of mutations through maternal lines. Also, the replication and distribution of mitochondrial DNA during cell division do not follow the nuclear mitotic cycle. Instead, there are contributions during cell division from the genes of various mitochondria to the progeny of dividing cells. The combination of a heteroplasmic state and the capricious dispersion of mitochondria to daughter cells (replicative segregation) explains the variable expression of mitochondrial mutations in different tissues and in different regions of the nervous system.

The genetic error in each of the mitochondrial diseases is most often a single-point mutation that leads to the alteration of a single amino acid, but there are also single or multiple deletions or duplications of mitochondrial genes that do not conform to maternal inheritance because they are caused by nuclear DNA defects. It is important to note that approximately 85 percent of the protein components of the respiratory chain are coded in nuclear DNA and are then imported into the mitochondrion; as mentioned above, this allows for a mitochondrial disease with a mendelian pattern of inheritance rather than a maternal one. Another of the general rules of mitochondrial inheritance is exemplified by an infantile myopathy (cytochrome oxidase deficiency) that is usually fatal but may also occur in a less severe form and have a later onset. In cases of earlier onset, there is less of the normal mitochondrial DNA than in the cases of later onset.

Because the unique function of mitochondria is the production of ATP by oxidative phosphorylation, it is not surprising that many of the genes contained in mitochondria code for proteins in the respiratory chain. However, there is not always concordance between the error in the mitochondrial genome and the enzymatic defect that leads to disease. Of the five complexes that make up the respiratory chain, cytochrome-*c* oxidase (complex IV) is the one most often disordered, and its deficient function gives rise to lactic acidosis, a feature common to many of the mitochondrial disorders (see further on). In keeping with the mutable nature of this class of disorders, it is thought that some cases of complex IV defect are autosomally transmitted. Complex I defects, which originate in mitochondrial mutations, are seen, for example, in Leber optic atrophy. A more complete account of the disorders of the mitochondrial respiratory chain can be found in the review by Leonard and Schapira.

As one would expect, aberrant function of the ubiquitous energy-producing mitochondria results in disease of many organs besides skeletal muscle (e.g., diabetes and other endocrinopathies and minor dysmorphic features are seen in several mitochondrial disorders). Nevertheless, most of the mitochondrial disorders affect the nervous system prominently and at times exclusively. Two characteristics traceable to mitochondrial abnormalities are particularly common; one is a special change in muscle fibers termed *ragged red fibers*, a clumping of mitochondria in muscle fibers described in more detail further on, and the other is a systemic lactic acidosis. Other than these, each of the mitochondrial diseases has distinctive features and in their main elements they do not resemble each other. The main syndromes are MELAS and MERRF (acronyms defined further on), Leber hereditary optic atrophy, progressive external ophthalmoplegia, and the Leigh syndrome. These diseases are described in detail in the last part of this chapter.

Diagnostic Features of Hereditary Metabolic Diseases

In clinical practice, one should consider the possibility of a hereditary metabolic disease when presented with the following lines of evidence:

1. A neurologic disorder of similar type in a sibling or close relative
2. Recurrent nonconvulsive episodes of impaired consciousness or intractable seizures in infants or young children or infantile spasms and progressive myoclonic seizures in the absence of neonatal hypoxia-ischemia
3. Some combination of unexplained symmetrical or generalized spastic weakness, cerebellar ataxia, extrapyramidal disorder, deafness, or blindness
4. Progression of a neurologic disease measured in months, or a few years
5. Developmental delay in an individual if there are no congenital somatic abnormalities or developmental delay in a sibling or close relative

In the face of such clinical information, one should obtain appropriate biochemical analyses of blood, urine, and cerebrospinal fluid (CSF); MRI of the brain; and, in certain instances, genetic studies.

In addition to the investigation of symptomatic individuals, the array of available genetic and biochemical tests has made practical the mass screening of newborns for inborn metabolic defects. Innovative tests have also led to the discovery of a number of previously unknown diseases and have clarified the basic biochemistry of old ones. As a consequence, the neurologist's role is changing. No longer must we wait until a disease of the nervous system has declared itself by conventional symptoms and signs, by which time the underlying lesion may have become irreversible. Now it is possible to find patients who, although asymptomatic, are at risk and to introduce dietary and other measures that may prevent injury to the nervous system. This is especially important to families who have already had an affected infant. To assume this new responsibility intelligently requires knowledge of genetics, biochemical screening methods, and public health measures.

The many clinical syndromes by which these inborn errors of metabolism declare themselves vary in accordance with the nature of the biochemical defect and the stage of maturation of the nervous system at which these metabolic alterations become apparent. In phenylketonuria, for example, there is a specific effect on the cerebral white matter, mainly during the period of active myelination; once the stages of myelinogenesis are complete as detailed in Chap. 28, the biochemical abnormality becomes relatively harmless. Even more important from the neurologist's point of view is the level of function that has been achieved by the developing nervous system when the disease strikes. A derangement of function in a neonate or infant, in whom much of the cerebrum is not fully developed, is much less obvious than one in an older child. Moreover, as the disease evolves, the clinical manifestations are always influenced by the ongoing maturation of the untouched elements in the nervous system. These interactions may give the impression of regression of attained neurologic function, lack of progress of development (developmental delay), or even improvement in function that is attributable to continuing maturation of the normal parts of the nervous system. The separation of metabolic-genetic from degenerative diseases (accorded a separate chapter) may disquiet the reader, for there are many overlaps between the two groups. The current division is tenable only until such time as all the degenerative diseases will have been shown to have a comprehensible pathogenesis.

Because of the overriding importance of the age factor and the tendency of certain pathologic processes to appear in particular epochs of life, it has seemed to the authors logical to group the inherited metabolic diseases not according to their major syndromes of expression, as we have done in other parts of the book, but in relation to the periods of life at which they are most likely to be encountered: the neonatal period, infancy (1 to 12 months), early childhood (1 to 4 years), late childhood, adolescence, and adult life. Only in the last two age periods do we return to the more clinically useful syndromic ordering of diseases.

In adopting this chronological subdivision, we realize that *certain hereditary metabolic defects that most typically manifest themselves at a particular period in life are not necessarily confined to that epoch and may appear, sometimes in variant form, at a later age*. Such variations are noted at appropriate points in the discussion.

METABOLIC DISEASES OF THE NEONATAL PERIOD

A small number of progressive metabolic diseases become evident in the first few days of life. The importance of these diseases relates not to their frequency (they constitute only a small fraction of diseases that compromise nervous system function in the neonate) but to the fact that they must be recognized promptly if the infant is to be prevented from dying or from suffering a lifelong severe developmental delay. This inherent threat introduces an element of urgency into neonatal neurology. Recognition of these diseases is also important for purposes of family and prenatal testing.

Two approaches to the neonatal metabolic disorders are possible—one, to screen every newborn, using a battery of biochemical tests of blood and urine, and the other, to undertake in the days following birth a detailed neurologic assessment that will detect the earliest signs of these diseases. Unfortunately, not all the biochemical tests have been simplified to the point where they can be adapted to a mass screening program, and many of the commonly used clinical tests at this age have yet to be validated as markers of disease. Moreover, many of the biochemical tests are costly, and practical issues, such as cost-effectiveness, insinuate themselves, to the distress of the pediatrician. The introduction of tandem mass spectrometry for the evaluation of blood and urine has allayed some of the latter concerns.

Neurologic Assessment of Neonates With Metabolic Disease

As pointed out in Chap. 28, the neonate's nervous system functions essentially at a brainstem–spinal level. The pallidum and visuomotor cortices are only beginning to be myelinated and their contribution to the totality of neonatal behavior cannot be very great. Neurologic examination, to be informative, must therefore be directed to evaluating diencephalic–midbrain, cerebellar–lower brainstem, and spinal functions. The integrity of these functions in the neonate is most reliably assessed by noting the following, as was also described in Chap. 28:

1. Control of respiration and body temperature; regulation of thirst, fluid balance, and appetite–hypothalamus–brainstem mechanisms
2. Certain elemental automatisms, such as sucking, rooting, swallowing, grasping—brainstem–cerebellar mechanisms
3. Movements and postures of the neck, trunk, and limbs, such as reactions of support, extension of the neck and trunk, flexion movements, and steppage—lower brainstem (reticulospinal), cerebellar, and spinal mechanisms
4. Muscle tone of limbs and trunk—spinal neuronal and neuromuscular function
5. Reflex eye movements—tegmental midbrain and pontine mechanisms (a modified optokinetic nystagmus can be recognized by the third day of life)
6. The state of alertness and attention (stimulus responsivity and capacity of the examiner to make contact) as well as sleep–waking and electroencephalographic patterns—mesencephalic–diencephalic mechanisms
7. Certain reflexive reactions such as the startle (Moro) response and placing reactions of the foot and hand—upper brainstem–spinal mechanisms with possible cortical facilitation

Derangements of these functions are manifest as impairments of alertness and arousal, hypotonia, disturbances of ocular movement (oscillations of the eyes, nystagmus, loss of tonic conjugate deviation of the eyes in response to vestibular stimulation, i.e., to rotation of the upright infant), failure to feed, tremors, clonic jerkings, tonic spasms, opisthotonos, diminution or absence of limb movements, irregular or chaotic breathing, hypothermia or poikilothermia, bradycardia, circulatory difficulties, poor color, and seizures.

In most instances of neonatal metabolic disease, the pregnancy and delivery proceed without mishap. Birth at full term is usual. The infant is of a size and weight expected for the duration of pregnancy, and there are no signs of a developmental abnormality (in a few instances the infant is somewhat small, and in G_{M1} gangliosidosis there may be a pseudo-Hurler appearance; see further on). Furthermore, function continues to be normal in the first few days of life. The first hint of trouble may be the occurrence of feeding difficulties: food intolerance, diarrhea, and vomiting. The infant becomes fretful and fails to gain weight and thrive—all of which should suggest a disorder of amino acid, ammonia, or organic acid metabolism.

The first definite indication of disordered nervous system function is likely to be the occurrence of seizures. These usually take the form of unpatterned clonic or tonic contractions of one side of the body or independent bilateral contractions, sudden arrest of respiration, turning of the head and eyes to one side, or twitching of the hands and face. Some of the ill-formed seizures may become generalized. They occur singly or in clusters and in the latter instance, are associated with unresponsiveness, immobility, and arrest of respiration.

The other clinical abnormalities in the motor realm, according to authorities such as Prechtl and Beintema, can be subdivided roughly into three groups, each of which constitutes a kind of syndrome: (1) hyperkinetic–hypertonic, (2) apathetic–hypotonic, or (3) unilateral or hemisyndromic. Prechtl and Beintema, from a study of more than 1,500 newborns, found that if clinical examination consistently discloses any one of the 3 syndromes, the chances are 2 in 3 that by the seventh year the child will be manifestly abnormal neurologically. They found also that certain neurologic signs—such as facial palsy, lack of grasping, excessive floppiness, and impairment of sucking—while sometimes indicative of serious disease of the nervous system, are less dependable; also, being rare, these signs will identify but few brain-damaged infants. It is not the single neurologic sign but groups of them that are held to be the most reliable indices of brain abnormality, and the 3 syndromes mentioned above are the important ones, even though their anatomic and physiologic bases are not completely known.

In cases of hypocalcemia-hypomagnesemia, the hyperkinetic–hypertonic syndrome prevails. Although most of the other diseases tend to induce the apathetic–hypotonic state, the hyperactive–hypertonic syndrome may represent the initial phase of the illness and always carries a less ominous prognosis than the apathetic–hypotonic state, which represents a more severe condition regardless of cause. The third putative group of unilateral abnormalities in the metabolic diseases is less common and more difficult to recognize. These syndromes frequently overlap and seizures may occur in all of them. The anatomic correlate for some of these neurologic abnormalities can be observed by MRI. Clearly what is needed is a more definitive neonatal neurologic semiology utilizing numerous stimulus–response tests, including those described by Andre Thomas and Dargassis.

Neonatal Metabolic Diseases and Their Estimated Frequency

In New England, screening of all newborns for metabolic disorders has been practiced for almost 50 years. Data on the diseases with neurologic implications were in the past collated by our colleague, H.L. Levy of Boston Children's Hospital, and are summarized in Table 37-1. Some of these disorders can be recognized by simple color reactions in the urine; these are listed in Table 37-2.

To this group should be added the inherited hyperammonemic syndromes and vitamin-responsive aminoacidopathies (such as pyridoxine dependency and biopterin deficiency), as well as certain nonfamilial metabolic disorders that make their appearance in the neonatal period—hypocalcemia, hypothyroidism and cretinism, hypomagnesemia with tetany, and hypoglycemia.

Table 37-1

METABOLIC DISORDERS DETECTED BY NEONATAL SCREENING IN NEW ENGLAND

DISORDERS	CASES PER 100,000
Biotinidase Deficiency	5.4
Galactosemia	1.5
Glutaric aciduria-I	0.4
Propionic aciduria	0.3
Methylmalonic aciduria-mutase	0.5
Cobalamin deficiency	1.3
Maple syrup urine disease	0.4
Isovaleric acidemia	0.8
Phenylketonuria	6.6
Homocystinuria	0.4
Tyrosinemia-type I	0.3
Ornithine transcarbamylase	0.8
Carnitine pamlityl transferase	0.1
Citrulinemia type I	0.3
Argininosuccinic aciduria	1.0
Glutaric Aciduria-Type II	0.6
Very long chain acyl CoA dehydrogenase	3.3
Carnitine palmitoyl transferase type 2	0.5
Long chain hydroxyacyl CoA dehydrogenase	0.8

Source: Courtesy of Dr. Inderneel Sahai, New England Newborn Screening Program, MA. Screening done by tandem mass spectrometry of dried blood spot. Abnormalities with no neurological significance or with extremely low rates are omitted.

Table 37-2

URINARY SCREENING TESTS FOR METABOLIC DEFECTS

DISEASE	FERRIC CHLORIDE	DNPH	BENEDICT REACTION	NITROPRUSSIDE REACTION
Phenylketonuria	Green	+	–	–
Maple syrup urine disease	Navy blue	+	–	–
Tyrosinemia	Pale green (transient)	+	–	+
Histidinemia	Green-brown	±	–	–
Propionic acidemia	Purple	+	–	–
Methylmalonic aciduria	Purple	+	–	–
Homocystinuria	–	–	–	+
Cystinuria	–	–	–	+
Galactosemia	–	–	+	–
Fructose intolerance	–	–	+	–

DNPH, diaminophenylhydrazine.

It is important to note that the three most frequently identified hereditary metabolic diseases—*phenylketonuria (PKU), hyperphenylalaninemia,* and *congenital hypothyroidism*—do not become clinically manifest in the neonatal period and are therefore discussed in a later portion of this chapter and in Chap. 40 (in the discussion of congenital hypothyroidism). This is fortunate, for it allows time to introduce preventive measures before the first symptoms appear. A number of other metabolic disorders, which can be recognized either by screening or by early signs, are synopsized below.

Vitamin-Responsive Aminoacidopathies

Included under this heading is a group of diseases that respond not to dietary restriction of a specific amino acid but to the oral supplementation of a specific vitamin. Some 30 vitamin-responsive aminoacidopathies are known (they are all rare, but the more frequent ones are listed in Table 41-3), and many of them result in injury to the central nervous system (CNS).

Pyridoxine-Dependent Seizures Pyridoxine dependency is the prototypic example of a genetic, vitamin-dependent biochemical disorder, albeit a rare disease. It is inherited as an autosomal recessive trait and is characterized by the early onset of convulsions, sometimes occurring in utero; failure to thrive; hypertonia–hyperkinesia; irritability; tremulous movements ("jittery baby"); exaggerated auditory startle (hyperacusis); and later, if untreated, by psychomotor retardation. The specific laboratory abnormality is an increased excretion of xanthurenic acid in response to a tryptophan load. There are decreased levels of pyridoxal-5-phosphate and gamma-aminobutyric acid (GABA) in brain tissue. The mutation is of the *ALDH7A1* gene.

The neuropathology has been studied in only a few cases. One patient of our colleague R.D. Adams, a 13.5-year-old boy affected in the neonatal period, was left in a state of mental retardation, with pale optic discs and spastic legs; the brain weight was 350 g below normal. There was a decreased amount of central white matter in the cerebral hemispheres and a depletion of neurons in the thalamic nuclei and cerebellum, with gliosis (Lott et al). Most importantly, in pyridoxine deficiency, the administration of 50 to 100 mg of vitamin B_6 suppresses the seizure state, and daily doses of 40 mg permit normal development.

Biopterin Deficiency

Some patients with increased concentrations of serum phenylalanine in the neonatal period are unresponsive to measures that lower phenylalanine. They are usually found to have a defect in biopterin metabolism. If this condition is unrecognized and not treated promptly, it leads to seizures of both myoclonic and, later, grand mal types, combined with a poor level of responsiveness and generalized hypotonia. Swallowing difficulty is another prominent symptom. Within a few months, developmental delay becomes prominent. Unlike in PKU, phenylalanine hydroxylase enzyme levels are normal, but there is a lack of tetrahydrobiopterin, which is a cofactor of phenylalanine hydroxylase. Treatment consists of administration of tetrahydrobiopterin in a dosage of 7.5 mg/kg/d in combination with a low-phenylalanine diet. It is important to recognize this condition early in life by the measurement of urine pterins and to institute appropriate therapy before irreversible brain injury occurs. A later onset form with diurnally fluctuating dystonia has also been described but its nature is not certain.

Galactosemia

Inheritance of this disorder is autosomal recessive. The biochemical abnormality consists of a defect in galactose-1-phosphate uridyl transferase (GALT), the enzyme that catalyzes the conversion of galactose-1-phosphate to uridine diphosphate galactose. Several forms of galactosemia have been described, based on the degree of completeness of the metabolic block and some of these are due to mutations in other galactose pathway genes. In the typical (severe) form, the onset of symptoms is in the first days of life, after the ingestion of milk; vomiting and diarrhea are followed by a failure to thrive. Drowsiness, inattention, hypotonia, and diminution in the vigor of neonatal automatisms then become evident. The fontanels may bulge, the liver and spleen enlarge, the skin becomes yellow (in excess of the common neonatal jaundice), and anemia develops. In a small number, there is thrombocytopenia with cerebral bleeding. Cataracts form as a result of the accumulation of galactitol in the lens. Studies of the outcome of surviving infants have shown delayed psychomotor development (IQ about 85), visual impairment, osteoporosis, ovarian failure, and residual cirrhosis, sometimes with splenomegaly and ascites. This seems to happen even with treatment. However, it is not known whether, in such patients, the treatment is always maintained through a critical developmental period. In one such patient, who died at age 8 years, the main change in the brain was slight microcephaly with fibrous gliosis of the white matter and some loss of Purkinje and granule cells in the cerebellum, and also gliosis (Crome). The diagnostic laboratory findings are an elevated blood galactose level, low glucose, galactosuria, and deficiency of GALT in red and white blood cells and in liver cells. The treatment is essentially dietary, using milk substitutes; if this is instituted early, the brain should be protected from injury.

A late-onset neurologic syndrome has also been observed by Friedman and colleagues in galactosemic patients who had survived the infantile disease. By late adolescence, they were cognitively delayed; some showed cerebellar ataxia, dystonia, and apraxia. One of these patients was middle-aged.

Organic Acidurias of Infancy

These have been divided into ketotic and nonketotic types. Among the *ketotic types,* the main one is *propionic acidemia.* This is an autosomal recessive disease caused by a primary defect in organic acid metabolism that is expressed clinically by episodes of vomiting, lethargy, coma, convulsions, hypertonia, and respiratory difficulty. The onset is in the neonatal or early infantile period; in time, psychomotor retardation becomes evident. Death usually occurs within a few months despite dietary treatment. Propionic acid, glycine, various forms of fatty acids, and butanone are elevated in the serum. As with other ketotic organic acidurias, high protein intake induces ketotic attacks. Marked restriction of dietary protein (specifically leucine) may prevent attacks of ketoacidosis and permit relatively good psychomotor development.

A number of other ketotic acidurias also occur in infancy. The most important of these are *methylmalonic acidemia, isovaleric acidemia, beta-keto acidemia,* and *lactic acidemia*. Each of these disorders can become manifest with profound metabolic acidosis and intermittent lethargy, vomiting, tachypnea, tremors, twitching, convulsions, and coma, with early death in about half the patients and developmental retardation in those who survive. Rare subtypes of methylmalonic acidemia respond to vitamin B_{12}. Isovaleric acidemia is characterized by a striking odor of stale perspiration, which has given it the sobriquet "sweaty foot syndrome." Numerous metabolic defects, most commonly of pyruvate decarboxylase and pyruvate dehydrogenase, are responsible for the accumulation of lactic and pyruvic acids. The enzymatic defect of isovaleric acidemia also has been demonstrated in a recurrent form of episodic cerebellar ataxia and athetosis and in a persistent form in mitochondrial encephalopathies (Leigh disease), as described further on in this chapter.

A separate and rare deficiency of aromatic L-amino acid decarboxylase has been described; the chemical signature is low levels of almost all catecholamines. This defect is associated with a peculiar movement disorder of oculogyric crises, dystonia and athetosis, and autonomic failure (see Swoboda et al).

A type II glutaric acidemia has also been observed in the neonatal period and causes episodes of acidosis with vomiting and hyperglycemia. Multiple congenital anomalies of brain and somatic structures and cardiomyopathy are conjoined. A diet low in the specific toxic amino acid and supplements of carnitine and riboflavin are recommended, but the effects are unclear.

In the *nonketotic form of hyperglycinemia*, there are high levels of glycine but no acidosis. The notable diagnostic finding is an elevation of the CSF glycine, several times higher than that of the blood. The effects on the nervous system are more devastating than in the ketotic form. In reported cases (the authors and our colleagues have seen several), the neonate is hypotonic, listless, and dyspneic, with dysconjugate eye movements, opisthotonic posturing, myoclonus, and seizures. A few such neonates survive to infancy but are extremely cognitively impaired and helpless. Spongy degeneration of the brain has been reported both in this disease and in the ketotic form (Shuman et al). No treatment has been effective in severe cases. In an atypical milder form, with neurologic abnormalities that appear in later infancy or childhood, reduction of dietary protein and administration of sodium benzoate in doses up to 250 mg/kg/d have been beneficial. The use of dextromethorphan, which blocks glycine receptors, is said to be effective in preventing seizures and coma.

Inherited Hyperammonemias

These are a group of six diseases caused by inborn deficiencies of the enzymes of the Krebs-Henseleit urea cycle; they are designated as N-*acetyl glutamate synthetase, carbamoyl phosphate synthetase* (CPS), *ornithine transcarbamylase* (OTC), *argininosuccinic acid synthetase (citrullinemia), argininosuccinase deficiency,* and *arginase deficiency*. Hyperornithinemia-hyperammonemia-homocitrullinemia (HHH) and intrinsic protein intolerance are closely related disorders. They are identified by the finding of a persistent or episodic elevation of ammonia levels in the blood. A detailed account of these inherited hyperammonemic syndromes is contained in the review by Brusilow and Horwich.

The pattern of inheritance of each of these disorders is autosomal recessive except for OTC deficiency, which is X-linked dominant. Their clinical manifestations are a common expression of an accumulation of ammonia or of urea cycle intermediates in the brain; they differ only in severity, in accordance with the degree of completeness of the enzymatic deficiency and with the age of the affected individual. The one exception is arginase deficiency, which commonly appears during later childhood as a progressive spastic paraplegia with mental retardation. Clinically, it has been convenient to divide the hyperammonemias into two groups—one that presents in the neonatal period and another that becomes evident in the weeks or months thereafter. This division is somewhat artificial, the clinical presentation being more in the nature of a continuous spectrum governed by the biologic factors mentioned above and even extending to rare cases that have their first symptoms during adulthood.

In the most severe forms of the hyperammonemic disorders, the infants are asymptomatic at birth and during the first day or two of life, after which they refuse their feedings, vomit, and rapidly become inactive and lethargic, soon lapsing into an irreversible coma. Profuse sweating, focal or generalized seizures, rigidity with opisthotonos, hypothermia, and hyperventilation have been observed in the course of the illness. These symptoms constitute a medical emergency, but even with measures to reduce serum ammonia, the disease is usually fatal.

In less severely affected infants, hyperammonemia develops some months later, when protein feeding is increased. There is a failure to thrive, and attempts to enforce feeding or during periods of constipation (both of which increase ammonia production in the bowel) may result in bouts of vomiting, lethargy, hyperirritability, and screaming. Respiratory alkalosis is a consistent feature. Other manifestations are periods of alternating hypertonia and hypotonia, seizures, ataxia, blurred vision, and of confusion, stupor, and coma. During episodes of stupor, often precipitated by dehydration, an alimentary protein load, or minor surgery, brain edema may be seen by CT and MRI; with repeated relapses, the brain edema gives way to atrophy, which appears as symmetrical areas of decreased attenuation in the cerebral white matter. Between attacks, some patients with partial deficiency may be normal or show only a slight hyperbilirubinemia (DiMagno et al; Rowe et al). With decompensation, the bilirubin rises, as does ammonia, but neither reaches exceedingly high levels. After repeated attacks, signs of developmental delay with motor and mental retardation become evident, and the patient is vulnerable to recurrent infections. Two adult male patients in our care, who were married (but with azoospermia, which is common) and working at technically demanding jobs, came to medical attention because of bouts of visual blurring followed by stupor that evolved over hours (Shih et al, 1999). They had displayed an aversion to protein and milk products as children; in later life, after meals high in protein, they became encephalopathic, one with severe brain swelling. There are few phenotypic differences among the late-onset hyperammonemias except for *argininosuccinic aciduria*, in which excessive dryness and brittleness of the hair (trichorrhexis nodosa) are notable features, and the aforementioned *arginase deficiency* with spastic diplegia.

Diagnosis is established by the finding of *hyperammonemia*, often as high as 1,500 mg/dL. The precise biochemical diagnosis requires testing of blood and urine for amino acids or assays for specific enzymes in red cells, liver, or jejunal biopsies. The primary hyperammonemias must be distinguished from the organic acidurias, including *methylmalonic aciduria* (see above), in which hyperammonemia can occur as a secondary metabolic abnormality.

In all the neonatal hyperammonemic diseases, the liver is often enlarged and liver cells appear to be inadequate in their metabolic functions, but how the enzymatic deficiencies or other disorders of amino acid metabolism affect the brain remains uncertain. It must be assumed that in some the saturation of the brain by ammonia impairs the oxidative metabolism of cerebral neurons, and when blood levels of ammonium increase (from protein ingestion, constipation, etc.), episodic coma or a more chronic impairment of cerebral functions occurs—as it does in adults with cirrhosis of the liver and portal-systemic encephalopathy. In the acutely fatal cases, the brain is swollen and edematous, and the astrocytes are diffusely increased in number and enlarged. The neurons are normal. Astrocytic swelling has been attributed to the accumulation of glutamate secondary to a suppression of glutamate synthetase. These changes have been reproduced in animals by the injection of ammonium chloride. When the hyperammonemia is abrupt in onset and severe, the resulting combination of encephalopathy, brain swelling, and respiratory alkalosis simulates the *Reye syndrome* (see "Reye-Johnson Syndrome" in Chap. 40).

As in all forms of liver disease, valproic acid and other hepatic toxins may cause hepatic coma by further impairing the urea cycle enzymes. Notable are a few cases of inherited hyperammonemia that come to light in childhood or adulthood only after the administration of one of these drugs.

Ornithine Transcarbamylase Deficiency and Argininosuccinic Aciduria Most cases present in the neonatal period with hyperammonemia but milder forms may appear later in life with episodic symptoms such as episodic stupor, ataxia, and seizures. The other features have been mentioned above.

Treatment of the Hyperammonemic Syndromes The *treatment* of acute hyperammonemic syndromes is directed at lowering ammonia levels by hemodialysis, exchange transfusions, and administration of arginine and certain organic acids. With subsidence of the acute symptoms, a systematic form of management should be undertaken, as outlined by Brusilow and colleagues and by Msall and colleagues. Sodium benzoate should be given in doses up to 250 mg/d, supplemented by sodium phenylacetate or sodium phenylbutyrate, which, on theoretical grounds, should divert nitrogen from the ureagenesis cycle. Arginine (50 to 150 mg/kg) should be added to the diet, as a deficiency of this substance may be responsible for the mental retardation and skin rashes. In more chronic cases, treatment consists of decreasing the ammonium load by the use of dietary protein restriction and by administration of oral antibiotics and lactulose. In infants with inborn errors of ureagenesis, there is a constant danger of recurrent episodes of hyperammonemia and coma, particularly in response to infections. In a few instances, careful management of the metabolic error has resulted in normal psychomotor development.

Liver transplantation may prove to be a therapeutic option.

Branched-Chain Aminoacidopathies (Maple Syrup Urine Disease)

These conditions are caused by a deficiency of α-keto acid dehydrogenase, resulting in the accumulation of the branched-chain amino acids leucine, isoleucine, and valine and the corresponding branched-chain α-keto acids. Maple syrup urine disease may be taken as the prototype. The pattern of inheritance is autosomal recessive. With the most-severe neonatal type, the infant appears normal at birth, but toward the end of the first week, poor feeding, intermittent hypertonicity, opisthotonos, and respiratory irregularities appear. These are followed by diminished neonatal automatisms, convulsions, severe ketoacidosis, and often coma and death toward the end of the second to fourth week. This disease is one of the causes of the malignant epileptic syndrome of early infancy (Brett). Four milder forms of the disease have been described. In these more chronic cases, feeding difficulties begin somewhat later in the early infantile period. They are manifest as recurrent infections, episodic acidosis, coma, and retarded growth and psychomotor development. Some of these patients, toward the end of the first year, may become quadriparetic or ataxic; or there may be only a nonspecific mental retardation. The disease derives its name from the maple syrup odor of the child's urine that tests positively for 2,4-dinitrophenylhydrazine (DNPH).

Other important laboratory findings are increased plasma and urine concentrations of leucine, isoleucine, valine, and keto acids. Secondary accumulation of a derivative of α-hydroxybutyric acid probably accounts for the maple syrup odor. The neuropathologic findings are uncertain. In the first acute case described, only interstitial edema was observed; but in more chronic cases, pallor and loss of myelin and gliosis of parts of the cerebral white matter that myelinate after birth may be found. This can be visualized in CT and MRI scans.

Treatment by restriction of foods containing branched-chain amino acids (leucine, isoleucine, and valine) allows reasonably normal mental development, but only if such restriction is begun in the neonatal period and maintained lifelong. A thiamine-responsive variant with a slightly different pattern of keto acids described by Prensky and Moser responds variably to 30 to 300 mg of thiamine. The acute episodes, which threaten life, may require peritoneal dialysis to remove the putative toxic metabolites; they respond to the administration of glucose amino acid mixtures that are free of branched-chain keto acids.

Other Organic Acidemias

In addition to maple syrup urine disease, there are a number of other metabolic disturbances, some of them of mitochondrial origin, that appear in the neonatal period or later and are marked by an organic acidemia. If they are severe, the infant develops a metabolic (lactic) acidosis soon after birth, with lethargy, feeding problems, rapid respirations, and vomiting. Or there may be irritability, jerky limb movements, and hypertonia. Later presentations take the form of feeding difficulties, repeated vomiting, hypotonia, and failure to thrive. With the passage of time, psychomotor retardation and drug-resistant seizures become evident. Metabolic stress—e.g., intercurrent infection or surgical procedures—may precipitate an episode of lactic or ketoacidosis.

Biochemical studies may disclose a biotinidase deficiency, methylmalonic aciduria, glutaric acidemia, methylglutaconic acidemia, or any number of other organic acid abnormalities. The precise abnormality is determined by measuring enzyme activity in white blood cells or cultured skin fibroblasts. As remarked above, some of these enzymes act in conjunction with a specific vitamin cofactor, so that exact diagnosis is imperative. The biotinidase deficiency may respond to 10 mg of biotin per day; the methylmalonic acidemia to 1 to 2 mg of vitamin B_{12} per day; maple syrup urine disease to 10 to 20 mg of thiamine per day; and glutaric acidemia types I and II to 300 mg of riboflavin per day. The administration of carnitine may increase the elimination of toxic metabolites.

The care of these patients during an acute illness is of extreme importance. See Lyon and colleagues for a more complete description.

Sulfite Oxidase Deficiency With or Without Molybdenum Cofactor Deficiency (See also "Sulfite Oxidase Deficiency")

These are extremely rare autosomal recessive disorders of sulfur metabolism, manifest clinically during the neonatal period by seizures, axial hypotonia, reduced level of responsivity, and spasms with opisthotonos. There may be added dislocation of lenses, blindness, coloboma, and enophthalmos in combination with severe mental retardation and dysmorphic facial features (widely spaced eyes, long face and philtrum, puffy cheeks). There are no differences between pure sulfite oxidase deficiency and that associated with molybdenum cofactor deficiency. With survival into infancy, episodic confusion and stupor give way to seizures, mental retardation, and ataxia. In one of our cases, described by Shih and colleagues (1977) a stroke-like syndrome of hemiplegia and aphasia appeared during a relapse at the age of 4.5 years, and in one case, subluxation of the lenses and choreoathetosis appeared at 8 months of age.

The biochemical abnormality is the accumulation of sulfite and possibly sulfatase as a result of the enzyme deficiency. Shih and colleagues (1977) have identified sulfite, thiosulfate, and *S*-sulfocysteine in the urine. Cerebral atrophy with loss and destruction of white matter and gray matter (cerebral cortex, basal ganglia, and cerebellar nuclei) was observed in one postmortem examination. Increasing the intake of molybdenum or lowering the dietary intake of sulfur amino acids is a therapeutic possibility not yet fully evaluated.

Diagnosis of Neonatal Metabolic Diseases

An important clue, of course, is provided by the history of a neonatal disease or unexplained death earlier in the same sibship or in a male maternal relative. A history that protein foods are rejected by the infant, or even a history among relatives of a dislike of protein or feeding difficulties in infancy, should raise the suspicion of an inherited hyperammonemic disorder or an organic acidemia. Measurements of blood ammonia and lactate and of the urine for ketones and reducing substances (that react with cupric sulfate) are the key laboratory tests. A wide-spectrum screening program may disclose a biochemical abnormality; this is the optimal state of affairs, especially when this type of screening provides the information before symptoms appear.

A number of nonhereditary metabolic diseases must be distinguished from the hereditary ones in this period of life. *Hypocalcemia* is one of the most frequent causes of neonatal seizures; tetany, spasms, and tremulous movements are usually present. Its cause is unknown, but the disorder is easily corrected, with excellent prognosis. Symptomatic *hypoglycemic reactions* are frequent in neonates. Premature infants are the most susceptible. Seizures, tremulousness, and drowsiness occur with blood sugar levels of less than 30 mg/dL in the mature infant, and less than 20 mg/dL in the premature. Maternal toxemia and diabetes mellitus also predispose to hypoglycemia. Other causes of hypoglycemia are adrenal insufficiency, galactosemia, an idiopathic pancreatic islet-cell hyperplasia, the treatable fatty-acid beta-oxidation disorders, and a congenital deficiency of CSF glucose transport—causing persistent hypoglycorrhachia and refractory seizures unless blood glucose levels are kept high. The damaging effects of untreated hypoglycemia were well documented by Koivisto and colleagues. Also now identified is a disorder of CSF serine transport causing failure to thrive, severe developmental disability with spasticity and intractable epilepsy. The diagnosis is made by measuring CSF amino acids; treatment is with high-dose oral serine. *Cretinism* and *idiopathic hypercalcemia* are other recognizable entities that appear during this age period.

Aicardi has described a neonatal myoclonic syndrome, and Ohtahara has described a malignant neonatal seizure disorder. In some of the cases, the neonatal syndrome merged later with the West type of infantile spasms and the Lennox-Gastaut syndrome (see Chap. 16). Some of the cases had developmental abnormalities of the cerebrum, and severe mental retardation was the outcome. In other cases of this type, a familial coincidence was a feature; a metabolic defect has been suspected in these cases but never proved.

The hereditary metabolic diseases must also be distinguished from a number of other catastrophic disorders that occur at or soon after birth, such as asphyxia, perinatal ventricular hemorrhage with the respiratory distress syndrome of hyaline membrane disease, other hypotensive–hypoxic states, erythroblastosis fetalis with kernicterus, neonatal bacterial meningitis, meningoencephalitis (herpes simplex, cytomegalic inclusion disease, listeriosis, rubella, syphilis, and toxoplasmosis), and hemorrhagic disease of the newborn. These are described in Chap. 38, on the developmental diseases.

HEREDITARY METABOLIC DISEASES OF INFANCY

The hallmark of all the hereditary metabolic diseases is *psychosensorimotor regression*. However, those that have their onset in the first year of life pose extraordinary problems in neurologic diagnosis. If the onset is in the first postnatal months, before the infant has had time to develop the normal complex repertoire of behavior, the first signs of disease may take the form of subtle delays in maturation rather than of psychomotor regression. Departures from normalcy include a lack of interest in the surroundings, a lack of visual engagement, poor head control, inability to sit up at the usual time, poor hand–eye coordination, and persistence of infantile automatisms. Of course, embryologic maldevelopment of the brain may have similar effects, and systemic diseases and other visceral malformations—such as cystic fibrosis, renal disease, biliary atresia and congenital heart disease, chronic infection, malnutrition, and seizures (with drug therapy)—may appear to impede psychomotor development. Diagnosis becomes somewhat easier in the second half of the first year, especially if development in the first half had proceeded normally. Then an observant mother, usually one with older children, can perceive a loss of certain early acquisitions, attesting to the progressive nature of a disease.

The most distinctive members of this category of neurologic disease are the *leukodystrophies* and the *lysosomal storage diseases*. The leukodystrophies are a group of inherited metabolic diseases of the nervous system characterized by progressive, symmetrical, and usually massive destruction of the white matter of the brain and sometimes of the spinal cord; each type of leukodystrophy is distinguished by a specific genetic defect in myelin metabolism. In the *lysosomal storage diseases*, there is a genetic deficiency of the enzymes (usually one or more of the acid hydrolases) necessary for the degradation of specific glycosidic or of peptide linkages in the intracytoplasmic lysosomes, causing nerve cells to become engorged with material that they would ordinarily degrade. These metabolites eventually damage the nerve cell or its myelin sheath.

Most of these diseases are classed as *sphingolipidoses*. Brady in 1966 made the observation that in each of these disorders an increased quantity of sphingolipid accumulated in the brain and other tissues. The sphingolipids are a class of intracellular lipids that all have ceramide as their basic structure, but each has a different attached oligosaccharide or phosphorylcholine. The rate of synthesis of the sphingolipids is normal and their accumulation results from a defect of a specific lysosomal enzyme that normally degrades each of the glycoproteins, glycolipids, and mucopolysaccharides by removing a monosaccharide or sulfate moiety. It is the type of enzyme deficiency and accumulated metabolite, as well as the tissue distribution of the nondegradable substrate, that impart a distinctive biochemical and clinical character to each of the diseases in this category.

The concept of lysosomal storage diseases, introduced by Hers in 1965, excited great interest at the time because it provided the potential for prenatal diagnosis and the detection of carriers. The diagnosis of this group of diseases has also been facilitated by the use of CT, MRI, and evoked response techniques, which confirm the existence of leukodystrophies and by the electron microscopic examination of skin, rectal, or conjunctival biopsies, circulating lymphocytes, and cultured amniotic fluid cells, which discloses the lysosomal storage material in nonneural cells.

There are now more than 40 lysosomal storage diseases in which the biochemical abnormalities have been determined. The main ones are listed in Table 37-3, which was adapted originally from the review of Kolodny and Cable and updated by our colleague, E. Kolodny. In addition to the sphingolipidoses, which are the lysosomal storage diseases most likely to be encountered in the first year of life, the table includes the storage diseases that may not appear clinically until a later age (in childhood and adolescence)—to be considered later in this chapter. The frequency of each of the various types, as detected in a comprehensive study of the Australian population, is given by Meikle and colleagues and generally accords with the ordering below. A broad perspective on the frequency of the lysosomal disorders can be appreciated from the report of the Australian national referral laboratory. There were 545 cases (75 detected prenatally) over a 16-year period, a calculated frequency of 1 case per 7,700 live births. This is close to the estimate in the United States, which is approximately 1 per 5,000 births.

The more frequent types of lysosomal storage diseases are as follows:

1. Tay-Sachs disease (G_{M2} gangliosidosis) and variants such as Sandhoff disease
2. Infantile Gaucher disease
3. Infantile Niemann-Pick disease
4. Infantile G_{M1} generalized gangliosidosis
5. Krabbe globoid-body leukodystrophy
6. Farber lipogranulomatosis
7. Pelizaeus-Merzbacher and other sudanophilic leukodystrophies
8. Spongy degeneration (Canavan-van Bogaert-Bertrand disease)
9. Alexander disease
10. Zellweger encephalopathy
11. Lowe oculorenal-cerebral disease

In the following descriptions, we have summarized the clinical and pathologic features of each of the diseases listed above and have italicized the characteristic clinical signs and corroborative laboratory tests. Leigh disease, which may appear in this age group, is described with the mitochondrial diseases, further on in this chapter.

Table 37-3

LYSOSOMAL STORAGE DISEASES[a]

DISORDER	PRIMARY DEFICIENCY	ACCUMULATED METABOLITE
Sphingolipidoses		
G_{M1} gangliosidosis	β-Galactosidase	G_{M1} ganglioside, galactosyl oligosaccharides, keratan sulfate
G_{M2} gangliosidosis		
Tay-Sachs disease	*N*-acetylhexosaminidase α subunit	G_{M2} ganglioside
Sandhoff disease	*N*-acetylhexosaminidase β subunit	G_{M2} ganglioside, oligosaccharides, glycosaminoglycans
Activator deficiency	G_{M2} activator	G_{M2} ganglioside
Metachromatic leukodystrophy	Arylsulfatase A (sulfatidase), sulfatide activator (saposin B)	Galactosylsulfatide, lactosylsulfatide
Krabbe disease	Galactocerebrosidase	Galactosylceramide
Fabry disease	α-Galactosidase A	Ceramide trihexoside
Gaucher disease	Glucocerebrosidase	Glucosylceramide, glycopeptides
Niemann-Pick disease		
Types A and B	Sphingomyelinase	Sphingomyelin, cholesterol
Type C	Cholesterol esterification	Free cholesterol, *bis*-monoacylglycerophosphate
Farber disease	Ceramidase	Ceramide
Schindler disease	α-Galactosidase B	α-*N*-acetylgalactosaminyl oligosaccharides and glycopeptides
Neuronal ceroid lipofuscinoses		
Infantile form (Haltia-Santavuori)	Palmitoyl-protein thioesterase	Granular osmiophilic deposits
Late infantile form (Jansky-Bielschowsky)	Tripeptidyl peptidase I	Curvilinear bodies, subunit C of mitochondrial ATP synthase
Juvenile form (Spielmeyer-Sjögren)	438-amino acid membrane protein	Curvilinear and laminated (fingerprint) bodies, subunit C of mitochondrial ATP synthase
Adult form (Kufs disease)	Unknown	Mixed-type osmiophilic deposits and lamellar inclusions
Glycoproteinoses		
Aspartylglycosaminuria	Aspartylglycosaminidase	Aspartylglycosamine
Fucosidosis	α-L-Fucosidase	Fucosyloligosaccharides, fucosylglycosphingolipids
Galactosialidosis	Protective protein (β-galactosidase and α-neuraminidase)	Sialyloligosaccharides, galactosyloligosaccharides
α-Mannosidosis	α-Mannosidase	α-Mannosyl oligosaccharides
β-Mannosidosis	β-Mannosidase	β-Mannosyl oligosaccharides
Mucolipidoses		
Sialidosis (mucolipidosis I)	α-Neuraminidase	Sialyloligosaccharides, sialylglycopeptides
Mucolipidosis II (I-cell disease)	UDP-*N*-acetylglucosamine: lysosomal enzyme, *N*-acetylglucosamine-1-phosphotransferase	Sialyloligosaccharides, glycoproteins, glycolipids
Mucolipidosis III (pseudo-Hurler polydystrophy)	Same phosphotransferase as above	Sialyloligosaccharides, glycoproteins, glycolipids
Mucolipidosis IV	Mucolipin-1	Gangliosides, phospholipids, mucopolysaccharides
Other lysosomal diseases		
Acid lipase deficiency		
Wolman disease	Acid lipase	Cholesterol esters, triglycerides
Cholesterol ester storage disease	Acid lipase	Cholesterol esters, triglycerides
Glycogenosis type II (Pompe disease)	α-Glucosidase (acid maltase)	Glycogen
Sialic acid storage disease		
Infantile form	Sialic acid transport	Free sialic acid
Salla disease	Sialic acid transport	Free sialic acid
Mucopolysaccharidoses (see Table 37-7)		

[a]See text for genetic designation.

Tay-Sachs Disease (G_{M2} Gangliosidosis, Hexosaminidase A Deficiency, HEXA Mutation)

This is an autosomal recessive disease, mostly of Jewish infants of eastern European (Ashkenazic) background. The first description came from Tay, a British ophthalmologist, in 1881, and Sachs, an American neurologist, in 1887; they called it amaurotic family idiocy. The disease becomes apparent in the first weeks and months of life, almost always by the fourth month. The first manifestations are a regression of motor activity and an abnormal startle to acoustic stimuli, accompanied by listlessness, irritability, and poor reactions to visual stimuli. These are followed by a progressive *delay in psychomotor development* or regression (by 4 to 6 months), with inability to roll over and sit. At first, axial hypotonia is prominent, but later spasticity and other corticospinal tract signs and visual failure become evident. Degeneration of the macular cells exposes the underlying red vascular choroid surrounded by a whitish gray ring of retinal cells distended with ganglioside. The resulting appearance is of the *cherry-red spot* with optic atrophy (Fig. 37-1). These are observed in the retinas in more than 90 percent of patients (but are also characteristics of other storage diseases—see Table 37-4). In the second year, there are tonic-clonic or minor motor seizures and an increasing size of the head and diastasis of sutures with relatively normal-size ventricles; in the third year, the clinical picture is one of dementia, decerebration, and blindness. Cachexia becomes increasingly severe and death occurs at 2 to 4 years. The electroencephalogram (EEG) becomes abnormal in the early stages (paroxysmal slow waves with multiple spikes). Occasionally, one can find basophilic granules in leukocytes and vacuoles in lymphocytes. There are no visceral, skeletal, or bone marrow abnormalities by light microscopy.

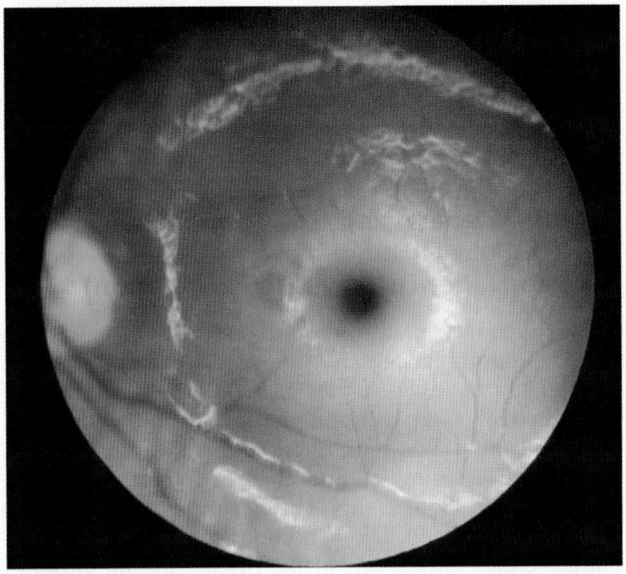

Figure 37-1. Retinal cherry-red spot in a patient with Tay-Sachs disease. The whitish ring surrounds the dark macula. In this dark-skinned child, the macular spot is dark rather than reddish. (Courtesy of Dr. Shirley Wray.)

Table 37-4

DISEASES DISPLAYING A CHERRY-RED MACULAR SPOT

G_{M1} gangliosidosis
G_{M2} gangliosidosis (Tay-Sachs and Sandhoff type)
Sialidosis
Niemann-Pick disease types A to D (not E and F); ring may be diffuse and indistinct
Farber lipogranulomatosis
Metachromatic leukodystrophy
Neuronal ceroid lipofuscinosis, late infantile form ("bull's-eye" maculopathy, not true cherry-red spot)

The basic enzymatic abnormality is a *deficiency of beta hexosaminidase A*, which normally cleaves the *N*-acetylgalactosamine from gangliosides. As a result of this deficiency, G_{M2} ganglioside accumulates in the cerebral cortical neurons, Purkinje cells, retinal ganglion cells, and, to a lesser extent, larger neurons of the brainstem and spinal cord. The enzymatic defect can be found in the serum, white blood cells, and cultured fibroblasts from the skin or amniotic fluid, the latter giving parents the option of abortion to prevent a presently untreatable and fatal disease. Testing for hexosaminidase A also permits the detection of heterozygote carriers of the gene defect. Detection of this enzyme defect is complicated by the fact that more than 50 mutations of the *HEXA* gene have been isolated, coding for alpha subunit of the beta hexosaminidases and the enzyme itself is normal in one form of activator enzyme deficiency. Fortunately, only three mutations account for 98 percent of the form that is common in individuals of Jewish ancestry.

The brain is large, sometimes twice the normal weight. In addition, there is a loss of neurons and a reactive gliosis; remaining nerve cells throughout the CNS are distended with glycolipid. Biopsies of the rectal mucosa disclose glycolipid distention of the ganglion cells of the Auerbach plexus, but the need for this procedure has been obviated by enzyme analysis of white blood cells. Under the electron microscope, the particles of stored material appear as membranous cytoplasmic bodies. Retinal ganglion cells are distended with the same material and, together with fat-filled histiocytes, cause the whitish gray rings around the fovea, where there are no nerve cells, as noted above.

Tay-Sachs disease is untreatable but can be prevented by testing all individuals of Jewish origin for the recessive trait. Where screening has been instituted the disease has become virtually extinct.

In *Sandhoff disease*, which affects infants of non-Jewish origins, there is a deficiency of both hexosaminidase A and B, moderate hepatosplenomegaly, and coarse granulations in bone marrow histiocytes. The clinical and pathologic picture is the same as in Tay-Sachs disease except for the additional signs of visceral lipid storage. Occasionally, these visceral organs are not enlarged.

In recent years numerous variants of hexosaminidase A and B deficiency have been identified. They differ clinically from Tay-Sachs disease in having a later onset, less-extensive brain involvement (cortical neurons relatively spared and intense affection of basal ganglia, as well as cerebellar and spinal neurons). Accordingly, the clinical expression of the variants appearing in childhood, adolescence, and adult life takes the form of athetosis, dystonia, ataxia, and motor neuron paralysis; mental function can be normal. The process has also been found in a few congenital cases in which there was a rapidly progressive decline of a microcephalic infant.

Infantile Gaucher Disease (Type II Neuronopathic Form, Glucocerebrosidase Deficiency, GBA Mutation)

This is an autosomal recessive disease without ethnic predominance, first described by Gaucher in 1882. The onset of the neuronopathic form is usually before 6 months and frequently before 3 months. The clinical course is more rapid than that of Tay-Sachs disease (most patients with infantile Gaucher disease do not survive beyond 1 year and 90 percent not beyond 2 years). Oculomotor apraxia and bilateral strabismus are early signs and are accompanied by rapid loss of head control, of ability to roll over and sit, and of purposeful movements of the limbs—along with apathy, irritability, frequent crying, and difficulty in sucking and swallowing. In some cases progression is slower, with acquisition of single words by the first year, bilateral corticospinal signs (Babinski signs and hyperactive tendon reflexes), *persistent retroflexion of the neck*, and *strabismus*. Laryngeal stridor and trismus, diminished reaction to stimuli, smallness of the head, rare seizures, normal optic fundi, *enlarged spleen* and slightly enlarged liver, poor nutrition, yellowish skin and scleral pigmentation, osteoporosis, vertebral collapse and kyphoscoliosis, and sometimes lymphadenopathy complete the clinical picture. The CSF is normal; the EEG is abnormal, but nonspecifically so.

The important laboratory findings are an *increase in serum acid phosphatase and characteristic histiocytes (Gaucher cells)* in marrow smears and liver and spleen biopsies. A *deficiency of glucocerebrosidase* in leukocytes and hepatocytes is diagnostic; glucocerebroside accumulates in the involved tissues. The characteristic pathologic feature is the Gaucher cell, 20 to 60 μm in diameter, with a wrinkled appearance of the cytoplasm and eccentricity of the nucleus. These cells are found in the marrow, lungs, and other viscera; neuronal storage is seldom evident. In the brain, the main abnormality is a loss of nerve cells—particularly in the bulbar nuclei, but also in the basal ganglia, cortex, and cerebellum—and a reactive gliosis that extends into the white matter.

In contrast to the type II form described above, type I Gaucher disease is a nonneuronopathic and relatively benign form. A less-frequent type III Gaucher disease is neuronopathic. It expresses itself in late childhood or adolescence by a slowly progressive mental decline, seizures, and ataxia, and, later, by spastic weakness and splenomegaly. Vision and retinae remain normal. Highly diagnostic is the defect in voluntary lateral gaze, with full movements on the oculocephalic ("doll's-head") maneuver. These signs help to differentiate Gaucher from Niemann-Pick disease, in which vertical eye movements are lost (see below). The nucleotide sequence of the cloned glucocerebrosidase gene of type I Gaucher disease was found by Tsuji and associates (1987) to be different from that of types II and III. There is no treatment for the latter types.

Infantile Niemann-Pick Disease (Sphingomyelinase Deficiency, NPC Mutation)

This is also an autosomal recessive disease. Two-thirds of the affected infants have been of Ashkenazi Jewish parentage. The onset of symptoms in the usual type A disease is between 3 and 9 months of age, frequently beginning with marked *enlargement of liver, spleen, and lymph nodes and infiltration of the lungs*; rarely, there is jaundice and ascites. Cerebral abnormalities are definite by the end of the first year, often earlier. The usual manifestations are loss of spontaneous movements, lack of interest in the environment, axial hypotonia with bilateral corticospinal signs, blindness and amaurotic nystagmus, and a macular cherry-red spot (in about one-quarter of the patients). Seizures may occur, but are relatively late. There is no acoustic-induced startle or myoclonus, and head size is normal or slightly reduced. Loss of tendon reflexes and slowed conduction in peripheral nerves have been recorded but are rare. Protuberant eyes, mild hypertelorism, slight yellowish pigmentation of oral mucosa, and dysplasia of dental enamel have also been reported but are rare. Most patients succumb to an intercurrent infection by the end of the second year.

Vacuolated histiocytes ("foam cells") in the bone marrow and vacuolated blood lymphocytes are the important laboratory findings. A *deficiency of sphingomyelinase* in leukocytes, cultured fibroblasts, and hepatocytes is diagnostic. Pathologic examination reveals a decrease in the number of neurons; many of the remaining ones are pale and ballooned and have a granular cytoplasm. The most prominent neuronal changes are seen in the midbrain, spinal cord, and cerebellum. The white matter is little affected. The retinal nerve cell changes are similar to those in the brain. The foamy histiocytes (Niemann-Pick cells) that fill the viscera contain sphingomyelin and cholesterol; the distended nerve cells contain mainly sphingomyelin.

There are also less-severe late infantile and juvenile forms of Niemann-Pick disease types C and D. These are discussed in a later section of this chapter.

Infantile Generalized G_{M1} Gangliosidosis (Type I, Beta-Galactosidase Deficiency, Pseudo-Hurler Disease, GLB1 Mutation)

This is probably an autosomal recessive disease without ethnic predominance. The infants appear abnormal at birth. They have *dysmorphic facial features*, like those of the mucopolysaccharidoses: depressed and wide nasal bridge, frontal bossing, hypertelorism, puffy eyelids, long upper lip, gingival and alveolar hypertrophy, macroglossia, and low-set ears. These features, with the bone changes mentioned below, account for the term *pseudo-Hurler*. Other indications of the disease are the onset of impaired awareness and reduced responsivity in the first days or weeks of life; lack of *psychomotor development* after 3 to 6 months; hypotonia, and later hypertonia with lively tendon reflexes and Babinski signs. Seizures are frequent. The head size is variable (microcephaly more often than macrocephaly). *Loss of vision, coarse nystagmus and strabismus, macular cherry-red spots* (in half the cases), flexion pseudocontractures of elbows and knees, kyphoscoliosis, and enlarged liver and sometimes enlarged spleen are the other important clinical findings. Radiographic abnormalities include subperiosteal bone formation, midshaft widening and demineralization of long bones, and hypoplasia and beaking of the thoracolumbar vertebrae. Vacuoles are seen in 10 to 80 percent of blood lymphocytes and foam cells in the urinary sediment.

A partial or complete deficiency of beta-galactosidase and accumulation of G_{M1} ganglioside in the viscera and in neurons and glia cells throughout the CNS are the specific biochemical abnormalities. In addition, the epithelial cells of renal glomeruli, histiocytes of the spleen, and liver cells contain a modified keratan sulfate and a galactose-containing oligosaccharide. The changes in the bone are also like those in the Hurler form of mucopolysaccharidosis. *The disease should be suspected in an infant having the facial features of mucopolysaccharidosis and severe early-onset neurologic abnormalities.*

A remarkably benign variant, also inherited as an autosomal recessive trait, begins later in childhood but may advance so slowly as to allow attainment of adult life. Dystonia, myoclonus, seizures, visual impairment, and macular red spots were features of the two cases described by Goldman and coworkers.

Globoid Cell Leukodystrophy (Krabbe Disease, Galactocerebrosidase Deficiency, GALC Mutation)

This is an autosomal recessive disease without ethnic predilection, first described by Krabbe, a Danish neurologist, in 1916. The onset is usually before the sixth month and often before the third month (10 percent after 1 year). Early manifestations are *generalized rigidity*, loss of head control, diminished alertness, frequent vomiting, irritability and bouts of inexplicable crying, and spasms induced by stimulation. With increasing muscular tone, *opisthotonic* recurvation of the neck and trunk develops. Later signs are adduction and extension of the legs, flexion of the arms, clenching of the fists, hyperactive tendon reflexes, and Babinski signs. Later still, the tendon reflexes are depressed or lost but Babinski signs remain, an indication that *neuropathy* is added to corticospinal damage. This finding, shared with some of the other leukodystrophies, is of diagnostic value. Blindness and optic atrophy supervene. Convulsions occur but are rare and difficult to distinguish from tonic spasms. Myoclonus in response to auditory stimuli is present in some cases. The head size is normal or, rarely, slightly increased. In the last stage of the disease, which may occur from one to several months after the onset, the child is blind and usually deaf, opisthotonic, irritable, and cachectic. Most patients die by the end of the first year and survival beyond 2 years is unusual, although a considerable number of cases of later onset have been reported (see below).

The EEG shows nonspecific slowing without spikes, and the CSF protein is usually elevated (70 to 450 mg/dL). Imaging shows symmetrical nonenhancing areas of increased signal in the internal capsules and basal ganglia.

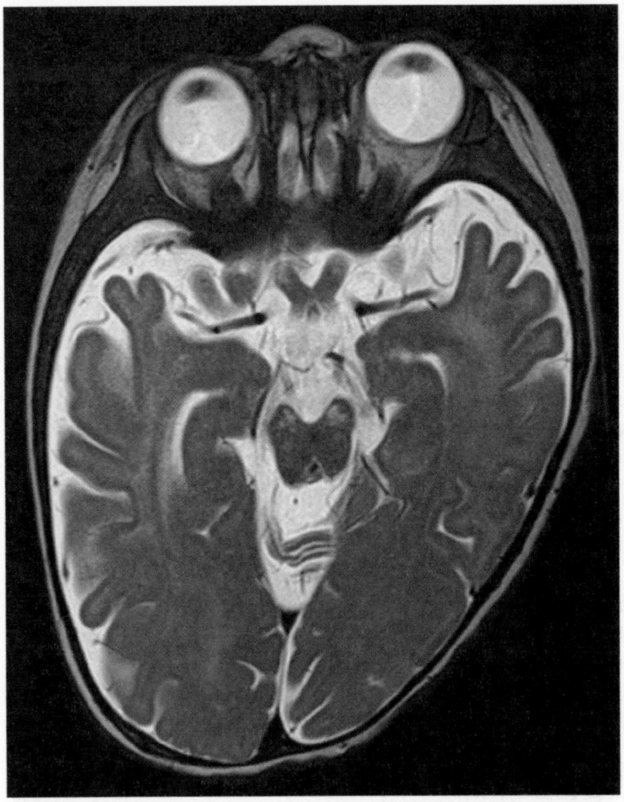

Figure 37-2. Krabbe disease. Axial T2-weighted MRI of a 6 month old with difficulty feeding, irritability, upper extremity hypertonia and lower extremity hypotonia, which began at 3 months. Laboratory testing confirmed low levels of leukocyte galactocerebrosidase activity. There is abnormal hyperintensity of the cerebral peduncles (corticospinal tract atrophy) as well as enlargement of the prechiasmatic optic nerves. Thalamic hypointensity, not shown here, is a common finding as well. (Image courtesy of Drs. Edward Yang and Sanjay Prabhu.)

As the disease advances, more of the cerebral white matter and brainstem become involved (Fig. 37-2). An additional feature in many cases is enlargement of the prechiasmatic optic nerves. Neuropathy is a feature in most cases, but clinical signs may be difficult to detect except for a decrease or loss of tendon reflexes; however, there is *evidence of denervation and slowed motor and sensory nerve conduction velocities*, reflecting a demyelinating polyneuropathy (see later comments on late-onset cases).

The deficient lysosomal enzyme in Krabbe disease is *galactocerebrosidase* (GALC; also called galactosylceramide beta-galactosidase); it normally degrades galactocerebroside to ceramide and galactose. The deficiency results in the accumulation of galactocerebroside; a toxic metabolite, psychosine, leads to the early destruction of oligodendrocytes and depletion of lipids in the cerebral white matter. The globoid cell reaction, however, indicates that impaired catabolism of galactosylceramide is also important. Gross examination of the brain discloses a marked reduction in the cerebral white matter, which feels firm and rubbery. Microscopically, there is widespread myelin degeneration, absence of oligodendrocytes, and astrocytic gliosis in the cerebrum, brainstem, spinal cord, and nerves. The characteristic globoid cells are large histiocytes containing the accumulated metabolite.

Schwann cells have tubular or crystalloid inclusions under electron microscopy.

About a dozen variants of globoid cell leukodystrophy have been reported, many of them allowing survival for years. In these, neurologic regression begins in the 2- to 6-year-old period. Visual failure with optic atrophy and a normal electroretinogram is an early finding. Later there is ataxia, as well as spastic weakness of the legs, mental regression, and finally decerebration. In three patients observed by R.D. Adams, a progressive quadriparesis with mild pseudobulbar signs, slowly progressive impairment of memory and other mental functions, dystonic posturing of the arms, and preserved sphincteric control constituted the clinical picture. The patients were alive at ages 9, 12, and 16 years. We have observed another rare variant, beginning in adult years, with spastic quadriparesis (asymmetrical) and optic atrophy. Mentation was essentially normal and, on imaging, the cerebral lesion was restricted. Unlike typical Krabbe disease, these CNS abnormalities are unaccompanied by any change in the spinal fluid. The nerve conduction velocities in the late-onset form may be either normal or abnormal.

Kolodny and colleagues reported 15 cases of even later onset (ages 4 to 73 years); pes cavus, optic pallor, progressive spastic quadriparesis, a demyelinating sensorimotor neuropathy, and symmetrical parietooccipital white matter changes (on imaging studies) were the main features. Galactocerebrosidase levels were not as reduced as in the infantile form; possibly these late-onset variants represent a structural mutation of the enzyme (see Farrell and Swedberg).

In this disease, as well as others described in this chapter, it has become clear that different mutations involving the same enzyme or metabolic pathway can produce strikingly different phenotypes and that there is a wide range in the age of onset in what had been considered, until relatively recently, a disease confined to infancy and early childhood.

Treatment

In what may be considered a possible breakthrough in the treatment of childhood metabolic disease, Escolar and colleagues reported the successful use of transplanted umbilical cord hematopoietic cells in asymptomatic babies with Krabbe disease. Patients who were treated after becoming symptomatic did not benefit, but 14 patients who had been diagnosed prenatally or very soon after birth demonstrated progressive myelination of the nervous system, normalization of blood galactocerebroside activity, and attained visual, developmental, and cognitive function. The donors were partially human leukocyte antigen (HLA)-matched and substantial antirejection medication was required.

Vanishing White Matter Disease

This more recently described and peculiarly named disease with variable age of onset is most typically manifest in this age group. After a period of normal development, and sometimes precipitated by infection or fever, there is a progressive encephalopathy punctuated by episodes of more rapid deterioration. The core syndrome is of irritability, loss of vision, seizures, ataxia, and coma, sometimes with recovery to a disabled state. The denominative feature is a symmetrical leukodystrophy with progressive disappearance of white matter and replacement by CSF or gliosis. The nature of this disease, metabolic, inflammatory, or genetic (mutations in *eIF2B*), has not been resolved despite tentative linkage to certain chromosomal regions. We include it in this section because exacerbation with fever, similar to the case in some mitochondrial diseases, is suggestive of a metabolic disorder (see Leegwater et al).

Lipogranulomatosis (Farber Disease, Ceramidase Deficiency)

This is a rare autosomal disorder that is based on a mutation in ASAH1. The onset is in the first weeks of life, with a hoarse cry because of fixation of laryngeal cartilage, respiratory distress, and sensitivity of the joints, followed by characteristic *periarticular and subcutaneous swellings* and *progressive arthropathy*, leading finally to ankylosis. Usually there is severe psychomotor delay, but a few patients have been neurologically normal. Inanition and recurrent infections lead to death in the first 2 years. The diagnostic abnormality is a *deficiency of ceramidase*, leading to accumulation of ceramide. There is widespread lipid storage in neurons, granulomas of the skin, and accumulation of periodic acid-Schiff (PAS)-positive macrophages in periarticular and visceral tissues.

Sudanophilic Leukodystrophies and Pelizaeus-Merzbacher Disease

These are a heterogeneous group of disorders that have in common a defective myelination of the cerebrum, brainstem, cerebellum, spinal cord, and peripheral nerves. Morphologic peculiarities and genetic features separate a certain group called *Pelizaeus-Merzbacher disease*; other types have been artificially delineated; as a result, a relatively meaningless terminology has been introduced.

Pelizaeus-Merzbacher Disease (PLP1 Mutation)

This is predominantly an X-linked disease of infancy, childhood, and adolescence, and includes other closely related pathologic entities with different modes of inheritance. The affected gene encodes proteolipid protein (PLP), one of the two myelin basic proteins. Koeppen and associates have provided evidence of a defective synthesis of this protein. While one group of PLP mutations causes Pelizaeus-Merzbacher disease, another set causes an infantile spastic paraplegia.

The onset of symptoms is most often in the first months of life; other cases begin later in childhood. The first signs are *abnormal movements of the eyes* (rapid, irregular, often asymmetrical pendular nystagmus), jerk nystagmus on extremes of lateral movements, upbeat nystagmus on upward gaze, and hypometric saccades (Trobe et al). There is spastic weakness of the limbs, optic atrophy (often with unexplained retention of pupillary light reflex), ataxia of limb movement and intention tremor, choreiform or athetotic movements of the arms, and slow psychomotor development with delay in sitting, standing, and walking. Seizures occur occasionally. In later-developing cases, pendular nystagmus, choreoathetosis, corticospinal signs, dysarthria, cerebellar ataxia, and mental deterioration are the major manifestations. There are milder cases of later onset with behavioral peculiarities and loss of tendon reflexes and, rarely, pure spastic paraparesis.

Imaging confirms the extensive and symmetrical white matter involvement. In the most severe cases, Seitelberger has observed an absence of oligodendrocytes and myelinated fibers. It is hypothesized that proteolipids accumulate in the endoplasmic reticulum of the oligodendrocytes, resulting in apoptosis. Patients may survive to the second and third decades. One group of cases resembles the Cockayne syndrome, with photosensitivity of skin, dwarfism, cerebellar ataxia, corticospinal signs, cataracts, retinitis pigmentosa, and deafness. Pathologically, islands of preserved myelin impart a tigroid pattern of degenerated and intact myelin in the cerebrum. Seitelberger has obtained pathologic verification of this lesion in cases beginning as late as adult years. *This disease and Cockayne syndrome are the only leukodystrophies in which nystagmus has been an invariable finding.*

Koeppen and Robitaille, in a thorough review of the subject of the pathogenesis of Pelizaeus-Merzbacher disease, summarized the evidence supporting the concept that misfolding of myelin proteins is the essential cause.

Unclassifiable Sporadic and Familial Sudanophilic Leukodystrophies

There are two types of such disorders, one with early and the other with late onset. In the former, the illness begins before 3 months of age, with survival of less than 2 years; in the latter, onset is between ages 3 and 7 years and the course is only slowly progressive to the point of being chronic. *Psychomotor regression; spastic paralysis; incoordination; blindness* and optic atrophy; seizures (rare); *severe microcephaly*; and absence of skeletal, visceral, and hematologic evidence of the metabolic abnormality are the main features. No characteristic laboratory abnormalities are known. Diffuse degeneration of myelinated fibers (visible by MRI) with phagocytosis of *sudanophilic degeneration products of myelin* and gliosis are the major changes. In two cases followed by R.D. Adams and T. Rabinowicz, a brother and sister living to adolescence, the destroyed white matter was widely cavitated.

Spongy Degeneration of Infancy (Canavan-van Bogaert-Bertrand or Canavan Disease, ASPA Mutation)

This is an autosomal recessive disease that was described in 1931 by Myrtelle Canavan as a form of Schilder disease (see Chap. 36), but later categorized as a special spongy degeneration of the brain by van Bogaert and Bertrand. Of 48 affected families reported by Banker and Victor, 28 were of Jewish ancestry. Onset is early, usually recognizable in the first 3 months of life and sometimes in the first neonatal weeks. There is either a lack of development or rapid *regression of psychomotor function, loss of sight and optic atrophy*, lethargy, difficulty in sucking, irritability, reduced motor activity, hypotonia followed by spasticity of the limbs with corticospinal signs, and an *enlarged head* (macrocephaly). There are no visceral or skeletal abnormalities but a variable sensorineural hearing loss has been found (Ishiyama et al). Seizures occur in some cases. An interesting but unexplored aspect of the disease is the occurrence of blond hair and light complexion in affected members, in contrast to the darker hair and complexion of their normal siblings (Banker and Victor).

The CSF is usually normal but the protein is slightly elevated in some cases. The disease is characterized by an increased urinary excretion of *N*-acetyl-L-aspartic acid (NAA), which may be used as a biochemical marker. It reflects the basic enzyme abnormality, a deficiency of aminoacylase II, which catalyzes the breakdown of NAA (Matalon et al). On CT there is *attenuation of cerebral and cerebellar white matter in an enlarged brain with relatively normal-size ventricles.* The MRI appearance (Fig. 37-3) is that of diffuse, somewhat uneven, high signal intensity on T2-weighted images. A leukodystrophy with behavioral regression, an enlarging head, a characteristic MRI abnormality, and a marked elevation of urinary NAA should leave little doubt about the diagnosis.

The characteristic pathologic changes are an increase in brain volume (and weight), spongy degeneration in the deep layers of the cerebral cortex and subcortical

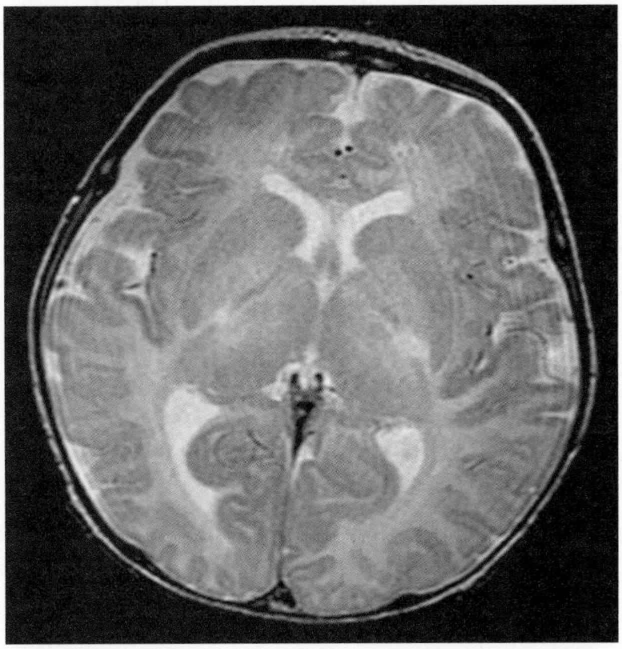

Figure 37-3. Spongy degeneration of infancy (Canavan-van Bogaert-Bertrand disease). Axial T2-weighted MRI of a 5-week old with hypertonia, nystagmus, and macrocephaly. There is abnormal hyperintensity in the globus pallidus, ventrolateral thalamus, and internal capsule. Abnormal white matter hyperintensity extends to the cortex without sparing of the arcuate fibers. MR spectroscopy (not shown) revealed a markedly elevated *N*-acetyl aspartate peak. (Image courtesy of Drs. Edward Yang and Sanjay Prabhu.)

white matter, widespread depletion of myelin involving the convolutional more than the central white matter, loss of Purkinje cells, and hyperplasia of Alzheimer type II astrocytes throughout the cerebral cortex and basal ganglia. Adachi and coworkers have demonstrated an abnormal vacuolar accumulation of fluid in astrocytes and between split myelin lamellae; they have suggested that the loss of myelin is secondary to these changes.

The enlargement of the brain in this disease must be distinguished clinically from G_{M2} gangliosidosis, Alexander disease, Krabbe disease, and nonprogressive megalocephaly and pathologically from a variety of disorders characterized by vacuolation of nervous tissue. There is no treatment.

Alexander Disease (GFAP Mutation)

This distinctive disease shares certain features with the leukodystrophies and also with gray matter diseases (poliodystrophies), both clinically and pathologically. The onset is in infancy with a *failure to thrive, psychomotor retardation, spasticity of the craniospinal musculature, and seizures*. An early and *progressive macrocephaly* has been a consistent feature. Alexander was the first to call attention to the enlargement of the brain, the extensive loss of cerebral white matter, and highly characteristic inclusions (the so-called Rosenthal fibers noted below) in astrocytes, and subpial and periventricular regions.

Pathologically, there are severe destructive changes in the cerebral white matter, most intense in the frontal lobes. Distinctive eosinophilic hyaline bodies, most prominent just below the pia and around blood vessels, are seen throughout the cerebral cortex, brainstem, and spinal cord. These have been identified as *Rosenthal fibers* and probably represent glial degradation products.

The astrocytic changes have been traced to a mutation in the glial fibrillary acidic protein (GFAP), as described by Gorospe and colleagues. It is usually inherited in an autosomal dominant pattern, and gives rise to the intermediate filament protein in astrocytes and, presumably, to the Rosenthal fiber inclusions. On the basis of this and related gene mutations, apparent milder forms of Alexander disease have been reported in juveniles and adults. They differed clinically in lacking the cerebral leukoencephalopathy. Instead, after a long period of constipation, sleep disorder, and orthostatic hypotension during adolescence, bulbar symptoms (dysarthria, dysphonia, and dysphagia), seizures, and in some cases ataxia gradually emerged during adult years. The myelin changes and atrophy of the medulla seen in MRI were confirmed by postmortem examination and the Rosenthal fibers; GFAP fibers were present in two autopsied cases.

Alpers Disease (POLG Mutation)

This is a progressive disease of the cerebral gray matter, known also as *progressive cerebral poliodystrophy or diffuse cerebral degeneration in infancy*. A familial form (probably autosomal recessive) as well many sporadic cases has been reported. In both groups there is a certain uniformity of clinical features—loss of smile and disinterest in the surroundings, sweating attacks, *seizures, and diffuse myoclonic jerks* beginning in early infancy and followed by incoordination of movements; progressive spasticity of limb, trunk, and cranial muscles; blindness and optic atrophy; growth retardation and *increasing microcephaly*; and finally virtual decortication. In some instances, the late onset of jaundice and fatty degeneration or cirrhosis of the liver have been described (Alpers-Huttenlocher syndrome); the hepatic changes are distinctive and probably not related to the use of anticonvulsant drugs, as had been hypothesized (Harding et al). By the age of 4 years, these patients are hypotonic, anemic, and thrombocytopenic. They also show fragile hair follicles that break at thickened nodes (trichorrhexis nodosa).

The nature of this combined hepatic–cerebral degeneration remains unexplained but some instances have been connected to the mitochondrial disorders, as noted below. EEG abnormalities, progressive atrophy (particularly occipital) on the CT, loss of visual evoked potentials, and abnormal liver function tests are diagnostically useful. Neuropathologic examination shows marked atrophy of the cerebral convolutions and cerebellar cortex, with loss of nerve cells and fibrous gliosis ("walnut brain"). The cerebral white matter and basal ganglia are relatively preserved. In some cases, the spongiform vacuolization of the gray matter of the brain resembles that seen in Creutzfeldt-Jakob disease. Hypoglycemic, hypoxic, and hypotensive encephalopathies must always be considered in the diagnosis but can usually be eliminated by knowledge of the clinical circumstances at the onset of the illness.

A number of biochemical abnormalities have been identified in patients with Alpers disease, including pyruvate dehydrogenase deficiency, decreased pyruvate utilization, dysfunction of the citric acid cycle, and decreased cytochromes a and aa_3. The biochemical and pathologic changes suggest a relationship to Leigh encephalomyelopathy and a mitochondrial transmission. Many authoritative texts classify it with the mitochondrial diseases, but its nosologic status is in our opinion still uncertain.

Congenital Lactic Acidosis

This uncommon disease of the neonatal period or early infancy has many biochemical etiologies. The symptoms have consisted of *psychomotor regression* and *episodic hyperventilation*, *hypotonia*, and *convulsions*, with intervening periods of normalcy. *Choreoathetosis* has been observed in a few cases. Death often occurs before the third year. The important laboratory findings are *acidosis with an anion gap and high serum lactate levels* and hyperalaninemia. Defects can be found in the pyruvate dehydrogenase complex of enzymes and the electron transport chain complexes, which function in the oxidative decarboxylation of pyruvate to acetyl coenzyme A (CoA), relating the disease to defects in the mitochondrial respiratory chain enzymes. Indeed, lactic acidosis is a feature of several of the mitochondropathies discussed later in this chapter. Cases examined postmortem have shown necrosis and cavitation of the globus pallidus and cerebral white matter. Possibly this is a variant of Leigh disease. It must be distinguished from the several diseases of infancy that are complicated secondarily by lactic acidosis, especially the organic acidopathies. Cases of benign transient infantile lactic acidosis have been reported, but their etiology is unclear.

Cerebrohepatorenal (Zellweger) Disease and the Peroxisomal Disorders (PEX1 and Other Mutations)

This disease, estimated to occur once in every 100,000 births, is inherited as an autosomal recessive trait. It has its onset in the neonatal period or early infancy and as a rule leads to death within a few months. Motor inactivity and hypotonia, *dysmorphic alterations of the skull and face* (high forehead, shallow orbits, hypertelorism, high arched palate, abnormal helices of ears, retrognathia), poor visual fixation, multifocal seizures, swallowing difficulties, fixed flexion posture of the limbs, cataracts, abnormal retinal pigmentation, optic atrophy, cloudy corneas, hepatomegaly, and hepatic dysfunction are the usual manifestations. *Stippled, irregular calcifications of the patellae and greater trochanters are highly characteristic.* Pathologically, there is dysgenesis of the cerebral cortex and degeneration of white matter as well as a number of visceral abnormalities—cortical renal cysts, hepatic fibrosis, intrahepatic biliary dysgenesis, agenesis of the thymus, and iron storage in the reticuloendothelial system.

As to the biochemical abnormality, Moser and coworkers (1984) demonstrated a fivefold increase of very-long-chain fatty acids, particularly hexacosanoic acid, in the plasma and cultured skin fibroblasts from 35 patients with Zellweger disease. A similar abnormality was found in cultured amniocytes of women at risk of bearing a child with Zellweger disease, thus permitting prenatal diagnosis. The findings of Moser and colleagues (1984) are in keeping with current notions about the basic abnormality in Zellweger syndrome, namely, that it is caused by a lack of liver peroxisomes (oxidase-containing, membrane-bound cytoplasmic organelles), in which the very-long-chain fatty acids are normally oxidized (Goldfischer et al).

Currently, a spectrum of at least 12 disorders of peroxisomal function is recognized, all of them characterized by deficiencies in the peroxisomal enzyme of fatty-acid oxidation. The most common form of Zellweger syndrome is due to a mutation in *PEX1*. However, the most widely recognized peroxisomal disorders are adrenoleukodystrophy and Refsum disease, but the Zellweger cerebrohepatorenal syndrome can be considered a prototype. Each variant can be identified by its characteristic profile of elevated long- and very-long-chain fatty acids, and the specific diagnosis can be confirmed by enzymology of cultured fibroblasts or amniocytes. Several of them become manifest at a later age and are discussed further on. For an authoritative discussion of peroxisomal biogenesis, the reader is referred to the article by Gould and Valle.

The Oculocerebrorenal (Lowe) Syndrome (OCRL1 Mutation)

Here the mode of inheritance is probably X-linked recessive, although sporadic cases have been reported in girls. The abnormal gene is located on chromosome Xq25.26. The clinical abnormalities comprise *bilateral cataracts* (which may be present at birth), glaucoma, large eyes with megalocornea and buphthalmos, corneal opacities and blindness, pendular nystagmus, hypotonia and absent or depressed tendon reflexes, corticospinal signs without paralysis, slow movements of the hands, tantrums and aggressive behavior, high-pitched cry, occasional seizures, and psychomotor regression. Later the frontal bones become prominent and the eyes sunken. The characteristic biochemical abnormality is a *renal tubular acidosis*, and death is usually from *renal failure*. Additional laboratory findings include demineralization of bones and typical rachitic deformities, anemia, metabolic acidosis, and generalized aminoaciduria. The neuropathologic changes are nonspecific; inconstant atrophy and poor myelination have been described in the brain and tubular abnormalities in the kidneys. The primary genetic defects are in the gene encoding inositol polyphosphate phosphatase of the Golgi complex. The main diagnostic distinction is from Zellweger disease. Treatment programs include anticonvulsant medication, correction of electrolyte disorders, and removal of cataracts.

Menkes Disease (Kinky- or Steely-Hair Disease; Trichopoliodystrophy, ATP7A Mutation)

This rare disorder is inherited as a sex-linked recessive trait. In most of the cases known to us, birth was premature. Poor feeding and failure to gain weight, instability of temperature (mainly *hypothermia*), and seizures become apparent in early infancy. The hair is normal at birth but the secondary growth is lusterless and depigmented and feels like steel wool; hairs break easily and under the microscope they appear twisted (*pili torti*). Radiologic examination shows *metaphysial spurring*, mainly of the femurs, and subperiosteal calcifications of the bone shafts. Arteriography discloses *tortuosity and elongation of the cerebral and systemic arteries* and occlusion of some. The combination of intracerebral hemorrhage and metaphysial bone spurs, which may be interpreted as "corner fractures," has led in some cases to the erroneous diagnosis of child abuse. There is no discernible neurologic development, and rarely does the untreated child survive beyond the second year. Three of our cases were examined postmortem (Williams et al). There was a diffuse loss of neurons in the relay nuclei of the thalamus, the cerebral cortex, and the cerebellum (granule and stellate cells) and of dendritic arborizations of residual neurons of the motor cortex and Purkinje cells.

The manifestations of this disease are attributable to one of numerous known mutations in a copper-transporting adenosine triphosphatase (ATPase), *ATP7A*, that is attributed to a *failure of absorption of copper from the gastrointestinal tract* and a profound deficiency of tissue copper (Danks et al). Furthermore, because copper fails to cross the placenta, a severe reduction of copper in the brain and liver is evident from birth. In this sense, the abnormality of copper metabolism is the opposite of that in Wilson disease. A relationship between Wilson and Menkes disease is nonetheless evident at a genetic level as they arise from genes encoding two different copper-transporting proteins that are both ATPases. The situation, however, may be more complex, as samples of intestinal tissue show a buildup of copper that indicates the problem is in mobilization of copper from the gut to the bloodstream. Other copper-dependent enzymes show impaired function, such as cytochrome oxidase. For the purposes of early diagnosis, Kaler and colleagues have taken advantage of the reduced activity of another copper-dependent enzyme, dopamine–β-hydroxylase, to detect increased plasma levels of its substrates (dopamine and dihydroxyphenylacetic acid [DOPAC]), as well as reduced levels of the enzyme products (norepinephrine and dihydroxyphenylglycol [DHPG]). The ratio of dopamine to norepinephrine and dihydroxyphenylacetic acid to dihydroxyphenylglycol proved, in their study, to be the most sensitive and specific for early detection. This has allowed the neonatal identification of cases in families with affected children and resulted in normal neurodevelopment in a few children who were treated with copper beginning in the first weeks of life. This same group has suggested that only those mutations in *ATP7A* that allow for some residual copper transport activity are associated with better outcomes.

Parenteral administration of cupric salts, usually in the form of copper histidine administered subcutaneously twice daily by the parents, restores the serum and hepatic copper and may allow normal development in a few children as noted above but it does not materially influence the neurologic symptoms if treatment is started later. However, even early treated cases showing limited neurodevelopment survive and show some neurologic advance, unlike the past experience in which few survived beyond 5 or 6 years.

Diagnosis of Inherited Metabolic Diseases of Infancy

It will be recognized from the foregoing synopses that many of the neurologic manifestations of the inherited metabolic diseases of infancy are nonspecific and are common to most or all of the diseases in this group. In general, in the early stages of all these diseases, there is a loss of postural tone and a paucity of movement without paralysis or loss of reflexes; later there is spasticity with hyperreflexia and Babinski signs. Equally nonspecific are features such as irritability and prolonged crying; poor feeding, difficulty in swallowing, inanition, and retarded growth; failure of fixation of gaze and following movements of the eyes (often misinterpreted as blindness); and tonic spasms, clonic jerks, and focal and generalized seizures.

The differentiation of the inherited metabolic diseases of infancy rests essentially upon four types of data: (1) a few highly characteristic neurologic and ophthalmic signs; (2) the presence of an enlarged liver and/or spleen; (3) special dysmorphic features of the face; and (4) the results of several relatively simple laboratory tests, such as images of the thoracolumbar spine, hips, and long bones; smears of the peripheral blood and bone marrow; CSF examination; and certain urinary tests and other biochemical estimations (serum lactate, glucose, ammonia, and urinary ketones, amino acids, and organic acids). For purposes of differential diagnosis, we have found the flowcharts constructed by our colleague, E. Kolodny, to be very useful. One such schematic, illustrated in Fig. 37-4, is based on the subdivision of patients into three groups: (1) dysmorphic, (2) visceromegalic, and (3) purely neurologic. Only rarely does an inherited metabolic disease fall into more than one of these categories. There is also considerable value in beginning the diagnostic process by classifying the syndrome as a leukodystrophy or a poliodystrophy (disease predominantly affecting neurons, see further on), although this distinction is easier to make in the older child. Once the major category of disease has been identified, correct diagnosis depends on particular clinical and laboratory features tabulated below (Tables 37-5 and 37-6).

Neurologic signs that are more or less specific for certain metabolic diseases are as follows:

1. Acousticomotor obligatory startle: Tay-Sachs disease
2. Abolished tendon reflexes with definite Babinski signs: globoid cell (Krabbe) leukodystrophy, occasionally Leigh disease, and (beyond infancy) metachromatic leukodystrophy
3. Peculiar eye movements, pendular nystagmus, and head rolling: Pelizaeus-Merzbacher disease, Leigh disease; later, hyperbilirubinemia and Lesch-Nyhan hyperuricemia (see below)
4. Marked rigidity, opisthotonos, and tonic spasms: Krabbe, Alpers disease, or infantile Gaucher disease (classic triad: trismus, strabismus, opisthotonos)
5. Intractable seizures and generalized or multifocal myoclonus: Alpers disease
6. Intermittent hyperventilation: Leigh disease and congenital lactic acidosis (also nonprogressive familial agenesis of vermis)
7. Strabismus, hypotonia, seizures, lipodystrophy: carbohydrate-deficient glycoprotein syndrome

Ocular abnormalities of specific diagnostic value in this age group are as follows:

1. Rapid pendular nystagmus: Pelizaeus-Merzbacher disease, rarely Krabbe leukodystrophy, Cockayne syndrome (later age)
2. Macular cherry-red spots: Tay-Sachs disease and Sandhoff variant, some cases of infantile Niemann-Pick disease, and rarely lipofuscinosis (see Table 37-4)
3. Corneal opacification: Lowe disease, infantile G_{M1} gangliosidosis; later, the mucopolysaccharidoses
4. Cataracts: galactosemia, Lowe disease, Zellweger disease (also congenital rubella)

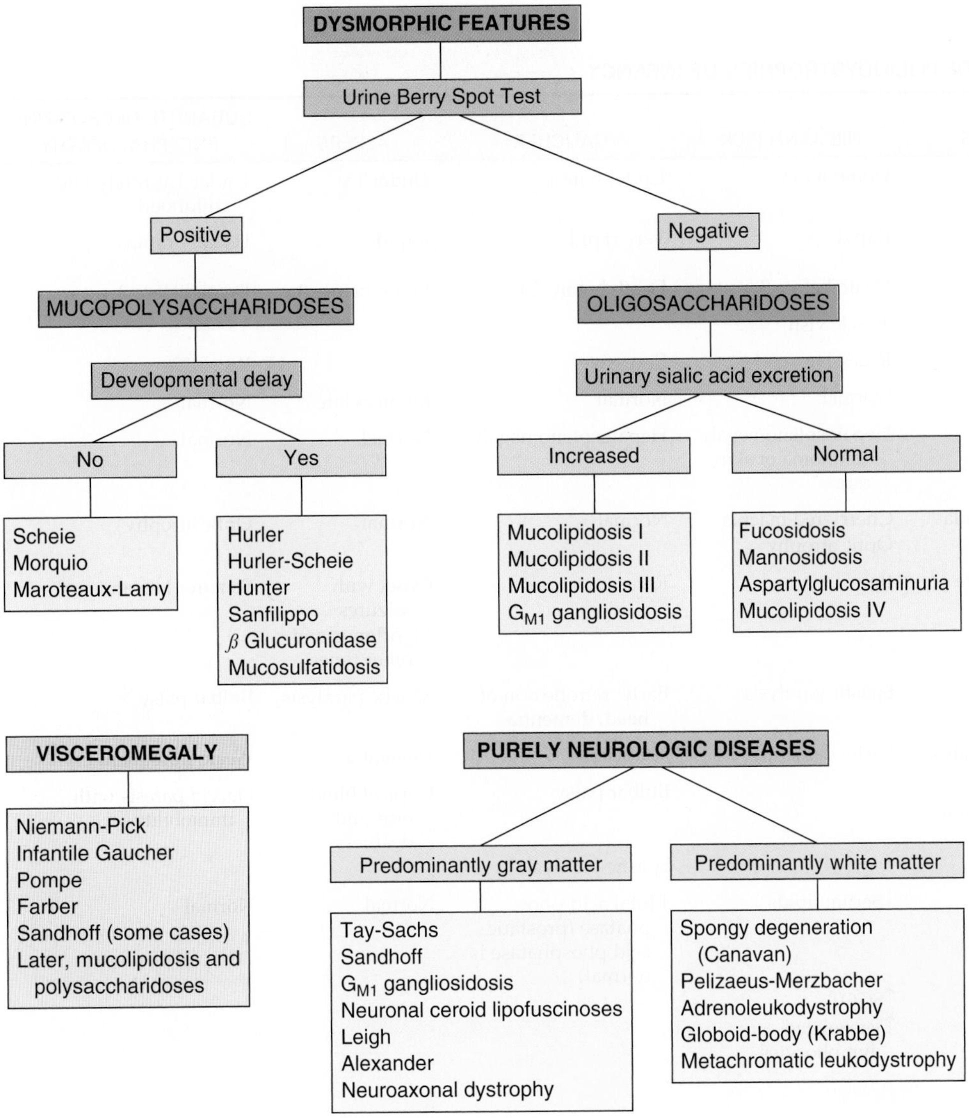

Figure 37-4. A schematic for diagnosis of the inherited metabolic diseases of infancy. (Courtesy of Dr. Edwin Kolodny.)

Several other medical findings are of specific diagnostic value:

1. Dysmorphic facies: generalized G_{M1} gangliosidosis, Lowe and Zellweger syndromes, and some early cases of mucopolysaccharidosis and mucolipidosis
2. Enlarged liver and spleen: infantile Gaucher disease and Niemann-Pick disease; one type of hyperammonemia; Sandhoff disease; later, the mucopolysaccharidoses and mucolipidoses
3. Enlarging head without hydrocephalus (macrocephaly): Canavan spongy degeneration of infancy, some cases of Tay-Sachs disease, Alexander disease
4. Beaking of vertebral bodies in radiographs: G_{M1} gangliosidosis (and, at a more advanced age, the mucopolysaccharidoses, fucosidosis, mannosidosis, and the mucolipidoses)
5. Multiple arthropathies and raucous dysphonia: Farber disease
6. Storage granules and vacuolated lymphocytes: Niemann-Pick disease, generalized G_{M1} gangliosidosis
7. Abnormal histiocytes in marrow smears: Gaucher cells, foamy histiocytes in Niemann-Pick disease, generalized G_{M1} gangliosidosis and closely related diseases, Farber disease
8. Colorless, friable hair: Menkes disease

INHERITED METABOLIC DISEASES OF EARLY CHILDHOOD

Included here are the diseases that become manifest between the ages of 1 and about 4 years. Diagnosis is less difficult than in the neonate and young infant. A pathologic process in the nervous system is reliably ascertained by the obvious progression of a neurologic disorder, such as a loss of ability to walk and to speak, which usually parallels a regression in other high-level (quasi-intellectual) functions. Embryologic anomalies, prenatal diseases, and birth injuries can be excluded with relative certainty if psychomotor development was normal in the

Table 37-5

DIFFERENTIAL DIAGNOSIS OF POLIODYSTROPHIES OF INFANCY

	TAY-SACHS	NIEMANN-PICK	GAUCHER	ALPERS	SUBACUTE NECROTIZING ENCEPHALOPATHY
Age of onset	4–6 mo	Under 6 mo	Under 6 mo	Under 1 y	Under 1 y, rarely late childhood
Rate of progression	Rapid	Rapid	Very rapid	Rapid	Usually rapid
	Death 2–3 y	Death before 3 y	Death before 2 y	Death before 3 y	Death before 3 y
Ethnic group	Almost all Jewish	50% Jewish			
Genetic	Recessive	Recessive	Recessive		Recessive
Head size	Enlarges late	Normal	Normal	Reduces late	Normal
Skin and/or systemic lesions	Normal	Hepatosplenomegaly xanthoma of skin, rare	Hepatosplenomegaly	Normal	Normal
Eye	Cherry-red macula Optic atrophy	Cherry-red macula Optic atrophy	Normal	Normal	Optic atrophy
Seizures	Frequent, but late	Rare	Rare	Onset with seizures Myoclonus and other types	Seizures late and rare
Neurologic signs	Early: flaccid paresis	Spastic paralysis	Early: retroflexion of head, dementia	Spastic paralysis	Bulbar palsy
	Late: spastic paralysis	Early: dementia	Strabismus	Dementia	Weak, infrequent cry
	Dementia: early hyperacusis with myoclonus		Bulbar palsy	Cortical blindness and deafness	Flaccid paresis with immobility
			Spastic paralysis		
Blood	Absent fructose 1-phosphate-aldolase	↑Serum lipids	↑Total acid phosphatase (prostatic acid phosphatase is normal)	Normal	Normal
	↑SGOT	↑SGOT ↑Vacuolated lymphocytes			
	↑Vacuolated lymphocytes				
Urine	Normal	Normal	Normal	Normal	Normal
CSF	Normal	Normal		Normal	Normal
Biopsy	Rectal	"Foam cells" in bone marrow	Gaucher cells in bone marrow		
X-ray		Diffuse pulmonary infiltrates Demineralization of bone			

Electroretinogram: normal.
Diagnostic biochemical abnormality: see text.

SGOT, serum glutamic-oxaloacetic transaminase.
Source: Adapted with permission from Drew AL Jr: The degenerative and demyelinating diseases of the nervous system, in Carter S, Gold AP (eds): *Neurology of Infancy and Childhood*. New York, Appleton-Century-Crofts, 1974, pp 57–89.

first year or two. Diseases characterized by seizures and myoclonus may prove more difficult to interpret, for the seizures may occur at any age from a variety of distant or immediate neurologic causes and, if frequent, may cause a significant impairment of psychomotor function. The effects of anticonvulsant medications may add to the impairment of cortical function. Unfortunately, most of the slowly advancing metabolic diseases of the second year may be so subtle in their effects that for a time the physician cannot be sure whether a regression of intellectual functions is taking place or mental retardation or autism is becoming apparent for the first time. An added difficulty arises when, for a number of years, the hereditary metabolic abnormality merely slows development. Repeated examinations and testing will usually settle the matter. Suspicion of a progressive encephalopathy is

Table 37-6

DIFFERENTIAL DIAGNOSIS OF LEUKODYSTROPHIES OF INFANCY

	KRABBE	METACHROMATIC LEUKODYSTROPHY	SPONGY DEGENERATION	PELIZAEUS-MERZBACHER	SCHILDER DISEASE; SUDANOPHILIC AND ADRENOLEUKODYSTROPHY
Age of onset	3–6 mo	1–2 y, rarely late childhood	0–4 mo	6–24 mo	5–10 y
Rate of progression	Rapid Death by 2 y Some later and slow	Slow Death by 3–5 y	Rapid Death by 3 y	Slow May survive to adult life	Abrupt onset Death in months to years
Sex or ethnic group			Mostly Jewish	Predominantly males	
Genetic	Recessive	Recessive	Recessive	Sex-linked recessive	Adrenoleukodystrophy form—X-linked recessive
Head size	Normal	Enlarges late	Enlarges early	Normal	Normal
Skin or systemic lesions	Normal	Normal	Normal	Normal	Bronzing with adrenal atrophy
Eye	Late: optic atrophy	Late: optic atrophy	Optic atrophy, blindness	Slow optic atrophy	Optic neuritis or optic atrophy
Seizures	Tonic spasms	Rare	Uncommon	Late	Rare, late
Neurologic signs	Spastic paralysis	Changes in gait	Hypotonia→ spastic diplegia→ decerebrate rigidity	Pendular nystagmus	Early spastic paralysis
	Nystagmus	Ataxia		Titubation of head and other cerebellar signs in early childhood	Dementia
	Head retraction	Combined upper and lower motor neuron signs			Late: cortical blindness, deafness, aphasia, pseudobulbar palsy
	Bulbar palsy Dementia		Late		
		Bulbar palsy		Spastic diplegia, late childhood	
		Blindness Deafness Dementia		Slow dementia	
Miscellaneous	Slowed nerve conduction (rare)	Slowed nerve conduction			EEG diffuse delta waves
Blood	Normal	Normal	↓*N*-acetyl-L-aspartic acid (NAA)	Normal	Normal or ↓cortisol
Urine	Normal	Metachromatic bodies	Normal	Normal	Normal
CSF	↑Protein (150–300 mg/dL)	Normal or ↑protein up to 200 mg/dL	↑Pressure ↑protein up to 200 mg/dL	Normal	Normal or ↑gamma globulin
Biopsy	Brain	Sural nerve	Brain		
X-ray		Nonfilling of gallbladder	Suture separation		

Diagnostic biochemical abnormality: see text.

Source: Adapted with permission from Drew AL Jr: The degenerative and demyelinating diseases of the nervous system, in Carter S, Gold AP (eds): *Neurology of Infancy and Childhood*. New York, Appleton-Century-Crofts, 1974, pp 57–89.

heightened by the presence of certain ocular, visceral, and skeletal abnormalities, as described below.

Once a neurologic syndrome is clearly established, there is a particular advantage in determining whether its main characteristics reflect a disorder of the cerebral white matter (oligodendrocytes and myelin) or of gray matter (neurons). Indicative of predominantly white matter affection (*leukodystrophy* or leukoencephalopathy) are early onset of spastic paralysis of the limbs, with or without ataxia, and visual impairment with optic atrophy but normal retinae. Seizures and intellectual deterioration are late events. MRI usually confirms the involvement of white matter. Indicative of gray matter disease (*poliodystrophy* or polioencephalopathy) are the early onset of seizures, myoclonus, blindness with retinal changes, and mental regression. Choreoathetosis and ataxia, spastic paralysis, and signs of sensorimotor tract involvement occur later. On MRI, only a generalized atrophy and ventricular enlargement may be seen.

Neuronal storage diseases, such as those described in the previous section, as well as neuroaxonal dystrophy and the lipofuscinoses, conform to the pattern of gray matter diseases (see Table 37-5). Metachromatic leukodystrophy, globoid-cell (Krabbe) disease, sudanophilic leukodystrophy, and spongy degeneration of infancy (Canavan disease) exemplify white matter diseases (see Table 37-6). Although this mode of categorization is helpful, there is some degree of overlap; for example, Tay-Sachs disease, a poliodystrophy, also causes white matter changes, and metachromatic leukodystrophy may be accompanied by some degree of neuronal storage.

The following are inherited metabolic diseases that become evident clinically in late infancy and early childhood:

1. Many of the milder disorders of amino acid metabolism
2. Metachromatic and other leukodystrophies
3. Late infantile G_{M1} gangliosidosis
4. Late infantile Gaucher disease and Niemann-Pick disease
5. Neuroaxonal dystrophy
6. The mucopolysaccharidoses
7. The mucolipidoses
8. Fucosidosis
9. The mannosidoses
10. Aspartylglycosaminuria
11. Ceroid lipofuscinosis (Jansky-Bielschowsky disease)
12. Cockayne syndrome

The Aminoacidopathies (Aminoacidurias)

In a group of 48 inherited aminoacidopathies tabulated by Rosenberg and Scriver, at least one-half were associated with recognizable neurologic abnormalities. Twenty other aminoacidopathies result in a defect in the renal transport of amino acids, some of which secondarily damage the nervous system. Usually, when the nervous system is involved, the only clinical manifestation is simply a lag in psychomotor development, which, if mild, does not become apparent until the second and third years or later. Like other inherited metabolic disorders, the aminoacidurias do not impair growth, development, or maturation in utero or interfere with parturition. (This is the result of the maternal blood supply, which defines the amino acid balance in utero.) No physical sign betrays their presence in the early months of life. The only possible means of detection is by the screening of all newborns. Table 37-1 indicates the relative frequency of these diseases and Table 37-2 summarizes the practical tests for their identification.

Three aminoacidopathies of the late infantile and early childhood period—PKU, tyrosinemia, and Hartnup disease—are described here because of their clinical importance and because they exemplify different types of biochemical defects. Reference is also made to certain other aminoacidurias, described in the first part of this chapter, which, like Hartnup disease, are associated with intermittent ataxia. Only passing comments are made about the other aminoacidurias, which are exceedingly rare or have only an uncertain effect on the nervous system. A detailed account of these disorders can be found in the monograph of Scriver and coworkers.

The Phenylketonurias (Phenylalanine Hydroxylase Deficiency)

Apart from being the most frequent of the aminoacidurias, this entity has a special historical significance. Since its discovery by Følling in 1934, it has remained the classic example of an aminoaciduria and illustrates three principles of medical genetics: first, it is inherited as an autosomal recessive trait; second, it exemplifies Garrod's cardinal principle of gene action, in which genetic factors specify chemical reactions as well as biochemical individuality; third, PKU is expressed only in an environment that contains an abundance of L-phenylalanine. Thus, as predicted by Galton, the ultimate phenotype is a product of "nature and nurture" (Scriver and Clow).

One must refer to the phenylketonurias in the plural, for there are (1) the usual type and several mild and severe variants thereof, in all of which mental retardation is invariable if the disease is not treated early in life; (2) other types, presumably allelic mutations, in which there is hyperphenylalaninemia without PKU and without effect on the nervous system; and (3) a rare adult type with a progressive spastic paraparesis or without neurologic manifestations. Also there are a small number of patients (3 percent in our series) in whom a lowering of the hyperphenylalaninemia does not prevent the progression of the neurologic lesion.

At birth, the typical PKU infant is believed to have a normal nervous system. The disease appears later, only after long exposure of the nervous system to phenylalanine (PA), because the homozygous infant lacks the means of protecting the nervous system. However, if the mother is homozygous with high PA levels in the blood during pregnancy, the CNS is damaged in utero and the heterozygous infant is mentally defective from birth.

In the classic form of PKU, the *impairment of psychomotor development* can usually be recognized in the latter part of the first year, when expected performance lags. By 5 to 6 years in an untreated child, when the IQ can be estimated, it is usually less than 20, occasionally 20 to 50, and exceptionally above 50. *Hyperactivity*, aggressivity, self-injurious behavior—including severe injury to the eyes, clumsy gait, fine tremor of the hands, poor coordination, odd posturings, *repetitious digital mannerisms* and other so-called rhythmias, and slight corticospinal tract signs stand out as the main clinical manifestations. Athetosis, dystonia, and frank cerebellar ataxia have been described but must be rare. Also, seizures occur in a small minority of severely affected patients, taking the form at first of flexor spasms and later of absence and grand mal attacks.

The majority of PKU patients are blue-eyed and fair in skin and hair color, and their skin is rough and dry and subject to eczema. A musty body odor (because of phenylacetic acid excretion) can often be detected. Two-thirds are slightly microcephalic. The fundi are normal, and there is no visceral enlargement or skeletal abnormality.

There are some people living in the community with asymptomatic PKU and normal intelligence. Instances of PKU in which the symptoms are of adult onset are rare but of interest because of the entirely unexpected diagnosis. The few such cases reported and summarized by Kasim and colleagues, with a case of their own, developed a progressive spastic paraparesis, some with mild dementia. The phenylalanine levels were at values that reflect total or partial enzyme deficiency.

The finding of *high levels of serum phenylalanine* (above 15 mg/dL) and of *phenylpyruvic acid in the blood, CSF, and urine* is diagnostic of PKU. The level is normal at birth and rises only after the first few days. But screening by the Guthrie (ferric chloride) test will reliably identify the patient at risk. The addition of 3 to 5 drops of 10 percent ferric chloride to 1 mL of urine is a simple and informative test. It yields an emerald-green color that reaches peak intensity in 3 to 4 min and fades in 20 to 40 min. In contrast, the green-brown color in the urine of patients with histidinemia is permanent. In maple syrup urine disease, the ferric chloride test gives a navy-blue color; propionic and methylmalonic acidemia and either ketones or salicylates in the urine yield a purple color.

The fundamental biochemical abnormality is a deficiency of the hepatic enzyme PA hydroxylase; the failure of conversion of PA to tyrosine results in the excretion of phenylpyruvic acid by affected individuals. The precise step that is faulty in the complex phenylalanine hydroxylating reaction is still unknown.

Pathologic examination shows poor staining of myelin in the cerebral hemispheres. This can be visualized by MRI in untreated children. Another instructive feature is that the pigmented nuclei (substantia nigra, locus ceruleus, dorsal vagal motor) fail to acquire dark coloration because of a block in the production of neuromelanin. Reduction in size of cortical neurons and their dendritic arborizations is said to be demonstrable in some cases.

Treatment If instituted in infancy, diets low but not totally lacking in PA can improve intellectual development (blood level should be maintained at 5 to 10 mg/dL). Careful dietary management may result in completely normal intellectual development. Once the neurologic picture unfolds, diet has little or no effect on the mental status but may improve behavior. Prolonged dietary treatment has many untoward effects and should be supervised by physicians and nutritionists experienced in its use; if too restricted, it may retard growth. This is particularly important, as it has been shown that intellectual impairment is greatest among children who were the earliest to abandon their diets, permitting the PA concentration to rise above 15 mg/dL, and least in children who maintained dietary control the longest (Holtzman et al). Continued dietary treatment is probably necessary, but the degree of restriction of PA may be relaxed once the nervous system is fully developed. The precise degree of allowed restriction of dietary PA restriction is not known but many children, having been raised on a low PA diet, will have little or no difficulty in maintaining the restrictions into adulthood.

With the widespread screening for PKU and the initiation of dietary control during early postnatal life, this metabolic brain disease has virtually disappeared in the New England states. Treated women who reach childbearing age should be particularly careful about dietary restriction, because high levels of phenylalanine are harmful to the normal fetus. Mild cases of PKU have been successfully treated with the cofactor tetrahydrobiopterin (Muntau et al).

The late forms of maple syrup urine disease, and hydroxyprolinemia evolve in much the same fashion as PKU and raise similar problems in diagnosis and therapy. Histidinemia can be detected by screening but is now considered a benign biochemical variant.

A small number of infants have a variant of PKU in which a restricted PA diet does not prevent neurologic involvement. In some such infants, a dystonic extrapyramidal rigidity ("stiff-baby syndrome") has appeared as early as the neonatal period, and, according to Allen and coworkers, it responds to biopterin. Such infants have normal levels of PA hydroxylase in the liver. The defect is a failure to synthesize the active cofactor tetrahydrobiopterin, because of either an insufficiency of dihydropteridine reductase or an inability to synthesize biopterin (see "Biopterin Deficiency"). The urinary metabolites of catecholamines and serotonin are reduced and are not responsive to low-PA diets. There is some evidence that the underlying neurotransmitter fault can be corrected by L-dopa and by 5-hydroxytryptophan (Scriver and Clow).

Hereditary Tyrosinemia (Oculocutaneous Tyrosinemia; Richner-Hanhart Disease)

This is a rare, predominantly dermatologic aminoacidopathy, but in approximately one-half of the infants there is a mild to moderate degree of mental retardation. Also, as in some other aminoacidopathies, there may be self-mutilation and incoordination of limb movements. Language defects are prominent. Toward the end of the first or second year of life, lacrimation, photophobia, and redness of the eyes (because of corneal erosions) appear. Neovascularization of the corneas and opacification follow. Palmar and plantar keratosis with hyperhidrosis and pain are frequently present as a result of an inflammatory reaction to deposits of crystalline tyrosine (also the cause of the corneal changes). Elevated tyrosine in the blood (>0.18 mM) and urine is diagnostic. The most severe form (type 1) is caused by a mutation in the gene (*FAH*) that codes for fumarylacetoacetate hydrolase, the final enzymatic step in tyrosine metabolism, a deficiency of which results in the accumulation of tyrosine and its metabolites.

A low-tyrosine and low-PA diet, optimized to allow growth and development, has resulted in rapid amelioration of symptoms but must be started early. Retinoids given orally improve the skin lesions. Neonatal tyrosinemia can cause liver failure and early death. This disease can be distinguished from the Cross syndrome (albinism with mental retardation, growth impairment, spastic weakness, and alkalosis) and from the Waardenburg ocular albinism syndrome (white forelock, hypertelorism, deafness). For a detailed discussion of the albinism syndromes, see the article by Oetting and King.

Tyrosine Hydroxylase Deficiency (TH Mutation)

This disease causes a progressive infantile encephalopathy; it is of special interest because tyrosine is the precursor of L-dopa and the other catecholamines. Levels of these chemical substances in the brain are greatly reduced. As a result, the encephalopathy takes the form mainly of fluctuating extrapyramidal signs in combination with ocular and vegetative symptoms. L-Dopa causes some improvement in the motor symptoms (see Hoffmann et al). This disease has similarities to juvenile dopa-responsive dystonia, which is exquisitely sensitive to L-dopa treatment (as discussed in Chap. 39) and to the deficiency of L-amino decarboxylase, described above, which also causes low levels of catecholamines and a movement disorder.

Hartnup Disease (SLC6A19 Mutation)

This amino acid disorder, named after the family in which it was first observed, is probably transmitted in an autosomal recessive pattern. The babies are normal at birth. The onset of symptoms is in late infancy or early childhood. The clinical features consist of an *intermittent red, scaly rash over the face, neck, hands, and legs*, resembling that of pellagra. It is often combined with an episodic personality disorder in the form of *emotional lability*, uncontrolled temper, and confusional-hallucinatory psychosis; *episodic cerebellar ataxia* (unsteady gait, intention tremor, and dysarthria); and, occasionally, spasticity, vertigo, nystagmus, ptosis, and diplopia. Attacks of disease are triggered by exposure to sunlight, emotional stress, and sulfonamide drugs and last for about 2 weeks, followed by variable periods of relative normalcy. The frequency of attacks diminishes with maturation, but some children suffer retarded growth and development with a mild persistent mental retardation.

The metabolic faults are the result of a transport error of neutral amino acids across renal tubules, with excretion of greatly increased amounts of these amino acids in the urine and feces. In particular, there is the excretion of large amounts of indicans, mainly indoxyl sulfate, particularly after oral L-tryptophan loading, and an abnormally high excretion of nonhydroxylated indole metabolites. Impaired intestinal transport of tryptophan and loss in the urine reduce its availability for the synthesis of niacin and accounts for the pellagrous skin changes. The pathologic basis of the disease is undetermined. It must be differentiated from the large number of intermittent and progressive cerebellar ataxias of childhood, described below.

Treatment consists of avoiding exposure to sunlight and to sulfonamide drugs. Because of the similarities between pellagra and Hartnup disease, the usual practice is to give nicotinamide in doses of 50 to 300 mg daily. The skin lesions disappear and there are reports of subsidence of ataxia and psychotic behavior. However, the results of treatment are inconsistent. Possibly a better response is obtained by the administration of L-tryptophan ethyl ester in doses of 20 mg/kg tid.

Other Metabolic Diseases With Episodic or Persistent Ataxia, Seizures, and Mental Retardation

In addition to Hartnup disease, a number of other metabolic diseases give rise to intermittent episodes of ataxia during early childhood. These are (1) mild forms of maple syrup urine disease and the congenital hyperammonemias (type II hyperammonemia, citrullinemia, argininosuccinic aciduria, hyperornithinemia), described in an earlier part of the chapter; (2) subacute necrotizing encephalomyelopathy (Leigh disease), described further on; (3) hyperalaninemia and hyperpyruvic acidemia (Lonsdale et al; Blass et al); and (4) autosomal dominant, acetazolamide-responsive ataxia that may have its onset in childhood but usually appears later; and (5) familial hypobetalipoproteinemia—Bassen-Kornzweig disease.

In all of these conditions, the ataxia, which is of cerebellar type, is variable from time to time and may follow a burst of seizures (such as occur in argininosuccinic aciduria). The seizures are treated with antiepileptic drugs, which may at first be held responsible for the ataxia. In time, however, it becomes apparent that the ataxia lasts a week or two and bears no relation to the anticonvulsant therapy. Indeed, seizures and ataxia are both a result of the common biochemical abnormality. Between attacks, in all the intermittent ataxias, the patient's movements are relatively normal, but most of the affected children have learning disabilities to a varying degree.

Progressive Cerebellar Ataxia of Early Childhood

The differentiation among the childhood ataxias is difficult. The problem is twofold—first, to be certain that ataxia exists and, second, to differentiate cerebellar ataxia from the sensory ataxia of peripheral nerve disease and from generalized tremor and polymyoclonus. Because cerebellar ataxia is more a disorder of voluntary than of postural movements, its presence usually cannot be determined with certainty until intentional (projected) movements become part of the child's repertoire of motor activity. As indicated in Chap. 28, the earliest signs become manifest in the arms when the infant reaches for an object and brings it to his mouth or transfers it from hand to hand. A jerky, wavering, tremulous movement then appears; in sitting, titubation of the head and a tremor of the trunk may be apparent. Once walking begins, apart from the usual clumsiness of the toddler, there is a similar incoordination of movement. Sensory ataxia is always difficult to distinguish but is rare at this age and usually accompanied by weakness and absence of tendon reflexes. By the fourth or fifth year, when more detailed sensory testing becomes possible, the presence or absence of a proprioceptive disturbance and a Romberg sign can be demonstrated.

The group of persistent and progressive cerebellar ataxias is heterogeneous and of varied etiology; some of them merge with Friedreich ataxia, Levy-Roussy neuropathy, and other adolescent–adult degenerative hereditary ataxias. These disorders are discussed in Chap. 39. There are many other childhood ataxias that probably belong in the category of degenerative disease, some in which cerebellar ataxia is the most prominent disorder and in which other neurologic abnormalities are more prominent. To describe each in detail would be impractical in a book on the principles of neurology; consequently, the non-Friedreich ataxias are only tabulated here.

1. Cerebellar ataxia with diplegia, hypotonia, and mental retardation (also called *atonic diplegia* of Foerster); this is a form of cerebral palsy.
2. Agenesis of the cerebellum: early cerebellar ataxia (with or without mental retardation) and episodic hyperventilation; this group included the selective agenesis of the vermis—Joubert syndrome.
3. Cerebellar ataxia with cataracts and oligophrenia: onset from childhood (mainly) to as late as adult years (Marinesco-Sjögren disease).
4. Familial cerebellar ataxia and retinal degeneration (Behr disease).
5. Familial cerebellar ataxia with cataracts and ophthalmoplegia or with cataracts and mental as well as physical retardation.
6. Familial cerebellar ataxia with mydriasis.
7. Familial cerebellar ataxia with deafness and blindness and a similar combination, called retinocochleodentate degeneration, involving the loss of neurons in these three structures.
8. Familial cerebellar ataxia with choreoathetosis, corticospinal tract signs, and mental and motor retardation.

In none of the syndromes mentioned above has a biochemical abnormality been established, so their metabolic nature is a matter of speculation. However, disorders of the electron transport chain can, on occasion, present as the Marinesco-Sjögren phenotype, mentioned above.

The persistent cerebellar ataxias of childhood in which a metabolic fault or gene defect has been demonstrated are as follows:

1. Refsum disease
2. Abetalipoproteinemia (Bassen-Kornzweig syndrome)
3. Ataxia-telangiectasia (See Chap. 38)
4. Galactosemia
5. Friedreich ataxia

Bassen-Kornzweig syndrome (onset more often in late than in early childhood) is described in the following section of this chapter. Ataxia-telangiectasia is described below.

Generally, it is not difficult to differentiate these diseases from the acquired postinfectious variety that occurs predominantly in children (see Chap. 36).

Metachromatic Leukodystrophy (MLD, Arylsulfatase Deficiency)

This is another of the lysosomal (sphingolipid) storage diseases (see Tables 37-3 and 37-6). The abnormality is the mutation of the gene for enzyme arylsulfatase A, which prevents the conversion of sulfatide to cerebroside (a major component of myelin) and results in an accumulation of the former. The disease is transmitted as an autosomal recessive trait and usually becomes manifest between the first and fourth years of life (variants have their onset in the congenital period, in late childhood, and even in adult life). Variability of gene mutation accounts for the different forms. The so-called O-type mutation causes a lack of active gene product and of the corresponding enzyme; the R-type mutation results in low levels. The infantile form is associated with two copies of the O gene, the juvenile form, with either O or R, and the adult form is usually from two copies of R. Another genetic classification system denominates I and A alleles and differentiates the types of diseases by age of onset and residual enzyme activity.

The disease in this age group is characterized clinically by progressive impairment of motor function (gait disorder, spasticity) in combination with reduced output of speech and mental regression. At first the tendon reflexes are usually brisk, but later, as the peripheral nerves become more involved, the tendon reflexes are decreased and eventually lost. Or, there may be variable hypotonia and areflexia from the beginning, or spasticity may be present throughout the illness, but with hyporeflexia and slowed conduction velocities. Signs of mental regression may be apparent from the onset or appear after the motor disorder has become established. Later there is impairment of vision, sometimes with squint and nystagmus; intention tremor in the arms and dysarthria; dysphagia and drooling; and optic atrophy (one-third of patients), sometimes with *grayish degeneration around the maculae*. Seizures are rare, and there are no somatic abnormalities. The head size is usually normal, but rarely there is macrocephaly. Progression to a bedridden quadriplegic state without speech or comprehension occurs over a 1- to 3-year period, somewhat more slowly in late-onset types. The CSF protein is elevated.

There is widespread degeneration of myelinated fibers in the cerebrum (Fig. 37-5), cerebellum, spinal cord, and peripheral nerves. The presence of metachromatic granules in glia cells and engorged macrophages is characteristic and enables the diagnosis to be made from a biopsy of a peripheral nerve. The stored material, *sulfatide*, stains brown-orange rather than purple with aniline dyes. Sulfatides are also PAS-positive in frozen sections.

The diagnostic laboratory findings, in addition to the MRI and histologic changes, are the *elevated CSF protein* (75 to 250 mg/dL) and a *marked increase in sulfatide in urine* and an *absence of arylsulfatase A* in white blood cells, in serum, and in cultured fibroblasts. Assays of arylsulfatase A activity in cultured fibroblasts and amniocytes permit the identification of carriers and prenatal diagnosis of the disease but a pseudodeficiency of the enzyme is known (the *Pd* allelic variant). In this condition, measured enzyme activity is 10 percent of normal, but no clinical manifestations result.

Treatment with enzyme replacement or bone marrow transplantation is being tried. Marrow transplant appears to be of less benefit once the patient becomes symptomatic, but it may be useful early in the disease and in the treatment of an asymptomatic sibling of an index case.

The differential diagnosis of this leukodystrophy includes neuroaxonal dystrophy (see below), cases of early-onset inherited polyneuropathy, late-onset Krabbe

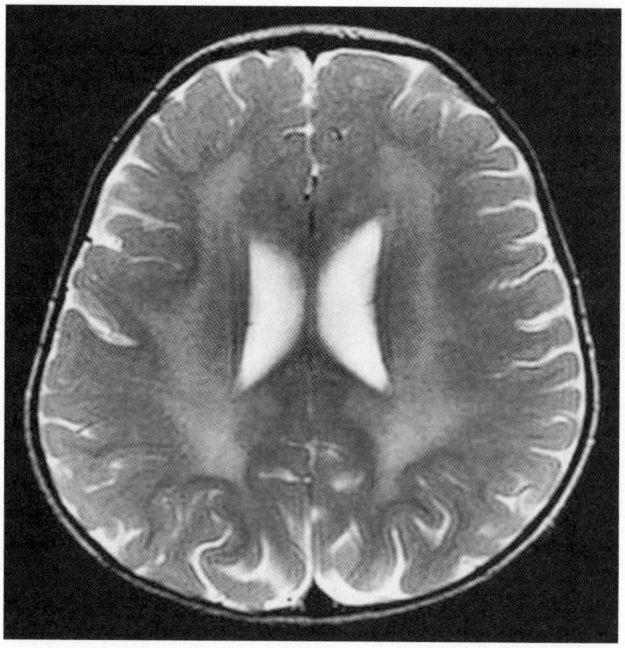

Figure 37-5. Metachromatic leukodystrophy. Axial T2-weighted MRI of a 2-year-old girl with developmental regression and EMG evidence of diffuse motor and sensory demyelination. There is abnormal symmetric central white matter hyperintensity with sparing of the subcortical arcuate fibers. (Image courtesy of Drs. Edward Yang and Sanjay Prabhu.)

disease, and childhood forms of Gaucher disease and Niemann-Pick disease. A *variant of metachromatic leukoencephalopathy*, caused by a deficiency of the isoenzymes of arylsulfatase A, B, and C, was described by Austin in 1973 and called *multiple sulfatase deficiency*. The neurologic manifestations resemble those of metachromatic leukodystrophy but, in addition, there are facial and skeletal changes similar to those of a mucopolysaccharidosis. Deafness, hepatic enlargement, ichthyosis, and beaking of lumbar vertebrae are additional findings in some cases. Metachromatic material is found in the urinary sediment. Pathologically, in addition to metachromasia of degenerating white matter in cerebrum and peripheral nerve, there may be storage material (sulfated glycolipids), like that found in the gangliosidoses in neurons as well as in liver, gallbladder, and kidney. Granules are demonstrable in neutrophilic leukocytes. There has also been described a state of "arylsulfatase pseudodeficiency," which exists as a polymorphism in approximately 7 percent of Europeans and makes the point that low enzyme levels alone are insufficient to be expressed as a phenotype of metachromatic leukodystrophy.

Forms of metachromatic leukodystrophy developing in adult years are discussed further on.

Neuroaxonal Dystrophy (Degeneration; PLA2G6 Mutation)

This is a rare disease, inherited as an autosomal recessive trait. In the largest group of cases (77 collected by Aicardi and Castelein), the onset was near the beginning of the second year in 50 patients and before the third year in all instances. The clinical constellation comprised psychomotor deterioration (loss of ability to sit, stand, and speak), marked hypotonia but brisk reflexes and Babinski signs, and progressive blindness with optic atrophy but normal retinae. Seizures, myoclonus, and extrapyramidal signs were rare. Loss of sensation was found later in some cases. Terminally, bulbar signs, spasticity, and decerebrate rigidity often supervened. The course was relentlessly progressive, with fatal issue in a decorticate state in 3 to 8 years. There were no abnormalities of the liver and spleen and no facial or skeletal changes.

Pathologic examination reveals eosinophilic spheroids of swollen axoplasm in the posterior columns and nuclei of Goll and Burdach and in the Clarke column, substantia nigra, subthalamic nuclei, central nuclei of brainstem, and cerebral cortex. There is cerebellar atrophy, affecting the granule cell layer predominantly, and increased iron-containing pigment in the basal ganglia (like that observed in the PANK mutation type of iron deposition discussed in a later section).

The CT and CSF are normal, and there are no biochemical or blood cell abnormalities. MRI may show decreased signal intensity of the pallidum bilaterally corresponding to iron deposition. Some reports are confusing in reporting an area of necrosis around a high signal that is characteristic of the aforementioned PANK mutation, with which it has overlapping clinical and pathologic features. After the age of 2 years, however, the EEG shows characteristic high-amplitude fast rhythms (16 to 22 Hz). Evoked responses may be abnormal. Nerve conduction velocities are normal despite EMG evidence of denervation. The diagnosis can be reliably established during life by electron microscopic examination of skin and conjunctival nerves, which show the characteristic spheroids within axons.

There is a later-onset form of the disease in which the course is more protracted and the neurologic manifestations (rigidity and spasticity, cerebellar ataxia, and myoclonus) are more pronounced. In these cases the mental regression is slow. Vision may be retained but retinal degeneration has been documented. Some of the late-onset cases are indistinguishable from Hallervorden-Spatz disease.

In early infantile forms there is a mutation in a lysosomal hydrolase. The primary mutation in the infantile form is in the *PLA2G6* gene.

Late Infantile and Early Childhood Gaucher Disease

As stated earlier, Gaucher disease usually develops in early infancy, but some cases, so-called Gaucher disease type III, may begin in childhood, between 3 and 8 years of age. The clinical picture is variable and combines features of infantile Gaucher disease—such as abducens palsies, dysphagia, trismus, rigidity of the limbs, and dementia—with features of the late childhood–early adult form, such as palsies of horizontal gaze, diffuse myoclonus, generalized seizures, and a chronic course. The diagnosis is established by the finding of splenomegaly, Gaucher cells, glucocerebroside storage, and deficient activity of glucocerebrosidase in leukocytes or cultured fibroblasts.

Late Infantile–Early Childhood Niemann-Pick Disease

Niemann-Pick disease is a subacute or chronic neurovisceral storage disease with early signs of hepatosplenomegaly and later signs (2 to 4 years) of neurologic involvement. These later-onset types have been termed C and D, and formerly, III and IV, to differentiate them from infantile forms discussed earlier. The neurologic disorder consists of progressive dementia, dysarthria, ataxia, rarely extrapyramidal signs (choreoathetosis), and *paralysis of horizontal and vertical gaze*, the latter being a distinguishing feature of the later-onset types. On attempting to look to the side, some of the patients make head-thrusting movements of the same type that one observes in ataxia-telangiectasia and the oculomotor apraxia of Cogan. Lateral eye movements are full on passive movement of the head (oculocephalic maneuver). Convergence is also deficient. A subtype called *juvenile dystonic lipidosis* is characterized by extrapyramidal symptoms and paralysis of vertical eye movements. The syndrome of the "sea-blue histiocyte" (liver, spleen, and bone marrow contain histiocytes with sea-blue granules)—in which there is retardation in mental and motor development, grayish macular degeneration, and, in rare cases, posterior column and pyramidal degeneration—may be another variant.

The diagnosis is made by bone marrow biopsy, which discloses vacuolated macrophages and sea-blue histiocytes, and by measuring the defect in cholesterol esterification in cultured fibroblasts.

Late Infantile–Childhood G_{M1} Gangliosidosis (GLB1 Mutation)

In type 2 or so-called juvenile G_{M1} gangliosidosis, the onset is between 12 and 24 months, with survival for 3 to 10 years. The first sign is usually *difficulty in walking*, with frequent falls, followed by awkwardness of arm movements, loss of speech, severe mental regression, gradual development of spastic quadriparesis and pseudobulbar palsy (dysarthria, dysphagia, drooling), and seizures. Retinal changes are variable—usually they are absent—but macular red spots may be seen at the age of 10 to 12 years; vision is usually retained, but squints (comitant) are common. There is a facial dysmorphism resembling that of the Hurler syndrome, and the liver and spleen are enlarged. Important laboratory findings are hypoplasia of the thoracolumbar vertebral bodies, mild hypoplasia of the acetabula, and the presence in the bone marrow of histiocytes with clear vacuoles or wrinkled cytoplasm. As noted in the discussion of Tay-Sachs disease, leukocytes and cultured skin fibroblasts show a *deficiency* or absence of *beta-galactosidase* activity. G_{M1} ganglioside accumulates in the cerebral neurons.

The Neuronal Ceroid Lipofuscinoses (Batten Disease)

Four types of lipofuscinoses have been identified, defined largely by the age of onset: Santavuori-Haltia Finnish infantile type, Jansky-Bielschowsky early childhood type, Vogt-Spielmeyer juvenile type, and Kufs adult type. All except a few adult cases are autosomal recessive. The storage material in neuronal cytoplasm consists of two pigmented lipids, presumably ceroid and lipofuscin, which are cross-linked polymers of polyunsaturated fatty acids and have the property of autofluorescence. At least 20 gene loci are implicated in the ceroid lipofuscinoses, for most of which the mutation has been identified. All the infantile forms and one of the juvenile forms of the disease are due to of mutations affecting the lysosomal enzyme palmitoyl–protein thioesterase. Other lysosomal enzymes are abnormal in the remaining juvenile and in the adult forms.

In the *Santavuori-Haltia form* of the disease, infants from 3 to 18 months of age, after a normal period of development, undergo psychomotor regression with ataxia, hypotonia, and *widespread myoclonus*. There are retinal changes with extinction of the electroretinogram, slowing of the EEG with spike and slow-wave discharges, and eventually an isoelectric record. Within a few years these patients become blind, develop spastic quadriplegia and microcephaly, and succumb.

In the *Jansky-Bielschowsky type*, the onset of symptoms is between 2 and 4 years, after normal or slightly slow earlier development, with survival to 4 to 8 years of age. Usually the first neurologic manifestations are seizures (petit mal or grand mal) and *myoclonic jerks* evoked by proprioceptive and other sensory stimuli, including voluntary movement and emotional excitement. Incoordination, tremor, ataxia, and spastic weakness with lively tendon reflexes and Babinski signs, deterioration of mental faculties, and dysarthria proceed to dementia and eventually to mutism. In patients with relatively late onset, a progressive dementia is the cardinal manifestation. Visual failure may occur early in some cases because of *retinal degeneration* (of rods and cones) with pigmentary deposits, but in others vision is normal. The electroretinogram becomes isoelectric if vision is affected. Abnormal inclusions (translucent vacuoles) are seen in 10 to 30 percent of circulating lymphocytes, and azurophilic granules in neutrophils. High-voltage EEG spikes are induced by photic stimuli. Only in early-onset cases is there microcephaly.

Pathologic examination shows neuronal loss in the cerebral and cerebellar cortices (granule and Purkinje cells), and curvilinear storage particles and osmophilic granules are visible in the remaining neurons. Inclusions are also observed in cutaneous nerve twigs and endothelial cells of blood vessels, findings that permit diagnosis during life by electron microscopy of skin, conjunctival, or rectal mucosal biopsies.

In many patients with lipofuscinoses, *diagnosis* can be confirmed by demonstrating the presence of one of several recently identified gene mutations. There are no definite markers for the group in blood or urine, but in some patients a structural component of mitochondria is excreted in excess (the so-called C-fragment).

In the differential diagnosis, one must consider late infantile G_{M1} gangliosidosis, idiopathic epilepsy, Alpers disease, and other forms of neuronal ceroid-lipofuscinosis.

The lipofuscinoses of later onset—the Vogt-Spielmeyer (juvenile) type and the Kufs (adult) type—are discussed further on. There is no treatment for the basic disease process but approaches involving gene therapy are being explored.

Mucopolysaccharidoses (Table 37-7)

This is a group of diseases in which the storage of lipid in neurons is combined with that of polysaccharides in connective tissues. As a consequence there is a conjunction of neurologic and skeletal abnormalities that is virtually unique. The nervous system may also be involved secondarily as a result of skeletal deformities and thickening and hyperplasia of connective tissue at the base of the brain, leading to obliteration of the subarachnoid space and obstructive hydrocephalus or compression of the cervical cord. The prevalence of mucopolysaccharides as a whole is approximately 1 per 8,000 births, according to Meikle and colleagues. Depending on the degree of visceral-skeletal and neurologic changes, at least 7 distinct clinical subtypes are recognized (see Table 37-7).

The basic abnormality is an enzymatic defect that prevents the degradation of acid mucopolysaccharides (now called *glycosaminoglycans*). The latter can be measured and are increased in serum, leukocytes, or cultured fibroblasts. The storage is, again, within lysosomes in the brain, spinal cord, heart, viscera, bone, and connective tissue. All forms of the disease except the Hunter syndrome, which is sex-linked, are inherited in an autosomal recessive pattern. The studies of Neufeld and Muenzer indicate that each type of mucopolysaccharidosis is caused by a defect in a different enzyme.

Hurler Disease (MPS I, IDUA Mutation)

This, the classic form, also known as MPS I, begins clinically toward the end of the first year. *Mental retardation* is severe, and *skeletal abnormalities* are prominent (dwarfism; gargoyle facies; large head with synostosis of longitudinal suture; kyphosis; broad hands with short, stubby fingers; flexion contractures at knees and elbows). Conductive deafness and corticospinal signs are usually present. Protuberant abdomen, hernias, *enlarged liver and spleen*, valvular heart disease, chronic rhinitis, recurrent respiratory infections, and *corneal opacities* complete the picture. The biochemical abnormalities consist of the accumulation of *dermatan* and *heparan sulfate* (glycosaminoglycans) in the tissues and their *excretion in the urine*, probably as a consequence of absence of activity of α-L-iduronidase. Also, there is an increase in the ganglioside content in nerve cells of the brains of these patients. In the milder Scheie (MPS V) variant of Hurler disease, intelligence and life span are normal.

Treatment Enzyme replacement therapy (laronidase) is now available. The enzymes are produced with recombinant technology and are successful where previous attempts with enzymes delivered by white cell or other infusions had been ineffective. Hematopoietic stem cell bone marrow transplantation (cord blood from unrelated donors) has also been used (see Staba et al). To be effective, treatment must commence before the accumulation of glycosaminoglycans and neurologic decline. The eye and bone deterioration associated with Hurler disease is not improved. In children with the milder *Scheie form* and those with CNS involvement, bone marrow transplantation is not helpful and enzyme replacement is recommended. Enzyme treatment is also being tried concurrently with bone marrow transplantation in early cases. These approaches have not been effective in the Hunter or the Sanfilippo diseases, discussed below.

Hunter Disease (MPS II, IDS Mutation)

Unlike the Hurler and other types, the Hunter form (MPS II) is transmitted as an *X-linked trait*. The Hurler

Table 37-7

CLASSIFICATION OF THE MUCOPOLYSACCHARIDOSES

NUMBER	EPONYM	CLINICAL MANIFESTATIONS	ENZYME DEFICIENCY	GLYCOSAMINOGLYCAN
MPS I[a]	Hurler	Corneal clouding, severe skeletal changes and MR, organomegaly, heart disease	α-L-Iduronidase	Dermatan sulfate, heparan sulfate
MPS II	Hunter	Dysostosis, normal corneas, MR, joint stiffness, hydrocephalus, short stature, organomegaly	Iduronate sulfatase	Dermatan sulfate, heparan sulfate
MPS III	Sanfilippo	MR, mild or absent somatic changes, hyperactivity, hepatosplenomegaly	Heparan *N*-sulfatase	Heparan sulfate
MPS IV	Morquio	Distinctive skeletal abnormalities, slight corneal clouding, odontoid hypoplasia, normal intelligence, hepatomegaly	Galactose 6-sulfatase	Keratan sulfate, chondroitin 6-sulfate
MPS V	No longer used			
MPS VI	Maroteaux-Lamy	Dysostosis, corneal clouding, normal intelligence, spinal cord compression, organomegaly	*N*-acetylgalactosamine, 4-sulfatase (arylsulfatase B)	Dermatan sulfate
MPS VII	Sly	Dysostosis, hepatosplenomegaly, wide range of severity, corneal clouding	β-Glucuronidase	Dermatan sulfate, heparan sulfate, chondroitin 4-sulfate

[a]Less-severe phenotypes are known as Scheie or Hurler-Scheie syndromes.
MR, mental retardation.
Source: Modified by permission from Neufeld and Muenzer.

and Hunter syndromes are clinically alike except that the Hunter form is milder: mental retardation is less severe than in the Hurler type, deafness is less common, and *corneal clouding is usually absent*. Probably there are two forms of the syndrome—a more severe one, in which the patients do not survive beyond their midteens, and a less severe form with relatively normal intelligence and survival to middle age. Excessive amounts of dermatan and heparan sulfate are excreted in the urine. The basic abnormality is a *deficiency of iduronate sulfatase*.

Sanfilippo Disease (MPS III, Several Genes Implicated)

This form, or MPS III, expresses itself clinically between 2 and 3 years of age, with progressive intellectual deterioration. The patients are of short stature, but in other respects the physical changes are fewer and less severe than in the Hunter and Hurler syndromes. Three and possibly four types of Sanfilippo disease, designated A, B, C, and D, are distinguished on the basis of their enzymatic defects (Neufeld and Muenzer). All subtypes are phenotypically similar, and all of them may excrete excessive amounts of heparan sulfate in the urine.

Morquio Disease (MPS IV, GALNS and GLB1 Mutations)

This form of the disease, MPS IV, is characterized by marked *dwarfism* and *osteoporosis*. Skeletal deformity and compression of the spinal cord and medulla are constant threats because of hypoplasia of the odontoid process and atlantoaxial dislocation and thickening of the dura around the cervical cord and inferior surface of the cerebellum. Intelligence is affected only slightly or not at all. *Corneal opacities may be present*. Patients excrete large amounts of keratan sulfate in the urine; two types of enzymatic deficiencies have been identified (Neufeld and Muenzer).

Maroteaux-Lamy Disease (MPS VI, ARSB Mutation)

This syndrome, MPS VI, includes severe skeletal deformities (short stature, anteriorly beaked vertebrae) but *normal intelligence*. Several patients observed by our colleagues have had a cervical pachymeningitis with spinal cord compression and hydrocephalus during adult life. Spinal cord function improved with cervical decompression and the hydrocephalus with ventriculoatrial shunting (Young et al). Hepatosplenomegaly is often present. Large amounts of dermatan sulfate are excreted in the urine, as a result of an *arylsulfatase B deficiency*.

β-Glucuronidase Deficiency (Sly Disease, MPS VII, GUSB Mutation)

This (MPS VII) is a rare type of mucopolysaccharidosis, the clinical features of which have yet to be sharply delineated. Short stature, progressive thoracolumbar gibbus, hepatosplenomegaly, and the bony changes of dysostosis multiplex (as in the Hurler type) are the main clinical features. There is excessive excretion of dermatan and heparan sulfate, the result of a deficiency of β-glucuronidase. Attempts to treat the mucopolysaccharidoses by enzyme replacement therapy, bone marrow transplantation, and gene transfer are in progress. None of these is far enough along to determine its efficacy.

Mucolipidoses and Other Diseases of Complex Carbohydrates (Sialidoses; Oligosaccharidoses) (See Table 37-3)

Several diseases have been described in which there is an abnormal accumulation of mucopolysaccharides, sphingolipids, and glycolipids in visceral, mesenchymal, and neural tissues, because of an α-*N*-acetylneuraminidase defect. In some types there is an additional deficiency of beta-galactosidase. All are autosomal recessive diseases that manifest many of the clinical features of Hurler disease, but—in contrast to the mucopolysaccharidoses—normal amounts of mucopolysaccharides are excreted in the urine. Frequently, G_{M1} gangliosidosis, described above, is also classified with the mucolipidoses. The other members of this category are synopsized below and in Table 37-3.

Mucolipidoses

At least three and possibly four closely related forms have been described. In mucolipidosis I (*lipomucopolysaccharidosis*), the morphologic features are those of gargoylism, with slowly progressive mental retardation. Cherry-red spots in the maculae, corneal opacities, and ataxia have been noted in some patients. Vacuolation of lymphocytes, marrow cells, hepatocytes, and Kupffer cells in the liver and metachromatic changes in the sural nerve have been described.

In *mucolipidosis II* (*I-cell disease*), the most common of the mucolipidoses, there is usually an early onset of psychomotor retardation, but in some cases this does not appear until the second or third decade of life. *Abnormal facies* and *periosteal thickening (dysostosis multiplex*, like that of G_{M1} gangliosidosis and Hurler disease) are characteristic. *Gingival hyperplasia* is prominent, and the *liver* and *spleen are enlarged*; but deafness is not found and corneal opacities are slower to develop. Tonic-clonic seizures are frequent in older patients. In most cases, death from heart failure occurs by the third to eighth year. There is a typical vacuolation of lymphocytes, Kupffer cells, and cells of the renal glomeruli. Bone marrow cells are also vacuolated and contain refractile cytoplasmic granules (hence the designation *inclusion-cell*, or *I-cell, disease*). A deficiency of several lysosomal enzymes required for the catabolism of mucopolysaccharides, glycolipids, and glycoproteins have been found.

In *mucolipidosis III* (*pseudo-Hurler polydystrophy*), the biochemical abnormalities are like those of I-cell disease, but there are clinical differences. In the pseudo-Hurler type, symptoms do not appear until 2 years of age or later and are relatively mild. Retardation of growth, fine corneal opacities, and valvular heart disease are the major manifestations.

Yet another variant, mucolipidosis IV, has been described (see Tellez-Nagel et al). Here, clouding of the corneas is noticed soon after birth, and profound developmental retardation is evident by 1 year of age. Skeletal deformities, enlargement of liver and spleen, seizures, or other neurologic abnormalities are notably lacking. Ultrastructural examination of conjunctival and skin fibroblasts has demonstrated lysosomal inclusions of material similar to lipids and mucopolysaccharides that remain to be further characterized.

Mannosidosis

This is another rare hereditary disorder with poorly differentiated symptomatology but with dysmorphic features of broad nose, depressed bridge, thick lips, and protruding tongue. The onset is in the first 2 years, with *Hurler-like facial* and *skeletal deformities, mental retardation*, and slight motor disability. Corticospinal signs, loss of hearing, variable degrees of gingival hyperplasia, and spoke-like opacities of the lens (but no diffuse corneal clouding) may be present. The liver and spleen are enlarged in some cases. Radiographs show beaking of the vertebral bodies and poor trabeculation of long bones. Vacuolated lymphocytes and granulated leukocytes are present and aid in diagnosis. The urinary mucopolysaccharides are normal. *Mannosiduria is diagnostic*, caused by a defect in α-mannosidase. Mannose-containing oligosaccharides accumulate in nerve cells, spleen, liver, and leukocytes (see Kistler et al).

Fucosidosis

This also is a rare autosomal recessive disorder, with neurologic deterioration beginning usually at 12 to 15 months and progressing to spastic quadriplegia, decerebrate rigidity, severe psychomotor regression, and death within 4 to 6 years. *Hepatomegaly*, splenomegaly, enlarged salivary glands, thickened skin, excessive sweating, normal or typical gargoyle facies, *beaking of the vertebral bodies*, and vacuolated lymphocytes are the main features. A variant of this disease has been described with slower progression and survival into late childhood and adolescence and even into adult life (Ikeda et al). The latter type is characterized by mental and motor retardation, along with the corneal opacities, coarse facial features, skeletal deformities of gargoylism, and dermatologic changes of Fabry disease (angiokeratoma corporis diffusum), but no hepatosplenomegaly. The basic abnormality in both types is a lack of lysosomal L-fucosidase, resulting in accumulation of fucose-rich sphingolipids, glycoproteins, and oligosaccharides in cells of the skin, conjunctivae, and rectal mucosa.

Aspartylglycosaminuria

This disease is characterized by the early onset of psychomotor regression; delayed, inadequate speech; severe behavioral abnormalities (*bouts of hyperactivity* mixed with apathy and hypoactivity or psychotic manifestations); progressive dementia; clumsy movements; corticospinal signs; corneal clouding (rare); retinal abnormalities and cataracts; coarse facies including low bridge of the nose, epicanthi, thickening of the lips and skin; enlarged liver; and abdominal hernias in some. Radiographs show minimal *beaking of the vertebral bodies*, and the blood lymphocytes are vacuolated.

The pattern of inheritance in this entire group of diseases, as already stated, is probably autosomal recessive. Diagnostic methods applicable to amniotic fluid and cells are being developed so that prenatal diagnosis will be possible, prompted often by the occurrence of the disease in an earlier child. Neurons are vacuolated rather than stuffed with granules, much like the lymphocytes and liver cells. The specific biochemical abnormalities, as far as they are known, are listed in Table 37-3.

Cockayne Syndrome

This disorder is probably inherited as an autosomal recessive trait. The onset is in late infancy, after apparently normal earlier development. The main clinical findings are *stunting of growth*, evident by the second and third years; *photosensitivity of the skin*; microcephaly; *retinitis pigmentosa, cataracts*, blindness, and pendular nystagmus; nerve deafness; *delayed psychomotor* and speech development; spastic weakness and *ataxia of limbs* and gait; occasionally athetosis; amyotrophy with abolished reflexes and reduced nerve conduction velocities; wizened face, sunken eyes, prominent nose, prognathism, anhidrosis, and poor lacrimation (resembling progeria and bird-headed dwarfism). Some cases show calcification of the basal ganglia. The CSF is normal, and there are no diagnostic biochemical findings.

Pathologic examination reveals a small brain, striatal and cerebellar calcifications, leukodystrophy like that of Pelizaeus-Merzbacher disease, and a severe cerebellar cortical atrophy. The peripheral nerve changes are those of a primary segmental demyelination.

It is now apparent that Cockayne syndrome, like ataxia-telangiectasia, is a consequence of mutations in genes that mediate DNA repair. At least three different forms of Cockayne syndrome have been identified, each with a different underlying gene defect.

Other Metabolic Diseases of Late Infancy and Early Childhood

Globoid cell leukodystrophy (Krabbe), subacute necrotizing encephalomyelopathy (Leigh), and Gaucher disease may also begin in late infancy or early childhood. They are described in the preceding section of this chapter. Familial striatocerebellar calcification (Fahr disease) and Lesch-Nyhan disease may also become manifest in this age period, but they usually have a later onset and are therefore described with the diseases of later childhood in the section that follows.

This group of metabolic disorders presents many of the same diagnostic problems as those of early infancy. The flow chart in Fig. 37-4, which divides these disorders into dysmorphic, visceromegalic, and purely neurologic groups, is equally useful in the differential diagnosis of both age groups. As with the early infantile diseases, certain clusters of neurologic, skeletal, dermal, ophthalmic, and laboratory findings are highly distinctive and often permit the identification of a particular disease. These signs are listed below:

1. Evidence of involvement of peripheral nerves (weakness, hypotonia, areflexia, sensory loss, reduced conduction velocities) in conjunction with lesions of the CNS—metachromatic leukodystrophy, Krabbe leukodystrophy, neuroaxonal dystrophy, and Leigh disease (rare)
2. Ophthalmic signs
   a. Corneal clouding—several of the mucopolysaccharidoses (Hurler, Scheie, Morquio, Maroteaux-Lamy), mucolipidoses, tyrosinemia, aspartylglycosaminuria (rare)
   b. Cherry-red macular spot—G_{M2} gangliosidosis, G_{M1} gangliosidosis (half the cases), lipomucopolysaccharidosis, occasionally Niemann-Pick disease
   c. Retinal degeneration with pigmentary deposits—Jansky-Bielschowsky lipid storage disease, G_{M1} gangliosidosis, syndrome of sea-blue histiocytes
   d. Optic atrophy and blindness—metachromatic leukodystrophy, neuroaxonal dystrophy
   e. Cataracts—Marinesco-Sjögren syndrome, Fabry disease, mannosidosis
   f. Ocular apraxia—ataxia-telangiectasia, Niemann-Pick disease
   g. Impairment of vertical eye movements—late infantile Niemann-Pick disease, juvenile dystonic lipidosis, sea-blue histiocyte syndrome, Wilson disease
   h. Jerky eye movements, limited abduction—late infantile Gaucher disease
3. Extrapyramidal signs—late-onset Niemann-Pick disease (rigidity, abnormal postures), juvenile dystonic lipidosis (dystonia, choreoathetosis), Rett, ataxia-telangiectasia (athetosis), Sanfilippo mucopolysaccharidosis, type I glutaric acidemia, Wilson disease, Segawa dopa-responsive dystonia
4. Facial dysmorphism—Hurler, Scheie, Morquio, and Maroteaux-Lamy forms of mucopolysaccharidosis, aspartylglycosaminuria, mucolipidoses, G_{M1} gangliosidosis, mannosidosis, fucosidosis (some cases), multisulfatase deficiencies (Austin), some mitochondrial disorders
5. Dwarfism, spine deformities, arthropathies—Hurler, Morquio, and other mucopolysaccharidoses, Cockayne syndrome
6. Enlarged liver and spleen—Niemann-Pick disease, Gaucher disease, all mucopolysaccharidoses, fucosidosis, mucolipidoses, G_{M1} gangliosidosis
7. Alterations of skin—photosensitivity (Cockayne syndrome and one form of porphyria); papular nevi and angiokeratoma (Fabry disease, fucosidosis); telangiectasia of ears, conjunctiva, chest (ataxia-telangiectasia); ichthyosis (Sjögren-Larsen disease, caused by fatty alcohol dehydrogenase deficiency); plaque-like lesions in Hunter syndrome
8. Beaked thoracolumbar vertebrae—all mucopolysaccharidoses, mucolipidoses, mannosidosis, fucosidosis; aspartylglycosaminuria, multiple sulfatase deficiencies
9. Deafness—mucopolysaccharidoses, mannosidosis, Cockayne syndrome
10. Hypertrophied gums—mucolipidoses, mannosidosis
11. Vacuolated lymphocytes—all mucopolysaccharidoses, mucolipidoses, mannosidosis, fucosidosis
12. Granules in neutrophils—all mucopolysaccharidoses, mucolipidoses, mannosidosis, fucosidosis, multiple sulfatase deficiencies

One of the most difficult diagnostic problems in this age period is distinguishing neuroaxonal dystrophy, metachromatic leukodystrophy, subacute necrotizing encephalomyelopathy (Leigh disease), some cases of lipofuscinosis, and the late form of G_{M1} gangliosidosis. In none of these diseases is the clinical picture entirely stereotyped. The clinician is aided in identifying neuroaxonal dystrophy by noting an onset, at 1 to 2 years of age, of severe hypotonia with retained reflexes and Babinski signs, early visual involvement without retinal changes, lack of seizures, normal CSF, physiologic evidence of denervation of muscles, fast-frequency EEG, normal CT, and *N*-acetylgalactosaminidase deficiency in cultured fibroblasts. Metachromatic leukodystrophy can be excluded if the CSF protein is normal and if nerve conduction velocities and enzymatic studies of leukocytes and fibroblasts are normal. Similar criteria enable one to rule out G_{M1} gangliosidosis. Mitochondrial disorders (Leigh disease) may begin at the same age; in many cases lactic acidosis and pyruvate decarboxylase defect will corroborate the diagnosis. Sequencing tests of the mitochondrial genome allow definitive diagnosis in most cases, as described in a later section. Also in Leigh disease, imaging of the brain may disclose hypodense lesions in the basal ganglia and brainstem, in contrast to the normal CT in neuroaxonal dystrophy. In metachromatic leukodystrophy, the cerebral white matter shows a diffusely decreased attenuation and the MR images are striking. Lipofuscinosis cannot always be diagnosed accurately; curvilinear bodies in nerve twigs and in the endothelial cells in skin biopsies and the recently discovered gene mutations are the most informative laboratory tests.

INHERITED METABOLIC ENCEPHALOPATHIES OF LATE CHILDHOOD AND ADOLESCENCE

Unavoidably, one must refer here to certain inherited metabolic diseases already described that permit survival into late childhood and adolescence, as well as to diseases that begin in adolescence or adult life after a normal childhood. There is a tendency for them to be less severe and less rapidly progressive, an attribute shared by many diseases with a dominant mode of inheritance. Nonetheless, there are diseases, such as Wilson disease, in which the onset of neurologic symptoms occurs after the tenth year and in rare instances after the thirtieth year, and the mode of inheritance is recessive in type. However, in the latter instance, the basic abnormality has existed since early childhood in the form of a ceruloplasmin deficiency with early cirrhosis and splenomegaly; only the neurologic disorder is of late onset. This brings us to another principle: The pathogenesis of the cerebral lesion may involve a factor or factors once removed from the underlying biologic abnormality.

Genetic heterogeneity poses another problem with respect to both the clinical and biochemical findings. It is well established that a single clinical phenotype, such as the one seen in Hurler disease, can be the expression of a number of different alleles of a given gene mutation. Conversely, a number of different clinical phenotypes may be based on different degrees of the same enzyme deficiency. One must, therefore, not rely solely on clinical appearances for diagnosis but always combine them with biochemical tests and molecular genetic studies for confirmation. No one of these lines of data, including genomics, is sufficient for classification of disease.

The diseases in this category are probably of greater interest to neurologists than the preceding ones, for they more consistently cause familiar neurologic abnormalities such as epilepsy, polymyoclonus, dementia, cerebellar ataxia, choreoathetosis, dystonia, tremor, spastic-ataxic paraparesis, blindness, deafness, and stroke. These manifestations appear much the same in late childhood and adolescence as they do in adult life, and the neurologist whose experience has been mainly with adult patients feels quite comfortable with them.

Diseases in this age period have a diversity of manifestations, yet each disease tends to have a certain characteristic pattern of neurologic expression, as though the pathogenetic mechanism were acting more selectively on particular systems of neurons. Such affinities between the disease process and certain anatomic structures raise the question of *pathoclisis*, i.e., specific vulnerability of particular neuronal systems to certain morbid agents. Stated another way, for each disease there is a common and relatively stereotyped clinical syndrome and a small number of variants; conversely, certain other symptoms and syndromes are rarely observed with a given disease. At the same time, however, it is clear that more than one disease may cause the same syndrome.

In deference to these principles, *the diseases in this section are grouped according to their most common mode of clinical expression,* as follows:

1. The progressive cerebellar ataxias of childhood and adolescence
2. The familial polymyoclonias and epilepsies
3. Extrapyramidal syndromes of parkinsonian type
4. The syndrome of dystonia and generalized choreoathetosis
5. The syndrome of bilateral hemiplegia, cerebral blindness and deafness, and other manifestations of focal cerebral disorder
6. Strokes in association with inherited metabolic diseases
7. Metabolic polyneuropathies
8. Personality changes and behavioral disturbances as manifestations of inherited metabolic diseases

It is advantageous to be familiar with these groupings. Like the age of onset and the distinctions between gray and white matter diseases of earlier onset, this scheme facilitates clinical diagnosis. One word of caution: It is a mistake to assume that the diseases in these categories affect one and only one particular part of the nervous system or to assume that they are exclusively neurologic. Once the biochemical abnormality is discovered, it is usually found to implicate cells of certain nonneurologic tissues as well; whether or not the effects of such involvement become symptomatic is often a quantitative matter. Also, one encounters mixed neurologic syndromes in which tremor, myoclonus, cerebellar ataxia, seizures, and choreoathetosis are present in various combinations; it is then difficult to decide whether a movement disorder is of one type or another.

The Progressive Cerebellar Ataxias of Late Childhood and Adolescence

In the preceding section it was pointed out that there is a large group of diseases, some with a known metabolic basis, in which an acute, episodic, or chronic cerebellar ataxia becomes manifest in early childhood. Here the discussion of the cerebellar ataxias is continued, with reference to those forms that begin in late childhood and adolescence. In these later age periods, the number of ataxias of proven metabolic type diminishes markedly. Most of them, of chronic progressive type, are part of the late-onset lipid storage diseases. Of the other cerebellar ataxias of late childhood and adolescence, only the Bassen-Kornzweig acanthocytosis, late-onset G_{M2} gangliosidosis, Refsum disease, ataxia-telangiectasia, and a genetic fault in vitamin E metabolism fall into the category of truly metabolic disease. Refsum disease is so clearly a polyneuropathy (cerebellar features only in exceptional cases) that it is presented in Chap. 46. Ataxia-telangiectasia is usually encountered in late childhood, but the ataxia may begin as early as the second year of life; therefore it has been described in the preceding section with the ataxias of early childhood.

There are many other conditions of metabolic type in which cerebellar ataxia figures in the clinical picture. Some of these are associated with polymyoclonus and cherry-red macular spots (mainly sialidosis or α-neuraminidase deficiency; see below). Cerebellar ataxia is a prominent feature of Unverricht-Lundborg (Baltic) disease and Lafora-body disease (see Chap. 16). The Cockayne syndrome and Marinesco-Sjögren disease persist into later childhood and adolescence or may even have their onset in this later period. In cerebrotendinous xanthomatosis (see further on), spastic weakness and pseudobulbar palsy are combined with cerebellar ataxia. Prader-Willi children have a broad-based gait and are clumsy in addition to being obese, genitally deficient, and diabetic. Several diseases associated with hyperuricemia implicate defective purine and pyrimidine metabolism and fit into this category; the enzymatic defect of Lesch-Nyhan disease is not present, however. Marsden and coworkers (1982) have observed cerebellar ataxia beginning in late childhood as an expression of adrenoleukodystrophy (see below). The familial syndrome of neuropathy, ataxia, and retinitis pigmentosa (NARP) caused by a mitochondrial genome mutation that impairs ATP synthase can cause ataxia and closely mimic the Marinesco-Sjögren syndrome.

Doubtless, many of the progressive forms of cerebellar ataxia now classified as degenerative and described in Chap. 39 will be proved to have an underlying biochemical or similar subcellular pathogenesis and will logically fall in place here, with the metabolic diseases. At present, when faced with a progressive ataxia of cerebellar type, even in a young adult, the reader should consult both this chapter and Chap. 39.

The *acute forms of cerebellar ataxia* that occur in late childhood and adolescence are essentially nonmetabolic, being traceable to postinfectious encephalomyelitis (see Chap. 36) or to postanoxic, postmeningitic, or posthyperthermic states and certain drug intoxications. With relatively pure cerebellar ataxias of this age period, postinfectious cerebellitis, cerebellar tumors (medulloblastomas, astrocytomas, hemangioblastomas, and ganglioneuromas of Lhermitte-Duclos) should be considered in the differential diagnosis. MRI establishes the correct diagnosis.

Bassen-Kornzweig Acanthocytosis (Abetalipoproteinemia)

Bassen and Kornzweig, in 1950, first described this rare metabolic disease of lipoproteins that causes ataxia, sensory neuropathy, and acanthocytic deformity of red cells. It excited great interest, for it gave promise of a breakthrough into a hitherto obscure group of "degenerative" disorders. The inheritance is autosomal recessive.

The initial symptoms, occurring between 6 and 12 years (range: 2 to 20 years), are weakness of the limbs with areflexia and ataxia of sensory (tabetic) type, to which a cerebellar component is added later (the first two aspects relating to a peripheral neuropathy are discussed in Chap. 46). Steatorrhea, raising the suspicion of celiac disease (sprue), often precedes the appearance of a weak and unsteady gait. Later, in more than half the patients, vision may fail because of retinal degeneration (similar to retinitis pigmentosa). Kyphoscoliosis, pes cavus, and Babinski signs are other elements in the clinical picture. The neurologic disorder is relatively slowly progressive—by the second to third decade, the patient is usually bedridden.

The diagnostic laboratory findings are spiky or thorny red blood cells (acanthocytes), low sedimentation rate, and a marked reduction in the serum of low-density lipoproteins (LDL cholesterol, phospholipid, and β-lipoprotein levels are all subnormal). Pathologic study has revealed the presence of foamy, vacuolated epithelial cells in the intestinal mucosa (causing absorption block); diminished numbers of myelinated nerve fibers in sural nerve biopsies, depletion of Purkinje and granule cells in all parts of the cerebellum; loss of fibers in the posterior columns and spinocerebellar tracts; loss of anterior horn and retinal ganglion cells and of muscle fibers and fibrosis of the myocardium. It has been proposed that the basic defect is an inability of the body to synthesize the proteins of cell membranes because of the impaired absorption of fat through the mucosa of the small intestine. Vitamin E deficiency may be a pathogenic factor, because the administration of a low-fat diet and high doses of vitamins A and E may prevent progression of the neurologic disorder, according to Illingworth and colleagues, but the pathophysiology appears to be more complex.

Often mentioned in the context of acanthocytosis is a related rare condition, McLeod syndrome, in which progressive muscular atrophy, seizures, involuntary movements, and elevated serum creatine kinase (CK) are combined in various configurations. The acanthocytosis in this disease is the result of an abnormality of the red cell surface Kell antigen (Kx, coding for the protein XK).

Familial Hypobetalipoproteinemia

This is another rare but well-defined disease resembling abetalipoproteinemia, in which there is hypocholesterolemia, acanthocytosis of red blood corpuscles, retinitis pigmentosa, and a pallidal atrophy (HARP syndrome). Inheritance is autosomal dominant, and heterozygotes may exhibit some part of the syndrome. Many cases are caused by mutations in the gene encoding β-lipoprotein B. Fat droplets may be seen in the jejunal mucosa, indicating malabsorption. Cases have been reported from Europe, Asia, and the United States. Treatment consists of restriction of dietary fat and supplements of vitamin E.

An adult form of acanthocytosis unrelated to the above several diseases is associated with hereditary chorea and dystonia but evidence of lipid malabsorption is lacking. This disease is described in Chap. 39.

Familial Polymyoclonus

As stated in Chap. 6, the term *myoclonus* is applied to many conditions that are not at all alike but share a single clinical feature—a multitude of exceedingly brief, random, arrhythmic twitches of parts of muscles, entire muscles, or groups of muscles. Myoclonic jerks differ from chorea by virtue of their brevity (15 to 50 ms). Notably, both phenomena are considered to be symptomatic of "gray matter" diseases ("polioencephalopathies").

Myoclonus or polymyoclonus may, in certain conditions, stand alone as a relatively pure syndrome. In most other cases, it is mixed with epilepsy or athetosis and dystonia, discussed further on. Most often, myoclonus is associated with cerebellar ataxia; thus it is being considered here, with the progressive cerebellar ataxias. The many acquired forms of polymyoclonus, such as subacute sclerosing panencephalitis, were mentioned in Chap. 6. This chapter is concerned only with those of known or presumed metabolic origin.

Myoclonic Encephalopathy of Infants (Infantile Opsoclonus-Myoclonus Syndrome)

Under this title, Kinsbourne originally described a form of widespread, continuous myoclonus (except during deep sleep) affecting male and female infants whose development had been normal until the onset of the disease at the age of 9 to 20 months. The myoclonus evolves over a week or less, affects all the muscles of the body, and interferes seriously with all the natural muscular activities of the child. The eyes are notably affected by rapid (up to 8/s), irregular conjugate movements ("dancing eyes" of an opsoclonic type). The child is irritable and speech may cease. All laboratory tests are normal.

Treatment Dexamethasone in doses of 1.5 to 4.0 mg/d suppresses the myoclonus and permits developmental progress. Some patients have recovered from the myoclonus but have been left mentally slow and mildly ataxic. Others have required corticosteroid therapy for 5 to 10 years, with relapse whenever it was discontinued. Ordinary anticonvulsants seem to have no effect. The pathology has not been determined.

A similar syndrome has been observed in conjunction with neuroblastoma in children and as a transient illness of unknown cause (probably viral or postinfectious) in young adults (Baringer et al; see Chap. 33). A similar condition is also known in adults as a paraneoplastic disease with ovarian, breast, gastric, and bronchogenic carcinomas and with other occult tumors.

In a broader survey of the pediatric opsoclonus-myoclonus syndrome, Pranzatelli and associates reported their experience with 27 cases, some with neural crest tumors, others with viral infections or hypoxic injury (intention myoclonus). In nearly all of their patients there was cerebellar ataxia and mental disorder, and 10 percent had seizures. The CSF was normal. The investigators have emphasized the pathogenetic heterogeneity and defined a rare serotoninergic type (low levels of 5-hydroxytryptophan and homovanillic acid in the CSF) that responds to 5-hydroxyindole acetic acid.

Familial Progressive Myoclonus

Five major categories of familial polymyoclonus of late childhood and adolescence have been delineated: (1) Lafora- or amyloid-body type, (2) juvenile cerebroretinal degeneration, (3) cherry-red spot myoclonus (sialidosis or α-neuraminidase deficiency), (4) mitochondrial encephalopathy, and (5) a more benign degenerative disease (dyssynergia cerebellaris myoclonica of Hunt). Familial myoclonus may also be a prominent feature of two other diseases—G_{M2} gangliosidosis and Gaucher disease—which occasionally have their onset in this age period.

Lafora-Body Polymyoclonus With Epilepsy This disease, which is inherited as an autosomal recessive trait, was first identified by Lafora in 1911 on the basis of the large basophilic cytoplasmic bodies that were found in the dentate, brainstem, and thalamic neurons. These inclusions have been shown by Yokoi and colleagues to be composed of a glucose polymer (polyglucosan) that is chemically but not structurally related to glycogen. Possibly some of the cases of familial myoclonus epilepsy reported by Unverricht and by Lundborg were of this type, but because these authors provided no pathologic data, one cannot be sure.

Beginning in late childhood and adolescence (11 to 18 years) in a previously normal individual, the disease announces itself by a seizure, a burst of myoclonic jerks, or both. In about half the cases there are focal (often occipital) seizures. The illness may at first be mistaken for ordinary epilepsy, but within a few months it becomes evident that something far more serious is occurring. The myoclonus becomes widespread and can be evoked as a startle by noise, an unexpected tactile stimulus (even the tap of a reflex hammer), and also by excitement, or certain sustained motor activities. An evoked train of myoclonic jerks may progress to a generalized seizure with loss of consciousness. As the disease advances, the myoclonus interferes increasingly with the patient's motor activities until voluntary function is seriously impaired. Speech may be marred, much as it is in chorea. Close examination may also reveal an alteration in muscle tone and a slight degree of cerebellar ataxia. At this time, or even before the onset of myoclonus and seizures, the patient may experience visual hallucinations or exhibit irritability, odd traits of character, uninhibited or impulsive behavior, and, ultimately, progressive failure in all cognitive functions. Deafness has been an early sign in a few cases. Rigidity or hypotonia, impaired tendon reflexes, acrocyanosis, and rarely corticospinal tract signs are late findings. Finally the patient becomes cachectic and bedfast and succumbs to intercurrent infection. Most do not survive beyond their twenty-fifth birthday. Nonetheless there are isolated reports of Lafora-body disease in which symptoms began as late as age 40 years, with death as late as age 50 years. These late cases may constitute a separate genetic type.

No abnormalities of the blood, urine, or CSF have been detected. The EEG shows diffuse slow waves and spikes as well as bursts of focal or multifocal discharges. Altered hepatocytes with homogeneous PAS-positive bodies that displace the nuclei have been observed in both the presymptomatic and symptomatic stages of the disease. These inclusions have been seen in skin and liver biopsies, even though liver function tests were normal. Neuropathologic examinations have shown a slight loss of granule and Purkinje cells and loss of neurons in the dentate nuclei, inner segment of globus pallidus, and cerebral cortex in addition to the Lafora bodies. The latter may also be seen in the retina, cerebral cortex, myocardium, and striated muscles. Anticonvulsant drugs, especially methsuximide and valproic acid, help in the control of the seizures but have no effect on the basic process.

Juvenile Ceroid Lipofuscinosis (Cerebroretinal Degeneration; Batten Disease) As stated earlier, this is one of the most variable forms of the lipidoses. The salient clinical features of the later-onset types are severe myoclonus, seizures, and visual loss. In the juvenile type, the first lesions are seen in the maculae; they appear as yellow-gray areas of degeneration and stand in contrast to the cherry-red spot and the encircling white ring of Tay-Sachs disease. At first, the particles of retinal pigment are fine and dust-like; later they aggregate to resemble more the bone-corpuscular shapes of retinitis pigmentosa. The liver and spleen are not enlarged and there are no osseous changes. The usual development of these and other manifestations of the disease were outlined by Sjögren, who studied a large number of the late infantile and juvenile types of cases in Sweden. He divided the illness into stages, the first of which was visual impairment, followed approximately sequentially by generalized seizures and myoclonus, often with irritability, poor control of emotions, and stuttering, jerky speech at 2 years, then gradual intellectual deterioration to which were added cerebellar ataxia and intention tremor, in this respect coming to resemble Wilson disease. Finally, the patient lies curled up in bed, blind and speechless, with strong extensor plantar reflexes, occasionally adopting dystonic postures. Life usually ends in 10 to 15 years.

In the early stages, the EEG pattern of random, high-voltage, triphasic waves is diagnostic; later, as the seizures and myoclonic jerks become less frequent and finally cease, only delta waves remain. The electroretinographic waveforms are lost once the retina is affected. The lateral ventricles are slightly dilated on CT and on MRI. The CSF is normal. Diagnosis can be confirmed by the appearance of inclusions of a curvilinear "fingerprint" pattern in electron microscopic study of biopsy material, particularly of the eccrine sweat glands of the skin. A defective membrane protein has been identified that forms the inclusion material in the most common, or classic, juvenile phenotype. The genetics of the lipofuscinoses have been reviewed by Mole.

Late Juvenile and Adult Ceroid Lipofuscinosis (Kufs-Parry or Kufs Disease)

The *type of ceroid lipofuscinosis that* develops later (15 to 25 years of age or older) is often unattended by visual or retinal changes and is even slower in its evolution. It is presented here for ease of exposition, but it becomes relevant mostly in relation to dementing illness in young adulthood. Personality change or dementia is one constellation, the other being myoclonic seizures with subsequent dementia and even later pyramidal and extrapyramidal signs. As the disease progresses, cerebellar ataxia, spasticity, rigidity or athetosis, or mixtures thereof, are combined with dementia. As a reflection of the variability of the clinical presentation, a recent patient of ours had vague visual difficulties at age 51 years and evolved a spastic quadriparesis with disinhibited behavior over 5 years. Additional comments regarding the unusual presentations of this disease can be found further on, under "Adult Forms of Inherited Metabolic Disease." van Bogaert pointed out to our colleague R.D. Adams that relatives of these patients may have retinal changes without neurologic accompaniments. The genetic defect for the adult form has been analyzed (see below).

Of all the lipidoses, these cerebroretinal degenerations had for decades defied unifying biochemical definition. Our understanding of these diseases is difficult because they embody both enzymatic defects and structural protein dysfunctions. In a few of the early childhood types, mutations of one of several lysosomal enzymes have been identified as summarized by Mole and by Wisniewski and colleagues. As mentioned earlier, Zeman and coworkers showed that the cytoplasmic inclusions are autofluorescent and give a positive histochemical reaction for both ceroid and lipofuscin, but this material is not different biochemically from the lipid substance that accumulates in aging cells. In addition to the presence of curvilinear bodies in the cytoplasm of neurons and other tissues, some in a fingerprint pattern, there is a reduction in type II synapses in the distal parts of the axon. All these changes precede nerve cell loss. The genetic defects have been tentatively determined for some of the subtypes of neuronal ceroid lipofuscinosis (see Wisniewski et al). These genes have been designated CLN 1 through 9 and they embody over 100 different mutations.

Childhood or Juvenile G_{M2} Gangliosidosis Instances of the recessive type of G_{M2} gangliosidosis rarely have their onset at the typical age period. Twenty-four such cases (from 20 kindreds) were collected from the medical literature by Meek and coworkers. Ataxia and dysarthria were frequently the presenting symptoms, followed by dementia, dysphagia, spasticity, dystonia, seizures, and myoclonus. Degeneration of anterior horn cells with progressive muscular atrophy may be a feature, although this is more characteristic of the adult-onset variety (see further on). Atypical cherry-red spots are observed in some patients. The biochemical abnormality, i.e., a deficiency of hexosaminidase A, is the same as in Tay-Sachs disease, but not as severe or as extensive. Progression of the disease is slow, over a period of many years.

Late Gaucher Disease With Polymyoclonus A type of Gaucher disease is occasionally encountered in which seizures, severe diffuse myoclonus, supranuclear gaze disorders (slow saccades, saccadic and pursuit horizontal gaze palsies), and cerebellar ataxia begin in late childhood, adolescence, or adult life. The course is slowly progressive. The intellect is relatively spared. The spleen is enlarged. The pathologic and biochemical abnormalities are the same as those of Gaucher disease of earlier onset.

Cherry-Red Spot-Myoclonus Syndrome (Sialidosis Type 1, α-Neuraminidase Deficiency) This is a genetically distinct class of disease characterized by the storage in nervous tissue of sialylated glycopeptides. It is caused by a neuraminidase deficiency. In some of the patients, the onset was in late childhood or adolescence, and in others, even later. In addition to the patients initially reported by Rapin and coworkers, 24 similar cases have appeared in the medical literature.

In the cases described by Rapin and colleagues the first findings were visual impairment with cherry-red macular spots, similar to those seen in Tay-Sachs disease and less consistently in G_{M1} gangliosidosis, Niemann-Pick disease, and metachromatic leukodystrophy. In one case, there was severe episodic pain in the hands, legs, and feet during hot weather, reminiscent of Fabry disease. Polymyoclonus followed within a few years and, together with cerebellar ataxia, disabled the patients. Mental function remained relatively normal. Liver and spleen were not enlarged, but storage material was found in the Kupffer cells, neurons of the myenteric plexus, and cerebral neurons, and presumably in cerebellar and retinal neurons.

The cases of Thomas and colleagues were young adults, all members of one generation, who had developed dysarthria, intention myoclonus, cerebellar ataxia, and cherry-red macular lesions. Like the cases of Rapin and coworkers, the heredity was autosomal recessive.

There was urinary excretion of sialylated oligosaccharides and a sialidase deficiency in cultured fibroblasts. The two patients described by Tsuji and associates (1982) are noteworthy in that they were of age 50 and 30 years. In addition to the macular lesions, polymyoclonia, and cerebellar ataxia, there were gargoyle-like facial features, corneal opacities, and vertebral dysplasia. These patients also had a neuraminidase (partial beta-galactosidase) deficiency.

Dentatorubral Cerebellar Atrophy With Polymyoclonus This progressive degeneration of the cerebellar-dental efferent system was originally described by Ramsay Hunt under the title of *dyssynergia cerebellaris myoclonica*. The onset is in late childhood; both sexes are vulnerable, and it probably has more than one cause. In Hunt's case, a progressive ataxia was accompanied by a striking degree of action myoclonus. Seizures are infrequent, and the intellect is relatively preserved. The neurons of the dentate nuclei and their ascending and descending brainstem axons gradually disappear. Berkovic and associates studied 84 cases of polymyoclonus, 13 of which conformed to the Hunt syndrome. Of these, 9 proved to have a mitochondrial encephalomyopathy. However, there are other reports (Tassinari et al) in which muscle biopsies showed no mitochondrial abnormalities. In the series of 30 cases reported by Marsden and coworkers (1990) the onset was usually before the age of 21 years. Cortical electrographic discharges were found to precede each myoclonic twitch (cortical myoclonus). A biochemically supported diagnosis could not be made in nearly half of their cases.

Extremely chronic forms of rhythmic myoclonus involving only the facial and bulbar muscles also occur. Although this benign familial polymyoclonia has not been associated with any biochemical abnormality, its association with cellular mitochondrial abnormalities in some cases justifies its inclusion in this chapter rather than with the degenerative diseases. Another mitochondrial disorder, the myoclonic epilepsy ragged red fiber (MERRF) disease, begins in the second decade or later with myoclonus and ataxia and enters into the differential diagnosis of this group of diseases. The mitochondrial diseases as a group are considered in the last part of this chapter.

Epilepsies of Hereditary Metabolic Disease

(See Chap. 16)

Convulsive seizures may complicate nearly all hereditary metabolic diseases. The seizures may occur at all ages but more frequently in the neonate, infant, or young child than in the older child or adolescent. The seizures take many forms, as discussed in Chap. 16. Most often they are generalized grand mal or partial types; typical petit mal probably does not occur. Some diseases may cause focal seizures, simple or complex partial, before becoming generalized. The combination of series of polymyoclonic jerks progressing to a generalized motor seizure is always highly suggestive of one of the hereditary metabolic diseases. Another highly significant form of presentation is with sensory evoked seizures. The subject of epilepsy and the hereditary metabolic diseases was reviewed by Sansaricq and colleagues.

EXTRAPYRAMIDAL SYNDROMES WITH HEREDITARY METABOLIC DISEASE

Parkinsonian Syndromes

In the typical parkinsonian syndrome, with features of rigidity, tremor, and bradykinesia, strength remains relatively intact and corticospinal signs are absent, but effectiveness of movement is nonetheless impaired by the patient's disinclination to use the affected parts (hypo- or akinesia), by slowness (bradykinesia), and by rigidity and tremor (see Chap. 4). Other clinical syndromes in this category include choreoathetosis, dystonia, and spasms of gaze.

When the parkinsonian syndrome or some component thereof has its onset in middle or late adult life, it usually indicates idiopathic Parkinson disease or related multisystem forms. The development of such an extrapyramidal motor disorder in late childhood and adolescence instead suggests Wilson disease, juvenile Huntington disease, Hallervorden-Spatz disease, and the Segawa type of L-dopa–responsive dystonia as well as other so-called parkin mutations (see Chap. 39).

Hepatolenticular Degeneration (Wilson Disease, Westphal-Strümpell Pseudosclerosis, ATP7B Mutation)

Wilson's description of "Progressive Lenticular Degeneration: A Familial Nervous Disease Associated with Cirrhosis of the Liver" appeared in 1912. A similar neurologic disorder had been described previously by Gowers (1906) under the title of "tetanoid chorea" and by Westphal (1883) and Strümpell (1898), as "pseudosclerosis." None of these authors, however, recognized the association with cirrhosis. The clinical studies of Hall (1921) and the histopathologic studies of Spielmeyer (1920), who reexamined sections from the liver and brain of Westphal's and Strümpell's cases, clearly established that the pseudosclerosis described by these authors was the same disease as the one that had been described by Wilson. Interestingly, none of these authors, including Wilson, noticed the golden-brown (Kayser-Fleischer) corneal ring, the one pathognomonic sign of the disease. Rumpell had demonstrated the greatly increased copper content of the liver and brain as early as 1913, but this discovery was generally ignored until Mandelbrote (1948) found, quite by chance, that the urinary excretion of copper was greatly increased in patients with Wilson disease and that it was increased even more after the intramuscular administration of the chelating agent British anti-Lewisite (BAL). In 1952, Scheinberg and Gitlin discovered that ceruloplasmin, the serum protein that binds copper, is reduced in this disease (see reviews by Scheinberg and Sternlieb for a full historical account and references). Denny-Brown demonstrated a recession of symptoms after prolonged treatment with BAL.

The prevalence of the disease cannot be stated exactly, but is on the order of 1 per 50,000 to 1 per 100,000 of the general population. The disease is transmitted as an autosomal recessive trait. The gene, called *ATP7B* (homologous with the *ATP7A* gene, which is defective in Menkes disease), codes for a membrane-bound, copper-binding ATPase. One of the curious aspects of the genetics of the disease is the multitude of mutations within this gene that give rise to the disease and no one mutation accounts for more than 30 percent of cases. Inadequate functioning of the ATPase enzyme in some way reduces excretion of copper in the bile. As noted further on, liver transplantation halts progression of the disease, indicating that the primary biochemical effect of the mutation is in the liver rather than the nervous system.

The mutation gives rise to two fundamental disturbances of copper metabolism: (1) a reduced rate of incorporation of copper into ceruloplasmin and (2) a reduction in biliary excretion of copper. The deposition of copper in tissues is the cause of virtually all the manifestations of the disease—cirrhosis, hemolytic anemia, renal tubular changes, Kayser-Fleischer rings, and, in all likelihood, the cerebral damage—as discussed below.

Clinical Features

The onset of neurologic symptoms is usually in the second, and less often in the third, decade, but rarely beyond that time. Half of patients are symptomatic by age 15 years, but exceptional cases, including two under our care, had their first clinical manifestations as late as their midfifties. In all instances the initial event is a deposition of copper in the liver, leading to an acute or chronic hepatopathy and eventually to multilobular cirrhosis and splenomegaly (Scheinberg and Sternlieb). In childhood, the liver disorder often takes the form of attacks of jaundice, unexplained hepatosplenomegaly, or hypersplenism with thrombocytopenia and bleeding. Rarely is there clear evidence of cirrhosis alone. The hepatic abnormalities may be asymptomatic (except for elevated serum transaminases), in which case the initial clinical presentation is neurologic. In some instances, a hemolytic anemia or, less often, renal tubular acidosis may first draw attention to the disease.

The first neurologic manifestations are most often extrapyramidal with a proclivity to affect the oropharyngeal musculature. The typical presentations are tremor of a limb or of the head and generalized slowness of movement (i.e., a parkinsonian syndrome); or slowness of movement of the tongue, lips, pharynx, larynx, and jaws, resulting in dysarthria, dysphagia, and hoarseness; or there may be slowness of finger movement and occasionally choreic movements or dystonic postures of the limbs. Often the mouth is held slightly open in the early stage of the disease. Exceptionally, an abnormality of behavior (argumentativeness, impulsiveness, excessive emotionality, depression, delusions) or a gradual impairment of intellectual faculties precedes other neurologic signs by a year or more (see Starosta-Rubinstein et al).

As the disease progresses, the "classic syndrome" evolves: dysphagia and drooling, rigidity and slowness of movements of the limbs; flexed limb postures; fixity of facial muscles with mouth constantly agape, giving an appearance of grinning or a "vacuous smile"; dysarthria or virtual anarthria (bulbar extrapyramidal syndrome); and a tremor in repose that increases when the limbs are outstretched to a coarse, "wing-beating" movement. Slowed saccadic eye movements and limitation of upgaze are also characteristic. *A notable feature is the tendency for the motor disorders to be concentrated in the bulbar musculature* and to spread caudally. Thus, the syndrome differs from classic parkinsonism. Usually elements of cerebellar ataxia and intention tremor of variable degree are added at some stage of the disease. Approximately 6 percent of patients develop seizures (Dening et al). Gradually the disability increases because of increasing rigidity and tremor. The patient becomes mute, immobile, extremely rigid, dystonic, and slowed mentally, the latter usually being a late and variable effect.

With progression of the neurologic disease, the *Kayser-Fleischer rings* become more evident (see Fig. 37-6). They take the form of a crescentic rusty-brown discoloration of the deepest layer of the cornea (Descemet membrane). In the purely hepatic stage of the disease, the rings may not be evident (in 25 percent of cases), but *they are virtually always present (if properly sought) once the neurologic signs become manifest.* A slit-lamp examination may be necessary for their early detection, particularly in brown-eyed patients, but in the majority of patients with neurologic signs the rings can be visualized with the naked eye or with the aid of an indirect ophthalmoscope focused on the limbus.

The diagnosis is virtually certain when there is a similar syndrome in a sibling or when an extrapyramidal motor disorder of this type is conjoined with liver disease and the corneal rings. Variants of the above syndrome that the authors have seen are an early choreoathetosis (like Sydenham chorea); prominent dystonic postures;

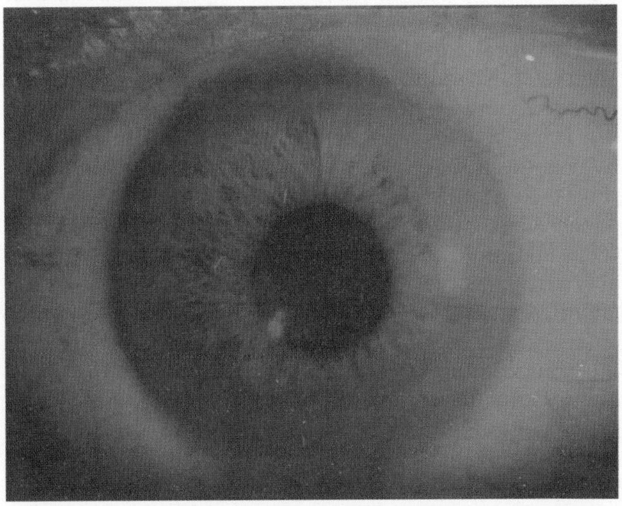

Figure 37-6. Kayser-Fleischer corneal ring in Wilson disease. Brown coloration is seen near the limbus of the cornea and represents copper deposition in Descemet's membrane. (Reproduced from Mackay D, Miyawaki E: Hyperkinetic Movement Disorders. ACP Medicine, Online S12C17, Topic ID 1271. © Decker Intellectual Properties. Courtesy of Drs. Edison Miyawaki and Donald Bienfang.)

a cerebellar ataxia with minimal rigidity; a syndrome of coarse action or action and intention tremor resembling that of dentatorubral degeneration; an immobile mute state with profound rigidity; and a dementia, character change, or psychosis with relatively few extrapyramidal signs. Action myoclonus as a prominent early manifestation has also been described. The parkinsonian features do not respond to L-dopa treatment.

Laboratory Findings In both the typical and variant forms of the disease, the finding of a low serum ceruloplasmin level (less than 20 mg/dL in 80 to 90 percent of patients), low serum copper (3 to 10 mM/L; normal 11 to 24 mM/L), and increased urinary copper excretion (more than 100 mg Cu/24 h) corroborate the diagnosis. Because 90 percent of copper is carried by ceruloplasmin and the latter is generally reduced in Wilson disease, serum copper values alone may be misleadingly normal. Early in the course of the illness, the most reliable diagnostic findings are a high copper content in a biopsy of liver tissue (more than 200 μg Cu/g dry weight) and a failure to incorporate labeled ^{64}Cu into ceruloplasmin. The latter test, however, fails to dependably differentiate asymptomatic carriers from affected individuals. Measurement of increased cupruresis after the administration of penicillamine has not been shown to be more sensitive than an unenhanced 24-h urine collection for copper. Persistent aminoaciduria, reflecting a renal tubular abnormality, is present in most but not all patients. Liver function tests are usually abnormal; some patients are jaundiced and other signs of liver failure may appear late in the illness. In these patients, the serum ammonia may be elevated and the symptomatology may worsen with increases in dietary protein. The cirrhosis is not always evident in a liver biopsy (some regenerative nodules are large, and the biopsy may be taken from one of them). On the other hand, the diagnosis in children may be revealed when a liver biopsy is taken for the evaluation of cirrhosis. As mentioned earlier, the large number of mutations that give rise to the disease makes it impractical to use genetic analysis for diagnosis, but once the gene abnormality has been established in a given family, linkage studies may be used to identify other affected sibs.

It has been established that copper deposition in the liver is the initial disturbance; over time it leads to cirrhosis, so that, as already mentioned, the hepatic stage of the disease precedes neurologic involvement. Cranial CT is abnormal even in the hepatic stage and are invariably so when the neurologic disorder supervenes. The lateral ventricles and often the third ventricle are slightly enlarged, the cerebral and cerebellar sulci are widened, the brainstem appears shrunken, and the posterior parts of the lenticular nuclei, red nuclei, and dentate nuclei become hypodense (Ropper et al). With treatment, these radiologic changes become less marked (Williams and Walshe). MRI is an even more sensitive means of visualizing the structural changes, particularly those in the subcortical white matter, midbrain, pons, and cerebellum (Starosta-Rubinstein et al). In the MRI survey by Saatci and colleagues, the putamen was involved most frequently (although not invariably), showing a symmetrical T2 signal change in a laminar pattern; there was also an increase in T1 signal throughout the basal ganglia, particularly in the pallidum. Signal changes are almost universally found in the claustrum and also in the midbrain (pars compacta of the substantia nigra), dentate nucleus of the cerebellum, pons, and thalami. We have been impressed with a glassy diffuse and confluent signal abnormality on T2-weighted and fluid-attenuated inversion recovery (FLAIR) images in the hemispheral white matter in some cases—findings that were mistaken for multiple sclerosis.

Neuropathologic Changes These vary with the rate of progress of the disease. Exceptionally, in the rapidly advancing and fatal form, there is frank cavitation in the lenticular (putaminal and pallidal) nuclei, as observed in Wilson's original cases. In the more chronic form, there is only shrinkage and a light-brown discoloration of these structures. Nerve cell loss and some degree of degeneration of myelinated fibers in lenticular nuclei, substantia nigra, and dentate nuclei are usually apparent. Subcortical myelin degeneration is found in some cases. More striking, however, is a marked hyperplasia of protoplasmic astrocytes (Alzheimer type II cells) in the cerebral cortex, basal ganglia, brainstem nuclei, and cerebellum, almost certainly a reaction to liver failure and hyperammonemia.

Treatment Ideally, treatment should be started before the appearance of neurologic signs; if this can be implemented, neurologic deterioration can be prevented to a large extent. Treatment consists of (1) reduction of dietary copper to less than 1 mg/d, which can usually be accomplished by avoidance of copper-rich foods (liver, mushrooms, cocoa, chocolate, nuts, and shellfish), and (2) administration of the copper chelating agent D-penicillamine (1 to 3 g/d) by mouth, in divided doses. Pyridoxine 25 mg/d should be added in order to prevent anemia. The use of D-penicillamine is associated with a number of problems. Sensitivity reactions to the drug (rash, arthralgia, fever, leukopenia) develop in 20 percent of patients and require a temporary reduction of dosage or a course of prednisone to bring them under control. Reinstitution of drug therapy should then be undertaken, using low dosages (250 mg daily) and, later, small, widely spaced increases. If the patient is still sensitive to D-penicillamine or if severe reactions (lupus-like or nephrotic syndromes or myasthenia gravis) occur, the drug should be discontinued and another chelating agent, triethylene tetramine (trientine) or ammonium tetrathiomolybdate may be substituted. Zinc, which blocks the intestinal absorption of copper, is also a suitable treatment, but ineffective alone. It is given as zinc acetate, 100 to 150 mg daily in 3 to 4 divided doses at least 1 h before meals (Hoogenraad et al). The appropriate drug must then be continued for the patient's lifetime. Some women report improvement in neurologic symptoms during pregnancy, although there is no apparent change in copper metabolism during this time. In most patients, neurologic signs improve in response to decoppering agents. The Kayser-Fleischer rings disappear and liver function tests may return to normal, although the abnormalities of copper metabolism remain unchanged. In moderately severe and advanced cases, clinical improvement may not begin for several months despite full doses of D-penicillamine, and it is important to resist discontinuing the drug during this latent period.

It is also well known that the institution of treatment with penicillamine may induce an abrupt worsening of neurologic signs, and we have witnessed several such instances, including one that culminated fatally from a cardiac arrhythmia. Furthermore, in many of these patients, the lost function is never retrieved. Presumably this deterioration is a result of the rapid mobilization of copper from the liver and its redistribution to the brain. The slow introduction of penicillamine may avoid this complication. The additional use of zinc or one of the newer agents mentioned above should be instituted as soon as neurologic deterioration becomes evident. In at least one reported case, new lesions of Wilson disease (shown by MRI) developed while the patient was receiving full doses of D-penicillamine and excellent decoppering of the liver had occurred (Brewer et al). In the few patients who develop seizures, they may become apparent soon after therapy is begun.

Many wilsonian patients with advanced liver disease have been subjected to liver transplantation, which is curative for the underlying metabolic defect. The degree of neurologic improvement varies; in some it has been remarkable and sustained, confirming that the hepatic defect is primary and that the brain is involved secondarily. According to Schilsky and coworkers, the main indication for transplantation is severe and progressive liver damage, but the operation has been used successfully in some patients with intractable neurologic deterioration and only mild signs of liver disease.

An important aspect of treatment is the screening of potentially affected relatives for abnormalities of serum copper and ceruloplasmin; if any relative is found to have the disease, penicillamine should be given indefinitely to prevent the emergence of neurologic symptoms. A full explanation of the dangers of ceasing the medication must be given, and compliance may have to be monitored.

Hereditary Deficiency of Ceruloplasmin (Aceruloplasminemia, CP Mutation)

This is a rare illness, similar to Wilson disease, occurring in patients with a recessively inherited deficiency of ceruloplasmin; it is not simply a heterozygous form of Wilson disease (the mutation involves a different gene). Cirrhosis and Kayser-Fleischer rings are not features of the disease but diabetes is common and extrapyramidal signs may or may not arise. Rather than copper, iron is deposited in the brain and liver (see discussion by Logan). Those few cases that have been well studied, mainly Japanese, show mainly an ataxic disorder (Miyajima et al).

Hyprocupric Myeloneuropathy

Noted briefly here and discussed more extensively in Chap. 44, is an idiopathic progressive posterior and lateral column myelopathy that closely simulates subacute combined degeneration of B_{12} deficiency. It is associated with low serum copper levels, usually idiopathic but sometimes caused by malabsorption or the intake of zinc as an over-the-counter supplement to prevent colds or to improve the senses of smell and taste; zinc inhibits absorption of copper from the gut.

Neurodegeneration With Brain Iron Accumulation (Formerly, Hallervorden-Spatz Disease, PANK Mutation)

This disease, recently renamed because of ignoble associations of the eponymous Hallervorden and Spatz, is also known as *pigmentary degeneration of the globus pallidus.* It is inherited as an autosomal recessive trait and is caused by, in all classic cases, a defect in the gene encoding pantothenate kinase 2 (*PANK2*), usually in the form of a missense mutation. The onset of symptoms is in late childhood or early adolescence with slow progression over a period of 10 or more years. The early signs are highly variable but are predominantly motor, both corticospinal (spasticity, hyperreflexia, Babinski signs) and extrapyramidal (rigidity, dystonia, and choreoathetosis). General deterioration of intellect is conjoined. In individual cases, ataxia and myoclonus have appeared at some phase of the illness. The spasticity and rigidity are most prominent in the legs, but in some instances they begin in the bulbar muscles, interfering with speech and swallowing, as happens in Wilson disease. We have observed patients who, over a period of years, exhibited only dystonia of the tongue, blepharospasm, or arching of the back. The relationship of this restricted form to the complete syndrome remains unsettled. Eventually, the patient becomes almost completely inarticulate and unable to walk or use his or her arms. Hayflick and colleagues found that only one-third of patients with atypical forms of the disease have mutations of the *PANK2* gene. Moreover, variant cases tended not to show the characteristic changes on MRI described below.

Reduced levels of PANK2 in the blood corroborate the diagnosis but this test is available only in research laboratories with an interest in the disease. The characteristic deposits of iron in the basal ganglia have not been associated with a demonstrable abnormality of serum iron or of iron metabolism. It has, however, been reported that there is increased uptake of radioactive iron in the region of the basal ganglia following intravenous injection of labeled ferrous citrate (Vakili et al; Szanto and Gallyas). CT reveals hypodense zones in the lenticular nuclei, resembling those of hepatolenticular degeneration (also of sulfite oxidase deficiency, glutaric acidemia and Leigh disease), although high-density lesions have been described in one autopsy-proven case of this disease (Tennison et al). The MRI findings are striking (Fig. 37-7). In T2-weighted images, the rim of the pallidum appears intensely black (iron deposition), with a small white area in its medial part that represents a zone of necrosis ("eye-of-the-tiger" sign; see also Savoiardo et al).

The neuropathologic features prove to be the most distinctive attributes of the disease. There is an intense brown pigmentation of the globus pallidus, substantia nigra (especially the anteromedial parts), and red nucleus. Granules and larger amorphous deposits of iron mixed with calcium stud the walls of small blood vessels or lie

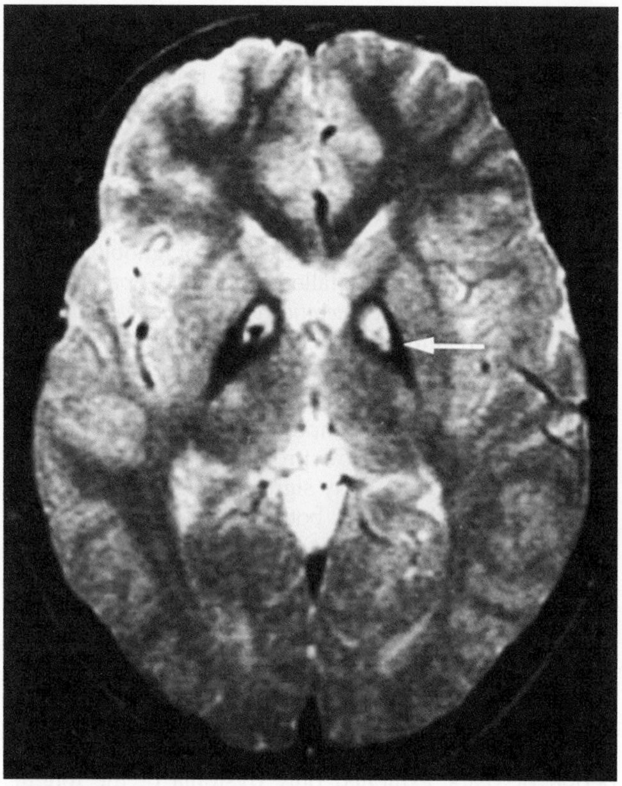

Figure 37-7. Pantothenate kinase-associated neurodegeneration (Hallervorden-Spatz disease). T2-weighted MRI showing areas of decreased signal intensity of the pallidum bilaterally (corresponding to iron deposition) and a central high signal area because of necrosis ("eye-of-the-tiger" sign). (Reproduced by permission from Lyon et al. Courtesy of Dr. C. Gillain.)

free in the tissue. A loss of neurons and medullated fibers occurs in the most affected regions. Another unique feature is the presence of swollen axon fragments, which resemble those of neuroaxonal dystrophy. The significance of iron deposition is difficult to judge. To some extent, there is an increase of iron in the basal ganglia in other degenerative diseases. In Parkinson disease and striatonigral degeneration, for example, the deposition of iron is two to three times normal, presumably the result of degeneration of those tissues that are known to be rich in iron.

No treatment is known to be effective. Some of our patients responded temporarily to L-dopa, but the effect was slight. The use of chelating agents to reduce iron storage has not helped.

Syndromes of Dystonia and Generalized Chorea and Athetosis

As indicated in Chap. 4, the differences between dystonia and choreoathetosis are not fundamental. If one examines many patients with these involuntary movements, every gradation between the two is seen, and often the quicker, unpatterned involuntary movements of mild ballismus are added. Even tremor and myoclonus may complicate the composite movement disorder. With reference to muscular tone in patients with athetosis and dystonia, there are unpredictable associations of hypertonia and hypotonia. A number of inherited metabolic diseases, all of them rare, express themselves by this syndrome of chorea, athetosis, and dystonia.

Lesch-Nyhan Syndrome (HPRT1 Mutation)

This rare metabolic disease is inherited as an X-linked recessive trait. Although it carries the names of Lesch and Nyhan, the occurrence of uricemia in association with spasticity and choreoathetosis in early childhood had been described earlier by Cateland Schmidt. Essentially, it is a hereditary choreoathetosis with self-mutilation and hyperuricemia. The affected children appear normal at birth and usually develop on schedule up to 3 to 6 months of age. Maturational delay then sets in, initially with hypotonia that later gives way to hypertonia. Also, the patient's behavior becomes abnormal, with aggressiveness and compulsive actions. The uncontrollable self-mutilation, mainly of the lips, occurs early (during the second and third year), and spasticity, choreoathetosis, and tremor come later. Most of the children learn to walk. Speech is delayed, and once attained, it is dysarthric and remains so throughout life. Mental retardation is moderately severe. In patients more than 10 years of age, gouty tophi appear on the ears, and there is increasing risk from gouty nephropathy. The serum levels of uric acid are in the range of 7 to 10 mg/dL.

A deficiency of the enzyme hypoxanthine-guanine-phosphoribosyl transferase (HPRT) has been found in all typical cases of this disease. The *HPRT* gene lies on the X chromosome (Xq 26-q 27), and accurate diagnosis of affected males and carriers can be made by DNA analysis. As a result of this deficiency, hypoxanthine is either excreted or catabolized to xanthine and uric acid. The details of the biochemical abnormality responsible for CNS dysfunction are unclear.

In the differential diagnosis, one must consider nonspecific mental retardation or autism with hand biting and other self-mutilations, athetosis from birth trauma, and encephalopathies with chronic renal disease. Hyperuricemia has also been reported in a family with spinocerebellar ataxia and deafness and in another with autism and mental retardation, neither of them with the enzymatic defect of Lesch-Nyhan disease. As mentioned earlier, there are several other disorders of purine and pyrimidine metabolism, some of them with hyperuricemia, that present with a neurologic syndrome like that of Lesch-Nyhan.

Treatment This is with the xanthine oxidase inhibitor allopurinol, which blocks the last steps of uric acid synthesis, reduces the uric acid in Lesch-Nyhan disease, and prevents the uricosuric nephropathy, but it seems to have no effect on CNS symptoms. Guanosine 5-monophosphate and inosine 5-monophosphate, both of which are deficient in Lesch-Nyhan disease, have been replaced without benefit to the patient. Transitory success has also been achieved by the administration of 5-hydroxytryptophan in combination with L-dopa. Fluphenazine (Prolixin) is reported to have suppressed the self-mutilation after haloperidol (Haldol) had failed to do so. Behavior modification programs may be of some value.

Calcification of Vessels in Basal Ganglia and Cerebellum

Ferrugination and calcification of vessels in the basal ganglia occur to a slight degree in many elderly persons (and in other mammals) who are otherwise normal. The widespread use of and MRI has brought the condition to light with increasing frequency (see Fig. 37-8). Usually it may be dismissed as an aging phenomenon of no clinical significance. When it occurs early in life and is of such degree as to be visible in plain films of the skull, it must always be regarded as abnormal.

Fahr Disease An adult case of this type was described by Fahr, so that his name is sometimes attached to this disorder. This is an idiopathic form of calcification of the basal ganglia and cerebellum in which choreoathetosis and rigidity are prominent acquired features. The clinical state may also take the form of a parkinsonian syndrome or bilateral athetosis. In two of our patients there was unilateral choreoathetosis, which was replaced gradually by a parkinsonian syndrome, and in another of our sporadic cases, the initial abnormality was a unilateral dystonia responsive to L-dopa. Some patients have been mentally retarded but most are intellectually intact. The serum calcium levels in the aforementioned diseases are usually normal and there is no explanation of the calcification. The gene(s) have not been identified at the time of this writing but there may be a locus on chromosome 14q.

Hypoparathyroidism In hypoparathyroidism (idiopathic or acquired) and pseudohypoparathyroidism (a rare familial disease, caused by end-organ insensitivity to parathyroid hormone with distinctive skeletal and developmental abnormalities), the diminution in ionized serum calcium induces not only tetany and seizures but also choreoathetosis. This last symptom is presumably a result of calcification of the basal ganglia, which occurs in about one-half of the patients but of unknown mechanism. Also, in some instances there are signs of a cerebellar lesion. Pseudopseudohypoparathyroidism is a disorder that imitates the bony abnormalities seen in pseudohypoparathyroidism but in which calcium metabolism is normal and there are no neurologic features.

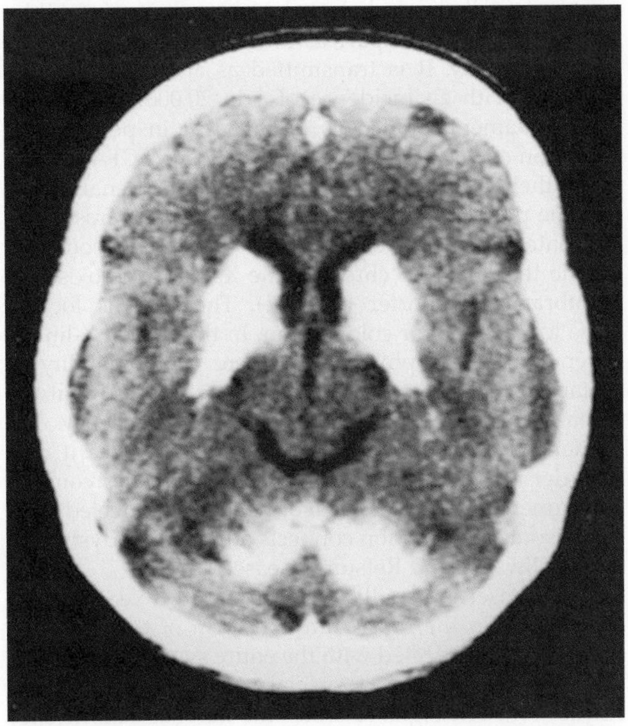

Figure 37-8. Idiopathic basal ganglionic and cerebellar calcification discovered 5 years after the onset of a slowly progressive rigid Parkinson syndrome in a 54-year-old woman.

Osteopetrosis

Sly and colleagues described the familial occurrence (21 cases in 12 families) of calcification in the caudate and lenticular nuclei, thalami, and frontal lobe white matter in association with osteopetrosis ("marble bones") and renal tubular acidosis. Clinically, there were multiple cranial nerve palsies—including optic atrophy as well as psychomotor delay and learning disabilities—but no extrapyramidal signs. The cranial nerve palsies, which are a result of bony encroachment in neural foramina, were much less severe than in the lethal form of osteopetrosis. The pattern of inheritance of this disease is autosomal recessive (rarely X-linked), and the basic abnormality was found to be a deficiency in carbonic anhydrase II in red blood corpuscles and probably in kidney and brain. Several types of disease have been associated with corresponding mutations, mostly in CLCN7.

Other Metabolic Disorders Associated With Choreoathetosis and Dystonia

We emphasize that acquired extrapyramidal disorders are much more common than metabolic ones. For example, athetosis may follow hypoxic encephalopathy of birth or follow kernicterus caused by Rh and ABO blood incompatibilities and erythroblastosis fetalis. The same is true of the Crigler-Najjar form of hereditary hyperbilirubinemia, in which kernicterus (with ataxia or athetosis) may rarely appear as late as childhood or adolescence, the defect being one of glucuronide-bilirubin conjugation. Later in life, the more common causes are medications, illicit drug use, focal cerebral lesions, hyperosmolar nonketotic state, antiphospholipid antibody syndrome, among many others discussed in Chap. 6. Furthermore, a number of other rare diseases, which can only be classified as heredofamilial degenerations, also figure in the differential diagnosis of choreoathetotic or dystonic syndromes and are discussed in Chap. 39. Torsion dystonia is the best-known example.

With regard to rarer metabolic causes, ceroid-lipofuscinosis of the Kufs type, G_{M1} gangliosidosis, late-onset metachromatic leukodystrophy, Niemann-Pick disease (type C), Hallervorden-Spatz disease, and Wilson disease may present with a syndrome of which dystonia or athetosis is an important component. Usually, there are other elements in the clinical picture as well, so that the correct diagnosis is seldom in doubt for long. dal Canto and colleagues have described a variant of neuronal ceroid-lipofuscinosis in which a boy and girl of unrelated non-Jewish parents developed severe choreoathetosis and dystonia at 6 to 7 years of age. Intellectual deterioration, gait abnormality, and seizures were added clinical features. Cerebral biopsy showed intraneuronal inclusions consisting of curvilinear bodies. These observations support the notion of nosologic heterogeneity among the nonglycolipid neuronal storage disorders.

Glutaric acidemia (type I) is another rare metabolic disorder, in which progressive choreoathetosis and dystonia are combined with intermittent acidemia. In some cases, ataxia of movement and a variable degree of mental retardation are also present. Glutaric acid is present in the urine, as are its metabolites 3-hydroxyglutarate and glutamate. The basic defect is in glutaryl CoA dehydrogenase, which has been found in leukocytes, hepatocytes, and fibroblasts. Neuropathologically, there is loss of neurons in the caudate, putamen, and pallidum, with gliosis. A spongy change is said to affect the white matter.

Infants with glutaric acidemia are often subject to sudden episodes of acidosis, coma, and flaccidity. There are signal changes on MRI, corresponding to the acute necrosis of nerve cells in the basal ganglia. These crises can be prevented and the infants can develop normally if the diagnosis is made before the development of neurologic signs, for example, in the sibling of an older affected child, and treatment is undertaken with a diet low in protein, particularly in tryptophan and lysine (Cho et al).

THE LEUKODYSTROPHIES: SYNDROMES OF BILATERAL HEMIPLEGIA, BLINDNESS, AND NEUROPATHY

Categorized here are late life manifestations of familial leukodystrophies. Of the several varieties of late-onset leukodystrophy, some are of unquestionable metabolic origin. The terms *metachromatic*, *sudanophilic*, *orthochromic*, etc., refer to the distinctive products of myelin degeneration and staining characteristics (or lack thereof) of the white matter in the individual leukodystrophies. As emphasized earlier, these are distinguished from the cerebral gray matter diseases (poliodystrophies), which have a different mode of presentation—seizures, myoclonus, chorea, choreoathetosis, and tremor being prominent. Instead, recognition of the entire group of leukodystrophies is based on symptoms and signs attributable to the interruption of tracts (corticospinal, corticobulbar, cerebellar peduncular, sensory) and visual pathways (optic nerve, optic tract, geniculocalcarine) and the infrequency or absence of seizures, myoclonus, and spike-and-wave abnormalities in the EEG. However, this distinction is not infallible, particularly in the later stages of the disease.

The syndrome of progressive spasticity and rigidity with spastic dysarthria and pseudobulbar palsy poses a difficult diagnostic problem. One's first impulse is to assume the presence of a corticospinal disorder, especially if tendon reflexes are brisk, but frequently the plantar reflexes are flexor and the facial reflexes are not enhanced ("pseudo-pseudobulbar palsy," a term we attribute to Marsden). In addition, unusual postures and a more plastic type of rigidity may occur, consistent with an extrapyramidal condition. Adrenomyeloneuropathy is another syndrome that combines reduced or absent tendon reflexes and Babinski signs, signifies a combination of corticospinal and peripheral nerve lesions, and is highly characteristic of metachromatic leukoencephalopathy.

The leukodystrophies that become apparent only in later life pose yet another problem: the clinical and radiologic differentiation from cerebral forms of multiple sclerosis. In identifying the metabolic diseases of myelin, one is helped by the relative symmetry and steady progression of the clinical signs; the early onset of cognitive impairment (which is uncharacteristic of multiple sclerosis); and the symmetrical and massive degeneration of the cerebral white matter (in distinction to the asymmetrical and often multiple lesions of demyelinative disease). At various times in life, particularly in young individuals, CADASIL (cerebral autosomal dominant arteriopathy with subcortical infarcts and leukoencephalopathy) enters into the differential diagnosis (see Chap. 34); late in life, distinguishing a metabolic disorder of myelin from the subcortical multiple infarctions of Binswanger disease and from the ubiquitous rarefaction of the periventricular regions of the cerebrum may be a problem. Differentiation from cerebral gliomatosis, brain lymphoma, toxic forms of leukodystrophy, and progressive multifocal leukoencephalopathy, all affecting deep cerebral or white matter structures, offers less difficulty.

Adrenoleukodystrophy (Sudanophilic Leukodystrophy, ABCD1 Mutation)

This combination of leukodystrophy and Addison disease, originally included under the rubric of Schilder disease, is now set apart as an independent metabolic encephalopathy. It is transmitted as an X-linked recessive trait with an incidence of 1 in 20,000 male births. The fundamental defect is impairment in peroxisomal oxidation of very-long-chain fatty acids (VLCFAs), leading to their accumulation in the brain and adrenal glands (see the publications of H.W. Moser and of Igarashi and associates). The deficient membrane protein, encoded by a gene that maps to chromosome X28, is a peroxisomal membrane transporter (*ABCD1*). The gene is located close to the gene for color vision. In the typical X-linked adrenoleukodystrophy (ALD), there is an inability to metabolize VLCFAs, but it came as a surprise that the disease was not caused by an enzyme deficiency. The modern classification of the disease categorizes it as a disorder of peroxisomes, subcellular organelles containing numerous enzymes, each of which is unaffected. This peroxisomal assignation connects adrenoleukodystrophy with Zellweger and Refsum disease.

The onset is usually between 4 and 8 years, sometimes later; in the most common form of this disorder, only males are affected with the entire syndrome (women carriers may display a special myelopathy discussed further on). The signs of either the adrenal insufficiency or the cerebral lesion may be the first to appear. In the case described by Siemerling and Creutzfeldt, the first recorded example of this disorder, bronzing of the skin of the hands appeared at 4 years of age; quadriparesis, with dysarthria and dysphagia (i.e., pseudobulbar palsy), became evident at 7 years; a single seizure occurred at 8 years; and by 9 years, shortly before death, the patient was *decerebrate* and unresponsive. In personally observed cases, the first abnormalities appeared at 9 to 10 years and took the form of episodic vomiting, decline in scholastic performance and change in personality with inappropriate giggling and crying. After a time, severe vomiting and an episode of circulatory collapse occurred, following which the gait became unsteady and arms ataxic with an intention tremor. Only then did the addisonian increase of pigmentation of the oral mucosa and the skin around nipples and over elbows, knees, and scrotum become evident. *Cortical blindness* follows in some instances. The late stages are marked by bilateral hemiplegia (at first asymmetrical), pseudobulbar paralysis, blindness, deafness, and impairment of all higher cerebral functions.

The severity of the disease varies. We are caring for two adult men in whom the cerebral symptoms have been mild, allowing for high-level cognitive achievement, albeit with peculiarities of personality, and with mild spastic gait, urinary difficulty, testicular insufficiency, and baldness. In each family there was a male sibling who died in childhood, ostensibly of adrenal insufficiency.

Griffin and coworkers have described a spinal-neuropathic form of the disease (adrenomyeloneuropathy [AMN]). In their patients, evidence of adrenal insufficiency had been present since early childhood, but only in the third decade of life did a progressive spastic paraparesis and a relatively mild polyneuropathy develop. It should be noted that the spasticity is occasionally asymmetrical, and the gait may have an ataxic component. This neurologic picture, in mild form and without adrenal insufficiency, is also the manner in which the disease may present in *female carriers of the gene abnormality* (see below). Like adrenoleukodystrophy, adrenomyeloneuropathy is typically inherited as an X-linked, male-specific trait. However, we have encountered a large family with adrenomyeloneuropathy in which males and females are both affected in a pattern that suggests dominant inheritance. The VLCFAs are modestly elevated in affected individuals, and there is no evidence of cerebral involvement.

Moser and colleagues (1980), using clinical and biochemical criteria, have identified the following subtypes of ALD:

1. A progressive degeneration of cerebral white matter in young males, often with cortical blindness—the classic type, accounting for half of all cases (Fig. 37-9)
2. An intermediate form in juvenile or young adult males with cerebral and spinal involvement (5 percent of cases)
3. A progressive spinal cord tract degeneration in adult males (25 percent of cases)
4. A chronic mild, nonprogressive spastic paraparesis in *heterozygous female carriers* (10 percent of cases)
5. Familial instances of Addison disease without neurologic involvement in males (10 percent of cases)
6. Possibly, in male infants, a form originating at birth (e.g., Zellweger disease)

Illustrating the variability in presentation among kindreds, Marsden and colleagues (1982) and, subsequently, Kobayashi and coworkers described a familial spinocerebellar syndrome, and Ohno and associates reported a sporadic instance of adrenoleukodystrophy presenting as olivopontocerebellar atrophy. Moser found cerebral forms alone in 30 percent, adrenomyeloneuropathy alone in 20 percent, and combined childhood cerebral and myelopathic forms in the remaining half.

Female Heterozygotes Neurologic manifestations develop in up to 50 percent of female carriers but in our experience with siblings of affected patients, the figure has been lower. The onset of a *spastic paraparesis* tends to occur later in life, usually in the third or fourth decade, and progression tends to be slow, but an explosive onset has been reported (see Chap. 44). As already mentioned, multiple sclerosis is the main consideration in differential diagnosis, particularly as 20 percent of heterozygotes have white matter changes on cerebral MRI. Overt adrenal insufficiency is rare in female carriers, but scalp hair may be scant as a subtle manifestation of adrenal hypofunction.

Pathologically in classic instances, massive degeneration of the myelin occurs, often asymmetrically in various parts of the cerebrum, brainstem, optic nerves, and sometimes spinal cord (see Fig. 37-9). Degradation products of myelin are visible in macrophages in recent lesions,

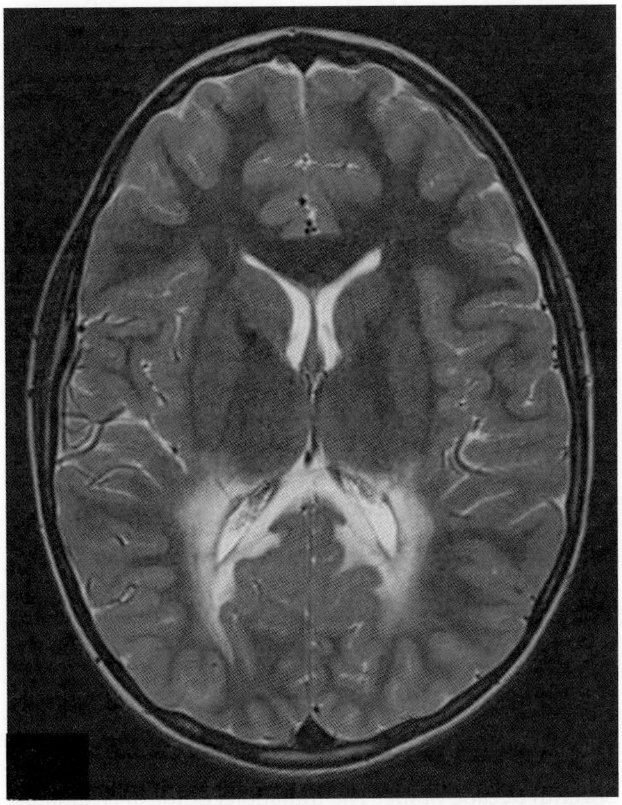

Figure 37-9. Adrenoleukodystrophy. Axial T2-weighted MRI of an 8-year-old boy with headache. There is abnormal posterior periventricular white matter hyperintensity extending across the splenium of the corpus callosum. Laboratory testing confirmed adrenal insufficiency. (Image courtesy of Drs. Edward Yang and Sanjay Prabhu.)

namely, sudanophilic demyelination. There is extensive astrocytic gliosis. Axons are damaged, but to a lesser degree. The cortex of the adrenal glands is atrophic, and the cells and invading histiocytes contain an abnormal lipid material. The testes show marked interstitial fibrosis and atrophy of the seminiferous tubules. Electron microscopically, the macrophages of the brain and adrenals and the Leydig cells of the testes contain characteristic lamellar cytoplasmic inclusions.

Laboratory Diagnosis The specific laboratory marker of the disease is an excess of VLCFAs, in particular three measurements are of value: the absolute level of hexacosanoic acid (C26), the ratio of C26 to C22 (docosahexanoic acid; C26:C22), and of C24 (tetracosanoic acid) to docosahexanoic acid (C24:C22) in plasma, erythrocytes, leukocytes, or cultured fibroblasts as detailed by Moser and colleagues (1999). This reflects the basic biochemical fault in this disease, namely defective fatty acid oxidation within the peroxisomes. If skin fibroblasts and plasma testing are both performed, 93 percent of female carriers will show the abnormal VLCFA. MRI of the brain is abnormal in the majority of patients with cerebral symptoms and in a proportion of others.

Other laboratory findings are low serum sodium and chloride levels and elevated potassium levels reflecting the atrophy of the adrenal glands. The latter results in reduced excretion of corticosteroids, low serum cortisol levels, and lack of rise in 17-hydroxyketosteroids after adrenocorticotropic hormone (ACTH) stimulation. The CSF protein may be elevated. As a research tool, Öz and colleagues have shown that magnetic resonance spectroscopy that measures the concentrations of several metabolites can be used as a guide to the progression of the disease and to gauge the effects of new therapies as they are introduced.

Treatment Adrenal replacement therapy prolongs life and occasionally effects a partial neurologic remission. A diet enriched with monounsaturated fatty acids and devoid of long-chain fatty acids has been said to slow the progress of the disease when administered before the age of 6 years. Bone marrow transplantation, to date performed in more than 50 children, has been the only treatment shown to stabilize the disease and reverse some of the MRI changes. The reviews by van Geel and colleagues, and the ones by Moser (1997 and 1999) the leading worker in the field, summarizing diagnosis and treatment, are recommended.

Juvenile and Adult Metachromatic Leukodystrophy

This form of leukodystrophy was described in relation to the inherited metabolic disorders of late infancy and early childhood in an earlier section. We mention it here to emphasize that the disease may have its onset at almost any age. Juvenile forms may begin between 4 and 12 years of age and adult forms between the midteens and the seventh decade of life. The mutations of the aryl sulfatase gene giving rise to these various forms are described in the earlier section on metachromatic leukodystrophy (MLD). Some of the sporadic cases reported in the adult probably were examples of cerebral multiple sclerosis, but we have seen, as have others, cases of MLD appearing as late as middle adult life. In almost all cases, the clinical picture, like those described by Turpin and Baumann, was one of slowly evolving intellectual decline or behavioral abnormality, followed by spastic weakness, hyperreflexia, Babinski signs, and stiff, short-stepped gait, with or without a polyneuropathy. Without manifest neurologic signs, misdiagnosis of psychiatric disease is common. As the disease progresses over a period of 3 to 5 years there may be a loss of vision and speech, then of hearing, and finally a state of virtual decerebration.

In some of these cases it is impossible to distinguish the white matter disease from that of Pelizaeus-Merzbacher and of Cockayne, described in the preceding section.

Orthochromatic Leukodystrophies

This refers to a heterogeneous group of disorders, also called nonmetachromatic leukodystrophy, in which no enzyme defect or special staining characteristic of degenerated white matter has been identified. Furthermore, most of them have been sporadic, obscuring the nosology of the process. One type is associated with cerebellar ataxia and dementia; other adult cases have been described in which epilepsy was associated with a frontal lobe type of dementia. A surprising feature, such as in the cases of Letournel and colleagues, has been normal MRI, even with the more sensitive FLAIR sequences.

Cerebrotendinous Xanthomatosis (CYP27A Mutation)

This rare disease is probably transmitted by an autosomal recessive gene. It usually begins in late childhood, with cataracts and xanthomas of tendon sheaths and lungs. As it progresses, difficulty in learning, impairment of retentive memory, and deficits in attention and visuospatial perception (the earliest neurologic manifestations) give way to dementia, ataxic or ataxic-spastic gait, dysarthria and dysphagia, and polyneuropathy. In the late stages (after 5 to 15 years), the patient becomes bedfast and helpless; death occurs at 20 to 30 years of age. In other cases, the clinical course is much more benign. Neuropathologic examination shows masses of crystalline cholesterol in the brainstem and cerebellum and sometimes in the spinal cord, with symmetrical destruction of myelin in the involved areas. The white matter lesions are visible by CT and MRI.

The basic defect is in the synthesis of primary bile acids, leading to an increased hepatic production of cholesterol and cholestanol, which accumulate in brain and tendons. The serum cholesterol levels are normal in most cases but may be as high as 450 mg/dL in others. The tendon xanthomas contain cholesterol, of which 4 to 9 percent is cholestanol (dihydrocholesterol) according to the studies of Moser and colleagues (1984). Cholestanol levels in the serum and red cells are increased. The same elevated levels are found in heterozygotes. The causative mutation is in CYP27A.

Treatment In response to long-term treatment with chenodeoxycholic acid, 750 mg daily, the corticospinal and cerebellar signs and dementia receded in 10 of 17 patients treated and followed by Berginer and coworkers. This drug corrects the defective synthesis of bile acids and restores the low level of chenodeoxycholic acid. Ideally, treatment should begin before the neurologic symptoms appear (Meiner et al).

STROKES IN ASSOCIATION WITH INHERITED METABOLIC DISEASES

In Chap. 34 it was remarked that strokes occur from time to time in children and young adults, often as a result of inherited disorders of the clotting system typified by protein C deficiency, but also of a number of other metabolic derangements, including the mitochondrial disorder MELAS (mitochondrial myopathy, encephalopathy, lactic acidosis, and stroke-like episodes). Among the many causes, three metabolic diseases must always be considered in the diagnosis of such cases: *homocystinuria*, *Fabry disease*, and *sulfite oxidase deficiency*. Other less-common ones are *Tangier disease* and *familial hypercholesterolemia*. Stroke in young persons is also a central feature of the mitochondrial disorder MELAS, discussed further on in this chapter, and of the genetically determined microvasculopathy CADASIL ("Familial Subcortical Infarction" discussed in Chap. 34).

Homocystinuria

This aminoaciduria is inherited as an autosomal recessive trait and simulates Marfan disease. Tall, slender habitus; great length of limbs, sometimes scoliosis and arachnodactyly (long, spidery fingers and toes); thin and rather weak muscles; knock-knees; highly arched feet; and kyphosis are the typical skeletal features. Sparse, blond, brittle hair; malar flush; and livedo reticularis are common dermal manifestations, and a dislocation of one or both lenses (usually downward) may occur, imparting a tremulous appearance to the irides (iridodonesis). The only neurologic abnormality is mental retardation, usually of mild degree, which sets this syndrome apart from Marfan disease, in which intellect is unimpaired. Several mutations in different genes have been implicated, the most common being in CBS that codes for cystathionine beta-synthase.

Blood vessel changes of thickening and fibrosis of the coronary, cerebral, and renal arteries tend to appear later in the illness. An abnormality of platelets favoring clot formation and thrombosis of cerebral arteries has been observed. Some patients have died of coronary occlusions during adolescence, and a myocardial lesion may be the source of emboli to cerebral arteries.

Homocysteine is elevated in the blood and CSF, and homocystine in the urine. This is because of an inherited cystathionine synthase deficiency that results in an inadequacy of cystathionine formation, a substance essential to many tissues including the brain. This may be the explanation of the developmental delay. Plasma methionine levels are also elevated. The infarcts in the brain are clearly related to thrombotic and embolic arterial occlusions. The administration of large doses (50 to 500 mg) of pyridoxine (a cystathionine synthase coenzyme), folate 5 mg daily and cobalamin (vitamin B_{12}) 1,000 μg daily, reduces the excretion of homocystine. If vascular lesions have occurred, anticoagulants probably prevent further occlusions.

Homocysteinemia and homocystinuria may also be expressions of 5,10-methylenetetrahydrofolate reductase deficiency. Again, the clinical manifestations consist of multiple cerebrovascular lesions, dementia, epilepsy, and polyneuropathy. The last is believed to be caused by a coincidental folic acid deficiency, but in some cases it may have been caused by chronic phenytoin administration (Nishimura et al).

Much milder elevations of serum homocystine have been recognized as contributing to the risk of coronary disease and stroke in otherwise normal individuals.

Fabry Disease (Anderson-Fabry Disease, GLA Mutation) (See also Chaps. 34 and 46)

This disease, also known as *angiokeratoma corporis diffusum*, is inherited as an X-linked recessive trait. It occurs in complete form in males and in incomplete form in female carriers. The primary deficit is in the enzyme alpha-galactosidase A, the result of which is the accumulation of ceramide trihexoside in endothelial, perithelial, and smooth muscle cells of blood vessels as well as in renal tubular and glomerular cells and other viscera and in nerve cells in many parts of the nervous system (hypothalamic and amygdaloid nuclei, substantia nigra, reticular and other nuclei of the brainstem, anterior and intermediolateral horns of the spinal cord, sympathetic and dorsal root ganglia).

The disease becomes manifest clinically in childhood or adolescence, with intermittent lancinating pains and dysesthesias of the extremities. A notable feature of these pains is their evocation by fever, hot weather, and vigorous exercise. Usually there is no sensory loss, but autonomic disturbances have been recorded in a series of our cases. Many years later there is a diffuse vascular involvement that leads to hypertension, renal damage, cardiomegaly, and myocardial ischemia. Thrombotic infarctions occur in the brain during early adult years. Occasional cases are discovered in adulthood with confluent cerebral white matter changes on MRI and progressive problems such as dysarthria.

The characteristic angiokeratomas tend to be most prominent periumbilically and resemble small angiomas that obliterate slightly with pressure. Desnick and colleagues have reviewed the neurologic, neuropathologic, and biochemical findings in this disease, and Cable and colleagues have written informatively on the autonomic aspects.

Treatment Enzyme replacement, given by infusion, is now available. The two main trials of this treatment, summarized in an editorial by Pastores and Thadhani, were each conducted quite differently. Both showed an improvement in kidney and other organ function but only one demonstrated a reduction in neuropathic pain, and neither studied the risk of stroke. Like enzyme replacement therapy for Gaucher disease, prolonged treatment is expensive; but some evidence from the trials cited above indicates that certain aspects of the disease are reversible.

The painful neuropathic features that have brought several cases to our attention are discussed with the polyneuropathies, in Chap. 46.

Sulfite Oxidase Deficiency

This disorder was discussed briefly with the neonatal metabolic disorders. The occurrence of stroke as a complication of this disorder was placed on record by our colleagues Shih et al (1977). A child 4.5 years of age, whose development had been retarded since birth (seizures and opisthotonos had been present), became hemiplegic. Another unrelated child, supposedly normal until 2 years of age, entered the hospital with fever, confusion, generalized seizures, right hemiplegia, and aphasia (infantile hemiplegia); subluxation of the lenses (upward) was discovered later. There was an increased level of sulfite and thiosulfate and an abnormal amino acid, *S*-sulfocysteine, in the blood. One child appeared to respond to a low-sulfur–amino-acid diet.

CHANGES IN BEHAVIOR AND INTELLECT AS MANIFESTATIONS OF INHERITED METABOLIC DISEASE

Certain metabolic diseases may be the cause of serious disturbances of cognitive function and behavior, even in the adolescent and early adult period. The diagnosis and management of these metabolic diseases are so unusual that some special remarks are appropriate. When they present later in adolescence and adult life they evolve more slowly than childhood forms. The most obvious and easily detectable of these derangements are in the cognitive sphere, i.e., memory, calculation, problem solving, and verbal skills. Impulsivity, loss of self-control, and antisocial behavior are the most troubling behavioral abnormalities. Each of these phenomena has its own cerebral anatomy, as pointed out in Chap. 22, and the state of dementia comprises various degrees and combinations of these abnormalities.

Intellectual functions are difficult to accurately assess in early childhood. Slowness in learning and in acquiring language functions become manifest in school and may then be interpreted loosely as mental retardation. Up until school age, these intellectual functions have not developed sufficiently to allow recognition of their regressive course. Only in late childhood do mental retardation and dementia become clearly distinguishable and measurable by standardized tests. Far less tangible are subtle changes in personality and behavior.

A useful principle in recognizing those adolescents with a metabolic brain disease is that sooner or later, such a condition will cause a *regression in cognitive and intellectual functions*. Bipolar disease, sociopathies, and character disorders do not result in the loss of neurologic function. The recognition of a metabolic cause of mental deterioration depends on the demonstration of failing memory, impaired thinking, inability to learn, and loss of verbal and arithmetic abilities, many of which are measured quantitatively by intelligence tests. The appearance of pyramidal signs, aphasia, apraxia, ataxia, or areflexia further sets them apart.

If one reviews all the diseases described in this chapter and selects those that may demonstrate *regression of cognitive function in association with personality change and alteration of behavior in an adult*—diseases that may for a time be unaccompanied by other neurologic abnormalities—the following metabolic disorders merit special consideration in approximate relative order of importance:

1. Wilson disease
2. Adrenoleukodystrophy
3. Metachromatic leukodystrophy
4. Hallervorden-Spatz pigmentary degeneration
5. Late-onset neuronal ceroid-lipofuscinosis (Kufs form)
6. Juvenile and adult Gaucher disease (type III)
7. Some of the mucopolysaccharidoses
8. Adult G_{M2} gangliosidosis
9. Mucolipidosis I (type I sialidosis)
10. Lafora-body myoclonic epilepsy
11. Nonwilsonian copper disorder (hereditary ceruloplasmin deficiency)

In each of these diseases, dementia and personality disorder may gradually develop and exist for many months, even a year or two, before other neurologic signs appear. One must look carefully for the earliest signs of movement disorders and other neurologic abnormalities, which greatly clarify the diagnostic problem. The common use of neuroleptic drugs, causing tardive dyskinesia and parkinsonian signs, is an obstacle to determining if there are neurologic features in these ostensibly psychiatric conditions.

ADULT FORMS OF INHERITED METABOLIC DISEASES

The increasing range and precision of biochemical and cytologic tests have brought to light a number of inherited metabolic diseases that sometimes have their onset in adult life. Such disorders, while uncommon, nevertheless are important because they must be considered in the differential diagnosis of degenerative diseases. Also to be considered in the differential diagnosis is an array of mitochondrial disorders, to be discussed further on in this chapter.

In the last three decades, the authors have personally observed or have otherwise come to know of examples of the following metabolic diseases, the onset of which was in adult life:

1. Metachromatic leukoencephalopathy
2. Adrenoleukodystrophy
3. Globoid body leukodystrophy (Krabbe disease)
4. Kufs form of neuronal ceroid lipofuscinosis
5. G_{M2} gangliosidosis
6. Wilson disease
7. Gaucher disease
8. Niemann-Pick disease
9. Carnitine palmityl transferase deficiency

10. Mucopolysaccharide encephalopathy
11. Mucolipidosis type I
12. Polyneuropathies (Andrade disease, Fabry disease, porphyria, Refsum disease)
13. Mitochondrial diseases, particularly progressive external ophthalmoplegia and Leigh disease

In the encephalopathic forms of the metabolic and mitochondrial diseases, the diagnosis is usually made only after symptoms have been present for months or years, the disease having been mistaken for some other condition, particularly depression or a degenerative dementia. Even a manifest psychosis may have occurred in relation to some of these disorders, but such occurrences are admittedly rare. For example, one of our patients with metachromatic leukodystrophy, a 30-year-old man, began failing in college years and was later unsuccessful in holding a job because of carelessness and mistakes in his work and indifference to criticism, irritability, and stubbornness (clearly traceable to a mild dementia). Only when Babinski signs and loss of tendon reflexes in the legs were detected was the correct diagnosis entertained for the first time. By then he had been ill for nearly 10 years. Bosch and Hart described a patient with the onset of dementia at 62 years of age and drew attention to 27 other similar cases of adult-onset metachromatic leukoencephalopathy (see also the 7 cases of Turpin and Baumann). Overt signs of neuropathy are usually lacking in these adult-onset cases, but EMG and sural nerve biopsy will disclose the characteristic abnormalities.

One of our adult patients with Wilson disease had been committed to a psychiatric hospital because of his paranoid tendencies and fighting with his family; the presence of a tremor and mild rigidity of the limbs had been attributed at first to phenothiazine drugs. In some of Griffin's cases of adrenomyeloneuropathy, a spastic weakness of the legs and sensory ataxia progressing over several years were the main clinical manifestations; a spinocerebellar degeneration was suspected. One of our patients with Kufs lipid storage disease began to deteriorate mentally in early adult life and only much later showed an increasing rigidity, with athetotic posturing of limbs and difficulty in walking; he succumbed to his disease after more than a decade of symptoms. Another recent patient with Kufs disease presented at age 51 with vague visual difficulty, which was followed by spasticity of the legs, behavioral disinhibition, and dementia spanning 6 years. Josephs and colleagues describe 2 of 5 patients with adult-onset type C Niemann-Pick disease who had a psychosis beginning at ages 61 and 27, respectively.

We have observed cerebellar ataxia, polymyoclonus, and progressive blindness in adolescents and adults with a variant of G_{M2} gangliosidosis; cherry-red macular spots provided the clue to diagnosis. Several such cases have been reported in the last decade, particularly among the Japanese (Miyatake et al). Nine cases of a spinocerebellar ataxia with dementia or psychosis of adult onset were described by Wilner and colleagues. Also in our service were 2 adult patients with progressive spinal muscular atrophy who proved to have this same G_{M2} hexosaminidase deficiency; the process was clinically almost indistinguishable from a very slowly progressive lower motor neuron form of motor neuron disease but they had no macular changes and displayed the additional features of ataxia and an intermittent and atypical psychosis. An asymmetrical corticospinal syndrome with areflexia had advanced so slowly in one of our cases of Krabbe disease that she became disabled only in her sixties.

Another of our patients, an adolescent with severe diffuse myoclonus and seizures and slight intellectual deterioration, was found after several years to have one of the rare variants of Gaucher disease. Another with dementia, rigidity, choreoathetosis, slight cerebellar ataxia, and Babinski signs had a variant of Niemann-Pick disease. Rarely, Gaucher disease may be associated with an early and severe parkinsonian syndrome. Cases of familial adult-onset Leigh disease have been described by Kalimo and colleagues. Adrenoleukodystrophy presenting in adult life as a spinocerebellar or olivopontocerebellar syndrome has already been mentioned.

These rare forms of inherited metabolic disease are notable for their chronicity and for the early prominence of a particular neurologic symptom or syndrome. Once the disease is established, however, there is nearly always evidence of involvement of multiple neuronal systems, reflected in a subtle or overt dementia, character disorder, or signs referable to corticospinal, cerebellar, extrapyramidal, visual, and peripheral nerve structures. *This multiplicity of neuronal system involvement is much more a feature of heritable metabolic disease than of degenerative disease and the finding of such involvement should provoke a search for an inherited metabolic disorder.*

To reiterate the clinical aspects, the aforementioned dictum that tract involvement (corticospinal, cerebellar, peduncular, sensory, optic nerve) indicates a leukodystrophy and that "gray matter" signs (seizures, myoclonus, dementia, retinal lesions) indicate a poliodystrophy is useful mainly in the early stages of a disease. Some of the lysosomal storage diseases affect both galactolipids (galactocerebrosides and sulfatides) and gangliosides; hence both white and gray matters are involved. The paper by Turpin and Baumann is of interest when this group of diseases is viewed from the strictly psychiatric point of view.

Certain outstanding clinical symptoms that are more often attributable to common diseases of the adult nervous system, such as multiple sclerosis and atherosclerosis, are sometimes the result of an inborn error of metabolism. These infrequent instances are categorized by their main features in Table 37-8, which is adopted from Grey et al.

Viewed from another perspective, patients are sometimes referred for the evaluation of diffuse white matter disease of the cerebrum that has been found with aiming studies. Multiple sclerosis and its variants come to mind immediately but, as discussed in Chap. 36, diseases other than MS are more likely to *cause diffuse, symmetric, and bilateral changes in the deep hemispheres*. These include CADASIL, Susac syndrome, infiltrative tumors such as lymphoma and gliomatosis cerebri, and autoimmune systemic conditions that secondarily affect the white matter,

Table 37-8

MAJOR SYNDROMES ADULT-ONSET INHERITED METABOLIC DISEASES

Dementia and psychosis
Kufs disease
Niemann-Pick disease type C
Wilson disease
Adrenoleukodystrophy
Metachromatic leukodystrophy
Aceruloplasminemia
Motor neuron disease
G_{M2} gangliosidosis
Polyglycosan disease
Choreoathetosis
Wilson disease
G_{M2} gangliosidosis
Niemann-Pick disease type C
Ataxia
Aceruloplasminemia
Abetalipoproteinemia
G_{M2} gangliosidosis
Hartnup disease
Sialidosis
Niemann-Pick disease type C
Leukodystrophy
Krabbe disease
Metachromatic leukodystrophy
Adrenoleukodystrophy
Orthochromatic leukodystrophy
Strokes
Fabry disease
Homocystinuria
MELAS

MELAS, mitochondrial encephalomyopathy, lactic acidosis, and stroke-like episodes.

perhaps by a mechanism of microvasculitis. However, the dysmyelinating leukodystrophies discussed in this chapter may manifest late in life and enter into the differential diagnosis of this imaging appearance. As a guide to evaluating such cases, Schiffmann and van der Knaap have provided an extensive listing of diseases and characterized them by the presence of the MRI characteristics, particularly the presence of *hypomyelination* in which the white matter is hyperintense or isointense to the cortex on T1-weighted images (and usually less T2 hyperintense than in other pathologic changes of white matter). They further divide the group that is not hypomyelinated by the feature of confluence of multifocal distribution. The algorithm they provide may guide the clinician in choosing an appropriate laboratory plan.

In concluding this discussion, which classifies the inherited monogenetic metabolic diseases in accordance with their clinical characteristics, the reader will appreciate its artificiality. Nearly every one of the diseases of each category may present some neurologic abnormality other than the ones we have emphasized, so that the potential number of variations is almost limitless. However, the plan presented here of thinking of these diseases in reference to age periods and syndromes, is of heuristic value and facilitates clinical study of this extremely difficult segment of neurologic medicine.

MITOCHONDRIAL DISORDERS

As with the metabolic disorders of the nervous system, the diseases included under this heading are so varied and may involve so many parts of the nervous system that the clinical entities by which they are identified cannot be easily addressed in any one part of this book. In their overlapping relationships, however, these diseases are unlike the more discrete clinical entities caused by nuclear genetic mutations. Their diversity is evident not only in the details of their clinical presentations but also in the age at which symptoms first become apparent and, what is most intriguing, sometimes in the abrupt onset of their neurologic manifestations. Most of this variability in presentation is understandable from the principles of mitochondrial genetics outlined in the introductory section of this chapter. Of particular importance is the mosaicism of the mitochondria within cells and from cell to cell and the crucial role the organelles play in the oxidative energy metabolism that supports the function of cells in all organs.

Fortunately for the clinician, the most important of these diseases are expressed in several recognizable core syndromes and in a few variants thereof. A number of acronyms derived from the initial letters of the main clinical features are used to designate the major mitochondrial syndromes: MERRF, MELAS, PEO, NARP, etc., as summarized in Table 37-9. The addition of certain subtle dysmorphic features including short stature; endocrinopathies, particularly diabetes; and a number of other systemic abnormalities such as lactic acidosis (discussed further on) aids in diagnosis of this class of disorder.

These diseases are the result of mutations in the mitochondrial genome, a ringed DNA of 16,569 base pairs and 37 genes contained within the organelle, or of mutations in a few nuclear genes that code for a component of the mitochondrion. To date, more than 100 point mutations and 200 deletions, insertions, and rearrangements have been identified. It is estimated that two-thirds of the point mutations affect the transfer RNA of the mitochondrion, one-third affect polypeptide units of the respiratory chain, and a small number affect mitochondrial ribosomal RNA. This corresponds approximately to the proportion of genes devoted to each of these functions. DiMauro and Schon wrote a thorough review of mitochondrial genomics and the most relevant diseases, which may be consulted by interested readers.

The first described and best-characterized member of this group of diseases is a symmetrical proximal myopathy that occurs as an isolated illness or in combination with any of the major mitochondrial syndromes. In 1966, Shy and coworkers described the histochemical and electron-microscopic abnormalities of the muscle mitochondria in a childhood myopathy, which they called *megaconial* (meaning marked enlargement of the mitochondria) or *pleoconial* (referring to an excessive number of mitochondria). Later this change came to be known as "ragged red fibers," so named because of the subsarcolemmal and intermyofibrillar collections of membranous

Table 37-9

THE MAJOR CATEGORIES OF MITOCHONDRIAL DISORDERS

SYNDROME	COMMON MITOCHONDRIAL GENE MUTATION	RAGGED RED FIBERS	LACTIC ACIDOSIS
Ragged red fiber polymyopathy	Point mutation at 3250	+	–
Progressive external ophthalmoplegia (PEO) and Kearns-Sayre variants	Heteroplasmic deletions or point mutation at 3243	–	–
Leigh syndrome, fatal lactic acidosis, and neuropathy with proximal weakness, ataxia, and retinitis pigmentosa (NARP)	Point mutation at 8993	–	+
Myoclonic-epilepsy and ragged red fibers in muscle (MERRF)	Point mutation at 8344	+ (usually)	±
Mitochondrial encephalomyopathy, lactic acidosis, and stroke-like episodes (MELAS)	Point mutation at 3243	+	+
Leber optic neuropathy	Point mutation at 3460, 4160, or 11778	–	–
Myoneural-gastrointestinal encephalopathy	Unknown (maternal inheritance)	+	–

+ = present; – = absent.

(mitochondrial) material in the type 1 (red) muscle fibers as visualized by the Gomori trichrome stain in sections of frozen muscle. This morphologic change may be an asymptomatic accompaniment of the mitochondrial disorders or, conversely, a mitochondrial disease of the CNS may exist without histologic or ultrastructural abnormalities in the muscle.

A second unifying feature of these diseases is an elevation of lactate concentration or of the lactate-to-pyruvate ratio in the blood and CSF; this is the result of the respiratory chain abnormalities. These elevations are most prominent after exercise, infection, fever, or alcohol ingestion and in some conditions are capable of inducing recurrent ketoacidotic coma, which may be the presenting manifestation of a mitochondrial disease. Leigh syndrome and MELAS particularly have a tendency to exhibit elevations of lactate; however, the diagnosis of either cannot be excluded in the presence of normal levels of this substance, even after provocation by exercise (see further on for a description of testing for elevated lactate). Using phosphorus MRI scans, one can compare levels of inorganic phosphate to phosphocreatine levels in muscle; in genetic muscle diseases of several types, this ratio increases, but it is highest in those of mitochondrial origin.

Although the mitochondrial diseases are considered here as a group, individual ones are of necessity mentioned in other chapters because of their outstanding characteristics. Thus the syndrome that combines epilepsy, deafness, and developmental delay with ragged red muscle fibers (myoclonic epilepsy with ragged red fibers, or MERRF) was discussed in Chap. 16, on epilepsy. The syndrome of progressive external ophthalmoplegia (PEO) has been included with other abnormalities of eye movements (see Chap. 50); lactic acidosis and stroke-like episodes (MELAS) were considered in Chap. 34, with the cerebrovascular diseases; and Leber hereditary optic neuropathy, with other causes of visual loss (see Chaps. 13 and 39). Leigh syndrome, a symmetrical subacute necrotizing encephalomyelopathy, usually with lactic acidosis, also has a number of complex presentations and is mentioned in the differential diagnosis of several diseases. For each of the aforementioned processes, wide clinical experience will bring to light an individual or a family in whom some odd syndrome has been linked to a mitochondrial disorder. Furthermore, two major syndromes may coexist in one individual and fragmentary subsyndromes are known to occur, having an onset any time from childhood to early adult life. Consequently, it serves little purpose to catalogue all of these associations. Only the best-characterized entities, listed in Table 37-9, are described here. The most common combinations of mitochondrial syndromes have been of Kearns-Sayre syndrome with MELAS or with MERRF, progressive ophthalmoplegia with MERRF, and MERRF with MELAS.

We prefer to avoid the issue of what defines a "mitochondrial disorder"—its genetic defect, the biochemical disorder, or the clinical syndrome. The clinician assigns this term to the combination of a mutation of mitochondrial DNA and certain clinical features that constitute a recognizable syndrome; the biochemical changes are taken as markers of the disordered energy-producing mechanisms of the mitochondrial machinery. Mitochondrial failure has also become a focus of interest in various degenerative neurologic conditions, such as Alzheimer and Parkinson diseases but none of the currently understood mutations of the mitochondrial genome is clearly implicated in these conditions.

Mitochondrial Myopathies

The mildest form of muscle disorder caused by mitochondrial disease is a benign and relatively static proximal weakness that tends to be more severe in the arms. Exercise intolerance alone is reported by more than half of these patients. There are adult-onset cases, but careful questioning usually reveals lifelong symptoms (weakness, poor endurance, discomfort, exertional dyspnea, and tachycardia), which may be so slight and slowly progressive that the patient leads a relatively normal life for decades. Less-frequent patterns of muscle disease include a fascioscapulohumeral or limb-girdle pattern of weakness as well as occasional episodes of exertional myoglobinuria. Some patients develop PEO several years after the limb weakness becomes evident. Several mutations are associated with a pure or predominant myopathic syndrome, the most common one being located at position 3250 of the mitochondrial genome. Rare variants, such as combined skeletal weakness and cardiomyopathy, are referable to other loci.

At the opposite end of the spectrum is an infantile myopathy in which weakness and lactic acidosis become evident in the first week of life and are fatal by 1 year. Many of these patients and some members of their families have a history of renal dysfunction combined with weakness of early onset. The muscle tissue shows numerous ragged red fibers, and cytochrome oxidase activity is virtually absent. DiMauro (1983) and others have described a remarkable partly reversible form, which, early on, requires ventilatory support and gastric feeding but improves clinically as the child ages; the lactic acidosis disappears by age 2 or 3 years. In these severe childhood cases, the deficiencies in cytochrome oxidase suggest a defect in mitochondrial genes, but the site has not been found.

As mentioned above, the histologic feature that unites mitochondrial myopathies is the presence of ragged red fibers. This finding points to the diagnosis of a mitochondrial disorder in any case where weakness is coupled with exercise intolerance and elevated serum lactate, particularly if there is a family history of similar problems. Also, the presence of ragged red fibers differentiates the mitochondrial myopathies from the glycogenoses but it bears emphasizing that ragged red fibers are rare in infants and young children, even in those with confirmed mitochondrial disease.

Progressive External Ophthalmoplegia and Kearns-Sayre Syndrome (See also Chap. 50)

The combination of progressive ptosis and symmetrical ophthalmoplegia is a common manifestation of mitochondrial disease. Usually there is no diplopia or strabismus or at most only transient diplopia, despite slightly dysconjugate gaze. Mitochondrial abnormalities are found in the extraocular muscles of these patients. We have been impressed at how long the illness can exist before it brings the patient to a physician. To be differentiated is myasthenia gravis, which is characterized by fatigable weakness and responsiveness to cholinergic medications, neither of which is a feature of mitochondrial disorders. In our experience, nearly all cases of PEO are because of mitochondrial disorders, but rarely the condition may be simulated by one of several genetically determined muscular dystrophies, including oculopharyngeal dystrophy and a type in which there are no other associated weaknesses but is, however, linked to facioscapulohumeral dystrophy (FSH; Chap. 50).

PEO bears a close relationship to the Kearns-Sayre syndrome of retinitis pigmentosa (onset before age 20 years), ataxia, heart block and other conduction defects, and elevated CSF protein; sensorineural deafness, seizures, or pyramidal signs may be added (see Chap. 50 for clinical description). The CNS syndromes of MELAS or MERRF (see further on) may also be combined with PEO.

Subacute Necrotizing Encephalomyelopathy (Leigh Disease)

This is a familial or sporadically occurring mitochondrial disorder with a wide range of clinical manifestations. Only some of the cases display a maternal pattern of inheritance. The onset of neurologic difficulty in more than half of these patients is in the first year of life, mostly before the sixth month; but late-onset forms, with great heterogeneity of presentation as late as early adulthood, are also known. Neurologic symptoms often appear subacutely or abruptly, sometimes precipitated by a febrile illness or a surgical operation. It has seemed to us that this rapid onset is more characteristic of Leigh disease than it is of the other mitochondrial disorders and the disease could reasonably be designated as "acute necrotizing encephalomyelopathy" (ANE), a term applied to a similar entity in Japan and China.

In infants, loss of head control and other recent motor acquisitions, hypotonia, poor sucking, anorexia and vomiting, irritability and continuous crying, generalized seizures, and myoclonic jerks constitute the usual clinical picture. If the onset is in the second year, there is delay in walking, ataxia, dysarthria, psychomotor regression, tonic spasms, characteristic respiratory disturbances (episodic hyperventilation, especially during infections, and periods of apnea, gasping, and quiet sobbing), external ophthalmoplegia, nystagmus, and disorders of gaze (like those of Wernicke disease), paralysis of deglutition, and abnormal movements of the limbs (particularly dystonia but also jerky and choreiform movements). Mild cases, showing mainly developmental delay, have been mistaken for cerebral palsy. Peripheral nerves are involved in some cases (areflexia, weakness, atrophy, and slowed conduction velocities of peripheral nerves); in a few, autonomic failure is the most prominent feature. In some children the disease is episodic; in others it is intermittently progressive and quite protracted, with exacerbation of neurologic symptoms in association with nonspecific infections. The CSF is usually normal but the protein content may be increased.

The pathologic changes take the form of bilaterally symmetrical foci of spongy necrosis with myelin degeneration, vascular proliferation, and gliosis in the thalami, midbrain, pons, medulla, and spinal cord. In cases of acute onset there may be minor hemorrhagic change. The basal ganglia are characteristically but not invariably affected. Also, there may be a demyelinative type of peripheral neuropathy. In their distribution and histologic appearance, the CNS lesions resemble those of Wernicke disease (caused by a deficiency of thiamine) except that the lesions of Leigh disease are more extensive—sometimes involving the striatum—and they spare the mammillary bodies. The lesions, particularly those of the lenticular nuclei and brainstem, may be seen in CT and are strikingly demonstrated by MRI. The histochemical appearance of muscle is normal, although electron microscopy may show an increased number of mitochondria.

The clinical boundaries of Leigh disease have not been defined precisely. A familial disorder of infancy and early childhood, referred to as *bilateral striatal necrosis* and associated with dystonia, visual failure, and other neurologic defects, is probably a variant. The same may be true of an obscure adult-onset syndrome of progressive dementia, caused by thalamic lesions, in the form of necrosis, vascular proliferation, and gliosis. A resemblance to what has recently been termed acute necrotizing encephalomyelopathy, arising in children after an infectious illness, was alluded to earlier.

The mitochondrial 8993 mutation associated with Leigh disease that explains 20 percent of cases is also discussed below in relation to the NARP syndrome. The close relationship between the two processes reemphasizes the point that several mitochondrial mutations rise to the clinical and pathologic picture of a necrotizing encephalopathy. However, it has been recently pointed out that many cases of Leigh disease are associated with nuclear mutations, including in *RANBP2* that codes for a component of the nuclear pore.

Neuropathy, Ataxia, Retinitis Pigmentosa Syndrome (NARP)

As just indicated, Leigh syndrome exemplifies to a remarkable degree the heterogeneity of abnormalities that may be associated with cytochrome oxidase deficiency caused by a single mitochondrial gene mutation. A minor transversion error, the substitution of one nucleotide in the mitochondrial DNA at position 8993, the same site implicated in Leigh syndrome, also gives rise to a maternally inherited syndrome of sensory NARP. The mutation creates a defective ATPase-6 of complex V of the mitochondrial respiratory chain. Included in some cases of NARP are developmental delay, seizures, and proximal muscle weakness.

The severity of the NARP syndrome corresponds to the amount of aberrant DNA in the mitochondrial genome; mutations involving more than 90 percent of mitochondrial DNA produce the more severe phenotype of the necrotizing encephalopathy.

Santorelli and colleagues found that 12 of 50 patients with Leigh syndrome from 10 families displayed the 8993 point mutation. Within one kindred, the mitochondrial aberration may vary from a mild developmental delay, to NARP, to the full-blown Leigh syndrome, or early death with lactic acidosis. These differences in severity are thought to result from the mosaicism of mitochondrial genetics and specifically to the protective effect of even small amounts of the normal mitochondrial genome. The first manifestations of disease may not appear until adulthood, although it only rarely begins after age 20 years.

Further confounding the clinical classification of this disease complex is the observation that many patients with the Leigh syndrome have a pyruvate dehydrogenase (usually X-linked) or pyruvate decarboxylase deficiency or a cytochrome oxidase deficiency. These are common to many mitochondrial disorders and inherited usually as an autosomal recessive trait. However, patients with Leigh syndrome and the 8993 mutation tend not to have these enzymatic deficiencies. Bridging these complex cases to the typical ones are instances with cytochrome oxidase deficiency with psychomotor retardation, slowed growth, and lactic acidosis, many without the striatal or brainstem spinal necroses of Leigh syndrome.

Congenital Lactic Acidosis and Recurrent Ketoacidosis

Certain types of organic acidemia occurring in early infancy and of unproved genetic etiology have already been mentioned. Here reference is made to those few cases that are associated with deletions of mitochondrial DNA. The syndrome consists of *psychomotor regression* and *episodic hyperventilation*, *hypotonia*, and *convulsions* with intervening periods of normalcy. Choreoathetosis or progressive ophthalmoplegia have been added in a few cases. Probably most cases of this type are caused by disorders of the mitochondrial respiratory chain, particularly of the pyruvate-decarboxylase complex. Some children are dysmorphic, with a broad nasal bridge, micrognathia, posteriorly rotated ears, short arms and fingers, and other similar but mild dysmorphic features. De Vivo and colleagues have written a synopsis of this disease. Death usually occurs before the third year. The important laboratory findings are acidosis with high lactate levels and hyperalaninemia. The few cases that have been examined postmortem are found to have necrosis and cavitation of the globus pallidus and cerebral white matter, as in subacute necrotizing encephalomyelopathy (SNE). The diagnosis can be made by the finding of ragged red fibers in muscle or by measurement of enzyme activity. The process must be distinguished from the several diseases of infancy that are complicated by lactic acidosis.

Myoclonic Epilepsy With Ragged Red Fibers (MERRF)

This disease presents as progressive myoclonic epilepsy or myoclonic ataxia. As was noted in Chap. 6, these cases must be differentiated from several similar clinical entities, such as juvenile myoclonic epilepsy, Unverricht-Lundborg disease, Lafora-body disease, Baltic myoclonus, and neuronal ceroid-lipofuscinosis, discussed earlier in this chapter. Tsairis and colleagues were the first to describe the connection between familial myoclonic epilepsy and mitochondrial changes in muscle, and numerous variants have been identified since their report.

Myoclonus in a child or young adult is the most typical feature and is elicited by startle or by voluntary movement of the limbs. The nature of the seizures varies but includes drop attacks, focal epilepsy, or tonic-clonic types, some of which are photosensitive. The ataxia tends to worsen progressively, replacing the myoclonus and seizures in some instances and remaining a minor feature in others. The myopathy usually produces inapparent or mild weakness, but the presence of mitochondrial muscle abnormalities is necessary for clinical diagnosis. To this constellation may be added any of the other elements of the mitochondrial diseases that have already been denoted, including deafness (present in our cases), mental decline, optic atrophy, ophthalmoplegia, cervical lipomas, short stature, or neuropathy.

Most cases are familial and display maternal inheritance, but the age of onset may vary and affected individuals have been reported with symptoms beginning as late as the sixth decade. Almost always the patients with later onset have the mildest disease, with only myoclonic epilepsy. Conversely, those with onset in the first decade tend to be more severely affected and die before the third decade. As with the other mitochondrial processes, the quantitative burden of mutant DNA bears some relationship to the time of onset and severity of the disease. Eighty percent of patients with MERRF have a point mutation of the mitochondrial genome at locus 8344, which codes for a transfer RNA and, conversely, most patients with this mutation will ultimately manifest some or all the clinical features of MERRF, including those with crossover features of the Leigh syndrome.

Mitochondrial Encephalomyopathy, Lactic Acidosis, and Stroke-Like Episodes (MELAS)

Patients with this syndrome have normal early development followed by poor growth, focal or generalized seizures, and recurrent acute episodes that resemble strokes or prolonged transient ischemic attacks. The stroke deficits often improve but in some cases lead to a progressive encephalopathy. Some have hemicranial headaches that cannot be distinguished from migraine, and others suffer repetitive vomiting or episodic lactic acidosis. If there is a characteristic feature it is the unusual clinical pattern of focal seizures, sometimes prolonged, which herald a stroke and produce an unusual radiographic pattern of infarction involving the cortex and immediate subcortical white matter. The CT may also show numerous low-density regions that have no clinical correlates. Most patients have ragged red fibers in muscle but only rarely is there weakness or exercise intolerance.

Approximately 80 percent of MELAS cases are related to a mitochondrial mutation occurring at the 3243 site of the mitochondrial gene or, in a few instances, at an alternative locus that also codes for a segment of transfer RNA. Maternal inheritance is common but sporadic cases are well known. In the survey conducted by Hammans and coworkers, only half of the cases of the 3243 mutation were associated with the MELAS syndrome. The finding of an abnormal mitochondrial genome in the endothelium and smooth muscle of cerebral vessels has been suggested as a basis for the strokes and migraine headaches.

The Diagnosis of Mitochondrial Disorders

The characteristic neurologic signs of a mitochondrial disorder fall into certain broad groups: (1) combinations of ataxia, seizures, and myoclonus, typified by the MERRF syndrome; (2) migraine-like headaches, recurrent small strokes, and preceding seizures, represented by the MELAS syndrome; (3) combinations of ophthalmoplegia (progressive external ophthalmoplegia), retinitis pigmentosa, polyneuropathy, or deafness (Kearns-Sayre syndrome); (4) optic atrophy (Leber type); and (5) a myopathy that is slowly progressive or fluctuating in severity. These may be combined with dementia, lactic acidosis, short stature, diabetes, ptosis, and cardiac conduction defects as well as with multiple symmetrical lipomas. Peripheral nerve involvement, although common in these disorders, is usually asymptomatic; autonomic failure may be a rare manifestation. A panoply of visceral dysfunctions are at times associated with the neurologic features including bone marrow changes of sideroblastic anemia, renal tubular defects, endocrinopathies (mainly diabetes mellitus, but also hypothyroidism or deficiency of growth hormone), hepatopathy, cardiomyopathy, and recurrent vomiting with intestinal pseudoobstruction. Diabetes has been a marker in several of the early-onset MELAS and MERRF cases that we have seen, but less often when the first manifestations appeared in adulthood.

The investigation of a suspected case of mitochondrial disease begins with an exploration of the family history for unusual childhood diseases including neonatal death, unexplained seizure disorders, and progressive neurologic deficits of the types already described. Unexplained deafness or diabetes in family members might also raise the level of suspicion of a mitochondrial disorder. The diagnosis should be suspected when a disorder with these characteristics occurs in a pattern that indicates maternal inheritance. However, one encounters families with mendelian patterns of inheritance due to nuclear gene defects as described in the introductory section of this chapter. Commercial tests are available for the more frequent mitochondrial point mutation sites (3243, 8993, and 8344) in leukocytes. Detection of deletions requires analysis of muscle tissue. They are useful for diagnosis but reveal abnormalities in only a modest number, estimated to be approximately 15 percent of cases that have the index aspect of this group of diseases, ragged red muscle fibers; the frequency is higher in cases with identifiable phenotypes such as MERRF and MELAS. Resting and postexercise lactate and pyruvate determinations are helpful, but this test of aerobic capacity has limitations. The more recent work of Taivassalo and colleagues, although showing a wide range of values, suggests that measurement of the partial pressure of oxygen in venous blood from the forearm after ischemic exercise (ischemic forearm test) may still be useful in distinguishing patients with mitochondrial disease from normal subjects. In the former there is a paradoxical rise in Po_2 from an average of 27 to 38 mm Hg, whereas normals show a decline in this value.

A muscle biopsy will disclose several basic abnormalities; ragged red fibers can be recognized by use of the modified Gomori stain on frozen material, and the absence of succinate dehydrogenase and cytochrome oxidase by appropriate histochemical staining. In cases of suspected Leigh syndrome or MELAS, the CT or MRI may show some of the characteristic cerebral lesions; in the other mitochondrial disorders, there are often focal nondescript hyperintensities on T2-weighted MRI as well as atrophy, lucencies, or calcification. Sampling of chorionic villi for prenatal diagnosis may reveal mutant mitochondrial DNA, but this information is not entirely dependable.

It should be evident from the foregoing discussion that normal findings in any of these tests, including the muscle biopsy, do not exclude mitochondrial disease. In the final analysis, it is the clinical syndrome, family history, and corroborating evidence of a mitochondrial disorder or its genetic representation that is diagnostic. Jackson and coworkers suggest that isolated phenomena, such as dementia, muscle weakness, epilepsy, nerve deafness, migraine with strokes, small stature, myoclonic epilepsy, and cardiomyopathy, should prompt consideration of a mitochondrial disorder when no other explanation is evident.

References

Adachi M, Torii J, Schneck L, Volk BW: Electron microscopic and enzyme histochemical studies of the cerebellum in spongy degeneration. *Acta Neuropathol* 20:22, 1972.

Adams RD, Prod'holm LS, Rabinowicz TH: Intrauterine brain death. *Acta Neuropathol* 40:41, 1977.

Agamanolis DP, Greenstein JI: Ataxia-telangiectasia. *J Neuropathol Exp Neurol* 38:475, 1979.

Aicardi J: Early myoclonic encephalopathy, in Roger J, Dravet C, Bureau M, et al (eds): *Epileptic Syndromes in Infancy, Childhood, and Adolescence*. New York, Demos, 1985, pp 13–23.

Aicardi J, Castelein P: Infantile neuroaxonal dystrophy. *Brain* 102:727, 1979.

Allen RJ, Young W, Bonacci J, et al: Neonatal dystonic parkinsonism, a "stiff-baby syndrome," in biopterin deficiency with hyperprolactinemia detected by newborn screening for hyperphenylalaninemia, and responsiveness to treatment. *Ann Neurol* 28:434, 1990.

Alpers BJ: Diffuse progressive degeneration of cerebral gray matter. *Arch Neurol Psychiatry* 25:469, 1931.

Auborg P, Scotto J, Richiciolli F: Neonatal adrenoleukodystrophy. *J Neurol Neurosurg Psychiatry* 49:77, 1986.

Austin J: Studies in metachromatic leukodystrophy: XII. Multiple sulfatase deficiency. *Arch Neurol* 28:258, 1973.

Banker BQ, Victor M: Spongy degeneration of infancy, in Goodman RM, Motulsky AG (eds): *Genetic Diseases Among Ashkenazi Jews*. New York, Raven Press, 1979, pp 210–216.

Baringer JR, Sweeney VP, Winkler GF: An acute syndrome of ocular oscillations and truncal myoclonus. *Brain* 91:473, 1968.

Bassen FA, Kornzweig AL: Malformation of the erythrocytes in a case of atypical retinitis pigmentosa. *Blood* 5:381, 1950.

Baumann RJ, Kocoshis SA, Wilson D: Lafora disease: Liver histopathology in presymptomatic children. *Ann Neurol* 14:86, 1983.

Berginer VM, Salen G, Shefer S: Long-term treatment of cerebrotendinous xanthomatosis with chenodeoxycholic acid. *N Engl J Med* 311:1649, 1984.

Berkovic SF, Andermann F, Carpenter S, et al: Progressive myoclonus epilepsies and specific causes and diagnosis. *N Engl J Med* 315:296, 1986.

Blass JP, Avigan J, Uhlendorf BW: A defect in pyruvate decarboxylase in a child with intermittent movement disorder. *J Clin Invest* 49:423, 1970.

Bosch EP, Hart MN: Late adult onset metachromatic leukodystrophy. *Arch Neurol* 35:475, 1978.

Brady RO: The sphingolipidoses. *N Engl J Med* 275:312, 1966.

Brett EM (ed): *Pediatric Neurology*, 3rd ed. New York, Churchill Livingstone, 1997.

Brewer GJ, Terry CA, Aisen AM, Hill GM: Worsening of neurologic syndrome in patients with Wilson's disease with initial penicillamine therapy. *Arch Neurol* 44:490, 1987.

Brusilow SW, Danney M, Waber LJ, et al: Treatment of episodic hyperammonemia in children with inborn errors of urea synthesis. *N Engl J Med* 310:1630, 1984.

Brusilow SW, Horwich AL: Urea cycle enzymes, in Scriver CR, Beaudet AL, Valle D, Sly WS (eds): *The Metabolic Basis of Inherited Disease*, 8th ed. New York, McGraw-Hill, 2001, pp 1909–1963.

Burton BK, Nadler HL: Clinical diagnosis of the inborn errors of metabolism in the neonatal period. *Pediatrics* 61:398, 1978.

Cable WJ, Kolodny EH, Adams RD: Fabry disease: Impaired autonomic function. *Neurology* 32:498, 1982.

Catel W, Schmidt J: On familial gouty diathesis associated with cerebral and renal symptoms in a small child. *Dtsch Med Wochenschr* 84:2145, 1959.

Cho CH, Mamourian AC, Filiano J, Nordgren RE: Glutaric aciduria: Improved MR appearance after aggressive therapy. *Pediatr Radiol* 25:484, 1995.

Cowen D, Olmstead EV: Infantile neuroaxonal dystrophy. *J Neuropathol Exp Neurol* 22:175, 1963.

Crocker AC, Farber S: Niemann-Pick disease: A review of 18 patients. *Medicine (Baltimore)* 37:1, 1958.

Crome L: A case of galactosaemia with the pathological and neuropathological findings. *Arch Dis Child* 37:415, 1962.

dal Canto MC, Rapin I, Suzuki K: Neuronal storage disorder with chorea and curvilinear bodies. *Neurology* 24:1026, 1974.

Danks DM, Cartwright E, Stevens BJ, Townley RRW: Menkes' kinky-hair disease: Further definition of the defect in copper transport. *Science* 179:1140, 1973.

Dening TR, Berrios GE, Walshe JM: Wilson's disease and epilepsy. *Brain* 111:1139, 1988.

Desnick RJ, Ioannou YA, Eng CM: α-Galactosidase A deficiency: Fabry disease, in Scriver CR, Beaudet AL, Valle D, Sly WS (eds): *The Metabolic and Molecular Bases of Inherited Disease*, 8th ed. New York, McGraw-Hill, 2001, pp 3733–3774.

De Vivo DC, Haymond MW, Obert KA, et al: Defective activation of the pyruvate dehydrogenase complex in subacute necrotizing encephalomyelopathy (Leigh disease). *Ann Neurol* 6:483, 1979.

DiMagno EP, Lowe JL, Snodgrass PJ, et al: Ornithine transcarbamylase deficiency: A cause of bizarre behavior in a man. *N Engl J Med* 315:744, 1986.

DiMauro S, Nicholson JF, Hays A, et al: Benign infantile mitochondrial myopathy due to reversible cytochrome *c* oxidase deficiency. *Ann Neurol* 14:226, 1983.

DiMauro S, Schon EA: Mitochondrial respiratory-chain diseases. *N Engl J Med* 348:2656, 2003.

Eldridge R, Anayiotos CP, Schlesinger S, et al: Hereditary adult-onset leukodystrophy simulating chronic progressive multiple sclerosis. *N Engl J Med* 311:948, 1984.

Elfenbein LB: Dystonic juvenile idiocy without amaurosis. *Johns Hopkins Med J* 123:205, 1968.

Escolar ML, Poe MD, Provenzale JM, et al: Transplantation of umbilical cord blood in babies with infantile Krabbe's disease. *N Engl J Med* 352:2069, 2005.

Fahr T: Idiopathische Verkalkung der Hirngefasse. *Zentralbl Allg Pathol* 50:129, 1930–1931.

Farrell DF, Swedberg K: Clinical and biochemical heterogeneity of globoid cell leukodystrophy. *Ann Neurol* 10:364, 1981.

Feero WG, Guttmacher AE, Collins FS: Genomic medicine—an updated primer. *N Engl J Med* 362:2001, 2010.

Følling A: Über Ausscheidung von Phenylbrenztraubensaure in den Harn als Stoffwechselanomalie in Verbindung mit Imbezilitat. *Hoppe Seylers Z Physiol Chem* 227:169, 1934.

Friedman JH, Levy HL, Boustany R-M: Late onset of distinct neurologic syndromes in galactosemic siblings. *Neurology* 39:741, 1989.

Frydman M, Bonne-Tamir B, Farber LA, et al: Assignment of the gene for Wilson disease to chromosome 13: Linkage to the esterase D locus. *Proc Natl Acad Sci USA* 82:1819, 1985.

Goldfischer S, Moore CL, Johnson AB, et al: Peroxisomal and mitochondrial defects in the cerebro-hepato-renal syndrome. *Science* 182:62, 1973.

Goldman JE, Katz O, Rapur I, et al: Chronic GM1 gangliosidosis presenting as dystonia: Clinical and pathological features. *Ann Neurol* 9:465, 1981.

Gorospe JR, Naidu S, Johnson AB, et al: Molecular findings in symptomatic and presymptomatic Alexander disease patients. *Neurology* 58:1494, 2002.

Gould SJ, Valle D: Peroxisome biogenesis disorders: Genetics and cell biology. *Trends Genet* 16:340, 2000.

Grey RGF, Preece MA, Green SH, et al: Inborn errors of metabolism as a cause of neurological disease in adults: An approach to investigation. *J Neurol Neurosurg Psychiatry* 69:5, 2000.

Griffin JW, Goren E, Schaumburg H, et al: Adrenomyeloneuropathy: A probable variant of adrenoleukodystrophy. *Neurology* 27:1107, 1977.

Griggs RC, Moxley RT, LaFrance RA, McQuillen J: Hereditary paroxysmal ataxia: Response to acetazolamide. *Neurology* 28:1259, 1978.

Hammans SR, Sweeny MG, Hanna MG, et al: The mitochondrial DNA transfer RNA Leu (44R) A G (3243) mutation: A clinical and genetic study. *Brain* 118:721, 1995.

Harding BN, Egger J, Portmann B, Erdohazi M: Progressive neuronal degeneration of childhood with liver disease. *Brain* 109:181, 1986.

Hayflick SJ, Westaway SK, Levinson B, et al: Genetic, clinical and radiographic delineation of Hallervorden-Spatz syndrome. *N Engl J Med* 348:33, 2003.

Hers HG: Inborn lysosomal diseases. *Gastroenterology* 48:625, 1965.

Hoffmann GF, Assmann B, Bräutigan C, et al: Tyrosine hydroxylase deficiency causes progressive encephalopathy and dopa-nonresponsive dystonia. *Ann Neurol* 54(Suppl 6):S56, 2003.

Holmes LB, Moser HW, Halldorsson S, et al: *Mental Retardation: An Atlas of Diseases with Associated Physical Abnormalities*. New York, Macmillan, 1972.

Holtzman NA, Kronmal RA, van Doorninck W, et al: Effect of age and loss of dietary control on intellectual performance and behavior of children with phenylketonuria. *N Engl J Med* 314:593, 1986.

Hoogenraad TU, Van Hattum J, Van Den Hamer CSA: Management of Wilson's disease with zinc sulfate: Experience in a series of 27 patients. *J Neurol Sci* 77:137, 1987.

Hunt JR: Dyssynergia cerebellaris myoclonica. *Brain* 44:490, 1921.

Igarashi M, Schaumburg HH, Powers J, et al: Fatty acid abnormality in adrenoleukodystrophy. *J Neurochem* 26:851, 1976.

Ikeda S, Kondo K, Oguchi K, et al: Adult fucosidosis: Histochemical and ultrastructural studies of rectal mucosa biopsy. *Neurology* 34:451, 1984.

Illingworth DR, Connor WE, Miller RG: Abetalipoproteinemia: Report of two cases and review of therapy. *Arch Neurol* 37:659, 1980.

Ishiyama G, Lopez I, Baloh R, Ishiyama A: Canavan's leukodystrophy is associated with defects in cochlear neurodevelopment and deafness. *Neurology* 60:1702, 2003.

Jackson MJ, Schaefer A, Johnson MA: Presentation and clinical investigation of mitochondrial respiratory chain disease. *Brain* 118:339, 1995.

Johns DR: Mitochondrial DNA and disease. *N Engl J Med* 333:638, 1995.

Johnson RC, McKean CM, Shah SN: Fatty acid composition of lipids in cerebral myelin and synaptosomes in phenylketonuria and Down syndrome. *Arch Neurol* 34:288, 1977.

Josephs KA, Van Gerpen MW, Van Gerpen JA: Adult onset Niemann-Pick disease type C presenting with psychosis. *J Neurol Neurosurg Psychiatry* 74:528, 2003.

Kaler SG, Goldstein DS, Holmes C, et al: Neonatal diagnosis and treatment of Menkes disease. *N Engl J Med* 358:605, 2008.

Kalimo H, Lundberg PO, Olsson Y: Familial subacute necrotizing encephalomyelopathy of the adult form (adult Leigh syndrome). *Ann Neurol* 6:200, 1979.

Kasim S, Moo LR, Zschocke J, et al: Phenylketonuria presenting in adulthood as progressive spastic paraparesis with dementia. *J Neurol Neurosurg Psychiatry* 71:795, 2001.

Kendall BE, Kingsley DPE, Leonard JV, et al: Neurological features and computed tomography of the brain in children with ornithine carbamyl transferase deficiency. *J Neurol Neurosurg Psychiatry* 46:28, 1983.

Kinsbourne M: Myoclonic encephalopathy in infants. *J Neurol Neurosurg Psychiatry* 25:271, 1962.

Kistler JP, Lott IT, Kolodny EH, et al: Mannosidosis. *Arch Neurol* 34:45, 1977.

Kobayashi T, Noda S, Umezaki H, et al: Familial spinocerebellar degeneration as an expression of adrenoleukodystrophy. *J Neurol Neurosurg Psychiatry* 49:1438, 1986.

Koeppen AH, Robitaille Y: Pelizaeus-Merzbacher disease. *J Neuropathol Exp Neurol* 61:747, 2002.

Koeppen AH, Ronca NA, Greenfield EA, Hans MB: Defective biosynthesis of proteolipid protein in Pelizaeus-Merzbacher disease. *Ann Neurol* 21:159, 1987.

Koivisto M, Blenco-Sequiros M, Krause U: Neonatal symptomatic hypoglycemia: A follow-up of 151 children. *Dev Med Child Neurol* 14:603, 1972.

Kolodny EH, Cable WJL: Inborn errors of metabolism. *Ann Neurol* 11:221, 1982.

Kolodny EH, Raghavan SS, Krivit W: Late-onset Krabbe disease (globoid cell leukodystrophy): Clinical and biochemical features in 15 cases. *Dev Neurosci* 13:232, 1991.

Koopman WJH, Willems PHG, Smeitink JAM: Monogenic Mitochondrial Disorders. *N Engl J Med* 366:1132, 2012.

Lance JW: Familial paroxysmal dystonic choreoathetosis and its differentiation from related syndromes. *Ann Neurol* 2:285, 1977.

Leegwater PA, Pronk JC, van der Knaap MS: Leukoencephalopathy with vanishing white matter: From magnetic resonance imaging pattern to five genes. *J Child Neurol* 18:639, 2003.

Leonard JV, Schapira AHV: Mitochondrial respiratory chain disorders I and II. *Lancet* 355:299, 389, 2000.

Lesch M, Nyhan WL: A familial disorder of uric acid metabolism and central nervous system function. *Am J Med* 36:561, 1964.

Letournel F, Etcharry-Bouyx F, Verny C, et al: Two clinicopathologic cases of a dominantly inherited adult onset orthochromatic leucodystrophy. *J Neurol Neurosurg Psychiatry* 74:671, 2003.

Levy HL: Screening of the newborn, in Tausch HW, Ballard RA, Avery ME (eds): *Diseases of the Newborn*. Philadelphia, Saunders, 1991, pp 111–119.

Logan JI: Hereditary deficiency of ferroxidase (aka ceruloplasmin). *J Neurol Neurosurg Psychiatry* 61:431,1996.

Lonsdale D, Faulkner WR, Price JW, Smeby RR: Intermittent cerebellar ataxia associated with hyperpyruvic acidemia, hyperalaninemia and hyperalaninuria. *Pediatrics* 43:1025, 1969.

Lott IT, Coulombe T, DiPaolo RV, et al: Vitamin B_6-dependent seizures: Pathology and chemical findings in brain. *Neurology* 28:47, 1978.

Lundborg H: *Die progressive Myoklonus-epilepsie* (*Unverricht's Myoklonie*). Uppsala, Sweden, Almqvist and Wiksell, 1903.

Lyon G, Kolodny EH, Pastores GM: *Neurology of Hereditary Metabolic Diseases of Children*, 3rd ed. New York, McGraw-Hill, 2006.

Maestri NE, Brusilow SW, Clissold DB, et al: Long-term treatment of girls with ornithine transcarbamylase deficiency. *N Engl J Med* 335:855, 1996.

Marsden CD, Harding AE, Obeso JA, Lu C-S: Progressive myoclonic ataxia (the Ramsay Hunt syndrome). *Arch Neurol* 47:1121, 1990.

Marsden CD, Obeso JA, Lang AE: Adrenoleukomyeloneuropathy presenting as spinocerebellar degeneration. *Neurology* 32:1031, 1982.

Matalon R, Michals K, Sebesta D, et al: Aspartoacylase deficiency and *N*-acetylaspartic aciduria in patients with Canavan disease. *Am J Med Genet* 29:463, 1988.

McFarlin DE, Strober W, Barlow M, et al: The immunological deficiency state in ataxia-telangiectasia. *Res Publ Assoc Res Nerv Ment Dis* 49:275, 1971.

McKusick VA: *Mendelian Inheritance in Man: A Catalog of Human Genes and Genetic Disorders*, 12th ed. Baltimore, MD, Johns Hopkins University Press, 1998.

Meek D, Wolfe LS, Andermann E, Andermann F: Juvenile progressive dystonia: A new phenotype of G_{M2} gangliosidosis. *Ann Neurol* 15:348, 1984.

Meikle PJ, Hopwood JJ, Clague AE, Carey WF: Prevalence of lysosomal storage diseases. *JAMA* 281:249, 1999.

Meiner V, Meiner Z, Reshef A, et al: Cerebrotendinous xanthomatosis: Molecular diagnosis enables presymptomatic detection of a treatable disease. *Neurology* 44:288, 1994.

Melchior JC, Benda CE, Yakovlev PI: Familial idiopathic cerebral calcifications in childhood. *Am J Dis Child* 99:787, 1960.

Miyajima H, Kono S, Takahashi Y, et al: Cerebellar ataxia associated with heteroallelic ceruloplasmin gene mutation. *Neurology* 57:2205, 2001.

Miyatake T, Atsumi T, Obayashi T, et al: Adult type neuronal storage disease with neuraminidase deficiency. *Ann Neurol* 6:232, 1979.

Moser AB, Kreiter N, Benzman L, et al: Plasma very long chain fatty acids in 3,000 peroxisome disease patients and 29,000 controls. *Ann Neurol* 45:100, 1999.

Moser AB, Singh I, Brown FR III, et al: The cerebrohepatorenal (Zellweger) syndrome. *N Engl J Med* 310:1141, 1984.

Moser HW: Adrenoleukodystrophy: Phenotype, genetics, pathogenesis and therapy. *Brain* 120:1485, 1997.

Moser HW, Dube P, Fatemi A: Progress in X-linked leukodystrophy. *Curr Opin Neurol* 17:263, 2004.

Moser HW, Moser AB, Kawamura N, et al: Adrenoleukodystrophy: Elevated C26 fatty acid in cultured skin fibroblasts. *Ann Neurol* 7:542, 1980.

Mount LA, Reback S: Familial paroxysmal choreoathetosis: Preliminary report on a hitherto undescribed clinical syndrome. *Arch Neurol Psychiatry* 44:841, 1940.

Msall M, Batshaw ML, Suss R, et al: Neurologic outcome in children with inborn errors of urea synthesis. *N Engl J Med* 310:1500, 1984.

Muntau AC, Röschinger W, Habich M, et al: Tetrahydrobiopterin as an alternative treatment for mild phenylketonuria. *N Engl J Med* 347:2122, 2002.

Neufeld EF, Muenzer J: The mucopolysaccharidoses, in Scriver CR, Beaudet AL, Valle D, Sly WS (eds): *The Metabolic and Molecular Bases of Inherited Disease*, 8th ed. New York, McGraw-Hill, 2001, pp 3421–3452.

Nishimura M, Yoshimo K, Tomita Y: Central and peripheral nervous system pathology due to methylenetetrahydrofolate reductase deficiency. *Pediatr Neurol* 1:375, 1985.

Nygaard TG, Marsden CD, Fahn S: Dopa-responsive dystonia: Long-term treatment response and prognosis. *Ann Neurol* 35:396, 1994.

Oetting WS, King RA: Molecular basis of albinism: Mutations and polymorphisms of pigmentation genes associated with albinism. *Hum Mutat* 13:99, 1999.

Ohno T, Tsuchida H, Fukuhara N, et al: Adrenoleukodystrophy: A clinical variant presenting as olivopontocerebellar atrophy. *J Neurol* 231:167, 1984.

Ohtahara S: Seizure disorders in infancy and childhood. *Brain Dev* 6:509, 1984.

Öz G, Tkác I, Charnas LR, et al: Assessment of adrenoleukodystrophy lesions by high field MRS in non-sedated pediatric patients. *Neurology* 64:434, 2005.

Pastores GM, Thadhani R: Enzyme-replacement therapy for Anderson-Fabry disease. *Lancet* 358:601, 2001.

Pavlakis SG, Phillips PC, DiMauro S, et al: Mitochondrial myopathy, encephalopathy, lactic acidosis, and stroke-like episodes: A distinctive clinical syndrome. *Ann Neurol* 16:481, 1984.

Prader A, Labhart A, Willi H: Ein Syndrom von Adipositas, Kleinwuchs, Kryptorchismus und Oligophrenie nach myatonieartigem Zustand im Neugeborenenalter. *Schweiz Med Wochenschr* 86:1260, 1956.

Pranzatelli MR, Huang Y, Tate E, et al: Cerebrospinal fluid 5-hydroxy indoleacetic acid in the pediatric opsoclonus-myoclonus syndrome. *Ann Neurol* 37:189, 1995.

Prechtl H, Beintema D: The Neurological Examination of the Full-Term *Newborn Infant*. London, Spastics Society, 1964.

Prensky AL, Moser HW: Brain lipids, proteo-lipids and free amino acids in maple syrup urine disease. *J Neurochem* 13:863, 1966.

Rapin I, Goldfischer S, Katzman R, et al: The cherry-red spot-myoclonus syndrome. *Ann Neurol* 3:234, 1978.

Robitaille Y, Carpenter S, Karpati G, et al: A distinct form of adult polyglucosan body disease with massive involvement of central and peripheral neuronal processes and astrocytes. *Brain* 103:315, 1980.

Ropper AH, Hatten HP, Davis KR: Computed tomography in Wilson disease: Report of two cases. *Ann Neurol* 5:102, 1979.

Rosenberg LE, Scriver CR: Disorders of amino acid metabolism, in Bondy PK, Rosenberg LE (eds): *Metabolic Control and Disease*, 8th ed. Philadelphia, Saunders, 1980, pp 583–776.

Rowe PC, Newman SL, Brusilow SW: Natural history of symptomatic partial ornithine transcarbamylase deficiency. *N Engl J Med* 314:541, 1986.

Saatci I, Topcu M, Baltaoglu FF, et al: Cranial MRI findings in Wilson's disease. *Acta Radiol* 38:250, 1997.

Salem M: Metabolic ataxias, in Vinken PJ, Bruyn GW (eds): *Handbook of Clinical Neurology*. Vol 21. Amsterdam, North-Holland, 1975, pp 573–585.

Sansaricq C, Lyon G, Kolodny EH: Seizures in hereditary metabolic disease: Evaluation of suspected hereditary metabolic disease in the etiology of seizures, in Kotogal P, Luders H (eds): *The Epilepsies: Etiologies and Prevention*. San Diego, CA, Academic Press, 1999, pp 457–464.

Santavuori P, Haltia M, Rapola J, Raitta C: Infantile type of so-called neuronal ceroid-lipofuscinosis: Part 1. A clinical study of 15 patients. *J Neurol Sci* 18:257, 1973.

Santorelli F, Shanske S, Macay A, et al: The mutation at nt 8993 of mitochondrial DNA is a common cause of Leigh's syndrome. *Ann Neurol* 34:827, 1994.

Savoiardo M, Halliday WC, Nardocci N, et al: Hallervorden-Spatz disease: MR and pathologic findings. *AJNR Am J Neuroradiol* 14:155, 1993.

Schapira AH, DiMauro S (eds): *Mitochondrial Disorders in Neurology*. Oxford, England, Butterworth-Heinemann, 1994.

Scheinberg IH, Gitlin D: Deficiency of ceruloplasmin in patients with hepatolenticular degeneration (Wilson's disease). *Science* 116:484, 1952.

Scheinberg IH, Sternlieb I: *Wilson's Disease: Major Problems in Internal Medicine*. Vol 23. Philadelphia, Saunders, 1984.

Schiffmann R, van der Knaap MS: An MRI-based approach to the diagnosis of white matter disorders. *Neurology* 72:750, 2009.

Schilsky ML, Scheinberg IH, Sternlieb I: Liver transplantation for Wilson's disease: Indications and outcome. *Hepatology* 19:583, 2001.

Scriver CR, Beaudet AL, Valle D, Sly WS (eds): *The Metabolic and Molecular Bases of Inherited Disease*, 8th ed. New York, McGraw-Hill, 2001.

Scriver CR, Clow CL: Phenylketonuria: Epitome of human biochemical genetics. *N Engl J Med* 303:1335, 1980.

Seitelberger F: Pelizaeus-Merzbacher disease, in Vinken PJ, Bruyn GW (eds): *Handbook of Clinical Neurology*. Vol 10. Amsterdam, North-Holland, 1970, pp 150–202.

Sethi KD, Ray R, Roesel RA, et al: Adult-onset chorea and dementia with propionic acidemia. *Neurology* 39:1343, 1989.

Shih VE, Abrams IF, Johnson JL, et al: Sulfite oxidase deficiency. *N Engl J Med* 297:1022, 1977.

Shih VE, Safran AP, Ropper AH, Tuchman M: Ornithine carbamoyl transferase deficiency: Unusual clinical findings and novel mutation. *J Inherit Metab Dis* 22:672, 1999.

Shuman RM, Leech RW, Scott CR: The neuropathology of the nonketotic and ketotic hyperglycinemias: Three cases. *Neurology* 28:139, 1978.

Shy GM, Gonatas NK, Perez M: Two childhood myopathies with abnormal mitochondria: I. Megaconial myopathy. II. Pleoconial myopathy. *Brain* 89:133, 1966.

Siemerling E, Creutzfeldt HG: Bronzekrankheit und sklerosierende encephalomyelitis (diffuse sklerose). *Arch Psychiatr Nervenkr* 68:217, 1923.

Sjögren T: Die juvenile amaurotische Idiotie: Klinische und erblichkeitsmedizinische Untersuchungen. *Hereditas* 14:197, 1931.

Sly WS, Whyte MP, Sunderam V: Carbonic anhydrase II deficiency in 12 families with the autosomal recessive syndrome of osteopetrosis with renal tubular acidosis with cerebral calcification. *N Engl J Med* 313:139, 1985.

Staba SL, Escolar ML, Poe M, et al: Cord-blood transplants from unrelated donors in patients with Hurler's syndrome. *N Engl J Med* 350:1960, 2004.

Starosta-Rubinstein S, Young AB, Kluin K, et al: Clinical assessment of 31 patients with Wilson's disease. *Arch Neurol* 44:365, 1987.

Strich SJ: Pathological findings in three cases of ataxia-telangiectasia. *J Neurol Neurosurg Psychiatry* 29:489, 1966.

Stumpf E, Masson H, Duquette A, et al: Adult Alexander disease with autosomal dominant transmission. *Arch Neurol* 60:1307, 2003.

Swoboda KJ, Saul JP, McKenna CE, et al: Aromatic L-amino acid decarboxylase deficiency. Overview of clinical features and outcomes. *Ann Neurol* 54(Suppl 6):S49, 2000.

Szanto J, Gallyas F: A study of iron metabolism in neuropsychiatric patients: Hallervorden-Spatz disease. *Arch Neurol* 14:438, 1966.

Tagawa A, Ono S, Shibata M, et al: A new neurological entity manifesting as involuntary movements and dysarthria with possible abnormal copper metabolism. *J Neurol Neurosurg Psychiatry* 71:780, 2001.

Taivassalo T, Abbott A, Wyrick P, et al: Venous oxygen levels during aerobic exercise: An index of impaired oxidative metabolism in mitochondrial myopathy. *Ann Neurol* 51:38, 2002.

Tassinari CA, Michelucci R, Genton P, et al: Dyssynergia cerebellaris myoclonica (Ramsay Hunt syndrome): A condition unrelated to mitochondrial encephalomyopathies. *J Neurol Neurosurg Psychiatry* 52:262, 1989.

Tellez-Nagel I, Rapin I, Iwamoto T, et al: Mucolipidosis IV. *Arch Neurol* 33:828, 1976.

Tennison MB, Bouldin TW, Whaley RA: Mineralization of the basal ganglia detected by CT in Hallervorden-Spatz syndrome. *Neurology* 38:155, 1988.

Thomas PK, Abrams JD, Swallow D, Stewart G: Sialidosis type I: Cherry-red spot-myoclonus syndrome with sialidase deficiency and altered electrophoretic mobilities of some enzymes known to be glycoproteins. *J Neurol Neurosurg Psychiatry* 42:873, 1979.

Trobe JD, Sharpe JA, Hirsch DK, Gebarski SS: Nystagmus of Pelizaeus-Merzbacher disease: A magnetic search-coil study. *Arch Neurol* 48:87, 1991.

Tsairis P, Engel WK, Kark P: Familial myoclonic epilepsy syndrome associated with skeletal muscle abnormalities. *Neurology* 23:408, 1973.

Tsuji S, Choudary PV, Martin BM, et al: A mutation in the human glucocerebrosidase gene in neuronopathic Gaucher's disease. *N Engl J Med* 316:570, 1987.

Tsuji S, Yamada T, Tsutsumi A, Miyatake T: Neuraminidase deficiency and accumulation of sialic acid in lymphocytes in adult type sialidosis with partial β-galactosidase deficiency. *Ann Neurol* 11:541, 1982.

Turpin JC, Baumann N: Manifestations psychiatriques ou cognitves inaugurales dans les neurolipidoses de l'adulte. *Rev Neurol* 159:637, 2003.

Vakili S, Drew AL, von Schuching S, et al: Hallervorden-Spatz syndrome. *Arch Neurol* 34:729, 1977.

van Bogaert L: Contribution clinique et anatomique a l'etude de la paralysie agitante juvenile primitive. *Rev Neurol* 2:315, 1930.

van Bogaert L: Le cadre des xanthomatoses et leurs differents types: Xanthomatoses secondaires. *Rev Med (Paris)* 17:433, 1962.

van Bogaert L, Bertrand I: Sur une idiotie famaliale avec dégénérescence spongieuse du neuraxe. *Acta Neurol Belg* 49:572, 1949.

van Geel MB, Assies J, Wanders RJ, Barth P'G: X linked adrenoleukodystrophy: Clinical presentation, diagnosis and therapy. *J Neurol Neurosurg Psychiatry* 63:4, 1997.

Vogt C, Vogt O: Zur Lehre der Erkrankungen des striaren Systems. *J Psychol Neurol* 25:627, 1920.

Walsh PJ: Adrenoleukodystrophy. *Arch Neurol* 37:448, 1980.

Williams FJB, Walshe JM: Wilson's disease: An analysis of the cranial computerized tomographic experiences found in 60 patients and the changes in response to treatment with chelating agents. *Brain* 104:735, 1981.

Williams RS, Marshall PC, Lott IT, et al: The cellular pathology of Menkes steely hair syndrome. *Neurology* 28:575, 1978.

Willvonseder R, Goldstein NP, McCall JT, et al: A hereditary disorder with dementia, spastic dysarthria, vertical eye movement paresis, gait disturbance, splenomegaly, and abnormal copper metabolism. *Neurology* 23:1039, 1973.

Wilner JP, Grabowski GA, Gordon RF, et al: Chronic G_{M2} gangliosidosis masquerading as atypical Friedreich's ataxia: Clinical, morphologic, and biochemical studies of nine cases. *Neurology* 31:787, 1981.

Wilson SAK: Progressive lenticular degeneration: A familial nervous disease associated with cirrhosis of the liver. *Brain* 34:295, 1912.

Wisniewski KE, Zhong N, Phillipart M: Pheno/genotypic correlations of neuronal ceroid lipofuscinosis. *Neurology* 57:576, 2001.

Yokoi S, Nakayama H, Negeshi T: Biochemical studies on tissues from a patient with Lafora disease. *Clin Chim Acta* 62:415, 1975.

Young RR, Kleinman G, Ojemann RG, et al: Compressive myelopathy in Maroteaux-Lamy syndrome: Clinical and pathological findings. *Ann Neurol* 8:336, 1980.

Zeman W, Donahue S, Dyken P, Green J: The neuronal ceroid-lipofuscinoses (Batten-Vogt syndrome), in Vinken PJ, Bruyn GW (eds): *Handbook of Clinical Neurology*. Vol 10. Amsterdam, North-Holland, 1970, pp 588–679.

38

Developmental Diseases of the Nervous System

This broad heading subsumes a large number of both genetically driven developmental malformations and diseases acquired during intrauterine or early neonatal periods of life. They number in the hundreds according to the tabulation of Dyken and Krawiecki although many, if not most, are rare. Taxonomically, they make up two broad categories. The first includes specific gene defects, either mutations, deletions, or duplications of parts of genes (copy number variation), or single nucleotide polymorphisms that give rise to developmental aberrations or delays. The second category comprises a variety of environmental and infectious agents acting at different times on the immature nervous system during embryonal, fetal, and perinatal periods of life.

GENERAL PRINCIPLES

Several points should be noted regarding the frequency of malformations. Jones, in the *Smith* monograph, has pointed out that a single minor malformation, usually of no clinical significance, occurs in 14 percent of newborns. Two malformations appear in 0.8 percent of newborns, and in this group, a major defect is five times more frequent than in the normal population. Three or more malformations are found in 0.5 percent of newborns, and in this latter group, more than 90 percent have one or more major abnormalities that seriously interfere with viability or physical well-being. The figures for major congenital malformations compiled by Kalter and Warkany are comparable but somewhat higher. What is most important for the neurologist is the fact that the nervous system is involved in most of infants with major malformations. Indeed, approximately 40 percent of deaths during the first postnatal year are in some manner related to prenatal malformations of the central nervous system.

Certain principles are applicable to the entire group of malformations. First, the abnormality of the nervous system is frequently accompanied by an abnormality of some other structure or organ (eye, nose, cranium, spine, ear, and heart), which relates them chronologically to a certain period of embryogenesis. Conversely, the presence of these malformations of nonnervous tissues suggests that an associated abnormality of the nervous system is developmental in nature. For example, the conjunction of cardiac, limb, gut, and bladder abnormalities with a neurologic disorder indicates the time at which the insult takes place: cardiac abnormalities occur between the fifth and sixth week; extroversion of the bladder at less than 30 days; duodenal atresia, before 30 days; syndactyly, before 6 weeks; meningomyelocele, before 28 days; anencephaly, before 28 days; cleft lip, before 36 days; syndactyly, cyclopia, and holoprosencephaly, before 23 days. Each is discussed in this chapter. This principle is not inviolable; in certain maldevelopments of the brain that must have originated in the embryonal period, all other organs are normal. One can only assume that the brain was more vulnerable than any other organ to prenatal as well as natal influences. Perhaps this occurs because the nervous system, of all organ systems, requires the longest time for its development and maturation, during which it is susceptible to disease. Low birth weight and gestational age, indicative of premature birth, increase the risk of cognitive or sensory developmental delay, seizures, and cerebral palsy.

A maldevelopment of whatever cause should be present at birth and remain stable thereafter, that is, be nonprogressive, in contrast to the majority of metabolic diseases of infancy discussed in the preceding chapter. However, this principle requires qualification: The abnormality may have affected parts of the brain that have not matured at birth, so that an interval of time must elapse postnatally before the defect can express itself.

Many of the teratologic conditions that cause birth defects pass unrecognized because they end in spontaneous abortions. For example, defects caused by chromosomal abnormalities occur in approximately 0.6 percent of live births, but such defects are found in more than 5 percent of spontaneous abortuses at 5 to 12 weeks gestational age.

Regarding the genetic causes of malformations and developmental delay, much has been learned in the past decade but a picture of the genetic influences on these conditions is still incomplete. For half a century, whole chromosome karyotyping allowed the recognition of conditions such as Down syndrome and its association with triplication of the entire chromosome 21. As more refined techniques became available, such as high-resolution banding, subtle changes such as small deletions in chromosomal architecture became apparent, as occur in Angleman and Prader-Willi syndrome and fragile-X syndrome.

What followed, by the use of linkage analysis and other genetic techniques, was the elucidation of single gene mutations that were obligatorily associated with malformations or developmental delays; most of the inherited metabolic disorders of infancy and childhood discussed in Chap. 37 are of this type but also certain gross malformations of the brain such as lissencephaly, discussed further on.

These were the forerunners of a completely different category of technical innovations, anchored by the original method of sequencing short lengths of part of a gene by the Sanger method and its derivatives. With the development of the polymerase chain reaction and automated methods, longer and longer sequences of genes could be studied. This has allowed large population studies, merged with statistical techniques that expose genes in affected individuals that may be responsible for disease and are not present in high frequency in the general populations. From there, the rapid evolution of technology that is able to analyze thousands of portions of DNA in parallel and compare numerous sequences to a reference library of DNA has revealed variants at the resolution of single base pairs, *single nucleotide polymorphisms* (SNPs). Most exploration of human disease has been, until recently, based on the "common disease–common variant" model, in which a disease is attributable to limited number variants that exist in more than 1 to 5 percent of a population. For example, five polymorphisms are each responsible for doubling or tripling the risk of macular degeneration. However, most of these variants are probably not themselves responsible for the disease.

These types of genetic changes do not appear to explain the majority of the various developmental diseases. A newer concept of duplication or deletion of portions of genes, "*copy number variation*" is emerging as possibly explanatory of some proportion of diseases such as autism as discussed further on. What is interesting about copy number variation is that they give rise to several phenotypes of similar disorder, quite unlike conventional mendelian mutations. This indicates that copy number variants, like SNPs, probably are not directly causative of a condition but instead modulate other functions that express proteins. This is the situation for many of the forms of developmental abnormalities such as generic cognitive developmental delay, autism, and certain psychiatric diseases.

A textbook on the principles of neurology cannot catalog all the hereditary and congenital developmental abnormalities that affect the nervous system. For such details, the interested reader should refer to several excellent monographs. Three that the authors consult are Brett's *Pediatric Neurology*, Berg's *Principles of Child Neurology*, and Lyon and Evrard's *Neuropediatrie*. These are supplemented by special atlases of congenital malformations mentioned further on. In this chapter, we sketch only the major groups and discuss in detail a few of the more common entities. The classification in Table 38-1 adheres to a *grouping in accordance with the main presenting abnormality*. Represented here are the common problems that lead families to seek consultation with the pediatric neurologist: (1) structural defects of the cranium, spine, and limbs, and of eyes, nose, ears, jaws, and skin; (2) disturbed motor function, taking the form of retarded development or abnormal movements; (3) epilepsy; and (4) developmental delay—mental retardation. The following discussion focuses on each of these clinical states.

Table 38-1

CLASSIFICATION OF CONGENITAL NEUROLOGIC DISORDERS

I. Neurologic disorders associated with craniospinal deformities
   A. Enlarged head (see also Table 38-2)
      1. Hydrocephalus
      2. Hydranencephaly
      3. Macrocephaly
   B. Craniostenoses
      1. Turricephaly
      2. Scaphocephaly
      3. Brachycephaly
   C. Disturbances of neuronal formation and migration
      1. Anencephaly
      2. Lissencephaly, holoprosencephaly, and gyral malformations
   D. Microcephaly
      1. Primary (vera)
      2. Secondary to cerebral disease
   E. Combinations of cerebral, cranial, and other anomalies
      1. Syndactylic craniocerebral anomalies
      2. Other craniofacial anomalies
      3. Oculoencephalic defects
      4. Oculoauriculocephalic anomalies
      5. Dwarfism
      6. Dermatocephalic anomalies
   F. Rachischisis
      1. Cephalic and spinal meningocele, meningoencephalocele, Dandy-Walker syndrome, meningomyelocele
      2. Chiari malformation
      3. Platybasia and cervical-spinal anomalies (see Chap. 44)
   G. Chromosomal abnormalities
II. The phakomatoses (see Table 38-4)
   A. Tuberous sclerosis
   B. Neurofibromatosis
   C. Cutaneous angiomatosis with central nervous system abnormalities
III. Restricted developmental abnormalities of the nervous system
   A. Focal cortical dysgenesis
   B. Möbius syndrome
   C. Congenital apraxia of gaze
   D. Other restricted congenital abnormalities (Horner syndrome, unilateral ptosis, anisocoria, etc.)
IV. Congenital abnormalities of motor function (cerebral palsy)
   A. Subependymal (matrix) hemorrhage
   B. Cerebral spastic diplegia
   C. Infantile hemiplegia, double hemiplegia, and quadriplegia
   D. Congenital extrapyramidal disorders (double athetosis; erythroblastosis fetalis and kernicterus)
   E. Congenital ataxias
   F. The flaccid paralyses
V. Prenatal and paranatal infections
   A. Rubella
   B. Cytomegalic inclusion disease
   C. Congenital neurosyphilis
   D. HIV infection
   E. Toxoplasmosis
   F. Other viral and bacterial infections
VI. Epilepsies of infancy and childhood
VII. Developmentally delayed

NEUROLOGIC DISORDERS ASSOCIATED WITH CRANIOSPINAL DEFORMITIES

A majority of the disorders in this group is the result of a genetic error, including those with a specific chromosomal abnormality. One has only to walk through an institution for the developmentally delayed to appreciate the remarkable number and diversity of dysmorphisms that attend abnormalities of the nervous system. Smith, in the third edition of his monograph on the patterns of human malformations, listed 345 distinctive syndromes; in the fourth edition (edited by K.L. Jones [1988]), many new ones were added. Indeed, a normal-appearing and severely cognitvely impaired individual stands out in such a crowd and will frequently be found to have an inherited metabolic defect or birth injury.

The intimate relationship between the growth and development of the cranium and that of the brain is likely responsible for many of the associations in maldevelopment. In embryonic life the most rapidly growing parts of the neural tube induce unique changes in, and at the same time are influenced by, the overlying mesoderm (a process termed *induction*); hence abnormalities in the formation of skull, orbits, nose, and spine are regularly associated with anomalies of the brain and spinal cord. During early fetal life the cranial bones and vertebral arches enclose and protect the developing brain and spinal cord. Throughout the period of rapid brain growth, as pressure is exerted on the inner table of the skull, the latter accommodates to the increasing size of the brain. This adaptation is facilitated by the membranous fontanels, which remain open until maximal brain growth has been attained; only then do they ossify (close). In addition, stature is apparently controlled by the nervous system, as shown by the fact that a majority of mentally retarded individuals are also stunted physically to a varying degree. Thus disorders of craniovertebral development assume importance not merely because of the physical disfigurement but also because they often reflect an abnormality of the underlying brain and spinal cord, whereby they become the main diagnostic signs of the maldevelopment.

Cranial Malformations at Birth and in Early Infancy

Certain alterations in size and shape of the head in the infant, child, or even the adult, always signify a pathologic process that affected the brain before birth or in early infancy. Because the size of the cranium reflects the size of the brain, the tape measure is one of the most useful tools in pediatric neurology—no examination in a neurologically affected child is complete without a measurement of the circumference of the head. Graphs of head circumference in males and females from birth to 18 years of age were compiled by Nellhaus and are commonly used by pediatricians. A newborn whose head circumference is below the third percentile for age and sex and whose fontanels are closed may be judged to have a developmental abnormality of the brain. A head that is normal in size at term but fails to keep pace with body length (microcephaly) reflects a later failure of growth and maturation of the cerebral hemispheres (microencephaly).

Enlargement of the Head (Macrocephaly)

This can be caused by factors extrinsic to the brain tissue, such as hydrocephalus and hydrancephaly (as defined below), or excessive brain growth (megalo- or macroencephaly; Table 38-2). The *hydrocephalic head* is distinguished by several features: frontal protuberance, or bossing; a tendency for the eyes to turn down so that the sclerae are visible between the upper eyelids and iris (sunset sign); thinning of the scalp and prominence of scalp veins; separation of the cranial sutures; and a "cracked pot" sound on percussion of the skull. Infantile hydrocephalus usually comes to medical attention because of an expanding cranium that exceeds normal dimensions for age. The usual causes are type II Chiari malformation, hereditary aqueductal stenosis, and prenatal infections, for example, toxoplasmosis. These disorders are discussed further on.

Hydranencephaly, defined as hydrocephalus and destruction or failure of development of parts of the cerebrum, is often associated with enlargement of the skull. When the cranium is transilluminated with a strong flashlight in a darkened room, the fluid-filled region of the cranium glows like a jack-o'-lantern. It can be caused by cerebral infarction from intrauterine vascular occlusion or by diseases such as toxoplasmosis and cytomegalovirus (CMV) disease, which destroy parts of each cerebral hemisphere. The lack of brain tissue reduces resistance to intraventricular pressure, permitting great enlargement of both lateral ventricles; it is especially marked if there is an added hydrocephalic state because of interference with cerebrospinal fluid circulation. This type of destruction of the cerebral mantle in the embryonal period may lead to the formation of huge brain defects with apposition of ventricular and pial surfaces (*porencephaly*) and subsequent failure of development of that part of the brain. Yakovlev and Wadsworth referred to the localized failure of evagination as *schizencephaly* and postulated that it was the result of a focal developmental defect in the wall of the cerebral mantle. They based their interpretation on the finding of malformed cortex in the margins of the defect but this might indicate only that the lesion preceded neuronal migration. Levine and coworkers

Table 38-2

CAUSES OF MACROCEPHALY

1. Hydrocephalus
2. Hydranencephaly
3. Macroencephaly (enlarged brain)
   a. Alexander disease
   b. Canavan disease
   c. Tay-Sachs disease
4. Agenesis of corpus callosum
5. Subdural hematoma
6. Constitutional (familial) macrocephaly
7. Hemimegalencephaly

attributed it to a destructive, possibly ischemic, lesion occurring in the first few weeks of gestation, at a time when neuronal migration was incomplete. However, at least some forms have been traced to genetic defects as detailed further on.

The *macrocephalic head* (a large head with normal or only slightly enlarged ventricles) may be indicative of an advancing metabolic disease that enlarges the brain, as in *Alexander disease*, *Canavan spongy degeneration of infancy*, and *later phases of Tay-Sachs disease*, all of which are described in Chap. 37. *Agenesis of the corpus callosum*, a common congenital defect, may be associated with macrocephaly and varying degrees of mental impairment, optic defects, and seizures. In a series of 56 patients with agenesis of the corpus callosum, Taylor and David reported the presence of epilepsy in 32 and varying degrees of developmental delay in 28; only 9 had no recognizable neurologic defects. Also noted was a high incidence of psychiatric disturbances in these patients. In such cases, CT and MRI reveal the characteristic "bat-wing" deformity of the ventricles. There is also asynchrony of electrical activity of the two cerebral hemispheres on the electroencephalogram (EEG). In a few of these patients, an autosomal dominant inheritance was found (Lynn et al). Agenesis of the corpus callosum is also part of the Aicardi syndrome (see further on) and the Andermann syndrome, and it has been noted, without explanation, in some cases of nonketotic hyperglycinemia.

Subdural hematomas also enlarge the child's head and cause bulging of the fontanels and separation of the sutures. The infant is usually irritable and listless, taking nourishment poorly. Infants and children with neurofibromatosis, osteogenesis imperfecta, and achondroplasia also have enlarged heads; in the last of these, some degree of hydrocephalus appears to be responsible. Ultrasonography, which can be performed in the prenatal and neonatal periods, is usually diagnostic in all these cranial enlargements. Also MRI and CT scanning will disclose the size of the ventricles and the presence of subdural blood or fluid (*hygroma*).

Apart from patients with these pathologic states, there are individuals whose heads and brains are enlarged but who are normal in all other respects. Many of them come from families with large heads. Schreier and colleagues, who traced this condition through three generations of several families, declared it to be an autosomal dominant trait. This group represented 20 percent of 557 children referred to a clinic because of cranial enlargement, according to Lorber and Priestley.

Hemimegalencephaly This term refers to a marked enlargement of one cerebral hemisphere as a result of a developmental abnormality. The cortical gray matter and sometimes the basal ganglia are greatly increased in volume and weight. The cerebellum, brainstem, and spinal cord retain their normal dimensions. The cranium may be misshapen or enlarged but is normal in size in some cases. Rarely, the face and body are enlarged on the side of the enlarged hemisphere. The cortex of the giant hemisphere is thick and disorganized. Neurons are in disarray and some are enlarged; in some places the natural lamination of the cortex is effaced. Nothing is known about causation, but clearly embryogenesis has been deranged at the stage of neuroblast formation.

Clinically, these individuals are cognitively delayed and some have epilepsy. A degree of hemiparesis may be present but severe hemispheral neurologic deficits are generally not reported. However, hemimegalencephaly has been discovered at autopsy in a few individuals who had no mental or neurologic deficits.

Craniostenoses

Some of the most startling cranial deformities are caused by premature closure of the cranial sutures (membranous junctions between bones of the skull). Such conditions are estimated to occur in 1 of every 1,000 births, with predominance in males (Lyon and Evrard). The growth of the cranium is inhibited in a direction perpendicular to the involved suture(s), creating a compensatory enlargement in other dimensions as allowed by the patent sutures. For example, when the lambdoid and coronal sutures are both affected, the thrust of the growing brain enlarges the head in a vertical direction (*tower skull*, or *oxycephaly*, also referred to as *turricephaly* and *acrocephaly*). The orbits are shallow, the eyes bulge, and skull films show islands of bone thinning (*lückenschädel*). When only the sagittal suture is involved, the head is long and narrow (*scaphocephalic*) and the closed suture projects, keel-like, in the midline. With premature closure of the coronal suture, the head is excessively wide and short (*brachycephalic*). The nervous system is usually normal in these restricted craniostenoses. If this condition is recognized before 3 months of age, the surgeon can make artificial sutures that may permit the shape of the head to become more normal (Shillito and Matson). Once brain growth has been completed, little can be done aside from complex reconstructive surgery. When several sutures (usually coronal and sagittal) are closed, so as to diminish the cranial capacity, intracranial pressure may increase, causing headache, vomiting, and papilledema. An operation is then needed to increase the capacity of the skull.

In acrocephalosyndactyly, or Apert syndrome, craniostenoses are combined with syndactyly (fused, or webbed, fingers or toes). There are often added complications: mental retardation, deafness, convulsions, and loss of sight secondary to papilledema. The so-called clover-shaped skull is the most severe and lethal of the craniostenoses because of the associated developmental anomalies of the brain (see further on).

Approximately one-quarter of affected children with craniostenoses will be found to have a single gene or chromosomal abnormality, most commonly in the *FGFR3* gene.

When, for any reason, an infant lies with the head turned constantly to one side (because of a shortened sternomastoid muscle or hemianopia, for example), the occiput on that side, over time, becomes flattened, as does the opposite frontal bone. The other occipital and frontal bones bulge, so that the maximum length of the skull is not in the sagittal but in the diagonal plane. This condition is called *plagiocephaly*, or *wry head*. Craniostenosis of one-half of a coronal suture may also distort the skull in this way.

Disturbances of Neuronal Migration and Cortical Development

Neuroembryologic studies have identified several milestones of neuroblast formation, migration, cortical organization, neuron differentiation, and connectivity. Certain developmental anomalies can be traced to one of these stages of cytogenesis and histogenesis in the first trimester of gestation and to the growth and differentiation that take place in the second and third trimesters. During the first trimester, postmitotic neurons that will ultimately reside in the cortex arise in the ventricular zone adjacent to the ventricles. They migrate along the scaffold of radial glia to form the multilayered cortex. It is interesting that neurons moving up the scaffold must pass through neurons that are already in position in the cortex, leading to an "inside-out" lamination in which the most recently born and arrived neurons reside on the outermost surface of the forming cortex.

Originally there is an excess of neurons, many of which degenerate during development—a process properly called *apoptosis*. There are recorded instances in which the full complement of neuroblasts and neurons fails to be generated. In the extreme, the emergence of two separate cerebral hemispheres may not occur (*holoprosencephaly*), or the bihemispheric brain may remain small (*microcephaly*). In other described instances, a diminished number of neurons are less obvious than their failure to migrate to the cortical surface; they remain scattered through the mantle zone in sheets and heterotopic aggregates. One type of focal band-shaped subcortical heterotopia is termed "double cortex." *Polymicrogyria* refers to an excessive number of abnormally small gyri. It is expressed by a syndrome of mental retardation, seizures, delayed speech, and motor abnormalities. The cortex may fail to become sulcated—that is, it is *lissencephalic* or may be defectively convoluted, forming microgyric and *pachygyric* (broad gyral) patterns. In yet other brains, neuronal migration is normal for the most part, but small groups of neurons in particular regions may lag or present in regional *heterotopias* (focal dysgeneses; Fig. 38-1). These migrational disorders, particularly heterotopias, are now being recognized more often by MRI and are found to have a functional significance in epilepsy but also possibly in such states as nonspecific developmental delay, and dyslexia. Finally, the cortex may be normally formed and structured but there is a failure of differentiation of intra- and intercortical and interhemispheral connections, the most obvious one being agenesis of the corpus callosum.

The timing of embryogenesis of the main visceral organs and of the coincident stages of neural tube closure were given in the introduction. With these elementary facts of neuroembryology in mind, the bases of the following clinical states are readily conceptualized: anencephaly, lissencephaly, holoprosencephaly, polymicrogyria and pachygyria, microcephaly, and special combinations of cranial and somatic abnormalities. Each is described below.

In regard to disorders of brain development, there are also special types of tumors that are the consequence of abnormal neuronal or glial development. These are

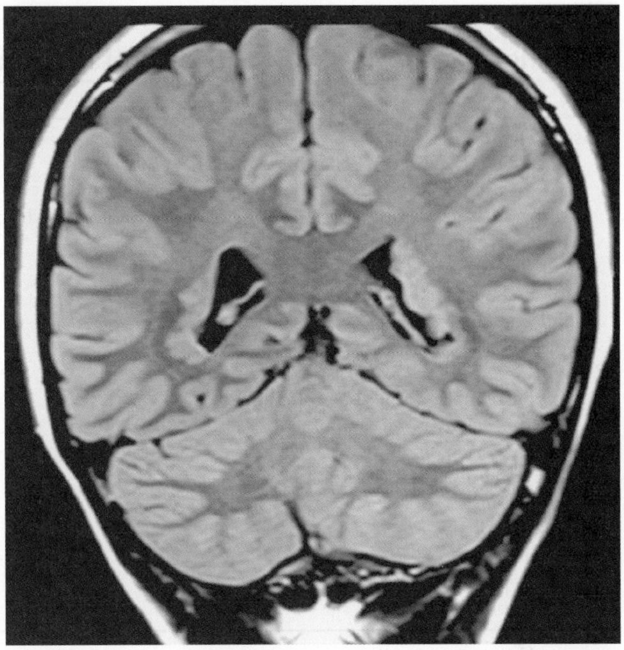

Figure 38-1. Focal cortical dysplasia. MRI in the coronal plane in a patient with seizures. Deep in the white matter, adjacent to the lateral ventricles, are multifocal heterotopic aggregates of gray matter, more apparent on the left.

variously termed gangliomas, or gangliocytomas, dysembryoplastic neuroepitheliomas (DNETs), and low-grade astrocytomas. Sometimes they become manifest in the first year of life or even before birth. Their relatively slow growth and benign character suggest that some of them represent hamartomas rather than true neoplasms (see Chap. 31). Among the ones we have encountered in adults is the Lhermitte-Duclos type of cerebellar gangliocytoma that is characterized by a "tigroid" appearance on MRI (see Fig. 31-15).

Genetics of Cerebral Disorders of Neuronal Migration (Table 38-3) Because each phase of cerebral development is under genetic control, it comes as no surprise that aberrant development might have a genetic basis. A singular advance in this field has been the identification in recent years of large numbers of genetic defects that underlie disorders of neuronal migration. These mutations, and what are known of their effects on the developing nervous system, were reviewed extensively by Mochida and Walsh, by Kato and Dobyn, and by Barkovich and colleagues; a summary is given in Table 38-3. The reader will notice that several quite different mutations may give rise to the same type of maldevelopment and that any given gene can cause malformations of varying severity but in most cases, the affected gene is active at a stage in brain development that makes the nature of the malformation understandable.

It should at the same time be noted that metabolic disturbances may also give rise to malformations of cerebral development. For example, in their review of the inborn errors of metabolism those are linked to cerebral dysgeneses. Nissenkorn and colleagues point out that disorders such as Zellweger syndrome and disorders

Table 38-3

MUTATIONS ASSOCIATED WITH DISORDERS OF NEURONAL MIGRATION AND CORTICAL MALDEVELOPMENT

DISEASE	GENE	GENE FUNCTION
Lissencephaly		
Lissencephaly with cerebellar hypoplasia	*RELN* (reelin)	Extracellular matrix protein
Lissencephaly (Miller-Dieker) or isolated lissencephaly	*LIS1*	Microtubule regulator
X-linked lissencephaly with hypogonadism (Partington syndrome)	*ARX* (aristaless)	Transcription factor
Muscle-eye-brain disease	*POMGNT1*	Glycosyltransferase
Walker-Warburg	*POMT1*	Glycosyltransferase
Holoprosencephaly	*SHH* (sonic hedgehog)	Transcription factor
Double cortex		
Double-cortex or X-linked lissencephaly	*DCX* (doublecortin)	Microtubule-associated protein
Heterotopias		
Periventricular nodular heterotopia	*FLNA* (filamin A)	Actin-binding protein
Tuberous sclerosis	*TSC1* (hamartin)	Tumor suppressor
Tuberous sclerosis	*TSC2* (tuberin)	Tumor suppressor
Fukuyama muscular dystrophy	*FCMD* (fukutin)	Possible glycosyltransferase
Schizencephaly		
Schizencephaly	*EMX2*	Transcription factor
Microcephaly		
Microcephaly	*MCPH1* (microcephalin)	? DNA repair
Microcephaly	*MCPH5 ASPM*	Mitotic/meiotic spindle

of fatty oxidation, phenylketonuria (PKU), hyperglycinemia, and pyruvate dehydrogenase deficiency cause aberrant neuronal migration and dysgenesis of the corpus callosum.

Anencephaly

This is one of the most frequent and also most appalling congenital malformations of the brain. Its incidence is 0.1 to 0.7 per all 1,000 births and females predominate in ratios ranging between 3:1 and 7:1 in different series. The concordance rate is low, both in identical and fraternal twins, but the incidence of the malformation is, nonetheless, several times the expected rate if one child in the sibship has been affected. Anencephaly has also been more frequent in certain geographic areas, for example, Ireland, for which various explanations of population genetics or environmental exposure have been postulated.

Missing in cases of anencephaly are large portions of scalp, cranial bones, and brain, including both cerebral cortex and white matter. All that remains is a hemorrhagic nubbin of nerve, glial, and connective tissue. Brainstem, cerebellum, and spinal cord are present but often, they too are malformed, as are the heart and other organs (15 to 40 percent of cases). In anencephalics who survive for a few days (65 percent die in utero and almost 100 percent before the end of the first postnatal week), startle reactions may be observed, as well as movements of limbs, spontaneous respirations, pupillary light reactions, ocular movements, and corneal reflexes. In a few, avoidance reactions, crying, and feeding reflexes can be elicited, indicating that only the rudimentary brain structures are required for these functions.

This condition, or a related one, can be anticipated if the mother's serum levels of alpha-fetoprotein and acetylcholinesterase are elevated—even more reliably anticipated if they are elevated in the amniotic fluid. Positive tests should lead to ultrasonograph imaging of the fetus. Hydramnios is common.

The causes of anencephaly are multiple and include chromosomal abnormalities, maternal hyperthermia, and, apparently, deficiencies of folate, zinc, and copper (see Medical Task Force on Anencephaly). Of these, there is fairly secure evidence that supplemental intake of folic acid during the first trimester of pregnancy (i.e., from the time of conception) reduces the incidence of anencephaly and of myelomeningocele. Additional comments on anencephaly are given further on in this chapter in the section on "Dysraphism, or Rachischisis" (lack of fusion of the neural tube).

Lissencephaly (Agyria), Holoprosencephaly, and Gyral Malformations

Included under this heading are several forms of defects of cerebral sulcation. In the lissencephalies, cortical convolutions may be absent altogether and there is morphologic evidence of several types of neuroblast deficiency. Such cases are of particular interest to neonatologists because of their associated physical abnormalities. The degree of impairment of neurologic function seldom allows longevity, so that relatively few affected individuals are found in institutions for the developmentally delayed. Seizures, poor temperature regulation, failure to accept nourishment, and apneic attacks combine to shorten life.

The failures of sulcation vary in severity. Neurons may fail to form or to migrate along glial projections to reach the more superficial layers of the cortex (a condition called in the past, Bielschowsky type); or the cortex, meninges, and eyes may fail to differentiate normally except for the dentate gyrus and hippocampus (Walker-Warburg type); or there may be other more minor focal derangements of cortical migrations and laminations with heterotopias of neurons in the white matter.

In the complete lissencephalies, the lateral and third ventricles enlarge because of a lack of the normal quantities of surrounding cerebral tissue (i.e., the aforementioned hydranencephaly). The cerebellar cortex is also abnormal. In some lissencephalic brains, there is slight sulcation presenting as abnormally broad or narrow convolutions, with thick, poorly laminated cortex; these are called *pachygyrias* or *microgyrias*, respectively, but the fundamental migratory abnormality is basically the same. The cerebellum is also abnormal, usually showing hypoplasia or aplasia involving the vermis or neocerebellum.

In the severe defects, the cranium is small at birth. In one type, which is inherited as an autosomal recessive trait, there are subtle craniofacial features (short nose, small mandible, ear abnormalities) as well as congenital heart disease. In another group, there is an associated familial congenital muscular dystrophy, placing the case between the Fukuyama and Walker-Warburg syndromes (see "Congenital Muscular Dystrophy" in Chap. 48).

Alobar and lobar *holoprosencephalies* are other examples of sulcation defects with craniofacial abnormalities in which development has gone awry in the fifth and sixth weeks of gestation (see Volpe, 1995). In these subtypes, the two cerebral hemispheres, either totally or only in part, form as a single telencephalic mass. In nearly all cases the cerebral defect is reflected by a single eye (cyclopia) and the absence of the nose, imparting an astonishing and diagnostic appearance.

Most of the severe disorders are sporadic, and the infants seldom survive for long. In a few of the malformations, a congenital infection with CMV or rubella has been implicated (Hayward et al).

The *Dandy-Walker syndrome* represents a more restricted form of migration and neural tube defect. There is cerebellar vermian hypoplasia with or without hydrocephalus and, in some cases, an added agenesis of the corpus callosum with cerebral cortical dysgeneses (Landrieu). This defect, which is identified by the cystic enlargement of the fourth ventricle, is discussed further on, with the dysraphic neural tube defects.

That some instances of lissencephaly have a genetic basis has already been mentioned (see Table 38-3). Two genes that modify microtubular function have been identified: *LIS1* and "doublecortin" or *DCX*. Large chromosomal deletions that span *LIS1* cause Miller-Dieker syndrome, in which lissencephaly is associated with distinctive facial abnormalities; small defects in the same gene cause only lissencephaly. Lissencephaly with cerebellar hypoplasia is caused by mutations in the human "reelin" gene (*RELN*), the analogue of the defective gene in reelin mice (which have a reeling gait and abnormal cortical neuronal lamination). Defects in the transcription factor ARX are associated with X-linked lissencephaly, agenesis of the corpus callosum, and hypogonadism. Periventricular nodular heterotopia is caused by another gene defect, filamin A gene on the X chromosome. Some cases of holoprosencephaly have been traced to mutations in the sonic hedgehog gene.

Microcephaly

In most of the above-described cerebral dysplasias, the cranium and brain are small, but there is also a primary form of hereditary microcephaly, called *microcephaly vera*, in which the head is astonishingly reduced in size (circumference less than 45 cm in adult life—i.e., 5 standard deviations below the mean). In contrast, the face is of normal size, the forehead is narrow and recedes sharply, and the occiput is flat. The brain often weighs less than 300 g (normal adult range: 1,100 to 1,500 g) and shows only a few primary and secondary sulci. The cerebral cortex is thick and unlaminated and grossly deficient in neurons. A few cases have an associated cerebellar hypoplasia or an infantile muscular atrophy. Stature is usually moderately reduced. Such individuals can be recognized at birth by their anthropoid appearance and later by their lumbering gait, extremely low intelligence, and lack of communicative speech. Vision, hearing, and cutaneous sensation are spared. In one of the cases studied by our colleagues, laborious effort using operant conditioning made it possible to teach the patient the shapes of simple figures. (His sister's brain, examined by R.D. Adams, was malformed and weighed only 280 g.) Skull films show that the cranial sutures are present, as are convolutional markings on the inner table.

Lesser degrees of microencephaly have been associated with progressive motor neuron disease and degeneration of the substantia nigra (Halperin et al). Evrard and associates have described another rare type of microcephaly, which they call "radial microbrain." The sulcal pattern is normal, and neuronal arrangements in the cerebral cortex are normal as well. The defect appears to be in the small number of neurons that are generated, not in their migration.

Disorders of the Pial Surface

This category of maldevelopment is characterized by inappropriate migration of neurons to the pial surface, leading to a nodularity of the surface described as a *cobblestone* appearance. In the three disorders with this pathologic finding, the clinical picture is one of developmental delay conjoined with congenital muscular dystrophy. Three identified gene defects are thought to alter the glycosylation of critical proteins in the brain and in skeletal muscle. These genes include the gene fukutin in Fukuyama muscular dystrophy (see "Congenital Muscular Dystrophy" in Chap. 48), the *POMGNT1* gene in muscle-eye-brain disease, and the *POMT1* gene in Walker-Warburg syndrome, as summarized in Table 38-3.

Combined Cerebral, Cranial, and Somatic Abnormalities

There are so many cerebrosomatic anomalies that one can hardly retain visual images of them, much less recall all the physicians' names by which they are known. There is great advantage in grouping these anomalies according to whether the extremities, face, eyes, ears, and skin are associated with a cerebral defect. The sheer number and variety of these anomalies permit only an enumeration of the more common ones and their most obvious physical characteristics. Unfortunately, apart from certain genetic linkages, no useful leads as to their origin have been forthcoming. Of necessity, one turns to atlases, one of the most thorough of which was compiled by Holmes and colleagues and is based on clinical material drawn in large part from the Fernald School and Eunice K. Shriver Center in Massachusetts. The reader may also turn to the texts by Gorlin and colleagues and by Jones for specific information. The older Ford's *Diseases of the Nervous System in Infancy, Childhood, and Adolescence* is still a valuable reference, as is Jablonski's *Dictionary of Syndromes and Eponymic Diseases*.

The Syndactylic–Craniocerebral Anomalies (Acrocephalosyndactyly)

Fusion of two fingers or two toes or the presence of a tab of skin representing an extra digit may be seen at birth in an otherwise normal individual. However, when syndactylism is more severe and is accompanied by premature closure of cranial sutures, the nervous system usually proves to be abnormal as well. The general term *acrocephalosyndactyly* is used to describe the several combinations of craniostenotic and facial deformities and fusion of digits. Several of these disorders are a consequence of mutations in genes encoding one of two fibroblast growth factors or proteins related to them. The following descriptions include only the major features; most have, in addition, distinctive malformations of the orbits, ears, and palate.

1. *Acrocephalosyndactyly types I and II (typical and atypical Apert syndrome).* Turribrachycephalic skull, syndactyly of hands and feet ("mitten hands," "sock feet"), moderate to severe mental retardation.
2. *Acrocephalosyndactyly III (Saethre-Chotzen syndrome).* Various types of craniostenoses, proximally fused and shortened digits, moderate degree of mental retardation. Transmission as an autosomal dominant trait.
3. *Acrocephalosyndactyly IV (Pfeiffer syndrome).* Turribrachycephaly; broad, enlarged thumbs and great toes; partially flexed elbows (radiohumeral or radioulnar synostoses); mild and variable mental retardation; autosomal dominant inheritance.
4. *Acrocephalopolysyndactyly V (Carpenter syndrome).* Premature fusion of all cranial sutures with acrocephaly, flat bridge of nose, medial canthi displaced laterally, excess digits and syndactyly, subnormal intelligence.
5. *Acrocephalosyndactyly with absent digits.* High, bitemporally flattened head; absent toes and syndactylic fingers; moderate mental retardation.
6. *Acrocephaly with cleft lip and palate, radial aplasia, and absent digits.* Microbrachycephaly because of craniostenosis, cleft lip and palate, absent radial bones, severe mental retardation.
7. *Dyschondroplasia, facial anomalies, and polysyndactyly.* Keel-shaped skull and ridge through center of forehead (metopic suture), short arms and legs, postaxial polydactyly and short digits, moderate mental retardation.

In all the foregoing types of syndactylism and cranial abnormalities, which may be regarded as variants of a common syndrome, the diagnosis can be made at a glance because of the deformed head, protuberant eyes, and abnormal hands and feet. The degree of cognitive delay proves to be variable, usually moderate to severe, but occasionally intelligence is normal or nearly so. The brain has been examined in only a few instances and not in a fashion to display fully the type and extent of this developmental abnormality.

Other Craniocephalic–Skeletal Anomalies

Members of this group have distinctive anomalies of the cranium, face, and other parts, but craniostenosis is not a consistent feature.

1. *Craniofacial dysostosis (Crouzon syndrome).* Variable degrees of craniosynostosis; broad forehead with prominence in the region of the anterior fontanel region; shallow orbits with proptosis; midline facial hypoplasia and short upper lip; malformed auditory canals and ears; high, narrow palate; moderate mental retardation. As noted above, a genetic defect in one of the fibroblast growth factor receptors is responsible for about one-third of cases that are not associated with other deformities (Moloney et al). Autosomal dominant inheritance is seen in most cases.
2. *Median cleft facial syndrome (frontonasal dysplasia; hypertelorism of Greig).* Widely spaced eyes, broad nasal root, cleft nose and premaxilla, V-shaped frontal hairline, heterotypic anterior frontal fontanel (midline cranial defect); mild to severe mental retardation.
3. *Chondrodystrophia calcificans congenita (chondrodysplasia punctata, Conradi-Hünermann syndrome).* Prominent forehead; flat nose; widely separated eyes; short neck and trunk with kyphoscoliosis; dry, scaly, atrophic skin; cicatricial alopecia; irregularly deformed vertebral bodies; mental retardation infrequent. Severe shortening of limbs is seen in some cases.
4. *Orofaciodigital syndrome.* All the patients are female; they have pseudoclefts involving the mandible, tongue, maxilla, and palate; hypertrophied buccal frenula; hamartomas of tongue; sparse scalp hair; subnormal intelligence in one-half of cases.
5. *Pyknodysostosis.* Large head and frontal-occipital bossing, underdeveloped facial bones, micrognathia, unerupted and deformed teeth, dense and defective long bones with shortened limbs, short and broad terminal digits of fingers and toes, mental retardation in one-quarter of the cases.
6. *Craniotubular bone dysplasias and hyperostoses.* Included under this title are several different genetic disorders of bone, characterized by modeling errors of tubular and cranial bones. Frontal and occipital hyperostosis, overgrowth of facial bones, and widening of long bones occur in various combinations. Hypertelorism, broad nasal root, nasal obstruction, seizures, visual failure, deafness, prognathism, and retardation of growth are the major features.

Oculoencephalic (Cranio-Ocular) Defects

In this category of anomalies, there is simultaneous failure or imperfect development of eye and brain.

One member of this group, the oculocerebrorenal syndrome of Lowe, has already been mentioned and, of course, many of the mucopolysaccharidoses are characterized by corneal opacities, skeletal changes, and psychomotor regression as considered separately in Chap. 37. Also, congenital syphilis, rubella, toxoplasmosis, and CMV inclusion disease may affect retina and brain; hypoxia at birth requiring treatment with oxygen may injure the brain and lead to *retrolental fibrodysplasia*. The true developmental defects in this group are as follows:

1. *Anophthalmia with mental retardation*. Sex-linked recessive. Absent eyes; orbits and maxillae remain underdeveloped, but adnexal tissues of eyes (lids) are intact; subnormal intelligence. Some cases of anophthalmia have been ascribed to genes encoding transcription factors that play a role in the development of the neuraxis (SOX2, RAX, RAX6).
2. *Norrie disease*. Also sex-linked recessive; some sight may be present at birth; later, eyes become shrunken and recessed (phthisis bulbi); some have short digits, outbursts of anger, hallucinations, and possibly regression of psychomotor function. A novel gene, norrin, on the X chromosome has been implicated.
3. *Oculocerebral syndrome with hypopigmentation*. Autosomal recessive with absence of pigment of hair and skin; small, cloudy, vascularized corneas and small globes (microphthalmia); marked mental retardation; athetotic movements of limbs.
4. *Microphthalmia with corneal opacities, eccentric pupils, spasticity, and severe mental retardation*.
5. *Aicardi syndrome with ocular abnormality*. Chorioretinopathy, retinal lacunae, staphyloma, coloboma of optic nerve, microphthalmos, mental retardation, infantile spasms and other forms of epilepsy, agenesis of corpus callosum, and cortical heterotopias. The "batwing" deformity of the third and lateral ventricles on MR images and asynchronous burst-suppression discharges and sleep spindles are diagnostic. The condition is found only in females.
6. *Lissencephaly of the Walker-Warburg type*. This anomaly has already been mentioned, as has its association with congenital muscular dystrophy. Inheritance is autosomal recessive. Ocular lesions are a regular feature but of variable type (retinal dysplasia, microphthalmia, coloboma, cataracts, corneal opacities). There may be hydrocephalus, and CT scans and MRI disclose the lack of cerebral sulci (lissencephaly). The abnormal eyes and orbits and absence of cerebellar vermis are diagnostic (see Table 38-3).
7. *Congenital tapetoretinal degeneration (Leber amaurosis)*. Visual loss from birth, moderate to severe mental retardation, and microcephaly. Early onset of blindness and absent electrical potentials on the electroretinogram (ERG) distinguish it from later-onset Leber optic atrophy, which is a mitochondrial disorder (see Chaps. 13 and 37).
8. *Septooptic dysplasia (de Morsier syndrome)*. Diminished visual acuity, small optic discs, absence of septum pellucidum, and precocious puberty. Varying degrees of pituitary insufficiency may be present, requiring endocrine replacement.

Oculoauriculocephalic Anomalies

These are less important from the neurologic standpoint, and mental retardation is present only in some cases.

1. *Mandibulofacial dysostosis (Treacher-Collins syndrome, Franceschetti-Zwahlen-Klein syndrome)*
2. *Oculoauriculovertebral dysplasia (Goldenhar syndrome)*
3. *Oculomandibulodyscephaly with hypotrichosis (Hallermann-Streiff syndrome)*

Dwarfism

Midgets are abnormally small but perfectly formed people of normal intelligence; they differ from dwarfs, who are not only very small but whose bodily proportions are markedly abnormal and who may or may not be cognitively normal. It should be commented that a majority of severely cognitively delayed patients fall below average for height and weight, but there is a small group whose fully attained height is well below 135 cm (4.5 ft) and who stand apart by this quality alone (see Jones for Smith's classification of dwarfs). The main types of dwarfism are as follows:

1. *Nanocephalic dwarfism (Seckel bird-headed dwarfism)*. The uncomplimentary term *bird head* has been applied to individuals with a small head, large-appearing eyeballs, beaked nose, and underdeveloped chin. Such a physiognomy is not unique to any disease, but when combined with dwarfism it includes a few more or less specific syndromes. Up to 1976, approximately 25 cases had been reported, some with other skeletal and urogenital abnormalities, such as medial curvature of middle digits; occasional syndactyly of toes; dislocations of elbow, hip, and knee; premature closure of cranial sutures; and clubfoot deformity. These individuals are short at birth and remain so, living until adolescence or adulthood. Retardation is severe. The cause is a homozygous or compound heterozygous mutation in RAD3-realted protein, which is also implicated in ataxia-telangectasia. At autopsy the brain is found to have a simplified convolutional pattern; one of our patients had a type of myelin degeneration similar to that of Pelizaeus-Merzbacher disease.
2. *Russell-Silver syndrome*. Possibly an autosomal dominant pattern of inheritance, with short stature of prenatal onset, craniofacial dysostosis, short arms, congenital hemihypertrophy (arm and leg on one side larger and longer), pseudohydrocephalic head (normal-sized cranium with small facial bones), abnormalities of genital development in one-third of cases, delay in closure of fontanels and in epiphyseal maturation, elevation of urinary gonadotropins. Some cases appear to be caused by a nonmutational modification of genes, which are nonetheless inherited (imprinting).
3. *Smith-Lemli-Opitz syndrome*. Autosomal recessive inheritance with microcephaly, broad nasal tip and anteverted nares, wide-set eyes, epicanthal folds, ptosis, small chin, low-set ears, enlarged alveolar maxillary ridge, cutaneous syndactyly, hypospadias in boys, short stature, subnormal neonatal activity, and normal amino acids and serum immunoglobulins.

Older survivors are bereft of language and are paraparetic, with increased reflexes and Babinski signs. The hips are usually dislocated. The responsible mutation is in *DHCR7*. The brain is small but has not been fully examined. Two of our patients are sibling girls.

4. *Rubinstein-Taybi syndrome*. Microcephaly but no craniostenosis, downward palpebral slant, heavy eyebrows, beaked nose with nasal septum extending below alae nasi, mild retrognathia, "grimacing smile," strabismus, cataracts, obstruction of nasolacrimal canals, broad thumbs and toes, clinodactyly, overlapping digits, excessive hair growth, hypotonia, lax ligaments, stiff gait, seizures, hyperactive tendon reflexes, absence of corpus callosum, mental retardation, and short stature. This dominantly inherited disease is a result of disruption of so-called CREB-binding protein, a nuclear protein necessary for gene expression that is modulated by cyclic adenosine monophosphate (cAMP).
5. *Pierre Robin syndrome*. Possible autosomal recessive pattern of inheritance with microcephaly but no craniostenosis, small and symmetrically receded chin, glossoptosis (tongue falls back into pharynx), cleft palate, flat bridge of nose, low-set ears, mental deficiency, and congenital heart disease in half the cases. Camptomelia (bent bones) and diastrophic dwarfism (short limbs) are common.
6. *DeLange syndrome (Cornelia DeLange syndrome)*. This phenotype shows some degree of variability but the essential diagnostic features are intrauterine growth retardation and stature falling below the third percentile at all ages, microbrachycephaly, generalized hirsutism and synophrys (eyebrows that meet across the midline), anteverted nostrils, long upper lip, and skeletal abnormalities (flexion of elbows, webbing of second and third toes, clinodactyly of fifth fingers, transverse palmar crease). All are moderately or, more often, severely retarded mentally, which, with the above craniofacial abnormalities, is diagnostic. It has been said, and it has been our experience, that many of these patients are prone to have a bad disposition, manifested by biting and spitting. Over half of cases are due to mutations in the *NAPBL* gene; the others involve *SMC1A* or *SMC3*.
7. *Smith-Magenis syndrome*. This is caused by deletions on chromosome 17, in which there is learning disability, severe behavioral problems (violence and self-injury), hyperactivity, deafness, and ocular abnormalities.

Neurocutaneous Anomalies With Mental Retardation

It is not surprising that skin and nervous system should share in pathologic states that impair development, as both have a common ectodermal derivation. Nevertheless, it is difficult to find a common theme in the diseases that affect both organs. In some instances, it is clear that ectoderm has been malformed from early intrauterine life; in others, a number of nondevelopmental acquired diseases of skin may have been superimposed. For reasons to be discussed later in this chapter, neurofibromatosis, tuberous sclerosis, and Sturge-Weber encephalofacial angiomatosis must be set apart in a special category of disease termed *phakomatoses*.

Hemangiomas of the skin are without doubt the most frequent cutaneous abnormalities present at birth, and usually they are entirely innocent. Many recede in the first months of life. However, an extensive vascular nevus located in the territory of the trigeminal nerve—and sometimes in other parts of the body as well—causes permanent disfigurement and usually portends an associated and topographically underlying cerebral lesion (Sturge-Weber syndrome).

Other neurocutaneous diseases are summarized below. A more complete review of these diseases will be found in the article by Short and Adams in Fitzpatrick's *Dermatology* and the 1987 monograph by Gomez. The importance of recognizing the cutaneous abnormalities relates to the fact that the nervous system is usually abnormal, and often the skin lesion appears before the neurologic symptoms are detectable. Thus the skin lesion becomes a predictor of potential neurologic involvement.

Basal-cell nevus syndrome. This condition is transmitted as an autosomal dominant trait and is characterized by superficial pits in the palms and soles; multiple solid or cystic tumors over the head, face, and neck appearing in infancy or early childhood; mental retardation in some cases; frontoparietal bossing; hypertelorism; and kyphoscoliosis.

Congenital ichthyosis, hypogonadism, and mental retardation. This disorder is inherited as a sex-linked recessive trait. Aside from the characteristic triad of anomalies, there are no special features.

Xeroderma pigmentosum. The genetic pattern of inheritance is autosomal recessive. Skin lesions appear in infancy, taking the form of erythema, blistering, scaling, scarring, and pigmentation on exposure to sunlight; old lesions are telangiectatic and parchment-like, covered with fine scales; skin cancer may develop later; loss of eyelashes, dry bulbar conjunctivae; microcephaly, hypogonadism, and mental retardation (50 percent of cases). Kanda and associates classify this disease with what in the past had been called DeSanctis-Cacchione syndrome of "xerodermic idiocy" and believe the basic mechanism to be a faulty repair of DNA. They described two young adults with low intelligence, evidence of spinal cord degeneration, and peripheral neuropathy. The peripheral nerve lesions resembled those of amyloidosis, Riley-Day syndrome, and Fabry disease in that there was a predominant loss of small fibers. Other variants are described.

Sjögren-Larsson syndrome. Autosomal recessive with congenital ichthyosiform erythroderma, normal or thin scalp hair, sometimes defective dental enamel, pigmentary degeneration of retinae, spastic legs, and mental retardation.

Poikiloderma congenitale (Rothmund-Thompson syndrome). Autosomal recessive heredity; appearance of skin changes from the third to sixth months of life; diffuse pink coloration of cheeks spreading to ears and buttocks, later replaced by macular and reticular pattern of skin atrophy mixed with striae, telangiectasia, and pigmentation; sparse hair in half of the cases; cataracts; small genitalia; abnormal hands and feet; short stature; and mental retardation.

Linear sebaceous nevus syndrome. Here there is a linear nevus of one side of face and trunk, lipodermoids on bulbar conjunctivae, vascularization of corneas, mental retardation, focal seizures, and spike and slow waves in the EEG. Genetics remain uncertain.

Incontinentia pigmenti (Bloch-Sulzberger syndrome). Only females are affected; appearance of dermal lesions in first weeks of life; vesicles and bullae followed by hyperkeratoses and streaks of pigmentation, scarring of scalp, and alopecia; abnormalities of dentition; hemiparesis; quadriparesis; seizures; mental retardation; and up to 50 percent eosinophils in blood. The status of this disease is uncertain.

Focal dermal hypoplasia. Also a disease limited to females. Areas of dermal hypoplasia with protrusions of subcutaneous fat, hypo- and hyperpigmentation, scoliosis, syndactyly in a few, short stature, thin body habitus. Intelligence is occasionally subnormal.

Other rare entities are neurocutaneous melanosis, neuroectodermal melanolysosomal disease with mental retardation, progeria, Cockayne syndrome, and ataxia-telangiectasia (see Chap. 37; also Gomez, 1987).

Dysraphism, or Rachischisis: Meningocele, Encephaloceles, and Spina Bifida

Included under this heading is the large number of disorders of fusion of dorsal midline structures of the primitive neural tube, a process that takes place during the first 3 weeks of postconceptual life. Exogenous factors are presumed to be operative in most cases but there are genetic forms. The most extreme form is anencephaly, as described earlier; it is characterized by the absence of the entire cranium at birth, and the undeveloped brain lies in the base of the skull, a small vascular mass without recognizable nervous structures.

An eventration of brain tissue and its coverings through an unfused midline defect in the skull is called an *encephalocele*. Frontal encephaloceles may deform the forehead or remain occult. Associated defects of the frontal cortex, anterior corpus callosum, and optic-hypothalamic structures, as well as cerebrospinal fluid (CSF) leakage into frontal or ethmoid sinuses, pose a risk of meningitis. Some of these children are relatively normal mentally. Far more severe are the posterior encephaloceles, some of which are enormous and are attended by grave neurologic deficits such as blindness, ataxia, and mental retardation. However, lesser degrees of the defect are well known and may be small or hidden, such as a *meningoencephalocele* connected with the rest of the brain through a small opening in the skull. Small nasal encephaloceles may cause no neurologic signs, but if they are mistaken for nasal polyps and snipped off, CSF fistulae result.

A failure of development of the midline portion of the cerebellum referred to earlier, forms the basis of the *Dandy-Walker syndrome* (Fig. 38-2). A cyst-like structure, representing the greatly dilated fourth ventricle, expands in the midline, causing the occipital bone to

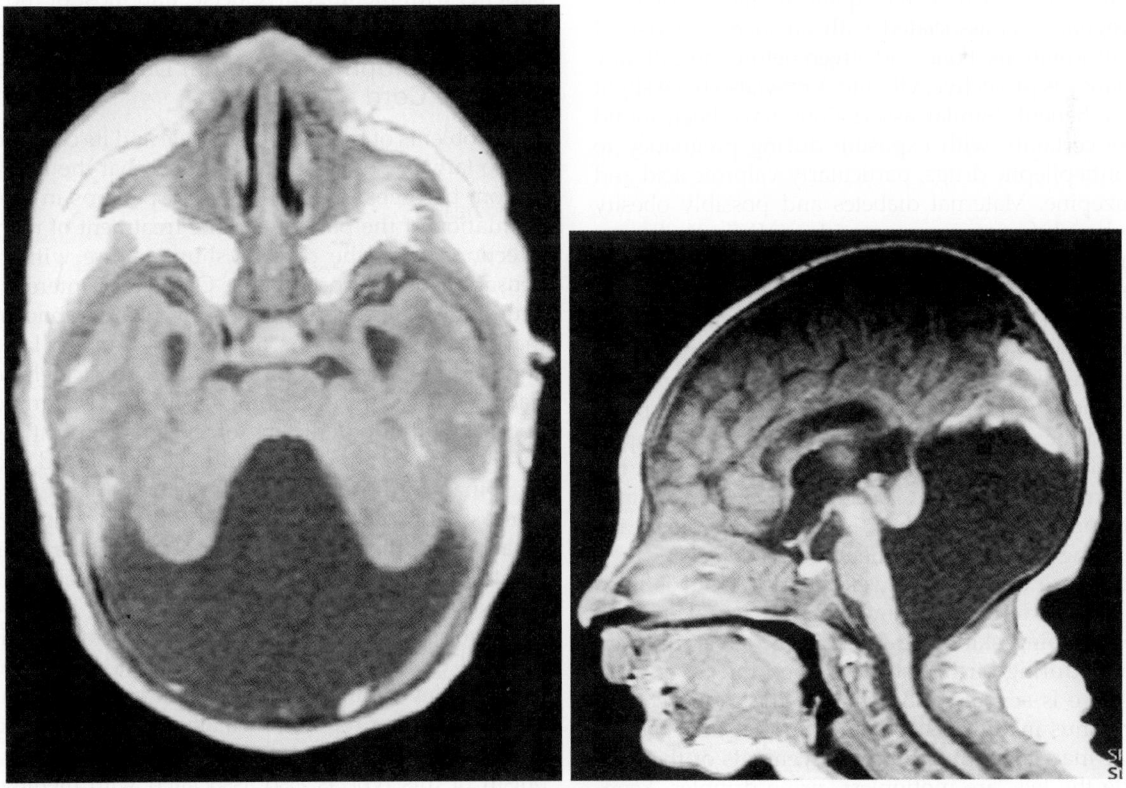

A B

Figure 38-2. Dandy-Walker syndrome. MRI showing agenesis of the midline cerebellum and large midline cyst, representing the greatly dilated fourth ventricle, which occupies almost the entire posterior fossa. *A.* Axial view. *B.* Sagittal view.

bulge posteriorly and displace the tentorium and torcula upward. In addition, the cerebellar vermis is aplastic, the corpus callosum may be deficient or absent, and there is dilatation of the aqueduct as well as the third and lateral ventricles.

Even more frequent are abnormalities of closure of the vertebral arches. These take the form of a *spina bifida occulta*, *meningocele*, and *meningomyelocele* of the lumbosacral or other regions. In *spina bifida occulta*, the cord remains inside the canal and there is no external sac, although a subcutaneous lipoma or a dimple or wisp of hair on the overlying skin may mark the site of the lesion. In *meningocele*, there is a protrusion of only the dura and arachnoid through the defect in the vertebral laminae, forming a cystic swelling usually in the lumbosacral region; the cord remains in the canal, however. In *meningomyelocele*, which is 10 times as frequent as meningocele, the cord (more often the cauda equina) is extruded also and is closely applied to the fundus of the cystic swelling.

The incidence of spinal dysraphism (myeloschisis), like that of anencephaly, varies widely from one locale to another, and the disorder is more likely to occur in a second child if one child has already been affected (the incidence then rises from 1 per 1,000 to 40 to 50 per 1,000).

Etiology Exogenous factors (e.g., potato blight in Ireland) were many times implicated in an increased rate of both myeloschisis and anencephaly, but the effects of starvation and vitamin deficiency could never be separated from the potential effect of a toxic factor. It has now been established by numerous case-control and randomized treatment trials that inadequate intake of folate in early pregnancy is associated with an increased risk of these malformations. Folic acid, given before the 28th day of pregnancy is protective; vitamin A may also have slight protective benefit. Similar associations have been found with less certainty with exposure during pregnancy to certain antiepileptic drugs, particularly valproic acid and carbamazepine. Maternal diabetes and possibly obesity have been risk factors in some epidemiologic studies, as summarized by Mitchell and colleagues. The greatest risk, however, almost 30-fold higher, attaches to a previous pregnancy affected with spina bifida in particular.

Diagnosis As with anencephaly, the diagnosis can often be inferred from the presence of alpha-fetoprotein in the amniotic fluid (sampled at 15 to 16 weeks of pregnancy) and the deformity confirmed by ultrasonography in utero. Blood contamination is a source of error in the fetoprotein test (Milunsky). Acetylcholinesterase immunoassay, done on amniotic fluid, is another reliable means of confirming the presence of neural tube defects.

In the case of meningomyelocele, the child is born with a large externalized lumbosacral sac covered by delicate, weeping skin. The defect may have ruptured in utero or during birth, but more often the covering is intact. There is severe dysfunction of the cauda equina roots or conus medullaris contained in the sac. Stroking of the sac may elicit involuntary movements of the legs. As a rule the legs are motionless, urine dribbles, keeping the patient constantly wet, there is no response to pinprick over the lumbosacral dermatomal zones, and the tendon reflexes are absent. In contrast, craniocervical structures are normal unless a Chiari malformation is associated, as it often is (see further on). Differences are noted in the neurologic picture depending on the level of the lesion. If the lesion is entirely sacral, bladder and bowel sphincters are affected but legs escape; if lower lumbar and sacral, the buttocks, legs, and feet are more impaired than hip flexors and quadriceps; if upper lumbar, the feet and legs are sometimes spared and ankle reflexes retained, and there may be Babinski signs. The two common complications of these severe spinal defects are meningitis and progressive hydrocephalus from a Chiari malformation (see below). The subject of spina bifida and neural tube defects was reviewed by Botto and colleagues and by Mitchell and coworkers.

Treatment Prevention by the administration of folate during pregnancy is obviously paramount. Opinions as to proper management of the established lesion vary considerably. Excision and closure of the coverings of the meningomyelocele in the first few days of life are advised if the objective is to prevent fatal meningitis. After a few weeks or months, as hydrocephalus reveals its presence by a rapid increase in head size and enlargement of the ventricles, a ventriculoperitoneal shunt is required. Less than 30 percent of such patients survive beyond 1 year and the long-term results of treating these patients have not been encouraging. Lorber and colleagues report that 80 to 90 percent of their surviving patients are developmentally delayed to some degree and are paraplegic. The decision to undertake rather formidable surgical procedures is being questioned more frequently. Exceptionally, patients with meningomyelocele, and most of those with lumbar meningocele, are mentally normal.

Other Developmental Spinal Defects Including Tethered Cord

The problems of meningomyelocele and its complications are so largely pediatric and surgical that the neurologist seldom becomes involved—except perhaps in the initial evaluation of the patient—in the treatment of meningeal infection, or in the case of shunt failure with decompensation of hydrocephalus. Of greater interest to the neurologist are a series of closely related abnormalities that produce symptoms for the first time in late childhood, adolescence, or even adult life. These include sinus tracts with recurrent meningeal infections, lumbosacral lipomas with low tethering of the spinal cord ("tethered cord") causing an early childhood or delayed radicular or spinal cord syndrome; diastematomyelia, cysts, or tumors with spina bifida and a progressive myeloradiculopathy; and the Chiari malformation and syringomyelia that first present in adolescence or adult life. These abnormalities are described below.

Another class of disorders involves an occult lumbosacral dysraphism that is not inherited but is a result of faulty development of the cell mass that lies caudal to the posterior neuropore (normally this undergoes closure by the 28th day of embryonic life). Occult spinal dysraphism of this type is also associated with meningoceles, lipomas, and sacrococcygeal teratomas. Another well-recognized anomaly is agenesis of the sacrum and sometimes the lower lumbar vertebrae (*caudal regression syndrome*).

Interestingly, in 15 percent of such cases, the mother is diabetic (Lyon and Evrard). Here there is flaccid paralysis of legs, often with arthrogrypotic contractures and urinary incontinence. Sensory loss is less prominent, mental function develops normally, and there is no hydrocephalus.

Sinus tracts in the lumbosacral or occipital regions are of importance, for they may be a source of bacterial meningitis at any age. They are often betrayed by a small dimple in the skin or by a tuft of hair along the posterior surface of the body in the midline. (The pilonidal sinus should not be included in this group.) The sinus tract may lead to a terminal myelocystocele and be associated with dermoid cysts or fibrolipomas in the central part of the tract. Cloacal defects (no abdominal wall and no partition between bladder and rectum) may be combined with anterior meningoceles. Evidence of sinus tracts should be sought in instances of unexplained meningitis, especially when there has been recurrent infection or the cultured organism is of nosocomial dermal origin.

Of great interest are *congenital cysts* and *tumors*, particularly lipoma and dermoid, that arise in the filum terminale and attach (tether) the cord to the sacrum. Progressive symptoms and signs are produced as the spine elongates during development, thereby stretching the caudally fixed cord (Fig. 38-3). Some of these children have bladder and leg weakness soon after birth. Others deteriorate neurologically at a later age (generally between 2 and 16 years, sometimes later—see below). Complex disturbances of bladder function that produce urgency and incontinence beginning in the second or third decade may be the only manifestation, or the bladder symptoms may be combined with impotence (in the male) and numbness of the feet and legs or foot-drop (Pang and Wilberger). Several of our adult patients have had unusual visceral reflex reactions, such as involuntary defecation or priapism with stimulation of the abdomen or perineum. According to most surgeons, it is not the myelolipoma but the tethering of the cord that gives rise to symptoms; removal of the tumor is of little benefit unless the cord is detached from the sacrum at the same time. This may be difficult, for the lipoma may be fused with the dorsal surface of the spinal cord.

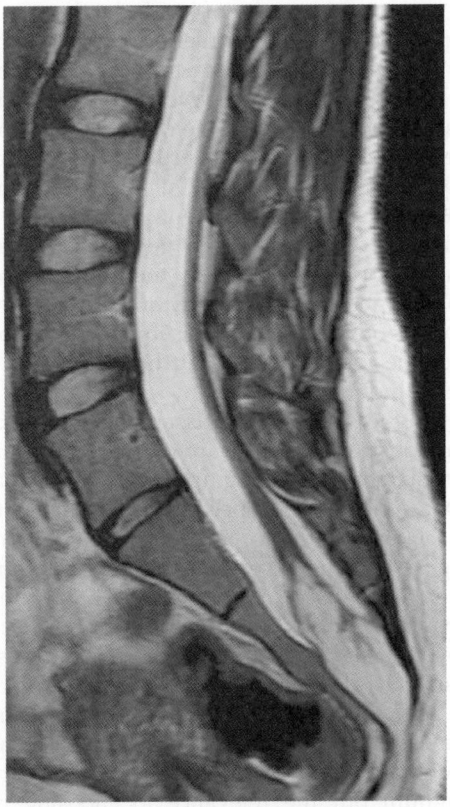

Figure 38-3. MRI of an adult with tethered cord and the typical lipoma at its caudal extent. No dysraphism is present. The main features were a flaccid bladder, asymmetrical weakness and atrophy of the forelegs, and a degree of spasticity in the legs.

Diastematomyelia is another unusual abnormality of the spinal cord often associated with spina bifida. Here a bony spicule or fibrous band protrudes into the spinal canal from the body of one of the thoracic or upper lumbar vertebrae and divides the spinal cord into halves for a variable vertical extent. In extreme examples, the division of the cord may be complete, each half with its own dural sac and complete set of nerve roots. This longitudinal fissuring and doubling of the cord are spoken of as *diplomyelia*. With body growth, the restriction created by the bone spicule leads to a *traction myelopathy*, presenting with pain and progressive sensory, motor, and bladder symptoms, sometimes as late as adult life. Removal of the fibrous-bony spicule and untethering of the spinal cord have been beneficial in some cases.

Syringomyelia (see also Chap. 44) is a developmental cavity within the cervical cord, extending a variable distance caudally or rostrally, and usually associated with an Arnold-Chiari malformation that is described below. There are a variety of other neurodevelopmental spinal abnormalities in the high cervical region, such as fusion of atlas and occiput or of cervical vertebrae (Klippel-Feil syndrome), congenital dislocation of the odontoid process and atlas, platybasia, and basilar impression. These abnormalities are discussed in Chap. 44, with other diseases of the spinal cord.

Chiari Malformation

Encompassed by this term are a constellation of related congenital anomalies at the base of the brain, the most consistent of which are (1) extension of a tongue of cerebellar tissue posterior to the medulla and cord that extends into the cervical spinal canal; (2) caudal displacement of the medulla and the inferior part of the fourth ventricle into the cervical canal; and (3) a frequent but not invariable association with syringomyelia or a spinal developmental abnormality. These and associated anomalies were first clearly described by Chiari (1891). Several translations of his original material have been made, but they have been criticized as inaccurate. Arnold's name is attached to the syndrome, but his contribution to our understanding of these malformations was relatively insignificant. Use of the double eponym *Arnold-Chiari malformation* is so entrenched that a dispute over its propriety serves little purpose. Chiari recognized four types of abnormalities. In recent years, the term has come to be restricted to Chiari's types I and II—that is, to cerebellomedullary descent without and with a meningomyelocele, respectively. Type III Chiari malformation is no more than a high cervical or occipitocervical meningomyelocele with cerebellar herniation, and type IV consists only of cerebellar hypoplasia.

The incidence among adults, acquired from autopsy series and more recently, from incidentally discovered descent of the cerebellar tonsils on imaging procedures, is about 0.6 percent of the population. It should be emphasized that a proportion of normal individuals have a small tongue of the posterior cerebellum protruding by a few millimeters below the lower lip of the foramen magnum; this is usually of no significance and does not justify inclusion as a Chiari malformation. A historical account of the clinical, pathologic, and imaging aspects of this malformation and the evolution of ideas concerning it has been given by Bejjani.

Several other morphologic features are characteristic of the true Chiari anomaly. The medulla and pons are elongated and the aqueduct is narrowed. The displaced tissue (medulla and cerebellum) occludes the foramen magnum; the remainder of the cerebellum, which is small, is also displaced so as to obliterate the cisterna magna. The foramina of Luschka and Magendie often open into the cervical canal, and the arachnoidal tissue around the herniated brainstem and cerebellum is fibrotic. All these factors are probably operative in the production of hydrocephalus, which is always associated. Just below the herniated tail of cerebellar tissue there is a kink or spur in the spinal cord, which is pushed posteriorly by the lower end of the fourth ventricle. In this fully expressed form of the malformation, a meningomyelocele is nearly always found. It should again be emphasized that *hydromyelia or syringomyelia of the cervical cord are commonly associated findings* and the main theories of causation of the latter are based on the change in CSF dynamics produced by the Chiari malformation.

Developmental abnormalities of the cerebrum, particularly polymicrogyria may infrequently coexist, and the lower end of the spinal cord may extend as low as the sacrum (i.e., a tethered cord). There are usually cranial bony abnormalities as well. The posterior fossa is small; the foramen magnum is enlarged and grooved posteriorly. Nishikawa and colleagues suggested that smallness of the posterior fossa with overcrowding is the primary abnormality leading to the brain malformation. Often the base of the skull is flattened or infolded by the cervical spine (basilar impression).

Clinical Manifestations

In type II Chiari malformation (with meningomyelocele), the problem becomes one of progressive hydrocephalus. Cerebellar signs cannot be discerned in the first few months of life. However, lower cranial-nerve abnormalities—laryngeal stridor, fasciculations of the tongue, sternomastoid paralysis (causing head lag when the child is pulled from lying to sitting), facial weakness, deafness, bilateral abducens palsies—may be present in varying combinations. If the patient survives to later childhood or adolescence, one of the syndromes that are more typical of the type I malformation may become manifest.

In the more common type I Chiari malformation (without meningocele or other signs of spinal dysraphism), neurologic symptoms may not develop until adolescence or adult life. The symptoms are those of (1) increased intracranial pressure, mainly headache, (2) progressive cerebellar ataxia, (3) progressive spastic quadriparesis, (4) downbeating nystagmus, or (5) the syndrome of cervical syringomyelia (segmental amyotrophy and sensory loss in the hands and arms, with or without pain). Or the patient may show a combination of disorders of the lower cranial nerves, cerebellum, medulla, and spinal cord (sensory and motor tract disorders), usually in conjunction with headache that is mainly occipital. This combination of symptoms is easily mistaken for multiple sclerosis or a tumor at the foramen magnum. The symptoms are usually chronic but may have an acute onset after sustained or forceful extension of the neck, as, for example, after a long session of dental work, hairdressing in women, or chiropractic manipulation. The physical habitus of such patients may be normal, but approximately 25 percent have signs of an arrested hydrocephalus, or a short "bull neck." When basilar impression (a congenital abnormality of the occipital bone that invaginates the posterior atlas into the cranial cavity) and a Chiari malformation coexist, it may be impossible to decide which of the two is responsible for the clinical findings.

The nature and severity of headache that are reasonably attributable to a Chiari malformation is somewhat unclear. Occipitonuchal pain with coughing, position change, or the Valsalva maneuver is the most dependable association, but even then, decompression may not relieve the symptoms. Exertional headache alone is a questionable association. Only large and genuine malformations, not minor descent of the tonsils should be considered causative. More generalized headaches may or may not be explained by the finding of a Chiari malformation and the advisability of a surgical treatment then depends on the degree of disability created by other aspects of the malformation. Further discussion of this subject is found in Chap. 10.

The tongue of cerebellar tissue and the kinked cervical cord obstruct the upward flow of CSF and give a highly characteristic imaging profile, particularly on sagittal MRI (Fig. 38-4). Inspection of the axial sections of scans at the level of the foramen magnum demonstrates crowding of the upper cervical canal by inferiorly displaced cerebellar tissue, but one must be aware of the variations in the normal position of the cerebellar tonsils at this level. A slight descent of the cerebellar tonsils that is reversible is also seen with low cerebrospinal fluid pressure and not indicative of a Chiari malformation. Recent inceptions in phase contrast MRI technology allow the imaging of CSF flow in the region of the foramen magnum but the relevance to choosing patients for surgical decompression has not been clarified (see summary by Menick). The CSF in Chiari malformation is usually normal but may show an elevated pressure and protein level in some cases for unexplained reasons.

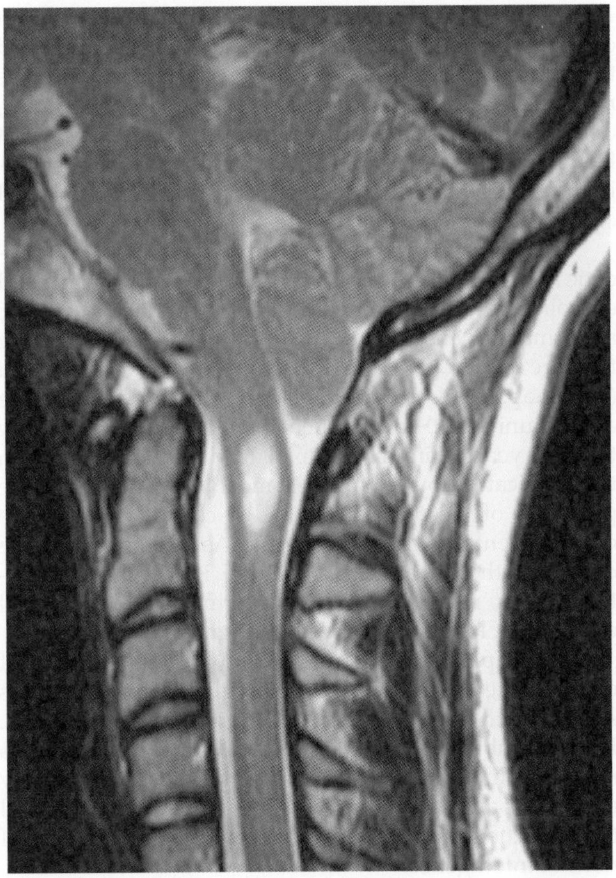

Figure 38-4. Chiari-type malformation and developmental syringomyelia. T2-weighted MRI of the low-lying cerebellar tonsils below the foramen magnum and behind the upper cervical cord and the syrinx cavity in the upper cord.

Treatment

The treatment of Chiari malformation and any associated basilar impression is far from satisfactory. If clinical progression is slight or uncertain, it is probably best to do nothing. If disability by way of spasticity, ataxia, pain in the shoulders or arms, or lower cranial-nerve disease is increasing, upper cervical laminectomy and enlargement of the foramen magnum are indicated. The proper course for patients that have headaches alone is uncertain but many such patients are operated upon if their cranial pain has been progressive, or if it is consistently and markedly worsened by cough or similar Valsalva actions, or if there is fainting or another associated symptom that can be reasonably related to the Chiari abnormality. The outcome of surgery, in our experience, has been less satisfactory when decompression was performed mainly for intractable headache, but there have been exceptions, especially when exertion or Valsalva maneuver elicits the symptoms.

The basic operation is suboccipital and C-1 decompression; various forms of shunting may be added if there is syringomyelia (the shunt is to the adjacent subarachnoid space) or hydrocephalus. The surgical procedure must be done cautiously. Opening of the dura and extensive manipulation of the malformation or excision of herniated cerebellum may aggravate the symptoms but is performed by some neurosurgeons to decompress the lower brainstem. Often, surgery halts the progress of the neurologic illness, arrests the hydrocephalus, or results in some other clinical improvement. The surgical series reported by Alzate and colleagues is representative. Emphasis was placed on proper patient selection, but the analysis of 66 cases, as in most other reports, was retrospective. (This reference is part of a very informative monograph). Most series report that a CSF leak follows surgery in about 5 percent of patients. The fate of an associated syringomyelia has been uncertain but most series report optimistic results.

As alluded to earlier, the role of phase-contrast MRI of CSF flow around the foramen magnum in selecting patients for decompression is unknown. The treatment of an associated syringomyelia and other developmental abnormalities in this region is discussed further in Chap. 44 under "Intramedullary Syringomyelic Syndrome." We are unable to comment on the use by a limited number of neurosurgeons of posterior fossa decompression for the treatment of chronic fatigue syndrome and all manner of other symptoms except to say that it is entirely illogical, even when a Chiari malformation is detected.

CHROMOSOMAL ABNORMALITIES (KARYOTYPIC CHROMOSOMAL DYSGENESES)

As mentioned in the introduction, mid-twentieth-century discovery of outstanding significance was the recognition of a group of developmental anomalies of the brain and other organs associated with a demonstrable abnormality of the karyotype of autosomal and sex chromosomes. Jacobs and Lejeune in 1959 almost simultaneously were the first to note a triplication of the 21st chromosome in Down syndrome, and there followed the discovery of a number of other trisomies as well as deletions or translocations of other autosomal chromosomes and a lack or excess of one of the sex chromosomes. Such an event must take place sometime after the formation of the oocyte, during the long period when it lies fallow in the ovary or during the process of conception or germination and first cell divisions. Thus, all the cells in the embryo may carry the changed chromosome, or only some of them may carry it, the latter condition being called *mosaicism*.

The precise manner in which triplication or some other imperfection of a chromosome is able to derail the pathways of ontogenesis is a mystery. In some instances, a chromosomal imperfection may result from the lack of a gene or a distortion or fragmentation of an unstable gene, as in the fragile X syndrome. These germ line alterations are to be distinguished from acquired partial duplications and deletions of parts of genes that occur as acquired somatic mutations in many tremors and from variations in copy number of segments of genes that are emerging as possible explanations for a number of diseases such as autism.

Certain chromosomal abnormalities are incompatible with life, and it has been found that the cells of many abortuses and stillborns show abnormal karyotypes. Conversely, the organism may survive and exhibit any one of many syndromes, of which the following are the most frequent: (1) Down syndrome (mongolism, trisomy 21); (2) one type of arrhinencephaly (trisomy 13, Patau syndrome); (3) trisomy 18 (Edwards syndrome); (4) cri-du-chat syndrome (deletion of short arm of chromosome 5); (5) monosomy 21 (so-called antimongolism); (6) ring chromosomes; (7) Klinefelter syndrome (XXY); (8) Turner syndrome (XO); (9) others (XXXX, XXX, XYY, YY, XXYY); (10) fragile X syndrome, the most common form of inherited mental retardation; (11) Williams syndrome; and (12) Prader-Willi and Angelman syndromes. There are numerous less-frequent types, some of which are also discussed below because they have special neurologic interest. The overall frequency of chromosomal abnormalities in live births is 0.6 percent (see the review by Kalter and Warkany). For a comprehensive account of the chromosome-linked disorders the reader is referred to the article by Lemieux and for speculations on the nature of genetic retardations, can be found in the article by Nokelainen and Flint.

Down Syndrome (Trisomy 21)

Described first in 1866 by Langdon Down, this is easily the best known of the chromosomal dysgeneses. Its frequency is 1 in 600 to 700 births, and it accounts for approximately 10 percent of all cases in every large series of cases of severe mental retardation. One cannot distinguish the Down syndrome with the common triplication of chromosome 21 from that caused by a translocation, and therefore duplication, of one arm, specifically the distal portion of the long arm that seems to contain the region responsible for the syndrome. Two genes have been of greatest interest in that region: *DYRK1A* and *DSCR1*.

Familiarity with the condition permits its recognition at birth, but the somatic appearance becomes more obvious with advancing age. The round head, open mouth, stubby hands, slanting palpebral fissures, and short stature impart an unmistakable appearance. The ears are low-set and oval, with small lobules. The palpebral fissures slant slightly upward and outward owing to the presence of medial epicanthal folds that partly cover the inner canthi (hence the old term *mongolism*). The bridge of the nose is poorly developed and the face is flattened (hypoplasia of the maxillae). The tongue is usually enlarged, heavily fissured, and protruded. Gray-white specks of depigmentation are seen in the irides (Brushfield spots). The little fingers are often short (hypoplastic middle phalanx) and incurved (clinodactyly). The fontanels are patent and slow to close. The hands are broad, with a single transverse (simian) palmar crease and other characteristic dermal markings. Lenticular opacities and congenital heart lesions (septal and other defects), as well as gastrointestinal abnormalities (stenosis of duodenum), are frequent. The patient with Down syndrome is slightly below average size at birth and is characteristically of short stature at later periods of life. The height attained in adult life seldom exceeds that of a 10-year-old child.

Hypotonia of the limbs is a prominent finding. At first, the Moro response is reduced or absent, and feeding is difficult. Most affected children do not walk until 3 to 4 years of age; their acquisition of speech is delayed, but over 90 percent talk by 5 years. The IQ is variable, and that of a large group follows a Gaussian curve with the median IQ being 40 to 50 and the range, 20 to 70. A placid, docile, and affectionate personality characterizes most Down patients. A high incidence of atlantoaxial instability puts these individuals at risk of traumatic spinal cord compression in athletic ventures.

An increased incidence of myelocytic and lymphocytic leukemia takes its toll. A number of patients have had embolic strokes and brain abscesses secondary to cardiac abnormalities and there is disproportionate occurrence of the rare cerebrovascular disorder known as moyamoya (see Chap. 34). Life expectancy is later shortened by the almost universal development of Alzheimer disease by the 40th year of life. This is explained by the presence on the duplicate copy of chromosome 21 of the gene for the precursor of the protein amyloid, a central factor in the development of Alzheimer disease. As Alzheimer disease develops, the usual clinical picture is marked by inattentiveness, reduced speech, impairment of visuospatial orientation, loss of memory and judgment, and seizures.

The triplication is found mostly in the offspring of older mothers, whereas the less-frequent translocation is found equally in the offspring of young and older women. In other subtypes of the Down syndrome, referred to as *mosaics*, some cells share in the chromosomal abnormality and others are normal. Affected individuals have atypical forms of the syndrome, and some such individuals are of normal intelligence.

The genetic changes that lead to cerebral maldevelopment and dysmorphic physical features are just beginning to be understood. A connection to genes that code for enzymes of folate has been suggested (among other mechanisms). The genetic aspects, as well as features pertaining to the medical care of these patients, are well summarized by Roizen and Patterson. They emphasize the high frequency of enteric sprue (celiac disease) and hypothyroidism and the need for screening for these conditions.

Laboratory and Pathologic Findings Brain weight is approximately 10 percent less than average. The convolutional pattern is rather simple. The frontal lobes are smaller than normal, and the superior temporal gyri are thin. There are claims of delayed myelination of cerebral white matter and also of immature and poorly differentiated cortical neurons. Alzheimer neurofibrillary changes and neuritic plaques are practically always found in Down patients who are older than 40 years of age, as mentioned.

It is possible to make the diagnosis of Down syndrome by demonstrating the chromosomal abnormalities in cells of the amniotic fluid. About one-third of pregnant mothers also have an abnormal elevation of serum alpha-fetoprotein in the second trimester of pregnancy. Other independent predictors of fetal Down syndrome are elevated serum chorionic gonadotropin and decreased estriol (Haddow et al). One can uncover a considerable proportion of the Down population by prenatal screening for these serum markers and by performing amniocentesis on women with positive tests to search for the chromosomal abnormality. Early detection is aided by the absence on imaging of a nasal bone between 11 and 14 weeks, at which time it is normally detected (Cicero et al).

Other Chromosomal Dysgeneses

These are listed here with brief descriptions of their main features.

1. *Trisomy 13 (Patau syndrome)*. Frequency 1 in 2,000 live births, more female than male, average maternal age 31 years, microcephaly and sloping forehead, microphthalmos, coloboma of iris, corneal opacities, anosmia, low-set ears, cleft lip and palate, capillary hemangiomata, polydactyly, flexed fingers, posterior prominence of heels, dextrocardia, umbilical hernia, impaired hearing, hypertonia, severe mental retardation, death in early childhood.
2. *Trisomy 18*. Frequency 1 in 4,000 live births, more in females, average maternal age 34 years, slow growth, occasional seizures, severe mental retardation, hypertonia, ptosis and lid abnormalities, low-set ears, small mouth, mottled skin, clenched fists with index fingers overlapping the third finger, syndactyly, rocker-bottom feet, shortened big toe, ventricular septal defect, umbilical and inguinal hernias, short sternum, small pelvis, small mandible, death in early infancy.
3. *Cri-du-chat syndrome* (deletion in short arm of chromosome 5). Abnormal cry, like a kitten, severe mental retardation, hypertelorism, epicanthal folds, brachycephaly, moon face, antimongoloid slant of palpebral fissures, micrognathia, hypotonia, strabismus.
4. *Ring chromosomes*. Mental retardation with variable physical abnormalities.
5. *Klinefelter syndrome (XXY)*. Only males affected. Eunuchoid appearance, wide arm span, sparse facial and body hair, high-pitched voice, gynecomastia, small testicles, usually developmentally delayed but not severely so; high incidence of psychosis, asthma, and diabetes.
6. *Turner syndrome (XO)*. Only females affected. Triangular face, small chin, occasionally hypertelorism and epicanthal folds, widely spaced nipples, clinodactyly, cubitus valgus, hypoplastic nails, short stature, webbed neck, delayed sexual development, mild developmental delay. The manner of inheritance of the X chromosome may have bearing on the patient's personality and level of functioning, as noted in Chap. 21.
7. *Colpocephaly*. A rare type of malformation of the brain consisting of marked dilatation of the occipital horns of the lateral ventricles, thickening of the overlying rim of cortical gray matter, and thinning of the white matter. The associated clinical picture comprises developmental delay, spasticity, seizures, and visual abnormalities (because of optic nerve hypoplasia). This disorder is probably of diverse causation, but it is listed here with the chromosomal abnormalities because some cases have been associated with the mosaicism for trisomy 8 (Herskowitz et al). The term *colpocephaly* is often used incorrectly to apply to all forms of ventricular enlargement (including hydrocephalus) associated with abnormal development of the brain.
8. *Fragile X syndrome* (see further on for additional clinical details in the section on developmental delay). This abnormality is among *the most common inherited forms of developmental delay*, estimated to occur in 1 of every 1,500 male live births and accounting for 10 percent of severe developmental delay in males. Females, with two X chromosomes, are affected about half as frequently, and then only to a slight degree. With the advent of new markers for the detailed structure of chromosomes, Lubs observed an unusual site of frequent breakage ("fragility") on the X chromosome and related it to a syndrome that included developmental delay, flaring ears, elongated facies, slightly reduced cranial perimeter, normal stature, and enlarged testes. More recently, rare *progressive ataxia* has been reported in adults who harbor the chromosomal abnormality and had displayed little or no cognitive deficiency.
9. The chromosomal fragility appears to be due to a heritable, unstable CGG repeating sequence in the X chromosome. Affected individuals have over 230 repeats and carriers have 60 to 230 repeats. The prolonged sequence inactivates a gene (*FMR1*) that codes for an RNA-binding protein of as yet an unknown connection to brain function. The genetics of this and other retardations was reviewed by Nokelainen and Flint. Rousseau and colleagues described a simple and sensitive test using DNA analysis for the diagnosis of the syndrome both prenatally and after birth. Because of mosaicism, the length of the triplet repeat does not directly relate to the degree of expression of retardation, and the fragile X alteration occasionally turns up in mentally normal males; in some instances, the male children of their daughters have the disease. In some of the cases we have observed, the intellectual deficit has been mild in degree and the main abnormalities have taken the form of troublesome behavior, logorrhea, an autistic type of gaze aversion, and asociality. These and other neurobehavioral features of the syndrome and its unique pattern of inheritance (it is neither recessive nor dominant) have been discussed by Shapiro.
10. *Williams syndrome*. Described by J.C.P. Williams and colleagues of Australia from the perspective of a supravalvular aortic stenosis and a year later by Beuren and colleagues, this unique combination of cerebral maldevelopment and cardiovascular abnormalities has been traced in most patients to a microdeletion on chromosome 7 in the region of the gene that codes for the protein elastin. Its frequency is 1 in 20,000 newborns. Further discussion of clinical features of this syndrome is found later in the chapter.
11. *Prader-Willi and Angelman syndromes*. The Prader-Willi syndrome was already mentioned in relation to the hyperphagia of hypothalamic disorders (adiposogenital dystrophy, Froehlich syndrome). It is not uncommon (1 in 20,000 births) and affects both sexes equally. Hypotonia (floppy infant), areflexia, small stature, dysmorphic facies, and hypoplastic genitalia are evident, and arthrogryposis may be present at birth. After the first year, developmental delay becomes obvious and obesity, due to hyperphagia, becomes prominent. Patients are identified by the "H3O" mnemonic, referring to hypomentia, hypotonia, hypogonadism, and obesity. The disorder is associated with a deletion at 15q11-q13 (a so-called microdeletion, as in Williams syndrome), which can

be identified by a combination of cytogenetic and DNA analyses. In 70 percent of cases the disease is caused by a noninherited deletion from the paternal X chromosome.

12. The Angelman syndrome, another cause of severe developmental delay, is associated with the identical chromosomal abnormality to that found in the Prader-Willi syndrome, but there is usually a maternally inherited single-gene defect. The difference in phenotype derives from a complex genetic phenomenon termed *spatially restricted imprinting*. The phenotype comprises severe developmental delay, microcephaly, refractory seizures, absence of speech, ataxia, inappropriate laughter, prominent jaw, thin upper lip, and prolonged tongue. Outstanding are an unusual marionette-like stance coupled with a persistent tendency to laugh and smile (hence the old name "happy puppet syndrome"; see also Chap. 37).
13. *Rett syndrome*, discussed more fully further on, is mentioned here because it is to the result of a dominant defect on the X chromosome. It affects 1 of every 10,000 to 15,000 girls. After 6 to 18 months of normal development, motor skills and mental abilities seem slowly to regress. Certain handwringing and other stereotyped hand movements appear as the disease progresses and are characteristic.

Several generalizations can be made about these chromosomal dysgeneses. First, the autosomal ones are often lethal (Rett syndrome is an exception), and they almost always have a devastating effect on cerebral growth and development, whether the infant survives or not. Anomalies of nonneural and a degree of externally visible dysmorphism structures are regularly present—an association so constant that one may safely predict that an otherwise normally formed infant will not have a detectable chromosomal defect. However, only in the Down syndrome and trisomy 13 (and possibly trisomy 18) are the physiognomy and bodily configuration highly characteristic. Surprisingly, some of the most grotesque disfigurements, such as anencephaly and multiple severe congenital anomalies, are not related to a morphologic abnormality of chromosomes. By contrast, an insufficiency of sex chromosomes induces only subtle effects on the brain, affecting intellect and personality; to some extent this is true of supernumerary sex chromosomes (XYY, for example).

The basic abnormality of the brain underlying the developmental delay in many of these chromosomal dysgeneses has not been ascertained. The cerebrum is slightly small, but only minor changes are seen in the convolutional pattern and cortical architecture in conventional microscopic preparations. Neurocellular methodologies to date are not sufficiently advanced to reveal the fundamental cerebral abnormality.

Teratologic Deformations of the Nervous System

A number of observations have repudiated the former belief that the human embryo is naturally shielded against exogenous causes of maldevelopment. Irradiation during the first trimester, rubella and CMV infections, severe hypothyroidism of the mother during this same period, and the action of alcohol, vitamin A, and thalidomide have all been observed, among a multitude of other agents, to give rise to serious disorders of development. Quite relevant to the neurologist, the offspring of mothers receiving anticonvulsant drugs during the early months of pregnancy have a slightly increased risk of developing birth defects (approximately 5 percent, compared to 3 percent for the general population—see "Teratogenic Effects of Antiepileptic Medications" in Chap. 16). Cleft lip and palate are the most common anomalies attributable to anticonvulsant drugs; other craniofacial defects, spina bifida, minor cardiac defects, and dysraphisms have also been reported at a slightly increased rate. Claims and counterclaims have been made concerning the pathogenicity of numerous other substances. Mainly, the data are from animals given amounts far in excess of any possible therapeutic doses in humans. The data from humans are so meager from a multitude of such substances that they are not discussed here. The reader may refer to the article by Kalter and Warkany for further information.

THE PHAKOMATOSES (CONGENITAL NEUROECTODERMOSES)

As stated earlier, there are two broad categories of neurocutaneous diseases. In one, the infant is born with a special type of skin disease or develops it in the first weeks of life; in the other forms, the cutaneous abnormality, although often present in minor degree at birth, later evolves as quasineoplastic disorders. The quasineoplastic disorders to which van der Hoeve in 1920 applied the term *phakomatoses* (from the Greek *phakos*, meaning "mother spot," "mole," or "freckle") are tuberous sclerosis, neurofibromatosis, and cutaneous angiomatosis with central nervous system (CNS) abnormalities, which have many features in common: hereditary transmission, involvement of organs of ectodermal origin (nervous system, eyeball, retina, and skin), slow evolution of lesions in childhood and adolescence, a tendency to form hamartomas (benign tumor-like formations because of maldevelopment), and a disposition to fatal malignant transformation. These disorders are discussed below and listed in Table 38-4.

Table 38-4

THE CONGENITAL NEUROECTODERMOSES

True phakomatoses
1. Tuberous sclerosis
2. Neurofibromatosis
Cutaneous angiomatosis with abnormalities of the central nervous system
1. Sturge-Weber syndrome
2. Dermatomal hemangiomas and spinal vascular malformations
3. Epidermal nevus (linear sebaceous nevus) syndrome
4. Osler-Weber-Rendu disease
5. von Hippel-Lindau disease
6. Ataxia-telangiectasia (Louis-Bar disease)
7. Fabry disease

Tuberous Sclerosis (Bourneville Disease)

Tuberous sclerosis is a congenital disease of hereditary type in which a variety of lesions, because of a limited hyperplasia of ectodermal and mesodermal cells, appear in the skin, nervous system, heart, kidney, and other organs. It is characterized by the triad of *adenoma sebaceum, epilepsy,* and *developmental delay*. Hypomelanotic skin macules ("ash-leaf" lesions) and the subepidermal fibrotic "shagreen patch" are diagnostic features.

It is stated that Virchow recognized scleromas of the cerebrum in the 1860s and that von Recklinghausen reported a similar lesion combined with multiple myomata of the heart in 1862, but Bourneville's articles, appearing between 1880 and 1900, presented the first systematic accounts of the disease and it was he who related the cerebral lesions to those of the skin of the face. Vogt (1890) fully appreciated the significance of the neurocutaneous relationship and formally delineated the triad of facial adenoma sebaceum, epilepsy, and developmental delay. "Epiloia," a term for the disease introduced by Sherlock in 1911, never gained general acceptance. These and other historical aspects are reviewed in Gomez's monograph.

Epidemiology

The disease has been described in all parts of the world and is equally frequent in all races and in both sexes. Heredity is self-evident in only a minority of cases—50 percent in some series and as little as 14 percent in the series of Bundag and Evans (cited by Brett). The disease is determined by two autosomal dominant genes (see below), but it has been estimated as 1 in 20,000 to 300,000. The disease is inherited in an autosomal dominant fashion but with variable penetrance. The abnormal gene may be in one of two sites—the long arm of chromosome 9, designated as *TSC 1* (hamartin), or in the short arm of chromosome 16, *TSC 2* (tuberin), which is common. A wide variety of mutations have been described and both alleles must be affected for expression of the disease ("loss of heterozygosity"). Approximately 15 percent of sporadic cases show no identifiable mutation and tend to have milder manifestations, perhaps on the basis of mosaicism. Hamartin and tuberin function as tumor suppressor proteins and interact to suppress cell growth. This may, in part, explain the proclivity to develop various growths and hamartomas. The cerebral lesions and two of the three associated skin lesions of tuberous sclerosis are of this type. Several hypotheses relating to neuronal migration or to excessive secretion of growth factors have been proposed to link the inactivation of these genes with the pathogenesis of the characteristic lesions. Much of the work in understanding the function of these two proteins and their role in tumor formation has been performed in *Drosophila* and are summarized in the extensive review by Crino and colleagues.

The disease involves many organs in addition to the skin and brain and it may assume a diversity of forms, the least severe of which (i.e., the *forme fruste*) is difficult to diagnose; hence, one cannot be precise about its incidence. Tuberous sclerosis accounts for about 0.66 percent of the developmentally delayed in institutions and 0.32 percent of epileptics. The medical literature contains a number of reports of patients whose mentality is preserved and who have never had convulsions.

Etiology and Pathogenesis

The cellular elements within the nodular cerebral lesions (called tubers; see below) are abnormal in number, size, and orientation. The tumor-like growths in different organs may include cells of more than one type (e.g., fibroblasts, cardiac myoblasts, angioblasts, glioblasts, and neuroblasts), and their number is locally excessive. Something appears to have gone awry with the proliferative process during embryologic development, yet it is kept under control, in the sense that only rarely do the growths undergo malignant transformation. Highly specialized cells within the lesions may attain giant size; neurons 3 to 4 times normal size may be observed in the cerebral scleroses. These facts emphasize the potentially blastomatous character of the process.

Surgically resected tubers show activation of a cell-size control pathway (mammalian target of rapamycin [mTOR]); this is in keeping with the effects of *TSC* mutations on this cascade and probably explains the giant neurons as mentioned further below.

Clinical Manifestations (Table 38-5)

The disease may be evident at the time of birth (the diagnosis has been made by CT scan in neonates), but more often the infant is judged at first to be normal. In approximately 75 percent of cases, attention is drawn to the disease initially by the occurrence of focal or generalized seizures or by slowed psychomotor development. As with any condition that leads to developmental delay, the first suspicion is raised by delay in reaching normal maturational milestones. Whatever the initial symptom, the convulsive disorder and developmental delay

Table 38-5

MANIFESTATIONS OF TUBEROUS SCLEROSIS

Cutaneous and ectodermal
Shagreen patch
Facial angiofibromas (adenoma sebaceum)
Ungular and subungual fibromas
Hypomelanotic skin macules (more than 3)
Multiple dental enamel pits
Bone cysts
Hamartomatous rectal polyps
Gingival fibromas
Retinal achromatic patch
Multiple renal cysts
Cardiac rhabdomyoma
Renal angiomyolipoma
Lymphangiomatosis
Neural
Seizures
Developmental delay
Cortical tubers
Subependymal nodules
Subependymal giant cell "astrocytoma"
Retinal hamartoma

become more prominent within 2 to 3 years. The facial cutaneous abnormality, adenoma sebaceum, appears later in childhood, usually between the fourth and tenth years, and is progressive thereafter.

As the years pass, the seizures change pattern. In the first year or two they take the form of massive flexion spasms with hypsarrhythmia (irregular dysrhythmic bursts of high-voltage spikes and slow waves in the EEG). As many as 25 percent of patients with these types of seizures have been found to have tuberous sclerosis. Later, the seizures change to more typical generalized motor and psychomotor attacks or atypical petit mal. Any one of the seizure types may be brief, especially if the patient is receiving anti-epileptic medication. Focal neurologic abnormalities, which one might expect to occur from the size and location of some of the lesions, are distinctly uncommon.

Mental function continues to deteriorate slowly. Exceptionally there is a spastic weakness or mild choreoathetosis of the limbs and in a few cases an obstructive hydrocephalus develops. As in any state of severe developmental delay, a variety of nonspecific motor peculiarities—such as constant crying, muttering, stereotypical rocking and swaying movements, and digital mannerisms—may be observed. In nearly half of the cases, affective and behavioral derangements, often of hyperkinetic and aggressive type, are added to the intellectual deficiency.

The lack of parallelism in the severity of the epilepsy, the mental deficit, and cutaneous abnormalities has been noted by all clinicians who have wide experience with this disease. Some patients are subject to recurrent seizures while retaining relatively normal mental function; in others, trivial skin lesions or a retinal phakoma (see below) may suggest the diagnosis in a mentally normal person with few seizures. In such cases, recognition may elude competent neurologists and dermatologists. As a general rule, early onset of seizures is predictive of developmental delay. Gomez and colleagues suggested that the seizures damage the brain, a point with which we tend to agree in part. However, it seems likely that both the epilepsy and developmental delay are the product of severe involvement of the brain by the lesions of tuberous sclerosis.

Limitation of space allows no more than a catalogue of the other visceral abnormalities in tuberous sclerosis. In about half the cases, gray or yellow plaques (in reality gliomatous tumors) may be found in the retina in or near the optic disc or at a distance from it. It is from this lesion, called a *phakoma*, that van der Hoeve derived the term that is applied to all neurocutaneous diseases of this class. About half of all benign rhabdomyomas of the heart are associated with tuberous sclerosis; if located in the wall of the atrium, they may cause conduction defects. Other benign tumors of mixed cell type (angiomyolipomas) have been found in the kidneys, liver, lungs, thyroid, testes, and gastrointestinal tract. Cysts of the pleura or lungs, bone cysts in digits, and zones of marbling or densification in bones are some of the less common abnormalities.

In approximately 90 percent of patients with tuberous sclerosis, congenital hypomelanotic macules—"ash-leaf" lesions—formerly mistaken for partial albinism or vitiligo, appear before any of the other skin lesions (Fitzpatrick et al). Gold and Freeman, as well as Fitzpatrick and colleagues, emphasized the frequency of these leukodermic lesions and their value in the diagnosis of tuberous sclerosis during infancy, before the appearance of the other characteristic cutaneous lesions. The hypomelanotic areas are arranged in linear fashion over the trunk or limbs and range in size from a few millimeters to several centimeters; their configuration is oval, with one end round and the other pointed, in the shape of an ash leaf. A Wood lamp, which transmits only ultraviolet rays, facilitates the demonstration of the ash-leaf lesions because of the absence of melanoblasts, which normally absorb light in the ultraviolet range (360-nm wavelength). These lesions become pink when rubbed and contain sweat glands; they are not usually present on the face or head. There is occasionally a white tuft of hair (poliosis). Electron microscopic examination of the hypomelanotic lesions shows a normal or reduced number of melanocytes, but their dopa reaction is reduced and melanosomes are small.

The well-developed facial lesions (adenomas of Pringle), pathognomonic of tuberous sclerosis, are present in 90 percent of patients older than 4 years of age. Although called "adenoma sebaceum," these nodules are actually angiofibromas; the sebaceous glands are only passively involved (Fig. 38-5). Typically they are red to pink nodules with a smooth, glistening surface, and they tend to be limited to the nasolabial folds, cheeks, and chin; sometimes they also involve the forehead and scalp. The earliest manifestation of facial angiofibromatosis may be a mild erythema over the cheeks and forehead that is intensified by crying. The occurrence of large plaques of connective tissue on the forehead is usually expressive of a severe form of the disease.

On the trunk, the diagnostic lesion is the "shagreen patch" (in reality a plaque of subepidermal fibrosis) found most often in the lumbosacral region. It appears as a flat, slightly elevated, flesh-colored area of skin 1 to 10 cm in

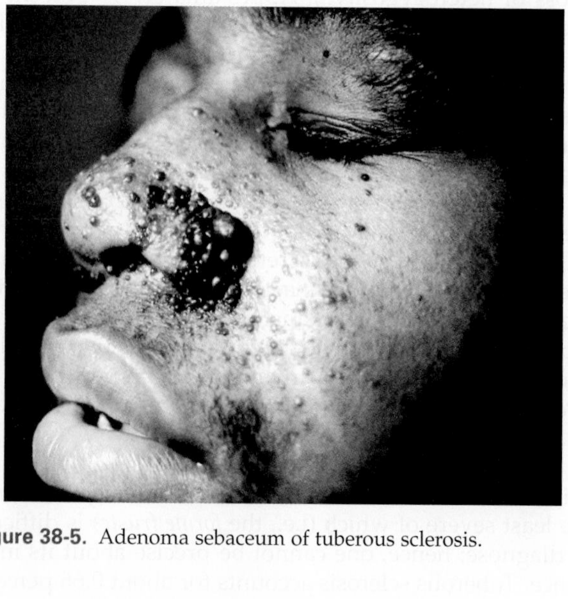

Figure 38-5. Adenoma sebaceum of tuberous sclerosis.

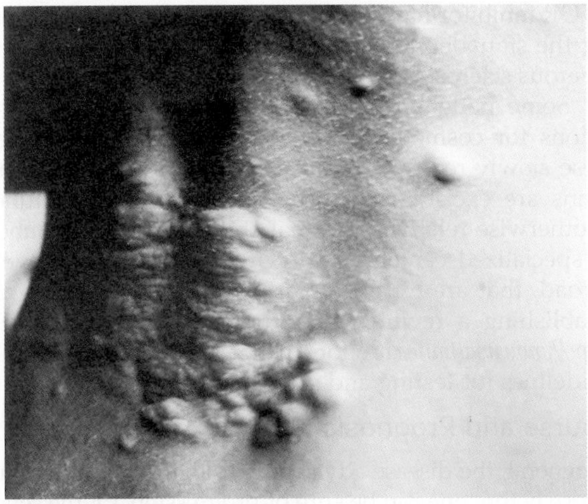

Figure 38-6. Shagreen patch on the skin of the lower back in a young patient with tuberous sclerosis.

diameter, with a "pigskin," "elephant hide," or "orange peel" appearance (Fig. 38-6). Another common site of fibromatous involvement is the nail bed; subungual fibromas usually appear at puberty and continue to develop with age. Other common skin changes, not in themselves diagnostic, include fibroepithelial tags (soft fibromas), café-au-lait spots, and port-wine hemangiomas.

Pathology

The brain exhibits a number of diagnostic anomalies. Broadening, unnatural whiteness, and firmness of parts of some of the cerebral convolutions are simulated by no other disease. These are the *tubers* after which the disease is named. On the surface of the brain, they range in width from 5 mm to 2 or 3 cm. Their cut surface reveals a lack of demarcation from cortex and white matter and the presence of white flecks of calcium; these, which are readily seen on CT and MRI, are called *brain stones* (see below and Fig. 38-7). The walls of the lateral ventricles may be encrusted with white or pink-white masses resembling candle gutterings. When calcified, they appear in radiographs as curvilinear opacities that follow the outline of the ventricle. Rarely, nodules of abnormal tissue are observed in the basal ganglia, thalamus, cerebellum, brainstem, and spinal cord.

Under the microscope the tubers are seen to be composed of interlacing rows of plump, fibrous astrocytes (much like an astrocytoma, though lacking in glial fibrillar protein). In the cerebral cortex and ganglionic structures, derangements of architecture result from the presence of abnormal-appearing cells: greatly enlarged "monstrous," or "balloon" neurons and glia cells—often difficult to distinguish from one another. Also, displaced normal-sized neurons contribute to the chaotic histologic appearance. Gliomatous deposits may obstruct the foramina of Monro or the aqueduct or floor of the fourth ventricle, causing hydrocephalus. Neoplastic transformation of abnormal glia cells, a not infrequent occurrence, usually takes the form of a large-cell astrocytoma, less often of a glioblastoma or meningioma. Recently, certain relationships have been drawn between the balloon cells of this disease and similar cells in focal cortical dysplasias (see Crino and colleagues for details).

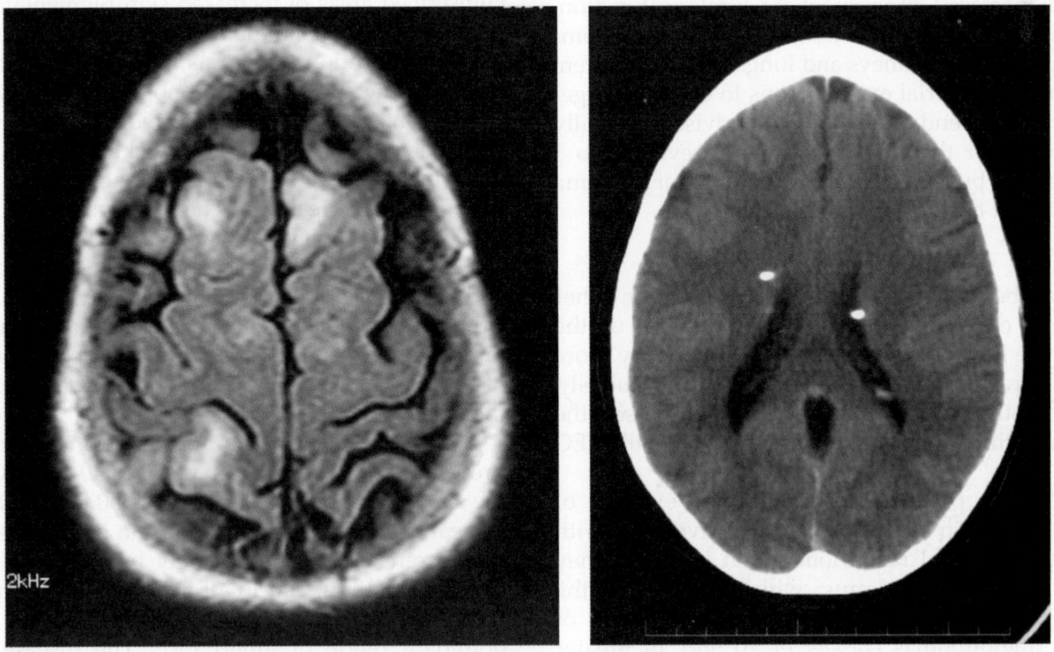

A B

Figure 38-7. Tuberous sclerosis. *A*. MRI showing multiple hamartomas. *B*. Subependymal nodules are demonstrated on CT, where their calcific nature has led them to be termed "brain stones."

The phakomas of the retina are also composed mainly of neuronal and glial components, but occasionally there is an admixture of fibrous tissue.

Diagnosis

When the full combination of seizures and mental and dermal abnormalities is conjoined, the diagnosis is self-evident. It is the early stage of the disease and the *formes frustes* that give trouble, and here the experienced dermatologist can be of great help. Epilepsy—that is, flexion spasms in infancy—and delay in psychomotor development are by no means diagnostic of tuberous sclerosis, as they occur in many diseases. It is in these cases, and also in every sizable population of the epileptic or developmentally delayed, especially when the family history is unrevealing, that a search for the dermal equivalents of the disease—the hypomelanotic ash-leaf spots, adenoma sebaceum, collagenous skin patch, phakoma of the retina, or subungual or gingival fibromas—is so rewarding. The finding of any one of these lesions provides confirmation of the partial and atypical case. Adenoma sebaceum may occasionally occur alone and is easily confused with acne vulgaris in the adolescent. The history of epilepsy or demonstration of developmental delay is helpful but neither is a requisite for the diagnosis of tuberous sclerosis (see the monograph by Gomez).

The most useful laboratory measures for corroborating the disease are the CT scan and MRI (see Fig. 38-7). The calcific tuber lesions tend to be periventricular and are particularly well shown on the CT scan, whereas MRI is more sensitive in detecting the hamartomatous giant cell subependymal and subcortical lesions. There is an absence of edema in the surrounding tissue. Roach and colleagues have indicated that an increasing number of cortical lesions demonstrated with MRI appear to correlate with an increased impairment of neurologic function. Clinics that treat large numbers of these patients recommend imaging of the kidneys and lungs and, in children, echocardiography. Serial examinations to detect enlargement of the subependymal tumors is advised annually for those younger than age 21 years and every 2 to 3 years thereafter, but the best course of action if a glioma emerges has not been clearly established.

Treatment

Nothing can be offered in the way of prevention other than genetic counseling. Antiepileptic therapy of the standard type suppresses the convulsive tendency more or less effectively and should be applied assiduously. Adrenocorticotropic hormone (ACTH) suppresses the flexor spasms in infancy and tends to normalize the EEG for a time.

It is usually pointless to attempt the excision of tumors, especially in severely affected individuals (with the exception of renal hamartomas that impair kidney function). However, sirolimus, which suppresses the mTOR signaling pathway, causes slight regression of the bodily angiolipomas (Bissler et al) and, of greater interest to the neurologist and neurosurgeon, the similar drug rapamycin has tentatively been shown in a report by Franz and colleagues to shrink subependymal giant cell astrocytomas in some patients. Everolimus, another mTOR inhibitor has been found to be useful in suppressing the status epilepticus associated with some cases of tuberous sclerosis (Krueger et al).

Some patients undergo dermabrasion of the facial lesions for cosmetic reasons, with the knowledge that these slowly regrow. To an increasing degree, neurosurgeons are excising single epileptogenic cortical tubers in otherwise relatively normal children. There are about 15 specialized centers in the United States, and several abroad, that are expert at caring for these patients and establishing a regimen of radiologic surveillance. (See *http://www.tsalliance.org* for further information including guidelines for testing and surveillance.)

Course and Prognosis

In general, the disease advances so slowly that years must elapse before one can be sure of progression. Of the severe cases, approximately 30 percent die before the fifth year, and 50 to 75 percent before attaining adult age. Worsening is mainly in the mental sphere. Status epilepticus accounted for many deaths in the past, but improved medication therapy has reduced this hazard. Neoplasias take their toll; the authors have had several such patients who died of malignant gliomas arising in striatothalamic regions.

Neurofibromatosis of von Recklinghausen (NF1 and NF2)

Neurofibromatosis (NF) is a comparatively common hereditary disease in which the skin, nervous system, bones, endocrine glands, and sometimes other organs are the sites of a variety of congenital abnormalities, often taking the form of benign tumors. The typical clinical picture, usually identifiable at a glance, consists of multiple circumscribed areas of increased skin pigmentation accompanied by dermal and neural tumors of various types.

The condition known as multiple idiopathic neuromas was the subject of a monograph by R.W. Smith in 1849; even at that time, he referred to examples recorded by other writers. It was von Recklinghausen, however, who, in 1882, gave the definitive account of its clinical and pathologic features. The subsequent studies of the disease by Yakovlev and Guthrie; Lichtenstein; Riccardi; and Martuza and Eldridge; and more recently by Créange and colleagues; and the comprehensive monographs of Crowe and colleagues and of Riccardi and Mulvihill are informative references that provide a complete analysis of the clinical, pathologic, and genetic data pertaining to the disease.

Epidemiology Crowe and associates calculated the prevalence of the disease to be 30 to 40 per 100,000, with the expectancy of 1 case in every 2,500 to 3,300 births over 50 years ago and these rates pertain in the all series from the current era. Approximately half of their cases had affected relatives, and in all instances the distribution of cases within a family was consistent with an autosomal dominant mode of inheritance. The disease has been observed in all races in different parts of the world, and males and females are about equally affected.

Cause and Pathogenesis The hereditary nature of NF has been appreciated for a century. More recently, it has been established that NF comprises two distinct disorders, the genes for which are located on different chromosomes. Both are inherited in an autosomal dominant pattern with a high degree of penetrance, but half the cases are a result of spontaneous mutations. The classic form of the disease with multiple neurofibromas, described below, is caused by a mutation located near the centromere on chromosome 17 in a gene called neurofibromin (Barker et al). The second type, in which the main feature is bilateral acoustic nerve neuromas, described further on, is caused by a mutation in the *merlin* gene (also called *schwannomin*). These two forms of NF have been loosely referred to as peripheral and central, respectively, but the terms *neurofibromatosis type 1 (NF1)* and *neurofibromatosis type 2 (NF2)* are less confusing (Martuza and Eldridge) and are used in the following discussion.

The large size of the *NF1* gene (60 exons) and the widely scattered mutations has made genetic testing complex but such testing is available. Virtually all families manifest different mutations and there have been no clear associations between specific mutations and phenotypic characteristics except that the rare complete deletion leads to early onset multiple neurofibromas, developmental delay, and facial dysmorphism.

The pathogenesis is less obscure now that the genes implicated in both diseases have been identified. Both involve tumor suppression. As with tuberous sclerosis, there is a suggestion of a disorder that allows low-grade ectodermal cell proliferation without tumor transformation. Cellular elements derived from the neural crest (i.e., Schwann cells, melanocytes, and endoneurial fibroblasts, the natural components of skin and nerves) proliferate excessively in multiple foci, and the melanocytes function abnormally. The hormones and growth factors involved in this proliferative process and the mechanism by which it occurs are as obscure as they are in tuberous sclerosis. It is known, however, that most of the numerous mutations in the *NF1* gene lead to premature termination of protein synthesis and a consequent "loss of function." This is in keeping with the tumor suppressor characteristics of the gene and the emergence of neoplasms in the presence of homozygous mutations.

Neurofibromatosis Type 1 (Classic, or Peripheral, NF) (Table 38-6)

In the majority of patients, spots of hyperpigmentation (café-au-lait lesions) and cutaneous and subcutaneous neurofibromatous tumors are the basis of clinical diagnosis. Pigmentary changes in the skin are nearly always present at birth, but neurofibromas are infrequent at that age. Both lesions increase in number and size during late childhood and adolescence. There may be a spurt of new lesions at puberty or during pregnancy. Exceptionally, a neurofibroma of a cranial nerve or a spinal root (sometimes with compression of the cord), disclosed during imaging of the spine or a neurosurgical intervention, may be the initial manifestation of the disease. In a large series of patients with neurofibromatosis (Crowe et al), approximately one-third were found to have only the cutaneous manifestations that were noted while being examined for symptoms of some other disease; that is to say, the NF was asymptomatic. Usually these are the patients with the slightest degree of cutaneous abnormality. Of the remaining two-thirds, most consulted a physician because of the disfigurement produced by the skin tumors or because some of the neurofibromas were producing neurologic symptoms.

The patches of cutaneous pigmentation, appearing shortly after birth and occurring anywhere on the body, constitute the most obvious clinical expression of the disease. They are approximately oval in shape and vary in size from a 1 to 2 mm to many centimeters, and in color from a light to dark brown (the term *café-au-lait* is applied) and are rarely associated with any other pathologic state (Fig. 38-8).

Table 38-6

MANIFESTATIONS OF NEUROFIBROMATOSIS TYPE 1

Cutaneous and ectodermal
Café-au-lait spots (generally 6 or more of >5 mm diameter prepubertal and >15 mm postpubertal)[a]
Axillary and integumentary freckling (Crowe sign)[a]
Lisch nodules (hamartomas of the iris)[a]
Bony lesions including sphenoid dysplasia or thinning of long bone cortex, pseudoarthroses[a]
Increased incidence of chronic myeloid leukemia, neurofibrosarcoma (malignant transformation of neurofibroma), rhabdomyosarcoma, pheochromocytoma
Short stature
Neural
Neurofibromas[a]
Cutaneous (most common)
Subcutaneous
Nodular plexiform
Diffuse plexiform
Seizures
Optic pathway glioma[a]
Risk of cerebral astrocytoma, brainstem glioma
Hypertension

[a]Denotes main diagnostic criteria, in addition to having an affected first-degree relative.

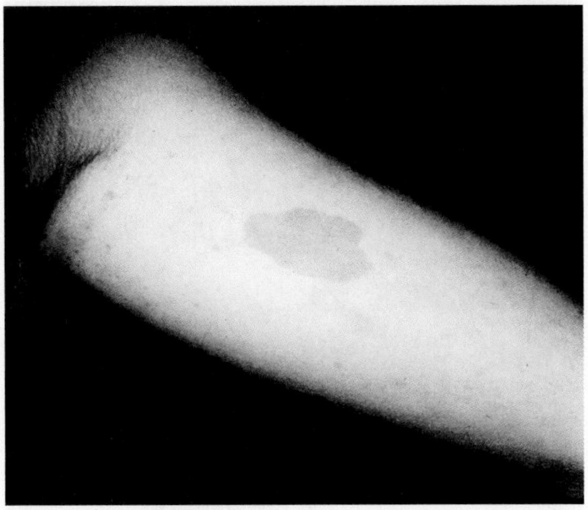

Figure 38-8. Typical large café-au-lait spot. The presence of 6 or more hyperpigmented lesions, each larger than 1.5 cm after puberty (>5 mm prepubertal), is diagnostic of neurofibromatosis type 1.

They do not appear to change in number as the patient ages, but they do enlarge during puberty and become more pigmented. In a survey of pigmented spots in the skin, Crowe and associates found that 10 percent of the normal population had one or more spots of this type; however, *anyone with more than 6 such spots, some exceeding 1.5 cm in diameter in postpubertal individuals (bigger than 0.5 mm in prepubertal ones), nearly always proved to have neurofibromatosis.* Of their 223 patients with NF, 95 percent had at least 1 spot and 78 percent had more than 6 large spots. Freckle-like or diffuse pigmentation of the axillae and other intertriginous areas (groin, under breast) and small, round, whitish spots are characteristic; when coupled with café-au-lait patches, they are together virtually pathognomonic of the disease.

The appearance of multiple cutaneous and subcutaneous tumors in late childhood or early adolescence is the other principal feature of the disease. The cutaneous tumors are situated in the dermis and form discrete soft or firm papules varying in size from a few millimeters to a centimeter or more (molluscum fibrosum; Fig. 38-9). They assume many shapes—flattened, sessile, pedunculated, conical, lobulated, and so on. They are flesh-colored or violaceous and often topped with a comedo. When pressed, the soft tumors tend to invaginate through a small opening in the skin, giving the feeling of a seedless raisin or a scrotum without a testicle. This phenomenon, spoken of as "buttonholing," is useful in distinguishing the lesions of this disease from other skin tumors, for example, multiple lipomas. A patient may have anywhere from a few of these dermal tumors to hundreds.

The subcutaneous neural tumors, which are also multiple, take two forms: (1) firm, discrete nodules attached to a nerve or (2) an overgrowth of subcutaneous tissue, sometimes reaching enormous size. The latter, which are called *plexiform neuromas* (also pachydermatocele, elephantiasis neuromatosis, *la tumeur royale*), occur most often in the face, scalp, neck, and chest, and may cause hideous disfigurement. When palpated, they feel like a bag of worms or strings; the bone underlying the tumor may thicken. Neurofibromas are easily distinguished from lipomas, which are soft, unattached to the skin or nerve, and not accompanied by any neurologic disorder. An exception to this last statement is the rare disease of multiple symmetrical lipomatosis with axonal polyneuropathy (Launois-Bensaude disease). As a rule, congenital neurofibromas tend to be highly vascular and invasive and are especially prominent in the orbital, periorbital, and cervical regions. They may be accompanied by hypertrophy of a segment of the body (a sign also seen in the arteriovenous malformation of Klippel-Trenaunay-Weber syndrome). When the hyperpigmentation lesion overlies a plexiform neurofibroma and extends to the midline, one should suspect an intraspinal neurofibroma tumor at that level.

Another unique finding is the Lisch nodule. This is a small whitish spot (actually a hamartoma) in the iris that was present in 94 percent of Riccardi's type 1 cases, but was not found in patients with NF2 or in normal individuals (Fig. 38-10 and below).

Headache, hydrocephalus, and tumors involving the optic pathways, meningiomas, gliomas, and malignant peripheral nerve tumors are common, even among adults, according to the survey of 158 patients by Créange and colleagues; also, pain was a common symptom in adults and often related to a malignant peripheral nerve sheath tumor.

Other abnormalities associated less consistently with type 1 (peripheral) NF include bone cysts, pathologic fractures (pseudoarthrosis), cranial bone defects with pulsating exophthalmos (sphenoid bone dysgenesis), bone hypertrophy, precocious puberty, pheochromocytoma, scoliosis, syringomyelia, nodules of abnormal glia cells in brain and spinal cord, and macrocephaly, rarely with obstructive hydrocephalus as a result of overgrowth of glial tissue around the sylvian aqueduct and fourth ventricle. Some degree of intellectual impairment is common; it was found in 40 percent of Riccardi's series of 133 patients. But in our experience, the figure is much lower and the impairment is usually not profound.

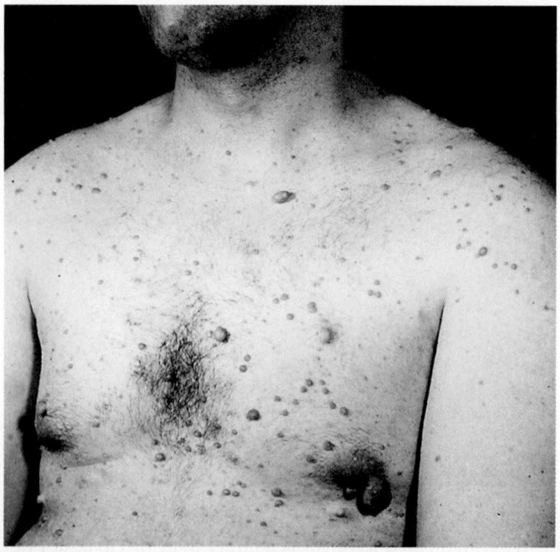

Figure 38-9. Molluscum fibrosum nonneural skin tumors of von Recklinghausen disease.

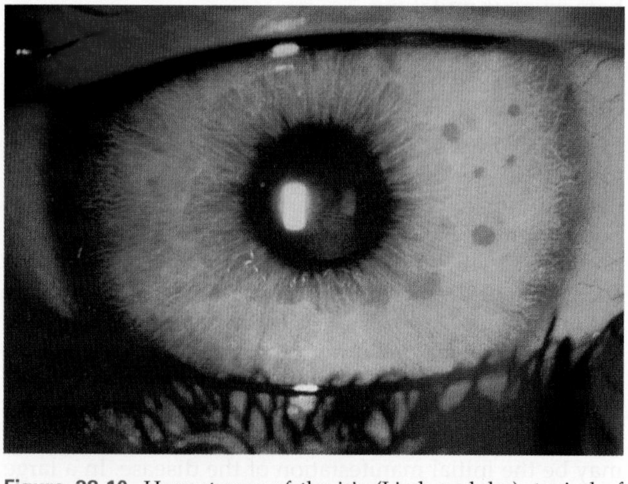

Figure 38-10. Hamartomas of the iris (Lisch nodules), typical of neurofibromatosis type 1. (Reproduced by permission from Damato BE, Spalton DJ: The uveal tract, in Spalton DJ, Hitchings RA, Hunter PA (eds): *Atlas of Clinical Ophthalmology*, 3rd ed. Oxford, Mosby Elsevier Ltd, 2005.)

Learning difficulty, developmental disorder, and hyperactivity have been more frequent abnormalities, occurring in almost 40 percent of patients. Rosman and Pearce have ascribed developmental delay in NF to congenital malformation of the cerebral cortex (cortical dysgenesis). The incidence of seizures is about 20 times higher than that in the general population, but these tend not to be a very frequent or intractable problem.

Exceptionally, NF is associated with peroneal muscular atrophy, congenital deafness, and partial albinism (Bradley et al).

In childhood, progressive blindness is a particularly dire complication from a tumor mass composed mainly of astrocytes (optic glioma). The tumor may involve one or both optic nerves. The diagnosis comes to mind at once in a child with any of the cutaneous manifestations of NF and this tumor. Uncertainty as to its nature arises from the fact that the neuropathologist may be unable to decide between a benign hamartoma and a grade 1 astrocytoma. Progressive enlargement in a succession of MRI scans may be needed to affirm its nature.

It needs to be stated that neurofibromas of the spinal roots occur regularly in patients without NF (see Chap. 44). Whether multiple such lesions implicate NF is not clear.

Neurofibromatosis Type 2 (Acoustic, or Central, NF)

This condition is considerably less frequent than NF1. Here there is an absence or paucity of cutaneous lesions. Progressive deafness and the demonstration by enhanced CT or MRI of *bilateral acoustic neuromas* afford accurate diagnosis (see Fig. 31-18). Also, an acoustic neuroma developing before age 30 years is suspect as being caused by NF2. Other cranial or spinal neurofibromas, meningioma (sometimes multiple), and glioma may be added to the syndrome of deafness or may occur prior to its emergence. Juvenile cataracts of the subcortical or capsular variety are seen in some affected patients.

Analysis for the *NF2* gene has become available from several laboratories. The genetics and affected protein (merlin or schwannomin) are discussed in "Cause and Pathogenesis" above.

Familial Schwannomatosis

As commented in Chap. 31 in the discussion of acoustic neuroma, it is now apparent that the propensity to develop multiple schwannomas can also be inherited as a dominant trait, without the vestibular tumors characteristic of NF2. This trait maps to a genetic locus on chromosome 22 that is distinct from the one for NF2. It has been estimated that 2 to 5 percent of schwannomas requiring resection are from this disease. The diagnostic criteria are based on the presence of two of more schwannomas without vestibular nerve tumors in an individual older than age 18 years, as summarized in a thorough review by MacCollin and colleagues, and more recently by Plotkin and colleagues. Pain is the dominant problem.

Pathology of NF1 and NF2

The cutaneous tumors are characterized by a rather thin epidermis whose basal layer may or may not be pigmented. The collagen and elastin of the dermis is replaced by a loose arrangement of elongated connective tissue cells. The lack of compactness of the normal dermal collagen allows the palpable opening in the skin. The pigmented (café-au-lait) lesions contain only the normal numbers of melanocytes; the dark color of the skin is instead the result of an excess of melanosomes in the melanocytes. Some of the abnormally large melanosomes measure up to several microns in diameter.

The nerve tumors are composed of a mixture of fibroblasts and Schwann cells (except the optic nerve tumors, which contain a combination of astrocytes and fibroblasts). Predominance of one or the other of these cells in the nerve is the basis of the diagnosis of neurofibroma or schwannoma. Palisading of nuclei and sometimes encircling arrangements of cells (Verocay bodies) are features of both (see Chap. 31). Occasionally, along spinal roots or sympathetic chains, one may find a tumor made up of partially or completely differentiated nerve cells, a typical ganglioneuroma. Clusters of abnormal glia cells may be found in the brain and spinal cord, and, according to Bielschowsky, they imply a link with tuberous sclerosis that has never been proved. Clinically and genetically, the two diseases are quite independent.

Malignant degeneration of the tumors is found in 2 to 5 percent of cases; peripherally they become sarcomas and centrally, astrocytomas or glioblastomas (Fig. 38-11).

Diagnosis

If skin tumors and café-au-lait spots are numerous and Lisch nodules are present in the iris, the identification of the disease as type 1 neurofibromatosis offers no difficulty. A history of the illness in antecedent and collateral family members makes diagnosis even more certain. Doubt arises most frequently in patients with bilateral acoustic neuromas or other cranial or spinal neurofibromas or schwannomas with no skin lesions or only a few random ones. The tendency for these forms of NF to have few skin lesions is well known, but differentiation of type 1 from type 2 may be uncertain unless genetic studies are undertaken. Plexiform neuromas with muscle weakness because of nerve involvement and abnormalities of underlying bone may be confused with other tumors, especially in young children, who tend to have few café-au-lait spots and few cutaneous tumors. Hypertrophy of a limb requires differentiation from other developmental anomalies including Klippel-Trenaunay-Weber syndrome.

As already mentioned, Crowe and coworkers expressed the view that 80 percent of patients with von Recklinghausen disease can be diagnosed by the presence of more than 6 café-au-lait spots. Of the remaining 20 percent, those older than 21 years of age will be found to have multiple cutaneous tumors, axillary freckling, and a few pigmented spots; in those younger than 21 years of age with no dermal tumors and only a few café-au-lait patches, a positive family history and radiographic demonstration of bone cysts will be helpful in some instances. Café-au-lait spots and cutaneous tumors should always be sought, for they may help the neurologist diagnose an otherwise obscure progressive spinal syndrome, a cerebellopontine angle syndrome, bilateral deafness, progressive

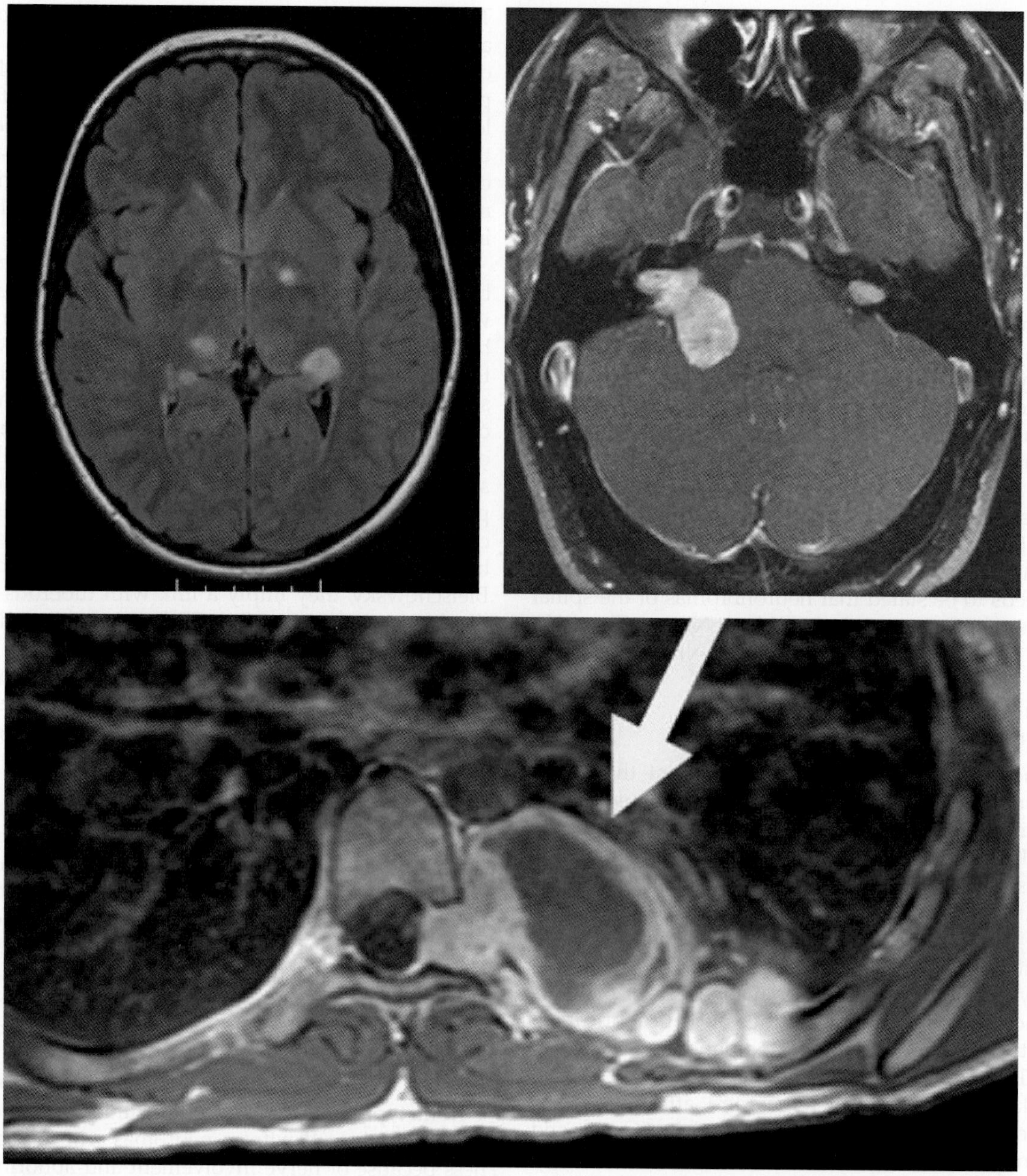

Figure 38-11. Neurofibromatosis. *Upper left*: T2-FLAIR MRI in the axial plane demonstrating multiple foci of hyperintensity, presumably hamartomas, in a patient with neurofibromatosis type 1. *Upper right*: Axial T1 MRI with gadolinium demonstrating bilateral (right larger than left) schwannomas in a patient with neurofibromatosis type 2. *Lower panel:* Axial T1 MRI with gadolinium of the thoracic spine showing a large left paraspinal schwannoma emanating from the neural foramen in a patient with schwannomatosis. Note the expansion and remodeling of the vertebral bones surrounding the lesion. (Images courtesy of Dr. Scott R. Plotkin.)

blindness, and an occasional case of precocious puberty, hydrocephalus, or developmental delay.

Because of the many potentially dangerous conditions that accompany classic NF, the initial clinical evaluation should be supplemented by a number of ancillary examinations that may include measurement of IQ, EEG, slit-lamp examination of irides, visual and auditory evoked responses, and CT scans or MRI of cranium and, sometimes, of the spine and mediastinum. In the series reported by Duffner and colleagues, 74 percent of cases had abnormal signals in T2-weighted images of the basal ganglia, thalamus, hypothalamus, brainstem, and cerebellum. The EEG was abnormal in 25 percent. If there is suspicion of a pheochromocytoma, 24-h urine should be tested for metabolites of epinephrine. Each of these tests not only is an aid to diagnosis but also is essential to the effective management of the illness.

Treatment

The skin tumors should not be excised unless they are cosmetically objectionable or show an increase in size, suggesting malignant change. The effects of radiotherapy on these lesions are so insignificant that they do not justify the risk of exposure. Plexiform neuromas about the face pose especially difficult problems. Here one must resort to plastic surgery, but the results are not always satisfactory because the growths may encompass distal branches of cranial nerves (with risk of greater paralysis after surgical excision) or alter the underlying bone, the latter being either eroded from pressure or hypertrophied from increased blood supply. Cranial and spinal neurofibromas are amenable to excision, and the gliomas and meningiomas usually demand surgical measures as well. Here the differentiation of hamartomas from gliomas of structures such as the optic nerves, hypothalamus, or pons may be difficult. Bilateral optic nerve gliomas are usually treated with radiation; unilateral ones are excised. Peripheral nerve tumors that have undergone malignant (sarcomatous) degeneration pose special surgical problems.

Affected individuals should be advised not to have children, a precaution that may not be necessary because fertility, especially in males, seems to be reduced by the disease. Prognosis varies with the grade of severity, being most favorable in those with only a few lesions. But the disease is always progressive, and the patient should remain under surveillance.

Other Cutaneous Angiomatoses With Abnormalities of the Central Nervous System

There are at least 7 additional diseases in which a cutaneous or ocular vascular anomaly is associated with an abnormality of the nervous system: (1) meningo- or encephalofacial (encephalotrigeminal) angiomatosis with cerebral calcification (Sturge-Weber syndrome); (2) dermatomal hemangiomas and spinal vascular malformations (sometimes with limb hypertrophy, as also occurs in Klippel-Trenaunay-Weber syndrome and in neurofibromatosis); (3) the epidermal nevus (linear sebaceous nevus) syndrome; (4) familial telangiectasia (Osler-Rendu-Weber disease); (5) hemangioblastoma of cerebellum and retina (von Hippel-Lindau disease); (6) ataxia-telangiectasia (Louis-Bar disease); and (7) angiokeratosis corporis diffusum (Fabry disease). The last three disorders are considered elsewhere: ataxia-telangiectasia and Fabry disease with the inherited metabolic disorders in Chap. 37, and von Hippel-Lindau disease below and with hemangioblastoma in Chap. 31.

Sturge-Weber Syndrome (Meningo- or Encephalofacial Angiomatosis with Cerebral Calcification)

This condition has been referred to as the Sturge-Weber syndrome, as it was W. Allen Sturge who, in 1879, described a child with sensorimotor seizures contralateral to a facial "port-wine mark," and Parkes Weber (1922, 1929), who gave the first radiographic demonstration of the atrophy and calcification of the cerebral hemisphere ipsilateral to the skin lesion. This eponym overlooks the important intervening contributions of Kalischer (1897, 1901), who first described the meningeal angioma in conjunction with the facial one; of Volland (1913), who demonstrated the intracortical calcific deposits; and of Dimitri (1923), who described the characteristic double-contoured radiographic shadows. Krabbe (1932, 1934) showed conclusively that the calcification lay not in the blood vessels (as Dimitri and many others had concluded), but in the second and third layers of the cortex (see Wohlwill and Yakovlev for historical review and bibliography).

A vascular nevus is observed at birth to cover a large part of the face and cranium on one side (in the territory of the ophthalmic division of the trigeminal nerve). In one-quarter of the cases the nevus is bilateral. The lesions vary in extent, the most limited being an involvement of only the upper eyelid and forehead, and the most extensive being the entire head and even other parts of the body. The skin lesion is deep red (port-wine nevus) and its margins may be flat or raised; soft or firm papules, evidently composed of vessels, cause surface elevations and irregularities. Orbital tissue, especially the upper eyelid, is almost invariably involved; congenital buphthalmos may enlarge the eye before birth and glaucoma may develop later in that eye, causing blindness. The choroid is implicated in some cases. The increased cutaneous vascularity may result in an overgrowth of connective tissue and underlying bone, giving rise to a deformity like that of the Klippel-Trenaunay-Weber syndrome. Indications of cerebral disease appear as early as the first year of life or later in childhood; the most frequent clinical manifestations are unilateral seizures followed by increasing degrees of spastic hemiparesis with smallness of the arm and leg, hemisensory defect, and homonymous hemianopia, all on the side contralateral to the trigeminal nevus. Skull films (usually normal just after birth) taken after the second year reveal a characteristic "tramline" calcification, which outlines the involved convolutions of the parietooccipital cortex. CT scanning and MRI show the abnormalities of the involved cortex at an earlier age (Fig. 38-12).

It is not the case that all cranial hemangiomas affect the cerebrum; the common facial nevi, especially the flat midline ones and the elevated strawberry nevi, are of no neurologic significance. And a cerebral–meningeal angiomatosis may be present without skin lesions. The involvement of the upper eyelid is of greatest importance since nearly all such cases are associated with cerebral lesions (Barlow). There seems to be a close correlation between the persistence or maldevelopment of the embryonic vascular plexus of the eyelid and forehead and that of the occipitoparietal parts of the brain. When the nevus lies entirely below the upper eyelid or high on the scalp, a cerebral lesion is usually absent, although in a few instances such an angioma has been associated with a vascular malformation of the meninges overlying the brainstem and cerebellum. In angiograms, the abnormal meningeal vessels, which are largely veins, are not well seen; thus they can be distinguished from true arteriovenous malformations. These purely meningeal venous nevi are rarely the source of subarachnoid or cerebral hemorrhage and they do not enlarge to form a mass. The cortical lesion is, however, destructive of cortical tissue, which is replaced by glial tissue that calcifies. One explanation holds that diversion of blood to the meninges during seizures causes progressive ischemia of the cerebral cortex. Barlow has stated that the seizures themselves

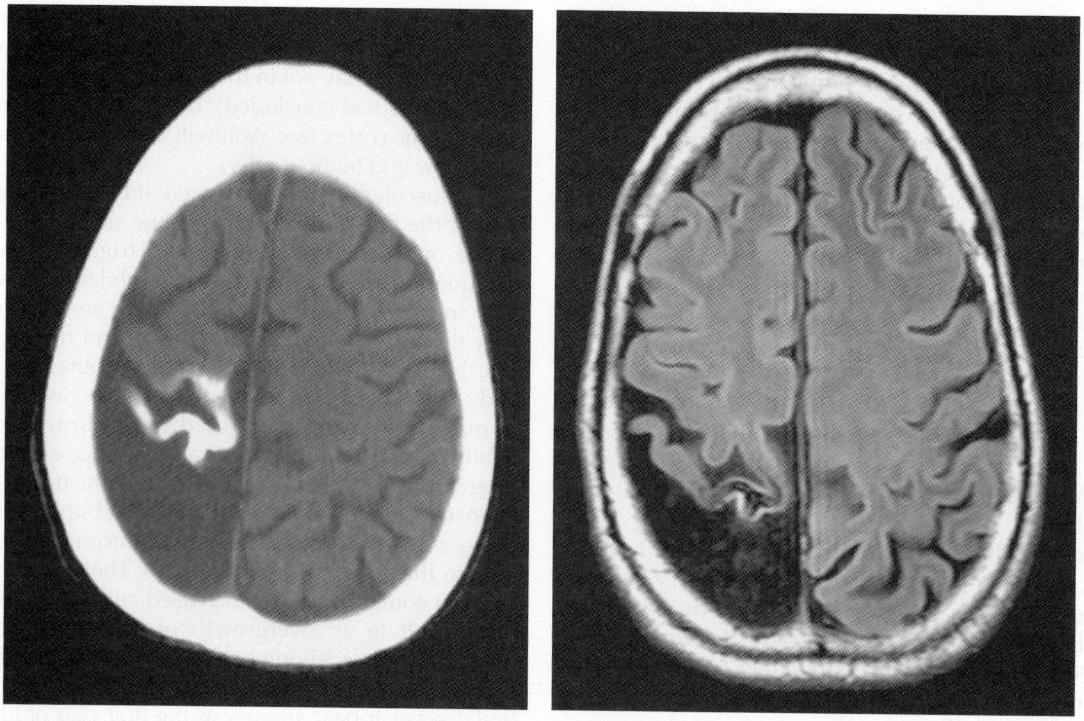

Figure 38-12. Sturge-Weber. *Left:* CT showing calcification of the vascular malformation and underlying cortical atrophy. *Right:* MRI, T2-FLAIR sequence, showing the pronounced atrophy in the same patient.

are responsible for the progressive neurologic deficits and that a special effort should be made to prevent them by carefully regulated medical therapy. Occasionally surgical excision of intractable discharging foci may be necessary, but often this may not be feasible in view of the magnitude of the cerebral lesion. Radiotherapy is unsuccessful in reducing the skin blemish; sensitive individuals usually try to hide it with cosmetics. There is little literature on treating the brain vascular malformation with endovascular techniques.

Although a heredofamilial trait has long been known, it was only recently that Shirley and colleagues found a polymorphism in the responsible gene, GNAQ, in almost 90 percent of individuals with the trait and in a similar number of patients with non-syndromic port-wine stains on the cranium. The variant may be of a mosaic type, being present only in affected tissues. This substitution in the gene activates extracellular signal-regulated kinase. Similar SNPs have been known to participate in other conditions that feature abnormal skin pigmentation.

Dermatomal Hemangiomas With Spinal Vascular Malformations

A hemangioma of the spinal cord may rarely be accompanied by a vascular nevus in the corresponding dermatome, as was first pointed out by Cobb. Such nevi are most frequent on the arm and trunk. When the cutaneous lesion involves an arm or leg, there may be enlargement of the entire limb or fingers in combination with underdevelopment of certain other parts (Klippel-Trenaunay-Weber syndrome). Some of these angiomatous syndromes combine a spinal or retinal-diencephalic arteriovenous malformation (AVM) with a nevus of the trunk or face, respectively. Such cases provide a link to the common AVMs described in Chap. 34.

Epidermal Nevus Syndrome

This is a closely related congenital neurocutaneous disorder in which a specific skin lesion (epidermal nevus or linear sebaceous nevus) is associated with a variety of hemicranial and neurologic abnormalities. The skull and brain abnormalities are ipsilateral to the nevus. One-sided thickening of the bones of the skull is characteristic. Developmental delay, seizures, and hemiparesis are the usual neurologic manifestations and have their basis in a wide variety of cerebral lesions—unilateral cerebral atrophy, porencephalic cyst, leptomeningeal hemangioma, arteriovenous malformation, and atresia of cerebral arteries and veins. The somatic and neurologic abnormalities of this syndrome have been comprehensively reviewed by Solomon and Esterley and by Baker and associates.

Hereditary Hemorrhagic Telangiectasia (Osler-Rendu-Weber Disease)

This vascular anomaly is transmitted as an autosomal dominant trait. To date, two mutant genes have been identified as causes of this disease: endoglin and novel kinase. The small arteriovenous malformations affect the skin, mucous membranes, gastrointestinal and genitourinary tracts, lungs, and occasionally the nervous system. The basic lesion is probably a defect in the vessel wall, and the main complication, bleeding, is thought to be a result of the mechanical fragility of the vessel. Located sparsely in the skin of any part of the body, these vascular lesions first appear during childhood, enlarge during adolescence, and may assume spidery forms, resembling the cutaneous telangiectases of cirrhosis in late adult life. The lesions range from the size of a pinhead to 3 mm or more, are bright red or violaceous, and blanch under pressure.

The significance of the lesions lies in their hemorrhagic tendency. During adult years they may give rise to severe and repeated epistaxis or gastric, intestinal, or urinary tract bleeding and result in an iron-deficiency anemia. Pulmonary fistulas constitute another important feature of the generalized vascular dysplasia; patients with such lesions are particularly subject to brain abscesses and less so to bland embolic strokes.

The angiomas of this disease may infrequently form in either the spinal cord or brain, where they can produce acute hemorrhage, or as in one of our patients, there may be an intermittently progressive focal thalamic syndrome resulting from enlargement of the vascular lesions or possibly from a succession of small hemorrhages. Repeated unexplained gastrointestinal, genitourinary, intracranial, or intraspinal hemorrhages warrant a search for small cutaneous lesions, which are easily overlooked. Satellite lesions tend to form after obliteration of an angioma.

von Hippel-Lindau Disease

This is a genetic disease of multiple neoplasms, specifically by the presence of a hemangioblastoma, sometimes multiple (these are discussed with other cerebral tumors in Chap. 31). The tumor is situated in the cerebellum in most cases, but may also arise in the brainstem or spinal cord. In addition to the characteristic cerebellar tumor with its nodule within a cyst, half of these patients have retinal hemangioblastomas and somewhat fewer develop renal cell cancer; an even smaller number have a pheochromocytoma, pancreatic tumors or cysts, or cystadenomas. Polycythemia vera is an interesting feature in a few cases. We have encountered rare cases that presented as subarachnoid hemorrhage.

The cerebellar hemangioblastoma typically develops in the fourth decade and causes symptoms of ataxia and headache. On imaging studies, the lesions have a striking appearance of a cyst with a nodule contained in its wall, and angiography demonstrates the highly vascular nature of the nodule, which represents the actual neoplasm (see Fig. 31-13). The other identifying features of the disease, retinal hemangiomas, are smaller but indistinguishable histologically from the craniospinal ones. They are multiple and bilateral, usually appearing earlier than the cerebellar lesions but remaining asymptomatic until they become extensive (retinal detachment is one feature). Their diagnosis is made by funduscopy, by which a large feeding vessel leading to an irregularly shaped ovoid tumor in the retina can usually be appreciated. Imaging studies of the cranium that use dye enhancement will reveal them as well.

Inheritance is autosomal dominant with variable but high penetrance by older age. The causative mutation is in the *VHL* gene located on chromosome 3. This is a tumor suppressor gene that is inactivated by the mutation and may induce oncogenesis by increasing the expression of vascular mitogenic factors such as vascular endothelial growth factor (VEGF) but the precise mechanisms are not known. Renal cell cancer is a serious component of the disease, occurring in up to 60 percent of cases, but the tumors, although multiple, tend initially to be small and of low grade. Nonetheless, renal cancer accounts for one-third of deaths from the disease, the remainder being largely the result of complications of the cerebellar neoplasm. An extensive review of the subject was written by Losner and colleagues.

Mentioned here is the cerebellar gangliocytoma of Lhermitte-Duclos disease. There are no cutaneous malformations but small vascular anomalies in the brain and elsewhere may accompany the cerebellar tumor as discussed in Chap. 31 (see Fig. 31-15).

Ataxia-Telangiectasia

This disease, also referred to as the *Louis-Bar syndrome*, was first described by Sylaba and Henner in 1926, long before Louis-Bar's report in 1941. It combines a progressive ataxia with humoral immune deficiency and telangiectasias. Like xeroderma pigmentosum and the Cockayne syndrome, ataxia-telangiectasia has been attributed to defective repair of DNA. The inheritance pattern is autosomal recessive and the clinical presentation is somewhat heterogeneous, with certain features predominating in a particular child and his siblings, as summarized by Boder and Sedgwick. An adult form may show few of the characteristic telangiectasias.

The disorder first presents as an ataxic-dyskinetic syndrome in children who appear to have been normal in the first few years of life. The onset of the disease coincides more or less with the acquisition of walking, which is awkward and unsteady. Later, by the age of 4 to 5 years, the limbs become ataxic, and choreoathetosis, grimacing, and dysarthric speech are added. The eye movements become jerky, with slow and long-latency saccades, and there is also apraxia for voluntary gaze (the patient turns the head but not the eyes on attempting to look to the side). This movement of the head and eyes in tandem is the most specific feature of the process. Optokinetic nystagmus is lost and reading becomes all but impossible. Severe cognitive developmental delay is infrequent, affecting perhaps 10 percent of children but in those affected, it is apparent by the age of 9 to 10 years; slight intellectual limitation is more common. Signs of mild polyneuropathy are evident at this age as well, appearing similarly the Charcot-Marie-Tooth phenotype. Seizures are not part of the syndrome.

Muscle power is reduced little if at all until late in the illness, but tendon reflexes may disappear. The characteristic telangiectatic lesions, which are mainly transversely oriented subpapillary venous plexuses, appear at 3 to 5 years of age or later (they are not apparent in some patients until approximately age 7) and are most apparent in the outer parts of the bulbar conjunctivae (Fig. 38-13), over the ears, on exposed parts of the neck, on the bridge of the nose and cheeks in a butterfly pattern, and in the flexor creases of the forearms. Vitiligo, café-au lait spots, loss of subcutaneous fat, and premature graying of hair are observed in some older patients. Many of the patients have endocrine alterations (absence

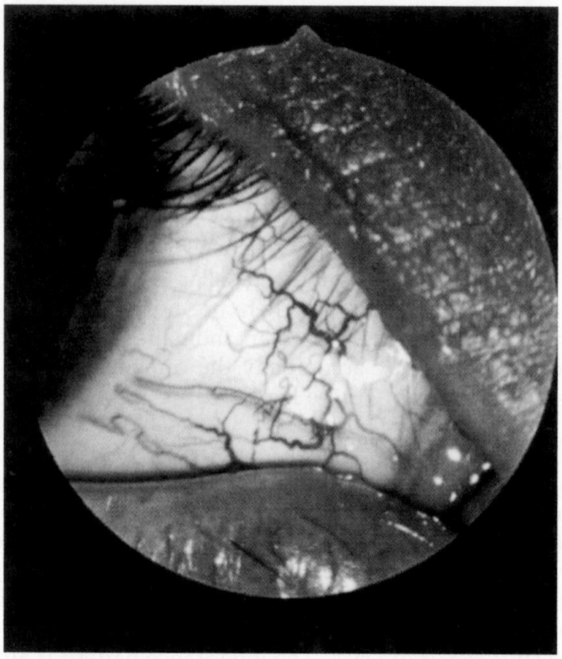

Figure 38-13. Ocular appearance of ataxia-telangectasia. (Reproduced by permission from Lyon G, Kolodny EH, Pastores GM: *Neurology of Hereditary Metabolic Diseases of Children*, 3rd ed. New York, McGraw-Hill, 2006.)

of secondary sexual development, glucose intolerance). The disease is progressive, and death may occur in the second decade from intercurrent bronchopulmonary infection or neoplasia—usually lymphoma, less often glioma, that develop in fewer one-third of patients.

As mentioned, the *adult form of ataxia-telangiectasia*, in which some of the deficient enzyme activity is retained (see below), manifests few telangiectasias but may be identified by an extrapyramidal syndrome in childhood and only later, with mild ataxia as summarized by Verhagen and colleagues; there may be a family history of cancers.

The significant abnormalities in the CNS are severe degeneration in the cerebellar cortex (visible on MRI scans); loss of myelinated fibers in the posterior columns, spinocerebellar tracts, and peripheral nerves; degenerative changes in the posterior roots and cells of the sympathetic ganglia; and loss of anterior horn cells at all levels of the spinal cord. In a few cases, vascular abnormalities, like the mucocutaneous ones, have been found scattered diffusely in the white matter of the brain and spinal cord, but they are of questionable significance. Also, there may be a loss of pigmented cells in the substantia nigra and locus ceruleus (a feature shared with PKU), and cytoplasmic inclusions (Lewy bodies) in the cells that remain (Agamanolis and Greenstein). During early development there are abnormalities of Purkinje cell migration and variations in nuclear size. Intranuclear inclusions and bizarre nuclear formations have also been found in the satellite cells (amphicytes) of dorsal root ganglion neurons (Strich).

There is an absence or decrease in several immunoglobulins—IgA, IgE and isotypes, IgG_2, IgG_4—in practically every patient. These deficiencies, shown by McFarlin and associates to be a result of decreased synthesis, are associated with hypoplasia of the thymus, loss of follicles in lymph nodes, failure of delayed hypersensitivity reactions, and lymphopenia. This immunodeficient state accounts for the striking susceptibility of these patients to recurrent pulmonary infections and bronchiectasis. Transplantation of normal thymus tissue into the patient and administration of thymus extracts have been of no therapeutic value.

The defective gene (designated *ATM*) is a kinase that is a transducer in the pathway for DNA repair that halts the cell cycle after DNA damage. For this reason, there is faulty repair of DNA after radiation and a greatly increased risk of lymphomas, leukemias, and other tumors as well as certain specific susceptibilities to the effects of cancer treatment. The protein is normally expressed ubiquitously and 90 percent of patients have no ATM protein, usually because of a stop codon in the mutated gene.

The only therapy centers on the control of infections. Free radical scavengers such as vitamin E have been recommended without proof of their effectiveness. Because of radiation sensitivity, even conventional diagnostic tests (dental, chest radiography) should be avoided unless there is a compelling reason for them.

RESTRICTED DEVELOPMENTAL ABNORMALITIES OF THE NERVOUS SYSTEM

In the course of clinical practice, one encounters a remarkable number of restricted disorders of the nervous system, many of which are transmitted from generation to generation as a mendelian, usually dominant, trait. Of the more severe ones, only a few of the more striking examples are described here. Milder and more restricted conditions, such as stuttering and dyslexia, that are pervasive in the population are described in Chap. 28. The reader may turn to books on genetics or teratology for an account of such oddities as hereditary unilateral ptosis, hereditary Horner syndrome, pupillary inequalities, jaw winking, and absence of a particular skeletal muscle.

Bifacial and Abducens Palsies (Möbius Syndrome)

The syndrome of congenital facial diplegia with convergent strabismus is referred to as *Möbius syndrome*, although Von Graefe had described it earlier. Its presence at birth is disclosed by the lack of facial movements and of full eye closure. A review of the subject in the English literature was written by Henderson, and a more recent analysis of 37 affected individuals was written by Harriëtte and colleagues. In Henderson's study of 61 cases of the congenital facial diplegia syndrome, there were 45 instances of associated abducens palsy,

15 of complete external ophthalmoplegia, 18 of lingual palsy, 17 of clubfeet, 13 of a brachial disorder, 6 of mental defect, and 8 of an absent pectoral muscle. Thus the overlap with other neuromuscular and CNS abnormalities is evident. Moreover, at least two configurations of brainstem dysfunction have been proposed, one because of a lack of the facial nerve nucleus and the other in the nerve, perhaps acquired in type, based on electrophysiologic studies, but we have no basis to judge the validity of this. Harriëtte and coworkers emphasize the frequency of hypoplastic or dysplastic tongue, palatal involvement, and general motor clumsiness. They suggest that the disorder represents a widespread form of brainstem maldevelopment.

Early in life the mouth hangs open, the lower lip is everted, and there is difficulty in sucking. Usually this syndrome can be distinguished from the facial palsy of forceps or birth injury by its bilaterality and the other associated weaknesses. Occasionally, more than one family member is affected (usually in a pattern suggesting autosomal dominant inheritance). The cause of this peculiar condition is not known. The few adequate pathologic studies have shown a paucity of nerve cells in the motor nuclei of the brainstem, changes that also characterize the Fazio-Londe type of muscular dystrophy discussed in Chap. 50. Rarely, there may be an aplasia of facial muscles. The Möbius syndrome is also referred to in Chap. 47 in relation to restricted palsies of myopathic and nuclear origin.

Partial paralysis of facial muscles that dates from birth and cannot be attributed to obstetric trauma is not infrequent. In a common type, the lower lip on one side remains immobile when the child smiles or cries; the lip on the unaffected side is drawn downward and outward, resulting in a prominent asymmetry of the lower face. Often it is not appreciated that the side that droops during crying is the normal side (Hoefnagel and Penry).

Congenital Lack of Lateral Gaze (Cogan Oculomotor Apraxia)

Children with this congenital defect are unable to turn their eyes to either side volitionally or on command. Attempting to look to the right, the child turns the head to the right (there is no associated apraxia of head turning), but the eyes lag and turn to the left. As a result, the patient has to overshoot the mark with the head in order to attain ocular fixation. Once the eyes fixate, the head returns to the primary position. To compensate for the deficiency of eye movements, the patient develops jerky thrusting movements of the head, which characterize all attempts at voluntary gaze. Caloric stimulation of the labyrinth causes tonic movement of the eyes but not nystagmus, as in the normal person. Also, optokinetic nystagmus cannot be induced. Vertical eye movements are normal. A similar ocular condition may occur in conjunction with ataxia-telangiectasia and in Gaucher disease. Children with oculomotor apraxia are slow to walk; Ford observed one such child whose sibling had an absence of the vermis of the cerebellum. Aside from this observation, the anatomic basis of the condition has not been studied.

CONGENITAL ABNORMALITIES OF MOTOR FUNCTION (CEREBRAL PALSY)

In this group of congenital disorders, a major disturbance of motor function, usually nonprogressive, has been present since infancy or early childhood. The popular terms for these conditions have been *infantile cerebral paralysis* (Freud) and *cerebral palsy*. The latter name is neither appropriate nor useful from the physician's viewpoint, collocating as it does diseases of widely differing etiologic and anatomic types, wherein the hereditary and acquired and the intrauterine, natal, and postnatal diseases lose their identity. But the name has been adopted as a slogan by fund-raising societies and for rehabilitation clinics throughout the United States, hence it will not soon disappear from medical terminology. The term, often abbreviated CP, is still being used indiscriminately to designate every conceivable cognitive and motor disorder of corticospinal, extrapyramidal, cerebellar, and even neuromuscular type in infants and children.

Etiology of the Congenital Cerebral Motor Disorders

Motor abnormalities that have had their onset early in life are numerous and diverse in their clinical manifestations. Marked prematurity is an associated factor in a large proportion of cases. Each year, approximately 50,000 infants weighing less than 1,500 g are born in the United States; approximately 85 percent survive. Of these, 5 to 15 percent have a motor disorder of cerebral origin and 25 to 30 percent are found to be mentally impaired at school age (Volpe, 1995; also Hack et al). It is helpful to categorize a given case according to the extent and nature of the motor abnormality. A careful history of prenatal, perinatal, or postnatal insults to the developing nervous system must be sought; certain correlations of these factors with the resulting pattern of neurologic deficit are outlined below. Most patients with these motor abnormalities reach adult years. Many but not all have epilepsy in addition to the motor abnormalities and there is an unavoidable overlap in considering the causes and mechanisms of these three clinical states.

The following discussion is given from the perspective of the three major etiologic syndromes: matrix hemorrhages in the immature infant, hypoxic-ischemic encephalopathy, and certain other developmental motor abnormalities including those due to intrauterine stroke.

Germinal Matrix (Subependymal) Hemorrhage in Premature Infants

In low-weight and premature immature infants (20 to 35 weeks' gestational age), there sometimes occurs, within a few days after birth, a catastrophic decline in cerebral function, usually preceded by respiratory distress (hyaline membrane disease) with spells of cyanosis and apnea. Also evident are deficiencies of brainstem automatisms (sucking and swallowing), bulging of the fontanels, and sanguineous CSF. If the infant becomes completely unresponsive, death usually ensues within a few days. Autopsy discloses a small lake of blood in each cerebral hemisphere (often asymmetrically distributed), occupying the highly cellular (subependymal) germinal matrix zone, near the caudate nucleus at the level of the foramen of Monro. This region is supplied by the lenticulostriate, choroidal, and Heubner recurrent arteries and is drained by deep veins, which enter the vein of Galen. In approximately 25 percent of cases, the blood remains loculated in the matrix zone, while in the majority it ruptures into the lateral ventricle or adjacent brain tissue. In a series of 914 consecutive autopsies in newborns, subependymal hemorrhage was found in 284 (31 percent); practically all of these neonates were of low birth weight, according to Banker and Bruce-Gregorios.

Lesser degrees of this cerebral hemorrhage are now being identified by ultrasonography (Fig. 38-14) and CT scans, and it is apparent that many infants with smaller hemorrhages survive. Some rapidly develop an obstructive hydrocephalus and require a ventricular shunt. In others, the hydrocephalus stabilizes and there is clinical improvement. Several series of surviving cases have now been followed for many years. Those in whom the hemorrhage was more extensive are often left with motor and intellectual handicaps.

Viewed from the perspective of cerebral palsy, just over half of the patients in the Swedish series of Hagberg and Hagberg with spastic diplegia had matrix hemorrhages, leukomalacia (see further on), or both. Congenital hemiplegia or quadriplegia was observed at a lower frequency. In another series of 20 cases of posthemorrhagic hydro-cephalus (Chaplin et al), 40 percent had significant motor deficits and more than 60 percent had IQ scores of less than 85. In an experience with 12 less severely affected surviving cases (mean birth weight 1.8 kg and gestational age of 32.3 weeks), R.D. Adams noted that only 1 had a residual spastic diplegia and 9 had IQs in the low-normal or normal range (personal communication).

The cause of matrix hemorrhage is not entirely clear. In all probability it is related to greatly increased pressure in the thin-walled veins of the germinal matrix coupled with a lack of adequate supporting tissue in these zones. During periods of unstable arterial or venous blood pressure that occur with the pulmonary disorders of immature infants, these thin-walled vessels rupture. These infants are also prone to the development of another characteristic lesion of the cerebral white matter (periventricular leukomalacia; see below), and the neurologic deficits resulting from these two lesions may be additive.

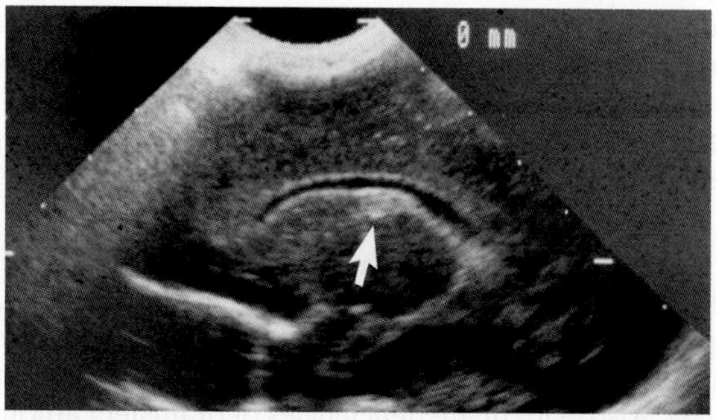

Figure 38-14. Ultrasonograph demonstration of subependymal matrix hemorrhage in a premature infant (*arrow*).

Treatment Control of the respiratory distress of prematurity may reduce the incidence of matrix hemorrhages and periventricular leukomalacia. Claims have been made that the administration of indomethacin ethamsylate, a drug that reduces capillary bleeding, and the intramuscular injection of vitamin E for the first 3 days after birth and possibly the use of betamethasone or other corticosteroids appears to be of value in reducing the incidence of periventricular hemorrhage (Benson et al; Sinha et al; see also Volpe [1989] for discussion of control of cerebral hemodynamics and effects of medications in the neonatal period). Acetazolamide and furosemide, which reduce the formation of spinal fluid, have been widely used in the treatment of posthemorrhagic hydrocephalus. However, in a large-scale controlled study, the effects were negligible and shunt placement was required to control worsening hydrocephalus (see International PHVD Drug Trial Group in the references).

Periventricular Leukomalacia

These are zones of necrosis of white matter in the deep territories of cortical and central arteries. They lie lateral and posterolateral to the lateral ventricles, in a position to involve the occipital radiations and the sensorimotor fibers in the corona radiata (first described by Banker and Larroche; see also Shuman and Selednik). The white matter lesions occur in about one-third of cases of subependymal hemorrhage as mentioned, but they may develop independently in both premature and full-term infants who have suffered hypotension and apnea. In a study of 753 preterm infants, those born at 28 weeks' gestation or less were at highest risk of this complication; the combination of intrauterine infection and premature rupture of membranes carried a 22 percent risk (Zupan et al). Survivors often manifest cerebral hemiplegia or diplegia and variable degrees of mental impairment. The motor disorder is usually more severe than the cognitive and language impairment. Increasingly, small lesions of this nature are being identified in term infants by cerebral imaging including ultrasound.

The mechanism of this type of periventricular infarction has been debated, and the terminology and clinical features, insofar as they overlap with germinal matrix hemorrhage, have been confusing. In recent years, most theories and experimental evidence converge on the notion that these represent regions of venous ischemia and infarction.

Hypoxic-Ischemic Damage and Neonatal Encephalopathy

It has been estimated that in the range of 1 to 6 of every 1,000 live births manifests a neonatal encephalopathy (as quoted in the review by Ferriero). The seriousness of the condition is further emphasized by the associated mortality rate of 20 percent in the newborn period and the 25 percent rate of neurodevelopmental disability in survivors. Little's conception of the hypoxic-ischemic form of "birth injury," enunciated in 1862, has been reconsidered over the years. Although it is evident that many newborns suffer some degree of perinatal asphyxia, relatively few seem to manifest brain damage. Moreover, many, if not most, infants with a variety of cerebral motor syndromes appear to have passed the parturitional (perinatal) period without mishap, indicating the greater importance of other prenatal and postnatal causative factors. Nonetheless, *severe neonatal asphyxia* of term or preterm babies can be an important cause of spastic, dystonic and ataxic syndromes, often accompanied by seizures and mental delay in development.

This field has been sullied by an unprecedented rise in malpractice litigation, spawned in part by the belief that early detection of asphyxia and rapid delivery would have prevented the motor, epileptic, and cognitive problems of birth injury. The fallacy of this assumption is highlighted both by the below comments and by the observation that the incidence of cerebral palsy has not changed in term infants over the past 30 years, despite the institution of fetal monitoring and more frequent cesarean sections.

One has the impression that the brain tolerates hypoxia and reduced blood flow in the immediate postnatal period better than at any other time in life. Indeed, animal experimentation supports this view. Not until the arterial oxygen tension is reduced dramatically to 10 to 15 percent of normal does brain damage occur, and even then the impaired function of other organs contributes to the damage. It is probably correct to think of the encephalopathy in terms of both hypoxia and ischemia, both of which usually occur in utero and are expressed postnatally by recognizable clinical syndromes.

Fenichel (1990), following the original work of Sarnat and Sarnat and of Levene and colleagues, has found it helpful to divide the encephalopathies that follow a complicated birth into three purely descriptive groups according to their severity, each having a prognostic value beyond that of the Apgar score: (1) In newborns with mild hypoxic-ischemic encephalopathy, the symptoms are maximal in the first 24 h and take the form of hyperalertness and tremulousness of the limbs and jaw (the "jittery baby") and a low threshold of the Moro reaction. The tone of the limbs is normal except for a mild increase in head lag during traction. The reflexes are brisk and there may be ankle clonus. The anterior fontanel is soft. The EEG is normal. Recovery is usually complete and the risk of handicap is low. (2) Newborns with moderate hypoxic-ischemic encephalopathy are lethargic, obtunded, and hypotonic, with normal movements. After 48 to 72 h, the neonate may improve (having passed through a jittery hyperactive phase) or worsen, becoming less responsive in association with convulsions, cerebral edema, hyponatremia, and hyperammonemia from liver damage. The EEG is abnormal. Fenichel associates epileptiform activity and voltage suppression with an unfavorable outcome. Abnormal visual and auditory evoked potentials are other poor prognostic signs. (3) In neonates with severe hypoxic-ischemic encephalopathy, stupor or coma is present from birth; respirations are irregular, requiring mechanical ventilation. There are usually convulsions within the first 12 h. The limbs are hypotonic and motionless even during attempts to elicit the Moro response. Sucking and swallowing are depressed or absent, but pupillary reactions and eye movements may at first be retained, only to be lost as the coma deepens.

It is in the second and third categories, that is, the states of moderate to severe encephalopathy, where correction of the respiratory insufficiency and the metabolic abnormalities permits survival, that a number of motor abnormalities (corticospinal, extrapyramidal, and cerebellar) and developmental delay eventually emerge. Included in the category of severe hypoxic-ischemic encephalopathy are also newborns with a variety of developmental anomalies of the brain and other organs. However, clouding the issue of causality is the absence of perinatal complications in a large number of children with cerebral palsy and the large number of normal babies who are born after complicated deliveries. Notably, only a few cases result from often blamed intrapartum factors such as forceps delivery, breech presentation, cord prolapse, abruptio placentae, and maternal fever.

In addition, such infants may have been exposed to certain prenatal risk factors (toxemia of pregnancy, antepartum uterine hemorrhage, maternal hypotension, and certain epidemiologic associations such as hypothyroidism or fertility treatment), or their growth may have been abnormal (small-for-date babies). Some of these babies are born at term; others are premature, and the birth process may or may not have been abnormal. One must then consider the possibility, originally pointed out by Sigmund Freud, that the abnormality of the birth process, instead of being causal, was actually the consequence of prenatal pathology. The latter might include preterm intrauterine hypoxia-ischemia.

Other evidence of multifactorial etiology in the "causation" of cerebral palsy has been provided by Nelson and Ellenberg, who found that maternal developmental delay, birth weight below 2,000 g, and fetal malformation were among the leading predictors. Breech presentation was another factor, and one-third of these cases also had some noncerebral malformation. Twenty-one percent of the 189 children in their series had also suffered some degree of asphyxia. Additional determinants were maternal seizures, a motor deficit in an older sibling, two or more prior fetal deaths, hyperthyroidism in the mother, preeclampsia, and eclampsia. In children with cerebral diplegia born at term, likely contributory factors that were operative in nearly half included toxemia of pregnancy, low birth weight for age, placental infarction, and intrauterine asphyxia.

The factors enumerated above are involved to different degrees in the outcome of pregnancies but are informative because they bring to light the significant proportion of cases of cerebral birth injury in which hypoxia-ischemia, matrix hemorrhages, and leukomalacia were not operative. In this group, can be included the symmetrical porencephalies and hydranencephalies.

Thus the complexity of assigning a cause for cerebral palsy is evident. In respect to the motor disorders discussed below, hypoxic-ischemic perinatal injury is still the most commonly specified cause of neonatal encephalopathy but is often unrelated to a permanent defect of cerebral palsy. This statement has been amply confirmed by a large and often cited study from Western Australia that detected neonatal encephalopathy in 3.8 of 1,000 live term births but was able to identify causative intrapartum factors alone in only 5 percent (Badawi et al). Furthermore, only 10 percent of all the infants with neonatal encephalopathy developed spastic quadriplegia, according to Evans and colleagues.

Imaging studies of cerebral palsy have increasingly appeared and it has even been suggested, perhaps with excessive enthusiasm, that all such children undergo scanning. Cowan and colleagues (2003) used MRI to determine the proportion of infants with a neonatal encephalopathy who had antenatal brain injury. Excluding those with major congenital malformations or obvious chromosomal abnormalities, 80 percent of cases had no established lesion or brain atrophy. In contrast, those with only seizures and no neonatal encephalopathy in 69 percent of cases had evidence of antenatal damage on MRI; infarctions because of thrombophilic disorders were most common. An MRI–clinical correlative study of children with cerebral palsy by Bax and colleagues in The European Cerebral Palsy Study came to similar conclusions but found that periventricular leukomalacia of prematurity was the most common MRI change, present in 42 percent of infants, followed in frequency by basal ganglionic damage (13 percent), cortical-subcortical lesions (9 percent), malformations (9 percent), and focal infarcts (7 percent). These authors found a correspondence between the clinical and MRI findings. These studies demonstrate the utility of MRI in identifying neonatal forms of encephalopathy and indicate that few are the result of obstetric accidents. Added difficulty is caused by the fact that the clinical signs of perinatal injury may emerge only when the maturational process of the nervous system exposes them at a later period of life. Woodward and coworkers suggested that the MRI pattern is predictive of developmental outcome in preterm infants, but this requires corroboration.

Treatment Much of the resources of neonatal intensive care is devoted to sustaining oxygenation and blood pressure, and reducing hyperbilirubinemia in premature and full-term but ill infants. Techniques such as the predelivery administration of corticosteroids in premature births to promote lung maturity, attempting to bring early births to 34 to 36 weeks' gestation, and the treatment of maternal infection have all contributed to improved outcomes in children.

The avoidance of the ostensible causes of cerebral palsy has been discussed in previous sections and endlessly in the medical literature. None of the usually assigned causes of birth injury, particularly perinatal hypoxia-ischemia, explains most cases. In addition, several trials have investigated the effects of induced hypothermia for severe neonatal encephalopathy from hypoxia but have given mixed results. Attempts to ameliorate brain injury by the use of hypothermia, a technique that has met with success in adult cardiac arrest, have given conflicting results. A randomized trial by Shankaran and colleagues using systemic hypothermia administered to infants with neonatal encephalopathy or a need for resuscitation showed a reduction in death or moderate to severe disability from 62 to 44 percent and a small benefit in IQ at age 7 that was not statistically significant. Hypothermia was applied soon after birth, at a mean of about 4 hours. The effects were seen mostly among infants with only moderate and not severe encephalopathy and none of the measures of mental and psychomotor disability was improved by cooling. Previous trials, such as the one reported by Azzopardi and colleagues, had shown no difference in outcomes but used different techniques, mainly selective cerebral cooling. Cooling appears promising but requires further study, and at the time of this writing, has not been widely adopted. It is also unclear if the short-term followup will be reflected at school age and beyond.

Clinical Syndromes of Congenital Spastic Motor Disorders

The most frequent motor disorder evolving from the four major categories of neonatal cerebral disease—matrix hemorrhage, periventricular leukomalacia, hypoxic-ischemic encephalopathy, kernicterus (discussed further on)—is spastic diplegia; that is, a motor disturbance that is severe in the lower limbs and mild in the upper, as discussed below. In addition, hypoxic-ischemic injury occurring in the term or preterm infant may take the form of a hemiplegia, double hemiplegia (quadriplegia), or a mixed pyramidal–extrapyramidal or spastic–ataxic syndrome.

A second form of motor disorder is characterized by the development of severe spastic quadriplegia and developmental delay. The major insult is usually intrapartum asphyxia and attendant fetal distress. Usually such infants will have required resuscitation and will have had low 5-min Apgar scores and seizures, which have important predictive value in this circumstance. The pathologic lesions of the brain in this second group consist of hypoxic-ischemic infarction in distal fields of arterial flow, primarily in the cortex and white matter of parietal and posterior frontal lobes, leaving a ulegyric sclerotic cortex.

A third group, discussed below, is characterized mainly by extrapyramidal abnormalities, combining athetosis, dystonia, and ataxia in various proportions. After reviewing the results of several large series of congenital and neonatal motor disorders, we have concluded that spastic diplegia occurs in 10 to 33 percent of cases, spastic quadriplegia in 19 to 43 percent, extrapyramidal forms in 10 to 22 percent, and mixed forms in 9 to 20 percent.

Spastic Diplegia ("Little Disease") The pattern of paralysis is more variable than the term *spastic diplegia* implies; actually, several subtypes may be distinguished: paraplegic, diplegic, quadriplegic, pseudobulbar, and generalized. Pure paraplegic and pseudobulbar types are relatively rare. The eponymic "Little disease" has been applied mainly to the spastic diplegic type, but it also has been attached to all forms of motor cerebral palsy in some older writings.

Usually all four extremities are affected, but the legs much more than the arms, which is the real meaning of *diplegia*. Hypotonia—with retained tendon reflexes and hypoactivity—is usually present initially. Only after the first few months will evident weakness and spasticity appear, first in the adductors of the legs. The plantar reflexes, which often take on ambiguous direction in the normal infant, here are clearly extensor, a finding that is pathologic at any later age. Also, stiff, awkward movements of the legs, which are maintained in an extended, adducted posture when the infant is lifted by the axillae, often do not attract attention until several weeks or months have passed. Seizures occur in approximately one-third of the cases, and it is not uncommon to observe a delay in all developmental sequences, especially those that depend on the motor system.

Once walking is attempted, usually at a much later date than usual, the characteristic stance and gait become manifest. The slightly flexed legs are advanced stiffly in short steps, each describing part of an arc of a circle; adduction of the thighs is often so strong that the legs may actually cross (scissors gait); the feet are flexed and turned in with the heels not touching the floor. In the adolescent and adult, the legs tend to be short and small, but the muscles are not markedly atrophic, as they are in spinal muscular atrophy. Passive manipulation of the limbs reveals spasticity in the extensors and adductors and slight shortening of the calf muscles. The arms may be affected only slightly or not at all, but there may be awkwardness and stiffness of the fingers and, in a few, pronounced weakness and spasticity. In reaching for an object, the hand may overpronate and a grasp may be difficult to release. Speech may be well articulated or noticeably slurred, and in some instances the face is set in a spastic smile. Scoliosis is frequent and may secondarily give rise to root compression and impaired respiratory function. As a rule, there is no disturbance of sphincteric function, although delay in acquiring voluntary bowel and bladder control is usual. Athetotic postures and movements of the face, tongue, and hands are present in some patients and may actually conceal the spastic weakness.

One subtype of spastic diplegia is associated with a relatively slight diminution in head size and of intelligence. As indicated above, there is no unifying neuropathology; the condition occurs independently of matrix hemorrhages and periventricular leukomalacia as well as with them. The frequency of cerebral spastic diplegia, which is closely related to the degree of prematurity, has declined significantly since the introduction of neonatal intensive care facilities, and there is reason to believe that genetic factors are of more importance.

Infantile Hemiplegia and Quadriplegia Hemiplegia is a common condition of infancy and early childhood. The functional difference between the two sides may be noticed soon after birth, but more often it is not perceived by the mother until after the first 4 to 6 months of life. In a second group, the child is in excellent health for a year or longer before the abrupt onset of hemiplegia (see below). In hemiplegia that dates from earliest infancy—that is, congenital hemiplegia—the parents first notice that movements of prehension and exploration are carried out with only one arm. A manifest hand preference at an early age should always raise the suspicion of a unilateral motor defect. The affection of the leg is usually recognized later, that is, during the first attempts to stand and walk. Sitting and walking are usually delayed by a few months. In the older child, there is evident hyperactivity of tendon reflexes and usually a Babinski sign. The arm is held flexed, adducted, and pronated, and the foot assumes an equinovarus posture. Sensory and visual field defects can be detected in some patients. A mental slowness may be associated with infantile hemiplegia but is less common and lesser in degree than with cerebral diplegia. There may also be speech delay, regardless of the side of the lesion; when this is present, there is usually developmental delay and bilaterality of motor abnormality. Convulsions occur in 35 to 50 percent of children with congenital hemiplegia, and these may persist throughout life. They may be generalized but are frequently unilateral and limited to the hemiplegic side (or the contralateral side if the hemiplegia is severe). After a series of seizures, the weakness on the affected side will be increased for several hours or longer (Todd paralysis). Gastaut and associates have described a hemiconvulsive–hemiplegic syndrome in which progressive paralysis and cerebral atrophy are attributed to the convulsions. As months and years pass, the osseous and muscular growth of the hemiplegic limbs is impeded, leading to an obvious hemiatrophy of the body.

With respect to the causation of congenital hemiplegia, it is generally agreed that perinatal asphyxia is only one of the possibilities. In the series of 681 children with "cerebral palsy" collected by Hagberg and Hagberg, there were 244 with hemiplegia of whom 189 were full-term babies and 55 were preterm. Prenatal risk factors were identified in only 45 percent, and mostly in the infants born prematurely. In nearly half of the cases, there was no clue as to the time in the intrauterine period when the cerebral lesion occurred.

In another group—*acquired infantile hemiplegia*—a normal infant or young child, usually between the ages of 3 and 18 months, develops a massive hemiplegia, with or without aphasia, within hours. The disorder often begins with seizures, and the hemiplegia may not be recognized until the seizures have subsided. In Banker's series of autopsy cases, there was arterial or venous thrombosis in some cases, but instances without vascular occlusions were found. Some of the latter cases, in which arteriography had been normal, may have been embolic, possibly of cardiac origin. In the recent era, imaging has shown a large area of cerebral infarction, consistent with a stroke in the territory of the middle cerebral artery (Fig. 38-15). If the stroke occurs at an early age, the recovery of speech may be complete, though reduced scholastic capacity remains. The degree of recovery of motor function varies. Often, as the deficit recedes, the arm becomes involved by athetotic, tremulous, or ataxic movements; there may be an interval of months or years between the hemiplegia and the athetosis.

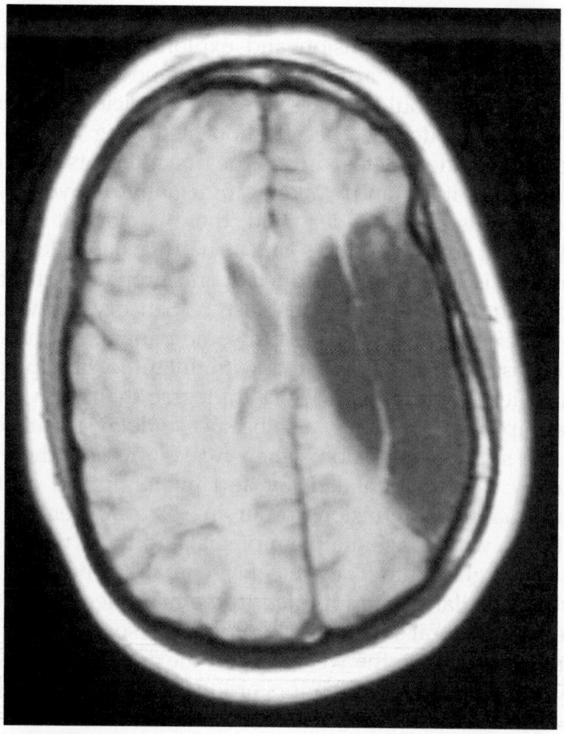

Figure 38-15. MRI of an adult with congenital hemiplegia. There is severe encephalomalacia mainly in the territory of the right middle cerebral artery.

Destructive lesions underlie most of the cases of infantile hemiplegia and some cases of bilateral hemiplegia (as well as many cases of seizures in the first few days of life). The pathologic change is essentially that of ischemic necrosis. In many cases, the lesions must have been acquired in utero. Precipitant delivery, fetal distress, and prepartum uterine hemorrhage may have been indications, more so than causes, of the process. What is most notable is that the ischemia tends to affect the tissues lying in arterial cortical border zones; there may also be venous stasis with congestion and hemorrhage occurring particularly in the deep central structures such as the basal ganglia and periventricular matrix zones. If they are purely hypoxic, the lesions should be bilateral. Myers has reproduced such lesions in the neonatal monkey by reducing the maternal circulation for several hours. As the lesions heal, the monkeys develop the same gliotic changes in the cortex and white matter of the cerebrum (lobar sclerosis) and the "marbling" (état marbré) that characterizes the brains of patients with spastic diplegia and double athetosis (see below).

The quadriplegic state differs from bilateral hemiplegias in that the bulbar musculature is often involved in the latter and developmental delay is more severe. The condition is relatively rare and is usually a result of a bilateral cerebral lesion. However, one should also be alert to the possibility of a high cervical cord lesion. In the infant, this is usually the result of a fracture dislocation of the cervical spine incurred during a difficult breech delivery. Similarly, in paraplegia, with weakness or paralysis limited to the legs, the lesion may be either a cerebral or a spinal one. Sphincteric disturbances and a loss of somatic sensation below a certain level on the trunk always point to a spinal localization. Congenital cysts, tumors, and diastematomyelia are more frequently causes of paraplegia than of quadriplegia. Another recognized cause of infantile paraplegia is spinal cord infarction from thrombotic complications of umbilical artery catheterization.

Extrapyramidal Syndromes

The spastic cerebral diplegias discussed above shade almost imperceptibly into the congenital extrapyramidal syndromes. These children are found in every cerebral palsy clinic, and, ultimately, they reach adult neurology clinics. Corticospinal tract signs may be absent and the student, familiar only with the syndrome of pure spastic diplegia, is always puzzled as to their classification. Some cases of extrapyramidal type are undoubtedly attributable to severe perinatal hypoxia and others to diseases such as erythroblastosis fetalis with kernicterus. To state the probable pathologic basis and future course of these illnesses, it is useful to separate the extrapyramidal syndromes of prenatal-natal origin (which usually become manifest during the first year of life) from the acquired or hereditary postnatal syndromes, such as familial athetosis, Wilson disease, dystonia musculorum deformans, and the hereditary cerebellar ataxias, which become manifest later.

Double Athetosis This is probably the most frequent of the congenital extrapyramidal disorders. Two types stand out—one that is caused by hyperbilirubinemia or Rh incompatibility (kernicterus; see below) and hypoxic-ischemic encephalopathy. With control of neonatal hyperbilirubinemia (by use of anti-Rh immune globulin, exchange transfusions, and phototherapy), kernicterus has almost disappeared, whereas the severe hypoxic-ischemic form regularly continues to be seen. Rarely, a congenital, nonhemolytic icterus or a glucose-6-phosphate dehydrogenase deficiency produces the same syndrome.

Like the spastic states, double athetosis may not be recognized at birth but only after several months or a year has elapsed. In some cases, the appearance of choreoathetosis is for unexplained reasons delayed for several years; it may seem to progress during adolescence and even early adult life. It must then be differentiated from some of the inherited metabolic and degenerative extrapyramidal diseases. Chorea and athetosis dominate the clinical picture, but bewildering combinations of involuntary movements—including dystonia, ataxic tremor, myoclonus, and even hemiballismus—may be found in a single case. At times, we have been unable to classify the movement disorder because of its complexity. It should be noted that practically all instances of double athetosis are also associated with a defect in voluntary movement.

Choreoathetosis in infants and children varies greatly in severity. In some, the abnormal movements are so mild as to be misinterpreted as restlessness or "the fidgets"; in others, every attempted voluntary act provokes violent involuntary spasms, leaving the patient nearly helpless. The clinical features of choreoathetosis and other involuntary movements are discussed in Chap. 4.

Early hypotonia, followed by delayed motor development, is the rule in these cases. Erect posture and walking may not occur until the age of 3 to 5 years and may never be attained in some patients. Tonic neck reflexes or fragments thereof tend to persist well beyond their usual time of disappearance. The plantar reflexes are usually flexor, although they may be difficult to interpret because of the continuous flexion and extension of the toes. Sensory abnormalities are not found. Because of the motor and speech impairment, patients are often erroneously thought to be mentally slow. In some, this conclusion is doubtless correct, but intellectual function is adequate in many others.

A variety of rehabilitative measures have been tried: physiotherapy, surgery, sensory integrative therapy, progressive patterned movement, and various undocumented forms of neuromuscular facilitation. We agree with Hur, who has critically reviewed this subject, that properly controlled studies provide no proof of the success of any of them. Surely, with growth and development, new postures and motor capacities are acquired. The less-severely affected patients make successful occupational adjustments. The more-severely affected children rarely achieve a degree of motor control that permits them to live independently. One sees some of these unfortunate persons bobbing and twisting laboriously as they make their way in public places.

Imaging studies are seldom of diagnostic value. Mild cerebral atrophy and loss of volume of the basal ganglia are seen in some cases, and cavitary lesions are present in some of the severe anoxic encephalopathies. The EEG is rarely helpful unless there are seizures.

The most frequent pathologic finding in the brain has been a whitish, marble-like appearance of the putamen, thalamus, and border zones of the cerebral cortex. These whitish strands represent foci of nerve cell loss and gliosis with condensation of bands of transversing myelinated fibers—so-called *status marmoratus (état marbré)*. This lesion does not develop if the insult occurs after infancy, that is, after myelination has completed its early developmental cycle.

Kernicterus This is now a rare cause of extrapyramidal motor disorder in children and adults. Such cases are the neurologic sequelae of erythroblastosis fetalis secondary to Rh and ABO blood incompatibilities or to a deficiency of the hepatic enzyme glucuronosyltransferase. The symptoms of kernicterus appear in the jaundiced neonate on the second or third postnatal day. The infant becomes listless, sucks poorly, develops respiratory difficulties as well as opisthotonos (head retraction), and becomes stuporous as jaundice intensifies. The serum bilirubin is usually greater than 25 mg/dL. In acidotic and hypoxic infants (e.g., those with low birth weight and hyaline membrane disease), the kernicteric lesions develop with much lower levels of serum bilirubin.

A proportion of infants with this disease die within the first week or two of life. Many of those who survive are developmentally delayed, deaf, hypotonic, and totally unable to sit, stand, or walk. There are exceptional patients, however, who are mentally normal or at most only slightly limited. They develop a variety of persistent neurologic sequelae—choreoathetosis, dystonia, and rigidity of the limbs—a picture not too different from that of cerebral spastic diplegia with involuntary movements. Kernicterus should always be suspected if an extrapyramidal syndrome is accompanied by bilateral deafness and paralysis of upward gaze. Later, in childhood there may be a greenish pigmentation of the dental enamel.

Neonates who die in the acute postnatal stage of kernicterus show a unique yellow staining (icterus) of nuclear masses at one time was called the "Kern nuclei" and gave the disease its name in the basal ganglia, brainstem, and cerebellum. In those surviving this postnatal insult, the pathologic changes consist of a symmetrically distributed nerve cell loss and gliosis in the subthalamic nucleus, the globus pallidus, the thalamus, and the oculomotor and cochlear nuclei; these lesions are the result of the hyperbilirubinemia. In more than 30 cases examined by R.D. Adams, the immature cerebral cortex including the hippocampus was spared. In the newborn, unconjugated bilirubin can pass through the poorly developed blood–brain barrier into these nuclei, where it is assumed to be directly toxic. Acidosis and hypoxia exacerbate the effect. Also in the newborn, the development of hyperbilirubinemia is enhanced by a transient deficiency of the enzyme glucuronosyltransferase, essential for the conjugation of bilirubin. *Hereditary hyperbilirubinemia*, caused by lack of this enzyme (*Crigler-Najjar syndrome*), may exhibit the same effects on the nervous system at a later period of infancy or childhood as hyperbilirubinemia because of Rh incompatibility.

Immunization, phototherapy, and exchange transfusions designed to prevent high levels of unconjugated serum bilirubin have been shown to protect the nervous system from the toxic effects of erythroblastosis fetalis. If the blood bilirubin level can be held to less than 20 mg/dL (10 mg/dL in premature infants), the nervous system may escape perinatal damage. The effective use of these measures has practically eradicated this disease.

Both kernicterus and ischemic état marbré must be differentiated clinically from hereditary choreoathetosis, the Lesch-Nyhan syndrome, and—later in life, from ataxia-telangiectasia and Friedreich ataxia.

Congenital and Neonatal Ataxias

In these patients, difficulty in standing and walking cannot be attributed to spasticity or paralysis. Hypotonia and poverty of movement are the initial motor abnormalities—as they are in athetoid cerebral palsy. The cerebellar deficit becomes manifest only later when the patient begins to sit, stand, and walk. There may or may not be a delay in reaching the normal motor milestones. Attempts to attain sitting balance early on reveal an unsteadiness that is not soon overcome, even with practice. Reaching for a proffered toy is accomplished by jerky, incoordinated movements. The first steps are unsteady, as would be expected, with many tumbles, but the gait remains clumsy. Instability of the trunk may be accompanied by similar, more or less rhythmic bobbing movements of the head—titubation. Despite the severity of the ataxia, the muscles are of normal size, and voluntary movements, although weak in some patients, are possible in all the limbs. The tendon reflexes are present, and the plantar reflexes are either flexor or extensor. In some cases, the ataxia is later associated with spasticity rather than hypotonia (spastic-ataxic diplegia). Relative improvement may occur in later years. In the older child, a cerebellar gait, ataxia of limb movements, nystagmus, and uneven articulation of words are readily distinguished from myoclonus, chorea, athetosis, dystonia, and tremor.

In only a few cases have the pathologic changes been studied. Aplasia or hypoplasia of the cerebellum has been observed, but sclerotic lesions of the cerebellum are more common. The CT scan or MRI verifies the cerebellar atrophy. However, in a few cases of a cerebellar-like tremor in adults under our care that had been attributed to neonatal injury the MRI did not show cerebellar atrophy. A cerebral and cerebellar lesion may coexist in patients with congenital ataxia, which is the reason for the term *cerebrocerebellar diplegia*.

Several risk factors have been identified in the congenital ataxias. Most importantly, cerebellar ataxia may be the most prominent or sole effect of neonatal ischemia-hypoxia. A genetic factor is operative in some cases (Hagberg and Hagberg). Mercury poisoning in utero is another cause of congenital ataxia. The many cases that are not the result of a degenerative condition, some of which are described just below, remain unexplained in our experience.

Pontocerebellar Hypoplasias and Joubert Syndrome Aside from the congenital ataxia described above, there are several rare familial forms in which a failure of cerebellar development is associated with developmental delay. What has now come to be called Joubert syndrome was reported in a family in which the central feature is dysgenesis of the vermis; developmental delay; episodic hyperpnea; irregular, jerky eye movements; and unsteady gait in 4 of 6 siblings. In other reports, choroidal-retinal colobomas, polydactyly, cryptorchidism, and prognathism have been mentioned. Detailed examination of the cerebra of such individuals has been lacking but the MRI has a characteristic configuration of a "molar tooth sign" that reflects a deep invagination caused by vermian hypoplasia with a narrow cleft separating the cerebellar hemispheres and thickening of the superior cerebellar peduncles. Several genetic loci have been implicated, most acting as recessive traits.

In the *Gillespie syndrome*, a combination of aniridia, cerebellar ataxia, and developmental delay is the denominating feature. In the *Paine syndrome*, a familial disorder with developmental delay and developmental delay, there is microcephaly, spasticity, optic hypoplasia, and myoclonic ataxia, the last presumably related to the cerebellar hypoplasia. These dysgeneses and the disequilibrium syndrome reported from Sweden are unified by the cerebellar ataxia; in the past, they were categorized as ataxic cerebral palsies. Imaging studies demonstrate the cerebellocerebral abnormality. Genetic factors are operative in some, but matters pertaining to etiology remain obscure (see the older monograph by Harding for details). One form of a pure nonprogressive congenital cerebellar hypoplasia has been mapped to a gene locus on chromosome Xq; it does not appear to be related to the fragile X syndrome, which may cause ataxia and tremor in adults as noted further on.

Differential Diagnosis of the Congenital Ataxias The congenital ataxias must be distinguished from the progressive hereditary ataxias. The latter are likely to begin at a later age than the congenital ones. Some hereditary ataxias are intermittent or episodic, one of which is responsive to acetazolamide and is the result of an abnormality of the calcium channel as discussed in Chaps. 5 and 37.

Also to be distinguished from the ataxias of congenital and neonatal origin is an *acute cerebellar ataxia of childhood*, which can usually be traced to a viral infection or postinfectious encephalitis, particularly after chickenpox. The *opsoclonus-myoclonus ("dancing eyes") syndrome* of Kinsbourne is another postinfectious disease peculiar to childhood (see Chaps. 14 and 39). The cerebellar ataxia in this disease may be overshadowed by polymyoclonus, which mars every attempted movement. With improvement, under the influence of corticosteroids, a cerebellar disorder of speech and movement becomes evident. A majority of the patients in which the disease became chronic (16 of the 26 cases followed by Marshall et al) were found later to be mentally slowed. The cause of the disease has never been established. An occult neuroblastoma or other tumor is uncovered occasionally. In the differential diagnosis of these acute forms of cerebellar ataxia, one must not overlook intoxication with phenytoin, barbiturates, or similar drugs.

The Flaccid Paralyses and the "Floppy Infant"

(Table 38-7; See also Chaps. 39 and 48)

The rare cerebral form of generalized flaccidity, first described by Foerster and called *cerebral atonic diplegia*, has already been alluded to in the discussion of cerebral palsy. It can usually be distinguished from the paralysis of spinal and peripheral nerve origin and congenital muscular dystrophy by the retention of postural reflexes (flexion of

Table 38-7

CAUSES OF CONGENITAL HYPOTONIA—THE FLOPPY INFANT SYNDROME

I. Cerebral
   A. Cerebral atonic diplegia (Foerster)
   B. Prader-Willi syndrome
   C. Idiopathic slackness
II. Spinal
   A. Werdnig-Hoffman spinal muscular atrophy
   B. Spinal cord natal injury
III. Myopathic
   A. Polymyopathies—central core, nemaline, rod-body, myotubular, fiber-type disproportion
   B. Infantile muscular dystrophy
   C. Myotonic dystrophy
   D. Polymyositis
IV. Neuropathic
   A. Inflammatory demyelinating neuropathy

(See also Chap. 48.)

the legs at the knees and hips when the infant is lifted by the axillae), preservation of tendon reflexes, and coincident failure of mental development. The Prader-Willi syndrome, discussed earlier in the chapter, also presents at first as a generalized hypotonia.

The syndrome of *infantile spinal muscular atrophy (Werdnig-Hoffmann disease)* is the leading example of flaccid paralysis of lower motor neuron type. Perceptive mothers may be aware of a paucity of fetal movements in utero; in most cases the motor defect becomes evident soon after birth or the infant is born with arthrogrypotic deformities. Several other types of familial progressive muscular atrophies have been described in which the onset is in early or late childhood, adolescence, or early adult life. Weakness, atrophy, and reflex loss without sensory change are the main features and are discussed in detail in Chap. 39. A few patients suspected of having infantile or childhood muscular atrophy prove, with the passage of time, to be merely inactive "slack" children, whose motor development has proceeded at a slower rate than normal. Others may remain weak throughout life, with thin musculature. These and several other congenital myopathies—*central core, rod-body, nemaline, mitochondrial, myotubular, and fiber-type disproportion and predominance*—are described in Chap. 52. Unlike Werdnig-Hoffmann disease, the effects of many of them tend to diminish as the natural growth of muscle proceeds. Rarely, polymyositis and acute idiopathic polyneuritis manifest themselves as a syndrome of congenital hypotonia.

Infantile muscular dystrophy and lipid and glycogen storage diseases may also produce a clinical picture of progressive atrophy and weakness of muscles. The diagnosis of *glycogen storage disease* (usually the Pompe form) should be suspected when progressive muscular atrophy is associated with enlargement of the tongue, heart, liver, or spleen. The motor disturbance in this condition may be related in some way to the abnormal deposits of glycogen in skeletal muscles, although it is more likely the result of degeneration of anterior horn cells that are also distended with glycogen and other substances. Certain forms of *muscular dystrophy* (myotonic dystrophy and several types of congenital dystrophy) may also be evident at birth or soon thereafter. The latter may have led to arthrogryposis and clubfoot (see Chap. 52 for an extensive discussion of the congenital neuromuscular disorders).

Brachial plexus palsies, well-known complications of dystocia, usually result from forcible extraction of the fetus by traction on the shoulder in a breech presentation or from traction and tipping of the head in a shoulder presentation. The effects of such injuries are sometimes lifelong. Their neonatal onset is betrayed later by the small size and inadequate osseous development of the affected limb. Either the upper brachial plexus (fifth and sixth cervical roots) or the lower brachial plexus (seventh and eighth cervical and first thoracic roots) suffer the brunt of the injury. Upper plexus injuries (Erb palsy) are about 20 times more frequent than lower ones (Klumpke palsy). Sometimes the entire plexus is involved. Further details are found in Chap. 46.

Facial paralysis, because of forceps injury to the facial nerve immediately distal to its exit from the stylomastoid foramen, is another common (usually unilateral) peripheral nerve affection in the newborn. Failure of one eye to close and difficulty in sucking make this condition easy to recognize. It must be distinguished from the congenital facial diplegia that is often associated with abducens palsy, that is, the Möbius syndrome discussed earlier in the chapter. In most cases of facial paralysis caused by physical injury, function is recovered after a few weeks; in some, the paralysis is permanent and may account for lifelong facial asymmetry.

Treatment

Once the motor features of cerebral palsy have been established, assistive devices, stretching therapy, and conventional orthopedic measures for joint stabilization and relief of spasticity are all useful. Injection of botulinum toxin for the relief of spasticity has gained wide favor and is now used early in the child's life to preempt deformities. Most published trials have been too small, however, to allow firm conclusions to be drawn about the durability of this treatment. Finally, hyperbaric oxygen treatment of children with cerebral palsy was ineffective in a randomized trial conducted by Collet and colleagues, despite periodic claims to the contrary.

In summary, it can be said that all these forms of disabling motor abnormalities rank high as important issues in neuropediatrics. In attempts at prevention, steps have been taken in most hospitals to identify and eliminate risk factors. Indeed, better prenatal care, reduction in premature births, and control of respiratory problems in critical care wards have reduced their incidence and prevalence. Physical and mental therapeutic measures appear to be helpful, but many of the methods have been difficult to evaluate in a nervous system undergoing maturation and development. The neurologist can contribute most by segregating groups of cases of identical pattern and etiology and in differentiating the congenital groups of delayed expressivity from the treatable acquired diseases of this age period. Woefully lacking are critical neuropathologic studies.

INTRAUTERINE AND NEONATAL INFECTIONS

Throughout the intrauterine period the embryo and fetus are subject to particular infections. Because the infective agent must reach the fetus through the placenta, it is evident that the permeability of the latter at different stages of gestation and the immune status of the maternal organism are determinative. We include a discussion of these intrauterine infections here because some of them may lead to malformations or destructive lesions of the brain and, later in life, must be distinguished from developmental abnormalities.

Until the third to fourth month of gestation, the large microbial organisms—such as bacteria, spirochetes, protozoa, and fungi—cannot invade the embryo, even if the mother harbors the infection. Viruses, however, may do so, specifically rubella, CMV, HIV, and possibly others. The rubella virus enters embryonal tissues during the first trimester, *Treponema pallidum* in the fourth to fifth post-conceptional months, and *Toxoplasma* after that period. Bacterial meningitis (except for that caused by *Listeria monocytogenes*, described below) is essentially a perinatal infection contracted during or immediately after parturition. Neonatal herpes simplex encephalitis, as a result of the type 2 (genital) virus, is also usually acquired by passage through an infected birth canal. Some cases of HIV infection may be acquired during delivery, but most are a result of transplacental transmission.

The main neonatal infections—toxoplasmosis, rubella, CMV, and herpes—have been commonly designated by the acronym TORCH (toxoplasmosis, other infections, rubella, cytomegalovirus, and herpes simplex). With the persistence of *Listeria*, the rise of AIDS infections, and a marked reduction in rubella infections, the mnemonic LATCH, which includes *Listeria* and AIDS, might be more appropriate. Infants with any of these infections share certain common features, such as low birth weight, prematurity, congenital heart disease, purpura, jaundice, anemia, microcephaly or hydrocephaly, cerebral calcifications, chorioretinitis, cataracts, microphthalmia, and pneumonitis; as a corollary, if any combination of these features is manifest, one should suspect one of these infectious agents and take measures to identify it. However, all these clinical manifestations are unlikely to be present in any one infant, and in the cases of rubella and CMV, only a small percentage of infected infants will show major systemic signs or symptoms. Nevertheless, on clinical grounds alone, certain infections can be identified and others excluded. For example, cerebral calcifications are present mainly in toxoplasmosis and CMV encephalopathy, being rare in rubella and absent in herpes simplex virus (HSV) encephalitis; the calcifications are widely disseminated in toxoplasmosis (Fig. 38-16) and have a periventricular distribution in CMV infection. Cardiac lesions are present only with rubella, and deafness occurs only with CMV and rubella. Thus, there are clinical signposts to guide the clinician in selecting the appropriate diagnostic tests. And importantly, in considering neonatal infections, one must also search for other, less-common infectious types (see Chaps. 32 and 33).

Added difficulty in the diagnosis of embryonal and fetal infections arises when the mother has been entirely asymptomatic. Isolation of the organism from fetal and neonatal tissues is possible, but usually they are inaccessible, and it may be impossible to demonstrate antibodies or other immune responses because of the early stage of the infection or limitations of the infant's immune response.

Congenital Rubella

Gregg, in 1941, first reported the association of maternal rubella and congenital cataracts in the neonate. His observations were quickly verified, and soon it became widely known that cataracts, deafness, congenital heart disease, and developmental delay constituted a kind of

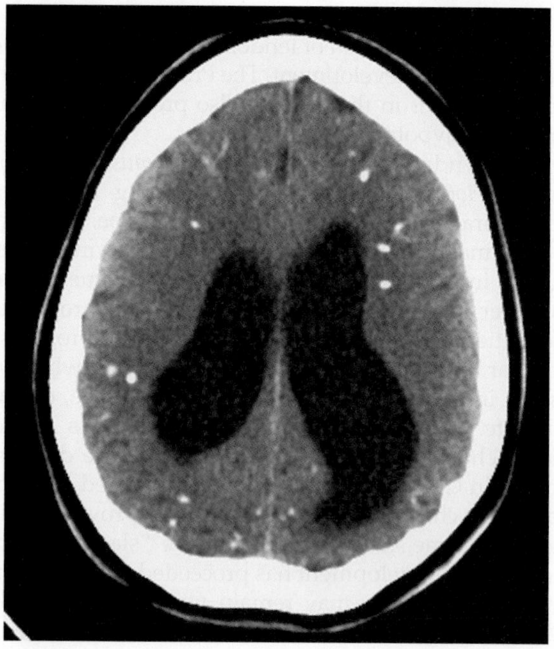

Figure 38-16. CT scan from a developmentally delayed adult with healed congenital toxoplasmosis. There is hydrocephalus and multiple calcifications in the white matter. Contrast this image with Fig. 38-7, which shows the periventricular calcifications of tuberous sclerosis.

tetrad diagnostic of this disease. That a virus could affect so many tissues, causing in essence a noninflammatory developmental disorder of multiple organs, was a novel concept, and it raised the interesting prospect that other viruses might have similar effects. Surprisingly, however, only CMV and possibly HSV have been incriminated in embryonal-developmental neuropathology. A large number of other viruses (e.g., influenza, Epstein-Barr, hepatitis) have been implicated in human teratogenesis, but in none is the relationship beyond doubt.

It is now well established that most instances of congenital rubella infection occur in the first 10 weeks of gestation and that the earlier the infection occurs, the greater the risk to the fetus. However, there may be some risk beyond the first trimester, up to the twenty-fourth week, according to Hardy.

Following the experience of the massive rubella epidemics of 1964 and 1965, the congenital rubella syndrome has been expanded to include low birth weight; sensorineural deafness, sometimes unilateral (the most common complication); microphthalmia; pigmentary degeneration of the retina (salt-and-pepper chorioretinitis); glaucoma, cloudy corneas, and cataracts of special type (the latter two abnormalities usually cause visual impairment); hepatosplenomegaly, jaundice, and thrombocytopenic purpura; and patent ductus arteriosus or interventricular septal defect. There may be one, a few, or many of these abnormalities, in various combinations. The developmental delay is severe and may be accompanied by seizures and motor defects such as hemiplegia or spastic diplegia and rarely by seizures. Psychiatric symptoms, some resembling autism, are said to occur.

Infection of the fetus after the first trimester results in a less impressive neonatal syndrome. The infant may seem lethargic and fail to thrive. The cranium is abnormally small. Only a cardiac abnormality, deafness, or chorioretinitis may provide clues to the diagnosis. The CSF later may show an increase of mononuclear cells and an elevated protein. The infection may persist for a year or longer. Foci of calcification are rare, and CT scanning and MRI are of little help in diagnosis. The maternal infection may be so mild that it is passed off as minor; but even when it is evident, the fetus is spared in approximately 50 percent of cases. Diagnosis can be verified in the neonate by demonstrating immunoglobulin (Ig) M antibodies to the virus or by the isolation of the virus from the throat, urine, stool, or CSF. Also, the virus has been obtained from cells in the amniotic fluid. In subsequent pregnancies, the fetus has been normal in our experience.

The neuropathology is of considerable interest. In the nervous system of fetuses exposed to maternal rubella in the first trimester, R.D. Adams found no visible lesions by light microscopy, even though the virus had been isolated from the brain by Enders (personal communications). At this period of development there is no inflammatory reaction because of the absence of polymorphonuclear leukocytes, lymphocytes, and other mononuclear cells in the fetus. At birth the brain is usually of normal size, and there may be no discernible lesions. There may be a mild meningeal infiltration of lymphocytes, and a few zones of necrosis and vasculitis with later calcification of vessels are seen, as are small hemorrhages, presumably related to the thrombocytopenia. Smallness of the brain and delay in myelination have been observed in children who died at 1 to 2 years of age. None of the brains in Adam's series was malformed. Rubella virus continues to be recoverable from the CSF for at least 18 months after birth. A form of delayed progressive rubella encephalitis in childhood is also known and is described in Chap. 33 under "Progressive Rubella Panencephalitis." Because there is no treatment for the active infection, the obvious approach to the problem of congenital rubella infection is to make sure that every woman of childbearing age has been vaccinated against rubella or has antibodies as a result of infection prior to pregnancy. The widespread use of rubella vaccine has reduced the chance of major outbreaks, but sporadic infections continue to be seen, and outbreaks of epidemic proportions continue to occur in developing countries.

Congenital Cytomegalovirus Infection

For many years it was known that there were swollen cells containing intranuclear and cytoplasmic inclusions in the tissues of some infants who died in the first weeks and months of life. This cytologic change seemed related to the fatalities. In 1956 and 1957, three different laboratories isolated what has come to be called the *human cytomegalovirus* (see Weller). This has proved to be the most frequent intrauterine viral infection, rivaled in the current era only by HIV.

CMV disease is widespread in the general population. Although cervicitis is common, the virus is probably transmitted to the fetus transplacentally. Infection of the fetus usually occurs in the first trimester of pregnancy, sometimes later, by way of an inapparent maternal viremia and infection of the placenta. The newborn can also be infected in the course of delivery or afterward by the mother's milk or by transfusions. However, only a small proportion of women known to harbor the virus give birth to infants with active infection. The likelihood of the fetus being infected is much greater if the seronegative mother becomes infected for the first time during pregnancy. In one study, 18 percent of infants born to such mothers were symptomatic at birth, and 25 percent became blind, deaf, or cognitively impaired within a few years (Fowler et al). In mothers with recurrent CMV infection, the infants were asymptomatic at birth, and only a few developed serious sequelae. Evidently, the presence of maternal antibodies before conception protects against congenital CMV infection.

Early infection of the fetus may result in a malformation of the brain; later, there is only inflammatory necrosis from encephalitis in parts of the normally formed brain. Disseminated inflammatory foci have been observed in the cerebrum, brainstem, and retinae. Here there were aggregates of lymphocytes, mononuclear cells, and plasma cells. The mononuclear histiocytes (microglia cells) contain inclusion bodies; some astrocytes are similarly affected. Granulomas form and later calcify, particularly in the periventricular regions. Often there is hydrocephalus. In the low-birth-weight or full-term infant, the clinical picture is one of jaundice, petechiae, hematemesis, melena, direct hyperbilirubinemia, thrombocytopenia, hepatosplenomegaly, microcephaly, mental defect, and convulsions. Cells in the urine may show cytomegalic changes. There is a pleocytosis and an increased protein in the CSF.

Congenital CMV infections pose a much greater problem than does rubella. There is no way of identifying the infected fetus prior to birth or to prevent inapparent infections in the pregnant woman. As indicated above, if the pregnant woman has measurable titers of antibodies to CMV at the time of conception, her infant is relatively protected. Moreover, some infected infants (with viruria) may appear normal at birth but develop neural deafness and developmental delay several years later. Viral replication in infected organs continues after the first year and health workers are at risk. A second child may be infected.

There is no known treatment. The difficulties in prenatal diagnosis of maternal infection preclude planned abortion. Routine serologic testing should be done on every young woman of childbearing age. Until an effective vaccine becomes available, pregnancy should be avoided if a sexual partner is infected.

Congenital HIV Infection and AIDS

In the United States, approximately 10 percent of cases of AIDS have occurred in women, almost all of them of childbearing age, and the rate of new cases is increasing at a faster rate among them than among men. The numbers are higher in many developing countries and particularly in parts of Africa. In children, practically all instances of AIDS come from an HIV-infected mother ("vertical transmission"). The infection may be acquired in utero, during delivery, or from breast-feeding. The relative importance of each of these modes of transmission has not been settled.

It is estimated that HIV infection and AIDS occur in 15 to 30 percent of infants born to HIV-seropositive mothers (see Prober and Gerson). Infected infants present special difficulties in diagnosis, and the infection runs a more accelerated course in them than in adults. In the perinatal period, infected and noninfected infants can only rarely be distinguished clinically, and laboratory diagnosis is hampered by the presence of maternally derived antibody to HIV. The initial clinical signs usually appear within a few months after birth; practically all infected infants become ill before their first birthday, and very few are asymptomatic beyond 3 years of age. Early signs consist of lymphadenopathy, splenomegaly, hepatomegaly, failure to thrive, oral candidiasis, and parotitis. In the European Collaborative Study, comprising 600 children born to HIV-infected mothers, 83 percent of infected children showed laboratory or clinical features of HIV infection by 6 months of age. By 12 months, 26 percent had clinical symptoms of AIDS and 17 percent had died of HIV-related diseases. Once AIDS is established in children, it does not differ materially from the syndrome in adults as described in Chap. 33.

There is often a delay in the attainment of psychomotor milestones. Or after a period of normal development, a psychomotor decline begins, with corticospinal or peripheral nerve signs, often with pleocytosis in the CSF. The typical giant cell AIDS encephalitis, neuritis, and myelitis are easily distinguished from CMV encephalitis and toxoplasmosis.

Infected children are also subject to a variety of opportunistic infections, including bacterial meningitis, toxoplasmosis, CMV encephalitis, fungal infections (cryptococcosis, aspergillosis, candidiasis), herpes simplex, syphilis, zoster, and mycobacterial meningitis. There may also be vascular lesions, with infarction or hemorrhage and lymphoid neoplasia. These are discussed in Chaps. 32 and 33. To date, there is little that one can do for these children, but this may be changing with the current use of 3-drug antiretroviral therapy.

Congenital Toxoplasmosis

This tiny protozoan *Toxoplasma gondii*, occurring freely or in pseudocyst form, is a frequent cause of meningoencephalitis in utero or in the perinatal period of life. The disease exists in all parts of the world but is more frequent in Western European countries, particularly in those with hot, humid climates, than it is in the United States. The mother is most often infected by exposure to cat feces, handling uncooked infected mutton or other meat, or eating partially cooked meat, but she is nearly always asymptomatic or has only a mild fever and cervical lymphadenopathy.

The precise times of placental and fetal invasion are unknown, but presumably they occur late in the gestational period. The clinical syndrome usually becomes manifest in the first days and weeks of postnatal life, when seizures, impaired alertness, hypotonia, weakness of the extremities, progressive hydrocephalus, and chorioretinitis appear. The retinal lesions consist of large pale areas of destroyed retina surrounded by deposits of pigment. If the infection is severe, the maculae are destroyed; optic atrophy and microphthalmos follow. We have several times observed hemiplegias in older infants, first on one side and then on the other, followed by tension hydrocephalus. The latter is present in about one-third of the cases.

The CSF contains a moderate number of white blood cells, mostly lymphocytes and mononuclear cells, and the protein content is in the range of 100 to 400 mg/dL (i.e., a higher protein content than all other neonatal infections except bacterial meningitis). The glucose values are normal. Fewer than 10 percent of infected children recover; the others are developmentally delayed to varying degrees, with seizures and paralysis. In those without symptoms of infection at birth, the outcome is better.

Granulomatous masses and zones of inflammatory necrosis abut the ependyma and meninges. The organisms, 6 to 7 mm in length and 2 to 4 mm in width, are visible in and near the lesions. Microcysts may also be found, lying free in the tissues without surrounding inflammatory reaction. The necrotic lesions calcify rapidly and, after several weeks or months, are readily visible in plain films of the skull. These appear in periventricular and other regions of the brain as multiple nodular densities (see Fig. 38-16).

In adults, often in association with AIDS, the disease takes the form of a rapidly evolving meningitis and multifocal encephalitis in conjunction with myocarditis, hepatitis, and polymyositis.

This syndrome is described in Chap. 32, as are the diagnostic tests and current treatment. In the infant, infections such as rubella, syphilis, CMV disease, and herpes simplex must be considered in the differential diagnosis. The most reliable means of diagnosis is the IgM indirect fluorescent antibody test, performed on umbilical cord blood. Passive transfer of IgG antibody from mother to fetus takes place, but its presence in the fetus is not proof of active infection.

In women who develop antibodies in the first 2 or 3 months of pregnancy, treatment with spiramycin (Rovamycine) prevents fetal infection. Once the fetus is infected, pyrimethamine and sulfadiazine must be used. A later second pregnancy is not affected.

Congenital Neurosyphilis

The clinical syndromes and pathologic reactions of congenital neurosyphilis of the newborn are similar to those of the adult, as described in Chap. 32. Such differences that exist are determined principally by the immaturity of the nervous system at the time of spirochetal invasion. The syphilitic infection may be transmitted to the fetus at any time from the fourth to the seventh months. The fetus may die, with resulting miscarriage or stillbirth, or may survive only to be born with florid manifestations of secondary syphilis. The dissemination of the spirochetes throughout the body, the time of appearance of the secondary manifestations, and the time of formation of antisyphilitic antibodies (reagin) in the blood are all governed by the same biologic principles that apply to adult syphilis.

At birth, the spirochetemia may not have had time to cause syphilitic antibodies to appear; hence a negative Venereal Disease Research Laboratory (VDRL) reaction in umbilical cord blood does not exclude congenital syphilis. In unselected groups of syphilitic mothers, 25 to 80 percent of fetuses have been infected, and in 20 to 40 percent of those infected, the CNS is invaded as judged by the finding of abnormal CSF. The types of congenital neurosyphilis (asymptomatic and symptomatic meningitis, meningovascular disease, hydrocephalus, general paresis, and tabes dorsalis) are the same as those in the adult except for the great rarity of tabes dorsalis. The classic Hutchinson triad (dental deformities, interstitial keratitis, and bilateral deafness) is infrequently observed in complete form.

The sequence of neurologic syndromes is also the same as in the adult, all stemming basically from chronic spirochetal meningitis. The infection may become symptomatic in the first weeks and months of postnatal life, meningovascular lesions and hydrocephalus reaching maximal frequency during the period from 9 months to 6 years. An early form of syphilitic meningoencephalitis may occur at 1 to 2 years and result in severe developmental delay. More often, a congenital paresis and tabes usually appear between the ninth and fifteenth years. The pathologic basis of the neurosyphilitic syndromes is discussed in Chap. 32.

Fewer cases of congenital neurosyphilis are being observed as the years pass, but there may be a recrudescence of the disease in HIV-infected patients. If the syphilitic mother is treated before the fourth month of pregnancy, the fetus will not be infected. The affected infant may be normal at birth or exhibit only mucocutaneous lesions, hepatosplenomegaly, lymphadenopathy, and anemia. In the neonatal period, there are no signs of meningeal invasion, or there may be only asymptomatic meningitis. If the latter is actively treated until the CSF is normal, vascular lesions of brain and spinal cord, hydrocephalus, general paresis, and tabes dorsalis will not develop.

Congenital syphilis must be considered a potential, albeit rare, cause of epilepsy and developmental delay. Once the syphilitic infection has been treated in early life and rendered inactive (acellular CSF, normal protein), the occurrence of a congenital infection can only be substantiated by an accurate history; the finding of the syphilitic stigmata in the eyes, teeth, and ears; or a positive serologic reaction in the CSF.

Treatment of syphilis in the child follows along the same lines as treatment of the syphilitic adult (see Chap. 32), with appropriate adjustment of dosage in accordance with the child's weight.

Other Viral and Bacterial Infections

Several other infections of late fetal life or the neonatal period are only mentioned here, for to describe them all would be excessive and would elucidate no new neurologic principles. Meningitis as a result of the small gram-positive rod *L. monocytogenes* may be acquired in the usual way, at the time of passage through an infected birth canal or in utero, as a complication of maternal and fetal septicemia because of this organism. In the latter case, it causes abortion or premature delivery. Neonatal bacterial meningitis with this organism is a particularly devastating and often fatal type of bacterial infection, not easily diagnosed unless the pediatrician is alert to the possibility of a silent meningitis in every case of neonatal infection. Coxsackievirus B, polioviruses, other enteroviruses, and arboviruses (western equine) seem to be able to cross the placental barrier late in pregnancy and cause encephalitis or encephalomyelitis in the near-term fetus, which is indistinguishable from the disease in the very young infant. Herpes zoster may occur in utero, leaving cutaneous scars and retarding development. Or zoster may appear soon after birth, the infection having been contracted from the mother. Only later in childhood can varicella induce an autoimmune perivenous demyelination and possibly a direct infection, affecting predominantly the cerebellum (see Chap. 33), or it may precede the now rare Reye syndrome.

Epstein-Barr virus is another frequent cause of meningoencephalitis. In some instances, it may present as aseptic meningitis or a Guillain-Barré type of acute polyneuritis. This infection tends to affect the nervous system of children rather than that of adults, but there are exceptions to this comment. It is estimated that approximately 2 percent of children and adolescents with this infection have some type of neurologic dysfunction; rarely will this be the only manifestation of the disease. Stupor, chorea, and aseptic meningitis were the main neurologic findings in the case reported by Friedland and Yahr, and acute cerebellar ataxia and deafness were observed in the case of Erzurum and associates (see also Chaps. 32 and 33).

EPILEPSIES OF INFANCY AND CHILDHOOD

The major types of seizure disorder have already been discussed in some detail in Chap. 16. In bringing them up here, attention is drawn to the fact that epilepsy is mainly a disease of infancy and childhood. Approximately 75 percent of epileptics fall into these age periods, and some of the most interesting and unique types of seizures are peculiar to these epochs of life. Epilepsies that are observed exclusively in infants and children are benign neonatal convulsions; benign myoclonic epilepsy of infancy; febrile seizures (both genetic and acquired); infantile spasms of West; absence seizures; the Lennox-Gastaut syndrome; rolandic and occipital paroxysms and other benign focal epilepsies; and the juvenile myoclonic epilepsies.

One principle that emerges is that the form taken by seizures in early life is in part age-linked. Neonatal seizures are predominantly partial or focal; infantile seizures take the form of myoclonic flexor (sometimes extensor) spasms; and the various forms of petit mal are essentially diseases of childhood (4 to 13 years). The motor phenomena of epilepsy in young children are often termed *myoclonic*, but this should not be confused with other, later-occurring epilepsies that are endowed with the same name. Furthermore, certain epileptic states tend to occur only during certain epochs of life—one type of febrile seizure from 6 months to 6 years, generalized or temporal spike-wave activity with benign motor and complex partial seizures from 6 to 16 years, and juvenile myoclonic epilepsy in the mid- and late-adolescent years. In general, idiopathic epilepsy, so called because the cause cannot be determined, is predominantly a pediatric neurologic problem. This is not to say that seizures of unknown cause do not occur for the first time in adult life but rather that the onset of such seizures is far more frequent in childhood and tends to diminish once adulthood is reached.

The clinical characteristics of infantile and childhood seizures, including those of genetic origin, are fully described in Chap. 16.

Developmental Delay Without Physical Morphologic Changes (Nondysmorphic Developmental delay)

Clinical Features

Two clinical types can be recognized based on the adequacy of motor skills that are acquired in parallel with cognitive skills. *In the first*, the essential characteristic is that, almost from birth, the infant is delayed in all aspects of development. There is a tendency to sleep more, to be less demanding of nourishment, to move less than normal, and to suck poorly and regurgitate. Parents comment on how good their baby is, how little he troubles them by crying. As the months pass, every expected achievement is late. The baby is usually more hypotonic and turns over, sits unsupported, and walks later than the normal infant. Yet despite these obvious motor delays, there is later no sign of paralysis, ataxia, chorea, or athetosis. These babies do not smile at the usual time and take little notice of the mother or other persons or objects in their environment. They are less attentive to visual, and often to auditory, stimuli, to the point where questions may be raised about blindness or deafness. Certain phases of normal development, such as hand regard, may persist beyond the sixth month, when they are normally replaced by other activities. Mouthing (putting everything in the mouth) and slobbering, which should end by 1 year of age, also persist. There are only fleeting signs of interest in toys, and the impersistence of attention becomes increasingly prominent. Vocalizations are scant, often guttural, piercing, or high-pitched and feeble. Babbling is not replaced by attempts at word formation at the usual time.

In the second type, early motor milestones (supporting the head, rolling over, sitting, standing, and walking) are attained approximately at their normal times, yet the infant is inattentive and slow in learning the usual nursery tricks. It seems as though motor development had somehow escaped the retardation process. There may, however, be aimless overactivity and persistence of rhythmic movements, grinding of the teeth (bruxism), and hypotonia.

Because the developmental sequence of motor function and speech may be normal, even to the point where the baby acquires a few words by the end of the first year, the examiner may be misled into thinking that the delayed infant was at first normal and had then deteriorated. In such infants it can even be shown that various test procedures yield lower scores with progressing age (from 3 years onward); this is not the result of a decline in ability but of the fact that the tests are not comparable at different times. In the early years, the tests are weighted toward sensorimotor functions and after that toward perception, memory, and concept formation. Interestingly, the development of language depends upon both groups of functions, needing a certain maturation of the auditory and motor apparatus at the start and highly specialized cognitive skills for continued development. These and other aspects of development of speech and language were considered earlier in this chapter and are commented on further in Chaps. 23 and 38.

Members of both groups of these mildly delayed individuals exhibit a number of noteworthy features that have medical and social implications. Although not overtly dysmorphic and having a normal or low-normal head circumference, they have a high incidence of minor congenital anomalies of the eyes, face, mouth, ears, and hands; they tend to be sickly, and the more severely affected among them have poor physiques and are often under-sized. Difficult behavior occurs frequently, most often taking the form of poor self-control and aggressiveness, especially pronounced in children with temporal lobe epilepsy. Other behavioral disturbances are restlessness, repetitive activity, explosive rage reactions and tantrums, stereotyped play, and the seeking of sensory experiences in unusual ways (Chess and Hassibi). Pica (the compulsive ingestion of nonnutritive substances) is a problem between ages 2 and 4 years of age, but is also seen in normal, neglected children.

An endless debate is centered on matters of causation—whether this category of mild delay is the product of genetic influence or of societal discrimination and lack of training and education coupled with the effects of malnutrition, infections, or other exogenous factors. Surely both factors are at work, with the genetic being dominant for the reasons discussed above, although the relative importance of each has proved difficult to determine (Moser et al).

A pathologic basis for most cases of mild developmental delay has not been established and new methodologies, perhaps relating to neuronal connectivity, will be needed if the brains of these individuals are to be differentiated from normal children. Differences might be expected in terms of the number of neurons in thalamic nuclei and cortex, in dendritic–axonal connectivity, or in synaptic surfaces, elements that are not being assayed by the conventional techniques of tissue neuropathology. The observations of Huttenlocher, who found a sparsity of dendritic arborization in Golgi-Cox preparations, and of Purpura, who found an absence of short, thick spines on dendrites of cortical neurons and other abnormalities of dendritic spines, are first steps in this direction but require confirmation.

Genetic Aspects of Nonsyndromic Developmental Delay

Sex linkage is a notable feature of some types of mild developmental delay. The fragile X syndrome, discussed later, is the most important of this group, predominating in males and accounting for approximately 10 percent of all cases of male developmental delay. These individuals may be physically normal except for large testicles. Renpenning and colleagues reported a series of 21 developmentally delayed males in three generations of a Canadian family, all free of any congenital malformations and with normal head size, and Turner and coworkers have described a similar Australian series. Other X-linked forms of developmental delay that have few or no dysmorphic features include the Partington, Lowe, Lesch-Nyhan, and Menkes syndromes and adrenoleukodystrophy, each with special characteristics in addition to developmental delay, as discussed in Chap. 37. Numerous other X-linked retardation syndromes with profound accompanying neurologic anomalies have been delineated; for example, the one caused by a mutation in the oligophrenin gene, in which there is epilepsy, and another involving cerebellar hypoplasia. The relationship of intelligence in general to the X chromosome is discussed in Chap. 21.

However, there is emerging information relating autosomal mutations, rather than X-linked ones, in genes that control synaptic function such as SYNGAP1, and non-dysmorphic developmental delay as detailed in the publication by Hamdan and coworkers. There are approximately 30 X-linked and 6 autosomal recessive genes associated with nonsyndromic developmental delay and more are sure to be found. Investigated from another perspective, de Ligt and colleagues sequenced the coding regions of over 21,000 genes in a series of 100 individuals with IQ below 50 and round that there were numerous de novo mutations that involved cerebral development of function. Together, all of the aforementioned genetic alterations, mutations, lesser polymorphisms and copy number variants, account for approximately 15 to 20 percent of cases of mild, moderate, and severe developmental delay and autism. Most are de novo mutations, making their discovery difficult. The challenge will be to elucidate the manner in which they disrupt cerebral development on a synaptic or subcellular level.

Diagnosis

Infants should be considered at risk for developmental delay when there is a family history of mental slowness, low birth weight in relation to the length of gestation (small-for-date babies), marked prematurity, maternal infection early in pregnancy (especially rubella), and toxemia of pregnancy. In the first few months of life, certain of the behavioral characteristics described above are of value in predicting developmental delay. Prechtl and associates have found that a low Apgar score (especially at 5 min after delivery, Table 28-3), flaccidity, underactivity, and asymmetrical neurologic signs are the earliest indices of subnormality in the infant. Slow habituation of orienting reactions to novel auditory and visual stimuli and the presence of "fine motor deficits" (as previously discussed under "Delays in Motor Development") are other early warnings of developmental delay.

In the first year or two of life, suspicion of developmental delay is based largely on clinical impression, but it should always be validated by psychometric procedures. Most pediatric neurologists use some of the criteria laid down by Gesell and Amatruda or the Denver Developmental Screening Scale, from which a DQ is calculated.

For testing of preschool children, the Wechsler Preschool and Primary Scale of Intelligence is used, and for school-age children, the Wechsler Intelligence Scale for Children is preferred. IQ tests for preschoolers must be interpreted with caution, as they have had less predictive validity for school success than the tests that are used after 6 years of age. In general, however, normal scores for age on any of these tests essentially eliminate developmental delay as a cause of poor school achievement and learning disabilities; special cognitive defects may, however, be revealed by low scores on particular subtests. Developmentally delayed children not only have low scores but exhibit more scatter of subtest scores. Also, like demented adults, they generally achieve greater success with performance than with verbal items. It is essential that the physician know the conditions of testing, for poor scores may be due to fright, inadequate motivation, lapses in attention, dyslexia, or a subtle auditory or visual defect rather than a developmental lag.

The EEG, in addition to exposing asymptomatic seizure activity, shows a high incidence of other abnormalities in the developmentally delayed child. Presumably this is because of a greater degree of immaturity of the cerebrum at any given age. However, a normal EEG is not infrequent and of relatively little help. Moreover, CT scanning and MRI have been singularly unhelpful in revealing abnormalities in this group of children.

In the diagnosis of milder grades of retardation, the possible effects of severe malnutrition, neglect and deprivation, chronic systemic disease, iodine deficiency, impaired hearing and vision, and possibly childhood psychosis should be considered. *Of particular importance is the differentiation of a group of patients who are normal for a variable period after birth and then manifest a progressive decline* from disease of the nervous system. This type of disorder is representative of the group of hereditary metabolic and degenerative diseases discussed in Chap. 37. Seizure disorders (and antiepileptic medications) can impair cerebral function, and several special childhood seizure disorders are associated with a progressive decline in mental function in this group of patients (see Chap. 16).

Management of Mild Developmental Delay

Because there is little or no possibility of restoring function to a nervous system that is developmentally or structurally damaged, the medical objective is to assist in planning for the patient's training, education, and social and occupational adjustments. As Voltaire remarked long ago, guidance is needed more than education. The parents must be guided in forming realistic attitudes and expectations. Psychiatric and social counseling may help the family to maintain gentle but firm support of the patient so that he can acquire, to the fullest extent possible, self-help skills, self-control, good work habits, and a congenial personality.

Most individuals with an IQ above 60 and no other handicaps can be trained to live an independent life. Special schooling enables such patients to realize their full potential. Social factors that contribute to underachievement must be eliminated if possible. Later, there is need for advice about possible occupational attainments. Great care must be exercised in deciding about institutionalization. Whereas severe degrees of retardation are all too apparent by the first or second year, less-severe degrees are difficult to recognize early. As stated above, psychologic tests alone are not trustworthy. The method of assessment suggested many years ago by Fernald still has a ring of soundness. It includes (1) physical examination, (2) family background, (3) developmental history, (4) school progress (grade achieved), (5) performance in schoolwork (tests of reading, arithmetic, etc.), (6) practical knowledge, (7) social behavior, (8) industrial efficiency, (9) moral reactions, and (10) intelligence as measured by psychologic tests. All these data except (5) and (10) can be obtained by a skillful physician during the initial medical and neurologic examination and are used to guide the family in its difficult decisions.

SEVERE FORMS OF DEVELOPMENTAL DELAY

The subject of developmental delay was introduced in Chap. 28, where it was pointed out that two major categories of this disorder have been delineated. In one, and by far the more common group, the mental limitation is relatively mild, allowing the individual to succeed with training and education; it is often familial and is featured by a lack of definite neurologic abnormalities (except possibly a slightly higher incidence of seizures) and the absence of neuropathologic changes. A large part of this group, falling between 2 and 3 standard deviations below the normal mean IQ, probably are the lower end of the Gaussian curve of intelligence, the converse of which is genius. This group is, however, contaminated with a small number of defined diseases of the nervous system occurring in a less-severe form. In a second group, the degree of developmental delay is usually more severe (IQ of 50 to 70), and yet more so in the third group (IQ less than 50 or not measurable because of limitations of cooperation or physical impediments). Most of the cases in the second and third groups are nonfamilial, and a wide variety of neuropathologic changes are in evidence. The subdivisions are not absolute, for there are a few metabolic and developmental diseases in which developmental delay is profound yet with no somatic or neurologic abnormalities and, most importantly, well-defined neuropathologic changes are lacking. Here we refer to conditions such as Rett syndrome, autism, and the X-linked developmental delay syndromes (Renpenning and fragile X types). In this chapter, these major types of *severe developmental delay* are described.

The overall frequency of severe developmental delay cannot be stated precisely. Rough estimates place the figure at 0.2 to 0.4 percent of the general population and at approximately 10 percent of the general developmentally delayed segment of society. It is important to emphasize that in a large proportion of individuals with severe developmental delay, a particular congenital abnormality or anomaly of development cannot at present be traced to any of the disorders reviewed in the preceding pages. More precisely stated, when groups of such severely impaired patients are studied clinically, a reasonably accurate etiologic determination of the underlying brain disease can be made in only slightly more than half. According to Penrose, chromosomal abnormalities account for 15 percent, single-gene disorders for 7 percent, and environmental agents for 20 percent. More recent studies of the subtelomeric parts of chromosomes reportedly find abnormalities in another 7 percent of severely retarded children (Knight et al). No cause is found for the remaining cases. Males outnumber females 3 to 1.

However, from the neuropathologic standpoint, *the examination of the brains of the severely developmentally delayed by conventional histopathologic methods discloses lesions in approximately 90 percent, and in fully three-quarters of the entire group, an etiologic diagnosis can be determined or tentatively assigned*. Many of the remaining 10 percent lack definite pathologic changes, but their brains are lighter in weight by 10 to 15 percent than age-matched normal brains. Interestingly, the proportion of vascular, hypoxic-ischemic, metabolic, and genetic lesions in this group of severely impaired individuals is much the same as is found in a group selected on the basis of "cerebral palsy."

Here it is important to repeat a point made earlier and in Chap. 28: A few of the severely disabled and a large majority of the mildly affected do not have a recognizable cerebral pathology or exhibit any of the familiar and conventional signs of cerebral disease. Although the milder forms of developmental delay tend to be familial, this does not by itself separate them from the severe forms of developmental delay. There are several types of hereditary developmental delay, in which the retardation may be severe and in some of which there may be maldevelopment of the cerebral cortex. These are discussed further on.

Clinical Characteristics of the Severely Developmentally Delayed

These cases can be broadly divided into four groups. In one large group, designated *dysmorphic retardation*, a variety of physical deformities, including microcephaly, is commonly present. In a second group, with *multiple-system retardation*, the developmental delay is linked to nonskeletal abnormalities (e.g., hepatosplenomegaly, hematologic and skin disorders), which provide reliable clues to the underlying somatic disease. In a third group, *neurologic retardation*, somatic abnormalities are lacking but a configuration of neurologic signs leads to the diagnosis. In the fourth group, and the most difficult one to clarify, that comprising *uncomplicated retardation*, there are no or minimal somatic, visceral, or neurologic abnormalities. One is then forced to turn to special features of the developmental delay itself for identification of the underlying disease. Table 38-8 elaborates a reasonable classification of the types of developmental delay.

The profoundly developmentally delayed infant with a virtually untestable IQ is identified early in life because he does not sit, stand, or walk. If any one of these motor activities is acquired, it appears late and is imperfectly performed. Language never develops; at most a few spoken words or phrases are understood and fewer are uttered, or the patient only vocalizes in a meaningless way. Such a person may not even indicate bodily needs for food, drink, excretion, and so on. Usually the patient is continuously idle and interacts little with people and objects. Only the most primitive emotional reactions are exhibited, often without connection to an appropriate stimulus. Physical growth is usually retarded, nutrition may be poor, and susceptibility to infections is increased. Sphincteric control may never be attained and, if attained, is precarious.

When the mental defect is less severe than described above, falling into the IQ ranges of 20 to 45, or 45 to 70, there may be somatic neurologic abnormalities. If specific motor defects do not coexist, then sitting, standing, and walking are achieved but not at the expected times. The existence of a mental defect is most clearly evidenced by a delay in psychomotor development and a failure to speak by the second or third postnatal year. The patient does not acquire the usual household and play activities as well as other children. However, delay in speech development must not, by itself, be taken as a mark of developmental delay, for in some children a unique delay in speech can be an isolated abnormality as described in Chap. 28, with subsequent normal development of speech and mental ability. Toilet training may be difficult to accomplish in the developmentally delayed child, but, again, bedwetting may be a problem in an otherwise normal child. Also, the deaf child may have to be considered separately; here the problem becomes apparent by an indifference to noise and reduced vocalization (stereotypy of babbling).

More thorough analyses of cognitive functions in the moderately cognitively impaired child have been undertaken by O'Connor and Hermelin, Pulsifer, and others. These authors measured the efficiency of visual and auditory perception, adequacy of communication, relations between language development and thought, crossmodal sensory encoding, alertness, attention, and memory. It was concluded that none of these functions was specifically impaired. Instead, the child could not properly encode new information because the memory systems and the stock of past assimilated knowledge were insufficient to provide a framework of items and categories with which new information could be integrated. Some patients also seemed unable, perhaps on the basis of this encoding problem, to extract from perceived material selective features that could be interpreted. Furthermore, they were unable to deal with an array of sensory experiences like normal children. The complexity of these mental operations, which we

Table 38-8

TYPES OF SEVERE DEVELOPMENTAL DELAY

I. Dysmorphic defect with somatic developmental abnormalities in nonnervous structures
   A. Those affecting cranioskeletal structures
      1. Microcephaly
      2. Macrocephaly
      3. Hydrocephalus (including myelomeningocele with Chiari malformation and associated cerebral anomalies)
      4. Down syndrome
      5. Cretinism (congenital hypothyroidism)
      6. Mucopolysaccharidoses (Hurler, Hunter, and Sanfilippo types)
      7. Acrocephalosyndactyly (craniostenosis) and other craniosomatic abnormalities
      8. Arthrogryposis multiplex congenita (in certain cases)
      9. Rare specific syndromes: De Lange
      10. Dwarfism, short stature: Russel-Silver dwarf, Seckel bird-headed dwarf, Rubinstein-Taybi dwarf, Cockayne-Neel dwarf, etc.
      11. Hypertelorism, median cleft face syndromes, agenesis of corpus callosum
   B. Those affecting nonskeletal structures
      1. Neurocutaneous syndromes: tuberous sclerosis, Sturge-Weber, neurofibromatosis
      2. Congenital rubella syndrome (deafness, blindness, congenital heart disease, small stature)
      3. Chromosomal disorders: Down syndrome, some cases of Klinefelter syndrome (XXY), XYY, Turner (XO) syndrome (occasionally), and others
      4. Laurence-Moon-Biedl syndrome (retinitis pigmentosa, obesity, polydactyly)
      5. Eye disorders: toxoplasmosis (chorioretinitis), galactosemia (cataract), congenital rubella
      6. Prader-Willi syndrome (obesity, hypogenitalism)
II. Nondysmorphic mental defect without somatic anomalies but with cerebral and other neurologic abnormalities
   A. Cerebral spastic diplegia
   B. Cerebral hemiplegia, unilateral or bilateral
   C. Congenital choreoathetosis or ataxia
      1. Kernicterus
      2. Status marmoratus
   D. Congenital ataxia
   E. Congenital atonic diplegia
   F. Syndromes resulting from hypoglycemia, trauma, meningitis, and encephalitis
   G. Associated with other neuromuscular abnormalities (muscular dystrophy, cerebellar ataxia, etc.)
   H. Cerebral degenerative diseases (lipidoses)
   I. Associated with inborn errors of metabolism (phenylketonuria, other aminoacidurias, organic acidurias, Lesch-Nyhan syndrome)
   J. Congenital infections (some cases of congenital syphilis, cytomegalic inclusion disease)
III. Genetic mental defect with minor or no signs of somatic abnormality or neurologic disorder
   A. Infantile autism, Renpenning, Williams, fragile X, Partington, and Rett syndromes

would reduce to a global failure of the normal processes of apperception and integration, was called by Piaget a "failure of assimilation and accommodation." However, within the spectrum of developmental delay, apart from cognitive impairments, there are curious differences in behavior and personality, even in those with more or less the same IQ. Some individuals with moderately severe retardation are pleasant and amiable and achieve a satisfactory social adjustment. This is particularly notable in patients with Down and Williams syndromes. At the opposite end of the behavioral scale are the syndromes of autism and that of Smith-Magenis and of DeLange, in which the individual fails to manifest normal interpersonal social contact, including communicative language. The phenylketonuric child is usually irritable, unaffectionate, and implacable, and the same is said of certain other forms of retardation, discussed earlier in the section on retardation with dwarfism.

Regarding differences in motor activity levels, many developmentally delayed individuals are slow, clumsy, and relatively akinetic. Others, as many as half, display an incessant hyperactivity characterized by a restless, seemingly inquisitive searching of the environment. When thwarted, they may exhibit a low frustration tolerance. They may be destructive and recklessly fearless and impervious to the risk of injury. Some exhibit a peculiar anhedonia that renders them indifferent to both punishment and reward. Other aberrant types of behaviors, such as violent aggressiveness and self-mutilation, are common.

Rhythmic rocking, head-banging, incessant arm movements—so-called *rhythmias* or *movement stereotypies*—are observed in the majority of those who are severely and moderately severely impaired. These movements are maintained hour after hour without fatigue and may be accompanied by breathing sounds, squeals, and other exclamations. A number of them tend to be particularly common in certain forms of retardation: hand-flapping in autism, handwringing in Rett syndrome, and hand-waving in Down syndrome and other disorders. Self-stimulation, even hurtful—such as striking the forehead or ears or biting the fingers and forearms—seems to be compulsive or perhaps to provide some sort of satisfaction. It is not that these rhythmias are by themselves abnormal, for some of them occur for brief periods in normal babies, but that they persist. Nevertheless, many moderately delayed persons, when assigned to a simple task such as putting envelopes in a box, can continue this activity under supervision for several hours.

In the least-severe types of retardation, all the mental activities are intact but subnormal. The point to be made is that all aspects of intellectual life, personality, and deportment are affected in slightly differing degrees and that these effects have a neurologic basis. There is more than a hint that in particular diseases, because of their anatomy, the cognitive experience, affective life, and behavior are affected in special ways.

The group of moderately delayed, like the severely affected ones, is divisible into groups with somatic systemic and neurologic abnormalities, although the proportions are not the same. There are fewer of the dysmorphic type and more of the nondysmorphic, nonneurologic group.

Etiology of Severe Developmental Delay

From Table 38-1 it is obvious that many diseases can blight the development and maturation of the brain. Some of these are acquired and some are congenital and hereditary. Some affect all parts of the organism, giving rise to associated dermal, skeletal, and visceral abnormalities, while others affect only the nervous system in particular patterns. With respect especially to the *milder degrees of developmental delay*, in all populations thus far studied, infants of extremely low birth weight are more likely to have disabilities, brain abnormalities, and poorer language development and scholastic achievement (see Chap. 28). Mild developmental delay also tends to correlate with lower social status, which must relate in some manner to biological factors, as pointed out in the Scottish Low-Birth-Weight Study. Viral and spirochetal infections and parturitional accidents are other common causes. They act acutely and are theoretically preventable.

The factor of malnutrition during the fetal or infantile period of life as a cause of severe developmental delay has received considerable attention because it is a worldwide problem. Animal experiments by Winick and others demonstrated that severe undernutrition in early life leads to behavioral abnormalities and biochemical and morphologic changes in the brain, which may be permanent (see Chap. 41). Galler studied a group of infants in Barbados who were severely malnourished during the first year of life and then given an adequate diet. These children were followed to adulthood and compared with normally nourished siblings. No effect was observed on physical growth, but there were persistent attention deficits in 60 percent of the undernourished group and in only 15 percent of controls. The IQ scores of the former were also lower. Unfortunately, genetic factors could not be completely controlled for. In general, it may be said that the data showing developmental delay to be caused by malnutrition, while suggestive, are far from convincing.

Severe protein-calorie malnutrition in the first 8 months of life, which induces kwashiorkor, has been reported to retard mental development. However, such patients are said to regain mental function when fed. The authors have been impressed with the ability of the nervous system to withstand the effects of nutritional deficiency, perhaps better than any other organ.

The action of exogenous toxins during pregnancy is another factor to be considered. Severe maternal alcoholism has been linked to a dysmorphic syndrome and developmental delay, but the findings of several studies have not been consistent (see Chap. 42); a similar problem attaches maternal exposure to anticonvulsant medications (see Chap. 16). Surprisingly, maternal addiction to opiates, while causing an opiate withdrawal in infants for weeks or even months (Wilson et al), seems not to result in permanent injury to the nervous system. The importance of exposure to extremely small amounts of environmental lead is also controversial.

The effect of psychologic deprivation on cognitive development has been of interest. Following the observations that complete isolation of young female monkeys had a devastating effect on their later sexual and nurturing behavior, the idea became popular that such deprivation might cause faulty mental development in humans. Orphaned and neglected babies were found to be inactive, apathetic, and backward in comparison with those who were constantly stimulated by caring mothers. But surprisingly, when nurtured properly at a later time, these babies soon caught up with their peers. This general idea of psychologic deprivation has been the basis of many interesting educational programs for poor and neglected children. To this day, however, it has not been proven that sensory, emotional, and psychologic deprivations of a degree observed in humans are the causes of severe developmental delay or repeated scholastic failure. The controversies regarding the effects of prematurity, maternal hypertension, and eclampsia, which are often associated with neonatal cerebral pathology and slowed psychomotor development, have been mentioned earlier in this chapter. The problem is complex and the argument's pro and con have been elaborated by Haywood and Wachs.

A Clinical Approach to Developmental Delay

As a particular guide to the pediatrician and neurologist who must assume responsibility for the diagnosis and management of backward children harboring a wide array of diseases and maldevelopments of the nervous system, the following clinical approach is suggested. First, as already described, there is an advantage in setting aside as one large group those who are only mildly developmentally delayed from those who have been severely delayed in psychomotor development since early life. With regard to the former group, having no obvious neurologic signs or physical stigmata, one should nevertheless initiate a search for the common metabolic, chromosomal, and infective diseases. In this large group, one must be sure that their deficit is a general one and not one of hearing, poor sight, or the special isolated language and attention deficits.

For patients with moderately severe and very severe cognitive deficits, one begins with a careful physical examination, searching specifically for somatic stigmata and neurologic signs. Abnormalities of eyes, nose, lips, ears, fingers, and toes are particularly important, as are head circumference and a variety of neurologic abnormalities, as outlined in Table 38-8. Data so obtained allow classification into one of three categories, as follows:

In those with somatic abnormalities (with or without obvious neurologic signs), one assumes the presence of a maldevelopment of the brain, possibly caused by a chromosomal abnormality. The psychomotor retardation is usually severe and often nongenetic and, as a rule, has a well-defined neuropathology. Diagnosis is determined by the gestalt of physical signs. The possible maldevelopments are numerous and diverse and are summarized in Tables 38-1 and 38-9; some of the main ones are described earlier in the chapter. Inevitably, one turns to the several atlases to denominate the syndromes (Holmes et al; Jones).

In the group in which the *abnormalities are confined to the nervous system*, attention is focused on a larger number of diseases, many caused by exogenous factors such as perinatal hypoxia-ischemia, pre- or postnatal infections, trauma, and so on. There are usually conspicuous neurologic signs. The degree of developmental delay is variable, depending on the location and extent of a demonstrable neuropathology. Usually the family history is negative, but careful questioning of parents regarding the pregnancy, delivery, and early postnatal period and examination of hospital records from birth may disclose the nature of the neurologic insult.

The third category is one in which *neither somatic anomalies nor focal neurologic signs* are present, or if present, they are minimal. The more severely delayed in cognitive development of this special group are represented by the following disease states: autism (Asperger-Kanner syndrome), the Rett and Williams syndromes, and the fragile X and Renpenning syndromes. All of these but autism are now known to have a genetic basis as noted earlier in the chapter and are described together below.

The practical importance of this clinical approach is that it directs the intelligent use of laboratory procedures for confirmation of the diagnosis. CT scanning and MRI are useful in clarifying maldevelopment and neurologic diseases but are seldom helpful in the third group of cases. EEG confirms seizure discharges when there is uncertainty as to the nature of episodic neural dysfunction. Karyotyping and genetic studies are useful in group 1 and rarely in group 2.

A major pitfall in this clinical approach is in mistaking a hereditary metabolic disease for a developmental one. Here one is helped by the fact that manifestations of the metabolic diseases are not usually present in the first days of life; they appear later and are progressive and often associated with specific visceral abnormalities. However, some metabolic diseases are of such slow progression that they appear almost stable, especially the late-onset ones, such as one type of metachromatic leukodystrophy, late-onset Krabbe leukodystrophy, adult adrenoleukodystrophy, and adult hexosaminidase deficiency (see Chap. 37).

Hereditary Developmental Delays

Fragile X Syndrome (See earlier discussion under "Other Chromosomal Dysgeneses")

There has been great interest in this syndrome, which some geneticists hold accountable at least in part for the preponderance of developmentally delayed males in whom an etiology could not be previously established. A large kindred in whom developmental delay was inherited in an X-linked pattern was first reported by Martin and Bell in 1943. It was in such a family, with X-linked developmental delay, that Lubs, in 1969, discovered a fragile site at the distal end of the long arm of the X chromosome; subsequently, it was established that there is an unstable inherited CGG repeating sequence at this site, which leads to breakage, as discussed previously. At first, it was assumed that the fragile X syndrome was only an example of the Renpenning syndrome (an X-linked hereditary developmental delay in males; see below) until it was pointed out that in this latter condition, stature was reduced, as was the cranial circumference, and further that the X chromosomes of the Renpenning patients were normal. The nature of chromosomal breakage that can be attributed to an expanded trinucleotide repeat sequence of the *FMR1* gene and a resultant loss of protein function were discussed earlier in "Other Chromosomal Dysgeneses."

In some series, fully 10 percent of developmentally delayed males have this fragile X chromosomal abnormality, although 2 to 4 percent is more accurate according to other series. Females are sometimes affected, but their mental function is only slightly reduced. Affected males have only mild dysmorphic features (large ears, broad forehead, elongated face, and enlarged testes) that may not become obvious until puberty. Others are somatically normal. Behavioral problems of one sort or another are almost universal. Pulsifer, whose review of the neuropsychologic aspects of developmental delay is recommended, lists self-injurious, hyperactive, and impulsive behaviors as the most common. The hand-flapping that is more characteristic of autism may be seen.

Fragile X Premutation Syndrome of Adults As discussed in Chap. 5, a curious form of progressive adult onset ataxia and tremor, previously thought to be of a degenerative type, has been discovered to be caused by a "premutation" of the fragile X gene (50 to 200 trinucleotide repeats). Some of these patients have characteristic symmetrical signal MRI changes in the middle cerebellar peduncles in the T2 sequence. Other unusual late presentations have been described, including a spastic paraparesis without ataxia or tremor (Cellini et al). A report by Grigsby and coworkers suggests that cognitive function may be diminished in these men, but only when adjusted for their level of education and not compared to normative data; the observation requires confirmation and any suggestions that a fragile X premutation is responsible for dementia in adults should be accepted cautiously. The permutation expansion may be manifest in women as premature ovarian failure. In contrast to the mutation that causes developmental delay, this disorder is thought to be related in some way to an excess of messenger RNA. Several papers suggest that the premutation may also be the cause of some cases of mild retardation and autistic-like behavior.

Rett Syndrome

This is yet another hereditary form of developmental delay, but one that affects girls. None of the cases in the extensive studies of Hagberg and coworkers (1983) was male. The responsible spontaneous mutation was shown to relate to a defect at chromosomal site Xq28, making it one of the X-linked developmental delays. A fatal outcome in boys because of a severe neonatal encephalopathy explains the expression of the disease only in girls, who are mosaics for the mutation. The involved gene, *MECP2*, is responsible for suppressing various other genes at critical stages of development (see Dunn and MacLeod). It has this effect by binding to methylated DNA. Defective function of the gene leads to an alteration in synaptogenesis and neural connectivity (Neul and Zoghbi). Severe inactivation of gene expression causes classic Rett syndrome, but it has become apparent that incomplete expression and mosaicism lead to a number of partial syndromes, including nonspecific developmental delay, tremor, psychiatric disturbances, and autism-like presentations.

Prevalence studies from Sweden indicate an occurrence of 1 per 10,000 girls; thus Rett syndrome is more common than phenylketonuria. Although most cases appear to be sporadic, there is a high familial incidence and some degree of concordance in twins (this is still uncertain).

The syndrome is usually marked by withdrawn behavior that simulates autism, dementia, ataxia, loss of purposeful hand movements, and respiratory irregularities. Highly characteristic is a period of 6 to 18 months of normal development followed by the rapid appearance and progression of all these signs, and then by relative stability for decades. Spasticity, muscle wasting, scoliosis, and lower limb deformities may become evident in the late stages of the illness. Handwringing and similar stereotypes are very typical features (and are different in subtle ways from the hand-flapping of autistic children).

Armstrong and Naidu, who have reviewed the neuropathology of Rett syndrome, have drawn attention to a number of subtle cortical abnormalities, most of which are consistent with disruption of the postnatal integrative phase of cerebral development; however, not all cases showed these abnormalities. There is generally a decrease in brain size, most marked frontally. Dendritic branching is reduced in several areas. The MRI scan is normal, but some patients show frontal or cerebellar atrophy in their teenage years.

Partington Syndrome

This is yet another X-linked type of developmental delay, which in its fully expressed form is associated with prominent dystonia of the hands and sometimes of the feet, or ataxia. Like Rett syndrome, discussed above, variations in gene expression appear to cause other syndromes including myoclonic epilepsy, West syndrome, autism, and nonspecific retardation, as well as lissencephaly. The mutated gene, termed Aristaless-related homeobox (*ARX*), is involved with regulation of protein-DNA interactions. The subject is reviewed by Sherr.

Renpenning Syndrome

A similar type of hereditary, male-sex-linked developmental delay was described by Renpenning and associates (and subsequently associated with Renpenning's name). The originally described family comprised 21 males in 2 generations of Mennonites in western Canada whose IQs ranged from 30 to 40. It has now been described in 15 families. As with the fragile X syndrome, female siblings may show slight degrees of retardation. Affected members were small in stature and slightly microcephalic but otherwise free of somatic and neurologic abnormalities. The mutated gene responsible is *PQBP1*, the polyglutamine binding protein of which produces the syndrome through unknown means.

Williams (Williams-Beuren) Syndrome

This inherited form of developmental delay is manifest in both males and females and was mentioned earlier. It is characterized by mild and variable developmental delay but with sometimes striking retention and even precocity or superiority of musical aptitude and social amiability. In some instances, a retained facility for writing permits the production of long, written descriptions; yet at the same time, these subjects are barely able to draw simple objects. The child is physically slow and has minor but distinctive somatic changes (wide mouth, almond-shaped eyes, short upturned nose, flat nasal bridge, long philtrum, delicate chin, and small pointed ears), together imparting an "elfin appearance" that is nonetheless variable and not as apparent in adulthood as the facial features coarsen. There is often an unusual sensitivity to auditory stimuli. The delay in acquisition of communicative speech and defects in visual, spatial, and motor skills make these children seem more deficient than they actually are. Striking sociability and empathy set them apart; they represent virtually the converse of autism in this respect. Memory for musical scores—such as memorizing parts of a complete symphony after one hearing—may be prodigious.

By the use of high-resolution cytogenetics, the disease was traced in over 90 percent of cases to a deletion on chromosome 7 in the *ELN* gene that controls the production of elastin (Nickerson et al). This is of interest because one index feature of these cases is supravalvular aortic stenosis and variations (but not necessarily deletions) in the same gene account for cases of familial supravalvular stenosis without developmental delay. This cardiovascular disease is the main cause of death in these individuals.

It is not known whether there is a characteristic brain pathology, but one 35-year-old patient examined by Golden and associates showed no cerebral abnormalities except for Alzheimer changes, mainly plaque formation in the entorhinal cortex and amygdala. The laboratory diagnosis can be established by the use of *ELN*-specific probes or other techniques that show only one allele of the gene. A most interesting related finding by Somerville and colleagues is that duplication at the same site on chromosome 7 implicated in Williams syndrome can cause a delay in the acquisition of expressive speech. The reader is referred to an extremely thorough clinical and genetic review of the syndrome by Pober.

Doublecortin Mutations

Among the disorders of cerebral sulcation, lissencephaly and the related disorder of subcortical band heterotopia are usually associated with severe defects in mental development. However, in female carriers, other mutations in the doublecortin gene (*DCX*) on the X chromosome have given rise to mild nondysmorphic developmental delay and cryptogenic epilepsy (see Guerrini and colleagues). Thus this disorder joins the group of X-linked developmental delays with minimal dysmorphic features and has implications for the understanding of X-chromosome inactivation in female carriers.

Autism (Kanner-Asperger Syndrome; Autistic Spectrum Disorders)

This condition was described almost simultaneously by Kanner in Baltimore (in 1943) and Asperger in Vienna (in 1944). Among a large group of developmentally delayed children, Kanner observed exceptional ones who appeared to be *asocial, lacking in communicative skills both verbal and nonverbal, and committed to repetitive ritualistic behaviors*. At the same time certain intellectual capacities—such as focused attention, retentive memory, skilled sensory and motor aptitudes, and capacity for visuospatial perception—were often retained or overly developed. In other words, the disorder pervaded only certain aspects of mental development.

It is the gestalt of negative and positive aptitudes that sets this syndrome apart from other types of delay. Kanner incorrectly ascribed the condition to psychosocial factors—such as a cold, aloof parent—and regarded it as a psychopathy. The implication that these children are literally "autistic"—that is, that they have a rich inner psychic life or dream world out of relation to reality—is an assumption wholly without foundation. Asperger, whose observations included somewhat older children who were less completely disabled, later ascribed the retardation (also incorrectly) to a metabolic disease, possibly related to hyperammonemia. Opinion varied as to the relationship between the severe Kanner syndrome and the less-severe Asperger syndrome. The authors have taken the more modern view that these forms of autism represent a single syndrome of varying severity, with similar pathologic underpinnings but possibly of multiple etiologies, including genetic. Some 1 percent of autistic children are of normal or superior intelligence.

In our opinion, the overarching issues in classification have become (1) the existence or embedding of autistic traits in a vast number of syndromes that are characterized by developmental delay; examples of this confluence include processes as divergent as fragile X syndrome, phenylketonuria, and tuberous sclerosis; and (2) the extent and margins of the diagnosis of "autistic spectrum disorder." If most socially awkward children are included, the disease begins to encroach on the spectrum personality structure and presents serious problems in diagnosis and the allocation of resources. With regard to the first issue of autistic elements that are part of another well-defined disease, it has become all too easy to ascribe genetic findings to that feature of the syndrome, confusing the problem of sorting out the true etiologies of a clearly identifiable clinical syndrome of autism alone. Baker takes another perspective in an article on the history of the definitions of the disorder that also comments on the DSM classification.

Despite many claims to the contrary, there is no evidence of a psychogenesis. However, as Rapin points out, behavioral modification and special education are beneficial for less-severely affected children.

The overall prevalence of the autistic state has been calculated at 4.5 to 20 per 10,000. Although there was said in the past to be no familial tendency, this is almost certainly incorrect; we have seen the disease in both identical twins and in brothers, and small familial subgroups are known to exist. Autistic traits, without the full syndrome, are being found with increasing frequency in sibs and other family members, suggesting a polygenic inheritance. DeMyer found that 4 of 11 monozygotic twins were concordant for autism and that siblings have a 50 times greater risk of developing the disorder than normal children. Bailey and associates and also LeCouteur and associates have reported a concordance rate in monozygotic twins of 71 percent for the autistic spectrum disorder (as defined below) and 92 percent for an even broader phenotype of disordered social communication and stereotypic or obsessive behaviors. DeLong has found an increased incidence of bipolar disease in the families of one group of autistic children and superior mathematical aptitudes in other family members.

The recent elucidation of microdeletions and microduplications within chromosome 16p by Weiss and the Autism Consortium is the first hint of a genetic locus for susceptibility to autism. Despite a high degree of penetrance in individuals with these changes, the importance of these findings is as a biologic direction for research as it explains no more than 1 percent of cases. Furthermore, certain polymorphisms, particularly in the SHANK3 may explain a small number of cases and this gene has variants that appear disproportionately often in schizophrenia, leading to speculation on common biologic processes. The reader is also referred to the discussion of genetic changes in mental retardation in the earlier sections of the chapter.

Clinical Features

The autistic child is ostensibly normal at birth and may continue to be normal in achieving early behavioral sequences until 18 to 24 months of age. Then an alarming regression occurs, sometimes fairly abruptly. In some instances, the abnormality appears even before the first birthday and the child is identified as different in some way by the mother; or, if there had been a previously autistic child, she recognizes the early behavioral characteristics of the disorder. The level of activity is reduced or increased. There may be less crying and an apparent indifference to surroundings. Toys are ignored or held tenaciously. Spinning toys or running water may hold a strange fascination for the child. Cuddling may be resisted. Motor developments, on the other hand, proceed normally and may even be precocious. Later there may be an unusual sensitivity to all modes of sensory stimulation. Occasionally the onset appears to have a relationship to an injury or an upsetting experience.

Regardless of the time and rapidity of onset, the autistic child exhibits a disregard for other persons; this is typically quite striking but can be subtle in milder cases. Little or no eye contact is made, and the child is no more interested in another person than in an article of furniture. Proffered toys may be manipulated cleverly, placed in lines, or rejected. Insistence on constancy of environment may reach a point where the patient becomes distraught if even a single one of his possessions has been moved from its original place and remains distressed until it is replaced. If speech develops at all, it is automatic (echolalic) and not used effectively to communicate. A repertoire of elaborate stereotyped movements—such as whirling of the body, manipulating an object, toe-walking, and particularly hand-flapping—are characteristic. It is important to point out, that in any sizable group of autistic children *there is a wide range of deficits in sociability, drive, affect, and communicative (verbal and gestural behavior) ability*, ranging from an averbal, completely isolated state to considerable language skill and some capacity for attachment to certain people as well as for scholastic achievement. However, the IQ of the majority is below 70 and in 20 percent it is below 35; 1 percent, however, have normal or superior intelligence. In this higher-functioning group, taken to typify the Asperger syndrome, the child may be unusually adept or even supernormal in reading, calculating, drawing, or memorizing ("idiot savant") while still having difficulty in adjusting socially and emotionally to others and in interpreting the actions of others. Many are clumsy and inept in athletic activities. The least degree of deficit allows success in a professional field but with handicap in the social sphere.

We take the current emphasis on the term *autistic spectrum disorders* to reflect a concept that each of the core elements of autism (in social, language, cognitive, and behavioral domains) may occur in widely varying degrees of severity. This view expands the diagnosis to many children who are highly functional except for a tendency to gaze aversion and other "soft signs," together called "pervasive developmental disorder" (Filipek). There is also crossover with a number of namable developmental delays as noted below.

Rapin, drawing on a large clinical experience, has carefully documented the linguistic, cognitive, and behavioral features of the syndrome. She uses the term *semantic-pragmatic disorder* to designate the characteristic problem with language and behavior and to distinguish it from other forms of developmental disorders and developmental delay. There is a striking ability to understand isolated facts but not to comprehend concepts or conceptual groupings; consequently, these children and adults seem to have difficulty generalizing from an idea. Temple Grandin, a patient with a high-functioning Asperger type of autism who has written of her experiences and has been described by Sacks, indicates that she thinks in pictures rather than in semantic language. She reports a curious comfort from being tightly swaddled and has a highly developed emotional sensibility to the experiences of cattle, which has allowed her success in reforming and designing abattoirs. According to Eisenberg, who reviewed many of Kanner's original cases and followed many other cases into adult life, one-third never spoke and remained social isolates, one-third acquired a rudimentary language devoid of communicative value, and the remainder were functional to various degrees, possessing an affected, stilted, colorless speech. It is in the latter group, representing the mildest degrees of autism, that one finds eccentrics, the mirthless, flat personalities, unable to adapt socially and habitually avoiding eye contact but sometimes possessing certain unusual aptitudes in memory, mathematics, factual knowledge, history, and science. Rutter, who has written extensively on the subject, says that the degree of language impairment and lowered intelligence predicts outcome; those who do not speak by 5 years of age will never learn to speak well.

As mentioned, elements of autism, but not the whole syndrome with its positive and negative attributes, may appear in other diseases that interfere with brain development, specifically fragile X and Rett syndromes, and fragmentary similarities are found in a few children with phenylketonuria, tuberous sclerosis, Angelman syndrome, and, rarely, Down syndrome—but these patients are easily distinguished from those with the far more common type of autism. Bolton and Griffiths have made the intriguing observation that autistic traits in patients with tuberous sclerosis correspond to the finding of tubers in the temporal lobe, and DeLong and Heinz point out that patients with seizures from bilateral (but not unilateral) hippocampal sclerosis may fail to develop (or may lose) language ability as well as failing to acquire social skills after a period of normal development, in a manner similar to autism.

Etiology and Pathology of Autism

The basis of childhood autism is as much a mystery today as it was when Kanner and Asperger described it. Most of these children are physically normal except for a slightly larger head size, on average, but with no other somatic anomalies. Despite instances in which the onset of mental and behavioral regression seems to be quite sudden, no environmental factors, including the often-mentioned measles-mumps-rubella (MMR) vaccination, mercury exposure, and food allergies, have been credibly connected to autism. The genetic microdeletions and microduplications described earlier have given few hints as to the biologic cause.

The EEG is normal, as is CT or MRI. The significance of cerebellar vermal changes, reported originally by Courchesne and colleagues, remains uncertain (Filipek). In the few brains examined postmortem, no lesions of any of the conventional types have been found. In 5 brains studied in serial sections by Bauman and Kemper, smallness of neurons and increased packing density were observed in the medial temporal areas (hippocampus, subiculum, entorhinal cortex), amygdala and septal nuclei, and mammillary bodies. In a subsequent review of the neuropathology, Kemper and Bauman concluded that three changes stood out: a curtailment of the normal development of neurons in the limbic system; a decrease in the number of Purkinje cells that appears to be congenital; and age-related changes in the size and number of the neurons in the diagonal band of Broca (located in the basal frontal and septal region), as well as in the cerebellar nuclei and inferior olive. The latter changes were inferred from studying the brains of autistic children who died at different ages, and they gave the appearance of a progressive or ongoing pathology that continues into adult life. These findings are in keeping with the concept of autism as a neurodevelopmental disorder, but they allow only speculation regarding the derivation of the clinical features of the disease. An increased concentration of platelet serotonin and low serum serotonin is detected in many but not all patients; also, serum oxytocin is reduced. The biologic significance of these findings is unclear.

Course, Treatment, and Prognosis

The disease is essentially nonprogressive although some patients, as they grow older, begin to manifest additional visuoperceptive or auditory defects. In the typical case, the outcome is bleak, although many less affected children show improvement in social relationships and schoolwork when given a serotonin reuptake inhibitor, sometimes in very small doses (DeLong; Filipek, personal communication). Administration of the peptide secretin had produced a number of anecdotal successes, but this could not be reproduced in controlled studies. Selective serotonin reuptake inhibitors (e.g., fluoxetine, citalopram) have also shown some benefit in managing repetitive behaviors and mood swings such that medications in this class are being widely prescribed to autistic children. In addition, serious behavioral changes such as self-injurious activities, aggression, and severe tantrums have been treated with drugs such as risperidone. These represent a therapeutic advance but, as pointed out by Hollander and colleagues in their review of the drug treatment of autism, the patients studied were selected for the severity and type of their symptoms for which reason these medications cannot be expected to be of help to all autistic individuals.

Management of Developmental Delay

Because there is little or no possibility of treating most of the diseases underlying developmental delay and there is no way of restoring function to a nervous system that is developmentally subnormal, the objective is to assist in planning for the patient's care, training, education, and social adjustment. The parents must be guided in forming realistic attitudes and expectations. Psychiatric and social counseling may help the family to maintain gentle but firm support of the patient so that he can acquire, to the fullest extent possible, good work habits and a congenial personality.

Most individuals with an IQ above 60 and no other handicaps can be trained to live an independent life; special schooling may enable them to learn skills useful in a vocation. Social factors that contribute to underachievement must be sought and eliminated if possible.

If the IQ is below 20, institutionalization is almost inevitable, for few families can provide the long-term custodial care that is needed. Well-run institutions are usually better than community homes because they offer many more facilities (medical, educational, recreational). Often institutional care is necessary for individuals with IQs of 20 to 50. Patients in this group, if stable in temperament and relatively well adjusted to society, can work under supervision, but they rarely become vocationally independent. For the more severely cognitively impaired, special training in hygiene and self-care is the most that can be expected.

Great care must be exercised in recommending institutionalization. Whereas the need will be all too apparent in the gravely impaired by the first or second year of life, the less-severely affected are difficult to evaluate at an early age. As stated earlier, psychologic tests alone are not altogether trustworthy. It is best to observe the patient over a period of time. As noted in Chap. 28, the method of evaluation suggested long ago by Fernald has a ring of soundness, albeit in quite dated terms. It should include observations of (1) the physical, medical, and neurologic findings; (2) family background; (3) developmental history; (4) school progress or lack thereof; (5) performance tests; (6) social behavior; (7) industrial efficiency; (8) behavioral disinhibition, which was called in Fernald's time "moral behavior"; and (9) intelligence as measured by psychologic tests.

References

Aicardi J: *Epilepsy in Children*. New York, Raven Press, 1986.

Aicardi J, LeFebvre J, Lerique-Koechlin A: A new syndrome: Spasm in flexion, callosal agenesis, ocular abnormalities. *Electroencephalogr Clin Neurophysiol* 19:609, 1965.

Alzate JC, Kothbauer KF, Jallo GI, et al: Treatment of Chiari type I malformation in patients with and without syringomyelia: A consecutive series of 66 cases. *Neurosurg Focus* 11(1): article 3, 2001.

Appozardi DV, Strohm B, Edwards AD, et al: Moderate hypothermia to treat perinatal asphyxial encephalopathy. *N Engl J Med* 361:1349, 2009.

Armstrong DD: Review of Rett syndrome. *J Neuropathol Exp Neurol* 56:843, 1997.

Asperger H: Die "Autistischen Psychopathen" im Kindesalter. *Arch Psychiatr Nervenkr* 117:76, 1944.

Badawi N, Kurinezuk J, Keogh J, et al: Antepartum risk factors for new born encephalopathy. *Br Med J* 317:1549, 1988.

Bailey A, LeCouteur A, Gottesman A, et al: Autism as a strongly genetic disorder: Evidence from a British twin study. *Psychol Med* 25:63, 1995.

Baker AP: Autism at 70—redrawing the boundaries. *N Engl J Med* 369:1089, 2013.

Baker RS, Ross PA, Bauman RJ: Neurologic complications of the epidermal nevus syndrome. *Arch Neurol* 44:227, 1987.

Banker BQ: Cerebral vascular disease in infancy and childhood: 1. Occlusive vascular disease. *J Neuropathol Exp Neurol* 20:127, 1961.

Banker BQ, Bruce-Gregorios J: A neuropathologic study of diseases of the nervous system in the first year of life, in Thompson GH, Rubin IL, Bilenker RM (eds): *Comprehensive Management of Cerebral Palsy*. New York, Grune & Stratton, 1982, pp 25–31.

Banker BQ, Larroche J-C: Periventricular leukomalacia of infancy. *Arch Neurol* 7:386, 1962.

Barker E, Wright K, Nguyen K, et al: Gene for von Recklinghausen neurofibromatosis in the pericentromeric region of chromosome 17. *Science* 236:1100, 1987.

Barkovich AJ, Kuzniecky RI, Jackson GD, et al: A developmental and genetic classification for malformations of cortical development. *Neurology* 65:1873, 2005.

Barlow CF: *Mental Retardation and Related Disorders*. Philadelphia, Davis, 1978.

Bauman M, Kemper TL: Histoanatomic observations of the brain in early infantile autism. *Neurology* 35:866, 1985.

Bax M, Tydeman C, Floodmark O: Clinical and MRI correlates of cerebral palsy, The European Cerebral Palsy Study. *JAMA* 296:1602, 2006.

Bejjani GK: Definition of the adult Chiari malformation: A brief historical overview. *Neurosurgery Focus* 11:1, 2001.

Benson JWI, Hayward C, Osborne J, et al: Multicentre trial of ethamsylate for prevention of periventricular hemorrhage in very low birth weight infants. *Lancet* 2:1297, 1986.

Berg BO (ed): *Principles of Child Neurology*. New York, McGraw-Hill, 1996.

Beuren AJ, Apitz J, Harmjanz D: Supravalvular aortic stenosis in association with mental retardation and a certain facial appearance. *Circulation* 26:1235, 1962.

Bielschowsky M: Über tuberose Sklerose and ihre Beziehungen zur Recklinghausenschen Krankheit. *Z Gesamte Neurol Psychiatr* 26:133, 1914.

Boder E, Sedgwick RP: Ataxia-telangiectasia: A familial syndrome of progressive cerebellar ataxia, oculocutaneous telangiectasia and frequent pulmonary infection. *Pediatrics* 21:526, 1958.

Bolton PF, Griffiths PD: Association of tuberous sclerosis of temporal lobes with autism and atypical autism. *Lancet* 349:392, 1997.

Botto LD, Moore CA, Khoury MJ, Erickson JD: Neural-tube defects. *N Engl J Med* 341:1509, 1999.

Bradley WG, Richardson J, Frew IJC: The familial association of neurofibromatosis, peroneal muscular atrophy, congenital deafness, partial albinism and Axenfeld's defect. *Brain* 97:521, 1974.

Brett EM (ed): *Paediatric Neurology*, 3rd ed. New York, Churchill Livingstone, 1997.

Cellini E, Forleo P, Ginestroni A, et al: Fragile X permutation with atypical symptoms at onset. *Arch Neurol* 63:1135, 2006.

Chaplin ER, Goldstein GW, Myerberg DZ, et al: Posthemorrhagic hydrocephalus in the preterm infant. *Pediatrics* 65:901, 1980.

Chapman PH: Congenital intraspinal lipomas: Anatomic considerations and surgical treatment. *Childs Brain* 9:37, 1982.

Chiari H: Uber Veränderungen des Kleinhirns infolge von Hydrocephalie des Grosshirns. *Dtsch Med Wochenschr* 17:1172, 1891.

Cicero S, Curcio P, Papageorgiou A, et al: Absence of nasal bone in fetuses with trisomy 21 at 11–14 weeks of gestation: An observational study. *Lancet* 358:1665, 2001.

Cobb S: Haemangioma of the spinal cord associated with skin naevi of the same metamere. *Ann Surg* 62:641, 1915.

Cogan DC: A type of congenital ocular motor apraxia presenting jerky head movements. *Trans Am Acad Ophthalmol* 56:853, 1952.

Collet JP, Vanasse M, Marios P, et al: Hyperbaric oxygen for children with cerebral palsy: A randomised multicentre trial. *Lancet* 357:582, 2001.

Courchesne E, Yeung-Courchesne R, Press GA, et al: Hypoplasia of cerebellar vermal lobules VI and VII in autism. *N Engl J Med* 318:1349, 1988.

Cowan F, Rutherford M, Groenendaal F, et al: Origin and timing of brain lesions in term infants with neonatal encephalopathy. *Lancet* 361:736, 2003.

Créange A, Zeller J, Rostaing-Rigattierei S, et al: Neurologic complications of neurofibromatosis type 1 in adulthood. *Brain* 122:473, 1999.

Crino P: Bourneville and Taylor: A developing story. *Ann Neurol* 52:6, 2002.

Crino PB, Nathanson KL, Henske EP: The tuberous sclerosis complex. *N Engl J Med* 355:1346, 2006.

Crowe FW: Axillary freckling as a diagnostic aid in neurofibromatosis. *Ann Intern Med* 61:1142, 1964.

Crowe FW, Schull WJ, Neel JV: *A Clinical, Pathological and Genetic Study of Multiple Neurofibromatosis*. Springfield, IL, Charles C Thomas, 1956.

de Ligt J, Wilmensen MH, van Born BWM, et al: Diagnostic exome sequencing in persons with severe intellectual disability. *N Engl J Med* 367:1921, 2012.

DeLong GR: Autism: New data suggest a new hypothesis. *Neurology* 52:911, 1999.

DeLong GR, Heinz ER: The clinical syndrome of early-life bilateral hippocampal sclerosis. *Ann Neurol* 42:11, 1997.

DeMyer MK: Infantile autism: Patients and families. *Curr Probl Pediatr* 12:1, 1982.

Dennis J: Neonatal convulsions: Aetiology, late neonatal status and long-term outcome. *Dev Med Child Neurol* 20:143, 1978.

Duffner PK, Cohen ME, Seidel G, Shucard DW: The significance of MRI abnormalities in children with neurofibromatosis. *Neurology* 39:373, 1989.

Dunn HG, MacLeod PM: Rett syndrome: Review of biological abnormalities. *Can J Neurol Sci* 28:16, 2001.

Dyken P, Krawiecki N: Neurodegenerative diseases of infancy and childhood. *Ann Neurol* 13:351, 1983.

Eisenberg L: The autistic child in adolescence. *Am J Psychiatry* 112:607, 1965.

Eldridge R: Central neurofibromatosis with bilateral acoustic neuroma, in Riccardi VM, Mulvihill JJ (eds): *Advances in Neurology*. Vol 29: Neurofibromatosis (Von Recklinghausen Disease). New York, Raven Press, 1981, pp 57–65.

Erzurum S, Kalavsky SM, Watanakunakorn C: Acute cerebellar ataxia and hearing loss as initial symptoms of infectious mononucleosis. *Arch Neurol* 40:760, 1983.

European Collaborative Study: Children born to women with HIV-1 infection: Natural history and risk of transmission. *Lancet* 337:253, 1991.

Evans K, Rigby AS, Hamilton P, et al: The relationships between neonatal encephalopathy and cerebral palsy: A cohort study. *J Obstet Gynaecol* 21:114, 2001.

Evrard PH, De Saint-Georges P, Kadhim H, et al: Pathology of prenatal encephalopathies, in French JH, Harel S, Casaer P (eds): *Child Neurology and Developmental Disabilities*. Baltimore, MD, Brookes, 1989, pp 153–176.

Fenichel GM: Hypoxic-ischemic encephalopathy in the newborn. *Arch Neurol* 40:261, 1983.

Fenichel GM: *Neonatal Neurology*, 3rd ed. New York, Churchill Livingstone, 1990.

Ferriero DM: Neonatal brain injury. *N Engl J Med* 351:1985, 2004.

Filipek PA: Quantitative magnetic resonance imaging in autism: The cerebellar vermis. *Curr Opin Neurol* 8:134, 1995.

Fitzpatrick TB, Szabo G, Hori Y, et al: White leaf-shaped macules, earliest visible sign of tuberous sclerosis. *Arch Dermatol* 98:1, 1968.

Ford FR: *Diseases of the Nervous System in Infancy, Childhood and Adolescence*, 6th ed. Springfield, IL, Charles C Thomas, 1973.

Fowler KB, Stagno S, Pass RF, et al: The outcome of congenital cytomegalovirus infection in relation to maternal antibody status. *N Engl J Med* 326:663, 1992.

Franz DN, Leonard J, Tudor C, et al: Rapamycin causes regression of astrocytomas in tuberous sclerosis complex. *Ann Neurol* 59:490, 2006.

Freud S: *Infantile Cerebral Paralysis*. Russin LA (trans). Coral Gables, FL, University of Miami Press, 1968.

Friedland R, Yahr MD: Meningoencephalopathy secondary to infectious mononucleosis: Unusual presentation with stupor and chorea. *Arch Neurol* 34:186, 1977.

Frith U (ed): *Autism and Asperger Syndrome*. Cambridge, England, Cambridge University Press, 1991.

Galler JR: Malnutrition: A neglected cause of learning failure. *Postgrad Med* 80:225, 1986.

Garcia CA, Dunn D, Trevor R: The lissencephaly (agyria) syndrome in siblings. *Arch Neurol* 35:608, 1978.

Gastaut H, Poirier F, Payan H, et al: HHE syndrome: Hemiconvulsion, hemiplegia, epilepsy. *Epilepsia* 1:418, 1960.

Gellis SB, Feingold M, Rutman JY: *Mental Retardation Syndromes*. Washington, DC, U.S. Department of Health, Education, and Welfare, 1968.

Gillberg C: Asperger syndrome in 23 Swedish children. *Dev Med Child Neurol* 31:520, 1989.

Gold AP, Freeman JM: Depigmented nevi, the earliest sign of tuberous sclerosis. *Pediatrics* 35:1003, 1965.

Golden JA, Nielsen GP, Pober BR, et al: The neuropathology of Williams syndrome: Report of a 35-year-old man with presenile beta/A4 amyloid plaques and neurofibrillary tangles. *Arch Neurol* 52:209, 1995.

Gomez MR: *Tuberous Sclerosis*. New York, Raven Press, 1979.

Gomez MR: *Neurocutaneous Disease (A Practical Approach)*. Boston, Butterworth, 1987.

Gomez MR, Kuntz NL, Westmoreland BF: Tuberous sclerosis, early onset of seizures, and mental subnormality: Study of discordant homozygous twins. *Neurology* 32:604, 1982.

Gorlin RS, Pindborg JJ, Cohen MM Jr: *Syndromes of the Head and Neck*. New York, McGraw-Hill, 1976.

Grandin T. *Thinking in Pictures: My Life With Autism*. Doubleday, New York, 1995.

Gregg NM: Congenital cataract following German measles in the mother. *Trans Ophthalmol Soc Austr* 3:35, 1941.

Grigsby J, Brega AG, Jacquemont S, et al: Impairment in the cognitive functioning of men with fragile X-associated tremor/ataxia syndrome (FXTAS). *J Neurol Sci* 248:227, 2006.

Guerrini R, Moro F, Andermann E, et al: Nonsyndromic mental retardation and cryptogenic epilepsy in women with *doublecortin* gene mutations. *Ann Neurol* 54:30, 2003.

Hack M, Taylor G, Klein N, et al: School-age outcomes in children with birth weight under 750 g. *N Engl J Med* 331:753, 1994.

Haddow JE, Palomaki GE, Knight GJ, et al: Prenatal screening for Down's syndrome with use of maternal serum markers. *N Engl J Med* 327:588, 1992.

Hagberg B: Rett syndrome: Clinical and biological mysteries. *Acta Paediatr* 84:971, 1995.

Hagberg B, Aicardi J, Dias K, et al: A progressive syndrome of autism, dementia, ataxia and loss of purposeful hand movements in girls: Rett's syndrome. *Ann Neurol* 14:471, 1983.

Hagberg B, Hagberg G: Prenatal and perinatal risk factors in a survey of 681 Swedish cases, in Stanley FJ, Alberman ED (eds): *The Epidemiology of the Cerebral Palsies*. Vol 10. London, Spastics International, 1984, pp 116–134.

Hagberg B, Hagberg G, Olow I: The changing panorama of cerebral palsy in Sweden, 1954–1976: II. Analysis of the various syndromes. *Acta Paediatr Scand* 64:193, 1975.

Halperin JJ, Williams RS, Kolodny EH: Microcephaly vera, progressive motor neuron disease and nigral degeneration. *Neurology* 32:317, 1982.

Hamdan FF, Gauhtier J, Spiegelman D, et al: Mutations in SYNGAP1 in autosomal nonsyndromic mental retardation. *N Engl J Med* 360:599, 2009.

Harding AE: *The Hereditary Ataxias and Related Disorders*. New York, Churchill Livingstone, 1984.

Hardy JB: Clinical and developmental aspects of congenital rubella. *Arch Otolaryngol* 98:230, 1973.

Harper JR: True myoclonic epilepsy in childhood. *Arch Dis Child* 43:28, 1968.

Harriëtte TF, van der Zwaag B, Cruysberg J, et al: Möbius syndrome redefined. A syndrome of rhombencephalic maldevelopment. *Neurology* 61:327, 2003.

Hayward JC, Titelbaum DS, Clancy RC, et al: Lissencephalypachygyria associated with congenital cytomegalovirus infection. *J Child Neurol* 6:109, 1991.

Haywood HC, Wachs TD: Intelligence, cognition and individual differences in Begab MJ, Haywood HC, Garber HL (eds): *Psychosocial Influences in Retarded Performance*. Vol I. Baltimore, MD, University Park Press, 1981, pp 95–126.

Henderson JL: The congenital facial diplegia syndrome: Clinical features, pathology and etiology. *Brain* 62:381, 1939.

Herskowitz J, Rosman P, Wheller CB: Colpocephaly: Clinical, radiologic and pathogenetic aspects. *Neurology* 35:1594, 1985.

Hoefnagel D, Penry JK: Partial facial paralysis in young children. *N Engl J Med* 262:1126, 1960.

Hollander E, Phillips AT, Yeh C: Targeted treatment for symptom domains in child and adolescent autism. *Lancet* 362:732, 2003.

Holmes LB, Moser HW, Halldórsson S, et al: *Mental Retardation: An Atlas of Diseases With Associated Physical Abnormalities*. New York, Macmillan, 1972.

Hur JJ: Review of research on therapeutic interventions for children with cerebral palsy. *Acta Neurol Scand* 91:427, 1995.

Huttenlocher PR, Hapke RJ: A follow-up study of intractable seizures in childhood. *Ann Neurol* 28:699, 1990.

Hutto C, Parks WP, Lai S, et al: A hospital-based prospective study of perinatal infection with human immunodeficiency virus type 1. *J Pediatr* 118:347, 1991.

International PHVD Drug Trial Group: International randomized controlled trial of acetazolamide and furosemide in posthemorrhagic ventricular dilatation in infancy. *Lancet* 352:433, 1998.

Jablonski S: *Dictionary of Syndromes and Eponymic Diseases*, 2nd ed. Malabar, FL, Krieger, 1991.

Johnson KP: Viral infections of the developing nervous system, in Thompson RA, Green JR (eds): *Advances in Neurology*. Vol 6. New York, Raven Press, 1974, pp 53–67.

Jones KL: *Smith's Recognizable Patterns of Human Malformation*, 6th ed. Philadelphia, Elsevier Saunders, 2006.

Kalter H, Warkany J: Congenital malformations: Etiologic factors and their role in prevention. *N Engl J Med* 308:424, 1983.

Kanda T, Oda M, Yonezawa M, et al: Peripheral neuropathy in xeroderma pigmentosum. *Brain* 113:1025, 1990.

Kanner L: Autistic disturbances of affective contact. *Nerv Child* 2:217, 1943.

Kato M, Dobyn WB: Lissencephaly and the molecular basis of neuronal migration. *Hum Mol Genet* 12(Suppl 1):89, 2003.

Kemper TL, Bauman M: Neuropathology of autism. *J Neuropathol Exp Neurol* 57:645, 1998.

Kinsbourne M: Myoclonic encephalopathy of infants. *J Neurol Neurosurg Psychiatry* 25:271, 1962.

Kline MW, Shearer WT: Impact of human immunodeficiency virus infection on women and infants. *Infect Dis Clin North Am* 6:1, 1992.

Knight SJ, Regan R, Nicod A, et al: Subtle chromosomal rearrangements in children with unexplained mental retardation. *Lancet* 354:1676, 1999.

Krishnamoorthy KS, Kuehnle KJ, Todres ID, DeLong GR: Neurodevelopmental outcome of survivors with posthemorrhagic hydrocephalus following grade II neonatal intraventricular hemorrhage. *Ann Neurol* 15:201, 1984.

Krueger DA, Wilfong AA, Holland-Bouley K, et al: Everolimus treatment of refractory epilepsy in tuberous sclerosis complex. *Ann Neurol* 2013. [Epub ahead of print]

Landrieu P: Approches de la pathologic cerebelleuse chronique chez l'enfant. *Rev Neurol (Paris)* 149:776, 1993.

LeCouteur A, Bailey A, Goode S, et al: A broader phenotype of autism: The clinical spectrum in twins. *J Child Psychol Psychiatry* 37:785, 1996.

Lemieux BG: Chromosome-linked disorders, in Swaiman K (ed): *Pediatric Neurology: Principles and Practice*, 2nd ed. St. Louis, Mosby, 1994, pp 357–419.

Levene MI, Grindulis H, Sands C, Moore JR: Comparison of two methods of predicting outcome in perinatal asphyxia. *Lancet* 1:67, 1986.

Levine DN, Fisher MA, Caviness VS Jr: Porencephaly with microgyria: A pathologic study. *Acta Neuropathol* 29:99, 1974.

Lewis EO: Types of mental deficiency and their social significance. *J Ment Sci* 79:298, 1933.

Lichtenstein BW: Neurofibromatosis (Von Recklinghausen's disease of the nervous system). *Arch Neurol Psychiatry* 62:822, 1949.

Lorber J: Spina bifida cystica: Results of treatment of 270 cases with criteria for selection in the future. *Arch Dis Child* 47:854, 1972.

Lorber J, Priestley BL: Children with large heads: A practical approach to diagnosis in 557 children with special reference to 109 children with megalencephaly. *Dev Med Child Neurol* 23:494, 1981.

Losner RR, Glenn GM, Walther M, et al: von Hippel-Lindau disease. *Lancet* 361:2059, 2003.

Louis-Bar D: Sur un syndrome progressif comprenant des télangiectasies capillaires cutanée et conjonctivales symetrique a disposition naevoide et des troubles cérébelleux. *Confin Neurol* 4:32, 1941.

Lubs HA: A marker X chromosome. *Am J Hum Genet* 21:231, 1969.

Lynn RB, Buchanan DC, Fenichel GM, Freeman FR: Agenesis of the corpus callosum. *Arch Neurol* 37:444, 1980.

Lyon G, Evrard PH: *Neuropediatrie*. Paris, Masson, 1987.

MacCollin M, Chicca EA, Evans DG, et al: Diagnostic criteria for schwannomatosis. *Neurology* 64:1838, 2005.

Marshall PC, Brett EM, Wilson J: Myoclonic encephalopathy of childhood (the dancing eye syndrome): A long-term follow-up study. *Neurology* 28:348, 1978.

Martin JP, Bell JA: A pedigree of mental defect showing sex linkage. *J Neurol Neurosurg Psychiatry* 6:154, 1943.

Martuza RL, Eldridge R: Neurofibromatosis 2 (bilateral acoustic neurofibromatosis). *N Engl J Med* 318:684, 1988.

Medical Task Force on Anencephaly: The infant with anencephaly. *N Engl J Med* 322:669, 1990.

Menick BJ: Phase-contrast magnetic resonance imaging of cerebrospinal fluid flow in the evaluation of patients with Chiari I malformation. *Neurosurg Focus* 11(1): article 5, 2001.

Milunsky A: Prenatal detection of neural tube defects: VI. Experience with 20,000 pregnancies. *JAMA* 244:2731, 1980.

Mitchell LE, Adzick NS, Melchionne J, et al: Spina bifida. *Lancet* 364:1885, 2004.

Mochida GH, Walsh CA: Genetic basis of developmental malformations of the cerebral cortex. *Arch Neurol* 61:637, 2004.

Moloney DM, Wall SA, Ashworth GJ, et al: Prevalence of Pro250Arg mutation of fibroblast growth factor receptor in coronal craniosynostosis. *Lancet* 349:1059, 1997.

Myers RE: Experimental models of perinatal brain damage: Relevance to human pathology, in Glueck L (ed): *Intrauterine Asphyxia and the Developing Fetal Brain*. Bethesda, MD, Year Book, 1977, pp 37–97.

Naidu S: Rett syndrome: A disorder affecting early brain growth. *Ann Neurol* 42:3, 1997.

Nellhaus G: Head circumference from birth to 18 years. *Pediatrics* 41:106, 1968.

Nelson KB, Ellenberg JH: Antecedents of cerebral palsy. *N Engl J Med* 315:81, 1986.

Neul JL, Zoghbi HY: Rett syndrome: A prototypical neurodevelopmental disorder. *Neuroscientist* 10:118, 2004.

Nickerson E, Greenberg F, Keating MT, et al: Deletions of the elastin gene at 7q11.23 occur in approximately 90% of patients with Williams syndrome. *Am J Hum Genet* 56:1156, 1995.

Nishikawa M, Sakamoto H, Hakura A, et al: Pathogenesis of Chiari malformation: A morphometric study of the posterior cranial fossa. *J Neurosurg* 86:40, 1997.

Nissenkorn A, Michelson M, Ben-Zeev B, Lerman-Sagie T: Inborn errors of metabolism. A cause of abnormal brain development. *Neurology* 56:1265, 2001.

Nokelainen P, Flint J: Genetic effects on human cognition: Lessons from the study of mental retardation syndromes. *J Neurol Neurosurg Psychiatry* 72:287, 2001.

O'Connor N, Hermelin B: Cognitive defects in children. *Br Med Bull* 27:227, 1971.

Ohtahara S: Seizure disorders in infancy and childhood. *Brain Dev* 6:509, 1984.

Ounsted C, Lindsay J, Richards P (eds): *Temporal Lobe Epilepsy, 1948–1986: A Biological Study*. London, Keith Press, 1987.

Pang D, Wilberger JE: Tethered cord syndrome in adults. *J Neurosurg* 57:32, 1982.

Penrose LS: *The Biology of Mental Defect*. New York, Grune & Stratton, 1949.

Piaget J: *The Origins of Intelligence in Children*. New York, International Universities Press, 1952.

Plotkin SR, Blakeley JO, Evans DG, et al: Update from the 2011 International Schwannomatosis Workshop: From genetics to diagnostic criteria. *Am J Med Genet* Part A 161A:405. 2013.

Pober BR: Williams-Beuren syndrome. *N Engl J Med* 362:239, 2010.

Prober CG, Gerson AA: Medical management of newborns and infants born to human immunodeficiency virus-seropositive mothers. *Pediatr Infect Dis J* 10:684, 1991.

Pulsifer MB: The neuropsychology of mental retardation. *J Int Neuropsychol Soc* 2:159, 1996.

Purpura DP: Normal and aberrant neuronal development in the cerebral cortex of human fetus and young infant, in Buchwald NA, Brazier MA (eds): *Brain Mechanisms in Mental Retardation*. New York, Academic Press, 1975, pp 141–171.

Rapin I: Autism. *N Engl J Med* 337:97, 1997.

Renpenning H, Gerard JW, Zaleski WA, et al: Familial sex-linked mental retardation. *Can Med Assoc J* 87:954, 1962.

Riccardi VM: Von Recklinghausen neurofibromatosis. *N Engl J Med* 305:1617, 1981.

Riccardi VM, Mulvihill JJ (eds): *Advances in Neurology*. Vol 29: Neurofibromatosis (Von Recklinghausen Disease). New York, Raven Press, 1981.

Roach ES, Williams OP, Laster DW: Magnetic resonance imaging in tuberous sclerosis. *Arch Neurol* 44:301, 1987.

Roizen HJ, Patterson D: Down's syndrome. *Lancet* 361:1281, 2003.

Rosman NP, Pearce J: The brain in neurofibromatosis. *Brain* 90:829, 1967.

Rousseau F, Heitz D, Biancalana V, et al: Direct diagnosis by DNA analysis of the fragile X syndrome of mental retardation. *N Engl J Med* 325:1674, 1991.

Rutter M: Infantile autism and other pervasive developmental disorders, in Rutter M, Taylor EA, Hersov LA (eds): *Child and Adolescent Psychiatry: Modern Approaches*, 3rd ed. Oxford, England, Blackwell, 1994, pp 563–593.

Sacks O: *An Anthropologist on Mars. Seven Paradoxical Tales.* New York, Alfred Knopf, 1995.

Sandler AD, Sutton KA, DeWeese J, et al: Lack of benefit of a single dose of synthetic human secretin in the treatment of autism and pervasive developmental disorder. *N Engl J Med* 341:1801, 1999.

Sarnat HB, Sarnat MS: Neonatal encephalopathy following fetal distress. *Arch Neurol* 33:696, 1976.

Schreier H, Rapin I, Davis J: Familial megalencephaly or hydrocephalus? *Neurology* 24:232, 1974.

Scottish Low Birthweight Study: II. Language attainment, cognitive status and behavioral problems. *Arch Dis Child* 67:682, 1992.

Shankaran S, Laptook A, Ehrenkranz RA, et al: Whole-body hypothermia for neonates with hypoxic-ischemic encephalopathy. *N Engl J Med* 353:1574, 2005.

Shapiro LR: The fragile X syndrome: A peculiar pattern of inheritance. *N Engl J Med* 325:1736, 1991.

Sherr EH: The ARX story (epilepsy, mental retardation, autism, and cerebral malformations): One gene leads to many phenotypes. *Curr Opin Pediatr* 15:567, 2003.

Shillito J Jr, Matson DD: Craniosynostosis: A review of 519 surgical patients. *Pediatrics* 41:829, 1968.

Shirley MD, Tang H, Gallione CJ, et al: Sturge-Weber syndrome and port-wine stains caused by somatic mutation in GNAQ. *N Engl J Med* 368:1971, 2013.

Short MP, Adams RD: Neurocutaneous diseases, in Fitzpatrick TB, Eisen AZ, Wolff K, et al (eds): *Dermatology in General Medicine*, 4th ed. New York, McGraw-Hill, 1993, pp 2249–2290.

Shuman RM, Selednik LJ: Periventricular leukomalacia. *Arch Neurol* 37:231, 1980.

Sinha S, Davies J, Toner N, et al: Vitamin E supplementation reduces frequency of periventricular hemorrhage in very premature babies. *Lancet* 1:466, 1987.

Solomon LM, Esterley NB: Epidermal and other congenital organoid nevi. *Curr Probl Pediatr* 6:1, 1975.

Somerville MJ, Mervis CB, Young EJ, et al: Severe expressive-language delay related to duplication of the Williams-Beuren locus. *N Engl J Med* 353:1694, 2005.

Taylor M, David AS: Agenesis of the corpus callosum: A United Kingdom series of 56 cases. *J Neurol Neurosurg Psychiatry* 64:131, 1998.

Thomas GH: High male:female ratio of germ line mutations: An alternative explanation for postulated gestational lethality in males with X-linked dominant disorders. *Am J Hum Genet* 58:1364, 1996.

van der Hoeve J: Eye symptoms of tuberous sclerosis of the brain. *Trans Ophthalmol Soc UK* 40:329, 1920.

Verhagen MM, Abdo WF, Willemsen MA, et al: Clinical spectrum of ataxia-telangiectasia in adulthood. *Neurology* 73:430, 2009.

Volkmar FR, Cohen DJ: Neurobiologic aspects of autism. *N Engl J Med* 318:1390, 1988.

Volpe JJ: Intraventricular hemorrhage in the premature infant: Current concepts, parts I and II. *Ann Neurol* 25:3, 109, 1989.

Volpe JJ: *Neurology of the Newborn*, 3rd ed. Philadelphia, Saunders, 1995.

Weber F, Parkes R: Association of extensive haemangiomatous naevus of skin with cerebral (meningeal) haemangioma, especially cases of facial vascular naevus with contralateral hemiplegia. *Proc R Soc Med* 22:25, 1929.

Weiss LA, Shen Y, Kom J, et al: Association between microdeletion and microduplication at 16p11.2 and autism. *N Engl J Med* 358:667, 2008.

Weller TH: The cytomegaloviruses: Ubiquitous agents with protean clinical manifestations. *N Engl J Med* 285:267, 1971.

Williams JC, Barratt-Boyes BG, Lowe JB: Supravalvular aortic stenosis. *Circulation* 24:1311, 1961.

Wilson GS, Desmond MM, Verniand W: Early development of infants of heroin-addicted mothers. *Am J Dis Child* 126:457, 1973.

Winick M: *Malnutrition and Brain Development*. New York, Oxford University Press, 1976.

Wohlwill FJ, Yakovlev PI: Histopathology of meningofacial angiomatosis (Sturge-Weber's disease). *J Neuropathol Exp Neurol* 16:341, 1957.

Woodward LJ, Anderson PJ, Austin NC, et al: Neonatal MRI to predict neurodevelopmental outcomes in preterm infants. *N Engl J Med* 355:685, 2006.

Wyburn-Mason R: *Vascular Abnormalities and Tumors of the Spinal Cord and Its Membranes*. St. Louis, Mosby, 1944.

Yakovlev PI, Guthrie RH: Congenital ectodermoses (neurocutaneous syndromes) in epileptic patients. *Arch Neurol Psychiatry* 26:1145, 1931.

Yakovlev PI, Wadsworth RC: Schizencephalies: A study of the congenital clefts in the cerebral mantle. *J Neuropathol Exp Neurol* 5:116, 169, 1946.

Zupan V, Gonzalez P, Lacaze-Masmonteil T, et al: Periventricular leukomalacia: Risk factors revisited. *Dev Med Child Neurol* 38:1061, 1996.

39

Degenerative Diseases of the Nervous System

The adjective *degenerative* has no great appeal to the modern neurologist. It is also not an entirely satisfactory term medically, as it implies an inexplicable decline from a previous level of normalcy to a lower level of function—an ambiguous conceptualization of disease that satisfies neither a clinician nor a scientist. Moreover, it gives no hint as to the fundamental causation of a process and in all likelihood combines a number of mechanisms under 1 nondescript term. It would be tempting to attribute all progressive disease of the nervous system that are of unknown cause to degeneration. The problem is that many degenerative diseases of mundane type are caused in a proportion of cases by germ line genetic changes. All are currently called *degenerative*, but this nosology may be a transitional method of holding a place while awaiting more refined understanding. What is lacking at the moment is a precise subcellular mechanism for cellular loss; that is knowledge that a protein aggregates within or between cells is not equivalent to understanding the cause of an illness.

Gowers in 1902 suggested the term *abiotrophy* to encompass the degenerative diseases, by which he meant a lack of "vital endurance" of the affected neurons, resulting in their premature death. This concept embodies an unproven hypothesis—that aging and degenerative changes of cells are based on the same process. Understandably, contemporary neuropathologists are reluctant to attribute to simple aging the diverse processes of cellular diseases that are constantly being revealed by ultrastructural and molecular genetic techniques. It is increasingly evident that many of the diseases included in this category depend on genetic factors. Some appear in more than one member of the same family, in which case they may be properly designated as *heredodegenerative*. Even more diseases, not differing in any fundamental way from the heredodegenerative ones, occur sporadically, that is as isolated instances but still, genetic factors such as single nucleotide polymorphisms and copy number variations are often involved in pathogenesis.

Degeneration is nonetheless used as a clinical and pathologic term that refers to a process of neuronal, myelin, or tissue breakdown, the degradative products of which evoke a reaction of phagocytosis and cellular astrogliosis. What characterizes the degenerative disease as much as the loss of cells is the concentration of damage in functionally related cells, or systems; for example the cerebral cortex, motor system, extrapyramidal apparatus, or cerebellum, which are representative of the structures that are the targets of damage in this class of disease.

The basis of aging changes is also explainable at the neuronal level, but the nature of these alterations is not understood. A fundamental problem is the distinction of these aging deteriorations from degenerative disease. When a degenerative neurological disease appears in adult life, one must assume that the clinical presentation is modified to some extent by life-cycle phenomena—the patient's function being a sum of both processes. However, their separation is of fundamental importance in diagnosis and therapeutics. One has to reconcile the fact that most degenerative diseases manifest themselves in later life, leading to the tentative conclusion that some aspect of the aging process is entwined with the cellular degenerations of disease. This creates a problem for the clinician, who may be inclined to attribute changes in a person's function to aging alone rather than searching for a disease that may allow for treatment or for specific prognostication and counseling. Moreover, a long-standing uncertainty pertains to certain degenerative conditions such as Alzheimer disease, which becomes so prevalent in later age as to offer the possibility that the disease is an invariable aspect of aging rather than an acquired perturbation in cellular function. For most degenerative diseases of the nervous system, however, this inevitability of occurrence with aging is clearly not the case. For example, the proportional incidence of Alzheimer pathologic change decreases continuously from age 70 to age 100 according to Savva and colleagues. This polemic regarding aging and degenerative disease is irresolvable and exposes difficulties with meaning of the term "disease." If the human being lived another 50 years beyond the current expectation, would all nervous structures show the changes of degenerative disease? The answer is probably "no," as there are distinctive cellular and subcellular features of degenerative diseases that are different from the uncomplicated, programmed loss of cells that is due to aging.

Much new and essential information has been gained regarding the biologic derangements that lead to neuronal death and dysfunction as a result of investigating the inherited forms of degenerative diseases. The application of the techniques of molecular genetics to these diseases has given stunning results. Even when the hereditary form of a degenerative condition is rare in comparison to the sporadic type, general principles have been exposed that are common to the mechanisms of both forms of the disorder. This approach holds promise for effective treatment of what heretofore have been considered progressive and incurable diseases.

It has been proposed that all degenerative diseases be classified according to their genetic and molecular abnormalities. However, when one notes the diversity of pathologic change that may accompany a single, seemingly unitary gene abnormality or, reciprocally, the diversity of genetic defects that may underlie a single phenotype, this type of classification does not prove immediately helpful to the clinician. In other words, the practice of creating new disease categories to encompass all the molecular and pathologic changes associated with a particular type of neuronal degeneration offers no great advantage in practice. For example, certain diseases are unified by the deposition of proteins such as tau and have been termed "tauopathies," "synucleinopathies," "amyloidopathies," and so forth. We endorse a more useful clinical approach that is based on an awareness of constellations of clinical features that relate to degeneration of neural systems. Until such time as the causation of the degenerative neurologic diseases is known, there must be a name and a place for a group of diseases that are united only by the common attribute of gradually progressive disintegration of a part or parts of the nervous system.

General Clinical Characteristics of Degenerative Diseases

The diseases included in the degenerative category have 2 outstanding characteristics: (1) *They affect specific parts or functional systems of the nervous system* and (2) *They begin insidiously, after a long period of normal nervous system function, and pursue a gradually progressive course.* Frequently, it is impossible to assign a date of onset. The patient or the patient's family may give a history of the abrupt appearance of disability, particularly if some injury, infection, surgical procedure, stroke, or other memorable event coincided with the initial symptoms. A skillfully taken history will reveal that there had been subtle symptoms for some time but had attracted little attention. Whether trauma or other stress can actually evoke or aggravate a degenerative disease is a question that cannot be answered with certainty; at present, evidence to this effect is largely anecdotal. Instead, these degenerative disease processes, by their very nature, appear to develop de novo, without relation to known antecedent events, and their symptomatic expressions are late events in the pathologic process, occurring only when the degree of neuronal loss exceeds the ability of a system to function at a clinically acceptable level. Irreversibility and steady progression of clinical manifestations when measured over periods of months or years is another feature common to the neurodegenerative conditions. However, several of these diseases sometimes display periods of relative stability.

Although most degenerative disease do not manifest expression in other members of the family, the *familial occurrence* of degenerative disease is of great importance both clinically and for scientific reasons as mentioned earlier, but such information is often difficult to obtain. The family may be small or widely scattered, so that the patient is unaware of the health of other members. The patient or the patient's relatives may be reluctant to acknowledge that a neurologic disease has affected another family member. Furthermore, it may not be realized that an illness is hereditary if other members of the family have a much more or much less severe, or a different form of the disorder than the patient. Or paternity may be in question. Even without clear familial occurrence, the patient's ethnicity may give clues to a propensity for certain diseases. Sometimes only the careful examination of other family members will disclose the presence of a hereditary disease. Also, it should be remembered that familial occurrence of a disease does not necessarily mean that it is inherited, but may indicate instead that more than one member of a family had been exposed to the same infectious or toxic agent.

Many symptoms of degenerative disease, while not currently curable, can be alleviated by skillful management. The physician's interest and advice are invaluable to the patient and his family by way of providing support, perspective, and information. This accords with the highest calling of the physician's abilities to relieve suffering.

General Pathologic and Pathogenic Features

Most of the degenerative diseases, as emphasized in the earlier general comments, are characterized by the *selective involvement of anatomically and physiologically related systems of neurons*. This feature is exemplified by amyotrophic lateral sclerosis (ALS), in which the pathologic process is virtually limited to motor neurons of the cerebral cortex, brainstem, and spinal cord, and by the progressive ataxias, in which only the Purkinje cells of the cerebellum are affected. Many other examples could be cited (e.g., Friedreich ataxia, Parkinson disease) in which discrete neuronal systems disintegrate, leaving others unscathed. Thus, these degenerative diseases had in the past been called *system atrophies*. The selective vulnerability of certain systems of neurons is not an exclusive property of the degenerative diseases; several different processes of known cause have similarly circumscribed effects on the nervous system. Contrariwise, in many degenerative diseases, the pathologic changes are somewhat less selective and eventually quite diffuse. Even then, there is an early tendency to involve special categories of neurons.

As one would expect of any pathologic process that is based on the slow wasting and loss of neurons, not only the cell bodies but also their dendrites, axons, and myelin sheaths disappear, unaccompanied by an intense tissue reaction or cellular response. The cerebrospinal fluid (CSF) shows little, if any, change, or at most a slight increase in protein content. Moreover, because these diseases invariably result in tissue loss, imaging examination shows either no change or only a volumetric reduction (atrophy) with a corresponding passive enlargement of the CSF compartments. These findings distinguish the neuronal atrophies from other large classes of progressive disease of the nervous system, namely, tumors, infections, and processes of inflammatory type.

At the cellular level, several processes characterize the death of individual cells. Among these mechanism is *apoptosis*, a term borrowed from embryology to specify the mechanisms that lead to neuronal degeneration. The original meaning of the term refers to a naturally occurring cell death during development that is driven by the expression of genes over a short period of time (i.e., "programmed" cell death), leaving no trace of a pathologic reaction. The process of neuronal degeneration is quite different in that it refers to a series of changes in mature neurons that occur over a protracted period of time, leading to cell death and often leaving a discrete glial scar, but not to regional tissue necrosis. In some models of degenerative disease, cell loss involves activation of specialized genes, although the time course and cellular morphology are not apoptotic in the original sense of the term. It is increasingly apparent that mechanisms other than programmed cell death will prove central to understanding the degenerative diseases, and that the clinical features of these conditions are manifest even before cellular destruction occurs. For example, interference with synaptic signaling and dysfunction of supporting glia cells are equally important to morphologic neuronal death.

It will become clear in the following discussion that the current theme in the study of degenerative diseases is that of aggregation within specific neurons of normal cellular proteins such as amyloid, tau, synuclein, ubiquitin, and huntingtin. In some cases, the protein is overproduced as a result of the simple fact of a triplication or overactivity of its corresponding gene. In other instances, enzymatic cleavage of a normal precursor protein yields a product with physical properties that lead to its aggregation (as happens with amyloid in Alzheimer disease) or, there may be failure of the normal mechanisms of protein removal, resulting in its excess accumulation. As mentioned above, this has resulted in the denomination of groups of diseases by the type of protein aggregate: tauopathy, synucleinopathy, etc. Even this is an uncertain or intermediate classification as it is not known in most cases if the protein is the cause or the result of cellular damage, and in any case, the fundamental mechanisms of cellular destruction are still being determined.

Another characteristic that has guided understanding of degenerative disease is the possible contiguous "spread" of protein aggregation from one to another region by synaptic connections. In some cases, this results in adjacent regions being affected sequentially and in others, circuits that are functionally integrated but not necessarily contiguous areas are affected. This geographic mechanism, proposed by Braak and Braak, conforms to certain pathologic observations such as the sequential appearance of synuclein in the olfactory system, thence in the Meissner-Auerbach plexus of the gut, followed by the vagus, to involvement of the vagal nuclei in the medulla, ascending trans-synaptically to the pons and midbrain nuclei. Whether this accounts for the selectivity of disease in areas such as the substantia nigra that is most affected in Parkinson disease, is not entirely known. In any case, the biologic and the physicochemical properties of these aggregated proteins have assumed great importance and the mechanisms by which they interfere with cellular function and potentially cause cell death are major areas of research in the degenerative diseases.

CLINICAL CLASSIFICATION

Because grouping of the degenerative diseases in terms of etiology is not entirely possible (except that a hereditary or genetic factor can be recognized in some), we resort for practical purposes to a division based on the presenting clinical syndromes and their pathologic anatomy. Although this is the most elementary mode of classification of naturally occurring phenomena, it is a necessary prelude to diagnosis and scientific study and preferable to a purely genetic or molecular classification. It is certainly an improvement on a haphazard listing of diseases by the names of the neurologists or neuropathologists who first described them. For reasons given in the introduction to this chapter, this approach remains the most effective in analyzing the problem presented by an individual patient. The main clinical categories are as follows:

I. Syndrome of progressive dementia, other neurologic signs absent or inconspicuous
   A. Alzheimer disease
   B. Some cases of Lewy-body disease
   C. Frontotemporal dementias—Pick disease, including behavioral variant, primary progressive aphasias (several types)
   D. Posterior cortical atrophy (visuospatial dementia)

II. Syndrome of progressive dementia in combination with other neurologic abnormalities
   A. Huntington disease (chorea)
   B. Lewy-body disease (parkinsonian features)
   C. Some cases of Parkinson disease
   D. Corticobasal ganglionic degeneration (rigidity, dystonia)
   E. Cortical-striatal-spinal degeneration (Jakob disease)
   F. Dementia-Parkinson-amyotrophic lateral sclerosis complex
   G. Cerebrocerebellar degeneration
   H. Familial dementia with spastic paraparesis, amyotrophy, or myoclonus
   I. Polyglucosan body disease (neuropathy)
   J. Frontotemporal dementia with parkinsonism or ALS

III. Syndrome of disordered posture and movement
   A. Parkinson disease
   B. Multiple system atrophy, MSA-P (striatonigral degeneration, Shy-Drager syndrome)
   C. Progressive supranuclear palsy
   D. Dystonia musculorum deformans
   E. Huntington disease (chorea)
   F. Acanthocytosis with chorea
   G. Corticobasal ganglionic degeneration
   H. Lewy-body disease
   I. Restricted dystonias, including spasmodic torticollis and Meige syndrome
   J. Essential tremor

IV. Syndrome of progressive ataxia
    A. Spinocerebellar ataxias
        1. Friedreich ataxia
        2. Non-Friedreich, early-onset ataxia (with retained reflexes, tremor, hypogonadism, myoclonus, and other disorders)
    B. Cerebellar cortical ataxias
        1. Holmes type of familial pure cerebellar-olivary atrophy
        2. Late-onset cerebellar atrophy
    C. Complicated hereditary and sporadic cerebellar ataxias (later-onset ataxia with brainstem and other neurologic disorders)
        1. Multiple system atrophies (MSA-C) including olivopontocerebellar degenerations (OPCA)
        2. Dentatorubral degeneration (Ramsay Hunt type)
        3. Dentatorubropallidoluysian atrophy (DRPLA)
        4. Machado-Joseph (Azorean) disease; SCA-3
        5. Other complicated late-onset, autosomal dominant ataxias with pigmentary retinopathy, ophthalmoplegia, slow eye movements, polyneuropathy, optic atrophy, deafness, extrapyramidal features, and dementia
V. Syndrome of slowly developing muscular weakness and atrophy
    A. Motor disorders with amyotrophy
        1. Amyotrophic lateral sclerosis
        2. Progressive spinal muscular atrophy
        3. Progressive bulbar palsy
        4. Kennedy syndrome and other hereditary forms of progressive muscular atrophy and spastic paraplegia
        5. Motor neuron disease with frontotemporal dementia
    B. Spastic paraplegia without amyotrophy
        1. Primary lateral sclerosis
        2. Hereditary spastic paraplegia (Strümpell-Lorrain)
VI. Sensory and sensorimotor disorders (neuropathies; see Chap. 46)
    A. Hereditary sensorimotor neuropathies—peroneal muscular atrophy (Charcot-Marie-Tooth); hypertrophic interstitial polyneuropathy (Dejerine-Sottas)
    B. Pure or predominantly sensory or motor neuropathic
    C. Riley-Day autonomic degeneration
VII. Syndrome of progressive blindness with or without other neurologic disorders (see Chap. 13)
    A. Pigmentary degeneration of retina (retinitis pigmentosa)
    B. Stargardt disease
    C. Age-related macular degeneration (ARMD)
VIII. Syndromes characterized by degenerative neurosensory deafness (see Chap. 15)
    A. Pure neurosensory deafness
    B. Hereditary hearing loss with retinal diseases
    C. Hereditary hearing loss with system atrophies of the nervous system

DISEASES CHARACTERIZED MAINLY BY PROGRESSIVE DEMENTIA

Alzheimer Disease

This is the most common and important degenerative disease of the brain, having an immense societal impact. Some aspects of the intellectual deterioration that characterize this disease were described in Chap. 21, under "The Neurology of Dementia," and the still ambiguous relationship of this disease to the aging process is mentioned above and in Chap. 29. There it was pointed out that some degree of shrinkage in size and weight of the brain, that is "atrophy," is an inevitable accompaniment of advancing age, but that these changes alone are of relatively slight clinical significance and uncertain structural basis (e.g., whether the loss of brain weight aging is the result of a simple depletion of neurons). By contrast, severe degrees of diffuse cerebral atrophy that evolve over a few years are associated with dementia, and the underlying pathologic changes in these cases most often prove to be those of Alzheimer disease. As also commented on in Chap. 29, the rate of cerebral atrophy, specifically of the hippocampus and medial parts of the temporal lobes, is accelerated in the early stages of Alzheimer disease, and longitudinal studies by magnetic resonance imaging can identify individuals who will subsequently develop the disease (Rusinick). Nevertheless, there is not a continuous increase in the deposition of plaques and tangles, the pathologic markers of Alzheimer disease, with increasing age. Therefore, Alzheimer changes are not an inevitable result of aging.

The now outdated practice of giving Alzheimer disease and senile dementia the status of separate diseases is attributable to the relatively young age (51 years) of the patient originally studied by Alois Alzheimer in 1907. Such a division is no longer tenable, as the 2 conditions, except for their age of onset, are clinically and pathologically indistinguishable. It is probably useful to consider as related but separable, the several heredofamilial forms of Alzheimer disease discussed below.

Epidemiology

Although Alzheimer disease has been described at every period of adult life, the majority of patients are in their sixties or older; a relatively small number have been in their late fifties or younger. It is one of the most frequent mental illnesses, making up a large proportion of persons in assisted living and skilled nursing facilities. The incidence of clinically diagnosed Alzheimer disease is similar throughout the world, and it increases with age, approximating 3 new cases yearly per 100,000 persons younger than age 60 years and a staggering 125 new cases per 100,000 of those older than age 60 years. The prevalence of the disease per 100,000 population is near 300 in the group aged 60 to 69 years; it is 3,200 in the 70- to 79-year-old group and 10,800 in those older than age 80. In the year 2008, there were estimated to be more than 2 million persons with Alzheimer disease in the

United States. (It should be borne in mind that these are not pathologically proven cases and, while probably correct as an approximation, are likely combined with other diseases.) Prevalence rates, which depend also on overall mortality, are 3 times higher in women, although the incidence of new cases is only slightly disproportionate in women. The survival of patients with Alzheimer disease is reduced to half the expected rate, mainly because of respiratory and cardiovascular causes and inanition, but also for other reasons that are not entirely clear.

Several putative epidemiologic risk factors for Alzheimer disease, such as birth order, mother's age at birth, and a family history of Down syndrome seem marginal at best and in some instances may be a result of selection bias. Depression and possibly head injuries do seem to confer a somewhat increased risk later in life. Whether low educational attainment is a risk factor for the development of Alzheimer disease or, conversely, whether cognitively demanding occupations or higher intelligence protects against dementia is still under discussion. Provocative data indicating that inherent intellectual endowment is important were presented in Chap. 21 (Katzman; Cobb et al). Finally, associations between diabetes or hyperglycemia and dementia, in general, have emerged from epidemiologic studies, for example, one reported by Crane and coworkers, but the ostensible mechanism by which this confers risk has not been established. In their report, a higher than average glucose level over the preceding 5 years conferred a slightly increased risk of dementia but not necessarily of Alzheimer disease.

The *familial occurrence* of Alzheimer disease has been well established. In less than 1 percent of such cases there is a dominant inheritance pattern with a high degree of penetrance and appearance of disease at a younger age (Nee et al; Goudsmit et al; see further). Reports of substantial familial aggregations of dementia without a specific pattern of inheritance also suggest the operation of more than one genetic factor. Many studies have documented an increase in the risk of ostensibly sporadic Alzheimer disease among first-degree relatives of patients with this disorder. Again, this risk is disproportionately greater in females, adding to the evidence that women in general are at slightly higher risk for Alzheimer disease (Silverman et al). Li and coworkers have provided evidence that patients with an earlier age of onset of Alzheimer disease (before age 70 years) are more likely to have relatives with the disease than are patients with later onset. Genetic studies are difficult to carry out because the disease does not appear at the same age in a given proband. Even in identical twins, the disease may develop at the age of 60 years in one of the pair and at 80 years in the other. Death from other causes may prevent its detection. The other genetic contributions to the occurrence of Alzheimer disease are discussed extensively further on.

Clinical Features (See also Chap. 21)

The onset of mental changes is usually so insidious that neither the family nor the patient can date the time of its beginning and most patients come to attention months or years after the decline began. Occasionally, however, the process becomes manifest by an unusual degree of confusion in relation to a febrile illness, an operation, mild head injury, or the institution of a new medication. Other patients have as their initial complaints dizziness, mental fogginess, nondescript headaches, or other vaguely expressed and changeable somatic symptoms.

The gradual development of forgetfulness is the major symptom. Small day-to-day happenings are not remembered. Seldom-used names become particularly elusive. Little-used words from an earlier period of life also tend to be lost. Appointments are forgotten and possessions misplaced. Questions are repeated again and again, the patient having forgotten what was just discussed. It is said that remote memories are preserved and recent ones lost (the Ribot law of memory), but this is only relatively true and it is difficult to check the accuracy of distant personal memories. For example, Albert and associates, who tested Alzheimer patients' recognition of dated political events and pictures of prominent people past and present, found that some degree of memory loss extends to all previous decades of the person's life (neuropsychologic testing is discussed further on).

Once the memory disorder has become pronounced in the prototypic disorder, other failures in cerebral function become increasingly apparent. The patient's speech is halting because of failure to access the needed word. The same difficulty interrupts writing. Vocabulary becomes restricted, and expressive language becomes stereotyped and inflexible. Comprehension of spoken words seems at first to be preserved, until it is observed that the patient does not carry out a complicated request; even then it is uncertain whether the request was not understood because of inattention or because it was forgotten. Almost imperceptible at first, these disturbances of language become increasingly apparent as the disease progresses. The range of vocabulary and the accuracy of spelling are reduced. Finally, after many years of illness, there is a failure to speak in full sentences; the finding of words requires a continuous search; and little that is said or written is fully comprehended. There is a tendency to repeat a question before answering it, and later there may be a rather dramatic repetition of every spoken phrase (*echolalia*). The deterioration of verbal skills has by then progressed beyond a groping for names and common nouns to an obvious anomic aphasia. Other elements of receptive and executive aphasia are later added, but discrete aphasias of the Broca or Wernicke type are characteristically lacking. In general, there is a paucity of speech and a quantitative reduction in mentation.

Skill in arithmetic suffers a similar deterioration. Faults in balancing the checkbook, mistakes in figuring the price of items and in making the correct change; all these and others progress to a point where the patient can no longer carry out the simplest calculations (*acalculia* or *dyscalculia*).

In some patients, visuospatial orientation becomes defective. The car cannot be parked; the arms do not find the correct sleeves of the jacket or shirt; the corners of the tablecloth cannot be oriented with the corners of the table; the patient turns in the wrong direction on the way home or becomes lost. The route from one place to another cannot be described, nor can given directions be understood. As this state worsens, the simplest of geometric forms and patterns cannot be copied.

Late in the course of the illness, the patient forgets how to use common objects and tools while retaining the necessary motor power and coordination for these activities. The razor is no longer correctly applied to the face; the latch of the door cannot be unfastened; and eating utensils are used awkwardly. Finally, only the most habitual and virtually automatic actions are preserved. Tests of commanded and demonstrated actions cannot be executed or imitated. *Ideational* and *ideomotor apraxia* are the terms applied to the advanced forms of this motor incapacity as described in Chaps. 3 and 22.

As these many amnesic, aphasic, agnostic, and apraxic deficits declare themselves, the patient at first seems unchanged in overall motility, behavior, temperament, and conduct. Social graces, whatever they were, are retained in the initial phase of the illness, but troublesome alterations may gradually appear in this sphere as well. Imprudent business deals may be made. Restlessness and agitation or their opposites—inertia and placidity—become evident. Dressing, shaving, and bathing are neglected. Anxieties and phobias, particularly fear of being left alone, may emerge. A disturbance of the normal day and night sleep patterns is prominent in some patients. A poorly organized paranoid delusional state, sometimes with hallucinations, may become manifest. The patient may suspect his elderly wife of having an illicit relationship or his children of stealing his possessions. A stable marriage may be disrupted by the patient's infatuation with a younger person or by sexual indiscretions, which may astonish the community. The patient's affect coarsens; he is more egocentric and indifferent to the feelings and reactions of others. A gluttonous appetite sometimes develops, but more often eating is neglected, resulting in gradual weight loss. Later, grasping and sucking reflexes and other signs of frontal lobe disorder are readily elicited (Neary et al), sphincteric continence fails, and the patient sinks into a state of relative akinesia and mutism, as described in Chap. 21.

Difficulty in locomotion, a kind of unsteadiness with shortened steps but with only slight motor weakness and rigidity, frequently supervenes. Elements of parkinsonian akinesia and rigidity and a fine tremor can be perceived in patients with advanced stages of the disease. Ultimately, the patient loses the ability to stand and walk, being forced to lie inert in bed and having to be fed and bathed, the legs curled into a fixed posture of paraplegia in flexion (in essence, a persistent vegetative state).

The symptomatic course of this illness is quite variable but usually extends over a period of 5 or more years, but judging from pathology studies, the pathologic course has a much longer asymptomatic duration. This concept of a preclinical stage is supported by the detailed studies of Linn and colleagues, who found that a lengthy period (7 years or more) of stepwise decline in memory and attention span preceded the clinical diagnosis. In the dominantly inherited forms of disease, careful studies of biomarkers in the spinal fluid and by imaging show that changes occur 15 years or longer before the clinical manifestations are apparent (Bateman et al). Throughout this period, corticospinal and corticosensory functions, visual acuity, ocular movements, and visual fields remain intact. If there is hemiplegia, homonymous hemianopia, and the like, either the diagnosis of Alzheimer disease is incorrect or the disease has been complicated by a stroke, tumor, or subdural hematoma. Exceptions to this statement are rare. The tendon reflexes are little altered and the plantar reflexes almost always remain flexor. There is no sensory or cerebellar ataxia. Convulsions are rare until late in the illness, when up to 5 percent of patients reportedly have infrequent seizures. Occasionally, widespread myoclonic jerks or mild choreoathetotic movements are observed late in the illness. Eventually, with the patient in a bedfast state, an intercurrent infection such as aspiration pneumonia or some other disease mercifully terminates life.

The sequence of neurologic disabilities may not follow this described order and one or another deficit may take precedence, presumably because the disease process, after becoming manifest in the memory cortex of the temporal lobes, affects a particular part of the associative cortex earlier or more severely in one patient than in another. This allows a relatively restricted deficit to become the source of early medical complaint, long before the full syndrome of dementia has declared itself.

There are at least 4 limited deficits that may represent the opening features of Alzheimer disease but each of which alone may be mild enough to qualify as *mild cognitive impairment* (MCI). According to Petersen, who developed this concept, the MCI syndrome is defined by the presence of cognitive difficulties in one or all spheres that are not severe enough to interfere with daily life.

The early presentation of Alzheimer disease may manifest mainly as one of the following syndromes with the first, memory dysfunction being the most common and, even as other aspects of the disease advance, it tends to remain the most prominent.

1. *Amnesia* The early stages of Alzheimer disease are usually dominated by a disproportionate failure of episodic (autobiographical) memory, with integrity of other cognitive abilities. This may be the sole difficulty for many years. In such patients, immediate memory (essentially a measure of attention), tested by the capacity to repeat a series of numbers or words, is intact; it is the short-and long-term (retentive) memory that fails. Memory may become impaired but as a business executive, for example, the individual may continue to make acceptable decisions if the work uses long-established habit patterns and practices.
2. *Dysnomia* The forgetting of words, especially proper names, may first bring the patient to a neurologist. Later the difficulty involves common nouns and progresses to the point where fluency of speech is seriously impaired. Every sentence is broken by a pause and search for the wanted word; if the desired word is not found, a circumlocution is substituted or the sentence is left unfinished. When the patient is given a choice of words, including the one that was missed, there may be a failure of recognition. Repetition of the spoken words of others, at first flawless, later brings out a lesser degree of the same difficulty. The defect in

naming is evident with even simple tests, for example, asking the patient to generate a list of farm animals or car brands—a test that may elicit only 3 or 4 responses. A more extensive examination entails asking the patient to name as many items as possible in each of 3 categories in 1 min—vegetables, tools, and clothing. Alzheimer patients fall well below a score of 50 items.

3. *Visuospatial disorientation* Parietooccipital functions are sometimes deranged in the course of Alzheimer disease and in a few cases may fail while other functions are relatively preserved. When it occurs in a pure form it is termed *posterior cortical atrophy,* as discussed in a later section (see Renner et al). As remarked above and in Chap. 22, prosopagnosia (impaired facial recognition), losing one's way in familiar surroundings or inability to interpret a road map, to distinguish right from left, or to park or garage a car, and difficulty in setting the table or dressing are all manifestations of a special failure to orient the schema of one's body with that of surrounding space. Exceptionally, there is a neglect of stimuli in one visual field. In the late states, some of these patients develop the Balint syndrome or Gerstmann syndrome (Tang-Wai et al; McMonagle et al).
4. *Paranoia and personality changes* Occasionally, at some point in the development of Alzheimer dementia, paranoia or bizarre behavior occasionally assumes prominence. This may appear before the more obvious memory or language defects announce themselves. The patient becomes convinced that relatives are stealing his possessions or that an elderly and even infirm spouse is guilty of infidelity. He may hide his belongings, even relatively worthless ones, and go about spying on family members. Hostilities arise, and wills may be altered irrationally. Many of these patients are constantly worried, tense, and agitated. Of course, paranoid delusions may be part of a depressive psychosis and of other dementias, but most of the elderly patients in whom paranoia is the presenting problem, seem not to be depressed, and their cognitive functions are for a time relatively well preserved. Social indiscretions, rejection of old friends, embarking on imprudent financial ventures, or an amorous pursuit that is out of character are examples of these types of behavioral change.
5. *Executive dysfunction* This may be the most disabling of the main aspects of the disease and when it appears early on, is not specific to Alzheimer dementia as it is a component of several other processes that affect the frontal lobes. These patients display early difficulties in coordinating and planning tasks and following complex conversations or instructions. They may become disinclined to participate in social activities and become withdrawn or quieter than usual. As the problem advances, simpler and formerly automatic actions such as driving become problematic for the patient; the degree of insight varies. Some are able to express that they feel "confused' but more often, it is the family that brings these changes to attention.

If one of the foregoing restricted deficits remains uncomplicated over a long period, one is justified in suspecting a cause other than Alzheimer disease, such as one of the lobar atrophies such as frontotemporal dementia (see further on), Binswanger disease, hydrocephalus, or embolic infarctions of the temporal or parietal lobes. Each of the restricted clinical disorders described above is only relatively pure. Careful testing of mental function—and this is of diagnostic importance—frequently discloses subtle abnormalities in several cognitive spheres. Initially, most patients have a disproportionate disorder of the temporoparietal cortices, reflected by an earlier impairment on the performance parts of the Wechsler Adult Intelligence Scale. Within a year or two, the more generalized aspects of mental deterioration become apparent, and the aphasic–agnosic–apraxic aspects of the syndrome become increasingly prominent. Although it is true that most patients with Alzheimer disease walk normally until relatively late in their illness, infrequently a short-stepped gait and imbalance draw attention to the disease and worsen slowly for several years before cognitive manifestations become evident. The general decrepitude in appearance that accompanies the middle and late stages of the disease in many patients is commented on in Chap. 21.

For research purposes and to establish certain inclusive and exclusive criteria for the diagnosis of Alzheimer disease, a working group of the National Institute of Neurological and Communicative Disorders and Stroke (NINCDS) and the Alzheimer's Disease and Related Diseases Association (ADRDA) had proposed the following criteria: (1) dementia defined by clinical examination, the Mini-Mental Scale (see Table 21-6), the Blessed Dementia Scale, or similar mental status examination; (2) patient older than age 40 years; (3) deficits in 2 or more areas of cognition and progressive worsening of memory and other cognitive functions, such as language, perception, and motor skills (praxis); (4) absence of disturbed consciousness; and (5) exclusion of other brain diseases (McKhann et al, 1984; Tierney et al, 1988). These criteria have essentially been reaffirmed by more recent consensus panels (see McKhann et al, 2011). Using these measures, the correct diagnosis is achieved in more than 85 percent of patients, but this is not surprising given that Alzheimer disease is overwhelmingly the most common cause of adult dementia. Most cases are identifiable without resorting to restrictive lists such as these, especially if the patient is observed serially over a period of months or years. There is strong interest in the addition of biomarkers to the diagnostic criteria for the disease but these have not reached the point of general clinical utility and the diagnosis remains predominantly a clinical one, aided by imaging and other tests.

Pathology

In the advanced stages of the disease, the brain presents a diffusely atrophied appearance and its weight is usually reduced by 20 percent or more. Cerebral convolutions are narrowed and sulci are widened. The third and lateral ventricles are symmetrically enlarged to varying degrees. Usually, the atrophic process involves the frontal, temporal, and parietal lobes, but cases vary considerably. The extreme atrophy of the hippocampus, the most prominent finding visible on MRI (mainly coronal images), is diagnostic in the proper clinical circumstances.

Microscopically, there is widespread loss of nerve cells. Early in the disease this is most pronounced in layer II of the entorhinal cortex. In addition to marked neuronal loss in the hippocampus, adjacent parts of the medial temporal cortex—namely, the parahippocampal gyri and subiculum—are affected. The anterior nuclei of the thalamus, septal nuclei, and diagonal band of Broca, amygdala, and particular brainstem parts of the monoaminergic systems are also depleted. The cholinergic neurons of the nucleus basalis of Meynert (the substantia innominata) and locus ceruleus are also reduced in number, a finding that has aroused great interest because of its putative role of the former in memory function (see below). In the cerebral cortex, the cell loss predominantly affects the large pyramidal neurons. Residual neurons are observed to have lost volume and ribonucleoprotein; their dendrites are diminished and crowd one another owing to the loss of synapses and neuropil. Astrocytic hypertrophy (more than proliferation) is in evidence as a compensatory or reparative process, most prominent in layers III and V.

Moreover, 3 microscopic changes give this disease its distinctive character: (1) The presence within the nerve cell cytoplasm of thick, fiber-like strands of silver-staining material, also in the form of loops, coils, or tangled masses (Alzheimer neurofibrillary changes or "tangles") (Fig. 39-1). These strands are composed of a hyperphosphorylated form of the microtubular protein, tau, and appear as pairs of helical filaments when studied ultrastructurally. (2) Spherical deposits of amorphous material scattered throughout the cerebral cortex and easily seen with periodic acid-Schiff (PAS); the core of the aggregates is the protein amyloid, surrounded by degenerating nerve terminals (*neuritic plaques*) that stains with silver. Amyloid is also scattered throughout the cerebral cortex in a nascent "diffuse" form, without organization or core formation and then is appreciated mainly by immunohistochemical methods, as well as deposition in the walls of small blood vessels near the plaques, so-called congophilic angiopathy. (3) *Granulovacuolar degeneration* of neurons, most evident in the pyramidal layer of the hippocampus. This last change is least important in diagnosis but there is uncertainty regarding its nature; it had been thought to be simply a reactive process but recent studies suggest it reflects a defect in phagocytosis of degraded proteins.

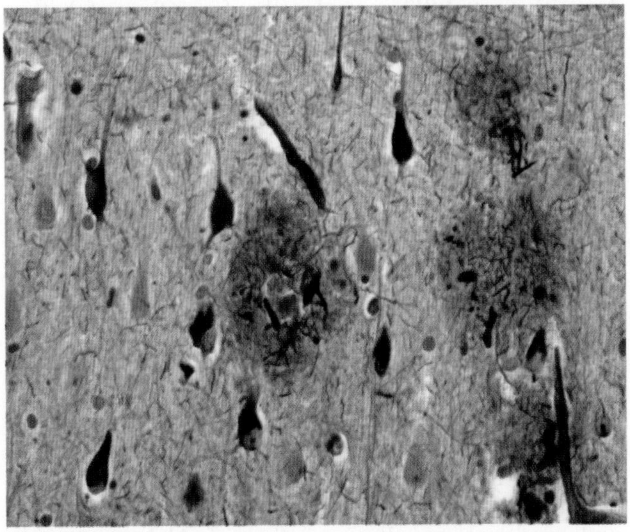

Figure 39-1. Photomicrograph of Alzheimer amyloid plaques and neurofibrillary tangles. Bielchowsky silver stain.

Neuritic plaques and neurofibrillary changes are found in all the association areas of the cerebral cortex, but it is the neurofibrillary tangles and quantitative neuronal loss, not the amyloid plaques, that correlate best with the severity of the dementia (Arriagada et al). If any part of the brain is disproportionately affected, it is the hippocampus, particularly the CA1 and CA2 zones (of Lorente de Nó) and the entorhinal cortex, subiculum, and amygdala. These parts have abundant connections with other parts of the temporal lobe cortex and dentate gyrus of the hippocampus and undoubtedly account for the amnesic component of the dementia. The associative regions of the parietal lobes are another favored site. Only a few tangles and plaques are found in the hypothalamus, thalamus, periaqueductal region, pontine tegmentum, and granule-cell layer of the cerebellum.

Experienced neuropathologists recognize a form of Alzheimer disease, particularly in older patients (75 years), in which there are senile plaques but few or no neuronal tangles (about 20 percent of 150 cases reported by Joachim et al). Increasingly, other pathologic changes are being appreciated in Alzheimer cases with fewer plaques and tangles than anticipated for the degree of dementia; Lewy bodies in particular are found by sophisticated techniques. Another problem for the neuropathologist is to distinguish between the normal-aged brain and that of Alzheimer disease. It is not unusual to find a scattering of senile plaques in individuals who were ostensibly mentally normal during life. Anderson and Hubbard studied 27 demented individuals aged 64 to 92 years and 20 age-matched nondemented controls. In the former, 3 to 38 percent of the hippocampal neurons contained neurofibrillary tangles; in all but 2 of the controls, the number of hippocampal neurons with tangles fell below 2.5 percent. Moreover, an increased number of tangles in the aged are associated with mild cognitive impairment and a higher likelihood of progression to Alzheimer disease.

Many demented individuals with clinical features of Alzheimer disease have sufficient neuronal loss and Lewy bodies in cortex and the substantia nigra to justify a diagnosis on histopathologic grounds of Parkinson disease (see further on). Leverenz and Sumi found that 25 percent of their Alzheimer patients showed the pathologic (and clinical) changes of Parkinson disease, a much higher incidence than can be attributed to chance. Similarly, of 11 patients with progressive supranuclear palsy (also discussed further on) reported by Gearing and coworkers, 10 were demented and 5 had the neuropathologic features of Alzheimer disease. These mixed cases present problems not only of classification but also in understanding the neurobiology of these degenerative diseases. This subject is discussed further in the section on Parkinson disease.

It is of historical interest that Alzheimer was not the first to describe plaques, one of the hallmarks of the pathologic state. Miliary lesions (*Herdchen*) had been observed in senile brains by Blocq and Marinesco in 1892 and were named *senile plaques* by Simchowicz in 1910. In 1907, Alzheimer described the case of a 51-year-old woman who died after a 5-year illness characterized by progressive dementia. Throughout the cerebral cortex he found the characteristic plaques, but he also noted, thanks to the use of Bielschowsky's newly devised silver impregnation method, a clumping and distortion of fibrils in the neuronal cytoplasm, the neurofibrillary change that now, appropriately, carries Alzheimer's name.

Pathogenesis

Analyses of the plaques and neuronal fibrillary changes have been undertaken in an attempt to elucidate the mechanism of Alzheimer disease, but so far, to little avail. Several histologic techniques assist in this endeavor, including refined methods for silver impregnation that stain both amyloid and its main constituent (beta-amyloid protein [Aβ]); immunostaining using antibodies specific to such proteins as ubiquitin, neuronal tau protein, and beta-amyloid protein; and visualization of β–pleated protein sheets using thioflavine S and Congo red with ultraviolet and polarized light. Tau (composed chemically of beta$_2$-transferrin) is a discrete cytoskeletal protein that promotes the assembly of microtubules, stabilizes their structure, and participates in synaptic plasticity in a yet to be defined manner. In the pathologic circumstances of Alzheimer disease, progressive supranuclear palsy, and frontotemporal dementia (see further on), tau is hyperphosphorylated and aggregates, resulting in paired helical filaments that make up the neurofibrillary tangles. Electrophoretically, tau moves with the β_2-globulins and is thought to function as a transferrin, that is it binds iron and delivers it to the cell. Its concentration can be measured in the CSF and serum, but this has not yet proven clearly to be useful as a diagnostic test.

The Aβ protein is a small portion of a larger entity, the *amyloid precursor protein* (APP), which is normally bound to neuronal membranes. As shown in Fig. 39-2, the Aβ protein is cleaved from APP by the action of proteases termed α, β, and γ secretase. One current hypothesis, developed by Selkoe and others, focuses on the manner in which APP is cleaved by these enzymes to give rise to different-length residues of Aβ. During normal cellular metabolism, APP is cleaved by either α or β secretase. The products of this reaction are then cleaved by the γ-secretase isoform of the enzyme. The sequential cleavage by α and then γ produces tiny fragments that are not toxic to neurons. However, cleavage by β and then γ results in a 40-amino-acid product, Aβ40, and a longer 42-amino-acid form. The latter Aβ42 form is toxic in several models of Alzheimer disease, and it has been proposed that the ratio of Aβ42 to Aβ40 is critical to the neuronal toxicity of amyloid.

Several pieces of evidence favor the view that elevation of the levels of Aβ42 leads to aggregation of amyloid

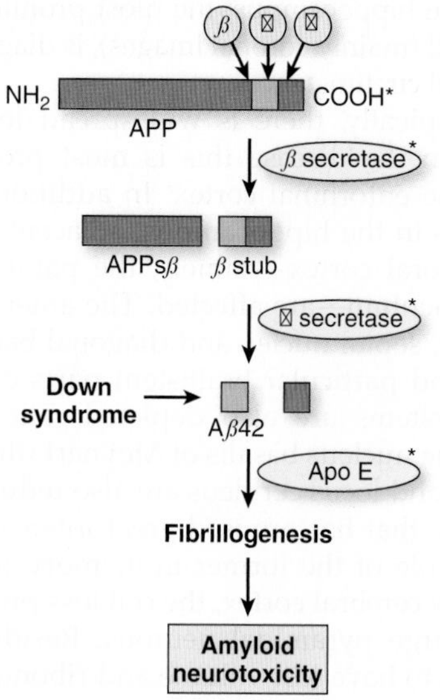

*Mutations in APP, β or ⊠ secretase, and the Apo E4 allele enhance toxicity.

Figure 39-2. Diagram of proteolysis of amyloid precursor protein (APP). When APP is cleaved sequentially by β secretase and then secretase, the resulting amyloid protein can be 40 (Aβ40) or 42 (Aβ42) amino acids in length. The latter favors the formation of aggregated fibrillary amyloid protein (fibrillogenesis) rather than normal APP degradation. The fibrillary form of amyloid is neurotoxic, a mechanism favored as the cause of cell damage in Alzheimer disease. Formation of Aβ42 is promoted by mutations, either in the *APP* gene itself or in the presenilins. In Down syndrome, excess production of APP and its product Aβ42 is caused by triplication of the long arm of chromosome 21, the location of the *APP* gene. The Apo E4 allele is associated with inadequate clearance of Aβ42 and is another mechanism that promotes fibrillogenesis. (Modified by permission from Sisodia SS, St. George–Hyslop PH: γ-Secretase, notch, Aβ and Alzheimer's disease: Where do the presenilins fit in? *Nat Rev Neurosci* 3:281–290, 2002.)

and then to neuronal toxicity. It appears that the diffuse deposition of Aβ42 precedes the formation of better-defined neurofibrils and plaques. The fact that the gene coding for APP is located on chromosome 21, one of the regions linked to one type of familial Alzheimer disease and the duplicated chromosome in Down syndrome, in which Alzheimer changes almost inevitably occur with aging (see further on), suggests that the overproduction of amyloid and all its Aβ residues are causative factors in the disease. Furthermore, the ratio of Aβ42 to Aβ40 is increased in Down syndrome. Another suggestive connection has been the finding that there are genetic defects in the genes encoding APP and in a pair of endosomal proteins termed *presenilin 1* and 2 in some familial forms of Alzheimer disease. The presenilins interact with, or may be a component of, γ secretase, the enzyme that produces the Aβ42 fragment. Mutations of presenilin 1 and 2 also increase the relative levels of Aβ42. It should be noted that mutations of the APP and presenilin genes explain a very small proportion of Alzheimer cases (Terry). Transgenic mice that express human Alzheimer disease-associated mutations in APP or presenilin genes develop plaques with Aβ42 but not neurofibrillary tangles. Many of the relationships and mechanisms depicted in Fig. 39-2 are derived from the understanding of genetic forms of Alzheimer disease; the extent to which they will be implicated in the idiopathic disease is unknown. However, some form of disruption in these mechanisms is likely to be involved in the sporadic disease.

It must be emphasized, however, that there is still uncertainty regarding the relationship of amyloid deposition to the loss of neurons and brain atrophy. Alternatively, soluble oligomers of Aβ amyloid may be the toxic agents, whereas the emphasis until now has been on the effects of visible assemblies of insoluble amyloid fibrils. Similarly, TDP-43, the product of inadequate functioning of the progranulin gene, is also deposited in neurons and may play a substantial role in the severity of expression of Alzheimer disease; this protein has been implicated in the pathogenesis of frontotemporal dementia and motor neuron disease, both discussed later in the chapter. Others have questioned the amyloid hypothesis and pointed to the imprecise relationship between amyloid deposition and neuronal loss, even suggesting that aggregated amyloid is in some way a protective mechanism of cells.

The importance of neurofibrillary tangles has also been questioned, and the manner in which amyloid deposition relates to tangle formation is unclear. Unexplained also is prominent senile plaque formation in some cases and neurofibrillary tangles in others. One prevalent view is that the tangles are a secondary phenomenon. In their review, Hardy and Selkoe, authoritative investigators in this field, pointed out that "Although the amyloid hypothesis offers a broad framework to explain AD pathogenesis, it is currently lacking in detail, and certain observations do not fit easily with the simplest version of the hypothesis." Nonetheless, the amyloid hypothesis is currently the strongest.

In recent years, some of the subcellular mechanisms that are deranged by the presence of intracellular or extracellular amyloid have been elucidated. The finding of a reduced number and enlargement of synapses in affected cortex early in the disease by DeKosky and Scheff and others could be interpreted as either the first sign of neuronal death or the result of the neuronal loss. Amyloid deposition would then be a later, secondary phenomenon. These are complex and uncertain connections but they are among the most promising findings in this field of research.

It was long ago established that Alzheimer disease is not caused by any of the usual types of arteriosclerosis. On the other hand, several studies have indicated that the presence of cerebral infarctions, small or large, and nondescript ischemic white matter disease accelerates the deposition of amyloid and the development of neurofibrillary tangles in the brains of Alzheimer patients (see further on); the mechanism of these interactions is not understood. Not surprisingly, cerebrovascular disease also exaggerates the rate of progression and degree of dementia. How this relates to the entity of *arteriosclerotic*, *multiinfarct*, or *vascular* dementia is entirely clear. Without doubt, as discussed in Chap. 34, multiple cerebral strokes cause increasing deficits that cumulatively qualify as a dementia. At least some of the focal lesions that contribute to the cognitive syndrome can be identified clinically and there is a stepwise decline in function that corresponds to strokes. Admittedly, this type of vascular dementia may be more difficult to recognize when a number of the infarcts are of the relatively silent lacunar type; the mental capacities of such patients may then appear to fail in a gradual and continuous fashion. Memory is relatively spared in the early stages and usually a pseudobulbar state or deterioration in gait accompanies the dementia. The subcortical white matter change of Binswanger disease causes similar diagnostic problems. We are inclined toward the view expressed in Chap. 21 and summarized in the commentary by Jagust that there is an undefined, and perhaps synergistic, interaction between strokes and progressive mental decline in patients with Alzheimer disease. Most often, in our experience, it is the degenerative condition of Alzheimer that explains the dementia. A similar relationship between Alzheimer disease and previous head injuries is tentative but has led to speculation that several types of brain injuries are conducive to the development of neurofibrillary tangles and amyloid deposition, perhaps as if they were part of a reparative response.

No relationship to premorbid personality traits earlier in life has been established, but an intriguing finding from what has become known as the "nun study" and several similar studies suggests that poorer linguistic capability early in life corresponded to the development of Alzheimer disease with aging (D.A. Snowden et al). In this study, the autobiographies of 93 nuns, written in their twenties, were rated for linguistic and ideational complexity. Of 14 sisters who died in late life, deterioration of cognitive function and neuropathologically proven Alzheimer disease occurred in 7 who had a low "idea density" in their writings and in none of 7 whose writings were cognitively more complex. Obviously this type of correlation is subject to several interpretations, but the general notion of "cognitive reserve" having either a protective property or simply hiding mental decline, has emerged from numerous other studies. Also, there has been a general perception confirmed by a few studies such as the one by Verghese and colleagues, that an active mental life may reduce the severity of mental decline with aging, but firm conclusions cannot be made from the available information.

Neurotransmitter Abnormalities Considerable interest was created in the late 1970s by the finding of a marked reduction in choline acetyltransferase (ChAT) and acetylcholine in the hippocampus and neocortex of patients with Alzheimer disease. This loss of cholinergic synthetic capacity was attributed to a reduction in the number of cells in the basal forebrain nuclei (mainly the nucleus basalis of Meynert), from which the major portion of neocortical cholinergic terminals originate (Whitehouse et al). However, a 50 percent reduction in ChAT activity has been found in regions such as the caudate nucleus, which shows neither plaques nor tangles (see review by Selkoe). The specificity of the nucleus basalis cholinergic changes has been questioned for other reasons as well. For one, Alzheimer brain also shows a loss of monoaminergic neurons and a diminution of noradrenergic, gabanergic, and serotonergic functions in the affected neocortex. The concentration of amino acid transmitters, particularly of glutamate, is also reduced in cortical and subcortical areas (Sasaki et al) and the concentration of several neuropeptide transmitters—notably substance P, somatostatin, and cholecystokinin are likewise low—but it has not been determined whether any of these biochemical abnormalities, including the cholinergic ones, are primary or secondary to heterogeneous neuronal loss. Nevertheless, the administration of cholinomimetics—either acetylcholine precursors (e.g., choline or lecithin), degradation inhibitors (e.g., physostigmine), or muscarinic agonists that act directly on postsynaptic receptors—have had a mild and unsustained therapeutic effect (see further under "Treatment").

Chase and associates have demonstrated a 30 percent reduction in cerebral glucose metabolism in Alzheimer disease, greatest in the parietal lobes, but this seems most likely to be secondary to tissue loss in these regions. Even if not of pathogenic significance, it finds value as a diagnostic marker of the disease. The role of aluminum in the genesis of neurofibrillary tangles, as was once proposed, has never been validated. It has been suggested that the use of estrogen by postmenopausal women or of antiinflammatory agents in men or women delayed the onset of the disease or reduced its occurrence, but neither of these have been corroborated by other studies.

Genetic Aspects of Alzheimer Disease (Table 39-1) Of great importance was the aforementioned series of discoveries in patients with inherited forms of Alzheimer disease, of defective genes that code for errant APPs localized to chromosome 21 near the *β*-amyloid gene (St. George-Hyslop et al). As mentioned, this also provided an explanation for the Alzheimer changes that characterize the brains of practically all patients with the trisomy 21 defect (Down syndrome) who survive beyond their twentieth year; they overproduce amyloid as a result of the triplication of the gene. But gene defects on chromosome 21 are responsible for only a small proportion of familial cases and a minuscule percentage of disease overall. Other kindreds with familial Alzheimer disease have been linked to rare dominant mutations of the presenilin genes on chromosome 14 (presenilin 1; Sherrington et al), accounting in some series for up to 50 percent of familial cases, and on chromosome 1 (presenilin 2), which may account for many of the remaining ones (Levy-Lahad et al). These are summarized in Table 39-1. The age of onset of the disease in these familial forms, as in the Down cases, is earlier than that in sporadic forms. These cohorts of patients have provided great insight into long duration between the appearance of amyloid in the brain, approximately a decade, and the onset of clinical disease, and they suggest the potential use of imaging of chemical biomarkers for the disease (The Dominantly Inherited Alzheimer Network; see Bateman et al).

It has been clear for some time that an excess or aberrant amyloid alone is an incomplete explanation for the disease. Certain sequence variants in normal genes confer an increased risk of the disease. The one first discovered was Apo E, a regulator of lipid metabolism that has an affinity for A*β* in Alzheimer plaques, has been found to modify the risk of acquiring Alzheimer disease. Of the several isoforms of Apo E, the presence of E4 (and its corresponding allele e4 on chromosome 19) is associated with a tripling of the risk of developing sporadic Alzheimer disease (Roses; Strittmatter et al; Polvikoski et al). This is the same allele that contributes to an elevated low-density lipoprotein fraction in the serum. Possession of two e4 alleles virtually assures the development of disease in those who survive to their eighties. The e4 allele also modifies the age of onset of some of the familial forms of the disease. In contrast, the e2 allele is underrepresented among Alzheimer patients. For these reasons it has been proposed that Apo E, by interacting with APP or tau protein in some way, modifies the formation of plaques. Indeed, possession of the e4 allele correlates with increased deposition of A*β* in the brain (McNamara). As pointed out by Hardy, Apo E appears to act at a point in the pathogenesis that is after the various genetic mutations have influenced the cellular pathology that ostensibly causes Alzheimer disease. However, these statistical relationships do not invariably connect an allele to the disease in a particular individual. In other words, the e4 allele does not act as a mendelian trait but as a susceptibility (risk) factor. It follows that many, if not most, individuals who develop Alzheimer disease do not

Table 39-1

MUTATIONS AND MODULATING FACTORS ASSOCIATED WITH ALZHEIMER DISEASE

GENE	PROTEIN	INHERITANCE	AGE	CLINICAL FEATURES
APP	Amyloid precursor protein	AD	Early	Rare but clinically simulates sporadic Alzheimer disease
PS1	Presenilin 1	AD	Early	As above
PS2	Presenilin 2	AD	Early	As above
Apo E	Apolipoprotein E	Haplotype	Late	Modifies susceptibility to Alzheimer disease; *ε*-4 allele represents risk
UBQLN1	Ubiquilin 1	SNP	Late	Familial cases only
TREM2	TREM2	SNP	Late	Modulating factor as for Apo E

AD, autosomal dominant; SNP, single nucleotide polymorphism.

have the risk allele. Moreover, many individuals with the e4 allele live into their seventies and eighties without developing Alzheimer disease. All that can be stated with certainty is that, on average, the presence of the e4 allele accelerates the appearance of Alzheimer disease by about 5 years.

Another polymorphism in TREM2 is quite rare in comparison to the aforementioned Apo E variants but confers an equivalent risk of Alzheimer disease that has been shown in several populations in (Guerreiro et al and Jonsson et al). In sporadic Alzheimer disease, the TREM2 polymorphism that is implicated in Alzheimer disease putatively causes inadequate phagocytic clearance of amyloid. Another rare modifying gene has been found in familial cases at the *UBQLN1* (ubiquilin 1) site, coding for a protein that interacts with PS1 and PS2 and participates in proteasomal degradation.

Diagnostic Studies

Studies with CT and MRI are useful, but not definitive ancillary tests (Fig. 39-3). In patients with advanced Alzheimer disease, the lateral and third ventricles are enlarged to about twice the normal size and the cerebral sulci are proportionately widened. Coronal MRI of the medial temporal lobes may reveal a disproportionate atrophy of the hippocampi and a corresponding enlargement of the temporal horns of the lateral ventricles. Early in the disease, however, the changes do not exceed those found in many mentally intact old persons. For this reason, one cannot rely solely on imaging procedures for diagnosis and CT and MRI are most valuable in excluding alternative causes of dementia such as brain tumor, subdural hematoma, cerebral infarction, and hydrocephalus. The EEG undergoes mild diffuse slowing, but only late in the course of the illness; it is useful again, in the exclusion of alternative causes of mental decline that manifest themselves in seizure activity or changes typical of metabolic encephalopathy. The CSF is also normal, although occasionally the total protein is slightly elevated. Using the constellation of clinical data, cerebral imaging in the context of the age of the patient and time course of the disease, the diagnosis of dementia of Alzheimer type is made correctly in 85 to 90 percent of cases.

Of considerable value have been studies of cerebral blood flow single-photon emission computed tomography [SPECT]) and metabolism (positron emission tomography [PET]), which early in the illness often, but not always, show diminished activity in the parietal association regions and the medial temporal lobes. In most cases, when such changes are evident, the diagnosis was already obvious on clinical grounds. Newer PET ligand agents that bind to amyloid, such as the "Pittsburgh compound" and tau-ligands are more sensitive in identifying and observing the course of Alzheimer disease. Their main utility may be in detecting changes before brain atrophy is evident and in identifying patients who have the earliest changes of Alzheimer disease, whose disease course may be amenable to alteration by medications.

Neuropsychologic tests in the typical case show disproportionate deterioration in memory and verbal access skills. Testing is particularly useful when there is a serial decline in ability. Certain aspects of attention and executive function in Alzheimer disease that also show changes in Alzheimer disease were reviewed by Perry and Hodges. The use of these examinations is described in Chap. 21.

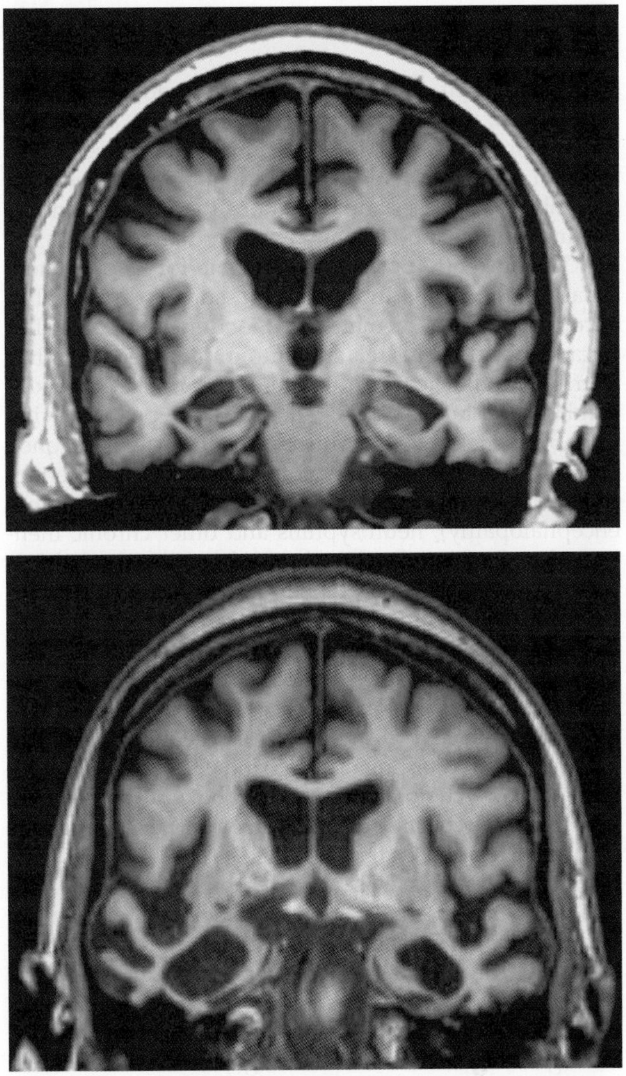

Figure 39-3. *Top:* Coronal T1-weighted MRI of a 74-year-old man with moderate Alzheimer-type dementia. Diffuse cerebral and hippocampal atrophy with ex vacuo ventricular and cortical sulcal dilation is noted. *Bottom:* Coronal T1-weighted MRI of a 70-year-old woman with behavioral variant frontotemporal lobar dementia. Atrophy of the right greater than left temporal lobes is out of proportion to atrophy of the frontal and parietal lobes.

There are no established biologic markers of Alzheimer disease with the possible exception of the ratio of Aβ42 to tau, in the cerebrospinal fluid (the ratio is low in Alzheimer disease). This test is used in some clinics, but may not be well enough validated for routine use (Maddalena et al). Schoonenboom and colleagues have shown that the incorporation of CSF phosphorylated tau (p-tau) with the typical CSF amyloid/tau ratio may provide additional specificity in distinguishing Alzheimer from other dementing diseases.

Differential Diagnosis of Alzheimer Disease

(See also Table 21-3)

Formerly, when virtually all forms of dementia were untreatable, there was little advantage to either the patient or the family in ascertaining the cause of the cerebral disease. There are now adequate treatments for a number of diseases and conditions that cause cognitive decline, putting a premium on proper diagnosis.

The currently potentially treatable forms of dementia are those caused by normal-pressure hydrocephalus; chronic subdural hematoma; the dementia of AIDS; paraneoplastic and related autoimmune encephalitis; nutritional deficiencies (thiamine—Wernicke-Korsakoff syndrome, Marchiafava-Bignami disease, pellagra, vitamin B_{12} deficiency); chronic intoxication (e.g., alcohol, sedatives); multiple cerebral infarctions; certain endocrine and metabolic disorders (myxedema, Hashimoto encephalopathy), neurosyphilis and other chronic meningitides, Cushing disease, chronic hepatic encephalopathy; frontal and temporal lobe tumors; vascular dementia, cerebral vasculitis; sarcoidosis; progressive multifocal leukoencephalopathy (PML), Whipple disease; multiple sclerosis; and sometimes neglected, the pseudodementia of depression. Exclusion of most of these diseases is readily accomplished by careful history, sequential clinical evaluations, and testing of blood and CSF, EEG, CT, MRI, and neuropsychologic testing can be undertaken. We have regularly but infrequently incorporated the results of metabolic brain imaging (both FDG-PET and amyloid-ligand imaging) as well as CSF amyloid-tau ratio. We anticipate that these tests or similar ones may find more frequent use. In exceptional situations, brain biopsy may be justified in the diagnosis of dementia, almost limited to rapidly progressive cases. A perspective, albeit from a sample that cannot be generalized to practice, has been given by Warren and colleagues of 90 consecutive brain biopsies performed between 1989 and 2003 for the evaluation of dementia. More than half provided a diagnosis, mostly Alzheimer, Creutzfeldt-Jakob disease, and inflammatory disorders. However, reasonable assurances must be given to the neurosurgeon that prion disease is unlikely.

One problem in differential diagnosis is the distinction between a late-life depression and a dementia, especially when some degree of both is present. Observation over several weeks or more, and the patient's demeanor, makes the distinction clearer. Multiinfarct dementia is usually not difficult to separate from Alzheimer dementia, as discussed further on. The dementia of normal-pressure hydrocephalus may also be confused with Alzheimer dementia (see Chap. 30). The problem of distinguishing Alzheimer disease from a more "benign" form of memory decline associated with aging comes up frequently in practice, as discussed further on. These treatable conditions are discussed in Chaps. 21, 30, and 34 and the important topic of depression is addressed in Chap. 52. Often we have been confident on clinical grounds that a patient had Alzheimer disease, only to have revealed at autopsy that progressive supranuclear palsy, Lewy-body disease, Pick disease, another non-Alzheimer degeneration of the frontal lobes, or cortical-basal-ganglionic degeneration was the cause. All are discussed later in this chapter.

Treatment

There is no evidence that any of the formerly proposed therapies for Alzheimer disease—cerebral vasodilators, stimulants, L-dopa, massive doses of vitamins B, C, and E, gingko biloba, hyperbaric oxygen, intravenous immunoglobulin, and many others—have any salutary effect. Trials of oral physostigmine, choline, and lecithin have yielded mostly negative or uninterpretable results.

The effect of the currently used cholinergic precursors and agonists and acetylcholinesterase inhibitors, such as donepezil, is modest. With regard to the latter group of drugs, several large trials have demonstrated a slight prolongation of the patient's ability to sustain an independent life, but such evidence generally requires that the medications be taken for 6 to 12 months. For example, a meta-analysis of the drugs collectively demonstrated a mean improvement of 2 to 3 points on the 70-point Alzheimer Disease Assessment Scale and a slight delay in progression. Despite some trials that have failed to demonstrate benefit (c.f., AD 2000 Collaborative Group), the balance of evidence favors the use of these medications in practice, but only in mildly or moderately affected patients.

Side effects of the aforementioned class of drugs may include nausea and less often, vomiting. The families of our patients report from time to time that the medication caused insomnia or increased confusion. It is worth mentioning that when the acetylcholine receptor antagonist succinylcholine is used prior to general anesthesia, its effects may be prolonged in patients taking the above drugs. The use of trazodone, haloperidol, thioridazine, risperidone, and related drugs may suppress some of the aberrant behavior and hallucinations when these are problems, making life more comfortable for both patient and family, but several trials suggest that their general application causes more problems than it solves and they must often be discontinued in response to adverse effects. The randomized trial conducted by Schneider and coworkers found that olanzapine, quetiapine, and risperidone for the treatment of psychosis, aggression, or agitation with Alzheimer disease were approximately as good as placebo in relieving these symptoms, but largely because the drugs were not tolerated. Olanzapine was slightly preferable in those who continued taking the medication. The clinician is left with little recourse but to use this class of medications or haloperidol to control unmanageable behavior. Small doses of diazepines, such as lorazepam, are useful when sleep is severely disturbed, but they often increase confusion as well.

The *N*-methyl-D-aspartate (NMDA) glutaminergic antagonists, specifically memantine (20 mg daily), have also been tried. In a study of memantine by Reisberg and colleagues of 252 patients (187 of whom completed the trial), there were better results on a few scales that reflected functional behavior compared to the use of placebo, but there was no change in 3 main measures of cognitive performance. Because the side effects were ostensibly minor, this drug has been approved for use in late-stage Alzheimer disease and in conjunction with cholinergic drugs. Nevertheless, hallucinations or agitation may occur and require discontinuation. The combination of memantine and donepezil in moderately to severely affected patients offered no benefit over either drug alone (Howard et al). The effects of these drugs in later stages of the disease are, in any case, minimal.

A provocative series of studies using a small molecule inhibitors of the enzyme γ-secretase (semagacestat; see Doody et al, 2013), and a monoclonal antibody directed at soluble forms of amyloid (solanezumab; see Doody et al, 2014) have failed to demonstrate clear benefit in early Alzheimer disease. The presumption is that such agents might be useful if started in the presymptomatic stages of disease.

A series of animal experiments that demonstrated the possibility of removal of plaques by immunization against amyloid has led to human studies with a similar vaccination. One trial was stopped because of the occurrence of an immune encephalitis in a small number of patients, but in autopsy material there were indications that this novel approach may have had the desired effect of reducing amyloid deposition (Orgogozo et al). Revised vaccines are being formulated for further testing of this approach.

Given the state of therapeutics for Alzheimer disease, always important is the general management of the demented patient, which should proceed along the lines outlined in Chap. 21, keeping in mind that the physician's counsel is often the family's main resource for important medical and social decisions.

Associated Pathologic States

As indicated earlier, the histologic changes of Alzheimer disease have a number of interesting associations. Amyloid plaques and tangle deposition are far more common in the brains of patients with Parkinson disease (20 to 30 percent) than in the brains of age-matched controls (Hakim and Mathieson). These findings partly explain the high incidence of dementia in patients with Parkinson disease (see further on). As mentioned, with the advance of Alzheimer disease, extrapyramidal features may emerge. In such cases, Burns and colleagues have found changes in the substantia nigra including accumulation of synuclein and tau representative of Lewy bodies. Another association between the 2 diseases is apparent in the *Guamanian Parkinson–dementia complex*, which is also discussed below. In this entity, the symptoms of dementia and parkinsonism are related to neurofibrillary changes in the cerebral cortex and substantia nigra, respectively; senile plaques and Lewy bodies are unusual findings. What can be deduced from the crossover syndromes is that multiple degenerative changes can occur in these diseases and give rise to heterogeneity in clinical presentation.

The finding of neurofibrillary tangles (and to a lesser extent of plaques) in boxers (*"punch-drunk" syndrome*, or *dementia pugilistica*) is another interesting ramification of the Alzheimer disease process in that trauma appears to be able to elicit one of the core features of the disease as discussed in Chap. 35. Some cases of *primary progressive aphasia* (see further on) have Alzheimer change and amyloid plaque deposition as the primary pathologic change. There are other unusual and meaningful associations, such as dementia with motor neuron disease or the cases of familial dementia with spastic paraplegia reported by Worster-Drought and by van Bogaert and their associates (see later in this chapter). Here, neurofibrillary change is the most prominent feature whereas amyloid plaques are negligible in number or absent.

Another provocative connection is the already mentioned interrelationship between cerebrovascular disease and Alzheimer disease. This is a complex area that at one time, considered the 2 processes to be intimately related and later, was rejected, only to now be resurrected with clearer focus, as discussed Chap 34.

Lobar Atrophies (Frontotemporal Lobar Degeneration, Posterior Lobar Degeneration)

This broad category of disease has evolved and the nosology is confusing because type of selective atrophy of a cerebral lobe may be caused by several different histopathologic changes. The notion of lobar atrophy was introduced in 1892 when Arnold Pick of Prague described a special form of cerebral degeneration in which the atrophy was circumscribed (most often in the frontal or temporal lobes), with involvement of both gray and white matter; hence the term he applied was *lobar* rather than *cortical* sclerosis. In 1911, Alzheimer presented the first careful study of the microscopic changes, followed by even more complete analyses of the pathologic changes by the prominent neuropathologists of the age. As mentioned the pathologic change associated may be any one of several types: Pick inclusion bodies, neurofibrillary tangles, other inclusions, or with no characteristic changes except for neuronal loss. Contrariwise, gliosis and mild spongiform changes in the superficial layers of cortex, and even typical plaque and tangle pathology, have all been associated with syndromes of gross atrophy of the frontal or temporal lobes. What has emerged since his work is that the most common and important of the lobar atrophies is a group of frontotemporal degenerations that have diverse clinical and pathologic profiles.

In contrast to Alzheimer disease, in which the atrophy is relatively diffuse, the pathologic change in lobar atrophy is circumscribed and often asymmetrical. The parietal lobes are involved less frequently than the frontal and temporal lobes. The affected gyri become paper thin, resembling, in the advanced stages, the kernel of a dried walnut. The cut surface reveals not only a marked narrowing of the cortical ribbon but a grayish appearance and reduced volume of the underlying white matter. The corpus callosum and anterior commissure share in the atrophy but almost certainly as secondary phenomena. The overlying pia-arachnoid is often thickened, and the ventricles are enlarged. The pre- and postcentral, superior temporal, and occipital convolutions are relatively unaffected and stand out in striking contrast to the wasted parts.

The more common frontotemporal lobar degenerations (FTLDs) (to which Pick's name was attached) may display any one of several pathologic changes and reflect different genetic causes. For example, the behavioral or the aphasic variants of FTD, which are described below, may be the result of the deposition of tau, progranulin, amyloid, or synuclein. It is not clear to us if the term "Pick disease" is worth retaining to denote a unique process aside from the unusual type that is due to deposition of argyrophilic intracytoplasmic inclusions (Pick bodies) and diffusely staining ballooned neurons (Pick cells). In other respects, it is simply one of the large group of FTLDs. It is the lobar atrophy and marked changes in the underlying white matter that provide the unifying elements of this group of diseases.

Clinical and Pathologic Features

The descriptive terms frontotemporal lobar atrophy and frontotemporal dementia are used by neurologists and neuropathologists to refer to a clinical syndrome that is associated with degeneration of the frontal and temporal lobes. Some of the clinical aspects of frontotemporal dementia were discussed in Chap. 21, but broadly speaking, there are 2 main types: a behavioral variant and a language variant, the latter being divided into semantic dementia, progressive nonfluent aphasia, and a logopenic variant, all described below.

Behavioral Variant FTLD Patients under consideration with behavioral changes present with personality and related abnormalities that include apathy, disinhibition, perseveration, poor judgment and limited ability for abstraction, loss of empathy, bizarre affect, eating disorders, and a general disengagement. Insight is almost always impaired and some subjects become euphoric or display repetitive compulsive behaviors. An initial diagnosis of depression has been common. Other psychiatric symptoms such as sociopathic and disinhibited behavior with aspects of hyperorality and hyperphagia may predominate late in the illness. Utilization behavior (the compulsive use of implements and tools put before the patient) is also displayed in advanced cases.

CT, MRI, and functional imaging demonstrate a disproportionate atrophy and hypofunction in the frontal lobes, usually asymmetric. A proportion of patients with this type of frontotemporal dementia have parkinsonian features. A form of motor neuron disease is also linked to frontotemporal dementia in a small number of cases. This is particularly the case in the Guamanian (now called *western Pacific*) variety and in the heredofamilial frontotemporal atrophy linked to a mutation on chromosome 17.

In some writings on this subject, the term frontotemporal dementia has come to be used in a highly restricted sense, being assigned to cases that show only tau-staining material in neurons. Most of the cases are sporadic, but the inherited variety linked to chromosome 17, in which parkinsonism is prominent, supports its distinction as a separate entity; it is in these cases that the intraneural deposition of tau is most striking, in both the frontotemporal cortex and the substantia nigra. In a few familial cases, this process is attributable to mutations in the gene on chromosome 17 that encodes the tau protein. These mutations alter the proportions of different isoforms of this protein and lead both to tau accumulation and its hyperphosphorylation. Indeed, many cases of frontotemporal dementia are associated with tau gene mutations. However, abnormal aggregates of tau have been identified in practically all neurodegenerative atrophies and, of course, form the main constituent of the paired helical filaments (neurofibrillary tangles) of Alzheimer disease, and in progressive supranuclear palsy where they are abundant, although of slightly different structure. From the observations of Brun and Passant and of Neary and associates, pure tau-reactive cases outnumber Pick disease when the latter is strictly defined by the cortical white matter degeneration and Pick inclusions.

Nonetheless, a frontotemporal dementia identical to that of the tau-reactive cases has been observed in others without any tau or synuclein staining of neurons. Many of the frontally predominant cases have shown deposition of the protein progranulin, consisting mainly of a ubiquitin neuronal inclusion consisting of TDP-43 (TAR DNA-binding protein), the result of PGRN mutations.

Primary Progressive Aphasias (PPA) Focal disturbances, particularly aphasia and apraxia, occur early and prominently in certain patients with lobar degenerations, indicating a lesion in the left frontal or temporal lobes. Viewed from another perspective, a prominent language disorder has been described in almost two-thirds of all patients with temporal lobe atrophy.

Several types of this disturbance have been delineated. In the first, *progressive nonfluent aphasia*, the patient initially speaks less and has word-finding difficulty (anomia), but language structure is intact (Mesulam, 1982); later, he may forget and misuse words and soon fails to understand much of what is heard or read. Sentences are short and telegraphed. Later, dysarthria and apraxia become apparent and finally, the patient is virtually mute, seemingly without impulse to speak, and with an inability to form words (Snowden et al, 1992).

A second type, *semantic dementia*, is characterized by early difficulty naming items, people, and words, followed by verbal perseveration, but fluency is retained. There is considerable difficulty in generating lists of words of a given category, such as animals. These individuals are quite aware that they are having trouble finding words. Eventually the patient loses not just the use of names of people and objects, but also their meaning, or the conceptual knowledge of the word. Some may develop severe prosopagnosia, especially if the atrophy is predominantly right sided. Memory for day-to-day events is preserved.

A third type has been proposed, *logopenic aphasia*, that shares most aspects of nonfluent aphasia but in which the meaning of words is retained.

According to Mesulam (2003), who has studied the condition extensively, 60 percent of these cases show no characteristic pathologic change, 20 percent have Pick bodies, and a similar proportion show the typical changes of Alzheimer disease in the affected cortical region. A clear familial tendency has not been found. Chapter 23 can be consulted for details of the aphasic disorders.

Posterior Cortical Atrophy This regional variant of lobar degeneration has been slightly less frequent than primary progressive aphasia in our practices. The fundamental feature is the progressive loss of the ability to understand and use visual information. The result is progressive and ultimately severe visuospatial difficulty with a relative preservation of memory. Prosopagnosia, achromatopsia, and dyslexia emerge, or, there may be difficulty with depth perception, reaching for objects and an inordinate sensitivity to bright light. Patients under our care have initially had a vague sense of visual disorientation followed over months by difficulty in seeing or recognizing objects in front of them. Many have alexia with agraphia while others have acalculia or the other elements of the Gerstmann syndrome. Several eventually become cortically blind. The syndrome is essentially that of an apperceptive visual disturbance that includes fragments of the Balint and the Gerstmann syndromes. The average age of onset is about 60 years. The most common pathologic change in most reports has been characteristic of Alzheimer disease.

Lewy-body Dementia (Diffuse Lewy-body Disease)

Next to Alzheimer disease, diffuse Lewy-body disease, or Lewy-body dementia, has been the most frequent pathologic diagnosis established in many series of globally demented patients. Reports of this condition have been increasing steadily since the original communication by Okazaki and colleagues in 1961 (see review by Kosaka). The disease is defined by the diffuse involvement of cortical neurons with Lewy-body inclusions and by an absence or inconspicuous number of neurofibrillary tangles and amyloid plaques. To some extent, increased recognition of this disorder is a result of improved histologic techniques, particularly the ability to detect ubiquitin and synuclein, main components of the Lewy body, by immunostaining. With this improved detection has come a better definition of the clinical syndrome and its distinctions from Alzheimer and other dementias. Because the Lewy bodies in cortical neurons are not surrounded by a distinct halo, as they are in the substantia nigra in cases of Parkinson disease (see further on for discussion and photomicrograph of a typical Lewy body) they were not readily appreciated. Aggreagated α-synuclein is the main component of the Lewy body an observation that will prove important in understanding both Parkinson disease and Lewy-body dementia.

Clinical Features

The disease in its typical form is marked by parkinsonian features, dementia, and a tendency to episodic delirium, especially nocturnally, and rapid eye movement (REM) sleep behavior disorder (described below and in Chap. 19). Diagnostic criteria have been offered by a working group, requiring 2 of 3 of the following: a parkinsonian syndrome (usually symmetric), fluctuations in behavior and cognition, and recurrent hallucinations (McKeith et al). The latest recursion of this group's criteria emphasizes the presence of the REM sleep behavior disorder and severe neuroleptic sensitivity.

In an analysis of 34 cases of diffuse Lewy-body disease, Burkhardt and colleagues, found that the most characteristic syndrome was one of progressive dementia in an elderly patient with the additional late onset of parkinsonism in many cases. In Lennox's summary of 75 cases, parkinsonism, particularly with limb and axial rigidity, was a prominent feature in 90 percent once the illness was fully developed, and almost half had tremor of the parkinsonian type (this is somewhat different from other series). Byrne and associates, as have many others, pointed out that episodic confusion, hallucinations, and paranoid delusions were features of Lewy-body dementia; such psychotic aspects are generally uncharacteristic of Alzheimer and lobar dementias, and only then, in advanced stages. In Lennox's review, one-third of patients had these swings in behavior, but as the illness advanced, amnesia, dyscalculia, visuospatial disorientation, aphasia, and apraxia differed little from those of Alzheimer disease. In the cases reported by Fearnley and coworkers, there was a supranuclear gaze palsy simulating that of progressive supranuclear palsy. These overlapping clinical features make diagnosis difficult unless the specific feature of episodic hallucinations is evident. Difficulty in diagnosis also arises because the parkinsonian disorder may be either mild or prominent and may occur as an early or a late manifestation.

The parkinsonian features can respond favorably to L-dopa, but only for a limited time and sometimes at the expense of causing an agitated delirium or hallucinations that would be uncharacteristic of early Parkinson disease (Hely et al); in others, the response to L-dopa is inconsistent or inapparent. Some patients also have orthostatic hypotension corresponding to cell loss and Lewy bodies in the intermediolateral cell column of the spinal cord or in the sympathetic ganglia, thereby simulating striatonigral degeneration or Shy-Drager syndrome (see further on). Others have commented on an extreme sensitivity of such patients to neuroleptic drugs, including increased confusion and greatly worsening parkinsonism or the development of the neuroleptic malignant syndrome.

In our experience with Lewy-body disease, the parkinsonian symptoms have been more prominent than they are in progressive supranuclear palsy, and the most characteristic feature besides the movement disorder and a slowly advancing dementia has been a vacuous, anxious state with intermittent psychotic or delirious behavior.

At least one randomized trial has described benefit from the anticholinesterase inhibitor, rivastigmine, in reducing delusions, hallucinations, and anxiety (McKeith and colleagues, 2000). With regard to diagnostic testing, the finding of reduced activity in the posterior parietal cortical regions on PET scans (as in Alzheimer disease) has been found as a relatively consistent, but not invariable, feature.

Other Degenerative Dementias

Argyrophilic Grain Disease

This obscure entity has been connected with a late-life dementia in which behavioral disturbances precede memory difficulty. Whether the finding of argyrophilic grains in the mediotemporal lobe, different from tau-laden neurofibrillary tangles and from the glial inclusions (putatively a defining feature of multiple system atrophy), constitutes a specific entity is not clear to the authors. The finding overlaps with the deposition of other materials that are more closely associated with dementing diseases such as phosphorylated tau and Lewy bodies. Probst and Tolnay remarked that these small argyrophilic inclusions are not found in nondemented individuals. It is unlikely that the condition can be identified in life; if it is a genuine entity, it must be rare. The interested reader may consult the review by Ferrer.

Neuroserpinopathy

There have been infrequent case reports of dominantly inherited, adult-onset dementia with a fulminant evolution suggestive of encephalopathy and the special feature of seizures. The distinctive feature has been the presence at autopsy of large eosinophilic, PAS-positive intraneuronal inclusions that contain aggregates of neuroserpin, thus the initial description of "familial encephalopathy with neuronal inclusion bodies." The serpins are a family of protease inhibitors that include neuroserpin, a protein expressed exclusively in neurons, and α_1-antitrypsin. The neuronal inclusions are densest in the deep layers of the cortex and in the substantia nigra. Missense mutations in the gene encoding neuroserpin have been identified as the cause. This entity is reviewed by Lomas and Carrell.

DEMENTING DISEASES IN WHICH OTHER NEUROLOGIC ABNORMALITIES ARE PROMINENT

Huntington Disease (Huntington Chorea)

This disease, distinguished by the triad of dominant inheritance, choreoathetosis, and dementia, commemorates the name of George Huntington, a medical practitioner of Pomeroy, Ohio. In 1872, his paper, read before the Meigs and Mason Academy of Medicine and published later that year in the *Medical and Surgical Reporter* of Philadelphia, gave a succinct and graphic account of the disease that was based on observations of patients that his father and grandfather had made in the course of their practice in East Hampton, Long Island. Reports of this disease had appeared previously (see DeJong for historical background) but they lacked the completeness of Huntington's description. In 1932, Vessie was able to show that practically all the patients with this disease in the eastern United States could be traced to about 6 individuals who had emigrated in 1630 from the tiny East Anglian village of Bures, in Suffolk, England. One remarkable family was traced for 300 years through 12 generations, in each of which the disease had expressed itself.

To quote Huntington, the rule has been that "When either or both of the parents have shown manifestations of the disease, one or more of the offspring invariably suffer of the disease, if they live to adult life. But if by any chance these children go through life without it, the thread is broken and the grandchildren and great grandchildren of the original shakers may rest assured that they are free from disease." Davenport, in a review of 962 patients with Huntington chorea, found only 5 who had descended from unaffected parents. Possibly, in these 5 patients, a parent had the trait, in very mild form, or parentage was in question, because spontaneous mutations are rare.

In university hospital centers, this is a regularly observed type of hereditary nervous system diseases and the main cause of progressive chorea at most ages. Its overall frequency is estimated at 4 to 5 per million, and 30 to 70 per million among whites of northern European ancestry. The usual age of onset is in the fourth and fifth decades, but 3 to 5 percent begin before the fifteenth year and some even in childhood, where it takes on special form. In approximately 30 percent, symptoms become apparent after 50 years. The progression of the disease is generally slower in older patients for reasons noted below. Once begun, the disease progresses relentlessly, until only a restricted existence is possible and a medical disease terminates life.

Exhaustive genealogic documentation many years ago established the cause to be an autosomal dominant gene with complete penetrance. Koller and Davenport made the observation that young patients usually inherit the disease from their fathers and older patients from their mothers. It has been observed beginning at almost the same age in identical twins.

The first important achievement in respect to the biologic understanding of Huntington disease was the discovery by Gusella and colleagues of a marker linked to the Huntington gene and localized to the short arm of chromosome 4. Subsequently, these investigators and others identified the mutation as an excessively long repeat of the trinucleotide CAG within the Huntington gene, the length (number) of which determines not only the presence of the disease, but also the age of onset, longer repeat lengths being associated with an earlier appearance of signs. At the Huntington gene locus there are normally 11 to 34 (median: 19) consecutive repetitions of the CAG triplet, each coding for glutamine. Individuals with 35 to 39 triplets may eventually manifest the disease but it tends to be late in onset and mild in degree, or limited to the below-mentioned "senile chorea." Those with more than 42 repeats almost invariably acquire the signs of disease if they live long enough. The rare alternative mutation, termed HDL2 (Huntington disease-like-2), is associated with CATCG repeat expansion of the juntophilin-3 gene, but it is so infrequent that few clinicians will encounter it (Margolis et al).

These discoveries have made possible the development of a genetic test for the measurement of the repeat length that confirms the diagnosis in symptomatic patients and allows screening of asymptomatic individuals. Because there is no treatment for the disease, testing raises certain ethical considerations that must be resolved before its widespread utilization.

Clinical Features

The *mental disorder* assumes several subtle forms long before the more obvious deterioration of cognitive functions becomes evident. In approximately half the cases, slight but annoying alterations of personality are the first to appear. Patients begin to find fault with everything, to complain constantly, and to nag other members of the family; they may be suspicious, irritable, impulsive, eccentric, untidy, or excessively religious, or they may exhibit a false sense of superiority. Poor self-control may be reflected in outbursts of temper, fits of despondency, slovenliness, alcoholism, or sexual promiscuity. Disturbances of mood, particularly depression, are common (almost half of the patients in some series) and may constitute the most prominent symptoms early in the disease. Invariably, sooner or later, the intellect begins to fail globally. The patient becomes less communicative and socially withdrawn. The emotional disturbances and changes in personality may reach such proportions as to constitute a virtual psychosis with persecutory delusions or hallucinations.

Diminished work performance, inability to manage household responsibilities, and disturbances of sleep may prompt medical consultation. There is difficulty in maintaining attention and concentration and in assimilating new material. Mental flexibility lessens. Simultaneously, there is loss of fine manual skills (see further on). The performance parts of the Wechsler Adult Intelligence Scale show greater loss than the verbal parts. Memory is relatively spared. This gradual dilapidation of intellectual function has been characterized as a "subcortical dementia," that is elements of aphasia, agnosia, and apraxia are observed only rarely and memory loss is not profound. Often the process is so slow, particularly in cases of late onset, that a fair degree of intellectual capacity seems to be retained for many years.

The *abnormality of movement* is subtle at first and most evident in the hands and face; often the patient is merely considered to be fidgety, restless, or "nervous." Slowness of movement of the fingers and hands, a reduced rate of finger tapping, and difficulty in performing a sequence of hand movements are early signs. Gradually these abnormalities become more pronounced until the entire musculature is implicated with chorea. The frequency of blinking is increased (the opposite of parkinsonism), and voluntary protrusion of the tongue, like other attempts at sustained posture, is constantly interrupted by unwanted darting movements. In the advanced stage of the disease the patient is seldom still for more than a few seconds. The choreic movements are slower than the brusque jerks and postural lapses of Sydenham chorea, and they involve many more muscles. They tend to recur in stereotyped patterns yet are not as stereotyped as tics. In advanced cases, they acquire an athetoid or dystonic quality. Muscle tone is usually decreased until late in the illness, when there may also be some degree of rigidity, tremor, and bradykinesia, elements suggestive of Parkinson disease. Parkinsonism with rigidity characterizes the Westphal or "rigid" variant, which is more common with a childhood onset, or the HDL2 genetic variant noted earlier. Tendon reflexes are exaggerated in one-third of patients, but only a few have Babinski signs. Voluntary movements are initiated and executed more slowly than normal, but there is no weakness and no ataxia, although speech, which becomes dysarthric and explosive because of incoordination between tongue and diaphragm, may convey the impression of a cerebellar disorder. Inability to hold the tongue protruded is characteristic. In late-onset cases there may be an almost constant rapid movement of the tongue and mouth, simulating the tardive dyskinesia that follows the use of neuroleptic drugs. These disorders of movement that characterize Huntington chorea are described more fully in Chap. 4.

Oculomotor function is subtly affected in most patients (Leigh et al; Lasker et al). Particularly characteristic are impaired initiation and slowness of both pursuit and volitional saccadic movements and an inability to make a volitional saccade without movement of the head. Excessive distractibility may be noticed during attempted ocular fixation. The patient feels compelled to glance at extraneous stimuli even when specifically instructed to ignore them. Upward gaze is often impaired as the illness progresses.

As Wilson stated, the relation of the choreic to the mental symptoms "abides by no general rule." Most often the mental symptoms precede the chorea but they may accompany or follow it, sometimes by many years. Once the movement disorder is fully established, there is nearly always some degree of cognitive abnormality. Exceptional cases have been reported in which the movement disorder existed for 10 to 30 years without mental changes (Britton et al); this would be most characteristic of patients with fewer CAG repeats. More typically after 10 to 15 years of symptoms, most patients deteriorate to a vegetative state, unable to stand or walk and eating little; in this late stage, a mild amyotrophy may appear. Noteworthy is the high suicide rate, as pointed out by Huntington himself (see also Schoenfeld et al). Because there is a higher-than-normal incidence of head trauma, chronic subdural hematoma is another common finding at autopsy.

The first signs of the disease may appear in childhood, before puberty (even younger than the age of 4 years), and several series of such early-onset cases have been described (Farrer and Conneally; van Dijk et al). Mental deterioration at this early age is more often accompanied by cerebellar ataxia, behavior problems, seizures, bradykinesia, rigidity, and dystonia than by chorea (Byers et al). However, this rigid form of the disease (Westphal variant) also occurs occasionally in adults as mentioned above, in some cases because of HDL2. Functional decline is much faster in children than it is in adults (Young et al).

The dementia is generally more severe in cases of early onset and with correspondingly longer repeat lengths (15 to 40 years of age) than in those of later onset (55 to 60 years of age). In adult patients with early onset, the emotional disturbance tends to be more prominent initially and precedes the chorea and intellectual loss by years; with older age of onset, choreiform features are more often the initial components; in the middle years, dementia and chorea have their onset at nearly the same age. At the other extreme of age, the first features may become evident in the eighties, with orofacial or other dyskinesias that are mistakenly attributed to an exposure to neuroleptic drugs or called "senile chorea" (see Chap. 4).

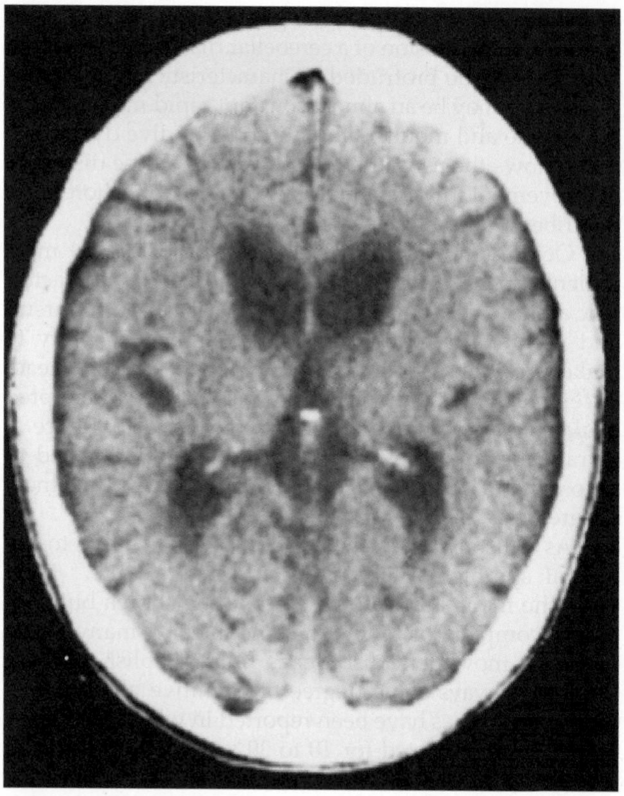

Figure 39-4. Axial CT from a 54-year-old mildly demented woman with a 10-year history of Huntington chorea. The bulge in the inferolateral border of the lateral ventricle, normally created by the head of the caudate nucleus, is obliterated. There is also diffuse enlargement of the lateral ventricles.

Pathology and Pathogenesis

Gross atrophy bilaterally of the head of the caudate nucleus and putamen is the characteristic abnormality, usually accompanied by a moderate degree of gyral atrophy in the frontal and temporal regions. The caudate atrophy alters the configuration of the frontal horns of the lateral ventricles in that the inferolateral borders do not show the usual bulge formed by the head of the caudate nucleus. In addition, the ventricles are diffusely enlarged (Fig. 39-4); in CT scans, the bicaudate-to-cranial ratio is increased, which corroborates the clinical diagnosis in the moderately advanced case.

The early articles of Alzheimer and Dunlap and the more recent one of Vonsattel and DiFiglia contain the most authoritative descriptions of the microscopic changes. The latter authors have graded the disease into early, moderately advanced, and far advanced stages. In 5 early but genetically verified cases, no striatal lesion was found, which suggests that the first clinical manifestations are based on a biochemical or infrastructural change. This view is supported by the observation that Huntington patients studied with PET show a characteristic decrease in glucose metabolism in the caudate nuclei, which precedes the volumetric loss of tissue (Hayden et al). The striatal degeneration begins in the medial part of the caudate nucleus and spreads, tending to spare the nucleus accumbens. Of the 6 cell types in the striatum (a differentiation based on size, dendritic arborizations, spines, and axon trajectories), the smaller neurons are affected before the larger ones. Loss of dendrites of the small spiny neurons has been an early finding, while the large cells are relatively preserved and exhibit no special alterations.

The anterior parts of the putamen and caudate are more affected than the posterior parts. Some observers have noted changes in the globus pallidus, subthalamic nucleus, red nucleus, cerebellum, and in the pars reticulata of the substantia nigra. In the cerebral cortex, there is slight neuronal loss in layers 3, 5, and 6, with replacement gliosis. Cases are reported with typical striatal lesions but normal cortices in which only chorea had been present during late life. Several neuropathologists have observed marked cell loss and gliosis in the subthalamic nuclei in Huntington-affected children or young adults with chorea and behavior disorders. However, Hadzi and colleagues have determined that the pathologic changes in the striatum and the cortex evolve differently and have separate relationships to the CAG repeat length.

Mechanism of Disease As mentioned above, there is a general relationship between the number of CAG repeats and the age of onset of symptoms. It has been found that it is the longer sequence on either of the 2 alleles that determines the age of onset, the size of the expansion of the normal allele exerting no influence (Lee et al, 2012). Earlier onset in successive generations (*anticipation*) is well described in the early writings on the subject and is now known to be attributable to increasing lengths of the CAG repeat sequence.

From the molecular perspective, the pathogenesis of this disease is a direct, but still poorly understood, consequence of the aforementioned expansion of the polyglutamine region of *huntingtin* (the protein product of the Huntington gene). It has been shown that the mutant huntingtin protein aggregates in the nuclei of neurons. Moreover, the protein accumulates preferentially in cells of the striatum and parts of the cortex affected in Huntington disease. Evidence, particularly that given by Wetz (cited in the review by Bates), suggests that these aggregates may be toxic to neurons, either directly or in their protofibrillary (unaggregated) form. The situation is, however, likely to be more complex, as the bulk of huntingtin deposition is found in cortical neurons, whereas the neuronal loss is predominantly striatal. One theory supports the concept that the polyglutamine complex renders certain cell types unduly sensitive to glutamate-mediated excitotoxicity. More recently, 2 mechanisms have been proposed based on an interruption of protein transcription by the binding of mutant huntingtin to transcription proteins or that mitochondrial dysfunction occurs directly or through the same transcriptional mechanism, as summarized by Greenamyre. Because polyglutamine expansions are implicated in several neurodegenerative diseases (reviewed in corresponding sections of this chapter), treatments that block their effects on cellular function may be broadly effective in several degenerative diseases.

Diagnosis

Once the disease has been observed in its fully developed form, its recognition requires no great clinical acumen. The main difficulty arises in patients who lack a family history but who display progressive chorea, emotional disturbance, and dementia. This problem has been largely overcome since the mutation was identified. It is now possible to confirm or exclude the diagnosis by analysis of DNA from a blood sample. The presence of more than 39 CAG repeats at the Huntington locus essentially confirms the disease and gives some indication of the expected time of onset; lesser numbers of repeat length leave room for equivocation and strings between 39 and 42 may not be manifest if the patient does not live long enough to express the illness.

Chorea that begins in late life with only mild or questionable intellectual impairment and without a family history of similar disease is a source of diagnostic difficulty. A few cases are the result of the earlier mentioned HDL2 mutation and others derive from alternative degenerative conditions discussed below. Referring to the problem as "senile chorea" does not solve the problem. Indeed, senile chorea has many causes. We have seen it appear with infections, hyperglycemia, drug therapy, strokes, and thyrotoxicosis, only to disappear after a few weeks. A few times we have been confronted with the problem of an older patient who displays orolingual dyskinesias that are most characteristic of exposure to neuroleptic drugs but in whom there was no such history of exposures; testing usually disclosed Huntington disease.

Chorea in early adult life always raises the question of a late form of Sydenham chorea, of lupus erythematosus with antiphospholipid antibodies, or of cocaine use, but neither familial occurrence nor mental deterioration is part of these processes. A "benign inherited chorea," transmitted as an autosomal dominant trait without prolongation of a triplet sequence, has been traced to chromosome 14q. It is differentiated from Huntington disease by onset before age 5 years, progressing little, and having no associated mental deterioration (Breedveld et al). Other progressive neurologic disorders inherited as autosomal dominant traits and beginning in adolescence or adult life (e.g., polymyoclonus with or without ataxia, acanthocytosis with progressive chorea, and dentatorubropallidoluysian degeneration) can closely mimic Huntington disease, as described further on; sometimes only the genetic and pathologic findings settle the matter. A midlife progressive chorea without dementia (after more than 25 years of followup) that does not display the Huntington genotype has been reported. In at least one family in which this clinical picture is dominantly inherited, the fundamental defect is a mutation in the gene encoding the light chain of ferritin (Curtis). Affected individuals have axonal changes in the pallidum with swollen, ubiquitin- and tau-positive aggregates; serum ferritin levels may be depressed. The implication of this mutation is that perturbations of iron metabolism may be toxic to neurons, a feature that also characterizes Hallervorden-Spatz disease.

Dentatorubropallidoluysian atrophy (DRPLA), sometimes mistaken clinically for Huntington chorea, was described in European families by Warner and associates and is discussed further on. The extrapyramidal manifestations include chorea, myoclonus, and rigidity. Adult-onset chorea and dementia has been described with *propionic acidemia*; propionic acid is elevated in the plasma, urine, and CSF. This disorder must be added to other metabolic diseases described in Chap. 37 as causes of childhood chorea and dyskinesia—such as glutaric acidemia, keratin sulfaturia, calcification of basal ganglia, phenylketonuria, and Hallervorden-Spatz disease, now called PANK (Hagberg et al).

Other problems in differential diagnosis include prion disease, Wilson disease (see Chap. 37), acquired hepatocerebral degeneration (see Chap. 40), paraneoplastic chorea (see Chap. 31), and most often and especially, tardive dyskinesia (see Chap. 41). Many drugs in addition to the toxic effects of L-dopa and antipsychotic medications occasionally cause chorea (amphetamines, cocaine, tricyclic antidepressants, lithium, isoniazid, linezolid). The hyperglycemic–hyperosmolar state is known for producing a variety of generalized or local movement disorders, prominent among them being chorea.

Treatment

The dopamine antagonist haloperidol, in daily doses of 2 to 10 mg, is effective partially in suppressing the movement disorder. Because of the danger of superimposing tardive dyskinesia on the chronic disorder, the chorea should be treated only if it is functionally disabling, using the smallest possible dosages. Haloperidol may also help alleviate abnormalities of behavior or emotional lability, but it does not alter the progress of the disease. The authors have not been impressed with the therapeutic effectiveness of other currently available drugs. Levodopa and other dopamine agonists make the chorea worse and, in the rigid form of the disease, evoke chorea. Drugs that deplete dopamine or block dopamine receptors—such as reserpine, clozapine, and particularly tetrabenazine, which has been validated in a controlled study (Huntington Study Group)—suppress the chorea to some degree, but their side effects (drowsiness, akathisia, and tardive dyskinesia) usually outweigh their desired effects. They may be tried in difficult cases. The juvenile (rigid) form of the disease is probably best treated with antiparkinsonian drugs. Preliminary studies of the transplantation of fetal ganglionic tissue into the striatum have achieved mixed results. The psychologic and social consequences of the disease require supportive therapy, and genetic counseling is essential. Antidepression drugs are widely implemented because of the high incidence of depression and suicidality but their efficacy is not clear. Huntington disease pursues a steadily progressive course and death occurs as mentioned, on average 15 to 20 years after onset, sometimes much earlier or later.

Acanthocytosis With Chorea

There are 2 categories of neurologic disease associated with red blood cell acanthocytosis; one with a defect in the red cell lipid membrane (represented by Bassen-Kornzweig disease and the HARP [hypobetalipoproteinemia, acanthocytosis, retinitis pigmentosa, and pallidal degeneration] syndrome [see Chap. 37]) and a second group that lacks a lipid abnormality. This latter type of neuroacanthocytosis enters into the differential diagnosis of Huntington chorea or unexplained progressive choreas and has the following characteristics: (1) onset in adolescence or early adult life of generalized involuntary movements (described as chorea but including dystonia and tics), usually beginning as an orofacial dyskinesia and spreading to other parts of the body and to other neural systems; (2) mild to moderate mental deterioration with behavioral disturbance in some but not all cases; (3) decreased or absent tendon reflexes and evidence of chronic axonal neuropathy and denervation atrophy of muscles; and (4) the defining feature of acanthocytosis (thorny or spiky appearance of erythrocytes). The main syndrome, and the one to which the term *neuroacanthocytosis* had for a long time been applied, is caused by an autosomal recessive mutation. However, there are now 4 additional subtypes, one dominantly transmitted and another X-linked (McLeod type), which is discussed below. These are all in distinction to Bassen-Kornzweig disease that is caused by an inherent defect in the lipid layer of the red cell membrane (see further on).

In the series of 19 cases reported by Hardie and colleagues, the manifestations included dystonia, tics, vocalizations, rigidity, and lip and tongue biting; more than half had cognitive impairment or psychiatric features. The average age of onset was 32 years; 7 of the 19 cases were sporadic. The disease has been linked in almost all families to chromosome 9q, where there is a mutation in the gene encoding a large (3,100-amino-acid) protein designated *chorein* that is involved in cellular protein sorting and trafficking (Rampoldi). Some of the families with dominantly inherited neuroacanthocytosis have mutations in the chorein gene. There is atrophy and gliosis of the caudate nuclei and putamens but no neuronal loss in the cerebral cortex or other parts of the brain.

According to Sakai and coworkers, the acanthocytosis is the result of an abnormal composition of covalently (tightly) bound fatty acids in erythrocyte membrane proteins (palmitic and docosahexenoic acids increased and stearic acid decreased). The cells should be examined in a fresh preparation of blood and isotonic saline; it is likely to be overlooked in a conventional Wright stain. More than 5 percent of the red cells have the characteristic structural abnormality in affected individuals. The acanthocytosis may also be detected by scanning electron microscopy. The latter may be necessary to undertake in cases of unexplained chorea that have the other features of this disease as genetic testing for the gene (see below) is not widely available.

McLeod disease, another disorder with acanthocytosis and the gradual development of chorea in middle to late life, is characterized by degeneration of the caudate and putamen and a myopathy (elevated serum creatine phosphokinase [CPK]). These individuals have fewer facial tics and orofacial features than those with neuroacanthocytosis. McLeod syndrome arises from mutations in a gene on the X-chromosome that encodes the KX protein, which binds to surface Kell antigens on red cells. In addition to the primary *KX* gene mutations, these individuals show diminished Kell antigen expression on the red-cell surface.

Corticostriatospinal Degenerations

Included in this category are a heterogeneous group of degenerative diseases in which the symptoms of parkinsonism and corticospinal degeneration are present in various combinations. Some of the diseases that make up this group have not been sharply delineated and are difficult to separate from one another.

Variants of this category of disease continue to appear, all rare. The authors have observed several patients in whom extreme rigidity, corticospinal signs but no dementia, have developed over a period of several years. In the later stages of the disease, the patient, while alert, is totally helpless and unable to speak, swallow, or move the limbs. Only eye movements are retained, and even these are hampered by supranuclear gaze palsies in advanced cases. Intellectual functioning appears to be better preserved than movement but is difficult to assess. Other bodily functions are intact. The course is slowly progressive and ends fatally in 5 to 10 years. There is no family history of similar disease, and there are no clues as to causation. Gilbert and colleagues have described similar cases with signs of Parkinson disease, motor neuron disease, and dementia; in their cases, there were no senile plaques or Lewy bodies. The concurrence of typical motor neuron disease and Parkinson disease may be coincidental, but Qureshi and colleagues described 13 patients in whom both clinical phenomena began within a short time and they considered them to be related. In the variant described by Tandan and colleagues, an autosomal dominant syndrome of Charcot-Marie-Tooth polyneuropathy was combined with ptosis, parkinsonism, and dementia, again without Lewy bodies or amyloid plaques. Other variants have been described by Schmitt and coworkers and by Mata and colleagues. Hudson reviewed 42 sporadic cases in which ALS-parkinsonism-dementia were combined.

Under the title "Spastic Pseudosclerosis," Jakob, in 1921, described a chronic disease of middle to late adult life, characterized by abnormalities of behavior and intellect; weakness, ataxia, and spasticity of the limbs (chiefly the legs); extrapyramidal symptoms such as rigidity, slowness of movement, tremors, athetotic postures, and hesitant, dysarthric speech; and normal spinal fluid. The pathologic changes were diffuse and consisted mainly of an outfall of neurons in the frontal, temporal, and central motor gyri, striatum, ventromedial thalamus, and bulbar motor nuclei. In one of Jakob's cases, there were also prominent changes in the anterior horn cells and corticospinal tracts in the spinal cord like those of ALS. The latter finding gave rise to Wilson's concept of the disease as a *corticostriatospinal degeneration*. Some restricted cases bear a resemblance to the type of frontotemporal dementia that occurs with motor neuron disease.

A degenerative and probably familial disorder that had been described earlier by Creutzfeldt was considered by Spielmeyer to be sufficiently similar to the one of Jakob to warrant the designation *Creutzfeldt-Jakob disease*. As discussed in Chap. 33, the disorder originally described by Creutzfeldt and Jakob has been a source of endless controversy because of its indeterminate character. It has been confused with the subacutely evolving myoclonic dementia, or subacute spongiform encephalopathy, which is now known to be an infection caused by a prion agent. The latter disease bears at best only a superficial resemblance to the one described by Creutzfeldt and Jakob, and the 2 disorders should be separated. Unfortunately, the use of the eponym for the prion-related disease is so entrenched that attempts to delete it are futile and probably unnecessary. However, the term *Jakob disease* has been used for the degenerative type of corticostriatospinal degeneration.

The *Guamanian Parkinson-dementia-ALS* complex deserves separate comment because there have been many carefully studied cases with almost uniform clinical and pathologic features. The disease occurs in the indigenous Chamorro peoples of Guam and the Mariana islands, predominantly in men between the ages of 50 and 60 years. Progressive parkinsonism and dementia are combined with upper or lower motor neuron disease (ALS is also common among the Chamorro) leading to death in 5 years. The pathologic changes, described by Hirano and associates, consist of severe cortical atrophy with neurofibrillary tangles and a depopulation of the substantia nigra, but notably no Lewy bodies or amyloid plaques, even with sensitive neurochemical staining. Cases with amyotrophy show a loss of anterior horn cells. The cause of the Guamanian multisystem degeneration is not known, although several studies have incriminated one or more putative neurotoxins in the food supply (see Chap. 43). There are some clinical and pathologic similarities to the form of frontotemporal dementia with motor neuron disease.

Familial Dementia With Spastic Paraparesis

Occasionally, the authors have encountered families in which several members developed a spastic paraparesis and a gradual failure of intellectual function during the middle adult years. The patient's mental horizon narrowed gradually, and the capacity for high-level thinking diminished; in addition, the examination showed exaggerated tendon reflexes, clonus, and Babinski signs. In one such family, the illness had occurred in 2 generations; in another, 3 brothers in a single generation were afflicted. Skre described 2 recessive types of hereditary spastic paraplegia in Norway, 1 with onset in childhood, the other with onset in adult life. In contrast to the dominant form (see further on), the recessive types displayed evidence of more widespread involvement of the nervous system, including dementia, cerebellar ataxia, and epilepsy. Also, Cross and McKusick have observed a recessive type of paraplegia accompanied by dementia beginning in adolescence. They named it the *Mast syndrome*, after the afflicted family.

Worster-Drought and others reported the pathologic findings in 2 cases of this type. In addition to plaques and neurofibrillary changes, there was demyelination of the subcortical white matter and corpus callosum and a "patchy but gross swelling of the arterioles," which gave the staining reactions for amyloid ("Scholz's perivascular plaques"). van Bogaert and associates published an account of similar cases that showed the characteristic pathologic features of Alzheimer disease.

Another interesting association of familial spastic paraplegia is with progressive cerebellar ataxia. Fully one-third of the cases that we have seen with such a spastic weakness were also ataxic and would fall into the category of spinocerebellar degenerations. Yet another variant of this group of diseases has been described by Farmer and colleagues; the inheritance in their cases was autosomal dominant, and the main clinical features were deafness and dizziness, ataxia, chorea, seizures, and dementia, evolving in that order. Postmortem examinations of 2 patients disclosed calcification in the globus pallidus, neuronal loss in the dentate nuclei, and destruction of myelinated fibers in the centrum semiovale.

Adult Polyglucosan Body Disease

Under this title, Robitaille and colleagues have described a progressive neurologic disease in adults characterized clinically by spasticity, chorea, dementia, and a predominantly sensory polyneuropathy that is reviewed in more detail in Chap. 39. Structures that closely resembled Lafora bodies and corpora amylacea were found in large numbers in both central and peripheral neural processes (mainly in axons) and also in astrocytes. These basophilic PAS-positive structures were composed of glucose polymers (polyglucosans) and were readily demonstrated in sural nerve biopsies and therefore probably best termed *polyglucosan bodies*. Some of these structures were also found in the heart and liver.

More recently, Rifal and associates reviewed the findings in 25 cases of this disease—one observed by them and 24 reported previously. The dementia was relatively mild, consisting of impairment of retentive memory, dysnomia, dyscalculia, and sometimes nonfluent aphasia and deficits of "visual integration"; this was overshadowed by rigidity and spasticity of the limbs and the peripheral nerve disorder. Bladder dysfunction has been an early sign in many patients including a middle-aged woman under our care who had only diffuse white matter changes in the cerebral MRI and a moderate sensory neuropathy. Nerve conduction velocities were diminished and the leg muscles were denervated. Moderate degrees of generalized cerebral atrophy, multifocal areas of white matter rarefaction, and degeneration of the corticospinal system, disclosed by MRI. Some cases simulate motor neuron disease. The finding of polyglucosan axonal inclusion in biopsied nerves confirms the diagnosis. The disease has sometimes been misinterpreted as adrenoleukodystrophy. The disorder appears to be a glycogenosis that is allied with Anderson disease, as discussed in Chaps. 38 and 48.

Adult forms of metachromatic leukodystrophy, adrenoleukodystrophy, Krabbe disease, and neuronal ceroid lipofuscinosis (Kufs disease) may be present with a similar clinical picture of progressive dementia (see Chap. 37) as may Whipple disease or the Wernicke-Korsakoff disease. Quite rare instances of the same syndrome with adult onset have proved to be caused by phenylketonuria or other aminoacidopathies (see Chap. 37).

DISEASES CHARACTERIZED BY ABNORMALITIES OF POSTURE AND MOVEMENT

Parkinson Disease

This common disease, known since ancient times, was first cogently described by James Parkinson in 1817. In his words, it was characterized by "involuntary tremulous motion, with lessened muscular power, in parts not in action and even when supported; with a propensity to bend the trunk forward, and to pass from a walking to a running pace, the senses and intellect being uninjured." Strangely, his essay contained no reference to rigidity or to slowness of movement and it stressed unduly the reduction in muscular power. The same criticism can be leveled against the term *paralysis agitans*, which appeared for the first time in 1841 in Marshall Hall's textbook *Diseases and Derangements of the Nervous System* and has fallen out of use, but was such a common term in the literature that it is included here.

The natural history of the disease is of interest. As a rule, it begins between 45 and 70 years of age, with the peak age of onset in the sixth decade. It is infrequent before 30 years of age, and most series contain a somewhat larger proportion of men. Trauma, emotional upset, overwork, exposure to cold, "rigid personality," and so on, were among many factors that had been suggested over the years as predisposing to the disease, but there is no evidence to support any such claims. Idiopathic Parkinson disease is observed in all countries, all ethnic groups, and all socioeconomic classes, although the incidence in African Americans is only one-quarter that in whites. There may be an increased incidence in rural compared to urban areas. In Asians, the incidence is one-third to one-half that in whites. The disease is frequent in North America, where there are approximately 1 million affected patients, constituting about 1 percent of the population over the age of 65 years. The incidence in European countries where vital statistics are kept is similar. A possible relationship to repeated cerebral trauma and to the "punch-drunk" syndrome (dementia pugilistica; chronic traumatic encephalopathy) has been particularly problematic and is unresolved despite several celebrated cases (Lees). A protective effect of smoking and coffee drinking has emerged in some epidemiologic studies but is marginal.

Clinical Features

A tetrad of hypo- and bradykinesia, resting tremor, postural instability, and rigidity are the core features of Parkinson disease. These are evident as an expressionless face, poverty and slowness of voluntary movement, "resting" tremor, stooped posture, axial instability, rigidity, and festinating gait. Much can still be gained from perusal of the often-cited study by Hoehn and Yahr, published in 1967 before the widespread use of L-dopa. Table 39-2 is reproduced from that paper. The manifestations of basal ganglionic disease are fully described in Chap. 4, and only certain diagnostic problems and variations of the clinical picture need be considered here.

Table 39-2

INITIAL SYMPTOMS IN PATIENTS WITH PARKINSON DISEASE

Tremor	70%
Gait disturbance	11%
Stiffness	10%
Slowness	10%
Muscle aches	8%
Loss of dexterity	7%
Handwriting disturbance	5%
Depression, nervousness, other psychiatric disturbance	4%
Speech disturbance	3%

Source: Adapted from Hoehn and Yahr's study of 183 idiopathic cases, 1967.

The early symptoms may be difficult to appreciate and are often overlooked by family members because they evolve slowly and tend to be attributed to the natural changes of aging. Speech becomes soft, monotonous, and cluttered. For a long time the patient may not be conscious of the inroads of the disease. At first the only complaints may be of aching of the back, neck, shoulders, or hips and of vague weakness. Slight stiffness and slowness of movement or a reduction in the natural swing of one arm during walking are ignored until one day it occurs to the physician or to a member of the family that the patient has the overall cast of Parkinson disease. Infrequency of blinking, as originally pointed out by Pierre Marie, is an early sign. The usual blink rate (12 to 20/min) is reduced in the parkinsonian patient to 5 to 10/min, and with it there is a slight widening of the palpebral fissures, creating a stare. A reduction in movements of the small facial muscles imparts the characteristic expressionless "masked" appearance (hypomimia). When seated, the patient makes fewer small shifts and adjustments of position than the normal person (hypokinesia), and the fingers straighten and assume a flexed and adducted posture at the metacarpophalangeal joints.

The characteristic tremor, which usually involves a hand, is often listed as the initial sign; but in at least half the cases observant family members will already have remarked on the patient's relative slowness of movement. In about one-quarter of cases the tremor is mild and intermittent, or evident in only one finger or one hand. The tremor of the fully developed case takes several forms, as was remarked in Chap. 6. The 4-per-second "pill-rolling" tremor of the thumb and fingers, although most characteristic, is seen in only about half the patients. It is typically present when the hand is motionless, that is not used in voluntary movement (hence the commonly used term *resting tremor*). Complete relaxation, however, reduces or abolishes the tremor, so that the term *tremor in the position of repose* is actually a more accurate description. Volitional movement dampens it momentarily. The rhythmic beat coincides with an alternating burst of activity in agonist and antagonist muscles in the electromyogram (EMG); hence the description *alternating tremor* is applied. The arm, jaw, tongue, eyelids, and foot are less often involved. Even the least degree of tremor is felt during passive movement of a rigid part (cogwheel phenomenon, or Negro sign, or at least this is the ostensible explanation for cogwheeling). The tremor shows surprising fluctuations in severity and is aggravated by walking and excitement, but its frequency remains constant (Hunker and Abbs). *It bears repetition that one side of the body is typically involved before the other with tremor and rigidity,* and the tremor in particular remains asymmetrical as the illness advances.

Lance and associates have called attention to the high incidence of a second essential type of tremor in Parkinson disease—a fine, 7- to 8-per-second, slightly irregular, action tremor of the outstretched fingers and hands. This tremor, unlike the slower one, persists throughout voluntary movement, is not evident with the limb in a resting position, and is more easily suppressed by relaxation. Electromyographically, it lacks the alternating bursts of action potentials seen in the typical tremor and resembles, if not equates with, essential tremor (see Table 6-1). It is subject to modulation by different medications than those used for the alternating Parkinson tremor. The patient may have either type of tremor or both.

Rigidity is less often an early finding. Once rigidity develops, it is constantly present and can be felt by the palpating fingers and as a salience of muscle groups even when the patient relaxes. When the examiner passively moves the limb, a mild resistance appears from the start (without the short free interval that characterizes spasticity) and it continues evenly throughout movement in both flexor and extensor groups, being interrupted to a variable degree only by the cogwheel phenomenon. Rigidity and its cogwheel component are elicited or enhanced by having the patient engage the opposite limb in a motor task requiring some degree of concentration, such as tracing circles in the air (termed *Froment sign*, or Noïka-Froment sign when the patient is asked to raise the other arm as high as possible, but this maneuver was actually utilized first to bring out cogwheeling in essential tremor) or touching each finger to the thumb. In the muscles of the trunk, postural hypertonus predominates in the flexor groups and confers on the patient the characteristic flexed posture. Other particulars of the parkinsonian appearance of muscle tone, stance, and gait are discussed in detail in Chaps. 4 and 7. There should be no pyramidal signs in Parkinson disease.

Here, a few additional points should be made regarding the quality of volitional and postural movements. The patient is slow and ineffective in attempts to deliver a quick hard blow; he cannot complete a rapid (ballistic) movement. On the EMG, the normal single burst of agonist–antagonist–agonist sequence of energizing activity is replaced by several sequential brief bursts, according to Hallett and Khoshbin. Alternating movements, at first successful, become progressively impeded if performed repetitively and, finally, they are blocked completely or adopt the rhythm of the patient's alternating tremor. The patient has great difficulty in executing 2 motor acts simultaneously. In the past the impaired facility of movement had been attributed to rigidity, but the observation that certain surgical lesions in the brain abolished rigidity without affecting movement refuted this interpretation. Thus slowness and lack of natural movements (bradykinesia and hypokinesia, respectively) are not derived from rigidity but are independent manifestations of the disease. The bradykinetic deficits underlie the characteristic poverty of movement, reflected also by infrequency of swallowing, slowness of chewing, a limited capacity to make postural adjustments of the body and limbs in response to displacement of these parts, a lack of small "movements of cooperation" (as in arising from a chair without first adjusting the feet), absence of arm swing in walking, and most of the other aspects of the parkinsonian countenance. Despite a perception of muscle weakness, the patient is able to generate normal or near-normal power, especially in the large muscles; however, in the small ones, strength is slightly diminished.

As the disorder of movement worsens, all customary activities show the effects. Handwriting becomes small (micrographia), tremulous, and cramped, as first noted by Charcot. Speech softens and seems hurried, monotonous, and mumbling (cluttered): The voice becomes less audible and, finally, the patient only whispers. Caekebeke and coworkers refer to the speech disorder as a *hypokinetic dysarthria* and attribute it to combined respiratory, phonatory, and articulatory dysfunctions. There is a failure to fully close the mouth. The consumption of a meal takes an inordinately long time. Each morsel of food must be swallowed before the next bite is taken.

Walking becomes reduced to a shuffle; the patient frequently loses balance, and in walking forward or backward seems to be "chasing" the body's center of gravity with a series of increasingly rapid short steps in order to avoid falling (festination). Defense and righting reactions are faulty. Falls do occur, but surprisingly infrequently given the degree of postural instability. Gait is improved by sensory guidance, as by holding the patient at the elbow. Obstacles such as door thresholds have the opposite effect, at times causing the patient to "freeze" in place. Getting in and out of a car or elevator or walking into a room or in a hall becomes particularly difficult. Difficulty in turning over in bed is a similarly characteristic feature as the illness advances, but the patient rarely volunteers this information. Several of our patients have fallen out of bed at a frequency that suggests a connection to their reduced mobility combined with slowed corrective or defensive postural movements. Shaving or applying lipstick becomes difficult, as the facial muscles become more immobile and rigid.

Persistent extension or clawing of the toes, jaw clenching, and other fragments of dystonia, often quite painful, may enter the picture and are sometimes early findings. (These are particularly resistant to treatment.)

A special problem of camptocormia occurs in some Parkinson patients wherein an extreme forward flexion of the spine and correspondingly severe stooping occur. It appears to be a type of axial dystonia when it occurs with Parkinson disease. The deformity resolves when the patient is supine or pushes upward on the handles of a walker. This symptom is associated with a variety of other diseases, some of them muscular. We have not been impressed that it is ameliorated by L-dopa. Why some patients with Parkinson disease are extremely bent over and others are not at all affected is unknown.

As noted above, these various motor impediments and tremors characteristically begin in one limb (more often the left) and spread to one side and later to both sides until the patient is quite helpless. Yet in the excitement of some unusual circumstance (as escaping from a fire, for example), the patient with all but the most advanced disease is capable of brief but remarkably effective movement (*kinesis paradoxica*).

Regarding elicitable neurologic signs, there is an inability to inhibit blinking in response to a tap over the bridge of the nose or glabella (Myerson sign) but grasp and suck reflexes are not present unless dementia supervenes and buccal and jaw jerks are rarely enhanced. Commonly there is an impairment of upward gaze and convergence; if prominent or noted early in the disease, this sign suggests more the possibility of progressive supranuclear palsy. Bradykinesia may extend to eye movements, in that there is a delay in the initiation of gaze to one side, slowing of conjugate movements (decreased maximal saccadic velocity), hypometric saccades, and breakdown of pursuit movements into small saccades.

There are no sensory findings, but a wide variety of paresthetic and other sensory complaints and discomforts are common. These affect mainly the calves and abdomen and are among the most distressing of the *nonmotor parkinsonian symptoms*. Drooling is troublesome; an excess flow of saliva has been assumed, but actually the problem is probably one of failure to swallow with normal frequency. Seborrhea and excessive sweating are claimed to be secondary as well, the former due to failure to cleanse the face sufficiently, the latter to the effects of the constant motor activity but this explanation seems lacking to us; an autonomic disturbance is more plausible. Other nonmotor features are mostly in the category of autonomic disturbances and include most prominently constipation, abdominal pains and cramps, erectile dysfunction, joint aches, and various other sensory experiences that may be difficult for the patient to describe. There is a tendency in some patients to have orthostatic hypotension and sometimes syncope; this has been attributed by Rajput and Rozdilsky to cell loss in the sympathetic ganglia. However, these features are not as prominent as in multiple system atrophy (Shy-Drager syndrome). It is worth mentioning that several of our younger Parkinson patients with recurrent syncope proved to have cardiac arrhythmias; hence other causes of fainting must be considered.

Postural instability is a core feature of the illness; it can be elicited by tugging at the patient's shoulders from behind and noting the lack of a small step backward to maintain balance often with a fall or the initiation of backward festination. The tendon reflexes vary, as they do in normal individuals from being barely elicitable to brisk. Even when parkinsonian symptoms are confined to one side of the body, the reflexes are usually equal on the two sides, and the plantar responses are flexor. Exceptionally, the reflexes on the affected side are slightly brisker, which raises the question of corticospinal involvement, but the plantar reflex remains flexor. In these respects, the clinical picture differs from that of corticobasal ganglionic degeneration, in which rigidity, hyperactive tendon reflexes, and Babinski signs are combined with apraxia (see further on).

As mentioned earlier, Parkinson disease may be complicated by dementia, a feature described by Charcot. The reported frequency of this combination varies considerably based on the selection of patients and type of testing. An estimate of 10 to 15 percent (Mayeux et al) is the generally accepted figure and matches our experience. The incidence increases with advancing age and duration of disease, approaching 65 percent in Parkinson patients older than 80 years of age, but mental decline may become apparent in patients in their late fifties. The pathologic basis of the dementia is discussed below.

The overall course of the disease is quite variable. In the majority of patients, the mean period of time from inception of the disease to a chairbound state is 7.5 years, but with a wide range (Hoehn and Yahr; Martilla and Rinne). As much as 10 percent of cases remain relatively mild and only very gradually progressive, and such patients may remain almost stable for 10 years or more. These trajectories have been altered somewhat by modern therapies.

Hemiparkinson–Hemiatrophy Syndrome Mentioned here is a rare syndrome described by Klawans and elaborated in a series of 30 patients by Wijemanne and Jankovic. The typical case shows atrophy in one or more body parts, including at times the face, often since childhood, and usually quite subtle. Signs of progressive parkinsonism or dystonia begin in midlife on the atrophic side and, for the most part, are responsive to L-dopa, but some, such as Klawans' original patients, are resistant. Several types of early life cerebral injury underlie the syndrome, but half of patients have no such lesion evident. Understanding of the idiopathic cases is limited. Those with deep brain lesions may be experiencing a slow degeneration of basal ganglia pathways.

Diagnosis

The 2 main difficulties are to distinguish typical Parkinson disease from the many parkinsonian syndromes caused by other degenerative conditions and by medications or toxins, and to distinguish the Parkinson tremor from other types, especially essential tremor. It is worth noting that Parkinson disease is far more common than any of the degenerative syndromes that resemble it. Bradykinesia and rigidity of the limbs and axial musculature are symptoms shared with other forms of parkinsonism, but it is mainly in Parkinson disease that one observes an early sign of "resting" alternating tremor that is more prominent in one arm.

When not all the typical signs are evident, there is no alternative but to reexamine the patient at several-month intervals until it is clear that Parkinson disease is present or until the characteristic features of another degenerative process become evident; these include early falls and vertical gaze impairment in progressive supranuclear palsy; dysautonomia with fainting, bladder, or vocal cord dysfunction in multiple system atrophy; early and rapidly evolving dementia or intermittent psychosis in Lewy-body disease; or apraxia in corticobasal ganglionic degeneration. Very symmetrical findings, particularly tremor, suggest an alternative to idiopathic Parkinson disease. Also, the constellation of features termed *"lower half parkinsonism"* consisting of difficulty purely with gait and stability, as discussed below and in Chap. 7, suggest a process other than Parkinson disease.

If the symptoms warrant, a beneficial and sustained response to levodopa or a dopamine agonist also gives a reasonably secure, although not entirely conclusive, indication of the presence of Parkinson disease (see further on). The other parkinsonian syndromes are for the most part changed only slightly or only for a few weeks or months by the drug. Conversely, although some experts disagree, we have adhered to the notion that complete resistance of the symptoms to L-dopa early in the illness makes the diagnosis unlikely. Furthermore, almost all patients with idiopathic Parkinson disease eventually acquire dyskinesias in response to L-dopa and the absence of this sign after approximately 3 to 5 years of use of the drug brings the diagnosis into question.

The epidemic of encephalitis lethargica (von Economo encephalitis) that spread over Western Europe and the United States after the First World War left great numbers of parkinsonian cases in its wake. No definite instance of this form of encephalitis had been recorded before the period 1914 to 1918, and very few have been seen since 1930; hence, this type of postencephalitic parkinsonism is no longer a diagnostic consideration. However, a Parkinson-like syndrome has been described following other forms of encephalitis, particularly with Japanese B virus, West Nile virus, and eastern equine encephalitis. In the few cases caused by these viruses that we have observed, there has been fairly symmetrical rigidity, hypokinesia, and little or no tremor.

An "arteriopathic" or "arteriosclerotic" form of Parkinson disease was at one time much diagnosed but we have never been entirely convinced of its reality, referring to damage to the substantia nigra as a result of vascular disease or to a syndrome that closely resembles Parkinson disease as a result of atherosclerotic white matter damage. Nonetheless, a number of authoritative clinicians are of the opinion that patients with a vascular cause have a predominantly "lower half" parkinsonism in which shuffling gait, stickiness on turning, and falling are disproportionate to other features. There is no tremor, and little or no response to L-dopa (see Winikates and Jankovic). MRI in such cases has shown substantial white matter changes in both cerebral hemispheres. In the few cases attributable to vascular parkinsonism that have come to our attention with autopsy material, there have been Lewy bodies in the appropriate locations. Pseudobulbar palsy from a series of lacunar infarcts or from Binswanger disease can cause a clinical picture that simulates certain aspects of Parkinson disease, but unilateral and bilateral corticospinal tract signs, hyperactive facial reflexes, spasmodic crying and laughing, and other characteristic features distinguish spastic bulbar palsy from Parkinson disease. Of course, the elderly parkinsonian patient is not impervious to cerebrovascular disease, and the 2 conditions overlap, but differentiating the predominantly gait or dementing disorders of widespread vascular brain damage from idiopathic Parkinson disease is not difficult.

Normal-pressure hydrocephalus can undoubtedly produce a syndrome resembling Parkinson disease, particularly in regard to gait and postural instability, and at times extending to bradykinesia; but rigid postures, slowness of alternating movements, hypokinetic ballistic movements, and resting tremor are not part of the clinical picture. The gait tends to be short-stepped but not shuffling and there is more of a tendency to retropulsion than there is in Parkinson disease. Sometimes a lumbar puncture gives surprising benefit, indicating hydrocephalus as the cause of the motor slowing and gait disorder.

Essential tremor is distinguished by its fine, quick quality, its tendency to become manifest during volitional movement and to disappear when the limb is in a position of repose, and the lack of associated slowness of movement or of flexed postures. Cogwheeling of minor degree may be associated. The head and voice are more often truly tremulous in essential tremor than in Parkinson disease. Some of the slower, alternating forms of essential tremor are difficult to distinguish from parkinsonian tremor; one can only wait to see whether it is the first manifestation of Parkinson disease. A markedly asymmetrical or unilateral tremor favors Parkinson disease. Also as noted, a faster oscillation is often mixed with the slow alternating Parkinson tremor, but the fast-frequency tremor is only occasionally an opening feature of the disease as discussed in Chap. 6.

Progressive supranuclear palsy (discussed in a section further on) is characterized by rigidity and dystonic postures of the neck and shoulders, a staring and immobile countenance, and a tendency to topple when walking—all of which are vaguely suggestive of Parkinson disease. Early and frequent falls are particularly suggestive of this disease, not being atypical of Parkinson disease until its late stages. Inability to produce vertical saccades and, later, paralysis of upward and downward gaze and eventual loss of lateral gaze with retention of reflex eye movements establish the diagnosis of PSP in most cases.

Paucity of movement, unchanging attitudes and postural sets, and a slightly stiff and unbalanced gait may be observed in patients with an anergic or hypokinetic type of depression. Because a fair proportion of parkinsonian patients are depressed, the separation of these 2 conditions is at times difficult. The authors have seen patients who were called parkinsonian by competent neurologists but whose movements became normal when antidepressant medication or electroconvulsive therapy was given. Several such patients have nonetheless insisted that levodopa helps them in some nondescript way.

The rapid onset of parkinsonism should suggest exposure to neuroleptic medications (used at times as antiemetics and gastric motility agents [metoclopramide]), a variant of Creutzfeldt-Jakob disease, an unusual postinfectious or paraneoplastic illness, or viral encephalitis. The implicated drugs may also evoke an inner restlessness, a "muscular impatience," an inability to sit still, and a compulsion to move about much like that which occurs at times in the parkinsonian patient (akathisia). Even the newer antipsychosis medications, favored specifically because of a putative lack of extrapyramidal effects, may be at fault.

Strict adherence to the diagnostic criteria for Parkinson disease also permits its differentiation from corticostriatospinal, striatonigral, and corticobasal ganglionic degeneration, calcification of the basal ganglia, Wilson disease, the acquired hepatolenticular degeneration of repeated hepatic coma, manganese poisoning, as well as Machado-Joseph disease, all of which are discussed in other parts of this chapter.

All in all, if one adheres to the standard definition of Parkinson disease—bradykinesia, hypokinesia "resting" tremor, postural changes and instability, cogwheel rigidity, and response to L-dopa—errors in diagnosis are few. Yet in a series of 100 cases, studied clinically and pathologically by Hughes and associates, the diagnosis was inaccurate in 25 percent. The ostensible explanation for this difficulty is that approximately one-quarter of Parkinson patients fail to display the characteristic tremor and approximately 10 percent are said to not respond to L-dopa. These authors noted that early dementia and autonomic disorder and the presence of ataxia or corticospinal signs were reliable guides to an alternate diagnosis.

Pathology and Pathogenesis

The most constant and pertinent finding in both idiopathic and postencephalitic Parkinson disease is a loss of pigmented cells in the substantia nigra and other pigmented nuclei (locus ceruleus, dorsal motor nucleus of the vagus). The substantia nigra is visibly pale to the naked eye; microscopically, the pigmented nuclei show a marked depletion of cells and replacement gliosis, and some of the remaining cells have reduced quantities of melanin, findings that enable one to state with confidence that the patient must have suffered from Parkinson disease. Also, many of the remaining cells of the pigmented nuclei contain eosinophilic cytoplasmic inclusions, surrounded by a faint halo, called *Lewy bodies* (Fig. 39-5). These are seen in practically all cases of idiopathic Parkinson disease. They were generally absent in postencephalitic cases, but there were neurofibrillary tangles within nigral cell in that disorder. Both these cellular abnormalities appear occasionally in the substantia nigra of aged, nonparkinsonian individuals. Possibly the individuals with Lewy bodies would have developed Parkinson disease had they lived a few more years. Many of the inherited forms of Parkinson disease also lack Lewy bodies.

Noteworthy is the finding by McGeer and colleagues that nigral cells normally diminish with age, from a maximal complement of about 425,000 to 200,000 at age 80 years.

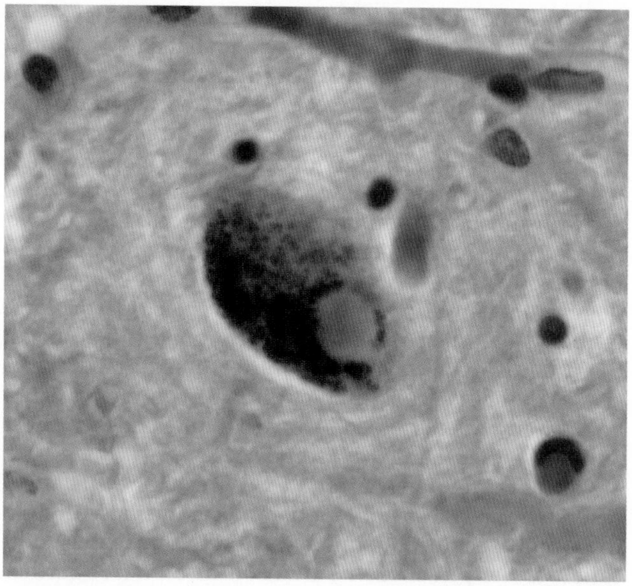

Figure 39-5. Photomicrograph of a round Lewy-body inclusion in the cytoplasm of a nigral neuron. (Hematoxylin and eosin [H&E] staining.) (Courtesy of Matthew Frosch, MD, PhD.)

Tyrosine-hydroxylase, the rate-limiting enzyme for the synthesis of dopamine, diminishes correspondingly. However, these authors and others have found that in patients with Parkinson disease the number of pigmented neurons is reduced to 30 percent or less of that in age-matched controls. Using more refined counting techniques, Pakkenberg and coworkers estimated the average total number of pigmented neurons to be 550,000 and to be reduced in absolute numbers by 66 percent in Parkinson patients. (The number of nonpigmented neurons was reduced in Parkinson cases by only 24 percent.) Thus aging contributes importantly to nigral cell loss, but the cell depletion is so much more marked in Parkinson disease that some factor other than aging must also be operative.

Other regions of neuronal loss are widespread as mentioned, but their significance is less clear. There is neuronal loss in the mesencephalic reticular formation, near the substantia nigra. These cells project to the thalamus and limbic lobes. In the sympathetic ganglia, there is slight neuronal loss and Lewy bodies are seen. This is also true of the pigmented nuclei of the lower brainstem as well as of neuronal populations in the putamen, caudatum, pallidum, and substantia innominata. On the other hand, dopaminergic neurons that project to cortical and limbic structures, to caudate nucleus and nucleus accumbens, and to periaqueductal gray matter and spinal cord are affected little or not at all. The lack of a consistent lesion in either the striatum or the pallidum is noteworthy. An alternative hypothesis offered by Braak and Tredici, mentioned in an earlier section of this chapter and attributed to Braak and Braak, is that the substantia nigra compacta is affected only late in the pathobiology of Parkinson disease. Their study found that the earliest changes in the brain occur in the dorsal glossopharyngeal-vagal and anterior olfactory nuclei, and only later did they appear in the midbrain nuclei. This theory accommodates a variety of clinical features and potential environmental triggers to the disease. Lang has suggested that this distribution of cell loss explains some of the nondopaminergic features of the disease and offers other avenues for therapy.

Statistical data relating Parkinson and Alzheimer diseases are difficult to assess because of different methods of examination from one series to another. Nevertheless, the overlap of the 2 diseases is more than fortuitous, as indicated earlier in this chapter. The majority of the demented Parkinson patients show some Alzheimer-type changes but there are some in whom few plaques or neurofibrillary changes can be found and instead display cortical neuronal loss accompanied by widespread distribution of Lewy bodies, marking the process as Lewy-body dementia and not Parkinson disease.

Of interest had been the observation, both in humans and in monkeys, that a neurotoxin (known as MPTP [1-methyl-4-phenyl-1,2,3,6-tetrahydropyridine]) produces irreversible signs of parkinsonism and selective destruction of cells in the substantia nigra. The toxin, an analogue of meperidine, which was self-administered by addicts, binds with high affinity to monoamine oxidase, an extraneural enzyme that transforms MPTP to a toxic metabolite, pyridinium MPP (1-methyl-4-phenylpyridinium). The latter is bound by the melanin in the dopaminergic nigral neurons in sufficient concentration to destroy the cells. The mechanism by which MPTP produces the clinical aspects of the Parkinson syndrome is unsettled. One hypothesis is that the inner segment of the globus pallidus is rendered hyperactive because of reduction of the influence of gamma-aminobutyric acid (GABA) of the subthalamic nucleus. The notion of some other environmental toxin as a cause of Parkinson disease has been stimulated by the MPTP findings (see Uhl et al; also the review by Snyder and D'Amato). For example, Parkinson disease is slightly more frequent in industrialized countries and in agrarian regions where organophosphates are commonly used, but its universal occurrence would argue against this hypothesis. Despite extensive study, no chemical toxin, heavy metal, or infection has been causally related to the disease. Some plausible theories hold that a toxin might be implicated only on a genetic background predisposing to the disease. The MPTP disease serves as a model for the neurophysiologic and neurochemical changes of Parkinson disease because of destruction of the substantia nigra, but in most other respects it does not reflect the naturally occurring disorder (including the absence of Lewy bodies).

Genetic Aspects

Considering its frequency, coincidence in a family on the basis of chance occurrence might be as high as 5 percent. However, careful epidemiologic studies suggest that a familial occurrence may be as high as 15 percent. A lack of concordance of Parkinson disease in twins was at first thought to negate the role of genetic factors, but a study of dopamine metabolism using PET scanning showed that 75 percent of asymptomatic twins of Parkinson patients had evidence of striatal dysfunction, whereas only a small portion of dizygotic twins showed these changes (Piccini et al). These data indicate a substantial role for inherited traits, even in cases of ostensibly sporadic Parkinson disease (see below regarding the better defined inherited forms). Some mutations and polymorphisms are more clearly modifying factors in producing the disease, but others act as dominant disease genes. These are summarized in Table 39-3. We have chosen to

Table 39-3

MAIN GENETIC DEFECTS ASSOCIATED WITH PARKINSON DISEASE

NOTATION	GENE (PROTEIN)	INHERITANCE	AGE OF ONSET	LEWY BODIES	SPECIAL FEATURES
Park1 & Park4	*SCNA* (α-synuclein)	AD	30–40 years	+	Two main mutations—A53T, A30P—promote oligomerization of α-synuclein.
Park2	*PARK2* (parkin)	AR	20–40 years	–	Accounts for 50% of early-onset inherited PD; 20% of "sporadic" early-onset cases.
Park3	*PARK3*	AD	Late onset	+	Resembles idiopathic PD.
Park5	*UCHL-1* (ubiquitin esterase)	SNP	50's	+	Two different polymorphisms confer risk of PD. Mutations decreased recycling of ubiquitin monomers.
Park6	*PINK1* (PTEN-induced putative kinase 1)	AR	Varies		Mitochondrial gene.
Park7	PARK7 (DJ-1)	AR	30's	?	Slow progression; gene plays role in cellular response to oxidative stress.
Park8	*LRRK2* (leucine-rich repeat kinase 2)	AD	Late	±	Ashkenazic Jews. Protein also called dardarin; related to Gaucher disease.
Park14	PLA2G6 (phospholipase A2)	?	Late	–	Dystonia-parkinsonism; late onset; other mutations cause neuroaxonal dystrophy.
NR4A2	*NURR1* (nuclear receptor related protein 1)	AD	Confers susceptibility to PD	?	Gene is implicated in the formation and identity of dopaminergic neurons.

AD, autosomal dominant; AR, autosomal recessive; PD, Parkinson disease.

retain the nomenclature of the *PARK* genes for ease of exposition but, as the genes are sequenced, their names have replaced this generic notation in many summaries of the genetics of the disease.

Numerous observations have implicated the nuclear and synaptic protein α-synuclein, the main component of Lewy bodies in both the sporadic and inherited forms of Parkinson disease, as well as in Lewy-body disease. Synuclein, a normal component of the synapse, exists in a soluble unfolded form, but in high concentrations it aggregates into filaments, which are the main (but not the only) constituent of the Lewy body. Immunostaining techniques disclose additional less-specific proteins, such as ubiquitin and tau within the Lewy bodies. Furthermore, in families with a rare autosomal dominant form of Parkinson disease, several different mutations on chromosome 4 code for an aberrant form of synuclein that decreases its stability and promotes its aggregation (Polymeropoulos et al). A family has also been described in which the cause of Parkinson disease is an extra nonmutant copy of the α-synuclein gene (Singleton et al), comparable to the circumstance or triplication of chromosome 21 in the Alzheimer disease of Down syndrome. Additionally, some cases of familial parkinsonism result from mutations that control the removal of α-synuclein from the cell via proteasomal pathways. Together, these findings indicate that instability or misfolding of α-synuclein or its deficient removal may be a primary defect in the disease. The protofibrillary form of the protein (i.e., a soluble protein in the cytosol) is also toxic to dopaminergic neurons. These processes are accelerated by defects in heat shock proteins that chaperone α-synuclein into and out of the cell. Curiously, Lewy bodies are not found in patients with most of the parkin mutations.

Parkin is a ubiquitin protein ligase that participates in the removal of unnecessary proteins from cells through the proteasomal system (Fig. 39-6). Attachment of parkin and ubiquitin to cytosolic proteins is understood to be an obligatory step in the disposal of proteins by proteasomes. Mutations in the parkin gene lead either to an inadequacy or misfolding of synuclein, resulting in its accumulation, or to the disruption of disposal of proteins in dopamine-producing cells. The importance of the ubiquitination pathway in this disease is further highlighted

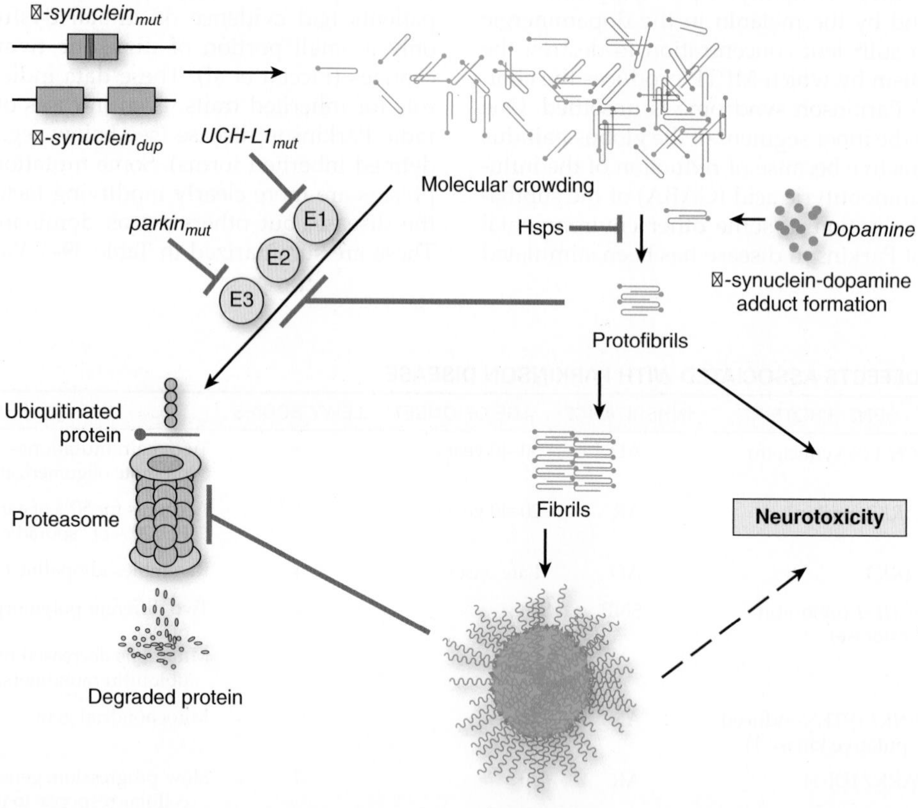

Figure 39-6. Schematic diagram of proposed mechanisms of α-synuclein toxicity in Parkinson disease. In this model, α-synuclein levels are elevated by (*a*) duplication of one copy of the α-synuclein gene; (*b*) point mutations in the α-synuclein gene that generate excessive accumulations of synuclein; or (*c*) mutations in parkin and *UCH-L1* genes that reduce normal removal of synuclein by the proteosomes. The excess of synuclein polymerizes to form protofibrils, a process that is enhanced by defects in heat shock proteins (Hsps) or by the action of dopamine, which binds to synuclein. In turn, this leads to formation of Lewy bodies. This model attributes the neurotoxicity to either the protofibrils or the Lewy bodies. (Adapted by permission from Eriksen JL, Dawson TM, Dickson DW, Petrucelli L: Caught in the act: α-Synuclein is the culprit in Parkinson's disease. *Neuron* 40:453–456, 2003.)

by the report that parkinsonian features are present in a family with mutations in ubiquitin carboxyterminal hydrolase L1 (*Park5, UCHL-1*; Table 39-3). Figure 39-6 illustrates these relationships and the processing of synuclein in the cell. It must be emphasized that most of the mechanisms illustrated are speculative or are derived from the molecular study of familial Parkinson disease and therefore may not apply to the sporadic process.

A mutation that has received much attention has been at the *LRRK2* (leucine-rich repeat kinase 2) site. It is implicated in both genetic and sporadic forms of the disease, particularly among those of Ashkenazic Jewish or North African origin. The LRRK2 protein (dardarin) is a cytoplasmic component that is widely distributed in the brain and peripheral nerves. It has been estimated that mutations in the gene (mainly one common one, G20195) are responsible for 1 percent of sporadic cases and are found in 5 to 8 percent of individuals with a first-degree relative who has the disease. The gene acts as a dominant trait but penetrance of the defect increases with age, being 85 percent at 70 years. Therefore, there may not be a family history. The clinical syndrome in most respects simulates the sporadic form of the disease according to Papapetropoulos and colleagues, but several other series have noted the absence of tremor. The genetics of this disorder, also called *Park8*, are reviewed by Brice.

Several other gene defects are of interest in familial parkinsonism. One is a dominantly inherited mutation in the gene *Nurr1*, whose normal function is to specify the identity of dopaminergic neurons. Another is in recessively inherited parkinsonism caused by defects in the gene *DJ-1*, a protein that is essential for the normal neuronal response to oxidative stress. Also, a disease-causing mutation in the gene termed *PINK*, corresponding to *Park6*, codes for a mitochondrial kinase, therefore implicating this cellular structure in some forms of Parkinson disease (Valente et al). Presumably, dopaminergic neurons are compromised in some manner by these defects.

There has also been emphasis on mutations on 1 of 12 exons in the so-called *Park2* gene, which codes for the protein parkin (see Table 39-3). The most common types are point mutations or deletions in exon 7, but abnormalities of the other exons evince similar syndromes. Homozygous mutations generally give rise to early-onset disease, but certain hemizygous changes (in exon 7) are associated with a later onset. The resultant syndromes have been termed *parkin disease* to distinguish them from the idiopathic variety. It has been estimated by Khan and colleagues that 50 percent of families that display an early onset of Parkinson disease and 18 percent of sporadic cases with early onset (before age 40 years) harbor mutations in this gene. Perhaps of greater clinical interest is finding that up to 2 percent of late-onset cases are associated with parkin mutations, and 1 percent due to changes in the aforementioned *LRRK2* gene. Sequencing of these genes is now available in commercial laboratories for the purposes of detecting mutations and polymorphisms.

From a clinical perspective, the presentation of the late-onset cases with parkin mutations has been quite variable. Collectively, they can often be identified by an extreme sensitivity to L-dopa, maintaining an almost complete suppression of symptoms over decades with only small doses of medication; also, they have a low threshold for dyskinesias induced by L-dopa. We can also corroborate from experience with our own patients an excellent response of tremor, postural changes, and bradykinesia to anticholinergic drugs. A second feature has been that most of these patients may enjoy a remarkable restorative benefit from sleep, which creates a diurnal pattern of symptoms. Several series, particularly those of Lohmann and associates and of Khan and colleagues, have indicated that there may be a wide variety of additional features: hyperreflexia, cervical, foot, or other focal dystonias, sometimes induced by exercise; and, less often, autonomic dysfunction, peripheral neuropathy, and psychiatric symptoms. The sensitivity to medication and sleep benefit have long been known as the distinguishing components of juvenile-onset parkinsonism with dopa-responsive dystonia (Segawa disease), which is discussed later in the chapter.

Of similar interest as a modulating factor in the development of the disease is strong association between mutations in the glucocerebrosidase gene (other mutations of which causes Gaucher disease) among Ashkenazi Jews (Sidransky et al), the same population predominantly affected by polymorphisms of LRRK2. Although population studies allow only limited conclusions about clinical correlations, the glucocerebrosidase mutation is present more often in patients with a family history of the disease, have an earlier onset that in patients with a normal gene and a lower incidence of resting tremor. Mutations have been present in 7 percent of Parkinson patients who had their genes fully sequenced, making it so far the most common genetic factor for the disease, and certainly in this ethnographic population.

It is hoped that the genetic mutations that give rise to Parkinson disease will expose the molecular pathophysiology of the disease. As discussed earlier, several sites are implicated in the familial forms of Parkinson disease, some related to the gene that codes for synuclein, the main component of the Lewy body.

Treatment

Although there is no current treatment that clearly halts or reverses the neuronal degeneration underlying Parkinson disease, methods are now available that afford considerable relief from symptoms. Treatment can be medical or surgical, although reliance is placed mainly on drugs, particularly on L-dopa (Table 39-4). The following sections are necessarily detailed so as to give the clinician a full comprehension of the use and side effects and interactions of these drugs.

L-Dopa and L-Dopa–Modifying Drugs At present, L-dihydroxyphenylalanine (L-dopa) is unquestionably the most effective agent for the treatment of Parkinson disease and the therapeutic results, even in those with

Table 39-4

DRUGS COMMONLY USED IN THE TREATMENT OF PARKINSON DISEASE

MEDICATION	STARTING DOSE	TARGET DOSE	MAIN BENEFIT	SIDE EFFECTS
L-Dopa				
Carbidopa-L-dopa	25/100 mg tid	Up to 50/250 mg q3h	Reduction of tremor and bradykinesia; less effect on postural difficulties	Nausea, dyskinesias, orthostatic hypotension, hallucinations, confusion
Controlled release carbidopa-L-dopa	25/100 mg tid	Up to 50/200 mg q4h	May prolong L-dopa effects	
Dopamine agonists				
Ropinirole	0.25 mg tid	9 to 24 mg/d	Moderate effects on all aspects; reduced motor fluctuations of L-dopa	Orthostatic hypotension, excessive and abrupt sleepiness, confusion, hallucinations
Pramipexole	0.125 mg tid	0.75 to 3 mg/d	As above	
Glutamate antagonist				
Amantadine	100 mg/d	100 mg bid–tid	Smoothing of motor fluctuations	Leg swelling, congestive heart failure, prostatic outlet obstruction, confusion, hallucinations, insomnia
Anticholinergics				
Benztropine	0.5 mg/d	Up to 4 mg/d	Tremor reduction, less effect on other features	Atropinic effects: dry mouth, urinary outlet obstruction, confusion, and psychosis
Trihexyphenidyl	0.5 mg bid	Up to 2 mg tid	As above	As above
COMT inhibitors				
Entacapone	200 mg with L-dopa		Prolonged effect of L-dopa	Urine discoloration, diarrhea, increased dyskinesias
MAO-inhibitors				
Rasagiline	0.5 mg	1 mg daily	Reduced "off" time, Potential neuroprotection	Hypertensive crisis with tyramine-rich foods and sympathomimetics
Selegiline	5 mg	5 mg bid	Potential neuroprotection	

far advanced disease, are much better than have been obtained with other drugs. The levodopa, or a dopamine agonist preparation as described below, is introduced when the symptoms begin to interfere with work and social life or falling becomes a threat, and then these drugs are used at the lowest possible dose. The theoretical basis for the use of this compound rests on the observation that striatal dopamine is depleted in patients with Parkinson disease but that the remaining diseased nigral cells are still capable of producing some dopamine by taking up its precursor, L-dopa. The number of neurons in the striatum is not diminished and they remain receptive to ingested dopamine acting through the residual nigral neurons. Over time, however, the number of remaining nigral neurons becomes inadequate and the receptivity to dopamine of the striatal target neurons becomes excessive, possibly as a result of denervation hypersensitivity; this results in both a reduced response to L-dopa and to paradoxical and excessive movements (dyskinesias) with each dose. The drug has an interesting history that includes many early trials that failed to persuade neurologists of its effectiveness; Barbeau's paper on this historical subject may be consulted by the interested reader.

Most patients tolerate the drug initially, experiencing few serious adverse effects and showing various degrees of improvement, sometimes dramatic, especially in hypokinesia and tremor after several days or sooner. However, the side effects and limitations of L-dopa become considerable as the drug therapy continues and the disease progresses, as discussed below.

By combining L-dopa with a decarboxylase inhibitor (carbidopa or benserazide), which is unable to penetrate the central nervous system (CNS), decarboxylation of L-dopa to dopamine is greatly diminished in peripheral tissues. This permits a greater proportion of L-dopa to reach nigral neurons and, at the same time, reduces the peripheral side effects of L-dopa and dopamine (nausea, hypotension, confusion). Combinations of carbidopa-levodopa are available in a 1:10 or 1:4 ratio and the benserazide-levodopa combination is available in a 1:4 ratio. The initial dose of carbidopa-levodopa is typically one-half to one of a 25/100-mg tablet given bid or tid and increased slowly until optimum improvement is achieved, usually up to 4 tablets administered 5 or more times daily as the disease advances, or a similar dose of the 25/250-mg combination.

A class of catechol-*O*-methyltransferase (COMT) inhibitors, typified by entacapone, extends the plasma half-life and the duration of L-dopa effect by preventing its breakdown (as opposed to increasing its bioavailability, as in the case of carbidopa). A combination of L-dopa, carbidopa, and a COMT inhibitor is available in a single pill.

Long-acting preparations of levodopa-carbidopa may provide slightly longer effect and reduce dyskinesias in some patients (Hutton and Morris) in the advanced stages of disease, but our experience with these drugs given earlier in the course of disease has given less-predictable results. The absorption of the long-acting drug, however, is approximately 70 percent and may be inconsistent, often necessitating a slight increase in total dose. To facilitate the treatment of morning rigidity and tremor, the long-acting tablet can be given late in the previous evening.

For patients who require very frequent but small doses of the drug because of severe motor fluctuations and dyskinesias, an oral suspension may be formulated that allows precisely measured doses to be delivered orally or through a nasogastric tube. The typical composition is 500 mg L-dopa (of carbidopa-L-dopa 10/100 or 25/100), 500 mg of ascorbic acid to stabilize the drug, and 250 mL of water, resulting in a concentration of L-dopa of 2 mg/mL, which is administered in small amounts. A gel preparation is also available for delivery through a duodenal tube.

Each patient requires empirical adjustment of the dose and timing of medication and then generally does well by maintaining a relatively regular medication schedule, supplemented by small intercalated doses when needed. The effect of L-dopa may be virtually immediate (i.e., after absorption, which occurs over 30 to 40 min) but there is a further cumulative effect over several days of consistent dosing. The principles that guide the adjustment of dosing (end-of-dose wearing off, dyskinesias, freezing, confusion) are discussed further on.

Dopamine Agonists These drugs have a direct dopaminergic effect on striatal neurons, thereby partially bypassing the depleted nigral neurons. They have found a place both as the initial treatment, replacing L-dopa in this role, and in modulating the effects of L-dopa later in the illness. However, dopamine agonists are consistently less potent than L-dopa in managing the main features of Parkinson disease and, in higher doses and in older individuals, they produce undesirable motor and cognitive side effects (see further on). They are favored because they are associated with fewer dyskinetic motor complications, or at least, delay the need for L-dopa and its dyskinetic effects. *Bromocriptine* and *lisuride* are synthetic ergot derivatives whose action in Parkinson disease is explained by their direct stimulating effect on dopamine (D_2) receptors located on striate neurons. The nonergot dopamine agonists *ropinirole* and *pramipexole* have a similar type and duration of effectiveness and are used more widely because of their minimal ergot-like effects. Pergolide and the related drug cabergoline are no longer used because of the risk of cardiac valvular damage, particularly at higher dose levels.

The dopamine agonists are introduced gradually. For example, the initial dose of pramipexole is 0.125 mg tid, following which the dosage is doubled weekly to a total of 3 to 4.5 mg/d if the medication is used without L-dopa. If an individual is already taking L-dopa, these drugs usually permit a gradual reduction in levodopa-carbidopa dose by approximately 50 percent. Their duration of action is slightly longer than that of L-dopa and they cause less nausea. These medications may be also useful in reducing the motor fluctuations of L-dopa.

Our experience is in general agreement with that of Marsden, who found that of 263 patients given dopamine agonists as the sole treatment, 181 had abandoned medication after 6 months because of lack of effect or adverse reactions. Nevertheless, the fact that a large enough proportion of patients continue to benefit for up to 3 to 5 years indicates that the initial use of dopamine agonists has merit (see also Rascol et al). A recent development of some interest is a transdermally absorbed dopamine agonist such as rotigotine. Several trials suggest that the transdermal system can maintain a stable plasma level of the drug. In the study by LeWitt and associates, the main effect was a doubling of "on" time without unwanted dyskinesias. The effects on the quality of life in Parkinson patients appear to be positive but minor in degree. Skin reactions are common and the sulfites used in the patch formulation can cause severe systemic reactions in sensitive individuals.

Even small doses of dopaminergic drugs, when first introduced, may induce orthostatic hypotension, but most patients are tolerant of them. They may also produce abrupt and unpredictable sleepiness, and patients should be warned of this possibility in relation to driving. In some individuals, particularly the elderly, dopamine agonists may produce hallucinosis or confusion; these problems are most profound in patients who are later determined to have Lewy-body disease (see further on). More data are required to judge the efficacy of the current trend of initiating therapy with a dopamine agonist rather than with L-dopa.

Many clinicians initiate treatment with small amounts of a dopamine agonist, at least as much for the putative delay of dyskinesias that they offer in comparison to starting L-dopa. Alternatively, carbidopa/L-dopa tid can be initiated and supplemented over a month with a dopamine agonist. The side effects and subtleties of dosing are explained in the sections above on each of these classes of drug. The issue of also starting an MAO inhibitor such as rasagiline early in the illness is discussed below.

Adjunctive Medications Because of the side effects of levodopa and of dopaminergic agents, some neurologists avoid pharmacotherapies if the patient is in the early phase of the disease and the parkinsonian symptoms are not troublesome. When the predominant manifestation is tremor, very satisfactory results can be obtained in some patients for up to several years with anticholinergic agents alone. The anticholinergic drugs have limited effect on the postural, hypokinetic, and other manifestations of disease. Koller's study, which quantified the effect of anticholinergic medication on tremor and compared it to L-dopa, concluded that there was considerable variability in response between patients but that L-dopa was on average more effective. Nonetheless, anticholinergic agents have long been in use for the treatment of tremor in younger patients and we still use them occasionally, either in conjunction with L-dopa or in patients who cannot tolerate the latter drug. The optimum dosage level is the point at which the greatest relief from tremor is achieved within the limits of tolerable side effects, mainly dry mouth. In older patients, one must be alert to changes in cognitive function, hallucinations, and urinary outflow obstruction.

Several synthetic preparations of anticholinergic drugs are available, the most widely used ones being trihexyphenidyl (beginning with 1 to 2 mg/d and increased up to 6 to 8 mg over several weeks) and benztropine mesylate (1 to 4 mg/d in divided doses). When it has been available, we have also had success with the related agent ethopropazine (50 to 200 mg daily in divided doses; but it has become difficult to obtain). The effects on tremor are cumulative and may not be evident for several days. To obtain maximum benefit from the use of these drugs, they should be given in gradually increasing dosage to the point where toxic effects appear: dryness of the mouth (which can be beneficial when drooling of saliva is a problem), blurring of vision from pupillary mydriasis, constipation, and urinary retention as mentioned (especially with prostatism). The presence of angle closure glaucoma is a contraindication to its use. Tremor abates in several days and most of our patients have become tolerant to the dry mouth after several weeks. Pyridostigmine, propantheline, or glycopyrrolate can be given to reduce the oral dryness.

With higher dose ranges, mental slowing, confusional states, hallucinations, and impairment of memory in elderly patients—specifically if there is already some degree of forgetfulness—are side effects that limit usefulness. Occasionally, further benefit may accrue from the addition of another antihistaminic drug, such as diphenhydramine or phenindamine.

The antiviral agent amantadine (100 mg bid) has mild or moderate benefit for tremor, hypokinesia, and postural symptoms. In some patients, it reduces L-dopa–induced dyskinesias (see further on). Its mechanism of action is unknown but antagonism of NMDA or release of stored dopamine has been proposed. It should be noted that amantadine commonly causes leg swelling, may worsen congestive heart failure, and can have an adverse effect on glaucoma, as well as exaggerate the cognitive changes associated with anticholinergic medications. The use of the centrally acting anticholinesterase, donepezil, is being explored for a possible effect on improving gait stability but requires further study. Finally, the monoamine oxidase inhibitors, described just below as putative neuroprotective agents, have a beneficial effect on motor fluctuations induced by L-dopa and may have a slight beneficial effect on the main Parkinson symptoms as described in several trials, such as the one reported by Rascol and colleagues.

Neuroprotective Agents An additional approach, still somewhat controversial, has been to initiate treatment early in the course of the disease with a monoamine oxidase-B inhibitor (MAO-B inhibitor), with the aim of reducing oxidative stress in dopaminergic neurons. The DTAATOP trial conducted by The Parkinson Study Group (1989) reported a slowing of disease progression but later followup showed little difference between treated and untreated groups. Other agents in this class, notably rasagiline, have given similar mixed results in brief studies including the ADAGIO trial reported by Olanow and coworker. The difficulty in assessing the benefit of these agents has to do with their mild but definite symptomatic benefit on motor function. A credible long-term study has reported that early initiation of treatment with bromocriptine (now little used) did not reduce mortality or motor disability over 14 years and that any reduction in motor complications was unsustained (Katzenschlager et al). Nonetheless, we institute one of these MAO-B inhibitors in many patients.

Following this same line of reasoning, several studies, most still disputed or unconfirmed, have suggested that ropinirole, pramipexole, and even L-dopa have "neuroprotective" effects in Parkinson disease. However, slowing of the progression of symptoms, as measured by a variety of scales, has not been corroborated. Technical problems in interpreting these results are discussed at length in the reviews by Wooten and by Clarke and Guttman. The uncertainties have to do with clinical grading systems, functional imaging techniques, and points of comparison to treatment with L-dopa.

The notion that the administration of L-dopa early in the disease might reduce the period over which it remains effective has been largely dispelled, but some neurologists continue to adhere to this idea. Cedarbaum and colleagues, who reviewed the course of the illness in 307 patients over a 7-year period, found no evidence that the early initiation of L-dopa treatment predisposed to the development of fluctuations in motor response or to dyskinesia and dementia. In fact, the findings of the "Elldopa" trial by The Parkinson Study Group (2004) were that functional and other measures were better in patients who had taken L-dopa for 40 weeks and then stopped the medications than in those who received no medication. Neuropathologic study of the substantia nigra in the brains of Parkinson patients and their medication histories also failed to corroborate a reduction in the number of pigmented neurons (Parkkinen et al). Also, the large multicenter study reported by Diamond and colleagues indicated that patients who were given L-dopa early in the disease actually survived longer and with less disability than those who began the medication late in the course; that is, L-dopa may have itself been neuroprotective. However, there have been many alternative interpretations of these data.

Finally, attempts to slow the disease by vitamin antioxidants such as vitamin E have met with mixed, but generally negative, results. A possible exception was the trial of coenzyme Q10 by Shults and colleagues. Massive doses of this agent, 1,200 mg/d, were found to offer marginal advantages on the progression over 6 to 18 months as measured by certain scores of overall daily function but not on most neurologic scales. Further study of this approach is advised.

Side Effects of Dopamine Treatment and Their Management The side effects of L-dopa are at times significant to the degree that its continuation cannot be tolerated. Some patients are at first troubled by nausea, although this can be mitigated by taking the medication with meals. Nausea usually disappears after several weeks of continued use or can be allayed by the specific dopaminergic chemoreceptor antagonist domperidone. A few have mild orthostatic hypotensive episodes.

The most troublesome effects of L-dopa as the disease advances, usually after several years of treatment, are end-of-dose reduction in efficacy and the induction of involuntary "dyskinetic" movements—restlessness, head wagging, grimacing, lingual-labial dyskinesia, blepharospasm, and especially, choreoathetosis and dystonia of the limbs, neck, and trunk. A decline in efficacy at the end of the dose interval, typically 2 to 4 h, may be treated by more frequent dosing, the addition of dopaminergic agonist, or a COMT inhibitor.

The *on–off* or *off phenomenon* is a rapid and sometimes unpredictable change—in a matter of minutes or from 1 h to the next—from a state of relative freedom from symptoms to one of nearly complete immobility. Both dyskinesias and severe "off" periods appear in approximately 75 percent of patients within 5 years. Few patients escape these opposing effects, forcing an increased frequency of administration and usually a reduction in dosage.

If involuntary dyskinetic movements are induced by relatively small doses of L-dopa, the problem may be suppressed to some extent by the addition of direct-acting dopaminergic agents or by the concurrent administration of amantadine, or by the use of an oral suspension of L-dopa as mentioned earlier. The use of lower doses of long-acting preparations of L-dopa may be helpful in reducing dyskinesias and the atypical antipsychotic medications have been said to be useful for this purpose but carry their own risks.

The onset of psychiatric symptoms coincident with the use of L-dopa or dopamine agonists may also present problems and is to be expected eventually in 15 to 25 percent of patients, particularly in the elderly. Confusion and outright *psychosis* (hallucinations and delusions) are seen in advanced cases of Parkinson disease when high doses of L-dopa are required and the disease has been present for many years. This may first be treated by reducing the dose of the drug. If this is not tolerated, the atypical neuroleptics olanzapine, clozapine, risperidone, or quetiapine may be given in low doses. The side effects of these drugs include sleepiness, orthostatic hypotension, and sialorrhea. As noted above, clozapine has been said to provide an additional benefit of suppressing dyskinesias in advanced Parkinson disease, but its hematologic risks have led to limited use. Although useful in the treatment of frankly psychotic patients, these drugs tend to be far less effective once dementia has supervened. The antiepileptic drug, valproate is also said to be useful in this circumstance, but it has not been as effective as clozapine and related drugs. Despite its lesser tendency to produce rigidity, olanzapine, and probably the other similar agents, in high doses may slightly worsen motor disability.

Depression, although frequent, is only occasionally a serious problem, even to the point of suicide. Delusional thinking may also occur in these circumstances. This combination of movement and psychiatric disorders is difficult to treat, and one is faced with instituting an antidepressant regimen or perhaps using one of the newer classes of antipsychotic medications that have the least extrapyramidal side effects (see below). While the selective serotonin reuptake inhibitors have been useful in cases of apathetic depression, they may cause slight worsening of parkinsonian symptoms. Trazodone has been helpful in treating depression and insomnia, the latter also being a major problem in some patients. Excitement and aggressiveness appear in a few. A return of libido may lead to sexual assertiveness. Other curious effects of excessive drive from L-dopa and dopamine agonists have been *pathologic gambling* (the same has been seen in treatment of restless legs syndrome) and *cross-dressing* (Quinn et al, 1983).

Anticholinergic agents or L-dopa should not be discontinued abruptly in advanced Parkinson disease. If abruptly discontinued, the patient may become totally immobilized by a sudden and severe increase of tremor and rigidity; rarely, a neuroleptic syndrome, sometimes fatal, has been induced by such withdrawal. Reducing the medication dose over a week or so is usually adequate.

With progressive loss of nigral cells, there is an increasing inability to store L-dopa and periods of drug effectiveness become shorter. In some instances, the patient becomes so sensitive to L-dopa that 50 to 100 mg will precipitate dyskinesias; if the dose is lowered by the same amount, the patient may develop disabling rigidity. With the end-of-dose loss of effectiveness and the on–off phenomenon, which with time become increasingly frequent and unpredictable, the patient may experience pain, respiratory distress, akathisia, depression, anxiety, and even hallucinations. Some patients function quite well in the morning and much less well in the afternoon, or vice versa. In such cases, and for end-of-dose and on–off phenomena, one must titrate the dose of L-dopa and use more frequent dosing during the 24-h day; combining it with a dopamine agonist or a long-acting preparation may be helpful. Sometimes temporarily withdrawing L-dopa and at the same time substituting other medications may reduce the on–off phenomenon.

Based on the principle that alimentary-derived amino acids compete for absorption of L-dopa, the use of a low-protein diet has been advocated as a means of controlling the motor fluctuations (Pincus and Barry). Symptoms can sometimes be reduced by the simple expedient of eliminating dietary protein from breakfast and lunch. Moreover, this dietary regimen may permit the patient to reduce slightly the total daily dose of L-dopa. Such dietary manipulation is worth trying in appropriate patients; it is not harmful, and most of our patients with advanced disease who have persisted with this diet have reported improvement in their symptoms or an enhanced effect of L-dopa. A novel observation by Pierantozzi and colleagues has been that the absorption of L-dopa may be influenced by the presence of gastric *Helicobacter pylori* infection and that eradication of the organism was associated with longer "on" time.

Surgical Measures

Until recently, success with L-dopa had replaced the use of the ablative surgical therapy pioneered by Cooper 50 years ago. The surgical approaches involved the placement of lesions in the globus pallidus, ventrolateral thalamus, or subthalamic nucleus, contralateral to the side of the body chiefly affected. The best results were obtained in relatively young patients, in whom unilateral tremor or rigidity rather than akinesia were predominant. The symptoms that responded least well to surgical therapy in Cooper's patients were postural imbalance and instability, paroxysmal akinesia, bladder and bowel disturbances, dystonia, and speech difficulties.

More recently, through the work of Laitinen, Leksell, and others, this mode of therapy has been revived as a stereotactically guided procedure and advanced by the newer technique of implanted electrodes (deep brain stimulation, DBS). For the treatment of Parkinson disease, the electrodes are placed in the posterior and ventral (medial) parts of the subthalamic nucleus or in the internal segment of the globus pallidus. Most patients who have DBS experience enhanced responsiveness to L-dopa and a reduction of drug-induced dyskinesias. Bilateral stimulation of the subthalamic nucleus has produced improvement in all features of the disease, including in bradykinesia, that is lost after several years, but there is generally little benefit for impaired gait and balance (Limousin et al; Weaver et al, who conducted a more extensive study but for only 6 months). A study by the Deep-Brain Stimulation for Parkinson's Disease Group demonstrated at least short-term benefit in motor fluctuations after the bilateral implantation of stimulating electrodes in the subthalamic nuclei and the durability of this effect with continued DBS in subsequent studies ranged from 2 to 7 years.

The ideal candidates for DBS are considered to be those in whom, after several years, there is a failure of medications to relieve symptoms but especially because of unmanageable dyskinesias that result from L-dopa. A randomized, blinded trial by Deuschl and colleagues confirmed this effect and demonstrated an overall improvement in the quality of life at 6 months. The benefit with bilateral stimulation of the globus pallidus has been essentially equivalent to results from subthalamic stimulation (Follett et al). Dystonia, when present as part of the native disease or as a result of medication, may also benefit from this treatment, perhaps more so with pallidal stimulation. Several groups have pointed out that cognitive function may decline slightly with DBS, but deterioration is not as prominent in some spheres of performance, such as speed of processing, with stimulation of the globus pallidus. Hemorrhage into the basal ganglia and local infection near the stimulator has occurred in a small number of patients so treated. Depression and suicides also appear as adverse events in some stimulation trials.

The typical patient who will derive benefit from deep-brain stimulation is considered to be one who, to maintain mobility, requires a dose of L-dopa that produces unacceptable dyskinesias and who is constantly cycling between on and off periods. More recently, DBS has been introduced earlier in the course of illness, when the patient is still largely responsive to L-dopa and before severe motor complications such as dyskinesias arise. These patients are, of course, younger and have had a shorter duration of disease. In a trial conducted by Schuepbach and coworkers, in patients with mean durations of illness of 7.5 years and 52 years of age, there was a significant and sustained benefit in quality of life measures, motor complications and on time, for subthalamic DBS.

The stimulator is inserted in a pouch that is created near the rostral pectoral muscle and inferior to the clavicle. An external controller allows the stimulator to be adjusted for which 4 electrodes on either side are activated and their polarity, voltage applied, frequency of pulses, and pulse duration are manipulated. All patients with implanted electrodes require frequent initial contact with a physician experienced in programming the stimulator. Some patients can make minor adjustments or even turn off the stimulator on their own with a small control device that has preset limits. The battery must be exchanged periodically, the duration of service depending on the voltage used over time and other parameters of use. A comprehensive review of the subject has been given by Okun, including comments on the controversies regarding the differences in cognitive disturbance and the reduction in L-dopa doses comparing stimulation of the globus pallidus with the subthalamic nucleus.

Presumably, the high-frequency electrical impulses cause a disruption of local neuronal activity that is the functional equivalent of an ablative lesion, but the effects of deep brain stimulation may be more complex by way of stimulating neurotransmitter release.

The cerebral implantation of fetal dopaminergic tissue provided a modest improvement in motor function for a limited period of time (Spencer et al; Freed et al). The study by Freed and colleagues found a small improvement on a global scale that measured functional, psychologic, and neurologic aspects only in younger patients but the effect waned by 1 year. These procedures are hampered by many difficulties, mainly in obtaining tissue and the failure of grafts to survive but also the problem of uncontrollable dyskinesias in some patients. Another provocative approach has been the delivery of neural trophic factors directly or in a viral vector through a small catheter; at least 2 trials have failed to show benefit. Similarly, the implantation of stem cells is being explored but has several obstacles.

Techniques of focused ultrasound energy to produce ablative lesions in deep nuclei are being developed. So far, they have found use for the treatment of essential tremor, such as in the trial conducted by Elias with thalamic lesions (ventral intermediate nucleus).

Ancillary Treatments In the management of the patient with Parkinson disease, one must not neglect the maintenance of general health and neuromuscular efficiency by a program of exercise, activity, and rest; physical therapy and exercises such as those performed in yoga may be of help in achieving these ends. Sleep may be aided by soporific antidepressants. Postural imbalance and falls can be greatly mitigated by the use of a cane or walking frame. A number of excellent exercise programs have been devised specifically for patients with Parkinson disease, and measures such as massage and yoga have their advocates. Among these mechanical therapies that have been studied systematically, tai chi has been found to improve balance and reduce falls as measured by objective criteria (Li et al), indicating that these approaches are of substantial value. Several of our patients have taken up dancing and report that their balance in daily circumstances is improved. Our position has been that any activity that keeps the patient moving and committed is of great value. Speech exercises help the motivated patient.

Hypotensive episodes respond to fludrocortisone or midodrine given each morning. Focal dystonias of the foot are partially treatable with local injections of botulinum toxin. In addition, the patient often needs emotional support in dealing with the stress of the illness, with the anxiety that seems to be an integral part of the disease in some patients, in comprehending the future, and in carrying on courageously in spite of it.

Multiple System Atrophy (Striatonigral Degeneration, Shy-Drager Syndrome, Olivopontocerebellar Degeneration)

As the name *multiple system atrophy* indicates, this depicts a group of disorders characterized by neuronal degeneration mainly in the substantia nigra, striatum, autonomic nervous system, and cerebellum. Following a report in 1964 by Adams and colleagues of what was then called *striatonigral degeneration*, many patients were recognized in whom the changes of striatonigral and olivopontocerebellar degeneration were combined and who had symptoms and signs of cerebellar ataxia and parkinsonian manifestations. The pathologic changes were found by chance in 4 middle-aged patients, in 3 of whom a parkinsonian syndrome had been described clinically, none with a family history of similar disease. Rigidity, stiffness, and akinesia had begun on one side of the body, then spread to the other, and progressed over a 5-year period but with minimal characteristic tremor of idiopathic Parkinson disease. A flexed posture of the trunk and limbs, slowness of all movements, poor balance, mumbling speech, and a tendency to faint when standing were other elements. There was an early-onset cerebellar ataxia in the fourth patient that was later obscured by a Parkinson syndrome.

The postmortem examinations disclosed extensive loss of neurons in the zona compacta of the substantia nigra, but notably, there were no Lewy bodies or neurofibrillary tangles in the remaining cells. Even more striking were the degenerative changes in the putamina and to a lesser extent in the caudate nuclei. Secondary pallidal atrophy (mainly a loss of striatopallidal fibers) was present. In the patient with ataxia there was, in addition, advanced degeneration of the pons, olives, and cerebellum (see below in the discussion of olivopontocerebellar degeneration).

Recognizing that the clinical and pathologic features of striatonigral degeneration, with or without autonomic failure, can coexist with olivopontocerebellar atrophy, Graham and Oppenheimer proposed the term *multiple system atrophy* (MSA), which has gained wide acceptance. Several large series of cases of this complex syndrome have been published, providing a perspective on the frequency and nature of its component syndromes. Either parkinsonism or cerebellar ataxia may predominate. In many writings they are categorized as MSA-P and MSA-C, respectively, depending on whether they display predominantly parkinsonism or cerebellar ataxia. More than half of the patients with striatonigral degeneration have *orthostatic hypotension*, which proves at autopsy to be associated with loss of intermediolateral horn cells and pigmented nuclei of the brainstem. This combined parkinsonian and autonomic disorder, formerly referred to as the Shy-Drager syndrome, was alluded to in Chaps. 18 and 26 and is now termed MSA-A, for multiple system atrophy with autonomic changes. In addition to orthostatic hypotension, other features of autonomic failure include erectile dysfunction loss of sweating, dry mouth, miosis, and urinary retention or incontinence. Vocal cord palsy is an important and sometimes initial manifestation of the disorder; it may cause dysphonia or stridor and airway obstruction requiring tracheostomy. A dusky discoloration of the hands as a sign of this disorder was ascribed to poor control of cutaneous blood flow by Klein and colleagues. A diagnostic problem arises in that orthostatic hypotension is also observed in up to 15 percent of patients with Parkinson disease, a feature that may be exaggerated by medications, but the degree of drop in blood pressure is far greater and more frequent in patients with this form of multiple system atrophy.

In the Brain Tissue Bank of the Parkinson Disease Society of Great Britain, MSA accounted for 13 percent of patients who had been identified during life as having idiopathic Parkinson disease. All the patients with MSA had one or more symptoms of autonomic failure (postural hypotension, urinary urgency or retention, urinary or fecal incontinence, erectile dysfunction) and dysphonia or stridor. Babinski signs were present in half the patients and cerebellar ataxia in one-third. Tremor was rare. Males were affected more often than females. In a comparable series of 100 patients (67 men and 33 women) studied by Wenning and coworkers (1994), the disease began with a striatonigral-parkinsonian syndrome in approximately half; often it was asymmetrical at the onset. Mild tremor was detected in some but in only a few was it of the "resting" Parkinson type. In nearly half, the illness began with autonomic manifestations; orthostatic hypotension occurred eventually in almost all patients, but it was disabling in only a few. Cerebellar features dominated the initial stages of the disease in only 5 percent, but ataxia was eventually obvious in half the larger group. This ataxic clinical presentation of multiple system atrophy will be elaborated further in the section on the degenerative cerebellar ataxias.

The extrapyramidal illness, on the whole, is more severe than in Parkinson disease, as more than 40 percent of patients are confined to a wheelchair or otherwise severely disabled within 5 years. These observations generally match the findings in the group described by Quinn and colleagues (1986), but they emphasized that pyramidal signs were present in 60 percent.

Colosimo and colleagues reviewed the clinical findings in 16 pathologically verified cases of MSA and found that several signs, namely, relative symmetry of the signs and rapid course, the lack of response to L-dopa, absence or minimal amount of tremor, and the early presence of autonomic disorders, reliably distinguished this syndrome from Parkinson disease. These observations are in keeping with our own and we would add that abnormalities of eye movement are not prominent in MSA. Additional features occurring occasionally in MSA are remarked upon in other series; anterocollis or dystonia of the lower facial muscles, for example, is striking in a few cases. It is noteworthy that levodopa has had little or no effect or has made these patients worse early in the disease but we have seen exceptions. The lack of L-dopa effect is probably attributable to the loss of striatal dopamine receptors.

The diagnosis of MSA, especially the form with ataxia, has been aided by imaging techniques. Both MRI and CT scanning frequently show atrophy of the cerebellum and pons in those with cerebellar features. The putamina are hypointense on T2-weighted MRI and may show an increased deposition of iron in the parkinsonian form. In the cerebellar form, a "hot cross bun" sign has been emphasized on MRI; it reflects atrophy of the pontocerebellar fibers that manifest high T2 signal intensity in an atrophic pons. Studies with PET have disclosed impairment of glucose metabolism in the striatum and to a lesser extent in the frontal cortex, a reflection, no doubt, of the loss of functioning neuronal elements in these parts.

Finally, despite the concurrence of striatonigral degeneration, olivopontocerebellar degeneration, and the Shy-Drager syndrome, *each of these disorders can occur in almost isolated clinical form*; we therefore retain their original designations.

Although the cause of this process is not known, and the majority of cases are sporadic, The Multiple System Atrophy Research Collaboration identified a mutation in the *COQ2* gene, coding for a protein involved in the synthesis of coenzyme Q_{10}, in both familial cases and a very small proportion of sporadic ones.

Pathology In recent years, attention has been drawn to the presence of abnormal staining material in the cytoplasm of astroglia and oligodendrocytes and in some neurons as well. These cytoplasmic aggregates have been referred to as *glial cytoplasmic inclusions* (Papp et al). Although they bear little resemblance morphologically to other discrete inclusions that have come to be accepted as characteristic of certain degenerative CNS diseases (e.g., Lewy bodies), they nonetheless contain α-synuclein (the main component of Lewy bodies). It is not clear to us whether these glial cytoplasmic accumulations represent a histopathologic hallmark of MSA as suggested by Chin and Goldman and by Lantos, as their presence is not specific; they have been identified in practically every degenerative disease that has been subjected to sensitive silver impregnation stains. Many types of inclusions are, of course, nonspecific, as, for example, α-synuclein–positive inclusions have been detected in several neurodegenerative syndromes. Appropriate control studies to determine whether the glial inclusions are found in *nondegenerative* lesions in brain (at the edge of an infarct, for example) are needed. Also lacking is information about the frequency of these cytoplasmic inclusions in relation to the aging brain.

Progressive Supranuclear Palsy

In 1963, Richardson, Steele, and Olszewski crystallized medical thought about a clinicopathologic entity—progressive supranuclear palsy (PSP)—to which there had been only ambiguous reference in the past. The condition is not rare. By 1972, when Steele reviewed the subject, 73 cases (22 with postmortem examinations) had been described in the medical literature. Rare familial clusters have been described in which the pattern of inheritance is compatible with autosomal dominant transmission (Brown et al; de Yébenes et al). Rojo and coworkers described 12 pathologically confirmed pedigrees and made note of the variable phenotypical expression of the disease even within a single pedigree. No toxic, encephalitic, racial, or geographic factor has been incriminated.

Clinical Features

The disease has its onset typically in the sixth decade (range: 45 to 75 years), with some combination of difficulty in balance, abrupt falls, visual and ocular disturbances (giving the syndrome its name), slurred speech, dysphagia, and sometimes vague changes in personality, including apprehensiveness and fretfulness suggestive of an agitated depression. The most common early complaint is unsteadiness of gait and unexplained falling without loss of consciousness. The patient has difficulty in describing his imbalance, using terms such as "dizziness," "toppling," or an ambiguous problem with walking. At first, the neurologic and ophthalmologic examinations may be unrevealing, and it may take a year or longer for the characteristic syndrome comprising supranuclear ophthalmoplegia, pseudobulbar palsy, and axial dystonia to develop fully.

Difficulty in voluntary vertical movement of the eyes, often downward but sometimes only upward, and later impairment of voluntary saccades in all directions are characteristic. A related but more subtle sign has been the finding of hypometric saccades in response to an optokinetic drum or striped cloth moving vertically in one direction (usually best seen with stripes moving downward). Later, both ocular pursuit and refixation movements are delayed and diminished in amplitude and eventually all voluntary eye movements are lost, first the vertical ones and then the horizontal ones as well. However, if the eyes are fixated on a target and the head is turned slowly, full movements can be obtained, demonstrating the supranuclear, nonparalytic character of paralysis of ocular pursuit. Other prominent oculomotor signs are sudden jerks of the eyes during fixation, "cogwheel" or saccadic choppiness of pursuit movements, and hypometric saccades of long duration (Troost and Daroff). The Bell phenomenon (reflexive upturning of eyes upon forced closure of the eyelids) and the ability to converge are also lost eventually, and the pupils become small but remain round and reactive to both light and to accommodative stimuli. The upper eyelids may be retracted, and the wide-eyed, unblinking stare imparts an expression of perpetual surprise. Blepharospasm and involuntary eye closure are prominent in some cases. In the late stages, the eyes may be fixed centrally and all oculocephalic and vestibular reflexes are lost. It should be emphasized, however, that *a proportion of patients do not demonstrate these eye signs for a year or more* after the onset of the illness. We have also followed several patients who had no disorder of eye movement during life but in whom the typical pathologic changes of PSP were nonetheless found. In one such patient, there was a subcortical type of dementia; in another, focal limb dystonia and parkinsonism. Furthermore, other degenerative conditions can manifest a supranuclear vertical gaze disorder, although never to the extent seen in PSP; these include corticobasal-ganglionic degeneration, Lewy-body disease, Parkinson disease, and Whipple disease.

The *gait disturbance* and *repeated falling* have proved difficult to analyze, as discussed in Chap. 7. Walking becomes increasingly awkward and tentative; the patient has a tendency to totter and fall repeatedly, but has no ataxia of gait or of the limbs and does not manifest a Romberg sign or orthostatic tremor. Some patients tend to lean and fall backward (retropulsion). One of our patients, a large man, fell repeatedly, wrecking household furniture as he went down, yet careful examination provided no clue as to the basic defect in this "toppling" phenomenon. Along with the oculomotor and balance disorders, there is a gradual stiffening and extension of the neck (in one of our patients it was sharply flexed in a manner consistent with camptocormia) but this is not an invariable finding. The face acquires a staring, "worried" expression with a furrowed brow (a result of the tonic contraction of the procerus muscle), made more striking by the paucity of eye movements. A number of our patients have displayed mild dystonic postures of a hand or foot, especially as the illness advanced but occasionally early on. The limbs may be slightly stiff and there are Babinski signs in a few cases.

The stiffness, slowness of movement, difficulty in turning and sitting down, and hypomimia may suggest a diagnosis of Parkinson disease. However, the facial expression of the PSP patient is more a matter of tonic grimace than of lack of movement, and the lack of tremor, the erect rather than stooped posture, and prominence of oculomotor abnormalities serve to distinguish the 2 disorders. The signs of pseudobulbar palsy are eventually prominent, and this feature, along with the eye movements, distinguishes the process most conspicuously from other degenerative conditions. The face becomes less expressive ("masked"), speech is slurred in a slowed spastic fashion, the mouth tends to be held open, and swallowing is difficult. Forced laughing and crying, said to be infrequent, have been present in about half of our cases late in the course. Many patients complain of sleep disturbances. The total sleep time and REM sleep are reduced, and spontaneous awakenings during the night are more frequent and longer than in normal individuals of the same age. Complaints of urinary frequency and urgency have also been frequent in advanced cases under our care.

The diagnosis often proves difficult to make if the main features are not outstanding. Other features, such as tremor, palilalia, myoclonus, chorea, orofacial dyskinesias, and disturbances of vestibular function, are observed in some cases. Finally the patient becomes anarthric, immobile, and quite helpless. Dementia of some degree is probably present in many cases, but is mild in most. Some patients do become forgetful and appear apathetic and slow in thinking; many others are irritable or at times euphoric. Dubois and colleagues proposed an "applause sign" as distinctive to this disease; the patient fails to stop clapping after being asked to do so only 3 times, but we are unable to corroborate this.

By MRI one can, in advanced cases, appreciate atrophy of the dorsal mesencephalon (superior colliculi, red nuclei) giving rise to a "mouse ears" configuration (Fig. 39-7), but these changes may not be evident early in the illness when diagnosis is most difficult. Several measurements of midbrain atrophy have been proposed as aiding diagnosis; for example, there is little overlap between PSP, multiple system atrophy, and Parkinson disease in the ratio of midbrain-to-pons cross-sagittal area, according to Oba and colleagues. The CSF remains normal. Nonetheless, the diagnosis continues to rest on the clinical features, mainly affecting eye movements.

Pathology *Postmortem examinations* have disclosed a bilateral loss of neurons and gliosis in the periaqueductal gray matter, superior colliculus, subthalamic nucleus,

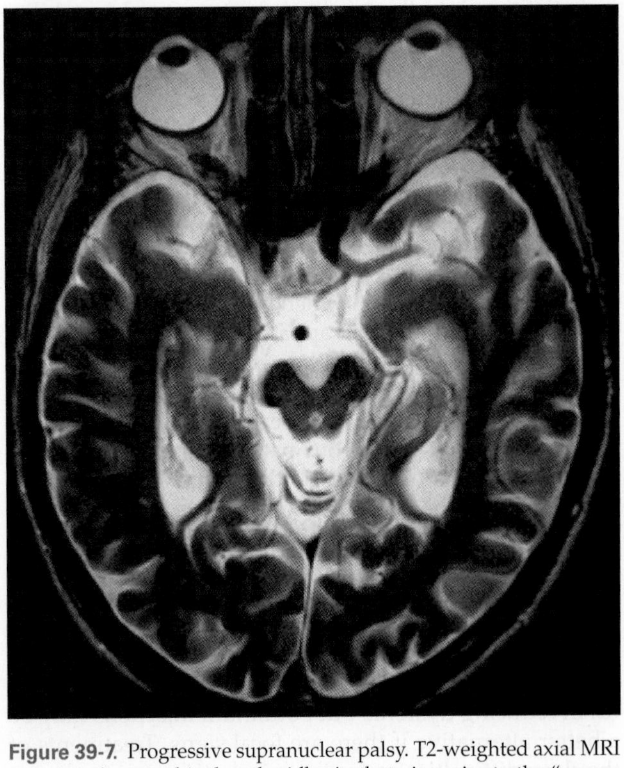

Figure 39-7. Progressive supranuclear palsy. T2-weighted axial MRI showing the atrophic dorsal midbrain that gives rise to the "mouse ears" (also "Mickey mouse") appearance.

red nucleus, pallidum, dentate nucleus, and pretectal and vestibular nuclei, and to some extent in the oculomotor nucleus. The expected loss of the myelinated fiber bundles arising from these nuclear structures has also been commented upon. The remarkable finding has been the neurofibrillary degeneration of many of the residual neurons. The neurofibrillary tangles are thick and often composed of single strands, either twisted or in parallel arrangement. The neurons of the cerebral cortex have been involved in some cases (shown by staining of tau protein), but these changes do not correlate with dementia. The cerebellar cortex is usually spared.

The cause and nature of this disease remain obscure. Though some clinical and pathologic heterogeneity is seen, the majority of cases of PSP conform to the typical pattern as we have just described. These interesting diagnostic and clinicopathologic aspects are summarized by Williams and Lees. Studies with PET demonstrate a decrease in blood flow, most marked in the frontal lobes, and a lesser extent of oxygen utilization in central structures (Leenders et al). Striatal dopamine formation and storage are significantly decreased when compared with control values. Much current interest has been directed to the neurofibrillary tangles and tau deposition in PSP and a potential link to the tau pathology displayed in frontotemporal dementia and in corticobasalganglionic degeneration (see below). As summarized by Golbe, certain tau gene haplotypes on chromosome 17p (the same site implicated in familial frontotemporal dementia) are more often associated with PSP than in unaffected individuals, but other factors, environmental or genetic, must also be involved. It is intriguing that the tau-gene haplotype of frontotemporal dementia is not found in PSP. A recent investigation into the mechanism of postural instability using functional imaging, showed a correlation between gait instability and decreased thalamic glucose metabolism and activation (Zwergal).

PSP should be suspected whenever an older adult inexplicably develops a state of imbalance, frequent falls with preserved consciousness, and variable extrapyramidal symptoms, particularly dystonia of the neck, ocular palsies, or a picture resembling pseudobulbar palsy. If the typical abnormalities of eye movements are present, the diagnosis is not difficult. When only a parkinsonian syndrome without tremor is apparent the main diagnostic consideration is striatonigral degeneration or the corticobasalganglionic syndrome, described below.

Treatment L-Dopa has been of slight and unsustained benefit in some of our patients, and combinations of L-dopa and anticholinergic drugs have been entirely ineffective in others. A marked response to these drugs should, of course, suggest the diagnosis of Parkinson disease. Recently, the drug zolpidem, a gabanergic agonist of benzodiazepine receptors, has been reported to ameliorate the akinesia and rigidity of PSP (Daniele et al); however, these observations require corroboration. Benztropine or trihexyphenidyl has been somewhat helpful in reducing dystonia but botulinum injections may be a better alternative if there are focal signs. Treatments of the sleep difficulties and urinary incontinence are of great assistance to the patient and family. A feeding tube becomes necessary in advanced cases. Observing the decline of these patients and the limitations of treatment is a frustrating ordeal for all involved.

Corticobasal Degeneration

Most neurologists have observed elderly patients in whom the essential abnormality was a progressive asymmetrical extrapyramidal rigidity combined with signs of corticospinal disease. Sometimes a mild postural action tremor beginning unilaterally and suggestive in some respects of Parkinson disease has been added. The parkinsonism is generally unresponsive to L-dopa. These cases have come to be known by the names *corticobasal-ganglionic* or *cortical-basal degeneration* and like sounding terms. The clinical relation of such cases is indeterminate to corticostriatospinal degeneration described earlier, and based on the finding of tau inclusions, to frontotemporal lobar degeneration and to progressive supranuclear palsy.

Wenning and colleagues (1998) described a series of such patients in whom the diagnosis was confirmed at postmortem examination. The most common early symptom was an asymmetrical clumsiness of the limbs, in half of the patients, with rigidity and, in one-fifth, with tremor; these features are now considered to be the most characteristic early features of the process. As the illness progressed, almost all the patients developed an asymmetric or unilateral akinetic-rigid syndrome, which may be considered the essential motor disorder of this disease and various forms of gait disorder and dysarthria. Stimulus-induced or spontaneous myoclonus and pyramidal signs, mentioned in other reports and frequent in our cases, were not prominent in their series; limitations of vertical gaze and frontal lobe release signs eventually became apparent in half.

Eventually, although able to exert considerable muscle power, these patients cannot effectively direct their voluntary actions. Attempts to move a limb to accomplish some purposeful act might result in a totally inappropriate movement, always with great enhancement of rigidity in the limb and in other affected parts, or the limb may drift off and assume an odd posture, such as a persistent elevation of the arm without the patient's awareness—a kind of catalepsy. The disorder of limb function has some of the attributes of a limb-kinetic or an ideomotor apraxia (see Chap. 3), but the hand postures, involuntary movements, and changes in tone are at times more of the type described as "alien hand." Some patients exhibit anosognosia, Babinski signs, impaired eyelid or ocular motion (upgaze paresis or abnormal saccadic movements), lingual dyskinesias, frontal release signs, myoclonus, or dysarthria.

Another distinct group has dementia as an early feature, as described by Grimes and colleagues, but mental deterioration is more often late and may not occur in all patients. There are also rare patients who present with behavioral disturbance or nonfluent aphasias as early features, which are difficult to distinguish from subtypes of frontotemporal dementia (Lee and colleagues, 2011). Occasionally, there is some involvement of lower motor neurons with resulting amyotrophy. Several of our patients had myoclonus as an early feature, one displaying it only on one side of the face, the other in an arm. The condition progresses for 5 years or more before some medical complication overtakes the patient.

Postmortem examination of patients, originally reported by Rebeiz and colleagues, disclosed a combination of findings that differentiated the disease process from other neurodegenerative conditions. Cortical atrophy (mainly in the frontal motor–premotor and anterior parietal lobes) was associated with degeneration of the substantia nigra and, in one instance, of the dentatorubrothalamic fibers. The loss of nerve cells was fairly marked, but there was no gross lobar atrophy, as occurs in Pick disease. The neuronal degeneration was more on one side of the brain than the other. There was moderate gliosis in the cortex and underlying white matter. The disease is now clearly considered to be related to tau deposition in specific brain structures; however, the original authors were more impressed with ballooned and chromatolytic neurons with eccentric nuclei, a state that was called *neuronal achromasia*. The presence of these achromatic cells in posterior frontal and parietal neurons continues to be considered an essential feature of the disease, although the rounded areas within neurons stain for tau and resemble globose tangles that are found occasionally in Alzheimer disease (corticobasal bodies); in this way, CBD is connected to the other tau-related neurodegenerative diseases, "*tauopathies*." In addition, adjacent glia are filled with various configurations of tau protein, thereby linking the disease to frontotemporal lobar degeneration and PSP. Our colleague Feany, with Dickson, has identified one type of these as "plaques" in the cortex that are composed of tau aggregates within the distal processes of astrocytes.

Both CT and MRI have demonstrated asymmetrical cerebral and pontine atrophy, and PET studies have revealed thalamoparietal metabolic asymmetries—a greater reduction of glucose metabolism on the side of the most extensive lesion (Riley et al).

There are no clues as to the pathogenesis of this disease. There are rare familial types but no definite genetic cause has been identified. No organ other than the CNS is affected. The progression is relentless. None of the drugs in common use for spasticity, rigidity, and tremor has been helpful.

Dystonic Disorders

Dystonia Musculorum Deformans (Torsion Dystonia)

Dystonia as a symptom was discussed in Chaps. 4 and 6. Here we are concerned with a disease or diseases of which dystonia is the major manifestation. Schwalbe's account, in 1908, of 3 siblings of a Jewish family who were afflicted with progressive involuntary movements of trunk and limbs probably represents the first description of a disease in which severe and progressive dystonia was the sole manifestation. In 1911, Oppenheim contributed other cases and coined the term *dystonia musculorum deformans* in the mistaken belief that the disorder was primarily one of muscle and always associated with deformity. Flatau and Sterling, in the same year, first suggested that the disease might have a hereditary basis and gave it the more accurate name *torsion dystonia of childhood*. At first the condition was considered by some to be a manifestation of hysteria; only later was it recognized as a neurologic entity with a predilection for individuals of Eastern European Jewish origin. Soon thereafter, a second hereditary form of torsion dystonia, affecting non-Jews, was observed. The recessive form begins in early childhood, is progressive over a few years, and is restricted to Jewish patients. The dominant form begins later, usually in late childhood and adolescence, progresses more slowly, and is not limited to any ethnic group.

As indicated in Chap. 6, most instances of idiopathic (primary) dystonias that come to our attention, particularly the segmental or restricted types, do not conform to the classic hereditary disorders as defined above, although some may represent limited variants of the disease. In general, these more restricted types have a later onset and a relatively milder, more slowly progressive course, with a tendency to involve an axial or a distal region alone. Only the paravertebral, cervical, or cranial muscles may be involved (focal dystonia including torticollis and writer's cramp), with little change from year to year. The clinical classification of the predominantly adult-onset dystonias is made more complex by the fact that both the restricted and generalized forms may be sporadic or genetic. Molecular genetic studies, although still incomplete, hold the promise of clarifying the classification of the heritable dystonias. More than 10 types have been distinguished by genetic mapping, as summarized by Németh. The most important of these is an abnormal gene (*DYT1*, also known as *TOR1A*) on chromosome 9q, which codes for the protein, torsin A in both Jewish and non-Jewish families. The most common *DYT1* mutation, causing deletion of a single glutamate from the torsin A peptide, is found in most cases of dystonia musculorum deformans. This disease is inherited in an autosomal dominant pattern. Although the penetrance of the clinical trait in these families is low, PET demonstrates hypermetabolism in the cerebellum, lenticular nuclei, and supplementary motor cortex in all carriers of the mutated gene.

The function of torsin A is not fully defined. It is present in neurons throughout the brain and has adenosine triphosphate (ATP) binding and nuclear localization. It may function as a chaperone protein that shuttles other proteins in and out of cells. A current speculation, shared with other degenerative disease, is that the absence of torsin A renders neurons unduly sensitive to oxidative stress (Walker and Shashidharan).

Although *DYT1* mutations account for the majority of inherited cases of generalized dystonia, they are also implicated in a small proportion of the more restricted dystonias, particularly blepharospasm (see further on). Some individuals in families affected with generalized dystonia will demonstrate only localized forms (e.g., writer's cramp or torticollis). The general rule stated above still holds, namely, that the inherited variety (dystonia musculorum deformans) related to *DYT1* manifests early in life and begins in one limb and then spreads to most muscles of the body, while in the common dystonias (mostly sporadic but some heritable) the disease remains confined to the craniocervical or another region, does not generalize, and has an adult onset.

Clinical Features The first manifestations of the generalized disease may be rather subtle. Intermittently, and usually after activity (late in the day), the patient (usually a child between 6 and 14 years of age, less often an adolescent) begins to invert one foot, to extend one leg and foot in an unnatural way, or to hunch one shoulder, raising the question of a nervous tic. As time passes, the motor disturbance becomes more persistent and interferes increasingly with the patient's activities. Soon the muscles of the spine and shoulder or pelvic girdle become implicated in involuntary spasmodic twisting movements. The cardinal feature of these severe dystonic muscle contractions is the simultaneous contraction of both agonists and antagonists at a joint. These cocontraction spasms are intermittent at first; in intervals that are free of the dystonia, muscular tone and volitional movements are normal. In some instances, the muscles are hypotonic. Gradually, the spasms become more frequent; finally, they are continuous and the body may become grotesquely contorted, as shown in Fig. 4-5*A*. Lateral and rotatory scoliosis uniformly results as secondary deformities. For a time, recumbency relieves the spasms, but later on position has no influence. The hands are seldom involved, although at times they may be held in a fisted posture. Cranial muscles do not escape, and in a few instances a slurring, staccato-type speech was the initial manifestation. Uncontrollable blepharospasm was the initial disorder in one of our patients; in two others, severe dysarthria and dysphagia were the first signs, caused by dystonia of the tongue, pharyngeal, and laryngeal muscles.

Other manifestations include torticollis, tortipelvis, dromedary gait, propulsive gait, action tremor, myoclonic jerks during voluntary movement, and mild choreoathetosis of the limbs. Excitement worsens the dystonia and sleep abolishes it. As the years pass the postural distortion may become fixed to the point where it does not disappear even in sleep. Tendon reflexes are normal, corticospinal signs are absent, and there is no ataxia, sensory abnormality, convulsive disorder, or dementia.

Pathology No agreement has been reached concerning the pathologic substrate of the disease. None of the features of symptomatic dystonia are found, such as the ferrocalcinosis of PKAN, the lesions of Wilson disease, kernicterus, état marbré of neonatal hypoxia, or the cavitation of familial striatal necrosis, lesions have been observed in the basal ganglia. However, in the hereditary forms of dystonia, which are the subject of this section, one cannot be certain of any specific lesions that would account for the clinical manifestations. The brain is grossly normal and ventricular size is not increased. According to Zeman, who reviewed all the reported autopsy studies up to 1970, there were no significant changes in the striatum, pallidum, or elsewhere. This means only that the techniques being used (qualitative analysis of random sections by light microscopy) are inadequate or the problem is subcellular. The report by McNaught and colleagues of perinuclear inclusions in periaqueductal neurons by the use of special immunostaining methods is provocative. There had been tentative interest in elevations of dopamine β-hydroxylase in patients with the autosomal dominant form of the disease, but the meaning of these findings is not clear.

Treatment Early in the course of the illness, several drugs including L-dopa, bromocriptine, carbamazepine, diazepam, and tetrabenazine seem to be helpful, but only in a few patients, and the benefit is not lasting. Intrathecal baclofen has been somewhat more successful in children. The rare hereditary form of dystonia-parkinsonism (described below) responds well to small doses of L-dopa and dopamine agonists and is exceptional in this respect. Burke and coworkers advocate the use of very high doses (up to 30 mg daily or more) of trihexyphenidyl (Artane). Apparently, dystonic children can tolerate these high doses if the medication is raised gradually, by 5-mg increments weekly. In adults, high-dose anticholinergic treatment is less successful but worthy of a trial. Clonazepam is beneficial in some patients with segmental myoclonus.

Impressive results were obtained in the past by the use of stereotactic techniques that made lesions in the ventrolateral nuclei of the thalamus or in the pallidum-ansa lenticularis region. Some frightfully disabled children, unable to sit or stand, were restored to near normalcy for a time. Approximately 70 percent of the patients in Cooper's series in the 1950s were moderately to markedly improved by unilateral or bilateral operations and, based on a 20-year followup study, the improvement was usually sustained. More recent studies report a somewhat less favorable but nonetheless clear improvement (see Tasker et al; Andrew et al). The main risk of the operation was a corticospinal tract lesion, produced inadvertently by damaging the internal capsule. Bilateral lesions have sometimes been disastrous, causing pseudobulbar palsy. The production of lesions has been supplanted, with success over long periods, by bilateral stimulation of the internal segments of the globus pallidus (Vidailhet and colleagues).

Hereditary Dystonia-Parkinsonism (Segawa Syndrome, Juvenile Dopa-Responsive Dystonia)

This process is discussed here because its main characteristic is a dystonia that is responsive to L-dopa, but most cases also have features of parkinsonism, which is why it was also mentioned in the earlier discussion of hereditary forms of Parkinson disease, especially in young patients. Following the description of the syndrome by Segawa and colleagues in 1976, others drew attention to this unique form of hereditary dystonia (Allen and Knopp; Deonna; Nygaard and Duvoisin). The pattern of inheritance is autosomal dominant and there is no ethnic predilection. Nygaard and colleagues found a linkage to the gene on chromosome 14q for the protein GTP cyclohydrolase 1 (*GCH1* gene) that is implicated in the synthesis of tetrahydrobiopterin, a cofactor for tyrosine hydroxylase. It is likely that the mutation impairs the generation of dopamine, a prediction that accords with responsiveness of the parkinsonian and dystonic features to L-dopa. In one autopsied case (an accidental death), there was a reduction in the amount of tyrosine hydroxylase in the striatum and depigmentation but no cell loss in the substantia nigra (Rajput et al). The affected enzyme was reduced in the striatum, as was the level of dopamine.

The dystonic manifestations usually become evident in childhood, usually between 4 and 8 years of age; females outnumber males in a ratio of 3:2. Often the legs are first affected by intermittent stiffening, with frequent falls and peculiar posturing, sometimes the feet assuming an equinovarus position. The arms become involved as well as the truncal muscles; retrocollis or torticollis may appear. Within 4 to 5 years, all parts of the body, including the bulbar muscles, are involved. Mild parkinsonian features (rigidity, bradykinesia, postural instability) can usually be detected early in the course of the illness, but more characteristically they are added to the clinical picture several years later. In our own patients, and in several of those of Deonna, there was rigidity of the limbs as well as slowness of movement and a tremor at rest, all aspects more parkinsonian than dystonic. In still others, the clinical picture has been one of cerebral spastic diplegia.

A remarkable feature is the disappearance or marked subsidence of the symptoms after a period of sleep and worsening as the day progresses. This diurnal variation is shared with many of the inherited forms of Parkinson disease listed in Table 39-3. Fluctuations of symptoms with exercise and menses and in the first month of pregnancy have been observed in some cases.

The special feature of this *juvenile dystonia-parkinsonism syndrome* is the dramatic response of both the dystonic and parkinsonian symptoms to treatment with L-dopa. As little as 10 mg/kg/d may eliminate the movement disorder and permit normal functioning. Unlike idiopathic Parkinson disease, the medication can be continued indefinitely without the development of tolerance, wearing-off effects, or dyskinesias. Segawa disease accounts for some cases that had in the past been reported as juvenile Parkinson disease.

Torticollis and Other Restricted Dyskinesias and Dystonias (See Chap. 6)

With advancing age, a large variety of focal or regional movement disorders come to light. Various neurophysiologic abnormalities, summarized in Chap. 6, have been implicated. In the common restricted dystonias, localized groups of adjacent muscles manifest arrhythmic cocontracting spasms (i.e., agonist and antagonist muscles are activated simultaneously). The patient's inability to suppress the dystonia and the recognition that it is for the most part beyond voluntary control distinguishes it from tics, habit spasms, and mannerisms described in Chap. 6. If the muscle contraction is frequent and prolonged, it is accompanied by an aching pain that may mistakenly be blamed for the spasm and the involved muscles may gradually undergo hypertrophy. Worsening under conditions of excitement and stress and improvement during quiet and relaxation are typical of this group of disorders and contributed in the past to the mistaken notion that the spasms had a psychogenic origin.

The most frequent and familiar type is *torticollis*, wherein an adult, more often a woman, becomes aware of a turning of the head to one side while walking. Usually this condition worsens gradually to a point where it may be more or less continuous, but in some patients it remains mild or intermittent for years on end. When followed over the years, the condition is observed to remain limited to the same muscles (mainly the scalene, sternocleidomastoid, and upper trapezius). Rarely, the torticollis is combined with dystonia of the shoulder, arm, and trunk; tremor; facial spasms; or dystonic writer's cramp.

Other restricted dyskinesias involve the neck in combination with facial muscles, the orbicularis oculi (*blepharospasm* and *blepharoclonus*), the throat and respiratory muscles (*spastic dysphonia, orofacial dyskinesia*, and *respiratory* and *phonatory spasms*), the hand in writer's cramp (*graphospasm*) or musician and other performing artist's dystonia, and proximal leg and pelvic-girdle muscles, where dyskinesia is elicited by walking. All these conditions and their treatments are discussed fully in Chap. 6.

Other Forms of Hereditary Dystonia

Several familial movement-induced (kinesogenic) dystonic syndromes and a type that is not kinesogenic and arises suddenly in adolescence, at times with parkinsonian features, have been described. There are other degenerative diseases that combine hereditary dystonia with neural deafness and intellectual impairment (Scribanu and Kennedy) and with amyotrophy in a paraplegic distribution (Gilman and Romanul). These are discussed in greater detail in Chap. 6.

Other important symptomatic dystonias that fall into the category of hereditary dystonia were described in Chap. 37. These are PKAN and calcification of the basal ganglia; of course, Wilson disease may have dystonia as a central feature. Many extrapyramidal diseases, including idiopathic Parkinson disease and progressive supranuclear palsy, may include fragmentary dystonias of the hand, foot, face, or periorbital muscles.

SYNDROME OF PROGRESSIVE ATAXIA

Wilson wrote that "the group of degenerative conditions strung together by the common feature of ataxia is one for which no very suitable classification has yet been devised," a statement that is not as appropriate today as when it was written 75 years ago. This topic was introduced in Chap. 5 and some of the congenital and acute acquired varieties are mentioned there. Here we consider the *chronic, progressive forms of cerebellar disease*. Although most of these are familial and are more or less confined to this part of the nervous system, a number of other systems may be involved to varying degrees. Most of the chronic progressive cerebellar diseases are subsumed under the "system atrophies," but no one classification designed to bring order to this category of diseases has proved satisfactory and a preferable genetic classification is emerging.

Setting aside those of congenital type and those caused by a metabolic disorder, Harding (1993) grouped the ataxias by age of onset, pattern of heredity, and associated features. A modification of the classifications of Greenfield and of Harding, which is included in the introductory listing of this chapter, still has clinical value. It divides the progressive cerebellar syndromes into 3 main groups: (1) the spinocerebellar ataxias, with unmistakable involvement of the spinal cord (Romberg sign, sensory loss, diminished tendon reflexes, Babinski signs); (2) the pure cerebellar ataxias, with no other associated neurologic disorders; and (3) the complicated cerebellar ataxias, with a variety of pyramidal, extrapyramidal, retinal, optic nerve, oculomotor, auditory, peripheral nerve, and cerebrocortical accompaniments including what is now referred to as multiple system atrophy.

Without doubt, the advances in molecular genetics of recent years have greatly altered our understanding of the inherited ataxias and have already disclosed a large number of unexpected relationships between mutations and other neural and nonneural disorders. These data are incorporated at appropriate points in the following discussion in Table 39-5, later in this section. Inherited ataxias of early onset (before the age of 20 years) are usually of recessive type; those of later onset are more likely to have a dominant pattern but may be autosomal recessive. Table 39-5 lists several types of ataxias that have a genetic basis. At the time of this writing, 29 types have been listed in the literature, many of limited clinical consequence and low incidence. We have included the main varieties that may be of interest to clinicians because they appear regularly or offer an insight into this class of disorders. At the same time, it should be emphasized that many patients with chronic progressive ataxia have no family history of an ataxia and may have had a spontaneous mutation; even then, the genetic aspects of many cases have not been elucidated.

Early-Onset Spinocerebellar Ataxias (Predominantly Spinal)

Friedreich Ataxia

This is the prototype of all forms of progressive spinocerebellar ataxias and accounts for about half of all cases of hereditary ataxias in most large case series (86 of 171 patients collected by Sjögren); its incidence among Europeans and North Americans is 1.5 cases per 100,000 per year. Friedreich, of Heidelberg, began in 1861 to report on a form of familial progressive ataxia that he had observed among nearby villagers. It was already known through the writings of Duchenne that locomotor ataxia was the prominent feature of spinal cord syphilis, that is tabes dorsalis, but it was Friedreich who demonstrated a nonsyphilitic hereditary type. This concept was greeted with skepticism, but soon Duchenne himself affirmed the existence of the new disease and other case reports appeared in England, France, and the United States. In 1882, in a thesis on this subject by Brousse of Montpelier, Friedreich's name was attached to the entity.

The pattern of inheritance is autosomal recessive. Genetic linkage studies led to the assignment of the gene mutation to chromosome 9q13-2 and subsequently, it was shown that in virtually all cases the mutation is an expansion of a GAA trinucleotide repeat within a gene that codes for the protein *frataxin*. (It is of interest that this mutation is within an intron). In a small proportion of cases, the mutation is a missense mutation rather than an expansion. In either case, the consequence of the mutation is a reduction in levels of frataxin and loss of its function. Cases in which the mutation allows the presence of some residual protein have a milder course. A current hypothesis is that frataxin is a mitochondrial matrix protein whose function is to prevent intramitochondrial iron overloading.

Clinical Features Ataxia of gait is nearly always the initial symptom. Difficulties in standing steadily and in running are early symptoms. The hands usually become clumsy months or years after the gait disorder, and dysarthric speech appears after the arms are involved (this is rarely an early symptom). Exceptionally the ataxia begins rather abruptly after a febrile illness, and one leg may become clumsy before the other. In some patients, pes cavus and kyphoscoliosis (scoliosis) are evident well before the neurologic symptoms; in others, they follow by several years. The characteristic foot deformity takes the form of a high plantar arch with retraction of the toes at the metatarsophalangeal joints and flexion at the interphalangeal joints (hammertoes).

A notable feature in more than half of patients is a cardiomyopathy. The myocardial fibers are hypertrophic and may contain iron-reactive granules (Koeppen). Many of the patients die as a result of cardiac arrhythmia or congestive heart failure. For this reason, it is essential that affected individuals have a cardiologic assessment including electrocardiography and echocardiography. The cardiomyopathy of Friedreich disease can develop insidiously but with fulminant consequences. Kyphoscoliosis and restricted respiratory function are additional important contributory causes of death. Harding observed that approximately 10 percent of these patients have diabetes mellitus and a higher proportion have impaired glucose tolerance; there is both insulin deficiency and peripheral insulin resistance.

In the fully developed syndrome, the abnormality of gait is of mixed sensory and cerebellar type, aptly called *tabetocerebellar* by Charcot. According to Mollaret, the author of an authoritative monograph on the disease, the cerebellar component predominates, but in our relatively small series we have been as impressed almost as much with the sensory (tabetic) aspect. The patient stands with feet wide apart, constantly shifting position to maintain balance. Friedreich referred to the constant teetering and swaying on standing as *static ataxia*. In walking, as with all sensory ataxias, the movements of the legs tend to be brusque, the feet resounding unevenly and irregularly as they strike the floor, and closure of the eyes causes the patient to fall (Romberg sign). This is one component of the spinal aspect (posterior columns) of the disease. Attempts to correct the imbalance may result in abrupt, wild movements. Often there is a rhythmic tremor of the head. Eventually, the arms are grossly ataxic, and both action and intention tremors are manifest. Speech is slow, slurred, explosive, and, finally, almost incomprehensible.

Table 39-5

GENETIC DEFECTS ASSOCIATED WITH SPINOCEREBELLAR ATAXIAS (SCA)

NOTATION	GENE (PROTEIN)	INHERITANCE	AGE OF ONSET	CLINICAL FEATURES IN ADDITION TO ATAXIA
Progressive				
Dentatorubropallidoluysian atrophy (DRPLA)	*ATN1* (atrophin1)	AD[a]	Childhood	Chorea, dystonia, seizures, dementia
SCA1	*ATXN1* (ataxin-1)	AD[a]	Variable	10–25% of dominant ataxias; spasticity, polyneuropathy, ophthalmoparesis, dementia
SCA2	*ATXN2* (ataxin-2)	AD[a]	Teens	Neuropathy, ophthalmoparesis, extrapyramidal features
SCA3 (Machado-Joseph)	*ATXN3* (ataxin-3)	AD[a]	Teens	25% of dominant ataxias, spasticity, neuropathy, extrapyramidal features
SCA6	*CACNA1A* (alpha$_{1A}$ calcium channel)	AD[a]	Adult	20% of dominant ataxias; dysarthria, nystagmus, posterior column signs (see episodic ataxia below; gene implicated in familial hemiplegic migraine)
SCA7	*ATXN7* (ataxin-7)	AD[a]	Late teens	Olivopontocerebellar atrophy and syndrome of retinal degeneration, hearing loss, ophthalmoplegia, spasticity; generational anticipation
			Infantile	Fulminant, with large CAG expansion
SCA8	*ATXN8* (ataxin-8; CTG repeat (noncoding)	AD, AR, sporadic	Adult	Slowly progressive sensory neuropathy, spasticity; known rapid infantile variant
SCA10	*ATTCT* repeat (ataxin-10)	AD	Teens–adult	Seizures, personality change
SCA11	*TTBK2* (serine/threonine kinase)	AD	Adult	Mild phenotype, nystagmus, cerebellar ataxia, neuropathy, dystonia
SCA12	*PPP2R2B* (protein phosphatase 2A), CAG repeat, noncoding	AD	Adult	Head and hand tremor
SCA13	*KCNC3* (Kv3.3 channel)	AD	Childhood	Developmental delay
SCA14	*PRKCG* (protein kinase C gamma)	AD	Teens–adult	Myoclonus, tremor
SCA15 & 16	*ITPR1* (ITPR1)	AD	Varies	Head and hand tremor, gaze palsy
SCA17	*TATA* (TATA box binding protein, TBP)	AD[a]	Variable	Cognitive decline, seizures, extrapyramidal features
SCA with tremor	Fibroblast growth factor 14	AD	Childhood	Tremor, cognitive defects, facial dyskinesia
Friedreich ataxia	*FXN* (frataxin)	AR	Teens	Spinocerebellar ataxia, neuropathy, cardiomyopathy, arrhythmia
Vitamin E deficiency	*TTPA* (vitamin E transfer protein)	AR	Childhood	Spinocerebellar ataxia, neuropathy, cardiomyopathy, arrhythmia
Episodic				
Episodic ataxia with myokymia (EA1, EAM))	*KCNA1* (Kv1.1)	AD	Teens	Limb stiffness, dizziness, visual blurring
Paroxysmal episodic ataxia (EA2)	*CACNA1A* (Cav2.1)	AD	Teens	Nystagmus, vertigo, weakness
Episodic ataxia (EA5)	*CACNB4* (calcium channel beta-subunit)	AD	Teens	Seizures, myoclonus, nystagmus

[a]CAG expansion. AD denotes autosomal dominant, AR autosomal recessive

Breathing, speaking, swallowing, and laughing may be so incoordinated that the patient nearly chokes while speaking. Holmes (1907a) remarked on an ataxia of respiration that causes "curious short inspiratory whoops." Facial, buccal, and arm muscles may display tremulous and sometimes choreiform movements.

Although mentation is generally preserved, emotional lability has been sufficiently prominent to provoke comment. Torsional and vertical nystagmus is rare but "square wave jerks" are seen in the early stages of disease. Horizontal nystagmus may be present late in the course of the illness, but not early, but it is slight in amplitude. Ocular movements usually remain full, and pupillary reflexes are normal. The facial muscles may seem slightly weak, and deglutition may become impaired. Amyotrophy occurs late in the illness and is usually mild, but it may be extreme in patients with an associated neuropathy (see below). The tendon reflexes are abolished in nearly every case; rarely, they may be obtainable when the patient is examined early in the illness (see below). Plantar reflexes are extensor and flexor spasms may occur even with complete absence of tendon reflexes (another manifestation of the spinal component). The abdominal reflexes are usually retained until late in the illness. Loss of vibratory and position sense is invariable from the beginning; later, there may be some diminution of tactile, pain, and temperature sensation as well. Sphincter control is usually preserved.

Variants of Friedreich Ataxia In one important *variant of Friedreich ataxia* the tendon reflexes are preserved or even hyperactive and the limbs may be spastic. It is the finding of the aberrant frataxin gene that links these unusual cases to Friedreich ataxia; some are associated with hypogonadism. Harding (1981) found 20 such cases among her 200 familial ataxias at the National Hospital, London. Nevertheless, the distinction between classic Friedreich ataxia and ataxia with retained tendon reflexes is an important one clinically, insofar as kyphoscoliosis and heart disease do not occur in the latter group and the prognosis is better. Two of our Friedreich patients had occasional seizures. There are many additional forms of spinocerebellar ataxia, most displaying mainly a cerebellar atrophy, that may simulate Friedreich disease, but due to different mutations. These are taken up below.

Laboratory Testing Laboratory tests of diagnostic value are the measurement of sensory nerve conduction velocities and amplitudes, which for the most part are normal because peripheral neuropathy is not a component of the process. Electrocardiography and echocardiography may demonstrate the heart block and ventricular hypertrophy. The CT and MRI seldom reveal a significant degree of cerebellar atrophy but the spinal cord is small. There is no consistent abnormality of blood or CSF and no biochemical abnormalities have been demonstrated. Genetic testing for the length of the GAA trinucleotide repeat segment is available.

Pathology The spinal cord is thin. The posterior columns and the corticospinal and spinocerebellar tracts are all depleted of myelinated fibers, and there is a mild gliosis that does not replace the bulk of the lost fibers. The nerve cells in the Clarke column and the large neurons of the dorsal root ganglia, especially lumbosacral ones, are reduced in number—but perhaps not to a degree that would fully explain the posterior column degeneration. The posterior roots are thin. Betz cells are also diminished in some cases, but the corticospinal tracts are relatively intact down to the medullary–cervical junction. Beyond this point, they are degenerated, but to a lesser degree than the posterior columns. The nuclei of cranial nerves VIII, X, and XII all exhibit a reduction of cells. Slight to moderate neuronal loss is seen also in the dentate nuclei, and the middle and superior cerebellar peduncles are reduced in size. Some depletion of Purkinje cells in the superior vermis and neurons in corresponding parts of the inferior olivary nuclei can be seen. Many of the myocardial muscle fibers degenerate and are replaced by fibrous connective tissue.

By way of exploring the anatomic basis of the clinical findings, pes cavus is not different from that seen in other neuromuscular diseases of early onset with mild hypertonus of the long extensors and flexors of the feet. There is also cause of amyotrophy of intrinsic foot muscles and foreshortening of the foot when the bones are still malleable. The kyphoscoliosis is probably a result of imbalance of the paravertebral muscles during development. The tabetic aspects of the disease are explained by the degeneration of large cells in the dorsal root ganglia and the large sensory fibers in nerves, dorsal roots, and the columns of Goll and Burdach. The loss of neurons in the sensory ganglia also causes abolition of tendon reflexes. Cerebellar ataxia is attributable to a combined degeneration of the superior vermis and the dentatorubral pathways but also the spinocerebellar tracts, in various combinations. Corticospinal lesions account for the weakness and Babinski signs and contribute to the pes cavus.

Diagnosis Friedreich disease and its variants must be distinguished from familial cerebellar cortical atrophy described next, and from familial spastic paraparesis with ataxia, as well as from peroneal muscular atrophy and the Levy-Roussy syndrome, which are discussed also with the hereditary neuropathies in Chap. 46. It is advisable to assay serum vitamin E levels, as a rare (except in North Africa) but treatable inherited deficiency of a vitamin E transport protein causes a spinocerebellar syndrome with areflexia in children that resembles Friedreich disease (see Chap. 41). The absence of dysarthria and of skeletal or cardiac abnormalities in the vitamin-deficiency illness may be helpful. Exceptionally, a cardiac disturbance has been seen in the vitamin deficiency. A form of chronic inflammatory demyelinating polyneuropathy has long since overtaken tabes dorsalis as the most frequent type of areflexic ataxia. It bears a superficial resemblance to Friedreich ataxia when the onset is in early life, but lacks dysarthria and Babinski signs. A form of spinocerebellar degeneration related to human T-cell lymphotrophic virus type I (HTLV-I), causing so-called tropical spastic paraparesis, as well as the vacuolar myelopathy of AIDS multiple sclerosis, syringomyelia, neuroacanthocytosis, and cervical spondylosis, must be included in the differential diagnosis of late-onset cases. Genetic testing settles the matter.

Treatment Not much can be said on this subject because there is little effective therapy. A double-blind crossover study by Trouillas and associates found that the administration of oral 5-hydroxytryptophan modified the cerebellar symptoms. This has not been tested in another study. Apart from this form of treatment, with which we have had no experience, no therapeutic measures are known to alter the course of the disease. In several small trials, idebenone, an antioxidant (the short-chain analogue of coenzyme Q10), reduced the progression of left ventricular hypertrophy, a risk factor for arrhythmias and sudden death in these patients, but this could not be confirmed in subsequent trials. These results are summarized in an article by Filla and Moss. Heart failure, arrhythmias, and diabetes mellitus are treated by the usual medical measures and it bears repetition that careful evaluation of the cardiac disorder may prevent premature death. Surgery for scoliosis and foot deformities may be helpful in selected cases.

Predominantly Cerebellar (Cortical, Holmes Type) Hereditary and Sporadic Ataxia

Soon after the publication of Friedreich's descriptions of a spinal type of hereditary ataxia, reports began to appear of somewhat different diseases in which the ataxia was related to degenerative changes in the cerebellum and brainstem rather than in the spinal cord. Claims of their independence from the spinal type were based largely on a later age of onset, a more definite hereditary transmission (usually of autosomal dominant type), the persistence or hyperactivity of tendon reflexes, and associations with ophthalmoplegia, retinal degeneration, and optic atrophy. Several of these clinical features, particularly briskness of tendon reflexes, are alien to the classic form of Friedreich ataxia.

By 1893, Pierre Marie thought it desirable to create a new category of hereditary ataxia that would embrace all of the non-Friedreich cases. He collated the familial cases of progressive ataxia that had been described by Fraser, Nonne, Sanger Brown, and Klippel and Durante (see both Greenfield and Harding [1993] for references) and proposed that all of them were examples of an entity to which he applied the name *hérédo-ataxie cérébelleuse*. Marie's proposition was based almost entirely on clinical observations not his own but those made by the aforementioned authors. Later, as members of these families died, postmortem examinations disclosed that Marie's hereditary cerebellar ataxia included not one but several disease entities. Indeed, as pointed out by Holmes (1907b) and later by Greenfield, in 3 of the 4 families the cerebellum showed no significant lesions at all. Yet there was by then no doubt of the existence of a separate class of predominantly cerebellar atrophies, some purely cortical and others associated with a variety of noncerebellar disorders.

Clinical Features

Holmes (1907a) described a family of 8 siblings, of whom 3 brothers and 1 sister were affected by a progressive ataxia, beginning with a reeling gait and followed by clumsiness of the hands, dysarthria, tremor of the head, and a variable nystagmus, but without additional features to implicate disease of the spinal cord or brainstem. It may be taken as the prototype of pure cerebellar cortical degeneration.

The ataxia begins insidiously, usually in the fourth decade but with wide variability in age of onset, and progresses slowly over many years. Ataxia of gait, instability of the trunk, tremor of the hands and head, and slightly slowed, hesitant speech is the usual clinical picture. Nystagmus is rare and intelligence is usually preserved. The patellar reflexes may be slightly increased but this may be apparent based on the pendular character of reflexes in cerebellar disease; the plantar reflexes are flexor and the ankle jerks are present but there are exceptions and probably mark the process as one of the other genetic ataxias.

This clinical syndrome probably can result from several genetically determined processes, some of which declare themselves as the illness progresses by displaying characteristic signs other than ataxia. The differential diagnosis in the nonfamilial cases is even broader, including many acquired types of ataxias discussed in Chap. 5 (see Table 5-1) and at the end of this section.

Pathology Postmortem examination of the Holmes-type cases discloses symmetrical atrophy of the cerebellum involving mainly the anterior lobe and vermis, the latter being more affected. Purkinje cells are absent in the lingula, centralis, and pyramis of the superior vermis and reduced in number in the quadrangularis, flocculus, biventral, and pyramidal lobes. The other cerebellar cortical neurons and granule cells and dorsal and medial parts of the inferior olivary nuclei are diminished less so. The white matter is slightly pale in myelin stains. The vermian atrophy and that of adjacent parts of the cerebellum can be visualized with clarity in MRIs (Fig. 39-8).

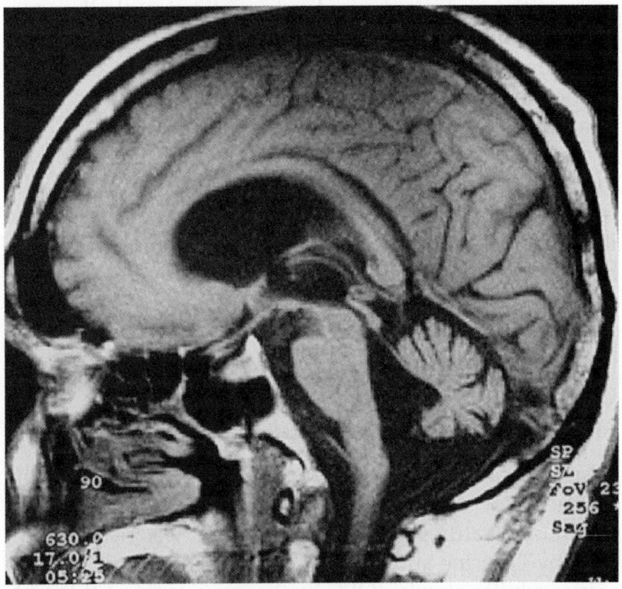

Figure 39-8. Familial cortical cerebellar atrophy. T1-weighted MRI in the sagittal plane showing marked atrophy of vermis and enlargement of fourth ventricle. The brainstem is only mildly atrophic and the posterior fossa is normal is size. Compare with Fig. 39-9 in which the cerebellum and pons are atrophic.

The vague similarity of the pathologic (and clinical) changes to those of *alcoholic cerebellar degeneration* is at once apparent and should raise the question of an alcoholic-nutritional cause in sporadic cases (see Chap. 41); in serious alcohol-nutritional disease, there usually is an accompanying polyneuropathy and reduced ankle reflexes.

Fragile X Tremor–Ataxic Premutation Syndrome

This type of developmental delay, caused by an unstable extended trinucleotide repeat sequence and breakage of the X-chromosome, is discussed in Chap. 38. Here we refer to an unusual variant of the degenerative process with onset in mid- or late adulthood, mainly but not exclusively in men, and consisting of gait or limb ataxia and mild tremor. The process affects carriers of a "premutation" who have 50 to 200 CGG repeat sequences in the *FMR1* gene. In contradistinction to the full mutation of over 200 repeats, there is apparently a buildup of messenger ribonucleic acid (mRNA) in the adult form that interferes in some way with cellular function. Aggregating several studies, the frequency of this genetic abnormality among otherwise unassignable adult ataxia cases is less than 10 percent.

The entire clinical spectrum has yet to be defined but our experience with 2 patients featured mild progressive gait ataxia in the sixth decade that was misattributed to normal-pressure hydrocephalus and an intermittent hand tremor that was probably ataxic in nature. Some reports have included a parkinsonian syndrome and more consistently, a mild frontal dementia, making the distinction from frontotemporal dementia difficult. Many cases have been confused with multiple system atrophy.

T2 hyperintensity in the cerebellar peduncles are characteristic of some cases, but this was not found in our patients, which showed only midline cerebellar atrophy. A family history of developmental delay or autistic spectrum disorder may be a hint to diagnosis and some proportion of individuals with the premutation also have a nonprogressive cognitive deficiency.

A study of the neuropathology by Greco and colleagues showed cerebral and cerebellar spongiform white matter changes and both intranuclear and astrocytic inclusions. Their report demonstrated a correspondence between the quantity of trinucleotide repeats and the number of inclusion bodies.

Familial and Sporadic Forms of Combined Cerebellar Atrophy With Brainstem and Extrapyramidal Features

A sporadically occurring disorder closely resembling the Holmes type of cortical cerebellar degeneration but with additional features of brainstem atrophy was described in 1900 by Déjérine and André-Thomas, who named it *olivopontocerebellar atrophy* (OPCA). As more cases of this type were collected, an autosomal dominant *hereditary pattern* was evident in some, and one or more long tracts in the spinal cord were found to have degenerated. About half the cases later developed the parkinsonism with degeneration of nigral cells and, in a few, of striatal cells, thereby marking the disease as a form of striatonigral degeneration that is essentially a type of *multiple system atrophy* (MSA-C) as discussed in detail in an earlier section and also below.

Notable findings in both the sporadic and the familial forms of many of the variants of cerebellar atrophy are extensive degeneration of the middle cerebellar peduncles, cerebellar white matter, and pontine, olivary, and arcuate nuclei; loss of Purkinje cells has been variable. Most likely this degeneration represents a "dying back" of axons of the cerebellar, pontine, and olivary nuclei with secondary myelin degeneration. Extreme atrophy of the medullary olivary nuclei, evident on MRIs (Fig. 39-9), identifies a special process that represents the aforementioned OPCA.

Although the associated features in each of the inherited cerebellar degenerations do not conform to newer genetic classifications, certain clinical constellations are nonetheless recognizable and clinically useful. Many texts use a genetic system exclusively to categorize these diseases. In the past, Konigsmark and Weiner subdivided them into several types, including a dominantly inherited OPCA (of Menzel); a recessive type (of Fickler-Winkler); a dominant type with retinal degeneration; one with spastic paraplegia and areflexia; and with dementia, ophthalmoplegia, and extrapyramidal signs. To these had been added cases of OPCA with neuropathy and slowed eye movements (Wadia type), of which we have seen 2 cases, and cases with dystonia and a variety of other clinical findings, most in single families (hemiballismus, athetosis, contractures of the legs, fixed pupils, ophthalmoplegia, ptosis, gaze palsy, deafness, retinal degeneration, mental retardation and epilepsy, claw foot and scoliosis, incontinence, parkinsonian symptoms and signs, plethora of presentations including a neonatal type). Some of these are detailed below.

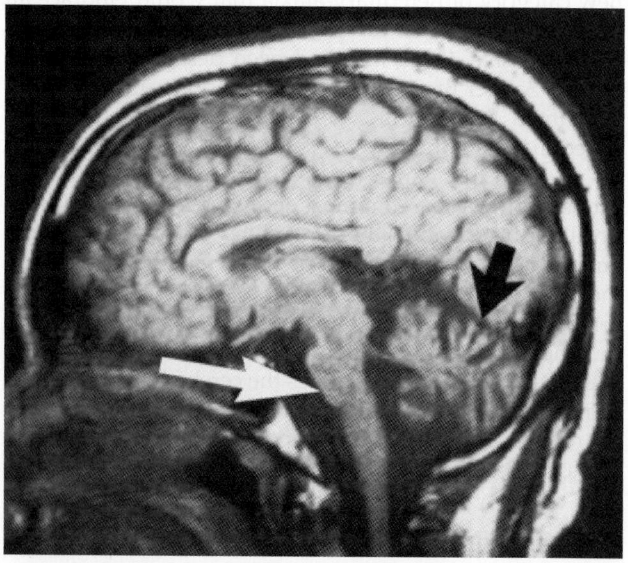

Figure 39-9. Olivopontocerebellar atrophy. MRI in the sagittal plane demonstrating both vermian atrophy (*black arrow*) and smallness of the pons (*white arrow*). (Reproduced by permission from Bisese JH: *Cranial MRI*. New York, McGraw-Hill, 1991.)

Cases of *sporadic olivopontocerebellar atrophy* are more common than the familial variety and tend to occur at an older age; nystagmus, optic atrophy, retinal degeneration, ophthalmoplegia, and urinary incontinence are generally not observed. However, there are numerous cases that include mild extrapyramidal and neuropathic signs, slow eye movements, dystonia, impairment of vertical saccadic eye movements (thus simulating progressive supranuclear palsy), vocal cord paralysis, all of which probably mark the process as multiple system atrophy (MSA-C) or Machado-Joseph-Azorean disease (SCA3, discussed below), and some cases with deafness. The relationship of olivopontocerebellar atrophy to MSA was discussed in under "Multiple System Atrophy," but we emphasize that OPCA occurs as often independently of extrapyramidal degeneration for which reason we retain a separate designation.

Cerebellar Atrophy With Prominent Basal Ganglionic Features

Machado-Joseph-Azorean Disease (SCA3)

A special form of hereditary ataxia with brainstem and extrapyramidal signs has been described in patients mainly, but not exclusively, of Portuguese-Azorean origin. The disorder is characterized by an autosomal dominant pattern of inheritance and by a slowly progressive ataxia beginning in adolescence or early adult life in association with hyperreflexia, extrapyramidal features, dystonia, bulbar signs, distal motor weakness, and ophthalmoplegia. There is usually no impairment of intellect and in the examples the authors have seen, the extrapyramidal symptoms were mainly rigidity and slowness of movement. Early Machado-Joseph disease characteristically demonstrates the finding of dysmetric horizontal and vertical saccades, even before the ataxia is obvious (Hotson et al). This conjunction of a parkinsonian syndrome with cerebellar ataxia is suggestive of MSA except for an earlier age of onset and the prominence in some cases of dystonia, amyotrophy, and ophthalmoplegia in Machado-Joseph. Postmortem examination discloses a degeneration of the dentate nuclei and spinocerebellar tracts and a loss of anterior horn cells and neurons of the pons, substantia nigra, and oculomotor nuclei. Cancel and colleagues found an unstable number of CAG repeating sequences in a gene, ataxin-3, and named the disorder spinocerebellar ataxia type 3 (SCA3).

An affected Azorean family named Joseph was described in 1976 by Rosenberg and colleagues under the name of *autosomal dominant striatonigral degeneration*. Using the term *Azorean disease of the nervous system* (now better known as *Machado-Joseph disease*), Romanul and colleagues described yet another family of Portuguese-Azorean descent, many members of which were affected by a syndrome comprising a progressive ataxia of gait, parkinsonian features, limitation of conjugate gaze, fasciculations, areflexia, nystagmus, ataxic tremor, and extensor plantar responses; the pathologic changes closely resembled those described by Woods and Schaumburg. Romanul and coworkers compared the genetic, clinical, and pathologic features of their cases with those described in other Portuguese-Azorean families and concluded that all of them represent a single genetic entity with variable expression. This concept of the disease has been corroborated by the further observations of Rosenberg and of Fowler who studied 20 patients with the Machado-Joseph-Azorean disease over a 10-year period and more recently by genetic testing.

The disease is not limited to Azoreans. Cases conforming to the above descriptions have now been observed among African American, Indian, and Japanese families (Sakai et al; Yuasa et al; Bharucha et al). There are no signs of polyneuropathy, which is the main feature of another disease in Portuguese emigrants caused by amyloid deposition, described by Nakano and colleagues as "Machado disease," this being the name of the progenitor of the afflicted family.

In fully developed cases, the MRI findings are of reduced width of the superior and middle cerebellar peduncles, atrophy of the frontal and temporal lobes, and smallness of the pons and globus pallidus (Murata et al). There is no treatment of proven value.

Multiple System Atrophy With Predominant Ataxia (See Section Multiple System Atrophy)

This entity has been discussed with the degenerative disorders of the basal ganglia earlier in the chapter. Here it is pointed out that a number of cases of sporadic progressive ataxia in mid- and late life are attributable to this process and have been termed MSA-C to signify the predominant cerebellar feature. The extrapyramidal, corticospinal, or autonomic aspects of the illness may or may not become evident only with continued observation or by pathologic examination. Some guidance as to the frequency of MSA as the cause of otherwise undifferentiated sporadic ataxia is given in the study by Abele and colleagues who found that it accounts for almost one-third of cases, but the precise number is open to question as pathologic examinations were not made.

Dentatorubropallidoluysian Atrophy (DRPLA)

This is a rare familial disorder, described mostly in Japan and in small European pockets, in which symptoms of cerebellar ataxia are coupled with those of choreoathetosis and dystonia and, in a few instances, parkinsonism, myoclonus, epilepsy, or dementia. Pathologically there is degeneration of the dentatorubral and pallidoluysian systems. The main consideration when chorea is a prominent feature is the separation of this disorder from Huntington disease. The gene defect in DRPLA is an unstable CAG trinucleotide repeat in the gene that codes for the protein atrophin. This same mutation has been defined in affected families from throughout the world (e.g., Warner et al). As with Huntington chorea (where the expanded polyglutamine tract is in the protein huntingtin), this disease is inherited as an autosomal dominant trait and shows an inverse correlation between the age of onset and the size of the gene expansion (anticipation). When chorea predominates early in the illness, there may be difficulty distinguishing DRPLA from Huntington disease. The diagnosis is confirmed by sequencing of the affected gene.

Dentatorubral Degeneration

This is a rare and still nebulous entity but it is probably distinct from the condition described above. There are several instructive features. In 1921, Ramsay Hunt published an account of 6 patients (2 of whom were twin brothers) in whom myoclonus was combined with progressive cerebellar ataxia. The age of onset in the 4 nonfamilial cases was between 7 and 17 years, and the cerebellar ataxia followed the myoclonus by an interval of 1 to 20 years. Hunt named the disorder *dyssynergia cerebellaris myoclonica*. There were signs of Friedreich ataxia in the twin brothers; postmortem examination of one showed cerebellar atrophy, degeneration of the posterior columns and spinocerebellar tracts but not of the corticospinal tracts. In 1947, Louis-Bar and van Bogaert reported a similar case and noted, in addition to the above findings, degeneration of the corticospinal tracts and loss of fibers in the posterior roots. Thus the pathology was identical to that of Friedreich ataxia except for the more severe atrophy of the dentate nuclei.

Earlier (1914), under the title *dyssynergia cerebellaris progressiva*, Hunt had drawn attention to a progressive disease in young individuals manifest by what he considered to be a pure cerebellar syndrome but one of his cases was revealed at autopsy to be Wilson disease. Hunt's reports emphasize the hazard of classifying cerebellar ataxias on the basis of clinical findings alone, a point made effectively by Holmes.

Paroxysmal Ataxias (See Chap. 5)

Two adult forms of hereditary cerebellar ataxia are paroxysmal in nature. In one (EA-2 for "episodic ataxia, type 2"), the episodes occur without explanation and last several hours; vertigo is the prominent feature of the attacks. Between attacks the patient is normal or has only minimal ataxia and nystagmus (Griggs et al). These ataxic episodes are prevented strikingly by the administration of oral acetazolamide. The disorder has been found to be a mutation of the calcium channel gene on chromosome 19 as listed in Table 39-5.

A similar but physiologically and genetically unrelated paroxysmal ataxia (EA-1) is characterized by episodes that may be precipitated by exercise and by the presence of muscle myokymia (rippling) between attacks. Vertigo does not occur and acetazolamide is less effective or not effective at all. The disorder is caused by an abnormality of the potassium channel gene on chromosome 12 (see Table 39-5). Both of these episodic ataxias are therefore "channelopathies" (see Chap. 50). Also of interest is spinocerebellar atrophy type 6, a progressive condition in which a mutation has been traced to same gene implicated in the EA-2 acetazolamide-responsive paroxysmal ataxia, but this disorder is not paroxysmal and results in progressive ataxia, dysarthria, and loss of proprioception.

Genetics of the Heredodegenerative Ataxias (See Table 39-5)

The many familial degenerative ataxic disorders described in the preceding pages are genetically distinct. As indicated, the *autosomal recessive* type of Friedreich ataxia is the result of an expanded GAA repeat in the frataxin gene (Campuzano et al), quite different from the large number of dominant forms of inherited ataxia. The direct molecular test for the GAA expansion is useful for diagnosis, particularly for atypical cases with late onset (Dürr et al). The rarer recessive spinocerebellar ataxia associated with vitamin E deficiency arises from mutations in the gene that encodes an alpha tocopherol (vitamin E) transport protein, as mentioned above.

Among the common *autosomal dominant* cerebellar ataxias of later onset, molecular and gene studies have identified numerous mutations. Of these autosomal dominant ataxias, many are known to be caused by expanded CAG-trinucleotide repeats (including SCA types 1, 3, 6, and 7, 12, 17, as well as DRPLA). Undoubtedly others will be discovered. However, the mechanisms by which the expanded polyglutamine molecule leads to neuronal cell death or dysfunction remain uncertain. It is likely that differences in the clinical manifestations of these disorders will reflect differences in the patterns of expression of the affected proteins; that is each is expressed in different populations of neurons and at different stages in development. This raises the possibility that the cascade of events that triggers neuronal degeneration is similar in each of the diseases with a CAG expansion and that a therapy might be discovered that is effective in all of them.

The special case of fragile X premutation that may cause ataxia and tremor in adults is addressed in Chap. 38. Table 39-5 summarizes the genes, terminology, related neural abnormalities, and clinical features of the cerebellar atrophies.

Differential Diagnosis of the Degenerative Ataxias in Adults (See also Table 5-1)

Sporadic forms of cerebellar ataxia in adults are in some instances traceable to strokes involving cerebellar pathways (Safe et al). These are, of course, of acute onset. Some cases of ataxia are alcoholic-nutritional in origin, and a few are related to excessive use of drugs or therapeutic medications, especially antiepileptic drugs, which may in a few cases cause a slowly progressive and permanent ataxia. Organic mercury induces subacute cerebellar degeneration, and adulterated heroin causes a more abrupt and severe ataxic syndrome. The paraneoplastic variety of cerebellar degeneration often enters into the differential diagnosis; it occurs mostly in women with breast or ovarian cancers and evolves much more rapidly than any of the heredodegenerative forms. The more rapid onset of ataxia and the presence of anti-Purkinje cell antibodies (anti-Yo; see "Paraneoplastic Cerebellar Degeneration" in Chap. 31) are central to identifying the nature of this disease. From time to time one observes a similar idiopathic variety of subacute cerebellar degeneration, particularly in women who have no neoplasm and lack the specific antibodies of the paraneoplastic disease (Ropper). Rare cases of ataxia have been associated with celiac disease and Whipple disease, and metronidazole as noted in Chap. 5. Ataxia may also be an early and prominent manifestation of Creutzfeldt-Jakob disease caused by a prion (see Chap. 33) or of an inherited metabolic disease (see Chap. 37). Of the latter, late-onset G_{M2} gangliosidosis may simulate cerebellar degeneration in adults (see Chap. 37). Rare cases of aminoacidopathy manifesting for the first time in adult life have also provoked a cerebellar syndrome (see Chap. 37).

Hereditary Polymyoclonus

The syndrome of quick, arrhythmic, involuntary single or repetitive twitches of a muscle or group of muscles was described in Chap. 6, where it was pointed out that the condition has many causes. Chapter 37 discusses those caused by hereditary metabolic diseases. Familial forms are known, one of which, associated with cerebellar ataxia, was discussed earlier (dyssynergia cerebellaris myoclonica of Ramsay Hunt). But there is another disease, known as *hereditary essential benign myoclonus*, that occurs in relatively pure form unaccompanied by ataxia (termed essential, or familial, myoclonus; see Chap. 6). In this condition, it is difficult to evaluate coordination because willed movement is interrupted by myoclonus that may be mistaken for intention tremor. Only by slowing the voluntary movement can the myoclonus be reduced or eliminated. This myoclonic disease is inherited as an autosomal dominant trait. It becomes manifest early in life; once established, it persists with little or no change in severity throughout life, often with rather little disability. It can, by its natural course, be differentiated from some of the hereditary metabolic diseases such as the Unverricht and Lafora types of myoclonic epilepsy, the lipidoses, tuberous sclerosis, and myoclonic disorders that follow certain viral infections and anoxic encephalopathy. Of interest is the response of this form of movement disorder to certain pharmacologic agents, notably clonazepam, valproic acid, and 5-hydroxytryptophan, the amino acid precursor of serotonin, particularly when these agents are used in combination (postanoxic myoclonus responds to the same medications).

Another form of nonprogressive myoclonus, dominantly inherited, is associated with dystonia, which is due to a mutation in a sarcoglycan gene, *SGCE*.

The main clinical distinctions are from juvenile myoclonic epilepsy (see Chap. 16), drug-induced myoclonus, particularly lithium and opiates; renal failure and other acquired metabolic disorders; asterixis; and from the startle responses and some of the diseases that have this sign as their main characteristic (see Chap. 6). Creutzfeldt-Jakob subacute spongiform encephalopathy may cause difficulty in diagnosis initially but the course of illness clarifies the situation rapidly. Myoclonus is also one component of the complex movement disorder in corticobasal-ganglionic degeneration that was described in an earlier section.

SYNDROME OF MUSCULAR WEAKNESS AND WASTING WITHOUT SENSORY CHANGES

Motor Neuron Disease

This general term designates a group of progressive degenerative disorders of motor neurons in the spinal cord, brainstem, and motor cortex, manifest clinically by muscular weakness, atrophy, and corticospinal tract signs in varying combinations. It is for the most part a disease of middle life and progresses to death in a matter of 2 to 5 years or longer in exceptional cases.

Customarily, motor system disease is subdivided into several subtypes on the basis of the grouping of symptoms and signs. The most frequent form, in which amyotrophy and hyperreflexia are combined, is *ALS* (*amyotrophy* is the term applied to denervation atrophy and weakness of muscles). Less frequent are cases in which weakness and atrophy occur alone, without evidence of corticospinal tract dysfunction; for these the term *progressive spinal muscular atrophy* is used. When the weakness and wasting predominate in muscles innervated by the motor nuclei of the lower brainstem (i.e., muscles of the jaw, face, tongue, pharynx, and larynx), it is customary to speak of *progressive bulbar palsy*). In a small proportion of patients, the clinical state is dominated by spastic weakness, hyperreflexia, and Babinski signs, with lower motor neuron aspects becoming apparent only at a later stage of the illness, or not at all. This is designated *primary lateral sclerosis*, an infrequent form of motor system disease in which the degenerative process remains confined to the corticospinal pathways (Pringle et al). The pure spastic paraplegias without amyotrophy may represent a special class of disease hence they are described separately. There are also relatively common familial forms of spastic paraplegia in which the disease is confined to the corticospinal tracts or, in some cases, combined with posterior column or other neurologic signs.

Furthermore, an important group of special spinal muscular atrophies occurs in infancy and childhood and are the leading cause of heritable infant mortality and, after cystic fibrosis, the most frequent form of serious childhood autosomal recessive disease (Pearn). The best known is the Werdnig-Hoffmann type of *infantile spinal muscular atrophy* (SMA type I); but there are other forms beginning in later childhood, adolescence, or early adult life (SMA types II and III, or the Wohlfart-Kugelberg-Welander type). Despite the clinical heterogeneity of the heritable childhood spinal muscular atrophies, they all derive from mutations in the *SMN* gene (see below; see Gilliam et al; Brzustowicz et al). This group of early-onset spinal muscular atrophies is separate genetically from a familial form of ALS.

Amyotrophic Lateral Sclerosis

History Credit for the original delineation of amyotrophic lateral sclerosis is appropriately given to Charcot. With Joffroy in 1869 and Gombault in 1871, he studied the pathologic aspects of the disease. In a series of lectures given from 1872 to 1874, he provided a lucid account of the clinical and pathologic findings. Although called Charcot disease in France, *amyotrophic lateral sclerosis* (the term recommended by Charcot) has been preferred in the English-speaking world. Duchenne had earlier (1858) described *labioglossolaryngeal paralysis*, a term that Wachsmuth in 1864 changed to *progressive bulbar palsy*. In 1869, Charcot called attention to the nuclear origin of progressive bulbar palsy, and in 1882 Déjérine established its relationship to ALS. Most authors credit Aran and Duchenne with the earliest descriptions of progressive spinal muscular atrophy, which they believed to be of myogenic origin. This interpretation was, of course, incorrect; Cruveilhier, a few years later, noted the slender anterior roots, and soon thereafter the disease was brought into line with ALS as a spinal muscular atrophy. The singular genetic discovery in relation to this disease has been of the mutation in the superoxide dismutase (*SOD1*) gene in familial cases of motor neuron disease.

Epidemiology This is a disease commonly encountered by neurologists, with an annual incidence rate of 0.4 to 1.76 per 100,000 population. Men are affected nearly twice as often as women. Most patients are older than age 45 years at the onset of symptoms, and the incidence increases with each decade of life (Mulder). The disease occurs in a random pattern throughout the world except for a dramatic clustering of patients among inhabitants of the Kii peninsula in Japan and in Guam, where ALS is often combined with dementia and parkinsonism. In approximately 10 percent of cases the disease is familial, being inherited as an autosomal dominant trait with age-dependent penetrance. The familial cases do not differ fundamentally in their symptoms and clinical course from nonfamilial ones, although as a group the former have an earlier age of onset, an equal distribution in men and women, and a slightly shorter survival. Unusual environmental associations are reported from time to time, for example, an increased incidence among Italian professional football players (Chio et al, 2005) and among soldiers who had served in various regions. All of these are questionable on methodologic grounds (they are retrospective case control epidemiologic studies) but further exploration is warranted.

Clinical Features In the most typical forms of disease, the onset is perceived by the patient as weakness in a distal part of one limb. This is noted first as an unexplained tripping from slight foot-drop, or by awkwardness in tasks requiring fine finger movements (handling buttons and automobile ignition keys), stiffness of the fingers, and slight weakness or wasting of the hand muscles on one side. In other words, features related to upper and to lower motor neuron degeneration (or both) may appear insidiously in one limb. Cramping beyond what seems natural and fasciculations of the muscles of the forearm, upper arm, and shoulder girdle may also arise. The earliest manifestation of the lower motor neuron component of this disease is sometimes volitional cramping—for example, leg cramps as the patient turns in bed during the early morning hours.

As the weeks and months pass, the other hand and arm become similarly affected with weakness, stiffness, slowness, atrophy or cramps. Before long, the triad of atrophic weakness of the hands and forearms, fasciculations, slight spasticity of the arms or legs, and generalized hyperreflexia—all in the absence of sensory change—leaves little doubt as to the diagnosis. Muscle strength and bulk diminish in parallel or there is a relative preservation of power early in the illness. Despite the amyotrophy, the tendon reflexes are notable for their liveliness. Babinski and Hoffmann signs are variably present; surprisingly, they may not appear even as the illness progresses. Abductors, adductors, and extensors of fingers and thumb tend to become weak before the long flexors, on which the handgrip depends, and the dorsal interosseous spaces become hollowed, giving rise to the "cadaveric" or "skeletal" hand. The muscles of the upper arm and shoulder girdles are typically involved later. There is a general tendency for adjacent areas to be involved before more distant ones. When an arm is the first limb affected, all this occurs while the thigh and leg muscles seem relatively normal, and there may come a time in some cases when the patient walks about with useless, dangling arms. Later the atrophic weakness spreads to the neck, tongue, pharyngeal, and laryngeal muscles, and eventually those in the trunk and lower extremities yield to the onslaught of the disease.

The affected parts may ache and feel cold, but true paresthesias, except from poor positioning and pressure on nerves, do not occur or are minor. Sphincteric control is well maintained even after both legs have become weak and spastic, but many patients acquire urinary and sometimes fecal urgency in the advanced stages of the disease. The abdominal reflexes may be elicitable even when the plantar reflexes are extensor. Extreme spasticity is rarely seen.

Coarse fasciculations are usually evident in the weakened muscles but may not be noticed by the patient until the physician calls attention to them. Fasciculations are almost never the sole presenting feature of ALS—a clinical truism with which one can reassure physicians and medical students who fear, on the basis of persistent focal muscle twitching in the thumb, face, foot, or forearm, that they are developing the disease.

The course of this illness, irrespective of its particular mode of onset and pattern of evolution, is progressive. There may be periods lasting weeks or months during which the patient observes no advance in symptoms but clinical changes can nonetheless be detected. Half the patients succumb within 3 years of onset and 90 percent within 6 years (Mulder et al). Several clinical variations that occur with regularity and have distinguishing clinical features are described below.

Other Patterns of Clinical Evolution In addition to the special configurations discussed further on, there are many patterns of neuromuscular involvement other than the one just described. A leg may be affected before the hands. A foot-drop with weakness and wasting of the pretibial muscles may be incorrectly attributed to peroneal nerve compression until weakness of the gastrocnemius and other muscles betray more widespread involvement of lumbosacral neurons. In our experience, this crural amyotrophy has been less frequent than the brachial-manual type. Another variant is early involvement of thoracic, abdominal, or posterior neck muscles, the last being one of the causes of head lolling and camptocormia (forward bending of the neck and trunk) in older individuals. Yet another pattern is of early diaphragmatic weakness; such cases come to attention because of respiratory failure. A symmetrical proximal limb or shoulder-girdle amyotrophy with onset at an early age is also known and simulates muscular dystrophy (Wohlfart-Kugelberg-Welander disease, discussed later in this chapter). On several occasions we have observed a pattern involving the arm and leg on the same side, first with spasticity and then with some degree of amyotrophy; this has been called the *hemiplegic* or *Mills variant*. However, this clinical pattern more often turns out to be a result of multiple sclerosis of compression of the spinal cord from laterally, as occurs with a neurofibroma.

The first and dominant manifestations of motor neuron disease may be a spastic weakness of the legs, in which case a diagnosis of primary lateral sclerosis is tentatively made (discussed further on); only after a year or two do the hand and arm muscles weaken, waste, and fasciculate, making it obvious that both upper and lower motor neurons are diseased. Early on, a spastic bulbar palsy with dysarthria and dysphagia, hyperactive jaw jerk and facial reflexes, but without muscle atrophy, may be the initial phase of disease.

As the disease advances, very mild distal sensory loss may be observed in the feet without explanation, but, if the sensory loss is a definite and early feature, the diagnosis must remain in doubt. Approximately 5 percent of cases of ALS are observed in conjunction with a frontotemporal dementia; less commonly, there is an association with a Parkinson syndrome.

Progressive Muscular Atrophy

This purely lower motor neuron syndrome is more common in men than in women, reportedly in a ratio of 4:1. It probably encompasses several diseases of the lower motor neuron, but most of which are manifestations of ALS.

These purely lower motor neuron amyotrophies tend to progress at a slower pace than the usual case of ALS, some patients surviving for 15 years or longer. Chio and colleagues (1985), who analyzed the factors affecting life expectancy in 155 patients with progressive muscular atrophy (PMA), found that younger patients had a more benign course: The 5-year survival was 72 percent in patients with an onset before age 50 years and 40 percent in patients with onset after age 50 years. Some of the most chronic varieties of PMA are familial. It has been revealed that the original report of a familial variety of this illness by William Osler described a family now known to have had a mutation in the *SOD1* gene, as discussed below. In about half the patients, the illness takes the form of a symmetrical (sometimes asymmetrical) wasting of intrinsic hand muscles, slowly advancing to the more proximal parts of the arms; less often, the legs and thighs are the sites of the initial atrophic weakness; or the proximal parts of the limbs are affected before the distal ones. Fascicular twitchings and cramping are variably present. Otherwise they differ from ALS only in that the tendon reflexes are diminished or absent, and signs of corticospinal tract disease cannot be detected. Nonetheless, many cases of ostensible PMA are found to have indications of corticospinal tract degeneration at autopsy (Ince et al).

The main disease to be distinguished from PMA is an immune-mediated motor neuropathy that occurs with or without multifocal block of electrical conduction (see Chap. 46), and various muscle diseases that produce a similar pattern of weakness, notably, inclusion body myopathy and polymyositis. The presence of a paraproteinemia, specifically immunoglobulin (Ig) M with antibodies against G_{M1} ganglioside, or the finding of focal conduction block or sensory nerve abnormalities on the EMG implies the presence of an autoimmune neuropathy disease rather than of a degenerative motor neuron type.

Progressive Bulbar Palsy

Here reference is made to a condition in which the first and dominant symptoms relate to weakness and laxity of muscles innervated by the motor nuclei of the lower brainstem, that is muscles of the jaw, face, tongue, pharynx, and larynx. This weakness gives rise to an early defect in articulation, in which there is difficulty in the pronunciation of lingual (*r, n, l*), labial (*b, m, p, f*), dental (*d, t*), and palatal (*k, g*) consonants. As the condition worsens, syllables lose their clarity and run together, until, finally, the patient's speech becomes unintelligible. In other patients, slurring is a result of spasticity of the tongue, pharyngeal, and laryngeal muscles; the speech sounds as if the patient were eating food that is too hot. Usually the voice is modified by a combination of atrophic and spastic weakness. Defective modulation with variable degrees of rasping and nasality is another characteristic. The pharyngeal reflex is lost, and the palate and vocal cords move imperfectly or not at all during attempted phonation. Mastication and deglutition become impaired; the bolus of food cannot be manipulated and may lodge between the cheek and teeth and the pharyngeal muscles do not force it properly into the esophagus. Liquids and small particles of food find their way into the trachea or nose. The facial muscles, particularly of the lower face, weaken and sag. Fasciculations and focal loss of tissue of the tongue are usually early manifestations; eventually the tongue becomes shriveled and lies useless on the floor of the mouth. The chin may also quiver from fascicular twitchings, but the diagnosis should not be made on the basis of fasciculations alone, in the absence of weakness and atrophy.

The jaw jerk may be present or exaggerated at a time when the muscles of mastication are markedly weak. In fact, spasticity of the jaw muscles may be so pronounced that the slightest tap on the chin will evoke clonus and blinking; rarely, attempts to open the mouth elicit a "bulldog" reflex (jaw snaps shut involuntarily). Spastic weakness of the oropharyngeal muscles may be the initial manifestation of bulbar palsy and may at times surpass signs of atrophic weakness; pseudobulbar signs (pathologic laughing and crying) may reach extreme degrees. This is the only common clinical situation in which spastic and atrophic bulbar palsy coexist. Strangely, the ocular muscles always escape.

As with other forms of motor system disease, the course of bulbar palsy is inexorably progressive. Eventually the weakness spreads to the respiratory muscles and deglutition fails entirely; the patient dies of inanition and aspiration pneumonia, usually within 2 to 3 years of onset. Approximately 25 percent of cases of motor system disease begin with bulbar symptoms, but rarely, if ever, does the sporadic form of progressive bulbar palsy run its course as an independent syndrome (pure heredofamilial forms of progressive bulbar palsy in the adult are known, e.g., Kennedy disease, discussed further on). In general, the earlier the onset of the bulbar involvement, the shorter the course of the disease.

Primary Lateral Sclerosis

This entity, like ALS, can be a form of motor neuron disease, although most cases appear to be examples of a unique degenerative process. Many patients in whom the signs of corticospinal tract degeneration suggest the presence of ALS will develop indications of lower motor neuron disease within 1 year, usually earlier. Approximately 20 percent, however, have a slowly progressive corticospinal tract disorder that begins with a pure spastic paraparesis; later, the arms and oropharyngeal muscles become involved and the disease remains one solely of the upper neurons. These cases have distinctive neuropathologic features and are designated as *primary lateral sclerosis* (PLS), a term originally suggested by Erb in 1875. A historical review of the subject appears in the article by Pringle and colleagues.

The typical case begins insidiously in the fifth or sixth decade with a stiffness in one leg, then in the other; there is a slowing of gait, with spasticity predominating over weakness as the years go on. Walking is still possible with the help of a cane for many years after the onset, but eventually this condition acquires the characteristic features of a severe spastic paraparesis. Over the years, finger movements become slower, the arms become spastic, and, if the illness persists for decades, speech takes on a pseudobulbar lilt. There are no sensory symptoms or signs. The legs are often found to be surprisingly strong, the difficulty in locomotion being attributable to rigid spasticity. About half the patients eventually acquire spasticity of the bladder. Pringle and associates suggest that a diagnostic criterion of the disease is progression for 3 years without evidence of lower motor neuron dysfunction.

Pathologic studies in a limited number of cases have disclosed a relatively stereotyped pattern of reduced numbers of Betz cells in the frontal and prefrontal motor cortex, degeneration of the corticospinal tracts, and preservation of motor neurons in the spinal cord and brainstem (Beal and Richardson; Fisher; Pringle et al). The corticospinal tract lesions are identical to those in typical ALS. Whether some of these cases are examples of late-onset familial spastic paraplegia (see further on) has not been extensively explored with molecular techniques.

Some patients who have only restricted bilateral signs of upper motor neuron disease prove to have multiple sclerosis, a slow compression of the spinal cord by spondylosis or meningioma, spinal dural arteriovenous fistula, or the myelopathic form of adrenoleukodystrophy (affected males or female carriers). In a few cases, tropical spastic paraplegia, HIV myelopathy, copper deficiency myelopathy, or a familial type of spastic paraplegia (described further on) will be uncovered. Exceptionally, progressive spastic paraparesis has been linked to an adult onset of phenylketonuria or other aminoacidopathies to vitamin B_{12} deficiency or to the fragile X premutation syndrome.

Laboratory Features of Motor Neuron Disease

Investigation provides useful confirmatory evidence even in the typical clinical syndrome. The EMG, as expected, displays widespread fibrillations (evidence of active denervation) and fasciculations and enlarged motor units (denoting reinnervation), and motor nerve conduction studies reveal only slight slowing, without focal motor conduction block. If the atrophic paresis is restricted to an arm or hand, raising the question of cervical spondylosis, evidence of denervation in many widely separated somatic segments favors the diagnosis of ALS. In questionable cases, it is good practice to insist that denervation be demonstrated in at least 3 limbs before concluding that the process is ALS. (The currently favored "El-Escorial" criteria that are used for the purposes of clinical research mandate that this finding be present.) Widespread denervation of the paraspinal muscles and of the genioglossus or facial muscles is also strongly suggestive of the disease but electromyographic testing of these muscles demands considerable experience and is uncomfortable for patients. A muscle biopsy is sometimes helpful in corroborating neurogenic denervation. Sensory nerve action potentials should be normal; tests of motor nerve conduction have a normal velocity, but the amplitudes become progressively lower as the disease progresses—in the earliest stages, they too may be normal. When in a typical case the amplitudes of sensory nerve action potentials are reduced, there is usually an underlying entrapment neuropathy, diabetes, or other late-life neuropathy. Sensory evoked potentials are mildly abnormal in a proportion of patients, but the explanation for this finding is unclear. (Sensory complaints and minimal sensory loss have been commented on above.)

The CSF protein is usually normal or marginally elevated. Serum creatine kinase is moderately elevated in patients with rapidly progressive atrophy and weakness, but it is just as often normal. Motor evoked potentials elicited from the cortex are also prolonged in patients with prominent corticospinal signs. In this group, the MRI may show slight atrophy of the motor cortices and wallerian degeneration of the motor tracts (Fig. 39-10). These changes may be diagnostically useful and appear as increased FLAIR and T2 signal intensity in the posterior limb of the internal capsule, descending motor tracts of the brainstem, and spinal cord, all of which are subtle and may be missed. All these laboratory findings, particularly the degeneration of the lateral columns of the cord and changes in the internal capsules, pertain also to primary lateral sclerosis with the notable exception of EMG findings of denervation and of elevations of creatine kinase (CK).

Pathology

The principal finding in ALS is a loss of nerve cells in the anterior horns of the spinal cord and motor nuclei of the lower brainstem. Large alpha motor neurons tend to be affected before small ones. In addition to neuronal loss, there is evidence of slight gliosis and proliferation of microglia cells. Many of the surviving nerve cells are small, shrunken, and filled with lipofuscin. It is not uncommon to detect ubiquitin inclusions in threads, skeins, or dense aggregates within the affected neurons by special stains. Occasionally, there is another ill-defined cytoplasmic inclusion that is present in neurons

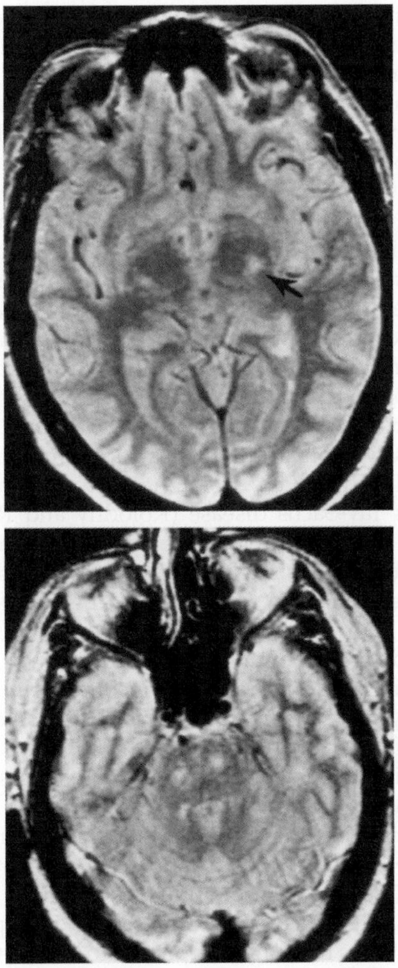

Figure 39-10. Axial T2-weighted MRI showing abnormal hyperintensity reflecting wallerian change in the corticospinal tracts at the level of the internal capsule (*top, arrow*) and the pons (*bottom*) in a patient with ALS.

and glia. Most studies indicate that these are made up of TDP-43 and ubiquitin as discussed in the alter section on "Pathogenesis". According to some reports, swelling of the proximal axon is an early finding, presumably antedating visible changes in the cell body itself. The anterior roots are thin, and there is a disproportionate loss of large myelinated fibers in motor nerves (Bradley et al). The muscles show typical denervation atrophy of different ages. Whitehouse and coworkers found a depletion of muscarinic, cholinergic, glycinergic, and benzodiazepine receptors in regions of the spinal cord where motor neurons had disappeared.

The corticospinal tract degeneration is most evident in the lower parts of the spinal cord, but it can be traced up through the brainstem to the posterior limb of the internal capsule and corona radiata by means of fat stains, which show the macrophages that accumulate in response to chronic myelin degeneration. There is a loss of Betz cells in the motor cortex; this is manifest as a slight frontal lobe atrophy on the MRI, but it is not a prominent finding in most cases of ALS (Kiernan and Hudson). Other fibers in the ventral and lateral funiculi are depleted, imparting a characteristic pallor in myelin stains. Some pathologists have interpreted this as evidence of involvement of nonmotor neurons and hence object to the term *motor system disease*. However, this condition of more diffuse pallor may be a result of a loss of collaterals of motor neurons that contribute to the lamina propria. One observes the same effect in long-standing poliomyelitis. In cases of familial ALS resulting from mutations in the *SOD1* gene, the nonmotor systems seem to be more affected (Cudkowicz et al).

Neuropathologic studies of cases of ALS with dementia are few in number. In addition to the usual loss of motor neurons, these cases have shown an extensive neuronal loss, gliosis, and vacuolation involving the frontal premotor area, particularly the superior frontal gyri and the inferolateral cortex of the temporal lobes. The histologic changes of Alzheimer or Pick disease have not been seen in our cases; neurofibrillary degeneration has been observed, but is inconsequential in comparison to that seen in the Guamanian Parkinson-dementia-ALS complex (Finlayson et al; Mitsuyama). Attempts to transmit this ALS–dementia syndrome to subhuman primates have been unsuccessful.

Diagnosis of ALS

The early clinical picture of motor system disease is closely simulated by a centrally placed cervical spondylotic bar or ruptured cervical disc, but with these conditions there is usually pain in the neck and shoulders, limitation of neck movements, and sensory changes, and the lower motor neuron changes are restricted to 1 or 2 spinal segments. The EMG is helpful if not decisive in differentiating these disorders. A mild hemiparesis or monoparesis because of multiple sclerosis may be, for a time, difficult to distinguish from early ALS and primary lateral sclerosis. Progressive spinal muscular atrophy may be differentiated from peroneal muscular atrophy (Charcot-Marie-Tooth neuropathy) by the lack of family history, the complete lack of sensory change, and different EMG patterns, as described in Chap. 46. Motor system disease beginning in the proximal limb muscles may be misdiagnosed as an inflammatory myopathy or a limb-girdle type of muscular dystrophy.

The main considerations in relation to progressive bulbar palsy are myasthenia gravis and, less often, inflammatory myopathy, muscular dystrophy, and especially the inherited (Kennedy) type of bulbospinal atrophy, which is discussed further on. The spastic form of bulbar palsy may suggest the pseudobulbar palsy of lacunar disease and can be a prominent part of the progressive supranuclear palsy described earlier in the chapter. A crural form of PMA may be confused with diabetic polyradiculopathy or polymyositis.

A major consideration is the differentiation of PMA from a chronic motor polyneuropathy, particularly the form that displays multifocal conduction block. Extensive nerve conduction studies and EMG examinations are necessary to distinguish the two; these neuropathic processes are discussed with the peripheral neuropathies in Chap. 46. The presence of an IgM monoclonal paraproteinemia or of specific antibodies directed against the G_{M1} ganglioside are usually indicative of the immune motor neuropathy, but in half of the cases these laboratory tests are negative. There is also a rare form of subacute poliomyelitis (possibly viral) in patients with lymphoma or carcinoma; it leads to an amyotrophy that progresses to death over a period of several months. Chapter 31 discusses this paraneoplastic variety of motor system disease in greater detail.

Because it may produce a motor-predominant radiculopathy, chronic Lyme infection is sometimes considered in the differential diagnosis of ALS. Some clinics screen for Lyme antibodies using both an enzyme-linked immunosorbent assay (ELISA) and the more sensitive and specific Western immunoblot, but we have never detected such a case and doubt there is much similarity. Infrequently, we have seen myelopathic motor findings and motor radiculopathy with vitamin B_{12} deficiency, and there are exceptional reports of myeloradiculopathy with lead poisoning; we sometimes include tests for these conditions. Another entity that may simulate ALS is inclusion body myositis (IBM), an atypical myopathy that begins asymmetrically and involves distal muscles, usually without much elevation of serum CPK levels. In a recent series of 70 patients with this condition, 13 percent were initially diagnosed as having ALS (Dabby et al). Features distinguishing the IBM cases included normal corticospinal function, preservation of deep tendon reflexes in weak muscles, and finger flexor weakness. One concludes from this series that a detailed, quantitative EMG and possibly a muscle biopsy are indicated in cases that display predominantly lower motor features. Fully developed ALS is difficult to confuse with these conditions. Acid maltase deficiency may also simulate ALS in causing fatigability and early respiratory failure.

Over the years, the authors have encountered young men with localized and asymmetrical amyotrophy of the leg or forearm that became arrested and did not advance over a decade or two. Several reports of such a partial cervical spinal amyotrophy have appeared in recent years (Hirayama et al; Moreno Martinez et al). In the type described by Hirayama and associates, young men are affected with progressive and asymmetrical amyotrophy of the forearm and hand that has been traced to ligamentous hypertrophy and buckling in the ventral spinal canal. This causes a compression of the cervical spinal cord gray matter, presumably by a chronic ischemic effect as discussed in detail in Chap. 44. In a familial variety of pure restricted amyotrophy, only the vocal cords became paralyzed over a period of years in adult life; only later were the hands affected.

Some patients who have recovered from paralytic poliomyelitis may develop progressive muscular weakness 30 or 40 years later; the nature of this relationship is obscure. We favor the explanation that atrophy of anterior horn cells with aging brings to light a critically depleted motor neuron population (see further on). It appears to progress little if at all.

An observation of interest is the finding of a form of progressive spinal muscular atrophy in patients with G_{M2} gangliosidosis, the storage disease that presents in infancy as Tay-Sachs disease (Kolodny and Raghavan). The onset is in late adolescence and early adult life and the atrophic paralysis is progressive, so that this condition is often mistaken for Wohlfart-Kugelberg-Welander disease or ALS. A number of cases of this type have been discovered in Ashkenazi Jews by the use of lysosomal enzyme analysis. The rare and incompletely characterized entity of polyglucosan disease, discussed in other sections of the book, has simulated ALS.

The differential diagnosis of the purely spastic state of primary lateral sclerosis is broad and has been listed earlier. An estimate of the frequency of all the aforementioned alternative diagnoses may be appreciated from a study of cases by Visser and colleagues that were initially presumed to be PMA but turned out to represent another process. In 17 of 89 patients the diagnosis proved to be anti-G_{M1} motor conduction block, chronic inflammatory demyelinating polyneuropathy, and various myopathies. This notwithstanding, ALS or the more discrete forms of motor system disease rarely offer any difficulty in diagnosis.

Pathogenesis

Insight into the sporadic form of the disease has been afforded by analyses of the approximately 10 percent of

Table 39-6

GENETIC DEFECTS ASSOCIATED WITH ALS

GENE	PROTEIN	INHERITANCE	AGE OF ONSET	CLINICAL FEATURES
SOD1	Superoxide dismutase 1	AD	Adult	Clinically and pathologically similar to sporadic ALS
FUS	Fused sarcoma	AD	Adult	ALS with frontotemporal dementia
TARDP5P		AD, rare recessive		
DCTN	Dynactin	AD	Adult	Slowly progressive with predominant bulbar features
CytoC	Cytochrome-*c* oxidase	Mitochondrial	Adult	Prominent spasticity
ALS2	GEF/alsin	AR	Juvenile	Very slowly progressive, predominantly corticospinal
SETX	Senataxin	AD	Juvenile	Very slowly progressive
VAPB	Vesicle-associated membrane protein	AD	Adult	Similar to sporadic ALS

AD autosomal dominant; AR autosomal recessive

ALS cases that are familial and caused by identifiable mutations. They are inherited mainly in an autosomal dominant pattern (Table 39-6). Of these inherited forms, approximately 40 percent are associated with a hexanucleotide expansion in the *C9orf72* gene, and provocatively, 4 to 8 percent of ostensibly sporadic cases have mutations in the gene. The mechanism of motor neuron death that results from this mutation is not known but may be associated with mishandling of RNA-binding proteins. Of similar interest are the *TARDBP* and *FUS* genes that each has an association with approximately 5 percent of familial cases and 2 percent of sporadic ones. These genetic and molecular influences are summarized by Andersen and Al-Chalabi. All 3 of the aforementioned genes have also been implicated in degenerative frontotemporal dementia and in the combination of this dementia with ALS. The *SOD1* mutation, the first to be found in familial ALS, codes for the cytosolic enzyme Cu-Zn superoxide dismutase (*SOD1*; Rosen et al); it has also been implicated in a small proportion of sporadic cases. There are yet other mutations in this group that have associations, not necessarily causal, with small numbers of both sporadic and inherited cases (Table 39-7).

What has emerged from these genetic studies is the common feature of the accumulation of the TDP-43 and FUS proteins in neurons. The mechanisms that lead to cell death as a result of any of these mutations or the protein deposition are being sought.

A rare and recessively inherited childhood form of motor neuron disease (affecting corticospinal more than spinal motor neurons) has been attributed to mutations in a gene whose protein (alsin) is a component of the neuronal cell-signaling pathways. Yet another rare childhood-onset form of disease arises from mutations in the senataxin gene, a DNA helicase that probably assists in chromatin folding and unfolding. (It is of interest that a recessively inherited mutation in the same gene transmits a recessive form of ataxia with oculomotor disorder.) In several families, a mutation has been detected in a protein that is involved in the transport of vesicles in neurons. Table 39-6 summarizes these various genetic forms of motor neuron disease.

Trauma, particularly traction injury of an arm, but also repetitive head and spine injury has been reported occasionally as an antecedent event in patients with ALS, but a causative relationship has not been established. Younger and coworkers have found a higher incidence of paraproteinemia in patients with motor system disease than can be accounted for by chance. Many other examples of disordered immune function have been described but a coherent explanation of ALS as an autoimmune disease has not emerged. It has never been proved that intoxication with heavy metals (lead, mercury, aluminum) can cause motor system disease, although there are reports of concurrent myelopathic and radicular motor signs in patients with lead intoxication. There is little evidence that such cases represent a reactivation of a virus or the presence of some other infectious agent. The progressive weakness that occurs some 30 to 40 years after recovery from polio should not be confused with PMA, as already indicated. Finally, we have had occasion to see patients who, many years after a severe electrical injury that passed through the region of the cord, developed a progressive and severe amyotrophy of the arms; other such extraordinary cases are known but the concordance is considered coincidental by most authorities (see Chap. 44).

Treatment

With the exception of riluzole, discussed below, there is no specific treatment for any of the motor neuron diseases. Supportive measures, however, are exceedingly important. In initial office visits, it has been our practice to give the patient some idea of the seriousness of the condition; but in early discussions we avoid the devastating statement that ALS is invariably fatal. Typically, patients and family members will ask explicitly about these matters in subsequent visits; such data as are appropriate to the patient's circumstances and character can be conveyed at that time, usually with the caveat that any individual may outlive the standard survival statistics.

The antiglutamate agent riluzole was shown by Bensimon and colleagues to slow the progression of ALS and improve survival in patients with disease of bulbar onset. However, it added only 3 months of life at best. This claim has been confirmed in several followup studies, although again the benefit has been marginal. Several additional agents are reported to have been effective in genetic models of ALS. These are presently undergoing study in ALS patients. Guanidine hydrochloride and injections of cobra venom, gangliosides, interferons, high-dose intravenous cyclophosphamide, and thyrotropin-releasing hormone are but some of a long list of agents that were said to arrest the disease process, but these claims have been discredited.

An attempt can be made to reduce the spasticity with medications, such as baclofen or tizanidine, or by subarachnoid infusions of baclofen via an implanted lumbar pump. Initial intrathecal test doses are given to predict a response to the pump infusions of baclofen, but this test may fail; consequently, in severe cases it may be advisable to proceed with a constant infusion for several days. Some degree of improved comfort from a reduction in the extreme rigidity is usually the most that can be expected. Partial relief from spasticity may also be afforded by the use of benzodiazepines or sometimes dantrolene. These approaches are most suitable for cases of primary lateral sclerosis, which can be expected to progress slowly and for a long period.

At all stages of ALS, physical therapy is useful in maintaining mobility, but overwork of the muscles leading to fatigue and cramps should be avoided. Physical therapy is invaluable, for example, for avoiding contractures of the fingers and shoulders. Occupational therapy is likewise helpful, particularly assessments of the patient's function in the home.

Important in the management of ALS is periodic monitoring of respiratory function. We typically perform pulmonary function tests every few months after the first year or so of illness. Our experience has been that the vital capacity in cubic centimeters can be estimated by multiplying the highest number to which a patient can count with one deep breath by 100. Thus, the ability to count to 25 with a full effort in a single breath corresponds to a vital capacity of approximately 2.5 L. Significant practical advances have been made in the respiratory management of ALS. The

Table 39-7

CLASSIFICATION OF THE SPINAL MUSCULAR ATROPHIES (SMA)

TYPE	INHERITANCE	AGE OF ONSET	CLINICAL FEATURES	PROGNOSIS
SMA I (infantile, Werdnig-Hoffmann)	Autosomal recessive Two copies of SMN 2	Preterm to 6 months	Neonatal hypotonia (floppy baby), weakness of sucking and swallowing, may have arthrogryposis, unable to sit	Few survive 1 year
SMA II (intermediate type; Dubowitz disease)	Autosomal recessive At least 3 copies of SMN 2	6 to 15 months	Proximal weakness, fasciculation, fine hand tremor, unable to stand	Variable; death from respiratory complications
SMA III (Wohlfart-Kugelberg-Welander)	Autosomal recessive or dominant At least 3 copies of SMN 2	1 year to adolescence	Delayed motor development, proximal leg weakness	Slowly progressive, variable outcome
SMA IV	Autosomal recessive At least 4 copies of SMN 2	After age 30	Proximal limb weakness and diaphragm	Slowly progressive; eventually wheelchair-bound but normal life expectancy
Kennedy syndrome (bulbospinal atrophy)	X-linked (CAG repeat expansion in the AR gene), less often autosomal dominant	Early adulthood	Scapuloperoneal or distal atrophy, oropharyngeal weakness, gynecomastia, oligospermia	Slowly progressive
Fazio-Londe disease	Autosomal recessive, rarely dominant, *SLC52A3* gene	Childhood to early adolescence	Progressive bulbar and respiratory failure	Survival for years, respiratory failure

introduction of bilevel positive airway pressure (BiPAP) has allowed patients to sleep better and reduce daytime somnolence. Many patients do not initially tolerate the device, usually because of maladjusted face masks or excessive applied airway pressures. Almost always, a seasoned pulmonary technologist can find solutions to these problems. It is appropriate to begin BiPAP at (or before) the earliest sign of carbon dioxide retention, a state that is heralded by disruption of sleep, nightmares, early morning headaches, and daytime drowsiness. With noninvasive respiratory assistance, it may be possible to defer tracheostomy for months or years. Ultimately, as the diaphragm fails, BiPAP is needed not only at night but also during the day. As BiPAP use approaches 20 to 24 h per day, patients must usually address the difficult question of tracheostomy and mechanical ventilation. We broach this subject early enough in the course of the disease to allow ample time for discussion and reflection. In practice, most patients elect not to undergo tracheostomy and full ventilation.

Another important issue regards nutrition. As oropharyngeal palsy progresses, food should be cut into small pieces and dry foods, such as toast should be avoided; milk shakes and preparations of the same consistency are ideal at this stage. Speech therapists are capable of teaching patients methods to adapt to declining bulbar function and at the same time minimizing aspiration. Ultimately, in our experience, most ALS patients will need a feeding tube to maintain normal hydration and caloric intake. Although we adopt a neutral position in discussions with patients regarding mechanical ventilation, we tend to urge patients to undergo placement of a feeding tube at the appropriate time. This presumably increases survival and improves quality of life by preventing dehydration and recurrent aspiration. Laparoscopic and radiologic technologies for the placement of a gastrostomy tube render the procedure swift and nearly painless. Some patients have tubes inserted as outpatients and then start gastric feeding within a day or two.

Other devices, often guided by the physical and occupational therapist, may be of great assistance to the patient and family as the disease progresses. These include a mechanized bed and structural accommodations in the home that facilitate entry of a wheelchair and the safe use of the bath or shower as well as thick-handled utensils. Ambulation aids, beginning with simple canes (first one, then two) followed by a walker (preferably with basket and seat) and then a wheelchair (manual or electric) are of value in maintaining a sense of independence and assuring safety.

The American Academy of Neurology has published explicit guidelines for management that have been of great aid to patients and physicians; they emphasize the complex and multidisciplinary needs of ALS patients (see Miller et al 2009a and 2009b).

Heredofamilial Forms of Progressive Muscular Atrophy

These diverse diseases are the concern mainly of child neurology. They are presented here because they fall within the category of system degenerations and are usually inherited.

Spinal Muscular Atrophy (Werdnig-Hoffman Disease)

The classic form of spinal muscular atrophy was described by Werdnig in 1891 and 1894, by Hoffmann in 1893 and, at about the same time, by Thomsen and Bruce. The cases described by these authors were all in infants. Further clinical analyses, however, indicated the inadequacy of this narrow grouping for the large group of spinal muscular atrophies. Brandt, in his study of 112 Danish patients, found that in about one-third the weakness was present at birth, and in 97 the onset was in the first year of life; in 9 patients, the disease was not recognized until after the first year of life. In 1956, Walton, and later Wohlfart and colleagues and Kugelberg and Welander (see below), identified milder forms of spinal muscular atrophy in which the onset was between 2 and 17 years and walking was still possible in adult life. Byers and Banker, in a study of 52 patients, subdivided them into 3 groups on the basis of age of onset; in one group the disease was recognized at birth or in the first month or two of life; in a second, between 6 and 12 months; and in a third, after the first year. In their last group, it was not unusual for the patient to survive into adolescence and adult life. In a few of the late-onset types, signs of corticospinal tract involvement are conjoined, and Bonduelle has also included some patients with areflexia, pes cavus, Babinski signs, choreiform movements, and developmental delay in this group. More recently, the designations SMA I, II, and III have been introduced, based largely on the age of onset (see Table 39-7).

Genetic Aspects of Spinal Muscular Atrophies Familial spinal muscular atrophy that begins in infancy and childhood is inherited mainly as an autosomal recessive trait. All the SMA phenotypes in children have been mapped to the same chromosome, 5q11.2-13.3 (Brzustowicz et al; Gilliam et al; Munsat et al). The mutations affect the gene at the "survival of motor neuron" (SMN) site. The SMN protein participates in forming protein-RNA complexes (small nuclear ribonucleoproteins and RNA) that are essential for gene splicing. Within the SMN locus there are 2 alleles: *SMN1*, which generates a full-length, fully functional form of SMN, and *SMN2*, which makes a truncated, partially functional SMN. The latter can partially compensate for the loss of SMN1. Making matters more complex, individuals vary in the number copies of *SMN2*. As a result, disease due to loss of both copies of *SMN1* causes very severe SMA in individuals who carry only one copy of *SMN2*, while those with multiple copies of *SMN2* have milder disease. Thus, the amount of SMN2 protein determines the severity and time of onset of disease.

Although affected siblings demonstrate very similar clinical patterns of disease, the same mutation may give rise to very different phenotypes in different families, so that additional modifying posttranscriptional or nongenetic attributes must be playing a role. Less often, autosomal dominant and X-linked patterns of inheritance have been found, resulting from mutations in UBA1, usually in adults. A rare autosomal dominant adult form is the result of mutations in VABP and a form that affects only the legs is associated with mutations in *DYNC1H1*.

Clinical Manifestations of Werdnig-Hoffmann Disease (SMA I) The most frequent form of these spinal muscular atrophies, the severe infantile type, is a common disease, occurring once in every 20,000 live births. After cystic fibrosis, it is also the most frequent cause of death from a recessively inherited disease. Characteristically the infant, usually born normally, is noted from birth to be unnaturally weak and limp ("floppy"). Some mothers report that fetal movement in utero had been less than expected or lacking altogether. In severe cases, arthrogryposis at the ankles and wrists or dislocation of the hips is noted at birth (arthrogryposis and its differential diagnosis is discussed in Chap. 48 in the section on the congenital neuromuscular disorders). The muscle weakness in these children is generalized from the beginning, and death comes early, usually within the first year. Other infants seem to develop normally for several months before the weakness becomes apparent. In these, the trunk, pelvic, and shoulder-girdle muscles are at first disproportionately affected, while the fingers and hands, toes and feet, and cranial muscles retain mobility. *Hypotonia* accompanies the weakness, and because passive displacement of articulated parts in testing muscle tone is easier to judge than power of contraction at this early age, it may be singled out as the dominant clinical characteristic. As a rule, the tendon reflexes are unobtainable. Volume of muscle is diminished but is difficult to evaluate in the infant because of the coverings of adipose tissue. Fasciculations are seldom visible except sometimes in the tongue. Perception of tactile and painful stimuli is undiminished, and emotional and social development measures up to age.

As the months pass, the weakness and hypotonia progress gradually and spread to all the skeletal muscles except the ocular ones. Intercostal paralysis with a degree of collapse of the chest is the rule. Respiratory movements become paradoxical (abdominal protrusion with chest retraction). The cry becomes feeble, and sucking and swallowing are less efficient. Such infants are unable to sit unless propped, and they cannot hold up their heads without support and cannot roll over or support their weight when placed on their feet. Their posture is characteristic: arms abducted and flexed at the elbow, legs in the "frog position" with external rotation and abduction at hips and flexion at hips and knees. If the effects of gravity are removed, all muscles continue to contract; that is there is paresis, not paralysis. Until late in the illness, these children appear bright-eyed, alert, and responsive.

Infants in whom the disease becomes apparent only after several months of life have a less-rapid decline than those affected in utero or at birth. Some of the former become able to sit and creep and even to walk with support; those with later onset may survive for several years and even into adolescence or early adult life, as already mentioned.

Laboratory data of confirmatory value are few. Muscle enzymes in the serum are usually normal or rarely elevated. The EMG, if performed at a late enough stage of development, displays fibrillations, proving the denervative basis of the weakness. Motor unit potentials are diminished in number and, in the more slowly evolving cases, some are larger than normal (giant or polyphasic potentials reflecting reinnervation). Motor nerve conduction velocities are normal or fall in the low-normal range (these are normally slower in infants than in adults). Electrophysiologic studies performed in the first few months of life may give ambiguous results.

Pathologic Findings Muscle biopsy after 1 month of age reveals a typical picture of group atrophy; shortly after birth this change is difficult to discern. Aside from denervative atrophy, the essential abnormalities are in the anterior horn cells in the spinal cord and the motor nuclei in the lower brainstem. Nerve cells are greatly reduced in number, and many of the remaining ones are in varying stages of degeneration; a few are chromatolytic and contain cytoplasmic inclusions. It is not unusual to see figures of neuronophagia. There is replacement gliosis and secondary degeneration in roots and nerves. Other systems of neurons, including the corticospinal and corticobulbar systems, are entirely unaffected.

Differential Diagnosis The major problem in diagnosis is to distinguish Werdnig-Hoffmann disease from an array of other diseases that cause hypotonia and delayed motor development in the neonate and infant. The list of disorders that imitates spinal muscular atrophy constitutes a large part of the differential diagnosis of the so-called *floppy infant*. The congenital myopathies (as described in Chap. 48), the glycogenoses, neonatal myasthenia gravis, Prader-Willi syndrome, and disorders of fatty acid metabolism frequently present in this way. The preservation of tendon reflexes and relative lack of progression of muscle weakness distinguish the latter disorders. Because of the gravity of the diagnosis, muscle biopsy should be performed if there is any suspicion of spinal muscular atrophy. If studied properly, the biopsy usually yields the correct diagnosis.

Clinical disorders more or less similar to the spinal muscular atrophies may be identified occasionally in certain hereditary metabolic diseases. For example, Johnson and coworkers have described a patient who began experiencing weakness of the legs, cramping, and fasciculations during adolescence in what proved to be a variant of hexosaminidase A (G_{M2}) deficiency, and biopsy of rectal mucosa showed nerve cells with the typical membranous cytoplasmic bodies of Tay-Sachs disease. Others have reported similar cases. A progressive motor neuron or motor nerve disorder has also been observed in glycogen storage disease affecting anterior horn cells. Motor nerve fibers also suffer damage in metachromatic and globoid body leukoencephalopathies.

Certain forms of muscular dystrophy, notably myotonic dystrophy, which is about twice as frequent as Werdnig-Hoffmann disease, may become manifest in the neonatal period and interfere with sucking and motor development (see Chap. 48). As a rule, the weakness is not as severe or diffuse as that in Werdnig-Hoffmann disease. The mother, but not the child, may display myotonia, either elicitable clinically or, if more subtle, with EMG recording. Also, a number of polyneuropathies may cause a serious degree of weakness in early childhood. Unfortunately, in respect to the latter, adequate sensory testing is not possible because of the patient's age, but the CSF protein is often elevated. Again, diagnosis is greatly facilitated by nerve-muscle biopsy and measurement of nerve conduction velocities. These velocities are reduced but must be interpreted with caution because of incomplete development of axons and of myelination in the first months of life. The needle EMG examination shows subtle signs of denervation that cannot be easily distinguished from the finding in the spinal muscular atrophies. Examination of parents and siblings may disclose a clinically inapparent neuropathy. Polymyositis of childhood may also simulate both muscular dystrophy and motor neuron disease. Finally nemaline and central core myopathy can manifest in infancy and early childhood and cause a floppy child syndrome.

Developmental delay with a flaccid rather than spastic weakness of the limbs is another major category of disease that must be distinguished. These include Down syndrome, cretinism, Prader-Willi syndrome, and achondrodysplasia. It should be commented that very sick children with celiac disease, cystic fibrosis, and other chronic diseases may be hypotonic to the point of simulating neuromuscular disease. Usually speech is not delayed and tendon reflexes are preserved in these purely medical states, and strength returns as the medical problem is corrected. Also, certain of the polioencephalopathies and leukodystrophies may weaken muscles and abolish tendon reflexes, but usually there is evidence of cerebral involvement.

There remains, after the assiduous study of the "floppy infant," a group of cases of hypotonia and motor underdevelopment that cannot be classified. The term *amyotonia congenita* (Oppenheim) was once applied to this entire group but is now obsolete. Walto proposed the term *benign congenital hypotonia* to designate patients who manifest limp and flabby limbs in infancy and a delay in sitting up and walking but who improve gradually, some completely and others incompletely. It is likely that among this group there are examples of congenital myopathy that await differentiation by application of modern histochemical, ultrastructural, and genetic techniques.

Chronic Childhood and Juvenile Proximal Spinal Muscular Atrophy (Wohlfart-Kugelberg-Welander Syndrome; SMA III) This is a somewhat different form of heredofamilial spinal muscular atrophy, which, as the name indicates, involves the proximal muscles of the limbs predominantly and is only slowly progressive. It was first separated from other forms of motor system disease and from muscular dystrophy by Wohlfart and by Kugelberg and Welander in the mid-1950s. In about one-third of the cases the onset is before 2 years of age, and in half, between 3 and 18 years. Males predominate, especially among patients with juvenile and adult onset. The usual form of transmission is by an autosomal recessive pattern; most cases result from mutations in the *SMN* gene; as mentioned, multiple copies of the *SMN2* gene partly rescue the loss of *SMN1* and lead to this milder form of disease. Families with dominant and sex-linked inheritance have also been described.

The disease begins insidiously, with weakness and atrophy of the pelvic girdle and proximal leg muscles, followed by involvement of the shoulder girdle and upper arm muscles. Unlike the sporadic form of spinal muscular atrophy, the Wohlfart-Kugelberg-Welander variety (also listed in other books and monographs as Kugelberg-Welander disease) is bilaterally symmetrical from the beginning, and fasciculations are observed in only half the cases. Ultimately the distal limb muscles are involved and tendon reflexes are lost. Bulbar musculature and corticospinal tracts are spared, although Babinski signs and an associated ophthalmoplegia (presumably neural) have been reported in rare instances.

The presence of fasciculations and the EMG and muscle biopsy findings—all of which show the characteristic abnormalities of neural atrophy—permit distinction from muscular dystrophy. Cases that have been examined postmortem have shown loss and degeneration of the anterior horn cells.

The disease progresses very slowly, and some patients survive to old age without serious disability. In general, the earlier the onset, the less favorable the prognosis; however, even the most severely affected patients retain the ability to walk for at least 10 years after the onset. Admittedly, it is difficult to make a sharp distinction between these cases of Wohlfart-Kugelberg-Welander disease and certain milder instances of Werdnig-Hoffmann disease with onset in late infancy and early childhood and prolonged survival (Byers and Banker).

A form that is intermediate between the severe Werdnig-Hoffman type and the milder Wohlfart-Kugelberg-Welander is termed Dubowitz syndrome and designated SMA II.

Kennedy Syndrome (X-Linked Bulbospinal Muscular Atrophy)

An unusual pattern of *distal muscular atrophy with prominent bulbar signs* and, less often, ocular palsies was described by Kennedy and coworkers. The onset has varied from childhood to adult age, but symptoms typically begin in the third decade. Most cases have shown an X-linked pattern of inheritance and a lesser number, an autosomal dominant pattern. The proximal shoulder and hip musculature are involved first by weakness and atrophy, followed in about half of patients by dysarthria and dysphagia. Muscle cramps or twitching often precedes weakness. Facial fasciculations and mild weakness are characteristic and may be striking. The tendon reflexes become depressed and may be absent; a mild sensory neuropathy is almost universal. In the family described by Kaeser, in which 12 members in 5 generations were affected, the pattern of weakness was shoulder-shank, that is scapuloperoneal; it may therefore be mistaken for muscular dystrophy. Two-thirds of patients have gynecomastia, a feature that may first identify affected men in a kindred; oligospermia and diabetes are additional associations; therefore, the presence of genuine progeny virtually excludes the disease in a male. The CK level is elevated, sometimes tenfold, and physiologic studies reveal denervation and reinnervation as well as indications of a mild sensory neuropathy.

As in Huntington disease and certain of the spinocerebellar atrophies, the genetic defect is a CAG expansion, in this case in the gene (AR) that codes for the androgen receptor on the short arm of the X-chromosome (La Spada et al; see Table 39-7). Indeed, the first reported polyglutamine disease was Kennedy syndrome. Lengthened sequences correlate with an earlier age of onset (anticipation, as in Huntington disease) but have no relation to the severity of disease. Androgen receptors have been found on motor neurons of the spinal cord; the subpopulation of motor neurons that is susceptible to both Kennedy syndrome and ALS express abundant surface androgen receptors, but it is not clear whether this finding has direct pathogenic significance. Neuronal inclusions have been described, composed of aggregations of the abnormally long polyglutamine protein sequences that correspond to the CAG expansion. A family with the bulbospinal phenotype but without the CAG expansion has also been reported (Paradiso et al). Other features, such as optic atrophy and sensory neuronopathy, were present in some members of this kindred but are not features of typical cases. The diagnosis can be confirmed by genetic testing for the lengthened trinucleotide sequence. Prenatal diagnosis and identification of female carriers are also possible by this method.

Progressive Bulbar Palsy of Childhood (Fazio-Londe Syndrome)

Fazio in 1892, and Londe in 1893, described the development of a progressive bulbar palsy in children, adolescents, and young adults. There is progressive paralysis of the facial, lingual, pharyngeal, laryngeal, and sometimes ocular muscles. The illness usually presents with stridor and respiratory symptoms, followed by facial diplegia, dysarthria, dysphagia, and dysphonia. These features become increasingly pronounced until the time of death some years later. In a few patients there is a late development of corticospinal signs and sometimes ocular palsies. Occasionally, jaw and oculomotor paresis appears, and in one case, there was progressive deafness. The disease is rare, only several dozen well-described examples had been recorded in the medical literature by 1992 (McShane et al). Inheritance may be autosomal dominant, as in Fazio's original case, and rarely X-linked, but it is more likely to be autosomal recessive. Pathologic examination has shown a loss of motor neurons in the hypoglossal, ambiguus, facial, and trigeminal motor nuclei. In a few cases, the nerve cells in the ocular motor nuclei also were diminished. This disease, the 2 times we have encountered it, had to be differentiated from myasthenia gravis, a pontomedullary glioma, and brainstem multiple sclerosis.

The cause of the disease is interesting in that it results from mutations in SLC52A3, a riboflavin transporter, and some beneficial effect is derived from the administration of riboflavin (vitamin B_2). The disease is allelic with *Brown-Vialetto-Van Laere syndrome*, another motor neuron degeneration, which includes deafness.

Hereditary Forms of Spastic Paraplegia

Hereditary Spastic Paraplegia (Strümpell-Lorrain Disease)

This disease was described by Seeligmuller in 1874 and later by Strümpell in Germany and Lorrain in France; it has now been identified in nearly every part of the world. The pattern of inheritance is usually autosomal dominant, less often recessive (one family has shown X-linked inheritance), and the onset may be at any age from childhood to the senium. Harding (1993) divided the disease

Table 39-8

GENETIC DEFECTS ASSOCIATED WITH HEREDITARY SPASTIC PARAPLEGIA (HSP)

HSP TYPE	GENE (PROTEIN)	GENETICS	AGE OF ONSET	CLINICAL AND MISCELLANEOUS FEATURES
3A	*ATL1* (atlastin)	AD	Childhood	Guanylate-binding protein
4	Spastin	AD	20's	40–50% of HSP; binds to microtubules
6	*NIPA1*	AD	Teens	Golgi membrane protein
10	*KIF5A* (kinesin-1)	AD	Childhood	Kinesin heavy chain–motor protein
13	*HSP* (heat shock protein)	AD	Adult	Located in mitochondrial matrix
17	*BSCL2* (seipin)	AD	Variable	Silver syndrome: HSP with wasting of hands, feet
7	*SPG7* (paraplegin)	AR	Adult	Mitochondrial chaperone and metalloprotease; optic atrophy, neuropathy, myopathy
	Spartin	AR		HSP with wasting of distal limbs, hands, feet
21	*SPG21* (maspardin)	AR	Late teens	Endosomal protein involved in protein transport
1	*L1CAM* (L1 cell adhesion molecule)	XR	Infancy	Developmental delay, hydrocephalus, callosal hypoplasia, spasticity
2	*PLP* (proteolipid protein)	XR	Infancy	Cognitive impairment, spasticity, ataxia

AD autosomal dominant; AR autosomal recessive; XR X-linked recessive

into 2 groups, the more common one beginning before age 35 with a very protracted course and the other with a late onset (40 to 60 years). The latter type often shows sensory loss, urinary symptoms, and action tremor.

The clinical picture is that of a gradual development of spastic weakness of the legs with increasing difficulty in walking. The tendon reflexes are hyperactive and the plantar reflexes extensor. In the pure form of the disease, sensory and other nervous functions are entirely intact. If the onset is in childhood, as many cases are, the foot arches become exaggerated, the feet are shortened, and there is a tightening (pseudocontracture) of calf muscles, forcing the child or adolescent to "toe-walk." This is a common orthopedic problem and may require surgical correction. In children, the legs appear to be underdeveloped, and in both children and adults they may become quite thin. Sometimes the knees are slightly flexed; at other times the legs are fully extended or hyperextended (genu recurvatum) and adducted. Weakness is variable and difficult to estimate. Sphincteric function is usually retained. Subtle sensory loss in the feet has been reported. The arms are variably involved. In some patients, the arms appear to be spared even though the tendon reflexes are lively. In others, the hands are stiff, movements are clumsy, and speech is mildly dysarthric. Conjoined findings such as nystagmus, ocular palsies, optic atrophy, pigmentary macular degeneration, ataxia (both cerebellar and sensory), sensorimotor polyneuropathy, ichthyosis, patchy skin pigmentation, epilepsy, and dementia have all been described in isolated families (see further on).

The few available pathologic studies have shown that, in addition to degeneration of the corticospinal tracts throughout the spinal cord, there is thinning of the columns of Goll, mainly in the lumbosacral regions, and of the spinocerebellar tracts, even when no sensory abnormalities had been detected during life. These were the pathologic findings described by Strümpell in his original (1880) report of 2 brothers with spastic paraplegia; one of them, in addition, had a cerebellar syndrome, but again, there were no sensory abnormalities. A reduction in the number of Betz and anterior horn cells has also been reported.

Genetic Aspects of Hereditary Spastic Paraplegia Numerous genetic mutations have given rise to this disease. As of this writing, there were 52 hereditary spastic paraplegia (HSP) loci many of which are shown in Table 39-8. The disease types have been renamed under the designation "SPG" (for spastic paraplegia) and numbered in order of discovery of the associated gene. The common uncomplicated autosomal dominant form of disease has been linked to mutations in many proteins, the most common being (proteins in parentheses) SPAST (spastin) and ALT1 (atlastin); and the common recessive varieties, are in SPG7 (paraplegin); and X-linked in L1CAM and PLP1 (proteolipid protein). The common spastin variety, associated with a mutation on chromosome 2p, results in great variability of clinical presentation within and among families (see Nielsen et al). A high frequency of partial deletions of the *SPAST* gene has been found. The possible subcellular mechanisms by which these mutations cause degeneration of the corticospinal tracts have been reviewed by Blackstone.

Differential Diagnosis In the diagnosis of this disorder, one should consider an indolent spinal cord or foramen magnum tumor, cervical spondylosis, a spinal from of multiple sclerosis (this was the clinical diagnosis in Strümpell's original cases), Chiari malformation, compression of the cord by a variety of congenital bony malformations at the craniocervical junction, and a number of chronic myelitides, among them, lupus erythematosus, sarcoidosis, AIDS, adrenomyeloneuropathy, primary lateral sclerosis (described earlier in this chapter), hypocupric myelopathy, spinal arteriovenous dural fistula, and especially, tropical spastic paraparesis (caused by the HTLV-1 virus as discussed in Chap. 33).

Variants of Familial Spastic Paraplegia

The literature contains a large number of descriptions of familial spastic paraplegia combined with other neurologic abnormalities. Some of the syndromes had developed early in life in conjunction with moderate degrees of mental retardation. In these, the rest of the neurologic picture appeared many years after birth and was progressive. Some idea of the number of these "hereditary paraplegia-plus" syndromes and the diverse combinations in which they may be present is conveyed in the review by Gout and colleagues. Again, it is hardly possible to describe each of these symptoms in any degree of detail. The list below includes the best-known entities but all are rare. But if the term *hereditary spastic paraplegia* is to have any neurologic significance, it should be applied only to the pure form of the progressive syndrome. The more common "atypical" or "syndromic" cases—with amyotrophy, cerebellar ataxia, tremors, dystonia, athetosis, optic atrophy, retinal degeneration, amentia, and dementia—should be put in separate categories and their identity retained for nosologic purposes until such time as additional biochemical and genetic data related to pathogenesis are forthcoming. The gene mutations found in some of the variant types have been summarized by Fink, but—as with all types of uncomplicated hereditary spastic paraplegia—the mechanisms of neuronal loss are not known. To be separated from these cases are all the congenital nonprogressive types of spastic diplegia and athetosis. The following list includes the best-known entities:

1. *Hereditary spastic paraplegia with ataxia (Ferguson-Critchley syndrome)* This syndrome is one of a collection of leg spasticity and generalized ataxia syndrome that may also be characterized by a disorder of gaze, or optic atrophy. Most impressive are the manifestations of spinocerebellar ataxia beginning during the fourth and fifth decades of life, accompanied by weakness of the legs, alterations of mood, pathologic crying and laughing, dysarthria and diplopia, dysesthesias of limbs, and poor bladder control. The tendon reflexes are lively, with bilateral Babinski signs. Sensation is diminished distally in the limbs. The whole picture resembles a chronic progressive form of multiple sclerosis. In other cases, running through several generations of a family, the extrapyramidal features were more striking; such cases overlap with the following syndromes. A dominant form of the disease is due to a mutation in *SAX1*.
2. *Hereditary spastic paraplegia with extrapyramidal signs* Action and static tremors, parkinsonian rigidity, dystonic tongue movement, and athetosis of the limbs have all been conjoined with spastic paraplegia. Gilman and Romanul have reviewed the literature on this subject. In the authors' experience, the picture of parkinsonism with spastic weakness and other corticospinal signs has been the most frequent combination.
3. *Hereditary spastic paraplegia with optic atrophy* This is known as *Behr syndrome* or *optic atrophy-ataxia syndrome*, since cerebellar signs are usually conjoined. Some patients also have athetosis. The syndrome is transmitted as an autosomal recessive trait, with onset in infancy and slow progression. The mutation is in *OPA3*. There may be a relationship to decreased excretion of 3-methylglutaconic aciduria of an optic atrophy and cataract syndrome (Costeff syndrome).
4. *Hereditary spastic paraplegia with macular degeneration (Kjellin syndrome)* Spastic paraplegia with amyotrophy, oligophrenia, and central retinal degeneration constitutes the syndrome described in 1959 by Kjellin. Although the developmental delay is stationary, the spastic weakness and retinal changes are of late onset and progressive. Mutations have been found in *SPG11* and *SPG15*.
5. *Hereditary spastic paraplegia with developmental delay or dementia* Many of the children with progressive spastic paraplegia either have been developmentally delayed since early life or have appeared to regress mentally as other neurologic symptoms developed. Examples of this syndrome and its variants are too numerous to be considered here but are contained in the review by Gilman and Romanul. The autosomal *recessive syndrome of Sjögren-Larsson*, with the onset in infancy of spastic weakness of the legs in association with developmental delay, stands somewhat apart from the others in this large group because of the associated ichthyosis. The mutation for the latter is in *ALDH3A2* that codes for fatty aldehyde dehydrogenase. This relates to both dry skin, itchy and discolored skin, and the myelinopathy that characterize Sjögren-Larsson syndrome.
6. *Hereditary spastic paraplegia with polyneuropathy* Our colleagues had observed several patients in whom a sensorimotor polyneuropathy was combined with unmistakable signs of corticospinal disease. The age of onset was in childhood or adolescence, and the disability progressed to the point where the patient was chairbound by early adult life. In two of the cases, a sural nerve biopsy revealed a typical hypertrophic polyneuropathy; in a third case there was only a depletion of large myelinated fibers. The syndrome resembles the myeloneuropathy of adrenoleukodystrophy.
7. *Spastic paraparesis with distal muscle wasting (Troyer syndrome)* This disorder is transmitted as an autosomal recessive trait in the Amish population. Onset is in childhood with amyotrophy of the hands, followed by spasticity and contractures of the lower limbs. Cerebellar signs (mild), athetosis, and deafness may be added. The mutation is in *SPG20*.

SYNDROME OF PROGRESSIVE BLINDNESS (See Chap. 13)

There are 2 main classes of progressive blindness in children, adolescents, and adults: progressive optic neuropathy and retinal degenerations (retinitis pigmentosa and tapetoretinal macular degeneration). Of course, there are many congenital anomalies and retinal diseases beginning in infancy that result in blindness and microphthalmia. Some of those of neurologic interest were described briefly in connection with the hereditary spastic paraplegias and in Chap. 13.

Leber Hereditary Optic Atrophy

Although familial amaurosis was known in the early eighteenth century, it was Leber, in 1871, who gave the definitive description of this disease and traced it through many genealogies. The family studies of Nikoskelainen and coworkers indicate that all daughters of carrier mothers become carriers themselves, a type of transmission that is determined by inheritance of defective mitochondrial DNA from the mother (Wallace et al). Common to all cases is the presence of a pathogenic mitochondrial DNA abnormality (Riordan-Eva et al), but the defect may occur at one of several sites as discussed in Chap. 37. Thus, Leber optic atrophy has been added to the growing list of mitochondrial diseases. Mutations in approximately 20 genes have been detected, together accounting for about half of cases.

In most patients, the visual loss begins between 18 and 25 years of age, but the range of age of onset is much broader. Usually the visual loss has an insidious onset and a subacute evolution, but it may evolve rapidly, suggesting a retrobulbar neuritis; moreover, in these latter instances, aching in the eye or brow may accompany the visual loss, just as it does in the demyelinative variety. Subjective visual phenomena are reported by some. Usually both eyes are affected simultaneously, although in some one eye is affected first, followed by the other after an interval of several weeks or months. In practically all cases, the second eye is affected within a year of the first. In the unimpaired eye, abnormalities of visual evoked potentials may antedate impairment of visual acuity (Carroll and Mastaglia).

Once started, the visual loss progresses over a period of weeks to months. Characteristically, central vision is lost before peripheral, and there is a stage at which bilateral central scotomata are readily demonstrated. Early on, perception of blue-yellow is deficient, while that of red and green is relatively preserved. In the more advanced stages, however, the patients are totally color-blind. Constriction of the fields may be added later. At first there may be swelling and hyperemia of the discs, but soon they become atrophic. Peripapillary vasculopathy, consisting of tortuosity and arteriovenous shunting, is the primary structural change; this has been present also in asymptomatic offspring of carrier females.

As visual symptoms develop, fluorescein angiography shows shunting in the abnormal vascular bed, with reduced filling of the capillaries of the papillomacular bundle. Although patients are left with dense central scotomata, it is of some importance that the visual impairment is seldom complete; in some patients, relative stabilization of visual function occurs. In a few, there may be a surprising improvement.

Examination of the optic nerve lesion shows the central parts of the nerves to be degenerated from papillae to the lateral geniculate bodies, that is the papillomacular bundles are particularly affected. Presumably axis cylinders and myelin degenerate together, as would be expected from the loss of nerve cells in the superficial layer of the retina. Both astrocytic glial and endoneurial fibroblastic connective tissue are increased. Tests for the 3 main mitochondrial mutations that give rise to the disorder are now available.

Congenital optic atrophy (of which recessive and dominant forms are known), retrobulbar neuritis, and nutritional optic neuropathy are the main considerations in differential diagnosis.

Retinitis Pigmentosa (See Chap. 13)

This remarkable retinal abiotrophy, known to Helmholtz in 1851, soon after he invented the ophthalmoscope, usually begins in childhood and adolescence. Unlike the optic atrophy of Leber, which affects only the third neuron of the visual neuronal chain, retinitis pigmentosa affects all the retinal layers, both the neuroepithelium and pigment epithelium (see Fig. 13-2). The incidence of this disorder is 2 or 3 times greater in males than in females. Inheritance is more often autosomal recessive than dominant; in the former, consanguinity plays an important part, increasing the likelihood of the disease by approximately 20 times. Sex-linked types are also known. It is estimated that 100,000 Americans are afflicted with this disease. Mutations in approximately 60 genes have been associated with the disorder but the most commonly affected in autosomal dominant cases is RHO; in recessive cases, USH2A, and in X-linked cases, RPGR and RP2.

The first symptom is usually an impairment of twilight vision (nyctalopia). Under dim light, the visual fields tend to constrict; but slowly, as the disease progresses, there is permanent visual impairment in all degrees of illumination. The perimacular zones tend to be the first and most severely involved, giving rise to partial or complete ring scotomata. Peripheral loss sets in later. Usually both eyes are affected simultaneously, but cases are on record where one eye was affected first and more severely. Ophthalmoscopic examination shows the characteristic triad of pigmentary deposits that assume the configuration of bone corpuscles, attenuated vessels, and pallor of the optic discs. The pigment is caused by clumping of epithelial cells that migrate from the pigment layer to the superficial parts of the retina as the rod cells degenerate. The pigmentary change spares only the fovea, so that eventually the world is perceived by the patient as though he were looking through narrow tubes.

The many and diverse syndromes to which retinitis pigmentosa may be linked include oligophrenia, obesity, syndactyly, and hypogonadism (Bardet-Biedl syndrome); hypogenitalism, obesity, and mental deficiency (Laurence-Moon syndrome); Friedreich and other types of spinocerebellar and cerebellar ataxia; spastic paraplegia and quadriplegia with Laurence-Moon syndrome; neurogenic amyotrophy, myopia, and color-blindness; polyneuropathy and deafness (Refsum disease); deaf mutism; Cockayne syndrome and Bassen-Kornzweig disease; and several mitochondrial diseases, particularly progressive external ophthalmoplegia and Kearns-Sayre syndromes.

Stargardt Disease

This is a bilaterally symmetrical, slowly progressive macular degeneration, differentiated from retinitis pigmentosa by Stargardt in 1909. In essence, it is a hereditary (usually autosomal recessive) tapetoretinal degeneration or dystrophy (the latter term being preferred by Waardenburg), with onset between 6 and 20 years of age, rarely later, and leading to a loss of central vision. The macular region becomes gray or yellow-brown with pigmentary spots, and the visual fields show central scotomata. Later the periphery of the retina may become dystrophic. The lesion is well visualized by fluorescein angiography, which discloses a virtually pathognomonic "dark choroid" pattern. Activity in the electroretinogram is diminished or abolished. Both recessively inherited Stargardt disease and the closely related cone-rod dystrophy have been linked to mutations of *ABCA4* or *ELOVL4* the former codes for a transporter protein (termed ABCR) of the photoreceptor.

This disease, with its selective loss of cone function, is in a sense the inverse of retinitis pigmentosa. According to Cohan and associates, it may be associated with epilepsy, Refsum syndrome, Kearns-Sayre syndrome, Bassen-Kornzweig syndrome, or Sjögren-Larsson syndrome, or with spinocerebellar and other forms of cerebellar degeneration and familial paraplegia.

SYNDROME OF CONGENITAL OR PROGRESSIVE DEAFNESS (See Chap. 15)

There is an impressive group of hereditary, progressive cochleovestibular atrophies that are linked to degenerations of the nervous system. These are the subject of an informative review by Konigsmark and are summarized below. Such neurotologic syndromes must be set alongside a group of 5 diseases that affect the auditory and vestibular nerves exclusively: dominant progressive nerve deafness; dominant low-frequency hearing loss; dominant midfrequency hearing loss; sex-linked, early-onset neural deafness; and hereditary episodic vertigo and hearing loss. The last of these is of special interest to neurologists because both balance and hearing are affected.

It should be pointed out that in 70 percent of cases of hereditary deafness, there are no other somatic or neurologic abnormalities. To date, 3 separate autosomal mutations have been identified that are associated with this pure "nonsyndromic" type of hereditary deafness, the most common of which is in the connexin gene, as discussed in Chap. 15. A number of mitochondrial disorders have been associated with deafness alone as well as with a number of the better-characterized mitochondrial syndromes (see Chap. 37). The age of onset of hearing loss in the pure forms has been variable, extending well into adulthood.

Hereditary Hearing Loss With Retinal Diseases

Konigsmark has separated this overall category into 3 subgroups: patients with typical retinitis pigmentosa, those with Leber optic atrophy, and those with other retinal changes. With respect to retinitis pigmentosa, 4 syndromes are recognized in which retinitis pigmentosa appears in combination: with congenital hearing loss (Usher syndrome); with polyneuropathy (Refsum syndrome); with hypogonadism and obesity (Alstrom syndrome); and with dwarfism, mental retardation, premature senility, and photosensitive dermatitis (Cockayne syndrome).

Hereditary hearing loss with optic atrophy forms the core of 4 special syndromes: dominant optic atrophy, ataxia, muscle wasting, and progressive hearing loss (Sylvester disease); recessive optic atrophy, polyneuropathy, and neural hearing loss (Rosenberg-Chutorian syndrome); optic atrophy, hearing loss, and juvenile diabetes mellitus (Tun-bridge-Paley syndrome); and opticocochleodentate degeneration with optic atrophy, hearing loss, quadriparesis, and developmental delay (Nyssen-van Bogaert syndrome).

Hearing loss has also been observed with other retinal changes, two of which are Norrie disease, with retinal malformation, hearing loss, and mental retardation (oculoacousticocerebral degeneration), and Small disease, with recessive hearing loss, mental retardation, narrowing of retinal vessels, and muscle atrophy. In the former, the infant is born blind, with a white vascularized retinal mass behind a clear lens; later the lens and cornea become opaque. The eyes are small, and the iris is atrophied. In the latter, the optic fundi shows tortuosity of vessels, telangiectases, and retinal detachment. The nature of the progressive generalized muscular weakness has not been ascertained.

In this group should be included Susac syndrome, ostensibly a microvasculopathy that causes characteristic changes in the white matter of the cerebral hemispheres, retinal vasculopathy, and progressive deafness as discussed in Chap. 34. The later onset and progressive nature of deafness in this and several other syndromes are distinguished from forms of congenital deafness that are typical of the group discussed below.

Hereditary Hearing Loss with Diseases of the Nervous System (See Table 15-1)

There are numerous conditions, mostly of childhood and including developmental abnormalities, in which congenital deafness accompanies disease of the peripheral or central nervous system. Those associated with mitochondrial encephalopathies have already been mentioned. The other main types with autosomal inheritance include the following:

1. *Hereditary hearing loss with epilepsy* The seizure disorder is mainly one of myoclonus. In one dominantly inherited form, photomyoclonus is associated with mental deterioration, hearing loss, and nephropathy (Hermann disease). In May-White disease, also inherited as an autosomal dominant trait, myoclonus and

ataxia accompany hearing loss. Congenital deafness and mild chronic epilepsy of recessive type have also been observed (Latham-Monro disease).

2. *Hereditary hearing loss and ataxia* Here Konigsmark was able to delineate 5 syndromes, the first 2 of which show a dominant pattern of heredity, the last 3 a recessive pattern: piebaldism, ataxia, and neural hearing loss (Telfer-Sugar-Jaeger syndrome); hearing loss, hyperuricemia, and ataxia (Rosenberg-Bergstrom syndrome); ataxia and progressive hearing loss (Lichtenstein-Knorr syndrome); ataxia, hypogonadism, mental deficiency, and hearing loss (Richards-Rundle syndrome); ataxia, mental retardation, hearing loss, and pigmentary changes in the skin (Jeune-Tommasi syndrome).
3. *Hereditary hearing loss and other neurologic syndromes* These include dominantly inherited sensory radicular neuropathy (Denny-Brown); progressive polyneuropathy, kyphoscoliosis, skin atrophy, eye defects (myopia, cataracts, atypical retinitis pigmentosa), bone cysts, and osteoporosis (Flynn-Aird syndrome); chronic polyneuropathy and nephritis (Lemieux-Neemeh syndrome); congenital pain asymbolia and auditory imperception (Osuntokun syndrome); and bulbopontine paralysis (facial weakness, dysarthria, dysphagia, and atrophy of the tongue with fasciculations) with progressive neural hearing loss. The onset of the last syndrome occurs at 10 to 35 years of age; the pattern of inheritance is autosomal recessive. The disease progresses to death. It resembles the progressive hereditary bulbar paralysis of Fazio-Londe except for the progressive deafness and loss of vestibular responses. Regrettably, in most of these syndromes, there are no data regarding labyrinthine function.

The details of these many syndromes are contained in Konigsmark's review, of course, in the era before the genetic underpinnings of these diseases were accessible. The main syndromes are listed in Table 15-1 and are summarized above so as to increase awareness of the large number of hereditary-degenerative neurologic diseases for which the clue is provided by the detection of impaired hearing and labyrinthine functions.

References

Abele M, Bûrk K, Schöls L, et al: The aetiology of sporadic adult-onset ataxia. *Brain* 125:961, 2002.

AD 2000 Collaborative Group: Long-term donepezil treatment in 565 patients with Alzheimer's disease (AD2000): Randomised double-blind trial. *Lancet* 363:2105, 2004.

Adams RD, van Bogaert L, van der Eecken H: Striato-nigral degeneration. *J Neuropathol Exp Neurol* 23:584, 1964.

Albert MS, Butters N, Brandt J: Patterns of remote memory in amnesic and demented patients. *Arch Neurol* 38:495, 1981.

Allen N, Knopp W: Hereditary parkinsonism-dystonia with sustained control by L-dopa and anticholinergic medication, in Eldridge R, Fahn S (eds): *Advances in Neurology*. Vol 14: Dystonia. New York, Raven Press, 1976, pp 201–215.

Alzheimer A: Uber eine eigenartige Erkrankung der Hirnrinde. *Allg Z Psychiatr* 64:146, 1907.

Alzheimer A: Uber eigenartige Krankheitsfalle des spateren Alters. *Z Gesamte Neurol Psychiatr* 4:356, 1911.

Anderson JM, Hubbard BM: Definition of Alzheimer disease. *Lancet* 1:408, 1985.

Andersen PM, Al-Chalabi A: Clinical genetics of amyotrophic lateral sclerosis: What do we really know? *Nature Rev Neurol* 7:603, 2011.

Andrew J, Fowler CJ, Harrison MJ: Stereotaxic thalamotomy in 55 cases of dystonia. *Brain* 106:981, 1983.

Arriagada PV, Growdon JH, Hedley-Whyte ET, Hyman BT: Neurofibrillary tangles but not senile plaques parallel duration and severity of Alzheimer's disease. *Neurology* 42:631, 1992.

Bannister R, Oppenheimer DR: Degenerative diseases of the nervous system associated with autonomic failure. *Brain* 95:457, 1972.

Barbeau A: L-Dopa therapy in Parkinson's disease. *Canad Med Assoc J* 101:59, 1969.

Bateman RJ, Xiong C, Benzinger TLS, et al: Clinical and biomarker changes in dominantly inherited Alzheimer disease. *N Engl J Med* 367:367, 2012.

Bates G: Huntingtin aggregation and toxicity in Huntington's disease. *Lancet* 361:1642, 2003.

Beal MF, Richardson EP Jr: Primary lateral sclerosis: A case report. *Arch Neurol* 38:630, 1981.

Behr C: Die komplizierte, hereditar-familiare Optikusatrophie des Kindesalters: Ein bisher nicht beschriebener Symptomkomplex. *Klin Monatsbl Augenheilkd* 47(Pt 2):138, 1909.

Bensimon G, Lacomblez L, Meininger V: A controlled trial of riluzole in amyotrophic lateral sclerosis: ALS/Riluzole Study Group. *N Engl J Med* 330:585, 1994.

Bharucha NE, Bharucha EP, Bhabha SR: Machado-Joseph-Azorean disease in India. *Arch Neurol* 43:142, 1986.

Blackstone C: Cellular pathways of hereditary spastic paraplegia. *Ann Rev Neurosci* 35:25, 2012.

Bonduelle M: Amyotrophic lateral sclerosis, in Vinken RT, Bruyn GW (eds): *Handbook of Clinical Neurology*. Vol 29. Amsterdam, North Holland, 1975, pp 281–338.

Braak H, Del Tredici K: Nervous system pathology in sporadic Parkinson disease. *Neurology* 70:1916, 2008.

Bradley WG, Good P, Rasool CG, et al: Morphometric and biochemical studies of peripheral nerves in amyotrophic lateral sclerosis. *Ann Neurol* 14:267, 1983.

Brandt S: *Werdnig-Hoffmann's Infantile Progressive Muscular Atrophy*. Thesis: Vol 22. Copenhagen, Munksgaard, 1950.

Breedveld GJ, Percy AK, MacDonald ME, et al: Clinical and genetic heterogeneity in benign hereditary chorea. *Neurology* 59:579, 2002.

Brice A: Genetics of Parkinson's disease: LRRK2 on the rise. *Brain* 128:2760, 2005.

Britton JW, Uitti RJ, Ahlskog JE, et al: Hereditary late-onset chorea without significant dementia. *Neurology* 45:443, 1995.

Brown J, Lantos P, Stratton M, et al: Familial progressive supranuclear palsy. *J Neurol Neurosurg Psychiatry* 56:473, 1993.

Brun A, Passant U: Frontal lobe degeneration of non-Alzheimer type: Structural characteristics, diagnostic criteria, and relation to frontotemporal dementia. *Acta Neurol Scand* 168:28, 1996.

Brzustowicz LM, Lehner T, Castilla LH, et al: Genetic mapping of chronic childhood-onset spinal muscular atrophy to chromosome 5q11.2-13.3. *Nature* 344:540, 1990.

Burke RE, Fahn S, Marsden CD: Torsion dystonia: A double-blind, prospective trial of high-dosage trihexyphenidyl. *Neurology* 36:160, 1986.

Burkhardt CR, Filley CM, Kleinschmidt-Demasters BK, et al: Diffuse Lewy body disease and progressive dementia. *Neurology* 38:1520, 1988.

Burns JM, Galvin JE, Roed CM, et al: The pathology of the substantia nigra in Alzheimer disease with extrapyramidal signs. *Neurology* 64:1397, 2005.

Byers RK, Banker BQ: Infantile muscular atrophy. *Arch Neurol* 5:140, 1961.

Byers RK, Gilles FH, Fung C: Huntington's disease in children: Neuropathologic study of four cases. *Neurology* 23:561, 1973.

Byrne EJ, Lennox G, Lowe J, Godwin-Austen RB: Diffuse Lewy body disease: Clinical features in 15 cases. *J Neurol Neurosurg Psychiatry* 52:709, 1989.

Caekebeke JFV, Jennekens-Schinkel A, van der Linden ME, et al: The interpretation of dysprosody in patients with Parkinson's disease. *J Neurol Neurosurg Psychiatry* 54:145, 1991.

Campuzano V, Montermini L, Moltò MD, et al: Friedreich's ataxia: Autosomal recessive disease caused by an intronic GAA triplet repeat expansion. *Science* 271:1423, 1996.

Cancel G, Abbas N, Stevanin G, et al: Marked phenotypic heterogeneity associated with expansion of a CAG repeat sequence at the spinocerebellar ataxia/3 Machado-Joseph disease locus. *Am J Hum Genet* 57:809, 1995.

Carroll WM, Mastaglia FL: Leber's optic neuropathy. *Brain* 102:559, 1979.

Caselli RN, Jack CR, Petersen RC, et al: Asymmetric cortical degenerative syndromes: Clinical and radiologic correlations. *Neurology* 42:1462, 1992.

Cedarbaum JM, Gandy SE, McDowell FH: "Early" initiation of levodopa treatment does not promote the development of motor response fluctuations, dyskinesias, or dementia in Parkinson's disease. *Neurology* 41:622, 1991.

Chase TN, Foster NL, Mansi L: Alzheimer's disease and the parietal lobe. *Lancet* 2:225, 1983.

Chawluk JB, Mesulam M-M, Hurtig H, et al: Slowly progressive aphasia without generalized dementia: Studies with positron emission tomography. *Ann Neurol* 19:68, 1986.

Chin SS-M, Goldman JE: Glial inclusions in CNS degenerative diseases. *J Neuropathol Exp Neurol* 55:499, 1996.

Chio A, Benzi G, Dossena M, et al: Severely increased risk of amyotrophic lateral sclerosis among Italian professional football players. *Brain* 128:472, 2005.

Chio A, Brignolio F, Leone M, et al: A survival analysis of 155 cases of progressive muscular atrophy. *Acta Neurol Scand* 72:407, 1985.

Clarke CE, Guttman M: Dopamine agonist monotherapy in Parkinson's disease. *Lancet* 360:1767, 2002.

Cobb JL, Wolf PA, Au R, et al: The effect of education on the incidence of dementia and Alzheimer's disease in the Framingham study. *Neurology* 45:1707, 1995.

Cohan SL, Kattah JC, Limaye SR: Familial tapetoretinal degeneration and epilepsy. *Arch Neurol* 36:544, 1979.

Cohen J, Low P, Feeley R: Somatic and autonomic function in progressive autonomic failure and multiple system atrophy. *Ann Neurol* 22:692, 1987.

Colosimo C, Albanese A, Hughes AJ, et al: Some specific clinical features differentiate multiple system atrophy (striatonigral variety) from Parkinson's disease. *Arch Neurol* 52:294, 1995.

Cooper IS: 20-year follow-up study of the neurosurgical treatment of dystonia musculorum deformans, in Eldridge R, Fahn S (eds): *Advances in Neurology*. Vol 14: Dystonia. New York, Raven Press, 1976, pp 423–453.

Crane PK, Walker R, Hubbard RA, et al: Glucose levels and risk of dementia. 369:540, 2013.

Creutzfeldt HG: Uber eine eigenartige herdformige Erkrankung des Zentralnervensystems. *Z Gesamte Neurol Psychiatr* 57:1, 1920.

Cross HE, McKusick VA: The mast syndrome. *Arch Neurol* 16:1, 1967.

Cudkowicz ME, McKenna-Yasek D, Chen C, et al: Limited corticospinal tract involvement in amyotrophic lateral sclerosis subjects with the A4V mutation in the copper/zinc superoxide dismutase gene. *Ann Neurol* 43:703, 1998.

Curtis AR, Fey C, Morris CM, et al: Mutation in the gene encoding ferritin light polypeptide causes dominant adult-onset basal ganglia disease. *Nat Genet* 28:350, 2001.

Dabby R, Lange DJ, Trojaborg W, et al: Inclusion body myositis mimicking motor neuron disease. *Arch Neurol* 58:1253, 2001.

Daniele A, Moro E, Bentivoglio AR: Zolpidem in progressive supra-nuclear palsy. *N Engl J Med* 341:543, 1999.

Davenport CB: Huntington's chorea in relation to heredity and eugenics. *Proc Natl Acad Sci U S A* 1:283, 1915.

de Bie RAM, de Haan RJ, Nijssen PCG, et al: Unilateral pallidotomy in Parkinson's disease: A randomized, single-blind multicentre trial. *Lancet* 354:1665, 1999.

Deep-Brain Stimulation for Parkinson's Disease Group: Deep-brain stimulation of the subthalamic nucleus or the pars interna of the globus pallidus in Parkinson's disease. *N Engl J Med* 345:956, 2001.

Déjérine J, André-Thomas: L'atrophie olivo-ponto-cérébélleuse. *Nouv Icon Salpét* 13:330, 1900.

DeJong RN: The history of Huntington's chorea in the United States of America, in Barbeau A, Klawans HL, Paulson GW, et al (eds): *Advances in Neurology*. Vol 1: Huntington's Chorea, 1872–1972. New York, Raven Press, 1973, pp 19–27.

DeKosky ST, Scheff SW: Synapse loss in frontal cortex biopsies in Alzheimer's disease: Correlation with cognitive severity. *Ann Neurol* 27:457, 1990.

Deonna T: DOPA-sensitive progressive dystonia of childhood with fluctuations of symptoms—Segawa's syndrome and possible variants. *Neuropediatrics* 17:81, 1986.

Deuschl G, Schade-Brittinger C, Krack P, et al: A randomized trial of deep-brain stimulation for Parkinson disease. *N Engl J Med* 355:896, 2006.

de Yébenes JG, Sarasa JL, Daniel SE, Lees AJ: Familial progressive supranuclear palsy. *Brain* 118:1095, 1995.

Diamond SG, Markham CH, Hoehn MM, et al: Multi-center study of Parkinson mortality with early versus late dopa treatment. *Ann Neurol* 22:8, 1987.

Doody RS, Raman R, Farlow M, et al: A phase 3 trial of semagacestat for treatment of Alzheimer's disease. *N Engl J Med* 369:341, 2013.

Doody RS, Thomas RG, Farlow M, et al: Phase 3 trials of solanezumab for treatment of mild to moderate Alzheimer's disease. *N Engl J Med*, 370:311, 2014.

Dubois B, Slachevsky A, Pillon B, et al: "Applause sign" helps to discriminate PSP from FTD and PD. *Neurology* 64:2132, 2005.

Dunlap CB: Pathologic changes in Huntington's chorea, with special reference to corpus striatum. *Arch Neurol Psychiatry* 18:867, 1927.

Dunnett SB, Björklund A: Prospects for the new restorative and neuroprotective treatments in Parkinson's disease. *Nature* 399 (Suppl 24):A32, 1999.

Dürr A, Cossee M, Agid Y, et al: Clinical and genetic abnormalities in patients with Friedreich's ataxia. *N Engl J Med* 335:1169, 1996.

Elias WJ, Huss D, Tiffini Voss NCS, et al: A pilot trial of focused ultrasound for essential tremor. *N Engl J Med* 369:640, 2013.

Emery AEH: The nosology of progressive muscular atrophy. *J Med Genet* 8:481, 1971.
Farmer TW, Wingfield MS, Lynch SA, et al: Ataxia, chorea, seizures, and dementia. *Arch Neurol* 46:774, 1989.
Farrer LA, Conneally M: Predictability of phenotype in Huntington's disease. *Arch Neurol* 44:109, 1987.
Feany MD, Dickson DW: Widespread cytoskeletal pathology characterizes corticobasal degeneration. *Am J Pathol* 146:1388, 1995.
Fearnley JM, Revesz T, Brooks DJ, et al: Diffuse Lewy body disease presenting with a supranuclear gaze palsy. *J Neurol Neurosurg Psychiatry* 54:159, 1991.
Ferrer I, Santpere G, van Leeuwen FW: Argyrophilic grain disease. *Brain* 131, 1416, 2008.
Figlewicz DA, Bird TD: "Pure" hereditary spastic paraplegias: The story becomes complicated. *Neurology* 53:5, 1999.
Figlewicz DA, Krizus A, Martolini MG, et al: Variants of the heavy neurofilament subunit are associated with the development of amyotrophic lateral sclerosis. *Hum Mol Genet* 3:1757, 1994.
Filla A, Moss AJ: Idebenone for treatment of Friedreich's ataxia. *Neurology* 60:1569, 2003.
Fink JK: Hereditary spastic paraplegia: Clinico-pathologic features and emerging molecular mechanisms. *Acta Neuropathol* 126:307, 2013.
Finlayson MH, Guberman A, Martin JB: Cerebral lesions in familial amyotrophic lateral sclerosis and dementia. *Acta Neuropathol* 26:237, 1973.
Fisher CM: Pure spastic paralysis of corticospinal origin. *Can J Neurol Sci* 4:251, 1977.
Flatau E, Sterling W: Progressiver Torsionsspasmus bei Kindern. *Z Gesamte Neurol Psychiatr* 7:586, 1911.
Follett KA, Weaver FM, Stern M, et al: Pallidal versus subthalamic deep-brain stimulation for Parkinson's disease. *N Engl J Med* 362:2077, 2010.
Fowler HL: Machado-Joseph-Azorean disease: A ten-year study. *Arch Neurol* 41:921, 1984.
Freed CR, Greene PE, Breeze RE, et al: Transplantation of embryonic dopamine neurons for severe Parkinson's disease. *N Engl J Med* 344:710, 2001.
Gearing M, Olson DA, Wattis RL, Mirra S: Progressive supranuclear palsy: Neuropathologic and clinical heterogeneity. *Neurology* 44:1015, 1994.
Gilbert JJ, Kish SJ, Chang LJ, et al: Dementia, parkinsonism, and motor neuron disease: Neurochemical and neuropathological correlates. *Ann Neurol* 24:688, 1988.
Gilliam TC, Brzustowicz LM, Castilla LH, et al: Genetic homogeneity between acute and chronic forms of spinal muscular atrophy. *Nature* 345:823, 1990.
Gilman S, Little R, Johanns J, et al: Evolution of sporadic olivopontocerebellar atrophy into multiple system atrophy. *Neurology* 55:527, 2000.
Gilman S, Romanul FCA: Hereditary dystonic paraplegia with amyotrophy and mental deficiency: Clinical and neuropathological characteristics, in Vinken PJ, Bruyn GW (eds): *Handbook of Clinical Neurology*. Vol 22. Amsterdam, North-Holland, 1975, pp 445–465.
Golbe LI, DiIorio G, Bonavita V, et al: A large kindred with autosomal dominant Parkinson's disease. *Ann Neurol* 27:276, 1990.
Goudsmit J, White BJ, Weitkamp LR, et al: Familial Alzheimer's disease in two kindreds of the same geographic and ethnic origin. *J Neurol Sci* 49:79, 1981.
Gout O, Fontaine B, Lyon-Caen O: Paraparesis spastique de l'adulte orientation diagnostiques. *Rev Neurol* 150:809, 1994.
Graham JG, Oppenheimer DR: Orthostatic hypotension and nicotine sensitivity in a case of multiple system atrophy. *J Neurol Neurosurg Psychiatry* 32:28, 1969.
Greco CM, Berman RF, Martin RM, et al: Neuropathology of fragile-X tremor/ataxia syndrome (FXTAS). *Brain* 129:243, 2006.
Greenamyre JT: Huntington's disease-making connections. *N Engl J Med* 356:518, 2007.
Greenfield JG: *The Spino-Cerebellar Degenerations*. Springfield, IL, Charles C Thomas, 1954.
Griggs RC, Moxley RT, LaFrance RA, et al: Hereditary paroxysmal ataxia: Response to acetazolamide. *Neurology* 28:1259, 1978.
Grimes DA, Lang AE, Bergeron CB: Dementia as the most common presentation of cortical-basal ganglionic degeneration. *Neurology* 53:1969, 1999.
Guerreiro R, Wojtas A, Bras J, et al: *TREM2* variants in Alzheimer's disease. *N Engl J Med* 368:117, 2013.
Gusella JF, Wexler NS, Conneally PM, et al: A polymorphic DNA marker, genetically linked to Huntington's disease. *Nature* 306:234, 1983.
Hadzi TC, Hendricks AE, Latourelle JC, et al: Assessment of cortical and striatal involvement in 523 Huntington brains. *Neurology* 79:1708, 2012.
Hagberg B, Kyllerman M, Steen G: Dyskinesia and dystonia in neurometabolic disorders. *Neuropadiatrie* 10:305, 1979.
Hakim AM, Mathieson G: Basis of dementia in Parkinson's disease. *Lancet* 2:729, 1978.
Hallett M, Khoshbin S: A physiological mechanism of bradykinesia. *Brain* 103:301, 1980.
Hardie RJ, Pullon HW, Harding AE, et al: Neuroacanthocytosis: A clinical, haematological, and pathological study of 19 cases. *Brain* 114(Pt 1A):13, 1991.
Harding AE: Early onset cerebellar ataxia with retained tendon reflexes: A clinical and genetic study of a disorder distinct from Friedreich's ataxia. *J Neurol Neurosurg Psychiatry* 44:503, 1981.
Harding AE: Clinical features and classification of inherited ataxias, in Harding AE, Deufel T (eds): *Inherited Ataxias*. New York, Raven Press, 1993, pp 1–14.
Hardy J: Alzheimer disease: Genetic evidence points to a single pathogenesis. *Ann Neurol* 54:143, 2003.
Hardy J, Selkoe DJ: The amyloid hypothesis of Alzheimer disease: Progress and problems on the road to therapeutics. *Science* 297:353, 2001.
Hayden MR, Martin WRW, Stoessi AJ, et al: Positron emission tomography in the early diagnosis of Huntington's disease. *Neurology* 36:888, 1986.
Hely MA, Reid WGJ, Halliday GM, et al: Diffuse Lewy body disease: Clinical features in nine cases without coexistent Alzheimer's disease. *J Neurol Neurosurg Psychiatry* 60:531, 1996.
Hirano A, Kurland LT, Krooth RS, Lessell S: Parkinsonism-dementia complex, an endemic disease on the Island of Guam: I. Clinical features. *Brain* 84:642, 1961.
Hirano A, Malamud M, Kurland LT: Parkinsonism-dementia complex on the Island of Guam: II. Pathological features. *Brain* 84:662, 1961.
Hirayama K, Tomonaga M, Kitano K, et al: Focal cervical poliopathy causing juvenile muscular atrophy of distal upper extremity: A pathological study. *J Neurol Neurosurg Psychiatry* 50:285, 1987.
Hoehn MM, Yahr MD: Parkinsonism: Onset, progression, and mortality. *Neurology* 17:427, 1967.
Hogan GW, Bauman ML: Familial spastic ataxia: Occurrence in childhood. *Neurology* 27:520, 1977.
Holmes GM: A form of familial degeneration of the cerebellum. *Brain* 30:466, 1907a.
Holmes GM: An attempt to classify cerebellar disease with a note on Marie's hereditary cerebellar ataxia. *Brain* 30:545, 1907b.
Hotson JR, Langston EB, Louis AA: The search for a physiologic marker of Machado-Joseph disease. *Neurology* 37:112, 1987.
Howard R, McShane R, Lindesay J, et al. Donepezil and memantine for moderate-to-severe Alzheimer's disease. *N Engl J Med* 366:893, 2012.

Hudson AJ: Amyotrophic lateral sclerosis and its associations with dementia, parkinsonism and other neurologic disorders. *Brain* 104:217, 1981.

Hughes AJ, Daniel SE, Kilford L, Less AJ: Accuracy of clinical diagnosis of idiopathic Parkinson's disease: A clinico-pathological study of 100 cases. *J Neurol Neurosurg Psychiatry* 55:181, 1992.

Hunker CJ, Abbs JH: Frequency of parkinsonian resting tremor in the lips, jaw, tongue, and index finger. *Mov Disord* 5:71, 1990.

Hunt JR: Dyssynergia cerebellaris progressiva: A chronic progressive form of cerebellar tremor. *Brain* 37:247, 1914.

Hunt JR: Progressive atrophy of the globus pallidus. *Brain* 40:58, 1917.

Hunt JR: Dyssynergia cerebellaris myoclonica—primary atrophy of the dentate system: A contribution to the pathology and symptomatology of the cerebellum. *Brain* 44:490, 1921.

Hunt JR: The striocerebellar tremor. *Arch Neurol Psychiatry* 8:664, 1922.

Huntington G: On chorea. *Med Surg Rep* 26:317, 1872.

Huntington Study Group: Tetrabenazine as antichorea therapy in Huntington disease. A randomized controlled trial. *Neurology* 66:366, 2006.

Hutton JT, Morris JL: Long-acting carbidopa-levodopa in the management of moderate and advanced Parkinson's disease. *Neurology* 42(Suppl 1):51, 1992.

Iizuka R, Hirayama K, Maehara K: Dentato-rubro-pallidoluysian atrophy: A clinico-pathological study. *J Neurol Neurosurg Psychiatry* 47:1288, 1984.

Ince PG, Evans J, Kropp M, et al: Corticospinal tract degeneration in the progressive muscular atrophy variant of ALS. *Neurology* 60:1252, 2003.

Jagust W: Untangling vascular dementia. *Lancet* 358:2097, 2001.

Jakob A: Uber eigenartige Erkrankungen des Zentralnervensystems mit bemerkenswertem anatomischen Befunde (Spastische Pseudosclerose-Encephalomyelopathie mit disseminierten Degenerationsherden). *Z Gesamte Neurol Psychiatr* 64:147, 1921.

Jakob A: Uber eine der multiplen Sklerose klinisch nahestehende Erkrankung des Zentralnervensystems (Spastische Pseudosklerose) mit bemerkenswertem anatomischen Befunde. *Med Klin* 17:382, 1921.

Jervis GA: Early senile dementia in mongoloid idiocy. *Am J Psychiatry* 105:102, 1948.

Joachim CL, Morris JH, Selkoe DJ: Clinically diagnosed Alzheimer disease: Autopsy results in 150 cases. *Ann Neurol* 24:50, 1988.

Johnson WG, Wigger J, Karp HR: Juvenile spinal muscular atrophy: A new hexosamine deficiency phenotype. *Ann Neurol* 11:11, 1982.

Jonsson T, Stefansson H., Steinberg S, et al: Variant of associated with the risk of Alzheimer's disease. *N Engl J Med* 368:107, 2013.

Kaeser HE: Scapuloperoneal muscular dystrophy. *Brain* 88:407, 1965.

Katzenschlager R, Head J, Schrag A, et al: Fourteen-year final report of the randomized PDRG-UK trial comparing three initial treatments in PD. *Neurology* 71:474, 2008.

Katzman R: Education and the prevalence of dementia and Alzheimer's disease. *Neurology* 43:13, 1993.

Kennedy WR, Alter M, Sung JH: Progressive proximal spinal and bulbar muscular atrophy of late onset: A sex-linked recessive trait. *Neurology* 18:617, 1968.

Kertesz A: Frontotemporal dementia and Pick's disease. *Ann Neurol* 54(Suppl 5): S3–S7, 2003.

Khan NL, Graham E, Critchley P, et al: Parkin disease: A phenotypic study of a large case series. *Brain* 126:1279, 2003.

Kiernan JA, Hudson AJ: Frontal lobe atrophy in motor neuron diseases. *Brain* 117:747, 1994.

Kirby R, Fowler C, Gosling J, Bannister R: Urethrovesical dysfunction in progressive autonomic failure with multiple system atrophy. *J Neurol Neurosurg Psychiatry* 49:554, 1986.

Kirshner HS, Tanridag O, Thurman L, Whetsell WO Jr: Progressive aphasia without dementia: Two cases with focal spongiform degeneration. *Ann Neurol* 22:527, 1987.

Kjellin KG: Hereditary spastic paraplegia and retinal degeneration (Kjellin syndrome and Barnard-Scholz syndrome), in Vinken PJ, Bruyn GW (eds): *Handbook of Clinical Neurology*. Vol 22. Amsterdam, North-Holland, 1975, pp 467–473.

Klawans HL: Hemiparkinsonism as a late complication of hemiatrophy: A new syndrome. *Neurology* 31:625, 1981.

Klein C, Brown R, Wenning G, et al: The "cold hands sign" in multiple system atrophy. *Mov Disord* 12:514, 1997.

Koeppen AH: The hereditary ataxias. *J Neuropathol Exp Neurol* 57:531, 1998.

Koller WC: Pharmacologic treatment of parkinsonian tremor. *Arch Neurol* 43:126. 1984.

Koller WC, Davenport J: Genetic testing in Huntington's disease. *Ann Neurol* 16:511, 1984.

Kolodny EH, Raghavan SS: G_{M2}-gangliosidosis hexosaminidase mutations not of the Tay-Sachs type produce unusual clinical variants. *Trends Neurosci* 6:16, 1983.

Konigsmark BW: Hereditary diseases of the nervous system with hearing loss, in Vinken PJ, Bruyn GW (eds): *Handbook of Clinical Neurology*. Vol 22. Amsterdam, North-Holland, 1975, pp 499–526.

Konigsmark BW, Weiner LP: The olivopontocerebellar atrophies: A review. *Medicine (Baltimore)* 49:227, 1970.

Kosaka K: Diffuse Lewy body disease in Japan. *J Neurol* 237:197, 1990.

Kugelberg E: Chronic proximal (pseudomyopathic) spinal muscular atrophy: Kugelberg-Welander syndrome, in Vinken PJ, Bruyn GW (eds): *Handbook of Clinical Neurology*. Vol 22. Amsterdam, North-Holland, 1975, pp 67–80.

Kugelberg E, Welander L: Heredofamilial juvenile muscular atrophy simulating muscular dystrophy. *Arch Neurol Psychiatry* 5:500, 1956.

Laitinen LV: Leksell's posteroventral pallidotomy in the treatment of Parkinson's disease. *J Neurosurg* 76:53, 1992.

Lance JW, Schwab RS, Peterson EA: Action tremor and the cogwheel phenomenon in Parkinson's disease. *Brain* 86:95, 1963.

Lang AE: The progression of Parkinson disease. A hypothesis. *Neurology* 68:948, 2007.

Lantos P: The definition of multiple system atrophy: A review of recent developments. *J Neuropathol Exp Neurol* 57:1099, 1998.

Lasker AG, Zee DS, Hain TC, et al: Saccades in Huntington's disease: Initiation defects and distractibility. *Neurology* 37:364, 1987.

La Spada AR, Wilson EM, Lubahn DB: Androgen receptor mutation in X-linked spinal and bulbar muscular atrophy. *Nature* 352:77, 1991.

Leber T: Ueber hereditare und congenital angelegte Sehnervenleiden. *Graefes Arch Clin Exp Ophthalmol* 17:249, 1871.

Lee J-M, Ramos EM, Lee- J-H, et al: CAG repeat expansion in Huntingon disease determines age at onset in a fully dominant fashion. *Neurology* 78:690, 2012.

Lee SE, Rabinovici GD, Mayo MC, et al: Clinicopathological correlations in corticobasal degeneration. *Ann Neurol* 70:327, 2011.

Leenders KL, Frackowiak SJ, Lees AJ: Steele-Richardson-Olszewski syndrome. *Brain* 111:615, 1988.

Lees AJ: Trauma and Parkinson's disease. *Rev Neurol* 153:541, 1997.

Leigh RJ, Newman SA, Folstein SE, et al: Abnormal ocular motor control in Huntington's disease. *Neurology* 33:1268, 1983.

Lennox G: Lewy body dementia. *Baillieres Clin Neurol* 1:653, 1993.

Leverenz J, Sumi SM: Parkinson's disease in patients with Alzheimer's disease. *Arch Neurol* 43:662, 1986.

Levy-Lahad E, Wasco W, Poorkaj P, et al: Candidate gene for the chromosome familial Alzheimer's disease locus. *Science* 269:973, 1995.

LeWitt PA, Lyons KE, Pahwa R, et al: Advanced Parkinson disease treated with rotigotine transdermal system. PREFER study. *Neurology* 68:1262, 2007.

Li F, Harmer P, Fitzgerald K, et al: Tai chi and postural stability in patients with Parkinson's disease. *N Engl J Med* 366:511, 2012.

Li G, Silverman JM, Smith CJ, et al: Age at onset and familial risk in Alzheimer's disease. *Am J Psychiatry* 152:424, 1995.

Limousin P, Krack P, Pollak P, et al: Electrical stimulation of the subthalamic nucleus in advanced Parkinson's disease. *N Engl J Med* 339:1105, 1998.

Linn RT, Wolf PA, Bachman DL: Preclinical phase of Alzheimer's disease. *Arch Neurol* 52:485, 1995.

Lippa CF, Cohen R, Smith TW, Drachman DA: Primary progressive aphasia with focal neuronal achromasia. *Neurology* 41:882, 1991.

Little BW, Brown PW, Rodgers-Johnson P, et al: Familial myoclonic dementia masquerading as Creutzfeldt-Jakob disease. *Ann Neurol* 20:231, 1986.

Lohmann E, Periquet M, Bonifati V, et al: How much phenotypic variation can be attributed to parkin genotype? *Ann Neurol* 54:176, 2003.

Lomas DA, Carrell RW: Serpinopathies and the conformational dementias. *Nat Rev Genet* 3:759, 2002.

Louis-Bar D, van Bogaert L: Sur la dyssynergie cérébelleuse myoclonique (Hunt). *Monatsschr Psychiatr Neurol* 113:215, 1947.

Maddalena A, Papassotiropoulos A, Muller-Tillmanns B, et al: Biochemical diagnosis of Alzheimer disease by measuring cerebrospinal fluid ratio of phosphorylated tau protein to beta-amyloid peptide42. *Arch Neurol* 60:1202, 2003.

Margolis RL, O'Hearn E, Rosenblatt A, et al: A disorder similar to Huntington's disease is associated with a novel CAG repeat expansion. *Ann Neurol* 50:373, 2001.

Marie P: Sur l'hérédo-ataxie cérébelleuse. *Semin Med* 13:444, 1893.

Marie P, Foix C, Alajouanine T: De l'atrophie cérébelleuse tardive à prédominance corticale. *Rev Neurol* 38:849, 1082, 1922.

Marsden CD: Parkinson's disease. *J Neurol Neurosurg Psychiatry* 57:672, 1994.

Martilla PJ, Rinne UK: Disability and progression in Parkinson's disease. *Acta Neurol Scand* 56:159, 1967.

Mata M, Dorvovini-Zis K, Wilson M, Young AB: New form of familial Parkinson dementia syndrome: Clinical and pathologic findings. *Neurology* 33:1439, 1983.

Mayeux R, Chen J, Mirabello E, et al: An estimate of the incidence of dementia in idiopathic Parkinson's disease. *Neurology* 40:1513, 1990.

McGeer PL, McGeer EG, Suzuki J, et al: Aging, Alzheimer disease and the cholinergic system of the basal forebrain. *Neurology* 34:741, 1984.

McKeith I, Del Ser T, Spano P, et al: Efficacy of rivastigmine in dementia with Lewy bodies: A randomised, double-blind, placebo-controlled international study. *Lancet* 356:2031, 2000.

McKeith LG, Dickson DW, Low J, et al: Diagnosis and management of dementia with Lewy bodies: Third report of the DLB Consortium. *Neurology* 65:1992, 2005.

McKhann G, Drachman D, Folstein M, et al: Clinical diagnosis of Alzheimer's disease. *Neurology* 34:939, 1984.

McKhann G, Knopman DS, Chertkow H, et al: The diagnosis of dementia due to Alzheimer's disease: Recommendations from the National Institute on Aging-Alzheimer's Association workgroups on diagnostic guidelines for Alzheimer's disease. *Alzheimers Dement* 7:263, 2011.

McMonagle P, Deering F, Berliner Y, et al: The cognitive profile of posterior cortical atrophy. *Neurology* 66:331, 2006.

McNamara MJ, Gomez-Isla T, Hyman BT: Apolipoprotein E genotype and deposits of Abeta40 and Abeta42 in Alzheimer disease. *Arch Neurol* 55:1001, 1998.

McNaught K, Kapustin A, Jackson T, et al: Brainstem pathology in DYT1 primary torsion dystonia. *Neurology* 56:540, 2004.

McShane MA, Boyd S, Harding B, et al: Progressive bulbar paralysis of childhood: A reappraisal of Fazio-Londe disease. *Brain* 115:1889, 1992.

Mendez MF, Adams NL, Lewandowski KS: Neurobehavioral changes associated with caudate lesions. *Neurology* 39:349, 1989.

Mendez MF, Mendez MA, Martin R, et al: Complex visual disturbances in Alzheimer's disease. *Neurology* 40:439, 1990.

Mesulam MM: Primary progressive aphasia—a language-based dementia. *N Engl J Med* 349:1535, 2003.

Mesulam MM: Slowly progressive aphasia without generalized dementia. *Ann Neurol* 11:592, 1982.

Miller RG, Jackson CE, Kasarskis EJ, et al: Practice parameter update: The care of the patient with amyotrophic lateral sclerosis: Multidisciplinary care, symptom management, and cognitive/behavioral impairment (an evidence-based review): Report of the Quality Standards Subcommittee of the American Academy of Neurology. *Neurology* 73:1227, 2009a.

Miller RG, Jackson CE, Kasarskis EJ, et al: Practice parameter update: The care of the patient with amyotrophic lateral sclerosis: Drug, nutritional, and respiratory therapies (an evidence-based review): Report of the Quality Standards Subcommittee of the American Academy of Neurology. *Neurology* 73:1218, 2009b.

Mitsuyama Y: Presenile dementia with motor neuron disease in Japan: Clinico-pathological review of 26 cases. *J Neurol Neurosurg Psychiatry* 47:953, 1984.

Mollaret P: *La Maladie de Friedreich*. Paris, Legrand, 1929.

Moreno Martinez JM, Garcia de la Rocha ML, Martin Araquez A: Monomelic segmental amyotrophy: A Spanish case involving the leg. *Rev Neurol (Paris)* 146:443, 1990.

Mulder DW, Kurland LT, Offord KP, Beard CM: Familial adult motor neuron disease: Amyotrophic lateral sclerosis. *Neurology* 36:511, 1986.

Multiple-System Atrophy Research Collaboration: Mutations in *COQ2* in familial and sporadic multiple-system atrophy. *N Engl J Med* 369:233, 2013.

Munsat TL, Skerry L, Korf B, et al: Phenotypic heterogeneity of spinal muscular atrophy mapping to chromosome 5q11.2-13.3 (SMA 5q). *Neurology* 40:1831, 1990.

Murata Y, Yamaguchi S, Kawakami H: Characteristic magnetic resonance imaging findings in Machado-Joseph disease. *Arch Neurol* 55:33, 1998.

Nakano KK, Dawson DM, Spence A: Machado disease: A hereditary ataxia in Portuguese emigrants to Massachusetts. *Neurology* 22:49, 1972.

Neary D: Non-Alzheimer's disease forms of cerebral atrophy. *J Neurol Neurosurg Psychiatry* 53:929, 1990.

Neary D, Snowden JS, Bowden DM: Neuropsychological syndromes in presenile dementia due to cerebral atrophy. *J Neurol Neurosurg Psychiatry* 49:163, 1986.

Nee LE, Eldridge R, Sunderland T, et al: Dementia of the Alzheimer type: Clinical and family study of 22 twin pairs. *Neurology* 37:359, 1987.

Németh AH: The genetics of primary dystonias and related disorders. *Brain* 125:695, 2002.

Nielsen JE, Krabbe K, Jennum P, et al: Autosomal dominant pure spastic paraplegia: A clinical, paraclinical and genetic study. *J Neurol Neurosurg Psychiatry* 64:61, 1998.

Nielsen SL: Striatonigral degeneration disputed in familial disorder. *Neurology* 27:306, 1977.

Nikoskelainen E, Savontaus ML, Wanne OP, et al: Leber's hereditary optic neuroretinopathy—a maternally inherited disease: A genealogic study in four pedigrees. *Arch Ophthalmol* 105:665, 1987.

Nygaard TG, Duvoisin RC: Hereditary dystonia-parkinsonism syndrome of juvenile onset. *Neurology* 36:1424, 1986.

Nygaard TG, Wilhelmsen KC, Risch NJ, et al: Linkage mapping of dopa-responsive dystonia (DRD) to chromosome 14q. *Nat Genet* 5:386, 1993.

Oba H, Yagashita A, Terada H, et al: New and reliable MRI diagnosis for progressive supranuclear palsy. *Neurology* 64:2050, 2005.

Okazaki H, Lipkin LE, Aronson SM: Diffuse intracytoplasmic ganglionic inclusions (Lewy type) associated with progressive dementia and quadriparesis in flexion. *J Neuropathol Exp Neurol* 20:237, 1961.

Okun MS: Deep-brain stimulation for Parkinson's disease. *N Engl J Med* 367:1529, 2012.

Olanow CW, Rascol O, Hauser R, et al: A double-blind delayed start trial of rasagiline in Parkinson's disease. *N Engl J Med* 361:1268, 2009.

Oppenheim H: *Textbook of Nervous Diseases* (A. Bruce, transl). Edinburgh, Schulze, 1911, p 512.

Orgogozo JM, Gilman S, Dartigues JF, et al: Subacute meningoencephalitis in a subset of patients with AD after Abeta42 immunization. *Neurology* 61:46, 2003.

Pakkenberg B, Moller A, Gundersen HJG, et al: The absolute number of nerve cells in substantia nigra in normal subjects and in patients with Parkinson's disease estimated with an unbiased stereological method. *J Neurol Neurosurg Psychiatry* 54:30, 1991.

Papp MI, Kahn JE, Lantos PL: Glial cytoplasmic inclusions in the CNS of patients with multiple system atrophy (striatonigral degeneration, olivopontocerebellar atrophy and Shy-Drager syndrome). *J Neurol Sci* 94:79, 1989.

Paradiso G, Micheli F, Taratuto AL, Parera IC: Familial bulbospinal neuronopathy with optic neuropathy: A distinct entity. *J Neurol Neurosurg Psychiatry* 61:196, 1996.

Parkkinen L, O'Sullivan SS, Kuoppamaki M, et al. Does levodopa accelerate the pathologic process in Parkinson disease brain? *Neurology* 77:1420, 2011.

Pearn J: Classification of spinal muscular atrophies. *Lancet* 1:919, 1980.

Perry RJ, Hodges JR: Attention and executive deficits in Alzheimer's disease. *Brain* 122:383, 1999.

Piccini P, Burn DJ, Ceravolo R, et al: The role of inheritance in sporadic Parkinson's disease: Evidence from a longitudinal study of dopaminergic function in twins. *Ann Neurol* 45:577, 1999.

Pick A: Uber die Beziehungen der senilen Hirnatrophie zur Aphasie. *Prager Med Wochenschr* 17:165, 1892.

Pierantozzi M, Pietroiosti A, Brusa L, et al: *Helicobacter pylori* eradication and L-dopa absorption in patients with PD and motor fluctuations. *Neurology* 66:1824, 2006.

Pillon B, Dubois B, Plaska A, Agid Y: Severity and specificity of cognitive impairment in Alzheimer's, Huntington's, and Parkinson's diseases and progressive supranuclear palsy. *Neurology* 41:634, 1991.

Pincus JH, Barry K: Influence of dietary protein on motor fluctuations in Parkinson's disease. *Arch Neurol* 44:270, 1987.

Polvikoski T, Sulkava R, Haltia M, et al: Apolipoprotein E, dementia, and cortical deposition of β-amyloid protein. *N Engl J Med* 333:1242, 1995.

Polymeropoulos MH, Lavedan C, Leroy E, et al: Mutation in the alpha-synuclein gene identified in families with Parkinson's disease. *Science* 276:2045, 1997.

Pringle CE, Hudson AS, Munoz DG, et al: Primary lateral sclerosis: Clinical features, neuropathology, and diagnostic criteria. *Brain* 115:495, 1992.

Probst A, Tolnay M: La maladie des grains argyrophiles: Une cause fréquente mais encore largement méconne de démence chez les personnes agées. *Rev Neurol* 158:155, 2002.

Quinn NP, Toone B, Lang AE, et al: Dopa dose-dependent sexual deviation. *Br J Psychiatry* 142:296, 1983.

Qureshi AI, Wilmot G, Dihenia B, et al: Motor neuron disease with Parkinsonism. *Arch Neurol* 53:987, 1996.

Rajput AH, Gibb WRG, Zhong XH, et al: Dopa-responsive dystonia: Pathological and biochemical observations in a case. *Ann Neurol* 35:396, 1994.

Rajput AH, Rozdilsky B: Dysautonomia in parkinsonism: A clinicopathologic study. *J Neurol Neurosurg Psychiatry* 39:1092, 1976.

Rampoldi L, Dobson-Stone C, Rubio JP, et al: A conserved sorting-associated protein is mutant in chorea-acanthocytosis. *Nat Genet* 28:119, 2001.

Rascol O, Brooks DJ, Korczyn AD, et al: A five-year study of the incidence of dyskinesias in patients with early Parkinson's disease who were treated with ropinirole or levodopa. *N Engl J Med* 342:1484, 2000.

Rascol O, Brooks DJ, Melamel E, et al: Rasagiline as an adjunct to levodopa in patients with Parkinson's disease and motor fluctuations: A randomized, double-blind, parallel-group trial. *Lancet* 365:947, 2005.

Rebeiz JJ, Kolodny EH, Richardson EP: Corticodentatonigral degeneration with neuronal achromasia. *Arch Neurol* 18:20, 1968.

Reisberg B, Doody R, Stoffler A, et al: Memantine in moderate-to-severe Alzheimer's disease. *N Engl J Med* 348:1333, 2003.

Renner JA, Burns JM, Hou CE, et al: Progressive posterior cortical dysfunction. *Neurology* 63:1175, 2004.

Richardson JC, Steele J, Olszewski J: Supranuclear ophthalmoplegia, pseudobulbar palsy, nuchal dystonia and dementia. *Trans Am Neurol Assoc* 88:25, 1963.

Rifal Z, Klitzke M, Tawil R, et al: Dementia of adult polyglucosan body disease. *Arch Neurol* 51:90, 1994.

Riley DE, Lang AE, Lewis A, et al: Cortical-basal ganglionic degeneration. *Neurology* 40:1203, 1990.

Riordan-Eva P, Sanders MD, Govan GG, et al: The clinical features of Leber's hereditary optic neuropathy defined by the presence of a pathogenic mitochondrial DNA mutation. *Brain* 118:319, 1995.

Ritchie K, Lovestone S: The dementias. *Lancet* 360:1759, 2002.

Robitaille Y, Carpenter S, Karpati G, Dimauro S: A distinct form of adult polyglucosan body disease with massive involvement of central and peripheral neuronal processes and astrocytes. *Brain* 103:315, 1980.

Rojo A, Pernaute RS, Fontan A, et al: Clinical genetics of familial progressive supranuclear palsy. *Brain* 122:1233, 1999.

Romanul FCA, Fowler HL, Radvany J, et al: Azorean disease of the nervous system. *N Engl J Med* 296:1505, 1977.

Ropper AH: Seronegative, non-neoplastic acute cerebellar degeneration. *Neurology* 43:1602, 1993.

Rosen DR, Siddique T, Patterson D, et al: Mutations in Cu-Zn super-oxide dismutase gene are associated with familial amyotrophic lateral sclerosis. *Nature* 362:59, 1993.

Rosenberg RN: DNA-triplet repeats and neurologic disease. *N Engl J Med* 335:1222, 1996.

Rosenberg RN, Nyhan WL, Bay C, Shore P: Autosomal dominant striatonigral degeneration: A clinical, pathologic and biochemical study of a new genetic disorder. *Neurology* 26:703, 1976.

Roses AD: Apolipoprotein E gene typing in the differential diagnosis, not prediction, of Alzheimer's disease. *Ann Neurol* 38:6, 1995.

Roussy G, Levy G: Sept cas d'un maladie familiale particulaire. *Rev Neurol* 1:427, 1926.

Rusinick H, De Santi S, Frid D, et al: Regional brain atrophy rate predicts future cognitive decline: 6-year longitudinal MR imaging study of normal aging. *Radiology* 229:691, 2003.

Safe AF, Cooper S, Windsor ACM: Cerebellar ataxia in the elderly. *Proc R Soc Med* 85:449, 1992.

Sakai T, Antoku Y, Iwashita H, et al: Chorea-acanthocytosis: Abnormal composition of covalently bound fatty acids of erythrocyte membrane proteins. *Ann Neurol* 29:664, 1991.

Sakai T, Ohta M, Ishino H: Joseph disease in a non-Portuguese family. *Neurology* 33:74, 1983.

Sasaki H, Muramoto A, Kanazawa I, et al: Regional distribution of amino acid transmitters in postmortem brains of presenile and senile dementia of Alzheimer type. *Ann Neurol* 19:263, 1986.

Savva GM, Wharton SB, Ince PC, et al: Age, neuropathology, and dementia. *N Engl J Med* 360:2302, 2009.
Schaumburg HH, Suzuki K: Non-specific familial presenile dementia. *J Neurol Neurosurg Psychiatry* 31:479, 1968.
Schmitt HP, Esmer W, Heimes C: Familial occurrence of amyotrophic lateral sclerosis, parkinsonism, and dementia. *Ann Neurol* 16:642, 1984.
Schneider LS, Tarlot PN, Dagerman KS, et al: Effectiveness of atypical antipsychotic drugs in patients with Alzheimer's disease. *N Engl J Med* 355:1525, 2006.
Schoenfeld M, Myers RH, Cupples LA, et al: Increased rate of suicide among patients with Huntington's disease. *J Neurol Neurosurg Psychiatry* 47:1283, 1984.
Schoonenboom NSM, Reesink FE, Verwey NA, et al: Cerebrospinal fluid markers for differential dementia diagnosis in a large memory clinic cohort. *Neurology* 78:47, 2012.
Schuepbach WMM, Rau J, Knudsen K, et al: Neurostimulation for Parkinson's disease with early motor complications. *N Engl J Med* 368:610, 2013.
Scribanu N, Kennedy C: Familial syndrome with dystonia, neural deafness and possible intellectual impairment: Clinical course and pathologic features, in Eldridge R, Fahn S (eds): *Advances in Neurology*. Vol 14: Dystonia. New York, Raven Press, 1976, pp 235–245.
Segawa M, Hosaka A, Miyagawa F, et al: Hereditary progressive dystonia with marked diurnal fluctuation. *Adv Neurol* 14:215, 1976.
Segawa M, Nomura Y, Tanaka S, et al: Hereditary progressive dystonia with marked diurnal fluctuation: Consideration on its pathophysiology based on the characteristics of clinical and polysomnographical findings. *Adv Neurol* 50:367, 1988.
Sherrington R, Rogaev EI, Liang Y, et al: Cloning of a gene bearing missense imitations in early-onset familial Alzheimer's disease. *Nature* 375:754, 1995.
Shults CW, Oakes D, Kieburtz K, et al: Effects of coenzyme Q10 in early Parkinson disease. Evidence of slowing of functional decline. *Arch Neurol* 59:1541, 2002.
Sidransky E, Nalls MA, Aasly JO, et al: Multicenter analysis if glucocerbroside mutations in Parkinson's disease. *N Engl J Med* 361:1651, 2009.
Silverman JM, Raiford K, Edland S, et al: The consortium to establish a registry for Alzheimer's disease (CERAD). *Neurology* 44:1253, 1994.
Singleton AB, Farrar M, Johnson J, et al: alpha-Synuclein locus triplication causes Parkinson's disease. *Science* 302:841, 2003.
Skre H: Hereditary spastic paraplegia in western Norway. *Clin Genet* 6:165, 1974.
Smith JK: Dentatorubropallidoluysian atrophy, in Vinken PJ, Bruyn GW (eds): *Handbook of Clinical Neurology*. Vol 21. Amsterdam, North-Holland, 1975, pp 519–534.
Snowden DA, Kemper SJ, Mortimer JA, et al: Linguistic ability in early life and cognitive function and Alzheimer's disease in late life: Findings from the Nun study. *JAMA* 275:528, 1996.
Snowden JS, Neary D, Mann DMA: Progressive language disorder due to lobar atrophy. *Ann Neurol* 31:174, 1992.
Snyder SH, D'Amato RJ: MPTP: A neurotoxin relevant to the pathophysiology of Parkinson's disease. *Neurology* 36:250, 1986.
Spatz H: Die Systematischen Atrophien. *Arch Psychiatry* 108:1, 1938.
Spencer DD, Robbins RJ, Naftolin F, et al: Unilateral transplantation of human fetal mesencephalic tissue into the caudate nucleus of patients with Parkinson's disease. *N Engl J Med* 327:1541, 1992.
Spielmeyer W: *Histopathologie des Nervensystems*. Berlin, Springer-Verlag, 1922, pp 223–229.
Stargardt K: Uber familiare, progressive Degeneration in der Maculagegend. *Graefes Arch Clin Exp Ophthalmol* 71:534, 1909.
Steele JC: Progressive supranuclear palsy. *Brain* 95:693, 1972.
St. George-Hyslop PH, Tanzi RE, Polinsky RJ, et al: The genetic defect causing familial Alzheimer's disease maps on chromosome 21. *Science* 235:885, 1987.
Strittmatter WJ, Saunders AM, Schmechel D, et al: Apolipoprotein E: High avidity binding to β-amyloid and increased frequency of type 4 allele in late-onset familial Alzheimer disease. *Proc Natl Acad Sci U S A* 90:1977, 1993.
Tandan R, Taylor R, Adesina A, et al: Benign autosomal dominant syndrome of neuronal Charcot-Marie-Tooth disease, ptosis, parkinsonism, and dementia. *Neurology* 40:773, 1990.
Tang-Wai DF, Graff-Radford NR, Boeve BF, et al: Clinical, genetic, and neuropathologic characteristics of posterior cortical atrophy. *Neurology* 63:1168, 2004.
Tasker RR, Doorly T, Yamashiro K: Thalamotomy in generalized dystonia. *Adv Neurol* 50:615, 1988.
Terry RD: The pathogenesis of Alzheimer disease: An alternative to the amyloid hypothesis. *J Neuropathol Exp Neurol* 55:1023, 1996.
Terry RD, Katzman R: Senile dementia of the Alzheimer type. *Ann Neurol* 14:497, 1983.
The Parkinson Study Group: Effect of deprenyl on the progression of disability in early Parkinson disease. *N Engl J Med* 321:1364, 1989.
The Parkinson Study Group: Levodopa and the progression of Parkinson's disease. *N Engl J Med* 351;2498, 2004.
Tierney MC, Fisher RH, Lewis AJ, et al: The NINCDS-ADRDA Work Group criteria for the clinical diagnosis of probable Alzheimer's disease: A clinicopathological study of 57 cases. *Neurology* 38:359, 1988.
Tierney MC, Snow WG, Reid DW, et al: Psychometric differentiation of dementia. *Arch Neurol* 44:720, 1987.
Troost BT, Daroff RB: The ocular motor defects in progressive supra-nuclear palsy. *Ann Neurol* 2:397, 1977.
Trouillas P, Serratrice G, Laplane D, et al: Levorotatory form of 5-hydroxytryptophan in Friedreich's ataxia. *Arch Neurol* 52:456, 1995.
Uhl JA, Javitch JA, Snyder SN: Normal MPTP binding in Parkinson substantia nigra. *Lancet* 1:956, 1985.
Valente EM, Abou-Sleiman PM, Caputo V, et al: Hereditary early-onset Parkinson's disease caused by mutations in PINK1. *Science* 304:1158, 2004.
van Bogaert L, van Maere M, Desmedt E: Sur les formes familiales precoces de la maladie d'Alzheimer. *Monatsschr Psychiatr Neurol* 102:249, 1940.
van Dijk JG, van der Velde EA, Roos RAC, et al: Juvenile Huntington's disease. *Hum Genet* 73:235, 1986.
van Mansvelt J: *Pick's disease: A syndrome of lobar cerebral atrophy: Clinicoanatomical and histopathological types*. Thesis, Utrecht, 1954.
Verghese L, Lipton RB, Katz MJ, et al: Leisure activities and the risk of dementia in the elderly. *N Engl J Med* 348:2508, 2003.
Verhagen Metman L, Del Dotto P, van den Munckhof P, et al: Amantadine as treatment for dyskinesias and motor fluctuations in Parkinson's disease. *Neurology* 50:1323, 1998.
Vessie PR: On the transmission of Huntington chorea for 300 years: The Bures family group. *J Nerv Ment Dis* 76:553, 1932.
Vidailhet M, Vercueil L, Houeto JL: Bilateral deep-brain stimulation of the globus pallidus in primary generalized dystonia. *N Engl J Med* 352:459, 2005.
Visser J, van den Berg-Vos RM, Franssen H, et al: Mimic syndromes in sporadic cases of progressive spinal muscular atrophy. *Neurology* 58:1593, 2002.
Vonsattel JP, DiFiglia M: Huntington disease. *J Neuropathol Exp Neurol* 57:369, 1998.
Waardenburg PJ: Uber familiar-erbliche Falle von seniler Maculade-generation. *Genetica* 18:38, 1936.
Wadia NH: A variety of olivopontocerebellar atrophy distinguished by slow eye movements and peripheral neuropathy. *Adv Neurol* 41:149, 1984.

Walker RH, Shashidharan P: Developments in the molecular biology of DYT1 dystonia. *Mov Disord* 18:1102, 2003.

Wallace DC, Singh G, Lott MT, et al: Mitochondrial DNA mutation associated with Leber's hereditary optic neuropathy. *Science* 242:1427, 1988.

Warner TT, Williams LD, Walker RW, et al: A clinical and molecular genetic study of dentatorubropallidoluysian atrophy in four European families. *Ann Neurol* 37:452, 1995.

Warren JD, Schott JM, Fox NC, et al: Brain biopsy in dementia. *Brain* 128:2016, 2005.

Weaver FM, Follett K, Stern M, et al: Bilateral deep brains stimulation vs best medical therapy for patients with advanced Parkinson disease. *JAMA* 301:63, 2009.

Wenning GK, Ben-Shlomo Y, Magalhaes M, et al: Clinical features and natural history of multiple system atrophy: An analysis of 100 cases. *Brain* 117:835, 1994.

Wenning GK, Ben-Shlomo Y, Magalhaes M, et al: Clinicopathologic study of 35 cases of multiple system atrophy. *J Neurol Neurosurg Psychiatry* 58:160, 1995.

Wenning GK, Litvan I, Jankcovic J, et al: Natural history and survival of 14 patients with corticobasal degeneration confirmed at postmortem examination. *J Neurol Neurosurg Psychiatry* 64:184, 1998.

Whitehouse PJ, Hedreen JC, White CL, et al: Basal forebrain neurons in the dementia of Parkinson disease. *Ann Neurol* 13:243, 1983.

Whitehouse PJ, Price DL, Clark AW, et al: Alzheimer disease: Evidence for loss of cholinergic neurons in nucleus basalis. *Ann Neurol* 10:122, 1981.

Wijemanne S, Jankovic J: Hemiparkinson's-hemiatrophy syndrome. *Neurology* 69:1585, 2007.

Williams DR, Lees AJ: Progressive supranuclear palsy: Clinicopathologic concepts and diagnostic challenges. *Lancet Neurol* 8:270, 2009.

Winikates J, Jankovic J: Clinical correlates of vascular parkinsonism. *Arch Neurol* 56:98, 1999.

Wohlfart G, Fex J, Eliasson S: Hereditary proximal spinal muscular atrophy: A clinical entity simulating progressive muscular dystrophy. *Acta Psychiatr Neurol Scand* 30:395, 1955.

Woodard JS: Concentric hyaline inclusion body formation in mental disease. Analysis of twenty-seven cases. *J Neuropathol Exp Neurol* 21:442, 1962.

Woods BT, Schaumburg HH: Nigro-spino-dentatal degeneration with nuclear ophthalmoplegia. A unique and partially treatable clinico-pathological entity. *J Neurol Sci* 17:149, 1972.

Wooten GF: Agonists vs levodopa in PD. *Neurology* 60:360, 2003.

Worster-Drought C, Greenfield JG, McMenemey WH: A form of familial progressive dementia with spastic paralysis. *Brain* 67:38, 1944.

Young AB, Shoulson I, Penney JB, et al: Huntington's disease in Venezuela: Neurologic features and functional decline. *Neurology* 36:244, 1986.

Young RR: The differential diagnosis of Parkinson's disease. *Int J Neurol* 12:210, 1977.

Younger DS, Rowland LP, Latov N, et al: Motor neuron disease and amyotrophic lateral sclerosis: Relation of high CSF protein content to paraproteinemia and clinical syndromes. *Neurology* 40:595, 1990.

Yuasa T, Ohama E, Harayama H, et al: Joseph's disease: Clinical and pathological studies in a Japanese family. *Ann Neurol* 19:152, 1986.

Zeman W: Pathology of the torsion dystonias (dystonia musculorum deformans). *Neurology* 20(No 11, Pt 2):79, 1970.

Zwergal A, la Fougere C, Lorenzl S, et al: Postural imbalance and falls in PSP correlate with functional pathology of the thalamus. *Neurology* 77:101, 2011.

40

The Acquired Metabolic Disorders of the Nervous System

An important segment of neurologic medicine, and one that is seen with great frequency in general hospitals, are disorders in which a global disturbance of cerebral function (encephalopathy) results from failure of some other organ system—heart and circulation, lungs and respiration, kidneys, liver, pancreas, and the endocrine glands. Unlike the diseases considered in Chap. 37, in which a genetic abnormality affects the metabolic functions of many organs and tissues including the brain, the cerebral disorders discussed in this chapter are strictly secondary to derangements of the visceral organs themselves. They stand at the interface of internal medicine and neurology.

Relationships of this type, between an acquired disease of some thoracic, abdominal, or endocrine organ and the brain, have rather interesting implications. In the first place, recognition of the neurologic syndrome may be a guide to the diagnosis of the systemic disease; indeed, the neurologic symptoms may be more informative and significant than the symptoms referable to the organ primarily involved. Moreover, these encephalopathies are often reversible if the systemic dysfunction is brought under control. Neurologists must therefore have an understanding of the underlying medical disorder, for this may provide the means of controlling the neurologic part of the disease. In other words, the therapy for what appears to be a nervous system disease lies squarely in the field of internal medicine—a clear reason why every neurologist should be well trained in internal medicine. Of more theoretical importance, the investigation of the acquired metabolic diseases provides new insights into the chemistry and pathology of the brain. Each visceral disease affects the brain in a somewhat different way and, because the pathogenic mechanism is not completely understood in any of them, the study of these metabolic diseases promises rich rewards to the scientist.

Table 40-1 lists the main acquired metabolic diseases of the nervous system according to their most common modes of clinical expression. Not included are the diseases caused by nutritional deficiencies and those caused by exogenous drugs and toxins, which can be considered metabolic in the broad sense; these are discussed in the following chapters.

DISEASES PRESENTING AS CONFUSION, STUPOR, OR COMA (METABOLIC ENCEPHALOPATHY)

The syndrome of impaired consciousness, its general features, the terms used to describe it, and the mechanisms involved are discussed in Chap. 17. There it was pointed out that metabolic disturbances are frequent causes of impaired consciousness and that their presence must always be considered when there are no focal signs of cerebral disease and both the imaging studies and the cerebrospinal fluid (CSF) are normal.

Intoxication with alcohol and other drugs figures prominently in the differential diagnosis. *The main features of the reversible metabolic encephalopathies are confusion, typified by disorientation and inattentiveness and accompanied in certain special instances by asterixis, tremor, and myoclonus, usually without signs of focal cerebral disease.* This state may progress in stages to one of stupor and coma. Slowing of the background rhythms in the electroencephalogram (EEG) reflects the severity of the metabolic disturbance. With few exceptions, usually pertaining to cerebral edema and certain cases of hepatic encephalopathy, imaging studies are normal. Seizures may or may not occur, most being associated with particular underlying causes of encephalopathy such as hyponatremia and hyperosmolarity.

Laboratory examinations are highly informative in the investigation of the acquired metabolic diseases. In patients with symptoms suggestive of a metabolic encephalopathy the following determinations are usually made: serum Na, K, Cl, Ca, Mg, glucose, HCO_3, renal function tests (blood urea nitrogen [BUN] and creatinine), liver function tests (aspartate aminotransferase [AST], alanine aminotransferase [ALT], bilirubin, NH_3), thyroid function tests (T_4 and thyroid-stimulating hormone [TSH]), and osmolality and, in certain cases, oxygen saturation and blood gas determinations. These are almost always supplemented by toxicology tests and measurement of the serum concentrations of relevant medications as discussed in the next chapter. Serum osmolality can be measured directly or calculated from

Table 40-1

CLASSIFICATION OF THE ACQUIRED METABOLIC DISORDERS OF THE NERVOUS SYSTEM IN ADULTS

I. Metabolic diseases presenting as a syndrome of confusion, stupor, or coma
   A. Ischemia-hypoxia
   B. Hypercapnia
   C. Hypoglycemia
   D. Hyperglycemia
   E. Hepatic failure
   F. Reye syndrome
   G. Azotemia
   H. Disturbances of sodium, water balance, and osmolality
   I. Hypercalcemia
   J. Other metabolic encephalopathies: acidosis due to diabetes mellitus or renal failure (see also inherited forms of acidosis, in Chap. 37); Addison disease
   K. Hashimoto disease steroid-responsive encephalopathy
   L. Myxedema

II. Metabolic diseases presenting as a progressive extrapyramidal syndrome
   A. Acquired hepatocerebral degeneration
   B. Hyperbilirubinemia and kernicterus
   C. Hypoparathyroidism

III. Metabolic diseases presenting as cerebellar ataxia
   A. Hypothyroidism
   B. Hyperthermia
   C. Celiac sprue disease

IV. Metabolic diseases causing psychosis, or dementia
   A. Cushing disease and steroid encephalopathy
   B. Hyperthyroid psychosis and hypothyroidism (myxedema)
   C. Hyperparathyroidism
   D. Pancreatic encephalopathy

the values of Na, glucose, and BUN (in mg/dL), using the following formula:

$$OSM = 2 \times Na + glucose/18 + BUN/3$$

Normal serum osmolality is 270 to 290 mOsm/L. When there is a discrepancy of greater than 10 mOsm/L between the calculated and the directly measured values (osmolal, or osmolar gap), it can be assumed that additional circulating ions are present. Most often they are derived from an exogenous toxin or drug such as mannitol, but renal failure, ketonemia, or an increase of serum lactate may result in the accumulation of small molecules that contribute to the measured serum osmolality.

A point to be remembered is that the brain may be damaged, even to an irreparable degree, by a disturbance of blood chemistry (e.g., hypoglycemia, hypoxia) that has vanished by the time the patient is examined.

Ischemic-Hypoxic Encephalopathy

Here the basic disorder is a lack of oxygen and of blood flow to the brain, the result of failure of the heart and circulation or of the lungs and respiration. Often, both are responsible and one cannot say which predominates; hence the dually ambiguous allusions in medical records to "ischemic-hypoxic" encephalopathy. This combined *encephalopathy* in various forms and degrees of severity is one of the most frequent and disastrous cerebral disorders encountered in every general hospital.

Reduced to the simplest formulation, a deficient supply of oxygen to the brain is either the result of a failure of cerebral perfusion (ischemia) or of a reduced amount of circulating arterial oxygen, of diminished oxygen saturation, or of insufficiency of hemoglobin (hypoxia). Although they are often combined, the neurologic effects of ischemia and hypoxia are subtly different. The medical conditions that most often lead to it are as follows:

1. A global reduction in cerebral blood flow (myocardial infarction, ventricular arrhythmia, aortic dissection, external or internal blood loss, and septic or traumatic shock)
2. Hypoxia from suffocation (drowning, strangulation, or aspiration of vomitus, food, or blood; from compression of the trachea by a mass or hemorrhage; tracheal obstruction by a foreign body, or a general anesthesia accident)
3. As a subset of the above, diseases that paralyze the respiratory muscles (Guillain-Barré syndrome, amyotrophic lateral sclerosis, myasthenia, and, in the past, poliomyelitis) or damages the medulla and leads to failure of breathing
4. The special case of carbon monoxide (CO) poisoning (nonischemic hypoxia)

The product of blood oxygen content and the cardiac output is the ultimate determinant of the adequacy of oxygen supply to the organs. When blood flow is stable, the most important element in the delivery of oxygen is the oxygen content of the blood. This is the product of hemoglobin concentration and the percentage of oxygen saturation of the hemoglobin molecule. At normal temperature and pH, hemoglobin is 90 percent saturated at an oxygen partial pressure of 60 mm Hg and still 75 percent saturated at 40 mm Hg; i.e., as is well known, the oxygen saturation curve is not linear.

Physiology of Ischemic and Hypoxic Damage

A number of physiologic mechanisms of a homeostatic nature protect the brain under conditions of both ischemia and hypoxia. Through a mechanism termed *autoregulation*, there is a compensatory dilatation of resistance vessels in response to a reduction in cerebral perfusion, which maintains blood flow at a constant rate, as noted in Chap. 34. When the cerebral blood pressure falls below 60 to 70 mm Hg, an additional compensation in the form of increased oxygen extraction allows normal energy metabolism to continue. In total cerebral ischemia, the tissue is depleted of its sources of energy in about 5 min, although longer periods are tolerated under conditions of hypothermia. Also, energy failure because of hypoxia is counteracted by an autoregulatory increase in cerebral blood flow; at a Po_2 of 25 mm Hg, the increase in blood flow is approximately 400 percent. A similar increase in flow occurs with a decrease in hemoglobin to 20 percent of normal.

In most clinical situations in which the brain is deprived of adequate oxygen, as already commented, there is a combination of ischemia and hypoxia, with one or the other predominating. The pathologic effects of ischemic brain injury from systemic hypotension differ from those caused by pure anoxia. Under conditions of transient ischemia, one pattern of damage takes the form of incomplete infarctions in the border zones between major cerebral arteries (Chap. 34). With predominant anoxia, neurons in portions of the hippocampus and the deep folia of the cerebellum are particularly vulnerable. More severe degrees of either ischemia or hypoxia, or the combination, lead to selective damage to certain layers of cortical neurons, and if more profound, to generalized damage of all the cerebral cortex, deep nuclei, and cerebellum. The nuclear structures of the brainstem and spinal cord are relatively resistant to anoxia and hypotension and stop functioning only after the cortex has been badly damaged.

The cellular pathophysiology of neuronal damage under conditions of ischemia is discussed in Chap. 34. One mechanism of injury is an arrest of the aerobic metabolic processes necessary to sustain the Krebs (tricarboxylic acid) cycle and the electron transport system. Neurons, if completely deprived of their source of energy, are unable to maintain their integrity and undergo necrosis. However, neuronal cell death occurs through more than one mechanism. The most acute forms of cell death are characterized by massive swelling and necrosis of neuronal and nonneuronal cells (cytotoxic edema). Short of immediate ischemic necrosis, a series of internally programmed cellular events may also propel the cell toward death in a delayed fashion, a process for which the term *apoptosis* has been borrowed from embryology. There is experimental evidence that certain excitatory neurotransmitters, particularly glutamate, contribute to the rapid destruction of neurons under conditions of anoxia and ischemia (Choi and Rothman); the pertinence of these effects to clinical situations is uncertain. Ultimately, this process may be affected by massive calcium influx through a number of different membrane channels, which activates various kinases that participate in the process of gradual cellular destruction. Free radical generation appears to play a role in membrane dissolution as a result of these processes. As shown in experimental models, one of the reasons for the irreversibility of ischemic lesions may be swelling of the endothelium and blockage of circulation into the ischemic cerebral tissues, the "no-reflow" phenomenon described by Ames and colleagues. There is also a poorly understood phenomenon of delayed neurologic deterioration after anoxia; this may be a result of the blockage or exhaustion of some enzymatic process during the period when brain metabolism is restored.

Clinical Features of Anoxic Encephalopathy

Mild degrees of hypoxia without loss of consciousness induce only inattentiveness, poor judgment, and incoordination; in our experience, there have been no lasting clinical effects in such cases, although Hornbein and colleagues found a slight decline in visual and verbal long-term memory and mild aphasic errors in Himalayan mountaineers who had earlier ascended to altitudes of 18,000 to 29,000 ft. These observations make the point that profound anoxia may be well tolerated if arrived at gradually. For example, we have seen several patients with advanced pulmonary disease who were fully awake when their arterial oxygen pressure was in the range of 30 mm Hg. This level, if it occurs abruptly, causes coma. *An important derivative observation is that degrees of hypoxia that at no time abolish consciousness rarely, if ever, cause permanent damage to the nervous system.*

In the circumstances of *severe global ischemia with prolonged loss of consciousness*, the clinical effects can be quite variable. Following cardiac arrest, for example, consciousness is lost within seconds but recovery can be complete if breathing, oxygenation, and cardiac action are restored within 3 to 5 min. Beyond 5 min there is usually permanent injury. Clinically, however, it is often difficult to judge the precise degree and duration of ischemia, because slight heart action or an imperceptible blood pressure may have served to maintain the circulation to some extent. Hence some individuals have made an excellent recovery after cerebral ischemia that apparently lasted 8 to 10 min or longer. Subnormal body temperatures, as might occur when the body is immersed in ice-cold water, greatly prolong the tolerable period of hypoxia. This has led to the successful application of moderate cooling after cardiac arrest as a technique to limit cerebral damage (see further on in Treatment of Hypoxic-Ischemic Encephalopathy section).

Generally speaking, anoxic patients who demonstrate intact brainstem function as indicated by normal pupillary light and ciliospinal responses, induced by passive head turning (doll's eye movements), and other vestibulo-ocular reflexes have a more favorable outlook for recovery of consciousness and perhaps of all mental faculties. Conversely, the absence of these brainstem reflexes even after circulation and oxygenation have been restored, particularly pupils that fail to react to light, implies a grave outlook as elaborated further on. If the damage is almost total, coma persists, decerebrate postures may be present spontaneously or in response to painful stimuli, and bilateral Babinski signs can be evoked. In the first 24 to 48 h, death may terminate this state in a setting of rising temperature, deepening coma, and circulatory collapse, or the syndrome of brain death intervenes, as discussed below.

Most patients who have suffered *severe but lesser degrees of hypoxia* will have stabilized their breathing and cardiac activity by the time they are first examined; yet they are comatose, with the eyes slightly divergent and motionless but with reactive pupils, the limbs inert and flaccid or intensely rigid, and the tendon reflexes diminished. Within a few minutes after cardiac action and breathing have been restored, generalized convulsions and isolated or grouped myoclonic twitches may occur. Either of these phenomena are poor prognostic signs. With severe degrees of injury, the cerebral and cerebellar cortices and parts of the thalami are partly or completely destroyed but the brainstem-spinal structures survive. Tragically, the individual may survive for an indefinite period in a state that is variously referred to as cortical death, irreversible coma, or *persistent vegetative state* (see discussion of these subjects in Chap. 17). Some patients remain mute, unresponsive, and unaware of their environment for weeks, months, or years. Long survival is usually attended by some degree of improvement but the patient appears to know nothing of his present situation and to have lost all past memories, cognitive function, and capacity for meaningful social interaction and independent existence (a *minimally conscious state,* actually a severe dementia; see Chap. 17). One has only to observe such patients and their families to appreciate the gravity of the problem, the family's anguish, and the tremendous expense of medical care. The only person who does not appear to suffer is the patient.

With *lesser degrees of anoxic-ischemic injury,* the patient improves after a period of coma lasting hours or less. Some of these patients quickly pass through this acute post-hypoxic phase and proceed to make a full recovery; others are left with varying degrees of permanent disability.

The findings on imaging studies vary. The most common early change in cases of severe injury is a loss of the distinction between the cerebral gray and white matter (Fig. 40-1); patients with this finding are invariably comatose and few awaken with a good neurologic outcome. With less severe and predominantly hypotensive-ischemic events such as cardiac arrest, watershed infarctions become evident in the border zones between the anterior, middle, and posterior cerebral arteries (Fig. 40-2). The clinical syndromes associated with watershed infarction are discussed below. Yet another pattern of brain destruction, seen at times also in CO poisoning, consists of striatal damage that is evident more by imaging than by clinical features (Fig. 40-3).

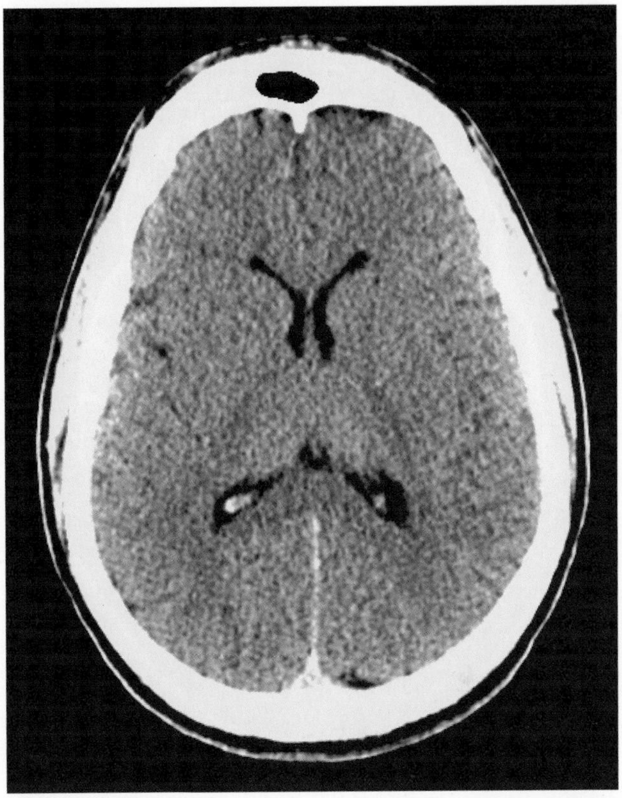

Figure 40-1. CT without contrast infusion after 1 day cardiac arrest demonstrating the loss of distinction between gray and white matter throughout the cerebral hemispheres. The patient remained comatose and became vegetative.

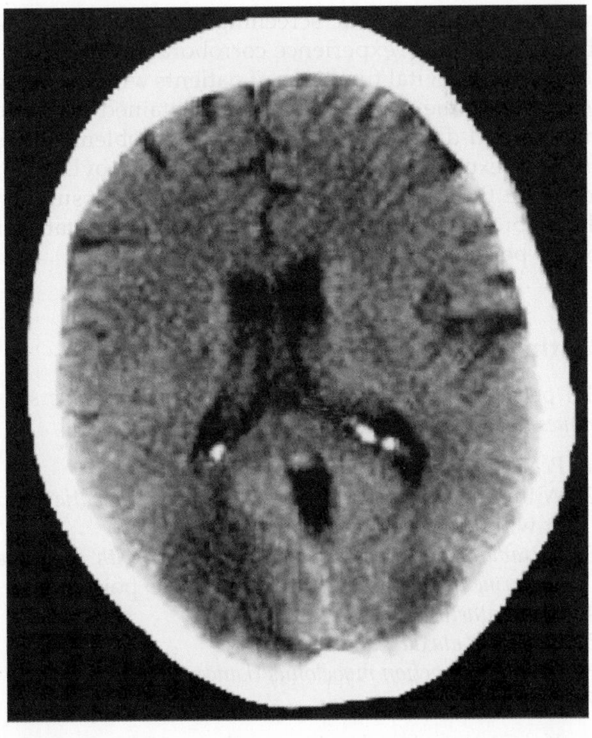

Figure 40-2. Watershed infarction between the middle and posterior cerebral arteries after brief cardiac arrest. The patient had Balint syndrome.

Brain Death Syndrome

(See Chap. 17 for a full discussion)

This represents the most severe degree of hypoxia, usually caused by circulatory arrest; it is manifest by a state of complete unawareness and unresponsiveness with abolition of all brainstem reflexes. Natural respiration cannot be sustained; only cardiac action and blood pressure are maintained. No electrical activity is seen in the EEG (it is isoelectric). At autopsy one finds that most, if not all, the gray matter of cerebral, cerebellar, and brainstem structures—and in some instances, even the upper cervical spinal cord—has been severely damaged.

One must always exercise caution in concluding that a patient has this form of irreversible brain damage, because anesthesia, intoxication with certain drugs, and hypothermia may also cause deep coma and an isoelectric EEG but permit recovery. Therefore it is often advisable to repeat the clinical and laboratory tests after an interval of a day or so, during which

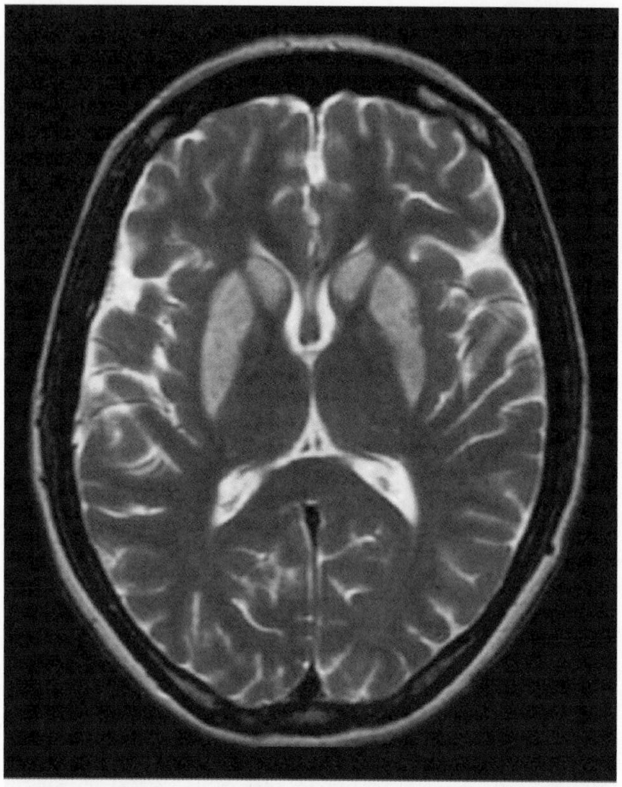

Figure 40-3. T2-weighted MRI of striatal damage after anoxia from hanging. The pallidum is spared, in contrast to typical cases of carbon monoxide poisoning (see Fig. 40-5).

time the results of toxic screening also become available. The authors' experience corroborates the general notion that the vital functions of patients with the brain death syndrome usually cannot be sustained for more than several days; in other words, the problem settles itself. In exceptional cases, however, the provision of adequate fluid, vasopressors, and respiratory support allows preservation of the body in a comatose state for longer periods.

Posthypoxic Neurologic Syndromes

The permanent neurologic sequelae or *posthypoxic syndromes* observed most frequently are as follows:

1. *Persistent coma or stupor,* described above
2. With lesser degrees of cerebral injury, *dementia* with or without extrapyramidal signs
3. *Extrapyramidal (parkinsonian) syndrome with cognitive impairment* (discussed in relation to CO poisoning)
4. *Choreoathetosis*
5. *Cerebellar ataxia*
6. *Intention or action myoclonus (Lance-Adams syndrome)*
7. *An amnesic state*

If *hypoperfusion* dominates, the patient may also display the manifestations of watershed infarctions that are situated between the end territories of the major cerebral vessels. The main syndromes that become evident soon after the patient awakens are:

1. *Visual agnosias including Balint syndrome and cortical blindness* (Anton Syndrome) (see Chap. 22), representing infarctions of the watershed between the middle and posterior cerebral arteries (see Fig. 40-2)
2. *Proximal arm and shoulder weakness*, sometimes accompanied by hip weakness (referred to as a "man-in-the-barrel" syndrome), reflecting infarction in the territory between the middle and anterior cerebral arteries. These patients are able to walk, but their arms dangle and their hips may be weak.

The two watershed syndromes may rarely coexist. The interested reader may consult the appropriate chapter in the text on neurologic intensive care by Ropper and colleagues for further details. There are also watershed areas in the spinal cord (Chap. 44).

Seizures may or may not be a problem, and they are often resistant to treatment. Well-formed motor convulsions are infrequent. Myoclonus is more common and may be intermixed with fragmentary convulsions. Myoclonus is a grave sign in most cases but it generally recedes after several hours or a few days. These movements are also difficult to suppress, as noted further on.

Delayed Postanoxic Encephalopathy and Leukoencephalopathy

This is a relatively uncommon and unexplained phenomenon. Initial improvement, which appears to be complete, is followed after a variable period of time (1 to 4 weeks in most instances) by a relapse, characterized by apathy, confusion, irritability, and occasionally agitation or mania. Most patients survive this second episode, but some are left with serious mental and motor disturbances (Choi; Plum et al). In still other cases, there appears to be progression of the initial neurologic syndrome with additional weakness, shuffling gait, diffuse rigidity and spasticity, sphincteric incontinence, coma, and death after 1 to 2 weeks. Exceptionally, there is yet another syndrome in which an episode of hypoxia is followed by slow deterioration, which progresses for weeks to months until the patient is mute, rigid, and helpless. In such cases, the basal ganglia are affected more than the cerebral cortex and white matter as in the case studied by our colleagues Dooling and Richardson. Instances have followed cardiac arrest, drowning, asphyxiation, and carbon monoxide poisoning.

The imaging features of the white matter disorder can be quite striking (Fig. 40-4). A mitochondrial disorder has been suggested, on uncertain grounds, as the underlying mechanism.

Prognosis of Hypoxic-Ischemic Brain Injury

(See also "Prognosis in Coma" in Chap. 17)

Several validated models have been developed to predict the outcome of anoxic-ischemic coma. All of them incorporate simple clinical features involving loss of motor, verbal, and pupillary functions in various combinations. The most often cited study of the prognostic aspects of coma following cardiac arrest is the one by Levy and colleagues

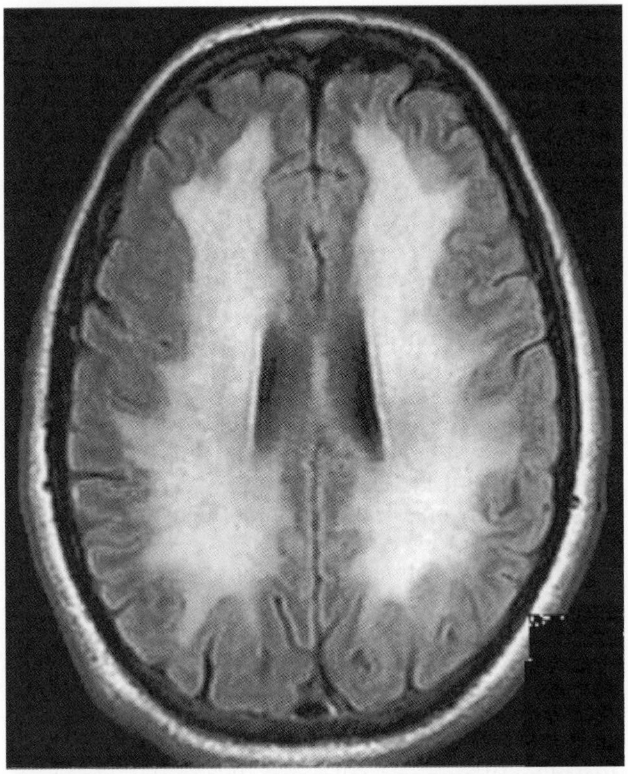

Figure 40-4. MRI fluid-attenuated inversion recovery (FLAIR) sequence of delayed postanoxic leukoencephalopathy in a patient who had recovered after drowning and deteriorated 2 weeks later.

of 210 patients, which provided the following guidelines: 13 percent of patients attained a state of independent function within 1 year; at the time of the initial evaluation, approximately 25 percent of patients had absent pupillary light reflexes, none of whom regained independent function; by contrast, the presence on admission of reactive pupils, eye movements, and any motor response, a configuration displayed in approximately 10 percent, was associated with a better prognosis in almost 50 percent of cases. The absence of neurologic function in any of these spheres at 1 day after cardiac arrest, unsurprisingly, was associated with an even poorer outcome. Similarly, Booth and colleagues analyzed previously published studies and determined that 5 clinical signs at 1 day after cardiac arrest predicted a poor neurologic outcome or death: (1) absent corneal responses, (2) absent pupillary reactivity, (3) no withdrawal to pain, and (4) the absence of any motor response. The use of somatosensory evoked potentials in the prognostication of coma is discussed in Chaps. 2 and 17.

Most workers in the field of coma studies have been unable to establish signs that confidently predict a good outcome. The role of somatosensory evoked potentials in prognosis of coma has been addressed in Chap. 17.

In any such case, concurrent intoxication must, of course, be excluded.

The question of what to do with patients in such states of protracted coma is a societal as much as a medical problem. The neurologist can be expected to state the level and degree of brain damage, its cause, and the prognosis based on his own and published experience. One prudently avoids heroic, lifesaving therapeutic measures once the nature of this state has been determined with certainty.

Treatment of Hypoxic-Ischemic Encephalopathy

Treatment is directed initially to the prevention of further hypoxic injury. A clear airway is secured, cardiopulmonary resuscitation is initiated, and every second counts in their prompt utilization. Oxygen may be of value during the first hours but is probably of little use after the blood becomes well oxygenated. Once cardiac and pulmonary function are restored, there is experimental and clinical evidence that reducing cerebral metabolic requirements by inducing hypothermia may have a slight beneficial effect on outcome and may prevent the delayed worsening referred to above, though a recent clinical trial brings this into question (see further on). The use of high-dose barbiturates has not met with the same success.

Much attention was drawn to the randomized trials conducted by Bernard and colleagues and by the Hypothermia After Cardiac Arrest Study Group, of mild hypothermia applied to unconscious patients immediately after cardiac arrest. They reduced the core temperature to 33°C (91°F) within 2 h of the arrest and sustained this level for 12 h in the first trial, and between 32°C and 34°C for 24 h in the second study. Both trials demonstrated improved survival and better cognitive outcome in survivors, compared to leaving the patient in a normothermic state and this led to the development of guidelines and a change in clinical practice in the U.S. and elsewhere after 2002. The outcomes were evaluated by coarse measures of neurologic function. Implementing and sustaining hypothermia, either by external cooling, infusion of cooled normal saline, or intravenous cooling devices is difficult, and the iatrogenic problems of hypotension, bleeding, ventricular ectopy and infection have sometimes arisen, although this mild degree of temperature reduction is usually well tolerated. A third larger trial conducted by Nielsen and colleagues compared temperature maintenance after cardiac arrest at 33°C to maintenance of 36°C and found no difference in the rate of death or in neurological outcome. The results of this third study are still being discussed and it is not clear if it should be interpreted as demonstrating that hypothermic treatment is ineffective or if the avoidance of even mild hyperthermia, observed in the control groups of previous trials, was the important factor in improving outcome. At the time of this writing, it seems to us that induced hypothermia is not obligatory after cardiac arrest but that attempts should be made to keep the body temperature from rising above normal.

Vasodilator drugs, glutamate blockers, opiate antagonists, and calcium channel blockers have been of no proven benefit despite their theoretical appeal and some experimental successes. Corticosteroids ostensibly help to allay brain (possibly cellular) swelling, but, again, their therapeutic benefit has not been evident in clinical trials.

Seizures should be controlled by the methods indicated in Chap. 16. If convulsions are severe, continuous, and unresponsive to the usual medications, continuous infusion of a drug such as midazolam or propofol, and eventually the suppression of convulsions with neuromuscular blocking agents may be required. Often the seizures cease after a few hours and are replaced by polymyoclonus. For the latter, clonazepam, 8 to 12 mg daily in divided doses may be useful but the commonly used antiepileptic drugs have little effect. A state of spontaneous and stimulus-sensitive myoclonus as well as persistent limb posturing usually presages a poor outcome. The striking disorder of delayed movement-induced myoclonus and ataxic tremor that appear after the patient awakens from an anoxic episode (Lance-Adams myoclonus) is a special issue, which is discussed in Chap. 6. Its treatment usually requires the use of multiple medications. Fever is treated with antipyretics or a cooling blanket combined with neuromuscular paralyzing agents.

Carbon Monoxide Poisoning

Strictly speaking, CO is an exogenous toxin, but it is considered here because it produces a characteristic cerebral injury and is frequently associated with delayed neurologic deterioration. The extreme affinity of CO for hemoglobin (more than 200 times that of oxygen) drastically reduces the oxygen content of blood and subjects the brain to prolonged hypoxia and acidosis. Cardiac toxicity and hypotension generally follow. Whether CO also has a direct toxic action on neuronal components is not settled. The effects on the brain for the most part simulate those caused by cardiac arrest. Neurologists are likely to encounter instances of CO poisoning in burn units and in patients who have attempted suicide or have been exposed accidentally to a faulty furnace or to car exhaust in a closed garage. A contemporary review of the subject has been given by Weaver.

Early symptoms include headache, nausea, dyspnea, confusion, dizziness, and clumsiness. These occur when the carboxyhemoglobin level reaches 20 to 30 percent of total hemoglobin. Exposure to relatively low levels of CO from faulty furnaces and gasoline engines should be suspected as the cause of recurrent headaches and confusion that clear upon hospitalization or other change of venue. A cherry-red color of the skin may appear, but is actually an infrequent finding; cyanosis is more common. At slightly higher levels of carboxyhemoglobin, blindness, visual field defects, and papilledema develop, and levels of 50 to 60 percent are associated with coma, decerebrate or decorticate posturing, seizures in a few patients, and generalized slowing of the EEG rhythms. The initial CT scanning is normal or shows mild cerebral edema; later scans may show a characteristic lesion in the pallidum, as described below. Only if there has been associated hypotension does one see the same types of vascular border-zone infarctions that appear after cardiac arrest.

Delayed neurologic deterioration 1 to 3 weeks (sometimes much longer) after CO exposure occurs more frequently than with other forms of cerebral hypoxia. In Choi's survey, this feature was observed in 3 percent of 2,360 cases of CO poisoning and in 12 percent of those ill enough to be admitted to a hospital. Extrapyramidal features (parkinsonian gait and bradykinesia) predominated. Three-quarters of such patients were said to recover within a year. Discrete lesions centered in the globus pallidus bilaterally and sometimes the inner portion of the putamina are characteristic of CO poisoning that had produced coma (Fig. 40-5), but similar focal destruction may be seen after drowning, strangulation, and other forms of anoxia. The common feature among the delayed-relapse patients is a prolonged period of pure anoxia (before the occurrence of ischemia). Basal ganglia lesions may be quite prominent on CT scans even when delayed neurologic sequelae do not occur but they are invariably present between 1 and 4 weeks in patients who develop the delayed extrapyramidal syndrome. In less-severely affected patients we have seen such lesions resolve entirely on CT and MRI and there is no resultant movement disorder.

The initial treatment for carbon monoxide exposure is with inspired oxygen. Because the half-life of CO (normally 5 h) is greatly reduced by the administration of hyperbaric oxygen at 2 or 3 atmospheres, this additional treatment is recommended when the carboxyhemoglobin concentration is greater than 40 percent or in the presence of coma or seizures (Myers et al). According to a trial conducted by Weaver and colleagues, this treatment reduces

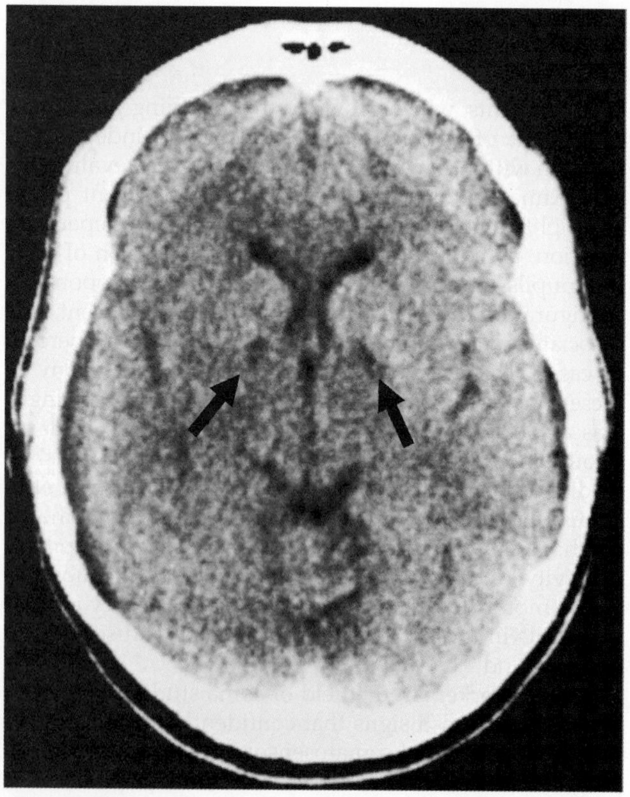

Figure 40-5. Unenhanced CT of the brain of a 30-year-old woman who attempted suicide by carbon monoxide inhalation. The only neurologic residua were a mild defect in retentive memory and areas of decreased attenuation in the pallidum bilaterally (*arrows*).

the incidence of cognitive sequelae from 46 to 25 percent. They administered 3 hyperbaric sessions in the first 24 h after exposure to CO.

High-Altitude (Mountain) Sickness

Acute mountain sickness is another special form of cerebral hypoxia. It occurs when a sea-level inhabitant abruptly ascends to a high altitude. Headache, anorexia, nausea and vomiting, weakness, and insomnia appear at altitudes above 8,000 ft; on reaching higher altitudes, there may be ataxia, tremor, drowsiness, mild confusion, and hallucinations. At 16,000 ft, according to Griggs and Sutton, 50 percent of individuals develop asymptomatic retinal hemorrhages, and it has been suggested that such hemorrhages also occur in the cerebral white matter. Extreme altitude sickness may result in fatal cerebral edema. The overexpression of vascular endothelial growth factor (VEGF), a protein originally noted for its effects on vascular permeability, has been implicated as the cause of cerebral edema in the experiments of Schoch and colleagues. With more prolonged exposure at these altitudes or with further ascent, affected individuals suffer mental impairment that may progress to coma. Hypoxemia at high altitudes is intensified during sleep, as ventilation normally diminishes and also by pulmonary edema, another manifestation of mountain sickness. Reference was made earlier to the observation of Hornbein and colleagues of a mild, but possibly lasting, memory impairment even in acclimated mountaineers who had been exposed to extremely high altitudes for several days. Hackett and Roach have reviewed the treatments for altitude illness.

Chronic mountain sickness, also called Monge disease (after the physician who described the condition in Andean Indians of Peru), is observed in long-term inhabitants of high-altitude mountainous regions. Pulmonary hypertension, cor pulmonale, and secondary polycythemia are the main features. There is usually hypercarbia as well, with the expected degree of mild mental dullness, slowness, fatigue, nocturnal headache, and, sometimes, papilledema (see below). Thomas and colleagues have called attention to a syndrome of burning hands and feet in Peruvians at high altitude, apparently a maladaptive response to chronic hypoxia.

Sedatives, alcohol, and a slightly elevated Pco_2 in the blood all reduce tolerance to high altitude. Dexamethasone and acetazolamide prevent and counteract mountain sickness to some extent. The most effective preventive measure is acclimatization by a 2- to 4-day stay at intermediate altitudes.

Hypercapnic Pulmonary Disease

Chronic obstructive pulmonary disease such as emphysema, fibrosing lung disease, neuromuscular weakness, and, in some instances, inadequacy of the medullary respiratory centers each may lead to persistent respiratory acidosis, with elevated of Pco_2 and reduced in arterial Po_2. The complete clinical syndrome of chronic hypercapnia described by Austen, Carmichael, and Adams comprises *headache, papilledema, mental dullness, drowsiness, confusion, stupor and coma, and asterixis*. More typically, only some of these features are found. Some patients have a fast-frequency tremor. The headache tends to be generalized, frontal, or occipital and can be quite intense, persistent, steady, and aching in type; nocturnal occurrence is a feature of some cases. The papilledema is bilateral but may be slightly greater in one eye than in the other, and hemorrhages may encircle the choked disc (a later finding). The tendon reflexes are lively and plantar reflexes may be extensor. Intermittent drowsiness, inattentiveness, reduction of psychomotor activity, inability to perceive all the items in a sequence of events, and forgetfulness constitute the more subtle manifestations of this syndrome and may prompt the family to seek medical help. Such symptoms may last only a few minutes or hours, and one cannot count on their presence at the time of a particular examination. In fully developed cases, the CSF is under increased pressure; Pco_2 may exceed 75 mm Hg, and the O_2 saturation of arterial blood ranges from 85 percent to as low as 40 percent. The EEG shows slow activity in the delta or theta range, which is sometimes bilaterally synchronous.

The mechanism of the cerebral disorder is from a direct CO_2 narcosis, but the biochemical details are not known. Normally the CSF is slightly acidotic in comparison to the blood and the Pco_2 of the CSF is about 10 mm Hg higher than that of the blood. With respiratory acidosis, the pH of the CSF falls (into the range of 7.15 to 7.25) and cerebral blood flow increases as a result of cerebral vasodilatation. However, the brain rapidly adapts to respiratory acidosis through the generation and secretion of bicarbonate by the choroid plexuses. Brain water content also increases, mainly in the white matter. In animal models of hypercarbia, blood and brain NH_3 is elevated, which may explain the similarity of the syndrome to that of hyperammonemic liver failure (Herrera and Kazemi).

The most effective therapeutic measures are positive-pressure ventilation, using oxygen if there is also hypoxia. Oxygen supplementation is, of course, used cautiously in these patients in order to avoid suppressing respiratory drive; marginally compensated patients treated with excessive oxygen have lapsed into coma. Treatment of heart failure, phlebotomy to reduce the viscosity of the blood, and antibiotics to suppress pulmonary infection may be necessary. Often these measures result in a surprising degree of improvement, which may be maintained for months or years.

Unlike pure hypoxic encephalopathy, prolonged coma because of hypercapnia is relatively rare and in our experience has not led to irreversible brain damage. Papilledema, myoclonus, and especially asterixis are important diagnostic features. If aminophylline is administered for the treatment of the underlying pulmonary airway disease, it may produce high blood levels and a tendency for it to produce seizures.

Hypoglycemic Encephalopathy

This condition is now relatively infrequent but is an important cause of confusion, convulsions, stupor, and coma; as such, it merits separate consideration as a metabolic disorder of the brain. The essential biochemical abnormality is a critical lowering of the blood glucose. At a level of about 30 mg/dL, the cerebral disorder takes the form of a confusional state and one or more seizures may occur; at a level of 10 mg/dL, there is coma that may result in irreparable injury to the brain if not corrected immediately by the administration of glucose. As with most other metabolic encephalopathies, the rate of decline of blood glucose is a factor in both the depression of consciousness and residual dementia.

The normal brain has a glucose reserve of 1 to 2 g (30 mmol/100 g of tissue), mostly in the form of glycogen. Because glucose is utilized by the brain at a rate of 60 to 80 mg/min, the glucose reserve may sustain cerebral activity for 30 min or less once blood glucose is no longer available. Glucose is transported from the blood to the brain by an active carrier system. Glucose entering the brain either undergoes glycolysis or is stored as glycogen. During normal oxygenation (aerobic metabolism), glucose is converted to pyruvate, which enters the Krebs cycle; with anaerobic metabolism, lactate is formed. The oxidation of 1 mole of glucose requires 6 mole of O_2. Of the glucose taken up by the brain, 85 to 90 percent is oxidized; the remainder is used in the formation of proteins and other substances, notably neurotransmitters and particularly gamma-aminobutyric acid (GABA).

When blood glucose falls, the central nervous system (CNS) can utilize nonglucose substrates to a variable extent for its metabolic needs, especially keto acids and intermediates of glucose metabolism, such as lactate, pyruvate, fructose, and other hexoses. In the neonatal brain, which has a higher glycogen reserve, keto acids provide a considerable proportion of cerebral energy requirements; this also happens after prolonged starvation. However, in the face of severe and sustained hypoglycemia, these alternative substrates are inadequate to preserve the structural integrity of neurons, and eventually adenosine triphosphate (ATP) is depleted as well. If convulsions occur, they usually do so during a period of confusion; the convulsions have been attributed to an altered integrity of neuronal membranes and to elevated NH_3 and depressed GABA and lactate levels (Wilkinson and Prockop).

The brain is the only organ besides the heart that suffers severe functional and structural impairment under conditions of severe hypoglycemia. Beyond what is described above, the pathophysiology of the cerebral disorder has not been fully elucidated. It is known that hypoglycemia reduces O_2 uptake and increases cerebral blood flow. As with anoxia and ischemia, there is experimental evidence that the excitatory amino acid glutamate is involved in the process. The levels of several brain phospholipid fractions decrease when animals are given large doses of insulin. However, the suggestion that hypoglycemia results in a rapid depletion and inadequate production of high-energy phosphate compounds has not been corroborated; some other glucose-dependent biochemical processes must be implicated.

Etiology

The most common causes of hypoglycemic encephalopathy are: (1) accidental or deliberate overdose of insulin or an oral diabetic agent; (2) islet cell insulin-secreting tumor of the pancreas; (3) depletion of liver glycogen, which occasionally follows a prolonged alcoholic binge, starvation, or any form of severe liver failure; (4) glycogen storage disease of infancy; and (5) an idiopathic hypoglycemia in the neonatal period and infancy; (6) subacute and chronic hypoglycemia from islet cell hypertrophy and islet cell tumors of the pancreas, carcinoma of the stomach, fibrous mesothelioma, carcinoma of the cecum, and hepatoma. Purportedly, an insulin-like substance is elaborated by these nonpancreatic tumors. In the past, hypoglycemic encephalopathy was a not infrequent complication of "insulin shock" therapy for schizophrenia. In functional hyperinsulinism, as occurs in anorexia nervosa and dietary faddism, the hypoglycemia is rarely of sufficient severity or duration to damage the CNS.

Clinical Features

The initial symptoms appear when the blood glucose has descended to about 30 mg/dL, nervousness, hunger, flushed facies, sweating, headache, palpitation, trembling, and anxiety. These gradually give way to confusion and drowsiness or occasionally, to excitement, overactivity, and bizarre or combative behavior. Many of the early symptoms relate to adrenal and sympathetic overactivity and some of the manifestations may be muted in diabetic patients with neuropathy. In the next stage, forced sucking, grasping, motor restlessness, muscular spasms, and decerebrate rigidity occur, in that sequence. Myoclonic twitching and convulsions develop in some patients. Rarely, there are focal cerebral deficits, the pathogenesis of which remains unexplained; according to Malouf and Brust, hemiplegia, corrected by intravenous glucose, was observed in 3 of 125 patients who presented with symptomatic hypoglycemia.

Blood glucose levels of approximately 10 mg/dL are associated with deep coma, dilatation of pupils, pale skin, shallow respiration, slow pulse and hypotonia, what had in the past been termed the "medullary phase" of hypoglycemia. If glucose is administered before this level has been attained, the patient can be restored to normal, retracing the aforementioned steps in reverse order. However, once this state is reached, and particularly if it persists for more than a few minutes, recovery is delayed for a period of days or weeks and may be incomplete as noted below.

The EEG is altered as the blood glucose falls, but the correlations are imprecise. There is diffuse slowing in the theta or delta range. During recovery, sharp waves may appear and coincide in some cases with seizures.

The major clinical differences between hypoglycemic and hypoxic encephalopathy lie in the setting and the mode of evolution of the neurologic disorder. The effects of hypoglycemia usually unfold more slowly, over a period of 30 to 60 min, rather than in a few seconds or minutes. The recovery phase and sequelae of the 2 conditions are quite similar.

A large dose of insulin, which produces intense hypoglycemia, even of relatively brief duration (30 to 60 min), is more dangerous than a series of less-severe hypoglycemic episodes from smaller doses of insulin, possibly because the former impairs or exhausts essential enzymes, a condition that cannot then be overcome by large quantities of intravenous glucose. Reflecting the benignity of repeated minor occurrences, the Epidemiology of Diabetes Interventions and Complications Study Research Group have demonstrated that recurrent hypoglycemic episodes in the course of treatment of diabetes over many years are very well tolerated and do not lead to cognitive decline.

A severe and prolonged episode of hypoglycemia may result in permanent impairment of intellectual function as well as other neurologic residua, like those that follow severe anoxia. We also have observed states of protracted coma, as well as relatively pure Korsakoff amnesia. However, one should not be hasty in prognosis, for we have observed slow improvement to continue for 1 to 2 years.

Recurrent hypoglycemia from an islet cell tumor may masquerade for some time as an episodic confusional psychosis or convulsive illness; diagnosis then awaits the demonstration of low blood glucose or hyperinsulinism in association with the neurologic symptoms. We saw a man in the emergency department whose main complaint was episodic inability to dial a touchtone telephone and a mild mental fogginess; he was found to have an insulinoma.

Functional or reactive hypoglycemia is the most ambiguous of all syndromes related to low blood glucose. This condition is usually idiopathic but may precede the onset of diabetes mellitus. The rise of insulin in response to a carbohydrate meal is delayed but then causes an excessive fall in blood glucose, to 30 to 40 mg/dL. The symptoms are malaise, fatigue, nervousness, headache and tremor, which may be difficult to distinguish from anxious depression. Not surprisingly, the term *functional hypoglycemia* has been much abused, being applied indiscriminately to a variety of complaints that would now be called chronic fatigue syndrome or an anxiety syndrome. In fact, a syndrome attributable to functional or reactive hypoglycemia is infrequent and its diagnosis requires the finding of an excessive reaction to insulin, low blood glucose during the symptomatic period, and a salutary response to oral glucose.

In all forms of hypoglycemic encephalopathy, the major damage is to the cerebral cortex. Cortical nerve cells degenerate and are replaced by microglia cells and astrocytes. The distribution of lesions is similar, although probably not identical to that in hypoxic encephalopathy. The cerebellar cortex is less vulnerable to hypoglycemia than to hypoxia. Auer has described the ultrastructural changes in neurons resulting from experimental hypoglycemia; with increasing duration of hypoglycemia and EEG silence, there are mitochondrial changes, first in dendrites and then in nerve cell soma, followed by nuclear membrane disruption leading to cell death.

Treatment of all forms of hypoglycemia obviously consists of correction of the hypoglycemia at the earliest possible moment. It is not known whether hypothermia or other measures will increase the safety period in hypoglycemia or alter the outcome. Seizures and twitching may not stop with antiepileptic drugs until the hypoglycemia is corrected.

Hyperglycemia

Two syndromes have been defined, mainly in diabetics: (1) hyperglycemia with ketoacidosis and (2) hyperosmolar nonketotic hyperglycemia.

In *diabetic acidosis*, the familiar picture is one of dehydration, fatigue, weakness, headache, abdominal pain, dryness of the mouth, stupor or coma, and Kussmaul type of breathing. Usually the condition has developed over a period of days in a patient known or proven to be diabetic. Often, the patient had failed to take a regular insulin dose. The blood glucose level is found to be more than 400 mg/dL, the pH of the blood less than 7.20, and the bicarbonate less than 10 mEq/L. Ketone bodies and β-hydroxybutyric acid are elevated in the blood and urine, and there is marked glycosuria. The prompt administration of insulin and repletion of intravascular volume correct the clinical and chemical abnormalities over a period of hours.

A small group of patients with diabetic ketoacidosis, such as those reported by Young and Bradley, develop deepening coma and cerebral edema as the elevated glucose is corrected. Mild cerebral edema is commonly observed in children during treatment with fluids and insulin (Krane et al). Prockop attributed this condition to an accumulation of fructose and sorbitol in the brain. The latter substance, a polyol that is formed during hyperglycemia, crosses membranes slowly, but once it does so, is said to cause a shift of water into the brain and an intracellular edema. However, according to Fishman (1974), the increased polyols in the brain in hyperglycemia are not present in sufficient concentration to be important osmotically; though they may induce other metabolic effects related to the encephalopathy. These are matters of conjecture, as the increase of polyols has never been found. The brain edema in this condition is probably a result of reversal of the osmolality gradient from blood to brain, which occurs with rapid correction of hyperglycemia.

The pathophysiology of the cerebral disorder in diabetic ketoacidosis is not fully understood. No consistent cellular pathology of the brain has been identified in the cases we have examined. Factors such as ketosis, tissue acidosis, hypotension, hyperosmolality, and hypoxia have not been identified. Attempts at therapy by the administration of urea, mannitol, salt-poor albumin, and dexamethasone are usually unsuccessful, though recoveries are reported.

In *hyperosmolar nonketotic hyperglycemia*, the blood glucose is extremely high, more than 600 mg/dL, but ketoacidosis does not develop, or if it does develop, it is mild. Osmolality is usually in excess of 330 mOsm/L. There is also hemoconcentration and prerenal azotemia. Appreciation of the neurologic syndrome is generally credited to Wegierko, who published descriptions of it in

1956 and 1957. Most of the patients are elderly diabetics but some were not previously known to have been diabetic. An infection, enteritis, pancreatitis, dehydration, or a drug known to upset diabetic control (thiazides, corticosteroids, and phenytoin) leads to polyuria, fatigue, confusion, stupor, and coma. Often the syndrome arises in conjunction with the combined use of corticosteroids and phenytoin (which inhibits insulin release), for example, in elderly patients with brain tumors. The use of osmotic diuretics enhances the risk.

Seizures and focal signs such as a hemiparesis, a hemisensory defect, choreoathetosis, or a homonymous visual field defect are more common than in any other metabolic encephalopathy and may erroneously suggest the possibility of a stroke. Fluids should be replaced cautiously, using isotonic saline and potassium. Correction of the markedly elevated blood glucose requires relatively small amounts of insulin, since these patients often do not have a high degree of insulin resistance.

Hepatic Stupor and Coma (Hepatic, or Portal–Systemic Encephalopathy)

Chronic hepatic insufficiency with portosystemic shunting of blood is punctuated by episodes of stupor, coma, and other neurologic symptoms—a state referred to as *hepatic stupor*, *coma*, or *encephalopathy*. It was clearly delineated by Adams and Foley over 50 years ago. This state complicates all varieties of liver disease and is unrelated to jaundice or ascites. Any form of shunting, even without hepatic disease, such as surgical portal–systemic shunt (Eck fistula) is attended by the same clinical picture (see further on). There are also a number of hereditary hyperammonemic syndromes, usually first apparent in infancy or childhood (discussed extensively in Chap. 37) that lead to episodic coma with or without seizures. In all these states, it is common for an excess of protein derived from the diet or from gastrointestinal hemorrhage to induce or worsen the encephalopathy. Additional predisposing factors are hypoxia, hypokalemia, metabolic alkalosis, excessive diuresis, use of sedative hypnotic drugs, and constipation. A special from of the syndrome in epilepsy patients exposed to valproate; confusion and ataxia may occur acutely or subacutely in these patients (Gomcelli et al). Reye syndrome following viral infections in children, now infrequent, was also associated with very high levels of ammonia in the blood and encephalopathy (see further on).

Clinical Features

The clinical picture of acute, subacute, or chronic hepatic encephalopathy consists of a derangement of consciousness, presenting first as mental slowing and confusion, occasionally with hyperactivity, followed by progressive drowsiness, stupor, and coma. The confusional state is combined with a characteristic intermittency of sustained muscle contraction; this phenomenon, which was originally described in patients with hepatic stupor by Adams and Foley and called *asterixis* (from the Greek *sterixis*, a "fixed position"). It is now recognized as a sign of various metabolic encephalopathies but is most prominent in this disorder (see Chap. 6). It is conventionally demonstrated by having the patient hold his arms outstretched with the wrists extended, but the same tremor can be elicited by any sustained posture, including that of the protruded tongue. We have seen patients in whom asterixis of the large antigravity muscles (e.g., iliopsoas or quadriceps) causes falling. A variable, fluctuating rigidity of the trunk and limbs, grimacing, suck and grasp reflexes, exaggeration or asymmetry of tendon reflexes, Babinski signs, and focal or generalized seizures round out the clinical picture in a few patients.

The EEG is a sensitive and reliable indicator of impending coma, becoming abnormal during the earliest phases of the disordered mental state. Foley, Watson, and Adams noted an EEG abnormality consisting of paroxysms of bilaterally synchronous slow or triphasic waves in the delta range, which at first predominate frontally and are interspersed with alpha activity and later, as the coma deepens, displace all normal activity (see Fig. 2-5*H*). A few patients show only random high-voltage asynchronous slow waves.

This syndrome of hepatic encephalopathy is remarkably diverse in its course and evolution. It usually appears over a period of days to weeks and may terminate fatally; or, with appropriate treatment, the symptoms may regress and then fluctuate in severity for several weeks or months. Persistent hepatic coma of the latter type proves fatal in about half of patients (Levy et al). In many patients, the syndrome is relatively mild and does not evolve beyond the stage of mental dullness and confusion, with asterixis and EEG changes. In yet others, a subtle disorder of mood, personality, and intellect may be protracted over a period of many months or even years; this chronic but nevertheless reversible mental disturbance need not be associated with overt clinical signs of liver failure (jaundice and ascites) or other neurologic signs. Characteristically in these patients, an extensive portal–systemic collateral circulation can be demonstrated (hence the term *portal–systemic encephalopathy*) and an association established between the mental disturbance and an intolerance to dietary protein as well as raised blood ammonia levels (Summerskill et al).

The diversion of blood from the portal system into the vena cava after ligation of the portal veins was first performed in dogs by Eck in 1877. Probably the first and certainly most striking example in man was the case of pure "Eck" fistula reported by McDermott and Adams, in which a portacaval shunt was created during the removal of a pancreatic tumor. The liver was normal. Episodic coma occurred thereafter whenever dietary protein increased. Consciousness was restored on a protein-free diet, and coma could be induced again by ammonium chloride. Postmortem examination 2 years later confirmed the normal liver and showed cerebral changes of hepatic encephalopathy, as described below.

Finally, there is a group of patients (most of whom have experienced repeated attacks of hepatic coma) in whom an *irreversible* mild dementia and a disorder of posture and movement (grimacing, tremor, dysarthria, ataxia of gait, choreoathetosis) gradually appear. This condition of *chronic acquired hepatocerebral degeneration* must be distinguished from other dementing and extrapyramidal syndromes (see further on). A few cases of isolated spastic paraplegia (so-called *hepatic myelopathy*, or more correctly *hepatic paraplegia*) have been described. Pant and Richardson attributed the syndrome to a loss of Betz cells in the frontal cortex; in other words, a restricted encephalopathy seen in some patients with portal-systemic encephalopathy. Indeed, the spasticity of the legs, increased tendon reflexes, and Babinski signs that are found with PSE, suggest that "hepatic paraparesis" is a common feature of the encephalopathy.

MRI in PSE often demonstrates high signal intensity in the globus pallidus, likely the result of manganese deposition.

The concentrations of blood NH_3, particularly if measured repeatedly in arterial blood samples, usually are well in excess of 200 mg/dL, and the severity of the neurologic and EEG disorders roughly parallels to the ammonia levels. With treatment, a fall in the NH_3 levels precedes clinical improvement.

Neuropathologic Changes

The striking finding by Adams and Foley in patients who died in a state of hepatic coma was a diffuse increase in the number and size of the protoplasmic astrocytes in the deep layers of the cerebral cortex, lenticular nuclei, thalamus, substantia nigra, cerebellar cortex, and red, dentate, and pontine nuclei, with little or no visible alteration in the nerve cells or other parenchymal elements. With periodic acid-Schiff (PAS) staining, the astrocytes were seen to contain glycogen inclusions. These abnormal glia cells are generally referred to as Alzheimer type II astrocytes, having been described originally in 1912 by von Hosslin and Alzheimer in a patient with Westphal-Strümpell pseudosclerosis (or Wilson disease). These astrocytes have been studied by electron microscopy in rats with surgically created portacaval shunts (Cavanagh; Norenberg); the cells show a number of striking abnormalities—swelling of their terminal processes, cytoplasmic vacuolation (distended sacs of rough endoplasmic reticulum), formation of folds in the basement membrane around capillaries, and an increase in both the number of mitochondria and enzymes that catabolize ammonia. Also, some degeneration in myelinated nerve fibers in the neuropil and an increase in the cytoplasm of oligodendrocytes are seen. In chronic cases, neuronal loss in the deep layers of the cerebral and cerebellar cortex and lenticular nuclei is found, as well as vacuolization of tissue (possibly astrocytic) resembling the lesions of Wilson disease.

The ubiquitous astrocytic alterations occur to some degree in all patients who die of progressive liver failure and the degree of glial abnormality corresponds generally to the intensity and duration of the neurologic disorder. Possibly, the astrocytic changes affect the synaptic activities of the neurons. The clinical and EEG features of hepatic encephalopathy as well as the astrocytic hyperplasia are more or less specific features of this metabolic disorder. Nevertheless, taken together in a setting of liver failure, they constitute a distinctive clinicopathologic entity.

Pathogenesis of Hepatic Encephalopathy

The most plausible hypothesis relates hepatic coma to an abnormality of nitrogen metabolism, wherein ammonia, which is formed in the bowel by the action of urease-containing organisms on dietary protein, is carried to the liver in the portal circulation but fails to be converted into urea because of hepatocellular disease, portal–systemic shunting of blood, or both. As a result, excess NH_3 reaches the systemic circulation, where it interferes with cerebral metabolism in a way that is not fully understood. The ammonia theory best explains the basic neuropathologic change. Because the brain is lacking in urea cycle enzymes, Norenberg has proposed that the hypertrophy of the astrocytic cytoplasm and proliferation of mitochondria and endoplasmic reticulum, as well as the increase in the astroglial glutamic dehydrogenase activity, all reflect heightened metabolic activity of these systems within astrocytes associated with ammonia detoxification. Removal of brain ammonia depends on the formation of glutamine, a reaction that is catalyzed by the ATP-dependent enzyme glutamine synthetase, which is compartmentalized to astrocytes. It has been shown in experimental animals that hyperammonemia leads to a depletion of ATP in midbrain reticular nuclei. Whether this is the primary cause of cerebral dysfunction has not been resolved.

Numerous alternative theories have been suggested. One is that CNS function in cirrhotic patients is impaired by phenols or short-chain fatty acids derived from the diet or from bacterial metabolism of carbohydrate. Another theory holds that biogenic amines (e.g., octopamine), which arise in the gut and bypass the liver, act as false neurotransmitters, displacing norepinephrine and dopamine (Fischer and Baldessarini). Zieve has presented evidence that mercaptans (methanethiol, methionine), which are also generated in the gastrointestinal tract and removed by the liver, act in conjunction with NH_3 to produce hepatic encephalopathy. This theory and others have been largely discounted; they are the subject of reviews by Butterworth and coworkers, by Zieve, by Rothstein and Herlong, and by Jones and Basile, to which the reader is referred for detailed information.

Also, manganese has emerged as a potential neurotoxin in the pathogenesis of hepatic encephalopathy (Kreiger et al; Pomier-Layrargues et al). In patients with chronic liver disease and with spontaneous or surgically induced portal–systemic shunts, manganese accumulates in the serum and in the brain, more specifically in the pallidum. This accumulation is readily discernible as a pallidal signal hyperintensity on T1-weighted MRI. Following liver transplantation, there is normalization of the MRI changes and of the associated extrapyramidal symptoms. The effects of manganese chelation on such patients have not been well studied and the mechanisms of accumulated manganese in the pathogenesis of hepatic encephalopathy are not known. It is clear, therefore, that any theory of hepatic encephalopathy must incorporate the cerebral effects of hyperammonemia.

For some time, it has been known that hepatic encephalopathy is associated with increased activity of the inhibitory transmitter GABA in the cerebral cortex. It has also been observed that increased gabanergic neurotransmission may result from substances that inhibit the binding of endogenous benzodiazepine-like compounds to their receptors (Basile et al). Furthermore, these antagonists are found to have some clinical effect—transient arousal in patients with hepatic encephalopathy. The actions of benzodiazepines are mediated by these receptors; hence the designation *GABA-benzodiazepine theory*. The practicality of using benzodiazepine receptor antagonists, which are short-acting and reversible (e.g., flumazenil) in the treatment of hepatic encephalopathy, remains to be determined (see Mullen), but they offer an interesting diagnostic test.

Until recently, the ammonia and the gabanergic-benzodiazepine hypotheses of the pathogenesis of hepatic encephalopathy had appeared to be unrelated. However, there is evidence, reviewed by Jones and Basile, that ammonia, even in the modestly elevated concentrations that occur in liver failure, inhibits metabolism of GABA by the astrocytes and enhances gabanergic neurotransmission—a concept that unifies hyperammonemia and the neurotransmitter change. Furthermore, the aforementioned glial abnormality may be the explanation for the disorder of the blood-brain barrier that leads to the brain swelling that is seen in some rapidly developing cases of PSE, the prototype for which is the now infrequent Reye syndrome. A parallel astrocytic dysfunction may lead to disruption of the blood–brain barrier and the brain swelling that is known to occur in cases of acute liver failure.

Treatment

Despite the incompleteness of our understanding of the role of disordered ammonia metabolism in the genesis of hepatic coma, an awareness of this relationship has provided the few effective means of treating this disorder: restriction of dietary protein; reduction of bowel flora by oral administration of neomycin or kanamycin, which suppresses the urease-producing organisms in the bowel; and the use of enemas. The mainstay of treatment has been oral lactulose, an inert sugar that is metabolized by colonic bacteria that produce hydrogen ions and shifts ammonia to ammonium, a nontoxic product that is eliminated in the stool. The past use of oral neomycin carried a risk of renal damage and ototoxicity and has therefore been replaced by rifaximin, a minimally absorbed antibiotic that has less risk. This antibiotic has also been shown by Bass and coworkers to be highly effective in preventing episodic hepatic encephalopathy in tenuously compensated patients. The salutary effect of these therapeutic measures, the common attribute of which is the lowering of the blood NH_3, further supports the theory of ammonia intoxication. Ultimately, in cases of intractable liver failure, transplantation becomes a treatment of last resort.

Other treatments with lesser value include bromocriptine, the aforementioned diazepine antagonist flumazenil, and keto analogues of essential amino acids. Theoretically, the keto analogues should provide a nitrogen-free source of essential amino acids (Maddrey et al), a treatment that has been largely abandoned, and bromocriptine, a dopamine agonist, should enhance dopaminergic transmission (Morgan et al) but its mechanism is not known. Administration of branched-chain amino acids may result in improvement in mental status but their effects have been variable and associated with an increased mortality (Naylor et al). The transient beneficial effect of the benzodiazepine antagonist flumazenil has already been mentioned; it is used as well as a diagnostic test.

Fulminant Hepatic Failure and Cerebral Edema

In *acute hepatitis*, confusional, delirious, and comatose states also occur but their mechanisms are still unknown. Blood NH_3 may be elevated but usually not to a degree that would be expected to cause encephalopathy. Severe acute hepatic failure may cause hypoglycemia, which contributes to the encephalopathy and often presages a fatal outcome but the levels of glucose typically detected do not provide an explanation for the encephalopathy.

Cerebral edema is a prominent finding in cases of fulminant hepatic failure and is the main cause of death in patients awaiting liver transplantation. The cerebral edema in these circumstances appears to be related to the rapidity of rise of blood ammonia, but it probably depends as well on additional metabolic derangements that complicate acute liver failure including glial cell failure with consequent incompetence of the blood-brain barrier. The combination of rapidly evolving hepatic failure and massive cerebral edema is similar to that observed in the Reye syndrome, described below.

CT and MRI are effective means of detecting cerebral edema in patients with fulminant hepatic failure, and according to Wijdicks and colleagues, the degree of cerebral swelling is roughly proportional to the severity of encephalopathy. Because patients with fulminant hepatic failure can survive liver transplantation with few or no neurologic deficits, it is important to recognize cerebral edema before the stage of stupor and increased intracranial pressure has been established. Short of transplantation, death in these cases may sometimes be prevented by monitoring the intracranial pressure (as outlined by Lidofsky et al) and administering osmotic diuretics and hyperventilation, as detailed in Chaps. 31 and 35 for the treatment of intracranial hypertension. Some survivors are nonetheless left with cerebral damage from raised intracranial pressure.

An additional issue that arises in assessing cerebral dysfunction in patients with liver disease is the possibility of adverse effects of medications. Individuals with hepatitis C who are treated with interferon-alpha may develop a spectrum of problems ranging from subtle cognitive impairment to a subacutely worsening headache, vomiting, altered consciousness, and focal neurologic findings. The milder syndromes are associated with no or few MRI-visible lesions but the severe ones are usually accompanied by signal changes in the white matter of the occipital lobes and elsewhere (posterior leukoencephalopathy; see Fig. 43-1).

Reye Syndrome (Reye-Johnson Syndrome)

This is a special type of nonicteric hepatic encephalopathy occurring in children and adolescents and characterized by acute brain swelling in association with fatty infiltration of the viscera, particularly the liver. Although individual cases of this disorder had been described for many years, its recognition as a clinical-pathologic entity dates from 1963, when a large series was reported from Australia by Reye and colleagues and from the United States by Johnson and coworkers. The disorder tended to occur in outbreaks (286 cases were reported to the Centers for Disease Control during a 4-month period in 1974). Mainly, these outbreaks were observed in association with influenza B virus and varicella infections, but a variety of other viral infections were implicated (influenza A, echovirus, reovirus, rubella, rubeola, herpes simplex, Epstein-Barr virus). Later it became apparent that the toxic or adjuvant effects of aspirin given during these infections played an important role in producing the disease. Today, only occasional instances of Reye syndrome are observed now that the association with aspirin administration has become widely known and its use in children with viral infections has been interdicted.

Most patients are children, boys and girls being equally affected, but rare instances are known in infants (Huttenlocher and Trauner) and young adults. In most cases, the encephalopathy is preceded for several days to a week by fever, symptoms of upper respiratory infection, and protracted vomiting. These are followed by the rapid evolution of stupor and coma, associated in many cases with focal and generalized seizures, signs of sympathetic overactivity (tachypnea, tachycardia, mydriasis), decorticate and decerebrate rigidity, and loss of pupillary, corneal, and vestibuloocular reflexes. One or two such cases were included in the series of acute "toxic encephalopathy" reported by Lyon and colleagues (see "Acute Toxic Encephalopathy" in Chap. 32). In infants, respiratory distress, tachypnea, and apnea are the most prominent features.

The liver may be greatly enlarged, often extending to the pelvis and providing an important diagnostic clue as to the cause of the cerebral changes. Initially there is a metabolic acidosis, followed by a respiratory alkalosis (rising arterial pH and falling Pco_2). The CSF is usually under increased pressure and is acellular; glucose values may be low, reflecting the hypoglycemia. The serum ALT, coagulation times, and blood ammonia are increased, sometimes to an extreme degree. The EEG is characterized by diffuse arrhythmic delta activity, progressing to electrocerebral silence in patients who fail to survive. CT and MRI show the cerebral swelling but are difficult to interpret in these young individuals, who lack any adult brain atrophy.

The major *pathologic findings* are cerebral edema, often with cerebellar herniation, and infiltration of hepatocytes with fine droplets of fat (mainly triglycerides); the renal tubules, myocardium, skeletal muscles, pancreas, and spleen are infiltrated to a lesser extent. There are no inflammatory lesions in the brain, liver, or other organs. There is not full agreement as to the pathogenesis of this disorder and the mechanism of aspirin toxicity but mitochondrial dysfunction has been implicated.

Prognosis and Treatment

In a series of children with blood ammonia levels greater than 500 mg/dL who were treated during the years 1967 to 1974, Shaywitz and colleagues reported a mortality of 60 percent. Once the child became comatose, death was almost inevitable. In more recent years, early diagnosis and initiation of treatment before the onset of coma have reduced the fatality rate to 5 to 10 percent. Treatment consists of the following measures: temperature control with a cooling blanket; nasotracheal intubation and controlled ventilation to maintain Pco_2 below 32 mm Hg; intravenous glucose covered by insulin to maintain blood glucose at 150 to 200 mg/dL; administration of lactulose, neomycin enemas, and hemodialysis to directly lower the NH_3 concentration; control of intracranial pressure by means of continual monitoring and the use of hypertonic solutions (see Chap. 30); and the maintenance of fluid and electrolyte balance (Trauner). Upon recovery, cerebral function returns to normal unless there had been deep and prolonged coma or protracted elevation of intracranial pressure.

Uremic Encephalopathy

Episodic confusion and stupor and other neurologic symptoms may accompany any form of severe renal disease—acute or chronic. The cerebral symptoms attributable to uremia (first described by Addison in 1832) are discerned in normotensive individuals in whom renal failure develops rapidly. Apathy, fatigue, inattentiveness, and irritability are usually the initial symptoms; later, there is confusion, dysarthria, tremor, and asterixis. Infrequently, this takes the form of a toxic psychosis, with hallucinations, delusions, insomnia, or catatonia (Marshall). These symptoms characteristically fluctuate from day to day, or even from hour to hour. In some patients, especially those who become anuric, symptoms may come on abruptly and progress rapidly to a state of stupor and coma. In others, in whom uremia develops more gradually, mild visual hallucinations and a disorder of attention may persist for several weeks in relatively pure form. The EEG becomes diffusely and irregularly slow and may remain so for several weeks after the institution of dialysis. The CSF pressure is normal and the protein is not elevated unless there is a uremic or diabetic neuropathy. In several reports, meningismus and a low-grade mononuclear pleocytosis have been mentioned (Merritt and Fremont-Smith), but we have not encountered this.

In acute renal failure, clouding of the sensorium is practically always associated with a variety of motor phenomena. These usually occur early in the course of the encephalopathy, sometimes when the patient is still mentally clear. The patient begins to twitch and jerk and may convulse. The myoclonic twitches involve parts of muscles, whole muscles, or entire limbs and are lightning-quick, arrhythmic, and asynchronous on the two sides of the body; they are incessant during both wakefulness and sleep. At times the movements resemble those of chorea or an arrhythmic tremor; asterixis is also readily evoked. The motor phenomena are often difficult to classify. Our predecessor authors described the condition as a *uremic twitch-convulsive syndrome*.

The resemblance of uremic encephalopathy to hepatic and other metabolic encephalopathies has been stressed by Raskin and Fishman, yet we are more impressed with differences than with similarities. When the twitch-convulsive syndrome is observed in association with other diseases such as widespread neoplasia, delirium tremens, diabetic coma, and lupus erythematosus, the causative factor of renal failure is usually discovered.

As the uremia worsens, the patient lapses into a quiet coma. Unless the accompanying metabolic acidosis is corrected, Kussmaul breathing appears and gives way to Cheyne-Stokes breathing and death.

Encephalopathy and coma in the patient with renal failure may, of course, be a result of disorders other than uremia itself. Because of the similarity of this syndrome to tetany, measurement should be made of serum calcium and magnesium—and, of course, hypocalcemia and hypomagnesemia do occur in uremia. But often the values for these ions are normal or near normal, and the administration of calcium and magnesium salts has little effect. The altered excretion of drugs leads to their accumulation, sometimes evoking excessive sedation. Subdural and intracerebral hemorrhages may complicate uremia (and dialysis) because of clotting defects and hypertension; and uremic patients are prone to infections, including meningitis.

Because chronic uremia is so frequently associated with hypertension, a major problem also arises in distinguishing the cerebral effects of uremia from those of severe and accelerated hypertension. Volhard was the first to make this distinction; he introduced the term *pseudouremia* to designate the cerebral effects of malignant hypertension and to separate them from true uremia. The preferable term, *hypertensive encephalopathy*, was first used by Oppenheimer and Fishberg. However, the myoclonic-twitch syndrome is not a component of hypertensive encephalopathy. The clinical picture of the latter disorder and its pathophysiology are discussed in "Hypertensive Encephalopathy and Eclampsia" in Chap. 34.

Pathogenesis

Opinions vary widely as to the biochemical basis of uremic encephalopathy and the twitch-convulsive syndrome. Restoration of renal function completely corrects the neurologic syndrome, attesting to the absence of structural change and a functional disorder of subcellular type. Whether caused by the retention of organic acids, elevation of phosphate in the CSF (claimed by Harrison et al), or the action of urea or other toxins, among them parathyroid hormone, has never been settled. The data supporting the causative role of urea itself are also ambiguous, just as they are for other putative endogenous agents (see Bolton and Young and the review by Burn and Bates). However, it can be stated that urea itself is not the sole inductive agent, as its infusion does not produce the syndrome in humans or animals.

It would appear that every level of the CNS is affected in uremia, from spinal cord to cerebrum. Cellular changes in the brain or spinal cord are limited to mild hyperplasia of protoplasmic astrocytes in some cases, but never of the degree observed in hepatic encephalopathy. Cerebral edema is notably absent. In fact, CT scans and MRI regularly show an element of cerebral shrinkage. A peripheral neuropathy is also a common complication of uremia and is considered in Chap. 46.

Treatment

Improvement of encephalopathic symptoms may not be evident for a day or two after institution of dialysis. Convulsions, which occur in about one-third of cases, often preterminally, may be resistant to treatment until the uremia is addressed. However, some seizures may be suppressed with relatively low plasma concentrations of antiepileptic drugs, the reason being that serum albumin is depressed in uremia, increasing the unbound, therapeutically active portion of a drug. If there are severe associated metabolic disturbances, such as hyponatremia, the seizures may be difficult to control. One must be cautious in prescribing any of a large number of drugs in the face of renal failure, for inordinately high, toxic blood levels may result. Examples that affect the nervous system are aminoglycoside antibiotics (vestibular damage); furosemide (cochlear damage); and nitrofurantoin, isoniazid, and hydralazine (peripheral nerve damage).

"Dialysis Disequilibrium" Syndrome

This term refers to a group of symptoms that may occur during and following hemodialysis or peritoneal dialysis as a byproduct of some degree of cerebral edema. The symptoms include headache, nausea, muscle cramps, nervous irritability, agitation, drowsiness, and convulsions. The headache, which may be bilateral and throbbing and resemble common migraine, develops in approximately 70 percent of patients, whereas the other symptoms are observed in 5 to 10 percent, usually in those undergoing rapid dialysis or in the early stages of a dialysis program. The symptoms tend to occur in the third or fourth hour of dialysis and last for several hours. Sometimes they appear 8 to 48 h after the completion of dialysis. Originally, these symptoms were attributed to the rapid lowering of serum urea, leaving the brain with a higher concentration of urea than the serum and resulting in a shift of water into the brain to equalize the osmotic gradient (*reverse urea syndrome*). Now it is believed that the shift of water into the brain is akin to water intoxication and is a result of the inappropriate secretion of antidiuretic hormone.

The symptoms of subdural hematoma, which in some series had in the past occurred in 3 to 4 percent of patients undergoing dialysis, now being less frequent, may be mistakenly attributed to the disequilibrium syndrome.

Dialysis Encephalopathy (Dialysis Dementia)

This is a subacutely progressive syndrome that in the past complicated chronic hemodialysis. Characteristically, the condition begins with a hesitant, stuttering dysarthria and aphasia, to which are added facial and then generalized myoclonus, focal and generalized seizures, personality and behavioral changes, and intellectual decline. The EEG is invariably abnormal, taking the form of paroxysmal and sometimes periodic sharp-wave or spike-and-wave activity (up to 500 mV and lasting 1 to 20 s), intermixed with abundant theta and delta activity. The CSF is normal except occasionally for increased protein.

At first the myoclonus and speech disorders are intermittent, occurring during or immediately after dialysis and lasting for only a few hours, but gradually they become more persistent and eventually permanent. Once established, the syndrome is usually steadily progressive over a 1- to 15-month period (average survival of 6 months in the 42 cases analyzed by Lederman and Henry). A characteristic feature is a transient improvement in speech with the administration of intravenous diazepines.

The neuropathologic changes are said to be subtle and consist of a mild degree of microcavitation of the superficial layers of the cerebral cortex. Although the changes are diffuse, they have been found in one study to be more severe in the left (dominant) hemisphere than in the right and more severe in the left frontotemporal operculum than in the surrounding cortex (Winkelman and Ricanati). The disproportionate affection of the left frontotemporal opercular cortex putatively explains the distinctive disorder of speech and language. In the one case we have studied carefully, we could not be certain of any microscopic changes.

The most plausible view of the pathogenesis of dialysis encephalopathy is that it represented a form of aluminum intoxication (Alfrey et al), the aluminum being derived from the dialysate or from orally administered aluminum gels. In recent years, this disorder has disappeared, the result, in all likelihood, of the universal practice of purifying the water used in dialysis and thereby removing aluminum from the dialysate. This subject has been reviewed by Parkinson and coworkers.

Complications of Renal Transplantation

The risk in immunosuppressed persons of developing a primary lymphoma of the brain or progressive multifocal leukoencephalopathy is well known and has been mentioned in previous chapters. An entirely different encephalopathy that is marked by widespread visual symptoms and edema of the cerebral white matter, evident on the MRI, but mainly occipital, occurs after the administration of cyclosporine and other immunosuppressant drugs. These imaging features of reversible posterior leukoencephalopathy or posterior reversible encephalopathy syndrome (PRES; see Chaps. 34 and 43), are not specific, being seen also in patients with hypertensive encephalopathy, eclampsia, intrathecal methotrexate administration, and other conditions (see Table 43-1 and Fig. 43-1) all of which are probably linked by endothelial dysfunction of cerebral vessels. Systemic fungal infections had in the past been found at autopsy in approximately 45 percent of patients who had had renal transplants and long periods of immunosuppressive treatment; in about one-third of these patients, the CNS was involved. *Cryptococcus*, *Listeria*, *Aspergillus*, *Candida*, *Nocardia*, and *Histoplasma* were the usual organisms. Recent experience suggests a far lower rate of infection but it remains a threat. Other CNS infections that have complicated transplantation are toxoplasmosis and cytomegalovirus (CMV) inclusion disease.

We have found examples of Wernicke-Korsakoff disease and central pontine myelinolysis in uremic patients. A bleeding diathesis may result in subdural or cerebral hemorrhage, as already mentioned.

Encephalopathy Associated with Sepsis and Burns ("Septic Encephalopathy")

Bolton and Young have drawn attention to the frequent occurrence, in severely septic patients, of a drowsy or confusional state that is reversible and not explained by hepatic, pulmonary, or renal failure, electrolyte imbalance, hypotension, drug intoxication, or a primary lesion of the brain. They called the condition "septic encephalopathy." According to their surveys, 70 percent of patients become disoriented and confused within hours of the onset of severe systemic infection; in a few cases, this state may progress to stupor and coma. Notably there are no signs of asterixis, myoclonus, or focal cerebral disorder but paratonia is common, as is the later development of a polyneuropathy. Rapid changes in water balance may occur, leading to the type of osmotic demyelination discussed below.

The encephalopathic state that occurs with severe systemic infection may also develop independently of sepsis, as a component of a syndrome of multiple organ failure and, according to some authors, a complication of widespread cutaneous burns (Aikawa et al). Others have questioned the validity of this last category and have instead found explanatory electrolyte disorders (particularly hyponatremia), sepsis, or multiple brain abscesses.

It has been useful in clinical work to distinguish these encephalopathies of infection and multiorgan failure from those caused by isolated hepatic or renal disease. The lack of a biochemical marker and the confounding effects of hypotension during sepsis (septic shock) leave doubt as to pathogenesis. Altered phenylalanine metabolism and circulating cytokines have been proposed as causes, without firm evidence. Of interest in two of our fatal cases was the presence of *brain purpura*, but this has otherwise been an infrequent finding. Here, the white matter of the cerebrum and cerebellum was speckled with myriad pericapillary hemorrhages and zones of adjacent necrosis. This pathologic reaction is nonspecific, having also been seen in cases of viral pneumonia, heart failure with morphine overdose, thrombotic thrombocytopenic purpura and arsenic poisoning.

Disorders of Sodium, Potassium, and Water Balance

Drowsiness, confusion, stupor, and coma, in conjunction with seizures and sometimes with other neurologic deficits, may have as their basis a more or less pure abnormality of electrolyte or water balance. Only brief reference is made here to some of these, such as hypocalcemia, hypercalcemia, hypophosphatemia, and hypomagnesemia, as they are considered in other parts of the text.

Hyponatremia and Syndrome of Inappropriate Antidiuretic Hormone

Hyponatremia is defined as a serum sodium level below 135 mEq/L. The hyponatremic state may be isotonic, hypertonic, or hypotonic, depending on the mechanism of reduced sodium concentration. The hypotonic variety is most common in neurologic practice but one also encounters cases of pseudohyponatremia caused by hyperlipidemia or hyperproteinemia (isotonic), hyperglycemic or mannitol-induced hyponatremia (hypertonic), and also cases of water intoxication. The last of these may be associated with systemic hypovolemic (blood loss, salt wasting), hypervolemic (edematous states such as renal, hepatic or heart failure), or isovolemic states (retention of free water).

Hypotonic isovolemic hypernatremia is most often a result of the *syndrome of inappropriate antidiuretic hormone secretion (SIADH)*. This state is of special importance because it complicates neurologic diseases of many types: head trauma, bacterial meningitis and encephalitis, cerebral infarction, subarachnoid hemorrhage, cerebral and systemic neoplasm, Guillain-Barré syndrome and the effects of certain medications. SIADH is the result of excretion of urine that is hypertonic relative to the plasma.

As the hyponatremia develops, there is a decrease in alertness, which progresses through stages of confusion to coma, often with convulsions. *As with many other metabolic derangements, the severity of the clinical effect is related to the rapidity of decline in serum Na.* Lack of recognition of this state may allow the serum Na to fall to dangerously low levels, 100 mEq/L or lower.

Treatment Most instances of hyponatremia have developed slowly, allowing for maintenance of brain volume by the extrusion from cells of various osmotic substances. Rapid correction of sodium in these circumstances risks a reversal of osmotic gradient and a reduction in brain volume. This, in turn, is associated with a special type of central nervous system demyelination ("osmotic demyelination" and central pontine myelinolysis) discussed below. One's first impulse is to administer NaCl intravenously, but this must be done cautiously to avoid these complications. Most cases of SIADH respond to the restriction of fluid intake—to 500 mL per 24 h if the serum Na is less than 120 mEq/L and to 1,000 mL per 24 h if less than 130 mEq/L. Even when the Na reaches 130 mEq/L, the fluid intake should not exceed 1,500 mL per 24 h. In extreme and rapidly developing (less than 48 h) hyponatremia with stupor or seizures, the mechanisms for maintaining cerebral cellular volume have not yet been engaged and therefore infusion of NaCl is necessary to prevent cerebral edema. The amount of NaCl to be infused can be calculated from the current and the target levels of serum Na by assuming that the infused sodium load is distributed throughout the total body water content (0.6 × weight in kilograms):

$$([\text{target Na} - \text{starting Na}] \times 0.6) \times \text{weight (kg)} = \text{infused Na load (mEq)}$$

The desired volume of normal saline can then be determined by keeping in mind that its sodium concentration is 154 mEq/L and that of 3 percent (hypertonic) saline solution is 513 mEq/L. If hypertonic saline is administered, it is usually necessary to simultaneously reduce intravascular volume with furosemide, beginning with a dose of 0.5 mg/kg intravenously, and to increase the dosage until a diuresis is obtained. (As a rule of thumb, 300 to 500 mL of 3 percent saline, infused rapidly intravenously, will increase the serum sodium concentration by about 1 mEq/L/h for 4 h.) Guidelines to prevent an overly rapid correction of Na are elaborated further on in relation to central pontine myelinolysis (no more rapidly than 10 mmol/L in the first 24 h). Although the syndrome of SIADH is usually self-limiting, it may continue for weeks or months, depending on the type of associated brain disease.

Not all patients with neurologic disorders who manifest hyponatremia have SIADH. Diuretic excess, adrenal insufficiency, and salt wasting also produce hypovolemic hyponatremia as a result of natriuresis. When renal salt wasting is seen in the context of a central neurologic disorder, the process has been termed "cerebral salt wasting" (Nelson et al). Sodium loss in these circumstances is attributable to the production by the heart or brain of a potent polypeptide natriuretic factor. As discussed in Chap. 34, under "Subarachnoid Hemorrhage," the distinction between SIADH and cerebral salt wasting is of more than theoretical importance, insofar as fluid restriction to correct hyponatremia may be dangerous in patients with salt wasting, particularly in those with vasospasm after ruptured intracranial aneurysms.

Arieff emphasized the hazards of *postoperative hyponatremia* in a series of 15 patients, all of them women, in whom *severe hyponatremia* followed elective surgery. About 48 h after these patients had recovered from anesthesia, their serum Na fell markedly, at which point generalized seizures occurred, followed by respiratory arrest. We are more familiar with acutely developing hyponatremia in the context of prostate surgery, where large amounts of hypotonic fluids are routinely administered both intravenously and intravascularly. A similar syndrome is known in instances of overly zealous fluid resuscitation in children with diabetic ketoacidosis. The mechanisms of neurologic deterioration in all of these cases is likely to be brain edema.

An important consideration in the management of severe hyponatremia, as mentioned earlier, is *the rapidity with which the abnormality is corrected and the danger of provoking central pontine myelinolysis* and related brainstem, cerebellar, and cerebral lesions (extrapontine myelinolysis; osmotic demyelination). These issues are considered below, in the section "Central Pontine Myelinolysis."

Hypernatremia

Hypernatremia (Na >155 mEq/L) and dehydration are observed in diabetes insipidus, the neurologic causes of which include head trauma with damage to the pituitary stalk (Chap. 27), and in nonketotic diabetic coma, protracted diarrhea in infants, and the deprivation of fluid intake in the stuporous patient. The last condition is usually associated with a brain lesion that impairs consciousness. Exceptionally, in patients with chronic hydrocephalus, the hypothalamic thirst center is rendered inactive and severe hypernatremia, stupor, and coma may follow a failure to drink. In hypernatremia from any cause, the brain volume is manifestly reduced. Retraction of the cerebral cortex from the dura has been known to rupture a bridging vein and cause a subdural hematoma.

As is true for hyponatremia, the degree of CNS disturbance in hypernatremia is generally related to the rate at which the serum Na rises. Slowly rising values, to levels as high as 170 mEq/L, may be surprisingly well tolerated. Rapid elevations of sodium shrink the brain, especially in infants. Extremely high levels cause impairment of consciousness with asterixis, myoclonus, seizures, and choreiform movements. In addition, muscular weakness, rhabdomyolysis, and myoglobinuria have been reported.

In hypernatremia with hyperosmolality, the brain retains its volume more effectively than do other organs by a compensatory mechanism that has been attributed to the presence of "idiogenic osmoles," possibly glucose, glucose metabolites, and amino acids. The impairment of neuronal function in this state is not understood. Theoretically one would expect neuronal shrinkage and possibly alteration of the synaptic surface of the cell.

Hypo- and Hyperkalemia

The main clinical effect of *hypokalemia* (≤2.0 mEq/L) is generalized muscular weakness (see Chap. 48). A mild confusional state had been alluded to in the literature but must be very infrequent. The electrolyte condition is readily corrected by adding K to intravenous fluid and infusing it at no more than 4 to 6 mEq/h. *Hyperkalemia* (>7 mEq/L) also may manifest itself by generalized muscle weakness, although the main effects are changes in the electrocardiogram (ECG), possibly leading to cardiac arrest.

Other Metabolic Encephalopathies

Limitation of space permits only brief reference to other metabolic disturbances that may present as episodic confusion, stupor, or coma. The most important members of this group are summarized below.

Hypercalcemia This is defined as an elevation of the serum calcium concentration greater than 10.5 mg/dL. If the serum protein content is normal, Ca levels greater than 12 mg/dL are required to produce neurologic symptoms. However, with low serum albumin levels, an increased proportion of the serum Ca is in the unbound or ionized form (upon which the clinical effects depend), and symptoms may occur with total serum Ca levels as low as 10 mg/dL.

In young persons, the most common cause of hypercalcemia is hyperparathyroidism (either primary or secondary); in older persons, osteolytic bone tumors, particularly meta-static carcinoma and multiple myeloma, are often causative. Less-common causes are vitamin D intoxication, prolonged immobilization, hyperthyroidism, sarcoidosis, and decreased calcium excretion (renal failure).

Anorexia, nausea and vomiting, fatigue, and headache are usually the *initial symptoms*, followed by confusion (rarely a delirium) and drowsiness, progressing to stupor or coma in untreated patients. A history of recent constipation is common. Diffuse myoclonus and rigidity occur occasionally, as do elevations of spinal fluid protein (up to 175 mg/100 mL). Convulsions are uncommon.

Hypocalcemia The usual manifestations are paresthesias, tetany, and seizures. With severe and persistent hypocalcemia, altered mental status in the form of depression, confusion, dementia, or personality change can occur. Anxiety to the point of panic attack is also known. Even coma may result, in which case there may be papilledema as a result of increased intracranial pressure. Aside from the raised pressure, the CSF shows no consistent abnormality. This increase in intracranial pressure may be manifest by headache and papilledema without altered mentation or with visual obscurations. Hypoparathyroidism is discussed again further on, under "Acquired Metabolic Diseases Presenting as Progressive Extrapyramidal Syndromes."

Other Electrolyte and Acid–Base Disorders Severe *metabolic acidosis* from any cause produces a syndrome of drowsiness, stupor, and coma, with dry skin and Kussmaul breathing. The CNS depression does not correlate with the concentration of ketones. Possibly, there are associated effects on neurotransmitters. It is often not possible to separate the effects of acidosis from those caused by an underlying condition or toxic ingestion.

In infants and children, acidosis may occur in the course of hyperammonemia, isovaleric acidemia, maple syrup urine disease, lactic and glutaric acidemia, hyperglycinemia, and other disorders, which are described in detail in Chap. 37. High-voltage slow activity predominates in the EEG, and correction of the acidosis or elevated ammonia level restores CNS function to normal provided that coma was not prolonged or complicated by hypoxia or hypotension. In uncomplicated acidotic coma, no recognizable neuropathologic change has been observed by light microscopy.

Encephalopathy as a consequence of *Addison disease* (adrenal insufficiency) may be attended by episodic confusion, stupor, or coma without special identifying features; it is usually precipitated in the addisonian patient by infection or surgical stress. Hemorrhagic destruction of the adrenals in meningococcal meningitis (Waterhouse-Friderichsen syndrome) is another cause. Hypotension and diminished cerebral circulation and hypoglycemia are the most readily recognized metabolic abnormalities; measures that correct these conditions reverse the adrenal crisis in some instances. Laureno (1993) reviewed the various neurologic syndromes that result from electrolytic disorders.

Central Pontine Myelinolysis and Other Patterns of Osmotic Demyelination

Adams, Victor, and Mancall observed a rapidly evolving quadriplegia and pseudobulbar palsy in a young alcoholic man who had entered the hospital 10 days earlier with symptoms of alcohol withdrawal. Postmortem examination several weeks later disclosed a large, symmetrical, essentially demyelinative lesion occupying the greater part of the base of the pons. Over the next 5 years, 3 additional cases (2 alcoholic patients and 1 with scleroderma) were studied clinically and pathologically, and in 1959 these 4 cases were reported by Adams and colleagues under the heading of *central pontine myelinolysis* (CPM). This term was chosen because it reflects both the main anatomic localization of the disease and its essential pathologic attribute: the remarkably dissolution of the sheaths of myelinated fibers and the sparing of neurons. Once attention was focused on this distinctive lesion, many other reports appeared and it became apparent that other areas of myelin in the brain could be similarly affected. The exact incidence of this disease is not known, but in a series of 3,548 consecutive autopsies in adults, the typical lesion was found in 9 cases, or 0.25 percent (Victor and Laureno).

Pathologic Features

One is compelled to define this disease in terms of its pathologic anatomy because this stands as its most characteristic feature, but it has been appreciated in recent years that the pons is not the only structure that may be affected. Transverse sectioning of the fixed brainstem discloses a grayish discoloration and fine granularity in the center of the base of the pons. The lesion may be only a few millimeters in diameter, or it may occupy almost the entire ventral pons. There is always a rim of intact myelin between the lesion and the surface of the pons. Posteriorly, it may reach and involve the medial lemnisci and, in the most advanced cases, other tegmental structures as well. Very rarely, the lesion encroaches on the midbrain but inferiorly it does not extend as far as the medulla. Identical extrapontine myelinolytic foci in the internal capsule, deep cerebral white matter and corpus callosum may occur independently ("extrapontine myelinolysis"). Exceptionally, symmetrically distributed lesions are found in the thalamus, subthalamic nucleus, striatum, amygdaloid nuclei, lateral geniculate body, white matter of the cerebellar folia (Wright et al).

Microscopically, the fundamental abnormality consists of destruction of the myelinated sheaths throughout the lesion, with relative sparing of the axons and intactness of the nerve cells of the pontine nuclei. These changes always begin and are most severe in the geometric center of the pons, where they may proceed to frank necrosis of tissue. Reactive phagocytes and glia cells are in evidence throughout the demyelinative focus, but oligodendrocytes are depleted. Signs of inflammation are conspicuously absent.

This constellation of pathologic findings provides easy differentiation of the lesion from infarction and the inflammatory demyelination of multiple sclerosis and postinfectious encephalomyelitis. Microscopically, the lesion resembles that of Marchiafava-Bignami disease (Chap. 41), with which it is rarely associated. In the chronic alcoholic, Wernicke disease is often associated with osmotic demyelination, but the lesions bear no resemblance to one another in terms of topography and histology.

Clinical Features

The two sexes are affected equally, and the patients do not fall into any one age period. Whereas the cases first reported had occurred in adults, there are now many reports of the disease in children, particularly in those with severe burns (McKee et al). More than half the cases have appeared in the late stages of chronic alcoholism, often in association with Wernicke disease and polyneuropathy. Most cases occur in the context of other serious medical conditions, and diseases with which osmotic demyelination has been conjoined are chronic renal failure being treated with dialysis, hepatic failure, advanced lymphoma, cancer, cachexia from a variety of other causes, severe bacterial infections, dehydration and electrolyte disturbances, acute hemorrhagic pancreatitis, and pellagra. The changes in serum sodium concentration, with which the process is closely aligned, are discussed below.

In many patients there are no symptoms or signs that betray the pontine lesion, presumably because it is so small, extending only 2 to 3 mm on either side of the median raphe and involving only a small portion of the corticopontine or pontocerebellar fibers. In others, its presence is obscured by coma from a metabolic or other associated disease. Prior to the inception of MRI only a minority of cases, exemplified by the first patient observed by Adams, Victor, and Mancall, were recognized during life. In this patient, a serious alcoholic with delirium tremens and pneumonia, there evolved, over a period of several days, a flaccid paralysis of all 4 limbs and an inability to chew, swallow, or speak (thus simulating occlusion of the basilar artery). Pupillary reflexes, movements of the eyes and lids, corneal reflexes, and facial sensation were spared. In some instances, however, conjugate eye movements are limited, and there may be nystagmus. With survival for several days, the tendon reflexes become more active, followed by spasticity and extensor posturing of the limbs on painful stimulation. Some patients are left in a state of mutism and paralysis with relative intactness of sensation and comprehension (pseudocoma, or locked-in syndrome).

The capacity of CT and especially MRI to visualize the pontine lesion has greatly increased the frequency of premortem diagnoses. The MRI discloses a characteristic "batwing" lesion of the pons in typical cases (Fig. 40-6), although this change may become evident only several days after the onset of symptoms. Brainstem auditory evoked responses also disclose the lesions that encroach upon the pontine tegmentum.

Variants of this syndrome are being encountered with increasing frequency. Two of our elderly patients, with confusion and stupor but without signs of corticospinal or pseudobulbar palsy, recovered; however, they were left with a severe dysarthria and cerebellar ataxia lasting many months. After 6 months, these patients' nervous system function was essentially restored to normal. In reference to the pathogenesis of this lesion, originally both patients had serum Na levels of 99 mEq/L, but information about the rate of correction of serum Na was not available. Another of our patients developed a typical locked-in syndrome after the rapid correction of a serum

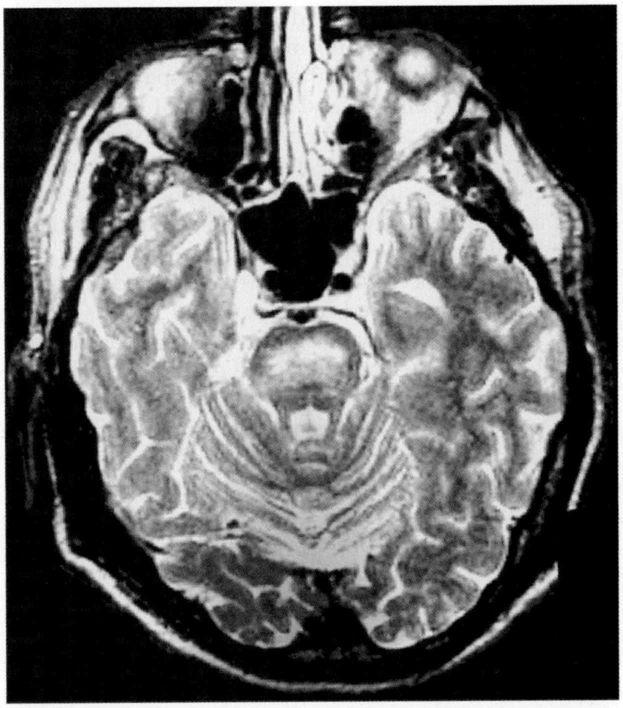

Figure 40-6. T2-weighted MRI showing the typical lesion of central pontine myelinolysis in an alcoholic patient.

sodium of 104 mEq/L. He showed large symmetrical lesions of the frontal cortex and underlying white matter but no pontine lesion (by MRI).

Brainstem infarction caused by basilar artery occlusion may be simulated by pontine myelinolysis. Sudden onset or step-like progression of the clinical state, asymmetry of long tract signs, and more extensive involvement of tegmental structures of the pons as well as the midbrain and thalamus are the distinguishing characteristics of vertebrobasilar thrombosis or embolism. On MRI studies, an evolving infarction shows signal changes on diffusion-weighted imaging, while the primary finding in osmotic demyelination is brightness of the T2-weighted images. Massive pontine demyelination in acute or chronic relapsing multiple sclerosis rarely produces a pure pontine syndrome. The clinical features and context provide the clues to correct diagnosis.

Etiology and Pathogenesis

As mentioned in the section on hyponatremia, a rapid rise in serum osmolality to normal or higher-than-normal levels is an almost obligate antecedent of this process. One encounters this most commonly in the rapid correction of hyponatremia. In cases related to the correction of hyponatremia, the initial serum sodium concentration is less than 130 mEq/L and usually much lower; this was the case in all the patients reported by Burcar and colleagues and by Karp and Laureno. Laureno (1983) demonstrated the importance of serum sodium in the pathogenesis of this disease experimentally. Dogs made severely hyponatremic (100 to 115 mEq/L) had the electrolyte disorder corrected rapidly by infusion of hypertonic (3 percent) saline; this led to spastic quadriparesis and pontine and extrapontine lesions were found at autopsy, indistinguishable in their distribution and histologic features from those of the human disease. Hyponatremia alone or slowly corrected hyponatremia (<15 mEq/dL in the initial 24 h) did not produce the disease.

McKee and colleagues adduced that in burn patients, extreme serum hyperosmolality was the important factor in the pathogenesis of demyelination. They found the characteristic pontine and extrapontine lesions in 10 of 139 severely burned patients who were examined after death. Each of their patients with CPM had suffered a prolonged, nonterminal episode of severe serum hyperosmolality, which coincided temporally with the onset of the lesion, as judged by its histologic features. Hyponatremia was not prominent and no other independent features could explain the changes. These observations suggest that rapidly rising osmolarity may be a cause of the osmotic demyelination syndromes.

At the present time all one can say is that specific myelinated regions of the brain, most often but not exclusively the center of the base of the pons, have a susceptibility to rapid increase in serum osmolality.

Karp and Laureno, on the basis of their experience and that of Sterns and colleagues, have suggested that the hyponatremia be corrected by no more than 10 mEq/L in the initial 24 h and by no more than about 21 mEq/L in the initial 48 h.

ACQUIRED METABOLIC DISEASES PRESENTING AS PROGRESSIVE EXTRAPYRAMIDAL SYNDROMES

These syndromes are usually of mixed type; i.e., they include a number of basal ganglionic and cerebellar symptoms in various combinations. They emerge as part of acquired chronic hepatocerebral degeneration or chronic hypoparathyroidism or as sequels to kernicterus, hypoxic, or hypoglycemic encephalopathy. The basal ganglionic–cerebellar symptoms that result from severe anoxia and hypoglycemia were described in the preceding section and in Chaps. 4 and 5. Kernicterus and calcification of the basal ganglia and cerebellum are considered in Chap. 37 and further on in this chapter. Acquired hypoparathyroidism may also lead to calcification of the basal ganglia and an extrapyramidal disorder. Choreiform movements are also observed in patients with hyperosmolar coma and with severe hyperthyroidism, ascribed by Weiner and Klawans to a disturbance of dopamine metabolism.

Chronic Acquired (Nonwilsonian) Hepatocerebral Degeneration

Patients who survive an episode or several episodes of hepatic coma are sometimes left with residual neurologic abnormalities such as tremor of the head or arms, asterixis, grimacing, choreic movements and twitching of the limbs, dysarthria, ataxia of gait, or impairment of intellectual function. These symptoms may worsen with repeated attacks of stupor and coma. In few patients with chronic liver disease, permanent neurologic abnormalities become manifest in the absence of discrete episodes of hepatic coma. Patients deteriorate neurologically over a period of months or years. Examination of their brains discloses foci of destruction of nerve cells and other parenchymal elements in addition to a widespread transformation of astrocytes, changes very much similar to those of Wilson disease.

Probably the first to describe this acquired type of hepatocerebral degeneration was van Woerkom, whose report appeared only 2 years after Wilson's original description of the familial form. A full account of the cases reported since that time as well as the extensive experience of our colleagues with this disorder is contained in the article by Victor, Adams, and Cole.

Clinical Features

The first symptom may be a tremor of the outstretched arms, fleeting arrhythmic twitches of the face and limbs (resembling either myoclonus or chorea), or a mild unsteadiness of gait with action tremor. As the condition evolves over months or years, a characteristic dysarthria, ataxia, wide-based, unsteady gait, and choreoathetosis, mainly of the face, neck, and shoulders, are joined in a syndrome. Mental function is slowly altered, taking the form of a dementia with a seeming lack of concern about the illness. A coarse, rhythmic tremor of the arms appearing with certain sustained postures, corticospinal tract signs ("hepatic paraplegia"), and diffuse EEG abnormalities complete the clinical picture. Other less-frequent signs are rigidity, grasp reflexes, tremor in repose, nystagmus, asterixis, and action or intention myoclonus. In essence, each of the neurologic abnormalities observed in patients with acute hepatic encephalopathy are also part of chronic hepatocerebral degeneration, the only difference being that the abnormalities are evanescent in the former and irreversible and progressive in the latter.

As a rule, all measurable hepatic functions are altered but the chronic neurologic disorder correlates best with an elevation of serum ammonia (usually >200 mg/dL). Unlike Wilson disease, where the cirrhosis usually remains occult for a long time, there is no question about its presence in the acquired syndrome; jaundice, ascites, and esophageal varices are manifest in most of the acquired cases. Wilson disease, which enters into the differential diagnosis, is usually not difficult to differentiate on clinical grounds, although the distinction in some cases requires the critical evidence of familial occurrence, Kayser-Fleischer rings (never found in the acquired type), and certain biochemical abnormalities (diminished serum ceruloplasmin, elevated serum copper, and elevated urinary copper excretion, discussed in Chap. 41).

Pathology

The cerebral lesions are localized more regularly in the cortex than is the case in Wilson disease. In some specimens an irregular gray line of necrosis or gliosis can be observed throughout both hemispheres and the lenticular nuclei may be shrunken and discolored. These lesions resemble hypoxic ones and may be concentrated in the vascular border zones but they tend to spare the hippocampus, globus pallidus, and deep folia of the cerebellar cortex, the sites of predilection in anoxic encephalopathy. Microscopically, a widespread hyperplasia of protoplasmic astrocytes is visible in the deep layers of the cerebral cortex and in the cerebellar cortex as well as in thalamic and lenticular nuclei and other nuclear structures of the brainstem. In the necrotic zones, the myelinated fibers and nerve cells are destroyed, with marginal fibrous gliosis; at the corticomedullary junction, in the striatum (particularly in the superior pole of the putamen) and in the cerebellar white matter, microcavitation may be prominent. Protoplasmic astrocytic nuclei contain PAS-positive glycogen granules. Some nerve cells appear swollen and chromatolyzed, taking the form of the Opalski cells usually associated with Wilson disease. The similarity of the lesions in the familial and acquired forms of hepatocerebral disease is striking.

Pathogenesis It is evident that a close relationship exists between the acute, transient form of hepatic encephalopathy and the chronic, largely irreversible hepatocerebral syndrome; frequently one blends imperceptibly into the other. The feature that ties these entities is the existence of portal–systemic shunting of blood. As noted above, this relationship is reflected in the pathologic findings as well. It appears that the parenchymal damage in the chronic disease simply represents the most severe degree of a pathologic process that in its mildest form is reflected in an astrocytic hyperplasia alone. Reducing the serum ammonia by the measures that are effective in acute hepatic encephalopathy will cause a recession of many of the chronic neurologic abnormalities—not completely, but to an extent that permits the patient to function better.

Hypoparathyroidism

This condition and pseudohypoparathyroidism were mentioned in relation to the hereditary metabolic disorders in Chap. 37. In the past, the usual cause was surgical removal of the parathyroid glands during subtotal thyroidectomy, although there continue to be idiopathic cases. With refinements in surgical technique and the use of radiation and drug therapy for thyroid disease, the number of surgically created cases has declined in proportion to nonsurgical ones. The condition in children may occur in pure form, presumably as an agenesis of the parathyroid glands, with unmeasurable levels of parathyroid hormone in the blood, or as part of the DiGeorge syndrome of agenesis of the thymus and parathyroid glands, organs that are embryologically derived from the third and fourth branchial clefts. Hypoparathyroidism is also part of a familial disorder in which a deficiency of thyroid, ovarian, and adrenal function, pernicious anemia, and other defects are combined, based presumably on autoimmune mechanisms. Other causes are intestinal malabsorption, pancreatic insufficiency, and vitamin D deficiency. In all instances the low levels of parathormone and normal responses to injected hormone permit the recognition of a primary defect of the parathyroid glands and distinguish it from all other conditions in which there is hypocalcemia and hyperphosphatemia.

The clinical manifestations, mainly attributable to the effects of hypocalcemia, are tetany, paresthesias, muscle cramps, laryngeal spasm, and convulsions. Children with this disease may be irritable and show behavioral changes. In adults with chronic hypocalcemia, calcium deposits occur in the basal ganglia, dentate nuclei, and cerebellar cortex. In such patients we have observed unilateral tremor, a restless choreoathetotic hand, bilateral rigidity, slowness of movement and flexed posture resembling Parkinson disease, and ataxia of the limbs and gait—in various combinations. Interestingly, the multiple skeletal and developmental abnormalities that characterize both pseudohypoparathyroidism (a failure of sensitivity to the hormone) and pseudopseudohypoparathyroidism (short stature, round face, short neck, stocky body build, shortening of metacarpal and metatarsal bones and phalanges from premature epiphyseal closure) are rarely seen in pure hypoparathyroidism.

A similar deposition of iron and calcium in the walls of small blood vessels of the lenticular and dentate nuclei, and to a lesser extent in other parts of the brain, is a common finding in normal older individuals (Fahr disease). It also occurs in animals. Occasionally, it reaches a degree of severity that destroys striatal or dentate neurons. In such cases, films of the skull and particularly CT scans will reveal the deposits (see Fig. 37-8), but the cause of the deposits is unknown. Apparently some protein in the capillary walls has an avidity for both calcium and iron.

ACQUIRED METABOLIC DISEASES PRESENTING AS CEREBELLAR ATAXIA

Cerebellar Ataxia with Myxedema

The association of myxedema and cerebellar ataxia has been mentioned sporadically in medical writings since the latter part of the nineteenth century. Jellinek and Kelly described 6 such cases; all showed gait ataxia; in addition, some degree of ataxia of the arms and dysarthria were present in 4, and nystagmus in 2. Cremer and coworkers reported a similar clinical experience based on a study of 24 patients with either primary or secondary hypothyroidism.

There are only a few reports of the pathologic changes. The myxedematous patient described by Price and Netsky had also been an alcoholic, and the clinical signs (ataxia of gait and of the legs) and pathologic changes (loss of Purkinje cells and gliosis of the molecular layer, most pronounced in the vermis) could be distinguished from those caused by alcoholism and malnutrition. Scattered throughout the nervous system of their case were unusual glycogen-containing bodies, similar but not identical to corpora amylacea. These structures, designated myxedema bodies by Price and Netsky, were also observed in the cerebellar white matter of a second case of myxedema; there were no other neuropathologic changes, however, and this patient had shown no ataxia during life. It is difficult to know whether these peculiar bodies have anything to do with myxedema. If they do, it should be possible to demonstrate them in more than 2 cases. Our colleagues did not see them in one carefully studied case of myxedema, nor have they been described by others. Serum creatine kinase (CK) is also slightly elevated in hypothyroidism, presumably because of its slowed metabolism. Thyroid medication corrects the defect in motor coordination and normalizes the CK, raising the possibility that this is the result of a subcellular mechanism.

Table 5-1 summarizes the various causes of cerebellar ataxia, including the metabolic ones. Notable metabolic disorders, some heritable, in which ataxia may be a leading manifestation include G_{M2} gangliosidosis, possibly sprue (discussed below), and a large number of neonatal and infantile aminoacidopathies.

Effects of Hyperthermia on the Cerebellum

The damaging effects of *hyperthermia*, like those of anoxia, involve the brain diffusely. In the case of hyperthermia, however, the changes are disproportionately severe in the cerebellum. The acute manifestations of profound hyperthermia are coma and convulsions, frequently complicated by shock and renal failure. Patients who survive the initial stage of the illness frequently show signs of widespread cerebral affection, such as confusion and pseudobulbar and spastic paralysis. These abnormalities tend to resolve gradually, leaving the patient with a more or less pure disorder of cerebellar function.

The most extensive account of the effects of hyperthermia is that of Malamud and colleagues. These authors studied 125 fatal cases of heat stroke but their observations are probably applicable to hyperthermia of other types. In patients who survived less than 24 h, the changes consisted mainly of a loss of some of the Purkinje cells and swelling, pyknosis, and disintegration of those that remained. In cases surviving beyond 24 h, there was almost complete degeneration of the Purkinje cells, with gliosis throughout the cerebellar cortex as well as degeneration of the dentate nuclei. The changes in the cerebellar cortex were equally pronounced in the hemispheres and vermis. The unanswered question is whether high temperature alone is an adequate cause or whether it must be combined with hypoxia and ischemia. It is of interest that this syndrome is not seen in patients with infective fevers, malignant hyperthermia, or the malignant neuroleptic syndrome—either the neuropathologic changes or the clinical cerebellar syndrome in survivors.

Cerebellar Syndromes Associated with Celiac Disease (Sprue, Gluten Sensitive Enteropathy)

Most often, the neurologic association with this disease has been a peripheral neuropathy, as described in Chap. 46. In addition, a progressive cerebellar ataxia of gait and limbs, sometimes with polymyoclonus in association with a gluten-sensitive enteropathy, has been the subject of several reports. The underlying cause of the enteropathy is an intestinal allergy to gluten in wheat that produces a villous atrophy of the intestinal mucosa. Between 0.5 and 1 percent of the white population are affected with the intestinal disorder. The classic features are diarrhea and malabsorption but many individuals are asymptomatic (see also Chap. 41).

The neurologic disorder may appear several years after onset of the enteropathy and, in addition to ataxia, usually includes signs of peripheral neuropathy and rarely, myelopathy or encephalopathy (dementia) or psychiatric symptoms (Hallert and Astrom; Hallert and Deerefeldt). A rare spinocerebellar syndrome was described by Cooke and Smith. According to Finelli and colleagues, neurologic abnormalities occur in approximately 10 percent of cases of adult celiac sprue. This subject was reviewed by Bhatia and colleagues and extensively by Hadjivassiliou and colleagues (1998, 2002). The latter authors emphasize the frequent occurrence of ataxia in patients with gluten sensitivity and, more specifically, antibodies to transglutaminase and endomysium, but, curiously, often without overt signs of bowel disease. There is also an association of sprue in more than 90 percent of patients with the HLA DQ2 and DQ8 genotypes. The few cases that have come to autopsy have shown severe cerebellar atrophy, a finding that may also be disclosed by MRI. Hadjivassiliou and colleagues (1998) observed lymphocytic infiltration and perivascular cuffing in the cerebellar cortex and peripheral nerves in one autopsied case but not in another, changes that they took to represent immunologic injury to these parts.

Despite these associations, some authors have been skeptical of a "gluten ataxia" (see the editorial by Cross and Golumbek and the contrary case for a valid connection by Hadjivassiliou et al [2002]). Reports of improvement in the ataxia following the institution of a gluten-free diet are conflicting.

The situation is further complicated by the finding that antigliadin antibodies (which are not autoantibodies but are directed against gluten, the offending agent), while not specific for celiac disease, do correspond to the presence of neurologic manifestations (ataxia and neuropathy); however, the more specific antiendomysium and antitransglutaminase autoantibody markers of sprue have little apparent relation to the presence of neurologic disease. Even more confusing is the claim that half of these patients will have one or another antibody but no clinical enteropathy, making it necessary to perform a small-bowel biopsy to detect villous atrophy.

A gluten-free diet is necessary, not only to reduce the enteropathy, if present, but also to reduce the chances of the later development of a bowel lymphoma. The medical issues relating to celiac disease and the use of antibody tests and bowel biopsy are reviewed by Farrell and Kelly.

We have sought evidence by antibody testing and bowel biopsy of sprue in numerous patients with an ataxia of obscure origin and have only once found it. Nevertheless, the evidence presented in the writings of several authors, particularly Hadjivassiliou, suggest that sprue may underlie some cases of subacute ataxia in adults. Paraneoplastic cerebellar degeneration and Creutzfeldt-Jakob disease should always be considered in the differential diagnosis of a case of subacute cerebellar ataxia. Vitamin E deficiency may induce a similar syndrome with features of spinocerebellar dysfunction.

Jejunoileal bypass operations, in addition to causing a chronic arthropathy, neuropathy, and vasculitic skin lesions, may give rise to an episodic confusion and cerebellar ataxia associated with a lactic acidosis and abnormalities of pyruvate metabolism. Overfeeding and fasting are provocative factors (Dahlquist et al).

ACQUIRED METABOLIC DISEASE PRESENTING AS PSYCHOSIS AND DEMENTIA

The point has been made that milder forms of metabolic diseases that cause episodic stupor and coma, if persistent, may have a protracted course and are then difficult to distinguish from the dementias (Chap. 21). Examples are associated with chronic hepatic encephalopathy and the syndromes of episodic hypoglycemia, chronic hypercalcemia (in multiple myeloma, metastatic cancer, and sarcoidosis), hyponatremia, and hypernatremia. Unlike the common types of dementia described in Chap. 21, the acquired metabolic diseases are nearly always accompanied by a degree of drowsiness and inattentiveness—attributes that usually allow an encephalopathic confusional state to be distinguished from a dementia. The presence of asterixis is also an aid. If the onset of the illness is abrupt rather than gradual and of brief duration, and if therapy reverses the condition, restoring full mental clarity, the conclusion is justified that one is dealing with a confusional state, but at any one time in the active phase of the disease, the clinical state may resemble dementia.

In general hospitals, an episodic confusional state lasting days and weeks in the course of a medical illness or following an operation should always raise the suspicion of one of the aforementioned metabolic derangements (*or an adverse effect of a drug*). Usually, however, if these causes can be excluded, one falls back on a rather unsatisfactory interpretation—that a combination of drugs, fever, toxemia, and unspecifiable metabolic disorders is responsible. The "septic encephalopathy" described earlier in this chapter conforms to this ambiguous notion.

In the endocrine encephalopathies described below, the clinical phenomena may take the form of a delirium. Confusional states may be combined with agitation, hallucinations, delusions, anxiety, and depression, and the time span of the illness may be in terms of weeks and months rather than days. Certain aspects of the endocrine psychoses are discussed further on.

Cushing Syndrome and Corticosteroid Psychoses

Derangements of mental function that follow administration of adrenocorticotropic hormone (ACTH) and of corticosteroids have become the prototypes of iatrogenic psychoses. The same disturbances of mental function may accompany Cushing disease (see "Corticosteroid and Adrenocorticotropic Hormone Psychosis" in Chap. 53). Experience with this neuropsychiatric condition came originally from observations of patients receiving ACTH and later from those receiving prednisone for a variety of neurologic and medical diseases. With low doses there is usually no psychic effect other than a sense of well-being and decreased fatigability. At higher doses (equivalent to 60 to 100 mg/d of prednisone), approximately 10 to 15 percent of patients become overly active, emotionally labile, and unable to sleep. Unless the dose is promptly reduced, a progressive shift in mood follows, usually toward euphoria and hypomania, but sometimes toward depression and then inattentiveness, distractibility, and mild confusion. The EEG becomes less-well modulated and slower frequencies appear. A minority of patients experience frank hallucinations and delusions, giving the illness a truly psychotic stamp and raising the suspicion of schizophrenia or bipolar disease. In nearly all instances, there is mixture of confusion and mood change, distinguishing the state from other mundane metabolic encephalopathies. Withdrawal of medication relieves the symptoms but full recovery may take several days to a few weeks, at which time, as with all confusional states and deliria, the patient has only a fragmentary recollection of events that occurred during the illness.

The neurologic basis of this condition is poorly understood. Its attribution to premorbid personality traits or a disposition to psychiatric illness is unconvincing. Critical studies of cellular or subcellular metabolism and morphologic changes are lacking. "Cerebral atrophy" (ventricular enlargement and sulcal widening) has been shown radiologically in patients with Cushing disease and after a prolonged period of corticosteroid therapy, but the basis of this change also is unclear (Momose et al). In most cases of brain shrinkage, withdrawal of steroids has led to a reduction in ventricular size, as documented on sequential imaging studies.

In patients with Cushing disease because of adrenal or basophilic pituitary tumors, mental changes suggestive of dementia and enlarged ventricles are unusual, especially by comparison to the incidence of these changes with exogenous corticosteroids. Here again, there is a peculiar combination of mood changes and impaired cognitive function. A frank psychosis may occur. This condition is described more completely in Chap. 53 and the attendant proximal myopathy, in Chap. 48.

Thyroid Encephalopathies

Hyperthyroidism

Allusions to psychosis in thyrotoxic patients are frequent in the medical literature. Mental confusion, seizures, manic or depressive attacks, and delusions occur singly or in combination. Action tremor is almost universal, and chorea occurs occasionally in various combinations with proximal muscular weakness. In descriptions of abnormal movements, it is often not clear whether it was chorea, tremor, myoclonus, or just fidgetiness that was observed. Treatment of the hyperthyroidism gradually restores the mental state to normal, leaving one with no explanation of what had happened to the CNS. The separate and special associations of hyperthyroidism with periodic paralysis and myasthenia are discussed in later chapters.

Thyroid crisis or "storm" refers to a fulminant increase in the symptoms and signs of thyrotoxicosis—extreme restlessness, tachycardia, fever, vomiting, and diarrhea—leading to delirium or coma. In the past, this was a not uncommon postoperative event in patients poorly prepared for thyroid surgery. Now it is seen mainly in patients with inadequately treated or untreated thyrotoxicosis complicated by serious medical or surgical illness.

Hashimoto Encephalopathy (Steroid-Responsive Encephalopathy Syndrome)

Brain and associates described an encephalopathy consisting of confusion, altered consciousness, and prominent myoclonus in patients with Hashimoto disease. The details were further elaborated by Shaw and colleagues and by Chong and associates. Some cases have had a relapsing course over months or years. It is important to note that most have had normal thyroid function. There are in these cases, however, high titers of several antithyroid antibodies, particularly antibodies against thyroid peroxidase and thyroglobulin; some affected individuals have more than one such antibody. Ferracci and colleagues found evidence of the production of these antibodies in the nervous system and of their presence in spinal fluid. One must be cautious, however, in interpreting the presence of antithyroid antibodies in the blood, as they are detected in many people without an encephalopathy, particularly older women, and in two-thirds of patients with Graves disease.

The most commonly observed syndrome is of confusion or stupor accompanied by multifocal myoclonus. Seizures—including myoclonic and rarely, nonconvulsive status epilepticus. Hemiparesis, ataxia, psychosis, and unusual tremors, including those of the palate, have been reported in individual cases as in the series reported by Castillo and colleagues; they found tremor, transient aphasia, myoclonus, ataxia and seizures to be present in that order of frequency. Many had liver function abnormalities and one-fifth showed inflammatory changes in the CSF. Some of the reports included children.

Often there are other members of the family with a different autoimmune disease. It has been the myoclonic aspect of the encephalopathy, a feature of all of the cases we have observed, which has usually led to consideration of this diagnosis. It is not uncommon for such cases to be mistaken for Creutzfeldt-Jakob disease (subacute spongiform encephalopathy). Early descriptions of the illness included a pleocytosis of the spinal fluid and white matter lesions, but we have not noted these abnormalities. What limited pathology there is, in a case studied after 5 months of illness, has shown only nonspecific activation of microglia cells (Perrot et al).

Treatment The encephalopathic symptoms and high titers of antithyroid antibodies respond well to steroid therapy (see Chong et al). In the case reported by Newcomer and associates, a rapid reversal of thyrotoxic coma (and corticospinal signs) was effected by plasma exchange, in parallel with a reduction in T_4 and T_3 levels, and similar results were reported by Boers and Colebatch. The circulating antibodies and the response to corticosteroids and plasma exchange implicate an immune pathogenesis, perhaps similar to paraneoplastic "limbic encephalitis" (see "Encephalomyelitis Associated with Carcinoma and Limbic Encephalitis" in Chap. 31) and to lupus, as well as to the rare encephalitis that may accompany thymoma or ovarian teratoma.

Hypothyroidism

As a rule, in the myxedematous patient, cognitive activity is slowed; in exceptional cases, there is a significant confusional state or stupor. When such changes have been observed, we have noted drowsiness, inattentiveness, and apathy as early features. In 2 cases observed by our colleagues, the somnolence was so extreme that the patients could not stay awake long enough to be fed or examined. They were in a state of hypothermic stupor but exhibited no other neurologic abnormality. In extreme form, the state progresses to "myxedema coma." This state is often precipitated by stresses, particularly surgery and sepsis, mainly in the elderly. Hypothermia, hyponatremia and elevation of serum creatine kinase (CK) concentration, hypoventilation, and elevation of the CSF protein can be expected. The clinical state and laboratory abnormalities are reversed within a few days by thyroid medication. The treatment of myxedema coma has several refined aspects, including the need to administer thyroid hormone cautiously; details can be found in *Harrison's Principles of Internal Medicine*.

Hypothyroidism is associated with a number of distinctive myopathic disturbances, which are discussed in Chap. 51. The ataxia and peripheral neuropathy that are sometimes observed in patients with myxedema were described earlier and in Chap. 46.

Cretinism and Neonatal Myxedema

This form of severe intrauterine hypothyroidism (in mother and fetus) or postnatally as a hereditary or acquired thyroid disease, is probably the most frequent and potentially preventable and correctable metabolic mental defect in the world. Table 37-1 provides a perspective on its relative frequency among neonatal metabolic disorders. Although the condition is most common in goitrous regions where there is a lack of iodine, it may also be the result of any of several genetically determined defects in thyroxin synthesis that have come to light in recent years (Vassart et al). In areas of endemic cretinism, additional factors may be operative, such as the widespread ingestion of cassava, which contains a toxic goitrogen that inhibits the uptake of iodine by the thyroid.

The symptoms and signs of congenital thyroid deficiency are not usually recognizable at birth but become apparent only after a few weeks; more often the diagnosis is first made between the sixth and twelfth months of life. Physiologic jaundice tends to have been severe and prolonged (up to 3 months), and this, along with widening of the posterior fontanelle and mottling of the skin, should raise suspicion of the disease.

Two types of early life hypothyroidism are recognized—sporadic and endemic. The sporadic type occurs occasionally in developed countries (less than once in 4,000 live births) and is a consequence of a congenital metabolic or anatomic disorder of the thyroid gland. At birth, the gland is either absent or represented by cysts, indicating a failure of development or a destructive lesion. In the sporadic form, in the latter part of the first year, stunting of growth and delay in psychomotor development become evident. Untreated, the child is severely retarded but placid and good natured; such children sleep contentedly for longer periods than normal children. Sitting, standing, and walking are delayed. Movements are slow, and if tendon reflexes can be obtained, their relaxation time is clearly delayed. The body temperature is low, and the extremities are cold and cyanotic. Although the head is small, the fontanelles may not close until the sixth or seventh year, and there is delayed ossification. This type of hypothyroidism is preventable by treatment with thyroid hormone.

Endemic cretinism is most common in developing countries, with an estimated incidence in some areas of 5 to 15 percent. DeLong and colleagues, on the basis of epidemiologic surveys mainly in western China, have distinguished two forms of endemic cretinism: neurologic and myxedematous. The occurrence of the two different types is governed by the timing, duration, and severity of the iodine deficiency (Thilly et al).

The *neurologic form of endemic cretinism* is characterized by varying degrees of deaf-mutism or lesser degrees of hearing loss, dysarthria, proximal limb and truncal rigid-spastic motor disorder involving mainly the lower extremities, and mental deficiency of a characteristic type. In the most severely affected, there is also strabismus, kyphoscoliosis, underdevelopment of leg muscles, and frontal lobe release signs. Bone age, head size, and height are normal and there are none of the coarse facial features of the myxedematous form. In the *myxedematous form of endemic cretinism*, short stature, microcephaly, coarse facial features, and retarded psychomotor development are the main features. There is no deafness or spastic rigidity of the limbs. In typical instances, the face is pale and puffy; the skin dry; the hair coarse, scanty, and dry; the eyelids thickened; the thickened lips parted by the enlarged tongue; the forehead low; and the base of the nose broad. There are fat pads above the clavicles and in the axillae. The abdomen is protuberant, often with an umbilical hernia, and the head is small.

DeLong and others attribute neurologic cretinism to a lack of available iodine in the mother and fetus during the second and third trimesters of pregnancy; neither mother nor fetus produces thyroxine. It is during the latter part of the second trimester, when the cochleas and the neuronal population of the cerebral cortex and basal ganglia are forming, that these structures suffer irreparable damage from lack of thyroid hormone. The effects of this midfetal hypothyroidism and iodine deficiency cannot be corrected by giving thyroid hormone at birth and thereafter. It can be prevented only by providing iodine therapy to the mother before and during the first trimester of pregnancy (Cao et al). The myxedematous form of cretinism is more likely to occur from lack of thyroid hormone in the late second and the third trimesters.

The congenital mental defect ranges from apathy and absence of social interaction to an alert, cooperative state but slowness in higher-order thinking and verbal facility is always evident. The status of the thyroid gland varies; among neurologic cretins, about half have goiters or have palpable glands; in the rest, the glands are atrophied; practically all myxedematous cretins are athyrotic. Although typical examples of neurologic and myxedematous hypothyroidism are readily distinguished, both types may exist in the same endemic area, and the stigmata of both forms may be recognized in the same individual. The QRS complex of the ECG is of low voltage; the EEG is slower than normal, with less alpha activity; the CSF contains an excess of protein (50 to 150 mg/dL); and the serum T_3 and T_4, protein-bound iodine, and radioactive iodine uptake are all subnormal. Serum cholesterol is increased (300 to 600 mg/dL).

At autopsy the brain of neurologic cretinism, although small, is normally formed, with all central and brainstem structures and cortical sulcation intact. A reduction in number of nerve cells was described by Marinesco, especially in the fifth cortical layer, but others have not confirmed this finding. The use of Golgi and other silver techniques has shown decreased interneuronal distances (packing density is increased, as in the immature cortex) where there is a deficiency of neuropil. The latter change is because of a poverty of dendritic branchings and crossings, and presumably there is a decrease of the synaptic surfaces of cells (Eayrs). Thyroid hormone appears to be essential, not for neuronal formation and migration but for dendritic–axonal development and organization.

There is substantial evidence that the administration of iodized salt or iodinated vegetable oil or iodide tablets to populations of women who are at risk of iodine deficiency, before and during the first trimester of pregnancy prevents sporadic and endemic cretinism. Treatment begun during the second trimester protects the fetal brain to a varying degree. Treatment that is started after the beginning of the third trimester does not improve the neurologic status, although head growth and statural development may improve slightly (Cao et al). In sporadic cretinism, if the condition is recognized at birth and treated consistently with thyroid hormones, height and mental development can be stimulated to normal or near-normal levels. The extent of recovery depends on the severity and duration of intrauterine hypothyroidism, i.e., its duration before treatment was begun and the adequacy of therapy. In most patients, some degree of mental deficiency persists throughout life.

"Pancreatic Encephalopathy"

This term was introduced by Rothermich and von Haam in 1941 to describe what they considered to be a fairly uniform clinical state in patients with acute abdominal symptoms referable to pancreatic disease, mainly pancreatitis. The encephalopathy, as they described it, consisted of an agitated, confused state, sometimes with hallucinations and clouding of consciousness, dysarthria, and changing rigidity of the limbs—all of which fluctuated over a period of hours or days. Coma and quadriplegia have been reported. At autopsy, a variety of lesions have been described; two cases have had central pontine myelinolysis and others have had small foci of necrosis and edema, petechial hemorrhages, and "demyelination" scattered through the cerebrum, brainstem, and cerebellum. These have been uncritically attributed to the action of released lipases and proteases from the action of pancreatic enzymes (see review of this subject by Sharf and Levy).

The term *pancreatic encephalopathy* is now more often applied to a depressive illness that seems to occur with disproportionate frequency before the symptoms of a pancreatic cancer become apparent. More common in our experience are numerous cases of pancreatic cancer and sequential cerebral emboli from nonbacterial thrombotic (marantic) endocarditis.

The status of pancreatic encephalopathy, in the authors' opinion, is uncertain. Pallis and Lewis also express reservations and suggest that before such a diagnosis can be entertained in a patient with acute pancreatitis, one must exclude delirium tremens, shock, renal failure, hypoglycemia, diabetic acidosis, hyperosmolality, and hypocalcemia or hypercalcemia—any one of which may complicate the underlying disease. Other cases conform to the encephalopathy of multiorgan failure, discussed earlier.

References

Adams RD, Foley JM: The neurological disorder associated with liver disease. *Res Publ Assoc Res Nerv Ment Dis* 32:198, 1953.

Adams RD, Victor M, Mancall EL: Central pontine myelinolysis. *Arch Neurol Psychiatry* 81:154, 1959.

Aikawa N, Shinozawa Y, Ishibiki K, et al: Clinical analysis of multiple organ failure in burned patients. *Burns Incl Therm Inj* 13:103, 1987.

Alfrey AC, Legendre GR, Kaehny WD: The dialysis encephalopathy syndrome: Possible aluminum intoxication. *N Engl J Med* 294:184, 1976.

Ames A, Wright RL, Kowada M, et al: Cerebral ischemia: II. The no-reflow phenomenon. *Am J Pathol* 52:437, 1968.

Arieff AI: Hyponatremia, convulsions, respiratory arrest, and permanent brain damage after elective surgery in healthy women. *N Engl J Med* 314:1529, 1986.

Auer RN: Progress review: Hypoglycemic brain damage. *Stroke* 17:699, 1986.

Austen FK, Carmichael MW, Adams RD: Neurologic manifestations of chronic pulmonary insufficiency. *N Engl J Med* 257:579, 1957.

Basile AS, Hughes RD, Harrison PM, et al: Elevated brain concentrations of 1,4-benzodiazepines in fulminant hepatic failure. *N Engl J Med* 325:473, 1991.

Bass NM, Mullen KD, Sanyal A, et al: Rifaximin treatment in hepatic encephalopathy. *N Engl J Med* 362:1071, 2010.

Bernard SA, Gray TW, Buist MD, et al: Treatment of comatose survivors of out-of-hospital cardiac arrest with induced hypothermia. *N Engl J Med* 346:557, 2002.

Bhatia MP, Brown P, Gregory R, et al: Progressive myoclonic ataxia associated with coeliac disease. *Brain* 118:1087, 1995.

Boers PM, Coers JG: Hashimoto's encephalopathy responding to plasma-pheresis. *J Neurol Neurosurg Psychiatr* 70:132, 2001.

Bolton CF, Young GB: *Neurological Complications of Renal Disease*. Boston, Butterworth, 1990.

Bolton C, Young GB, Zochodne DW: The neurological complications of sepsis. *Ann Neurol* 33:94, 1993.

Booth CM, Boone RH, Tomlinson G, Detsky AS: Is this patient dead, vegetative, or severely impaired? *JAMA* 291:870, 2004.

Brain L, Jellinek EH, Ball K: Hashimoto's disease and encephalopathy. *Lancet* 2:512, 1966.

Burcar PJ, Norenberg MD, Yarnell PR: Hyponatremia and central pontine myelinosis. *Neurology* 27:223, 1977.

Burn DJ, Bates D: Neurology and the kidney. *J Neurol Neurosurg Psychiatry* 65:810, 1998.

Butterworth RF, Giguiere JF, Michaud J, et al: Ammonia: Key factor in the pathogenesis of hepatic encephalopathy. *Neurochem Pathol* 6:1, 1987.

Cao X-Y, Jian GX-M, Dou Z-H, et al: Timing of vulnerability of the brain to iodine deficiency in endemic cretinism. *N Engl J Med* 331:1739, 1994.

Castillo P, Woodruff B, Caselli R, et al: Steroid-responsive encephalopathy associated with autoimmune thyroiditis. *Arch Neurol* 63:197, 2006.

Cavanagh JB: Liver bypass and the glia. *Res Publ Assoc Res Nerv Ment Dis* 53:13, 1974.

Choi DW, Rothman SM: The role of glutamate neurotoxicity in hypoxic-ischemic neuronal death. *Annu Rev Neurosci* 13:171, 1990.

Choi IS: Delayed neurologic sequelae in carbon monoxide intoxication. *Arch Neurol* 40:433, 1983.

Chong JY, Rowland LP, Utiger RD: Hashimoto encephalopathy: Syndrome or myth? *Arch Neurol* 60:164, 2003.

Cooke WT, Smith WT: Neurologic disorders associated with adult coeliac disease. *Brain* 89:683, 1966.

Cremer GM, Goldstine NP, Paris J: Myxedema and ataxia. *Neurology* 19:37, 1969.

Cross AH, Golumbek PT: Neurologic manifestations of celiac disease. *Neurology* 60:1566, 2003.

Dahlquist NR, Perrault J, Callaway CW: D-Lactic acidosis and encephalopathy after jejunoileostomy: Response to overfeeding and to fasting in humans. *Mayo Clin Proc* 59:141, 1984.

DeLong GR, Stanbury JB, Fierro-Benitez R: Neurological signs in congenital iodine-deficiency disorder (endemic cretinism). *Dev Med Child Neurol* 27:317, 1985.

Diabetes Control and Complications Trial/Epidemiology of Diabetes Interventions and Complications (DCCT/EDIC) Study Research Group, The Long-term effect of diabetes and its treatment on cognitive function. *N Engl J Med* 356:1842, 2007.

DiMauro S, Tonin P, Servidei S: Metabolic myopathies, in Rowland LP, DiMauro S (eds): *Handbook of Clinical Neurology*. Vol 18. New York, Elsevier, 1992, pp 479–526.

Dooling EC, Richardson EP Jr: Delayed encephalopathy after strangling. *Arch Neurol* 33:196, 1976.

Eayrs JT: Influence of the thyroid on the central nervous system. *Br Med Bull* 16:122, 1960.

Farrell RJ, Kelly CP: Celiac sprue. *N Engl J Med* 346:180, 2002.

Ferracci F, Morett OG, Candeago RM, et al: Antithyroid antibodies in the CSF. Their role in the pathogenesis of Hashimoto's encephalopathy. *Neurology* 60:712, 2003.

Finelli PF, McEntee WJ, Ambler M, Kestenbaum D: Adult celiac disease presenting as cerebellar syndrome. *Neurology* 30:245, 1980.

Fischer JE, Baldessarini RJ: Pathogenesis and therapy of hepatic coma, in Popper H, Schaffner F (eds): *Progress in Liver Disease*. New York, Grune & Stratton, 1976, pp 363397.

Fishman RA: Cell volume, pumps and neurologic function: Brain's adaptation to osmotic stress. *Res Publ Assoc Res Nerv Ment Dis* 53:159, 1974.

Fishman RA: *Cerebrospinal Fluid in Diseases of the Nervous System*, 2nd ed. Philadelphia, Saunders, 1992.

Foley JM, Watson CW, Adams RD: Significance of the electroencephalographic changes in hepatic coma. *Trans Am Neurol Assoc* 51:161, 1950.

Gomcelli YB, Kutku L, Cavdar L, et al: Different clinical manifestations of hyperammonemic encephalopathy. *Epilepsy Behav* 10:583, 2007.

Griggs RC, Sutton JR: Neurologic manifestations of respiratory diseases, in Asbury AK, McKhann GM, McDonald WI (eds): *Diseases of the Nervous System*, 2nd ed. Philadelphia, Saunders, 1992, pp 14321441.

Hackett PH, Roach RC: High-altitude illness. *N Engl J Med* 345:107, 2001.

Hadjivassiliou M, Grünewald RA, Chatopadhyay AK, et al: Clinical, radiological, neurophysiological, and neuropathological characteristics of gluten ataxia. *Lancet* 352:1582, 1998.

Hadjivassiliou M, Grünewald RA, Davies-Jones GA: Gluten sensitivity as a neurological illness. *J Neurol Neurosurg Psychiatry* 72:560, 2002.

Hallert C, Astrom J: Psychic disturbances in adult celiac disease: II. Psychological findings. *Scand J Gastroenterol* 17:21, 1982.

Hallert C, Deerefeldt T: Psychic disturbances in adult celiac disease: I. Clinical manifestations. *Scand J Gastroenterol* 17:17, 1982.

Harrison TR, Mason MF, Resnick H: Observations on the mechanism of muscular twitchings in uremia. *J Clin Invest* 15:463, 1936.

Herrera L, Kazemi H: CSF bicarbonate regulation in metabolic acidosis: Role of HCO_3 formation in CSF. *J Appl Physiol* 49:778, 1980.

Hornbein TF, Townes BD, Schoene RB, et al: The cost to the central nervous system of climbing to extremely high altitude. *N Engl J Med* 321:1714, 1989.

Huttenlocher P, Trauner D: Reye's syndrome in infancy. *Pediatrics* 62:84, 1978.

Hypothermia After Cardiac Arrest Study Group: Mild therapeutic hypothermia to improve the neurologic outcome after cardiac arrest. *N Engl J Med* 346:549, 2002.

Jellinek EH, Kelly RE: Cerebellar syndrome in myxedema. *Lancet* 2:225, 1960.

Johnson GM, Scurletis TD, Carroll NB: A study of sixteen fatal cases of encephalitis-like disease in North Carolina children. *N C Med J* 24:464, 1963.

Jones EA, Basile AS: Does ammonia contribute to increased GABA-ergic neurotransmission in liver failure? *Metab Brain Dis* 13:351, 1998.

Karp BI, Laureno R: Pontine and extrapontine myelinolysis: A neurologic disorder following rapid correction of hyponatremia. *Medicine (Baltimore)* 72:359, 1993.

Krane EJ, Rockoff MA, Wallman JK, Walsdorf HU: Subclinical brain swelling in children during treatment of diabetic ketoacidosis. *N Engl J Med* 312:1147, 1985.

Kreiger D, Kreiger S, Jansen O, et al: Manganese and chronic hepatic encephalopathy. *Lancet* 346:270, 1995.

Lance JW, Adams RD: The syndrome of intention or action myoclonus as a sequel to hypoxic encephalopathy. *Brain* 87:111, 1963.

Laureno R: Central pontine myelinolysis following rapid correction of hyponatremia. *Ann Neurol* 13:232, 1983.

Laureno R: Neurologic syndromes accompanying electrolyte disorders, in Goetz CG, Tanner CM, Aminoff MKl (eds): *Handbook of Clinical Neurology*. Vol 63. Amsterdam, Elsevier, 1993, pp 545573.

Lederman RS, Henry CE: Progressive dialysis encephalopathy. *Ann Neurol* 4:199, 1978.

Levy DE, Caronna JJ, Singer BH, et al: Predicting outcome from hypoxic-ischemic coma. *JAMA* 253:1420, 1985.

Lidofsky SD, Bass NM, Prager MC, et al: Intracranial pressure monitoring and liver transplantation for fulminant hepatic failure. *Hepatology* 16:1, 1992.

Lyon G, Dodge PR, Adams, RD: The acute encephalopathies of obscure origins in infants and children. *Brain* 84:680, 1961.

Maddrey WC, Weber FL Jr, Coulter AW, et al: Effects of keto analogues of essential amino acids in portal-systemic encephalopathy. *Gastroenterology* 71:190, 1976.

Malamud N, Haymaker W, Custer RP: Heat stroke: A clinicopathologic study of 125 fatal cases. *Mil Surg* 99:397, 1946.

Malouf R, Brust JCM: Hypoglycemia: Causes, neurological manifestations, and outcome. *Ann Neurol* 17:421, 1985.

Marinesco G: Lesions en myxoedeme congenitale avec idiotie. *Encephale* 19:265, 1924.

Marshall JR: Neuropsychiatric aspects of renal failure. *J Clin Psychiatry* 40:181, 1979.

McDermott W, Adams RD: Episodic stupor associated with an Eck fistula in the human with particular reference to the metabolism of ammonia. *J Clin Invest* 33:1, 1954.

McKee AC, Winkelman MD, Banker BQ: Central pontine myelinolysis in severely burned patients: Relationship to serum hyperosmolality. *Neurology* 38:1211, 1988.

Merritt HH, Fremont-Smith F: *The Cerebrospinal Fluid*. Philadelphia, WB Saunders, 1938, p 212.

Momose KJ, Kjellberg RN, Kliman B: High incidence of cortical atrophy of the cerebral and cerebellar hemisphere in Cushing's disease. *Radiology* 99:341, 1971.

Morgan MY, Jakobovits AW, James IM, Sherlock S: Successful use of bromocriptine in the treatment of chronic hepatic encephalopathy. *Gastroenterology* 78:663, 1980.

Mullen KD: Benzodiazepine compounds and hepatic encephalopathy. *N Engl J Med* 325:509, 1991.

Myers RAM, Snyder SK, Emhoff TA: Subacute sequelae of carbon monoxide poisoning. *Ann Emerg Med* 14:1163, 1985.

Naylor CD, O'Rourke K, Detsky AS, Baker JP: Parenteral nutrition with branched-chain amino acids in hepatic encephalopathy: A meta-analysis. *Gastroenterology* 97:1033, 1989.

Nelson PB, Seif SM, Maroon JC, Robinson AG: Hyponatremia in intracranial disease: Perhaps not the syndrome of inappropriate secretion of antidiuretic hormone (SIADH). *J Neurosurg* 55:938, 1981.

Newcomer J, Haire W, Hartman CR: Coma and thyrotoxicosis. *Ann Neurol* 14:689, 1983.

Nielsen N, Wetterslev J, Cronberg T, et al: Targeted temperature management at 33°C versus 36°C after cardiac arrest. *N Engl J Med* 369:2197, 2013.

Norenberg MD: Astroglial dysfunction in hepatic encephalopathy. *Metab Brain Dis* 13:319, 1998.

Oppenheimer BS, Fishberg AM: Hypertensive encephalopathy. *Arch Intern Med* 41:264, 1928.

Pallis CA, Lewis PD: *The Neurology of Gastrointestinal Disease*. London, Saunders, 1974.

Pant SS, Rebeiz J, Richardson EP: Spastic paraparesis following portacaval shunt. *Neurology* 18:134, 1968.

Parkinson IS, Ward MK, Kerr DNS: Dialysis encephalopathy, bone disease and anemia: The aluminum intoxication syndrome during regular hemodialysis. *J Clin Pathol* 34:1285, 1981.

Perrot X, Firaud P, Biacabe A-G, et al: Encephalopathie d'Hashimoto: Une observation anatomo-clinique. *Rev Neurol* 158:461, 2002.

Plum F, Posner JB, Hain RF: Delayed neurological deterioration after anoxia. *Arch Intern Med* 110:18, 1962.

Pomier-Layrargues G, Rose C, Spahr L, et al: Role of manganese in the pathogenesis of portal-systemic encephalopathy. *Metab Brain Dis* 13:311, 1998.

Price TR, Netsky MG: Myxedema and ataxia: Cerebellar alterations and "neural myxedema bodies." *Neurology* 16:957, 1966.

Prockop LD: Hyperglycemia: Effects on the nervous system, in Vinken PJ, Bruyn BW (eds): *Handbook of Clinical Neurology*. Vol 27: Metabolic and Deficiency Diseases of the Nervous System. Part I. Amsterdam, North-Holland, 1976, pp 7999.

Raskin NH, Fishman RA: Neurologic disorders in renal failure. *N Engl J Med* 294:143, 204, 1976.

Reye RDK, Morgan G, Baral J: Encephalopathy and fatty degeneration of the viscera: A disease entity in childhood. *Lancet* 2:749, 1963.

Ropper AH, Gress DR, Diringer MN, et al: Hypoxic-ischemic cerebral injury, in *Neurological and Neurosurgical Intensive Care*, 4th ed. Philadelphia, Lippincott Williams & Wilkins, 2004, pp 260-277.

Rothermich NO, von Haam E: Pancreatic encephalopathy. *J Clin Endocrinol* 1:872, 1941.

Rothstein JD, Herlong HF: Neurologic manifestations of hepatic disease. *Neurol Clin* 7:563, 1989.

Schoch HJ, Fischer S, Marti HH: Hypoxia-induced vascular endothelial growth factor expression causes vascular leakage in the brain. *Brain* 125:2549, 2002.

Sharf B, Levy N: Pancreatic encephalopathy, in Vinken PJ, Bruyn GW, Klawans H (eds): *Handbook of Clinical Neurology*. Vol 27: Metabolic and Deficiency Diseases of the Nervous System. Part I. Amsterdam, North-Holland, 1976, pp 449458.

Shaw PJ, Walls TJ, Neman MB, et al: Hashimoto's encephalopathy: A steroid-responsive disorder associated with high antithyroid antibody titers—report of 5 cases. *Neurology* 41:228, 1991.

Shaywitz BA, Rothstein P, Venes JL: Monitoring and management of increased intracranial pressure in Reye syndrome: Results in 29 children. *Pediatrics* 66:198, 1980.

Sterns RH, Riggs JE, Schochet SS: Osmotic demyelination syndromes following correction of hyponatremia. *N Engl J Med* 314:1535, 1986.

Summerskill WHJ, Davidson EA, Sherlock S, Steiner RE: The neuropsychiatric syndrome associated with hepatic cirrhosis and extensive portal collateral circulation. *Q J Med* 25:245, 1956.

Thilly CH, Bourdoux PP, Due DT, et al: Myxedematous cretinism: An indicator of the most severe goiter endemias, in Medeiros-Neto G, Gaitan E (eds): *Frontiers in Thyroidology*. New York, Plenum Press, 1986, pp 10811084.

Thomas PK, King RH, Feng SF, et al: Neurological manifestations in chronic mountain sickness: The burning feet–burning hands syndrome. *J Neurol Neurosurg Psychiatry* 69:447, 2000.

Trauner DA: Treatment of Reye syndrome. *Ann Neurol* 7:2, 1980.

van Woerkom W: La cirrhose hepatique avec alterations dans les centres nerveux evoluant chez des sujets d'age moyen. *Nouv Iconogr Salpétrière* 27:41, 1914.

Vassart G, Dumont JE, Refetoff S: Thyroid disorders, in Scriver CR, Beaudet AL, Sly WS, Valle D (eds): *The Metabolic and Molecular Bases of Inherited Diseases*, 7th ed. New York, McGraw-Hill, 1995, pp 28832928.

Victor M, Adams RD, Cole M: The acquired (non-Wilsonian) type of chronic hepatocerebral degeneration. *Medicine (Baltimore)* 44:345, 1965.

Victor M, Laureno R: Neurologic complications of alcohol abuse: Epidemiologic aspects, in Schoenberg BS (ed): *Advances in Neurology*. Vol 19. New York, Raven Press, 1978, pp 603617.

Victor M, Rothstein J: Neurologic manifestations of hepatic and gastrointestinal diseases, in Asbury AK, McKhann GM, McDonald WI (eds): *Diseases of the Nervous System*, 2nd ed. Philadelphia, Saunders, 1992, pp 14421455.

Volhard F: Clinical aspects of Bright's disease, in Berglund H, Medes G, Huber CG, et al (eds): *The Kidney in Health and Disease*. Philadelphia, Lea & Febiger, 1935, pp 665673.

von Hosslin C, Alzheimer A: Ein Beitrag zur Klinik und pathologischen Anatomie der Westphal-Strumpellschen Pseudosklerose. *Z Gesamte Neurol Psychiatr* 8:183, 1912.

Weaver LK: Carbon monoxide poisoning. *N Engl J Med* 360:1217, 2009.

Weaver LK, Hopkins RO, Chan KJ, et al: Hyperbaric oxygen for acute carbon monoxide poisoning. *N Engl J Med* 347:1057, 2002.

Wegierko J: Typical syndrome of clinical manifestations in diabetes mellitus with fatal termination in coma without ketotic acidemia: So-called third coma. *Pol Tyg Lek (Wars)* 11:2020, 1956.

Weiner WJ, Klawans HL: Hyperthyroid chorea, in Vinken PJ, Bruyn BW (eds): *Handbook of Clinical Neurology*. Vol 27: Metabolic and Deficiency Diseases of the Nervous System. Part I. Amsterdam, North-Holland, 1976, pp 279281.

Wijdicks EFM, Plevak DJ, Rakela J, Wiesner RH: Clinical and radiologic features of cerebral edema in fulminant hepatic failure. *Mayo Clin Proc* 70:119, 1995.

Wilkinson DS, Prockop LD: Hypoglycemia: Effects on the nervous system, in Vinken PJ, Bruyn BW (eds): *Handbook of Clinical Neurology*. Vol 27: Metabolic and Deficiency Diseases of the Nervous System. Part I. Amsterdam, North-Holland, 1976, pp 5378.

Wilson SAK: Progressive lenticular degeneration: A familial nervous disease associated with cirrhosis of the liver. *Brain* 34:295, 1912.

Winkelman MD, Ricanati ES: Dialysis encephalopathy: Neuropathologic aspects. *Hum Pathol* 17:823, 1986.

Wright DG, Laureno R, Victor M: Pontine and extrapontine myelinolysis. *Brain* 102:361, 1979.

Young E, Bradley RF: Cerebral edema with irreversible coma in severe diabetic ketoacidosis. *N Engl J Med* 276:665, 1967.

Zieve L: Pathogenesis of hepatic encephalopathy. *Metab Brain Dis* 2:147, 1987.

41

Diseases of the Nervous System Caused by Nutritional Deficiency

Among nutritional disorders, those of the nervous system occupy a position of special interest and importance. The early studies of beriberi at the turn of the twentieth century were largely responsible for the discovery of thiamine and consequently for the modern concept of deficiency disease. A series of notable achievements in the science of nutrition followed the discovery of vitamins. Despite such progress, a number of diseases caused by nutritional deficiency, and particularly those of the nervous system, continue to represent a worldwide health problem of serious proportions. In some communities, where the diet consists mainly of highly milled rice, there is still a significant incidence of beriberi. In some developing countries, deficiency diseases are endemic, the result of chronic dietary deprivation. And the ultimate effects on the nervous system of intermittent mass starvation, involving large portions of the African continent, are alarming to contemplate.

It comes as a surprise to many physicians that deficiency diseases still occur in the United States and other parts of the developed world. To some extent this is attributable to the prevalence of alcoholism. Relatively less common causes are dietary faddism and impaired absorption of dietary nutrients, which occurs in patients with celiac sprue, pernicious anemia, or surgical exclusion of portions of the gastrointestinal tract for treatment of obesity, and the wasting syndromes of cancer and AIDS. Finally, there are iatrogenic deficiencies induced by the use of vitamin antagonists or certain drugs, such as isonicotinic acid hydrazide (INH), which is used in the treatment of tuberculosis and interferes with the enzymatic function of pyridoxine or methotrexate.

General Considerations

The term *deficiency* is used throughout this chapter in its strictest sense to designate disorders that result from *the lack of an essential nutrient or nutrients in the diet or from a conditioning factor that increases the need for these nutrients.* The most important of these are the vitamins, more specifically, members of the B group—thiamine, nicotinic acid, pyridoxine, pantothenic acid, riboflavin, folic acid, and cobalamin (vitamin B_{12}). However, some deficiency diseases cannot be related to the lack of a single vitamin. Usually the effects of several vitamin deficiencies can be recognized (thiamine deficiency causing Wernicke disease and subacute combined degeneration [SCD] of the cord, as a result of vitamin B_{12} deficiency, are notable exceptions that are due to single deficiencies).

Furthermore, nutritional diseases of the nervous system are not simply a matter of vitamin deprivation. The general signs of undernutrition, such as circulatory abnormalities and loss of subcutaneous fat and muscle bulk, are usually associated and conversely, a total lack of vitamins, as in starvation, is rarely associated with the classic deficiency syndromes of beriberi or pellagra. In other words, a certain amount of food is necessary to produce them. In a similar way, excessive intake of carbohydrates relative to the supply of thiamine favors the development of a thiamine-deficiency state. All deficiency diseases, including those of the nervous system, are influenced by factors such as exercise, growth, pregnancy, neoplasia, and systemic infection, which increase the need for essential nutrients, and by disorders of the liver and the gastrointestinal tract, which may interfere with the synthesis and absorption of these nutrients.

As already mentioned, alcoholism is an important factor in the causation of nutritional diseases of the nervous system. Alcohol acts mainly by displacing food in the diet but also by adding carbohydrate calories (alcohol is burned almost entirely as carbohydrates), thus increasing the need for thiamine. There is some evidence as well that alcohol impairs the absorption of thiamine and other vitamins from the gastrointestinal tract.

In infants and young children, a reduction in protein and caloric intake (so-called protein-calorie malnutrition [PCM]) has a devastating effect on body growth. Whether or not PCM also hinders the growth of the brain, with consequent effects on intellectual and behavioral development, cannot be answered as readily. The data bearing on this matter are discussed in the last part of this chapter.

Characteristic of the nutritional diseases is the potential for involvement of both the central and peripheral nervous systems, an attribute shared only with certain metabolic disorders. In addition, there are several distinctive neurologic disorders in which nutritional deficiency may play a role, although this has not been proved. These include (1) "alcoholic" cerebellar degeneration, (2) Marchiafava-Bignami disease (degeneration of the corpus callosum), and (3) central pontine and extrapontine myelinolysis, which are more closely aligned with the rapid correction of hyponatremia, as discussed in Chap. 40.

Some comments will also be made in this chapter about PCM, the neurologic disorders consequent to intestinal malabsorption, and the rare hereditary vitamin-responsive diseases. Deficiencies of trace elements, because of their rarity, are not discussed; only iodine deficiency (cretinism) is of much importance in humans, and it was discussed in Chap. 40 on acquired metabolic diseases.

WERNICKE-KORSAKOFF SYNDROME (THIAMINE [B_1] DEFICIENCY)

Wernicke disease and the Korsakoff amnesic state are common neurologic disorders that have been recognized since the 1880s. *Wernicke disease* is characterized by nystagmus, abducens and conjugate gaze palsies, ataxia of gait, and mental confusion. These symptoms develop acutely or subacutely and may occur singly or, more often, in combination. Wernicke disease is specifically the result of a deficiency of thiamine and is observed mainly, although far from exclusively, in alcoholics.

The *Korsakoff amnesic state* (Korsakoff psychosis) is a mental disorder in which retentive memory is impaired out of proportion to all other cognitive functions in an otherwise alert and responsive patient. This amnesic disorder, like Wernicke disease, is most often associated with the thiamine deficiency of alcoholism and malnutrition, but it may be a symptom of various other non-nutritional diseases that have their basis in structural lesions of the medial thalami or the hippocampal portions of the temporal lobes, such as infarction in the territory of branches of the posterior cerebral arteries, hippocampal damage after cardiac arrest, third ventricular tumors, and herpes simplex encephalitis. An almost equivalent type of memory disturbance may also follow acute lesions of the basal septal nuclei of the frontal lobe. Transient impairments of retentive memory of the Korsakoff type may be the salient manifestations of temporal lobe epilepsy, concussive head injury, and a unique disorder known as transient global amnesia. The anatomic basis of the Korsakoff amnesic syndrome is described in Chap. 21.

In the nutritionally deficient patient, Korsakoff amnesia is usually associated with and immediately follows the occurrence of Wernicke disease. For this reason and others elaborated in the following text, the term *Wernicke disease* or *Wernicke encephalopathy* is applied to a symptom complex of ophthalmoparesis, nystagmus, ataxia, and an acute apathetic–confusional state. If an enduring defect in learning and memory results, as it often does, the symptom complex is designated as the *Wernicke-Korsakoff syndrome.*

It is perhaps in part due to the emphasis in previous editions of this book that alcoholism has been inordinately associated with this disease complex. The disease arises in many other clinical settings. One of Wernicke's original cases, for example, occurred in a woman with hyperemesis gravidarum and such instances are still found. However, bariatric surgery, cancer chemotherapy, inanition in AIDS and from anorexia nervosa, and even in the frailty of older age, in nutritionally susceptible persons, starvation for economic and social reasons all may give rise to thiamine deficiency. Even the elderly and frail who subsist for years on "tea and toast" can acquire the disease. In addition, there are common medical circumstances in which a subclinical thiamine deficiency becomes manifest. Perhaps the most important of these is a carbohydrate load, particularly the administration of intravenous glucose to a malnourished individual; other precipitants are unbalanced intravenous hyperalimentation, refeeding syndrome, thyrotoxicosis, and hypomagnesemia.

The presence of this disease must be constantly emphasized. As summarized in the review by Sechi and Serra of published series from several countries, there is a discrepancy between the detection of the process in autopsy series, 0.5 to 3 percent, and the prevalence of the clinical diagnosis, 0.04 to 0.13 percent, indicating that *approximately three-quarters of cases are not recognized during life.*

Historical Note In 1881, Carl Wernicke first described an illness of sudden onset characterized by paralysis of eye movements, ataxia of gait, and mental confusion. His observations were made in 3 patients, of whom 2 were alcoholics and 1 was a young woman with persistent vomiting following the ingestion of sulfuric acid. In each of these patients there was progressive stupor and coma culminating in death. The pathologic changes described by Wernicke consisted of punctate hemorrhages affecting the gray matter around the third and fourth ventricles and aqueduct of Sylvius; he considered these changes to be inflammatory in nature and confined to the gray matter, hence his designation "polioencephalitis hemorrhagica superioris." In the belief that Gâyet had described an identical disorder in 1875, the term *Gâyet-Wernicke* is used frequently by French authors. Such a designation is hardly justified insofar as the clinical signs and pathologic changes in Gâyet's patients differed from those of Wernicke's patients in all essential details.

The first comprehensive account of this disorder was given by the Russian psychiatrist S.S. Korsakoff in a series of articles published between 1887 and 1891 (for English translation and commentary, see reference by Victor and Yakovlev). Korsakoff stressed the relationship between "neuritis" (a term used at that time for all types of peripheral nerve disease) and the characteristic alcoholic disorder of memory, which he believed to be "2 facets of the same disease" and which he called "psychosis polyneuritica." But he also made the points that neuritis need not accompany the amnesic syndrome and that both disorders could affect nonalcoholic as well as alcoholic patients. His clinical descriptions were remarkably complete and have not been surpassed to the present day. It is of interest that the relationship between Wernicke disease and Korsakoff polyneuritic psychosis was appreciated neither by Wernicke nor by Korsakoff. Murawieff, in 1897, first postulated that a single cause was responsible for both. The intimate clinical relationship was established by Bonhoeffer in 1904, who stated that in all cases of Wernicke disease he found neuritis and an amnesic psychosis. Confirmation of this relationship on pathologic grounds came much later. For further details the reader is referred to the extensive monograph by Victor, Adams, and Collins.

Clinical Features

The incidence of the Wernicke-Korsakoff syndrome cannot be stated with precision, but it had been a common disorder as noted in the introductory comments. At the Cleveland Metropolitan General Hospital, for example, in a consecutive series of 3,548 autopsies in adults (for the period 1963 to 1976), our colleague M. Victor (1990) found the pathognomonic lesions in 77 cases (2.2 percent). The disease affects males slightly more often than females and the age of onset is fairly evenly distributed between 30 and 70 years. In the past few decades, the incidence of the Wernicke-Korsakoff syndrome has fallen in the alcoholic population, but it is being recognized with increasing frequency among nonalcoholic patients in a variety of clinical settings that are prone to include malnutrition, including iatrogenic ones.

The triad of clinical features described by Wernicke of ophthalmoplegia (with nystagmus), ataxia, and disturbances of mentation and consciousness is still clinically useful provided that the diagnosis is suspected and the signs are carefully sought. Often, the disease begins with ataxia, followed in a few days or weeks by mental confusion; or there may be confusion alone, or the more or less simultaneous onset of ataxia, nystagmus, and ophthalmoparesis with or without confusion. In approximately one-third of cases, one component of this triad may be the sole manifestation of the disease. Timely treatment with thiamine prevents the permanent Korsakoff-amnesic component of the disease. A schematic representation of the various features is shown in Fig. 41-1, adapted from the series of 131 autopsied proved cases described by Harper, Giles, and Finlay-Jones. The notable aspects are that all 3 of the typical signs were present in only 16 percent; 1 sign in 31 percent, usually confusion alone; 2 signs in 28 percent; and no signs reported or detected during life in 19 percent. A description of each of the major manifestations follows.

Oculomotor Abnormalities The diagnosis of Wernicke disease is made most readily on the basis of the ocular signs. These consist of (1) nystagmus that is both horizontal and vertical and mainly evoked by gaze; this is the most common feature, (2) weakness or paralysis of the lateral rectus muscles, and (3) weakness or paralysis of conjugate gaze. Usually there is some combination of these abnormalities (see Chap. 14).

Next to nystagmus, the most frequent ocular abnormality is lateral rectus weakness, which is bilateral but not necessarily symmetrical and is accompanied by diplopia and internal strabismus. With complete paralysis of the lateral rectus muscles, nystagmus is absent in the abducting eyes and it becomes evident as the weakness improves under treatment. The palsy of conjugate gaze varies from merely a paretic nystagmus on extreme gaze to a complete loss of ocular movement in horizontal or vertical movements, abnormalities of the former being more frequent. An isolated paralysis of downward gaze

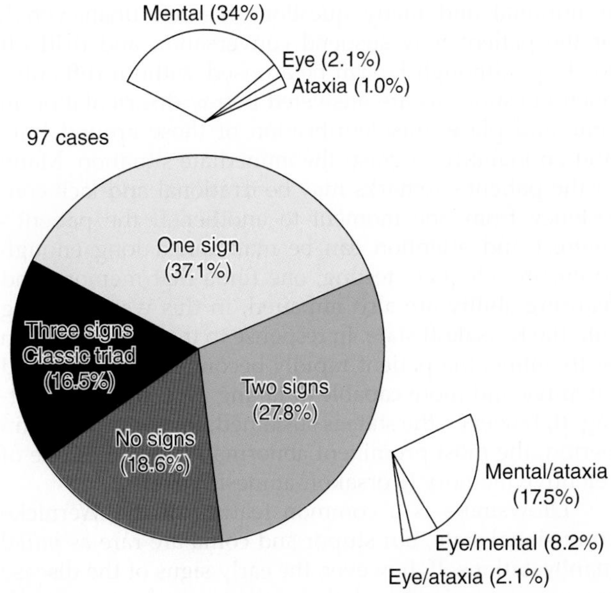

Figure 41-1. Clinical features of Wernicke-Korsakoff disease in a series of 131 autopsy proved cases. (Reprinted with permission from Harper CG, Giles M, and Finlay-Jones R: *J Neurol Neurosurg Psychiatry* 49:341–345, 1986.)

does occur but is an unusual manifestation, and a pattern that simulates internuclear ophthalmoplegia has been seen. In advanced stages of the disease there may be a complete loss of ocular movements and the pupils, which are otherwise usually spared, may become miotic and nonreacting. Ptosis, small retinal hemorrhages, involvement of the near–far focusing mechanism, and evidence of optic neuropathy occur occasionally, but neither we nor our colleagues have observed papilledema that was included in Wernicke's original description. These ocular signs are highly characteristic of Wernicke disease and disappearance of nystagmus and an improvement in ophthalmoparesis within hours or a day of the administration of thiamine confirms the diagnosis.

Ataxia Essentially the ataxia is one of stance and gait; in the acute stage of the disease it may be so severe that the patient cannot stand or walk without support. Lesser degrees are characterized by a wide-based stance and a slow, uncertain, short-stepped gait; the mildest degrees are apparent only in tandem walking. In contrast to the gross disorder of locomotion is a relative infrequency of limb ataxia and of intention tremor; when present, they are more likely to be elicited by heel-to-knee than by finger-to-nose testing. Dysarthric, cerebellar-type scanning speech is present only rarely.

Disturbances of Consciousness and Mentation These occur in some form in all but 10 percent of patients who have clinical signs. From Fig. 41-1 it can also be appreciated that when there is only one sign of Wernicke disease, it is usually a confusional state. Several related types of disturbed mentation and consciousness are recognized. By far the most common disturbance is a *global confusional state*. The next following in frequency is memory loss discussed as follows. The patient is apathetic, inattentive, and indifferent to his surroundings. Spontaneous speech is minimal and many questions are left unanswered, or the patient may suspend conversation and drift off to sleep, although he can be aroused without difficulty. Such questions as are answered betray disorientation in time and place, misidentification of those around him, and an inability to grasp the immediate situation. Many of the patient's remarks may be irrational and lack consistency from one moment to another. If the patient's interest and attention can be maintained long enough to ensure adequate testing, one finds that memory and learning ability are also impaired, in this way blending into the Korsakoff state. In response to the administration of thiamine, the patient rapidly becomes more alert and attentive and more capable of taking part in mental testing. If, however, the state is sustained, for some uncertain period, the most prominent abnormality becomes one of retentive memory (Korsakoff-amnesic state).

Drowsiness is a common feature of the Wernicke confusional state, but stupor and coma are rare as *initial* manifestations. If, however, the early signs of the disease are not recognized and the patient remains untreated, a progressive depression of the state of consciousness occurs with stupor, coma, and death in a matter of a week or two, just as occurred in Wernicke's original cases. Autopsy series of Wernicke disease are heavily weighted with cases of the latter type, often undiagnosed during life (Harper; Torvik et al).

Some patients are alert and responsive from the time they are first seen and already show the characteristic features of the Korsakoff amnesic state. In a small number of such patients, the amnesic state is the only manifestation of the syndrome, and no ocular or ataxic signs (other than possibly nystagmus) can be discerned.

The Amnesic State As indicated in Chap. 21, the core of the amnesic disorder is a defect in learning (*anterograde amnesia*) and a loss of past memories (*retrograde amnesia*). The defect in learning can be remarkably severe. The patient may be incapable, for example, of committing to memory the simplest of facts (such as the examiner's name, the date, and the time of day) despite countless attempts; the patient can repeat each fact as it is presented, indicating that he understands what is wanted of him and that "registration" is intact, but by the time the third fact is repeated, the first may have been forgotten. However, certain nonverbal learning may take place; for example, with repeated trials, the patient may learn complex tasks such as mirror writing or how to negotiate a maze, despite no recollection of ever having been confronted with these tasks.

Anterograde amnesia is always coupled with a disturbance of past or remote memory (retrograde amnesia). The latter disorder is usually severe in degree, although not complete, and covers a period that antedates the onset of the illness by up to several years. A few isolated events and information from the past are retained, but these are related without regard for the intervals that separated them or for their proper temporal sequence. Usually the patient "telescopes" events into a brief period of time; sometimes the opposite occurs. This aspect of the memory disorder becomes prominent as the initial confusional stage of the illness subsides.

It is probably true that memories of the recent past are more severely impaired than those of the remote past (the rule of Ribot); language, computation, knowledge acquired in school, and all habitual actions are preserved. This is not to say that all remote memories are intact. As discussed in Chap. 21, these are not as readily tested as more recent memories, making the two difficult to compare. It is our impression that there are gaps and inaccuracies in memories of the distant past in practically all cases of the Korsakoff amnesic state, and serious impairments in many.

The cognitive impairment of the Korsakoff patient is not exclusively one of memory loss. Psychologic testing discloses that certain cognitive and perceptual functions that depend little or not at all on retentive memory are also impaired. As a rule, the Korsakoff patient has no insight into his illness and is characteristically apathetic and inert, lacking in spontaneity and initiative, and indifferent to everything and everybody around him. However, the patient has a relatively normal capacity to reason with data immediately before him.

Confabulation has generally been considered to be a specific feature of Korsakoff psychosis, but the validity of this view depends largely on how one defines confabulation, and there is no uniformity of opinion on this point. The observations of our colleague Victor and his colleagues (1959) do not support the oft-repeated statement that the Korsakoff patient fills the gaps in his memory with confabulation. In the sense that gaps in memory exist and that whatever the patient supplies in place of the correct answers fills these gaps, the statement is incontrovertible. It is hardly explanatory, however. The implication that confabulation is a deliberate attempt to hide the memory defect, out of embarrassment or for other reasons, is incorrect. In fact, the opposite seems to pertain: As the patient improves and becomes more aware of a defect in memory, the tendency to confabulate diminishes. Furthermore, confabulation can be associated with both phases of the Wernicke-Korsakoff syndrome: The initial one in which profound general confusion dominates the disease, and the convalescent phase in which the patient recalls fragments of past experience in a distorted fashion. Events that were separated by long intervals are juxtaposed or related out of sequence, so that the narrative has an implausible or fictional aspect. In the chronic state of the disease, confabulation is usually absent. These and other aspects of confabulation are discussed fully in the monograph by Victor and colleagues (1959).

Other Clinical Abnormalities Approximately 15 percent of patients show signs of alcohol withdrawal, that is, hallucinations and other disorders of perception, confusion, agitation, tremor, and overactivity of autonomic nervous system function. These symptoms are evanescent in nature and usually mild.

Signs of *peripheral neuropathy* are found in more than 80 percent of patients with the Wernicke-Korsakoff syndrome. In most, the neuropathic disease is mild and does not account for the disorder of gait, but it may be so severe and particularly painful that stance and gait cannot be tested. In a small number, retrobulbar optic neuropathy is added. Despite the frequency of peripheral neuropathy, overt signs of beriberi heart disease are rare.

However, indications of disordered cardiovascular function such as tachycardia, exertional dyspnea, postural hypotension, and minor electrocardiographic abnormalities are frequent; occasionally, the patient dies suddenly following only slight exertion. These patients may show an elevation of cardiac output associated with low peripheral vascular resistance, abnormalities that revert to normal after the administration of thiamine. *Postural hypotension* and syncope are common findings in Wernicke disease and are probably a result of impaired function of the autonomic nervous system, more specifically to a defect in the sympathetic outflow (Birchfield). There may be mild *hypothermia*, loss of libido, and erectile dysfunction.

Patients with the Korsakoff amnesic state may have a demonstrably *impaired olfactory discrimination*. This deficit, like the notable apathy present in most Wernicke's patients, is probably attributable to a lesion of the mediodorsal nucleus of the thalamus and its connections, and not to a lesion of the peripheral olfactory system (Mair et al). Vestibular function, as measured by the response to standard ice-water caloric tests, is universally impaired in the acute stage of Wernicke disease (Ghez), but vertigo is not a complaint. This vestibular paresis probably accounts for the severe disequilibrium in the initial stage of the illness.

Laboratory Findings

The acute lesions of the Wernicke-Korsakoff syndrome in the mammillary bodies, and other medial thalamic and periaqueductal areas can be demonstrated in most cases by magnetic resonance imaging (MRI) (Donnal et al; Varnet et al). The changes are most apparent on the fluid-attenuated inversion recovery (FLAIR), T2, and diffusion-weighted sequences (if there is hemorrhage), but they may also enhance as shown in Fig. 41-2. It is not clear to what extent gradient-echo MRI images can be expected to consistently reveal the small hemorrhagic lesions of the diencephalon and periventricular areas. Imaging is particularly useful in patients in whom stupor or coma has supervened or in whom ocular and ataxic signs are otherwise inevident (Victor, 1990), but in milder cases a normal MRI does not preclude the diagnosis. The typical MRI changes are observed in only 58 percent of cases according to Weidauer and colleagues. In the chronic state, the mammillary bodies may be shrunken if measured by volumetric techniques (Charness and DeLaPaz).

The cerebrospinal fluid (CSF) in uncomplicated cases of the Wernicke-Korsakoff syndrome is normal or shows only a modest elevation of the protein content. Protein values greater than 100 mg/dL or a pleocytosis indicates the presence of a complicating illness such as subdural hematoma, meningeal infection, or encephalitis.

Measurements of serum thiamine and red blood cell transketolase have been explored as aids to diagnosis but are not sufficiently sensitive for clinical use and they are not readily available. Before treatment with thiamine, patients with Wernicke disease show a marked reduction in transketolase. Restoration of these values and of thiamine di- and triphosphate toward normal occurs within a few hours of the administration of thiamine, and completely normal values are usually attained within 24 h.

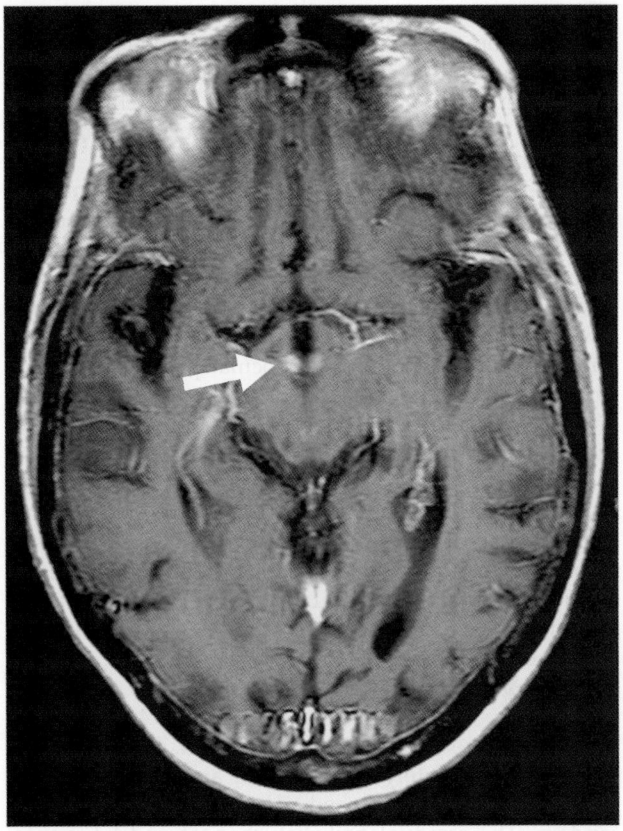

Figure 41-2. Axial T1-postgadolinium image of a 63-year-old woman with Wernicke encephalopathy showing abnormal enhancement of the mammillary bodies (arrow).

There are suggestions that there is a hereditary factor in the susceptibility of Wernicke-Korsakoff disease and possibly explains why only a small proportion of nutritionally deficient alcoholics develop this disease. Candidates for this variability have been proposed to be in transketolase activity or in the thiamine transporter gene, possibly on an epigenetic basis, but other genetic regions have been studied and to our reading, there is no clarity on this subject.

Approximately half of patients with Wernicke-Korsakoff disease show electroencephalographic (EEG) abnormalities, consisting of diffuse mild to moderate slow activity. Total cerebral blood flow and cerebral oxygen and glucose consumption may be reduced in the acute stages of the disease and may still be present after several weeks of treatment (Shimojyo et al). These observations indicate that significant reductions in brain metabolism need not be reflected in EEG abnormalities or in depression of the state of consciousness and that the latter is more a function of the location of the lesion than of the overall degree of metabolic defect.

Course of the Illness

The mortality rate in the acute phase of Wernicke disease was 17 percent in the series of patients collected by Victor, Adams, and Collins (1989) many decades ago.

The fatalities were attributable mainly to hepatic failure and infection (pneumonia, pulmonary tuberculosis, and septicemia being at that time the most common). Some deaths were undoubtedly a result of the cerebral or cardiac effects of thiamine deficiency that had reached an irreversible stage.

Most patients respond in a fairly predictable manner to the administration of thiamine, as detailed further on. The most dramatic improvement is in the ocular manifestations. Recovery often begins within hours or sooner after the administration of thiamine and practically always within several days. This effect is so constant that a failure of the nystagmus and ocular palsies to respond to thiamine should raise doubts about the diagnosis of Wernicke disease. Horizontal nystagmus sometimes disappears in minutes. Sixth-nerve palsies, ptosis, and vertical gaze palsies recover *completely* within a week or two in most cases, but vertical nystagmus may sometimes persist for several months. Horizontal gaze palsies recover completely as a rule, but in 60 percent of cases a fine horizontal nystagmus remains as a permanent sequela. In this respect, horizontal nystagmus is unique among the ocular signs.

In comparison with the ocular signs, improvement of ataxia is delayed. Approximately 40 percent of patients recover completely from ataxia. The remaining recover incompletely or not at all and are left with a slow, shuffling, wide-based gait and inability to walk tandem. The residual gait disturbances and horizontal nystagmus provide a means of identifying obscure and chronic cases of dementia as alcoholic-nutritional in origin. Vestibular function improves at about the same rate as the ataxia of gait, and recovery is usually but not always complete.

The early symptoms of apathy, drowsiness, and global confusion invariably recede, and as they do the defect in memory and learning stands out more clearly. However, the memory disorder, once established, recovers completely or almost completely in only 20 percent of patients. The remainder is left with varying degrees of permanent Korsakoff amnesia.

It is apparent from the foregoing account that Wernicke disease and Korsakoff amnesia are not separate diseases, but that *the ocular and ataxic signs and the transformation of the global confusional state into an amnesic syndrome are successive stages in a single disease process*. Of 186 patients in the series of Victor, Adams and Collins (1989) who survived the acute illness, 157 (84 percent) showed this sequence of clinical events. As a corollary, a survey of alcoholic patients with Korsakoff amnesia in a psychiatric hospital disclosed that in most patients the illness had begun with the symptoms of Wernicke disease and that approximately 60 percent of them still showed some ocular or cerebellar stigmata of Wernicke disease many years after the onset. The same continuum cannot be invoked to explain alcoholic-nutritional cerebellar degeneration that arises as an independent illness and is not as a residual of the ataxia of Wernicke disease (see further on).

Neuropathologic Findings

Patients who die in the acute stages of Wernicke disease show symmetrical lesions in the paraventricular regions of the thalamus and hypothalamus, mammillary bodies, periaqueductal region of the midbrain, floor of the fourth ventricle (particularly in the regions of the dorsal motor nuclei of the vagus and vestibular nuclei), and superior cerebellar vermis. Lesions are consistently found in the mammillary bodies and less consistently in other areas. The microscopic changes are characterized by varying degrees of necrosis of parenchymal structures. Within the area of necrosis, nerve cells are lost, but usually some remain; some of these are damaged but others are intact. Myelinated fibers are more affected than neurons. These changes are accompanied by a prominence of the blood vessels, although in some cases there appears to be a primary endothelial proliferation and evidence of recent or old petechial hemorrhage. In the areas of parenchymal damage there is astrocytic and microglial proliferation. Discrete hemorrhages were found in only 20 percent of Victor's (1989) cases, and many appeared to be agonal in nature. The cerebellar changes consist of degeneration of all layers of the cortex, particularly of the Purkinje cells; usually this lesion is confined to the superior parts of the vermis, but in advanced cases the cortex of the most anterior parts of the anterior lobes is involved as well. Of interest is the fact that the lesions of Leigh encephalomyelopathy, a mitochondrial disorder implicating pyruvate metabolism, bear a resemblance to those of Wernicke disease but have a slightly different distribution and histologic characteristics.

The ocular muscle and gaze palsies are attributable to lesions of the sixth- and third-nerve nuclei and adjacent tegmentum, and the nystagmus to lesions in the regions of the vestibular nuclei. The latter are also responsible for the loss of caloric responses and probably for the gross disturbance of equilibrium that characterizes the initial stage of the disease. The lack of significant destruction of nerve cells in these lesions accounts for the rapid improvement and the high degree of recovery of oculomotor and vestibular functions. The persistent ataxia of stance and gait is caused by the lesion of the superior vermis of the cerebellum; ataxia of individual movements of the legs is attributable to an extension of the lesion into the anterior parts of the anterior lobes. Hypothermia, which occurs sometimes as an early feature of Wernicke disease, is probably attributable to lesions in the posterior and posterolateral nuclei of the hypothalamus (experimentally placed lesions in these parts have been shown to cause hypothermia or poikilothermia in monkeys).

The topography of the neuropathologic changes in patients who die in the chronic stages of the disease, when the amnesic symptoms are established, is much the same as the changes in the acute stages of Wernicke disease. Apart from the expected differences in age of the glial and vascular reactions, the only important difference has to do with the involvement of the medial dorsal and anterior nuclei of the thalamus. The medial parts of these nuclei were consistently involved in the patients who had shown the Korsakoff amnesic state during life; they were not affected in patients who had had no persistent amnesic symptoms in the series of Victor, Adams, and Collins (1989). The mammillary bodies were affected in all the patients, both those with the amnesic defect and those without. These observations suggest that the lesions responsible for the memory disorder are those of the thalami, predominantly of parts of the medial dorsal nuclei (and their connections with the medial frontal and temporal lobes and amygdaloid nuclei), and not those of the mammillary bodies, as is frequently stated. It is notable that the hippocampal formations, the site of damage in most other types of Korsakoff memory loss, are intact.

Treatment of the Wernicke-Korsakoff Syndrome

Wernicke disease constitutes a medical emergency; its recognition (or even the suspicion of its presence) requires the *administration of thiamine*. The prompt use of thiamine prevents progression of the disease and reverses those lesions that have not yet progressed to the point of fixed structural change. As emphasized earlier, in patients who show only ocular signs and ataxia, the administration of thiamine is crucial in preventing the development of an irreversible amnesic state.

Although 2 to 3 mg of thiamine may be sufficient to modify the ocular signs, much larger doses are needed to sustain improvement and replenish the depleted thiamine stores—initially, 50 to 200 mg intravenously and a similar dose mg intramuscularly—the latter being repeated each day until the patient resumes a normal diet. Certain writings indicate that initial doses of 500 mg are necessary to fully reverse the manifestations of Wernicke disease and prevent progression to the point of a Korsakoff syndrome. It appears that these higher doses, given for several days parenterally, are needed to replete vitamin levels in alcoholic and nutritionally deprived patients (see the articles by Thomson et al), but the need for high-dose regimens to reverse Wernicke disease is based on less-persuasive data. Nonetheless, current guidelines from the Royal College of Physicians, given by Thomson, promote high-dose regimens and seem advisable. The risks of administering parenteral thiamine have probably been overstated; anaphylactic reactions occurred in 0.1 percent of the series of Wrenn and colleagues and minor reactions in 1 percent.

To avoid precipitating Wernicke disease, it has become standard practice in emergency departments to administer 100 mg or more of thiamine in malnourished or alcoholic patients if intravenous fluids that contain glucose are being infused. Magnesium is given as well because it is required as cofactor for thiamine activity. It is similarly advisable to give B vitamins to alcoholic patients who are seen for other reasons in the emergency department so as to raise body stores of thiamine and other vitamins. The chronic alcoholic (or the nonalcoholic with persistent vomiting) exhausts thiamine in a matter of 7 or 8 weeks, during which time the administration of glucose may serve to precipitate Wernicke disease or cause an early form of the disease to progress rapidly. The further management of Wernicke disease involves the use of a balanced diet and all the B vitamins, as the patient is usually deficient in more than thiamine alone.

A different problem in management may arise once the patient has recovered from Wernicke disease and the amnesic syndrome becomes prominent. Only a minority of such patients (fewer than 20 percent in Victor's series) recover entirely; moreover, the time of recovery may be delayed for several weeks or even months, and then it proceeds very slowly over a period of many months. The extent to which the amnesic symptoms will recover cannot be predicted during the acute stages of the illness. Interestingly, the alcoholic Korsakoff patient, once more or less recovered, seldom demands alcohol but will drink it if it is offered.

Infantile Wernicke–Beriberi Disease

This designates an acute and frequently fatal disease of infants, which until recently was common in rice-eating communities of the Far East. It affects only breast-fed infants, usually in the second to the fifth months of life. Acute cardiac symptoms dominate the clinical picture, but neurologic symptoms (aphonia, strabismus, nystagmus, spasmodic contraction of facial muscles, and convulsions) have been described in many of the cases. This syndrome can be reversed dramatically by the administration of thiamine, so that some authors prefer to call it *acute thiamine deficiency in infants*. In the few neuropathologic studies that are available, changes like those of Wernicke disease in the adult have been described. Occasionally, there are outbreaks of this condition due to inadequately formulated baby foods that lack thiamine.

Infantile beriberi bears no consistent relationship to beriberi in the mother. Infants of mothers with overt signs of beriberi may be quite normal. The absence of beriberi in the mothers of affected infants suggests that infantile beriberi might be due to the result of a toxic factor in breast milk, but such a factor, if it exists, has never been isolated. The levels of thiamine in the breast milk of such mothers have not been measured, however.

Rarely, the clinical manifestations of beriberi in infancy represent an inherited (autosomal recessive) thiamine-dependent state, responding to the continued administration of massive doses of thiamine (Mandel et al; see also Table 41-3, further on).

NUTRITIONAL POLYNEUROPATHY (NEUROPATHIC BERIBERI)

(See also Chap. 46)

Most physicians in the Western world have only a dim notion about beriberi, which they recall as an ill-defined, predominantly cardiac disorder occurring among people whose diet was dominated by polished rice. The milling process, or "polishing," removes the husk that contains most of the vitamin nutrients. In fact, beriberi is a distinct clinical entity that is not confined to any particular part of the world. Essentially, it is a disease of the heart and of the peripheral nerves (which may be affected separately), with or without edema, the latter feature providing the basis for the old division into "wet" and "dry" forms. The cardiac manifestations range from tachycardia and exertional dyspnea to acute and rapidly fatal heart failure, the latter being the most dramatic but uncommon manifestation of beriberi. Here we emphasize the peripheral neuropathy, or *neuropathic beriberi.*

That beriberi is essentially a disorder of the peripheral nerves was established in the late nineteenth century by the studies of the Dutch investigators Eijkman, Pekelharing and Winkler, and Grijns. Only after beriberi gained acceptance as a nutritional disease (this followed Funk's discovery of vitamins in 1911) was it suspected that the neuropathy of alcoholics was also nutritional in origin. The similarity between beriberi and alcoholic neuropathy was commented upon by several authors, but it was Shattuck, in 1928, who first seriously discussed the relationship of the 2 disorders. He suggested that "polyneuritis of chronic alcoholism was caused chiefly by failure to take or assimilate food containing a sufficient quantity B vitamins and might properly be regarded as true beriberi." Convincing evidence that "alcoholic neuritis" is not a result of the neurotoxic effect of alcohol was supplied by Strauss. He allowed 10 patients to continue their daily consumption of whiskey while they consumed a well-balanced diet supplemented with yeast and vitamin B concentrates; the peripheral nerve symptoms improved in every case. The observations made by Victor (1984) support Strauss's contention that alcoholic polyneuropathy is essentially a nutritional disease.

Clinical Features

The symptomatology of nutritional polyneuropathy is diverse. In fact, many patients are asymptomatic and evidence of peripheral nerve disease is found only by clinical or electromyographic examination. The mildest neuropathic signs are thinness and tenderness of the leg muscles, loss or depression of the Achilles reflexes and perhaps of the patellar reflexes and at times, a patchy blunting of pain and touch sensation over the feet and shins.

Most patients, however, are symptomatic and have weakness, paresthesias, and pain as the usual complaints. The symptoms are insidious in onset and slowly progressive, but occasionally they seem to evolve or to worsen rapidly over a matter of days. The initial symptoms are usually referred to the distal portions of the limbs and progress proximally if the illness remains untreated. The feet are always affected earlier and more severely than the hands. Usually some aspect of motor disability is part of the chief complaint, but in about one-third of the patients the main complaints are pain and paresthesias. It is this painful syndrome that has been the most prominent feature in the patients we have encountered in recent years. The discomfort takes several forms: a dull, constant ache in the feet or legs; sharp and lancinating pains, momentary in duration, like those of tabes dorsalis; sensations of cramping or tightness in the muscles of the feet and calves; or band-like feelings around the legs. Coldness of the feet is a common complaint but is not corroborated by palpation. Far more distressing are feelings of heat or "burning" affecting mainly the soles, less frequently the dorsal aspects of the feet. These dysesthesias fluctuate in severity and characteristically are worsened by contactual stimuli, sometimes to the point where the patient cannot walk or bear the touch of bedclothes, despite the relative preservation of motor power (allodynia). The term *burning feet* has been applied to this syndrome, but it is not particularly apt, as the patient also complains of other types of paresthesias, dysesthesias, and pain, and these symptoms may involve the hands as well as the feet.

Examination discloses varying degrees of motor, sensory, and reflex loss. As the symptoms suggest, the signs are symmetrical, and more severe in distal than in proximal portions of the limbs, and often confined to the legs. In some cases, the disproportionate affection of motor power may be striking, taking the form of a foot- and wrist-drop, but the proximal muscles are usually affected as well (indicated, for example, by climbing stairs or by difficulty in arising from a squatting position). In a few patients, the weakness appears to be most severe in the proximal muscles. Absolute paralysis of the legs had been observed in the past only rarely; immobility caused by contractures at the knees and ankles in neglected patients was a more common occurrence. Tenderness of muscles on deep pressure is a highly characteristic finding, elicited most readily in the muscles of the feet and calves. In the arms, tendon reflexes are sometimes retained despite a loss of strength in the hands. In patients in whom pain and dysesthesias are prominent and motor loss is slight, the reflexes at knee and ankle may be retained or even of greater than average briskness. This attests to the predominant affection of the small nerve fibers.

Excessive sweating of the soles and dorsal aspects of the feet and of the volar surfaces of the hands and fingers is a common manifestation of alcohol-induced nutritional neuropathy. Postural hypotension is sometimes associated, all symptoms indicative of involvement of the peripheral sympathetic nerve fibers.

Sensory loss or impairment may involve all the modalities, although one may be affected out of proportion to the others, usually pain and temperature. One cannot predict from the patient's symptoms which mode of sensation might be affected disproportionately. In patients with impairment of superficial sensation (i.e., touch, pain, and temperature), the border between impaired and normal sensation is not sharp but shades off gradually over a considerable vertical extent of the limbs.

Patients in whom pain is the outstanding symptom do not constitute a distinct group in terms of their neurologic signs. Pain and dysesthesias may be prominent in patients with either severe or slight degrees of motor, reflex, and sensory loss. The term *hyperesthetic* is used commonly to designate the exquisitely painful form of neuropathy but is not well chosen; as pointed out in Chap. 8, one is usually able, by using finely graded stimuli, to demonstrate an elevated threshold to painful, thermal, and tactile stimuli in the "hyperesthetic" zone. Once the stimulus is perceived, however, it has a painful and diffuse, unpleasant quality (hyperpathia).

Tactile evocation of pain or burning is an example, as mentioned, of allodynia.

In most patients with nutritional polyneuropathy, only the limbs are involved and the abdominal, thoracic, and bulbar muscles are usually spared; however, we have encountered 2 cases in which there was sensory loss in the pattern of an escutcheon over the anterior thorax and abdomen. In the most advanced instances of neuropathy, hoarseness and weakness of the voice and dysphagia as a result of degeneration of the vagus nerves may be added to the clinical picture.

Some idea of the incidence of the motor, reflex, and sensory abnormalities and the combinations in which they occur can be obtained from Table 41-1, which is based on Victor's (1984) examination of 189 nutritionally depleted alcoholic patients. Noteworthy is the fact that only 66 (35 percent) of the 189 patients showed the clinical picture of polyneuropathy in its entirety, that is, a symmetrical impairment or loss of tendon reflexes, sensation, and motor power affecting legs more than the arms and the distal more than the proximal segments of the limbs. In the remaining patients, the motor-reflex-sensory signs occurred in various combinations.

Stasis edema and pigmentation, glossiness, and thinness of the skin of the lower legs and feet are common findings in patients with any severe form of neuropathy. Major dystrophic changes, in the form of perforating plantar ulcers and painless destruction of the bones and joints of the feet ("Charcot forefeet"), have been described but are rare. Repeated trauma to insensitive parts and superimposed infection are thought to be responsible for the neuropathic arthropathy, as discussed in Chaps. 8 and 46.

The CSF is usually normal, although a modest elevation of protein content is found in a small number. Findings of nerve conduction studies include mild to moderate degrees of slowing of motor and sensory conduction and a marked reduction in the amplitudes of sensory action potentials; the motor conduction velocities in distal segments of the nerves may be reduced, while conduction in proximal segments is normal. Denervated muscles show fibrillation potentials in a pattern that is consistent with more severe involvement peripherally.

Table 41-1

CLINICAL FINDINGS IN NUTRITIONAL POLYNEUROPATHY

NEUROPATHIC ABNORMALITY	LEGS (189 CASES)	ARMS (57 CASES)
Loss of reflexes alone	45 (24)[a]	6 (10)[b]
Loss of sensation alone	10 (5)	10 (18)
Weakness alone	—	5 (9)
Weakness and sensory loss	2 (1)	10 (18)
Reflex and sensory loss	40 (21)	2 (3)
Sensory, motor, and reflex loss	66 (35)	17 (30)
Data incomplete	26 (14)	7 (12)

[a]Figures in parentheses indicate percent of 189 cases.
[b]Figures in parentheses indicate percent of 57 cases.

Pathologic Features

The essential change is one of axonal degeneration, with destruction of both axon and myelin sheath. Segmental demyelination occurs only in a small proportion of fibers. The most pronounced changes are observed in the distal parts of the longest and largest myelinated fibers in the crural and, to a lesser extent, brachial nerves. In advanced cases, the changes extend into the anterior and posterior nerve roots. The vagus and phrenic nerves and paravertebral sympathetic trunks may be affected in advanced cases. Anterior horn and dorsal root ganglion cells undergo chromatolysis, indicating axonal damage. Secondary changes in the posterior columns are seen in some cases.

Pathophysiology

The nutritional factor(s) responsible for the neuropathy of alcoholism and beriberi has not been defined precisely. Because of the difficulty in producing peripheral neuropathy in mammals by means of a thiamine-deficient diet, the idea that thiamine is the antineuritic vitamin was questioned in the past. Very few of the animal experiments undertaken to settle this point were satisfactory from a nutritional and pathologic point of view. Nevertheless, several studies in birds and humans do indeed indicate that uncomplicated thiamine deficiency may result in peripheral nerve disease. The necessity of either accepting or rejecting the specific role of thiamine became less urgent when it was demonstrated, in both animals and humans; a deficiency of pyridoxine or of pantothenic acid could also result in degeneration of the peripheral nerves (Swank and Adams).

The question of whether polyneuropathy in the alcoholic patient might be a result of the direct toxic effects of alcohol and not of a nutritional deficiency has been raised from time to time (see the preceding text and Denny-Brown and Behse and Buchthal). The evidence for this view is not compelling, either on clinical or on experimental grounds, as already mentioned (see reference to Strauss, in introductory section on nutritional neuropathy). The data presented more recently by Koike and colleagues, ostensibly in favor of the existence of a true alcoholic neuropathy, in our view present no convincing support of a direct toxic effect of alcohol. In the end, we view alcoholic–beriberi neuropathy as a multiple B-vitamin deficiency. The interested reader will find a detailed critique of this subject in the chapters by Victor and by Windebank in the second and third editions, respectively, of *Peripheral Neuropathy*, edited by Dyck and coworkers.

Treatment and Prognosis

The first consideration is to supply adequate nutrition over a long period in the form of a balanced diet supplemented with B vitamins (equally important is to make certain that the patient follows the prescribed diet). If persistent vomiting or other gastrointestinal complications prevent the patient from eating, parenteral feeding becomes necessary; the vitamins may be given intramuscularly or added to intravenous fluids.

Where pain and sensitivity of the feet are the major complaints, the pressure of bedclothes may be avoided by placing a cradle support over the legs. Aching of the limbs may be related to their immobility, in which case they should be moved passively on frequent occasions. Aspirin or acetaminophen is usually sufficient to control hyperpathia and allodynia; occasionally codeine or methadone must be added. Obviously, opiates and addicting synthetic analgesics should be avoided if possible, but we have resorted to fentanyl patches for short periods in a few severely affected patients. Some of our patients with severe burning pain (similar to causalgia) in the feet had in the past been helped temporarily by blocking the lumbar sympathetic ganglia or by epidural injection of analgesics. The response to phenytoin, carbamazepine, and gabapentin has been inconsistent, but they are widely used. Adrenergic-blocking medication has been of little value and mexiletine, in our experience, of uncertain benefit.

The regeneration of peripheral nerves, which may take many months, will be of little avail if the muscles have been allowed to undergo contracture and the joints to become fixed. In cases of severe paralysis, molded splints should be applied to the arms, hands, legs, and feet during periods of rest. Pressure on the heels and elbows can be avoided by padding the splints and by turning the patient frequently or by asking the patient to do so. As function returns, more vigorous physiotherapeutic measures can be undertaken.

Recovery from nutritional polyneuropathy is a slow process. In the mildest cases there may be a considerable restoration of motor function in a few weeks. In severe forms of the disease, many months may pass before the patient is able to walk unaided. The sensory features and pain in particular may be slower to recover, having taken over a year in one of our recently observed patients. The slowness of recovery creates a special problem for the alcoholic patient, in whom the great danger to continued recovery is the resumption of drinking and inadequate diet.

Riboflavin Deficiency (Vitamin B_2 Deficiency)

Whether or not riboflavin deficiency leads to neurologic symptoms has been controversial. In the past, there were claims that glossitis, cheilosis, and neuropathy were caused by riboflavin deficiency, but its effects were never isolated. It is a component of general malnutrition, making it difficult to separate the cause of various disorders. Night blindness seems, however, to be caused by B_2 deficiency. Antozzi and coworkers reported that a metabolic disorder similar to the Reye syndrome can be caused by riboflavin deficiency and is correctable by administration of riboflavin alone. The affected infants in their studies were hypoglycemic, hypotonic, and episodically weak and unresponsive. Generally, 15 mg per day in divided doses is used for replacement, but restoration of a normal diet is paramount.

Antozzi and colleagues also recorded instances of disease in older children and adults, manifesting as a type of lipid storage polymyopathy as a result of either a deficiency or malabsorption of riboflavin. Presumably, a disorder of flavin metabolism had caused an impairment of both beta-oxidation of fatty acids and respiratory chain I and II complexes. Serum creatine phosphate was normal in these individuals, but carnitine was reduced. The oral administration of 200 mg of riboflavin and 4 g of carnitine per day relieved the symptoms. We have had no experience with such cases.

PELLAGRA (NIACIN, NICOTINIC ACID, B_3 DEFICIENCY)

In the early 1900s, pellagra attained epidemic proportions in the southern United States and in the alcoholic population of large urban centers. Since 1940, it has diminished greatly because of the general practice of enriching bread with niacin. Nevertheless, among the vegetarian, maize-eating people of underdeveloped countries, and among the black population of South Africa, pellagra is still a common disease (Bomb et al; Shah et al; Ronthal and Adler). In developed countries, pellagra is practically confined to alcoholics (Ishii and Nishihara; Spivak and Jackson; Serdaru et al).

Clinical Features

In its fully developed form, pellagra affects the skin, alimentary tract, and hematopoietic and nervous systems. The early symptoms may be mistaken for those of a psychiatric disorder. Insomnia, fatigue, nervousness, irritability, and feelings of depression are common complaints; taken together they have the character of neurasthenia. Examination discloses mental dullness, apathy, and a mild impairment of memory. Sometimes an acute confusional psychosis dominates the clinical picture. Untreated, these symptoms may progress to a dementia. Pellagra may not only produce mental impairment but occasionally result from it, by virtue of anorexia and refusal of food. The dermatologic feature, often the aspect that permits one to make a confident diagnosis, is a *scaly dermatitis in sun-exposed areas*, followed by hyperpigmentation of these areas. Diarrhea and glossitis or other forms of mucous membrane disorder may be accompaniments (hence the alliterative triad dementia-dermatitis-diarrhea; the "3 Ds"). The *spinal cord* manifestations have not been clearly delineated, but in general, the signs are referable to both posterior and lateral columns, predominantly the former, and thereby simulating SCD. Signs of *peripheral neuropathy* are relatively less common and are indistinguishable from those of neuropathic beriberi.

Pathologic Changes

These are most readily discerned in the large cells of the motor cortex (Betz cells), and to a lesser extent in the smaller pyramidal cells of the cortex, the large cells of the basal ganglia, the cranial motor and cerebellar dentate nuclei, and the anterior horn cells of the spinal cord. The affected neurons are swollen and rounded, with eccentric nuclei and loss of the Nissl bodies that have the appearance of a secondary axonal reaction. However, in the pathologic material presented by Hauw and associates, these chromatolytic changes were most pronounced in the brainstem nuclei (upper reticular and pontine) and not in the Betz cells. They concluded that the neuronal changes were not caused by a retrograde axonal lesion but did not comment on the status of the spinal cord or nerves. The few studies of the peripheral nerves in pellagra have disclosed changes like those in alcoholics and other patients with nutritional deficiency.

The spinal cord lesions in pellagra take the form of a symmetrical degeneration of the dorsal columns, especially of Goll, and to a lesser extent of the corticospinal tracts. The posterior column degeneration is likely to be secondary to degeneration of the dorsal root ganglion cells or posterior roots. The reason for the corticospinal tract degeneration is not clear.

Etiology

It has been known since 1937, when Elvehjem and coworkers showed that nicotinic acid cured black tongue, a pellagra-like disease in dogs, that this vitamin is effective in the treatment of pellagra. Many years before, Goldberger had demonstrated the curative effects of dietary protein and proposed that pellagra was caused by a lack of specific amino acids (see Terris). Now it is known that pellagra may result from a deficiency of either nicotinic acid or tryptophan, the amino acid precursor of nicotinic acid. One milligram of nicotinic acid is formed from 60 mg of tryptophan, a process for which pyridoxine is essential. The relationship of niacin to tryptophan metabolism explains the frequent occurrence of pellagra in persons who subsist mainly on corn, which contains only small amounts of tryptophan and niacin, some of the niacin being in bound form and unavailable for absorption.

It should be pointed out that in experimental subjects, only the cutaneous-gastrointestinal-neurasthenic manifestations of pellagra have been produced by diets that are tryptophan or niacin deficient; neurologic abnormalities have not resulted from these diets (Goldsmith). As a corollary, only the dermal, gastrointestinal, and neurasthenic manifestations respond to treatment with niacin and tryptophan; neurologic disturbances in pellagrins have proved to be recalcitrant to prolonged treatment with the vitamin, although the peripheral nerve disorder may subsequently respond to treatment with thiamine. In monkeys, degeneration of peripheral nerves and the cerebrocortical changes of pellagra were induced by a deficiency of pyridoxine (Victor and Adams, 1956). Swank and Adams described degeneration of the peripheral nerves in pyridoxine- and pantothenic acid-deficient swine, and Vilter and colleagues produced polyneuropathy in human subjects rendered pyridoxine deficient; these subjects also showed seborrheic dermatitis and glossitis (indistinguishable from that of niacin deficiency) and the cheilosis and angular stomatitis that are usually attributed to riboflavin deficiency. The foregoing observations indicate that certain lingual and cutaneous manifestations of pellagra may be produced by a deficiency of pyridoxine or other B vitamins, and that the neurologic manifestations of pellagra are most likely caused by pyridoxine deficiency.

In the special case of Hartnup disease in infants (which resembles pellagra in most respects including the dermatitis), a secondary niacin deficiency is believed to result from the high excretion of indicans and indole metabolites (see Chap. 37).

Treatment

The administration of niacin 500 mg per day for approximately 3 weeks reverses the process. If the patient is unable to take oral medications, intravenous doses of 100 mg per day for 5 to 7 days are utilized. If the patient is simultaneously deficient in pyridoxine, as for example when INH is used for tuberculosis treatment, the pyridoxine must also be replaced in order to allow the conversion of dietary tryptophan to endogenous niacin.

Nicotinic Acid-Deficiency Encephalopathy

Under this title, Jolliffe and coworkers, in 1940, described an acute cerebral syndrome in alcoholic patients consisting of clouding of consciousness, progressing to extrapyramidal rigidity and tremors ("cogwheel" rigidity) of the extremities, uncontrollable grasping and sucking reflexes, and coma. Some of their patients showed overt manifestations of nutritional deficiency, such as Wernicke disease, pellagra, scurvy, and polyneuropathy. These authors concluded that the encephalopathy represented an acute form of nicotinic acid deficiency, as most of their patients recovered when treated with a diet of low vitamin B content supplemented by intravenous glucose and saline and large doses of nicotinic acid. Sydenstricker and colleagues (1938) had previously reported the salutary effects of nicotinic acid on the unresponsive state observed in elderly undernourished patients, and Spillane (1947) described a similar syndrome and response to nicotinic acid in the indigent Arab population of the Middle East.

The status of this syndrome and its relation to pellagra are uncertain. The clinical, nutritional, and pathologic features were never delineated precisely. Serdaru and associates reported 22 presumed examples of this syndrome in the alcoholic population of the Salpêtriére clinic in Paris, all diagnosed retrospectively after the finding in postmortem material of pellagra-like changes in nerve cells. The prominent features were confusional states, paratonic rigidity, ataxia, and polymyoclonia, a picture somewhat like that described by Jolliffe and coworkers. Skin lesions were absent. We have not encountered identical cases among the undernourished patients in the alcoholic population.

Pyridoxine (Vitamin B_6) Deficiency

Pyridoxine deficiency or excess has been associated with a sensory polyneuropathy. The occurrence of neuropathy caused by INH was recognized in the early 1950s, soon after the introduction of this drug for the treatment of tuberculosis. It was characterized by paresthesia and burning pain of the feet and legs, followed by weakness of these parts and loss of ankle reflexes. Rarely, with continued use of the drug, the hands were affected as well. The nature of INH-induced neuropathy was clarified by Biehl and Vilter who found that isoniazid causes a marked excretion of pyridoxine and that the administration of pyridoxine in conjunction with INH prevents the development of neuropathy. Because of this simple preventive measure, very few examples of INH-induced neuropathy are now observed. Hydralazine, closely related in structure to INH, when used in the past caused the formation of pyridoxal-isoniazid complexes (hydrazones), which make pyridoxal (the main form of vitamin B_6) unavailable to the tissues. The neuropathy responds favorably to discontinuation of the drug and the administration of pyridoxine.

Pyridoxine deficiency also leads to homocystinemia because the vitamin is a coenzyme for the conversion of homocystine to cystathionine. Vascular thrombosis may result from the excess homocystine.

Severe pyridoxine deficiency in animals and humans also causes *seizures*. This was first observed in swine by Swank and Adams, and later in infants who were maintained on a milk formula lacking in pyridoxine. A pyridoxine-responsive seizure disorder (pyridoxine dependency) of the neonatal period is discussed in Chap. 16.

Treatment

For pyridoxine deficiency caused by malnutrition, the treatment is 50 mg per day orally for several weeks, followed by 2 mg per day and resumption of a normal diet. When the deficiency results from a pyridoxine antagonist such as INH, penicillamine, hydralazine, or cycloserine, the treatment is 50 mg per day, only when the antagonist is in use. Treatment for the inherited form with convulsions is discussed in the section on neonatal seizures in Chap. 16. Lifelong supplementation is required after the seizures are aborted with a large intravenous dose of the vitamin.

Pyridoxine Toxicity

Paradoxically, the *consumption of large amounts of pyridoxine* (mainly by vitamin faddists) may also cause a sensory peripheral neuropathy or ganglionopathy (Schaumburg et al; Albin et al). There is no weakness; the symptoms, including ataxia and areflexia, are purely sensory and can be quite disabling. Symptoms may extend to the trunk, scalp, and face. Improvement is the rule when the drug is withdrawn. This disorder is probably a direct toxic effect of pyridoxine on dorsal root ganglion cells.

Folate (B_9 Deficiency)

Despite the frequency of folic acid deficiency and its hematologic effects, its role in the pathogenesis of nervous system disease has not been established beyond doubt (see reviews by Crellin et al and by Carney). However, folate antagonists such as methotrexate are known to cause a neuropathy that is probably predicated on the vitamin deficiency. The polyneuropathy that occasionally complicates the chronic administration of phenytoin has also been attributed, on uncertain grounds, to folate deficiency. Botez and colleagues have described a group of 10 patients with sensorimotor polyneuropathy (4 also had spinal cord disease) presumably because of intestinal malabsorption; all the patients improved over several months while receiving large doses of folic acid. This experience is unique, however. The possible role of folate deficiency in the pathogenesis of spinal cord disease was mentioned previously in relation to vitamin B_{12} deficiency, and its putative role in psychiatric disease has been discussed by Carney. In such cases of folate deficiency, if subacute combined degeneration or mental changes occur, they must be rare.

The folate deficiency of pregnancy is a special case that is known to increase the incidence of neural tube defects.

For nutritional folate deficiency, difficult to separate from the lack of other vitamins, replacement is with 1 mg per day. In pregnant women, higher doses are used, separately from a multivitamin preparation in order to avoid vitamin A toxicity. When a folate antagonists is the underlying cause, folinic acid (leukovorin, citrovorum factor) 15 mg orally is given every 6 h for 10 doses starting after methotrexate infusion.

Pantothenic Acid Deficiency

A predominantly sensory neuropathy also has been induced, again in swine, by Swank and Adams, and later in humans by a deficiency of pantothenic acid (a constituent of coenzyme A [CoA]), as reported by Bean and colleagues. In some patients, the administration of pantothenic acid has reportedly reversed the painful dysesthesias of the "burning foot" syndrome.

VITAMIN B_{12} (COBALAMIN) DEFICIENCY (SUBACUTE COMBINED DEGENERATION)

The spinal cord, brain, optic nerves, and peripheral nerves are all affected by vitamin B_{12} (cobalamin) deficiency, giving rise to a classic neurologic syndrome. The spinal cord is usually affected first and often exclusively. The term *subacute combined degeneration* (SCD) is customarily reserved for the spinal cord lesion of vitamin B_{12} deficiency and serves to distinguish it from other types of spinal cord diseases that happen to involve the posterior and lateral columns (loosely referred to as *combined system disease*). Whether a peripheral neuropathy is a primary component of the disease or is secondary to damage of the posterior root fibers of entry in the dorsal cord has been debated, but the available pathologic evidence favors the latter, except perhaps for a few advanced cases, in which other nutritional deficiencies could have been responsible.

The hematologic effects of vitamin B_{12} deficiency, when they result from *pernicious anemia*, are distinctive insofar as they usually result not from a dietary lack of vitamin B_{12} but from the failure to transfer minute amounts of this nutrient across the intestinal mucosa, "starvation in the midst of plenty," as Castle aptly put it.

This failure derives from the chronic absence of an intrinsic factor, which is secreted (along with hydrochloric acid) by the parietal cells of the gastric mucosa and transports cobalamin ("extrinsic factor") to the ileum, where it is absorbed into the portal venous system. This is referred to as a *conditioned deficiency*, as it is conditional on the lack of an intrinsic factor. Minot and Murphy's clinical experiment that showed the cure of the neurologic process by the feeding of liver, or parenteral liver extract that contained an "extrinsic factor" later found to be cobalamin, was a remarkable feat of translational medicine. A movie can be seen depicting this work at: http://bloodjournal.hematologylibrary.org/content/107/12/4970.1/suppl/DC1. It was Castle, experimenting on himself, who isolated the "intrinsic factor" that facilitates absorption of the vitamin.

The hematologic and neurologic manifestations of vitamin B_{12} deficiency often complicate many of the malabsorptive disorders, including poor nutrition in the elderly, especially those with atrophic gastritis, but also individuals of any age with celiac sprue; gastric or ileal resections; overgrowth of intestinal bacteria in "blind loops," anastomoses, diverticula, and other conditions resulting in intestinal stasis; and infestation with cobalamin-metabolizing fish tapeworm (*Diphyllobothrium latum*). Uncommon instances of vitamin B_{12} deficiency are observed in lactovegetarians and in infants nursed by mothers deficient in vitamin B_{12}; vitamin B_{12} deficiency may also be a result of a rare genetic defect of methylmalonyl-CoA mutase as discussed further on.

It should be further commented that interference with methionine synthetase, a methylcobalamin-dependent enzyme, can be produced by exposure to nitrous oxide. Chronic exposure can produce the entire subacute combined syndrome but more often, an individual is marginally deficient, often but not always elderly, and even short exposure may then induce symptoms. A megaloblastic anemic state, as well as the neurologic features of SCD, is thereby induced by the gas. This illness, cleverly named "anesthesia paresthetica" by Kinsella and Green, arises in operating room personnel (we have seen it in several anesthesia nurses), occasionally in dentists, and in abusers of the gas (whippets) to obtain a "high." Their serum B_{12} levels are usually in the low-normal range, and measurements of methylmalonic acid are greatly elevated (see further on).

Clinical Manifestations

Symptoms of nervous system disease occur in the majority of patients with pernicious anemia and in most with B_{12} deficiency of other sources. The patient first notices mild general weakness and paresthesias consisting of tingling, "pins and needles" feelings, or other vaguely described sensations. The paresthesias involve the hands and feet, more often and first in the hands, and tend to be constant and steadily progressive and the source of much distress. As the illness progresses, the gait becomes unsteady and stiffness and weakness of the limbs, especially of the legs, develop. If the disease remains untreated, an ataxic paraplegia evolves with variable degrees of spasticity.

Early in the course of the illness, when only paresthesia is present, there may be no objective sign. Later, examination discloses a disorder of the posterior and lateral columns of the spinal cord, predominantly of the former. *Loss of vibration sense is the most consistent sign*; it is more pronounced in the feet and legs than in the hands and arms and frequently extends over the trunk. Position sense is usually impaired in parallel. The motor signs, usually limited to the legs, include a mild symmetrical loss of strength in proximal limb muscles, spasticity, enhanced tendon reflexes, clonus, and extensor plantar responses. At first, the patellar and Achilles reflexes are diminished as frequently as they are increased; they may even be absent. This is most likely the result of a neuropathy due to multiple vitamin deficiencies as cases of pure cobalamin loss, for example due to nitrous oxide, almost never obliterate the tendon reflexes. This controversy regarding the presence of a polyneuropathy as a component of SCD has already been alluded to. The gait at first is predominantly ataxic, later ataxic and spastic.

Loss of superficial sensation below a segmental level on the trunk should suggest an alternative diagnosis involving the spinal cord. However, 2 of our patients have described a band-like sensation around the thorax. A defect of cutaneous sensation may take the form of impaired tactile, pain, and thermal sensation over the limbs in a distal distribution, implicating the small fibers of the peripheral nerves or the spinothalamic tracts, but such findings are relatively uncommon. The Lhermitte phenomenon (paresthesia down the spine or across the shoulders induced by rapid flexion of the neck) may be found if sought but is a sign more often allied with multiple sclerosis. The nervous system involvement in SCD is roughly symmetrical and distal, and sensory disturbances precede the motor ones; predominantly motor involvement from the beginning and a definite asymmetry of motor or sensory findings maintained over a period of weeks or months or prominent truncal or facial symptoms should always cast doubt on the diagnosis.

Cognitive symptoms and signs are frequent, ranging from irritability, apathy, somnolence, suspiciousness, and emotional instability to a marked confusional or depressive psychosis or dementia. Lindenbaum and coworkers have reported cases in which neuropsychiatric symptoms, responsive to vitamin B_{12}, were present without spinal cord or peripheral nerve abnormalities. In our clinical material, symptoms of dementia or psychosis have not been frequent and always followed the spinal cord disorder. Perhaps a slight degree of mental illness is all that is seen in early stages.

Visual impairment caused by optic neuropathy occasionally may be an early or sole manifestation of pernicious anemia; examination discloses roughly symmetrical centrocecal scotomata and optic atrophy in the most advanced cases. That visually evoked potentials may be abnormal in vitamin B_{12}-deficient patients without clinical signs of visual impairment suggests that the visual pathways are affected more often than is evident from the neurologic examination alone. A small number of patients have symptoms of autonomic dysfunction, including urinary sphincteric symptoms and impotence.

The CSF is usually normal; in some cases there is a moderate increase in protein. The nerve conduction studies may show slowing of sensory conduction or reduced-amplitude sensory potentials, but they are as often normal in early cases. Frequently, according to Hemmer and colleagues, somatosensory evoked potentials are delayed or absent; these changes are known to recover with treatment. Quite remarkable in corresponding to the locus of pathologic change, as these and other authors have indicated, is the finding on MRI of a T2 hyperintensity that demarcates the posterior columns of the cord and sometimes the lateral columns, as shown in Fig. 41-3. In a few of our patients these have taken the form solely of well-defined linear changes over a long extent of the posterior columns of the cervical cord.

Neuropathologic Changes

The pathologic process takes the form of a diffuse, although uneven, degeneration of white matter of the spinal cord and occasionally of the brain. The earliest histologic event is swelling of myelin sheaths, characterized by the formation of intramyelinic vacuoles and separation of myelin lamellae. This is followed by a coalescence of small foci of tissue destruction into larger ones, imparting a vacuolated, sieve-like appearance to the tissue, an appearance also observed in the myelopathy of AIDS and rarely in lupus erythematosus. The myelin sheaths and axis cylinders are both involved in the degenerative process, the former more obviously and perhaps earlier and more severely than the latter. There is relatively little fibrous gliosis in the early lesions, but in more chronic ones, particularly those in which considerable tissue is destroyed, the gliosis is pronounced. The changes begin in the posterior columns of the lower cervical and upper thoracic segments of the cord and spread from this region up and down the cord as well as forward into the lateral and anterior columns. The lesions are not limited to systems of fibers within the posterior or lateral columns but are scattered irregularly through the white matter, thereby representing a myelinopathy.

In rare instances, foci of spongy degeneration are found in the optic nerves and chiasm and in the central white matter of the brain (Adams and Kubik). The peripheral nerves may show a loss of myelin, but there is no unequivocal evidence that axons are significantly affected.

Agamanolis and colleagues (1978) showed that monkeys sustained on a vitamin B_{12}-deficient diet for a prolonged period develop neuropathologic changes indistinguishable from those of SCD in humans. The time required for the production of nervous system changes in monkeys, 33 to 45 months, is comparable to the time required to deplete the vitamin B_{12} stores of patients with pernicious anemia in whom parenteral vitamin B_{12} therapy had been discontinued. It is noteworthy that vitamin B_{12}-deprived monkeys do not become anemic despite the prolonged period of vitamin B_{12} deficiency. Also in

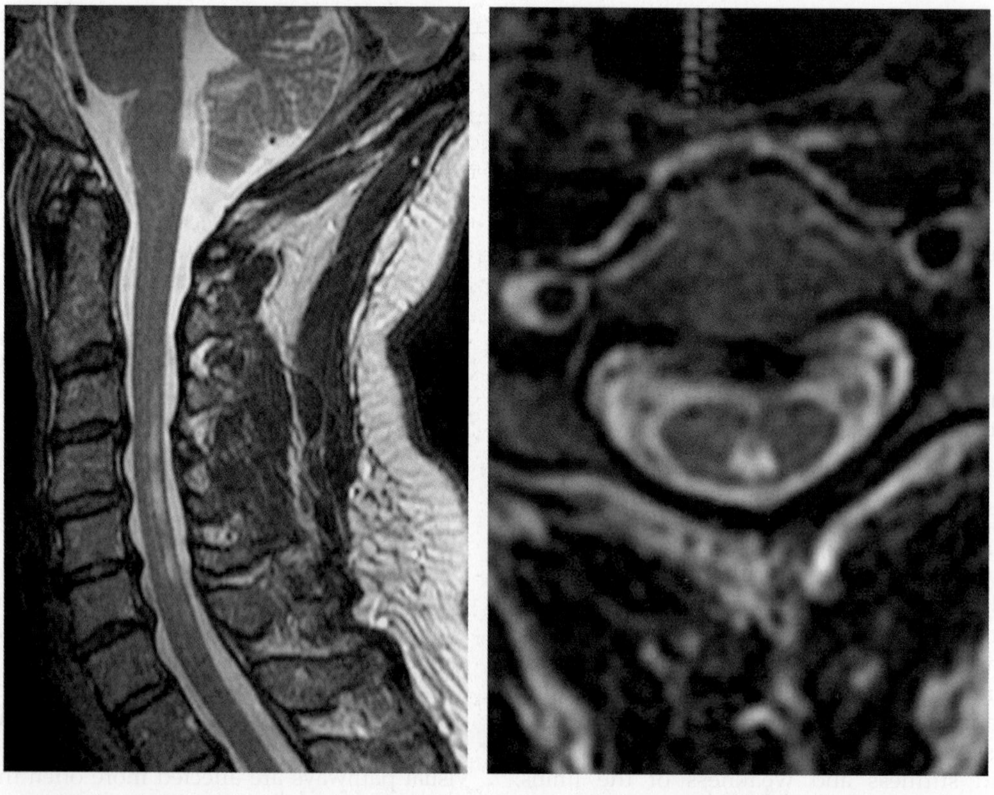

Figure 41-3. Sagittal (*left image*) and axial (*right image*) T2 MRI in subacute combined degeneration (SCD) showing abnormal hyperintensity in the posterior columns. The patient had markedly reduced vibration and position sense and a Romberg sign; the tendon reflexes were preserved and there were no corticospinal tract or peripheral nerve signs.

distinction to the human condition, involvement of the optic nerves is particularly severe in the monkey and probably precedes the degeneration of the spinal cord. The optic nerve lesions appear first in the papillomacular bundles, in the retrobulbar portions of the nerves; it subsequently spreads beyond the confines of this bundle and caudally in the optic nerves, chiasm, and tracts. These changes are much the same as those of "Tobacco–Alcohol Amblyopia" (see the section on this subject further on). The peripheral nerves are not affected in the experimentally produced vitamin B_{12} deficiency.

Paresthesia, impairment of deep sensation, and ataxia are caused by lesions in the posterior columns. Weakness, spasticity, increased tendon reflexes, and Babinski signs depend on involvement of the corticospinal tracts. The spinothalamic tracts may rarely be involved in the pathologic process, which explains the rare finding of a sensory level for pain and temperature on the trunk. The distal and symmetrical impairment of superficial sensation and loss of tendon reflexes that occur in advanced cases, however, may be explained by involvement of peripheral nerves and are then reflected in nerve conduction studies (see further on, under "Diagnosis").

Pathogenesis

Methylcobalamin is an essential cofactor in the conversion of homocysteine to methionine. An impairment of this reaction caused by a deficiency of cobalamin is thought to cause a failure of DNA synthesis, accounting for the hematologic abnormalities, particularly for the production of megaloblasts. However, because neurons do not divide, this sequence of chemical events does not explain the central nervous system abnormalities. One of the better-understood functions of vitamin B_{12} is its role as a coenzyme in the methylmalonyl-CoA mutase reaction. In this reaction, which is a key step in propionate metabolism, methylmalonyl-CoA is transformed to succinyl-CoA, which subsequently enters the Krebs cycle. A lack of the cobalamin-dependent enzyme methylmalonyl-CoA mutase leads to the accumulation of methylmalonyl-CoA and its precursor, propionyl-CoA. According to this mechanism, propionyl-CoA displaces succinyl-CoA, which is the usual primer for the synthesis of even-chain fatty acids; this results in the anomalous insertion of odd-chain fatty acids into membrane lipids, such as are found in myelin sheaths. Conceivably, this biochemical abnormality underlies the lesions of myelinated fibers that characterize the disease. However, Carmel and associates described a hereditary form of cobalamin deficiency in which methylmalonyl-CoA mutase activity was normal, despite the presence of typical neurologic abnormalities. In their view, the primary failure is one of methylation of homocysteine to methionine, that is, a failure of the methionine synthetase reaction, for which the coenzyme methylcobalamin is necessary.

Evidence for the latter view comes also from the observations, mentioned earlier, that prolonged administration of nitrous oxide (N_2O) may produce not only megaloblastic changes in the marrow (Amess et al), but also a sensorimotor polyneuropathy, often combined with signs of involvement of the posterior and lateral columns of the spinal cord (Layzer). Probably N_2O produces its effects by inactivating the methylcobalamin-dependent enzyme, methionine synthetase. These and other hypotheses are discussed by Jandl, Carmel and colleagues, and Beck (1988).

The role of *folate deficiency* in the genesis of SCD is less certain. One known clinical mistake has been to treat pernicious anemia by giving folic acid; this corrects the anemia but may worsen or even evoke the spinal cord lesions. Nevertheless, there have been a few reported examples of cerebral and spinal cord lesions indistinguishable from those caused by vitamin B_{12} deficiency in patients with defective folate metabolism, both in adults with acquired deficiency (Pincus) and in children with an inborn metabolic error (Clayton et al). The current view, however, is that folate deficiency alone does not produce SCD.

Diagnosis

The main differential diagnostic considerations of the combined sensory and motor features are cervical spondylosis (see Chaps. 11 and 44), multiple sclerosis of the cervical cord (see Chap. 36), rarities such as the female carrier state of adrenoleukodystrophy (see Chap. 37), and, most importantly, non-B_{12}-deficient combined system disease caused by low levels of serum copper (see Chap. 44). The last of these refers to a myelopathic process that affects the posterior and lateral columns subacutely in a manner identical to that of subacute combined degeneration but unassociated with any form of B_{12} deficiency or related enzyme derangement. Somewhat to our surprise, the copper disorder has been as frequent as the classic type caused by B_{12} deficiency in our clinics. This entity is described more extensively in Chap. 44. One remarkable circumstance, with which we have had experience, is the creation of severe SCD including paralysis in a B_{12}-deficient patient whose myelopathic symptoms were misattributed to cervical spondylosis and who had an operation for spondylosis in which spondylosis in nitrous oxide was used as anesthesia.

The chief obstacle to *early diagnosis* of SCD is the lack of parallelism that may exist between the hematologic and neurologic signs, particularly in patients who have taken dietary or medicinal folate. Anemia may also at times be absent, sometimes for many months, even in patients who have not taken folate. For example, in a retrospective study of 141 patients with neuropsychiatric abnormalities caused by cobalamin deficiency, there were 19 patients in whom both the hematocrit and mean red blood cell volume were normal (Lindenbaum et al); in these patients, subtle morphologic abnormalities such as hypersegmented polymorphonuclear leukocytes and megaloblastosis in bone marrow smears were almost always found if carefully sought.

Laboratory Diagnosis

Serum cobalamin should be measured whenever the diagnosis of vitamin B_{12} deficiency is in question. Microbiologic assay (using *Euglena gracilis*) is the most accurate measurement, but the method is time-consuming and cumbersome and has been replaced by a commercial radioisotope dilution assay (the inexpensive chemiluminescence assay is an alternative but slightly less dependable). With the radioassay, a serum B_{12} level below 100 pg/mL is usually associated with neurologic symptoms and signs of vitamin B_{12} deficiency. A level below 200 pg/mL that is unassociated with symptoms calls for further investigation of cobalamin deficiency. However, even serum levels of 200 to 300 pg/mL may still be associated (in 5 to 10 percent of cases) with cobalamin deficiency. High serum concentrations of cobalamin metabolites, methylmalonic acid (normal range, 73 to 271 nmol/L), and homocysteine (normal range 5.4 to 16.2 mmol/L) are additional reliable indicators of an intracellular cobalamin deficiency and can be used to corroborate the diagnosis in cases of low-mid-range B_{12} levels (Allen et al; Lindenbaum et al). It must be emphasized that the serum cobalamin level is not a measure of total-body cobalamin. In a patient who stops absorbing ingested cobalamin, the serum levels may remain in the normal range for months or years despite decreasing tissue reserves. In patients who have received vitamin B_{12} parenterally, the 2-stage Schilling test is a more reliable indicator of cobalamin deficiency because it uncovers a defect in absorption of the vitamin; however, the Schilling test has been largely supplanted for routine diagnosis by the measurement of antibodies to intrinsic factor and parietal cells.

Achlorhydria is almost invariably present in patients with pernicious anemia; its presence can be inferred by measuring the serum gastrin level. Antibodies to gastric parietal cells are also present in as many as 90 percent of patients with cobalamin deficiency, specifically in those with pernicious anemia as opposed to those with diminished B_{12} intake, but this test, although diagnostically specific, is positive in only 60 percent of cases. A relationship between helicobacter gastritis and autoimmunity against gastric parietal cells is being explored.

Low cobalamin levels with or without the clinical signs of deficiency may occur in patients with atrophic gastritis or after subtotal gastrectomy as mentioned. The malabsorption in such cases is thought to be because of a failure to extract cobalamin from food rather than a failure of the intrinsic factor mechanism ("food-cobalamin malabsorption"). Because the absorption of free cobalamin is normal, the Schilling test is unimpaired (Carmel, 1990). Infection of the gastric mucosa with *Helicobacter pylori* has been implicated in some cases. There are also rare inherited defects in the gene for intrinsic factor that render it ineffective.

The results of nerve conduction tests have varied in vitamin B_{12}-deficient patients. Early in the course of SCD, nerve conduction may be normal, but some patients have slowing of distal sensory conduction; others have found reduced amplitudes and minor signs of denervation, suggestive of axonal change. This again raises the controversy regarding the presence of a peripheral nerve disorder in uncomplicated B12 deficiency. Authoritative texts indicate that a neuropathy is present but certainly, such involvement is not integral to the disease as many patients with prominent neurological manifestations, particularly early in the course, have normal nerve conduction studies. In patients with normal peripheral nerve studies, the somatosensory evoked potentials usually show abnormalities attributable to central conduction delays, implicating the posterior columns as the cause of the sensory symptoms (Fine and Hallett). In advanced cases, motor conduction and late responses may be affected to a slight degree. These ambiguities reflect the inconsistent and poorly understood role of the peripheral neuropathic component of this disease.

The MRI lesions in the posterior columns were described earlier; they extend through the cervical and upper thoracic cords and, less often, to the lateral columns. The frequency of these findings, however, is not known, and their absence cannot be considered evidence against the diagnosis.

Treatment

The diagnosis of pernicious anemia demands the administration of vitamin B_{12} and the continuation of treatment for the rest of the patient's life. In cases of pernicious anemia, the patient is given 1,000 μg of cyanocobalamin or hydroxocobalamin intramuscularly each day for several days. The usual approach is to repeat the injection weekly for a month and then monthly for an indefinite period. Although most of the injected cobalamin is excreted, these patients must be flooded with the vitamin because the repletion of cobalamin tissue stores is a direct function of the dose.

In recent years, the notion that all forms of B_{12} deficiency must be circumvented by parenteral administration of the vitamin has been questioned and the use of oral cobalamin 500 to 1,000 μg daily has been used as an alternative, particularly for maintenance treatment. Several studies have indicated the effectiveness of this approach in elderly patients with poor B_{12} absorption and in persons with restricted diets, such as vegans, but we would express reservation regarding the use of oral replacement in the treatment of manifest subacute combined degeneration with neurologic manifestations until further studies have been published.

The most important factor influencing the response to treatment is the duration of symptoms; age, sex, and the degree of anemia are of lesser importance. The greatest improvements occur in patients whose disturbance of gait has been present for less than 3 months and recovery is usually complete if therapy is instituted within a few weeks after the onset of symptoms. All neurologic symptoms and signs may improve, mostly during the first 3 to 6 months of therapy, and then at a slower tempo during the ensuing year or even longer. In practically all instances, there is some degree of improvement after treatment, although in cases of longest duration, the best that can be accomplished is an arrest of progression.

DISORDERS CAUSED BY DEFICIENCIES OF FAT-SOLUBLE VITAMINS

Vitamin E Deficiency

This occurs in 2 types: a defect in intestinal absorption and an inherent hepatic enzyme deficiency that blocks incorporation of vitamin E into lipoprotein. A rare neurologic disorder of childhood, sometimes later in life, consisting essentially of spinocerebellar degeneration in association with polyneuropathy and pigmentary retinopathy, has been attributed to a deficiency of vitamin E consequent to prolonged intestinal fat malabsorption (Muller et al; Satya-Murti et al). The same mechanism has been proposed to explain the neurologic disorders that sometimes complicate abetalipoproteinemia (see Chap. 37), fibrocystic disease (Sokol et al), celiac sprue disease, and extensive intestinal resections (Harding et al). Vitamin E deficiency has also been observed in young children with chronic cholestatic hepatobiliary disease (Rosenblum et al).

Ataxia, loss of tendon reflexes, ophthalmoparesis, proximal muscle weakness with elevated serum creatine kinase, and decreased sensation are the usual manifestations of vitamin E deficiency. These symptoms are referable to parts of the nervous system and musculature that are found to be diseased in animals deprived of vitamin E: degeneration of Clark columns, spinocerebellar tracts, posterior columns, nuclei of Goll and Burdach, and sensory roots (Nelson et al). Local differences in the natural concentration of vitamin E in various parts of the nervous system and musculature are believed to account for the distribution of the lesions. In affected children, neurologic function improves after long-term daily supplementation with high doses of vitamin E.

In recent years there have been reports of a form of spinocerebellar degeneration attributable to an inherited but conditioned deficiency of vitamin E that may closely mimic the phenotype of Friedreich ataxia ("familial isolated vitamin E deficiency" as discussed in Chap. 39). The onset is usually in early adolescence, but there is variability, particularly among different families. In these patients, absorption and transport of vitamin E to the liver is normal, but hepatic incorporation of tocopherol (the active form of vitamin E) into very-low-density lipoproteins is defective (Traber et al). The abnormality has been traced to a mutation in *TTPA*, the gene encoding α-tocopherol transfer protein (Gotoda et al). In a sense, this is a vitamin deficiency conditioned by a genetic mutation. An important feature of these cases is that chronic oral administration of large doses of vitamin E can halt and even reverse progression of the ataxia (Gabsi et al).

Vitamins A and D Deficiencies

Neurologic disorders caused by a lack or excess of these fat-soluble vitamins have been reported, but they are rare. Vitamin A deficiency sometimes occurs with malabsorption syndromes, causing impairment of vision. *Excess of vitamin A* in children or adults may result in the syndrome of *pseudotumor cerebri* (see Chap. 30). Vitamin D deficiency is associated with hypoparathyroidism or a malabsorption state that leads to hypocalcemia, proximal muscle weakness, and rickets.

NUTRITIONAL SYNDROMES OF UNCERTAIN ETIOLOGY

Several related conditions of nutritional deficiency overlap in their presentations and have in common an uncertainty as to the primary cause. In all likelihood, there is a combination of factors, perhaps conditioned by genetic susceptibility. Here we refer especially to a syndrome of spastic ataxia, blindness, and a severe painful neuropathy with glossitis but there are other derivative syndromes that we discuss in this section.

Nutritional Spinal Spastic and Ataxic Syndrome

This syndrome is observed occasionally in nutritionally depleted alcoholics. The main clinical signs are spastic weakness of the legs, with absent abdominal and increased tendon reflexes, clonus, extensor plantar responses, and a loss of position and vibratory senses. In our experience, this syndrome has usually been associated with other nutritional disorders such as Wernicke disease and peripheral and optic neuropathy. In prisoner-of-war camps, the "spastic syndrome" was observed in association with mental and emotional changes and dimness of vision, and at times with widespread muscular rigidity, confusion, coma, and death. The latter syndrome has never been studied pathologically, so that it is impossible to state whether the lesions are the same as or different from those of pellagra or from Strachan syndrome, described further on.

The syndromes of tropical spastic paraparesis and of lathyrism, another form of spastic paraplegia common in India and certain parts of Africa, were for many years suspected of being nutritional in origin but are now known to be caused by a virus and a toxin, respectively. These and other types of tropical spastic paraplegia are discussed in greater detail with the spinal cord diseases (see Chap. 44). A chronic tropical disease of the peripheral nerves, called "ataxic neuropathy of Nigeria," has been attributed to the ingestion of inadequately detoxified cassava (Osuntokun). Another form of spastic ataxia, called "konzo," has been attributed to the production of cyanide by an ingested toxic glycoside in individuals who are protein deficient. The differential diagnosis of progressive spastic ataxia is quite broad and includes multiple sclerosis.

Nutritional Optic and Peripheral Neuropathy, "Tobacco–Alcohol Amblyopia," and Strachan Syndrome (See also Chap. 13)

These terms refer to a characteristic form of visual impairment that results from nutritional deficiency. The defect in vision is the result of a lesion of the optic nerves, more or less confined to the region of the papillomacular bundle. Typically, the patient complains of dimness or blurring of vision for near and distant objects, evolving gradually over a period of several days or weeks. Examination discloses a reduction in visual acuity because of the presence of central or centrocecal scotomata, which are larger for colored than for white test objects. Pallor of the temporal portion of the optic disc is observed in some cases. These abnormalities are bilateral and roughly symmetrical and, if untreated, may progress to blindness and irreversible optic atrophy. With normal diet and vitamin supplements improvement occurs in almost all cases but the most chronic ones; the degree of recovery depends on the severity of the amblyopia and particularly on its duration before therapy is instituted.

Although the precise deficiency responsible for this disease cannot be determined, its nutritional basis was established beyond doubt during World War II and the Korean War, when innumerable instances were observed in prisoners of war who had been confined for prolonged periods under conditions of severe dietary deprivation. Fisher described the optic nerve lesions in 4 such patients who had died of unrelated causes between 8 and 10 years after the onset of amblyopia. In each case, there was a loss of myelin and axis cylinders restricted to the region of the papillomacular fibers. Of the 4 cases, 3 also showed demyelination of the posterior columns of the spinal cord, no doubt an expression of the associated sensory polyradiculopathy.

In the Western world, a visual disorder indistinguishable clinically and pathologically from that observed in prisoners of war is observed infrequently, mainly among undernourished alcoholics. For many years this had been referred to as *tobacco–alcohol amblyopia*, with the implication that the visual loss is a result of the toxic effects of alcohol, tobacco, or both. Actually, the evidence is overwhelming that so-called tobacco–alcohol amblyopia is caused by nutritional deficiency and not by toxic exposure. A specific nutrient has not been identified, however. There are data in humans and animals that under certain conditions a deficiency of one or more of the B vitamins: thiamine, vitamin B_{12}, and perhaps riboflavin, may cause degenerative changes in the optic nerves, a situation that pertains in the peripheral nerves as well. Part of the confusion in delineating a specific cause has been sporadic outbreaks of optic neuropathy in underdeveloped countries that may have been caused by a disseminated ingested toxin as described further on.

In the 1960s, a popular theory held that the combined effects of vitamin B_{12} deficiency and chronic poisoning by cyanide (generated in tobacco smoke) were responsible for "tobacco amblyopia." Vitamin B_{12} deficiency is a rare but undoubted cause of optic neuropathy, as noted further on, but the notion that cyanide or other substances in tobacco smoke have a damaging effect on the optic nerves is unsupported (see reviews of Potts and of Victor [1970]). Instances of Leber hereditary optic atrophy, a mitochondrial disorder, may be also mistaken for "tobacco–alcohol amblyopia," an error that should be made less often because Leber disease disorder can now be identified by mitochondrial DNA testing.

Recent outbreaks of an apparently nutritional or perhaps toxic optic neuropathy occurred in Cuba during the period 1991 to 1993 and in Tanzania. In both instances the optic neuropathy was frequently associated with peripheral neuropathy. The association of this epidemic with widespread dietary deprivation and the salutary response of both optic and peripheral nerve symptoms to treatment with B vitamins suggests a nutritional causation (see Centers for Disease Control and Prevention and the report of the Cuba Neuropathy Field Investigation Team), but a toxic cause could not be excluded. Shortly thereafter, Plant and colleagues reported on a similar outbreak of optic and peripheral neuropathy from Tanzania.

There remains to be considered a neuropathic syndrome that almost certainly is nutritional in origin but does not conform clinically to beriberi or pellagra, the classic deficiency diseases. This syndrome was originally observed by Strachan in 1897 among Jamaican sugarcane workers. The main symptoms in his patients were pain, numbness, and paresthesias of the extremities; objectively there was ataxia of gait, weakness, wasting, and loss of deep tendon reflexes and sensation in the limbs. Dimness of vision and impairment of hearing were common findings, as were soreness and excoriation of the mucocutaneous junctions of the mouth. This disorder, originally known as "Jamaican neuritis," was quickly recognized in other parts of the world, particularly in the undernourished populations of tropical countries. Subsequently, many cases of this syndrome were observed in the besieged population of Madrid during the Spanish Civil War and during World War II among prisoners of war in North Africa and the Far East.

The clinical descriptions from these varied sources are not entirely uniform, but certain features are common to all of them and occur with sufficient frequency to allow the delineation of the neurologic syndrome; it appears to be almost identical to the one described by Strachan. The core disorder is combined optic and peripheral neuropathy. The latter consists mainly of sensory symptoms and signs, and the former of the subacute evolution of failing vision, which, if untreated, progresses to complete blindness and pallor of the optic discs. Deafness and vertigo are uncommon, but in some outbreaks among prisoners of war, these symptoms were frequent enough to earn the epithet "camp dizziness." In all these respects, the syndrome differs from beriberi. Along with the neurologic signs there may be varying degrees of stomatoglossitis, corneal degeneration, and genital dermatitis (the orogenital syndrome). The mucocutaneous lesions are unlike those of pellagra and riboflavin deficiency.

There have been only a few neuropathologic studies of this syndrome. Aside from the changes in the papillomacular bundle of the optic nerve, which are similar to the deficiency amblyopia discussed previously, the most consistent abnormality has been a loss of myelinated fibers in each column of Goll adjacent to the midline. Fisher interpreted this change to indicate a degeneration of the central processes of the bipolar sensory neurons of the dorsal root ganglia (i.e., the dorsal roots). The fact that the primary sensory neuron is the main site of the neuropathic disorder is consistent with the predominantly sensory symptomatology. The present authors find it difficult to draw a sharp dividing line between the nutritional peripheral (and optic) neuropathy described previously and the Strachan syndrome.

"Alcoholic" Cerebellar Degeneration

This term refers to a common and uniform type of degeneration of the vermian and anterior lobes of the cerebellum in alcoholics. Its incidence was in the past about twice that of Wernicke disease, and like the latter, it is considerably more frequent in men than in women. It is characterized clinically by a wide-based stance and gait, varying degrees of instability of the trunk, and ataxia of the legs, the arms being affected to a lesser extent and often not at all. Nystagmus and dysarthria are infrequent. In addition to an ataxic (intention) tremor, there may be a tremor of the fingers or hands resembling 1 of the 2 types of parkinsonian tremor, but appearing only when the limbs are placed in certain sustained postures. Mauritz and coworkers demonstrated that the instability of the trunk in these cases consists of a specific 3-Hz rhythmic swaying in the anteroposterior direction; by contrast, patients with lesions of the cerebellar hemispheres show only slight postural instability without directional preponderance.

In most cases, the cerebellar syndrome evolves over a period of several weeks or months, after which it remains unchanged for many years. In others, it develops more rapidly or more slowly, but in these cases also the disease eventually stabilizes. Occasionally, the cerebellar disorder progresses in a saltatory manner, the symptoms worsening in relation to a severe infectious illness or an attack of delirium tremens.

The *pathologic changes* consist of a degeneration of all the neurocellular elements of the cerebellar cortex but particularly of the Purkinje cells in the anterior and superior aspects of the vermis. The cerebellar atrophy is readily visualized by CT (Fig. 41-4) and MRI.

Two particular forms of this syndrome have not been emphasized sufficiently. In one, the clinical abnormalities are limited to an instability of station and gait, individual movements of the limbs being unaffected. The pathologic changes in such cases are restricted to the anterosuperior portions of the vermis. A second type is strikingly acute but transient. Here, except for their reversibility, the cerebellar symptoms are identical to those that characterize the chronic, fixed form of the disease. In this transient type, the derangement is only one of function ("biochemical lesion") and has probably not progressed to the point of fixed structural changes. These forms of cerebellar disease, and particularly the restricted and reversible varieties, cannot be distinguished from the cerebellar manifestations of Wernicke disease either on pathologic or on clinical grounds. It is our opinion that the cerebellar ataxia of Wernicke disease and that referred to as *alcoholic cerebellar degeneration* are based on the same disease process, the former term being applicable when the cerebellar abnormalities are associated with ocular and mental signs and the latter when the cerebellar syndrome stands alone and becomes persistent. Alcoholic cerebellar degeneration is in all likelihood a result of nutritional deficiency and not of the toxic effects of alcohol, for reasons already indicated. Insofar as the cerebellar ataxia usually improves to some extent under the influence of thiamine alone (see earlier, under "Wernicke-Korsakoff Syndrome [Thiamine (B_1) Deficiency]"), it is likely that a deficiency of this vitamin is in whole or part responsible for the cerebellar lesion, but this has not been proven.

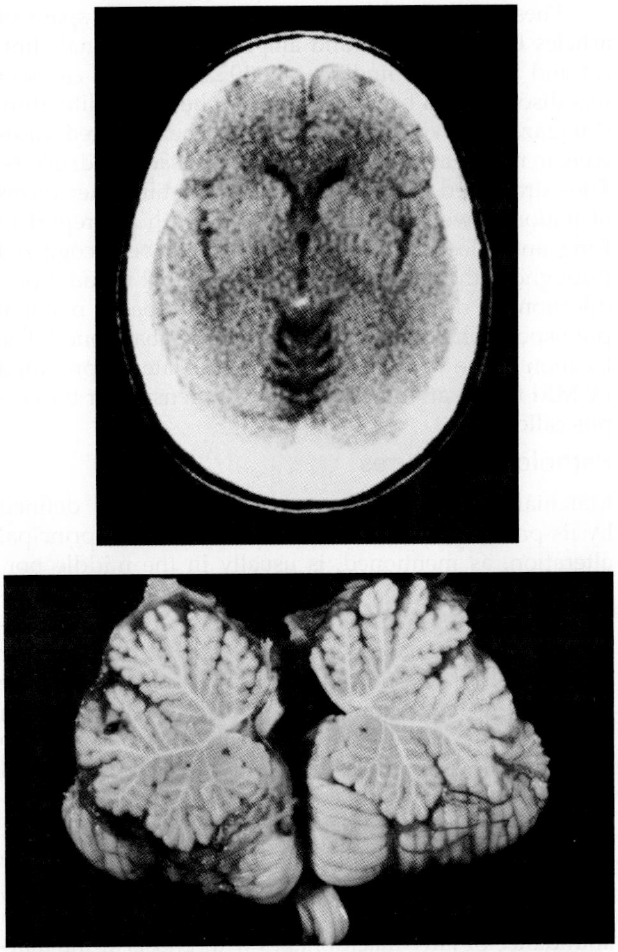

Figure 41-4. CT from a 60-year-old alcoholic patient showing prominence of midline cerebellar sulci (*upper image*). A broad-based gait and ataxia of the legs had been present for many years. Death was from myocardial infarction. The cerebellum, cut in the midsagittal plane (*lower image*), shows folial atrophy of the anterosuperior vermis, characteristic of alcoholic cerebellar degeneration.

Marchiafava-Bignami Disease (Degeneration of the Corpus Callosum)

In 1903, the pathologists Marchiafava and Bignami described a unique alteration of the corpus callosum in 3 alcoholic patients. In each case, coronal sectioning of the fixed brain disclosed a pink-gray discoloration of the central portion of the corpus callosum throughout the longitudinal extent of this structure. Microscopically, the lesion proved to be confined to the middle lamina (which makes up about two-thirds of the thickness of the corpus callosum), in which there was a loss of myelin and, to some degree, of the axis cylinders; macrophages were abundant in the altered zone, and astrocytic proliferation had followed. The clinical observations in these patients were few and incomplete. In 1907, Bignami described a case in which the corpus callosum lesion was accompanied by a similar lesion in the central portion of the anterior commissure.

These early reports were followed by a spate of articles that confirmed and amplified the original clinical and pathologic findings. By 1922, about 40 cases of this disorder had been described in the Italian literature (Mingazzini). With 1 exception, all the reported cases were in males, and all these men were insatiable drinkers. They drank red wine for the most part, but other forms of liquor as well. Beginning in 1936, with the report of King and Meehan, the disease came to be recognized throughout the world, and the notions that it had a predilection for drinkers of red wine and a special national predisposition or geographic locale were abandoned. The location of the white matter lesion was later appreciated by MRI to be variable with only a propensity for the corpus callosum.

Pathologic Features

Marchiafava-Bignami disease is more readily defined by its pathologic than its clinical features. The principal alteration, as mentioned, is usually in the middle portion of the corpus callosum, which on gross examination appears rarefied and sunken and reddish or gray-yellow in color, depending on its age. In the anterior portion of the corpus callosum, the lesion tends to be more severe in the midline than in its lateral parts; in the splenium, however, the opposite may pertain. The most chronic lesion takes the form of a centrally placed gray cleft or cavity, with collapse of the surrounding tissue and reduction in thickness of the corpus callosum. Microscopically, corresponding to the gross lesions, one observes clearly demarcated zones of demyelination, with variable involvement of the axis cylinders and an abundance of fatty macrophages with gliosis at the margins. Inflammatory changes are absent.

Infrequently, lesions of a similar nature are found in the central portions of the anterior and posterior commissures and the brachia pontis. These zones of myelin destruction are surrounded by a rim of intact white matter. The predilection of this disease process for commissural fiber systems has been stressed, but it is certainly not confined to these fibers. Symmetrically placed lesions have been observed in the columns of Goll, superior cerebellar peduncles, and cerebral hemispheres, involving the centrum semiovale and extending, in some cases, into the adjacent convolutional white matter. As a rule, the internal capsule and corona radiata, subcortical arcuate fibers, and cerebellum are spared. In several cases, the lesions of deficiency amblyopia (see earlier) have been added; in others, the lesions of Wernicke disease.

Many of the reported cases, as first pointed out by Jequier and Wildi, have involved cortical lesions of a special type: The neurons in the third layer of the frontal and temporal lobe cortices had disappeared and were replaced by a fibrous gliosis. Morel, who first described this *cortical laminar sclerosis*, did not observe its association with Marchiafava-Bignami disease. However, when Jequier and Adams reviewed his original cases (unpublished), all had Marchiafava-Bignami disease. In a subsequent report by Delay and colleagues comprising 14 cases of cortical laminar sclerosis, the cortical lesion was also consistently associated with a corpus callosum lesion. We believe the cortical lesions are best explained as secondary to the callosal degeneration.

Clinical Features

The disease affects persons in middle and late adult life. With few exceptions, the patients have been males and severe chronic alcoholics. The clinical features of the illness are otherwise quite variable, and a clear-cut syndrome has not emerged. Many patients have presented in a state of terminal stupor or coma, precluding a detailed neurologic assessment. In others, the clinical picture was dominated by the manifestations of chronic inebriation and alcohol withdrawal, namely tremor, seizures, hallucinosis, and delirium tremens. In some of these patients, following the subsidence of the withdrawal symptoms, no signs of neurologic disease could be elicited, even in the end stage of the disease, which lasted for several days to weeks. In yet another group, a progressive dementia has been described, evolving slowly over a year before death. Emotional disorders, dysarthria, slowing and unsteadiness of movement, transient sphincteric incontinence, hemiparesis, and apractic or aphasic disorders have been reported. The last stage of the disease is characterized by physical decline, seizures, stupor, and coma. An impressive feature of these varied neurologic deficits in some patients has been their tendency toward remission when nutrition was restored.

In 2 cases that have come to our attention, the clinical manifestations were essentially those of bilateral frontal lobe disease: motor and mental slowness, apathy, prominent grasping and sucking reflexes, gegenhalten, incontinence, and a slow, hesitant, wide-based gait. In both these cases, the neurologic abnormalities evolved over a period of about 2 months, and both patients recovered within a few weeks of hospitalization. Death occurred several years later as a result of liver disease and subdural hematoma, respectively. In each case, autopsy disclosed an old lesion typical of Marchiafava-Bignami disease confined to the central portion of the most anterior parts of the corpus callosum, but one had to look closely to see the gray line of gliosis.

In view of the great variability of the clinical picture and the obscuration in many patients of subtle mental and neurologic abnormalities by the effects of chronic inebriation and other alcoholic neurologic disorders, the diagnosis of Marchiafava-Bignami disease is understandably difficult. In fact, it is rarely made during life, but the CT and MRI have disclosed typical but unsuspected examples (see Kawamura et al). In some cases studied sequentially, MRI has disclosed demyelination, swelling, and necrosis of the corpus callosum with extension toward the subcortical white matter. In a few cases these findings have reversed over time after vitamin therapy, leaving residual callosal atrophy (Gambini et al). The occurrence, in a chronic alcoholic, of a frontal lobe syndrome or a symptom complex that points to a diagnosis of frontal or corpus callosum tumor but in whom the symptoms remit should suggest the diagnosis of Marchiafava-Bignami disease. The image appearance may be easily mistaken for multiple sclerosis, gliomatosis cerebri, or progressive multifocal leukoencephalopathy.

Pathogenesis and Etiology

Originally, Marchiafava-Bignami disease was attributed to the toxic effects of alcohol, but this is an unlikely explanation in view of the prevalence of alcoholism and the rarity of corpus callosum degeneration. Furthermore, the distinctive callosal lesions have not been observed with other neurotoxins. Very rarely, undoubted examples of Marchiafava-Bignami disease have occurred in abstainers, so that alcohol cannot be an indispensable factor. A nutritional etiology has been invoked, but the putative factor that is deficient has not been determined. This view is underscored by reports of improvement in a few, but not all, cases following administration of thiamine. The mechanisms involved in the selective demyelination and noninflammatory necrosis of particular areas of white matter remain to be elucidated. Perhaps, when its mechanism becomes known, Marchiafava-Bignami disease, like central pontine myelinolysis (which it resembles histologically), will have to be considered in a chapter other than one on nutritional disease.

PROTEIN-CALORIE MALNUTRITION AND DEVELOPMENTAL DELAY

(See also Chap. 38)

There is increasing evidence that severe dietary deprivation during critical phases of brain development may result in permanent impairment of cerebral function and in developmental delay. Inasmuch as there are an estimated 100 million children in the world who are undernourished and suffer from varying degrees of protein, calorie, and other dietary inadequacies, this is one of the most pressing problems in medicine and society.

The literature is too large to review here, but excellent critiques have been provided by Winick, Birch and coworkers, Latham, and Dodge and colleagues. In contrast to the devastating effect of protein-calorie malnutrition (PCM) on body growth, brain weight is only slightly reduced. Nevertheless, on the basis of experiments in dogs, pigs, and rats, it is evident that prenatal and early postnatal malnutrition retards cellular proliferation in the brain. All cells are affected, including oligodendroglia, with a proportional reduction in myelin. Also, the process of dendritic branching may be retarded by early malnutrition. A limited number of studies in humans suggest that PCM has a similar effect on the brain during the first 8 months of life. In animals, varying degrees of recovery from the effects of early malnutrition are possible if normal nutrition is reestablished during the vulnerable periods. Presumably this is true for humans as well, although proof is difficult to obtain. In every series of severely undernourished infants and young children who have been observed for a period of many years, a variable proportion has been developmentally delayed to a modest degree; the majority recovers, however (Galler). Unfortunately, the neurologic and intellectual consequences of PCM have defied accurate assessment because of the difficulty of isolating the effects of severe malnutrition from those of infection, social deprivation, genetic mechanisms, and other factors.

Nutritional Deficiencies Secondary to Malabsorption

The vitamins known to be essential to the normal functioning of the central and peripheral nervous systems cannot be synthesized by the human organism. Each is ingested as an essential part of the normal diet and absorbed in certain regions of the gastrointestinal tract. Impairment or failure of absorption caused by diseases of the gastrointestinal tract gives rise to several malabsorption syndromes, some of which have already been referred to, for example, malabsorptive vitamin E deficiency. In these diseases, the site of the block in transport from the intestinal lumen varies; it may be at the surface of the enterocytes or at their interface with the lymphatic channels and portal capillaries.

Table 41-2, which is modified from Pallis and Lewis, lists the main malabsorptive diseases and their relationships to the intestinal abnormalities. Of all these diseases, celiac sprue (gluten enteropathy) is the most common. The neurologic complications of this disorder, in our experience, have taken the form of a symmetrical, predominantly sensory polyneuropathy, as described in Chap. 46. However, other complications have been described, notably a progressive cerebellar syndrome with cortical, dentatal, and olivary cell loss. The cerebellar changes may be coupled with a symmetrical demyelination of the posterior columns, producing a spinocerebellar disorder similar to that of vitamin E deficiency, but in the latter case, vitamin E supplementation has no consistent effect. Others have remarked on a high incidence of depression and other psychiatric disturbances in adult patients with celiac sprue, as also discussed in Chap. 40. Unexplained seizures are also said to occur.

Polyneuropathy and SCD of the spinal cord manifesting themselves many years after gastrectomy are encountered only rarely. The neurology of gastrointestinal disease has also been reviewed by Perkin and Murray-Lyon.

INHERITED VITAMIN-RESPONSIVE NEUROLOGIC DISEASES

(See Table 41-3 and Chap. 37)

Although humans lack the capacity to synthesize essential vitamin molecules, they are nonetheless able to use them in a series of complex chemical reactions involved in intestinal absorption, transport in the plasma, entry into the organelles of many organs, activation of the vitamin into coenzyme, and, finally, their interaction with certain specific apoenzyme proteins. This compels consideration of another aspect of nutrition wherein one or more of these steps in vitamin utilization may be defective because of a genetic abnormality. Under

Table 41-2

MECHANISMS WHEREBY MALABSORPTION MAY BE RELATED TO NEUROLOGIC DISEASE

GASTROINTESTINAL DEFECT	SUBSTANCE MALABSORBED	ASSOCIATED NEUROLOGIC DISORDER
Localized gastric lesions:		
Pernicious anemia	Vitamin B_{12}	Myelopathy, optic neuropathy, etc.
Congenital lack of intrinsic factor	Vitamin B_{12}	Myelopathy, neuropathy, etc.
Partial gastrectomy	Vitamin B_{12}	Myelopathy, neuropathy, etc.
	Vitamin D	Osteomalacic myopathy
Lesions of small intestine:		
Predominantly proximal	? Water-soluble vitamins	? Hypovitaminosis B
	Vitamin D	? Osteomalacic myopathy
	Folic acid	Probably none
Predominantly distal	Vitamin B_{12}	Neuropathy, myelopathy, etc.
Diffuse		Myoclonus, ataxia, etc.
Bacterial contamination of small bowel (jejunal diverticulosis, blind-loop syndrome, strictures)	Vitamin B_{12}	Neuropathy, myelopathy, etc.
Congenital absorptive defect	"Neutral" amino acids	Hartnup disease
	Tryptophan	"Blue diaper" syndrome
	Methionine	"Oast-house" urine disease
	Folic acid	Mental retardation, seizures, ataxia, choreoathetosis
	Vitamin B_{12}	Neuropathy, myelopathy
Transmucosal transport disorders associated with steatorrhea:	Fat-soluble vitamins	Xerophthalmia
		Keratomalacia
Endocrine causes		? Osteomalacic myopathy
Postirradiation		
Drug induced		
Defective synthesis of chylomicrons with prolonged intestinal malabsorption	Vitamin E (carrier lipoprotein not synthesized in liver)	Bassen-Kornzweig disease, spinocerebellar degeneration with polyneuropathy
Infiltration of villous cores	Fats (defective chylomicron release)	Encephalopathy of Whipple disease
Competition for essential nutrients (e.g., fish tapeworm)	Vitamin B_{12}	Neuropathy, myelopathy

Source: Reproduced by permission from Pallis and Lewis.

these circumstances, the signs of vitamin deficiency result not from vitamin deficiency in the diet but from a genetically deranged control mechanism. In some instances the defect is only quantitative, and by loading the organism with a great excess of the vitamin in question, the biochemical abnormality can be overcome. The aforementioned special type of vitamin E deficiency that results from an inherited inability to incorporate the vitamin into lipoproteins falls into this category, the diseases of which, being of hereditary type, have already been described in Chap. 37. Rosenberg has listed the most important of these hereditary vitamin-responsive diseases, which we have abstracted for the reader in Table 41-3.

Table 41-3

VITAMIN-RESPONSIVE INHERITED DISORDERS AFFECTING THE NERVOUS SYSTEM

VITAMIN	DISORDER	THERAPEUTIC DOSE	ENZYMATIC DEFECT	NEUROLOGIC MANIFESTATIONS
Thiamine (B_1)	Branched-chain ketoaciduria	5–20 mg	Branched-chain ketoacid decarboxylase	Lethargy, coma
	Lactic acidosis	5–20 mg	Pyruvate carboxylase	Mental retardation
	Pyruvic acidemia	5–20 mg	Pyruvate dehydrogenase	Cerebellar ataxia
	Anemia	50 mg	—	Same as thiamine-deficient beri-beri of infancy and childhood
Pyridoxine (B_6)	Homocystinuria	>25 mg	Cystathionine synthase	Mental retardation, cerebrovascular accidents, psychoses
	Infantile convulsions	10–50 mg	Glutamic acid decarboxylase	Seizures
	Xanthurenic aciduria	5–10 mg	Kynureninase	Mental retardation
Cobalamin (B_{12})	Methylmalonic aciduria	1,000 g	Methylmalonyl-CoA mutase apoenzyme	Lethargy, coma, psychomotor retardation
	Methylmalonic aciduria and homocystinuria	>500 g	Defects in synthesis of adenosylcobalamin and methylcobalamin	Developmental arrest, cerebellar ataxia
Folic acid	Megaloblastic anemia	<0.05 mg	Folate deficiency	Mental retardation
	Formiminotransferase deficiency	>5 mg	Intestinal malabsorption of formiminotransferase	Mental retardation
	Homocystinuria and hypomethioninemia	>10 mg	N^5, N^{10}-Methylenetetrahydrofolate reductase	Schizophrenic syndrome
Biotin	*β*-Methylcrotonylglycinuria	↑5–10 mg	*β*-Methylcrotonyl-CoA carboxylase	Mental retardation
	Propionic acidemia	↑5–10 mg	Propionyl-CoA carboxylase	Lethargy, coma
Nicotinamide	Hartnup disease	>400 mg	Intestinal malabsorption of tryptophan	Cerebellar ataxia

Source: Adapted from Rosenberg and from Matsui et al.

References

Adams RD, Kubik CS: Subacute degeneration of the brain in pernicious anemia. *N Engl J Med* 231:2, 1944.

Agamanolis DP, Chester EM, Victor M, et al: Neuropathology of experimental vitamin B_{12} deficiency in monkeys. *Neurology* 26:905, 1976.

Agamanolis DP, Victor M, Harris JW, et al: An ultrastructural study of subacute combined degeneration of the spinal cord in vitamin B_{12} deficient rhesus monkeys. *J Neuropathol Exp Neurol* 37:273, 1978.

Albin RL, Albers JW, Greenberg HS, et al: Acute sensory neuropathy-neuronopathy from pyridoxine overdosage. *Neurology* 37:1729, 1987.

Allen RH, Stabler SP, Savage DG, Lindenbaum J: Diagnosis of cobalamin deficiencies: I. Usefulness of serum methylmalonic acid and total homocysteine concentrations. *Am J Hematol* 34:90, 1990.

Amess JAL, Burman JF, Nancekievill DG, Mollin DL: Megaloblastic haemopoiesis in patients receiving nitrous oxide. *Lancet* 2:339, 1978.

Antozzi C, Garavaglia B, Mora M, et al: Late-onset riboflavin-responsive myopathy with combined multiple acyl coenzyme A dehydrogenase and respiratory chain deficiency. *Neurology* 44:2153, 1994.

Bean WB, Hodges RE, Daum KE: Pantothenic acid deficiency induced in human subjects. *J Clin Invest* 34:1073, 1955.

Beck WS: Cobalamin and the nervous system. *N Engl J Med* 318:1752, 1988.

Beck WS: Neuropsychiatric consequences of cobalamin deficiency. *Adv Intern Med* 36:33, 1991.

Behse F, Buchthal F: Alcoholic neuropathy: Clinical, electrophysiological, and biopsy findings. *Ann Neurol* 2:95, 1977.

Biehl JP, Vilter RW: The effect of isoniazid on vitamin B_6 metabolism and its possible significance in producing isoniazid neuritis. *Proc Soc Exp Biol Med* 85:389, 1954.

Bignami A: Sulle alterazione del corpo calloso e della commissura anteriore ritrovate in un alcoolista. *Policlinico [Prat]* 14:460, 1907.

Birch HG, Pineiro C, Alcade E, et al: Relation of kwashiorkor in early childhood and intelligence at school age. *Pediatr Res* 5:579, 1971.

Birchfield RE: Postural hypotension in Wernicke's disease: A manifestation of autonomic nervous system involvement. *Am J Med* 36:404, 1964.

Blass JP, Gibson GE: Abnormality of a thiamine-requiring enzyme in patients with Wernicke-Korsakoff syndrome. *N Engl J Med* 297:1367, 1977.

Bomb BS, Bedi HK, Bhatnagar LK: Post-ischaemic paresthesiae in pellagrins. *J Neurol Neurosurg Psychiatry* 40:265, 1977.

Botez MI, Peyronnard J, Charron L: Polyneuropathies responsive to folic acid therapy, in Botez MI, Reynolds EH (eds): *Folic Acid in Neurology, Psychiatry, and Internal Medicine*. New York, Raven Press, 1979, pp 401–412.

Carmel R: Subtle and atypical cobalamin deficiency states. *Am J Hematol* 34:108, 1990.

Carmel R, Watkins D, Goodman SI, Rosenblatt DS: Hereditary defect of cobalamin metabolism (cb1G mutation) presenting as a neurologic disorder in adulthood. *N Engl J Med* 318:1738, 1988.

Carney MWP: Neuropsychiatric disorders associated with nutritional deficiencies. *CNS Drugs* 3:279, 1995.

Carton H, Kayenbe K, Kabeya, et al: Epidemic spastic paraparesis in Bandundu (Zaire). *J Neurol Neurosurg Psychiatry* 49:620, 1986.

Centers for Disease Control and Prevention: Epidemic neuropathy—Cuba, 1991–1994. *MMWR Morb Mortal Wkly Rep* 43:183, 189, 1994.

Charness ME, DeLaPaz RL: Mamillary body atrophy in Wernicke's encephalopathy: Antemortem identification using magnetic resonance imaging. *Ann Neurol* 22:595, 1987.

Chopra JS, Dhand UK, Mehta S, et al: Effect of protein calorie malnutrition on peripheral nerves. *Brain* 109:307, 1986.

Clayton PT, Smith I, Harding B, et al: Subacute combined degeneration of the cord, dementia, and parkinsonism due to an inborn error of metabolism. *J Neurol Neurosurg Psychiatry* 49:920, 1986.

Cooke WT, Smith WT: Neurological disorders associated with adult coeliac disease. *Brain* 89:683, 1966.

Crellin R, Bottiglieri T, Reynolds EH: Folate and psychiatric disorder: Clinical potential. *Drugs* 45:623, 1993.

Cuba Neuropathy Field Investigation Team: Epidemic optic neuropathy in Cuba—clinical characterization and risk factors. *N Engl J Med* 333:1176, 1995.

Delay J, Brion S, Escourolle R, Sanchez A: Rapports entre la degenerescence du corps calleux de Marchiafava-Bignami et la sclerose laminaire corticale de Morel. *Encephale* 49:281, 1959.

Denny-Brown DE: The neurological aspects of thiamine deficiency. *Fed Proc* 17(Suppl 2):35, 1958.

Dodge PR, Prensky AL, Feigin R: *Nutrition and the Developing Nervous System*. St. Louis, Mosby, 1975.

Donnal JF, Heinz ER, Burger PC: MR of reversible thalamic lesions in Wernicke syndrome. *AJNR Am J Neuroradiol* 11:893, 1990.

Dreyfus PM, Moniz R: The quantitative histochemical estimation of transketolase in the nervous system of the rat. *Biochim Biophys Acta* 65:181, 1962.

Elvehjem CA, Madden RJ, Strong FM, Woolley DW: Relation of nicotinic acid and nicotinic acid amide to canine black tongue. *J Am Chem Soc* 59:1767, 1937.

Fine EJ, Hallett M: Neurophysiological study of subacute combined degeneration. *J Neurol Sci* 45:331, 1980.

Fisher CM: Residual neuropathological changes in Canadians held prisoners of war by the Japanese. *Can Serv Med J* 11:157, 1955.

Gabsi S, Gouider-Khouja N, Belal S, et al: Effect of vitamin E supplementation in patients with ataxia with vitamin E deficiency. *Eur J Neurol* 8:477, 2001.

Galler JR: Malnutrition—a neglected cause of learning failure. *Postgrad Med* 80:225, 1986.

Gambini A, Falini A, Moiola L, et al: Marchiafava-Bignami disease: Longitudinal MR imaging and MR spectroscopy study. *AJNR Am J Neuroradiol* 24:249, 2003.

Ghez C: Vestibular paresis: A clinical feature of Wernicke's disease. *J Neurol Neurosurg Psychiatry* 32:134, 1969.

Goldsmith GA: Niacin-tryptophan relationships in man and niacin requirement. *Am J Clin Nutr* 6:479, 1958.

Gotoda T, Arita M, Arai H, et al: Adult-onset spinocerebellar dysfunction caused by a mutation in the gene for the α-tocopherol-transfer protein. *N Engl J Med* 333:1313, 1995.

Green R, Kinsella LJ: Current concepts in the diagnosis of cobalamin deficiency. *Neurology* 45:1435, 1995.

Hallert C, Astrom J: Psychic disturbances in adult celiac disease: II. Psychological findings. *Scand J Gastroenterol* 17:21, 1982.

Hallert C, Deerefeldt T: Psychic disturbances in adult celiac disease: I. Clinical manifestations. *Scand J Gastroenterol* 17:17, 1982.

Harding AE, Mathews S, Jones S, et al: Spinocerebellar degeneration associated with a selective defect of vitamin E absorption. *N Engl J Med* 313:32, 1985.

Harper C: The incidence of Wernicke's encephalopathy in Australia—a neuropathological study of 131 cases. *J Neurol Neurosurg Psychiatry* 46:593, 1983.

Harper CG, Giles M, Finlay-Jones R: Clinical signs in the Wernicke-Korsakoff complex: A retrospective analysis of 131 cases diagnosed at necropsy. *J Neurol Neurosurg Psychiatry* 49:341, 1986.

Hauw J-J, deBaecque C, Hausser-Hauw C, Serdaru M: Chromatolysis in alcoholic encephalopathies: Pellagra-like changes in 22 cases. *Brain* 111:843, 1988.

Hemmer B, Glocker FX, Schumacher M, et al: Subacute combined degeneration: Clinical, electrophysiologic, and magnetic resonance imaging findings. *J Neurol Neurosurg Psychiatry* 65:822, 1998.

Ishii N, Nishihara Y: Pellagra among chronic alcoholics: Clinical and pathological study of 20 necropsy cases. *J Neurol Neurosurg Psychiatry* 44:209, 1981.

Jandl JH: Cobalamin deficiency, in Jandl JH (ed): *Blood: Textbook of Hematology*, 2nd ed. Boston, Little, Brown, 1996, pp 259–270.

Jequier M, Wildi E: Le syndrome de Marchiafava-Bignami. *Schweiz Arch Neurol Psychiatr* 77:393, 1956.

Jolliffe N, Bowman KM, Rosenblum LA, Fein HD: Nicotinic acid deficiency encephalopathy. *JAMA* 114:307, 1940.

Kawamura M, Shiota J, Yagishita T, Hirayama K: Marchiafava-Bignami disease: Computed tomographic scan and magnetic resonance imaging. *Ann Neurol* 18:103, 1985.

King LS, Meehan MC: Primary degeneration of the corpus callosum (Marchiafava's disease). *Arch Neurol Psychiatry* 36:547, 1936.

Kinsella LJ, Green R: "Anesthesia paresthetica": Nitrous oxide-induced cobalamin deficiency. *Neurology* 45:1608, 1995.

Koike H, Iijima M, Sugiura M, et al: Alcoholic neuropathy is clinicopathologically distinct from thiamine-deficiency neuropathy. *Ann Neurol* 54:19, 2003.

Kopelman MD: Two types of confabulation. *J Neurol Neurosurg Psychiatry* 50:1482, 1987.

Latham MC: Protein-calorie malnutrition in children and its relation to psychological development and behavior. *Physiol Rev* 54:541, 1974.

Layzer RB: Myeloneuropathy after prolonged exposure to nitrous oxide. *Lancet* 2:1227, 1978.

Leventhal CM, Baringer JR, Arnason BG, Fisher CM: A case of Marchiafava-Bignami disease with clinical recovery. *Trans Am Neurol Assoc* 90:87, 1965.

Lindenbaum J, Healton EB, Savage DG, et al: Neuropsychiatric disorders caused by cobalamin deficiency in the absence of anemia or macrocytosis. *N Engl J Med* 318:1720, 1988.

Mair RG, Capra C, McEntee WJ, Engen T: Odor discrimination and memory in Korsakoff's psychosis. *J Exp Psychol* 6:445, 1980.

Mandel H, Bernat M, Hazani A, Naveh Y: Thiamine-dependent beriberi in the thalamic-responsive anemia syndrome. *N Engl J Med* 311:836, 1984.

Marchiafava E, Bignami A: Sopra un alterazione del corpo calloso osservata in soggetti alcoolisti. *Riv Patol Nerv Ment* 8:544, 1903.

Matsui SM, Mahoney MJ, Rosenberg LE: The natural history of inherited methylmalonic acidemias. *N Engl J Med* 308:857, 1983.

Mauritz KH, Dichgans J, Hufschmidt A: Quantitative analysis of stance in late cortical cerebellar atrophy of the anterior lobe and other forms of cerebellar ataxia. *Brain* 102:461, 1979.

Mingazzini G: *Der Balken*. Berlin, Springer-Verlag, 1922.

Morel F: Une forme anatomo-clinique particuliere de l'alcoolisme chronique: Sclerose corticale laminaire alcoolique. *Rev Neurol* 71:280, 1939.

Muller DPR, Lloyd JK, Wolff OH: Vitamin E and neurological function. *Lancet* 1:225, 1983.

Nelson JS, Fitch CD, Fisher VW, et al: Progressive neuropathologic lesions in vitamin E deficient rhesus monkey. *J Neuropathol Exp Neurol* 40:166, 1981.

Osuntokun BO: Cassava diet, chronic cyanide intoxication and neuropathy in the Nigerian Africans. *World Rev Nutr Diet* 36:141, 1981.

Pallis CA, Lewis PD: *The Neurology of Gastrointestinal Disease*. Philadelphia, Saunders, 1974.

Perkin CD, Murray-Lyon I: Neurology and the gastrointestinal system. *J Neurol Neurosurg Psychiatry* 65:291, 1998.

Pincus JH: Folic acid deficiency: A cause of subacute combined system degeneration, in Botez MI, Reynolds EH (eds): *Folic Acid in Neurology, Psychiatry, and Internal Medicine*. New York, Raven Press, 1979, pp 427–433.

Plant GT, Mtanda AT, Arden GB, Johnson GJ: An epidemic of optic neuropathy in Tanzania: Characterization of the visual disorder and associated peripheral neuropathy. *J Neurol Sci* 145:127, 1997.

Potts AM: Tobacco amblyopia. *Surv Ophthalmol* 17:313, 1973.

Ronthal M, Adler H: Motor nerve conduction velocity and the electromyograph in pellagra. *S Afr Med J* 43:642, 1969.

Rosenberg LE: Vitamin-responsive inherited diseases affecting the nervous system, in Plum F (ed): *Brain Dysfunction in Metabolic Disorders*. Vol 53. New York, Raven Press, 1974, pp 263–270.

Rosenblum JL, Keating JP, Prensky AL, Nelson JS: A progressive neurologic syndrome in children with chronic liver disease. *N Engl J Med* 304:503, 1981.

Satya-Murti S, Howard L, Krohel G, Wolf B: The spectrum of neurologic disorder from vitamin E deficiency. *Neurology* 36:917, 1986.

Schaumburg H, Kaplan J, Windebank A, et al: Sensory neuropathy from pyridoxine abuse: A new megavitamin syndrome. *N Engl J Med* 309:445, 1983.

Sechi G, Serra A: Wernicke's encephalopathy: new clinical settings and recent advances in diagnosis and management. *Lancet Neurol* 6:442, 2007.

Serdaru M, Hausser-Hauw C, Laplane D, et al: The clinical spectrum of alcoholic pellagra encephalopathy. *Brain* 111:829, 1988.

Shah DR, Singh SV, Jain IL: Neurological manifestations in pellagra. *J Assoc Physicians India* 19:443, 1971.

Shattuck GC: Relation of beriberi to polyneuritis from other causes. *Am J Trop Med Hyg* 8:539, 1928.

Shimojyo S, Scheinberg P, Reinmuth OM: Cerebral blood flow and metabolism in the Wernicke-Korsakoff syndrome. *J Clin Invest* 46:849, 1967.

Sokol RJ, Butler-Simon N, Neubi JE, et al: Vitamin E deficiency neuropathy in children with fat malabsorption: Studies in cystic fibrosis and chronic cholestasis. *Ann N Y Acad Sci* 570:156, 1989.

Spillane JD: *Nutritional Disorders of the Nervous System*. Baltimore, Lippincott Williams & Wilkins, 1947.

Spivak JL, Jackson DL: Pellagra: An analysis of 18 patients and a review of the literature. *Johns Hopkins Med J* 140:295, 1977.

Strachan H: On a form of multiple neuritis prevalent in the West Indies. *Practitioner* 59:477, 1897.

Strauss MB: Etiology of "alcoholic" polyneuritis. *Am J Med Sci* 189:378, 1935.

Swank RL, Adams RD: Pyridoxine and pantothenic acid deficiency in swine. *J Neuropathol Exp Neurol* 7:274, 1948.

Sydenstricker VP, Schmidt HL Jr, Fulton MC, et al: Treatment of pellagra with nicotinic acid: Observations in 45 cases. *South Med J* 31:1155, 1938.

Terris M (ed): *Goldberger on Pellagra*. Baton Rouge, Louisiana State University Press, 1964.

Thomson AD, Cook CC, Touquet R, et al: The Royal College of Physicians report on alcohol: guidelines for managing Wernicke's encephalopathy in the accident and emergency department. *Alcohol Alcohol* 37:513, 2002.

Torvik A, Lindboe CF, Rogde S: Brain lesions in alcoholics: A neuropathological study with clinical correlations. *J Neurol Neurosurg Psychiatry* 56:233, 1982.

Traber MG, Sokol RJ, Burton GW, et al: Impaired ability of patients with familial isolated vitamin E deficiency to incorporate α-tocopherol into lipoproteins secreted by the liver. *J Clin Invest* 85:397, 1990.

Varnet O, De Seze J, Soto-Ares G, et al: Encéphalopathie de Gayet-Wernicke: Intérêt diagnostique et pronostique de l'Imagerie par Résonance Magnétique. *Rev Neurol* 158:1181, 2002.

Victor M: MR in the diagnosis of Wernicke-Korsakoff syndrome. *AJNR Am J Neuroradiol* 11:895, 1990.

Victor M: Polyneuropathy due to nutritional deficiency and alcoholism, in Dyck PJ, Thomas PK, Lambert EH, Bunge R (eds): *Peripheral Neuropathy*, 2nd ed. Philadelphia, Saunders, 1984, pp 1899–1940.

Victor M: Tobacco amblyopia, cyanide poisoning and vitamin B_{12} deficiency: A critique of current concepts, in Smith JL (ed): *Miami Neuro-ophthalmology Symposium*. Vol 5. Hallandale, FL, Huffman, 1970, pp 33–48.

Victor M, Adams RD: Neuropathology of experimental vitamin B_6 deficiency in monkeys. *Am J Clin Nutr* 4:346, 1956.

Victor M, Adams RD: On the etiology of the alcoholic neurologic diseases with special reference to the role of nutrition. *Am J Clin Nutr* 9:379, 1961.

Victor M, Adams RD, Collins GH: *The Wernicke-Korsakoff Syndrome and Related Neurologic Disorders Due to Alcoholism and Malnutrition*, 2nd ed. Philadelphia, Davis, 1989.

Victor M, Adams RD, Mancall EL: A restricted form of cerebellar degeneration occurring in alcoholic patients. *Arch Neurol* 1:577, 1959.

Victor M, Mancall EL, Dreyfus PM: Deficiency amblyopia in the alcoholic patient: A clinicopathologic study. *Arch Ophthalmol* 64:1, 1960.

Victor M, Yakovlev PI: S.S. Korsakoff's psychic disorder in conjunction with peripheral neuritis: A translation of Korsakoff's original article with brief comments on the author and his contribution to clinical medicine. *Neurology* 5:394, 1955.

Vilter RW, Mueller JF, Glazer HS, et al: The effect of vitamin B_6 deficiency induced by deoxypyridoxine in human beings. *J Lab Clin Med* 42:335, 1953.

Weidauer S, Nichtweiss M, Lanfermann H, et al: Wernicke's encephalopathy: MR findings and clinical presentation. *Eur Radiol* 13:1001, 2003.

Windebank AJ: Polyneuropathy due to nutritional deficiency and alcoholism, in Dyck PJ, Thomas PK, et al (eds): *Peripheral Neuropathy*, 3rd ed. Philadelphia, Saunders, 1993, pp 1310–1321.

Winick M: *Malnutrition and Brain Development*. New York, Oxford University Press, 1976.

Wrenn KD, Murphy F, Slovis CM: A toxicity study of parenteral thiamine hydrochloride. *Ann Emerg Med* 18:867, 1989.

42

Alcohol and Alcoholism

Intemperance in the use of alcohol creates many problems in modern society, the importance of which can be judged by the emphasis it has received in contemporary writings, both literary and scientific. These problems may be divided into three categories: psychologic, medical, and sociologic. The main psychologic issue regards why a person drinks excessively, often with full knowledge that such action will result in physical injury and even death. The medical problem embraces all aspects of alcoholic addiction and habituation as well as the diseases that result from the abuse of alcohol. The sociologic problem encompasses the effects of sustained drinking on the patient's work, family, and community. Some idea of the enormity of these problems can be gleaned from figures supplied by the secretary of Health and Human Services, which indicate that up to 40 percent of medical and surgical patients have alcohol-related problems and that these patients account for 15 percent of all healthcare costs. Several surveys have suggested a rate of alcohol dependence of 3 to 5.5 percent of adults. A minimum of 3 percent of deaths in the United States are attributable to alcohol-related causes. More striking, but not at all surprising, is the fact that alcohol intoxication is responsible for approximately 45 percent of fatal motor vehicle accidents and 22 percent of boating accidents. It requires little imagination to conceive the havoc wrought by alcohol in terms of suicide, accidents, crime, mental and physical disease, and disruption of family life. Finally, the problems engendered by excessive drinking cannot easily be separated from one another.

Etiology of Alcoholism

The cause of alcoholism as an addiction remains as obscure as it is for other forms of dependence and addiction, although environmental, cultural, and genetic factors are clearly implicated. No single personality type has been shown to predict reliably who will become addicted to alcohol. Similarly, no particular aspect of alcohol metabolism has been found to account for the development of addiction, with the possible exception of aldehyde dehydrogenase (see further on). Some persons drink excessively and become alcoholic in response to a profoundly disturbing personal or family problem, but most do not. Alcoholism may develop in response to a depressive illness, more so in women than in men, but far more often depression is a consequence of drinking. Social and cultural influences are undoubtedly important in the genesis of alcoholism as evidenced, for example, by the remarkably high incidence of alcoholism and drinking problems in the American Indian and Eskimo populations and by the disparity in the prevalence of alcoholism, within a single community, among various ethnic groups. However, no ethnic or racial group and no social or economic class are exempt.

The importance of genetic factors in alcoholism has been amply identified. Goodwin and coworkers studied adopted Danish men whose biologic parents were alcoholic and control subjects whose biologic parents were not alcoholic. All of the subjects had been adopted before the age of 5 weeks and had no knowledge of their biologic parentage. Twenty percent of the offspring of biologic alcoholic parents, but only 5 percent of the control subjects, had become alcoholics by the age of 25 to 29 years. A Swedish adoption study (Bohman) and one in the United States (Cadoret et al) corroborate these findings. Family studies disclose a three- to fourfold increased risk for alcoholism in sons and daughters of alcoholics, and twin studies show a twofold higher concordance rate for alcoholism in monozygotic than in dizygotic pairs. Details of these studies can be found in the comprehensive reviews of the genetics of alcoholism by Grove and Cadoret and by Schuckit. The search goes on for a biologic trait, or marker, that would identify those who are genetically vulnerable to the development of alcoholism, but none has proved to be sufficiently practical or sensitive to identify all such persons (Reich).

Pharmacology and Physiology of Alcohol

Ethyl alcohol, or ethanol, is the active ingredient in beer, wine, whiskey, gin, brandy, and other alcoholic beverages. The stronger spirits contain enanthic ethers, which provide flavor but have no important pharmacologic properties. In some preparations, impurities such as amyl alcohol (fusel oil) and acetaldehyde act like alcohol but are more toxic.

Alcohol is metabolized chiefly by oxidation, less than 10 percent being excreted chemically unchanged in the urine, perspiration, and breath. The energy liberated by the oxidation of alcohol (7 kcal/g) can be utilized as completely as that derived from the metabolism of other carbohydrates. However, calories from alcohol are empty of nutrients such as proteins and vitamins and cannot be used in the repair of damaged tissue. All ingested alcohol, except that metabolized by alcohol dehydrogenase in the stomach wall, is carried by the portal system to the liver. Here several enzyme systems independently oxidize alcohol to acetaldehyde. The most important of these, accounting for 80 to 90 percent of ethanol oxidation in vivo, are alcohol dehydrogenase (ADH) and its isoenzymes. This reaction leads to the formation of acetaldehyde and the reduction of nicotinic acid dehydrogenase (NAD) to nicotinamide adenine dinucleotide (NADH). A second pathway of lesser importance involves catalase, which is located in the peroxisomes and mitochondria; a third uses the "microsomal ethanol oxidizing system" (MEOS), located mainly in the microsomes of the endoplasmic reticulum. The details of the process by which acetaldehyde is metabolized are still not settled. Most likely it is converted by aldehyde dehydrogenase to acetate. Acetaldehyde has a number of unique biochemical effects that are not produced by alcohol alone. Persons who flush easily after ingestion of alcohol (Chinese, Japanese, and other Asians) differ from "nonflushers" with respect to the metabolism of acetaldehyde rather than to the metabolism of alcohol. The flushing reaction has been traced to a deficiency of aldehyde dehydrogenase activity (Harada et al). The low rate of alcoholism among Asians is said to be related to the flushing reaction (which is, in effect, a modified alcohol–disulfiram reaction; see further on), but this can hardly be the case, as North American Indians, a group with a high incidence of alcoholism, show the same reaction.

A scale relating various degrees of functional impairment to blood alcohol levels in *nonhabituated* persons was constructed many years ago by Miles. At a blood alcohol level of 30 mg/dL, a mild euphoria was detectable, and at 50 mg/dL, mild incoordination. At 100 mg/dL, ataxia was obvious; at 200 mg/dL, there was confusion and a reduced level of mental activity; at 300 mg/dL, the subjects were stuporous; and a level of 400 mg/dL—accompanied by deep anesthesia—was potentially fatal. These figures are valid provided that the alcohol content in the blood rises steadily over a 2-h period.

For all practical purposes, once the absorption of alcohol has ended and equilibrium has been established with the tissues, *ethanol is oxidized at a constant rate, independent of its concentration in the blood* (about 150 mg alcohol per kilogram of body weight per hour, or about 1 oz of 90-proof whiskey per hour). Actually, slightly more alcohol is metabolized per hour when the initial concentrations are very high, and repeated ingestion of alcohol may facilitate its metabolism, but these increments are of little clinical significance. In contrast, the rate of oxidation of acetaldehyde does depend on its concentration in the tissues. This fact is of importance in connection with the drug disulfiram (Antabuse), which acts by raising the tissue concentration necessary for the metabolism of a certain amount of acetaldehyde per unit of time. The patient taking both disulfiram and alcohol will accumulate an inordinate amount of acetaldehyde, resulting in nausea, vomiting, and hypotension, sometimes so pronounced in degree as to be fatal. Certain other drugs—notably the sulfonylureas, metronidazole, and furazolidone—have effects like those of disulfiram but are less potent.

Alcohol acts directly on neuronal membranes in a manner akin to that of the general anesthetics. These agents, as well as barbiturates and benzodiazepines, are lipid-soluble and are thought to dissolve in the cell membranes (in direct relation to the degree of their lipid solubility). With continued ingestion of alcohol, the neuronal membranes ostensibly "rigidify" and become resistant to the fluidizing effect of alcohol (Chin and Goldstein; Harris et al). It is unlikely, however, that these changes in the physical properties of cell membranes are in themselves sufficient to alter cell function. Probably of equal importance are the effects of alcohol on membrane receptor systems that regulate ion channels, particularly the chloride and calcium channels. One likely site that relates to the acute intoxicating effects of alcohol is a receptor for the inhibitory neurotransmitter gamma-aminobutyric acid (GABA) and its associated chloride-ion channel. Benzodiazepine antagonists appear to block the potentiation by alcohol of GABA-induced chloride flux. Like the GABA-chloride channel, the *N*-methyl-D-aspartate (NMDA) receptors, which transduce signals carried by glutamate (the major excitatory transmitter in the brain), are sensitive to extremely low concentrations of alcohol. There is also evidence that alcohol selectively potentiates serotonin receptor-ion currents, and the activity of this receptor has been implicated in alcohol- and drug-seeking behavior and addiction.

The effect of chronic administration of alcohol is to increase the number of neuronal calcium channels in the cell membrane. Moreover, calcium channel blockers, given during chronic administration, prevent both the increase in neuronal calcium channels and the development of tolerance to alcohol (Dolin and Little). The significance of these findings has been demonstrated by Little and colleagues, who showed that calcium channel blockers, given to chronically intoxicated animals after withdrawal, prevent withdrawal convulsions.

The molecular mechanisms involved in alcohol intoxication and tolerance are obviously more complex than the foregoing remarks would indicate (see reviews by Charness and by Samson and Harris). There is now a vast literature on this subject, much of it contradictory and a unified concept of the role of neurotransmitters and their receptors and modulators in the production of alcohol intoxication and tolerance has yet to emerge. The part played by internal cellular messengers, which have attracted much attention in the field of addiction, is also currently under investigation.

Alcohol Tolerance A scale of blood concentrations such as the one previously described has virtually no value in the chronic alcoholic patient, as it does not take into account the phenomenon of tolerance. It is common knowledge that a habituated person can drink more and show fewer effects than the moderate drinker or abstainer. This phenomenon accounts for the surprisingly large amounts of alcohol that the chronic drinker can consume without showing significant signs of drunkenness. Sober-appearing alcoholics may have blood alcohol levels of 400 to 500 mg/dL. This aspect of tolerance must be considered in judging the significance of a single estimation of the blood alcohol concentration as an index of functional capacity. The mechanisms that underlie tolerance and addiction are just beginning to be understood. There is little evidence that an enhanced rate of alcohol metabolism can adequately account for the degree of tolerance observed in alcoholics. An increase of neuronal adaptation to alcohol is a more likely explanation. Theoretically, the factors that are operative in this adaptation are the increasing resistance of neuronal membranes to the effects of alcohol and an increase in the number of neuronal calcium channels in the cell membrane.

CLINICAL EFFECTS OF ALCOHOL ON THE NERVOUS SYSTEM

Alcohol functions as a central nervous system (CNS) depressant. Some of the early effects of alcohol, such as garrulousness, aggressiveness, excessive activity, and increased electrical excitability of the cerebral cortex—all of them suggestive of cerebral stimulation—are thought to be caused by the inhibition of certain subcortical structures (possibly the high brainstem reticular formation) that ordinarily modulate cerebrocortical activity. Similarly, the initial hyperactivity of tendon reflexes may represent a transitory escape of spinal motor neurons from higher inhibitory centers. With increasing amounts of alcohol, however, the depressant action involves the cortical as well as other brainstem and spinal neurons. All manner of motor functions—whether the simple maintenance of a standing posture, the control of speech and eye movements, or highly organized and complex motor skills—are adversely affected by alcohol. The movements involved in these acts are not only slower than normal but also more inaccurate and random in character and therefore less well adapted to the accomplishment of specific ends.

Alcohol also impairs the efficiency of mental function by interfering with the speed of perception and the ability to persist in mental processing. The learning process is slowed and rendered less effective. Facility in forming associations, whether of words or of figures, and the ability to focus, sustain attention, and concentrate are reduced. Finally, alcohol impairs the faculties of judgment and discrimination and, all in all, the ability to think and reason clearly.

A number of neurologic disorders are characteristically associated with alcoholism. The factor common to all of them, of course, is the abuse of alcohol, but the mechanism by which alcohol produces its effects varies widely from one group of disorders to another and in many cases, the essential problem is one of nutritional deficiency as discussed in the preceding chapter. The classification that follows is based for the most part on known mechanisms.

I. Alcohol intoxication—drunkenness, coma, paradoxical excitement ("pathologic intoxication"), "blackouts"
II. Abstinence or withdrawal syndrome—tremulousness, hallucinosis, seizures, delirium tremens
III. Nutritional diseases of the nervous system accompanying alcoholism (see Chap. 41)
   A. Wernicke-Korsakoff syndrome
   B. Polyneuropathy
   C. Optic neuropathy ("tobacco-alcohol amblyopia")
   D. Pellagra
IV. Diseases of uncertain pathogenesis associated with alcoholism
   A. Cerebellar degeneration
   B. Marchiafava-Bignami disease
   C. Central pontine myelinolysis
   D. "Alcoholic" myopathy and cardiomyopathy
   E. Alcoholic dementia
   F. Cerebral atrophy
V. Fetal alcohol syndrome
VI. Neurologic disorders resulting from cirrhosis and portal–systemic shunts (see Chap. 40)
   A. Hepatic stupor and coma
   B. Chronic hepatocerebral degeneration
VII. Traumatic brain lesions acquired during intoxication—subdural hematoma, cerebral contusion

Alcohol Intoxication and Related Disorders

The usual manifestations of alcohol intoxication are so commonplace that they require little elaboration. They consist of varying degrees of exhilaration and excitement, loss of restraint, irregularity of behavior, loquacity and slurred speech, incoordination of movement and gait, irritability, drowsiness, and, in advanced cases, sleepiness, stupor, and coma. There are several *complicated* types of alcohol intoxication, which are considered below.

As has been indicated, the symptoms of alcoholic intoxication are the result of the depressant action of alcohol on cerebral and spinal neurons. In this respect alcohol acts on nerve cells in a manner akin to the general anesthetics and can cause coma. Unlike the anesthetics, however, the margin between the dose of alcohol that produces surgical anesthesia and that which dangerously depresses respiration is a narrow one, a fact that adds an element of urgency to the diagnosis and treatment of alcoholic coma. One must also be alert to the possibility that other sedative-hypnotic drugs may have potentiated the depressant effects of alcohol. Another treacherous situation is that of traumatic brain injury that is complicated by intoxication, a circumstance that is prone to misinterpretation because of uncertainty as to the main cause of stupor or coma.

Pathologic Intoxication

Despite what has been said earlier, on rare occasions, alcohol has an exclusively excitatory rather than a sedative effect. This reaction has been referred to in the past as *pathologic*, or *complicated*, *intoxication* and as *acute alcoholic paranoid state*. Because all forms of intoxication are pathologic, *atypical intoxication* or *idiosyncratic alcohol intoxication* are more appropriate designations. Nevertheless, the term *pathologic intoxication* is still widely used. The boundaries of this syndrome have never been clearly drawn. In the past, variant forms of delirium tremens and epileptic phenomena, as well as psychopathic and criminal behavior, were indiscriminately included. Now the term is generally used to designate an outburst of blind fury with assaultive and destructive behavior. Often the patient is subdued only with difficulty. The attack terminates with deep sleep, which occurs spontaneously or in response to parenteral sedation; on awakening, the patient has no memory of the episode. Lesser degrees are also known wherein the patient, after several drinks, repeatedly commits gross social indiscretions. Allegedly this reaction may follow the ingestion of a small amount of alcohol, but in some of the patients we have observed the amount has often been substantial. Unlike the usual forms of alcohol intoxication and withdrawal, the atypical form has not been produced in experimental subjects, and the diagnosis depends upon the aforementioned arbitrary criteria.

Pathologic intoxication has been ascribed to many factors, but there are no meaningful data to support any of them. However, an analogy may be drawn between pathologic intoxication and the paradoxical reaction that occasionally follows the administration of barbiturates or other sedative drugs. The few patients we have seen, mostly young men of college age or slightly older, have been docile and seemingly well adjusted when not drinking. Usually, they have avoided alcohol after a first episode of this sort, but there have been exceptions.

The main disorders to be distinguished from pathologic intoxication are temporal lobe seizures that occasionally take the form of outbursts of rage and violence and the explosive episodes that characterize the behavior of certain sociopaths. The diagnosis in these cases may be difficult and depends on eliciting the other manifestations of temporal lobe epilepsy or sociopathy. *Pathologic intoxication* may require the use of restraints and the parenteral administration of diazepam (5 to 10 mg) or haloperidol (2 to 5 mg), repeated once after 30 to 40 min if necessary.

Alcoholic "Blackouts"

In the language of the alcoholic, the term *blackout* refers to an interval of time, during a period of severe intoxication, for which the patient later has no memory—even though the state of consciousness, as observed by others, was not grossly altered during that interval. However, a systematic assessment of mental function during the amnesic period has usually not been made. A few observations indicate that it is short-term (retentive) memory rather than immediate or long-term memory that is impaired; this feature and the subsequent amnesia for the episode are vaguely reminiscent of the disorder known as *transient global amnesia* (see Chap. 21) but without the incessant repetitive questioning and competence in nonmemory mental activities that characterize the latter.

Blackouts may occur at any time in the course of alcoholism, even during the first drinking experience, and they certainly have happened in persons who never became alcoholic. The salient facts are that there is a degree of intoxication that interferes with the registration of events and the formation of memories during the period of intoxication and that the amount of alcohol consumed in moderate social drinking will rarely produce this effect.

Treatment of Severe Alcohol Intoxication

Coma caused by alcohol intoxication represents a medical emergency. The main objective of treatment is to prevent respiratory depression and its complications as described in Chap. 17. One would like to lower the blood alcohol level as rapidly as possible. The previously favored administration of fructose or of insulin and glucose for this purpose is now known to be of little value. Analeptic drugs such as amphetamine and various mixtures of caffeine and picrotoxin are antagonistic to alcohol only insofar as they are overall nervous system excitants but they do not hasten the oxidation of alcohol and are not clinically useful. The use of hemodialysis should be considered in comatose patients with extremely high blood alcohol concentrations (>500 mg/dL), particularly if accompanied by acidosis, and in those who have concurrently ingested methanol or ethylene glycol or some other dialyzable drug.

Methyl, Amyl, and Isopropyl Alcohols and Ethylene Glycol

Poisoning with alcohols other than ethyl alcohol is a rare but catastrophic occurrence. *Amyl alcohol* (fusel oil) and *isopropyl alcohol* are used as industrial solvents and in the manufacture of varnishes, lacquers, and pharmaceuticals; in addition, isopropyl alcohol is readily available as a rubbing alcohol. Intoxication may follow the ingestion of these alcohols or inhalation of their vapors. The effects of both are much like those of ethyl alcohol, but much more toxic. They also have in common the generation of acidosis, usually with an anion gap and if a sample of serums obtained soon after the ingestion, an osmolar gap that represents the molecules of the circulating alcohol.

Methyl alcohol (methanol, wood alcohol) is a component of antifreeze and many combustibles and is used in the manufacture of formaldehyde, as an industrial solvent, and as an adulterant of alcoholic beverages, the latter being the most common source of methyl alcohol intoxication. The oxidation of methyl alcohol to formaldehyde and formic acid proceeds relatively slowly; thus, signs of intoxication do not appear for several hours or may be delayed for a day or longer. Many of the toxic effects are like those of ethyl alcohol, but in addition severe methyl alcohol poisoning may produce serious degrees of acidosis (with an anion gap). The characteristic features of this intoxication, however, are damage to retinal ganglion cells—giving rise to scotomata and varying degrees of blindness, dilated unreactive pupils, and retinal edema—and bilateral degeneration of the putamens, readily visible on CT scans. Survivors may be left blind or, less often, with putamenal necrosis and dystonia or Parkinson disease (McLean et al). The most important aspect of treatment is the intravenous administration of large amounts of sodium bicarbonate to reverse acidosis. Hemodialysis and 4-methylpyrazole (see later) may be useful adjuncts because of the slow rate of oxidation of methanol.

Ethylene glycol, an aliphatic alcohol, is a commonly used industrial solvent and the major constituent of antifreeze. In the latter form, it is sometimes consumed by skid-row alcoholics (5,000 cases of poisoning annually in the United States) and in suicide attempts with disastrous results. At first the patient merely appears drunk, but after a period of 4 to 12 h, hyperventilation and severe metabolic acidosis develop, followed by confusion, convulsions, coma, and renal failure and death in rapid succession. Cerebrospinal fluid lymphocytosis is a common but not invariable feature. The metabolic acidosis is a result of the conversion of ethylene glycol by alcohol dehydrogenase into glycolic acid, thus *producing an anion gap* that reflects the presence of this additional substance in the blood. (The anion gap has been defined in different ways, but the most convenient is the difference between the positive ion Na^+ and the sum of negative ions, Cl^- plus HCO_3^- [venous CO_2 is used for the latter]; a value greater than 12 is considered a gap.) The cause of the renal toxicity is less clear—probably it is a result of the formation of oxalate from glycolate and the deposition of oxalate crystals in renal tubules. (One of our recent patients had hippurate crystals in the urine, a finding that is more characteristic of toluene ingestions.) These crystals appear in the urine and sometimes in the cerebrospinal fluid (CSF) and aid in diagnosis.

Treatment of Nonethanol Alcohol Intoxication

The treatment of ethylene glycol poisoning has, until relatively recently, consisted of hemodialysis and the intravenous infusion of sodium bicarbonate and ethanol, the latter serving as a competitive substrate for alcohol dehydrogenase. However, the use of ethanol in this regimen is problematic. Baud and colleagues, and more recently Brent and colleagues and Jacobsen, have advocated the use of intravenous 4-methylpyrazole (fomepizole), which is a far more effective inhibitor of alcohol dehydrogenase than is alcohol. They recommend this form of treatment for methanol poisoning as well. Information from the American Academy of Toxicology is cited in a review of the use of fomepizole by Brent, which is recommended to the interested reader. Generally, for either methanol of ethylene glycol, a plasma level of the alcohol above 20 mg/dL, or above 10 mg/dL when combined with an osmolal gap over 10 is considered appropriate to institute the drug. In the case of ethylene glycol, oxaluria and acidosis are additional factors that may precipitate treatment. Dialysis remains an essential therapy if cerebral and renal damage is not too advanced.

Some patients who recover from the acute renal and metabolic effects are left with multiple cranial nerve defects, particularly of the seventh and eighth nerves. The latter abnormalities develop 6 to 18 days after the ingestion of ethylene glycol and have been attributed to the deposition of oxalate crystals along the subarachnoid portions of the affected nerves (Spillane et al).

The Alcohol Abstinence, or Withdrawal, Syndrome

This is the well-known symptom complex of tremulousness, hallucinations, seizures, confusion, and psychomotor and autonomic overactivity. Although a sustained period of chronic inebriation is the most obvious factor in the causation of these symptoms, they become manifest

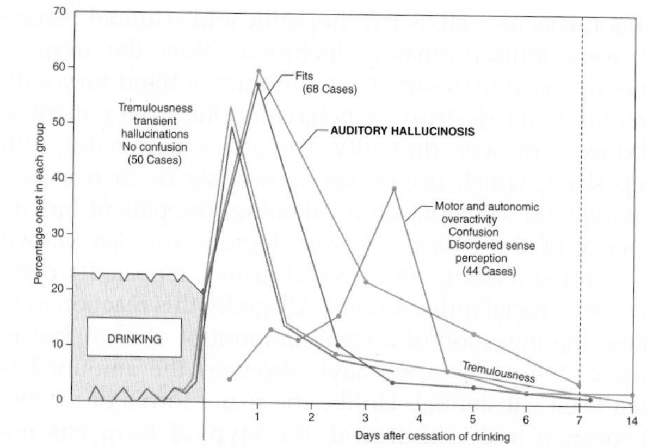

Figure 42-1. Relation of acute neurologic disturbances to cessation of drinking. The shaded drinking period is greatly foreshortened and not intended to be quantitative. The periodic notching in the baseline represents the tremulousness, nausea, and so on that occur following a night's sleep. The time relations of the various groups of symptoms to withdrawal are explained in the text. (Adapted from Victor M, Adams RD: The effect of alcohol on the nervous system. *Res Publ Assoc Res Nerv Ment Dis* 32:526, 1953, by permission.)

only after a *period of relative or absolute abstinence* from alcohol—hence the designation *abstinence*, or *withdrawal*, syndrome. Figure 42-1 illustrates this concept. Each of the major manifestations of the withdrawal syndrome may occur in more or less pure form and are so described below, but usually they occur in combination. Major withdrawal symptoms are observed mainly in the binge, or periodic, drinker, although the steady drinker is not immune if for some reason he stops drinking, such as during a hospital admission for surgery or a medical illness. The full syndrome, depicted further on, is called *delirium tremens*.

Tremulousness

The most common single manifestation of the abstinence syndrome is tremulousness, often referred to as "the shakes" or "the jitters," combined with general irritability and gastrointestinal symptoms, particularly nausea and vomiting. These symptoms first appear after several days of drinking, usually in the morning after a night's abstinence. The patient "quiets his nerves" with a few drinks and is then able to drink for the rest of the day without undue distress. The symptoms return on successive mornings with increasing severity. The symptoms then become augmented, reaching their peak intensity 24 to 36 h after the complete cessation of drinking. *Generalized tremor* is the most obvious feature. It is of fast frequency (6 to 8 Hz), slightly irregular, and variable in severity, tending to diminish when the patient is in quiet surroundings and to increase with motor activity or emotional stress. The tremor may be so violent that the patient cannot stand without help, speak clearly, or eat without assistance. Sometimes there is little objective evidence of tremor, and the patient complains only of being "shaky inside."

Within a few days, flushed facies, anorexia, tachycardia, and tremor characteristic of the mild withdrawal syndrome subside to a large extent, but overalertness, tendency to startle easily, and jerkiness of movement may persist for a week or longer. Feelings of uneasiness may not leave the patient completely for 10 to 14 days. According to Porjesz and Begleiter, certain electrophysiologic abnormalities (diminished amplitudes of sensory evoked potentials and prolonged latencies and conduction velocities of auditory brainstem potentials) remain altered long after the clinical abnormalities have subsided.

Hallucinations

Symptoms of disordered perception occur in about one-quarter of withdrawing hospitalized tremulous patients. The patient may complain of "bad dreams"—nightmarish episodes associated with disturbed sleep—which he finds difficult to separate from real experience. Sounds and shadows may be misinterpreted, or familiar objects may be distorted and assume unreal forms (illusions). There may also be more overt hallucinations, which are purely visual in type, mixed visual and auditory, tactile, or olfactory, in this order of frequency. There is little evidence to support the popular belief that certain visual hallucinations (bugs, pink elephants) are specific to alcoholism. Actually, the hallucinations comprise the full range of visual experience. They are more often animate than inanimate; persons or animals may appear singly or in panoramas, shrunken or enlarged, natural and pleasant, or distorted, hideous, and frightening. The hallucinosis may be an isolated phenomenon lasting for a few hours, and it may later be attended by other withdrawal signs.

Acute and Chronic Auditory Hallucinosis

A special type of alcoholic psychosis consisting of a more or less pure auditory hallucinosis has been recognized for many years. Kraepelin referred to it as the "hallucinatory insanity of drunkards," or "alcoholic mania." A report of 75 such cases was made by Victor and Hope. The central feature of the illness, in the beginning, is the occurrence of auditory hallucinations despite an otherwise clear sensorium during the withdrawal period; i.e., the patients are not disoriented or obtunded, and they have an intact memory. The hallucinations may take the form of unstructured sounds such as buzzing, ringing, gunshots, or clicking (the elementary hallucinations of Bleuler), or they may have a musical quality, like a low-pitched hum or chant. The most common hallucinations, however, are human voices. When the voices can be identified, they are often attributed to the patient's family, friends, or neighbors—rarely to God, radio, or television. The voices may be addressed directly to the patient, but more frequently, they discuss him in the third person. In the majority of cases, the voices are maligning, reproachful, or threatening in nature and are disturbing to the patient; a significant proportion, however, are not unpleasant and leave the patient undisturbed. To the patient, the voices are clearly audible and intensely real, and they tend to be exteriorized; i.e., they come from behind a radiator or door, from the corridor, or through a wall, window, or floor. Another feature of auditory hallucinosis is that the patient's response is more or less understandable in light of the hallucinatory content. The patient may call on the police for protection or erect a barricade against invaders; he may even attempt suicide to avoid what the voices threaten. The hallucinations are most prominent during the night, and their duration varies greatly: they may be momentary, or they may recur intermittently for days on end and, in exceptional instances, for weeks or months.

While hallucinating, most patients have no appreciation of the unreality of their hallucinations. With improvement, the patient begins to question the inauthenticity and may be reluctant to talk about them and may even question his own sanity. Full recovery is characterized by the realization that the voices were imaginary and by the ability to recall, sometimes with remarkable clarity, some of the abnormal thought content of the psychotic episode.

A unique feature of this alcoholic psychosis is its evolution, in a small proportion of the patients, to a state of *chronic auditory hallucinosis*. The chronic disorder begins like the acute one, but after a short period, perhaps a week or two, the symptomatology begins to change. The patient becomes quiet and resigned, even though the hallucinations remain threatening and derogatory. Ideas of reference and influence and other poorly systematized paranoid delusions become prominent. At this stage the illness may be mistaken for paranoid schizophrenia and indeed was so identified by Bleuler. There are, however, important differences between the two disorders: the alcoholic illness develops in close relation to a drinking bout and the past history rarely reveals schizoid personality traits. Moreover, alcoholic patients with hallucinosis are not distinguished by a high incidence of schizophrenia within their families (Schuckit and Winokur; Scott), and a large number of such patients, whom our colleagues Victor and Adams evaluated long after their acute attacks, did not show signs of schizophrenia. There is some evidence that repeated attacks of acute auditory hallucinosis render the patient more susceptible to the chronic state.

Withdrawal Seizures ("Rum Fits")

In the setting of alcohol withdrawal either as relative or absolute abstinence following a period of chronic inebriation, convulsive seizures are common. More than 90 percent of withdrawal seizures occur during the 7- to 48-h period following the cessation of drinking, with a peak incidence between 13 and 24 h. During the period of seizure activity, the electroencephalogram (EEG) is usually abnormal, but it reverts to normal in a matter of days, even though the patient may go on to develop delirium tremens. During the period of seizure activity and for days afterwards, the patient is unusually sensitive to stroboscopic stimulation; almost half the patients respond with generalized myoclonus or a convulsive seizure (photoparoxysmal response).

Seizures occurring in the abstinence period have a number of other distinctive features. There may be only a single seizure, but in the majority of cases the seizures occur in bursts of 2 to 6 over a day, occasionally even more; only 2 percent of patients studied by Victor (1968) developed status epilepticus. The seizures are grand mal in type, i.e., generalized, tonic-clonic convulsions with loss of consciousness. Focal seizures should always suggest the presence of a focal brain lesion (most often traumatic) in addition to the effects of alcohol. Twenty-eight percent of Victor's patients with generalized withdrawal seizures went on to develop delirium tremens (the percentage has been less in other series); almost invariably, the seizures preceded the delirium. The postictal confusional state may blend imperceptibly with the onset of the delirium, or the postictal state may have cleared over several hours or even a day or longer before the delirium sets in. Seizures of this type typically occur in a patient whose drinking history has extended over a period of many years and must be distinguished from other forms of seizures that have their onset in adult life. The term *rum fits*, or *whiskey fits*—the names sometimes used by alcoholics—is reserved for seizures with the attributes described here. This serves to distinguish them from seizures that occur in the interdrinking period, long after withdrawal has been accomplished.

It is important to note that the common idiopathic or posttraumatic forms of epilepsy are also influenced by alcohol. In these types of epilepsy, a seizure or seizures may be precipitated by only a short period of drinking (e.g., a weekend, or even one evening of heavy social drinking); perhaps unsurprisingly in these circumstances, the seizures occur not when the patient is intoxicated but usually the morning after, in the "sobering-up" period. Except for the transient dysrhythmia in the withdrawal period, the incidence of EEG abnormalities in patients who have had rum fits is no greater than in normal persons, in sharp contrast to the EEGs of nonalcoholic patients with recurrent seizures.

Treatment and Prevention of Withdrawal Seizures

Most patients during withdrawal do not require antiepileptic drugs, as the entire episode of seizure activity—whether a single seizure or a brief flurry of seizures—may have terminated before the patient is brought to medical attention. The parenteral administration of diazepam or sodium phenobarbital early in the withdrawal period does, however, prevent withdrawal fits in patients with a previous history of this disorder, as well as in those who might be expected to develop seizures on withdrawal of alcohol. This approach has been supported by the observations of D'Onofrio and colleagues that intravenous lorazepam (2 mg in 2 mL of normal saline) was highly effective in preventing *recurrent seizures* after a first seizure in the same withdrawal period. Only 3 of 100 patients so treated had a second seizure within 48 h, compared to 21 of 86 untreated patients. The long-term administration of anticonvulsants is neither necessary nor practical: if such patients remain abstinent, they will be free of seizures; if they resume drinking, they usually abandon their medications. Furthermore, it is not certain that continued administration of anticonvulsants dependably prevents abstinence seizures. The rare instances of status epilepticus should be managed like status of any other type (see Chap. 16). In alcoholics with a history of idiopathic or posttraumatic epilepsy, the goal of treatment should be abstinence from alcohol, because of the tendency of even short periods of drinking to precipitate seizures. Such patients need to be maintained on anticonvulsant drugs.

Delirium Tremens and Related Disorders

This is the most dramatic and grave of all the acute alcoholic illnesses. It is characterized by profound confusion, delusions, vivid hallucinations, tremor, agitation, and sleeplessness, as well as by the signs of increased autonomic nervous system activity—i.e., dilated pupils, fever, tachycardia, and profuse perspiration. The clinical features of delirium are presented in detail in Chap. 20 as they relate to delirium tremens (DTs) and to other illnesses that simulate it.

Delirium tremens develops in one of several settings. The patient, an excessive and steady drinker for many years, may have been admitted to the hospital for an unrelated illness, accident, or operation and, after 2 to 4 days, occasionally even later, becomes delirious. Or, following a prolonged drinking binge, the patient may have experienced several days of tremulousness and hallucinosis or one or more seizures and may even be recovering from these symptoms when delirium tremens develops, rather abruptly as a rule.

As to the frequency of delirium tremens, Foy and Kay reported an incidence of 0.65 percent of all patients admitted for other reasons to a large general hospital. Among 200 consecutive alcoholics admitted to a city hospital, Ferguson and colleagues reported that 24 percent developed delirium tremens; of these, 8 percent died—figures that are considerably higher than those recorded in our hospitals (see below). Of course, the reported incidence of delirium tremens will vary greatly, depending on the population served by a particular hospital.

In the majority of cases, delirium tremens is benign and short-lived, ending as abruptly as it begins. Consumed by relentless activity and wakefulness for several days, the patient falls into a deep sleep and then awakens lucid, quiet, and exhausted, with virtually no memory of the events of the delirious period. Less commonly, the delirious state subsides gradually with intermittent episodes of recurrence. In either event, when delirium tremens occurs as a single episode, the duration is 72 h or less in more than 80 percent of cases. Less frequently still, there may be one or more relapses, several episodes of delirium of varying severity being separated by intervals of relative lucidity—the entire process lasting for several days or occasionally for as long as 4 to 5 weeks.

In the past, approximately 15 percent of cases of delirium tremens ended fatally, but the figure now is closer to 5 percent. In many of the fatal cases there is an associated infectious illness or injury, but in others, no complicating illness is discernible. Many of the patients die in a state of hyperthermia; in some, death comes so suddenly that the nature of the terminal events cannot be determined. Reports of series of cases with a negligible mortality rate in delirium tremens can usually be traced to a failure to distinguish between delirium tremens and the minor forms of the withdrawal syndrome, which are far more common and practically never fatal.

We make note here of our experience with delirium following the withdrawal of barbiturates (Romero et al), which is almost identical to the DTs, including the abrupt cessation of symptoms, as discussed in the section on "Barbiturate Abstinence, or Withdrawal, Syndrome" in Chap. 43.

There are also alcohol withdrawal states, closely related to delirium tremens and about as frequent, in which one facet of the delirium tremens complex assumes prominence, to the virtual exclusion of the other symptoms. The patient may simply exhibit a transient state of quiet confusion, agitation, or peculiar behavior lasting several days or weeks. Or there may be a vivid hallucinatory–delusional state and abnormal behavior consistent with the patient's false beliefs. Unlike typical delirium tremens, the atypical states usually present as a single circumscribed episode without recurrences, are only rarely preceded by seizures, and do not end fatally.

Pathologic examination is singularly unrevealing in patients with delirium tremens. Edema and brain swelling have been absent in the authors' pathologic material except when shock or hypoxia had occurred terminally. There have been no significant light microscopic changes in the brain, which is what one would expect in a disease that is essentially reversible. The EEG findings have been discussed in relation to withdrawal seizures.

Pathogenesis of the Tremulous-Hallucinatory-Delirious Disorders

Prior to 1950, it was the common belief that these symptoms represented the most severe forms of alcohol intoxication—an idea that fails to satisfy the simplest clinical logic. The symptoms of toxicity—consisting of slurred speech, uninhibited behavior, staggering gait, stupor, and coma—are in themselves distinctive and, in a sense, the opposite of the symptom complex of tremor, fits, and delirium. It is evident, from observations in both humans and experimental animals, that the most important and the one obligate factor in the genesis of delirium tremens and related disorders is the withdrawal of alcohol following a period of sustained chronic intoxication. Furthermore, the emergence of withdrawal symptoms depends on a rapid *decline* in the blood alcohol level from a previously higher level and not necessarily upon the complete disappearance of alcohol from the blood.

The mechanisms by which the withdrawal of alcohol produces symptoms are incompletely understood. In all but the mildest cases, the early phase of alcohol withdrawal is attended by a drop in serum magnesium concentration and a rise in arterial pH—the latter on the basis of respiratory alkalosis (Wolfe and Victor). Possibly the compounded effect of these two factors, both of which are associated with hyperexcitability of the nervous system, is responsible in part for seizures and for other symptoms that characterize the early phase of withdrawal. However, these factors alone are not explanatory. The molecular mechanisms that are thought to be operative in the genesis of alcohol tolerance and withdrawal have been mentioned earlier. The gabaergic system has been most strongly implicated, in part because the receptors for this inhibitory transmitter are downregulated by chronic alcohol use, but the situation is not nearly so simple, insofar as the excitatory glutaminergic system is also inhibited by alcohol.

Laboratory Findings Rarely, blood glucose is seriously depressed in the alcohol withdrawal states. Ketoacidosis with normal blood glucose is another infrequent finding. Disturbances of electrolytes are of varying frequency and significance. Serum sodium levels are altered infrequently and are more often increased than decreased. The same is true for chloride and phosphate. Serum calcium and potassium are lowered in about one-quarter of patients. Most patients show some degree of hypomagnesemia, low Pco_2, and high arterial pH—abnormalities that are probably important in the pathogenesis of withdrawal symptoms (see later). Abnormalities of the CSF occur unpredictably (it is usually normal), as do changes on CT scanning or MRI; they may indicate the presence of some medical or surgical complication. Enlargement of the third and lateral ventricles is a common finding (see later). The MRI is normal unless there is an incipient Wernicke disease, in which case lesions in the periaqueductal region and subthalami may be evident, as described in the previous chapter.

Treatment of Delirium Tremens and Minor Withdrawal Symptoms (See Chap. 20)

The treatment of delirium tremens begins with a search for associated injuries (particularly head injury with cerebral lacerations or subdural hematoma), infections (pneumonia or meningitis), pancreatitis, and liver disease. Because of the frequency and seriousness of these complications, chest films and a CT scan should be obtained in most instances, and lumbar puncture should be performed if there is suspicion of meningitis. In severe forms of delirium tremens, the temperature, pulse, and blood pressure should be measured at frequent intervals in anticipation of peripheral circulatory collapse and hyperthermia, which, added to the effects of injury and infection, are the usual causes of death in this disease. In the case of hypotension, one must act quickly, using intravenous fluids and, if called for, vasopressor drugs. The occurrence of hyperthermia demands the use of a cooling mattress or evaporative cooling in addition to specific treatment for any infection that may be present.

An additional important element in treatment is the correction of fluid and electrolyte imbalance, particularly hypokalemia and severe hypomagnesemia. Severe degrees of agitation and perspiration may require the administration of up to 5 L of fluid daily, of which at least 1,500 to 2,000 mL should be normal saline. The specific electrolytes and the amounts that must be administered are governed by the laboratory values for these electrolytes. If the serum sodium is extremely low, one must be cautious in raising the level lest a central pontine myelinolysis be induced (see Chap. 40). In the rare case of hypoglycemia, the administration of glucose is an urgent matter. Patients who present with severe alcoholic ketoacidosis and normal or only slightly elevated blood glucose concentrations usually recover promptly, without the use of insulin.

It must be emphasized, as it was in Chap. 41, that a *special danger attends the use of glucose solutions in alcoholic patients*. The administration of intravenous glucose may serve to consume the last available reserves of thiamine and precipitate Wernicke disease. Typically, these patients have subsisted on a diet disproportionately high in carbohydrate (in addition to alcohol, which is metabolized entirely as carbohydrate) and low in thiamine, and their body stores of B vitamins may have been further reduced by gastroenteritis and diarrhea. For this reason it is good practice to add B vitamins, specifically thiamine (which may also be supplemented by intramuscular injection), in all cases requiring parenterally administered glucose—even though the alcoholic disorder under treatment, e.g., delirium tremens, is not primarily caused by vitamin deficiency.

With respect to the use of medications to treat the withdrawal syndromes, it is important to distinguish between mild symptoms, which are essentially benign and responsive to practically any sedative drug, and full-blown delirium tremens. There is no certain way to predict whether a patient with the early signs of withdrawal will progress to delirium tremens. In the latter state, the object of therapy is to blunt the psychomotor and autonomic overactivity, prevent exhaustion, and facilitate the administration of parenteral fluid and nursing care; one should not attempt to suppress agitation "at all costs," as doing so requires an amount of drug that might depress respiration.

A wide variety of drugs are effective in controlling withdrawal symptoms. The more popular ones have been chlordiazepoxide (Librium), diazepam (Valium), and the ancillary medications, clonidine and beta-adrenergic blockers, and a number of both older and newer anticonvulsant drugs such as gabapentin, which may reduce the requirement for sedative drugs. There is little to choose among the primary sedative drugs in respect to their therapeutic efficacy. More importantly, there are few data to indicate that any one of them can prevent hallucinosis or delirium tremens, or shorten the duration, or alter the mortality rate of the latter disorder (Kaim et al). A contemporary summary of the medication management of withdrawal has been given by Kosten and O'Connor. In general, phenothiazine drugs should be avoided because they may reduce the threshold to seizures. Probably, the use of any of the diazepine medications is as effective as a single dose of lorazepam in prophylactically suppressing seizures (see earlier discussion).

If parenteral medication is necessary, we still prefer 10 mg of diazepam or chlordiazepoxide given intravenously and repeated once or twice at 20- to 30-min intervals until the patient is calm but awake; we also favor midazolam in closely controlled circumstances when hyperactivity and hallucinosis are extreme. Beta-adrenergic–blocking agents, such as propranolol, labetalol, and atenolol, are helpful in reducing heart rate, blood pressure, and the tremor to some extent. Lofexidine, an $alpha_2$-agonist that blocks autonomic outflow centrally, and clonidine are similarly effective in reducing the severity of most of the withdrawal symptoms, but they are not recommended as the sole treatments. Corticosteroids have no place in the treatment of the withdrawal syndrome and more potent agents such as propofol are usually not necessary.

Wernicke-Korsakoff Syndrome and Alcoholic–Nutritional Diseases

(See Chap. 41)

Alcoholism provides the ideal setting for the development of nutritional diseases of the nervous system. Although only a small proportion of alcoholics develop nutritional diseases, the overall number of these diseases is substantial because of the frequency of alcoholism. The importance of the alcohol-induced deficiency diseases relates to the fact that they are preventable and, if neglected, may lead to permanent disability. These illnesses, particularly the Wernicke-Korsakoff syndrome, are discussed fully in Chap. 41. Contrary to popular opinion with regard to the prevention of Wernicke disease, the content of B vitamins in American beer and other liquors is so low as to have little nutritional value (Davidson).

Disorders of Uncertain Pathogenesis Associated With Alcoholism

Also discussed in Chap. 41 are *alcoholic cerebellar degeneration* and *Marchiafava-Bignami disease*. The former is almost certainly of nutritional origin; in the latter a nutritional–metabolic etiology seems likely but has not been established. Central pontine myelinolysis, although frequently observed in alcoholics, is more appropriately considered with the acquired metabolic disorders, usually the too rapid correction of hyponatremia (see Chap. 40). Certain disorders of skeletal and cardiac muscle associated with alcoholism (*acute alcoholic myopathy* and *cardiomyopathy*) are described in Chap. 51, with the myopathies caused by drugs and toxins. There remain to be discussed several diverse disorders that have been attributed to alcoholism but whose causal relationship to alcohol abuse, nutritional deficiency, or some other relevant factor is not clear.

Alcoholic Dementia and Cerebral Atrophy

The term *alcoholic dementia* is used widely and often indiscriminately to designate a presumably distinctive form of dementia that is attributable to the chronic, direct effects of alcohol on the brain. Unfortunately, a syndrome subsumed under the title of *alcoholic dementia* and its many synonyms that appear in the older literature (*alcoholic deteriorated state, chronic alcoholic psychosis, chronic or organic brain syndrome due to alcohol*) has never been delineated satisfactorily, either clinically or pathologically. In the *Comprehensive Textbook of Psychiatry*, it has been defined as "a gradual disintegration of personality structure, with emotional lability, loss of control, and dementia" (Sadock and Sadock). Purported examples of this state show a remarkably diverse group of symptoms, including jealousy and suspiciousness; coarsening of moral fiber and other personality and behavioral disorders; deterioration of work performance, personal care, and living habits; and disorientation, impaired judgment, and defects of intellectual function, particularly of memory.

There have been many attempts to redefine alcoholic dementia. Cutting, as well as Lishman, expressed the view that the term *Korsakoff psychosis* should be limited to patients with a fairly pure disorder of memory of acute onset and that patients with more global symptoms of intellectual deterioration, of gradual evolution, be considered to have alcoholic dementia. These are rather weak diagnostic criteria. As pointed out in Chap. 41, *Korsakoff psychosis* may have an insidious onset and gradual progression, and patients with this disorder, in addition to an amnesic defect, characteristically show disturbances of cognitive functions that depend little or not at all on memory. More importantly, in none of the patients designated by these authors as having alcoholic dementia was there a neuropathologic examination, without which the clinical assessment must remain arbitrary and imprecise.

The pathologic changes that purportedly underlie primary alcoholic dementia are even less precisely defined than the clinical syndrome. Courville, whose writings have been quoted most frequently in this respect, described a series of cerebral cortical changes that he attributed to the toxic effects of alcohol. Some of them turn out on close inspection to be quite nonspecific, reflecting nothing more than the effects of aging or the insignificant artifacts of tissue fixation and staining. Harper and Blumbergs, and subsequently Harper and Kril, reported that the mean brain weight is decreased in alcoholics and the pericerebral space is increased in volume—findings that do no more than confirm the brain shrinkage that is demonstrable by CT scans in many alcoholics and is to some extent reversible with sustained abstinence (see later).

The majority of cases that come to autopsy with the label of *alcoholic dementia* prove simply to have the lesions of the Wernicke-Korsakoff syndrome. Traumatic lesions of varying degrees of severity are commonly added. Other cases show the lesions of Marchiafava-Bignami disease, hepatic encephalopathy, subdural hematomas, or an unrelated communicating hydrocephalus, Alzheimer disease, ischemic necrosis, or some other disease quite unrelated to alcoholism. Practically always in our material, the clinical state can be accounted for by one or a combination of these disease processes and there has been no need to invoke a hypothetical toxic effect of alcohol on the brain. This has also been the experience of Torvik and associates; with a few exceptions, such as coincidental Alzheimer disease, all their cases that had been diagnosed as having alcoholic dementia turned out, on neuropathologic examination, to have the chronic lesions of Wernicke-Korsakoff disease.

In brief, the most serious flaw in the concept of a primary alcoholic dementia is that it lacks a distinctive, well-defined pathology. Until such time as the morphologic basis is established, its status must remain ambiguous. A more detailed discussion of this subject and of so-called alcoholic cerebral atrophy (see later) can be found in the review by Victor (1994).

Alcoholic cerebral atrophy likewise does not constitute a well-defined entity. The concept was the product originally of pneumoencephalographic studies. Relatively young alcoholics, some with and some without symptoms of cerebral disease were often found to have enlarged cerebral ventricles and widened sulci, mainly of the frontal lobes (see, e.g., reports of Brewer and Perrett and of Haug). Similar findings have been reported in chronic alcoholics examined by CT scanning and MRI (see review by Carlen et al). The clinical correlates of these radiologic findings are unclear. Wilkinson demonstrated that in clinically normal alcoholics, the radiologic measures of "brain atrophy" were age related; once the age factor was removed, the CT findings in these subjects did not differ significantly from those in nonalcoholic controls. However, from the studies by Harper and colleagues (1982 and 1985) it may indeed be the case that chronic exposure to alcohol induces cerebral atrophy, but this requires confirmation. The idea of alcoholic atrophy is open to criticism mainly on the grounds that dilated ventricles have in fact been reversible to a considerable extent when abstinence is maintained (Carlen et al; Lishman; Zipursky et al; Schroth et al).

Fetal Alcohol Syndrome

That parental alcoholism may have an adverse effect on the offspring has been a recurrent theme in medical writings. Probably the first allusion to such a relationship was that of Sullivan in 1899, who reported that the mortality among the children of drunken mothers was more than two times greater than that among children of nondrinking women of "similar stock." This increased mortality was attributed by Sullivan and later by Haggard and Jellinek to postnatal influences such as poor nutrition and a chaotic home environment, rather than to the intrauterine effects of alcohol. The idea that maternal alcoholism could damage the fetus was generally rejected and relegated to the category of superstitions about alcoholism or the claims of temperance ideologues.

In the late 1960s, the effects of alcohol abuse on the fetus were rediscovered, so to speak. Lemoine and associates in France, and then Ulleland and Jones and Smith in the United States, described a distinctive pattern of abnormalities in infants born of severely alcoholic mothers. They stated that the affected infants are small in length in comparison to weight, and most of them fall below the third percentile for head circumference. They are distinguished also by the presence of short palpebral fissures (shortened distance between inner and outer canthi) and epicanthal folds; maxillary hypoplasia, micrognathia, indistinct philtrum, and thin upper lip; and longitudinally oriented palmar creases, flexion deformities of the fingers, and a limited range of motion of other joints. Minor anomalies (usually spontaneously closing cardiac septal defects), anomalous external genitalia, and cleft lip and palate are much more frequent than in the general population. All of these features have similarities to the syndrome described in a proportion of infants whose mothers had taken anticonvulsants during pregnancy, the "fetal anticonvulsant syndrome" (see Chap. 16). The newborn infants suck and sleep poorly, and many of them are irritable, restless, hyperactive, and tremulous; these last symptoms resemble those of alcohol withdrawal except that they persist.

The first long-term study of children with what has come to be called *fetal alcohol syndrome* (FAS) was reported by Jones and coworkers. Among 23 infants born to alcoholic mothers, there was a neonatal mortality of 17 percent; among the infants who survived the neonatal period, almost half failed to achieve normal weight, length, and head circumference or remained backward mentally to a varying degree, even under optimal environmental conditions. Several large groups of severely affected children have now been observed for 20 years or longer (see Streissguth). Distractibility, inattentiveness, hyperactivity, and impairment of fine motor coordination are prominent features in early childhood. Most such children fall into the category of attention-deficit hyperactivity disorder. Slow growth of head circumference is a consistent finding throughout infancy and childhood. The physical stigmata of the syndrome become less distinctive after puberty, but practically all adolescents are left with some degree of mental retardation and behavioral abnormalities.

The pathologic changes that underlie the syndrome have been studied in a small number of cases and no uniform change has emerged. Of some interest are observations such as those of Ikonomidu and coworkers that demonstrate a profound effect of alcohol exposure on the deletion of millions of neurons in the developing rat brain by a mechanism of apoptosis. The main vulnerability occurs during periods of synaptogenesis, which in humans extends from the sixth month of gestation onward.

It is noteworthy that infants born to nonalcoholic mothers who had been subjected to severe dietary deprivation during pregnancy (during World War II) were small and often premature, but these infants did not show the pattern of malformations that characterizes FAS. Alcohol readily crosses the placenta in humans and animals; in the mouse, rat, chick, miniature swine, and beagle dog, alcohol has been shown to have both embryotoxic and teratogenic effects. Thus, the evidence to date favors a toxic effect of alcohol, although a possible toxic effect of acetaldehyde and smoking and a possible contributory role for nutritional deficiency have not been totally excluded.

Unequivocal cases of FAS observed to date have occurred only in infants born to severely alcoholic mothers (many of them with delirium tremens and liver disease) who continued to drink heavily throughout pregnancy. It is important to state that a relationship to lesser degrees of alcohol intake is far less secure. Data derived from the collaborative study sponsored by the National Institutes of Health indicate that about one-third of the offspring of women who are heavy drinkers have FAS. Abel and Sokol have estimated that the worldwide incidence of FAS is 1.9 per 1,000 live births and have pronounced it the leading known cause of mental retardation in the western world. The degree of maternal alcoholism that is necessary to produce the syndrome and the critical stage in gestation during which it occurs are still vague. The various teratogenic effects described earlier are estimated to occur in the embryonic period, i.e., in the first 2 months of fetal life. Other nonteratogenic effects appear to be related to periods during gestation when the fetus is exposed to particularly high alcohol levels.

A comprehensive and not outdated account of alcohol-related birth defects and the controversial issues surrounding this subject is contained in a special issue of *Alcohol Health and Research World*, published by the National Institutes of Health (Vol. 18, 1994).

Neurologic Complications of Alcoholic Cirrhosis and Portal–Systemic Shunts

This category of alcoholic disease is discussed in Chap. 40, in connection with the acquired metabolic disorders of the nervous system.

TREATMENT OF ALCOHOL DEPENDENCE

Following recovery from the acute medical and neurologic complications of alcoholism, the patient still must face the underlying problem of alcohol dependence. To treat only the medical complications and leave the management of the drinking problem to the patient alone is shortsighted. Almost always, drinking is resumed, with a predictable recurrence of medical illness. For this reason the medical profession must be prepared to deal with the addiction or at least to initiate treatment.

The problem of excessive drinking is formidable but not nearly as hopeless as it is generally made out to be (see review of O'Connor and Schottenfeld). A common misconception among physicians is that specialized training in psychiatry and an inordinately large amount of time are required to deal with the addictive drinker. Actually, a successful program of treatment can be initiated by any interested physician, using the standard techniques of history taking, establishing rapport with the patient, and setting up a schedule of frequent visits, although not necessarily for prolonged periods. Our position on this matter was reinforced by a controlled study of problem drinkers in whom treatment was equally successful whether carried out by general practitioners or by specialists (Drummond et al). O'Connor and Schottenfeld summarize the various approaches to the patient who has a drinking problem but is not yet alcohol dependent. They favor brief and focused interventions that point out the problem in unambiguous terms and offer empathetic advice; the physician is often the central person in this interaction.

It appears that the requisite for successful treatment is total abstinence from alcohol; for all practical purposes, this represents the only permanent solution. There are alcohol addicts who have been able to reduce their intake of alcohol and eventually to drink in moderation, but they represent only a small proportion of the addicted population. Alcoholic patients must be made fully aware of the medical and social consequences of continued drinking. They must also be made to understand that because of some constitutional peculiarity (like that of the diabetic, who cannot handle sugar) they are incapable of drinking in moderation. These facts should be presented in much the same way as one would explain the essential features of any other disease; there is nothing to be gained from adopting a punitive or moralizing attitude. Yet patients should not be given the idea that they are in no way to blame for their illness; there appears to be an advantage in making them feel that they are responsible for doing something about their drinking.

A number of methods have proved valuable in the short- and long-term management of alcoholic patients. The more important of these are admission to a detoxification or special hospital unit, rehabilitative therapy, aversion treatment, the use of disulfiram (Antabuse), and the participation in self-help organizations for recovery from alcoholism. Detoxification clinics and special hospital units for the treatment of alcoholism are now widely available. The physician should be aware of all the community resources available for the management of this problem and should be prepared to take advantage of them in appropriate cases. Most inpatient programs include individual and group counseling, didactics about the illness and recovery, and family intervention. Outpatient treatment (of individuals or groups) is widely available, either from specialized facilities or from specialized therapists in general mental health facilities; family counseling is usually offered as well and is often beneficial. Most professional alcoholism treatment in the United States includes an introduction to the methods and utilization of Alcoholics Anonymous (AA; see below).

Disulfiram, less used in recent years, interferes with the metabolism of alcohol, so that a patient who takes both alcohol and disulfiram accumulates an inordinate amount of acetaldehyde in the tissues, resulting in nausea, vomiting, and hypotension, sometimes pronounced in degree. It is no longer considered necessary to demonstrate these effects to patients; it is sufficient to warn them of the severe reactions that may result if they drink while they have the drug in their bodies.

The opioid antagonist naltrexone (50 mg/d orally) or a long-acting injectable formulation has also been used for this purpose, with overall favorable results in numerous trials. The depot injectable form has the advantage of improving compliance in this population that is difficult to treat and to retain in clinical trials. The relevant trials and clinical implementation of naltrexone for alcohol dependence are summarized by Anton (2008). In Europe, modest success has been achieved with the GABA and glutamate modulator acamprosate (2,000 mg daily), but this drug is not yet available in the United States and some trials have shown it to be ineffective. Putatively, a novel approach has been to block the addicting effects of alcohol on the mesolimbic dopaminergic system by the use of anticonvulsants such as topiramate. Johnson and colleagues were able to demonstrate a reduction in alcoholic intake in patients taking this drug, in comparison to placebo, albeit over only a 12-week period. The use of these medications and the possible reasons for conflicting results between studies are given in a review by Swift. A complex randomized trial conducted by Anton and colleagues (2006) compared naltrexone, cognitive-behavioral therapy, and both, and found that abstinence was most likely, in the short period of 4 months, with the drug alone or when combined with the psychologic therapy; those who received the cognitive therapy but neither naltrexone or a placebo pill did somewhat worse.

Treatment with disulfiram is instituted only after the patient has been sober for several days, preferably longer. It should never be given to patients with cardiac or advanced liver disease. Should the patient drink while taking disulfiram, the ensuing reaction is usually severe enough to require medical attention, and a protracted spree can thus be prevented. Disulfiram may cause a polyneuropathy if continued over months or years, but this is a rare complication.

Alcoholics Anonymous, an informal fellowship of recovering alcoholics, has proven to be the single most effective force in the rehabilitation of alcoholic patients. The philosophy of this organization is embodied in its "12 Steps," a series of principles for sober living that guide the patient to recovery. The AA approach stresses in particular the practice of making restitution, the necessity to help other alcoholics, trust in a higher power, the group confessional, and the belief that the alcoholic alone is powerless over alcohol. Although accurate statistics are lacking, it is said that about one-third of the members who express more than a passing interest in the program attain a state of long-sustained or permanent sobriety. The methods used by AA are not acceptable to every patient, but most who persist in its activities appear to benefit; in particular, the physician should not accept a patient's initial negative reaction as reason to abandon AA as a mode of treatment.

Finally, it should be noted that alcoholism is very frequently associated with psychiatric disease of other types, particularly sociopathy and affective illness (the term "dual diagnosis" is used by psychiatrists to denote this combination of psychopathologies). In the latter case, the prevailing mood is far more often one of depression than of mania and is more often encountered in women, who are more apt to drink under these conditions than are men. In these circumstances, expert psychiatric help should be sought, preferably from someone who is also familiar with addictive diseases.

The role of physicians in caring for patients with alcohol problems has been outlined by several governmental agencies and is summarized in the review article by O'Connor and Schottenfeld.

References

Abel EL, Sokol RJ: Incidence of fetal alcohol syndrome and economic impact of FAS-related anomalies. *Drug Alcohol Depend* 19:51, 1987.

Anton RF: Naltrexone for the management of alcohol dependence. *N Engl J Med* 359:715, 2008.

Anton RF, O'Malley SS, Ciraulo DA, et al: Combined pharmacotherapies and behavioral interventions for alcohol dependence. *JAMA* 295:2003, 2006.

Baud FJ, Galliot M, Astier A, et al: Treatment of ethylene glycol poisoning with intravenous 4-methylpyrazole. *N Engl J Med* 319:97, 1988.

Bohman M: Some genetic aspects of alcoholism and criminality. *Arch Gen Psychiatry* 35:269, 1978.

Brent JB: Fomepizole for ethylene glycol and methanol poisoning. *N Engl J Med* 360:2216, 2009.

Brent J, McMartin K, Phillips S, et al: Fomepizole for the treatment of ethylene glycol poisoning. *N Engl J Med* 340:832, 1999.

Brewer C, Perrett L: Brain damage due to alcohol consumption: An air-encephalographic, psychometric and electroencephalographic study. *Br J Addict* 66(3):170, 1971.

Cadoret RJ, Cain C, Grove WM: Development of alcoholism in adoptees raised apart from alcoholic biologic relatives. *Arch Gen Psychiatry* 37:561, 1980.

Carlen PL, Wortzman G, Holgate RC, et al: Reversible cerebral atrophy in recently abstinent chronic alcoholics measured by computed tomography scans. *Science* 200:1076, 1978.

Charness ME: Molecular mechanisms of ethanol intoxication, tolerance, and physical dependence, in Mendelson JH, Mello NK (eds): *Medical Diagnosis and Treatment of Alcoholism*. New York, McGraw-Hill, 1992, pp 155–199.

Chin JH, Goldstein DB: Drug tolerance in biomembranes: A spin label study of the effects of ethanol. *Science* 196:684, 1977.

Clarren SK, Alvord EC Jr, Sumi SM, et al: Brain malformations related to prenatal exposure to ethanol. *J Pediatr* 92:64, 1978.

Courville CB: *Effects of Alcohol on the Nervous System of Man*. Los Angeles, San Lucas Press, 1955.

Cutting J: The relationship between Korsakov's syndrome and "alcoholic" dementia. *Br J Psychiatry* 132:240, 1978.

Davidson CS: Nutrient content of beers and ales. *N Engl J Med* 264:185, 1961.

Dolin SJ, Little HJ: Are changes in neuronal calcium channels involved in ethanol tolerance? *J Pharmacol Exp Ther* 250:985, 1989.

D'Onofrio G, Rathlev NK, Ulrich AS, et al: Lorazepam for the prevention of recurrent seizures related to alcohol. *N Engl J Med* 340:915, 1999.

Drummond DC, Thom B, Brown C, et al: Specialist versus general practitioner treatment of problem drinkers. *Lancet* 336:915, 1990.

Ferguson JA, Suelzer CJ, Ecjert GJ, et al: Risk factors for delirium tremens development. *J Gen Intern Med* 11:410, 1996.

Foy A, Kay J: The incidence of alcohol-related problems and the risk of alcohol withdrawal in a general hospital population. *Drug Alcohol Rev* 14:49, 1995.

Frezza M, Di Padova C, Pozzato G, et al: High blood alcohol levels in women: The role of decreased gastric alcohol dehydrogenase activity and first-pass metabolism. *N Engl J Med* 322:95, 1990.

Gessner PK: Drug therapy of the alcohol withdrawal syndrome, in Majchrowicz E, Noble EP (eds): *Biochemistry and Pharmacology of Ethanol*. Vol 2. New York, Plenum Press, 1979, pp 375–435.

Goldstein DB: *Pharmacology of Alcohol*. New York, Oxford University Press, 1983.

Goodwin DW, Schulsinger F, Moller N, et al: Drinking problems in adopted and nonadopted sons of alcoholics. *Arch Gen Psychiatry* 31:164, 1974.

Grant BF, Harford TC, Choup P, et al: Prevalence of DSM-III-R alcohol abuse and dependence: United States, 1988. *Alcohol Health Res World* 15:91, 1991.

Grove WM, Cadoret RJ: Genetic factors in alcoholism, in Kissin B, Begleiter H (eds): *The Biology of Alcoholism*. Vol 7. The Pathogenesis of Alcoholism. New York, Plenum Press, 1983, pp 31–56.

Haggard HW, Jellinek EM: *Alcohol Explored*. Garden City, NY, Doubleday Doran, 1942.

Harada S, Agarwal DP, Goedde HW: Aldehyde dehydrogenase deficiency as cause of facial flushing reaction to alcohol in Japanese. *Lancet* 2:982, 1981.

Harper CG, Blumbergs PC: Brain weights in alcoholics. *J Neurol Neurosurg Psychiatry* 45:838, 1982.

Harper CG, Kril JJ: Brain atrophy in chronic alcoholic patients: A quantitative pathologic study. *J Neurol Neurosurg Psychiatry* 48: 211, 1985.

Harris RA, Baxter DM, Mitchell MA, et al: Physical properties and lipid composition of brain membranes from ethanol tolerant-dependent mice. *Mol Pharmacol* 25:401, 1984.

Haug JO: Pneumoencephalographic evidence of brain damage in chronic alcoholics: A preliminary report. *Acta Psychiatr Scand* 203(Suppl):135, 1968.

Ikonomidu C, Bittigan P, Ishimaru M, et al: Ethanol-induced apoptotic neurodegeneration and fetal alcohol syndrome. *Science* 287:1058, 2000.

Isbell H, Fraser HF, Wikler A, et al: An experimental study of the etiology of "rum fits" and delirium tremens. *Q J Stud Alcohol* 16:1, 1955.

Jacobsen D: New treatment for ethylene glycol poisoning. *N Engl J Med* 340:879, 1999.

Johnson BA, Ait-Daoud N, Bowden CL, et al: Oral topiramate for treatment of alcohol dependence: A randomised controlled trial. *Lancet* 361:1677, 2003.

Jones KL, Smith DW: Recognition of the fetal alcohol syndrome in early infancy. *Lancet* 2:999, 1973.

Jones KL, Smith DW, Streissguth AP, Myrianthopoulos NC: Outcome in offspring of chronic alcoholic women. *Lancet* 1:1076, 1974.

Kaim SC, Klett CJ, Rothfeld B: Treatment of acute alcohol withdrawal state: A comparison of four drugs. *Am J Psychiatry* 125:1640, 1969.

Kosten TR, O'Connor PG: Management of drug and alcohol withdrawal. *N Engl J Med* 348:1786, 2003.

Kril JJ, Harper CG: Neuronal counts from four cortical regions in alcoholic brains. *Acta Neuropathol* 79:200, 1989.

Lemoine P, Harousseau H, Borteyru JP, Menuet JC: Les enfants de parents alcooliques: Anomalies observées à propos de 127 cas. *Ouest-Med* 25:477, 1968.

Lishman WA: Cerebral disorder in alcoholism: Syndromes of impairment. *Brain* 104:1, 1981.

Little HJ, Dolin SJ, Halsey MJ: Calcium channel antagonists decrease the ethanol withdrawal syndrome. *Life Sci* 39:2059, 1986.

McLean DR, Jacobs H, Mielke BW: Methanol poisoning: A clinical and pathological study. *Ann Neurol* 8:161, 1980.

Miles WR: Psychological effects of alcohol and man, in Emerson H (ed): *Alcohol and Man*. New York, Macmillan, 1932, p 224.

O'Connor PG, Schottenfeld RS: Patients with alcohol problems. *N Engl J Med* 338:592, 1998.

Peiffer J, Majewski F, Fischbach H, et al: Alcohol embryo- and fetopathy: Neuropathology of 3 children and 3 fetuses. *J Neurol Sci* 41:125, 1979.

Porjesz B, Begleiter H: Brain dysfunction and alcohol, in Kissin B, Begleiter H (eds): *The Biology of Alcoholism*. Vol 7: The

Pathogenesis of Alcoholism. New York, Plenum Press, 1983, pp 415–483.
Reich T: Biologic-marker studies in alcoholism. *N Engl J Med* 318:180, 1988.
Romero CE, Barohn JD, Knox AD, et al: Barbiturate withdrawal following Internet purchase of Fioricet. *Arch Neurol* 61:1111, 2004.
Sadock BJ, Sadock VA (eds): *Kaplan and Sadock's Comprehensive Textbook of Psychiatry*. Philadelphia, Lippincott Williams & Wilkins, 2000.
Samson HH, Harris RA: Neurobiology of alcohol abuse. *Trends Pharmacol Sci* 13:206, 1992.
Schroth G, Naegele T, Klose U, et al: Reversible brain shrinkage in abstinent alcoholics, measured by MRI. *Neuroradiology* 30:385, 1988.
Schuckit MA, Winokur G: Alcoholic hallucinosis and schizophrenia: A negative study. *Br J Psychiatry* 119:549, 1971.
Scott DF: Alcoholic hallucinosis: An aetiological study. *Br J Addict* 62:113, 1967.
Secretary of Health and Human Services. *Ninth Special Report to the U.S. Congress on Alcohol and Health*. NIH publication no. 97-4017. Washington, DC: Government Printing Office, 1997.
Spillane L, Roberts JR, Meyer AE: Multiple cranial nerve deficits after ethylene glycol poisoning. *Ann Emerg Med* 20:208, 1991.
Streissguth AP: A long-term perspective of FAS. *Alcohol Health Res World* 18:74, 1994.
Sullivan WC: A note on the influence of maternal inebriety on the offspring. *J Mental Sci* 45:489, 1899.
Swift RM: Drug therapy for alcohol dependence. *N Engl J Med* 340:1482, 1999.
Torvik A, Lindboe CF, Rogde S: Brain lesions in alcoholics. *J Neurol Sci* 56:233, 1982.
Ulleland C: The offspring of alcoholic mothers. *Ann N Y Acad Sci* 197:167, 1972.
Victor M: Alcoholic dementia. *Can J Neurol Sci* 21:88, 1994.
Victor M: Introductory remarks. *Ann N Y Acad Sci* 215:210, 1973.
Victor M: The pathophysiology of alcoholic epilepsy. *Res Publ Assoc Res Nerv Ment Dis* 46:431, 1968.
Victor M, Adams RD: The effect of alcohol on the nervous system. *Res Publ Assoc Res Nerv Ment Dis* 32:526, 1953.
Victor M, Adams RD, Collins GH: *The Wernicke-Korsakoff Syndrome and Other Disorders Due to Alcoholism and Malnutrition.* Philadelphia, Davis, 1989.
Victor M, Hope J: The phenomenon of auditory hallucinations in chronic alcoholism. *J Nerv Ment Dis* 126:451, 1958.
Wilkinson DA: Examination of alcoholics by computed tomographic scans: A critical review. *Alcohol Clin Exp Res* 6:31, 1982.
Wolfe SM, Victor M: The relationship of hypomagnesemia and alkalosis to alcohol withdrawal symptoms. *Ann N Y Acad Sci* 162:973, 1969.
Zipursky RB, Lim KO, Pfefferbaum A: MRI study of brain changes with short-term abstinence from alcohol. *Alcohol Clin Exp Res* 13:664, 1989.

43

Disorders of the Nervous System Caused by Drugs, Toxins, and Chemical Agents

Subsumed under this title is a diverse group of disorders of the nervous system that result from drugs and other injurious or poisonous substances. The neurologist must be concerned with the myriad of chemical agents that have no therapeutic utility but may adversely affect the nervous system; they abound in the environment as household products, insecticides, industrial solvents and other poisons, as well as substances that may have therapeutic value but are used for their "recreational" psychotropic effects, or are conventional medications with known toxic effects and may be accidentally ingested. These constitute the field of neurotoxicology. Also among the neurotoxins are those generated by bacteria and other infectious organisms, as well as toxins several found in nature, such as marine toxins.

It would hardly be possible within one chapter to discuss the innumerable drugs and toxins that affect the nervous system. The interested reader is referred to a number of comprehensive monographs and references listed at the end of this chapter. In addition, a current handbook of pharmacology and toxicology is a useful part of the library of every physician.

The scope of this chapter is also limited because the therapeutic and adverse effects of many drugs are considered elsewhere in this volume in relation to particular symptoms and diseases. Thus, the toxic effects of ethyl, methyl, amyl, and isopropyl alcohol, as well as ethylene and diethylene glycol, are discussed in Chap. 42. The adverse effects of antibiotics on cochlear and vestibular function and on neuromuscular transmission are discussed in Chaps. 15 and 49, respectively. Many of the undesirable side effects of the common drugs used in the treatment of extrapyramidal motor symptoms, pain, headache, seizure and sleep disorders, psychiatric illnesses, and so forth are also considered in the chapters dealing with each of these disorders and in the chapters that cover psychiatric diseases. Cyanide and carbon monoxide poisoning are discussed in relation to anoxic encephalopathy (see Chap. 40). A number of therapeutic agents that predictably damage the peripheral nerves (e.g., cisplatin, disulfiram, vincristine) are mentioned in this chapter but are discussed further in Chap. 46, and those that affect muscle are included in Chap. 48, "Diseases of Muscle."

The presentation of this subject is introduced by some general remarks on the action of drugs on the nervous system and is followed by discussion of the main classes of agents that affect nervous function. The references at the end of the chapter are listed in relation to each of these categories:

1. Opiates and synthetic analgesics
2. Sedative-hypnotic drugs
3. Antipsychosis drugs
4. Antidepressant drugs
5. Stimulants
6. Psychoactive drugs
7. Bacterial toxins
8. Plant poisons, venoms, bites, and stings
9. Heavy metals
10. Industrial toxins
11. Antineoplastic and immunosuppressive agents
12. Antibiotics
13. Cardioactive agents

GENERAL PRINCIPLES OF NEUROTOXICOLOGY

The rational use of any drug requires knowledge of the best route of administration, the drug's absorption characteristics, its distribution in the nervous system and other organs, and its biotransformations and excretion (*pharmacokinetics*). Because every drug, if given in excess, has some adverse effects, therapeutics and toxicology are inseparable.

All systems of neurons are not identical; each has its own vulnerabilities to particular drugs and toxic agents. This principle, originally enunciated by Oskar and Ceclie Vogt in their theory termed *pathoclisis* is now embodied as "selective vulnerability." For example, selective vulnerability explains the production of parkinsonism by the neurotoxin 1-methyl-4-phenyl-1,2,3,6-tetrahydropyridine (MPTP), in which a synthetic toxin affects a progressive loss of melanin-bearing dopaminergic nigral neurons (see Chap. 39). Another example is the preferential effects of anesthetics on the neurons of the upper brainstem reticular formation. Not only may certain groups of nerve cells be selectively destroyed by a particular agent but particular parts of their structure may be altered. Drugs may be targeted even to the terminal axons, dendrites, neurofilaments, or receptors on pre- and postsynaptic surfaces of neurons or to certain of their metabolic activities, whereby they synthesize and release neurotransmitters or maintain their cellular integrity by the synthesis of RNA, DNA, and other proteins. An intriguing but not yet fully established extension of this theme relates to the manner in which certain drugs or toxins affect individuals differently with a genetic disposition by way of single nucleotide polymorphisms; this is the emerging field of pharmacogenetics.

The same mechanisms by which drugs and toxins act on particular steps in the formation, storage, release, uptake, catabolism, and resynthesis of neurotransmitters such as dopamine, serotonin, norepinephrine, acetylcholine, and other catecholamines cannot be separated from their toxic effects. Johnston and Gross have summarized views of how these transmitters and modulating agents, by attaching to receptors at neuronal synapses, are able to increase or decrease the permeability of ion channels and stimulate or inhibit second cytoplasmic messengers (cyclic adenosine monophosphate [cAMP] and G-proteins). For example, drugs such as L-dopa, tryptophan, and choline enhance the synthesis of dopamine, serotonin, and acetylcholine, respectively, and may impart toxic effects through these same mechanisms. Baclofen modulates the release of gamma-aminobutyric acid (GABA), the main inhibitory transmitter in the central nervous system (CNS). Botulinum toxin prevents the release of acetylcholine in the neuromuscular junction and tetanus toxin does the same on GABA in Renshaw cells of the spinal cord. Benzodiazepines, bromocriptine, and methylphenidate are viewed as receptor agonists; the phenothiazines and anticholinergics act as receptor antagonists. Certain drugs enhance the activity of neurotransmitters by inhibiting their reuptake as, for example, the class of antidepressant drugs that has a relatively selective influence on the reuptake of serotonin. Others deplete existing neurotransmitters, as reserpine does for norepinephrine and another class of drugs promotes the release of preformed synaptic transmitters; amphetamines and modafinil are examples in this class. Amantadine, an antiviral agent, may promote the release of dopamine. One must not assume that these are the exclusive modes of action of each of these drugs; for example, cocaine acts as a direct stimulant and through the inhibition of reuptake of catecholamines.

Bioavailability

A majority of drugs that act on the nervous system are ingested; factors that govern their intestinal absorption must therefore be taken into account. Small molecules usually enter the plasma by diffusion, larger ones by pinocytosis. The substances with which the drugs are mixed; the presence of food, other drugs, or intestinal diseases; and the age of the patient all influence the rate of absorption and blood concentrations. Different calculations are necessary for intramuscular, subcutaneous, and intrathecal routes of administration. To some extent, the solubilities of drugs (in lipid or water) determine the routes by which they can be given; some drugs, such as morphine, can be administered by numerous routes. Carried in the blood, the drug (or toxin) reaches many tissues, including the nervous system; protein binding in the plasma has an important influence on distribution. Many drugs and toxic substances bind to serum albumin and other serum proteins, limiting the availability of the ionized form. The common drug and toxin transformations involve hydroxylation, deamination, oxidation, and dealkylation, which enhance their solubility and elimination mainly by the kidney. Most of these catalytic processes occur in liver cells and utilize multiple enzymes.

To enter the extracellular compartment of the nervous system, a drug or toxic agent must transgress the tight capillary–endothelial barrier (blood–brain barrier) and the barrier between the blood and cerebrospinal fluid (blood–CSF barrier). Intrathecal injection circumvents these barriers, but then the agent tends to concentrate in the immediate subpial and subependymal regions. The process of movement from plasma to brain is by diffusion through capillaries or by facilitated transport. The solubility characteristics of the drug determine its rate of diffusion.

In the following discussion on neurotoxins, the reader will appreciate a number of phenomena: *tolerance* (lessening effect of increasing dose), *dependence* and *addiction* (insatiable need), *habituation*, *drug-seeking behaviors*, and *abstinence* with its associated *withdrawal effects*. These were described in Chap. 42 regarding alcoholism and are further elaborated in sections below. Particularly difficult in reference to drugs such as nicotine is the separation of habituation from addiction, i.e., of psychologic dependence from physical dependence (see further on).

The few examples given earlier are intended to provide a glimpse of the complex interactions between chemical agents and the cells of the nervous system. For more specific information, the reader is referred to *The Biochemical Basis of Neuropharmacology* by Cooper, Bloom, and Roth, a text that we have consulted through its many editions and to *Goodman and Gilman's The Pharmacological Basis of Therapeutics*.

OPIATES AND SYNTHETIC ANALGESIC DRUGS

The opiates, or opioids, strictly speaking, include all the naturally occurring alkaloids in opium, which is prepared from the seed capsules of the poppy *Papaver somniferum*. For clinical purposes, the term *opiate* refers only to the alkaloids that have a high degree of analgesic activity, i.e., morphine. The terms *opioid* and *narcotic-analgesic* designate drugs with actions similar to those of morphine. Compounds that are chemical modifications of morphine include diacetylmorphine, or heroin, hydromorphone (Dilaudid), codeine, hydrocodone, oxycodone (OxyContin), and from the Victorian era and later, laudanum and paregoric. A second class of opioids comprises the purely synthetic analgesics: meperidine (Demerol) and its congeners, notably fentanyl, methadone, levorphanol, propoxyphene (Darvon), loperamide (the active ingredient in Imodium), and diphenoxylate (the main component of Lomotil). The synthetic analgesics are similar to the opiates in both their pharmacologic effects and patterns of abuse, the differences being mainly quantitative.

Opioids activate G-coupled transmembrane receptors, meaning they influence neuronal activity through the intermediate of cAMP; the receptor types are denominated as mu, delta, and kappa. An understanding of the clinical effects of opioids is clarified by the knowledge that these receptors are concentrated in the thalamus and dorsal root ganglia (mu receptors, pain), amygdala (affect) and brainstem raphe (alertness), and Edinger-Westphal nuclei (pupillary miosis). Receptors in the brainstem, also of the mu type, are involved in modulating respiratory responses to hypoxia and hypercarbia (respiratory suppression). Receptors are also widely distributed in neural components of other organs, particularly the gastrointestinal tract, accounting for the constipation that is an effect of the administration of this class of drugs.

The clinical effects of the opioids are considered from two points of view: acute poisoning and addiction.

Opioid Overdose

Because of the common, and particularly the illicit, use of opioids, poisoning is a frequent occurrence. This happens also as a result of ingestion or injection accidentally or with suicidal intent, errors in the calculation of dosage, the use of a substitute or contaminated street product, or unusual sensitivity. Children exhibit an increased susceptibility to opioids, so that relatively small doses may prove toxic. This is true also of adults with myxedema, Addison disease, chronic liver disease, and pneumonia. Acute poisoning may also occur in persons who are unaware that opioids available from illicit sources vary greatly in potency and that tolerance for opioids declines quickly after the withdrawal of the drug; upon resumption of the habit, a formerly well-tolerated dose can be fatal.

Unresponsiveness, shallow respirations, slow respiratory rate (e.g., 2 to 8 per min) or periodic breathing, pinpoint pupils, bradycardia, and hypothermia are the well-recognized clinical manifestations of acute opioid poisoning. In the most advanced stage, the pupils dilate, the skin and mucous membranes become cyanotic, and the circulation fails. Later in the course, pulmonary edema may arise, or aspiration pneumonia may become evident as summarized the review of opioid overdose by Boyer. The immediate cause of death is usually respiratory depression with consequent asphyxia. Patients who suffer a cardiorespiratory arrest are sometimes left with all the known residua of anoxic encephalopathy (see Chap. 40). Mild degrees of intoxication are reflected by anorexia, nausea, vomiting, constipation, and loss of sexual interest. Toxicology screens for opiates may be useful but action must be taken before the results of these tests are completed.

Treatment of Overdose

This consists of the support of ventilation and administration of naloxone (Narcan), or the longer-acting nalmefene, both specific antidotes to the opiates and also to the synthetic analgesics. The dose of naloxone in adults is usually 0.05 mg and repeated in larger increments (the second dose is typically 2 mg) every 2 min to a dose of 15 mg *intravenously* as outlined by Boyer. For children, a higher initial dose of 0.1 mg/kg is recommended. The improvements in circulation and respiration and reversal of miosis are usually dramatic. Failure of naloxone to produce such a response should cast doubt on the diagnosis of opioid intoxication. If an adequate respiratory and pupillary response to naloxone is obtained, the patient should nonetheless be observed for up to 24 h and further doses of naloxone (50 percent higher than the ones previously found effective) can be given *intramuscularly* as often as necessary. An intravenous infusion of naloxone has been recommended if a long-acting narcotic is the cause of overdose. (It is well to inspect the patient for the presence of unnoticed fentanyl patches and establish if a long-acting drug has been available for abuse.)

Naloxone has less direct effect on consciousness, however, and the patient may remain drowsy for many hours. This is not harmful provided respiration is well maintained. Although nalmefene has a plasma half-life of 11 h, compared to 60 to 90 min for naloxone, it has no clear advantage in emergency practice. Gastric lavage is a useful measure if the drug was taken orally. This procedure may be efficacious many hours after ingestion, as one of the toxic effects of opioids is ileus, which causes some of the drug to be retained in the stomach. Concerns of precipitating opioid withdrawal by giving naloxone are generally unfounded.

Once the patient regains consciousness, complaints such as pruritus, sneezing, tearing, piloerection, diffuse body pains, yawning, and diarrhea may appear. These are the recognizable symptoms of the opioid abstinence, or withdrawal, syndrome described later. Consequently, an antidote must be used with great caution in an addict who has taken an overdose of opioid, because in this circumstance, it may precipitate withdrawal phenomena. Nausea and severe abdominal pain, presumably because of pancreatitis (from spasm of the sphincter of Oddi), are other troublesome symptoms of opiate use or withdrawal. Seizures are rare.

Opioid Addiction

Just 50 years ago there were an estimated 60,000 persons addicted to narcotic drugs in the United States, exclusive of those who were receiving drugs because of incurable painful diseases. This represented a relatively small public health problem in comparison with the abuse of alcohol and barbiturates. Moreover, opioid addiction was of serious proportions in only a few cities—New York, Chicago, Los Angeles, Washington, DC, and Detroit. Since the late 1960s, a remarkable increase in opioid (mainly heroin) addiction has taken place. The precise number of opioid addicts is unknown but is currently estimated by the Drug Enforcement Administration to be well more than 500,000 (a disproportionate number in large cities). The problem assumes enormous importance when one recognizes that one-quarter of addicts are seropositive for HIV and are the chief source of transmission of AIDS to newborns and to the heterosexual nonaddicted population.

Etiology and Pathogenesis

A number of factors—socioeconomic, psychologic, and pharmacologic—contribute to the genesis of opioid addiction. The most susceptible subjects are young men living in the economically depressed areas of large cities but significant numbers are found in suburbs and in small cities. The onset of opioid use is usually in adolescence, with a peak at 17 to 18 years; fully two-thirds of addicts start using the drugs before the age of 21. Almost 90 percent engage in criminal activity to obtain their daily ration of drugs but most of them have a history of arrests or convictions predating their addiction. Also, many of them have psychiatric disturbances, conduct disorder and sociopathy being the most common ("dual-diagnosis," in psychiatric jargon). Monroe and colleagues, using the Lexington Personality Inventory, examined a group of 837 opioid addicts and found evidence of antisocial personality in 42 percent, emotional disturbance in 29 percent, and thought disorder in 22 percent; only 7 percent were free of such disorders. Vulnerability to addiction was not confined to one personality type.

Association with addicts is the apparent explanation for becoming addicted. In this sense, opioid addiction is contagious, and partly as a result of this pattern, opioid addiction has attained epidemic proportions. A small, almost insignificant proportion of addicts are introduced to drugs by physicians in the course of an illness. Thus there has been a regrettable tendency not to prescribe opiates to patients with acute or chronic pain (e.g., cancer pain) because of the risk of addiction.

Opioid addiction consists of three recognizable phases: (1) intoxication, or "euphoria," (2) pharmacogenic dependence or drug-seeking behavior (addiction), and (3) the propensity to relapse after a period of abstinence. Some of the symptoms of opioid intoxication have already been considered. In patients with severe pain or pain-anticipatory anxiety, the administration of opioids produces a sense of unusual well-being, a state that has traditionally been referred to as *morphine euphoria*. It should be emphasized that only a negligible proportion of such persons continue to use opioids habitually after their pain has subsided. The vast majority of potential addicts are not suffering from painful illnesses at the time they initiate opioid use, and the term *euphoria* is probably not an apt description of the initial effects. These persons, after several repetitions, recognize a "high," despite the subsequent recurrence of unpleasant, or *dysphoric*, symptoms (nausea, vomiting, and faintness as the drug effect wanes).

The repeated self-administration of the drug is the most important factor in the genesis of *addiction*. Regardless of how one characterizes the state of mind that is produced by episodic injection of the drug, the individual quickly discovers the need to increase the dose in order to obtain the original effects (*tolerance*). Although the initial effects may not be fully recaptured, the progressively increasing dose of the drug does relieve the discomfort that arises as the effects of each injection wear off. In this way a new *pharmacogenically induced* need is developed, and the use of opioids becomes self-perpetuating. At the same time a marked degree of *tolerance* is produced, so that enormous amounts of drugs, e.g., 5,000 mg of morphine daily, can eventually be administered without the development of toxic symptoms.

The pharmacologic (in contrast to psychologic) criteria of addiction, as indicated in Chap. 42 in regards to alcoholism, are *tolerance* and *physical dependence*. The latter refers to the symptoms and signs that become manifest when the drug is withdrawn following a period of continued use. These symptoms and signs constitute a specific clinical state, termed *the abstinence* or *withdrawal syndrome* (see later). The mechanisms that underlie the development of tolerance and physical dependence are not fully understood. However, it is known that opioids activate an opioid antinociceptive system (enkephalins, dynorphins, endorphins), which are opioid receptors and are located at many different levels of the nervous system (these were referred to earlier and are described in Chap. 8; see also the review of Fields). The desensitization of opioid receptors, probably mainly the mu type, accounts for tolerance through a mechanism of uncoupling of the receptor from the G-protein complex.

The Opioid Abstinence Syndrome

The intensity of the *abstinence* or *withdrawal* syndrome depends on the dose of the drug and the duration of addiction. The onset of abstinence symptoms in relation to the last exposure to the drug, however, is related to the pharmacologic half-life of the agent. With morphine, the majority of individuals receiving 240 mg daily for 30 days or more will show moderately severe abstinence symptoms following withdrawal. Mild signs of opiate abstinence can be precipitated by narcotic antagonists in persons who have taken as little as 15 mg of morphine or an equivalent dose of methadone or heroin tid for 3 days.

The abstinence syndrome that occurs in the morphine addict may be taken as the prototype. The first 8 to 16 h of abstinence usually pass asymptomatically. At the end of this period, yawning, rhinorrhea, sweating, piloerection, and lacrimation are manifest. Mild at first, these symptoms increase in severity over a period of several hours and then remain constant for several days. The patient may be able to sleep during the early abstinence period but is restless, and thereafter insomnia remains a prominent feature. Dilatation of the pupils, recurring waves of "gooseflesh," and twitching of the muscles appear. The patient complains of aching in the back, abdomen, and legs and of "hot and cold flashes"; he frequently asks for blankets. At about 36 h the restlessness becomes more severe, and nausea, vomiting, and diarrhea usually develop. Temperature, respiratory rate, and blood pressure are slightly elevated. All these symptoms reach their peak intensity 48 to 72 h after withdrawal and then gradually subside. The opioid abstinence syndrome is rarely fatal (it is life-threatening only in infants). After 7 to 10 days, the clinical signs of abstinence are no longer evident, although the patient may complain of insomnia, nervousness, weakness, and muscle aches for several more weeks, and small deviations of a number of physiologic variables can be detected with refined techniques for up to 10 months (protracted abstinence).

Habituation, the equivalent of emotional or psychologic *dependence*, refers to the substitution of drug-seeking activities for all other aims and objectives in life. It is this feature that fosters relapse to the use of the drug long after the physiologic ("nonpurposive") abstinence changes seem to have disappeared. The cause for relapse is not fully understood. Theoretically, fragments of the abstinence syndrome may remain as a conditioned response, and these abstinence signs may be evoked by the appropriate environmental stimuli. Thus, when a "cured" addict returns to a situation where narcotic drugs are readily available or in a setting that was associated with the initial use of drugs, the incompletely extinguished drug-seeking behavior may reassert itself.

The characteristics of addiction and of abstinence are qualitatively similar with all drugs of the opiate group as well as the related synthetic analgesics. The differences are quantitative and are related to the differences in dosage, potency, and length of action. Heroin is 2 to 3 times more potent than morphine but the heroin withdrawal syndrome encountered in hospital practice is usually mild in degree because of the low dosage of the drug in the street product. Dilaudid (hydromorphone) is more potent than morphine and has a shorter duration of action; hence the addict requires more doses per day, and the abstinence syndrome comes on and subsides more rapidly. Abstinence symptoms from codeine, while definite, are less severe than those from morphine. The addiction liabilities of propoxyphene, a weak opioid, are negligible. Abstinence symptoms from methadone are less intense than those from morphine and do not become evident until 3 or 4 days after withdrawal; for these reasons methadone can be used in the treatment of morphine and heroin dependency (see further on). Meperidine addiction is of particular importance because of its high incidence among physicians and nurses. Tolerance to the drug's toxic effects is not complete, so that the addict may show tremors, twitching of muscles, confusion, hallucinations, and sometimes convulsions. Signs of abstinence appear 3 to 4 h after the last dose and reach their maximum intensity in 8 to 12 h, at which time they may be worse than those of morphine abstinence.

As to the biologic basis of addiction and physical dependence, our understanding is still very limited. Experiments in animals have provided insights into the neurotransmitter and neuronal systems involved. As a result of microdialyzing opiates and their antagonists into the central brain structures of animals, it has been tentatively concluded that mesolimbic structures, particularly the nucleus accumbens, ventral tegmentum of the midbrain, and locus ceruleus are activated or depressed under conditions of repeated opiate exposure. Thus, chronic opiate usage increases the levels of intracellular messengers (G-proteins) as noted earlier that drive cAMP activity in the locus ceruleus and in the nucleus accumbens; blocking the expression of these proteins markedly increases the self-administration of opiates by addicted rats. As in alcoholism, certain subtypes of the serotonin and dopamine receptors in limbic structures have been implicated in the psychic aspects of addiction and habituation. These same structures are conceived as a common pathway for the impulse to human drives such as sex, hunger, and psychic fulfillment. Camí and Farré reviewed the neurochemical mechanism of addiction.

The *diagnosis* of addiction is usually made when the patient admits to using and needing drugs. Should the patient conceal this fact, one relies on collateral evidence such as miosis, needle marks, emaciation, abscess scars, or chemical analyses. Meperidine addicts are likely to have dilated pupils and twitching of muscles. The finding of morphine or opiate derivatives (heroin is excreted as morphine) in the urine is confirmatory evidence that the patient has taken or has been given a dose of such drugs within 24 h of the test. The diagnosis of opiate addiction is also at once apparent when the treatment of acute opiate intoxication precipitates a characteristic abstinence syndrome.

Treatment of the Opioid Abstinence Syndrome

Views on the nature of drug addiction and appropriate methods of treatment are as much national and sociologic as they are biologic. Berridge has reviewed some of these historically based factors in reference overall "harm reduction" by using heroin itself to treat heroin addiction. One approach that has achieved some degree of success over the past 40 years has been the substitution of methadone for opioid, in the ratio of 1 mg methadone for 3 mg morphine, 1 mg heroin, or 20 mg meperidine. Because methadone is long acting and effective orally, it needs to be given only twice daily by mouth—10 to 20 mg per dose being sufficient to suppress abstinence symptoms. After a stabilization period of 3 to 5 days, this dosage of methadone is reduced and the drug is withdrawn over a similar period. An alternative but probably less effective method has been the use of clonidine (0.2 to 0.6 mg bid for a week), a drug that counteracts most of the noradrenergic withdrawal symptoms; however, the hypotension that is induced by this drug may be a problem (Jasinski et al).

In Europe, addicts who could not be detoxified and kept free of drugs by any other means have been given diacetylmorphine, the active ingredient in heroin, with some success when compared in clinical trials to methadone (see Oviedo-Joekes et al). Special settings that are capable of medical reversal of overdose are required but the notion of overall reduction in personal and societal harm seems to be attained by even this seemingly extreme measure.

A rapid detoxification regimen that is conducted under general anesthesia was popular in a number of centers as a means of treating opiate addiction has now been largely abandoned for reasons of safety but it could be resurrected if other more conventional approaches continue to be futile. The technique consisted of administering increasing doses of opioid receptor antagonists (naloxone or naltrexone) over several hours while the autonomic and other features of the withdrawal syndrome were suppressed by the infusion of propofol or a similar anesthetic, supplemented by intravenous fluids. Medications such as clonidine and sedatives were also given in the immediate postanesthetic period. There are substantial risks involved in this procedure and several deaths have occurred for which reason it has been all but abandoned. Furthermore, a number of patients continue to manifest signs of withdrawal after the procedure and require continued hospitalization.

Treatment of Opiate Habituation This is in some ways far more demanding than the treatment of opioid withdrawal and can be best accomplished in special facilities and programs that are devoted wholly to the problem. These are available in most communities. The most effective ones have been the ambulatory methadone maintenance clinics, where more than 100,000 former heroin addicts are participating in rehabilitation programs approved by the FDA. Methadone, in a dosage of 60 to 100 mg daily (sufficient to suppress the craving for heroin), is given under supervision day by day (less often with long-acting methadone) for months or years. Various forms of psychotherapy and social service counseling often administered by former heroin addicts are integral parts of the program.

The results of methadone treatment are difficult to assess and vary considerably from one program to another. Even the most successful programs suffer an attrition rate of approximately 25 percent when they are evaluated after several years. Of the patients who remain, the majority achieves a degree of social rehabilitation, i.e., they are gainfully employed and no longer engage in criminal behavior or prostitution.

The usual practice of methadone programs is to accept only addicts older than age 16 years with a history of heroin addiction for at least 1 year. This leaves many adolescent addicts untreated. The number of addicts who can fully withdraw from methadone and maintain a drug-free existence is very small. This means that the large majority of addicts now enrolled in methadone programs are committed to an indefinite period of methadone maintenance and the effects of such a regimen are uncertain.

An alternative method of ambulatory treatment of the opiate addict involves the use of narcotic antagonists, of which naloxone and naltrexone are the best known. The physical effects of abusing narcotics are thereby partially blocked, and there may be some degree of aversive conditioning if withdrawal symptoms are produced. Naltrexone is favored because it has a longer effect than naloxone, is almost free of agonist effects, and can be administered orally. Similar results have also been achieved with cyclazocine in a small number of highly motivated patients; this drug is administered orally in increasing amounts until a dosage of 2 mg/70 kg body weight is attained. The drug is taken bid (for 2 to 6 weeks) and is then withdrawn slowly.

More recently, interest has centered on the use of sublingual buprenorphine for the treatment of heroin (and cocaine) abuse; this drug has both opioid agonist and antagonist properties; it mutes the effect of withdrawal, also serves as an aversive agent, and its abuse potential is relatively low. A randomized trial conducted by Fudala and colleagues has demonstrated the superiority over methadone of a combination of buprenorphine and naloxone combined with brief counseling in keeping opioid addicts in treatment and abstinent of abused drugs. This approach has been available in Europe for many years and has been adopted in the United States under a Department of Health–supervised program for primary care offices. In addition, there is evidence, based on animal experiments and experience with small numbers of addicts, that it may be useful for the treatment of dual dependence on cocaine and opiates (see Mello and Mendelson), but this has not been confirmed in other clinical trials.

Medical and Neurologic Complications of Opioid Use

In addition to the toxic effects of the opioid itself, the addict may suffer a variety of neurologic and infectious complications resulting from the injection of contaminated adulterants (quinine, talc, lactose, powdered milk, and fruit sugars) and of various infectious agents (injections administered by unsterile methods). The most important of these is HIV infection, but septicemia, endocarditis, and viral hepatitis may also occur. Particulate matter that is injected with heroin or a vasculitis that is induced by chronic heroin abuse may cause stroke by an incompletely understood *occlusion of cerebral arteries*, with hemiplegia or other focal cerebral signs. *Amblyopia*, probably as a result of the toxic effects of quinine in the heroin mixtures, has been reported, as well as *transverse myelopathy* and several types of *peripheral neuropathy*. The spinal cord disorder expresses itself clinically by the abrupt onset of paraplegia with a level on the trunk below which motor function and sensation are lost or impaired and by urinary retention. Pathologically, there is an acute necrotizing lesion involving both gray and white matter over a considerable vertical extent of the thoracic and occasionally the cervical cord. In some cases, a myelopathy has followed the first intravenous injection of heroin after a prolonged period of abstinence. We have also seen two cases of cervical myelopathy from heroin-induced stupor and a prolonged period of immobility with the neck hyperextended over the back of a chair or sofa.

In addition, we have observed several instances of a subacute progressive cerebral leukoencephalopathy after heroin use, similar to ones that occurred in Amsterdam in the 1980s, the result of inhalation of heroin or an adulterant (Wolters et al; Tan et al). Most instances of this leukoencephalopathy are the result of inhalation of heated heroin vapor in a practice known as "chasing the dragon." The clinical presentation has varied but generally includes stupor, coma, and death, after a latent period of hours or days. In one of our patients, the white matter changes were concentrated in the posterior regions of the hemispheres and in the internal capsules and, in one striking case, in the cerebellar white matter. The MRI is fairly characteristic and the white matter is vacuolated, sparing U-fibers, as indicated by Ryan and colleagues, with an appearance that some authors have indicated simulates the spongiform change of prion disease. The pathophysiology is unknown but adulterants or mitochondrial damage has been suggested.

A similar leukoencephalopathy has also been reported in cocaine users, although a hypertensive encephalopathy or an adrenergic-induced vasculopathy may have played a role in these cases.

Damage to single peripheral nerves at the site of injection of heroin and from compression is a relatively common occurrence. However, bilateral compression of the sciatic nerves, the result of sitting or lying for a prolonged period in a stuporous state or in the lotus position, has occurred in several of our patients. In sciatic compression of this type, the peroneal branch has been more affected than the tibial, causing foot-drop with less weakness of plantar flexion. More difficult to understand in heroin abusers is the involvement of other individual nerves, particularly the radial nerve, and painful affection of the brachial plexus, apparently unrelated to compression and remote from the sites of injection. Possibly in some instances there was a vasculitis affecting peripheral nerves.

An acute generalized *myonecrosis* with myoglobinuria and renal failure has been ascribed to the intravenous injection of adulterated heroin. Brawny edema and fibrosing myopathy (Volkmann contracture) are the sequelae of venous thrombosis resulting from the administration of heroin and its adulterants by the intramuscular and subcutaneous routes. Occasionally, there may be massive swelling of an extremity into which heroin had been injected subcutaneously or intramuscularly; infection and venous thrombosis appears to be involved in its causation.

The diagnosis of drug addiction always raises the possibility of an assortment of infectious complications: AIDS, syphilis, abscesses and cellulitis at injection sites, septic thrombophlebitis, hepatitis, and periarteritis from circulating immune complexes. Tetanus, endocarditis (mainly caused by *Staphylococcus aureus*), spinal epidural abscess, meningitis, brain abscess, and tuberculosis have occurred less frequently.

SEDATIVE-HYPNOTIC DRUGS

This class of drugs consists of two main groups. The first includes the barbiturates, meprobamate, and chloral hydrate. These drugs are now little used, having been largely replaced by a second group, the *benzodiazepines*, the most important of which are chlordiazepoxide (Librium), lorazepam (Ativan), alprazolam (Xanax), clonazepam (Klonopin), and diazepam (Valium). Closely related are the nonbenzodiazepine hypnotics, typified by zolpidem. The advantages of the benzodiazepine drugs are their *relatively* low toxicity and addictive potential and their minimal interactions with other drugs.

Barbiturates

In the past, about 50 barbiturates were marketed for clinical use, but now only a few are encountered with any regularity: pentobarbital (Nembutal), secobarbital (Seconal), amobarbital (Amytal), thiopental (Pentothal), and phenobarbital. The first three were the ones most commonly abused. Barbiturates are also a component of combination preparations for the treatment of migraine (e.g., butalbital in Fiorinal).

Mechanism of Action

All the common barbiturates are derived from barbituric acid; the differences among them depend on variations in the side chains of the parent molecule. The potency of each drug is a function of the ionization constant and lipid solubility. The higher its lipid solubility, the greater the drug's central nervous system potency and the quicker and briefer its action. The lowering of plasma pH increases the rate of entry of the ionized form into the brain. The action of barbiturates is to suppress neuronal transmission, presumably by enhancing GABA inhibition at pre- and postsynaptic receptor sites, and to reduce excitatory postsynaptic potentials. The major points of action in the CNS are similar to those of alcohol and other coma-producing drugs; impaired consciousness or coma relates to inactivation of neurons in the reticular formation of the upper brainstem. The liver is the main locus of drug metabolism and the kidney is the method of elimination of the metabolites. The clinical problems posed by the barbiturates are different depending on whether the intoxication is acute or chronic.

Acute Barbiturate Intoxication

The symptoms and signs vary with the type and amount of drug as well as with the length of time that has elapsed since it was ingested. Pentobarbital and secobarbital produce their effects quickly and recovery is relatively rapid. Phenobarbital induces coma more slowly and its effects tend to be prolonged. In the case of long-acting barbiturates, such as phenobarbital and barbital, the hypnotic-sedative effect lasts 6 h or more after an average oral dose; with the intermediate-acting drugs such as amobarbital, 3 to 6 h; and with the short-acting drugs, secobarbital and pentobarbital, less than 3 h. Most fatalities follow the ingestion of secobarbital, amobarbital, or pentobarbital. The ingestion by adults of more than 3 g of these drugs at one time will prove fatal unless intensive treatment is applied promptly. The potentially fatal dose of phenobarbital is 6 to 10 g. The lowest plasma concentration associated with lethal overdosage of phenobarbital or barbital has been approximately 60 mg/mL and that of amobarbital and pentobarbital, 10 mg/mL.

Severe intoxication occurs with the ingestion of 10 to 20 times the oral hypnotic dose. The patient cannot be roused by any means, i.e., the patient is comatose. Respiration is slow and shallow or irregular, and pulmonary edema and cyanosis may be present. The tendon reflexes are usually, but not invariably, absent. Most patients show no response to plantar stimulation, but in those who do, the responses are extensor. With deep coma, the corneal and gag reflexes may also be abolished. Ordinarily the pupillary light reflex is retained in severe intoxication and is lost only if the patient is asphyxiated; but in advanced cases, the pupils become miotic and poorly reactive, simulating opiate intoxication. At this point respiration is greatly depressed and oculocephalic and oculovestibular reflex responses are usually abolished. In the early hours of coma, there may be a phase of flexor or extensor posturing or rigidity of the limbs, hyperactive reflexes, ankle clonus, and extensor plantar signs; persistence of these signs indicates that anoxic damage has been added. The temperature may be subnormal, the pulse is faint and rapid, and the blood pressure is greatly reduced. Failure of respiration to quicken on painful stimulation is an ominous sign.

There are few conditions other than barbiturate intoxication that cause a flaccid coma with small reactive pupils, hypothermia, and hypotension. A pontine hemorrhage may do so, but a hysterical trance or catatonic stupor does not present a problem in differential diagnosis. The use of gas and high-pressure liquid chromatography provides a reliable means of identifying the type and amount of barbiturate in the blood. A patient who has also ingested alcohol may be comatose with relatively low blood barbiturate concentrations. Contrariwise, the barbiturate addict may show only mild signs of intoxication with very high blood barbiturate concentrations.

Management In mild or moderate intoxication, recovery is the rule and special treatment is not required except to prevent aspiration. If the patient is unresponsive, special measures must be taken to maintain respiration and prevent infection. An endotracheal tube should be inserted, with suctioning as necessary. Any risk of respiratory depression or underventilation requires the use of a positive-pressure respirator.

Hemodialysis or hemofiltration with charcoal may be used in comatose patients who have ingested long-acting barbiturates and these treatments are particularly advisable if anuria or uremia has developed. Occasionally, in the case of a barbiturate addict who has taken an overdose of the drug, recovery from coma is followed by the development of abstinence symptoms, as described later.

Barbiturate Abstinence, or Withdrawal, Syndrome

Immediately following withdrawal, the patient seemingly improves over a period of 8 to 12 h, as the symptoms of intoxication diminish. Then a new group of symptoms develops, consisting of nervousness, tremor, insomnia, postural hypotension, and weakness. With chronic phenobarbital or barbital intoxication, withdrawal symptoms may not become apparent until 48 to 72 h after the final dose or it does not occur at all because of the slow metabolism and long half-life of these drugs. Generalized seizures with loss of consciousness may occur, usually between the second and fourth days of abstinence, but occasionally as long as 6 or 7 days after withdrawal. There may be a single seizure, several seizures, or, rarely, status epilepticus. Characteristically, in the withdrawal period, there is a greatly heightened sensitivity to photic stimulation, to which the patient responds with myoclonus or a seizure accompanied by paroxysmal changes in the EEG. The convulsive phase may be followed directly by a delusional-hallucinatory state or, as occurred in one of our cases (Romero et al), a full-blown delirium indistinguishable from delirium tremens. Death has been reported under these circumstances. The abstinence syndrome may occur in varying degrees of completeness; some patients have seizures and recover without developing delirium, and others have a delirium without preceding seizures.

Chloral Hydrate

This is the oldest and one of the safest, most effective, and most inexpensive of the sedative-hypnotic drugs. After oral administration, chloral hydrate is reduced rapidly to trichloroethanol, which is responsible for the depressant effects on the CNS. A significant portion of the trichloroethanol is excreted in the urine as the glucuronide, which may give a false-positive test for glucose.

Tolerance and addiction to chloral hydrate develop only rarely; for this reason, it was in the past commonly used for insomnia. Poisoning with chloral hydrate is a rare occurrence and resembles acute barbiturate intoxication except for the finding of miosis, which is said to characterize the former. Treatment follows along the same lines as for barbiturate poisoning. Death from poisoning is because of respiratory depression and hypotension; patients who survive may show signs of liver and kidney disease. Combining alcohol and chloral hydrate, the popular "Mickey-Finn" of detective stories in the mid-last century, produced severe intoxication and amnesia.

Paraldehyde, another member of this group of sedative drugs, is no longer being manufactured in the United States, and chloral hydrate is now available mainly as an elixir for pediatric use.

Benzodiazepines

With the introduction of chlordiazepoxide in 1960 and the benzodiazepine drugs that followed (particularly diazepam), the older sedative drugs (barbiturates, paraldehyde, chloral hydrate) have become virtually obsolete. Indeed, the benzodiazepines are among the most commonly prescribed drugs in the world today. According to Hollister (1990), 15 percent of all adults in the United States use a benzodiazepine at least once yearly and about half this number use the drug for a month or longer.

The benzodiazepines have been prescribed frequently for the treatment of anxiety and insomnia, and they are especially effective when the anxiety symptoms are severe. Also, they have been used to control overactivity and destructive behavior in children and the symptoms of alcohol withdrawal in adults. Diazepam is particularly useful in the treatment of delirious patients who require parenteral medication. The benzodiazepines possess anticonvulsant properties, and the intravenous use of diazepam, lorazepam, and midazolam is an effective means of controlling status epilepticus, as described in Chap. 16. Diazepam in massive doses has been used with considerable success in the management of muscle spasm in tetanus and in the "stiff man" syndrome (see Chap. 50). Alprazolam has a central place in the treatment of panic attacks and other anxiety states, and as an adjunct in some depressive illnesses. It seems, however, to create more dependence than some of the others in its class.

Other important benzodiazepine drugs are lorazepam (Ativan), flurazepam (Dalmane), triazolam (Halcion), clorazepate (Tranxene), temazepam (Restoril), oxazepam (Serax), alprazolam (Xanax) and other newer varieties, all widely used in the treatment of insomnia (see Chap. 19), and clonazepam (Klonopin), which is useful in the treatment of myoclonic seizures (see Chap. 16) and intention myoclonus (see Chaps. 6 and 40). Midazolam (Versed), a short-acting parenteral agent, is given frequently to achieve the brief sedation required for procedures such as MRI or endoscopy and is useful in the treatment of status epilepticus. Many other benzodiazepine compounds have appeared in recent years, but a clear advantage over the original ones remains to be demonstrated (Hollister, 1990).

The benzodiazepine drugs, like barbiturates, have a depressant action on the CNS by binding to specific receptors on GABA inhibitory systems. The newer nonbenzodiazepine sleeping medication differs from the benzodiazepines structurally but is pharmacologically similar in binding to similar gabaergic receptors. The benzodiazepines act in concert with GABA to open chloride ion channels and hyperpolarize postsynaptic neurons and reduce their firing rate. The primary sites of their action are the cerebral cortex and limbic system, which accounts for their anticonvulsant and anxiolytic effects.

While quite safe in the recommended dosages, they are far from ideal. They frequently cause unsteadiness of gait and drowsiness and at times syncope, confusion, and impairment of memory, especially in the elderly. If taken in large doses, the benzodiazepines can depress the state of consciousness, resembling that of other sedative-hypnotic drugs, but with less respiratory suppression and hypotension.

Flumazenil, a specific pharmacologic antagonist of the CNS effects of benzodiazepines, rapidly but briefly reverses most of the symptoms and signs of benzodiazepine overdose. It acts by binding to CNS diazepine receptors and thereby blocking the activation of inhibitory gabanergic synapses. Flumazenil also may be diagnostically useful in cases of coma of unknown etiology and in hepatic encephalopathy.

Signs of physical dependence and true addiction, although relatively rare, undoubtedly occur in chronic benzodiazepine users, even in those taking therapeutic doses. The withdrawal symptoms are much the same as those that follow the chronic use of other sedative drugs (anxiety, jitteriness, insomnia, seizures) but may not appear until the third day after the cessation of the drug and may not reach their peak of severity until the fifth day (Hollister, 1990). In chronic benzodiazepine users, the gradual tapering of dosage over a period of 1 to 2 weeks minimizes the withdrawal effects. However, we have observed numerous cases over the years in which the cessation of moderate doses of chronically used diazepines has resulted in one or more seizures. This is likely to happen when the patient is hospitalized for other reasons and the accustomed sleeping or anxiolytic medication is omitted.

Buspirone

A class of antianxiety agents, exemplified by the selective 5-HT_{1A} receptor serotonergic agonist buspirone, is chemically and pharmacologically different from the benzodiazepines, barbiturates, and other sedatives. Its distinctive nature is confirmed by the observation that it does not block the withdrawal syndrome of other sedative-hypnotic drugs. Because of its apparently reduced potential for abuse and tolerance, it is not included in the list of controlled pharmaceutical substances in the United States but adverse interactions with monoamine oxidase (MAO) inhibitors are known. Its use with other psychotropic drugs is still under investigation (see Chap. 52).

ANTIPSYCHOSIS DRUGS

In the mid-1950s, a large series of pharmacologic agents, originally referred to as tranquilizers (later, as psychotropic or neuroleptic drugs), came into prominent use, mainly for the control of schizophrenia, psychotic states associated with "organic brain syndromes," and affective disorders (depression and bipolar disease). The mechanisms by which these drugs ameliorate disturbances of thought and affect in psychotic states are not fully understood, but presumably they act by blocking the postsynaptic mesolimbic dopamine receptors of which there are four subtypes, termed D1 through D4 on neuronal membranes (see Table 4-2, and discussion of dopamine receptor subtypes). The D2 receptors are located mainly in the frontal cortex, hippocampus, and limbic cortex, and the D1 receptors are in the striatum, as discussed in Chap. 4. The blockade of dopamine receptors in the striatum is probably responsible for the parkinsonian side effects of this entire class of drugs, and the blockade of another dopaminergic (tuberoinfundibular) system, for the increased prolactin secretion by the pituitary. These drugs also produce some adrenergic blocking effect. The newer "atypical" antipsychotic drugs, exemplified by clozapine, apparently achieve the same degree of D2 and D3 blockade in the temporal and limbic lobes while exhibiting substantially less antagonistic activity in the striatum—accounting also for their lesser parkinsonian side effects. These drugs also block subsets of serotonin receptors.

Since the introduction in the 1950s of the phenothiazine chlorpromazine as an anesthetic agent and the serendipitous discovery of its antipsychotic effect on schizophrenia, a large number of antipsychotic drugs have been marketed for clinical use. No attempt is made here to describe or even list all of them. Some have had only an evanescent popularity and others have yet to prove their value. Chemically, these compounds form a heterogeneous group. Eight classes of them are of particular clinical importance: (1) the phenothiazines; (2) the thioxanthenes; (3) the butyrophenones; (4) the rauwolfias alkaloids; (5) an indole derivative, loxapine, and a unique dihydroindolone, molindone; (6) a diphenylbutylpiperidine, pimozide; (7) dibenzodiazepines, typified by clozapine and olanzapine; and (8) a benzisoxazole derivative, risperidone. Molindone and loxapine are about as effective as the phenothiazines in the management of schizophrenia and their side effects are similar, although claims have been made that they are less likely to induce tardive dyskinesias and seizures. Their main use is in patients who are not responsive to the older drugs or who suffer intolerable side effects from them.

The antipsychotic agents in the class of clozapine (which is less used than other agents in the class because of cases of aplastic anemia) have attracted great interest, because—as already mentioned—they are associated with relatively fewer extrapyramidal side effects. For this reason, they are particularly favored in controlling the confusion and psychosis of parkinsonian patients. The other new class of drugs, of which risperidone is the main example, also has fewer extrapyramidal side effects than the phenothiazines and a more rapid onset of action than the traditional antipsychotic medications. All of these newer medications produce the "metabolic syndrome" of weight gain, adverse lipid changes, and glucose intolerance. Pimozide may be useful in the treatment of haloperidol-refractory cases of Gilles de la Tourette syndrome (see Chap. 6); its main danger is its tendency to produce cardiac arrhythmias.

Phenothiazines

This group comprises chlorpromazine (Thorazine), promazine (Sparine), triflupromazine (Vesprin), prochlorperazine (Compazine), perphenazine (Trilafon), fluphenazine (Permitil, Prolixin), thioridazine (Mellaril), mesoridazine (Serentil), and trifluoperazine (Stelazine). In addition to their psychotherapeutic effects, these drugs have a number of other actions, so that certain members of this group are used as antiemetics (prochlorperazine) and antihistaminics (promethazine).

The phenothiazines have had their widest application in the treatment of the major psychoses, namely schizophrenia and, to a lesser extent, bipolar psychosis. Under the influence of these drugs, many patients who would otherwise have been hospitalized were able to live at home and even work productively. In the hospital, the use of these drugs has facilitated the care of hyperactive, delirious, and combative patients (see Chaps. 52 and 53 for details of this clinical use).

Side effects of the phenothiazines are frequent and often serious. All of them may cause a cholestatic type of jaundice, agranulocytosis, seizures, orthostatic hypotension, skin sensitivity reactions, mental depression, and, most importantly, immediate or delayed extrapyramidal motor disorders. The neuroleptic malignant syndrome is the most extreme complication and is discussed separately further on and in Chap. 53. The following types of extrapyramidal symptoms, also discussed in Chap. 6, have been noted in association with all of the phenothiazines as well as the butyrophenones, and to a lesser extent with metoclopramide and pimozide, which block dopaminergic receptors. These are summarized in Table 53-1.

1. A *parkinsonian syndrome* is the most common complication—masked facies, slight symmetric tremor, reduced blinking, generalized rigidity, shuffling gait, and slowness of movement. These symptoms may appear after several days of drug therapy but more often after several weeks. Suppression of dopamine in the striatum (similar to the effect of loss of dopaminergic nigral cells that project to the striatum) is presumably the basis of the parkinsonian signs.
2. *Acute dyskinetic and dystonic reactions*, taking the form of involuntary movements of lower facial muscles (mainly around the mouth) and protrusion of the tongue (buccolingual or oral-masticatory syndrome), dysphagia, torticollis and retrocollis, oculogyric crises, and tonic spasms of a limb. These complications usually occur early in the course of administration of the drug, sometimes after the initial dose, in which case they recede dramatically upon immediate discontinuation of the drug and the intravenous administration of diphenhydramine hydrochloride or benztropine.
3. *Akathisia*, which is an inner restlessness reflected by a persistent shifting of the body and feet and an inability to sit still, such that the patient paces the floor or jiggles the legs constantly (see Chap. 6). Of all the phenothiazines, molindone has a tendency to cause akathisia. This disorder often responds to oral propranolol.
4. *Tardive dyskinesias* are a group of *late and persistent complications* of neuroleptic therapy, which may continue after removal of the offending drug, that comprises lingual-facial-buccal-cervical dyskinesias, choreoathetotic and dystonic movements of the trunk and limbs, diffuse myoclonus (rare), perioral tremor ("rabbit" syndrome), and dysarthria or anarthria. Snyder postulated that the movements are because of hypersensitivity of dopamine receptors in the basal ganglia, secondary to prolonged blockade of the receptors by antipsychotic medication. Baldessarini estimates that as many as 40 percent of patients receiving long-term antipsychotic medication develop tardive dyskinesia of some degree. The effect is likely a result of subcellular pathophysiologic alterations in the basal ganglia. Treatment is discussed later.
5. The *neuroleptic malignant syndrome* is discussed separately later because of its gravity and requirement for specific treatment.

Butyrophenones

Haloperidol (Haldol) is the only member of this group approved for use as an antipsychotic in the United States. It has much the same therapeutic effects as the phenothiazines in the management of acute psychoses and shares the same side effects as the phenothiazines, but exhibits little or no adrenergic blocking action. It is an effective substitute for the phenothiazines in patients who are intolerant of the latter drugs, particularly of their autonomic effects. It is also one of the main drugs for the treatment of Gilles de la Tourette syndrome (the other being pimozide; see Chap. 6) and the movement disorder of Huntington chorea.

Treatment of Neuroleptic Side Effects

As indicated earlier, acute dystonic spasms usually respond to cessation of the offending drug and to the administration of diphenhydramine. Administration of antiparkinsonian drugs of the anticholinergic type (trihexyphenidyl, procyclidine, and benztropine) may hasten recovery from some of the acute symptoms. The purely parkinsonian syndrome usually improves as well, but the tardive dyskinesias stand apart because they may persist for months or years and may be permanent.

Oral, lingual, and laryngeal dyskinesias of the tardive type are affected relatively little by any antiparkinsonian drugs. Amantadine in doses of 50 to 100 mg tid has been useful in a few of the cases of postphenothiazine dyskinesia. Other drugs such as benztropine have been tried in the treatment of regional and more generalized tardive dyskinesia with uncertain results. Nevertheless, there is a tendency for most of the obstinate forms to subside slowly even after several years of unsuccessful therapy. Once a tardive syndrome has been identified, several authoritative clinicians recommend a gradual reduction in the dose of the antipsychosis medication to the minimum necessary for the control of psychotic symptoms. Some reports favor the substitution of one of the newer "atypical" antipsychotic medications but no systematic study of their effectiveness has been undertaken.

For severe and recalcitrant cases, particularly those involving axial dystonias and similar disabling features, Fahn recommends administration of the dopamine-depleting drug tetrabenazine (similar but faster in action and less toxic than reserpine). This medication is given in doses of 75 to 300 mg/d. Jankovic and Beach report an 83 percent success rate using this approach for tardive dyskinesias. The medication is not easily available in the United States.

Neuroleptic Malignant Syndrome

This is the most dreaded complication of phenothiazine and haloperidol use; rare instances have been reported after the institution or the withdrawal of L-dopa and similar dopaminergic agents, as well as a few instances reported with the newer antipsychosis drugs. Its incidence has been calculated to be only 0.2 percent of all patients receiving neuroleptics (Caroff and Mann) but its seriousness is underscored by a mortality rate of 15 to 30 percent if not recognized and treated promptly. It may occur days, weeks, or months after neuroleptic treatment is begun.

The syndrome consists of hyperthermia, rigidity, stupor, unstable blood pressure, diaphoresis, and other signs of sympathetic overactivity, high serum creatine kinase (CK) values (up to 60,000 units), and, in some cases, renal failure because of myoglobinuria. The syndrome was first observed in patients treated with haloperidol, but since then other neuroleptic drugs have been incriminated, particularly the highly potent thioxanthene derivatives and the phenothiazines—chlorpromazine, fluphenazine, and thioridazine—but also, on rare occasions, the less potent drugs that are used to control nausea, such as promethazine. It has become evident that the newer antipsychotic drugs, and specifically olanzapine, are also capable of inducing the syndrome but the risk in comparison to the first generation of antipsychotic drugs has not been established.

If treatment of the neuroleptic malignant syndrome is started early, when consciousness is first altered and the temperature is rising, bromocriptine in oral doses of 5 mg tid (up to 20 mg tid) will terminate the condition in a few hours. If oral medication can no longer be taken because of the patient's condition, dantrolene, 0.25 to 3.0 mg intravenously, may be lifesaving. Once coma has supervened, shock and anuria may prove fatal or leave the patient in a vegetative state. The rigors during high fever may cause muscle damage and myoglobinuria, and shock may lead to hypoxic-ischemic brain injury.

One pitfall is to mistake neuroleptic malignant syndrome for worsening of the psychosis and inadvisably administer more antipsychosis medication. Meningitis, heat stroke, lithium intoxication, catatonia, malignant hyperthermia, and acute dystonic reactions figure in the differential diagnosis. Of course, neuroleptic medication must be discontinued as soon as any of the severe extrapyramidal reactions are recognized. It has been common practice to avoid future administration of the offending neuroleptic but the risk of using another class of antipsychotic agents has not been fully addressed.

The neuroleptic malignant syndrome bears an uncertain relationship to *malignant hyperthermia* by way of its clinical aspects but also in its response to bromocriptine and dantrolene (see later). Malignant hyperthermia in susceptible individuals is triggered by inhalation anesthetics and skeletal muscle relaxants (see Chap. 53). This disorder was described before the introduction of neuroleptic drugs, and in a small proportion of cases, has been related to a mutation of the ryanodine receptor gene. A genetic factor may underlie a small number of cases of the neuroleptic malignant syndrome (a polymorphism in the D2 receptor gene; see Suzuki et al) possibly provoked by fatigue and dehydration. There is no evidence that the occurrence of one of these syndromes confers a susceptibility to the other.

ANTIDEPRESSION MEDICATIONS

Four classes of drugs—the MAO inhibitors, the tricyclic compounds, the serotonergic drugs, and lithium—are particularly useful in the treatment of depressive illnesses. The adjective *antidepressant* refers to their therapeutic effect and is employed here in deference to common clinical practice. *Antidepressive* or *antidepression* drugs would be preferable, as the term *depressant* still has a pharmacologic connotation that does not necessarily equate with the therapeutic effect.

Monoamine Oxidase Inhibitors

The observation that iproniazid, an inhibitor of MAO, had a mood-elevating effect in tuberculous patients initiated a great deal of interest in compounds of this type and led quickly to their exploitation in the treatment of depression. Iproniazid proved exceedingly toxic to the liver, as were several subsequently developed MAO inhibitors; but other drugs in this class, much better tolerated, are still available. These include isocarboxazid (Marplan), phenelzine (Nardil), and tranylcypromine (Parnate), the latter two being the more frequently used. Tranylcypromine, which bears a close chemical resemblance to dextroamphetamine, may produce unwanted stimulation, but the most common adverse effect of all the MAO inhibitors is postural hypotension. Also, interactions with a wide array of other drugs and ingested substances may induce severe hypertension.

Monoamine oxidase is located on the outer surface of the mitochondria in neurons and is used in the catabolism of catecholamines (Coyle). In the gut and liver, the isoenzyme MAO-A normally serves to deaminate phenethylamine, tyramine, and tryptamine—all of which are products of protein catabolism. Inhibition of MAO-A allows these dietary amines, which have an amphetamine-like action, to enter the systemic circulation in increased quantities, thus releasing norepinephrine from sympathetic nerve endings and increasing heart rate and blood pressure. Most antidepressant medications are of this class. Medications used in Parkinson disease (see Chap. 39) inhibit the MAO-B isoenzyme, which deaminates phenylethylamine and trace amines, with a correspondingly lower risk of causing hypertension.

More relevant to their action as antidepressants, the MAO inhibitors have in common the ability to block the intraneuronal oxidative deamination of naturally occurring amines (norepinephrine, epinephrine, dopamine, and serotonin) and it has been suggested that the accumulation of these substances is responsible for the antidepressant effect. However, many enzymes other than monoamine oxidase are inhibited by MAO inhibitors, and the latter drugs have numerous actions unrelated to enzyme inhibition. Furthermore, many agents with antidepressant effects like those of the MAO inhibitors do not inhibit MAO. Therefore, one cannot assume that the therapeutic effect of these drugs has a direct relation to MAO inhibition in the brain.

The MAO inhibitors must be dispensed with caution and awareness of their potentially serious side effects. They may at times cause excitement, restlessness, agitation, insomnia, and anxiety, occasionally with the usual dose but more often with an overdose. Mania and convulsions may occur (especially in epileptic patients). Other side effects are muscle twitching and involuntary movements, urinary retention, skin rashes, tachycardia, jaundice, visual impairment, enhancement of glaucoma, impotence, sweating, muscle spasms, paresthesias, and a serious degree of orthostatic hypotension.

Patients taking MAO-A inhibitors must be warned against the use of phenothiazines, CNS stimulants, and tricyclic and serotoninergic antidepressants (see later), as well as sympathomimetic amines and tyramine-containing foods. The combination of an MAO inhibitor and any of these drugs or amines may induce hypertension, atrial and ventricular arrhythmia, pulmonary edema, stroke, or death. Sympathomimetic amines are contained in some commonly used cold remedies, nasal sprays, nose drops, and certain foods—aged cheese, beer, red wine, pickled herring, sardines, sausages, and certain preserved meat or fish. Exaggerated responses to the usual dose of meperidine (Demerol) and other narcotic drugs have also been observed sporadically; in these cases, respiratory function may be depressed to a serious degree, and hyperpyrexia, agitation, and pronounced hypotension may occur as well, sometimes with fatal issue. Unpredictable side effects may also accompany the simultaneous administration of barbiturates and MAO inhibitors. The abrupt occurrence of severe occipital headache, nausea, vomiting, pupillary dilatation, or visual blurring should suggest a hypertensive crisis. Treatment is with intravenous phentolamine 5 mg, nitroprusside, labetalol, or a calcium channel blocker administered slowly to prevent hypotension. Overdosage of MAO inhibitors may lead to coma, for which there is no treatment other than supportive care.

The therapeutic use of MAO inhibitors for depression is discussed in Chaps. 51 and 52, and for Parkinson disease, in Chap. 39.

Tricyclic Antidepressants

Soon after the first successes with MAO inhibitors, another class of tricyclic compounds appeared. The mode of action of these agents is not fully understood, but there is evidence that they block the reuptake of amine neurotransmitters, both norepinephrine and serotonin. Blocking this amine pump mechanism (called the presynaptic plasma transporter), which ordinarily terminates synaptic transmission, permits the persistence of neurotransmitter substances in the synaptic cleft and does no more than support the hypothesis that endogenous depression is associated with a deficiency of noradrenergic or serotonergic transmission.

These medications have been divided into classes of tertiary amines (imipramine, amitriptyline and doxepin, trimipramine), which have activity as reuptake inhibitors of norepinephrine and serotonin, and the secondary amines (desipramine, amoxapine, maprotiline, nortriptyline, protriptyline), which have a preferential effect on reuptake of norepinephrine. Subsequently, a number of additional antidepressant drugs were introduced. A full account of these drugs, which will not be attempted here, can be found in the chapters by Baldessarini listed in the references.

The tricyclic antidepressants and the serotonergic drugs discussed in the next section, are presently the most effective drugs for the treatment of patients with depressive illnesses, the former being particularly useful for those with anergic depressions, early morning awakening, and decreased appetite and libido. The side effects of the tricyclic drugs are less frequent and far less serious than those of the MAO inhibitors.

The tricyclic compounds are also potent anticholinergic agents, which accounts for their most prominent and bothersome side effects—orthostatic hypotension, urinary bladder weakness, drowsiness, confusion, blurred vision, and dry mouth. They may also occasionally produce CNS excitation—leading to insomnia, agitation, and restlessness—but usually these effects are readily controlled by small doses of benzodiazepines given concurrently or in the evenings.

As indicated earlier, the tricyclic drugs should not be given with an MAO inhibitor; serious reactions have occurred when small doses of imipramine were given to patients who had discontinued the MAO in the previous days or week. Both the MAO inhibitors and the tricyclic antidepressants are dangerous drugs when taken in excess.

Tricyclic compounds are a cause of accidental poisoning and suicide of depressed patients. It is common for the intoxicated patient to have taken several drugs, in which case chemical analyses of the blood and urine are particularly helpful in determining the drugs involved and in sorting out therapeutic and toxic concentrations. Mortality from overdose is mostly a result of cardiac rhythm disturbances, particularly tachyarrhythmias, and impaired conduction (atrioventricular block). Treatment consists of gastric aspiration and instillation of activated charcoal and the addition of physostigmine to reverse serious arrhythmias; the short duration of action of physostigmine requires that frequent doses be given. Dialysis is of no value because of the low plasma concentrations of the drug.

Serotonin Reuptake Inhibitors and Related Drugs

The selective serotonin reuptake inhibitors (SSRIs) constitute a newer class of antidepressants; paroxetine (Paxil), fluoxetine (Prozac), and sertraline (Zoloft) are common examples but they continue to be developed at a rapid pace. Of the several related drugs such as venlafaxine (Effexor), nefazodone (Serzone), mirtazapine (Remeron), citalopram (Celexa), trazodone (Desyrel) and bupropion (Wellbutrin), each has a novel structure that is not analogous to that of the other categories of antidepressants. They are believed to act similarly to the SSRI class by inhibiting the reuptake of serotonin and norepinephrine. This results in a potentiation of the actions of these neurotransmitters.

Because they do not bind as avidly as tricyclic drugs to the muscarinic and adrenergic receptors in the brain, they produce fewer side effects, but some patients complain of anxiety or insomnia when they are first introduced. These drugs share the same side effects to varying degrees, including the danger of concomitant MAO inhibitor administration.

The risk of seizures related to the taking of certain of these medications has been much discussed. For the most part, the risk is quite small but there is little information to guide their use in known epileptics. Several studies suggest that the frequency of convulsions may increase in such patients. Bupropion has been particularly associated with seizures in about 0.5 percent of patients treated at higher dose levels (over 400 mg/d) and this drug should not be used in individuals with a history of seizures.

The SSRI drugs are well tolerated, may be effective in a shorter time than the tricyclic agents, and are very popular at the moment, but their long-term therapeutic usefulness in comparison with their predecessors remains to be determined (see review of Richelson). Fluoxetine has also been used with benefit in a group of autistic children (see "Course, Treatment, and Prognosis" under "Autism" in Chap. 38). Constipation, dry mouth, and reduced sexual potency are to be expected to some, but varying degrees. Hyponatremia is a rare complication.

Serotonin Syndrome

The symptoms of a "serotonin syndrome" that results from excessive intake of the above listed drugs or from the concurrent use of MAO inhibitors include confusion and restlessness, tremor, tachycardia, hypertension, clonus and hyperreflexia, shivering, and diaphoresis, as summarized by Boyer and Shannon. The long list of other medications, when used concurrently with SSRIs can produce the syndrome (including "triptans" for migraine), are noted in this reference.

The treatment is by discontinuation of the medication, reduction of temperature and hypertension, benzodiazepines to control agitation, and in severe cases, the addition of cyproheptadine, a 5-HT_{2A} receptor blocker. The typical dose is 4 to 8 mg every 4 to 6 h (or a higher initial dose); tablets are crushed and administered by nasogastric tube. Atypical antipsychosis agents with similar serotonin antagonist activity have also been used as treatment (olanzapine, chlorpromazine).

Lithium

The discovery of the therapeutic effects of lithium salts in mania has led to its widespread use in the treatment of bipolar disease (bipolar disorder). The drug has proved relatively safe and blood levels are easily monitored. Its value is much more certain in treatment of the manic phase of bipolar disorder and prevention of recurrences of cyclic mood shifts than it is in treatment of anxiety and depression. Guidelines for the clinical use of lithium are given in Chap. 52. Its mechanism of action is unclear but there is experimental evidence that lithium blocks the stimulus-induced release of norepinephrine and dopamine and enhances the reuptake of this amine—the opposite in a sense, of what occurs with the other classes of antidepressants.

With blood levels of lithium in the upper therapeutic range (therapeutic 0.6 to 1.2 mEq/L), it is not uncommon to observe a fast-frequency action tremor or asterixis, together with nausea, loose stools, fatigue, polydipsia, and polyuria. These symptoms usually subside with time. Above a level of 1.5 to 2 mEq/L, particularly in patients with impaired renal function or in those taking a thiazide diuretic, serious intoxication becomes manifest—clouding of consciousness, confusion, delirium, dizziness, nystagmus, ataxia, stammering, diffuse myoclonic twitching, and nephrogenic diabetes insipidus. Vertical (downbeating) nystagmus and opsoclonus (see Chap. 14) may also be prominent. A variety of skin problems is common including worsening of acne vulgaris. An uncommon toxic effect is the development of goiter but most patients remain euthyroid although the thyroid-stimulating hormone (TSH) levels may increase slightly. The goiter usually requires no treatment but it is possible to administer thyroid hormone so as to cause the thyroid enlargement to regress.

The myoclonic state, particularly when combined with confusion and sharp waves in the EEG, may mimic Creutzfeldt-Jakob disease (see Chap. 33) but there should be no problem in diagnosis if the setting of the illness and the administration of lithium are known. At blood lithium concentrations above 3.5 mEq/L, these symptoms are replaced by stupor and coma, sometimes with convulsions, and may prove fatal.

Discontinuing lithium in the intoxicated patient, which is the initial step in therapy, does not result in immediate disappearance of toxic symptoms. This may be delayed by a week or two, and the diabetes insipidus may persist even longer. Fluids, sodium chloride, aminophylline, and acetazolamide promote the excretion of lithium. Lithium coma may require hemodialysis, which has proved to be the most rapid means of reducing the blood lithium concentration.

STIMULANTS

Drugs that act primarily as CNS stimulants assume clinical importance for several reasons, mainly in their use for sleep disorders and attention deficit disorder. Some members of this group, the amphetamines, are much abused and others are not infrequent causes of poisoning. Their main mechanism of action is the release of endogenous catecholamine from vesicles in the presynaptic terminals.

Amphetamines and Related Agents

The *amphetamines (d-amphetamine, d,l-amphetamine, pemoline, methamphetamine, methylphenidate)* are analeptics (CNS stimulants) and in addition have significant hypertensive, respiratory-stimulant, and appetite-depressant effects. They are effective in the management of narcolepsy but have been more widely and sometimes indiscriminately used for the control of obesity, the abolition of fatigue, and the treatment of hyperactivity in children (see Chap. 37 for full discussion). Undoubtedly, they are able to reverse fatigue, postpone the need for sleep, and elevate mood but these effects are not entirely predictable and the user must compensate for the period of wakefulness with even greater fatigue and often with depression that follows. The intravenous use of a high dose of amphetamine produces an immediate feeling of ecstasy.

Because of the popularity of the amphetamines and the ease with which they can be procured, instances of acute and chronic intoxication are frequently seen. Methamphetamine is the most frequently abused in this category, as intravenous "crystal" or smoked as "ice." The toxic signs are essentially an exaggeration of the activating effects—restlessness, excessive speech and motor activity, tremor, and insomnia. Severe intoxication gives rise to hallucinations, delusions, and changes in affect and thought processes—a state that may be indistinguishable from paranoid schizophrenia. An amphetamine-associated vasculopathy and intracerebral and subarachnoid hemorrhage are well recognized but rare complications of chronic or acute intoxication (Harrington et al and Chap. 34). Similar cerebrovascular complications may appear with sympathomimetic agents contained in over-the-counter cold medications and in dieting aids. Phenylpropanolamine has been implicated most often but ephedrine, cocaine (see below), and similar agents rarely have the same effects and induce a vasculopathy. The pathogenesis of the vascular lesion is unknown (both vasospasm and arteritis have been reported).

Chronic use of amphetamines can lead to a high degree of tolerance and psychologic dependence. Withdrawal of the drug after sustained oral or intravenous use is regularly followed by a period of prolonged sleep (a disproportionate amount of which is rapid eye movement [REM] sleep), from which the patient awakens with a ravenous appetite, muscle pains, and feelings of profound fatigue and depression. Treatment consists of discontinuing the use of amphetamine and administering antipsychosis drugs. Hypertension may need to be treated until the effect of the drug has waned.

Cocaine

The conventional use of cocaine as a local anesthetic has for many years been overshadowed by its illicit and widespread use as a stimulant and mood elevator. Cocaine is abused intranasally ("snorted"), smoked, or injected intravenously or intramuscularly. There has been an alarming escalation in the use of cocaine, mainly because a relatively pure and inexpensive form of the free alkaloid base ("crack") became readily available in the 1980s. This form of cocaine is heat-stable and therefore suitable for smoking. According to the National Household Survey on Drug Abuse, there are an estimated 600,000 frequent cocaine users in the United States. (Frequent use was arbitrarily defined as use on 51 or more days during the preceding year.) The number of occasional users (less than 12 days in the preceding year) was 2.4 million. These figures are probably subject to significant underreporting.

A sense of well-being, euphoria, loquacity, and restlessness are the familiar effects. Pharmacologically, cocaine is thought to act like the tricyclic antidepressants; i.e., it blocks the presynaptic reuptake of biogenic amines, thus producing vasoconstriction, hypertension, and tachycardia and predisposing to generalized tremor, myoclonus, seizures, and psychotic behavior. It has an additional weaker action, similar to amphetamines, of causing the release of endogenous monoamines. The cocaine abuser readily develops psychologic dependence and habituation, i.e., an inability to abstain from frequent compulsive use. The manifestations of physical dependence are more subtle and difficult to recognize. Nevertheless, abstinence from cocaine following a period of chronic abuse is regularly attended by insomnia, restlessness, anorexia, depression, hyperprolactinemia, and signs of dopaminergic hypersensitivity—a symptom complex that constitutes an identifiable withdrawal syndrome.

With the increasingly widespread use of cocaine, a variety of new complications continues to emerge. The symptoms of severe intoxication (overdose), noted above, may lead to coma and death and require emergency treatment in an intensive care unit, along the lines indicated for the management of other forms of coma. Seizures often occur in this setting and are treated more effectively with benzodiazepines than with standard anticonvulsant drugs. Spontaneous subarachnoid or intracerebral hemorrhage and cerebral infarction have rarely followed the intranasal use and smoking of cocaine (Levine et al). These complications could be the result of acute hypertension induced by the sympathomimetic actions of cocaine and the incidence of vascular malformations appears to be higher in those patients who have a cerebral hemorrhage (see Chap. 34). Cocaine and amphetamines also, on occasion, produce a state of generalized vasospasm leading to multiple cortical infarctions and posterior white matter changes that are evident on imaging studies, essentially a form of hypertensive encephalopathy (see Chap. 34). Roth and colleagues have described 39 patients who developed acute rhabdomyolysis after cocaine use; 13 of these had acute renal failure, severe liver dysfunction, and disseminated intravascular coagulation and 6 of them died. Some reports indicate that cocaine use during pregnancy may cause fetal damage, abortion, or persistent signs of toxicity in the newborn infant.

Anxiety, paranoia, and other manifestations of psychosis may develop within several hours of cocaine use. These complications are best treated with antipsychosis drugs, particularly haloperidol.

Khat and Cathionine Stimulants

The psychostimulant khat is used widely in certain countries, mainly in the Far East. The khat leaf is chewed to release cathionine that produces euphoria by an amphetamine-like effect. A chemically designed congener, the *N*-methyl analog of cathionine, or methcathinone ("Jeff," "Cat," "mulka," and other street names), is manufactured from over-the-counter cold medications such as ephedrine, pseudoephedrine, and phenylpropanolamine and is frequently abused. In Russia and some other countries, potassium permanganate is used to reduce the basic substances and is a source of a manganese-induced extrapyramidal syndrome. Furthermore, entirely synthetic cathinones, often called "bath salts," although they have no relation to that original product, are amphetamine-like substances that are taken orally or nasally and produce rapid activation of behavior and sympathetic hyperactivity.

HALLUCINOGENS

Included in this category is a heterogeneous group of drugs, the primary effect of which is to alter perception, mood, and thinking out of proportion to other aspects of cognitive function and consciousness. This group of drugs comprises lysergic acid diethylamide (LSD), *phenylethylamine derivatives* (mescaline or peyote), *psilocybin, certain indolic derivatives, cannabis* (marijuana), *phencyclidine* (PCP), and a number of less important compounds. They are also referred to as psychoactive or psychotomimetic drugs or as hallucinogens and psychedelics. The problems raised by the nontherapeutic use of these drugs, which has declined somewhat but is still of serious proportions, have been reviewed by Nicholi and by Verebey and their associates.

Marijuana

During the past three decades, the prevalence of marijuana use in the United States has declined by about half but it is still the most commonly used illicit drug in the United States. The effects, when taken by inhaling the smoke from cigarettes or pipe, are prompt in onset and evanescent. With low doses, the symptoms are like those of mild alcohol intoxication (drowsiness, euphoria, dulling of the senses, and perceptual distortions). With increasing amounts, the effects are similar to those of LSD, mescaline, and psilocybin (see later); they may be quite disabling for many hours. With even larger doses, severe depression and stupor may occur, but death is rare (for a full account, see Hollister [1988]). No damage to the nervous system has been found after chronic use.

As summarized by Iverson, this agent activates the CB_1 receptor, mainly on gabanergic neurons in the hippocampus, amygdala, and cortex. Activation of the receptor inhibits the release of oligopeptide neurotransmitters and monoamines. They also have complex electrophysiologic effects on neurons.

Reverse tolerance to marijuana (i.e., increasing sensitization) may be observed initially, but on continued use, tolerance to the euphoriant effects develops. In one of the few experimental studies of chronic marijuana use, the subjects reported feeling "jittery" during the first 24 h after abrupt cessation of smoking marijuana, although no objective withdrawal signs could be detected. Chronic intoxicated users demonstrate reduced cognitive performance, but according to Iverson, a persistent cognitive decline has not been shown definitely.

The mild antiemetic effects of marijuana coupled with euphoria have led to its use. Putative effects on spasticity and on neuropathic pain have not been adequately substantiated.

Synthetic Cannabinoids

With the cathionines discussed above, this is a new class of synthetic drugs; they go by the names of "Spice," "K2," " K4," and others. These agents bind even more avidly to cannabinoid receptors than does the original drug and produce a heightened stimulant effect. Agitation, delusions, and paranoia result, a veritable psychosis, and some patients we have admitted have been physically almost uncontrollable, only to awaken and have entirely normal affect and cognition. Because the synthetic agents are chemically quite different from cannabis, they do not appear on conventional toxicology-drug screens. Treatment of intoxication is by diazepines and haloperidol but often to little avail until the drug is metabolized.

Mescaline, LSD, and Psilocybin

These drugs produce much the same clinical effects if given in comparable amounts. The perceptual changes are the most dramatic: the user describes vivid visual hallucinations, alterations in the shape and color of objects, unusual dreams, and feelings of depersonalization. An increase in auditory acuity has been described but auditory hallucinations are rare. Cognitive functions are difficult to assess because of inattention, drowsiness, and inability to cooperate in mental testing. The somatic symptoms consist of dizziness, nausea, paresthesia, and blurring of vision. Sympathomimetic effects—pupillary dilatation, piloerection, hyperthermia, and tachycardia—are prominent, and the user may also show hyperreflexia, incoordination of the limbs, and ataxia.

Tolerance to LSD, mescaline, and psilocybin develops rapidly, even on a once-daily dosage. Furthermore, subjects tolerant to any one of these three drugs are cross-tolerant to the other two. Tolerance is lost rapidly when the drugs are discontinued and no characteristic signs of physical dependence ensue. In this sense, addiction does not develop, although users may become psychologically dependent upon the drugs.

These drugs are taken by "drugheads" (a colorful term we have retained from the previous authors to describe individuals who use any agent that alters consciousness) and by many college and high school students for a way of socializing, for conformity, or for reasons that even they cannot ascertain. There is some evidence that marijuana is a "gateway" drug that engenders further experimentation with more dangerous substances.

The use of these drugs may be attended by a number of serious adverse reactions taking the form of acute panic attacks ("bad trip"), long-lasting psychotic states resembling paranoid schizophrenia, and flashbacks (spontaneous recurrences of the original LSD experience, sometimes precipitated by smoking marijuana and accompanied by panic attacks). Serious physical injury may follow upon impairment of the user's critical faculties. Numerous claims have been made that LSD and related drugs are effective in the treatment of mental disease and a wide variety of social ills, and that they have the capacity to increase one's intellectual performance, creativity, and self-understanding. To date, no acceptable studies validate any of these claims.

Phencyclidine ("Angel Dust") and "Ecstasy"

During the early 1970s, the abuse of phencyclidine (PCP) and its analogues was a significant problem. The popularity of these drugs has dropped, but some illicit use continues because they are relatively cheap, easily available, and quite potent. (Their manufacture as a veterinary anesthetic was stopped in 1979.) Phencyclidine is taken in the form of a granular powder, frequently mixed with other drugs, and is smoked or snorted. It is usually classified as a hallucinogen, although it also has stimulant and depressant properties. The effects of intoxication are like those of LSD and other hallucinogens, and resemble those of an acute schizophrenic episode, which may last several days to a week or longer. After the ingestion of a large amount (10 mg or more) of phencyclidine, it is present in the blood and urine for only a few hours sometimes making its detection difficult.

Toxicity from the illicit use of "ecstasy" (methylenedioxymethamphetamine [MDMA]) during parties ("raves") has increased as a result of its ill-founded reputation for safety. It appears to cause a release of both serotonin and dopamine in the brain, and produces an elated state similar to the effects of cocaine. Seizures, cerebral hemorrhages, and psychosis have been reported in previously healthy individuals (Verebey et al).

DISORDERS CAUSED BY BACTERIAL TOXINS

The most important diseases in this category are *tetanus, botulism,* and *diphtheria*. Each is caused by an extraordinarily powerful bacterial toxin that acts primarily on the nervous system.

Tetanus

The cause of this disease is the anaerobic, spore-forming rod *Clostridium tetani*. The organisms are found in the feces of some humans and many animals, particularly horses, from which they readily contaminate the soil. The spores may remain dormant for many months or years, but when they are introduced into a wound, especially if a foreign body or purulent bacteria are present, they are converted into their vegetative forms, which produce the exotoxin *tetanospasmin*. In developing countries, tetanus is still a common disease, particularly in newborns, in whom the spores are introduced via the umbilical cord (*tetanus neonatorum*). In the United States, the incidence rate of tetanus is about 1 per million people per year. Injection of contaminated heroin is a significant cause. Approximately 67 percent of all injuries leading to tetanus occur from deep scratches and puncture wounds in the home, and approximately 20 percent from deep scratches and puncture wounds in gardens and on farms.

Since 1903, when Morax and Marie proposed their theory of centripetal migration of the tetanus toxin, it has been taught that spread to the nervous system occurs via the peripheral nerves, the toxin ascending in the axis cylinders or the perineural sheaths. Modern studies, using fluorescein-labeled tetanus antitoxin, have disclosed that the toxin is also widely disseminated via blood or lymphatics, probably accounting for the generalized form of the disease. However, in local tetanus (see Chap. 50), the likely mode of spread to the CNS is indeed by retrograde axonal transport.

Mode of Action of Tetanus Toxin

Like botulinum toxin, the tetanus toxin is a zinc-dependent protease. It blocks neurotransmitter release by cleaving surface proteins of the synaptic vesicles, thus preventing the normal exocytosis of neurotransmitter.

The toxin interferes with the function of the reflex arc by the blockade of inhibitory transmitters, mainly GABA, at presynaptic sites in the spinal cord and brainstem. The Renshaw cell, the source of recurrent inhibition of spinal and brainstem motor neurons, is preferentially affected. Elicitation of the jaw jerk, for example, is normally followed by the abrupt suppression of motor neuron activity, manifested in the electromyogram (EMG) as a "silent period" (see further on). In the patient with tetanus, there is a failure of this inhibitory mechanism, with a resulting increase in activation of the neurons that innervate the masseter muscles (*trismus*, or lockjaw). Of all neuromuscular systems, the masseter innervation seems to be the most sensitive to the toxin. Not only do afferent stimuli produce an exaggerated effect, but they also abolish reciprocal innervation, allowing both agonists and antagonists to contract, giving rise to the characteristic muscular spasm of tetanus (see below). In addition to its generalized effects on the motor neurons of the spinal cord and brainstem, there is evidence that the toxin acts directly on skeletal muscle at the point where the axon forms the endplate (accounting perhaps for localized tetanus) and also upon the cerebral cortex and the sympathetic nervous system in the hypothalamus.

The incubation period varies greatly, from a day or two to a month or longer. Long incubation periods are associated with mild and localized types of the disease.

Clinical Features

There are several clinical types of tetanus, usually designated as local, cephalic, and generalized.

Generalized Tetanus This is the most common form. It may begin as local tetanus that becomes generalized after a few days, or it may be diffuse from the beginning. Trismus is frequently the first manifestation. In some cases this is preceded by a feeling of stiffness in the jaw or neck, slight fever, and other general symptoms of infection. The localized muscle stiffness and spasms spread quickly to other bulbar muscles as well as those of the neck, trunk, and limbs. A state of unremitting rigidity develops in all the involved muscles: the abdomen is board-like, the legs are rigidly extended, and the lips are pursed or retracted (*risus sardonicus*); the eyes are partially closed by contraction of the orbicularis oculi, or the eyebrows are elevated by spasm of the frontalis. Superimposed on this persistent state of enhanced muscle activity are paroxysms of tonic contraction or spasm of muscles (tetanic seizures or "convulsions"), which occur spontaneously or in response to the slightest external stimulus. They are agonizingly painful. Consciousness is not lost during these paroxysms. The tonic contraction of groups of muscles results in opisthotonos or in forward flexion of the trunk, flexion and adduction of the arms, clenching of the fists, and extension of the legs. Spasms of the pharyngeal, laryngeal, or respiratory muscles carry the constant threat of apnea or suffocation. Fever and pneumonia are common complications. Large swings in blood pressure and heart rate as well as profuse diaphoresis are typical, mainly in response to the intense muscular contractions but they may also be related to the action of the toxin on the CNS. Death is usually attributable to asphyxia from laryngospasm, to heart failure, or to shock, the latter resulting from the action of the toxin on the hypothalamus and sympathetic nervous system.

Generalized spasms and rigidity of trunk and limbs developing in a neonate a few days after birth should always suggest the diagnosis of tetanus. This form of tetanus occurs when there has been inadequate sterile treatment of the umbilical cord stump in a neonate born to an unimmunized mother.

Local Tetanus This is the most benign form. The initial symptoms are stiffness, tightness, and pain in the muscles in the neighborhood of a wound, followed by twitchings and brief spasms of the affected muscles. Local tetanus occurs most often in relation to a wound of the hand or forearm, rarely in the abdominal or paravertebral muscles. Gradually, some degree of continuous involuntary spasm becomes evident. There is sustained tautness of the affected muscles and resistance of the part to passive movement. Superimposed on this background of more or less continuous motor activity are brief, intense spasms, lasting from a few seconds to minutes and occurring spontaneously or in response to all variety of stimulation (Struppler et al). Early in the course of the illness there may be periods when the affected muscles are palpably soft and appear to be relaxed. A useful diagnostic maneuver at this stage is to have the patient perform some repetitive voluntary movements, such as opening and closing the hand, in response to which there occurs a gradual increase in the tonic contraction and spasms of the affected muscles, followed by spread to neighboring muscle groups (recruitment spasm). Even with mild localized tetanus there may be slight trismus, a useful diagnostic sign.

Symptoms may persist in localized form for several weeks or months. Gradually the spasms become less frequent and more difficult to evoke, and they finally disappear without residue. Complete recovery is to be expected, as there are no pathologic changes in muscles, nerves, spinal cord, or brain, even in the most severe generalized forms of tetanus.

Cephalic Tetanus This form of tetanus follows wounds of the face and head. The incubation period is short, 1 or 2 days as a rule. The affected muscles (most often facial) are weak or paralyzed. Nevertheless, during accessions of tetanic spasm, the palsied muscles are seen to contract. Apparently, the disturbance in the facial motoneurons is sufficient to prevent voluntary movement but insufficient to prevent the strong reflex impulses that elicit facial spasm. The spasms may involve the tongue and throat, with persistent dysarthria, dysphonia, and dysphagia. Ophthalmoparesis is known to occur but is difficult to verify because of severe blepharospasm. In a strict sense, these cephalic forms of tetanus are examples of local tetanus that frequently becomes generalized. Many cases prove fatal.

Diagnosis

This is made from the clinical features and a history of preceding injury. The latter is sometimes disclosed only after careful questioning, the injury having been trivial, forgotten and entirely healed. The organisms may or may not be recovered from the wound by the time the patient receives medical attention; other laboratory tests, apart from the EMG, are of little value. Serum CK may be moderately elevated if the rigidity is generalized. The EMG recorded from muscles in spasm shows continuous discharges of normal motor units like those recorded from a forceful voluntary muscle contraction. Most characteristic of tetanus, as mentioned earlier, is a loss of the physiologic silent period that occurs 50 to 100 ms after reflex contraction. This pause, normally produced by the recurrent inhibition of Renshaw cells, is blocked by tetanus toxin. In generalized tetanus the loss of the silent period can almost always be demonstrated in the masseter, and it is found in a muscle affected by local tetanus. Interestingly, the silent period is preserved in the stiff man syndrome (see Chap. 50).

Tetany caused by hypocalcemia, the spasms of strychnine poisoning or black widow spider bite, trismus as a result of painful conditions in and around the jaw, the dysphagia of rabies, hysterical spasms, rigidity and dystonic spasms caused by neuroleptic drugs, and the spasms of the stiff man syndrome all resemble the spasms of tetanus but should not be difficult to distinguish when all aspects of these disorders are considered. Nonetheless, the diagnosis is difficult to bring to mind in a nonendemic area.

The death rate from tetanus is approximately 50 percent overall; it is highest in newborns, heroin addicts, and patients with the cephalic form of the disease. The patient usually recovers if there are no severe generalized muscle spasms during the course of the illness or if the spasms remain localized.

Treatment

This is directed along several lines. At the outset, a single dose of antitoxin (3,000 to 6,000 U of tetanus immune human globulin) should be given along with a 10-day course of penicillin (1.2 million U of procaine penicillin daily), metronidazole (500 mg q6h intravenously or 400 mg rectally), or tetracycline (2 g daily). These drugs are effective against the vegetative forms of *C. tetani*. Immediate surgical treatment of the wound (excision or debridement) is imperative, and the tissue around the wound should be infiltrated with antitoxin.

Survival depends on expert and constant nursing in an intensive care unit and may be necessary for weeks. Tracheostomy is a requisite in all patients with recurrent generalized tonic spasms and should not be delayed until apnea or cyanosis has occurred. The patient must be kept as quiet as possible to avoid stimulus-induced spasms. This requires a darkened, quiet room and the judicious use of sedation. The benzodiazepines are the most useful drugs for both sedation and muscle relaxation; diazepam 120 mg/d or more can be given in frequent divided doses if ventilatory support is available; alternatively midazolam or propofol can be used in a continuous intravenous infusion. Short-acting barbiturates and chlorpromazine may also be useful, as may be morphine. Intrathecal baclofen and continuous atropine infusions have been used with success in severe cases, and intramuscular injections of botulinum toxin may be used for trismus and local spasm. The aim of therapy is to suppress muscle spasms and to keep the patient drowsy to avoid the horrible discomfort of the spasms. All treatments and manipulations should be kept to a minimum and coordinated so that the patient may be sedated beforehand.

Failure of these measures to control the tetanic paroxysms requires that intravenous administration of neuromuscular blocking agents such as pancuronium or vecuronium be used to abolish all muscle activity; appropriate sedative medication is instituted for as long as necessary, breathing being maintained by a positive-pressure respirator. Many intensive care units favor the use of neuromuscular paralytic drugs in all but the mildest cases. Further details concerning treatment can be found in the review by Farrar and colleagues.

All persons should be immunized against tetanus and receive a booster dose of toxoid every 10 years—a practice that is frequently neglected in the elderly. Injuries that carry a threat of tetanus should receive toxoid if the patient has not received a booster injection in the preceding year, and a second dose of toxoid is needed 6 weeks later. If the injured person has not received a booster injection since the original immunization, he should receive an injection of both toxoid and human antitoxin; the same applies to the injured person who has never been immunized. An attack of tetanus does not confer permanent immunity and persons who recover should be actively immunized.

Diphtheria

Diphtheria, an acute infectious disease caused by *Corynebacterium diphtheriae*, is now quite rare in the United States and Western Europe. The faucial-pharyngeal form of the disease, which is the most common clinical type, is characterized by the formation of an inflammatory exudate of the throat and trachea; at this site, the bacteria elaborate an exotoxin, which affects the heart and nervous system in approximately 20 percent of cases.

The involvement of the nervous system follows a predictable and biphasic pattern (Fisher and Adams). It begins locally, with *palatal paralysis* (nasal voice, regurgitation, and dysphagia) between the fifth and twelfth days of illness. At this time or shortly afterward, other cranial nerves (trigeminal, facial, vagus, and hypoglossal) may also be affected. *Ciliary body paralysis* with loss of accommodation and blurring of vision but with preserved light reaction usually appears in the second or third week (the opposite of the Argyll Robertson reaction). Rarely, the extraocular muscles are weakened. The cranial nerve signs may clear without further involvement of the nervous system, or a delayed sensorimotor polyneuropathy may develop between the fifth and eighth weeks of the disease. The latter varies in severity from a mild, predominantly distal polyneuropathy of the limbs to a rapidly evolving, ascending paralysis, like that of the Guillain-Barré syndrome; CSF findings are similar as well (acellular fluid with elevated protein). The neuropathic symptoms progress for a week or two, and if the patient does not succumb to respiratory paralysis or cardiac failure (cardiomyopathy), these conditions stabilize and then improve slowly and more or less completely.

The early oropharyngeal symptoms, the ciliary paralysis with relatively retained pupillary response to light, and subacute evolution of a delayed symmetrical sensorimotor peripheral neuropathy distinguish diphtheria from other forms of polyneuropathy. The long latency between the initial infection and the involvement of the nervous system has no clear explanation. In experimental animals, Waksman and colleagues demonstrated that the toxin reaches the Schwann cells in the most vascular parts of the peripheral nervous system within 24 to 48 h of infection but its metabolic effect on cell membranes extends over a period of weeks. The toxin produces demyelination in the proximal parts of spinal nerves, in dorsal root ganglia, and in spinal roots. The cardiac musculature and the conducting system of the heart undergo mild focal necrosis.

The source of diphtheritic infection may be extrafaucial—a penetrating wound, skin ulcer, or infection of the umbilicus in the neonate. The systemic and neurologic complications of faucial diphtheria can also be observed in the extrafaucial form of the disease (wound infection) after a similar latent period. It is probable, therefore, that the toxin reaches neural sites via the bloodstream; but in addition, some action is exerted locally, as evidenced by palatal paralysis in faucial cases and by initial weakness and sensory impairment in the neighborhood of the infected wound.

There is no specific treatment for the neurologic complications of diphtheria. It is generally agreed that the administration of antitoxin within 48 h of the earliest symptoms of the primary diphtheritic infection lessens the incidence and severity of the peripheral nerve complications. The polyneuropathy of diphtheria is discussed further in Chap. 46.

Botulism

Botulism is a rare form of food-borne illness caused by the exotoxin of *Clostridium botulinum*. Outbreaks of poisoning are most often caused by ingested bacteria contained in home-preserved than in commercially canned products, and vegetables and home-cured ham are incriminated more commonly than are other food products. Very rarely, a contaminated wound is the source of infection. Although the disease is ubiquitous, five western states (California, Washington, Colorado, New Mexico, and Oregon) account for more than half of all reported outbreaks in the United States. *Neonatal and infantile forms* of the disease have been reported. These are a result of absorption of the toxin formed by germination of ingested spores (rather than ingestion of preformed toxin), an important source of which is contaminated natural (raw) honey. A few adult cases may have a similar source.

It is now well established on the basis of observations in both animals and humans that the primary site of action of toxin is at a neuromuscular junction, more specifically on the presynaptic membrane. The toxin interferes with the release of acetylcholine from peripheral motor nerves at the neuromuscular synapse. The physiologic defect is similar to the one that characterizes the myasthenic syndrome of Lambert-Eaton (see Chap. 53) but different from that of myasthenia gravis.

Symptoms usually appear within 12 to 36 h of ingestion of the tainted food. Anorexia, nausea, and vomiting occur in most patients. As a rule, blurred vision and diplopia are the initial neural symptoms; their association with ptosis, strabismus, and extraocular muscle palsies, particularly of the sixth nerve, may at first suggest a diagnosis of myasthenia gravis. In botulism, however, accommodation is lost and the pupils are often unreactive to light. Other symptoms of bulbar involvement—nasality of voice, hoarseness, dysarthria, dysphagia, and an inability to phonate—follow in quick succession. These, in turn, are followed by progressive weakness of the muscles of the face, neck, trunk, and limbs, and by respiratory insufficiency. Despite the oropharyngeal weakness, it is not unusual for the gag reflex to be retained. Tendon reflexes are lost in cases of severe generalized weakness. These symptoms and signs evolve rapidly, over 2 to 4 days as a rule, and may be mistaken for those of the Guillain-Barré syndrome. Sensation remains intact, however, and the spinal fluid shows no abnormalities. Severe constipation is characteristic of botulism, perhaps as a result of paresis of smooth muscle of the intestine. Consciousness is retained throughout the illness unless severe degrees of anoxia develop as a result of respiratory failure. In the past, the mortality was greater than 60 percent, but it has declined greatly in recent decades, with improvements in the intensive care of acute respiratory failure and the effectiveness of *C. botulinum* antitoxins.

The clinical diagnosis can be confirmed by electrophysiologic studies. Specifically, there is reduced amplitude of evoked muscle potentials and an increase in amplitude with rapid repetitive nerve stimulation (the opposite of what is found in myasthenia gravis). In patients who recover, improvement begins within a few weeks, first in ocular movement, then in other cranial nerve functions. Complete recovery of paralyzed limb and trunk musculature may take many months.

The three types of botulinum toxins—A, B, and E—cannot be distinguished by their clinical effects alone, so that the patient should receive the trivalent antiserum as soon as the clinical diagnosis is made. This antitoxin can be obtained from the Centers for Disease Control and Prevention, Atlanta, Georgia. An initial dose of 10,000 U is given intravenously after intradermal testing for sensitivity to horse serum, followed by daily doses of 50,000 U intramuscularly until improvement begins. Penicillin or metronidazole are given to eradicate the organism in a wound (but are not as useful if the exogenous preformed toxin has been ingested).

Guanidine hydrochloride (50 mg/kg) has been somewhat useful in reversing the weakness of limb and extraocular muscles. Antitoxin and guanidine probably change the course of the illness relatively little and recovery depends on the effectiveness of respiratory care, maintenance of fluid and electrolyte balance, prevention of infection, and so on.

The therapeutic injection of small quantities of botulinum toxin into a muscle affected by dystonia or spasticity will weaken or paralyze it for weeks to months (see Chap. 6). Mild symptoms of botulism can occur with relatively large doses, mainly affecting the oropharyngeal and ciliary muscles.

POISONING CAUSED BY PLANTS, VENOMS, BITES, AND STINGS

Ergotism

Ergotism is the name applied to poisoning with ergot, a drug derived from the rye fungus *Claviceps purpurea*. Ergot is used therapeutically to control postpartum hemorrhage caused by uterine atony; one of its alkaloids, ergotamine, is used in the treatment of migraine (see Chap. 10), and a class of dopamine agonists used in the treatment of Parkinson disease has ergot activity (see Chap. 39). Chronic and repeated use of the drug is the usual cause of ergotism; acute overdosage in the postpartum state or in the treatment of migraine may cause an alarming rise in blood pressure.

Two types of ergotism are recognized: *gangrenous*, which is caused by a vasospastic, occlusive process in the small arteries of the extremities, and *convulsive*, or *neurogenic*, ergotism. The latter is characterized by fasciculations, myoclonus, and spasms of muscles, followed by seizures. In nonfatal cases, a tabes-like neurologic syndrome may develop, with loss of knee and ankle jerks, ataxia, and impairment of deep and superficial sensation. The pathologic changes consist of degeneration of the posterior columns, dorsal roots, and peripheral nerves, but they have been poorly described. The relation of these changes to ergot poisoning is not clear, because most of the cases occurred in areas where malnutrition was endemic. The authors have had no experience with this condition.

Lathyrism

Lathyrism is a neurologic syndrome characterized by the relatively acute onset of pain, paresthesia, and weakness in the lower extremities, progressing to a permanent spastic paraplegia. It is a serious medical problem in India and in some North African countries and is probably caused by a toxin contained in the chickling vetch pea, *Lathyrus*, a legume that is consumed in excess quantities during periods of famine. This disorder is discussed further with the spinal cord diseases (see Chap. 44).

Mushroom Poisoning

The gathering of wild mushrooms, a popular pastime in late summer and early fall, always carries with it the danger of poisoning. As many as 100 species of mushrooms are poisonous. Most of them cause only transient gastrointestinal symptoms but some elaborate toxins that can be fatal. The most important of these toxins are the cyclopeptides, which are contained in several species of *Amanita phalloides* and *muscaria* and account for more than 90 percent of fatal mushroom poisonings. These toxins disrupt RNA metabolism, causing hepatic and renal necrosis. Symptoms of poisoning with *Amanita* usually appear between 10 and 14 h after ingestion and consist of nausea, vomiting, colicky pain, and diarrhea, followed by irritability, restlessness, ataxia, hallucinations, convulsions, and coma. There may be added evidence of a neuromyopathy presenting as flaccid areflexic paralysis, high serum CK, diminished EMG potentials, and fiber necrosis.

Other important mushroom toxins are methylhydrazine (contained in the *Gyromitra* species) and muscarine (*Inocybe* and *Clitocybe* species). The former gives rise to a clinical picture much like that caused by the cyclopeptides. The symptoms of muscarine poisoning, which appear within 30 to 60 min of ingestion, are essentially those of parasympathetic stimulation—miosis, lacrimation, salivation, nausea, vomiting, diarrhea, perspiration, bradycardia, and hypotension. Tremor, seizures, and delirium occur in cases of severe poisoning.

The mushroom toxins have no effective antidotes. If vomiting has not occurred, it should be induced with ipecac, following which activated charcoal should be administered orally in order to bind what toxin remains in the gastrointestinal tract. A local poison control center may help identify the poisonous mushroom and its toxin. Even more important, the gathering and ingestion of field varieties of mushrooms should be left to those absolutely certain of their identity.

Buckthorn Poisoning

A rapidly progressive and sometimes fatal paralysis follows the ingestion of the small fruit of the buckthorn shrub that is indigenous to northern Mexico and the neighboring southwestern parts of the United States. The responsible toxin causes a predominantly motor polyneuropathy, probably of axonal type. Except for a normal spinal fluid protein concentration, the disorder closely resembles Guillain-Barré syndrome and tick paralysis (see later), and its recognition depends on awareness of ingestion of the fruit in endemic areas.

Neurotoxin Fish Poisoning (Ciguatera)

Ingestion of marine toxins that block neural sodium channels is a common form of poisoning throughout coastal areas and islands of the world. It results from eating fish that have fed on toxin-containing microscopic dinoflagellates. Reef fish and shellfish ingest high concentrations of these organisms during periodic upswings in the population of the dinoflagellates. They may be so profuse as to color the surrounding water (red tide).

Although the toxins differ (tetrodotoxin—puffer fish; ciguatoxin—snails; saxitoxin and brevetoxin—shellfish), the neurologic and gastrointestinal symptoms that follow the ingestion of poisoned fish are similar. The initial symptoms are diarrhea, vomiting, or abdominal cramps coming on minutes to hours after the ingestion. These are followed by paresthesias that begin periorally and then involve the limbs distally. Hot and cold sensory stimuli (e.g., ice cream) are characteristically associated with electrical-like or burning paresthesias in the mouth. Muscle aches and shooting pains are also mentioned by most patients. In puffer fish poisoning, and in advanced stages of poisoning from other fish, weakness occurs, and there have been a few reports of coma and of respiratory failure.

The recognition of this type of fish poisoning is straightforward in endemic areas, in some of which there is a seasonal clustering of cases. In tourists returning home from endemic areas, and in persons consuming imported fish, the illness may be mistaken for Guillain-Barré syndrome. Prominent perioral paresthesias should suggest the correct diagnosis. Supportive treatment is all that is required but treatment with intravenous mannitol is said to hasten recovery.

Pearn has reviewed the biochemistry and physiologic and clinical effects of the various marine toxins and points out a form of chronic intoxication that is apparently endemic in certain island communities. The main chronic effects are severe fatigue and asthenic weakness. The problem of distinguishing this syndrome from depression is acknowledged by the author and the cases on which we have consulted locally almost always fall into the psychiatric category. One of our patients developed chronic paresthesias.

Venoms, Bites, and Stings

Although relatively rare, they are nonetheless important causes of mortality. The venoms of certain species of snakes, lizards, spiders (especially the black widow spider, see Chap. 50), and scorpions contain neurotoxins that may cause a fatal depression of respiration and curare-like paralysis of neuromuscular transmission. In the United States, there are approximately 8,000 poisonous snake bites per year. Some, such as the coral snake envenomation, are neurotoxic, producing pupillary dilatation, ptosis, ocular palsies, ataxia, and respiratory paralysis. Others (rattlesnakes, water moccasin snakes) cause tissue necrosis and circulatory collapse. These are reviewed by Gold and colleagues. The serious effects of *Hymenoptera stings* (bees, wasps, hornets, and fire ants) are mainly the result of hypersensitivity and anaphylaxis. Several instances of cerebral and myocardial infarction have been reported after bee and wasp stings (Crawley et al). A substantial inception has been the development of an antivenom for scorpion stings that can be administered in parallel with diazepines to children and results in more rapid resolution of paralysis and respiratory failure (Boyer and colleagues). All of these disorders are discussed in detail in *Harrison's Principles of Internal Medicine*.

Tick Paralysis

This rare condition is the result of a toxin secreted by the gravid tick. In Canada and the northwestern United States, the wood tick *Dermacentor andersoni* is mainly responsible; in the southeastern United States it is *Dermacentor variabilis*, a dog tick (the tick in Australia is the *Ixodes holocyclus*), but various other ticks occasionally may have the same effect. Most cases occur in children because their small body mass renders them susceptible to the effects of relatively small amounts of the toxin. The illness arises almost exclusively in the spring when the mature gravid ticks are most plentiful. The illness is more common and is generally more severe in cases on the Australian continent than it is in North America. Clinical manifestations require that the tick be attached to the skin for several days.

The neurotoxin causes a generalized, flaccid, areflexic paralysis, appearing over 1 or 2 days and thereby mimicking the Guillain-Barré syndrome. In a few cases, several days of ataxia and areflexia precede the paralysis but sensory loss tends to be minimal. External ophthalmoplegia, which occurred in 5 of the 6 children described by Grattan-Smith and colleagues, is exceptional, judging by other reports; internal ophthalmoplegia and pharyngeal weakness are also known to occur, and while not typical, raise the possibility of botulism or diphtheria. The CSF is normal and electrophysiologic studies show reduction in the amplitude of the muscle action potentials but normal or only slightly slowed nerve conduction. Prominent ptosis and neck weakness may also raise the question of a neuromuscular process, but repetitive stimulation testing is normal or evokes only a slight decrement or increment in some cases.

The ticks tend to attach to the hairlines or in the matted hair of the scalp, neck, and pubis, where a careful search will reveal them (for which reason nurses and electroencephalography technicians often are most likely to find them; see Felz et al). The diagnosis is much in the awareness of clinicians in endemic areas during the tick season, for they are gratified with rapid and dramatic improvement when the tick is removed. The paralysis has been reported to become transiently worse after tick removal in some of the Australian cases.

From a neurologic point of view, *Lyme disease* is a far more common tick-borne disorder. The causative agent is *Borrelia burgdorferi*, a spirochetal organism. The disorder is discussed fully with other infectious diseases in Chap. 32 and in Chap. 46, with the neuropathies.

HEAVY METALS

Lead

The causes and clinical manifestations of lead poisoning are quite different in children and adults.

Lead Poisoning in Children

In the United States, this disease has been identified most often in 1- to 3-year-old children who inhabit urban slum areas where old, deteriorated housing prevails. (Lead paint was used in most houses built before 1940 and in many built before 1960.) The chewing of leaded paint is promoted by compulsive ingestion (pica) from windowsills and painted plaster walls. The development of an acute encephalopathy is the most serious complication, resulting in death in 5 to 20 percent of cases and in permanent neurologic and mental deficits in more than 25 percent of survivors.

Clinical Manifestations These develop over a period of 3 to 6 weeks. The child becomes anorectic, less playful and less alert, and more irritable. These symptoms may be misinterpreted as a behavior disorder or a manifestation of mental retardation. Intermittent vomiting, vague abdominal pain, clumsiness, and ataxia may be added. If these early signs of intoxication are not recognized and the child continues to ingest lead, more flagrant signs of acute encephalopathy may develop—most frequently in the summer months, for reasons that are not understood. Vomiting becomes more persistent, apathy progresses to drowsiness and stupor interspersed with periods of hyperirritability, and, finally, seizures and coma supervene. This syndrome may evolve in a period of a week or less, most rapidly in children younger than 2 years of age; in older children, it is more likely to develop in recurrent and less severe episodes. This clinical syndrome must be distinguished from tuberculous meningitis, viral meningoencephalitis, and the various conditions causing acute increased intracranial pressure. Usually, in lead encephalopathy, the CSF is under increased pressure with manifest papilledema, and there may be a slight lymphocytic pleocytosis and elevated protein but normal glucose values. It follows that lumbar puncture should be done with caution and only if it is essential for diagnosis.

Diagnosis Because the symptoms of plumbism are nonspecific, the diagnosis depends on an appreciation of the potential causative factors and the results of certain laboratory tests. Lead lines at the metaphyses of long bones and basophilic stippling of red cells are seen but are too inconstant to be relied on, but basophilic stippling of bone marrow erythroblasts is uniformly increased. Impairment of heme synthesis, which is exquisitely sensitive to the toxic effects of lead, results in the increased excretion of urinary coproporphyrin (UCP) and of Δ-aminolevulinic acid (ALA). These urinary indices and the lead concentrations in the serum bear an imperfect relationship to the clinical manifestations. In the test for UCP, which is readily performed in the clinic and emergency department, a few milliliters of urine are acidified with acetic acid and shaken with an equal volume of ether; if coproporphyrin is present, the ether layer will reveal a reddish fluorescence under a Wood lamp. This test is strongly positive when the whole blood concentration of lead exceeds 80 mg/dL. The diagnosis can be confirmed by promoting lead excretion with calcium disodium edetate ($CaNa_2$ ethylenediaminetetraacetic acid [EDTA]), given in three doses (25 mg/kg) at 8-h intervals. Excretion of over 500 mg in 24 h is indicative of plumbism. The measurement of zinc protoporphyrin (ZPP) in the blood is another reliable means of determining the presence and degree of lead exposure. The binding of erythrocyte protoporphyrin to zinc occurs when lead impairs the normal binding of erythrocyte protoporphyrin to iron. Elevated ZPP can also be induced when access to iron is limited by other conditions, such as iron deficiency anemia.

At blood lead concentrations of 70 mg/dL symptoms may be minimal, but acute encephalopathy may occur abruptly and unpredictably, for which reason the child should be hospitalized for chelation therapy (see below). Some children with a blood lead level of 50 mg/dL may have symptoms of severe encephalopathy, whereas others may be asymptomatic. In the latter case, an attempt should be made to discover and remove the source of lead intoxication and the child should be reexamined at frequent intervals. The seriousness of lead encephalopathy is indicated by the fact that most of the children who become stuporous or comatose remain mentally retarded despite treatment. The physician's aim, therefore, is to institute treatment before the severe symptoms of encephalopathy have become manifest.

Pathology In children who die of acute lead encephalopathy, the brain is massively swollen, with herniation of the temporal lobes and cerebellum, multiple microscopic ischemic foci in the cerebrum and cerebellum, and endothelial damage and deposition of proteinaceous material and mononuclear inflammatory cells around many of the small blood vessels. There are also hyperplastic changes in arteries and arterioles and in some places, perivascular infiltrates of lymphocytes and mononuclear cells. In the territories of some of these vessels there are foci of ischemic necrosis with surrounding glial reaction appropriate for the age of the lesion. Similar changes are present in the kidney.

Treatment The plan of therapy includes the establishment of urinary flow, following which intravenous fluid therapy is restricted to basal water and electrolyte requirements. In cases of acute encephalopathy, combined chelation therapy with 2,3-dimercaptopropanol (British anti-Lewisite [BAL]; 12 to 24 mg/kg) and $CaNa_2$ EDTA (0.5 to 1.5 g/m^2 body surface area) for 5 to 7 days. This is followed by a course of oral penicillamine (40 mg/kg, not exceeding 1 g/d). In acute cases the goal is to reduce the serum lead levels below 40 mg/dL. Once the absorption of lead has ceased, chelating agents remove lead only from soft tissues and not from bone, where most of the lead is stored. Any intercurrent illness may result in a further mobilization of lead from bones and soft tissues and an exacerbation of symptoms of lead intoxication.

Repeated doses of mannitol may be used for relief of cerebral edema. Microcytic hypochromic anemia is treated with iron once the chelating agents have been discontinued. Seizures are best controlled with intravenous diazepam or midazolam.

Prevention The prevention of reintoxication (or initial intoxication) demands that the child be removed from the source of lead. Although this is axiomatic, it is often difficult to accomplish, despite the best efforts of local health departments and hospital and city social workers. Nevertheless, an attempt to eliminate the environmental factor must be made in each case. Such attempts, among other things, have resulted in a marked decrease in the incidence of acute lead encephalopathy in the past two decades. Although florid examples of this encephalopathy are now uncommon, undue exposure to lead (blood levels greater than 30 mg/dL) remains inordinately prevalent and a continuing source of concern to public health authorities.

As to the levels that pose a danger to the child, there is still some uncertainty. Rutter, who reviewed all of the evidence up to 1980, concluded that persistent blood levels above 40 mg/dL may cause slight cognitive impairment and, less certainly, an increased risk of behavioral difficulties. More recently, Canfield and colleagues reported, from a prospective study of 172 children, that even lower levels may induce a decline in IQ at 3 and 5 years of age. These data require confirmation before general acceptance. Further compounding the problem of interpreting low-level lead exposure in children with blood lead concentrations below 45 g/dL is the observation by Rogan and colleagues that treatment with succimer, while successful in reducing lead levels, did not improve cognitive or behavioral function.

The oral lead chelator succimer is approved for outpatient treatment of asymptomatic children with blood lead levels higher than 45 mg/dL. A 3-week course of treatment is given, with weekly monitoring of blood lead levels to identify lead mobilization from bones and soft tissues (Jorgensen).

In 1988, on the basis of epidemiologic and experimental studies in the United States, Europe, and Australia, the Agency for Toxic Substances and Disease Registry set a much lower threshold for neurobehavioral toxicity (10 to 15 mg/dL). It estimated that 3 to 4 million American children have blood levels in excess of this amount. Needleman and colleagues studied the long-term effects of low doses of lead in asymptomatic children, 132 of whom had had demonstrable levels of lead in the dentin of shed teeth (average 24 mg/dL). Eleven years later, the children were found to have behavioral abnormalities proportionate to their early lead levels. In comparison to a normal population, more had dropped out of school and more had lower vocabulary and grammatical reasoning scores, more reading difficulty, poorer hand–eye coordination performance, slower finger-tapping rates, and longer reaction times. The authors claimed to have eliminated other confounding variables such as lower social class and genetic factors. These findings are similar to those of the long-term studies of Baghurst and colleagues (see also Mahaffey). There are no adequate pathologic or MRI studies of such cases.

Lead Intoxication in Adults

Lead intoxication in adults is much less common than in children. The hazards to adults are the result of inhaling the dust of inorganic lead salts and the fumes from the burning of objects containing lead or involvement in processes that require the remelting of lead. Painting, printing, pottery glazing, lead smelting, welding, and storage battery manufacturing are the industries in which these hazards are likeliest to occur. In the past, miners and brass foundry and garage workers (during automobile radiator repair, when soldered joints were heated) were the ones most at risk. Currently, other, sometimes idiosyncratic, sources are more common. For example, the authors have encountered a striking case of lead encephalopathy in a man of Indian origin who was taking large amounts of an Ayurvedic herbal remedy for arthritis. The first manifestation was a series of generalized seizures followed by a fluctuating encephalopathy. His serum lead level was 70 mg/dL, and 24-h urine collection contained 1,550 mg of lead (normal being less than 400 mg). There was a T2-weighted hyperintensity in the cerebral cortex. Whitfield and colleagues reviewed 23 instances of lead encephalopathy in adults. At the time of their report most cases were caused by moonshine (homemade whiskey from lead-lined stills). More recently, most cases have been from various herbal medications, as already mentioned. Combined lead and arsenic poisoning from herbal compounds is also known.

The usual manifestations of lead poisoning in adults are colic, anemia, and peripheral neuropathy. Encephalopathy of the type described above is decidedly rare. Lead colic, frequently precipitated by an intercurrent infection or by alcohol intoxication, is characterized by severe, poorly localized abdominal pain, often with rigidity of abdominal muscles but without fever or leukocytosis. The pain responds to the intravenous injection of calcium salts, at least temporarily, but responds poorly to morphine. Mild anemia is common. A black line of lead sulfide may develop along the gingival margins. Peripheral neuropathy, usually a bilateral wrist drop, is a rare manifestation and is discussed in Chap. 46.

The diagnostic tests for plumbism in children are generally applicable to adults, with the exception of bone films, which are of no value in the latter. Also, the treatment of adults with chelating agents follows the same principles as in children.

Intoxication with tetraethyl and tetramethyl (organic) lead, used as additives in gasoline, is caused by inhalation of gasoline fumes. It occurs most often in workers who clean gasoline storage tanks. Insomnia, irritability, delusions, and hallucinations are the usual clinical manifestations, and a maniacal state may develop. The hematologic abnormalities of inorganic lead poisoning are not found, and chelating agents are of no value in treatment. Organic lead poisoning is usually reversible, but fatalities have been reported. The pathologic changes have not been well described.

Arsenic

In the past, medications such as Fowler solution (potassium arsenite) and the arsphenamines, used in the treatment of syphilis, were frequent causes of intoxication, but now the most common cause is the suicidal or accidental ingestion of herbicides, insecticides, or rodenticides containing copper acetoarsenite (Paris green) or calcium or lead arsenate. In rural areas, arsenic-containing insecticide sprays are a common source of poisoning. Arsenic is used also in the manufacture of paints, enamels, and metals; as a disinfectant for skins and furs; and also in galvanizing, soldering, etching, and lead plating. Occasional cases of poisoning are reported in relation to these occupations. Arsenic is still contained in some topical creams and oral solutions that are used in the treatment of psoriasis and other skin disorders and in some herbal remedies.

Arsenic exerts its toxic effects by reacting with the sulfhydryl radicals of certain enzymes necessary for cellular metabolism. The effects on the nervous system are those of an encephalopathy or peripheral neuropathy. The latter may be the product of chronic poisoning or may become manifest between 1 and 2 weeks after recovery from the effects of acute poisoning. It takes the form of a distal axonopathy that is described in Chap. 46. In cases of arsenical polyneuropathy we have cared for, a distal sensorimotor areflexic syndrome developed subacutely. At autopsy there was a dying back pattern of myelin and axons with macrophage and Schwann cell reactions and chromatolysis of motor neurons and sensory ganglion cells. The CNS appeared normal.

The symptoms of encephalopathy (headache, drowsiness, mental confusion, delirium, and convulsive seizures) may also occur as part of acute or chronic intoxication. In the latter case, they are accompanied by weakness and muscular aching, hemolysis, chills and fever, mucosal irritation (in patients exposed to arsine gas), diffuse scaly desquamation, and transverse white lines, 1 to 2 mm in width, above the lunula of each fingernail (Mees lines). Acute poisoning by the oral route is associated with severe gastrointestinal symptoms, shock and death in a large proportion of patients. The CSF is normal. Examination of the brain in such cases discloses myriads of punctate hemorrhages in the white matter. Microscopically, the lesions consist of capillary necrosis and of pericapillary zones of degeneration, which, in turn, are ringed by red cells (brain purpura). These neuropathologic changes are not specific for arsenical poisoning, but have been observed in such diverse conditions as pneumonia, gram-negative bacillary septicemia from urinary tract infections, sulfonamide and phosgene poisoning, dysentery, disseminated intravascular coagulation, and others.

The diagnosis of arsenical poisoning depends on the demonstration of increased levels of arsenic in the hair and urine. Arsenic is deposited in the hair within 2 weeks of exposure and may remain fixed there for long periods. Concentrations of more than 0.1 mg arsenic per 100 mg hair are indicative of poisoning. Arsenic also remains within bones for long periods and is slowly excreted in the urine and feces. Excretion of more than 0.1 mg arsenic per liter of urine is considered abnormal; levels greater than 1 mg/L may occur soon after acute exposure. We would caution, however, that individuals who consume fish on a regular basis, as occurs in coastal regions, may have slightly or moderately elevated levels of arsenic and that various conditions such as neuropathy and amyotrophic lateral sclerosis (ALS) may be mistakenly attributed to this innocuous finding. The levels return to normal within a few months of abstaining from fish.

The CSF protein level may be raised (50 to 100 mg/dL).

Treatment Acute poisoning is treated by gastric lavage, vasopressor agents, dimercaprol (BAL), maintenance of renal perfusion, and exchange transfusions if massive hemoglobinuria occurs. Once polyneuropathy has occurred, it is little affected by treatment with BAL, but other manifestations of chronic arsenical poisoning respond favorably. There has been a gradual recovery from the polyneuropathy under our care.

Manganese

Manganese poisoning results from the chronic inhalation and ingestion of manganese particles and occurs in miners of manganese ore and in workers who separate manganese from other ore. Several clinical syndromes have been observed. The initial stages of intoxication may be marked by a prolonged confusional-hallucinatory state. Later, the symptoms are predominantly extrapyramidal. They are often described as parkinsonian in type, but in the patients seen by the authors, the resemblance was not close: an odd gait ("cock" walk), dystonia and rigidity of the trunk, postural instability, and falling backward were features seen in two South American miners. Others, however, have reported stiffness and awkwardness of the limbs, often with tremor of the hands, "cogwheel" phenomenon, gross rhythmic movements of the trunk and head, and retropulsive and propulsive gait. Corticospinal and corticobulbar signs may be added. Progressive weakness, fatigability, and sleepiness as well as psychiatric symptoms (manganese madness) are other clinical features. Rarely, severe axial rigidity and dystonia, like those of Wilson disease, are said to have been the outstanding manifestations. The emergence of an extrapyramidal syndrome from the use of illicit drugs that are synthesized with potassium permanganate has already been mentioned in relation to the cathionine stimulants.

Neuronal loss and gliosis, affecting mainly the pallidum and striatum but also the frontoparietal and cerebellar cortex and hypothalamus, have been described, but the pathologic changes have not been carefully studied.

Treatment

The neurologic abnormalities have not responded to treatment with chelating agents. In the chronic dystonic form of manganese intoxication, dramatic and sustained improvement has been reported with the administration of L-dopa; patients with the more common parkinsonian type of manganese intoxication have shown only slight, if any, improvement with L-dopa.

Mercury

Mercury poisoning arises in two forms, one caused by inorganic compounds (elemental or mercury salt) and the other, more dangerous, caused by organic mercury. The sources of potential exposure are reviewed by Clarkson. Among the *organic compounds*, methylmercury gives rise to a wide array of serious neurologic symptoms that may be delayed for days or weeks after exposure, including tremor of the extremities, tongue, and lips; mental confusion; and a progressive cerebellar syndrome, with ataxia of gait and arms, intention tremor, and dysarthria. Choreoathetosis and parkinsonian facies have also been described. Changes in mood and behavior are prominent, consisting at first of subjective weakness and fatigability and later of extreme depression and lethargy alternating with irritability. This *delayed form of subacute mercury poisoning* has been reported in chemical laboratory workers after exposure to methyl mercury compounds. These agents, particularly dimethylmercury, are extremely hazardous because they are absorbed transdermally and by inhalation, allowing severe toxicity to occur with even brief contact. In a fatal case of a chemist reported by Nierenberg and colleagues, a rapidly progressive ataxia and stupor progressing to coma developed 154 days after exposure. Cerebellar function was most severely impaired, and visual function was affected.

The pathologic changes are characterized by a striking degeneration of the granular layer of the cerebellar cortex, with relative sparing of the Purkinje cells and neuronal loss and gliosis of the calcarine cortex and to a lesser extent of other parts of the cerebral cortex, similar to the Minamata disease cases described later.

The chronic form of *inorganic mercury poisoning* occurs in persons exposed to large amounts of the metal used in the manufacture of thermometers, mirrors, incandescent lights, x-ray machines, and vacuum pumps. Because mercury volatilizes at room temperature, it readily contaminates the air and then condenses on the skin and respiratory mucous membranes. Nitrate of mercury, used formerly in the manufacture of felt hats ("mad hatters"), and phenyl mercury, used in the paper, pulp, and electrochemical industries, are other sources of intoxication. Paresthesias, lassitude, confusion, incoordination, and intention tremor are characteristic, and, with continued exposure, a delirious state occurs. Headache, various bodily pains, visual and hearing disorders, and corticospinal signs may be added, but their pathologic basis is unknown. The term *erethism* was coined to describe the timidity, memory loss, and insomnia that were said to be characteristic of chronic intoxication. If the exposure is more than a minimal degree over a long period, gastrointestinal disturbances are prone to occur (anorexia, weight loss), as well as stomatitis and gingivitis with loosening of the teeth.

Acute exposure to inorganic mercury in larger amounts is even more corrosive to the gastrointestinal system and produces nausea, vomiting, hematemesis, abdominal pain, and bloody diarrhea, as well as renal tubular necrosis.

Isolated instances of *polyneuropathy* associated with exposure to mercury have also been reported (Albers et al; Agocs et al) and may be responsible for the paresthesias that accompany most cases, as well as the acrodynic syndrome described below. The polyneuropathy associated with mercury poisoning is discussed in Chap. 46.

The presence of mercury in industrial waste has contaminated many sources of water supply and fish, which are ingested by humans and cause mercurial poisoning. So-called Minamata disease is a case in point. Between 1953 and 1956, a large number of villagers living near Minamata Bay in Kyushu Island, Japan, were afflicted with a syndrome of chronic mercurialism, traced to the ingestion of fish that had been contaminated with industrial wastes containing methylmercury. Concentric constriction of the visual fields, hearing loss, cerebellar ataxia, postural and action tremors, and sensory impairment of the legs and arms and sometimes of the tongue and lips were the usual clinical manifestations. The syndrome evolved over a few weeks. Pathologically there was diffuse neuronal loss in both cerebral and cerebellar cortices, most marked in the anterior parts of the calcarine cortex and granule cell layer of the cerebellum. CT scans in survivors, years after the mass poisoning, disclosed bilaterally symmetrical areas of decreased attenuation in the visual cortex and diffuse atrophy of the cerebellar hemispheres and vermis, especially the inferior vermis (Tokuomi et al).

A painful neuropathy of children (acrodynia) has been traced to mercury exposure from interior latex paint, to calomel (mercurous chloride), to teething powders, and to a mercuric fungicide used in washing diapers (Agocs et al; Clarkson). Albers and colleagues observed the appearance of symptoms (mild decrease in strength, tremor, and incoordination) 20 to 35 years after exposure to elemental mercury. These authors believed that the natural neuronal attrition with aging had unmasked the neurologic disorder, a theory that we cannot validate.

The authors believe it worth mentioning that there is no convincing evidence linking typical dietary ingestion of fish containing metallic compounds such as mercury and any neurologic or developmental disease. The inhalation of vaporized mercury as a result of extensive dental work, or simply the presence of a large number of fillings ("amalgam illness"), is alleged to affect the peripheral nerves or to cause fatigue, but the connection is also highly doubtful as is the alleged relationship between vaccines containing mercury preservatives (thiomersal) and autism.

Treatment In the *treatment* of chronic mercury poisoning, penicillamine has been the drug of choice, because it can be administered orally and appears to chelate mercury selectively, with less effect on copper, which is an essential element in many metabolic processes. Dimercaptosuccinic acid (succimer), which is also given orally and has few side effects, will probably prove to be a superior form of treatment (Clarkson). Because it increases the concentration of mercury in the brain, BAL is an unsuitable chelating agent.

Phosphorus and Organophosphate Poisoning

Nervous system function may be deranged as part of acute and frequently fatal poisoning with inorganic phosphorus compounds (found in rat poisons, roach powders, and match heads). More important clinically is poisoning with organophosphorus compounds, the best known of which is triorthocresyl phosphate (TOCP).

Organophosphates are widely used as *insecticides*. Since 1945, approximately 15,000 individual compounds in this category have come into use. Certain ones, such as tetraethylpyrophosphate, have been the cause of major outbreaks of neurologic disorder, especially in children. These substances have an acute anticholinesterase effect but no delayed neurotoxic action. Chlorophos, which is a 1-hydroxy-2,2,2-trichlorethylphosphonate, is an exception; it has both an acute and delayed action, as does TOCP.

The *immediate* anticholinesterase effect manifests itself by headache, vomiting, sweating, abdominal cramps, salivation, wheezing (secondary to bronchial spasm), miosis, and muscular weakness and twitching. Most of these symptoms can be reversed by administration of atropine and pralidoxime. The *delayed effect* manifests 2 to 5 weeks following acute organophosphorus insecticide poisoning. This takes the form of a distal symmetrical sensorimotor (predominantly motor) polyneuropathy, progressing to muscle atrophy (see Chap. 46). Recovery occurs to a variable degree and then, in patients poisoned with TOCP, signs of corticospinal damage become detectable. The severity of paralysis and its permanence vary with the dosage of TOCP. Whether a polyneuropathy can arise without the preceding symptoms of cholinergic toxicity is debated; however, based on a review of the subject and a study of 11 patients exposed to these agents, 3 of whom later acquired sensory neuropathy, Moretto and Lotti express the view that such an occurrence must be rare.

In addition to the acute and delayed neurotoxic effects of organophosphorus, an *intermediate syndrome* has been described (Senanayake and Karalliedde). Symptoms appear 24 to 96 h after the acute cholinergic phase and consist of weakness or paralysis of proximal limb muscles, neck flexors, motor cranial nerves, and respiratory muscles. Respiratory paralysis may prove fatal. In patients who survive, the paralytic symptoms last for 2 to 3 weeks and then subside. The intermediate and delayed symptoms do not respond to atropine or other drugs.

Several striking outbreaks of TOCP poisoning have been reported. During the latter part of the prohibition era and to a lesser extent thereafter, outbreaks of so-called jake paralysis were traced to drinking an extract of Jamaica ginger that had been contaminated with TOCP. Adams had examined several "ginger jake" patients many years later and related to us that he found only signs of corticospinal disease. Presumably in the early stage of this disease they were obscured by the neuropathy. Another outbreak occurred in Morocco in 1959, when lubricating oil containing TOCP was used deliberately to dilute olive oil. Several other outbreaks have been caused by the ingestion of grain and cooking oil that had been stored in inadequately cleaned containers previously used for storing TOCP.

The effect of TOCP on the peripheral nervous system has been studied extensively in experimental animals. In cats, there occurs a dying back from the terminal ends of the largest and longest medullated motor nerve fibers, including those from the annulospiral endings of the muscle spindles (Cavanagh and Patangia). The long fiber tracts of the spinal cord show a similar dying-back phenomenon. Abnormal membrane-bound vesicles and tubules were observed by Prineas to accumulate in axoplasm before degeneration. These effects have been traced to the inhibitory action of TOCP on esterases. There is still uncertainty as to the details of these reactions, and no treatment for the prevention or control of the neurotoxic effects has been devised.

Thallium

In the late nineteenth century, thallium was used medicinally in the treatment of venereal disease, ringworm, and tuberculosis, and later in rodenticides and insecticides. Poisoning was fairly common. Sporadic instances of poisoning still occur, usually as a result of accidental or suicidal ingestion of thallium-containing rodenticides and rarely from overuse of thallium-containing depilatory agents. Patients who survive the effects of acute poisoning develop a rapidly progressive and painful sensory polyneuropathy, optic atrophy, and occasionally ophthalmoplegia—followed, 15 to 30 days after ingestion, by diffuse alopecia (see Chap. 46). The latter feature should always suggest the diagnosis of thallium poisoning, which can be confirmed by finding this metallic element in the urine. Two of our patients had a severe sensory and mild motor polyneuropathy and alopecia, from which they were recovering months later. It is not uncommon for the neuropathy to have a painful component involving acral regions. The condition can end fatally. The use of potassium chloride by mouth may hasten thallium excretion.

Other Metals

Iron, antimony, tin, aluminum, zinc, barium, bismuth, copper, silver, gold, platinum, and lithium may all produce serious degrees of intoxication. The major manifestations in each case are gastrointestinal or renal, but certain neurologic symptoms—notably headache, irritability, confusional psychosis, stupor, coma, and convulsions—may be observed in any of these if the poisoning is severe, often as a terminal event.

Gold preparations, which are still used occasionally in the treatment of arthritis, may, after several months of treatment, give rise to focal or generalized myokymia and a rapidly progressive, symmetrical polyneuropathy (Katrak et al). The adverse effects of *platinum* are discussed later, with the antineoplastic agents. *Lithium* was discussed earlier.

Mentioned here is a novel but quite rare *cobalt-chromium metallosis* due to the leaching of metals from prosthetic hips into surrounding tissues. A painful sensorimotor polyneuropathy has been reported, in some patients accompanied by hearing loss. Although only a few cases have been documented, the process has attracted considerable attention and our only encounter with it has been the ill-advised revision of hip implants for nondescript sensory symptoms, similar to the peculiar obsession with removing dental fillings for erroneously diagnosed mercury poisoning.

Attention already has been drawn to the possible causative role of *aluminum intoxication* in so-called dialysis dementia or encephalopathy (see Chap. 43). Removal of aluminum from the water used in renal dialysis has practically eliminated this disorder. It should be noted that the neuropathologic changes in experimental aluminum intoxication (see later) are not those observed in dialysis dementia. Perl and colleagues have reported the accumulation of aluminum in tangle-bearing neurons of patients with Alzheimer disease and in the Guamanian Parkinson–dementia–ALS complex. However, analysis of neuritic plaques by nuclear microscopy, without using chemical stains, failed to demonstrate the presence of aluminum (Landsberg et al). The significance of these findings remains to be determined. Longstreth and colleagues described a progressive neurologic disorder consisting of intention tremor, incoordination, and spastic paraparesis in 3 patients who had worked for more than 12 years in the same pot room of an aluminum smelting plant. Similar cases clearly attributable to aluminum intoxication have not been reported, however.

Organic compounds of *tin* may seriously damage the nervous system. Diffuse edema of the white matter of the brain and spinal cord has been produced experimentally with *triethyltin*. Presumably, this was the basis of the mass poisoning produced by a triethyltin-contaminated drug called Stalinon. The illness was characterized by greatly elevated intracranial pressure and by a spinal cord lesion in some cases (Alajouanine et al). *Trimethyltin* intoxication is much rarer; seizures are the main manifestation. Experimental studies in rats have shown neuronal loss in the hippocampus, largely *sparing* the Sommer sector, with later involvement of neurons in the pyriform cortex and amygdala (see review by LeQuesne).

A stereotyped episodic encephalopathy has been associated with *bismuth intoxication*, usually arising from the ingestion of bismuth subgallate. Large outbreaks have been reported in Australia and France (Burns et al; Buge et al). The onset of the neurologic disturbance is usually subacute, with a mild and fluctuating confusion, somnolence, difficulty in concentration, tremulousness, and sometimes hallucinations and delusions. With continued ingestion of bismuth, there occurs a rapid (24 to 48 h) worsening of the confusion and tremulousness, along with diffuse myoclonic jerks, seizures, ataxia, and inability to stand or walk. These symptoms regress over a few days to weeks when the bismuth is withdrawn, but some patients have died of acute intoxication. High concentrations of bismuth were found in the cerebral and cerebellar cortices and in the nuclear masses throughout the brain. These concentrations can be recognized as hyperdensities in the CT scan (Buge et al).

Industrial Toxins

Some of these, the heavy metals, already have been considered. In addition, a large number of synthetic organic compounds are widely used in industry and are frequent sources of toxicity, and the list is constantly being expanded. The reader is referred to the references at the end of the chapter, particularly to the most current text, edited by Spencer and Schaumburg, for details concerning these compounds. Here we can do little more than enumerate the most important ones: chlorinated diphenyls (e.g., dichlorodiphenyltrichloroethane [DDT]) or chlorinated polycyclic compounds (Kepone), used as insecticides; diethylene dioxide (Dioxane); carbon disulfide; the halogenated hydrocarbons (methyl chloride, tetrachloroethane, carbon tetrachloride, trichloroethylene, and methyl bromide); naphthalene (used in moth repellants); benzine (gasoline); benzene and its derivatives (toluene, xylene, nitrobenzene, phenol, and amyl acetate [banana oil]); and the hexacarbon solvents (*n*-hexane and methyl-*n*-butyl ketone).

With a few exceptions, the acute toxic effects of these substances are much the same from one compound to another. In general, the primary effect is on nonneurologic structures. Neural symptoms consist of varying combinations of headache, restlessness, drowsiness, confusion, delirium, coma, and convulsions, which, as a rule, occur late in the illness or preterminally. Some of these industrial toxins (carbon disulfide, carbon tetrachloride and tetrachloroethane, acrylamide, *n*-hexane, and diethylene glycol [Sterno; see Rollins]) may cause polyneuropathy, which becomes evident with recovery from acute toxicity.

Extrapyramidal symptoms may result from chronic exposure to carbon disulfide. A syndrome of persistent fatigue, lack of stamina, inability to concentrate, poor memory, and irritability has also been attributed to chronic exposure to solvents, but these symptoms are quite nonspecific, and evidence for such a syndrome is unsupported by convincing experimental or epidemiologic studies.

Of the aforementioned industrial toxins, the ones most likely to cause neurologic disease are *toluene* (methyl benzene) and the *hexacarbons*. The chronic inhalation of fumes containing toluene (usually in glue, contact cement, or certain brands of spray paint) may lead to severe and irreversible tremor and cerebellar ataxia, affecting movements of the eyes (opsoclonus, ocular dysmetria) and limbs, as well as stance and gait. Cognitive impairment is usually associated; corticospinal tract signs, progressive optic neuropathy, sensorineural hearing loss, and hyposmia occur in some patients. Generalized cerebral atrophy and particularly cerebellar atrophy are evident in CT scans (Fornazzari et al; Hormes et al). Also, it has become apparent that acute toluene intoxication is an important cause of seizures, hallucinations, and coma in children (King et al).

The prolonged exposure to high concentrations of *n*-hexane or methyl-*n*-butyl ketone may cause a sensorimotor neuropathy, so-called glue-sniffer's neuropathy (see Chap. 46). These solvents are metabolized to 2,5-hexanedione, which is the agent that damages the peripheral nerves. The neuropathy may result from exposure in certain industrial settings (mainly the manufacture of vinyl products) or, more often, from the deliberate inhalation of vapors from solvents, lacquers, glue, or glue thinners containing *n*-hexane (see also Chap. 46). Impure trichloroethylene, through its breakdown product dichloroacetylene, has a predilection for the trigeminal nerve, which can be damaged selectively.

Hydrogen peroxide poisoning, usually by accidental ingestion, causes multiple small cerebral infarcts through a mechanism of gas embolus (Ijichi et al). Most cases have been reversible. According to Humberson and colleagues (cited by Ijichi et al) 120 mL of 35 percent hydrogen peroxide releases 14 L of oxygen on contact with organic tissue. The lung is involved, and the unmistakable brain lesions consist of tiny gas bubbles concentrated in parasagittal watershed areas.

ANTINEOPLASTIC AND IMMUNOSUPPRESSIVE AGENTS

The increasing use of potent antineoplastic agents has given rise to a diverse group of neurologic complications, the most important of which are summarized here. A more detailed account of these agents—as well as the neurologic complications of corticosteroid therapy, immunosuppression, and radiation—can be found in the monograph edited by Rottenberg and in the review of Tuxen and Hansen and in appropriate chapters of the book. The neurotoxic effects of certain agents used in the treatment of brain tumors are specifically considered in Chap. 31.

Vincristine

This drug is used in the treatment of acute lymphoblastic leukemia, lymphomas, and some solid tumors. Its most important toxic side effect, and the one that limits its use as a chemotherapeutic agent, is a peripheral neuropathy. Paresthesias of the feet, hands, or both may occur within a few weeks of the beginning of treatment; with continued use of the drug, a progressive symmetrical neuropathy evolves (mainly sensory with reflex loss). Cranial nerves are affected less frequently, but ptosis and lateral rectus, facial, and vocal cord palsies have been observed. Autonomic nervous system function may also be affected: constipation and impotence are frequent complications; orthostatic hypotension, atonicity of the bladder, and adynamic ileus are less frequent. The polyneuropathy caused by vincristine is described more fully in Chap. 46. Inappropriate antidiuretic hormone secretion and seizures have been reported but are uncommon.

Although rarely noted in the literature, the authors have seen an instance of reversible posterior leukoencephalopathy with cortical blindness and headache after a single dose of vincristine, identical to the syndrome reported with the use of calcineurin inhibitors (see further on).

The neural complications of *vinblastine* are similar to those of vincristine but are usually avoided because bone marrow suppression limits the dose of the drug that can safely be employed. *Vinorelbine* is a more recently introduced semisynthetic vinca alkaloid. It has much the same antitumor activity as vincristine but is supposedly less toxic.

Cisplatin

Cisplatin, a heavy metal that inhibits DNA synthesis, is effective in the treatment of gonadal and head and neck tumors, as well as carcinoma of the bladder, prostate, and breast. The dose-limiting factors in its use are nephrotoxicity and vomiting and a peripheral neuropathy (see Chap. 46). The latter manifests itself by numbness and tingling in fingers and toes, sometimes painful—symptoms that are being observed with increasing frequency. This toxic manifestation appears to be related to the total amount of drug administered, and it usually improves slowly after it has been discontinued. Biopsies of peripheral nerve have shown a primary axonal degeneration. Approximately one-third of patients receiving this drug also experience tinnitus or high-frequency hearing loss or both. Ototoxicity is also dose related, cumulative, and only occasionally reversible. Retrobulbar neuritis occurs rarely. Seizures associated with drug-induced hyponatremia and hypomagnesemia have been reported.

Paclitaxel and Docetaxel

Taxol (paclitaxel) and Taxotere (docetaxel) are newer anticancer drugs derived from the bark of the western yew. Both are particularly useful in the treatment of ovarian and breast cancer, but they have a wide range of antineoplastic activities. A purely or predominantly sensory neuropathy is a common complication. These drugs are thought to cause neuropathy by their action as inhibitors of the depolymerization of tubulin, thereby promoting excessive microtubule assembly within the axon. The neuropathy is dose-dependent, occurring with doses greater than 200 mg/m^2 of paclitaxel and at a wide range of dose levels for docetaxel (generally greater than 600 mg/m^2). Symptoms may begin 1 to 3 days following the first dose and affect the feet and hands simultaneously. Autonomic neuropathy (orthostatic hypotension) may occur as well. The neuropathy is axonal in type, with secondary demyelination, and is at least partially reversible after discontinuation of the drug.

Procarbazine

This drug, originally synthesized as an MAO inhibitor, is now an important oral agent in the treatment of Hodgkin disease and other tumors. It has also proved to be especially effective in the treatment of oligodendrogliomas. Neural complications are infrequent and usually take the form of somnolence, confusion, agitation, and depression. Diffuse aching pain in proximal muscles of the limbs and mild symptoms and signs of polyneuropathy occur in 10 to 15 percent of patients treated with relatively high doses. A reversible ataxia has also been described. Procarbazine, taken in conjunction with phenothiazines, barbiturates, narcotics, or alcohol, may produce serious degrees of oversedation. Other toxic reactions, such as orthostatic hypotension, are related to its inhibition of MAO.

L-Asparaginase

This enzymatic inhibitor of protein synthesis is used in the treatment of acute lymphoblastic leukemia. Drowsiness, confusion, delirium, stupor, coma, and diffuse EEG slowing are the common neurologic effects and are dose related and cumulative. They may occur within a day of onset of treatment and clear quickly when the drug is withdrawn, or they may be delayed in onset, in which case they persist for several weeks. These abnormalities are at least in part attributable to the systemic metabolic derangements induced by L-asparaginase, including liver dysfunction.

In recent years, increasing attention has been drawn to cerebrovascular complications of L-asparaginase therapy, including ischemic and hemorrhagic infarction and cerebral venous and dural sinus thrombosis. Fineberg and Swenson analyzed the clinical features of 38 such cases. These cerebrovascular complications are attributable to transient deficiencies in plasma proteins that are important in coagulation and fibrinolysis.

5-Fluorouracil

This is a pyrimidine analogue, used mainly as a secondary treatment of cancer of the breast, ovary, and gastrointestinal tract. A small proportion of patients receiving this drug develop dizziness, cerebellar ataxia of the trunk and the extremities, dysarthria, and nystagmus—symptoms that are much the same as those produced by cytarabine (ara-C; see below). These abnormalities must be distinguished from metastatic involvement of the cerebellum and paraneoplastic cerebellar degeneration. The drug effects are usually mild and subside within 1 to 6 weeks after discontinuation of therapy. The basis of this cerebellar syndrome is unknown.

Methotrexate (See also Chap. 31)

Administered in conventional oral or intravenous doses, methotrexate (MTX) is not usually neurotoxic. However, given intrathecally to treat meningeal leukemia or carcinomatosis, MTX commonly causes aseptic meningitis, with headache, nausea and vomiting, stiff neck, fever, and cells in the spinal fluid. Very rarely, probably as an idiosyncratic response to the drug, intrathecal administration results in an acute paraplegia that may be permanent. The pathology of this condition has not been studied.

The most serious and more common of the neurologic problems associated with systemic MTX chemotherapy is leukoencephalopathy or leukomyelopathy, especially when it is given in combination with cranial or neuraxis radiation therapy. This develops several months after repeated intrathecal or high systemic doses of the drug, and a few milder cases are known to have occurred without radiation treatments, i.e., with oral or intravenous MTX alone, such as the case reported by Worthley and McNeil. We have seen one such instance in a woman receiving oral MTX for a systemic vasculitis; no alternative explanation for widespread white matter changes and mild dementia could be discerned. Nonetheless, this must be quite uncommon. The full-blown syndrome consists of the insidious evolution of dementia, pseudobulbar palsy, ataxia, focal cerebral cortical deficits, or paraplegia. Milder cases show only radiographic evidence of a change in signal intensity in the posterior cerebral white matter ("posterior leukoencephalopathy") that is similar to the

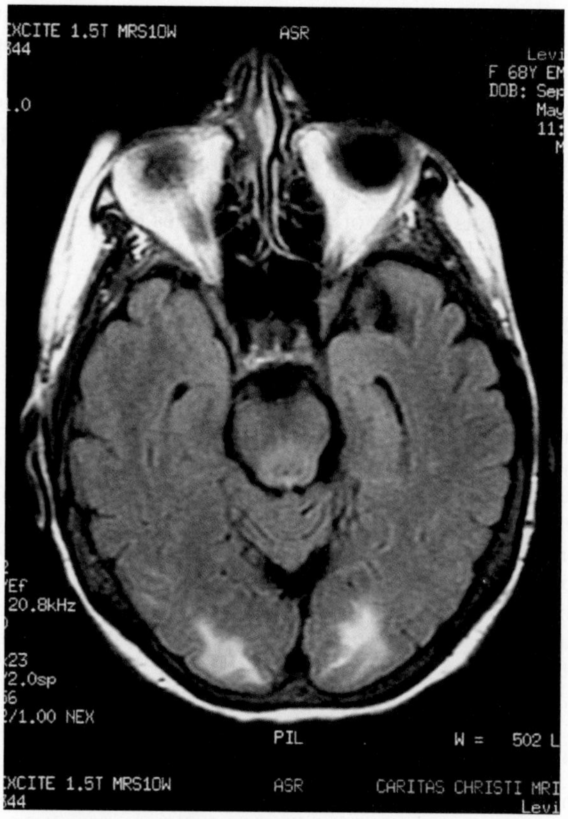

Figure 43-1. Toxic reversible posterior leukoencephalopathy. Axial fluid-attenuated inversion recovery (FLAIR) MRI in a patient with cortical blindness and severe headache days after receiving vincristine. This syndrome and radiographic findings are more typical following the use of cyclosporine, FK-506, and other chemotherapies. Compare this image to the similar conditions of hypertensive encephalopathy and toxemia shown in Fig. 34-29.

imaging findings that follow cyclosporine use (see further on) and hypertensive encephalopathy (Fig. 43-1). In severe cases, the brain shows disseminated foci of coagulation necrosis of white matter, usually periventricular, which can be detected with CT and MRI.

Mineralizing microangiopathy (fibrosis and calcification of small vessels, mainly in the basal ganglia) is yet another complication of MTX therapy. It may occur with MTX treatment or with cranial irradiation but is particularly common when both forms of treatment are combined. The present authors have the impression that the severe necrotic lesions possess features comparable to (and therefore may be the result of) the coagulative necrosis of radiation encephalopathy.

The Nitrosoureas

Carmustine (BCNU) and lomustine (CCNU) are nitrosoureas used to treat malignant cerebral gliomas. They are not neurotoxic when given in conventional intravenous doses, but intracarotid injection of the drugs may cause orbital, eye, and neck pain, focal seizures, confusion, and possibly focal neurologic deficits. Postmortem examinations of patients who had been treated with intravascular BCNU have disclosed a diffuse vasculopathy characterized by fibrinoid necrosis and microthrombi and diffuse foci of swollen axis cylinders and myelin vacuolization (Burger et al; Kleinschmidt-de Masters).

Cytarabine (Ara-C)

This drug, long used in the treatment of acute nonlymphocytic leukemia, is not neurotoxic when given in the usual systemic daily doses of 100 to 200 mg/m^2. The administration of very high doses (up to 30 times the usual dose) induces remissions in patients' refractory to conventional treatments. It also may produce, however, a severe degree of cerebellar degeneration in a considerable proportion of cases (4 of 24 reported by Winkelman and Hines). Ataxia of gait and limbs, dysarthria, and nystagmus develop as early as 5 to 7 days after the beginning of high-dose treatment and worsen rapidly. Postmortem examination has disclosed a diffuse degeneration of Purkinje cells, most marked in the depths of the folia, as well as a patchy degeneration of other elements of the cerebellar cortex. Other patients receiving high-dose ara-C have developed a mild, reversible cerebellar syndrome with the same clinical features. Because patients older than 50 years of age are said to be far more likely to develop cerebellar degeneration than those younger than 50 years of age, the former should be treated with a lower dosage (Herzig et al).

Calcineurin Inhibitors (Cyclosporine, Tacrolimus, Sirolimus)

These immunosuppressive drugs are used to prevent transplant rejection and to treat aplastic anemia and certain intrinsic immune diseases. Tremor is perhaps the most frequent side effect and myoclonus may be added. Sometimes these impart a stuttering character to speech. Headache and insomnia are common. Seizures may be a manifestation of toxicity, but the cause may lie with the other complications of organ transplantation and immunosuppression. Wijdicks has reviewed the neurologic effects of these drugs.

A posterior leukoencephalopathy syndrome (PRES, see Chap. 34) resembling hypertensive encephalopathy—headache, vomiting, confusion, seizures, and visual loss (cortical blindness)—may follow the use of either drug and with an expanding list of other agents including some of the new monoclonal antibodies used in the treatment of cancer and autoimmune diseases (Table 43-1). There does not seem to be a consistent dose-response effect, drug levels often being in the therapeutic range.

The appearance on CT scans and MRI of symmetrical signal and density changes mainly in the posterior white matter likewise conform to the pattern that is seen in hypertensive encephalopathy (reversible posterior leukoencephalopathy [RPLE] or PRES). Lesions may also appear subcortically in the frontal and parietal lobes. Interferon treatment for malignant melanoma and a number of other chemotherapeutic agents have been associated with the same condition. Hinchey and colleagues have described several such cases and suggested that cyclosporine alters the blood–brain barrier and that the fluid overload and hypertension which accompanies the use of cyclosporine underlies the radiologic changes. A variety of psychotic syndromes with delusions, paranoia, and visual hallucinations also have been ascribed to the use of these drugs (see Wijdicks).

Table 43-1

NON-VASCULAR CAUSES OF REVERSIBLE POSTERIOR LEUKOENCEPHALOPATHY (SEE ALSO CHAP. 34)
Methotrexate (intravenous and rarely oral)
Calcineurin inhibitors (cyclosporine, tacrolimus, sirolimus)
Cyclophosphamide
Interferon (intravenous)
L-Asparaginase
Vincristine
Cisplatin
Cytarabine
Gemcitabine
Doxorubicin
Etopiside
Intravenous immunoglobulin
Granulocyte colony stimulating factor
Erythropoetin
Rituximab
Surafinib
Sunitinib
Bevicziumab
Combination chemotherapies, particularly those including cyclophosphamide or cytarabine

Thalidomide

Despite the catastrophic effects of thalidomide on the developing fetus (following its introduction as a soporific in 1957), this drug has now found several specific uses in the treatment of immunologic, neoplastic, and infectious diseases. It is effective in the treatment of leprosy, erythema nodosum, and the oral ulcerations of AIDS and Behçet disease. Experimental uses include suppression of graft-versus-host reactions and inhibition of blood vessel proliferation in vascular tumors such as renal cell cancer. A dose-dependent sensory neuropathy is the limiting factor in its use, and serial electrophysiologic testing is recommended if the medication is to be prescribed for protracted periods. Of course, it must not be given to a woman who is or might be pregnant.

Antibiotics and Other Medications

Numerous antibiotics, cardioactive medications, and other drugs may have adverse effects on the central or peripheral nervous system. Some of the latter are addressed in Chap. 46. Here we mention mainly that penicillin and its derivatives such as imipenem, and to a lesser degree, the cephalosporins, are capable of causing seizures when high serum concentrations are attained. This is favored in most instances by concomitant renal failure.

Other important examples of antibiotic toxicity are optic neuropathy caused by ethambutol toxicity; ototoxicity and neuromuscular blockade from aminoglycoside and fluoroquinolone antibiotics (see Chap. 41); peripheral neuropathy, encephalopathy, and an Antabuse-like reaction to alcohol in patients taking metronidazole; a metronidazole-induced polyneuropathy, isoniazid (INH) neuropathy and optic neuropathy, and possibly a peripheral neuropathy caused by chloramphenicol.

Woodruff and colleagues, as well as others, reported a curious and reversible cerebellar syndrome caused by *metronidazole* with MRI signal changes in the dentate nuclei, or more widespread signal changes in other parts of the brainstem and cerebral white matter as noted by Kim and coworkers, who carried out an MIR study of 7 patients. Dysarthria, confusion, and gait ataxia seem to form the core of the clinical syndrome but imaging changes may be found coincidentally as well.

The most notorious toxic consequences with this group of drugs were seen with *clioquinol*, which was sold as Entero-Vioform and was used in many parts of the world to prevent traveler's diarrhea and as a treatment for chronic gastroenteritis. In 1971, clinical observations began to appear in medical journals of a subacute myelo-opticoneuropathy (SMON). During the 1960s, more than 10,000 cases of this disease were collected in Japan by Tsubaki and colleagues. Usually the illness began with ascending numbness and weakness of the legs, paralysis of sphincters, and autonomic disorder. Later, vision was affected. The onset was acute in about two-thirds of the cases and subacute in the remainder. The occurrence of these neurologic complications was found to be related to the prolonged use of clioquinol. In Japan, the drug was withdrawn from the market, and the incidence of SMON immediately fell, supporting the theory that it was caused by the drug. Recovery was usually incomplete.

Also mentioned here, because neurologists are often asked to consult on these cases, is a curious effect of the anesthetic propofol. Seizures and myoclonic-like movements have been seen in a small number of individuals, presumably as an idiosyncratic effect. Sometimes these take the form of less-organized twitching, opisthotonus, or involuntary movements. Some inhaled anesthetics such as enflurane can cause seizures in susceptible patients. In our own experience, the seizures have occurred in the first hour after emergence from anesthesia, but as many cases are reported with seizures occurring during induction, emergence, and after the use of the drug (see Walder).

References

General

Cooper JR, Bloom FE, Roth RH: *The Biochemical Basis of Neuropharmacology*, 7th ed. New York, Oxford University Press, 1996.
Dickey W, Morrow JI: Drug-induced neurological disorders. *Prog Neurobiol* 34:331, 1990.
Enna SJ, Coyle JT: *Pharmacological Management of Neurological and Psychiatric Disorders*. New York, McGraw-Hill, 1998.
Fahn S: A therapeutic approach to tardive dyskinesia. *J Clin Psychiatry* 46:19, 1985.
Goldfrank LR, Flomenbaum N, Lewin N, et al (eds): *Goldfrank's Toxicologic Emergencies*, 8th ed. Beverly Farms, MA, OEM Press, 2006.
Harbison RD (ed): *Hamilton and Hardy's Industrial Toxicology*, 5th ed. St. Louis, Mosby, 1998.
Hardman JG, Limbird LE, Molinoff PB, et al (eds): *Goodman and Gilman's The Pharmacological Basis of Therapeutics*, 10th ed. New York, McGraw-Hill, 2001.
Hollister LE: *Clinical Pharmacology of Psychotherapeutic Drugs*, 3rd ed. New York, Churchill Livingstone, 1990.
Jankovic J, Beach J: Long-term effects of tetrabenazine in hyperkinetic movement disorders. *Neurology* 48:358, 1997.
Johnston MV, Gross RA: Fundamentals of drug therapy in neurology, in Johnston MV, Gross RA (eds): *Principles of Drug Therapy in Neurology*, 2nd ed. Oxford, UK, Oxford University Press, 2008, pp 3–32.
Klaassen CD (ed): *Casarett and Doull's Toxicology: The Basic Science of Poisons*, 6th ed. New York, McGraw-Hill, 2001.
Levy BS, Wegman DH: *Occupational Health: Recognizing and Preventing Work-Related Disease and Injury*, 4th ed. Philadelphia, Lippincott Williams & Wilkins, 1999.
Rom WN (ed): *Environmental and Occupational Medicine*, 3rd ed. Philadelphia, Lippincott-Raven, 1998.
Rosenberg NL: *Occupational and Environmental Neurology*. Boston, Butterworth-Heinemann, 1995.
Spencer PS, Schaumburg HH (eds): *Experimental and Clinical Neurotoxicology*, 2nd ed. New York, Oxford, 2000.

Opiates and Synthetic Analgesics

American Psychiatric Association: Practical guidelines for the treatment of substance use disorders. *Am J Psychiatry* 152(Suppl):1, 1995.
Ball J, Ross A: *The Effectiveness of Methadone Maintenance Treatments*. New York, Springer Verlag, 1991.
Boyer EW: Management of opioid analgesic overdose. *N Engl J Med* 367:2, 2012.
Camí J, Farré M: Drug addiction. *N Engl J Med* 349:975, 2003.
Fields HL: *Pain*. New York, McGraw-Hill, 1987.
Fudala PJ, Bridge TP, Herbert S, et al: Office-based treatment of opiate addiction with a sublingual-tablet formulation of buprenorphine and naloxone. *N Engl J Med* 349:949, 2003.
Jasinski DR, Johnson RE, Kocher TR: Clonidine in morphine withdrawal. *Arch Gen Psychiatry* 42:1063, 1985.
Mello NK, Mendelson JH: Buprenorphine treatment of cocaine and heroin abuse, in Cowan A, Lewis JW (eds): *Buprenorphine: Combatting Drug Abuse With a Unique Opioid*. Wilmington, DE, Wiley-Liss, 1995, pp 241–287.
Monroe JJ, Ross WF, Berzins JI: The decline of the addict as "psychopath": Implications for community care. *Int J Addict* 6:601, 1971.
Oviedo-Joekes E, Brissette S, Marsh DC, et al: Diacetylmorphine versus methadone for the treatment of opioid addiction. *N Engl J Med* 361:777, 2009.
Tan TP, Algra PR, Valk J, Wolters EC: Toxic leukoencephalopathy after inhalation of poisoned heroin: MR findings. *AJNR Am J Neuroradiol* 15:175, 1994.
Wikler A: *Opioid Dependence: Mechanisms and Treatment*. New York, Plenum Press, 1980.

Wolters EC, Van Wijngaarden GK, Stam FC, et al: Leukoencephalopathy after inhaling "heroin" pyrolysate. *Lancet* 2:1233, 1982.

Barbiturates, Benzodiazepines, Antidepressants, and Neuroleptic Drugs

Baldessarini RJ: Drugs and the treatment of psychiatric disorders: Psychosis and anxiety, in Hardman JG, Limbrin LE, Gilman AG, et al (eds): *Goodman and Gilman's The Pharmacological Basis of Therapeutics*, 10th ed. New York, McGraw-Hill, 2001, pp 447–484.

Baldessarini RJ: Drugs and the treatment of psychiatric disorders: Depression and mania, in Hardman JG, Limbrin LE, Gilman GA, et al (eds): *Goodman and Gilman's The Pharmacological Basis of Therapeutics*, 10th ed. New York, McGraw-Hill, 2001, pp 485–520.

Baldessarini RJ, Frankenburg FR: Clozapine: A novel antipsychotic agent. *N Engl J Med* 324:746, 1991.

Bloomer HA, Maddock RK Jr: An assessment of diuresis and dialysis for treating acute barbiturate poisoning, in Mathew H (ed): *Acute Barbiturate Poisoning*. Amsterdam, Excerpta Medica, 1971, pp 76–91.

Boyer EW, Shannon M: The serotonin syndrome. *N Engl J Med* 352:1112, 2005.

Caroff SN, Mann SC: Neuroleptic malignant syndrome. *Med Clin North Am* 77:185, 1993.

Charney DS, Mihic SJ, Harris RA: Hypnotics and sedatives, in Hardman JG, Limbrin LE, Gilman GA (eds): *Goodman and Gilman's Pharmacologic Basis of Therapeutics*, 10th ed. New York, McGraw-Hill, 2001, pp 349–428.

Coyle JT: Psychiatric disorders, in Johnston MV, Gross RA (eds): *Principles of Drug Therapy in Neurology*, 2nd ed. Oxford, UK, Oxford University Press, 2008, pp 387–400.

Enna SJ, Coyle JT: *Pharmacological Management of Neurological and Psychiatric Disorders*. New York, McGraw-Hill, 1998.

Isbell H, Altschul S, Kornetsky CH, et al: Chronic barbiturate intoxication: An experimental study. *Arch Neurol Psychiatry* 64:1, 1950.

Krisanda TJ: Flumazenil: An antidote for benzodiazepine toxicity. *Am Fam Physician* 47:891, 1993.

Marks J: *The Benzodiazepines: Use, Overuse, Misuse, Abuse*, 2nd ed. Boston, MTP Press, 1985.

Richelson E: Pharmacology of antidepressants—Characteristics of the ideal drug. *Mayo Clin Proc* 69:1069, 1994.

Romero CE, Baron JD, Knox AP, et al: Barbiturate withdrawal following Internet purchase of Fioricet. *Arch Neurol* 61:1111, 2004.

Snyder SH: Receptors, neurotransmitters and drug responses. *N Engl J Med* 300: 465, 1979.

Suzuki A, Kondo T, Otani K, et al: Association of the TagIA polymorphism of the dopamine (D2) receptor gene with predisposition to neuroleptic syndrome. *Am J Psychiatry* 158:1714, 2001.

Stimulants (Including Cocaine and Amphetamines) and Psychomimetic Drugs

Altura BT, Altura BM: Phencyclidine, lysergic acid diethylamide and mescaline: Cerebral artery spasms and hallucinogenic activity. *Science* 212:1051, 1981.

Baldessarini RJ: Drugs and the treatment of psychiatric disorders: Psychosis and anxiety, in Hardman JG, Limbrin LE, Molinoff PB, et al (eds): *Goodman and Gilman's The Pharmacological Basis of Therapeutics*, 9th ed. New York, McGraw-Hill, 1996, pp 399–430.

Cregler LL, Mark H: Medical complications of cocaine abuse. *N Engl J Med* 315:1495, 1986.

Gawin FH, Ellinwood FH: Cocaine and other stimulants: Actions, abuse, and treatment. *N Engl J Med* 318:1173, 1988.

Greenblatt DJ, Harmatz JS, Zinny MA, Shader RI: Effect of gradual withdrawal on the rebound sleep disorder after discontinuation of triazolam. *N Engl J Med* 317:722, 1987.

Harrington H, Heller A, Dawson D: Intracerebral hemorrhage and oral amphetamine. *Arch Neurol* 40:503, 1983.

Hollister LE: Cannabis. *Acta Psychiatr Scand* 78(Suppl 345):108, 1988.

Hollister LE: *Clinical Pharmacology of Psychotherapeutic Drugs*, 3rd ed. New York, Churchill Livingstone, 1990.

Hollister LE, Csernansky JG: Drug-induced psychiatric disorders and their management. *Med Toxicol* 1:428, 1986.

Iverson L: Cannabis and the brain. *Brain* 126:1252, 2003.

Levine SR, Brust JCM, Futrell N, et al: Cerebrovascular complications of the use of the "crack" form of alkaloidal cocaine. *N Engl J Med* 323:699, 1990.

Mendelson JH, Mello NK: Management of cocaine abuse and dependence. *N Engl J Med* 334:965, 1996.

Nicholi AM: The nontherapeutic use of psychoactive drugs. *N Engl J Med* 308:925, 1983.

O'Brien CO: Drug addiction and drug abuse, in Hardman JG, Limbrin LE, Gilman AG, et al (eds): *Goodman and Gilman's The Pharmacological Basis of Therapeutics*, 10th ed. New York, McGraw-Hill, 2001, pp 621–642.

Peroutka SJ, Newman H, Harris H: Subjective effects of 3-4 methyl-enedioxymethamphetamine in recreational users. *Neuropsychopharmacology* 1:273, 1988.

Peterson RC, Stillman RC: Phencyclidine: An overview, in Peterson RC, Stillman RC (eds): *Phencyclidine (PCP) Abuse, Research*. Monograph Series 21. Washington, DC, National Institute on Drug Abuse, 1978, pp 19–28.

Roth D, Alarcon FJ, Fernandez JA, et al: Acute rhabdomyolysis associated with cocaine intoxication. *N Engl J Med* 319:673, 1988.

Verebey K, Alrazi J, Jaffe JH: Complications of "ecstasy" (MDMA). *JAMA* 259:1649, 1988.

Tetanus

Farrar JJ, Yen LM, Cook T, et al: Tetanus. *J Neurol Neurosurg Psychiatry* 69:292, 2000.

Griffin JW: Bacterial toxins: Botulism and tetanus, in Kennedy PGE, Johnson RT (eds): *Infections of the Nervous System*. London, Butterworth, 1987, pp 83–92.

Sanford JP: Tetanus—forgotten but not gone. *N Engl J Med* 332:812, 1995.

Struppler A, Struppler E, Adams RD: Local tetanus in man. *Arch Neurol* 8:162, 1963.

Weinstein L: Current concepts: Tetanus. *N Engl J Med* 289:1293, 1973.

Diphtheria

Fisher CM, Adams RD: Diphtheritic polyneuritis: A pathological study. *J Neuropathol Exp Neurol* 15:243, 1956.

McDonald WI, Kocen RS: Diphtheritic neuropathy, in Dyck PJ, Thomas PK, Griffin JW, et al (eds): *Peripheral Neuropathy*, 3rd ed. Philadelphia, Saunders, 1993, pp 1412–1423.

Pappenheimer AM: Diphtheria toxin. *Annu Rev Biochem* 46:69, 1977.

Waksman BH, Adams RD, Mansmann HC: Experimental study of diphtheritic polyneuritis in the rabbit and guinea pig. *J Exp Med* 105:591, 1957.

Botulism

Ferrari ND, Weisse ME: Botulism. *Adv Pediatr Infect Dis* 10:81, 1995.

Griffin JW: Bacterial toxins: Botulism and tetanus, in Kennedy PGE, Johnson RT (eds): *Infections of the Nervous System*. London, Butterworth, 1987, pp 76–92.

Hatheway CL: Botulism: The present status of disease. *Curr Top Microbiol Immunol* 195:55, 1995.

Jankovic J: Botulinum toxin in movement disorders. *Curr Opin Neurol* 7:358, 1994.

Mayer RF: The neuromuscular defect in human botulism, in Locke S (ed): *Modern Neurology*. Boston, Little, Brown, 1969, pp 169–186.

Roblot P, Roblot F, Fauchere JL, et al: Retrospective study of 108 cases of botulism in Poitiers, France. *J Med Microbiol* 40:379, 1994.

Mushroom Poisoning

Koppel C: Clinical symptomatology and management of mushroom poisoning. *Toxicon* 31:1513, 1993.
Mushroom poisoning. *Med Lett Drugs Ther* 26:67, 1984.

Marine Toxins

Pearn J: Neurology of ciguatera. *J Neurol Neurosurg Psychiatry* 70:4, 2001.

Venoms, Bites, and Stings

Boyer LV, Theodorous AA, Berg, RA, et al: Antivenom for critically ill children with neurotoxicity from scorpion stings. *N Engl J Med* 360:2090, 2009.
Crawley F, Schon F, Brown M: Cerebral infarctions: A rare complication of wasp sting. *J Neurol Neurosurg Psychiatry* 66:550, 1999.
Felz MW, Smith CD, Swift TR: A six-year-old girl with tick paralysis. *N Engl J Med* 342:90, 2000.
Garcia-Monco JC, Benach J: Lyme neuroborreliosis. *Ann Neurol* 37:691, 1995.
Gold BS, Dart RC, Barish RA: Bites of venomous snakes. *N Engl J Med* 347:347, 2002.
Grattan-Smith PJ, Morris JG, Johnston HM, et al: Clinical and neurophysiological features of tick paralysis. *Brain* 120:1975, 1997.
Rahn D, Evans J (eds): *Lyme Disease*. Philadelphia, American College of Physicians, 1998.

Metals and Industrial Agents—General

Dyck PJ, Thomas PK, Griffin JW, et al (eds): Neuropathy associated with industrial agents, metals, and drugs, in *Peripheral Neuropathy*, 3rd ed. Vol 2. Philadelphia, Saunders, 1993, pp 1533–1581.

Lead

Agency for Toxic Substances and Disease Registry: *The Nature and Extent of Lead Poisoning in Children in the United States: A Report to Congress*. Atlanta, GA, Department of Health and Human Services, 1988.
Baghurst PA, McMichael AJ, Wigg NR, et al: Environmental exposure to lead and children's intelligence at the age of seven years—the Port Pirie Cohort Study. *N Engl J Med* 327:1279, 1992.
Canfield RL, Henderson CR, Cery-Slechata DA, et al: Intellectual impairment in children with blood lead concentrations below 10 g per deciliter. *N Engl J Med* 348:1517, 2003.
Goldman RH, Baker EL, Hannan M, Kamerow DB: Lead poisoning in automobile radiator mechanics. *N Engl J Med* 317:214, 1987.
Jorgensen FM: Succimer: The first approved oral lead chelator. *Am Fam Physician* 48:1496, 1993.
Mahaffey KR: Exposure to lead in childhood. *N Engl J Med* 327:1308, 1992.
Mahaffey KR, Annest JL, Roberts J, Murphy RS: National estimates of blood lead levels: United States, 1976–1980. *N Engl J Med* 307:573, 1982.
Mortensen ME, Walson PD: Chelation therapy for childhood lead poisoning. The changing scene in the 1990s. *Clin Pediatr (Phila)* 32:284, 1993.
Needleman HL: Childhood lead poisoning. *Curr Opin Neurol* 7:187, 1994.
Needleman HL, Schell A, Bellinger D, et al: The long-term effects of exposure to low doses of lead in childhood: An 11-year follow-up report. *N Engl J Med* 322:83, 1990.
Rogan WJ, Dierich KN, Ware JH, et al: The effect of chelation therapy with succimer on neuropsychological development in children exposed to lead. *N Engl J Med* 344:1421, 2001.
Rutter M: Raised lead levels and impaired cognitive/behavioural functioning: A review of the evidence. *Dev Med Child Neurol* 22(Suppl 42):1, 1980.
Whitfield CL, Chien L, Whitehead JD: Lead encephalopathy in adults. *Am J Med* 52:289, 1972.

Arsenic

Heyman A, Pfeiffer JB Jr, Willett RW, Taylor HM: Peripheral neuropathy caused by arsenical intoxication. *N Engl J Med* 254:401, 1956.
Jenkins RB: Inorganic arsenic and the nervous system. *Brain* 89:479, 1966.
Moyer TP: Testing for arsenic. *Mayo Clin Proc* 68:1210, 1993.

Manganese

Calne DB, Chu NS, Huang CC, et al: Manganism and idiopathic parkinsonism: Similarities and differences. *Neurology* 44:1583, 1994.
Mena I, Marin O, Fuenzalida S, Cotzias GC: Chronic manganese poisoning: Clinical picture and manganese turnover. *Neurology* 17:128, 1967.

Mercury

Agocs MM, Etzel RA, Parrish RG, et al: Mercury exposure from interior latex paint. *N Engl J Med* 323:1096, 1990.
Albers JW, Kallenbach LR, Fine LJ, et al (The Mercury Workers Study Group): Neurological abnormalities associated with remote occupational elemental mercury exposure. *Ann Neurol* 24:651, 1988.
Clarkson TW: The toxicology of mercury—current exposures and clinical manifestations. *N Engl J Med* 349:1731, 2003.
Harada M: Minamata disease: Methylmercury poisoning in Japan caused by environmental pollution. *Crit Rev Toxicol* 25:1, 1995.
Kark RAP, Poskanzer DC, Bullock JD, Boylen G: Mercury poisoning and its treatment with *N*-acetyl-*dl*-penicillamine. *N Engl J Med* 285:10, 1971.
Nierenberg DW, Nordgren RE, Chang MB, et al: Delayed cerebellar disease and death after accidental exposure to dimethylmercury. *N Engl J Med* 338:1672, 1998.
Tokuomi H, Uchino M, Imamura S, et al: Minamata disease (organic mercury poisoning): Neuroradiologic and electrophysiologic studies. *Neurology* 32:1369, 1982.

Organophosphates

Cavanagh JB, Patangia GN: Changes in the central nervous system of the cat as a result of tri-*o*-cresyl phosphate poisoning. *Brain* 88:165, 1965.
Jamal GA: Long term neurotoxic effects of organophosphate compounds. *Adverse Drug React Toxicol Rev* 14:85, 1995.
Moretto A, Lotti M: Poisoning by organophosphorus insecticides and sensory polyneuropathy. *J Neurol Neurosurg Psychiatry* 64:463, 1998.
Prineas J: The pathogenesis of the dying-back polyneuropathies. *J Neuropathol Exp Neurol* 28:571, 1969.
Senanayake N, Karalliedde L: Neurotoxic effects of organophosphate insecticide. *N Engl J Med* 316:761, 1987.
Sherman JD: Organophosphate pesticides—neurological and respiratory toxicity. *Toxicol Ind Health* 11:33, 1995.

Thallium

Bank WJ, Pleasure DE, Suzuki D, et al: Thallium poisoning. *Arch Neurol* 26:456, 1972.
Desenclos JC, Wilder MH, Coppenger GW, et al: Thallium poisoning: An outbreak in Florida, 1988. *South Med J* 85:1203, 1992.

Gold

Katrak SM, Pollock M, O'Brien CP, et al: Clinical and morphological features of gold neuropathy. *Brain* 103:671, 1980.

Aluminum

Landsberg JP, McDonald B, Watt F: Absence of aluminum in neuritic plaque cores in Alzheimer's disease. *Nature* 360:65, 1992.

LeQuesne PM: Toxic substances and the nervous system: The role of clinical observation. *J Neurol Neurosurg Psychiatry* 44:1, 1981.

Longstreth WT, Rosenstock L, Heyer NJ: Potroom palsy? Neurologic disorder in three aluminum smelter workers. *Arch Intern Med* 145:1972, 1985.

Perl DP, Brody AR: Alzheimer's disease: X-ray spectrometric evidence of aluminum accumulation in neurofibrillary tangle-bearing neurons. *Science* 208:297, 1980.

Perl DP, Gajdusek DC, Garruto RM, et al: Intraneuronal aluminum accumulation in amyotrophic lateral sclerosis and parkinsonism-dementia of Guam. *Science* 217:1053, 1982.

Tin

Alajouanine TH, Derobert L, Thieffry S: Etude clinique d'ensemble de 210 cas d'intoxication par les sels organiques d'étain. *Rev Neurol (Paris)* 98:85, 1958.

LeQuesne PM: Metal neurotoxicity, in Asbury AK, McKhann GM, McDonald WI (eds): *Diseases of the Nervous System*, 2nd ed. Philadelphia, Saunders, 1992, pp 1250–1258.

Bismuth

Buge A, Supino-Viterbo V, Rancurel G, Pontes C: Epileptic phenomena in bismuth toxic encephalopathy. *J Neurol Neurosurg Psychiatry* 44:62, 1981.

Burns R, Thomas DQ, Barron VJ: Reversible encephalopathy possibly associated with bismuth subgallate ingestion. *Br Med J* 1:220, 1974.

Mendelowitz PC, Hoffman RS, Weber S: Bismuth absorption and myoclonic encephalopathy during bismuth subsalicylate therapy. *Ann Intern Med* 112:140, 1990.

Industrial Toxins and Solvents

Editorial: Hexacarbon neuropathy. *Lancet* 2:942, 1979.

Elofsson SA, Gamberale F, Hindmarsh T, et al: Exposure to organic solvents. *Scand J Work Environ Health* 6:239, 1980.

Fornazzari L, Wilkinson DA, Kapur BM, Carlen PL: Cerebellar, cortical and functional impairment in toluene abusers. *Acta Neurol Scand* 67:319, 1983.

Hormes JT, Filley CM, Rosenberg NL: Neurologic sequelae of chronic solvent vapor abuse. *Neurology* 36:698, 1986.

Ijichi T, Iton T, Sakai R, et al: Multiple brain gas embolism after ingestion of concentrated hydrogen peroxide. *Neurology* 48:277, 1997.

King MD, Day RE, Oliver JS, et al: Solvent encephalopathy. *Br Med J* 283:663, 1981.

Rollins YD, Filley CM, McNut JT, et al: Fulminant ascending paralysis as a delayed sequela of diethylene glycol (Sterno) ingestion. *Neurology* 59:1460, 2002.

Spencer PS, Schaumburg HH: Organic solvent neurotoxicity. *Scand J Work Environ Health* 11(Suppl 1):53, 1985.

Antineoplastic and Immunosuppressive Agents and Antibiotics

American Academy of Pediatrics Committee on Drugs: Clioquinol (iodochlorhydroxyquin, Vioform) and iodoquinol (diiodohydroxyquin): Blindness and neuropathy. *Pediatrics* 86:797, 1990.

Burger PC, Kamenar E, Schold SC, et al: Encephalomyelopathy following high-dose BCNU therapy. *Cancer* 48:1318, 1981.

Filley CM, Kleinschmidt-DeMasters BK: Toxic leukoencephalopathy. *N Engl J Med* 345:425, 2001.

Fineberg WM, Swenson MR: Cerebrovascular complications of L-asparaginase therapy. *Neurology* 38:127, 1988.

Herzig RH, Hines JD, Herzig GP: Cellular toxicity with high-dose cytosine-arabinoside. *J Clin Oncol* 5:927, 1987.

Hinchey J, Chaves C, Appigani B, et al: A reversible posterior leukoencephalopathy syndrome. *N Engl J Med* 334:494, 1996.

Kaplan RS, Wiernik PH: Neurotoxicity of antineoplastic drugs. *Semin Oncol* 9:103, 1982.

Kim E, Na DG, Kim EY, et al: MR imaging of metronidazole-induced encephalopathy: lesion distribution and diffusion-Weighted imaging findings. *AJNR* 28:1652, 2007.

Kleinschmidt-de Masters BK: Intracarotid BCNU leukoencephalopathy. *Cancer* 57:1276, 1986.

Postma TJ, Vermorken JB, Liefting AJ, et al: Paclitaxel-induced neuropathy. *Ann Oncol* 6:489, 1995.

Rottenberg DA (ed): *Neurological Complications of Cancer Therapy*. Boston, Butterworth-Heinemann, 1991.

Ryan A, Molloy FM, Farrell MS, et al: Fatal toxic leukoencephalopathy: Clinical, radiological, and necropsy findings in two patients. *J Neurol Neurosurg Psychiatry* 76:1014, 2005.

Tsubaki T, Honmay Y, Hoshl M: Neurological syndrome associated with clioquinol. *Lancet* 1:696, 1971.

Tuxen MK, Hansen SW: Neurotoxicity secondary to antineoplastic drugs. *Cancer Treat Rev* 20:191, 1994.

Walder B, Tramer MR, Seeck M: Seizure-like phenomena and propofol. A systematic review. *Neurology* 58:1327, 2002.

Wijdicks EFM: Neurologic manifestations of immunosuppressive agents, in Wijdicks EFM (ed): *Neurologic Complications in Organ Transplant Recipients*. Boston, Butterworth-Heinemann, 1999.

Winkelman MD, Hines JD: Cerebellar degeneration caused by high-dose cytosine arabinoside: A clinicopathological study. *Ann Neurol* 14:520, 1983.

Woodruff BK, Wijdicks EF, Marshall WF: Reversible metronidazole-induced lesions of the cerebellar dentate nuclei. *N Engl J Med* 346:68, 2002.

Worthley SG, McNeil JD: Leukoencephalopathy in a patient taking low dose oral methotrexate therapy for rheumatoid arthritis. *J Rheumatol* 22:335, 1995.

PART 5

DISEASES OF SPINAL CORD, PERIPHERAL NERVE, AND MUSCLE

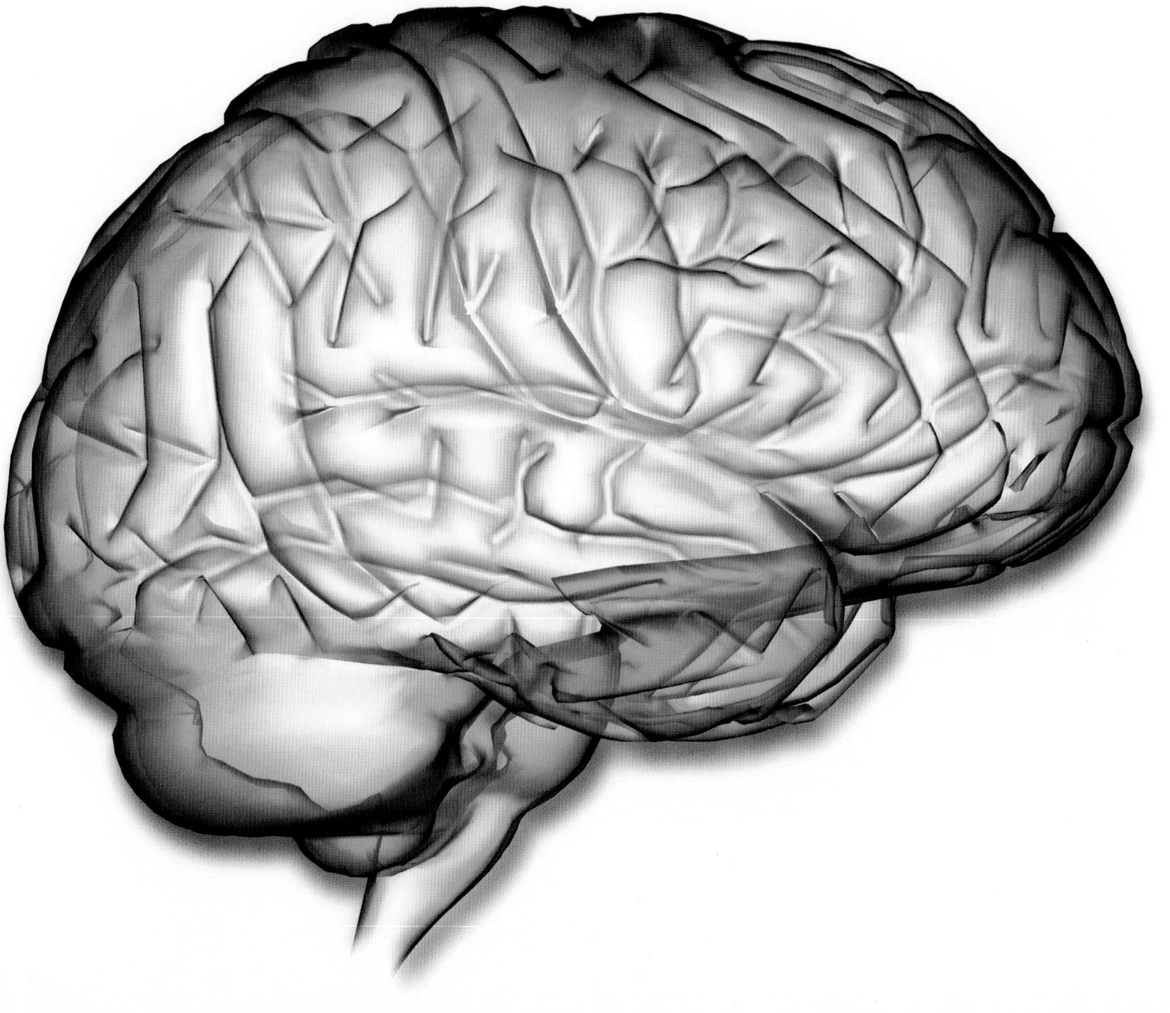

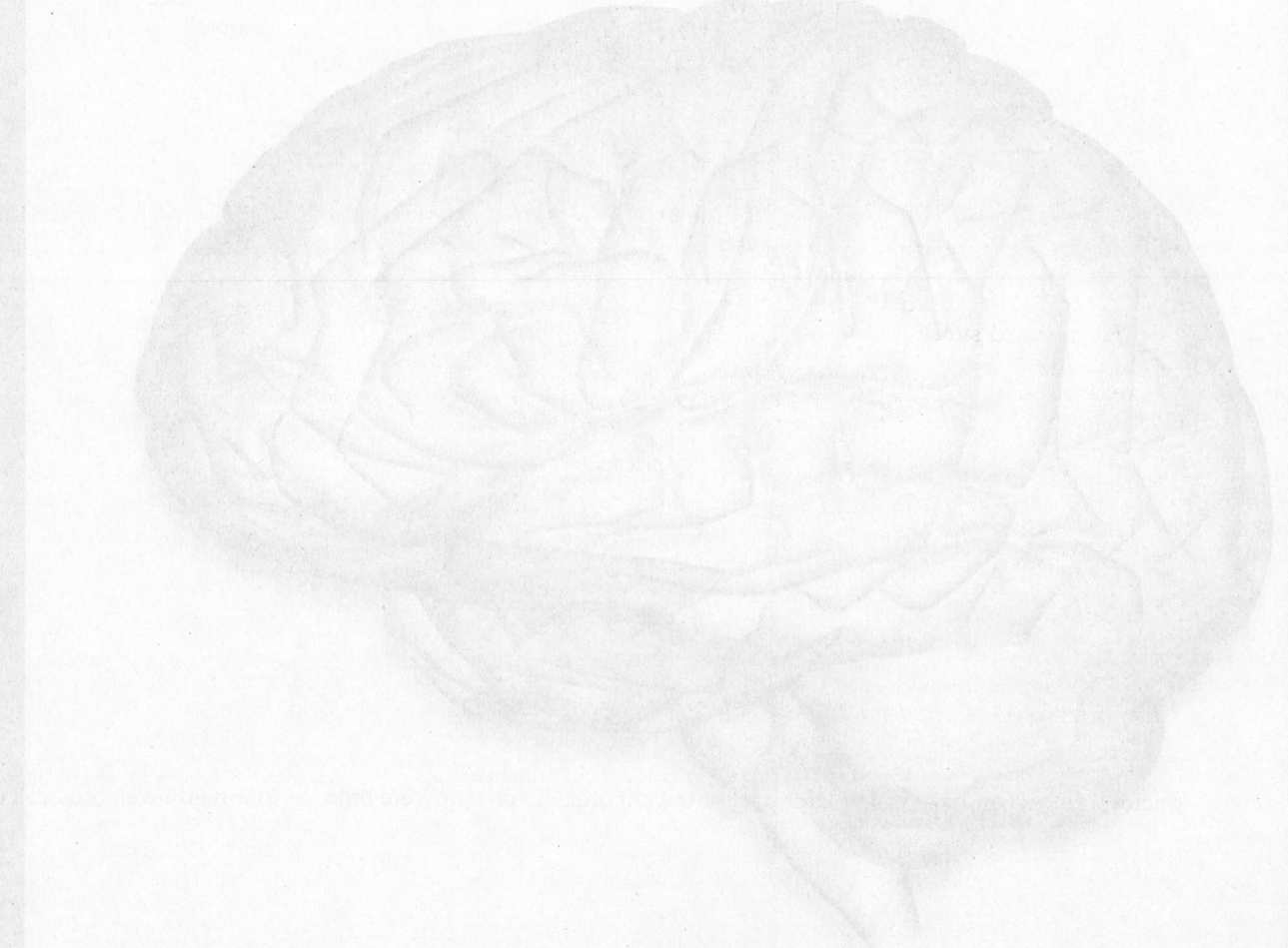

44

Diseases of the Spinal Cord

Diseases of the nervous system may be confined to the spinal cord where they produce a number of distinctive syndromes. These relate to the special anatomic features of the cord, such as its prominent function in sensorimotor conduction and relatively primitive reflex activity; its long, cylindrical shape; its small cross-sectional size; the peripheral location of myelinated fibers next to the pia; the special arrangement of its blood vessels; and its intimate relationship to the vertebral column. Woolsey and Young estimated that approximately 30 diseases are known to affect the spinal cord, of which half are seen with regularity. These processes express themselves in a number of readily recognized ways and, as will be evident, certain diseases preferentially produce special syndromes. This syndromic grouping of the spinal cord disorders, which is in keeping with the general plan of this book, greatly facilitates clinical diagnosis.

The main syndromes considered in this chapter are (1) a complete or almost complete sensorimotor myelopathy that involves most or all of the ascending and descending tracts (transverse myelopathy); (2) a combined painful radicular and transverse cord syndrome; (3) the hemicord (Brown-Séquard) syndrome; (4) a ventral cord syndrome, sparing posterior column function; (5) a high cervical–foramen magnum syndrome; (6) a central cord or syringomyelic syndrome; (7) a syndrome of the conus medullaris; and (8) a syndrome of the cauda equina. In addition, an important distinction is made between lesions within the cord (*intramedullary*) and those that compress the cord from without (*extramedullary*). Some of the anatomic and physiologic considerations pertinent to an understanding of disorders of the cord and of the spine can be found in Chaps. 3, 9 (Figs. 9-5 and 9-7), and Chap. 11, on motor paralysis, somatic sensation, and back pain, respectively. The typical spinal cord syndromes are represented most perfectly by tumor compression that originates in an adjacent vertebral body; this important process is therefore described as a model in the introductory section and again in a later part of the chapter.

THE SYNDROME OF ACUTE PARAPLEGIA OR QUADRIPLEGIA CAUSED BY TRAUMATIC AND OTHER PHYSICAL FACTORS (TRANSVERSE MYELOPATHY)

This syndrome is best considered in relation to trauma, its most frequent cause, but it occurs also as a result of other acute damage including infarction or hemorrhage and with rapidly advancing compressive, necrotizing, demyelinative, or inflammatory lesions. Each of these categories of acute spinal cord disease is discussed in the following pages. For convenience we have included in this group radiation myelopathy, which is transverse but evolves subacutely.

Traumatic Injuries of the Spine and Spinal Cord

Throughout recorded medical history, advances in the understanding of spinal cord disease have coincided largely with periods of warfare. The first thoroughly documented study of the effects of sudden total cord transection was by Theodor Kocher in 1896, based on his observations of 15 patients. During World War I, Riddoch, and later Head and Riddoch, gave what are now considered the classic descriptions of spinal transection in humans; Lhermitte and Guillain and Barré are credited with refining those observations. Little could be done for patients in that era and fully 80 percent died in the first few weeks (from infections); survival was possible only if the spinal cord lesion was partial. World War II marked a turning point in the understanding and management of spinal injuries. The advent of antibiotics and the ability to control skin, bladder, and pulmonary infections permitted the survival of unprecedented numbers of soldiers with cord injuries and provided the opportunity for long-term observation. In special centers, and the care and rehabilitation of the paraplegic patient were brought to a high level. Studies conducted in these centers greatly enhanced our knowledge of the functional capacity of the chronically isolated spinal cord. Kuhn, Munro, Martin and Davis, Guttmann, Pollock, and Pollock and associates made particularly important contributions to this subject.

Mechanisms of Spinal Injury

The usual circumstances of spinal cord injury, in approximate order of frequency in civilian practice are motor vehicle and motorcycle accidents, falls (sometimes during a state of alcoholic intoxication), gunshot or stab wounds, diving accidents, crushing industrial injuries, and birth injury. In the United States, the annual incidence of spinal cord injury has been given as 5 cases per 100,000 population; males predominate (4:1). Each year approximately 3,500 persons die in relation to their spinal injury, and another 5,000 are left with complete or nearly complete loss of spinal cord function.

Although trauma may involve the spinal cord alone, the vertebral column is almost invariably injured at the same time. Often there is an associated cranial injury as pointed out in Chap. 35.

A useful classification of *vertebral column injuries* divides them into fracture–dislocations, pure fractures, and pure dislocations. The spinal cord that is situated beneath any of these injuries is traumatized by direct compression as a result of dislocation of spinal bones, or by buckling of the ligaments inside the spinal canal. The relative frequency of the three types is about 3:1:1. Except for bullet, shrapnel, and stab wounds, a direct blow to the spine is a relatively uncommon cause of serious spinal cord injury. In civilian life, most fractures and dislocations of the spinal column are the result of force applied at a distance from the site of the disruption of the spinal column. Specifically, all three types of spinal injury are typically produced by a vertical compression of the spinal column, to which either anteroflexion or retroflexion (hyperextension) is added. The most important variables in the mechanics of vertebral injury are the structure of the bones and ligaments at the level of the injury and the intensity, direction, and point of impact of the force. The main elements of the spine are illustrated in Chap. 11.

In keeping with the mechanism of force applied at a distance, blows to the head may result in cervical spinal injuries. If a hard object at high velocity strikes the cranium, a skull fracture occurs, the force of the injury being absorbed mainly by the elastic quality of the skull. If the traumatizing force is relatively soft yet unyielding, or is applied more slowly, the spine, and particularly its most mobile (cervical) portion, will be the part injured. If the neck happens to be rigid and straight and the force is applied quickly to the head, the atlas and the odontoid process of the axis may fracture.

In the case of *cervical flexion injury*, the head has usually been bent sharply forward when the force is applied. The cervical vertebrae are forced together at the level of maximum stress, driving the anteroinferior edge of the upper vertebral body into the one below, sometimes splitting it in two. The posterior part of the fractured body is displaced backward and compresses the cord. Concomitantly, there is tearing of the interspinous and posterior longitudinal ligaments. Less severe degrees of anteroflexion injury produce only dislocation of adjacent cervical vertebrae at one of several levels. Vulnerability to the effects of anteroflexion (and to some extent to retroflexion injuries) is increased by the presence of cervical spondylosis or ankylosing spondylitis or by a congenital narrowness of the spinal canal.

In *cervical hyperextension injuries*, the mechanism is one of vertical compression with the head in an extended position. Stress is mainly on the posterior elements (the laminae and pedicles) of the midcervical vertebrae (C4 to C6), or sometimes at higher levels (see the named fractures below), which may be fractured unilaterally or bilaterally, and on the anterior ligaments. This dual disruption in the spinal architecture allows for displacement of one vertebral body upon the adjacent one and compresses the cord between the laminae of the lower vertebra and the body of the one above.

However, spinal cord trauma may also occur from hyperextension injury without apparent damage or misalignment of the vertebrae. In these instances, the spinal cord damage, which can be nonetheless profound and permanent, is considered to be caused by a sudden inward bulge of the ligamentum flavum or by transient vertebral dislocation that is permitted because of ligamentous disruption; when viewed with imaging studies, the vertebral bodies are found to have spontaneously realigned. In such cases, rupture of the supporting ligamentous elements and spinal instability can be revealed by gentle flexion and extension of the neck under radiologic observation, which demonstrates movement of the vertebra in relation to an adjacent one. CT and plain lateral spine films are satisfactory means of demonstrating the vertebral injury but the tearing and bulging of ligaments from vertebral dislocation are more dependably demonstrated by MRI.

Another potential mechanism of cord and spinal root injury involving extremes of extension and flexion of the neck is so-called whiplash or recoil injury, most often the result of an automobile accident. When a vehicle is struck sharply from behind, the head of the occupant is flung back uncontrollably, or if a fast-moving vehicle stops abruptly, there is sudden forward flexion of the neck, followed by retroflexion. Under these conditions the occipitonuchal and sternocleidomastoid muscles and other supporting structures of the neck and head are affected much more often than the spinal cord or roots. Nevertheless, in rare instances, quadriparesis, temporary or permanent, results from a violent whiplash injury. The exact mechanism of neural injury in these circumstances is not clear; perhaps there is a transient posterior dislocation of a vertebral body, a momentary buckling of the ligamentum flavum, or retropulsion of the intervertebral disc into the spinal canal. Other ostensible results of whiplash, such as dizziness, are highly controversial and are discussed in Chap. 11. However, the main comment to be made regarding whiplash is that all manner of neurologic symptoms have been uncritically and inappropriately attributed to it, often with implications for medicolegal and disability determinations.

The presence of a congenitally narrow cervical spinal canal or of acquired spinal diseases such as cervical spondylosis, rheumatoid arthritis, or ankylosing spondylitis adds greatly to the hazard of damage to the cord or roots. Neck trauma of almost any configuration may in particular aggravate preexisting spondylotic symptoms. There are in addition examples of spinal cord compression that result from prolonged static hyperextension of the cervical spine during a protracted period of stupor. This accounts for some cases of quadriplegia following a period of sustained unresponsiveness due to opiate or sedative drug overdose (Ell et al). Arterial hypotension may be an added factor in some instances.

A special type of spinal cord injury, occurring most often in wartime, is one in which a high-velocity missile penetrates the vertebral canal and damages the spinal cord directly. In some cases the missile strikes the vertebral column without entering the spinal canal but disrupts and virtually shatters the intradural contents or produces lesser degrees of spinal cord dysfunction. Or, the transmitted shock wave from a bullet passing nearby the vertebral column causes paralysis of spinal cord function that is largely reversible in a day or two (*spinal cord concussion*, which is described further on).

Acute traumatic paralysis may also be the indirect consequence of a vascular mechanism, mainly through infarction from fibrocartilaginous emboli arising in an intervertebral disc that has ruptured into a radicular artery or vein of the cord. Or a traumatic dissecting aneurysm of the aorta may occlude the segmental arteries of the spinal cord, as in the cases reported by Weisman and Adams and by Kneisley. One striking variant of this type of vascular injury is infarction of the upper cervical cord, resulting in hemi-, tri-, or tetraplegia, from dissection of one or both vertebral arteries and occlusion of their tributary anterior spinal arteries at the cervicomedullary junction.

Vertebral fracture and dislocation An analysis from a former era of 2,000 cases of spinal injury collected from the medical literature by Jefferson up to 1927 is still valid and showed that most vertebral injuries occurred at the levels of the first and second cervical, fourth to sixth cervical, and eleventh thoracic to second lumbar vertebrae. Industrial accidents most often involved the thoracolumbar vertebrae. Impact to the head with the neck flexed or sharply retroflexed, as mentioned earlier, was the main cause of injuries to the cervical region. These are not only the most mobile portions of the vertebral column but also the regions in which the cervical and lumbar enlargements of the cord greatly reduce the space between neural and bony structures. The thoracic cord is relatively small and its spinal canal is capacious; additional protection is provided by the high and overlapping articular facets, making dislocation difficult, and limitations in anterior displacement of vertebral bodies imposed by the thoracic cage.

Several configurations of vertebral fractures are common enough that they are designated by eponyms or descriptive terms. The knowledgeable clinician has some familiarity with them. They are summarized in Table 44-1. They include the Jefferson fracture, hangman's fracture, the Chance fracture, atlanto-axial (C1-C2) and the more common atlanto-occipital fracture-dislocation, including fracture of the dens of C-2. Regarding hangman's fracture, contrary to the popular notion, most penal hangings do not cause vertebral bony disruption and death is instead by strangulation; a more common mechanism for hangman's fracture is an elderly person who falls and strikes the chin, causing hyperextension of the neck. The majority of fatal cases of cervical spine injury are from fracture–dislocations of the upper cervical spine (C1 to C3 vertebrae, thus encompassing atlanto-occipital and atlanto-axis dislocations with sudden respiratory paralysis).

Acute Evaluation of the Spine-Injured Patient

The level of the spinal cord damage and, by implication, the level of disruption of the spinal column, can be determined from clinical findings. Diaphragmatic paralysis occurs with lesions of the upper three cervical segments (transient arrest of breathing from brainstem paralysis is common in severe head injury). Complete paralysis of the arms and legs usually indicates a fracture or dislocation at the fourth to fifth cervical vertebrae. If the legs are paralyzed and the arms can still be abducted and flexed, the lesion is likely to be at the fifth to sixth cervical vertebrae. Paralysis of the legs and only the hands indicates a lesion at the sixth to seventh cervical level. Below the cervical region, the spinal cord segments and roots are not directly opposite their similarly numbered vertebrae (Fig. 44-1). The spinal cord ends at the first lumbar vertebra, usually at its rostral border. Vertebral column lesions below this point give rise predominantly to cauda equina syndromes; these carry a better prognosis than injuries to the lower thoracic vertebrae, which involve both cord and multiple roots.

The level of sensory loss on the trunk, as determined by perception of pinprick, is an accurate guide to the level of the lesion, with a few qualifications. (See Figs. 9-1, 9-3, and 9-4 for maps of the sensory dermatomes.) Lesions of the lower cervical cord, even if complete, may spare sensation down to the nipple line because of the contribution of the C3 and C4 cutaneous branches of the cervical plexus, which variably innervate skin below the clavicle. Or a lesion that involves only the outermost fibers of the spinothalamic pathways results in a sensory level (to pain and temperature) well below the level of the lesion. In all cases of spinal cord and cauda equina injury, the prognosis for recovery is more favorable if any movement or sensation is elicitable during the first 48 to 72 h.

If the spinal column can be examined safely, it should be inspected and palpated for angulations or irregularities and gently percussed to detect underlying bony injury. Collateral injury of the thorax, abdomen, and long bones should be sought and cranial injury is a concern if the mechanism of direct spinal impact is not known from the history.

Table 44-1

MAJOR VERTEBRAL FRACTURES AND DISLOCATIONS

NOMENCLATURE	MECHANISM	IMAGING	STABILITY	CLINICAL EFFECTS[a]
Atlanto-occipital dislocation	Rotatory force to head	Displacement of occipital condyles in relation to lateral masses of C1	Unstable	Common in children; fatal if severe
Atlanto-axial dislocation	Rotatory mechanism common in children; flexion in adults	Dislocation of C1-C2 facet	Unstable	Varies from asymptomatic to severe myelopathy
Jefferson fracture (C1)	Axial downward force on vertex of head	Bilateral anterior and posterior arch fractures	Stable	Usually asymptomatic; transverse ligament may be disrupted
Odontoid (dens) fractures (C2)	Hyperflexion	Fracture through C2[b]: Type 1: tip of dens Type 2: base of dens Type 3: body of C2	Type 2 most "unstable" and unlikely to heal spontaneously	Varies from asymptomatic to tetraparesis
Hangman's fracture (C2)	Hyperextension with axial loading	Fractures through pedicles of C2	Usually stable	Most are asymptomatic
Subaxial fracture-dislocation	Severe flexion	Dislocation (perched or jumped) of facets with reversal of normal "shingled" appearance	Poor	Occurs at any level C3 to T1; common cause of traumatic tetra- and quadriplegia; vertebral artery dissection
Burst fracture (thoracolumbar)	Axial loading	Fracture through vertebral body with loss of height	Variable	Root compression from retropulsion of bone fragment
Chance fracture (thoracolumbar)	Flexion of lower thoracic spine —"seat-belt" injury	Same as burst fracture but includes fractures through facets and posterior elements	Variable	Commonly asymptomatic
Compression (wedge) fracture (thoracolumbar)	Hyperflexion	Wedging of anterior vertebral body, no loss of height and no subluxation	Usually stable	Local pain, rarely neurologic deficit

[a]Pain at the site of the fracture or dislocation is common to all these injuries.
[b]These features are in addition to local pain over the site of the vertebral injury.

A neurologic examination with recording of motor, sensory, and sphincter function is necessary to follow the clinical progress of spinal cord injury. A common practice is to define the injury according to the standards of the American Spinal Injury Association and to assign the injury to a point on the ASIA Impairment, or AIS (a derivative of the formerly used Frankel scale). A paraphrased version that we have found useful is presented here with comments regarding functional ability from the Frankel scale:

A. *Complete*: no sensory or motor function below the level of the lesion including in the sacral segments
B. *Sensory incomplete*: sensory function is preserved but motor function is lost below the zone of injury
C. *Motor incomplete* (first grade): motor function is reduced in *more than half* of key muscles below the level of the lesion; this usually renders the patient unable to walk. (Reduced motor function is defined as active movement in a full range of motion only if gravity is eliminated.)
D. *Motor incomplete* (second grade): motor function is reduced in *fewer than half* of key muscles below the level of the lesion; this usually allows standing and walking
E. *Normal*: reflexes may be abnormal

Obviously, groups C, D, and E have a more favorable prognosis for recovery of ambulation than does groups A and B.

In cases of suspected spinal injury, the immediate concern is that movement (especially flexion) of the cervical spine be avoided. The patient should ideally be placed supine on a firm, flat surface (with one person assigned, if possible, to keeping the head and neck immobile) and should be transported by a vehicle that can accept the litter. The board may be placed under the patient, gently

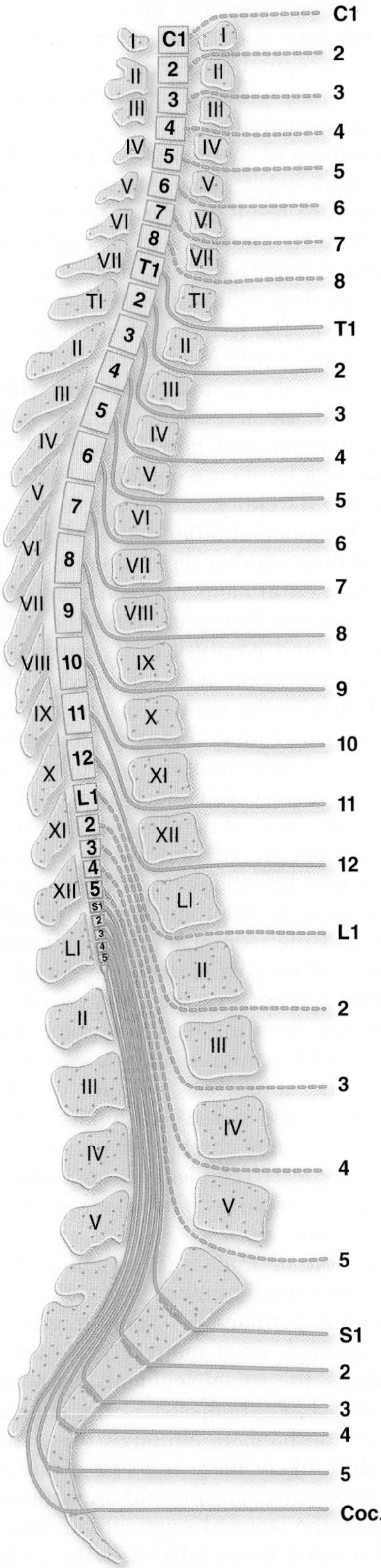

Figure 44-1. The relationship of spinal segments and roots to the vertebral bodies and spinous processes. The cervical roots (except C8) exit through foramina above their respective vertebral bodies, and the other roots issue below these bodies. (From Haymaker and Woodhall: *Peripheral Nerve Injuries*, 2nd ed. Philadelphia, Saunders, 1953, by permission.)

rolling him to one side with the head, neck, and body held in alignment. If moving the patient is not feasible, the neck may be immobilized in place with a form collar or an equivalent device that is contrived at the scene, or even the examiner's hands held firmly along the cervical spine. The patient should ideally be transported by an ambulance equipped with spine boards, to which the head is fixed by straps. This provides a more effective means of immobilization than sandbags or similar objects placed on each side of the head and neck. On arrival at the hospital, it is prudent to have the cervical spine remain immobilized until a lateral film or a CT or MRI of the cervical spine can been obtained, with the qualifications below.

Several schemes have been devised for determining which patients may require imaging; these are comparable to "rules" for the use of imaging in head injury that are discussed in Chap. 35. The two more widely cited ones for spinal injury are those of the NEXUS group (Hoffman et al) and the "Canadian C-spine Rule" (Stiell et al). The former identifies those at low risk for spinal cord injury on the basis of the absence of posterior midline cervical-spine tenderness, no evidence of intoxication, a normal level of alertness (thereby allowing accurate reporting of the circumstances of injury and the presence of neck pain, and suggesting there has not been serious brain injury), no focal neurologic deficit, and no other painful injuries that distract the patient from reporting neck pain. The Canadian rule has been found to be slightly more sensitive and specific (this has been disputed); it is based on three high-risk criteria: age older than 65 years, a dangerous mechanism of injury, and limb paresthesias; and on any of six features that are associated with low-risk of cord injury: simple rear-end motor vehicle collision, sitting position in the emergency department, being ambulatory at any time after injury, delayed (not immediate) onset of neck pain, absence of midline cervical-spine tenderness, coupled with the ability to turn the head 45 degrees in both directions without pain.

Pathology of Traumatic Spinal Cord Injury

As a result of squeezing or shearing of the spinal cord, there is destruction of gray and white matter and a variable amount of hemorrhage, chiefly in the more vascular central parts. These changes, designated as *traumatic necrosis* of the cord, are maximal at the level of injury and at one or two segments above and below it. Rarely is the cord cut in two, and seldom is the pia-arachnoid lacerated. Separation of the components of traumatic necrosis, such as hematomyelia, concussion, contusion, and hematorrhachis (bleeding into the spinal canal) is not of great value either clinically or pathologically. As the lesion heals, it leaves a gliotic focus or cavitation with variable amounts of hemosiderin and iron pigment. Progressive cavitation (*traumatic syringomyelia*) may develop after an interval of months or years and, as the cavity enlarges beyond the main lesion, lead to a delayed central or incomplete transverse cord syndrome. In some instances, the lesion is virtually restricted to the centrally situated gray matter, giving rise to segmental weakness and sensory loss in the arms with few long tract signs. This is the *central cervical cord syndrome*, also called the *Schneider syndrome* (see further on). Fragments of the central cord syndrome commonly occur as transient phenomena that reverse over several days.

Experimental Spinal Cord Injury

Investigation of the pathophysiology of acute spinal cord injury dates from the experimental studies of Allen in the early 1900s. His method consisted of dropping graded weights onto the dura-covered thoracic cord of surgically prepared animals. The technique was refined over the years by precise measurements of the velocity, force, and direction of the dropped weights. This type of impact on the cord, of sufficient severity to render the animal immediately paraplegic and abolish sensory-evoked responses from structures below the lesion, indicates that action potentials can no longer be conducted across the injured spinal cord segment. No histologic changes, by either light or electron microscopy, can be detected for several minutes after impact. The earliest tissue alterations consist of hyperemia and small hemorrhages in the central gray matter. By 1 h, the microscopic hemorrhages coalesce and become macroscopically visible. Tissue oxygen saturation is diminished in the region. Within 4 h, the central part of the cord swells and a spreading edema pervades the surrounding white matter; however, necrosis may not be evident for up to 8 h, an observation that has led to numerous strategies designed to spare the neurons and long tracts. Surgical intervention to minimize white matter edema—such as laminectomy and myelotomy—spinal cord cooling, hyperbaric exposure, and the administration of pharmacologic measures have been tried but, for the most part, have had no meaningful effects on the evolving lesion.

Certain mechanisms that are thought to be operative in the death of cerebral neurons exposed to ischemia or to traumatic forces have also been invoked in spinal cord injury but with limited evidence to support this commonality. These include release of excitotoxins such as glutamate and exposure of neurons to calcium and free radicals. Despite early experiments implicating neurotransmitters or opioid-like substances, later work failed to substantiate this or other similar secondary mechanisms. One problem with all the experimental work is that it only imperfectly reproduces spinal injury in humans. Most recent work in the field of spinal cord injury has been on regeneration of spinal tissue across gaps in the cord using stem cells, gene therapy, and tissue scaffolding made of artificial or in vitro cell structures. None has yet proved satisfactory for clinical implementation.

Clinical Effects of Spinal Cord Injury

When the spinal cord is suddenly and severely impacted, three disorders of function are at once evident: (1) all voluntary movement in parts of the body below the lesion is immediately lost; (2) sensation from the lower parts of the body is abolished; and (3) reflex functions in segments of the isolated spinal cord are suspended. The last effect, termed *spinal shock*, involves tendon as well as autonomic reflexes. This state is of variable duration (1 to 6 weeks but sometimes far longer) and is so dramatic that Riddoch used it as a basis for dividing the clinical effects of spinal cord transection into two stages, that of spinal shock with areflexia followed by a stage of heightened reflex activity.

The separation of these stages is not as sharp as this statement might imply. Less complete or less sudden lesions of the cord result in little or no spinal shock. The features of complete functional spinal cord transection are now presented in detail because of their practical value and the special place they occupy in classic neurology.

Spinal Shock The loss of motor function at the time of injury, tetraplegia with lesions of the fourth to fifth cervical segments or above, and paraplegia with lesions of the thoracic cord, are accompanied by immediate atonic paralysis of bladder and bowel, gastric atony, loss of sensation below a level corresponding to the spinal cord lesion, muscular flaccidity, and almost complete suppression of spinal segmental reflex activity below the lesion. As a result of their sudden separation from higher levels of control, the neural elements below the lesion essentially fail to perform their normal function. As dramatic as this state of reflex paralysis is, its physiologic basis is incompletely understood. Also impaired in the segments below the lesion is the control of autonomic function. Vasomotor tone, sweating, and piloerection in the lower parts of the body are temporarily abolished. As a result, there may be severe systemic hypotension that itself contributes to spinal cord damage. The lower extremities lose heat if left uncovered, and they swell if dependent. The skin over time becomes dry and pale, and ulcerations may develop over bony prominences. The sphincters of the bladder and the rectum remain contracted to some degree because of the loss of the normal inhibitory influence of higher centers, but the detrusor of the bladder and smooth muscle of the rectum become atonic. Urine accumulates until the intravesicular pressure is sufficient to overcome the sphincters, causing overflow incontinence. There is also passive distention of the bowel, retention of feces, and absence of peristalsis (paralytic ileus). Genital reflexes (penile erection, bulbocavernosus reflex, contraction of dartos muscle) are abolished or profoundly depressed.

The duration of the stage of spinal shock varies considerably. In a small number (5 of Kuhn's 29 patients, for example) it is permanent, or only fragmentary reflex activity is regained, even many years after the injury. In such patients, the spinal segments below the level of transection may have themselves been injured, perhaps by a vascular mechanism, although this explanation is unproven. More likely there is a loss of the brainstem–spinal facilitatory mechanisms and an increase in inhibitory activity in the isolated segments. In other patients, minimal genital and flexor reflex activity can be detected within a few days of the injury and minimal reflex activity appears within a period of 1 to 6 weeks. Usually the bulbocavernosus reflex is the first to return. Contraction of the anal sphincter can be elicited by plantar or perianal stimulation, and other genital reflexes reappear at about the same time. The F-waves, electrophysiologic responses that reflect the functioning of the motor neurons of the isolated segment of the cord, are suppressed until spasticity supervenes, at which time they become overly easy to elicit. Noxious stimulation of the plantar surfaces evokes a tremulous twitching and brief flexion or extension movements of the great toes.

The explanation of spinal shock, which is brief in sub-mammalian animals and more lasting in higher mammals, especially in primates, is believed to be the sudden interruption of suprasegmental descending fiber systems that normally keep the spinal motor neurons in a continuous state of readiness. In the cat and monkey, Fulton found the facilitatory tracts in question to be the reticulospinal and vestibulospinal. Subsequent studies showed that in monkeys, some degree of spinal shock could result from interruption of the corticospinal tracts alone. This is probably not a significant factor, however, at least in humans, because spinal shock does not result from acute cerebral and brainstem lesions that interrupt the corticospinal tracts.

Stage of Heightened Reflex Activity This is the more familiar condition of spasticity that emerges some time after spinal injury and is also typical of most of the nontraumatic subacute myelopathies that have developed more slowly than traumatic injuries and have not had a period of spinal shock. A few weeks after an acute traumatic injury, all reflex responses, which are initially minimal and unsustained, become stronger and more easily elicitable and as time passes, come to include additional and more proximal muscles. Gradually, the typical pattern of heightened flexion reflexes emerges: dorsiflexion of the big toe (Babinski sign); fanning of the other toes; and later, flexion or slow withdrawal movements of the foot, leg, and thigh with contraction of the tensor fascia lata muscle (the last several features referred to as "triple flexion"). Tactile stimulation of the foot may suffice as a stimulus, but a painful stimulus is more effective. The Achilles reflexes and then the patellar reflexes return. Retention of urine becomes less complete, and at irregular intervals urine is expelled by spontaneous contractions of the detrusor muscle. Reflex defecation also begins. After several months the withdrawal reflexes become greatly exaggerated, to the point of flexor spasms, and they may be accompanied by profuse sweating, piloerection, and automatic emptying of the bladder (occasionally of the rectum). This is the "mass reflex," which can be evoked by stimulation of the skin of the legs or by some interoceptive stimulus, such as a full bladder. Varying degrees of heightened flexor reflex activity may last for years, or indefinitely. Heat-induced sweating is defective, but reflex-evoked ("spinal") sweating may be profuse (see Kneisley). In such cases the lateral horn cells in much of the thoracic cord are still viable and have been disinhibited. Above the level of the lesion, thermoregulatory sweating may be exaggerated in order to compensate for the loss of evaporative cooling of lower segments, and there is cutaneous flushing, hypertension that causes pounding headache and reflex bradycardia. This syndrome ("autonomic dysreflexia") is episodic and occurs in response to a certain stimuli, such as a distended bladder or rectum. It has been ascribed to the reflex release of adrenaline from the adrenal medulla and of norepinephrine from the disinhibited sympathetic terminals caudal to the lesion but is exaggerated by defective baroreceptor compensatory reflexes as discussed in Chap 27.

Extensor reflexes and tone eventually develop in most cases (18 of 22 of Kuhn's patients who survived more than 2 years), but their appearance does not lead to the abolition of the exaggerated flexor reflexes. The overactivity of extensor muscles may appear as early as 6 months after the injury, but this only happens, as a rule, after the flexor responses are fully developed. Extensor responses are at first manifest in certain muscles of the hip and thigh and later of the leg. In a few patients, extensor reflexes are organized into support reactions sufficient to permit *spinal standing*. Kuhn observed that extensor movements were at first provoked most readily by a sudden shift from a sitting to a supine position and later by proprioceptive stimuli (squeezing of the thigh muscles) and tactile stimuli from wide areas. Marshall, in a study of 44 patients with chronic spastic paraplegia of spinal origin, found all possible combinations of flexor and extensor reflexes; the type of reflex obtained was determined by the intensity and duration of the stimulus (a mild prolonged noxious stimulus evoked an ipsilateral extensor reflex; an intense brief stimulus, a flexor response).

From these observations one would suspect that the ultimate posture of the legs—flexion or extension—does not depend solely on the completeness or incompleteness of the spinal cord lesion, as originally postulated by Riddoch. The development of *paraplegia in flexion* (extreme flexion of the hips and knees, as in a fetal position) relates also to the level of the lesion, being seen most often with cervical lesions and progressively less often with more caudal ones. Greatly troubling to the spinal patient are repeated flexor spasms, which are more frequent with higher lesions of the cord, and the ensuing contractures ultimately produce a fixed flexor posture. Furthermore, reduction of flexor spasms by elimination of nociceptive stimuli (infected bladder, decubitus, etc.) favors an extensor posture of the legs (*paraplegia in extension*). According to Guttmann, the positioning of the limbs during the early stages of paraplegia influences their ultimate posture. Thus, prolonged fixation of the paralyzed limbs in adduction and semiflexion favors subsequent paraplegia in flexion. Placing the patient prone or placing the limbs in abduction and extension facilitates the development of predominantly extensor postures. Nevertheless, strong and persistent extensor postures are usually observed only with partial lesions of the spinal cord.

A number of sensory phenomena are expected after functional cord transection. The main one, of course, is the loss of all sensibility below the lesion, i.e., the sensory level. Of some interest is the fact that many patients report sensory symptoms in segments of the body below the level of their transection. Thus, a tactile stimulus above the level of the lesion may be felt below the transection (a type of synesthesia). Patients describe a variety of paresthesias, the most common being a dull, burning pain in the lower back and abdomen, buttocks, and perineum. We have encountered several patients in whom aching testicular or rectal pain was a very distressing problem. The pain may be intense and last for a year or longer, after which it gradually subsides. It persists after rhizotomy but can be abolished by anesthetizing the stump of the proximal (upper) segment of the spinal cord, according to Pollock and coworkers. Transmission of sensation over splanchnic afferents to levels of the spinal cord above the lesion, the conventional explanation, is therefore not the most plausible one.

The overactivity of sensory systems in the isolated segments of the spinal cord has several explanations. One assumes that suprasegmental inhibitory influences have been removed by the transection, so that afferent sensory impulses evoke exaggerated nocifensive and phasic and tonic myotatic reflexes. But isolated neurons also become hypersensitive to neurotransmitters. Since the early experiments of Cannon and Rosenblueth, it has been known that section of sympathetic motor fibers leaves the denervated structures hypersensitive to epinephrine and to acetylcholine.

Various combinations of residual deficits (of lower and upper motor neurons and sensory neurons) are to be expected. High cervical lesions, for example, may result in extreme and prolonged tonic spasms of the legs as a result of release of tonic myotatic reflexes. Under these circumstances, attempted voluntary movement may excite intense contraction of all flexor and extensor muscles lasting for several minutes. Segmental damage in the low cervical or lumbar gray matter, destroying inhibitory Renshaw neurons, may release activity of remaining anterior horn cells, leading to spinal segmental spasticity.

Any residual symptoms persisting after 6 months are likely to be permanent, although in a small proportion of patients some return of function (particularly sensation) is possible after this time. Loss of motor and sensory function above the lesion, coming on years after the trauma, is the result of an enlarging cavity in the proximal segment of the cord (see further on, under "Syringomyelia [Syrinx]").

Transient Cord Injury (Spinal Cord Concussion)

These terms refer to a transient loss of motor sensory function of the spinal cord that recovers within minutes or hours but may persist in mild form for days or more. In most instances, the symptoms are rapidly diminishing and few neurologic abnormalities are found at the time of the first examination. There are a number of such transient syndromes: bibrachial weakness; quadriparesis (occasionally hemiparesis); paresthesias and dysesthesias in a similar distribution to the weakness; or sensory symptoms alone ("burning hands syndrome"). In the first and last of these, transient dysfunction of the central gray matter of the cervical cord is implicated. It is assumed that the cord undergoes some form of elastic deformation when the cervical spine is compressed or hyperextended; however, the same effects can be produced by direct blows to the spine or forceful falls flat on the back and occasionally, by a sharp fall on the tip of the coccyx. Little is known of the physiologic mechanisms that underlie these reversible syndromes.

Spinal cord concussion from direct impact is observed most frequently in athletes engaged in contact sports (football, rugby, and hockey). An incomplete and reversible myelopathy is referable to the site and level of the injury. A congenitally narrow cervical canal is thought to predispose to spinal cord concussion and to increase the risk of recurrence. As with cerebral concussion, particularly if there have been previous concussions, a difficult decision arises—whether or not to allow resumption of competitive sports. There are no reliable data on which to base this decision, only guidelines that tentatively allow continued participation, after an unspecified period of rest, if the deficit has been brief. It is, however, advisable in most cases to be certain that spinal instability has not been induced by the injury. This can be ascertained from flexion and extension X-ray images of the affected spinal region. The subject is reviewed by Zwimpfer and Bernstein. In athletic contact injury, unilateral arm and hand paresthesias are more common than symptoms of both arm, but they are usually from stretching of the brachial plexus on one side (a "stinger"), rather than from a cord injury.

Central Cord ("Schneider") Syndrome and Cruciate Paralysis A special from of acute cervical cord injury implicates mainly central cord damage, resulting in the loss of motor function solely or more severely in the upper limbs than in the lower ones, and it particularly affects the hands. Bladder dysfunction with urinary retention occurs in some cases and sensory loss is often slight (hyperpathia over the shoulders and arms may be the only sensory abnormality). Many of these instances are reversible but damage to the centrally situated gray matter may leave an atrophic, areflexic paralysis of the arms and hands and a segmental loss of pain and thermal sensation from interruption of crossing pain and thermal fibers. Retroflexion injuries of the head and neck are the ones most often associated with the central cord syndrome, but other causes include hematomyelia, fibrocartilaginous embolism, and infarction from dissection of the vertebral artery in the medullary-cervical region as mentioned earlier in the chapter (see Morse for further discussion).

According to Dickman and colleagues, approximately 4 percent of patients who survive injuries of the very rostral cervical cord demonstrate a very limited form of the central cord syndrome, recognized by Nielson and named by Bell, "cruciate paralysis." The weakness is very selective, being practically limited to the arms, a feature that is attributable to the segregation within the pyramidal decussation of corticospinal fibers to the arms (being rostral) and to the legs (more caudally situated). The arm weakness may be asymmetrical or even unilateral and sensory loss is inconsistent. The patients described have had contusions of the C1-C2 region. Whether the lesion lies strictly within the decussating corticospinal tract or involves central gray matter is not always clear; MRI findings have implicated the latter, as described by Inamasu et al.

Management of Spinal Injury

For some time, many centers administered methylprednisolone in high dosage (bolus of 30 mg/kg followed by 5.4 mg/kg every hour), beginning within 8 h of the injury and continued for 23 h. This measure, according to the multicenter National Acute Spinal Cord Study (Bracken et al, 1990) resulted in a slight improvement in both motor and sensory function. The therapeutic value of this measure has since been questioned after reanalysis of the data (Nesathurai; Hurlbert) and it is no longer considered essential. Hypotension is treated with infusions of normal saline and may require the transient use of pressor agents. The use of hypothermia with cooling blankets or the infusion of cooled saline is under investigation to protect spinal tissue but has not been validated.

Next, imaging examinations are undertaken to determine the alignment of vertebrae and pedicles, fracture of the pedicle or vertebral body, compression of the spinal cord or cauda equina as a consequence of malalignment, or bone debris in the spinal canal, and the presence of tissue damage within the cord. MRI is ideally suited to display these processes, but if it is not available, myelography with CT scanning is an alternative. Instability of the spinal elements can often be inferred from dislocations or from certain fractures of the pedicles, pars articularis, or transverse processes, but gentle flexion and extension of the injured areas must sometimes be undertaken and plain films obtained in each position.

If a cervical spinal cord injury is associated with vertebral dislocation, traction on the neck may be necessary to secure proper alignment and maintain immobilization. Depending on the nature of the injury, this is accomplished by use of a halo brace, which, of all the appliances used for this purpose provides the most rigid external fixation of the cervical spine. This type of fixation is usually continued for 4 to 6 weeks, after which a rigid collar may be substituted.

Concerning the early surgical management of spinal cord injury, there have traditionally been two perspectives. One, represented by Guttmann and others, advocated reduction and alignment of the dislocated vertebrae by traction and immobilization until skeletal fixation is obtained, and then rehabilitation. The other approach, represented by Munro and later by Collins and Chehrazi, proposed early surgical decompression, correction of bony displacements, and removal of herniated disc tissue and intra- and extramedullary hemorrhage; often the spine is fixed at the same time by a bone graft or other form of stabilization. The issue of acute decompressive surgery remains contentious to the present day. The MRI has altered these empirical approaches by allowing the early demonstration of hematomas and other sources of compression that may be amenable to surgery. With clinical evidence of a complete spinal cord lesion, most surgeons do not favor early surgery.

The results of the conservative and aggressive surgical plans of management for incomplete cord injuries have been difficult to compare and have not been evaluated with modern neurologic techniques. Collins, a participant in the National Institutes of Health (NIH) study of acute management of spinal cord injury 20 years ago, concluded that the survival rate was increased as a result of early surgical stabilization of fractures and fixation of the spine. Others, however, have not been able to document a reduction in neurologic disability and have increasingly been inclined toward nonoperative management of both complete and partial spinal cord lesions (see, for example, Clark; Murphy et al). Many North American neurosurgeons take the less aggressive stance, delaying operation or operating only on patients with compound wounds or those with progression or worsening of the neurologic deficit despite adequate reduction and stabilization. In each case, the approach is guided by the specific aspects of the injuries; ligamentous disruption, presence of hematoma, misalignment-displacement of spinal segments, instability of the injury, and fracture type.

The greatest risks to the patient with spinal cord injury occur in the first 10 days when gastric dilatation, ileus, shock, and infection are threats to life. According to Messard and colleagues, the mortality rate falls rapidly after 3 months; beyond this time, 86 percent of paraplegics and 80 percent of quadriplegics will survive for 10 years or longer. In children, the survival rate is even higher according to DeVivo and colleagues, who found that the cumulative 7-year survival rate in spinal cord–injured children (who had survived at least 24 h after injury) was 87 percent. Advanced age at the time of injury and being rendered completely quadriplegic were the worst prognostic factors.

The aftercare of patients with paraplegia, in addition to substantial psychological support to allow accommodation to new limitations while encouraging a productive life, is concerned with management of bladder and bowel disturbances, care of the skin, prevention of pulmonary embolism, and maintenance of nutrition. Decubitus ulcers can be reduced by frequent turning to avoid pressure necrosis, use of special mattresses, and meticulous skin care. Deep decubitus lesions require debridement and full-thickness grafting. At first, continual catheterization is necessary; then, after several weeks, the bladder can be managed by intermittent catheterization once or twice daily, using a scrupulous aseptic technique. Close surveillance is needed for bladder infection, which is treated promptly should it occur. Bacteriuria alone is common and does not require treatment with antibiotics unless there is associated pyuria. Morning suppositories and periodically spaced enemas are effective means of controlling fecal incontinence. Chronic pain (present in 30 to 50 percent of cases) requires the use of nonsteroidal antiinflammatory medication, injections of local anesthetics, and transcutaneous nerve stimulation. A combination of carbamazepine or gabapentin and either clonazepam or tricyclic antidepressants may be helpful in cases of burning leg and trunk pain. Remaining pain may require more aggressive therapy, such as epidural injections of analgesics or corticosteroids or an implanted spinal cord stimulator that is applied to the dorsal columns or an analgesic pump, but often even these measures are ineffective. Fentanyl transcutaneous patches may be tried. Spasticity and flexor spasms may be troublesome; oral baclofen, diazepam, or tizanidine may provide some relief. In permanent spastic paraplegia with severe stiffness and adductor and flexor spasms of the legs, intrathecal baclofen, delivered by an automated pump in doses up to 400 mg/d, has also been helpful. The drug is believed to act at the synapses of spinal reflexes (Penn and Kroin). Selective injection of botulinum toxin may provide relief of some spastic deformities and of spasms. One must always be alert to the threat of pulmonary embolism from deep-vein thrombi, although the incidence is surprisingly low after the first several months. Physical therapy, muscle reeducation, and the proper use of braces are all important in the rehabilitation of the patient. All this is best carried out in special centers.

Radiation Injury of the Spinal Cord

Delayed necrosis of the spinal cord and brain are recognized sequela of radiation therapy for tumors in the thorax and neck. Mediastinal irradiation for Hodgkin disease or for other lymphomas is a typical setting for the development of these complications up to decades later. A lower motor neuron syndrome, presumably a result of injury to the gray matter of the spinal cord, may also follow radiation therapy in which the cord was inside the zone of treatment, as described below.

Transient Radiation Myelopathy

An "early" type of radiation myelopathy (appearing 3 to 6 months after radiotherapy) is characterized mainly by spontaneous uncomfortable sensations in the extremities. The paresthesias may be evoked by neck flexion (Lhermitte symptom). In one of our patients there was impairment of vibratory and position sense in the legs, but no weakness or signs of spinothalamic tract damage. The sensory abnormalities disappear after a few months and, according to Jones, are not followed by the delayed progressive radiation myelopathy described below. The pathology of the early and transient radiation myelopathy has not been fully elucidated, but there is a spongy appearance of the white matter with demyelination and depletion of oligodendrocytes.

Delayed Progressive Radiation Myelopathy

This is one of the most dreaded complications of radiation therapy. It is a progressive myelopathy that follows, after a variable latent period, the radiation of malignant lesions in the vicinity of the spinal cord. The incidence of this complication is difficult to determine because many patients die of their malignant disease before the myelopathy has fully evolved but it is estimated to be between 2 and 3 percent (Palmer). According to Douglas and colleagues, patients who have undergone hyperthermia as an adjunctive treatment for cancer are particularly vulnerable to radiation myelopathy.

Clinical Features The neurologic disorder first appears 6 months or more after the course of radiation therapy, usually between 12 and 15 months (latent periods as long as 60 months or longer have been reported). The onset is insidious, usually with sensory symptoms—paresthesias and dysesthesias of the feet or a Lhermitte phenomenon, and similar symptoms in the hands in cases of cervical cord damage. Weakness of one or both legs usually follows the sensory loss. Initially, local pain is absent, in distinction to the effects of spinal metastases. In some cases, the sensory abnormalities are transitory as in the syndrome described above; more often, additional signs make their appearance and progress, at first rapidly and then more slowly and irregularly, over a period of several weeks or months, with involvement of the corticospinal and spinothalamic pathways. The neurologic disturbance may take the form of a Brown-Séquard syndrome, but with progression it is usually overtaken by a transverse myelopathy.

Reagan and coworkers, who have had considerable experience with this condition, described yet another myelopathic radiation syndrome, namely, a slowly evolving amyotrophy, with weakness and atrophy of muscles and areflexia in parts of the body supplied by anterior horn cells of the irradiated spinal segments. Most patients with this form of the disease die within a year of onset. Knowledge of the pathology is incomplete. This syndrome is reminiscent of the delayed motor neuron myelopathy following electrical or lightning injury described in the next section. There is also an unusual paraneoplastic variety of poliomyelopathy and an even less common necrotic myelopathy, mentioned below and in Chap. 31.

The CSF in delayed progressive radiation transverse myelopathy is normal except for a slight elevation of protein content in some cases. MRI of the affected segments of cord demonstrates abnormal signal intensity, decreased in T1-weighted and increased in T2-weighted images. Early in the course of the myelopathy the cord may be swollen, and there is often heterogeneous enhancement with gadolinium infusion. The location of the lesion corresponds to the irradiated portal, which can be identified by the radiation effect on the marrow of the overlying vertebral bodies. The spinal cord lesion tends to be more extensive in rostral–caudal dimension than the usual vascular or demyelinative myelopathy. These are important points to establish, because a mistaken diagnosis of intraspinal tumor or of a dural arteriovenous fistula may lead to an unnecessary operation or further irradiation.

Pathologic Findings Corresponding with the level of the radiated area and extending over several segments, there is an irregular zone of coagulation necrosis involving both white and gray matter, the former to a greater extent than the latter. Varying degrees of secondary degeneration are seen in the ascending and descending tracts. Vascular changes—necrosis of arterioles or hyaline thickening of their walls and thrombotic occlusion of their lumens—are prominent in the most severely damaged portions of the cord. Most neuropathologists have attributed the parenchymal lesion to the blood vessel changes; others believe that the degree of vascular change is insufficient to explain the necrosis (Malamud et al; Burns et al). Certainly, the most severe changes in the cord are consistent with infarction, but the insidious onset and slow, steady progression of the disorder and the coagulative nature of the necrosis would then have to be explained by a steady succession of vascular occlusions. Exceptional instances, in which a transverse myelopathy has developed within a few hours of radiation treatment (as described by Reagan et al), are more readily explained by thrombotic occlusion of a large spinal artery.

Neurologists associated with cancer treatment centers are sometimes confronted with a patient who exhibits the late development (up to 10 to 15 years after radiation) of a slowly progressive sensorimotor paralysis of only one limb (motor weakness predominates) or one region of the body. This usually represents damage in the peripheral nervous system. Examples that we have encountered are multiple cranial neuropathies after radiation of nasopharyngeal tumors, cervical and especially brachial neuropathies after laryngeal and breast cancers, and lumbosacral plexopathies and cauda equina damage with pelvic radiation. These are discussed further in Chap. 46, on diseases of the peripheral nerves.

Treatment and Prevention Kagan and colleagues have determined the tolerance of the adult human spinal cord to radiation, taking into account the volume of tissue irradiated, the duration of the irradiation, and the total dose. They reviewed all of the cases in the literature up to 1980 and concluded that radiation injury could be avoided if the total dose was kept below 6,000 cGy and was given over a period of 30 to 70 days, provided that each daily fraction did not exceed 200 cGy and the weekly dose was not in excess of 900 cGy. It is noteworthy that in the cases reported by Sanyal and associates, the amount of radiation surpassed these limits. Forewarned with this knowledge, radiation specialists have the impression that the incidence of this complication is decreasing. Of course, if the underlying neoplasm is likely to be imminently fatal, palliative radiation can exceed these limits.

A number of case reports remark on temporary improvement in neurologic function after the administration of corticosteroids. This therapy should be tried because in some patients it appears to arrest the process short of complete destruction of all sensory and motor tracts. Claims have also been made of regression of early symptoms in response to the administration of heparin split products and of hyperbaric oxygen, but most have not been confirmed.

Spinal Cord Injury Caused by Electric Currents and Lightning

Among acute physical injuries to the spinal cord, those caused by electric currents and lightning, despite their rarity, are of great interest because they produce unusual clinical syndromes. Electrical forces can also injure the brain and peripheral nerves. These effects are noted only briefly here, because they are infrequent. It is the spinal cord that is most consistently and severely damaged.

Electrical Injuries

In the United States, inadvertent contact with an electric current causes approximately 1,000 deaths annually and many more nonfatal but serious injuries. About one-third of the fatal accidents result from contact with household currents.

The factor that governs the damage to the nervous system is the amount of current, or amperage, with which the victim has contact, not simply the voltage, as is generally believed. In any particular case, the duration of contact with the current and the resistance offered by the skin to current (greatly reduced if the skin is moist or a body part is immersed in water) are of importance. The physics of electrical injuries is much more complex than these brief remarks indicate (for a full discussion, see the reviews by Panse and by Winkelman).

Any part of the peripheral or central nervous system may be injured by electric currents and lightning. The effects may be immediate, which is understandable, but of greater interest are the instances of neurologic damage that occur after a delay of 1 day to 6 weeks (1 week on average) and a rarer syndrome of anterior horn cell damage that arises after many years. The immediate effects are the result of direct heating of the nervous tissue, but the pathogenesis of the delayed effects is not well understood. They have been attributed to vascular occlusive changes induced by the electric current, a mechanism proposed to underlie the similar delayed effects of radiation therapy (see earlier). However, the latent period is measured in many months or a few years rather than in days and the course is more often progressive than self-limited. Moreover, the few postmortem studies of myelopathy as a consequence of electrical injury have disclosed a widespread demyelination of long tracts, to the point of tissue necrosis in some segments, and relative sparing of the gray matter, but no abnormalities of the blood vessels. There may also be spinal fracture from the vigorous muscle contraction.

The extraordinary syndrome of focal muscular atrophy occurring with a delay of weeks to years after an electric shock has been described by Panse under the title *spinal atrophic paralysis*. It occurs when the path of the current, usually of low voltage, is from arm to arm (across the cervical cord) or from an arm to leg. When the head is one of the contact points, the patient becomes unconscious or suffers tinnitus, deafness, or headache for a short period following the injury. Pain and paresthesias occur immediately in the involved limb but these symptoms are transient. Mild weakness, also unilateral, is immediate, followed in several weeks or months by muscle wasting, most often taking the form of segmental muscular atrophy. The syndrome simulates a regional form of amyotrophic lateral sclerosis (ALS) or transverse myelopathy (most patients have some degree of weakness and spasticity of the legs). However, we have encountered cases of asymmetric and profound atrophic weakness of the arms that began almost two decades after the shock and progressed over many years without long tract signs, both with a previously presumed diagnosis of amyotrophic lateral sclerosis. In contrast to injuries caused by high current, which affects mainly the spinal white matter (see earlier), it is the gray matter that is injured in cases of spinal atrophic paralysis, at least as judged from the clinical effects.

In a small number of surviving patients, after an asymptomatic interval of days to months, there has been an apoplectic onset of hemiplegia with or without aphasia or a striatal or brainstem syndrome, presumably because of thrombotic occlusion of cerebral vessels with infarction of tissue, but this condition has not been well studied.

The separate issue of the relationship of electrical shock exposure and the later development of typical ALS is quite controversial. Most series are hampered by retrospective acquisition of data about the shock. Although we have encountered a few remarkable instances of this association, including two who developed severe amyotrophy of the limb that was in contact with the electrical source many years before, a relationship to typical motor neuron disease has been considered coincidental.

Lightning Injuries

The factors involved in injuries from lightning are less well defined than those from electric currents, but the effects are much the same. Direct strikes are often fatal; nearby strikes produce neurologic damage as described below. Topographic prominences such as trees, hills, and towers are struck preferentially, so these should be avoided; a person caught in the open should curl up on the ground, lying on one side with legs close together.

Arborescent red lines or burns on the skin indicate the point of contact of the energy generated by direct or nearby lightning. The path through the body can be approximately deduced from the clinical sequelae. Death is a result of ventricular fibrillation or of the effects of intense desiccating heat on the brain. Lightning that strikes the head is particularly dangerous, proving fatal in 30 percent of cases. Most persons struck by lightning are initially unconscious, irrespective of where they are struck. In those who survive, consciousness is usually regained rapidly and completely. Rarely, unconsciousness or an agitated-confusional state may persist for a week or two. Persistent seizures are surprisingly rare.

There is usually a disturbance of sensorimotor function of a limb or all the limbs, which may be pale and cold or cyanotic. As a rule, these signs are also evanescent, but in some instances they persist, or an atrophic paralysis of a limb or part of a limb makes its appearance after a symptom-free interval of several months as in the case of electrical injury.

A severe, predominantly motor polyneuropathy has been reported to appear after a variable interval and, while it bears similarities to the motor neuron disorder ostensibly associated with electrical injury discussed in the section above, there is a more persuasive relationship to the less common event of lightning. There are also a few cases on record of recovery from generalized polyneuropathy after lightning injury, but our experience with one case was of profound generalized axonal damage with little recovery (see Chap. 46).

Myelopathy Following Spinal Anesthesia

This subject is introduced here with the other forms of spinal cord injury for want of a better way to categorize it. A transient and often asymmetric paraparesis is known to occur following prolonged spinal anesthesia but this is probably the result of a temporary effect of the injected agents on the cauda equina roots (see Chap. 46). A more serious and permanent injury has been caused by inadvertent injection of anesthetic directly into the conus medullaris (see Hamandi et al; Wilkinson et al). The patient reports leg weakness and numbness on one side immediately with the injection or upon awakening if sedation has been used. The MRI reveals an eccentrically placed traumatic lesion within the caudal spinal cord. Although this complication is rare, it has occurred even when experienced anesthesiologists perform the procedure; misidentification of the L3-L4 spinal interspace has been cited as the problem. Flat-tipped needles are as likely to cause injury to the conus as are ones with sharp beveled tips. Arachnoiditis from irritative agents, no longer used to any great extent, in the past caused a myelopathy (see Chap. 11).

MYELITIS (INFLAMMATORY MYELOPATHIES)

In the nineteenth century, almost every disease of the spinal cord was labeled myelitis. Morton Prince, writing in *Dercum's Textbook of Nervous Diseases* in 1895, referred to traumatic myelitis, compressive myelitis, and so on, obviously giving a rather imprecise meaning to the term. Gradually, knowledge of neuropathology advanced, and one disease after another was removed from this category until only the verifiably inflammatory ones remained.

The spinal cord is known to be the locus of a limited number of infective and noninfective inflammatory processes, some causing selective destruction of neurons, others affecting primarily white matter (tracts), and yet another group involving the meninges and white matter or leading to a necrosis of both gray and white matter. Other special terms, qualifying *myelitis*, are used to indicate more precisely the distribution of the process: if confined to gray matter, the proper expression is *poliomyelitis;* if to white matter, *leukomyelitis*. If approximately the whole cross-sectional area of the cord is involved at one or more levels, the process is said to be a *transverse myelitis* (although the term is still used more broadly for many myelitides); if the lesions are multiple and widespread over a long vertical extent, the modifying adjectives *diffuse* or *disseminated* are used and recently *longitudinally extensive myelopathy* has been introduced to denote a special form of necrotic myelopathy that is associated in most cases with particular circulating autoantibodies (see Chap, 36). The term *meningomyelitis* refers to combined inflammation of meninges and spinal cord and *meningoradiculitis* to combined meningeal and root involvement. An inflammatory process limited to the spinal dura is called *pachymeningitis*, and if infected material collects in the epidural or subdural space, it is called *epidural* or *subdural spinal abscess* or *granuloma*, as the case may be. The adjectives *acute*, *subacute*, and *chronic* denote the tempo of evolution of myelitic symptoms—namely, more or less within days, 2 to 6 weeks, or more than 6 weeks, respectively. The main causes of myelitis are listed below.

Classification of Inflammatory Diseases of the Spinal Cord

I. Viral myelitis (Chap. 33)
   A. Enteroviruses (groups A and B Coxsackievirus, poliomyelitis, others)
   B. Herpes zoster
   C. Myelitis of AIDS
   D. Epstein-Barr virus (EBV), cytomegalovirus (CMV), herpes simplex
   E. Rabies
   F. Arboviruses-Flaviviruses (Japanese, West Nile, etc.)
   G. HTLV-I (human T-cell lymphotropic virus type I; tropical spastic paraparesis)
II. Myelitis secondary to bacterial, fungal, parasitic, and primary granulomatous diseases of the meninges and spinal cord (Chap. 32)
   A. *Mycoplasma pneumoniae*
   B. Lyme disease
   C. Pyogenic myelitis
      1. Acute epidural abscess and granuloma
      2. Abscess of spinal cord
   D. Tuberculous myelitis (Chap. 32)
      1. Pott disease of the spine with secondary cord compression
      2. Tuberculous meningomyelitis
      3. Tuberculoma of spinal cord
   E. Parasitic and fungal infections producing epidural granuloma, localized meningitis, or meningomyelitis and abscess, especially certain forms of schistosomiasis (Chap. 32)
   F. Syphilitic myelitis (Chap. 32)
      1. Chronic meningoradiculitis (tabes dorsalis)
      2. Chronic meningomyelitis
      3. Meningovascular syphilis
      4. Gummatous meningitis including chronic spinal pachymeningitis
   G. Sarcoid myelitis (Chap. 32)
III. Myelitis of noninfectious inflammatory type (Chap. 36)
   A. Postinfectious and postvaccinal myelitis
   B. Acute and chronic relapsing or progressive multiple sclerosis (MS)
   C. Subacute necrotizing myelitis, neuromyelitis optica (NMO, Devic disease; longitudinally extensive myelopathy) due to antibodies against aquaporin (Chap. 36)
   D. Myelopathy with lupus or other forms of connective tissue disease and antiphospholipid antibody
   E. Paraneoplastic myelopathy and poliomyelitis (Chap. 31)

From this outline it is evident that many different and totally unrelated diseases are under consideration and that a general description cannot possibly encompass such a diversity of processes. Overall, myelitis caused by multiple sclerosis and postinfectious processes are the most common causes in practice. This was the case in the series collected by de Seze and colleagues (2001a); Nowak and coworkers reported a similar distribution. Many of the myelitides are considered elsewhere in this volume in relation to the diseases of which they are a part. Here it is only necessary to comment on the principal categories and to describe a few of the common subtypes.

Viral Myelitis (See also Chap. 33)

The enteroviruses, of which Coxsackie and poliomyelitis are examples, herpes zoster, arboviruses such as West Nile and the equine encephalitic viruses, and HIV are the important members of this category. The enteroviruses in particular have an affinity for neurons of the anterior horns of the spinal cord and the motor nuclei of the brainstem (i.e., they are neuronotropic and cause a disease that can be generically termed *poliomyelitis*), and herpes zoster virus has a clear affinity for the dorsal root ganglia; hence the disturbances of function are in terms of motor and sensory neurons, respectively, not of spinal tracts. We have cared for several patients who have had destruction of anterior horn cells as a consequence of an enterovirus other than poliomyelitis virus (see further on). West Nile virus shows the same proclivity to damage anterior horn cells. The onset of these conditions is acute and takes the form of a febrile meningomyelitis. Although there are fever, systemic symptoms, and sometimes, cutaneous features (in the case of zoster), it is the nervous system disorder that is most significant. The patient suffers the immediate effects of nerve cell destruction, and some degree of improvement nearly always follows as some neurons recover. Later in life, possibly as the neuronal loss of aging reduces the number of anterior horns, there may be an apparent increased loss of strength in muscles originally weakened by poliomyelitis ("postpolio" syndrome).

Relatively infrequent examples of a more or less transverse myelitis caused by herpes simplex virus (HSV types 1 and 2), varicella-zoster virus (VZV), CMV, EBV, any of the hepatitis viruses, and SV70 virus (causing epidemic conjunctivitis) have been reported, some in patients with immunodeficiency states, mainly AIDS. The situation is complex clinically, as most of these agents may also elicit a postinfectious variety of myelitis, described further on in this chapter and in Chaps. 33 and 36. HSV type 2 and CMV infections may also produce an acute lumbosacral radiculitis with urinary retention (Elsberg syndrome). A few cases of zoster myelitis have shown evidence of extensive inflammatory necrosis of the spinal cord with involvement of sensory and motor tracts, causing acute paraplegic and tetraplegic transverse syndromes. Pleocytosis in the cerebrospinal fluid and isolation of the viral DNA from the cerebrospinal fluid confirm the diagnosis of a primary viral infection as discussed in Chap. 33.

There are other rare forms of poliomyelitic reactions of unknown, possibly viral etiology. One such condition presents as an acute febrile or afebrile meningomyelitis and leaves all the limbs paralyzed and flaccid, sparing the brainstem and affecting the diaphragm to a variable extent. Several such patients have harbored a cancer or Hodgkin disease, and the pathology was more typical of a poliomyelitic viral infection rather than of the usual paraneoplastic syndromes (Chap. 31). Involvement of the white matter with sensory and motor paralysis below the level of a lesion has also been reported in so-called "dumb" rabies (in contrast to the usual form of "mad" or "furious" rabies encephalitis), and in an infection transmitted by the bite of a monkey, called the *B virus*. These are decidedly rare. More common are the viral myelopathy of HIV-AIDS and of HTLV-I infection. With these exceptions, one may say that myelitis that expresses itself mainly by dysfunction of motor and sensory tracts will usually prove not to be viral in origin but rather to one of the disease processes in category III (noninfectious, inflammatory) of the preceding classification, for example, multiple sclerosis. The unique myelopathies of HIV and of human HTLV infections are described below.

Vacuolar Myelopathy With HIV

(See also "AIDS Myelopathy" in Chap. 33)

As the neurology of AIDS has been elucidated, the clinical and pathologic characteristics of a viral myelopathy have been studied in detail. The frequency of this condition is impressive—it was present in 20 of 89 successive cases of AIDS on whom a postmortem examination was performed by Petito and colleagues. Often, the clinical symptoms and signs of spinal cord disease are obscured by a neuropathy or one or more of the cerebral disorders that complicate AIDS either because of HIV or due to an opportunistic infection (CMV, toxoplasmosis, progressive multifocal leukoencephalopathy [PML]). In 5 cases of severe vacuolar myelopathy in the aforementioned series, there was leg or leg and arm weakness, often asymmetrical and developing over a period of weeks, to which the signs of sensory tract involvement and sphincteric disorder were added. A sensory ataxia has also been a common early feature in our experience. The CSF shows a small number of lymphocytes, a slight elevation of protein, and, occasionally, bizarre giant cells.

The white matter of the spinal cord is vacuolated, by which is meant a ballooning within myelin sheaths of the long tracts. The changes are most severe in thoracic segments with the posterior and lateral columns are affected diffusely. Axons are involved to a lesser degree, and lipid-laden macrophages are present in abundance. Similar vacuolar lesions may be seen in the brain in some cases. The lesions in the spinal cord resemble those of subacute combined degeneration but levels of vitamin B_{12} and folic acid are normal. (A similar lesion was found in one of our patients with myelopathy from chronic lupus erythematosus.)

The antiretroviral drugs that slow the progress of AIDS, with the exception of a few cases, seem to have little effect on the myelopathy and one can only resort to symptomatic treatment of spasticity.

Tropical Spastic Paraparesis Caused by Human T-Cell Lymphotropic Virus Type I (HTLV-I)

This disease was brought to the attention of neurologists 50 years ago through the observations and writings of Cruickshank. However, it is only more recently that a chronic infective-inflammatory disease of the spinal cord caused by the retrovirus HTLV-I has been discovered and its connection to what had been called tropical myelitis, appreciated. The implications of this discovery are potentially broad and extend even to the demyelinative and possibly the degenerative diseases.

Spinal cord disease of this type has been reported from the Caribbean islands, southeastern United States, southern Japan, South America, and Africa. The clinical picture is one of a slowly progressive paraparesis with increased tendon reflexes and Babinski signs; disorder of sphincteric control is usually an early feature but symmetric paresthesias, reduced vibratory and position senses, and ataxia follow over several months or years. A few patients have had an associated polyneuropathy, as in Cruickshank's early cases. The upper extremities are usually spared (except for lively tendon reflexes), as are cerebral and brainstem functions.

The CSF contains small numbers of T-lymphocytes (10 to $50/mm^3$), normal concentrations of protein and glucose, and an increased content of immunoglobulin (Ig) G with antibodies to HTLV-I. The diagnosis is confirmed by the detection in the serum of the antibodies to the virus. Thinness of the spinal cord is evident on MRI and subcortical cerebral white matter lesions may be seen as well. Neuropathologic study has documented an inflammatory myelitis with focal spongiform, demyelinative, and necrotic lesions, perivascular and meningeal infiltrates of inflammatory cells, and focal destruction of gray matter. The posterior columns and corticospinal tracts are the main sites of disease, most evident in the thoracic cord.

Because of slow evolution, the clinical picture can easily be confused with that of progressive spastic paraplegia of the heredofamilial variety, sporadic motor neuron disease, or the chronic phase of multiple sclerosis. There are also similarities with the AIDS myelopathy described earlier, but the other features of HIV infection are absent. There are reports of improvement with intravenous administration of gamma globulin but these have not been consistent and had no effect in two of our patients.

Myelitis Secondary to Bacterial, Fungal, Parasitic, and Granulomatous Diseases

(See also Chap. 32)

With few exceptions, this class of spinal cord disease seldom offers difficulty in diagnosis. The CSF usually holds the clue to causation. In most cases, the inflammatory reaction in the meninges is only one manifestation of a generalized (systemic) disease process. The spinal lesion may involve primarily the pia-arachnoid (leptomeningitis), the dura (pachymeningitis), or the epidural space, e.g., taking the form of a compressive abscess or granuloma; or it may reside in the adjacent spinal bones. In some acute forms both the spinal cord and meninges are simultaneously affected, or the cord lesions may predominate. Chronic spinal meningitis may involve the pial arteries or veins; and as the inflamed vessels become thrombosed, infarction (myelomalacia) of the spinal cord results. Chronic meningeal inflammation may provoke a progressive constrictive pial fibrosis (spinal arachnoiditis) that virtually strangulates the spinal cord. In certain cases, spinal roots become progressively damaged, especially the lumbosacral ones, which have a long meningeal exposure. Posterior roots, which enter the subarachnoid space near arachnoidal villi (where CSF is resorbed) tend to suffer greater injury than anterior ones (as happens in tabes dorsalis). Interestingly, there are cases of chronic cerebrospinal meningitis that remain entirely without symptoms until the spinal cord or roots become involved.

The infrequent but curious bacterial myelitis caused, or in some way precipitated, by the atypical pneumonia agent *M. pneumoniae* has come to be viewed as a postinfectious immune disease, as discussed in Chap. 32. However, portions of the DNA from this organism have been found in the spinal fluid early in the course of illness in some cases, suggesting the possibility of a direct bacterial infection of the spinal cord. It is not known whether antibiotic treatment alters the course of the illness.

Syphilitic myelitis is also discussed in Chap. 32. *Bacterial abscess of the spinal cord* is rare, especially in comparison to epidural spinal abscess, and it is recognized by MRI. At times, it stands as a single pyogenic metastasis from a distant infection and subsequent bacteremia, but more often there has been spread from a contiguous infected surgical site or a fistulous connection with a superficial paraspinal abscess. Vertebral osteomyelitis is addressed further on in relation to epidural abscess.

Sarcoid Myelitis (See also "Sarcoidosis" in Chap. 32)

Sarcoid granulomas may occur as one or more intramedullary spinal cord masses, as in the cases reported by Levivier and colleagues. In our experience, the granulomatous lesion, which may be focal or multifocal, simulates demyelinative disease with respect to its tendency to relapse and remit and in its response to corticosteroids. An asymmetrical ascending paraparesis and bladder disturbance have been the main features in our patients. Usually there is evidence of systemic sarcoidosis and the CSF is abnormal (increase in cells and protein; glucose usually normal), but we have encountered a few instances of sarcoid restricted to the spinal cord before it was evident in the mediastinum (i.e., thoracic CT failing to demonstrate hilar adenopathy or diffuse parenchymal lung disease). Elevation of the spinal fluid IgG concentration and oligoclonal bands may be found, but they are not consistent features; often there are activated histiocytes in the CSF.

The use of angiotensin-converting enzyme levels in the CSF to distinguish sarcoidosis from multiple sclerosis suffers from the lack of normative values for this test, but it is reported in some small series to be elevated in two-thirds of patients. The MRI is abnormal and the conus or other portions of the cord reveal intramedullary lesions. The most characteristic finding, however, is a multifocal-subpial nodular enhancement of the meninges adjacent to a lesion within the cord or nerve roots—a picture that resembles neoplastic meningeal infiltration. The diagnosis can be confirmed by mediastinal lymph node biopsy or by the far less desirable method of biopsy of the spinal meninges, spinal roots and affected subpial cord.

On occasion, a number of other rare granulomatous conditions cause an intrinsic or, more often, extrinsic compressive myelopathy; these, include brucellosis, xanthogranulomatosis, and eosinophilic granuloma. The diagnosis may be suspected if the systemic disease is apparent at the time but usually, only the histology of a surgical specimen reveals the underlying process.

Spinal Epidural Abscess

This condition is worthy of emphasis because the diagnosis is often missed or mistaken for another disease, sometimes with disastrous results. Children or adults may be affected. Infection of the epidural space has a wide variety of sources. *Staphylococcus aureus* is the most frequent etiologic agent, followed in frequency by streptococci, gram-negative bacilli, and anaerobic organisms. An injury to the back, often trivial at the time, furunculosis or other skin or wound infection, or a bacteremia may permit seeding of the spinal epidural space or of a vertebral body. This gives rise to osteomyelitis with extension of the purulent process to the epidural space. Occasionally, the spread is from an infected disc. Another source is bacteremia in a drug addict following the use of nonsterile needles or the injection of contaminated drugs.

Organisms may be introduced into the epidural space during spinal surgery or rarely via a lumbar puncture needle during epidural or spinal anesthesia or from epidural injections of steroid or other therapeutic agents; the localization is then over the lumbar and sacral roots. In these cases of *cauda equina epidural abscess*, back pain may be severe but neurologic symptomatology is minimal unless the infection extends upward to the upper lumbar and thoracic segments of the spinal cord. It must be acknowledged that some, even fulminant, cases have no clear source in the body for the bacterial abscess.

At first, the purulent process in the cervical or thoracic region is accompanied only by low-grade fever and aching local back pain, usually intense, in most cases followed within a day or several days by radicular pain. Headache and nuchal rigidity are sometimes present; more often there are just persistent pain and a disinclination to move the back. After several days, there may be a rapidly progressive paraparesis associated with sensory loss in the lower parts of the body and sphincteric paralysis. Percussion of the spine elicits considerable tenderness over the site of the infection. Examination discloses all the signs of a complete or partial transverse cord lesion, including at times the elements of spinal shock if paralysis has evolved rapidly.

Diagnosis The diagnosis can usually be ascertained from MRI (Fig. 44-2) but care must be taken to obtain images from levels rostral and caudal enough to detect the infected collection. There may be enhancement of the margins of the purulent collection after several days.

If a diagnostic spinal puncture is performed, the CSF usually contains white cells but of surprisingly small number (fewer than 100/mm^3), both polymorphonuclear leukocytes and lymphocytes, unless of course, the needle

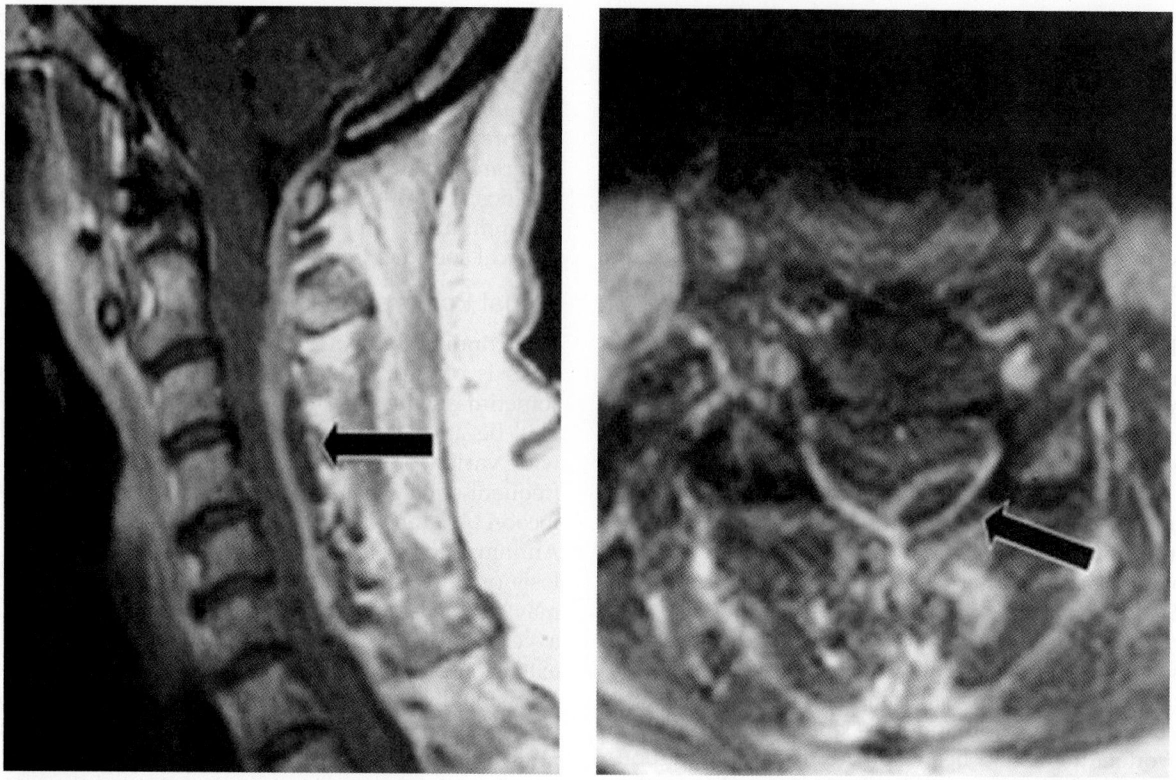

Figure 44-2. MRI of spinal epidural abscess compressing the dorsolateral cervical spinal cord. Sagittal (*left*) and axial (*right*) T1 gadolinium-enhanced images show the peripherally enhancing pyogenic collection (*arrows*) which extends over several vertebral segments.

penetrates the abscess, in which case pus is obtained. The CSF protein content is high, (100 to 400 mg/100 mL or more) but the glucose is normal. Elevation of the sedimentation rate, C-reactive protein, and peripheral neutrophilic leukocytosis are additional indicators to the diagnosis. The last of these tests is abnormal in two-thirds of cases. Blood cultures demonstrate the organism in a similar proportion. Cultures from the CSF are infrequently positive. The decades old series reported by Baker and colleagues is still a valuable reference, as is the more recent discussion by Darouiche. The differential diagnosis includes other forms of spinal cord compression and, in cases with areflexic spinal shock, tetraparesis and respiratory failure, Guillain-Barré syndrome.

Treatment The foregoing clinical findings call for MRI to be performed relatively quickly or CT myelography if MRI is not possible, to demonstrate the mass of the abscess and to determine its level. If not treated surgically by laminectomy and drainage before the onset of paralysis, the spinal cord lesion, which is probably partly a result of venous ischemia, becomes more or less irreversible. Broad-spectrum antibiotics in large doses must be given initially and the choice of treatment is then refined based on cultures from the abscess or the blood, or on a presumed source of bacteria, usually found to be staphylococcus.

When osteomyelitis of a vertebral body is the primary abnormality, the epidural extension may implicate only a few spinal sensory and motor roots, leaving long tracts and other intramedullary structures intact. In some cases with cervical epidural abscesses, stiff neck, fever, and deltoid-biceps weakness are the main neurologic abnormalities. Having emphasized the urgency of treatment, there are instances of small epidural abscesses that do not compress the cord and are limited to one or at most two levels for which we have avoided surgery by administering antibiotics alone. Also, lumbar epidural abscess and cauda equina compression without neurologic signs may be, in some cases, treated solely with antibiotics, although many surgeons favor drainage, which must be undertaken in any case, if osteomyelitis develops. Antibiotics are continued for several weeks, and the patient should be examined at regular intervals and have sequential MRI scans of the affected region.

Even after apparently successful drainage and antibiotic treatment of an epidural abscess, there may be a slowly progressive and then static syndrome of partial spinal cord compression. This is the result of formation of a fibrous and granulomatous reaction at the operative site. Distinguishing this sterile inflammatory mass from residual epidural abscess is quite difficult, even with enhanced MRI, but persistent fever, leukocytosis, and an elevated sedimentation rate, C-reactive and peripheral white blood cell count suggest that surgical drainage of the abscess was incomplete.

Spinal subdural abscess due to bacterial infections also occur and, clinically, are virtually indistinguishable from epidural ones on clinical grounds. The MRI will usually clarify the situation but a clue is provided by the CT myelogram, in which the subdural lesion has a less sharp margin and usually, a greater vertical extent. The epidural and subdural infections, if they smolder owing to delayed diagnosis or inadequate therapy, may also evolve into a local chronic adhesive meningomyelitis.

Subacute pyogenic infections and *granulomatous infections* (tuberculous, fungal) may also arise in the spinal epidural space, as noted below.

Spinal Cord Abscess

Purulent collections within the substance of the cord was first described by Hart in 1830 and, although it is rare, 73 cases had been reported by 1994 (Candon and Frerebeau). In some instances, the patient was known to have had systemic bacterial infection, septicemia, or endocarditis; in others, there was a contiguous abscess in the skin or subcutaneous tissues with a fistula to the spinal cord through an intervertebral foramen. Spinal cord abscess is a rare complication of spinal dysraphism or of a developmentally open dorsal fistulous tract. The symptoms are indistinguishable from those of epidural abscess, namely, spinal and radicular pain followed by sensory and motor paralysis; the CSF findings are also the same. Woltman and Adson described a patient in whom surgical drainage of an encapsulated intramedullary abscess led to recovery, and Morrison and associates reported a similar case caused by *Listeria monocytogenes*, which was successfully drained and the meningeal infection suppressed by ampicillin and chloramphenicol. There was no way to be certain of the diagnosis prior to the availability of MRI.

Vertebral Bacterial Osteomyelitis

This process is presented in juxtaposition to epidural abscess, with which it is closely aligned. As with other forms of osteomyelitis, vertebral infection is typically due to hematogenous implantation of bacteria during episodes of bacteremia or, it is associated with the exogenous introduction of bacteria during spinal surgery, particularly if catheters or other devices, including for spinal stabilization, are incorporated. In the case of postsurgical infection, coagulase-negative staphylococci or propionibacterium are almost always implicated, whereas with bacteremia, a number of low-virulence organisms including staphylococcus are found and multiple organisms may be involved. The source of bacteremia may be urinary infection, endocarditis, or intravenous drug abuse but many affected individuals also have diabetes, are immunosuppressed, or receiving dialysis for renal failure. In the group of immunocompromised patients, unusual or endemic organisms such as Brucella may be found. However, in almost half of patients who have not had surgery, no source is identified. Approximately one-fifth of cases have an associated epidural abscess, as discussed above. This is often indicated by an increase in local back pain or extremely severe pain from the onset.

The lumbar spine is the region most affected. The typical presentation is relatively nondescript with back pain, elevated white blood cell count and see-reactive protein level. Fever, however, is inconsistent. Several types of imaging studies may be used to demonstrate the infection, however, MRI more dependably than CT shows edema within the bone marrow and, if there is destruction of the disc adjacent to an effective vertebral body, infection is almost certain. Technetium bone scans were popular for the demonstration of osteomyelitis in general but the findings may be nonspecific. A well-known adage is that neoplasms affecting the vertebral body do not cross the disc space.

A point of contention has been the need for biopsy of the affected bone when blood cultures are negative and no obvious source of infection in the body can be found. This procedure is generally suggested although extension of the infection from the vertebral body to the paravertebral or epidural spaces may also be performed under CT guidance.

Initiating therapy with oral fluoroquinolones, with or without rifampin, has been suggested as a broad approach while the specific infecting bacteria are identified. Therapy is generally continued for at least 4 to 6 weeks, if not longer but no clear guidance is available on the appropriate duration. Surgical removal of infected bone is generally not undertaken unless the osteomyelitis is the result of implanted hardware during previous spinal surgery. Almost invariably, this hardware must be removed. Surveillance for persistent infection after treatment is probably appropriate but the MRI has not proven useful for this purpose. Inflammatory markers in the blood are apparently more dependable. A thorough review of this subject can be found in the clinical practice article by Zimmereli.

Tuberculous Spinal Osteomyelitis (Pott Disease)

Tuberculous osteomyelitis of the spine with kyphosis (Pott disease) is well known in regions of endemic tuberculosis. Children and young adults are most often affected. The osteomyelitis is the result of reactivation of tuberculosis at a site previously established by hematogenous spread. An infectious endarteritis causes bone necrosis and collapse of a thoracic or upper lumbar (less often cervical) vertebral body resulting in a characteristic angulated kyphotic deformity (Fig. 44-3); any degree of additional rotary instability allows the emergence of a gibbus deformity. Most patients have some active tuberculous infection as evidenced by fever, night sweats, and other constitutional symptoms; the sedimentation rate is invariably elevated but the degree may be slight. A compressive myelopathy occurs in some cases as a result of the spinal deformity, but it is infrequent and an epidural tuberculous abscess is a more common cause of cord compression (see below). What is surprising to us about Pott disease is the excellent result that may be obtained by external stabilization of the spine and long-term antituberculous medication. A recent young patient of ours was saved from an operation by the intercession by telephone of his father, a physician from India. Although there is some controversy regarding spinal surgery, it is certainly required in the presence of severe deformities or a compressive myelopathy as noted in Chap. 32.

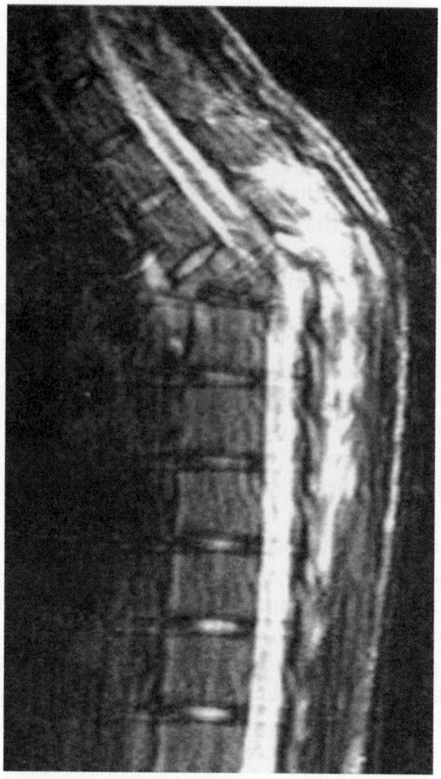

Figure 44-3. Sagittal T2-weighted MRI in Pott tuberculous spine disease. The angulated deformity of the thoracic spine is highly characteristic. (Courtesy of Dr. Randall Edgell, New York University Medical Center.)

Tuberculous Myelitis and Epidural Abscess

Solitary tuberculoma of the spinal cord as part of a generalized infection is a rarity. More often, pus or caseous granulation tissue extrudes from an infected vertebra and gives rise to an epidural compression of the cord (Pott paraplegia, as distinct from Pott disease). Occasionally tuberculous meningitis may result in pial arteritis and spinal cord infarction. The paraplegia may appear before the tuberculous meningitis is diagnosed. All these forms of tuberculosis are infrequent in the United States and Western Europe, but we see a new case every several years in a patient who had spent his earlier life in India or Africa. Additional comments can be found in Chap. 32.

Meningomyelitis Caused by Fungus and Parasitic Diseases

A wide variety of fungal and parasitic agents may involve the spinal meninges. Such infections are rare, and some do not occur at all in the United States or are limited to certain geographic areas, particularly among immigrant populations. *Actinomyces*, *Blastomyces*, *Coccidioides*, and *Aspergillus* may invade the spinal epidural space via intervertebral foramina or by extension from a vertebral osteomyelitic focus. *Cryptococcus*, which causes meningoencephalitis and, rarely, a cerebral granuloma, in our experience, seldom causes spinal lesions. Hematogenous metastases to the spinal cord or meninges may occur in both blastomycosis and coccidioidomycosis. Occasionally an echinococcal infection of the posterior mediastinum may extend to the spinal canal (epidural space) via intervertebral foramina and compress the spinal cord.

Schistosomiasis (bilharziasis) is a recognized cause of myelitis in the Asia, Africa, and South America. The spinal cord is a target for all three common forms of *Schistosoma*: *S. haematobium*, *S. japonicum*, and *S. mansoni*, but most particularly the last of these (see "Schistosomiasis" in Chap. 32). The schistosomal ova evoke an intense granulomatous myelomeningoradiculitis. The lesions are destructive of gray and white matter, with ova in arteries and veins leading to vascular obstruction and ischemia (Scrimgeour and Gajdusek). Less often, a localized granuloma gives rise to a cord syndrome and, rarely, the disease takes the form of an acute transverse myelitis with massive necrosis of cord tissue (Queiroz et al). A pruritic "swimmer's itch" at the site of entry of the parasite is reported by many patients in the days prior to the myelopathy. In the often cited review by Scrimgeour and Gajdusek, the latency between exposure and symptoms was 38 days to several years. We have cared for several patients over the years in whom the spinal cord in the low thoracic and lumbar region was infected approximately 3 weeks after they swam in contaminated water during an east African vacation and then returned home to the United States The CSF showed only a slight elevation of protein, but in almost all cases there is a pronounced pleocytosis ranging from 5 to 500 lymphocytes/mm^3 and the glucose is normal or minimally reduced. Systemic and CSF eosinophilia are variable so are not dependable for diagnosis. The diagnosis is confirmed by the finding of elevated titers of antibody directed against the schistosome in the CSF or blood. There are usually oligoclonal bands of IgG in the CSF as well. The parasite can sometimes be found in biopsies of the rectosigmoid mucosa. The administration of praziquantel arrested the course of the illness, but all but one of our patients was left disabled.

Myelitis of Noninfectious Inflammatory Type (Multiple Sclerosis and Acute and Subacute Transverse Myelitis) (See Chap. 36)

The spinal cord disorders that make up this category take the form of a leukomyelitis based on either demyelination or necrosis of portions of the spinal cord. The critical factor in their pathogenesis appears to be a disordered immune response, in some cases, as a response to an infection, and in others such as multiple sclerosis an idiopathic immune disorder. Varied clinical syndromes are produced, and the basic disease is classified in textbooks under headings such as *acute transverse myelitis*, *postinfectious myelitis*, *postvaccinal myelitis*, *acute MS*, *neuromyelitis optica*, and *necrotizing myelitis*. While each of these conditions may affect other parts of the nervous system (most often the optic nerves and brain), often the only manifestations are spinal. The aforementioned myelopathies are characterized by various degrees of inflammatory destruction, usually with lymphocytes congregating around venules in the cord, but they are sufficiently distinct to justify their separate classification. Nonetheless, transitional cases sharing the clinical and pathologic attributes of more than one disease are encountered in any large clinical practice and pathologic collection.

Postinfectious and Postvaccinal Myelitides

The characteristic features of these diseases are their temporal relationship following a viral infection or vaccination with the delayed development of neurologic signs over the period of a few days, and a monophasic course, i.e., a single attack with variable degrees of recovery and no recurrence. These processes may involve the brain as well as the spinal cord, in which case the process is properly designated as *acute disseminated encephalomyelitis* (ADEM). On the basis of the clinical features of disseminated postinfectious encephalomyelitis and the animal model of experimental allergic encephalomyelitis (EAE), postinfectious myelitis is presumed to be immunologic in nature, reflecting an attack that is more or less confined to spinal cord myelin as described in more detail in Chap. 36.

The usual history in these cases is of weakness and numbness of the feet and legs (less often of the hands and arms), which typically develop over a few days, and for the sensory symptoms to ascend from the feet to the trunk. Paresthesias in the feet and legs, which simulate a polyneuropathy, are common early symptoms. Sphincteric disturbances and backache are also common in the first days but as often arise later. A slight asymmetry of the symptoms and signs, a sensory level on the trunk, or a Babinski sign clearly marks the disease as a myelopathy and serves to distinguish it from a rapidly progressive polyneuropathy such as the Guillain-Barré syndrome. Back pain of varying degree and headache and stiff neck may or may not be present. In about half of cases the patient can identify a recent infectious illness, usually a mundane upper respiratory syndrome, but the fever has usually abated when the neurologic symptoms begin. The illness evolves over several days, sometimes a single day or on the other extreme, over 1 or 2 weeks. Despite the term *transverse myelitis*, fewer than half of cases demonstrate a truly "transverse" involvement of the cord; more often there is an incomplete corticospinal and spinothalamic syndrome affecting one side more than the other. As discussed further on, it is usually not possible to distinguish an acute episode of postinfectious myelitis from the first attack of multiple sclerosis, but a well-defined preceding infection with certain organisms favors the former process. The latency between infection and myelitis is an uncertain matter but there are well-documented instances in which the febrile episode blends into the neurologic syndrome and others in which the latency has been 2 weeks; considerably longer intervals make the association suspect.

Almost invariably, the CSF contains lymphocytes and other mononuclear cells in the range of 10 to 50/mm^3 (sometimes higher), with slightly raised protein and normal glucose content. However, there may be only 3 or 4 cells/mm^3, or none, making the inflammatory aspect less clear. Oligoclonal bands are usually absent. In most instances that have come under our care, the MRI has shown slight T2 signal abnormalities and minimal gadolinium enhancement extending over 2 or 3 spinal segments. Although the cord may be swollen in these regions (Fig. 44-4), several of our patients with mild and partial myelitis have had normal MRI studies.

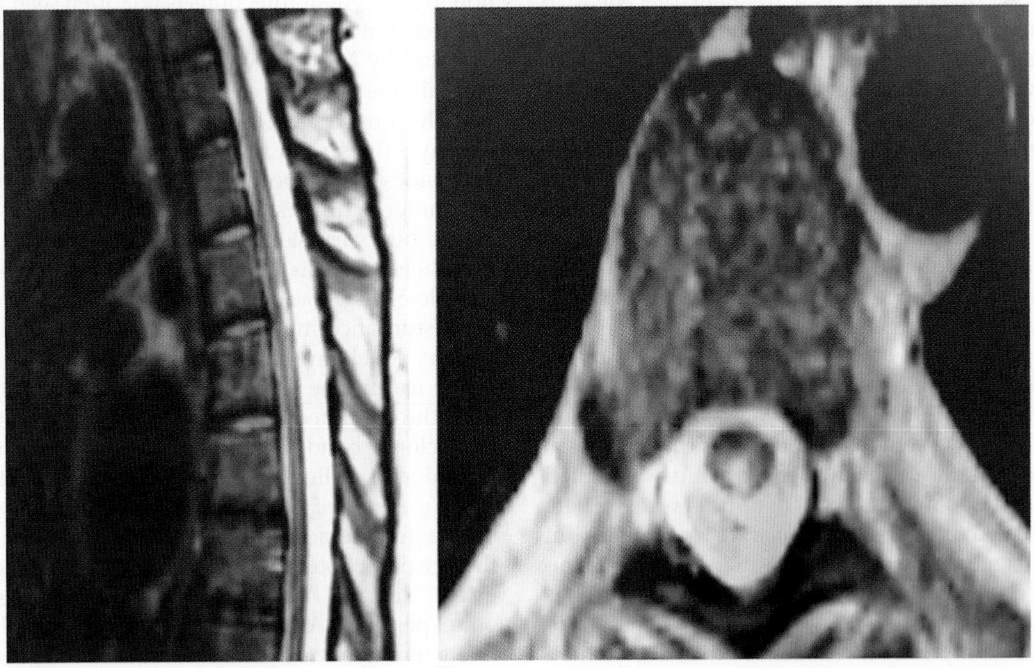

Figure 44-4. T2-weighted MRI of acute postinfectious myelitis in the sagittal (*A*) and axial (*B*) planes. There is abnormal T2 hyperintensity within the dorsal spinal cord and the cord is mildly enlarged. Mild enhancement following gadolinium infusion was noted (not shown).

Clinical variants of this syndrome are frequent in our experience; including an almost pure paresthetic illness with posterior column dysfunction and the converse; a symmetrical paraparesis with analgesia below a level on the trunk but without involvement of deep sensation (a syndrome more typically associated with infarction in the territory of the anterior spinal artery); a syndrome of variable sensory loss involving the leg and groin on one side or both; a purely lumbosacral or sacral myelopathy (conus syndrome with saddle analgesia and sphincter disturbances); and a partial Brown-Séquard syndrome.

In the past, postinfectious myelitis was most often observed in relation to the common exanthems (rubella, rubeola, varicella). The neurologic signs appeared as the rash was fading, often with a slight recrudescence of fever. Practically all human viruses have at one time or another been found to have preceded acute myelitis; however, the DNA viruses such as Epstein-Barr and cytomegalovirus are most common, and hepatitis B, varicella, and entero- and rhinoviruses have been detected from time to time. *Mycoplasma* is almost unique in being a bacterial trigger of the disease, but as noted earlier, there is some uncertainty regarding its ability to cause direct infection rather than a postinfectious immune reaction. Our interpretation of the existing information still favors a postinfectious etiology. In most instances of postinfectious myelitis, the connection to a preceding infection is presumed but cannot be proved. Only the associations with EBV, CMV, and *Mycoplasma* seem fairly certain based on the regularity of their occurrence, but it may simply reflect the relative ease with which a recent infection can be documented by serologic tests. The list of antecedent infections is otherwise much the same as for the Guillain-Barré syndrome with the notable difference of *Campylobacter jejuni*, which has not led to myelitis and is a frequent precedent to acute polyneuropathy. It can be reasonably assumed that, for example, pharyngitis, respiratory infection, and conjunctivitis, with or without fever, was a likely trigger for myelitis and the finding of abnormal liver function tests or severe pharyngitis with cervical adenopathy usually indicates EBV or, less often, CMV infection.

More difficult to understand are the large number of cases of myelitis, including autopsy-proven ones, in which the disease develops without an apparent antecedent infection. There is understandable uncertainty in such cases as to whether the illness is the opening phase of multiple sclerosis of the type described below under "Acute Demyelinating Myelitis of Multiple Sclerosis." In the numerous cases of transverse myelitis under our care, fewer than half have shown other signs of MS after 10 to 20 years (this is a far lower incidence than disseminated multiple sclerosis following a bout of optic neuritis). There is also an isolated form of *relapsing myelitis*, sometimes but not always triggered by an infection that does not manifest lesions elsewhere in the neuraxis and therefore has an ambiguous relationship to MS. Further discussion of acute transverse myelitis in relation to other demyelinating diseases can be found below and in Chap. 36.

The *pathologic changes* in postinfectious myelitis take the form of numerous subpial and perivenular zones of demyelination, with perivascular and meningeal infiltrations of lymphocytes and other mononuclear cells, and para-adventitial pleomorphic histiocytes and microglia. Taken in isolation, these pathologic changes cannot be distinguished from those of MS.

Treatment Once symptoms begin, it is not clear if any treatment is of consistent value. One's first impulse, assuming the mechanism to be autoimmune, is to administer high doses of corticosteroids, a practice we have followed but without conviction. Perhaps it is advisable to do so, but there is as yet no evidence that this alters the course of the illness. We have also used plasma exchange or intravenous immune globulin in several patients with uncertain results, although this approach was seemingly helpful in a few patients who had an explosive clinical onset.

The prognosis of this illness is better than the initial symptoms might suggest. Invariably, the myelitic disease improves, sometimes to a surprising degree, but there are examples in which the sequelae have been severe and permanent. Pain in the midthoracic region or an abrupt, severe onset usually indicates a poor prognosis (Ropper and Poskanzer). The authors have several times given a good prognosis for long-term recovery and assurance that no relapse will occur, only to witness a recrudescence of other symptoms at a later date, indicating that the original illness was probably multiple sclerosis.

Acute Demyelinating Myelitis of Multiple Sclerosis (Chap. 36)

The lesions of acute MS share many of the features of the postinfectious type as noted above. However, the clinical manifestations of the former tend to evolve more slowly, over a period of 1 to 3 weeks or even longer. Also, a relation to antecedent infections is not often seen in MS. Only the occurrence of subsequent attacks or additional lesions revealed by MRI or evoked potentials indicates that the basic illness is one of chronic recurrent demyelination.

The most typical of clinical expression of demyelinating myelitis is with numbness that spreads over one or both sides of the body from the sacral segments to the feet, anterior thighs, and up over the trunk, with coincident but variable and usually asymmetric weakness and then paralysis of the legs. As this process becomes complete, the bladder is also affected. The sensorimotor disturbance may extend to involve the arms, and a sensory level can be demonstrated on the upper parts of the trunk. The CSF may show a mild lymphocytosis, as in the postinfectious variety, but it is as often normal. Oligoclonal bands may be absent with the first attack. Bakshi and colleagues have suggested that in myelitis as a result of MS, the changes seen on MRI occupy only a few adjacent spinal segments in comparison to the postinfectious lesions, which have a longer vertical extent, but this has not been a consistent distinction in our experience. As a general rule, acute spinal MS is relatively painless and without fever, and the patient usually improves, with variable residual signs. The differential diagnosis of demyelinating myelitis is considered more fully in Chap. 36.

Treatment Corticosteroids, as outlined for the treatment of MS in Chap. 36, may lead to a regression of symptoms, sometimes with relapse when the medication is discontinued (after 1 to 2 weeks). Other patients, however, show no apparent response, and a proportion of cases have even continued to worsen while the medication was being given. Plasma exchange and intravenous immune globulin have reportedly been beneficial in individual cases, particularly in those with an explosive onset (see later). The results in our patients have been too variable to interpret.

Neuromyelitis Optica, Acute and Subacute Necrotizing Myelitis, and Devic Disease

(See discussion in Chap. 36)

In every large center, examples of this disorder are found among the many patients who present with a subacute paraplegia or quadriplegia, sensory loss, and sphincter paralysis. The neurologic signs may erupt so precipitously that a vascular lesion is assumed. In most other cases, the disease evolves at a slower and usually stepwise pace, over several months or years. Necrotizing myelopathy is distinguished from the more common types of transverse myelitis by a persistent and profound flaccidity of the legs (or arms if the lesion is cervical), areflexia, and atonicity of the bladder—all reflecting a widespread necrosis that involves both the gray and white matter of the spinal cord over a considerable vertical extent. This clinical picture is unexpected for a spinal cord lesion and, therefore, is often mistakenly attributed to spinal shock or to a completely different process such as Guillain-Barré syndrome.

This combination of spinal cord necrosis and optic neuritis corresponds to the syndrome described by Devic in 1894 and named by him *neuromyelitis optica* (Devic disease). Nearly all neurologists agree that a similar clinical syndrome involving the optic nerve and spinal cord (usually without necrosis) may also be caused by postinfectious encephalomyelitis or by MS, however, the finding by Lennon and colleagues of a specific serum IgG antibody in half of cases of Devic disease was a notable advance. The antibody is directed against the aquaporin channel in capillaries of the brainstem and cerebellum and its role in the pathogenesis of the disease partially resolves the decades old uncertainty regarding a distinction between Devic disease and forms of multiple sclerosis, in which the antibody is not present.

In both the isolated necrotic myelopathy and in Devic disease, a few or up to several hundred mononuclear cells per cubic millimeter and increased protein may be found in the CSF but oligoclonal banding is usually absent. Some cases show only an elevated protein concentration. More so than with postinfectious transverse myelitis, the MRI reveals extensive signal changes and gadolinium enhancement, usually occupying several contiguous spinal segments; called a "longitudinally extensive" lesion (Fig. 44-5). Imaging studies performed weeks or more later show atrophy of the involved segments of cord. Persistent swelling of the affected region is more suggestive of spinal cord tumor or another type of inflammation, but the permissible duration of cord swelling may extend for weeks. The electromyogram (EMG) often shows denervation of several contiguous myotomes, reflecting damage to the gray matter of those segments.

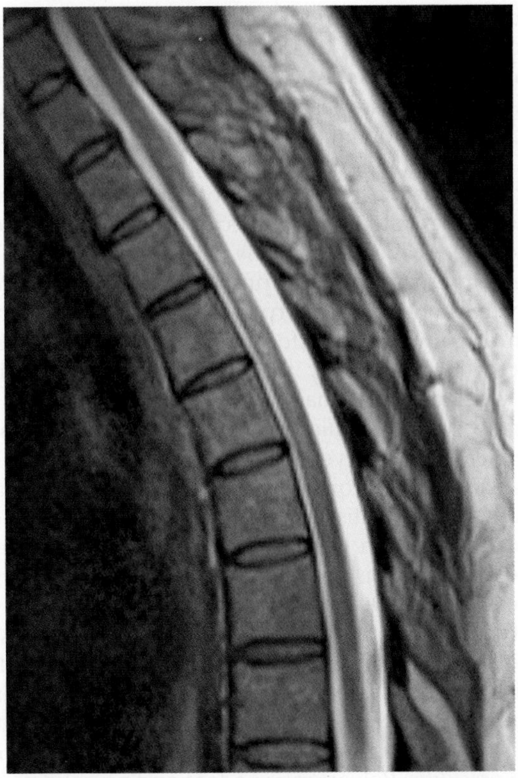

Figure 44-5. MRI of necrotic myelopathy in a patient with neuromyelitis optica. Note the long extent of the lesion and thinning of the cord as the acute illness subsides.

In cases coming to postmortem examination at variable times after the onset of symptoms, the lesion has proved to be a necrotizing myelitis with widespread loss of spinal cord tissue. The pattern of tissue destruction appears, at least in part, infarctive, i.e., not respecting the borders of gray and white matter. However, areas of residual inflammation and demyelination are often detected at the edges of the destructive lesions. Older lesions leave the spinal cord cavitated or collapsed over a vertical extent of 5 to 20 cm, with conical extensions of necrosis into the gray matter above and below the area of transverse damage. Probably many of these cases would now be categorized as part of the neuromyelitis family with aquaporin autoantibodies.

Subacute Necrotic Myelopathy and Foix-Alajouanine Myelopathy

Under the title "Subacute Necrotic Myelitis," Foix and Alajouanine, and later Greenfield and Turner, and later, Hughes, described a disorder mainly of adult men characterized by amyotrophic paraplegia that ran a progressive course over several months. The defining feature, one that still gives rise to lively polemical discussions, is severe necrosis of both gray and white matter in the lumbosacral region and a marked increase in the number of small vessels, their walls thickened, cellular, and fibrotic ("angiodysplastic"), yet without vascular occlusion. The veins are also thickened and surrounded by lymphocytes, mononuclear cells, and macrophages.

These findings have been difficult to interpret and their relationship to the group of arteriovenous malformations and fistulas, discussed later, has been unclear but we are inclined to the view of Antoni and others who were impressed with the prominence of large arteries and veins and have reinterpreted this pathologic process as an arteriovenous malformation. In many other cases of necrotic myelopathy that are not associated with a true vascular malformation, the vascular changes simply reflect a neovascular response to necrosis or may be examples of neuromyelitis optica.

A similar syndrome is produced by a rare idiopathic necrotizing vasculitis that is confined to the spinal cord (Caccamo et al). In these cases, there is a persistent and marked pleocytosis and some clinical stabilization with corticosteroids. One of our young male patients with this type of subacute necrotizing myelitis, responsive to corticosteroids, had mononuclear cells in the spinal fluid persistently over a year and died as a result of fulminant inflammatory cerebral hemorrhages. There were multiple occlusions of small vessels surrounding the spinal cord and a *vasculitis*. Polyarteritis nodosa and necrotizing arteritis only rarely involve the spinal cord. Schistosomiasis, as mentioned earlier, may also produce a necrotizing myelitis of the lumbosacral region.

Myelitis (Myelopathy) With Connective Tissue Disease

A rapidly evolving or subacute myelopathy occurs in association with systemic lupus erythematosus. The process is presumed to arise from a microvasculitis or an autoantibody. Propper and Bucknall presented such a case and reviewed 44 others in which patients with lupus developed a transverse myelitis over a period of days. There was back pain at the level of sensory loss (the cases we have seen have been painless), and pleocytosis and elevation of CSF protein were characteristic. The MRI revealed segmental swelling of the spinal cord. Postmortem examinations of similar cases have disclosed widespread vasculopathy of small vessels with variable inflammation and myelomalacia, and, rarely, a vacuolar myelopathy.

Some but not all cases also have circulating antiphospholipid antibody; the relationship of these antibodies to the myelopathy and to microvascular occlusion is uncertain (see also "Antiphospholipid Antibody Syndrome" in Chap. 34 and further discussion in Chap. 36). The incidence of lupus myelopathy is not known, but one such case is admitted to our service, in a hospital with an active rheumatology division, about every year.

Sjögren Syndrome Myelopathy

In addition to a well-described posterior root ganglionopathy and sensory neuritis, an inflammatory myelitis is associated with Sjögren syndrome. In most instances, the patient has had overt symptoms of Sjögren disease including, the sicca complex, and in others, the association has been established through serologic testing or by the finding of inflammatory infiltration of minor salivary glands (obtained by biopsy). In many reported cases, the myelopathy has simulated the myelitis of MS, even to the extent of including episodes of optic neuritis as in the cases described by Williams and colleagues and by de Seze and coworkers. The myelitis has been in different cases acute, chronic, or relapsing and displayed MRI changes in the cord that would otherwise be considered to be postinfectious or demyelinating myelitis. The spinal fluid formula has also varied but generally does not contain oligoclonal bands. Treatment with prednisone and cyclophosphamide or methotrexate has been suggested and was seemingly successful in several of our patients.

The authors cannot comment authoritatively on this entity. There is little pathologic material on which to judge the association, but the presence of other inflammatory lesions of the central and peripheral nervous system in Sjögren disease makes the existence of myelitis plausible. Antibody tests (anti-SS-A [Ro] and SS-B [La]) and possibly a biopsy of the minor salivary glands (at the junction of mucosa and epidermis of the lower lip) are justified in patients with unusual myelopathies or in those with sicca symptoms; however, screening in this manner of all cases that otherwise suggest MS or postinfectious myelitis may be excessive. This subject is also reviewed in Chap. 36, in relation to multiple sclerosis.

There is also the rare occurrence of nondescript myelitis with scleroderma as mentioned above (systemic sclerosis). The authors of most reports acknowledge the difficulty in distinguishing between the myelopathies of various connective tissue diseases. There may be some response to corticosteroids and other immunosuppressive medications. Myopathy and neuropathy, particularly trigeminal neuritis, are more common manifestations of scleroderma.

Paraneoplastic Myelitis (See also Chap. 31)

A subacute necrotic myelitis developing in conjunction with bronchogenic carcinoma was first brought to notice by Mancall and Rosales in 1964. Several dozen cases have since been recorded in association with lymphomas and carcinomas, but the disease must be rare. Actually, in cancer patients, intramedullary metastasis, quite infrequent to begin with, is more common as a cause of intrinsic myelopathy and, of course, a compressive lesion is far more frequent than either of these conditions.

The clinical syndrome consists of a progressive painless loss of motor and then sensory function, usually with sphincter disorder, over weeks. Imaging studies demonstrate an area of T2 signal change in the cord, occupying one or several contiguous segments, similar to neuromyelitis optica (Devic disease); some have slight enhancement with gadolinium or rarely, imaging may be normal. This is in distinction to the nodular enhancing appearance of an intramedullary metastasis or of extradural metastatic disease with cord compression.

The CSF may contain a few mononuclear cells and a slightly increased protein, or it may be normal. The lesions are essentially of necrotic type and respect neither gray nor white matter, but the latter is more affected. There is little or no evidence of an infective-inflammatory or ischemic lesion, for the blood vessels, apart from a modest cuffing with mononuclear cells, are normal. No tumor cells are visible in the CSF, meninges, or spinal cord tissue, and no virus has been isolated. Unlike the situation in most of the paraneoplastic neurologic disorders, there are no diagnostic markers by way of specific antineural antibodies. In particular, this myelopathy does not seem to be a component of the anti-Hu–associated encephalitis-neuropathy spectrum.

In some cases of paraneoplastic myelopathy, the pathologic changes have been more chronic, confined to the posterior and lateral columns, and associated with a diffuse loss of cerebellar Purkinje cells. This latter syndrome may have a special association with ovarian carcinoma but has been observed with carcinoma of other types and with Hodgkin disease as discussed in Chap. 31. Most of the reported cases of these types have ended fatally. Steroids and plasma exchanges have been of no clear value. Treatment of the underlying systemic tumor or immunosuppression has also failed in most cases to alter the myelopathy according to Flanagan and colleagues. A rare variety of anterior horn cell destruction that resembles motor neuron diseases is known to occur with certain lymphomas; it is also discussed with the paraneoplastic syndromes in Chap. 31.

Subacute Spinal Neuronitis (Propriospinal Myoclonus)

Two distinct entities seem to be encompassed under this name, both rare; a progressive myelopathy and a regional disorder, mainly of the abdominal muscles. Whitely and colleagues drew attention to the process characterized clinically by tonic rigidity and intermittent myoclonic jerking of the trunk and limb muscles and by painful spasms of these muscles evoked by sensory or emotional stimuli. Their cases were progressive and eventually involved the limbs.

In the few well-studied cases of this type, the brunt of the pathologic process has fallen on the cervical portion of the spinal cord. Widespread loss of internuncial neurons with relative sparing of the anterior horn cells, reactive gliosis and microglial proliferation, conspicuous lymphocytic cuffing of small blood vessels, and scanty meningeal inflammation have been the main findings. Involvement of the white matter is less marked. The pathophysiology of the rigidity in these cases is presumed to be because of the impaired function (or destruction) of Renshaw cells, with the release of tonic reflexes (Penry et al). The painful spasms and dysesthesias relate in some way to neuronal lesions in the posterior horns of the spinal cord and dorsal root ganglia. Whitely and Lhermitte and their coworkers proposed that these cases probably represent an obscure form of viral myelitis.

The cases we have observed have been of the type that remained confined to several contiguous spinal segments, usually the upper abdomen and lower thorax as described by Brown and colleagues. Some patients report a premonitory sensation before the abdominal jerking, or there is worsening with the supine position. Whether these represent the same disease as the one noted above is unclear but the segmental, abdominal variety is now a firmly established entity, albeit also idiopathic, as described in a series by Roze et al and discussed under "Spinal or Segmental Myoclonus" in Chap. 6. The CSF may be normal or show a mild lymphocytosis and increase in protein content.

Myoclonic jerking of the trunk and limbs in a focal or segmental distribution is probably a result of neuronal damage of this same type that is limited to a few segments of the spinal cord. Clonazepan, various antiepileptic and antispasticity drugs in combination may partially suppress the myoclonus, and local injection of botulinum toxin has improved the symptoms in some. A similar syndrome in a few cases has followed vertebral or spinal artery angiography (see later). A paraneoplastic variety usually associated with breast cancer has been proposed, as in the case described by Roobol and colleagues, but its nature has not been fully elucidated.

VASCULAR DISEASES OF THE SPINAL CORD

In comparison with the brain, the spinal cord is an uncommon site of vascular disease. Blackwood, in a review of 3,737 necropsies at the National Hospital for Nervous Diseases, London, during the period 1903 to 1958, found only 9 cases of spinal cord infarction, but in general hospitals, the incidence (judged on clinical grounds in our hospital) is higher. The spinal arteries tend not to be susceptible to atherosclerosis, and emboli rarely lodge there. Of all the vascular disorders of the spinal cord, infarction as a result of aortic disease, dural fistula, bleeding, and arteriovenous malformation are the only ones that are encountered with any regularity, but even taken together, they are infrequent in comparison to demyelinating myelitis or compression of the cord by tumor. In current practice, most cases of infarction have developed in relation to operations on the aorta, usually the thoracic portion, where the vessel must be clamped for some period. The dural arteriovenous fistulas that cause spinal cord swelling are being recognized increasingly as their clinical syndromes are exposed and vascular imaging of small spinal arteries becomes more sophisticated. They have probably overtaken in frequency cord infarction in this category of disease. An understanding of these disorders requires knowledge of the blood supply of the spinal cord.

Vascular Anatomy of the Spinal Cord

The blood supply of the spinal cord is derived from a series of segmental vessels arising from the aorta and from branches of the subclavians and internal iliac arteries. The most important branches of the subclavian are the vertebral arteries, small branches of which give rise to the rostral origin of the anterior spinal artery and to smaller posterolateral spinal arteries that together constitute the major blood supply to the cervical cord. The thoracic and lumbar cord is nourished by segmental arteries arising from the aorta and internal iliac arteries. Segmental branches of the lateral sacral arteries supply the sacral cord.

A typical segmental artery divides into an anterior and a posterior ramus (Fig. 44-6). Each posterior ramus gives rise to a spinal artery, which enters the vertebral foramen, pierces the dura, and supplies the spinal ganglion and roots through its anterior and posterior radicular branches. Most anterior radicular arteries are small and some never reach the spinal cord, but a variable number (4 to 9), arising at irregular intervals, are much larger and supply most of the blood to the spinal cord. Tributaries of the radicular arteries supply blood to the vertebral bodies and surrounding ligaments. The venous drainage is into the posterior veins forming the spinal plexus. Their importance relates to the pathogenesis of fibrocartilaginous embolism (see further on).

Lazorthes, in his thorough review of the circulation of the spinal cord, divides the radiculomedullary arteries into three groups: (1) upper or cervicothoracic, which are derived from the anterior spinal arteries and branches of the thyrocervical and costovertebral arteries; (2) intermediate or middle thoracic (T3 to T8 cord segments), usually from a single T7 radicular artery; and (3) lower or thoracolumbar, from a large T10 or L1 anterior radicular artery, better known as the *artery of Adamkiewicz.* This artery supplies the lower two-thirds of the cord, but in any individual the precise area supplied by this or any other anterior radiculomedullary artery varies greatly and one cannot predict what portion or proportion of cord will be infarcted if one of these vessels is occluded. The junction between the vertebral spinal and aortic circulations typically lies at the T2-T3 spinal segment, but most ischemic lesions lie well below this level.

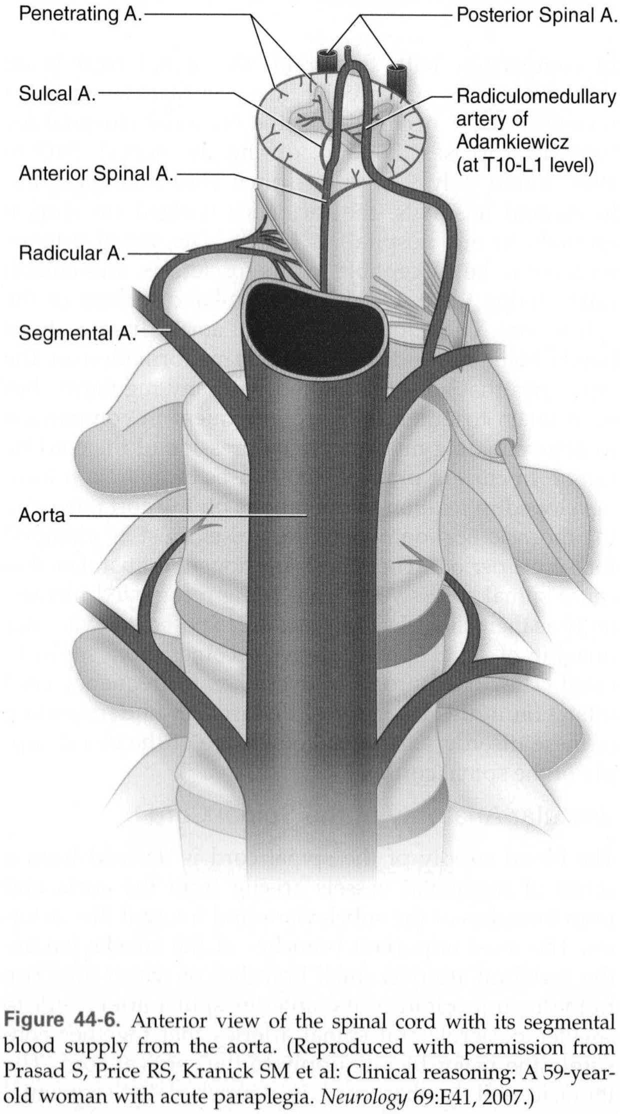

Figure 44-6. Anterior view of the spinal cord with its segmental blood supply from the aorta. (Reproduced with permission from Prasad S, Price RS, Kranick SM et al: Clinical reasoning: A 59-year-old woman with acute paraplegia. *Neurology* 69:E41, 2007.)

The anterior medullary arteries form the single anterior spinal artery, which runs the full length of the cord in its anterior sulcus and gives off direct penetrating branches via the central (sulcocommissural) arteries. These penetrating branches supply most of the anterior gray columns and the ventral portions of the dorsal gray columns of neurons (see Fig. 44-6). The peripheral rim of white matter of the anterior two-thirds of the cord is supplied from a pial radial network, which also originates from the anterior median spinal artery. *Thus, the branches of the anterior median spinal artery supply roughly the ventral two-thirds of the spinal cord.* Infarction of the region supplied by this artery give rise to an anterior spinal cord syndrome that consists of loss of pain and temperature and paralysis below the level of the lesion, but with sparing of proprioception and vibration sense that correspond to transaction of the spinothalamic and corticospinal tracts but not of the posterior columns.

The posterior medullary arteries form the paired posterior spinal arteries that supply the dorsal third of the cord by means of direct penetrating vessels and a plexus of pial vessels (similar to that of the ventral cord, with which it anastomoses freely). Within the cord substance, then, there is a "watershed" area of capillaries where the penetrating branches of the anterior spinal artery meet the penetrating branches of the posterior spinal arteries and the branches of the circumferential pial network. All spinal segments, because of the variable size of collateral arteries, do not have the same abundance of circulatory protection.

Normally there are 8 to 12 anterior medullary veins and a greater number of posterior medullary veins arranged fairly close to one another at every segmental level. They drain into radicular veins. In addition, a network of valveless veins extends along the vertebral column from the pelvic venous plexuses to the intracranial venous sinuses without passing through the lungs (Batson plexus) and is considered a route for metastatic disease from the pelvis.

Infarction of the Spinal Cord

Ischemic infarction of the spinal cord usually involves the territory of the anterior spinal artery, i.e., a variable vertical extent of the ventral two-thirds of the spinal cord. Infarctions in this territory are relatively uncommon as already mentioned, representing 1.2 percent of all strokes (Sandson and Friedman). The resulting clinical abnormalities are generally referred to as the *anterior spinal artery syndrome,* described by Spiller in 1909. Atherosclerosis and thrombotic occlusion of the anterior spinal artery is quite uncommon, as noted, and infarction in the territory of this artery is more often secondary to disease of the extravertebral collateral artery or to disease of the aorta, either advanced atherosclerosis, a dissecting aneurysm, or intraoperative surgical occlusion—which compromises the important segmental spinal arteries at their origins. An ischemic myelopathy has been reported in cocaine users, preceded sometimes by episodes of cord dysfunction resembling transient ischemic attacks. Cardiac and aortic surgery, which requires clamping of the aorta for more than 30 min, and aortic arteriography may also be complicated by infarction in the territory of the anterior spinal artery; more often in these circumstances damage to central neuronal elements is greater than that to anterior and lateral funiculi, as described below.

Rarely, polyarteritis nodosa may cause occlusion of a spinal medullary artery. Systemic cholesterol embolism arising from a severely atheromatous aorta may have the same effect. This latter type of embolism is prone to occur after surgical procedures, angioplasty, or cardiopulmonary resuscitation. For unexplained reasons, the spinal cord infarction sometimes follows one of the aforementioned procedures by up to 3 weeks, as emphasized in Dahlberg's series of cases. In almost all such patients, other evidence of widespread embolism can be expected. Infarction may also result from systemic hypotension, the most vulnerable part being of the thoracic segments of the cord. One of our patients had cord infarction during a bout of diabetic coma.

Among the most curious causes of cervical cord infarctions is *dissection of the extracranial vertebral arteries,* either unilateral or bilateral. The resultant ischemia in the territories of the anterior spinal arteries causes anterior and central cervical cord ischemia. In two cases of this nature that have been brought to our attention, there were an asymmetric brachial diplegia and a suspended sensory loss, preceded by intense radicular and neck pain. The patients reported by Weidauer and colleagues are representative, and there are numerous other case reports although the cause of the vertebral artery dissections has not always been clear. A few patients have vertigo at the onset, directing attention to the vertebral artery damage. We have also encountered instances of myelomalacia in adolescents and young adults in whom no aortic or spinal arterial disease could be demonstrated. Possibly, some of these were because of embolization of disc material (nucleus pulposus) into the local vasculature (see further on).

A quite different progressive ischemic necrosis of the cord can occur in the neighborhood of an arteriovenous malformation or dural fistula and is considered later in this chapter (see also the subacute necrotic myelitis of Foix and Alajouanine, described earlier).

Despite the elucidation of these causes of spinal cord infarction, a large group in any series has no identifiable cause; for example, an etiology could be established in only 7 of 27 consecutive cases in the series from Novy and colleagues. The clinical manifestations of spinal arterial occlusion will, of course, vary with the level and portions of the cord that are infarcted, but common to practically all cases of infarction in the territory of the anterior spinal artery is pain in the neck or back and the development of paralysis and loss of pain and thermal sensations below the level of the lesion, accompanied by paralysis of sphincteric function. Except in high cervical lesions, the sensory changes are dissociated, i.e., pain and temperature sensations are lost (because of interruption of the spinothalamic tracts), but vibration and position sense are unimpaired (a result of sparing of posterior columns).

Rarely, infarction is preceded by *spinal transient ischemic attacks* as has been emphasized in cases related to cocaine use. The symptoms may develop instantaneously or, more often in our experience, over an hour or two; in any case, more rapidly than in the inflammatory myelitides. Radicular pain corresponding to the upper level of the lesion is sometimes a complaint. Paralysis is usually bilateral, occasionally unilateral, and rarely complete. Also reported is a bibrachial paralysis as a fragment of the anterior spinal artery syndrome, as mentioned earlier. In cases that cause a complete transverse myelopathy, the limbs are initially flaccid and areflexic, as in spinal shock from traumatic lesions, followed after several weeks by the development of spasticity and the return of a degree of voluntary bladder control (unless sacral segments have been infarcted). Many patients regain a substantial degree of motor function, mainly in the first month but extending over a year (see Sandson and Friedman; Cheshire et al; Novy et al).

Infarction in the territory of the posterior spinal arteries is uncommon and the corresponding syndrome is not stereotyped; only 2 of 27 cases from the series by Novy and colleagues had this pattern. It may occur with surgery or trauma of the spine or rarely with vertebral artery dissections.

Some, but not all, spinal cord infarctions are detected by MRI. After a few days, there are obvious lesions on the T2 sequences, presumably reflecting edema that extends over several levels. There may be slight enhancement after infusion of gadolinium. It is notable, however, that the MRI taken in the first hours or day is often normal. The reason for the delay in the appearance of the imaging findings is not known. In the chronic stages, the infarcted region collapses and has an attenuated signal on MRI. Whether diffusion weighted sequences can dependably demonstrate these infarctions is not clear.

Dissecting aneurysm of the aorta, which is characterized by intense interscapular and/or chest pain (occasionally it is painless), widening of the aorta, and signs of impaired circulation to the legs or arms and various organs, gives rise to a number of myelopathic syndromes. The neurologic picture was first described by Kalischeri in 1914 and the aortic lesion leading to dissection, according to Erdheim, was a medionecrosis. The spinal syndromes of aortic dissection according to Weisman and Adams are (1) paralysis of the sphincters and both legs with sensory loss below T6; (2) ischemic infarction of the cord confined to the gray matter, in which case there is an abrupt onset of muscle weakness or myoclonus and spasms in the legs but no pain or sensory loss; (3) obstruction of the origin of a common carotid artery with hemiplegia; and, less commonly, (4) obstruction of a brachial artery with a sensorimotor neuropathy of the limb.

With regard to *aortic aneurysm surgery*, paraplegia is uncommon after procedures performed on the infrarenal segment but occurs as frequently as 5 to 10 percent following repair of thoracoabdominal aneurysms. Again emphasized here is the not easily explained observation that up to a quarter of these myelopathies do not appear for several days postoperatively (8 days in one of our patients). The article by Lintott and colleagues may be consulted for further details.

In the past, aortography was sometimes complicated by an acute myelopathy; we had observed a number of such cases and Killen and Foster reviewed 43 examples of this accident. The most striking examples, fortunately rare, are now the result of complications of vertebral angiography, resulting in high cervical infarction, similar in most ways to the aforementioned spinal infarction from extracranial dissection of the vertebral artery. The onset of sensorimotor paralysis is immediate, and the effects are often permanent. The syndrome of painful segmental spasms, spinal myoclonus, and rigidity, mentioned earlier, has also been observed under these conditions. It was presumed that vascular spasm and occlusion resulted in infarct necrosis. The frequency of this complication was greatly reduced by the introduction of less toxic contrast media.

Treatment Whether the acute effects of spinal infarction can be modified by high-dose corticosteroids, agents that increase blood flow, or anticoagulation is not known. There are case reports of improvement in paraplegia following aortic dissection by the use of CSF drainage, for example, as in the cases reported by Blacker and colleagues and by Killen and associates, but other factors may have contributed. Many surgical services insert a spinal drain prior to aortic procedures in order to reduce spinal fluid pressure, ostensibly reducing the incidence of cord infarction. There may be gradual improvement after spinal cord infarction, as Robertson and colleagues have reported in perhaps the largest series available, but most patients remain with substantial difficulties.

Surfer's Myelopathy

This unusual nontraumatic athletic problem has been described by Thompson and colleagues from Hawaii. It mainly affecting novice surfers who were prone for prolonged times on the surfboard and then engaged in vigorous movements, followed by assuming a standing position. Within an hour of surfing, there was characteristic severe upper lumbar or thoracic pain after, followed by progressive paraparesis or paraplegia, and urinary retention. In several reports, MRI showed signal changes in a long extent of the thoracic spinal cord and when the proper imaging sequences have been performed, some cases have restricted diffusion in the affected region. On the basis of the latter finding and preservation of proprioception some patients (implicating ischemia of the anterior portion of the spinal cord), a vascular mechanism has been proposed. In the series reported by Chang and colleagues, improvement was inconsistent.

Hemorrhage of the Spinal Cord (Hematomyelia) and Canal

Hemorrhage into the spinal cord is rare compared with the frequency of cerebral hemorrhage. The apoplectic onset of symptoms that involve spinal tracts (motor, sensory, or both), associated with blood and xanthochromia in the spinal fluid are the identifying features of *hematomyelia*. Aside from trauma, hematomyelia is usually traceable to a vascular malformation or a bleeding disease and particularly to the administration of anticoagulants. Actually, most vascular malformations of the spinal cord do not cause hemorrhage, but instead produce a progressive, presumably ischemic myelopathy as described later and mentioned in the earlier section on the Foix-Alajouanine type of subacute necrotic myelopathy.

The same causes (anticoagulation, blood dyscrasia with coagulopathy, and arteriovenous malformation [AVM]) may underlie bleeding into the epidural or subdural space and give rise to a rapidly evolving compressive myelopathy. In some cases, as in those of Leech and coworkers, one cannot ascertain the source of the bleeding, even at autopsy. Epidural or subdural bleeding, like epidural abscess, represents a neurologic emergency and calls for immediate radiologic localization and, in most cases, surgical evacuation.

Advances in the techniques of selective spinal angiography and microsurgery have permitted the visualization and treatment of vascular lesions that cause bleeding with a precision not imaginable a few decades ago. These procedures make it possible to distinguish among the several types of vascular malformations, arteriovenous fistulas, and vascular tumors, such as hemangioblastomas, and to localize them accurately to the spinal cord, epidural or subdural space, or vertebral bodies. This subject is discussed further on.

Vascular Malformations and Fistulas of the Spinal Cord and Dura

These lesions cause both ischemic and hemorrhagic lesions. Some are true arteriovenous malformations (AVMs), implying a congenital connection between the two sides of the circulation and others are more limited fistulas in the dura, probably mostly acquired for various reasons. The distinction is in the size of the nidus of communication between an artery and a vein and the size and location of feeding and draining vessels. The classification of spinal AVMs is confusing, in part because the enlarged draining veins by which the lesions were formerly identified are probably secondary features. A more useful categorization reflects the appearance and location of the malformation: (1) arteriovenous malformations that are strictly intramedullary or that also involve the meninges and surrounding structures, such as the vertebral bodies, to a limited extent; (2) a variety of intradural perimedullary fistulas that lie on the pial and subpial surface of the cord (these probably conform most closely to the lesion described by Foix and Alajouanine discussed in the earlier section "Subacute Necrotic Myelopathy and Foix-Alajouanine Myelopathy"); and (3) dural fistulas. There is insufficient pathologic material to determine whether these represent distinct pathologic entities or simply differing degrees and configurations of a common developmental process but, as mentioned, the last of these types may be acquired from local venous occlusions and the other types do not originate in this way. Once recognized, treatment of a spinal cord malformation of any type may be an urgent matter, especially in cases with rapid clinical deterioration and impending paralysis.

Dural Arteriovenous Fistula The entity is addressed first because it has emerged as the most common type, at least in our practices. Fistulas within the dura that overlies the spinal cord are capable of causing a myelopathy, sometimes several segments distant from the vascular lesion. Most are situated in the region of the low thoracic cord or the conus and have a limited venous draining system. Some are in a dural root sleeve and drain into the normal perimedullary coronal venous plexus. Men seem to be affected disproportionately.

The presenting clinical features in our patients have included slowly progressive bilateral but asymmetric leg weakness with variable sensory loss. According to Jellema and colleagues, who studied 80 patients with spinal dural fistulas, the most common initial symptoms were gait imbalance, numbness, and paresthesias. As the process progressed, the majority developed urinary problems, leg weakness, and numbness in the legs and buttocks. The degree of leg weakness varied greatly and back pain in their series was infrequent and has not been a consistent feature in the patients under our care.

The myelopathy may have a subacute or saltatory evolution, presumably from fluctuating venous congestion within the cord. A claudicatory syndrome has also been reported. Characteristically, activities that increase venous pressure (Valsalva maneuver, exercise) transiently amplify the symptoms or produce irreversible, stepwise worsening. One remarkable such case involved a baritone opera singer whose legs gave way repeatedly while singing (Khurana et al). A few of our patients have reported transient symptoms upon standing. Many cases occur, however, without a stepwise progression or elicitable worsening. As mentioned, many reported cases have been painless, although most of our patients have had a moderate spinal ache or sciatica. In contrast to the larger parenchymal arteriovenous lesions, these bleed only rarely. The spinal fluid is normal or shows a slight elevation of protein.

The disease can be inferred from the MRI appearance of a characteristic swelling of one or a few adjacent segments of the cord that represents venous congestion and edema as discussed further on.

Intramedullary AVM The true AVM, previously referred to as *angioma racemosum venosum* or *dorsal extramedullary arteriovenous malformation*, is typically located on the dorsal surface of the lower half of the spinal cord and occurs most often in middle-aged and elderly men (23 of 25 of Logue's patients were male). However, this lesion may occur at any age and at any location in the cord and may be quite widespread. In a few cases has there been an overlying dermatomal nevus.

The clinical picture was well described by Wyburn-Mason. Acute cramp-like, lancinating pain, sometimes in a sciatic distribution, is often a prominent early feature. It may occur in a series of episodes over a period of several days or weeks; sometimes it is worse in recumbency. Almost always there is weakness or paralysis of one or both legs and numbness and paresthesias in the same distribution with a highly variable duration of evolution; an abrupt apoplectic onset is known or the neurologic signs may appear over months, most cases conforming to the middle of these extremes. Wasting and weakness of the legs may introduce the disease in some instances, with uneven progression, sometimes in a series of abrupt episodes. Severe disability of gait is usually present within 6 months, and half of the patients described by Aminoff and Logue were chair-bound within 3 years; the average survival in the past was 5 to 6 years, but the disorder has rarely been fatal in our patients. These lesions only infrequently give rise to intramedullary or subarachnoid hemorrhage. The spinal fluid shows high protein but little or no cellular reaction.

When viewed directly, the dorsal surface of the lower cord may be covered with a tangle of veins, some involving roots and penetrating the surface of the cord. The progression of symptoms is presumably a result of chronic venous hypertension and secondary intramedullary ischemic changes, and the abrupt episodes of worsening are attributed to the thrombosis of vessels, all on uncertain grounds because angiographic studies sometimes show only a single or a few such dilated draining vessels. Furthermore, there is insufficient pathologic material to determine whether some of the more prominent venous anomalies represent true venous angiomas (probably they do not).

Intradural Perimedullary and Subpial AVM The pial fistulous arteriovenous communication that involves the superficial aspect of the cord to a variable extent is the least frequent in this category but probably of a similar nature to the dural type; it may be related (or identical) to the vascular lesion in the earlier discussed Foix-Alajouanine process. In contrast to dorsal arteriovenous malformations, these fistulas tend to involve the lower thoracic and upper lumbar segments or the anterior parts of the cervical enlargement. The patients are often younger and the sexes are equally affected. The clinical syndrome may take the form of slow spinal cord compression, sometimes with a sudden exacerbation, or the initial symptoms may be apoplectic in nature, either because of thrombosis of a vessel or of a hemorrhage from an associated draining vein that dilates to aneurysmal size and bleeds into the subarachnoid space or cord (hematomyelia and subarachnoid hemorrhage); the latter complication occurred in 7 of 30 cases reported by Wyburn-Mason.

Diagnosis These lesions—dural or parenchymal—may be apparent on MRI or CT myelography by the presence of one or more enlarged and serpiginous draining vessels in the subarachnoid space; just as often, they are not visualized by these methods (Jones et al). For this reason, the possibility should come to mind that an otherwise unexplained myelopathy with signs of congestion of the cord on MRI may be the result of a vascular malformation. However, several studies, such as the one by Toossi and colleagues, have suggested that the absence of both T2 hyperintensity and flow voids on MRI makes the presence of a dural fistula unlikely and spares the patient from the need for angiography.

Imaging features that have been emphasized with dural fistulas include enlargement of the spinal cord at the level of the lesion and T2 bright signal of the swollen cord over several segments, but these are not invariable. Infrequently, the draining surface vessels are evident on MRI (Fig. 44-7A). Because of the slow blood flow within the vascular lesion, the affected region may have a hypointense T1 signal. Hurst and Grossman have commented on the presence of peripherally located regions of T2 hypointense signal changes. Many of these changes are reversed by surgical or endovascular interventions that ablate the malformation. There is no enhancement although, with increasingly improved MRI techniques, more fistulas are becoming apparent. Some remarkable ones appear as a multiple small enhancing areas that are like hairs standing on end, coating the cord over several levels.

The diagnosis is usually established through selective angiography, which shows the fistula in the dura overlying the cord or on the surface of the cord itself but the most conspicuous finding is often the associated early draining vein (Fig. 44-7B). Demonstration of the fistula requires the injection of feeding vessels at numerous levels above and below the suspected lesion, because the main artery of origin is often some distance away from the malformation. The small angiodysplastic vessels of the Foix-Alajouanine lesion may not be opacified with angiography. In rare instances, the fistula or high-flow arteriovenous malformation lies well outside the cord, for example, in the kidney, and gives rise to a myelopathy, presumably by raising venous pressures within the cord.

Other Rare Vascular Anomalies of the Cord In the *Klippel-Trenaunay-Weber syndrome*, a sometimes extensive vascular malformation of the spinal cord is associated with a cutaneous vascular nevus overlying the AVM or in a limb supplied by the affected cord level; when the malformation lies in the low cervical region, there may be enlargement of finger, hand, or arm (the hemangiectatic hypertrophy of Parkes Weber; neurofibromatosis is another cause of limb enlargement). Spinal segmental and tract lesions may occur at any age, but the patients we have observed were young adults. Vascular occlusion

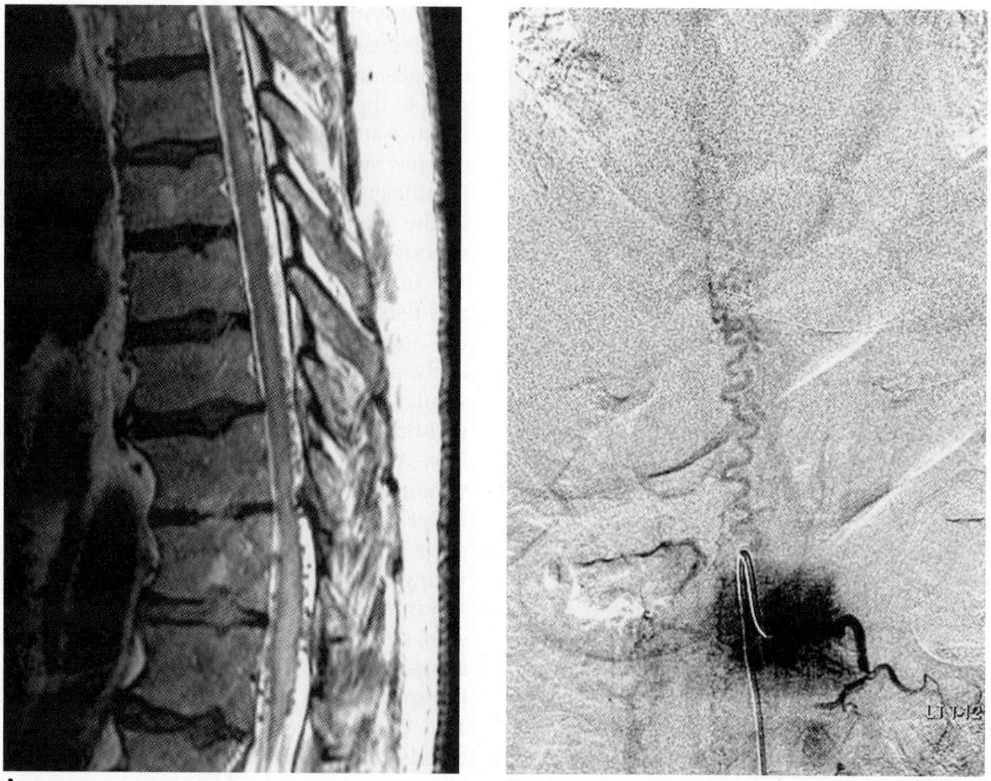

Figure 44-7. Dural arteriovenous fistula of the cord. *A.* Sagittal T2-weighted MRI of the lower spinal cord of a 50-year-old man with progressive myelopathy. Cord edema (T2 hyperintensity at the conus medullaris) and multiple vascular flow voids surrounding the spinal cord and extending up to the mid-thoracic vertebral levels are seen, both the result of the arterio-venous fistula. *B.* Angiographic injection of the left T12 radicular artery from the patient whose MRI is shown in *A*, demonstrating abnormal early filling of veins surrounding the spinal cord, confirming the presence of an arterio-venous fistula. The fistula was repaired and the patient's symptoms partially improved.

or hemorrhage was responsible for the myelopathy. Some of these vascular lesions have been treated by defining and ligating their feeding vessels. In a few reported cases it has been possible to extirpate the entire lesion, especially if it occupied the surface of the cord.

Other rare vascular anomalies of the spinal cord include *aneurysm of a spinal artery with coarctation of the aorta* and *telangiectasia of the cord*, which may or may not be associated with the hereditary hemorrhagic type of Osler-Rendu-Weber. Over the years, the authors have had under their care patients with the latter disease who developed acute hemorrhagic lesions of the spinal cord. We have also observed several *cavernous hemangiomas of the spinal cord*. In two of our patients, an angiographically negative solitary cavernous angioma was the source of an acute partial transverse myelopathy. The lesions were clearly demonstrable only in the T2-weighted MR images. McCormick and associates have reported similar cases. Characteristically, the angiomas cause partial syndromes and are followed by considerable recovery of function just as when they occur in the brain. There may or may not be blood in the CSF. Rarely, the same disease is responsible for one or more hemorrhagic lesions of the brain. The association of cavernous angiomas with arteriovenous fistulas of the lung is a rare finding, and the latter may be a source of brain abscess. In *coarctation of the aorta*, the circulation to the lower part of the spinal cord may be deficient, with resultant paresis of the legs, sensory loss, and sphincteric impairment. Or there may be intracranial subarachnoid hemorrhage from a ruptured saccular aneurysm, an associated condition in a small number of cases.

Treatment The rate of progression of the myelopathy from these various lesions varies greatly. In some cases, as already noted, it may become a matter of some urgency to reverse the venous congestion and avoid infarction of the cord. Other lesions require a more measured approach. By occluding the feeding artery of a spinal AVM or fistula, which is often single, and thereby eliminating the excess pressure in veins, the course of disease can be arrested and any pain reduced (Symon et al). In most of our patients, there has been postoperative improvement in the neurologic deficit over a few weeks or months. In cases of the larger racemose AVMs, stripping the enlarged veins along the dorsal cord is no longer considered necessary and may be dangerous. Increasingly, one resorts to obliteration of a fistula or a reduction of the AVM by the use of endovascular techniques and various types of embolic particles. The procedure is long and painstaking, for the operator must identify and embolize all the feeding vessels of the malformation; general anesthesia is required in most cases.

This approach has certain drawbacks; recanalization occurs months later in many instances, as does distal occlusion of the venous drainage system with worsening of the myelopathy. For these reasons, surgical ligation of the arterial supply is still preferred as the initial procedure for larger AVMs. Some surgeons advise a staged approach in which the size of the malformation is first reduced by endovascular techniques, thereby making the surgery less complicated. Intradural fistulas are usually treated by endovascular methods but they can be excised if visualized intraoperatively. Interventional techniques have also been used to advantage in the intramedullary malformations, either as the sole treatment or in combination with surgery. Focused radiation has been tried but the results have been difficult to evaluate.

Fibrocartilaginous Embolism

Naiman and coworkers described the case of an adolescent boy who died of sudden paralysis after a fall in a seated position. Postmortem examination revealed extensive myelomalacia as a result of occlusions of numerous spinal vessels by emboli of nucleus pulposus material. The clinical picture is essentially one of spinal apoplexy; after spinal trauma of even mild degree the patient experiences the abrupt onset of pain in the back or neck, accompanied by the signs of a transverse cord lesion affecting all sensory, motor, and sphincteric functions and evolving over a period of a few minutes to an hour or more. Occasionally, the syndrome spares the posterior columns, thus simulating an anterior spinal artery occlusion. The CSF is normal. As with other types of cord infarction, the changes may not appear on MRI for a day or more.

In some of the reported instances there was said to have been no excessive activity or spinal trauma preceding the spinal cord symptoms. However, this has not been true of our patients, most of whom had been participating in some strenuous activity, but often earlier in the day rather than at the time of the paraplegia. Others had fallen and injured themselves on preceding days; a direct blow to the back during contact athletic sports was the antecedent event in several others and is the easiest-to-understand cause.

At autopsy, numerous small arteries and veins within the spinal cord are occluded by fibrocartilage, with necrosis of the spinal cord over 1 or 2 segments. A ruptured disc of the usual type is usually not found in these patients, but high-resolution radiographs have exposed a discontinuity of the cortical bone of the vertebral body adjacent to a collapsed disc and herniation of disc tissue into a vertebral body in a few instances (Tosi et al). The explanation suggested by Yogananden and colleagues is that the high intravertebral pressure forces nucleus pulposus material into venules and arteries of the marrow of the vertebral body, and thence into the adjacent radicular vessels. This mechanism has probably been overlooked in some otherwise unexplained cases of acute ischemic myelopathy.

Caisson Disease (Decompression Sickness, "Bends")

This extraordinary myelopathy, which is well known to the scuba diving community, is observed in persons who are subjected to high underwater pressure and then ascend too rapidly. It affects mainly the upper thoracic spinal cord as a result of nitrogen bubbles that form and are trapped in spinal vessels. There may be little or no involvement of the brain. Haymaker, who has provided the most complete account of the neuropathologic changes, observed ischemic lesions mainly in the white matter of the upper thoracic cord; the posterior columns were more affected than lateral and anterior ones. We have encountered instances in which an almost complete transverse myelopathy was evident soon after the patient resurfaced but the syndrome then improved, leaving the patient with an asymmetrical and incomplete albeit permanent residual deficit. The smallest degree of damage is manifest as a minor myelopathy that affects the anterior or the posterior funiculi, leaving either spasticity or numbness of the legs. Immediate treatment consists of recompression in a hyperbaric chamber; later treatment is symptomatic, with antispasticity drugs and physical therapy.

Spinal Subdural Hemorrhage

This is an unusual process but we have reported cases that presented with excruciating thoracic back pain of such severity as to cause a bizarre, almost psychotic, reaction (Swann et al). The neck becomes slightly stiff and there may be a headache, suggesting subarachnoid hemorrhage. However, signs of a myelopathy do not appear, indicating that the bleeding is confined to the pliable subdural spaces surrounding the cord, thereby allowing the blood to spread over several segments.

Lumbar puncture yields a distinctive dark yellow-brown spinal fluid that resembles, to us, used motor oil. The color is imparted by methemoglobin and reflects the presence of an adjacent, decomposing walled-off clot. Usually there are also red blood cells in the CSF, suggesting seepage into the subarachnoid space from the adjacent collection. MRI or CT myelography shows a subdural collection, with characteristically smooth borders. When drained operatively, this is found to be clotted blood. Usually, no vascular malformation is demonstrable and the cause remains obscure. Trauma or anticoagulation underlies a few cases but many are spontaneous. The symptoms resolve in 1 or 2 weeks after removal of the subdural hematoma. Small collections may be managed without surgery, in which case corticosteroids may be helpful in reducing the pain.

The syndrome of spinal subarachnoid hemorrhage has been mentioned earlier and is also covered in Chap. 34 under "Other Causes of Intracranial Bleeding and Multiple Cerebral Hemorrhages."

SYNDROME OF SUBACUTE OR CHRONIC SPINAL PARAPARESIS WITH OR WITHOUT ATAXIA

The gradual development of weakness of the legs is the common manifestation of many diseases of the spinal cord. A syndrome of this type, including ataxia of gait beginning insidiously in late childhood or adolescence and progressing steadily, is usually indicative of hereditary spinocerebellar degeneration (Friedreich ataxia) or one of its variants (see Chap. 39). In early adult life, MS is the most frequent cause and AIDS myelopathy is being increasingly recognized; syphilitic meningomyelitis, formerly of great importance, is now quite uncommon. In middle and late adult life, cervical spondylosis, subacute combined degeneration of the cord (vitamin B_{12} deficiency), combined system degeneration of the nonpernicious anemia type, some associated with low levels of serum copper, radiation myelopathy, tropical spastic paraplegia, spinal arachnoiditis, and thoracic spinal tumor, particularly meningioma, are the important diagnostic considerations for the slowly progressive cord syndrome. In most forms of subacute and chronic spinal cord disease, spastic paraparesis is more prominent than posterior column ataxia, Friedreich ataxia and the myelopathy caused by vitamin B_{12} deficiency being notable exceptions.

Spinal Multiple Sclerosis

(See earlier under "Acute Demyelinating Myelitis of Multiple Sclerosis" and also Chap. 36 for a discussion of multiple sclerosis.)

Ataxic paraparesis is among the most common manifestations of MS. Asymmetrical involvement of the limbs and signs of cerebral, optic nerve, brainstem, and cerebellar involvement usually provide confirmatory diagnostic evidence. Nevertheless, purely spinal involvement may occur, no lesions being found outside the spinal cord even at autopsy. A frequent problem in diagnosis is posed by the older woman who was not known to have had MS in earlier life, previous episodes having been absent, asymptomatic, or forgotten. A secondary progressive stage of spinal multiple sclerosis is the consequence of recurrent demyelinating attacks. There is another group, however, in which slowly advancing neurologic deterioration represents the primary manifestation of the disease. The National Hospital Research Group examined 20 cases of the secondary progressive type of spinal MS and 20 of the primary type by gadolinium-enhanced MRI of the spinal cord and brain and found new lesions in only 3 of each group (Kidd et al). They suggest that the progression correlates better with progressive atrophy of the spinal cord than with recurrent demyelinative lesions.

This clinical state must be differentiated from cervical disc disease, spondylosis, and tumor. The main aids in diagnosis are the CSF findings (minor pleocytosis and oligoclonal IgG abnormalities), present in 70 to 90 percent of cases, the demonstration by MRI of other unsuspected white matter lesions in the spinal cord and brain.

Cervical Spondylosis With Myelopathy (Spondylitic Myelopathy) (See also Chap. 11)

It has been stated, correctly in our opinion, that this is the most frequently observed myelopathy in general practice. It is a degenerative disease of the spine involving the lower and midcervical vertebrae that narrows the spinal canal and intervertebral foramina and causes progressive injury of the spinal cord, roots, or both.

Historical Note Key, in 1838, probably gave the first description of a spondylotic bar, or ossified protrusion into the spinal canal. In 2 cases of compressive myelopathy with paraplegia, he found "a projection of the inter-vertebral substance and posterior ligament of the spine, which was thickened and presented as a firm ridge that had lessened the diameter of the canal by nearly a third." The ligament, where it passes over the posterior surface of the intervertebral substance, was found to be "ossified." In 1892, Horsley performed a cervical laminectomy on such a patient, removing a "transverse ridge of bone" compressing the spinal cord at the level of the sixth cervical vertebra. Thereafter, operations were performed in many cases of this sort, and the tissues removed at operation were repeatedly misidentified as benign cartilaginous tumors or "chondromata." In 1928, Stookey described the pathologic effects upon the spinal cord and roots of these "ventral extradural chondromas." Peet and Echols, in 1934, were probably the first to suggest that the so-called chondromata represented protrusions of disc material. But this idea never gained wide credence until the publication, in the same year, of the classic article on the ruptured intervertebral disc by Mixter and Barr. Although their names are associated with the lumbar disc syndrome, 4 of their original 19 cases were instances of cervical disc disease. It was C.S. Kubik who identified the extruded material as nucleus pulposus from surgical specimens obtained by Mixter and Barr's.

Also of importance is Gowers' account, in 1892, of *vertebral exostoses*, in which he described osteophytes that protrude from the posterior surfaces of the vertebral bodies and encroach upon the spinal canal, causing slow compression of the cord as well as bony overgrowth in the intervertebral foramina, giving rise to radicular pain. Gowers correctly predicted that these lesions would offer a more promising field for the surgeon than would other kinds of vertebral tumors.

For some reason, there was little awareness of the frequency and importance of spondylotic myelopathy for many years after these early observations had been made. All the interest was in the acute ruptured disc. Finally, it was Russell Brain who, in 1948, put cervical spondylosis on the neurologic map, so to speak. He drew a distinction between acute rupture and protrusion of the cervical disc (often traumatic and more likely to compress the nerve roots than the spinal cord) and chronic spinal cord and root compression consequent to disc degeneration and associated osteophytic outgrowths (*hard disc*), as well as changes in the surrounding joints and ligaments. In 1957, Payne and Spillane documented the importance of a developmentally smaller-than-normal spinal canal in the genesis of myelopathy in patients with cervical spondylosis. These reports were followed by a spate of articles on the subject (see Wilkinson). Rowland's review of the natural history of cervical spondylosis and the results of surgical therapy is a useful modern reference, as is that by Uttley and Monro.

Symptomatology

The characteristic syndrome consists of combinations of the following in varying degrees: (1) painful, stiff neck or pain in the neck, shoulders, and upper arms (brachialgia) that may be aching or radicular (stabs of sharp and radiating pain evoked by movement), asymmetric or unilateral; (2) numbness and paresthesias of the hands; and (3) spastic leg weakness with Babinski signs, unsteadiness of gait, and a Romberg sign. The numbness and paresthesias are occasionally the earliest symptoms and typically involve the distal limbs, especially the hands. Variations of these symptoms are elaborated below. Each of the components may occur separately, or they may occur in combination and various sequences.

With reference to the most common of these symptoms, the neck and shoulder pain, in any sizable group of patients older than 50 years of age, approximately 40 percent will be found at times to have some clinical abnormality of the neck, usually crepitus or pain, with restriction of lateral flexion and rotation (less often of extension). Pallis and colleagues, in a survey of 50 patients, all of them older than 50 years of age and none with neurologic complaints, found that 75 percent showed radiologic evidence of narrowing of the cervical spinal canal as a result of osteophytosis of the posterior vertebral bodies or of narrowing of the intervertebral foramina because of osteoarthropathy at the apophyseal joints; thickening of the ligaments (both the ligamentum flavum posteriorly and the posterior longitudinal ligament anteriorly) adds to the narrowing of the canal. However, only half of the patients with radiologic abnormalities showed physical signs of root or cord involvement such as changes in the tendon reflexes in the arms, briskness of reflexes and impairment of vibratory sense in the legs, and sometimes Babinski signs. The occasional finding of a Babinski sign in older individuals who had never had a stroke or complained of neurologic symptoms is often explained by an otherwise inevident cervical osteophyte (Savitsky and Madonick).

The pain is usually centered at the base of the neck or higher, often radiating to an area above the scapula. When brachialgia is also present, it takes several forms: a sharp pain in the pre- or postaxial border of the limb, extending to the elbow, wrist, or fingers; or a persistent dull ache in the forearm or wrist, sometimes with a burning sensation. Discomfort may be elicited by coughing, Valsalva maneuver, or neck extension, or neck flexion may induce electrical feelings down the spine (Lhermitte symptom). Rarely, the pain is referred substernally.

As to the sensory features (which may occasionally be absent), numbness, tingling, and prickling of the hands and soles of the feet and around the ankles are the most frequent complaints. Some patients complain of numbness or paresthesias, most often in one or two digits, a part of the palm, or a longitudinal band along the forearm. Slight clumsiness or weakness of a hand is another complaint. A feeling as if "wearing gloves," "swollen," or the hands "coated with glue" are common descriptions. Several of our patients have complained of paresthesias in the distal limbs and trunk for years before there was any indication of motor involvement. In advanced cases, there may be a vague sensory level at or just above the clavicles. Impaired vibratory sensation and diminished position sense in the toes and feet (all indicative of a lesion of the posterior columns), as well as the Romberg sign, are the most conspicuous sensory findings. This imparts a "tabetic" unsteadiness to the gait. Sensory defects tend to be asymmetrical. (It is noteworthy that symmetric sensory symptoms and signs of identical type are seen with subacute combined degeneration as a result of vitamin B_{12} deficiency.) Rarely, the sensorimotor pattern takes the form of a Brown-Séquard syndrome. Less frequently, paresthesias and dysesthesias in the lower extremities and trunk may be the principal symptoms; even less often there are sensory complaints on the face, ostensibly corresponding to compression of the trigeminal sensory tract in the upper cervical cord.

The third part of the typical syndrome, spastic legs from a compressive myelopathy, most often manifests as a complaint of weakness of a leg or of getting up stairs and slight unsteadiness of gait. The entire leg or the quadriceps feels stiff and heavy and gives out quickly after exercise. Mobility of the ankle may be reduced, and the advancing toe of the shoe scrapes the floor. On examination, slight hypertonicity of the legs is usually more evident than weakness, and the tendon reflexes are increased (ankle jerks may not share in this change in the elderly). Although the patient may believe that only one leg is affected, it is commonly found that both plantar reflexes are extensor, the one on the side of the stiffer leg being more clearly so. Less often, both legs are equally affected. As the compression continues, walking becomes unsteady because of the addition of sensory ataxia.

The biceps and brachioradial reflexes on one or both sides may be depressed, sometimes in association with an increase in the triceps and finger reflexes. The hand or forearm muscles may undergo slight atrophy; in a few cases, the atrophy of hand muscles is severe. In such cases, the spondylotic compression, as judged by MRI or CT myelography, may be confined to the high cervical cord, well above the levels of the motor neurons that innervate these muscles. In patients with sensory loss, pain and thermal sensation often appear to be affected more than tactile sense. An unexpected Babinski sign has already been mentioned and a few fasciculations may be seen, especially in proximal arm muscles. Another unusual feature in advanced stages of cervical cord compression is the appearance of *mirror movements* of the hands, in which effortful attempts to make refined movements of the fingers of one hand, causes the opposite hand to move similarly.

As the myelopathy progresses, sometimes intermittently, both legs become weaker and more spastic. Sphincteric control may then be altered; slight hesitancy or precipitancy of micturition are the usual complaints; frank incontinence is infrequent. In the more advanced form of this condition, walking requires the aid of a cane or canes or a walker; in some cases, all locomotion ultimately becomes impossible, especially in the elderly patient. Abrupt worsening, even paraplegia or quadriplegia, may follow forceful traumatic flexion or extension injuries of the neck, as indicated later.

Pathologic Changes

The fundamental spinal lesion is generated initially by a fraying of the annulus fibrosus with extrusion of disc material into the spinal canal. The disc becomes covered with fibrous tissue or partly calcified, thereby forming a transverse osteophytic "spondylitic bar" or there may be simply central bulging of the annulus without extrusion of nuclear material. The latter, unlike ruptured discs that occur mainly at the C5-C6 or C6-C7 interspace, often involve higher interspaces and may occur at several adjacent levels. The dura may be thickened and adherent to the posterior longitudinal ligament at affected levels. The underlying pia-arachnoid is also thickened and the adjacent ligamentous hypertrophy contributes to compression of the cord or the nerve roots. This series of pathologic changes is often ascribed to a type of hypertrophic osteoarthritis. However, osteophyte formation and ridging are so frequently observed in patients who have no other signs of arthritic disease that this explanation is surely not totally correct. Subclinical trauma in persons who are structurally susceptible to spondylosis is more likely to be the cause of bar formation, in the authors' opinion.

When a cervical nerve root is compressed by lateral osteophytic overgrowth, the dural sleeve is thickened and truncated and the root fibers are damaged. Usually the fifth, sixth, or seventh cervical roots are affected in this way, both the anterior and posterior, or only the anterior, on one or both sides. A small neuroma may rarely appear proximal to the site of anterior root compression.

The dura is ridged and the underlying spinal cord is flattened. The root lesions may lead to secondary wedge-shaped areas of degeneration in the lateral parts of the posterior columns at higher levels. The most marked changes in the spinal cord are at the level(s) of compression. There are zones of demyelination or focal necrosis at the points of attachment of the dentate ligaments (which tether the spinal cord to the dura) and areas of rarefaction in the posterior and lateral columns, as well as loss of nerve cells. Ventral gray matter lesions, often asymmetrical, are attributed by Hughes to ischemia.

Pathogenesis

The vulnerability of the cervical spine to degenerative change has no ready explanation. Most likely it is related in some way to the high degree of mobility of the lower cervical vertebrae, which is accentuated by their location next to the relatively immobile thoracic spine.

The mechanism of spinal cord injury would seem to be one of simple compression and ischemia. When the spinal canal is developmentally narrow in its anteroposterior dimension at one or several points, the space available for the spinal cord becomes insufficient. A small canal certainly makes an individual more subject to the compressive effects of spondylosis. The range acquired of narrowing of the canal that produces symptomatic cervical spondylosis is generally from 7 to 12 mm (normal canal diameter: 17 to 18 mm). Consequently, one must consider several additional mechanisms by which the cord might be damaged. The effects of the natural motions of the spinal cord during flexion and extension of the neck are probably important in this respect. Adams and Logue confirmed the observation of O'Connell that, during full flexion and extension of the neck, the cervical cord and dura move up and down. The spinal cord is literally dragged over protruding osteophytes and hypertrophied ligaments; conceivably it is this type of intermittent trauma that causes progressive injury.

It has also been shown that the spinal cord, displaced posteriorly by osteophytes, is compressed by the infolding of the posterolateral ligamentum flavum each time the neck is extended (Stoltmann and Blackwood). Segmental ischemic necrosis resulting from intermittent compression of spinal arteries or from compression of the anterior spinal artery has also been postulated. Most neuropathologists favor the idea of intermittent cord compression between osteophytes anteriorly and ligamentum flavum posteriorly, with an added vascular element accounting for the scattered lesions deep in the cord. Trauma from sudden extreme extension, as in a fall, severe whiplash injury, or chiropractic manipulation, or from a lesser degree of retraction of the head during myelography, tooth extraction, or a tonsillectomy may be operative in individual cases, particularly in patients with congenitally narrow canals. The lateral extension of the osteophyte and hypertrophy of the adjacent facet joint together compress the nerve root as it is entering its spinal foramen. Sometimes these are the main changes and cause only a radiculopathy, as discussed in Chap. 11.

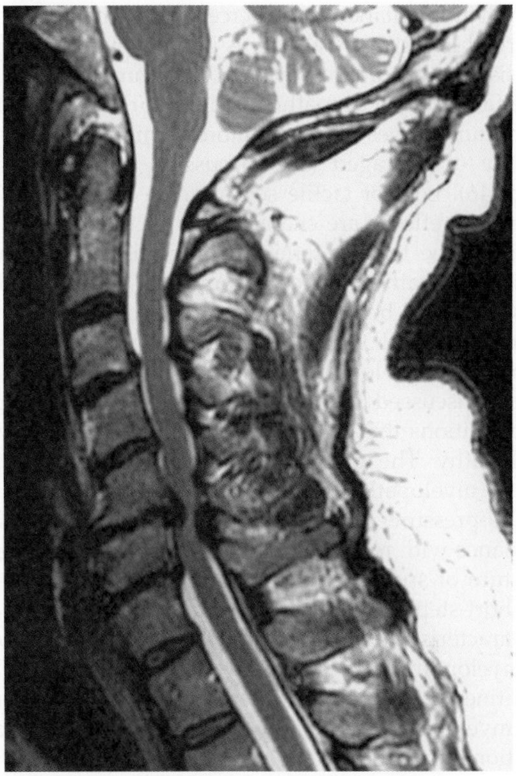

Figure 44-8. Sagittal T2 MRI in a patient with symptomatic cervical spondylosis. The spinal cord is severely compressed at the C5-C6 intervertebral disc space. Faint abnormal T2 hyperintensity of the spinal cord can be seen at the point of compression. Following surgical decompression, the patients myelopathic symptoms partially improved.

Diagnosis

When pain and stiffness in the neck, brachialgia, either in the form of aching or a more distinctive radicular pain, and sensorimotor-reflex changes in the arms are combined with signs of myelopathy, there is little difficulty in diagnosis. When the neck and arm changes are inconspicuous or absent, the diagnosis becomes more difficult. The myelopathy must then be distinguished from the late, progressive form of spinal multiple sclerosis. Because posterior vertebral osteophytes and other bony alterations are frequent in the sixth and seventh decades of life, the question that must be answered in any given case is whether the vertebral changes are adequately severe to cause the neurologic abnormality. The finding of some degree of sensorimotor or reflex change corresponding only to the level of the spinal abnormalities is a point that always favors spondylotic myelopathy. A lack of such corresponding changes and the presence of oligoclonal bands and signs of lesions in the optic nerves and brain indicate demyelinating myelopathy.

The detailed findings on both MRI and CT myelography become critical in such cases (Fig. 44-8). The MRI may overestimate the degree of cord compression by an osteophyte, but clear deformation of the cord into the shape of a kidney bean and obliteration of the surrounding CSF spaces in the transverse image support the diagnosis of spondylotic compression. To confidently attribute neurologic symptoms to spondylosis there should be considerable encroachment on and obliteration of the circumferential CSF space at that level, not simply an impingement or slight deformation of the normal oval shape of the cord. Signal changes within the body of the cord underlying or within a half segment of the compression are seen in advanced cases and usually indicate a degree of irreversibility of at least the sensory symptoms. Curiously, these signal changes may be one or two levels above or below the site of main compression. However, serious symptoms may occur even without changes in the intrinsic MRI signal. Contrast myelography with the patient supine and lateral views taken during flexion and extension of the neck are useful diagnostic procedures in uncertain cases.

It has been stated that spondylotic myelopathy may simulate amyotrophic lateral sclerosis (amyotrophy of arms and spastic weakness of the legs). This has seldom been a diagnostic problem. Although brachial and shoulder fasciculations with muscle atrophy may be combined with hyperreflexia in spondylosis, the widespread denervation and progressive course of ALS are not in evidence. We have observed only a few patients with spondylotic myelopathy who exhibited an absolutely pure motor syndrome, i.e., one in which there was no cervical or brachial pain and no sensory symptoms in the arms or impairment of vibratory or position sense in the legs. Likewise, a pure spastic paraparesis is more likely to be a manifestation of MS, hereditary spastic paraplegia, motor neuron disease (primary lateral sclerosis type), HTLV-I myelopathy, or the carrier state of adrenoleukodystrophy or other intrinsic myelopathy.

When imbalance, both perceived by the patient and observed in tests of walking, is a major symptom, spondylosis must be differentiated from a number of acquired large-fiber polyneuropathies, particularly inflammatory or immune types and the more benign sensory neuropathy of the aged (see discussion of this entity in Chap. 46). Loss of tactile sensation in the feet and loss of tendon reflexes are characteristic of the latter; examination of the tendon reflexes distinguishes neuropathy from myelopathy. Subacute combined degeneration of the spinal cord because of vitamin B_{12} deficiency or low serum copper, AIDS and HTLV-I myelopathy, ossification of the posterior longitudinal ligament, and spinal cord tumor (discussed further on) are usually listed among the conditions that might be confused with spondylotic myelopathy. The gait abnormality produced by spondylotic myelopathy may also be mistaken for that of normal-pressure hydrocephalus; a marked increase of imbalance with removal of visual cues (Romberg sign) is a feature of spondylosis but not of hydrocephalus, and the short-stepped and magnetic quality of walking that is characteristic of hydrocephalus is not seen in cervical myelopathy (see Chap. 31 for discussion of NPH). Incontinence occurs only in advanced cases of spondylotic myelopathy but usually follows soon after gait deterioration in hydrocephalus.

The special problems of spondylotic radiculopathy, which may accompany or occur independently of the myelopathy, are discussed in Chap. 11.

Treatment

The slow, intermittently progressive course of cervical myelopathy with long periods of relatively unchanging symptomatology makes it difficult to evaluate the effects of treatment. Assuming that the prevailing view of the mechanism of cord and root compression is correct, the use of a soft collar to restrict anteroposterior motions of the neck seems reasonable. This form of immobilization may be sufficient to reduce discomfort in the neck and arms; only exceptionally in our experience, however, has arm and shoulder pain alone been sufficiently severe and persistent to require surgical decompression unless there is in addition a laterally protruded disc or osteophytic constriction of a root foramen. Many patients have been dissatisfied with the results of this passive approach and are unable to wear a collar for prolonged periods.

If osteophytes have narrowed the spinal canal at several interspaces, a posterior decompressive laminectomy with severance of the dentate ligaments helps to prevent further injury. The results of such a procedure in relieving symptoms are fairly satisfactory (Epstein and Epstein); in fully two-thirds of the patients, improvement in the function of the legs occurs, and in most of the others, progression of the myelopathy is halted. The operation carries some risk; rarely, an acute quadriplegia—presumably a result of manipulation of the spinal cord and damage to spinal arteries—has followed the surgical procedure. When only one or two interspaces are the site of osteophytic compression, their removal by an anterior approach (anterior cervical discectomy, or "ACD") has given better results and carries less risk. Braakman has reviewed the surgical methods and their relative advantages.

Even with modern surgical techniques, most series indicate that once symptomatic, the outcome varies and that a significant proportion of patients, even after adequate decompression and initial improvement, have persistent symptoms or undergo some degree of later functional deterioration (see also Chap. 11). This creates a conundrum for the physician in advising the patient about the correct time to undertake surgical decompression. Nonetheless, certain clinical observations pertain and may be used as guides to treatment. Any degree of spasticity, sphincter disturbance, or loss of sensation in the hands will not improve, and indeed usually worsens over months, without surgery. Hand weakness and muscular atrophy that is the result of radicular compression will improve with decompression of the appropriate root by one of several surgical approaches, but weakness that is from central cord damage requires decompression to halt the process and probably should not be delayed more than a few weeks once it is apparent that this is the problem. Usually, such patients have MRI signal changes within the substance of the cervical cord in apposition to an osteophytic bar.

Lumbar Stenosis (See Chap. 11)

This is another spondylotic abnormality seen with particular frequency in older individuals, especially men. Usually it declares itself by numbness and weakness of the legs, sometime with poor control of sphincters. Many texts state that there may be little or no pain or only a spinal ache that fluctuates from day to day but in our experience the majority of patients have constant backache and sciatica. A notable feature is the induction or aggravation of the neurologic symptoms upon standing and walking (neurologic claudication). This topic is discussed in "Lumbar Stenosis" in Chap. 11, which should be consulted for a detailed discussion.

Ankylosing Spondylitis

This condition of the spine is a result of inflammation at the sites of ligamentous insertions into bone that leads to an intense calcification. The sacroiliac joints and lumbar spine are most affected, as discussed in Chap. 11, but as the disease advances, the entire spine becomes fused and rigid. The biomechanics of the rigid spine make it susceptible to fracture. The most common complication is a spinal stenosis and cauda equina syndrome. Bartleson and associates described 14 patients (and referred to 30 others in the medical literature) who, years after the onset of spondylitis, developed sensory, motor, reflex, and sphincteric disorders referable to L4, L5, and the sacral roots. Surprisingly, the spinal canal was not narrowed but instead the caudal sac was actually dilated. Confavreux and coworkers presented evidence that enlargement of the lumbar dural sac is caused by a defect in resorption of the CSF. There are usually arachnoidal diverticula on the posterior root sleeves, but no other explanation can be given for the radicular symptoms and signs. Surgical decompression has not benefited most patients, nor has corticosteroid therapy.

This condition occasionally occurs at higher levels and gives rise to a myelopathy. Our experience includes several cases with symptoms related to the cervical roots.

The most hazardous complication of ankylosing spondylitis is compression of the cord from seemingly minor trauma that has resulted in fracture-dislocation of the cervical (or lumbar) vertebrae. Fox and colleagues treated 31 such patients in a 5-year period; the majority of unstable fractures that required surgical fixation were in the cervical region, and several patients had fracture–dislocations at two levels. The instability at the upper spinal levels may be difficult to detect radiologically, and caution should be observed in allowing patients to resume full activity after a neck injury if the cervical spine is involved by ankylosing spondylitis. Careful flexion and extension radiograph views usually, but not always, demonstrate the instability.

As mentioned briefly earlier, multiple arachnoid cysts in the thoracic or lumbar region are associated with ankylosing spondylitis (and with *Marfan syndrome*).

Rheumatoid Arthritis of the Spine

The spinal changes of rheumatoid arthritis differ somewhat from those of ankylosing spondylitis although the latter too may be a cause of atlantoaxial dislocation (see further on under "Anomalies at the Craniocervical Junction"). The ligaments that attach the odontoid to the atlas and to the skull and the joint tissue are weakened by the destructive inflammatory process. The subsequent dislocation of the atlas on the axis may remain mobile or become fixed and give rise to an intermittent or persistent paraparesis or quadriparesis. Similar effects may result from a forward subluxation of C4 on C5 (see Nakano et al). Atlantoaxial dislocation is known to be a cause of collapse and sudden death. If the upper cervical cord is compressed, the odontoid process must be removed and C1-C2 decompressed and stabilized. Other levels of the spine are less frequently affected.

Ossification of the Posterior Longitudinal Ligament (OPLL)

Compressive cervical myelopathy caused by this process occurs almost exclusively in patients of Japanese extraction and has been demonstrated to us as an almost mundane finding by colleagues in Hawaii. The clinical signs are much the same as those of cervical spondylosis, but the radiologic appearance of cancellous bone along a segment of the posterior longitudinal ligament is unique. The ligamentous calcification can be seen on plain films, CT scan, and MRI and may be mistaken for spondylotic change. The ossified areas may enlarge enough to form islands of bone marrow. Laminoplasty with enlargement of the spinal canal has been successful.

Cervical Dural Sac Myelopathy (Hirayama Disease)

This unusual myelopathy has usually been considered in discussions of the motor neuron disorders because of its characteristic features of chronic wasting of one or both hands and forearms without sensory changes or long tract signs. It appears, however, that the damage in this disease is from intermittent compression of the lower cervical cord and gradual deterioration of the motor neurons in the anterior grey matter. Hirayama pointed out that in the young men who were affected, the mechanism of cord damage is a buckling of the dorsal dural sac and an intermittent anterior displacement and ligamentous compression of the cord during flexion of the neck.

The muscles innervated by C7, C8, and T1, encompassing mainly the hand and forearm, are affected on one side or bilaterally, but asymmetrically. There are few or no fasciculations and no sensory changes; the painless loss of power and muscle bulk proceeds smoothly over several years, giving the impression of a degenerative condition. MRI or CT myelogram performed with the neck flexed, as described by Hirayama and Tokumaru, shows the cervical cord to be atrophic with signal changes in the anterior parts of the cord and confirms the diagnosis of compression by the buckled dura. We have examined several such patients and can corroborate their claim from observation of MRI with the patient placed in a flexed-neck position. Presumably, this configuration causes ischemia of the anterior gray matter, but this has not been proved. Others have reported the syndrome in the absence of this structural configuration (Willeit et al). Two of our young male patients had long swan-like necks. What is most important about this process is the degree of recovery afforded by ligamentous sectioning and by similar surgical approaches that accomplish decompression of the lower cervical cord.

Paget Disease of the Spine (Osteitis Deformans)

Enlargement of the vertebral bodies, pedicles, and laminae in Paget disease may result in narrowing of the spinal canal. The clinical picture is one of cord compression. The plasma alkaline phosphatase concentration is high, and the typical bone changes are seen in radiographs. Usually, several adjacent vertebrae of the thoracic spine are affected but other parts of the skeleton are also involved (see later), which facilitates diagnosis. Posterior surgical decompression leaving the pedicles intact is indicated if there is sufficient stability of the vertebral bodies to prevent collapse. Medical management includes the use of nonsteroidal antiinflammatory drugs for persistent pain; calcitonin to reduce pain and plasma levels of alkaline phosphatase; and cytotoxic drugs such as plicamycin and etidronate disodium to reduce bone resorption.

Other Spinal Abnormalities With Myelopathy

The spinal cord is obviously vulnerable to any vertebral maldevelopment or disease that encroaches upon the spinal canal or compresses its nutrient arteries. Some well-known abnormalities are listed here.

Congenital Anomalies at the Craniocervical Junction

Of these, congenital *fusion of the atlas and foramen magnum* is the most common. McCrae, who described the radiologic features of more than 100 patients with bony abnormalities at the craniocervical junction, found this partial or complete bony union of the atlas and occipital bone in

28 cases. He also noted that whenever the anteroposterior diameter of the canal behind the odontoid process was less than 19 mm, there were signs of spinal cord compression. Fusion of the second and third cervical vertebrae is a common associated anomaly but does not seem to be of clinical significance. There is considerable crossover with the foreshortened neck of the Klippel-Feil syndrome mentioned below.

Abnormalities of the Odontoid Process These were found in 17 cases of McCrae's series. There may be complete separation of the odontoid from the axis or chronic *atlantoaxial dislocation* (atlas displaced anteriorly in relation to the axis). These abnormalities may be congenital or the result of injury and are known causes of acute or chronic spinal cord compression and stiffness of the neck.

In all the congenital anomalies of the foramen magnum and the upper cervical spine there is a high incidence of syringomyelia. McCrae found that 38 percent of all patients with syringomyelia and syringobulbia showed such bony anomalies, but this is considerably higher than in our experience. All patients whose symptoms might be explained by a lesion in the cervicocranial region (particularly patients in whom MS and foramen magnum tumor are suspected) require careful radiologic examination.

In mucopolysaccharidosis IV, or the Morquio syndrome (Chap. 37), a typical feature is the absence or severe hypoplasia of the odontoid process. This abnormality, combined with laxity or redundancy of the surrounding ligaments, results in atlantoaxial subluxation and compression of the spinal cord. Affected children refuse to walk or develop spastic weakness of the limbs. Early in life they excrete an excess of keratan sulfate, but this may no longer be detectable in adult life. In certain of the mucopolysaccharidoses, we have also seen a true pachymeningopathy with great thickening of the dura in the basal cisterns and high cervical region with spinal cord compression. Surgical decompression and spinal immobilization have been curative.

Achondroplasia This dominantly inherited form of dwarfism is caused by a mutation in one of the fibroblastic growth factors, which causes a failure of conversion of fetal cartilage to bone at the growth plate. It occasionally results in great thickening of the vertebral bodies, neural arches, laminae, and pedicles because of increased periosteal bone formation. The spinal canal is narrowed in the thoracolumbar region, often with kyphosis, leading sometimes to a progressive spinal cord or cauda equina syndrome. Another complication, which results from a small foramen magnum, is hydrocephalus (or markedly widened subarachnoid spaces). In young children, a syndrome of central apnea and spasticity of the legs is characteristic. These complications may require ventricular shunting. Narrowing of the lumbar canal tends to present later in life.

Platybasia and Basilar Invagination *Platybasia* refers to a flattening of the base of the skull (the angle formed by intersection of the plane of the clivus and the plane of the anterior fossa is greater than 135 degrees). *Basilar impression* or *invagination* has a somewhat different meaning, namely, an upward bulging of the occipital condyles; if the condyles, which bear the thrust of the spine, are displaced above the plane of the foramen magnum, basilar invagination is present. Each of these abnormalities may be congenital or acquired (as in Paget disease); frequently they are combined. They give rise to a characteristic shortness of the neck and a combination of cerebellar and spinal signs. A normal-pressure hydrocephalus may also develop.

In the *Klippel-Feil syndrome* there is fusion of the upper cervical vertebrae or of the atlas to the occiput. The anomaly is easily identified by substantial foreshortening of the neck. Affected individuals are susceptible to compression of the cervical cord after minor trauma. Many such patients demonstrate mirror movements of their hands, comparable to those described earlier in cervical spondylosis.

Tethered Cord This developmental anomaly is discussed more fully and illustrated in Chap. 38. A progressive cauda equina syndrome with prominent urinary difficulties and varying degrees of spasticity are the usual presentations.

Syphilitic Meningomyelitis

Here, as in multiple sclerosis, the degree of ataxia and spastic weakness is variable. A few patients have an almost pure state of spastic weakness of the legs, requiring differentiation from motor system disease and familial spastic paraplegia. Such a syndrome, formerly called Erb spastic paraplegia and attributed to meningovascular syphilis, is now recognized as being nonspecific and more often caused by demyelinating disease. In a minority of chronic syphilitic patients, sensory ataxia and other posterior column signs predominate. Ventral roots are involved in the chronic meningeal inflammation, giving rise to signs of segmental amyotrophy—hence the term *syphilitic amyotrophy* of the upper extremities with spastic paraplegia. Confirmation of this now infrequent diagnosis depends on finding a lymphocytic pleocytosis, an elevated protein and gamma globulin, and a positive serologic reaction in the CSF. Other aspects of this disease and treatment are discussed under "Spinal Syphilis" in Chap. 32. Tabes dorsalis is, of course, another important form of syphilitic myelitis.

Subacute Combined Degeneration of the Spinal Cord (See Chap. 41)

This form of nutritional spinal cord disease is caused by vitamin B_{12} deficiency and is fully described in Chap. 41. Almost invariably it begins with bilateral symptoms and signs of posterior column involvement in the hands (paresthesias and reduced touch, pressure, and joint sensibility), which, if untreated, is followed within a matter of several weeks or months by progressive spastic paraparesis because of involvement of the corticospinal tracts to which a vague sensory level on the trunk may be added. Particular importance attaches to the fact that this is a treatable disease and that the degree of reversibility is dependent upon the duration of symptoms before specific treatment is begun.

Copper Deficiency Myelopathy (Combined System Disease of Nonpernicious Anemia Type)

This refers to a metabolic disease of the spinal cord caused by low copper, affecting the posterior and lateral columns, in this sense, also a combined system degeneration. The clinical syndrome and potential causes were elegantly elaborated by Kumar and colleagues. A homologous disease exists as "swayback" in lambs. A deficiency of vitamin B_{12} is not causative, but may coexist in some cases, probably on the basis of a shared inadequacy of dietary intake. Women are more often affected than men. Imbalance is the most common presenting complaint. Posterior column signs and gait ataxia tend to predominate but a degree of spasticity is usually conjoined and there may be Babinski signs and reduced ankle reflexes. The problem is typically one of impaired absorption of copper, for example, after gastric bypass or bowel surgery, which together account for half of cases. Of importance in causation in some patients is excess zinc intake in the form of health supplements, coin swallowing, and denture creams (see Nations et al).

There is an associated hypocupremic anemia with ringed sideroblasts and leukopenia with vacuolated myeloid precursors in the marrow that may be mistaken for a myelodysplastic process. The idiopathic variety has certain similarities to the disorder of copper mobilization in Menkes disease, but the disordered enzyme responsible in the latter has been normal. As reported by others, in a recent case on our service without explanation for the discovered copper deficiency, MRI of the cervical cord revealed distinctive signal changes in both the posterior and lateral columns identical to those of B_{12} deficiency, and these were no longer present after copper treatment. The majority of affected patients have abnormal somatosensory evoked potentials with delays in central conduction.

Treatment Oral copper supplementation, 2 mg/d for at least several months, seems effective in most patients, but some do not improve and the appropriate duration of treatment is unknown. Some patients relapse after an initial improvement even with continued administration or when copper supplementation is stopped. The gluconate, sulfate, or chloride preparations of copper may be used, although there has been concern about the bioavailability of the first-named compound. Intravenous therapy as a way of initially replenishing copper stores has been introduced but the need for such treatment is uncertain. Zinc supplements must, of course, be discontinued, as they lower copper levels.

There remains a group of subacute ataxic-spastic myelopathies that are not caused by multiple sclerosis or by B_{12} or copper deficiency. Progressive spastic or spastic-ataxic paraparesis of a chronic, irreversible type may also develop in conjunction with chronic, decompensated liver disease; with AIDS; in cases of adrenoleukodystrophy, particularly in the symptomatic female heterozygote; in tropical spastic paraplegia (HTLV-I); radiation myelopathy; and adhesive spinal arachnoiditis, which is discussed immediately below.

Spinal Arachnoiditis (Chronic Adhesive Arachnoiditis) (See Chap. 11)

This is now a relatively uncommon spinal cord disorder that was introduced in relation to the subject of low back pain in Chap. 11. It is characterized by a combination of painful root and spinal cord symptoms that may mimic intraspinal tumor. There is opacification and thickening of the arachnoidal membranes and adhesions between the arachnoid and dura—the result of proliferation of connective tissue. The subarachnoid space is unevenly obliterated. In this sense, the term *arachnoiditis* is not entirely appropriate, although it seems likely that the connective tissue overgrowth is a reaction to an antecedent arachnoidal inflammation. Some forms of arachnoiditis were traced to syphilis or to a subacute, therapeutically resistant meningitis of another type. Most others in the past followed the introduction of a variety of substances, most no longer used, into the subarachnoid space for diagnostic or therapeutic purposes or following spinal anesthesia, soon afterward or after an interval of weeks, months, or even years. This complication was eventually traced to a detergent that had contaminated vials of procaine.

More pernicious, however, is a delayed meningomyelopathy that developed within a few months or years of the inciting event, causing a spastic paralysis, sensory loss, and incontinence of sphincters. There are also cases on record in which an epidural or similar catheter has accidentally penetrated the cord and caused a traumatic partial myelopathy as mentioned earlier. Still seen regularly is a restricted form of arachnoiditis that complicates a series of operations for lumbar discs or the spinal injection of methylene blue. Less convincing are cases attributed to closed spinal injuries. In many cases, no provocative factor can be recognized. A familial form was reported by Duke and Hashimoto, but we have had no experience with it.

Clinical Manifestations Symptoms may occur in close temporal relation to an acute arachnoidal inflammation or may be delayed for weeks, months, or even years as indicated above. The most common mode of onset is with pain in the distribution of one or more sensory nerve roots, first on one side, then on both, in the lumbofemoral regions. The pain has a burning, stinging, or aching quality and is persistent. Abnormalities of tendon reflexes are common, but weakness and atrophy, the results of damage to anterior roots, are less frequent. In thoracic lesions, symptoms of root involvement may antedate those of cord compression by months or years. Sooner or later, however, there is involvement of the spinal cord, manifest by a slowly progressive spastic ataxia with sphincter disturbances.

The localized lumbar arachnoiditis associated with repeated disc surgery (the common variety seen in pain clinics) is characterized by back and or leg pain with other inconstant signs of radiculopathy (loss of tendon reflexes, weakness, and variable degrees of sensory loss), usually bilateral.

The CSF is abnormal during the acute stage in practically all cases that ultimately result in adhesive arachnoiditis. In some there is a moderate lymphocytic pleocytosis, occurring soon after the inciting event. In the localized lumbar arachnoiditis, referred to earlier, the CSF may be normal or show only a slight increase in protein content. The prominent finding with imaging is a partial or complete obliteration of the spinal subarachnoid space. The loculated myelographic appearance of arachnoiditis is characteristic (patchy dispersion of the column of dye and a "candle-guttering" appearance that was most evident with oil-based contrast media); MRI reveals a loss of the normal ring of CSF or localized loculations of CSF (see Fig. 11-5).

Treatment In the early stages of arachnoiditis, corticosteroids have been given to control the inflammatory reaction and to prevent progress of the disease, but their value is questionable. Surgery may be effective in the case of localized "cyst" formation and cord compression. Severe radicular pain can be effectively relieved by posterior rhizotomy, but there is a strong tendency for the pain to return after an interval of several months or a year or two so that this approach has been all but abandoned. For chronic adhesive lumbar arachnoiditis in which diffuse back and limb pain is the most distressing symptom, there is little effective surgical or medical treatment, although relief has reportedly been provided in isolated instances by painstaking microsurgical dissection of the lumbar roots. In some cases, the loculations return. Administration of corticosteroids, systemic and epidural, has not been consistently beneficial but may be tried. Immune-suppressant medication such as azathioprine or interferons have been tried but not studied systematically. Transcutaneous stimulator treatment and gabapentin have also been used with inconsistent results.

Herniation of the Cord Through a Dural Tear

Violent trauma to the spinal canal or skull such as a fall or blow to the back can cause arachnoidal and dural tears. The associated neural injury dominates the picture and the dural tear may require repair so as to minimize the development of meningitis. More difficult to understand is the occurrence of spinal cord herniation through a spontaneous rent in the adjacent dura with no preceding injury. In view of the fact that we have encountered five such instances in a decade, without trauma having occurred, it is probably not rare.

In the typical case, a vertically oriented tear of limited extent occurs in the ventral dura overlying the mid- or high-thoracic region, and a segment of the spinal cord protrudes through it into the epidural space. The result is a painless, subacute, and incomplete spinal cord syndrome, which reaches a plateau and leaves the patient with an asymmetrical spastic paraparesis and variable sensory loss. There are reports of a Brown-Séquard hemi-cord syndrome and variations of it as described in the small series by Watters and colleagues. Orthostatic headache of low-CSF pressure is not usually part of the syndrome. MRI or CT myelopathy demonstrates the protruded segment of the cord where it buckles through the dura. Presumably the herniation creates a sufficient degree of local ischemia or mechanical disturbance to account for the myelopathic symptoms. Surgical restoration of the cord to its proper position and repair of the tear, have resulted in partial or complete return of neurologic function (Vallee et al).

As to the cause of this condition, a congenital duplication of the dura membranes combined with herniation through the inner layer has been observed in some cases at operation. The abnormal configuration of the membrane has been proposed as a cause of the propensity for the fibers to separate and create an aperture.

Intraspinal Tumors

Compression of the spinal cord by a metastatic tumor in the vertebral column is a common occurrence in many types of cancers. Primary tumors of the spinal cord are considerably less frequent. In the Mayo Clinic series of 8,784 primary tumors of the CNS, only 15 percent were intraspinal (Sloof et al). In contradistinction to brain tumors, the majority of intraspinal ones is benign and produces effects mainly by compression of the spinal cord rather than by invasion. Thus, a proportion of intraspinal tumors are amenable to surgical removal, and their early recognition, before irreversible neurologic changes have occurred, becomes a matter of utmost importance.

General Considerations (See also Chap. 31)

Neoplasms and other space-occupying lesions within the spinal canal can be divided into two groups: (1) those that arise within the substance of the spinal cord, either as a primary neural neoplasm or as a metastasis, and invade and destroy tracts and central gray structures (*intramedullary*) and (2) those arising outside the spinal cord (*extramedullary*), either from vertebral bodies and epidural tissues (*extradural*) or in the leptomeninges or roots (*intradural*). In a general hospital, the relative frequency of spinal tumors in these different locations is approximately 5 percent intramedullary, 40 percent intradural–extramedullary, and 55 percent extradural, the majority of the latter being metastatic cancers, as already mentioned. This percentage of extradural lesions is higher than that encountered in more specialized neurosurgical services (e.g., Elsberg's figures of 7, 64, and 29 percent, respectively), probably because the latter do not include as many patients with extradural lymphomas, metastatic carcinomas, and the like, as are seen in general hospitals.

Intraspinal Tumors The most common *primary extramedullary* tumors are the neurofibromas and meningiomas, which together constitute approximately half of all intraspinal neoplasms. They are more often intradural than extradural. Neurofibromas have a predilection for the lumbar and thoracic region, whereas meningiomas are more evenly distributed over the vertical extent of the cord (Fig. 44-9). The other primary extramedullary tumors are sarcomas, vascular tumors, chordomas, and epidermoid and similar tumors, in that order of frequency.

Primary intramedullary tumors of the spinal cord have the same cellular origins as those arising in the brain (Chap. 31), although the proportions of particular cell types differ. Ependymomas, some of which arise from the filum terminale, make up 60 percent of the spinal cord cases and astrocytomas make up approximately

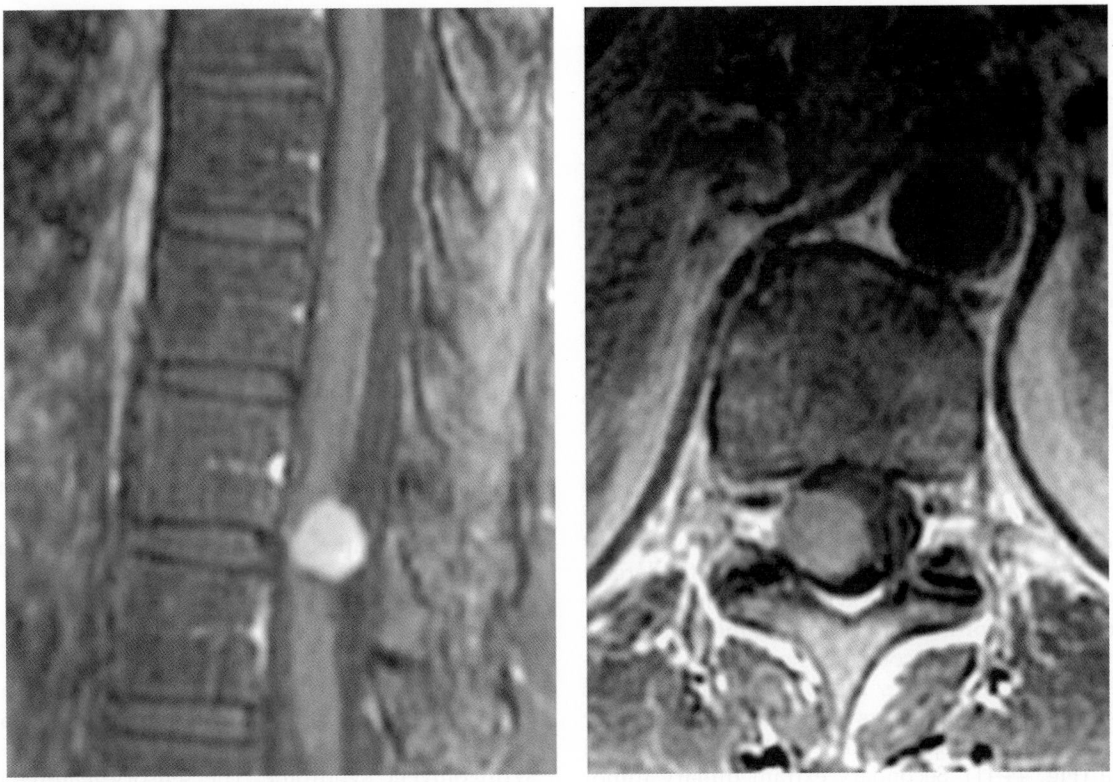

Figure 44-9. Sagittal (*left*) and axial (*right*) gadolinium-enhanced T1-weighted MRI of an intraspinal meningioma that displaced and compressed the spinal cord, causing incontinence and leg weakness. As in intracranial meningiomas, homogenous contrast enhancement and a dural attachment are seen.

25 percent. The astrocytoma is the most common intramedullary tumor if one excludes tumors arising in the filum terminale (Fig. 44-10). Oligodendrogliomas are much less common. The remainder (approximately 15 percent) consists of a diverse group of nongliomatous tumors: lipomas, epidermoids, dermoids, teratomas, hemangiomas, hemangioblastomas, chordomas, schwannomas, and intraspinal metastatic carcinomas. The cavernous hemangioma may be a source of spontaneous hematomyelia. As indicated further on, there is a frequent association between intramedullary tumors (both gliomatous and nongliomatous) and syringomyelia. The basis of this relationship remains obscure.

Spinal ependymomas arise from ependymal lining of the central canal of the spinal cord. The myxopapillary type originates from clusters of ependymal cells in the filum terminale. The myxopapillary ependymoma that originates in the filum terminale causes a special syndrome referable to both lumbar roots (cauda equina) and conus. As commented in Chap. 31, a combination of asymmetric or bilateral sciatic or anterior thigh pain, sphincter difficulty, and upper motor neuron signs is typical. These spinal tumors occur in adults as often as in children, quite different from intracranial ependymomas, which are mainly childhood tumors. Although they are considered to be benign, intraspinal spread can occur and local recurrence after resection occurs in 10 percent of cases, even decades after surgery as described by Rezai and colleagues. Treatment is with surgical removal and selective

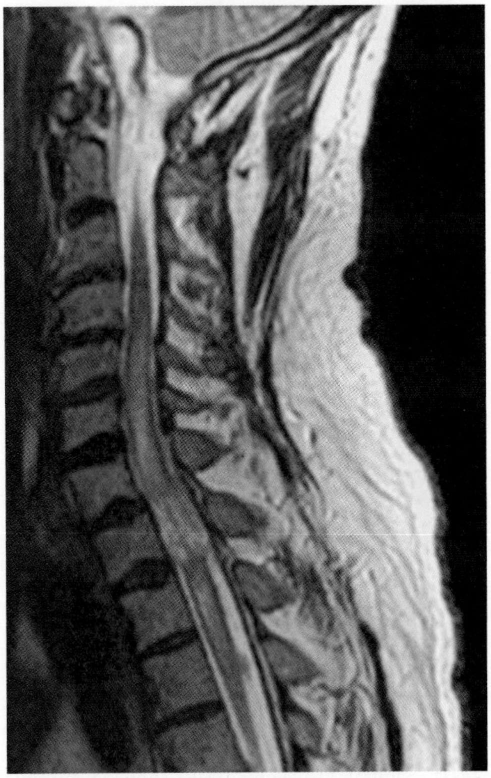

Figure 44-10. Sagittal T2-weighted MRI of a primary glioma of the thoracic spinal cord in a middle-aged man. Note the expansion of the spinal cord.

radiation if there has not been gross total removal and long-term survival is the rule. The main differential diagnosis is a spinal schwannoma (neurofibroma).

Intramedullary growths invade as well as compress and distort fasciculi in the spinal cord white matter. As the cord enlarges from the tumor growing within it or is compressed by a tumor from without, the free space around the cord is eventually consumed, and the CSF below the lesion becomes isolated or loculated from the remainder of the circulating fluid above the lesion. This is marked by Froin syndrome (xanthochromia and clotting of CSF from greatly elevated protein content) and an interruption of flow of contrast medium in the subarachnoid space. The most informative diagnostic procedure is an MRI, which demonstrates both the intramedullary extent of the tumor and the effect on the surrounding subarachnoid space.

Secondary spinal cord tumors can also be subdivided into intramedullary and extramedullary types. *Extradural metastases (carcinoma, lymphoma, myeloma) are the most common of all spinal tumors.* They account for the largest group of patients who develop symptoms of myelopathy while being cared for in hospital and are therefore likely to be encountered in the course of neurologic consultations. Extradural metastases arise from hematogenous deposits or extend from tumors of the vertebral bodies or from a paraspinal tumor extending via the intervertebral foramina (Fig. 44-11). Secondary extramedullary tumor growths are far more often extradural than intradural. The intradural type takes the form of a meningeal carcinomatosis or lymphomatosis and the rare primary melanoma of the meninges, which are considered in Chap. 31.

Intramedullary metastases are not as rare as is generally believed. In a retrospective autopsy study of 627 patients with systemic cancer, Costigan and Winkelman found 153 cases with central nervous system (CNS) metastases, in 13 of which the metastases were located within the cord. In 9 of the 13 cases, the metastasis was deep in the cord, unassociated with leptomeningeal carcinomatosis; in 4 cases, the neoplasm seemed to extend from the pia. Bronchogenic carcinoma was the main source. Diagnosis is difficult but is aided greatly by MRI with gadolinium infusion; there is generally extensive contiguous edema (Fig. 44-12). Differentiation is from meningeal carcinomatosis, radiation myelopathy, and paraneoplastic necrotizing myelopathy, which is the least common of these entities. Treatment is usually ineffective unless radiation therapy is begun before paraplegia supervenes (Winkelman et al).

Symptomatology

Patients with spinal cord tumors are likely to present with one of three clinical syndromes: (1) a sensorimotor spinal tract syndrome, (2) a painful radicular-spinal cord syndrome, or (3) least often, an intramedullary syringomyelic syndrome. The sensory features of these syndromes are depicted in Fig. 9-7.

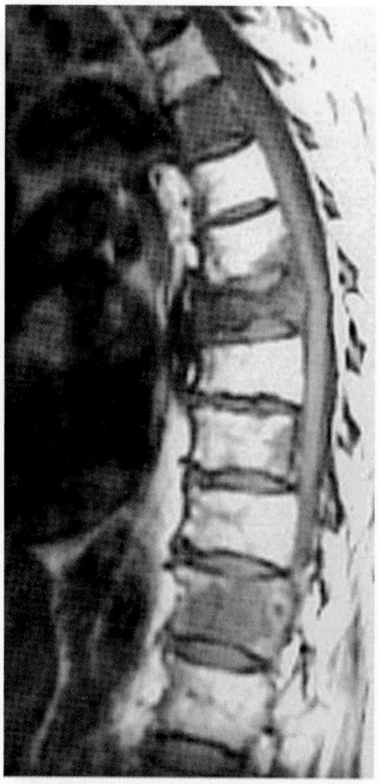

Figure 44-11. Sagittal T1-weighted MRI showing multiple spinal metastases from carcinoma of the lung. The metastases exhibit low signal intensity due to tumor replacement of bone marrow, which is normally T1 hyperintense.

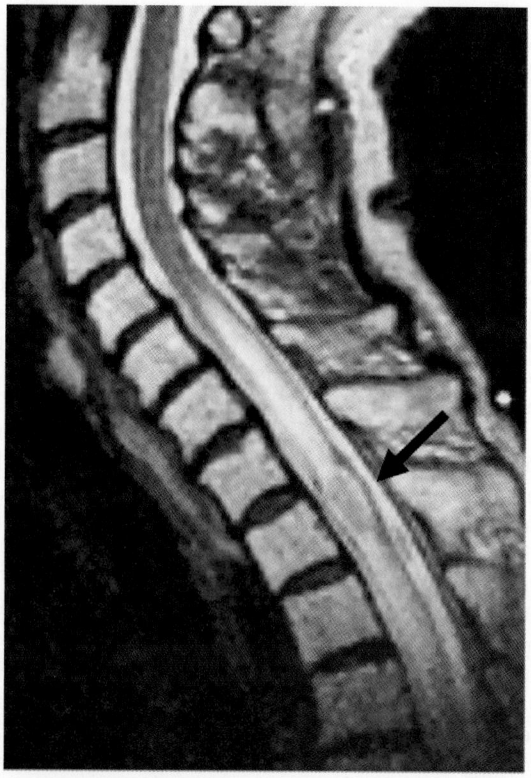

Figure 44-12. Sagittal T2 MRI of an intramedullary metastasis from breast cancer. The expansile lesion is at the T2 vertebral level (*arrow*) and the adjacent edema extends superiorly and inferiorly over a great length of the spinal cord.

Pain and stiffness of the back may antedate signs of spinal cord disease or dominate the clinical picture in some cases of extramedullary tumor. The back pain is usually worse when the patient lies down or may become worse after several hours in the recumbent position and be improved by sitting up. *In children*, severe back pain associated with spasm of paravertebral muscles is often prominent initially; scoliosis and spastic weakness of the legs come later. Because of this somewhat unusual clinical presentation and the rarity of intraspinal lesions in childhood, spinal cord tumors in this age group may be overlooked.

Sensorimotor Spinal Tract Syndrome The clinical picture is related predominantly to compression and less often to invasion and destruction of spinal cord tracts. The signs of compression consist of a combination of (1) an asymmetrical spastic weakness of the legs with thoracolumbar lesions and of the arms and legs with cervical lesions, (2) a sensory level on the trunk below which perception of pain and temperature is reduced or lost, (3) posterior column signs, and (4) a spastic bladder under weak voluntary control. The onset of the compressive symptoms is usually gradual and the course progressive over a period of weeks and months, frequently with back pain. With extradural tumors, paralysis usually develops over a period of days to several weeks, but the tempo of progression may be more rapid or more leisurely. The initial disturbance may be of motor or sensory function and the distribution may be asymmetrical. High cervical or foramen magnum lesions produce special clinical syndromes, as described in Chap. 3 and below. With thoracic lesions, one leg usually becomes weak and stiff before the other one. Subjective sensory symptoms of the dorsal column type (tingling paresthesias) assume similar distributions. Pain and thermal senses are more likely to be affected than tactile, vibration, and position senses. Nevertheless, the posterior columns are frequently involved as the process progresses. Initially, the sensory disturbance is contralateral to the maximum motor weakness, but a sharply defined Brown-Séquard hemicord syndrome is rarely observed. The bladder and bowel usually become paralyzed coincident with paralysis of the legs. If the compression is relieved, there is recovery from these sensory and motor symptoms, often in the reverse order of their appearance; the first part affected is the last to recover, and sensory symptoms tend to disappear before motor ones.

Radicular-Spinal Cord Syndrome Here the syndrome of spinal cord compression is combined with radicular pain, i.e., pain in the distribution of a sensory nerve root. The discomfort is described as knife-like or as a dull ache with superimposed sharp stabs of pain, which radiate in a distal direction, i.e., away from the spine, and are intensified by coughing, sneezing, or straining. Segmental sensory changes (paresthesias, impaired perception of pinprick and touch) or motor disturbances (cramp, atrophy, fascicular twitching, and loss of tendon reflexes) and an ache in the spine, in addition to the radicular pain, are the usual manifestations. Tenderness of the spinous processes over the tumor is found by percussion in about half the patients. The segmental changes, particularly the sensory radicular ones, often precede the signs of spinal cord compression by months if the lesion is benign.

Intramedullary Syringomyelic Syndrome No single symptom is unique to the *intramedullary tumors*. Some degree of pain, sometimes minor, is common and is almost invariably present with tumors of the filum terminale. Ependymomas and astrocytomas, the two most common intramedullary tumors, usually give rise to a mixed sensorimotor tract syndrome. When the intramedullary tumor involves the central gray matter, a central cord, or *syringomyelic syndrome* may result. The main features are segmental or dissociated sensory loss, amyotrophy, early incontinence, and late corticospinal weakness. Sacral sparing of sensation may be found as described in Chap. 9 on the sensory syndromes but is of less value in distinguishing intramedullary from extramedullary lesions. A dissociation of thermal pain and tactile sensory loss over several contiguous segments on the trunk is a more dependable sign of an intramedullary lesion. Rarely, an extramedullary tumor may give rise to a syringomyelic sensory syndrome, possibly by causing vascular insufficiency in the central portion of the cord.

Special Spinal Syndromes Unusual clinical syndromes may be found in patients with *tumors in the region of the foramen magnum*, as discussed in Chap. 3. They produce quadriparesis with pain in the back of the head and stiff neck, weakness and atrophy of the hands and dorsal neck muscles, marked imbalance, and variable sensory changes or, if they spread intracranially, there may be signs of cerebellar and lower cranial nerve involvement. Slowly growing tumors in this region, such as meningiomas, characteristically produce an "around the clock" progression of weakness beginning in one limb and proceeding to the adjacent one in a clockwise or counterclockwise direction. Lesions at the level of the lowermost thoracic and the first lumbar vertebrae may result in mixed cauda equina and spinal cord symptoms. A Babinski sign indicates that the spinal cord is involved above the fifth lumbar segment.

Lesions of the cauda equina alone, always difficult to separate from those of the lumbosacral plexuses and multiple nerves, are usually attended in the early stages by sciatic and other root pain and lumbar ache, which are variously combined with a bilaterally asymmetrical, atrophic, areflexic paralysis, radicular sensory loss, and sphincteric disorder. These must be distinguished from *lesions of the conus medullaris* (lower sacral segments of the spinal cord), in which there are early disturbances of the bladder and bowel (urinary retention and constipation), back pain, symmetrical hypesthesia or anesthesia over the sacral dermatomes, a lax anal sphincter with loss of anal and bulbocavernosus reflexes, impotence, and sometimes weakness of leg muscles. Sensory abnormalities may precede motor and reflex changes by many months. Very rarely, for unclear reasons, tumors of the thoracolumbar cord (intramedullary, as a rule) are associated with markedly elevated spinal fluid protein and hydrocephalus; these respond to shunting and removal of the spinal tumor (Feldman et al). Less often, these tumors are associated with a pseudotumor cerebri syndrome.

Differential Diagnosis

Several problems arise in the diagnosis of spinal cord tumors in addition to several previously mentioned. In the early stages, neoplastic compression or invasion of the cord must be distinguished from other diseases that cause pain over certain segments of the body, e.g., diseases affecting the gall-bladder, pancreas, kidney, stomach and intestinal tract, pleura. Localization of the pain to a dermatome; its intensification by sneezing, coughing, and straining, and sometimes by recumbency; and the finding of segmental sensory changes and minor alterations of motor, reflex, or sensory function in the legs will usually provide the clues to the presence of a spinal cord–radicular lesion. MRI will settle the diagnosis in most instances. The pain of tumor or blood clot in the retroperitoneal space may cause an orthostatic and nocturnal back pain that is similar to that of spinal tumor.

There is then the problem of locating the segmental level of the lesion. At first, the sensory and motor deficits may be most pronounced in those parts of the body farthest removed from the lesion, i.e., in the feet or lumbosacral segments. Later the levels of the sensory and motor deficits ascend, but they may still be at a level several segments below the lesion. In determining the level of the lesion, the location of back pain, root pain, and atrophic paralysis are of greater help than the upper level of hypoalgesia.

Once vertebral and segmental levels of the lesion are settled, there remains the necessity of determining whether the lesion is extradural, intradural–extramedullary, or intramedullary and whether it is neoplastic. If there is a visible or palpable spinal deformity or radiographic evidence of vertebral destruction, one may confidently assume an extradural localization. Even without these changes, one still suspects an extradural lesion if root pain developed early and is bilateral, if pain and aching in the spine are prominent and percussion tenderness is marked, if motor symptoms below the lesion preceded sensory ones, and if sphincter disturbances were late. However, to distinguish between intradural–extramedullary lesions and intramedullary lesions on clinical grounds alone is often difficult. The findings of segmental amyotrophy and sensory loss of dissociated type (loss of pain and temperature and preservation of tactile sensation) point to an intramedullary lesion.

Extradural tumors, both primary and secondary, must be differentiated from cervical spondylosis, tuberculous granuloma, sarcoidosis, arteriovenous malformations of the cord, spinal dural fistulas, and certain chronic pyogenic or fungal granulomatous lesions, as well as from lipomas in patients receiving corticosteroids for prolonged periods and from the necrotizing myelopathy associated with occult tumors or occurring independently of them. A number of rarer conditions of the vertebral bodies such as bone cysts, chondromas, eosinophilic granuloma, chordomas and giant cell tumors must also be considered; these are summarized by Ropper and coworkers (2011). In the thoracic region, a ruptured disc or eventration of the cord through a dural tear is always a possibility. In the region of the lower back, i.e., over the cauda equina, one must also distinguish between tumor and protruded inter-vertebral disc. Here, an extradural tumor may produce mainly sciatic and low back pain with little or no motor, sensory, reflex, or sphincteric disturbances. With intradural–extramedullary lesions, the important diagnostic considerations are meningioma, neurofibroma, meningeal carcinomatosis, cholesteatoma, and teratomatous cyst, a meningomyelitic process, or adhesive arachnoiditis. Intramedullary lesions are usually gliomas, ependymomas, or vascular malformations or, in the context of a known carcinoma, intramedullary metastases. The definition of vascular malformations by means of selective spinal angiography was discussed in an earlier section. Normal protein in the CSF and negative MRI effectively exclude an intramedullary tumor.

Treatment

The main consideration in the management of epidural metastases is the need for early diagnosis, at a stage when only back pain is present and before neurologic symptoms and signs have appeared. Once these signs appear, especially sphincter disturbances, the results of treatment are less successful but may still result in good limb and bladder function. Epidural growths of carcinoma and lymphoma are best managed by administration of high to moderate doses of corticosteroids and radiation of the region of tumor. This may be supplemented by endocrine therapy (for carcinoma of breast and prostate), and of antineoplastic drugs (for certain lymphomas and myelomas. Pain relief is sometimes difficult to attain and requires narcotics. Only infrequently is operation necessary as a first resort. Gilbert and associates presented evidence that patients who receive high-dose corticosteroids (16 to 60 mg of dexamethasone) and fractionated radiation (500 cGy on each of the first 3 days and then spaced radiation up to 3,000 cGy) do as well as those who have surgical decompression.

However, laminectomy and decompression are necessary to prevent irreversible compressive effects and infarction of the cord for rapidly growing tumors that have caused recent and severe loss of function below the level of compression, Cases that have been allowed to progress should be operated on if paraplegia has occurred within one or perhaps two days or less and the overall state of the patient's cancer makes survival likely for at least several weeks. If the maximal safe radiation dosage had previously been applied to the spinal column, or the diagnosis can only be made from tissue obtained from the site of spinal compression, surgical palliation is also usually undertaken.

Intradural–extramedullary tumors should generally be removed if this can be accomplished safely, and this applies to benign extradural tumors that are symptomatic as well. Laminectomy, decompression, excision in isolated cases, and radiotherapy constitute the treatment of intramedullary gliomas. Such patients may improve and lead useful lives for a decade or longer. Constantini and colleagues, based on a large experience with intramedullary lesions, mainly gliomas in children and young adults, recommend a radical excision of the tumor, but this approach has not been subjected to a trial.

Other Causes of Spinal Cord Compression

Epidural fat deposition (*epidural lipomatosis*) with spinal cord compression occurs in Cushing disease and after the long-term use of corticosteroids, but also in the absence of these disorders. The clinical picture may suggest discogenic disease (Lipson et al). Copious amounts of normal adipose tissue are found at laminectomy and removal of this tissue is curative. Lowering the dose of steroid and caloric restriction may help mobilize the fat and relieve the symptoms. An intra-spinal lipoma is also a component of the developmentally tethered cord, but in this process the essential problem is a conus medullaris myelopathy from stretching of the cord, rather than compression (see Chap. 38 and Thomas and Miller.)

Arachnoid diverticula—intra- or extradural outpouchings from the posterior nerve root—are rare causes of a radicular-spinal cord syndrome, first described by Bechterew in 1893. They tend to occur in the thoracic or lumbosacral regions. The symptoms, in order of decreasing frequency, are pain, radicular weakness and sensory disorder, gait disorder, and sphincteric disturbances, as described by Cilluffo et al. The frequent association of arachnoid diverticula with osteoporosis, ankylosing spondylitis, and arachnoiditis makes it difficult to interpret the role of the diverticula themselves. Surgical obliteration of the pouches has yielded unpredictable results. They have attained clinical importance more often as the source of spontaneous CSF leaks and a low-pressure syndrome (see Chap. 30).

Spinal cord compression with paraplegia may be caused by *extramedullary hematopoiesis* in cases of myelosclerosis, thalassemia, cyanotic heart disease, myelogenous leukemia, sideropenic anemia, and polycythemia vera. A similar phenomenon occurs with ossification of the posterior longitudinal ligament, as described earlier.

Solitary *osteochondromas* of vertebral bodies and *multiple exostoses* of hereditary type are other reported causes of spinal cord compression. In the case reported by Buur and Morch, the clinical syndrome was one of pure spastic paraparesis of several months' progression.

Lathyrism (See also Chap. 43)

From the interesting historical review of Dastur, one learns that this disease was known to Hippocrates, Pliny, and Galen in Europe, to Avicenna in the Middle East, and to the ancient Hindus. The term *lathyrism* was applied by Cantani, in Italy, because of its recognized relationship to the consumption of *Lathyrus sativus* (chickling vetch, vetch pea, or grass pea).

The disease is still common in some parts of India and Africa. In these districts, during periods of famine when wheat and other grains are in short supply, the diet may for months consist of flour made of the grass pea. In individuals so exposed, a gradual weakening of the legs accompanied by spasticity and cramps occurs. Paresthesias, numbness, formication in the legs, and frequency and urgency of micturition, erectile dysfunction, and sphincteric spasms are added. The upper extremities may exhibit coarse tremors and involuntary movements. These symptoms, once established, are more or less permanent but not progressive, and most of the patients live out their natural life span.

Only two reports on the neuropathology of lathyrism were known to Dastur, one by Buzzard and Greenfield in England, the other by Filiminoff in Russia. Both of their patients had been in a stationary paraplegic state for years. Greenfield noted a loss of ascending and descending tracts in the spinal cord, particularly the corticospinal and direct spinocerebellar tracts. Filiminoff observed a loss of myelinated fibers in the lateral and posterior columns. Unlike the cases of Spencer and colleagues, there had been a loss of pain and thermal sensation in the upper extremities. The larger Betz cells had disappeared, while anterior horn cells were unaffected. Gliosis and thickening of blood vessels was seen in the degenerated tracts.

The toxic nature of this disease, long suspected, was confirmed by Spencer and colleagues. They extracted a neuroexcitatory amino acid, beta-*N*-oxalylaminoalanine (BOAA), from grass peas and were able to induce corticospinal dysfunction in monkeys by giving this substance with a nutritious diet. Subsequently, Hugon and coworkers produced a primate model of lathyrism by feeding monkeys a diet of *L. sativus* in addition to an alcoholic extract of this legume. These findings tend to negate the importance of several other factors that had been thought to be causative, namely, malnutrition, ergot contamination, and toxins derived from *Vicia sativa*, the common vetch that grows alongside the lathyrus species.

The African acute spastic paraplegia called *konzo* has a similar toxic pathogenesis; it is caused by cyanide-like compounds in flour made from cassava.

Dysraphic Syndromes (Spina Bifida) and Tethered Cord

These are described in Chap. 38 but should be considered in cases of chronic and progressive syndromes of the cauda equina and conus medullaris.

Familial Spastic Paraplegia (See Chap. 39)

There are several familial forms of progressive spastic paraplegia, some beginning in childhood, others in adult life. The pattern of inheritance in almost all our adult cases has been autosomal dominant. A lack of sensory symptoms and signs and sparing of sphincteric function until late in the illness are important diagnostic features. A number of adult cases are "complicated" in the sense that the spastic paraplegia is associated with cerebellar ataxia or dementia. By contrast, *primary lateral sclerosis*, a sporadic form of degenerative disease of the motor system, is characterized by a pure spastic paraplegia and bulbar spastic palsy either initially or with progression, the result of changes that are confined to the corticospinal pathways. These disorders are discussed extensively with the heredodegenerative diseases in Chap. 39, and the myelopathy associated with adrenoleukodystrophy, in Chap. 37.

SYRINGOMYELIC SYNDROME OF SEGMENTAL SENSORY DISSOCIATION WITH BRACHIAL AMYOTROPHY

This syndrome is most often attributable to developmental syringomyelia, i.e., a central cavitation of the spinal cord of undetermined cause, but a similar clinical syndrome may be observed in association with other pathologic states such as intramedullary cord tumors, traumatic myelopathy, postradiation myelopathy, infarction (myelomalacia), bleeding (hematomyelia), and, rarely, with extramedullary tumors, cervical spondylosis, spinal arachnoiditis, and cervical necrotizing myelitis.

Syringomyelia (Syrinx) (See also Chap. 38)

Syringomyelia (from the Greek *syrinx*, "pipe" or "tube") is defined as a chronic progressive degenerative or developmental disorder of the spinal cord, characterized clinically by painless weakness and wasting of the hands and arms (brachial amyotrophy) and segmental sensory loss of dissociated type (loss of thermal and painful sensation with sparing of tactile, joint position, and vibratory sense, as described later). The cause is a cavitation of the central parts of the spinal cord, usually in the cervical region, but extending upward in some cases into the medulla and pons (syringobulbia) or downward into the thoracic and even into the lumbar segments. Frequently, there are associated developmental abnormalities of the vertebral column (thoracic scoliosis, fusion of vertebrae, or Klippel-Feil anomaly), of the base of the skull (platybasia and basilar invagination), and there is a special relationship to developmental deformations of the cerebellum and brainstem (particularly type I Chiari malformation). A large proportion of cases of developmental syringomyelia have type I Chiari malformation, consisting of a descent of cerebellar tonsils below the foramen magnum as discussed in Chap. 38. There is also a group of less frequent but well-described syringomyelias that derives from the acquired processes mentioned earlier such as intramedullary tumor (astrocytoma, hemangioblastoma, ependymoma) and from preceding traumatic or hemorrhagic necrosis of the spinal cord.

Wider experience with the pathology of developmental syringomyelia has led to the following classification, modified from Barnett and colleagues that unfortunately creates some confusion because it simulates the Roman numeral classification of the Chiari malformations, with which it is sometimes allied:

- Type I. Syringomyelia with obstruction of the foramen magnum and dilatation of the central canal (developmental type)
  - A. With type I Chiari malformation
  - B. With other obstructive lesions of the foramen magnum, usually bony anomalies
- Type II. Syringomyelia without obstruction of the foramen magnum (idiopathic developmental type)
- Type III. Syringomyelia with other diseases of the spinal cord (acquired types)
  - A. Spinal cord tumors (usually intramedullary, especially hemangioblastoma)
  - B. Traumatic myelopathy
  - C. Spinal arachnoiditis and pachymeningitis
  - D. Secondary myelomalacia from cord compression (tumor, spondylosis), infarction, hematomyelia
- Type IV. Pure hydromyelia (developmental dilatation of the central canal), with or without hydrocephalus

Historical Note Although pathologic cavitation of the spinal cord was recognized as early as the sixteenth century, the term *syringomyelia* was first used to describe this process in 1827 by Ollivier d'Angers (cited by Ballantine et al). Later, following recognition of the central canal as a normal structure, it was assumed by Virchow (1863) and by Leyden (1876) that cavitation of the spinal cord had its origin in an abnormal expansion of the central canal, and they renamed the process *hydromyelia*. Cavities in the central portions of the spinal cord, unconnected with the central canal, were recognized by Hallopeau (1870); Simon suggested in 1875 that the term *syringomyelia* be reserved for such cavities and that the term *hydromyelia* be restricted to simple dilatation of the central canal. Thus, a century ago, the stage was set for an argument about pathogenesis that has not been settled to the present day.

Clinical Features

The clinical picture varies in the four pathologic types previously listed, the differences depending not only on the extent of the syrinx but also on the associated pathologic changes, particularly those related to the Chiari malformation. In the type I developmental syrinx (idiopathic, Chiari-associated developmental syringomyelia), symptoms usually begin in early adult life (20 to 40 years). Males and females are equally affected. Rarely, some abnormality is noted at birth, but usually the first symptom appears in late childhood or adolescence. The onset is usually insidious and the course irregularly progressive. In many instances, the symptoms or signs are discovered accidentally, for example, as a result of painless burn or atrophy of the hand, and the patient cannot say when the disease began. Rarely, there is an almost apoplectic onset or worsening; there are cases on record of an aggravation of old symptoms or the appearance of new symptoms after a violent strain or paroxysm of coughing. Trauma is a less certain precipitant. Once the disease is recognized, some patients remain much the same for years, even decades, but more often there is intermittent progression to the point of being chair-bound within 5 to 20 years. This extremely variable course makes it difficult to evaluate therapy.

The precise clinical picture at any given point in the evolution of the disease depends on the cross-sectional and longitudinal extent of the syrinx, but certain clinical features are so common that the diagnosis can hardly be made without them. These traditionally cited elements are: (1) *segmental weakness and atrophy of the hands and arms*, (2) *loss of some or all tendon reflexes in the arms*, and (3) *segmental anesthesia of a dissociated type* (loss of pain and thermal sense and preservation of the sense of touch) over the neck, shoulders, and arms. The last of these leads to one of the most characteristic features of syringomyelia: painless injuries and burns of the hands. Finally, there are in cases of extensive cavitation weakness and ataxia of the legs from involvement of the corticospinal tracts (possibly at their decussation) and posterior columns in the cervical region.

Kyphoscoliosis is added in many of the cases and in nearly one-quarter of them there is an overt cervicooccipital malformation (short neck, low hairline, odd posture of the head and neck, fused or missing cervical vertebrae, i.e., Klippel-Feil abnormality).

The particular muscle groups that are affected on the two sides may vary. Exceptionally, motor function is spared, and the segmental dissociated sensory loss and/or pain are the only marks of the disease. In a few of the cases, especially those with the Chiari malformation, the reflexes in the arms are preserved or even hyperactive, as might be expected with upper rather than lower motor neuron involvement. Or the shoulder muscles may be atrophic and the hands spastic. In the lower extremities the weakness, if present, is of a spastic (corticospinal) type.

The characteristic segmental sensory dissociation is usually bilateral but a unilateral pattern affecting only one hand and arm is not unknown, and this is true of the amyotrophy as well. The sensory loss is distributed in a "cape" or hemicape pattern, often extending to back of the head or the face and onto the trunk. Although tactile sensation is usually preserved, there are cases in which it is impaired, usually in the region of the densest analgesia over the trunk or hand. Exceptionally there is no sensory loss in the presence of amyotrophy, and cases have been recorded in which only a hydrocephalus and hydromyelia were present with spastic paraparesis. If tactile sensation is affected in the arms, joint position and vibratory sense tend also to be impaired. In the lower extremities and over the abdomen there may be some loss of pain and thermal sensation proximally, but more often there is a loss of vibratory and position sense, which is indicative of a posterior column lesion and is the basis of ataxia. A Horner syndrome may result from ipsilateral involvement of the intermediolateral cell column at the C8, T1, and T2 levels.

Pain has been a symptom in about half of our patients with developmental types of syringomyelia. The pain is usually unilateral or more marked on one side of the neck, shoulder, and arm; it is of a burning, aching quality, mostly in or at the border of areas of sensory impairment. In a few patients, it involves the face or trunk. An aching pain at the base of the skull or posterior cervical region that is intensified by coughing, sneezing, or stooping (brief exertional pain) is often present, but, as Logue and Edwards point out, pain of this type may be a feature of Chiari malformation without syringomyelia and in that case is probably attributable to compression or stretching of cervical roots.

Syringobulbia is the lower brainstem equivalent of syringomyelia. Usually the two coexist and the brainstem cavity is simply an extension of one in the upper cord, but occasionally the bulbar manifestations precede the spinal ones or, rarely, occur independently. The glial cleft or cavity is located most often in the lateral tegmentum of the medulla, but it may extend into the pons and, rarely, even higher. The symptoms and signs are characteristically unilateral and consist of nystagmus, analgesia, and thermoanesthesia of the face (numbness); wasting and weakness of the tongue (dysarthria); and palatal and vocal cord paralysis (dysphagia and hoarseness). Diplopia, episodic vertigo, trigeminal pain or facial sensory loss, and persistent hiccough are less common symptoms. For understandable reasons, the diagnosis of brainstem MS is often raised. The clinical and pathologic features of syringobulbia have been described in great detail by Jonesco-Sisesti.

When a Chiari malformation is associated with syringomyelia and syringobulbia, it may be difficult to separate the effects of the two disorders. A typical example is shown in Fig. 38-4. Clinical features that favor the predominance of Chiari malformation are nystagmus, cerebellar ataxia, exertional head and neck pain, prominent corticospinal and sensory tract involvement in the lower extremities, hydrocephalus, and craniocervical malformations. In syringomyelia without a Chiari malformation but with some other type of obstructive lesion at the foramen magnum, the clinical picture is much the same, and the nature of the foramen magnum lesion can be determined only by MRI or surgical exploration.

The association of syringomyelia with an intramedullary tumor (type III) should be suspected when there is a disassociated sensorimotor abnormality extending over many segments of the body. With von Hippel-Lindau disease, the diagnosis hinges on the finding of the characteristic hereditary hemangioblastoma in the syrinx and retinal and cerebellar vascular malformations. In the posttraumatic cases, necrosis of the spinal cord that has been stable for months or years begins to cause pain and spreading sensory or motor loss, recognizable only in segments above the original lesion (Schurch et al). This occurred in approximately 3 percent of the traumatic myelopathy cases of Rossier and coworkers, more often in quadriplegics than in paraplegics. The posttraumatic syrinx is not as well defined anatomically as the usual forms of syringomyelia but consists instead of several contiguous areas of glia-lined myelomalacia with differing degrees of cavitation. In some instances of progressive spinal cord symptoms occurring several years after spinal surgery, the lesion has proved to be one of arachnoiditis and cord atrophy and not a syrinx (Avrahami et al).

Hydromyelia

This refers to a dilatation of the central canal that is distinct from developmental syringomyelia. The relationship between hydromyelia and syringomyelia has been the source of endless debate, in part the result of the lack of a coherent pathophysiologic explanation for either process. At least one hypothesis for the origin of syringomyelia includes an initial dilatation of the central canal (see later). Our impression is that a relatively nonprogressive, well-defined, cylindrical enlargement of the central canal over a few thoracic segments is a frequent enough occurrence in the absence of clinical changes that it represents an independent entity. In the few cases of symptomatic hydromyelia that have come to our attention, there had usually been a long-standing congenital hydrocephalus complicated years later by progressive weakness and atrophy of the shoulders and the muscles of the arms and hands. More often, there is no associated obstruction at the upper cord and no hydrocephalus for which reason it is our impression that most cases are benign and relatively nonprogressive. Proof of the existence of pure hydromyelia in the past has been based on necropsy demonstration of an enormously widened central canal, with or without hydrocephalus. Now, hydromyelia is easily diagnosable by MRI and numerous asymptomatic cases are being discovered, causing unnecessary concern and neurologic consultation.

Pathogenesis

Experimental work in animals has indicated that there is a normal flow of CSF from the spinal subarachnoid space through perivascular spaces to the parenchyma of the cord and possibly into the central canal. It has been suggested that impediments to flow might explain dilatation of the central canal, or the creation of a parallel or attached syrinx cavity.

One theory of the pathogenesis of developmental syringomyelia, of which Gardner was the main advocate, is that the normal flow of CSF from the central canal to the fourth ventricle and its outlets is prevented by an obstruction of the foramina of Luschka and Magendie. As a result, a pulse wave of CSF pressure that is generated by systolic pulsations of the choroid plexuses is transmitted into the cord from the fourth ventricle through the central canal. According to this theory, the syrinx consists essentially of a greatly dilated central canal with a diverticulum that ramifies from the central canal and dissects along gray matter and adjacent fiber tracts. The frequency with which syringomyelia is linked to malformations at the craniocervical junction, i.e., to Chiari and other lesions that could interfere with normal flow of CSF, lends credence to this theory.

There are many instances, however, in which Gardner's hydrodynamic theory could not explain syringomyelia. In some cases, for example, the foramina of Luschka and Magendie are found to be patent, and other abnormalities of the posterior fossa or foramen magnum that block CSF flow are not in evidence. Furthermore, in many cases, including several we have inspected, serial histologic sections have failed to demonstrate a connection between the fourth ventricle and the syrinx in the spinal cord or of a widening of the central canal above the syrinx (see also Hughes). Gardner's theory has been questioned on other grounds. Ball and Dayan calculated the pulse-pressure wave transmitted into the cord to be of such low amplitude as to be unlikely to produce a syrinx. In their view, the CSF around the cervical cord, under increased pressure during strain or physical effort because of subarachnoid obstruction at the craniocervical junction, tracks into the spinal cord along the Virchow-Robin spaces or other subpial channels. Over a prolonged period, abetted perhaps by traumatic lesions, small pools of fluid coalesce to form a syrinx. In their view, originally the syrinx forms independently of the central canal, but eventually the two may become connected, allowing secondary enlargement of the canal (hydromyelia ex vacuo). The findings of Heiss and colleagues lend support to this theory. They found that progression of syringomyelia is produced by the compressive effect of the cerebellar tonsils, which partially occlude the subarachnoid space at the foramen magnum and create pressure waves that compress the spinal cord from without and not from within; the pressure waves propagate syrinx fluid caudally with each heartbeat. This hardly exhausts the list of hypotheses that have been offered over the years but none of them has been confirmed.

The authors favor the type of hydrodynamic mechanism as postulated originally by Gordon Holmes and elaborated by Ball and Dayan. In this view, a relationship exists between basal cranial, cervical spine, the cerebellospinal Chiari malformation, syringomyelia, and disturbed hydrodynamics of perispinal CSF. Logue and Edwards documented several cases of syringomyelia in which the foramen magnum was obstructed by a lesion other than a Chiari formation, e.g., by dural cyst, localized arachnoiditis, atlantoaxial fusion, simple cerebellar cyst, and basilar invagination (see Williams for a review of the numerous hypotheses of causation).

Irrespective of its mode of origin, the syrinx first occupies the central gray matter of the cervical portion of the spinal cord, usually independent of the central canal but sometimes extending into it. It interrupts the crossing pain and temperature fibers in the anterior commissure at several successive cord segments. As the cavity enlarges, it extends symmetrically or asymmetrically into the posterior and anterior horns and eventually into the lateral and posterior funiculi of the cord. It may enlarge the spinal cord. The cavity is lined with astrocytic glia and a few thick-walled blood vessels, and the fluid in the cavity is clear and in our patients, has had relatively low protein content, like intracranial CSF.

The cavitation nearly always arises in the cervical portion of the cord and can only reach the thoracic and lumbar portions by its extension from the cervical region, sometimes by a small, flat and thin, eccentrically placed. Either a cavity or a glial septum may extend asymmetrically into the medulla, usually in the vicinity of the descending tract of the fifth cranial nerve to create a syringobulbia.

Diagnosis

The clinical picture of syringomyelia is so characteristic that diagnosis is seldom in doubt. Now one can obtain

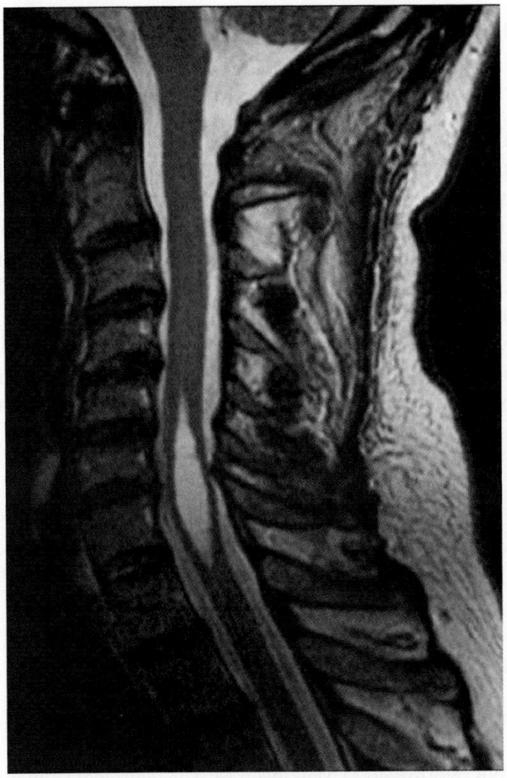

Figure 44-13. Sagittal T2-weighted MRI showing a developmental syringomyelia without Chiari malformation. The cervical spinal cord is greatly expanded but there were only signs of spinothalamic sensory loss over the arms.

spectacular demonstrations of the syrinx, either traumatic or developmental (Fig. 44-13), Chiari malformations, and other foramen magnum lesions by MRI of the sagittal planes of the brain and spinal cord (see Fig. 38-4). Also, hours after a CT myelogram, contrast material fills the syrinx and the central canal directly, possibly by diffusion from the surface of the cord.

Certain rare polyneuropathies (amyloid, Tangier disease, and Fabry disease) that preferentially affect small fibers in the nerves of the upper extremities can reproduce the dissociated sensory loss that is characteristic of a syrinx ("pseudosyringomyelic" deficit), but motor abnormalities are not prominent in these neuropathic cases. These diseases are discussed in Chap. 46.

Treatment

The only therapy of lasting value for type I syringomyelia (related to Chiari malformation) is surgical decompression of the foramen magnum and upper cervical canal. Headache and neck pain are helped most; ataxia and nystagmus tend to persist, but these are related to the Chiari process. The cavity tends to cease enlarging. Radiation therapy, which was formerly recommended, is of no benefit. The operation advised by Gardner, of plugging the connection between the fourth ventricle and the central canal of the cervical cord, has been abandoned. There were complications of this operative procedure, and the results were no better than those obtained from simple decompression. The decompression operation also carries some risk, especially if there is an attempt to excise the tonsillar projections of the cerebellum. In the series of Logue and Edwards, comprising 56 cases of type I syringomyelia, the occipitocervical pain was relieved by decompression in most patients, but the shoulder-arm pain usually persisted. Upper motor neuron weakness of the legs and sensory ataxia were often improved, whereas the segmental sensory and motor manifestations of the syringomyelia were not. Hankinson, in the past, had reported good results from decompression in 75 percent of type I cases of syringomyelia. In the retrospective review of 141 adult patients by Stevens and colleagues, good surgical outcome was achieved in 50 percent of those with minor degrees of descent of the cerebellar tonsils, but in only 12 percent of those with major cerebellar ectopia. A distended syrinx also led to a more favorable outcome. Whether the long-term course of these diseases is altered has not been determined. Other surgical series of Chiari-syrinx are discussed and cited in Chap. 38.

Syringotomy or shunting of the cavity has been performed in type I and some of the type II (idiopathic) cases, but the results have been unpredictable. Love and Olafson, who performed this procedure in 40 patients of both types (mainly type II), stated that 30 percent had an excellent outcome. Schurch and coworkers obtained improvement of pain and motor weakness in five of their seven cases by stabilization of the spine and syringotomy with placement of a T-tube within the syrinx. In a more recent and comprehensive study of 73 patients with a developmental syrinx operated by Sgouros and Williams (1995), one-half remained clinically stable for a 10-year period; 15 percent had serious complications from the surgery, however. Our experience with this procedure has not persuaded us of its lasting value; most of these patients, even those who reported some improvement originally, soon relapsed to their preoperative state, and the disease then progressed in the usual way. An enlarged cervical cord with progressive clinical worsening may nonetheless justify an attempt to shunt the cavity. Other comments are found in Chap. 38.

Surgery for the *posttraumatic cases* has given only slightly more favorable results. With incomplete myelopathy, syringotomy relieved the pain in all 10 patients of Shannon and associates. Where they found the myelopathy to be complete, the cord was transected and the upper stump excised. Sgouros and Williams (1996) studied 57 such patients and recommend decompressive laminectomy and reconstruction of the subarachnoid space as the most effective of the several procedures used in the management of traumatic cavities. An extensive review of surgical approaches to syringomyelia can be found in the article by Brodbelt and Stoodley, who tentatively recommend lysis of arachnoidal adhesions as preferable to shunting or filleting of the cord, but acknowledge that the current state of treatment is unsatisfactory.

In the cases of syringomyelia with tumor, in which the cyst fluid may be high in protein and viscid (unlike the low-protein fluid of the usual syrinx), the tumor should be excised if possible. This has been done successfully with hemangioblastomas of the posterior columns and occasionally with ependymomas.

The infrequent case of symptomatic purely hydromyelic may benefit from ventriculoperitoneal shunts of hydrocephalus, and a few excellent results are reported. This procedure has also been attempted in type I developmental cases, with unimpressive results unless there is an associated hydrocephalus. Draining the central canal by amputation of the tip of the sacral cord has been unsuccessful and can be harmful. Most patients with hydromyelia do not require treatment.

CONCLUDING REMARKS ON DISEASES OF THE SPINAL CORD

It is always well to remind oneself that of the more than 30 diseases of the spinal cord, effective means of treatment are available for many of the common ones: spondylosis, extramedullary spinal cord tumors, epidural abscess, hematoma and granuloma (tuberculous, fungal, sarcoidosis), myelitis, syringomyelia, and subacute combined degeneration and other forms of nutritional myelopathy. Many of the inflammatory myelopathies respond well to immune-modulating measures. The physician's major responsibility is to determine whether the patient has one of these treatable diseases.

References

Adams CBT, Logue V: Studies in cervical spondylotic myelopathy. *Brain* 94:557, 569, 1971.

Allen AR: Surgery of experimental lesions of the spinal cord equivalent to crush injury of fracture dislocation of the spinal column: A preliminary report. *JAMA* 57:878, 1911.

American Spinal Injury Association: *Standards for Neurological Classification of Spinal Injury Patients*. Chicago, American Spinal Injury Association, 1984.

Aminoff MJ, Logue V: The prognosis of patients with spinal vascular malformations. *Brain* 97:211, 1974.

Antoni N: Spinal vascular malformations (angiomas) and myelomalacia. *Neurology* 12:795, 1962.

Avrahami E, Tadmor R, Cohn DF: Magnetic resonance imaging in patients with progressive myelopathy following spinal surgery. *J Neurol Neurosurg Psychiatry* 52:176, 1989.

Baker AS, Ojemann RG, Swartz MN, Richardson EP Jr: Spinal epidural abscess. *N Engl J Med* 293:463, 1975.

Bakshi R, Kinkel PR, Mechtler LL, et al: Magnetic resonance imaging findings in 22 cases of myelitis: Comparison between patients with and without multiple sclerosis. *Eur J Neurol* 5:35, 1998.

Ball MJ, Dayan AD: Pathogenesis of syringomyelia. *Lancet* 2:799, 1972.

Ballantine HT, Ojemann RG, Drew JH: Syringohydromyelia, in Krayenbuhl H, Maspes PE, Sweet WH (eds): *Progress in Neurological Surgery*. Vol 4. New York, Karger, 1971, pp 227–245.

Barnett JHM, Foster JB, Hudgson P: *Syringomyelia*. Philadelphia, Saunders, 1973.

Bartleson JO, Cohen MD, Harrington TM: Cauda equina syndrome secondary to long-standing ankylosing spondylitis. *Ann Neurol* 14:662, 1983.

Bell HS: Paralysis of both arms from injury of the upper portion of the pyramidal decussation" "cruciate paralysis." *J Neurosurg* 33:376, 1970.

Blacker DJ, Wijkicks EFM, Rama Krishna G: Resolution of severe paraplegia due to aortic dissection after CSF drainage. *Neurology* 61:142, 2003.

Blackwood W: Discussion of vascular disease of the spinal cord. *Proc R Soc Med* 51:543, 1958.

Braakman R: Management of cervical spondylotic myelopathy and radiculopathy. *J Neurol Neurosurg Psychiatry* 57:257, 1994.

Bracken MR, Shepard MJ, Collins WF, et al: A randomized controlled trial of methylprednisolone or naloxone in treatment of acute spinal cord injury. *N Engl J Med* 322:1405, 1990.

Bracken MR, Shepard MJ, Collins WF, et al: Methylprednisolone or naloxone treatment after acute spinal cord injury: 1-year follow-up data. *J Neurosurg* 76:23, 1992.

Brain WR: Discussion on rupture of the intervertebral disc in the cervical region. *Proc R Soc Med* 41:509, 1948.

Brain WR, Northfield D, Wilkinson M: The neurological manifestations of cervical spondylosis. *Brain* 75:187, 1952.

Brodbelt AR, Stoodley MA: Posttraumatic syringomyelia: A review. *J Clin Neurosci* 10:401, 2003.

Brown P, Thompson PD, Rothwell JC, et al: Axial Myoclonus of propriospinal origin. *Brain* 114:197, 1991.

Burns RJ, Jones AN, Robertson JS: Pathology of radiation myelopathy. *J Neurol Neurosurg Psychiatry* 35:888, 1972.

Buur T, Morch MM: Hereditary multiple exostoses with spinal cord compression. *J Neurol Neurosurg Psychiatry* 46:96, 1983.

Caccamo DV, Garcia JH, Ho K-L: Isolated granulomatous angiitis of the spinal cord. *Ann Neurol* 32:580, 1992.

Campbell AMG, Garland H: Subacute myoclonic spinal neuronitis. *J Neurol Neurosurg Psychiatry* 19:268, 1956.

Candon E, Frerebeau P: Abcés bacteriens de la moelle épinière. *Rev Neurol* 150:370, 1994.

Cannon WB, Rosenblueth A: *The Supersensitivity of Denervated Structures*. New York, Macmillan, 1949.

Chang CWJ, Donovan DJ, Liem LK, et al: Surfer's myelopathy. Neurology 79:2171, 2012.

Cheshire WP, Santos CC, Massey EW, Howard JF: Spinal cord infarction: Etiology and outcome. *Neurology* 47:321, 1996.

Cilluffo JM, Gomez MR, Reese DF, et al: Idiopathic (congenital) spinal arachnoid diverticula. *Mayo Clin Proc* 56:93, 1981.

Clark K: Injuries to the cervical spine and spinal cord, in Youmans JR (ed): *Neurological Surgery*, 2nd ed. Philadelphia, Saunders, 1982, pp 2318–2337.

Collins WF, Chehrazi B: Concepts of the acute management of spinal cord injury, in Mathews WB, Glaser GH (eds): *Recent Advances in Clinical Neurology*. London, Churchill Livingstone, 1983, pp 67–82.

Confavreux C, Larbre J-P, Lejeune E, et al: Cerebrospinal fluid dynamics in the tardive cauda equina syndrome of ankylosing spondylitis. *Ann Neurol* 29:221, 1991.

Constantini S, Miller DC, Allen JC, et al: Radical excision of intramedullary spinal cord tumors: Surgical morbidity and long-term follow-up evaluation in 164 children and young adults. *J Neurosurg* 93:183, 2000.

Costigan DA, Winkelman MD: Intramedullary spinal cord metastasis. *J Neurosurg* 62:227, 1985.

Creed RS, Denny-Brown D, Eccles JC, et al: *Reflex Activity of the Spinal Cord*. Oxford, UK, Clarendon Press, 1932, p 154.

Cruickshank EK: A neuropathic syndrome of uncertain origin. *West Indian Med J* 5:147, 1956.

Dahlberg PJ, Frecentese DF, Cogbill TH: Cholesterol embolism: Experience with 22 histologically proven cases. *Surgery* 10:737, 1989.

Darouiche RO: Spinal epidural abscess. *N Engl J Med* 355:2012, 2006.

Dastur DK: Lathyrism. *World Neurol* 3:721, 1962.

de Seze J, Stojkovic T, Breteau G, et al: Acute myelopathies. Clinical, laboratory and outcome profiles in 79 cases. *Brain* 124:1509, 2001a.

de Seze J, Stojkovic T, Hachulla E, et al: Myélopathies et syndrome de Gougerot-Sjögren: Étude clinique, radiologique et profil évolutif. *Rev Neurol* 157:6, 2001b.

DeVivo MJ, Kartus PT, Stover SI: Seven-year survival following spinal cord injury. *Arch Neurol* 44:872, 1987.

Dickman CA, Hadley NM, Pappas CTE, et al: Cruciate paralysis: A clinical and radiologic analysis of injuries to the cervicomedullary spine. *J Neurosurg* 73:850, 1990.

Douglas MA, Parks LC, Bebin J: Sudden myelopathy secondary to therapeutic total-body hyperthermia after spinal-cord irradiation. *N Engl J Med* 304:583, 1981.

Duke RJ, Hashimoto S: Familial spinal arachnoiditis. *Arch Neurol* 30:300, 1974.

Ebersold MJ, Pare MC, Quast LM: Surgical treatment for cervical spondylotic myelopathy. *J Neurosurg* 82:745, 1995.

Elkington J St C: Arachnoiditis, in Feiling A (ed): *Modern Trends in Neurology*. New York, Hoeber-Harper, 1951, pp 149–161.

Ell JJ, Uttley D, Silver JR: Acute myelopathy in association with heroin addiction. *J Neurol Neurosurg Psychiatry* 44:448, 1981.

Elsberg CA: *Surgical Diseases of the Spinal Cord, Membranes and Nerve Roots: Symptoms, Diagnosis and Treatment*. New York, Hoeber-Harper, 1941.

Epstein JA, Epstein NE: The surgical management of cervical spinal stenosis, spondylosis, and myeloradiculopathy by means of the posterior approach, in Cervical Spine Research Society (ed): *The Cervical Spine*. Philadelphia, Lippincott, 1989, pp 625–669.

Feldman E, Bromfield E, Navia B, et al: Hydrocephalic dementia and spinal cord tumor. *Arch Neurol* 43:714, 1986.

Filiminoff IN: Zur pathologisch-anatomischen Charakteristik des Lathyrismus. *Z Ges Neurol Psychiatry* 105:76, 1926.

Flanagan EP, McKeon A, Lennon VA, et al: Paraneoplastic isolated myelopathy: clinical course and neuroimaging clues. *Neurology* 76:2089, 2011.

Foix C, Alajouanine T: La myelite necrotique subaigue. *Rev Neurol* 2:1, 1926.

Folliss AGH, Netzky MG: Progressive necrotic myelopathy, in Vinken PJ, Bruyn GW (eds): *Handbook of Clinical Neurology*. Vol 9. Amsterdam, North-Holland, 1970, pp 452–468.

Fox MW, Onofrio BM, Kilgore JE: Neurological complications of ankylosing spondylitis. *J Neurosurg* 78:871, 1993.

Fulton JF: *Physiology of the Nervous System*. London, Oxford University Press, 1943.

Gardner WJ: Hydrodynamic mechanism of syringomyelia: Its relationship to myelocele. *J Neurol Neurosurg Psychiatry* 28: 247, 1965.

Gilbert RW, Kim J-H, Posner JB: Epidural spinal cord compression from metastatic tumor: Diagnosis and treatment. *Ann Neurol* 3:40, 1978.

Greenberg HS, Kim JH, Posner JB: Epidural spinal cord compression from metastatic tumor. *Ann Neurol* 8:361, 1980.

Greenfield JG, Turner JWA: Acute and subacute necrotic myelitis. *Brain* 62:227, 1939.

Guttmann L: *Spinal Cord Injuries: Comprehensive Management and Research*. Oxford, UK, Blackwell, 1976.

Hamandi K, Mottershead J, Lewis T, et al: Irreversible damage to the spinal cord following spinal anesthesia. *Neurology* 59:624, 2002.

Hankinson J: Syringomyelia and the surgeon, in Williams D (ed): *Modern Trends in Neurology*. Vol 5. Oxford, Butterworth, 1970, pp 127–148.

Haymaker W: Decompression sickness, in Scholz W (ed): *Handbuch der Speziellen Pathologischen Anatomie und Histologie*. Vol XIII/1B. Berlin, Springer-Verlag, 1957, pp 1600–1672.

Head H, Riddoch G: The automatic bladder: Excessive sweating and some other reflex conditions in gross injuries of the spinal cord. *Brain* 40:188, 1917.

Heiss JD, Patronas N, DeVroom HL, et al: Elucidating the pathophysiology of syringomyelia. *J Neurosurg* 91:553, 1999.

Herrick M, Mills PE Jr: Infarction of spinal cord. *Arch Neurol* 24:228, 1971.

Hirayama K, Tokumaru Y: Cervical dural sac and spinal cord in juvenile muscular atrophy of distal upper extremity. *Neurology* 54:1922, 2000.

Hoffman JR, Mower WR, Wolfson AB, et al: Validity of a set of clinical criteria to rule out injury to the cervical spine in patients with blunt trauma. *N Engl J Med* 343:94, 2000.

Holmes G: On the spinal injuries of warfare: Goulstonian lectures. *Br Med J* 2:769, 1915.

Howell DA, Lees AJ, Toghill PJ: Spinal internuncial neurones in progressive encephalomyelitis with rigidity. *J Neurol Neurosurg Psychiatry* 42:773, 1979.

Hughes JT: *Pathology of the Spinal Cord*, 2nd ed. Philadelphia, Saunders, 1978.

Hugon J, Ludolph A, Roy DN, et al: Studies on the etiology and pathogenesis of motor neuron diseases: II. Clinical and electrophysiologic features of pyramidal dysfunction in macaques fed *Lathyrus sativus* and IDPN. *Neurology* 38:435, 1988.

Hurlbert RJ: Methylprednisolone for acute spinal cord injury: An inappropriate standard of care. *J Neurosurg* 93:1, 2000.

Hurst RW, Grossman RI: Peripheral spinal cord hypointensity on T2-weighted MR images: A reliable imaging sign of venous hypertensive myelopathy. *AJNR Am J Neuroradiol* 21:781, 2000.

Inamasu J, Hori S, Ohsuga F, et al: Selective paralysis of the upper extremities after odontoid fracture: Acute central cord syndrome or cruciate paralysis? *Clin Neurol Neurosurg* 103:238, 2001.

Jefferson G: Discussion on spinal injuries. *Proc R Soc Med* 21:625, 1927.

Jellema K, Canta LR, Tijssen CC, et al: Spinal dural arteriovenous fistulas: Clinical features in 80 patients. *J Neurol Neurosurg Psychiatry* 74:1438, 2003.

Jones A: Transient radiation myelitis. *Br J Radiol* 37:727, 1964.

Jones BV, Ernst RJ, Tomsick TA, et al: Spinal dural arteriovenous fistulas: Recognizing the spectrum of magnetic resonance imaging findings. *J Spinal Cord Med* 20:43, 1997.

Jonesco-Sisesti N: *Syringobulbia: A Contribution to the Pathophysiology of the Brainstem*. Translated into English, edited, and annotated by RT Ross. New York, Praeger, 1986.

Kagan RA, Wollin M, Gilbert HA, et al: Comparison of the tolerance of the brain and spinal cord to injury by radiation, in Gilbert HA, Kagan RA (eds): *Radiation Damage to the Nervous System*. New York, Raven Press, 1980.

Khurana VG, Perez-Terzic CM, Petersen RC, Krauss WE: Singing paraplegia: A distinctive manifestation of a spinal dural arteriovenous malformation. *Neurology* 58:1279, 2002.

Kidd D, Thorpe JW, Kiendall BE, et al: MRI dynamics of brain and spinal cord in progressive multiple sclerosis. *J Neurol Neurosurg Psychiatry* 60:15, 1996.

Killen DA, Foster JH: Spinal cord injury as a complication of contrast angiography. *Surgery* 59:962, 1966.
Killen DA, Weinstein C, Reed W: Reversal of spinal cord ischemia resulting from aortic dissection. *J Thorac Cardiovasc Surg* 119:1049, 2000.
Kneisley LW: Hyperhydrosis in paraplegia. *Arch Neurol* 34:536, 1977.
Kocher T: Die Wirletzungen der Virbelsäule zugleich als Beitrag zur Physiologie des menschlichen Ruckenmarcks. *Mitt Grenzgeb Med Chir* 1:415, 1896.
Kuhn RA: Functional capacity of the isolated human spinal cord. *Brain* 73:1, 1950.
Kumar N, Crum B, Petersen RC, et al: Copper deficiency myelopathy. *Arch Neurol* 61:762, 2004.
Lazorthes G: Pathology, classification and clinical aspects of vascular diseases of the spinal cord, in Vinken PJ, Bruyn GW (eds): *Handbook of Clinical Neurology*. Vol 12. Amsterdam, North-Holland, 1972, pp 492–506.
Leech RW, Pitha JV, Brumback RA: Spontaneous haematomyelia: A necropsy study. J Neurol Neurosurg Psychiatry 54:172, 1991.
Lennon VA, Wingerchuk DM, Kryzer RJ, et al: A serum autoantibody marker for neuromyelitis optica: Distinction from multiple sclerosis. *Lancet* 364:2106, 2004.
Levivier M, Baleriaux D, Matos C, et al: Sarcoid myelopathy. *Neurology* 41:1529, 1991.
Lhermitte F, Chain F, Escourolle R, et al: Un nouveau cas de contracture tetaniforme distinct du stiff-man syndrome. *Rev Neurol* 128:3, 1923.
Lintott P, Hafez HM, Stansby G: Spinal cord complications of thoracolumbar aneurysm surgery. *Br J Surg* 85:5, 1998.
Lipson SJ, Naheedy MH, Kaplan MH: Spinal stenosis caused by epidural lipomatosis in Cushing's syndrome. *N Engl J Med* 302:36, 1980.
Logue V: Angiomas of the spinal cord: Review of the pathogenesis, clinical features, and results of surgery. *J Neurol Neurosurg Psychiatry* 42:1, 1979.
Logue V, Edwards MR: Syringomyelia and its surgical treatment: An analysis of 75 cases. *J Neurol Neurosurg Psychiatry* 44:273, 1981.
Love JG, Olafson RA: Syringomyelia: A look at surgical therapy. *J Neurosurg* 24:714, 1966.
McCormick PC, Michelsen WJ, Post KD, et al: Cavernous malformations of the spinal cord. *Neurosurgery* 23:459, 1988.
McCrae DL: Bony abnormalities in the region of the foramen magnum: Correlation of the anatomic and neurologic findings. *Acta Radiol* 40:335, 1953.
Malamud N, Boldrey EB, Welch WK, Fadell EJ: Necrosis of brain and spinal cord following x-ray therapy. *J Neurosurg* 11:353, 1954.
Mancall EL, Rosales RK: Necrotizing myelopathy associated with visceral carcinoma. *Brain* 87:639, 1964.]
Marshall J: Observations on reflex changes in the lower limbs in spastic paraplegia in man. *Brain* 77:290, 1954.
Martin J, Davis L: Studies upon spinal cord injuries: Altered reflex activity. *Surg Gynecol Obstet* 86:535, 1948.
Messard L, Carmody A, Mannarino E, Ruge D: Survival after spinal cord trauma: A life table analysis. *Arch Neurol* 35:78, 1978.
Mixter WJ, Barr JS: Rupture of the intervertebral disc with involvement of the spinal canal. *N Engl J Med* 211:210, 1934.
Morrison RE, Brown J, Gooding RS: Spinal cord abscess caused by *Listeria monocytogenes*. *Arch Neurol* 37:243, 1980.
Morse SD: Acute central cervical spinal cord syndrome. *Ann Emerg Med* 11:436, 1982.
Munro D: The rehabilitation of patients totally paralyzed below the waist. *N Engl J Med* 234:207, 1946.
Murphy KP, Opitz JL, Cabanela ME, Ebersold MJ: Cervical fractures and spinal cord injury: Outcome of surgical and nonsurgical management. *Mayo Clin Proc* 65:949, 1990.
Naiman JL, Donahue WL, Pritchard JS: Fatal nucleus pulposus embolism of spinal cord after trauma. *Neurology* 11:83, 1961.
Nakano KK, Schoene WC, Baker RA, Dawson DM: The cervical myelopathy associated with rheumatoid arthritis: Analysis of 32 patients, with 2 postmortem cases. *Ann Neurol* 3:144, 1978.
Nations SP, Boyer PJ, Love LA, et al: Denture cream. An unusual source of excess zinc, leading to hypocupremia and neurologic disease. *Neurology* 71:639, 2008.
Nesathurai S: Steroids and spinal cord injury: Revisiting the NASCIS 2 and NASCIS 3 trials. *J Trauma* 45:1088, 1998.
Novy J, Carruzzo A, Maeder P, Bogousslavsky J: Spinal cord ischemia. Clinical and imaging patterns, pathogenesis, and outcomes in 27 patients. *Arch Neurol* 63:1113, 2006.
Nowak DA, Mutzenbach S, Fuchs HH: Acute myelopathy. Retrospective clinical, laboratory, MRI and outcome analysis in 49 patients. *J Clin Neurosci* 11:145, 2004.
O'Connell JEA: The clinical signs of meningeal irritation. *Brain* 69:9, 1946.
Osame M, Matsumoto M, Usuku K, et al: Chronic progressive myelopathy associated with elevated antibodies to human T-lymphotropic virus type I and adult T-cell leukemia-like cells. *Ann Neurol* 21:117, 1987.
Pallis C, Jones AM, Spillane JD: Cervical spondylosis. *Brain* 77:274, 1954.
Palmer JJ: Radiation myelopathy. *Brain* 95:109, 1972.
Panse F: Electrical lesions of the nervous system, in Vinken PJ, Bruyn GW (eds): *Handbook of Clinical Neurology*, Vol 7. Amsterdam, North-Holland, 1970, pp 344–387.
Payne EE, Spillane JD: The cervical spine: An anatomicopathological study of 70 specimens (using a special technique) with particular reference to the problem of cervical spondylosis. *Brain* 80:571, 1957.
Peet MM, Echols DH: Herniation of nucleus pulposus: Cause of compression of spinal cord. *Arch Neurol Psychiatry* 32:924, 1934.
Penn RD, Kroin JS: Continuous intrathecal baclofen for severe spasticity. *Lancet* 2:125, 1985.]
Penry JK, Hoefnagel D, Vanden Noort S, Denny-Brown D: Muscle spasm and abnormal postures resulting from damage to interneurones in spinal cord. *Arch Neurol* 3:500, 1960.
Petito CK, Navia BA, Cho ES, et al: Vacuolar myelopathy pathologically resembling subacute combined degeneration in patients with AIDS. *N Engl J Med* 312:874, 1985.
Pollock LJ: Spasticity, pseudospontaneous spasm, and other reflex activities late after injury to the spinal cord. *Arch Neurol Psychiatry* 66:537, 1951.
Pollock LJ, Brown M, Boshes B, et al: Pain below the level of injury of the spinal cord. *Arch Neurol Psychiatry* 65:319, 1951.
Propper DJ, Bucknall RC: Acute transverse myelopathy complicating systemic lupus erythematosus. *Ann Rheum Dis* 48:512, 1989.
Queiroz L de S, Nucci A, Facure NO, Facure JJ: Massive spinal cord necrosis in schistosomiasis. *Arch Neurol* 36:517, 1979.
Reagan TJ, Thomas JE, Colby MY: Chronic progressive radiation myelopathy. *JAMA* 203:106, 1968.
Rezai AR, Woo HL, Lee M, et al: Disseminated ependymomas of the central nervous system. *J Neurosurg* 85:618, 1996.
Riddoch G: The reflex functions of the completely divided spinal cord in man, compared with those associated with less severe lesions. *Brain* 40:264, 1917.
Robertson CE, Brown RD, Wijdicks EFM, Rabenstein AA: recovery after spinal cord infarcts. *Neurology* 78:114, 2012.
Roobol TH, Kazzaz BA, Vecht CJ: Segmental rigidity and spinal myoclonus as a paraneoplastic syndrome. *J Neurol Neurosurg Psychiatry* 50:628, 1987.
Ropper AE, Cahill KS, Hanna JW, et al: Primary vertebral tumors: A review of epidemiologic, histologic, and imaging findings, Part I: Benign tumors. Neurosurgery 69:1171, 2011.

Ropper AH, Poskanzer DC: The prognosis of acute and subacute transverse myelitis based on early signs and symptoms. *Ann Neurol* 4:51, 1978.

Rose E, Bounolleau P, Ducreux D, et al: Priopriospinal Myoclonus revisited. *Neurology* 72:1301, 2009.

Rossier AB, Foo D, Shillito J: Posttraumatic cervical syringomyelia. *Brain* 108:439, 1985.

Rowland LP: Surgical treatment of cervical spondylotic myelopathy: Time for a controlled study. *Neurology* 42:5, 1992.

Sandson TA, Friedman SH: Spinal cord infarction: Report of 8 cases and review of the literature. *Medicine (Baltimore)* 68:282, 1989.

Sanyal B, Pant GC, Subrahmaniyam K, et al: Radiation myelopathy. *J Neurol Neurosurg Psychiatry* 42:413, 1979.

Savitsky N, Madonick MJ: Statistical control studies in neurology: Babinski sign. *Arch Neurol Psychiatry* 49:272, 1943.

Schneider RC, Cherry G, Pantek H: The syndrome of acute central cervical spinal cord injury. *J Neurosurg* 11:546, 1954.

Schurch B, Wichmann W, Rossier AB: Posttraumatic syringomyelia (cystic myelopathy): A prospective study of 449 patients with spinal cord injury. *J Neurol Neurosurg Psychiatry* 60:61, 1996.

Scrimgeour EM, Gajdusek DC: Involvement of the central nervous system in *Schistosoma mansoni* and *S. haematobium* infection. *Brain* 108:1023, 1985.

Sgouros S, Williams B: A critical appraisal of drainage in syringomyelia. *J Neurosurg* 82:1, 1995.

Sgouros S, Williams B: Management and outcome of posttraumatic syringomyelia. *J Neurosurg* 85:197, 1996.

Shannon N, Simon L, Logue V: Clinical features, investigation, and treatment of posttraumatic syringomyelia. *J Neurol Neurosurg Psychiatry* 44:35, 1981.

Sloof JH, Kernohan JW, MacCarty CS: *Primary Intramedullary Tumors of the Spinal Cord and Filum Terminale*. Philadelphia, Saunders, 1964.

Spencer PS, Roy DN, Ludolph A, et al: Lathyrism: Evidence for role of the neuroexcitatory amino acid BOAA. *Lancet* 2:1066, 1986.

Spiller WG: Thrombosis of the cervical anterior median spinal artery: Syphilitic acute anterior poliomyelitis. *J Nerv Ment Dis* 36:601, 1909.

Stiell IG, Clement CM, McKnight RD, et al: The Canadian C-spine rule versus the NEXUS low-risk criteria in patients with trauma. *N Engl J Med* 349:2510, 2003.

Stevens JM, Serva WA, Kendall BE, et al: Chiari malformation in adults: Relation of morphologic aspects to clinical features and operative outcome. *J Neurol Neurosurg Psychiatry* 56:1072, 1993.

Stoltmann HF, Blackwood W: The role of the ligamenta flava in the pathogenesis of myelopathy in cervical spondylosis. *Brain* 87:45, 1964.

Stookey B: Compression of the spinal cord due to ventral extradural cervical chondromas. *Arch Neurol Psychiatry* 20:275, 1928.

Swann KW, Ropper AH, New PFJ, Poletti CE: Spontaneous spinal subarachnoid hemorrhage and subdural hematoma. *J Neurosurg* 61:975, 1984.

Symon L, Kuyama H, Kendall B: Dural arteriovenous malformations of the spine: Clinical features and surgical results in 55 cases. *J Neurosurg* 60:238, 1984.

Thomas JE, Miller RH: Lipomatous tumors of the spinal canal. *Mayo Clin Proc* 48:393, 1973.

Thompson TP, Pearce J, Chong G, et al: Surfer's myelopathy. *Spine* 29:E353, 2004.

Toossi S, Josephson SA, Hetts SW, et al: Utility of MRI in spinal arteriovenous fistula. *Neurology* 79:25, 2012.

Tosi L, Rigoli G, Beltramello A: Fibrocartilaginous embolism of the spinal cord: A clinical and pathogenetic consideration. *J Neurol Neurosurg Psychiatry* 60:55, 1996.

Uttley D, Monro P: Neurosurgery for cervical spondylosis. *Br J Hosp Med* 42:62, 1989.

Vallee B, Mercier P, Menei P, et al: Ventral transdural herniation of the thoracic cord: Surgical treatment in four cases and review of the literature. *Acta Neurochir (Wien)* 141:907, 1999.

Wadia NH: Myelopathy complicating congenital atlantoaxial dislocation (a study of 28 cases). *Brain* 90:449, 1967.

Watters MR, Stears JC, Osborn AG, et al: Transdural spinal cord herniation. *AJNR* 19:1337, 1998.

Weidauer S, Nichtweiss M, Lanfermann H, et al: Spinal cord infarction: MR imaging and clinical features in 16 cases. *Neuroradiology* 44:851, 2002.

Weisman AD, Adams RD: The neurological complications of dissecting aortic aneurysm. *Brain* 67:69, 1944.

Westenfelder GO, Akey DT, Corwin SJ, et al: Acute transverse myelitis due to *Mycoplasma pneumoniae* infection. *Arch Neurol* 38:317, 1981.

Whitely AM, Swash M, Urich H: Progressive encephalomyelitis with rigidity. *Brain* 99:27, 1976.

Wilkinson M: *Cervical Spondylosis*, 2nd ed. Philadelphia, Saunders, 1971.

Wilkinson PA, Valentine A, Gibbs JM: Intrinsic spinal cord lesions complicating epidural anaesthesia and analgesia: Report of three cases. *J Neurol Neurosurg Psychiatry* 72:537, 2002.

Willeit J, Kiechl S, Kiechl-Kohlendarfer U, et al: Juvenile asymmetric segmental spinal muscular atrophy (Hirayama's disease): Three cases without evidence of "flexion myelopathy." *Acta Neurol Scand* 104:320, 2001.

Williams B: The cystic spinal cord. *J Neurol Neurosurg Psychiatry* 58:649, 1995.

Williams CS, Butler E, Roman GC: Treatment of myelopathy in Sjögren syndrome with a combination of prednisone and cyclophosphamide. *Arch Neurol* 59:815, 2001.

Winkelman MD: Neurological complications of thermal and electrical burns, in Aminoff MJ (ed): *Neurology and General Medicine*. New York, Churchill Livingstone, 1994, pp 915–929.

Winkelman MD, Adelstein DJ, Karlins NL: Intramedullary spinal cord metastases: Diagnostic and therapeutic considerations. *Arch Neurol* 44:526, 1987.

Woltman HW, Adson AW: Abscess of the spinal cord. *Brain* 49:193, 1926.

Woolsey RM, Young RR (eds): *Neurologic Clinics: Disorders of the Spinal Cord*. Philadelphia, Saunders, 1991.

Wyburn-Mason R: *Vascular Abnormalities and Tumors of the Spinal Cord and Its Membranes.* St. Louis, Mosby, 1944.

Yogananden N, Larson SJ, Gallagher M: Correlation of microtrauma in the spine with intraosseous pressure. *Spine* 19:435, 1994.

Zimmerili W: Vertebral osteomyelitis. *N Engl J Med* 362:1022, 2010.

Zwimpfer TJ, Bernstein M: Spinal cord compression. *J Neurosurg* 72:894, 1990.

45

Electrophysiologic and Laboratory Aids in the Diagnosis of Neuromuscular Disease

The clinical suspicion of neuromuscular disease, disclosed by any of the symptoms or syndromes in the succeeding chapters, finds ready confirmation in the laboratory. The intelligent selection of ancillary examinations requires knowledge of the biochemistry and physiology of nerve action potentials, neuromuscular transmission, and muscle fiber contraction. These basic subjects, with the relevant anatomy, serve as an introduction to the descriptions of the laboratory methods and the subject matter of the chapters on the diseases of muscle and nerve that follow.

ELECTROLYTES AND NEUROMUSCULAR ACTIVITY

Since the early studies of Hodgkin (1951) and of Hodgkin and Huxley (1952), tomes have been written on the subject of the conduction of electrical impulses in neural tissues. Such conduction in nerve and muscle depends first on the maintenance of a fluid internal environment that is distinctly different from the external or interstitial medium. The main intracellular constituents are potassium (K), magnesium (Mg), and phosphorus (P), whereas those outside the cell are sodium (Na), calcium (Ca), and chloride (Cl). In both nerve and muscle the intracellular concentrations of these ions are held within a narrow range by both passive electrical and active chemical forces, which maintain the membranes in an electrochemical equilibrium termed the resting membrane potential. These forces are the result of selective permeability of the membranes to various ions and to the continuous expulsion of intracellular Na through specific channels by a pump mechanism (the sodium pump). The function of the sodium pump is dependent on the enzyme Na-K-ATPase (adenosine triphosphatase), which is localized in the membranes.

This resting membrane potential is the result of the differential concentrations of K and Na. The interior of the cell is some 30 times richer in K than the extracellular fluid, and the concentration of Na is 10 to 12 times greater in the extracellular fluid. In the resting state, the chemical forces that promote diffusion of K ions out of the cell (down their concentration gradient) are counterbalanced by electrical forces, the internal negativity, that opposes further diffusion of K to the exterior of the cell. The situation of Na ions in the equilibrium state is the opposite; they tend to diffuse into the cell, both because of their concentration gradient and because of the relative negativity inside the cell. Because the membrane at rest is less permeable to Na than to K, the amount of K leaving the cell exceeds the amount of Na entering the cell, thus creating the difference in electrical charge across the membrane. This discrepancy creates an electrical potential across the membrane such that, in the resting state, the intracellular compartment is 70 to 90 mV negative relative to the extracellular space (the resting membrane potential). The actions of the Na:K pump and the presence of impermeant, negatively charged intracellular proteins, contribute to maintaining this negative potential.

From this resting potential, any electrical discharge of neural and muscular tissue is predicated on the special property of excitable membranes; namely, the permeability of the cell to Na is linked to the electrical potential across the membrane by voltage-gated (i.e., voltage sensitive or voltage triggered) ion channels. Any depolarization of the membrane by a slight electrical or chemical change, creates an increased permeability to Na through the sodium channels and a consequent inward movement of sodium. Subsequently, K moves outward and repolarizes the membrane and thereby reduces its permeability to Na. If a greater degree of depolarization occurs, a situation arises in which the outward movement of K is unable to stabilize the membrane potential. The membrane then becomes even more depolarized and progressively more permeable to Na, and an "explosive," or regenerative Na current develops in which Na rushes down its chemical and electrical gradients into the cell. With the elevation in Na permeability, the Na ions continue to depolarize the intracellular compartment to about +40 mV (the Nernst equilibrium potential for Na). It is this depolarization of the intracellular compartment, lasting a few milliseconds, that constitutes the action potential.

However, an equilibrium at this level is not established because there is a rapid (within 5 ms) fall in membrane Na permeability back to baseline levels. This fall in Na permeability occurs because the depolarization inactivates Na conductance. The transient depolarization at the same time activates an increase in membrane permeability to K. The combined effects of the resulting efflux of K and a diminishing influx of Na repolarizes the membrane back to its resting level. During a brief period immediately after repolarization, the nerve and muscle fibers are refractory, at first absolutely then relatively, to another depolarizing stimulus. The duration of the refractory period is determined largely by the duration of the inactivation of the Na channel.

Conduction, or propagation, of the action potential along nerve or muscle, occurs as the current created by depolarization of a small segment of membrane flows into the contiguous membrane, which, in turn, becomes depolarized. When the depolarization reaches the threshold for development of an action potential, a new zone of increased Na permeability is created. In this manner, the action potential spreads in an "all-or-none" fashion, down the length of the nerve or muscle membrane. The action potentials in individual nerve fibers are too small and brief to be detected by conventional nerve conduction techniques, but a summated volley of all the fibers within a nerve is large enough to be recorded, and it is this electrical potential and the one it produces in the muscle that it innervates that is utilized to study nerve function.

As nerve impulses pass centrifugally from the axon into its terminal branches, transmission may "break down," especially if impulses arrive too frequently at branch points; they then fail to reach the neuromuscular junction of these fibers; or there may be failure of conduction at the neuromuscular junction, which is the characteristic feature of myasthenia gravis.

In large motor and sensory nerves, contiguous spread of action potentials along a fiber eventually decays over long distances. Conduction is aided by the structure and configuration of the myelin sheaths surrounding the axon. The sodium channels, which generate the action potential, are concentrated at short exposed segments of the axon, the nodes of Ranvier, lying between longer segments of myelinated axon, the internodes. In contrast, the internodes covered by myelin remain electrically insulated. This creates "flux lines" that converge on the nodes and allows current to be regenerated at each gap in the myelin. The speed of electrical conduction, which jumps in a "saltatory" fashion from node to node, is many times faster than conduction through an unmyelinated axon. The largest-diameter fibers have the thickest myelin sheaths and longest internodal distances, conferring on them the fastest conduction times.

Conventional laboratory studies of nerve conduction generally measure the speed of these fastest-conducting fibers. This dependence of nerve conduction on large, heavily myelinated fibers explains a number of electrophysiologic abnormalities that are a consequence of nerve disease. One common result, is a mild slowing of nerve conduction because of a dependence on the remaining smaller diameter, slower conducting axons. When myelin destruction is the prominent feature of a neuropathy (*demyelinating neuropathy*), conduction velocity is greatly slowed because of delays in regenerating the sodium current at nodes of Ranvier, or there may be total block of electrical conduction. An intermediate state of partial demyelination slows and desynchronizes the electrical volley, leading to temporal dispersion of the action potentials that reach the muscle. The cumulative effect of any of these changes is to reduce the number of nerve fibers that are capable of conducting an electrical volley, leading to a graduated reduction in the amplitude of the muscle action potential over longer segments of nerve. This reduction in amplitude of the compound motor action potential (CMAP) as the stimulating electrode is moved proximally is termed *conduction block* (discussed under "Studies of Nerve Conduction" further on). Blocked conduction of this restricted nature is a reliable marker of an acquired demyelinating neuropathy; of all the electrophysiologic changes, it also corresponds most closely to the degree of muscle weakness (see further on).

In contrast to these effects of demyelination of peripheral nerve, loss of axon fibers (*axonal neuropathy*) results in a reduction of the amplitude of summed electrical activity of the action potential in muscles uniformly all along the nerve, and to atrophic denervation of muscle as described further on.

THE NEUROMUSCULAR JUNCTION (MOTOR ENDPLATE)

This is the interface between the finely branched nerve fiber and the muscle fiber, where the electrical activity of the motor nerve is translated into muscle action (Fig. 45-1). The nerve fiber contacts the muscle membrane in a trough-like junctional space of 50 mm—the *synaptic* cleft—between the axolemma and sarcolemma (see Fig. 49-1). Within the nerve terminal, a relatively fixed number of packets, or quanta, of acetylcholine (ACh), each packet containing about 10,000 molecules, are liberated through an exocytotic process that is triggered by the arrival of axonal action potentials. Arrival of the electrical impulse opens calcium channels in the presynaptic neural membrane, which serves to bind packets of ACh to the membrane and govern their release. Molecules of ACh diffuse into the synaptic cleft and attach to receptor sites on the postsynaptic membrane. Each impulse triggers the release of approximately 20 to 50 quanta of ACh and produces a depolarization of sufficient size to initiate an action potential in the postsynaptic muscle membrane through the same mechanism of a regenerative sodium current described earlier. Botulinum toxin interferes with exocytosis of ACh at the release site by cleaving "synaptic protein 25." There is also a nonquantal release of ACh through continuous leakage. This appears to play a role in the trophic influence of nerve on muscle.

The ACh molecule binds to the postsynaptic ACh receptor, a complex of 5 proteins that constitute the postsynaptic ion channel. Binding of ACh by this receptor causes a conformational change in the receptor that leads to a local increase in the conductance of Na and K and other small ions. This produces a depolarization known as the *endplate potential*. Small (miniature) endplate potentials (MEPPs) are continuously formed

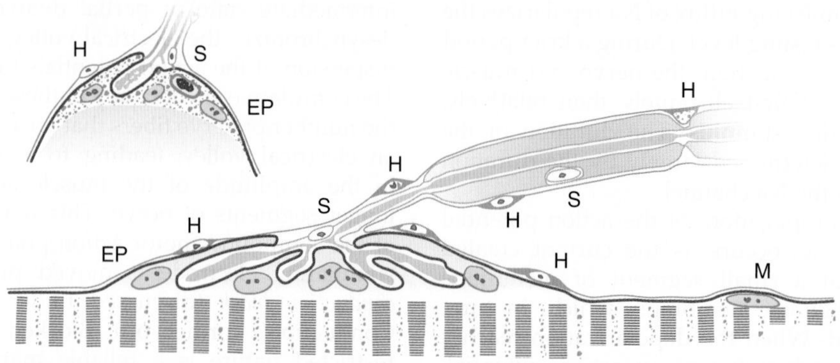

Figure 45-1. Motor endplate showing relationship between various structures in nerve and muscle. Last segment of myelin, with Schwann nucleus (*S*), terminates abruptly, leaving axis cylinder covered by sheaths of Schwann and Henle. Endplate nuclei (*EP*) of muscle fiber lie embedded in sarcoplasm and have same staining reactions as sarcolemmal nuclei (*M*). Ramifications of axis cylinder (telodendria) lie in grooves or pouches in granular sarcoplasm, each lined by spiny "subneural apparatus" of Couteaux, which is continuous with membranous sarcolemma and also Schwann membrane. Nucleus (*S*) of sheath of Schwann commonly lies near point of branching of axon. Sheath of Henle has small nuclei (*H*) and fuses with endomysial sheath of muscle fiber.

and regenerated as the membranes repolarize, much as in the process of passive decay previously described. These potentials are too small to be recorded by routine electromyography (EMG) testing or to trigger an action potential, although fortuitous needle placement adjacent to a synapse may detect them.

The bound ACh is hydrolyzed by cholinesterase, a glycoprotein enzyme that exists in free form in the neuromuscular junction clefts. Its main function is to terminate the action potential and permit the sequential activation of muscle. The postsynaptic membrane, once depolarized, is refractory to another action potential until it is repolarized.

The calcium that entered the presynaptic nerve terminal is sequestered and then extruded, and the choline from the hydrolyzed ACh enters the nerve terminal, where it is resynthesized to ACh near the release sites.

The analysis of a rapid series of electrically of voluntarily elicited muscle contractions is used to test the function of the neuromuscular junction by stressing conduction across the junction. In general, a decrement in the amplitude of serial muscle action potentials is typical of postsynaptic failure, and an increment in the amplitude from a train of stimuli is a reflection of presynaptic failure.

Myasthenia gravis is the principal disease affecting the neuromuscular junction and represents a failure of postsynaptic function (see Chap. 49). In this process, the fundamental defect is not a deficiency of ACh or its release, but rather a failure of ACh to attach to the postsynaptic receptor, as a result of blockade by an antibody at the receptor site or of destruction of the membrane by antibody attack. There are several quite different synaptic disorders caused by botulism, aminoglycoside antibiotics, and the antibodies of the Lambert-Eaton myasthenic syndrome, which impede presynaptic release of ACh.

A number of pharmacologic agents also interfere with neuromuscular transmission by combining with the cholinergic (nicotinic) receptor on the postsynaptic membrane, thereby competitively blocking the transmitter action of ACh. The curariform drugs, derived from curare and termed *nondepolarizing neuromuscular blockers* because they do not alter the postsynaptic membrane potential are the main examples. Other drugs, notably succinylcholine and decamethonium, cause neuromuscular blockage by producing direct depolarization of the endplate and adjacent sarcoplasmic membrane (*depolarizing neuromuscular blockers*). Agents that inactivate cholinesterase have the opposite effect, i.e., they enhance the action of ACh. The ones in clinical use for the treatment of myasthenia gravis are the carbamates neostigmine, physostigmine, and pyridostigmine, the effects of which are reversible. The organophosphates are irreversible blockers of cholinesterase function, for which reason they are feared weapons of chemical warfare. Because the potent cholinergic antagonist atropine is active only at muscarinic sites, it has no effect at the neuromuscular junction.

BIOCHEMISTRY OF MUSCLE CONTRACTION

The sarcolemma, the transverse tubules, and the sarcoplasmic reticulum each play a role in the control of the activity of muscle fibers. Figure 45-2 illustrates the structural components involved in excitation, contraction, and relaxation of muscle. Following nerve stimulation, an action potential is transmitted by the sarcolemma from the motor endplate region to both ends of the muscle fiber. Depolarization spreads quickly to the interior of the fiber along the walls of the transverse tubules, probably by a conducted action potential. The transverse tubules and the terminal cisternae of the sarcoplasmic reticulum come into close proximity at points referred to as *triads*. Here, depolarization of the transverse tubules alters the conformation of a voltage-sensitive calcium channel in the transverse tubule membrane. This causes a large

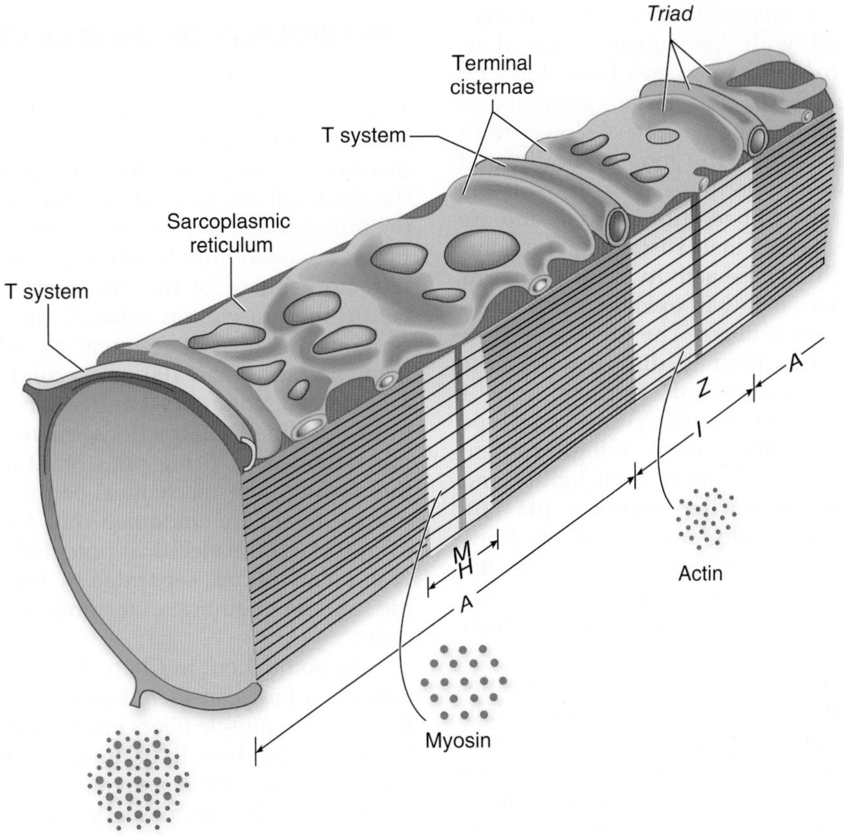

Figure 45-2. Schematic of the major subcellular components of a myofibril. The transverse (*T*) system, which is an invagination of the plasma membrane of the cell, surrounds the myofibril midway between the *Z* lines and the center of the *A* bands; the *T* system is approximated to, but apparently not continuous with, dilated elements (terminal cisternae) of the sarcoplasmic reticulum on either side. Thus, each sarcomere (the repeating *Z*-line-to-*Z*-line unit) contains two "triads," each composed of a pair of terminal cisternae on each side of the *T* tubule. (From Peter, by permission.)

protein (the ryanodine receptor) in the membrane of the adjacent sarcoplasmic reticulum (SR) to open an internal calcium pore, allowing stored calcium to exit the SR and flood into the cytoplasm. The released calcium binds to the regulatory protein *troponin*, thereby removing the inhibition exerted by the troponin–tropomyosin system upon the contractile protein *actin*. This allows an interaction to occur between the actin molecules of the thin filaments and the cross-bridges of the myosin molecules in the thick filaments and enables myosin ATPase to split adenosine triphosphate (ATP) at a rapid rate, thereby providing the energy for contraction. This chemical change allows the filaments to slide past each other, thereby shortening the muscle fiber. Relaxation occurs as a result of active (energy-dependent) Ca reuptake by the sarcoplasmic reticulum.

The pyrophosphate bonds of ATP, which supply the energy for muscle contraction, must be replenished constantly by a reaction that involves interchanges with the muscle phosphagen creatine diphosphate, where high-energy phosphate bonds are stored. These interactions, in both contraction and relaxation, require the action of creatine kinase (CK).

Myoglobin, another important muscle protein, functions in the transfer of oxygen, and a series of oxidative enzymes are involved in this exchange. The intracellular Ca, as noted earlier, is released by the muscle action potential and must be reaccumulated within the cisternae of the sarcoplasmic reticulum before actin and myosin filaments can slide back past one another in relaxation. This reuptake of Ca requires the expenditure of considerable energy. When there is defective generation of ATP, for example, from an enzyme deficiency, the muscle remains shortened, as in the *contracture* of phosphorylase deficiency (McArdle disease) or of phosphofructose kinase deficiency. The same sort of shortening contracture occurs under normal conditions in some of the "catch muscles" of certain mollusks and is the basis of rigor mortis in mammals.

Many glycolytic and other enzymes (transaminases, aldolase, CK) are utilized in the metabolic activity of muscle, particularly under relatively anaerobic conditions. Muscle fibers differ from one another in their relative content of oxidative and glycolytic enzymes; the latter determine the capacity of the muscle fiber to sustain anaerobic metabolism during periods of contraction with inadequate blood flow. Muscle cells rich in oxidative enzymes (type 1 fibers) contain more mitochondria and larger amounts of myoglobin (therefore appearing red), have slower rates of contraction and relaxation, fire more tonically, and are less fatigable than muscle fibers poor in oxidative enzymes. The latter (type 2 fibers) fire in bursts and are used in quick phasic, rather than sustained, reactions. The amount of myosin ATPase activity, which governs the speed of contraction, is low in oxidative-rich fibers and high in glycolytic-rich fibers. The myosin ATPase stain at pH 9.4 has been used to differentiate these two types of fibers in microscopic sections. Type 1 fibers have a low content of myosin ATPase, and type 2 (phosphorylative-rich) fibers have a high content of this enzyme; hence type 1 fibers stain lightly and type 2 darkly (the reverse reaction occurs at pH 4.6). All the fibers within one motor unit are of the same type, a feature that is used to advantage to identify the reinnervation of muscle fibers by a single motor neuron after adjacent neurons have died and denervated their constituent muscle fibers (fiber-type grouping).

The chemical energy required to maintain the various activities of the muscle cell is derived mainly from the metabolism of carbohydrate (blood glucose, muscle glycogen) and from fatty acids (plasma-free fatty acids, esterified fatty acids, and ketone bodies). There is a lesser contribution to energy from branched-chain and other amino acids, but their activity increases during prolonged exercise.

The most readily available source of muscular energy is glycogen, which is synthesized and stored in muscle cells. It provides more than 90 percent of the energy needs of muscle under conditions of high work intensity and during the early stages of submaximal exercise. Blood glucose and free fatty acids supplement intracellular glycogen as exercise proceeds. The free fatty acids are obtained from endogenous triglycerides (found mostly in type 1 fibers), from the triglycerides released by circulating lipoproteins, and from the lipolysis of adipose tissue. Most of the energy needs of resting muscle are provided by fatty acids.

The enzymatic reactions involved in the transport of these substrates into muscle cells and their intracellular synthesis and degradation during anaerobic and aerobic cell conditions have been thoroughly investigated and most of the participating enzymes have been identified. This subject is too extensive to be presented in a textbook of neurology, but enough is known about these matters to state that there are diseases that impair the contractile functions of muscle without destroying the fiber. In particular, specific enzymatic deficiencies alter carbohydrate utilization (myophosphorylase, debrancher enzyme, phosphofructokinase, and phosphoglyceromutase deficiencies), fatty acid utilization (carnitine and carnitine palmitoyl transferase deficiencies), pyruvate metabolism, and cytochrome oxidase activity (in the mitochondrial muscle diseases). These diseases are discussed in later chapters.

PHYSIOLOGY OF MUSCLE CONTRACTION

The contraction of a muscle fiber may be viewed as a series of electrochemical events that culminate in a mechanical effect. The mechanical change far outlasts the electrical one and extends through the period when the muscle fiber is refractory to another action potential. When a second muscle action potential arrives after the refractory phase of the previous action potential, but before the muscle has relaxed, the contraction will be prolonged. Thus, at frequencies of anterior horn cell firing of more than 100 per second, twitches fuse into a sustained voluntary contraction or *fused tetanus*. In most sustained contractions, there is incomplete tetanus, attained by firing rates of 40 to 50 per second. In this fashion, the mechanical contractions of individual muscle fibers are smoothed into a continuous process, even though the electrical potentials present as a series of depolarizations, separated by intervals during which the muscle membrane resumes its resting polarized state.

As pointed out in Chap. 3, the physiology of muscle activity is best considered in terms of motor units, i.e., the group of muscle fibers innervated by a single anterior horn cell. The strength of muscle contraction is in turn a function of the number and rates of firing of many adjacent motor units. The smoothness of contraction depends on the integrated and sequential enlistment of motor units of increasing size. The electrical signal of this summated contraction, the compound motor action potential, or CMAP, as recorded at the skin surface overlying a muscle is the main feature of the surface EMG and serves as the basis for quantifying the size of the motor nerve potential in the nerve conduction examinations.

The CMAP can be visualized on the screen of an oscilloscope or a computer and its onset used to measure the speed of motor nerve conduction (conduction velocity) as well as the summated amplitudes produced by all the innervating nerve fibers. It can also be converted into an audible noise. Further study involves the insertion into the muscle of a coaxial needle, which samples several motor units in the vicinity of the electrode. When elicited by a sustained voluntary contraction, the flurry of electrical activity from many muscle fibers at different distances from the electrodes is referred to as an *interference pattern* (see further on, under "Studies of Nerve Conduction" and "Needle Examination of Muscle [Electromyography]").

Various biochemical changes may cause not only an impairment of muscular activity (paresis, paralysis) but also excessive irritability, tetany, spasm, and cramp. In these instances, spontaneous discharges may occur from instability of axon polarization; hence a single nerve impulse may initiate a train of action potentials in nerve and muscle, as in the tetany of hypocalcemia. The common cramps of calf and foot muscles (painful, sustained contractions with motor unit discharges at frequencies up to 200 per second) may be a result of increased excitability (or unstable polarization) of the motor axons. Quinine, procainamide, diphenhydramine, and warmth reduce the irritability of nerve and muscle fiber membranes, as do a number of antiepileptic drugs that act by blocking sodium channels, thereby limiting spontaneous membrane discharges.

The muscle fiber, which is wholly dependent on the nerve for its stimulus to contract, may be physiologically activated or paralyzed in a number of ways that are explained by the principles described above. The main disturbances of nerve, muscle, and neuromuscular function occur when the motor nerve cell or its axon is injured or inexcitable, in which case the muscle cannot be stimulated; or, the nerve cell in the anterior horn of the spinal cord may be disinhibited, permitting the discharge of continuous action potentials, as in tetanus and the "stiff man" syndrome (see Chap. 48); the nerve fiber may fail to conduct impulses (demyelinating neuropathies) or the number of fibers may be inadequate to produce a fused and sustained contraction (axonal neuropathies); the distal axon may not distribute the nerve impulse simultaneously to all parts of the motor unit; ACh may not be released at the presynaptic region of the neuromuscular junction (as occurs in botulism and in the Eaton-Lambert syndrome) or, once released, ACh may not be inactivated by cholinesterase (physostigmine, organophosphates); the receptor zone on the postsynaptic membrane may be destroyed or blocked by antibodies or pharmacologic agents (myasthenia gravis or curariform drugs); and, finally, the metabolic or contractile elements of the muscle may not react or, once contracted, may not relax. One type of this last category is due to genetically determined abnormalities of voltage-gated ion channels, the "channelopathies," that are the subject of Chap. 50.

Similarly, there may be an unstable polarization of the nerve fibers, as in tetany and in dehydration with salt depletion, or hyperirritability of the motor unit, as in amyotrophic lateral sclerosis. The threshold of mechanical activation or electrical reactivation of the sarcolemmal membrane may be reduced, as occurs in myotonia, or impairment of an energy mechanism within the fiber may slow the contractile process, as in hypothyroidism; or a deficiency of phosphorylase, which deprives muscle of its carbohydrate energy source, may prevent relaxation, as in the contracture of McArdle disease. Lesions of the most peripheral branches of nerves, which allow nerve regeneration, may give rise to continuous activity of motor units. This is expressed clinically as a rippling of muscle, or *myokymia.*

In recent years, special techniques have made it possible to study each of the proteins and channels involved in neuromuscular transmission and the excitation-contraction-relaxation of muscle fibers. The amino acid composition of these proteins has also been determined. This information is being increasingly applied to the analysis of genetic diseases of muscle in the normal state and under conditions of disease. Pertinent comments and references to this subject are found in the chapters that follow.

EFFECTS ON MUSCLE OF SERUM ELECTROLYTES

Diffuse muscle weakness or muscle twitching, spasms, and cramps should always raise the question of uremia or an abnormality in serum electrolytes. These disorders reflect the concentrations of electrolytes in the intra- and extracellular fluids. If the plasma concentration of *K falls below 2.5 mEq/L or rises above 7 mEq/L,* weakness of extremity and trunk muscles results; below 2 mEq/L or above 9 mEq/L, there is almost always flaccid paralysis of these muscles and later, of the respiratory ones as well; only the extraocular and other cranial muscles are spared. In addition, the tendon reflexes are diminished or absent. The normal reaction of muscle to direct percussion is also reduced or abolished, suggesting impairment of transmission along the sarcolemmal membranes themselves. *Hypocalcemia of 7 mg/dL or less* (as in rickets or hypoparathyroidism) or relative reduction in the proportion of ionized calcium (as in hyperventilation) causes increased muscle irritability and spontaneous discharge of sensory and motor nerve fibers (i.e., tetany) and sometimes convulsions from similar effects upon cerebral neurons; frequent repetitive and prolonged spontaneous discharges grouped in couplets or triplets appear in the EMG. *Hypercalcemia* with Ca levels above 12 mg/dL (as occurs in vitamin D intoxication, hyperparathyroidism, carcinomatosis, sarcoidosis, and multiple myeloma) causes weakness perhaps on a central basis, and lethargy. Extreme *hypophosphatemia,* observed most often with intravenous hyperalimentation or bone tumor, can cause acute areflexic paralysis with nerve conduction abnormalities. *Reduction in the plasma concentration of magnesium* also results in tremor, muscle weakness, tetanic muscle spasms, and convulsions; a considerable *increase in magnesium levels* leads to muscle weakness and depression of central nervous function. The weakness of muscle in hypermagnesemia may also be partly a result of reduced release of ACh at the motor endplate.

The electrocardiogram (ECG) also becomes abnormal with many of these systemic electrolyte derangements as a result of alterations of the intracellular levels of electrolytes in the myocardium; ECG patterns are most sensitive to extreme changes in serum K levels.

CHANGES IN SERUM LEVELS OF ENZYMES ORIGINATING IN MUSCLE CELLS

In all diseases that cause extensive damage to striated muscle fibers, intracellular enzymes leak out of the fibers and enter the blood. Those measured routinely are the transaminases, lactic acid dehydrogenase, aldolase, and, especially, CK. The concentration of CK in serum has proved to be the most consistent and most sensitive measure of skeletal muscle damage. Because high concentrations of this enzyme are found in heart muscle and brain, raised serum values may be a result of myocardial or cerebral infarction, as well as of the necrotizing diseases of striated muscle (polymyositis, muscle trauma, muscle infarction, and the more rapidly advancing muscular dystrophies). For serum CK levels to be interpretable, one has to be certain that the enzyme released into the serum is not derived from heart or brain. This can be determined by the quantitation of serum isoenzymes of CK, referred to as MB, MM, and BB (M, muscle; B, brain); their measurement provides a means for the detection of damage to myocardium (MB), skeletal muscle (MM), and nervous tissue (BB), respectively.

The MM form of CK is found in highest concentration in striated muscle, but these muscles also contain 5 to 6 percent MB isoform. Myocardial tissue contains 17 to 59 percent MB; hence, the diagnosis of myocardial infarction requires that the CK-MB fraction be greater than 6 percent (or that troponin, which is overrepresented in heart muscle, be elevated in the serum). Embryonic and regenerating muscle contains more CK-MB than mature normal muscle. In patients with destructive lesions of striated muscle, serum values of CK often exceed 1,000 U/L and may reach 50,000 U or more (the upper limit of normal varies from 65 to 300 U/L, depending on the method of measurement). It is notable that in some black men the level may normally be in the range of 500 U/L in the absence of muscle or nerve disease (see below). The serum of the healthy adult contains only the MM isoenzyme, but in healthy children, as much as 25 percent of serum CK may be derived from the MB fraction.

As interesting is the rise in serum enzyme concentration in some children with progressive muscular dystrophy before there is enough destruction of fibers for the disease to be clinically manifest, at least as judged by the relatively crude test of muscle strength. Moreover, the unaffected female carrier of Duchenne dystrophy may be identified by an elevated serum level of CK; these changes reflect a "leaky" membrane that allows the transgression of the large enzyme molecules. Alterations of serum enzyme levels are, however, nonspecific as they occur in all types of disease that damage the muscle fiber. Moreover, in the more slowly evolving types of dystrophy, the serum levels of CK may be normal.

It would be expected that enzyme values would be normal in paralysis due to denervation with secondary muscular atrophy, but elevations are sometimes observed in patients with progressive spinal muscular atrophy and amyotrophic lateral sclerosis, particularly if there is relatively rapid progression of the disease. Even vigorous exercise or surgical operations involving muscle elevate CK, sometimes with the MB fraction exceeding 6 percent.

Idiopathic "HyperCKemia" In some normal individuals, CK may be persistently elevated without evidence of muscle or other disease. There is a particularly high incidence of this finding, albeit of mild degree, in African American men. An unexplained alteration of the sarcolemma with elevated serum CK occurs in hypothyroidism and in alcoholism. Toxic myopathies, for example, the type caused by the cholesterol-lowering drugs (statins), are another common cause of elevation in CK in current practice. Among the causes of persistently elevated CK are numerous underlying genetically determined muscle defects, usually one of the varieties of abnormal dystrophin or another membrane protein. Detailed examination may reveal slight proximal weakness and perhaps minimal calf enlargement characteristic of the mildest forms of Becker dystrophy. Closely related is the finding of CK elevations that occur in females who are asymptomatic carriers of Duchenne or Becker dystrophies. These diseases are described in Chap. 48.

Several nondystrophic muscle diseases also present as elevated CK levels in the blood, including polymyositis and dermatomyositis, carnitine palmityl transferase deficiency, some of the mitochondrial myopathies, McArdle disease, central core disease, multicore disease, and some forms of inclusion body myopathy. Finally, the rapid denervation of muscle that accompanies some cases of ALS may cause CK elevation.

If other sources of persistently elevated CK levels have been excluded, particularly those caused by exercise, trauma, and by drug-induced muscle damage, it is appropriate to follow the patient over time so that mild weakness may be detected, or to perform a biopsy to resolve the issue of an inflammatory myopathy or a mild muscular dystrophy. Because treatment would likely be withheld until weakness or pain arises, in idiopathic cases of raised enzyme levels, it seems prudent to delay biopsy unless the enzyme levels are massively elevated.

An isolated elevation of aldolase, the serum enzyme other than CK that is derived predominantly from skeletal muscle, generally has less clinical significance. Measurement in the serum of various transaminases or lactate dehydrogenase is not particularly useful for the diagnosis of muscle disease because of the ubiquitous distribution of these enzymes in many mammalian tissues. Nevertheless, the neurologist should be aware that unexplained elevations in all of the muscle-derived enzymes (CK, lactate dehydrogenase [LDH], serum glutamic-oxaloacetic transaminase [SGOT], aldolase) can be caused by inevident muscle trauma and by many other processes that damage the muscle membrane. As mentioned, cardiac muscle-specific enzyme, troponin, is not expressed in skeletal muscle and therefore is not found in the serum in cases of muscle disease, except in unusual circumstances in which regenerating muscle fibers in muscular dystrophies may transiently express the enzyme (the T, but the I, isotype) as noted in the series reported by Jaffe and colleagues. More often, elevations or troponin in these muscular diseases reflects a parallel myocardial disorder that accompanies several varieties of dystrophy.

MYOGLOBINURIA

The red pigment myoglobin, responsible for much of the color of muscle, is an iron-protein compound present in the sarcoplasm of striated skeletal and cardiac fibers. Of the hematin compounds, approximately 25 percent are in muscle and the remainder are in red blood corpuscles and other cells. Destruction of striated muscle, regardless of the cause liberates myoglobin, and because of its relatively small size, the molecule filters through the glomeruli and appears in the urine, imparting to it a burgundy-red color. Because of the low renal threshold for myoglobin, excretion of the pigment is so rapid that the serum remains uncolored. In contrast, the high renal threshold for hemoglobin colors both the serum and the urine if there is destruction of red blood corpuscles. Myoglobinuria should thus be suspected when the urine is deep red and the serum is normal in color. It is estimated that 200 g of muscle must be destroyed to color the urine visibly (Rowland).

As with hemoglobinuria, the guaiac and benzidine tests performed on urine are positive if myoglobin is present. However, the colored urine does not fluoresce, as it does in porphyria. On spectroscopic analysis, myoglobin shows an absorption band at 581 nm but the most sensitive method for measuring myoglobin in the urine and serum is by radioimmunoassay. Some years ago, the measurement of creatine and creatinine in blood and urine was a standard method of estimating damage to striated muscle. This technique is now seldom used, having been replaced by the measurement of CK and its isoenzymes. However, measurement of urine creatinine in large-volume samples of urine that have been collected for other testing assures that an adequate amount of renal excretion is being captured in the sample.

ENDOCRINE MYOPATHIES

In a number of disorders of the endocrine glands, muscle weakness may be a prominent feature, and occasionally may be the chief complaint. These diseases are discussed in detail in Chap. 48 but it should be noted here that such metabolic causes of muscle weakness, acute or chronic, may occur in the absence of changes in serum electrolytes or enzymes. Specific hormone assays are then necessary for diagnosis. This is particularly true of patients with thyrotoxicosis or Cushing disease, and of those receiving prolonged corticosteroid therapy. In thyrotoxicosis, muscle weakness may appear without the signs of Graves disease.

ELECTRODIAGNOSIS OF NEUROMUSCULAR DISEASE (NERVE CONDUCTION AND ELECTROMYOGRAPHY)

It was long ago discovered that muscle would contract when a pulse of electric current was applied to the skin, near the point of entrance of the muscular nerve (*the motor point*). The electrical pulse required is brief, less than a millisecond, and is most effectively induced by rapidly alternating (faradic) current. *If there has been muscle denervation*, an electrical pulse of several milliseconds induced by a constant electrical (galvanic) stimulus is required to produce the same response. This change, in which the galvanic stimulus remains effective after the faradic one has failed, was the basis of the "Erb reaction" of degeneration, and varying degrees of this change were formerly plotted in the form of strength-duration curves. For decades, this was the standard electrical method for evaluating denervation of muscle. Although still valid, it was replaced by nerve conduction studies and by the needle electrode examination. The latter test, based on the sherringtonian concept of the "motor unit" described in Chap. 3, is accomplished by the insertion into muscle of needle electrodes to measure spontaneous and voluntarily evoked muscle fiber activity. The terms *electromyography* and *electromyogram* were used originally to describe the needle electrode examination but are now a common shorthand designation for the entire electrodiagnostic evaluation, including the *nerve conduction studies.*

Studies of Nerve Conduction

The main laboratory technique for the study of peripheral nerve function involves the transcutaneous stimulation of motor or sensory nerves and recording of the elicited action potentials in the muscle (CMAP) and the sensory nerve action potential (SNAP). The results of these *motor and sensory nerve conduction studies*, expressed as amplitudes, conduction velocities, and distal latencies, yield certain quantitative information and additional qualitative observations regarding the waveform and dispersion of electrical neural and muscular impulses.

Hodes and coworkers, in 1948, were the first to describe nerve conduction studies in patients, and the techniques used currently are not much changed. An accessible nerve is stimulated through the skin by surface electrodes, using a stimulus that is large enough to recruit (cause a discharge in) all the available nerve fibers. The resulting action potential is recorded by electrodes on the skin (1) over the muscle distally in the case of motor fibers stimulated in a mixed or motor nerve (CMAP), (2) over the nerve more distally, using antidromic techniques for sensory nerve conduction studies (this has technical advantages over orthodromic techniques), and (3) over the nerve more proximally for mixed (sensory and motor) nerve conduction studies (Fig. 45-3). These techniques are the ones used most often in clinical work. An alternative but much more demanding technique uses "near-nerve" needle electrodes to record action potentials as they course through the nerve. The main characteristics of the conventional nerve conduction studies are described below.

Distal (Terminal) Latencies, Conduction Times, and Conduction Velocities

The conduction times from the most distal stimulating electrode to the recording site over a muscle, in milliseconds, as determined by the latency from the stimulus artifact to the onset and to the peak of the CMAP, are termed the *distal* (or terminal) and *peak* motor latencies, respectively (see Fig. 45-3). The former is the one used more often as a reflection of conduction time in routine work. A stimulus may then be applied to the nerve at a second

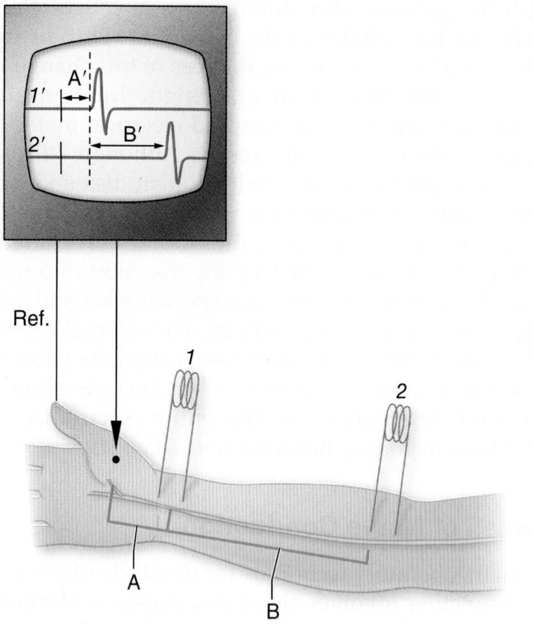

Figure 45-3. The median nerve is stimulated percutaneously (1) at the wrist and (2) in the antecubital fossa with the resultant compound muscle action potential recorded as the potential difference between a surface electrode over the thenar eminence (*arrow*) and a reference electrode (*Ref.*) more distally. Sweep 1′ on the display depicts the stimulus artifact followed by the compound muscle action potential. The distal latency, A′, is the time from the stimulus artifact to the take-off phase of the compound muscle action potential and corresponds to conduction over distance A. The same is true for sweep 2′, where stimulation is at 2 and the time from the artifact to the response is A′ + B′. The maximum motor conduction velocity over segment B is calculated by dividing distance B by the time B′.

site more proximally (or if recording electrodes can be placed more proximally in the case of sensory fibers), and a conduction time can be measured over a longer segment of nerve. When the distance (in millimeters) between the two sites of stimulation is divided by the difference in conduction times (in milliseconds), one obtains a *conduction velocity* (in meters per second), which describes the maximal velocity of propagation of the action potentials in the largest-diameter and fastest-conducting nerve fibers. These velocities in normal subjects vary from a minimum of 40 or 45 m/s to a maximum of 65 to 75 m/s, depending upon which nerve is studied (e.g., slower in the legs than in the arms; Table 45-1). Values are lower in infants, reaching the adult range by the age of 2 to 4 years, and declining again slightly with advancing age. Conduction velocity also is diminished with exposure to cold, a potentially important factor if these recordings are taken when the patient's skin is cool; consequently, measurement of skin temperature is routinely done prior to performing the nerve conduction tests.

Normal values have been established for distal latencies from the usual sites of stimulation on various mixed nerves to the appropriate muscles. Stimulating the median nerve at the wrist, for example (see electrode 1 and segment A in Fig. 45-3), has a latency for motor conduction through the carpal tunnel to the median-innervated thenar muscles of less than approximately 4.5 ms in healthy adults. Similar normal values have been compiled for orthodromic and antidromic sensory conduction velocities and for distal latencies in all the main peripheral nerves (see Table 45-1).

Disease processes that preferentially injure the fastest-conducting, large-diameter fibers in peripheral nerves reduce the maximal conduction velocity because the remaining thinner fibers conduct more slowly. In most neuropathies, all of the axons are affected either by a fairly uniform "dying-back" phenomenon or by wallerian degeneration as described in Chap. 46, and nerve conduction velocities are then less informative. This is true, for example, in typical alcoholic-nutritional, carcinomatous, uremic, diabetic, and other metabolic neuropathies, in which conduction velocities range from the low-normal range to mildly slowed. In these "axonal neuropathies," the motor and sensory nerve amplitudes are diminished.

By contrast, demyelinating neuropathies of the acute (Guillain-Barré) and chronic types, such as chronic inflammatory, metachromatic leukodystrophy, and the common type of Charcot-Marie-Tooth disease, show marked slowing of conduction and, in the case of the acquired demyelinating diseases, there is also dispersion of the motor action potential and a highly characteristic conduction block (see later).

Amplitude of the Compound Muscle Action Potential

In addition to the study of distal latency and conduction velocity, the amplitude of the evoked muscle action potential (CMAP) yields valuable information about peripheral nerve function. These amplitudes are a semi-quantitative measure of the number of nerve fibers that respond to a maximal stimulus (and of the innervated volume of muscle). Demyelinative lesions affecting the large, fast-conducting fibers are detected by the finding of differential slowing among various caliber fibers that causes a dispersal of the CMAP response. Reduction in motor and sensory amplitudes is a more specific and sensitive indicator of axonal loss than is slowing of conduction velocity or prolongation of distal latencies. Conversely, prolonged distal latencies and slowed motor conduction velocities, as well as conduction blocks and dispersed responses (described below), are the hallmarks of demyelinative lesions. Table 45-1 shows the range of normal amplitudes for the CMAPs that are elicited by stimulation of the main motor nerves.

It is usually possible to obtain a reliable motor conduction study as long as some functioning nerve fibers remain intact. The conduction velocities then reflect the status of the surviving axons, and the velocity may be normal or nearly so despite widespread axonal degeneration. This is most apparent following incomplete transection of a nerve; the maximal motor conduction velocity may be normal in the few remaining fibers, although the muscle involved is almost paralyzed and the compound muscle potential recorded from it is very low.

Table 45-1

NORMAL VALUES FOR REPRESENTATIVE NERVE CONDUCTION VALUES AT VARIOUS SITES OF STIMULATION (MEAN VALUES ± 2 SD FOR ADULTS 16 TO 65 YEARS OF AGE)

Motor Nerve Conduction Studies

NERVE	DISTAL STIMULATION SITE	OTHER STIMULATION SITES	RECORDING SITE	ONSET LATENCY (ms)	AMP (mv)	CV (M/S)	DISTANCE (cm)	F-WAVE LATENCY (ms)
Median	Wrist	Elbow	APB	<4.2	>4.4	>49	6–8	<31
Ulnar	Wrist	BG, AG	ADM	<3.4	>6.0	>49	5.5–7.5	<32
Radial	Forearm	Elbow, SG	EIP	<5.2	>4.0	>50	10	NA
Peroneal	Ankle	BFH, AFH	EDB	<5.8	>2.0	>42	6–11	<58
Peroneal	BFH	AFH	TA	<3.0	>5.0	>42	10	NA
Tibial	Ankle	PF	AH	<6.5	>3.0	>41	6–8	<59[a]

Sensory Nerve Conduction Studies[b]

NERVE	DISTANCE STIMULATION SITES	RECORDING SITE	ONSET LATENCY (ms)	PEAK LATENCY (ms)	AMP (μv)	CV (M/S)	DISTANCE (cm)
Median	Wrist	Dig2	<2.5	<3.5	>20	>52	13
Ulnar	Wrist	Dig5	<2.1	<3.0	>15	>52	11
Radial	Forearm	Wrist	<1.9	<2.8	>20	>48	10
Sural	Calf	Ankle	<3.2	<4.4	>6	>42	14

ADM, adductor digiti minimi; AFH, above fibular head; AG, above ulnar groove; AH, abductor hallucis; APB, abductor pollicis brevis; BFH, below fibular head; BG, below ulnar groove; EDB, extensor digitalis brevis; EIP, extensor indicis proprius; PF, popliteal fossa; SG, spiral groove; TA, anterior tibialis.

[a]Tibial H reflexes: latency <35 ms; side-to-side difference <1.4 ms.

[b]Sensory studies are performed antidromically; amplitudes are measured from baseline to negative peak of nerve potential.

Sensory Nerve Action Potentials

When motor fibers in a mixed nerve are stimulated, an amplified CMAP of many hundreds of microvolts can easily be recorded from electrodes on the skin over the muscle. However, when one attempts to measure sensory potentials, where activity must be recorded from nerve fibers themselves, the "amplification" provided by many motor units is not available and electronic amplification is required. Sensory potentials are sometimes very small or absent even when powerful computer-averaging techniques are used, and sensory conduction measurements may then be difficult to determine. Table 45-1 gives the range of normal values for sensory nerve action potential amplitudes and velocities.

Conduction Block

By stimulating a motor nerve at multiple sites along its course, it is possible to demonstrate segments in which conduction is partially "blocked" or is differentially slowed. From such data one infers the presence of a multifocal demyelinative process in motor nerves. This contrasts with the findings in certain of the inherited and metabolic demyelinating neuropathies, in which all parts of the nerve fiber are altered to more or less the same degree, i.e., there is uniform slowing and reduction in amplitude and no conduction block.

As a technical matter, conduction block is demonstrated by a reduction in the amplitude of the CMAP elicited from the proximal site along the motor nerve, compared to stimulation at a distal site. Generally, a 40 percent reduction in amplitude over a short distance of nerve, or 50 percent over a longer distance, qualifies as a block, one possible exception being along the tibial nerve, in which there is some degree of physiologic dispersion (it is also difficult to stimulate all the motor nerve fibers of this nerve in obese patients); therefore a slight drop in amplitude over the length of the nerve is normally expected. It is important to be sure that any reduction in amplitude along the course of the nerve is not solely a result of dispersion of the waveform. The presence of a conduction block can also be inferred from the finding of poor recruitment of muscle action potentials and the concurrent absence of active denervation (see further on). The finding of conduction block is a main feature of a number of acquired immune demyelinating neuropathies including Guillain-Barré syndrome, chronic inflammatory demyelinating neuropathy, and multifocal conduction block associated with the G_{M1} antibody, which are discussed in Chap. 46.

Focal conduction block may be caused simply by nerve compression at certain common sites (fibular head, across the elbow, flexor retinaculum at the wrist, etc.) rather than to an intrinsic disease of the peripheral nerves. *Focal compression of nerve*, as occurs in these entrapment syndromes, produces localized slowing or blocks in conduction, perhaps because of segmental demyelination, only at the site of compression. The demonstration of such localized changes of conduction affords ready confirmation of nerve entrapment; for example, if the distal latency of the median nerve (see *A*, Fig. 45-3) exceeds 4.5 ms while that of the ulnar nerve remains normal, compression of the median nerve in the carpal tunnel is likely. Similar focal slowing or partial block of conduction may be recorded from the ulnar nerve at the elbow and from the peroneal nerve at the fibular head.

Electrodiagnostic Studies of Nerve Roots and Spinal Segments (Late Responses, Blink Responses, Evoked Responses)

H Reflex

Information about the conduction of impulses through the proximal segments of a nerve is provided by the study of the H reflex and the F wave. In 1918, Hoffmann, after whom the H reflex was named, showed that submaximal stimulation of mixed motor–sensory nerves, insufficient to produce a direct motor response, nonetheless induces a muscle contraction (H wave) after a latency that is far longer than that of the direct motor response. This reflex is based on the activation of afferent fibers from muscle spindles (the same axons that conduct the afferent volley of the tendon reflex), and the long delay reflects the cumulative time required for the impulses to reach the spinal cord via the sensory fibers, synapse with anterior horn cells, and to be transmitted along motor fibers to the muscle (see Fig. 3-1). Thus the H reflex is the electrical representation of the tendon reflex circuit and is a useful measure because the impulse traverses both the posterior and anterior spinal roots. The H reflex is particularly helpful in the diagnosis of S1 radiculopathy and of polyradiculopathies. Its status generally parallels that of the clinically elicited Achilles reflex. However, it is difficult to obtain an H reflex from nerves other than the tibial. Stimuli of increasing frequency but low intensity cause a progressive depression and finally obliteration of H waves. The latter phenomenon has been used to study spasticity, rigidity, and cerebellar ataxia, in which there are differences in the frequency-depression curves of H waves. In parallel with the Achilles tendon reflex, the H-reflex is transiently obliterated in spinal shock (see Chap. 44).

F Response (Wave)

The F response, so named because it was initially elicited in the feet, was first described by Magladery and McDougal in 1950. It is evoked by a supramaximal stimulus of a mixed motor–sensory nerve. After a latency that is longer than for the direct motor response (latencies of 28 to 32 ms in arms, 40 to 59 ms in legs), a second small muscle action potential is recorded. This F wave is the result of the impulses that travel antidromically in motor fibers to the anterior horn cells, a small number of which are activated and produce an orthodromic response that is recorded in a distal muscle. The F response is a more reliable test than the H wave of proximal motor nerve and root conduction in that the F wave traverses only the ventral root and can be elicited from a number of muscles. The combination of a normal F response and an absent H reflex is found in diseases of sensory nerves and roots. Both of these "late responses" find their main use as corroborative tests that are interpreted in the context of the entire nerve conduction examination (see Wilbourn). As with the H reflex, the F wave may be absent in the state of spinal shock (see Chap. 44). Table 45-1 gives the normal F wave response latencies.

Blink Responses

This special nerve conduction test is not in frequent clinical use but it serves a purpose in the diagnosis of certain demyelinating neuropathies and in any process that affects the trigeminal or facial nerve. The supraorbital (or infraorbital) nerve is stimulated transcutaneously and the reflex closure of both orbicularis oculi muscles is recorded with surface electrodes. Two CMAP bursts are observed: the first (R1) appears ipsilaterally 10 ms after the stimulus and the second (R2), ipsilaterally at 30 ms and contralaterally up to 5 ms later. The amplitudes of the responses vary considerably and are not in themselves clinically important. The first response is not visible as a muscular contraction but may serve some preparatory function by shortening the blink reflex delay. R1 is mediated by an oligosynaptic pontine circuit consisting of one to three neurons located in the vicinity of the main sensory nucleus; R2 uses a broader and less-well-defined reflex pathway in the pons. It has been established that R1 and R2 are generated by the same facial motor neurons.

The elicitation of blink reflexes establishes the integrity of the afferent trigeminal nerve, the efferent facial nerve, and the interneurons in the pons (R1) and caudal medulla (related to the bilateral R2 response). The test may also be helpful in identifying a demyelinating neuropathy when the facial and oropharyngeal muscles are affected and those of the limbs are relatively spared, thereby leaving conventional nerve studies normal. In such cases, the blink responses are delayed ipsilaterally and contralaterally as a result of conduction block in the proximal facial nerve. Direct facial nerve stimulation often fails to demonstrate this block because only the distal segment of the nerve is amenable to study. Although the blink responses are rarely necessary for diagnosis, most patients with hereditary neuropathy have blink response abnormalities. In Bell's palsy there is a delay or absence of R1 and R2 responses only on the affected side. Large acoustic neuromas (vestibular schwannomas) may interfere with the afferent trigeminal portion of the pathway and give rise to abnormal responses on the affected side. Diseases of the brainstem have yielded inconsistent responses. It is noteworthy that the test is normal in patients with trigeminal neuralgia.

Segmental Motor, Cranial, and Somatosensory Evoked Potentials (See also Chap. 2)

These techniques find use in diseases that affect the spinal roots and in studying central pathways.

By applying a magnetic stimulus, which induces an electrical impulse, or by a directly delivered electrical stimulus over the lower cervical or lumbar spine, it is possible to activate the motor (anterior) roots and to measure the time required to elicit a muscle contraction (see review by Cros and Chiappa). These root stimulation tests can be quite uncomfortable for the patient as a result of the contraction of muscles surrounding the stimulation site.

Transcranial magnetic stimulation of the cerebral cortex permits measurement of the latency of muscle contraction after excitation of motor neurons in the cortex. Thus, the integrity of the entire corticospinal system, from the cortical motor neurons through spinal tracts, anterior horn cells, and the peripheral motor nerve can be determined. By combining this technique with the above-described root stimulation, it becomes possible to measure central and peripheral motor conduction times. These forms of motor testing have their main use in the study of multiple sclerosis, amyotrophic lateral sclerosis (ALS), and related disorders.

As described in Chap. 2, by applying repetitive electrical stimuli to a peripheral nerve, the sensory evoked responses can be recorded from sites along the nerve and plexus as well as in central pathways (the thalamus and somatosensory cortex). These somatosensory evoked potential tests find their main use in the diagnosis of multiple sclerosis and in disorders of the sensory nerve roots as discussed in Chaps. 2 and 36. Discussion of magnetic stimulation, collision techniques, and quantitative EMG, among other topics, can be found in several monographs, such as the ones by Kimura, by Aminoff, and by Brown and Bolton.

Repetitive Motor Nerve Stimulation

(See also Chap. 49)

This test of the neuromuscular junction is based on Jolly's observation in 1895 that in myasthenia gravis the strength of muscular contractions progressively declines in response to a train of stimuli. By adjusting the amplitude of a stimulus over a nerve to the supramaximal range, a maximal CMAP may be obtained for each stimulus. With repeated stimuli, each response will have the same waveform and amplitude until normal fatigue supervenes. In a healthy individual, a muscular response follows each stimulus with rates of stimulation up to 25 per second for periods of 60 s or more before a decrement of the CMAP appears. In certain disorders, notably myasthenia gravis, a train of 4 to 10 stimuli at rates of 2 to 5 per second (optimally 2 to 3 per second), the amplitude of the motor potentials decreases and then, after four or five further stimuli, may increase slightly (Fig. 45-4*A*). A progressive reduction in amplitude is most likely to be found in proximal muscles, but these are not easily stimulated for which reason the locations most commonly used for clinical testing are the accessory nerve in the posterior triangle of the neck (trapezius), the ulnar nerve (hypothenar muscle), the median nerve at the wrist (thenar muscle), and the facial nerve (orbicularis oculi muscle). A decrement of 10 percent or more denotes a failure of a proportion of the neuromuscular junctions.

The sensitivity of the procedure is improved by first exercising the tested muscle for 30 to 60 s; a form of posttetanic potentiation. (The full procedure consists of testing the muscle with a train of stimuli before and immediately after exercise [or maximal voluntary contraction] and at 30-s intervals for several minutes. The posttetanic potentiation partially compensates for the depletion of ACh during slow rates of stimulation; this is followed by a decrease in the excitability of the neuromuscular junction during the approximately 2 to 4 min after exercise.) The induced failure of neuromuscular transmission in myasthenia is similar to the one produced by curare and other nondepolarizing neuromuscular blocking agents, and both cases can be partially corrected with anticholinesterase drugs such as neostigmine and edrophonium. Similar but lesser decremental responses may occur in poliomyelitis, ALS, and certain other diseases of the motor unit or motor nerve, particularly those resulting in the growth of reinnervating nerve twigs.

The Lambert-Eaton myasthenic syndrome, often associated with oat cell carcinoma of the lung, as discussed in Chap. 49, is characterized by a presynaptic blockage of acetylcholine release and produces the opposite defect of neuromuscular transmission to the one recorded in myasthenia gravis. During tetanic stimulation (20- to 50-per-second repetitive stimulation of nerve), the muscle action potentials, which are small or practically absent with the first stimulus, increase in voltage with each successive response until a more nearly normal amplitude is attained (see Fig. 45-4*B*). Exercising the muscle for 10 s before stimulation will cause a similar posttetanic facilitation in patients with the Lambert-Eaton syndrome (200-fold increases are not uncommon). A less important decremental response to slow stimulation may occur, but it is difficult to discern because of the greatly diminished amplitude of the initial responses. Neostigmine has little effect on this phenomenon, but it is reversed by guanidine and 3,4-diaminopyridine, which stimulate the presynaptic release of ACh. The effects of botulinum toxin and of aminoglycoside antibiotics are similar, i.e., being active at the presynaptic membrane, they produce an incremental response at high rates of stimulation.

The single-fiber EMG, discussed in a later section, is an even more sensitive method of detecting failure of the neuromuscular junction.

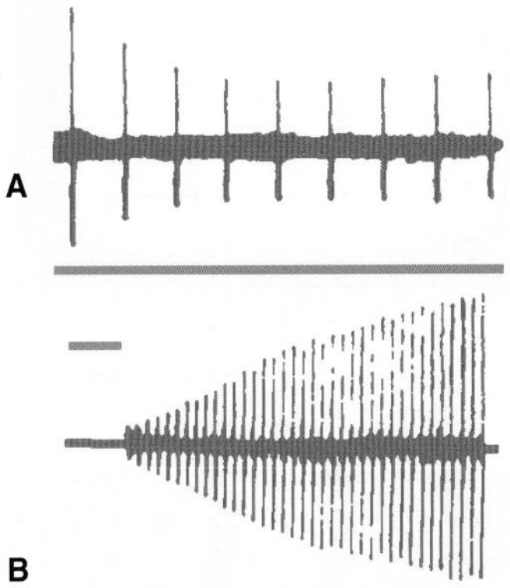

Figure 45-4. Compound action potentials evoked in hypothenar muscles by electrical stimulation of the ulnar nerve at the wrist. *A*. Patient with myasthenia gravis—typical pattern of decrement in first four responses followed by slight increment. At this rate of stimulation (4 per second), the decrement in response does not continue to zero. *B*. Patient with Lambert-Eaton syndrome and oat cell carcinoma—typical marked increase toward normal amplitude with rapid repetitive stimulation (20 per second). Horizontal calibration: 250 ms.

Needle Examination of Muscle (Electromyography)

This technique requires the use of monopolar or concentric bipolar needle electrodes, which are inserted into the body of the muscle to record the electrical activity generated by contraction. With concentric electrodes, the tip of the wire that runs in the hollow of the needle is in proximity to many muscle fibers belonging to several different overlapping motor units; this is the active recording electrode. The shaft of the needle, in contact over most of its length with intercellular fluid and many other muscle fibers, serves as the reference electrode. Monopolar electrodes use the uninsulated needle tip as the active electrode, while the reference electrode may be another monopolar needle electrode placed elsewhere in subcutaneous tissue or a surface electrode on the skin overlying the muscle. Patients almost invariably find this portion of the test uncomfortable and should be prepared by a description of the procedure. Rapid and brief needle insertion by the skilled examiner makes the test more tolerable.

As the electrical impulse travels along the surface of the muscle toward the recording electrode, a positive potential is recorded on the oscilloscope, i.e., the recorded signal is deflected downward by convention (at *A* in Fig. 45-5). When the depolarized zone moves under the recording electrode, it becomes relatively negative and the beam is deflected upward (at *B*). As the depolarized zone continues to move along the sarcolemma, away from the recording electrode, the current begins to flow outward through the membrane toward the distant depolarized region, and the recording electrode becomes relatively positive again (at C). There is then a return to the resting isopotential position. The net result is a triphasic action potential, as in Fig. 45-5. This configuration is typical of the firing of a single fiber.

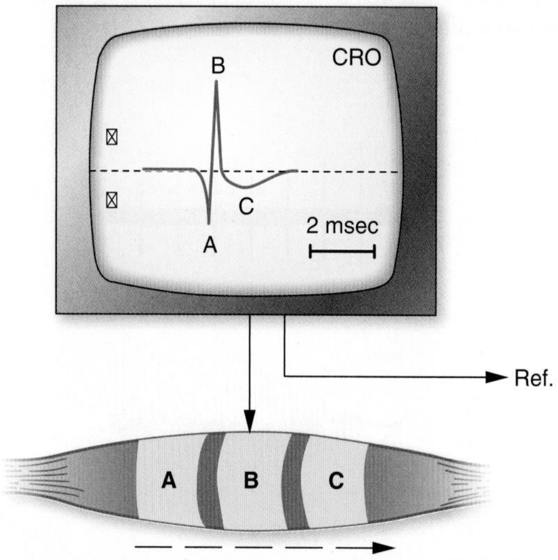

Figure 45-5. The shaded area represents the zone of the action potential, which is negative to all other points on the fiber surface. It is shown at three points in its course (*from left to right*) along the fiber. At each point, the correspondingly lettered portion of the triphasic muscle action potential displayed on the display screen reflects the potential difference between the active (*vertical arrow*) and reference (*Ref.*) electrodes. Polarity in this and subsequent figures is negative upward as depicted. The time calibration is on the screen.

The electrical activity of various muscles is recorded both at rest and during active contraction by the patient. As indicated earlier, muscle fibers do not normally discharge until activated together in motor unit activity. This involves the almost simultaneous contraction of all the muscle fibers innervated by a single anterior horn cell. Although the typical configuration of a motor unit potential (MUP) is triphasic, up to 10 percent of normal MUPs consist of four or more phases (*polyphasic potentials*); however, an excess of polyphasic potentials beyond this is pathologic.

Normal muscle in the resting state should be electrically silent; the small tension spoken of as muscle tone has no EMG equivalent. There are, however, two closely related types of normal spontaneous activities and another that is induced by the insertion of the needle itself. One is a low-amplitude, 10- to 20-μV monophasic (negative) potential of very brief (0.5 to 1 ms) duration. These represent single or synchronized miniature end plate potentials (MEPPs) because of the small number of ACh quanta that are being released all the time. They are normally sparse but are most evident when the recording needle electrode is placed near a motor endplate ("endplate noise"). Fortuitous placement of the needle electrode very close to or in contact with the endplate gives rise to a second type of normal spontaneous activity. That is characterized by irregularly discharging high-frequency (50- to 100-Hz) biphasic spike discharges, 100 to 300 μV in amplitude (i.e., large enough to cause an isolated muscle action potential). These potentials have been termed *endplate spikes* and represent discharges of single muscle fibers excited by spontaneous activity in nerve terminals. They must be distinguished from fibrillation potentials (see later). Finally, insertion of the needle electrode into the muscle injures and mechanically stimulates a number of fibers, causing a burst of potentials of short duration (300 ms). This is referred to as normal *insertional activity*, but the extent of this activity is greatly raised in certain pathologic states as noted below.

When a muscle is voluntarily contracted, the action potentials of motor units begin to appear. One can observe a pattern of force build up by watching the progressive recruitment of MUPs; the initial ones, representing smaller motor units, firing at rates of 5 to 10 per second. With increased force of contraction, there is recruitment of larger, previously inactive motor units as well as an increased rate of firing (40 to 50 per second; Fig. 45-6*A*). Because individual MUPs can no longer be distinguished during maximal voluntary contraction, this activity is referred to as a *complete interference pattern* (Fig. 45-6*A*, *right*). This is seen not only as a summated signal pattern but is also heard as a mixed high-frequency clicking when the electrical activity is made audible. As muscles relax, an increasing number of units drop out. If a muscle is weakened by denervation or if electrical conduction is blocked, there obviously will be fewer MUPs, but the firing rate is still rapid (*reduced recruitment*; see

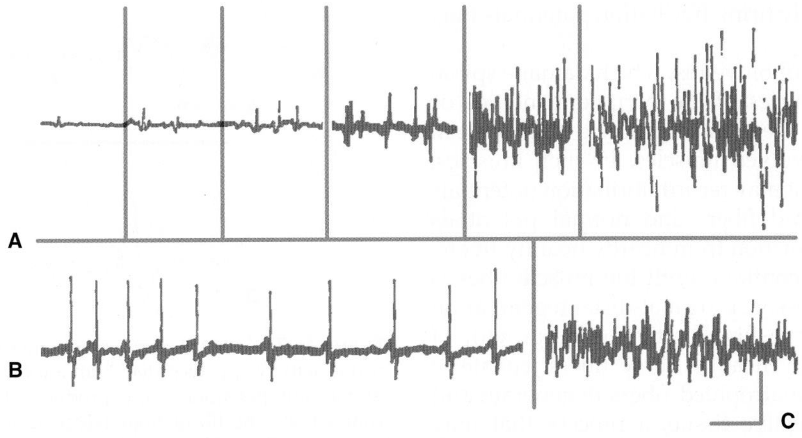

Figure 45-6. Patterns of motor unit recruitment. *A*. Normal. With each increment of voluntary effort, more and larger units are brought into play until, with full effort at the extreme right, a complete "interference pattern" is seen in which single units are no longer recognizable. *B*. After denervation, only a single motor unit is recorded despite maximal effort. It is seen to fire repetitively. *C*. With myopathic diseases, a normal number of units are recruited on minimal effort, though the amplitude of the pattern is reduced. Calibrations: 50 ms (horizontal) and 1 mV in *A* and *B*; 200 μV in C (vertical).

Fig. 45-6*B*). In contrast, with poor voluntary effort and with upper motor neuron lesions, the MUPs fire in decreased numbers, at slower rates, and often in an irregular pattern (termed *poor activation*).

In the usual EMG examination, a plan for the study is made based on detailed knowledge of muscular innervation and focusing on the regions affected by weakness. In some patients, as in those with motor neuron diseases or polymyositis, a wider sampling of muscles is required to detect changes in asymptomatic regions.

The Abnormal Electromyogram

Clinically important deviations from the normal EMG include (1) increased or decreased activity upon insertion of the needle; (2) the occurrence of abnormal "spontaneous" activity during the relaxed state (fibrillation potentials, positive sharp waves, fasciculation potentials, cramp potentials, myotonic discharges, myokymic potentials); (3) abnormalities in the amplitude, duration, and shape of single MUPs; (4) a decrease in the number of MUPs and changes in their firing pattern; (5) variation in amplitude and number of phases of MUPs during voluntary contraction; and (6) the demonstration of special phenomena, such as electrical silence during shortening of the muscle (physiologic contracture and states of continuous muscle fiber activity).

Insertional Activity At the moment the needle is inserted into muscle, there is a brief burst of action potentials that ceases once the needle is stable, provided that it is not in a position to irritate a nerve terminal. Increased insertional activity is seen in most instances of denervation as well as in many forms of primary muscle disease and in disorders that dispose to muscle cramps. In cases of advanced denervation or myopathy, in which muscle fibers have been largely replaced by connective tissue and fat, insertional activity may be decreased and there is a palpable increase in the mechanical resistance to the insertion of the needle.

Abnormal "Spontaneous" Activity With the muscle at rest, spontaneous activity of single muscle fibers and of motor units, known respectively as *fibrillation* potentials and *fasciculation* potentials, is abnormal. The two phenomena are often confused. *Fibrillation* is the spontaneous contraction of a *single muscle fiber*. It occurs when the muscle fiber has lost its nerve supply and is ordinarily not visible through the skin (but may be visible in the tongue). *Fasciculation* represents the spontaneous firing of an entire motor unit, causing contraction of a group of muscle fibers, and may be visible through the skin. The irregular firing of a number of motor units, seen as a rippling of the skin, is called *myokymia*.

Fibrillation Potentials Destruction of a motor neuron or interruption of its axon causes the distal part of the axon to degenerate, a process that takes several days or more. The muscle fibers formerly innervated by the branches of the dead axon—that is, the motor unit—are thereby disconnected from the nervous system. By mechanisms that are still obscure, the chemosensitive region of the sarcolemma at the motor endplate "spreads" after denervation to involve the entire surface of the muscle fiber. Then, 10 to 25 days after death of the axon, the denervated fibers develop spontaneous activity; each fiber contracts at its own rate and without relation to the activity of neighboring fibers. This spontaneous activity is associated with a random conglomeration of brief di- or triphasic fibrillation potentials (Fig. 45-7*A*) having a duration of 1 to 5 ms and rarely exceeding 300 μV in amplitude. When brief spontaneous fibrillation potentials of this sort are observed firing regularly at two or three different locations (outside the endplate zone) of a resting muscle, one may conclude that the fibers are denervated. Usually, fibrillation potentials discharge at an almost regular rate. In some early lesions (less than

6 to 8 weeks), irregularly firing fibrillation potentials may be observed.

Diseases such as poliomyelitis, which damage spinal motor neurons, or injuries of the peripheral nerves or anterior spinal roots, frequently produce only partial denervation of the involved muscles. In such muscles, one electrode placement may record fibrillation potentials at rest from denervated fibers and normal potentials during voluntary contraction from nearby healthy fibers. Fibrillation potentials continue until the muscle fiber is reinnervated by progressive proximal-distal regeneration of the interrupted nerve fiber or by the outgrowth of new axons from nearby healthy nerve fibers (collateral sprouting), or until the atrophied fibers degenerate and are replaced by connective tissue, a process that may take many years. In addition, fibrillation potentials may take the form of positive sharp waves, i.e., spontaneous, initially positive diphasic potentials of longer duration and slightly greater amplitude than the spikes of fibrillation potentials (see Fig. 45-7*A*).

Fibrillation potentials, while characteristic of neurogenic denervation, are not altogether specific; for example, they are seen in muscle diseases such as polymyositis and inclusion body myopathy which presumably damage the muscle fiber and make its membrane electrically unstable.

Fasciculation Potentials As stated earlier, a fasciculation is the spontaneous or involuntary contraction of a motor unit or part of a motor unit. Such contractions may cause a visible dimpling or twitching under the skin, although ordinarily they are of insufficient force to move a joint. Large distal fasciculations can briefly displace a finger or toe. They occur irregularly and infrequently, and prolonged inspection of the skin overlying a muscle may be necessary to detect them. The accompanying electrical form of an individual fasciculation potential is relatively constant. Typically, a fasciculation potential will have 3 to 5 phases (i.e., they are "polyphasic" as described later, in contrast to normal biphasic muscle activity), a duration of 5 to 15 ms (longer than normal but somewhat less in the facial muscles), and an amplitude of several millivolts (see Fig. 45-7*B*). Fasciculation potentials are evidence of motor nerve fiber irritability. Thus, the combination of fibrillations and fasciculations indicates active denervation combined with more chronic reinnervation of muscle.

The precise source of fasciculation is still contested. Forster and colleagues challenged the original belief that the discharge originated in anterior horn cells by demonstrating that fasciculations persisted after nerve block in ALS and ceased only with the appearance of fibrillation potentials, signifying wallerian (axonal) degeneration. These observations favored a distal site of generation. Other physiologic and pharmacologic evidence pointed to the first segment of the motor axon, or to the distal axon, or even to the motor point (the site of insertion of the nerve into muscle), involving elements of the postsynaptic muscle membrane (particularly in the case of benign fasciculations) as the source of the spontaneous electrical activity. It seems that several regions of the axon are capable of spontaneous impulse generation, depending on the underlying disease. Most of the diseases that produce fasciculations involve the anterior horn cell or the motor root, but more distal sites in the motor axon are spontaneously active in cases of nerve compression and polyneuropathy.

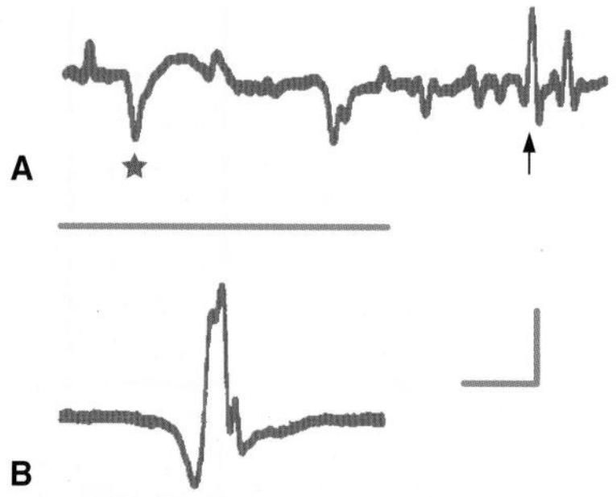

Figure 45-7. *A*. Fibrillations and positive sharp waves. This spontaneous activity was recorded from a totally denervated muscle—no motor unit potentials were produced by attempts at voluntary contraction. The fibrillations (*above arrow*) are 1 to 2 ms in duration, 100 to 300 mV in amplitude, and largely negative (upward) in polarity following an initial positive deflection. A typical positive sharp wave is seen above the star. *B*. Fasciculation. This spontaneous motor unit potential was recorded from a patient with amyotrophic lateral sclerosis. It has a serrated configuration and it fired once every second or two. Calibrations: 5 ms (horizontal) and 200 mV in *A*; 1 μV in *B* (vertical).

Occasional fasciculation potentials, particularly in the calves, hands, and periocular or paranasal muscles, occur in many normal persons. They can be almost constant for days or weeks on end, or even for years in some individuals, without weakness or wasting; therefore they need not be taken as evidence of disease ("benign fasciculations"). Certain quantitative features of fasciculations, such as brief duration and a consistent pattern and location of firing, favor benign over pathologic discharges. Shivering induced by low temperature and twitchings associated with low serum calcium levels are other forms of fasciculatory activity.

Fasciculation potentials occur with great frequency in chronic, slowly advancing, destructive diseases of the anterior horn cells, such as ALS and progressive spinal muscular atrophy. In these diseases, both voluntary MUPs and fasciculation potentials may be of long duration (more than 15 ms) and of increased amplitude, indicating chronic denervation and reinnervation. They are seen often in the early stages of poliomyelitis but only occasionally in the chronic phase of the disease, perhaps because the affected cells die rapidly. When anterior horn cells degenerate once again in older individuals who had had poliomyelitis (postpolio syndrome), fasciculations may return. Occasionally, they are seen in one muscle as a result of a compressive anterior root lesion, such as those caused by a protruded intervertebral disc. Large numbers of axons may be affected in this case, with the result that the fasciculations (or even cramps) may be even more prominent than with disease of anterior horn cells but they are restricted to the territory of innervation of the root or nerve. Fasciculation potentials in lesser numbers are also observed with chronic nerve entrapments, e.g., ulnar neuropathy at the elbow and other peripheral nerve lesions and some polyneuropathies. In all these cases, the damaged neuron or its axon seems to leave intact axons in a state of hyperirritability. The blocking of axon conduction by local anesthesia does not abolish fasciculations, but curare-like drugs do so.

Other Types of Spontaneous and Elicited Electrical Activity (See Chaps. 48 and 50) These various phenomena, including some discussed above, can be classified according to their generating source. The muscle fibers themselves are the source of fibrillations, positive sharp waves, and complex repetitive discharges (CRDs). The motor axons produce fasciculation potentials, myokymic discharges, neuromyotonia, and cramp syndromes; and the central nervous system is the source of complex ensembles of continuous motor activity such as occur in the stiff man syndrome.

The common phenomenon of complex repetitive discharges, referred to in the past as bizarre high-frequency discharges, consists of repetitive spontaneous potentials created by numerous single muscle fibers that fire in near synchrony; there is often an erratic configuration and abrupt starting and stopping of the discharges. They are seen in some myopathies, in hypothyroidism, and in certain denervating disorders, and are a mark of chronicity (lesions more than 6 months old). High-frequency coupling of action potentials into doublets, triplets, or higher multiples of single units, indicating instability in repolarization of the nerve fiber to a muscle, occurs in tetany and in the early stages of myokymia.

Myokymia is a persistent quivering and rippling of muscles at rest (colloquially called "live flesh"). The EMG picture is distinctive. The spontaneously firing MUPs are called *myokymic potentials,* or *discharges* and consist of groups of repetitive discharging units, each firing at its own rate, quasirhythmically, usually several times per second, followed by a briefer period of silence. The small motor unit discharges may occur singly or as doublets, triplets, or multiplets.

The site of generation of this activity has been contested, possibly because it may arise from several sites along the motor nerve. The discharge corresponds to an alteration in the calcium concentration in the microenvironment of the axon. Spontaneous discharges arising in large myelinated fibers have been implicated in the genesis of myokymia; indeed, demyelinating polyneuropathies are among the conditions that give rise to this phenomenon. Myokymia is also caused by peripheral nerve hyperexcitability because of both K channel mutations and antibodies against the channels. This activity may be blocked by lidocaine infusion around the peripheral nerve and may be diminished by carbamazepine or phenytoin. Central forms of myokymia also occur, as in multiple sclerosis; the mechanism is similar to the peripheral form, namely irritation or demyelination of the motor nerve, but in its fascicular (central) course.

Focal and *segmental myokymias* differ in small ways from the generalized form of myokymia with regard to the timing and duration of the discharges. The focal types refer mainly to facial myokymia, seen most often in multiple sclerosis, Guillain-Barré syndrome, large cerebellopontine angle tumors, or compression of the facial nerve by a small aberrant blood vessel, but it may follow any peripheral nerve injury and regeneration. The EMG patterns are complex, either high-frequency (30- to 100-Hz) recurrent bursts or brief lower-frequency bursts. Segmental myokymia is a common occurrence in demyelination and in radiation injuries of the brachial plexus. The EMG bursts tend to be longer and less frequent than in generalized myokymia, and the interburst frequency is highly variable. The origin of these discharges is probably in the distal peripheral nerve, where activity of afferent fibers, possibly via ephaptic transmission, irregularly excites distal motor terminals. *Segmental myokymia* refers to similar activity in the distribution of one or more adjacent motor roots again, usually related in some way to demyelination. This activity persists during sleep and general anesthesia.

The phenomenon of generalized *myotonia,* or neuromyotonia denotes a failure of voluntary relaxation of muscle because of sustained firing of the muscle membrane (see Chaps. 48 and 50), is characterized by high-frequency repetitive discharges generally having a positive sharp waveform. These myotonic discharges wax and wane in amplitude and frequency, producing a "dive-bomber" sound on the audio monitor. The discharges can be elicited mechanically by percussion of the muscle or movement of the needle electrode and are also seen following voluntary contraction or electrical stimulation of the muscle via its motor nerve. The MUPs may appear normal during voluntary contraction, but they are not followed by the silence that normally occurs on relaxation; instead, there is a "prolonged afterdischarge" consisting of long trains of fibrillation-like potentials that may take as long as several minutes to subside (Fig. 45-8*A*). These EMG findings can be seen with any myotonic disorder. If the muscle is activated repeatedly at short intervals, the late discharge becomes briefer and briefer and eventually disappears (see Fig. 45-8*B*), as the patient becomes able to relax the exercised muscle ("warmup" effect).

In *paradoxical myotonia* the myotonia worsens after each of a succession of voluntary contractions. This is the converse of what happens in myotonia congenita (Thomsen disease). As shown by single-fiber EMG studies, myotonia is generated by single muscle fibers and the mechanism of the membrane instability, at least in some forms, seems to involve changes in the chloride conductance. These disorders are discussed in subsequent chapters.

The *cramp-like contracture* of McArdle disease and phosphofructokinase deficiency is associated with electrical silence of contracting muscle. This feature is an important part of the definition of true physiologic muscle contracture (as distinguished from chronic shortening of a muscle and its tendon which, strictly speaking, is a pseudocontracture).

In the *syndrome of continuous muscle fiber activity or Isaacs syndrome* (see Chap. 50), which is a generalized form of myokymia, the EMG discloses high-frequency (up to 300-Hz) repetitive discharges of varying waveforms.

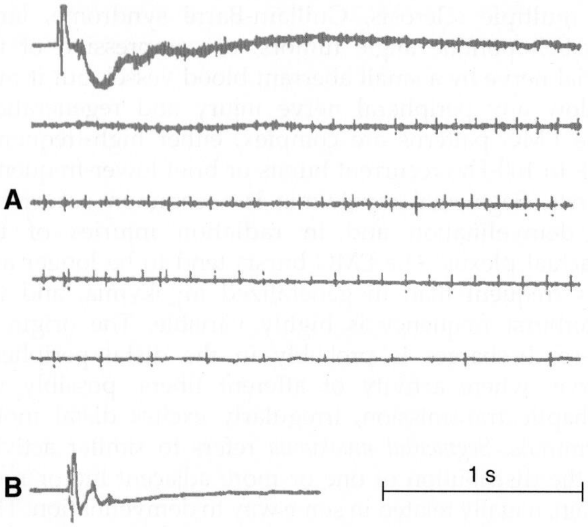

Figure 45-8. *A*. Myotonia congenita (Thomsen disease). The five lines are a continuous record of activity in the biceps brachii following a tap on the tendon. The initial response is within normal limits, but it is followed by a prolonged burst of rapid activity, gradually subsiding over a period of many seconds or minutes. *B*. Same electrode placement as in *A*. Response to the fifth of a series of tendon taps. "Warmup" has occurred, and the characteristic prolonged myotonic activity is no longer evident. (See Chap. 48 for a description of the disease.)

In the *stiff man syndrome*, painful muscle spasms and stiffness are generated by a spinal mechanism; the EMG potentials resemble normal motor units but are abnormal by virtue of continuous firing at rest (see Chap. 50).

Abnormalities in Amplitude, Duration, and Shape of Motor Unit Potentials

Figures 45-9 (schematically) and 45-10 depict the ways in which disease processes affect the motor unit and the appearance of the MUP in the EMG.

Motor Unit Potentials in Denervation Early in the course of denervation, many motor units with functional connections to the spinal cord are unaffected, and although the number of MUPs appearing during contraction is reduced, the configurations of the remaining ones are quite normal. In time, the remaining MUPs often increase in size and in electrical amplitude, perhaps two to three times normal, and become longer in duration and sometimes *polyphasic* (more than four phases).

Such large and sometimes *giant polyphasic potentials* (see Figs. 45-9*C* and 45-10*B*) arise from motor units containing more than the usual number of muscle fibers that are spread out over a greatly enlarged territory within the muscle. Presumably, new nerve twigs have sprouted from nodal points and terminals of undamaged axons and have reinnervated previously denervated muscle fibers, thus adding them to their own motor units. Soon after reinnervation, the MUPs generated will be low in amplitude, extremely prolonged, and polyphasic, findings that constitute a transitional configuration of early reinnervation. These amplitudes disappear as the motor unit is reestablished. Increased amplitude is usually associated with very chronic, proximal axon

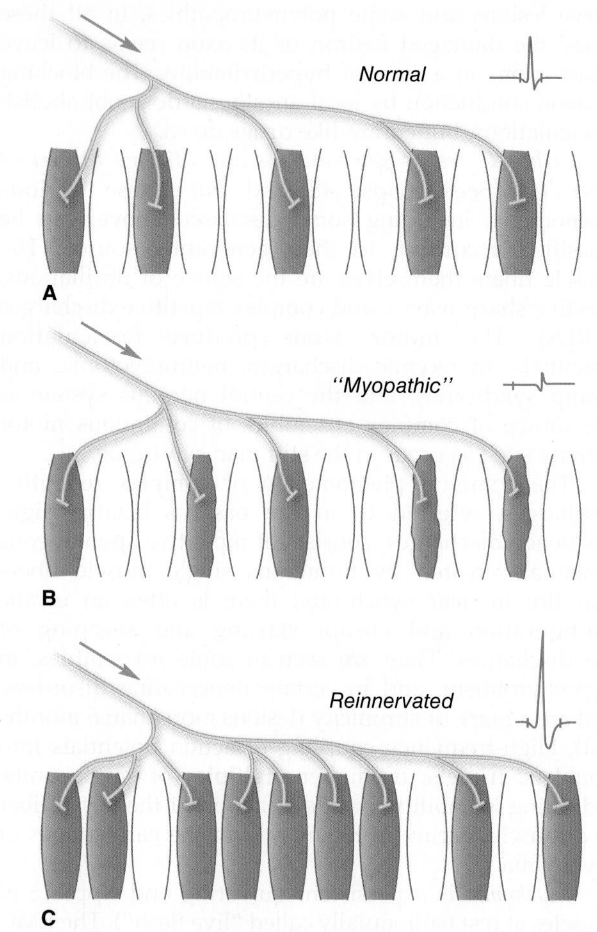

Figure 45-9. The *colored* muscle fibers are functional members of one motor unit, whose axon enters from the upper left and branches terminally to innervate the appropriate muscle fibers. The action potential produced by each motor unit is seen in the upper right: its duration is measured between the two vertical lines. The normal-appearing but *uncolored* fibers belong to other motor units. *A*. Hypothetical situation, with five muscle fibers in the active unit. *B*. In this myopathic unit, only two fibers remain active; the other three (shrunken) were affected by one of the primary muscle diseases. *C*. Four fibers that originally belonged to other motor units and had been denervated are now reinnervated by terminal sprouting from an undamaged axon. Both the motor unit and its action potential are now larger than normal. Note that only under these abnormal circumstances do fibers in the same unit lie next to one another.

loss, for example, with remote poliomyelitis and chronic radiculopathy. These MUPs are to be differentiated from (1) polyphasic potentials of normal duration, which, as has been mentioned, make up as much as 10 percent of the total number of MUPs in normal muscle, and (2) polyphasic MUPs of short duration and low amplitude, which are characteristic of most myopathies and of myasthenia gravis and other disorders of neuromuscular transmission.

The Motor Unit Potential in Myopathy As Fig. 45-9*B* shows, diseases such as polymyositis, the muscular dystrophies, and other myopathies that

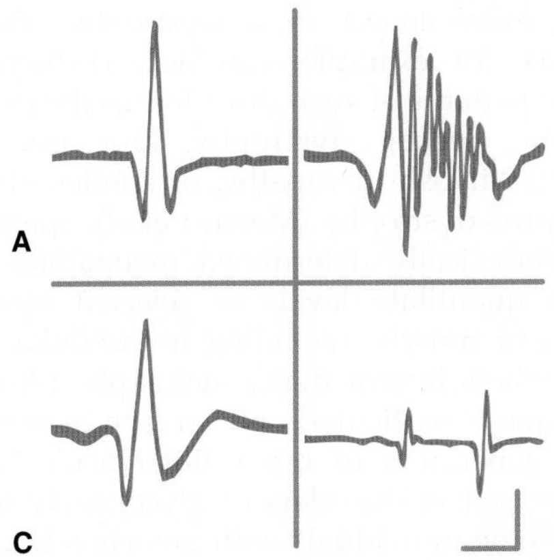

Figure 45-10. Single voluntary motor unit potentials. *A*. Normal. *B*. Prolonged polyphasic potential seen with reinnervation. *C*. "Giant unit"—normally shaped but of much greater amplitude than normal. *D*. Brief, low-amplitude "myopathic" units. Calibrations: 5 ms (horizontal) and 1 mV in *A* and *B*; 5 mV in *C*; 100 mV in *D* (vertical).

randomly destroy muscle fibers or render them nonfunctional, and obviously reduce the population of muscle fibers per motor unit. Therefore, when such a unit is activated, its potential is of lower voltage and shorter duration than normal, and it may also appear polyphasic as the compound MUP becomes fragmented into its constituent single-fiber potentials. Slowing of the propagated muscle fiber action potential in affected muscle fibers also contributes to the changes in the "myopathic" MUP. When most of the muscle fibers are affected, the MUPs are very small and of short duration and are recruited out of proportion to the tension generated, so-called *early recruitment*. Both types of alterations produce a characteristic high-pitched crackling sound from the audio monitor that has been likened to rain falling on a tin roof. They occur in all forms of chronic myopathies. Identical MUP changes are seen occasionally with other processes that cause disintegration of the motor unit, for example, early Guillain-Barré syndrome (because of conduction block along some of the terminal nerve fibers), and rarely with disorders of neuromuscular transmission (myasthenia gravis, other myasthenic syndromes), but they are most characteristic of primary muscle disease.

As mentioned earlier, fibrillation potentials, while typical of denervation, are sometimes seen in the myositides, and the rapidly progressive muscular dystrophies, perhaps because the muscle membrane has been made unstable; in the past the finding was attributed to isolation of a segment of the fiber from its nerve supply. In myasthenia gravis, where transmission of impulse fails at the neuromuscular junction, a single MUP may vary in amplitude during sustained weak contraction and some fibers cease to function. Electromyographic recordings of single muscle fibers belonging to the same motor unit disclose varying interpotential intervals on successive discharges; this phenomenon is called "jitter" and increases to the point of actual block, with deficits in neuromuscular transmission within a motor unit (see below and Chap. 50).

Abnormalities of the Interference Pattern Diseases that reduce the population of functional motor neurons or axons within the peripheral nerve decrease the number of motor units that can be recruited in the affected muscles. The decreased number of motor units available for activation produces a low-amplitude interference pattern with only a few remaining units firing at a moderate to rapid rate. A severe reduction in the interference pattern may result in the recruitment of only a single unit (see Fig. 45-6*B*). Structural damage to nerve, as well as demyelinating block, can produce this pattern of reduced recruitment; indeed, a reduced recruitment pattern coupled with the absence of denervation indicates a conduction block.

If muscle power is reduced in diseases such as polymyositis or muscular dystrophy, in which individual muscle fibers are affected, there may be little or no reduction in the number of motor units available for recruitment until the process is far advanced and entire MUPs have been lost as a result of random loss of all their constituent muscle fibers. Nonetheless, each motor unit will consist of fewer muscle fibers than normal, so more motor units must be activated to reach a certain degree of force. A modest effort can thus produce a full interference pattern despite marked weakness (increased recruitment). Because fewer muscle fibers are firing, the amplitude of the pattern will be reduced from normal. This type of full, highly complex interference pattern of less-than-usual amplitude in the face of dramatic weakness is the hallmark of myopathy (see Fig. 45-6*C*).

Motor Unit Quantification

This experimental technique, developed by McComas and colleagues estimates the size of motor units and is thus exquisitely sensitive to changes of denervation and reinnervation. It is carried out by applying a weak stimulus to a motor nerve or motor point and increasing it gradually as the evoked muscle response is recorded. Each quantal increase in the compound-evoked response is presumed to be caused by the addition of a single motor unit. In reinnervated muscles, the additional units are reduced in number and are abnormally large. The technique is used mainly for the investigation of motor neuron disorders. When a normal number and configuration of motor units is found, it has been helpful in distinguishing benign fasciculations from those of serious diseases.

Single-Fiber Electromyography

This is a special technique for the recording of single-muscle-fiber action potentials that has found utility in measuring muscle fiber density and in detecting so-called jitter in disease of the neuromuscular function, particularly myasthenia gravis. *Fiber density* is an index of the number and distribution of muscle fibers within a motor unit. *Jitter* is the variability of the interpotential interval of successive discharges of two single muscle fibers belonging to the same motor unit. This phenomenon is largely a result of the very slight variability of delay at the branch points in the distal axon and by synaptic delay at the neuromuscular junction, especially in myasthenia gravis where it has found its main clinical use. Fiber density and jitter may, however, also be increased in neuropathic disorders that cause denervation with reinnervation. Both are usually normal or only slightly increased in myopathic disorders.

Testing for jitter is carried out by having the patient voluntarily contract a muscle to the slightest degree possible so as to activate only one motor unit (requiring a great deal of cooperation by the patient) or by stimulating an intramuscular nerve twig (requiring great patience on the part of the examiner). The EMG needle is advanced until two muscle fibers from the same motor unit are recorded. If the oscilloscope sweep is triggered by the firing of the first fiber, a fluctuating latency of the second fiber potential can be seen on the screen as a movement (jitter) of the second peak. The degree of jitter can be quantitated by measuring the interval between the activation of the two muscle fibers (the result of slightly differing lengths of the terminal axons) from which a mean interpeak interval is determined. Approximately 20 fiber pairs are sampled, and an average of the mean consecutive intervals can be derived. In a muscle such as the extensor digitorum communis, the average variation should be no more than 34 ms. The acceptable average is lower for large proximal muscles. Also, in disease of the neuromuscular junction, one muscle fiber in a pair may fail to fire intermittently as a result of a blocking of conduction. Further details of this technique and its clinical applications are discussed by Stålberg and Trontelj.

Imaging of Muscle and Nerve

Imaging techniques—CT, MRI, and ultrasonography—enable one to measure muscle volume and to recognize qualitative changes in muscle structure (see review of DeVisser and Reimers). Such methods are finding some clinical and research use in the diagnosis of disorders of muscle and in gauging the effects of treatment. CT scans of dystrophic muscle show foci of decreased attenuation, representing masses of fat cells. The fatty masses spread gradually from multiple foci and eventually replace muscle fibers. The original shape of the muscle is retained; indeed, an enlarged weak muscle containing mostly fat confirms the clinical impression of pseudohypertrophy. In denervative atrophy, the muscles are obviously small and contain multiple punctate areas of decreased attenuation, which represent interstitial fat. Eventually, large portions of chronically denervated muscle may be replaced by fat. Blood, blood products, and calcium deposits are expressed by increased attenuation in CT. This may be helpful in the diagnosis of muscle trauma, myositis ossificans, and dermato- and polymyositis.

Fat and bone marrow have a high signal intensity in MR images, whereas fascia, ligaments, and cortical bone lack signal intensity. In T1-weighted images, normal muscle has a low signal and dystrophic muscle, a slightly increased signal; in T2-weighted images, dystrophic muscle has a slightly enhanced signal. Given its sensitivity to these dystrophic changes in muscle, MRI is particularly effective in determining the distribution of muscle involvement in a dystrophy. Transverse MR sections, for example, can help distinguish the topographic patterns of such disorders as the proximally predominant Becker dystrophy and the distally predominant Miyoshi myopathy, or subtle subtypes of Emery-Dreifuss dystrophy (Mercuri et al). Spectroscopic MRI in metabolically determined myopathies has the capacity to quantitate levels of selected biochemical constituents of muscle, including intracellular pH and levels of metabolic intermediates such as phosphocreatine. This technique is particularly effective in demonstrating subnormal generation of intracellular acidosis after a limb is exercised in disorders of glycogenolysis and of glycolysis. Some individuals with mitochondrial disease of muscle will demonstrate rapid depletion of energy supplies and profound delays in recovery that can be quantified and used as an end point for treatments.

New magnetic resonance techniques are also being developed that allow the imaging of nerves. This may be an aid in assessing traumatic nerve injury and in demonstrating neuromas, hypertrophy or atrophy of a nerve trunk, as well as neural tumors.

BIOPSIES OF MUSCLE AND NERVE

Muscle Biopsy

Muscle biopsy can be of great diagnostic value, but both surgical and microscopic techniques must be exacting. The muscle chosen for study should be accessible; there should be evidence that it has been affected but not totally destroyed by the disease in question; and it should not have been the site of a recent injection or EMG study, since the trauma of the needles produces focal necrotizing and inflammatory lesions. Muscle biopsy is helpful in distinguishing the following basic disorders in patients with neuromuscular disease.

1. *Denervation atrophy*. Reduction in the size of muscle fibers with an accompanying enlargement of intact motor units (because of collateral reinnervation) and degenerative changes in some fibers are the main changes of denervation atrophy. *Group atrophy* denotes enlarged motor units where all the fibers in the group are reduced to the same size; this is typical of progressive denervation. Normally, the fibers of each motor unit are not clustered, so that when grouping occurs it means that some fibers of a denervated unit have been adopted by an adjacent intact motor unit. This change typifies axonal neuropathies and many spinal cord diseases that affect the anterior horn cell. A related change is particularly well shown in histochemical stains for ATPase, phosphorylase, and oxidases, where the normal mosaic pattern of fiber types is altered. The use of these stains reveals *fiber type grouping*, the most specific histologic evidence of denervation and reinnervation. Here, muscle fibers of similar histochemical type form groups of 15 or more fibers as a result of reinnervation by a single motor neuron. The diagnosis of denervation atrophy

can usually be made from the clinical and EMG examinations; seldom is biopsy necessary for this purpose, but it is still used in cases of possible ALS, for example, where the diagnosis remains uncertain after other testing.

2. *Segmental necrosis of muscle fibers with myophagia and various manifestations of regeneration*. These are the typical changes in idiopathic polymyositis (in combination with infiltrates of inflammatory cells), and infective polymyositis (e.g., in the presence of *Trichinella* or *Toxoplasma*). These changes may also be observed in more limited form in Duchenne and other rapidly progressive muscular dystrophies.
3. *Inflammation and vasculitis*. Lymphocytic infiltration of the endomysium is most characteristic of polymyositis and in dermatomyositis it is predominantly perivascular and perimysial. The lymphocytic infiltrate may be florid in these processes but, as often, it is less intense and scattered. Inclusion body myopathy is characterized by inflammation but has additional diagnostic features. Lesser degrees of inflammation are common in the myopathies associated with Sjögren syndrome, mixed connective tissue disease, and scleroderma. Numerous other processes, including the infections mentioned earlier and some dystrophies (especially the fascioscapulohumeral type)—may be associated with an inflammatory reaction. There is usually acute myofibrillar destruction in regions of maximal lymphocytic infiltration.
4. *Vasculitis*. The muscle is a site of inflammatory vascular destruction in systemic diseases such as polyarteritis nodosa, and for this reason it is often useful to obtain a small sample of muscle adjacent to a nerve biopsy. The finding of a granulomatous myopathy may indicate the presence of systemic sarcoidosis.
5. *Alterations in the protein and histochemical composition of muscle fibers* are shown by special stains for enzymes, glycogen, and structural proteins that are implicated in disease. It has become possible to detect the absence or deficiency of specific structural proteins of the muscle membrane that define each of the muscular dystrophies: dystrophin, sarcoglycan, laminin, dysferlin, and others as discussed in Chap. 48. These tests require rapid freezing (in a cryostat) rather than formalin fixation. Also, a number of enzymatic deficiencies and intrafiber glycogen storage that lead to weakness and muscle fatigue may be detected by appropriate histochemical staining (see Chap. 48).
6. *Unusual changes of muscle fibers*. Included here are sarcoplasmic masses and disorganized ring or serpentine collections of myofibrils and myofilaments (*Ringbinden*) in myotonic dystrophy; glycogen masses in glycogen storage diseases, rods (nemaline), central cores, aggregates of lipid bodies, and other cytoplasmic changes in certain congenital myopathies; and nuclear and cytoplasmic inclusions that characterize but are not isolated to inclusion-body myositis. Application of histochemical methods and electron microscopy are the important techniques in the diagnosis of these disorders. These are discussed in relation to each of these specified diseases in the following chapters.
7. *Abnormalities of mitochondria*. Several distinctive abnormalities are readily visualized in muscle biopsies and are virtually diagnostic of an entire class of mitochondrial diseases. Light microscopy of frozen sections of muscle stained with the Gomori trichrome stain show the main feature, so-called ragged red fibers, which are accumulations of subsarcolemmal mitochondria.
8. *Disorders of the neuromuscular junctions*. Here, an abnormality may be revealed by performing the demanding procedure of motor point biopsy (to include the motor endplate), and the use of electron microscopy and special staining techniques for nerve terminals, cholinesterase, and the outlining of acetylcholine receptors. Myasthenia gravis, botulism, Lambert-Eaton syndrome, and myasthenic syndrome with motor endplate cholinesterase deficiency fall into this category. Biopsy is rarely necessary for the diagnosis of these disorders, but it has added considerably to our understanding of them.

As a rule, the muscle biopsy procedure requires no more than a small cleanly excised block of muscle, 1.0 to 2.0 cm, which is prevented from contracting by a clamp or by tying at full length to a tongue depressor. As an alternative to the standard surgical technique, percutaneous needle biopsies are now being done routinely in neuromuscular clinics and may be adequate for the diagnosis of certain muscle dystrophies and for their study over time and for a number of other muscle diseases and denervation atrophy. Unfortunately, the erratic distribution of lesions in many of the common disorders of muscle lessens the diagnostic yield of all types of biopsies, but in general the needle biopsy is less satisfactory than an open biopsy. The study of the muscle biopsy requires special care in removal, transport, and fixation techniques. These are discussed in detail by Engel (1994b).

Nerve Biopsy

Nerve biopsies are processed for study by conventional histologic methods and by thin-section phase and electron microscopy. These methods, sometimes supplemented by study of teased fiber preparations and immunologic studies, can provide valuable histopathologic data. With ordinary microscopy and staining, one may find evidence of focal inflammation, demyelination, axon destruction, vasculitis, amyloidosis, leprosy, or sarcoidosis. As mentioned in reference to certain guidelines cited below, these procedures are most valuable in the diagnosis of inflammatory, vasculitic, and amyloid neuropathies. In children, the nerve biopsy may reveal the histologic features of metachromatic or globoid leukodystrophy, giant axonopathy, or neuroaxonal dystrophy. However, nerve biopsy is relatively unhelpful in most other polyneuropathies and should be used prudently because the procedure is not without complications, including the occasional occurrence of wound infections, painful stump neuromas, persistent dysesthesias of the lateral foot or heel, and thrombophlebitis. Guidelines given by England and associates from a review of the literature up to 2009, has suggested that nerve biopsy is useful in cases of mononeuropathy multiplex, suspected amyloidosis, and unusual forms of chronic inflammatory demyelinating neuropathy, all the subjects of discussion in Chap. 46, but not clearly useful in nondescript distal peripheral sensorimotor neuropathies.

Representative of the results of nerve biopsies in a neuromuscular clinic is a prospective study of 50 consecutive cases of sural nerve samples reported by Gabriel and colleagues in which nerve biopsy served only to confirm the clinical diagnosis in 70 percent of cases and altered the clinical diagnosis in only 14 percent. Nevertheless, in some instances of idiopathic polyneuropathy that are not clarified by clinical and electrophysiologic testing, and particularly if a treatable chronic inflammatory polyneuropathy is suspected, many neuromuscular experts resort to sural nerve biopsy as a final diagnostic step. Although the sural nerve is typically chosen for biopsy, the superficial peroneal nerve and the adjacent peroneus brevis muscle gives a higher yield in cases of vasculitis (see Collins et al).

In diseases that involve only the motor nerves, it is sometimes useful to sample a fascicle of the superficial radial nerve or the nerve to the extensor digitorum brevis, which may be taken with the muscle itself and leaves little or no clinical deficit. Chronic inflammatory neuropathy and vasculitic neuropathy may be disclosed by this selective biopsy technique when the sural nerve is unaffected. In selected circumstances we have undertaken biopsy of small radicles of upper lumbar roots (L1 or L2) to establish the diagnosis of an infiltrative lymphoma. Little deficit occurs from the removal of nerves from these sites if the procedure is done by an experienced surgeon.

Additional techniques that are used in the study of muscle biopsies and specific pathologic findings that characterize the many individual diseases, of both muscle and peripheral nerve, are discussed in the chapters that follow.

Other Laboratory Tests in the Study of Muscle and Nerve Disease

None of the diagnostic procedures previously described may be taken as an infallible diagnostic index of a specific disease of muscle or nerve. Each procedure is subject to technical error and the findings to misinterpretation. A biopsy specimen may be taken from an unaffected muscle or portion of an affected muscle, and such an error causes the sample to be normal in the face of obvious clinical evidence of disease. This is particularly true of the inflammatory myopathies that affect muscle in heterogeneous and spotty manner.

Rough excision and improper fixation and staining produce artifacts that may be misinterpreted as marks of disease when, in fact, the muscle (and nerve) is microscopically normal. Similarly, EMG study may fail to record fibrillations in obviously denervated muscle, particularly in slowly progressive disorders. Also, in some of the muscles of the feet, fibrillations and fasciculations may be found in normal asymptomatic older individuals (Falck and Alaranta). As in the study of all disease, laboratory data have significance only if evaluated in the light of the clinical findings.

References

Aminoff MJ: *Electrodiagnosis in Clinical Neurology,* 5th ed. New York, Elsevier Churchill Livingstone, 2005.

Brown WE, Bolton CF: *Clinical Electromyography,* 2nd ed. Boston, Butterworth-Heinemann, 1993.

Buchthal F, Kamieniecka Z: Diagnostic yield of quantified electromyography and quantified muscle biopsy in neuromuscular disorders. *Muscle Nerve* 5:265, 1982.

Collins MP, Mendell JR, Periquet MI, et al: Superficial peroneal nerve/peroneus brevis muscle biopsy in vasculitic neuropathy. *Neurology* 55:636, 2000.

Cros D, Chiappa K: Cervical magnetic stimulation. *Neurology* 40:1751, 1990.

Denny-Brown D, Nevin A: The phenomenon of myotonia. *Brain* 64:1, 1941.

DeVisser M, Reimers CD: Muscle imaging, in Engel AG, Franzini-Armstrong C (eds): *Myology: Basic and Clinical,* 2nd ed. New York, McGraw-Hill, 1994, pp 795–806.

Elmquist D, Lambert EH: Detailed analysis of neuromuscular transmission in a patient with the myasthenic syndrome associated with bronchogenic carcinoma. *Mayo Clin Proc* 43:689, 1968.

Engel AG: The neuromuscular junction, in Engel AG, Franzini-Armstrong C (eds): *Myology: Basic and Clinical,* 2nd ed. New York, McGraw-Hill, 1994(a), pp 261–302.

Engel AG: The muscle biopsy, in Engel AG, Franzini-Armstrong C (eds): *Myology: Basic and Clinical,* 2nd ed. New York, McGraw-Hill, 1994(b), pp 822–831.

England JD, Gronseth GS, Franklin G, et al: Practice parameter: Evaluation of distal symmetric polyneuropathy: Role of autonomic testing, nerve biopsy, and skin biopsy (an evidence-based review). Report of the American Academy of Neurology, American Association of Neuromuscular and Electrodiagnostic Medicine, and American Academy of Physical Medicine and Rehabilitation. Neurology 72:177, 2009.

Falck B, Alaranta H: Fibrillation potentials, positive sharp waves and fasciculations in the intrinsic muscles of the foot in healthy subjects. *J Neurol Neurosurg Psychiatry* 46:681, 1983.

Forster FM, Borkowski WJ, Alpers BJ: Effects of denervation on fasciculations in human muscle. *Arch Neurol Psychiatry* 56:276, 1976.

Franzini-Armstrong C: The sarcoplasmic reticulum and transverse tubules, in Engel AG, Franzini-Armstrong C (eds): *Myology: Basic and Clinical,* 2nd ed. New York, McGraw-Hill, 1994, pp 176–199.

Gabriel CM, Howard R, Kinsella N, et al: Prospective study of the usefulness of sural nerve biopsy. *J Neurol Neurosurg Psychiatry* 69:442, 2000.

Hodes R, Larrabee MG, German W: The human electromyogram in response to nerve stimulation and conduction velocity of motor axons: Studies on normal and on injured peripheral nerves. *Arch Neurol Psychiatry* 60:340, 1948.

Hodgkin AL: Ionic basis of electrical activity in nerve and muscle. *Biol Rev* 26:339, 1951.

Hodgkin AL, Huxley AF: Currents carried by sodium and potassium ions through the membranes of the giant axon of Loligo. *J Physiol* 116:449, 1952.
Huxley HE: Molecular basis of contraction in cross-striated muscles, in Bourne GH (ed): *The Structure and Function of Muscle*, 2nd ed. Vol 1. Structure. New York, Academic Press, 1972, pp 301–387.
Jaffe AS, Vasile VC, Milone M, et al: A noncardiac source of increased circulating concentrations of cardiac troponin T. *J Am Coll Cardiol* 58:1819, 2011.
Kakulas BA, Adams RD: *Diseases of Muscle: Pathological Foundations of Clinical Myology*, 4th ed. New York, Harper & Row, 1985.
Katz B: *Nerve, Muscle and Synapse*. New York, McGraw-Hill, 1966.
Kimura J: *Electrodiagnosis in Diseases of Nerve and Muscle: Principles and Practice*, 3rd ed. Oxford, UK, Oxford University Press, 2001.
Magladery JW, McDougal DB: Electrophysiological studies of nerve and reflex activity in normal man. *Johns Hopkins Med J* 86:265, 1950.
McComas AJ, Fawcett PR, Campbell MJ, et al: Electrophysiologic estimation of the number of motor units within a human muscle. *J Neurol Neurosurg Psychiatry* 34:121, 1971.
Mercuri E, Counsell S, Allsop J, et al: Selective muscle involvement on magnetic resonance imaging in autosomal dominant Emery-Dreifuss muscular dystrophy. *Neuropediatrics* 33:10, 2002.
Newham DJ, Jones DA, Edwards RHT: Large delayed CK changes after stepping exercise. *Muscle Nerve* 6:380, 1983.
Nielsen VK, Friis ML, Johnsen T: Electromyographic distinction between paramyotonia congenita and myotonia congenita: Effect of cold. *Neurology* 32:827, 1982.
Peter JB: Skeletal muscle: Diversity and mutability of its histochemical, electron-microscopic, biochemical and physiologic properties, in Pearson CM, Mostofi FK (eds): *The Striated Muscle*. Baltimore, MD, Williams & Wilkins, 1973, pp 1–18.
Rowland LP: Myoglobinuria. *Can J Neurol Sci* 11:1, 1984.
Stålberg E, Trontelj JV: *Single Fiber Electromyography*. Old Woking, Surrey, UK, Miraville Press, 1979.
Wilbourn AJ: The value and limitations of electromyographic examination in the diagnosis of lumbosacral radiculopathy, in Hardy RW (ed): *Lumbar Disc Disease*. New York, Raven Press, 1982, pp 65–109.
Wilbourn AJ, Aminoff MJ: AAEE Minimonograph 32: The electrophysiologic examination in patients with radiculopathies. *Muscle Nerve* 11:1099, 1988.

46

Diseases of the Peripheral Nerves

In this single chapter, an attempt is made to provide an overview of the very large and difficult subject of peripheral nerve disease. Because the structure and function of the peripheral nervous system are relatively simple, one might suppose that our knowledge of its diseases would be fairly complete. Such is not the case. For example, when a group of patients with chronic polyneuropathy were investigated intensively in a highly specialized center for the study of peripheral nerve diseases several decades ago, a suitable explanation for their condition could not be found in 24 percent (Dyck et al, 1981) and even more discouraging figures prevail in our clinics today. Moreover, the physiologic basis of many neuropathic symptoms continues to be elusive and in several of the neuropathies the pathologic changes have not been fully determined.

There has, however, been a surge of interest in diseases of the peripheral nervous system (PNS), which promises to change this state of affairs. Rapidly advancing techniques in the fields of immunology and molecular genetics are now clarifying entire categories of neuropathic disease. Also, in recent years, effective forms of treatment for several peripheral neuropathies have been introduced, making accurate diagnosis imperative. For these reasons, clinicians now find the peripheral neuropathies among the most challenging and gratifying categories of neurologic disease.

GENERAL CONSIDERATIONS

It is important to have a clear concept of the extent of the PNS and the mechanisms by which it is affected by disease. The PNS includes all neural structures lying outside the pial membrane of the spinal cord and brainstem with the exception of the optic nerves and olfactory bulbs, which are special extensions of the brain. The nerves within the spinal canal and attached to the ventral and dorsal surfaces of the cord are the *spinal roots*; those attached to the ventrolateral surface of the brainstem are the *cranial nerve roots*, or cranial nerves.

The dorsal, or posterior (afferent, or sensory), spinal roots consist of central axonal processes of the sensory and cranial ganglia. On reaching the spinal cord and brainstem, the roots extend for variable distances into the dorsal horns and posterior columns of the cord and into the spinal trigeminal and other tracts in the medulla and pons before synapsing with secondary sensory neurons, as described in Chaps. 8 and 9 that are devoted to the neurology of pain and sensation. The peripheral axons of the dorsal root ganglion cells are the sensory nerve fibers. They terminate as freely branching or specialized corpuscular endings—i.e., the sensory receptors—in the skin, joints, and other tissues. The sensory nerve fibers vary greatly in size and in the thickness of their myelin covering; based on these dimensions, they are classified as type A, B, or C, as discussed in Chap. 8.

The ventral, or anterior (efferent, or motor), roots are composed of the emerging axons of anterior and lateral horn cells and motor nuclei of the brainstem. Large, heavily myelinated fibers terminate on muscle fibers and smaller unmyelinated ones terminate in sympathetic or parasympathetic ganglia. From these autonomic ganglia issue the axons that terminate in smooth muscle, heart muscle and conducting system, and glands. Traversing the subarachnoid space, where they lack well-formed epineurial sheaths, the cranial and spinal roots (both sensory and motor) are bathed in and are susceptible to substances in the cerebrospinal fluid (CSF), the lumbosacral roots having the longest exposure (Fig. 46-1).

The vast extent of the peripheral ramifications of cranial and spinal nerves is noteworthy, as are their thick protective and supporting sheaths of perineurium and epineurium that are endowed with a vascular supply through longitudinal arrays of richly anastomosing nutrient arterial branches. The perineurium comprises the connective tissue sheaths that surround and separate each bundle of nerve fibers (fascicles) of varying size, each fascicle containing several hundred axons. The sheath that binds and surrounds all the fascicles of the nerve is the epineurium. As the nerve root approaches the cord, the epineurium blends with the dura (see Fig. 46-1). The fine connective tissue covering of individual nerve fibers is the endoneurium. Longitudinally oriented and widely anastomotic endoneural vessels also nourish the nerve fibers and are susceptible to disease.

The nerves traverse narrow foramina (intervertebral and cranial) and a few pass through tight channels peripherally in the limbs (e.g., the median nerve between the carpal ligament and tendon sheaths of flexor forearm

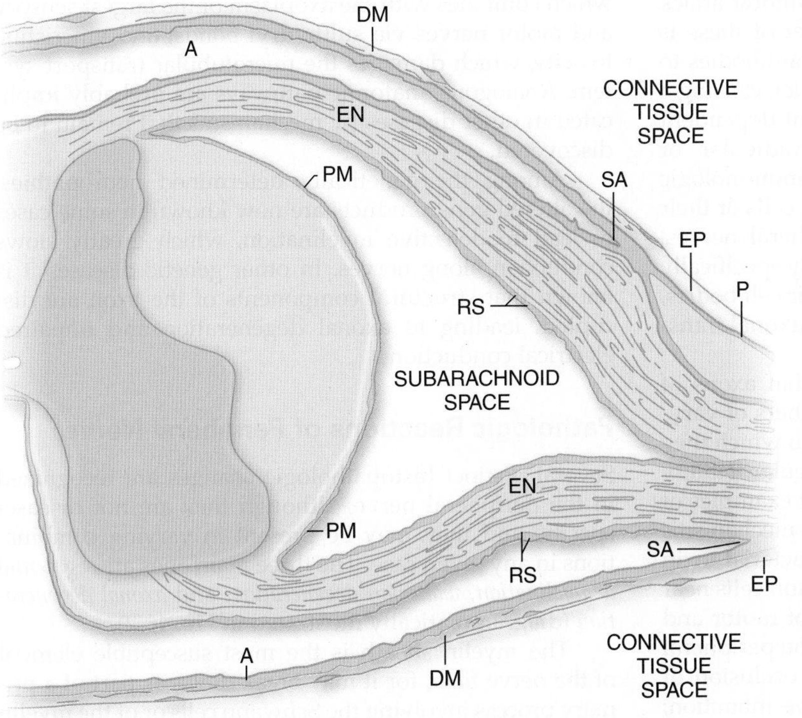

Figure 46-1. Diagram showing the relationships of the peripheral nerve sheaths to the meningeal coverings of the spinal cord. The epineurium (*EP*) is in direct continuity with the dura mater (*DM*). The endoneurium (*EN*) remains unchanged from the peripheral nerve and spinal root to the junction with the spinal cord. At the subarachnoid angle (*SA*), the greater portion of the perineurium (*P*) passes outward between the dura mater and the arachnoid (*A*), but a few layers appear to continue over the nerve root as part of the root sheath (*RS*). At the subarachnoid angle, the arachnoid is reflected over the roots and becomes continuous with the outer layers of the root sheath. At the junction with the spinal cord, the outer layers of the root sheath become continuous with the pia mater (*PM*). (From Haller FR, Low FM: The fine structure of the peripheral nerve root sheath in the subarachnoid space in the rat and other laboratory animals. *Am J Anat* 131:1, 1971, by permission.)

muscles that make up the carpal tunnel; the ulnar nerve in the cubital tunnel). These anatomic features explain the sites of susceptibility of certain nerves to compression and entrapment and also to ischemic damage.

The axons themselves contain a complex internal microtubular apparatus for maintaining the integrity of their membranes and for transporting substances such as neurotransmitters over long distances between the nerve cell body and the distant reaches of the nerve fiber. As discussed in Chap. the long axons of sensory nerves can properly be considered to be dendrites but we use the term "axon" in this and other chapters to denote all the neuronal processes of peripheral enrves. Nerve fibers (axons) are coated with short segments of myelin of variable length (250 to 1,000 μm), each of which is enveloped by a Schwann cell and its membrane that constitute the myelin sheath. In fact, the PNS may be accurately defined as the part of the nervous system that is invested by the cytoplasm and membranes of Schwann cells. Each myelin segment and Schwann cell has a symbiotic relationship to the axon but is morphologically independent. The structure of the axonal membrane in the gaps between segments of the myelin sheaths (nodes of Ranvier) is specialized, containing a high concentration of sodium channels and permitting the saltatory electrical conduction of nerve impulses as described in Chap. 45. Unmyelinated fibers, more numerous in peripheral nerves than myelinated ones, also arise from cells in dorsal root and autonomic ganglia. Small bundles of these naked (unmyelinated) axons are enveloped by a single Schwann cell; delicate tongues of Schwann cell cytoplasm partition these bundles and separate individual axons. Each sensory nerve fiber terminates in a specialized ending which is designed to be especially sensitive to certain natural stimuli as discussed in Chaps. 8 and 9.

Pathogenic Mechanisms in Peripheral Nerve Disease

The features described previously enable one to conceptualize the possible avenues by which disease may affect the peripheral nerves. Pathologic processes may be directed at any one of the several groups of nerve cells whose axons constitute the nerves, i.e., the cells of the anterior or lateral horns of the spinal cord, the dorsal root ganglia, or the sympathetic and parasympathetic ganglia. Each of these cell types exhibits specific vulnerabilities to disease, and if destroyed—as, for example, the motor nerve cells in poliomyelitis—there is secondary degeneration of the axons and myelin sheaths of the peripheral fibers of these cells. Neuropathic symptoms are also induced by alterations of function and structure of the ventral and dorsal columns of the spinal cord, which contain the fibers of exit and entry of anterior horn and dorsal root ganglion cells, respectively. The myelin of these centrally located fibers is constituted differently from that of the peripheral nerves, being enveloped by oligodendrocytes rather than Schwann cells and the nerve fibers are supported by astrocytes rather than fibroblasts.

Because of the intimate relation of the nerve roots to the CSF and to specialized arachnoidal cells (the arachnoidal villi), a pathologic process in the CSF or leptomeninges may damage the exposed spinal roots. Diseases of the connective tissues affect the peripheral nerves that lie within their sheaths. Diffuse or localized arterial diseases may injure nerves by occluding their nutrient arteries. In a large category of immune-mediated neuropathies, the damage is the result of a cellular or humoral attack on various components of myelin. A subset of these is characterized by the binding of circulating antibodies to the specialized regions at the nodes of Ranvier, causing a block of electrical conduction. A complement-dependent humoral immune reaction against the radicular or peripheral axon is also known. Toxic or immunologic agents that selectively damage the Schwann cells or their membranes cause demyelination of peripheral nerves, leaving axons relatively intact, or a toxin may specifically affect axons and dendrites by poisoning their cell bodies, the axolemma, or the lengthy and complex axonal transport apparatus.

Finally, one might correctly suppose that axons of the motor or sensory nerves, sympathetic fibers of varying diameter and length, or the end organs to which they are attached would each have its own particular liability to disease. At present we can cite only a few examples of diseases that cause disease through these mechanisms exclusively: e.g., diphtheria, in which the bacterial toxin acts directly on the membranes of the Schwann cells near the dorsal root ganglia and adjacent parts of motor and sensory nerves (the most vascular parts of the peripheral nerve); polyarteritis nodosa, which causes occlusion of vasa nervorum, resulting in multifocal nerve infarction; tabes dorsalis, in which there is a treponemal meningoradiculitis of the posterior roots (mainly of the lumbosacral segments); doxorubicin toxicity, wherein protein synthesis of dorsal root ganglion cells is blocked with subsequent neuronal destruction; poisoning by arsenic, which combines with the axoplasm of the largest sensory and motor nerves via sulfhydryl bonds; and vincristine toxicity, which damages the microtubular transport system. Analogous anatomic pathways are probably implicated in other diseases by mechanisms that remain to be discovered.

Among the genetically determined neuropathies, the altered gene products are now known in some cases to lead to defective myelination, which greatly slows conduction along nerves. In other genetic diseases it is known that structural components of the axon are disrupted, leading to axonal degeneration and impaired electrical conduction.

Pathologic Reactions of Peripheral Nerve

Several distinct histopathologic changes are recognized in the peripheral nerve, although they are not disease-specific and they may be present in varying combinations in any given case. The three main ones are *segmental demyelination*, *wallerian degeneration*, and *axonal degeneration* (diagrammatically illustrated in Fig. 46-2).

The myelin sheath is the most susceptible element of the nerve fiber, for it may break down as part of a primary process involving the Schwann cells or of the myelin itself, or it may be damaged secondarily as a consequence of disease affecting its axon. Focal degeneration of the myelin sheath with sparing of the axon is called *segmental demyelination*. The characteristic change of segmental demyelination is the disappearance of the sheath over

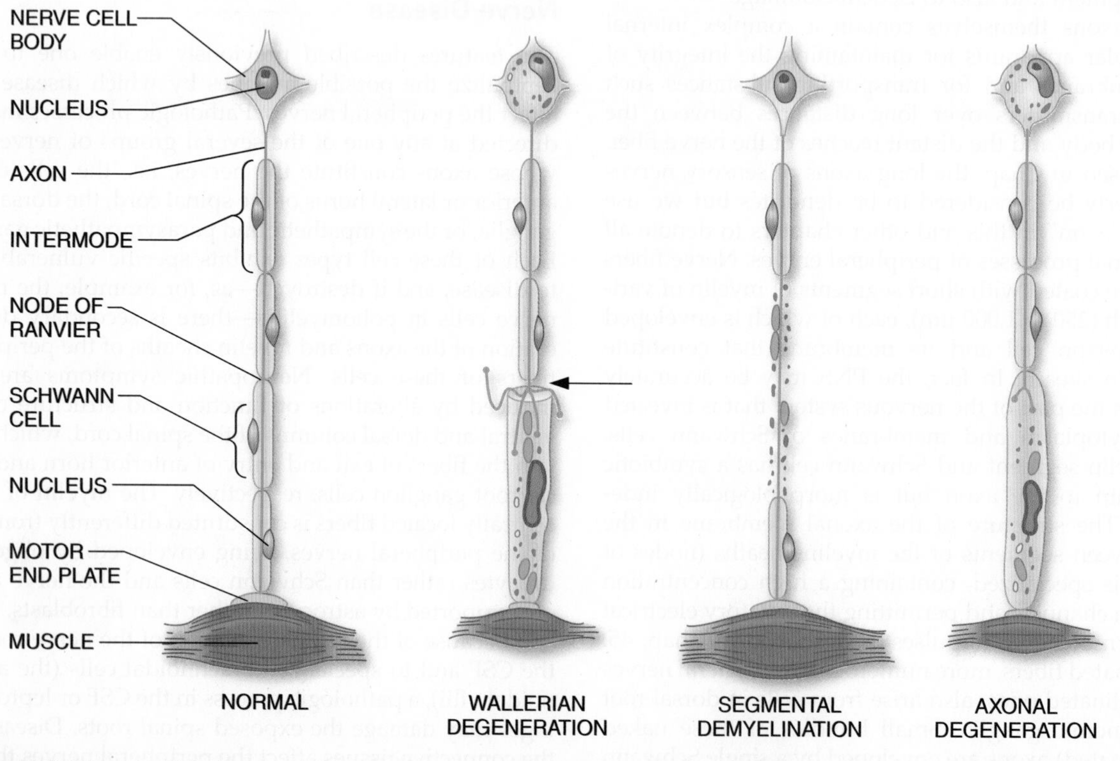

Figure 46-2. Diagram of the basic pathologic processes affecting peripheral nerves. In wallerian degeneration, there is degeneration of the axis cylinder and myelin distal to the site of axonal interruption (*arrow*) and central chromatolysis. In segmental demyelination, the axon is spared. In axonal degeneration, there is a distal degeneration of myelin and the axis cylinder as a result of neuronal disease. Both wallerian and axonal degeneration cause muscle atrophy. Further details are found in the text. (Courtesy of Dr. Arthur Asbury.)

segments of variable length, bounded on each end by one side of a node of Ranvier and an adjacent preserved segment of myelin. This exposes long segments of the axon to the interstitial environment. Myelin may also degenerate from axonal disease in a general process that may occur either proximal or distal to the site of axonal interruption.

Common to many lesions of the peripheral nerve is *wallerian degeneration*, a reaction of both the axon and myelin *distal to* the site of disruption of an axon. Wallerian degeneration might be described as "dying forward," a process in which the nerve degenerates from the point of axonal damage outward. In contrast, when the axon degenerates as part of a "dying-back" phenomenon in a more generalized metabolically determined polyneuropathy, it is termed *axonal degeneration*. Here, the axon is affected progressively from the distal-most site to the proximal, with dissolution of myelin that occurs roughly in parallel with the axonal change. One possible explanation for this process is that the primary damage is to the neuronal cell body, which fails in its function of synthesizing proteins and delivering them to the distal parts of the axon. Certain toxic and metabolic processes affect axons uniformly along their length or impair anterograde axonal transport to the periphery; the functional impairment is then proportional to the size and length of the blocked axons.

Destruction of a proximal spinal motor root results in a gradual dissolution of the distal motor nerve and its myelin sheath (a form of wallerian degeneration). The neuronal motor cell body that gives rise to the motor fiber undergoes characteristic retrograde morphologic changes described below but does not die. Similar destruction of the dorsal spinal root produces secondary wallerian degeneration of the posterior columns of the spinal cord, but not of the peripheral sensory nerve because the dorsal root ganglion cell maintains the integrity of the distal axon. In other words, destruction of axons results within several days in wallerian degeneration of the myelin distal to the point of injury but not transgressing the neuronal cell body. The myelin breaks down into blocks or ovoids in which lie fragments of axons (digestion chambers of Cajal). The myelin fragments are then converted, through the action of macrophages, into neutral fats and cholesterol esters and carried by these cells to the bloodstream.

Certain diseases affect the neuron primarily rather than the axon and cause either a motor or sensory *neuronopathy*. In the former case, the anterior horn cell is affected by a disease process (motor neuron disease, or motor neuronopathy) and in the latter, the sensory ganglion cell (ganglionopathy) is destroyed. A type of wallerian distal degeneration of the respective nerve fibers follows.

Some of these pathologic reactions are more easily understood if one considers certain features of cytoskeletal structure and function of nerve cells and their axons. The axon contains longitudinally oriented neurofilaments and microtubules, which are separated but interconnected by cross-bridges. Their main function involves the transport of substances from nerve cell body to axon terminal (anterograde transport) and from the distal axon back to the cell body (retrograde transport). Thus, when the axon is severed, organelles cannot be transmitted to the distal axon for the purpose of renewing membrane and neurotransmitter systems. By means of retrograde axonal transport, the cell bodies receive signals to increase their metabolic activity and to produce growth factors and other materials needed for axonal regeneration. In an incompletely defined way, the axon also creates a local environment that allows the Schwann cell to maintain the integrity of the adjacent myelin sheath. Loss of this trophic influence leads to dissolution of the myelin sheath, but not of the Schwann cell itself.

There are also highly characteristic histopathologic changes in the nerve cell body termed *chromatolysis* as a secondary consequence of axonal interruption. These retrograde changes consist of swelling of the cell cytoplasm and marginalization and dissolution of the Nissl substance. The important point again is that despite the destructive changes in the nerve fibers, the nerve cells, while altered in histologic appearance, are left intact with preservation of the apparatus required for recovery.

In segmental demyelination, recovery of function may be rapid because the intact but denuded axon needs only become remyelinated. The newly formed internodal segments are initially thinner than normal and of variable length. By contrast, recovery is much slower with wallerian or axonal degeneration, often requiring months to a year or more because the axon must first regenerate and then reinnervate the muscle, sensory organ, or blood vessel before function returns. When the regenerating axon first becomes myelinated, the internodal myelin segments are short, the length of one normal internode being replaced by three or four shorter new ones. Recurrent demyelination and remyelination lead to "onion bulb" formations and enlargement of nerves, the result of proliferating Schwann cells and fibroblasts that encircle the axon and its thin myelin sheath. If nerve cells are destroyed, no recovery of function is possible except by collateral regeneration of axons from intact nerve cells. Interruption of a nerve fiber by severing or by crude destruction usually prevents continuity from being reestablished. Regenerating axon filaments take aberrant courses and, with fibroblastic scar formation, they may form a disorganized clump of tissue termed pseudoneuroma.

These relatively few pathologic reactions do not, in themselves, differentiate the many dozens of diseases of the peripheral nerves, but when they are considered in relation to the selective effects on various types and sizes of fibers, the topography of the lesions, and the time course of the process, they furnish criteria for fairly accurate diagnosis. Moreover, the identification of these basic reactions is of great value in the inspection of pathologic material obtained from biopsy or autopsy.

There are additional special pathologic changes, not specifically neural in nature that characterize certain diseases of the peripheral nervous system. These involve inflammatory or vascular changes or deposition of material in the interstitium of the nerve. For example, acute demyelinative polyneuritis of the Guillain-Barré type is characterized by endoneurial infiltrations of lymphocytes and other mononuclear cells in the nerves, roots, and sensory and sympathetic ganglia. Deposition of amyloid in the endoneurial connective tissue and walls of vessels affecting the nerve fibers are the distinctive features of inherited and acquired amyloid polyneuropathy. Diphtheritic polyneuropathy is typified by the demyelinative character of the nerve fiber change, the location of this change in and around the roots and sensory ganglia, the subacute course, and the lack of inflammatory reaction. A number of neuropathies are characterized by the deposition of antibodies and complement on the myelin sheath or on elements of the axon. These changes can be demonstrated by immunohistopathologic techniques. Many other polyneuropathies (paraneoplastic, nutritional, porphyric, arsenical, and uremic) are topographically symmetrical and represent forms of axonal degeneration but cannot be easily distinguished from one another on histopathologic grounds.

Concerning the pathology of the *mononeuropathies*, our knowledge is somewhat more complete. Compression of nerve or nerve roots, local or segmental ischemia, stretch, and laceration of nerves are understandable mechanisms and their pathologic changes can be reproduced experimentally. Tumor infiltration and importantly, vasculitis with ischemic infarction of nerve account for a proportion of cases. Of infections and granulomas localized to single nerves, leprosy, sarcoid, and herpes zoster represent identifiable disease states. For most of the acute mononeuropathies that are a result of transient compression, the pathologic changes have yet to be fully defined, as they are usually reversible states that provide no opportunity for complete pathologic examination. Experimental models of nerve compression indicate disruption of tubular transport and local demyelination. The common symptoms of compression such as paresthesias are explained, as discussed further on, by exposure of sodium channels along denuded axons and spontaneous and ectopic electrical discharges.

SYMPTOMATOLOGY OF PERIPHERAL NERVE DISEASE

There are a number of motor, sensory, reflex, autonomic, and trophic symptoms and signs that are typical of peripheral nerve disease. Grouping them into syndromes based on their temporal and topographic features has proved to be of great value in clinical diagnosis. Although motor, sensory, reflex, and trophic changes are taken together to determine specific diagnosis, each element of the neuropathic diseases is first given in detail further on.

Impairment of Motor Function

It is not surprising that weakness in various patterns and degrees is a feature of almost all neuropathies. The degree of weakness is proportional to the number of axons or motor neurons affected. *Polyneuropathies* that are the result of axonal damage are characterized foremost by a relatively symmetric distribution of weakness that is, moreover, distal because the pathologic changes begin in the far distal parts of the largest and longest nerves and advance along the affected fibers toward their nerve cell bodies (dying-back neuropathy, or "distal axonopathy"). The muscles of the feet and legs are typically affected earlier and more severely than those of the hands and forearms. In milder forms of axonal disease, only the feet and lower legs are involved. Truncal and cranial muscles are usually the last to yield, and then only in severe cases. This represents the "length-dependent" pattern that is typical of axonal degeneration. The nutritional, metabolic, and toxic neuropathies assume this predominantly distal "axonal" pattern. An exception is porphyria, an axonal process in which there may be mainly proximal weakness. By contrast, in *demyelinating polyneuropathies*, the multifocal nature of lesions and blockage of electrical conduction often leads to weakness of proximal limb and facial muscles before or at the same time as distal parts are affected.

Another pattern of neuropathic weakness is one in which all the muscles of the limbs, trunk, and neck are involved almost simultaneously, often including respiratory paralysis, therefore making it impossible to determine if the axons or myelin, or both, have been damaged. The best characterized of these processes is the Guillain-Barré syndrome (GBS). Less common causes of *generalized paralysis* include diphtheria, tick paralysis, and certain toxic polyneuropathies. Fatalities, when they occur, are usually a result of respiratory failure.

A predominantly *bibrachial paralysis* is an unusual presentation of neuropathic disease but may occur in the inflammatory-demyelinating polyneuropathies, as well as in Sjögren syndrome, chronic immune or paraneoplastic neuropathies, lead neuropathy, Tangier disease, and in a familial type of brachial neuritis. (A more frequent cause of bibrachial palsy is disease of the motor neurons themselves namely, motor system disease, or a lesion placed centrally in the cervical cord that damages these same neurons.) *Paraparesis* is not typical of the generalized polyneuropathies, but it is observed with infections and inflammations of the cauda equina, as occurs with Lyme disease, cytomegalovirus, herpes simplex, and with neoplastic infiltration of the nerve roots. Bifacial and other cranial nerve paralyses are likely to occur in GBS, neoplastic invasion, with connective tissue diseases, HIV and herpes virus infection, sarcoidosis, Lyme disease, or one of the rare metabolic neuropathies (Refsum, Bassen-Kornzweig, Tangier, and Riley-Day). These are discussed in Chap. 47 on diseases of the cranial nerves and in respective chapters on infections and metabolic diseases of the nervous system.

Atrophy of weak or paralyzed muscles is characteristic of chronic disease of the motor neuron or motor axon and conversely, demyelinating neuropathies relatively spare muscle bulk because of the absence of denervation. Atrophy proceeds slowly over several weeks and months, the degree being proportional to the number of damaged motor nerve fibers. The maximum degree of denervation atrophy after an acute injury to the axons occurs in 90 to 120 days and reduces muscle volume by 75 to 80 percent. Atrophy may also be a consequence of disuse; it occurs over many weeks but in itself does not reduce muscle volume by more than 25 to 30 percent. In chronic axonal neuropathies, the degrees of paralysis and atrophy tend to correspond. As mentioned previously, atrophy does not coincide with weakness in acute paralysis caused by the demyelinative neuropathies in which the nerve fiber is relatively less affected than is the myelin. Ultimately in muscle atrophy, there is degeneration and loss of the denervated muscle fibers. This process begins in 6 to 12 months; in 3 to 4 years, most of the denervated fibers will have degenerated. If reinnervation takes place within a year or so, motor function and muscle volume may be restored.

Tendon Reflexes

As a rule, neuropathies are associated with a reduction or loss of tendon reflexes. Most often, this is the result of an interruption of the afferent (sensory) portion of the monosynaptic reflex arc. The reflexes may be diminished if muscular function is impaired, but this occurs mainly in the case of extreme atrophy, in which there are too few muscle fibers to manifest a contraction. There are, of course, many other processes that reduce the tendon reflexes, but it is the neuropathies with which loss of reflexes is most closely associated. An exception is the group of *small-fiber neuropathies*, in which tendon reflexes may be retained, even with marked loss of perception of painful stimuli. This discrepancy is attributable to the dependence of the afferent component of the tendon reflex arc on the large, heavily myelinated fibers that originate in muscle spindles. Conversely, in neuropathies that affect the largest diameter, heavily myelinated fibers, the tendon reflexes are diminished early and disproportionately to weakness. Slowing of conduction in sensory fibers may also abolish the reflex by dispersing the afferent volley of impulses initiated by the tendon tap. There is generally a concordance between areflexia and a loss of proprioceptive and joint-position senses; i.e., the large nerve fibers from spindle afferents are of the same type and size as those mediating these forms of sensation. Furthermore, loss of sensory functions that are dependent on these large fibers in the presence of preserved reflexes implicates the central projections of the sensory ganglion cells i.e., a lesion in the posterior columns of the spinal cord that does not interrupt the afferent tendon reflex arc. Regional loss of a reflex is usually a sign of a radiculopathy.

Sensory Loss (See also "Sensory Syndromes" in Chap. 9)

Most polyneuropathies cause impairment of both motor and sensory functions, but one is often affected more than the other. In the toxic and metabolic neuropathies, sensory loss usually exceeds weakness. These differences are emphasized in the descriptions of individual peripheral nerve diseases in later parts of the chapter.

In the axonal polyneuropathies, sensation is affected symmetrically in the distal segments of the limbs and more in the legs than in the arms, owing to the length-dependent nature of most diseases that affect peripheral nerves. In most types, all sensory modalities (touch-pressure, pain and temperature, vibratory and joint position senses) are impaired or eventually lost, although one modality is affected disproportionately to the others, or pain and temperature sensation (small afferent fibers) may be impaired more than joint position and vibration (larger fibers). As an axonal neuropathy worsens, there is spread of sensory loss from the distal to more proximal parts of the limbs and eventually, to the anterior abdomen, thorax, and the face. An "escutcheon" pattern of sensory loss over the abdomen and thorax in severe axonal neuropathy may be mistaken for the sensory level of a spinal cord lesion. Another characteristic form of sensory loss affects the trunk, scalp, and face; this is the pattern of a sensory ganglionopathy that is the result of simultaneous dysfunction of all parts of the sensory nerve.

Most often, *universal sensory loss* is attributable to an acquired disease affecting the sensory ganglia (sensory neuronopathy); a paraneoplastic process, certain toxic or immune diseases are usually responsible (e.g., Sjögren disease, scleroderma).

Paresthesias, Pain, and Dysesthesias

These symptoms were described in Chaps. 8 and 9. Sensory symptoms tend to be especially marked in the hands and feet. "Pins and needles," "falling asleep," "stabbing," "tingling," "prickling," "electrical," and "Novocain-like" are the adjectives chosen by patients to describe these positive sensory experiences. In some neuropathies, paresthesias and numbness are the only symptoms and objective sensory loss is lacking or minimal. Certain neuropathies characteristically cause pain, which is described as burning, aching, sharp and cutting, or crushing and at times may resemble the lightning pains of tabes dorsalis. Perversion of sensation (allodynia) is also commonplace in some polyneuropathies—e.g., tingling, burning, stabbing pain, or just an uncomfortable dysesthesia is induced by tactile stimuli. Under these conditions a stimulus induces not only an aberrant sensation but also one that radiates to adjacent areas and persists after the stimulus is withdrawn. As remarked in Chap. 9, the reactions of a patient with allodynia may seem to indicate hypersensitivity ("hyperesthesia"), but more often the sensory threshold is actually raised and it is the sensory experience or response that is exaggerated (*hyperpathia*).

Painful paresthesias and dysesthesias are particularly common in diabetic, alcoholic–nutritional, and amyloid neuropathies. Mainly they affect the feet ("burning feet") and less often the hands. In herpes zoster, they are confined to dermatomal regions of the body. A particularly intense form of burning pain typifies the *causalgia* of a partial nerve lesion (usually traumatic) of the ulnar, median, posterior tibial, peroneal, or occasionally some other nerve (see Chap. 8 and further on in this chapter).

The mechanism of thermal and painful dysesthesias is not fully understood. It has been theorized that a loss of large touch-pressure fibers disinhibits the pain-receiving nerve cells in the posterior horns of the spinal cord. An argument against this explanation is the lack of pain in Friedreich ataxia, in which the larger neurons degenerate, and also in certain purely sensory polyneuropathies, where only the perception of tactile stimuli (large fibers) is lost. A more likely explanation, supported by microneurographic recordings, is that dysesthetic pain results from ectopic discharges arising at many sites along surviving intact or regenerating nerve fibers or their terminal receptors. It has been postulated, on uncertain grounds, that the deep, aching neuropathic pain of sciatica or brachial neuritis (nerve trunk pain) arises from irritation of the normal endings (nervi nervorum) in the sheaths of the nerve trunks themselves (Asbury and Fields). These considerations are discussed in Chap. 8.

Sensory Ataxia and Tremor

Proprioceptive deafferentation with retention of a reasonable degree of motor function may give rise to ataxia of gait and of limb movement as discussed in Chap. 9. Dysfunction of the spinocerebellar fibers of the peripheral nerves is probably the source of the ataxia. Some of the most severe ataxias of this type occur with sensory ganglionopathy, as commented further on.

Ataxia without weakness is also characteristic of tabes dorsalis, a purely posterior root disease, but this syndrome is duplicated by diabetic polyneuropathy, which may affect posterior roots (diabetic pseudotabes) and by a variant of GBS (termed Fisher syndrome). The ataxia is indistinguishable from that caused by cerebellar diseases, but other features of cerebellar dysfunction such as dysarthria and nystagmus are lacking. Characteristic of the sensory-ataxic gait are brusque, flinging, slapping movements of the legs. Loss of proprioception may also give rise to small wavering, fluctuating movements of the outstretched fingers—called *pseudoathetotic*, or "dancing fingers."

An action tremor of fast-frequency type may also appear during certain phases of a polyneuropathy; Shahani and coworkers had the impression that it is a result of loss of input from the muscle-spindle afferents. Corticosteroid therapy enhances this fast tremor. A particularly severe form of slower action tremor is combined with clumsiness of movement in the neuropathies caused by the autoimmune, anti-myelin-associated glycoprotein (anti-MAG) polyneuropathy and in some cases of chronic inflammatory demyelinating polyneuropathy (CIDP). The tremor may be so coarse as to resemble the intention tremor of cerebellar disease and all movements are rendered useless. However, a tremor at rest is not found in these afferent-sensory neuropathies. The neuropathic type of tremor is also discussed in Chap. 6.

Deformity and Trophic Changes

In a few of the chronic polyneuropathies, the feet, hands, and even the spine may become progressively deformed. This is most likely to occur when the disease begins during childhood. Austin pointed out that foot deformity is found in 30 percent of patients with hereditary polyneuropathy, and spine curvature is found in 20 percent. In early life, the feet are pulled into a position of talipes equinus (plantar deviation) because of disproportionate weakness of the pretibial and peroneal muscles and the unopposed action of the calf muscles. Weakness of the intrinsic foot muscles during the period of life when the bones are forming allows the long extensors of the toes to dorsiflex the proximal phalanges and the long flexors to shorten the foot, heighten the arch, and flex the distal phalanges. The result is the *claw foot—le pied en griffe*—or pes cavus (high arches) when the process is less severe. These changes in the structure of the foot are valuable diagnostic indicators that a neuromuscular disease originated in early childhood or during intrauterine development. A congenital claw hand has a similar implication. Unequal weakening of the paravertebral muscles on the two sides of the spine during early development leads to kyphoscoliosis.

Denervation atrophy of muscle can be considered the main trophic disturbance resulting from interruption of the motor nerves. However, there are numerous other changes. Analgesia of distal limb parts makes them susceptible to burns, pressure sores, and other forms of injury that are easily infected and heal poorly. In an anesthetic and immobile limb, the skin becomes tight and shiny, the nails curved and ridged, and the subcutaneous tissue thickened ("trophic changes"). Hair growth is diminished in denervated areas. If the autonomic fibers are also interrupted, the limb becomes warm and pink. Repeated injuries and chronic subcutaneous and osteomyelitic infections result in a painless loss of digits and the formation of plantar ulcers (*mal perforant du pied*). These are prominent features of the recessive form of hereditary sensory neuropathy and we have observed them in dominant forms as well. In tabes dorsalis and syringomyelia as well as certain familial and other chronic polyneuropathies analgesic joints, when chronically traumatized, may first become deformed and then actually disintegrate in a process called Charcot arthropathy ("Charcot joint").

Apart from analgesia, a critical factor in these trophic changes may be aberrant neural regulation of the distal vasculature, which interferes with normal tissue responses to trauma and infection. Ali and colleagues have related the ulcer formation to loss of C fibers, which mediate both pain and autonomic reflexes. However, paralyzed limbs, even in hysteria, if left dependent, are often cold, swollen, and pale or blue. These are probably secondary effects of immobilization, as pointed out long ago by Lewis and Pickering. Erythema and edema, burning pain, and cold sensations surely can be evoked by peripheral nerve irritation, particularly of C and A-δ fibers as discussed in Chap. 8.

Autonomic Dysfunction

Anhidrosis and orthostatic hypotension, two of the most frequent manifestations of autonomic failure, predominate in certain types of polyneuropathies. They occur frequently in amyloidosis and in other small-fiber polyneuropathies, especially diabetic, and in several congenital types. These are also the main features of an acute autonomic polyneuropathy called *pandysautonomia* (Young et al; Adams et al; Low et al) and can be prominent in some cases of GBS. The neuropathic dysautonomic conditions are described in detail in Chap. 26 and later in this chapter.

Other manifestations of autonomic paralysis are small or medium-sized unreactive pupils that are unusually sensitive to certain drugs (see Chap. 14); lack of sweat, tears, and saliva; erectile dysfunction; weak bowel and bladder sphincters with urinary retention or overflow incontinence; and weakness and dilation of the esophagus and colon. As a result of vagal and other parasympathetic dysfunction, the normal variability of heart rate with respiration (sinus arrhythmia) is lost and there may be paralytic ileus or dyscoordinated peristalsis, as well as achlorhydria and hyponatremia. Some of these abnormalities are found in diabetic and amyloid polyneuropathy. They correspond to degeneration of small unmyelinated autonomic fibers in the peripheral nerves.

In any neuropathy involving sensory nerves, there is loss of autonomic function in the same zones as sensory loss. *This is not true of radicular diseases* because the autonomic fibers join the spinal nerves from the sympathetic chain and parasympathetic ganglia more distally. Changes in sweating and cutaneous blood flow may be demonstrated by a number of special tests described in Chap. 26.

Fasciculations, Cramps, and Spasms (See also Chap. 48)

Fasciculations and cramps are not prominent features in most polyneuropathies and in this respect there is a difference from diseases of the anterior horn cells where they are important features. There are exceptions, however. Chronic spinal motor root compression leads to fasciculations or painful spasms in the innervated muscles. Occasionally one observes a state of mild motor polyneuropathy that, upon recovery, leaves the muscles in a state variably referred to as myokymia, continuous muscular activity, and neuromyotonia as discussed in Chaps. 45 and 50. The affected muscles ripple and quiver and occasionally cramp. Use of the muscles increases this activity and there is a reduction in their contractile efficiency, which the patient senses as a stiffness and heaviness. In some instances this apparently constitutes the entire neuropathic syndrome and may be relieved by carbamazepine or phenytoin.

Other closely related phenomena are spasms or involuntary movements of the toes and feet. The latter, when the sole manifestation of disease, was referred to by Spillane and colleagues as the syndrome of *painful legs and moving toes.* It has been attributed by Nathan to ectopic discharges in sensory roots, ganglia, or nerves, evoking both pain and organized movements. This is but one of many causes of the nocturnal restless leg syndrome, but it does not explain the more common type of idiopathic restless leg nocturnal syndrome described in Chap. 19. Other possible mechanisms for cramps and spasms are ephaptic cross-transmission between adjacent axons denuded of myelin, segmental hyperactivity from deafferentation, and neuronal sprouting during reinnervation. Infrequently, the muscle activity induces odd postures or slow writhing movements that Jankovic and van der Linden have likened to dystonia. The pathophysiology of these asynchronous activities of motor neurons is not known. Stimulation of a motor nerve in these cases, instead of causing a brief burst of action potentials in the muscle, results in a prolonged or dispersed series of potentials lasting several hundred milliseconds. Evidently, branched axons involved in collateral innervation have unstable polarization that may last for years.

APPROACH TO THE PATIENT WITH PERIPHERAL NEUROPATHY

The clinician is faced initially with several problems that can be solved sequentially when dealing with this group of diseases: (1) establishing the existence of disease of the peripheral nervous system and differentiating it from a process of the central nervous system, neuromuscular junction or the muscles; (2) distinguishing by clinical examination which of the main topographic syndromes it being displayed; (3) determining by examination and nerve conduction studies) if the problem is predominantly of a motor or sensory or autonomic in nature or is of mixed type and whether the myelin sheath, the axon, or cell body (motor or sensory neurons) is the target of disease; and (4) assessing if the neuropathy is acquired or hereditary in nature. When taken together, these features limit the likely etiologic diagnoses from a vast list of possibilities.

Topographic and Clinical Patterns of Neuropathy (Table 46-1)

At the outset it must be determined whether the neurologic findings correspond to one of the following syndromic patterns:

1. Polyneuropathy
2. Radiculopathy or polyradiculopathy
3. Neuronopathy—motor or sensory
4. Mononeuropathy
5. Multiple mononeuropathies (mononeuropathy multiplex)
6. Plexopathy (involvement of multiple nerves in a plexus)

A discussion of these patterns is given in Chap. 9, but the main facts are repeated here.

In *polyneuropathy*, a generalized process affecting the peripheral nerves, weakness is relatively symmetrical from the beginning and progresses bilaterally; reflexes are lost in affected parts but particularly at the ankles; sensory complaints and loss of sensation are most pronounced distally, and in the feet before the hands in most cases.

Polyradiculopathy, a disease of multiple spinal roots, differs from polyneuropathy in that the neurologic signs are asymmetrical, with an erratic distribution that may, for example, be proximal in one limb and distal in another. Weakness and zones of sensory loss correspond to involvement of one or more spinal or cranial roots. Pain in the sensory distribution of the roots is a common feature. The common *single radiculopathy*, most often the result of root compression by disease of the spinal column, is identified by pain, sensory, motor, and reflex change solely in the distribution of one nerve root. The distinction from mononeuropathy (see later) is not always apparent and one must resort to a reference or to memorized knowledge of the motor and sensory innervation patterns

Table 46-1

ACTIONS OF THE PRINCIPAL MUSCLES AND THEIR NERVE ROOT SUPPLY

ACTION TESTED	ROOTS[a]	NERVES	MUSCLES
Cranial			
Closure of eyes, pursing of lips, exposure of teeth	Cranial 7	Facial	Orbicularis oculi Orbicularis oris
Elevation of eyelids, movement of eyes	Cranial 3, 4, 6	Oculomotor, trochlear, abducens	Levator palpebrae, extraocular
Closing and opening of jaw	Cranial 5	Motor trigeminal	Masseters Pterygoids
Protrusion of tongue	Cranial 12	Hypoglossal	Lingual
Phonation and swallowing	Cranial 9, 10	Glossopharyngeal, vagus	Palatal, laryngeal, and pharyngeal
Elevation of shoulders, anteroflexion and turning of head	Cranial 11 and upper cervical	Spinal accessory	Trapezius, sternomastoid
Brachial			
Adduction of extended arm	*C5*, C6	Brachial plexus	Pectoralis major
Fixation of scapula	C5, C6, C7	Brachial plexus	Serratus anterior
Initiation of abduction of arm	*C5*, C6	Brachial plexus	Supraspinatus
External rotation of flexed arm	*C5*, C6	Brachial plexus	Infraspinatus
Abduction and elevation of arm up to 90°	*C5*, C6	Axillary nerve	Deltoid
Flexion of supinated forearm	C5, C6	Musculocutaneous	Biceps, brachialis
Extension of forearm	C6, *C7*, C8	Radial	Triceps
Extension (radial) of wrist	C6	Radial	Extensor carpi radialis longus
Flexion of semipronated arm	C5, *C6*	Radial	Brachioradialis
Adduction of flexed arm	C6, *C7*, C8	Brachial plexus	Latissimus dorsi
Supination of forearm	C6, C7	Posterior interosseous	Supinator
Extension of proximal phalanges	*C7*, C8	Posterior interosseous	Extensor digitorum
Extension of wrist (ulnar side)	*C7*, C8	Posterior interosseous	Extensor carpi ulnaris
Extension of proximal phalanx of index finger	*C7*, C8	Posterior interosseous	Extensor indicis
Abduction of thumb	*C7*, C8	Posterior interosseous	Abductor pollicis longus and brevis
Extension of thumb	*C7*, C8	Posterior interosseous	Extensor pollicis longus and brevis
Pronation of forearm	C6, C7	Median nerve	Pronator teres
Radial flexion of wrist	C6, C7	Median nerve	Flexor carpi radialis
Flexion of middle phalanges	C7, *C8*, T1	Median nerve	Flexor digitorum superficialis
Flexion of proximal phalanx of thumb	C8, *T1*	Median nerve	Flexor pollicis brevis
Opposition of thumb against fifth finger	C8, *T1*	Median nerve	Opponens pollicis
Extension of middle phalanges of index and middle fingers	C8, *T1*	Median nerve	First, second lumbricals
Flexion of terminal phalanx of thumb	*C8*, T1	Anterior interosseous nerve	Flexor pollicis longus
Flexion of terminal phalanx of second and third fingers	C8, T1	Anterior interosseous nerve	Flexor digitorum profundus
Flexion of distal phalanges of ring and little fingers	C7, *C8*	Ulnar	Flexor digitorum profundus
Adduction and opposition of fifth finger	C8, *T1*	Ulnar	Hypothenar
Extension of middle phalanges of ring and little fingers	C8, *T1*	Ulnar	Third, fourth lumbricals
Adduction of thumb against second finger	C8, *T1*	Ulnar	Adductor pollicis
Flexion of proximal phalanx of thumb	*C8*, Tl	Ulnar	Flexor pollicis brevis
Abduction and adduction of fingers	C8, *T1*	Ulnar	Interossei

(Continued)

Table 46-1

ACTIONS OF THE PRINCIPAL MUSCLES AND THEIR NERVE ROOT SUPPLY (*CONTINUED*)

ACTION TESTED	ROOTS[a]	NERVES	MUSCLES
Crural			
Hip flexion from semiflexed position	***L1, L2,*** L3	Femoral	Iliopsoas
Hip flexion from externally rotated position	L2, L3	Femoral	Sartorius
Extension of knee	L2, ***L3, L4***	Femoral	Quadriceps femoris
Adduction of thigh	***L2, L3,*** L4	Obturator	Adductor longus, magnus, brevis
Abduction and internal rotation of thigh	***L4, L5,*** S1	Superior gluteal	Gluteus medius
Extension of thigh	***L5, S1,*** S2	Inferior gluteal	Gluteus maximus
Flexion of knee	L5, ***S1,*** S2	Sciatic	Biceps femoris
			Semitendinosus
			Semimembranosus
Dorsiflexion of foot (medial)	***L4,*** L5	Peroneal (deep)	Anterior tibial
Dorsiflexion of toes (proximal and distal phalanges)	***L5,*** S1	Peroneal (deep)	Extensor digitorum longus and brevis
Dorsiflexion of great toe	***L5,*** S1	Peroneal (deep)	Extensor hallucis longus
Eversion of foot	L5, S1	Peroneal (superficial)	Peroneus longus and brevis
Plantar flexion of foot	***S1,*** S2	Tibial	Gastrocnemius, soleus
Inversion of foot	L4, ***L5***	Tibial	Tibialis posterior
Flexion of toes (distal phalanges)	L5, ***S1, S2***	Tibial	Flexor digitorum longus
Flexion of toes (middle phalanges)	***S1, S2***	Tibial	Flexor digitorum brevis
Flexion of great toe (proximal phalanx)	S1, S2	Tibial	Flexor hallucis brevis
Flexion of great toe (distal phalanx)	L5, ***S1, S2***	Tibial	Flexor hallucis longus
Contraction of anal sphincter	S2, S3, S4	Pudendal	Perineal muscles

[a]Predominant root(s) supplying a particular muscle are indicated in bold italic type.

of roots and nerves as given in Figs. 9-1, 9-2, and 9-3 and on the overleafs. Most helpful is the limitation of sensory loss to one of the dermatomes, but it so happens that there is overlap between adjacent dermatomes and such a pattern is not easily discerned.

Mononeuropathy is the most circumscribed form of peripheral nerve disease. It is reflected by weakness and sensory loss in the territory of a single peripheral nerve. Specific features serve to differentiate mononeuropathy from a radiculopathy—for example, weakness in dorsiflexion and eversion of the foot is referable either to the peroneal nerve or to the L5 nerve root; however, if there is weakness of inversion of the foot, innervated by the tibial nerve, the fault must be with the L5 root, not with the peroneal nerve. Conversely, if inversion is spared in a foot drop, the lesion ins in the peroneal nerve. The distribution of sensory loss also aids in distinguishing the two processes; for example, in the aforementioned case the region of sensory change corresponding to the L5 root extends almost up to the knee on the anterior surface of the foreleg whereas it ends a limited distance above the ankle in the case of a peroneal nerve lesion (see the sensory maps in Figs. 9-1, 9-2, and 9-3).

At times, particularly in advanced stages, the accumulation of multiple mononeuropathies, termed *mononeuropathy multiplex*, may be difficult to differentiate from polyneuropathy as discussed further on.

Plexopathies (brachial or lumbosacral) create the most confusing patterns of motor and sensory involvement; only one limb is affected, but the motor, sensory, and reflex loss does not conform to a pattern of several adjacent nerve roots or nerves. Knowledge of the innervation of the involved muscles at the level of the plexus usually clarifies the situation.

In *sensory neuronopathy*, the ganglion cells rather than the peripheral sensory nerves are predominantly affected. This gives rise to symptoms and signs of sensory loss in both a proximal and distal distribution, including the scalp, thorax, abdomen, and buttocks as well as the extremities; sensory ataxia is a common accompaniment. There is no weakness, but movements may be awkward as a result of a sensory ataxia. *Motor neuronopathy* is essentially the obverse condition, a disorder of the anterior horn causing weakness, fasciculations, and atrophy in a widespread distribution and, therefore, not properly included as a process of the peripheral nerves.

The apparent complexity of peripheral nerve disease is greatly simplified by recognizing that, of the multitude of diseases, each manifests itself by one or another of above-described topographic and sensory-motor patterns for which reason *the pattern of neuropathy sets limits on the etiologic possibilities.*

In the analysis of a *polyneuropathy*, it is of further value to determine whether the process is predominantly motor with less sensory involvement or the converse, or purely sensory, motor, or mainly autonomic. The *time course* of the disease also informs diagnosis. An acute onset (i.e., rapid evolution) is nearly always an inflammatory, immunologic, toxic, or vascular polyneuropathy. The other extreme, a polyneuropathy evolving over many years, is indicative of a hereditary or, rarely, a metabolic disease. Most of the toxic, nutritional, and systemic diseases of nerve develop subacutely over several weeks and months. In addition to the patient's report of the progress of symptoms, signs such as muscle atrophy signify a process of relatively long-standing, at least several months in duration.

The etiologic diagnosis of polyneuropathy is next guided by deducing whether the myelin sheath or the axon is primarily involved (i.e., *demyelinating* or *axonal neuropathy*). The neurologic examination alone may be sufficient to make this distinction, but greater precision is attained from nerve conduction studies and needle examination of muscles (EMG). The latter test also helps separate primary disorders of muscle (myopathies) and neurogenic denervation of muscle or neuromuscular block (myasthenia). The electrical examinations of nerve and muscle described in Chap. 45 greatly reduce the number of possible diagnoses. These EMG and nerve conduction abnormalities may be so characteristic as to virtually define a neuropathy, e.g., chronic demyelinative motor neuropathy with multifocal conduction block.

Other useful laboratory procedures are (1) biochemical tests to identify metabolic, nutritional, or toxic states; (2) CSF examination (increase in protein and in cells that indicate radicular or meningeal involvement); (3) nerve, and occasionally accompanying muscle biopsy (the latter aids in the diagnosis of vasculitic causes of neuropathy); (4) measurement of immunoglobulins and antineural antibodies that relate to immune-mediated neuropathies; and (5) genetic testing for several of the inherited neuropathies. These are discussed in the context of each of the main diseases of nerve and in the later parts of Chap. 45.

Once having established that the patient has a disease of the peripheral nerves and having ascertained its clinical and electrophysiologic pattern and time course, one is usually able to determine its cause. This is accomplished most readily by allocating the case in question to one of the categories listed in Table 46-2, which classifies the peripheral nerve diseases syndromically according to their mode of evolution and clinical presentation. Our use of the terms *acute*, *subacute*, and *chronic* neuropathy must be explained. By *acute*, we mean evolution in terms of days, and by *subacute*, evolution in terms of weeks. *Chronic* is divided into two groups: one in which the neuropathy has progressed for a period of several months

Table 46-2

THE PRINCIPAL NEUROPATHIC SYNDROMES AND THEIR CAUSES

I. Syndrome of acute motor paralysis with variable disturbance of sensory and autonomic function
  A. Guillain-Barré syndrome (GBS; acute inflammatory demyelinating polyneuropathy [AIDP]); see also Table 46-3
  B. Acute axonal form of GBS (AMAN)
  C. Acute sensory neuropathy and neuronopathy syndrome
  D. Diphtheritic polyneuropathy
  E. Porphyric polyneuropathy
  F. Certain toxic polyneuropathies (thallium, triorthocresyl phosphate)
  G. Rarely, paraneoplastic
  H. Acute pandysautonomic neuropathy
  I. Tick paralysis
  J. Critical illness polyneuropathy
II. Syndrome of subacute sensorimotor paralysis
  A. Symmetrical polyneuropathies
    1. Deficiency states: alcoholism (beriberi), pellagra, vitamin B_{12} deficiency, chronic gastrointestinal disease (see Chap. 41)
    2. Poisoning with heavy metals and solvents: arsenic, lead, mercury, thallium, methyl *n*-butyl ketone, *n*-hexane, methyl bromide, ethylene oxide, organophosphates (TOCP, etc.), acrylamide (see Chap. 43)
    3. Drug toxicity: isoniazid, ethionamide, hydralazine, nitrofurantoin and related nitrofurazones, disulfiram, carbon disulfide, vincristine, cisplatin, paclitaxel, chloramphenicol, phenytoin, pyridoxine, amitriptyline, dapsone, stilbamidine, trichloroethylene, thalidomide, clioquinol, amiodarone, adulterated agents such as L-tryptophan
    4. Uremic polyneuropathy (see Chap. 40)
    5. Subacute inflammatory polyneuropathy
    6. Paraneoplastic polyneuropathy
    7. HIV
  B. Asymmetrical neuropathies (mononeuropathy multiplex)
    1. Diabetes
    2. Polyarteritis nodosa and other inflammatory angiopathic neuropathies (Churg-Strauss, hypereosinophilic, rheumatoid, lupus, Wegener granulomatosis, isolated peripheral nervous system vasculitis); see also Table 46-3
    3. Mixed cryoglobulinemia

(Continued)

Table 46-2

THE PRINCIPAL NEUROPATHIC SYNDROMES AND THEIR CAUSES (*CONTINUED*)

4. Sjögren-sicca syndrome
5. Sarcoidosis
6. Ischemic neuropathy with peripheral vascular disease
7. Lyme disease
8. HIV
9. Diabetes
10. Multifocal motor neuropathy (MMN)
11. Multifocal conduction block (MADSAM)

C. Unusual sensory neuropathies
1. Wartenberg migrant sensory neuropathy
2. Sensory perineuritis

D. Meningeal based nerve root disease (polyradiculopathy)
1. Neoplastic infiltration
2. Granulomatous and infectious infiltration: Lyme, sarcoidosis
3. Spinal diseases: osteoarthritic spondylitis
4. Idiopathic polyradiculopathy

III. Syndrome of early chronic sensorimotor polyneuropathy
A. Paraneoplastic: carcinoma, lymphoma, myeloma, and other malignancies
B. Chronic inflammatory demyelinating polyneuropathy (CIDP)
C. Paraproteinemias
D. Uremia (occasionally subacute)
E. Nutritional beriberi (usually subacute)
F. Diabetes
G. Connective tissue diseases
H. Amyloidosis
I. Leprosy
J. Hypothyroidism
K. Benign sensory form in the elderly

IV. Syndrome of more chronic (late) polyneuropathy, genetically determined forms (see Table 46-6)
A. Inherited polyneuropathies of predominantly sensory type
1. Dominant mutilating sensory neuropathy in adults
2. Recessive mutilating sensory neuropathy of childhood
3. Congenital insensitivity to pain
4. Other inherited sensory neuropathies, including those associated with spinocerebellar degenerations, Riley-Day syndrome, and the universal anesthesia syndrome

B. Inherited polyneuropathies of mixed sensorimotor types
1. Peroneal muscular atrophy (Charcot-Marie-Tooth; CMT types 1 [demyelinating] and 2 [axonal] and CMTX [X-linked])
2. Hypertrophic polyneuropathy of Dejerine-Sottas, adult and childhood forms (CMT3)
3. Roussy-Lévy polyneuropathy
4. Polyneuropathy with optic atrophy, spastic paraplegia, spinocerebellar degeneration, or dementia
5. Hereditary liability to pressure palsy (HNPP)

C. Inherited polyneuropathies with a recognized metabolic disorder (see Chap. 37)
1. Refsum disease
2. Metachromatic leukodystrophy
3. Globoid-body leukodystrophy (Krabbe disease)
4. Adrenoleukodystrophy
5. Amyloid polyneuropathy
6. Porphyric polyneuropathy
7. Anderson-Fabry disease
8. Abetalipoproteinemia (Bassen-Kornzweig)
9. Tangier disease

V. Neuropathy associated with mitochondrial diseases (see Chap. 37)

VI. Syndrome of recurrent or relapsing polyneuropathy
A. Porphyria
B. Chronic inflammatory demyelinating polyneuropathy
C. Certain forms of mononeuritis multiplex
D. Beriberi or intoxications
E. Refsum disease
F. Tangier disease
G. Repeated toxic exposures

VII. Syndrome of mononeuropathy or plexopathy
A. Brachial plexus neuropathies
B. Brachial mononeuropathies

Table 46-2

THE PRINCIPAL NEUROPATHIC SYNDROMES AND THEIR CAUSES (*CONTINUED*)

C. Causalgia
D. Lumbosacral plexopathies
E. Crural mononeuropathies
F. Migrant sensory neuropathy
G. Entrapment neuropathies

to a few years and another in which progression is over many years, most of which prove to have a genetic cause. It can be restated that these temporal properties are, with the topographic pattern, the main determinants in the categorization of neuropathy.

Diseases of the peripheral nerves are considered in a more comprehensive fashion in the two-volume *Peripheral Neuropathy*, edited by Dyck and colleagues and in the text by Amato and Russell cited in the references. Also recommended are more concise monographs by Schaumburg and associates and by Asbury and Thomas, and the atlas on the pathology of peripheral nerve by King.

SYNDROME OF ACUTE MOTOR PARALYSIS WITH VARIABLE DISTURBANCE OF SENSORY AND AUTONOMIC FUNCTION

A number of differences separate the polyneuropathies in this category: (1) acute inflammatory demyelinating or axonal polyneuropathy (GBS), (2) vasculitic polyneuropathies, (3) porphyria, (4) certain toxic polyneuropathies, and (5) acute sensory and autonomic polyneuropathies. Of these various acute polyneuropathic diseases, the Guillain-Barré demyelinative syndrome, because of its frequency and gravity, is most demanding of the physician's attention.

Guillain-Barré Syndrome (Landry-Guillain-Barré-Strohl Syndrome, Acute Inflammatory Demyelinating Polyneuropathy, AIDP)

This is the most common cause of acute or subacute generalized paralysis in practice. (During certain past epochs it was exceeded in frequency by polio.) GBS occurs in all parts of the world and in all seasons, affecting children and adults of all ages and both sexes. A mild respiratory or gastrointestinal infection or immunization precedes the neuropathic symptoms by 1 to 3 weeks in approximately 60 percent of cases. Typical is a nondescript upper respiratory infection, but almost every known febrile infection and immunization has at one time or another been reported to precede GBS (some probably coincidentally). In recent years, it has been appreciated from serologic studies that the enteric organism *Campylobacter jejuni* is the most frequent identifiable antecedent infection, but it accounts for only a relatively limited proportion of cases. Other common antecedent events or associated illnesses include viral exanthems in children and numerous other viral illnesses in adults and children, particularly the large viruses of the herpes family (cytomegalovirus [CMV], Epstein-Barr virus [EBV], HIV), and less often, bacterial infections other than *Campylobacter* (*Mycoplasma pneumoniae*, Lyme disease). There are less certain associations with lymphoma (particularly Hodgkin disease) and with the systemic autoimmune diseases.

Historical Background

The earliest description of an afebrile generalized paralysis is probably that of Wardrop and Ollivier, in 1834. Important landmarks were Landry's report (1859) of an acute, ascending, predominantly motor paralysis with respiratory failure leading to death among peasants on his land; Osler's (1892) description of "febrile polyneuritis"; and the account by Guillain, Barré, and Strohl (1916) of a benign polyneuritis with albuminocytologic dissociation in the CSF (increase in protein without cells). The first comprehensive account of the pathology of GBS was that of Haymaker and Kernohan (1949), who stressed that edema of the nerve roots was an important change in the early stages of the disease. Subsequently, Asbury and colleagues (1969) established that the essential lesion, from the beginning of the disease, was perivascular mononuclear inflammatory infiltration of the roots and nerves. More recently, it has been found that complement deposition on the myelin surface may be the earliest immunologic event. For details of the historical and other aspects of this disease, see the monographs by Ropper and colleagues (1991) and by Hughes (1990).

Incidence

The incidence rate of GBS has varied between 0.4 and 1.7 cases per 100,000 persons per year; the median taken from several studies is 1.1 and may be most dependable. It is generally a nonseasonal and nonepidemic disease, but outbreaks have been recorded in rural China following exposure of children to *C. jejuni* through chicken feces deposited in rice paddies. Women appear to be slightly more susceptible. The age range in our series has been 8 months to 81 years, with attack rates highest in persons 50 to 74 years of age. Cases are known in infants and in the very aged.

In addition to a seasonal increase in incidence after natural influenza outbreaks, the administration of the A/New Jersey (swine) influenza vaccine, given in the United States in late 1976, brought attention to a slight increase in the incidence of GBS and several, but not most subsequent influenza vaccination programs have been associated with a marginal increase in cases. Representative was the widely publicized worldwide H1N1 vaccination program that was studied in Quebec, where the calculated risk of developing GBS after vaccination was in the range 2 cases per 1 million doses of vaccine, barely above the baseline rate and appearing mostly in individuals over 50 years (De Wals et al). GBS appears in temporal relationship to almost all other vaccinations, but the association in these instances may be idiosyncratic and infrequent. Trauma and surgical operations may precede the neuropathy, but a causal association to them also remains uncertain.

Symptomatology

The typical case is readily identified. Paresthesias and slight numbness in the toes and fingers are the earliest symptoms; only infrequently are they absent throughout the illness. The major clinical manifestation is weakness that evolves more or less symmetrically over a period of several days to a week or two, or somewhat longer. The proximal as well as distal muscles of the limbs are involved, usually the lower extremities before the upper (thus the older term *Landry ascending paralysis*); the trunk, intercostal, neck, and cranial muscles may be affected later. Weakness progresses in approximately 5 percent of patients to total motor paralysis with respiratory failure within a few days. In severe cases, the ocular motor nerves are paralyzed and even the pupils may be unreactive.

More than half of the patients complain of pain and an aching discomfort in the muscles, mainly those of the hips, thighs, and back. These symptoms precede weakness and may be mistaken for lumbar disc disease, back strain, and orthopedic diseases. A few patients describe burning in the fingers and toes, and if this appears as an early symptom, it may become a persistent problem. Sensory loss is variable during the first days and may initially be barely detectable so that the typical case has the character of a predominantly motor neuropathy. By the end of a week, vibration and joint position sense in the toes and fingers are usually reduced; when such loss is present, deep sensibility (touch-pressure-vibration) tends to be more affected than superficial (pain-temperature).

Reduced and then absent tendon reflexes are consistent findings. Only the ankle reflexes may be lost during the first week of illness. At an early stage, the arm muscles are usually stronger than the leg muscles, and in a few cases, they are spared almost entirely. Facial diplegia occurs in more than half, sometimes bilaterally at the same time or sequentially over days. Other cranial nerve palsies, if they occur, usually come later, after the arms and face are affected; they are the initial signs in a variant pattern of disease as described further on. At the onset, there is no fever, and if lymphadenopathy or splenomegaly occurs, they are related to a preceding viral infection.

Disturbances of autonomic function include sinus tachycardia and, less often, bradycardia, facial flushing, fluctuating hypertension and hypotension, loss of sweating, or episodic profuse diaphoresis; one or more are common in minor form and infrequently do they become pronounced or persist for more than a week. Urinary retention occurs in approximately 15 percent of patients soon after the onset of weakness, but catheterization is seldom required for more than a few days. Numerous medical complications follow in severe cases as a result of immobilization and respiratory failure, as discussed further on under "Treatment."

The archetypical illness described in the preceding paragraphs is typically a result of the widespread inflammatory-demyelinating process within peripheral nerves. This is contrasted with an axonal form of GBS described just below.

Acute Axonal Form of Guillain-Barré Syndrome

Attention was drawn by Feasby and colleagues (1986) to an acute areflexic polyneuropathy clinically similar to typical GBS but characterized pathologically by widespread and severe axonal degeneration. In their initial report they described 5 patients with a rapid evolution of polyneuropathy and slow and poor recovery. Unlike the common form of demyelinating GBS, muscle atrophy became apparent relatively early in the axonal form (within weeks). The defining feature was the presence of numerous electrically inexcitable motor nerves and signs of extensive denervation. This finding could also signify a distal demyelinating block from which complete recovery is possible (Triggs et al). Nevertheless, most cases of abrupt and severe denervating paralysis, particularly if postinfectious, are caused by the axonal form of GBS (Ropper, 1986b).

Postmortem examinations have disclosed severe axonal degeneration in nerves and roots with minimal inflammatory changes and little demyelination, even early in the disease. Based on the deposits of complement and the presence of macrophages in the periaxonal space, a humoral antibody directed against some component of the axolemma was postulated by Griffin and associates (1995). Visser and colleagues reported similar findings in a series of acute motor polyneuropathies. The outbreaks of motor neuropathy that occur seasonally in rural China have many of the same characteristics. These cases appear to be triggered largely by *C. jejuni* infections. Some, but not all, sporadic instances of acute axonal GBS have been preceded by the same infection. It is noteworthy that infection with the same bacteria can also induce a typical demyelinating form of GBS.

A proportion of axonal cases, perhaps up to one-fifth, are associated with circulating antibodies to the G_{M1} ganglioside of peripheral nerve, and some of these reflect recently preceding infection with *C. jejuni*. The acronyms AMAN (acute motor) and AMSAN (acute motor-sensory axonal neuropathy) are equivalents to axonal GBS. Another variant of this illness, of which we have seen several instances, has been an acute multifocal neuropathy with electrophysiologic motor conduction block that leaves the reflexes unaltered and has high titers of anti-G_{M1} antibody (Capasso et al). Most experience with the generalized axonal form of GBS indicates that recovery is prolonged and incomplete.

Table 46-3

VARIANTS OF GUILLAIN-BARRÉ SYNDROME

Regional
Fisher syndrome of ophthalmoplegia, ataxia, and areflexia
Cervico-brachial-pharyngeal weakness, often with ptosis
Oculopharyngeal weakness
Predominant paraparesis
Bilateral facial or abducens weakness with distal paresthesias
Ophthalmoplegia with GQ_1b autoantibodies
System specific
Generalized ataxia without dysarthria or nystagmus
Pure sensory
Pure motor
Pandysautonomia
Axonal (AMAN)

Variants of Guillain-Barré Syndrome
(Table 46-3)

Portions of the clinical picture of GBS appear in isolated or abortive form and are a source of diagnostic confusion. Whereas in most patients the paralysis ascends from legs to trunk, to arms, and then to cranial regions, and reaches a peak of severity within 10 to 14 days, the *pharyngeal-cervical-brachial* muscles may be affected first or constitute the entire illness, causing difficulty in swallowing with neck and proximal arm weakness (Ropper, 1986a). Ptosis, often with ophthalmoplegia, may be added. The differential diagnosis then includes myasthenia gravis, diphtheria, and botulism and a lesion affecting the central portion of the cervical spinal cord and lower brainstem.

A syndrome comprising virtual or *complete ophthalmoplegia with ataxia* and areflexia represents a variant of GBS described by Fisher (and is called *Fisher syndrome*). A *purely ophthalmoplegic* form also exists; it may be coupled with the pharyngeal-cervical-brachial pattern mentioned earlier. Ophthalmoplegia, whether occurring alone or with weakness or ataxia of other parts, is almost uniformly associated with a specific antineural antibody, anti-GQ_1b. The ophthalmoplegic pattern raises the diagnostic possibilities of myasthenia gravis, botulism, diphtheria, tick paralysis, and basilar artery occlusion. Bilateral but asymmetrical facial and abducens weakness coupled with distal paresthesias or with proximal leg weakness is other variants in our experience (Ropper, 1994). The tendon reflexes may be absent only at the ankles or at the knees. Lyme disease and sarcoidosis are then considerations in diagnosis. Whether bifacial palsy alone represents a variant of GBS is uncertain, but almost every case in our experience has had an alternative explanation.

Paraparetic, *ataxic*, and *purely motor* or *purely sensory* forms of the illness have also been observed. Less difficulty attends the correct diagnosis of GBS if paresthesias in the acral extremities, progressive reduction or loss of reflexes, and relative symmetry of weakness appear after several days. The laboratory tests, particularly nerve conduction studies that affirm the diagnosis of typical GBS, give similar but generally milder abnormalities if they are carefully sought in all these variant forms. In a few patients, the weakness continues to evolve for 3 to 4 weeks or longer. From this group, a chronic form of demyelinative neuropathy (CIDP) may emerge and an intermediate group that progresses for 4 to 8 weeks and then improves can be identified (see further on).

Laboratory Findings

The most important laboratory aids are the electrodiagnostic studies and CSF examination. The CSF is under normal pressure and is acellular or contains only a few lymphocytes in all but 10 percent of patients; in the latter group, 10 to 50 cells (rarely more) per cubic millimeter, predominantly lymphocytes, may be found. The number of cells then decreases in a matter of 2 to 3 days; persistent pleocytosis suggests an alternative or additional process producing aseptic meningitis such as neoplastic infiltration, HIV, sarcoidosis, or Lyme infection. We have been unable to relate pleocytosis in the spinal fluid with any of the clinical features of GBS or to the severity of illness. The protein content is usually normal during the first few days of illness, but then it rises, reaching a peak in 4 to 6 weeks and persisting at a variably elevated level for many weeks. The increase in CSF protein is probably a reflection of widespread inflammatory disease of the nerve roots, but high values have had no clinical or prognostic significance in our material, apart from a few exceptional cases of pseudotumor cerebri (Ropper and Marmarou). In a few patients (fewer than 10 percent), the CSF protein values remain normal throughout the illness. From our experience, there is a higher proportion of patients with normal or only slightly elevated protein values among those with Fisher syndrome and other restricted or axonal forms of GBS.

Abnormalities of nerve conduction are early and dependable diagnostic indicators of GBS. In cases with a typical clinical and EMG/NCS presentation, one can probably dispense with the CSF analysis as a confirmatory test. The most frequent early electrodiagnostic findings are a reduction in the amplitude of muscle action potentials, slowed conduction velocity, and conduction block in motor nerves, singly or in combination (see Chap. 45). Prolonged distal latencies and reduced distal amplitudes (reflecting distal conduction block) and prolonged or absent F responses (indicating involvement of proximal parts of motor nerves and roots) are other important diagnostic findings, all reflecting focal areas of demyelination. The H reflex is almost always much delayed, or more often absent, but this does little more than confirm the loss of ankle reflexes. Although a limited electrodiagnostic examination may be normal early in the illness, a thorough study, which includes measurement of late responses, invariably shows disordered conduction in an affected limb within days of the first symptom. Features that indicate widespread axonal damage portend a poor and protracted recovery in both young and old patients as discussed above.

The clinical, CSF, and electrodiagnostic criteria for GBS were assessed by Asbury and Cornblath and are discussed in detail in the monograph by Ropper and colleagues.

Many patients with acute GBS have shown gadolinium enhancement of the cauda equina roots on magnetic resonance imaging (21 of 24 patients in our study) and this may serve as a useful test in complicated cases (Gorson et al, 1996).

Beyond the close association between autoantibodies to GQ 1b and Fisher syndrome or other variants that include ophthalmoplegia as mentioned previously other anti-ganglioside antibodies have become of interest in GBS. The acute motor axonal variety has a tendency to be associated with antibodies to GM1 or GD1a and the pharyngeal-cervical-brachial syndrome, to GT1a. Much of this work comes from the laboratory of Yuki, and his review article with Hartung is recommended for further explanations of potential autoimmune mechanisms.

Abnormalities of liver function occur in fewer than 10 percent of patients, probably reflecting a recent or ongoing viral hepatitis, usually as a result of CMV or EBV infections (rarely one of the hepatitis viruses). T-wave and other electrocardiographic changes of minor degree are reported frequently but tend to be evanescent. The sedimentation rate is normal unless there is an additional process of infectious, neoplastic, or autoimmune nature, any of which can occasionally coexist with GBS. Hyponatremia occurs in a proportion of cases after the first week, but particularly in ventilated patients. This is usually attributable to the syndrome of inappropriate antidiuretic hormone secretion (SIADH), but a natriuretic type also occurs, from an excess of atrial natriuretic factor (Wijdicks et al). Transient diabetes insipidus is a rare and unexplained complication. With regard to proteinuria due to glomerulonephritis reported by several groups in cases of GBS, we have found it infrequently.

Pathologic Findings

These have had a relatively consistent pattern and form. Even when the disease is fatal within a few days, most cases show endoneural perivascular (mainly perivenous) lymphocytic infiltrates. Later, there is segmental demyelination and a variable degree of wallerian degeneration. The cellular infiltrates are scattered throughout the cranial nerves, ventral and dorsal spinal roots, dorsal root ganglia, and along the entire length of the peripheral nerves. Swelling of nerve roots at the site of their dural exit has been emphasized by some authors and theorized to cause root damage.

Variations of this pattern have been observed, each perhaps representing a different immunopathology. For example, there may be widespread demyelinative changes and only a paucity of perivascular lymphocytes (Ropper and Adelman). In patients whose electrophysiologic tests display severe axonal damage early in the illness as discussed earlier the pathologic findings corroborate the predominantly axonal nature of the disease with secondary myelin damage and usually little inflammatory response. An occasional case has shown an inflammatory process with primary axonal damage rather than demyelination (Honovar et al).

Pathogenesis and Etiology

Most evidence supports a cell-mediated immunologic reaction directed at peripheral nerves. Waksman and Adams demonstrated that experimentally induced peripheral nerve disease (experimental allergic neuritis [EAN]), clinically and pathologically indistinguishable from GBS, develops in animals 2 weeks after immunization with peripheral nerve homogenates. Brostoff and colleagues suggested that the antigen in this reaction is a basic protein, designated P2, found only in peripheral nerve myelin. Subsequent investigations by these authors indicated that the neuritogenic factor might be a specific peptide in the P2 protein. However, it has become evident that there is no dominant antigen–antibody reaction in GBS and it is likely that any number of myelin and axonal elements may be involved in inciting the immune reaction. Figure 46-3 diagrammatically illustrates the pathologic steps in this proposed reaction. As noted further on, complement also seems to be a necessary factor in the initial attack on myelin.

Although the transmission of EAN by T cells sensitized to myelin is strong evidence of their role in GBS, antimyelin antibodies are probably involved in the initial part in the disease. The serum from patients with GBS damages myelin in tissue cultures and induces a characteristic ("vesicular") form of myelin destruction. Subepineural injection of serum from GBS patients into the sciatic nerve of rats leads to local demyelination and electrical conduction block. The studies by Koski and associates of complement-dependent myelin damage by immunoglobulin (Ig) M antimyelin antibodies in GBS provided evidence that antimyelin antibodies are able to initiate myelin destruction even through T cells and that macrophages are the ultimate effectors of the damage. Indeed, the very earliest change that could be detected by Hafer-Macko and colleagues was the deposition of complement on the inner layer of myelin.

As mentioned earlier, circulating autoantibodies directed at components of nerve ganglioside are detected but only inconsistently in patients with GBS, the most important being anti-GQ_1b, which is found in almost all patients with ophthalmoplegia. Approximately one-fifth of patients have anti-G_{M1} antibodies early in their course, corresponding in most instances to a predominantly motor presentation and to axonal damage, the highest titers being associated with cases that follow *Campylobacter* infections. Antibodies directed against GD_1a or GT_1b are associated in some cases with the pharyngeal-brachial-cervical variant. Thus it would seem that casting GBS exclusively as a humoral or as a cellular immune process is an oversimplification.

An unanswered question is what incites the immune reaction isolated to peripheral nerves in humans. All attempts to identify a virus or microbial agent within nerves have failed and it is likely that a variety of agents—viral, bacterial (particularly *C. jejuni*), certain vaccines, and perhaps neural injury itself—are each capable, in susceptible individuals, of precipitating an immune response against components of autologous peripheral nerve. The occurrence of GBS in patients with AIDS or with EBV or CMV infections simply indicates that these agents too

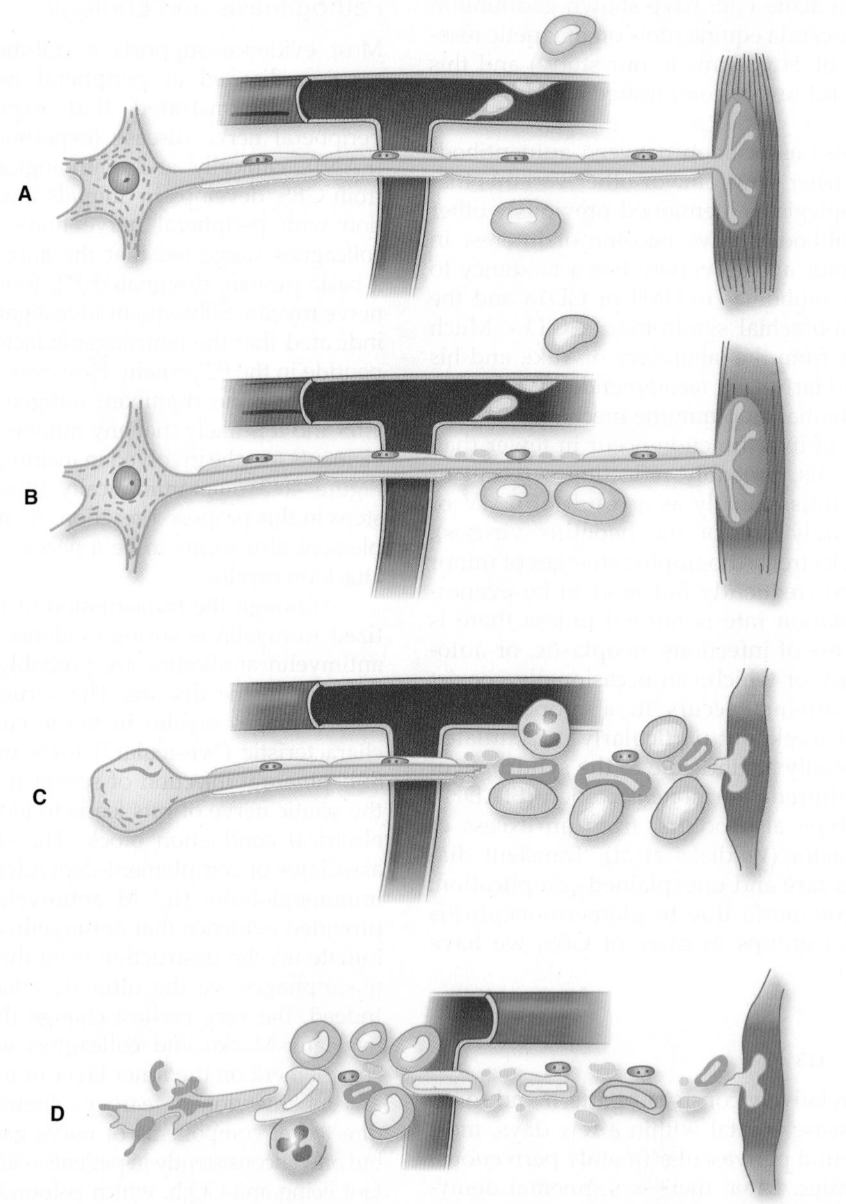

Figure 46-3. Diagram of probable cellular events in acute inflammatory polyneuropathy (Guillain-Barré syndrome). *A*. Lymphocytes attach to the walls of endoneurial vessels and migrate through the vessel wall, enlarging and transforming as they do so. At this stage no nerve damage has occurred. *B*. More lymphocytes have migrated into the surrounding tissue. The first effect on the nerve is breakdown of myelin, the axon being spared (segmental demyelination). This change appears to be mediated by the mononuclear exudate, but the mechanism is uncertain. *C*. The lesion is more intense, polymorphonuclear leukocytes being present as well as lymphocytes. There is interruption of the axon in addition to myelin sheath damage; as a result, the muscle undergoes denervation atrophy and the nerve cell body shows central chromatolysis. If the axonal damage is distal, the nerve cell body will survive, and regeneration and clinical recovery are likely. If, as in *D*, axonal interruption has occurred proximally because of a particularly intense root or proximal nerve lesion, the nerve cell body may die and undergo dissolution. In this situation, there is no regeneration, only the possibility of collateral reinnervation of muscle from surviving motor fibers. (From Asbury et al [1969], by permission.)

induce such an autoimmune response without implicating a direct viral infection of nerve. The observation that only one of many individuals who are infected with a particular pathogen go on to develop GBS suggests that host factors are significant (there is, however, little consistency of human leukocyte antigen [HLA] types in GBS patients). Whether the aforementioned antibodies against various gangliosides of peripheral nerve are pathogenically active is also uncertain.

Several animal diseases—namely coonhound paralysis of dogs, Marek disease of chickens (a viral neuritis), and cauda equina neuritis of horses—resemble GBS superficially but do not share its main clinical or pathologic features.

Differential Diagnosis

GBS is not only the most frequent acute generalized polyneuropathy seen in general hospitals but also the most rapidly evolving and potentially fatal form. Any polyneuropathy that brings the patient to the brink of death or to respiratory failure within a few days will usually be of this variety. Most cases, however, are of the more limited variety with paresthesias, limb weakness, and areflexia. Several other conditions must be considered. The immediate problem is to differentiate GBS from acute spinal cord disease marked by sensorimotor paralysis with a defined spinal level and prominent sphincter disturbances. There may be diagnostic difficulty in the case of an acute lesion of the cord in which tendon reflexes are initially lost (spinal shock), or with necrotizing myelopathy, where a permanent loss of tendon reflexes follows extensive destruction of spinal gray matter. Early and transient urinary retention occurs in a proportion of patients with GBS and causes diagnostic confusion with spinal disease. Several features are useful in distinguishing GBS from a cervical myelopathy: in GBS, the facial and respiratory muscles are usually involved if there is generalized paralysis; the fingertips should be paresthetic once sensory symptoms have ascended to the level of the midcalves; marked sensory loss proximal to the hands or feet or only of the trunk is unusual early in the illness; and tendon reflexes are almost invariably lost in limbs that are too weak to resist gravity. Of course, careful testing of sensation on the trunk and limbs will expose the cause of paralysis as spinal in origin.

Tick paralysis, a disease of children in the United States but affecting both children and adults in Australia and elsewhere, may be nearly impossible to distinguish from GBS unless one finds the tick (see Chap. 43). In addition to an ascending generalized paralysis, both may cause ataxia and may paralyze eye movements, but sensory loss is not usually a feature of tick paralysis and the CSF protein is normal. Episodes of painful paralytic porphyria also bear a superficial resemblance to GBS. Predominant motor features in comparison to sensory ones is the major characteristic of GBS, for which reason the differential diagnosis also includes poliomyelitis, caused by the West Nile virus and by enteroviruses other than the polio agent. In these infectious cases, the illness is marked by fever, meningoencephalitic symptoms, early pleocytosis in the spinal fluid, and purely motor and usually asymmetrical areflexic paralysis, all unusual in GBS.

Several times we were misled by cases of carcinomatous meningitis with polyradiculopathy that caused a painless, subacute, and fairly symmetric but mainly distal weakness, similar to GBS. An irregular distribution of weakness between proximal and distal parts, the absence of facial weakness, and the appearance of symptoms sequentially in one limb after another suggest the presence of this type of neoplastic polyradiculopathy. Sciatica may occur as an early feature with either process but radicular pain in the arms is unusual in GBS. Examination of the spinal fluid usually settles the matter.

Another problem arises in distinguishing generalized GBS with ophthalmoparesis or the Fisher variant from basilar artery thrombosis. The presence of reactive pupils, areflexia, and F-wave abnormalities in GBS, and of lively reflexes and Babinski signs in the case of brainstem infarction, dependably separate the disorders. Ptosis and oculomotor weakness in GBS causes confusion with myasthenia gravis, but there are no sensory symptoms and the tendon reflexes are unimpaired in the latter disease. The mandibular muscles remain relatively strong in GBS, whereas the exercised jaw hangs open in myasthenia. Botulism also simulates this cranial variant of GBS, but pupillary reflexes are lost early in botulism (pupillary paralysis occurs mainly in advanced cases of GBS) and there is usually a bradycardia, which is unusual for GBS. Ingestion of shellfish or reef fish contaminated with saxitoxin, ciguatoxin, or tetrodotoxin (ciguatera, neurotoxic shellfish poisoning) is another cause of facial-brachial paresthesias, weakness, tachypnea, and iridoplegia lasting up to a few days—symptoms that resemble the cranial nerve variants of GBS.

A number of neuromuscular disorders in critically ill patients with systemic medical conditions are difficult to distinguish from GBS. These include the polyneuropathy of critical illness (see further on in the chapter); an accelerated neuropathy of renal failure that is seen mainly in diabetic patients receiving peritoneal dialysis (both discussed further on); acute hypophosphatemia induced by hyperalimentation; polymyopathy produced by the administration of high-dose corticosteroids; and the prolonged effects of neuromuscular blocking drugs, resulting in the accumulation of their metabolites in patients under conditions of renal failure and acidosis.

Treatment

General Medical Care In severe cases, respiratory assistance and assiduous nursing are paramount, because the disease remits naturally and the outlook for recovery is favorable in the majority of patients. About one-quarter of our patients have required mechanical ventilation. Because a patient's condition may deteriorate unpredictably and rapidly in the first days of illness, virtually all but the mildest cases should be admitted to the hospital for observation of respiratory, autonomic, and motor function. The comments that follow are applicable to most other forms of acute and subacute neuromuscular respiratory failure, including myasthenia gravis and high spinal cord injury.

Measurement of maximal inspiratory force and expiratory vital capacity suffices for the bedside estimation of diaphragmatic strength and respiratory function. The trend of these measurements is a guide to the likelihood of respiratory failure. As had been observed in poliomyelitis, the strength of the neck muscles and trapezii, which share the same segmental innervation as the diaphragm, tends to parallel diaphragmatic power. A rough estimate of breathing capacity may be obtained by having the patient count quickly on one deep breath. The ability to reach 20 generally corresponds to a vital capacity of greater than 1.5 L. If a downward trend in these measurements is recognized and the vital capacity diminishes to below about 10 mL/kg, endotracheal intubation and mechanical ventilation are usually necessary (see further on). However, a fairly severe impairment of ventilation may occur before the first sign of dyspnea appears and before there is elevation of arterial carbon dioxide content. Incipient respiratory failure may be evident by tachypnea and a decrease in arterial oxygen tension (Po_2 less than 85 mm Hg) reflecting pulmonary atelectasis. When respiratory failure arises gradually as the patient weakens over days, there is slight tachycardia, diaphoresis, restlessness, and tachypnea. Attempts to forestall intubation and positive-pressure ventilation by using negative-pressure cuirass-type devices have been unsatisfactory in our experience. Patients with oropharyngeal weakness require intubation even earlier so as to prevent aspiration, but full mechanical ventilation is not always necessary at the same time. Patients in these circumstances should obviously be admitted to an intensive care unit staffed by personnel skilled in maintaining ventilation and airway patency.

The other major aspects of the treatment in severely affected patients involve the management of *autonomic instability* and the prevention of the many *general medical problems* that attend any immobilizing critical illness. Hypotension from *dysautonomia*, which occurs in approximately 10 percent of paralyzed patients and a smaller proportion with lesser degrees of weakness, is treated by intravenous infusions of saline and by the use of vasopressor agents for brief periods. Extremes of hypertension are managed by short-acting and titratable antihypertensive medications, such as intravenous labetalol. The choice and dosing of an antihypertensive drug is important, as episodes of hypertension may be rapidly succeeded by precipitous declines in pressure. Severe autonomic problems are difficult to anticipate, but provocative maneuvers such as ocular pressure to elicit heart block are used in some units to identify patients at risk.

In patients who are bedbound, prevention of electrolyte imbalances, gastrointestinal hemorrhage, and particularly pulmonary embolism (by the use of subcutaneous heparin or pneumatic compression boots) requires careful attention. Adynamic ileus is a problem in some cases, manifest by abdominal pain coincident with nasogastric tube feeding and by bloating; it may lead to bowel perforation even if feeding is discontinued. As mentioned, a number of patients become hyponatremic, usually from SIADH but occasionally from a natriuresis, and the drop in sodium is exaggerated by positive-pressure mechanical ventilation. The distinction between the two conditions that cause hyponatremia determines the course of treatment: fluid restriction in the case of SIADH or salt replacement in the case of sodium loss. Many patients have bizarre waking dreams or hallucinations after weeks of immobilization (oneiric hallucinations). A dependable mode of communication should be established by the nursing staff, preferably before the patient is intubated. A Plexiglas or opaque board with letters and phrases is useful for this purpose.

Failure to effectively clear the tracheobronchial airways and the need for prolonged mechanical ventilation are the usual indications for tracheostomy. In most cases, this procedure can be postponed until the third week of intubation. However, patients who become rapidly quadriplegic and ventilator-dependent benefit from tracheostomy earlier. Once tracheostomy is performed, careful tracheal toilet and treatment of pulmonary and urinary tract infections by the use of appropriate antibiotics are required; prophylactic antibiotic treatment is not recommended. With tracheostomy and intensive care, the mortality from the disease can be reduced to approximately 3 percent (Ropper and Kehne; see further on under "Prognosis").

The decisions to wean and then discontinue respiratory aid and to remove the endotracheal or tracheostomy tube are based on the degree and timing of recovery of respiratory function. The weaning process generally begins when the vital capacity reaches approximately 10 mL/kg and comfortable breathing can be sustained for a few minutes. The relative merits of the numerous methods of delivering positive-pressure volume-cycled ventilation and its gradual withdrawal are not covered here, but there is little to favor one over the other and the reader is referred to the monograph *Neurological and Neurosurgical Intensive Care* by Ropper and colleagues.

Physical therapy (passive movement and positioning of limbs to prevent pressure palsies and, later, mild resistance exercises) can begin once they can be comfortably undertaken.

Plasma Exchange and Immune Globulin Specific treatment of the presumed immune disorder that underlies GBS includes plasma exchange and IVIg. Our practice has been to observe patients who are still able to walk unaided rather than institute treatment immediately. If the patient becomes unable to walk, shows a reduction in vital capacity, or signs of oropharyngeal weakness, plasma exchange or IVIg is instituted promptly. This typically occurs at the fifth to tenth day after the appearance of the first symptoms, but may be as early as 1 day or as late as 3 weeks.

Three large randomized trials comprising more than 500 patients have established the efficacy of *plasma exchange* administered during the evolving phase of GBS. In patients who are treated within 2 weeks of onset, there is an approximate halving of the period of hospitalization, of the duration of mechanical ventilation, and of the time required to achieve independent ambulation. However, in the largest trial, if the first plasma exchange was delayed for 2 weeks or longer after the onset of the disease, the procedure was of little value. Nonetheless, if a patient continues to progress in the third or fourth week of illness, it is probably still appropriate to institute the exchanges. The most important predictors of responsiveness to plasma exchange treatment are the same as for the overall prognosis, namely the patient's age (responders are younger) and the preservation of motor compound muscle action potential amplitudes prior to instituting treatment (McKhann et al). One study has found that the condition of patients was better at 6 and 12 months after treatment as compared to untreated patients; other studies have been equivocal on this point and demonstrated mainly accelerated improvement.

The advised regimen of plasma exchange removes a total of 200 to 250 mL/kg of plasma in 4 to 6 treatments on alternate days, or over a shorter period if there is no coagulopathy. The replacement fluid is saline combined with 5 percent albumin. The need for large-bore venous access usually requires the insertion of a double-lumen subclavian or internal jugular catheters and this may be the main source of complications (pneumothorax, infection, hemorrhage). In some patients, treatment can be instituted, and sometimes the entire course completed, through the antecubital veins. During and after the procedure, hypotension, hypoprothrombinemia with bleeding and cardiac arrhythmias may occur. Some units measure the level of fibrinogen, which is greatly reduced by exchanges, before the next exchange to gauge to the risk of potential hemorrhage. Reactions to the citrate that is used to prevent blood from clotting in the plasma exchange machine are common but can be obviated by the cautious addition of calcium to the intravenous return line. Hepatitis and AIDS are not risks if plasma is replaced with albumin and saline rather than with pooled plasma.

As effective as plasma exchange is, IVIg (0.4 g/kg per day for 5 consecutive days) is both easier to administer and probably safer because there is no need for large intravenous access. The results of the first trial conducted by van der Meché and colleagues were corroborated in an international study led by Hughes, in which we participated (see Plasma Exchange/Sandoglobulin Guillain-Barré Syndrome Trial Group). That trial compared plasma exchange to IVIg and also evaluated their use sequentially. There was a tenuous trend toward a better outcome in patients who received plasma exchange and results were perhaps slightly better in a group who were treated with plasma exchange followed immediately by 5 days of immune globulin infusions; in both instances, however, the differences failed to attain statistical significance and the three modes of treatment were said to be equivalent. Renal failure, proteinuria, and aseptic meningitis, manifested most often by severe headache, are infrequent complications of IVIg. The only serious reactions we have encountered have been in a very few patients who congenitally lacked IgA and in whom pooled gamma globulin caused anaphylaxis, and a few cases of inflammatory local venous thrombosis in the region of the infusion site. The pharmacokinetics of IVIg are highly variable among individuals and some groups have found an association between a high rate of clearance of agent and poorer clinical outcome (see Kuitwaard and colleagues). This group has suggested that patients who show only a small increment in serum IgG levels might benefit from higher doses or a second course of IVIg.

After the use of either plasma exchange or IVIg, 5 to 10 percent of patients who initially improve will have a relapse that becomes apparent several days or up to 3 weeks after completion of treatment. If there had been a response to the initial therapy, the same treatment may be repeated or the alternative treatment may be tried; either can be successful. A few such patients relapse repeatedly and have the course of chronic inflammatory demyelinating polyneuropathy (see further on). In some patients under our care, this form of the disease stabilized after several months in response to the administration of corticosteroids, with very gradual tapering of the dose over several months, or in combination with repeated courses of IVIg or plasma exchanges.

The clinical improvement that follows the administration of IVIg or plasma exchange usually cannot be readily discerned in an individual patient; i.e., it is apparent only by comparing large groups of treated and untreated patients. For this reason it is not possible to judge that a patient who fails to improve or who worsens through the period of treatment has derived no benefit from therapy. The question nevertheless arises regarding further plasma exchanges or continued infusion of immune globulin in cases of continued worsening or lack of improvement. Further complicating the matter are the limited expectations for early improvement in cases of axonal GBS. Our advice has been to repeat either of the two immune treatments if a patient is clearly declining, particularly if there is evidence of demyelinating neuropathy on the NCS, and if the illness is not much longer than 4 weeks in duration. Performing plasma exchanges after the use of IVIg does not make sense to us (but this notion has not been tested); therefore, we either follow a series of exchanges with IVIg or, more often, repeat a course of IVIg as suggested by Farcas and colleagues.

The value of corticosteroids alone in the treatment of GBS has been disputed for decades. Many clinicians were persuaded of their benefit; however, two randomized controlled trials, one with conventional-dose prednisolone and the other with high-dose methylprednisolone, have failed to demonstrate beneficial effect (Hughes et al, 1991). Although corticosteroids can no longer be recommended as routine treatment for acute GBS, we have observed a few instances in which the administration of intravenous high-dose corticosteroids seemingly halted the progress of an acute case.

Prognosis

As already indicated, approximately 3 to 5 percent of patients do not survive the illness, even in the best equipped hospitals. In the early stages, death is most often a result of cardiac arrest, sometimes related to dysautonomia, adult respiratory distress syndrome, pneumo- or hemothorax, or some type of accidental machine failure. Later in the illness, pulmonary embolism and infectious complications of prolonged immobilization and respiratory failure are the main causes of death.

The majority of patients recover with mild motor deficits or sensory complaints in the feet or legs. In approximately 10 percent, however, the residual disability is pronounced; this occurs in those with the most severe and rapidly evolving form of the disease, when there has been evidence of widespread axonal damage and in those requiring early and prolonged mechanical ventilatory assistance. A fairly consistent predictor of residual weakness and muscle atrophy is the finding of greatly reduced amplitudes of muscle action potentials and widespread denervation, both indicative of axonal damage.

In patients with respiratory failure, the average period of machine-assisted respiration has been 22 days and the period of hospitalization approximately 50 days (these were twice as long prior to the introduction of plasma exchange and IVIg). As a rule, older adults recover more slowly than younger ones and children and have more residual weakness.

The most common remaining difficulties are weakness of the lower leg muscles, numbness of the feet and toes, and mild bifacial weakness. A few patients are left with sensory ataxia that tends to be severe and quite disabling. Distal neuropathic pain and persistent autonomic problems occur but are also infrequent. All manner of other late symptoms are attributed with little evidence to the illness and should be addressed on their own merits—fatigue and asthenia, muscle cramps, dizziness, pain, and breathlessness. Depression has not been frequent.

The speed of recovery varies, but its pace is steady. Often, it occurs within a few weeks or months; however, if axons have been damaged, their regeneration may require 6 to 18 months or longer. In our experience, little improvement can be expected in disabilities that have lasted 2 or more years.

Some 5 to 10 percent of patients encounter one or more recurrences of the acute polyneuropathy. An illness that in the beginning appeared to be an acute inflammatory polyradiculoneuropathy may fail to stabilize and continue to progress steadily, or there may be an incomplete remission followed by a chronic, fluctuating, slowly progressive neuropathy. These more chronic forms of inflammatory neuropathy are described in a later section of this chapter.

Critical Illness Polyneuropathy

An acute or subacute symmetrical polyneuropathy is a frequent development in critically ill and septic patients, particularly in those with failure of multiple organs (Zochodne et al). This neuropathy causes difficulty in weaning a patient from the ventilator, even as the underlying critical illness comes under control. The neuropathic process, predominantly of motor type, varies in severity from an electrophysiologic abnormality without overt clinical signs, to quadriparesis with respiratory failure. Sensory symptoms and signs are variable but tend to be mild. Usually the cranial nerves are spared and there are few or no dysautonomic manifestations. In general, this type of polyneuropathy appears after several days or more of bacterial sepsis or other overwhelming infection (now called *systemic inflammatory response syndrome [SIRS]*) and multiple organ failure, and is preceded in most instances by a confusional state or a depressed state of consciousness ("septic encephalopathy").

The EMG and NCS findings of a primary axonal process with early denervation and a normal CSF distinguish this entity from the typical demyelinative form of GBS. Autopsy material has usually disclosed little or no inflammatory changes in the peripheral nerves. Differentiating critical illness polyneuropathy from critical illness myopathy (see just below) and from the axonal form of GBS is difficult and depends on the context in which the illness occurs. All of these processes that occur in the intensive care unit, when extreme, can eliminate the motor nerve action potentials and when this configuration is found, the problem is most often attributed to the neuropathy, although this is not always correct. The toxic effects of drugs and antibiotics and nutritional deficiency must be considered in causation, but rarely can they be established. The many systemic mediators of sepsis are toxic to the peripheral nervous system; tumor necrosis factor has been proposed as one such endogenous toxin in causing neuropathy.

Critical illness polyneuropathy must also be distinguished from a poorly understood *acute quadriplegic myopathy* (critical illness myopathy) that also complicates critical illness (see Chap. 48). High doses of corticosteroids, particularly in combination with neuromuscular blocking agents, have been implicated. The acute myopathy, which affects both distal and proximal muscles, is sometimes heralded by an elevation in the serum creatine kinase (CK) concentration (at times up to several thousand units) and myopathic potentials in the EMG, and a unique degeneration of myofilaments in all the muscles is found. This illness is described in more detail in Chap. 48.

Acute Uremic Polyneuropathy

In addition to the well-known chronic sensory polyneuropathy associated with chronic renal failure that is discussed later in the chapter, there is a more rapid ("accelerated") process that has not been widely appreciated as a cause of acute and subacute weakness. Most patients in our series were diabetics with stable end-stage renal failure who had been treated by peritoneal dialysis for their long-standing kidney disease (Ropper, 1993). In contrast to the better characterized and less severe chronic uremic neuropathy, generalized weakness and distal paresthesias progress over 1 or more weeks until a bedbound state is reached. The illness simulates subacute GBS. More aggressive dialysis or a change to hemodialysis has little immediate effect, although kidney transplantation is curative. Electrophysiologic studies show demyelinating features (slowing of conduction velocity), but usually not a conduction block. There is raised CSF protein concentration (not unexpectedly, for there is usually an element of diabetic neuropathy). A few reported cases have responded to plasma exchange or gamma globulin. As with the more common chronic uremic neuropathy, the cause of the acute form is unknown.

Acute Sensory Neuronopathy (Acute Sensory Ganglionopathy)

Attention was initially drawn to this entity by Sterman and colleagues in a report of 3 adult patients with rapidly evolving sensory ataxia, areflexia, numbness, and pain, beginning in the face and spreading to involve the entire body. In each instance, the symptoms began within 4 to 12 days following the institution of penicillin therapy for a febrile illness (antibiotics were subsequently shown not to be associated). Proprioception was profoundly reduced, but there was no weakness or muscle atrophy, despite generalized areflexia. The sensory deficit attained its maximum severity within a week, after which it stabilized and improved very little.

Electrophysiologic studies showed absent or slowed sensory conduction, but there were no abnormalities of motor nerve conduction or signs of denervation. In two patients, the CSF protein content was elevated to 126 and 175 mg/dL. Followup observations (for up to 5 years) disclosed no neoplastic or immunologic disorder, the usual identifiable causes of such a sensory neuronopathy. Lacking pathologic material, it was assumed from the permanence of the condition that sensory neurons were destroyed (*sensory neuronopathy*). A subsequent series of 42 patients reported by Windebank and colleagues emphasized an asymmetrical and brachial pattern of symptoms in some patients and initial involvement of the face in others. In contrast to Sterman's cases, the CSF was usually normal and most patients had some improvement or a spontaneous resolution of symptoms. These authors viewed the process as a sensory neuropathy. In this and subsequent reports, as mentioned, antibiotics were not implicated.

This clinical pattern should be viewed as a syndrome rather than as a disease. There are two main presentations: with limb ataxia that does not have accompanying dysarthria or nystagmus, thus distinguishing it from a cerebellar disorder; and with generalized facial and truncal numbness that involves proximal and distal sensory areas and may include the top of the head, trunk, buttocks, scrotum, and oral mucosal membranes. The latter syndrome must be delineated from an evolving polyneuropathy, the early proximal symptoms being the most salient identifying feature for a ganglionopathy as mentioned in the introductory sections of this chapter. All the just described processes are accompanied by areflexia, but this may not be fully developed in the case of ganglionopathy for several days or longer.

Probably, most instances are immune and postinfectious in nature. The same pattern of sensory loss evolving in a subacute or chronic manner is well known to occur as a paraneoplastic illness, described further on in this chapter, or in association with the Sjögren syndrome, scleroderma, lupus erythematosus, paraproteinemia, HIV and human T-cell lymphotropic virus type I (HTLV-I) infection. Certain drugs and other agents, especially cisplatin and excessive intake of pyridoxine, are also causes of a sensory neuronopathy. These are discussed again later, under "Drug-Induced Neuropathies and Neuronopathies" A rare form of GBS involves solely the large sensory fibers and produces ataxia, thereby simulating an acute sensory neuronopathy. In GBS, however, there is usually some degree of proximal weakness and the sensory changes do not extend to the face and trunk.

Diphtheritic Polyneuropathy

The neurotoxic effects of *Corynebacterium diphtheriae* and the mode of action of the exotoxin elaborated by the bacillus are described in Chap. 43. Local action of the exotoxin may paralyze pharyngeal and laryngeal muscles (dysphagia, nasal voice) within 1 or 2 weeks after the onset of the infection and shortly thereafter may cause blurring of vision because of paralysis of accommodation, but these and other cranial nerve symptoms may be overlooked. At this stage, the cranial neuropathy must be distinguished from that of GBS, botulism, and most of all, from myasthenia gravis.

A polyneuropathy, appearing 5 to 8 weeks later, takes the form of an acute or subacute limb weakness with paresthesias and distal loss of vibratory and position sense. The weakness characteristically involves all extremities at the same time or may descend from arms to legs. The patient may be unable to stand or walk and occasionally the paralysis is so extensive as to impair respiration. The CSF protein is usually elevated (50 to 200 mg/dL). Deaths that occur after the pharyngeal infection has subsided are a result of cardiomyopathy or, less often, of severe polyneuropathy with respiratory paralysis. This type of polyneuropathy, now quite rare, should be suspected in the midst of an outbreak of diphtheritic infection, as occurred in Russia (Logina and Donaghy).

The important pathologic change is one of segmental demyelination without inflammatory reaction of spinal roots, sensory ganglia, and adjacent spinal nerves. Anterior horn cells, axons, peripheral nerves distally, and muscle fibers remain normal (Fisher and Adams).

Treatment Diphtheria antitoxin, given within 48 h of the onset of the infection, reduces the incidence and severity of neuropathic complications. Antitoxin is probably of little value once the polyneuropathy begins. Thereafter, treatment is purely symptomatic, along the lines indicated for GBS. The prognosis for full recovery is excellent once respiratory paralysis is circumvented.

Porphyric Polyneuropathy

A severe, rapidly advancing, more or less symmetrical and mainly motor polyneuropathy—often with abdominal pain, psychosis (delirium or confusion), and convulsions—may be a manifestation of *acute intermittent porphyria*. This type of porphyria is inherited as an autosomal dominant trait and is not associated with cutaneous sensitivity to sunlight. The metabolic defect is in the liver and is marked by increased production and urinary excretion of porphobilinogen and of the porphyrin precursor Δ-aminolevulinic acid. The peripheral and central nervous systems may also be affected in another hepatic type of porphyria (the variegate type). In the latter, the skin is markedly sensitive to light and trauma, and porphyrins are at all times found in the stools. Both of these *hepatic* forms of porphyria must be distinguished from the rarer *erythropoietic (congenital photosensitive)* porphyria, in which the nervous system is not affected.

The classic study of acute intermittent porphyria was made by Waldenstrom in 1957. The initial and often the most prominent symptom is moderate to severe colicky abdominal pain. It may be generalized or localized and is unattended by rigidity of the abdominal wall or tenderness. Constipation and intestinal distention (ileus) are frequent. Attacks last for days to weeks and repeated vomiting may lead to inanition. In latent forms, the patient may be asymptomatic or complain only of slight dyspepsia.

The disease can be identified after some time by its characteristic recurrent attacks, often precipitated by drugs such as sulfonamides, griseofulvin, estrogens, barbiturates, phenytoin, and the succinimide anticonvulsants. The possibility of sensitivity to these drugs must always be kept in mind when convulsions are being treated in the porphyric patient. The first attack rarely occurs before puberty, and the disease is most likely to threaten life during adolescence and early adulthood. In contrast, acute polyneuropathy that appears for the first time in mid- or late adult life is not likely to be porphyric.

The neurologic manifestations are usually those of an acute polyneuropathy involving the motor nerves more severely than the sensory ones; less often, both sensory and motor nerves are affected more or less equally and sometimes autonomic nerves as well. The symptoms may begin in the feet and legs and ascend, or they may begin in the hands and arms (sometimes asymmetrically) and spread in a few days to the trunk and legs. Often, the weakness predominates in the proximal muscles of the limbs and limb girdle muscles, in which case there is loss of knee jerks with preservation of reflexes at the ankles. Sensory loss, often extending to the trunk, is present in half the cases. Facial paralysis, dysphagia, and ocular palsies are features of only the most severe cases. The CSF protein content is normal or slightly elevated.

The course of the polyneuropathy is variable. In mild cases the symptoms regress in a few weeks. Severe cases may progress to a fatal respiratory or cardiac paralysis in a few days, or the symptoms may advance in a saltatory fashion over several weeks, resulting in a severe sensorimotor paralysis that improves only after many months.

A disturbance of cerebral function (confusion, delirium, visual field defects, and convulsions) is likely to precede the severe, but not always the mild, forms of polyneuropathy, or there may be none of these central features. Cerebral manifestations subside in a few days or weeks, although one of our patients was left with a lasting homonymous hemianopia. Tachycardia and hypertension are frequent in the acute phase of the disease and fever and leukocytosis may occur in severe cases. In general, the prognosis for recovery is excellent, although relapse of the porphyria may result in cumulative damage to the peripheral nervous system (see discussion further on under "Diagnosis of Recurrent or Relapsing Polyneuropathy").

In summary, the most characteristic features of porphyric neuropathy are the relapsing nature, acute onset, abdominal pain, psychotic symptoms, predominant motor neuropathy, often with an early bibrachial distribution of weakness, truncal sensory loss, and tachycardia. Rarely, the neuropathy develops without other symptoms.

The pathologic findings in the peripheral nervous system vary according to the stage of the illness at which death occurs. In the first few days, the myelinated fibers may appear entirely normal, despite almost complete paralysis. If symptoms had been present for weeks, degeneration of both axons and myelin sheaths are found in most of the peripheral nerves. The relation between the abnormality of porphyrin biosynthesis in the liver and nervous dysfunction has never been explained satisfactorily.

The diagnosis is confirmed by the demonstration of large amounts of porphobilinogen and Δ-aminolevulinic acid in the urine. The urine turns dark when standing as a consequence of the formation of porphobilin, an oxidation product of porphobilinogen.

Treatment The use of intravenous glucose and intravenous hematin (4 mg/kg daily for 3 to 14 days) is recommended as the most effective therapy. Other aspects of treatment include respiratory support, use of beta-blocking agents (labetalol) if tachycardia and hypertension are severe, continued intravenous glucose to suppress the heme biosynthetic pathway, and pyridoxine (100 mg bid) on the supposition that vitamin B_6 depletion has occurred. Attempted *prevention* is of the utmost importance, since attacks can be precipitated by the aforementioned drugs as well as numerous others that are porphyrinogenic.

Acute Toxic Polyneuropathies

As indicated in Chap. 43, the peripheral nerves may be affected by a wide variety of toxins including metals, drugs, organophosphates, and industrial solvents. As a rule, the neuropathies induced by these agents fall into the subacute and chronic categories (to be discussed further on). However, certain drugs—notably triorthocresyl phosphate (TOCP) and other organophosphates (see Chap. 40), thallium and rarely, arsenic—produce a polyneuropathy that may be fatal in a matter of days. It should be stressed that organophosphate neuropathy can be identified in almost all instances by the severe anticholinergic effects that are apparent immediately after exposure. Severe and permanent motor paralysis is caused by TOCP; this ultimately proves to be a result of involvement of both upper and lower motor neurons.

Thallium salts, when taken in sufficient amount, produce a clinical picture resembling that of GBS or an acute sensory polyneuropathy. If the salts are taken orally, there is first abdominal pain, vomiting, and diarrhea, followed within a few days by pain and tingling in the toes and fingertips and then rapid weakening of muscles of the limbs, initially the distal ones. As the weakness progresses, the tendon reflexes diminish. Pain sensation is reduced more than tactile, vibratory, and position sense. Persistent acral pain with allodynia has been a major feature in 3 of the 5 patients we have examined; in 2 of our patients there was no weakness, only sensory loss and ataxia. All cranial nerves except the first and eighth may be affected; facial palsies, ophthalmoplegia, nystagmus, optic neuritis with visual impairment, and vocal cord palsies are additional abnormalities but only in the most severely affected patients. The CSF protein rises to more than 100 mg. Death may occur in the first 10 days as a result of cardiac arrest. The early onset of painful paresthesias, sensory loss, and pain localized to joints, back, and chest, as well as *rapid loss of hair* (after a week or two), all serve to differentiate this neuropathy from GBS, porphyria, and other acute polyneuropathies. Relative preservation of reflexes is noteworthy and rapidly evolving complete alopecia is a striking feature. Patients with lesser degrees of intoxication may recover completely within weeks or months. Thallium salts act like potassium and a high intake of potassium chloride hastens the excretion of thallium. Chelating agents are of unproven value but are usually included in treatment.

Some cases of *arsenical* and possibly *mercurial* polyneuropathy may also develop acutely. More often these conditions evolve subacutely, for which reason they are discussed further on. As alluded to earlier and in Chap. 43, certain other toxic neuropathies, such as those related to organophosphate or diethylene chloride (Sterno) poisoning, may have an acute onset and progress over days.

In regard to this category of polyneuropathy, many instances are imputed to toxins by both patients and unskeptical physicians with little substantiation. Before making such an attribution, it is useful to ask whether the clinical features are compatible with the known neurotoxicity of an environmental agent or drug; whether the severity of symptoms is consistent with degree of presumed exposure (real or imagined); whether the associated systemic signs of an intoxication are present; if other individuals similarly exposed are affected; and whether symptoms stabilize or improve once the patient is removed from the presumed source of exposure. Failure to satisfy these precepts generally signifies some other disorder.

Other Acute Polyneuropathies

On occasion, a vasculitic polyneuropathy as an isolated process or associated with lupus erythematosus, polyarteritis nodosa, and related disorders may develop as rapidly as GBS and careful clinical and electrophysiologic testing are needed to distinguish them. Three of our patients with polyarteritis and one with Churg-Strauss disease became completely paralyzed within a week and one died of intestinal perforation. However, most cases of neuropathy caused by vasculitis evolve more slowly, with the syndrome assuming an asymmetrical and multifocal distribution, for which reason it is described in the next section. There is no doubt that paraneoplastic neuropathies, discussed further in the subacute category, can evolve more rapidly than is typical for this process and thereby simulate GBS.

We have observed a few patients with alcoholism, occult carcinoma, Hodgkin disease, and renal transplantation develop an acute polyneuropathy, as rapid in its evolution as GBS, and acute episodes of this type have also been described in patients with Refsum disease.

Acute Autonomic Polyneuropathy ("Pure Pandysautonomia")

Since the first description of such a case by Young and colleagues and Adams and associates, a number of others have been recorded and summarized by Low and colleagues. The condition, probably a type of postinfectious polyneuropathy in the category of GBS, is described in detail in Chap. 26. Some success has been achieved by treatment with IVIg. A subacute and more chronic form, also immune in nature, is described later under "Idiopathic Autonomic Neuropathy" and a paraneoplastic variety is known.

SYNDROME OF SUBACUTE SENSORIMOTOR PARALYSIS FROM PERIPHERAL NEUROPATHY

Placed in this category are neuropathies that evolve over several weeks to months and, after reaching their peak of severity, tend to persist for a variable period. Admittedly, the dividing line between such cases and those that evolve over somewhat shorter or longer periods is indistinct; there are many diseases of nerve that overlap both the acute and the early chronic categories. In contrast to the acute polyneuropathies, however, most that are subacute have prominent sensory features and are of axonal type. The main exception is a subacute inflammatory–demyelinative type, essentially a slow form of GBS, evolving over 4 to 8 weeks, as described by Hughes and coworkers. Similarly, some instances of diphtheritic neuropathy evolve subacutely. Despite these qualifications, in the end, a symmetrical polyneuropathy syndrome of *subacute type* most often proves to be caused by nutritional deficiency, (often complicated by alcoholism) by a remote effect of cancer (paraneoplastic, as described later), by poisoning with arsenic, lead, or by the toxic effects of any number of drugs used for therapeutic purposes (cisplatin, nitrofurantoin, isoniazid, etc.). Occasionally other drugs, metals, and industrial solvents are incriminated; these are discussed in Chap. 43.

Nutritional Deficiency Neuropathy

(See Chap. 41)

In the Western world, nutritional polyneuropathy is usually associated with chronic alcoholism. As indicated in earlier discussions, all data point to the identity or at least close relationship between alcoholic neuropathy and neuropathic beriberi. A nutritional factor is responsible for both, although in any given case it remains unclear whether the deficiency is one of thiamine, nicotinic acid, pyridoxine, pantothenic acid, folic acid, or a combination of these B vitamins. Our colleague M. Victor, who devoted considerable attention to this subject, was never persuaded of the existence of a form of polyneuropathy attributable solely to the toxic effect of alcohol, although claims of such an entity continue to be made and the perception persists among most physicians that alcohol is directly damaging to nerves. Nutritional neuropathy and other neurologic complications of deficiency disorders (Strachan syndrome, pellagra, vitamin B_{12} deficiency, and malabsorption syndromes) are described fully in Chap. 41. A predominantly sensory neuropathy with burning pain is typical of most forms of severe nutritional deprivation.

Paraneoplastic Polyneuropathy and Sensory Ganglionopathy (See Chap. 31)

Although capable of producing diverse clinical presentations, most often the remote effect of cancer takes the form of a predominantly distal, symmetrical sensory, or sensorimotor polyneuropathy. Weakness and atrophy, ataxia, and sensory loss of the limbs may advance over several weeks or months to the point where the patient is confined to a wheelchair or bed; usually the CSF protein concentration is mildly elevated. All these symptoms may occur months or even a year or longer before a malignant tumor is found, although usually the tumor is apparent and most often is a lung cancer.

In most series, a mixed sensorimotor polyneuropathy has been 4 to 5 times more frequent than a purely sensory one. However, the latter is a more specific syndrome identified with lung cancer (described originally by Denny-Brown); it is characterized by a loss of all modalities of sensation spreading from the distal to the proximal segments of the limbs and eventually to the trunk and face. There is loss of tendon reflexes, but motor power may be retained. It has also been appreciated that the sensory loss in the beginning may have a multifocal distribution. Another variety is characterized by initial sensory ataxia, similar to that discussed in the earlier section "Acute Sensory Neuronopathy (Sensory Ganglionopathy)." The illness reaches its peak in a few weeks or months and in a very few instances the development has been as rapid as that of GBS.

The pathologic changes are those of an inflammatory and destructive *sensory neuropathy and neuronopathy* (ganglionitis) and are sometimes part of a more widespread disorder of the nervous system related to the anti-Hu antibody (also termed *antinuclear neuronal antibody type 1 (ANNA-1)*; see Chap. 31). This polyneuropathy has proven to be most typical of small cell cancer of the lung. In a series of 71 patients with paraneoplastic sensory neuronopathy reported by Dalmau and colleagues, more than half were associated with symptomatic inflammatory lesions in the temporal lobes (limbic encephalitis), the brainstem, and, rarely, the anterior horn neurons of the spinal cord. Other distinctive paraneoplastic syndromes such as cerebellar degeneration and Lambert-Eaton myasthenic syndrome were combined with polyneuropathy in isolated cases and there were signs of dysautonomia in 28 percent. Our experience has been that most cases of the Lambert-Eaton syndrome have occurred in isolation, but there are many cases that exist in parallel with various neoplasms, including some of our patients with lymphomas of various types.

The CSF protein is mildly elevated but usually acellular. Sensory potentials are usually absent in all nerves after a few weeks, but may be spared early on. The localization of anti-Hu antibody to the several affected regions of the nervous system and to the tumor itself has led to speculation that the lung tumors are typically small or inevident because the antibody suppresses tumor growth. Almost all cases of paraneoplastic sensory neuropathy and a proportion of the more nondescript sensory predominant or sensorimotor paraneoplastic polyneuropathies also demonstrate anti-Hu antibodies, making this testing useful in distinguishing paraneoplastic varieties of sensory neuropathy and neuronopathy from those caused by postinfectious or immune disorders such as Sjögren syndrome and HIV infection. The finding of high antibody titers should lead to chest imaging and, in appropriate cases, bronchoscopic or positron emission tomography (PET) examinations to detect an underlying cancer. A rare vasculitic mononeuropathy multiplex that occurs with cancer is discussed further on.

An unusual assortment of polyneuropathies has been associated with non-Hodgkin lymphomas of both T- and B-cell types and with several related conditions, such as Castleman disease (angiofollicular lymphoid hyperplasia), intravascular T-cell lymphoma (and the related lymphomatoid granulomatosis; see Chap. 31), hypersensitivity lymph node hyperplasia (angioimmunoblastic or immunoblastic lymphadenopathy), and Kimura disease (lymphoid hyperplasia with eosinophilia mainly involving skin). In most of these neuropathies, particularly the one associated with Castleman disease, there is a paraproteinemia, often polyclonal, thereby relating this group to the paraproteinemic neuropathies and to osteosclerotic myeloma, discussed later. In several of our patients, the neuropathic manifestations appeared simultaneously with lymph node enlargement in the groin, axilla, or thorax. Clinically, the illness may take the form of GBS, chronic demyelinating polyneuropathy, subacute motor polyneuropathy or anterior horn cell disease, lumbar and brachial plexopathy, or a polyradiculopathy—each occurring as a paralymphomatous condition clearly separable from cases of meningeal and neural infiltration by tumor. Corticosteroids have been helpful in some of our patients with the lymphoid diseases; in others, the neuropathy resolves spontaneously or with radiation of the lymph nodes but otherwise progresses for months. Vallat and colleagues have summarized their experience with the more conventional types of neuropathy accompanying non-Hodgkin lymphoma. Intravascular lymphoma, a widespread neoplastic and vascular disease (described in Chap. 31), may infiltrate the peripheral nerves in a multiple mononeuropathy pattern.

The various forms of paraneoplastic polyneuropathy are manifest clinically in 2 to 5 percent of patients with malignant disease. The figures are higher if one includes the neuropathies accounted for by malnutrition and pressure palsies that occur in the later stages of cancer and those identified by EMG in asymptomatic patients (Henson and Urich). Carcinoma of the lung accounts for approximately 50 percent of the cases of paraneoplastic sensorimotor polyneuropathy and for 75 percent of those with pure sensory neuropathy (Croft and Wilkinson); nevertheless, these neuropathies may be associated with neoplasms of all types.

Although anti-Hu binds to the peripheral nerve, the *immunopathology* of the paraneoplastic polyneuropathies has not been completely defined. In the purely sensory type, there is not only a loss of nerve cells in the dorsal root ganglia but also an inflammatory reaction (Horwich et al)—much the same changes as occur with the sensory neuronopathy of Sjögren syndrome. In the mixed sensorimotor polyneuropathy, degeneration is greater in the distal than it is in the proximal segments of the peripheral nerves, but it extends into the roots in advanced cases. Dorsal root ganglion cells may be reduced in number in both types. If the histologic examination is performed early in the course of the neuropathy, sparse infiltrates of lymphocytes are observed distributed in foci around blood vessels. No tumor cells are seen in the nerves or spinal ganglia, unlike the rare instances of carcinomatous and lymphomatous mononeuropathy multiplex, in which tumor cells actually infiltrate nerves. Degeneration of the dorsal columns and chromatolysis of anterior horn cells are secondary to changes in the peripheral nerves and roots.

The *prognosis* of the paraneoplastic neuropathies is poor. Even though the polyneuropathy may stabilize or even remit to some extent on its own or with therapy, most patients succumb to the underlying tumor within a year.

Treatment If the tumor can be treated effectively, the neuropathy may improve, the exception being pure sensory neuronopathy, which rarely does so. Treatment with plasma exchange, gamma globulin, or immunosuppression has had only a minimal effect, but there are anecdotal reports of success with each of these treatments applied early in the course. In the report by Uchuya and colleagues, only 1 of 18 patients with a subacute sensory neuropathy improved and another became dependent for sustained improvement on immune globulin; most of the others stabilized or worsened and the authors concluded that treatment was of doubtful value. Corticosteroids have not been tested in a systematic way for paraneoplastic neuropathy and there is little clinical evidence to support their use.

Subacute Toxic Neuropathies

Arsenical Polyneuropathy

Of the neuropathies caused by metallic poisoning, that caused by arsenic is particularly well characterized. In cases of chronic poisoning, the neuropathic symptoms develop rather slowly, over a period of several weeks or months and have the same sensory and motor distribution as the nutritional polyneuropathies. Gastrointestinal symptoms, the result of ingestion of arsenic compounds, may precede the polyneuropathy, which is nearly always associated with anemia, jaundice, brownish cutaneous pigmentation, hyperkeratosis of palms and soles, and later with white transverse banding of the nails (Mees lines). The disease is accompanied by an excess of arsenic in the urine and hair. Pathologically, this form of arsenical neuropathy is categorized as of the dying-back (axonal degeneration) type.

In patients who survive the ingestion of a single massive dose of arsenic, a more rapidly evolving polyneuropathy may appear after a period of 8 to 21 days as discussed earlier. Diagnosis and treatment of arsenical poisoning are discussed further in Chap. 43. Here it is emphasized that the ingestion of fish in many areas of the industrialized world gives high levels of blood and urine arsenic, but the metal is in the form of arsenobetaine, which has low toxicity and does not cause neuropathy.

Lead Neuropathy (Plumbism)

This is an uncommon disorder. In adults, it occurs following chronic exposure to lead paint or fumes (from smelting industries or burning batteries) or from ingestion of liquor distilled in lead pipes. Its most characteristic presentation is a motor mononeuropathy in the distribution of the radial nerves (wrist and finger drop). In a few personally observed patients this was the main abnormality, but there was also a sensory loss in the radial territory of the hand. Less commonly, there is foot-drop occurring alone or in combination with weakness of the proximal arm and shoulder girdle muscles. As pointed out in Chap. 43, lead neuropathy seldom occurs in children, in whom poisoning usually results in an encephalopathy. Although the neuropathy has been known since ancient times, details of the pathobiology are still obscure. Axonal degeneration with secondary myelin change and swelling and chromatolysis of anterior horn cells has been described. Lead accumulates in the nerve and may be toxic to Schwann cells or to endothelial capillary cells, causing edema.

The diagnosis is established by the history of lead exposure, the predominant and restricted motor involvement, associated medical findings (anemia, basophilic stippling of red blood cell precursors in the bone marrow, a "lead line" along the gingival margins, colicky abdominal pain, and constipation), and the urinary excretion of lead and coproporphyrins. Blood lead levels of more than 70 μg/dL are always abnormal. In patients with lower levels, doubling of the 24-h urinary lead excretion following an infusion of the chelating agent $CaNa_2$ ethylenediaminetetraacetic acid (EDTA) indicates a significant degree of lead intoxication. Coproporphyrin in the urine is abnormal in any amount, but it may also be found in porphyria, alcoholism, iron deficiency, and other disorders as well as in lead intoxication.

Treatment consists of terminating the exposure to lead and eliminating lead from the bloodstream and the bones by chelation as discussed in Chap. 43. For this purpose, penicillamine, which is generally safe and can be administered orally, is preferable to dimercaprol (British anti-Lewisite [BAL]) or EDTA.

Other Metals and Industrial Agents

Chronic poisoning with *thallium* and sometimes with *lithium*, *gold*, *mercury*, and *platinum* (in the antineoplastic agents cisplatin and carboplatin as discussed further on) produces a sensorimotor polyneuropathy; these intoxications are discussed in Chap. 43 and the acute form was addressed earlier in the chapter. A predominantly motor neuropathy is induced by occupational exposure to metallic mercury and mercury vapor but any connection to the mercury content in dental amalgam has little credibility. Exposure to manganese, bismuth, antimony, zinc, and copper may give rise to systemic signs of poisoning; some of them affect the central nervous system (CNS) but one cannot be certain that any of them specifically involves peripheral nerves. The devastating encephalopathy of organic mercury toxicity does not, to our knowledge, cause neuropathy.

As mentioned in Chap. 43, a predominantly motor polyneuropathy has been reported as a rare complication of *gold* therapy for rheumatoid arthritis. Most often the cumulative dose of gold had exceeded 1 g but in a few instances the neuropathy occurred with 0.5 g. Painful distal burning is the initial complaint with weakness and wasting following. The onset of weakness, although usually insidious, can be abrupt enough to simulate GBS. There have been trigeminal, facial, and oculomotor palsies. One of the unusual features, not shared with most other toxic neuropathies, is a marked rise in CSF protein concentration.

A distal, symmetrical sensorimotor (predominantly sensory) neuronopathy may follow exposure to certain hexacarbon industrial solvents. These include n-*hexane* (found in contact cements, thus affecting "glue sniffers" who inhale the vapors); *methyl* n-*butyl ketone* (used in the production of plastic-coated and color-printed fabrics); dimethylaminopropionitrile (DMAPN), used in the manufacture of polyurethane foam); the fumigant *methyl bromide*; and the gas sterilant *ethylene oxide*. Operating room nurses may be affected by the latter when the agent is absorbed through the skin, leaving a characteristic rash at exposed sites (usually the wrists, where a surgical gown ends). A mild peripheral neuropathy and CNS changes of memory loss and headaches have been reported from this agent by Brashear and colleagues. Nurses are also subject to a risk of *nitrous oxide* neurotoxicity and this usually takes the form of a myelopathy similar to that seen with cobalamin deficiency. Most cases are caused by repeated use of the gas to induce euphoria. As with vitamin B-12 deficiency, the syndrome may be mistaken for a neuropathy but nerve conduction studies fail to demonstrate one. The associated macrocytic anemia is reversed by the administration of B_{12}, but the neurologic illness may be less responsive as discussed in Chap. 41.

Triorthocresyl phosphate and *acrylamide* are potent peripheral nerve toxins. Both of these drugs cause a dying-back polyneuropathy with axonal degeneration and have been used experimentally to produce this effect. *Vacor*, a phenylnitrosourea rodenticide, taken as a suicidal agent, gives rise to a profound sensory and autonomic neuropathy with abdominal pain and hyperglycemia caused by acute pancreatitis.

Detailed accounts of the clinical and experimental neurotoxicology of these agents can be found in the monograph by Spencer and colleagues.

Drug-Induced Neuropathies and Neuronopathies

A large number of medications are potential sources of polyneuropathy of predominantly sensory type. Most are dose-dependent and are therefore more or less predictable after large cumulative doses of the drug have been given (e.g., in cancer chemotherapy) or after prolonged administration for other reasons. A more complete list than can be compiled here can be found in the review by England and Asbury.

Antineoplastic Drugs (See also Chap. 43.) Among chemotherapeutic agents in current use, particularly *cisplatin, carboplatin,* and *bortezomib,* are known to evoke a dose-dependent, predominantly sensory polyneuropathy, which begins several weeks after completion of therapy in at least half of the patients. Proprioception and vibratory sensation are most severely impaired. Some patients develop acrodynia and episodic color changes in the fingertips and toes suggesting that autonomic nerves are also involved; in severe cases there is sensory ataxia and pseudoathetosis. The severity of histopathologic changes in the peripheral nervous system corresponds to the concentration of platinum in these tissues, the highest being found in dorsal root ganglia. Secondary degeneration in the posterior columns is the basis for a Lhermitte symptom reported by some patients.

The taxanes *paclitaxel* and the more potent *docetaxel,* both cited as inhibitors of the depolymerization of neurotubules, are used mainly in the treatment of ovarian cancer. They produce a sensory polyneuropathy similar to that of cisplatin. The nerve lesion regresses slowly with a reduction in dosage. Pathologic studies have shown a neuronopathy and distal axonopathy affecting mainly large fibers.

For decades it has been known that peripheral neuropathy commonly complicates the use of *vincristine,* an antineoplastic agent most widely used in treatment of the lymphomas and leukemia. Paresthesias are the most common early symptom, and loss of ankle jerks is an early sign. Some degree of weakness usually precedes objective sensory loss; the extensor muscles of the fingers and wrists are affected; later the dorsiflexors of the toes and feet causing foot-drop or, more often in our experience, foot-drop may appear first. With the dose regimens currently used, the weakness is usually mild, but in the past, some patients became quadriparetic and bedbound. Adults are more severely affected than are children, as are persons with preexisting polyneuropathies. The neuropathy is strictly dose-related and reduction in dosage is followed by improvement of neuropathic symptoms although this may take several months. Many patients are then able to tolerate vincristine in low dosage, such as 1 mg every 2 weeks, for many months. Thalidomide produces a similar sensory neuropathy. It is finding use in the treatment of inflammatory conditions such as Behçhet disease, graft versus host reactions, erythema nodosum, lepromatous eruptions, aphthous stomatitis in AIDS patents and highly vascular tumors certain tumors such as renal cell cancer.

Antimicrobial Drugs As mentioned in Chap. 43, *isoniazid* (INH)-induced polyneuropathy was a common occurrence in the early 1950s when this drug was first used for the treatment of tuberculosis. Symptoms of neuropathy appeared between 3 and 35 weeks after treatment was begun and affected approximately 10 percent of patients receiving therapeutic doses in the upper range (10 mg/kg daily). The initial symptoms are symmetrical numbness and tingling of the toes and feet spreading, if the drug is continued, to the knees and occasionally to the hands. Aching and burning pain in these parts then becomes prominent. In addition to sensory loss, examination usually discloses a loss of tendon reflexes and weakness in the distal muscles of the legs. Severe degrees of weakness and loss of deep sensation are observed only rarely.

Isoniazid produces its effects on the peripheral nerves by interfering with pyridoxine metabolism, perhaps by inhibiting the phosphorylation of pyridoxine (the collective name for the B_6 group of vitamins) and decreasing the tissue levels of its active form, pyridoxal phosphate. The administration of 150 to 450 mg of pyridoxine daily in conjunction with the isoniazid completely prevents the neuropathy. The same mechanism is probably operative in the neuropathies that occasionally complicate the administration of the isoniazid-related substances such as *ethionamide*, used sometimes in the treatment of tuberculosis and the now little-used antihypertensive agent *hydralazine*. Paradoxically, the taking of *extremely high doses of pyridoxine* over a prolonged period may actually cause a disabling, predominantly sensory ganglionopathy (Schaumburg et al, 1983).

A relatively mild sensory neuropathy (acral paresthesia) associated with optic neuropathy occasionally complicates *chloramphenicol* therapy. The chronic administration of *metronidazole* may have the same effect (and can produce lesions in the deep cerebellum). The newer antimicrobial, linezolid, has been associated with a fairly severe sensory neuropathy in a few cases after prolonged use. A predominantly motor neuropathy has been reported with the chronic administration of *dapsone*, a sulfone used to treat leprosy and certain dermatologic conditions. *Stilbamidine*, used in the treatment of kala azar, may also induce a purely sensory neuropathy with a propensity to affect the trigeminal nerves.

The introduction, in 1952, of *nitrofurantoin* for the treatment of bladder infections was soon followed by reports of neurotoxicity attributable to the drug. The earliest symptoms are pain and tingling paresthesias of the toes and feet, followed shortly by similar sensations in the fingers. If the drug is not discontinued, the disorder progresses to a severe, symmetrical sensorimotor polyneuropathy. Patients with chronic renal failure are particularly prone to neurotoxicity from nitrofurantoin because of diminished drug excretion resulting in high tissue levels. To make matters more complex, the uremic state itself may be responsible for a polyneuropathy so that the distinction between uremic and nitrofurantoin neuropathy may be impossible. The neuropathologic studies of Lhermitte and colleagues disclosed an axonal degeneration in peripheral nerves and sensory roots.

Cardiac Drugs *Amiodarone*, a drug used for treating recalcitrant ventricular tachyarrhythmias, induces a motor-sensory neuropathy in about 5 percent of patients after several months of treatment. It may also cause a toxic myopathy. *Perhexiline maleate* for the treatment of angina pectoris may also cause a generalized, predominantly sensory polyneuropathy in a small proportion of patients. Hydralazine as a neurotoxic agent has already been mentioned. Affected persons show a striking neuronal lipidosis. Patients taking *niacin* to lower blood cholesterol levels may experience distal and truncal paresthesias, but an associated neuropathy has been identified.

Other Pharmaceutical Agents Causing Polyneuropathy The development of a sensorimotor neuropathy similar to that produced by INH may be associated with the chronic use of disulfiram in the treatment of alcoholism. Its neurotoxic effects have been attributed to the action of *carbon disulfide*, which is produced during the metabolism of the drug, and is known to cause polyneuropathy and sometimes an optic neuropathy in workers in the viscose rayon industry. Pathologic data, although scant, tend to discredit this notion, insofar as disulfiram evokes a wallerian type of axonal degeneration, whereas carbon disulfide neuropathy is characterized by swollen (giant) axons that are filled with neurofilaments (Bouldin et al).

Some patients who have taken *phenytoin* for decades may lose ankle and patellar reflexes and acquire mild distal symmetrical impairment of sensation, slowed conduction velocity in the peripheral nerves of the legs and rarely, weakness of the distal musculature. The mechanism and frequency of this complication are not clear. The cholesterol-lowering *statin* drugs have been tentatively implicated in a painful, paresthetic distal axonal polyneuropathy with retained reflexes (Gaist et al). More often the problem with statins is one of a toxic myopathy. The frequency of polyneuropathy is low but, if no other explanation is identified, it may be advisable to discontinue the drug. *Colchicine* has long been known to cause a myopathy, but a few cases of predominantly axonal sensory neuropathy have also been reported (*neuromyopathy*).

Among various other agents that cause neuropathy are hydroxychloroquine and colchicine are known to cause a toxic neuropathy. The anesthetic agent *trichloroethylene*, as with the aforementioned stilbamidine, has a predilection for cranial nerves, particularly the fifth. The neurotoxicity is apparently caused by dichloroacetylene, formed as a product of trichloroethylene. The neuropathic potential of nitrous oxide has already been mentioned. Most of the group of TNF-alpha (TNF-α) inhibitors may cause a polyneuropathy, but this category of agents do not appear to have a direct toxic effect on nerves but instead alter immune function in some way that results in a process that simulates chronic inflammatory demyelinating polyneuropathy (see further on).

Residual effects of polyneuropathy were seen in patients with the toxic eosinophilia-myalgia syndrome; the problem was traced to the ingestion of *adulterated* L-*tryptophan*, which had been used in nonprescription drugs for insomnia. One patient under our care suffered permanent areflexic quadriplegia. There may be an eosinophilic infiltrate in nerves, but the neuropathy is probably the result of a direct toxic mechanism. A sensory neuropathy, resulting from excessive *pyridoxine* ingestion alluded to earlier, is still seen among individuals who take huge doses of vitamin supplements. *Amitriptyline* is capable of producing paresthesias, but the effect seems to be idiosyncratic and infrequent.

Diabetic Neuropathy

Diabetes mellitus is the most common cause of polyneuropathy in general clinical practice, for which reason it is accorded a separate section. We are referring mainly to a generalized, predominantly sensory syndrome, but several focal or regional forms of peripheral nerve disease also result from diabetes and for convenience of exposition, are included here. In recent years, attention has also been directed to a possible association between a nondescript sensory polyneuropathy and impaired glucose tolerance, even without manifest diabetes, persistent hyperglycemia, or an elevation of hemoglobin A_{1c}. The survey by Sumner and colleagues makes a case for such an association, but we remain uncertain about the relationship between glucose intolerance alone and polyneuropathy. By statistically adjusting for relevant factors such as glycemic control and glycosylated hemoglobin, Tesfaye and colleagues have suggested that some cardiovascular risk factors subsumed under the term "metabolic syndrome" (triglyceride levels, body mass, hypertension) are themselves risk factors for diabetic polyneuropathy.

Approximately 15 percent of patients with diabetes have symptoms and signs of polyneuropathy, but nearly 50 percent of cross-sectional population samples have evidence of peripheral nerve damage as judged by nerve conduction abnormalities. The duration of diabetes is perhaps the most important factor. Fewer than 10 percent of patients have clinically evident polyneuropathy at the time of discovery of diabetes, but this figure rises to 50 percent after 25 years. The presence of diabetic retinopathy is associated with higher incidences of neuropathy. It is not surprising, therefore, that neuropathy is most common in diabetics older than 50 years; it is infrequent in those younger than age 30 years and is rare in childhood. Dyck and colleagues (1993) studied diabetics in Rochester, Minnesota, and found that 54 percent with type 1 (insulin-deficient) and 45 percent with type 2 (insulin-resistant) had polyneuropathy. The percentages were lower when patients were selected on the basis of clinical symptoms alone rather than on the presence of changes in nerve conduction; close to 15 percent at the time of diagnosis in both groups. In the syndromes described further on, both type 1 and type 2 diabetic patients are susceptible, the duration of diabetes being a major factor.

Several fairly distinct clinical syndromes of diabetic neuropathy have been delineated: (1) the most common as noted is a distal, symmetrical, primarily sensory polyneuropathy affecting feet and legs in a chronic, slowly progressive manner; the others are (2) acute ophthalmoplegia that affects the third, and less often the sixth, cranial nerve on one side; (3) acute mononeuropathy of limbs or trunk including a painful thoracolumbar radiculopathy; (4) an acute or subacute painful, asymmetrical, predominantly motor, multiple neuropathy affecting the upper lumbar roots and the proximal leg muscles ("diabetic amyotrophy"); (5) a more symmetrical, proximal motor weakness and wasting, usually without pain and with variable sensory loss, pursuing a subacute or chronic course; and (6) an autonomic neuropathy involving bowel, bladder, sweating and circulatory reflexes. These forms of neuropathy often coexist or overlap, particularly the autonomic and distal symmetrical types and the subacute proximal neuropathies.

Most of the syndromes listed here are likely to be a result of ischemia or infarction of nerves or nerve fascicles, because of a diabetic microvasculopathy. All but the first are special types of *mononeuropathy multiplex*. The polyneuropathy is associated with occlusion of small endoneurial blood vessels (vasonervorum) but possibly also incorporate a poorly understood metabolic abnormality; however, other theories of causation abound. In recent years, an inflammatory process has been postulated as yet another mechanism of peripheral nerve damage. These aspects are discussed further on.

Distal Sensory Diabetic Polyneuropathy

The *distal, symmetrical, primarily sensory form* of polyneuropathy is the most common type. It is usually a chronic process, sometimes unnoticed by the patient. The main complaints are persistent and often distressing numbness and tingling, usually confined to the feet and lower legs and worse at night. The ankle jerks are absent and, sometimes, the patellar reflexes as well. As a rule, sensory loss is confined to the distal parts of the lower extremities, but in severe cases the hands are involved and the sensory loss may even spread to the anterior trunk, simulating a sensory level of spinal cord disease (Said et al, 1983). Trophic changes in the form of deep ulcerations and neuropathic degeneration of the joints (Charcot joints) are encountered in the most severe and long-standing cases, presumably as a result of sensory analgesia, trophic changes, and repetitive injury. (Foot ulcerations are more common simply as a result of the microvascular disease of skin in diabetic patients.) Muscle weakness is usually mild, but in some patients a distal sensory neuropathy is combined with a proximal weakness and wasting of the types mentioned earlier. Treatment of the acral pain may be a major problem and is discussed further on.

In another group of patients with diabetic polyneuropathy the clinical picture may be dominated instead by loss of deep sensation, ataxia, and atony of the bladder, with only slight weakness of the limbs, in which case it resembles tabes dorsalis (hence the term *diabetic pseudotabes*). The similarity to tabes dorsalis is even closer if lancinating pains in the legs, unreactive pupils, abdominal pains, and neuropathic arthropathy are present.

Acute Diabetic Mononeuropathies

Among these, *diabetic ophthalmoplegia* is a common occurrence, usually in a patient with well-established diabetes. It commonly presents as isolated, painful third nerve palsy with sparing of pupillary function. In the first autopsied patient reported by Dreyfus and colleagues, there was an ischemic lesion in the center of the retroorbital portion of the third nerve. Subsequently, a similar case was described by Asbury and colleagues (1970). Slightly less often, the sixth nerve on one side is involved. The disorder was described earlier in Chap. 14.

Isolated involvement of practically all the major peripheral nerves has been described in diabetes, but the ones most frequently affected are the *femoral*, *sciatic*, and *peroneal nerves*, in that order. Rarely is a nerve in the upper extremity affected. As mentioned, the acute mononeuropathies, both cranial and peripheral, are presumably a result of infarction of the nerve, but it is only in pathologic studies of the third nerve that this basis has been established. Recovery is the rule but may take many months.

Diabetic Multiple Mononeuropathies and Radiculoplexus Neuropathy (Diabetic Lumbar Plexopathy; Diabetic Amyotrophy; Garland Syndrome)

This category overlaps with the mononeuropathies. A syndrome of painful unilateral or asymmetrical multiple neuropathies tends to occur in older patients with relatively mild or even unrecognized diabetes. Multiple nerves are affected in a random distribution (mononeuropathy multiplex). The mononeuropathies often emerge during periods of transition in the diabetic illness, for example, after an episode of hyper- or hypoglycemia, when insulin treatment is initiated or adjusted, or when there has been rapid weight loss.

The most characteristic syndrome affects the lumbar roots. Pain, which can be severe, begins in the low back or hip and spreads to the thigh and knee on one side; the discomfort has a deep, aching character with superimposed lancinating jabs and there is a propensity for pain to be most severe at night. Weakness and later atrophy are evident in the pelvic girdle and thigh muscles, although the distal muscles of the leg may also be affected. The patellar reflex is lost on the affected side. Curiously, we have found the opposite patellar reflex to be absent in some patients without explanation. Deep and superficial sensation may be intact or mildly impaired, conforming to either a multiple nerve or multiple adjacent root distribution (i.e., L2 and L3, or L4 and L5). The pain lasts for several days and then gradually abates. Motor recovery is the rule although months and even years may elapse before it is complete. The same syndrome may recur after an interval of months or years in the opposite leg. The EMG shows denervation in the lumbar and sometimes adjacent myotomes.

This form of neuropathy has been referred to as *diabetic amyotrophy*, a term that draws attention to one facet of the syndrome. Garland's name (also Bruns's) has been attached to this diabetic lumbar radiculoplexopathy based on his thorough report (but he mistakenly attributed the condition to a spinal cord lesion). Clinical experience has shown that an identical painful lumbofemoral neuropathy may develop in nondiabetics; possibly this form is also vasculopathic or vasculitic. While lumbar disc herniation, retroperitoneal hematoma compressing upper lumbar roots, carcinomatous meningeal seeding, and neoplastic and sarcoid infiltration of the proximal lumbar plexus enter into the differential diagnosis, the diabetic type is usually so distinctive as to permit recognition on clinical grounds alone. In one of the most informative reexaminations of this syndrome, Barohn and colleagues (1991) point out that there is considerable overlap between the chronic polyneuropathy of diabetes and this rapidly evolving regional disorder. They also point out a high incidence of involvement of the L5 root, but this is difficult to reconcile with the frequent finding of hip flexor and quadriceps weakness. As with the diabetic mononeuropathies, the upper extremities are only rarely affected by this process.

Also observed in diabetic patients is a relatively painless syndrome of proximal symmetrical leg weakness, wasting, and reflex loss of more insidious onset and gradual evolution as discussed by Pascoe and colleagues. The iliopsoas, quadriceps, and hamstrings are involved in varying degrees. The muscles of the scapulae and upper limbs, usually the deltoid and triceps, are affected less frequently. Sensory changes, if present, are distal, symmetrical, and usually mild.

In an attempt to delineate these types of proximal diabetic neuropathies, it must be emphasized that they overlap and that distal parts of a limb may be involved to a mild degree and the evolution of symptoms varies. Whether the proximal and distal syndromes should be distinguished on pathologic or electrophysiologic grounds is not clear.

A syndrome of *thoracoabdominal radiculopathy* characterized by severe pain and dysesthesia is also well described. Almost always the diabetes has been of long standing (Kikta et al). The pain is distributed over one or several adjacent segments of the chest or abdomen; it may be unilateral, or less often bilateral, and, as with the lumbar radiculoplexopathy, sometimes follows a period of recent weight loss. Superficial sensory loss can be detected over the involved area in most patients. The pathology of this state is not known, but it is presumed to be an ischemic radiculopathy. The EMG changes consist of fibrillations of the paraspinal and abdominal muscles in one or more adjacent myotomes, corresponding to the painful area. With control of the diabetes, or perhaps spontaneously, recovery eventually occurs but it may be protracted. The differential diagnosis includes preeruptive herpes zoster, sarcoid infiltration of nerve roots, and thoracic disc rupture.

In all forms of diabetic polyneuropathy the CSF protein may be elevated from 50 to 150 mg/dL and sometimes higher. The protein concentration is usually normal in cases of diabetic mononeuropathy. Whether a slight elevation of CSF protein, discovered incidentally, can be attributed to diabetes in the absence of a polyneuropathy is uncertain.

Autonomic Diabetic Neuropathy

Symptoms of *autonomic involvement* include any combination of pupillary and lacrimal dysfunction, impairment of sweating and vascular reflexes, nocturnal diarrhea, atonicity of the gastrointestinal tract (gastroparesis) and bladder dilation, erectile dysfunction, and postural hypotension. The most striking examples in our experience include severe abdominal and limb pain in young type 1 diabetics, symptoms comparable to the crises of tabes dorsalis that required narcotics to control.

The basis of this type of autonomic involvement is not well understood. Duchen and associates, who studied the sympathetic ganglia in diabetic patients with autonomic symptoms, described vacuoles and granular deposits in sympathetic neurons and little if any neuronal degeneration; there was also a loss of myelinated nerve fibers in the vagus and splanchnic nerves and the rami communicantes, as well as changes in neurons of the intermediolateral columns of the spinal cord.

Pathology and Pathophysiology of the Diabetic Neuropathies

In the typical symmetrical diabetic distal sensory polyneuropathy, loss of myelinated nerve fibers is the most prominent finding. In addition, segmental demyelination and remyelination of remaining axons are apparent in teased nerve fiber preparations. The latter findings are probably too severe and widespread to be simply a reflection of axonal degeneration. Occasionally, repeated demyelination and remyelination lead to onion-bulb formations of Schwann cells and fibroblasts, as it does in the relapsing inflammatory neuropathies. Unmyelinated fibers are also reduced in number in most specimens. Similar scattered lesions are found in the posterior roots and posterior columns of the spinal cord, and in the rami communicantes and sympathetic ganglia. Under the electron microscope, the basement membranes of intraneural capillaries are thickened and duplicated. There are changes in the microvasculature of the nerves as well, similar to what is seen in other organs and in the skin of diabetics.

As can be surmised from this discussion, uncertainties persist about the pathogenesis of the diabetic neuropathies. Both the cranial and peripheral mononeuropathies, as well as the painful, asymmetrical, predominantly proximal neuropathy of sudden onset, have been considered by most neuropathologists to be ischemic in origin, secondary to a vasculopathy of the vasa nervorum. Obliterative microvascular lesions were well illustrated by Raff and coworkers and corresponding multiple small infarcts were found in the nerve trunks in other studies. The observations of Dyck (1986b) and of Johnson and their associates also suggested that all forms of diabetic neuropathy had the same microvascular basis. The latter authors described multiple foci of fiber loss throughout the length of the peripheral nerves, beginning in the proximal segments and becoming more frequent and severe in the distal. This pattern of change differs from that observed in diffuse metabolic disease of Schwann cells and in the dying-back type of neuropathy. Fagerberg had earlier noted that the fascicular capillaries and epineural arterioles have thickened and hyalinized basement membranes, similar to the microvascular changes seen in the retina, kidney, and other organs. But occlusion of vessels and frank infarction of nerve has not been observed in most cases of polyneuropathy for which reason a vascular pathogenesis remains unsettled.

An alternative view has been offered, based largely on the work of Dyck and colleagues and of Said and coworkers (2003). They have found areas of perivascular inflammation and adjacent damage to nerve fascicles in the proximal radicular plexus syndrome. These findings, if valid, have implications for possible treatment with anti-inflammatory drugs.

Several biochemical findings implicated in diabetic polyneuropathy and their interpretations were reviewed by Brown and Greene, who advanced the idea that persistent hyperglycemia inhibits sodium-dependent myoinositol transport. Low levels of intraneural myoinositol reduce phosphoinositide metabolism and sodium-potassium adenosine triphosphatase (ATPase) activity. Others have emphasized a deficiency of aldose reductase and an elevation of polyols (particularly sorbitol) as being causally important. The role of factors other than hyperglycemia that are subsumed under the "metabolic syndrome" mentioned earlier is also unclear. In reviewing these studies, one can only conclude that a convincing biochemical pathogenesis for neuropathy in diabetes has yet to be formulated.

Another group of novel findings holds that there is a reduction in trophic factors within diabetic nerves (nerve growth factor [NGF], vascular endothelial growth factor [VEGF], erythropoietin); partial reversal of the polyneuropathy has been obtained in animals by replacement of these factors through gene therapy. Trials addressing this mode of treatment are noted later.

Treatment The only preventive treatment for diabetic neuropathy is the maintenance of blood glucose concentration at close to normal range. The prevailing view, derived from long-term human studies, is that there is a relationship between peripheral nerve damage and inadequate regulation of the diabetes. This is supported by the findings of the National Diabetic Complications Trial, in which 715 patients with type 1 diabetes were followed for 6 to 10 years. There was a relation between strict glucose control by means of an intravenous insulin infusion system and a reduction or delay in the occurrence of painful neuropathic symptoms, retinopathy, and nephropathy. However, this came at the price of a threefold increase in hypoglycemic reactions (see also Samanta and Burden). Whether similar protective effects of glucose control apply to type 2 diabetes is not known, but for most patients rigid control is impractical. A number of small trials have been conducted with aldose reductase inhibitors based on theoretical considerations of the above-discussed metabolic changes. Some recent interest has also been directed at the therapeutic use of gangliosides, which are normal components of neuronal membranes and can be administered exogenously. These approaches have not entered routine practice.

Treatment using gene transfer had been pursued by our group. In experimental models of diabetic neuropathy, the intramuscular administration of VEGF has had a beneficial effect on several measures of nerve conduction and on the histologic changes of diabetic nerve damage in the treated limb (Ropper et al, 2009). Whether this was mediated by a trophic influence on nerves and Schwann cells, or is the result of angiogenesis, is not known. With similar intentions, two trials of NGF injections in almost 500 patients conducted by Apfel and colleagues gave equivocal results, the first being positive and the followup study not showing improvement. VEGF has resulted in improvement of sensory symptoms but not of nerve conduction or of the sensory examination in a trial we conducted.

The distressing paresthesias of the distal extremities can be managed with amitriptyline, other tricyclic antidepressants, or one of the newer generation of antidepressants, duloxitine, gabapentin, or pregablain but the response is usually incomplete. Shooting, stabbing pain also responds to some degree to anticonvulsant drugs but only modest effects can be expected. Gabapentin may give reasonable results, perhaps in part because high doses are tolerated (Gorson et al, 1999). Topical creams with capsaicin, lidocaine or other substances, or compounds with several of these (including ketorolac, gabapentin, ketamine) have been found helpful by a few patients. Nerve blocks and epidural injections have been helpful in very few patients. In the proximal asymmetrical, truncal, or ophthalmoplegic neuropathies, the severe pain usually lasts for only a short period and requires the judicious use of analgesics, as outlined in Chap. 8. The *course* in patients with the distal, symmetrical sensory neuropathy is generally of slow progression, but in the other types improvement and eventual recovery may be expected over a period of months or years.

ASYMMETRICAL AND MULTIFOCAL POLYNEUROPATHIES (MONONEUROPATHY, OR MONONEURITIS MULTIPLEX) (Table 46-4)

In addition to diabetes, several systemic conditions are accompanied by acute or subacute involvement of *multiple individual nerves* serially or almost simultaneously. This configuration gives rise to the distinctive clinical picture of mononeuropathy multiplex. The most notable examples of this syndrome are associated with the vasculitides that produce nerve infarction, polyarteritis nodosa and other vasculitides and particularly a form of idiopathic vasculitis that is confined to the peripheral nervous system, from which the associated term *mononeuritis multiplex* is derived. The distinctive features of the multiple mononeuropathy syndromes are the acute or subacute evolution of complete or almost complete sensorimotor paralysis in the distribution of single peripheral nerves. In addition to vasculitis or the nerves, sarcoidosis, forms of HIV-related neuropathy, Leprosy and Lyme disease may become manifest in this fashion, probably from infiltration or inflammation of nerves rather than infarction. The diabetic mononeuropathies were addressed in the preceding section.

Table 46-4

CAUSES OF MONONEUROPATHY MULTIPLEX

Common
Polyarteritis nodosa
Microscopic polyangiitis
Churg-Strauss disease
Leprosy[a]
Wegener granulomatosis
Diabetes
Hereditary liability to preserve palsies
Cryoglobulinemia
Sarcoidosis
Lyme disease
HIV
Less Common
Paraneoplastic
Amyloidosis
Systemic lupus
Rheumatoid arthritis
Leukemia-lymphoma infiltration
Intravascular lymphoma
Sjögren syndrome

[a]Leprosy is the most common cause of this syndrome worldwide but infrequent in areas in which it is not endemic.

Vasculitic Neuropathies

More than half of all cases of mononeuropathy multiplex can be traced to a *systemic vasculitis* involving *the vasa nervorum*. These are the main causes of mononeuritis multiplex. Included in this category are polyarteritis nodosa, the Churg-Strauss syndrome (allergic bronchial asthma and eosinophilia), rheumatoid arthritis, lupus erythematosus, scleroderma, cryoglobulinemia, Wegener granulomatosis, and the aforementioned idiopathic variety of vasculitis that is confined to the peripheral nerves and has no systemic manifestations. In Said's series of 425 cases of vasculitis (2005) affecting the peripheral nerves, 24 percent were associated with polyarteritis nodosa, 23 percent with rheumatoid arthritis, and about 32 percent with other connective tissue diseases; in 21 percent there were no signs of vasculitis beyond the peripheral nerves. Elevation of the sedimentation rate, C-reactive protein and other serologic abnormalities are typical features but not invariable of this group. The most recent addition to the diagnostic list has been a microscopic polyangiitis that is different from the vasculitis of medium-sized vessels that characterizes the remainder of the group. This subject has been reviewed by Collins, who summarizes guidelines for diagnosis.

Polyarteritis Nodosa

Almost 75 percent of cases of polyarteritis nodosa include involvement of the small nutrient arteries of peripheral nerves (these figures come from autopsy series), but a symptomatic form of neuropathy develops in about half this number. Nonetheless, involvement of the peripheral nerves may be the principal or first sign to the diagnosis, before the main components of the clinical picture—abdominal pain, hematuria, fever, eosinophilia, hypertension, vague limb pains, and asthma—had not fully declared themselves or had been misinterpreted.

Although characteristically a disease of multiple discrete mononeuropathies, the syndrome associated with polyarteritis nodosa may appear more or less generalized and symmetrical as a result of the accumulation of many small nerve infarctions; i.e., it can simulate a polyneuropathy. In these cases, careful clinical and electrophysiologic examinations disclose elements of mononeuritis that have been engrafted on an otherwise generalized process. For example, an asymmetrical foot- or wrist-drop or a disproportionate affection of one nerve in a limb, such as ulnar palsy with relative sparing of function of the adjacent median nerve, are clues to the multifocal nature of the process. More often it takes form throughout its course of random infarctions of two or more individual nerves.

The onset is usually abrupt with symptoms of pain or numbness at a focal site along a nerve or in the distal distribution of an affected nerve, followed in hours or days by motor or sensory loss in the distribution of that nerve and then by involvement in a saltatory fashion of other peripheral nerves. Both the spinal and cranial nerves may be affected but far less often than the nerves in the limbs. Virtually no two cases are identical.

The CSF is usually normal. Nerve biopsy, usually taken from the sural nerve, will in most cases show the necrotizing arteritis in medium-size vessels (fibrinoid necrosis of all 3 coats of the vessel walls), with infiltrating eosinophils and occlusion of vessels. Muscle biopsy may also show perivascular inflammation and necrosis, but the diagnostic yield is less than for biopsy of a nerve, particularly an affected one. On the basis of the smaller size of affected vessels and the presence of perinuclear antinuclear cytoplasmic autoantibodies (p-ANCA), Lhote and colleagues have differentiated a "microscopic" polyarteritis. Rapidly progressive glomerulonephritis and lung hemorrhage are the additional features of the latter disease, neuropathy occurring somewhat less frequently than in typical polyarteritis.

Treatment Based on the response to the systemic vasculitides with ANCA activity, mononeuritis multiplex caused by vasculitis has been treated with corticosteroids and either rituximab 375 mg/m^2 weekly for 4 weeks, or cyclophosphamide 1 g/m^2 intravenously once a month for several months, but other equivalent regimens have been suggested. For the corticosteroid regimen, we have used intravenous methylprednisolone, 1.5 mg/kg, for several days, followed by oral corticosteroid treatment. It appears from clinical experience that corticosteroids alone are often inadequate, but some clinicians have taken this approach initially. Azathioprine is a reasonable alternative if cyclophosphamide is not tolerated. Treatment must be continued for at least several months. In intractable cases and in those with systemic involvement, treatment with methotrexate may be indicated, or this may be used initially. Spontaneous remission and therapeutic arrest are known, but many cases have a fatal outcome from kidney and systemic complications. The infarctive nerve palsies and sensory loss of the mononeuropathies generally persist to a large degree even when the systemic disease is brought under control.

Churg-Strauss and Hypereosinophilic Syndrome

These closely related systemic illnesses involve multiple individual peripheral nerves, much as in polyarteritis. A characteristic feature is the excess of circulating and tissue eosinophils (more so than in polyarteritis) and a tendency of the vasculitis to involve the lungs and skin, in contrast to the renal and bowel infarctions of polyarteritis nodosa. There is considerable degree of pathologic and clinical overlap between both polyarteritis and Churg-Strauss necrotizing vasculitis with the more benign hypereosinophilic syndrome that is less aggressive and has a greater tendency for eosinophilic infiltration of other tissues. One medication (zafirlukast) that is used in Europe to treat asthma has precipitated several cases of Churg-Strauss disease. Rarely, the overall illness has apparently been preceded by treatment with a macrolide antibiotic (e.g., azithromycin), estrogen, or carbamazepine, but these associations are uncertain and most cases are idiopathic.

In Churg-Strauss disease, rhinitis or asthma may be present for years and only later is there marked eosinophilia and organ infiltration, particularly an eosinophilic pneumonitis. The neuropathy that then develops in approximately three-quarters of patients is usually preceded by fever and weight loss and takes the form of an acute, painful mononeuritis multiplex. A granular cytoplasmic pattern of antineutrophil cytoplasmic autoantibodies (c-ANCA) of the same type that occurs in Wegener granulomatosis is found in more than half of cases. The histologic feature in nerve biopsies is similar to polyarteritis nodosa, but the eosinophilic infiltration tends to be more intense. We have seen other types of cutaneous diseases with vasculitic mononeuritis, the most impressive being a massive leukocytoclastic vasculitis of the skin (necrotic polymorphonuclear cells surrounding venules) resulting in large confluent hemorrhagic lesions.

The *idiopathic eosinophilic syndrome* comprises a heterogeneous group of disorders, the common features of which are a persistent and extreme degree of eosinophilia and eosinophilic infiltration of many organ systems. Neuropathy occurs in fewer than half of the cases, taking the form of a painful diffuse sensorimotor syndrome with axonal damage or of a mononeuritis multiplex (see Moore et al). The pathologic appearance is one of diffuse infiltration of the nerves by eosinophils rather than a vasculitis. The neuropathic effects are attributable to the infiltration itself or to a postulated tissue-damaging effect of the eosinophilic cell.

Treatment Both the Churg-Strauss and the idiopathic hypereosinophilic syndrome are treated initially with high doses of corticosteroids, with which the peripheral eosinophilia, as well as tissue damage, may abate in several weeks or months. Further immunosuppressive treatment in the forms of rituximab as discussed previously, azathioprine, methotrexate, or cyclophosphamide has been used in fulminant or refractory cases, which includes most of the ones that we have seen.

Wegener Granulomatosis

This disorder gives rise to asymmetrical multiple mononeuropathy indistinguishable from the other angiopathic neuropathies described earlier and, probably based on the same mechanism, mononeuropathies of the lower cranial nerves directly as they exit the skull and pass through the retropharyngeal tissues. The frequency of peripheral nerve involvement in Wegener disease is much lower than in the other of classic vasculitides and the affected vessels are of a smaller caliber than in polyarteritis nodosa. Nonetheless, DeGroot and colleagues emphasized in a prospective analysis of 128 patients with Wegener disease that 25 had evidence of mononeuritis multiplex, with the peroneal nerve most often involved, and an even greater number had distal polyneuropathy; however, the proportion of their cases in which neuropathy was the presenting or sole manifestation of disease was higher than in other series. The finding of circulating c-ANCA is relatively specific for Wegener granulomatosis and for Churg-Strauss disease, as mentioned earlier (Specks et al), and helps to differentiate it from polyarteritis (which may be associated with p-ANCA) and from retropharyngeal carcinoma, chordoma, sarcoidosis, and herpes zoster. Wegener vasculitis as it affects the lower cranial nerves is discussed in Chap. 47.

Treatment is along the lines of corticosteroids and rituximab or cyclophosphamide as already discussed.

Essential Mixed Cryoglobulinemia

This process may be associated with a vasculitic mononeuritis multiplex as well as a more generalized polyneuropathy. In many cases, glomerulonephritis, arthralgia, and purpura are conjoined, reflecting the systemic nature of the vasculopathy, but the mononeuritis may occur in isolation. The evolution in the cases under our care has been slower than in the typical vasculitic neuropathies, sometimes taking weeks or months between attacks of mononeuropathy. The neurologic disorder may become quiescent for long periods, during which time considerable improvement may occur. There is no evident relationship between the mode of onset or severity of the neuropathy and the concentration of cryoprecipitable proteins in the serum. These proteins can be detected by cooling the serum and demonstrating a precipitation of IgG and IgM proteins that redissolve upon warming to 37°C (98.6°F). To demonstrate this phenomenon the blood sample must be carefully transported to the laboratory in a warm water bath. An association of cryoglobulinemia with hepatitis C is well known, but many patients have had polyneuropathy from cryoglobulins but without the infection.

Treatment Garcia-Bragado and colleagues suggested that the neuropathy can be stabilized by corticosteroids and cyclophosphamide, but rituximab has been increasingly employed rather than cyclophosphamide and plasma exchange; the comparison between approaches has not been systematically tested. If the underlying problem is hepatitis C infection, pegylated alpha-interferon and ribavirin are usually administered as antiviral agents, with rituximab if the neuropathy is severe. It is too early to judge if the new protease inhibitors for the treatment of hepatitis C will reduce the occurrence and degree of polyneuropathy. Other aspects of the condition are discussed further under "Polyneuropathy Associated with Paraproteinemia" and "Other Vasculitic Neuropathies."

Rheumatoid Arthritis

Some 1 to 5 percent of patients with rheumatoid arthritis have vasculitic involvement of one or more nerves at some time in the course of their disease, apart from more mundane pressure neuropathies as a result of thickened tendons and destructive joint changes. The arteritis is of small-vessel fibrinoid type and immune globulins are demonstrable in the walls of vessels. Most of the affected patients under our care have had severe rheumatic disease for many years and were strongly seropositive. In addition to the neuropathy, such patients often have rheumatoid nodules, skin vasculitis, weight loss, and fever. There are rarer forms of chronic progressive polyneuropathy that complicate rheumatoid arthritis; they are described further on.

Systemic Lupus Erythematosus

Approximately 10 percent of patients with lupus exhibit symptoms and signs of peripheral nerve involvement, but only a negligible number occur before the established and more advanced stages of the disease (i.e., rarely has it been the initial presentation). In our several patients, the polyneuropathy has taken the form of a symmetrical, progressive sensorimotor paralysis, beginning in the feet and legs and extending to the arms, evolving over a period of several days or weeks, thereby simulating GBS. In a few, weakness and areflexia were more prominent than the sensory loss; the latter involved mainly vibratory and position senses. A more common syndrome in our experience has been a progressive or relapsing disease that cannot be distinguished clinically from chronic inflammatory demyelinating polyneuropathy (discussed further on). Multiple mononeuropathies have also been reported, as has involvement of the autonomic nervous system. An elevation of CSF protein that is found in some instances suggests nerve root involvement. Sural nerve biopsies may show vascular changes consisting of endothelial thickening and mononuclear inflammatory infiltrates in and around the small vessels for which reason the disease is included here with the other vasculitic neuropathies. Axonal degeneration is the most common change, but a chronic demyelinating pathology has also been described (Rechthand et al). Vascular injury from deposition of immune complexes is the proposed mechanism of nerve damage.

Isolated (Nonsystemic) Vasculitic Neuropathy

In contrast to the aforementioned disorders, which involve several tissues and organs in addition to the peripheral nerves, necrotizing vasculitis may be limited to the nerves. Cases of this type appear as often as all the other systemic vasculitic types together. This restricted form of mononeuritis multiplex usually presents as a subacute symmetrical or asymmetrical polyneuropathy with superimposed mononeuropathies or solely with multiple mononeuritis. Circulating antineutrophil cytoplasmic antibody (ANCA) is found in a few cases, but other tests for inflammatory and connective tissue diseases are negative. In the series reported by Collins and colleagues (2003), the sedimentation rate was mildly elevated, the mean being 38 mm/h, with only one-quarter having values greater than 50 mm/h. The main diagnostic difficulty in diagnosis arises when the EMG performed early in the course of illness shows conduction block that simulates a demyelinating polyneuropathy. Nerve biopsy should then settle the issue.

Treatment The neuropathy tends to be less aggressive (and nonlethal) than the systemic forms of vasculitic neuropathy and has usually responded to corticosteroids without treatment with cyclophosphamide (Dyck et al, 1987). However, in the aforementioned series reported by Collins, the use of cyclophosphamide for 6 months with corticosteroids resulted in a more rapid remission and fewer relapses. An expert group has provided guidelines for treatment specifically of this condition that approximates this approach by adding an immunosuppressive agent to corticosteroids only if the disease behaves aggressively (Collins et al, 2010).

Other Vasculitic Neuropathies

In the past, administration of pooled serum for the treatment of various infections led to brachial plexus neuritis or to an immune mononeuropathy multiplex, presumably from deposition of antibody–antigen complexes in the walls of the vasa nervorum. A similar "serum sickness" reaction occurred after certain viral infections associated with arthritis, rash, and fever. The neuropathy that arises with hepatitis C infection may be of this type, perhaps mediated by the frequently associated cryoglobulinemia as mentioned earlier. Interferon, which has been effective in treating the hepatitis, may also ameliorate the neuropathy,but greater success has been achieved with cyclophosphamide. Pooled immunoglobulin for the treatment of diverse neuromuscular diseases such as Guillain-Barré syndrome and myasthenia gravis has not, to our knowledge, led to a serum-sickness neuropathy, but one of our patients with Churg-Strauss disease developed a fulminating vasculitic skin eruption while being treated with IVIg.

In 2 cases of severe systemic vasculitis related to administration of hydralazine, we observed no neuropathic features; whether this applies to other drug-induced vasculitides is not known. Minocycline is another drug that has been associated in rare instances with a vasculitis, including mononeuropathies. The increasing appearance of vasculitic neuropathy with *HIV infection*, including a type that is independent of CMV infection, has already been mentioned; such cases have tended to improve spontaneously or with corticosteroid therapy. In about half of these cases the CSF contains polymorphonuclear cells. From time to time a patient with a lymphoproliferative disorder such as Hodgkin disease will develop mononeuritis multiplex that is found by biopsy to be caused by vasculitis. (A chronic demyelinating, nonvasculitic polyneuropathy is more common with lymphomas of any type as discussed earlier.)

A rare *paraneoplastic variety of vasculitic neuropathy* has also been described. Oh reported 2 of his patients and reviewed 13 previous ones. The most common underlying cancer was of the small oat cell lung type. Anti-Hu antibodies that are typical of paraneoplastic neurologic diseases from this cancer are generally not detected (see Chap. 31). Other solid tumors (renal, gastric, gynecologic) have been associated with a similar neuropathy but only in a few instances. Almost all have had slightly elevated protein concentration in the CSF but few showed a pleocytosis. At autopsy, the vasculitis was limited to nerve and muscle.

The role of an obscure small-vessel vasculitis in otherwise idiopathic axonal polyneuropathies of elderly patients has been reported, but is, in our view, controversial. We have not found, as did Chia and colleagues, an unexpected vasculitis in the nerve biopsies of such patients. The vasoocclusive and infiltrative condition of intravascular lymphoma often includes a syndrome of multiple painless mononeuropathies as part of a larger multifocal illness of the central and peripheral nervous system.

Neuropathy of Critical Limb Ischemia

A few patients with severe atherosclerotic ischemic disease of the iliac or leg arteries will be found to have localized sensory changes or diminished reflexes. Usually, the other effects of ischemia—claudication and pain at rest, absence of distal pulses and trophic skin changes—are so prominent that the neurologic changes are minor by comparison. In experimental studies, combined occlusion of the aorta and multiple limb vessels are required to produce neural ischemia because of the profusely ramifying vasculature. In our experience of 12 patients with a critically ischemic leg, there was a neuropathy with a pronounced distal predominance; sensory loss in the feet was worse than the symptoms might suggest and there was mild weakness of the toes and depression or loss of the ankle reflex (Weinberg et al). Although paresthesias, numbness, and deep aching pain at rest were characteristic, the patients were more limited by symptoms of their vascular claudication than by the neuropathic ones. Restoration of circulation to the limb by surgical or other means resulted in some improvement of the regional neuropathy. Reviews of the literature on this subject can be found in the writings of Eames and Lange.

A poorly understood but presumably localized ischemic neuropathy occurs in the region of arteriovenous shunts that have been placed for the purpose of hemodialysis. Complaints of transient diffuse tingling of the hand are not uncommon soon after creation of the shunt but only a few patients develop persistent forearm weakness, numbness and burning in the fingers, reflecting variable degrees of ulnar, radial, and median nerve, and possibly also muscle, ischemia. The role of an underlying uremic polyneuropathy in facilitating this neuropathy has not been studied.

A progressive, symmetrical polyneuropathy as a result of systemic cholesterol embolism has been described by Bendixen and colleagues. An inflammatory and necrotizing arteritis surrounds embolic cholesterol material within small vessels and appears to account for the progression of symptoms. This neuropathic process is more often discovered at autopsy than it is in the clinic, being eclipsed during life by the cerebral manifestations of cholesterol embolism. The peripheral part of the illness simulates the polyneuropathy of a small-vessel polyarteritis.

Sarcoid Neuropathies

The generalized granulomatous disease of sarcoidosis infrequently produces subacute or chronic polyneuropathy, polyradiculopathy, or mononeuropathies. A painful, small-fiber sensory neuropathy has also been described by Hoitsma and colleagues. Any of the neuropathies may be associated with granulomatous lesions in muscles (polymyositis) or with signs of CNS involvement, most often of the stalk of the pituitary with diabetes insipidus or a myelopathy (see Chap. 44).

Involvement of a single nerve with sarcoid most often implicates the facial nerve (facial palsy), but sometimes multiple cranial nerves are affected in succession (see Chap. 47). Next in frequency is weakness and reflex and sensory loss, appearing sequentially (polyradiculopathy), in the distribution of several spinal nerves or roots. The occurrence of large, irregular zones of sensory loss over the trunk is said to distinguish the neuropathy of sarcoidosis from other forms of mononeuropathy multiplex. This pattern particularly when accompanied by pain, resembles diabetic radiculopathy (see earlier in "Diabetic Multiple Mononeuropathies and Radiculoplexus Neuropathy").

Unlike the cases of sarcoid polyneuropathy we have reported (Zuniga et al), in the series of 11 patients with sarcoid neuropathy studied by Said and colleagues (2002), only 2 were known to have pulmonary granulomas before the onset of neuropathic symptoms; 6 had a focal or multifocal neuropathic syndrome (including 1 with a clinical and electrophysiologic pattern that simulated multifocal conduction block). The remainder had a nonspecific symmetric polyneuropathy, 1 of which had an acute onset. Facial diplegia was common, as is well known. The pathologic changes in nerve and muscle biopsy specimens consisted mainly of epineurial granulomas and endoneurial inflammatory infiltrates, but there were indications of necrotizing vasculitis in 7 cases. Among the cases we studied, 6 of 10 had a subacute or chronic sensorimotor polyneuropathy. It is notable that in only 2 of Said's patients were levels of angiotensin-converting enzyme elevated in the serum.

Lyme Neuropathies (See also Chap. 32)

The neuropathy that develops in 10 to 15 percent of patients with this disease takes several forms. Cranial nerve involvement is well known, uni- or bilateral facial palsy being by far the most frequent manifestation. Other cranial nerves may also be affected as may almost any of the spinal roots, mostly in the cervical or lumbar region. Even phrenic nerve palsy has been attributed to Lyme disease in a few cases. A concurrent mild or moderate aseptic meningoradiculitis (10 to 100 mononuclear cells/mm^3) is characteristic (although this may also occur in HIV and CMV and other forms of neuritis). The CSF glucose is usually normal but has been slightly depressed in a few cases with multiple radiculopathies. Some of the CSF cells may have immature features suggesting a lymphomatous infiltration. (See further on and Chap. 32 for further details of the laboratory diagnosis.) There may be radicular pain not unlike that of cervical or lumbar disc or plexus disease.

The triad of cranial nerve palsies, radiculitis, and aseptic meningitis is most characteristic of Lyme disease during its disseminated phase, i.e., from 1 to 3 weeks after the tick bite or from the appearance of the typical rash. The disease tends to be seasonal in the period of maximal tick exposure. The special polyradiculitis form of Lyme is discussed further on.

Besides the just described cranial neuropathies, the following are the main neuropathic syndromes of Lyme disease: (1) multiple mononeuropathies (involvement of a single major nerve in the limbs, resulting in an isolated foot- or wrist-drop—a distinctly rare pattern); (2) lumbar or brachial plexopathy (the latter being well described but rare); (3) a predominantly sensory polyneuropathy in which paresthesias and loss of superficial sensation in the feet and legs are coupled with loss of ankle jerks; (4) a generalized axonal polyneuropathy (Loggigian et al), mainly sensory and sometimes accompanied by a mild encephalopathy; and (5) acute GBS (we have encountered only 2 such cases in more than 400 patients with Guillain-Barré but the syndrome appears to be more common in Europe following *Borrelia* infection).

Electrophysiologic testing indicates that the various peripheral nerve syndromes frequently overlap. All of the preceding processes excepting the one that resembles GBS usually occur as subacute or late complications of Lyme disease, several months or, rarely, years after the initial infection (in untreated cases). These late neuropathic syndromes respond less favorably to treatment than do the acute ones, and have a less certain connection to the infection (see further on). As the disease is not fatal, there are few adequate pathologic studies of the peripheral nerves in Lyme disease. The infective agent has not been demonstrated in nerve tissue, but perivascular inflammation and vasculitic changes are found in small vessels within the nerves.

Lyme Polyradiculitis and Bannwarth Syndrome This is perhaps the best characterized, but not the most common, group of Lyme neuropathies. A painful lumbosacral polyradiculitis has long been known in Europe by the term *Bannwarth syndrome* (in France as Garin-Bujadoux syndrome). The pathogen in Europe is a *Borrelia* spirochete slightly different from the one that causes Lyme disease in North America. In Bannwarth syndrome there is an intense inflammatory reaction in the cauda equina, giving rise to sciatic and buttock pain and bladder dysfunction. Less frequently, a cervical polyradiculopathy occurs with shoulder and arm pain that cannot be distinguished on clinical grounds from brachial neuritis. Cases of Bannwarth syndrome from North American Lyme under our care have progressed subacutely over days or weeks and involved the L2-L3-L4 roots, first one leg, then the other, and, subsequently, the midcervical roots on one or both sides. Sparing of a proximal or distal part of a limb while the adjacent part is weakened gives rise to a striking syndrome. One or more thoracic radiculopathies may be added and cause local discomfort.

The nerve conduction tests show preservation of sensory potentials, which marks the process as radicular. Headache and a marked pleocytosis (over 100 mononuclear cells/mm^3) in the spinal fluid may accompany the pain and usually precedes the radiculopathies by days. Polymerase chain reaction for the detection of the organism in the CSF gives variable results, especially after several days of neurologic illness. A value above unity of CSF to serum anti-Lyme antibodies is probably a dependable indicator of acute or subacute disease, but there have been few systematic studies of this measurement. Oligoclonal bands in the CSF are common as a reflection of these antibodies.

A similar syndrome of lumbar polyradiculitis may also be caused by the herpes and Epstein-Barr viruses or more often by an opportunistic CMV infection in a patient with AIDS.

Diagnosis This is both aided and at times confused by serologic testing (see Chap. 32). The enzyme-linked immunosorbent assay (ELISA) is not altogether satisfactory because it frequently yields false-positive and, occasionally, false-negative results. Western blot testing of CSF is more specific. Information to the effect that the patient has lived in or visited an endemic area is useful, but far more compelling is evidence of a tick bite followed by the characteristic rash, or a well-defined history of nonneurologic manifestations of Lyme disease (cardiac, arthritic). Bifacial palsy in any of these clinical contexts also favors the diagnosis of Lyme.

Treatment Treatment of the Lyme neuropathic syndromes is with intravenous antibiotics, preferably ceftriaxone 2 g daily for 1 month. More prolonged or intravenous treatment has not been shown to be superior. Corticosteroids have an uncertain role in the painful radicular syndromes, but we have used them in low doses and they relieved pain. In most series, there is recovery or virtually complete resolution of radicular symptoms in approximately 90 percent of patients, although this may take months. Facial palsies also tend to improve, but with a lower rate of complete resolution. It has been stated that many of the peripheral and cranial neuropathies improve even without treatment, but this has not been studied systematically.

Sjögren Disease–Associated Neuropathies

This is a chronic, slowly progressive autoimmune disease characterized by lymphocytic infiltration of the exocrine glands, particularly the parotid and lacrimal glands, that results in keratoconjunctivitis sicca and xerostomia (dry eyes and mouth). These core features may be combined with arthritis or with a wide range of other abnormalities, notably lymphoma, vasculitis, IgM paraproteinemia, renal tubular defects (renal tubular acidosis), and, quite often, a predominantly sensory polyneuropathy (see review by Kaplan et al). In the series collected by Grant and colleagues, the neuropathy was the presenting problem in 87 percent of 54 patients with Sjögren disease. The sicca symptoms are often mild and reported only upon specific inquiry. A symmetrical sensory polyneuropathy or a sensory ganglionopathy are the most common patterns. Sensorimotor polyneuropathy, polyradiculoneuropathy, autonomic neuropathy, or mononeuropathy (most often of the trigeminal nerve, as described by Kaltrieder and Talal) are less common. We have observed yet another neuropathic syndrome taking the form of asymmetrical sensory loss, mostly of position sense and involving the upper limbs predominantly, in association with tonic pupils and trigeminal anesthesia that is probably a variant of the ganglionopathy.

The sensory polyneuropathies of the Sjögren syndrome are of particular interest to neurologists, as they will encounter most cases before other physicians (Griffen et al). More than 80 percent of affected patients are older women. The polyneuropathic syndrome often begins with paresthesias of the feet, usually mild in degree. The main clinical features are subacute and widespread sensory loss that may include the trunk and sometimes, profoundly diminished kinesthetic sense, giving rise to sensory ataxia of the limbs and of gait that reflect a ganglionitis. Loss of pain and temperature sensation is variable; tendon reflexes are abolished. A nondescript large- or small-fiber distal sensory neuropathy is also known, for which reason testing for Sjögren-related serum antibodies is included in the general evaluation of polyneuropathies in older patients, and the heterogeneity of sensory neuropathy presentation has been emphasized by several authors. In time, some patients develop autonomic abnormalities such as bowel atony, urinary retention, loss of sweating, and pupillary changes. There is usually little or no pain, but there have been exceptions.

Diagnosis Sjögren disease–associated neuropathy or ganglionopathy should be suspected in an older woman with sensory neuropathy or neuronopathy, particularly if sicca symptoms are present. There may be telangiectasias over the bridge of the nose, on the lips, and fingers. The evaluation is aided by the Schirmer and Rose Bengal tests, which usually demonstrate a reduction of tearing. Even without this confirmatory test, we have found it advisable to perform a biopsy of the lip (at the epithelial–mucosal juncture) to detect inflammatory changes in the small salivary glands. This is a minor office procedure in most instances. The diagnosis of Sjögren syndrome from the biopsy requires at least 2 collections of 50 or more lymphocytes in a 4-mm^2 specimen. Some patients have serologic abnormalities such as antinuclear antibodies (anti-Ro, also termed *SS-A*, and anti-La, or *SS-B*) or monoclonal immunoglobulins, particularly of the IgM subclass. The frequency of specific Sjögren-specific antibodies varies between series; they may be useful as screening tests, but the lip biopsy appears to be more sensitive. In our series of 20 cases with minor salivary gland biopsies that demonstrated inflammatory changes diagnostic of the syndrome, only 6 had serologic evidence of the disease and 2 had positive serologic tests but a negative biopsy (Gorson and Ropper, 2003). The sedimentation rate in our patients was often slightly elevated; however, only 5 of our 20 had a value greater than 40 mm/min and many have had normal or only slightly elevated C-reactive protein levels. The main differential diagnostic entity, if the neuropathy appears subacutely, is a paraneoplastic sensory ganglionitis.

Mellgren and also Leger and their colleagues have stressed that a proportion of unexplained polyneuropathies in middle and late life are putatively caused by Sjögren syndrome. The latter authors found typical Sjögren abnormalities in the lip biopsies of 7 of 32 patients with chronic axonal polyneuropathy that could not otherwise be classified. Several other studies have corroborated this finding of inflammatory disruption of the minor salivary glands in obscure neuropathies, particularly in older women and in some men. The diagnosis in our clinics has not been nearly as frequent in this group. Nonetheless, a search for Sjögren disease may be revealing in otherwise obscure sensory neuropathies.

Nerve biopsies have variably revealed necrotizing vasculitis, inflammatory cell infiltrates, and focal nerve fiber destruction. Usually, the CSF protein is normal and there is no cellular reaction. The few times a dorsal root ganglion has been examined in autopsy material; there were infiltrates of mononuclear cells and lymphocytes and destruction of nerve cells.

Treatment Corticosteroids in doses of approximately 60 mg daily of prednisone, cyclophosphamide (100 mg per day), and rituximab (1,000 mg per day, 2 weeks apart) have been used when the neuropathy is severe and are indicated when there is vasculitis involving renal and pulmonary structures. We have initially administered prednisone 60 mg daily, sometimes in tandem with intermittent plasma exchange, but with little evidence of response, before adding a second immunosuppressive agent.

The review of the neurologic manifestations of Sjögren syndrome by Lafitte and by Berkowitz and colleagues are recommended.

Idiopathic Sensory Ganglionopathy (Chronic Ataxic Neuropathy)

In addition to the subacute pansensory syndrome described previously and paraneoplastic, postinfectious, and toxic processes, there is a yet another more chronic idiopathic syndrome characterized by severe global sensory loss and ataxia. We have encountered several such patients resembling the cases described by Dalakas. The numbness and sensory findings progressed over months and spread to proximal parts of the arms and legs and then to the trunk. The face and top of the scalp were finally involved. Despite ataxia and complete areflexia, muscular power remained normal and pain was not a problem. There are reports of fasciculations in a few patients, but not in the ones we have seen. Within a year, most of these patients became completely disabled from the ataxia, unable to walk or even feed themselves. Autonomic failure was another feature in a few and one of our patients became deaf. Extensive examinations for an occult cancer, paraproteinemia, Sjögren disease, Refsum disease, autoimmune diseases, and all potential causes of an ataxic neuropathy proved to be frustratingly negative. Of course, it is possible that some patients had an as yet undiscovered tumor. Yet other instances have had all the features of a truncal–limb sensory neuropathy, with little or no ataxia and only muted reflexes; these have had a more benign course but still no cause was found (Romero et al). Illa and colleagues (2001), in a review of 17 patients with idiopathic sensory ataxic neuropathy, found antibodies against the ganglioside GD_1 in only 1 case and concluded that the majority was not caused by an immunologic mechanism.

The motor nerve conduction studies have been normal or slightly impaired, while the sensory potentials were eventually lost (but they may at first be normal). A puzzling feature in 2 patients has been an unexpected preservation of many sensory nerve potentials even after a year of illness. In these cases, the process presumably lay in the dorsal roots rather than in the ganglia. In a few instances the MRI has shown a change in the posterior columns of the spinal cord, certainly as a secondary phenomenon from the root disease. The spinal fluid has generally contained a slightly elevated protein concentration with few or no cells, up to $18/mm^3$ in our cases.

Pathologic examination of the sensory ganglia in a few cases has disclosed an inflammatory process identical to that of Sjögren disease. Our attempts at treatment using plasma exchanges, IVIg, corticosteroids, and immunosuppressive agents have been mostly unsuccessful.

Also mentioned here is a subacute or chronic *idiopathic small-fiber ganglionopathy* that affects function primarily. These patients complain of pain and burning in proximal body parts, including the face, tongue, and scalp with reduced sensation of pinprick in affected areas. The reflexes may be preserved and vibration sensory perception may be preserved. Our experience with such patients and anecdotal responses to treatment was summarized by Gorson and colleagues (2008). Whether such aberrant proximal sensory complaints as "burning mouth syndrome" (see Chap. 10) are allied with this entity is not clear but they may occur together.

Idiopathic Autonomic Neuropathy

Under this term is collected a group of subacute and chronic dysautonomias that on extensive evaluation cannot be attributed to diabetes, amyloidosis, autoimmune disease, Fabry disease, HIV, toxin exposure, or another systemic disease. A few cases will be found to be due to one of several rare mutations in genes, of which four sites have been described so far (SPTLC1, HSN2, IKBKAP, NTRK1).

A number of such cases, almost half in the series of Suarez and colleagues (1994), have been acute in onset and conform most closely to the "pure pandysautonomia" condition described by Young and colleagues, discussed earlier as a variant of Guillain-Barré syndrome. The others follow a subacute or chronic course and about one-fourth of these have a serum antibody that is directed against the acetylcholine receptor of sensory ganglia (Klein et al). Orthostatic hypotension is the leading feature; in those with the previously mentioned antibody, pupillary changes and difficulty with accommodation, dry mouth and dry eyes, and gastrointestinal paresis were the most common findings according to Sandroni and colleagues. Perhaps a subgroup is in some way related to Sjögren syndrome as sicca symptoms are prominent, but these later features could just as well be a component of the autonomic failure. There is not enough information to determine if all these cases are accounted for by one process or to judge the effects of various immune treatments.

Migratory Sensory Neuritis (Wartenberg Syndrome)

The defining features of this unusual syndrome are searing and pulling sensations involving small cutaneous areas, that are evoked by extending or stretching the limb, as happens when reaching for an object, kneeling, or pointing with the foot. The pain is momentary but leaves in its wake a patch of circumscribed numbness. Cutaneous sensory nerves must be involved in some way and are irritated during such mechanical maneuvers. The areas involved are usually proximal to the most terminal sensory distribution of nerves encompassing, for example, a patch on the lateral side of the hand and the proximal fifth finger or a larger region over the patella (these were the sites affected in 3 of our patients). Recovery of the area of numbness takes several weeks, but it may persist if the symptoms are induced repeatedly. Except for these patches of cutaneous analgesia, the clinical examination is normal. Selected sensory nerves may show abnormalities in conduction, but nerve conduction studies are for the most part normal. Matthews and Esiri have listed the many areas that may be affected in a single patient and have described an increase in the endoneurial connective tissue in a biopsied sural nerve. The syndrome may come in episodes over many years, without symptoms between attacks. A spurious diagnosis of multiple sclerosis is often made. The pathology is not certain, but some form of fibrosis or inflammation of cutaneous nerves has been suggested, perhaps similar to the condition of perineuritis described below.

Sensory Perineuritis

Under this title, Asbury and colleagues (1972) described a patchy, burning, painful, partially remitting distal cutaneous sensory neuropathy. The pathologic picture was one of inflammatory scarring restricted to the perineurium, with compression of the contained nerve fibers. As with the Wartenberg syndrome above, reflexes and motor function were unaffected. Digital nerves, as well as the medial and lateral branches of the superficial peroneal nerve, were the ones most often involved. Matthews and Squier have described a trigeminal and occipital distribution of painful sensory symptoms and 1 of the patients of Asbury and coworkers (1972) also had symptoms on the scalp. A Tinel sign is characteristically elicited by tapping the skin overlying the involved cutaneous nerves and is indicative of partial nerve damage and regeneration.

The differential diagnosis includes numerous other forms of painful sensory neuropathy, but the patchy and painful, and often burning, quality of symptoms distinguishes this process. The diagnosis can only be established with certainty by biopsy of a distal cutaneous branch of a sensory nerve. Perhaps some of the large group of patients with "burning" feet may have a small-fiber neuropathy that affects intradermal nerve fibers in a similar way (see further on).

Since the original report, the fibrosing perineurial pathologic changes that characterize perineuritis have been described in a number of polyneuropathies, mainly in diabetic patients but also in those with cryoglobulinemia, nutritional diseases, and malignancies (Sorenson et al). However, these patients displayed diverse clinical patterns of neuropathy, mainly mononeuritis multiplex and demyelinating neuropathy. Nonetheless, the pathologic feature of perineuritis may be less specific than initially thought but a perineuritis clinical syndrome is still a useful concept. A proportion of the idiopathic cases seem to respond to corticosteroids.

Celiac-Sprue Neuropathy

Among the multitude of odd neurologic manifestations attributed to this disease, the best known ones are cerebellar ataxia and myoclonus. In addition, Hadjivassiliou and colleagues have reported patients with a range of neuromuscular disorders in whom the neurologic symptoms antedated the diagnosis of the bowel disorder. A nondescript sensorimotor neuropathy was the most frequent, but one patient had mononeuropathy multiplex and Chin and colleagues have reported a multifocal neuropathy pattern. In a small prospective survey of treated celiac disease, Luostarinen and colleagues found 23 percent with evidence of a polyneuropathy by nerve conduction testing, but the clinical findings were scant. Antigliadin antibodies (simple antibodies directed against gluten), as well as more specific anti-transglutaminase antibodies and histologic examination of a duodenal biopsy are confirmatory of the diagnosis. Luostarinen and colleagues suggested that a search be made for these antibodies in patients with polyneuropathies of obscure origin. It is not clear how many of their cases could be attributed to nutritional deficiency. We have not encountered a definite instance despite attempts to detect the special sprue antibodies in the evaluation of over 200 cases of otherwise obscure polyneuropathy.

Neuropathies Associated With AIDS (See also Chap. 33)

Patients infected with HIV are prone to several types of neuropathies, including a predominantly sensory type that may be painful, a lumbosacral polyradiculopathy, cranial (mainly facial nerve) and limb mononeuropathies, CIDP, GBS, and a vasculitic mononeuritis multiplex—none of which differs from the idiopathic or conventional varieties except that there is often a pleocytosis in the spinal fluid. Almost unique and common patterns in this group are the CMV cauda equina neuritis syndrome and an acute or subacute painful infiltrative lymphocytic neuropathy—the diffuse infiltrative lymphocytosis syndrome (DILS; Moulingier et al). Polyneuropathy may also be induced by antiviral agents that are used in the treatment of HIV infection, as discussed in Chap. 33.

SYNDROME OF POLYRADICULOPATHY (WITH AND WITHOUT MENINGEAL INFILTRATION)

These are among the most clinically complex diseases of the peripheral nerves. Involvement of multiple spinal nerve roots produces a distinctive or sometimes confusing constellation of findings, usually quite different from those of polyneuropathy and from multiple mononeuropathies. As described earlier, muscle weakness caused by polyradiculopathy is characteristically asymmetrical and variably distributed in proximal and distal parts of the limbs, reflecting a pattern of muscles that share common root innervations (e.g., the combination of weakness in hamstring and gastrocnemius, or of iliopsoas, quadriceps, and obturator). However, muscles with similar innervation are not necessarily affected to the same degree because of the disproportionate contribution of a given root to each muscle. Sensory loss tends also to be patchy and to involve both the proximal and distal aspects of a dermatome. Pain is common in a radicular pattern, but sometimes only in the distal distribution of the root or in the back. The sensory findings tend to be less prominent than the motor ones. In keeping with nerve root pattern, certain tendon reflexes may be spared; a normal ankle jerk combined with an absent knee jerk, or the opposite, are particularly suggestive of a polyradiculopathy (or a lumbar plexopathy). Pain often takes the form of sharp jabs projected into the innervated zone of the involved root. As with mononeuritis multiplex, the cumulative effect of multiple root lesions can simulate a polyneuropathy in which case the tendency for polyradiculopathy to involve proximal muscles is the most helpful distinguishing feature.

A special pattern of polyradiculopathy occurs wherein all the sensory roots are involved, simulating tabes dorsalis. The clinical state is similar to that of a sensory ganglionopathy described earlier. Large- and small-fiber sensory loss is combined with ataxia while power is normal and there is no atrophy. A prominent feature is shooting and burning pain. We have occasionally found sensory loss over the anterior abdomen and thorax in these cases, a finding more typical of chronic dying-back axonal polyneuropathy.

Some of the diseases that affect nerve roots predominantly already have been discussed. They can be grouped into three broad categories: (1) diseases of the spinal column that compress adjacent roots; (2) infiltrative diseases of the meninges that secondarily involve the roots as they course through the subarachnoid space, mainly neoplastic of granulomatous infiltrations such as sarcoid; and (3) intrinsic neuropathies, inflammatory, infectious, or diabetic, that have a predilection for the radicular portion of the nerves. An elevated CSF protein and a pleocytosis usually accompany neoplastic or inflammatory meningeal diseases; the others show variable formulas in the spinal fluid.

Often what appears to be a polyneuropathy on clinical grounds will be found to have an electrophysiologic pattern of root disease at multiple spinal levels. McGonagle and colleagues estimated that polyradiculopathies accounted for 5 percent of all cases referred to their EMG laboratory and our experience approximates this. Consequently, careful EMG and nerve conductions testing is the most useful ancillary examination in cases of complex neuropathic syndromes because the pattern of muscle denervation can be ascertained with greater certainty than by clinical means and a common root pattern can then be logically derived. Of great confirmatory value is the preservation of sensory potentials in nerves that innervate regions of sensory loss and supply weak and denervated muscles. This proves that the lesion is located proximal to the dorsal root ganglion and spares the peripheral sensory axons. Loss of the F and H late responses is also typical of polyradiculopathies. The proximal location of the lesion can be further corroborated by early evidence of weakness and denervation in the paraspinal, gluteal, or rhomboid muscles, which are supplied by nerves that arise very proximally from the roots. In axonal cases of neuropathy, these proximal muscles are the last to be involved.

Among the acute and subacute meningeal radiculopathies, neoplastic infiltration (carcinomatous and lymphomatous) is the most common. Others are Lyme disease, sarcoidosis, herpes virus, arachnoiditis, AIDS-related cauda equina neuritis of CMV infection, or independently, EBV meningoradiculitis. In the past, meningeal syphilis of course was a common cause (tabes dorsalis).

Diseases of the spine, exemplified by lumbar and cervical spondylosis, commonly impinge on nerve roots, as discussed in Chap. 11. Metastatic carcinoma of the vertebral bodies may compress one or several adjacent roots by encroaching on posterolateral recesses of the canal and proximal neural foramina. Among rare causes of polyradiculopathy is a chronic lumbosacral syndrome associated with dural eventrations surrounding nerve roots, which may complicate ankylosing spondylitis.

However, one is often confronted by a pattern of subacute or chronic polyradiculopathy and abnormal CSF formula for which extensive examination fails to identify any of the diseases enumerated above. This idiopathic form of polyradiculopathy comes to our attention several times yearly. Some will turn out to have a lymphomatous infiltration at autopsy for which reason we have on occasion asked a neurosurgeon to remove a midlumbar (L2 or L3) motor rootlet for examination. Also particularly difficult diagnostically is a polyradiculopathy that involves the motor roots exclusively or predominantly and is indistinguishable from motor neuron disease except for the absence of widespread denervation or of progressive upper motor neuron signs and differing from the immune motor neuropathies discussed further on by the absence of conduction block.

SYNDROME OF CHRONIC SENSORIMOTOR POLYNEUROPATHY

In these common syndromes, reduced sensation, weakness, muscular atrophy, and loss of tendon reflexes progress over a period of months or years. Within this large category, two groups are distinguished. In the first and *less chronic* of the two, the neuropathy appears over months or a year or two. Comprising this group are *acquired* processes such as certain metabolic and immune-mediated polyneuropathies. Paraneoplastic neuropathies may also fall into this category, although they are more often subacute in onset, being almost fully developed in a matter of weeks. Leprous neuritis is the one infectious member of this group and also the one exception to the rule that all chronic neuropathies are more or less symmetrical in pattern. The polyneuropathies that make up the second group are *far more chronic* than the first, evolving insidiously over many years or decades; these are mainly the *heredodegenerative* diseases of the peripheral nervous system caused by specific genetic mutations.

Acquired Forms of Chronic Polyneuropathy

Polyneuropathy Associated With Paraproteinemia

The occurrence of a chronic sensorimotor polyneuropathy in association with an abnormality of serum immunoglobulins is recognized with increasing frequency, but its boundaries are still not well established as will be apparent in the following discussion. The excess blood protein, called a *paraprotein* or "M-spike," is usually in the form of a monoclonal immunoglobulin. It may be an isolated abnormality or a by-product of a plasma cell malignancy, specifically multiple myeloma, plasmacytoma, or Waldenström macroglobulinemia. Several lines of evidence suggest that a pathogenetically active antibody against components of myelin or axon is present in at least some of these cases. Special forms of neuropathy are also associated with amyloidosis. Both the acquired and genetic forms of amyloidosis are discussed further on.

Neuropathy With Monoclonal Gammopathy of Undetermined Significance (MGUS, Benign Monoclonal Gammopathy) The association of a nonneoplastic IgM monoclonal protein and a neuropathy was first described by Forssman and colleagues and was treated as coincidental until Kahn established a compelling statistical association between the two conditions. A more direct relationship was established by the finding of antiperipheral nerve antibodies in some patients who had such a protein in their blood. This category of polyneuropathy is associated with a monoclonal or sometimes polyclonal excess of immunoglobulin (IgG, IgM, or IgA, rarely others, mainly with a kappa light chain components; see Kyle and Dyck). These cases are far more common than those caused by a malignant plasma cell disorder. In our experience, monoclonal proteins underlie the largest group of otherwise unexplained neuropathies in adults.

The polyneuropathy associated with monoclonal gammopathy affects mainly, but not exclusively, males in the sixth and seventh decades of life. The onset is insidious over weeks and months or more, with numbness and paresthesias of the feet and then of the hands, followed by a relatively symmetrical weakness and slight wasting of these muscles. In some patients, sensory signs predominate. The tendon reflexes, eventually lost or diminished, may be preserved in the early phases of the illness. The course is usually slowly progressive, sometimes static after a year or so, and rarely remitting and relapsing. The CSF typically shows an elevation of the protein in the range of 50 to 100 mg/dL, and this is not due to passive diffusion of the excess paraprotein into the CSF.

The majority of cases of polyneuropathy with monoclonal gammopathy have a demyelinating or mixed axonal–demyelinating pattern on the EMG and nerve conduction study, but once the illness is well established, most will have predominantly axonal features. With few exceptions we have been unable to distinguish the axonal and demyelinating groups on clinical grounds or by their response to therapy (Gorson et al, 1997). Sural nerve biopsies show a loss of myelinated fibers of all sizes; unmyelinated fibers are mostly spared; hypertrophic changes, reflecting cycles of demyelination and remyelination with fibrosis are present in about half the cases according to Smith and colleagues. They found the monoclonal IgM antibody bound to surviving myelin sheaths and Latov and coworkers have shown that the serum IgM fraction often displays antimyelin activity.

Typically, the monoclonal protein in the blood is present in a concentration much less than 2 g/dL and there is no evidence of multiple myeloma or other malignant blood dyscrasia. It should be emphasized that routine serum protein electrophoresis (SPEP) fails to detect the majority of these paraproteins; immunoelectrophoresis (IEP) or the more sensitive immunofixation testing is required. The bone marrow aspirate shows a normal or only mildly increased proportion of plasma cells, which are the source of the paraprotein and the plasma cells are not morphologically atypical as they are in myeloma. Insofar as myeloma becomes manifest in perhaps one-quarter of patients many years after the gammopathy has been recognized, the condition is termed *monoclonal gammopathy of undetermined significance* (MGUS), although the older term *benign monoclonal gammopathy* is less cumbersome.

The importance of excess immunoglobulin as a cause of neuropathy can be appreciated by noting that 6 percent of patients referred to the Mayo Clinic with chronic polyneuropathy of unknown cause and as many as 20 percent in our clinical material and in other series have proved to have a monoclonal paraproteinemia (of course, the majority of patients with a blood paraprotein do not develop neuropathy).

Despite the fact that IgG is the most frequent paraprotein in adults, a polyneuropathy is associated somewhat more often with the IgM class. Combining three large series of patients with neuropathy and monoclonal paraproteinemias (62 patients of Yeung et al, Gosselin et al, and our patients as reported by Simovic et al), 60 percent had IgM, 30 percent IgG, and 10 percent with IgA subclass paraproteins. An identical but infrequent condition exists in which only the light chain component of an immunoglobulin is overproduced by the plasma cells and is found exclusively in the urine (similar to the Bence Jones protein of multiple myeloma).

Four-fifths of patients have had a *kappa* light chain component, as mentioned previously, although *lambda* light chain has special significance as discussed further on in relation to plasmacytoma and the polyneuropathy, organomegaly, endocrinopathy, M protein, and skin changes (POEMS) syndrome. In our experience and in that of others, patients with IgM paraprotein more often have severe sensory findings and a demyelinative type of nerve conduction abnormality when compared with the IgG group. However, with the exception of the special anti-MAG syndrome (see later), we have not found the extent of difference in clinical features and response to treatment between the immunoglobulin subclasses that has been reported by others (Simovic et al).

Although more than a dozen specific antibodies against myelin and other components of nerve have been identified among the paraproteins, the ones that give rise to the most distinctive clinical syndromes, present in 50 to 75 percent of patients with IgM-associated neuropathies, are those that react with a MAG, related glycolipids, or sulfatide components of myelin (the latter are referred to as sulfate-3-glucuronyl paragloboside [SGPG] and related sulfatides). Proprioceptive sensory loss with gait imbalance, tremor, and the Romberg sign are typical findings in the group with anti-MAG activity, while weakness and atrophy tend to appear later in the illness. Other IgM antineural antibodies have a more tentative connection to polyneuropathy. It is reasonable to assume that IgG monoclonal gammopathies are also capable of causing chronic neuropathies, but the evidence is less compelling and based mainly on the frequency of their presence in cases of otherwise unexplained polyneuropathy. Indeed, it has been suggested that in many reported instances the association with neuropathy with IgG paraproteinemia is coincidental. The anti-MAG illnesses are relentlessly progressive at various rates in most patients at various rates but in about 15 percent of our patients with anti-MAG antibody the illness has been mild and static for years at a time, even without treatment.

Because of the risk of myeloma or Waldenström disease, bone marrow examination is generally performed some time in the course and particularly if the concentration of the paraprotein exceeds 3 g/dL or climbs progressively over years, or if other hematologic changes such as unexplained anemia or thrombocytopenia develop.

TREATMENT In most cases of uncomplicated monoclonal gammopathy with polyneuropathy that are associated with IgG or IgA paraproteins, particularly if not of long standing, plasma exchange may produce transient improvement for several weeks to months (Dyck et al, 1991). The treatment regimen generally is a total volume of approximately 200 to 250 mL/kg exchanged in each of 4 to 6 treatments over about 10 days and the removed plasma replaced with a mixture of albumin and saline.

In patients who have IgM serum activity against specific components of myelin (particularly anti-MAG), the results of treatment have been inconsistent and generally less favorable. Plasma exchange alone has effected transient improvement in half of cases but sustained improvement in only 10 to 20 percent of our patients. Series of plasma exchanges every 2 to 4 months has sometimes resulted in transient responses. According to some reports, the response to immunosuppression with intravenous cyclophosphamide or fludarabine, mycophenolate, or oral chlorambucil, when coupled with plasma exchanges, has been somewhat better, at times allowing a reduction in the frequency of exchanges but our experience has generally not affirmed this. Rituximab, which has the appeal of having a preferential effect on the B-cell lymphocyte population, after initial enthusiasm based on small series, has given conflicting and generally negative results in several trials but may be reasonable to try in intractable cases. A listing of the applicable trials that have been reported up to 2009 has been given by Brannigan.

Improvement with high-dose infused immune globulin (IVIg) has been transiently effective in half of our cases with typical paraproteinemia and in 20 percent of those with anti-MAG neuropathy but the illness nonetheless progresses in most patients. In almost all instances, immunosuppression and plasma exchanges or IVIg, if used, must be repeated indefinitely at intervals of 1 to several months as determined by the clinical course. An indwelling catheter is then usually required to allow repeated venous access. This group of neuropathies responds poorly or not at all to corticosteroids.

POEMS Syndrome, Osteosclerotic Myeloma, and Multiple Myeloma A neuropathy associated with *multiple myeloma* has already been mentioned; it complicates 13 to 14 percent of cases of multiple myeloma and has a disproportionately high association with the osteosclerotic form of the disease. An abnormal monoclonal globulin (mainly with the *kappa* light chain component in multiple myeloma but *lambda* in the osteosclerotic type) is found in the serum of more than 80 percent of patients with myelomatous neuropathy.

In a special and small group of patients with osteosclerotic myeloma, there is a predominantly demyelinating sensorimotor *p*olyneuropathy and systemic disease termed *POEMS* (i.e., polyneuropathy of moderate severity is associated with organomegaly, *e*ndocrinopathy, elevated *M* protein, and *s*kin changes, mainly hypertrichosis and skin thickening). The same process has been referred to as the Crow-Fukase syndrome in Japan, where the disease is prevalent. In many cases there is lymphadenopathy attributable to the angiofollicular hyperplasia of Castleman disease. Another characteristic feature of the osteosclerotic-related polyneuropathy is a greatly elevated CSF protein.

The presence of the disease can be suspected from the presence of demyelinating features on the nerve conduction studies, an immunoglobulin spike in the blood, sometimes polyclonal or biclonal rather than monoclonal and, as mentioned, possessing a lambda light chain component. The diagnosis requires the demonstration of one or more osteosclerotic lesions by a radiographic survey of the long bones, pelvis, spine, and skull as well as a PET study, which usually shows the osteosclerotic lesions as highly active (a bone scan is insensitive) and a bone marrow examination, which shows a moderate increase in the number of well-differentiated plasma cells. In most of our patients there have been several discrete bone lesions concentrated in the ribs and spine; the skull and long bones may harbor such lesions as well, or there may be a single lesion, which is often situated in the spinal column. Biopsy of a bone lesion is justified. The organomegaly and skin changes are apparently the result of high levels of circulating VEGF that is produced by the tumor and is useful in confirming the diagnosis.

TREATMENT OF POEMS The neuropathy that complicates a solitary plasmacytoma may improve markedly following irradiation of the bone lesion. Multiple lesions, including those in the POEMS syndrome, when treated with chemotherapy (melphalan and prednisone) or focused radiation, may lead to some improvement or stabilization in the neuropathy. Treatment with plasma exchange has yielded uncertain but generally positive short-term results in our patients. Autologous stem cell transplantation or bevacizumab (a monoclonal antibody directed against VEGF) have been tried with mixed results (Kuwabara et al, 2008).

Waldenström Macroglobulinemia *Macroglobulinemia* was the term applied by Waldenström to a systemic condition occurring mainly in older persons and characterized by fatigue, weakness, and a bleeding diathesis. Immunoelectrophoretic examination of the blood disclosed a marked and mostly monoclonal increase in the IgM plasma fraction. About half of patients with Waldenström disease and polyneuropathy will have specific anti-MAG antibodies, similar to the approximately one-third of patients with nonmalignant IgM paraproteins. (An uncertain proportion of patients with a "benign" IgM paraprotein will, over the years, develop Waldenström disease.) A few patients with Waldenström hyperproteinemia have a hyperviscosity state manifest by diffuse slowing of the retinal and cerebral circulations, giving rise to episodic confusion, coma, impairment of vision, and sometimes strokes (*Bing-Neel syndrome*). Most reports attribute this syndrome to infiltration of neural by malignant plasma cells rather than to hyperviscosity.

The polyneuropathy, when present, evolves over months or longer and may be asymmetrical, particularly at the onset, but becomes bilateral, mainly sensory, and distal. The pattern in our patients has been very slowly progressive, and initially limited to the feet and legs with sensory ataxia and loss of knee and ankle jerks. The CSF protein is usually elevated and the globulin fraction increased. In a case recorded by Rowland and colleagues, the polyneuropathy was purely motor and simulated motor neuron disease. Treatment is discussed further on.

Cryoglobulinemia As mentioned in the section on vasculitic neuropathies, *cryoglobulin*, a serum protein that precipitates on cooling, is usually of the IgG or IgM type and most often polyclonal. While cryoglobulinemia may occur without any apparent associated condition (essential cryoglobulinemia), it also accompanies a wide variety of disorders such as multiple myeloma, lymphoma, connective tissue disease, chronic infection, and particularly, hepatitis C. Peripheral neuropathy occurs in a small proportion both of the essential and symptomatic cases. Occasionally the neuropathy evolves over a period of a few days and remits rapidly. More often it takes the form of a distal symmetrical sensorimotor loss, which develops insidiously (76 percent of the cases in the series reported by Gemignani et al) in association with the Raynaud phenomenon and purpuric eruptions of the skin. Initially, the neuropathic symptoms may consist only of pain and paresthesias that may be precipitated by exposure to cold (as often, there is no cold sensitivity). Later, weakness and wasting develop, more in the legs than in the arms, and more or less in the same distribution as the vascular changes. In some cases there may be a mononeuropathy multiplex with severe denervation in the territory of the involved nerves (9 percent of the series reported by Gemignani et al; see also Garcia-Bragado et al). In a few cases, the two neuropathic syndromes have been combined. As remarked earlier, detection of cryoglobulin requires special handling of the blood sample. The specimen should be carried to the laboratory in a bath of warm water to prevent precipitation of the protein.

Any of the paraproteinemic states may be associated with an amyloid polyneuropathy, a subject accorded a separate section later in the chapter.

The pathology of the cryoglobulinemic and macroglobulinemic neuropathies has been incompletely studied and the mechanisms by which these disorders cause neuropathy are uncertain. One presumes that some component of the paraprotein acts as an antineural antibody or that deposition of the protein is in some way toxic to the nerves or to the endoneurial vessels. In our most thoroughly autopsied case, there was widespread distal axonal degeneration of nonspecific type without amyloid deposition or inflammatory cells; yet in other reported cases, amyloid has been found in the nerve and the neuropathy has been attributed directly to it. Immune deposits of IgM had impregnated the inner layers of the perineurium in the case reported by Ongerboer de Visser and colleagues. Dalakas and Engel (1981b) have made similar observations. In yet other instances, the neuropathy of cryoglobulinemia is a result of the intravascular deposition of cryoglobulins, causing a more acute vasculitic mononeuropathy multiplex, as discussed earlier (Chad et al).

Treatment In the macroglobulinemic neuropathies, the use of prednisone, the alkylating agent chlorambucil, cyclophosphamide, and repeated plasma exchange has at times led to improvement both in the systemic and neuropathic symptoms, although recovery has been incomplete. The monoclonal antibody rituximab has been effective in small studies. The optimal treatment of cryoglobulinemic neuropathy has not been settled. We have used plasma exchange and added immunosuppression in the vasculitic variety of this disease.

Acquired Primary (Nonfamilial, AL) Amyloid Neuropathy

A heredofamilial type of amyloidosis (familial amyloidosis [FA]) is well known and is described further on. In addition, there are numerous sporadic instances of a peripheral neuropathy caused by amyloid deposition. As in the familial variety, the heart, kidneys, and gastrointestinal tract may be involved. This acquired type of amyloid disease has also been called *primary systemic amyloidosis* to distinguish it from the variety associated with chronic diseases. The term is misleading in that in most cases the amyloid is derived from a circulating paraprotein, but the proportion of "benign" and malignant plasma cell sources of the protein varies from one report to another. For example, in the large series collected by Kyle and Bayrd, only 26 percent of patients with primary amyloidosis had a malignant plasma cell dyscrasia. This agrees with our own experience, but other series have found rates of myeloma as high as 75 percent. In any case, 90 percent of primary amyloidosis is the result of a monoclonal protein in the blood (rarely polyclonal). Macrophage enzymes cleave the larger immunoglobulin molecules and the light chains aggregate to form amyloid deposits in tissue, or the plasma cells may produce light chains directly ("light chain disease"). Lambda light chain predominates in the idiopathic variety of amyloidosis and kappa light chain is more common in myeloma. In a few cases, the light chain is found only in the urine (as Bence Jones protein).

In primary amyloidosis there is no evidence of preceding or coexisting disease (except the association with paraproteinemia or multiple myeloma). *Secondary amyloidosis (AA)*, an infrequent occurrence nowadays, is the result of chronic infection or other chronic disease outside the nervous system and, as a rule, is not associated with neuropathy (e.g., it is not cited in the large recent series by Lachmann and colleagues [2007]). In contrast, *familial amyloidosis*, a third variety, is almost invariably associated with neuropathy but is associated with a paraprotein in only a small proportion of cases and the amount of immunoglobulin is small (see "Inherited [Familial Amyloidosis] Amyloid Neuropathies" later).

Primary amyloidosis is mainly a disease of older men, the median age at the time of diagnosis being 65 years. In our clinical material, the majority of the patients have had peripheral neuropathy, but this may reflect a referral bias as in other series, less than one-third were so affected (Kyle et al). The neuropathic symptoms and signs are similar to those of hereditary amyloid polyneuropathy discussed further on, but the progress of the disease is considerably more rapid.

The initial syndrome is primarily sensory—numbness, paresthesias, and very often, acral pain—signs that are mainly characteristic of involvement of small-diameter sensory fibers (loss of pain and thermal sensation). It is the painful aspect and the autonomic features discussed later that distinguish this disease from the other paraproteinemic neuropathies and indeed, from most other polyneuropathies. Weakness follows, initially limited to the feet but becoming more extensive as the disease progresses and eventually spreads to the hands and arms. Only later is there loss of mainly large fibers that mediate sensations of touch, pressure, and proprioception. Twenty-five percent of patients have carpal tunnel syndrome from infiltration of the flexor retinaculum. Exceptionally, patterns other than the painful and sensory predominant polyneuropathy have been associated with amyloidosis; preferential involvement of motor nerves, lumbar roots, plexopathy, and amyloidomas involving single nerves (sciatic, facial, trigeminal) have been reported. Unusual cases of mononeuritis multiplex are difficult to explain.

Autonomic involvement can be severe in amyloid neuropathy (familial or primary) and may become evident early in the course of the illness; several of our patients presented with disturbances of gastrointestinal motility such as episodic diarrhea and orthostatic dizziness or erectile dysfunction and bladder disturbances. The pupils may show a slow reaction to light, or there may be a reduction in sweating. An infiltrative *amyloid myopathy* also occurs as a rare complication of the disease; it presents as an enlargement and induration of many muscles, particularly those of the tongue (macroglossia), pharynx, and larynx.

Progression of the illness is relatively rapid, the mean survival being 12 to 24 months. An indolent neuropathy that evolves over years is unlikely to be a result of amyloidosis, although we have seen such a case. Death is a result of the renal, cardiac, or gastrointestinal effects of amyloid deposits, the manifestations of which are already evident in more than half of the patients who present with neuropathy. A nephrotic syndrome is also characteristic.

Analysis of the serum and urine, searching for an abnormal paraprotein, is the most useful screening test for amyloid neuropathy. Next in value is a microscopic examination of a biopsy of the abdominal fat pad, gingiva, or rectal mucosa for deposition of amyloid in tissue or blood vessels. Biopsy of the sural nerve or of the involved viscera has a high diagnostic yield; muscle tissue gives variable results. The liver biopsy is positive in virtually all cases of primary amyloid and the kidney shows amyloid infiltration in 85 percent. In several of our patients with a clinical syndrome typical of amyloid neuropathy but in whom amyloid was absent in the sural nerve, the diagnosis was established only after sequential biopsy of numerous sites (fat pad, kidney, liver). If the sural nerve is severely depopulated of nerve fibers, the amount of congophilic staining and the characteristic amyloid birefringence may be meager and yield a spuriously negative result. It is also critical to ensure the accuracy of congophilic staining by comparison with positive and negative control tissue from the same laboratory. The CSF has a normal or mildly elevated protein concentration, but this does not distinguish the neuropathic process from many others.

Lachmann and colleagues (2002) emphasized that 10 percent of patients who appear by all the usual criteria to have primary amyloidosis will be found to have a genetic type. However, as mentioned, only a small proportion of the latter group has a monoclonal gammopathy and it tends to be of low concentration (it has been estimated to occur in one-quarter of familial cases but we have not encountered it). This difference and the rapid progression of the primary acquired form assist in distinguishing it from the genetic type that is discussed further on.

In addition to the more slowly evolving familial types, the differential diagnosis of acquired amyloid neuropathy includes the myelomatous varieties, toxic and nutritional small-fiber neuropathies, diabetic polyneuropathy, paraneoplastic polyneuropathy, Sjögren disease, and an idiopathic small-fiber sensory neuropathy, all of which cause pain and which we have encountered more frequently than amyloidosis.

TREATMENT OF AMYLOID NEUROPATHY The prognosis of primary amyloidosis and its associated neuropathy are dismal. Attempts at immunomodulation, immunosuppression (which may help the renal disease), or removal of amyloid by plasma exchange have been marginally effective. Another approach has been bone marrow suppression with high doses of melphalan followed by stem cell replacement (previously harvested from the patient). Several such patients have survived for years with marked improvement in the neuropathy. Recently, several small molecules designed to prevent the aggregation of amyloid fibrils have shown preliminary benefit as evidenced by biologic markers and in some clinical features. (In the familial type due to a transthyretin mutation discussed further on, liver transplantation has stabilized the process in the majority of patients, particularly those with the Val30Met mutation.)

Pain is a serious problem in the amyloid neuropathies that may be treated with transcutaneous fentanyl patches or with oral narcotic medications. Orthostatic hypotension responds to the use of leg stockings, midodrine, and mineralocorticoids, as well as sleeping with the bed elevated at the head so that the patient's entire body is angled down toward the feet.

Chronic Inflammatory Demyelinating Polyradiculoneuropathy

This form of polyneuropathy was separated from acute inflammatory polyradiculopathy, or GBS, by Austin in

1958 on the basis of a prolonged and relapsing course, enlargement of nerves, and responsiveness to corticosteroids. Excluding the duration of evolution, the acute and chronic forms are similar in many ways. Both are widespread polyradiculoneuropathies, usually with cytoalbuminologic dissociation of the CSF (raised protein concentration with few or no cells); both exhibit nerve conduction abnormalities characteristic of a demyelinating neuropathy (reduced conduction velocity and partial conduction block in motor nerves), and pathologically, both show similar multifocal perivenous inflammatory infiltrates. But there are also important differences, the most evident of which are the modes of evolution, responses to treatment, and prognosis. As a rule, chronic inflammatory demyelinating polyradiculoneuropathy (CIDP) begins insidiously and evolves slowly, either in a steadily progressive or stepwise manner, attaining its maximum severity after several months. From the beginning it may be asymmetrical or involve the arms predominantly. However, in a small proportion of patients (16 percent in the series of McCombe et al [1987b] and a smaller proportion in our own series) the disease at first emerges from a mild or moderate case of GBS, in which case the illness becomes relapsing or simply worsens slowly and progressively.

An antecedent infection is usually not identified in patients with CIDP as it is in GBS. Furthermore, CIDP may be distinct immunologically from GBS, insofar as certain HLA antigens occur with greater frequency in patients with CIDP than they do in the normal population, whereas there are no clear HLA propensities in patients with GBS. Finally, in contrast to acute GBS, many cases of CIDP respond favorably to the administration of prednisone. An ambiguity is introduced here because, as mentioned in the section on GBS, Hughes (1992) has described a group of patients with polyneuritis in whom weakness progressed steadily for 4 to 12 weeks and who responded to corticosteroids (subacute GBS), in such cases, blurring the distinction between GBS and CIDP.

Chronic symmetric sensorimotor loss and areflexia coupled with nerve conduction findings of demyelination essentially defines the illness. Elevated spinal fluid protein concentration is so frequent that it might be added as a diagnostic criterion. The typical findings in nerve conduction studies are of multifocal conduction block as described in Chap. 45; prolonged distal latencies ("distal block"); nerve conduction slowing to less than 80 percent of normal values in several nerves; loss of late responses; and dispersion of the compound muscle action potentials—all reflecting demyelination in motor nerves. One or several of these changes have been present in 75 percent of our patients (Gorson et al, 1997). In the early stages of the disease, demyelinating features must be carefully sought by testing multiple nerves at several sites along their courses. After several months there is often some degree of axonal change (30 percent of our series), but the fundamental process continues to be one of multiple foci of demyelination. A fairly dependable finding is the absence of denervation changes early in the illness despite weakness and reduced amplitude of the motor action potential (indicative of a demyelinating block to conduction at a proximal site).

Several large series of CIDP cases are available for review. Dyck and colleagues (1975) studied 53 patients in whom the neuropathy progressed for more than 6 months. The clinical course was monophasic and slowly progressive in about one-third, stepwise and progressive in another third, and relapsing in the remaining third. The periods of worsening or improvement were measured in weeks or months. Weakness of the limbs, particularly of the proximal leg muscles, or numbness, paresthesias, and dysesthesias of the hands and feet were the initial symptoms. In 45 of the 53 patients, the signs were those of a mixed sensorimotor polyneuropathy with weakness of the shoulder, upper arm, and thigh muscles in addition to motor and sensory loss in the distal parts of the limbs. In 5 patients the neuropathy was purely motor, and in 3, purely sensory. Cranial nerve abnormalities were distinctly unusual. Enlarged, firm nerves were found in 6 patients. Not emphasized in their series is the common occurrence of a cerebellar-like tremor in cases of long standing.

In the series reported by McCombe et al (1987b) comprising 92 patients, two major subgroups were recognized: *relapsing* (corresponding to the relapsing and stepwise progressive cases of Dyck et al [1975]) and *nonrelapsing* ones. In our own series of now over 100 patients, we have been impressed with several variant patterns of clinical presentation. In approximately 10 percent, numbness and weakness of the hands preceded involvement of the feet, which is unusual in other polyneuropathies, and a sensory ataxic form, a purely motor form, and mononeuropathies superimposed on a mild generalized polyneuropathy each accounted for approximately 5 percent.

As mentioned earlier, a small proportion of cases began as acute GBS but continue to progress or relapse in the following months (Gorson et al, 1997). Other comprehensive accounts of the disease have been given by Barohn, Cornblath, Dyck (1975), and Hughes and their associates. All of these studies have included cases with clinical progression for longer than 8 or 12 weeks; thus CIDP has come to be defined in part by a progressive polyneuropathy of this duration.

As might be imagined from the experience with GBS, there are variant syndromes that align with CIDP but have special clinical characteristics. The best characterized of these is *multifocal conduction block* (called multifocal acquired demyelinating sensory and motor neuropathy; *MADSAM*), but these are also described a polyradicular process that presents as an ataxic illness with large fiber attributable sensory loss and spared sensory nerve action potentials (see Sinnreich et al), and a slowly progressive distal neuropathy (*distal acquired demyelinating symmetrical neuropathy; DADS*). Regarding the last of these, there are distal sensory and sometimes motor, disturbances and greatly prolonged distal latencies in most patients, and two-thirds have an associated IgM monoclonal gammopathy with kappa light chain component; the illness responds poorly to treatment, aligning it clinically in some respects with the anti-MAG neuropathies but in most clinical and electrophysiologic features appearing to be a variant of CIDP (see Katz et al).

The status of a predominantly *axonal* polyneuropathy that clinically simulates CIDP and responds to some extent to the same immunomodulating treatments has been described by Uncini and colleagues and by Gorson and Ropper. The present authors have the impression that it is an immune-mediated neuropathy comparable to CIDP but with preferential destruction of axons rather than of myelin. Its frequency as a cause of acquired polyneuropathy is unknown, but we see several new cases every year.

Also recognized is the frequency (up to 25 percent of the patients in some series, less often in our experience) with which there was a parallel systemic condition such as paraproteinemia, lymphoma, an undifferentiated reactive adenopathy or lupus, in association with an inflammatory demyelinating polyneuropathy (even aside from the rare DADS process mentioned above). These associations create problems in nosology that can be reconciled by labeling a given instance as, for example, "CIDP with paraproteinemia" or "CIDP with lupus," thus separating such cases from the idiopathic variety. These symptomatic inflammatory polyneuropathies respond to corticosteroids, albeit unpredictably, and to treatment of the underlying disease.

Laboratory Features The CSF protein is elevated in more than 80 percent of patients with CIDP, typically in the range of 75 to 250 mg/dL. In rare instances there is papilledema and a pseudotumor cerebri syndrome (see Chap. 30) in relation to extremely high levels of CSF protein (usually >1,000 mg/dL). Elevation of the CSF gamma globulin fraction and a mild lymphocytic pleocytosis are found in 10 percent of patients (often in those who are HIV-seropositive), a considerably higher percentage than in our series.

In sural nerve biopsy material, half are found to have interstitial and perivascular infiltrates of inflammatory cells, although one expects that most nerves would show these changes if a sufficient number could be sampled. Some specimens show only demyelination, or in cases of long standing, severe depletion of all nerve fibers. As in GBS, the demyelination appears to be affected by T cells and macrophages within the endoneurium and perineurium. The loss of myelinated fibers is variable and many of the remaining fibers are seen to be undergoing wallerian degeneration or show changes of segmental demyelination or demyelination-remyelination. Onion-bulb formations are conspicuous in recurrent and relapsing cases. The few adequate autopsy studies have shown only minimal or patchy inflammation and a considerable degree of axonal damage, probably reflecting the long duration of illness before examination. The presence of endoneurial and subperineurial edema has been emphasized by Prineas and McLeod.

Treatment Several trials have shown a short-term benefit from the intravenous infusion of high doses of gamma globulin (IVIg, total 2 g/kg in divided infusions over 2 to 5 days). More than half of our patients have responded to this treatment, albeit for only several weeks or months, after which the infusions must be repeated to maintain clinical improvement. A desire to spare patients the side effects of indefinite prednisone administration (see later) makes this mode of therapy a reasonable alternative, in some cases for almost 10 years without ill effects. Patients who require treatment at such short intervals as to be impractical have benefited from the addition of small doses of prednisone or of an immunosuppressive drug as described below. The main drawbacks of IVIg are its expense and the several hours required for its infusion. Rare instances of nephrotic syndrome, aseptic meningitis, serum sickness, thrombolic venous, or arterial occlusion, including stroke and hypotension, have been reported, particularly if the infusion is too rapid.

Half of patients with CIDP also respond well to plasma exchanges. In a prospective double-blinded trial, Dyck and colleagues (1986a) found that plasma exchange administered twice weekly for 3 weeks had a beneficial effect on both neurologic disability and nerve conduction. The response to plasma exchange in our patients has been comparable to that obtained with IVIg and with steroids, but we have discerned that some patients respond to one type of treatment and not another. The effects of plasma exchanges in most patients subside in 10 to 21 days, or even less; in some, the response lasts longer as found by Dyck and colleagues (1986a) and in the series reported by Hahn and colleagues (1996a). For these reasons we prefer to try plasma exchange or immune globulin before committing a patient to long-term treatment with prednisone. The relative ease of administering IVIg favors its use first, followed by a series of plasma exchanges if there is no improvement. When there is a clear response, 3 or 4 brief series of plasma exchanges or repeated infusions of immune globulin may suffice to bring the patient to an improved level of function. These treatments can be supplemented by small doses of prednisone when frequent infusions or exchanges become impractical. It has been our experience that in about one-third of cases, IVIg and plasma exchange cease to have benefit after repeated use for 1 or more years.

Corticosteroids were formerly the mainstay of therapy, but many patients become dependent on the medication and correspondingly suffer side effects. Our approach has been to use corticosteroids as an adjunct to one of the previously mentioned treatments, but other centers use them first. The usual regimen begins with 60 to 80 mg of prednisone daily that is tapered over months to the lowest effective dose, typically 25 to 40 mg. Without substantiation by a controlled trial, we have found that corticosteroids can be withdrawn without relapse in some patients by slow tapering over many months or a year. Attempts to withdraw the steroids more quickly have led to further cycles of relapse.

A number of patients will have no response to corticosteroids within the first 1 or 2 months but will improve if treatment is continued. Barohn and colleagues (1989) have found that the earliest improvement occurs only after 2 months of treatment and is maximal at approximately 6 months. In addition to all the well-known side effects, the drug may produce tremor or exaggerate the tremor caused by the neuropathy. Long remissions lasting several years have been reported with the use of pulses of orally administered high-dose or daily corticosteroids, for example, by Eftimov and colleagues, who used dexamethasone 40 mg per day for 4 days, repeated for 6 cycles, or daily prednisolone, 60 mg for 6 weeks. Should a sustained trial of prednisone therapy prove unsuccessful, a course of azathioprine (for at least 3 months), 3 mg/kg in a single daily dose, has been recommended (Dalakas and Engel, 1981a), but a controlled trial has failed to show benefit from this combination and we have had little success with it.

When the preceding measures prove unsatisfactory, cyclophosphamide, mycophenolate, rituximab, or another similar immunosuppressive medication can be added, but we have been unable to draw any firm conclusions as to the effectiveness of these combined regimens.

Some patients who have failed to benefit from the aforementioned treatments have seemingly improved in response to the administration of alpha-interferon; however, in larger trials, interferon allowed an increase in the interval between infusions of IVIg but was not an effective primary therapy. High-dose cyclophosphamide has proven helpful in several cases under our care, although it has often failed (see Brannagan et al and the review by Brannagan that lists the applicable clinical trials). The usual regimen is 50 mg/kg IV daily for 4 days followed by granulocyte-stimulating factor beginning on the tenth day until the absolute neutrophil count recovers. Individual reports of successful treatment by autologous stem cell transplantation after high-dose chemotherapy have appeared but 1 patient relapsed after 5 years (Vermuelen and van Oers). This may become an option in severe and treatment-resistant cases. We have no explanation for the remarkable improvement and continued good health of a few of our patients after a severe toxic bacterial infection (Ropper, 1996).

One of the most difficult problems in this field is the lack of useful clinical measurements to guide treatment with IVIg and plasma exchange and even the proper adjustment of the dose of corticosteroid. Often, one may be influenced by the patient's fear of losing any ground and even slight changes in sensory or motor symptoms.

It has been stated that patients with discrete relapses have a better prognosis than those with a progressive course. In McCombe's series (1987b), 73 percent were said to have eventually recovered, but the long-term outcome has generally been poor. In fewer than 10 percent of patients has the disease finally remitted; additionally, unexplained remission occurs occasionally. The 5-year followup of 38 patients by Kuwabara and colleagues gives a figure of 49 percent with full or partial remission, far higher than in our series.

Multifocal Motor Neuropathy and Multifocal Conduction Block

Several polyneuropathies that share many of the features of CIDP have been delineated on the basis of unique clinical, immune, or electrophysiologic attributes. These include particularly *multifocal motor neuropathy (MMN)* and *multifocal conduction block* (also called *MADSAM* as mentioned earlier). The latter has as its main feature a block of mixed nerve conduction at focal sites in a limited number of nerves as described earlier. In multifocal motor neuropathy, only blocks in motor nerve conduction are evident.

The distinction between these two entities has been difficult. There are similarities in clinical features and response to treatment (see Delmont et al), but there is utility in separating them. Multifocal motor neuropathy, but not multifocal conduction block, is associated in half of cases with a particular IgM antibody, anti-G_{M1}, directed against a ganglioside component of peripheral myelin (Pestronk et al). For this reason, some view this illness as belonging to the class of paraproteinemic neuropathies (see earlier and Simmons et al) and it is certainly distinctive enough clinically to be categorized separately. Its importance as a clinical entity lies in the similarity of the clinical picture to a purely lower motor neuron type of amyotrophic lateral sclerosis (ALS) and, unlike ALS, its potential responsiveness to treatment. The pathophysiologic role of anti-G_{M1} antibodies is further displayed by a case of transplacental transmission of a motor neuropathy to a neonate (Attarian et al).

Multifocal motor neuropathy and motor conduction block predominate in men. They usually begin with an acute or subacute motor mononeuropathy, manifest, for example, as weakness of the wrist or foot-drop, and are often joined insidiously by another focal motor palsy. The process is painless, unlike vasculitic mononeuritis multiplex, involves the nerve incompletely, and, in its usual form, is unaccompanied by any sensory symptoms such as paresthesias or numbness. Despite the initially demyelinating character of the disorder, there is almost always atrophy of the weakened muscle within months and there may be a few fasciculations, thus simulating ALS. Nevertheless, the weakness tends to be disproportionate to atrophy. Usually, the tendon reflex is lost or muted in an affected region, but for unexplained reasons, some patients have one or more brisk reflexes. Our experience has been that this latter reflex change does not reach the point of appearing "pathologic" and that clonus and Babinski signs are categorically not part of the illness, as they are in ALS.

When there is an association of the motor features with sensory symptoms or sensory loss and there is slowing of sensory conduction in regions of motor conduction block (multifocal conduction block), the acronym MADSAM (multifocal acquired demyelinating sensory and motor neuropathy) has been used as noted earlier, but the disorder, while similar to multifocal conduction block, more resembles CIDP. This conforms to what has been called Lewis-Sumner syndrome based on the description by these authors and their colleagues of subacute, painless asymmetric, distal multiple mononeuropathies. The ulnar and median nerves were involved in their patients and there was motor conduction block and sensory slowing in affected nerves. Curiously, 2 of their 5 original patients had optic neuritis, a feature not reported subsequently. The disease is not directly connected to antibodies against G_{M1}, but a few patients with the sensorimotor disorder will display them.

Treatment For multifocal motor conduction block and motor neuropathy, with or without anti-GM1 antibodies, IVIg infusions have been effective, albeit temporarily, in more than half of patients. Some authoritative clinicians favor the early addition of rituximab in treatment-resistant cases or when the frequency of infusions is unsustainable and if that fails, cyclophosphamide. Other immune-modulating drugs have been tried in small series with various results. There is no response to corticosteroids. The MADSAM illness responds similarly to corticosteroids, IVIg, or plasma exchange, similar to the effects of these approaches in CIDP.

Uremic Polyneuropathy

Polyneuropathy is among the most common complications of chronic renal failure. Robson has estimated that neuropathy complicates end-stage renal failure in two-thirds of patients who are about to begin dialysis therapy. Bolton's figures are much the same; 70 percent of his patients being dialyzed regularly had polyneuropathy and in 30 percent of all his patients, it was moderate or severe in degree. As described originally by Asbury and associates (1963), the neuropathy takes the form of a painless, progressive, symmetrical sensorimotor paralysis of the legs and then of the arms. In some patients, the syndrome begins with burning dysesthesias of the feet or with sensations of creeping, crawling, and itching of the legs and thighs, which tend to be worse at night and are relieved by movement (comparable to "restless legs" syndrome described in Chap. 19). Renal failure that is accompanied by diabetes gives rise to a particularly severe form of polyneuropathy.

The combination of muscle weakness and atrophy, areflexia, sensory loss, and the graduated, distally predominant distribution of the neurologic deficit in the limbs leaves little doubt about the neuropathic nature of the disorder. Usually the neuropathy evolves slowly over many months. Infrequent instances of a more acute sensorimotor polyneuropathy that have been reported occur mainly in diabetic patients receiving peritoneal dialysis as discussed earlier (Ropper, 1993; Asbury et al, 1963). A rare uremic polymyositis with hypophosphatemia has also been described (Layzer). The neuropathy has been observed with all types of chronic kidney diseases. More important to the development of chronic neuropathy than the nature of the renal lesion are the duration and severity of the renal failure and symptomatic uremia.

With long-term hemodialysis, the neuropathic symptoms and signs stabilize but improve in relatively few patients. In fact, rapid hemodialysis may worsen the polyneuropathy (or perhaps its symptoms) temporarily. Peritoneal dialysis appears to be more successful than hemodialysis in improving the neuropathy, but this observation has not been firmly established. Complete recovery, occurring over a period of 6 to 12 months, usually follows successful renal transplantation for reasons given later.

The pathologic findings are those of a nonspecific and noninflammatory axonal degeneration. In rapidly progressive cases, there is a tendency for the large fibers to be more affected; this is evident particularly on electrophysiologic testing that shows slowing of nerve conduction velocities, but there is no conduction block as occurs in other acquired demyelinating polyneuropathies. In all types of uremic polyneuropathies, pathologic changes are most intense in the distal segments of the nerves with the expected chromatolysis of their cell bodies.

The cause of uremic polyneuropathy is unknown. What has been called the "middle molecule" theory is plausible. The end stage of renal failure is associated with the accumulation of toxic substances in the range of 300 to 2,000 kDa molecular weight. Furthermore, the concentration of these substances, which include methyl guanidine and myoinositol, has been shown to correlate with the degree of neurotoxicity (Funck-Brentano et al). These toxins (and the clinical signs of neuropathy) are not greatly reduced by hemodialysis. In contrast, the transplanted kidney effectively eliminates substances of wide-ranging molecular weights, which would account for the almost invariable improvement of neuropathy after transplantation. As is the case with uremic encephalopathy, urea alone given to experimental animals and in controlled studies of humans, does not seem capable of inducing a metabolic neuropathy.

Alcoholic–Nutritional Polyneuropathy

As described at length in Chap. 41, in virtually all patients with alcoholic–nutritional polyneuropathy who for some reason remain untreated with vitamin and protein restoration, the weakness and atrophy of the legs, and to a lesser extent the arms, may reach an extreme degree. Thus this disease, although subacute in its evolution as described earlier in the chapter, becomes a frequent cause of chronic polyneuropathy. There are usually prominent sensory features and considerable acral pain and allodynia. Certain cases of diabetic neuropathy behave similarly.

Leprous Polyneuritis

This is the best example of an infectious neuritis, caused by the direct invasion of nerves by the acid-fast *Mycobacterium leprae*. The disease is still frequent in India and Central Africa and there are many lesser endemic foci, including parts of South America and Florida, Texas, and Louisiana, which border the Gulf of Mexico. Limited outbreaks have been reported during treatment for AIDS, with armadillos as the probable intermediate host.

The initial lesion in leprosy is an innocuous-appearing skin macule or papule, which is often hypopigmented and lacking in sensation; it is caused by the invasion of cutaneous nerves by *M. leprae*. In patients with a degree of immunologic resistance to infection, the disease progresses no further than this stage, which is spoken of as *indeterminate leprosy*, or it may evolve in several ways, depending mainly upon the resistance of the host. The bacilli may be locally invasive, producing a circumscribed epithelioid granuloma that involves cutaneous and subcutaneous nerves and results in a characteristic hypopigmented patch of superficial numbness and sensory loss (*tuberculoid leprosy*). The underlying subcutaneous sensory nerves may be palpably enlarged. If a large nerve in the vicinity of the granuloma is invaded (the ulnar, median, peroneal, posterior auricular, and facial nerves are most frequently affected), a sensorimotor deficit in the distribution of that nerve is added to the patch of cutaneous anesthesia.

In contrast to the limited tuberculoid variety of leprosy, lack of resistance to the organism permits the proliferation and hematogenous spread of bacilli and the diffuse infiltration of skin, ciliary bodies, testes, lymph nodes, and nerves (*lepromatous leprosy*). Widespread invasion of the cutaneous nerves produces a symmetrical pattern of pain and temperature loss involving the pinnae of the ears (earlobes) and nose, as well as the dorsal surfaces of hands, elbows, forearms, and feet and anterolateral aspects of the legs—a distribution that is determined by the relative coolness of these parts of the skin. This *temperature-dependent pattern* is the most characteristic feature of the disease, as pointed out by our colleague T. Sabin. The sensory maps he has drawn (Fig. 46-4) are typical of established cases. The process evolves over years. Eventually, the anesthesia spreads to involve most of the cutaneous surface. Extensive sensory loss is followed by impaired motor function owing to invasion of muscular nerves where they lie closest to the skin (the ulnar nerve is the most vulnerable). There is loss of sweating in areas of sensory loss but otherwise the autonomic nervous system is unaffected. In distinction to other polyneuropathies, tendon reflexes are usually preserved in leprosy despite widespread sensory loss. Probably this is the result of sparing of most of the muscular and larger sensory nerves. Because of widespread anesthesia, injuries may pass unrecognized, with resultant infections, trophic changes, and loss of tissue. Variations in host immunity result in patterns of disease having both tuberculoid and lepromatous characteristics (dimorphous leprosy). Erythema nodosum occurs in a few cases. The diagnosis can be made from a skin scraping or biopsy, but multiple samples are often required.

The findings on nerve conduction studies are varied, but they usually include findings that are consistent with a generalized but heterogeneous sensorimotor polyneuropathy that includes features of demyelination such as slowed nerve conduction velocities, temporal dispersion and occasionally, conduction block.

Treatment All forms of leprosy require long-term treatment with sulfones (dapsone being the most commonly used), rifampin, and clofazimine. The skin lesions of lepromatous leprosy are responsive to thalidomide, which itself may cause a sensory neuropathy (Barnhill and McDougall). Reactivation of disease, or a conversion from the tuberculoid to the lepromatous pattern, may occur during times of reduced immunity.

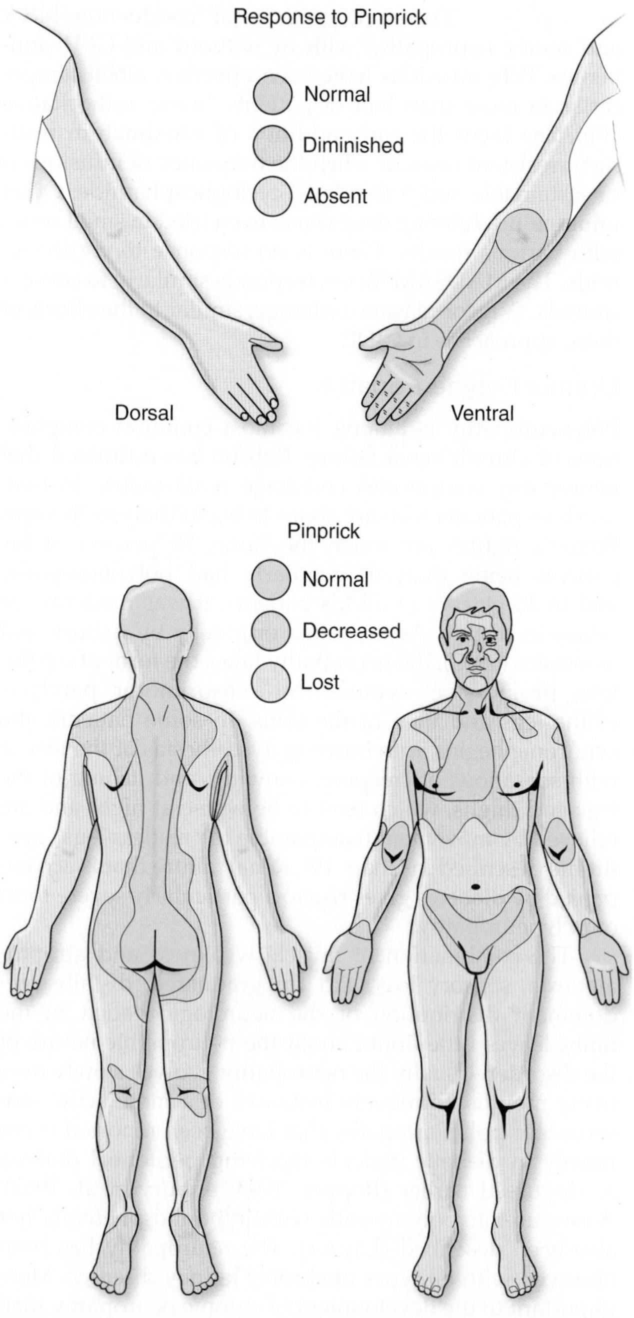

Figure 46-4. Patterns of sensory loss in leprosy. The localization of these areas to cooler portions of the body is unique to this disorder. There is almost universal analgesia but sparing of warmer regions such as the midline of the back, popliteal and antecubital spaces, lower abdomen and groin, and the head and neck. (From Sabin TD: Preservation of sensation in a cutaneous vascular malformation in lepromatous leprosy. *N Engl J Med* 282:1084, 1970, with permission.)

Polyneuropathy With Hypothyroidism

The status of this disorder is uncertain and the authors have not encountered a definite case. Although characteristic disturbances of skeletal muscle are known to complicate hypothyroidism, the demonstration of a definite polyneuropathy has been infrequent. However, a number of elderly myxedematous patients complain of weakness and numbness of the feet, legs, and, to a lesser extent, hands, for which no other explanation can be found. Loss of reflexes, diminution in vibratory, joint-position, and touch-pressure sensations, and weakness in the distal parts of the limbs are the usual findings. The neuropathic manifestations are seldom severe. Nerve conduction velocities are slowed and the protein content of the CSF is usually increased to more than 100 mg/dL. Possibly the latter finding is a reflection of the increased protein content of the serum in the hypothyroid state. The subjective improvement and complete or near-complete reversibility of neuropathic signs following treatment with thyroid hormones provides evidence of a hypothyroid etiology. In biopsies of nerve, an edematous protein infiltration of the endoneurium and perineurium, a kind of metachromatic mucoid material, has been seen. Dyck and Lambert (who should be credited for drawing attention to this neuropathy) noted segmental demyelination in teased fiber preparations. In electron-microscopic sections, a slight increase in glycogen, acid mucopolysaccharides, and aggregates of glycogen and cytoplasmic laminar bodies in Schwann cells have been observed by others.

Polyneuropathy of sensorimotor type has also been observed in association with a syndrome of chronic lymphocytic thyroiditis and alopecia (Hart et al).

Idiopathic Small-Fiber Sensory Polyneuropathy (Numb, Burning Feet Syndrome)

This, of course, does not have the status of a single entity, but all neurologists encounter numerous cases of a relatively nonprogressive idiopathic sensory polyneuropathy, mainly in older patients. Paresthesias of feet and lower legs, sensory loss, and absent ankle reflexes are the usual findings. The hands may be mildly affected, but leg weakness and imbalance are absent or minor. A painful variety is also known (see later).

The most common situation in our experience has been one that affects elderly women with slowly progressive (over years) *burning and numbness of the feet*, ascending to the ankles or midcalves. There are few findings on examination. Often, there is only mild loss of pinprick and thermal sensation; ankle reflexes may or may not be reduced. There is little progression over the years. Most of these cases are idiopathic, but there is a broad differential diagnosis, including the diseases mentioned earlier, as outlined by Mendell and Sahenk (Table 46-5 is adapted from their discussion).

Electrophysiologic tests are likewise normal or virtually so; a few show diminished sural nerve potentials and minor changes of motor amplitudes. When the causes listed in the table have been excluded, a substantial group of patients is left and are in need of symptomatic relief. Some have been helped by gabapentin or by antidepressants and analgesic cream applied nightly to the soles and toes. A few of the more severe cases have apparently responded to gamma globulin infusions, but these observations require corroboration (Gorson and Ropper, 1995). In a number of cases of burning feet, the intradermal sensory nerves in skin biopsy specimens are depleted, but the meaning of this finding is not certain (Periquet et al) and the clinical diagnosis of a small-fiber neuropathy in affected older patients can be inferred without this procedure.

Identifiable causes for painful sensory neuropathy in the elderly include mainly diabetes, alcoholic–nutritional deficiency states, connective tissue disease, amyloidosis, and vasculitis. Presumably, in the idiopathic cases, there is a similar small-fiber neuropathy, but the common clinical situation is that an etiology cannot be found. An alternative cause in these neuropathies that are characterized mainly by painful burning is that there is an abnormality of the sodium channel that renders the sensory neurons or fibers hyperexcitable. In the experience of the group from Maastricht, 8 of 28 patients in whom no etiologic diagnosis for small-fiber neuropathy could be found, there were mutations in the gene (*SCN9A*) encoding voltage-gated sodium channel $Na_v1.7$. The mutation caused a gain of function in this gene and allowed dorsal root ganglion neurons to become hyperexcitable (Faber at al). Yet another rare cause of this syndrome has been the finding of antibodies to peripherin, which is a dominantly inherited trait (Stogbauer et al).

Table 46-5

CAUSES OF PAINFUL SENSORY NEUROPATHY

Common
Nutritional
Idiopathic in the elderly
Diabetes
Vasculitis
Residue of Guillain-Barré syndrome
Renal failure
Connective tissue disease, especially Sjögren disease
Human immune deficiency virus
Less common
Amyloidosis, familial and primary
Voltage gated sodium channel mutation
Paraneoplastic
Sarcoidosis
Toxic neuropathy, esp. arsenic poisoning
Fabry disease
Perineuritis

Source: Adapted from Mendell and Sahenk.

GENETIC FORMS OF CHRONIC POLYNEUROPATHY

A polyneuropathy that advances slowly over 10 years or more is almost invariably genetic in origin. The neuropathic disease may be remarkably restricted, as in familial analgesia with foot ulcers, or extensive, as in familial peroneal muscular atrophy. The time of onset of these very chronic neuropathies is usually in early life but often cannot be dated with certainty by the patient or family. In infants, the condition may be mistaken for muscular dystrophy or infantile muscular atrophy until sensory testing becomes possible. In the developing child, whose musculature naturally increases in power and volume with age, it may be difficult to decide whether the disease is progressive but typically, there is trouble running or walking making it difficult to keep up with other children, repeated ankle injuries, toe catching, labeled as "clumsiness," or falls. Strongly indicative of one of these conditions at any age are pes cavus, hammertoes, and, in extreme forms, talipes equinus. One of these deformities is commonly detected in most cases of inherited polyneuropathy. In later life, some of the inherited neuropathies are manifest as trophic changes of skin and bone in distal parts of the limbs indicate involvement of small (pain) fibers and the presence of deformed and degenerated joints (Charcot joint). The mutilating effects are the result of repeated injury to analgesic parts and to a lack of autonomic vascular reflexes. Atrophy of muscle and trophic changes in the skin are generally more marked than in the acquired forms of polyneuropathy.

The CSF protein content may be mildly or moderately elevated over a period of years. Charcot-Marie-Tooth (CMT) disease (type 1) shows slowed nerve conduction as a consequence of a disorder of myelin. A distinctive feature of hereditary neuropathy is the uniformity of the electrophysiologic changes, e.g., a similar degree of slowing of nerve conduction velocity in all the nerves, a feature that distinguishes this group from most acquired neuropathies. The distinction between the demyelinating and axonal types of inherited neuropathies is based on the motor nerve (typically ulnar or median nerve) conduction velocities in the arms, with slowing to velocities below 38 m/s defining the demyelinating category.

To the reader not immersed in neuromuscular diseases, the classification, nomenclature, and number of genes that give rise to this group of diseases is dizzying. One approaches the affected patient, however, in a more circumscribed way by noting that the dominantly inherited demyelinating types are designated CMT1 and the dominant axonal types, as CMT2. The group of myelinopathies with onset in infancy (also called Dejerine-Sottas disease or congenital hypomyelinating neuropathy), are subsumed under CMT3, whereas most recessively inherited neuropathies (both axonal and demyelinating) are termed CMT4. There are, in addition, forms with intermediate degrees of conduction slowing that are not easily classified. An older nomenclature uses the term hereditary motor-sensory neuropathies, or HMSNs, for the main CMT types. The hereditary sensory neuropathies (HSNs) and the hereditary sensory autonomic neuropathies (HSANs) are considered separate entities. This category includes a variety of metabolic neuropathies and types that do not fit into the CMT classification.

Recent genetic findings have in some ways simplified the matter of classification and have permitted the creation of a nosology that more or less parallels the clinical one. The systems in Tables 46-2 and 46-6 represent an attempt to conciliate the clinical and genetic data.

Of this large and varied group, only the sensorimotor Charcot-Marie-Tooth type is the one likely to be seen with any regularity by neurologists and general physicians. This group has become quite large as more individual mutations are discovered, but a small number accounts for the majority of cases. The commonly encountered varieties are indicated in italics in Table 46-6. The major forms of hereditary neuropathy are designated as subcategories of CMT disease, grouped by patterns of inheritance and described in more detail further on.

Inherited Polyneuropathies of Mixed Sensorimotor-Autonomic Types

Charcot-Marie-Tooth Disease Types 1 (Demyelinating) and 2 (Axonal) and Related Neuropathies (See Table 46-6)

Clinical Features These are the most common forms of inherited peripheral neuropathy and, indeed, among the most common of all inherited neurologic diseases. The early symptoms of childhood clumsiness and athletic imprecision are listed previously, to which are added foot deformities of high arches and hammer toes. There may have been ankle fractures, foot-drop, medical plantar foot calluses and a need for podiatric treatment at an early age, painless or foot ulcers. In adolescence, an "inverted champagne bottle" appearance of the forelegs may become apparent. The typical case of CMT has its onset during late childhood or adolescence, although neurologists are increasingly aware that some cases, particularly type 2, may not attract attention until middle life. CMT1 cases usually make their appearance during the first decade while the peak age of onset of CMT2 is in the second decade or even later. Both motor and sensory signs are said to be more severe in the first type (Harding and Thomas, 1980). Adult patients have difficulty dating the onset of symptoms, so much so that with milder forms, they may not even be aware of having a neuropathic illness. In some cases, the widespread nerve conduction changes only come to light when this test is performed for the diagnosis of an unrelated problem or when a parent becomes aware of their own neuropathy after their child proves to have the disease. Some types that present in adulthood may even have a subacute or seemingly acute presentation, particularly the myelin protein zero (MPZ) and the PMP22 deletion (hereditary liability to pressure palsies) types.

Because the clinical description was provided in 1886 almost simultaneously by Tooth in England and by Charcot and Marie in France, all of their names have been attached to it, even though similar cases had been recorded earlier by Eulenberg (1856), Friedreich (1873), Ormerod (1884), and Osler (1880). The two important advances in our understanding of this disease since the original descriptions have been the separation of the main subtypes on the basis of their electrophysiologic (EMG) features and the discovery of genetic mutations that cause most of these diseases.

The frequency of the disease cannot be stated with precision because of its clinical heterogeneity, but the usually quoted prevalence is 1 in 2,500 of the population, the most frequent subtype occurring in 1 in 4,000. This class of neuropathies is characterized clinically, as discussed previously, by the pattern of heredity, the speed of motor nerve conduction, and special clinical characteristics including the age of onset of symptoms such as difficulty walking and certain appended neuropathic syndromic findings such as hearing loss. From a genetic perspective, the classification is based on the gene that is affected and the nature of the mutation; deletions and duplications are the most common, but many single nucleotide polymorphisms have also been identified.

Table 46-6

CLASSIFICATION OF THE INHERITED PERIPHERAL NEUROPATHIES[a]

	PATHOLOGY	ONSET	GENE	CLINICAL AND THERAPEUTIC FEATURES
I. Charcot-Marie-Tooth (CMT) and Related Disorders				
1. CMT1 (demyelinating, dominantly inherited)				
*CMT1A**	demyelinating	c	PMP22 duplication	Early areflexia, distal weakness, sensory loss
*CMT1B**	demyelinating	c, a	Myelin protein P0 (MPZ)	Early areflexia, distal weakness, sensory loss
CMT1C	demyelinating	a	Lipopolysaccharide-induced TNF-α (LITAF)	
CMT1D, CMT4E	demyelinating	c, a	Transcription factor EGR2	May be severe and congenital
CMT1F, CMT2E	demyelinating, axonal	c, a	Neurofilament light subunit (NEFL) or PMP22 point mutation	
Congenital hypomyelination	demyelinating	c	Rho guanine exchange factor	Mild or asymptomatic
2. CMT2 (axonal, dominantly inherited)				
*CMT2A**	axonal	c, a	Kinesin KIF1Bβ motor protein	
CMT2A2 (alt)	axonal	c, a	Mitofusin (MFN2)	
CMT2B	axonal	a	GTP-binding protein RAB7	
CMT2C	axonal	c, a	TRPV4	Vocal cord, diaphragm paralysis
CMT2D	axonal	a	Glycyl t-RNA synthetase (GARS)	
CMT2F	axonal	c, a	Heat shock protein (BSPB1)	Slow, motor predominant
3. AR-CMT2—(recessively inherited axonopathy)				
AR-CMT2A	axonal		Nuclear membrane lamin (LMNA)	
4. CMT3 (Dejerine-Sottas disease)	demyelinating	inf	PMP22 most common; also P0, EGR2 (see above)	
5. CMT4 (recessively inherited myelin-axonopathy)				
CMT4A	demyelinating	c	Ganglioside-induced differentiation protein (GDAP1)	May be rapidly progressive
CMT4B	demyelinating	c	Myotubularin-related protein (MTMR2)	Focally folded myelin
CMT4B 2	demyelinating	c, a	SET-binding factor (MTMR13))	
CMT4C	demyelinating	c	SHT3TC2	Early scoliosis
CMT4D	demyelinating	c	Schwann cell protein Nm-ycDRG1 (NDRG1)	Neuropathy + hearing loss
CMT4F	demyelinating	c	Nuclear membrane protein (periaxin; PRX)	Early onset, severe
6. *CMT1 X (X-linked demyelinating)**	demyelinating	c, a	GJB1	Similar to CMT1A
7. Recurrent brachial plexopathy (AD)	axonal	c, a	Unknown	Focal, painful brachial plexitis
8. *HNPP**	axonal	c	*PMP22* gene deletion	Focal entrapments, chronic neuropathy
II. Hereditary Sensory and Autonomic Neuropathy (HSAN)				
1. HSAN1 (AD)	axonal	a	Serine palmitoyl transferase	Small-fiber sensory and distal motor deficits
2. HSAN2 (AR)	axonal	inf	Novel neuronal protein	
3. HSAN3 (Riley-Day, AR)	axonal	inf	Kinase-associated protein (IKBKAP)	

(*Continued*)

Table 46-6

CLASSIFICATION OF THE INHERITED PERIPHERAL NEUROPATHIES[a] (*CONTINUED*)

	PATHOLOGY	ONSET	GENE	CLINICAL AND THERAPEUTIC FEATURES
4. HSAN4 (AR)	axonal	inf	TrkA/NGF receptor	Congenital SN with anhidrosis
5. HSAN5 (AR)	axonal	inf	Nerve growth factor-beta	Absent pain
III. Familial Amyloid Polyneuropathies (AD)				
1. Type 1—Portuguese	axonal	a	Transthyretin	Liver transplant may be beneficial
2. Type 2—Indiana/Swiss	axonal	a	Transthyretin	Liver transplant may be beneficial
3. Type 3—Van Allen	axonal	a	Apolipoprotein A1	
4. Type 4—Finnish	axonal	a	Gelsolin	Lax skin and "bloodhound" face; corticospinal, posterior column deficits
IV. Hereditary Disorders of Lipid Metabolism Causing Neuropathy (AR)				
1. Metachromatic leukodystrophy	demyelinating	inf-a	Arylsulfatase A and B	
2. Krabbe disease	demyelinating, axonal	inf-a	β-galactosidase	Early bone marrow transplant may be beneficial
3. Fabry disease	axonal	c	α-galactosidase	Heat-induced pain, macular rash
4. Adrenomyeloneuropathy (XR/XD)	demyelinating, axonal	inf-a	ABCD1 transporter	Early bone marrow transplant may be beneficial
5. Refsum disease	demyelinating	inf-a	Phytanoyl-αCoA-hydroxylase	Dietary restriction may ameliorate the disease
6. Tangier disease	axonal	a	ABC1	Small-fiber neuropathy, facial weakness, very low HDL
7. Bassen-Kornzweig	axonal	c	MTP	Acanthocytosis, cerebellar ataxia
V. Miscellaneous Inherited Neuropathies				
1. Giant axonal neuropathy (AR)	axonal	c	Gigaxonin	
2. Porphyria (AR)	axonal	c, a	Porphobilinogen deaminase	May respond to hematin, glucose
3. "Mitochondrial" neuropathies (NARP)	axonal			Retinitis pigmentosa
4. Severe PNS, CNS demyelination (AD)	demyelinating	inf, c	Myelin transcription factor SOX10	CNS, PNS hypomyelination

[a]*Italicized* types with an asterisk are the most common in practice. CMT1A accounts for approximately 40 percent of cases with an identifiable mutation; CMT1B and HNPP approximately 6 percent each, and CMT1X approximately 6 percent of affected males.
a, adult onset; c, childhood onset; inf, infantile onset.

As a guide to the frequency of various types, Saporta and colleagues in a study of over 1,000 patients from neuromuscular clinics found that two-thirds of patients had a mutation detected by conventional means. When combined with the mode of inheritance, the most common type was the typical demyelinating variety of Charcot-Marie-Tooth disease (CMT1A), and fewer than 10 percent each had X-linked CMT1X, hereditary liability to pressure palsies (HNPP), CMT1B, or the main axonal type, CMT2A; together, these implicated only 4 genes and all other forms, derived from about 30 other mutations, accounted for under 1 percent each. This is informative in guiding genetic testing in clinical circumstances. Still, almost one-third of patients with a clear history of heredofamilial neuropathy had none of the currently detectable mutations.

The chronic degeneration of peripheral nerves and roots results in distal muscle atrophy beginning in the feet and legs and later involving the hands. The extensor hallucis and digitorum longus, the peronei, and the intrinsic muscles of the feet are affected early in life and this muscle imbalance produces the bony changes of pes cavus and *pied en griffe* (high arches and hammertoes). Later, all muscles of the legs and sometimes the lower third of the thigh become weak and atrophic. The thin legs have been likened to those of a stork or, if the lower thigh muscles are affected, to an inverted champagne bottle. Eventually the nerves to the calf muscles degenerate and the ability to plantar flex the feet is lost. After a period of many years, atrophy of the hand and forearm muscles develops in some cases. The hands later become clawed. The wasting seldom extends above the elbows or above the middle third of the thighs. Paresthesias and cramps are present but only to a slight degree and there is always some impairment, usually also mild, of deep and superficial sensation in the feet and hands, shading off proximally. Rarely, the sensory loss is severe and perforating ulcers appear as they do in the pure sensory varieties of inherited neuropathy. The tendon reflexes are absent in the involved limbs. The illness progresses very slowly over decades, giving the impression of stabilization for long periods.

Walking difficulty, which is ultimately the main disability, is caused by a combination of sensory ataxia and weakness. Foot-drop and instability of the ankles are additional handicaps. The feet and legs may ache after use and cramps may be troublesome as mentioned, but otherwise pain is unusual; the feet may become cool, swollen, and blue, secondary to inactivity of the muscles of the feet and legs and their dependent position. There is usually no disturbance of autonomic function. Fixed pupils, optic atrophy, and nystagmus and endocrinopathies, epilepsy, and spina bifida, which have been reported occasionally in association with peroneal muscular atrophy, probably represent coincidental congenital disorders. The only distinguishing clinical feature between types 1 and 2, and this is present in only a minority of cases, is perhaps enlargement of the nerves in type 1, most easily appreciated by palpation of the greater auricular and peroneal nerves. The clinical heterogeneity of CMT disease has been alluded to in the previous discussion and is evident in the numerous mutations that give rise to similar chronic polyneuropathies. Restricted forms are known to affect only the peroneal and pectoral or scapular muscles (scapuloperoneal form).

The *differential diagnosis* involves the distal muscular dystrophies, late forms of familial motor system disease, Friedreich ataxia, Roussy-Lévy syndrome (see later) and other familial polyneuropathies, and, in adult onset cases, CIDP and the paraproteinemic neuropathies, discussed earlier.

Electrophysiologic Features Dyck and Lambert (1975) and Harding and Thomas (1980) are credited with subdividing CMT into the two broad types based on the speed of motor nerve conduction in the ulnar or median nerves, as mentioned, slow (mean conduction velocity less than 38 m/s but often in the range of 20 m/s) in type 1, and normal or near-normal conduction in type 2. Electromyographers appropriately refer to these, respectively, as the demyelinating and axonal types. In both, the compound muscle action potentials and sensory potentials are greatly reduced in amplitude, but in type 2 there are findings of denervation in the EMG. In type 1 there is severe and widespread slowing of nerve conduction, but the electrical conduction block that characterizes acquired demyelinating neuropathies is not found and, in distinction to almost most all acquired diseases of peripheral nerves, the electrophysiologic findings, particularly the pronounced slowing of conduction in CMT1, are uniform throughout the peripheral nervous system.

Genetic Features and Genetic Testing Aspects of the genetic causes of these diseases were addressed in the introductory comments and here it is emphasized that a few basic principles apply. First, only a small number of cases of Charcot-Marie-Tooth disease arise as de novo mutations (Hoogendijk et al). Second, different mutations in the same gene can give rise to more than one type of disease. Third, only four genes (*PMP22, MPZ, GJB1,* and *MFN2*) account for 92 percent of cases of CMT and this allows efficient testing in practice.

The most prevalent form of the disease is CMT1A, which displays an autosomal dominant pattern of inheritance with almost complete penetrance; it is due to duplication of PMP 22 on chromosome 17 p11. Less often, CMT1 is autosomal recessive and even less frequently, X-linked dominant or X-linked recessive (see Table 46-6). Two common mutations in chromosomes 1 or 17 cannot be easily distinguished from one another on clinical grounds, but they have distinctive EMG features. The condition of *hereditary liability to pressure palsies* (HNPP) also displays an aberration on chromosome 17, but in the form of a deletion rather than a duplication of the gene for PMP22. This disease is discussed further on under "Brachial Plexus Neuropathies." The X-linked variant is the result of a mutation of the gene for connexin-32, another component of myelin. In a large proportion of CMT2 cases, the genetic basis cannot be established with current clinically available genetic testing. Undoubtedly, further studies of genes and gene products will continue to advance our understanding of the inherited neuropathies. For example, the study by Lupski and colleagues using whole genome sequencing has identified heretofore unknown compound heterozygous alleles that produce CMT phenotypes, most rare, but demonstrating that the frequency of unidentified mutations will be continuously be reduced.

Based on the finding that only a few mutations are implicated in the majority of cases of CMT, various algorithms have been designed, taking into account the degree of slowing of motor nerve conduction velocity and clinical features. For example, PMP22 testing is a reasonable first step if the patient has the typical clinical appearance of CMT1A and motor nerve conductions are slower than 38 m/s. If this shows no mutation and there is male-to-male transmission, screening for CMT1X is performed, or if autosomal inheritance, for MPZ mutations (CMT1B). If these are unrevealing, a third step may be screening for point mutations in PMP22, SIMPLE, and EGR2. If the nerve conduction velocities are severely slowed, below 15 m/s, PMP22 duplication or MPZ mutations are likely to be present. Those with intermediate conduction velocities, between 35 and 45 m/s are likely to have CMT1X or CMT1B and mutations in the corresponding genes. It is worth again noting that only a third of CMT2 cases will have mutations found by current methods. These prescriptions for testing will change as new sequencing methods are introduced

Pathologic Findings Degenerative changes in the nerves result in depletion of the population of large sensory and motor fibers, leaving only the condensed endoneurial connective tissue. As far as one can tell, axons and myelin sheaths are both affected, the distal parts of the nerve more than the proximal ones. In type I, the nerves may be enlarged, with "onion-bulb" formations of Schwann cells and fibroblasts, as in Dejerine-Sottas disease (CMT3; type III HMSN in the Dyck classification). This change can often be seen in sural nerve biopsies. Anterior horn cells are slightly diminished in number and some are chromatolyzed as a secondary change. Dorsal root ganglion cells suffer a similar fate. The disease involves sensory posterior root fibers with degeneration of the posterior columns of Goll more than of Burdach. The autonomic nervous system remains relatively intact. The muscles contain large fields of atrophic fibers (group atrophy). Some of the larger fibers have a target appearance and may show degenerative changes. All these muscle changes are typical of neurogenic denervation. Former claims of a coincidental myelopathy and degeneration of spinocerebellar and corticospinal tracts probably indicate that the associated disease was really Friedreich ataxia or some other combination of chronic myelopathy and neuropathy.

Treatment No specific treatment is known. Stabilizing the ankles by arthrodeses is indicated if foot-drop is severe and the disease has reached the point where it is not progressing. Pediatric orthopedic specialists have experience with several techniques to stabilize the joints of weakened limbs. Regular exercise, but avoiding excessive weight training, is usually prescribed. In mild and early cases, fitting the legs with light braces and the shoes with springs to overcome foot-drop can be helpful.

Hereditary Neuropathy With Pressure Palsies

This unusual but distinctive process of multiple recurrent local neuropathies, first reported by Earl and colleagues, is caused by a deletion of the *PMP22* gene, the one that is duplicated in the previously described CMT1A. In both CMT1A and hereditary neuropathy with pressure palsies (HNPP), the *PMP22* gene is functionally normal and these disorders arise because the total amount of the protein is abnormal. In CMT1A the gene is duplicated on one chromosome, thereby increasing the total PMP22 protein; by contrast, in HNPP, the gene is deleted so that the PMP22 protein is at approximately half-normal levels. HNPP is transmitted as a dominant trait. In these individuals, the focal neuropathies and plexopathies are generally not painful (in contrast with related conditions of hereditary neuralgic amyotrophy discussed further on). Focal nerve lesions are often provoked by slight or even brief compression. In addition to recurrent focal nerve palsies, most individuals with HNPP have an underlying chronic but slowly progressive demyelinating sensorimotor neuropathy that is mild on clinical examination (e.g., not all cases show areflexia). Electrophysiologic studies are abnormal, but may be only subtly so, with some slowing of conduction and distal motor and sensory nerve abnormalities, particularly across sites of compression. Nerve biopsies from these patients are most remarkable for the presence of localized nerve sheath thickening with duplication of the myelin lamellae (so-called tomaculae, meaning sausage shaped).

Hypertrophic Neuropathy of Infancy (Dejerine-Sottas Disease, Congenital Hypomyelination, CMT3)

This relatively rare but striking neuropathy is inherited as an autosomal recessive trait. It begins in childhood or infancy, earlier than the typical form of peroneal muscular atrophy. Walking is delayed in onset and then progressively impaired. Pain and paresthesias in the feet are early symptoms, followed by the development of symmetrical weakness and wasting of the distal portions of the limbs. Talipes equinovarus postures with clawfeet and later clawhands are common. All modalities of sensation are impaired in a distal distribution, and the tendon reflexes are absent. Miotic, unreactive pupils, nystagmus, and kyphoscoliosis have been observed in some cases. The trunk and other cranial nerves are spared. The ulnar, median, radial, posterior tibial and peroneal nerves stand out like tendons and are easily followed with the gently roving finger. The enlarged nerves are not tender. Unlike other forms of hereditary neuropathy, the CSF protein is persistently elevated in Dejerine-Sottas disease, in all likelihood because the spinal roots are enlarged. Nerve conduction velocities are markedly reduced, even when there is little or no functional impairment. Patients are usually more disabled than those with peroneal muscular atrophy and are confined to wheelchairs at an early age. Treatment is purely symptomatic.

It is important to emphasize that the occurrence of hypertrophic neuropathy is not confined to this particular inherited disease. If one groups all patients in whom the nerves are diffusely enlarged (incorrectly called "hypertrophic" as it is mainly a nonspecific reaction of the epineural and perineural connective tissue that contributes to the bulk of the nerves), several diseases, both genetic and acquired, are included. The identifying histologic lesion in these cases is the "onion bulb," which consists of a whorl of overlapping, intertwined, attenuated Schwann cell processes that encircle naked or finely myelinated axons and of endoneurial fibrofilaments. Enlarged nerves have been described in cases of recurrent demyelinating polyneuritis (CIDP), familial amyloidosis, Refsum disease, CMT type I, and other diseases. As was first pointed out by Thomas, any pathologic process that causes recurrent segmental demyelination and subsequent repair and remyelination may have this effect. In some patients with a history of early childhood hereditary polyneuropathy, the nerves are not yet palpably enlarged, but the characteristic Schwann cell abnormalities are revealed in biopsy material from a cutaneous nerve.

Phenotype-Genotype Correlations in the Inherited Sensorimotor Polyneuropathies

As the molecular basis of the inherited polyneuropathies has been elucidated, it has become clear that diverse mutations and molecular defects can give rise to the same clinical phenotype. From a neurobiologic perspective, it is intriguing that both Dejerine-Sottas and Roussy-Lévy syndromes are linked to a recessively inherited loss of the myelin protein P0, and that the salient clinical features of this disorder are manifestations of defective nerve myelination. However, it has also become apparent that nearly identical clinical syndromes are associated with mutations in the genes for PMP22 and for the Schwann cell DNA-binding protein EGR2. Moreover, while some mutations in the P0 gene cause infantile onset neuropathies with the Dejerine-Sottas and Roussy-Lévy phenotypes, other mutations in the same gene cause adult onset neuropathies. Although the early-onset cases show marked slowing of nerve conduction, the adult ones have conduction velocities that are typically above 35 m/s. The infancy-onset cases reveal major disruptions of folding of compact myelin, whereas in the adult-onset cases subtle alterations in the myelin protein PO lead to a slow, predominantly axonal degeneration in adult life. Many other insights into the genetic and structural alterations of this vast category of disease have been revealed and can be appreciated from reading subspecialty texts on the subject, including the chapters by Amato and Russell and the monograph by Klein, Xuan and Shy, and the study by Saporta and coworkers, which are recommended.

Inherited Polyneuropathies of Predominantly Sensory Type

Common to the diseases comprising this group are insensitivity to pain, lancinating pains, and ulcers of the feet and hands, leading to osteomyelitis, osteolysis, stress fractures, and recurrent episodes of cellulitis. Because similar symptoms and signs occur in syringomyelia, leprosy, and tabes dorsalis, there is considerable uncertainty in older writings on this subject as to whether the reported cases were examples of one of these diseases or of hereditary neuropathy. According to Dyck and Lambert (1975), it was Leplat in 1846, who first described plantar ulcers (*mal perforant du pied*).

Mutilating Hereditary (Dominant) Sensory Polyneuropathy in Adults (Hereditary Sensory and Autonomic Neuropathy Type 1)

The characteristic features of this group of polyneuropathies are an autosomal dominant mode of inheritance and onset of symptoms in the second decade or later. Characteristically this begins with subtle loss of sensation for painful stimuli in the feet (e.g., inability to feel the hot sand or hot water in a tub). As the disease evolves, there is involvement of the feet with calluses of the soles and, later, episodes of blistering, ulceration, and lymphangitis followed by osteomyelitis and osteolysis, shooting pains, distal sensory loss with greater affection of pain and thermal sensation than of touch and pressure, loss of sweating, diminution or absence of tendon reflexes, and only slight loss of muscle power. Over time, loss of pain sensation in the fingers leads to fingertip ulcerations, osteomyelitis, and amputations.

The plantar ulcer overlying the head of a metatarsal bone is the most dreaded complication, because it often leads to osteomyelitis. Infection of the pulp of the fingers and paronychias are uncommon. Some patients have a mild pes cavus and weakness of the peroneal and pretibial muscles, with foot-drop and steppage gait. Lancinating pains may occur in the legs, thighs, and shoulders, and, exceptionally, the pain may last for days or longer and be as disabling as that of tabes dorsalis; however, in the majority of patients there is no pain whatsoever. Neural deafness was present in one of Denny-Brown's patients. In that case, which was studied postmortem, there was a loss of small nerve cells in the lumbosacral dorsal root ganglia; the dorsal roots were thin, and the fibers in the posterior columns of the spinal cord and those in the peripheral nerves were diminished in number. Myelinated and unmyelinated fibers were both affected. Both axonal degeneration and segmental demyelination have been demonstrated in teased nerve preparations. Sensory nerve conduction may be absent or is uniformly slowed in every nerve tested.

It must be emphasized that despite its categorization as a "sensory and autonomic neuropathy," the most common, dominantly inherited form, termed *HSAN1*, also entails progressive, disabling, distal motor weakness, a consequence of ongoing axonopathy and denervation. HSAN1 is a consequence of a loss of function of the enzyme serine palmitoyltransferase, which is the rate-limiting step in the biosynthesis of sphingolipids.

Recessive Mutilating Sensory Polyneuropathy of Childhood

Here the pattern of inheritance is autosomal recessive. Onset is in infancy and early childhood and walking is delayed; there is pes cavus deformity and the first movements are ataxic. Ulcerations of the tips of toes and fingers and repeated infections of these parts result in the formation of paronychias and whitlows. The tendon reflexes are absent, but power is well preserved. All sensory modalities are impaired (touch-pressure somewhat more than pain-temperature), mainly in the distal parts of the limbs but also over the trunk. In addition, there are reports of several sibships in which multiple members had a sensory neuropathy manifest by a generalized insensitivity to pain of the type described later. The lesions and electrophysiologic findings are similar to those in the dominantly inherited sensory neuropathy described previously.

In all types of hereditary sensory neuropathies, measures must be taken to prevent stress fractures, acral mutilation, and infection. This is more difficult in the small child who does not understand the problem.

It is also now evident that some of the infantile hereditary sensory neuropathies are a result of a disruption of molecular signaling pathways for neurotropic substances, such as nerve growth factor, that are critical to neural development.

Congenital Insensitivity to Pain

In *congenital insensitivity or indifference to pain*, a syndrome in which the patient throughout life is unreactive to the pain of injury, there is no loss of the ability to distinguish pinprick and other noxious stimuli from nonnoxious ones. Furthermore, the nervous system of such individuals seems to be normal. There is another variety characterized by universal analgesia (Swanson et al). This latter type is inherited as an autosomal recessive trait and at least one form involves the gene for a nerve growth factor receptor located on chromosome 1q immediately adjacent to the site of the mutation for Charcot-Marie-Tooth disease type 1B (see Table 46-6). During childhood, one of the patients of Swanson and colleagues had high fever when the environmental temperature was raised and the other had orthostatic hypotension. One of the patients died in his twelfth year and was found to have an absence of small neurons in the dorsal root ganglia, an absence of Lissauer tracts, and a decrease in size of the descending spinal tracts of the trigeminal nerves. Sweat glands were present in the skin but were not innervated.

Multiple Symmetrical Lipomas With Sensorimotor Polyneuropathy

Whereas the usual cutaneous lipomas have no neurologic accompaniments, this clinical curiosity, known as Launois-Bensaude disease, consists of symmetrical lipomas of the neck and shoulders that are associated with polyneuropathy and sometimes, deafness. A mitochondrial disorder of similar genetic origin as the MERRF syndrome (see Chap. 37) has been identified (see Neumann's review for clinical details).

Polyglucosan Disease

This interesting process was mentioned in Chap. 39 in relation to dementia in which it is pointed out that there is a multisystem neurologic disease characterized by the widespread deposition in nervous tissue of corpora amylacea, in this disease termed *polyglucosan bodies*. The main presentation of this disorder is of slowly progressive motor and pronounced sensory loss in the legs due to an axonal polyneuropathy, neurogenic bladder, and a degree of upper motor neuron signs that may also be evident. It is the early appearance of the urinary difficulties or the upper motor neuron features that mark the illness as unusual in relation to other polyneuropathies. Biopsy of the sural nerve demonstrates profuse deposition of the polyglucosan bodies in the endoneurium. When dementia occurs, either with the neuropathy or in isolation, the corpora amylacea are found throughout the cerebrum. The process is detailed by Robitaille and colleagues and an upper motor neuron presentation that simulates amyotrophic lateral sclerosis, by McDonald and coworkers.

The bodies are made up largely of glucose polymers that are well known to occur in the aging brain and, when present in small numbers, have been assigned an innocuous meaning. In the usual type of polyglucosan disease, which is found in individuals of Ashkenazic Jewish origin, there is a deficiency in glycogen branching enzyme (GBE) that is shared with glycogenosis type IV, and infantile recessive process, Anderson disease. As such, it could be considered with the other neuropathies that have an identifiable metabolic cause, discussed as a group further on. However, a proportion of cases do not have the inherited GBE enzyme abnormality.

Riley-Day Familial Dysautonomia

(See also Chap. 26)

This disorder, inherited as an autosomal recessive trait, affects predominantly children of Ashkenazic Jewish heritage. Familial dysautonomia is usually manifested soon after birth (poor sucking, failure to thrive, unexplained fever, episodes of pneumonia). Hyporeflexia and impairment or loss of pain and temperature sensation, with relative preservation of pressure and tactile sense, are the main manifestations. Motor fibers are probably involved as well, but only to a slight degree; this is shown more effectively by reduced motor conduction velocity in peripheral nerves than it is by weakness. At a later age, the neuropathy becomes overshadowed by other manifestations of the disease, notably repeated infections and abnormalities of the autonomic nervous system—lack of tears, corneal ulceration, fixed pupils, blotchiness of the skin, defective temperature control, cold hands and feet, excessive sweating, lability of blood pressure, postural hypotension, difficulty in swallowing, esophageal and intestinal dilation, emotional instability, recurrent vomiting, and stunted growth. The tongue lacks fungiform papillae.

Nerve biopsy reveals a diminution of small myelinated and unmyelinated fibers, which explains the impairment of pain and temperature sensation. In autopsy material, sympathetic and parasympathetic ganglion cells and, to a lesser extent, nerve cells in the sensory ganglia are diminished in number. Patients excrete increased amounts of homovanillic acid and decreased amounts of vanillylmandelic acid and methoxyhydroxyphenylglycol. Weinshilboum and Axelrod demonstrated a decrease in serum dopamine β-hydroxylase, the enzyme that converts dopamine to norepinephrine. The disease is caused by a mutation in a gene that expresses a kinase-associated protein (see HSAN3 in Table 46-6). There is no treatment for the disease except to provide symptomatic relief of gastrointestinal symptoms and orthostatic fainting.

Other examples of congenital polyneuropathy with absence of autonomic function, probably differing from the Riley-Day dysautonomia, have been reported. Some of these develop transient episodes of reflex sympathetic dystrophy. A congenital failure of development of neural elements derived from the neural crest has been postulated.

Ataxia-telangiectasia and Chédiak-Higashi disease are other genetic diseases with a recognized metabolic abnormality that may cause a polyneuropathy. They are described in Chap. 37, with the hereditary metabolic disorders.

Other Forms of Inherited Sensory Neuropathy

Included here are numerous disorders similar to the ones described in the preceding pages but caused by different mutations; neuropathy with cerebellar degeneration; and the neuropathies in which there are recognized metabolic abnormalities, including familial amyloidosis. Some years ago a young man and woman with universal anesthesia affecting head, neck, trunk, and limbs came to attention (Adams et al); all forms of sensation were absent. The patients were areflexic but retained nearly full motor power; their movements were ataxic. Autonomic functions were impaired but not abolished. In a sural nerve biopsy, nearly all fibers—large and small, myelinated and unmyelinated—had disappeared. Surprisingly, there were no trophic changes of any kind. Donaghy and coworkers and others have described a variant of the recessively inherited form of sensory neuropathy in which there was an associated neurotrophic keratitis and a selective loss of small myelinated fibers in sural nerve biopsies. We continue to observe variant and unclassifiable cases of purely motor, sensory, or mixed types in which genetic testing does not reveal a mutation such as these every year.

Hereditary Areflexic Dystasia (Roussy-Lévy Syndrome)

In 1926, Roussy and Lévy reported 7 cases of a dominantly inherited ataxic and neuropathic malady that had not previously been described. Its close relation to Friedreich ataxia and the amyotrophy of Charcot-Marie-Tooth disease was recognized. On the basis of molecular genetic testing, these relationships been clarified. Most classifications group it with CMT1 on the basis of the causative mutations and nerve conduction studies.

The condition is a sensory ataxia with pes cavus and areflexia, affecting mainly the lower legs and progressing later to involve the hands. Some degree of sensory loss, mainly of vibratory and position sense, is described in all cases. Atrophy of the muscles of the legs and postural tremor eventually become prominent, but the patients do not have signs of cerebellar disease (dysarthria, tremor, nystagmus). Kyphoscoliosis, a feature typical of Friedreich disease, has been described in several cases. Although the feet may be cold or slightly discolored, no autonomic defects are documented and the nerves are not palpably enlarged. Electrocardiographic abnormalities similar to those of Friedreich ataxia have been noted in one family but are not usual. The onset in many patients is during infancy, possibly dating from birth, and the course is relatively benign; all descendants of the original Roussy-Lévy family were still able to walk during their seventh decade of life.

On clinical and pathologic grounds, Dyck and Lambert (1975) placed the Roussy-Lévy kinships within the category of the demyelinating type of Charcot-Marie-Tooth disease (CMT1). The mode of inheritance of the two syndromes, their benign course, pattern of neurologic signs, slow nerve conduction, and biopsy features (demyelination of nerve fibers with onion-bulb formation) are much the same. This view has been reinforced by the genetic findings reported by Planté-Bordeneuve and colleagues. In affected members of the original Roussy-Lévy family, these investigators identified a point mutation in the domain of the myelin protein gene PO, the same gene that is implicated in Dejerine-Sottas disease. Most currently studied cases (there are few) have point mutations in PMP22 or MPZ. Based on limited pathologic study, there is no cerebellar degeneration; nevertheless, the shared clinical features with Friedreich ataxia are unmistakable and create diagnostic confusion before genetic testing.

Polyneuropathy With Cerebellar Degeneration

(See "Predominantly Cerebellar Forms of Hereditary and Sporadic Ataxia" in Chap. 39)

Several such cases of adult onset have come to our attention over the years. Unlike Friedreich disease, the ataxia is mild and there is no kyphoscoliosis, but pes cavus or hammer-toe deformities are found, attesting to the early onset of the neuropathy. The lower legs become atrophic and findings characteristic of CMT such as absent ankle reflexes and mild to moderate loss of distal deep sensibility are present. There is no Romberg sign and no Babinski signs. The outstanding feature is a profound atrophy of the cerebellar hemispheres, and to some extent of the vermis, on MRI. Although the illness is slowly progressive, our patients, like those with Roussy-Lévy disease, have remained highly functional into late age, having difficulty mostly with maintaining balance when dancing or wearing high-heeled shoes. The EMG is consistent with CMT2. The electrocardiogram has been normal. Several, but not all, such patients have had a family history of a similar process, but the available genetic testing has failed to reveal the site of a mutation. As mentioned, the process can simulate Friedreich ataxia in some respects. The genetic basis is uncertain and various genotypes have been reported in single families.

Polyneuropathy With Spastic Paraplegia

From time to time we have observed children and young adults with unmistakable progressive spastic paraplegia superimposed on a sensorimotor polyneuropathy of extremely chronic evolution. Sural nerve biopsy in 2 of our cases disclosed a typical "hypertrophic" polyneuropathy. In another case, only loss of nerve fibers was found. Cavanaugh and colleagues and Harding and Thomas (1984) reported similar patients. Our patients were severely disabled, being barely able to stand on their atrophic legs. An even more ambiguous form of disease was described by Vucic and colleagues in which there is typical CMT but with brisk reflexes. There were Babinski signs in half the patients and spastic dysphonia in a few others. The mutation is not known.

Although few in number, some cases of chronic polyneuropathy are combined with optic atrophy, with or without deafness or retinitis pigmentosa, and Dyck and Lambert (1975) classed these in a separate group. Jaradeh and Dyck have also described a hereditary motor-sensory polyneuropathy with the later development of a parkinsonian or a choreic-dystonic syndrome that responded to L-dopa. Most cases of this type have had an autosomal recessive inheritance.

Hereditary Recurrent Brachial Plexopathy (Hereditary Neuralgic Amyotrophy)

This entity, mentioned earlier in relation to hereditary neuropathy with pressure palsies because of the implication of a similar genetic locus, is discussed in the later section under "Brachial Neuritis, Brachial Plexitis (Neuralgic Amyotrophy, Parsonage-Turner Syndrome)."

Inherited Polyneuropathies with a Recognized Metabolic Disorder

Refsum Disease (HMSN IV)

This rare disorder, named after Refsum who made the first clinical observations, is inherited as an autosomal recessive trait and has its onset in late childhood, adolescence, or early adult life. It is slowly progressive but may be punctuated by acute or subacute worsening.

Diagnosis is based on a combination of clinical manifestations—retinitis pigmentosa, ataxia, and chronic polyneuropathy—coupled with the metabolic marker of the disease, an increase in blood phytanic acid. Phytanic acid accumulates because of a deficiency of the peroxisomal enzyme, phytanoyl-coenzyme A (CoA) hydroxylase. The deficiency is caused by mutations in one of two disparate genes. Cardiomyopathy and neurogenic deafness are present in most patients, and pupillary abnormalities, cataracts, and ichthyotic skin changes (particularly on the shins) are added features in some. Anosmia and night-blindness (nyctalopia) with constriction of the visual fields may precede the neuropathy by many years. The polyneuropathy is sensorimotor, distal, and symmetrical in distribution, affecting the legs more than the arms. All forms of sensation are reduced, often deep sensation more so than pain and thermal sense, and tendon reflexes are lost. The CSF protein is increased, sometimes markedly. Usually, the polyneuropathy develops gradually, although in some patients it has a subacute onset or, after being established for some time, a tendency to worsen fairly abruptly.

Although the nerves may not be palpably enlarged, "hypertrophic" changes with onion-bulb formation are invariable pathologic features. The metabolic defect has been discovered to be in the utilization of dietary phytol; a failure of oxidation of phytanic acid—a branched-chain tetramethylated 16-carbon fatty acid—that accumulates in the absence of activity of the enzyme phytanoyl-CoA-hydroxylase. The relation between the increased phytanic acid and the polyneuropathy is uncertain.

Clinical diagnosis is confirmed by the finding of increased phytanic acid in the blood of a patient with a chronic, mainly sensory neuropathy; the normal level is less than 0.3 mg/dL but in patients with this disease, it constitutes 5 to 30 percent of the total fatty acids of the serum lipids. Urinary phytanic acid concentration is also raised. Genetic testing reveals the mutation.

Treatment Diets low in phytol may be beneficial but this is difficult to judge, because after an acute attack there is sometimes a natural remission. The claimed effects of plasma exchange have also been difficult to interpret. In some patients there is a very slow progression of the disease, and in others, a more rapid progression with death from cardiac complications.

Mitochondrial Neuropathy

Like the cases of mitochondrial disease with neuropathy reported by Tuck and McLeod, we have observed several in which the clinical picture was almost identical to that of Refsum disease, but elevations in phytanic acid were not present. Mild ichthyosis, sensorineural deafness, ataxia of mixed tabetic-cerebellar type, areflexia, and retinitis pigmentosa were the main findings, conforming to the NARP syndrome described in Chap. 37. None of our cases had a family history of a similar disorder. Sural nerve biopsy showed loss of large fibers. There was an identifiable mitochondrial disorder in most of the recently studied cases, as described in Chap. 37. It should be remarked that most mutations of mitochondrial DNA cause a myopathy with multisystem disease, but not a neuropathy. The onset of the disease is in childhood or adolescence with slow progression.

Abetalipoproteinemia (Bassen-Kornzweig Syndrome) (See also Chap. 37)

This rare autosomal recessive childhood disorder was described in Chap. 37 with the inherited metabolic disorders of the nervous system and commented upon with neuroacanthocytosis in Chap. 39, although there is no relationship between the two processes. It is mentioned here because the brunt of the neurologic disorder falls upon the peripheral nerves. *Acanthocytosis* of red blood cells is its identifying feature. The earliest neurologic finding is usually diminution or absence of tendon reflexes, detected as early as the second year of life. Later, when the child is first able to cooperate in sensory testing, a loss of vibratory and position sense is found in the legs. Cerebellar signs (ataxia of gait, trunk, and extremities; titubation of the head; and dysarthria), muscle weakness, ophthalmoparesis, Babinski signs, and loss of pain and temperature sense are the other characteristic neurologic abnormalities, in more or less this order of frequency. Developmental delay, usually mild, occurs in some patients. Irregular progression occurs over a few years, and many patients are unable to stand and walk by the time they reach adolescence.

Skeletal abnormalities include pes cavus and kyphoscoliosis, which are secondary to the early onset neuropathy. Constriction of the visual fields and ring scotomata are manifestations of the macular degeneration and retinitis pigmentosa in some cases. Cardiac enlargement and congestive failure are serious late complications.

Neuropathologic findings consist of demyelination of peripheral nerves and degeneration of nerve cells in the spinal gray matter and cerebellar cortex. Diagnosis is confirmed by the finding of red blood cell acanthocytes, low serum cholesterol, and β (low-density)-lipoproteins. The disease is caused by defects in a triglyceride transfer protein, as discussed in Chap. 37. A deficiency of vitamin E, as a result of malabsorption, may be a factor, and large doses of the vitamin should be tried as therapy.

A closely related disease, also with familial hypobetalipoproteinemia, was described by van Buchem and coworkers. It, too, is associated with malabsorption syndrome, ill-defined weakness, ataxia, dysesthesia of the legs, and Babinski signs. There is no sensory loss.

Tangier Disease

This is a rare, familial, small-fiber neuropathy of which we have seen a few cases, inherited as an autosomal recessive trait. It is named for the island off the Virginia coast where the first-described patients resided. The mutation eliminates the function of the adenosine triphosphate (ATP)-cassette transporter protein. It results in a deficiency of high-density lipoprotein, extremely low serum cholesterol, and high triglyceride concentrations in the serum. Perhaps on the basis of these abnormalities, the patients are disposed to early and severe atherosclerosis. The presence of enlarged, yellow-orange (cholesterol-laden) tonsils is said to be a frequent manifestation (of course, previous tonsillectomies obviate this sign). About half of the reported cases have had neuropathic symptoms, taking the form of an asymmetrical sensorimotor neuropathy that fluctuates in severity.

The sensory loss is predominantly for pain and temperature and extends over the entire body; at times it is limited to the face and upper extremities, simulating syringomyelia ("pseudosyringomyelia"). Tactile and proprioceptive sensory modalities tend to be preserved. The polyneuropathy may come in attacks—that is to say, it simulates a recurrent process. Muscular weakness, if present, affects either the lower or upper extremities or both, particularly the hand muscles, which may undergo atrophy and show denervation by EMG. In a small number of patients there has been facial diplegia out of proportion to weakness elsewhere. In one of our patients, the pain and temperature loss was restricted to the head, neck, and arms. Tendon reflexes are often lost or diminished. Transient ptosis and diplopia have been reported. Nerve conduction is slowed.

Fat-laden macrophages are present in the bone marrow and elsewhere. No complete pathologic studies are available. There is no known treatment but dietary measures to reduce triglycerides may help, particularly in preventing atherosclerosis but the influence on the neuropathy is uncertain.

Fabry Disease (Anderson-Fabry Disease)

(See also Chap. 37)

The genetic and metabolic aspects of this sex-linked disorder caused by deficiency of alpha-galactosidase A were considered with the inherited metabolic diseases. Here we offer some additional remarks about the painful neuropathic component. It bears commenting that 10 percent of heterozygous women display neuropathic symptoms, but usually of later onset and lesser degree than in males.

The pain, which is usually the initial symptom in childhood and adolescence, often has a burning quality or occurs in brief lancinating jabs, mostly in the fingers and toes, and may be accompanied by paresthesias of the palms and soles. Changes in environmental temperature and exercise may induce pain in "crises," an identifying feature. These abnormalities are a result of the accumulation of glycolipid (ceramide trihexoside) in peripheral nerves, both perineurally and intraneurally, as well as in cells of the spinal ganglia and the anterior and intermediolateral horns of the spinal cord. Ohnishi and Dyck demonstrated a preferential loss of small myelinated and unmyelinated fibers and small neurons of dorsal root ganglia, and Cable and colleagues reported autonomic changes in other cases. Involvement of the sensory ganglia and the associated degenerative changes in the afferent fibers are thought to be the likely cause of the thermally induced painful sensory phenomena (Kahn).

Later in the illness there is progressive impairment of renal function and cerebral and myocardial infarction. The characteristic dermal feature is the presence of numerous dark red macules and papules (angiokeratomas), up to 2 mm in diameter, over the trunk and limbs, most closely clustered over the thighs and lower trunk and around the umbilicus (*angiokeratoma corporis diffusum*). The comprehensive review by Brady and Schiffman is recommended.

Treatment Phenytoin, carbamazepine, gabapentin, or amitriptyline may be helpful in alleviating the pain and dysesthesias. As discussed in Chap. 37, enzyme replacement therapy has become available and seems to lead to partial remission of many of the features including the neuropathic ones.

Polyneuropathy of Acromegaly and Gigantism

Nerve entrapment, particularly of the median nerve, is a well-known feature of acromegaly. Pickett and colleagues identified carpal tunnel syndrome in 56 percent of acromegalics. Also recognized as a complication of acromegaly, but not because of multiple nerve entrapments, is *polyneuropathy* characterized by paresthesia, loss of tendon reflexes in the legs, and atrophy of slight degree in the distal leg muscles. Sometimes there are enlarged nerves. In the case reported by Stewart, the enlargement was the result of hypertrophic changes in the endoneurial and perineurial tissues, similar to those that occur in other so-called hypertrophic neuropathies of inflammatory or heredofamilial origin. In cases of extreme gigantism, a more severe polyneuropathy has sometimes been reported, to the point of causing Charcot joints (Daughaday).

Mentioned here is a case we have observed in which a severe and slowly progressive relatively symmetric motor neuropathy occurred in a patient with Pyle disease, a metaphyseal dysplasia that resembles acromegaly.

Metachromatic Leukodystrophy (See also Chap. 37)

In this metabolic disease, the congenital absence of the degradative enzyme sulfatase leads to massive accumulation of sulfatide throughout the central and peripheral nervous systems and to a lesser extent in other organs. The abnormality is transmitted as an autosomal recessive trait. Progressive cerebral deterioration is the most obvious clinical feature, but hyporeflexia, muscular atrophy, and diminished nerve conduction velocity reflect the presence of a neuropathy. Early in the course of the illness, the weakness, hypotonia, and areflexia may suggest Werdnig-Hoffmann disease; in older children there may be a complaint of paresthesias and demonstrable sensory loss. Bifacial weakness has been reported but must be rare. Sensory and motor conduction velocities are greatly slowed similarly in all nerves. Metachromatically staining granules accumulate in the cytoplasm of Schwann cells in nerves as well as in the cerebral white matter. There is loss of peripheral myelinated fibers. The measurement of arylsulfatase A activity in peripheral leukocytes or urine and biopsies of sural nerves are used to establish the diagnosis, even early in the course of the illness.

Inherited (Familial Amyloidosis, TTR Amyloidosis) Amyloid Neuropathies

(See Table 46-6)

As noted earlier in the discussion of acquired (primary) amyloidosis, *amyloid* is a descriptive term for any of the proteins that are deposited in filamentous beta-pleated sheets; it can be derived from a number of precursor protein sources. Peripheral neuropathy is a common and often the most prominent manifestation of amyloidosis. The polyneuropathies are of two main types—those associated with familial amyloidosis (referred to as FA) and the other associated with primary (nonfamilial) systemic deposition of amyloid (termed AL), which is derived from a circulating monoclonal protein. The acquired type has been discussed earlier. The most notable difference between these two types is the absence of a significant amount of paraprotein in the inherited forms (see further on). The amyloidosis that is secondary to chronic infectious or inflammatory disease, referred to as AA, is an increasingly rare condition and, in any case, does not affect the nerves.

In the following described most common familial amyloidoses, the amyloid is derived from an inherited abnormality of serum protein transthyretin (TTR, formerly called "prealbumin"). Several different amino acid substitutions have been identified in each type of amyloidosis. In the originally described Andrade type, methionine replaces valine at amino acid 30; therefore this has been referred to as *transthyretin amyloidosis* and as the *TTR met 30 type*. However, there are over 100 variants in the transthyretin gene that can give rise to amyloidosis.

The familial amyloid polyneuropathies comprise several distinct groups, as enumerated in Table 46-6. The pattern of inheritance in all types is autosomal dominant; males and females are affected with equal frequency. Although a descriptive classification based on the ethnic or geographic origin of affected families is still in use and is retained in the narrative categorization below, it is now possible to categorize the diseases according to their genetic causes and the corresponding chemical structure of the amyloid protein that is deposited in tissue. The recent cloning of many of the amyloid protein genes has made possible not only the detection of the common transthyretin mutation but also DNA tests for some of the other types of familial amyloidoses. Lachmann and colleagues emphasize the high frequency of genetic defects in amyloid precursor proteins and the finding in one-quarter of cases of a low-level monoclonal gammopathy. Characteristic of all the amyloid polyneuropathies is the preferential involvement of small-diameter sensory and autonomic nerves and deposition of amyloid in various organs. Sensory loss, therefore, dominates the picture and pain and autonomic changes are prominent in most varieties of the disease.

The following are the main recognized types of *familial amyloid neuropathies*.

1. **The Portuguese (Andrade) type.** Andrade, in 1939, recognized that a chronic familial illness known as "foot disease" among the inhabitants of Oporto, Portugal, was a special type of amyloid polyneuropathy. He was not the first to have seen amyloid in degenerating nerve but deserves credit for identifying the disease as one of the heredofamilial polyneuropathies. By 1969 he had studied 148 sibships, comprising 623 individuals, among whom there were 249 with polyneuropathy. Descendants of this family have been traced to Africa, France, and Brazil. Other foci of the disease have been reported in Japan (Araki et al; Ikeda et al), the United States (Kantarjian and DeJong), Germany (Delank et al), Poland, Greece, Sweden, and northwest Ireland (Staunton et al). As far as one can tell, these are separate, unrelated probands in different ethnic groups.

   The age of onset of this form of familial amyloid polyneuropathy is between 25 and 35 years. The disease progresses slowly and terminates fatally in 10 to 15 or more years. The initial symptoms are usually numbness, paresthesias, and sometimes pain in the feet and lower legs. Weakness is minimal, and the tendon reflexes, although diminished, may be retained early in the course of the illness. Pain and thermal sense are reduced more than tactile, vibratory, and position sense (a "pseudosyringomyelic") pattern. Autonomic involvement is another important characteristic—loss of pupillary light reflexes and miosis, anhidrosis, vasomotor paralysis with orthostatic hypotension, alternating diarrhea and constipation, and erectile dysfunction. These autonomic changes tend to be more extensive than the sensory ones. Difficulty in walking also develops and has its basis in a combination of faulty position sense and mild muscle weakness. Later, tendon reflexes are abolished and the legs become thin. The nerves are not enlarged. Cranial nerve involvement (facial weakness and numbness, loss of taste) is a late manifestation and occurs in only a few cases.

   The clinical details vary somewhat from case to case, even within a family. Cardiac enlargement and irregularities in cardiac rhythm as a result of bundle-branch or atrioventricular (AV) block occur early in some and late in others. A few patients have had severe amyloid cardiomyopathy from the onset (Ikeda et al). Weight loss may be pronounced owing to anorexia and disordered bowel function and the later development of a malabsorption syndrome. The liver may become enlarged (as it may in the acquired form). Vitreous opacities (veils, specks, and strands) may progress to blindness but this has been rare; in a few, there has been an impairment of hearing. Involvement of the CNS—manifest as behavioral abnormalities, cerebellar ataxia, and bilateral corticospinal signs—has also been reported in a few cases but their nature and pathologic basis is controversial (Ikeda et al). A nephrotic syndrome and uremia terminate life in some patients. The CSF may be normal or the protein content may be increased (50 to 200 mg/dL); the blood is normal except for anemia caused by amyloidosis of the bone marrow. This is probably the most common transthyretin mutation–derived amyloidosis.
2. **Familial amyloidosis with carpal tunnel syndrome (Swiss type).** Falls and coworkers, in 1955, and later Rukavina and associates described a large group of patients of Swiss stock living in Indiana who developed, in their fourth and fifth decades, a syndrome of acroparesthesias in the hands as a result of deposition of amyloid in the connective tissues and beneath the carpal ligaments. Similar kindreds of German descent were recognized in Maryland. There were sensory loss and atrophic muscle weakness in the distribution of the median nerves, which were compressed. Section of the carpal ligaments relieved the symptoms. In some of the patients, other nerves of the arms were said to have become involved later.

Vitreous deposits have been observed frequently in this form of the disease. As with the Portuguese type, an abnormal transthyretin is the basis of the deposition of amyloid.

3. **Iowa type.** In 1969, van Allen described an Iowa kindred with onset, in their thirties, of a fairly severe sensorimotor neuropathy, involving the legs and then the arms. There was amyloid deposition in the testes, adrenal glands, and kidneys (the usual cause of death), as well as a high incidence of peptic ulcer disease. The amyloid in this disease is derived from a mutated apolipoprotein A1, in which there is an amino acid substitution.
4. **Cranial neuropathy with corneal lattice dystrophy and facial palsies.** This unusual form of amyloid neuropathy was first described in three Finnish families by Meretoja, hence the label "Finnish type." Subsequently, it was reported from several different parts of the world in families of non-Finnish heritage. The disease usually begins in the third decade with lattice corneal dystrophy. Vitreous opacities are not observed, and visual acuity is little affected. Peripheral neuropathy may not be evident until the fifth decade, at which time the facial nerves, particularly their upper branches, become affected. The nerves of the limbs are involved even later and to a much lesser extent than in other amyloid neuropathies. In advanced cases there is a distinctive appearance of excessive skin folds about the face, facial diparesis, dysarthria, spasticity, and dense loss of posterior column function. At postmortem examination, deposits of amyloid are found in virtually every organ, mainly in the kidneys and blood vessels and in the perineurium of affected nerves.

The amyloid fibrils are derived from the protein gelsolin. The latter is normally an actin-binding protein, but it is also an important constituent of basement membranes, which may explain the deposition of amyloid in the cornea and skin.

Diagnosis of Familial Amyloid Neuropathy When the characteristic painful small-fiber type of sensory disturbance and autonomic changes are coupled with a family history of the same constellation, the diagnosis is not difficult. As noted in the earlier section on the acquired paraproteinemic neuropathy, the presence of a monoclonal (rarely polyclonal) immunoglobulin in the blood is found in only a limited number of patients with familial amyloid cases and it is usually just above the upper limit of normal for the immunoglobulin subclass. Otherwise the two types of amyloid diseases, FA and AL, are quite similar and, indeed, approximately 10 percent of cases considered by history and examination to be acquired will be found to have the genetic disorder (Lachmann et al). The situation has been clarified by the availability of commercial gene sequencing to detect mutations in transthyretin that are related to amyloidosis.

Pathologic Findings Amyloid deposits are demonstrable in the walls of blood vessels, the interstitial (endoneurial) tissues of the peripheral somatic and autonomic nerves, and in the spinal and autonomic ganglia and roots. There is a loss of nerve fibers, the unmyelinated and small myelinated fibers being more depleted than the large myelinated ones. The anterior horn and sympathetic ganglion cells are swollen and chromatolyzed because of involvement of their axons, and the posterior columns of the spinal cord degenerate, also on a secondary basis.

The pathogenesis of the fiber loss in familial amyloidosis, as in the acquired type, is not fully understood. On the basis of their findings in a sporadic case of amyloid polyneuropathy with diabetes mellitus, Kernohan and Woltman suggested that amyloid deposits in the walls of the small arteries and arterioles interfered with the blood supply in the nerves and that amyloid neuropathy is essentially an ischemic process. In other cases, however, the vascular changes are relatively slight and the degeneration of the nerve fibers appears to be related to their compression and distortion by the endoneurial deposits of amyloid or, alternatively, there may be a direct toxic effect of the embedded amyloid. Amyloid also deposits in the tongue, gums, heart, gastrointestinal tract, kidneys, and many other organs, where it may act as a tissue toxin or has a mechanically disrupting effect on cells.

Treatment In recent years, liver transplantation has proved curative of some of the familial amyloid polyneuropathies, but obviously it has no role in the acquired forms. According to Herlenius and colleagues, more than 500 patients at the time of their writing had received liver transplants with a 77 percent rate of survival, equivalent to liver transplantation for other diseases. Two novel approaches, a small molecule, tafamidis, that prevents the aggregation of amyloid fibrils by stabilizing it in a tetrameric form (Coelho et al, 2012) and interfering RNA therapy (RNAi) that are delivered in lipid nanoparticles that reduces the production of mutant amyloid (Coelho et al, 2013) are both promising.

Problems in Diagnosis of the Chronic Polyneuropathies

This is the group of peripheral nerve diseases that has given the present authors the most difficulty. The cause of acute and many of the subacute and relapsing forms of nerve disease usually can be established by widely available clinical and laboratory methods. It is the early and late chronic polyneuropathies that continue to baffle the neurologist and general physician, despite the respectable advances that have been made in the field of genetic testing.

Diagnosis of Early Chronic Polyneuropathy

A *sensorimotor paralysis*, which evolves over several weeks (subacutely) or more slowly, over many months or a year or two, and involves legs more than arms and distal parts more than proximal should lead to a search for diabetes, occult neoplasia (carcinoma, lymphoma, multiple myeloma, or plasmacytoma), HIV infection, paraproteinemia (including amyloid neuropathy), systemic autoimmune disease, and CIDP. In our experience, the *subacute and chronically evolving demyelinating neuropathies* (over months) that have slowed motor conduction velocities, conduction block, and relatively normal needle EMG studies generally turn out to be variants of CIDP, some with a paraproteinemia. Marked weakness and reduced muscle action potential amplitudes in the face of minimal denervation, even if present in only a few nerves, also indicate the presence of focal demyelination. Most of the mixed axonal–demyelinating cases in which one eventually arrives at a diagnosis will also be related to an immune (paraproteinemic) or inflammatory (CIDP) process. In exceptional cases, a neoplastic process may remain hidden for as long as 2 or 3 years after the onset of neuropathy. An environmental toxin, endocrine disorder (except for diabetes), or nutritional cause is seldom identified, despite the frequent attribution of obscure polyneuropathies to such causes. Nonetheless, history of exposure to industrial or hobbyist toxins, sociopathy or psychopathy that would lead to toxin ingestion, or foreign travel should be sought and the evaluation should include testing for heavy metals in obscure cases. Unusual causes of nutritional deficiency such as celiac-sprue and other malabsorption syndromes (Whipple disease, Crohn disease, chronic hepatic disease, and particularly intestinal bypass surgery) have usually been obvious enough when present, so that the experienced clinician rarely overlooks them. Perhaps sprue is able to cause a neuropathy with minimal gastrointestinal symptoms. Vitamin B_{12} deficiency should be sought in cases of large-fiber neuropathy. A difficult problem is that of an older person with a mild, nonprogressive sensorimotor polyneuropathy in whom there is evidence of mild hypothyroidism, marginally low vitamin B_{12} and folic acid levels in the blood, a somewhat unbalanced diet, perhaps an excessive alcohol intake, and an abnormal glucose tolerance response. It is easy to propose but hard to prove that any of these factors is relevant. Vitamin replacement should be undertaken nonetheless if no other cause is found.

In the *purely or predominantly sensory polyneuropathies not caused by diabetes*—some painful, some not, and some with marked ataxia—an association with occult carcinoma, an IgM or other paraproteinemia, primary and familial amyloidosis, or Sjögren syndrome are the primary considerations. The problem of a mild sensory neuropathy in an elderly patient with or without burning feet was discussed earlier. When the symptoms are confined to the feet and legs, hereditary sensory neuropathy must always be considered if the condition is long standing. Intoxications with pyridoxine or metals account for a few chronic sensory neuropathies. Despite all these considerations, we still regularly encounter patients in whom the cause is not disclosed by any of the available tests. We have watched helplessly as some of these patients were reduced to a bed and wheelchair existence and others suffered from pain until they became dependent on opiates.

Table 46-7 lists the laboratory tests that are useful in the investigation of this group of neuropathies, with electrophysiology being most valuable.

Table 46-7

LABORATORY TESTS FOR THE INVESTIGATION OF SUBACUTE AND CHRONIC POLYNEUROPATHIES

Distal Symmetric Polyneuropathies[a]
Serum glucose, glucose tolerance test, hemoglobin A_{1c}
Anti-Hu antibody
Immunoelectrophoresis of serum and urine
Antimyelin-associated glycoprotein (MAG) and SGPG
Anti-G_{M1} antibody (if evidence of multifocal motor conduction block)
Vitamin B_{12} and methylmalonic acid levels
Human immune deficiency virus antibody
Lyme antibody Western blot
Heavy metal concentrations in blood and tissue
Blood urea nitrogen
Anti-gliadin and anti-transglutaminase antibodies
Vitamin E levels
Genetic testing for Charcot-Marie-Tooth disease and related hereditary neuropathies as indicated in text
Mononeuropathy Multiplex
Sedimentation rate, C-reactive protein
p-ANCA, c-ANCA
Cryoglobulins
Hepatitis serologies
HIV
Angiotensin converting enzyme (ACE) and chest imaging for sarcoid
CMV
PMP22 deletion in appropriate circumstances
Consider nerve biopsy
Sensory Ganglionopathy
Sedimentation rate, C-reactive protein
Anti-SSA/SSB
Anti-Hu and related paraneoplastic antibodies
Pyridoxine level if appropriate
Consider biopsy of minor salivary gland of lip
Small-Fiber Painful Neuropathy
Serum glucose, glucose tolerance test, hemoglobin A_{1c}
HIV
Transthyretin (TTR) mutation
Above listed testing pertaining to rheumatologic diseases
Heavy metal concentrations
Vitamin B levels and carotene
Alpha-galactosidase A concentration (Fabry disease)
Voltage-gated sodium channel sequencing (1.7)
Consider autonomic testing and skin biopsy for nerve fiber quantification
Consider abdominal fat pad biopsy for amyloidosis
Consider nerve biopsy for microscopic vasculitis

[a]Testing for each category of neuropathy is determined for Sjogren disease by clinical circumstances and results of electrophysiologic studies. See England et al, 2009.

Diagnosis of Late Chronic Polyneuropathy

The majority of these (evolving over years) prove to be heredofamilial or one of the infrequent sporadic mutations of the genes that are responsible for the inherited types. The observations of Dyck and coworkers (1981), referred to in the introduction to this chapter, are of interest in this respect. In a series of 205 patients who were referred to the Mayo Clinic with neuropathies of unknown cause, 86 were found to have an inherited form of disease. With appropriate genealogic data, the diagnoses of the peroneal muscular atrophy of Charcot-Marie-Tooth disease can usually be made on clinical grounds alone (high arches, distal foreleg atrophy, chronicity, etc.). Sporadic cases are more difficult. Some of the patients who have consulted us in adulthood for an obscure polyneuropathy report having had operations on their feet and toes for these reasons, but the connection to a genetic neuropathy had not been previously made. Additional hints are frequent sprained ankles and the need to tape the ankles during adolescence in order to run or participate in sports. Dyck and associates found that direct examinations of the patients' siblings, children, parents, and other close relatives were often successful in revealing a hereditary basis for the neuropathy. Sometimes, the absence of ankle reflexes or foot deformities in their relatives discloses the diagnosis.

DNA testing for the main forms of Charcot-Marie-Tooth disease is available from commercial laboratories and has increased the diagnostic certainty. A comment has already been made regarding the utility of such testing and the small number of mutations that give rise to over one-third of cases of inherited sensorimotor neuropathy. As already alluded to, individuals with a chronic demyelinating neuropathy, pes cavus or hammer toes, and a likely autosomal dominant pattern of inheritance probably have CMT1A and sequencing for PMP22 duplication may be undertaken. If there is male-to-male transmission, CMT1X is likely and the *GJB1* gene may be investigated. If both genes lack causative mutations in a demyelinating case, CMT1B is possible, especially if motor nerve conduction velocities are very slow (below 15 m/s), and the *MPZ* gene is suspect. Whether testing beyond this, which would include the *SIMPLE*, *PMP22*, and *EGR2* genes that occur in low frequency with CMT1A, is worthwhile depends on the clinical circumstances. Some cases of axonal, CMT2, will have one of several very low-frequency mutations that have been delineated. Numerous easily accessible algorithms for genetic testing have been published, similar to the guidance in the article by Saporta and colleagues, that are based on inheritance, nerve conduction velocity, and clinical features and we have not reproduced them here.

Slowly progressive polyneuropathy with features of central nervous system degeneration, particularly cerebellar ataxia, most often has a genetic basis, but a small number are found to be the result of a genetic metabolic disorder such as a leukodystrophy.

In contrast, a few young patients have come to our attention in whom a gradually progressive polyneuropathy that evolved over almost a decade turned out to be an acquired chronic inflammatory demyelinating condition rather than the expected genetic type. The absence of a family history of neuropathy and of high arches and heterogeneous slowing of both nerve conduction velocities and reductions in motor amplitudes on the nerve conduction studies provided hints to the acquired nature of the condition.

Finally, it should be conceded again that even after the most assiduous clinical and laboratory investigation, a substantial proportion of chronic neuropathies remain unexplained.

Diagnosis of Recurrent or Relapsing Polyneuropathy

Several types of neuropathies are particularly prone to recurrence: CIDP, Refsum disease, Tangier disease, and porphyria, the last of which may display attacks that recur spontaneously or are precipitated by the administration of various drugs. Repeated exposure to environmental toxins can do the same. Approximately 2 percent of patients with GBS have one or more relapses, in which the clinical and pathologic changes differ little between episodes. Some instances of mononeuritis multiplex, especially when associated with cryoglobulinemia, are also characterized by remissions and relapses over many years, although the remissions are incomplete. A common cause of relapse is the withdrawal of corticosteroids in CIDP patients who are dependent on these drugs; similarly, lapses in the treatment of paraproteinemic neuropathies cause similar fluctuations in symptoms. Enlargement of nerves may occur with repeated attacks from any of these diseases. It is self-evident that patients who have recovered from an episode of alcoholic–nutritional or toxic polyneuropathy will develop a recurrence if they again subject themselves to intoxication or nutritional deficiency.

Neuropathic symptoms that fluctuate in relation to environmental factors such as cold (cryoglobulinemia), heat (Fabry and Tangier diseases), or intermittent exposure to heavy metal or other type of poisoning may simulate an inherently relapsing polyneuropathy.

MONONEUROPATHY, MONONEUROPATHY MULTIPLEX, AND PLEXOPATHY

The diagnosis of this group of neuropathies rests on the finding of motor, reflex, and sensory changes confined to the territory of a single nerve; of several individual nerves affected in a random manner (*mononeuritis* or *mononeuropathy multiplex*); or of a plexus of nerves or part of a plexus (*plexopathy*). Certain neuropathies of this type—traceable mainly to polyarteritis nodosa or other vasculitides, leprosy, sarcoid, or diabetes—have already been discussed and are the main causes of the multiple mononeuropathy pattern. In addition to the signs of mononeuropathy multiplex, pain overlying the site of nerve infarction or distally is characteristic. The CSF protein is usually normal or slightly elevated, and in certain of these diseases there is a CSF pleocytosis (e.g., HIV, Lyme disease). Inflammatory neuropathy and the multifocal motor neuropathy caused by antibodies to G_{M1} also may be considered, because of their clinical similarity, in this group.

In identifying a process as caused by single or multiple mononeuropathies, the reader can refer to Table 46-1, which lists the roots, nerves, and muscles that are involved in particular movements, and to Table 46-4, which gives the main etiologies of mononeuropathy multiplex.

Brachial Plexus Neuropathies

Brachial plexus neuropathies, or brachial plexopathies, comprise an interesting group of neurologic disorders. Most develop without apparent cause and manifest themselves by sensorimotor derangements ascribable to one or more of the cords of the plexus. Some are a result of infiltration by tumor, compression, obscure infections (possibly viral), and the delayed effects of radiotherapy. Of obvious cause are those that result from trauma, in which the arm is hyperabducted or the shoulder violently separated from the neck. Difficult births are an important source of such traction injuries to the plexus, but their nature is also evident. Rarely, the brachial plexus or other peripheral nerves may be damaged at the time of an electrical injury, either from lightning or from a household or industrial source (see "Electrical Injuries" in Chap. 44). Direct compression of parts of the plexus by adjacent skeletal anomalies (cervical rib, fascial bands, narrowed thoracic outlet) represents another, still somewhat controversial, category of brachial plexus injury. A subcutaneous or intramuscular injection of vaccine or foreign serum was in the past sometimes followed by a brachial plexopathy, usually partial. There are also plexus lesions of presumed toxic nature, such as those following heroin injection. Granulomatous diseases such as sarcoid and secondary inflammatory processes related to lymphoma may implicate a plexus and an ischemic condition resulting from thrombosis of the subclavian artery or vein (Paget-Schrötter syndrome) is known.

More common, however, is an idiopathic *brachial plexus neuritis* of obscure origin, also called *Parsonage-Turner syndrome,* discussed further on. It stands apart as a special clinical entity, often difficult to distinguish from other types of brachial and axillary pain. Some of these cases, surprisingly, are familial; others occur in small outbreaks, but most are sporadic.

In assessing the type and degree of plexus injury, electrophysiologic testing is of particular importance. Early after a traumatic injury or other acute disease of the plexus, the only electrophysiologic abnormality may be an absence of late responses (F wave). After 7 to 10 days or more, as the process of wallerian degeneration proceeds, sensory potentials are progressively lost and the amplitudes of compound muscle action potentials are variably reduced. Fibrillation potentials, indicative of denervation, then begin to appear in the corresponding muscles. Even later, usually after several weeks, signs of reinnervation can be detected. In more chronic cases, all of these features are evident when the patient is first studied. The pattern of denervated muscles allows a distinction to be made between a plexopathy, radiculopathy, and mononeuritis multiplex based on the known patterns of muscle innervation (see Table 46-1). If denervation changes are found in the paraspinal muscles, the source of weakness and pain is in the intraspinal roots, proximal to the plexus. In this case, the sensory potentials are retained. MRI may expose metastatic deposits of the plexus, but small nodular lesions may escape detection and one then defers to the clinical data if the circumstances suggest an infiltrative or compressive lesion.

The anatomic plan of the brachial (and lumbosacral) plexus and their relations to blood vessels and bony structures (Fig. 46-5) and one of the detailed monographs on the peripheral nerves should be consulted. We often resort to the illustrations of individual nerves and plexuses that are well demonstrated in the monograph published by the Guarantors of Brain.

For orientation, it is enough to remember that the brachial plexus is formed from the anterior and posterior divisions of cervical roots 5, 6, 7, and 8 and thoracic nerve root 1. The fifth and sixth cervical roots merge into the upper trunk, the seventh root forms the middle trunk, and the eighth cervical and first thoracic roots form the lower trunk. Each trunk divides into an anterior and posterior division. The posterior divisions of each trunk unite to form the posterior cord of the plexus. The anterior divisions of the upper and middle trunks unite to form the lateral cord. The anterior division of the lower trunk forms the medial cord. Two important nerves emerge from the upper trunk (dorsal scapular nerve to the rhomboid and levator scapulae muscles, and long thoracic nerve to the anterior serratus). The posterior cord gives rise mainly to the radial nerve. The medial cord gives rise to the ulnar nerve, medial cutaneous nerve to the forearm, and medial cutaneous nerve to the upper arm. This cord lies in close relation to the subclavian artery and apex of the lung and is the part of the plexus most susceptible to traction injuries and to compression by tumors that invade the costoclavicular space. The median nerve is formed by the union of parts of the medial and lateral cords.

Lesions of the Entire Brachial Plexus

In this case, the entire arm is paralyzed and hangs uselessly at the side; the sensory loss is complete below a line extending from the shoulder diagonally downward and medially to the middle third of the upper arm. Biceps, triceps, radial, and finger reflexes are abolished. The usual cause is vehicular trauma, especially motorcycle injury.

Upper Brachial Plexus Paralysis

This is a result of injury to the distal fifth and sixth cervical roots, the most common causes of which are forceful separation of the head and shoulder during difficult delivery, pressure on the supraclavicular region during anesthesia, immune reactions to injections of foreign serum or vaccines, and idiopathic brachial plexitis (see later). The muscles affected are the biceps, deltoid, supinator longus, supraspinatus and infraspinatus, and, if the lesion is very proximal, the rhomboids. The arm hangs at the side, internally rotated and extended at the elbow. Movements of the hand and forearm are unaffected. The prognosis for spontaneous recovery is generally good, although this may be incomplete. Injuries of the upper brachial plexus and spinal roots incurred at birth (termed in older literature as Erb-Duchenne palsy) usually persist throughout life.

Lower Brachial Plexus Paralysis

This is commonly the result of traction on the abducted arm in a fall or during an operation on the axilla, infiltration or compression by tumors extending from the apex of the lung (superior sulcus or Pancoast syndrome), or compression by cervical ribs or bands. Injury may occur during birth, particularly with breech deliveries

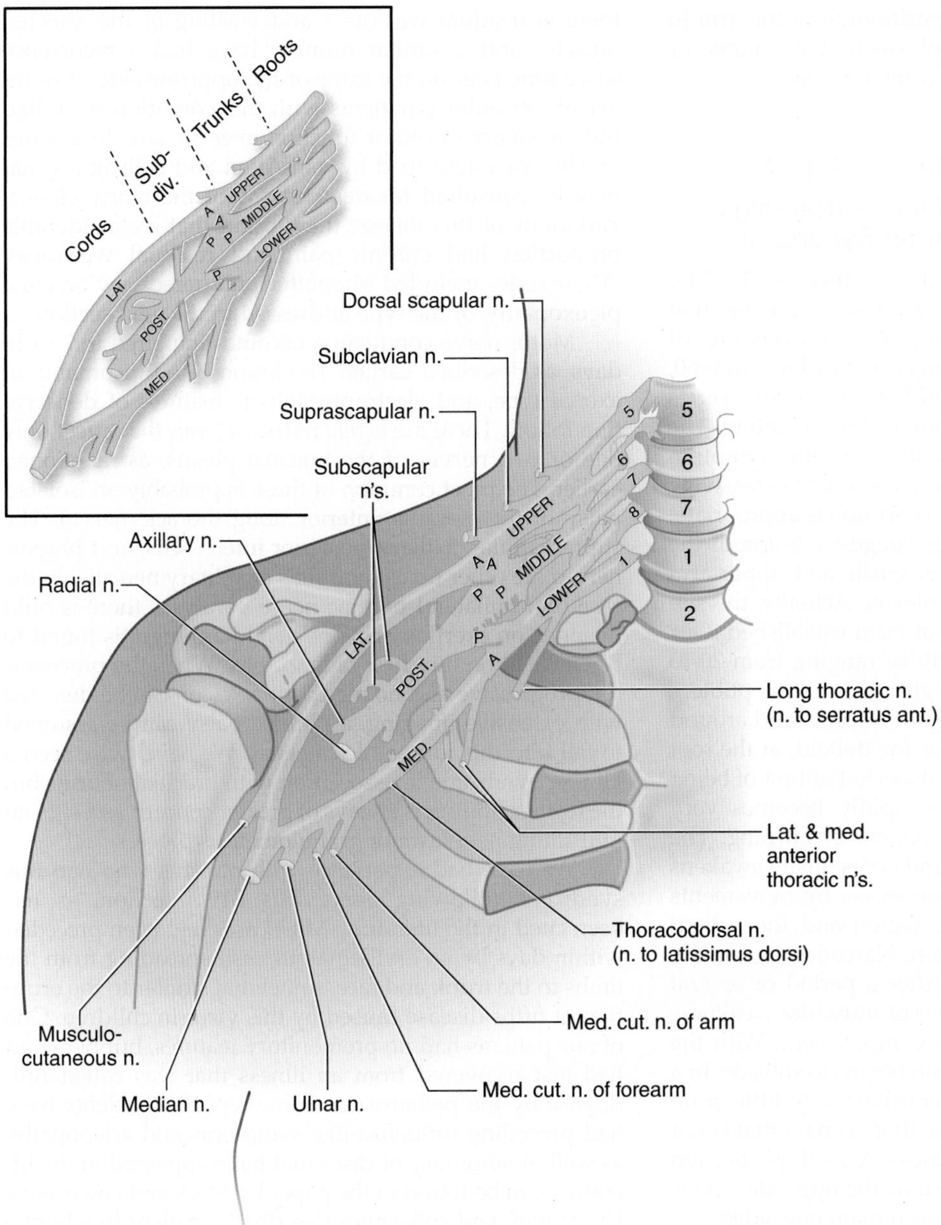

Figure 46-5. Diagram of the brachial plexus: the components of the plexus have been separated and drawn out of scale. Note that peripheral nerves arise from various components of the plexus: roots (indicated by cervical roots *5, 6, 7, 8*, and thoracic root *1*); trunks (upper, middle, lower); divisions (anterior and posterior); and cords (lateral, posterior, and medial). The median nerve arises from the heads of the lateral and medial cords. (From Haymaker and Woodhall, *Peripheral Nerve Injuries*, 2nd ed. Philadelphia, Saunders, 1953, by permission.)

(termed Dejerine-Klumpke paralysis). There is weakness and wasting of the small muscles of the hand and a characteristic clawhand deformity. Sensory loss is limited to the ulnar border of the hand and the inner forearm; if the first thoracic motor root is involved, there may be an associated paralysis of the cervical sympathetic nerves with a Horner syndrome. Invasion of the lower plexus by tumors is usually painful; postradiation lesions are more likely to cause paresthesias without pain (Lederman and Wilbourn, 1984).

Infraclavicular Lesions Involving Cords of the Brachial Plexus (See Fig. 46-5)

A lesion of the *lateral cord* causes weakness of the muscles supplied by the musculocutaneous nerve and the lateral root of the median nerve; it manifests mainly as a weakness of flexion and pronation of the forearm. The intrinsic muscles of the hand innervated by the medial root of the median nerve are spared. A lesion of the *medial cord* of the plexus causes weakness of muscles supplied by the medial root of the median nerve and the ulnar nerve. The effect is that of a combined median and ulnar nerve palsy. A lesion of the *posterior cord* results in weakness of the deltoid muscle, extensors of the elbow, wrist, and fingers, and sensory loss on the outer surface of the upper arm.

One group of infraclavicular injuries, often iatrogenic, results from damage to the subclavian or axillary vessels and the formation of pseudoaneurysms or hematomas. Small puncture wounds—as might occur with catheterization of the subclavian vein, anesthetic block of the brachial plexus, or transaxillary arteriography—are likely to produce this type of injury. As mentioned earlier, thrombosis of the vessels of the neurovascular subclavian bundle are a rare cause. Other frequent causes of injury to the cords are dislocation of the head of the humerus, direct axillary trauma (stab wounds), and supraclavicular compression during awkward positioning of the arm in an operation. Any cords of the plexus may be injured or they may be affected in various combinations.

Thoracic Outlet Syndrome

This subject is discussed extensively in Chap. 11.

Brachial Neuritis, Brachial Plexitis (Neuralgic Amyotrophy, Parsonage-Turner Syndrome)

This illness develops abruptly in an otherwise healthy individual; it may also complicate an infection, an injection of vaccine or antibiotic, childbirth, surgical procedures of any type, or the use of heroin. Magee and DeJong, in 1960, and Tsairis and coworkers, in 1972, reported large series of cases and amplified a well-known clinical picture. The term *neuralgic amyotrophy* was applied to this symptom complex by Parsonage and Turner, who wrote extensively on the subject. Their term for the condition is appropriate, as the clinical and EMG findings suggest a lesion of the peripheral nerves of the shoulder girdle and upper arm rather than in the cords of the plexus. Actually, the site of the pathologic changes has not been established. Our patients have nearly all been adults, ranging from 20 to 65 years of age. Males may be slightly more susceptible.

Beginning as an ache or deep burning in and around the shoulder that is centered over the deltoid, at the root of the neck or in the axilla, and suspected at first of being only a muscle strain, the pain rapidly becomes very intense and may include a component of burning. The onset can be remarkably abrupt and occasionally awakens the patient from sleep. It is made worse by movements that involve the muscles in the region and the patient searches for a comfortable position. Narcotics are usually required to suppress the pain. After a period of several days there is a rapid development of muscular weakness and thereafter, sensory and reflex impairment. With the development of weakness, the pain begins to subside. In a few cases, the neurologic disorder occurs with little or no antecedent pain. Possibly in some there is pain that is not followed by demonstrable weakness. A small proportion of cases are bilateral at the outset, or the opposite side is affected weeks later but most cases remain one-sided.

Unlike restricted radicular lesions, which almost never cause complete paralysis of a muscle, certain muscles involved in brachial neuritis, such as the serratus anterior, deltoid, biceps, or triceps, may be totally or almost paralyzed, sometimes in isolation (see later). Rarely are all the muscles of the arm involved (4 of 99 cases of Tsairis et al). Most of the neurologic deficits in our patients have been localized around the shoulder and upper arm. Either the biceps or triceps reflex may be abolished. In a few cases there has been an additional median, radial, anterior, or posterior interosseous nerve palsy that can be detected and isolated by EMG to a site distal to the plexus (see later). Affected patients usually have no fever, leukocytosis, or increased sedimentation rate. Occasionally there is a mild pleocytosis (10 to 50 white blood cells/mm^3) and slightly increased protein in the CSF, but most cases have a normal formula and sampling of CSF is not necessary for diagnosis.

Recovery of paralysis and restoration of sensation are usually complete in 6 to 12 weeks, but sometimes not for a year or longer. In approximately 10 percent of cases there is residual weakness and wasting of the affected muscles and a similar number have had a recurrence some time later on the same or the opposite side. A number of our elderly patients with this condition have had little recovery of motor function over 5 years. In a series of 246 cases described by van Alfen and colleagues that may be consulted for descriptions of the many clinical variations of this illness, they found that a considerable proportion had chronic pain and residual weakness. (Their series included idiopathic and hereditary brachial pleoxopathy, of the type addressed in the next section.

Motor nerve conduction becomes impaired in 7 to 10 days, as described earlier. The lesions are presumably of axonal type, and electrophysiologic features of denervation follow. There are *highly restricted forms* that affect only one or two nerves of the brachial plexus, as mentioned earlier. The most common of these is probably an isolated palsy of the serratus anterior (long thoracic nerve). The suprascapular, axillary, posterior interosseus, and phrenic nerves are other occasional sites of solitary neuritis. In the case of a unilateral phrenic nerve paralysis, there is mild dyspnea on exertion and one hemidiaphragm is found to be elevated on the chest radiographs. When the process is not progressive and no mediastinal lesion can be detected with extensive imaging, a phrenic palsy can be assumed to fall into this idiopathic category. We have twice seen a Horner syndrome in association with brachial neuritis but the former finding is always of greater concern as a sign an infiltrating neoplasm or granulomatous process.

We have had experience with patients who had this syndrome following parvovirus B19 infection, as has been cited in the literature. Most cases had been preceded within days by an erythematous rash spreading from the limbs to the trunk and face, somewhat similar to the eruption of fifths disease caused by this virus in children. One of our patients had no premonitory features, but her child had just recovered from an illness that was called fifth disease by the pediatrician. Some reported patients have had preceding influenza-like symptoms and adenopathy as well. A summary of cases that have appeared in the literature can be found in the paper by Maas and coworkers. Duchowny and colleagues described a patient in whom a typical brachial neuritis occurred as part of a febrile illness that proved to be caused by a CMV infection and the same has been observed (albeit rarely) in patients with AIDS. A few outbreaks of brachial neuritis have been recorded and prompted the suggestion that the Coxsackievirus was the cause. Whether Lyme infection can cause brachial neuritis is unsettled, but we have seen at least one instance that was more of a cervical radiculopathy—there was a pleocytosis in the CSF. The therapeutic use of interleukin-2 and interferon has apparently precipitated a few cases. In the past, when animal antisera were in common use, this entity was frequent; in the modern era it has been seen rarely after injection of tetanus toxoid, typhoid-paratyphoid vaccine, and triple vaccine (pertussis, diphtheria, and tetanus).

Plexitis also occurs as an uncommon idiopathic complication of the *postpartum state* (Lederman and Wilbourn, 1996). Some of these are repetitive or bilateral and some are familial, but otherwise the plexopathy has no distinguishing features from the idiopathic type. The heredofamilial variety is described later.

One must differentiate idiopathic brachial plexitis from the following conditions: (1) spondylosis or ruptured disc with root compression, particularly the C5 and C6 roots, in which paralysis is rarely as severe as it is in plexitis; (2) brachialgia from bursitis, labral tear, or rotator cuff syndrome; (3) polymyalgia rheumatica; (4) entrapment neuropathies, particularly of the subscapular or dorsal scapular nerve; (5) carcinomatous plexopathy; (6) radiation plexopathy; and (7) sarcoid and other granulomatous infiltrations. Dissection of the vertebral artery may rarely simulate the pain and weakness of brachial neuritis (Berrior et al).

Pathologic data are sparse, but Suarez and coworkers (1996) have reported collections of intense mononuclear inflammation in fascicles of the plexus obtained by biopsy. Perivascular lymphocytes were found in the endoneurial space and, less so, in the epineurium.

Therapy is purely symptomatic, but we have usually embarked on a course of steroids and, in a few cases, other immunosuppressants, when the illness continued to advance over many weeks. Corticosteroids sometimes have a beneficial effect on pain and have also been successful in some cases of lumbosacral plexitis. Uncontrolled observations by van Eijk and coworkers on the of the use of prednisolone in 50 patients has suggested that pain relief and motor outcome were better than in untreated patients.

Heredofamilial Brachial Plexopathy (Hereditary Neuralgic Amyotrophy)

Rarely, an acute and painful *recurrent brachial neuropathy* occurs in a familial pattern. The inheritance is autosomal dominant and the attacks, which are painless, occur most commonly in the second and third decades of life. The authors have observed this syndrome in 3 generations of a family, some members having had 5 attacks at ages ranging from 3 to 45 years. We have had experience with the contemporaneous onset of brachial plexitis in an adult brother and sister who shared the same household but had no family history of a similar problem. A shared exposure to viral or environmental agents was suspected. Lower cranial nerve involvement and mononeuropathies in other limbs are conjoined in some instances (see Taylor). Attacks may be spontaneous or precipitated by compression, slight stretching, or minor trauma to the region of the plexus. In one family, attacks have been triggered by events that activate the immune system (fevers, infections, surgical procedures). In several such families, there are subtle characteristic facial features including narrowed and horizontally positioned eyes and a long nasal bridge (Modigliani face). Cleft palate and unusual skin folds and creases have been observed in other kindreds (Jeannet et al).

The clinical course is usually benign with good recovery of each episode, but residual deficits may accumulate after recurrent attacks. In Dutch families affected by the disease, Alfen and colleagues have pointed out that some patients experience a more chronic and undulating course rather than discrete attacks.

Madrid and Bradley examined the sural nerves from two patients with familial recurrent brachial neuropathy. In teased single nerve fibers they found sausage-like segments of thickened myelin and redundant loops of myelin with secondary constriction of the axon. In addition, nerve fibers showed a considerable degree of segmental demyelination and remyelination. They called this aberration of myelin formation "tomaculous" neuropathy (from *tomaculum*, "sausage"), changes that are now appreciated as valid but relatively nonspecific.

The genetic basis for this is a mutation of SEPN1. Another cause of recurrent brachial palsy, or of derivative syndromes involving nerves in the arms, is HNPP, discussed in the earlier section on inherited neuropathies and due to a deletion in the *PMP22* gene ("Hereditary Neuropathy With Pressure Palsies"). As commented there, the gene defect is also on chromosome 17, but it is not the one associated with familial brachial neuritis (see Chance et al). Some confusion has arisen because CMT1A, HNPP, and the familial brachial palsy disease all have chromosome 17 defects. Pressure palsies in HNPP are painless and there is usually an underlying and slowly advancing polyneuropathy. In some families, such as the one reported by Thomas and Ormerod, the distinction between hereditary neuralgic amyotrophy (HNA) and HNPP was unclear as the recurrent brachial plexopathies were painful (consistent with the former), but there was also a painless multifocal sensory neuropathy (consistent with the latter).

Brachial Neuropathy following Radiation Therapy

This is usually a complication of irradiation of the axilla for carcinoma of the breast. Stoll and Andrews studied a group of 117 such patients who were treated with high-voltage, small-field therapy and had received either 6,300 or 5,775 cGy in divided doses. Of those receiving the larger dose, 73 percent developed weakness and sensory loss in the hand and fingers between 4 and 30 months after treatment, most of them after 12 months. In 1 autopsied case, the brachial plexus was ensheathed in dense fibrous tissue; distal to this zone, both myelin and axons had disappeared (wallerian degeneration), presumably as a result of entrapment of nerves in fibrous tissue; possibly a vascular factor was also operative.

Kori and coworkers, who analyzed the brachial plexus lesions in 100 patients with cancer, also found that doses exceeding 6,000 cGy were associated with radiation damage. Usually the upper plexus was involved and was sometimes associated with a painless lymphedema. Myokymic discharges and fasciculations are particularly suggestive of radiation damage. In patients who received lower doses, the development of brachial plexopathy usually indicated tumor infiltration; these lesions affected the lower plexus more than the upper; they were often painful and accompanied by Horner syndrome (see Lederman and Wilbourn, 1984). Rarely, radiation may give rise many years later to a malignant tumor of nerve or the surrounding connective tissue, a sarcoma in 2 cases familiar to us.

Herpes Zoster Plexitis, Neuritis, and Ganglionitis (See Chap. 33)

This organism is perhaps the best defined infectious cause of the above listed syndromes, but its identification is usually obvious on the basis of the skin eruption of shingles. Cases are known in which radicular pain precedes the eruption by many days or in which shingles do not appear, thereby simulating a herniated disc (zoster sine herpete). These conditions are discussed with the other viral infections of the nervous system in Chap. 33.

Brachial Mononeuropathies (See Table 46-1)

Long Thoracic Nerve (of Bell)

This nerve is derived from the fifth, sixth, and seventh cervical nerves and supplies the serratus anterior muscle, which fixates the lateral scapula to the chest wall. Paralysis of this muscle results in an inability to raise the arm over the head and winging of the medial border of the scapula when the outstretched arm is pushed forward against resistance. The nerve is injured most commonly by carrying heavy weights on the shoulder or by strapping the shoulder to the operating table. As stated earlier, the neuropathy may be the only affected nerve in a brachial plexus neuropathy of either the inherited or idiopathic variety (Phillips).

Suprascapular Nerve

This nerve is derived from the fifth (mainly) and sixth cervical nerves and supplies the supraspinatus and infraspinatus muscles. Lesions may be recognized by the presence of atrophy of these muscles and weakness of the first 15 degrees of abduction (supraspinatus) and of external rotation of the arm at the shoulder joint (infraspinatus). The latter muscle is tested by having the patient flex the forearm and then, pinning the elbow to the side, asking him to swing the forearm backward against resistance. This nerve is often involved as a result of a herniated C5-C6 disc (see Chap. 11), or as part of a brachial plexus neuropathy of either the sporadic or inherited type. It may be affected during infectious illnesses and may be injured in gymnasts, or as a result of local pressure from carrying heavy objects on the shoulder ("meatpacker's neuropathy"). An entrapment syndrome has also been reported; it is characterized by pain and weakness on external rotation of the shoulder joint with atrophy of the infraspinatus muscle (Table 46-8). Decompression of the nerve where it enters the spinoglenoid notch relieves the condition.

Axillary Nerve

This nerve arises from the posterior cord of the brachial plexus (mainly from the C5 root, with a smaller contribution from C6) and supplies the teres minor and deltoid muscles. It may be involved in dislocations of the shoulder joint, fractures of the neck of the humerus, disc protrusion, and brachial neuritis; in other instances, no cause may be apparent. The anatomic diagnosis depends on recognition of paralysis of abduction of the arm (in testing this function, the angle between the side of the chest and the arm must be greater than 15 degrees and less than 90 degrees), wasting of the deltoid muscle, and slight impairment of sensation over the outer aspect of the shoulder.

Musculocutaneous Nerve

The origin of this nerve is from the fifth and sixth cervical roots. It is a branch of the lateral cord of the brachial plexus and innervates the biceps brachii, brachialis, and coracobrachialis muscles. Lesions of the nerve result in wasting of these muscles and weakness of flexion of the supinated forearm. Sensation may be impaired along the radial and volar aspects of the forearm (lateral cutaneous nerve). Isolated lesions of this nerve are usually the result of fracture of the humerus.

Table 46-8

ENTRAPMENT NEUROPATHIES

NERVE	SITE OF ENTRAPMENT
Suprascapular	Spinoglenoid notch
Lower trunk or medial cord of branchial plexus	Cervical rib or band at thoracic outlet
Median	
Wrist	Carpal tunnel
Elbow	Between heads of pronator teres (pronator syndrome)[a]
Ulnar	
Wrist	Guyon's canal (ulnar tunnel)
Elbow	Bicipital groove, cubital tunnel
Posterior interosseous nerve	Radial tunnel—at point of entrance into supinator muscle (arcade of Frohse)[a]
Lateral femoral cutaneous (meralgia paresthetica)	Inguinal ligament
Obturator	Obturator canal[a]
Posterior tibial	Tarsal tunnel; medial malleolus–flexor retinaculum[a]
Interdigital plantar (Morton metatarsalgia)	Plantar fascia: heads of third and fourth metatarsals

[a]These are not well-defined syndromes and may be subject to overdiagnosis. Alternative diagnoses should be considered. For example, multifocal motor neuropathy and brachial neuritis account for cases that may be incorrectly attributed to radial tunnel syndrome and cases of distal sensory neuropathy may be attributed to tarsal tunnel syndrome.

Radial Nerve

This nerve is derived from the sixth to eighth (mainly the seventh) cervical roots and is the distal extension of the posterior cord of the brachial plexus. It innervates the triceps, brachioradialis, and supinator muscles, and continues below the elbow as the posterior interosseous nerve, which innervates the extensor muscles of the wrist and fingers, the main abductor of the thumb (the abductor pollicis longus, which is easier to isolate than the median nerve innervated abductor pollicis brevis), and the extensors of the fingers at both joints. A complete proximal radial nerve lesion results in paralysis of extension of the elbow, flexion of the elbow with the forearm midway between pronation and supination (a result of paralysis of the brachioradialis muscle), supination of the forearm, extension of the wrist and fingers, and extension and abduction of the thumb in the plane of the palm. If the lesion is confined to the posterior interosseous nerve, only the extensors of the wrist and fingers are affected. Sensation is impaired over the posterior aspects of the forearm and over a small area on the radial aspect of the dorsum of the hand.

The radial nerve may be compressed in the axilla ("crutch" palsy), but more frequently at a lower point, where the nerve winds around the humerus (see Table 46-8); pressure palsies incurred during an alcoholic stupor and fractures of the humerus commonly injure the nerve at the site of injury. It is susceptible to lead intoxication and is frequently involved as part of brachial neuritis and mononeuritis multiplex.

Median Nerve

This nerve originates from the fifth cervical to the first thoracic roots but mainly from the sixth cervical root and is formed by the union of the medial and lateral cords of the brachial plexus. It innervates the pronators of the forearm, long finger flexors, and abductor and opponens muscles of the thumb and is a sensory nerve to the palmar aspect of the hand. Complete interruption of the median nerve results in inability to pronate the forearm or flex the hand in a radial direction, paralysis of flexion of the index finger and terminal phalanx of the thumb, weakness of flexion of the remaining fingers, weakness of opposition and abduction of the thumb in the plane at a right angle to the palm (abductor and flexor pollicis brevis), and sensory impairment over the radial two-thirds of the palm and dorsum of the distal phalanges of the index and third fingers. The nerve may be injured in the axilla by dislocation of the shoulder and in any part of its course by stab, gunshot, or other types of wounds, and like the radial nerve, is often a component of the mononeuritis multiplex syndrome. Incomplete lesions of the median nerve between the axilla and wrist may result in causalgia (see further on).

Carpal Tunnel Syndrome (See also Chap. 11.) Compression of the median nerve at the wrist (*carpal tunnel syndrome*) is the most common disorder affecting the median nerve and the most frequent nerve entrapment syndrome. The problem arises usually as a result of excessive use of the hands and occupational microtrauma. Infiltration of the transverse carpal ligament with amyloid (as occurs in multiple myeloma and amyloidosis) or thickening of connective tissue in rheumatoid arthritis, acromegaly, mucopolysaccharidosis, and hypothyroidism are less commonly identified causes. It is also common for the condition to make its appearance during pregnancy. In elderly individuals, the cause of the carpal tunnel syndrome is often not apparent. According to Kremer and colleagues, it was McArdle, in 1949, who first suggested that the cause of this syndrome was compression of the median nerve at the wrist and that the symptoms would be relieved by division of the flexor retinaculum forming the ventral wall of the carpal tunnel. Dysesthesias and pain in the fingers, referred to for many years as "acroparesthesia" came to be recognized as a syndrome of median nerve compression only in the early 1950s.

The syndrome is essentially a sensory one; the loss or impairment of superficial sensation affects the palmar aspect of the thumb and the index and middle fingers (especially the index finger) and may or may not split the ring finger (splitting does not occur with a plexus or root lesion). The paresthesias are characteristically worse during the night. As pointed out in Chap. 11, the pain in carpal tunnel syndrome may radiate into the forearm and even into the region of the biceps and rarely, to the shoulder. Weakness and atrophy of the abductor pollicis brevis and other median-innervated muscles occur in only advanced cases of compression. Electrophysiologic testing confirms the diagnosis by demonstrating prolonged sensory conduction across the wrist and explains cases in which operation has failed (see the review by Stevens).

Several provocative tests are useful. The Phalen maneuver consists of hyperflexion of the wrist for 30 to 60 s—usually performed by opposing the outer surfaces of the hands with the wrists flexed. The Tinel sign is elicited by lightly tapping the volar aspect of the wrist at the transverse carpal ligament (distal to the first wrist crease). Both of these tests are meant to elicit pain or paresthesias over the digits innervated by the median nerve. The sensitivity of these tests is close to 50 percent, but their specificity is considerably higher. Other tests involving prolonged pressure over the median nerve have been devised, but they are of uncertain value, e.g., Durken's test of the Phalen maneuver combined with digital compression of the nerve.

TREATMENT Surgical division of the carpal ligament with decompression of the nerve is curative but is required only in severe and protracted cases. Splinting of the wrist to limit flexion almost always relieves the discomfort but denies the patient the full use of the hand for some time. It is a useful temporizing measure for a few weeks, as is the injection of hydrocortisone into the carpal tunnel. Studies of oral corticosteroids give conflicting results. Treatment of an underlying condition such as arthritis, hypothyroidism and possibly diabetes, is often helpful. Some patients have benefited, paradoxically, from the stopping of corticosteroids or estrogen. Also, some practitioners favor the use of nonsteroid antiinflammatory medication, but we have been generally unimpressed with the results. Most often, splinting and local steroid injections are very satisfactory in the short-term, especially if the symptoms are of recent onset.

Another less common site of compression of the median nerve is at the elbow, where the nerve passes between the two heads of the pronator teres, or just above that point behind the bicipital aponeurosis. It gives rise to the "pronator syndrome," in which forceful pronation of the forearm produces an aching pain (see Table 46-8). There is weakness of the abductor pollicis brevis and opponens muscles and numbness of the first three digits and palm.

Ulnar Nerve

This nerve is derived from the eighth cervical and first thoracic roots. It innervates the ulnar flexor of the wrist, the ulnar half of the deep finger flexors, the adductors and abductors of the fingers, the adductor of the thumb, the third and fourth lumbricals, and muscles of the hypothenar eminence. Complete ulnar paralysis is manifest by a characteristic clawhand deformity; wasting of the small hand muscles results in hyperextension of the fingers at the metacarpophalangeal joints and flexion at the interphalangeal joints. The flexion deformity is most pronounced in the fourth and fifth fingers, as the lumbrical muscles of the second and third fingers, supplied by the median nerve, counteract the deformity. Sensory loss occurs over the fifth finger, the ulnar aspect of the fourth finger, and the ulnar border of the palm.

The ulnar nerve is vulnerable to pressure in the axilla from the use of crutches, but it is most commonly injured at the elbow by fracture or dislocation involving the joint. *Delayed ("tardive") ulnar palsy* may occur many months or years after an injury to the elbow that had resulted in a cubitus valgus deformity of the joint. Because of the deformity, the nerve is stretched in its groove over the ulnar condyle and its superficial location renders it vulnerable to compression. A shallow ulnar groove, quite apart from abnormalities of the elbow joint, may expose the nerve to compressive injury from more innocuous situations such as prolonged resting of the arm on the side of a chair or even excessive flexion of the elbow. Anterior transposition of the ulnar nerve is a simple and effective form of treatment for these types of ulnar palsies. Compression of the nerve may occur just distal to the medial epicondyle, where it runs beneath the aponeurosis of the flexor carpi ulnaris (*cubital tunnel*). Flexion at the elbow causes a narrowing of the tunnel and constriction of the nerve. This type of ulnar palsy is treated by incising the aponeurotic arch between the olecranon and medial epicondyle. Yet another site of ulnar nerve compression is in the ulnar tunnel at the wrist. Prolonged pressure on the ulnar part of the palm may result in damage to the deep palmar branch of the ulnar nerve, causing weakness of small hand muscles but no sensory loss. This site is most often implicated in patients who hold tools or implements tightly in the hand for long periods (we have seen it in machinists and professional cake decorators). The lesion is localizable by nerve conduction studies.

A syndrome of burning pain (causalgia) and associated symptoms (causalgia) may follow incomplete lesions of the ulnar nerve (or other major nerves of the limbs) and is described further on.

Lumbosacral Plexus and Crural Neuropathies

The twelfth thoracic, first to fifth lumbar, and first, second, and third sacral spinal nerve roots compose the lumbosacral plexuses and innervate the muscles of the lower extremities (Fig. 46-6 and Table 46-1). The following are the common plexus and crural nerve palsies.

Lumbosacral Plexus Lesions

Extending as it does from the upper lumbar area to the lower sacrum and passing near several lower abdominal and pelvic organs, this plexus is subject to a number of special injuries and diseases. The cause may be difficult to ascertain because the primary disease is often not within reach of the palpating fingers, either from the abdominal side or through the anus and vagina; even refined radiologic techniques may not reveal it. Diagnosis involves exclusion of spinal root (cauda equina) lesions by EMG, examination of CSF if root disease is likely, and MRI of the plexus. The clinical findings help to focus studies on the appropriate part of the lumbosacral plexus.

The main effects of upper lumbar plexus lesions are weakness of flexion and adduction of the thigh and

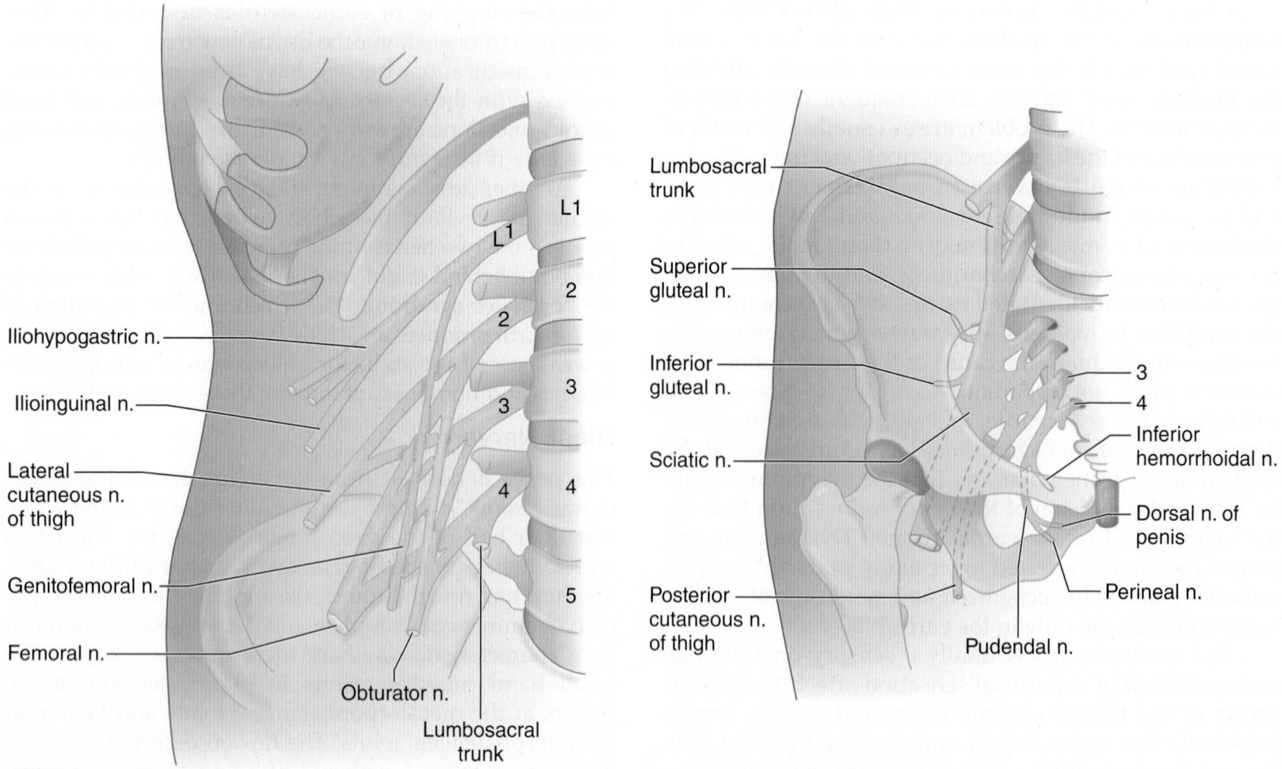

Figure 46-6. Diagram of the lumbar plexus (*left*) and the sacral plexus (*right*). The lumbosacral trunk is the liaison between the lumbar and the sacral plexuses. (From Haymaker and Woodhall, *Peripheral Nerve Injuries*, 2nd ed. Philadelphia, Saunders, 1953, by permission.)

extension of the leg, with sensory loss over the anterior thigh and leg; these effects must be distinguished from the symptoms and signs of femoral neuropathy (see later). Lower plexus lesions weaken the posterior thigh, leg, and foot muscles and abolish sensation over the first and second sacral segments (sometimes the lower sacral segments also). Lesions of the entire plexus, which occur infrequently, cause weakness or paralysis of all leg muscles with atrophy, areflexia, and anesthesia from the toes to the perianal region and autonomic loss with warm, dry skin.

The types of lesions that involve the lumbosacral plexus are rather different from those affecting the brachial plexus. Cancer, diabetes, and an idiopathic variety (Dyck et al) have dominated our material. Trauma is a rarity except with massive pelvic, spinal, and abdominal injuries because the plexus is so well protected. Occasionally, a pelvic fracture will damage the sciatic nerve as it issues from the plexus. In contrast, some part of the plexus may be damaged during surgical procedures on abdominal and pelvic organs, often for reasons that may not be entirely clear. For example, hysterectomy has on a number of occasions led to neurologic consultation in our hospitals because of numbness and weakness of the anterior thigh. Either the cords of the upper part of the plexus or the femoral nerve were compressed by retraction against the psoas muscle, or in vaginal hysterectomy (when thighs are flexed, abducted, and externally rotated) the femoral nerve was compressed against the inguinal ligament. A similar injury may be associated with vaginal delivery (see further on). Lumbar sympathectomy has also been associated with upper plexus lesions, of which the most disabling sequelae are burning pain and hypersensitivity of the anterior thigh. Appendectomy, pelvic explorations, and hernial repair may injure branches of the upper plexus (ilioinguinal, iliohypogastric, and genitofemoral nerves), with severe pain and slight sensory loss in the distribution of one of these nerves. The pain may last for months or a year or more.

The lumbar plexus may be compressed by an aortic atherosclerotic aneurysm. Usually there is pain that radiates to the hip, the anterior thigh, and occasionally the flank. Slight weakness in hip flexion and altered sensation over the anterior thigh are found on examination. Plexus involvement with tumors is commonplace and presents special difficulties in diagnosis. Carcinoma of either the cervix or prostate may seed along the perineurial lymphatics and cause pain in the groin, thigh, knee, or back without much in the way of sensory, motor, or reflex loss. The pain is more often unilateral than bilateral. The CSF and spinal canal (by MRI) are normal. Testicular, uterine, ovarian, and colonic tumors or retroperitoneal lymphomas, by extending along the paravertebral gutter, implicate various parts of the lumbosacral plexus. Instances of endometriosis that involve the plexus have also been reported, in which case pain fluctuates in parallel with the menstrual cycle (a similar condition exists that implicates only the sciatic nerve. The neurologic symptoms are projected at a distance in the leg and may or may not be confined to the territory of any one nerve. Pelvic and rectal examinations may be negative, and CT scanning and MRI may be necessary to show such lesions. If all these examinations are negative, exploratory laparotomy may have to be undertaken.

In cancer patients, it is sometimes difficult to distinguish the effects of radiation on the lumbosacral plexus from those of metastatic tumor, as is the case in relation to the brachial plexus. Again, the earliest symptom in metastatic lumbosacral plexopathy is usually pain, whereas in radiation plexopathy it is weakness (Thomas et al). Plexopathy from metastatic tumor is usually unilateral and detectable by CT scanning; radiation plexopathy is as often bilateral and changes are not evident in CT or MRI scans. Fasciculations and myokymia are more likely to be seen in patients with radiation plexopathy, which seemingly occurs more frequently in patients with diabetic neuropathy.

Sarcoidosis is another cause and may be responsive to corticosteroids.

Reference has already been made to femoral nerve injury during parturition, but other *puerperal complications* are also observed. Back pain in the latter part of pregnancy is, of course, common, but there are instances in which the patient complains of severe pain in the back of one or both thighs during labor and after delivery has numbness and weakness of the leg muscles with diminished ankle jerks. *Parturitional lumbosacral plexus injuries* occur with a frequency of 1 per 2,000 deliveries. This injury is usually unilateral and is manifest by pain in the thigh and leg and symptoms and signs of involvement of the superior gluteal and sciatic nerves (Feasby et al). The attribution of these symptoms to pressure of the fetal head on the sacral plexus(es) is conjectural. A limited plexopathy, occurring after difficult vaginal delivery, mainly impairs sensation in the perineum and sphincteric function (Ismael et al). The perineal muscles may show signs of denervation. Protrusion of an intervertebral disc may also occur during delivery and simulate plexus injury.

Idiopathic Lumbosacral Plexitis In addition to the diabetic type detailed earlier in the chapter, an idiopathic *neuralgic amyotrophy* or *lumbosacral plexitis*, analogous to the brachial variety, has been observed. Bradley and coworkers have recorded such cases and their paper can be referred to for the clinical details. After causing widespread unilateral or bilateral sensory, motor, and reflex changes in a leg, lumbosacral plexitis may leave the patient with dysesthesias as troublesome as those that follow herpes zoster (which also may occur at this level). Loss of sweating and warmth of the feet indicate interruption of autonomic fibers by lesions in peripheral nerves rather than in roots. The sedimentation rate may be elevated. Dyck and colleagues inferred an autoimmune basis from biopsy material and immunosuppressant drugs were possibly beneficial in 4 of 6 cases reported by Bradley and coworkers. The outcome is variable with complete recovery being uncommon.

Diabetic amyotrophy caused by involvement of the lumbar plexus and roots was discussed in an earlier section ("Diabetic Multiple Mononeuropathies and Radiculoplexus Neuropathy").

Lateral Cutaneous Nerve of the Thigh (Meralgia Paresthetica)

This sensory nerve originates from the second and third lumbar roots and supplies the anterolateral aspect of the thigh from the level of the inguinal ligament almost to the knee. The nerve penetrates the psoas muscle, crosses the iliacus, and passes into the thigh by coursing between the attachments of the lateral part of the inguinal ligament to just anterior to the anterior superior iliac spine. Compression (entrapment) may occur at the point where it passes between the two prongs of attachment of the inguinal ligament.

Compression of the nerve results in uncomfortable paresthesias and sensory impairment in its cutaneous distribution, a common condition known as *meralgia paresthetica* (*meros*, "thigh"). Usually numbness and mild sensitivity of the skin are the only symptoms, but occasionally there is a persistent distressing burning pain. Perception of touch and pinprick are reduced in the territory of the nerve; there is no weakness of the quadriceps or diminution of the knee jerk. The symptoms are characteristically worsened in certain positions and after prolonged standing or walking. Occasionally, for an obese person, sitting is the most uncomfortable position. Obesity, pregnancy, and diabetes mellitus may be contributory factors. Most often the neuropathy is unilateral, but Ecker and Woltman found 20 percent of their patients to have bilateral symptoms.

Most of our patients with meralgia paresthetica request no treatment once they learn of its benign character. Weight loss and adjustment of restrictive clothing or correction of habitual postures that might compress the nerve are sometimes helpful. A few with the most painful symptoms have demanded a neurectomy or section of the nerve, but it is always wise to perform a lidocaine block first, so that the patient can decide whether the persistent numbness is preferable. In one specimen of nerve obtained at operation, we found a discrete traumatic neuroma. Corticosteroid injections at the point of entrapment may have helped in a few cases, but this has not been studied in a systematic way.

Obturator Nerve

This nerve arises from the third and fourth and to a lesser extent the second lumbar roots. It supplies the adductors of the thigh and contributes to the innervation of the internal and external rotators. The adductors have the added function of contributing to flexing the hip. The nerve may be injured by the fetal head or forceps during the course of a difficult labor or compressed by an obturator hernia. Rarely, it is affected with diabetes, polyarteritis nodosa, and osteitis pubis and by retroperitoneal spread of carcinoma of the cervix, uterus, and other tumors (Rogers et al).

Femoral Nerve

This nerve is formed from the second, third, and fourth lumbar roots. Within the pelvis it passes along the lateral border of the psoas muscle and enters the thigh beneath the Poupart ligament, lateral to the femoral artery. Branches arising within the pelvis supply the iliacus and psoas muscles. Just below the Poupart ligament the nerve splits into anterior and posterior divisions. The former supplies the pectineus and sartorius muscles and carries sensation from the anteromedial surface of the thigh; the posterior division provides the motor innervation to the quadriceps and the cutaneous innervation to the medial side of the leg from the knee to the internal malleolus. The distinction between femoral neuropathy and a third lumbar root lesion is made by detecting weakness of the hip adductor (innervated by the obturator nerve) in the case of the root lesion.

Following injury to the femoral nerve, there is weakness of extension at the knee, wasting of the quadriceps muscle, and failure of fixation of the knee. The knee jerk is abolished. If the nerve is injured proximal to the origin of the branches to the iliacus and psoas muscles, there is additionally weakness of hip flexion.

The most common cause of femoral neuropathy is diabetes. The nerve may also be involved by pelvic tumors. Not uncommon is injury to the nerve during pelvic operations. Usually this is the result of improper placement of retractors, which may compress the nerve directly or indirectly by undue pressure on the psoas muscle. Bleeding into the iliacus muscle or the retroperitoneum, observed in patients receiving anticoagulants and in hemophilia patients, is a relatively common cause of isolated femoral neuropathy (Goodfellow et al). The presenting symptom of iliacus hematoma is pain in the groin spreading to the lumbar region or thigh, in response to which the patient assumes a characteristic posture of flexion and lateral rotation of the hip. A palpable mass in the iliac fossa and the signs of femoral nerve compression (quadriceps weakness and loss of knee jerk) follow in a day or two. Infarction of the nerve may occur in the course of diabetes mellitus and polyarteritis nodosa. Not infrequently acute femoral neuropathy is of indeterminate cause.

Sciatic Nerve (See also Chap. 11)

This nerve is derived from the fourth and fifth lumbar and first and second sacral roots, for which reason a ruptured disc at any of these levels may simulate sciatic neuropathy (sciatica). The sciatic nerve supplies motor innervation to the hamstring muscles and all the muscles below the knee through its two divisions, the tibial and peroneal nerves (see later); the sciatic nerve conveys sensory impulses from the posterior aspect of the thigh, the posterior and lateral aspects of the leg, and the entire sole. In complete sciatic paralysis, the knee cannot be flexed and all muscles below the knee are paralyzed. Weakness of gluteal muscles and pain in the buttock and posterior thigh point to nerve involvement in the pelvis. Lesions beyond the sciatic notch spare the gluteal muscles but not the hamstrings. Partial compressive lesions are more common and tend to involve peroneal-innervated muscles more than tibial ones, giving the impression of a peroneal palsy.

Rupture of one of the lower lumbar intervertebral discs is the most common cause of sciatica, although it does, of course, not directly involve the sciatic nerve. The associated motor and sensory findings allow localization of the root compression (L4-L5 disc compressing L5 root: pain in posterolateral thigh and leg with numbness over the inner foot and weakness of dorsiflexion of the foot and toes; L5-S1 disc compressing S1 root: pain in posterior thigh and leg, numbness of lateral foot, weakness of foot plantar flexion and loss of ankle jerk), as discussed in Chap. 11.

The sciatic nerve is commonly injured by fractures of the pelvis or femur, fracture/dislocation of the hip, gunshot wounds of the buttock and thigh, and the injection of toxic substances into the lower gluteal region. Total hip arthroplasty is another cause. Tumors of the pelvis (sarcomas, lipomas) or gluteal region may compress the nerve. Sitting for a long period with legs flexed and abducted (lotus position) under the influence of narcotics or barbiturates or lying flat on a hard surface in a sustained stupor may severely injure one or both sciatic nerves or branches thereof. The nerve may be involved by neurofibromas and infections and by ischemic necrosis in diabetes mellitus and polyarteritis nodosa. Cryptogenic forms of sciatica occur and in a referral practice are more frequent than those of identifiable cause. Partial lesions of the sciatic nerve occasionally result in causalgia (see further on).

The common Morton neuroma, typically between the third and fourth metatarsals, causes interdigital or intermetatarsal pain and can be detected by MRI. It is subject to surgical section. Also mentioned here is a distressingly painful compression of the plantar branches of the sciatic nerve.

Common Peroneal (Fibular) Nerve

Just above the popliteal fossa the sciatic nerve divides into the tibial nerve (*medial*, or *internal*, *popliteal nerve*) and the common peroneal nerve (*lateral*, or *external*, *popliteal nerve*). The latter swings around the head of the fibula to the anterior aspect of the leg, giving off the *superficial peroneal nerve* that provides musculocutaneous branches (to the peroneal muscles) and to the *deep peroneal nerve* (formerly called *anterior tibial nerve*). Branches of the latter supply the dorsiflexors of the foot and toes (anterior tibialis, extensor digitorum longus and brevis, and extensor hallucis longus muscles) and carry sensory fibers from the dorsum of the foot and lateral aspect of the lower half of the leg. There was weakness of dorsiflexion of the foot (foot-drop) in all of the 116 cases of common peroneal neuropathy reported by Katirji and Wilbourn, and numbness of the dorsum of the foot was present in most cases. Weakness of eversion of the foot is usually demonstrable; because inversion is a function of the L5 root and the tibial nerve, it is spared in peroneal palsy, thereby allowing a distinction between foot-drop at the two sites. (Foot eversion should be tested with the ankle passively dorsiflexed.) Pain is variable.

Pressure during an operation or sleep or from tight plaster casts, obstetric stirrups, habitual and prolonged crossing of the legs while seated, and tight knee boots are the most frequent causes of injury to the common peroneal nerve. The point of compression of the nerve is where it passes over the head of the fibula. Emaciation in patients with cancer or AIDS increases the incidence of these types of compressive injuries. The nerve may also be affected in diabetic neuropathy and injured by fractures of the upper end of the fibula. A Baker cyst, which consists of inflamed synovium extending into the retropopliteal space, may compress the nerve, and it may be damaged by muscle swelling or small hematomas behind the knee in asthenic athletes. The prognosis is generally good in cases of partial paralysis.

Tibial Nerve

This, the other of the two divisions of the sciatic nerve (it divides in the popliteal fossa), supplies all of the calf muscles—i.e., the plantar flexors and invertors of the foot and toes—after which it continues as the posterior tibial nerve. This nerve passes through the tarsal tunnel, an osseofibrous channel that runs along the medial aspect of the calcaneus and is roofed by the flexor retinaculum. The tunnel also contains the tendons of the tibialis posterior, flexor digitorum longus, and flexor hallucis longus muscles and the vessels to the foot. The posterior tibial nerve terminates under the flexor retinaculum and divides into medial and lateral plantar nerves (supplying the small muscles of the foot).

Complete interruption of the tibial nerve results in a calcaneovalgus deformity of the foot, which can no longer be plantar-flexed and inverted. There is loss of sensation over the plantar aspect of the foot.

The posterior tibial nerve may be compressed in the *tarsal tunnel* (an entrapment syndrome as discussed below) by thickening of the tendon sheaths or the adjacent connective tissues or by osteoarthritic changes. Neuromuscular experts have expressed concern that this is one of the over diagnosed entrapment syndromes. Tingling pain and burning over the sole of the foot develop after standing or walking for a long time. Pain in the ankle or foot is added in some cases and the pain may be referred proximally along the sciatic nerve. Pressure over the nerve in the inferior malleolar region produces pain, which radiates to the terminal distributions of the nerve. Usually there is no motor deficit. Relief is obtained by severing the flexor retinaculum.

Entrapment Neuropathies

Reference has been made in several places in the preceding pages to the most frequently encountered entrapment neuropathies. A nerve passing through a tight canal is trapped and subjected to constant movement or pressure, forces not applicable to nerves elsewhere. The epineurium and perineurium become greatly thickened, strangling the nerve, with the additional possibility of demyelination. Function is gradually impaired, sensory more than motor, and the symptoms fluctuate with activity and rest. The most frequently compressed nerves are the median, ulnar, peroneal, tibial, and plantar in approximately that order. It is well to keep in mind the systemic processes that enhance pressure palsies by infiltration of the nerve or surrounding tissues. The main ones are hypothyroidism, amyloid, pregnancy, and hereditary liability to pressure palsies.

Table 46-8 lists the common entrapment neuropathies and the locations of compression. Detailed accounts of these disorders are contained in the monographs of Dawson and colleagues and of Asbury and Gilliat.

Complex Regional Pain Syndrome; Causalgia, Reflex Sympathetic Dystrophy

(See Chaps. 8 and 11)

One unfortunate result of partial injury to a peripheral nerve is the delayed appearance of severe pain roughly in the distribution of the affected nerve. This complex problem, which consists of burning pain termed *causalgia* and associated local trophic and autonomic changes that are subsumed under the term *reflex sympathetic dystrophy*, is discussed further in Chap. 8 in the context of other pain syndromes and in Chap. 11.

Traumatic Interruption of Nerves

Although the management of such lesions is best delegated to specialized neurosurgeons, several aspects involve the neurologist. Surgical advances have allowed the successful apposition of severed nerve ends. The current recommendation is that end-to-end suturing of the stumps within 72 h should be undertaken to repair a sharp and clean division. In cases where the nerve is found on exploration to be bluntly severed with ragged ends, most surgeons recommend tacking the free ends to adjacent connective tissue planes and attempting the repair in 2 to 4 weeks. Most injuries, however, are blunt and retain some continuity of the nerve. If such continuity across the traumatized region can be demonstrated by electrophysiologic examination, operation is unnecessary. In the absence of improvement in the clinical and electrophysiologic features after several months (up to 6 months for plexus lesions), surgical repair may facilitate limited healing. Pain that appears months or years after injury suggests the development of a neuroma at the site of nerve section; a Tinel sign at that site aids in identifying this problem.

References

Adams RD, Shahani BT, Young RR: A severe pansensory familial neuropathy. *Trans Am Neurol Assoc* 98:67, 1973.

Alfen N, Van Engelen BG, Reinders JW, et al: The natural history of hereditary neurologic amyotrophy in the Dutch population. Two distinct types? *Brain* 12:718, 2000.

Ali Z, Carroll M, Robertson KP, Fowler CJ: The extent of small fibre sensory neuropathy in diabetics with plantar foot ulceration. *J Neurol Neurosurg Psychiatry* 52:94, 1989.

Amato AA, Russell JA: *Neuromuscular Disorders*. New York, McGraw-Hill, 2008.

American Academy of Neurology AIDS Task Force: Research criteria for diagnosis of chronic inflammatory demyelinating polyneuropathy (CIDP). *Neurology* 41:617, 1991.

Andrade C, Canijo M, Klein D, Kaelin A: The genetic aspect of the familial amyloidotic polyneuropathy: Portuguese type of paramyloidosis. *Humangenetik* 7:163, 1969.

Apfel SC, Schwartz S, Adornato BT, et al: Efficacy and safety of recombinant human nerve growth factor in patients with diabetic polyneuropathy: A randomized controlled trial. rhNGF Clinical Investigator Group. *JAMA* 284:2215, 2000.

Araki S, Mawatari S, Ohta M, et al: Polyneurotic amyloidosis in a Japanese family. *Arch Neurol* 18:593, 1968.

Asbury AK, Aldredge H, Hershberg R, et al: Oculomotor palsy in diabetes mellitus. A clinicopathologic study. *Brain* 93:555, 1970.

Asbury AK, Arnason BGW, Adams RD: The inflammatory lesion in acute idiopathic polyneuritis. *Medicine (Baltimore)* 48:173, 1969.

Asbury AK, Cornblath DR: Assessment of current diagnostic criteria for Guillain-Barré syndrome. *Ann Neurol* 27:S21, 1990.

Asbury AK, Fields HL: Pain due to peripheral nerve damage: An hypothesis. *Neurology* 34:1587, 1984.

Asbury AK, Gilliat RW (eds): *Peripheral Nerve Disorders*. London, Butterworth, 1984.

Asbury AK, Picard EH, Baringer JR: Sensory perineuritis. *Arch Neurol* 26:302, 1972.

Asbury A, Thomas PK: *Peripheral Nerve Disorders*, 2nd ed. London, Butterworth & Heinemann, 1995.

Asbury A, Victor M, Adams RD: Uremic polyneuropathy. *Arch Neurol* 8:113, 1963.

Attarian S, Azulay J, Chabrol B, et al: Neonatal lower motor neuron syndrome associated with maternal neuropathy with anti-G_{M1} IgG. *Neurology* 63:379, 2004.

Austin JH: Observations on the syndrome of hypertrophic neuritis (the hypertrophic interstitial radiculoneuropathies). *Medicine (Baltimore)* 35:187, 1956.

Barnhill RL, McDougall AC: Thalidomide: Use and possible mode of action in reactional lepromatous leprosy and in various other conditions. *J Am Acad Dermatol* 7:317, 1982.

Barohn RJ, Kissel JT, Warmolts JR, Mendell JR: Chronic inflammatory polyradiculoneuropathy: Clinical characteristics, course, and recommendations for diagnostic criteria. *Arch Neurol* 46:878, 1989.

Barohn RJ, Sahenk Z, Warmolts JR, Mendell JR: The Bruns-Garland syndrome (diabetic amyotrophy). Revisited 100 years later. *Arch Neurol* 48:1130, 1991.

Bendixen BH, Younger DS, Hair LS, et al: Cholesterol emboli neuropathy. *Neurology* 42:428, 1992.

Berroir S, Sarazin M, Amarenco P: Vertebral artery dissection presenting as neuralgic amyotrophy. *J Neurol Neurosurg Psychiatry* 72:522, 2002.

Bolton CF: Peripheral neuropathies associated with chronic renal failure. *Can J Neurol Sci* 7:89, 1980.

Bouldin TW, Hall CO, Krigman MR: Pathology of disulfiram neuropathy. *Neuropathol Appl Neurobiol* 6:155, 1980.

Bradley WG, Chad D, Verghese JP, et al: Painful lumbosacral plexopathy, with elevated sedimentation rate: A treatable inflammatory syndrome. *Ann Neurol* 15:457, 1984.

Brady RO, Schiffman R: Clinical features of and recent advances in therapy for Fabry disease. *JAMA* 284:2771, 2000.

Brannagan TH: Current treatments of chronic immune-mediated demyelinating polyneuropathies. *Muscle Nerve* 39:563, 2009.

Brannagan TH, Pradhan A, Heiman-Patterson T, et al: High-dose cyclophosphamide without stem-cell rescue for refractory CIDP. *Neurology* 58:1856, 2002.

Brashear A, Unverzaght FW, Farber MO, et al: Ethylene oxide neurotoxicity: A cluster of 12 nurses with peripheral and central nervous system toxicity. *Neurology* 46:992, 1996.

Brostoff SW, Levit S, Powers JM: Induction of experimental allergic neuritis with a peptide from myelin P2 basic protein. *Nature* 268:752, 1977.

Brown MJ, Greene DA: Diabetic neuropathy: Pathophysiology and management, in Asbury AK, Gilliat RW (eds): *Peripheral Nerve Disorders*. Boston, Butterworth, 1984, pp 126–153.

Cable WJ, Kolodny EH, Adams RD: Fabry disease: Impaired autonomic function. *Neurology* 32:498, 1982.

Capasso M, Caporale CM, Pomilio F, et al: Acute motor conduction block neuropathy. Another Guillain-Barré variant. *Neurology* 61:617, 2003.

Cavanaugh NPC, Eames RA, Galvin RJ, et al: Hereditary sensory neuropathy with spastic paraplegia. *Brain* 102:79, 1979.

Chad D, Periser K, Bradley WG, et al: The pathogenesis of cryoglobulinemic neuropathy. *Neurology* 32:725, 1982.

Chance PF, Lensch MW, Lipe H, et al: Hereditary neuralgic amyotrophy and hereditary neuropathy with liability to pressure palsies: Two distinct entities. *Neurology* 44:2253, 1994.

Chia L, Fernandez A, Lacroix D, et al: Contribution of nerve biopsy findings to the diagnosis of disabling neuropathy in the elderly. A retrospective review of 100 consecutive patients. *Brain* 119:1091, 1996.

Chin RL, Tseng VG, Green PH, et al: Multifocal axonal polyneuropathy in celiac disease. *Neurology* 66:1923, 2006.

Coelho T, Adams D, Silva A, et al: Safety and efficacy of RNAi therapy for transthyretin amyloidosis. *N Engl J Med* 369:819, 2013.

Coelho T, Maia L Cotto F, Silva AM, et al. Tafamidis for transthyretin familial amyloid polyneuropathy. *Neurology* 79:785, 2012.

Collins MP: The vasculitic neuropathies: An update. *Curr Opin Neurol* 25:573, 2012.

Collins MP, Dyck PJ, Gronseth GS, Guillevin et al: Peripheral Nerve Society Guideline on the classification, diagnosis, investigation, and immunosuppressive therapy of non-systemic vasculitic neuropathy: Executive summary. *J Peripher Nerv Syst* 15:176, 2010.

Collins MP, Periquet MI, Mendell JR, et al: Nonsystemic vasculitic neuropathy: Insights from a clinical cohort. *Neurology* 61:623, 2003.

Cornblath DR, McArthur JC, Kennedy PGE, et al: Inflammatory demyelinating peripheral neuropathies associated with human T-cell lymphotropic virus type III infection. *Ann Neurol* 21:32, 1987.

Croft PB, Wilkinson M: The incidence of carcinomatous neuromyopathy in patients with various types of carcinoma. *Brain* 88:427, 1965.

Dalakas MC: Chronic idiopathic ataxic neuropathy. *Ann Neurol* 19:545, 1986.

Dalakas MC, Engel WK: Chronic relapsing (dysimmune) polyneuropathy: Pathogenesis and treatment. *Ann Neurol* 9:134, 1981a.

Dalakas MC, Engel WK: Polyneuropathy with monoclonal gammopathy: Studies of 11 patients. *Ann Neurol* 10:45, 1981b.

Dalmau J, Graus F, Rosenbaum MK, Posner JB: Anti-Hu–associated paraneoplastic encephalomyelitis/sensory neuropathy: A clinical study of 71 patients. *Medicine (Baltimore)* 71:59, 1992.

Daughaday WH: Extreme gigantism: Analysis of growth velocity and occurrence of severe peripheral neuropathy with neuropathic joints. *N Engl J Med* 297:1267, 1977.

Dawidenkow S: Über die neurotische Muskelatrophie Charcot-Marie: Klinisch-genetische Studien. *Z Neurol* 107:259; 108:344, 1927.

Dawson DM, Hallett M, Wilbourn, AJ: *Entrapment Neuropathies*, 3rd ed. Boston, Lippincott-Raven, 1999.

DeGroot K, Schmidt DK, Arlt AC, et al: Standardized neurologic evaluation of 128 patients with Wegener granulomatosis. *Arch Neurol* 58:1215, 2001.

Delank HW, Koch G, Kohn G, et al: Familiare amyloid Polyneuropathie typus Wohlwill-Corino Andrade. *Arztl Forsch* 19:401, 1965.

Delmont E, Azulay JP, Giorgi R, et al: Multifocal motor neuropathy with and without conduction block. *Neurology* 67:592, 2006.

Denny-Brown D: Hereditary sensory radicular neuropathy. *J Neurol Neurosurg Psychiatry* 14:237, 1951.

De Wals P, Deceuninck G, Toth E, et al: Risk of Guillain-Barré syndrome following H1N1 influenza vaccination in Quebec. *JAMA* 308:175, 2012.

Donaghy M, Hakin RN, Bamford JM, et al: Hereditary sensory neuropathy with neurotrophic keratitis. Description of an autosomal recessive disorder with a selective reduction of small myelinated nerve fibres and a discussion of the classification of the hereditary sensory neuropathies. *Brain* 110:563, 1987.

Dreyfus PM, Hakim S, Adams RD: Diabetic ophthalmoplegia: Report of a case with postmortem study and comments on vascular supply of human oculomotor nerve. *AMA Arch Neurol Psychiatry* 77:337, 1957.

Duchen LW, Anjorin A, Watkins PJ, Mackay JD: Pathology of autonomic neuropathy in diabetes mellitus. *Ann Intern Med* 92:301, 1980.

Duchowny M, Caplan L, Siber G: Cytomegalovirus infection of the adult nervous system. *Ann Neurol* 5:458, 1979.

Dyck PJ, Daube J, O'Brien P, et al: Plasma exchange in chronic inflammatory demyelinating polyneuropathy. *N Engl J Med* 314:461, 1986a.

Dyck PJ, Karnes JL, O'Brien P, et al: The spatial distribution of fiber loss in diabetic polyneuropathy suggests ischemia. *Ann Neurol* 19:440, 1986b.

Dyck PJ, Karnes JL, O'Brien P, Rizza R: Fiber loss is primary and multifocal in sural nerves in diabetic polyneuropathy. *Ann Neurol* 19:425, 1986c.

Dyck PJ, Kratz KM, Karnes JL, et al: The prevalence by staged severity of various types of diabetic neuropathy, and nephropathy, in a population based cohort. *Neurology* 43:817, 1993.

Dyck PJ, Lais AC, Ohta M, et al: Chronic inflammatory polyradiculoneuropathy. *Mayo Clin Proc* 50:621, 1975.

Dyck PJ, Lambert EH: Lower motor and primary sensory neuron disease with peroneal muscular atrophy. *Arch Neurol* 18:603, 1968.

Dyck PJ, Lambert EH: Polyneuropathy associated with hypothyroidism. *J Neuropathol Exp Neurol* 29:631, 1970.

Dyck PJ, Lambert EH: Inherited neuronal degeneration and atrophy affecting peripheral motor, sensory, and autonomic neurons, in PJ Dyck, PK Thomas, EH Lambert (eds): *Peripheral Neuropathy*. Philadelphia, Saunders, 1975, pp 825–867.

Dyck PJ, Low PA, Windebank AJ, et al: Plasma exchange in polyneuropathy associated with monoclonal gammopathy of undetermined significance. *N Engl J Med* 325:1482, 1991.

Dyck PJ, Oviatt KF, Lambert EH: Intensive evaluation of referred unclassified neuropathies yields improved diagnosis. *Ann Neurol* 10:222, 1981.

Dyck PJB, Engelstad J, Norell J, Dyck PJ: Microvasculitis in nondiabetic lumbosacral radiculoplexus neuropathy (LSRPN): Similarity to the diabetic variety (DLSRPN). *J Neuropathol Exp Neurol* 59:525, 2000.

Eames RA, Lange LS: Clinical and pathologic study of ischaemic neuropathy. *J Neurol Neurosurg Psychiatry* 30:215, 1967.

Earl CJ, Fullerton PM, Wakefield GS, Schutta HS: Hereditary neuropathy with liability to pressure palsies. *Q J Med* 33:481, 1964.

Ecker AD, Woltman WH: Meralgia paresthetica: A report of one hundred and fifty cases. *JAMA* 110:1650, 1938.

Eftimov F, Veremuelen M, Doorn PA, et al: Long-term remission of CIDP after pulsed dexamethasone or short-term prednisolone treatment. *Neurology* 78:1079, 2012.

Ekbom KA: Restless legs syndrome. *Neurology* 10:858, 1960.

England AC, Denny-Brown D: Severe sensory changes and trophic disorders in peroneal muscular atrophy (Charcot-Marie-Tooth type). *AMA Arch Neurol Psychiatry* 67:1, 1952.

England JD, Asbury AK: Peripheral neuropathy. *Lancet* 363:2151, 2004.

England JD, Gronseth GS, Franklin G, et al: Evaluation of distal symmetric polyneuropathy: The role of laboratory and genetic testing (an evidence-based review). *Muscle Nerve* 39:116, 2009.

Faber CG, Hoeijmakers JG, Ahn HS, et al: Gain of function $Na_v1.7$ mutations in idiopathic small fiber neuropathy. *Ann Neurol* 71:26, 2012.

Fagerberg SE: Diabetic neuropathy: A clinical and histological study on the significance of vascular affections. *Acta Med Scand* 164(Suppl 345):1, 1959.

Falls HF, Jackson JH, Carey JG, et al: Ocular manifestations of hereditary primary systemic amyloidosis. *Arch Ophthalmol* 54:660, 1955.

Farcas P, Avnum L, Frisher S, et al: Efficacy of repeated intravenous immunoglobulin in severe unresponsive Guillain-Barré syndrome. *Lancet* 350:1747, 1997.

Feasby TE, Burton SR, Hahn AF: Obstetrical lumbosacral plexus injuries. *Muscle Nerve* 15:937, 1992.

Feasby TE, Gilbert JJ, Brown WF, et al: An acute axonal form of Guillain-Barré polyneuropathy. *Brain* 109:1115, 1986.

Fisher CM: An unusual variant of acute idiopathic polyneuritis (syndrome of ophthalmoplegia, ataxia and areflexia). *N Engl J Med* 255:57, 1956.

Fisher CM, Adams RD: Diphtheritic polyneuritis: A pathological study. *J Neuropathol Exp Neurol* 15:243, 1956.

Forrester C, Lascelles RG: Association between polyneuritis and multiple sclerosis. *J Neurol Neurosurg Psychiatry* 42:864, 1979.

Forssman O, Bjorkman G, Hollender A, Englund NE: IgM-producing lymphocytes in peripheral nerve in a patient with benign monoclonal gammopathy. *Scand J Haematol* 11:332, 1973.

French Cooperative Group: Efficiency of plasma exchange in Guillain-Barré syndrome. *Ann Neurol* 22:753, 1987.

Funck-Brentano JL, Cueille GF, Man NK: A defense of the middle molecule hypothesis. *Kidney Int* 13(Suppl 8):S31, 1978.

Gaist D, Jeppesen U, Andersen M, et al: Statins and risk of polyneuropathy: A case control study. *Neurology* 58:1333, 2002.

Garcia-Bragado F, Bernandez JM, Navarro C, et al: Peripheral neuropathy in essential mixed cryoglobulinemia. *Arch Neurol* 45:1210, 1988.

Garland H: Diabetic amyotrophy. *Br Med J* 2:1287, 1955.

Gemignani F, Brindani F, Alferi S, et al: Clinical spectrum of cryoglobulinemic neuropathy. *J Neurol Neurosurg Psychiatry* 76:1410, 2005.

Goodfellow J, Fearn CB, Matthews JM: Iliacus haematoma: A common complication of haemophilia. *J Bone Joint Surg Br* 49B:748, 1967.

Gorson KC, Allam G, Ropper AH: Chronic inflammatory demyelinating polyneuropathy: Clinical features and response to treatment in 67 consecutive patients with and without monoclonal gammopathy. *Neurology* 48:321, 1997.

Gorson KC, Herrmann DN, Thiagarajan R, et al: Non-length dependent small fibre neuropathy/ganglionopathy. *J Neurol Neurosurg Psychiatry* 79:163, 2008.

Gorson KC, Ropper AH: Axonal neuropathy associated with monoclonal gammopathy of undetermined significance. *J Neurol Neurosurg Psychiatry* 63:163, 1997.

Gorson KC, Ropper AH: Idiopathic distal small fiber neuropathy. *Acta Neurol Scand* 92:376, 1995.

Gorson KC, Ropper AH: Positive salivary gland biopsy, Sjögren syndrome and neuropathy: Clinical implications. *Muscle Nerve* 28:553, 2003.

Gorson KC, Ropper AH, Mureillo M, Blair R: Prospective evaluation of MRI lumbosacral root enhancement in acute Guillain-Barré syndrome. *Neurology* 47:813, 1996.

Gorson KC, Ropper AH, Weinberg DH: Upper limb predominant, multifocal inflammatory demyelinating neuropathy. *Muscle Nerve* 22:758, 1999.

Gorson KC, Ropper AH, Weinberg DH, Weinstein R: Treatment experience in patients with anti-myelin-associated glycoprotein neuropathy. *Muscle Nerve* 24:778, 2001.

Gorson KC, Schott C, Rand WM, et al: Gabapentin in the treatment of painful diabetic neuropathy: A placebo-controlled, double-blind, crossover trial. *J Neurol Neurosurg Psychiatry* 66:251, 1999.

Gosselin S, Kyle RA, Dyck PJ: Neuropathy associated with monoclonal gammopathy of undetermined significance. *Ann Neurol* 30:54, 1991.

Grant I, Hunder GG, Homburger HA, Dyck PJ: Peripheral neuropathy associated with sicca complex. *Neurology* 48:855, 1997.

Griffin JW, Cornblath DR, Alexander B, et al: Ataxic sensory neuropathy and dorsal root ganglionitis associated with Sjögren's syndrome. *Ann Neurol* 27:304, 1990.

Griffin JW, Li CY, Ho TW, et al: Guillain-Barré syndrome in northern China: The spectrum of neuropathological changes in clinically defined cases. *Brain* 118:577, 1995.

Guarantors of Brain: *Aids to the Examination of the Peripheral Nervous System*, 2nd ed. London, Baillière-Tindall, 1986.

Guillain-Barré Study Group: Plasmapheresis and acute Guillain-Barré syndrome. *Neurology* 35:1096, 1985.

Hadjivassiliou M, Chattopadhyay AK, Davies-Jones GA, et al: Neuromuscular disorder as presenting feature of coeliac disease. *J Neurol Neurosurg Psychiatry* 63:770, 1997.

Hafer-Macko CE, Sheikh KA, Li CY, et al: Immune attack on the Schwann cell surface in acute inflammatory demyelinating polyneuropathy. *Ann Neurol* 39:625, 1996.

Hahn AF, Bolton CF, Pillay N, et al: Plasma exchange therapy in chronic inflammatory demyelinating polyneuropathy. *Brain* 119:1055, 1996a.

Hahn AF, Bolton CF, Zochodne D, Feasby TE: Intravenous immunoglobulin treatment in chronic inflammatory demyelinating polyneuropathy. *Brain* 119:1067, 1996b.

Hahn AF, Hartung HP, Dyck PJ: Chronic inflammatory demyelinating polyradiculoneuropathy, in Dyck PJ, Thomas PK, et al (eds): *Peripheral Neuropathy*, 4th ed. Philadelphia, Elsevier Saunders, 2005, pp 2221–2253.

Harding AE, Thomas PK: Peroneal muscular atrophy with pyramidal features. *J Neurol Neurosurg Psychiatry* 47:168, 1984.

Harding AE, Thomas PK: The clinical features of hereditary motor and sensory neuropathy: Types I and II. *Brain* 103:259, 1980.

Hart ZH, Hoffman W, Winbaum E: Polyneuropathy, alopecia areata, and chronic lymphocytic thyroiditis. *Neurology* 29:106, 1979.

Hartung H-P, Reiners K, Schmidt B, et al: Serum interleukin-2 concentrations in Guillain-Barré syndrome and chronic idiopathic demyelinating polyneuropathy: Comparison with other neurological diseases of presumed immunopathogenesis. *Ann Neurol* 30:48, 1991.

Haymaker W, Kernohan JW: The Landry-Guillain-Barré syndrome: Clinicopathologic report of fifty fatal cases and critique of the literature. *Medicine (Baltimore)* 28:59, 1949.

Henson RA, Urich H: *Cancer and the Nervous System*. Oxford, UK, Blackwell, 1982, pp 368–405.

Herlenius G, Wilczek HE, Larsson M, et al: Ten years of international experience with liver transplantation for familial amyloidotic polyneuropathy: Results from the Familial Amyloidotic Polyneuropathy World Transplant Registry. *Transplantation* 77:64, 2004.

Hoitsma E, Marziniak M, Faber GC, et al: Small fibre neuropathy in sarcoidosis. *Lancet* 359:2085, 2002.

Honovar M, Tharakan JK, Hughes RAC, et al: A clinico-pathological study of Guillain-Barré syndrome: Nine cases and literature review. *Brain* 114:1245, 1991.

Hoogendijk JE, Hensels GW, Gabreel S, et al: De novo mutation in hereditary motor and sensory neuropathy, type 1. *Lancet* 339:1081, 1992.

Horwich MS, Cho L, Porro RS, Posner JB: Subacute sensory neuropathy: A remote effect of carcinoma. *Ann Neurol* 2:7, 1977.
Hughes R, Sanders E, Hall S, et al: Subacute idiopathic demyelinating polyradiculoneuropathy. *Arch Neurol* 49:612, 1992.
Hughes RAC: *Guillain-Barré Syndrome*. London, Springer–Verlag, 1990.
Hughes RAC: Ineffectiveness of high-dose intravenous methylprednisolone in Guillain-Barré syndrome. *Lancet* 338:1142, 1991.
Ikeda S-I, Hanyu N, Hongo M, et al: Hereditary generalized amyloidosis with polyneuropathy: Clinicopathological study of 65 Japanese patients. *Brain* 110:315, 1987.
Illa I, Graus F, Ferrer I, Enriquez J: Sensory neuropathy as the initial manifestation of primary biliary cirrhosis. *J Neurol Neurosurg Psychiatry* 52:1307, 1989.
Illa I, Rojas R, Gallardo E, et al: Chronic idiopathic sensory ataxic neuropathy: Immunological aspects of a series of 17 patients. *Rev Neurol* 157:517, 2001.
Ismael SS, Amarenco G, Bayle B, Kerdraon J: Postpartum lumbosacral plexopathy limited to autonomic and perineal manifestations: Clinical and electrophysiologic study of 19 patients. *J Neurol Neurosurg Psychiatry* 68:771, 2000.
Jankovic J, Van der Linden C: Dystonia and tremor induced by peripheral trauma: Predisposing factors. *J Neurol Neurosurg Psychiatry* 51:1512, 1988.
Jaradeh S, Dyck PJ: Hereditary motor sensory neuropathy with treatable extrapyramidal features. *Arch Neurol* 49:175, 1992.
Jeannet PY, Watts GD, Bird TD, Chance PF: Craniofacial and cutaneous findings expand the phenotype of hereditary neuralgic amyotrophy. *Neurology* 57:1963, 2001.
Johnson PC, Doll SC, Cromey DW: Pathogenesis of diabetic neuropathy. *Ann Neurol* 19:450, 1986.
Kahn P: Anderson-Fabry disease: A histopathological study of three cases with observations on the mechanism of production of pain. *J Neurol Neurosurg Psychiatry* 36:1053, 1973.
Kahn SN, Riches PG, Kohn J: Paraproteinemia in neurological disease: Incidence, association and classification of monoclonal immunoglobulins. *J Clin Pathol* 33:617, 1980.
Kaltrieder HB, Talal N: The neuropathy of Sjögren's syndrome: Trigeminal nerve involvement. *Ann Intern Med* 70:751, 1961.
Kantarjian AD, DeJong RN: Familial primary amyloidosis with nervous system involvement. *Neurology* 3:399, 1953.
Kaplan JG, Rosenberg R, Reinitz E, et al: Invited review: Peripheral neuropathy in Sjögren's syndrome. *Muscle Nerve* 13:573, 1990.
Katirji MB, Wilbourn AJ: Common peroneal mononeuropathy: A clinical and electrophysiologic study of 116 lesions. *Neurology* 38:1723, 1988.
Katz JS, Saperstein DS, Gronseth D, et al: Distal acquired demyelinating symmetric neuropathy. *Neurology* 54:615, 2000.
Kelly JJ, Adelman LS, Berkman E, Bhan I: Polyneuropathies associated with IgM monoclonal gammopathies. *Arch Neurol* 45:1355, 1988.
Kemler MA, Bareudse GA, Van Kleef M, et al: Spinal cord stimulation in patients with chronic reflex sympathetic dystrophy. *N Engl J Med* 343:618, 2000.
Kennett RP, Harding AE: Peripheral neuropathy associated with the sicca syndrome. *J Neurol Neurosurg Psychiatry* 49:90, 1986.
Kernohan JW, Woltman HW: Amyloid neuritis. *Arch Neurol Psychiatry* 47:132, 1942.
Kikta DG, Breuer AC, Wilbourn AJ: Thoracic root pain in diabetes: The spectrum of clinical and electromyographic findings. *Ann Neurol* 11:80, 1982.
King R: *Atlas of Peripheral Nerve Pathology*. London, Arnold, 1999.
Klein CJ, Duan X, Shy ME: Inherited neuropathies: Clinical overview and update. AANEM Monograph. *Muscle Nerve* 48:604, 2013.
Klein CM, Vernino S, Lennon VA, et al: The spectrum of autoimmune autonomic neuropathies. *Arch Neurol* 53:752, 2003.
Kori SH, Foley KM, Posner JB: Brachial plexus lesions in patients with cancer: 100 cases. *Neurology* 31:45, 1981.
Koski CL, Gratz E, Sutherland J, et al: Clinical correlation with anti-peripheral nerve myelin antibodies in Guillain-Barré syndrome. *Ann Neurol* 19:573, 1986.
Kremer M, Gilliatt RW, Golding JSR, Wilson TG: Acroparaesthesiae in the carpal-tunnel syndrome. *Lancet* 2:590, 1953.
Kuitwaard K, de Gelder J, Tio-Gillen AP, et al: Pharmacokinetics of intravenous immunoglobulin and outcome in Guillain-Barré syndrome. *Ann Neurol* 66:597, 2009.
Kuwabara S, Misawa S, Kanai K, et al: Neurologic improvement after peripheral blood stem cell transplantation in POEMS syndrome. *Neurology* 71:1691, 2008.
Kuwabara S, Misawa S, Mori M, et al: Long-term prognosis of chronic inflammatory demyelinating polyneuropathy—a five-year follow-up of 38 cases. *J Neurol Neurosurg Psychiatry* 77:66, 2006.
Kyle RA, Bayrd ED: Amyloidosis: Review of 236 cases. *Medicine (Baltimore)* 54:271, 1975.
Kyle RA, Dyck PJ: Neuropathy associated with the monoclonal gammopathies, in Dyck PJ, Thomas PK, et al (eds): *Peripheral Neuropathy*, 4th ed. Philadelphia, Elsevier Saunders, 2005, pp 2255–2276.
Kyle RA, Kelly JJ, Dyck PJ: Amyloidosis and neuropathy, in Dyck PJ, Thomas PK, et al (eds): *Peripheral Neuropathy*, 4th ed. Philadelphia, Elsevier Saunders, 2005, pp 2427–2451.
Lachmann HJ, Booth DR, Booth SE, et al: Misdiagnosis of hereditary amyloidosis as AL (primary) amyloidosis. *N Engl J Med* 346:1786, 2002.
Lachmann HJ, Goodman HJ, Gilbertson JA, et al: National history and outcome in systemic AA amyloidosis. *N Engl J Med* 356:2361, 2007.
Lafitte C: Manifestations neurologique du syndrome de Gougerot-Sjögren primitif. *Rev Neurol* 154:658, 1998.
Latov N, Gross RB, Kastelman J, et al: Complement-fixing antiperipheral nerve myelin antibodies in patients with inflammatory polyneuritis and with polyneuropathy and paraproteinemias. *Neurology* 31:1530, 1981.
Layzer RB: *Neuromuscular Manifestations of Systemic Disease: Contemporary Neurology Series*. Vol 25. Philadelphia, Davis, 1984.
Lederman RJ, Wilbourn AJ: Brachial plexopathy: Recurrent cancer or radiation? *Neurology* 34:1331, 1984.
Lederman RJ, Wilbourn AJ: Postpartum neuralgic amyotrophy. *Neurology* 47:1213, 1996.
Leger JM, Bouche P, Cervera P, Hauw JJ: Primary Sjögren syndrome in chronic polyneuropathy presenting in middle or old age. *J Neurol Neurosurg Psychiatry* 59:1276, 1995.
Lewis RA, Sumner AJ, Brown MJ, Asbury AK: Multifocal demyelinating neuropathy with persistent conduction block. *Neurology* 32:958, 1982.
Lewis T, Pickering GW: Circulatory changes in the fingers in some diseases of the nervous system with special reference to the digital atrophy of peripheral nerve lesions. *Clin Sci* 2:149, 1936.
Lhermitte F, Fritel D, Cambier J, et al: Polynevrites au cours de traitements par la nitrofurantoine. *Presse Med* 71:767, 1963.
Lhote F, Cohen P, Genereau T, et al: Microscopic polyangiitis: Clinical aspects and treatment. *Ann Med Interne (Paris)* 147:165, 1996.
Llewelyn JG, Tomlinson DR, Thomas PK: Diabetic neuropathies, in Dyck PJ, Thomas PK, et al (eds): *Peripheral Neuropathy*, 4th ed. Philadelphia, Elsevier Saunders, 2005, pp 1951–1991.
Loggigian EL, Kaplan RF, Steere AC: Chronic neurologic manifestations of Lyme disease. *N Engl J Med* 323:1438, 1990.
Logina I, Donaghy M: Diphtheritic polyneuropathy: A clinical study and comparison with Guillain-Barré syndrome. *J Neurol Neurosurg Psychiatry* 67:433, 1999.

Low PA, Dyck PJ, Lambert EH: Acute panautonomic neuropathy. *Ann Neurol* 13:412, 1983.

Luostarinen L, Himanen S-L, Luostarinen M, et al: Neuromuscular and sensory disturbances in patients with well treated coeliac disease. *J Neurol Neurosurg Psychiatry* 74:490, 2003.

Lupski JR, Reid JG, Gonzaga-Jauregui C, et al: Whole-genome sequencing in a patient with Charcot-Marie-Tooth neuropathy. *N Engl J Med* 362:1181, 2010.

Maas JJ, Beersma MFC, Haan J, et al: Bilateral brachial plexus neuritis following parvovirus B19 and cytomegalovirus infection. *Ann Neurol* 40:928, 1996.

Madrid R, Bradley WG: The pathology of neuropathies with focal thickening of the myelin sheath (tomaculous neuropathy). *J Neurol Sci* 25:415, 1975.

Magee KR, DeJong RN: Paralytic brachial neuritis. *JAMA* 174:1258, 1960.

Marquez S, Turley JJ, Peters WJ: Neuropathy in burn patients. *Brain* 116:471, 1993.

Matthews WB, Esiri M: The migrant sensory neuritis of Wartenberg. *J Neurol Neurosurg Psychiatry* 46:1, 1983.

Matthews WB, Squier MV: Sensory perineuritis. *J Neurol Neurosurg Psychiatry* 51:473, 1988.

McCombe PA, McLeod JG, Pollard JD, et al: Peripheral sensorimotor and autonomic polyneuropathy associated with systemic lupus erythematosus. *Brain* 110:533, 1987a.

McCombe PA, Pollard JD, McLeod JG: Chronic inflammatory demyelinating polyradiculoneuropathy: A clinical and electrophysiological study of 92 cases. *Brain* 111:1617, 1987b.

McDonald TD, Faust PL, Bruno C, et al: Polyglucosan body disease simulating amyotrophic lateral sclerosis. *Neurology* 43:785, 1993.

McGonagle TK, Levine SR, Donofrio PD, Albers JW: Spectrum of patients with EMG features of polyradiculopathy without neuropathy. *Muscle Nerve* 13:63, 1990.

McKhann GM, Griffin JW, Cornblath DR, et al: Plasmapheresis and Guillain-Barré syndrome: Analysis of prognostic factors and the effect of plasmapheresis. *Ann Neurol* 23:347, 1988.

Mellgren SI, Conn DL, Stevens JC, Dyck PJ: Peripheral neuropathy in primary Sjögren's syndrome. *Neurology* 39:390, 1989.

Mendell JR, Sahenk Z: Painful sensory neuropathy. *N Engl J Med* 348:1243, 2003.

Meretoja J: Familial systemic paramyloidosis with lattice dystrophy of the cornea, progressive cranial neuropathy, skin changes and various internal symptoms: A previously unrecognized heritable syndrome. *Ann Clin Res* 1:314, 1969.

Moore PM, Harley JB, Fauci AS: Neurologic dysfunction in the idiopathic hypereosinophilic syndrome. *Ann Intern Med* 102:109, 1985.

Moulignier A, Authier F-J, Baudrimont M, et al: Peripheral neuropathy in human immunodeficiency virus-infected patients with the diffuse infiltrative lymphocytosis syndrome. *Ann Neurol* 41:438, 1997.

Nathan PW: Painful legs and moving toes: Evidence on the site of the lesion. *J Neurol Neurosurg Psychiatry* 41:934, 1978.

Naumann M, Schalke B, Klopstock T, et al: Neurological multisystem manifestation in multiple symmetric lipomatosis: A clinical and electrophysiologic study. *Muscle Nerve* 18:693, 1995.

Oh S: Paraneoplastic vasculitis of the peripheral nervous system. *Neurol Clin* 15:849, 1997.

Ohnishi A, Dyck PJ: Loss of small peripheral sensory neurons in Fabry disease. *Arch Neurol* 31:120, 1974.

Ongerboer de Visser BW, Feltkamp-Vroom TM, Feltkamp CA: Sural nerve immune deposits in polyneuropathy as a remote effect of malignancy. *Ann Neurol* 14:261, 1983.

Osterman PO, Fagius J, Safwenberg J, et al: Early relapses after plasma exchange in acute inflammatory polyradiculoneuropathy. *Lancet* 2:1161, 1986.

Pallis CA, Scott JT: Peripheral neuropathy in rheumatoid arthritis. *Br Med J* 1:1141, 1965.

Parsonage MJ, Turner JWA: Neuralgic amyotrophy: The shoulder girdle syndrome. *Lancet* 1:973, 1948.

Pascoe MK, Low PA, Windebank AJ, Litchy WJ: Subacute diabetic proximal neuropathy. *Mayo Clin Proc* 72:1123, 1997.

Periquet MI, Novak V, Collins MP, et al: Painful sensory neuropathy: Prospective evaluation using skin biopsy. *Neurology* 52: 1641, 1999.

Pestronk A, Chaudhry V, Feldman EL, et al: Lower motor neuron syndromes defined by patterns of weakness, nerve conduction abnormalities, and high titers of antiglycolipid antibodies. *Ann Neurol* 27:316, 1990.

Phillips LH: Familial long thoracic nerve palsy: A manifestation of brachial plexus neuropathy. *Neurology* 36:1251, 1986.

Pickett JBE, Layzer RB, Levin SR, et al: Neuromuscular complications of acromegaly. *Neurology* 25:638, 1975.

Planté-Bordeneuve V, Guichon-Mantel A, Lacroix C, et al: The Roussy-Lévy family: From the original description to the gene. *Ann Neurol* 46:770, 1999.

Plasma Exchange/Sandoglobulin Guillain-Barré Syndrome Trial Group. Randomised trial of plasma exchange, intravenous immunoglobulin, and combined treatments in Guillain-Barré syndrome. *Lancet* 349:225, 1997.

Prineas JW, McLeod JG: Chronic relapsing polyneuritis. *J Neurol Sci* 27:427, 1976.

Raff MC, Sangalang V, Asbury AK: Ischemic mononeuropathy multiplex associated with diabetes mellitus. *Arch Neurol* 18:487, 1968.

Rechthand E, Cornblath DR, Stern BJ, Meyerhoff JO: Chronic demyelinating polyneuropathy in systemic lupus erythematosus. *Neurology* 34:1375, 1984.

Refsum S: Heredopathia atactica polyneuritiformis: A familial syndrome not hitherto described. *Acta Psychiatr Scand Suppl* 38:1, 1946.

Robitaille Y, Carpenter S, Karpati G, Dimauro S: A distinct form of adult polyglucosan body disease with massive involvement of central and peripheral neuronal processes and astrocytes. *Brain* 103:315, 1980.

Robson JS: Uraemic neuropathy, in Robertson RF (ed): *Some Aspects of Neurology*. Edinburgh, UK, Royal College of Physicians, 1968, pp 74–84.

Rogers LR, Borkowski JW, Albers KH, et al: Obturator mononeuropathy caused by pelvic cancer: Six cases. *Neurology* 43:1489, 1993.

Romero CE, Jacobs BJ, Ropper AH: Clinical characteristics of a mild sensory-fasciculatory syndrome. *Neurology* 62(Suppl 5):A519, 2004.

Ropper AH: Accelerated neuropathy of renal failure. *Arch Neurol* 50:536, 1993.

Ropper AH: Chronic demyelinating polyneuropathy: Improvement after sepsis. *Neurology* 46:848, 1996.

Ropper AH: Further regional variants of acute immune polyneuropathy. *Arch Neurol* 51:671, 1994.

Ropper AH: Severe acute Guillain-Barré syndrome. *Neurology* 36:429, 1986b.

Ropper AH: The Guillain-Barré syndrome. *N Engl J Med* 326:1130, 1992.

Ropper AH: Unusual clinical variants and signs in Guillain-Barré syndrome. *Arch Neurol* 43:1150, 1986a.

Ropper AH, Adelman L: Early Guillain-Barré syndrome without inflammation. *Arch Neurol* 49:979, 1992.

Ropper AH, Gorson KC: Neuropathies associated with paraproteinemias. *N Engl J Med* 338:1601, 1998.

Ropper AH, Gorson KC, Gooch CL, et al: Vascular endothelial growth factor gene transfer for diabetic polyneuropathy: A randomized, double-blinded trial. *Ann Neurol* 65:386, 2009.

Ropper AH, Gress DR, Diringer MN, Green DM, Mayer SA, Bleck TP (eds): *Neurological and Neurosurgical Intensive Care*, 4th ed. Philadelphia, Lippincott Williams & Wilkins, 2004.

Ropper AH, Kehne SM: Guillain-Barré syndrome: Management of respiratory failure. *Neurology* 35:1662, 1985.

Ropper AH, Marmarou A: Mechanism of pseudotumor in Guillain-Barré syndrome. *Arch Neurol* 41:259, 1984.

Ropper AH, Wijdick EFM, Truax BT: *Guillain-Barré Syndrome*. Philadelphia, Davis, 1991.

Rowland LP, Defendini R, Sheman W, et al: Macroglobulinemia with peripheral neuropathy simulating motor neuron diseases. *Ann Neurol* 11:532, 1982.

Rukavina JG, Block WD, Jackson CE, et al: Primary systemic amyloidosis: A review and an experimental genetic and clinical study of 29 cases with particular emphasis on the familial form. *Medicine (Baltimore)* 35:239, 1956.

Sabin TD: Temperature-linked sensory loss: A unique pattern in leprosy. *Arch Neurol* 20:257, 1969.

Said G: Perhexiline neuropathy: A clinicopathologic study. *Ann Neurol* 3:259, 1978.

Said G, Elgrably F, Lacroix C, et al: Painful proximal diabetic neuropathy: Inflammatory nerve lesions and spontaneous favorable outcome. *Ann Neurol* 41:762, 1997.

Said G, Lacroix C: Primary and secondary vasculitic neuropathy. *J Neurol* 252:633, 2005.

Said G, Lacroix C, Lozeram P, et al: Inflammatory vasculopathy in multifocal diabetic neuropathy. *Brain* 126:376, 2003.

Said G, Lacroix C, Planto-Bordenevue U, et al: Nerve granulomas and vasculitis in sarcoid peripheral neuropathy. *Brain* 125:264, 2002.

Said G, Slama G, Selva J: Progressive centripetal degeneration of axons in small fiber type diabetic polyneuropathy: A clinical and pathological study. *Brain* 106:791, 1983.

Samanta A, Burden AC: Painful diabetic neuropathy. *Lancet* 1:348, 1985.

Sandroni P, Vernino S, Klein CM, et al: Idiopathic autonomic neuropathy. Comparison of cases seropositive and seronegative for ganglionic acetylcholine receptor antibody. *Arch Neurol* 61:44, 2004.

Saporta, ASD, Sottile SL, Miller LJ, et al: Charcot-Marie-Tooth disease subtypes and genetic testing strategies. *Ann Neurol* 69:22, 2011.

Saraiva MJM, Costa PP, Goodman DS: Genetic expression of a transthyretin mutation in typical and late-onset Portuguese families with familial amyloidotic polyneuropathy. *Neurology* 36:1413, 1986.

Schaumburg HH, Berger AR, Thomas PK: *Disorders of Peripheral Nerves*, 2nd ed. Philadelphia, Davis, 1992.

Schaumburg HH, Kaplan J, Windebank A, et al: Sensory neuropathy from pyridoxine abuse. *N Engl J Med* 309:445, 1983.

Shahani BT, Young RR, Adams RD: Neuropathic tremor: Evidence on the site of the lesion. *Electroencephalogr Clin Neurophysiol* 34:800, 1973.

Shy ME, Lupski JR, Chance PF, et al: Hereditary motor and sensory neuropathies, in Dyck PJ, Thomas PK, et al (eds): *Peripheral Neuropathy*, 4th ed. Philadelphia, Elsevier Saunders, 2005, pp 1623–1658.

Simmons Z, Albers JW, Bromberg MB, Feldman EL: Long-term follow-up of patients with chronic demyelinating polyradiculoneuropathy without and with monoclonal gammopathy. *Brain* 118:359, 1995.

Simovic D, Gorson KC, Ropper AH: Comparison of IgM-MGUS and IgG-MGUS polyneuropathy. *Acta Neurol Scand* 97:194, 1998.

Sinnreich M, Klein CJ, Daube JR, et al: Chronic immune sensory polyradiculopathy. *Neurology* 63:1662, 2004.

Skjeldal OH, Nyberg-Hansen R, Stokke O: Neurological disorders and phytanic acid metabolism. *Acta Neurol Scand* 78:324, 1988.

Smith IS, Kahn SN, Lacey BW, et al: Chronic demyelinating neuropathy associated with benign IgM paraproteinemia. *Brain* 106:169, 1983.

Sorenson EJ, Sima AAF, Blaivas M, et al: Clinical features of perineuritis. *Muscle Nerve* 20:1153, 1997.

Specks U, Wheatley CL, McDonald TJ, et al: Anticytoplasmic autoantibodies in the diagnosis and follow-up of Wegener's granulomatosis. *Mayo Clin Proc* 64:28, 1989.

Spencer PS, Schaumburg HH, Ludolph AC (eds): *Experimental and Clinical Neurotoxicology*. New York, Oxford University Press, 1999.

Spillane JW, Nathan PW, Kelly RE, Marsden CD: Painful legs and moving toes. *Brain* 94:541, 1971.

Staunton H, Dervan P, Kale R, et al: Hereditary amyloid polyneuropathy in northwest Ireland. *Brain* 110:1231, 1987.

Sterman AB, Schaumberg HH, Asbury AK: The acute sensory neuropathy syndrome: A distinct clinical entity. *Ann Neurol* 7:354, 1980.

Stevens JC: The electrodiagnosis of the carpal tunnel syndrome. *Muscle Nerve* 12:99, 1987.

Stewart BM: The hypertrophic neuropathy of acromegaly: A rare neuropathy associated with acromegaly. *Arch Neurol* 14:107, 1966.

Stogbauer F, Young P, Kuhlenbaumer G, et al: Autosomal dominant burning feet syndrome. *J Neurol Neurosurg Psychiatry* 67:78, 1999.

Stoll BA, Andrews JT: Radiation induced peripheral neuropathy. *Br Med J* 1:834, 1966.

Suarez CM, Fealy RD, Camilleri M, Low PA: Idiopathic autonomic neuropathy. Clinical, neurophysiologic, and follow-up studies on 27 patients. *Neurology* 44:1675, 1994.

Suarez GA, Giannini C, Bosch EP, et al: Immune brachial plexus neuropathy: Suggestive evidence for inflammatory-immune pathogenesis. *Neurology* 46:559, 1996.

Sumner CJ, Sheth S, Griffin JW, et al: The spectrum of neuropathy in diabetes and impaired glucose tolerance. *Neurology* 60:108, 2003.

Sun SF, Steib EW: Diabetic thoracoabdominal neuropathy: Clinical and electrodiagnostic features. *Ann Neurol* 9:75, 1981.

Swanson AG, Buchan GC, Alvord EC Jr: Anatomic changes in congenital insensitivity to pain: Absence of small primary sensory neurons in ganglia, roots and Lissauer's tract. *Arch Neurol* 12:12, 1965.

Symonds CP, Shaw ME: Familial clawfoot with absent tendon jerks: A "forme-fruste" of the Charcot-Marie-Tooth disease. *Brain* 49:387, 1926.

Taylor RA: Heredofamilial mononeuritis multiplex with brachial predilection. *Brain* 83:113, 1960.

Tesfaye S, Chaturvedi N, Easton SE, et al: Vascular risk factors and diabetic neuropathy. *N Engl J Med* 352:341, 2005.

Thévenard A: L'acropathie ulcero-mutilante familiale. *Rev Neurol* Q74:193, 1942.

Thomas JE, Cascino TL, Earle JD: Differential diagnosis between radiation and tumor plexopathy of the pelvis. *Neurology* 35:1, 1985.

Thomas PK, Ormerod IE: Hereditary neurologic amyotrophy associated with a relapsing multifocal sensory neuropathy. *J Neurol Neurosurg Psychiatry* 56:107, 1993.

Thomas PK, Willison JH: Paraproteinemic neuropathy, in McLeod JG (ed): *Inflammatory Neuropathies: Bailliére's Clinical Neurology*. Vol 3. London, Bailliére-Tindall, 1994, p 129.

Triggs WJ, Cros D, Gominak SC, et al: Motor nerve inexcitability in Guillain-Barré syndrome. *Brain* 115:1291, 1992.

Tsairis P, Dyck PJ, Mulder DW: Natural history of brachial plexus neuropathy: Report on 99 cases. *Arch Neurol* 27:109, 1972.

Tuck RR, McLeod JG: Retinitis pigmentosa, ataxia, and peripheral neuropathy. *J Neurol Neurosurg Psychiatry* 46:206, 1983.

Uchuya M, Graus F, Vega F, et al: Intravenous immunoglobulin treatment in paraneoplastic neurological syndromes with anti-neuronal antibodies. *J Neurol Neurosurg Psychiatry* 60:388, 1996.

Uncini A, Sabatelli M, Mignogna T, et al: Chronic progressive steroid responsive axonal polyneuropathy: A CIDP variant or a primary axonal disorder. *Muscle Nerve* 19:365, 1996.

Vallat JM, DeMascarel A, Bordessoule D, et al: Non-Hodgkin malignant lymphomas and peripheral neuropathies C13 cases. *Brain* 118:1233, 1995.

van Alfen N, van Engelen BGM: the clinical spectrum of neuralgic amyotrophy in 246 cases. *Brain* 129:438, 2006.

van Allen MW, Frohlich JA, Davis JR: Inherited predisposition to generalized amyloidosis. *Neurology* 19:10, 1969.

van Buchem FSP, Pol G, De Gier J, et al: Congenital β-lipoprotein deficiency. *Am J Med* 40:794, 1966.

van der Meché FGA, Schmitz PIM, the Dutch Guillain-Barré Study Group: A randomized trial comparing intravenous immune globulin and plasma exchange in Guillain-Barré syndrome. *N Engl J Med* 326:1123, 1992.

van Eijk JJJ, van Alfen N, Berrevoets M, et al: Evaluation of prednisolone treatment in the acute phase of neuralgic amyotrophy: an observational study. *J Neurol Neurosurg Psychiatr* 80:1120, 2008.

Verhalle D, Löfgren A, Nelis E, et al: Deletion in the CMT1A locus on chromosome 17 p11.2 in hereditary neuropathy with liability to pressure palsies. *Ann Neurol* 35:704, 1994.

Vermuelen M, Van Oers MH: Relapse of chronic inflammatory demyelinating polyneuropathy 5 years after autologous stem cell transplantation. *J Neurol Neurosurg Psychiatry* 78:1154, 2007.

Visser LH, Van der Meché FGA, Van Doorn PA, et al: Guillain-Barré syndrome without sensory loss (acute motor neuropathy). *Brain* 118:841, 1995.

Vucic S, Kennerson M, Zhu D, et al: CMT with pyramidal features. *Neurology* 60:696, 2003.

Waksman BH, Adams RD: Allergic neuritis: An experimental disease of rabbits induced by the injection of peripheral nervous tissue and adjuvants. *J Exp Med* 102:213, 1955.

Waldenstrom J: The porphyrias as inborn errors of metabolism. *Am J Med* 22:758, 1957.

Wartenberg R: *Neuritis, Sensory Neuritis, and Neuralgia*. New York, Oxford University Press, 1958, pp 233–247.

Weinberg DH, Simovic D, Ropper AH, Isner J: Chronic ischemic monomelic neuropathy. *Neurology* 57:1008, 2001.

Weinshilboum RM, Axelrod J: Reduced plasma dopamine-hydroxylase activity in familial dysautonomia. *N Engl J Med* 285:938, 1971.

Wijdicks EF, Ropper AH, Nathanson JA: Atrial natriuretic factor and blood pressure fluctuations in Guillain-Barré syndrome. *Ann Neurol* 27:337, 1990.

Williams IR, Mayer RF: Subacute proximal diabetic neuropathy. *Neurology* 26:108, 1976.

Windebank AJ, Blexrud MO, Dyck PJ, et al: The syndrome of acute sensory neuropathy: Clinical features and electrophysiologic and pathologic changes. *Neurology* 40:584, 1990.

Wulff CH, Hansen K, Strange P, Trojaborg W: Multiple mononeuritis and radiculitis with erythema, pain, elevated CSF protein, and pleocytosis: Bannwarth's syndrome. *J Neurol Neurosurg Psychiatry* 46:485, 1983.

Yeung KB, Thomas PK, King RHM, et al: The clinical spectrum of peripheral neuropathies associated with benign monoclonal IgM and IgA paraproteinemias. *J Neurol* 238:383, 1991.

Young RR, Asbury AK, Corbett JL, Adams RD: Pure pan-dysautonomia with recovery. *Brain* 98:613, 1975.

Yuki N, Hartung H-P: Guillain-Barré syndrome. *N Engl J Med* 366:2294, 2012.

Zochodne DW, Bolton CF, Wells GA: Critical illness polyneuropathy: A complication of sepsis and multiple organ failure. *Brain* 110:819, 1987.

Zuniga G, Ropper AH, Frank J: Sarcoid peripheral neuropathy. *Neurology* 41:1558, 1991.

47

Diseases of the Cranial Nerves

The cranial nerves are susceptible to a number of special diseases, some of which do not affect the spinal peripheral nerves. For this reason alone they are considered separately. Certain of the cranial nerves and their disorders have already been discussed: namely, disorders of olfaction in Chap. 12; of vision and extraocular muscles in Chaps. 13 and 14; of cochlear and vestibular function in Chap. 15; and craniofacial pain in Chap. 10. There remain to be described the disorders of the facial (VII) nerve and of the lower cranial nerves (IX to XII), as well as certain diseases that affect the trigeminal (V) nerve. These are considered here.

The Fifth, or Trigeminal, Nerve

Anatomic Considerations

The fifth nerve (Fig. 47-1) is a mixed sensory and motor nerve. It conducts sensory impulses from the greater part of the face and head; from the mucous membranes of the nose, mouth, and paranasal sinuses; and from the cornea and conjunctiva. It also provides the sensory innervation of the dura in the anterior and middle cranial fossae. The cell bodies of the sensory part of the nerve lie in the *gasserian*, or semilunar, *ganglion*. This, the largest sensory ganglion in humans, lies in the inferomedial part of the middle cranial fossa in a recess called Meckel's cave. The central axons of the ganglion cells form the sensory root of the nerve. These fibers, on entering the lateral mid pons, divide into short ascending and long descending branches. The former are concerned mainly with tactile and light pressure sensation and synapse with second-order neurons in the principal sensory nucleus. Proprioceptive afferents from facial muscles and the masseter also ascend to terminate in the mesencephalic nucleus. The fibers that mediate pain and temperature sensation do not end in these nuclei but form long descending branches of the spinal trigeminal tract. This pathway, which contains both facilitatory and inhibitory fibers, together with its adjacent nucleus, extends from the junction of the pons and medulla to the uppermost segments (C2 or C3) of the spinal cord (as evidenced by the relief of facial pain after medullary trigeminal tractotomy).

The spinal trigeminal nucleus in the upper cervical cord is a continuation of the spinal tract of Lissauer and substantia gelatinosa; the main trigeminal sensory nucleus in the pons and medulla is a continuation of the nucleus of the medial lemniscus. From all parts of the principal sensory and spinal trigeminal nuclei, second-order fibers cross to the opposite side and ascend to the thalamus. They come to lie in the most medial part of the spinothalamic tract and lateral part of the medial lemniscus. These systems of fibers are called the *trigeminothalamic tract*. In addition, the secondary trigeminal neurons project to the facial and hypoglossal nuclei bilaterally, the salivatory nuclei, the cuneate nuclei of the upper cervical segments, and other cranial nerve nuclei. The principal sensory and spinal trigeminal nuclei receive fibers from the reticular formation, the thalamus, the nucleus tractus solitarius, and the somatosensory cortex.

The peripheral branches of the gasserian ganglion form the three sensory divisions of the nerve. The first (ophthalmic) division passes through the cavernous sinus and superior orbital fissure; the second (maxillary) division also passes through the cavernous sinus and leaves the middle fossa through the foramen rotundum; and the third (mandibular), does not traverse the cavernous sinus and instead exits Meckel's cave inferiorly through the foramen ovale.

The motor portion of the fifth nerve, which supplies the masseter and pterygoid muscles, has its origin in the trigeminal motor nucleus in the mid pons; the exiting fibers pass underneath (but not through) the gasserian ganglion and become incorporated into the mandibular nerve. The masseter and pterygoid muscles are used in chewing and are implicated in a number of brainstem reflexes, the best known of which is the jaw jerk. Tapping the chin with the jaw muscles relaxed stimulates proprioceptive afferents that terminate in the mesencephalic nucleus of the midbrain, which sends collaterals to the motor nucleus of the fifth nerve and causes the masseters to contract. This reflex is enhanced in spastic bulbar (pseudobulbar) palsy. Another pontine reflex that uses afferent trigeminal sensory nerves is the blink reflex. Tapping of the brow or bridge of the nose evokes bilateral blink through activation of the orbicularis oculi muscles (facial nerve efferents). Touching the eyelids and cornea (corneal reflex) does the same.

Because of their wide anatomic distribution, complete interruption of both the motor and sensory fibers of the trigeminal nerve is rarely observed. In contrast,

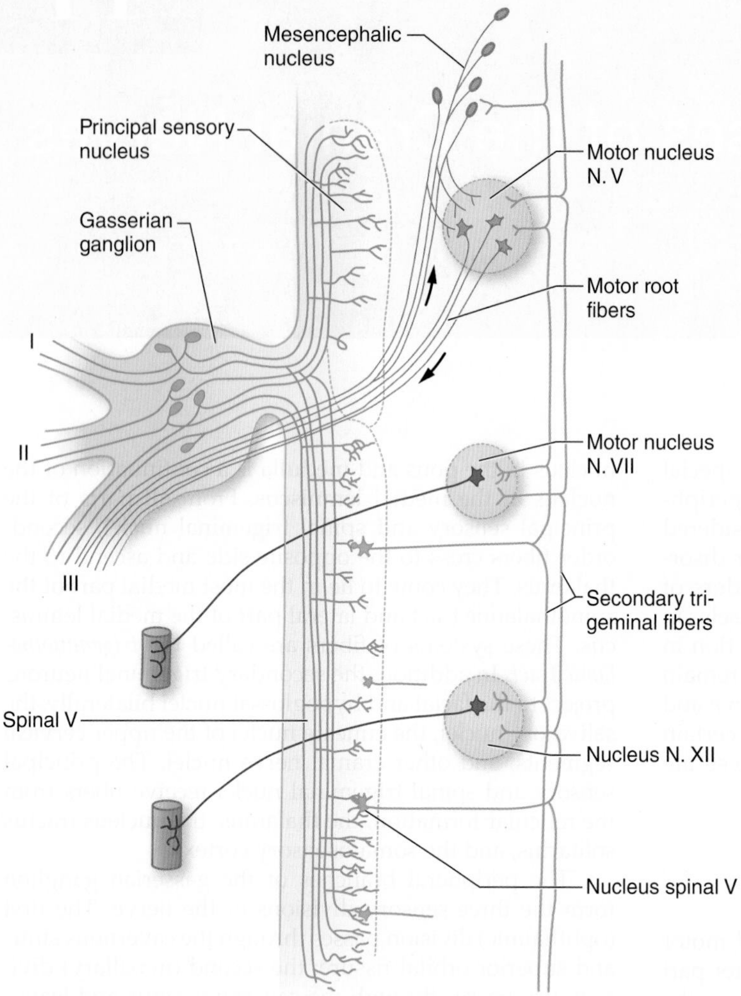

Figure 47-1. Scheme of the trigeminal nuclei and some of the trigeminal reflex arcs. I, ophthalmic division; II, maxillary division; III, mandibular division. (Originally from Ramon y Cajal S: *La Textura del Sistema Nervista del Hombre y los Vertebrados*, Madrid, Moya, as adapted from Carpenter MB, Sutin J: *Human Neuroanatomy*, 8th ed. Baltimore, Williams & Wilkins, 1982, by permission.)

partial dysfunction of the trigeminal nerve, particularly of the sensory part, is common, the main symptoms being facial numbness and pain. The various cranial nerve and brainstem syndromes in which the fifth nerve is involved are listed in Tables 47-1, 31-5, and 34-3, the last in relation to stroke syndromes of the brainstem that affect the nerve in its fascicular course or in its nucleus.

Diseases Affecting the Fifth Nerve

A variety of diseases may affect the peripheral branches of the trigeminal nerves, the gasserian ganglion, and the roots (sensory and motor). Hughes has summarized them and the main ones are described below. The role of the nerve in migraine is discussed in Chap. 10.

Trigeminal Neuralgia (See also "Trigeminal Neuralgia" in Chap. 10) The most frequent and at the same time the most elusive disease of the fifth nerve from the standpoint of its pathologic basis is *trigeminal neuralgia (tic douloureux)*. This condition has been known since ancient times, having been described by Arateus in the first century A.D., by John Locke in 1677, by Nicolaus Andre in 1756, and by John Fothergill in 1776 (according to Katusic et al). The overall incidence rate for both sexes combined is 4.3 per 100,000 persons per year, but it is higher for women than for men (in a ratio of 3:2) and is much higher in the elderly. The mean age of onset is 52 to 58 years for the idiopathic form and 30 to 35 years for the symptomatic forms, the latter being caused by trauma or vascular, neoplastic, and demyelinative diseases. In the last decade it has become apparent, mainly from the work of Jannetta, that a proportion of cases is a result of compression and secondary demyelination of trigeminal nerve rootlets by small branches of the basilar artery (see Love and Coakham).

The paroxysmal nature of the facial pain, its unilaterality, the tendency to involve the second and third divisions of the trigeminal nerve, an intensity that makes the patient grimace or wince (tic), the presence of a trigger point on the face, the lack of demonstrable sensory or motor deficit, and its response in more than half of the cases to antiepileptic drugs are characteristic. The diagnosis of "idiopathic" trigeminal neuralgia and its differentiation from other forms of intermittent facial pain described below—as well as from cluster headache, dental neuralgia, temporomandibular joint pain, and

Table 47-1

EXTRAMEDULLARY CRANIAL NERVE SYNDROMES

SITE	CRANIAL NERVES INVOLVED	EPONYMIC SYNDROME	USUAL CAUSE
Sphenoidal fissure	III, IV, ophthalmic, V, VI	Foix	Invasive tumors of sphenoid bone, aneurysms
Lateral wall of cavernous sinus	III, IV, ophthalmic (occasionally maxillary), V, VI	Tolosa-Hunt	Aneurysms or thrombosis of cavernous sinus; invasive tumors from sinuses and sella turcica; sometimes recurrent, benign granulomatous reactions, responsive to steroids
Retrosphenoidal space fossa	II, III, IV, V, VI	Jaccoud	Large tumors of middle cranial
Apex of petrous bone	V, VI	Gradenigo	Petrositis, tumors of petrous bone
Internal auditory meatus	VII, VIII		Tumors of petrous bone (dermoids, etc.), vestibular schwannoma
Pontocerebellar angle	V, VII, VIII, and sometimes IX		Vestibular schwannomas, meningiomas
Jugular foramen	IX, X, XI	Vernet	Tumors (glomus jugulare), venous sinus thrombosis, and aneurysms
Posterior laterocondylar space	IX, X, XI, XII	Collet-Sicard	Tumors of parotid gland, carotid body; secondary and lymph node tumors, tuberculous adenitis, carotid artery dissection
Posterior retroparotid space	IX, X, XI, XII, and Horner syndrome	Villaret	Same as above, and granulomatous lesions (sarcoid, fungi)
Posterior retroparotid space	X and XII, with or without XI	Tapia	Parotid and other tumors of, or injuries to, the high neck

(See also Tables 31-5 and 34-3.)

atypical facial pain—is usually not difficult, especially if there is a trigger point and no demonstrable evidence of sensory or motor impairment. Furthermore, the vascular compressive form is difficult to diagnose without high-resolution neuroimaging or exposure at operation and most such cases are therefore characterized as idiopathic until revealed as vascular in causation.

In rare instances, trigeminal neuralgia is preceded or accompanied by hemifacial spasm, a combination that Cushing called *tic convulsif*. This may be indicative of a tumor (cholesteatoma), an aneurysmal dilatation of the basilar artery or one of its branches, or an arteriovenous malformation that compresses both the trigeminal and facial nerves. Trigeminal neuralgia and glossopharyngeal neuralgia (pain in the tonsillar region) may also be combined in these conditions.

Trigeminal Neuropathies and Neuritis Of the conditions that damage the branches of the trigeminal nerve, facial and cranial injuries, and fractures are probably the most common, but they do not usually come to the attention of neurologists. The most superficial branches of the nerve—the supratrochlear, supraorbital, and infraorbital—are the ones usually involved by trauma. The sensory loss is present from the time of the injury, and partial regeneration may be attended by constant pain.

Of the various inflammatory and infectious diseases that affect the trigeminal nerves or ganglia, *herpes zoster* ranks first. Persistent pain after herpetic infection of the fifth nerve is a serious problem, not responding well to any type of treatment. This subject is discussed in Chap. 10 with other forms of facial pain. Middle ear infections and osteomyelitis of the apex of the petrous bone may spread to the ganglion and root, also implicating the sixth cranial nerve (*Gradenigo syndrome*). HIV infection has not been clearly implicated in infection of the fifth nerve (as it has in the seventh nerve), but reactivation of latent herpes zoster is seen with AIDS.

The trigeminal root may be compressed or invaded by intracranial meningiomas, vestibular schwannomas, trigeminal schwannomas, cholesteatomas, and chordomas and by tortuous branches of the basilar artery. Sinus tumors and metastatic disease may also infiltrate the nerve, causing pain and a gradually progressive sensory loss. Demyelination at the trigeminal root entry point into the pons is another well-characterized cause in cases of multiple sclerosis (Fig. 47-2).

The ophthalmic division of the fifth nerve may be involved in the wall of the cavernous sinus in combination with the third, fourth, and sixth nerves by a variety of processes, including thrombosis of the cavernous sinus. Tumors of the sphenoid bone (myeloma, metastatic carcinoma, squamous cell carcinoma, and lymphoepithelioma of the nasopharynx) may involve branches of the trigeminal nerve at their foramina of entry or exit. An unusual perineural infiltration of superficial branches of the nerve by squamous cell skin cancers of the face is discussed further on under "Multiple Cranial-Nerve Palsies." The mandibular division of the nerve may be compressed by the roots of an impacted third molar (wisdom) tooth. Well known to clinicians is a sign of numbness of the chin and lower lip from infiltration of the mental nerve as the first indication of metastatic carcinoma of the breast, prostate, or multiple myeloma. Massey and colleagues have described the details of 19 such cases of the "numb-chin" sign.

Neurologists also encounter instances of slowly evolving unilateral or bilateral trigeminal neuropathy in which sensory impairment is confined to the territory

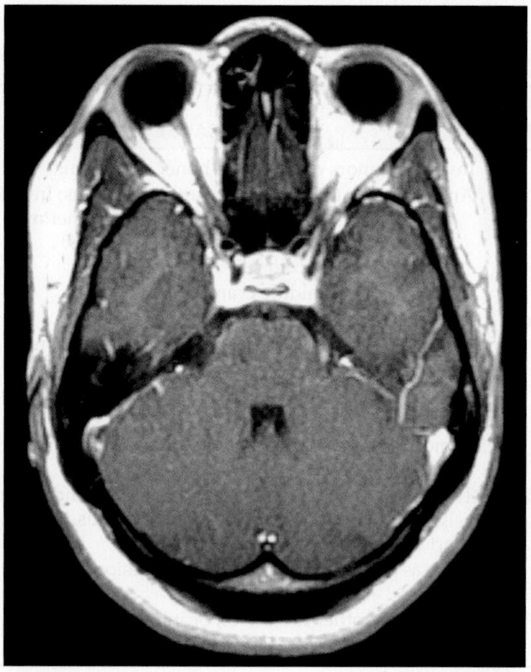

Figure 47-2. Left-sided facial sensory loss due to demyelination of the trigeminal root entry zone in a patient with multiple sclerosis. Abnormal enhancement of the nerve root is seen on T1 postgadolinium MRI.

of the trigeminal nerve, sometimes associated with pain, paresthesias, or disturbances of taste. This type of loss of facial sensation can also occur as part of a widespread sensory neuropathy or ganglionopathy that occurs as a paraneoplastic effect of cancer (see Chap. 31) or with Sjögren disease.

As common is an association between *isolated trigeminal neuropathy* and immune-mediated connective tissue diseases. Of 22 such cases described by Lecky and colleagues, 9 had either scleroderma or mixed connective tissue disease, and a similar number had either organ- or nonorgan-specific serum autoantibodies. Several specific antibody tests are used to establish the diagnosis of scleroderma. The symptoms may involve the other side of the face years later. Hughes has also described cases of trigeminal neuropathy with scleroderma, lupus erythematosus, and Sjögren disease. We have seen several patients with Sjögren disease in whom the trigeminal neuropathy and the associated antibodies or inflammation of the minor salivary glands were evident well before the characteristic sicca syndrome or other systemic manifestations of the disease. The condition may remain troublesome for years. Pathologic data are limited but point to an inflammatory lesion of the trigeminal ganglion or sensory root. Stilbamidine and trichloroethylene are known to cause sensory loss, tingling, burning, and itching exclusively in the trigeminal sensory territory.

Spillane and Wells, many decades ago, discussed an isolated trigeminal neuropathy (it had been called *Spillane's trigeminal neuritis*). Four of their 16 patients had an associated paranasal sinusitis, but subsequent reports have failed to substantiate a causal relationship between sinusitis and cranial neuritis. One wonders how many of these individuals had connective tissue disease. A less common form of idiopathic trigeminal sensory neuropathy with which we have limited experience has an acute onset and a tendency to resolve completely or partially, in much the same manner as Bell's palsy, with which it is sometimes associated (Blau et al). A recurrent variety of acute trigeminal symptoms of uncertain origin has been reported in the dental literature. We have had experience with two patients whose facial numbness was a component of an upper cervical disc syndrome that included numbness on the same side of the body; presumably the cervical spinal trigeminal nucleus or tract was compressed. Facial numbness, of course, also occurs with diverse conditions such as syringomyelia that affect the spinal nucleus of the trigeminal nerve but there are additional signs of brainstem or upper cervical cord disease.

An idiopathic pure unilateral *trigeminal motor neuropathy* is known but is a clinical rarity. Chia described five patients in whom an aching pain in the cheek and unilateral weakness of mastication were the main features. Electromyography (EMG) showed denervation changes in the ipsilateral masseter and temporalis muscles. The outcome was favorable.

In most cases of trigeminal neuropathy, except those caused by tumor, herpes zoster, and demyelination, the results of gadolinium-enhanced MRI are normal, as is the cerebrospinal fluid (CSF). The function of the nerve may be studied by the recording of blink reflexes. A few laboratories have developed an evoked potential test specifically of the trigeminal nerve.

The Seventh, or Facial, Nerve

Anatomic Considerations

The seventh nerve is mainly a motor nerve, supplying all the muscles concerned with facial expression on one side.

The sensory component is small (the nervus intermedius of Wrisberg); it conveys taste sensation from the anterior two-thirds of the tongue and, variably, cutaneous sensation from the anterior wall of the external auditory canal. The taste fibers at first traverse the lingual nerve (a branch of the trigeminal mandibular) and then join the chorda tympani, which conveys taste sensation via the facial nerve to the nucleus of the tractus solitarius. Secretomotor fibers originate in the superior salivatory nucleus and innervate the lacrimal gland through the greater superficial petrosal nerve and the sublingual and submaxillary glands through the chorda tympani (Fig. 47-3).

Several other anatomic facts are worth noting. The motor nucleus of the seventh nerve lies ventral and lateral to the abducens nucleus, and the intrapontine fibers of the facial nerve partly encircle and pass dorsolaterally to the abducens nucleus before emerging from the lower pons, just lateral to the corticospinal tract. The impression made by these looping fibers of the seventh nerve is visible in the floor of the upper fourth ventricle as a protuberance, the *facial colliculus*. In this region of the pons, infiltrative lesions affect the sixth and seventh nerves simultaneously.

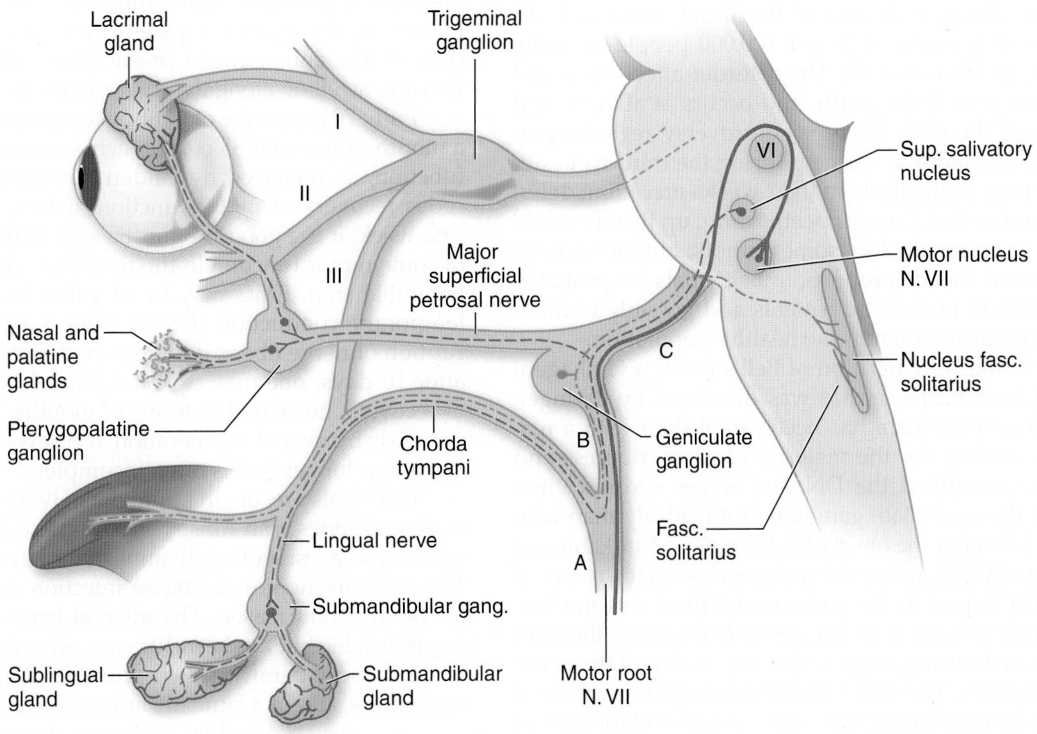

Figure 47-3. Scheme of the seventh cranial (facial) nerve. The motor fibers are represented by the *heavy blue line*. Parasympathetic fibers are represented by *regular dashes*; special visceral afferent (taste) fibers are represented by *long dashes and dots*. *A*, *B*, and *C* denote lesions of the facial nerve at the stylomastoid foramen, distal to the geniculate ganglion, and proximal to the geniculate ganglion. Disturbances resulting from lesions at each of these sites are described in the text. (From Carpenter MB, Sutin J: *Human Neuroanatomy*, 8th ed. Baltimore, Williams & Wilkins, 1982, by permission.)

The facial nerve enters the internal auditory meatus with the vestibulocochlear nerve bundle and then bends sharply forward and downward around the anterior boundary of the vestibule of the inner ear. At this angle (*genu*) lies the sensory ganglion (named *geniculate* because of its proximity to the genu). The nerve continues in its own bony channel, the facial canal, within which, just distal to the geniculate ganglion, it provides a branch to the pterygopalatine ganglion, i.e., the greater superficial petrosal nerve, which exits the skull through the vidian canal and innervates the lacrimal, nasal, and palatine glands. Somewhat more distally, it gives off a small motor branch to the stapedius muscle and is then joined by the chorda tympani, which projects to the submandibular ganglion and in turn, the submandibular and sublingual glands. The motor root of the facial nerve exits the skull at the stylomastoid foramen and then passes through the parotid gland and subdivides into five branches that supply the facial muscles, the stylomastoid muscle, the platysma, and the posterior belly of the digastric muscle.

A complete interruption of the facial nerve at the stylomastoid foramen paralyzes all muscles of facial expression on the same side. The corner of the mouth droops, the creases and skin folds are effaced, the forehead is unfurrowed, the palpebral fissure is widened and the eyelids will not close completely. Upon attempted closure of the lids, both eyes roll upward (Bell phenomenon), but the one on the paralyzed side remains visible because of lack of eyelid closure. The lower lid sags also, and the punctum falls away from the conjunctiva, permitting tears to spill over the cheek. (In contrast, the paralyzed frontalis muscle in patients of Asian origin sometimes lowers the eyelid and makes the palpebral fissure appear narrowed.) Food and secretions collect between the teeth and cheek, and saliva may dribble from the corner of the mouth. The patient complains of heaviness or numbness and sometimes an aching pain in the face, but sensory loss can usually not be demonstrated. Taste, however, is intact because the chorda tympani has separated from the main trunk of the facial nerve proximal to the stylomastoid foramen.

If the lesion is in the facial canal above the junction with the chorda tympani but below the geniculate ganglion, all the preceding symptoms are present but in addition, taste is lost over the anterior two-thirds of the tongue on the same side. The nerve to the stapedius muscle is also usually involved with a lesion at this site and there is *hyperacusis* (sensitivity to sudden loud sounds). If the geniculate ganglion or the motor root proximal to it is damaged, lacrimation and salivation may be reduced. Lesions at this point may also affect the adjacent eighth nerve, causing deafness, tinnitus, or dizziness.

Bell's Palsy

The most common disease of the facial nerve is Bell's palsy (incidence rate of 23 per 100,000 people annually according to Hauser et al). The disorder affects men and women more or less equally and occurs at all ages and all times of the year. There is controversy regarding an increased incidence in women during the third trimester of pregnancy, particularly in the 2 weeks preceding delivery and in the first 2 weeks postpartum; up to a threefold increase has been cited by some authors, but others have failed to find this disproportion. Bell's palsy is probably more common in diabetic patients and possibly in those with hypertension than in the healthy population.

Regarding the causation of Bell's palsy, a viral agent has long been suspected, as was discussed by Baringer, any such a mechanism has been established with a reasonable certainty for the majority of cases. Burgess and colleagues identified the DNA of herpes simplex virus (HSV) in the geniculate ganglion of an elderly man who died 6 weeks after the onset of Bell's palsy. Murakami and coworkers (1996), using the polymerase chain reaction, found HSV type I in the endoneurial fluid surrounding the seventh nerve in 11 of 14 cases of Bell's palsy; the fluid was obtained during surgical decompression of the nerve in severe cases. The same investigators produced facial paralysis by inoculating HSV into the ears and tongues of mice; virus antigens were then found in the facial nerve and geniculate ganglion. Varicella zoster virus (VZV) was not found in any of their patients but was isolated from patients with the Ramsay Hunt syndrome, which overtly follows shingles (see further on). Patients with fracture or other infections of the temporal bone yielded neither *HSV* nor *VZV* gene sequences. In the light of these findings, the term *idiopathic facial paralysis*, until now the accepted synonym for Bell's palsy, is not entirely appropriate. As one might expect, the opportunity to examine the facial nerve in the course of Bell's palsy occurs very rarely. Only a handful of such cases are on record, all showing varying degrees of degeneration of nerve fibers. One case was said to show inflammatory changes, but these may have been misinterpreted (see Karnes).

The onset of Bell's palsy is acute; about one-half of cases attain maximum paralysis in 48 h and practically all within 3 or 4 days. Pain behind the ear may precede the paralysis by a day or two and in a few patients is intense and persistent. Although a report by the patient of fullness or numbness in the face is common, in a small number there is hypesthesia in one or more branches of the trigeminal nerve. The explanation of this finding is not clear. Impairment of taste is present in most patients but it rarely persists beyond the second week of paralysis. This indicates that the lesion has extended proximal to the point at which the chorda tympani joins the facial nerve. Hyperacusis or distortion of sound is then experienced in the ipsilateral ear and, as mentioned, indicates paralysis of the stapedius muscle.

The facial nerve in Bell's palsy often displays abnormal signal on gadolinium-enhanced MRI although this may be difficult to appreciate in axial sections if the change is in the vertical part of the facial canal. There is a mild increase of lymphocytes and mononuclear cells in the CSF in a few instances. Cases with more pronounced contrast enhancement of the facial nerve apparently have a worse prognosis (Kress). The enhancement presumably reflects inflammation and swelling along the course of the facial nerve.

Fully 70 percent of patients recover completely within a month or two and 85 percent achieve near-normal facial function, as reviewed by Gilden. Recovery of taste precedes recovery of motor function; if taste returns in the first week, it is a good prognostic sign. But early recovery of some motor function in the first 5 to 7 days is the most favorable sign. EMG may be of value in distinguishing temporary conduction defects from a pathologic interruption of nerve fibers; if there is evidence of denervation after 10 days, one may expect a long delay in the onset of recovery, measured in terms of months. Recovery then proceeds by axonal regeneration, a process that may take 2 years or longer and is often incomplete.

Bell's palsy recurs in approximately 8 percent of cases in several series (van Amstel and Devriese; Pitts et al), presumably as a result of reactivation of the latent herpes virus. The palsy reemerges during an infection or pregnancy, or for no apparent reason. The interval between episodes is unpredictable but has been 10 years, on average. Recurrent forms of facial paralysis also occur with Lyme disease and sarcoidosis, and in a familial variety as mentioned below.

Treatment Protection of the eye during sleep is generally employed in the management of Bells' palsy. There is no evidence that surgical decompression of the facial nerve is effective, and it may be harmful. The administration of prednisone (40 to 60 mg/d, or an equivalent corticosteroid) during the first week to 10 days after onset has been beneficial in several trials. These medications are thought to decrease the possibility of permanent paralysis from swelling of the nerve in the tight facial canal.

The finding of viral genome surrounding the seventh nerve suggested that antiviral agents might be useful in the management of Bell's palsy but most evidence from large randomized trials, particularly the one conducted by Sullivan and colleagues, fails to support the use of these drugs alone or in combination with steroids The numerous earlier studies suggesting benefit from the combined antiviral and steroid treatments must be viewed in the context of these larger prospective trials. In appropriate circumstances, testing should be undertaken for infectious causes that would require alternative therapy (e.g., Lyme, HIV, and perhaps mycoplasma) but this is not routinely required. The treatment of facial palsy caused by VZV (Ramsay Hunt syndrome) with antiviral drugs is discussed later.

Other Causes of Facial Palsy

Lyme disease commonly involves the facial nerve, as indicated in Chap. 32. The mechanism is uncertain but there is, so far, no evidence of direct spirochetal infection of the nerve. The diagnosis is likely when there has been a tick bite with well-documented erythema migrans or arthritis. Several of our Lyme-infected patients have had almost simultaneous facial palsy and mild distal sensory polyneuropathy. HIV infection is another well-known infectious cause of facial palsy. The facial palsy of both

Lyme and HIV infections is associated with a pleocytosis in the spinal fluid, for which reason serologic and CSF examination may be useful if there is suspicion of either process. Rarely, chicken pox in children may be followed in 1 to 2 weeks by facial paralysis. Tuberculous infection of the mastoid and middle ear or of the petrous bone is a cause of facial paralysis in parts of the world where this infection is particularly common. Facial palsy may occur during or soon after infectious mononucleosis and was observed occasionally in poliomyelitis. The facial nerve is also frequently involved in leprosy. Bilateral involvement of the facial nerve is commented on below. The nerve is often involved in sarcoidosis, where the lesion is probably in the meninges as discussed in the following section.

The *Ramsay Hunt syndrome*, caused by herpes zoster of the geniculate ganglion, consists of a facial palsy associated with a vesicular eruption in the external auditory canal, other parts of the cranial integument, and mucous membrane of the oropharynx. This infection may be initially indistinguishable from Bell's palsy as the vesicles may not become apparent for days, or they never appear. Often the eighth cranial nerve is affected as well, causing nausea, vertigo, and deafness. Murakami and colleagues (1998) showed that the virus can be detected even before the emergence of typical vesicles by collecting exudate from the skin of the pinna on a Schirmer strip (otherwise used to quantitate tearing) and applying polymerase chain reaction (PCR) techniques. In this way, in a matter of a few hours, they documented VZV infection in 71 percent of patients with Ramsay Hunt syndrome without vesicles. Currently, treatment with acyclovir, valacyclovir, or famciclovir is recommended, and there is no clear role for corticosteroids. The randomized trial by Whitley et al and review by Sweeney and Gilden are recommended to the interested reader.

Tumors of the parotid gland or ones that invade the temporal bone (carotid body, cholesteatoma, and dermoid) or granulomatosis including the earlier mentioned sarcoidosis, or pachymeningitis at the base of the brain may produce a facial palsy; the onset is insidious and the course progressive. Fracture of the temporal bone (usually with damage to the middle or internal ear), otitis media, and middle ear surgery are uncommon causes. The orientation of the petrous fracture determines the prognosis (see discussion in Chap. 35). Acoustic neuromas, neurofibromas, glomus jugulare tumors, and aneurysmal dilatations of the vertebral or basilar artery may involve the facial nerve. Pontine lesions, most often vascular or neoplastic, cause facial palsy, usually in conjunction with other neurologic signs. Weakness of only a portion of the facial musculature, associated with numbness in the same region, may be the result of perineural tumor invasion by squamous cell or other skin cancers (see further on under "Multiple Cranial-Nerve Palsies"). An autosomal dominant syndrome of facial palsy, multiple truncal café-au-lait spots and mild developmental delay was described by Johnson and colleagues.

Bilateral Facial Palsy

Bell's palsy may be bilateral, but only rarely is the involvement on the two sides simultaneous. The truly contemporaneous appearance of *bilateral facial paralysis* (facial diplegia) is most often a manifestation of the Guillain-Barré syndrome (GBS) and may also occur in Lyme disease and rarely, with HIV infection. There are numerous other causes of bilateral facial palsy, all of them infrequent. Keane (1994) listed the idiopathic (now presumably mainly viral) variety, GBS, and meningeal infiltration by tumor as the most common causes, but also found two cases of syphilis among 43 patients. The bilateral syndrome has been reported in approximately 7 of every 1,000 patients with sarcoidosis, although our impression is that it is more frequent. When acute in onset and associated with parotid gland swelling from sarcoidosis, it has been referred to as *uveoparotid fever*, or *Heerfordt syndrome*. In typical cases of sarcoidosis, the paralysis on each side tends to be temporally separated by weeks or more. Mononucleosis may affect both sides of the face almost simultaneously; this is probably a form of GBS. Bifacial palsy is also a feature of the developmental disorder, Möbius syndrome (see Chap. 38).

Less common is the *Melkersson-Rosenthal syndrome*, consisting of the triad of *recurrent facial paralysis*, facial (particularly labial) edema, and less constantly, plication of the tongue. The syndrome begins in childhood or adolescence and may be familial. Biopsy of the lip or skin may reveal a granulomatous inflammation. The cause is not known and, despite the cardinal feature of angioneurotic edema, complement levels are normal. A series of biopsied cases has been reported by Elias and colleagues.

Kennedy syndrome, causes bifacial weakness in addition to bulbar palsy as the disease progresses; preceding facial fasciculations are characteristic. Facioscapulohumeral muscular dystrophy, as the name implies, incorporates facial weakness but would not be mistaken for Bell's palsy (see Chap. 48). The same is true for the rare form of amyloidosis associated with crystal lattice deposits in the cornea that typically involves both facial nerves.

Causes of *recurrent Bell's palsy* have been listed earlier and are summarized by Pitts and colleagues.

Facial Hemiatrophy (Parry-Romberg Syndrome)

This obscure disorder occurs mainly in females and is characterized by a disappearance of fat in the dermal and subcutaneous tissues on one or both sides of the face, giving the appearance of facial paresis. It usually begins in adolescence or early adulthood and is slowly progressive. In its advanced form, the affected side of the face is gaunt and the skin thin, wrinkled, and rather dark; the hair may turn white and fall out, and the sebaceous glands become atrophic; the muscles and bones are not involved as a rule. The condition is a form of *lipodystrophy*, but the localization within a myotome suggests the operation of some neural factor (possibly a growth factor) of unknown nature. A variegated coloration of the iris and a congenital oculosympathetic paralysis are found in some cases. Rarely, certain central nervous system abnormalities referable to the ipsilateral hemisphere (mainly focal seizures, migraine, trigeminal neuralgia, and ventricular dilatation), are conjoined (Hosten). The significance of these associations is unclear. Wilson and Hoxie have pointed out the frequent coexistence of facial asymmetry in adults with congenital or early onset superior oblique palsy and compensatory head tilt or torticollis.

Aberrant Effects of Recovery from Facial Nerve Palsy

If a peripheral facial paralysis has existed for some time and return of motor function has begun but is incomplete, a contracture with diffuse myokymic activity may appear. The palpebral fissure becomes narrowed, and the nasolabial fold deepens. Spasms of facial muscles may develop and persist indefinitely, being initiated by any facial movement. With the passage of time, the corner of the mouth and even the tip of the nose may become pulled to the affected side. This is a special acquired form of hemifacial spasm, the more common variety of which is described below.

Anomalous or aberrant regeneration of the seventh nerve fibers, following Bell's palsy or other injury, may result in other curious disorders that represent limited types of synkineses. The most common is the "jaw-winking" phenomenon (also called *Wartenberg* or *inverse Marcus-Gunn sign*), in which jaw movements, especially lateral movements (engaging the pterygoid muscle), cause an involuntary closure of the eyelid ipsilateral to the movement. If regenerating fibers originally connected with the orbicularis oculi become connected with the orbicularis oris, closure of the lids may cause a retraction of the corner of the mouth; or if visceromotor fibers originally innervating the salivary glands later come to innervate the lacrimal gland, anomalous tearing (crocodile tears) occurs whenever the patient salivates. A similar mechanism explains gustatory sweating of the cheek and upper lip.

Hemifacial Spasm

The facial muscles on one side may be involved in painless irregular clonic contractions of varying degree (*hemifacial spasm*). This condition usually develops in the fifth and sixth decades, affects women more than men, and often proves to be caused by a compressive lesion of the facial nerve, usually by a tortuous branch of the basilar artery that lies on the ventral surface of the pons and forms a loop under the proximal seventh nerve. Less often the cause of compression is a fusiform basilar artery aneurysm or a vestibular schwannoma or meningioma. Multiple sclerosis is another rare cause.

The spasm usually begins in the orbicularis oculi muscle and gradually spreads to other muscles on that side of the face, including the platysma. Paroxysms may be induced or aggravated by voluntary and reflexive movements of the face.

The pathophysiology of the spasm is believed to be focal demyelination at the site of nerve root compression by the vessel. The demyelinated axon is presumed to activate adjacent nerve fibers by ephaptic transmission ("artificial" synapse of Granit et al). Another possible source of the spasm is spontaneous ectopic excitation arising in injured fibers. Nielsen and Jannetta have shown that ephaptic transmission disappears after the nerve is decompressed.

Treatment Jannetta has attributed virtually all cases to a compression of the root of the facial nerve by an aberrant looped blood vessel. Microsurgical decompression of the root with the interposition of a pledget between the vessel and the facial nerve relieved the facial spasm in most of his operative patients. These results were corroborated by Barker and associates in a series of 705 patients followed postoperatively for an average period of 8 years; 84 percent achieved an excellent result. An even higher rate of benefit was obtained in a prospective series by Illingworth and colleagues (cure of 81 of 83 patients).

Surgical decompression of the aforementioned vascular loop, which involves exploration of the posterior fossa, however, carries some risk. The facial muscles may be weakened, sometimes permanently. Another complication has been deafness as a result of injury of the adjacent eighth nerve. Also, there is a risk of recurrence of the spasms, usually within 2 years of the operation (Piatt and Wilkins). Tight dural closure is required to prevent CSF leakage from the posterior fossa.

We suggest that patients with idiopathic hemifacial spasm should first be treated medically. Alexander and Moses noted that carbamazepine in doses of 600 to 1,200 mg/d controls the spasm in two-thirds of the patients. Baclofen or gabapentin can be tried if carbamazepine fails. Some patients cannot tolerate these drugs, have only brief remissions, or fail to respond; they may be treated with botulinum toxin injected into the orbicularis oculi and other facial muscles. The hemifacial spasms are relieved in this way for 4 to 5 months and injections can be repeated without danger. Some patients have been injected repeatedly for more than 5 years without apparent adverse effects. Failing these conservative measures, surgery may be appropriate.

Other Disorders of the Facial Nerve

Facial myokymia is a fine rippling activity of all the muscles of one side of the face mentioned earlier and in Chap. 48. It develops most often in the course of multiple sclerosis or a brainstem glioma, and can be seen in some disorders of the neuromuscular junction (e.g., neuromyotonia). It has also occurred after other diseases of the facial nerve, e.g., in GBS, in which case it is usually bilateral. We have seen it more often in the recovery stage than in the early phase of GBS. The fibrillary nature of the involuntary movements and their arrhythmicity tend to distinguish them from the coarser intermittent facial spasms and contracture, tics, tardive dyskinesia, and clonus. The EMG pattern is one of spontaneous asynchronous discharge of adjacent motor units, appearing singly or in doublets or triplets at a rate varying from 30 to 70 cycles per second. Demyelination of the intrapontine part of the facial nerve and possibly supranuclear disinhibition of the facial nucleus, have been the postulated mechanisms. But the observation of facial myokymia in GBS informs us that the abnormal movement may have its origin in a lesion at any point along the nerve.

A clonic or tonic contraction of one side of the face may be the sole manifestation of a cerebral cortical seizure. Involuntary recurrent spasm of both eyelids (*blepharospasm,* as discussed in Chaps. 6 and 14) may occur with almost any form of dystonia, but is most frequent in elderly persons as an isolated phenomenon, and there may be varying degrees of spasm of the other facial muscles (see Chap. 6). Although relaxant and tranquilizing drugs are of little help in this disorder, injections of botulinum toxin into the orbicularis oculi muscles give temporary or lasting relief. A few of our patients have been helped (paradoxically) by L-dopa; baclofen, clonazepam, and tetrabenazine in increasing doses may be helpful as well. In the past, failing these measures, the periorbital muscles were destroyed by injections of doxorubicin or surgical myectomy. With the advent of botulinum treatment, there is no longer a need to resort to these extreme and irreversible measures. In some cases, blepharospasm subsides spontaneously. Rhythmic unilateral myoclonus, akin to palatal myoclonus (actually a tremor as noted in Chap. 6), may be restricted to facial, lingual, or laryngeal muscles.

Hypersensitivity of the facial nerve occurs in hypocalcemic tetany; spasm of the facial muscles is elicited by tapping in front of the ear (Chvostek sign) but this phenomenon is seen in many normal individuals.

The Ninth, or Glossopharyngeal, Nerve

Anatomic Considerations

This nerve arises from the lateral surface of the medulla by a series of small roots that lie just rostral to those of the vagus nerve. The glossopharyngeal, vagus, and spinal accessory nerves leave the skull together through the jugular foramen and are then distributed peripherally. The *ninth nerve* is mainly sensory, with cell bodies in the inferior, or petrosal, ganglion (the central processes of which end in the nucleus solitarius) and the small superior ganglion (the central fibers of which enter the spinal trigeminal tract and nucleus). Within the nerve are afferent fibers from baroreceptors in the wall of the carotid sinus and from chemoreceptors in the carotid body. The baroreceptors are involved in the regulation of blood pressure, and chemoreceptors are responsible for the ventilatory responses to hypoxia. The somatic efferent fibers of the ninth nerve are derived from the nucleus ambiguus, and the visceral efferent (secretory) fibers, from the inferior salivatory nucleus. These fibers contribute in a limited way to the motor innervation of the striated musculature of the pharynx (mainly of the stylopharyngeus, which elevates the pharynx), the parotid gland, and the glands in the pharyngeal mucosa. A discussion of its role in swallowing is found in Chap. 26.

It is commonly stated that this nerve mediates sensory impulses from the faucial tonsils, posterior wall of the pharynx, and part of the soft palate as well as taste sensation from the posterior third of the tongue. However, an isolated lesion of the ninth cranial nerve is a rarity and therefore the effects are not fully known. In one personally observed case of bilateral surgical interruption of the ninth nerves, verified at autopsy, there had been no demonstrable loss of taste or other sensory or motor impairment. This suggests that the tenth nerve may be responsible for these functions, at least in some individuals. The role of the ninth nerve in the reflex control of blood pressure and ventilation has been alluded to earlier but referable clinical manifestations from damage of this cranial nerve are infrequent except perhaps for syncope as noted below.

One may occasionally observe glossopharyngeal palsy in conjunction with vagus and accessory nerve involvement because of a tumor in the posterior fossa or an aneurysm or intracranial dissection of the vertebral artery, or thrombosis of the sigmoid sinus or internal jugular vein. The nerves may be compressed as they pass through the jugular foramen. Hoarseness as a result of vocal cord paralysis, some difficulty in swallowing, deviation of the soft palate to the sound side, anesthesia of the posterior wall of the pharynx, and weakness of the upper trapezius and sternomastoid muscles make up the clinical picture (see Table 47-1, jugular foramen syndrome). On leaving the skull, the ninth, tenth, and eleventh nerves lie adjacent to the cervical internal carotid artery, where they can be damaged (presumably made ischemic) by a dissection of that vessel.

Glossopharyngeal Neuralgia (See additional discussion of this subject in Chap. 10)

This disorder, first described by Weisenburg in 1910, resembles trigeminal neuralgia in many respects except that the unilateral stabbing pain is localized to one side of the root of the tongue and throat. It is far less common than trigeminal neuralgia. Sometimes the pain overlaps the vagal territory beneath the angle of the jaw and external auditory meatus. It may be triggered by coughing, sneezing, swallowing, and pressure on the tragus of the ear. Temporary blocking of the pain by anesthetizing the tonsillar fauces and posterior pharynx with 10 percent lidocaine spray is diagnostic. Rarely, herpes zoster may involve the glossopharyngeal nerve. Fainting as a manifestation of vagoglossopharyngeal neuralgia is described in Chap. 10.

The same antiepileptic and other drugs that are helpful in the treatment of tic douloureux may be used to treat glossopharyngeal neuralgia, but their efficacy is difficult to judge. Regarding vascular compression of the nerve as a cause of glossopharyngeal neuralgia, Resnick and colleagues have reported the results of microvascular decompression of the ninth nerve in 40 patients; in 32 of these, relief of symptoms was complete and was sustained during an average followup of 4 years; 3 patients remained with permanent weakness of structures ostensibly innervated by the ninth nerve. A similar high rate of success has been achieved by others. If syncope is associated with the pain, it can be expected to cease with abolition of the attacks of pain. Syncope can also occur when the ninth nerve is involved by tumors of the parapharyngeal space; most of these are squamous cell carcinomas and both the ninth and tenth nerves are implicated. Section of rootlets of the ninth nerve has reportedly reduced or abolished the episodes of fainting in these cases.

The Tenth, or Vagus, Nerve

Anatomic Considerations

This nerve has an extensive sensory and motor distribution and important autonomic functions. It has two ganglia: the *jugular*, which contains the cell bodies of the somatic sensory nerves (innervating the skin in the concha of the ear), and the *nodose*, which contains the cell bodies of the afferent fibers from the pharynx, larynx, trachea, esophagus, and thoracic and abdominal viscera. The central processes of these two ganglia terminate in relation to the nucleus of the spinal trigeminal tract and the tractus solitarius, respectively. The motor fibers of the vagus are derived from two nuclei in the medulla—the nucleus ambiguus and the dorsal motor nucleus. The former supplies somatic motor fibers to the striated muscles of the larynx, pharynx, and palate; the latter supplies visceral motor fibers to the heart and other thoracic and abdominal organs. The distribution of vagal fibers is illustrated in Fig. 47-4, and their participation in swallowing is described in Chap. 26, which the reader is encouraged to consult.

Complete interruption of the intracranial portion of one vagus nerve results in a characteristic pattern of paralysis. The soft palate droops on the ipsilateral side and does not rise in phonation. The uvula deviates to the normal side on phonation, but this is an inconstant sign in disease. There is loss of the gag reflex on the affected side and of the *curtain movement* of the lateral wall of the pharynx, whereby the faucial pillars move medially as the palate rises in saying "ah." The voice is hoarse, often nasal, and the vocal cord on the affected side lies immobile in a "cadaveric" position, i.e., midway between abduction and adduction. With partial lesions, movements of abduction are affected more than those of adduction (Semon's law). There may be a loss of sensation at the external auditory meatus and back of the pinna. Usually no change in visceral function can be demonstrated with a unilateral lesion except by special autonomic testing. If the pharyngeal branches of both vagi are affected, as in diphtheria, the voice has a nasal quality, and regurgitation of liquids through the nose occurs during the act of swallowing.

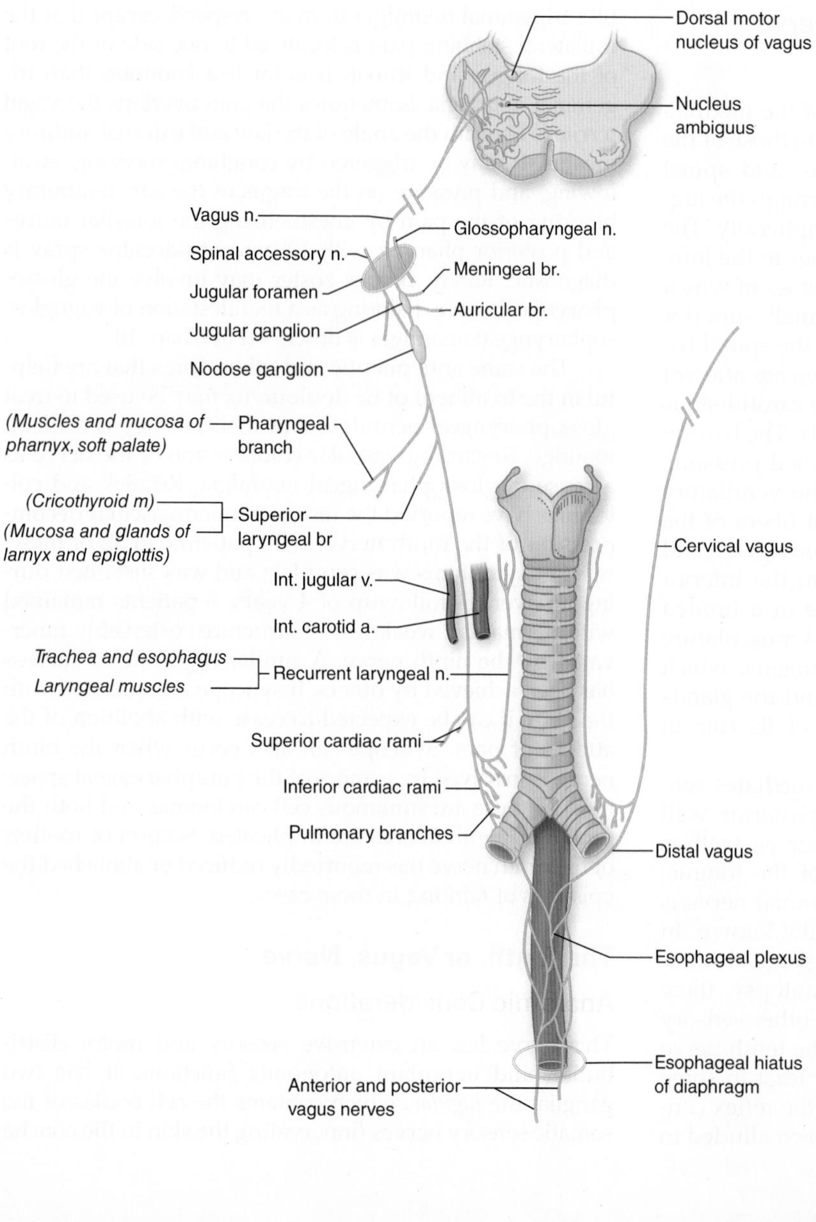

Figure 47-4. Anatomic features of the vagus nerve. Note the relationship to the spinal-accessory and glossopharyngeal nerves at the jugular foramen and the long course of the left recurrent laryngeal nerve, which is longer than the right and hooks around the aortic arch (not shown).

Diseases Affecting the Vagus

Complete bilateral paralysis is said to be incompatible with life, and this is probably true if the nuclei are entirely destroyed in the medulla by poliomyelitis or some other disease. However, in the cervical region, both vagi were blocked with procaine in the treatment of intractable asthma in past days without mishap. Of interest in this regard, Johnson and Stern reported a case of bilateral vocal cord paralysis in association with familial hypertrophic polyneuropathy, and Plott relates three brothers with congenital laryngeal abductor paralysis caused by bilateral dysgenesis of the nucleus ambiguus. Bannister and Oppenheimer have called attention to defects of phonation and laryngeal stridor as early features of autonomic failure in multiple system atrophy (see Chap. 39). We have seen several such patients in whom stridor was a prominent feature of the illness, in one patient for almost a year before other features of the degenerative disease became evident.

The vagus nerve may be implicated at the meningeal level by tumors neoplastic meningitis, and infectious processes and within the medulla by vascular lesions (e.g., the lateral medullary syndrome of Wallenberg, as described in Chap. 34), by motor neuron disease, and occasionally by sarcoid. Herpes zoster may attack this nerve, either alone or together with the ninth nerve as part of a jugular foramen syndrome. The vagus is often affected along with the glossopharyngeal nerve in spontaneous dissection of the carotid artery at the base of the skull. The nerves may be damaged in the course of thyroid surgery and may be involved in cases of advanced alcoholic or diabetic neuropathy. A fact of some importance is that the left recurrent laryngeal nerve, because of its long course under the aortic arch, is damaged as a result of thoracic disease. There is no dysphagia with lesions at this point in the nerve because the branches to the pharynx (but not to the larynx) have already been given off. For this reason, an aneurysm of the aortic arch, an enlarged left atrium, mediastinal lymph nodes from bronchial carcinoma, and a mediastinal or superior sulcus lung tumor are more frequent causes of an isolated (left) vocal cord palsy than are intracranial diseases. Finally, the vagus is compressed by lesions of the jugular foramen as part of a multiple cranial nerve syndrome as summarized in Table 47-1; metastatic tumors such as from the prostate or breast and jugular vein thrombosis are typical causes.

It is estimated that in one-quarter to one-third of all cases of paralysis of the recurrent laryngeal nerve no cause can be established, i.e., they are idiopathic. The highest incidence is in the third decade, and males are more susceptible than females. Of the 21 cases reported by Blau and Kapadia, 5 recovered completely and 5 partially within a few months; no other disease appeared in the 8-year period that followed. Berry and Blair described palsies of the superior and recurrent laryngeal nerves, occurring as part of isolated vagal neuropathies. A few were bilateral and, again, the majority of the cases were idiopathic and had much the same prognosis as isolated palsies of the recurrent laryngeal nerve.

Laryngeal neuralgia is a rare entity in which paroxysms of pain are localized over the upper portion of the thyroid cartilage or hyoid bone on one or both sides. The pain may be evoked by coughing, yawning, talking, or sneezing. In the case reported by Brownstone and coworkers, the symptoms were relieved by carbamazepine.

Neurologic Diagnosis of Vocal Cord Paralysis

When confronted with a case of vocal cord palsy, the physician is advised to determine the site of the lesion. If intramedullary, there are usually ipsilateral cerebellar signs, loss of pain and temperature sensation over the ipsilateral face and contralateral arm and leg, and an ipsilateral Bernard-Horner syndrome (see Table 34-3). If the lesion is extramedullary but intracranial, the glossopharyngeal and spinal accessory nerves are frequently involved as well (jugular foramen syndrome; see Table 47-1). If extracranial in the posterior lateral condylar or retroparotid space, there may be a combination of ninth, tenth, eleventh, and twelfth cranial-nerve palsies and a Horner syndrome. Combinations of these lower cranial-nerve palsies, which have a variety of eponymic designations (see Table 47-1) are caused by various tumors, both primary and metastatic, or by chronic inflammations or granulomas involving lymph nodes at the base of the skull. If there is no palatal weakness and no pharyngeal or palatal sensory loss, the lesion is below the origin of the pharyngeal branches, which leaves the vagus nerve high in the cervical region. The usual site of disease is then the mediastinum.

The Eleventh, or Spinal Accessory, Nerve

Anatomic Considerations

This is a purely motor nerve, of spinal rather than cranial origin. Its fibers arise from the anterior horn cells of the upper four or five cervical segments and enter the skull through the foramen magnum. Intracranially, the accessory nerve travels for a short distance with the part of the tenth nerve that is derived from the caudalmost cells of the nucleus ambiguus; together, the two roots are referred to as the *vagal-accessory nerve* or the *cranial root of the accessory nerve*. The two roots together leave the skull through the jugular foramen. The vagus fibers then rejoin the main trunk of the vagus. The motor fibers derived from the upper cervical segments of the spinal cord form an "external ramus" and innervate the ipsilateral sternocleidomastoid and trapezius muscles. Only the somatic motor fibers constitute the accessory nerve in the strict sense. In patients with torticollis, however, division of the upper cervical motor roots or the spinal accessory nerve has often failed to ablate completely the contraction of the sternocleidomastoid muscle. This suggests a wider innervation of the muscle, perhaps by fibers of apparent vagal origin that join the accessory nerve for passage through the jugular foramen.

A complete lesion of the accessory nerve results in weakness of the sternocleidomastoid muscle and upper part of the trapezius (the lower part of the trapezius is innervated by the third and fourth cervical roots through the cervical plexus). Weakness can be demonstrated by asking the patient to shrug his shoulders; the affected side will be found to be weaker, and there will often be evident atrophy of the upper part of the trapezius. With the arms at the sides, the shoulder on the affected side droops and the scapula is slightly winged; the latter defect is accentuated with lateral movement of the arm (with serratus anterior weakness, winging of the scapula is more prominent and occurs on forward elevation of the arm). When the patient turns his head forcibly against the examiner's hand, preferably starting with the head deviated to the opposite side, the sternocleidomastoid of the opposite side does not contract firmly beneath the fingers. This muscle can be further tested by having the patient press his head forward against resistance or lift his head from the pillow.

Motor neuron disease, poliomyelitis, syringomyelia, and spinal cord tumors may involve the cells of origin of the spinal accessory nerve. In its intracranial portion, the nerve is usually affected along with the ninth and tenth cranial nerves by herpes zoster or by lesions of the jugular foramen (glomus tumors, neurofibromas, metastatic carcinoma, internal jugular vein thrombosis). Tumors at the foramen magnum may also damage the nerve. In the posterior triangle of the neck, the eleventh nerve can be damaged during surgical operations and by external compression or injury. Compressive-invasive lesions of this nerve may be visualized by CT or MRI of the posterior cervical space.

A benign disorder of the eleventh nerve, akin to Bell's palsy, has been described by Spillane and by Eisen and Bertrand. It begins with pain in the low lateral neck that subsides in a few days and is followed by weakness and atrophy in the distribution of the nerve. Also, a recurrent form of spontaneous accessory neuropathy has been described (Chalk and Isaacs). About one-quarter to one-third of eleventh nerve lesions are estimated to be of this idiopathic type; most, but not all, of the patients recover.

Bilateral sternocleidomastoid and trapezius palsy, which occurs with primary disease of muscles—e.g., polymyositis and muscular dystrophy—may be difficult to distinguish from a bilateral damage to the accessory nerves or the motor nuclei (progressive bulbar palsy). The supranuclear innervation of the spinal accessory nuclei is apparently mainly ipsilateral as evidenced by contraversive turning of the head during a seizure, the result of contraction of the ipsilateral sternocleidomastoid muscle. Whether this is attributable to a direct ipsilateral tract, or to double crossing of the supranuclear tracts, is not known.

The Twelfth, or Hypoglossal, Nerve

Anatomic Considerations

This is also a pure motor nerve, which supplies the somatic musculature of the tongue. It arises as a series of rootlets that issue from the ventral medulla between the pyramid and inferior olivary complex. The nerve leaves the skull through the hypoglossal foramen and innervates the genioglossus muscle, which acts to protrude the tongue; the styloglossus, which retracts and elevates its root; and the hypoglossus, which causes the upper surface to become convex. Complete interruption of the nerve results in paralysis of one side of the tongue. The tongue curves slightly to the healthy side as it lies in the mouth, but on protrusion it deviates to the affected side, owing to the unopposed contraction of the healthy genioglossus muscle. By pushing against the tongue in the cheek, one can judge the degree of weakness. The tongue also cannot be moved with natural facility, causing difficulty with handling food in the mouth as well as mild but characteristic *lingual dysarthria*. The denervated side becomes wrinkled and atrophied, and fasciculations can be seen.

Isolated lesions of the hypoglossal nerve roots are rare. Occasionally an intramedullary lesion, usually a stroke, damages the emerging fibers of the hypoglossal nerve, corticospinal tract, and medial lemniscus (see Table 34-3). The result is paralysis and atrophy of one side of the tongue, together with spastic paralysis and loss of vibration and position sense in the opposite arm and leg. Poliomyelitis and motor neuron disease may destroy the hypoglossal nuclei. The latter is the most common cause of a bilaterally atrophic and fasciculating tongue. Lesions of the basal meninges and of the occipital bones (tumor invasion, platybasia, invagination of the occipital condyles, Paget disease) may involve the nerve in its extramedullary course, and it is sometimes damaged in operations on the neck including carotid endarterectomy. Goodman and coworkers showed a dissecting aneurysm of the carotid artery to have compressed the hypoglossal nerve, with resultant weakness and atrophy of the tongue. Rare instances of temporal arteritis and Takayasu arteritis affecting the carotid artery and adjacent twelfth nerve have been described. Lance and Anthony have described the simultaneous occurrence of nuchal-occipital pain and ipsilateral numbness of the tongue, provoked by the sudden, sharp turning of the head and termed it the *neck–tongue syndrome*. The phenomenon has been attributed to compression in the atlantoaxial space of the second cervical root, which carries some of the sensory fibers from the tongue, via the hypoglossal nerve, to the C2 segment of the spinal cord.

It is worth mentioning here that the tongue is often red and smooth in vitamin-deficiency states. *Glossodynia* (burning mouth syndrome discussed in Chap. 10), a condition most frequently seen in the elderly and in young women, may or may not be accompanied by redness and dryness, but not by lingual weakness. A habit of tongue-thrusting and teeth-clenching is often associated. The ascription of these motor abnormalities to a psychogenic mechanism does not agree with the authors' experience (see Quinn).

SYNDROME OF BULBAR PALSY

This syndrome is the result of weakness or paralysis of muscles that are supplied by the motor nuclei of the lower brainstem, i.e., the motor nuclei of the fifth, seventh, and ninth to twelfth cranial nerves. (Strictly speaking, the motor nuclei of the fifth and seventh nerves lie outside the "bulb," which is the old name for the medulla oblongata.) Involved are the muscles of the jaw and face; the sternocleidomastoids and upper parts of the trapezii; and the muscles of the tongue, pharynx, and larynx. If weakness develops rapidly, as may happen in GBS, diphtheria, or poliomyelitis, there is no time for muscle atrophy.

Myasthenia gravis, inclusion body myopathy, and polymyositis on rare occasions may produce such a picture, but motor neuron disease is the most common cause. When the latter disease is isolated to the bulbar muscles, it has been called *progressive bulbar palsy*. The more chronic diseases—e.g., progressive bulbar palsy and Kennedy bulbospinal atrophy (forms of motor neuron disease) and the childhood form of Fazio-Londe disease—result in marked wasting and fasciculation of the facial, tongue, sternocleidomastoid, and trapezius muscles. All of these disorders must be differentiated from pseudobulbar palsy that is discussed in Chaps. 23 and 25.

MULTIPLE CRANIAL-NERVE PALSIES

As one can readily understand, several cranial nerves may be affected by a single disease process. The first clinical problem that arises is whether the lesion lies within or outside the brainstem. Lesions lying on the surface of the brainstem, infiltrating the meninges, or situated at the base of the skull are characterized by involvement of adjacent cranial nerves (often occurring in succession and sometimes painful) and by late and only slight, if any, involvement of the long sensory and motor pathways. These are discussed later and listed in Table 47-1 by their eponymic designations. The opposite is true of intramedullary, intrapontine, and intramesencephalic lesions; lesions within the brainstem that involve cranial nerves often produce a crossed-sensory or motor paralysis (cranial nerve signs on one side of the body and tract signs on the opposite side). In this way, a number of distinctive brainstem syndromes, to which eponyms have been attached, are produced. These are listed in Table 34-3 because they are most often the result of brainstem stroke. An extramedullary lesion is more likely to cause bone erosion seen radiographically. The special problems of multiple cranial-nerve palsies of the ocular motor nerves are addressed in Chap. 14.

Involvement of multiple cranial nerves outside the brainstem may be the result of trauma; localized infections such as herpes zoster (subacute onset); Lyme disease as reported by Schmutzhard and colleagues; cytomegalovirus (CMV) infection in an HIV patient; Wegener granulomatosis, sarcoidosis, or other types of granulomatous diseases or compression by tumors and saccular aneurysms (more chronic development with pain). *The sequential painless affection of contiguous or noncontiguous nerves over several days or weeks is particularly characteristic of meningeal carcinomatosis or lymphomatosis.* In the series of 79 cases accumulated by Keane (2005), tumor was by far the most common underlying cause of multiple cranial-nerve palsies particularly schwannomas, metastases, and meningiomas; trauma, infection, and vascular disease followed in frequency after neoplasm. The eighth nerve is commonly incorporated in these neoplastic meningeal infiltrations. Among the solid tumors that cause local compression of nerves, neurofibromas, schwannomas, meningiomas, cholesteatomas, carcinomas, chordomas, and chondromas have all been observed. Nasopharyngeal carcinoma (Schmincke tumor or lymphoepithelioma) may implicate several cranial nerves in succession by invading the base of the skull (mainly the fifth and sixth but also higher nerves; Fig. 47-5), as do basilar invagination and Chiari malformation. Several lower cranial nerves may be involved on one side by a carotid artery dissection. In France, a successive involvement of all cranial nerves on one side has been called the *Garcin syndrome*, or hemibasal syndrome. It has been reported in chondromas and chondrosarcomas of the clivus, but may occur with nasopharyngeal carcinomas. Table 47-2 lists the main causes of multiple cranial-nerve palsies of extramedullary origin in our experience.

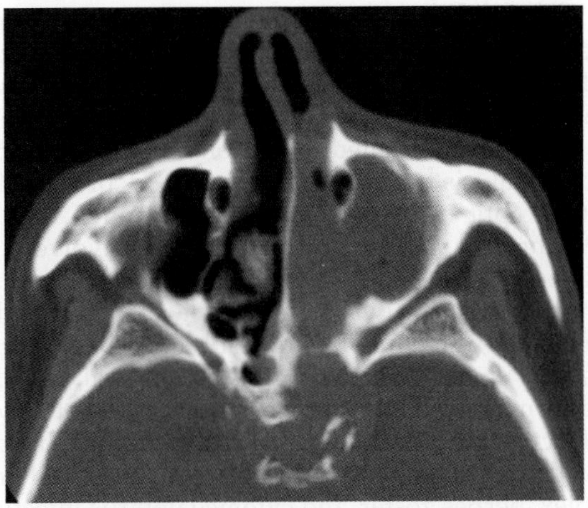

Figure 47-5. Nasopharyngeal carcinoma invading the anterior right side of the base of the skull and causing third and fifth nerve palsies. Axial CT windowed for bones.

Table 47-2

CAUSES OF EXTRAMEDULLARY MULTIPLE CRANIAL NERVE PALSIES

Meningeal processes
Carcinomatous and lymphomatous meningitis
Sarcoidosis and Wegener granulomatosis
Infectious radiculitis (tuberculous, fungal, syphilitic, Lyme)
Idiopathic pachymeningitis
Lesions affecting nerves at the skull base
Metastasis of solid tumor or lymphomatous infiltration
Local spread from nasopharyngeal tumor, chordoma, sarcoma
Trauma
Vascular occlusion or dissection (carotid artery dissection, jugular vein thrombosis)
Paget disease, basilar invagination, Arnold-Chiari, and other bony disorders
Processes within nerves
Perineural invasion of spindle cell, basal cell, parotid, and squamous cell cancer
Granulomas and infectious diseases (Listeria, sarcoid, Wegener granulomatosis, diphtheria, HIV, Lyme disease, CMV infection in AIDS, Sjögren syndrome, idiopathic)
Herpes zoster and other viral and postinfectious inflammatory lesions (GBS)
Mixed connective tissue disease
Idiopathic
Tolosa-Hunt–like syndrome affecting nonorbital nerves
Post- and parainfectious

Multiple or single cranial-nerve palsies of abrupt onset may precede or accompany infectious mononucleosis and sometimes other viral or mycoplasmal diseases. DeSimone and Snyder assembled a series of 20 such cases associated with mononucleosis; bilateral facial paralysis was the most common presentation, bilateral optic neuritis the next most common, and in 3 cases, three or four cranial nerves were involved. The prognosis is excellent. The question of *viral infections of cranial nerves* is always raised by acute neuropathies of the facial, trigeminal, and vestibulocochlear nerves, especially when the condition is bilateral, involves several nerves in combination, or is associated with a pleocytosis in the spinal fluid. Actually, the only proved viral etiologies in this group of cases are herpes simplex, herpes zoster, and cytomegalovirus infections. Because neural deafness, vertigo, and other cranial-nerve palsies have been observed in conjunction with the postinfectious encephalomyelitides of *Mycoplasma*, varicella, measles, rubella, mumps, and scarlet fever, they probably share an immune-mediated mechanism. Some cases formerly thought to be postinfectious in nature may be true infections of the nerve. The same may be said of the single and multiple cranial-nerve palsies that are sometimes associated with HIV and CMV infections. Treatment of the parainfectious cases is symptomatic; the prognosis for recovery is good in many cases. The main causes of bilateral facial palsy were discussed earlier in the chapter. A purely motor disorder of the facial and oropharyngeal muscles without atrophy always raises the question of myasthenia gravis or a muscular dystrophy.

Quite often one observes an acute or subacute form of *multiple cranial neuropathy of undetermined cause*. Juncos and Beal reported on 14 cases of this type, incorporating 6 well-documented cases of the Tolosa-Hunt orbitocavernous sinus syndrome with oculomotor palsies. In the group that was not attributable to Tolosa-Hunt, the onset was with facial pain and headache (temporofrontal), followed within days by abducens palsy (12 of 14), oculomotor palsy (6 of 14), trigeminal palsy (5 of 14), and facial weakness (4 of 14), and less often by involvement of the eighth, ninth, and tenth cranial nerves (unilaterally in most instances). Increased CSF protein and pleocytosis occurred in several. The prompt relief of pain upon administration of steroids was similar to that obtained in the Tolosa-Hunt syndrome. The mode of recovery, which usually occurred within a few months, was also much the same in the two groups of patients. Juncos and Beal concluded that the clinical features of the two groups overlapped and that their separation into two syndromes was arbitrary. We have seen a relapsing form of this illness in young adults, responsive on each occasion to steroids and stabilizing after several years. Numerous tests of the CSF by polymerase chain reaction revealed no viruses. Conceivably, some of these cases represent variant forms of GBS, inasmuch as they may be preceded by a nonspecific infection and may at times be accompanied by areflexia or evanescent paresthesias and elevated CSF protein without pleocytosis. Others probably are examples of the entity described by Juncos and Beal, possibly reflecting a granulomatous process in the pachymeninges.

As a more chronic affliction, we have observed numerous cases in which cranial nerves were affected sequentially over a period of many years (*polyneuritis cranialis multiplex*). Two were later found to have tuberculosis of cervical lymph nodes (presumably tuberculous scrofula), and three had sarcoidosis. No cause was determined in the rest. Symonds had similar experience. It is usually worth obtaining a biopsy of an enlarged cervical lymph node in these circumstances.

Chapter 14 discusses the special case of painful multiple oculomotor palsies. The main causes are GBS, botulism, myasthenia gravis, thyroid ophthalmopathy, and diphtheria. In cases of chronic evolution, oculopharyngeal dystrophy and mitochondrial myopathy (progressive external ophthalmoplegia) must also be considered.

In cases of *Tolosa-Hunt* syndrome in which the orbital or cavernous sinus has been biopsied, a nonspecific granuloma has been found as discussed in Chap. 14. *Sarcoid* and *tuberculosis* have been the causes of a few cases, as noted earlier. In *Wegener granulomatosis*, multiple cranial-nerve palsies, usually lower ones, are reported. The administration of cyclophosphamide has led to remission.

The *cavernous sinus syndrome*, discussed in Chaps. 32, and 34 and elsewhere in the book, consists of various combinations of oculomotor palsies and upper trigeminal sensory loss, usually accompanied by signs of increased pressure or inflammation of the venous sinus. The third, fourth, fifth, and sixth cranial nerves are affected first on one side only, but any of the processes that infiltrate or obstruct the sinus may spread to the other side. The main causes are septic or aseptic thrombosis of the venous sinus due to trauma, hypercoagulable states, or adjacent infections in adjacent structures, carotid artery aneurysm, carotid-cavernous fistulae, and neoplastic infiltration. Keane (1996) summarized his experience with an astonishing 151 instances of cavernous sinus syndrome and found trauma and surgical procedures to be the most common causes, followed by neoplasms (specifically those originating in the nasopharynx), pituitary tumors, metastases, and lymphomas; our experience has tended more toward local infectious causes in diabetic patients and hypercoagulable states.

A special cause of multiple cranial-nerve palsies that has been brought to our attention is an infiltration along the distal nerves in the skin and subcutaneous tissues by squamous cell carcinomas of the face, especially by spindle cell and other atypical varieties of tumor. A variant of malignant melanoma, "lentigo maligna" may do the same but has more of a tendency to infiltrate along larger nerves to the base of the skull and cause larger areas of loss of facial sensation and pain, vertigo, and deafness. This type of perineural spread first causes very restricted unilateral palsies and sensory loss related to the superficial branches of the fifth and seventh cranial nerves in one region of the face and then extends to the base of the skull and to the ventral brainstem. According to Clouston and colleagues, who have presented five cases in detail, the initial symptoms are usually pain and numbness in the area underlying the skin lesion and facial weakness confined to the same regions of the face; this pattern is a result of the proximity of fifth and seventh nerve branches in the skin and subcutaneous tissues. Various combinations of oculomotor palsies may follow as a result of tumor entry into the orbit via the infraorbital branch of the maxillary nerve. Occasionally there is no pain. We have also observed a similar regional pattern of extracranial involvement of trigeminal and facial nerves with an infiltrative mixed-cell tumor of the parotid gland.

References

Alexander GE, Moses H: Carbamazepine for hemifacial spasm. *Neurology* 32:286, 1982.

Bannister R, Oppenheimer DR: Degenerative diseases of the nervous system associated with autonomic failure. *Brain* 95:457, 1972.

Baringer JH: Herpes simplex virus and Bell palsy. *Ann Intern Med* 124:63, 1996.

Barker FG, Jannetta PJ, Bissonette DJ, et al: Microvascular decompression for hemifacial spasm. *J Neurosurg* 82:201, 1995.

Berry H, Blair RL: Isolated vagus nerve palsy and vagal mononeuritis. *Arch Otolaryngol* 106:333, 1980.

Blau JN, Harris M, Kennet S: Trigeminal sensory neuropathy. *N Engl J Med* 281:873, 1969.

Blau JN, Kapadia R: Idiopathic palsy of the recurrent laryngeal nerve: A transient cranial mononeuropathy. *Br Med J* 4:259, 1972.

Brodal A: *The Cranial Nerves*. Springfield, IL, Charles C Thomas, 1959.

Brownstone PK, Ballenger JJ, Vick NA: Bilateral superior laryngeal neuralgia. *Arch Neurol* 37:525, 1980.

Burgess RC, Michaels L, Bale JF Jr, Smith RJ: Polymerase chain reaction amplification of herpes simplex viral DNA from the geniculate ganglion of a patient with Bell's palsy. *Ann Otol Rhinol Laryngol* 103:775, 1994.

Chalk C, Isaacs H: Recurrent spontaneous accessory neuropathy. *J Neurol Neurosurg Psychiatry* 53:621, 1990.

Chia L-G: Pure trigeminal motor neuropathy. *BMJ* 296:609, 1988.

Clouston PD, Sharpe DM, Corbett AJ, et al: Perineural spread of cutaneous head and neck cancer: Its orbital and central neurologic complications. *Arch Neurol* 47:73, 1990.

De Diego JI, Prim MP, De Sarria MJ, et al: Idiopathic facial paralysis: A randomized, prospective, and controlled study using single-dose prednisone versus acyclovir three times daily. *Laryngoscope* 108:573, 1998.

DeSimone PA, Snyder D: Hypoglossal nerve palsy in infectious mononucleosis. *Neurology* 28:844, 1978.

Devinsky O, Feldmann E: *Examination of the Cranial and Peripheral Nerves*. New York, Churchill Livingstone, 1988.

Eisen A, Bertrand G: Isolated accessory nerve palsy of spontaneous origin: A clinical and electromyographic study. *Arch Neurol* 27:496, 1972.

Elias MK, Mateen FJ, Weller CR, et al: The Melkersson-Rosenthal syndrome: A retrospective series of biopsied cases. *J Neurol* 260:138, 2013.

Gilden DH: Bell's palsy. *N Engl J Med* 351:1323, 2004.

Goodman JM, Zink WL, Cooper DF: Hemilingual paralysis caused by spontaneous carotid artery dissection. *Arch Neurol* 40:653, 1983.

Granit R, Leskell L, Skogland CR: Fibre interaction in injured or compressed region of nerve. *Brain* 67:125, 1944.

Hauser WA, Karnes WE, Annis J, Kurland LT: Incidence and prognosis of Bell's palsy in the population of Rochester, Minnesota. *Mayo Clin Proc* 46:258, 1971.

Hosten N: MR of brain involvement in progressive facial hemiatrophy (Romberg disease): Reconsideration of a syndrome. *AJNR Am J Neuroradiol* 15:145, 1994.

Hughes RAC: Diseases of the fifth cranial nerve, in Dyck PJ, Thomas PK, Lambert EH, et al (eds): *Peripheral Neuropathy*, 3rd ed. Philadelphia, Saunders, 1993, pp 801–817.

Illingworth RD, Porter DG, Jakubowski J: Hemifacial spasm: A prospective long-term follow up of 83 patients treated by microvascular decompression. *J Neurol Neurosurg Psychiatry* 60:73, 1996.

Jannetta PJ: Posterior fossa neurovascular compression syndromes other than neuralgias, in Wilkins RH, Rengachary SS (eds): *Neurosurgery*, 2nd ed. New York, McGraw-Hill, 1996, pp 3227–3233.

Johnson JA, Stern LZ: Bilateral vocal cord paralysis in a patient with familial hypertrophic neuropathy. *Arch Neurol* 38:532, 1981.

Johnson VP, McMillin JM, Aceto T, Bruins G: A newly recognized neuroectodermal syndrome of familial alopecia, anosmia, deafness, and hypogonadism. *Am J Med Genet* 15:497, 1983.

Juncos JL, Beal MF: Idiopathic cranial polyneuropathy. *Brain* 110:197, 1987.

Karnes WE: Diseases of the seventh cranial nerve, in Dyck PJ, Thomas PK, Lambert EH, et al (eds): *Peripheral Neuropathy*, 3rd ed. Philadelphia, Saunders, 1993, pp 818–836.

Katusic S, Beard CM, Bergstralh E, Kurland LT: Incidence and clinical features of trigeminal neuralgia, Rochester, Minnesota, 1945–1984. *Ann Neurol* 27:89, 1990.

Keane JR: Bilateral seventh nerve palsy: Analysis of 43 cases and review of the literature. *Neurology* 44:1198, 1994.

Keane JR: Cavernous sinus syndrome: Analysis of 151 cases. *Arch Neurol* 53:967, 1996.

Keane JR: Multiple cranial nerve palsies: Analysis of 79 cases. *Arch Neurol* 62:1714, 2005.

Kress B, Griesbeck F, Stippich C, et al: Bell's palsy: Quantitative analysis of MR imaging data as a method of predicting outcome. *Radiology* 230:504, 2004.

Lance JW, Anthony M: Neck-tongue syndrome on sudden turning of the head. *J Neurol Neurosurg Psychiatry* 43:97, 1980.

Lecky BRF, Hughes RAC, Murray NMF: Trigeminal sensory neuropathy. *Brain* 110:1463, 1987.

Love S, Coakham HB: Trigeminal neuralgia. Pathology and pathogenesis. *Brain* 124:2347, 2001.

Massey EW, Moore J, Schold SC Jr: Mental neuropathy from systemic cancer. *Neurology* 31:1277, 1981.

Mayo Clinic Department of Neurology: *Clinical Examinations in Neurology*, 7th ed. St. Louis, Mosby-Year Book, 1998.

Murakami S, Honda N, Mizobuchi M, et al: Rapid diagnosis of varicella zoster virus in acute facial palsy. *Neurology* 51:1202, 1998.

Murakami S, Mizobuchi M, Nakashiro Y, et al: Bell palsy and herpes simplex virus: Identification of viral DNA in endoneurial fluid and muscle. *Ann Intern Med* 124:27, 1996.

Nielsen VK, Jannetta PJ: Pathophysiology of hemifacial spasm: Effects of facial nerve decompression. *Neurology* 34:891, 1984.

Piatt JH, Wilkins RH: Treatment of tic douloureux and hemifacial spasm by posterior fossa exploration: Therapeutic implications of various neurovascular relationships. *Neurosurgery* 14:462, 1984.

Pitts DB, Adour KK, Hilsinger RL: Recurrent Bell's palsy analysis of 140 patients. *Laryngoscope* 98:535, 1988.

Plott D: Congenital laryngeal-abductor paralysis due to nucleus ambiguus dysgenesis in three brothers. *N Engl J Med* 271:593, 1964.

Quinn JH: Glossodynia. *J Am Dent Assoc* 70:1418, 1965.

Resnick DK, Jannetta PJ, Bissonette D, et al: Microvascular decompression for glossopharyngeal neuralgia. *Neurosurgery* 36:64, 1995.

Schmutzhard E, Stanek G, Pohl P: Polyneuritis cranialis associated with *Borrelia burgdorferi*. *J Neurol Neurosurg Psychiatry* 48:1182, 1985.

Silverman JE, Liu GT, Volpe NJ, Galetta SL: The crossed paralyses. *Arch Neurol* 52:635, 1995.

Spillane JD: Isolated unilateral spinal accessory nerve palsy of obscure origin. *Br Med J* 2:365, 1949.

Spillane JD, Wells CEC: Isolated trigeminal neuropathy: A report of 16 cases. *Brain* 82:391, 1959.

Sullivan FM, Swan IR, Donnan PR, et al: Early treatment with prednisolone or acyclovir in Bell's palsy. *N Engl J Med* 357:1598, 2007.

Sweeney CJ, Gilden DH: Ramsay Hunt syndrome. *J Neurol Neurosurg Psychiatry* 71:149, 2001.

Sweet WH: The treatment of trigeminal neuralgia (tic douloureux). *N Engl J Med* 315:174, 1986.

Symonds C: Recurrent multiple cranial nerve palsies. *J Neurol Neurosurg Psychiatry* 21:95, 1958.

van Amstel AD, Devriese PP: Clinical experience with recurrences of Bell's palsy. *Arch Otorhinolaryngol* 245:302, 1998.

Whitley RJ, Weiss H, Gnann JW, et al: Acyclovir with and without prednisone for the treatment of herpes zoster: A randomized, placebo-controlled trial. *Ann Intern Med* 125:376, 1996.

Wilson ME, Hoxie J: Facial asymmetry in superior oblique muscle palsy. *J Pediatr Ophthalmol Strabismus* 30:315, 1993.

48

Diseases of Muscle

Skeletal, or voluntary, muscle constitutes the principal organ of locomotion, as well as a vast metabolic reservoir. Disposed in more than 600 separate muscles, this tissue makes up as much as 40 percent of the weight of adult human beings. An intricacy of structure and function undoubtedly accounts for its diverse susceptibility to disease, for which reason the main anatomic and clinical facts are provided as an introduction to the muscle diseases.

A single muscle is composed of thousands of muscle fibers that extend for variable distances along its longitudinal axis. Each fiber is a relatively large and complex multinucleated cell varying in length from a few millimeters to several centimeters (34 cm in the human sartorius muscle) and in diameter from 10 to 100 μm. Some fibers span the entire length of the muscle; others are joined end to end by connective tissue. Each muscle fiber is enveloped by an inner plasma membrane (the sarcolemma) and an outer basement membrane. The multiple nuclei of each fiber, which are oriented parallel to its longitudinal axis and may number in the thousands, lie beneath the plasma membrane (sarcolemma); hence they are termed *subsarcolemmal*, or *sarcolemmal nuclei*.

The cytoplasm (sarcoplasm) of the cell is abundant, and it contains myofibrils and various organelles such as mitochondria and ribosomes. Each myofibril is enveloped in a membranous net, the sarcoplasmic reticulum (SR; see Fig. 45-2). Extensions of the plasma membrane into the fiber form the transverse tubular system (T tubules), which are extracellular channels of communication with the intracellular sarcoplasmic reticulum. The SR and T tubules are anatomically independent but functionally related membrane systems. The junctional gap between the T tubules and SR is occupied by protein formations that are attached to the SR and are referred to as *junctional feet*; the latter have been identified as ryanodine receptors and are responsible for the release of calcium from the SR, which is a critical step in exciting the muscle (see Franzini-Armstrong).

The myofibrils themselves are composed of longitudinally oriented interdigitating filaments (myofilaments) of contractile proteins (actin and myosin), additional structural proteins (titin and nebulin), and regulatory proteins (tropomyosin and troponin). The series of biochemical events by which these proteins, under the influence of calcium ions, accomplish the contraction and relaxation of muscle is described in Chap. 45. Droplets of stored fat, glycogen, various proteins, many enzymes, and myoglobin, the latter imparting the red color to muscle, are contained within the sarcoplasm or its organelles.

The individual muscle fibers are surrounded by delicate strands of connective tissue (endomysium), which provide their support and permit unity of action. Capillaries, of which there may be several for each fiber, and nerve fibers lie within the endomysium. Muscle fibers are bound into groups or *fascicles* by sheets of collagen (perimysium), which also bind together groups of fascicles and surround the entire muscle (epimysium). The latter connective tissue tunics are richly vascularized, different types of muscle having different arrangements of arteries and veins. The muscle fibers are attached at their ends to tendon fibers, which, in turn, connect with the skeleton. By this means, muscle contraction maintains posture and imparts movement.

Other notable characteristics of muscle are its natural mode of contraction, that is, through neural innervation—and the necessity of intact innervation for the maintenance of its normal tone and trophic state. Each muscle fiber receives a nerve twig from a motor nerve cell in the anterior horn of the spinal cord or nucleus of a cranial nerve; the nerve twig joins the muscle fiber at the *neuromuscular junction* or *motor endplate*. As was pointed out in Chaps. 3 and 45, groups of muscle fibers with a common innervation from one anterior horn cell constitute the *motor unit*, which is the basic physiologic unit in all reflex, postural, and voluntary activity.

Embedded in the surface membrane are several types of ion channels that are responsible for maintaining the electrical potential and propagating depolarizing currents across the muscle membrane. Diseases of these channels are discussed in Chap. 50. Also constituting a large part of the membrane is a series of anchoring structural proteins, the nature of which have been thoroughly elucidated in the past few decades. These are described in detail in relation to the muscular dystrophies.

In addition to motor nerve endings, muscle contains several types of sensory endings, all of them mechanoreceptors: Free nerve endings subserve the sensation of deep pressure-pain; Ruffini and pacinian corpuscles are pressure sensors; and the Golgi tendon organs and muscle spindles are tension receptors and participate in the maintenance of muscle tone and reflex activity. The Golgi receptors are located mainly at the myotendon junctions; pacinian corpuscles are localized in the tendon but are also found sparsely in muscle itself. Muscle spindles are specialized groups of small muscle fibers that regulate muscle contraction and relaxation, as described in Chap. 45. All of these receptors are present in highest density in muscles that are involved in fine movements.

Muscles are not equally susceptible to disease, despite the apparent similarity of their structure. In fact, practically no disease affects all muscles in the body and each pathologic entity has a characteristic topography within the musculature. The topographic differences between diseases provide incontrovertible evidence of structural or physiologic differences between muscles that are not presently disclosed by the light or electron microscope, that is, the factors responsible for the selective vulnerability of certain muscles are not known but several hypothetical explanations come to mind. One may relate simply to fiber size; consider, for example, the large diameter and length of the fibers of the glutei and paravertebral muscles in comparison with the smallness of the ocular muscle fibers. The number of fibers composing a motor unit may also be of significance; in the ocular muscles, a motor unit contains only 6 to 10 muscle fibers (some even fewer), but a motor unit of the gastrocnemius contains as many as 1,800 fibers. Also, the eye muscles have a much higher metabolic rate and a richer content of mitochondria than the large trunk muscles. Differences in patterns of vascular supply may permit some muscles to withstand the effects of vascular occlusion better than others. Histochemical studies of skeletal muscles have disclosed that within any 1 muscle, there are subtle metabolic differences between fibers, certain ones (type 1 fibers) being richer in oxidative and poorer in glycolytic enzymes and others (type 2 fibers) having the opposite distribution. The distribution of certain structural proteins may alter the topography of disease expression; for example, the eye muscles do not contain dystrophin, a submembrane protein that is deficient in Duchenne muscular dystrophy, which explains the muscles' lack of involvement in this disease. The endomysial fibroblasts of eye muscles contain an abundance of glycosaminoglycans, which renders them susceptible to thyroid diseases. Diseases of the neuromuscular junction show a distribution of weakness in relation to the density of these junctions in different muscles. Doubtless other differences will be discovered.

Normal muscle is endowed with a population of embryonic muscle precursor cells, known as satellite cells, and, as a result, it possesses a remarkable capacity to regenerate, a point often forgotten. It has been estimated that enough new muscle can be generated from a piece of normal muscle the size of a pencil eraser to provide normal musculature for a 70-kg adult. However, with complete destruction of the muscle fiber, this regenerative capacity is greatly impaired. Inflammatory and metabolic destructive processes are usually followed by fairly complete restoration of the muscle cells, provided that some part of each fiber has survived and the endomysial sheaths of connective tissue have not been severely disrupted. Unfortunately, many pathologic processes of muscle are chronic and unrelenting. Under such conditions, any regenerative activity fails to keep pace with the disease and the loss of muscle fibers becomes permanent. The bulk of the muscle is then replaced by fat and collagenous connective tissue, typical, for example, of the muscular dystrophies.

The Development and Aging of Muscle (See also Chap. 29)

The accepted view of the embryogenesis of muscle is that muscle fibers form by fusion of myoblasts soon after the latter differentiate from somatic mesodermal cells. Muscle connective tissue derives from the somatopleural mesoderm. After fusion of the myoblasts, a series of cellular events including the sequential activation of myogenic transcription factors leads to myofibril formation. The newly formed fibers are thin, centrally nucleated tubes (appropriately called *myotubes*) in which myofilaments begin to be produced from polyribosomes. As myofilaments become organized into myofibrils, the nuclei of the muscle fiber are displaced peripherally to a subsarcolemmal position. Once the nuclei assume a peripheral position, the myofiber is fully formed. The detailed mechanisms whereby myoblasts seek one another, the manner in which each of a series of fused nuclei contributes to the myotube, the formation of actin and myosin fibrils, Z-discs, and the differentiation of a small residue of satellite cells on the surface of the fibers are reviewed by Rubenstein and Kelly.

The mechanisms that determine the number and arrangement of fibers in each muscle are not as well understood. Presumably the myoblasts themselves possess the genetic information that controls the program of development, but within any given species there are wide individual variations that account for obvious differences in the size of muscles and their power of contraction.

The number of fibers assigned to each muscle is probably attained by birth, and growth of muscle thereafter depends mainly on the enlargement of fibers. Although the nervous system and musculature develop independently, muscle fibers continue to grow after birth only when they are active and under the influence of nerve. Measurements of muscle fiber diameters from birth to old age show the growth curve ascending rapidly in the early postnatal years and less rapidly in adolescence, reaching a peak during the third decade. After puberty, growth of muscle is less in females than in males, and such differences are greater in the arm, shoulder, and pelvic muscles than in the leg; growth in ocular muscles is about equal in the 2 sexes. At all ages, disuse of muscle decreases fiber size by as much as 30 percent, and overuse increases the size by about the same amount (work hypertrophy). Normally, type 1 (oxidative enzyme-rich) fibers are slightly smaller than type 2 (phosphorylative enzyme-rich) fibers; the numerical proportions of the 2 fiber types vary in different muscles in accordance with the natural functions of that muscle. The exercising of young animal muscle causes a hypertrophy of high-oxidative type 1 fibers and an increase in the proportion of low-oxidative type 2 fibers; aging muscle lacks this capacity; exercise produces only an increase in the proportion of type 2 fibers (Silbermann et al). No such data are available in humans, but clinical observation suggests that with aging, the capacity of muscle to respond to intense, sustained exercise is diminished.

During late adult life, the number of muscle fibers diminishes and variation in fiber size increases as mentioned in Chap. 29 on aging. The variations are of 2 types: *group atrophy*, in which clusters of 20 to 30 fibers are all reduced in diameter to about the same extent, and *random single-fiber atrophy*. Also, muscle cells, like other cells of postmitotic type, are subject to aging changes (lipofuscin accumulation, autophagic vacuolization, enzyme loss) and to death. Group atrophy, present to a slight degree in the gastrocnemii of almost all individuals older than 60 years, represents denervation effect from an aging-related loss of lumbar motor neurons and peripheral nerve fibers. Further comments regarding muscle and aging can be found in the work of Tomlinson and colleagues and in Chap. 29.

Denervation from spinal motor neuron or nerve disease at every age has roughly the same effect; namely, atrophy of muscle fibers (first in random distribution, then in groups) and later, degeneration. Muscle necrosis at all ages excites a regenerative response from sarcolemmal and satellite cells in any intact parts of the fibers. If this occurs repeatedly, the regenerative potential wanes, with ultimate death of the fiber leading to permanent depopulation of fibers with the expected muscle weakness.

APPROACH TO THE PATIENT WITH MUSCLE DISEASE

The number and diversity of diseases of striated muscle greatly exceed the number of symptoms and signs by which they express themselves clinically; thus, different diseases share certain common symptoms and syndromes. To avoid excessive repetition in the description of individual diseases, we discuss here, in one place, the broad clinical manifestations of muscle disease.

The physician is initially put on the track of a myopathic disease by eliciting complaints of muscle weakness or fatigue, pain, limpness or stiffness, spasm, cramp, twitching, or a muscle mass or change in muscle volume. Of these, the symptom of weakness is by far the most frequent and at the same time the most elusive. As remarked in Chap. 24, when speaking of weakness, the patient often means excessive fatigability and poor endurance. Although fatigability in the strict sense of gradually reduced power with ongoing use of a muscle may be a feature of muscle diseases, particularly those affecting the neuromuscular junction such as myasthenia gravis, it is far more frequently a complaint of patients with chronic systemic disease or with anxiety or depression. As stated in Chap. 24, fatigue is an abstruse symptom, always requiring analysis and interpretation. When not attended by manifest reduction in muscle power, it is usually nonmuscular in origin. It may, on medical investigation, prove to be a systemic manifestation of infection, metabolic or endocrine disorder, severe anemia, reduced cardiopulmonary function, or neoplasia. More often, when expressed as a feeling of poor endurance, weariness, and disinclination to undertake or sustain mental and physical activity, it is indicative of neurasthenia, a psychiatric manifestation common to states of chronic anxiety and depression. An elusive syndrome of lifelong exercise intolerance, often accompanied by muscle cramps during exercise, has been traced in a limited number of cases to mutations in the cytochrome *b* gene of the mitochondrial DNA (Andreu et al), but these are rare. The subject of fatigue as a physiologic phenomenon and as a clinical feature of many psychiatric and medical diseases, including those that are predominantly myopathic, is considered fully in Chap. 24.

Evaluation of Muscle Weakness and Paralysis

Rather than relying on the patient's report to distinguish between fatigability and weakness, it is more informative to observe the patient during the performance of certain common activities such as walking, climbing stairs, and arising from a sitting, kneeling, squatting, or reclining position or using the arms over the head. Difficulty in performing these tasks signifies weakness rather than fatigue. Sometimes the weakness of a group of muscles becomes manifest only after a period of activity; for example, the feet and legs may "drag" only after the patient has walked a long distance. The physician, upon being told this by the patient, should attempt to conduct the examination under circumstances that duplicate the complaints. Of course, these impairments of muscle function may be caused by a neuropathic or central nervous system (CNS) disturbance rather than of a myopathic one, but usually these conditions can be separated by the basic methods indicated further on in this chapter and in Chaps. 3 and 24.

Reduced strength of muscle contraction—manifest by diminished power of single contractions against resistance (peak power) and during the sustained performance of prolonged or repetitive movements (i.e., endurance)—are the indubitable signs of muscle or neuromuscular disease. In such testing, the physician may encounter difficulty in enlisting the patient's cooperation. The tentative, hesitant performance of the asthenic or suggestible individual, or the hysteric or malingerer, poses difficulties that can be surmounted by experience and by the techniques described in Chap. 3. In infants and small children, who cannot follow commands, one assesses muscle power by the resistance to passive manipulation or by observing performance while the child is engaged in natural activities. The patient may be reluctant to fully contract the muscles in a painful limb; indeed, pain itself causes a reflex diminution in the power of contraction (*algesic paresis*). Estimating the strength of isometric contractions that do not require the painful part to be moved is a way around this difficulty.

Ascertaining the extent and severity of muscle weakness requires a systematic examination of the main groups of muscles. The patient is asked to contract each group with as much force as possible, while the examiner opposes the movement and offers a graded resistance in accordance with the degree of residual power (isokinetic contraction). Alternatively, the patient is asked to produce a maximal contraction and the examiner estimates power by the force needed to overcome or "break" it (isometric contraction or maximum voluntary isometric contraction). If the weakness is unilateral, one has the advantage of being able to compare it with the strength on the normal side. If it is bilateral, the physician must refer to his concept of what constitutes normalcy based on experience in muscle testing. With practice, one can distinguish true weakness from unwillingness to cooperate, feigned or neurasthenic weakness, and inhibition of movement by pain.

To quantitate the degree of weakness, a rating scale may be required. Widely used is the one proposed by the Medical Research Council (MRC) of Great Britain, which recognizes 6 grades of muscle strength as follows:

0—Complete paralysis
1—Minimal contraction
2—Active movement only with gravity eliminated
3—Full movement against gravity but cannot offer resistance to manual muscle opposition
4—Active movement against gravity and resistance but can be overcome by manual muscle opposition
5—Normal strength

Further gradations may be added, specified as 4+ for barely detectable weakness and 4 for easily detected weakness, 3+ and 3, and so on, allowing for 10 grades of power.

The ocular, facial, lingual, pharyngeal, laryngeal, cervical, shoulder, upper arm, lower arm and hand, truncal, pelvic, thigh, and lower leg and foot muscles are examined sequentially. In the case of muscle disease, it is most convenient to test the same muscle from each side. To fully and properly use tools such as the MRC scale and to detect mild weakness, muscles such as the neck flexors and extensors must be tested with the patient in the prone and supine positions. The anatomic significance of each of the actions tested, that is, what roots, nerves, and muscles are involved, can be determined by referring to Table 46-1. A practiced examiner can survey the strength of these muscle groups in 2 to 3 min.

A word of caution is in order: In manually resisting the patient's attempts to contract the large and powerful trunk and girdle muscles, the examiner may fail to detect slight degrees of weakness, particularly in well-muscled individuals. These muscle groups are best examined by having the patient use the muscle groups for their intended purposes: squat and kneel and then assume the erect posture, arise from and, walk on toes and heels, and lift a heavy object (e.g., *Harrison's Principles of Internal Medicine*) over his head. The strength of muscles of the hand can be quantified with a dynamometer; for research purposes, similar but more sophisticated devices exist for other muscle groups (see Fenichel et al). Nonetheless, the examiner should not dismiss the patient's complaint of weakness simply if it cannot be substantiated by the examination.

Changes in the Contractile Process and Definition of Terms

In the *myasthenic states* there is a rapid failure of contraction in the affected muscles during sustained or repetitive activity. For instance, after the patient looks upward at the ceiling for a few minutes, the eyelids progressively droop; closing the eyes and resting the levator palpebrae muscles causes the ptosis to lessen or disappear. Similarly, holding the eyes in a far lateral position will induce diplopia and strabismus. These effects, in combination with restoration of power by the administration of neostigmine or edrophonium, are the most valuable clinical criteria for the diagnosis of myasthenia gravis, as described in Chap. 49.

The opposite of the myasthenic phenomenon, an increment in power with a series of several voluntary contractions is a feature of the *Lambert-Eaton myasthenic syndrome*, which is associated in approximately 50 percent of cases with small cell carcinoma of the lung. The same increment occurs in botulism. In both instances there is an increase in the amplitude of compound muscle action potentials on the nerve conduction studies obtained following brief exercise (10 to 15 sec), or at high rates of repetitive nerve stimulation (20 to 50 Hz), as described in Chap. 45.

Other abnormalities may be discovered by observing the speed and efficiency of contraction and relaxation during one or a series of maximal actions of a group of muscles. In myxedema, for example, stiffness and slowness of contraction in a muscle such as the quadriceps may be seen on change in posture (*contraction myoedema*) and by direct percussion of a muscle, and there is an associated prolonged duration of the tendon reflexes. Slowness in relaxation of muscles is another feature of hypothyroidism, accounting for the complaint of uncomfortable tightness of proximal limb muscles. A curious *rippling phenomenon* in muscles may be the result of several processes and occurs as an inherited autosomal dominant trait. After a period of relaxation, stiffening and rippling occurs in the contracting or stretched muscles.

A prolonged failure of relaxation following contraction of a muscle is characteristic of *myotonia*, which typifies certain diseases: myotonia congenita, myotonic dystrophy, and paramyotonia congenita. True myotonia, with its prolonged discharge of membrane action potentials, requires strong contraction to elicit, is more evident after a period of relaxation, and tends to disappear with repeated contractions as discussed further in relation to the ion channel disorders in Chap. 50. This persistence of contraction is demonstrable also by tapping a muscle (*percussion myotonia*), a phenomenon easily distinguished from the electrically silent local bulge (*myoedema*) induced by tapping the muscle of a myxedematous or cachetic patient and from the brief fascicular contraction that is induced by tapping a normal or partially denervated muscle; the latter is referred to as *idiomuscular contraction*. In paramyotonia congenita one observes *paradoxical myotonia*, which refers to an increase in the degree of myotonia during a series of contractions (the reverse of what happens in the usual type of myotonia).

The effect of cold on muscle contraction may also prove informative; either paresis or myotonia, lasting for a few minutes, may be evoked or enhanced by cold. This is most prominent in the paramyotonia of Eulenburg, but it may occur to some degree in all the other myotonic disorders. Also, a cold pack applied to a ptotic eyelid of myasthenia will often reduce the weakness.

Myotonia and myoedema must also be distinguished from the recruitment and spread of involuntary spasm induced by strong and repeated contractions of limb muscles in patients with mild or localized tetanus, with the "stiff man" syndrome and with dystonias of various types. These are not primary muscle phenomena but are neural in origin, a result of an abolition of inhibitory mechanisms and also taken up in Chap. 50.

In practice, the term *contracture* is applied (somewhat indiscriminately as discussed previously) to all states of fixed muscle shortening. Several distinct types can be recognized. In *true physiologic contracture* a group of muscles, after a series of strong contractions, remain shortened for many minutes because of failure of the metabolic mechanism necessary for relaxation. In this shortened state, the electromyogram (EMG) remains relatively silent, in contrast to the high-voltage, rapid discharges observed with cramp, tetanus, and tetany. True physiologic contracture occurs in McArdle disease (phosphorylase deficiency), phosphofructokinase deficiency, and possibly in another condition, as yet undefined, where phosphorylase seems to be present. Yet another type of exercise-induced contracture, described originally by Brody, has been attributed by Karpati and coworkers to an autosomal recessive deficiency of calcium adenosine triphosphatase in the sarcoplasmic reticulum in type 2 muscle fibers. True contracture needs to be distinguished from paradoxical myotonia (see earlier) and from cramp, which in certain conditions (dehydration, tetany, pathologic cramp syndrome, amyotrophic lateral sclerosis [ALS]) can also be initiated by one or a series of strong voluntary muscle contractions.

It is appropriate here to comment on *pseudocontracture (myostatic or fibrous contracture)*, for which the term *contracture* is used in general medicine. This is the common form of muscle and tendon shortening that follows prolonged fixation and inactivity of the normally innervated muscle (as occurs in a broken limb immobilized by a cast or flaccid weakness of a limb that is allowed to remain immobile). Here the shortened state of the muscle and tendons has no clearly established anatomic, physiologic, or chemical basis. Fibrosis of muscle, a state following chronic fiber loss and immobility of muscle, is another cause of muscle shortening. Depending on the predominant position, certain muscles are both weakened and shortened. Flexor fibrous contracture of the arms is a prominent feature of the Emery-Dreifuss form of muscular dystrophy. It also accounts for the rigidity and kyphoscoliosis of the spine, which are so frequently a part of myopathic diseases. The latter state is distinguished from *ankylosis* by the springy nature of the resistance, coincident with increased tautness of muscle and tendon during passive motion, and from *Volkmann contracture*, in which there is fibrosis of muscle and surrounding tissues as a result of ischemic injury, usually after a fracture of the elbow.

Arthrogryposis is another form of fibrous contracture that is found in newborns, involving multiple muscle groups; it occurs in association with several diseases that have two features in common: an onset during intrauterine life and an alteration of the neural or muscular apparatus that results in muscular weakness. In other words, contractures and fixity of the limbs in arthrogryposis are the result of reduced mobility of the developing joints, consequent upon muscle weakness during fetal development. Most often the cause is a loss or failure of development of anterior horn cells, as in Werdnig-Hoffman disease, but the abnormality may be in the nerve roots, peripheral nerves, or motor endplates, or in the muscle itself. The *rigid spine syndrome* (RSS) in children is yet another form of fibrous contracture, presumably the result of an unusual axial muscular dystrophy.

Notably, few of the primary muscle diseases are painful. When pain is prominent and continuous during rest and activity, there will usually be evidence of disease of the peripheral nerves, as in alcoholic–nutritional neuropathy, or of adjacent joints and ligaments (rheumatoid arthritis, polymyalgia rheumatica). Pain localized to a group of muscles is more a feature of torticollis and dystonias. Pain tends not to be prominent in polymyositis and dermatomyositis, but there are exceptions, as commented below. Pain tends to be more definite in polyneuritis, poliomyelitis, and polyarteritis nodosa than it is in polymyositis, various forms of dystrophy, and other myopathies. If pain is present in polymyositis, it usually indicates coincident involvement of connective tissues and joint structures. Hypothyroidism, hypophosphatemia, and hyperparathyroidism are other sources of a myalgic myopathy. Certain drugs produce muscle aches in susceptible individuals. They include the "statin" lipid-lowering drugs, clofibrate, captopril, lithium, colchicine, beta-adrenergic blocking drugs, penicillamine, cimetidine, suxamethonium, and numerous others (see the table contained in the review by Mastaglia and Laing).

There are probably a limited number of mechanisms of muscle pain. Prolonged and sustained contraction gives rise to a deep aching sensation. Contraction under ischemic conditions—as when the circulation is occluded by a tourniquet or from atherosclerotic vascular disease—induces pain; the pain of intermittent claudication is presumably of this type and is not accompanied by cramp. It was postulated that lactic acid or some other metabolite accumulates in muscles and activates pain receptors, but there is also evidence to the contrary. The delayed pain, swelling, and tenderness that occur after sustained exercise of unconditioned muscles are evidently a result of fiber necrosis (Armstrong).

Muscle biopsy infrequently reveals the cause of these painful syndromes, but it may be undertaken in cases of suspected metabolic or dystrophic muscle disease. In their retrospective series, Filosto and colleagues determined that the biopsy was most likely to be helpful if there was exercise-induced muscle pain and the creatine kinase (CK) concentration was greatly elevated; even then two-thirds of the entire group had either normal or nonspecific findings on the biopsy.

Having listed all these causes of proximal pains, all physicians are aware that arthritic and mundane musculoskeletal complaints are more common causes of discomfort.

Benign fasciculations, a common finding in otherwise normal individuals, can be identified by the lack of muscular weakness and atrophy and by the small-size muscle fascicles involved and repetitive appearance in only or regions. The recurrent twitches of the eyelid or muscles of the thumb experienced by most normal persons are often referred to inaccurately as "live flesh" or myokymia but are benign fasciculations of this type. Individuals with truly benign fasciculations have normal EMGs (i.e., they have no fibrillations) as demonstrated in a large series of such patients studied and followed for many years by Blexrud and colleagues. *Myokymia* is a less common condition, in which there are repeated twitchings and rippling of a muscle at rest.

Muscle cramps, despite their common occurrence, are a poorly understood phenomenon. They occur at rest or with movement (action cramps), and they are frequently reported in motor system disease, tetany, dehydration after excessive sweating and salt loss, metabolic disorders (uremia and hemodialysis, hypocalcemia, hypothyroidism, and hypomagnesemia), and certain muscle diseases (e.g., rare cases of Becker muscular dystrophy and congenital myopathies). Gospe and colleagues reported a familial (X-linked recessive) type of myalgia and cramps associated with a deletion of the first third of the dystrophin gene, which is the one implicated in Duchenne dystrophy; strangely, there was no weakness or evidence of dystrophy. Lifelong, severe cramping of undetermined type has also been seen in a few families. The dramatic Satoyoshi syndrome is characterized by continuous, painful leg cramps, alopecia universalis, and diarrhea.

Far more frequent than all these types of cramping, and experienced at one time or another by most normal persons, is the benign form (*idiopathic cramp syndrome*) in which no other neuromuscular disturbance can be found. Most often benign cramps occur at night and affect the muscles of the calf and foot, but they may occur at any time and involve any muscle group. Some patients state that cramps are more frequent when the legs are cold and daytime activity has been excessive. In others, the cramps are provoked by the abrupt stretching of muscles, are very painful, and tend to wax and wane before they disappear. The EMG counterpart is a high-frequency discharge. Although of no pathologic significance, the cramps in extreme cases are so persistent and readily provoked by innocuous movements as to be disabling. Cramps of all types need to be distinguished from *sensations of cramp* without muscle spasm. The latter is a dysesthetic phenomenon in certain polyneuropathies. The disorders that simulate cramps, such as stiff-man syndrome and other forms of continuous muscle fiber activity that have various bases, is discussed in Chap. 50.

Contrasted to cramp is the already described physiologic contracture, observed in McArdle disease and related metabolic myopathies, in which increasing muscle shortening and pain gradually develop during muscular activity. Unlike cramping, it does not occur at rest, the pain is less intense, and the EMG of the contracted muscle at the time is relatively silent. Continuous spasm intensified by the action of muscles and with no demonstrable disorder at a neuromuscular level is a common manifestation of localized tetanus and also follows the bite of the black widow spider. There may also be difficulty distinguishing cramps and spasms from the early stages of a dystonic illness.

Altered structure and function of muscle are not accurately revealed by palpation. Of course, the difference between the firm, hypertrophied muscle of a well-conditioned athlete and the slack muscle of a sedentary person is as apparent to the palpating fingers as to the eye, as is also the persistent contraction in tetanus, cramp, contracture, fibrosis, and extrapyramidal rigidity. The muscles in dystrophy are said to have a "doughy" or "elastic" feel, but we find this difficult to judge. In the Pompe type of glycogen storage disease, attention may be attracted to the musculature by an unnatural firmness and increase in bulk. The swollen, edematous, weak muscles in acute rhabdomyolysis with myoglobinuria or severe polymyositis may feel taut and firm but are usually not tender. Areas of tenderness in muscles that otherwise function normally, a state called *myogelosis*, have been attributed to fibrositis or fibromyositis, but their nature has not been divulged by biopsy.

Topography and Patterns of Myopathic Weakness

In almost all the diseases under consideration, some muscles are affected and others spared, each disease displaying its own pattern. Restated, the topography or distribution of weakness tends to be alike in all patients with the same disease. The pattern of weakness is as important a diagnostic attribute of muscular disease as for the various diseases of the peripheral nervous system discussed in Chap. 46, but the configurations differ in important ways. *As a general rule, muscle diseases are identified by a predominantly proximal weakness that is symmetric.*

The following patterns of muscle involvement constitute a core of essential clinical knowledge in this field. Subacute and chronic evolution of weakness is distinguished in each category from more acute causes.

Ocular Palsies Presenting as Ptosis, Diplopia, and Strabismus Primary diseases of muscle do not involve the pupil, and in most instances their effects are bilateral.

In lesions of the third, fourth, or sixth cranial nerves, a neural origin is disclosed by the pattern of ocular muscle palsies, abnormalities of the pupil, or both. When weakness of the orbicularis oculi (muscles of eye closure) is added to weakness of eye opening (levator palpebrae; ptosis), it nearly always signifies myasthenia gravis and occasionally, a rare primary disease of muscle (progressive external ophthalmoplegia [PEO]). Other causes of *subacute and chronic* development of *relatively pure* weakness of the muscles of eye movement are oculopharyngeal dystrophy, and exophthalmic (hyperthyroid) ophthalmopathy. In PEO, the muscles, including the levators of the eyelids, become paralyzed almost symmetrically over a period of years. In most cases, this disorder is a form of mitochondrial myopathy. Oculopharyngeal dystrophy involves primarily the levators of the eyelids and, to a lesser extent, other eye muscles and pharyngeal-upper esophageal striated muscles. It begins in middle or late adult life and later, and—like PEO—tends only decades later to involve girdle and proximal limb muscles.

There are several other less common chronic myopathies in which external ophthalmoplegia is associated with involvement of other muscles or organs, namely, the congenital ophthalmoplegia of the Goldenhar-Gorlin syndrome (see Aleksic et al); the Kearns-Sayre syndrome (retinitis pigmentosa, heart block, short stature, generalized weakness, and ovarian hypoplasia); other congenital myotubular and mitochondrial myopathies; and nuclear ophthalmoplegia with bifacial weakness (Möbius syndrome). Rarely, eye muscle weakness may occur at a late stage in a few other dystrophies and ptosis has a wider diagnostic range that includes myotonic dystrophy. Although not a regular feature of the disease, ophthalmoparesis can occur in the Lambert-Eaton myasthenic syndrome.

Ptosis is variable in all of these conditions. When present in infantile myopathic disease, it is frequently a marker of the congenital myasthenic syndromes. Trichinosis is a rare cause, associated also with periorbital edema.

Bifacial Palsy Presenting as an Inability to Smile, to Expose the Teeth, and to Close the Eyes Varying degrees of bifacial weakness are observed in myasthenia gravis, usually conjoined with ptosis and ocular palsies. On occasion, weakness of facial muscles may be combined with myasthenic weakness of the masseters and other bulbar muscles without involvement of ocular muscles. Facial weakness and ptosis are features of myotonic dystrophy. More severe or complete facial palsy occurs in facioscapulohumeral dystrophy, sometimes presenting several years before weakness of the shoulder girdle muscles. Bifacial weakness is also a feature of certain congenital myopathies (centronuclear, nemaline), Kennedy type of degenerative bulbospinal motor neuron disease, and the Möbius syndrome of the absence of the facial nuclei (in combination with abducens palsies).

Advanced scleroderma, Parkinson disease, or a pseudobulbar state can immobilize the face to the point of simulating myopathic or neuropathic paralysis, but always in a context that makes the cause obvious.

Bulbar (Oropharyngeal) Palsy Presenting as Dysphonia, Dysarthria, and Dysphagia With or Without Weakness of Jaw or Facial Muscles Myasthenia gravis is the most frequent cause of this syndrome and must also be considered whenever a patient presents with the solitary finding of a hanging jaw or fatigue of the jaw while eating or talking; usually, however, ptosis and ocular palsies are conjoined. Dysphagia and dysphonia may be early and prominent signs of polymyositis, as well as inclusion body myositis (IBM), and may appear in patients with myotonic dystrophy, because of upper esophageal atonia.

Combinations of these palsies are not typically of muscular or neuromuscular origin but instead are observed as an *acute syndrome* in botulism, in brainstem stroke, and at the outset of Guillain-Barré syndrome. Diphtheria and bulbar poliomyelitis are now rare diseases that may present in this way. Progressive bulbar palsy (motor neuron disease) may be the basis of this syndrome (see Chap. 39); the last of these diagnoses is most obvious when the tongue is withered and twitching. Syringobulbia, basilar invagination of the skull, and certain types of Chiari malformation may reproduce some of the findings of bulbar palsy by involving the lower cranial nerves. Rare cases of progressive aphonia include the X-linked Kennedy syndrome of bulbospinal atrophy.

Cervical Palsy Presenting With Inability to Hold the Head Erect or to Lift the Head From the Pillow ("Hanging, or Dropped, Head" Syndrome, "Camptocormia") This is caused by weakness of the posterior neck muscles and of the sternocleidomastoids and other anterior neck muscles. In advanced forms of this syndrome, the head may hang with chin on chest unless the patient holds it up with the hands. There may be difficulty differentiating the condition from a dystonic anterocollis; in the latter there is palpable tonic spasm of the sternomastoid and posterior neck muscles. A pattern of neck and spine extensor weakness also occurs in advanced Parkinson disease. A common error in all these cases is to attribute the problem to structural disease of the cervical spine.

This topographic pattern occurs most often in idiopathic polymyositis and IBM, in which cases it is often combined with mild dysphagia, dysphonia, and weakness of girdle muscles. The same symptom may be a feature of motor neuron disease and is infrequently the presenting feature of that process. Myasthenic patients commonly complain of an inability to hold up their heads late in the day; both flexors and extensors of the neck are found to be weak. Occasionally, this pattern of weakness is observed in patients with nemaline rod myopathy. Cases of hanging head have appeared many years after local radiation of the neck and thorax for Hodgkin disease as described by Rowin and colleagues and with syringomyelia (Nalini and Ravishankar).

There is, in addition, a poorly characterized local myopathic process isolated to the cervical paraspinal muscles, which has no distinguishing histopathologic or histochemical features but has accounted for many of the cases of neck extensor weakness that we have encountered. The condition is observed in elderly persons, in some series mainly men, but our experience has included as many women. There is severe but relatively nonprogressive weakness of the neck extensors and only mild weakness of shoulder girdle and proximal arm muscles. Katz and colleagues have suggested the designation "isolated neck extensor myopathy" in preference to dropped head syndrome. What has been referred to as a *bent spine syndrome* (for which the term *camptocormia* is also used) is probably the same entity and may follow after years of the condition affecting the neck, or it may surface independently. These conditions of cervical weakness are reviewed by Umapathi and colleagues and by Azher and Jankovic. Several recent series have suggested that mutations in RYR1 that encodes for ryanodine receptor may be a common cause of late onset axial myopathy and neck extensor weakness-bent spine syndrome (Løseth et al). Mutations in RYR1 are more commonly associated with the central core congenital myopathy or malignant hyperthermia as noted in a later section.

The major types of progressive muscular dystrophies, when advanced, usually affect the anterior neck muscles severely. Syringomyelia, spinal accessory neuropathy, some form of meningoradiculitis, and loss of anterior horn cells in conjunction with systemic lymphoma or carcinoma may differentially paralyze the various neck muscles.

Weakness of Respiratory and Trunk Muscles Usually the diaphragm, chest, and trunk muscles are affected in association with shoulder and proximal limb muscles, but occasionally, isolated weakness of the respiratory muscles is the initial or the dominant manifestation of a muscle disease. Dyspnea and diminished vital capacity first bring the patient to the pulmonary clinic. The main causes are motor neuron disease, myasthenia gravis and less often because of their rarity, glycogen storage disease (acid maltase deficiency—Pompe disease), mitochondrial myopathies, and nemaline myopathy. Polymyositis may cause respiratory weakness, but pulmonary difficulty is more often the result of interstitial lung disease. Unilateral paralysis of the diaphragm may result from compression of the phrenic nerve in the thorax by tumor or aortic aneurysm; an idiopathic or postinfectious variety may be related to brachial plexitis (see Chap. 46). The diaphragm and accessory muscles may be severely affected in some types of muscular dystrophies, but usually in association with pelvocrural and shoulder muscle weakness. Nocturnal dyspnea, sleep apnea, and respiratory arrest may occur, particularly in myasthenics and in patients with glycogen storage myopathies, and respiratory failure may threaten life in severe myasthenia gravis, Guillain-Barré syndrome, and poliomyelitis.

As a general observation, in the acute neuromuscular paralyses, the cervical and shoulder muscles and the diaphragm, all of which share a common innervation, show a similar degree of weakness. Asking the patient to count aloud on 1 maximal breath can help detect diaphragmatic weakness (counting to 20 equates with a vital capacity of approximately 2 L). Paradoxical inward movement of the abdomen with inspiration is another sign of diaphragm weakness. Disorders of breathing and ventilation are discussed in Chaps. 26 and 46 in relation to its most dramatic presentation in the Guillain-Barré syndrome.

Bibrachial Palsy and the Dangling-Arm (Flail-Arm) Syndrome Weakness, atrophy, and fasciculations of the hands, arms, and shoulders characterize the common form of motor neuron disease, ALS. Primary diseases of muscle hardly ever weaken these parts disproportionately. A diffuse weakness of both arms and the shoulder muscles may occur in the early stages of Guillain-Barré syndrome, paraneoplastic neuropathy, and amyloid polyneuropathy, in special forms of immunoglobulin (Ig) M-related paraproteinemic, or in inflammatory polyneuropathy (e.g., brachial neuritis) and porphyric polyneuropathy. A lesion affecting the central portion of the spinal cord in the cervical region produces this same pattern, but in that case there is an associated loss of pain and thermal sensation in the upper limbs and shoulders, signs that exclude disease of muscle.

Proximal Limb-Girdle Palsies Presenting as Inability to Raise the Arms or to Arise From a Squatting, Kneeling, or Sitting Position This is the common pattern of a number of myopathies. Polymyositis, IBM, dermatomyositis, and the muscular dystrophies most often manifest themselves in this fashion. The endocrine and the acquired metabolic myopathies (e.g., Cushing disease, hyperthyroidism, and steroid or statin administration) are other typical causes. Proximal limb weakness is a feature of myasthenia but almost always after the development of ocular or pharyngeal involvement. The childhood Duchenne, Becker, and limb-girdle types of dystrophies tend first to affect the muscles of the pelvic girdle, gluteal region, and thighs, resulting in a lumbar lordosis and protuberant abdomen, a waddling gait, and difficulty in arising from the floor and climbing stairs without the assistance of the arms. Climbing up by placing the hands on the thighs (Gower sign) is particularly characteristic of the dystrophies. Facioscapulohumeral dystrophy affects the muscles of the face and shoulder girdles foremost, and it is manifest by incomplete eye closure, inability to whistle and to raise the arms above the head, winging of the scapulae, and thinness of the upper arms with preserved forearm bulk ("Popeye" effect). Certain early or mild forms of dystrophy may selectively involve only the peroneal and scapular muscles. In milder forms of polymyositis, weakness may be limited to the neck muscles or to the shoulder or pelvic girdles.

A number of other diseases of muscle may express themselves by a disproportionate weakness of girdle and proximal limb musculature. An intrinsic metabolic myopathy, such as the adult form of acid maltase deficiency and the familial types of periodic paralysis, may affect only this region. The congenital myopathies (central core, nemaline, myotubular) cause a relatively nonprogressive weakness of girdle muscles more than distal ones. Proximal muscles are occasionally implicated in spinal muscular atrophy or late onset type and in Kennedy bulbospinal atrophy.

Bicrural Palsy Presenting as Lower Leg Weakness With Inability to Walk on the Heels and Toes, or as Paralysis of All Leg Muscles With the exception of certain distinctive distal types of muscular dystrophies, this pattern, usually due to weakness of peroneal, anterior tibial, and thigh muscles, is usually not a result of myopathy.

Symmetrical weakness of the lower legs is more often caused by polyneuropathy. In cases of total leg and thigh weakness, one first considers a spinal cord disease. Motor neuron disease may begin in the legs, asymmetrically and distally as a rule, and affect them disproportionately to other parts of the body. Thus the differential diagnosis of distal or generalized leg weakness involves more diseases than are involved in the restricted paralyses of other parts of the body.

Isolated Quadriceps Femoris Weakness *Isolated quadriceps femoris weakness* may be the expression of several diseases. In adults, the most common cause is IBM (where it may be unilateral or asymmetrical) or, a restricted form of Becker muscular dystrophy. In thyrotoxic and steroid myopathies, the major effects are on the quadriceps muscles. If unilateral or bilateral with loss of patellar reflex and sensation over the inner leg, this condition is most often the result of a femoral neuropathy, as occurs from diabetes, or of an upper lumbosacral plexus lesion. Injuries to the hip and knee cause rapid disuse atrophy of the quadriceps muscles. A painful condition of infarction of the muscle on 1 side is seen in diabetic patients.

Distal Bilateral Limb Palsies Presenting as Foot-Drop with Steppage Gait (With or Without Pes Cavus), Weakness of All Lower Leg Muscles, and Later Wrist-Drop and Weakness of Hands The principal cause of this syndrome is a familial polyneuropathy, mainly of the Charcot-Marie-Tooth type (see Chap. 46); the course is over decades. Chronic nonfamilial polyneuropathies, particularly paraproteinemic and inflammatory ones with motor conduction block and exceptionally, some forms of familial progressive muscular atrophy and distal types of progressive muscular dystrophy, and sarcoid myopathy may also present in this way. In myotonic dystrophy, there may be weakness of the leg muscles as well as the forearms, sternocleidomastoids, face, and eyes. With these exceptions, the generalization that *girdle weakness without sensory changes is indicative of myopathy and that distal weakness is indicative of neuropathy is clinically useful.*

Generalized or Universal Paralysis: Limb (but Usually Not Cranial) Muscles, Involved Either in Attacks or as a Chronic Persistent, Progressive Deterioration When acute in onset and *episodic*, this syndrome is usually a manifestation of familial or acquired hypokalemic or hyperkalemic periodic paralysis. One variety of the hypokalemic type is associated with hyperthyroidism, another with hyperaldosteronism. Attacks of porphyric neuropathy and of Refsum disease with generalized weakness have an episodic nature. Widespread paresis (rather than paralysis) that has an acute onset and lasts many weeks is at times a feature of a severe form of idiopathic or parasitic (trichinosis) polymyositis and, rarely, of the toxic effects of certain pharmaceutical agents, particularly those used to treat hypercholesterolemia. Idiopathic polymyositis and, rarely, IBM may involve all limb and trunk muscles, but usually spare the facial and ocular muscles, whereas the weakness in trichinosis is mainly in the ocular and lingual muscles. In infants and young children, a chronic and persistent generalized weakness of all muscles, except those of the eyes, always raises the question of Werdnig-Hoffman spinal muscular atrophy or, if milder in degree and relatively nonprogressive, of one of the congenital myopathies or polyneuropathies. In these diseases of infancy, paucity of movement, hypotonia, and retardation of motor development may be more obvious than weakness, and there is arthrogryposis at birth.

Paralysis of Single Muscles or a Group of Muscles This is usually neuropathic, less often spinal or myopathic. Muscle disease does not need to be considered except in certain instances of pressure-ischemic necrosis of muscle as a result of local pressure or infarction, as in monoplegic alcoholic myopathy or in diabetic muscle infarction. The weakness of IBM has a preference for certain sites, specifically parts of the quadriceps, or of the forearm muscles, particularly the long finger flexors (flexor digitorum profundus), and also therefore enters into consideration.

From this exposition of the topographic aspects of weakness, one can appreciate that each neuromuscular disease exhibits a predilection for particular groups of muscles. Apart from these patterns that suggest certain possibilities of disease and exclude others, diagnosis depends on the age of the patient at the time of onset and tempo of progression, the coexistence of medical disorders, certain laboratory findings (serum concentrations of muscle enzymes, EMG, and biopsy findings), and genetic determinants.

The symptoms and signs of muscle disease are considered in this chapter mainly in connection with the age of the patient at the time of onset, their mode of evolution, and the presence or absence of familial occurrence. Because many muscle diseases are hereditary, a careful family history is important. The pattern of inheritance has diagnostic significance and, if genetic counseling or prenatal diagnosis is a consideration, a detailed genealogic tree becomes essential. When historical data are insufficient, it is often necessary to examine siblings and parents of the proband. The molecular genetics and other genetic aspects of the heritable muscle diseases, subjects of intense interest in recent years, are discussed at appropriate points in the chapter.

In summary, the clinical recognition of myopathic diseases is facilitated by a prior knowledge of a few topographic syndromes, the age of the patient at the onset of the illness, a familial occurrence of the same or similar illnesses, and of the medical setting in which weakness evolves. Diagnostic accuracy is aided by the intelligent use of the laboratory examinations discussed in Chap. 45, particularly the muscle enzymes, EMG, and muscle biopsy.

THE INFECTIOUS MYOPATHIES

The discovery that striated skeletal muscle and that cardiac muscle could be the sole targets of a number of infectious agents came about during the era of the development of microbiology and occupied the attention of many prominent clinicians, including Osler. As these diseases were being characterized, however, a number of other inflammatory states affecting muscle were found for which there was no infectious cause. Later, an autoimmune mechanism was postulated, but even today this is not securely established. This group of idiopathic inflammatory myopathies figures so prominently in clinical myology that we devote a separate section to the subject. First, the infections of muscle are described.

Parasitic Myositis

Included here are trichinosis, toxoplasmosis, parasitic and fungal infections, and a number of viral infections. The related but unclassifiable entity of sarcoid myopathy is addressed in a later section of this chapter.

Trichinosis

This parasitic disease is caused by the nematode *Trichinella spiralis*. Its general features are discussed in Chap. 32. Regarding the myopathic aspect of the illness, the authors have been most impressed with the ocular muscle weakness, which results in strabismus and diplopia; with weakness of the tongue, resulting in dysarthria; and with weakness of the masseter and pharyngeal muscles, which interferes with chewing and swallowing. Any weakness of limb muscles is usually mild and more severe proximally than distally. However, the diaphragm may be involved, as well as the myocardium. The affected muscles are slightly swollen and tender in the acute stage of the disease. Often, there is conjunctival, orbital, and facial edema, sometimes accompanied by subconjunctival and subungual splinter hemorrhages. As the trichinae become encysted over a period of a few weeks, the symptoms subside and recovery is complete. Many, perhaps the majority, of infected patients are asymptomatic throughout the invasive period, and as much as 1 to 3 percent of the population in certain regions of the country will be found at autopsy to have calcified trichinella cysts in their muscles with no history of parasitic illness. Heavy infestations have been known to end fatally, usually from cardiac and diaphragmatic involvement. In these more massive infections, the brain also may be involved, probably by emboli that arise in the heart from an associated myocarditis.

Diagnosis Clinically, one should suspect the disease in a patient who presents with a puffy face and tender muscles. Eosinophilia is practically always present in the peripheral blood (>700 cells/mm^3), although the sedimentation rate is often normal. The CK level is moderately elevated. A skin test using *Trichinella* antigen is available, but it is unreliable. The enzyme-linked immunosorbent assay (ELISA) blood test is more accurate, but it becomes positive only after 1 or 2 weeks of illness. Biopsy of almost any muscle (usually the deltoid or gastrocnemius), regardless of whether it is painful or tender, is probably the most reliable confirmatory test. More than 500 mg of muscle may be required to demonstrate larvae, but smaller specimens will almost invariably show an inflammatory myopathy. Muscle fibers undergo segmental necrosis, and the interstitial inflammatory infiltrates contain a predominance of eosinophils. This accounts for the edema, pain, and tenderness of heavily infested muscles. The capsules of the larvae gradually thicken in the first month of the infection and then calcify. The EMG may exhibit profuse fibrillation potentials, a phenomenon attributed on theoretical grounds to the disconnection of segments of muscle fibers from their motor endplates (Gross and Ochoa).

Treatment No treatment is required in most cases. In patients with severe weakness and pain, a combination of thiabendazole, 25 to 50 mg/kg daily in divided doses for 5 to 10 days, and prednisone, 40 to 60 mg/d, is recommended. Albendazole, in a single oral dose of 400 mg daily, is equally effective but is not available in the United States except by special request (from Smith Kline Beecham). Recovery, as mentioned, is complete as a rule, except in rare patients with cerebral infarcts. Other aspects of this parasitic infestation are discussed in Chap. 32.

Toxoplasmosis

This is an acute or subacute systemic infection caused by the encephalitozoon *Toxoplasma gondii*. Most *Toxoplasma* infections in immunocompetent patients, which occur in up to 10 to 30 percent of the population, are asymptomatic, but there may be fever and varying degrees of involvement of the skin, lymph nodes, retina, myocardium, liver, brain, and muscle. In one such case studied by our colleagues, *Toxoplasma* organisms and pseudocysts were detected in skeletal muscle (Kass et al); wherever a parasitic pseudocyst had ruptured, there was focal inflammation. Some muscle fibers had undergone segmental necrosis, but this was not prominent (one contained the organism), accounting for the relative paucity of muscle symptoms. With the emergence of AIDS, many more toxoplasmic infections of the brain, but also including those of skeletal muscle, were seen (Gherardi et al). However, physicians who see many cases of AIDS have indicated to us that a primary AIDS myopathy and treatment-related muscle diseases are more common (see later). Again, in this population, brain infestation with *Toxoplasma* is many times more common than is myositis. The subject of AIDS and toxoplasmic infection is discussed in greater detail in Chap. 32.

The myopathy, which occurs with variable fever, lymphopenia, and failure of other organs, consists of weakness, wasting, myalgia, and elevated CK levels. Presumably, the immunocompromised patient is unable to respond to protozoan infections, allowing latent infections to be reactivated. Sulfadiazine in combination with pyrimethamine or trisulfapyrimidine, which act synergistically against the toxoplasmic trophozoites, improves the muscle symptoms and reduces serum CK. Folic acid is given in addition.

Other Parasitic and Fungal Infections of Muscle

Echinococcosis, cysticercosis, trypanosomiasis (Chagas disease), sparganosis, toxocariasis, and actinomycosis have all been known to affect skeletal muscle on occasion, but the major symptoms relate more to involvement of other organs. Only cysticercosis may first claim the attention of the clinical myologist because of a dramatic pseudohypertrophy of thigh and calf muscles. Hydatids infest the paravertebral and lumbar girdle muscles in 5 percent of cases and may lead to their enlargement. Coenurosis and sparganosis are causes of movable lumps in the rectus abdominis, thigh, calf, and pectoralis muscles. Protozoan infections of muscle—microsporidiosis, African and American trypanosomiasis—which occurred only rarely until a decade ago, are now being observed in immunodeficient (HIV-infected) individuals in endemic areas. The reader who seeks more details may refer to the chapter on parasitic myositis by Banker (2004).

Viral Infections of Muscle

HIV and Human T-Lymphotropic Virus Type I Myositis

HIV and human T-lymphotropic (or leukemia) virus type I (HTLV-I) are increasingly common causes of viral myositis (Engel and Emslie-Smith). Moreover, as discussed further on, zidovudine (ZVD), a drug included in many regimens to treat HIV infections, may itself induce a myopathy with myalgia and weakness that is, at times, indistinguishable from HIV myopathy (Dalakas et al).

An inflammatory, and presumed infectious, myopathy may develop early in the course of HIV infection but is rarely the initial manifestation. The pattern is like that of idiopathic polymyositis with painless weakness of the girdle and proximal limb muscles. Reflexes are diminished in most cases, but this is difficult to interpret in view of the high incidence of concomitant polyneuropathy. Serum CK is elevated, and the EMG shows an active myopathy with fibrillations, brief polyphasic motor units, and complex repetitive discharges.

The myopathologic changes in AIDS are also like those of idiopathic polymyositis described further on. Additionally, in some cases electron microscopy discloses the presence of nemaline (rod) bodies within type 1 fibers, similar to those observed in the congenital form of nemaline myopathy discussed further on. As implied earlier, the pathogenesis of the AIDS myopathy has not been firmly established as there is scant evidence of a direct viral infection of the muscle fibers. An immune basis has been suggested in view of a response to corticosteroids, plasma exchange, and gamma globulin, comparable to the beneficial effects in the idiopathic variety of polymyositis. Corticosteroids in doses similar to those used in the treatment of idiopathic polymyositis are effective in ameliorating the weakness, but they entail special risks in immunocompromised patients.

The clinical features of putative ZVD-induced myopathy are much the same as those of HIV myopathy except that moderate pain is said to be characteristic of the drug-induced variety. The myopathy has been attributed to the mitochondrial toxicity of the drug, which may account for the presence of "ragged red" fibers in biopsy specimens. The onset of symptoms appears to be related to the sustained administration of high doses of the drug (1,200 mg daily for a year or longer). Cessation or reduction in dosage of the drug diminishes the muscular discomfort within weeks, but strength recovers more slowly.

A myopathy caused by HTLV-I infection also simulates polymyositis in its clinical and histologic features. The illness occurs most often in endemic areas but is less common than the myelopathy that is associated with the virus.

Distinguished from the HIV- and ZVD-related inflammatory myopathies is the severe generalized muscle wasting that characterizes advanced, cachectic AIDS. Muscle enzymes are normal and strength is affected little, especially considering the loss of muscle bulk. Histologically, there is atrophy of type 2 fibers. The pathogenesis of this cachectic syndrome is uncertain; it has been attributed to a multiplicity of systemic factors, including circulating catabolic cytokines, just as in other wasting syndromes such as cancer.

Other Viral Myopathies

In most patients with pleurodynia (epidemic myalgia, Bornholm disease), muscle biopsies disclose no abnormalities and there is no clear explanation of the pain. However, group B Coxsackie virus has been isolated from striated muscle of a few patients with this disorder. A necrotizing myositis has been suspected in a number of patients with influenza; under the electron microscope, some muscle fibers contain structures with the features of influenza virions. Malaise, myalgia, and slight weakness and stiffness were the clinical manifestations. Because of the myalgia, it is difficult to know how much of the weakness is only apparent. Recovery has been complete within a few weeks. In 1 patient with generalized myalgia and myoglobinuria, the influenza virus was isolated from muscle (Gamboa et al). These observations suggest that the intense muscle pain in certain viral illnesses might be the result of a direct viral infection of muscle. However, there are many cases of influenzal myalgia, mainly of the calves and thighs, such as those reported by Lundberg and by Antony and coworkers, in which it was not possible to establish that there was a muscular disorder at all. In the condition described as *epidemic neuromyasthenia* (benign myalgic encephalomyelitis, Icelandic disease), in which influenza-like symptoms were combined with severe pain and weakness of muscles, a viral cause was postulated, but an organism was never isolated. The illness has been absorbed into the large and indistinct category of chronic fatigue syndrome (discussed in Chap. 24).

Despite these ambiguities, viral myositis is an established entity in myopathology. Echo 9, adenovirus 21, herpes simplex, Epstein-Barr virus, coxsackievirus, and *Mycoplasma pneumoniae* have all been cited by Mastaglia and Ojeda and by others as causes of sporadic myositis with rhabdomyolysis. In these infections the nonmyopathic aspects of the disease usually predominate; in some of them, the evidence of invasion of muscle has not been fully substantiated, as in many instances a nonspecific (Zenker-type) degeneration could have explained the muscle findings. The existence of a postinfectious type of polymyositis is also unsettled.

IMMUNE-INFLAMMATORY MYOPATHIES (POLYMYOSITIS, DERMATOMYOSITIS, INCLUSION BODY MYOSITIS, NECROTIZING MYOPATHY)

These are common diseases that affect primarily the striated muscle and skin and sometimes connective tissues. The term used to describe the disease reflects the tissues involved. If the inflammatory changes are restricted clinically to the striated muscles, the disease is called *polymyositis* (PM); if, in addition, the skin is involved, it is called *dermatomyositis* (DM), although the two diseases are now understood to be immunopathologically distinct. Either may be associated with a connective tissue disorder, in which case the designation is PM or DM with rheumatoid arthritis, rheumatic fever, lupus erythematosus, scleroderma, Sjögren syndrome, or mixed connective tissue disease, as the case may be. There is also an important but inconsistent relationship of these myositides and systemic carcinoma, as discussed further on.

Both diseases have been known since the nineteenth century. Polymyositis was first described by Wagner in 1863 and 1887, and DM was established as an entity by Unverricht in a series of articles written from 1887 to 1891. A modern classification introduced in the monograph of Walton and Adams included categories associated with neoplasia and with connective tissue diseases. References to the original articles and a survey of the literature since that time can be found in the monograph of Kakulas and Adams and in the chapters on the PM and DM syndromes by Engel and colleagues.

It is emphasized further on that there is disagreement regarding the frequency of PM as an independent entity. Amato and Griggs have expressed the opinion that many cases so classified are a result of DM, an immune necrotizing myopathy commented on below, or IBM, or are related to an underlying connective tissue disease. Even other cases are examples of muscular dystrophy with secondary inflammatory changes. The main point of controversy has been the proposal they favor, that isolated PM is rare and overdiagnosed (see van der Muelen et al).

Inflammatory myopathy coexists with numerous systemic diseases as discussed, and some authors consider it to be a syndrome rather than a disease. The current authors continue to see a few well-studied and convincingly documented cases of "classic" PM that are unassociated with other disease.

Recently added to the traditional group of inflammatory myopathies is an increasingly recognized *immune-mediated necrotizing myopathy* (IMNM); instances of myopathy that were previously classified as either dermato- or polymyositis are now recognized as being the result of antibodies to anti-signal recognition particle (SRP), and some cases of necrotizing myopathy that are due to statins are similarly caused by antibodies directed at HMGCoA reductase, and not a direct toxic effect of the medication. This process emphasizes that clinicians should conduct a careful evaluation before concluding that a patient has idiopathic polymyositis.

Polymyositis

This is an idiopathic *subacute or chronic and symmetrical weakness of proximal limb and trunk muscles without dermatitis*. The onset is usually insidious and the course progressive over a period of several weeks or months. It may develop at almost any age and in either sex; however, the majority of patients are 30 to 60 years of age, and a smaller group shows a peak incidence at 15 years of age; women predominate in all age groups. A febrile illness or benign infection may precede the weakness, but in most patients the first symptoms develop in the absence of these or other apparent initiating events.

The usual mode of onset is with mainly painless weakness of the proximal limb muscles, especially of the hips and thighs and to a lesser extent the shoulder girdle and neck muscles. Often, the patient cannot easily determine the time of onset of weakness. Certain actions—such as arising from a deep or low chair or from a squatting or kneeling position, climbing or descending stairs, walking, putting an object on a high shelf, or combing the hair—become increasingly difficult. Pain of an aching variety in the buttocks, calves, or shoulders is experienced by approximately 15 percent of patients, and it may indicate a combination of PM and rheumatoid arthritis, tendonitis, or other connective tissue disorder.

When the patient is first seen, many of the muscles of the trunk, shoulders, hips, upper arms, and thighs are usually involved. The posterior and anterior neck muscles (the head may loll) and the pharyngeal, striated esophageal, and laryngeal muscles (dysphagia and dysphonia) may be involved as well. In restricted forms of the disease, only the neck or paraspinal muscles (camptocormia) may be implicated. Ocular muscles are not affected in PM, but there are rare instances of combined PM and myasthenia gravis. The facial, tongue, and jaw muscles are only occasionally affected, and the distal muscles, namely the forearm, hand, leg, and foot are spared in 75 percent of cases. The respiratory muscles are weakened to a minor degree and in only an exceptional case is there dyspnea, the cause of which is revealed only by an intercostal muscle biopsy (Thomas and Lancaster). Occasionally, the early symptoms predominate in one proximal limb before becoming generalized. As emphasized further on, onset after age 50 years, normal CK, or aberrant patterns of weakness, such as early wrist or finger flexor, quadriceps, or ankle dorsiflexor involvement, are indicative of IBM.

The muscles are usually not tender, and atrophy and reduction in tendon reflexes, although sometimes present, are far less pronounced than they are in patients with chronic denervation atrophy, IBM, or Lambert-Eaton myasthenic syndrome (the last of these is discussed in Chap. 49). As the weeks and months pass, the weakness and muscle atrophy progress unless treatment is initiated. Without physical therapy, fibrous contracture of muscles eventually develops. Some elderly individuals with a particularly chronic form of the disease may present with severe atrophy and fibrosis of muscles; the response to treatment in such cases is poor.

In both PM and DM, there may be involvement of organs other than muscle. In a surprising number of our cases of PM (and DM), cardiac abnormalities have been observed and in a small proportion of these, sudden death has occurred. The cardiac manifestations have taken the form of relatively minor electrocardiographic (ECG) changes, but several patients have had arrhythmias with clinical consequences. Among the fatal cases, about half have shown necrosis of myocardial fibers at autopsy, usually with only modest inflammatory changes. Interstitial lung disease is another known association in a few cases; its frequency ranges from 5 to 47 percent in different series (see further on under "Laboratory Diagnosis of PM and DM"), but the lower figure is probably correct. Exceptionally, there is a low-grade fever, especially if joint pain coexists.

Dermatomyositis

The presentation of muscle weakness is similar to that of polymyositis, but the denominative feature is a rash. Most often, the skin changes precede the muscle syndrome and take the form of a localized or diffuse erythema, maculopapular eruption, scaling eczematoid dermatitis, or exfoliative dermatitis. Sometimes, skin and muscle changes evolve together over a period of 3 weeks or less. A characteristic form of the skin lesions are patches of a scaly roughness over the extensor surfaces of joints (elbows, knuckles, and knees) with varying degrees of pink-purple coloration. Red, raised papules may be present over exposed surfaces such as the elbows, knuckles, and distal and proximal interphalangeal joints (Gottron papules); these are particularly prominent in DM of childhood. Also typical is a lilac-colored (heliotrope) change in the skin over the eyelids, on the bridge of the nose, on the cheeks, and over the forehead; it may have a scaly component. Itching may be a troublesome symptom in regions of the other skin eruptions. A predominance of rash over the neck and upper shoulders has been termed the *V sign*, while rash over the shoulders and upper arms, the *shawl sign*. This distribution suggests that the skin changes reflect heightened photosensitivity (a feature shared with pellagra). Periorbital and perioral edema are additional findings but mainly in fulminant cases. Skin changes may be transient and in some instances are restricted to 1 or more patches of dermatitis; they are difficult to appreciate in dark-skinned individuals. Evanescent and restricted skin manifestations are emphasized because they are frequently overlooked and provide clues to diagnosis. In the healing stage, the skin lesions leave whitened atrophic scars with a flat, scaly base.

In contrast to PM, DM affects children and adults about equally. Among adults, DM is more frequent in females whereas in childhood, males and females are affected equally.

Other physical signs include periarticular and subcutaneous calcifications that are common in the childhood form. Signs of associated connective tissue disease are more frequent than in pure PM (see further on). The Raynaud phenomenon has been reported in nearly one-third of the patients and a similar number have dilated or thrombosed nail fold capillaries. Whether this signifies the presence of a systemic autoimmune tissue disease has not been clarified. Others subsequently develop a mild form of scleroderma, and an associated esophageal weakness is demonstrated by fluoroscopy in up to 30 percent of all patients. The superior constrictors of the pharynx may be involved, but cinefluoroscopy may be necessary to demonstrate the abnormality.

Carcinoma With Adult Polymyositis or Dermatomyositis At one time this was a controversial subject and in some respects it remains so because of widely varying incidences of concurrence between systemic malignancy with PM and DM (see Engel et al and Buchbinder and Hill). In the large series reported by Sigurgeirsson and colleagues, 9 percent of 396 patients with PM were found to have carcinoma, either at the time of diagnosis of the muscle disease or within 5 years. DeVere and Bradley reported that 29 percent of their overall group of DM patients had an associated carcinoma; this figure rose to 40 percent if the patient was older than 40 years, and to 66 percent if the patient was both male and older than 40 years. This, however, is higher than reported in most other series. The relationship between myositis and malignancy is not understood; nonetheless, the connection appears valid, even if of uncertain frequency.

The neoplastic processes linked most often with myositis are lung and colon cancer in men and breast and ovarian cancer in women; however, tumors have been reported in nearly every organ of the body. In about half the cases, myositis antedates the clinical manifestations of the malignancy, sometimes by 1 to 2 years, a duration that then brings the association into question. The morbidity and mortality of patients with this combination is usually determined by the nature of the underlying tumor and its response to therapy. Occasionally, excision of the tumor is attended by remission of the myositis, but information on this point comes mostly from sporadic reports.

Dermatomyositis of Childhood

Idiopathic myositis occurs in children, but less frequently than in adults. Some cases tend to be relatively benign but otherwise do not differ from the syndrome in adults. More frequently, there is a distinctive illness, described by Banker and Victor, which differs in some respects from the usual adult form of the disease. In these children and adolescents, there is greater involvement of blood vessels in the connective tissue of multiple organs, as well as in skin and muscle. This childhood form of DM begins, as a rule, with typical skin changes accompanied by anorexia and fatigue. Erythematous discoloration of the upper eyelids (the previously noted heliotrope rash), frequently with facial edema, is another characteristic early sign. The erythema spreads to involve the periorbital regions, nose, malar areas, and upper lip as well as the skin over the knuckles, elbows, and knees. Cuticular overgrowth, subungual telangiectasia, and ulceration of the fingertips may be found. Capillary prominence in the nail beds and avascular regions in the cuticle are said to be characteristic but need to be sought with a magnifying lens or ophthalmoscope (these signs are also seen in the "CREST" [calcinosis cutis, Raynaud phenomenon, esophageal motility disorder, sclerodactyly, telangiectasia] form of scleroderma).

Symptoms of weakness, stiffness, and pain in the muscles usually follow but may precede the skin manifestations. The weakness is generalized but always more severe in the muscles of the shoulders and hips and proximal portions of the limbs. A tiptoe gait, the result of fibrous contractures of flexors of the ankles, is a common late abnormality. Tendon reflexes are depressed or abolished, but only commensurate with the degree of muscle weakness. Intermittent low-grade fever, substernal and abdominal pain (like that of peptic ulcer), melena, and hematemesis from bowel infarction may occur, the result of an accompanying systemic vasculitis.

The mode of progression of DM of childhood, like that of the adult form, is variable. In fulminant cases, the weakness appears rapidly, involving all the muscles including those of chewing, swallowing, talking, and breathing and leading to total incapacitation. Perforation of the gastrointestinal tract from bowel infarction may be the immediate cause of death, as it has been in two of our patients. In others, there is slow progression or arrest of the disease and, in a small number, there is a remission of weakness. Flexion contractures at the elbows, hips, knees, and ankles and subcutaneous calcification and ulceration of the overlying skin, with extrusion of calcific debris are manifestations in the late, untreated stages of the disease.

Systemic Autoimmune (Connective Tissue) Diseases With Polymyositis and Dermatomyositis

In both PM and DM, the inflammatory changes are often not confined to muscle but are associated with systemic autoimmune diseases such as rheumatoid arthritis, scleroderma, lupus erythematosus, or combinations thereof (mixed connective tissue disease); the same muscle changes are associated less often with the Sjögren syndrome. Conversely, in the aforementioned immune diseases, inflammatory muscle changes are frequently found but in only a limited number of muscles and often asymptomatically. The incidence of these "crossover" or overlap cases cannot be stated with certainty. A true necrotizing–inflammatory myopathy has been reported in up to 8 percent of cases of lupus erythematosus (far higher than in our experience), and an even smaller proportion of cases of systemic sclerosis, rheumatoid arthritis, and Sjögren syndrome. The treatment of rheumatoid arthritis with d-penicillamine increases the incidence of, or perhaps independently precipitates, a myositis.

Also notable is the sporadic concurrence of myositis with other autoimmune diseases such as myasthenia gravis and Hashimoto thyroiditis and less often, with a monoclonal paraprotein in the blood; it is not clear whether these are coincidental, but it is likely that they reflect an underlying genetic propensity to autoimmune disease.

In the overlap syndromes that incorporate autoimmune disease and myositis, there is usually greater muscular weakness and atrophy than can be accounted for by the muscle changes alone. Inasmuch as arthritis or periarticular inflammation may limit motion because of pain, result in disuse atrophy, and also at times cause a vasculitic polyneuropathy, the interpretation of diminished strength in these autoimmune diseases is not simple. Malaise, aches, and pains are common and attributable mostly to the systemic disease. Sometimes the diagnosis of myositis must depend on muscle biopsy, EMG findings, and measurements of muscle enzymes in the serum. In these complicated cases, myositis may accompany the connective tissue disease or occur many years later.

It is worth noting that PM may occur during pregnancy and that rarely the fetus is affected (most often the fetus and neonate are normal) with elevated CK levels for months postpartum (Messina et al).

Laboratory Diagnosis of PM and DM

In the majority of patients, serum levels of CK and other muscle enzymes, such as aldolase, are elevated. Serum CK levels tends to be higher in PM than in DM because of the widespread single-fiber necrosis in the former (as described in the following section on pathologic changes). However, in DM, if there are infarcts in muscle, CK levels will be moderately elevated as well. The sedimentation rate is normal or mildly elevated in both diseases.

It has been appreciated that some cases of PM and DM are associated with autoantibodies in the blood. Some of these are undoubtedly nonspecific markers of an autoimmune or inflammatory state, but others may be of pathogenetic significance or are markers for syndromes with multiorgan damage that extends beyond muscle. Tests for circulating rheumatoid factor or antinuclear antibody (ANA) are positive in fewer than half of cases. A high titer of ANA, in conjunction with elevated antiribonuclear antibodies, suggests the coexistence of systemic lupus or mixed connective tissue disease. It must be emphasized, however, that absent or low-titer ANA and a normal sedimentation rate do not exclude the diagnosis of PM, a fact that limits their diagnostic usefulness. Other antibodies can be found on occasion that are directed against constituents of a nucleolar protein complex (PM-Scl) and ribonucleoproteins (Ro/SS-A and La/SS-B).

Of greater interest are the findings that perhaps 20 percent of patients with PM and DM have antibodies against various cellular components of muscle, in particular, antibodies directed against cytoplasmic transfer ribonucleic acid (tRNA) synthetases (anti-Jo1), or against the tRNA itself. These are fairly specific to PM and, less frequently, to DM; they are found when the myositis is coupled with an expanded illness that involves other organs or connective tissues. The clinical disorders associated with these antibodies usually combine myositis with (1) interstitial lung disease but also (2) arthritis, (3) Raynaud syndrome, and (4) thickening of the skin of the hands ("mechanic's hands"). Following from the designation of the main type of antibody, these have been termed *synthetase syndromes*. Furthermore, an unexpectedly high proportion of cases of PM and DM show myositis-specific antibodies that are directed against a cytoplasmic ribonucleoprotein complex (SRP), or against a protein complex that is a nuclear helicase (Mi-2). The former is found in approximately 10 percent of cases of PM, and of DM (and with inclusion body myopathy; see further on), and in some series has carried a heightened risk of cardiac muscle inflammatory involvement. Although these various autoantibodies, with the possible exception of anti-Jo1, have not been especially useful as primary diagnostic tools, they do have a role in refining diagnosis. For example, a positive Jo1 antibody, although too uncommon to use as a screening test, precludes the diagnosis of inclusion body myopathy (which has been associated with a different set of autoantibodies as discussed further on) and its presence raises concern about the later development of interstitial lung disease. The presence of these antibodies also underscores the role for the humoral immune system in the pathogenesis of PM and raises opportunities for investigation discussed as follows.

Myoglobinuria can be detected in the majority of patients with most forms of myositis, particularly a necrotizing form, provided that a sensitive immunoassay procedure is used, but this test is not routinely performed.

The EMG is quite helpful in diagnosis but has been normal in a small proportion of our patients, even when many muscles are sampled. A typical "myopathic pattern is disclosed," that is, many abnormally brief action potentials of low voltage in addition to numerous fibrillation potentials, trains of positive sharp waves, occasional polyphasic units, and myotonic activity—all but the brief potentials possibly reflecting irritability of the muscle membranes (see Chap. 45). These findings are most apparent in weak muscles and are almost always seen when proximal weakness is well developed but they also may be observed in clinically unaffected areas. Indolent and chronic cases in which fibrosis of muscle and wasting have supervened may show polyphasic units that simulate denervation–reinnervation changes, juxtaposed with myopathic motor units. The EMG is also helpful in choosing a muscle for biopsy sampling but care must be taken not to obtain tissue from precisely the same site as a recent EMG needle insertion as a spurious histopathologic appearance of muscle damage may be obtained in this region (see the following text). Our approach has been to perform the needle EMG examination on one side of the body and biopsies on the other side.

As stated earlier, the ECG is abnormal in some cases and this finding may suggest the need for vigilance regarding cardiac symptoms and arrhythmias.

The results of magnetic resonance imaging (MRI) of muscle have been interesting and may aid the clinician in that abnormalities in T1, T2 and STIR signal intensity define regions of increased water content and inflammation and spectroscopic studies demonstrate regional deficits in energy production. Although MRI cannot at this time replace a biopsy for diagnosis, it can refine the distribution of lesions and aid in targeting the muscle biopsy, as well as provide a useful index of the efficacy of drug therapy. In some cases, MRI can distinguish IBM from either PM or metabolic muscle disease (see Lodi et al and also Dion et al).

Pathologic Changes in PM and DM

Because of the scattered distribution of inflammatory lesions and destructive changes, only part (or none) of the complex of pathologic changes may be divulged in any single biopsy specimen. Because of this limitation, more than one site of biopsy or multiple samples through one incision is advisable.

The principal changes in idiopathic PM consist of widespread destruction of segments of muscle fibers with an inflammatory reaction, that is, phagocytosis of muscle fibers by mononuclear cells and infiltration with a varying number of lymphocytes and lesser numbers of other mononuclear and plasma cells. Evidence of regenerative activity of muscle, mainly in the form of proliferating sarcolemmal nuclei, basophilic (RNA-rich) sarcoplasm, and new myofibrils, is evident in damaged regions. Many of the residual muscle fibers are small, with increased numbers of sarcolemmal nuclei. Some of the small fibers are found in clusters, the result of splitting of regenerating fibers. Either the degeneration of muscle fibers or an infiltration of inflammatory cells may predominate in any given biopsy specimen, although both types of changes are in evidence at autopsy.

In a single section from a biopsy sample, there may be only necrosis and phagocytosis of individual muscle fibers without infiltrates of inflammatory cells, or the reverse may be observed. However, in serial sections, muscle necrosis is shown to be adjacent to inflammatory infiltrates. Repeated attacks of a necrotizing myositis exhaust the regenerative potential of the muscles so that fiber loss, fibrosis, and residual thin and large fibers in haphazard arrangement may eventually impart a dystrophic appearance. For all these reasons, the pathologic picture can be correctly interpreted only in relation to clinical and other laboratory data. Guidelines for the interpretation of the muscle biopsy reflecting these comments, a critical step in correct diagnosis of the inflammatory myopathies, are given in the review by Dalakas and Hohlfeld.

In DM, there are several other distinctive histopathologic changes. In contrast to the evident necrosis of single fibers of PM, DM is characterized by perifascicular muscle fiber atrophy (referring to changes at the periphery of a fascicle, for reasons noted below). Moreover, the inflammatory infiltrates in DM predominate in the perimysial connective tissue, whereas in PM they are scattered throughout the muscle and are most prominent in relation to the muscle fiber membrane and the endomysium. The muscle lesions in dermatomyositis of childhood are similar to those of the adult form, only greatly accentuated. In a biopsy sample, the diagnosis can be inferred from the perifascicular pattern of degeneration and atrophy of muscle fibers.

Even more distinctive of DM are microvascular changes in muscle. Endothelial alterations (tubular aggregates in the endothelial cytoplasm) and occlusion of vessels by fibrin thrombi may be appreciated, with associated zones of infarction. The same vascular changes underlie the lesions in the connective tissue of skin, subcutaneous tissue, and gastrointestinal tract when they are present. The perifascicular muscle fiber atrophy had in the past been attributed to an ischemic process set up by capillary occlusion, but recent evidence suggests otherwise (see Greenberg and Amato).

Etiology and Pathogenesis

PM and DM are idiopathic. All attempts to isolate an infective agent have been unsuccessful. Several electron microscopists observed virus-like particles in muscle fibers, but a causative role has not been proved. A polymyositic illness has not been induced in animals by injections of affected muscle as it has in models of several other inflammatory neurologic conditions. Nevertheless, the notion that an autoimmune mechanism is operative in PM and DM is supported by the association of these disorders with a number of the more clearly established autoimmune diseases enumerated earlier in this chapter. Further evidence of an autoimmune nature is given by the presence of specific autoantibodies in nearly half of cases, as also described earlier.

Immunopathologic studies have partially substantiated an autoimmune mechanism and suggested that PM and DM can be distinguished from one another on the basis of their immunopathologic characteristics. In DM, immune complexes, IgG, IgM, complement (C3), and membrane-attack complexes are deposited in the walls of venules and arterioles, indicating that the immune response is directed primarily against intramuscular blood vessels (Whitaker and Engel; Kissel et al). Such a response is lacking in PM (and in IBM, discussed further on). Engel and Arahata have demonstrated a difference between the two disorders on the basis of the subsets and locations of lymphocytes that make up the intramuscular inflammatory aggregates. However, the deposition of these complexes may be a secondary event as our colleagues Greenberg and Amato propose. In PM, there are a large number of activated T cells, mainly of the CD8 class, whereas B cells are sparse. Moreover, T cells, accompanied by macrophages, enclose and invade nonnecrotic muscle fibers. In DM, very few fibers are affected in this manner, and the percentage of B cells at all sites is significantly higher than it is in PM. Engel and Arahata interpreted these differences as indicating that the effector response in DM is predominantly humoral, whereas in PM the response is composed of cytotoxic T cells, clones of which have been sensitized to a yet undefined antigen on the muscle fiber.

Treatment

Most clinicians agree that corticosteroids (prednisone, 1 mg/kg, as a single daily dose orally, or intravenously) are a reasonable first line of therapy for both PM and DM. The response to treatment is monitored by careful testing of strength and measurement of CK (not by following the erythrocyte sedimentation rate [ESR]). In patients who respond, the serum CK decreases before the weakness subsides; with relapse, the serum CK rises before weakness returns. Once the CK level normalizes and strength improves, typically several weeks or longer, the dosage may be reduced gradually—by no more than 5 mg every 2 weeks—toward 20 mg daily. It is then appropriate to attempt to control the disease with an alternate-day schedule with double this amount (i.e., prednisone, 40 mg every other day) so as to reduce the side effects of the drug. After cautious reduction of prednisone over a period of 6 months to 1 year or longer, the patient can usually be maintained on doses of 7.5 to 20 mg daily, with the aim of eventual discontinuation of the drug. Corticosteroids should not be discontinued prematurely, for the relapse that may follow is often more difficult to treat than the original illness.

In acute and particularly severe cases, treatment may be facilitated by the use initially of high-dose methylprednisolone (1 g infused over 2 h each day for 3 to 5 days). This form of treatment should be regarded as a temporary measure until oral prednisone becomes effective.

Alternatively, or sometimes in tandem with this approach, intravenous immunoglobulin (IVIg) or plasma exchanges may be instituted. In patients with DM who respond poorly to corticosteroids and other immunosuppressants or are severely affected early on, the addition of IVIg infusions often proves helpful, although several courses of treatment at monthly intervals may be required to achieve sustained improvement. In several controlled studies of small numbers of patients with DM, practically all showed improvement in muscle strength and in skin changes, and a reduction in CK concentration (see Dalakas; Mastaglia et al). PM has also been reported to respond favorably to treatment with IVIg, but the evidence is less certain. Further controlled studies are required to corroborate these reports and to establish, in both PM and DM, the optimal doses and modes of administration. It is noteworthy from our experience that IVIg has seldom been effective in PM or DM when used alone or as initial therapy. The proper use of these treatments in crossover cases with connective tissue disease has not been established.

Some patients who cannot tolerate, or are refractory to, prednisone may respond favorably to oral *azathioprine* with care being taken to avoid severe leukopenia. *Methotrexate* is currently favored by many groups over azathioprine as an adjunct to steroids (5 to 10 mg/week in 3 divided oral doses, increased by 2.5 mg/week, to a total dose of 20 mg weekly). Methotrexate or azathioprine should generally be given along with the lowest effective doses (15 to 25 mg) of prednisone. Although 1 study failed to show efficacy (Oddis et al), in cases that have been refractory to corticosteroids and methotrexate, we and our colleagues have had success rituximab intravenously, 750 mg/m^2, repeated in 2 weeks and sometimes required every 6 to 18 months. Some clinicians favor, from the beginning, a combination of prednisone in low dosage and one of these immunosuppressant drugs, and this approach is generally necessary when myocarditis or interstitial pneumonitis is coupled with DM. Mycophenolate mofetil has also been introduced and has allowed a reduction in steroid dose within several months in both PM and DM, according to a number of anecdotal reports, but has not proven clearly effective in a randomized trial; the reasons for this failure are being actively discussed and we have not abandoned its use. *Cyclosporine* has also been used in recalcitrant cases; it has few advantages over other immunosuppressant drugs and has a number of potentially serious side effects, including nephrotoxicity. *Cyclophosphamide*, which is a useful drug in the treatment of Wegener granulomatosis, polyarteritis, and other vasculitides, is said to be of lesser value in PM, but it may be useful in refractory cases and has perhaps the highest toxicity of the immunosuppressive medications that are used for inflammatory myopathies; we no longer use it with any regularity.

Prognosis

Except for patients with malignancy, the prognosis in adult PM and DM is generally favorable. Only a small proportion of patients with PM succumb to the disease and then usually from a secondary pulmonary complication or from myocarditis as already mentioned. Several of our patients have had severe aspiration pneumonias as a result of their dysphagia. The period of activity of disease varies considerably but is typically 2 to 3 years in both the child and adult. As indicated earlier, the majority improves with corticosteroid therapy, but many are left with varying degrees of weakness of the shoulders and hips. Approximately 20 percent of our patients have recovered completely after steroid therapy and long-term remissions have been achieved after withdrawal of medication in about an equal number. The extent of recovery is roughly proportional to the acuteness and severity of the disease and the duration of symptoms prior to institution of therapy. Patients with acute or subacute PM in whom treatment is begun soon after the onset of symptoms have the best prognosis. In the series collected by DeVere and Bradley, in which patients were treated early, there was remission in more than 50 percent of cases, whereas Riddoch and Morgan-Hughes reported a far lower rate in patients who were treated more than 2 years after onset of the disease. Those patients who have come to our attention after a long period of proximal weakness and with substantial muscle atrophy have not recovered completely, although some improvement occurred over years.

Even in patients who have a coexistent malignancy, muscle weakness may lessen and serum enzyme levels decline in response to corticosteroid therapy, but weakness returns after a few months and may then be resistant to further treatment. As already stated, if the tumor is successfully removed, muscle symptoms may remit, but even this experience has not been uniform.

The overall mortality after several years of illness had in the past approximated 15 percent, being higher in childhood DM, in PM with connective tissue diseases, and, of course, when a malignancy is found. Recent figures give more optimistic results.

Inclusion Body Myositis

Inclusion body myositis (IBM) is the third major form of inflammatory myopathy and, depending on the care taken with histologic diagnosis, is the most common inflammatory myopathy in patients older than 50 years. Its defining features, intracytoplasmic and intranuclear inclusions, were first described in 1965 by Adams and colleagues, who also drew attention to a number of clinical attributes now considered characteristic. By 1994, only 240 sporadic cases had been recorded in the medical literature (Mikol and Engel), but the diagnosis is now made so frequently that this low number almost certainly reflects the misidentification of IBM as PM in the past. Garlepp and Mastaglia concluded that more than one-third of cases of inflammatory myopathy, especially in men, are IBM. Moreover, the majority of myopathies in patients over 50 years, not attributable to medication toxicity, are due to IBM. A set of clinical and pathologic diagnostic criteria for the disease have been proposed by Griggs and coworkers and are useful for research purposes. A source of confusion has been the entirely separate entity of *inclusion body myopathy*, a largely hereditary, pauci-inflammatory process, and displays a different pattern of weakness from IBM. The myositis, as alluded to earlier, predominates in males (in a ratio of 3:1) and has its onset in middle or late adult life. Diabetes, any one of a variety of autoimmune diseases, and a relatively mild polyneuropathy are associated in approximately 20 percent of sporadic cases of IBM, but associations with malignancy or systemic autoimmune disease have not been established.

Clinical Manifestations

The illness is more variable but generally more focal in presentation than is PM and DM. It is characterized by a steadily progressive, painless muscular weakness and modest atrophy, which is usually distal in the arms and both proximal and distal in the legs. In approximately 20 percent of cases, the disease begins with focal weakness of the quadriceps, finger or wrist flexors, or lower leg muscles on one or both sides, and gradually spreads to other muscle groups after many months or years. Selective weakness of the flexor pollicis longus is a particularly characteristic pattern of involvement, and isolated quadriceps weakness or neck extensor weakness should also bring the diagnosis to mind, although IBM is not the exclusive cause of these patterns. In most patients, the deltoids are spared and the thumb flexors are weak, the opposite pattern to PM and DM. The tendon reflexes are normal initially but diminish in about half the patients, especially the knee jerks, as the disease progresses. Interestingly, the knee jerks may be depressed or lost even without much in the way of quadriceps weakness; this is not the case in PM, in which the reflexes are spared until the muscle is extremely weak. These clinical features are well displayed in the series reported by Amato and colleagues. Dysphagia is common (Wintzen et al). Selective or asymmetric involvement of distal muscles, when it occurs, erroneously suggests the diagnosis of motor neuron disease (the reflexes are not, however, enhanced as they are in ALS).

Laboratory and Muscle Biopsy Features

The CK is normal or slightly elevated, generally showing lower levels than in cases of PM with comparable amounts of weakness. EMG abnormalities are much like those found in PM, as discussed earlier. In addition, a small proportion of IBM patients display a more typically neuropathic EMG pattern, mainly with long-duration polyphasic potentials because of the chronicity of the disease, in the distal limb muscles. However, the EMG changes tend to be restricted to weakened muscles, a distinction from ALS.

The diagnosis depends on the clinical features and is supported by the muscle biopsy. There are structural abnormalities of muscle fibers and inflammatory changes. The latter are identical to but usually of lesser severity than those observed in idiopathic PM. (The infiltrating cells are mainly T cells of the CD8 type.) The denominative finding is of intracytoplasmic, subsarcolemmal vacuoles and eosinophilic inclusions in both the cytoplasm and nuclei of degenerating muscle fibers. The vacuoles contain, and are rimmed by, basophilic granular material "rimmed vacuoles. Special stains, particularly Gomori trichrome on frozen sections, and extensive inspection of biopsy specimens are required to disclose the rimmed vacuoles, for they are infrequent, widely dispersed, and easily overlooked. The inclusions may be congophilic, and may stain for TDP-43, p62, SM1-31, and, particularly, beta amyloid. As noted in subsequent sections similar inclusions are found in a number of other muscle diseases and are not in and of themselves diagnostic, especially without the destructive and mildly inflammatory changes of IBM. Moreover, the clinical context of these other diseases usually causes little difficulty in identifying the inclusions as ancillary and minor abnormalities on the biopsy.

Of clinical utility has been the recent introduction of testing for the earlier mentioned cytosolic antibodies (anti-cN1; NT5C1A) that are found in two-thirds of patients with IBM. They appear to be specific and assist in particular by differentiating this disease from the other inflammatory myopathies and in its detection when there is an unusual pattern of weakness that is not typically of an inflammatory myopathy. Testing other antibodies such as anti-Jo is probably suited to confirming cases that have the elements of a larger syndrome that includes, for example, interstitial lung disease.

Ultrastructural studies show that the protein inclusions accumulate at or near foci of abnormal tubulofilamentous structures in both the nuclei and cytoplasm. The nature of these diverse changes is obscure. The tubulofilamentous inclusions suggested to earlier investigators a viral origin, but an agent has never been isolated and serologic studies have failed to substantiate an infectious causation.

Treatment

IBM has not responded in any consistent fashion to treatment with corticosteroids or other immunosuppressive drugs. Indeed, the disease should be suspected in recalcitrant cases of apparent PM. The level of CK and the degree of leukocyte infiltration of muscle often diminish with corticosteroid treatment despite a lack of clinical improvement. On this basis, Barohn and coworkers suggested that the inflammatory response is not a primary cause of muscle destruction. In a few cases there has been brief improvement in response to IVIg, especially in weakened muscles involved in swallowing, but the gains have been unsustained and serial histopathologic examinations have detected no change. Two controlled trials have failed to show a benefit of IVIg. Plasma exchange and leukocytapheresis have also been tried, with generally discouraging results.

The disease in most patients is relentlessly progressive over many years, sometimes very slowly, and no method of treatment has so far altered the long-term prognosis. Sometimes, the process remains fairly restricted in scope or severity for up to a decade, thereby creating less disability than in cases that become generalized.

Problems in Diagnosis of Inflammatory Myopathy

The main issue here is differentiation from inclusion body myopathy, a subject introduced in the next section. The specific problem of determining which patients with DM or PM should have an extensive evaluation for a systemic malignancy and for connective tissue disease has been partially settled. We have adopted the practice of careful inspection of the chest radiograph, routine blood tests and stool examination for blood for all patients, and of undertaking a more extensive evaluation in patients older than 55 years and in smokers of any age. The evaluation of patients over 55 and smokers includes chest and abdominal computed tomographic (CT) scans, colonoscopy, pelvic ultrasound, cancer antigen (CA)-125, carcinoembryonic antigen (CEA), as well as other tests. In patients with recent weight loss, anorexia, or other symptoms suggestive of malignancy, we have included upper endoscopy and resorted to a body positron emission tomography scanning.

In addition to these main issues of distinguishing PM and DM from IBM, currently aided by antibody testing for the latter, we call attention to the following problems that we have encountered in connection with *diagnosis*:

1. *The patient with proximal muscle weakness is incorrectly diagnosed as having progressive muscular dystrophy (actually, the opposite pertains more often).* Points in favor of myositis are (1) lack of family history (although many dystrophies have recessive inheritance); (2) older age at onset; (3) rapid evolution of weakness; (4) evidence, past or present, of other connective tissue diseases; (5) high serum CK values (again, can be high in certain dystrophies; (6) marked degeneration and regeneration in muscle biopsy; and, finally, if there is still doubt, (7) unmistakable improvement with corticosteroid therapy.
2. *The patient with a systemic autoimmune disease (rheumatoid arthritis, scleroderma, lupus erythematosus, Sjögren syndrome) is suspected of having PM in addition.* Pain in these conditions prevents strong exertion (algesic pseudoparesis). Points against the coexistence of myositis are (1) the inability to document weakness out of proportion to muscle atrophy and the presence of pain on passive movement of the limbs; (2) normal EMG; (3) normal serum CK; and (4) normal muscle biopsy except possibly for areas of infiltration of chronic inflammatory cells in the endomysial and perimysial connective tissue (interstitial myositis).
3. *When muscle pain is a prominent feature, polymyalgia rheumatica must be differentiated.* This latter syndrome

is characterized by pain, stiffness, and tenderness in the muscles of the neck, shoulders, and arms, and sometimes of the hips and thighs; even passive motion of the limbs causes pain because of the periarticular locus of this disease. A high sedimentation rate, usually above 65 mm/h, is a diagnostic feature, but more typically the value is close to 100 mm/h, levels higher than in myositis. Biopsy of the temporal artery frequently discloses a giant cell arteritis. CK levels—and, of course, muscle biopsy—are normal. Rapid disappearance of pain with administration of small doses of prednisone is also diagnostic of polymyalgia rheumatica (see Chap. 11).

4. *The patient has restricted muscle weakness.* Weakness or paralysis of the posterior neck muscles, with inability to hold up the head, restricted bilateral quadriceps weakness, and other limited pelvocrural palsies are examples. Most often, the head-hanging or head-lolling syndrome proves to be caused by PM, and the other syndromes are caused by restricted forms of dystrophy or by motor neuron disease. IBM is the main alternative consideration in cases of neck or quadriceps weakness, particularly if the latter weakness is asymmetric; muscle enzymes in the serum are normal or slightly elevated. EMG and biopsy are helpful in diagnosis.
5. *The patient has diffuse myalgia and fatigability.* Most such patients have proved to be depressed and only rarely to have a myopathy. A few will be found to be caused by a toxic myopathy, particularly from one of the statin class of drugs. Hypothyroidism, McArdle disease, hyperparathyroidism, steroid myopathy, adrenal insufficiency, and early rheumatoid arthritis must be excluded by appropriate studies. Features that virtually exclude a myositis are (1) lack of reduced peak power of contraction and (2) normal EMG, serum enzymes, and muscle biopsy.
6. *Trichinosis, toxoplasmosis, HIV, and other infectious causes of myositis* can simulate acute immune myositis as described in the early parts of this chapter. Occasionally, the diagnosis of sarcoidosis is made from the muscle biopsy, but the myopathic features (weakness and pain) tend to be minor.

Other Inflammatory Myopathies

There are a large number of unrelated myositides and rare forms of focal myositis or relatively minor changes in muscle that occur in the course of inflammatory diseases of blood vessels or systemic infections and, curiously, with certain tumors such as thymoma. Most of these do not warrant extensive consideration and are described in detail in monographs devoted to muscle disease (see Banker). We are uncertain how to place the newly described and undoubtedly rare entity of myositis with abundant macrophage infiltration and aluminum hydroxide crystalline deposits. A type of fasciitis that is characterized by pronounced infiltration of macrophages has been related to vaccinations that contain the aluminum compound, but the myositis does not seem to be related to this aforementioned entity (see Bassez et al).

Three inflammatory myopathic diseases, however, are distinctive and of interest to neurologists: (1) eosinophilic myositis, fasciitis, and myalgia syndrome, (2) orbital myositis, and (3) sarcoidosis of muscle.

Eosinophilic Myositis and Fasciitis

This term has been applied to 4 overlapping clinical entities: (1) eosinophilic fasciitis, (2) eosinophilic monomyositis (sometimes multiplex), (3) eosinophilic PM, and (4) the eosinophilia-myalgia syndrome.

Eosinophilic Fasciitis This condition, mistakable for PM, was reported by Shulman in 1974. He described 2 men with a scleroderma-like appearance of the skin and flexion contractures at the knees and elbows associated with hyperglobulinemia, elevated sedimentation rate, and eosinophilia. Biopsy revealed greatly thickened fascia, extending from the subcutaneous tissue to the muscle and infiltrated with plasma cells, lymphocytes, and many eosinophils; the muscle itself appeared normal and the skin lacked the characteristic histologic changes of scleroderma. One of Shulman's patients recovered in response to prednisone.

The many reports that followed have substantiated and amplified Shulman's original description. The disease predominates in men in a ratio of 2:1. Symptoms appear between the ages of 30 and 60 years and are often precipitated by heavy exercise (Michet et al). There may be low-grade fever and myalgia followed by the subacute development of diffuse cutaneous thickening and limitation of movement of small and large joints. In some patients, proximal muscle weakness and eosinophilic infiltration of muscle can be demonstrated (Michet et al). Repeated examinations of the blood disclose an eosinophilia in most but not all patients. The disease usually remits spontaneously or responds well to corticosteroids. A small number relapse and do not respond to treatment and some have developed aplastic anemia and lympho- or myeloproliferative disease.

Eosinophilic Monomyositis Painful swelling of a calf muscle or, less frequently, some other muscle has been the chief characteristic of this disorder. Biopsy discloses inflammatory necrosis and edema of the interstitial tissues; the infiltrates contain large but variable numbers of eosinophils. The disorder was typified by 1 of our patients, a young woman who developed such an inflammatory mass first in 1 calf and, 3 months later, in the other. The response to prednisone was dramatic; the swelling and pain subsided in 2 to 3 weeks and her power of contraction was then normal. When the connective tissue and muscle are both damaged, a chaotic regeneration of fibroblasts and myoblasts may result, forming a pseudotumorous mass that may persist indefinitely.

Eosinophilic Polymyositis Layzer and associates described an eosinophilic disorder that they classified as "subacute polymyositis." Their patients were adults in whom predominantly proximal weakness evolved over several weeks. The features of the muscle disorder were typical of PM except that the inflammatory infiltration was predominantly eosinophilic and the muscles were swollen and painful. Moreover, the muscle disorder was part of a widespread systemic illness typical of the *hypereosinophilic syndrome*. The systemic manifestations included a striking eosinophilia (20 to 55 percent of the white blood cells), cardiac involvement (conduction disturbances and congestive failure), vascular disorder (Raynaud phenomenon, subungual hemorrhages), pulmonary infiltrates, strokes, anemia, neuropathy, and hypergammaglobulinemia. There was a favorable response to corticosteroids in 2 patients, but in a third the outcome was fatal in 9 months. Layzer and coworkers noted that a lack of necrotizing arteritis distinguished this process from polyarteritis nodosa and Churg-Strauss disease. No infective agent was isolated. An allergic mechanism seems possible, and in the present authors' view one cannot exclude an angiitis as a cause of the muscle lesions.

The last two of these previously mentioned syndromes (eosinophilic monomyositis and polymyositis) have overlapping features as shown by Stark's cases, in which a monomyositis was accompanied by several of the systemic features described by Layzer and colleagues. An uncertain proportion of cases are attributable to mutations in CAPN3, the gene for calpain-3 (Krahn et al). Moreover, some cases of eosinophilic polymyositis without systemic features have been found to be limb-girdle muscular dystrophy 2A, also due to a calpain mutation (i.e., both are considered to be "calpainopathies"). Patients with the dystrophic process, who also have a peripheral eosinophilia, probably have eosinophilic myositis.

Eosinophilia-Myalgia Syndrome Beginning in 1980, sporadic reports documented a lingering systemic illness characterized by severe generalized myalgia and eosinophilia of the peripheral blood following the ingestion of contaminated L-tryptophan. In late 1989 and early 1990, an outbreak occurred of this eosinophilia-myalgia syndrome, as the illness came to be called. More than 1,200 cases were reported to the Centers for Disease Control and Prevention (Medsger) and we examined several of them. The outbreak was ultimately traced to the use of nonprescription L-tryptophan tablets used as a sleep aid supplied by a single manufacturer and contaminated by ethylidene-bis-tryptophan and methyltetrahydro-beta-carboline-carboxylic acid, both close chemical relatives of L-tryptophan (Mayeno et al, 1990, 1992).

The onset of the muscular illness was relatively acute, with fatigue, low-grade fever, and eosinophilia (>1,000 cells/mm^3). Muscle pain and tenderness, cramps, weakness, paresthesias of the extremities, and induration of the skin were the main clinical features. A severe axonal neuropathy with slow and incomplete recovery was associated in some cases. Biopsies of the skin fascia, muscle, and peripheral nerve disclosed a microangiopathy and an inflammatory reaction in connective tissue structures; changes like those observed in scleroderma, eosinophilic fasciitis, and in the *toxic oil syndrome*. The latter syndrome, caused by the ingestion of contaminated rapeseed oil, occurred in an outbreak in Spain in 1981 and gave rise to a constellation of clinical and pathologic changes that were essentially identical to those caused by contaminated l-tryptophan (Ricoy et al; see also Chap. 46). The two toxins are also closely linked chemically and there have been other more limited outbreaks of the toxic neuropathy, usually from adulterated cooking oil.

The cutaneous lesions and eosinophilia of this syndrome responded to treatment with prednisone and other immunosuppressive drugs, but other symptoms persisted. Severe axonal neuropathy in our patients improved incompletely over several years, leaving one chair-bound with severe distal atrophic weakness after 15 years. Although no longer a problem that is likely to be seen by physicians, it serves as a model for future peculiar myopathic syndromes from adulterated drugs that otherwise would seem innocuous.

Acute Orbital Myositis

Among the many cases of orbital inflammatory disease (pseudotumor of the orbit and Tolosa-Hunt syndrome, as described in Chap. 14), there is a small group in whom the inflammatory process appears to be localized to the extraocular muscles. To this group, the term *acute orbital myositis* has been applied. The abrupt onset of orbital pain that is made worse by eye motion, redness of the conjunctiva adjacent to the muscle insertions, diplopia caused by restrictions of ocular movements, lid edema, and mild proptosis are the main clinical features and, admittedly, the distinctions from orbital pseudotumor are not clear. It may spread from one orbit to the other. The ESR is usually elevated and the patient may feel generally unwell, but only rarely can the ocular disorder be related to a systemic autoimmune disease or any other specific systemic disease. CT and MRI have proved to be particularly useful in demonstrating the swollen ocular muscles or muscle, and in separating orbital myositis from the other remitting inflammatory orbital and retroorbital conditions (Dua et al). As a rule, acute orbital myositis resolves spontaneously in a matter of a few weeks, although it may recur in the same or the opposite eye. Administration of steroids appears to hasten recovery.

Sarcoid Myopathy, Granulomatous Myositis, and Localized Nodular Myositis

There are undoubted examples of muscle involvement in patients with sarcoidosis, but they seem to be less frequent and less certain than would appear from the medical literature. In some cases, sarcoid myopathy becomes evident as a slowly progressive, occasionally fulminant, painless proximal or distal weakness. The CK levels are elevated. Muscle biopsy discloses numerous noncaseating granulomas. However, such lesions may also be found in patients with sarcoidosis who have no weakness. Treatment with moderate doses of corticosteroids (prednisone, 25 to 50 mg daily) is usually effective in symptomatic cases, but an additional immunosuppressive agent, such as cyclosporine, may have to be instituted if improvement is not evident in several weeks.

Much more puzzling have been cases of myopathy with the clinical features of idiopathic polymyositis and the presence of noncaseating granulomas in the muscle biopsy but with no evidence of sarcoidosis of the nervous system, lungs, bone, skin, or lymph nodes. Such cases call into question the validity of a muscle granuloma as a criterion of sarcoidosis, but the matter cannot be settled until we have a better definitions and etiology for sarcoidosis. These cases are presently classified as *granulomatous myositis* and, if limited to one or a small group of muscles, *localized nodular myositis* (Cumming et al). In a syndrome described by Namba and colleagues, this type of myositis was combined with myasthenia gravis, myocarditis, and thyroiditis. The muscle process has, on a few occasions, also been associated with Crohn disease. Electron microscopy has disclosed muscle fiber invasion by lymphocytes, suggesting a cell-mediated immune reaction. Very rarely, a granulomatous myositis may complicate tuberculosis or syphilis.

THE MUSCULAR DYSTROPHIES

(Tables 48-1 through 48-3)

The muscular dystrophies are a group of progressive hereditary degenerative diseases of skeletal muscles. The intensity of the degenerative changes in muscle and the cellular response and nature of the regenerative changes distinguish the dystrophies histologically from other diseases of muscle and also have implications regarding their pathogenesis. The category of more benign and relatively nonprogressive myopathies—each named from its special histopathologic appearance, such as central core, nemaline, mitochondrial, and centronuclear diseases—present greater difficulty in classification. Like the dystrophies, they are primarily diseases of muscle and are often heredofamilial in nature, but they are placed in a separate category because of a nonprogressive or slowly progressive course and their distinctive histochemical and ultrastructural features.

The current clinical classification of the muscular dystrophies is based mainly on the distribution of the dominant muscle weakness; however, several of the classical types have retained their eponymic designations: Duchenne, Becker, Emery-Dreifuss, Landouzy-Dejerine, Miyoshi, Welander, Fazio-Londe, and Bethlem are among the ones that still have utility in shorthand. To these are added myotonic dystrophy and a group of so-called congenital muscular dystrophies, usually severe in degree.

The extraordinary depth of information regarding the molecular nature of the dystrophies is one of the most gratifying developments of modern neuroscience.

Table 48-1

DUCHENNE/BECKER, EMERY-DREIFUSS, LIMB-GIRDLE, AND RELATED MAJOR MUSCULAR DYSTROPHIES

INHERITANCE TYPE	GENE OR CHROMOSOME	ONSET DECADE	CK ELEVATION	REGIONS AFFECTED
X-linked recessive				
Duchenne/Becker	Dystrophin	1st	10–50 ×	Proximal, then distal muscles
				Cardiac muscle
Emery-Dreifuss	Emerin	2nd–3rd	5 ×	Proximal muscles, joint contractures; cardiac arrhythmias
Scapuloperoneal	*FHL1*			Scapular-peroneal
Autosomal dominant				
LGMD 1A	Myotilin	3rd–4th	2 ×	Distal greater than proximal weakness, vocal cords, pharynx; allelic with myofibrillar myopathy
LGMD 1B	Lamin A/C	1st–2nd	3–5 ×	Resembles Emery-Dreifuss disease
				Proximal muscles and heart, joint contractures
LGMD 1C	Caveolin-3	1st	4–25 ×	Proximal muscles
LGMD 1D	6p	3rd–5th	2–4 ×	Proximal muscles; cardiomyopathy
LGMD 1E	Desmin	1st	Nl	Proximal muscles
Autosomal recessive				
LGMD 2A	Calpain-3	1st–2nd	3–15 ×	Proximal and distal muscles
LGMD 2B	Dysferlin	2nd–3rd	10–50 ×	Proximal and distal muscles
				Allelic to Miyoshi myopathy
LGMD 2C–F	α, β, γ, δ-sarcoglycans	1st–3rd	5–40 ×	Phenotype of Becker dystrophy
LGMD 2G	Telethonin	2nd	3–17 ×	Proximal greater than distal muscles
LGMD 2H	*TRIM32*	1st–3rd	2–25 ×	Proximal greater than distal muscles
LGMD 2I	*FKRP*	1st–3rd	10–30 ×	Proximal greater than distal muscles
				FKRP defects also cause CMD
LGMD 2J	Titin	1st–3rd	2 ×	Proximal and sometimes distal muscles
LGMD 2M	*POMGNT1**	Birth		Mutations also associated with muscle-eye-brain diseases

CK, creatine kinase; CMD, childhood muscular dystrophy; FKRP, fukutin-related protein; LGMD, limb-girdle muscular dystrophy; Nl, normal.

Table 48-2

SELECTED MUSCULAR DYSTROPHIES[a]

TYPE	GENE OR CHROMOSOME	ONSET DECADE	CK ELEVATION	REGIONS AFFECTED
Myotonic dystrophy (DM1)	Expanded intronic CTG repeat in myotonin kinase	1st–2nd	1–2 ×	Distal weakness, myotonia, cataracts Testicular atrophy, balding, cardiac arrhythmias
Proximal myotonic myopathy (DM2)	Expanded intronic CCTG repeat in zinc finger protein	1st–2nd	1–2 ×	Resembles myotonic dystrophy with prominent proximal muscle weakness but no infancy onset; less facial weakness
Facioscapulohumeral dystrophy	Multigene dysregulation at 4q telomere	1st–4th	1–2 ×	Facial, scapular, anterior tibial muscles Hearing loss, ocular telangiectasias
Oculopharyngeal dystrophy	Exonic GCG expansion (alanine) in poly-A binding protein	6th–7th	1–2 ×	Oculopharyngeal and levator palpebrae muscles
Bethlem myopathy	Collagen VI, subunits α 1-3	1st–3rd	1–4 ×	Proximal weakness Contractures in fingers, elbows, knees May present as CMD
Myofibrillar myopathy	Myotilin, desmin, $\alpha\beta$-crystallin	2nd–4th	1–5 ×	Allelic with LGMD-1A

[a]All inherited in an autosomal dominant pattern.
CCTG, cytosine, cytosine, thymine, guanidine; CMD, childhood muscular dystrophy; CTG, cytosine, thymine, guanidine; GCG, guanidine, cytosine, guanidine; LGMD, limb-girdle muscular dystrophy.

Table 48-3

DISTAL MUSCULAR DYSTROPHIES

INHERITANCE DISORDER	GENE OR PROTEIN DEFICIENCY	ONSET DECADE	CK ELEVATION	REGIONS AFFECTED
Autosomal recessive				
Miyoshi myopathy	Dysferlin	2nd–3rd	10–50 ×	Begins in gastrocnemius muscles, rarely, in anterior tibial muscles Identical genetic defects may cause LGMD-2B Involves multiple muscle groups, spares heart
Nonaka myopathy with rimmed vacuoles (familial IBM)	GNE kinase–epimerase UDP-*N*-acetylglucosamine-2-epimerase/*N*-mannosamine kinase	2nd–3rd	3–10 ×	Distal more than proximal weakness Quadriceps sparing Spares heart
Autosomal dominant				
Welander distal dystrophy	Unknown	4th–5th	2–3 ×	Weakness begins in hands Slow progression Spares cardiac muscle
Tibial muscular dystrophy	Titin	4th–8th	2–4 ×	Onset in tibial distribution No cardiac involvement
Scapuloperoneal dystrophy	X-linked (see Table 48-1)	3rd–6th	2–10 ×	Scapuloperoneal weakness Hyaline bodies in muscle Early onset of foot-drop
Desmin myopathy	Desmin	3rd–4th	2–3 ×	Onset of distal weakness, slowly progressive Cardiac arrhythmias (sometimes fatal)
Gower-Laing	*MYHC-1 (MYH7)*	2nd–3rd	3 ×	Anterior tibial (early foot-drop)
Markesbery-Griggs	*ZASP*	2nd–3rd	2 ×	Anterior tibial Cardiomyopathy common

IBM, inclusion body myopathy.

The majority of the dystrophies are caused by changes in structural elements of the muscle cell, mainly in its membrane, but other important mechanisms also are being identified, such as altered messenger RNA (mRNA). In keeping with the outlook expressed throughout the book, we adhere to a clinical orientation in describing the muscular dystrophies but make clear that treatment in the future could be determined based on understanding of molecular mechanisms. Each of the muscular dystrophies is described in accordance with this scheme.

The differentiation of dystrophic diseases of muscle from those secondary to neuronal degeneration was an achievement of neurologists of the second half of the nineteenth century. Isolated cases of muscular dystrophy had been described earlier, but no distinction was made between neuropathic and myopathic disease. In 1855, the French neurologist Duchenne described the progressive muscular atrophy of childhood that now bears his name. However, it was not until the second edition of his monograph in 1861 that the "hypertrophic paraplegia of infancy" was recognized as a distinct syndrome. By 1868 he was able to write a comprehensive description of 13 cases and recognized that the disease was muscular in origin and restricted to males. Gowers in 1879 gave a masterful account of 21 personally observed cases and called attention to the characteristic way in which such patients arose from the floor (Gowers sign). Erb, in 1891, crystallized the clinical and histologic concept of a group of diseases caused by primary degeneration of muscle, which he named *muscular dystrophies*. The first descriptions of facioscapulohumeral dystrophy were published by Landouzy and Déjerine in 1894; of progressive ocular myopathy by Fuchs in 1890; of myotonic dystrophy by Steinert and by Batten and Gibb in 1909; of distal dystrophy by Gowers in 1888, Milhorat and Wolff in 1943, Welander in 1951, and Miyoshi and colleagues in 1986; and of oculopharyngeal dystrophy by Victor and associates in 1962. References to these and other writings of historical importance can be found in the works of Kakulas and Adams, of Walton and colleagues, and of Engel and Franzini-Armstrong, and most recently of Amato and Russell.

In the more recent history of the dystrophies, the most notable event was the discovery by Kunkel, in 1986, of the dystrophin gene and its protein product. Since then there has been an extraordinary accumulation of molecular-genetic, ultrastructural, and biochemical information about the muscular dystrophies, which has greatly broadened our understanding of their mechanisms. It has also clarified a number of uncertainties as to their clinical presentations and has necessitated a revision of an older classification.

Duchenne Muscular Dystrophy

This is the most frequent and best known of the early-onset muscular dystrophies. It begins in early childhood and runs a relatively rapid, progressive course. The incidence is in the range of 13 to 33 per 100,000 yearly or about 1 in 3,300 live male births. There is a strong familial liability as the disease is transmitted as an X-linked recessive trait, occurring almost exclusively in males. However, careful examination of the mothers of affected boys shows slight muscle involvement in as many as half of them, as pointed out by Roses and coworkers (a frequency higher than in our limited experience). Approximately 30 percent of patients have no family history of the disease and these represent spontaneous mutations.

Rarely, a severe proximal Duchenne-type muscular dystrophy occurs in young girls. This may have several explanations. The female may have only 1 X chromosome, as occurs in the Turner (XO) syndrome, and that chromosome carries the Duchenne gene, or the Lyon principle may be operative; that is, there is inactivation of the unaffected paternal X chromosome allowing expression of the mutated Duchenne protein from the maternal chromosome in a large proportion of embryonic cells (mosaicism). It so happens that most childhood dystrophies in girls prove to be of an entirely different type that is caused by an autosomal recessive mutation causing a limb-girdle dystrophy as discussed further on.

Clinical Features

Duchenne muscular dystrophy is usually recognized by the third year of life and almost always before the sixth year. Nearly half of children show evidence of disease before beginning to walk. Many of them are slightly backward in other ways (mild mental retardation) and the muscle weakness may at first be overlooked. A greatly elevated CK may be the clue. In another group of young children, an indisposition to walk or run normally at the expected time brings them to medical attention or, having achieved these motor milestones, they appear less active than expected and are prone to falls. Increasing difficulty in walking, running, and climbing stairs, excessive lumbar lordosis, and waddling gait become more obvious as time passes. The iliopsoas, quadriceps, and gluteal muscles are involved initially; then the pretibial muscles weaken (foot-drop and toe walking). Muscles of the pectoral girdle and upper limbs are affected after the pelvicrural ones; the serrati, lower parts of pectorals, latissimus dorsi, biceps, and brachioradialis muscles are affected, more or less in this order.

Enlargement of the calves and certain other muscles is progressive in the early stages of the disease but most of the muscles, even the ones that are originally enlarged, eventually decrease in size; only the gastrocnemii, and to a lesser extent the lateral vasti and deltoids, are consistently large and this peculiarity may attract attention before the weakness becomes evident. The enlarged muscles have a firm, resilient ("rubbery") feel and are slightly weaker and more hypotonic than healthy ones. Thus the muscle enlargement is a pseudohypertrophy. Rarely, all muscles are at first large and strong, even the facial muscles, as in one of Duchenne's cases (from the marble statue, Farnese Hercules); histologically, this is a true muscle hypertrophy.

Muscles of the pelvic girdle, lumbosacral spine, and shoulders become weak and wasted, accounting for certain clinical peculiarities. Weakness of abdominal and paravertebral muscles accounts for a lordotic posture and protuberant abdomen when standing and the rounded back when sitting. Weakness of the extensors of the knees and hips interferes with equilibrium and with activities such as climbing stairs or rising from a chair or from a stooped posture. In standing and walking, the patient places his feet wide apart so as to increase his base of support. To rise from a sitting position, he first flexes his trunk at the hips, puts his hands on his knees, and pushes the trunk upward by working the hands up the thighs. In rising from the ground, the child first assumes a four-point position by extending the arms and legs to the fullest possible extent and then works each hand alternately up the corresponding thigh (the sign traditionally attached to Gowers' name). In getting up from a recumbent position, the patient turns his head and trunk and pushes himself sideways to a sitting position. S.A.K. Wilson used an alliterative phrase to describe the characteristic abnormalities of stance and gait: The patient "straddles as he stands and waddles as he walks." The waddle is the result of bilateral weakness of the gluteus medius. Many affected boys have a tendency to walk on their toes as a consequence of contractures in the gastrocnemii muscles. Calf pain is frequent. Weakening of the muscles that fix the scapulae to the thorax (serratus anterior, lower trapezius, rhomboids) causes winging of the scapulae, and the scapular angles can sometimes be seen above the shoulders when one is facing the patient.

Later, weakness and atrophy spread to the muscles of the legs and forearms. The muscles that are preferentially affected among these are the neck flexors, wrist extensors, brachioradialis, costal part of the pectoralis major, latissimus dorsi, biceps, triceps, and anterior tibial and peroneal muscles. The ocular, facial, bulbar, and hand muscles are usually spared, although weakness of the facial and sternocleidomastoid muscles and of the diaphragm occurs in the late stages of the disease. As the trunk muscles atrophy, the bones stand out like those of a skeleton. The space between the lower ribs and iliac crests diminishes with atrophy and weakness of the abdominal muscles.

The limbs are usually loose and slack, but as the disability progresses, fibrous contractures appear as a result of the limbs remaining in one position and the imbalance between agonists and antagonists. Early in the ambulatory phase of the disease, the feet assume an equinovarus position as a result of shortening of the posterior calf muscles, which act without the normal opposition of the pretibial and peroneal muscles. Later, the hamstring muscles become permanently shortened because of a lack of counteraction of the weaker quadriceps muscles. Similarly, contractures occur in the hip flexors because of the relatively greater weakness of hip extensors and abdominal muscles. This leads to a pelvic tilt and compensatory lordosis to maintain standing equilibrium. The consequences of these contractures account for the habitual posture of the patient with Duchenne dystrophy: lumbar lordosis, hip flexion and abduction, knee flexion, and plantar flexion. As they become severe, these contractures contribute importantly to the eventual loss of ambulation. Scoliosis, as a result of unequal weakening of the paravertebral muscles, and flexion contractures of the forearms appear, usually after walking is no longer possible.

The tendon reflexes are diminished and then lost as muscle fibers disappear, the ankle reflexes being the last to go. The bones are thin and demineralized, and the appearance of ossification centers is delayed. Smooth muscles are spared, but the heart is affected by various types of arrhythmias. The ECG shows prominent R waves in the right precordial leads and deep Q waves in the left precordial and limb leads, the result of cardiac fiber loss and replacement fibrosis of the basal part of the left ventricular wall (Perloff et al).

Death is usually the result of pulmonary infections and respiratory failure and sometimes, of cardiac decompensation. Patients with Duchenne dystrophy usually survive until late adolescence, but not more than 20 to 25 percent live beyond the twenty-fifth year. The last years of life are spent in a wheelchair; finally the patient becomes bedfast.

Mild degrees of developmental delay, which is nonprogressive, are observed in many cases. The average IQ is 85 and approximately one-quarter have an IQ below 70, but the range has been 40 to 130.

As mentioned earlier, Roses and colleagues have studied the female carriers of the disease (i.e., the mothers of affected boys) and described slight weakness and enlargement of the calves as well as elevated CK values and abnormalities of the electromyelogram (EMG) and muscle biopsy, all slight in degree, in more than half; as mentioned, this is far higher than in our experience and that of our colleagues. A small number of female carriers manifest a moderate myopathy that may mimic limb-girdle dystrophy (see further on). The muscle fibers of such patients (referred to as *manifesting* or *symptomatic* carriers) show a mosaic immunostaining pattern mentioned earlier, some fibers containing dystrophin and others lacking it (Hoffman et al, 1988). This diagnostic information is particularly helpful in genetic counseling.

The serum CK values are 25 to 200 times normal, which, with the EMG and muscle biopsy findings, help exclude spinal muscular atrophy. The EMG shows fibrillations, positive waves, low-amplitude and brief polyphasic motor unit potentials, and, sometimes, high-frequency discharges. The female carrier may occasionally display the same abnormalities, but to a much milder degree. The molecular and genetic bases of the disease are discussed further on.

Becker Muscular Dystrophy

This milder dystrophy is closely related to the Duchenne type clinically, genetically, and ultrastructurally. It had long been noted that mixed with the Duchenne group were certain relatively benign cases. In 1955, Becker and Keiner proposed that the latter be separated as a distinct entity, now called Becker muscular dystrophy. The incidence is difficult to ascertain, but it has been estimated as 3 to 6 per 100,000 male births. Like the Duchenne form, it is an X-linked disorder, practically limited to males and transmitted by females. It causes weakness and hypertrophy in the same muscles as Duchenne dystrophy, but the onset is much later (mean age: 12 years; range: 5 to 45 years). While boys with Duchenne dystrophy are usually dependent on a wheel-chair by early in the second decade, it is not uncommon for those with Becker dystrophy to walk well into adult life. In comparison to Duchenne dystrophy, those with Becker and intermediate types retain their ability to raise the head fully off the bed. We have, for example, encountered patients who served in the military with the disease undetected. If maternal uncles are affected by the disease and are still walking, the diagnosis is relatively easy. Mentation is usually normal and cardiac involvement is far less frequent than in Duchenne dystrophy, but there are cases that present with a cardiomyopathy and we have been made aware of 2 brothers who had cardiac transplantation before the disease was detected. Kuhn and associates have reported a genealogy in which early myocardial disease and cramping myalgia were prominent features.

Pathology of Duchenne and Becker Dystrophies

In the early stages of Duchenne dystrophy, the most distinctive features are prominent segmental degeneration and phagocytosis of single muscle fibers or groups of fibers and evidence of regenerative activity (basophilia of sarcoplasm, hyperplasia and nucleation of sarcolemmal nuclei, and the presence of myotubes and myocytes). The necrosis excites a regenerative or restorative process, which explains the forking of fibers and clustering of small fibers with prominent nuclei. The necrotic sarcoplasm and sarcolemma are removed by mononuclear phagocytic (macrophage) cells. There may also be a few T lymphocytes in the region, suggesting inflammation. There is a hyalinization of the sarcoplasm of many degenerating and nondegenerating fibers. In longitudinal sections these are seen as "contraction bands," expressive of the irritability of dystrophic muscle. This phenomenon may be present before there is any significant degree of degeneration and is more extensive in Duchenne than in any of the other dystrophies. Eventually, there are histologic changes that are common to all types of advanced muscular dystrophies: loss of muscle fibers, residual fibers of larger and smaller size than normal, all in haphazard arrangement, and the secondary reaction of an increase in lipocytes and fibrosis.

Hypertrophy of muscle is apparently the result of work-induced enlargement of the remaining sound fibers in the face of adjacent fiber injury. However, examples of true hypertrophy of entire muscles prior to the first sign of weakness also occur and are difficult to explain. In these cases, large fibers may be present when at most there are only a few degenerating fibers. The more common feature of pseudohypertrophy is a result of lipocytic replacement of degenerated muscle fibers, but in its earlier stages, the presence of many enlarged fibers may contribute to the enlargement of muscle. Thus a true hypertrophy appears to give way to pseudohypertrophy. In the late stage of the dystrophic process, only a few scattered muscle fibers remain, almost lost in a sea of fat cells. It is notable that the late, or burned-out, stage of chronic polymyositis resembles muscular dystrophy in that the fiber population is depleted, the residual fibers are of variable size, and fat cells and endomysial fibrous tissue are increased; lacking only are the hypertrophied fibers of dystrophy. This resemblance confirms that many of the typical changes of muscular dystrophy are nonspecific, reflecting mainly the chronicity of the myopathic process.

Etiology of Duchenne and Becker Dystrophies

The most important development in our understanding of the Duchenne and Becker muscular dystrophies was the discovery by Kunkel of the mutation on the X chromosome and of its gene product, *dystrophin* (Hoffman et al, 1987). The protein is expressed in skeletal, cardiac, and smooth muscle, as well as in brain. To date, the dystrophin gene is the largest one known in humans, spanning more than 2 Mb of DNA. This is in part the explanation for the observation that one-third of affected boys have a spontaneous mutation in the gene. The biochemical assay of dystrophin and its histochemical demonstration near the sarcolemma have made possible the accurate diagnosis of the Duchenne and Becker phenotypes and have clarified the relationship between these two disorders. Whereas dystrophin is absent in patients with the Duchenne phenotype, it is present but structurally abnormal in the Becker type. Moreover, phenotypes that fall between the classic Duchenne and Becker forms exist and are characterized by a lower-than-normal amount of dystrophin. The Duchenne and Becker dystrophies and their intermediate forms are spoken of as *dystrophinopathies*.

A slightly different form of dystrophin, originating in a different part of the gene, is found in neurons of the cerebrum and brainstem and in astrocytes, Purkinje cells, and Schwann cells at nodes of Ranvier (Harris and Cullen). A deficiency of cerebral dystrophin may in some yet unexplained way account for the mild cognitive developmental delay. It will be interesting to learn how such a deficiency might impair brain development and whether there is any connection to some cases of mental deficiency without muscular dystrophy.

Figure 48-1 schematically represents the structural basis of the dystrophinopathies and certain of the limb-girdle and congenital dystrophies described further on. In normal skeletal and cardiac muscle, dystrophin is localized to the cytoplasmic surface of the sarcolemma, where it interacts with F-actin of the cytoskeleton (the filamentous reinforcing structure of the muscle cell). Dystrophin is also tightly bound to a complex of sarcolemmal proteins known as dystrophin-associated proteins (DAPs) and to dystrophin-associated glycoproteins (DAGs). Of special biologic importance in this complex are these proteins and a 156-kDa glycoprotein called *dystroglycan*. The latter actually lies just outside the muscle cell and links the sarcolemmal membrane to the extracellular matrix (the inner portion of the basement membrane) by binding with merosin, a subunit of laminin. The dystrophin–glycoprotein complex functions in this scheme as a transsarcolemmal structural link between the subsarcolemmal cytoskeleton and the extracellular matrix. Moreover, each of these membrane-binding proteins (adhalin, merosin, and laminin) is implicated in specific muscular dystrophies, as discussed later in this chapter.

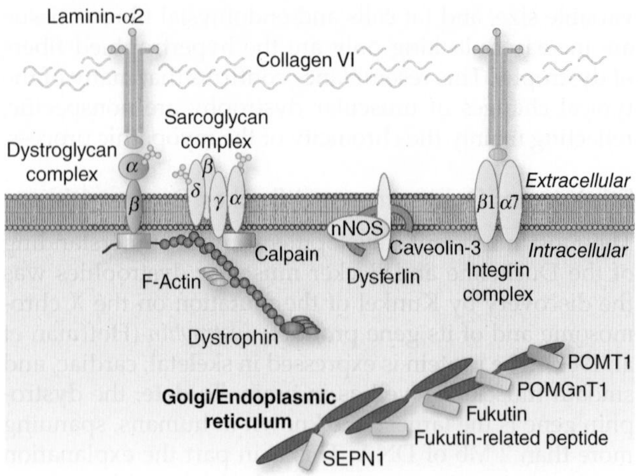

Figure 48-1. The molecular organization of the dystrophin-glycoprotein complex in the membrane and sarcolemma and endoplasmic reticulum-Golgi apparatus. These proteins are related to Duchenne, limb-girdle, Miyoshi, and certain congenital dystrophies. Details in text.

The loss of dystrophin leads to a parallel loss of DAPs and to disruption of the dystroglycan–protein complex. This change renders the sarcolemma susceptible to breaks and tears during muscle contraction, a hypothesis proposed first by Mokri and Engel and entirely consistent with the ultrastructural abnormalities that characterize Duchenne dystrophy. These authors demonstrated defects of the plasma membrane (sarcolemma) in a large proportion of nonnecrotic hyalinized muscle fibers, allowing ingress of extracellular fluid and calcium. The entrance of calcium is speculated to activate proteases and to increase protein degradation. The membrane defects and the associated alterations in the underlying region of the fiber represent the earliest and most basic pathologic change in Duchenne dystrophy and account for the leakage into the serum of CK and other enzymes of muscle.

Diagnosis of Duchenne and Becker dystrophies

The identification of dystrophin has made possible a number of highly refined tests for the diagnosis of Duchenne and Becker dystrophies, as well as for the carrier state. Analysis of the dystrophin gene in DNA obtained from white blood cells or from 50 mg of skeletal muscle can demonstrate the gene mutations in Duchenne and Becker patients and discriminate between these diseases. Also, immunostaining of muscle for dystrophin makes possible the differentiation of Duchenne, Becker, the carrier state, and other muscle disorders. An alternative method, developed by Byers and colleagues, uses an ELISA to measure the dystrophin levels in muscle biopsy samples. This testing is a rapid and relatively inexpensive tool for establishing the diagnosis of Duchenne and Becker muscular dystrophies and distinguishing them from unrelated disorders.

Other Rarer Dystrophinopathies

Testing for the dystrophin protein has also brought to light several much rarer types of dystrophin abnormalities. One, described by Gospe and coworkers, takes the form of a familial X-linked *myalgic-cramp-myoglobinuric syndrome*, resulting from the deletion of the first third of the dystrophin gene. The muscle changes are mild and relatively nonprogressive. Another dystrophinopathy takes the form of an *X-linked cardiomyopathy* characterized by progressive heart failure in young persons without clinical evidence of skeletal muscle weakness; biopsy of skeletal muscle reveals reduced immunoreactivity to dystrophin (Jones and de la Monte). In yet another type, a glycerol-kinase deficiency is associated with varying degrees of adrenal hypoplasia, mental retardation, and myopathy.

Emery-Dreifuss Muscular Dystrophy

This is a highly diverse group of disorders that encompasses at least six different genetic types, the most common probably being an X-linked muscular dystrophy characterized by the special feature of muscle contractures. That process is relatively benign in comparison with the Duchenne dystrophy. It was described originally by Emery and Dreifuss and subsequently by Hopkins and by Merlini and their colleagues. The primary gene defect is a deficiency of the protein emerin, a constituent of the nuclear membrane, encoded by a gene on the X chromosome (Fig. 48-2). However, also described are autosomal dominant forms with mutations in the gene for laminin A/C (called LGMD 1B, obviously affecting both girls and boys), an additional X-linked form due to mutations in FHL-1 as well as sporadic and dominant mutations of other genes encoding for entirely disparate proteins. Making a complete understanding of this syndrome even more complex is the recent appreciation that many of cases have none of these mutations.

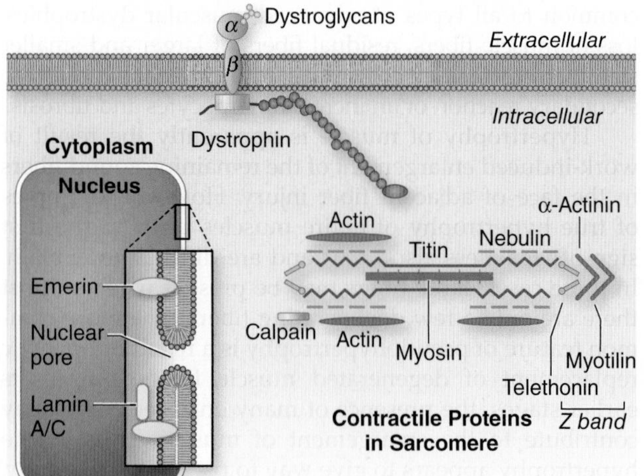

Figure 48-2. Expanded schematic of the nuclear and contractile proteins of the muscle. These proteins are referable to Emery-Dreifuss dystrophy and a number of the distal and the congenital dystrophies, as well as several of the limb-girdle dystrophies. Details in text.

The age of onset varies from childhood to late adolescence or adulthood. Weakness affects first the upper arm and pectoral girdle musculature and later the pelvic girdle and the distal muscles in the lower extremities. The distinguishing feature of the disease is the early appearance of contractures in the flexors of the elbow, extensors of the neck, and posterior calf muscles. Facial muscles are affected occasionally. There is no hypertrophy or pseudohypertrophy, and mentation is unaffected. However, severe cardiomyopathy with variable sinoatrial and atrioventricular conduction defects is a common accompaniment.

The course of the myopathy is generally benign, more like that of Becker dystrophy, but weakness and contractures are severe in some cases and sudden cardiac death is a not infrequent occurrence. For this reason, close monitoring by a cardiologist and the prophylactic insertion of a pacemaker at the appropriate time may be lifesaving.

The less common types of Emery-Dreifuss dystrophy, as mentioned, may have a *scapuloperoneal* (*FHL-1* gene) or *humeroperoneal* (laminin mutation).

Facioscapulohumeral Muscular Dystrophy (Landouzy-Dejerine Muscular Dystrophy)

This is a slowly progressive dystrophy involving primarily the musculature of the face and shoulders, often with long periods of nearly complete arrest. The pattern of inheritance is usually autosomal dominant. Almost all are of the facioscapulohumeral muscular dystrophy 1 (FSHD1) type; 5 to 10 percent are designated FSHD2, for which the mutation has recently been identified. The clinical presentations are very similar.

Although less common than the Duchenne and myotonic dystrophies, FSHD is not rare (an estimated yearly incidence rate of 5:100,000) and we have seen 1 or more cases yearly. The age of onset is usually between 6 and 20 years, but cases beginning in early adult life are occasionally encountered. Weakness and atrophy of the involved muscles are the major physical findings; pseudohypertrophy occurs only rarely and is slight. As a rule, the first manifestations are difficulty in raising the arms above the head and winging of the scapulae, although bifacial weakness may have initially attracted attention, even in early childhood. There is involvement especially of the orbicularis oculi, the zygomaticus, and the orbicularis oris, whereas the masseters, as well as the temporalis, extraocular, pharyngeal, and respiratory muscles are spared. There is an inability to close the eyes firmly, to purse the lips, and to whistle; the lips have a peculiar looseness and tendency to protrude. The lower parts of the trapezius muscles and the sternal parts of the pectorals are almost invariably affected. By contrast, the deltoids may seem to be unusually large and strong, an appearance that may be mistaken for pseudohypertrophy. The advancing atrophic process involves the sternocleidomastoid, serratus magnus, rhomboid, erector spinae, latissimus dorsi, and eventually the deltoid muscles as well. The bones of the shoulders become prominent; the scapulae are winged and elevated ("angel-wing" appearance), and the clavicles stand out. The anterior axillary folds slope down and out as a result of wasting of the pectoral muscles. Usually the biceps waste less than the triceps, and the brachioradialis muscles even less, so that the upper arm may be thinner than the forearm ("Popeye" effect). Pelvic muscles are involved later and to a milder degree, giving rise to a slight lordosis and pelvic instability. The pretibial muscles weaken, and foot-drop is added to the waddling gait. The Beevor sign, an upward movement of the umbilicus on flexing the neck as a result of weakness of the lower abdominal muscles, is reportedly common (Awerbuch et al), but we have not seen it in early cases.

Initially, and even throughout the course, the muscular weakness may be asymmetrical (winging of only one scapula). Many of the patients with milder degrees of this form of dystrophy are unaware that they have the disease. This was true of nearly half of the large series of patients described by Tyler and Stephens in the Utah Mormon population. At any point, the disease may become virtually arrested. Nevertheless, 15 to 20 percent of patients eventually require a wheelchair (Tawil et al).

An interesting feature of this group of diseases is the occasional congenital absence of a muscle (amyoplasia of one pectoral, brachioradialis, or biceps femoris) or part of a muscle in patients who later develop the typical features of the disease. The external ocular muscles are known to occasionally become affected late in the illness. Although cardiac involvement is rare, in a few cases tachycardia, cardiomegaly, and arrhythmias have occurred. Mental function is normal. Serum CK values are normal or slightly elevated.

At a molecular level, FSHD1 has been found to have a consistent association with deletions of variable size on the tip of chromosome 4q. This disorder is a consequence of alterations of a noncoding portion of DNA. Deletions in a repeated segment interfere with the structure of chromatin and allow the expression of normally inactive genes such as DUX4. Only patients with an allele that contains a repeat segment FSHD2 (called D4Z4 repeats) are susceptible to the disease. An entirely different mutation in a gene that maintains the structural integrity of chromatin accounts for the less common FSHD2; this change results in hypomethylation of the D4Z4 segments (an epigenetic mechanism) and is therefore also dependent on the permissive repeat allele.

A variant in which only the shoulder and arm muscles are affected, sparing the face, and a form with bilateral foot-drop are known (Krasnianski et al). In some cases, usually with severe deletions at the FSH locus on chromosome 4, there is an early-onset, relatively rapid progression and an association with facial diplegia, sensorineural deafness, and, sometimes, exudative retinal detachment (Coats disease). Using fluorescein angiography, Fitzsimmons and others have found a variety of other retinal abnormalities: telangiectasia, occlusion, leakage, and microaneurysms; in the majority of cases, suggesting that these retinal abnormalities are an integral part of the disease. Less common manifestations of FSHD include isolated scapular winging or other focal weakness such as foot drop, sparing of facial muscles, a variant with limb-girdle weakness, and rare instances of PEO.

Scapuloperoneal Muscular Dystrophy

Beginning with Brossard in 1886, there were numerous reports of a distinctive pattern of progressive muscular weakness and wasting that involved the muscles of the neck, shoulders, and upper arms, and of the anterior tibial and peroneal groups, causing severe foot-drop. The nature of this disorder has been a matter of controversy, some writers claiming it to be a progressive muscular dystrophy and others, a muscular atrophy of spinal or neuropathic type. Probably both are correct in that either process can produce more or less the same pattern of weakness. Davidenkow, who wrote extensively on this subject, described a form of familial scapuloperoneal weakness and atrophy associated with areflexia and distal sensory loss (a spinal-neuronopathic form) that was later found to have a mutation in the desmin gene, and others have confirmed these findings (see discussions of Thomas et al [1972, 1975] and of Munsat and Serratrice). Nevertheless, Thomas and colleagues (1975) firmly established the existence of a purely myopathic form and the mutation is in the *FHL-1* gene on the X-chromosome (see Table 48-1). The onset of symptoms in their 6 patients was in early or middle adult life, with difficulty in walking because of bilateral foot-drop; symptoms referable to scapulohumeral involvement came later. Progression was slow, and none of the patients became severely incapacitated.

Limb-Girdle Muscular Dystrophies (Scapulohumeral and Pelvifemoral Muscular Dystrophies, Erb Dystrophy) (See Table 48-1)

There is a large group of patients with muscular dystrophy who do not fit into the Duchenne/Becker, facioscapulohumeral, or scapuloperoneal categories. Children of both sexes in this group lack the hypertrophy of calves and other muscles; adults with late-onset forms have either pelvic or shoulder girdle involvement or both, and their facial muscles are spared. Because Wilhelm Erb first called attention to these types of dystrophy, they were classified by Walton and Nattrass as the "limb-girdle dystrophies of Erb." This clinically based grouping has been problematic from the time it was proposed because, like the scapuloperoneal group, it is heterogeneous, the only unifying feature being the presence of limb-girdle weakness with sparing of the facial muscles. The inheritance is variable, but the autosomal recessive forms are the most common. Either the shoulder girdle or pelvic girdle muscles may be first affected (traditionally these forms had been referred to as the Erb juvenile atrophic and Leyden-Möbius types, respectively). Weakness and atrophy may become evident during either late childhood or early adult life and spread from shoulders to hips or vice versa.

The status of this group of limb-girdle muscular dystrophies (LGMDs) as a clinical–genetic entity is being steadily revised. The delineation of the progressive spinal muscular atrophies and the congenital and metabolic myopathies has considerably narrowed the category of limb-girdle dystrophies as originally described. During the past decade, with the application of molecular genetic techniques, progress in this direction has accelerated greatly. The now well-populated class of limb-girdle dystrophies is classified as LGMD1 for the autosomal dominant types, and LGMD2 for the recessive types, and further subclassified based on the specific genotype. At the time of this writing, at least 19 forms of autosomal recessive (LGMD type 2A-2S) and 6 forms of autosomal dominant (LGMD type 1A-1E) limb-girdle dystrophies have been defined, most with an identifiable mutation and a protein that in most cases is a constituent of the sarcolemmal, sarcomeric, or nuclear membrane structural protein (Bushby). The later the onset of these disorders, the more likely that the course will be benign. In these lesser-affected patients the EMG is myopathic and the CK values are only moderately elevated and may be normal. More severe cases can have greatly elevated CK levels. Cardiac involvement occurs but is infrequent (mainly in the group classified as myofibrillar dystrophies), and mental function is normal, but there are exceptions including in cases of laminin A/C mutations (type 1B), *FKRP* (fukutin-related protein mutation) mutations (type 2I), and in the sarcoglycanopathies.

This information is summarized in Table 48-2 and discussion of the better-characterized types follows.

Limb-Girdle Muscular Dystrophy 2I (Fukutin-Related Protein Mutation)

The discovery of the "fukutin-related protein" initially came about because mutant forms caused a severe congenital muscular dystrophy (CMD). It later became apparent that certain mutations also cause a common type of later onset limb-girdle dystrophy. As the designation "2" indicates, it is transmitted in an autosomal recessive manner. This is the most common form of limb-girdle dystrophy in patients of Northern European descent. In a series of 16 patients from 14 families, Poppe and colleagues characterized the main features as having an onset of proximal girdle weakness in the second to fourth decades of life (but as early as age 2 years). The majority of patients eventually had respiratory failure and several displayed varying degrees of congestive heart failure, features that also accompany some of the other limb-girdle dystrophies. In most other ways, this disease reflects the heterogeneity of clinical presentation of the other subtypes of limb-girdle disease. A period of stabilization lasting several to 35 years is common, followed by a decade or more of progression that eventually involves the shoulder muscles. Most patients, particularly those with later onset, remained able to walk into their forties. Other features are variable, for example, dysphagia and ptosis; however, distal weakness is not seen and intelligence is normal.

The defective *FKRP* gene is related in function to 4 other muscle genes in addition to fukutin (hence its name). All 5 of these genes are glycosyl transferases that attach sugar groups to proteins such as alpha-dystroglycan. The severity of the clinical phenotype is inversely related to the levels of glycosylation of alpha-dystroglycan. Defects in any of the 5 genes can cause developmental lesions in the brain in addition to muscle disease, although those associated with FKRP mutations are less common and less severe.

Severe Childhood Autosomal Recessive Muscular Dystrophy (Sarcoglycanopathies; LGMD 2C, D, E, and F)

These entities comprise the best-defined group of limb-girdle dystrophy. Clinically they resemble severe Duchenne dystrophy in practically all respects, including the presence of calf hypertrophy, cardiomyopathy, and marked elevation of CK in the early stages of the illness. The obvious distinction from Duchenne dystrophy is the autosomal recessive pattern of inheritance (affection of both girls and boys in the same sibship). The largest and best-studied group of this severe, recessive pelvic-pectoral dystrophy (99 children in 28 families) has come from Tunisia (Ben Hamida et al). It also occurs commonly in other Arab countries and has been observed repeatedly in Brazil, but less so in Europe and North America.

The basic defect is in 1 of 4 dystrophin-associated glycoproteins (DAGs)—α-, β-, γ- and δ-sarcoglycan (see Fig. 48-1); α-sarcoglycan (designated 50 DAG) is also called adhalin, from the Arabic word *adhal*, meaning muscle. A primary deficiency of adhalin has been traced to a defective gene on chromosome 17q21 (Roberds et al). A primary defect in β-sarcoglycan (43 DAG) has been mapped to chromosome 4q12, of γ-sarcoglycan (35 DAG) to the pericentromeric region of chromosome 13q, and of β-sarcoglycan (43 DAG) to chromosome 5q. Primary defects in 25 DAG may also lead to a deficiency of adhalin, but the latter is incomplete and represents a secondary effect, possibly explained by the proximity of the defective genes to the adhalin gene.

Because of clinical similarities, there may be difficulty in distinguishing limb-girdle dystrophies (formerly termed severe childhood autosomal recessive muscular dystrophy [SCARMD]) from a dystrophinopathy (except that the former occur in females). In addition to the difference in inheritance, they can be readily diagnosed by showing a loss of sarcolemmal immunostaining for any of the dystrophin-associated glycoproteins but with preservation of staining for dystrophin itself. However, it is not possible on clinical grounds to distinguish one sarcoglycanopathy from another; this can be accomplished only by specific immunostaining.

Autosomal Recessive Muscular Dystrophy (LGMD 2A and B; Calpain-3 and ANO-5 Mutations)

These forms of limb-girdle dystrophies have been described in large kindreds, in Indiana (among the Amish people), on the island of Réunion in the Indian Ocean, in Brazil, Great Britain, Italy and Spain, and elsewhere, affecting males and females equally. Both the shoulder and pelvic girdles are involved. The degree of weakness has varied considerably. In one form of the disease, called LGMD 2A, the abnormal gene codes for a calcium-activated neutral protease, or calpain (see Fig. 48-2). This "calpainopathy" is currently believed to account for approximately 40 percent of patients with LGMD. Frequently, and early in the course of disease, there are Achilles tendon contractures and very high serum CK levels (at least 10 times normal), features that may permit distinction from the sarcoglycanopathies.

Yet another fairly common recessive limb-girdle dystrophy of slow progression is caused by a mutation in the gene for the protein dysferlin, which localizes to the muscle fiber membrane. Noteworthy is the fact that this same protein is involved in the distal form of Miyoshi muscular dystrophy described further on. Early involvement of the gastrocnemius muscle (inability to walk on tiptoe) and extraordinarily high levels of CK, as in calpainopathy, are clues to the latter disease.

Autosomal Dominant Limb-Girdle Dystrophies (LGMD 1A-1E)

Several dystrophies with the LGMD phenotype are inherited as autosomal dominant traits. For example, LGMDA 1A is an autosomal dominant limb-girdle dystrophy of late onset that was described in a large North Carolina family (49 affected members in a pedigree of 218 persons). The mean age at onset was 27 years. Proximal leg weakness, with or without proximal arm weakness, and elevated CK values were the main clinical characteristics. Speer and colleagues have documented that the primary defect is in a gene encoding the protein *myotilin* (see Fig. 50-2). LGMDA 1A is allelic to a form of myofibrillar myopathy.

LGMD 1B is a dominantly inherited disorder arising from mutations in the gene encoding the nuclear membrane protein *lamin A/C* (see Fig. 50-2). Mercuri and colleagues note that the phenotypes of these mutations vary widely. The muscle disorders range from severe cases that mimic CMD to milder ones with features of limb girdle dystrophy or Emery-Dreifuss muscular dystrophy. The diverse, nonmuscular manifestations of lamin A/C mutations include a cardiomyopathy, a form of lipodystrophy, a syndrome of accelerated aging (Hutchinson-Gilford progeria), and a recessively inherited axonal neuropathy.

Progressive External Ophthalmoplegia (Kearns-Sayre Syndrome) (See also "Progressive External Ophthalmoplegia [PEO] and Kearns-Sayre Syndrome" in Chap. 37)

This has proved to be a confusing group of processes characterized by slowly progressive myopathy primarily involving and often limited to the extraocular muscles. Usually, the levators of the eyelids are the first to be affected, causing ptosis, followed by progressive balanced ophthalmoparesis. This disorder usually begins in childhood, sometimes in adolescence, and rarely in adult life (as late as 50 years).

Several types have been described. The most common one arises from either deletions or point mutations in mitochondrial DNA and are discussed in Chap. 37

with other metabolic disorders. However, when the foregoing progressive external ophthalmoplegia (PEO) categories are eliminated, there remains a distinctly different category of dominantly inherited PEO. Males and females are equally affected; the pattern of inheritance is autosomal dominant in some and recessive or uncertain in others. Once started, the disease progresses relentlessly until the eyes are motionless. Simultaneous involvement of all extraocular muscles permits the eyes to remain in a central position, so that strabismus and diplopia are uncommon (in rare instances, one eye is affected before the other). The pupillary responses and accommodation are normal. As the patient attempts to raise his eyelids and to see under them, the head is thrown back and the frontalis muscle is contracted, wrinkling the forehead (hutchinsonian facies). The eyelids are abnormally thin due to atrophy of the levator muscles. The orbicularis oculi muscles are frequently involved in addition to the extraocular muscles. Thus, in PEO, as in myasthenia gravis and myotonic dystrophy, there can be a characteristic combination of weakness of eye closure and eye opening, a combination that is nearly always myopathic. Other facial muscles, masseters, sternocleidomastoids, deltoids, or peronei are variably weak and wasted in approximately 25 percent of cases. The characteristic feature of PEO is that ptosis and ocular paralysis precede involvement of other muscles by many years.

Given that there is considerable clinical overlap between the mitochondrial syndrome and dominantly inherited PEO, it is not surprising that some of the dominantly inherited gene defects causing PEO result in disturbances in mitochondrial DNA. Mutations in three nuclear genes have been implicated. (These are twinkle, a mitochondrial DNA binding protein; *ANT1*, an adenine nucleotide transporter in the intermembrane space in the mitochondrion; and *POLG*, a subunit of the mitochondrial DNA polymerase.) There are also recessively inherited instances of familial PEO, one of which involves a nuclear gene.

Oculopharyngeal Dystrophy (See Table 48-2)

Oculopharyngeal dystrophy is inherited as an autosomal dominant trait and is unique in its late onset (usually after the forty-fifth year) and the restricted muscular weakness, manifest mainly as a bilateral ptosis and dysphagia. E.W. Taylor first described the disease in 1915 and assumed that it was caused by a nuclear atrophy (oculomotor-vagal complex). However, Victor and colleagues, in 1962, showed that the descendants of Taylor's cases had a late-life dystrophy (myopathic EMG and biopsy). One of the families described by Victor, Hayes, and Adams was subsequently traced by Barbeau through 10 generations to an early French-Canadian immigrant, who was the progenitor of 249 descendants with the disease. Other families showing a dominant (rarely recessive) pattern of inheritance and a number of sporadic cases have been observed in many parts of the world.

Difficulty in swallowing and change in voice are associated with slowly progressive ptosis. Swallowing becomes so difficult that food intake is limited, resulting in cachexia, which can be ameliorated by cutting the cricopharyngeus muscles, or, if that fails, by a gastrostomy or nasogastric tube. Later in the disease, in some families the external ocular muscles and shoulder and pelvic muscles become weakened and atrophic to a varying extent. In the few autopsied cases, a loss of fibers of modest proportions was widespread in these and many other muscles. Rimmed vacuoles in the sarcoplasm and, by electron microscopy, intranuclear tubular filaments are characteristic but not specific histologic findings (these features are seen in other myopathies, particularly in inclusion body myositis). The brainstem nuclei and cranial nerves are normal. As in the other mild and restricted muscular dystrophies, the serum CK and aldolase levels are normal and the EMG is altered only in the affected muscles.

The gene product is a protein that binds to RNA (poly-A binding protein). The defect is an expansion of a string of alanines. Normally, there are 6 repeats; in dominantly inherited oculopharyngeal dystrophy, there are 8 to 13 repeats; in the recessively inherited form there are 7 repeats on each allele. Thus this represents one of the most subtle nucleotide expansion diseases yet discovered.

Myotonic Dystrophy Types 1 and 2

There are 2 types of myotonic dystrophies (DM1 and DM2/PROMM). Type 1 (DM1) is the most common adult muscular dystrophy. It was described in 1909 by Steinert, who considered it to be a variant of congenital myotonia (Thomsen disease; see Chap. 50) and in the same year by Batten and Gibb, who recognized it as a unique clinical entity.

DM1 is distinguished by an autosomal dominant pattern of inheritance with a high level of penetrance, special topography of the muscle atrophy, associated obvious myotonia, and occurrence of dystrophic changes in nonmuscular tissues (lens of eye, testicle and other endocrine glands, skin, esophagus, heart, and, in some cases, the cerebrum). Certain muscles, the levator palpebrae, facial, masseter, sternocleidomastoid, and forearm, hand, and pretibial muscles, are consistently involved in the dystrophic process. It is possible that Gowers' famous case of an 18-year-old youth with weakened and wasted anterior tibial and forearm muscles and sternocleidomastoids, in conjunction with paresis of the orbicularis and frontalis muscles, was an example of this disease.

Despite some clinical variability of myotonic dystrophy, the defective gene in the first type has been the same in every population that has been studied. At this locus on chromosome 19q there is a specific molecular defect, an unstable trinucleotide sequence (CTG) in the *DMPK* gene that is longer in affected individuals than it is in healthy siblings or unaffected subjects. Whereas healthy individuals will have 5 to 30 CTG repeats, patients with myotonic dystrophy have 50 to 2,000. Longer sequences are associated with more severe disease, and they increase in size through successive generations lead to earlier occurrence (genetic anticipation). The CTG repeats reside within the myotonin protein kinase gene. It is of considerable interest that these CTG repeating segments do not code for a protein (i.e., they are intronic), quite unlike conditions such as Huntington disease in which the triplet expansion codes for amino acid sequences within a protein.

The milder type 2 myotonic dystrophy (DM2) is caused by an expanded triplet repeat in the *CNBP* gene on chromosome 3, as discussed further on under "Proximal Myotonic Myopathy (PROMM, DM2)." A critical element in the pathogenesis of this disease in both types is the intranuclear accumulation of the expanded RNA sequences; these disrupt the regulation of alternative splicing of mRNA and perturb the expression of many genes, thus the multiple systems affected clinically.

Clinical Features of DM1

In most instances of myotonic dystrophy, the weakness and muscular wasting do not become evident until early adult life, but they may present in childhood, usually with facial weakness and ptosis. Also, a severe *neonatal (congenital) form* of the disease is well known and is described separately further on.

In the common early adult form of the disease, the small muscles of the hands along with the extensor muscles of the forearms are often the first to become atrophied. In other cases, ptosis of the eyelids and thinness and slackness of the facial muscles may be the earliest signs, preceding other muscular involvement by many years. Atrophy of the masseters leads to narrowing of the lower half of the face, and the mandible is slender and malpositioned so that the teeth do not occlude properly. This, along with the ptosis, frontal baldness, and wrinkled forehead, imparts a distinctive physiognomy that, once seen, can be recognized at a glance ("hatchet" face). The sternocleidomastoids are almost invariably thin and weak and are associated with an exaggerated forward curvature of the neck ("swan neck"). Atrophy of the anterior tibial muscle groups, leading to foot-drop, is an early sign in some families.

Pharyngeal and laryngeal weakness results in a weak, monotonous, nasal voice. The uterine muscle may be weakened, interfering with normal parturition, and the esophagus is often dilated because of loss of muscle fibers in the striated as well as smooth muscle parts. Megacolon occurs in some patients. Diaphragmatic weakness and alveolar hypoventilation, resulting in chronic bronchitis and bronchiectasis, are common late features, as are cardiac abnormalities; the latter are most often a result of disease of the conducting apparatus, giving rise to bradycardia and a prolonged P-R interval. Patients with extreme bradycardia atrial tachyarrhythmia or high degrees of atrioventricular block may die suddenly; for such individuals, insertion of a pacemaker is often recommended (Moorman et al; Groh et al). Mitral valve prolapse and left ventricular dysfunction (cardiomyopathy) are less frequent abnormalities. In this disorder, as in Emery-Dreifuss dystrophy, careful assessment by a knowledgeable cardiologist is required.

The disease progresses slowly, with gradual involvement of the proximal muscles of the limbs and muscles of the trunk. Tendon reflexes are lost or much reduced. Contracture is rarely seen, and the thin, flattened hands are consequently soft and pliable. Most patients are confined to a wheelchair or bed within 15 to 20 years of the first signs, and death occurs before the normal age from pulmonary infection, heart block, or heart failure.

The phenomenon of *myotonia*, which expresses itself in prolonged idiomuscular contraction following brief percussion or electrical stimulation and in delay of relaxation after strong voluntary contraction, is the third striking attribute of the disease (the other two being the facial, ptotic, and limb weakness, and the cardiac-autoimmune features). Not as widespread or severe as in myotonia congenita, it is, nonetheless, easily elicited in the hands and tongue in almost all cases, and in the proximal limb muscles in half of the cases. Gentle movements do not evoke it (eye blinks, movements of facial expression, and the like are not impeded), whereas strong closure of the lids and clenching of the fist are followed by a long delay in relaxation.

Myotonia may precede weakness by several years. Indeed, Maas and Paterson have claimed that many cases diagnosed originally as myotonia congenita eventually proved to be examples of myotonic dystrophy. Of interest is the fact that in congenital or infantile cases of myotonic dystrophy, the myotonic phenomenon is not elicited until later in childhood, after the second or third year of life (see later). The child often becomes accustomed to the myotonia and does not complain about it. The relation of myotonia to the dystrophy is not direct. Certain muscles that show the myotonia best (tongue, flexors of fingers) are seldom weak and atrophic. Moreover, there may be little or no myotonia in certain families that show the other characteristic features of myotonic dystrophy. The muscle hypertrophy that is characteristic of myotonia congenita is not a feature of myotonic dystrophy.

The fourth major characteristic of the disease is the dystrophic change in nonmuscular tissues. The most common of these is lenticular opacities, found by slit-lamp examination in 90 percent of patients. At first dust-like, they then form small, regular opacities in the posterior and anterior cortex of the lens just beneath the capsule; under the slit lamp they appear blue, blue-green, and yellow, and are highly refractile. Microscopically, the crystalline material (probably lipids and cholesterol, which cause the iridescence) lies in vacuoles and lacunae among the lens fibers. In older patients, a stellate cataract slowly forms in the posterior cortex of the lens.

Mild to moderate degrees of developmental cognitive delay are common in DM1, and the brain weight in several of our patients was 200 g less than that in normal individuals of the same age. Late in adult life, some patients become suspicious, argumentative, and forgetful. In some families, a hereditary sensorimotor neuropathy may be added to the muscle disease (Cros et al). Other nonspecific abnormalities, such as hyperostosis of the frontal bones and calcification of the basal ganglia, both readily discerned by CT, seem to be more common in patients with myotonic dystrophy than they are in healthy persons.

Progressive frontal alopecia, beginning at an early age, is a characteristic feature in both men and women with this disease. Testicular atrophy with androgenic deficiency, reduced libido or impotence, and sterility are additional frequent manifestations. In some patients gynecomastia and elevated gonadotropin excretion are found. Testicular biopsy shows atrophy and hyalinization of tubular cells and hyperplasia of Leydig cells. (Thus all the clinical characteristics of the Klinefelter syndrome may be present but without the "sex chromatin" mass [Barr body].) Ovarian deficiency occasionally develops in the female patient, but it is seldom severe enough to interfere with menstruation or fertility. The prevalence of clinical or chemical diabetes mellitus is slightly increased in patients with myotonic dystrophy, but an increased insulin response to a glucose load has proved to be a common abnormality. Numerous surveys of other endocrine functions have yielded little of significance.

We have been impressed with the variability of clinical expression. In many patients, intelligence has been unimpaired and the myotonia and muscle weakness have been so mild that the patients were unaware of any difficulty. Pryse-Philips and associates emphasized these features in their description of a large Labrador kinship in which 27 of 133 patients had only a partial syndrome and only minor muscle symptoms at the time of examination.

Pathologic Features

In addition to displaying most of the common findings of muscular dystrophy, there are several highly unusual myopathologic features. Peripherally placed sarcoplasmic masses and circular bundles of myofibrils (ringbinden) are found. There is hypertrophy of type 1 fibers with centrally placed nuclei (this may be a marked finding) and many atrophic fibers show nuclear clumping. In many of the muscle spindles there is an excess of intrafusal fibers (particularly in the congenital form; see later). Many of the terminal arborizations of the peripheral nerves are unusually elaborate and elongated.

Congenital Myotonic Dystrophy

Brief reference was made earlier to this inherited, distinctive and potentially lethal form of myotonic dystrophy. Harper's (1975) study of 70 personally observed patients and 56 others gathered from the medical literature suggests this disease exists in every pediatric neurology service. Profound hypotonia and facial diplegia at birth are the most prominent clinical features; myotonia is notably absent. Drooping of the eyelids, the tented upper lip ("carp" mouth), and the open jaw impart a characteristic appearance, which allows immediate recognition of the disease in the newborn infant and child. Difficulty in sucking and swallowing, bronchial aspiration (because of palatal and pharyngeal weakness), and respiratory distress (because of diaphragmatic and intercostal weakness and pulmonary immaturity) are present in varying degrees; the latter disorders are responsible for a previously unrecognized group of neonatal deaths (24 such deaths among siblings of affected patients in Harper's study). In surviving infants, delayed motor and speech development, swallowing difficulty, mild to moderately severe mental retardation, and talipes or generalized arthrogryposis are common. Once adolescence is attained, the disease follows the same course as the later form. As stated earlier, clinical myotonia in the congenital form of the disease becomes evident only later in childhood, although EMG study may disclose myotonic discharges in early infancy. The diagnosis may be suspected by the simple test of eliciting myotonia in the mother. ECG changes occur in one-third of the patients.

In the congenital form of this disease the affected parent is always the mother with type 1 (DM1) myotonic dystrophy, in whom the disease need not be severe. Electrophysiologic testing will bring out the myotonia in the mother if it is inevident on percussion of muscle. (In cases of adult onset, transmission is maternal or paternal.) These data suggest that in addition to inheriting the myotonic dystrophy gene, the congenital cases also receive some maternally transmitted factor, possibly methylation of DNA that allows expansion of the trinucleotide repeat in oocytes. The prenatal diagnosis of myotonic dystrophy is readily accomplished by examination for CTG repeats in the amniotic fluid or in a biopsy of chorionic villi. However, it is not possible to predict whether a fetus with an expanded mutation will have congenital myotonic dystrophy or later-onset myotonic dystrophy.

Proximal Myotonic Myopathy (PROMM, DM2)

Under this name, Ricker and colleagues (1994, 1995) described a myopathy characterized by autosomal dominant inheritance, proximal muscle weakness, myotonia, and cataracts. Seventeen families containing 50 affected members were studied by these authors. Onset was between 20 and 40 years of age, with intermittent myotonic symptoms of the hands and proximal leg muscles, followed by a mild, slowly progressive weakness of the proximal limb muscles without significant atrophy. In contrast to DM1, cataracts developed in one-half of their patients and cardiac arrhythmias in only two. Onset in infancy, ptosis, weakness of facial, jaw, and distal limb muscles, and mental abnormalities were notably absent, further distinguishing PROMM from the conventional (DM1) form of myotonic dystrophy.

Histologically, there are many fibers with multiple (5 to 10 or more) internalized nuclei, without ringbinden or subsarcolemmal masses. In addition, there are atrophic fibers with nuclear clumps. Analysis of leukocyte and muscle DNA discloses no expansion of the CTG component of the myotonic dystrophy gene. Rather, the gene defect for this disease has been mapped to the *CNBP* gene on chromosome 3q where there is an expansion of a CCTG repeats. Like the expanded CTG repeat in myotonic dystrophy, the CCTG expansion in PROMM is associated with intranuclear accumulation of the expanded RNA transcript, and like the CTG repeats of myotonic dystrophy, the CCTG segments do not code for a protein.

Distal Muscular Dystrophies (Welander, Miyoshi, and Other Types) (See Table 48-3)

Included in this group are several slowly progressive distal myopathies with onset principally in adult life. Weakness and wasting of the muscles of the hands, forearms, and lower legs, especially the extensors, are the main clinical features. Although such cases had been reported by Gowers and others, their differentiation from myotonic dystrophy and peroneal muscular atrophy was unclear until relatively recently. Several types of distal dystrophies are inherited as *autosomal dominant* traits.

A different dominantly inherited distal dystrophy was described by Welander in a study of 249 patients from 72 Swedish pedigrees (not to be confused with the Kugelberg-Welander juvenile spinal muscular atrophy affecting proximal muscles; see Chap. 39). Weakness developed first in the small hand muscles and then spread to the distal leg muscles, causing a steppage gait. Fasciculations, cramps, pain, sensory disturbances, and myotonia were notably absent. Some patients have a low-grade sensory neuropathy, suggesting that pathology in this disorder may not be exclusively in muscle. Cataracts appeared after the age of 70 years in 3 patients and can be discounted as having special significance. No endocrine disorders were detected. Dystrophic changes were demonstrated in 3 autopsies and 22 biopsy specimens. Some muscle biopsy material has shown rimmed vacuoles and inclusions that are similar to inclusion body myopathy. Progression of the disease was very slow; after 10 years or so, some wasting of proximal muscles was seen in a few of the patients. Welander dystrophy has been linked to mutations in T1A1 on chromosome 2p13, near the locus for the below described Miyoshi myopathy.

Markesbery and colleagues reported a late-onset distal myopathy in which weakness began in the distal leg muscles (tibialis anterior) and later spread to the hands; there was also cardiomyopathy and heart failure. A mutation in the *ZASP* gene has been found. Very similar distal myopathies have been described in Finnish patients by Udd and colleagues and caused by dominant mutations in the "titin" gene. A form beginning in childhood described by Laing and colleagues was shown to be caused by a mutation in the gene (*MYHC7*) that codes for myosin heavy chain 1 protein. The characteristic feature in all these cases is progressive bilateral foot-drop.

Miyoshi Dystrophy

A type of distal dystrophy characterized by *autosomal recessive* pattern of inheritance is particularly prevalent in Japan (Miyoshi et al), but numerous cases exist in all parts of the world. The Miyoshi myopathy is the one we have encountered most often among the distal muscular dystrophies. Onset of the disease is in early adult life, with weakness and atrophy of the leg muscles most prominent in the peroneal or the gastrocnemius and soleus muscles. Over many years the weakness extends to the thighs, gluteal muscles, and arm muscles, including the proximal ones. Serum CK concentrations are greatly increased in the early stages of the disease. In this type of dystrophy the mutation leads to an absence of the muscle protein *dysferlin*, a membrane protein that does not interact with any of the dystrophin-binding elements. Whereas dystrophin and its binding partners are believed to confer tensile strength, dysferlin and its associated proteins (e.g., the annexins) function in calcium-mediated membrane repair (Lennon). As mentioned earlier, limb-girdle dystrophy 2B has been linked to the same chromosomal locus and it also lacks the dysferlin protein. It is also striking that different family members with the same dysferlin mutation can have disease onset in either a proximal (LGMD) or distal (Miyoshi) pattern, suggesting that additional factors modify the pattern of weakness produced by dysferlin deficiency. We have encountered 1 family in which 2 individuals with dysferlin mutations had proximal weakness at onset while a sibling with the same disease had anterior tibial weakness.

An apparently separate form of distal myopathy with autosomal dominant inheritance and onset before 2 years of age has been described by Magee and DeJong and by van der Does de Willebois and coworkers. Whether these infantile-onset cases represent a true muscular dystrophy has not been established. Several even rarer distal myopathies with linkage to specific genetic sites are summarized in the review by Illa, but most are not well-enough characterized to require elaboration here. A discussion can be found in the text from our colleagues Amato and Russell.

Congenital Muscular Dystrophy (Fukuyama, Walker-Warburg, Merosin Deficient, Rigid Spine, and Other Types) (Table 48-4)

Early in the twentieth century there were scattered reports of congenital myopathy, but the status of this condition was difficult to evaluate. Some cases may have represented congenital myotonic dystrophy or one of the congenital myopathies described later. In 1957, Banker and associates described 2 patients (siblings), 1 dying 1.5 h after birth and the other dying at the age of 10 months of a congenital muscular dystrophy (CMD) with arthrogryposis. The pathologic changes consisted of muscle fiber degeneration, variation in fiber size, fibrosis, and fat cell replacement. The central and peripheral nervous systems were intact. The severity of the degenerative changes was such that a developmental disorder of muscle could be excluded. Pearson and Fowler, in 1963, reported a brother and sister with similar clinical and pathologic findings, and Walton and colleagues described yet another patient, 4 years of age. By 1967, Vassella and colleagues were able to collect 27 cases from the medical literature and to add 8 cases of their own. The high incidence of sibling involvement pointed to an autosomal recessive inheritance.

Preceding the modern genetic findings, in 1976, Bethlem and van Wijngaarden described an autosomal dominant, early-onset limb-girdle dystrophy in 28 members of 3 unrelated Dutch families. Flexion contractures of the elbows, ankles, and hyperextensible interphalangeal joints of the fingers were present from the beginning stages of weakness, but neither the weakness nor the contractures were disabling. Also unlike Emery-Dreifuss dystrophy, contractures of the neck and spine were not present. Uniformity of clinical expression, slow progression with long periods of arrest, and normal longevity are other important features of the illness. Mohire and coworkers have proposed the designation *Bethlem myopathy*. A milder

Table 48-4

CONGENITAL MUSCULAR DYSTROPHIES

DISORDER	GENE OR PROTEIN DEFICIENCY	CK ELEVATION	REGIONS AFFECTED
Merosin deficiency	Merosin	5–35 ×	Hypotonia, diffuse weakness, slow motor development Cognitive function largely spared
Fukutin CMD[a]	Fukutin	10–50 ×	Hypotonia, diffuse weakness, slow motor development Mental retardation, seizures common MRI: hypomyelination, hydrocephalus
FKRP CMD	*FKRP*	10–50 ×	Hypotonia, diffuse weakness, slow motor development Cognitive function largely spared
Muscle-eye brain disease	*N*-acetyl-glucosaminyl-transferase *POMGnT1*	5–20 ×	Hypotonia, diffuse weakness, slow motor development Mental retardation, seizures common Cataracts, retinal dysplasias, retinitis, glaucoma Hypoplasia of optic nerve MRI: hypomyelination, hydrocephalus, lissencephaly
Walker-Warburg disease	*O*-Mannosyl-transferase 1 *POMT1*	5–20 ×	Hypotonia, diffuse weakness, slow motor development Mental retardation, seizures common Cataracts, retinal dysplasias, retinitis, glaucoma MRI: hypomyelination, hydrocephalus, lissencephaly
Rigid spine syndrome	Selenoprotein *SEPN1*	Nl	Hypotonia, restricted flexion of the neck and spine Contractures at multiple joints, normal heart Cognitive function largely spared
Integrin CMD	Integrin *α-7*	1–2 ×	Hypotonia, diffuse weakness, slow motor development Slowed motor development ± mental retardation
LARGE CMD	*LARGE*	Nl	Profound mental retardation, cerebral white matter changes

[a]Allelic with LGMD-2L.

form that is allelic with the Bethlehem type is termed *Ulrich myopathy*; many of these patients survive into their fifties because of the slow progression of disease.

Defined as a muscle dystrophy already present at birth, often with contractures of proximal muscles and trunk, the severity of the weakness and degree of progression have varied widely. Of the 8 cases reported by Rotthauwe and colleagues, 1 had a benign course, but the others all had weakness and hypotonia at birth, and difficulty in sucking and swallowing had interfered with nutrition. Their oldest patients, 14 and 23 years of age, and several others had walked, but at a late age. In the Finnish series of Donner and associates, congenital dystrophy accounted for 9 percent of the 160 cases of neuromuscular disease seen at their hospital over a decade. The weakness and hypotonia were generalized, and 3 had ECG abnormalities. The CK values were elevated and the EMGs were myopathic.

This group of dystrophies began to come into focus in the 1960s with a series of articles from Japan relating the details in more than 100 patients with congenital dystrophy (Fukuyama et al). Although it is the second most common muscular dystrophy in Japan, it is rare elsewhere. The special feature of these cases was the coexistence of severe mental retardation and developmental anomalies of the cerebral cortex. Hyperlucency in the periventricular white matter (by CT) was frequently observed. In another group of cases, CMD was associated with lissencephaly as well as cerebellar and retinal malformations (Walker-Warburg syndrome; see Dobyns et al). In a series reported by Santavuori and coworkers, CMD was associated with retinal degeneration and optic atrophy, hydrocephalus, pachygyria-polymicrogyria, and hypoplastic or absent septum pellucidum and corpus callosum ("muscle-eye-brain" [MEB] disease). Lebenthal and colleagues later described a large Arab pedigree with CMD and patent ductus arteriosus. Some patients had contractures at birth; in others, contractures developed at a later age. The EMG disclosed a myopathic pattern and CK levels were moderately elevated.

In recent years, the classification and relationships of the congenital muscular dystrophies have been clarified to some extent by a number of genetic studies (see Table 48-4). Remarkably, the major congenital muscular dystrophies share an important biologic attribute: each involves either an abnormality of a protein that binds to the dystrophin complex (e.g., laminin α_2 or merosin) or an abnormality of a protein in the Golgi apparatus that is important in processing proteins (such as the dystroglycans and sarcoglycans) that interact with the dystrophin complex (see Figs. 50-1 and 50-2).

The most frequent congenital dystrophy in the white population is the "Occidental" type, so called because it is characterized exclusively by muscle involvement. There are only occasionally abnormal white matter signals on MRI. Tomé and colleagues showed that in approximately 50 percent of such patients, merosin is completely absent ("merosin-negative" cases). Merosin, the predominant isoform of α-laminin in the basement membrane of the muscle fiber, is closely bound to alpha-dystroglycan, which in turn is bound to the dystrophin cytoskeleton (see Fig. 50-1). An absence of merosin interrupts this linkage and leads to muscle degeneration. The diagnosis of merosin deficiency can be made prenatally by immunostaining chorionic villi cells, and postnatally by staining skeletal muscle biopsy material. In most cases that are merosin deficient, the disorder is genetically linked to the merosin (laminin α_2) gene that either alters or prevents expression of the protein. An additional member of the group of merosin-positive congenital muscular dystrophies is termed *rigid spine syndrome* (RSS). The term first proposed by Dubowitz and the clinical syndrome, as outlined by Flanigan and coworkers, consists of (1) infantile hypotonia with early weakness of neck muscles and poor head control; (2) stabilization with only slight decrease in muscle strength but marked loss of muscle bulk; (3) prominent contractures of spinal muscles resulting in scoliosis and rigidity in flexion and, to a lesser extent, contractures of limb joints; (4) respiratory insufficiency with onset before adolescence; and (5) normality of intellectual and cardiac function. This unusual CMD with RSS (CMD-RSS) arises from mutations in a gene encoding a so-called selenoprotein.

In the Fukuyama type of CMD, as noted previously, fukutin is one of 5 genes whose mutations alter protein glycosylation, deranging function of both muscle and brain. Thus, the genes for MEB and the Walker-Warburg syndrome are also glycosyltransferases (respectively, *POMGnT1* and *POMT1*), as is the aforementioned fukutin-related peptide. It has been shown that another form of CMD follows mutations of another glycosylation gene (known as *LARGE*).

Myofibrillar Myopathy

The field of chronic and congenital myopathies has been muddied by a plethora of reports describing curious inclusions in muscle fibers under a bewildering array of terms: *myopathy with inclusion bodies, atypical myopathy with myofibrillar aggregates; cytoplasmic body myopathy; spheroid body myopathy; myopathy with characteristic sarcoplasmic bodies and skeleton (desmin) filaments; and others.* Implied by these reports is the notion that each of these structural abnormalities represented a new and distinctive myopathy. More recently, in a careful light microscopic evaluation of published reports and their own cases, Nonaka and Engel and Ozawa and their colleagues have demonstrated that most of these changes are the consequence of a single pathologic process, a focal dissolution of myofibrils, followed by an accumulation of degradative products. These authors proposed the term *myofibrillar myopathy* to encompass the entire spectrum of these pathologic changes. Most authorities now consider this to be a muscular dystrophy because mutations have been found in muscle constituent proteins.

Mutations of one of the proteins that relate to the Z-disc (the connection between adjacent sarcomeres, which are the structural units of the myofibril) of muscle seem to be the unifying feature. Some of these abnormalities can be traced to a dominant mutation in the genes coding for the filament proteins myotilin, also implicated in one of the limb-girdle dystrophies, in desmin, and in the chaperone protein $\alpha\beta$-crystallin, as described in the review by Selcen and colleagues. Presumably, mutations in either gene predispose to protein aggregation, the former by destabilizing desmin and the latter by altering the capacity of the $\alpha\beta$-crystallin to facilitate normal desmin folding.

The diagnosis of myofibrillar myopathy is usually made in adult life by muscle biopsy. Men and women are equally affected. Slowly progressive weakness of the muscles of limbs and trunk is the main clinical feature. Both proximal and distal muscles are affected, more in the legs than in the arms. Hyporeflexia is usual. Cardiac involvement, usually abnormalities of conduction, is present in approximately 25 percent of the patients. The pattern of inheritance is most often autosomal dominant, but autosomal recessive and X-linked patterns also have been described. An astonishing 63 patients were studied by Selcen and associates; their article can be consulted for further details.

Genetically there is considerable heterogeneity. At the time of writing, more than 9 chromosomal loci for myofibrillar myopathy have been documented (desmin, myotilin, ZASP, $\alpha\beta$-crystallin, BAG3, filamin C, DNAJB6, TNP03) and more are likely to exist (Engel and Franzini-Armstrong).

Problems in Diagnosis of the Muscular Dystrophies

The following are some of the common problems that arise in the diagnosis of muscular dystrophy:

1. *The diagnosis of muscular dystrophy in a child who has just begun to walk or in whom walking is delayed.* Tests of peak power on command cannot be used with reliability in small children. The most helpful points in identifying Duchenne dystrophy are (1) unusual difficulty in climbing stairs or arising from a crouch or from a recumbent position on the floor, showing greater weakness at the hips and knees than at the ankles; (2) unusually large, firm calves; (3) male sex; (4) high serum CK, aldolase, and myoglobin levels; (5) myopathic EMG; (6) biopsy findings; and (7) special methods of testing for dystrophin protein (see previous discussion).
2. *The adult patient with diffuse or proximal muscle weakness of several months' duration, raising the question of polymyositis versus dystrophy.* Even biopsy may be misleading in showing a few inflammatory foci in an otherwise dystrophic picture. As a rule, polymyositis evolves

more rapidly than dystrophy. It may be associated with higher CK and aldolase values than most of the dystrophies except the Duchenne and distal Miyoshi types. With these points in mind, if immunostaining of a muscle biopsy fails to reveal the diagnosis of a dystrophy, there may still be uncertainty, in which instance a trial of prednisone may be indicated for a period of 6 months. Unmistakable improvement favors polymyositis; questionable improvement (physician's and patient's judgment not in accord) leaves the diagnosis unsettled but suggests inclusion of body myositis or a dystrophy. Pompe disease, a treatable metabolic glycogen storage myopathy discussed elsewhere in this chapter, may simulate Becker or limb-girdle dystrophy in an adult or child. Clues to the diagnosis are early respiratory involvement, myotonic or pseudomyotonic discharges in the EMG. Muscle biopsy with immunohistochemistry establishes the diagnosis, but the standard stains may be unrevealing.

3. *An adult with a very slowly evolving proximal weakness.* In addition to facioscapular and limb-girdle dystrophies, myositis and inclusion body myopathy, several of the congenital polymyopathies may begin to cause symptoms or to worsen in adult years. These include central core and nemaline myopathy. Examples have been reported in the adult of mild forms of acid maltase or debrancher enzyme deficiency with glycogenosis, progressive late-stage hypokalemic polymyopathy, mitochondrial myopathy, the abovementioned Pompe disease, and carnitine myopathy. Muscle biopsy and histochemical staining of the muscle usually provide the correct diagnosis.
4. *The occurrence of subacute or chronic symmetrical proximal weakness in a child or adolescent that raises the question of spinal muscular atrophy as well as of polymyositis and muscular dystrophy.* EMG and muscle biopsy settle the matter by distinguishing neuropathic from myopathic changes. Some of the same problems arise in an adult with distal dystrophy.
5. *Weakness of a shoulder or one leg with increasing atrophy.* This is usually a result of a radiculopathy or mononeuritis, the beginning of motor system disease (progressive spinal muscular atrophy), but rarely may be the early stage of a muscular dystrophy. The first two diseases may develop silently, in mild form, and attract notice only when wasting begins (denervation atrophy takes 3 to 4 months to reach its peak). Points in favor of these acquired diseases are (1) acute or subacute onset and pain; (2) confinement of the disease to muscles originally affected and sparing of other muscles; and (3) an EMG showing denervation effects. Facioscapulohumeral dystrophy may begin with asymmetrical shoulder weakness. Biopsy is seldom performed under such circumstances, because, by temporizing, the problem eventually settles itself. Invariably muscle dystrophy becomes bilateral and symmetrical; mononeuritis stabilizes or recovers; motor neuron disease declares itself by the presence of fasciculations and relatively rapid progression of weakness.
6. *The distinctions, in the child or adolescent, between dystrophy and one of the congenital or metabolic myopathies are considered later in this chapter.*

Treatment of the Muscular Dystrophies

There has, until recently, been no specific treatment for any of the muscular dystrophies. The physician is forced to stand by and witness the unrelenting progression of weakness and wasting. The various vitamins, amino acids, testosterone, and drugs, such as penicillamine, recommended in the past, have all proved to be ineffective. The administration of prednisone appears to slightly retard the tempo of progression of Duchenne dystrophy for a period of up to 3 years (Fenichel et al). The optimal dose is 0.75 mg/kg given daily, but it must often be reduced because of intolerable side effects (weight gain, behavioral and gastrointestinal disorders).

In recent years, there has been interest in three novel approaches to treatment of Duchenne dystrophy in particular. The first is the injection of human myoblasts, stem cells, or satellite dells that contain a full complement of dystrophin and other structural elements into the muscles of patients with muscular dystrophy. The preclinical aspects of this strategy have been summarized by Blau and are being slowly implemented in patients. There is an analogous effort to use the technology of viral-mediated gene delivery to allow gene and protein replacement in the recessively inherited dystrophies. The difficulties of injecting every dystrophic muscle are obvious.

With another remarkable approach, it was possible to cause the skipping of selected exons during splicing of pre-mRNA and to correct the open reading frame in mutated dystrophin. van Deutekom and colleagues have been able to elicit expression of normal dystrophin in the anterior tibialis at the site of injection of an antisense oligonucleotide that accomplishes the exon skipping. The same oligonucleotide administered subcutaneously for five weeks was shown by Goermans and coworkers of the same group that performed local injections, to produce dystrophin expression and modestly improve the ability of patients to accomplish a standardized 6-minute walk test.

Respiratory failure occurs in virtually all patients affected with Duchenne dystrophy after they become wheelchair-bound, as well as in some of the other dystrophic diseases. It may be so insidious as to become evident only as sleep apnea, as retention of carbon dioxide that causes morning headache, or as progressive weight loss that reflects the excessive work of breathing. If there are frequent episodes of oxygen desaturation, some improvement in daytime strength and alertness can be attained by assisting ventilation at night. This may be accomplished in the early stages of disease by a negative-pressure cuirass-type of device that expands the chest wall periodically or, more conveniently, by nasal-positive pressure (NIPPV [noninvasive positive-pressure ventilation] or BiPAP [bilevel positive airway pressure]). Later, positive-pressure ventilation through a fenestrated tracheostomy is required that allows nighttime ventilation but leaves the patient free to speak and breathe during the day. With regard to earlier or anticipatory treatment, in patients free of respiratory failure with vital capacities between 20 and 50 percent of predicted values, a randomized trial of nasal mechanical ventilation failed to demonstrate improvement or prolonged survival (Raphael et al). There has been a clinical impression that even more severely affected patients can be managed at home for prolonged periods with respiratory assistance. Needless to say, the common complications of muscular dystrophy—pulmonary infections and cardiac decompensation—must be treated symptomatically. Surgical management of cataracts is indicated when they become mature.

As noted earlier, a vital element in the care of patients with certain of the dystrophies is monitoring for early evidence cardiac arrhythmias. In disorders such as myotonic dystrophy, Emery-Dreifuss dystrophy, the myofibrillar myopathies, and some of the mitochondrial disorders, it is imperative that cardiac status should be evaluated on a regular basis (typically yearly) with ECG and echocardiography and periodically with 24-h rhythm monitoring if the ECG is abnormal or the patient reports episodic symptoms referable to an arrhythmia such as lightheadedness, palpitations, or dyspnea. The timely use of cardiac pacemakers or defibrillators, implemented at the earliest sign of arrhythmia or prophylactically, is often needed in this patient population to reduce the chance of sudden death.

Mexiletine has been shown to reduce myotonia, especially in DM2 and the nondystrophic myotonias as demonstrated in the trial reported by Statland and coworkers but, like quinine that caused rare cardiac arrhythmias, is also now not entirely in favor by some clinicians. Further discussion of myotonia and its treatment can be found in Chap. 50. Testosterone has been found to increase muscle mass in patients with myotonic dystrophy, but was of no value in preserving strength or lessening myotonia (Griggs et al, 1989).

Vignos, who reviewed the studies that evaluated muscle-strengthening exercises, has offered evidence that maximal resistance exercises, if begun early, can strengthen muscles in Duchenne, limb-girdle, and facioscapulohumeral dystrophies. In the study he conducted, none of the muscles was weaker at the end of a year than at the beginning. Cardiorespiratory function after endurance exercise was not significantly improved. Contractures were reduced by passive stretching of the muscles 20 to 30 times a day and by splinting at night. If contractures have already formed, fasciotomy and tendon lengthening are indicated in patients who are still ambulating, but this is not recommended early in the course of the disease. Maintenance of ambulation and upright posture will delay scoliosis. In general, preventive measures are more successful than restorative ones.

From such observations it may be concluded that two factors are of importance in the management of patients with muscular dystrophy: avoiding prolonged bed rest and encouraging the patient to maintain as full and normal a life as possible. These help prevent the rapid worsening associated with inactivity and conserve a healthy attitude of mind. Obesity should be avoided; this requires careful attention to diet. Swimming is a useful exercise. Massage and electrical stimulation are probably worthless. The education of children with muscular dystrophy should continue, with the aim of preparing them for a sedentary occupation.

Prevention by prenatal counseling is available for most dystrophies, but proper diagnosis is essential. Special centers provide the genetic and psychological services necessary to carry this out properly.

THE METABOLIC MYOPATHIES

Two main classes of metabolic diseases of muscle are recognized—one is traceable to a primary, or hereditary, metabolic abnormality of the muscle itself; another in which the myopathy is secondary to a disorder of endocrine function, that is, to disease of the thyroid, parathyroid, pituitary, or adrenal gland. Yet a third group of myopathies is the result of a large variety of myotoxic drugs and other chemical agents; they are addressed separately.

The hereditary metabolic myopathies are of special interest because they reveal certain aspects of the complex chemistry of muscle fibers. Indeed, each year brings to light some new genetically determined enzymopathy of muscle. As a consequence, a number of diseases formerly classified as dystrophic or degenerative have been added to the enlarging list of metabolic myopathies. There are now so many of them that only the most representative can be presented in a textbook of neurology. Complete accounts of this subject can be found in the section on metabolic disorders in Engel and Franzini-Armstrong and in DiMauro and colleagues (1992).

Primary Metabolic Disorders of Muscle

The chemical energy for muscle contraction is provided by the hydrolysis of adenosine triphosphate (ATP) to adenosine diphosphate (ADP); ATP is restored by phosphocreatine and ADP acting in combination. These reactions are particularly important during brief, high-intensity exercise. During periods of prolonged muscle activity, rephosphorylation requires the availability of carbohydrates, fatty acids, and ketones, which are catabolized in mitochondria. Glycogen is the main sarcoplasmic source of carbohydrate, but blood glucose also moves freely in and out of muscle cells as needed during sustained exercise. The fatty acids in the blood, derived mainly from adipose tissue and intracellular lipid stores, constitute the other major source of energy. Carbohydrate is metabolized during aerobic and anaerobic phases of metabolism; the fatty acids are metabolized only aerobically.

Resting muscle derives approximately 70 percent of its energy from the oxidation of long-chain fatty acids. As stated earlier, the circumstances during exercise are somewhat different. During a short period of intense exercise, the muscle uses carbohydrate derived from glycogen stores; myophosphorylase is the enzyme that initiates the metabolism of glycogen. With longer aerobic exercise, blood flow to muscle and the availability of glucose and fatty acids are increased. At first, glucose is the main source of energy during exercise; later, with exhaustion of glycogen stores, energy is provided by oxidation of fatty acids. Thus, muscle failure at a certain phase of exercise is predictive of the type of energy failure. A rising blood concentration of β-hydroxybutyrate reflects the increasing oxidation of fatty acids, and an increase in blood lactate reflects the anaerobic metabolism of glucose. The cytochrome oxidative mechanisms are essential in both aerobic and anaerobic muscle metabolism; these mechanisms are considered in Chap. 37 in relation to the mitochondrial diseases in which muscle tissue is prominently involved, and they are referred to here only briefly.

It follows from these observations that the efficiency and endurance of muscular contraction depend on a constant supply of glycogen, glucose, and fatty acids, and on the adequacy of the enzymes committed to their metabolism. Biochemical derangements in the storage, breakdown, or utilization of these substrates give rise to a large number of muscle disorders, the most important of which are elaborated in the following pages.

Glycogen Storage Myopathies

An abnormal accumulation of glycogen in the liver and kidneys was described by von Gierke in 1929; shortly thereafter, Pompe (1932) reported a similar disorder involving cardiac and skeletal muscle. Major contributions to our understanding of glycogen metabolism were made by McArdle, by Cori and Cori, and by Hers, who discovered the deficiency of acid maltase in Pompe disease and enunciated the concept of inborn lysosomal diseases (see Chap. 37). Since then, many nonlysosomal enzyme deficiencies of muscle and other organs have been identified and have become the basis of the classification presented in Table 48-5. These enzymatic deficiencies alter the metabolism of many cells, but most strikingly those of the liver, heart, and skeletal muscle. In about half of affected individuals, a chronically progressive or intermittent myopathic syndrome is the major manifestation of the disease. It is a curious fact, that with the exception of the rare phosphoglycerate kinase deficiency (X-linked recessive inheritance), *all the glycogenoses are inherited as autosomal recessive traits*. The most impressive and common of these glycogen storage diseases from the standpoint of the clinical neurologist are 1,4-glucosidase (acid maltase) and myophosphorylase deficiencies.

Acid Maltase Deficiency (Glycogenosis Type II; Pompe Disease and Related Disorders)

A deficiency of the enzyme acid maltase (also called acid alpha-glucosidase and due to mutations in the *GAA* gene) takes three clinical forms, of which the first (Pompe disease) is the most serious. Pompe disease typically develops in *infancy*, between 2 and 6 months; dyspnea and cyanosis call attention to enlargement of the heart, and the liver may be enlarged as well. The skeletal muscles are weak and hypotonic, although their bulk may be increased. The tongue may be enlarged, giving the infant a cretinoid appearance. Hepatomegaly, while often present, is not pronounced. Exceptionally, the heart is normal in size and the CNS and muscles bear the brunt of the disorder. The clinical picture then resembles infantile spinal muscular atrophy (Werdnig-Hoffmann disease) and, to add to difficulty in differential diagnosis, there may be fasciculations. The infantile disease is rapidly progressive and ends fatally in a few months. The EMG shows myopathic changes, but there are, in addition, fibrillation potentials, heightened insertional activity, and pseudomyotonia. Large amounts of glycogen accumulate in muscle, heart, liver, and neurons of the spinal cord and brain. All tissues lack acid maltase (also called alpha-glucosidase) because of a mutation in its gene.

In the second *(childhood) form*, onset is during the second year, with delay in walking and slowly progressive weakness of shoulder, pelvic girdle, and trunk muscles. The toe walking, waddling gait, enlargement of calf muscles, and lumbar lordosis resemble those of Duchenne dystrophy. Cardiomyopathy is exceptional, hepatomegaly is less frequent than in the infantile form, and mental retardation is present in a minority (DiMauro et al, 1992). Death occurs between 3 and 24 years of age, usually from ventilatory failure and recurrent pulmonary infections.

In the third, *or adult, form* there is a more benign truncal and proximal limb myopathy that is slowly progressive over many years, and death is usually the result of weakness of respiratory muscles. At times, the only severe weakness is of the diaphragm, as in the case reported by Sivak and colleagues, making adult acid maltase deficiency part of a select group of neuromuscular disorders that may present in this way (along with motor neuron disease, nemaline myopathy, and myasthenia gravis). The liver and heart are not enlarged. CK values can be normal or slightly increased. The EMG discloses a number of abnormalities—brief motor unit potentials, fibrillation potentials, positive waves, bizarre high-frequency discharges, and occasional myotonic discharges (without clinical evidence of myotonia). The disease must be differentiated from other chronic adult myopathies, including polymyositis and the endocrine myopathies, and from motor neuron disease.

Aside from the elevation of the muscle-derived enzymes CK and of aldolase, blood studies are normal. A simply implemented dried blood spot screening test for alpha-glucosidase has been developed and, if it shows that there is no enzyme detectable, a biopsy can be omitted and the clinician can proceed to genetic testing. This screening test is particularly important in babies with suspected disease, as they are susceptible to general anesthesia that may be used to accomplish a biopsy.

The diagnosis of acid maltase deficiency in early-onset cases is readily confirmed by muscle biopsy, but later onset cases may show only nonspecific changes. The main features, when found, are vacuoles containing periodic acid-Schiff (PAS)–positive diastase-digestible material; they stain intensely for acid phosphatase. The glycogen particles lie in aggregates; electron microscopy shows some of them to occupy lysosomal vesicles and others, to lie free. The myofibrils are disrupted and some muscle fibers degenerate. Glycogen accumulation is more pronounced in type 1 fibers. The earlier mentioned blood-spot test is useful in cases, particularly those of late

Table 48-5

THE GLYCOGENOSES AFFECTING SKELETAL MUSCLE[a]

GLYCOGENOSIS TYPE (PROPER NAME)	DEFECTIVE ENZYME	ONSET OF DISEASE[b]	HYPOTONIA	EXERCISE INTOLERANCE (MYALGIA, CRAMPS, STIFFNESS, ± MYOGLOBINURIA)	EARLY FATIGUE AND SECOND WIND	MYOPATHY ± ATROPHY	SEVERE RESPIRATORY MUSCLE WEAKNESS	CONTRACTURES
II (Pompe)	Acid maltase	I	+			+	+	
II	Acid maltase	C				+	+	
II	Acid maltase	A				+	+	
III (Cori-Forbes)	Debrancher	C-A	+			+		+
IV (Andersen)	Branching	I-C	+			+		+
V (McArdle)	Myophosphorylase	C, Ad, A		+	+	+		+
VII (Tarui)	Phosphofructokinase	C-A		+	+	+		+
VIII	Phosphorylase B kinase	I, C, Ad, A	+	+		+		
IX	Phosphoglycerate kinase	I, C-A		+		+		
X	Phosphoglycerate mutase	A		+				
XI	Lactic dehydrogenase	Ad-A		+	+			

[a]All types: elevated creatine kinase (CK); myopathic electromyogram, with increased irritability and myotonia.
[b]A, adult; Ad, adolescence; C, childhood; I, infancy.
Additional features (not charted above): feeding difficulties, II Pompe; retarded growth, III; neurologic abnormalities, II Pompe, IX; seizures, VIII, IX; hypoglycemic seizures, III; jaundice, VII, IX; cirrhosis, IV; generalized scaling erythema, XI; firm consistency of muscle, II Pompe; elevated serum aspartate aminotransferase and lactic dehydrogenase, II; elevated serum bilirubin, VII, IX; failure of lactate dehydrogenase to rise proportionally to elevation of CK, XI; fasting hypoglycemia, III; hemolytic anemia and reticulocytosis, VII, IX; hemoglobinuria, IX; excessive rise in serum pyruvates during ischemic exercise test, XI.

ORGANOMEGALY	MYOGLOBINURIA	POSITIVE ISCHEMIC EXERCISE TEST	ENZYME-DEFICIENT CELLS FOR ASSAY	MEMBRANE-LINED VACUOLES WITH GLYCOGEN	INCREASED GLYCOGEN IN SUBSARCOLEMMA AND INTER-MYOFIBRILLAR AREAS	INTRA-AND EXTRA-VACUOLAR ACID PHOSPHATASE	AMYLOPECTIN DEPOSITS	HISTO-CHEMISTRY
+			Muscle, WBC, chorionic villus, amniotic fluid	+	+	+		
			Muscle	+	+	+		
			Muscle	+	+	+		
±	+		Muscle, WBC, fibroblasts		+			
+			Muscle, WBC fibro-blasts amniotic fluid		+	+	+	
	+	+	Muscle, WBC		+			Absence of myophos-phorylase
	+	+	Muscle, RBC		+		+	Absence of phospho-fructokinase
+	+	+	Muscle		+			
+	+	+	Muscle, RBC		±			
	+	+	Muscle		+			
	+	+	Muscle		+			

onset, that have the typical characteristics of disease but display only nonspecific histopathologic changes.

As indicated earlier, in the more severe infantile form of acid maltase deficiency, heart muscle and the large neurons of the spinal cord and brainstem may also accumulate glycogen and degenerate. The difference in severity between infant and adult forms relates to the completeness of enzyme deficiency, but possibly other factors are also at work as more than one of the three types may occur in the same family.

Treatment The adult who is threatened by respiratory failure should be observed frequently with measurements of vital capacity and blood gases. Umpleby and coworkers reported that a low-carbohydrate, high-protein diet may be beneficial. A few of our patients died unexpectedly during sleep. Respiratory support (rocking bed, nasal positive pressure, cough-assist devices, and negative-pressure cuirass) may prolong life.

Enzyme replacement therapy is available to treat Pompe disease. Recombinant acid alpha-glucosidase has been shown to prolong survival in the typical infantile Pompe case, but the benefits are modest in later-onset cases, although walking was improved and pulmonary function stabilized in one series (van er Ploeg et al). The agent is injected intravenously every 2 weeks.

Myophosphorylase Deficiency (Type V Glycogenosis; McArdle Disease) and Phosphofructokinase Deficiency (Type VII Glycogenosis; Tarui Disease)

These disorders are considered together because they are clinically virtually identical and both express themselves by the development of muscle cramps after exercise (actually true physiologic contractures, as described in Chap. 45). In both diseases, an otherwise normal child, adolescent, or adult begins to complain of weakness and stiffness and sometimes pain on using the limbs. Muscle contraction and relaxation are normal when the patient is in repose, but strenuous exercise, either isometric (carrying heavy weights) or dynamic (climbing stairs or walking uphill), causes the muscles to shorten (contracture), a result of their inability to relax. After vigorous exercise, episodes of myoglobinuria are common, in some cases resulting in renal failure. With mild sustained activity, the patient experiences progressive muscle fatigue and weakness, which diminish following a brief pause. The patient can then resume his activities at the original pace ("second-wind" phenomenon). During the second-wind phase, the patient copes with his symptoms by increasing cardiac output and substituting free fatty acids and blood-borne glucose for muscle glycogen (Braakhekke et al).

The primary abnormality in *McArdle disease* is a deficiency of myophosphorylase, which prevents the conversion of glycogen to glucose-6-phosphate. Phosphofructokinase deficiency (*Tarui disease*) interferes with the conversion of glucose-6-phosphate to glucose-1-phosphate; the defect in the latter condition is also present in red blood cells (Layzer et al). The mutations for the conditions are located on different chromosomes and analysis of DNA from the patient's leukocytes can be used for genetic diagnosis. The muscle (M) subunit of the phosphofructokinase protein in Tarui disease is at fault. This defect predominates in Ashkenazi Jewish men.

Clinical variations of these disorders, particularly in severity and age of onset, are well known. Some patients, with no previous symptoms of cramps or myoglobinuria, develop progressive weakness of limb muscles in the sixth or seventh decade. One of these older patients came to our attention because of chronically elevated levels of CK and mild muscle cramping after climbing stairs. In others, rapidly progressive weakness became evident in infancy, with early death from respiratory failure. Curiously, these extreme forms are not directly related to severity of the enzyme deficiencies.

The contracted muscles, unlike muscles in other involuntary spasms, no longer use energy and they are more or less electrically silent (i.e., no electrical activity is recorded from maximally contracted muscle during the cramps). Moreover, the muscle does not produce lactic acid. The shortened state is spoken of as *physiologic contracture* as discussed in the introductory sections of this chapter. Ischemia contributes to this condition by denying glucose to the muscle, which then cannot function adequately on fatty acids and nonglucose substrates. These features are the basis of the *forearm ischemic exercise test*, which, although controversial in its use and sensitivity, may be helpful if performed carefully. An indwelling catheter is placed in the antecubital vein and a basal blood sample is obtained. Above the elbow, a sphygmomanometer cuff is inflated to exceed arterial pressure. After 1 min of vigorous hand exercise (30 hand closures against an ergometer), blood samples are obtained at 1 and 3 min. Normal individuals show a 3- to 5-fold increase in blood lactate. In patients with either McArdle or Tarui disease, the lactate fails to rise. This procedure has reportedly caused a localized rhabdomyolysis (Meinck et al), for which reason Griggs and associates recommend that the test be carried out *without* a blood pressure cuff. Problems with consistency in conducting the test and in processing blood samples for lactate limit its validity unless it is performed by experienced individuals and laboratories. Definitive diagnosis depends more on the histochemical stains of biopsied muscle, which reveal an absence of phosphorylase activity (in McArdle disease) or of phosphofructokinase activity (in Tarui disease). Genetic analysis, mentioned previously, can be used to corroborate the diagnosis, but it is unnecessary if the histochemical tests are definitive.

Treatment The main treatment is a planned reduction and intermittency in physical activity. Sucrose, taken as 75 g in a beverage, has been shown by Vissing and Haller to cause a short-lived improvement in exercise tolerance, and they propose that exercise-induced rhabdomyolysis can be avoided by a well-timed drink. Fructose and creatine taken orally are also said to be helpful in some cases, but the reported results are not as impressive as they are for sucrose. Improvement has also been described after the administration of glucagon (Kono et al) and with a high-protein diet (Slonim and Goans), but these effects are not consistent.

Other Forms of Glycogenosis (See Table 48-5)

Of the remaining glycogen storage diseases, type III (*debranching enzyme deficiency; Cori-Forbes disease*) affects muscle but only inconsistently. The childhood form is characterized mainly by a benign hepatopathy, sometimes accompanied by diminished muscle strength and tone. An adult form beginning in the third and fourth decades presents with proximal and distal myopathy. The course is slowly progressive and may be associated with wasting of the leg and hand muscles. In the series reported by DiMauro and colleagues (1992), several patients who developed weakness during adult life complained of rapid fatigue and aching of muscles, occurring with exertion and first noticed at an early age. Serum CK values were elevated and the EMG showed a myopathic picture as well as increased insertional activity, pseudomyotonic discharges, and fibrillation potentials. Rarely in the adult form, glycogen also accumulates in the peripheral nerves, giving rise to mild symptoms of polyneuropathy. The enzymatic defect is one of amylo-1,6-glucosidase deficiency.

Disturbance of skeletal muscle is even less prominent in type IV glycogenosis (*branching enzyme deficiency*, or *Andersen disease*, which is also implicated in the polyglucosan disease that causes a special neuropathy discussed in Chap. 46, a motor system disease with flaccid bladder, or a leukoencephalopathy with dementia). This is a progressive disease of infancy and early childhood, characterized by cirrhosis and chronic hepatic failure, usually with death in the second or third year. Hepatomegaly as a result of accumulation of an abnormal polysaccharide is a universal finding. Muscle weakness and atrophy, hypotonia, and contractures occur less regularly and are overshadowed by the liver disease. The diagnostic hallmark of the myopathy is the presence of basophilic, intensely PAS-positive polysaccharide granules in skin and muscle.

The remaining nonlysosomal glycogenoses (types VIII through XI) need only be mentioned briefly. They are all rare and clinically heterogeneous, and a myopathy—characterized by intolerance to exercise, cramps, myoglobinuria, elevated CK, and, sometimes, renal failure—has been observed in a small proportion of them. Phosphoglycerate kinase deficiency (type IX glycogenosis) differs in that it is inherited as a sex-linked recessive trait localized to chromosome Xq13. Hemolytic anemia—becoming evident soon after birth—mental retardation, seizures, and tremor are other features that set this glycogenosis apart from the others. The myopathic features of the lysosomal and nonlysosomal glycogenoses are listed in Table 48-5 and detailed accounts can be found in the monographs by Griggs and associates and of Engel and Franzini-Armstrong (chapters by DiMauro and Tsujino and by Engel and Hirschhorn).

Disorders of Lipid Metabolism Affecting Muscle (Lipid Myopathies)

Although it has long been known that lipids are an important source of energy in muscle metabolism (along with glucose), it was only in 1970 that W.K. Engel and associates reported the abnormal storage of lipid in muscle fibers attributable to a defect in the oxidation of long-chain fatty acids. The subjects of their report were twin sisters who had experienced intermittent cramping of muscles associated with myoglobinuria after vigorous exercise. In 1973, A.G. Engel and Angelini described a young woman with progressive myopathy, lipid storage predominantly in type 1 muscle fibers, and a deficiency of muscle carnitine, a cofactor required for the oxidation of fatty acids. Since that time, highly sophisticated biochemical techniques have greatly expanded the study of fatty acid metabolism and the identification of many of the primary defects.

Carnitine (β-hydroxy-gamma-*N*-trimethylamino-butyrate), derived from lysine and methionine, plays a central role in the metabolism of fatty acids. Approximately 75 percent of carnitine comes from dietary sources (red meat and dairy products); the remainder is synthesized in the liver and kidneys. Practically all of the body carnitine is stored in muscle, where it has two main functions: (1) transporting long-chain fatty acylcoenzyme As (CoAs) from the cytosol compartment of the muscle fiber into the mitochondria, where they undergo beta-oxidation, and (2) preventing the intramitochondrial accumulation of acyl-CoAs, thus protecting the muscle cell from the membrane-destabilizing effects of these substances.

To be oxidized, the long-chain fatty acids undergo a series of biochemical transformations. First they are activated to corresponding acyl-CoA esters by acyl-CoA synthetase, which is located on the outer mitochondrial membrane. Because the inner mitochondrial membrane is impermeable to acyl-CoA esters, they are transferred into the mitochondria as acylcarnitine esters. This is accomplished by carnitine palmitoyltransferase I (CPT I), also located on the outer mitochondrial membrane. A second carnitine palmitoyltransferase (CPT II), bound to the inner face of the inner mitochondrial membrane, reconverts the acylcarnitines to fatty acyl-CoAs, which undergo beta-oxidation within the mitochondrial matrix. The steps in the transport of long-chain fatty acids into the mitochondrial matrix (the carnitine cycle) are described in detail in the reviews of DiMauro and colleagues (1973), and DiDonato and Taroni. Isoforms of CPT are critically involved in this process at the inner and outer membranes of the mitochondria.

Despite the many biochemical abnormalities that have been identified in the fatty acid metabolic pathways, there are essentially 3 clinical patterns by which these defects are expressed:

1. One constellation of symptoms referred to as the *encephalopathic* syndrome has its onset in infancy or early childhood. Its very first manifestation may be sudden death (sudden infant death syndrome [SIDS]), or there may be vomiting, lethargy and coma, hepatomegaly, cardiomegaly, muscular weakness, and hypoketotic hypoglycemia, with prominent hyperammonemia, that is, a Reye-like syndrome. Undoubtedly, instances of this syndrome have not been recognized as abnormalities of fatty acid metabolism but have been designated incorrectly as the Reye syndrome or as SIDS. They are discussed in Chap. 37 with other inherited metabolic disorders.

2. A second (*myopathic*) syndrome appears in late infancy, childhood, or adult life and takes the form of a progressive myopathy, with or without cardiomyopathy. The myopathy may follow episodes of hypoketotic hypoglycemia or may develop de novo.
3. The third syndrome is one that usually begins in the second decade of life and is induced by a sustained period of physical activity or fasting. It is characterized by repeated episodes of *rhabdomyolysis* with or without myoglobinuria.

Summarized in the following text are the main disorders of fatty acid metabolism that affect skeletal muscle; these are rare but interesting diseases.

Primary Systemic Carnitine Deficiency

To date, this is the only form of carnitine deficiency that can be considered primary (see further on for discussion of the secondary types). Its main clinical features are progressive lipid storage myopathy and cardiomyopathy, sometimes associated with the signs of hypoketotic hypoglycemia. There is no dicarboxylic aciduria, in distinction to the secondary beta-oxidation defects, in all of which dicarboxylic aciduria is present. The cardiomyopathy, which is fatal if untreated, responds to oral administration of l-carnitine, 2 to 6 g/d. This disorder is inherited as an autosomal recessive trait. In these families there is frequently a history of sudden unexplained death in siblings, so that early identification of affected children is essential.

Carnitine Palmitoyltransferase Deficiency

This disease is also inherited as an autosomal recessive trait and the gene encoding carnitine palmitoyltransferase (CPT) has been identified. There are three types: types I, IIA, and IIB. Type I is the most common. It affects males predominantly, beginning in the second decade of life. Attacks of myalgia, cramps, and muscle weakness, "tightness," and stiffness are precipitated by sustained (although not necessarily intense) exercise and less often by a prolonged period of fasting. Fever, anesthesia, drugs, emotional stress, and cold have been additional but rare precipitating events. The attacks vary greatly in frequency. They are usually accompanied by myoglobinuria, with resultant renal failure in about one-fourth of cases (DiMauro et al, 1973). Rest does not abort the attacks and, once initiated, there is no second-wind phenomenon. There are no warning signs of an impending attack. Any muscle group may be affected. Persistence of weakness after an attack is uncommon. Serum CK rises to high levels not only during attacks but also after vigorous exercise without myoglobinuria. A mild form is more likely to occur in females.

In type I deficiency, necrosis of muscle fibers, particularly type I fibers, occurs during attacks, followed by regeneration. Between attacks, the muscle appears normal. In type IIA, lipid bodies accumulate in the liver, and in type IIB, excess lipid is detected in heart, liver, kidneys, and skeletal muscle.

CPT is either undetectable or greatly reduced in muscle, and assays are now available for the measurement of CPT I and II in circulating lymphocytes and cultured fibroblasts.

Treatment A high-carbohydrate, low-fat diet, ingestion of frequent meals, and additional carbohydrate before and during exercise appear to reduce the number of attacks. Patients need to be instructed about the risks of prolonged exercise and skipped meals. Recently, the use of bezafibrate, a drug used for dyslipidemia, has been helpful in patients with mild CPT II.

Secondary Systemic Carnitine Deficiency

This is occasionally the result of severe dietary deprivation or impaired hepatic and renal function. Such instances have been observed in patients with alcoholic–nutritional diseases and kwashiorkor, in premature infants receiving parenteral nutrition, in patients with chronic renal failure undergoing dialysis, and rarely, as a complication of valproate therapy. However, most cases of systemic carnitine deficiency are a result of defects of beta-oxidation, described as follows.

Other Lipid Myopathies

Carnitine Acylcarnitine Translocase Deficiency This condition causes muscular weakness, cardiomyopathy, hypoketotic hypoglycemia, and hyperammonemia, which develop in early infancy and usually lead to death in the first month of life.

Long-Chain Acyl-CoA Dehydrogenase Deficiency The presentation is in infancy, with recurrent episodes of fasting hypoglycemic coma, muscle weakness, and myoglobinuria, and sometimes sudden death. Survivors may develop a progressive myopathy. Administration of carnitine improves the cardiac disorder and prevents metabolic attacks.

Medium-Chain Acyl-CoA Dehydrogenase Deficiency This is a cause of SIDS and a Reye-like syndrome. About half of survivors develop a lipid-storage myopathy in childhood or adult life. The abnormal gene has been mapped to chromosome 1p31. Oral L-carnitine may be of therapeutic value.

Short-Chain Acyl-CoA Dehydrogenase Deficiency This myopathy in a limb-girdle distribution may appear initially in older children and adults, or it may follow episodic metabolic disorders in infancy.

Long-Chain Hydroxyacyl-CoA Dehydrogenase Deficiency This is a disease of infancy marked by episodes of Reye-like syndrome, hypoketotic hypoglycemia, lipid storage myopathy, cardiomyopathy, and sometimes sudden death.

Short-Chain Hydroxyacyl-CoA Dehydrogenase Deficiency This presents as an episodic disorder such as the one described previously, long-chain hydroxyacyl-CoA dehydrogenase deficiency (HAD), but its onset is in adolescence. Recurrent attacks may be associated with myoglobinuria.

Multiple Acyl-CoA Dehydrogenase Deficiency; Glutaric Aciduria Type II Some cases are caused by a deficiency of electron transfer flavoprotein (ETF) and others by a deficiency of electron transfer flavoprotein-ubiquinone oxidoreductase (ETF-QO). In the severest form of multiple acyl-CoA dehydrogenase deficiency (MADD), infants are born prematurely and many die within the first week of life; added to the common metabolic abnormalities are multiple congenital defects and a characteristic "sweaty feet" odor. In less severe cases, the congenital anomalies are absent. In the least severe form, the onset may be in late infancy (with episodic metabolic disturbances) or in childhood or adult life (with a lipid storage myopathy and a deficiency of serum and muscle carnitine). The prenatal diagnosis of glutaric aciduria type II (GA II) is suggested by the finding of large amounts of glutaric acid in the amniotic fluid. In the milder forms of the disease, oral riboflavin (100 to 300 mg/d) may be helpful.

Muscle Coenzyme Q10 Deficiency This condition presents as a slowly progressive lipid storage myopathy from early childhood. The basic defect is in coenzyme Q10 in the respiratory chain of muscle mitochondria. The administration of coenzyme Q10 has improved the myopathic weakness.

Neutral Lipid Storage Diseases (Chanarin disease) These abnormalities of lipid metabolism are distinct from the beta-oxidation defects; they occur in 2 forms, Chanarin disease, which is characterized by ichthyosis, and a form without skin changes. A progressive myopathy is combined with neurologic manifestations, such as developmental delay, ataxia, neurosensory hearing loss, and microcephaly. The lipid material is stored in muscle as triglyceride droplets that are nonlysosomal and non-membrane-bound.

ENDOCRINE MYOPATHIES

Thyroid Myopathies

Several myopathic diseases are related to alterations in thyroid function: (1) chronic thyrotoxic myopathy; (2) exophthalmic ophthalmoplegia (infiltrative orbital ophthalmopathy—Graves disease); (3) myasthenia gravis associated with thyrotoxicosis; (4) periodic paralysis associated with thyrotoxicosis; and (5) muscle hypertrophy and slow muscle contraction and relaxation associated with myxedema and cretinism. Although they are not common, we have encountered up to several examples of these diseases in a single year in our general hospital.

Chronic Thyrotoxic Myopathy

This disorder, first noted by Graves and Basedow in the early nineteenth century, is characterized by progressive weakness and wasting of the skeletal musculature, occurring in conjunction with overt or covert ("masked") hyperthyroidism. The thyroid disease is usually chronic and the goiter is usually of the nodular rather than the diffuse type. Exophthalmos and other classic signs of hyperthyroidism are often present but need not be. This complication of hyperthyroidism is most frequent in middle age, and men are more susceptible than women. Some degree of myopathy has been found when sought in more than 50 percent of thyrotoxic patients, although the manifestations may be subtle. The onset is insidious, and the weakness progresses over weeks and months. The muscular disorder as noted is most often mild in degree, but it may be so severe as to suggest progressive spinal muscular atrophy (motor system disease). Muscles of the pelvic girdle and thighs are weakened more than others (Basedow paraplegia), although all are affected to some extent, even the bulbar muscles and, albeit rarely, the ocular ones. However, the shoulder and hand muscles show the most conspicuous atrophy (not an obligatory feature). Tremor and twitching during contraction may occur, but we have not seen fasciculations. The tendon reflexes are of average briskness, possibly more lively than normal. Both the contraction and relaxation phases of the tendon reflexes are shortened, but usually this cannot be detected by the clinician.

Serum concentrations of muscle enzymes are not increased and may be reduced. The EMG is typically normal although the action potentials may be abnormally brief or polyphasic. Biopsies of muscle, except for slight atrophy of both types 1 and 2 fibers and an occasional degenerating fiber, have been normal. Muscle power and bulk are gradually restored when thyroid hormone levels are reduced to normal levels.

Exophthalmic Ophthalmoplegia (Graves Ophthalmopathy) (See discussion in Chap. 14)

This refers to the cooccurrence of weakness of the ocular muscles and exophthalmos in patients with Graves disease (pupillary and ciliary muscles are always spared). The exophthalmos varies in degree, sometimes being absent at an early stage of the disease, and it is not in itself responsible for the muscle weakness. Often there is some degree of orbital pain. Both the exophthalmos and the weakness of the extraocular muscles may precede the signs of hyperthyroidism, be associated with the other classic features of hyperthyroidism (tachycardia, weight loss, tremor), or may follow effective treatment of the disorder.

The eye signs, both ocular paresis and exophthalmos, become apparent over days or weeks and may occasionally be unilateral, especially at the onset. Any of the external eye muscles may be infiltrated, usually one more than others, accounting for strabismus and diplopia; the inferior and medial recti are the most frequently affected, but upward movements are usually limited as well. The typical but not invariable sign of lid retraction imparts a staring appearance. Subtle exophthalmos can be appreciated by standing above and behind the seated patient and observing the relative positions of the lids and the eyelashes. Conjunctival edema and vascular engorgement over the insertions of the medial and lateral rectus muscles can be appreciated by inspecting and palpating the globe in its extreme lateral positions. These swollen muscles are easily visible on orbital ultrasonography, CT, and MRI. The differential diagnosis of this imaging appearance is from orbital pseudotumor, a usually painful condition, which is discussed in Chap. 14.

Examination of the eye muscles in biopsy and autopsy material has shown prominent fibroblasts, many degenerated fibers, and infiltrations of lymphocytes, mononuclear leukocytes, and lipocytes; hence the term *infiltrative ophthalmopathy*. These histopathologic findings are suggestive of an autoimmune disease—a hypothesis supported by the finding of serum antibodies that react (inconsistently) with extracts of eye muscles (Kodama et al). Possibly the antibodies target glycosaminoglycans of the orbital fibroblasts. A sensitivity of muscle fibers to beta-adrenergic activity caused by excessive thyroid hormone has also been postulated. Other factors are almost certainly involved, such as the small size of oculomotor motor units, the absence of dystrophin, and the rich mitochondrial content.

Treatment Because the ophthalmoparesis often runs a self-limited course, as does the exophthalmos, therapy is difficult to evaluate. Certainly the maintenance of a euthyroid state seems desirable (Dresner and Kennerdell). If the exophthalmos is slight, topical applications of adrenergic blocking agents (guanethidine eye drops, 5 percent) and ophthalmic ointment to prevent corneal drying are adequate. Severe exophthalmos, marked by periorbital and conjunctival edema, and the extraocular muscle weakness may be partially controlled by high doses of corticosteroids (about 80 mg/d prednisone). Because of the hazards of protracted corticosteroid therapy, this approach should be reserved for patients who would otherwise require surgical intervention to decompress the contents of the orbit. In a number of such cases, it has been possible for the patient treated with corticosteroids to weather the crisis for several weeks or more and avoid the damaging effects of extreme exophthalmos and risks of surgery. Exophthalmos of a degree that threatens to injure the cornea or cause blindness requires tarsorrhaphy or decompression by removal of the roof of the orbit.

Thyrotoxic Hypokalemic Periodic Paralysis

This disorder closely resembles familial hypokalemic periodic paralysis (as described in Chap. 50). It consists of attacks of mild to severe weakness of the muscles of the trunk and limbs; usually the cranial muscles are spared. The weakness develops over a period of a few minutes or hours and lasts for part of a day or longer. In some series of patients with periodic paralysis, as many as half have had hyperthyroidism and most of them have been Asian males. Unlike the typical hypokalemic form, thyrotoxic periodic paralysis is not a familial disorder and its onset is usually in early adult life. Nevertheless, in most of the thyrotoxic cases, the serum potassium levels have been low during the attacks of weakness and the administration of 100 to 200 mg of potassium chloride has terminated the episodes. Propranolol in doses of 160 mg daily in divided doses is also helpful in preventing the episodes. More importantly, effective treatment of the hyperthyroidism abolishes the periodic attacks of weakness in more than 90 percent of cases. A mutation in the potassium channel, Kir2.6, has been found to confer susceptibility to the disease. Other aspects of periodic paralysis are discussed in Chap. 50.

Myasthenia Gravis with Hyperthyroidism

Myasthenia is discussed fully in Chap. 49. Here only a few remarks are made on its special relationship to thyrotoxicosis. Myasthenia gravis in its typical autoimmune, anticholinesterase-responsive form may accompany hyperthyroidism or rarely, hypothyroidism, which are also autoimmune in nature. Approximately 5 percent of patients with myasthenia have hyperthyroidism and the frequency of myasthenia gravis in patients, while low, is 20 to 30 times higher in hyperthyroidism than in the general population. Either condition may appear first, or they may coincide. The weakness and atrophy of chronic thyrotoxic myopathy may be added to that of the myasthenia without appearing to affect the requirement for or response to anticholinesterase medications. By contrast, hypothyroidism, even of mild degree, seems to aggravate the weakness of myasthenia gravis, greatly increasing the need for pyridostigmine and at times inducing a myasthenic crisis. In these cases, thyroxine is beneficial and, with respect to myasthenia, restores the patient to the status that existed before the onset of thyroid insufficiency. The myasthenia should probably be regarded as an autoimmune disease independent of the thyroid disease and each must be treated separately.

Hypothyroid Myopathy

Abnormalities of skeletal muscle consisting of diffuse myalgia and increased volume, stiffness, and slowness of contraction and of relaxation are common manifestations of hypothyroidism, whether in the form of myxedema or cretinism. These changes probably account for the relatively large tongue and dysarthria that one observes in myxedema. Weakness, however, is not a prominent feature. The presence of action myospasm and myokymia (both of which are rare) and of percussion myoedema and slowness of both the contraction and relaxation phases of tendon reflexes assists the examiner in making a bedside diagnosis. The administration of thyroxine corrects the muscle disturbance.

Cretinism in association with these muscle abnormalities is known as the *Kocher-Debré-Semelaigne syndrome*, and myxedema in childhood or adult life with muscle hypertrophy is the *Hoffmann syndrome*; the latter simulates hypertrophia musculorum vera and myotonia congenita. In neither cretinism nor myxedema, however, is there evidence of true myotonia, either by clinical testing or by EMG, although muscle action potentials are myopathic and often show bizarre high-frequency discharges. Serum transaminase values are normal but CK levels are usually elevated, often markedly so. Muscle biopsies have disclosed only the presence of large fibers or an increase in the proportion of small fibers (either type 1 or 2) and slight distention of the sarcoplasmic reticulum and subsarcolemmal glycogen (probably all a result of disuse atrophy).

Pathogenesis of the Thyroid Myopathies

How thyroid hormone affects the muscle fiber is still a matter of conjecture. Clinical data indicate that thyroxine influences the contractile process in some manner but does not interfere with the transmission of impulses in the peripheral nerve across the myoneural junction or along the sarcolemma. In hyperthyroidism an undefined functional disorder enhances the speed of the contractile process and reduces its duration, the net effect being fatigability, weakness, and loss of endurance of muscle action. In hypothyroidism, muscle contraction is slowed, as is relaxation, and its duration is prolonged.

The speed of the contractile process is related to the quantity of myosin adenosine triphosphatase (ATPase), which is increased in hyperthyroid muscle and decreased in hypothyroid muscle. The speed of relaxation depends on the rate of release and reaccumulation of calcium in the endoplasmic reticulum. This is slowed in hypothyroidism and increased in hyperthyroidism (Ianuzzo et al). The myopathic effects of hypothyroidism need to be distinguished from those of a neuropathy, which may rarely complicate hypothyroidism (see Chap. 46).

Corticosteroid Myopathies

The widespread use of adrenal corticosteroids has created a class of muscle diseases similar to the one that occurs in the Cushing disease as described many decades ago by Müller and Kugelberg. A deficiency of corticosteroids, as occurs in Addison disease, also causes generalized weakness and asthenia, but without an identifiable muscle disease.

Corticosteroid and Cushing Disease Myopathy

The prolonged use of corticosteroids causes the proximal limb and girdle musculature to become weak to the point of causing difficulty in elevating the arms and arising from a sitting, squatting, or kneeling position; walking up stairs may also be hampered. Some individuals seem to be more susceptible than others. The problem often arises of distinguishing an iatrogenic steroid-induced myopathy from the weakness produced by a primary neuromuscular disorder that is being treated with these medications such as one of the myositides or myasthenia. In some of our myasthenic patients, the use of high-dose corticosteroids has resulted in a selective, rapid, and severe weakness of the hip flexors.

The EMG is normal or mildly myopathic, with small and abundant action potentials but no fibrillations. Biopsies disclose only a slight variation in fiber size with atrophic fibers, mainly of type 2b, but little or no fiber necrosis and no inflammatory cells. Under electron microscopic examination there are aggregates of mitochondria, accumulations of glycogen and lipid, and slight myofibrillar loss that suggest more disuse atrophy than they do a primary muscle disorder. The serum CK and aldolase are usually normal. These changes are the same in Cushing disease and an otherwise unexplained proximal myopathy with these features suggests that diagnosis (Cushing disease and Cushing syndrome).

There is and imprecise correlation between the total dose of corticosteroid administered and the severity of muscle weakness. Nevertheless, in patients who develop this type of myopathy, the corticosteroid dosage has usually been high and sustained over a period of months or years. All corticosteroids may produce the disorder, although fluorinated ones, on uncertain evidence, are said to be more culpable than others. Discontinuation or reduction of corticosteroid administration leads to gradual improvement and recovery; alternate-day regimens may be also allow recovery, albeit gradually.

As the foregoing discussion implies, the mechanism by which corticosteroids cause muscle weakness is not known. In corticosteroid-treated animals, there is a measurable decrease in the uptake of amino acids and protein synthesis by muscle, but the underlying pathways have not been elucidated. This has even greater bearing on the next discussed subject.

Critical Illness Myopathy (Acute Steroid Myopathy; Acute Quadriplegic Myopathy)

In addition to the proximal myopathy induced by the long-term use of steroids, an acute and far more severe myopathy has been recognized in critically ill patients. It was described initially with cases of severe asthma in patients who were exposed to high doses of steroids for treatment. Subsequently this acute myopathy has been recognized with all types of critical systemic diseases and organ failure, again, usually in the context of the administration of high doses of corticosteroids but in a few cases, with sepsis and shock without exposure to this class of medication. Moreover, the use of neuromuscular blocking agents appears to play an important complementary role in the genesis of the myopathy, being reported as a factor in more than 80 percent of cases; it is uncertain whether these agents alone, without sepsis or organ failure, can produce a similar process (see reviews by Gorson and Ropper, Lacomis et al, and Barohn et al).

Patients who acquire this problem may have been exposed to high doses of corticosteroids for only brief periods. Exceptional instances have been reported in which the myopathy was induced by doses as low as 60 mg prednisone administered for 5 days, but we have not encountered such a case. The degree and type of simultaneous exposure to neuromuscular blocking agents have varied, but the doses have generally also been quite high, falling in the range of a total dose of 500 to 4,000 mg of pancuronium or an equivalent, over several days.

The severe generalized muscle weakness usually becomes evident when the systemic illness subsides, often as attempts are made to wean the patient from the ventilator. The tendon reflexes are normal or diminished, and there may be confounding features of a "critical illness polyneuropathy," which is discussed in Chap. 46. Most of our patients with acute myopathy have recovered over a period of 6 to 12 weeks after the corticosteroid agent has been greatly reduced in dose or withdrawn, but a few have remained weak for as long as a year.

Serum CK is elevated, at least early in the process. The EMG discloses the characteristic features of a myopathy; often there are fibrillations as well, theorized to be a result of separation of the motor endplate region from intact segments of muscle fibers. A concurrent polyneuropathy and any residual effects of neuromuscular blockade can be excluded by appropriate electrophysiologic studies. Muscle biopsy shows varying degrees of necrosis and vacuolation affecting mainly type 2 fibers. The identifying histologic feature is a striking loss of thick (myosin) filaments. Severe degrees of muscle necrosis occur and have been accompanied by massively elevated CK levels and by myoglobinuria with renal failure.

Several experimental observations may explain the apparent additive effect on muscle of corticosteroids and neuromuscular blocking agents. Animals exposed to high doses of steroids soon after experimental denervation of a muscle display a selective loss of myosin, the characteristic finding of acute steroid myopathy. Myosin depletion is reversed by reinnervation but not by withdrawal of the corticosteroids. Furthermore, denervation of muscle has been found to induce an increase in glucocorticoid receptors on the surface of the muscle. On this basis, Dubois and Almon have postulated that exposure to neuromuscular blocking agents creates a functional denervation, rendering the muscle fiber vulnerable to the damaging effects of steroids. It is curious that this myopathy has not been seen after high-dose corticosteroid administration for neurologic diseases such as multiple sclerosis, but the observation of Panegyres and colleagues of a patient with myasthenia who developed a severe, myosin-depleted myopathy following high doses of methylprednisolone supports such a dual action of denervation (at the postsynaptic membrane) and glucocorticoids. Whether it also explains the more common circumstance of clinical worsening of myasthenia gravis that sometimes accompanies the initial administration of corticosteroid treatment is also not clear.

Adrenocortical Insufficiency

Generalized weakness and fatigability are characteristic of adrenocortical insufficiency, whether *primary* in type, that is, because of *Addison disease* (infectious, neoplastic, or autoimmune destruction of the adrenal glands or adrenal hemorrhage), or secondary to a pituitary deficiency of adrenocorticotropic hormone (ACTH). The weakness and fatigability, however, are probably related to mostly water and electrolyte disturbances and hypotension, not to a primary disorder of muscle. Perhaps there is also an element of reduced central drive of motor activity. Biopsy has not disclosed any abnormalities of muscle and postmortem examination in one case showed no changes. Likewise, the EMG is normal, and the tendon reflexes are retained. Addisonian weakness responds (as does hyperkalemic paralysis) to glucocorticoid and mineralocorticoid replacement.

Primary Aldosteronism

Production of excess aldosterone by adrenal adenomas has been the subject of many articles, one of the earliest and most notable being that of Conn muscular weakness has been observed in 75 percent of the reported cases of hyperaldosteronism. In nearly half of those with muscle weakness there was either hypokalemic periodic paralysis or tetany. Chronic potassium deficiency may express itself either by periodic weakness or by a chronic myopathic weakness. An associated severe alkalosis causes the tetany. As in the weakness of Addison disease, there is no structural disorder of muscle, except perhaps for vacuolation, which is the result of severe hypokalemia.

Diseases of Parathyroid Glands and Vitamin D Deficiency

A proportion of patients with *parathyroid adenomas* complain of weakness and fatigability. Vicale described the first example of this disorder and remarked on the muscular atrophy and weakness and the pain on passive or active movement. The tendon reflexes were retained. A few scattered muscle fibers had undergone degeneration, but claims for a denervative muscle process are disputed. We have not been impressed with either a myopathy or neuropathy in this disease.

In *hypoparathyroidism*, muscle cramping is prominent, but there are no other neuromuscular manifestations. In both hypoparathyroidism and pseudohypoparathyroidism—the latter with characteristic skeletal abnormalities and, in some instances, mental slowness—the most important muscle abnormality is *tetany*. This is a result of low ionized serum calcium, which depolarizes axons more than muscle fibers (see Chap. 45 for a discussion of the effects of electrolytes on muscle function).

Osteomalacia, as a result of vitamin D deficiency and disorders of renal tubular absorption, often includes muscle weakness and pain as common complaints, similar to those in patients with primary hyperparathyroidism and with uremia (see Layzer for further comment).

More striking than any of the foregoing disturbances, in our view, has been a chronic proximal myopathy in conjunction with *hypophosphatemia associated with solitary bone cysts*. In two of our patients, removal of the cyst restored serum phosphorus levels and cured the generalized muscle weakness. Also known is an uncommon syndrome of severe hypophosphatemia and generalized bone pain in association with usually benign mesenchymal tumors of soft tissue and bone (*oncogenic hypophosphatemia*). These tumors express a fibroblast growth factor that induces renal wasting of phosphorous. *Hypophosphatemic myopathic weakness* has been noted in our and other critical care units, precipitated by hyperalimentation solutions; the onset of weakness can be so abrupt in this circumstance, as to simulate the Guillain-Barré syndrome. The oral administration of phosphates to raise serum phosphorus cures the nonneoplastic cases. Presumably phosphorus depletion limits the phosphorylation reactions and the synthesis of ATP in muscle.

Diseases of the Pituitary Gland

Proximal muscle weakness and atrophy have been recorded as late developments in many *acromegalic* patients. Formerly thought to be caused by neuropathy, these symptoms in acromegaly have been convincingly shown by Mastaglia and colleagues to be the result of a generalized myopathy. The serum CK is slightly elevated in some cases, and myopathic potentials are observed in the EMG. Biopsy specimens have shown atrophy and reduced numbers of type 2 fibers, but necrosis of only a few fibers. Treatment of the pituitary adenoma and correction of the hormonal changes restores strength. A mild peripheral neuropathy of sensorimotor type has also been reported in a few patients with acromegaly but is far less frequent than carpal tunnel syndrome and other focal entrapments in this disease.

MITOCHONDRIAL MYOPATHIES

(See Chap. 37)

The genetic aspects of mitochondrial diseases and the diverse and overlapping clinical syndromes that constitute this category—including the myopathic ones—are discussed in Chap. 37. The histologic change termed *ragged red fibers* reflects the mitochondrial changes of this class of diseases and is common to many of them, even without manifest symptoms of muscle disease.

MYOPATHIES CAUSED BY DRUGS AND TOXINS; RHABDOMYOLYSIS (Table 48-6)

A vast number of drugs and other chemical agents have been identified as myotoxic. In 1989, Curry and colleagues found reports (in the English literature alone) of approximately 100 drugs that had caused rhabdomyolysis and myoglobinuria, mostly acting in an idiosyncratic manner, and the list continues to grow. Additional myotoxic agents that can be expected to appear as new drugs are introduced. Because it is impractical to describe all the implicated drugs and toxins individually, they are broadly categorized and their main features listed in Table 48-6.

Exogenous agents may produce myopathic changes in several ways. They may act directly on muscle cells, either diffusely or locally, as occurs with intramuscular injections, or the muscle damage can be a result of diverse secondary factors—electrolyte disturbances (hypokalemia), renal failure, excessive energy requirements of muscle (as occur with drug-induced seizures and malignant hyperthermia), or inadequate delivery of oxygen and nutrients. Of course, there is a derivative category of drug-induced coma with compressive-ischemic injury to muscle. However, the most important group is that of direct toxic effects on the muscle membrane on the internal apparatus of the cell.

Several clinical features mark a myopathy as toxic in nature: lack of preexisting muscular symptoms; a predictable delay in onset of symptoms after exposure to a putative toxin; the lack of any other cause for the myopathy; and often, complete or partial resolution of symptoms after withdrawal of the toxic agent. Pathologically, this group of disorders is characterized by nonspecific myopathic changes, which in most severe degrees take the form of myonecrosis (rhabdomyolysis) and resultant myoglobinuria. This necrotizing muscle syndrome is the most frequent and serious myotoxic syndrome.

In any disease that results in rapid destruction of striated muscle fibers (rhabdomyolysis), myoglobin and other muscle proteins enter the bloodstream and appear in the urine. The latter is "cola"-colored (burgundy red or brown), much like the urine in hemoglobinuria. In hemoglobinuria, however, the serum is pink, because hemoglobin (but not myoglobin) is bound to haptoglobin, and this complex is not excreted in the urine as readily as myoglobin; also in addition, the hemoglobin molecule is three times as large as the myoglobin molecule. (The hemoglobin–haptoglobin complex is removed from the blood plasma over a period of hours and haptoglobin may be depleted, so that hemoglobinuria is present without grossly evident hemoglobinemia.) Differentiation of the two pigments in urine is difficult; both are guaiac-positive and may be detected by the "dipstick" test that can be used to advantage at the bedside in appropriate circumstances. Only small differences are seen on spectroscopic examination. The most sensitive means of detecting myoglobin is by radioimmunoassay. It should be mentioned that porphyrins are another cause of discoloration of the urine. The clinical picture in porphyria is one of a polyneuropathy and not a myopathy.

Many of the causes of myonecrosis have already been mentioned in this chapter, including acute inflammatory myopathy, several types of glycogenoses, CPT deficiency, and as a result of poisoning or therapeutic use of a vast array of drugs (including the combination of steroids and pancuronium in critically ill patients, discussed earlier), environmental toxins, and venoms (see Table 48-6). Myoglobinuria is an important feature of many other medical conditions: crush injury; extensive infarction of muscle that occurs in cases of vascular disease and of diabetes; in cases of severe acute alcohol intoxication, excessive use or repeated injury to muscles in status epilepticus, generalized tetanus, malignant hyperthermia, malignant neuroleptic syndrome, prolonged marching, electrical and lightning injuries; or simply excessive exercise—although muscle necrosis after exercise suggests an underlying metabolic disease of muscle.

Regardless of the cause of the rhabdomyolysis, the affected muscles become painful and tender within a few hours and their power of contraction is diminished. Sometimes the skin and subcutaneous tissues overlying the affected muscles (nearly always of the limbs and sometimes of the trunk) are swollen and congested. There is a marked elevation of CK in the serum and there may be a low-grade fever and a reactive leukocytosis. If myoglobinuria is mild, recovery occurs within a few days and there is only a residual albuminuria. When severe, renal damage may ensue and lead to anuric renal failure requiring dialysis. The mechanism of the renal damage is not entirely clear; it is not simply a mechanical obstruction of tubules by precipitated myoglobin (although this does occur).

Table 48-6

FEATURES OF TOXIN-INDUCED MYOPATHIES

MYOPATHIC SYNDROME	AGENT	CLINICAL FEATURES	PATHOLOGY	LABORATORY FINDINGS[a]
Necrotizing myopathy (rhabdomyolysis)	1. Statin drugs-immune mechanism 2. Alcohol excess 3. Clofibrate, gemfibrozil 4. Amphetamine derivatives	Acute/subacute painful proximal myopathy; tendon reflexes usually preserved	Necrosis, regeneration	CK ↑↑, myoglobinuria +/−
	5. Hypervitaminosis E	5. Painless	5. Paracrystalline inclusion bodies	
	6. Organophosphates			
	7. Snake venoms	7. Severe, acute intoxication		
	8. High-dose corticosteroids in critical illness	8. Neuromuscular blockers implicated		
	9. Mushroom poisoning (*Amanita phalloides*)		9. Loss of myosin	
	10. Cocaine			
Steroid myopathy	1. Acute (high IV steroid doses, ventilated patients on pancuronium) 2. Myasthenics	Severe proximal and distal weakness	1. Necrosis of mainly type 2 fibers; loss of myosin; vacuolar changes	CK ↑↑, myoglobinuria +
	3. Chronic	2 and 3. Proximal atrophy, weakness	2. Type 2 fiber atrophy	Blood lymphocytosis
Hypokalemic myopathy	1. Diuretics 2. Laxatives 3. Licorice, carbenoxolone 4. Amphotericin B, toluene 5. Alcohol abuse	Weakness may be periodic, reflexes may be depressed or absent, rarely severe myoglobinuria	Necrosis, regeneration, vacuolization	CK ↑↑, myoglobinuria +/−, hypokalemia
Amphiphilic cationic drug myopathy (lysosomal storage, "lipidosis")	1. Chloroquine (>500 mg), hydroxychloroquine, quinacrine, plasmocid 2. Amiodarone 3. Perhexiline	Proximal muscle pain and weakness, sensorimotor neuropathy, cardiomyopathy	Chloroquine: vacuole formation, optically dense structures	CK ↑
Impaired protein synthesis	Ipecac syrup, emetine	Myalgia, proximal weakness, cardiomyopathy	Focal mitochondrial loss, vacuoles	CK ↑
Antimicrotubular myopathy	1. Colchicine 2. Vincristine	Proximal weakness, peripheral neuropathy; CK may be normal	Vacuolar myopathy (rimmed vacuoles)	CK ↑
Inflammatory myopathy	1. D-Penicillamine 2. Procainamide 3. Cimetidine? Ciguatera toxin?	Proximal muscle pain, weakness, skin changes possible	Inflammation, necrosis, regeneration	CK ↑, myoglobinuria +/−
Fasciitis, perimyositis, microangiopathy	1. Toxic oil syndrome 2. Eosinophilia-myalgia syndrome	Myalgia, skin changes, peripheral neuropathy, other systems also affected	Vasculitis, connective tissue infiltration	Eosinophilia
Mitochondrial myopathy	1. Zidovudine 2. Germanium	Proximal myalgia and weakness	Ragged red fibers, necrosis, regeneration	CK normal or ↑
Various	1. Cyclosporine 2. Labetalol			
	3. Anthracycline antibiotics	3. Humans: only cardiomyopathy		
	4. Rifampin, amiodarone			
Local myopathy due to IM injections	1. Acute: IM injection of various drugs—e.g., cephalothin, lidocaine, diazepam	Local pain, swelling, sometimes abscess formation	Focal necrosis	CK ↑
	2. Chronic: Repeated IM injections—e.g., pethidine, pentazocine, intravenous drug abuse, antibiotics (in children)	Induration and contracture of injected muscles	Marked fibrosis and myopathic changes	Normal

[a]CK (serum creatinine kinase): ↑ (mild), ↑↑ (moderate), ↑↑↑ (marked) elevations; myoglobinuria: +/− (may be present).

Source: Adapted from Sieb JP: Myopathies due to drugs, toxins, and nutritional deficiency, in Engel AG, Franzini-Armstrong C (eds): *Myology*, 3rd ed. New York, McGraw-Hill, 2004, pp 1693–1712, by permission (originally from Victor and Sieb).

Treatment of Myoglobinuria Alkalinization of the urine by ingestion or infusion of sodium bicarbonate is said to protect the kidneys by preventing myoglobin casts, but in severe cases it is of doubtful value and the sodium may actually be harmful if anuria has already developed. Diuresis induced by mannitol or by loop diuretics such as furosemide and by the administration of intravenous fluids reduces the chances of anuric renal failure if given in time. Therapy is much the same as for the anuria that follows shock (see *Harrison's Principles of Internal Medicine*). In cases of focal muscle injury, for example, as occurs in diabetics or from vascular occlusion, surgical decompression of the overlying fascia and skin may be necessary to prevent ongoing ischemia, the "compartment syndrome."

Statin-Induced Myopathy

With the widespread use of these lipid-lowering medications, myotoxicity has become a well-described but possibly overrated idiosyncratic problem. Symptoms range in severity from mild muscular aches with slightly elevated CK concentrations in the serum to a rare but potentially fatal rhabdomyolytic syndrome. The first generation of these drugs were fungal metabolites (lovastatin, pravastatin, simvastatin) and were infrequently implicated in muscle damage, but the newer synthetic ones (atorvastatin, fluvastatin, cerivastatin) are more frequently toxic, especially when given with gemfibrozil (which has reportedly led to a small number of deaths from myoglobinuric renal failure and has been removed from the market). Few cases are this dramatic. The subject has been reviewed by Thompson and associates. Drugs in the statin class with higher lipid solubility appear to have a greater potential for toxicity as a result of their increased muscle penetration.

In addition to the direct toxicity, there is an autoantibody syndrome directed against HMGCo-A reductase, which is rarely induced by statins and may cause necrotizing myopathy as discussed in an earlier section.

The mechanism of directly toxic muscle damage is not well understood, but it is likely that inherent enzymatic defects are present in a proportion of the severe cases (see the brief review by Farmer). A novel insight derived from genome-wide screening has been that variants in a gene (*SLCO1B1*) that codes for an organic anion-transporting polypeptide confers a risk of statin myopathy (4.5-fold for a heterozygous state and 17 times for the homozygous state; see the study by The SEARCH Collaborative Group). In addition, the chronic use of statin drugs reduces levels of both ubiquinone and small guanosine triphosphate (GTP)–binding proteins, also plausible factors in statin-induced muscle toxicity.

A clinical problem arises when the CK level is elevated, but the patient taking one of these medications has no muscular symptoms. It has been our general practice to continue the medication if the elevation of CK is in the low range and does not rise over time, and if the medication is considered necessary. If alternative and safe means of lowering the lipid level are available, they should be tried in lieu of a statin, but each patient's circumstances differ. In a small series, Phillips and colleagues have called attention to a similarly vexing and not uncommon problem: myopathic symptoms such as muscle stiffness, tenderness, and weakness with normal CK concentrations in patients taking a drug in this class. A trial of discontinuing the medication might be appropriate. Finally, we have encountered a number of patients whose CK levels have remained high for months or longer after the medications have been stopped. In a few, CK elevations have remained over years, but we have had no way to ensure that the test was not abnormal before taking the statin. Noted in Chap. 46 is a polyneuropathy in which statin drugs have been tentatively implicated.

Colchicine Myoneuropathy

This condition is included here as much for its curious histopathologic features as for its clinical interest. The drug, used widely in the treatment of gout, often gives rise to a mild subacute proximal muscular weakness but has also produced an acute necrotizing myopathy. Most instances of the latter have occurred in patients with a degree of renal failure, which allows accumulation of the drug (even though the drug is metabolized predominantly by the liver). In rare instances the myopathy has affected the cranial musculature and the diaphragm. Many cases also show clinical or electrophysiologic evidence of a polyneuropathy, as pointed out by Kuncl and colleagues, leading to the term *colchicine myoneuropathy*. The reflexes are diminished and there is mild distal sensory loss. Rare cases of colchicine-induced hypokalemic periodic paralysis and also of myotonia have been reported.

The serum CK concentration may be elevated or normal. The muscle biopsy shows elements of both myopathic and neuropathic disease, with the special feature in muscle of rimmed vacuoles on the Gomori trichrome stain that are more central in the muscle fibers than those seen with inclusion body myositis. The mechanism of the muscle damage is unknown but is probably attributable to the drug's interference with tubulin, a protein required for the polymerization of microtubules in muscle and nerve. Weakness resolves in a matter of days or weeks when the drug is discontinued, but the neuropathic features may remain.

Other drugs that cannot be compactly summarized but may produce a toxic myopathy or neuromyopathy include *amiodarone*, *chloroquine*, and *hydroxychloroquine* as mentioned in Chap. 43.

Alcohol Myopathy

Several forms of muscle weakness have been ascribed to alcoholism. In one type, a painless and predominantly proximal weakness develops over a period of several days or weeks in the course of a prolonged drinking bout and is associated with severe degrees of *hypokalemia* (serum levels <2 mEq/L). The urinary excretion of potassium is not significantly increased, and depletion is probably the result of vomiting and diarrhea. In addition, serum levels of liver and muscle enzymes are markedly elevated. Biopsies from severely weakened muscles show single-fiber necrosis and vacuolation. Treatment consists of the administration of potassium chloride intravenously (about 120 mEq daily for several days), after which oral administration suffices. Strength returns gradually in 7 to 14 days, and enzyme levels return to normal concomitantly.

A more dramatic myopathic syndrome, occurring acutely at the height of a prolonged drinking bout and appropriately termed *acute alcoholic myopathy*, is manifest by severe pain, tenderness, and edema of the muscles of the limbs and trunk, accompanied in severe cases by renal damage (see Hed et al). Hypokalemia is not implicated. The myonecrosis is generalized in some patients, and remarkably focal in others. A swollen, painful, tender limb or part of a limb may give the appearance of a deep venous thrombosis or lymphatic obstruction. Myonecrosis is reflected by high serum levels of CK and aldolase and the appearance of myoglobin in the urine, leading in the most severe cases to fatal myoglobinuric renal failure. Indeed, in a general hospital, alcoholism is one of the most common causes of rhabdomyolysis and myoglobinuria, rivaled only by status epilepticus and trauma. Some patients recover within a few weeks, but others require several months, and relapse during another drinking spree occurs frequently. Restoration of motor power occurs with muscle regeneration but may be hindered by polyneuropathy and other syndromes of neuromuscular disability associated with alcoholism. Haller and Drachman have produced rhabdomyolysis in rats by subjecting the animals to a brief fast following a 2- to 4-week exposure to alcohol, suggesting that a similar mechanism may be operative in alcoholic individuals.

Perkoff and his associates described what is presumably a third form of acute muscular disorder in alcoholics, characterized by severe muscular cramps and diffuse weakness in the course of a sustained drinking bout. They noted a number of biochemical abnormalities in these patients, as well as in asymptomatic alcoholics who had been drinking heavily for a sustained period before admission to the hospital: elevated serum levels of CK, myoglobinuria, and a diminished rise in blood lactic acid in response to ischemic exercise. The status of this syndrome and its relation to the conventional acute alcoholic myopathy are unclear to us.

From time to time in alcoholics one observes the subacute or chronic evolution of painless weakness and atrophy of the proximal muscles of the limbs, especially of the legs, with only minimal signs in the distal segments of the legs and feet. Cases such as these have been referred to as *chronic alcoholic myopathy*, implying a direct toxic effect of alcohol on muscle, but the data are insufficient to warrant such an assumption. Some of these cases have shown necrosis of individual muscle fibers and other signs of polymyositis; most cases seen by the authors have proved to be neuropathic in nature. This has been the experience of others as well (Faris and Reyes; Rossouw et al). Treatment follows along the lines indicated for nutritional-alcoholic neuropathy, and complete recovery can be expected if the patient abstains from alcohol and maintains adequate nutrition.

THE CONGENITAL MYOPATHIES

Included under this section are two sizable groups of muscle diseases: one is an assemblage of congenital deformities that involve muscle and the other is a unique class of congenital myopathies. Insofar as all of the disorders comprising these categories are congenital, it may be helpful by way of introduction to refer briefly the main facts about the natural development and aging of muscle in the introductory section of this chapter. These diseases are of particular importance in pediatric neurology, for most of them attract notice at an early age.

Congenital Deformities of Muscle

Arthrogryposis (Table 48-7)

This disorder of multiple congenital contractures, now referred to as *arthrogryposis* (literally, curved joints), has been estimated to occur once in 3,000 births. The deformities result from a lack of movement during fetal development and are therefore produced by any disorder that immobilizes the developing embryo, whether from a lack of anterior horn cells, peripheral nerves, the motor end plate (as in an infant born to a myasthenic mother), or diseases of muscle. Often, there are associated developmental defects of the nervous system and somatic structures, low-set ears, wide and flat nose, micrognathia, and high-arched palate; less often, there are short neck, congenital heart disease, hypoplasia of the lungs, and cryptorchidism.

Of the many conditions that underlie arthrogryposis, developmental abnormalities of the anterior horn cells, mainly *Werdnig-Hoffmann disease* as discussed in Chap. 39, is by far the most common. A failure in development of anterior horn cells results in an uneven smallness and paresis of limb muscles. The unopposed contraction of relatively normally innervated muscles sets the fixed deformities. In a less common group of myopathic causes of arthrogryposis, the nervous system is usually intact and the disease is that of a congenital myopathy or congenital dystrophy. It has been observed that in the myopathic variety the limbs are fixed in a position of flexion at the hips and knees and adduction

Table 48-7

THE MAIN CAUSES OF ARTHROGRYPOSIS
Werdnig-Hoffmann motor neuron disease
Myotonic dystrophy
Congenital myasthenia (see Chap. 49)
Congenital myopathy
Congenital muscular dystrophy
Neonatal neuropathy
Prader-Willi syndrome
Amyoplasia (focal arthrogryposis)

of the legs, in contrast to the variable postures of the myelopathic (anterior horn cell) form. In addition to these two well-recognized causes of arthrogryposis, occasional cases are attributable to a neonatal neuropathy, neonatal myasthenia gravis, or to the Prader-Willi syndrome (causing intrauterine hypotonia).

An infant with arthrogryposis should be evaluated with an EMG that is interpreted by an experienced electromyographer, and by a biopsy of muscle for the detection of group atrophy and of the congenital myopathies described further on in this chapter. Both these tests are difficult to interpret in the incompletely formed nervous system of the premature infant. In many circumstances, it is valuable to delay the tests until several weeks of postterm development when the results are usually clearer. Sometimes, the electrophysiologic and biopsy tests may have to be repeated after several weeks or more to give a definitive diagnosis. If the initial evaluations are unrevealing, an imaging study of the brain to detect cerebral malformations and high-resolution banding of chromosome structure (or sequencing of chromosome 5 for Prader-Willi syndrome) may prove useful.

Congenital Focal Fibrous Contractures

This term refers to a fixation of limb posture as a result of a developmental lack or destruction of muscles, with shortening and fibrosis of supporting tissue and ligaments. A surprising number of deformities in infants and children are traceable to this type of defect. The most common are congenital clubfoot (talipes), congenital torticollis (*wryneck*), congenital elevation of the scapula (Sprengel deformity), and congenital dislocation of the hips. In all these conditions, the postural distortion is produced and maintained either by a weakened, fibrotic muscle or by a normal one that is contracted and shortened because of the absence of a countervailing antagonist. Trauma to a muscle during intrauterine life or at birth may lead to fibrosis and to fibrous contracture in some cases.

Congenital Clubfoot Here the deformity may be one of plantar flexion of the foot and ankle (talipes equinus), inversion (talipes varus or clubfoot), eversion (talipes valgus or splayfoot), or dorsiflexion of foot at the ankle (talipes calcaneus). Approximately 75 percent of cases are of the equinovarus clubfoot variety (i.e., the foot turns downward and inward). Usually both feet are affected. Multiple incidences may occur in one family. Several explanations of cause and pathogenesis have been offered: fetal malposition, an embryonic abnormality of tarsal and metatarsal bones, a primary defect in nerves or anterior horn cells of the spinal cord, or a congenital dystrophy of muscle. No one theory explains all cases, and available pathologic data exclude a single cause and pathogenesis. In some instances, clubfoot is the only recognizable congenital abnormality, but as often it occurs as a manifestation of generalized arthrogryposis (see later) and is an indicator of a more widespread intrauterine involvement of the CNS. (See Kakulas and Adams and also Banker for pertinent literature on the subject.)

Congenital Torticollis (Wryneck) This disorder begins during the first months of life and, unlike the torticollis of adults discussed in Chap. 6, it is not the result of a dystonia but instead is caused by congenital shortening of the sternocleidomastoid muscle, which is firm and taut. The head is inclined to one side and the occiput slightly rotated to the side of the affected muscle. This disorder is nonfamilial and is ascribed to injury to the sternocleidomastoid at birth. Whether the injury is a purely mechanical one to the muscle itself or is caused by ischemia stemming from arterial or venous occlusion (or an entirely different cause) is not clear. Congenital torticollis often gives rise to a sternocleidomastoid enlargement (a pseudotumor) that appears, on exploration, as a pale, spindle-shaped swelling of the muscle belly. The histologic findings are similar to those of Volkmann contracture, that is, replacement of the muscle fibers by relatively acellular connective tissue, suggesting that an ischemic mechanism underlies the defect in at least some cases.

Congenital Absence of Muscles (Amyoplasia)

It is well known that some individuals are born without certain individual muscles. This pertains not only to certain inconstant and functionally unimportant muscles, such as the palmaris longus, but also to more substantial ones. The muscles found to be absent most frequently are the pectoralis, trapezius, serratus anterior, and quadriceps femoris, but many single muscles may be missing in isolated cases.

Congenital absence of muscle is usually associated with congenital anomalies of neighboring nonmuscular tissues. For example, congenital absence of the pectoral muscle is accompanied by aplasia or hypoplasia of the mammary structures or of syndactyly and microdactyly. Agenesis of the pectoral muscle may also be associated with scoliosis, webbed fingers, and underdevelopment of the ipsilateral arm and hand (Poland syndrome). Another unusual constellation consists of congenital absence of portions of the abdominal muscles ("prune belly"), often in association with arthrogryposis and a defect of ureters, bladder, and genital organs. Amyoplasia also occurs in a few cases of facioscapulohumeral dystrophy.

Restricted Nuclear Amyotrophies

In another group of restricted palsies, the essential abnormality is in the CNS (nuclear amyotrophies). One of the most frequent is congenital ptosis as a result of an inborn defect of the innervation of the levator palpebrae muscles. Complete paralysis of all muscles supplied by the oculomotor nerve, apparently a result of hypoplasia of the third nerve nuclei, may be observed in several members of a family and occasionally in only one member. Bilateral abducens palsy is often associated with bifacial palsy in the newborn and is known as the *Möbius syndrome*; this usually nonfamilial anomaly, the cause of which is thought to be a nuclear hypoplasia or aplasia, is discussed with the developmental disorders in Chap. 38. In these familial nuclear amyotrophies, the muscles develop independently of the nervous system but have no prospect of surviving because of failure of innervation. It is, therefore, a kind of congenital denervation hypotrophy. Of course, a primary dystrophy may also give rise to bifacial weakness, as in FSHD.

CONGENITAL STRUCTURAL MYOPATHIES (Table 48-8)

Beginning in 1956, with the account by Shy and Magee of a patient whose muscle fibers showed a peculiar central densification of sarcoplasm ("cores"), a new class of hereditary diseases of muscle was delineated. The more common and better-defined members of this group are the *central core*, *nemaline* (rod-body), myotubular, and *centronuclear myopathies.* A variety of other types of congenital myopathy have been described, but they are relatively uncommon and some are of dubious specificity; they are mentioned only briefly. As the names imply, in each of these diseases there is no loss of muscle fibers, but within each fiber there is a distinctive morphologic abnormality. These processes usually express themselves early in life by a lack of muscle bulk, hypotonia, weakness of the limbs, and often, with additional but subtle dysmorphic features of other parts of the body.

Further study has revealed that the diseases of this group are not confined to infancy and early childhood and some of them, especially those present at birth, are not as benign as their early descriptions implied. Each of the entities mentioned earlier has been observed at a later age, even in middle adult life. Indeed, if the disease is mild, there is often no way of deciding whether it has been present since birth.

The characteristic feature of most of these myopathies, in addition to usual early onset, is *lack of progression* or *extremely slow progression*, in contrast to the more rapid pace of many muscular dystrophies, Werdnig-Hoffmann disease, and of other forms of hereditary motor system disease of childhood and adolescence. Exceptionally, an example of more rapid progression of a congenital myopathy has been reported, and prior to the use of histochemical and electron microscopic techniques such patients were usually considered to have a "benign muscular dystrophy." Familial occurrence has also been established in some types, so the clinical line of separation between this group of diseases and some of the more slowly progressive muscular dystrophies may in certain cases remain ambiguous. There is no specific treatment for any of the congenital myopathies.

The characteristic lesions in the congenital myopathies are revealed most clearly by the systematic application of histochemical stains to frozen sections of muscle biopsy tissue and by phase and electron microscopy. Some of the abnormalities are also disclosed by the conventional stains used in light microscopy, but as a group their identification has been the product of newer histologic techniques.

A word of caution is in order about the specificity of some of the morphologic changes and the classifications of the congenital myopathies based on these changes. It is inadvisable to assume that a change in a single organelle or a subtle change in the sarcoplasm of a muscle fiber can be relied on to characterize a pathologic process. Indeed, as more careful studies have been made of this class of disease, the specificity of some of the changes has come to

Table 48-8

THE MAIN CONGENITAL MYOPATHIES

TYPE	GENETICS	GENE OR CHROMOSOME	ONSET DECADE	CK ELEVATION	REGIONS AFFECTED
Central core disease	AD, AR	Ryanodine receptor	1st–2nd	1–10 ×	Diffuse myopathy presenting in infancy
					Proximal myopathy beginning in adolescence
					Risk of malignant hyperthermia
					May include mental retardation
Nemaline rod myopathy	AD, AR	α-Tropomyosin	1st–2nd	1–2 ×	Diverse phenotypes
		Nebulin			May present as severe congenital myopathy or as childhood-onset myopathy
		Coflin-2			
		β-Tropomyosin			May include facial weakness, high-arched palate, and high pedal arches
		Ryanodine receptor			
		Troponin T1			
		α-Actin			
Myotubular myopathy	X-linked	Myotubularin	1st	1–4 ×	Proximal and distal weakness
	AD, AR,	Dynamin-2			May include facial weakness, ophthalmoparesis, ptosis
		MYF6			

AD, autosomal dominant; AR, autosomal recessive; CK, creatine kinase.

be questioned. For example, central cores are sometimes found in the same muscle as nemaline bodies, and so on, and each of the denotative lesions has been reported in association with other systemic diseases and even as a result of certain medications. Nevertheless, the prominence of the morphologic change in any individual case, along with certain characteristic clinical features, permits an accurate diagnosis to be made.

Central Core Myopathy

In the original family described by Shy and Magee, 5 members (4 males) in 3 successive generations were affected, suggesting an autosomal dominant pattern of inheritance. The youngest was 2 years old; the oldest, 65 years. In each there was weakness and hypotonia soon after birth (again, "floppy infant") and a general delay in motor development, particularly in walking, which was not achieved until the age of 4 to 5 years. These patients had difficulty in rising from a chair, climbing stairs, and running. The weakness was greater in proximal than in distal muscles, although the latter did not escape, and shoulder-girdle muscles were affected less than those of the pelvic girdle. Facial, bulbar, and ocular muscles were spared. The tendon reflexes were hypoactive and symmetrical. Muscle atrophy was not a prominent feature, although poor muscular development was present in 1 patient and has since been reported in others. There were no fasciculations, cramps, or myotonia, but cramps following exercise have been described in other families. The ECGs were normal.

The disease is rare, but as additional cases have been discovered, milder forms have come to be recognized, and in some of them the symptoms first appeared in adult life. Originally these patients were thought to have limb-girdle dystrophy because of the disproportionate involvement of proximal muscles. In other families, such as the one reported by Patterson and colleagues, the disease was first recognized in middle adult life with the rapid evolution of a proximal myopathy. Dislocation of the hips, pes cavus or pes planus, and kyphoscoliosis has been found in a few children, but arthrogryposis is rare. In the majority of cases, the progress of the disease is extremely slow, with slight worsening over many years. These represent the two extremes of the process.

The EMG reveals brief, small-amplitude motor unit potentials with a normal interference pattern. Serum concentration of CK is normal or only slightly elevated, as it is in all the congenital myopathies.

The disease has another remarkable attribute in that every patient is a potential candidate for the development of *malignant hyperthermia* and should wear a bracelet or be otherwise identified to indicate vulnerability to this anesthetic-induced complication. A mutation for central core disease has been mapped to the ryanodine receptor, RYR1, on chromosome 19q13.1, a mutation of which is also implicated in the causation of a small number of cases of malignant hyperthermia (see Chap. 50) and of the rare recessively inherited condition of *minicore disease* (multiple, or multi-minicore), a congenital myopathy that may include ophthalmoplegia.

Pathologically, the majority of the muscle fibers appears normal in size or enlarged, and no focal destruction or loss of fibers can be found. The unique feature of the disease is the presence in the central portion of each muscle fiber of a dense, amorphous condensation of myofibrils or myofibrillar material. This altered zone characteristically lacks mitochondria and other organelles and gives a reduced positive PAS reaction and a dark blue coloration with the Gomori trichrome stain, contrasting with the normal blue-green color of the peripheral myofibrils. Within the core, there is a lack of phosphorylase and oxidative enzymes. Most of the cores are in type 1 fibers, which predominate in muscle biopsies. These cores run the length of the muscle fiber, thus differing from the multiple cores or minicores that are seen in oculopharyngeal and multiminicore myopathy.

Nemaline (Rod-Body) Myopathy

This disorder also expresses itself by hypotonia and impaired motility in infancy and early childhood, but unlike the case in central core disease, the muscles of the trunk and limbs (proximal greater than distal), as well as the facial, lingual, and pharyngeal muscles, are strikingly thin and hypoplastic. Several forms have been observed. One is congenital, with generalized weakness in the neonatal period, making breathing and feeding difficult. The limbs are flaccid and flexic (again "floppy" infant). Pneumonia and death occur within weeks to months. In forms that permit longer survival, the weakness is less severe, involving mainly the proximal muscles. Tendon reflexes are diminished or absent. The young child with this disease usually suffers from inanition and frequent respiratory infections, which may shorten life. Strength slowly improves with growth, the latter process evidently counteracting the advance of the disease.

A slender appearance, narrow face, open mouth, narrow, arched palate, and kyphoscoliosis are regular but not invariable accompaniments of nemaline myopathy. These dysmorphic features are not typical of the other congenital polymyopathies. Pes cavus or clubfoot may be added. Some of the milder cases reach adulthood, at which time a cardiomyopathy may threaten life. A.G. Engel, as well as W.K. Engel and Reznick, observed individuals who first showed signs of the disease in middle age; the weakness was mainly in proximal muscles and the dysmorphic and skeletal abnormalities of the childhood form were lacking. The EMG is "myopathic," and serum enzymes are normal or only slightly elevated.

Cases of nemaline myopathy have come to attention during adulthood because of disproportionate involvement of the *respiratory muscles*, a feature shared with the adult appearance of acid maltase deficiency. Usually these patients have had a history of poor physical performance throughout their earlier life.

An unexplained accompanying monoclonal gammopathy has appeared in case reports of late-onset nemaline myopathy and probably represents a separate process that is more than chance occurrence. In the series of late-onset cases described by Chahin and colleagues, 7 of 14 cases had an abnormal blood protein and these authors suggested that the prognosis may be less favorable than in those lacking the protein. The patients who have been shown with this combination of adult proximal weakness and monoclonal protein had no dysmorphic features, suggesting that these cases are different from the typical genetically determined nemaline myopathy described as follows.

Nemaline myopathy appears to be genetically heterogeneous. The pattern of inheritance is most often autosomal dominant with variable penetrance. In some families there has been an autosomal recessive or an X-linked pattern of inheritance. Studies of the various gene defects have begun to clarify the uncertainties about inheritance and explain the relationships between the different forms of the disease. The genes implicated in nemaline myopathy include those for alpha-tropomyosin, beta-tropomyosin, alpha-actin, nebulin, troponin, coflin-1, and the ryanodine receptor (the last of these is more commonly implicated in central core disease, as mentioned just above).

The disease is so named for the rods or coils of thread-like structures in pathology material. Frozen muscle tissue stained with Gomori trichrome discloses the characteristic lesion, which can be seen under the light microscope. Myriads of bacillus-like rods, singly and in small packets, are seen beneath the plasma membrane of the muscle fiber. They are composed of material that resembles that of Z bands under the electron microscope, and often actin filaments are attached, just as they are to Z bands. The type 1 fibers, which usually predominate, are smaller than normal, as in central core disease. The size of the motor neurons has been reported to be reduced. Weakness is probably related to a smallness and reduction in the number of muscle fibers and possibly to focal interruption of their cross-striations, particularly of the Z bands.

Centronuclear (Myotubular) Myopathy

In this familial disease, hypotonia and weakness become manifest soon after birth or in infancy or early childhood. In the mildest form, the diagnosis does not become evident until adult years. All the striated skeletal muscles are involved to some degree, but distinctive features are ptosis and ocular palsies combined with weakness of facial, masticatory, lingual, pharyngeal, laryngeal, and cervical muscles in most of the infants with this disease, but not in adults. In the limbs, distal weakness keeps pace with proximal weakness. The limbs remain thin and are flexic throughout life. Motor development is secondarily slowed, though some improvement with maturation can occur. Later, however, motor functions that had been acquired may be lost as the disease slowly advances. Several patients have shown signs of cerebral abnormality with seizures and an abnormal electroencephalogram (EEG), but it is not clear whether this is truly part of the disease. Needle EMG examination shows the usual myopathic pattern as well as both positive sharp waves and fibrillation potentials in some cases. Abundant spontaneous activity should suggest the diagnosis of centronuclear myopathy (Griggs et al).

Heckmatt and colleagues classified this disorder into three types, based on severity, mode of presentation, and genetic pattern: (1) a severe neonatal X-linked recessive type, now known to be associated mainly with mutations in myotubularin, MTM1; (2) a less severe early infantile, late-infantile, or childhood autosomal recessive type associated with BIN1, RYR1, or titin; and (3) a still milder late childhood–adult autosomal dominant type associated in some cases with mutations in DYN2 (dynamin) or MYF6, a helix-loop-helix protein that appears to function as a myogenic transcription factor.

The outstanding pathologic features of the disease are the smallness of muscles and their constituent fibers and central nucleation. In one group of centronuclear myopathies, there is hypotrophy of type 1 fibers (Bethlem et al; Karpati et al). Surrounding most of the centrally placed nuclei is a clear zone, in which there is a lack of organization of contractile elements. Because of central nucleation, the disease has incorrectly been referred to as *myotubular myopathy*, implying an arrest in development of muscle at the myotubular stage. Actually, the nature of the pathologic process is obscure. The small, centrally nucleated fibers do not really resemble typical myotubes. There is evidence from electron microscopic studies of changes in the central parts of the fibers (lack of enzymatic activity in the clear zones surrounding the nuclei), leading in all probability to fiber loss. Such changes argue against a purely developmental abnormality.

Myopathy With Tubular Aggregates

The accumulation of tubular aggregates in the subsarcolemmal or more interior regions of muscle fibers was first observed in patients with hypokalemic periodic paralysis and myotonia congenita, and later with a number of diverse conditions, such as chronic drug intoxication, hypoxia, and congenital myasthenic syndromes. However, tubular aggregates are also the defining feature of several rare and purely myopathic syndromes: (1) a slowly progressive muscular weakness, in a limb-girdle distribution, with onset in childhood or early adult life; inheritance is either autosomal dominant or recessive in type; (2) a childhood onset of proximal weakness, easy fatigability, and myasthenic features; heredity is autosomal recessive. This syndrome may respond to pyridostigmine; and (3) muscle pain, cramps, and stiffness induced by exercise; the cases to date have been sporadic.

The histologic changes are readily overlooked in paraffin sections. Frozen sections show masses of material that is basophilic with hematoxylin and eosin and bright red with Gomori trichrome and shows an intense reaction with reduced form of nicotinamide adenine dinucleotide (NADH) dehydrogenase. By electron microscopy, the bundles of tubular aggregates are sharply demarcated from myofibrils.

Other Congenital Myopathies

The foregoing congenital myopathies—central core, nemaline, centronuclear, and tubular aggregate types—are fairly well-defined clinicopathologic entities. Other less common types have been described, each named according to a distinctive morphologic alteration of organelles in muscle fibers in histochemical and electron microscopic preparations. In none of these additional types has the pattern of inheritance or the gene locus been identified. Some of these myopathies (*multicore [minicore], fingerprint body, sarcotubular*) have been reported in only a few cases, quite insufficient to allow their categorization as disease entities. Two other types, *congenital fiber type disproportion* and *congenital fiber type predominance*, originally designated as congenital myopathies, have proved to be nonspecific histochemical alterations observed in many infants and children with congenital developmental abnormalities, delays in motor development, and other conditions. Other putative congenital myopathies include so-called *reducing body*, *trilaminar*, and *cap disease; zebra body*; and *familial myopathy with lysis in type 1 fibers*, among others. They most likely also represent nonspecific reactions in muscle or fixation artifacts; as yet there is no evidence that any one of them represents a clinicopathologic entity.

Myofibrillar Myopathy

This entity, more a group of myopathies, was formerly included among the congenital myopathies but now clearly belongs in the category of dystrophies and is discussed in an earlier section on that class of diseases.

As stated in the introductory section, there is currently no treatment for any of the congenital myopathies.

THE SPINAL MUSCULAR ATROPHIES OF INFANCY AND CHILDHOOD (See Chap. 39)

Obviously this important group of diseases, appearing as they do in the same periods of life as the congenital myopathies and of certain of the congenital muscular dystrophies, must figure in the differential diagnosis of early-onset muscle weakness, hypotonia, and of arthrogryposis. Indeed, they represent the main problems faced by the clinician studying neuromuscular diseases of the infant. Their hereditary nature, their progression to fatal outcome or delayed motor attainments, and their tendency in certain instances to produce disabling contractures are shared with the primary muscle diseases. The proper application of current laboratory techniques sets them apart in most instances. In deference to their neuronal origin, we have placed them with the other degenerative diseases in Chap. 39.

DISORDERS OF MUSCLE CHARACTERIZED BY CRAMP, SPASM, PAIN, AND LOCALIZED MASSES (See also Chap. 50)

Quite apart from spasticity and rigidity, which are caused by a disinhibition of spinal motor mechanisms, there are forms of muscular stiffness and spasm that can be traced to abnormalities of the lower motor neuron and its spinal inhibitory mechanisms or to the sarcolemma of the muscle fiber. Muscles may go into spasm because of an unstable depolarization of motor axons, sending volleys of impulses across neuromuscular junctions—as occurs in myokymia, hypocalcemic tetany, and pseudohypoparathyroidism. In other states, the innervation of muscle is normal, but contraction persists despite attempts at relaxation (myotonia). Or, after one or a series of contractions, the muscle may be slow in decontracting, as occurs in paradoxical myotonia and hypothyroidism. In the contracture of McArdle phosphorylase deficiency and phosphofructokinase deficiency, muscle, once contracted, lacks the energy to relax. In yet another type of muscle stiffness, the muscle may ripple or respond to percussion by mounding and rapidly contrasting and relaxing. Cramping should also be differentiated from restless leg syndrome (see Chap. 19), which is primarily a nocturnal disorder but may carry over into the daytime hours.

Each of these conditions evokes the complaint of cramp or spasm, which is variably painful and interferes with free and effective voluntary activity. Each condition has its own identifying clinical and EMG characteristics and most of them respond favorably to therapy.

MUSCLE CRAMP

This subject was introduced at the beginning of this chapter, where it is pointed out that everyone at some time or other experiences muscle cramps. Cramps often occur during the night, after a day of unusually strenuous activity; less frequently they occur during the day, either during a period of relaxation or occasionally after a strong voluntary contraction or postural adjustment. A random restless or stretching movement may induce a hard contraction of a single muscle (most frequently of the foot or leg) that cannot be voluntarily relaxed. The muscle is visibly and palpably taut and painful, and the condition is readily distinguished from an illusory cramp, in which the sensation of cramp is experienced with little or no contraction of muscle. The latter phenomenon may occur in normal persons as well as in those with peripheral nerve diseases. Massage and vigorous stretch of the cramped muscle will cause the spasm to yield, although for a time the muscle remains excitable and subject to recurrent cramps. Visible fasciculations may precede and follow the cramp, indicating excessive excitability of the terminal branches of motor neurons supplying the muscle. Sometimes the cramp is so intense that the muscle is injured; it remains sore to touch and painful upon use for a day or longer. Cramps of precordial chest muscles or diaphragm may arouse fear of heart or lung disease. In the EMG, the cramp is marked by bursts of high-frequency, high-voltage action potentials, and the precramp phase shows runs of activity in motor units. Why cramps should be painful is not known; probably the demands of the overactive muscle exceed metabolic supply, causing a relative ischemia and accumulation of metabolites. Overwork of muscle with or without impairment of circulation is also painful. Between cramps, the muscles are normal clinically and electromyographically.

Cramps are known to increase in frequency under certain conditions and with certain diseases. They are common during pregnancy for reasons not fully understood. Dehydration and excessive sweating predispose to cramping and are a constant threat to athletes. Exertional cramps are elicited more easily than usual in motor system disease, hypothyroidism, and in chronic polyneuropathies. Focal cramping occurs after partial nerve or root injury. For example, the calf muscle on one side is subject to severe recurrent cramps after decompression of the S1 root for lumbar disc disease; in extreme cases, the muscle hypertrophies after long periods of intermittent cramping. Patients undergoing hemodialysis are subject to cramps, which can be suppressed by intravenous hypertonic saline or hypertonic glucose.

The mechanism of muscle cramping is obscure. Several enzymes have been implicated, among them, myoadenylate. This enzyme, which is present in high concentration in muscle, is thought to function primarily during aerobic exercise and facilitate the regeneration of ATP from ADP through the action of adenylate kinase. However, low levels of this enzyme are not specific, occurring in such unrelated disorders as hypokalemic periodic paralysis and spinal muscular atrophy (see Layzer for details).

Quinine sulfate (300 mg at bedtime and repeated in 4 h if necessary, or 300 mg tid for idiopathic diurnal cramping) had been an effective medication but is no longer widely used because of a low risk of ventricular arrhythmia. Some patients, nonetheless, seek relief from the use of quinine water, some brands of which still contain the chemical. Diphenhydramine hydrochloride (Benadryl) 50 mg or procainamide 0.5 to 1.0 g are alternatives. Phenytoin, carbamazepine, and other antiepileptic drugs, and clonazepam may be useful in alleviating repeated daytime cramping.

Tetany, Pseudotetany, and Related Cramp Syndromes

As pointed out earlier, a reduction in ionizable calcium and magnesium is associated with involuntary cramp-like spasms; in their mildest form they appear as distal carpopedal spasms, but they may involve any of the muscles except the extraocular ones. Under these circumstances, stimulation of a muscle through its nerve at high frequencies (15 to 20 times per second) reproduces spasms, and hyperventilation and ischemia increase the tendency. Indeed, the Trousseau sign—carpal spasms with occlusion of the blood supply to the arm—takes advantage of the latter phenomenon. Hypocalcemic tetany is attributable to an unstable depolarization of the axonal membrane of the nerve fiber. This mechanism is affirmed by (1) the sensitivity of nerve to percussion (e.g., tapping over the facial nerve near its foramen of exit induces a facial twitch, or Chvostek sign), (2) fast-frequency doublets and triplets of motor unit potentials in the EMG indicating excessive neural excitability, (3) evocation of spasm by application of a tourniquet to proximal parts of a limb (causing ischemia of segments of nerve beneath the tourniquet), and (4) the associated tingling, prickling paresthesias from excitation of sensory nerve fibers. Hypocalcemia also causes a lesser change in the muscle fibers themselves; hence nerve block does not completely eradicate tetany. We comment here that the Chvostek sign is found in some normal individuals, without obvious explanation.

The previously described idiopathic benign cramps resemble tetany but without measurable hypocalcemia (*pseudotetany*). Just as in tetany, in about half of cases of benign cramp, stimulation of nerve at 15 or more times per second produces repetitive discharges. Biopsies have disclosed no abnormalities of the muscle fibers except for a few ringbinden (circumferential bands of myofibrils encircling a normal core of longitudinally oriented myofibrils). Calcium and diazepam are of no therapeutic value, but some patients respond to phenytoin, quinine (no longer widely used because of the risk of arrhythmia), procainamide, or chlorpromazine.

A familial (autosomal dominant) form of the benign cramp syndrome was reported by Jusic and coworkers; the cramps affected the distal limb muscles, began in childhood and adolescence, and persisted throughout life. Another such family with cramps beginning somewhat later in life and affecting the anterior neck, arm, and abdominal muscles as well as those of the thigh and calf was described by Ricker and Moxley. Also, a familial myalgic-cramp syndrome alluded to early in this chapter has been associated with deletion of part of the dystrophin gene (but with little or no dystrophic weakness). A tendency to cramp and pain has also been noted in a number of the congenital myopathies and in some families with Duchenne and Becker dystrophies.

Satoyoshi Syndrome

Satoyoshi described a group of patients who, in addition to widespread and severe cramping of muscle, developed universal alopecia, amenorrhea, intestinal malabsorption with frequent diarrhea, and some developed epiphyseal destruction and retarded growth. Most Japanese patients he described were younger than 20 years, but the 2 cases we have observed in whites were middle-aged. The serum calcium in these patients is normal, and the EMG shows only high-frequency discharges that are characteristic of cramps. A patient of ours with this condition had decades of chronic diarrhea, alopecia, and continuous, extremely painful calf cramps that had the gross appearance of fasciculations. This triad virtually identifies the disease. The cause of the disorder is obscure but is tentatively presumed to be autoimmune. Glucocorticoids, particularly in high doses over short periods, have been tried with some success; dantrolene has also been used and we had the impression that plasma exchange may have been helpful in one case.

Continuous Muscle Fiber Activity Due to Disorders of Nerve And Distal Axons

(See Chap. 50)

While the main manifestations of this group of disorders, muscular cramps, would seem to belong in this chapter on muscle diseases, they are, in fact, related to disorders of motor nerves, axons, and their terminal arborizations. For this reason, they appear in Chap. 50 on channelopathies and in Chap. 46, with disorders of the peripheral nerves.

MYALGIC STATES

Many of the muscle diseases described previously are associated with aching and discomfort. These are particularly prominent in conditions that are accompanied by cramp and biochemical contracture (phosphorylase and phosphofructokinase deficiency). Ischemia of muscle—that is, intermittent claudication—is also painful, as is dystonia in some cases. Muscle weakness that imposes persistent abnormal postures on the limbs may cause stretch injury to muscles and tendons. This is observed in a number of the congenital myopathies and dystrophies. In all these conditions, clinical study will usually disclose the source or sources of the pain.

Diffuse muscle pain, which merges with malaise, is a frequent expression of a large variety of systemic infections—for example, influenza, brucellosis, dengue, Colorado tick fever, measles, malaria, relapsing fever, rheumatic fever (in which it was called "growing pains"), salmonellosis, toxoplasmosis, trichinosis, tularemia, and Weil disease. When the pain is intense, especially if it is localized to one side of the lower chest and abdomen, the most likely diagnostic possibility is epidemic myalgia (also designated as *pleurodynia*, "devil's grip," and *Bornholm disease* caused by Coxsackievirus infection). Poliomyelitis may be accompanied by intense pain at the onset of neurologic involvement, and later the paralyzed muscles may ache. This is true also of the Guillain-Barré syndrome, in which the pain may precede weakness by several days. Little is known about the pathologic basis of the muscular pain in these diseases; it is not a result of muscle inflammation and is probably produced by circulating cytokines that are common to most systemic infections. Mild muscle pain is a frequent but not a necessary accompaniment of polymyositis and dermatomyositis.

Polymyalgia Rheumatica (See Chap. 11)

The major consideration in elderly and middle-aged patients with pain in proximal muscles of the limbs is polymyalgia rheumatica. This subject is mentioned briefly in other sections of this book in relation to back and extremity pain (see Chap. 11) and to temporal arteritis, to which it is closely connected (see Chap. 10). The muscular soreness may be diffuse or asymmetrical, particularly in the proximal arms and shoulders. Every movement is reported as stiff and painful. The periarticular tissues and their muscular attachments are affected primarily and may be tender, but this is difficult to interpret, because tenderness in these regions may be found in healthy individuals. The sedimentation rate is elevated in the majority of patients, and a 48-h trial of prednisone, by completely alleviating muscle pain, confirms the diagnosis. In the context of muscle pain, systemic symptoms such as weight loss, headache, and fatigue, as well as mild anemia, are particularly suggestive of polymyalgia rheumatica.

Fibromyalgia

This would appear, by definition, to represent an inflammation or other affection of the fibrous tissues of the muscles, fascia, and aponeuroses. Unfortunately, the pathologic basis of this state remains obscure. Only some clinical facts can be stated. During the first movements after a period of inactivity, a muscle or group of muscles may become painful and tender, particularly after exposure to cold, dampness, or minor trauma, but often for no reason that can be discerned. One looks in vain for signs of tendinous, muscular, or arthritic disease. The neck and shoulders are the most common sites. Tender areas, up to several centimeters in diameter, can be palpated within the muscles ("fibrositic nodules" by experts), and active contraction or passive stretching of the involved muscles increases the pain—points said to be of diagnostic value, but disputed. Often, symptoms such as mental and physical fatigue, insomnia, and headache are associated and raise the suspicion of an anxiety state or depression. In a few instances the condition clears up in a few weeks; local heat and massage and local injections of anesthetics or steroids are found to give comfort while symptoms are present, but most often it becomes a chronic condition.

The chronic form of fibromyalgia presents far greater problems, usually disabling the patient and causing a change in accustomed habits and employment as discussed in Chap. 11. It has become one of the prime diagnoses made by rheumatologists and physiatrists, but the patient may first come to the attention of a neurologist. Most definitions of the syndrome have been circular or somewhat arbitrary. Those now in general use are similar to the one proposed by a committee of the American College of Rheumatology. The basis for diagnosis is the presence of widespread pain, including focal areas of pain (trigger points) that can be produced by 4 kg of digital pressure in 11 of 18 typical locations over muscles, tendons, or bone—these are concentrated around the shoulders and paraspinal regions—and there is no requirement for the presence of the several common systemic complaints that accompany the illness in most patients (fatigue, difficulty concentrating, sleeping difficulty, or anxiety). In the past, similar pains were associated with cases of irritable bowel or irritable bladder syndromes, dysmenorrhea, chronic headache, and cold intolerance. Depending on how broad a definition one allows for the widespread pain and painful trigger points, most or all patients in our experience manifest many of the same complaints as those with the chronic fatigue syndrome, which is discussed in Chap. 24. Writers on the subject, however, have pointed out that in the majority of patients, formal assessment by modern criteria fails to confirm the presence of depression, and that when depression coexists with the muscular complaints, the two are discordant temporally and in severity. While we acknowledge that antidepressants often give disappointing results and that in our practice there have been a number of patients with fibromyalgia who appeared to be psychologically sound and lacked depression, they have been the exceptions. The literature eschews the use of corticosteroids for treatment of the pain, but we have had occasion to see patients whose symptoms were relieved when these medications were used for other purposes.

Fibromyalgia remains a problematic illness, defined largely by a pattern of pain that justifies its name. Despite attempts to objectify the physical symptoms, psychiatric factors should not be overlooked. This condition is a favorite illness with physiotherapists, who claim that their physical measures are helpful, as they may well be. Rarely, a similar syndrome is the forerunner of what proves, after some days, with the onset of neurologic signs, to be a radiculitis, brachial neuritis, or outbreak of herpes zoster (see Goldenberg).

Other Myalgic States

An impressive polymyalgia follows excessive exercise. Often, the patient observes that aching pain occurs not at the time of activity but some hours or even a day or two later, resembling the discomfort following the excessive use of unconditioned muscles. The muscles are sore and there is an intolerance of exercise and physical exertion. The serum CK concentration is mildly to moderately elevated. This is a natural phenomenon and is self-limiting. When such a state persists indefinitely and a program of conditioning exercises does not alleviate the pain, it represents a special category of disease. In a few instances an increased sedimentation rate or other laboratory aids may clarify the diagnosis, and muscle biopsy may reveal a nonspecific interstitial nodular myositis or the giant cell arteritis associated with polymyalgia rheumatica. Whether or not patients on lipid-lowering statin medications are particularly susceptible to this problem is not clear. A few individuals go on to have the features of the previously described fibromyalgic syndrome. However, this cluster of symptoms most often occurs without explanation, and one can only suspect an obscure infection or a subtle aberration of muscle metabolism, presently impossible to demonstrate. Reference has been made in the literature to the controversial finding of a *myoadenylate deaminase deficiency* in some of these cases. There is also a group of patients who have idiopathic leg pain during rest after activity. Some families afflicted in this way are forced to live a sedentary existence. The condition does not respond to analgesics. In 2 cases, a deficiency of calcium ATPase was found and reportedly alleviated by a calcium channel blocker such as verapamil, 120 mg (Walton; Taylor et al). It must be distinguished from the syndromes of painful legs and moving toes, and from the restless leg syndrome discussed in Chap. 19.

Before dismissing vague muscle aches as an excessive somatic concern, hypothyroidism, hyperparathyroidism, and renal tubular acidosis, hypophosphatemia, hypoglycemia, and the intrinsic phosphorylase or phosphofructokinase defects should be considered. Patients with these latter diseases often complain of soreness, stiffness, and lameness after strenuous muscular effort. According to Mills and Edwards, *the most valuable screening tests are the sedimentation rate and serum CK concentration*. Some patients probably have an obscure metabolic myopathy, presently undiagnosable. In every reported series, such as that of Serratrice and coworkers, half of the cases with diffuse myalgia are of this uncertain type. This coincides with, or is more optimistic than, our own experience.

LOCALIZED MUSCLE MASSES

Masses may be found in one or many muscles in a variety of clinical settings, and the clinical findings in each one have a different significance.

Muscle or tendinous rupture is usually caused by a violent strain attended by an audible snap and then a bulge, which appears when the muscle contracts. A very focal weakening in contractile power and mild discomfort are usually noted by the patient. The biceps brachii and soleus muscles are most often affected. Treatment is by surgical repair; if that is delayed, little can be done for the condition.

Hemorrhage into muscle may occur as a consequence of trauma, as a complication of the use of anticoagulants, in hematologic diseases, in severe myotonia, or after a minor trauma to a patient with Zenker degeneration of muscle who is convalescing from typhoid fever or some other infection. Runners may acquire painful localized hematomas in leg muscles.

Tumors of muscle include *desmoid tumor* (a benign massive growth of fibrous tissue observed most often in parturient women and after surgery), *rhabdomyosarcoma* (a highly malignant tumor with strong liability to local recurrence and metastasis), *liposarcoma*, and *angioma*. Large neurofibromas or neurofibrosarcomas beneath large muscles such as the hamstring may be difficult to differentiate by physical examination or MRI from masses within the muscle. *Pseudotumorous* growths, sometimes massive, may follow injury to a muscle. Interlacing regenerating muscle fibers and fibroblasts compose the mass. Excision of the entire muscle had been undertaken in several cases in the belief that the growth was a rhabdomyosarcoma, whereas it is actually a benign reaction to trauma (Kakulas and Adams). Metastasis to muscle occurs, most often lymphomatous in our experience.

Thrombosis of arteries or, more often, of *veins* causes congestion and infarction of muscle. A special type of *muscle infarction* occurs in patients with complicated and poorly controlled diabetes mellitus (Banker and Chester). Usually it involves the anterior thigh, and occasionally other muscles of the lower limb. The symptoms are the sudden onset of pain and swelling of the thigh, with or without the formation of a tender, palpable mass. Recurrent infarction of the same or opposite thigh is characteristic. The stereotypical clinical picture and the striking MRI appearance obviate the need for diagnostic muscle biopsy. Extensive infarction of muscle is due to the occlusion of many medium-sized muscular arteries and arterioles, most likely the result of embolization of atheromatous material from eroded plaques in the aorta or iliac arteries. Recognition of this complication and immobilization of the limb are of prime practical importance, as muscle biopsy and early ambulation may cause serious hemorrhage into the infarcted tissue.

The *pretibial*, or *compartment syndrome*, also well recognized, follows direct trauma or excessive activity (marching, exercising of unconditioned muscles) or ischemic infarction due to arterial occlusion. There is swelling of the extensor hallucis longus, extensor digitorum longus, and anterior tibial muscles. Being tightly enclosed by the bones and pretibial fascia, the swelling leads to ischemic necrosis and myoglobinuria. Permanent weakness of this group of muscles can be prevented by incising the pretibial fascia and thereby decompressing the affected muscles. A similar compartment syndrome can occur in the forearm.

Myositis Ossificans

This condition involves the deposition of bone within the substance of a muscle. Two types are recognized. One is a localized form that appears in a single muscle or group of muscles after trauma, and the other is a progressive, widespread ossifying process, entirely unrelated to trauma, in many muscles of the body.

Localized (Traumatic) Myositis Ossificans After a muscle tear, a single blow to the muscle, or repeated minor trauma, a painful area develops in the muscle. It is gradually replaced by a mass of cartilaginous consistency, and within 4 to 7 weeks a solid mass of bone can be felt and seen in CT or radiographs. This most frequently happens in vigorous adult men. The inner thigh muscles (in those who ride horses) and to a lesser extent the pectoralis major and biceps brachii are the most frequent locations. The mass tends to subside after several months if the patient desists from the activity that produced the trauma.

Generalized Myositis Ossificans This disease, first described by Munchmeyer in 1869, has since been referred to by his name or as *myositis ossificans progressiva*. It is rare, although Lutwak, in 1964, was able to collect 264 cases from the literature. The cause is unknown, but the disease is probably inherited as an autosomal dominant trait. It consists of widespread bone formation along the fascial planes of muscles and has its onset in infancy and childhood in 90 percent of cases. Biopsies of indurated swellings have revealed extensive proliferation of interstitial connective tissue in which little inflammatory cell reaction is found. Within a few weeks, the connective tissue becomes less cellular and retracts, compressing the adjacent muscle fibers. Osteoid and cartilage formation occur at a later stage, developing in the connective tissue and enclosing relatively intact muscle fibers.

Nearly 75 percent of all reported cases have been associated with congenital anomalies, the most frequent of which is a failure of development of the great toes or thumbs and less often, other digits. Less frequently, there is hypogenitalism, deafness, and an absence of upper incisors. The first symptom is often a firm swelling and tenderness in a paravertebral or cervical muscle. There is, in addition, a mild discomfort during muscle contraction, and the overlying skin may be reddened and slightly swollen. Trauma may be recalled as the initiating factor, but as the months pass, other muscles not injured in any recognizable way become similarly involved. At first, radiographs reveal no important changes, but within 6 to 12 months, calcium deposits are observed, and one can feel stony-hard masses within the muscles. As the disease advances, limitation of movement and deformities become increasingly evident. Calcified bridges between adjacent muscles and across joints lead to rigidity of the spine, jaw, and limbs; scoliosis; and limited expansion of the thorax. Ultimately, the patient is virtually "changed to stone." A genetic basis for one type, fibrodysplasia ossificans progressiva, has been determined.

The principal problem in diagnosis is to differentiate generalized myositis ossificans from *calcinosis universalis*. The latter usually occurs in relation to scleroderma or polymyositis and is characterized by calcium deposits in the skin, subcutaneous tissues, and connective tissue sheaths around the muscles; in myositis ossificans, there is actual bone formation within the muscles. The pathologic data are often too meager to justify this sharp distinction. The prolonged ingestion of large doses of vitamin D may also result in the deposition of masses of calcium salts around muscles, joints, and subcutaneous tissue.

Calcific deposits, perhaps true ossification, may occur in the soft tissues around the hips and knees of paraplegics and rarely following a hemiplegia ("paralytic myositis ossificans") or other causes of prolonged immobilization such as casting.

Myositis ossificans may undergo spontaneous remissions and may stabilize for many years, during which the patient is capable of adequate function. In other cases, progression leads to marked debilitation and respiratory embarrassment, the final illness often being a terminal pneumonia or other infection.

The molecular basis for myositis ossificans is unknown, but it has been suggested that one causative defect is the overexpression of bone morphogenic protein. In mice, the forced expression of this protein induces heterotopic bone formation. It is likely that the primary problem arises either because of inappropriate expression of one element of the protein or of excessive binding between signaling proteins and their receptors (Glaser et al).

Treatment

The administration of a diphosphonate (ethane-1-hydroxy-1,1-diphosphate [EHDP], 10 to 20 mg/kg orally), a compound that inhibits the deposition of calcium phosphate, has been said to cause regression of new swellings and to prevent calcification (Russell et al). Some of the calcium deposits in calcinosis universalis have receded in response to prednisone, and because of the unclear relationship of this disease to generalized myositis ossificans, it is probably advisable to try this form of therapy as well. Excision of bony deposits may be undertaken if it is certain that they are the cause of particular disabilities.

References

Adams RD: Thayer lectures: I. Principles of myopathology: II. Principles of clinical myology. *Johns Hopkins Med J* 131:24, 1972.

Adams RD, Kakulas BA, Samaha FA: A myopathy with cellular inclusions. *Trans Am Neurol Assoc* 90:213, 1965.

Aleksic S, Budzilovich C, Choy A: Congenital ophthalmoplegia in oculoauriculovertebral dysplasia hemifacial microsomia (Golden-har-Gorlin syndrome). *Neurology* 26:638, 1976.

Amato AA, Griggs RC: Unicorns, dragons, polymyositis, and other mythological beasts. *Neurology* 61:288, 2003.

Amato AA, Gronseth GS, Jackson CE, et al: Inclusion body myositis: Clinical and pathological boundaries. *Ann Neurol* 40:581, 1996.

Amato AA, Russell J: *Neuromuscular Disease*. New York, McGraw-Hill, 2008.

André-Thomas, Chesni Y, Saint-Anne Dargassies S: The neurological examination of the infant, in MacKeith RC, Polani PE, Clayton-Jones E (eds): *Little Club Clinics in Developmental Medicine*, No. 1. London, National Spastics Society, 1960.

Andreu AL, Hanna MG, Reichman H, et al: Exercise intolerance due to mutations in the cytochrome b gene of mitochondrial DNA. *N Engl J Med* 341:1037, 1999.

Antony JH, Procopis PG, Ouvrier RA: Benign acute childhood myositis. *Neurology* 29:1068, 1979.

Arahata K, Ishiura S, Ishiguro T, et al: Immunostaining of skeletal and cardiac muscle surface membrane with antibody against Duchenne muscular dystrophy peptide. *Nature* 333:861, 1988.

Armstrong RB: Mechanisms of exercise-induced, delayed onset muscular soreness: A brief review. *Med Sci Sports Exerc* 16:529, 1984.

Aslanidis C, Jansen G, Amemiya C, et al: Cloning of the essential myotonic dystrophy region and mapping of the putative defect. *Nature* 355:548, 1992.

Awerbuch GI, Nigro MA, Wishnow R: Beevor's sign and facioscapulohumeral dystrophy. *Arch Neurol* 47:1208, 1990.

Azher SN, Jankovic J: Camptocormia. Pathogenesis, classification, and response to therapy. *Neurology* 65:355, 2005.

Banker BQ: Congenital deformities, in Engel AG, Franzini-Armstrong C (eds): *Myology*, 3rd ed. New York, McGraw-Hill, 2004, pp 1931–1962.

Banker BQ: Dermatomyositis of childhood: Ultrastructural alterations of muscle and intramuscular blood vessels. *J Neuropathol Exp Neurol* 34:46, 1975.

Banker BQ: Other inflammatory myopathies, in Engel AG, Franzini-Armstrong C (eds): *Myology*, 2nd ed. New York, McGraw-Hill, 1994, pp 1461–1486.

Banker BQ: Parasitic myositis, in Engel AG, Franzini-Armstrong C (eds): *Myology*, 3rd ed. New York, McGraw-Hill, 2004, pp 1419–1444.

Banker BQ, Victor M: Dermatomyositis (systemic angiopathy) of childhood. *Medicine (Baltimore)* 45:261, 1966.

Banker BQ, Victor M, Adams RD: Arthrogryposis multiplex due to congenital muscular dystrophy. *Brain* 80:319, 1957.

Barbeau A: The syndrome of hereditary late onset ptosis and dysphagia in French Canada, in Kuhn EE (ed): *Progressive Muskeldystrophies, Myotonie, Myasthenie*. New York, Springer-Verlag, 1966.

Barohn RJ, Amato AA, Sahenk Z, et al: Inclusion body myositis: Explanation for poor response to immunosuppressive therapy. *Neurology* 45:1302, 1995.

Barohn RJ, Jackson CE, Rogers SJ, et al: Prolonged paralysis due to non-depolarizing neuromuscular blocking agents and corticosteroids. *Muscle Nerve* 17:647, 1994.

Bassez G, Authier FJ, Lechat-Zakman E, et al: Inflammatory myopathy with abundant macrophages (IMAM). A condition sharing similarities with cytophagic histiocytic panniculitis and distinct from macrophagic myofasciitis. *J Neuropathol Exp Neurol* 62:464, 2003.

Batten FE, Gibb HP: Myotonia atrophica. *Brain* 32:187, 1909.

Becker PE, Keiner F: Eine neue X-chromosomale muskeldystrophie. *Arch Psychiatr Nervenkr Z Gesamte Neurol Psychiatr* 193:427, 1955.

Ben Hamida M, Fardeau M, Attia N: Severe childhood muscular dystrophy affecting both sexes and frequent in Tunisia. *Muscle Nerve* 6:469, 1983.

Bethlem J, Arts WF, Dingemans KP: Common origin of rods, cores, miniature cores, and focal loss of cross-striations. *Arch Neurol* 35:555, 1978.

Bethlem J, van Wijngaarden GK: Benign myopathy with autosomal dominant inheritance: A report on three pedigrees. *Brain* 99:91, 1976.

Blau HM: Cell therapies for muscular dystrophy. *N Engl J Med* 359:1403, 2008.

Blexrud MD, Windebank AJ, Daube JR: Long-term follow-up of 121 patients with benign fasciculations. *Ann Neurol* 34:622, 1993.

Braakhekke JP, De Bruin MI, Stegeman DF, et al: The second wind phenomenon in McArdle's disease. *Brain* 109:1087, 1986.

Brody I: Muscle contracture induced by exercise: A syndrome attributable to decreased relaxing factor. *N Engl J Med* 281:187, 1969.

Brouwer R, Hensgstman GJD, Egberts WV, et al: Autoantibody profiles in the sera of European patients with myositis. *Ann Rheum Dis* 60:116, 2001.

Buchbinder R, Hill CL: Malignancy in patients with inflammatory myopathy. *Curr Rheumatol Rep* 4:415, 2002.

Bushby KMD: Making sense of the limb girdle muscular dystrophies. *Brain* 122:1403, 1999.

Buxton J, Shelbourne P, Davies J, et al: Detection of an unstable fragment of DNA specific to individuals with myotonic dystrophy. *Nature* 355:547, 1992.

Byers TJ, Neumann PE, Beggs AH, Kunkel LM: ELISA quantitation of dystrophin for the diagnosis of Duchenne and Becker muscular dystrophies. *Neurology* 42:570, 1992.

Campbell KP: Three muscular dystrophies: Loss of cytoskeleton-extra cellular matrix linkage. *Cell* 80:675, 1995.

Chahin N, Selcen D, Engel AG: Sporadic late onset nemaline myopathy. *Neurology* 65:1158, 2005.

Chakrabarti A, Pearse JMS: Scapuloperoneal syndrome with cardiomyopathy: Report of a family with autosomal dominant inheritance and unusual features. *J Neurol Neurosurg Psychiatry* 44:1146, 1981.

Cori GT, Cori CF: Glucose-6-phosphatase of the liver in glycogen storage disease. *J Biol Chem* 199:661, 1952.

Cros D, Harnden P, Pouget J, et al: Peripheral neuropathy in myotonic dystrophy: A nerve biopsy study. *Ann Neurol* 23:470, 1988.

Cumming WJK, Weiser R, Teoh R, et al: Localized nodular myositis: A clinical and pathological variant of polymyositis. *Q J Med* 46:531, 1977.

Curry SC, Chang D, Connor D: Drug- and toxin-induced rhabdomyolysis. *Ann Emerg Med* 18:1068, 1989.

Dalakas MC: Intravenous immune globulin therapy for neurological diseases. *Ann Neurol* 126:721,1997.

Dalakas MC, Hohlfeld R: Polymyositis and dermatomyositis. *Lancet* 362:971, 2003.

Dalakas MC, Illa I, Pezeshkpour GH, et al: Mitochondrial myopathy caused by long-term zidovudine therapy. *N Engl J Med* 322:1098, 1990.

Davidenkow S: Scapuloperoneal amyotrophy. *Arch Neurol Psychiatry* 41:694, 1939.

DeVere R, Bradley WG: Polymyositis, its presentation, morbidity and mortality. *Brain* 98:637, 1975.

DiDonato S, Taroni F: Disorders of lipid metabolism, in Engel AG, Franzini-Armstrong C (eds): *Myology*, 3rd ed. New York, McGraw-Hill, 2004, pp 1587–1622.

DiMauro S, Melis-DiMauro P: Muscle carnitine palmitoyltransferase deficiency and myoglobinuria. *Science* 182:929, 1973.

Dion E, Cherin P, Payan C, et al: Magnetic resonance imaging criteria for distinguishing between inclusion body myositis and polymyositis. *J Rheumatol* 29:1897, 2000.

Dobyns WB, Pagon R, Armstrong D, et al: Diagnostic criteria for Walker-Warburg syndrome. *Am J Med Genet* 32:195, 1989.

Donner M, Rapola J, Somer H: Congenital muscular dystrophy: A clinicopathological and follow-up study of 13 patients. *Neuropediatrie* 6:239, 1975.

Dresner SC, Kennerdell JS: Dysthyroid orbitopathy. *Neurology* 35:1628, 1985.

Dua HS, Smith FW, Singh AK, Forrester JV: Diagnosis of orbital myositis by nuclear magnetic resonance imaging. *Br J Ophthalmol* 71:54, 1987.

Dubois DC, Almon RR: A possible role for glucocorticoids in denervation atrophy. *Muscle Nerve* 4:370, 1981.

Dubowitz V: Rigid spine syndrome: A muscle syndrome in search of a name. *Proc R Soc Med* 66:219, 1973.

Edwards RHT: New techniques for studying human muscle function, metabolism and fatigue. *Muscle Nerve* 7:599, 1984.

Emery AEH, Dreifuss FE: Unusual type of benign X-linked muscular dystrophy. *J Neurol Neurosurg Psychiatry* 29:338, 1966.

Engel AG: Myofibrillar myopathy. *Ann Neurol* 46:681, 1999.

Engel AG, Angelini C: Carnitine deficiency of human skeletal muscle with associated lipid storage myopathy: A new syndrome. *Science* 179:899, 1973.

Engel AG, Angelini C, Gomez MR: Fingerprint body myopathy. *Mayo Clin Proc* 47:377, 1972.

Engel AG, Arahata K: Mononuclear cells in myopathies: Quantitation of functionally distinct subsets, recognition of antigen-specific cell-mediated cytotoxicity in some diseases and implications for the pathogenesis of the different inflammatory myopathies. *Hum Pathol* 17:704, 1986.

Engel AG, Emslie-Smith AM: Inflammatory myopathies. *Curr Opin Neurol Neurosurg* 2:695, 1989.

Engel AG, Franzini-Armstrong C (eds): *Myology*, 3rd ed. New York, McGraw-Hill, 2004.

Engel AG, Hohlfeld R, Banker BQ: The polymyositis and dermatomyositis syndromes, in Engel AG, Franzini-Armstrong C (eds): *Myology*, 3rd ed. New York, McGraw-Hill, 2004, pp 1321–1366.

Engel AG, Ozawa E: Dystrophinopathies, in Engel AG, Franzini-Armstrong C (eds): *Myology*, 3rd ed. New York, McGraw-Hill, 2004, pp 961–1026.

Engel WK, Reznick JS: Late onset rod-myopathy: A newly recognized, acquired, and progressive disease. *Neurology* 16:308, 1966.

Engel WK, Vick NK, Glueck J, Levy RI: A skeletal muscle disorder associated with intermittent symptoms and a possible defect in lipid metabolism. *N Engl J Med* 282:697, 1970.

Faris AA, Reyes MG: Reappraisal of alcoholic myopathy: Clinical and biopsy study on chronic alcoholics without muscle weakness or wasting. *J Neurol Neurosurg Psychiatry* 34:86, 1971.

Farmer JA: Learning from the cerivastatin experience. *Lancet* 358:1383, 2001.

Fenichel GM, Cooper DO, Brooke MH (eds): Evaluating muscle strength and function: Proceedings of a workshop. *Muscle Nerve* 13(Suppl):S1:57, 1990.

Fenichel GM, Florence JM, Pestronk A, et al: Long-term benefit from prednisone therapy in Duchenne muscular dystrophy. *Neurology* 41:1874, 1991.

Filosto M, Tonin P, Vattemi et al: The role of muscle biopsy in investigating isolated muscle pain. *Neurology* 68:181, 2007.

Fitzsimmons RB, Gurwin EB, Bird AC: Retinal vascular abnormalities in facioscapulohumeral muscular dystrophy. *Brain* 110:631, 1987.

Flanigan KM, Kerr L, Bromberg MB, et al: Congenital muscular dystrophy with rigid spine syndrome: A clinical, pathological, and genetic study. *Ann Neurol* 47:152, 2000.

Franzini-Armstrong C: The membrane systems of muscle cells, in Engel AG, Franzini-Armstrong C (eds): *Myology*, 3rd ed. New York, McGraw-Hill, 2004, pp 232–256.

Fukuyama Y, Osawa M, Saito K (eds): *Congenital Muscular Dystrophies*. Amsterdam, Elsevier, 1997.

Gamboa ET, Eastwood AB, Hays AP, et al: Isolation of influenza virus from muscle in myoglobinuric polymyositis. *Neurology* 29:556, 1979.

Garlepp MJ, Mastaglia FL: Inclusion body myositis. *J Neurol Neurosurg Psychiatry* 60:251, 1996.

Gherardi R, Baudrimont M, Lionnet F, et al: Skeletal muscle toxoplasmosis in patients with acquired immunodeficiency syndrome: A clinical and pathological study. *Ann Neurol* 32:535, 1992.

Gilchrist JM, Leshner RT: Autosomal dominant humeroperoneal myopathy. *Arch Neurol* 43:734, 1986.

Goermans NM, Tulinius M, van der Akker JT, et al: Systemic administration of PRO051 in Duchenne's muscular dystrophy. *N Engl J Med* 364:1513, 2011.

Gorson KC, Ropper AH: Generalized paralysis in the intensive care unit: Emphasis on the complications of neuromuscular blocking agents and corticosteroids. *J Int Care Med* 11:219, 1996.

Gospe SM, Lazaro RP, Lava NS, et al: Familial X-linked myalgia and cramps: A nonprogressive myopathy associated with a deletion in the dystrophin gene. *Neurology* 39:1277, 1989.

Gowers WR: A lecture on myopathy, a distal form. *Br Med J* 2:89, 1902.

Gowers WR: *Pseudohypertrophic Muscular Paralysis*. London, Churchill Livingstone, 1879.

Greenberg SA, Amato AA: Uncertainties in the pathogenesis of adult dermatomyositis. *Curr Opin Neurol* 17:359, 2004.

Griggs RC, Askanas V, DiMauro S, et al: Inclusion body myositis and myopathies. *Ann Neurol* 38:705, 1995.

Griggs RC, Mendell JR, Miller RG: *Evaluation and Treatment of Myopathies*. Philadelphia, Davis, 1995.

Griggs RS, Pandya S, Florence JM, et al: Randomized controlled trial of testosterone in myotonic dystrophy. *Neurology* 39:219, 1989.

Groh WJ, Groh MR, Saha C, et al: Electrocardiographic abnormalities and sudden death in myotonic dystrophy type 1. *N Engl J Med* 358:2688, 2008.

Gross B, Ochoa J: Trichinosis: A clinical report and histochemistry of muscle. *Muscle Nerve* 2:394, 1979.

Haller RG, Drachman DB: Alcoholic rhabdomyolysis: An experimental model in the rat. *Science* 208:412, 1980.

Harley HG, Brook JD, Rundle SA, et al: Expansion of an unstable DNA region and phenotypic variation in myotonic dystrophy. *Nature* 355:545, 1992.

Harper PS: Congenital myotonic dystrophy in Britain. *Arch Dis Child* 50:505, 514, 1975.

Harper PS: *Myotonic Dystrophy*. Philadelphia, Saunders, 1979.

Harris JB, Cullen MJ: Ultrastructural localization and possible role of dystrophin, in Kakulas BA, Howell JM, Rosas AD (eds): *Duchenne Muscular Dystrophy*. New York, Raven Press, 1992.

Hart MN, Linthicum DS, Waldschmidt MM, et al: Experimental autoimmune inflammatory myopathy. *J Neuropathol Exp Neurol* 46:511, 1987.

Heckmatt JZ, Sewry CA, Hodes D, Dubowitz V: Congenital centronuclear (myotubular) myopathy. *Brain* 108:941, 1985.

Hed R, Lundmark C, Fahlgren H, Orell S: Acute muscular syndrome in chronic alcoholism. *Acta Med Scand* 171:585, 1962.

Henderson JL: The congenital facial diplegia syndrome: Clinical features, pathology and aetiology. *Brain* 62:381, 1939.

Hengstman GJD, van Engelen BGM, van Egberts WTMV, et al: Myositis-specific autoantibodies: Overview and recent developments. *Curr Opin Neurol* 13:476, 2001.

Hers HG: Alpha-glucosidase deficiency in generalized glycogen storage disease (Pompe's disease). *Biochem J* 86:11, 1963.

Hoffman EP, Arahata K, Minetti C, et al: Dystrophinopathy in isolated cases of myopathy in females. *Neurology* 42:967, 1992.

Hoffman EP, Brown RH Jr, Kunkel LM: Dystrophin: The protein product of the Duchenne muscular dystrophy locus. *Cell* 51:919, 1987.

Hoffman EP, Fischbeck KH, Brown RH, et al: Characterization of dystrophin in muscle-biopsy specimens from patients with Duchenne's or Becker's muscular dystrophy. *N Engl J Med* 318:1363, 1988.

Hopkins LC, Jackson JA, Elias LJ: Emery-Dreifuss humeroperoneal muscular dystrophy: An X-linked myopathy with unusual contractures and bradycardia. *Ann Neurol* 10:230, 1981.

Ianuzzo D, Patel P, Chen V, et al: Thyroidal trophic influence on skeletal muscle myosin. *Nature* 270:74, 1977.

Illa I: Distal myopathies. *J Neurol* 247:169, 2000.

Illingworth B, Cori GT: Structure of glycogens and amylopectins: III. Normal and abnormal human glycogen. *J Biol Chem* 199:653, 1952.

Illingworth B, Larner J, Cori GT: Structure of glycogens and amylopectins: I. Enzymatic determination of chain length. *J Biol Chem* 199:631, 1952.

Jones HR, de la Monte SM: Case records of the Massachusetts General Hospital: Case 22-1998. *N Engl J Med* 339:182, 1998.

Kakulas BA, Adams RD: *Diseases of Muscle: Pathological Foundations of Clinical Myology*, 4th ed. Philadelphia, Harper & Row, 1985.

Karpati G, Carpenter S, Nelson RF: Type 1 muscle fiber atrophy and central nuclei. *J Neurol Sci* 10:489, 1970.

Karpati G, Charuk J, Carpenter S, et al: Myopathy caused by a deficiency of Ca-adenosine triphosphatase in sarcoplasmic reticulum (Brody's disease). *Ann Neurol* 20:38, 1986.

Kass EH, Andrus SB, Adams RD, et al: Toxoplasmosis in the human adult. *Arch Intern Med* 89:759, 1952.

Katz JS, Wolfe GI, Burns DK, et al: Isolated neck extensor myopathy: A common cause of dropped head syndrome. *Neurology* 46:917, 1996.

Kearns TP, Sayre GP: Retinitis pigmentosa, external ophthalmoplegia and complete heart block. *Arch Ophthalmol* 60:280, 1958.

Kissel JT, Mendell JR, Rammohen KW: Microvascular deposition of complement membrane attack complex in dermatomyositis. *N Engl J Med* 314:329, 1986.

Kodama K, Sikorska H, Bandy-Dafoe P, et al: Demonstration of circulating autoantibody against a soluble eye-muscle antigen in Graves' ophthalmopathy. *Lancet* 2:1353, 1982.

Kono N, Mineo I, Sumi S, et al: Metabolic basis of improved exercise tolerance: Muscle phosphorylase deficiency after glucagon administration. *Neurology* 34:1471, 1984.

Krahn M, de Munain AL, Streichenberger N, et al: CAPN3 mutations in patients with idiopathic eosinophilic myositis. *Ann Neurol* 59:905, 2006.

Krasnianski M, Eger K, Neudeckers S, et al: Atypical phenotypes in patients with facioscapulohumeral muscular dystrophy 4q35 deletion. *Arch Neurol* 60:1421, 2003.

Kugelberg E, Welander L: Heredofamilial juvenile muscular atrophy simulating muscular dystrophy. *Arch Neurol Psychiatry* 75:500, 1956.

Kuhn E, Fiehn W, Schroder JM, et al: Early myocardial disease and cramping myalgia in Becker type muscular dystrophy: A kindred. *Neurology* 29:1144, 1979.

Kuncl RW, Duncan G, Watson D, et al: Colchicine myopathy and neuropathy. *N Engl J Med* 316:1562, 1987.

Kunkel LM: Analysis of deletions in DNA from patients with Becker and Duchenne muscular dystrophy. *Nature* 322:73, 1986.

Lacomis D, Giuliani MJ, Van Cott A, Kramer DJ: Acute myopathy of intensive care: Clinical, electromyographic, and pathological aspects. *Ann Neurol* 40:645, 1996.

Layzer RB: *Neuromuscular Manifestations of Systemic Disease*. Philadelphia, Davis, 1985.

Layzer RB, Rowland LP, Ranney HM: Muscle phosphofructokinase deficiency. *Arch Neurol* 17:512, 1967.

Layzer RB, Shearn MA, Satya-Murti S: Eosinophilic polymyositis. *Ann Neurol* 1:65, 1977.

Lebenthal E, Shochet SR, Adam A, et al: Arthrogryposis multiplex congenita: 23 cases in an Arab kindred. *Pediatrics* 46:891, 1970.

Lennon N, Kho A, Bacskai BJ, et al: Dysferlin interacts with annexins A1 and A2 and mediates sarcolemmal wound healing. *J Biol Chem* 278(50):50466, 2003.

Lodi R, Taylor DJ, Tabrizi SJ, et al: Normal in vivo skeletal muscle oxidative metabolism in sporadic inclusion body myositis assessed by ^{31}P-magnetic resonance spectroscopy. *Brain* 121:2119, 1998.

Løseth S, Voermans NC, et al. A novel late-onset axial myopathy associated with mutations in the skeletal muscle ryanodine receptor (RYR1) gene. *J Neurol* 260:1504, 2013.

Lotz BP, Engel AG, Nishino H, et al: Inclusion body myositis: Observations in 40 patients. *Brain* 112:727, 1989.

Lundberg A: Myalgia cruris epidemica. *Acta Paediatr Scand* 46:18, 1957.

Maas O, Paterson AS: Myotonia congenita, dystrophia myotonica, and paramyotonia. *Brain* 73:318, 1950.

Markesbery WR, Griggs RC, Leach RP, Lapham LW: Late onset hereditary distal myopathy. *Neurology* 23:127, 1974.

Mastaglia FL, Barwich DD, Hall R: Myopathy in acromegaly. *Lancet* 2:907, 1970.

Mastaglia FL, Laing NG: Investigation of muscle disease. *J Neurol Neurosurg Psychiatry* 60:256, 1996.

Mastaglia FL, Ojeda VJ: Inflammatory myopathies. *Ann Neurol* 17:278, 317, 1985.

Mastaglia FL, Phillips BA, Zilko PJ: Immunoglobulin therapy in inflammatory myopathies. *J Neurol Neurosurg Psychiatry* 65:107, 1998.

Matsuda C, Akoi M, Hayashi YK, et al: Dysferlin is a surface membrane-associated protein that is absent in Miyoshi myopathy. *Neurology* 53:1119, 1999.

Mayeno AN, Belongia EA, Lin F, et al: 3-(phenylamino)alanine, a novel aniline derived amino acid associated with the eosinophilia-myalgia syndrome: A link to the toxic oil syndrome? *Mayo Clin Proc* 67:1134, 1992.

Mayeno AN, Lin F, Foote CS, et al: Characterization of "peak E," a novel amino acid associated with eosinophilia-myalgia syndrome. *Science* 250:1707, 1990.

McArdle B: Myopathy due to a defect in muscle glycogen breakdown. *Clin Sci* 10:13, 1951.

Medsger TA Jr: Tryptophan-induced eosinophilia-myalgia syndrome. *N Engl J Med* 322:926, 1990.

Meinck HM, Goebel HH, Rumpf KW, et al: The forearm ischaemic work test—hazardous to McArdle patients? *J Neurol Neurosurg Psychiatry* 45:1144, 1982.

Mercuri E, Pope M, Quinlivan R. et al: Extreme variability of phenotype in patients with an identical missense mutation in the lamin A/C gene. *Arch Neurol* 61:690, 2004.

Merlini L, Granata C, Dominici P, Bonfiglioli S: Emery-Dreifuss muscular dystrophy: Report of five cases in a family and review of the literature. *Muscle Nerve* 9:481, 1986.

Messina S, Fagiolari G, Lamperti C, et al: Women with pregnancy-related polymyositis and high serum CK levels in the newborn. *Neurology* 58:482, 2002.

Michet CJ Jr, Doyle JA, Ginsburg WW: Eosinophilic fasciitis: Report of 15 cases. *Mayo Clin Proc* 56:27, 1981.

Mielke U, Ricker K, Emser W, Boxler K: Unilateral calf enlargement following S1 radiculopathy. *Muscle Nerve* 5:434, 1982.

Milhorat AT, Wolff HG: Studies in diseases of muscle: XIII. Progressive muscular dystrophy of atrophic distal type; report on a family; report of autopsy. *Arch Neurol Psychiatry* 49:655, 1943.

Miyoshi K, Kawai H, Iwasa M, et al: Autosomal recessive distal muscular dystrophy as a new type of progressive muscular dystrophy. *Brain* 109:31, 1986.

Mohire MD, Tandan R, Fries TJ, et al: Early-onset benign autosomal dominant limb-girdle myopathy with contractures (Bethlem myopathy). *Neurology* 38:573, 1988.

Mokri B, Engel AG: Duchenne dystrophy: Electron microscopic findings pointing to a basic or early abnormality in the plasma membrane of the muscle fiber. *Neurology* 25:1111, 1975.

Moorman JR, Coleman RE, Packer DL, et al: Cardiac involvement in myotonic muscular dystrophy. *Medicine (Baltimore)* 64:371, 1985.

Müller R, Kugelberg E: Myopathy in Cushing's syndrome. *J Neurol Neurosurg Psychiatry* 22:314, 1959.

Munsat TL, Serratrice G: Facioscapulohumeral and scapuloperoneal syndromes, in Vinken PJ, Bruyn GW, Klawans H (eds): *Handbook of Clinical Neurology*. Vol 18 (new series). Amsterdam, Elsevier Science, 1992, pp 161–176.

Nakano S, Engel AG, Waclawik AJ, et al: Myofibrillar myopathy with abnormal foci of desmin positivity: I. Light and electron microscopy analysis of 10 cases. *J Neuropathos Exp Neurol* 55:549, 1996.

Nalini A, Ravishankar S: "Dropped head syndrome" in syringomyelia: Report of two cases. *J Neurol Neurosurg Psychiatry* 76:290, 2005.

Namba T, Brunner MG, Grog N: Idiopathic giant cell polymyositis: Report of a case and review of the syndrome. *Arch Neurol* 31:27, 1974.

Neville HE, Baumbach LL, Ringel SP, et al: Familial inclusion body myositis: Evidence for autosomal dominant inheritance. *Neurology* 42:897, 1992.

Nevin S: Two cases of muscular degeneration occurring in late adult life with a review of the recorded cases of late progressive muscular dystrophy (late progressive myopathy). *J Med* 5:51, 1936.

Nonaka I, Sunohara N, Satoyoshi E, et al: Autosomal recessive distal muscular dystrophy: A comparative study with distal myopathy with rimmed vacuole formation. *Ann Neurol* 17:52, 1985.

Oddis CV, Reed AM, Aggarwal R, et al: Rituximab in the treatment of refractory adult and juvenile dermatomyositis and adult polymyositis: a randomized, placebo-phase trial. *Arthritis Rheum* 65:314, 2013.

Pachman LM: An update on juvenile dermatomyositis. *Curr Opin Rheumatol* 7:437, 1995.

Panegyres PK, Squier M, Mills KR, Newsom-Davis J: Acute myopathy associated with large parenteral dose of corticosteroid in myasthenia gravis. *J Neurol Neurosurg Psychiatry* 56:702, 1993.

Patterson VH, Hill TRG, Fletch PJH, Heron JR: Cental core disease: Clinical and pathological progression within a family. *Brain* 102:581, 1979.

Pearson CM, Fowler WG: Hereditary nonprogressive muscular dystrophy inducing arthrogryposis syndrome. *Brain* 86:75, 1963.

Perkoff GT, Hardy P, Velez-Garcia E: Reversible acute muscular syndrome in chronic alcoholism. *N Engl J Med* 274:1277, 1966.

Perloff JK, Roberts WC, DeLeon AC, et al: The distinctive electrocardiogram of Duchenne's muscular dystrophy. *Am J Med* 42:179, 1967.

Phillips PS, Haas RH, Banny KHS, et al: Statin-associated myopathy with normal creatine kinase levels. *Ann Intern Med* 137:581, 2002.

Poppe M, Cree L, Bourke J, et al: The phenotype of limb-girdle muscular dystrophy type 2I. *Neurology* 60:1248, 2003.

Pryse-Philips W, Johnson GJ, Larsen B: Incomplete manifestations of myotonic dystrophy in a large kinship in Labrador. *Ann Neurol* 11:582, 1982.

Raphael JC, Chevret S, Chastang C, et al: Randomised trial of preventive nasal ventilation in Duchenne muscular dystrophy. French Multicentre Cooperative Group on Home Mechanical Ventilation Assistance in Duchenne de Boulogne Muscular Dystrophy. *Lancet* 343:1600, 1994.

Ricker K, Koch MC, Lehmann-Horn F, et al: Proximal myotonic myopathy: A new dominant disorder with myotonia, muscle weakness, and cataracts. *Neurology* 44:1448, 1994.

Ricoy JR, Cabello A, Rodriguez J, Tellez I: Neuropathological studies on the toxic syndrome related to adulterated rapeseed oil in Spain. *Brain* 106:817, 1983.

Riddoch D, Morgan-Hughes JA: Prognosis in adult polymyositis. *J Neurol Sci* 26:71, 1975.

Roberds SL, Leturcq F, Allamand V, et al: Missense mutation in the adhalin gene linked to autosomal recessive muscular dystrophy. *Cell* 78:625, 1994.

Roe CR, Ding J: Mitochondrial fatty acid oxidation disorders, in Scriver CR, Beaudet AL, Valle D, Sly WS (eds): *The Metabolic and Molecular Bases of Inherited Disease*, 8th ed. New York, McGraw-Hill, 2001, pp 2297–2326.

Roses MS, Nicholson MT, Kircher CS, Roses AD: Evaluation and detection of Duchenne's and Becker's muscular dystrophy carriers by manual muscle testing. *Neurology* 27:20, 1977.

Rotthauwe HW, Mortier W, Beyer H: Neuer Typ einer recessiv X-chromosomal verebten Muskeldystrophie: Scapulohumerodistale Muskeldystrophie mit fruhzeitigen Kontrakturen und Herzrhythmusstorungen. *Humangenetik* 16:181, 1972.

Rowin J, Cheng G, Lewis SL, Meriggoli MN: Late appearance of dropped head syndrome after radiotherapy for Hodgkin's disease. *Muscle Nerve* 34:666, 2006.

Rubenstein NA, Kelly AM: The diversity of muscle fiber types and its origin during development, in Engel AG, Franzini-Armstrong C (eds): *Myology*, 3rd ed. New York, McGraw-Hill, 2004, pp 87–103.

Santavuori P, Somer H, Sainio A, et al: Muscle-eye-brain disease (MEB). *Brain Dev* 11:147, 1989.

SEARCH Collaborative Group, The. SLCO1B1 variants and statin-induced myopathy—a genomewide study. *N Engl J Med* 359:789, 2008.

Seitz D: Zur nosologischen Stellung des sogenannten scapulo-peronealen syndroms. *Dtsch Z Nervenheilkd* 175:547, 1957.

Selcen D, Ohno K, Engel AG: Myofibrillar myopathy—clinical, morphological and genetic studies in 63 patients. *Brain* 127:439, 2004.

Shulman LE: Diffuse fasciitis with hyperglobulinemia and eosinophilia: A new syndrome? *J Rheumatol* 1(Suppl):46, 1974.

Shy GM, Gonatos NK, Perez M: Two childhood myopathies with abnormal mitochondria. *Brain* 89:133, 1966.

Shy GM, Magee KR: A new congenital non-progressive myopathy. *Brain* 79:610, 1956.

Sigurgeirsson B, Lindelof B, Edhag O, Allander E: Risk of cancer in patients with dermatomyositis or polymyositis. *N Engl J Med* 326:363, 1992.

Silbermann M, Finkelbrand S, Weiss A, et al: Morphometric analysis of aging skeletal muscle following endurance training. *Muscle Nerve* 6:136, 1983.

Sivak ED, Salanga VD, Wilbourn AJ, et al: Adult onset acid maltase deficiency presenting as diaphragmatic paralysis. *Ann Neurol* 9:613, 1981.

Slonim AE, Goans PJ: Myopathy in McArdle's syndrome. Improvement with a high-proten diet. *N Engl J Med* 312:355, 1985.

Slonim AE, Weisberg MD, Benke P: Reversal of debrancher deficiency myopathy by the use of high protein nutrition. *Ann Neurol* 11:420, 1982.

Spector RH, Carlisle JA: Minimal thyroid ophthalmopathy. *Neurology* 37:1803, 1987.

Speer MC, Yamaoka LH, Gilchrist JH, et al: Confirmation of genetic heterogeneity in limb-girdle muscular dystrophy: Linkage of an autosomal dominant form to chromosome 5q. *Am J Hum Genet* 50:1211, 1992.

Stark RJ: Eosinophilic polymyositis. *Arch Neurol* 36:721, 1979.

Statland JM, Bundy BN, Wang Y, et al for the Consortium for Clinical Investigation of Neurologic Channelopathies: Mexiletine for symptoms and signs of myotonia in nondystrophic myotonia: a randomized controlled trial. *JAMA* 308:1357, 2012.

Steinert TH: Über das klinische und anatomische Bild des Muskelschwunds der Myotoniker. *Dtsch Z Nervenheilkd* 37:58, 1909.

Swash M, Heathfield KWG: Quadriceps myopathy: A variant of the limb-girdle dystrophy syndrome. *J Neurol Neurosurg Psychiatry* 46:355, 1983.

Tawil R, Figlewicz DA, Griggs RC, et al: Facioscapulohumeral dystrophy: A distinct regional myopathy with a novel molecular pathogenesis. *Ann Neurol* 43:279, 1998.

Thomas MR, Lancaster R: Polymyositis presenting with dyspnea, greatly elevated muscle enzymes but no apparent muscular weakness. *Br J Clin Pract* 44:378, 1990.

Thompson PD, Clarkson P, Karas RH: Statin-associated myopathy. *JAMA* 289:1681, 2003.

Tomé FMS, Evangelista T, Leclerc A, et al: Congenital muscular dystrophy with merosin deficiency. *C R Acad Sci III* 317:351, 1994.

Tomlinson BF, Walton JN, Rebeiz JJ: The effects of aging and cachexia upon skeletal muscle: A histopathologic study. *J Neurol Sci* 8:201, 1969.

Tonin P, Lewis P, Servidei S, DiMauro S: Metabolic causes of myoglobinuria. *Ann Neurol* 27:181, 1990.

Tyler FH, Stephens FE: Studies in disorders of muscle: II. Clinical manifestations and inheritance of facioscapulohumeral dystrophy in large family. *Ann Intern Med* 32:640, 1950.

Udd B, Partanen J, Halonen P, et al: Tibial muscular dystrophy. Late adult-onset distal myopathy in Finnish patients. *Arch Neurol* 50:604, 1993.

Umapathi T, Chaudry V, Cornblath D, et al: Head drop and camptocormia. *J Neurol Neurosurg Psychiatry* 73:1, 2002.

Umpleby AM, Wiles CM, Trend PS, et al: Protein turnover in acid maltase deficiency before and after treatment with a high protein diet. *J Neurol Neurosurg Psychiatry* 50:587, 1987.

van der Kooi AJ, Ledderhof TM, De Voogt WG, et al: A newly recognized autosomal dominant limb girdle muscular dystrophy with cardiac involvement. *Ann Neurol* 39:363, 1996.

van der Kooi AJ, Van Meegan M, Ledderhof TM, et al: Genetic localization of a newly recognized autosomal dominant limb-girdle muscular dystrophy with cardiac involvement (LGMD 1B) to chromosome 1q11-21. *Am J Hum Genet* 60:891, 1997.

van der Muelen MFG, Bronner IM, Hoogendijk JE, et al: Polymyositis: An overdiagnosed entity. *Neurology* 61:316, 2003.

van der Ploeg AT, Clemens PR, Corzo D, et al: A randomzied study of alglucosidase alfa in late-onset Pompe's disease. *N Engl J Med* 362:1396, 2010.

van Deutekom, Janson AA, Ginjaar IB, et al: Local dystrophin restoration with antisense oligonucleotide PRO051. *N Engl J Med* 357:2677, 2007.

Vassella F, Mumenthaler M, Rossi E, et al: Congenital muscular dystrophy. *Dtsch Z Nervenheilkd* 190:349, 1967.

Vicale CT: The diagnostic features of a muscular syndrome resulting from hyperparathyroidism, osteomalacia owing to renal tubular acidosis, and perhaps to related disorders of calcium metabolism. *Trans Am Neurol Assoc* 74:143, 1949.

Victor M, Hayes R, Adams RD: Oculopharyngeal muscular dystrophy: A familial disease of late life characterized by dysphagia and progressive ptosis of the eyelids. *N Engl J Med* 267:1267, 1962.

Vignos PJ: Physical models of rehabilitation in neuromuscular disease. *Muscle Nerve* 6:323, 1983.

Vissing J, Haller RG: The effect of oral sucrose on exercise tolerance in patients with McArdle's disease. *N Engl J Med* 349:2503, 2003.

Walton JN: The idiopathic inflammatory myopathies and their treatment. *J Neurol Neurosurg Psychiatry* 54:285, 1991.

Walton JN, Adams RD: *Polymyositis*. London, Livingstone, 1958.

Walton JN, Karpati G, Hilton-Jones D (eds): *Disorders of Voluntary Muscle*, 6th ed. Edinburgh, UK, Churchill Livingstone, 1994.

Walton JN, Nattrass FS: On the classification, natural history and treatment of myopathies. *Brain* 77:169, 1954.

Welander L: Myopathia distalis tarda hereditaria. *Acta Med Scand* 141(Suppl 265):1, 1951.

Whitaker JN, Engel WK: Vascular deposits of immunoglobulin and complement in idiopathic inflammatory myopathy. *N Engl J Med* 286:333, 1972.

Wintzen AR, Bots GTH, DeBakker HM, et al: Dysphagia in inclusion body myositis. *J Neurol Neurosurg Psychiatry* 51:1542, 1988.

Wohlfart G, Fex J, Eliasson S: Hereditary proximal spinal muscle atrophy simulating progressive muscular dystrophy. *Acta Psychiatr Neurol Scand* 30:395, 1955.

49

Myasthenia Gravis and Related Disorders of the Neuromuscular Junction

Included under this title is a group of diseases affecting the neuromuscular junction, the most important of which is myasthenia gravis. Most of these disorders exhibit the characteristic and striking features of fluctuating weakness and fatigability of muscle. Some degree of weakness is usually present at all times but it is made worse by activity. The weakness and fatigability reflect physiologic abnormalities of the neuromuscular junction that are demonstrated by clinical signs and by special electrophysiologic testing. As an aid to understanding the diseases discussed in this chapter, the reader should consult the discussion of the structure and function of the neuromuscular synapse given in Chap. 45.

MYASTHENIA GRAVIS

The cardinal feature of myasthenia gravis, usually referred to simply as myasthenia, is fluctuating weakness of voluntary (skeletal) muscles, particularly those innervated by motor nuclei of the brainstem, i.e., ocular, masticatory, facial, deglutitional, and lingual. Manifest weakening during continued activity, quick restoration of power with rest, and dramatic improvement in strength following the administration of anticholinesterase drugs such as neostigmine are the other notable characteristics. Myasthenia is an immune disease in which circulating antibodies against components of the motor postsynaptic membrane and subsequent structural changes in that membrane explain virtually all the features of the disease.

Historical Note Several students of medical history affirm that Willis, in 1672, gave an account of a disease that could be none other than myasthenia gravis. Others give credit to Wilks (1877) for the first description and for having noted that the medulla was free of disease, in distinction to other types of bulbar paralyses. The first reasonably complete accounts were those of Erb (1878), who characterized the disease as a bulbar palsy without an anatomic lesion, and of Goldflam (1893); for many years thereafter, the disorder was referred to as the *Erb-Goldflam syndrome.* Jolly (1895) was the first to use the name *myasthenia gravis*, to which he added the term *pseudoparalytica* to indicate the lack of structural changes at autopsy. Also it was Jolly who demonstrated that myasthenic weakness could be reproduced in affected patients by repeated faradic stimulation of the motor nerve and that the "fatigued" muscle would still respond to direct galvanic stimulation of its membrane. Interestingly, he suggested the use of physostigmine as a form of treatment but there the matter rested until Reman, in 1932, and Walker, in 1934, demonstrated the therapeutic value of the drug. The relationship between myasthenia gravis and tumors of the thymus gland was first noted by Laquer and Weigert in 1901, and in 1949, Castleman and Norris gave the first detailed account of the pathologic changes in the gland.

In 1905, Buzzard published a careful clinicopathologic analysis of the disease, commenting on both the thymic abnormalities and the infiltrations of lymphocytes (called *lymphorrhages*) in muscle. In 1973 and subsequently, the autoimmune nature of myasthenia gravis was established through a series of investigations by Patrick and Lindstrom, Fambrough, Lennon, and A.G. Engel (1977) and their colleagues (see further on). These and other references to the historical features of the disease can be found in the reviews by Viets and by Kakulas and Adams; A.G. Engel's monograph (1999) is an excellent comprehensive reference.

Clinical Manifestations

Myasthenia gravis, as the name implies, is a muscular weakness formerly with a grave prognosis. As mentioned, repeated or persistent activity of a muscle group exhausts contractile power, leading to a progressive paresis, and rest restores strength, at least partially. These are the identifying attributes of the disease and their demonstration, assuming that the patient cooperates fully, is usually enough to establish the diagnosis.

The special vulnerability of the neuromuscular junctions in certain muscles gives myasthenia a highly characteristic clinical appearance. Usually the eyelids and the muscles of eye movement, and somewhat less often, of the face, jaws, throat, and neck, are the first to be affected. Infrequently the initial complaint is referable to the limbs or to breathing. Specifically, weakness of the levator palpebrae or extraocular muscles is the initial manifestation of the disease in about half the cases, and these muscles are involved eventually in more than 90 percent of cases. Ocular palsies and ptosis are usually accompanied by weakness of eye closure, a combination that is virtually always indicative of the disease although it may be observed in certain muscular dystrophies. Diplopia is common in myasthenia, but it does not correspond to the innervatory pattern of a nerve; instead, it is the result of asymmetrical weakness of several muscles in both eyes. As the disease advances, it spreads insidiously from the cranial to the limb and axial muscles, but there are instances of fairly rapid development, sometimes initiated by an infection, usually respiratory. In rare cases, the distal extremity muscles may be involved, such as the "myasthenic hand" described by Janssen and colleagues. Symptoms may first appear during pregnancy or, more commonly, during puerperium or in response to drugs used during anesthesia.

In addition to certain circulating autoantibodies, inflammatory *thymic abnormalities* of several types are closely connected with the disease, as elaborated further on, and weakness may begin months or years before or after removal of a thymoma.

Particular ocular signs are highly characteristic of myasthenia. For example, sustained upgaze for 30 or more seconds will usually induce or exaggerate ptosis and may uncover myasthenic ocular motor weakness. Cogan described a twitching of the upper eyelid that appears a moment after the patient moves the eyes from a downward to the primary position ("lid-twitch" sign). Or, after sustained upward gaze, one or more twitches may be observed upon closure of the eyelids or during horizontal movements of the eyes. Repeated ocular versions when tracking a target or by an optokinetic stimulus may disclose progressive paresis of the muscles that carry out these movements. Unilateral painless ptosis without either ophthalmoplegia or pupillary abnormality in an adult will most often prove to be a result of myasthenia. Usually, there is subtle ptosis of the other eye that can be revealed by manually elevating the more affected eyelid. Attempts by the patient to overcome ptosis may impart a staring expression of the opposite eye. Bright sunlight is said to aggravate the ocular signs and cold to improve them. The application of an ice pack over the eye often relieves the ptosis for a brief period.

Muscles of facial expression, mastication, swallowing, and speech are affected in 80 percent of patients at some time in the illness, and in 5 to 10 percent, these are the first or only muscles to be involved. Less frequent is early involvement of the flexors and extensors of the neck, muscles of the shoulder girdle, and flexors of the hips. (This pattern may be associated with a special autoantibody as discussed later.) Of the trunk muscles, the erector spinae are the most frequently affected. In the most advanced cases, all muscles are weakened, including the diaphragmatic, abdominal, and intercostal, and even the external (skeletal muscle) sphincters of the bladder and bowel. As the disease progresses, the involvement of any group of muscles closely parallels their degree of weakness early in the disease. The clinical rule also holds that the proximal muscles are far more vulnerable than distal ones, as they are in most other forms of myopathy.

Another characteristic and understandable feature of myasthenic weakness is its tendency to increase as the day wears on or with repeated use of an affected muscle group but curiously, patients seldom volunteer this information. A few patients report paradoxical worsening on awakening, especially if they have not taken medication during the night. In general terms, therefore, myasthenia gravis may be conceived as a fluctuating and fatigable oculofaciobulbar palsy.

Other features conform to the topography and fatigability of the disease. The natural smile becomes transformed into a snarl; the jaw may sag, so that it must be propped up by the patient's hand; chewing tough food may be difficult and the patient may have to terminate a meal because of inability to masticate and swallow. It may be more difficult to eat after talking, and the voice fades and becomes nasal after sustained conversation. Women may complain of inability to fix their hair or makeup because of fatigue of the shoulders, or of difficulty in applying lipstick because they are unable to purse and roll their lips. Weakness of the neck muscles causes fatigue in holding up the head. In cases with generalized weakness, there is difficulty in retaining flatus because of weakness of the external rectal sphincter.

A peculiarity of myasthenic muscle contraction that may be observed occasionally is a sudden lapse of sustained posture or interruption of movement resulting in a kind of irregular tremor, similar to that of normal muscle nearing the point of exhaustion. A dynamometer demonstrates the rapidly waning power of contraction of a series of hand grips, and repetitive stimulation of a motor nerve at slow rates while recording muscle action potentials shows the same decremental strength in a quantitative fashion (see Fig. 45-4*A* and further on).

Weakened muscles in myasthenia gravis undergo atrophy to only a minimal degree or not at all. Tendon reflexes are seldom altered. Even repeated tapping of a tendon does not usually tax muscles to the point where contraction fails. Smooth and cardiac muscles are not involved and other neural functions are preserved. Weakened muscles, especially those of the eyes and back of the neck, may ache, but pain is seldom an important complaint. Paresthesias of the face, hands, and thighs are reported infrequently but are not accompanied by demonstrable sensory loss. The tongue may display one central and two lateral longitudinal furrows (trident tongue), as pointed out originally by Buzzard; the tongue may be atrophic in the MuSK (muscle-specific tyrosine kinase) form of disease (see further on).

Certain *epidemiologic features* of the disease are of clinical interest. Its prevalence is variously estimated to be from 43 to 84 per million persons and the annual incidence rate is approximately 1 per 300,000. The disease may begin at any age, but onset in the first decade is relatively rare (only 10 percent of cases begin in children younger than 10 years of age). The peak age of first symptoms is between 20 and 30 years in women and between 50 and 60 years in men. Under the age of 40, females are affected two to three times as often as males whereas in later life, the incidence in males is higher (3:2). Of patients with thymomas, the majority is older (50 to 60 years) and males predominate.

Familial occurrence of myasthenia is known, but it is rare. Many such cases prove to have one of the genetically determined myasthenic syndromes and not the acquired autoimmune form of disease (see further on). More common is a family history of one of the autoimmune diseases enumerated earlier. For example, in the series reported by Kerzin-Storrar and associates 30 percent had a maternal relative with a connective tissue disease, suggesting that myasthenia gravis patients inherit a susceptibility to autoimmune disease. Two of our patients have sisters with lupus. There have also been reports of the concurrence of myasthenia and multiple sclerosis, but this association is less certain. There is an increased representation of HLA-B8 and -DR3 haplotypes, as occurs in other autoimmune diseases, which is discussed further on.

Clinical Grading To facilitate clinical staging of therapy and prognosis, the classification introduced by Osserman remains useful; it can be found in his monograph cited in the references and in previous editions of this book. This system has been replaced by a scheme suggested by a task force of the Myasthenia Gravis foundation (see Jaretzki et al) as reproduced here.

Class I Any ocular muscle weakness
May have weakness of eye closure
All other muscle strength is normal

Class II Mild weakness affecting other than ocular muscles
May also have ocular muscle weakness of any severity

IIa Predominantly affecting limb, axial muscles, or both
May also have lesser involvement of oropharyngeal muscles

IIb Predominantly affecting oropharyngeal muscles, respiratory muscles, or both
May also have lesser or equal involvement of limb, axial muscles, or both

Class III Moderate weakness affecting other than ocular muscles
May also have ocular muscle weakness of any severity

IIIa Predominantly affecting limb, axial muscles, or both
May also have lesser involvement of oropharyngeal muscles

IIIb Predominantly affecting oropharyngeal muscles, respiratory muscles, or both
May also have lesser or equal involvement of limb, axial muscles, or both

Class IV Severe weakness affecting other than ocular muscles
May also have ocular muscle weakness of any severity

IVa Predominantly affecting limb and/or axial muscles
May also have lesser involvement of oropharyngeal muscles

IVb Predominantly affecting oropharyngeal muscles, respiratory muscles, or both
May also have lesser or equal involvement of limb, axial muscles, or both

Class V Intubation, with or without mechanical ventilation, except when employed during routine postoperative management. The use of a feeding tube without intubation places the patient in class IVb.

Others, for example, Compston and colleagues, have proposed a classification based on a constellation of the age of onset, presence or absence of thymoma, antibody level against acetylcholine receptor (AChR), and association with human leukocyte antigen (HLA) haplotypes. Their system is as follows: (1) myasthenia gravis with thymoma—no sex or HLA association, high AChR antibody titer; (2) onset before age 40, no thymoma—female preponderance and an increased association with HLA A1, B8, and DRW3 antigens; (3) onset after age 40, no thymoma—male preponderance, increased association with HLA A3, B7, and DRW2 antigens, low AChR antibody titer. The last group includes a proportion of older men with purely ocular symptoms (formerly Osserman type I). Classifications such as these are meant to capture certain types and contexts of myasthenia more than to convey the severity of illness.

Course and Prognosis

The *course of the illness* is extremely variable. Rapid spread from one muscle group to another occurs in some, but in others the disease remains unchanged for years before progressing or there is no progression. Remissions may take place without explanation, usually in the first years of illness, but these happen in less than half the cases and seldom last longer than a month or two. If the disease remits for a year or longer and then recurs, it then tends to be steadily progressive. Relapse may also be occasioned by the same events that in some cases preceded the onset of the illness, especially infections.

In Simpson's opinion, and this coincides with our observations, the danger of death from generalized myasthenia gravis is greatest in the first year after onset of the disease. A second period of danger in progressive cases is from 4 to 7 years after onset. After this time, the disease tends to stabilize and the risk of severe relapse diminishes. Fatalities relate mainly to the respiratory complications of pneumonia and aspiration. The mortality rate in the first years of illness, formerly in excess of 30 percent, is now less than 5 percent and with appropriate therapy virtually all patients lead productive lives.

An aspect of interest is the timing and frequency of conversion from ocular and restricted oropharyngeal patterns of weakness to more widespread involvement including the diaphragm. Bever and coworkers have confirmed the general impression that an increasing duration of purely ocular myasthenia is associated with a decreasing risk of late generalization of weakness. In a retrospective study of 108 patients, these authors found that only 15 percent of the observed instances of generalization occurred more than 2 years after isolated ocular manifestations.

A later age at onset was also associated with a higher incidence of fatal respiratory crises. In general, patients whose disease begins at a younger age run a more benign course. Grob and colleagues, who recorded the course of an astonishing 1,036 patients for a mean duration of 12 years, found that the clinical manifestations remained confined to the extraocular muscles and orbicularis oculi in 16 percent. Their data further indicated that localized ocular myasthenia present for only a month was associated with a 60 percent likelihood that the disease would generalize, but in those cases that remained restricted for more than a year, only 16 percent became generalized. In contrast, of 37 consecutive cases carefully studied by Weinberg with only ocular signs, 17 had more widespread weakness within a period of 6 years. Also informative in Grob's series was that in 67 percent the disease attained its maximum severity within a year of onset, and in 83 percent, within 3 years. It has been stated that the progression of symptoms is more rapid in male than in female patients.

It is not widely recognized that isolated muscle groups may occasionally remain *permanently weak* even when the ocular and generalized weakness has resolved. The muscles most often affected in this way are the anterior tibialis, triceps, and portions of the face.

The long-term outlook for *children with myasthenia* is better than it is for adults, and their life expectancy is only slightly reduced. Rodriguez and colleagues followed a group of 149 children for an average of 17 years; 85 of them had thymectomies, one of the main treatments for myasthenia as discussed further on. Approximately 30 percent of the nonthymectomized and 40 percent of the thymectomized patients underwent remission and were free of symptoms, usually in the first 3 years of illness. Those children with bulbar symptoms and no ocular or generalized weakness had the most favorable outcome.

Thymic and Systemic Disorders Associated With Myasthenia

A nonneoplastic lymphofollicular hyperplasia of the thymic medulla occurs in 65 percent or more of cases of myasthenia and *thymic tumors* occur in 10 to 15 percent. Thymomas with malignant characteristics may spread locally in the mediastinum and to regional lymph nodes but they rarely metastasize beyond these structures; when they do, the lungs and liver are usually affected. It should be emphasized that thymic enlargement and tumors may be missed in plain films of the chest and should be sought by CT scanning.

A striking degree of hyperplasia of the medulla of the thymus characterized by lymphoid follicles with active germinal centers is found in the majority of cases. Hyperplasia is even more frequent in younger patients in the third and fourth decades. The cells in the centers of the follicles are histiocytes surrounded by helper T lymphocytes, B lymphocytes, and plasma cells; immunoglobulin G (IgG) is elaborated in the germinal follicles. These resemble the cellular reaction observed in the thyroid tissue of Hashimoto thyroiditis. Because the latter disease has been reproduced in animals by injecting extracts of thyroid with Freund adjuvants, it had long ago been suggested that the so-called thymitis of myasthenia gravis is the result of a similar autoimmune sensitization but the inciting events for this process are entirely unknown. Immunosuppression with steroids causes involution of the thymus.

With regard to thymic tumors, two forms have been described: one composed of histiocytic cells like the reticulum cells in the center of the follicles, and the other predominantly lymphocytic and considered to be lymphosarcomatous. Some of the tumors have a high proportion of spindle-shaped cells. Overlapping types have been common. Thymic tumors may be unattended by myasthenia, though myasthenia has eventually developed in all of the cases under our observation, sometimes 15 to 20 years after the tumor was removed surgically. According to Bril and colleagues, the severity of myasthenic symptoms is no different in patients with thymoma than it is from that in patients without a tumor, but our impression has been that patients with tumors, particularly children, often have a peculiar clinical course. For example, we have observed unexpected sudden remissions and severe relapses, as well as resistance to medications.

Many contemporary studies, including more than 40 autopsies at our hospitals, have confirmed Erb's original contention that myasthenia gravis is a disease without a central nervous system lesion. The brain and spinal cord are normal unless damaged by hypoxia and hypotension from cardiorespiratory failure. Furthermore, the *muscle fibers* are generally intact, although in fatal cases with extensive paralysis, isolated fibers of esophageal, diaphragmatic, and eye muscles may undergo segmental necrosis with variable regeneration (Russell). Scattered aggregates of lymphocytes (lymphorrhages) are also observed, as originally noted by Buzzard, but none of these changes in muscle explains the widespread and severe weakness.

The main ultrastructural alterations occur in the *motor endplate*. These changes, elegantly demonstrated by A.G. Engel and associates (1976, 1977, 1987), consist of a reduction and simplification in the surface area of the postsynaptic membrane (sparse, shallow, abnormally wide, or absent secondary synaptic clefts) and a widening of the synaptic cleft (Fig. 49-1). The number and size of the presynaptic vesicles and their quanta of acetylcholine (ACh) are normal. The observation of regenerating axons near the junction, the many simplified junctions, and the absence of nerve terminals supplying some postsynaptic regions suggested to Engel and coworkers (1976, 1977, 1987) that there was an active process of degeneration and repair of the neuromuscular junction, particularly of the postsynaptic side.

Although not directly relevant to myasthenia, it is of interest that a number of curious neurologic disorders occur in association with thymoma. Among our own patients were 2 with "limbic encephalitis" with memory loss and confusion that could not be differentiated from the paraneoplastic variety of encephalitis (see Chap. 31), 1 case of midbrain encephalitis, 1 of Morvan's fibrillary chorea (discussed in Chap. 50), and 1 of aplastic anemia. Some of these neurologic processes are associated with antibodies directed against voltage-gated potassium channels (VGKC). Such cases appear in the literature, and all are considered to have a humoral immune basis.

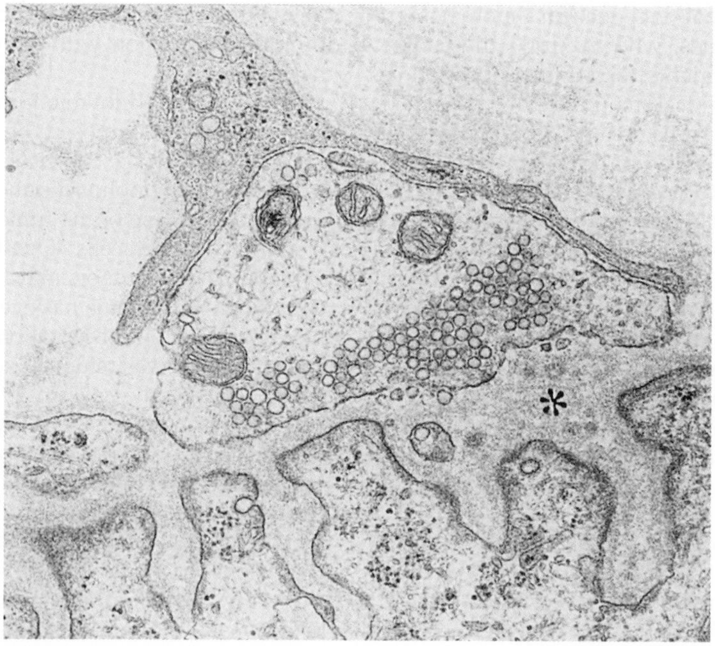

A

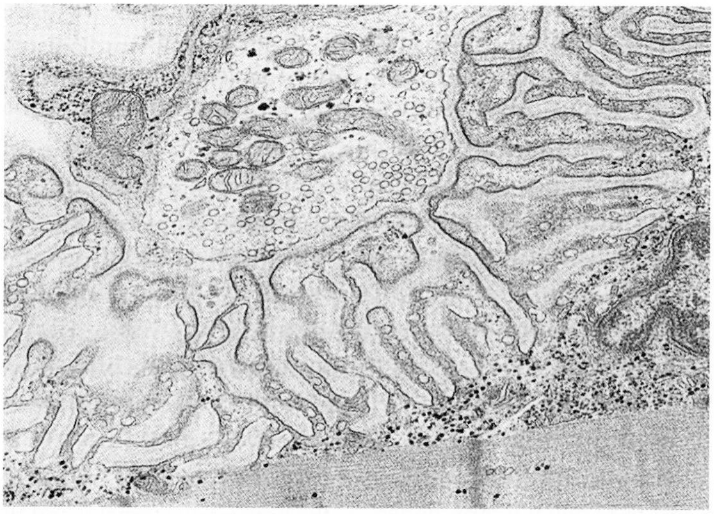

B

Figure 49-1. *A.* Endplate from a patient with myasthenia gravis. The terminal axon contains abundant presynaptic vesicles, but the postsynaptic folds are wide and there are few secondary folds. The loose junctional sarcoplasm is filled with microtubules and ribosomes. The synaptic cleft (*asterisk*) is widened. (From Santa et al by permission.) *B.* Normal endplate for comparison. (Courtesy of Dr. A.G. Engel.)

Of biologic and even greater clinical importance is the coexistence of myasthenia gravis and other autoimmune diseases. *Thyrotoxicosis* with periodic paralysis (5 percent of myasthenic patients; see further on and Chap. 50), lupus erythematosus, rheumatoid arthritis, Sjögren syndrome, mixed connective tissue disease, anticardiolipin antibody, and (curiously) polymyositis have all been associated with myasthenia more often than can be explained by chance. A proportion of young women with myasthenia have moderately elevated titers of antinuclear antibody without the clinical manifestations of systemic lupus.

Etiology and Pathogenesis

The clear demonstration of an *immunologic mechanism* operative at the neuromuscular junction was the most significant development in our understanding of myasthenia gravis. Patrick and Lindstrom discovered that repeated immunization of rabbits with AChR protein obtained from the electric eel caused a muscular weakness (contrary to what is stated in some books, their discovery was not accidental). Lennon and colleagues recognized this model as being similar to that of myasthenia gravis. Soon thereafter, Fambrough and coworkers demonstrated that the basic defect in myasthenia gravis was a marked reduction in the number of ACh receptors on the postsynaptic membrane of the neuromuscular junction. These observations were followed by the creation of an experimental model of the disease and the demonstration that experimentally induced myasthenia had clinical, pharmacologic, and electrophysiologic properties identical with those of human myasthenia gravis (Engel et al, 1976). It was also shown that humoral antibodies directed against protein components of AChR could transfer the myasthenic weakness to normal animals, and that the weakness as well as the physiologic abnormalities could be reversed by the administration of anticholinesterase drugs. Thus, the accumulated evidence satisfied the criteria for the diagnosis of an autoantibody-mediated disorder (Drachman, 1990).

The present view is that myasthenic weakness and fatigue are a result of the failure of effective neuromuscular transmission on the postsynaptic side. The greatly reduced number of receptors and the competitive activity of anti-AChR antibodies (see later) produce postsynaptic potentials of insufficient amplitude to discharge some muscle fibers. Blocked transmission at many endplates results in a reduction in the contractile power of the muscle. This deficiency is reflected first in the ocular and cranial muscles that are both the most continuously active and have the fewest AChRs per motor unit. Fatigue is understandable as the result of the normal decline in the amount of ACh released with each successive impulse.

Antibodies to AChR protein are present in more than 85 percent of patients with generalized myasthenia and in 60 percent of those with ocular myasthenia (Newsom-Davis). The presence of receptor antibodies has proved to be a reasonably sensitive and reliable test of the disease, as discussed later. The manner in which the antibodies that are directed against proteins in the intracellular compartment (such as anti-MuSK discussed later) causes weakness is not known.

Neuromuscular transmission is therefore impaired in several ways: (1) the antibodies block the binding of ACh to the AChR; (2) serum IgG from myasthenic patients has been shown to induce an increase in the degradation rate of AChR. This may be the result of the capacity of antibodies to cross-link the receptors; (3) antibodies cause a complement-mediated destruction of the postsynaptic folds (Engel and Arahata).

Although the evidence that an autoimmune mechanism is responsible for the functional disorder of muscle in myasthenia gravis is incontrovertible, the source of the autoimmune response has not been established. Because most patients with myasthenia have thymic abnormalities and a salutary response to thymectomy, it is logical to implicate the lymphoid reaction in this gland in the pathogenesis of the disease. Both T and B cells from the myasthenic thymus are particularly responsive to the AChR, more so than analogous cells from peripheral blood. Moreover, the thymus contains "myoid" cells (resembling striated muscle) that bear surface AChR. It is not known with certainty that thymic myoid cells are the source of immunologic stimulation in myasthenia gravis. The most obvious objection is that such cells are even more abundant in the normal than in the myasthenic thymus (according to Schluep et al). Another suggested pathogenesis, yet unconfirmed, is that a virus with a tropism for thymic cells might alter such cells and induce antibody formation. A viral infection might at the same time have a potential for oncogenesis, accounting for thymic tumors, but this is all speculative. Scadding and associates have suggested a different mode of thymic involvement; they have shown that thymic lymphocytes from patients with myasthenia gravis can synthesize anti-AChR antibody, both in culture and spontaneously.

Diagnosis

In patients who present with a changeable, specifically fatigable, diplopia or ptosis and the typical myasthenic facies—unequally drooping eyelids, relatively immobile mouth turned down at the corners, a smile that looks more like a snarl, a hanging jaw supported by the hand—the diagnosis can hardly be overlooked. However, only a few patients display this fully developed syndrome. Ptosis, diplopia, difficulty in speaking or swallowing, or weakness of the limbs is at first mild and inconstant and may be mistaken for a cerebrovascular disease. However, the finding that sustained activity of small cranial muscles results in weakness (e.g., increasing droop of eyelids while looking at the ceiling or diplopia when fixating in lateral or vertical gaze or reading for 2 to 3 min) and that contraction improves after a brief rest is virtually diagnostic, even in the early stages of the disease. Any other affected group of muscles may be tested in similar fashion. The characteristic ocular signs have already been described. For confirmation, the measurement of specific antibody (anti-AChR), electromyography, and certain pharmacologic tests described below are necessary. Several special clinical problems and associated conditions are summarized further on.

Electrophysiologic Testing Characteristic of myasthenia is a rapid reduction in the amplitude of compound muscle action potentials during a series of repetitive stimulations of a peripheral nerve at a rate of 3 per second (*decrementing response* as shown in Fig. 45-4*A*). Reversal of this response by neostigmine or edrophonium has been a reliable confirmatory finding in most cases. A decremental response to stimulation can usually be obtained most often from the proximal limb muscles followed by the facial and, to a lesser extent, the hand muscles, which may or may not be clinically weak. During a progressive phase of the disease or during corticosteroid therapy, a slight initial incrementing response may be obtained, not to be confused with the marked incrementing response after voluntary contraction that characterizes the Lambert-Eaton syndrome (see further on).

Single-fiber electromyography (EMG) represents an even more sensitive method of detecting the defect in neuromuscular transmission. This technique demonstrates an inconstancy of the normally invariant interval between the firing of muscle fibers connected to the same motor unit ("jitter"—see "Single-Fiber Electromyography" in Chap. 45) or complete blocking of successive discharges from single muscle fibers belonging to the same motor unit. The test requires a great deal of cooperation from the patient and that contraction of a muscle be sustained at just the right amplitude in order to isolate single muscle fibers from the same unit. It is also possible to detect such pairs of fibers by electrical stimulation of a nerve. Nerve conduction velocities and distal motor latencies are normal unless there is a coincident polyneuropathy.

Neostigmine Test Almost as valuable as electrophysiologic testing is testing with the anticholinesterase inhibitors neostigmine and in the past, edrophonium a more rapidly acting agent. These drugs prolong and exaggerate the effects of ACh in the synapse and thereby produce an increment in muscle power in the patient with myasthenia. Edrophonium is not easily available in the United States at the time of this writing but neostigmine affords a longer time for observation, as noted in the next paragraph. The tests are performed in the following manner. After the estimation of strength in a cranial (usually the levator palpebrae or an extraocular muscle) or limb muscle (by dynamometry), or vital capacity, neostigmine is injected intramuscularly in a dose of 1.5 mg. Atropine sulfate (0.8 mg) should be given several minutes in advance to counteract the unpleasant muscarinic effects of neostigmine (salivation, sweating bronchorrhea, borborygmi, bowel cramps and, sometimes, diarrhea). Neostigmine may alternatively be given intravenously in a dose of 0.5 mg, but its effect is often too brief to be as useful. After intramuscular injection of neostigmine, objective improvement occurs within 10 to 15 min, reaches its peak at 20 min, and lasts up to 1 h, allowing for careful verification of the neurologic improvement. Many neurologists perform this test twice, once with an injection of saline as a control.

Alternatively, 1 mg (0.1 mL) of edrophonium is given intravenously; if this dose is tolerated and no definite improvement in strength occurs after 45 s, another 4 to 9 mg is injected. A total dose of 10 mg is rarely necessary. Most patients who respond do so after 3 to 5 mg has been administered. The mild muscarinic effects of edrophonium are blocked by pretreatment with atropine 0.8 mg subcutaneously as for neostigmine. The clinical effect of improved ptosis, extraocular movements, oropharyngeal function, arm and shoulder abduction, or vital capacity persists for no more than 5 min with edrophonium and 60 min with neostigmine.

One caution: with either drug, some patients deteriorate immediately, but briefly, as a result of an increase in pulmonary secretions. A positive test consists of visible (objective) improvement in muscle contractility, fusion of diplopia, or resolution of fatigable ptosis. Dynamometry and measurement of forced vital capacity serve as more objective markers of improvement, or lack of effect. The report of subjective improvement alone is not dependable and one must be distrustful of equivocal test results, which may occur with ocular palsies due to tumors, thyroid disease, Guillain-Barré syndrome (GBS), progressive supranuclear palsy, or carotid aneurysms (pseudoocular myasthenia).

A negative test with an anticholinesterase agent does not entirely exclude myasthenia gravis but is a strong point against the diagnosis. In a small number of patients with periodic and purely ocular symptoms who later prove to have myasthenia gravis, the edrophonium and neostigmine tests (and electrophysiologic studies and AChR antibody measurements) may be entirely normal during the first or even after several acute episodes. Only later, for inexplicable reasons, do these tests become positive. Finally, the anticholinesterase-inhibiting drugs carry a small risk of inducing ventricular fibrillation and cardiac arrest so that testing should be carried out where emergency support is accessible.

Measurement of Receptor Antibodies in Blood The detection of *anti-AChR antibodies* provides a reasonably sensitive and highly specific test for the diagnosis of myasthenia. The radioimmunoassay method of detection is accurate and widely used. Serum antibodies are found in 80 to 90 percent of patients with generalized myasthenia gravis and in approximately 60 percent of those whose symptoms are restricted to the ocular muscles (Vincent and Newsom-Davis). For the most part, adults with myasthenia whose sera are persistently negative for AChR antibodies do not differ clinically or electromyographically from those with antibodies with the exception noted below. Persistently negative AChR antibody tests are more frequently found in patients with ocular myasthenia than in patients with generalized weakness. Patients with a thymoma and severe generalized myasthenia are practically always seropositive. Interestingly, the antibody titers usually remain elevated during clinical remissions.

Instances of "seronegative" disease are sometimes due to antibody production against unusual muscle epitopes that are located on or near the acetylcholine receptor; their detection requires a special panel of tests. However, the majority of such cases have been ascribed to IgG antibodies directed against an intracellular *muscle-specific kinase* (MuSK). This enzyme plays a role in supporting the normal structure of the postsynaptic membrane and in the arrangement of AChR but its main function may be in developmental synaptic differentiation. Scuderi and colleagues and others have proposed that patients with MuSK antibody, mostly women, have a special clinical syndrome of prominent oculobulbar weakness, often with severe disease and respiratory crises (see also Evoli et al). Others have reported a different pattern of mainly neck and proximal weakness that simulates a typical myopathy. Many of these patients are inadequately responsive to anticholinesterase treatment. Also of interest, but not currently used in routine diagnosis, is the presence of *antibodies directed against striated muscle* in almost half of myasthenic patients and an even higher incidence (stated to be 85 percent) in patients who also have a thymoma.

Each of the commonly used diagnostic tests, electrophysiology, edrophonium, and antibodies, proves to be about equally reliable. Kelly and coworkers obtained positive results with single-muscle-fiber recording in 79 percent, with the antireceptor antibody test in 71 percent, and with the edrophonium test in 81 percent. Combined, they confirmed the diagnosis in 95 percent of clinically suspected cases. Presumably, had the anti-MuSK receptor antibody test been available, the sensitivity of serologic diagnosis would have been higher.

In keeping with the observation of some myasthenic patients that their weakness improves in the cold, a test has been devised in which an ice pack is placed over a ptotic eyelid for 2 min or to the limit of the patient's tolerance. Sethi and colleagues found that ptosis was diminished in 8 of 10 patients. In our patients, this effect has not been as consistently evident, but it may be a useful adjunctive test.

Other diagnostic tests performed routinely in essentially all patients with myasthenia gravis include CT of the chest (for the detection of thymic enlargement or thymoma), tests of thyroid function for reasons discussed further on, and in cases of uncertain diagnosis, magnetic resonance imaging of the cranium and orbits to exclude compressive and inflammatory lesions of the cranial nerves and ocular muscles.

Special Diagnostic Problems

We have encountered the following clinical problems in myasthenia:

1. *The concurrence of myasthenia gravis and thyrotoxicosis.* Thyrotoxicosis may produce a characteristic ocular myopathy and there is a tentative relation to periodic paralysis as indicated in Chap. 50. There is no certain evidence that thyrotoxicosis aggravates myasthenia gravis; some have even observed an inverse relationship between the severity of the two conditions. Hypothyroidism, however, does worsen the myasthenic symptoms. The ophthalmoplegia of thyrotoxicosis can usually be distinguished by the presence of an associated exophthalmos (early in the disease, exophthalmos may be absent), lack of ptosis, and the lack of definitive response to neostigmine. Polymyositis and inclusion body myopathy are differentiated from myasthenia by lack of involvement of extraocular muscles, but they may affect oropharyngeal muscles, as does myasthenia. Finding the signs of these diseases in combination with those of myasthenia indicates a concurrence of two independent autoimmune diseases.
2. *The neurasthenic or depressed patient who complains of weakness when actually referring to fatigability.* There is no ptosis, strabismus, or dysphagia, though an anxious individual may complain of diplopia (usually of momentary duration when drowsy) and also of tightness in the throat (globus hystericus). A number of such patients claim improvement with neostigmine but objective and reversal is always uncertain. Conversely, myasthenia is as often mistaken for hysteria or other emotional illness, mainly because the physician is unfamiliar with myasthenia (or with hysteria) and has been overly impressed with the precipitation of the illness by an emotional crisis. Furthermore, fatigability is a feature of all of these conditions, but only in the psychiatric ones does it extend to the sphere of mental endurance. Those with myasthenia do not usually complain of fatigue of the mind, whereas these are frequent complaints in psychiatric conditions. A similar problem arises frequently on our services in judging breathlessness due to anxiety or cardiopulmonary disease in a patient with presumed myasthenia. Careful appraisal of the breathing pattern and determination of the vital capacity or other spirometric measurements are helpful here.
3. *Progressive external ophthalmoplegia and other restricted myopathies, including the congenital myasthenic states.* These may be mistaken for long-established myasthenia gravis. It should be emphasized that the extraocular muscles and levator palpebrae may be permanently damaged by myasthenia and cease to respond to neostigmine. Another possibility is that restricted ocular myasthenia may not respond to anticholinesterase drugs from the beginning and the diagnosis of myasthenia is erroneously excluded. One must then turn to other muscles for clinical and electromyographic and serologic confirmation of the diagnosis.
4. *Myasthenia with dysarthria and dysphagia, but without ptosis or obvious strabismus.* These may be confused with multiple sclerosis, polymyositis, inclusion body myopathy, stroke, motor neuron disease, or some other neurologic disease. Testing with an anticholinesterase inhibitor, single-fiber and repetitive stimulation recording, and measurement of antibodies usually clarifies the matter.
5. *The initial manifestations of botulism*—blurred vision, diplopia, ptosis, strabismus, and ophthalmoparesis—may be mistaken for myasthenia gravis of acute onset. In botulism, however, the pupils are usually large and unreactive, and the eye signs are followed in rapid succession by involvement of bulbar, trunk, and limb muscles.

   Similarly, the *oculopharyngeal-brachial* and *variants of Guillain-Barré syndrome (GBS)* in the early stages have many of the features of myasthenia, including ptosis, that may be partially responsive to anticholinesterase drugs. The loss of tendon reflexes, acral paresthesias and areflexia, or the development of ataxia in the limbs make the diagnosis of GBS at once apparent and detailed electrophysiologic testing distinguishes the two conditions.
6. *Intoxication with organophosphate insecticides,* because of their capacity to induce a cholinergic crisis, may be confused with a myasthenic crisis (see further on).

Certain other small clinical points may be helpful in differentiating myasthenia from other diseases that affect the cranial musculature. A hanging jaw and hanging head are indicative of myasthenia, whereas complete or asymmetric facial paresis is typical of GBS. Botulism usually affects the pupillary convergence reaction, and GBS does so only when there is complete internal and external ophthalmoplegia; diphtheria affects mainly the accommodative reaction early on. The question of midbrain stroke as a consequence of basilar artery occlusion arises in a case with total ophthalmoplegia; it should be recalled that the level of consciousness is usually reduced if vertical gaze and pupillary reactions are lost in cases of basilar artery stroke; such is not the case in neuromuscular diseases. The myasthenic syndrome of Lambert-Eaton, discussed further on, only occasionally affects the ocular muscles, but is identified by its other clinical and electrophysiologic features. Ocular paresis, as may occur in nemaline polymyopathy, oculopharyngeal dystrophy, and thyrotoxic ophthalmic disease, come on too slowly in most cases to be confused with myasthenia gravis. On occasion, the eye movements in myasthenia simulate an internuclear ophthalmoplegia or other "central" sign, even to the extent of including nystagmus in an abducting eye.

Treatment

The treatment of this disease involves the careful use of two groups of drugs—anticholinesterases and immunosuppressants including corticosteroids and in special acute circumstances, plasma exchange and intravenous immune globulin. An elective thymectomy is appropriate in many patients as discussed below.

Anticholinesterase Drugs The two drugs that give the best results in ameliorating myasthenic weakness are neostigmine (Prostigmin) and pyridostigmine (Mestinon), the latter being preferred by most clinicians and patients. The usual dose of pyridostigmine is 30 to 90 mg given every 6 h (typically a 60-mg pill is tried first); the oral dose of neostigmine ranges from 7.5 to 45 mg given every 2 to 6 h. Extended-action forms of both drugs are available but are given at bedtime mainly to patients who complain of weakness during the night or early morning hours. The dosage of these drugs and their frequency of administration vary considerably from patient to patient, but we agree with Drachman (2003) that the maximal useful dosage of pyridostigmine rarely exceeds 120 mg given every 3 h. Table 49-1 lists the approximate dose-equivalents of these various drugs.

For mild cases, for patients in partial remission after thymectomy, and for purely ocular myasthenia, the use of anticholinesterase drugs may be the only form of therapy necessary for some period of time (ocular myasthenia often responds well to small doses of corticosteroids as noted further on). Although these drugs seldom relieve symptoms completely (the response of ocular symptoms is typically incomplete), most such patients are able to function well.

Corticosteroids For the patient with moderate to severe generalized weakness who is responding inadequately to anticholinesterase drugs, the long-term administration of corticosteroids is the most consistently effective form of treatment, as described in a large series of patients by Pascuzzi and colleagues. Small doses of corticosteroids (prednisone 15 to 25 mg daily) alone or in combination with azathioprine (see later) are also often adequate to control ocular myasthenia. However, one must be prepared to contend with the side effects of long-term corticosteroid therapy and we hesitate to undertake such a program in children or patients with severe diabetes or other diseases that are likely to be aggravated. Because recent experience with the newer immunosuppressive agents was not incorporated into most prior series, the uniform use of steroids might not be correct.

The usual form of corticosteroid therapy is prednisone (or corresponding doses of prednisolone), beginning with 15 to 20 mg/d and increasing the dose gradually until a satisfactory clinical response is obtained or until a daily dose of 50 to 60 mg is reached. *With higher doses or more rapid elevations of the doses, worsening of weakness in the first weeks may occur* and hospitalization and careful observation for respiratory difficulty may be advisable. Improvement after the initiation of corticosteroids occurs over a few weeks. Once the maximal effect from prednisone has been attained, the dosage can be reduced gradually over months to the lowest point at which it is still effective. Our practice has been to then attempt to institute an alternate-day schedule, which diminishes the side effects; some patients have done better with a modest difference in dose from one day to the next, rather than omitting a dose entirely on alternate days. Potassium supplements and antacids should be prescribed liberally if needed, as with any chronic corticosteroid regime and consideration should be given to prophylaxis with antibiotics for *Pneumocystis* infection, and bisphosphonate for osteoporosis if long-term treatment is anticipated. At the outset of steroid therapy, anticholinesterase drugs are given simultaneously; as the patient improves, the dosage of the latter may be adjusted downward.

Azathioprine and Other Immunosuppressive Drugs *Azathioprine* is a useful adjunct to steroids in patients who cannot tolerate or fail to respond to prednisone. It has been possible to manage the disease reasonably well in a few of patients with azathioprine alone, but there is no study to support this practice (see Palace et al, 1998). Treatment typically begins with 50 mg (1 tablet) bid for a few days; if this is tolerated, the dosage is raised to 2 to 3 mg/kg/d (150 to 250 mg daily). However, improvement occurs much more slowly than with corticosteroids and a significant response may not be evident for many months to a year (Witte et al). Liver function tests and blood cell count should be checked regularly. The Myasthenia Gravis Clinical Study Group found that the most severe forms of the disease, particularly those resistant to either prednisone or azathioprine alone, benefit from the combination of the two medications. Azathioprine is a prodrug of mercaptopurine, which is metabolized principally by thiopurine methyltransferase (TPMT). Approximately 3 per 100,000 persons are deficient in the enzyme, for which reason, some clinicians measure its level before initiating azathioprine in order to avoid bone marrow toxicity; it has not been our practice to do so. There are many variant alleles of TPMT and a larger number of patients have partial deficiency of the enzyme or even excessive enzyme activity but it has not been clear how to utilize

Table 49-1

DOSE-EQUIVALENTS FOR DRUGS USED IN THE TREATMENT OF MYASTHENIA GRAVIS

	DOSE EQUIVALENT	ONSET	TIME TO MAXIMUM RESPONSE
Pyridostigmine (Mestinon)	60 mg (oral)	40 min	1 h
Neostigmine oral (Prostigmin)	15 mg	1 h	1.5 h
Neostigmine IM	1.5 mg	30 min	1 h
Neostigmine IV	0.5 mg	Immediate	20 min

this information in myasthenia. Azathioprine interacts with other drugs such as allopurinol and warfarin.

Cyclosporine is another immunosuppressive drug that has shown benefit in clinical trials (Tindall et al). It is given in 2 divided doses daily, to a total of 6 mg/kg, but not often used currently because of serious side effects (hypertension, nephrotoxicity) and its high cost. Because of the success of alternative regimens, we have had occasion over the years to use cyclosporine only once for myasthenia.

Mycophenolate is currently being used as an adjunct to corticosteroids and has been beneficial in several small trials but failed to demonstrate similar effect in larger controlled studies. The clinical improvement, when it does occur, has generally occurred sooner than it does with azathioprine (Meriggioli et al). Diarrhea was the main adverse effect. Several experts in the field believe that mycophenolate is preferable to most of the adjunctive medications and in some milder cases may be effective alone, but reconciling this view with recent failed trials is vexing.

De Feo and coworkers have used *cyclophosphamide* administered in intravenous pulses; they were able to remove 5 of their 12 patients from steroids, but the appropriate use of this potent agent is not clear and we have resorted to it infrequently. Drachman and colleagues (2003), as well as others, describe a regimen of high-dose cyclophosphamide (50 mg/kg/d for 4 consecutive days) followed by granulocyte-stimulating factor to "reboot" the immune system in refractory cases. This approach has risks but may be justified if all other measures have failed. Liver function and white blood cell count require monitoring. On the basis of pilot trials, many other drugs, for example, tacrolimus as reported by Ponseti and colleagues, rituximab, and etanercept have come into use in patients who are dependent on or resistant to corticosteroids, including those with antibodies to MuSK (Diaz-Manero et al).

Plasma Exchange and Intravenous Immune Globulin For severe myasthenia that is refractory to treatment with anticholinesterase drugs and prednisone, or during an acute period of worsening, one must resort to other measures. Striking temporary remissions (2 to 8 weeks) may be obtained by the use of *plasma exchange*. This form of treatment may be lifesaving during a myasthenic crisis. It also finds use before and after thymectomy and at the start of immunosuppressive drug therapy. Plasma exchange is also helpful in limiting the aforementioned weakness that is often induced by the institution of high-dose corticosteroids. The number and volume of exchanges required in these circumstances is somewhat arbitrary but they tend to be less than those required for GBS; several exchanges of 2 to 3.5 L each (totaling approximately 125 mL/kg) performed over a week usually suffice. The removed plasma is replaced with albumin and saline. It has been estimated that a 2-L exchange will remove 80 percent of circulating antibodies and that this will be reflected in reduced ACh antibody levels in 3 to 5 days. There is only an approximate correlation between a reduction in the titer of anti-AChR antibody and the degree of clinical improvement. In a crisis requiring plasma exchanges and mechanical ventilation, it has been our practice to discontinue or curtail the use of anticholinesterase drugs and resume them as the patient is being weaned from the ventilator. Also, it may be that sensitivity to these drugs may be enhanced in the hours after an exchange so that their dosages must be adjusted accordingly.

A small number of patients respond so well to plasma exchange and find the side effects of steroids so intolerable that they choose to be maintained with two to three exchanges every several weeks or months. Immunoadsorption, a technique similar to plasma exchange that removes antibodies and immune complexes by passing blood over a tryptophan column, is less cumbersome than conventional plasma exchange and has been effective, but experience with this procedure is limited.

Intravenous immune globulin is similarly useful in the short-term control of acutely worsening myasthenia. The usual dose is 2 g/kg given in divided doses over 3 to 5 days. Several small series suggest that the effect is equivalent to a series of plasma exchanges. However, plasma exchange and immune globulin have been subjected to only limited systematic study or comparison and, while these treatments are invaluable in deteriorated patients or those in crisis, they offer only short-term benefit. In two separate small studies, Gajdos and colleagues and Barth et al found no difference between intravenous immune globulin (IVIg) and plasma exchange (1997) and no difference between IVIg 1 g/kg/d given for 1 or 2 days (2005) in myasthenic exacerbations, most cases of which were less severe than typical crisis.

Thymectomy This operation, first introduced by Blalock, despite the absence of proof in trials, is considered an appropriate procedure for many patients with generalized myasthenia gravis between puberty and 55 years of age. The surgery is performed electively and not during an acute deterioration of myasthenia. The remission rate after thymectomy is approximately 35 percent provided that the procedure is done in the first year or two after onset of the disease, and another 50 percent will improve to some extent (Buckingham et al). The remission rate is progressively lower, but not negligible, if the operation is postponed beyond this time. In patients with myasthenia restricted to the ocular muscles for a year or longer, the prognosis is so good that thymectomy is unnecessary. The response to thymectomy is not evident for several months and is maximal in most cases by 3 years. In favorably responding cases, levels of circulating receptor antibody are reduced or disappear entirely. If possible, thymectomy should be postponed until puberty because of the importance of the gland in the development of the immune system, but juvenile myasthenia is also quite responsive. The results are not as predictable in patients who harbor a thymoma.

A suprasternal approach for removal of the gland has been developed and results in less postoperative pain and morbidity than occurs with a transsternal thoracotomy but the transsternal operation may be preferable because it assures a more complete removal of thymic tissue. Thymectomy is best performed in a hospital where there is close collaboration between the thoracic surgeon and the neurologist. If the patient is weak preoperatively, a course of plasma exchange or immune globulin may be given preceding the surgical procedure. Large "stress doses" of corticosteroids seem to be unnecessary in most patients who have been taking these medications chronically. After operation, respiratory assistance must be available if needed. Neostigmine intramuscularly, may be given every 3 to 6 h postoperatively. Usually the dose requirement is about 75 percent of that taken before surgery. As improvement occurs, oral medications are resumed as remission is not anticipated for many months or longer as noted above.

Thymectomy may also be a safe and effective treatment in elderly patients with myasthenia. In 12 such individuals, Olanow and associates reported complete remission in 9 and clinical improvement in the remainder. The improvement in older patients is less convincing than it is in the younger group, in part because the thymus is atrophic. Nonetheless, some of our patients who were older than age 60 years did benefit.

Removal of the thymus gland is also indicated in practically all patients in whom *thymoma* is detected by CT scanning of the chest. The tumor can be locally invasive but rarely metastasizes. The operative approach is through the anterior thorax, with adequate exposure to remove all the tumor tissue. If the tumor cannot be removed completely, the remaining tissue should be treated with focused radiation. Local spread and lymph node invasion have been treated with combinations of chemotherapy including cisplatin, but it is not very satisfactory. Park and colleagues concluded from a large retrospective study of metastatic cases that chemotherapy offers some benefit in terms of survival, but this remains controversial.

Despite this endorsement of thymectomy for generalized myasthenia, it has remained an unproven therapy by a modern trial and attempts to recruit patients for such an endeavor have been difficult.

Myasthenic and Cholinergic Crisis

A rapid and severe deterioration of the myasthenia itself, termed *myasthenic crisis,* can bring the patient to the brink of respiratory failure and quadriparesis in a matter of hours. A respiratory infection or excessive use of sedative medications or drugs with a potential for blocking neuromuscular transmission may precede the myasthenic crisis. We have encountered numerous cases in which oropharyngeal weakness has led to aspiration pneumonia, which, in turn, precipitated a crisis. Just as often, a precipitating event is not evident. Rarely, a respiratory arrest is the first manifestation of crisis. Such events may occur at any time after the diagnosis of myasthenia, but half are evident within 12 to 18 months. In an experience with 53 patients in myasthenic crisis at the Columbia-Presbyterian Medical Center, pneumonia was the most frequent precipitating event, but no cause could be determined in almost one-third of cases (Thomas et al).

Incipient respiratory failure is usually marked by a reduction of vital capacity, often accompanied by restlessness, anxiety, diaphoresis, or tremor. Once the diaphragm fails, movements of the chest wall and abdomen become paradoxical (the abdomen moves inward during inspiration) or there may be shallow excursions of the chest, alternating with paradoxical movements as discussed in Chap. 26 where the characteristics of neuromuscular respiratory failure are described. In an emergency, after clearing of the airway, such a patient can be supported briefly by a tight-fitting face mask and manual bag (Ambu) breathing. The chest wall will be very compliant as a result of muscular weakness.

Management of the crisis entails timely and careful intubation followed by mechanical ventilation in a critical care unit that is equipped to attend to the medical and neurologic needs of such patients. Respiratory failure in a few patients can be managed by the use of bilevel positive airway pressure (BIPAP) according to Rabinstein and Wijdicks, but in our experience, this has not been consistently effective in avoiding endotracheal intubation. One must cope with both the oropharyngeal weakness and secretions that endanger the airway, and the diaphragmatic weakness. Anticholinesterase drugs, which exaggerate secretions, are best withdrawn at the time of intubation. A useful maneuver is to allow the patient to remain off cholinergic drugs for several days while on a ventilator; there is often a heightened response to the reinstitution of medications after this period. The use of plasma exchange or intravenous gamma globulin as described earlier, is equivalently effective in hastening improvement and weaning from the ventilator. Some of our colleagues have used high-dose corticosteroid infusions in these circumstances but this measure has not been particularly successful in our unit and, in the short run, carries the risk of inducing worsening of the weakness (Panegyres et al).

Patients generally respond equivalently to plasma exchange or immunoglobulin infusions in 1 or 2 days, but more often a week or more is required for recovery after a full course of 4 to 5 exchanges or 3 to 5 g/kg IVIg given in divided daily doses. Whether the previously mentioned studies (e.g., Gajdos et al) comparing the two treatments and comparing doses of IVIg in myasthenic exacerbations are pertinent to crisis is unknown but we almost always institute one or the other soon after it as it is apparent that respiratory failure is imminent or worsening.

It is generally best to wait 2 or 3 weeks before committing a patient to tracheostomy. When weaning from the ventilator is anticipated, anticholinesterase agents are reintroduced slowly, and treatment with corticosteroids can be instituted if necessary. *Oral doses of 60 mg pyridostigmine or 15 mg neostigmine are roughly equivalent to 0.5 to 1 mg neostigmine intravenously and 1.5 to 2 mg intramuscularly,* as noted in Table 49-1. The management of the critically ill patient with myasthenia is reviewed in the monograph by Ropper and colleagues.

Most patients with myasthenic crisis take several weeks to recover, and a few of our patients have remained ventilator-dependent for months. In the extensive experience of 53 patients from Columbia-Presbyterian, half of the patients could be safely extubated within 2 weeks and three-quarters by a month (Thomas et al). There were 7 deaths among 53 patients, reflecting the gravity of this syndrome even in the modern era of intensive care. Atelectasis, severe anemia, congestive heart failure, and clostridial diarrhea (associated with antibiotic use) portend a prolonged period of generalized weakness and intubation. From time to time, one encounters a patient in whom respiration and ambulation do not improve for many months after a myasthenic crisis. In our experience these have been middle-aged or older patients, usually women, in whom an element of hyperthyroidism or hypothyroidism may have been operative. They become wasted as the proximal limb and axial muscles, including the diaphragm, fail to recover their power, even though the ocular and oropharyngeal muscles improve. The role of corticosteroids in producing a concomitant proximal myopathy is a consideration that can be solved by careful electrophysiologic examination.

If the response to anticholinesterase drugs is poor and progressively larger doses are not relieving symptoms, there is always the danger of a *cholinergic crisis.* In our own experience with more than 60 patients of severe myasthenia in an intensive care unit, we have been persuaded of the occurrence of a cholinergic crisis only rarely. This consists of a relatively rapid increase in muscular weakness, usually coupled with the adverse muscarinic effects of the anticholinesterase drug (nausea, vomiting, pallor, sweating, salivation, bronchorrhea, colic, diarrhea, miosis, bradycardia). An impending cholinergic effect is betrayed by constriction of pupils. If the blood pressure falls with bradycardia, 0.6 mg atropine sulfate should be given slowly by the intravenous route. Neostigmine or repetitive stimulation may be used to determine whether or not weakness is to the result of an excess of anticholinesterase medications. However, this test has been misleading and undoubtedly has contributed to an overestimation of the frequency and importance of the cholinergic crisis. Infection, or the natural course of the disease, has been far more common causes of acutely worsening weakness and respiratory failure.

The only recourse in cases of long-standing and severe myasthenia is to continue an average dose of corticosteroids, immunosuppressive, and anticholinesterase medications with intermittent trials of immune globulin or plasma exchanges. This is also a desperate situation in which high-dose cyclophosphamide followed by granulocyte-stimulating factor, as mentioned earlier, may result in slow improvement. Other agents such as rituximab may be tried.

Management of Anesthesia and Pregnancy in the Myasthenic Patient

These represent special problems. Surgical procedures of any type are often sufficiently stressful to produce decompensation of the disease. If the patient is unable to take medications orally, anticholinesterase agents may be given intramuscularly (approximately one-thirtieth of the oral dose of pyridostigmine and one-tenth the oral dose of neostigmine listed in Table 49-1). If corticosteroids were being used they may be continued and the dose generally left unchanged; large "stress" doses are generally unnecessary, as mentioned earlier in the discussion of thymectomy. Neuromuscular blocking agents of the noncompetitive type may have a very prolonged effect in these patients and should be avoided as part of the anesthetic regimen. If they are necessary for some reason, a period of mechanical ventilation should be anticipated. In contrast, the dose of succinylcholine (which is not recommended) required to produce muscle relaxation may be larger than usual. Any drug, the use of which is contemplated in anesthetic and postsurgical management, should be checked against the list of agents that are capable of exaggerating myasthenic weakness (see further on).

Pregnancy is usually uncomplicated in patients with myasthenia but some women who are partially treated for myasthenia and have generalized weakness may have difficulty in assisting with vaginal delivery. However, the use of intravenous cholinesterase inhibitors is contraindicated because of the possibility of inducing uterine contractions, and cytotoxic drugs are generally avoided during pregnancy because of the potential for fetal abnormalities. Also, magnesium is not recommended for the treatment of eclampsia because its neuromuscular blocking effects may worsen myasthenic weakness. Delivery usually proceeds normally, and breast-feeding is not thought to be a problem with regard to the transmission of AChR antibodies. Almost half of women with myasthenia have an exacerbation of varying degree in the several weeks postpartum. A rapidly dropping level of alpha-fetoprotein has been implicated as this protein inhibits binding of antiacetylcholine antibodies to postsynaptic receptors. The issues of neonatal myasthenia and of reduced intrauterine movements with arthrogryposis are considered later.

OTHER DISORDERS OF NEUROMUSCULAR TRANSMISSION (Table 49-2)

Considered here are several disorders of neuromuscular transmission characterized clinically by muscular weakness and fatigability but differing in mechanism from autoimmune myasthenia gravis. The Lambert-Eaton myasthenic syndrome, neonatal myasthenia, the congenital myasthenic syndromes, and the myasthenic syndromes induced by drugs and toxins are the main disorders in this group. Two additional important diseases—botulism and organophosphate poisoning—are described elsewhere in the book.

The Myasthenic-Myopathic Syndrome of Lambert-Eaton (Lambert-Eaton Syndrome)

This special form of myasthenia, observed most often in patients with oat cell carcinoma of the lung, was first described by Lambert, Eaton, and Rooke in 1956 and further by Eaton and Lambert in 1957. Unlike myasthenia gravis, the muscles of the trunk, shoulder girdle, pelvic girdle, and lower extremities are the ones that become weak and fatigable. The first symptoms are difficulty in arising from a chair, climbing stairs, and walking; the shoulder muscles are usually affected later. Although ptosis, diplopia, dysarthria, and dysphagia may occur, presentation with these symptoms is distinctly unusual. Increasing weakness after exertion stamps the condition as myasthenic, but in direct contrast to myasthenia gravis, *there may be a temporary increase in muscle power*

Table 49-2

MAJOR DISORDERS OF THE NEUROMUSCULAR JUNCTION

MYASTHENIC SYNDROMES	CAUSAL AGENT OR GENE DEFECT	ONSET DECADE	TREATMENT	CLINICAL FEATURES
	ACQUIRED MYASTHENIC SYNDROMES			
Presynaptic				
Botulism (Chap. 43)	Peptide toxin from *Clostridium botulinum*	Any	Supportive; ventilation	Blurred vision, dysphagia, limb weakness
Lambert-Eaton myasthenic syndrome	Autoimmune reduction in calcium-mediated quantal release	Midlife	3,4-DAP Possibly IVIg	Truncal weakness, dysautonomic features Two-thirds have cancer
Synaptic				
Insecticides (Chap. 43)	Organophosphates (inhibits AChE)	Any	Remove toxins Atropine	Miosis, diarrhea, cramps, weakness Delayed sensorimotor neuropathy
Postsynaptic				
Myasthenia gravis	Autoimmune attack on postsynaptic membrane Antibodies to AChR or MuSK protein	Adult	AChE inhibitors, IVIg Other immunosuppressants	Diplopia, ptosis Limb weakness with exertion
Snake venom toxins (Chap. 43)	Multiple peptide toxins that lyse muscle, bind Na channels, K channels (acting both post- and presynaptically)	Any	Supportive Possibly AChE inhibitors	Acute weakness

during the first few contractions. The tendon reflexes are often diminished but complete abolition of the reflexes should raise the question of an associated carcinomatous polyneuropathy. Fasciculations are not seen.

One of the most instructive reviews of this disease is that by O'Neill and colleagues: In 50 well-studied cases they described proximal leg weakness in all, arm weakness in 39, diplopia in 25, ptosis in 21, and dysarthria in 12. Other complaints were paresthesias, aching pain (suggesting arthritis), and a number of autonomic disturbances, such as dryness of the mouth, constipation, difficult micturition, and impotence. This latter group of symptoms gives the syndrome an unmistakable stamp as discussed further on under "Diagnosis." One should not be surprised to find other neurologic manifestations of neoplasia (e.g., polyneuropathy, polymyositis or dermatomyositis, multifocal leukoencephalopathy, cerebellar degeneration, as discussed in Chap. 31).

The onset of weakness is subacute and the course, variably progressive. Males are affected far more often than females (5:1). The weakness may precede discovery of the tumor by months or years. Approximately 60 percent of cases are associated with small cell lung cancer, but small numbers have also occurred with carcinoma of the breast, prostate, stomach, and rectum, and with lymphomas; in about one-third of patients, no tumor is found. Some cases are associated with other autoimmune diseases, but most are paraneoplastic or idiopathic. The condition may occur in children, usually with no relation to tumor. In the tumor cases, death usually occurs in a few months or years from the effect of the neoplasm; the idiopathic ones fluctuate over years.

The response to neostigmine and pyridostigmine is poor or at least unpredictable, and this finding in a myasthenic patient should bring the diagnosis of Lambert-Eaton syndrome to mind. In contrast, *d*-tubocurarine, suxamethonium chloride, gallamine, and other muscle relaxants have a deleterious effect and may cause fatality, just as in myasthenia gravis.

Conventional electrodiagnostic studies show no abnormality in the peripheral nerves. A single stimulus of nerve may evoke a low-amplitude muscle action potential (in contrast to myasthenia gravis, in which it is normal or nearly so) whereas at fast rates of stimulation (50 per s as shown in Fig. 45-4*B*) or following strong voluntary contraction (for 15 s or longer) there is a marked increase in the amplitude of action potentials (incrementing response hence the term "inverse myasthenia," which has been applied to Lambert-Eaton syndrome [LEMS]). Single-fiber recordings show an increase in "jitter" as in myasthenia gravis, as described in Chap. 45.

Elmquist and Lambert, from a series of studies of excised muscle, deduced that there is a defect in the release of ACh quanta from the *presynaptic* nerve terminals, akin to the effects of botulinum toxin, magnesium excess, and neomycin. The presynaptic vesicles themselves appear to be normal in morphology and content. Also in contrast to myasthenia gravis, the surface area of the postsynaptic receptor membrane in this syndrome is actually increased (A.G. Engel, 1976).

The physiologic mechanism in Lambert-Eaton myasthenic syndrome is a loss of voltage-gated calcium channels on the presynaptic motor nerve terminal. The calcium channels become cross-linked and aggregated by IgG autoantibodies, ultimately reducing the number of functioning channels (Fukunaga et al). These antibodies against a specific component of the *presynaptic* membrane have the effect of reducing the presynaptic release of ACh, virtually the opposite of myasthenia gravis.

A serologic test for these antibodies is available and is performed to confirm the diagnosis. Even in patients without detectable antibodies against voltage-gated calcium channels, passive transfer experiments indicate the presence of a circulating factor with similar activity. Muscle biopsy is normal or shows only the same slight, nonspecific changes as in myasthenia gravis. The thymus is, of course, normal.

Recognition of the Lambert-Eaton syndrome should lead to a search for an occult tumor, particularly of the lung. A positron emission tomography (PET) scan of the body may be useful for this purpose, although CT of the lungs is usually adequate. If found, it should be treated; this alone may result in improvement in the neurologic syndrome. If none is found, the search should be repeated at regular intervals, as the tumors at first are small and may be inapparent even at autopsy. Numerous cases of the more typical paraneoplastic syndromes discussed in Chap. 31, such as cerebellar degeneration, may coexist with the Lambert-Eaton syndrome, most of them are a result of small cell lung cancer (see Mason and colleagues) while others a result of idiopathic antibodies to the calcium channels.

Treatment

Most patients with this disease benefit from administration of 3,4-diaminopyridine (3,4-DAP), an agent that blocks potassium channels in the distal motor terminal, thus prolonging depolarizations and enhancing the release of ACh vesicles. The drug is given as 20 mg, up to five times a day, either alone or in conjunction with pyridostigmine (Lundh et al). It is not approved by the FDA in the United States and must be obtained from specialty pharmacies but nonetheless, has replaced the formerly used guanidine hydrochloride that had hematologic and renal toxicity with long-term use. With regard to long-term relief, numerous regimens have been tried and favored by different groups. Streib and Rothner were able to achieve improvement with prednisone. Dau and Denys have claimed the best results in nontumor cases with repeated courses of plasmapheresis in combination with prednisone and azathioprine. Intravenous immune globulin has also been effective in a few reported cases. Bain and coworkers indicate that the benefit is a result of reduction in calcium channel autoantibodies, but the mechanism whereby intravenous immune globulin produces this effect could not be established. Many clinicians prefer alternate-day administration of prednisone and azathioprine (prednisone 25 to 60 mg/d, and azathioprine 2 to 3 mg/kg body weight daily) supplemented intermittently as needed by intravenous immune globulin. The response to treatment tends to be slow, over a period of months and sometimes up to a year. Some patients recover fully; in others, restoration of power is incomplete.

Diagnosis

A syndrome of symmetrical weakness and fatigability of proximal muscles coupled with dry mouth, sphincter disturbances, aching muscles, and diminished reflexes are diagnostic. The illnesses with which it might be confused are myasthenia gravis, inclusion body myopathy, and polymyositis. There is a superficial resemblance to hysterical paralysis, where the patient may do better with encouragement on making a succession of voluntary contractions, and arthritis, where pain hampers the first movements more than the successive ones. Then the electrodiagnostic and specific serologic tests are of value.

Neonatal Myasthenia Gravis

An estimated 10 to 20 percent of babies born to mothers with myasthenia show transient signs of myasthenia (hypotonia, weak cry and suck). This transitory phenomenon is apparent at birth and has a mean duration of about 2 to 5 weeks; recovery is usually complete within 2 months of birth (rarely longer), without later relapse. Uncommonly, the mother with myasthenia reports reduced intrauterine movements, suggesting a dangerous degree of myasthenia in the fetus. A few of these children will be born with arthrogryposis, the result of a sustained period of intrauterine immobility, and this complication tends to recur in subsequent births.

It has long been assumed that neonatal myasthenia is a result of the passive transplacental transfer of AChR antibodies. This explanation is not entirely satisfactory insofar as maternal AChR antibodies are transferred from mother to fetus in all AChR antibody-positive pregnancies and the incidence and severity of neonatal myasthenia gravis do not correlate with the severity or duration of the mother's illness or with the serum level of the maternal AChR antibody. In fact, neonatal myasthenia may occur when the mother is in remission.

Administration of plasma exchange and anticholinesterase drugs to the infant may be useful in hastening recovery from neonatal myasthenia.

Congenital Myasthenic Syndromes

(See Table 49-3)

Sporadically in the medical literature, there have appeared reports of a benign congenital myopathy in which myasthenic features could be recognized in the neonatal period or soon thereafter. The affected infants had been born to mothers who did not have myasthenia and were in the past described under headings such as "Myasthenia Gravis in the Newborn" and "Familial Infantile Myasthenia" (Greer and Schotland; Robertson et al) to distinguish the condition from passively transmitted neonatal myasthenia.

Table 49-3

HEREDITARY AND CONGENITAL MYASTHENIC SYNDROMES

Presynaptic				
Episodic apnea	Choline acetyltransferase	1st	AChE inhibitors Apnea monitor	Mild episodes of weakness; recurrent apnea Ptosis common
Paucity of synaptic vesicles	Unknown	1st	AChE inhibitors	Recurrent, sometimes pronounced weakness
Reduced quantal release of acetylcholine	Unknown	1st	AChE inhibitors and 3,4-aminopyridine	Wasting, respiratory failure, dysmorphism
Synaptic				
AChE deficiency	AChE Collagen tail for AChE	1st	None Avoid AChE inhibitors	Diffuse weakness, ptosis
DOK-7 "synopathy"	DOK-7 mutation	1st	None	Limb-girdle, ptosis
Postsynaptic				
Slow channel syndrome	AChR subunits	1st to 6th	Quinidine, AChE inhibitors Avoid 3,4-DAP	Ptosis, diffuse weakness, delayed motor milestones Often show atrophy of dorsal forearms
Fast channel syndrome	AChR subunits	1st	3,4-DAP	Ptosis, recurrent weakness, motor development delays
Primary AChR deficiency	AChR subunits	1st	AChE inhibitors, 3,4-DAP	Ptosis, recurrent weakness, motor development delays
Rapsyn deficiency	Rapsyn	1st	AChE inhibitors, 3,4-DAP	Ptosis, recurrent weakness
Plectin deficiency	Plectin	1st	3,4-DAP	Myasthenic features, epidermolysis bullosa
Escobar syndrome	Defective fetal γ-AChR subunit	In-utero	Maturity with replacement of γ- with ε-AChR subunit	Arthrogryposis, respiratory failure, pterygium (webbing of skin)

AChE, acetylcholinesterase; AChR, acetylcholine receptor; DAP, diaminopyridine; IVIg, intravenous immune globulin; MuSK, muscle-specific kinase.

In the 1970s and 1980s, after the autoimmune basis of myasthenia gravis was established and its morphologic and physiologic features defined, the differences between this disease and the familial infantile forms became evident. Since then, at least eight distinct and rare congenital myasthenic syndromes have been delineated on the basis of their electrophysiologic and ultrastructural features, and a number of others have been partially characterized.

As indicated in Table 49-3, the congenital myasthenic syndromes are inherited defects in components of the presynaptic, synaptic, or postsynaptic junctional apparatus. Broadly speaking, the defects involve resynthesis or packaging of ACh or a paucity of synaptic vesicles (presynaptic); deficient quantal release; a deficiency of endplate ACh esterase (synaptic); or kinetic abnormalities in the AChR channels, or AChR deficiency (postsynaptic). It has been estimated that in three-fourths of the cases, the defect is postsynaptic.

These disorders are distinguished by neonatal onset, fluctuating and sometimes progressive weakness that may be quite severe, sometimes pronounced muscle hypotrophy, persistent ptosis, and seronegativity for anti-AChR and anti-MuSK antibodies. Moreover, heritability (typically autosomal recessive) is suggested by familial occurrence of the disorders among siblings. The most important clue to the disease in the neonate is an increase in ptosis and in bulbar and respiratory weakness with crying. Later in infancy these symptoms, as well as fluctuating ocular palsies and abnormal fatigability, are brought out by other types of sustained activities. Motor milestones may be delayed. In some cases, the myasthenic weakness and fatigability do not become evident until the second and third decades of life. Testing with anticholinesterase drugs is inconsistently positive in a few forms of congenital myasthenia as mentioned further on, but it usually is negative.

Two of the congenital myasthenic diseases—*fast channel syndrome* and *slow channel syndrome*—are consequences of mutations in AChR subunits that accelerate (fast channel) and slow (slow channel) the kinetics of gating of receptor channel (Croxen et al). Another well-characterized type, usually causing arthrogryposis and recurrent apneic spells but occasionally having an adult onset (as late as 48 years) has been traced to mutations in the "rapsyn" gene. The rapsyn protein plays a role in maintaining the integrity of the postsynaptic membrane (see Burke et al). Deficiency of the enzyme required to synthesize and package ACh in vesicles (choline acetyltransferase) causes a congenital myopathy with episodes of stress-induced apnea. In another type, the synaptic vesicles form poorly and are reduced in number. Being largely presynaptic defects, both of these disorders respond to acetylcholine esterase (AChE) inhibitors. In comparison, children with congenital myasthenia as a result of deficiency of AChE deteriorate markedly if given AChE inhibitors. Three disorders affecting postsynaptic structures (the fast-channel syndrome, AChR deficiency, and the myasthenic syndromes associated with deficiencies of rapsyn and plectin) also respond to AChE inhibition and 3,4-DAP, although both agents are hazardous in individuals with the slow-channel syndrome.

Another recently discovered congenital myasthenia is caused by a recessive mutation in *DOK-7* that causes a simplified structure of the synapse but no alteration in acetylcholine receptors (Beeson et al). The clinical features as described by Palace and colleagues (2007) are of a limb-girdle pattern of weakness that causes a delay in walking after the child has reached other normal motor milestones and of ptosis from an early age.

A further category of congenital syndromes of defects in the presynaptic quantal release of acetylcholine have been described by Milone and colleagues and an intriguing prenatal myasthenic disease called *Escobar syndrome* (arthrogryposis, pterygia, and respiratory distress) has been traced to mutations in the gamma subunit of the acetylcholine receptor, a component expressed only in fetal life and replaced with maturity by the epsilon subunit (see Hoffman and coworkers).

The studies of A.G. Engel have systematically defined and classified these disorders in a series of extensive investigations of more than 100 cases. A detailed account of this work can be found in his review with Ohno and Sine and in the chapter on the subject in his monograph *Myasthenia Gravis and Myasthenic Disorders*.

Myasthenic Weakness Caused by Antibiotics and Other Drugs and by Natural Environmental Toxins (See Chap. 43 and Table 49-2)

Many drugs can cause a myasthenic syndrome or a worsening of myasthenia gravis by their action on pre- or postsynaptic structures. In the case of a nonmyasthenic patient, this is most likely to happen in the presence of hepatic or renal disease that allows excessive accumulation of the causative agent. The myasthenic state in these conditions is acute and lasts hours or days, with full recovery provided that the patient does not succumb to respiratory failure. The ocular, facial, and bulbar muscles are involved, just as in native myasthenia. The treatment is to provide respiratory support, discontinue the offending drug, and attempt to reverse the conduction block at the motor endplate by infusions of calcium gluconate, potassium, and anticholinesterases, along the lines suggested by Argov and Mastaglia.

There are more than 30 drugs in current clinical use (other than anesthetic agents) that may, under certain circumstances, interfere with neuromuscular transmission in otherwise normal individuals. Of these, the most important are the aminoglycoside and quinolone antibiotics. Myasthenic weakness has been reported with 18 different antibiotics but particularly neomycin, kanamycin (less so with gentamicin), colistin, streptomycin, polymyxin B, and certain tetracyclines (McQuillen et al; Pittinger et al). It has been shown that these drugs impair transmitter release by interfering with calciumion fluxes at nerve terminals. The fluorinated quinolones (fluoroquinolones)—typified by ciprofloxacin—affect both pre- and postsynaptic activity. They are especially hazardous when given to patients with myasthenia but they may be used if necessary to treat infections in patients who are already receiving ventilatory support.

Other agents—particularly the organophosphate insecticides and nerve gases—cause paralysis by binding to cholinesterase and blocking the hydrolysis of ACh. The endplate remains depolarized and is refractory to neural stimuli. The most notable of these agents are (1) botulinum toxin, which binds to cholinergic motor endings, blocking quantal release of ACh; (2) black widow spider venom, which causes a massive release of ACh, resulting in muscular contraction and then paralysis from a lack of ACh; (3) *d*-tubocurarine, which binds to AChR; (4) suxamethonium and decamethonium, which also bind to AChR; (5) organophosphates, which bind irreversibly to AChE; and (6) malathion and parathion, which inhibit AChE. The actions of all these agents except for the organophosphate "nerve gases" are transitory.

The administration of *d*-penicillamine has also caused an unusual type of myasthenia. The weakness is typical in that rest increases strength—as do neostigmine and edrophonium—and the electrophysiologic findings are also the same. In such cases, Vincent and associates (1978) found anti-AChR antibodies in the serum; hence, one must assume that this is a form of induced autoimmune myasthenia gravis. In these respects it differs from the weakness caused by aminoglycosides (see review by Swift). Rarely, typical autoimmune myasthenia gravis develops as part of a chronic graft-versus-host disease in long-term (2- to 3-year) survivors of allogeneic marrow transplants.

A large group of naturally occurring environmental neurotoxins are known to act at the neuromuscular junction and to induce muscle paralysis of a pattern like that of myasthenia gravis. Venoms of certain snakes, spiders, and ticks are common and well-known animal poisons, as are ciguatera and related toxins (from fish that have ingested certain dinoflagellates), curare (from plants), and *Clostridium botulinum*—all of which are discussed in other parts of this book, particularly Chap. 43. Poisoning by these natural neurotoxins constitutes an important public health hazard in many parts of the world. This class of disorders of neuromuscular transmission has been reviewed by Senanayake and Roman.

References

Argov Z, Mastaglia FL: Disorders of neuromuscular transmission caused by drugs. *N Engl J Med* 301:409, 1979.

Bain PG, Motomura M, Newsom-Davis J, et al: Effects of intravenous immunoglobulin on muscle weakness and calcium channel auto-antibodies in the Lambert-Eaton myasthenic syndrome. *Neurology* 47:678, 1996.

Barth D, Nabavi Nouri M, Ng E, et al: Comparison of IVIg and PLEX in patients with myasthenia gravis. *Neurology* 76:2017, 2011.

Beeson D, Higuchi O, Palace J, et al: Dok-7 mutations underlie a neuromuscular junction synaptopathy. *Science* 313:1975, 2006.

Bever CT Jr, Aquino AV, Penn AS, et al: Prognosis of ocular myasthenia. *Ann Neurol* 14:516, 1983.

Bril V, Kojic J, Dhanani A: The long-term clinical outcome of myasthenia gravis in patients with thymoma. *Neurology* 51:1198, 1998.

Buckingham JM, Howard FM Jr, Bernatz PE, et al: The value of thymectomy in myasthenia gravis: A computer-assisted matched study. *Ann Surg* 184:453, 1976.

Burke G, Cossins J, Maxwell S, et al: Rapsyn mutation in hereditary myasthenia. Distinct early and late phenotypes. *Neurology* 61:826, 2003.

Buzzard EF: The clinical history and postmortem examination of 5 cases of myasthenia gravis. *Brain* 28:438, 1905.

Cogan DG: Myasthenia gravis: A review of the disease and a description of lid twitch as a characteristic sign. *Arch Ophthalmol* 74:217, 1965.

Cohen MS, Younger D: Aspects of the natural history of myasthenia gravis: Crisis and death. *Ann N Y Acad Sci* 377:670, 1981.

Compston DAS, Vincent A, Newsom-Davis A, Batchelor JR: Clinical, pathological, HLA antigen, and immunological evidence for disease heterogeneity in myasthenia gravis. *Brain* 103:579, 1980.

Croxen R, Hattan C, Shellay C, et al: Recessive inheritance and variable penetrance of slow-channel congenital myasthenic syndromes. *Neurology* 59:162, 2002.

Dau PC, Denys EH: Plasmapheresis and immunosuppressive therapy in the Eaton-Lambert syndrome. *Ann Neurol* 11:570, 1982.

De Feo LG, Schottlender J, Martelli NA, et al: Use of intravenous pulsed cyclophosphamide in severe generalized myasthenia gravis. *Muscle Nerve* 26:31, 2002.

Diaz-Manera J, Matinez-Hernandez E, Querol L, et al: Long-lasting effect of rituximab in MuSK myasthenia. *Neurology* 78:189, 2012.

Drachman DB: How to recognize an antibody-mediated autoimmune disease: Criteria. *Res Publ Assoc Res Nerv Ment Dis* 68:183, 1990.

Drachman DB: Myasthenia gravis. *N Engl J Med* 298:136, 186, 1978.

Drachman DB: Myasthenia gravis. *N Engl J Med* 330:1797, 1994.

Drachman DB, Jones RJ, Brodsky RA: Treatment of refractory myasthenia: "Rebooting" with high dose cyclophosphamide. *Ann Neurol* 53:29, 2003.

Eaton LM, Lambert EH: Electromyography and electric stimulation of nerves and diseases of motor unit: Observations on myasthenic syndrome associated with malignant tumors. *JAMA* 163:1117, 1957.

Elmquist D, Lambert EH: Detailed analysis of neuromuscular transmission in a patient with the myasthenic syndrome, sometimes associated with bronchial carcinoma. *Mayo Clin Proc* 43:689, 1968.

Engel AG: Congenital myasthenic syndromes, in Engel AG (ed): *Myasthenia Gravis and Myasthenic Disorders.* New York, Oxford University Press, 1999, pp 251–297.

Engel AG (ed): *Myasthenia Gravis and Myasthenic Disorders.* New York, Oxford University Press, 1999.

Engel AG, Lambert EH, Howard FM: Immune complexes (IgG and C3) at motor end-plate in myasthenia gravis. *Mayo Clin Proc* 52:267, 1977.

Engel AG, Lambert EH, Santa T: Study of long-term anticholinesterase therapy. *Neurology* 23:1273, 1973.

Engel AG, Tsujihata M, Lambert EH, et al: Experimental autoimmune myasthenia gravis: A sequential and quantitative study of the neuromuscular junction ultrastructure and electrophysiologic correlations. *J Neuropathol Exp Neurol* 35:569, 1976.

Engel AG, Tsujihata M, Lindstrom JM, Lennon VA: The motor end plate in myasthenia gravis and in experimental autoimmune myasthenia gravis. *Ann N Y Acad Sci* 274:60, 1976.

Engel AG, Ohno K, Sine SM: Congenital myasthenic syndromes: Progress over the past decade. *Muscle Nerve* 27:4, 2003.

Engel AL, Arahata K: The membrane attack complex of complement at the endplate in myasthenia gravis. *Ann N Y Acad Sci* 505:326, 1987.

Evoli A, Tonali P, Padua L, et al: Clinical correlates with anti-MuSK antibodies in generalized seronegative myasthenia gravis. *Brain* 126:2304, 2003.

Fambrough DM, Drachman DB, Satyamurti S: Neuromuscular junction in myasthenia gravis: Decreased acetylcholine receptors. *Science* 182:293, 1973.

Fukunaga H, Engel AG, Osane M, et al: Paucity and disorganization of presynaptic membrane active zones in the Lambert-Eaton myasthenic syndrome. *Muscle Nerve* 5:686, 1982.

Gajdos P, Chevret S, Clair B, et al: Clinical trial of plasma exchange and high-dose intravenous immunoglobulin in myasthenia gravis. *Ann Neurol* 41:789, 1997.

Gajdos P, Tranchant C, Clair B, et al: Treatment of myasthenia gravis exacerbation with intravenous immunoglobulin: A randomized double-blind clinical trial. *Arch Neurol* 62:1689, 2005.

Greer M, Schotland M: Myasthenia gravis in the newborn. *Pediatrics* 26:101, 1960.

Grob D, Brunner NG, Namba T: The natural course of myasthenia gravis and effect of therapeutic measures. *Ann N Y Acad Sci* 377:652, 1981.

Hoffmann K, Muller JS, Stricker S, et al: Escobar syndrome is a prenatal myasthenia caused by disruption of the acetylcholine receptor fetal gamma subunit. *Am J Hum Genet* 79:303, 2006.

Janssen JC, Larner AJ, Harris J, et al: Myasthenic hand. *Neurology* 51:913, 1998.

Jaretzki A., Barohn RJ, Ernstoff RM, et al: Myasthenia gravis. Recommendations for clinical research standards. *Neurology* 55:16, 2000.

Kakulas BA, Adams RD: *Diseases of Muscle: Pathological Foundations of Clinical Myology*, 4th ed. Philadelphia, Harper & Row, 1985.

Kelly JJ, Daube JR, Lennon VA: The laboratory diagnosis of mild myasthenia gravis. *Ann Neurol* 12:238, 1982.

Kerzin-Storrar L, Metcalfe RA, Dyer PA: Genetic factors in myasthenia gravis: A family study. *Neurology* 38:38, 1988.

Lambert EH, Eaton LM, Rooke ED: Defect of neuromuscular transmission associated with malignant neoplasm. *Am J Physiol* 187:612, 1956.

Lambert EH, Lindstrom JM, Lennon VA: End-plate potentials in experimental autoimmune myasthenia gravis in rats. *Ann N Y Acad Sci* 274:300, 1976.

Lennon VA: Immunologic mechanisms in myasthenia gravis—a model of a receptor disease, in Franklin E (ed): *Clinical Immunology Update—Reviews for Physicians.* New York, Elsevier/North-Holland, 1979, pp 259–289.

Lennon VA, Lindstrom JM, Seybold ME: Experimental autoimmune myasthenia gravis in rats and guinea pigs. *J Exp Med* 141:1365, 1975.

Lindstrom JM, Lambert EH: Content of acetylcholine receptor and antibodies bound to receptor in myasthenia gravis, experimental autoimmune myasthenia gravis, and Eaton-Lambert syndrome. *Neurology* 28:130, 1978.

Lundh H, Nilsson O, Rosen I: Treatment of Lambert-Eaton syndrome: 3,4-Diaminopyridine and pyridostigmine. *Neurology* 34:1324, 1984.

Mason WP, Graus F, Land B, et al: Small-cell lung cancer, paraneoplastic cerebellar degeneration and Lambert-Eaton myasthenic syndrome. *Brain* 120:1279, 1997.

Mayer RF, Williams IR: Incrementing responses in myasthenia gravis. *Arch Neurol* 31:24, 1974.

McQuillen MP, Cantor HE, O'Rourke JR: Myasthenic syndrome associated with antibiotics. *Arch Neurol* 18:402, 1968.

Meriggioli MN, Ciafaloni E, Al-Hayk KA, et al: Mycophenolate mofetil for myasthenia gravis. *Neurology* 61:1438, 2003.

Meyers KR, Gilden DH, Rinaldi CF, Hansen JL: Periodic muscle weakness, normokalemia, and tubular aggregates. *Neurology* 22:269, 1972.

Milone M, Fukada T, Shen XM, et al: Novel congenital myasthenic syndromes associated with defect in quantal release. *Neurology* 66:1223, 2006.

Mossman S, Vincent A, Newsom-Davis J: Myasthenia gravis without acetylcholine receptor antibody: A distinct disease entity. *Lancet* 1:116, 1986.

Myasthenia Gravis Clinical Study Group: A randomized clinical trial comparing prednisone and azathioprine in myasthenia gravis: Results of the second interim analysis. *J Neurol Neurosurg Psychiatry* 56:1157, 1993.

Nastuk WL, Plescia OJ, Osserman KE: Changes in serum complement activity in patients with myasthenia gravis. *Proc Soc Exp Biol Med* 105:177, 1960.

Newsom-Davis J: Diseases of the neuromuscular junction, in Asbury AK, McKhann GM, McDonald WI (eds): *Diseases of the Nervous System,* 2nd ed. Philadelphia, Saunders, 1992, pp 197–212.

Olanow CW, Lane RJM, Roses AD: Thymectomy in late-onset myasthenia gravis. *Arch Neurol* 39:82, 1982.

O'Neill JH, Murray NM, Newsom-Davis J: The Lambert-Eaton myasthenic syndrome. A review of 50 cases. *Brain* 14:577, 1988.

Osserman KE: *Myasthenia Gravis.* New York, Grune & Stratton, 1958.

Palace J, Lashley D, Newsom-Davis J, et al: Clinical features of the DOK-7 neuromuscular junction synaptopathy. *Brain* 130:1507, 2007.

Palace J, Newsom-Davis J, Lecky B: A randomized double-blind trial of prednisolone alone or with azathioprine in myasthenia gravis. *Neurology* 50:1778, 1998.

Panegyres PM, Squier M, Mills KR, Newsom-Davis J: Acute myopathy associated with large parenteral dose of corticosteroid in myasthenia gravis. *J Neurol Neurosurg Psychiatry* 56:702, 1993.

Park HS, Shin DM, Lee JS, et al: Thymoma. A retrospective study of 87 cases. *Cancer* 73:2491, 1994.

Pascuzzi RM, Coslett HB, Johns TR: Long-term corticosteroid treatment of myasthenia gravis: Report of 116 cases. *Ann Neurol* 15:291, 1984.

Patrick J, Lindstrom JP: Autoimmune response to acetylcholine receptor. *Science* 180:871, 1973.

Patrick J, Lindstrom JP, Culp B, McMillan J: Studies on purified eel acetylcholine receptor and antiacetylcholine receptor antibody. *Proc Natl Acad Sci U S A* 70:3334, 1973.

Perez MC, Buot WL, Mercado-Donguilan C: Stable remissions in myasthenia gravis. *Neurology* 31:32, 1981.

Pittinger CB, Eryase Y, Adamson R: Antibiotic-induced paralysis. *Anesth Analg* 49:487, 1970.

Ponsetti JM, Azem J, Fort JM, et al: Long-term results of tacrolimus in cyclosporine- and prednisone-dependent myasthenia gravis. *Neurology* 64:1641, 2005.

Rabinstein A, Wijdicks EFM: BiPAP in acute respiratory failure due to myasthenic crisis may prevent intubation. *Neurology* 59:1647, 2002.

Reman L: Zur pathogenese und therapie der myasthenia gravis pseudoparalytica. *Dtsch Z Nervenheilkd* 128:66, 1932.

Reuther P, Fulpius BW, Mertens HB, Hertel G: Anti-acetylcholine receptor antibody under long-term azathioprine treatment in myasthenia gravis, in Dau PC (ed): *Plasmapheresis and the Immunobiology of Myasthenia Gravis.* Boston, Houghton Mifflin, 1979, pp 329–348.

Robertson WC, Chun RWM, Kornguta SE: Familial infantile myasthenia. *Arch Neurol* 37:117, 1980.

Rodriguez M, Gomez MR, Howard FM: Myasthenia gravis in children: Long-term followup. *Ann Neurol* 13:504, 1983.

Ropper AH, Gress DR, Diringer MN, et al (eds): *Neurological and Neurosurgical Intensive Care*, 4th ed. Baltimore, Lippincott Williams Wilkins, 2004, pp 299–311.

Russell DS: Histological changes in myasthenia gravis. *J Pathol Bacteriol* 65:279, 1953.

Santa T, Engel AG, Lambert EH: Histometric study of neuromuscular junction ultrastructure: I. Myasthenia gravis. *Neurology* 22:71, 1972.

Scadding GK, Vincent A, Newsom-Davis J, Henry K: Acetylcholine receptor antibody synthesis by thymic lymphocytes: Correlation with thymic histology. *Neurology* 31:935, 1981.

Schluep M, Willcox N, Vincent A, et al: Acetylcholine receptors in human thymic cells in situ: An immunohistological study. *Ann Neurol* 22:212, 1987.

Scuderi F, Marino M, Colonna L, et al: Anti-p110 autoantibodies identify a subtype of "seronegative" myasthenia gravis with prominent oculobulbar involvement. *Lab Invest* 82:1139, 2002.

Senanayake N, Roman GC: Disorders of neuromuscular transmission due to natural environmental toxins. *J Neurol Sci* 107:1, 1992.

Sethi KD, Rivner MH, Swift TR: Ice pack test for myasthenia gravis. *Neurology* 37:1383, 1987.

Simpson JA: Myasthenia gravis: A new hypothesis. *Scott Med J* 5:419, 1960.

Streib EW, Rothner D: Eaton-Lambert myasthenic syndrome: Long-term treatment of 3 patients with prednisone. *Ann Neurol* 10:448, 1981.

Swift TR: Disorders of neuromuscular transmission other than myasthenia gravis. *Muscle Nerve* 4:334, 1981.

Thomas CE, Mayer SA, Gungor Y, et al: Myasthenic crisis: Clinical features, mortality, complications, and risk factors for prolonged intubation. *Neurology* 48:1253, 1997.

Tindall RSA, Phillips JT, Rollins JA, et al: A clinical therapeutic trial of cyclosporine in myasthenia gravis. *Ann N Y Acad Sci* 681:539, 1993.

Viets HR: A historical review of myasthenia gravis from 1672 to 1900. *JAMA* 153:1273, 1953.

Vincent A, Newsom-Davis J: Acetylcholine receptor antibody as a diagnostic test for myasthenia gravis: Results in 153 validated cases and 2967 diagnostic assays. *J Neurol Neurosurg Psychiatry* 48:1246, 1985.

Vincent A, Newsom-Davis J, Martin V: Antiacetylcholine receptor antibodies in *d*-penicillamine associated myasthenia gravis. *Lancet* 1:1254, 1978.

Vincent A, Wray D (eds): *Neuromuscular Transmission. Basic and Applied Aspects.* New York, Manchester Press, 1990.

Walker MB: Treatment of myasthenia gravis with physostigmine. *Lancet* 1:1200, 1934.

Weinberg DH, Rizzo JF, Hayes MT, et al: Ocular myasthenia gravis: Predictive value of single-fiber electromyography. *Muscle Nerve* 22:1222, 1999.

Witte AS, Cornblath DR, Parry GJ, et al: Azathioprine in the treatment of myasthenia gravis. *Ann Neurol* 15:602, 1984.

Yamamoto T, Vincent A, Ciulla TA, et al: Seronegative myasthenia gravis: A plasma factor inhibiting agonist-induced acetylcholine receptor function copurifies with IgM. *Ann Neurol* 30:550, 1991.

50

The Myotonias, Periodic Paralyses, Cramps, Spasms, and States of Persistent Muscle Fiber Activity

This chapter considers a category of disorders that is characterized by disturbances of the electrical excitability of the skeletal muscle membrane. Although the main manifestations are episodes of generalized paralysis and myotonia, there are many others. Another related group of diseases are unified by spontaneous and persistent muscle fiber activity and these are addressed in a later part of this chapter. The myotonias have been historically categorized as a special group of muscle diseases unified by the clinical sign of myotonia and were aligned in older classifications with the muscular dystrophies. This view was based on myotonia as it was understood in the classic form of myotonic dystrophy, a subject discussed in Chap. 48. Similarly, before fundamental knowledge of their mechanism was revealed, the periodic paralyses (better called *episodic paralysis*) were considered to be metabolic diseases of muscle. However, it has become evident that most diseases that feature prominent myotonia and the processes that cause episodic muscular paralysis are neither degenerative nor dystrophic. Clinical and electrophysiologic studies show that myotonia is an elemental feature of many nondystrophic conditions, foremost among them are the hyperkalemic form of periodic paralysis and myotonia congenita. Most of these diseases are caused by mutations in genes that code for chloride, sodium, calcium, or potassium ion channels in the muscle membrane, and they are referred to as *ion channel diseases*, or as "channelopathies" (see Ryan and Ptácek). Within this group there are also instances of muscle conditions that display no myotonia but only periodic paralysis.

Given that these are disorders of muscle membrane excitability, it is not surprising that the primary defects are in voltage-dependent ion channels. By analogy, it was anticipated that ion channelopathies would be implicated in two other categories of disease in which there is altered membrane excitability, namely the epilepsies and certain cardiac arrhythmias and indeed, this has proven to be the case (see discussion in Chap. 16 on the epilepsies). In the process, several new forms of nondystrophic myotonia have been defined. Molecular studies, notably those of Rüdel, Lehmann-Horn (2004), and Ricker and their associates, identified the fundamental defects in the myotonias and episodic paralyses and clarified their relationships. The biology of the ion channels and their disease-related mutations are reviewed by Hanna and colleagues, by Cannon, and by Heatwole and colleagues.

Table 50-1 summarizes the main features of the ion channel diseases affecting muscle and the individual members of the group are described as follows.

CHLORIDE CHANNEL DISEASES

Myotonia Congenita (Thomsen Disease)

This is an uncommon disease of skeletal muscle that begins in early life and is characterized by myotonia, muscular hypertrophy, nonprogressive course, and dominant inheritance. It is distinctly different from myotonic dystrophy, which is characterized by a progressive degeneration of muscle fibers and has a different genetic basis. Thomsen disease is caused by one of several inherited molecular defects in the voltage-dependent chloride channel gene (*CLCN1*), as first demonstrated by Jentsch and associates (see Koch et al). It is interesting that most mutations behave as dominant traits, whereas others have either a dominant or recessive pattern of inheritance (see Table 50-1). The physiologic mechanism whereby these mutations alter ion fluxes across the muscle membrane and cause myotonia is described further on.

History

The disorder was first brought to the attention of the medical profession in 1876 by Julius Thomsen, a Danish physician who himself suffered from the disease, as did 20 members of his family over 4 generations. His designation of *ataxia muscularis* was not correct, but his description left no doubt as to the nature of the condition in that it featured "tonic cramps in voluntary muscles associated with an inherited psychical indisposition." The latter aspect of the condition was not borne out by subsequent studies and is now thought to be his erroneous speculation as to causality. In 1881, Strümpell assigned the name *myotonia congenita* to the disease and in 1883, Westphal referred to it as *Thomsen's disease*. Erb provided the first description of its pathology and called attention to two additional unique features: muscular hyperexcitability and hypertrophy. In 1923, Nissen, Thomsen's great-nephew, extended the original genealogy to 35 cases in 7 generations, and in 1948, Thomasen updated the subject in a monograph that is still a useful clinical reference.

Table 50-1

THE MAIN INHERITED MYOTONIAS AND PERIODIC PARALYSES (THE CHANNELOPATHIES)

CHANNEL AFFECTED	CHLORIDE	CHLORIDE	SODIUM	SODIUM	CALCIUM	CALCIUM	POTASSIUM
Disease	Myotonia congenita (Thomsen)	Generalized myotonia (Becker)	Hyperkalemic periodic paralysis	Paramyotonia congenita (Eulenburg)	Hypokalemic periodic paralysis	Malignant hyperthermia	Andersen disease
Inheritance	Dominant	Recessive	Dominant	Dominant	Dominant	Dominant	Dominant
Gene	*CLCN1*	*CLCN1*	*SCN4A*	*SCN4A*	*DHP* receptor	*RYR1*	*KCNJ2*
Channel protein	CLC1	CLC1	Alpha subunit	Alpha subunit	Dihydropyridine receptor	Ryanodine receptor	Inward rectifying K channel
Myotonia (electrical)	++	++	+/–	++	—	—	—
Myotonia (clinical)	++	+++	+/–	—	—	—	—
Paramyotonia (clinical)	—	—	+/–	+++	—	—	—
Episodic paralysis	—	—	+++	+/–	+++	—	+
Onset	Congenital to late childhood	Late childhood or earlier	First decade	Paramyotonia at birth	Late childhood to third decade	All ages	Childhood
Precipitating factors							
Increases with exercise	—	—	—	+++	—	—	+
Appears after exercise	++	++	++	—	++	—	—
Fasting	—	—	+	—	—	—	—
Carbohydrate load	—	—	—	—	+	—	—
Potassium load	—	—	++	+/–	—	—	—
Cold	+	+	+	+++	+	—	—
Pregnancy	+	+	++	++	+	—	?
"Warmup" phenomenon	++	++	+	—	+	—	—
Involvement of cranial muscles	+	+	+	++	—	—	++
Muscle hypertrophy	++	+	—	—	—	—	—
Permanent myopathy	—	+	++	—	++	—	+
Serum CK during attack	Normal to border-line	Increased 2 to 3 times	Increased	Increased 5 to 10 times	Normal to slightly increased	Markedly increased	Normal
Serum K during attack	Normal	Normal	Increased	Normal	Decreased	Normal	High, low, or normal
Serum K between attacks	Normal	Normal	Normal	Normal	Normal	Normal	Normal
Significant myopathology (vacuolar myopathy)	—	—	++	—	++	Rhabdomyolysis, cores	Tubular aggregates
Treatment	Mexiletine if required for myotonia	Mexiletine if required for myotonia	During attack, glucose and calcium; for prevention, acet-azolamide CHO, low-K diet	Mexiletine if needed for myotonia	KCl during and acetazolamide between attacks	Intravenous dantrolene	Acetazolamide

CHO, carbohydrates; +, mild; ++, moderate; +++, severe.

Clinical Features

Myotonia, a tonic spasm of muscle after forceful voluntary contraction, stands as the cardinal feature and is best represented in this disease. As emphasized in Chap. 45, this phenomenon reflects electrical hyperexcitability of the muscle membrane. It is most pronounced after a period of inactivity. Repeated contractions "wear it out," so to speak, and the later movements in a series become more swift and effective. Rarely, the converse is observed—where only the later movements of a series induce myotonia (*myotonia paradoxica*); usually this is a feature of another condition, cold-induced paramyotonia congenita (see further on). Unlike cramp, the myotonic spasm is painless but after prolonged activity, nocturnal myalgia (a pinching-aching sensation in the overactive muscles) may develop and prove distressing. Close observation reveals a softness of the muscles during rest and the initial contraction appears not to be significantly slowed.

The disease as mentioned above is usually inherited as a dominant trait so that most often, other members of the family have been affected. Its congenital nature may be evident even in the crib, where the infant's eyes are noted to open slowly after it has been crying or sneezing and its legs are conspicuously stiff as the child tries to take its first steps. In other cases, the myotonia becomes evident only later in the first or second decade. The muscles are generously proportioned and may become hypertrophied but seldom to the degree observed in the recessive form of the disease described further on.

Despite their muscular appearance, these patients are inept in athletic pursuits as a result of the myotonia. When severe, myotonia affects all skeletal muscles but is especially prominent in the lower limbs. Attempts to walk and run are impeded to the extent that the patient stumbles and falls. Other limb and trunk muscles are also thrown into spasm, as are those of the face and upper limbs. One of the characteristic features is grip myotonia in which the patient is unable to release a handshake and must slowly open the fingers one at a time. Occasionally a sudden noise or fright may cause generalized stiffness and falling. Small, gentle movements such as blinking or elicitation of a tendon reflex do not initiate myotonia, whereas strong closure of the eyelids, as in a sneeze, sets up a spasm that may prevent complete opening of the eyes for many seconds. Spasms of extraocular muscles occur in some instances, leading to strabismus. If the patient has not spoken for a time, there is sometimes a striking dysarthria. Arising at night, the patient cannot walk without first moving the legs for a few minutes. After a period of rest, the patient may have difficulty in arising from a chair or climbing stairs. Loosening of one set of muscles after a succession of contractions does not prevent the appearance of myotonia in another area, nor in the same ones if used in another pattern of movement. Smooth and cardiac muscles are not affected and intelligence is normal. Lacking also are the narrow face, frontal balding, cataracts, and endocrine changes typical of myotonic dystrophy that is discussed in Chap. 48. Myotonia that is evident in infancy is far more likely to represent myotonia congenita than myotonic dystrophy, in which myotonia rarely has its onset in the first few years of life.

Myotonia can also be induced in most cases by tapping a muscle belly with a percussion hammer (percussion myotonia). Unlike the lump or ridge produced in hypothyroid or cachectic muscle (myoedema), the myotonic contraction involves an entire fasciculus or an entire muscle and, unlike the phenomenon of idiomuscular irritability (contraction of a fascicle in response to striking the muscle), it persists for several seconds. If tapped, the tongue shows a similar reaction. An electrical stimulus delivered to the motor point in a muscle induces a prolonged contraction (Erb myotonic reaction). In Thomsen disease, as in virtually all forms of myotonia, the stiffness is somewhat exaggerated in cold. On a cold day, affected individuals may have a prolonged grimace with closed eyes after a sneeze. We encountered two brothers with this disorder who described diving into a cool swimming pool on a hot summer day and having to lie nearly motionless at the bottom of the pool for several seconds until the muscle stiffness abated enough to allow them to swim to the top. However, as mentioned, prominent cold-induced myotonia, is more characteristic of paramyotonia congenita (see later).

Biopsy reveals no abnormality other than enlargement of muscle fibers, and this change occurs only in hypertrophied muscles. As often happens in fibers of increased volume, central nucleation is somewhat more frequent than it is in normal muscle. The large fibers contain increased numbers of normally structured myofibrils. In well-fixed biopsy material examined under the electron microscope, Schroeder and Adams discerned no significant morphologic changes.

Myotonia levior was the name applied by DeJong to a dominantly inherited form of myotonia congenita in which the symptoms are milder and of later onset than those of Thomsen disease. In 2 patients of a myotonia levior family, Lehmann-Horn and coworkers (1995) identified a mutation of the same chloride ion channel (*CLCN1*) that is implicated in Thomsen's disease. Thus it appears that myotonia levior is simply a mild form of Thomsen disease.

Diagnosis

In patients who complain of spasms, cramping, and stiffness, myotonia must be distinguished from several of the disorders of persistent muscle activity described in Chap. 48. None of these disorders displays percussion myotonia or the typical electromyogram (EMG) abnormality of myotonic discharge. The only possible exceptions are the Schwartz-Jampel syndrome of hereditary stiffness combined with short stature and muscle hypertrophy, and stiff-man syndrome which are discussed in Chap. 48.

Uncertainty in diagnosis arises in patients who have *only myotonia* in early life and later prove to have classic (type 1) myotonic dystrophy or who notice myotonia in adulthood with mild proximal weakness and are found to have type 2 myotonic dystrophy (see later). The myotonia in myotonic dystrophy is usually mild and in several families that we have followed, some degree of weakness and the typical facies of myotonic dystrophy could be appreciated even in early childhood. This is not the case in the less-frequent type 2 myotonic dystrophy in which there are no dysmorphic features (also called proximal myotonic myopathy [PROMM]; see Chap. 48 and further on). In paramyotonia congenita there is also myotonia of early onset, but, again, it tends to be mild, involving mainly the orbicularis oculi, levator palpebrae, and tongue; the diagnosis of paramyotonia is seldom in doubt because of the worsening with continued activity and prominent cold-induced episodes of myotonia and paralysis.

In patients with very large muscles, one must consider not only myotonia congenita but also familial hyperdevelopment, hypothyroid myopathy, the Bruck-de Lange syndrome (congenital hypertrophy of muscles, mental retardation, and extrapyramidal movement disorder), Becker myotonia (see later), Duchenne dystrophy, and most of all, hypertrophic myopathy (hypertrophia musculorum vera); this last disease is of interest because the aberrant protein (myostatin) and gene defect have been characterized. Muscle hypertrophy is not, of course, a feature of myotonic dystrophy. The demonstration of myotonia by percussion and EMG study usually resolves the problem, although in exceptional cases of Thomsen disease, the persistence of contraction may be difficult to demonstrate. In hypothyroidism, the EMG may show bizarre high-frequency (pseudomyotonic) discharges; however, true myotonia does not occur, myoedema is prominent, and, along with other signs of thyroid deficiency, there is slowing of contraction and relaxation of tendon reflexes not seen in myotonia congenita.

Treatment

Quinine is effective in reducing myotonia but is now used infrequently because of the (low) risk of causing torsade de pointes. Procainamide, 250 to 500 mg qid, and mexiletine, 100 to 300 mg tid, are beneficial in relieving the myotonia. Phenytoin, 100 mg tid, is useful in some cases. The cardiac antiarrhythmic drug tocainide (1,200 mg daily) has also proved effective, but it sometimes causes agranulocytosis and is no longer recommended.

Generalized Myotonia (Becker Disease)

This is a second form of myotonia congenita, inherited as an autosomal recessive trait. Like the dominant Thomsen form, it is caused by an allelic mutation of the gene encoding the chloride ion channel of the muscle fiber membrane. The clinical features of the dominant and recessive types are similar except that myotonia in the recessive type does not become manifest until 10 to 14 years of age, or even later, and tends to be more severe in the dominantly inherited variety. The myotonia appears first in the lower limbs and spreads to the trunk, arms, and face. Hypertrophy is invariably present. There may be associated mild distal weakness and atrophy; this was found in the forearms in 28 percent of Becker's 148 patients and in the sternocleidomastoids in 19 percent. Dorsiflexion of the feet was limited and fibrous contractures were common. Weakness may also be present in the proximal leg and arm muscles. The most troublesome aspect of the disease is the transient weakness that follows initial muscle contraction after a period of inactivity. Progression of the disease continues to about 30 years of age, and according to Sun and Streib, the course of the illness thereafter remains unchanged. In contrast to Thomsen disease, the creatine kinase (CK) may be elevated. Testicular atrophy, cardiac abnormality, frontal baldness, and cataracts—the features that characterize myotonic dystrophy—are conspicuously absent.

SODIUM CHANNEL DISEASES

The main diseases in this category are *hyperkalemic periodic paralysis* and *paramyotonia congenita*. The derivative disorders *normokalemic periodic paralysis*, *acetazolamide-responsive myotonia*, *myotonia fluctuans*, and *myotonia permanens* are variants of hyperkalemic periodic paralysis. All of them are caused by mutations in the gene encoding the alpha subunit of the membrane-bound voltage-gated sodium channel in skeletal muscle (*SCN4A*).

Hyperkalemic Periodic Paralysis

The essential features of this disease are episodic generalized weakness of fairly rapid onset and a rise in serum potassium during attacks. Weakness appearing after a period of rest that follows exercise is particularly characteristic. This type of periodic paralysis was first described and distinguished from the more common (hypokalemic) form by Tyler and colleagues in 1951. Five years later, Gamstorp described two additional families with the disorder and named it *adynamia episodica hereditaria*. As further examples were reported, it was noted that in many of them there were minor degrees of myotonia, which brought the condition into relation with paramyotonia congenita (see further on). Hyperkalemic periodic paralysis is associated with a defect in the alpha subunit of the sodium channel gene (Fontaine et al, 1990). It is now appreciated that there are distinct variants of hyperkalemic periodic paralysis that are genetically distinct. All are associated with membrane hyperexcitability because of delays in sodium channel inactivation following membrane depolarization, as discussed later.

Clinical Manifestations

The pattern of inheritance is autosomal dominant as noted, with an onset usually in infancy and childhood. Characteristically, attacks of weakness occur before breakfast and later in the day, particularly when resting following exercise. In the latter case, the weakness appears after 20 to 30 min of becoming sedentary. The patient notes difficulty that begins in the legs, thighs, and lower back and spreads to the hands, forearms, and shoulders over minutes or more. Only in the severest attacks are the neck and cranial muscles involved; respiratory muscles are usually spared. As the muscles become inexcitable, tendon reflexes are diminished or lost. Attacks usually last 15 to 60 min, and recovery can be hastened by mild exercise. After an attack, mild weakness may persist for a day or two.

In severe cases, the attacks may occur every day; during late adolescence and the adult years, when the patient becomes more sedentary, the attacks may diminish and even cease entirely. In certain muscle groups, if myotonia coexists, it is difficult to separate the effects of weakness from those of myotonia. Indeed, when an attack of paresis is prevented by continuous movement, firm, painful lumps may form in the calf muscles. Usually, however, the presence of myotonia can only be detected electromyographically. Some patients with repeated attacks may be left with a permanent weakness and wasting of the proximal limb muscles.

During the attack of weakness serum K rises, often, but not always, up to 5 to 6 mmol/L. This is associated with increased amplitude of T waves in the electrocardiogram (ECG) and a fall in the serum Na level (because of entry of Na into muscle). With increased urinary excretion of K, the serum K falls and the attack terminates. Between attacks serum K is usually normal or only slightly elevated.

The attacks of paralysis are virtually alike in all clinical variants of the disease. In the paramyotonic form discussed below, the attacks are associated with paradoxical myotonia (myotonia induced by exercise and also by cold).

The *provocative test*, undertaken under careful supervision when the patient is functioning normally, consists of the oral administration of 2 g of KCl in a sugar-free liquid repeated every 2 h for 4 doses, if that many are necessary to provoke an attack. The test is given in the fasting state, ideally just after exercise. The weakness typically has a latency of 1 to 2 h after the administration of K. The patient must be carefully monitored by ECG and frequent serum estimations of serum potassium. The test should never be undertaken in the presence of an attack of weakness, or when there is reduced renal function, or in those with diabetes requiring insulin.

The *treatment* of this syndrome is the same as that for paramyotonia congenita, described further on.

Normokalemic Periodic Paralysis This form of episodic paralysis resembles the hyperkalemic form in practically all respects except that serum potassium does not increase out of the normal range, even during the most severe attacks. However, some patients with normokalemic periodic paralysis are sensitive to potassium loading (Poskanzer and Kerr); other kindreds are not (Meyers et al). The disorder is also transmitted as an autosomal dominant trait and the basic defect has proved to stem from the same mutation as that of hyperkalemic periodic paralysis of which it may be considered a variant.

Paramyotonia Congenita (Eulenburg Disease)

In this disease, attacks of periodic paralysis are associated with myotonia, which may be paradoxical in type—that is, developing during exercise and worsening as the exercise continues. In addition, a widespread myotonia, often coupled with weakness, is induced by exposure to cold. In some patients, the myotonia can be elicited even in a warm environment. The weakness may be diffuse, as in hyperkalemic periodic paralysis, or limited to the part of the body that is cooled. As commented in the earlier sections, cold exaggerates many types of myotonia to some extent, but this property is most characteristic of paramyotonia and it is in this condition that cold-induced weakness persists for up to several hours once started, even after the body is rewarmed. Percussion myotonia can be evoked in the tongue and thenar eminence. According to Haass and colleagues, myotonia that is constantly present in a warm environment diminishes with repeated contraction, whereas myotonia induced by cold increases with repeated contraction (paradoxical myotonia).

Like hyperkalemic periodic paralysis, paramyotonia congenita is transmitted in an autosomal dominant manner and both diseases have been linked to the same gene (*SCN4A*), which encodes the alpha subunit of the muscle membrane sodium channel; the two mutations are allelic.

Laboratory Findings

In both hyperkalemic periodic paralysis and paramyotonia congenita, the serum K is usually above the normal range during bouts of weakness, but paralysis has been observed at levels of 5 mEq/L and lower. Each patient appears to have a critical level of serum K, which, if exceeded, will be associated with weakness. (This has led some authors to term the periodic paralysis as *potassium dependent*.) The administration of KCl, raising serum K to above 7 mEq/L, a level that has no effect on normal individuals, invariably induces an attack. As mentioned earlier, the ECG must be monitored during such provocative testing. The EMG shows myotonic discharge in all muscles, even at normal temperatures. The CK may be elevated.

In vitro studies of muscle from patients with cold-induced stiffness and weakness have shown that as temperature is reduced, the muscle membrane is progressively depolarized to the point where the fibers are inexcitable (Lehmann-Horn et al, 1987). A sodium channel blocker (tetrodotoxin) prevents the cold-induced depolarization. In patients with paramyotonia, but not in those with hyperkalemic periodic paralysis, Subramony and colleagues observed a diminution of the compound muscle action potential in response to the cooling of muscle, largely settling the argument as to whether the two syndromes (hyperkalemic paralysis and paramyotonia) are the same or different.

Some patients with paramyotonia, like those with certain other forms of periodic paralysis, may in later life slowly develop a myopathy that causes persistent weakness. In some cases this is sufficiently severe that it mimics the pattern of late-onset limb-girdle muscular dystrophy. However, in the case of paramyotonia there are relatively few histologic changes, primarily vacuoles in some of the muscle fibers and minimal evidence of myofiber degeneration.

Treatment

Most patients with hyperkalemic periodic paralysis and its variants benefit from prophylactic use of the carbonic anhydrase inhibitor acetazolamide, 125 to 250 mg bid or tid (paradoxically, as it has a tendency to produce potassium retention). Acetazolamide reduces the frequency of attacks and may provide some relief from myotonia. There are no controlled studies of acetazolamide in these disorders, but a trial of the related carbonic anhydrase inhibitor dichlorphenamide demonstrated a reduced frequency of paralytic spells in both hyper- and hypokalemic forms of periodic paralysis (Tawil et al). However, in some patients the attacks of hyperkalemic paralysis and of paramyotonia congenita are too infrequent, too brief, or too mild to require continuous treatment.

The administration of diuretics such as hydrochlorothiazide (0.5 g daily), keeping the serum K below 5 mEq/L, also prevents attacks but risks inducing dangerous degrees of hypokalemia. When the myotonia is more troublesome than the weakness, mexiletine 200 mg tid is perhaps the best alternative, because it prevents both cold- and exercise-induced myotonia but it does not influence frequency of acute attacks. Some additional benefit may be gained by adding inhaled beta-adrenergic agonists such as albuterol or salbutamol. Some studies suggest that one agent in this class, clenbuterol, may have a direct effect in blocking the sodium channel, independent of its activation of adrenergic receptors. Procainamide or the lidocaine derivative tocainide, in doses of 400 to 1,200 mg daily, is also useful for the myotonia (tocainide carries a small risk of agranulocytosis).

For the treatment of an acute and severe episode, intravenous calcium gluconate (1 to 2 g) often restores power. If after a few minutes this treatment is unsuccessful, intravenous glucose or glucose and insulin and hydrochlorothiazide should be tried so as to reduce the serum potassium concentration.

Other Sodium Channel Disorders

Several other clinical presentations of hereditary periodic paralysis have been linked to mutations of the gene encoding the alpha subunit of the skeletal muscle sodium channel and probably represent variants of the disease. One of these, described by Ricker and colleagues, has been designated *myotonia fluctuans*, because muscle stiffness fluctuated in severity from day to day. In other respects the clinical features resemble those of myotonia congenita, including provocation of attacks of myotonia by exercise. The muscle stiffness is only slightly sensitive to cold but is markedly aggravated by the ingestion of potassium and, interestingly, never progresses to muscular weakness or paralysis. *Myotonia permanens* is the name given to a severe, persistent myotonia and marked hypertrophy of muscles, particularly of the neck and shoulders. The EMG discloses continuous muscle activity. This disease was discovered in the course of genotyping a patient who earlier had been reported by Spaans and associates as an example of "myogenic" Schwartz-Jampel syndrome, but it affects the same channel as in hyperkalemic periodic paralysis.

Trudell and colleagues studied 14 patients from a large kindred with autosomal dominant myotonia, the main feature of which was periodic worsening of myotonia accompanied by muscle pain and stiffness, most severe in the face and hands. The symptoms were enhanced by cold (suggesting paramyotonia) and severe stiffness and palpable rigidity followed within 15 min of the ingestion of potassium but neither of these measures provoked muscle weakness. Muscle biopsy disclosed a normal ratio of types 1, 2A, and 2B fibers, further distinguishing this disorder from typical myotonia congenita, where 2B fibers may be reduced in number. All patients in this family who were treated with the carbonic anhydrase inhibitor acetazolamide had a dramatic resolution of symptoms within 24 h, hence the name *acetazolamide-responsive myotonia*. This disorder has been linked to the same molecular alteration of the sodium channel gene as occurs in hyperkalemic periodic paralysis (Ptácek et al, 1994b).

Rosenfeld and coworkers described yet another form of *painful congenital myotonia* attributable to a novel mutation in the sodium channel alpha-subunit gene (*SCN4A*). Affected members of this family experienced debilitating pain, particularly severe in the intercostal muscles. Also, the pain was resistant to treatment with acetazolamide and other antimyotonic drugs (mexiletine and tocainamide) and could not be provoked by ingestion of potassium-rich foods, differing in these ways from the patients described by Trudell and Ptácek (1994a) and their associates.

Finally, in regard to disorders of the sodium channel, it should be mentioned that the marine toxins (ciguatoxin, tetrodotoxin, saxitoxin), discussed in Chap. 43, produce their effects on the peripheral and central nerves by blocking sodium channels, but have little obvious effect on muscle function.

Pathophysiology of Myotonia and Hyperkalemic Periodic Paralysis

(See also Chap. 45)

In both myotonia congenita and hyperkalemic paralysis, the absence of major morphologic changes and the prominence of the myotonic phenomenon in individual muscle fibers is consistent with a disorder of the sodium channel. This is also compatible with the observation that myotonia persists after the administration of curare, thereby exonerating neural input as the source of myofiber hyperexcitability.

The electromyographic pattern of a myotonic muscle reveals highly characteristic discharges that persist following the cessation of voluntary contraction. The tension of the myotonic muscle fibers is slow to diminish as a result of these greatly prolonged trains of muscle action potentials (see Fig. 45-8). Some of these afterdischarge potentials are the size of fibrillations, but others are as large as normal motor units. Thus myotonia can be distinguished electrophysiologically from contracture (e.g., that encountered in McArdle disease, in which the muscle is electrically silent). In experiments conducted in the 1940s, Denny-Brown and Foley, stimulating single muscle fibers directly, found that myotonic discharges could be elicited only by a volley of stimuli and not by a single stimulus. They also noted that the series of myotonic potentials progressively diminished in size. Percussion elicits myotonia by imparting a brief but relatively intense repetitive excitation of the muscle membrane.

The biophysical basis of myotonia is now well understood in terms of the functioning of chloride and sodium channels in the muscle membrane and internal structures. The correspondence between mathematical models of the electrical properties of the membrane and the clinical features of the myotonic and periodic paralyses is quite remarkable. During the normal action potential in all neural and muscular tissue, membrane depolarization is terminated by two events: the depolarization-induced inactivation of the sodium channel (which ends the inward sodium current) and the subsequent action of the outward potassium current. In muscle, the termination of an action potential requires an additional factor. Because of its large size, excitation of the muscle fiber involves depolarization that propagates not only along the cell surface but also radially into the center of the muscle cell through the transverse tubules (T tubules). The tubules are very narrow structures whose internal spaces are in continuity with the extracellular space. When the repolarizing outward potassium current is activated, potassium ions flood into the tubules from the muscle cytoplasm. By itself, this tubular K accumulation would depolarize the muscle membrane and prolong excitation. Normally, this does not occur because there is a large opposing chloride conductance in the tubules that counteracts the influence of potassium accumulation.

The first clues to the importance of the chloride channel in this electrical stabilizing process were obtained by Bryant who performed in vitro studies of myotonic goat muscle and found a reduced chloride conductance in the transverse tubular system. Subsequent studies of muscle from patients with myotonia congenita by Lipicky and Bryant (1971) demonstrated a similarly low chloride conductance. That a mutation in a muscle chloride channel could produce myotonia was confirmed in a mouse model by Jentsch and Steinmeyer and colleagues (see Koch et al), who subsequently also described the first human chloride channel (*CLCN1*) mutations.

As indicated, an essential event for normal repolarization of an excitable membrane is the rapid inactivation of the inward sodium current. This process of rapid, complete sodium channel inactivation is impaired by the sodium channel mutations implicated in hyperkalemic periodic paralysis. The mutations cause imperfect inactivation of the channel and lead to aberrant and early reopenings. Repolarization is then incomplete, rendering the muscle cell more readily re-excited; it is this hyperexcitability that causes the myotonia of hyperkalemic periodic paralysis. The problem becomes self-reinforcing because, as the membrane fails to repolarize fully, its electrolytic inactivation becomes increasingly less effective. If this process is not aborted, the result is such excessive depolarization that the muscle cell ultimately becomes unexcitable—a state that corresponds to the paralytic phase of hyperkalemic periodic paralysis. These features are evident in hyperkalemic muscle in vitro (Cannon) and can be recapitulated in computer simulations of aberrant channels. Presumably, over several hours, a variety of compensatory mechanisms (e.g., activation of Na-K adenosine triphosphatase [ATPase] pumps) restores the baseline excitability of the muscle membrane.

CALCIUM CHANNEL DISEASES

Hypokalemic Periodic Paralysis

This is the best-known form of periodic paralysis. The history of the disease is difficult to trace, but the first unmistakable account was probably that of Hartwig in 1874, followed by the accounts of Westphal (1885) and Oppenheim (1891). Goldflam (in 1895) first called attention to the remarkable vacuolization of the muscle fibers that is characteristic of the process. In 1937, Aitken and associates described the occurrence of low serum potassium during attacks of paralysis and reversal of the paralysis by the administration of potassium, thus setting the stage for subsequent differentiation from the hyperkalemic forms of periodic paralysis. For English-speaking readers, Talbott's monograph serves as the best historical review of the subject and includes all cases that had been reported prior to 1941; the more contemporary reviews by Layzer and by Lehmann-Horn and their associates (2004) bring the subject largely up-to-date.

The usual pattern of inheritance is autosomal dominant with reduced penetrance in women (male-to-female ratio of 3 or 4:1). Fontaine and coworkers (1990, 1994) localized the mutation to a region containing the gene that encodes the alpha subunit of the calcium channel of skeletal muscle and the gene has now been determined. The subunit, which is part of the dihydropyridine receptor complex, is located in the transverse tubular system. This region is believed to act both as a voltage sensor that controls calcium release from the sarcoplasmic reticulum, thus mediating muscle excitation–contraction coupling, and as a calcium-conducting pore. How precisely the reduced calcium channel function relates to hypokalemia-induced attacks of muscle weakness is not fully known. Approximately 10 percent of cases, however, are due to a mutation in the earlier discussed sodium channel, SCN4A.

Clinical Manifestations

In our experience, this disease has become clinically apparent after adolescence and has been much more severe in males. We note, however, that in Talbott's review of 152 cases, there were 40 in which symptoms began before the tenth year of life and 92 before the sixteenth year. The typical attack comes on during the second half of the night or the early morning hours, after a day of unusually strenuous exercise; a meal rich in carbohydrates favors its development. Excessive hunger or thirst, dry mouth, palpitation, sweating, diarrhea, nervousness, and a sense of weariness or fatigue are mentioned as prodromata but do not necessarily precede an attack. Usually, the patient awakens to discover a mild or severe weakness of the limbs. However, diurnal attacks also occur, especially after a nap that follows a large meal. The attack evolves over minutes to several hours; at its peak, it may render the patient so helpless as to be unable to call for assistance. Once established, the weakness lasts a few hours if mild or several days if severe.

The distribution of the paralysis varies. Limbs are affected earlier and often more severely than trunk muscles, and proximal muscles are possibly more susceptible than distal ones. The legs are often weakened before the arms, but exceptionally the order is reversed. The muscles most likely to escape are those of the eyes, face, tongue, pharynx, larynx, diaphragm, and sphincters, but on occasion even these may be involved. When the attack is at its peak, tendon reflexes are reduced or abolished and cutaneous reflexes may also disappear. As the attack subsides, strength generally returns first to the muscles that were last to be affected. Headache, exhaustion, diuresis, and occasionally diarrhea may follow the attack. Myotonia is not seen; indeed, clinical or EMG evidence of myotonia essentially excludes the diagnosis of hypokalemic periodic paralysis.

Attacks of paralysis tend to occur every few weeks and tend to lessen in frequency with advancing age. Rarely, death may occur from respiratory paralysis or derangements of the conducting system of the heart. Mainly, such fatal cases were reported in the era before modern intensive care.

Atypical forms include weakness of one limb or certain groups of muscles, bibrachial palsy (inability to lift one's arms or to comb one's hair), and transient weakness during accustomed activities such as walking. Some of our patients had a talipes deformity from early life. During middle adult life, a number of patients have developed a severe, slowly progressive proximal myopathy, with vacuolated and degenerated fibers and myopathic action potentials, in some instances long after attacks of periodic paralysis had ceased.

Laboratory Findings

The attacks are accompanied by reduction in serum K levels, as low as 1.8 mEq/L, but usually at levels that would not be associated with muscle weakness in normal subjects. The fall in serum K is associated with little or no increase in urinary K excretion. Presumably, large quantities of K enter the muscle fibers during an attack but this explanation may not be complete. Some episodes occur with near-normal levels of K, and weakness persists for a time after the serum level has been restored. The serum K levels return to normal during recovery. Although the shifts in K are of undoubted importance in the pathogenesis of muscle weakness, the marked sensitivity to small reductions of serum K suggests that other factors are operative and that the fall in K may be a secondary phenomenon.

As in hyperkalemic paralysis, the muscular weakness in this disease is associated with a decrease in the amplitude, and eventual loss, of muscle action potentials and there is failure of excitation by supramaximal stimulation of peripheral nerve or by strong voluntary effort. A decline in strength precedes the loss of motor unit potentials and the failure of propagation of action potentials over the surface of the fiber. The polarization potentials of muscle fibers measured by intracellular recordings are initially normal despite the failure of impulse propagation by the sarcolemma. One would expect the muscle fiber to be hyperpolarized as K moves into it, but it actually becomes depolarized. Rüdel and associates attribute the latter change to an increased Na conductance. The ECG changes also begin at levels of K that are slightly below normal (about 3 mEq/L); they consist of prolonged PR, QRS, and QT intervals and flattening of T waves.

Diagnosis at a time when the patient is normal may be facilitated by *provocative tests*. With the patient carefully monitored, including the use of ECG, the oral administration of 50 to 100 g of glucose or loading with 2 g of NaCl every hour for 7 doses, followed by vigorous exercise, brings on an attack, which then can be terminated by 2 to 4 g of oral KCl (the opposite of what pertains in hyperkalemic periodic paralysis).

Pathologic Changes

The muscle fibers are uniformly somewhat large but the most striking change, particularly in the late degenerative phases of the disease, is vacuolization of the sarcoplasm. The myofibrils are separated by round or oval vacuoles containing clear fluid, presumably water, and a few periodic acid-Schiff (PAS)-positive granules. There are pathologic changes in myofibrils and mitochondria as well, and focal increases in muscle glycogen. Isolated muscle fibers may undergo segmental degeneration. Electron microscopic studies have shown that the vacuoles arise as a result of proliferation and degeneration of membranous organelles within the sarcoplasmic reticulum and transverse tubules (A.G. Engel).

Treatment

A low-sodium diet (less than 160 mEq/d), avoidance of large meals and of exposure to cold, and acetazolamide 250 mg tid may be helpful in preventing attacks. That acetazolamide reduces attacks is somewhat surprising as it is kaluretic, but it may work through the production of acidosis; a few patients have worsened with the drug. Patients who are unresponsive to acetazolamide may be treated with the more potent carbonic anhydrase inhibitor, dichlorphenamide, 50 to 150 mg/d, or with the potassium-sparing diuretics spironolactone or triamterene (both in doses of 25 to 100 mg/d), but caution must then be exercised with the simultaneous administration of oral potassium supplements. The daily administration of 5 to 10 g of KCl orally in an unsweetened aqueous solution prevents attacks in many patients and apparently, this program can be maintained indefinitely. If this approach fails, a low-carbohydrate, low-salt, high-K diet combined with a slow-release K preparation may be effective.

For an *acute attack*, 0.25 mEq KCl/kg should be given orally or, if this is not tolerated, some other K salt may be tried. This dose may be insufficient and if there is no improvement in 1 or 2 h, KCl may have to be given intravenously: 0.05 to 0.1 mEq/kg initially in a bolus at a safe rate, followed by 20 to 40 mEq KCl in 5 percent mannitol, avoiding glucose or NaCl as the carrier solution. For the late-progressive polymyopathy that follows many severe attacks of periodic paralysis, Dalakas and Engel report successful restoration of strength by the long-term administration of dichlorphenamide. Regular exercise (not too strenuous) to keep the patient fit is desirable.

Secondary Kalemic Periodic Paralyses

In addition to the hereditary kalemic paralyses described earlier, transitory episodes of weakness are associated with a number of acquired derangements of potassium metabolism (mainly hypokalemia); these include thyrotoxicosis, aldosteronism, 17α-hydroxylase deficiency (Yazaki et al), barium poisoning (Lewi and Bar-Khayim), glycyrrhizic acid ingestion (a substance in licorice that has mineralocorticoid activity), and abuse of thyroid hormone (Layzer). Other forms of secondary hypokalemic weakness have been observed in patients suffering from chronic renal and adrenal insufficiency or disorders caused by a loss of potassium, as occurs with excessive use of diuretics or laxatives (the most common cause in practice). (Renal failure with hyperkalemia can also induce considerable weakness.)

Thyrotoxicosis With Periodic Paralysis

This is a special form of secondary hypokalemic periodic paralysis and occurs mainly in young adult males (despite the higher incidence of thyrotoxicosis in women), with a strong predilection for those of Japanese and Chinese origin (Pothiwala). In Japan, Okinaka and associates found that 8.9 percent of males with thyrotoxicosis had periodic paralysis, but this was the case in only 0.4 percent of females; in China, the corresponding figures were 13.0 and 0.17 percent (McFadzean and Yeung). The paralytic disorder is unrelated to the severity of the hyperthyroidism. In patients with the familial forms of periodic paralysis, the induction of hyperthyroidism is said not to increase the frequency or intensity of attacks. Therefore, it seems likely that thyrotoxicosis has unmasked another type of hereditary periodic paralysis, although a familial occurrence in the thyrotoxic cases is exceptional. Clinically, the attacks of paralysis are much the same as those of familial hypokalemic type except for a greater liability to cardiac irregularity. As in the familial form, the paralyzed muscles are electrically inexcitable. Potassium chloride restores power in paralytic attacks, and treatment of the hyperthyroidism prevents their recurrence (see "Myasthenia Gravis With Hyperthyroidism" in Chap. 49).

Hypokalemic Weakness in Primary Aldosteronism (Conn Syndrome)

Hypokalemic weakness because of hypersecretion of the major adrenal mineralocorticoid aldosterone was first described by Conn and associates in 1955. In *primary aldosteronism*, the cause of the hypersecretion is in the adrenal gland itself, usually an adrenal cortical adenoma, less often adrenal cortical hyperplasia. Although the disorder is uncommon (occurring in approximately 1 percent of unselected hypertensive patients), its recognition is essential for effective treatment. Persistent aldosteronism is frequently associated with hypernatremia, polyuria, and alkalosis, which predispose to attacks of tetany as well as to hypokalemic weakness. Conn and associates (1964), in an analysis of 145 patients with primary aldosteronism, found that persistent muscular weakness was a major complaint in 73 percent; intermittent attacks of paralysis occurred in 21 percent; and tetany in another 21 percent. These manifestations were much more frequent in women than in men, in contrast to the preponderance of men among patients with hypokalemic periodic paralysis of familial type. Rarely, as already noted, primary aldosteronism is produced by the chronic ingestion of licorice; this is due to its content of glycyrrhizic acid, a potent mineralocorticoid (Conn et al, 1968).

The muscle fibers of patients with primary aldosteronism show necrosis and vacuolation. Ultrastructurally, the necrotic areas are characterized by dissolution of myofilaments with degenerative vacuoles; nonnecrotic fibers contain membrane-bound vacuoles and show dilatation of the sarcoplasmic reticulum and abnormalities of the transverse tubular system, suggesting that vulnerability of the latter structures may be responsible for the muscle fiber necrosis (Atsumi et al).

Malignant Hyperthermia

This dramatic syndrome is observed during general anesthesia in susceptible individuals, some of whom clearly have a channelopathy. It is characterized by rapidly rising body temperature, extreme muscular rigidity, and a high mortality rate. Since the original report by Denborough and Lovell in 1960, as larger experience was gained with this entity, it proved in some cases to be a metabolic myopathy inherited as a dominant trait, rendering the individual vulnerable to any volatile anesthetic agent, particularly halothane, and to the muscle relaxant succinylcholine. The fundamental cause in a large proportion of cases is an aberration in a component of the ryanodine calcium channel. Malignant hyperthermia has been estimated to occur approximately once in the course of every 50,000 administrations of general anesthesia.

The full clinical picture is striking but anesthesiologists have become adept at detecting its earliest stages and aborting the process. As halothane or a similar inhalational anesthesia is induced, or succinylcholine is given for muscular relaxation, the jaw muscles unexpectedly become tense rather than relaxed and soon rigidity extends to all of the muscles. Thereafter, the body temperature rises to 42°C or 43°C and there is tachypnea and tachycardia. Blood pH may fall to 7 or below. There may be gross myoglobinuria and serum CK reaches extraordinarily high levels. Circulatory collapse and death may ensue in approximately 10 percent of cases, or the patient may survive with gradual recovery. In some cases there is the same sequence of events (increased temperature and acidosis) without muscular spasm. In cases of early death, the muscle may appear normal by light microscopy. With survival for several days, samples of muscle reveal scattered segmental necrosis and phagocytosis of sarcoplasm without inflammation. Patients with a particular congenital myopathy (central core myopathy), and those with King-Denborough syndrome mentioned later, have a propensity to malignant hyperthermia as noted in Chap. 48.

Pathophysiology and Etiology

The pathogenesis of malignant hyperthermia has been the subject of numerous investigations. During the rigor phase, oxygen consumption in muscle increases threefold and serum lactate, 15- to 20-fold. Muscle from most affected individuals is abnormally sensitive to caffeine, which induces contracture in vitro. It has been postulated that halothane acts in a manner similar to caffeine—that is, to release calcium from the sarcoplasmic reticulum and prevent its reaccumulation, thus interfering with relaxation of the muscle. The essential physiologic change is one of increased intracellular calcium.

Insight into the disease has been gained from a breed of pigs, inbred for muscular development, in which muscle spasm (true contracture) and hyperthermia follow the administration of anesthetic agents. These swine have an inherited defect in the ryanodine receptor, a protein component of the calcium channel of the sarcoplasm that is sensitive to both caffeine and ryanodine. However, one of several similar defects in ryanodine is found in somewhat fewer than 20 percent of people with the susceptibility to malignant hypothermia. It is presumed that other yet unidentified allelic mutations of this receptor protein or another that controls the structure of the calcium channel account for the remainder of cases. The cause of the high fever is unknown; it is probably caused by the muscle spasm, but an effect of the anesthetic on heat-regulating centers has not been excluded.

Clues as to which patients are at risk for this condition come from several sources. Other members of the family may have difficulties or have died during anesthesia. Some susceptible individuals exhibit myopathic and musculoskeletal abnormalities (Isaacs and Barlow). One such dysmorphic constellation consists of short stature, ptosis, strabismus, highly arched palate, dislocated patellae, and kyphoscoliosis, which have been present in several families (King-Denborough syndrome). As mentioned just above and in Chap. 48 on the congenital myopathies, central core (sometimes called multicore) myopathy is frequently complicated by malignant hyperthermia. This is understandable insofar as both disorders have been linked to the gene encoding the ryanodine receptor; the two diseases are a result of allelic variations (Quane et al). It has been pointed out that another rare muscle disease (Evans myopathy, named after the affected family) may also be a predisposing condition. It is inherited as an autosomal trait and may be asymptomatic until the anesthetic reaction but some patients have wasting of the distal thigh muscles and an elevation of serum CK concentration (see Harriman et al).

Diagnostic Testing

Various tests for susceptibility to malignant hyperthermia have undergone phases of popularity. The only currently valid one involves in vitro exposure of a muscle biopsy specimen to halothane and to caffeine and the detection of muscle contracture with both agents. This is performed only in a few centers, which are listed at *http://www.mhaus.org*. The review by Denborough may be consulted for further details on the testing and clinical aspects of the disease.

Treatment

This consists of discontinuation of anesthesia at the first hint of masseter spasm or rise of temperature. The intravenous administration of dantrolene, which inhibits the release of calcium from the sarcoplasmic reticulum, may be lifesaving. An infusion of 1 mg/kg is given initially and increased slowly until symptoms subside, the total dosage not exceeding 10 mg/kg. Other measures should include body cooling, intravenous hydration, sodium bicarbonate infusion to correct acidosis, and mechanical hyperventilation to decrease acidosis. Thereafter, halothane and other volatile anesthetic agents and succinylcholine should be avoided in such individuals and surgical procedures, if necessary, should be done with other agents, such as propofol, nitrous oxide, fentanyl, thiopental (or other barbiturate), or local anesthesia. Intravenous dantrolene (2.5 mg/kg given slowly 1 h prior to anesthesia) prevents the syndrome, but this is not a preferred option in patients with the disorder.

Neuroleptic Malignant Syndrome

This state, in which hyperthermia occurs as an idiosyncratic reaction to neuroleptic drugs, is also accompanied by widespread myonecrosis. It shares some features with malignant hyperthermia but is a distinct entity, as discussed in Chap. 43.

POTASSIUM CHANNEL DISEASES

The discovery of several types of seizure disorders based on inherited defects of the potassium channel has elicited considerable interest and only recently was it appreciated that one form of periodic paralysis, Andersen disease, is associated with the voltage-gated potassium channel.

Andersen Disease

Andersen and coworkers first drew attention to a distinct form of potassium-sensitive periodic paralysis characterized by the triad of periodic potassium-sensitive weakness, ventricular dysrhythmias with long QT syndrome, and dysmorphic features (micrognathia, short stature, scaphocephaly, hypertelorism, broad nose, low-set ears, and short index fingers). From a study of 5 kindreds, Sansone and colleagues have pointed out that attacks of paralysis can be associated with hypo-, normo-, or hyperkalemia, and that a prolonged QT interval is an integral feature of the disease (and sometimes the only sign in a given family). Plaster and colleagues demonstrated that most cases of Andersen disease are a consequence of dominant-negative mutations in the gene *KCNJ2* that encodes a type of K channel. In vitro studies indicate that the mutation impairs the ability of preformed channels to migrate to the membrane surface and also impedes the current-carrying capacity of the potassium channel system. This defect would be expected to impair repolarization of the muscle membrane, thereby making both skeletal and cardiac muscle hyperexcitable.

Morvan Fibrillary Chorea (Chorée Fibrillaire)

This oddly named disease is included in this chapter because an abnormality of voltage-gated potassium channels (VGKC) or circulating antibodies against the channel has been discovered in many patients. It is characterized by continuous muscle fiber activity sometimes referred to as "neuromyotonia" and therefore may also be considered among similar disorders of constant muscle activity that are discussed further in the chapter. Hyperhidrosis, weight loss, insomnia, and hallucinations may occur, and most cases so far described have ended fatally in a matter of months (Serratrice and Azulay). Plasma exchange reversed the syndrome in the case described by Ligouri and colleagues. Some cases have an associated thymoma and its removal may be curative. Weak oligoclonal bands are sometimes found in the spinal fluid. Whether the antibodies are responsible for the cerebral symptoms is unknown, but the connection is plausible.

An interesting category of disease has emerged as being caused by antibodies to the voltage-gated potassium channel (Thieben et al), sometimes parallel to an idiopathic or paraneoplastic "limbic" encephalitis, which is described in Chap. 31.

OTHER DISEASES AFFECTING MUSCLE MEMBRANE EXCITABILITY

In addition to the above disorders, various seizure syndromes (see Chap. 16) and a category of spinocerebellar ataxias are also attributable to mutations of ion channels and are addressed in other sections of the book. Also mentioned here for completeness are several diseases that result from secondary dysfunction of these same ion channels. Most of these conditions are acquired and autoimmune in nature, for example, the Lambert-Eaton myasthenic syndrome that results from an autoimmune attack on calcium channels (see Chap. 49), the Isaac syndrome that results from an autoimmune attack on potassium channels, producing neuromyotonia (see Chap. 45), anti-voltage-gated potassium channel and anti-NMDA encephalitis (see Chap. 31), and erythromelalgia that implicates a sodium channel (see Chap. 11). Thus, ion channels, being ubiquitous in all excitable tissues, might be expected to produce a large variety of diseases that affect central and peripheral nervous structures. Despite this, each of the genetic and acquired processes has remarkably specific features that are pertinent only to the channel as expressed in a single tissue.

Muscle Contracture, Pseudomyotonia, Tetanus, and Related States

Many of these states were discussed in Chap. 48 on diseases of muscle. They are reintroduced here in relation to specific diseases with which they are associated.

Physiologic Contracture Caused by Phosphorylase Deficiency (McArdle Disease) and Phosphofructokinase Deficiency (Tarui Disease)

Contractures are examples of an entirely different type of painful shortening and hardness of muscle. In both these diseases, an otherwise healthy child, adolescent, or adult begins to complain of weakness and stiffness and sometimes pain on using the limbs. Muscle contraction and relaxation are normal when the patient is in repose, but strenuous activity, especially under conditions of ischemia, causes the muscles to shorten gradually, because of a failure of relaxation. The contracted muscles in these disorders—unlike muscles in cramp, continuous muscular activity syndromes, or myotonia and other involuntary spasms—no longer use energy for which reason they are almost silent electrically in the EMG. This condition is spoken of as *physiologic contracture*. McArdle and Tarui diseases are discussed more fully in a later section.

Pseudomyotonia

This phenomenon is observed in *hypothyroidism*, where the muscle fibers contract and relax slowly, a response readily demonstrated in the tendon reflexes, particularly the Achilles reflex. The muscles are large and subject to myoedema. When contracted, they may show waves of slow contraction. The basis of this disorder appears to be slowness in the reaccumulation of calcium ions in the endoplasmic reticulum and in the disengagement of actin and myosin filaments. The EMG may show afterpotentials following voluntary contraction, but they do not resemble the typical waning discharges ("myotonic runs") of true myotonia.

A closely related syndrome, wherein painless contracture is induced by exercise, has been described by Lambert and Goldstein, and by Brody. Muscle contraction is normal but the relaxation phase becomes increasingly slow during exercise. Lambert and Goldstein referred to it as an unusual type of myotonia, and Brody, as a decrease of "relaxing factor"; the slow relaxation has also been attributed to a decreased uptake of calcium by the sarcoplasmic reticulum. In some cases, the disease is transmitted as a recessive trait with a mutation that impairs the function of a sarcoplasmic reticular calcium adenosine triphosphatase (ATPase). In other instances, the disease is transmitted as a dominant trait that is not genetically linked to calcium ATPase. This latter process may be more closely aligned with the muscular dystrophies and is mentioned in Chap. 48 under that heading.

Tetanus (See "Tetanus" in Chap. 43)

This toxic disorder is characterized by persistent spasms of skeletal muscles, owing to the effect of the tetanus toxin on spinal neurons (Renshaw and other cells), the natural function of which is to inhibit the motor neurons. As the condition develops, activities that normally excite the neurons (i.e., voluntary contraction and startle from visual and auditory stimulation) all evoke involuntary spasms. Sleep tends to quiet them, and they are suppressed by spinal anesthesia and curare. The EMG shows the expected interference pattern of muscle action potentials. Once the muscle is involved in persistent contraction, it is said that the shortened state is not abolished by procaine block or severance of nerve (in animals), but this type of *myostatic contracture* has not been demonstrated in humans.

The effect of tetanus toxin on the spinal inhibitory neurons is analogous to that of strychnine. There is also an action of the toxin at the neuromuscular junction, which has been more difficult to evaluate in the face of its powerful central action. Having injected this toxin locally in animals, Price and associates demonstrated its localization at motor endplates. It binds with ganglioside in the axon membrane and is transported by retrograde flow to the spinal cord, where it induces local tetanus effects. Neurons that innervate slow-twitch type 1 muscle fibers are more sensitive than those supplying fast-twitch type 2 fibers. Presynaptic vesicles increase in number, acetylcholine (ACh) is blocked, and terminal axon injury may paralyze muscle fibers. Fibrillation potentials and axonal sprouting follow. The similarities to stiff man syndrome are mentioned further on.

Black Widow Spider Bite

The toxin produced by this spider within a few minutes of the bite leads to a striking syndrome of cramps and spasms and then a painful rigidity of abdominal, trunk, and leg muscles. The spasms are followed by weakness. There is also vasoconstriction, hypertension, and autonomic hyperactivity. If death does not occur in the first 24 to 48 h, recovery is complete.

The spider venom has a presynaptic localization and rapidly releases quanta of ACh. The vesicles became depleted. There is some evidence that the venom prevents endocytosis of the vesicles by inserting itself into the presynaptic membranes, causing a disturbance of ionic conductance channels (Swift).

Treatment consists of calcium gluconate infusions and diazepine. Intravenous magnesium sulfate also helps to reduce the release of ACh and control the convulsions that sometimes occur. There is antiserum that is available in regions where such envenomation is frequent; it shortens the illness considerably.

Metal or other type of poisoning may simulate an inherently relapsing polyneuropathy.

States of Persistent Muscle Activity

This is an interrelated group of clinical states, all characterized by some degree of regional continuous muscular activity that in some cases cannot be fully differentiated from one another. From a clinical perspective we have found it is useful to categorize them in groups that are caused by (1) hyperexcitability of the peripheral motor nerves (fasciculations and myokymia), (2) centrally mediated hyperexcitability of motor output (Isaacs syndrome, stiff man syndrome), and (3) nonmyotonic hyperexcitability of muscle (rippling muscle disease, Schwartz-Jampel syndrome).

Hyperexcitability of Peripheral Nerve

This comprises a set of disorders in which peripheral motor nerve activity is augmented such that there are excessive, sometimes sustained contractions of the motor unit. Its mildest manifestation is benign fasciculation. In more severe form the manifestations include neuromyotonia, Isaacs disease, and a disease of potassium-gated ion channels (Morvan disease, or Morvan fibrillary chorea discussed below) that may also involve the brain. These processes are not generally familial and several lines of investigation suggest an acquired autoimmune nature (Newsom-Davis). For example, all but benign fasciculations are associated more often than might be expected with other autoimmune diseases such as myasthenia gravis and some respond to autoimmune therapies such as plasmapheresis, the patient's serum possesses antibodies to either voltage-gated potassium channels as mentioned or, less frequently, to nicotinic acetylcholine (ACh) receptors (Vernino and Lennon).

Benign Fasciculations

A few random fasciculations in the muscles of the calf, small muscles of the hand or of the face, or elsewhere are seen in most normal individuals. They are of little significance but can be a source of worry to physicians and patients who have read that fasciculations are an early sign of amyotrophic lateral sclerosis. A simple clinical rule is that fasciculations in relaxed muscle are not indicative of motor system disease unless there is associated weakness, atrophy, or reflex change.

Healthy individuals experience intermittent twitching of a muscle (or even part of a muscle), such as one of the muscles of the thenar eminence, eyelids, calves, or orbicularis oculi. They may continue for days. Electromyographically, benign fasciculations tend to be more constant in location and more frequent and rhythmic than the ominous fasciculations of amyotrophic lateral sclerosis but such distinctions are not entirely reliable. Quantitative study of the motor unit size may be helpful in these circumstances by demonstrating normally modeled units in the benign form and abnormally large units because of reinnervation in the case of motor neuron disease.

Occasionally, benign fasciculations are widespread and may last for months or even years. In several of our patients they have recurred in bouts separated by months and lasting several weeks. No reflex changes, sensory loss, nerve conduction, EMG abnormality (other than fasciculations), or increase in serum muscle enzymes is found. Low energy and fatigability in some of these patients may suggest an endogenous depressive illness yet the fasciculations are not explained by this mechanism. Patients commonly report a sense that the muscles affected by the twitching are weak but this cannot be confirmed by testing and several of our patients, curiously most of whom have been physicians, complained of equally troubling migratory zones of paresthesias. Pain of aching or burning type may increase after activity and cease during rest. Fatigue and a sense of weakness are frequent complaints. We suspect that this fasciculatory state reflects a disease of the terminal motor nerves, for a few of our patients have shown slowing of distal latencies, and Cöers and associates have found degeneration and regeneration of motor nerve terminals in similar cases. However, most such cases are of benign nature and settle down in a matter of weeks or months. In the cases reported by Hudson and colleagues, the condition, even after years, did not progress to spinal muscular atrophy, polyneuropathy, or amyotrophic lateral sclerosis. This conforms to our experience and to that reported from the Mayo Clinic where 121 patients with benign fasciculations, followed in some cases for more than 30 years, showed no progression of symptoms and did not acquire motor neuron disease or neuropathy (Blexrud et al). It should be acknowledged, however, that there are infrequent patients with seemingly benign fasciculations in whom the EMG shows some abnormal features (e.g., rare fibrillations) in numerous muscles and who later develop the other features of motor neuron disease. Carbamazepine, and to a lesser extent phenytoin, has been helpful in reducing the fasciculations and sensations of weakness in a proportion of cases and numerous other medications have been reportedly helpful.

Cramp-Fasciculation Syndrome

This is probably a variant of the above-described benign entity in which fasciculations are conjoined with cramps, stiffness, and systemic features such as exercise intolerance, fatigability, and muscle aches. Although affected individuals may be to some degree disabled by these symptoms, the prognosis is good. The salient finding on physiologic studies is that stimulation of peripheral nerves results in sustained muscle firing due to prolonged trains of action potentials in the distal motor nerve. This phenomenon may be brought out in special electrophysiologic testing, as described by Tahmoush and colleagues. In effect, this is a mild form of neuromyotonia, which is described further on. In a small number of patients with cramp-fasciculation syndrome it is possible to demonstrate the presence of autoantibodies directed against voltage-gated axonal potassium channels. Carbamazepine or gabapentin may be beneficial.

There are, in addition to these benign states, several syndromes of abnormal muscle activity. The main ones are *myokymia*, a state of successive contractions of motor units imparting an almost continuous undulation or rippling of the overlying body surface, and several syndromes of *continuous muscle fiber activity described below*.

Myokymia This state of abnormal rippling muscle activity may be generalized or limited to one part of the body such as the muscles of the shoulders or of the lower extremities. It is observed most often with demyelination of peripheral nerve following injury, and thus it is neuropathic in nature. The common underlying conditions are multiple sclerosis or Guillain-Barré syndrome affecting the facial nerve and radiation damage to the brachial or lumbar plexus. In the EMG, myokymic discharges consist of repetitive firing of one motor unit, firing at 5 to 60 Hz and recurring regularly at 0.2- to 10-s intervals. The driving impulses arise in the most peripheral parts of the axon of chronically damaged nerves. In some patients cramping is associated, and those muscles about to cramp may twitch or show premonitory spontaneous rippling contractions; the cramping may be associated with sweating. Thus, myokymia, fasciculation, and cramping seem to be related but not clinically identical conditions.

Continuous Muscle Fiber Activity (Isaacs Syndrome)

The relation of myokymia to the state called *continuous muscle fiber activity* is ambiguous. Sporadically in the neurologic literature there have been descriptions of patients whose muscles at some point begin to "work" continuously (see Isaacs). Terms such as *neuromyotonia* and *widespread myokymia with delayed muscle relaxation* are additional names that have been applied to what is essentially the same condition. At the moment, there is little reason to distinguish one from another except in gradations of severity. In each case the excessive and spontaneous activity can be attributed to hyperexcitability of terminal parts of motor nerve fiber, possibly as a result of a partial loss of motor innervation and compensatory collateral sprouting of surviving axons (Cöers et al; Valli et al). Twitching, spasms, and rippling of muscles (myokymia) are evident, the latter being the main clinical sign. In advanced cases there is generalized muscle stiffness and a sense of weakness. Complaints of muscle aching are usual, but severe myalgia is uncommon. The tendon reflexes may be reduced or abolished. Any muscle group may be affected. The stiffness and slowness of movement make walking laborious ("armadillo" syndrome); in extreme cases, all voluntary movement is blocked. The muscle activity persists throughout sleep. The continuous visible and painful cramps of the above-described Satoyoshi disease may be difficult to distinguish from myokymia clinically, but they represent a different phenomenon.

General and spinal anesthesia do not always suppress the muscular activity but curare does; nerve block usually has no effect or may reduce the activity, as in the case described by Lütschg and colleagues. The EMG findings are much the same as those described earlier.

Special types of myokymia arise in childhood or adult life, sometimes in association either with a polyneuropathy or rarely with an inherited type of episodic ataxia that is variably responsive to acetazolamide or remits spontaneously (see Chap. 5). An inherited form of continuous muscle fiber activity has been traced to a mutation of the peripheral nerve K channel (Gutmann and Gutmann). In addition to the association with polyneuropathy, a state of continuous muscular activity has also been described in association with lung cancer and thymoma in which cases an immune mechanism has been inferred (see reviews by Thompson and by Newsom-Davis and Mills and the discussion of paraneoplastic syndromes in Chap. 31).

Treatment Phenytoin or carbamazepine often abolish the continuous muscular activity and cause a return of reflexes. Acetazolamide has been helpful in other cases (Celebisoy et al). Many of the idiopathic cases will improve spontaneously after several years, however, plasma exchange may be tried if the symptoms are intractable.

Centrally Mediated Motor Hyperexcitability and Stiff Man (Stiff Person) Syndrome

This is a condition of persistent and intense spasms, particularly of the proximal lower limbs and lumbar paraspinal muscles. It was originally described by Moersch and Woltman in 1956 as stiff man syndrome. Since then, many examples have been reported all over the world and the term *stiff person syndrome* has been used to indicate its occurrence in both women and men. For lack of a better place in the book to discuss it, it is included here with other processes that cause muscular spasms and cramps.

The onset is insidious, usually in middle life. No genetic predisposition is known. At first the stiffness and spasms are intermittent, then gradually they become more or less continuously active in the proximal leg and axial trunk muscles and increasingly painful. The spasms impart a robotic appearance to walking and an exaggerated lumbar lordosis. Attempts to move an affected part passively yield an almost rock-like immobility, perceptibly different from spasticity, paratonia, or extrapyramidal rigidity. Muscles of respiration and swallowing and those of the face may be involved in advanced cases, but trismus, a common feature of tetanus, does not occur. We have observed brief periods of cyanosis and respiratory arrest during episodes of intense spasm, and one of our patients died during such an episode. The eye muscles are rarely affected.

As the illness progresses, any noise or other sensory stimulus or attempted passive or voluntary movement may precipitate painful spasms of all the involved musculature. The tendon reflexes are normal if they can be tested. The affected muscles, particularly the lumbar paraspinals and glutei, are extremely taut when palpated and eventually they become hypertrophied. It is this axial spasm that is most characteristic of the disease and gives rise to a characteristic lumbar lordosis. We have experience with one unusual instance of this disease that caused the obverse, namely, flexion spasm of the abdominal musculature with a bent-over camptocormia.

A similar stiffness of one limb (*"stiff limb" syndrome*) has been differentiated from the generalized variety by Barker and colleagues and others (see Saiz et al; Brown et al), but most of the localized cases have antibodies to glutamic acid decarboxylase, as described below. The limited form of the condition begins in one leg and spreads to its opposite, but remains isolated to the lower extremities, similar to localized tetanus.

A central origin of the muscle spasms is indicated by their disappearance during sleep, during general anesthesia, and with proximal nerve block. The electrophysiologic features differ from those of myokymia and continuous muscle fiber activity syndrome in that the EMG in stiff man syndrome consists entirely of activated but normally configured motor units, with no evidence of distal motor nerve disturbance.

Of interest is the finding that about two-thirds of the cases of stiff man syndrome display circulating autoantibodies that are reactive with glutamic acid decarboxylase (GAD), the synthesizing enzyme for gamma-aminobutyric acid (GABA; Solimena et al). On several occasions the test for this antibody has become positive after samples taken over 2 years were negative. An antibody to the glycine receptor (GlyR) has been identified in a subset of patients with stiff man syndrome with anti-GAD antibodies (McKeon and colleagues). The GlyR antibody, mainly expressed in the brain stem and spinal cord, has also been associated with progressive encephalomyelitis with rigidity and myoclonus, but appears to be highly specific for stiff man syndrome in patients who have anti-GAD antibodies.

Reduced spinal GABA presumably creates an imbalance between the spinal inhibitory (gabanergic) input and the excitatory input to alpha motor neurons. This interpretation is supported by the fact that the spasms worsen under the influence of drugs that enhance aminergic activity, thereby facilitating long-latency spinal reflexes, or that inhibit catecholaminergic or gabanergic transmitters. An autoimmune mechanism is further suggested by the high incidence of insulin-dependent diabetes (present eventually in almost all the cases under our care) with detectable antibodies to islet cells; a few patients have thyroiditis, pernicious anemia, or immune-mediated vitiligo.

There are rare paraneoplastic varieties of stiff man syndrome, mostly accompanying breast cancer and associated in some cases with circulating antibodies directed against amphiphysin or gephyrin, proteins associated with synaptic GABA receptors. Some of the cases related to the antiamphiphysin antibodies also display more conventional types of paraneoplastic neurologic disorder such as encephalopathy or opsoclonus (see Chap. 31).

The stiff man syndrome must be distinguished from tetanus (see "Tetanus" in Chap. 43 and further on), Isaacs syndrome, and the rare syndrome of subacute myoclonic spinal neuronitis, described in Chaps. 33 and 44. In both the stiff man syndrome and myoclonic spinal neuronitis, the intense spasms and stiffness of muscles are a result of disinhibition of interneurons in the gray matter of the spinal cord.

The syndromes of continuous muscle activity are usually distinguishable clinically and electromyographically from extrapyramidal and corticospinal abnormalities such as dystonia, dyskinesia, and rigidity, although early phases of axial dystonic disorders and stiff man syndrome have similarities.

Treatment In the stiff man syndrome, diazepam in doses of up to 50 to 250 mg/d, increased gradually, is most effective; clonazepam, vigabatrin, or baclofen is sometimes effective as well. In keeping with the presumed autoimmune mechanism of most cases, plasma exchange, high-dose corticosteroids, or intravenous gamma globulin are helpful in some patients, albeit for only several weeks or months before another infusion is required. Several of our patients have required intravenous gamma globulin for several years at intervals of 6 to 12 weeks but nevertheless became disabled if the dose of diazepam was reduced below 100 mg/d. A small randomized trial of intravenous immune globulin conducted by Dalakas and colleagues has demonstrated the efficacy of this treatment; in their study, the benefits varied in duration from 6 weeks to 1 year. The typical dose is 0.4 mg/kg daily for 4 or 5 consecutive days. Immunosuppression with rituximab is being used increasingly, on the basis of numerous case reports and small series but a small randomized trial has been negative.

Congenital Neonatal Rigidity

A "stiff infant" syndrome, observed by Dudley and colleagues in four families of mixed heritage, probably should be included in this general category. The condition came to medical attention because of respiratory distress as the result of a generalized muscular rigidity beginning at about 2 months of age. The rigidity spread slowly from cervical muscles to those of the trunk and limbs, and, as it persisted, slight hypertrophy developed. The use of respiratory aid and a feeding gastrostomy enabled the infants to survive. The rigidity slowly diminished in the second year of life. The clinical course was unlike that of tetanus. In fatal cases there were zones of fiber loss, with fibrosis in skeletal and cardiac muscles, and a greater than normal variation in fiber size. Altered Z lines were observed with electron microscope in some fibers.

Primary Hyperexcitability of Muscle

At least three varieties of primary muscle disorder are known, not myotonic in nature, that produce continuous muscle activity. The first described below is because of a defect in the muscle membrane; the second has been found to be a disease of the extracellular matrix of muscle. The third disorder, Brody disease, is only mentioned here for completeness as it is quite rare, even in comparison to the other unusual disorders in this section.

"Rippling Muscle Disease"

Ricker and Burns and their associates described a rare familial disorder (autosomal dominant) in which muscles display an unusual sensitivity to stretch, manifest by rippling waves of muscle contraction. Percussion of muscles yields a pronounced and painful local mounding. The activation is a type of myokymia. Similar familial and sporadic cases have been traced to a defect in caveolin, a protein otherwise implicated in one of the muscular dystrophies (Vorgerd). An autoimmune process was implicated in some other cases (Ashok Muley and Day). The EMG discloses neither myotonic discharges nor the action potentials of cramp, indicating that the basic abnormality is in the muscle membrane.

Schwartz-Jampel Syndrome

A syndrome characterized by continuous muscle fiber activity with stiffness and blepharospasm, accompanied by obvious dysmorphic features (dwarfism, pinched face with low-set ears, blepharophimosis, high-arched palate, receding chin, diffuse metaphyseal and epiphyseal bone dysplasia with flattened vertebrae), was described by Schwartz and Jampel in 1962. It has been reported under other names including *myotonic chondrodystrophy*. There may be percussion myotonia. Intelligence is usually preserved. The stiff muscles disturb gait most obviously.

The muscle stiffness is the result of frequent, almost continuous muscle activity with a combination of normal motor units and high-frequency discharges and afterdischarges similar to those seen in Isaacs syndrome. The discharges can be demonstrated to arise from muscle fibers themselves as the activity is not obliterated by curare. Agents such as procainamide, which block sodium channels in muscle, inhibit the discharges, just as they do in some other myotonic disorders. However, Spaans and associates, who have reviewed the clinical, EMG, and histologic features of 30 cases of this syndrome, report a diminished chloride conductance by the sarcolemma, which can be suppressed by procainamide or even better by mexiletine.

The disorder is usually inherited as an autosomal recessive trait that is caused by mutations in perlecan, a heparin-sulfate proteoglycan that is bound to the basement membranes of skeletal muscle and cartilage. Loss of function of the protein perturbs the organization of the basement membrane leading to an altered clustering of ACh esterase and abnormal expression of ion channels. Electron microscopic studies of muscle have yielded inconsistent findings: dilated T system, Z-band streaming, and dilatation of mitochondria; in addition, in the patient reported by Fariello and colleagues, muscle biopsy disclosed signs of denervation (group atrophy). In the latter case, treatment with procainamide, phenytoin, diazepam, and barbiturates was ineffective.

The condition, described by Aberfeld and coworkers, of two siblings in whom myotonia was combined with dwarfism, diffuse bone disease, and unusual ocular and facial abnormalities, and thought by them to represent a unique disorder, is probably a variant of the Schwartz-Jampel syndrome.

References

Aberfeld DC, Hinterbuchner LP, Schneider M: Myotonia, dwarfism, diffuse bone disease, and unusual ocular and facial abnormalities (a new syndrome). *Brain* 88:313, 1965.

Aitken RS, Allot EN, Casteldon LI, Walker M: Observations on a case of familial periodic paralysis. *Clin Sci* 3:47, 1937.

Andersen ED, Krasilnikoff PA, Overvad H: Intermittent muscular weakness, extrasystoles, and multiple developmental anomalies. *Acta Paediatr Scand* 60:559, 1971.

Ashok Muley S, Day JW: Autoimmune rippling muscle. *Neurology* 61:869, 2003.

Atsumi T, Ishikawa S, Miyatake T, Yoshida M: Myopathy and primary aldosteronism: Electron microscopic study. *Neurology* 29:1348, 1979.

Barker RA, Reeves T, Thom M, et al: Review of 23 patients affected by the stiff man syndrome: Clinical subdivision into stiff trunk (man) syndrome, stiff limb syndrome, and progressive encephalomyelitis with rigidity. *J Neurol Neurosurg Psychiatry* 65:633, 1998.

Becker PE: Genetic approaches to the nosology of muscle disease: Myotonias and similar diseases: Part 7. Muscle, in Bergsma D (ed): *The Clinical Delineation of Birth Defects*. Baltimore, MD, Williams & Wilkins, 1971.

Blexrud MD, Windebank AJ, Daube JR: Long term follow-up of 121 patients with benign fasciculations. *Neurology* 34:622, 1993.

Brody IA: Muscle contracture induced by exercise: A syndrome attributable to decreased relaxing factor. *N Engl J Med* 281:187, 1969.

Brown P, Rothwell PJ, Marsden CD: The stiff leg syndrome. *J Neurol Neurosurg Psychiatry* 62:31, 1997.

Bryant SH: Cable properties of external intercostal muscle fibers from myotonic and nonmyotonic goats. *J Physiol* 204:539, 1969.

Burns RJ, Bretag AH, Blumbergs PC, Harbord MG: Benign familial disease with muscle mounding and rippling. *J Neurol Neurosurg Psychiatry* 57:344, 1994.

Cannon SC: An expanding view for the molecular basis of familial periodic paralysis. *Neuromuscul Disord* 12:533, 2002.

Cannon SC, Brown RH Jr, Corey DP: Theoretical reconstruction of myotonia and paralysis caused by incomplete inactivation of sodium channels. *Biophys J* 65:270, 1993.

Celebisoy N, Cologlu Z, Akbaba Y, et al: Continuous muscle fibre activity: A case treated with acetazolamide. *J Neurol Neurosurg Psychiatry* 64:256, 1998.

Cöers C, Telerman-Toppet N, Durda J: Neurogenic benign fasciculations, pseudomyotonia, and pseudotetany. *Arch Neurol* 38:282, 1981.

Conn JW, Knopf RF, Nesbit RM: Clinical characteristics of primary aldosteronism from an analysis of 145 cases. *Am J Surg* 107:159, 1964.

Conn JW, Rovner DR, Cohen EL: Licorice-induced pseudoaldosteronism: Hypertension, hypokalemia, aldosteronopenia and suppressed plasma renin activity. *JAMA* 205:492, 1968.

Dalakas MC, Engel WK: Treatment of "permanent" muscle weakness in familial hypokalemic periodic paralysis. *Muscle Nerve* 6:182, 1983.

Dalakas MC, Fugii M, Li M, et al: High dose intravenous immune globulin for stiff-person syndrome. *N Engl J Med* 345:1870, 2001.

DeJong JGY: Myotonia levior, in Kuhn E (ed): *Progressive Muskeldystrophie-Myotonie-Myasthenie*. Heidelberg, Springer, 1966, pp 255–259.

Denborough MA: Malignant hyperthermia. *Lancet* 352:1131, 1998.

Denborough MA, Forster JF, Lovell RR: Anaesthetic deaths in a family. *Br J Anaesth* 1962:34, 395.

Denny-Brown D, Foley JM: Evidence of a chemical mediator in myotonia. *Trans Assoc Am Physicians* 62:187, 1949.

Denny-Brown D, Nevin S: The phenomenon of myotonia. *Brain* 64:1, 1941.

Engel AG: Evolution and content of vacuoles in primary hypokalemic periodic paralysis. *Mayo Clin Proc* 45:774, 1970.

Fariello R, Meloff K, Murphy EG, et al: A case of Schwartz-Jampel syndrome with unusual muscle biopsy findings. *Ann Neurol* 3:93, 1978.

Fontaine B, Khurana TS, Hoffman EP, et al: Hyperkalemic periodic paralysis and the adult muscle sodium channel alpha-subunit gene. *Science* 250:1000, 1990.

Fontaine B, Vale Santos JM, Jurkat-Rott JK, et al: Mapping of hypokalemic periodic paralysis (hypo PP) to chromosome 1q31-q32 by a genome-wide search in three European families. *Nat Genet* 6:267, 1994.

Frank JP, Harati Y, Butler JJ, et al: Central core disease and malignant hyperthermia syndrome. *Ann Neurol* 7:11, 1980.

Gamstorp I: Adynamia episodica hereditaria. *Acta Paediatr Scand* 45(Suppl 108):1, 1956.

Gutmann L, Gutmann L: Axonal channelopathies: An evolving concept in the pathogenesis of peripheral nerve disorders. *Neurology* 47:18, 1996.

Haass A, Ricker K, Rüdel R, et al: Clinical study of paramyotonia congenita with and without myotonia in a warm environment. *Muscle Nerve* 4:388, 1981.

Hanna MG, Wood NW, Kullmann DM: Ion channels and neurological disease: DNA based diagnosis is now possible, and ion channels may be important in common paroxysmal disorders. *J Neurol Neurosurg Psychiatry* 65:427, 1998.

Harriman DGF, Summer DW, Ellis FR: Malignant hyperthermia myopathy. *Q J Med* 42:639, 1973.

Heatwole CR, Statland JM, Logigian EL: The diagnosis and treatment of myotonic disorders. *Muscle Nerve* 47:632, 2013.

Hudson AJ, Brown WF, Gilbert JJ: The muscular pain-fasciculation syndrome. *Neurology* 28:1105, 1978.

Isaacs H: Continuous muscle fibre activity in an Indian male with additional evidence of terminal motor fibre abnormality. *J Neurol Neurosurg Psychiatry* 30:126, 1967.

Isaacs H, Barlow MB: Malignant hyperpyrexia. *J Neurol Neurosurg Psychiatry* 36:228, 1973.

Koch MC, Steinmeyer K, Lorenz C, et al: The skeletal muscle chloride channel in dominant and recessive human myotonia. *Science* 257:797, 1992.

Lambert EH, Goldstein NP: An unusual form of "myotonia." *Physiologist* 1:51, 1957.

Layzer RB: *Neuromuscular Manifestations of Systemic Disease*. Philadelphia, Davis, 1985.

Lehmann-Horn F, Mailänder V, Heine R, George AL: Myotonia levior is a chloride channel disorder. *Hum Mol Genet* 4:1397, 1995.

Lehmann-Horn F, Rüdel R, Jurkat-Rott K: Nondystrophic myotonias and periodic paralyses, in Engel AG, Franzini-Armstrong C (eds): *Myology*, 3rd ed. New York, McGraw-Hill, 2004, pp 1257–1300.

Lehmann-Horn F, Rüdel R, Ricker K: Membrane defects in paramyotonia congenita (Eulenburg). *Muscle Nerve* 10:633, 1987.

Lewi Z, Bar-Khayim Y: Food poisoning from barium carbonate. *Lancet* 2:342, 1964.

Ligouri R, Vincent A, Clover L, et al: Morvan's syndrome: Peripheral and central nervous system and cardiac involvement with antibodies to voltage-gated potassium channels. *Brain* 124:2417, 2001.

Lipicky RJ, Bryant SH: Ion content, potassium flux, and cable properties of myotonic, human, external intercostal muscle. *Trans Am Neurol Assoc* 96:34, 1971.

Lipicky RJ, Bryant SH: Sodium, potassium, and chloride fluxes in intercostal muscle from normal goats and goats with hereditary myotonia. *J Gen Physiol* 50:89, 1966.

Lütschg J, Jerusalem F, Ludin HP, et al: The syndrome of "continuous muscle fiber activity." *Arch Neurol* 35:198, 1978.

McFadzean AJS, Yeung R: Periodic paralysis complicating thyrotoxicosis in Chinese. *Br Med J* 1:451, 1967.

McKeon B, Martinez-Hernandez E, Lancaster E, et al: Glycine receptor autoimmune spectrum with stiff-man syndrome phenotype. *JAMA Neurol* 70:44, 2013.

Meyers KR, Gilden DH, Rinaldi CF, Hansen JL: Periodic muscle weakness, normokalemia, and tubular aggregates. *Neurology* 22:269, 1972.

Mills KR, Edwards RHT: Investigative strategies for muscle pain. *J Neurol Sci* 58:73, 1983.

Moersch FP, Woltman HW: Progressive fluctuating muscular rigidity ("stiff-man syndrome"): Report of a case and some observations in 13 other cases. *Mayo Clin Proc* 31:421, 1956.

Newsom-Davis J: Neuromyotonia. *Rev Neurol* 160:85, 2004.

Newsom-Davis J, Mills KR: Immunological associations of acquired neuromyotonia (Isaacs' syndrome). *Brain* 116:453, 1993.

Nissen K: Beiträge zur Kenntnis der Thomsen'schen Krankheit (Myotonia congenita), mit besonderer Berücksichtigung des hereditären Momentes und seinen Beziehungen zu den Mendelschen Vererbungsregeln. *Z Klin Med* 97:58, 1923.

Okinaka S, Shizume K, Iinos S, et al: The association of periodic paralysis and hyperthyroidism in Japan. *J Clin Endocrinol Metab* 17:1454, 1957.

Plaster NM, Tawil R, Tristani-Firouzi M, et al: Mutations in Kir2.1 cause the developmental and episodic electrical phenotypes of Andersen's syndrome. *Cell* 105:511, 2001.

Poskanzer DC, Kerr DNS: A third type of periodic paralysis with normokalemia and favorable response to NaCl. *Am J Med* 31:328, 1961.

Pothiwala P, Levine SN: Thyrotoxic periodic paralysis: A review. *J Intensive Care Med* 25:71, 2010.

Ptácek LJ, Fu YH: Channelopathies: Episodic disorders of the nervous system. *Epilepsia* 42(Suppl 5):35, 2001.

Ptácek LJ, Tawil R, Griggs RC, et al: Dihydropyridine receptor mutations cause hypokalemic periodic paralysis. *Cell* 77:863, 1994a.

Ptácek LJ, Tawil R, Griggs RC, et al: Sodium channel mutations in acetazolamide-responsive myotonia congenita, paramyotonia congenita, and hyperkalemic periodic paralysis. *Neurology* 44:1500, 1994b.

Price DL, Griffin JW, Peck K: Tetanus toxin: Evidence for binding at presynaptic nerve endings. *Brain Res* 121:379, 1977.

Quane KA, Healy JMS, Keating KE, et al: Mutations in the ryanodine receptor gene in central core disease and malignant hyperthermia. *Nat Genet* 5:51, 1993.

Ricker K, Moxley RT, Heine R, Lehmann-Horn F: Myotonia fluctuans: A third type of muscle sodium channel disease. *Arch Neurol* 51:1095, 1994.

Ricker K, Moxley RT, Rohkamm R: Rippling muscle disease. *Arch Neurol* 46:405, 1989.

Rosenfeld J, Sloan-Brown K, George AL: A novel muscle sodium channel mutation causes painful congenital myotonia. *Ann Neurol* 42:811, 1997.

Rüdel R, Lehmann-Horn F, Ricker K, et al: Hypokalemic periodic paralysis: In vitro investigation of muscle fiber membrane parameters. *Muscle Nerve* 7:110, 1984.

Ryan DP, Ptácek LJ: Episodic neurological channelopathies. *Neuron* 68:282, 2010.

Saiz A, Graus F, Valldeoriola F, et al: Stiff-leg syndrome: A form of stiff-man syndrome. *Ann Neurol* 43:400, 1998.

Sansone V, Griggs RC, Meola G, et al: Andersen's syndrome: A distinct periodic paralysis. *Ann Neurol* 42:305, 1997.

Satoyoshi E: A syndrome of progressive muscle spasm, alopecia and diarrhea. *Neurology* 28:458, 1978.

Schröder JM, Adams RD: The ultrastructural morphology of the muscle fiber in myotonic dystrophy. *Acta Neuropathol* 10:218, 1968.

Schwartz O, Jampel R: Congenital blepharophimosis associated with a unique generalized myopathy. *Arch Ophthalmol* 68:52, 1962.

Serratrice G, Azulay JP: Que reste-t-il de la chorée fibrillaire de Morvan? *Rev Neurol (Paris)* 150:257, 1994.

Solimena M, Folli F, Aparisi R, et al: Autoantibodies to GABA-ergic neurons and pancreatic beta cells in stiff-man syndrome. *N Engl J Med* 322:1555, 1990.

Spaans F, Theunissen P, Reekers AD, et al: Schwartz-Jampel syndrome: 1. Clinical, electromyographic, and histologic studies. *Muscle Nerve* 13:516, 1990.

Stevens JR: Familial periodic paralysis, myotonia, progressive amyotrophy, and pes cavus in members of a single family. *Arch Neurol Psychiatry* 72:726, 1954.

Streib EW: Paramyotonia congenita: Successful treatment with tocainide: Clinical and electrophysiologic findings in seven patients. *Muscle Nerve* 10:155, 1987.

Streib EW: Successful treatment with tocainide of recessive generalized congenital myotonia. *Ann Neurol* 19:501, 1986.

Subramony SH, Wee AS, Mishra SK: Lack of cold sensitivity in hyperkalemic periodic paralysis. *Muscle Nerve* 9:700, 1986.

Sun SF, Streib EW: Autosomal recessive generalized myotonia. *Muscle Nerve* 6:143, 1983.

Swift TR: Disorders of neuromuscular transmission other than myasthenia gravis. *Muscle Nerve* 4:334, 1981.

Tahmoush AJ, Alonso RJ, Tahmoush GP, et al: Cramp-fasciculation syndrome: A treatable hyperexcitable peripheral nerve disorder. *Neurology* 41:1021, 1991.

Talbott JH: Periodic paralysis: A clinical syndrome. *Medicine (Baltimore)* 20:85, 1941.

Tawil R, McDermott MP, Brown RH Jr, et al: Randomized trials of dichlorphenamide in the periodic paralyses. Working Group on Periodic Paralysis. *Ann Neurol* 47:46, 2000.

Thieben MJ, Lennon VA, Askanit AJ, et al: Potentially reversible autoimmune limbic encephalitis with neuronal potassium channel antibody. *Neurology* 62:1177, 2004.

Thomasen E: *Myotonia, Thomsen's Disease, Paramyotonia, Dystrophia Myotonica*. Aarhus, Denmark, Universitetsforlaget i Aarhus, 1948.

Thomsen J: Tonische Krämpfe in willkürlich beweglichen Muskeln in Folge von ererbter psychischer disposition (Ataxia muscularis?). *Arch Psychiatr Nervenkr* 6:706, 1876.

Thompson PD: Stiff muscles. *J Neurol Neurosurg Psychiatry* 56:121, 1993.

Trudell RG, Kaiser KK, Griggs RC: Acetazolamide-responsive myotonia congenita. *Neurology* 37:488, 1987.

Tyler FH, Stephens FE, Gunn FD, Perkoff GT: Studies on disorders of muscle: VII. Clinical manifestations and inheritance of a type of periodic paralysis without hypopotassemia. *J Clin Invest* 30:492, 1951.

Valli G, Barbieri S, Stefano C, et al: Syndromes of abnormal muscular activity: Overlap between continuous muscle fiber activity and the stiff-man syndrome. *J Neurol Neurosurg Psychiatry* 46:241, 1983.

Vernino S, Lennon VA: Ion channel and striational antibodies define a continuum of autoimmune neuromuscular hyperexcitability. *Muscle Nerve* 26:702, 2002.

Vorgerd M, Ricker K, Ziemssen W, et al: A sporadic case of rippling muscle disease caused by a de novo caveolin-3 mutation. *Neurology* 57:2273, 2001.

Yazaki K, Kuribayashi T, Yamamura Y, et al: Hypokalemic myopathy associated with a 17α-hydroxylase deficiency: A case report. *Neurology* 32:94, 1982.

PART 6

PSYCHIATRIC DISORDERS

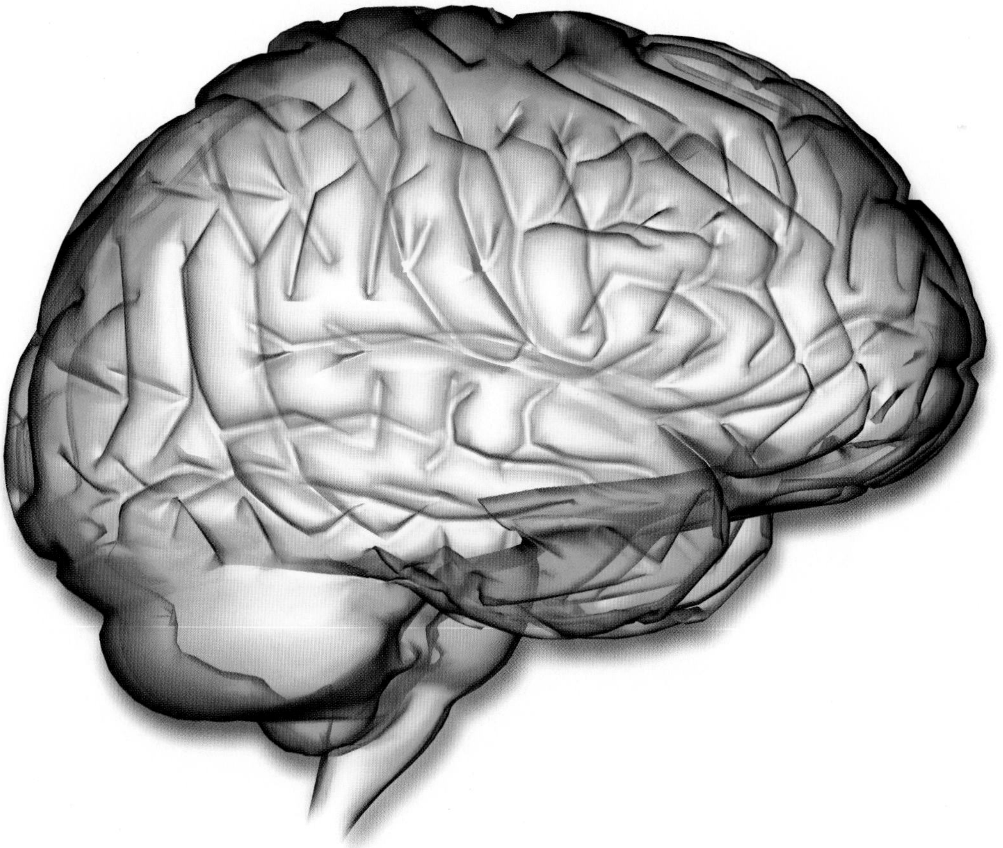

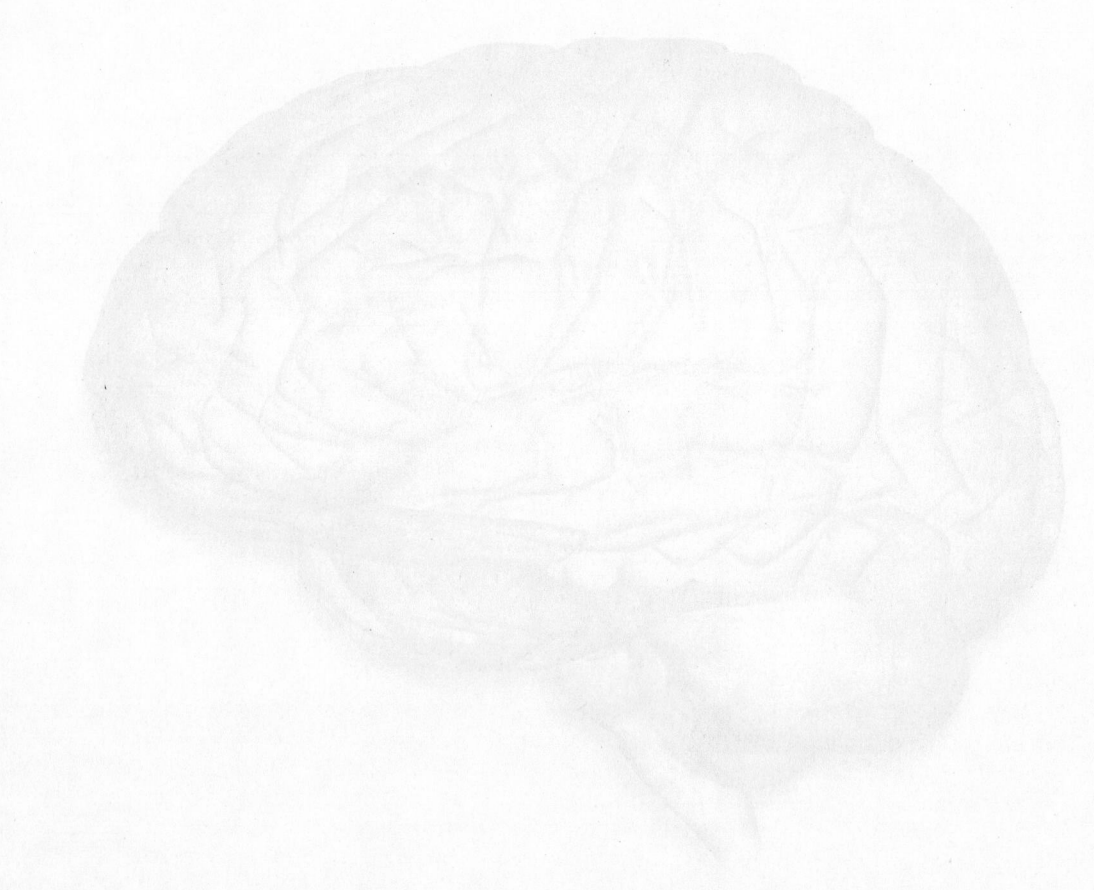

51

Anxiety Disorders, Hysteria, and Personality Disorders

The relationship between psychiatry and neurology, at one time unified specialties, has been problematic for over half a century. With the emergence of numerous theories of the nature of mental life and of the mind, came corresponding systems for the treatment of psychiatric disease. Most of these systems, typified by psychoanalysis, seemed to have little in common with neurologic ideas about the structure and function of the brain. Freed from the archetype of the main mental disease that was the result of structural damage to the brain, syphilitic general paresis, psychiatry was able to turn to matters that were less anchored in medicine. With the emergence of a new "biologic psychiatry" based on neurochemistry, genetics, and functional imaging of the brain, it would seem that the gap between diseases of the mind and of the brain is closing. However, neurologists should view some of these modern ideas with at least some skepticism. For example, the observation of brain function by the use of imaging methods, and disruption of that function in disease, is not the equivalent of the disease itself and certainly cannot capture the experience through which mental disease is manifest. To dissociate an individual's personal history and experiences, aspects of life that probably cannot be quantified or visualized, from diseases of the mind remains an artifice now, as it was in the time of the classic philosophers. Moreover, the separation of quirks of personality and character traits, probably reflecting the biologic diversity of the development of the brain, from genuine disease will remain eternally problematic. Even the margins between the disease and mental dysfunction have been disputed and have given rise to numerous "shadow syndromes" of psychologic origin that are subject to change with popular culture and fashion. This serves as an appropriate introduction to a chapter on what was formerly termed the "neuroses."

In every society, there are many troubled individuals who are neither mentally ill nor developmentally impaired. They differ from other people in being plagued by feelings of inferiority or self-doubt, suspicion about the motives of others, low energy, inexplicable fatigue, shyness, irritability, moodiness, sense of guilt, and unreasonable worries and fears. They suffer as a result of these feelings or they behave in ways that are upsetting to those around them and to society at large. Yet none of these conditions precludes partaking in the everyday life, such as attending school, working, marrying, and raising a family. As these conditions were more carefully documented in the early part of the last century, they came to be called *psychoneuroses,* and later, *neuroses*, and those that created societal difficulties were called *psychopathies,* and more recently, personality disorders and *sociopathies.*

The question of the purity and homogeneity of these mental states creates an ongoing polemic in psychiatry. The neuroses as a group appeared to be so diverse as to require subdivision in serial editions of the *Diagnostic and Statistical Manual of Mental Disorders* (DSM) into no less than seven different types. In this and in subsequent chapters we refer to the DSM, now in its fifth edition (DSM-5), but have chosen not to use it as a dominant guide in discussing psychiatric disease. We take this position not out of iconoclasm but because the definitions in that system are changed frequently, are subject to considerable controversy, and often do not accord with neurobiologic ideas of brain function. In any case, readers may wish to consult DSM-5 where appropriate, to gain insight into the thinking of the psychiatric community.

Originally, Freud referred to the neuroses as psychoneuroses and the subject became enmeshed in psychoanalytic theory. The assumption was that an undercurrent of anxiety arising from unconscious conflict explained all the different types of neuroses as well as the psychopathies. Later, psychiatrists uncommitted to psychoanalytic theory attributed these states to social forces leading to maladaptive behavior from childhood. These notions were not acceptable to biologically oriented physicians, with the result that the term *psychoneurosis* was expunged from later editions of the DSM, and even *neurosis* was replaced by *anxiety disorders*, *phobic states*, and *obsessive-compulsive disorder*. These terms are at present applied to mental disorders with the following characteristics: (1) symptoms that are distressing to the affected individual and regarded by the person as unacceptable or alien; (2) intactness of reality testing (the patient's evaluation of the relationship between himself and the outside world); (3) symptomatic behavior that does not seriously violate social norms, although personal functioning may be considerably impaired; (4) a disturbance that has its onset early in life and is enduring—not a transitory reaction to stress; and (5) the absence of a discernible medical cause or structural disease of the brain. The foregoing definition of anxiety and its allied disorders has the virtue of being descriptive without committing one to any theory of causation.

The genesis of the anxiety, phobic, and obsessive states remains elusive. It is generally conceded that they do not arise de novo. The antecedents are thought in some quarters to be abnormalities in personality development, strongly influenced by genetic factors and molded by stressful events in the life of the individual (Noyes et al). Traits of this nature undoubtedly arise in several individuals from the same family. Thus any discussion requires a brief digression into the origins of normal personality development and departures from it. Even if one is not certain of a relationship between development and psychologic disorders in the broad category of neurosis, it is clear from the interactions of daily life that minor forms of anxiety contribute to the makeup of the normal personality.

PERSONALITY DISORDERS

Chapter 28 introduced the concept of *personality* and its development. There it was pointed out that the term embraces the totality of a person's mental attributes, observable behavior, and reportable subjective experience—the sum of which distinguishes one individual from all others. Thus it includes elements of what might be called the individual's character and includes intelligence, drives, temperament, and sentiments—in short, all forces from within the organism that determine a person's reactions to the prevailing environment. The term *character* is almost synonymous with personality but is less useful in medicine because of its emphasis on interpersonal and ethical aspects and its moralistic connotation.

Pertinent to this subject matter is the assumption that in approximately 15 percent of the general population, certain personality traits are so pronounced as to be distressing to the individual and disturbing to others, even though the patient is not manifestly sociopathic or psychotic.

The roots of personality features such as boldness and timidity, novelty seeking and excitability, level of energy and motor activity, fearfulness and fearlessness, social adaptability and rigidity or stubbornness are already evident in the first months of life. Monozygotic twins are alike (but not absolutely identical) in these respects, even when reared apart. Gesell and his colleagues, in their studies of infants (see Chap. 28), observed individual differences that are clearly innate; each of these characteristics is likely to be genetically determined, like intelligence. The personalities that result are as individualistic as fingerprints. One example of a biologic and genetic basis of a human personality trait, albeit to a limited degree, has been found in the expression of thrill seeking, exploration, and excitability. According to the early work of Cloninger and colleagues (1996), polymorphisms of a dopamine receptor gene on chromosome 11 accounts in small measure for the genetic variability of this personality type. Findings such as these have been reproduced for similar polymorphisms that contribute to the traits of timidity, anxiety, and obsessiveness. The notion, expressed by authors such as Kandel, that genetics will explain a large part of mental function and mental illness sounds reasonable enough, but the data to establish this are far from complete.

The interesting and related construct of a "national character" is embedded in social discourse but has not been extensively studied. It is mentioned here to allow for a more complete picture of the concept of character. A fascinating survey by Terracciano and colleagues indicates that mean personality traits in 49 cultures do not correspond to general stereotypes and are therefore probably simply contrivances for maintaining national identity. Similar comments can be proffered regarding sex differences in personality that are embedded in cultural stereotypes but these latter personality profiles have more data to suggest a degree of uniformity and validity in differences between men and women in all cultures.

An unsolved problem is whether each of the personality types accepted by the American Psychiatric Association is predictive or determinative of a later mental disorder. In this regard, two broad groups of personality disorders can be recognized. In one group—comprising the paranoid, schizoid, cyclothymic, and obsessive-compulsive personality types—there are obvious similarities to major types of psychiatric illness. Thus, among patients who develop paranoid schizophrenia, a considerable number will have had the attributes described under "paranoid personality type." Similarly, among patients who develop schizophrenia of another type, the history will frequently disclose a preexistent "schizoid" personality. In fact, it may be difficult to judge where the personality disorder leaves off and the schizophrenic illness began. Similarly, it seems clear from several family studies that the cyclothymic personality is related to bipolar disease. Obsessive-compulsive personality is related not only to obsessive-compulsive neurosis, as one might expect, but also to depressive disease.

Recently, the notion of clusters of personality traits has been introduced and may be more useful in clinical work than are the discrete personality types (see Tyrer).

Perhaps most problematic in classification but seen regularly in psychiatric practice is the "borderline personality disorder." As with other personality types, the pattern of behaviors is pervasive and lifelong in the affected individual. An ensemble of poorly regulated emotions, impulsive and aggressive actions, and repeated self-injury form the core aspects of the disorder. These patients typically express a range of profound emotional "pains" and a sense of dysphoria, often rapidly changing from one mood to another without provocation. There may be additional nonpsychotic problems that border on paranoia with feelings of low self-esteem. Interpersonal relationships are made unstable as a result of fear of being left alone combined with argumentativeness. These are among the most distressing individuals for families and physicians to deal with and little success has been achieved in treatment. The potential biologic roots of the borderline personality disorder were reviewed by Lieb and colleagues and the clinical features, by Gunderson, who emphasizes the difficulties in treating these people, currently limited mainly to various types of insight-oriented psychotherapies.

The defining features of the personality disorders therefore fall short of meeting the diagnostic criteria for more serious mental illness. Yet, an understanding of these personal peculiarities and their less obtrusive traits may be of great help to the physician. This knowledge makes it possible to appreciate their role as sources of perennial complaint, self-concern, and family discord, and to explain a patient's reactions that have interfered with diagnostic and therapeutic procedures during a medical illness. It is, however, quite common for extremes of personality to create depression and anxiety, either of which is amenable to medical and psychotherapeutic treatment. As a final comment, one should never underestimate the power of maturation to ameliorate the turmoil of adolescence and to settle the young mind.

ANXIETY DISORDERS

Although considered to be the most frequent of mental disturbances, the anxiety disorders are among the least understood. They were established as clinical entities in the late nineteenth century, but there are still major unresolved issues with respect to their nature, classification, and etiology. Descriptively, they are meant to include (1) anxiety disorder; (2) phobic disorder, which includes phobia of illness, social phobia, and agoraphobia; (3) obsessive-compulsive states; (4) hysteria; and (5) hypochondriasis. Former classifications included additional types called neurasthenia (dysthymia or depressive neurosis), which is now considered with the depressive illnesses, and "depersonalization neurosis" (dissociative disorders), which is a form of hysterical neurosis. Although each of these syndromes is clinically separable when occurring in pure form, experience shows that most patients suffer from symptoms of more than one type and thus are said to have "mixed neuroses." In the most recent classifications, all of the neuroses have been again subsumed in three broad categories: (1) *anxiety disorders* (which include panic states, with and without agoraphobia, and the phobic and obsessive-compulsive neuroses); (2) *somatoform disorders* (comprising hysterical neurosis, or conversion disorder, and hypochondriasis); and (3) *dissociative disorders*.

An interesting view of the relative frequency of mental disorders of the day was provided by an analysis of 1,045 consecutive psychiatric consultations at the New England Center Hospital during the years 1955 and 1956 in which the dominant psychiatric syndrome in approximately 20 percent of patients was an anxiety state. Other epidemiologic studies have also disclosed a strikingly high incidence of anxiety disorders in the general population (see the review of Winokur and Coryell). Lifetime prevalence figures indicate that at least 11 percent of the population is so affected—i.e., some 25 million persons in the United States. Such information as is available suggests that the incidence of the neuroses is much the same in an urban population (midtown New York) as it is in a rural one (Stirling County, Nova Scotia), indicating that socioeconomic, racial, and cultural factors are of limited importance. Furthermore, in times of calamity, such as the bombing of London, the incidence of neurotic symptoms was said not to have increased. Thus, it is probably an oversimplification to view neuroses as merely by-products of life in civilized society or reactions to environmental stress (see also Chap. 24). This raises the issue alluded to earlier and discussed more extensively further on: namely, the role of background personality traits in promoting extreme and persistent anxiety after a traumatizing event (PTSD; see Chap. 24).

The symptoms of the anxiety disorders typically arise in late childhood, adolescence, or early adult life. Admittedly, symptoms may be recognized for the first time after this age, but a good clinical rule is to suspect any mental illness that appears for the first time after the age of about 40 years to be either a depression or a dementia.

ANXIETY DISORDER AND PANIC ATTACKS

As mentioned, the term *anxiety neurosis* was introduced by Freud to describe a syndrome of general irritability, anxious expectation, anxiety attacks, somatic accompaniments or equivalents of anxiety (breathlessness, chest pain, asthenia), and nightmares. In anxiety neurosis, this symptom complex constitutes the entire illness. However, parts of this constellation also appear with many other psychiatric diseases—bipolar disease, schizophrenia, hysteria, and phobic neurosis. Its closest link is with depression, which it resembles in another respect, namely, *a strong hereditary factor*, as pointed out by Mandel Cohen and Paul Dudley White in 1940.

Clinical Presentation

Anxiety disorder is a chronic state, some would say a disease, punctuated by recurrent attacks of acute anxiety or panic. The acute attacks are the hallmark of the disease and some psychiatrists are reluctant to make a diagnosis of anxiety neurosis in their absence. Because of the clinical features of panic attacks and particularly their episodic nature, simulating an acute medical condition, they are of special interest to neurologists and general physicians. While anxiety may be inferred from observing the activities of young children, and is reported as a form of nervousness by older children and adolescents, more often there are physical complaints at times of transition or stress during the day or year.

Panic attacks in their full form are prone to begin after this age and are almost as dramatic as seizures. They begin with distressing feelings of dread and foreboding. The patient is assailed by a sense of strangeness, as though his body had changed or the surroundings were unreal. He is frightened, sometimes by the prospect of imminent death (*angor animi*) or of losing his mind or self-control. There may be a feeling of smothering. "I am dying" or "I can't breathe" are the characteristic expressions of alarm and panic. The heart races, breathing comes in rapid gasps, the pupils may be dilated, and the patient may sweat or tremble. The palpitation and breathing difficulties are so prominent that a cardiologist is often consulted. Some of our psychiatric colleagues identify breathlessness or a suffocating feeling as central to the diagnosis of panic (and attribute psychologic meaning to the symptom), but this is not sustained in our observations of affected patients. The symptoms abate spontaneously after 15 to 30 min, leaving the patient shaken, tense, perplexed, and often embarrassed. There is no confusion, and after the episode there is full memory of the event.

Most anxiety attacks are of lesser severity with complaints of apprehension, slight faintness, palpitations, or a feeling of postural instability referred to by the patient as dizziness. Breathlessness, vague chest or upper abdominal discomfort, a palpitating sensation as if the heart were beating too hard, and a generalized "washed out" feeling (asthenia) are other common symptoms. More than 50 years ago Cohen and White listed the following symptoms in order of frequency in the patients they observed: palpitation, 97 percent; easy fatigue, 93 percent; breathlessness, 90 percent; nervousness, 88 percent; chest pain, 85 percent; sighing, 79 percent; dizziness, 78 percent; apprehensiveness, 61 percent; headache, 58 percent; paresthesias, 58 percent; weakness, 56 percent; insomnia, 53 percent; unhappiness, 50 percent. What is evident from this listing is that the experience of anxiety is conjoined with a polysymptomatic physical syndrome. (This, indeed, was the James-Lang theory of emotion—that the sensory experience was all there was to emotion.) It is not surprising, therefore, that many patients with chronic or recurrent symptoms first consult a physician not with a complaint of "anxiety" but with symptoms referable to the cardiorespiratory system or gastrointestinal system (dyspepsia, loss of appetite, or "irritable colon").

Many patients experience a constant uneasiness that the spells may reoccur, especially in public; hence the patient may be fearful of leaving home lest help not be available should an attack occur (agoraphobia). Except in minor details, it is notable that the attacks are alike in any one individual. Between attacks, most patients feel relatively well but many complain of the symptoms of anxiety and asthenia in lesser but persistent fashion.

Hyperventilation is a special, although not invariable, feature of the anxiety attack. Hyperventilation itself, by reducing the Pco_2, will cause giddiness, paresthesias of the fingers, tongue, and lips, and, at times, frank tetany. However, contrary to what is stated in some textbooks, in only a minority of patients does a 3-min period of deep breathing reproduce the symptoms of an anxiety or panic attack. Nonetheless, this maneuver may be used to assist the patient in describing certain aspects of an attack.

Attacks in minor form, without the full force of the physical accompaniments may occur at infrequent intervals or several times a day. Much to the patient's surprise, they usually occur in situations where there are no easily recognizable sources of fear, as when the patient is sitting quietly at home or has just awakened from sleep. In other instances, a trying or upsetting experience induces an attack, which is nonetheless excessive for the condition that provoked it. In some patients, attacks are brought on consistently by confinement to a closed space (claustrophobia)—an elevator, for example—or by crowded surroundings, as in a church, restaurant, or theater. An anxiety state frequently follows an accident and then may, according to Modlin, be a source of ongoing disability, a condition more akin to posttraumatic stress disorder. Similar spells of anxiety are also a prominent feature of the postconcussive and posttraumatic stress syndromes.

From the patient's life history, two patterns of anxiety neurosis are discernible. In one, there is a nearly lifelong history of poor exercise tolerance, little stamina, and inability to do heavy physical work or participate in vigorous sports, tenseness, nervousness, and intolerance of crowds, i.e., what had in the past been called neurasthenia. When these symptoms arose during military service, they were designated, since the American Civil War as *neurocirculatory asthenia*, "irritable heart," or "soldier's heart." In the other pattern of onset, the patient is vigorous and symptom-free before the anxiety state begins in adulthood.

The course of anxiety neurosis is variable. A 20-year followup study by Wheeler and associates showed that symptoms were still present in 88 percent but persisted in being moderately or severely disabling in only 15 percent. Most affected patients were able to work and to enjoy a reasonably normal family and social life. Their only liability to further psychiatric illness was to later anxious depression, whereas so-called psychosomatic illnesses and other psychiatric illnesses did not occur more frequently than in the general population. Those with uncomplicated anxiety neurosis rarely commit suicide.

Etiology and Pathogenesis

Anxiety disorder has been attributed to a genetic abnormality, to a "constitutional weakness" of the nervous system, to social and psychologic factors, and to physiologic and biochemical derangements; but none of these factors provides a completely satisfactory explanation of the primary problem.

The onset of both acute and chronic anxiety is rare before age 18 years or after 35 to 40 years of age (average age of onset 25 years). The condition in some series is twice as frequent in women as in men and there is clearly a high familial incidence. In one study (Wheeler et al) there was a prevalence of 49 percent among the grown children of patients with anxiety neurosis, compared with 5 percent in the general population. Slater and Shields found that there was a concordance rate of 40 percent in identical twins, compared with 4 percent in dizygotic twins. Among the relatives of index cases, the mothers suffered from anxiety neurosis more often than did the fathers; in the latter, alcoholism was more frequent than in the population at large (Modlin). A clear pattern of inheritance has not been established, but it approximates that of autosomal dominance with incomplete penetrance. The psychodynamic theories that attempt to provide a unified explanation of these diverse anxiety states were reviewed by Nemiah and we do not dismiss them but cannot comment authoritatively.

The symptoms of an anxiety attack resemble those of fear in many ways, although nearly always the former are longer in duration and less distinct. The most important difference, however, is that the cause of fear is known to the patient, whereas that of anxiety is not. The most extreme but not inconceivable interpretation of anxiety is the James-Lange theory of emotion, mentioned earlier, which attributes the psychologic experience entirely to the accompanying physical symptoms.

On the physiologic and biochemical side, it has been observed that anger provokes an excessive secretion of norepinephrine, whereas fear is accompanied by increased secretion of epinephrine. Actually, fear activates the autonomic nervous system as a whole and the increase in epinephrine is more than counterbalanced by a parasympathetic discharge. Attention has been focused on overactivity of the locus ceruleus and upper brainstem nuclei as the possible anatomic substrates of anxiety (Judd et al). Other studies have implicated serotonergic centers. Evidently, the responsiveness of the autonomic nervous system in these patients remains heightened and a number of stimuli (cold, pain, muscular effort) may produce abnormal responses in pulse, respiration, oxygen consumption, and work performance. Another interesting abnormality (first noted by Cohen et al) is that the blood lactic acid levels in response to exercise are higher than normal. The presence of these changes does not necessarily mean that they are causal; they are as likely secondary to other factors such as poor physical condition and apprehension associated with the syndrome. Nevertheless, some investigators have found that infusions of lactic acid can trigger panic attacks in persons with anxiety neurosis (Liebowitz et al). Subsequently, numerous other theories of causation have been proposed based on the reported provocation of panic attacks by a number of different substances—carbon dioxide, yohimbine, gamma-aminobutyric acid (GABA), isoproterenol, and others. None provides a comprehensive biologic explanation.

Studies correlating cerebral function and blood flow indicate that when panic is induced by an intravenous injection of sodium lactate, there is an immediate increase in blood flow to the cortex of both temporal lobes. In states of fear, the tips of the temporal lobes and the amygdaloid nuclei are known to become activated. In the relaxed period between panic attacks, the right limbic system and the parahippocampal gyrus are abnormally active in some studies. As with the aforementioned biochemical models, these seem to be more reflections of brain activity in response to the psychic experience than they are explanations. Nevertheless, parts of the limbic system are presumably involved in a germinal way in the production and perpetuation of anxiety and its related states.

The discovery that the benzodiazepines bind to specific sites of the GABA receptor complex and that the sedative and amnesic effects (α_1 subunit) of these drugs seem to be separable from their anxiolytic effects (α_2 subunit) raises the possibility that abnormalities of the GABA system directly underlie anxiety. However, there is only indirect evidence for this mechanism. Of potentially greater importance is the finding of genetic polymorphisms that relate statistically to the presence of anxiety states, such as one in the serotonin transporter gene (Lesch et al). It has been estimated that allelic differences on the chromosome contribute perhaps 10 percent to the overall anxiety tendency. One presumes that there are numerous additional genes that participate in a similar way. Others have not found this particular association or have found it only in patients with generalized anxiety and not in those with panic attacks. Consequently, the precise relationship of genetic polymorphisms to anxiety states cannot be stated at this moment, but a heritable component is undoubted.

Differential Diagnosis

Shorn of the psychologic components of apprehension and fear, the anxiety attack consists essentially of an excessive autonomic discharge. Some of the autonomic symptoms are therefore duplicated by chromaffin tumors, hyperthyroidism, and the menopause. The prominence of chest discomfort and respiratory distress during an acute anxiety attack may be mistaken for myocardial ischemia, in which case the patient is often subjected to a series of studies of cardiac function. Another form of the illness—in which nondescript dizziness, vague difficulty with visual clarity, and fear of losing consciousness are the most prominent features—may be mistaken for an otologic problem (see "Nonvertiginous Types of Dizziness" in Chap. 15) or for epilepsy. In contrast, headache is (surprisingly) a relatively infrequent experience in our patients and the diagnosis should be suspect if it is a prominent feature. Other medical diseases that may be brought to mind by isolated elements of an anxiety state are pulmonary embolism, cardiac arrhythmias, hypoglycemia, hypoparathyroidism, alcohol, drug, nicotine withdrawal, and, especially, complex partial seizures. In regard to seizures as imitators of anxiety, however, loss of consciousness, incontinence, and clonic or myoclonic movements do not occur. Adherence to the diagnostic criteria of these disease states readily permits their differentiation from acute anxiety, but diagnosis may be difficult if the symptoms are brief.

Of equal importance is the relationship of anxiety to depression. A large proportion of patients with depression have symptoms of anxiety. Indeed, some psychiatrists believe that anxiety neurosis is accounted for mainly by a variant of depression. As has been mentioned, an anxiety state appearing for the first time after the fortieth year usually proves to be primarily a depression, although it may be that a predisposing personality trait is involved. The presence of symptoms such as overwhelming fatigue, self-deprecation, and feelings of hopelessness and, of course, ideas of self-destruction makes depression the fundamental diagnosis, with anxiety an associated feature (anxious depression). As mentioned, a very small number of patients with a condition diagnosed as pure anxiety neurosis have committed suicide, but this does not hold if depression is the central illness.

Schizophrenia may also begin with prominent anxiety symptoms. Here the diagnosis rests on finding the characteristic thought disorder of schizophrenia, which may emerge only after several interviews. Hysteria may include anxiety symptoms, though they are seldom prominent, and phobic and obsessive-compulsive neuroses constantly create an anxious state in affected patients, but each has distinguishing attributes.

Treatment

Certain medications, particularly anxiolytics and antidepressants, are effective in suppressing panic attacks and creating a sense of well-being. Among these, the benzodiazepine alprazolam (2 to 6 mg/d) is favored by some psychiatrists, but lorazepam and clonazepam are almost as effective and are considered slightly less likely to cause dependence. They are all effective within hours. In mild cases, the benzodiazepines may be used intermittently rather than several times daily, but they tend to be less useful once a panic attack has become established. Panic attacks tend to recur when the medications are discontinued, even after prolonged (6 to 12 months) administration. Any reduction in the amount of these medications should be gradual.

Tricyclic antidepressants and drugs that raise serotonin concentrations in the nervous system (selective serotonin reuptake inhibitors [SSRIs]) are also effective in the prevention of panic attacks and agoraphobia, but their onset of action is delayed for weeks. They become useful for symptoms of anxiety that recur or persist for more than several months. The doses are similar to those used to treat depression, and small differences between them do not seem to be clinically important (see Chap. 52). Buspirone, a specific serotonin 5-HT_2 agonist, has been promoted as effective in the treatment of anxiety and as a surrogate for benzodiazepines, but to us its benefit has seemed to be slight. *It is important to point out that during the initial weeks of administration of antidepressants, the underlying anxiety symptoms may worsen and an anxiolytic is usually required* until the antidepressant becomes effective. Propranolol, 10 to 20 mg tid, or a long-acting form of adrenergic blocker, reduces many of the autonomic accompaniments of anxiety and is useful to many patients. Psychiatric consultation is, of course, invaluable. With regard to psychotherapy, behavioral therapy (progressive exposure of the patient to panic-provoking situations) is said to be beneficial, particularly if agoraphobia is a major symptom. Relaxation activities, including biofeedback and meditation, help many patients, although persistence is required in performing these exercises at least once daily and they are less helpful once a panic attack has begun. Cognitive-behavioral psychotherapy, which is discussed in relation to the treatment of depression in Chap. 52, also appears to be useful in the treatment of panic disorder, according to Andreasen and Black.

A cardiac consultation and some simple tests (electrocardiogram, chest films) are often needed to reinforce to the patient the benign nature of the cardiac and respiratory symptoms and to alleviate fear of heart disease. These and other concepts of the treatment of anxiety are discussed by Goodwin and Guze. Anxiety symptoms arising in relation to a particular threatening event in a nonneurotic individual carry the best prognosis, but the symptoms may be prolonged, a feature of posttraumatic stress disorder.

PHOBIC DISORDER

In this state, patients are overwhelmed by an intense and irrational fear of some animal, object, social situation, or disease. Although acknowledging that there are no grounds for a particular fear (hence it is not a delusion) and that such provocative stimuli are for the most part innocuous, the patient is nonetheless powerless to suppress it. This disorder was known to Hippocrates, who drew a distinction between normal and morbid fears. Westphal, in 1871, was the first to give morbid fears the status of a disease. Women are affected slightly more often than are men.

Unlike an anxiety attack, such a phobia always focuses on a specific object or situation. The patient is chronically fearful of a particular animal or situation and becomes extremely anxious or panic stricken and incapacitated when placed in a situation that evokes the phobia. These situations are avoided at all costs. As a result, it may be impossible for the patient to leave the house or neighborhood unaccompanied or at all, mingle in a crowd, walk across a bridge, or travel by air. This fear of being in places or situations from which escape might be difficult or extremely embarrassing is spoken of as *agoraphobia*. (Agoraphobia, however, is a secondary feature of other psychiatric disorders, the most frequent being anxiety with panic attacks as already mentioned.) The most common phobia—and one that is not disabling for the most part—is claustrophobia, the fear of being confined in a close space such as an elevator or a magnetic resonance scanner. Other phobias are those of open (agoraphobia), closed, or high places, dogs, cats, insects, dirt, sprays and other contaminants, air travel, AIDS, cancer, insanity, and death. Feelings of helplessness, pessimism, and despondency, the hallmarks of a depressive illness, result after years of phobic suffering. Often there are obsessive-compulsive tendencies as well, and some patients are hypochondriacal. Phobias are essentially *obsessive fears* and are somehow allied with this latter category of neurosis. The present authors have observed a number of patients whose phobic (or obsessive-compulsive) neurosis became greatly exaggerated as an endogenous depression developed. Recovery from the depression returned them to their earlier and milder phobic state.

OBSESSIVE-COMPULSIVE DISORDER

Like the pure phobic states, a state dominated by obsessions and compulsions is relatively rare, occurring in less than 5 percent of patients seeking help in a psychiatric outpatient clinic, but it can be extremely disabling. Minor compulsions (e.g., not stepping on cracks in the sidewalk), like minor phobias, are common in children, cause little or no distress, and tend to disappear in later life. A few, such as rechecking a locked door or a gas stove, may persist throughout life. Also, certain habits and rigid, obsessional ways of thinking, stubbornness, extreme punctuality, and excessive attention to detail may be persistent but excite little attention medically unless they interfere with a diagnostic procedure or the treatment of a medical disease.

Obsessive-compulsive disorder begins in adolescence or early adult years, although treatment may not be sought until middle age. The two sexes are equally affected. The onset is usually gradual and often cannot be accurately dated, but in some cases it is precipitated by a particular event in the patient's life, such as the death of a relative. The family history often discloses a high incidence of obsessional or phobic personality in other members. There is usually a prevailing undercurrent of insecurity and anxiety.

Obsessions are defined as imperative and distressing thoughts and impulses that persist in the patient's mind despite a desire to resist and to get rid of them. They take various forms; the most common are *intellectual obsessions*, in which phrases, rhymes, ideas, or vivid images (these are often absurd, blasphemous, obscene, and sometimes frightening) constantly intrude into consciousness; *impulsive obsessions*, in which the mind is dominated by an impulse to kill oneself, to stab one's children, or to perform some other objectionable act; and *inhibiting obsessions*, in which every act must be ruminated upon and analyzed before it is carried out—a state that is cleverly called *doubting mania*. Every effort at distraction fails to rid the patient of the obsessive thought. It engulfs the individual's mind, rendering the person dysphoric and, often, inefficient. Probably the most disturbing obsessions are the impulsive ones, in which patients constantly struggle with the fear that they will put some terrible thought into action. Even as they tell of the obsession, they reveal a severe underlying anxiety and seek reassurance that they will not yield to it. Fortunately, such patients rarely obey their pathologic impulses. Phobias, as mentioned earlier, are considered by some authorities to be essentially obsessive fears and are included in this category of neurosis.

Compulsions are acts that result from obsessions. These are single acts or a series of acts (rituals) that the patient must carry out in order to put his mind at ease. Examples are repeated checking of the gas jets or the locks on doors, adjusting articles of clothing, repeated hand washing, using a clean handkerchief to wipe objects that have been touched by others, tasting foods in specific ways, and touching or arranging objects in a particular sequence. The most common of these obsessions and compulsions center around contamination concerns that lead to repeated hand washing or bathing. Other obsessions and compulsions can be identified as clusters of thoughts that derive from the above-mentioned concern about harm to oneself or to others and consequent checking on others. Less common clusters involve excessive focus on symmetry, precision, and ordering, and on saving and hoarding.

Certain motor disturbances—namely, habit spasms or tics—are, in a sense, *motor compulsions*. They consist of repetitious movements of the shoulders, arms, hands, and certain of the facial muscles (see Chap. 6). One feature that separates quasivoluntary tics from involuntary movements of extrapyramidal type is the patient's feeling that the tics must be carried out to relieve an inner tension. Unlike compulsions, however, tics are not usually based directly on obsessive thoughts—except perhaps the Gilles de la Tourette syndrome, in which multiple tics are combined with compulsive utterances, often offensive ones (see later).

In all these obsessions and compulsions and in the phobias, patients recognize the irrationality of their ideas and behaviors, yet are powerless to control them. It is this insight into the obsessional experience and the struggle against it that distinguish obsessions from delusions.

After the condition has persisted for a time, they may become depressed and suffer from typical anxiety attacks.

Mechanisms of Obsessive Disorder

For many years, a number of psychoanalytic dynamic conceptualizations held sway of obsessional states as the product of intrapsychic conflicts. Only relatively recently has a more reasonable neurobiologic model been advanced. These are largely derived from the findings of functional imaging, which have been quite consistent in demonstrating increased metabolic activity in the orbitofrontal cortex, cingulate, and, to a lesser extent, striatum. The orbitofrontal cortex and amygdala were reported to be shrunken in other cases. In a study of 13 patients who developed elements of obsessiveness and compulsive disorder after incurring focal brain lesions, Berthier and colleagues found lesions in diverse loci, including the cingulate, frontal, and temporal cortices, as well as the basal ganglia. Two of the most accurately localized lesions in their series were a hamartoma of the right parahippocampal gyrus and an infarction in the posterior putamen. The presence of brain injuries and seizure disorders in other of their patients made precise localization less certain.

Additional insight into obsessive-compulsive disorder may be obtained from the many cases in which acquired striatal damage may be linked to obsessional behavior. One such entity is a poststreptococcal tic disorder termed *PANDAS* (pediatric autoimmune neuropsychiatric disorders associated with streptococcal infections), discussed in Chap. 6. This disorder is presumably related to another extrapyramidal condition, Sydenham chorea, in which tics and similar movement disorders, as well as obsessive behavioral abnormalities, have long been known to coexist. Functional imaging studies in patients with PANDAS have yielded variable findings, but generally there has been increased activity in the caudate nucleus and orbitofrontal cortex in association with the patient's compulsive thoughts.

The *Gilles de la Tourette syndrome* of multiple tics, including vocal ones, beginning in childhood or adolescence and lasting more than a year, has a strong component of obsessive-compulsive disorder in more than half of patients. Both disorders occur in a pattern of inheritance that is close to an autosomal dominant trait with incomplete penetrance (Kurlan). Because dopamine antagonists are beneficial in the management of the Tourette syndrome, a number of etiologic hypotheses revolve around serotonergic and dopaminergic neurotransmitter systems (Baxter). The neurochemical alterations in obsessive-compulsive disorder have been based in part on the responses to medications, notably to the serotonin reuptake inhibitors, as noted further on. These agents are found to be of therapeutic benefit, as are stereotactic neurosurgical lesions in the cingulate gyri (see further on). More extensive comments on the Gilles de la Tourette syndrome are found in Chap. 6.

Treatment

This is best left to the experienced psychiatrist. At the least there should be a trial of therapy using behavioral modification techniques. In the case of phobic neurosis, the aim is to reduce the patient's fear to the extent that exposure to the phobic situation can be tolerated. A popular form of therapy is *systematic desensitization*, which consists of increasing and graded exposure of the patient to the object or situation that arouses the fear. Psychotherapy, if undertaken, need not be intensive, consisting instead of repeated explanation, reassurance, and guidance in dealing with symptoms. As with phobic neurosis, several reports have indicated that compulsive rituals can often be abolished by the techniques of behavior therapy. Much in vogue is cognitive-behavioral psychotherapy discussed in Chap. 52.

Certain medications, particularly the SSRI types such as fluoxetine, are considered to be effective in reducing obsessions and compulsions in more than half of patients. The less selective agent, clomipramine, is also highly effective, as were the commonly used tricyclic antidepressants in the past, but clomipramine is not nearly as well tolerated as are the conventional SSRI drugs (see review by Stein).

In the past, cingulotomy produced symptomatic improvement in both phobic and obsessional neuroses and was considered a reasonable procedure. This measure is largely outdated as the implantation of electrical stimulating electrodes (direct brain stimulation) in this region or in the subthalamic nucleus has proved effective for intractable and disabling obsessive compulsive disorder but without affecting the degree of anxiety and at the expense of a moderate number of surgical complications (Mallet et al).

HYSTERIA (BRIQUET DISEASE; SOMATIZATION DISORDER; PSYCHOGENIC NEUROLOGIC DISEASE)

This subject is of great importance to neurologists and general physicians because of its frequency. Although hysteria has been known since ancient times, many writers credit the first description of the syndrome to the French physician Briquet in 1859. Charcot later elaborated certain manifestations of the disease, particularly those with a theatrical aspect, and thereby interested Freud and Janet in the problem. Charcot demonstrated that the symptoms could be produced and relieved by hypnosis (mesmerism). Janet postulated a *dissociative state* of mind to account for certain features, such as trances and *fugue* states, a term that has reappeared in modern psychiatry. Freud and his acolytes conceived of hysterical symptoms as a product of "ego defense mechanisms" in which psychic energy, generated by unconscious sexual conflicts, was "converted" into physical symptoms. This latter concept was widely accepted, to the point where the term *conversion* became incorporated into the nomenclature of the neuroses and the terms *conversion symptoms* and *conversion reaction* came to be equated with the disease hysteria. In the present authors' opinion, the term *conversion*, if it is used at all, should refer only to certain unexplained symptoms, such as amnesia, paralysis, blindness, and aphonia that mimic neurologic disease. We see no merit in the dichotomy, based on unsubstantiated psychodynamic theory, of a conversion type as separate from a dissociative type of hysteria, as claimed by the DSM classification. Nemiah, who is in other respects partial to the psychoanalytic interpretation, agrees. The term *hysteria* is probably best reserved for a *disease* that is largely confined to women and is characterized by a distinctive age of onset, natural history, and certain somatic symptoms and signs, which typically include conversion symptoms, dissociative reactions, or states of "multiple personality." We use the term "psychogenic" in this chapter and throughout the book as an etiologic term broadly attached to dramatic neurologic signs and symptoms that are not explicable on the basis of a lesion of the nervous system.

In clinical neurology one encounters two types of psychogenic neurologic signs, both identified as having no possibility of explanation in disease of the nervous system: (1) a chronic illness marked by multiple and often dramatically presented symptoms and somatic abnormalities of "classic hysteria," almost limited to girls and women and (2) an illness predominantly of men but also of women who develop physical symptoms or remain inexplicably disabled for the purpose of obtaining compensation, influencing litigation, avoiding military duty or imprisonment, or for the manipulation of some other interpersonal or societal situation. This latter state is called *compensation neurosis*, *compensation hysteria*, or *hysteria with sociopathy*, in other words, *malingering*.

Classic Hysteria (Briquet disease)

This accounts for 1 to 2 percent of admissions to a neurologic service and a greater number of outpatient visits. It usually has its onset in the teens or early twenties, almost exclusively in young women; a very few cases begin before puberty. Once established, the symptoms recur intermittently, although with reduced frequency, throughout the adult years even to an advanced age. No doubt there are cases of lesser severity in which symptoms occur only a few times or perhaps only once, just as there are mild forms of other diseases. The patient may be seen for the first time during middle life or later, and the earlier history may not at first be forthcoming. Careful probing almost invariably reveals that the earliest manifestations of the illness had appeared before the age of about 25 years.

Other important data are also revealed by eliciting a careful past history. During late childhood and adolescence, the normal activities of the patient, including education, had often been interrupted by periods of ill-defined illness. In the past, rheumatic fever, and in the current era, chronic fatigue, Lyme disease, sick building syndrome, or multiple environmental allergy may be carried as explanatory diagnoses from other physicians or the patient's research on the Internet. Later in life, problems in work adjustment and marriage are frequent. Notable in many cases is a high incidence of marital incompatibility, separation, and divorce. The patient's life history is punctuated by symptoms that do not conform to recognizable patterns of medical and surgical disease. For these ailments, many forms of therapy including surgical operations may have been performed.

In the past, rarely had adult life been reached without at least one abdominal operation for vague abdominal pain, persistent nausea and vomiting, or an obscure gynecologic complaint. Often the indications for the surgical procedures were unclear; moreover, the same symptoms or others often recurred to complicate the convalescence. The biographies of these patients are replete with disorders that center about menstrual, sexual, and procreative functions. Menstrual periods may be painfully prostrating, irregular, or excessive. Sexual intercourse may be painful or unpleasant. Pregnancies may be exceedingly difficult; the common vomiting of the first trimester may persist all through the gestational period, with weight loss and prostration; labor may be unusually difficult and prolonged, and all manner of unpredictable complications are said to have occurred during and after parturition.

Hysteria is a polysymptomatic disorder, involving almost every organ system. In a study of 50 unmistakable cases of hysteria (as compared with a control group of 50 healthy women), the most frequent symptoms reported by Purtell and colleagues included headache, blurred vision, lump in the throat, loss of voice, dyspnea, palpitation, anxiety attacks, anorexia, nausea and vomiting, abdominal pain, unusual food allergies, severe menstrual pain, urinary retention, painful intercourse, paresthesias, dizzy spells, nervousness, and easy crying.

The mental examination of the patient with hysteria demonstrates a lack of precision in relating the details of the illness. Questions regarding the chief complaint usually elicit a narration of a series of incidents or problems, many of which prove to have little or no relevance to the question. Memory defects (amnesic gaps) are apparent while the history is being taken; the patient appears to have forgotten important segments of the history, some of which he had clearly described in the past and are part of the medical record. The description of symptoms is dramatic and not in accord with the facts as elicited from other members of the family. Often, a rather casual demeanor is manifest, the patient insisting that everything in her life is quite normal and controlled, when, in fact, her medical record is checkered with instances of dramatic and unexplained illness. This calm attitude toward a turbulent illness and seemingly disabling physical signs is so common that it has been singled out as an important characteristic of hysteria, *la belle indifference*. Other patients, however, are obviously tense and anxious and report frank anxiety attacks. Emotional reactions are superficial and scenes that are disturbing to others are quickly forgotten. Claims of early life sexual abuse are common and often prove to be true, or sometimes are not valid; when present, they may play a role in the genesis of some cases (see further on).

There are no pathognomonic findings. Although many in the past have commented on the rather youthful, girlish appearance and coquettish ("seductive") manner of the patients, these by no means characterize most patients in the current era. The abdomen may be diffusely and exceedingly tender but without other signs of abdominal disease. The so-called stigmata of hysteria—i.e., corneal anesthesia; absence of gag reflex; spots of pain and tenderness over the scalp, sternum, breasts, lower ribs, and ovaries—are often suggested by the examiner and are too inconsistent to be of much help in diagnosis. The variation and pleomorphism of the physical signs are limited only by the patient's ability to produce them by voluntary effort. Accordingly, symptoms and signs that are beyond volitional control should not be accepted as manifestations of hysteria. Sometimes the patient's physical signs are an imitation of those of another member of the family ("folie à deux") or are evoked by a stressful event in the patient's personal life. However, this may not be disclosed at the time of the first examination.

Neurologic Syndromes of Psychogenic Origin

A few hysterical syndromes occur with regularity that every physician may expect to encounter them. Most are neurologic in nature. They constitute some of the most puzzling diagnostic problems in medicine.

Hysterical Pain

This may involve any part of the body; generalized or localized headache, "atypical facial pain," vague abdominal pain, and chronic back pain with camptocormia are the most frequent and troublesome. In many of these patients the response to analgesic drugs has been unusual or excessive, and some of them are addicted. The hysterical patient may respond readily to a placebo as though it were a potent drug, but it should be pointed out that this is a notoriously unreliable means of distinguishing hysterical pain from that of other diseases. A greater error is to mistake the pain of osteomyelitis or visceral tumor—before other symptoms have developed—for a manifestation of hysteria. There are several helpful diagnostic features of hysterical pain: (1) the patient's inability to give a clear, concise description of the type of pain; (2) the location of the pain does not conform to the pattern of pain in the familiar medical syndromes; (3) the dramatic elaborations of its intensity (speaking in inflated metaphors—"like a giant knife stabbing") and its effects on the body ("tearing my limb off"); (4) its persistence, either continuous or intermittent, for long periods of time; (5) the assumption of bizarre postures; and, most important, (6) the coexistence of other clinical features or previous attacks of hysterical nature.

Hysterical Vomiting

This is often combined with pain and tenderness in the lower abdomen and results in unnecessary appendectomies and removal of pelvic organs in adolescent girls and young women. The vomiting often occurs after a meal, leaving the patient hungry and ready to eat again; it may be induced by unpleasant circumstances. Some of these patients can vomit at will, regurgitating food from the stomach like a ruminant animal. Vomiting may persist for weeks with no cause being found. Weight loss may occur, but seldom to the degree anticipated. As remarked earlier, the usual first-trimester vomiting of pregnancy may continue throughout the entire 9 months, and occasionally pregnancy will be interrupted because of it. Anorexia may be a prominent associated symptom and must be differentiated from anorexia nervosa–bulimia, another closely related disease of young women.

Psychogenic Seizures (PNES), Trances, and Fugues (See also Chap. 16)

These conditions seem to be no less frequent than in the days of Charcot, when *la grande attaque d'hysterie* was often exhibited before medical audiences, but it is quite familiar to all neurologists and one of the main concerns of epileptologists. To witness an attack is of great assistance in diagnosis but electroencephalogram (EEG) monitoring is often required for certainty. The lack of an aura, initiating cry, hurtful fall, or incontinence; the presence of peculiar movements such as grimacing, squirming, thrashing and flailing of the limbs, side-to-side motions of the head, and striking at or resisting those who offer assistance; the retention of consciousness during a motor seizure that involves both sides of the body; a long duration of the seizure, its abrupt termination by strong sensory stimulation, lack of postictal confusion, and failure to produce a rise in creatine kinase—are all typical of the psychogenic attack. Sometimes hyperventilation will initiate an attack and is therefore a useful diagnostic maneuver. Both epilepsy, particularly of frontal-lobe type, and hysteria may occur in the same patient, a combination that invariably causes difficulty in diagnosis as discussed in Chap. 16.

Hysterical trances or fugues, in which the patient wanders about for hours or days and carries out complex acts may simulate temporal lobe epilepsy or any of the conditions that lead to confusional psychosis. The most reliable point of differentiation comes from observation of the patient, who, if hysterical, is likely to indicate a degree of alertness and promptness of response not seen in temporal lobe seizures or confusional states. Following the episode, an interview with the patient—under the influence of hypnosis, strong suggestion, or midazolam (formerly used was amobarbital [Amytal])—will often reveal memories of what happened during the episode. This helps to exclude the possibility of an epileptic spell.

Hysterical Paralyses, Gait, Sensory Loss, and Tremors (See also Chaps. 3, 6, 7, and 9)

Hysterical palsies may involve an arm, a leg, one side of the body, or both legs. If the affected limb can be moved at all, muscle action is weak and tremulous. Movements are slow, tentative, and poorly sustained; often it can be demonstrated that the strength of voluntary movement is proportional to the resistance offered by the examiner, thus imparting a "give-way" character, as noted in the discussion of these signs in Chap. 3. One can detect by palpation that agonist and antagonist muscles are contracting simultaneously, thereby holding the limb in place rather than opposing the examiner, and when the resistance is suddenly withdrawn, there is no follow-through or rebound, as is normally the case. Many other signs have been devised to demonstrate inconsistencies with normal physiologic principles and a purposive lack of cooperation. These are elaborated upon in the articles by Stone and associates (2002b and 2013). The discrepancies are usually found by testing an agonist, antagonist, or fixator movement while the patient is focused on making an effort with another group of muscles (e.g., the Hoover sign; see Chap 3). Muscular tone in the affected limbs is usually normal but slight resistance may sometimes be found. A seeming lack of effort and the absence of full compliance with the examiner's requests during the testing of muscle strength, while common in hysterical patients, are not confined to them; one encounters such findings not infrequently during the examination of suggestible but nonhysterical patients who harbor a neurologic disease and in those with a painful condition in an adjacent joint.

Walking and standing may be impossible (astasia-abasia) or the gait may be bizarre with collapsing legs that bring the patient to a squat, or a "skating" gait in which one foot is pushed ahead of the body. Other forms—some quite absurd, as noted in Chap. 7—are easily recognized as inconsistent with the makings of the nervous system in disease. Weakness and poor balance are combined elements in both the quadriparetic and hemiparetic forms. In Keane's informative series of 60 cases of hysterical gait, the hemiparetic and monocrural forms were twice as frequent as the quadriparetic. The gait disorder is sometimes difficult to describe because of its variability. Sudden falls without voluntary protective movements and inconsistencies of balance are helpful features. Difficulty in walking and moving the legs while seated is, of course, not unique to hysteria; it also occurs in so-called frontal lobe gait apraxia and in ataxia from midline cerebellar lesions and in hydrocephalus.

In a most remarkable and recalcitrant form of psychogenic movement disorder, maintenance of the limbs in a rigid or dystonic posture for a long time may result in a bed-bound, crippled state with severe flexion pseudocontractures of the limbs. We have seen 1 such case of 18 years' duration. The tendon reflexes are usually normal if they can be tested, but with hysterical rigidity and muscular contractures, the abdominal and plantar reflexes may be suppressed.

Anesthesia or hypesthesia is almost always inadvertently suggested by the physician's examination.

Seldom is sensory loss a spontaneous complaint, although "numbness" and paresthesias are not uncommon in hysterics. The sensory loss may involve one or more limbs below a sharp line (stocking and glove distribution), or may involve precisely one half of the body, or vibratory sense may be lost over precisely one-half of the skull (a test favored to demonstrate hysterical hemianesthesia). Touch, pain, taste, smell, vision, and hearing may all be affected on that side, which is an anatomic impossibility from a single lesion. Other aspects of psychogenic sensory disturbance are discussed in Chap. 9. The closest syndrome is that produced by a thalamic infarction but this, too, is easily distinguishable from psychogenic hemianesthesia.

The sometimes-stated notion that hysterical paralysis and sensory deficits are more common on the left side is untrue, according to Stone and colleagues (2002a).

The features of hysterical tremor and other movement disorders are described in Chap. 6. Emphasized here are the cessation of tremor with distracting tasks—e.g., complex finger movement patterns on the side opposite the tremor (such as touching the fourth, second, and fifth fingers in sequence rapidly), or refixation of the eyes on a target, or walking on the outside of the heels. The ability of the examiner to "chase" the tremor to proximal or distal parts of the limb by holding and immobilizing one part is highly characteristic. A fairly dependable sign is worsening of a tremor with loading that is accomplished by placing a heavy object in the patient's hand (most basal ganglionic and cerebellar tremors are muted by this maneuver).

Some general characteristics of psychogenic movement disorders that ring true to our experiences with patients are summarized in a review by Hinson and Haren; they include a typically acute onset and rapid progression of the movements, distractibility, variability and the simultaneous occurrence of various abnormal movements and of unexplainable paralysis, sensory loss, or pain. Needless to say the movements are not explainable by conventional characteristics of organic brain diseases, but as with all forms of hysteria, it is not on this feature alone that the diagnosis can rest. They point out, paradoxically, that an associated depressive or anxiety disorder is a good prognostic aspect.

Hysterical Blindness (See also Chap. 13)

This dramatic event may affect one or both eyes and may be coupled with hemiparesis or appear in isolation. The symptoms usually develop suddenly, often after an altercation or other emotionally charged event. The patient stares straight ahead blandly when undisturbed, but may squint or move the head as if straining to see when asked to view an object. Some such individuals can reduce reflexive blinking in response to a visual threat. The psychic nature of the problem may be recognized by a nurse who observes the patient reaching for a cup or for the phone. The preservation of vision is confirmed by the presence of normal pupillary reflexes and of optokinetic nystagmus, although one occasionally encounters a patient who has learned to suppress the latter response as well. A mirror passed slowly in the patient's central vision often engages eye movements. Other similar maneuvers are favored by different examiners. The presence of visual evoked responses also confirms the intactness of retino-occipital connections. The patient expresses little concern about the condition, which is usually short-lived. Cortical blindness and variants of the Balint syndrome are the main diagnostic considerations (see Chap. 22).

Convergence spasm, occurring as an isolated phenomenon, is practically always of hysterical nature.

A related phenomenon involves the *self-administration of mydriatic eyedrops* by healthcare personnel. The patient arrives on the emergency ward complaining of reduced vision (expected) or with headache and claiming to have an intracranial mass. This behavior is perhaps more sociopathic (or malingering) than hysterical.

Hysterical Amnesia

Patients brought to a hospital in a state of amnesia, not knowing their own identity, are usually hysterical females or sociopathic males involved in a crime. Usually, after a few hours or days, with encouragement, they divulge their life history. Epileptic patients or victims of a concussion, transient global amnesia, or acute confusional psychosis do not come to a hospital asking for help in establishing their identity. Moreover, the complete loss of memory for all previous life experiences by patients who are otherwise able to comport themselves normally is not observed in any other condition.

In the *Ganser syndrome* (amnesia, disturbance of consciousness, and hallucinations) patients pretend to have lost their memory or to have become insane. They may act in an absurd manner, simulating the way they believe that an insane or demented person would act, and give senseless or only approximate answers to every question asked of them (calling the color red *blue* or answering 5 for 2 + 2).

Malingering (See also further on under Sociopathy)

As stated earlier, symptoms of the same nature as those in hysteria occur in men, most often in those trying to avoid legal difficulties or military service or attempting to obtain disability or compensation following injury. Sociopaths often present with this type of illness. Unless such a motivating factor can be identified, the diagnosis of hysteria in the male should be made with caution. In compensation neurosis, as in the classic form of hysteria, multiple symptoms are reported; many of the symptoms are the same as those listed under female hysteria. Or the patient may be monosymptomatic (e.g., "seizures") and the symptoms, particularly chronic pain, may be confined to the neck, head, arm, or low back. The description of symptoms tends to be lengthy and circumstantial, and the patient fails to give details that are necessary for diagnosis. A tangible gain from the illness may be discovered by simple questioning. This is usually in the form of monetary compensation, which, surprisingly, is sometimes less than that which the patient could earn if he returned to work. Most such patients are actively engaged in litigation when first seen. Another interesting feature is the frequency with which the patient expresses extreme dissatisfaction with the medical care given him; he is often hostile toward the physicians and nurses. Many of these patients have already been subjected to an excessive number of hospitalizations and rather dramatic mishaps have allegedly occurred in carrying out diagnostic and therapeutic procedures. The majority of these patients were previously suspected of malingering.

Women who suffer injury at work or are involved in auto accidents may exhibit the same symptoms and signs of compensation neurosis as men, but in our experience, do so infrequently or at least less overtly.

Etiology and Pathogenesis

Psychoanalytic theory, which held that both conversion and dissociative symptoms are based on particular psychodynamic mechanisms, is impossible to affirm or refute. Although subject to some question of fabricated recall, we have been impressed at the high rate of childhood sexual abuse reported by women with severe monosymptomatic cases of hysteria or fugue states. This conforms to some extent with psychoanalytic views. An acknowledged history of childhood abuse related by the patient alerts the physician to the possibility of hysteria. Sociologic and educational factors may be important, for it has been observed that hysterical women as a group tend to be less intelligent and less educated than nonhysterical women but there are many exceptions. A genetic causation must also be considered since family studies have disclosed that approximately 20 percent of first-degree relatives of female hysterics have the same illness, an incidence 10 times that in the general population. This supports, in some views, the idea that hysteria is a disease and not merely a surfacing of a basic personality disorder (see Goodwin and Guze).

Whether conversion symptoms are consciously produced by the patient or arise unconsciously, without the patient's awareness, is a question that has been debated endlessly without resolution. Babinski attributed the symptoms to *hypersuggestibility*. In fact, he defined hysteria as an illness whose symptoms could be induced (and removed) by suggestion. There is strong evidence to support this idea, as most patients can be readily hypnotized and their symptoms temporarily eliminated by this procedure or by an interview and examination under the influence of midazolam. The present authors place great credence on this notion of hypersuggestibility, in keeping with older studies that emphasized these patients' unusual susceptibility to hypnosis and suggestion. Fascinating in this regard were the observations of Charcot's students that on their wards, the patients' symptoms disappeared in his absence.

Some insights can be obtained from studies of functional imaging in hysterical paralysis (see also Chap. 3). In general, the contralateral prefrontal cortex is suppressed when the patient with hysteria attempts to move a limb, suggesting to Spence and colleagues a "choice" of an active attempt not to move the limb. The pattern of activation was quite different from volunteers who purposefully feigned paralysis and who did not demonstrate such reduced prefrontal activity. When the hysteric with unilateral sensory loss is stimulated on the affected limb, there is no activation of the contralateral sensory cortex but bilateral stimulation results in activation of the appropriate regions in both hemispheres (Ghaffar et al). Some of the recent findings using functional imaging in hysterical states are reviewed by Carson and colleagues.

As pointed out by Carothers and by Guze and colleagues, hysteria and sociopathy may be closely related. Hysteria is a disease of women and sociopathy mainly of men. As restated by Cloninger and colleagues (1975), they may constitute expressions of a single underlying variable. This relationship is also supported by family studies. First-degree male relatives of hysterical women have an increased incidence of sociopathy and alcoholism; among first-degree female relatives of convicted male felons, there is an increased prevalence of hysteria. Moreover, careful histories of sociopathic girls reveal that many of them develop the full syndrome of hysteria. Women felons often present a mixed picture of hysteria and sociopathy, according to Cloninger and Guze.

Diagnosis

The characteristic age of onset; the longitudinal history of recurrent multiple complaints as outlined earlier; the attitude of the patient and the manner of presenting her symptoms; the incongruity of affect and clinical state; the discrepancy between the neurologic deficit and the signs on examination; the impossibility of explaining the patient's signs on an anatomic or physiologic basis; and the absence of symptoms and signs of other medical and surgical disease will permit an accurate diagnosis in the majority of cases. Certain tests designed to reveal normal functioning of a limb, of vision, and of gait already have been mentioned.

There is a significant overlap of hysteria and other medical and neurologic diseases. On record are numerous studies in which patients with an initial diagnosis of hysteria by general physicians were followed for many years. Up to one-third of them (far less in most series) turned out eventually to have an "organic condition" that, in retrospect, explained the initial symptoms (Couprie et al). This emphasizes that the original clinical diagnosis of hysteria is sometimes erroneous, although numerous other surveys emphasize the opposite, as noted below. When the diagnostic criteria in these cases are closely analyzed, it becomes apparent that the diagnosis was made solely by the "discrepancy method"—i.e., the patient's symptoms or signs were not deemed to be credible manifestations of disease, based mainly on the clinical experience of the examiner. Of course, this assumes that the examiner has a wide experience; unfortunately for the novice, many syndromes are unknown or incomprehensible.

However, when diagnosis is based on the totality of the clinical picture and not on the "discrepancy method," it can be quite accurate. The physician can be further reassured that in followup studies of patients with so-called conversion disorder (exclusive of pseudoseizures), virtually none develops a neurologic lesion that in retrospect was related to the initial episode as, for example, in the study by Stone and colleagues (2003). It is of interest that in the series cited, most patients had persistent functional disability from their conversion symptoms, even a decade later.

So-called projective tests (the Rorschach and Thematic Apperception Tests), which for a time were popular with dynamic psychiatrists, are not helpful in diagnosis and are now used very little. The presence of extreme suggestibility and the tendency to dramatize symptoms as measured by one part of the Minnesota Multiphasic Personality Inventory and other psychometric tests is helpful in diagnosis but not pathognomonic; these traits appear under certain conditions in individuals who never develop hysteria.

Finally, it should be emphasized that single bouts of isolated hysterical paresis, blindness, and anesthesia are quite common in neurologic practice and do not presage a chronic hysterical illness. The same is true for transient neurologic signs exhibited during the course of the examination, mainly pertaining to unusual or drifting sensory loss or asthenic weakness of a limb.

Treatment of Hysteria and Hysterical Symptoms

Here, opinions differ. Treatment may be considered from two aspects: the amelioration of the long-standing basic personality defect and relieving the recently acquired physical symptoms. Little or nothing can be done about the former. Psychotherapists have attempted to modify it by long-term reeducation, but their results are uninterpretable and there are no control studies for the few reports of therapeutic success. Many psychiatrists are inclined to regard the female with hysteria who has a lifelong history of ill health as having a severe personality disorder—i.e., sociopathy. In other less severe cases and especially in those in whom hysterical symptoms have appeared under the pressure of a major crisis, explanatory and supportive psychotherapy appears to be helpful, and the patients have been able thereafter to resume their places in society.

The acute symptoms can usually be mitigated by persuasion and demonstration. One tactic is to treat the patient as though she has had an illness and is now in the process of recovering. The earlier this is done after the development of symptoms, the more likely they are to be relieved. Sometimes a single symptom such as hemiparesis or tremor can be halted by a particular maneuver and this demonstration suffices to begin recovery. In chronically bedridden patients, strong pressure to get out of bed and resume function must be applied. Stone and Edwards, who have thought considerably about this subject, have suggested showing the patient objective evidence of the functional nature of weakness, such as Hoover sign, by way of demonstrating the correctness of the diagnosis and demonstrating its potential reversibility.

Several approaches to discussing the symptomatology with the patient have been suggested. At one extreme is a confrontative approach in which the patient is told the symptoms are psychologic, or "in your head." We have found this to be counterproductive and almost always provokes an angry response that does not aid clinical improvement. At the other extreme is complete avoidance on the part of the physician, an approach that is almost as unproductive. We prefer to ask the patient if the symptoms can in some way be the result of "stress" or an upsetting recent experience. On occasion, in private, we will inquire about childhood sexual abuse and often get an affirmative response from the patient, with later confirmation by a spouse or sibling. Very powerful is nonjudgmental but firm reassurance that there is no serious disease. We have found it useful to list the diseases that have been excluded by examination and testing: brain tumor, stroke, amyotrophic lateral sclerosis, multiple sclerosis, etc. This often evokes an acknowledgment by the patient that one of the diseases had been a preoccupying concern. We then indicate, without using psychologic terms, that the brain may at times adopt certain patterns of behavior that do not reflect structural damage, and, furthermore, that these patterns can be unlearned with physical therapy and time, as described below.

That the patient's response to these conversations varies widely is not surprising. One group seems not to mind and to be relieved by the expression of concern and reassurance that there is no dangerous disease at the root of the problem. They can be sent to a physical therapist and may do well in the short run. Another group is indignant and unlikely to consult the physician again; several in the past have refused to pay the doctor's bill. Some have objected to the explanation based on their own view, often derived from research on the Internet and with similarly afflicted persons, that Lyme disease, chronic viral infection, environmental toxins, allergies, etc., are to blame. A few of these cases have the flavor of a delusion. All that the physician can offer here is an openness to see and reexamine the patient in several months; "cure" has no meaning in these instances and there is a high likelihood that such individuals will see a long line of doctors.

Some of our better results have been obtained by indicating that the neurologic symptoms are a "pattern of brain circuits" or "constitutional" weakness that can be overcome by physical and other therapies. Once the current neurologic disorder has disappeared, it may be helpful to counsel the patient in ways to prevent its recurrence. Family members can be given the same explanation. A regimen of physical therapy should be instituted, using an experienced therapist and setting simple goals for success. Every subsequent illness in such patients should be evaluated objectively, so as not to overlook any medical or surgical disease, which may strike a hysterical patient just as it does any other person.

The success of this program over a long period is unknown. The eradication of recently acquired hysterical symptom is relatively easy. The real test is whether it enables the patient to adjust satisfactorily to family and society and to perform daily activities effectively, and whether it prevents addiction, unnecessary medical treatments, and operations. Estimates of the recurrence rate of hysterical symptoms vary widely from 12 to 80 percent. In the series reported by Gatfield and Guze and by Merskey, the recurrence of somatic symptoms of similar or of other types was as high as in sociopathies. We have seen a few patients with monosymptomatic hysteria (paraparesis, bizarre gait, crippling dystonia) that persisted for years on end regardless of treatment. The long-term poor prognosis for well-established symptoms in several series was alluded to earlier. The use of a wheelchair for more than several days has been a bad prognostic sign in these cases.

Hypochondriasis

This is the preoccupation with bodily functions or physical signs and sensations, leading to the fear or belief of having serious disease. Hallmarks of this condition are the failure of repeated examinations to disclose any physical basis for the patient's symptoms and the failure of reassurance to affect either the patient's symptoms or his conviction of being sick. It is estimated that 85 percent of hypochondriasis is secondary to other mental disorders, chiefly depression, but also schizophrenia and anxiety neuroses. In approximately 15 percent of cases, however, there appears to be no associated illness (*primary hypochondriasis*). Most patients in this latter category are habitués of medical outpatient clinics, who are passed from specialist to specialist, perplexing and angering doctors along the way, because their symptoms defy both satisfactory diagnosis and cure.

Related to hypochondriasis, but probably more delusional are young adults who present with a fixed somatic belief regarding a peculiar symptom such as that the tongue is swollen, the jaw is not properly aligned, or the penis is ulcerated, when in fact no such abnormalities are present. The troubling aspect to the family and physician of such an illness is the persistence of the symptom and disability that extends for years, all tests having been negative. Probably these patients should be treated like schizophrenics, which many of them probably are. What to do with patients who are less severely affected but who have an unshakable belief that they have Lyme disease or environmental "allergies" depends on the context, but the likelihood of dissuasion is almost as poor as for the worst hypochondriac patients.

The treatment of primary hypochondriasis is difficult unless the physician keeps in mind the personality of the patient and the therapeutic goals. A psychodynamic outlook would suggest that these patients need to retain their symptoms, so that the usual concept of "curing" is inapplicable. The presence of symptoms provides the context for a relationship with a physician and it is the continuation of this relationship, which is often the only dependable contact in the patient's life, that is the motivation for some hypochondriac patients. Such patients are best managed by general physicians who realize that these are patients who do not necessarily want or expect a cure, and who are content with small gains and the avoidance of unnecessary surgery.

SOCIOPATHY

Of all the abnormal personality types listed in Table 51-1, the antisocial is the best defined and the one most likely to cause trouble in the family and community. It had been

Table 55-1

PERSONALITY DISORDERS

TYPE	CHARACTERISTICS
Paranoid	Chronic wariness, suspiciousness, litigiousness, hypersensitivity, jealousy, envy; lack of insight or humor, tendency to blame others; sense of self-importance and entitlement
Cyclothymic	Recurring periods of depression (low energy, pessimism, hopelessness, despair) and elation (high energy, ambition, enthusiasm, optimism) not readily explained by circumstances
Schizoid	Isolation, seclusiveness, secretiveness, discomfort in relationships; often eccentric and lacking in energy; few friends; detachment; inability to express ideas and feelings, especially anger
Explosive	Outbursts of rage and aggression not in keeping with usual personality, often in response to minor provocation; sense of loss of control followed by regret
Obsessive-compulsive (anankastic)	Chronic worries about standards; excessive concern about self-image; tension in relationships, leading to isolation; inability to relax and excessive inhibitions; overly meticulous, conscientious, and perfectionist; predisposition to depression and obsessive-compulsive neurosis
Hysterical	Immaturity, histrionic behavior, excitability, emotional instability, sexualization of relationships, low frustration tolerance, and shallow interpersonal ties; dependency
Asthenic	Chronic weakness, easy fatigability, sense of vulnerability, oversensitive to physically and emotionally taxing situations, little ambition or aggression; low energy level; anhedonia
Passive-aggressive	Obstructive behavior, stubborness, intentional errors or omissions; intolerance of authority with struggles over control, often creating difficulties in medical settings; externalization of conflicts and blaming others for untoward events
Inadequate	Chronic inability to meet ordinary life demands in the absence of mental retardation; severe dependency on others; tendency to become institutionalized or to become dependent on institutions
Antisocial	Unsocialized or antisocial behavior in conflict with society; selfishness, callousness, impulsiveness, lack of loyalty, and little guilt; low frustration tolerance; tendency to blame others, long history of interpersonal and social difficulties and arrests
Passive-dependent	Lack of self-confidence, indecisiveness, tendency to cling to and seek support from others
Immature	Ineffectual responses to social, psychologic, and physical demands; lack of stamina; poor adaptation to ordinary situations; a "loser"
Borderline	Poorly regulated emotions, self-injury, dysphoria, unstable interpersonal relationships
Narcisstic	Grandiosity, fantasies of power, success, idealized love, and belief that he or she is special or unique and can only be understood by or associate with others of high status

defined (in DSM) as a state in which the individual *"is always in trouble, profiting not from experience or punishment, unable to empathize with family or friends or to maintain loyalties to any person, group, or code. He is likely to be shallow, callous, and hedonistic, showing marked emotional immaturity with lack of sense of responsibility, lack of judgment, and an ability to rationalize his behavior so that it appears warranted, reasonable and justified."*

Since Prichard, in 1835, first described this condition under the term *immoral insanity*, there have been many attempts to give it a more precise definition and to avoid using it as a psychiatric wastebasket. At the turn of the century, Koch introduced the term *psychopathic inferiority*, implying that it was a constitutionally determined deviation in personality. Later the term *psychopathic personality* came into common use. In the past, many authors used this last term indiscriminately to embrace all forms of deviant personality. Subsequently, the term came to be used in a more restricted sense to define a subgroup of antisocial or aggressive psychopaths (*antisocial personality disorder* in DSM-IV). Aubrey Lewis has given a lucid account of the history of the concept of sociopathy. By far the best modern study of sociopathy is that of L.N. Robins, based on a 30-year followup study of 524 cases from a child guidance clinic and 100 controls. Other investigations of note are those of Cleckley, of McCord and McCord, and of Guze and coworkers, who studied psychiatric illness in large numbers of felons and their first-degree relatives. More recently, the descriptor, "callous youth" has become part of the syndrome. The following material and the preceding quotation are taken largely from these writings and from those of Reid.

Clinical Description

This condition, unlike the majority of psychiatric disorders, is manifest by the age of 12 to 15 years and frequently earlier. The manifestations of sociopathic behavior in children and adults are 5 to 10 times more frequent in males than they are in females. It consists essentially of deviant behavior in which individuals seem driven to cause difficulty in everything they do or behave in a way that most societies identify as grossly criminal. Codes imposed by family, school, religion, and society are broken. Seemingly, the sociopath acts on impulse, but after committing the unsocial act, he shows no remorse. The most frequent antisocial activities are theft, truancy, running away, associating with undesirable characters, indiscriminate sexual relations, repeated fighting, recklessness and impulsivity, lying without cause, vandalism, abuse of drugs and alcohol, and, later, inability to work steadily or keep a job. Criminality is intimately associated. Fire setting and cruelty to animals are particularly associated with future sociopathy according to several authors (the "callous youth" alluded to above). In the study by Robins, of children or adolescents who exhibited 10 or more antisocial symptoms, 43 percent were categorized as sociopaths in adulthood. If only 8 or 9 of these traits were present, 29 percent were so grouped; if 6 or 7, 25 percent; and 3 to 5, 15 percent. Conversely, not a single adult sociopath was observed who did not manifest antisocial symptoms in earlier life. Interestingly, a number of other problems of childhood and adolescence—such as enuresis, dirty appearance, sleepwalking, irritability, nail biting, oversensitivity, poor eating habits, nervousness, being withdrawn or seclusive, unhappiness, tics, and fears—were not predictive of adult sociopathy. None of Robins' patients was mentally retarded.

At the same time, it should be noted that more than half the disturbed children in Robins' study (even those with 10 or more antisocial manifestations) had lost most of their sociopathic traits by adulthood. This does not mean that they remained psychiatrically normal. Of those who did not become adult sociopaths, the large majority developed other adult psychiatric illnesses, particularly addiction to alcohol. Only in the group of children with fewer than three antisocial symptoms did a reasonable number (one-third) remain entirely well from a psychiatric point of view in adult life. Because sociopathic behavior in children may terminate spontaneously or evolve into other disorders, it is advised that the diagnosis of antisocial personality disorder be reserved for adults; the same behavior pattern in children is designated as *conduct disorder*.

Also of interest are Robins' findings that sociopaths showed an unusually high incidence of "conversion" symptoms (we would substitute "malingering" as discussed further on), as well as depressive symptoms and anxiety, and that these symptoms are in proportion to the sociopathic ones. Among women with sociopathic behavior there was a high incidence of hysterical manifestations—evidence that female hysteria may be the counterpart of male sociopathy. In Robins' series, a search for evidence of encephalitis, often postulated in the past as the basis of sociopathy, was not revealing, nor was there any proof of other brain damage. In the current era, head trauma is often imputed as the cause of troublesome behavior in adolescents and young adults, but there is no basis for this view.

EEG abnormalities, taking the form of mild to moderate bilateral slowing, are more frequent in criminals and sociopaths than they are in the normal population in some series, but the validity of this finding is uncertain.

Other findings suggest a strong genetic predisposition to antisocial personality. In a Danish study of criminals by Christiansen, "inappropriate nonpsychotic impulse-ridden behavior" was found five times more frequently in first-degree biologic relatives than it was in the general population. Criminality was two times more frequent in monozygotic twins than it was in dizygotic twins. His study also confirmed an association between hysteria and sociopathy. More direct evidence of a genetic factor was provided by Cadoret's study of adoptees who were separated at birth from antisocial biologic parents. A higher incidence of antisocial behavior was present in the adoptees than were in controls. His study also suggested that excessive childhood hyperactivity and classic female hysteria were phenotypic manifestations of an antisocial personality genotype, but this is by no means confirmed.

There is no information as to the best methods of treatment and the role of the medical profession has never been clear.

Treatment Most psychiatrists have been discouraged by the results of psychotherapy, but whether behavioral therapy, psychoanalysis, or drugs have more to offer cannot be determined from available data. Medical efforts should be directed to evaluating the patient's neurologic status, assessing his intelligence, and explaining the nature of the disorder to parents and social agencies, tasks best performed by a psychiatrist.

Malingering

This problem arises frequently in connection with both hysteria and sociopathy, and the physician should know how to deal with it. The term *malingering* refers to the *conscious and deliberate feigning of illness or disability in order to attain a desired goal.* It does not appear as an isolated phenomenon, and its occurrence must be interpreted as a sign of a serious personality disturbance, often one that prevents effective work or military service, as a means of obtaining recompense for an alleged injury, although noteworthy exceptions to this statement can be found.

In the malingerer one may observe pain, hyperesthesia, anesthesia, limping gait, tremor, contracture, paralysis, amaurosis, deafness, stuttering, mutism, amnesia, pseudoconvulsions and fugues, jumping of limbs with touch, and unexplained skin lesions—in short, the same array of symptoms and signs, singly or in combination, as in the patients with hysteria. Certainly there is a similarity between hysteria and malingering, but the nature of the relationship is nebulous and there may be great difficulty in establishing a clinical differentiation. As Jones and Llewellyn have observed:

> *Nothing...resembles malingering more than hysteria; nothing, hysteria more than malingering. In both alike we are confronted with the same discrepancy between fact and statement, objective sign and subjective symptom—the outward aspect of health seemingly giving the lie to all the alleged functional disabilities. We may examine the hysterical person and the malingerer, using the same tests, and get precisely the same results in one case as the other.*

The following have been cited as the main points of difference between the two conditions: (1) the conscious or unconscious quality of the motivation, which seems more unconscious in the hysteria patient and more conscious in the malingerer; (2) the influence of persuasion, which is usually effective in hysteria and not in the malingerer; and (3) the attitude of the patient. The patient with hysteria appears more genuinely ill and invites examination; the malingerer seems less ill and evades examination. Most of the more obvious cases of malingering seen by the present authors have been in sociopaths, for which reason discussions of the two conditions have been juxtaposed here.

A particular form of sociopathy or malingering, which consists essentially of systematically and specifically deceiving the medical profession, has been described as *Munchausen's syndrome*—named (not altogether aptly) after a seventeenth-century German soldier, Baron von Munchausen, who invented incredible tales of adventure and daring. Ireland and colleagues, who analyzed 59 cases (45 men, 14 women), listed the following characteristic features, which will be recognized at once by all neurologists with extensive hospital experience: feigned severe illness of a dramatic and emergency nature; factitious evidence of disease, surreptitious interference with diagnostic procedures, or self-mutilation; a history of many hospitalizations (sometimes more than 100); extensive travel or visits to innumerable physicians; and, finally, regular departure from the hospital against medical advice. Unlike the usual forms of compensation hysteria, an ulterior motive is not readily discernible and the psychopathology of this syndrome is obscure. It has been regarded by various experts as a form of sociopathy, malingering, or compensation hysteria, but the distinctions between them are too ambiguous to be of clinical value. Probably the medical profession has placed too great a reliance on degree of conscious awareness of deception. In such unstable and immature individuals, the terms *conscious*, *unconscious*, and *deception* are too uncertain to be useful.

Intermittent Explosive Disorder

Designated by this title is an uncommon disorder, the characteristic feature of which is the occurrence of repetitive, unpredictable outbursts of violent, aggressive behavior disproportionate to the provoking situation. This condition needs to be set apart from the uncontrollable outbursts that sometimes are associated with dementia, mental retardation, schizophrenia, drug addiction, or alcoholism, or those that follow serious head injuries or other brain diseases. Neurologic opinions have been solicited on our services for patients afflicted with this condition, the question usually being one of seizures as a cause of the aberrant behavior. Some persons with intermittent explosive disorder have, from early childhood, reacted to frustration with a loss of self-control, striking out in blind rage at anyone who crossed them (*episodic dyscontrol syndrome*); as adults, they may inflict serious injury or kill. Lesser degrees are recognized as expressions of "hot temper." Sometimes such behavior appears to be a continuation of the temper tantrums of earlier childhood. What is surprising in some of our patients has been a discrepancy between this episodic behavior and a pleasant and concerned demeanor at other times. Such patients are aware of the inappropriate nature of their behavior and its impact on others; they express remorse and may seek medical assistance to mute the outbursts. Others, of course, have no such insight and their anger episodes are simply an extension of their sociopathy.

The causes of aggressive violence are poorly understood. There appears to be a heritable tendency (Cadoret et al, 1997); males predominate and a sex-linked form extending over several generations has been described. Polymorphisms of the androgen receptor have been implicated in several preliminary studies. In only a very small number of patients, a seizure disorder can be identified, particularly temporal lobe epilepsy, but the majority still appear to be constitutional in nature. A state of adrenergic hyperactivity has been suggested and supported to some extent by these patients' response to propranolol but this is not explanatory of the behavior (Elliott; Jenkins et al; also see Chap. 25's discussion of the limbic system). Most instances probably represent a variant of sociopathy. Intense outbursts of anger and physical violence are also features of the diagnostic category of *borderline personality disorder*, the other manifestations of which include "a pervasive pattern of instability of mood, interpersonal relationships, and self-image." Besides propranolol, lithium, carbamazepine, and phenytoin have been found to be helpful in controlling and preventing the explosive attacks. We have noted the recent increased use by psychiatrists of serotonergic antidepressants in these patients, but have no way to judge their effect.

ANOREXIA NERVOSA AND BULIMIA

Anorexia nervosa is a behavioral disorder of previously healthy girls and young women living in affluent societies, mainly from upper and middle social classes, who become emaciated as a result of voluntary starvation. It is rare in Asian and African American women, and very uncommon in males. Herzog and Becker remind us that it was Richard Morton who first described the condition in 1649, under the title of "nervous phthisis," a "nervous consumption" resulting from "sadness and anxious cares"—a title that embodied enigmatic roots in psychologic derangements. Bulimia (literally ox-hunger), to which it is closely related, was not identified as an eating disorder until the latter part of the nineteenth century.

As a rule, anorexia nervosa begins shortly after puberty—sometimes later, but seldom after 30 years of age. Some of the patients were overweight in childhood, especially in the prepubertal period. Dieting is much talked about and may have been encouraged, especially by mothers who want their daughters to be more attractive. In epochs such as the current one, where dieting and female thinness are considered normative and desirable, the illness seems to be more common and lesser but transient forms of the disorder are rampant in high school- and college-age young women. Sometimes there appears to be a precipitating event, such as leaving home, disruption of family life, or other stress. Whatever the provocation, it leads to an obsessive refusal to eat. What is more important, the abnormal eating habits persist even when the patient has become painfully thin, and when counseled to eat normally she will use every artifice to starve herself. Food is hidden instead of being eaten, vomiting may be provoked after a meal, or the bowel may be emptied by laxatives. The patient shows no concern about her obvious emaciation and remains active. If left alone, these patients waste away, and approximately 5 percent have succumbed to some intercurrent infection or other medical complication, placing it among the most lethal of psychiatric conditions.

One is struck with the degree of emaciation; it exceeds that of most of the known wasting diseases. Often 30 percent or more of the body weight will have been lost by the time the patient's family insists on medical consultation. Bradycardia and hypotension are indicators for hospitalization. A fine lanugo covers the face, body, and limbs. The skin is thin and dry, without its normal elasticity, and the nails are brittle. The dental enamel is eroded. Pubic hair and breast tissue (except for loss of fat) are normal, and, in this respect, anorexia nervosa is unlike hypopituitary cachexia (Simmonds disease). Surprisingly, however, there are no neurologic signs of nutritional deficiency. The patient is alert and cheerfully indifferent to her condition. Any suggestion that she is unattractively thin or seriously depleted is rejected.

Amenorrhea is practically always present and may precede the extreme weight loss. Luteinizing hormone (LH) concentrations are reduced to pubertal or prepubertal levels. Clomiphene citrate fails to stimulate a rise in LH, as it does normally. Administration of gonadotropic-releasing factor raises the LH and follicle-stimulating hormone (FSH) levels, suggesting a hypothalamic disorder. The basal metabolic rate is low; triiodothyronine (T_3) and thyroxine (T_4) are low, while levels of physiologically inactive 3,3,5-triiodothyronine (reverse T_3) are normal or increased. Plasma thyrotropin (thyroid-stimulating hormone [TSH]) and growth hormone levels are normal. Serum cortisol levels are usually normal; excretion of 17-hydroxysteroids is slightly reduced. In sum, there is evidence of hypothalamic–pituitary dysfunction, but this is probably secondary to starvation, as indicated by the study of Scheithauer and colleagues who found no definite changes in the pituitary gland in 12 fatal cases. These endocrine abnormalities, most of which are probably secondary effects of weight loss, are summarized in the review by Becker and colleagues. Brain imaging shows slight to moderate enlargement of the lateral and third ventricles, which return to normal size when the illness subsides.

The etiology of anorexia nervosa is unknown, although there is no lack of hypotheses. Holland and coworkers reported a high concordance in monozygotic twins as compared with dizygotic twins. Earlier signs of hysterical tendencies, obsessional personality traits, and depression are mentioned as being frequent in some series, but not in others. Certain polymorphisms in the serotonin transporter gene, of types different from those that have been tentatively attached to anxiety and to obsessive traits, have also been reported. These findings are difficult to interpret. A functional imaging study has shown activation of the left insula, amygdala, and cingulate when high-calorie drinks were imbibed by anorectic women (Ellison et al), but this conceivably may have reflected anxiety that the authors termed *calorie fear* rather than a specific biologic feature of the disease.

Reports concerning the percentage of first-degree relatives of anorectic patients with bipolar disease are also inconsistent. An increased prevalence of neurosis or alcoholism has been noted in other members of the family. However, psychiatrists seem to agree that the patient does not have symptoms that conform to any of the major neuroses or psychoses. Certainly loss of appetite, lack of self-esteem and interest in personal appearance, and self-destructive behavior—common features of anorexia nervosa—are also symptoms of depressive illness, yet most of the patients do not look or admit to being dejected. Moreover, endogenous depression affects both sexes. The pathologic fear of becoming fat and the obsession with weight might be interpreted as a phobic or obsessional neurosis.

That anorexia nervosa is practically confined to females must figure in any acceptable explanation of the syndrome. Among psychiatric disorders, only hysteria has this sex predilection. Probably important is that anorexia nervosa has its onset in relation to menarche, at a time when the female exhibits rather large fluctuations in appetite and weight. This has suggested to some an imbalance between the satiety center, believed to lie in the ventromedial hypothalamus, and the feeding center, in the lateral hypothalamus.

An association of *anorexia* with structural disease involving the appetite centers has not been established, although the cases of acquired anorexia reported by Lewin and colleagues and of White and Hain are informative. Martin and Reichlin, in citing these rare cases, attribute the anorexia and cachexia to lesions of the lateral hypothalamus. A disorder of infants described under the title of "diencephalic syndrome" causes progressive and ultimately fatal emaciation ("failure to thrive") despite normal food intake in an otherwise alert and cheerful infant. The causative lesion has usually proved to be a low-grade astrocytoma of the anterior hypothalamus or optic nerve region (Burr et al). Also interesting is a case in which profound and long-standing anorexia nervosa resolved after a left thalamic stroke (Dusoir et al). See Chap. 27 for further discussion and references.

Treatment Treatment at the moment consists of winning the patient's confidence, supportive psychotherapy, assignment of one individual to sit with the patient as each meal is eaten, and a gradual increase of a balanced diet (Anderson). Extreme cases require hospitalization. If the patient refuses to eat, tube feeding is the only alternative. As weight is gained over several weeks, the patient usually becomes more normal in her attitude toward eating and will continue to recover on this regimen at home. The menses do not return until considerable weight has been gained (approximately 10 percent above the weight at the time of the menarche). Our colleagues report better success with such a regimen when imipramine or fluoxetine is added. Others have found these drugs to be ineffective except in patients with prominent symptoms of depression.

Becker and colleagues emphasized the potentially devastating medical complications to which severely anorectic patients are prone and the need to evaluate and treat these problems at the same time that nutritional therapy is undertaken. In particular, an electrocardiogram is essential in order to exclude a prolonged QT interval—the presence of which contraindicates the use of tricyclic antidepressants and increases the risk of ventricular tachycardia.

On average, 50 percent of patients recover completely or almost completely (Steinhausen and Seidel). In the remainder, the outcome is quite unfavorable. They either relapse after an initial period of improvement or remain chronically anorectic. Many patients are said to lapse into a chronic dysfunctional state characterized by a persistent preoccupation with food, weight, and dieting. It is not generally appreciated that chronic anorexia nervosa significantly shortens life; after a mean followup period of 12 years, 11 percent of a group of 84 patients had died (Deter and Herzog), and 15 percent after 20 years (Ratnasuriya et al). Suicide is a major contributor to this high mortality rate (Sullivan). The addition of antidepression drugs to a behavioral regimen has been tried with generally disappointing results.

The few adolescent boys who we have seen with this syndrome recovered on antidepressant medication. Cases caused by tumors within the hypothalamus were mentioned earlier and in Chap. 27.

In general, the therapeutic benefit of these drugs is considerably greater in cases of bulimia than it is in anorexia nervosa. A review of the problem of bulimia nervosa, binge eating followed by purging, is given by Mehler. The medical complications of either component disorder may be seen but particularly hypokalemia and alkalosis.

References

Anderson AE: *Practical Comprehensive Treatment of Anorexia Nervosa and Bulimia*. Baltimore, Johns Hopkins University Press, 1985.

Andreasen NC, Black DW: *Introductory Textbook of Psychiatry*, 3rd ed. Washington, DC, American Psychiatric Press, 2001.

Arlington VA: American Psychiatric Association: *Diagnostic and Statistical Manual of Mental Disorders*, 5th ed (DSM-5). American Psychiatric Publishing, 2013.

Baxter LR: Neuroimaging in obsessive-compulsive disorder: Seeking the mediating neuroanatomy, in Jenike MA, Baer L, Minichiello WE (eds): *Obsessive-Compulsive Disorders: Theory and Management*, 2nd ed. Chicago, Mosby-Year Book, 1990, pp 167–188.

Becker AE, Grinspoon SK, Klibanski A, Herzog DB: Eating disorders. *N Engl J Med* 340:1092, 1999.

Berthier ML, Kulisevsky J, Gironell A, et al: Obsessive-compulsive disorder associated with brain lesions: Clinical phenomenology, cognitive function and anatomic correlates. *Neurology* 47:353, 1996.

Briquet P: *Traite Clinique et Therapeutique a l'Hysterie*. Paris, Ballière, 1859.

Burr IM, Slonim AE, Danish RK: Diencephalic syndrome revisited. *J Pediatr* 88:429, 1976.

Cadoret RJ: Psychopathology in adopted-away offspring of biologic parents with antisocial behavior. *Arch Gen Psychiatry* 35:176, 1978.

Cadoret RJ, Cain C, Crowe RR: Evidence for gene-environment interaction in the development of adolescent antisocial behavior. *Behav Genet* 13:301, 1983.

Cadoret RJ, Leve LD, Devor E: Genetics of aggressive and violent behavior. *Psychiatr Clin North Am* 20:301, 1997.

Cannon WB: *Bodily Changes in Pain, Hunger, Fear and Rage*, 2nd ed. New York, Appleton, 1920.

Carothers JC: Hysteria, psychopathy and the magic word. *Mankind Q* 16:93, 1975.

Carson AJ, Brown R, David AS, et al: Functional (conversion) neurological symptoms: Research since the millennium. *J Neurol Neurosurg Psychiat* 83:842, 2013.

Christiansen KO: Crime in a Danish twin population. *Acta Genet Med Gemellol (Roma)* 19:323, 1970.

Cleckley H: *The Mask of Sanity*. St. Louis, Mosby, 1955.

Cloninger CR, Adolfsson R, Svrakic NM: Mapping genes for human personality. *Nat Genet* 12:3, 1996.

Cloninger CR, Guze SB: Psychiatric illness and female criminality: The role of sociopathy and hysteria in the antisocial woman. *Am J Psychiatry* 127:303, 1970.

Cloninger CR, Reich T, Guze SB: The multifactorial model of disease transmission: III. Familial relationship between sociopathy and hysteria (Briquet's syndrome). *Br J Psychiatry* 127:23, 1975.

Cohen ME, White PD: Life situations, emotions, and neurocirculatory asthenia (anxiety neurosis, neurasthenia, effort syndrome). *Res Publ Assoc Res Nerv Ment Dis* 29:832, 1949.

Cohen ME, White PD, Johnson RE: Neurocirculatory asthenia, anxiety neurosis or the effort syndrome. *Arch Intern Med* 81:260, 1948.

Couprie W, Wijdicks EFM, Rooijmans HGM, Van Gijn J: Outcome in conversion disorder: A follow-up study. *J Neurol Neurosurg Psychiatry* 58:750, 1995.

Deter H-C, Herzog W: Anorexia nervosa in a long-term perspective: Results of the Heidelberg-Mannheim study. *Psychosom Med* 56:20, 1994.

Dusoir H, Owens C, Forbes RB, et al: Anorexia nervosa remission following left thalamic stroke. *J Neurol Neurosurg Psychiatry* 76:144, 2005.

Elliott FA: Propranolol for the control of belligerent behavior following acute brain damage. *Ann Neurol* 1:489, 1977.

Ellison Z, Foong J, Howard R, et al: Functional anatomy of calorie fear in anorexia nervosa. *Lancet* 352:1192, 1998.

Gatfield PD, Guze SB: Prognosis and differential diagnosis of conversion reactions: A follow-up study. *Dis Nerv Syst* 23:623, 1962.

Ghaffar O, Staines R, Feinstein A: Unexplained neurologic symptoms: An fMRI study of sensory conversion disorder. *Neurology* 67:2036, 2006.

Glueck S, Glueck E: *Criminal Careers in Retrospect*. New York, Commonwealth Fund, 1943.

Goodwin DW, Guze SB: *Psychiatric Diagnosis*, 5th ed. New York, Oxford University Press, 1996.

Gunderson JG: Borderline personality disorder. *N Engl J Med* 364:2037, 2011.

Guze S: The role of follow-up studies: The contribution to diagnostic classification as applied to hysteria. *Semin Psychiatry* 2:392, 1970.

Guze SB, Goodwin DW, Crane JB: Criminal recidivism and psychiatric illness. *Am J Psychiatry* 127:832, 1970.

Herzog DB, Becker AE: Eating disorders, in Nicholi AM (ed): *The New Harvard Guide to Psychiatry*, 3rd ed. Cambridge, MA, Belknap Harvard University Press, 1999, pp 400–414.

Hinson VK, Haren WB: Psychogenic movement disorders. *Lancet Neurol* 5:695, 2006.

Holland AJ, Sicotte N, Treasure J: Anorexia nervosa: Evidence for a genetic basis. *J Psychosom Res* 32:561, 1988.

Ireland P, Sapira JD, Templeton B: Munchausen's syndrome. *Am J Med* 43:579, 1967.

Jenkins SC, Maruta T: Therapeutic use of propranolol for intermittent explosive disorders. *Mayo Clin Proc* 62:204, 1987.

Jones AB, Llewellyn LJ: *Malingering*. Philadelphia, Lippincott, 1918.

Judd FK, Brurrows GD, Norman TR: The biological basis of anxiety: An overview. *J Affect Disord* 9:271, 1985.

Kandel ER: A new intellectual framework for psychiatry. *Am J Psychiatry* 155:457, 1998.

Keane JR: Hysterical gait disorders: 60 cases. *Neurology* 39:586, 1989.

Kurlan R: Tourette's syndrome: Current concepts. *Neurology* 39:1625, 1989.

Lazare A: Conversion symptoms. *N Engl J Med* 305:745, 1981.

Lesch K-P, Bengel D, Heils A, et al: Association of anxiety-related traits with polymorphism in the serotonin transporter gene regulatory region. *Science* 274:1527, 1996.

Levine SB: Paraphilias, in Sadock BJ, Sadock VA (eds): *Kaplan and Sadock's Comprehensive Textbook of Psychiatry*, 7th ed. Philadelphia, Lippincott Williams & Wilkins, 2000, pp 1631–1646.

Lewin K, Mattingly D, Mills RR: Anorexia nervosa associated with hypothalamic tumor. *Br Med J* 2:629, 1972.

Lewis A: Psychopathic personality: A most elusive category. *Psychol Med* 4:133, 1974.

Lieb K, Zanarini MC, Schmal C, et al: Borderline personality disorder. *Lancet* 364:453, 2004.

Liebowitz MR, Fryer AJ, Goerman JM, et al: Lactate provocation of panic attacks. *Arch Gen Psychiatry* 41:764, 1984.

Mallet L, Polosan M Jaafari N, et al: Subthalamic nucleus stimulation in severe obsessive compulsive disorder. *N Engl J Med* 359:2121, 2008.

Martin JB, Reichlin S: *Clinical Neuroendocrinology*, 2nd ed. Philadelphia, Davis, 1987.

McCord W, McCord J: *The Psychopath*. Princeton, NJ, Van Nostrand, 1964.

Mehler PS: Bulimia nervosa. *N Engl J Med* 349:875, 2003.

Merskey H: *The Analysis of Hysteria*. London, Ballière Tindall, 1979.

Modlin HC: Postaccident anxiety syndrome: Psychosocial aspects. *Am J Psychiatry* 123:1008, 1967.

Nemiah JC: The psychodynamic basis of psychopathology, in Nicholi AM Jr (ed): *The Harvard Guide to Psychiatry*. Cambridge, MA, Belknap Harvard University Press, 1999, pp 203–219.

Noyes R, Clarkson C, Crowe R, et al: A family study of generalized anxiety disorder. *Am J Psychiatry* 144:1019, 1987.

Pauls DL, Leckman JF: The inheritance of Gilles de la Tourette's syndrome and associated behaviors: Evidence for autosomal dominant transmission. *N Engl J Med* 315:993, 1986.

Pope HG, Hudson JI, Jones JM, et al: Bulimia treated with imipramine: A placebo-controlled double-blind study. *Am J Psychiatry* 140:554, 1983.

Purtell JJ, Robins E, Cohen ME: Observations on clinical aspects of hysteria. *JAMA* 146:902, 1951.

Raskin M, Talbott JA, Meyerson AT: Diagnosis of conversion reactions: Predictive value of psychiatric criteria. *JAMA* 197:530, 1966.

Ratnasuriya RH, Eisler I, Szmukler GJ, Russell GFM: Anorexia nervosa: Outcome and prognostic factors after 20 years. *Br J Psychiatry* 158:495, 1991.

Reid W (ed): *The Psychopath: A Comprehensive Study of Antisocial Disorders and Behaviors*. New York, Brunner-Mazel, 1978.

Robins E, Purtell JJ, Cohen ME: Hysteria in men. *N Engl J Med* 246:677, 1952.

Robins LN: *Deviant Children Grown Up: A Sociological and Psychiatric Study of Sociopathic Personality*. Huntington, NY, Krieger, 1974.

Scheithauer BW, Kovacs KT, Jariwala LK, et al: Anorexia nervosa: An immunohistochemical study of the pituitary gland. *Mayo Clin Proc* 63:23, 1988.

Slater B, Shields J: Genetical aspects of anxiety, in Lader MH (ed): *Studies of Anxiety*. London, Royal Medico-Psychological Association, 1969, pp 62–71.

Slater E: A heuristic theory of neurosis. *J Neurol Neurosurg Psychiatry* 7:48, 1944.

Spence SA, Crimlisk HL, Cope H, et al: Discrete neurophysiological correlates in prefrontal cortex during hysterical and feigned disorder of movement. *Lancet* 355:1243, 2000.

Stein DJ: Obsessive-compulsive disorder. *Lancet* 360:397, 2002.

Steinhausen HC, Seidel R: The Berlin follow-up study of eating disorders in adolescence, Part 2: Intermediate-term catamnesis after 4 years. *Nervenarzt* 65:26, 1994.

Stone J, Edwards M: Trick or treat? Showing patients with functional (psychogenic) motor symptoms their physical signs. *Neurology* 79:282, 2013.
Stone J, Reuber M, Carson A: Functional symptoms in neurology. *Pract Neurol* 13:104, 2013.
Stone J, Sharpe M, Carson A, et al: Are functional motor and sensory symptoms really more common on the left? A systematic review. *J Neurol Neurosurg Psychiatry* 73:578, 2002a.
Stone J, Sharpe M, Rothwell PM, et al: The 12 year prognosis of unilateral functional weakness and sensory disturbance. *J Neurol Neurosurg Psychiatry* 74:591, 2003.
Stone J, Zeman A, Sharpe M: Functional weakness and sensory disturbance. *J Neurol Neurosurg Psychiatry* 73:241, 2002b.
Sullivan PE: Mortality in anorexia nervosa. *Am J Psychiatry* 152:1073, 1995.
Terracciano A, Abdel-Khalek AM, Ádám N, et al: National character does not reflect mean personality trait levels in 49 cultures. *Science* 310:96, 2005.
Tyrer P: New approaches to the diagnosis of psychopathy and personality disorder. *J R Soc Med* 97:371, 2004.
Von Korff M, Eaton W, Keyl P: The epidemiology of panic attacks and panic disorder. *Am J Epidemiol* 122:970, 1985.
Wheeler EO, White PD, Reed EW, Cohen ME: Neurocirculatory asthenia (anxiety neurosis, effort syndrome, neurasthenia): A twenty year follow-up study of one hundred and seventy-three patients. *JAMA* 142:878, 1950.
White LF, Hain RF: Anorexia in association with a destructive lesion of the hypothalamus. *Arch Pathol* 68:275, 1959.
Winokur G, Coryell W: Anxiety disorders: The magnitude of the problem, in Coryell W, Winokur G (eds): *The Clinical Management of Anxiety Disorders*. New York, Oxford University Press, 1991, pp 3–9.

52

Depression and Bipolar Disease

Psychosis, in its broadest definition, refers to any major derangement in mental function in which the individual's ability to perceive and interact with the environment is impaired. Hallucinations are a frequent accompaniment but do not alone define this category of illness. From a neurologic perspective, there are four major categories of psychosis: (1) confusional-delirious states, (2) psychoses associated with focal or multifocal cerebral lesions, (3) affective disorders (bipolar and depressive psychoses), and (4) schizophrenia. The first two categories are discussed in Chaps. 20 and 22. The latter two are the subject of this and the following chapter.

Depression is perhaps the cause of more grief and misery than any other single disease to which humankind is subject. This view, expressed by Kline more than 40 years ago, is still shared by everyone in the field of mental health. The several forms of depression taken together are the most frequent of all psychiatric illnesses. In a general hospital, as indicated in the previous chapter, depression accounted for an estimated 50 percent of psychiatric consultations and 12 percent of all admissions. Although depression has been known for more than 2,000 years (melancholia is described in the writings of Hippocrates), there is still uncertainty as to its medical status as a disease state (kraepelinian concept) or as a type of psychologic reaction (meyerian concept). In other words, is it basically a biologic derangement or a response to psychosocial stress? An eclectic position is that both are correct—i.e., that there are two basic forms of depression: exogenous (an apparent cause) and endogenous (with no overt external cause), and that there may be both an interplay between them and biologic susceptibility to either one.

In respect to endogenous depression and the related condition of bipolar disease, genetic and neurochemical data cited further on support the kraepelinian view of a disease state. Nonetheless, a lay concept persists, perpetuated perhaps by some process-oriented psychiatrists, that events in one's life, either distant or current, underlie all types of depressive illnesses. An unfortunate consequence of this view is the assumption that an inability to deal with these stresses represents a personal failure of sorts and this in turn may inhibit the acceptance of psychiatric help.

Of considerable consequence for clinical work, depressive states are often associated with obscure physical symptoms. For this reason they are likely to come first to the attention of general physicians than are other psychiatric entities. All fields of medical specialty, however, have depressive equivalents; the physical symptoms frequently are mistakenly attributed to anemia, low or high blood pressure, hypothyroidism, migraine, tension headaches, chronic pain syndrome, or chronic infection, or are casually attributed to emotional problems, worry, and stress. Neurologists are most likely to encounter depressed patients who complain of fatigue and weakness, chronic headache, and difficulty in thinking or remembering. Depression masquerading as a chronic pain or a fatigue state or some other medical condition had been called *masked depression* or *depressive equivalent*, terms we still find appropriate and useful in explaining certain symptoms to patients.

There are numerous reasons for separating the problem of endogenous depression from bipolar disease but the distinction clinically may be difficult because bipolar disease may be dominated by depressions, with manic or hypomanic episodes appearing as only a minor or background problem. Foremost among the reasons to consider them separately, however, are differences in response to treatment. In keeping with modern notions, endogenous depression and bipolar disorder are presented separately in this chapter but an understanding of either one is incomplete without knowledge of the other.

Another important reason why all physicians should be knowledgeable about depressive illness in all its forms is the danger of suicide, which may be attempted and successfully accomplished before the depression is recognized. Timely diagnosis may prevent such a tragedy—one that is all the more regrettable as most depressive illnesses can be successfully treated.

ENDOGENOUS DEPRESSION

As remarked in Chap. 24, the term *depression* embraces more than a feeling of sadness and unhappiness. It stands for *a complex of disturbed feelings* (called *mood*, or *affective, disorder*)—which may include aspects of despair, hopelessness, sense of worthlessness, and thoughts of self-harm—associated with decreased energy and libido, loss of interest in personal affairs, impaired concentration, various abnormalities of behavior and appearance, and prominent physical complaints—the most important of which may include anxiety, insomnia, anorexia or overeating, headache, and various types of regional pain. At one extreme are depressive symptoms of psychotic proportions including paranoid or somatic delusions, which create chaos in the lives of the patient and those close to him. At the other extreme are the common feelings of unhappiness, anhedonia (loss of pleasurable responses), discouragement, and resentment that may occur in almost everyone as a reaction to the disappointments of everyday life such as loss of employment, failure to gain recognition, or unsuccessful sexual or social adjustment.

The place in this nosology of the special case of postpartum depression has not been clear, and it is discussed in this chapter as well in the in the next one, as it is sometimes difficult to differentiate it from postpartum psychosis, a more dramatic and well-defined disorder discussed in the next chapter. Some modern authors question the existence of a primary biologic depression that is tied to the postpartum period (see summary by Brockington) but this diverges markedly from the general experience, in which varying degrees of depression are quite common in the weeks after delivery and cannot simply be attributed to psychosocial factors or sleep deprivation.

As a purely phenomenological observation, an abnormally elevated mood, or *mania*, is about one-third as frequent as depression. It may develop as a relatively pure, recurrent clinical state, or more often may alternate or be intertwined with depression, in which case it was referred to as *manic-depressive disease* (now, *bipolar disorder* in the classification of the *Diagnostic and Statistical Manual of Mental Disorders*. *Hypomania* and *cyclothymic disorder* are the names given to milder forms of mania and bipolar disorder, respectively. The DSM classifications also acknowledge the existence of a mixed *schizoaffective state* in which attributes of depression and schizophrenia are combined. Distinguishing these various types of depressive illnesses is of therapeutic as well as theoretical importance insofar as a particular type may respond better to one form of treatment than to another. Finally, the neurologist should always bear in mind the possibility of an incipient dementia presenting as a depression, although the reverse, a masked depression causing difficulty with thinking and memory (pseudodementia) is more common.

Reactive Depressions and Depressions with Medical and Neurologic Diseases

Patients reacting to a medical or neurologic illness seldom express feelings of sadness or despair without mentioning physical accompaniments such as easy fatigability, anxiety, headaches, dizziness, loss of appetite, reduced interest in life and love, trouble in falling asleep, or premature awakening. It follows that whenever these symptoms become manifest in the course of medical disease, they should arouse suspicion of a depressive reaction (Table 52-1).

Table 52-1

DEPRESSION SECONDARY TO NEUROLOGIC, MEDICAL, AND SURGICAL DISEASES AND DRUGS

1. Neurologic diseases
   a. Neuronal degenerations—Alzheimer, Huntington, frontotemporal dementia, Lewy-body disease, Parkinson disease, and multiple system atrophy
   b. Focal CNS disease—strokes, brain tumors and trauma, multiple sclerosis
2. Metabolic and endocrine diseases
   a. Corticosteroids, excess or withdrawal
   b. Hypothyroidism, rarely thyrotoxicosis
   c. Cushing syndrome
   d. Addison disease
   e. Pernicious anemia (vitamin B_{12} deficiency)
3. Myocardial infarction, open heart surgery, and other operations
4. Infectious diseases
   a. Brucellosis
   b. Viral hepatitis, influenza, pneumonia
   c. Infectious mononucleosis
   d. Whipple disease
   e. Creutzfeldt-Jakob disease
5. Cancer, particularly pancreatic and metastatic
6. Parturition
7. Medications
   a. Corticosteroids and ACTH
   b. Interferons
   c. Analgesics and anti-inflammatory agents (other than steroids)—indomethacin, phenacetin
   d. Amphetamines (when withdrawn)
   e. Antibiotics, particularly cycloserine, ethionamide, griseofulvin, isoniazid, nalidixic acid, and sulfonamide
   f. Antihypertensive drugs—clonidine, propranolol (and certain other beta-adrenergic blockers)
   g. Cardiac drugs—digitalis, procainamide
   h. Disulfiram
   i. L-Dopa
   j. Methysergide
   k. Oral contraceptives
8. Alcoholism

ACTH, adrenocorticotropic hormone; CNS, central nervous system.

Chronic pain is a particularly frequent somatic manifestation of depression. The pain may be based on an attendant disease but is prolonged, disabling, sometimes vague in nature, and recalcitrant to straightforward medical and surgical approaches. Furthermore, depressed mood exacerbates and prolongs pain of any type. All patients with chronic pain syndromes should be evaluated psychiatrically, as pointed out in Chap. 8.

In a number of major medical illnesses depressive symptoms occur with such frequency as to become almost part of the disease. Contrariwise, in certain chronic and occult diseases, symptoms such as lassitude and fatigue may resemble and be mistaken for a depressive reaction. Hypothyroidism, infectious mononucleosis, hepatitis, lymphoma, myeloma, metastatic carcinoma, malnutrition, polymyalgia rheumatica, and frontal lobe tumors, especially meningiomas, may simulate depression for weeks or months before the diagnosis becomes evident. A special relationship to occult pancreatic or other abdominal cancers has been suggested but is difficult to understand. Sedative drugs, beta-adrenergic blocking agents, beta-interferons used for the treatment of multiple sclerosis and hepatitis, and the phenothiazines may also evoke a depressive reaction; corticosteroids can induce a peculiar psychiatric state in which confusion, insomnia, and either an elevation of mood or depression are combined, even to the point of psychoses. A depressed mood may also emerge during the tapering-off period of corticosteroid medication or during their initial use (a hypomanic state is more common).

Of particular significance is the reactive depression that occurs on learning of a serious medical or neurologic disease. Often such an emotional reaction, which the physician may tend to ignore, is the dominant manifestation of a disease that threatens the life pattern and independence of the patient. Recognition by the patient that he has suffered a stroke or that he has cancer, multiple sclerosis, amyotrophic lateral sclerosis, or Parkinson disease, is almost always followed by some degree of reactive depression, often with an element of anxiety. A prime example is the depression that follows myocardial infarction (Wishnie et al). Usually it begins toward the end of the patient's stay in the hospital and attracts little attention. Once the patient is home, fatigability that approaches exhaustion is the main complaint and interferes with accustomed activities and rehabilitation. It may be described as weakness and falsely attributed to heart failure. Symptoms of irritability, anxiety, and despondency are next in order of frequency, followed by insomnia and feelings of aimlessness and boredom. Although most of these patients ultimately recover without medical assistance the depression exacts a high toll in terms of mental suffering.

Depression Following Stroke and with Degenerative Neurologic Disease An analogous depressive reaction occurs in some patients after a stroke. Some studies have indicated that patients with left anterior cerebral lesions, involving predominantly the lateral frontal cortex or basal ganglia, have a greater frequency and severity of depression than do patients with lesions in other locations (Starkstein et al, 1987; Robinson). According to these authors, lesions of the right hemisphere do not show this correlation with depression but have a higher association with pathologic cheerfulness or mania. However, House and colleagues, in a British community-based study of stroke survivors, failed to confirm these findings, perhaps because the infarcts were small in size (more than half the patients had never been admitted to hospital) and many patients were examined for the first time only at 6 and 12 months after their strokes. Our colleagues Levine and Finkelstein have reported the occurrence of psychotic depression with hallucinations and delusions in patients with right temporoparietal infarcts. Our own experience suggests an unsurprising relationship between the degree of motor and language disability and the severity of poststroke depression, but a less predictable relationship to the location of the lesion. The possible predisposing effects of minor previous episodes of depression, family history of depressive illness, and medications have not been studied systematically. These issues are also incorporated into Chap. 34.

With regard to emotional reactions in degenerative brain diseases, Parkinson disease is complicated by a depressive reaction in approximately one-quarter of cases. Weakness and fatigability, already aspects of the motor syndrome, are added to the principal psychologic manifestations and the resulting therapeutic problem becomes formidable. Another hazard in Parkinson and in Lewy-body disease is the tendency for L-dopa itself to provoke a depression in a limited number of patients, sometimes with suicidal tendencies, paranoid ideation, and psychotic episodes. Huntington chorea is quite often associated with depression, even before the movement disorder and dementia become conspicuous. In one series, 10 of 101 patients with Huntington disease either committed suicide or attempted it, and this outcome is commented on in almost all large series of that disease. Alzheimer disease may be accompanied by depressive symptoms, in which instance it is difficult or impossible early in the illness to evaluate the relative contributions of the mood disorder and the dementia. In later stages, the overt signs of depression usually abate.

Depression during and after Pregnancy The main risk for depression during pregnancy is a history of previous depressions. Certain epidemiologic factors also come into play including a family history of depression, single motherhood, cigarette smoking, low income, youth, and domestic violence. The implications, however, of depression during pregnancy are great in that the fetus is at risk of suffering due to inadequate prenatal care and an increased rate of miscarriage. Several pieces of controversial evidence suggested that maternal depression may affect fetal growth and infant temperament. Furthermore, postpartum depression is also more common in women with prenatal depression and may lead to similar difficulties with infant care.

The treatment of depression during pregnancy has attracted considerable attention because of the potential risks to the fetus of the modern class of serotonin reuptake inhibitors. This is discussed in a later section. The clinical aspects of depression during pregnancy have been summarized by Stewart.

Clinical Presentation

Fully developed endogenous depression may evolve within a few days, or, more often, it emerges more gradually, on a background of vague prodromal symptoms that had been present for months. Chapter 24 provides a detailed description of the symptoms and signs of depression. Here it need only be repeated that the patient, when asked, or spontaneously expresses feelings of sadness, unhappiness, discouragement, hopelessness, and despondency, with loss of self-esteem. Reduced energy and activity, typically expressed as mental and physical exhaustion, is almost always present, to the point of catatonia in the most severe cases. Indeed, as emphasized in Chap. 24, the most common cause of symptoms relating to reduced psychic and physical energy and drive (conation) is depression. There is heightened irritability, usually reported by a spouse or friends, as well as a lack of interest in most activities that formerly were pleasurable.

According to DSM, the essential diagnostic criteria of endogenous depression ("major depressive syndrome") consist of a dysphoric mood or loss of interest or pleasure in all usual activities (including sexual activity) in combination with at least four of the following seven symptoms: (1) disturbance of appetite and change in weight; (2) sleep disorder; (3) psychomotor retardation or agitation; (4) decreased energy and fatigue; (5) self-reproach, feelings of worthlessness or guilt; (6) indecisiveness, complaints of memory loss and difficulty in concentrating; and (7) thoughts of death or suicide or actual suicide attempts. In this diagnostic scheme, each of the four diagnostic symptoms should have been present for at least 2 weeks. This is a useful listing but simply recapitulates the well-described emotional, conative, and physical aspects of endogenous depression. The formalized diagnostic criteria have been devised for both screening and diagnosis of major depression (Table 52-2). These codify the clinical features discussed in previous paragraphs but separate major depression from bipolar disorder by requiring the absence of elements that suggest a manic or hypomanic episode and further exclude depression that is plausibly connected to personal distress or grieving due to a loss, or the effects of a drug or toxic substance.

The depressed patient tends to move slowly, sighing is frequent, and speech is reduced. The mental life of such an individual may narrow to a single-minded concern about physical or mental health. In dialogue, the patient's responses become so stereotyped that the listener can soon predict exactly what is going to be said. There is a poverty of ideation and sometimes a notable absence of insight. Consciousness is clear, and although there is no evidence of a schizophrenic type of thought disorder, delusional ideas, and less often hallucinations, may be prominent in some patients, justifying the term *depressive psychosis*. The delusions are generally congruent with the patient's mood and are not as fixed or bizarre as those of schizophrenia or paranoia. In our experience, delusions are more common in older patients and tend to appear only after weeks or months of more typical symptoms of depression. Hallucinations, when they occur, are usually transitory, vocal, and vaguely accusatory; their presence should always raise the possibility of an associated structural brain disease, drug intoxication, or alcoholic auditory hallucinosis.

Frequently, agitation or irritability rather than physical inactivity and mental slowness are the principal behavioral abnormalities. The source of the agitation appears usually to be an underlying anxiety state. Pacing the floor and wringing the hands, particularly in the early morning hours, are characteristic. Such patients tend to be overly talkative and vexed in their manner of expression, irritable, short-tempered, impatient, and intolerant of minor problems—changes noted mainly by family members. Attempts at reassurance may meet with initial success, only to be dispelled in the next rush of doubts. These patients remain impervious to reason and logic with respect to their symptoms, even though they are reasonable and logical in other areas of their lives. At its worst, the illness takes the form of a depressive stupor; the patient becomes mute, indifferent to nutritional needs, and neglectful even of bowel and bladder functions (anergic depression). The condition in this extreme form is a *catatonic depression*. Such patients must be fed and their other needs attended to until therapy (usually electroconvulsive therapy [ECT]) brings about improvement.

The most important concern in patients with mid- and late-life depression is suicide, a topic addressed again further on. Because many of these individuals have reputations for being sound, dependable, and stable and deny being depressed, one's inclination is to doubt the possibility of self-destruction. *Such patients should nonetheless be questioned forthrightly on this subject*: Do they feel that life is not worthwhile? Have there been thoughts of suicide? Do they think themselves capable of committing suicide? Have they made such plans or made suicide attempts before? Is there a family history of suicide? Do they own a firearm? Are they fearful of dying? Do they have a strongly held religious view that proscribes suicide? These questions relate to features that have been shown to put depressed individuals at risk of suicide. If, from their answers, they are judged to carry an imminent risk of suicide, they should be directed to a psychiatrist and generally admitted to a hospital. In recent years, it has come to be appreciated that the elderly are increasingly prone to suicide and that older white men have the highest rates of completed suicides (mainly with firearms).

In some depressions, hypochondriacal preoccupation with bowel and digestive functions accounts for repeated visits to the physician. In one study, 21 of 120 such

Table 52-2

DIAGNOSTIC CRITERIA FOR MAJOR DEPRESSIVE EPISODE TAKEN FROM DSM[a]

Five more of the following symptoms are required during the same 2-week period with at least one of the first two included:
Depressed mood most of the day, nearly everyday
Markedly diminished interest or pleasure in all, or almost all, activities most of the day, nearly everyday
Significant weight loss without diet, or weight gain of more than 5% of body weight in a month, or decrease or increase in appetite nearly everyday
Insomnia or hypersomnia nearly everyday
Psychomotor agitation or retardation nearly everyday
Fatigue or loss of energy nearly everyday
Feelings of worthlessness or excessive or inappropriate guilt nearly everyday
Diminished ability to think or concentrate or indecisiveness nearly everyday
Recurrent thoughts of death, recurrent suicidal ideas without a specific plan, or suicide attempt or specific plan for committing suicide

[a]Appropriate exclusions are made for manic episodes that would mark the illness as bipolar, and special forms of depression due to grief, significant personal or social distress, and drugs or toxic substances are discussed in the text.

patients were subsequently diagnosed as being depressed. Persistent insomnia may be the major complaint of the depressed patient. Early awakening is typical, and the morning hours are then the worst period of the day for the low emotional state. Other patients have difficulty falling asleep, especially if there is an associated anxiety state. A complaint in the male of loss of libido and erectile dysfunction is another monosymptomatic presentation; only with probing inquiry about other disturbances common to depression will the diagnosis become evident.

Adherence to the aforementioned diagnostic criteria (see Table 52-1) undoubtedly facilitates diagnosis, but not infrequently a single one of these symptoms so dominates the clinical picture as to suggest the diagnosis of another disease state and obscure the presence of an underlying depression. As mentioned earlier, depressed patients who are referred to the neurologist tend to complain inordinately of physical and cognitive symptoms and to minimize or deny the purely affective ones. Complaints of fatigue, weakness, malaise, or widespread aches and pains, for example, suggest a variety of medical diseases, such as anemia, Addison disease, hypothyroidism, chronic infection, polymyositis, or early rheumatoid arthritis. Quite often the fatigue state is misinterpreted as muscular weakness, and this directs a medical search for neuromuscular disease. Similarly, complaints of persistent headache may suggest the presence of intracranial disease. Complaints of poor memory, inability to concentrate, and other cognitive impairments raise the question of a dementia until it is found, by careful examination, that mental competence belies the patient's appraisal of his own defects.

A number of psychologic testing scales are used to detect and score the severity of depression. Although they are of value mainly for clinical studies, several of them can be helpful in clinical work since they are sensitive to one or another aspect of depression. They do not supplant the clinical examination in determining if an individual is depressed or suicidal but they may be helpful in differentiating depression from dementia and in detecting depression in cases where physical complaints are more prominent than psychic ones. The tests most familiar to neurologists are the Hamilton and the Beck scales, but several others are as valid and widely used.

BIPOLAR DISEASE AND MANIA

Bipolar disease is a disorder of mood consisting of prolonged episodes of depression, interrupted by, or coexistent with episodes of mania. It was given the name manic-depressive disease by Kraepelin in 1896, and it was with him that our current clinical concept of this disorder originated. He viewed the manic and depressive attacks as opposite poles of the same underlying process and pointed out that, unlike dementia praecox (his name for schizophrenia), bipolar psychosis entails no intellectual deterioration with recurrent episodes. A traditional view of this disease was that of a periodic or cyclic condition in which one major mood swing was followed by an equal but opposite excursion. This is seldom the case, however. Episodes of depression are more than twice as frequent as manic ones, and according to current experts, the most common form of the illness is characterized by episodic depression alone and many patients have several episodes of depression before their first period of mania.

Recurrence of episodes of pure mania without interspersed episodes of depression is known but relatively uncommon. As a consequence, bipolar psychosis has been divided into two subtypes: the *unipolar group*, in which only an endogenous depressive illness occurs, and a *bipolar group*, in which one or more bouts of mania occur with or without depression. The bipolar variety occurs in approximately 10 percent of patients with affective disorder. The biologic accuracy of this classification has not been critically determined. There has been an arbitrary further subdivision of *bipolar I* to denote at least one episode of full mania, and *bipolar II* when the process entails an episode of hypomania.

In addition, there are *mixed affective states*, in which symptoms of both depression and mania occur within a single episode of the illness. A so-called "rapid-cycling" form of bipolar disease has also been recognized in which four or more circumscribed episodes occur in a year. Like other variants of the disease, it tends to have an aberrant or unpredictable response to medication. Still other patients with affective elements of depression present with atypical features; for example, instead of anorexia, weight loss, and insomnia, they sleep and eat excessively.

The prevalence of bipolar disease cannot be stated with precision, mainly because of varying criteria used for diagnosis. Certainly depression and depressive episodes are ubiquitous and mania is less common. The apparent increase of the disease in the past 50 years probably reflects a growing awareness of the condition among both physicians and the laity. Studies of large groups of patients from isolated areas of Iceland and the Danish islands of Bornholm and Samsø indicate that 5 percent of men and 9 percent of women will develop symptoms of major depression, mania, or both at some time during their lives (Goodwin and Guze). Some recent studies, such as the one conducted by the National Comorbidity Survey, report lifetime prevalence for bipolar disorder in the United States as 4.5% (Merikangas et al).

Bipolar disease occurs most frequently in middle and later adult years, with a peak age of onset between 55 and 65 for both sexes. However, a significant proportion of patients experience the first attack in childhood, adolescence, or early adult life. Depression is also a major problem in the elderly. Blazer and Williams, who studied 997 persons older than age 65 years in North Carolina, found symptoms of a major depressive illness in 3.7 percent. The disease was two or three times more frequent among women. There is no known explanation for this gender difference, but some have speculated that just as many men are depressed, only they deny it or turn to alcohol. Patients in the bipolar group have an earlier age of onset, more frequent and shorter cycles of illness, and a greater prevalence of affective disorder among their relatives than do patients with unipolar depression (Winokur).

Clinical Presentation

The *manic state* is, in most ways, the opposite of the depressed state, being characterized by a flight of ideas, motor and speech hyperactivity, and an increased appetite and sex urge. When such a state is fully developed, it qualifies as a psychosis. After a minimum of sleep, the patient awakes with enthusiasm and expectation. The manic individual appears to possess great drive and confidence yet lacks the ability to carry out plans. Often headstrong, impulsive, socially intrusive behavior is characteristic. Judgment may be so impaired that reckless investments are made; fortunes are spent in gambling or on extravagant shopping sprees. Setbacks do not perturb the patient, but rather act as goads to new activities. Euphoria and expansiveness sometimes bubble over into delusions of power and grandeur, which, in turn, may make the patient offensively aggressive. Up to a point, the patient's mirth and good spirits may be contagious, and others may join in; however, if the patient is thwarted, the warmth and good humor can suddenly change to anger. Irritability rather than elation may become the prevailing mood. The threshold for paranoid thinking is low, which makes the patient sensitive and suspicious. Personal neglect may reach the point of dishevelment and poor hygiene. In its most advanced form, a condition described as "delirious mania," the patient becomes totally incoherent and altogether disorganized in behavior. At this stage visual and auditory hallucinations and paranoid delusions may be rampant.

Hypomania describes a milder degree of the disorder but this term is also used loosely to depict behavior in a normally functioning individual who is unusually energetic and active. In this latter sense, hypomania is a personality trait found in many talented and productive persons and need not arouse concern unless it is excessive and out of character for the individual. As Belmaker noted, a number of highly creative individuals have had bipolar disorders, but full-blown mania is uniformly destructive of careers and personal relationships. Such individuals are actually more creative when treated with appropriate medications.

First attacks of either depression or mania last an average of 6 months if untreated, although the duration varies greatly. With treatment, this can be reduced by more than half in most patients. Although most attacks of bipolar disease subside in a matter of months, a significant number, unipolar patients more than bipolar ones, remain chronically ill for long periods. According to Winokur and colleagues, 14 percent of their bipolar patients had not recovered after 2 years and 5 percent had not recovered after 5 years. Comparative figures for primary unipolar patients were 19 and 12 percent, respectively. The majority of depressed patients have one or more recurrences. Variables that are predictive of an unfavorable outcome are high degrees of anxiety, strongly positive family history of a similar psychiatric illness, and presence of depression-provoking circumstances (Hirschfeld et al). Perhaps most important is the duration of illness before treatment, i.e., earlier treatment is generally associated with a more favorable prognosis.

Mania Presenting as an Encephalopathy The manic patient may be disoriented and slightly agitated, with a clouded sensorium. This extreme is not frequently encountered but we have several times admitted patients to the neurology service with mania that presented in a manner suggesting an encephalopathy and global confusional state. The patient conducted himself pleasantly, without psychosis, pressured speech or overactive motor behavior but with an inattentive, confusion as the dominant feature. Conditions such as herpes encephalitis, alcohol or drug withdrawal, stroke, and paraneoplastic encephalitis were considered until the patient began filling notebooks with writing, manifesting insomnia, and making connections between ideas and events that were individually valid but just outside the realm of likelihood. One insisted that one of us was also his wife's cardiologist and another, that one of the authors had scored a winning touchdown at a college football game at which he was present. Stories about public figures were factually correct but attached to the wrong person. The patient sat near the door to his hospital room and incessantly but pleasantly attracted our attention to speak to him every time one of us was in sight. At the same time, performance on orientation, arithmetic, and language tasks were normal.

Special Problems in Patient with Depressive Illness

In our experience, the following are some of the common and troublesome clinical situations in which it may prove difficult to recognize an underlying depression:

1. *Patients with chronic pain*. The association of chronic pain and depression has long been appreciated. This is far from a homogeneous group. The special case of chronic headache, confronted often by neurologists, is discussed below and in Chap. 10. In some patients with chronic pain, the symptoms and signs of depression are quite apparent. If the pain has been present for less than a year and had its onset at the same time as other depressive symptoms, response to antidepressant treatment is likely to be favorable. Far more difficult to understand, and to manage, are patients with persistent pain as the only complaint; the head, face, and lower back are the most common loci. Weeks or months of unremitting daily tension-type headaches in the context of a normal examination are highly suggestive of depression at any age. If an exhaustive search for the source of the pain proves unsuccessful, the conclusion is finally reached that the pain is "psychogenic." This attribution of pain to some obscure psychologic mechanism is hardly helpful. Nevertheless, in a fair proportion of such patients, that pain will be alleviated by antidepressant drugs is suggestive of a linkage of the pain and depression. The problem may have been made even more difficult by repeated surgical operations as well as dependency on analgesic drugs, which in themselves deplete energy and have other adverse effects. Such patients are to be found among those disabled after multiple operations for ruptured intervertebral disc or arthritic hips or those with atypical facial pain.

2. *Depression and alcoholism.* These are commonly associated, and it is important to determine which is primary and which is secondary. A depressive syndrome developing for the first time on a background of alcoholism is a common clinical occurrence. In a large series of alcoholic patients studied by Cadoret and Winokur, a secondary depression occurred in 30 of 61 females and in 41 of 112 males; moreover, once the alcoholism was established, depression became evident much earlier in the women than in the men. The opposite occurrence (i.e., the development of alcoholism on the background of a primary depression) is less common. Again, women are disproportionately affected. As mentioned earlier, these differences may be spurious; Winokur's family studies (1991) suggest that the same genetic predisposition leads to depression in females and alcoholism and sociopathy in men.
3. *Depression in childhood and adolescence.* We have observed depressive states in children and they have often been misdiagnosed by both pediatricians and psychiatrists. The common manifestations have been chronic headache, refusal to go to school, withdrawal from social activities, anorexia, vomiting and weight loss, and scholastic failure. Puberty is a time of onset in many cases, but we have seen depressive disease in late childhood and it is frequent in high school and college students. It is a tragic mistake not to appreciate this fact and to treat the patient for some presumed nonaffective nervous symptoms, only to have the patient commit suicide.
4. *Anxiety, hypochondriasis, and pseudodementia.* These are clinical circumstances in which an underlying depressive illness may not be immediately apparent but must be suspected, as discussed in detail in Chap. 51. The complaint of severe chronic fatigue without medical explanation should raise the same suspicion (see Chap. 24). An elderly person with seemingly early signs of dementia may, on closer examination, turn out to have a severe depressive illness.

Etiology of Depression

The following are the main theories, not mutually exclusive, that have been proposed to explain the origin of depression; for a detailed review of the subject, the reader is referred to the review by Belmaker and Agam.

Genetic Factors

The capacity to experience sadness and depression is common to all people but there is no question that some individuals are more liable to depression than others who are subjected to similar psychosocial forces. It has been estimated, using various genetic techniques, that as much as 40 percent of the risk of depression is heritable (lower than for schizophrenia and bipolar disease). Adopted children whose biologic parents had affective disorder are at greater risk of developing this disease than are adoptees whose biologic parents were not affected (Mendlewicz and Rainer; Cadoret). The frequency of these illnesses is greatly increased in the relatives of affected patients (prevalence rate of 14 to 25 percent in first-degree relatives). Similarly, the risk of depression among first-degree relatives is increased (15 percent, in comparison to 1 to 2 percent risk in the general population). If several twin studies are taken together, 72 percent of monozygotic twins are concordant for bipolar disease, compared with 14 percent of same-sex dizygotic twins; comparative figures for unipolar disease are 40 percent and 11 percent, respectively (see Goodwin and Guze). All of these findings indicate a strong genetic factor. The genes for bipolar disease remain to be discovered, and current thinking holds that several are likely to be involved. One indication that specific genes may alter the susceptibility to depression has been presented by Ogilvie and colleagues; they and others have found allelic variations in the serotonin transporter gene (the main target of the selective serotonin antidepressants) that were associated with a sevenfold increased risk of major depression. Not all studies agree on these points. This result has been reinforced by Caspi and colleagues who reported that a variant in the serotonin transporter correlates with an increase in depression in response to stress. Other hypotheses have postulated susceptibility loci on chromosomes 18, 21, and X. Again, a single gene locus seems unlikely (see Sanders et al).

Anatomic Correlates

Several lines of study, including those employing functional imaging, indicate that a few select regions of the brain are implicated in the pathogenesis of the complex symptomatology of depression (Drevets). Hypometabolism in the left frontal cortex is among the most consistent findings. Also prominent in many studies are metabolic changes in the cingulate and orbitofrontal cortices, related parts of the medial limbic system, and the hippocampus.

An intriguing observation, and one that does not entirely accord with the above, has been made by Bejjani and colleagues in the course of deep brain stimulation for the treatment of Parkinson disease. One of their patients displayed transient but dramatic manifestations of depression only when high-frequency stimulation was delivered to the left substantia nigra. Positron emission tomography imaging during stimulation showed activation in the left orbitofrontal cortex and, less consistently, in the left amygdala, globus pallidus, thalamus, and right parietal lobe. In two other cases with no prior psychiatric symptoms, deep brain stimulation of the subthalamic nucleus induced a reversible manic state (Herzog et al; Kulisevsky et al). Fisher noted a hypomanic episode in the early stages of herpes encephalitis, and numerous cases of temporary secondary mania have been reported after stroke and after brain trauma, the latter affecting most often the right temporal lobe.

On histologic level, several studies have shown a depletion of and changes in the pyramidal neurons of the CA3 region of the hippocampus in both depression and stress, but the meaning of these findings is unclear (Sapolsky). They are referred to later in relation to neurogenesis (the appearance in adults of new neurons) in the temporal lobe and recovery from depression. These ideas regarding neurogenesis, which are still speculative, are discussed in Chap. 29. Interestingly, in a rodent model of depression, neurogenesis was required for the beneficial effects of antidepressants to take place (Santarelli). Based in part on this observation, a relationship has been suggested between depressive illness and the later development of dementia. The reviews of Starkstein (1987, 1991) and Robinson and their colleagues, and that of Belmaker and Agam mentioned earlier, may be consulted for further information on anatomic lesions that cause changes in affect.

Biochemical Theories

It has been evident for several years that the biogenic monoamines (norepinephrine, serotonin, and dopamine) are in some way involved in the biology of depression. However, most of the neurochemical theories of depression suffer from the weakness that they have been the result of backward reasoning from the effects of antidepressants on various neurotransmitters to the putative mechanisms of the disease. Following the observations that the tricyclic antidepressants and the monoamine oxidase (MAO) inhibitors exerted their effect by increasing norepinephrine and serotonin at central adrenergic receptor sites in the limbic system and hypothalamus and that depression-provoking drugs (such as reserpine) deplete biogenic amines at these sites, it was proposed that naturally occurring depressions might be associated with a deficiency of these substances. Furthermore, depressed patients and their first-degree relatives, as well as healthy individuals, develop a depressed mood after dietary depletion of the monoamine precursor tryptophan and concentrations of 3-methoxy-4-hydroxyphenylglycol (MHPG), a metabolite of norepinephrine, are reduced in the cerebrospinal fluid during endogenous depression and the levels are elevated in manic states. Some neurochemical imaging studies corroborate these findings and others do not. Along similar lines, 5-hydroxyindoleacetic acid (5-HIAA), a deaminated metabolite of serotonin, is reduced in the cerebrospinal fluid of depressed patients (Carroll et al).

Certain of the newer antidepressants act as selective serotonin reuptake inhibitors (SSRIs) and apparently produce their salutary effects by increasing the amount of serotonin that is functionally active in the synapse (they also raise the concentrations of norepinephrine). For these reasons, serotonin and its neuronal pathways are also currently implicated in the genesis of depression. However, the reader should be reminded that only two decades ago it was widely held that depletion of norepinephrine fulfilled this role. It is also not yet clear which neurochemical alterations are primary and which modulate other systems. For example, reports suggest that substance P plays an important role in the causation of depression (Kramer et al) and that blockade of substance P receptors has antidepressant effects. Why there is a delay of several weeks in the improvement of depression related to the taking of the various antidepressants is unexplained by any of the neurochemical models.

Another set of observations that has continued to capture interest for more than a decade implicates a disorder of hypothalamic–pituitary–adrenal axis function (summarized by Schlesser et al). It had been found several decades ago that the parenteral administration of 1 to 2 mg of dexamethasone failed to suppress serum cortisol secretion while the patient was ill with endogenous depression, but did so after recovery. In a comparable series of reactive depressions, there was a normal suppression of cortisol secretion. Originally, the dexamethasone suppression test was believed to separate the two large groups of depressed patients and to predict the response to drug therapy. However, subsequent studies have shown that the specificity of this test was far less than earlier reports had indicated (Amsterdam et al; Insel et al). Accumulated evidence indicates that 50 percent of severely depressed patients do not show suppression of cortisol secretion, and a positive test can be obtained in a significant number of patients with other psychiatric disorders.

The failure of dexamethasone suppression has been attributed to hyperactivity in the hypothalamic pituitary axis and a corresponding increase in secretion of corticotropin-releasing hormone, adrenocorticotropic hormone (ACTH), and glucocorticoids. Elevated levels of glucocorticoids have been theorized to impede neurogenesis in the medial temporal lobe, and perhaps to explain or exaggerate the loss of hippocampal neurons demonstrated in some studies of the brains of deceased depressed patients. A proposal that ECT acts by elevating levels of neurotrophic factors is at least consistent with this view and with the hypothesis that one component of recovery from depression is in some way associated with restoration of normal neuronal architecture in regions of the hippocampus and the hypothalamus (Chen). Although highly speculative, perhaps some of these changes explain the delay in improvement after the administration of antidepression drugs.

At the present time, it must also be conceded that there is no reliable biologic test for depression. One must resort to clinical analysis not only for diagnosis but also for the differentiation of special types of depressive reactions.

Psychosocial Theories

Many experienced psychiatrists have emphasized the importance of psychosocial factors in the genesis of depressive illness. Among patients with primary depressive disorders, life events of a stressful nature were found to have occurred more frequently in the months preceding the onset of depression than in matched control groups. In the study by Thomson and Hendrie, this was equally true of patients with a positive family history of depression and of those without such a history. Nor did patients with endogenous depression differ in this respect from those with reactive depression. Left unanswered is the question of why some individuals are subject to a reactive depression. Are they predisposed by psychologic, personality, or genetically transmitted factors of heightened vulnerability to the effects of psychosocial stress? One is tempted to conclude that many depressions attributed to psychosocial stress are contaminating a group of endogenous depressions. Psychiatrists have also failed to find a consistent correlation between depressive illness and personality type or a particular psychodynamic mechanism.

Treatment of Depression

The use of medications for depression is now so widespread that all physicians should be familiar with them. Those untrained in psychiatry would, however, be unwise to undertake the management of bipolar disease or a serious endogenous depression without the advice or assistance of a psychiatrist. On the other hand, if the symptoms are primarily neurologic (e.g., chronic headache, generalized weakness, and fatigability) and if there is a low risk of suicide, it is appropriate for the neurologist or generalist to institute treatment with antidepressant medication.

Antidepressant Medication

In the management of bipolar and depressive disease, six main categories of drugs are in general use—the tricyclic antidepressants, the "atypical" or nontricyclic group of compounds, the MAO inhibitors, serotonin agonists (reuptake inhibitors), antiepileptic drugs, and lithium. The pharmacologic properties and modes of action of these drugs were considered in Chap. 43. Additional points of therapeutic interest are mentioned here. It should also be stated that meta-analyses of several large studies on the therapeutic effects of antidepressants suggest that clinical improvement attributable to the drugs themselves occurs in approximately 50 percent of patients; remarkably, an additional improvement in up to 25 percent is attributable to a placebo effect or, more likely, to the natural course of the disease. The remainder fails to improve in a timely manner or relapse while on medication. The incremental value of certain forms of psychotherapies is discussed further on.

Most psychiatrists currently prefer to begin treatment with one of the functional serotonin agonists (SSRIs)—fluoxetine (Prozac), sertraline (Zoloft), paroxetine (Paxil), citalopram (Celexa), escitalopram (Lexapro), and others, or one of a related group, exemplified by venlafaxine (Effexor) and nefazodone (Serzone). New drugs of similar type are appearing yearly. These drugs have less sedating and anticholinergic effects than the tricyclic antidepressants discussed below, and may have a slightly faster onset of effect against depression. Fluoxetine has a tendency to produce insomnia and weight loss, making it particularly useful in the treatment of depressions that are characterized by overeating and hypersomnia. Some female patients have experienced an opposite effect, i.e., weight gain. Patients with anorexia, insomnia, and high levels of anxiety may do better with a more sedating medication, such as amitriptyline. Fluoxetine would be a reasonable choice for patients in whom lethargy is a prominent complaint. Certain side effects such as loss of libido and erectile dysfunction occur in a proportion of patients and are difficult to differentiate from the signs of depression. Other side effects occur in a proportion of patients, including gastrointestinal upset, increased anxiety as discussed in Chap. 51, blurred vision, dizziness, among many (see Chap. 43).

The contentious issues of (1) inducing mania, (2) precipitating suicide soon after the institution of these medications, and (3) the use of these drugs in children are important issues that can only be addressed here cursorily. Ryan summarizes these problems and points out that the overall rates of suicide among adolescents are decreasing at the time of increasing use of SSRI agents. The precipitation of a manic episode by serotonergic antidepressants in some patients with bipolar disorder seems a regular enough occurrence that it is no longer a point of contention. Also to be emphasized is an increased risk of pulmonary hypertension in the babies of mothers exposed to SSRI during the pregnancy.

The tricyclic antidepressants comprise amitriptyline, imipramine, desipramine, doxepin, clomipramine, and trimipramine, and the closely related drugs nortriptyline and protriptyline. Among this group, most psychiatrists start with imipramine or amitriptyline because of their relative safety. In general, all of these drugs are equally effective, although an individual patient may have a better response or tolerance to one than to another. The starting dose for amitriptyline or imipramine is 25 mg/d, which is then raised by 25 mg q3–4d as needed up to 150 mg/d. These drugs, taken at bedtime, are also very helpful in alleviating the insomnia that accompanies depression. The therapeutic effect of tricyclic medication is generally not evident for 2 to 4 weeks after treatment has been initiated, and it is important that this be explained to the patient and family. Common side effects are orthostatic hypotension, dry mouth, constipation, tachycardia, urinary hesitancy or retention (especially in patients with prostatic hypertrophy), tremor, and drowsiness. Closed-angle glaucoma may decompensate. Caution should be exercised in elderly patients with cardiac disorders of all types because of the possibility of causing heart block or arrhythmia. For such patients, the serotonin drugs or one of a newer group of nontricyclic antidepressant drugs—bupropion and trazodone—may be preferable, but the latter causes orthostatic hypotension and sedation in doses required for consistent antidepression effects. The latter drugs appear to be as effective as the tricyclic agents in the treatment of depression without the adverse anticholinergic and cardiotoxic effects.

If one of the SSRI or tricyclic and related drugs, given in full doses for 4 to 6 weeks, does not produce the desired effect, or, as often happens, if the patient is intolerant of the given drug, another one from an alternative group, e.g., an MAO inhibitor, may be tried. In one of the many new "effectiveness" trials sponsored by the National Institutes of Mental Health, as distinguished from "efficacy" in controlled and randomized trials, failure of citalopram to accomplish remission of depression (about half of patients, as expected), changing to bupropion, sertraline, or venlafaxine had equivalent effects and were successful in 25 percent of cases (Rush et al). In the case of SSRIs, *there must be a drug-free interval of 1 to 2 weeks before instituting an MAO inhibitor*. Some studies suggest that MAO inhibitors are superior in depression with atypical features such as increased appetite. Phenelzine, isocarboxazid, and tranylcypromine are in this category, of which the first is said to be the least likely to produce serious side effects. The usual starting dose is 15 mg tid, which is gradually increased as needed to a maximum of 45 mg tid. The most serious risk of MAO inhibitors is the occurrence of a hypertensive crisis; consequently, these drugs should be dispensed with caution in patients with hypertension and with cardiovascular or cerebrovascular disease. Patients taking these drugs should avoid foods with a high tyramine content (aged cheese, many pickled foods, chicken liver, beer, wines, yeast extract) as well as medications containing sympathomimetic agents or L-dopa (decongestants, amphetamines, caffeine) and the aforementioned serotonin agonists. The use of the MAOI (monoamine oxidase inhibitor)-B drugs for Parkinson disease (see Chap. 39) is also interdicted.

Supplementation of antidepressants with the administration of an antiepileptic medication is a popular approach with many psychiatrists. Valproate or gabapentin are used, but also used are carbamazepine or phenytoin. There are few credible studies by which to judge the value of this strategy, but these drugs may provide some additional benefit as "mood stabilizers," if only as antianxiety agents. More persuasive are the data suggesting that antiepileptic drugs are useful in treatment of the manic state.

Because many depressed patients are responsive to one of the tricyclic drugs, MAO inhibitors, or serotonin agonists but not to all of them, the clinician is greatly aided by information regarding which of these drugs has been helpful in past episodes. As mentioned, response to antidepressant drugs is not expected for several weeks. Treatment, if successful, should be continued for 6 to 9 months and generally combined with some type of psychotherapy. The premature discontinuation of medications is a major source of relapse. The dosage of medication may then be reduced slowly over a period of weeks. Rapid reduction may result in withdrawal symptoms (nausea, vomiting, malaise, and muscular pains). If depressive symptoms recur upon withdrawal, the effective dose should be gradually reinstituted. Mann (2005) provides a thorough review of the medical treatment of depression; the side effects of each are given in tabular form and adapted for Table 52-3.

Treatment of Bipolar Disease

Lithium Carbonate

This has for decades, until very recently, been the drug of choice in treating the manic phase of bipolar disease and it is useful in preventing relapses of depression in some patients. Certain of the newer antipsychotic drugs, discussed in the next chapter, have overtaken lithium for the treatment of bipolar disease, with little evidence that they are superior. During an acute manic attack, hospitalization may be required to protect the manic patient from impulsive and aggressive behavior that might cause personal and interpersonal difficulty or jeopardize a career. Haloperidol (Haldol), or one of the newer antipsychosis agents discussed in Chap. 53—or ECT if these drugs are ineffective—can be used to control the mania until lithium carbonate becomes effective, usually a matter of 4 or 5 days. The usual dosage of lithium is 1,200 to 2,400 mg daily in divided oral doses, which produces a desired serum level of 0.9 to 1.4 mEq/L. The serum level of lithium must be checked frequently, both to ensure that a therapeutic dose is being taken and to guard against toxicity (see later).

The side effects of lithium are nausea and vomiting, diarrhea (especially if the dose is increased too rapidly), a feeling of mental dullness, action tremor, weakness, ataxia, slurred speech, blurred vision, dizziness, nystagmus (especially vertical or down beating), stupor, and coma. A confusional psychosis with polymyoclonus and ataxia-simulating Creutzfeldt-Jakob disease (including periodic sharp waves in the electroencephalogram) may occur at toxic levels. In patients who do not tolerate lithium, carbamazepine, valproate, or another antiepileptic may be substituted. A combination of lithium and a tricyclic or SSRI medication at the lowest effective level has been one of the best long-term preventive therapies for bipolar disease, and the same combination is useful for patients with mixed bipolar disorder in which depressive and manic manifestations occur within a single episode of illness.

Antipsychotic Drugs and Mood Stabilizers

Perhaps the most marked change in the treatment of bipolar disease is to initiate one of the approved antipsychotic medications (quetiapine, fluoxetine) rather than lithium to bring both the depression and episodic cycling into mania under control. Failing this, a "mood stabilizing" drug such as lamotrigine or divalproex has been used. As mentioned earlier, there is scant evidence that these approaches are superior to lithium but the point to be made is that the use of conventional antidepressants is currently less popular because of the risk of worsening depression to the point of a suicidal state or of inducing mania or hypomania. Other combinations have been used such as olanzapine with a serotonergic antidepressant (e.g., fluoxetine). These are ably summarized in the review by Frye but taken together the effectiveness of these new approaches serve to emphasize the importance of proper diagnosis of bipolar disease in contrast to unipolar depression. Haloperidol may be necessary to control a dangerous manic episode while one of these newer medications becomes effective.

Electroconvulsive Therapy and Transcranial Magnetic Stimulation

What used to be called infelicitously "electroshock" therapy continues to be a highly effective treatment for severe endogenous depression and can also be used to interrupt manic episodes. The technique is relatively simple and, in properly supervised clinics, quite safe. The patient is anesthetized by an intravenous injection of a short-acting

Table 52-3

CLASSIFICATION AND SIDE EFFECTS OF ANTIDEPRESSANTS

	SIDE EFFECTS						
FUNCTIONAL CLASSIFICATION	INSOMNIA AND AGITATION	SEDATION	HYPOTENSION	ANTICHOLINERGIC EFFECTS	NAUSEA OR GASTROINTESTINAL EFFECTS	SEXUAL DYSFUNCTION	WEIGHT GAIN
Reuptake inhibitors							
Selective serotonin reuptake inhibitors (SSRIs)							
Fluoxetine	++	−/+	−/+	−/+	++	++	+
Paroxetine	++	−/+	−/+	+	++	++	+
Sertraline	++	−/+	−/+	−/+	++	++	+
Fluvoxamine	++	+	−/+	−/+	++	++	+
Citalopram	++	−/+	−/+	−/+	++	++	+
Escitalopram	++	−/+	−/+	−/+	++	++	+
Nonselective norepinephrine reuptake inhibitors							
Desipramine	+	−/+	++	+	−/+	+	+
Nortriptyline	+	+	+	+	−/+	+	+
Maprotiline	+	−/+	+	+	−/+	+	++
Mixed or dual-action reuptake inhibitors							
Older agents (TCAs)							
Amitriptyline	−/+	++	++	+++	−/+	+	++
Dothiepin	−/+	++	++	++	−/+	+	++
Imipramine	++	+	++	++	−/+	+	++
Newer agents (non-TCAs)							
Venlafaxine	++	−/+	−/+	−/+	++	++	−/+
Bupropion	++	−/+	−/+	+	+	−/+	−/+
Duloxetine	−/+	+	−/+	+	+	−/+	−/+
MAOIs							
Phenelzine	++	+	++	+	+	++	+
Tranylcypromine	++	+	++	+	+	++	+
Isocarboxazid	++	−/+	++	+	+	++	++
Selegiline	+	−/+	+	+	+	+	+
Mixed-action newer agents							
Mirtazapine	−/+	+++	+	−/+	−/+	−/+	+++
Nefazodone	−/+	++	+	+	+	−/+	+
Trazodone	−/+	+++	+	−/+	+	++	+

−, none; +, mild; ++, moderate; +++, severe; DRI, dopamine reuptake inhibitor; MAOI, monoamine oxidase inhibitor; TCA, tricyclic antidepressant.
Source: Adapted from Mann (2005).

barbiturate, benzodiazepine, or propofol, and is also medicated with a muscle relaxant (succinylcholine). In the conventional method, an electrode is placed over each temple and a current of about 400 mA and 70 to 120 V is passed between them for 0.1 to 0.5 s. The machine itself has as the essential element a large capacitor that is discharged to produce an electrographic seizure. The succinylcholine prevents strong and injurious muscle spasms. The patient is awake within 5 to 10 min and is up and about in 30 min. The mechanism by which ECT produces its effects is unknown. Treatments are usually given every other day for 6 to 14 sessions. The only absolute contraindication is the presence of increased intracranial pressure, as may occur with a neoplasm or intracranial hematoma. Whether epilepsy is precipitated or worsened by ECT is still debated. This treatment should also be used cautiously in the presence of uncontrolled systemic hypertension or with a known sensitivity to the anesthetic agents that are used as premedication, particularly malignant hyperthermia.

The major drawback of ECT is the production of a transient impairment of recent memory for the period of treatment and for the days that follow, the degree of impairment related to the number of treatments given. Placing both electrodes on the nondominant side (unilateral ECT) or using lower amounts of current and a briefer pulse rather than a sine wave produces less memory disturbance and has been adopted because it is almost as effective against the depression.

With the recognition that transcranial magnetic motor stimulation sometimes produced an elevation of mood, its use as a substitute for ECT is being introduced. The magnetic technique has the advantage of being free of any but minor physical effects, and because it produces no loss of consciousness, anesthesia and neuromuscular paralysis are not needed. Brief pulses of high-frequency stimuli are used. Few controlled studies have as yet been performed and this technique could conceivably replace ECT, but the initial sense is that it is not as effective against severe or prolonged depressions and probably not at all for catatonia.

Until the advent of the antidepressant drugs, ECT was the treatment of choice for the agitated depression of middle and late life and for catatonia. Following a course of 6 to 14 treatments, close to 90 percent of patients recovered within 2 months or less. Prior to the use of ECT, this type of depression might last for 2 years or longer before remission or suicide occurred. In cases of catatonia or severe psychotic depression most psychiatrists favor the initial use of one of the newer antipsychosis agents, followed by a trial of an antidepressant before resorting to ECT. Following ECT therapy, maintenance therapy with an antidepressant, or lithium is necessary to prevent relapse. Deep brain stimulation is under study for refractory depression.

Psychotherapy

In all patients with depression or bipolar disease, careful explanations of the patient's illness, reassurance that the illness is self-limited, and encouragement and instruction of the family are of value in helping both the patient and family to understand the illness and cope with it. At the same time, there should be vigilance for suicidality, admittedly a difficult task given its unpredictability. As a general rule, bipolar illness is best managed by a physician who is willing to follow the patient over a long period of time and who is known to the family. He should be available to reevaluate the patient on suspicion of a relapse. Although the prognosis for any individual attack is relatively good, it is wise to arrange for a plan of action that will be set in operation at the first hint of a recurrence.

Tomes have been written about various psychodynamic approaches to psychotherapy and the authors are unable to comment authoritatively on them. A structured and problem-oriented approach to psychotherapy using "cognitive-behavioral" and "interpersonal" strategies has gained considerable popularity since its introduction in the 1970s by Beck. It draws to a limited extent on psychoanalytic and other psychodynamic theories and has been used in patients with depression and in those with anxiety chronic pain, and other disorders. According to Blenkiron, cognitive-behavioral therapy is most effective in patients with mild to moderate (not chronic) depression, generalized anxiety and panic disorder, and obsessive-compulsive and phobic disorders. Essentially, in the short term, the therapist provides the patient with information on the nature of the illness, its common symptoms, and the active interventions that are to be undertaken by the patient with the aid of the therapist to alter the specific misperceptions and the dysfunctional behaviors that spring from them. In difficult chronic forms of depression, Keller and colleagues compared an antidepression drug (nefazodone), cognitive-behavioral therapy, or the combination, and found remissions in approximately 50 percent of each of the first two groups and in 85 percent of the combined treatment cohort by 12 weeks. This stands as one of the better demonstrations of the value of modern, result-oriented psychotherapy. The interested reader can find discussion of this subject in the current edition of *Kaplan and Sadock's Comprehensive Textbook of Psychiatry* (Sadock and Sadock). Noteworthy is the opinion of Gabbard that behavioral-cognitive psychotherapy has been shown to be no better or worse than other forms of psychotherapy, but it has the virtues of relative brevity, uniformity of application, and straightforwardness that avoids blaming the patient, family, environment, or other external forces.

Suicide

Some 30,000 suicides are recorded annually in the United States, and attempted suicides exceed this number by approximately 10 times. All psychiatrists agree that these are conservative figures. Suicide is the eighth leading cause of death among adults in the United States and the second leading cause among persons between the ages of 15 and 24 years, figures that emphasize the importance of recognizing depression that has a high potential for self-destruction. Every physician should be familiar with the few clues we possess to identify those patients who intend to end their lives. Some of the questions that may be broached in the interview regarding depression were listed earlier, but particularly, "Do you think of hurting yourself or taking your own life?" and the follow-through query, "Do you have a plan?" Physicians should also be aware that the majority of suicides are accomplished by taking an overdose of prescribed medications, for which reason caution needs to be exercised in their distribution and administration in depressed patients.

Some views, summarized by Mann (1998), are that suicidal intent represents a special form of depression, or an important variant of it, and that certain individuals are by nature susceptible as a result of biologic factors. In other words, suicide is not simply a cognitive response to extreme stress or despondency. There is no way for the authors to judge this view, but it seems correct and proponents have pointed to particular indices of serotonin function that differ between depressed individuals who attempt suicide and those who do not. It has also been observed that the inception of modern antidepressant medications has not greatly altered the rate of suicide among depressed patients. Bipolar illness, endogenous depression, depression resulting from a debilitating disease (particularly Huntington disease, cancer, and AIDS), pathologic grief, and depression in an alcoholic or schizophrenic, all carry the risk of suicide. In bipolar disease and endogenous depression, the risk of suicide over the lifetime of the patient is approximately 15 percent (Guze and Robins). In Robins' series of 134 patients who committed suicide, 47 percent had a known depressive illness and 25 percent were alcoholic. Other series have recorded even higher rates of depression, alcoholism, and drug abuse (see Andreasen and Black).

Most suicides are planned, not impulsive. Furthermore, the intention of committing suicide is more often than not communicated to someone significant in the patient's life. The message may be in the form of a direct verbal statement of intent, or it may be indirect, such as giving away a treasured possession or revising a will. It is known that successful suicide is three times more common in men than in women and particularly common among men older than 40 years of age. Patients with a history of suicide in either mother or father carry a higher risk than those without such a history. A previous suicide attempt adds to the risk. As alluded to earlier, important deterrents to suicide are devout Catholicism or comparable religious belief (suicide is a sin), concern about the suffering it would cause the family, and fear of death sincerely expressed by the patient. However, no single one of these attributes stands out as entirely predictive of suicide. As a consequence, one is left with clinical judgment and an index of suspicion as the main guides. The only rule of thumb is that all suicidal threats are to be taken seriously and all patients who threaten to kill themselves should be evaluated quickly by a psychiatrist.

For the depressed patient with terminal disease, the authors have taken the personal position of providing comfort by all possible means, but not in assisting the patient to commit suicide.

References

American Psychiatric Association: *Diagnostic and Statistical Manual of Mental Disorders*, 5th ed (DSM-5). Washington, DC, APA, 2013.

Amsterdam JD, Winokur G, Caroff SN, et al: The dexamethasone suppression test in outpatients with primary affective disorder and healthy control subjects. *Am J Psychiatry* 139:287, 1982.

Andreasen NC, Black DW: *Introductory Textbook of Psychiatry*, 2nd ed. Washington, DC, American Psychiatry Press, 1995.

Beck AT: *Cognitive Therapy and the Emotional Disorders*. New York, International Universities Press, 1976.

Bejjani B-P, Damier P, Arnulf I, et al: Transient acute depression induced by high-frequency deep-brain stimulation. *N Engl J Med* 340:1476, 1999.

Belmaker RH: Bipolar disorder. *N Engl J Med* 351:476, 2004.

Belmaker RH, Agam G: Major depressive disorder. *N Engl J Med* 358:55, 2008.

Blazer D, Williams CD: Epidemiology of dysphoria and depression in an elderly population. *Am J Psychiatry* 137:439, 1980.

Blenkiron P: Who is suitable for cognitive behavioural therapy. *J R Soc Med* 92:222, 1999.

Brockington I: Postpartum psychiatric disorders. *Lancet* 363:303, 2004.

Cadoret RJ: Evidence for genetic inheritance of primary affective disorder in adoptees. *Am J Psychiatry* 135:463, 1978.

Cadoret RJ, Winokur G: Depression in alcoholism. *Ann N Y Acad Sci* 233:34, 1974.

Carroll BJ, Feinberg M, Greden JF, et al: A specific laboratory test for the diagnosis of melancholia. *Arch Gen Psychiatry* 38:15, 1981.

Caspi A, Sugden K, Morritt TE, et al: Influence of life stress on depression: Moderation by a polymorphism in the 5-HTT gene. *Science* 301:386, 2003.

Cassidy WL, Flanagan NB, Spellman M, Cohen ME: Clinical observations in manic-depressive disease. *JAMA* 164:1535, 1957.

Chen B, Dowlatshahi D, MacQueen GM, et al: Increased hippocampal BDNF immunoreactivity in subjects treated with antidepressant medication. *Biol Psychiatry* 50:260, 2001.

Drevets WC: Neuroimaging and neuropathological studies of depression: Implications for the cognitive-emotional features of mood disorders. *Curr Opin Neurobiol* 11:240, 2001.

Fisher CM: Hypomanic symptoms caused by herpes simplex encephalitis. *Neurology* 47:1374, 1996.

Freud S: Mourning and melancholia, in Jones E (ed): *The Complete Psychological Works of Sigmund Freud*. Vol 14. London, Hogarth, 1957, pp 237–258.

Frye MA: Bipolar disease—A focus on depression. *N Engl J Med* 364:51, 2011.

Gabbard GD: Mood disorders: Psychodynamic aspects, in Sadock BJ, Sadock VA (eds): *Kaplan and Sadock's Comprehensive Textbook of Psychiatry*, 7th ed. Philadelphia, Lippincott Williams & Wilkins, 2000, pp 1328–1338.

Goodwin DW, Guze SB: *Psychiatric Diagnosis*, 5th ed. New York, Oxford University Press, 1996.

Guze SB, Robins E: Suicide and primary affective disorders. *Br J Psychiatry* 117:437, 1970.

Herzog J, Reiff J, Krack P, et al: Manic episode with psychotic symptoms induced by subthalamic nucleus stimulation in a patient with Parkinson's disease. *Mov Disord* 18:1382, 2003.

Hirschfeld RMA, Klerman GL, Andreasen NC, et al: Psycho-social predictors of chronicity in depressed patients. *Br J Psychiatry* 148:648, 1986.

House A, Dennis M, Warlow C, et al: Mood disorders after stroke and their relation to lesion location. *Brain* 113:1113, 1990.

Insel TR, Kalin NH, Guttmacher LB, et al: The dexamethasone suppression test in patients with primary obsessive-compulsive disorder. *Psychiatry Res* 6:153, 1982.

Keller MB, McCullough JP, Klein DN, et al: A comparison of nefazodone, the cognitive behavioral-analysis system of psychotherapy, and their combination for the treatment of chronic depression. *N Engl J Med* 342:1462, 2000.

Kline N: Practical management of depression. *JAMA* 190:732, 1964.

Kramer MS, Cutler N, Feighner J, et al: Distinct mechanisms for anti-depressant activity by blockade of central substance P receptors. *Science* 281:1640, 1998.

Kulisevsky J, Berthier ML, Gironell A, et al: Mania following deep brain stimulation for Parkinson's disease. *Neurology* 59:1421, 2002.

Levine DN, Finkelstein S: Delayed psychosis after right temporoparietal stroke or trauma. *Neurology* 32:267, 1982.

Lewis A: Melancholia: A historical review, in *The State of Psychiatry: Essays and Addresses*. New York, Science House, 1967, pp 71–110.

Lindemann E: Symptomatology and management of acute grief. *Am J Psychiatry* 101:141, 1944.

Mann JJ: The medical management of depression. *N Engl J Med* 353:1819, 2005.

Mann JJ: The neurobiology of suicide. *Nat Med* 4:25, 1998.

Mendlewicz J, Rainer JD: Adoption study supporting genetic transmission in manic-depressive illness. *Nature* 268:327, 1977.

Merikangas KE, Akisaki HS, Angst J, et al: Lifetime and 12-month prevalence of bipolar spectrum disorder in the National Comorbidity Survey replication. *Arch Gen Psychiatry* 64:543, 2007.

Ogilvie AD, Battersby S, Bubb VJ, et al: Polymorphism in serotonin transporter gene associated with susceptibility to major depression. *Lancet* 346:731, 1996.

Pirodsky DM, Cohn JS: *Clinical Primer of Psychopharmacology: A Practical Guide*, 2nd ed. New York, McGraw-Hill, 1992.

Robins E: *The Final Months: A Study of the Lives of 134 Persons Who Committed Suicide*. Oxford, UK, Oxford University Press, 1981.

Robinson RG: Mood disorders secondary to stroke. *Semin Clin Neuropsychiatry* 2:244, 1997.

Rush AJ, Trivedi MH, Wisniewski R, et al: Bupropion-SR, sertraline, or venlafaxine-XR after failure of SSRIs for depression. *N Engl J Med* 354:1231, 2006.

Ryan ND: Treatment of depression in children and adolescents. *Lancet* 366:933, 2005.

Sadock BJ, Sadock VA (eds): *Kaplan and Sadock's Comprehensive Textbook of Psychiatry*, 7th ed. Philadelphia, Lippincott Williams & Wilkins, 2000.

Sanders AR, Detera-Wadleigh SD, Gershon ES: Molecular genetics of mood disorders, in Charney DS, Nestler EJ, Bunney BS (eds): *Neurobiology of Mental Illness*. New York, Oxford University Press, 1999, pp 299–316.

Santarelli L, Saxe M, Gross C, et al: Requirement of hippocampal neurogenesis for the behavioral effects of antidepressants. *Science* 301:805, 2003.

Sapolsky RM: Glucocorticoids and hippocampal atrophy in neuropsychiatric disorders. *Arch Gen Psychiatry* 57:925, 2000.

Schlesser MA, Winokur G, Sherman BM: Hypothalamic-pituitary-adrenal axis activity in depressive illness. *Arch Gen Psychiatry* 37:737, 1980.

Starkstein SE, Fedoroff P, Berthier ML, Robinson RG: Manic-depressive and pure manic states after brain lesions. *Biol Psychiatry* 29:149, 1991.

Starkstein SE, Robinson RG, Price TR: Comparison of cortical and subcortical lesions in the production of poststroke mood disorders. *Brain* 110:1045, 1987.

Stewart DE: Depression during pregnancy. *N Engl J Med* 365:1605, 2011.

Thomson KC, Hendrie HC: Environmental stress in primary depressive illness. *Arch Gen Psychiatry* 26:130, 1972.

Winokur G: *Mania and Depression: A Classification of Syndrome and Disease*. Baltimore, MD, Johns Hopkins University Press, 1991.

Winokur G, Cadoret RJ: The irrelevance of the menopause to depressive disease, in Sachar EJ (ed): *Topics in Psychoendocrinology*. New York, Grune & Stratton, 1975, pp 59–66.

Winokur G, Coryell W, Keller M, et al: A prospective follow-up of patients with bipolar and primary unipolar affective disorder. *Arch Gen Psychiatry* 50:457, 1993.

Wishnie HA, Hackett TP, Cassem NH: Psychological hazards of convalescence following myocardial infarction. *JAMA* 215:1292, 1971.

53

Schizophrenia, Delusional and Paranoid States

SCHIZOPHRENIA

Schizophrenia is among the most serious of all unsolved diseases. This was the opinion expressed 60 years ago in *Medical Research: A Mid-Century Survey*, sponsored by the American Foundation. Because of a worldwide lifetime prevalence of approximately 0.85 percent and particularly because of its onset early in life, its chronicity, and the associated social, vocational, and personal disabilities, the same conclusion is justified today (see Carpenter and Buchanan).

Neurologists and psychiatrists currently accept the idea that schizophrenia comprises a group of closely related disorders characterized by a particular type of disordered thinking, affect, and behavior. The syndrome by which these disorders manifest themselves differs from those of delirium, confusional states, dementia, and depression in ways that will become clear in the following pages. Unfortunately, the diagnosis of schizophrenia depends on the recognition of characteristic psychologic disturbances largely unsupported by physical findings and laboratory data. This inevitably results in a certain degree of diagnostic imprecision. In other words, any group classified as schizophrenic will include patients with diseases that only resemble schizophrenia, whereas variant or incomplete cases of schizophrenia may not have been included. Moreover, there is not full agreement as to whether all the conditions that are called schizophrenic are the expression of a single disease process. In the United States, for example, *paranoid schizophrenia* is usually considered to be a subtype of the common syndrome, whereas in some parts of Europe it is thought to be a separate disease.

Historical Background

Present views of the disease now called schizophrenia originated with Emil Kraepelin, a Munich psychiatrist, who first clearly separated it from bipolar psychosis. He called it *dementia praecox* (adopting the term introduced earlier by Morel) to refer to a deterioration of mental function at an early age, from a previous level of normalcy. At first, Kraepelin believed that "catatonia" and "hebephrenia," which had previously been described by Kahlbaum and by Hecker, respectively, as well as the paranoid form of schizophrenia, were separate diseases, but later, by 1898, he had concluded that several subtypes were a single disease. He emphasized an onset in adolescence or early adult life and a chronic course, often ending in marked deterioration of personality as the defining attributes of all forms of the disease. Early in the twentieth century, the Swiss psychiatrist Eugen Bleuler substituted the term *schizophrenia* for dementia praecox. This was an improvement insofar as the term *dementia* was already being used to specify the clinical effects of another category of disease; unfortunately, however, the new name implied a "split personality" or "split mind." By the "splitting" of psychic functions, Bleuler meant the lack of correspondence between ideation and emotional display—the inappropriateness of the patient's affect in relation to his thoughts and behavior. In contrast, in bipolar disease, the patient's mood and affect accurately express his morbid thoughts. Bleuler also introduced the term *autism* ("thinking divorced from reality") as an aspect of the thought disorder.

Bleuler believed that all the schizophrenic syndromes were composed of primary or basic symptoms, summarized by subsequent authors as the "four A's" (loose *a*ssociations, flat *a*ffect, *a*mbivalence, and *a*utism) and of secondary or "partial phenomena" such as delusions, hallucinations, negativism, and stupor. However interesting this formulation proved to be, the psychologic abnormalities are so difficult to define precisely that these divisions have come to be of only mnemonic value.

Meyer, who introduced the "psychobiologic approach" to psychiatry, sought the origins of schizophrenia, as well as other psychiatric syndromes, in the personal and medical history of patients, emphasizing particularly their habitual reactions to life events. Freud viewed schizophrenia as a manifestation of a "weak ego" and an inability to control anxiety and instinctual forces—the result of a fixation of libido at an early ("narcissistic") stage of psychosexual development. None of these theories has been corroborated, and none ever gained wide acceptance.

A contemporary approach to schizophrenia, summarized below, has involved the isolation of its many pervasive mental and behavioral features into three clusters: (1) *negative symptoms* of diminished psychomotor activity (poverty of speech and spontaneous movement, flatness of affect); (2) a "disorganization" syndrome, or *thought disorder* (fragmentation of ideas, loosening of associations, tangentiality, and inappropriate emotional expression); and (3) *reality distortion*, comprising hallucinations and delusions, or positive symptoms (see Liddle). The separation of behaviors into "positive" and "negative" symptoms was believed to be useful in distinguishing among the types of schizophrenias and perhaps to align the mental status with conventional physiologic analysis, but this view is an oversimplification, as pointed out by Andreasen. Although there is disagreement as to whether each of these features is primary or secondary, positive or negative, they have the value of lending themselves to objective study.

Epidemiology

Schizophrenia has been found in every racial and social group so far studied. On average, 35 new cases per 100,000 population appear annually (Jablensky). As indicated earlier, studies of prevalence suggest that at any given time 0.85 percent of the world population is suffering from schizophrenia and expectancy rates are estimated to be as high as 1 chance in 100 that a person will manifest the condition during his or her lifetime. The incidence of schizophrenia has remained more or less the same over the past several decades. Males and females are affected with equal frequency. For unknown reasons, the incidence is higher in social classes showing high mobility and disorganization. It has been suggested that this is a by-product of "downward drift"—a result of deteriorating function in those with the disease that forces them into the lowest socioeconomic stratum where one finds poverty, crowding, limited education, and associated handicaps—and the same data have been used to support the idea that schizophrenia can be caused by such social factors.

Schizophrenic patients occupy about half the beds in mental hospitals—more hospital beds than are allocated to any other single disease—and they constitute 20 to 30 percent of all new admissions to psychiatric institutions (100,000 to 200,000 new cases per year in the United States). The age of admission generally is between 20 and 40 years, with a peak between 28 and 34 years. The economic burden created by this disease is enormous—the direct and indirect costs in the United States have been estimated to be over $50 billion.

Clinical Syndrome of Schizophrenia

The central abnormalities in schizophrenia are hallucinations and a special disorder in the perception of one's self in relation to the external world. It is unlike the condition that prevails in delirium and other confusional states, dementia, and depression. Some patients with chronic schizophrenia, before the onset of a flagrant psychosis or when in remission, show none of the usual symptoms and—during brief testing of mental status—might even pass for normal. But on longer observation, they are vague and preoccupied with their own thoughts. They seem unable to think in the abstract, to understand fully figurative statements, or are able to separate relevant from irrelevant data. There is what has been called a circumstantiality and tangentiality about their thinking and remarks. They fail to communicate their ideas clearly. Their thinking no longer respects the logical limits of time and space so that parts of ideas are confused with the whole or are clustered together or condensed in an illogical way. In an analysis of a problem or a situation, there is a tendency to be overinclusive rather than underinclusive (as happens in dementia). In conversation and in writing, the trend of an argument or thought sequence is often interrupted abruptly, with a resulting disorder of verbal communication. Such disorders of thinking are reflected in the patient's behavior. Over time there is a general deterioration in functioning, social withdrawal and bizarre actions, self-absorption, and aimlessness.

In more severely affected schizophrenic patients, thinking is even more disintegrated. They appear to be totally preoccupied with their inner psychic life (thus the early use of the term *autism*) and may do no more than utter a series of meaningless phrases or neologisms, or their speech may be reduced to a nonsensical "word salad." They are unable to attend to any task or to concentrate, and their performance is interrupted by sudden "blocking" or by insertion of some extraneous idea or inexplicable act, somewhat like that observed in a severely confused or delirious patient. At times these patients are talkative and exhibit odd behavior; at other times they are quiet and idle. In the extreme, the patients are mute or assume and maintain imposed postures or remain immobile (catalepsy). With remission, they may remember much of what has happened or may have only fragmentary memories of events that occurred.

Typical of schizophrenia is the patient's expression of remarkably unusual experiences and ideas. The patient may express the thought that his body is somehow separated from his mind, that he does not feel like himself, that his body belongs to someone else, or that he is unsure of his own identity or even sex. These experiences have been called *depersonalization*. *Thought insertion*, wherein it seems to the patient that an idea has been implanted into his mind, or *thought withdrawal*, wherein an idea has been extracted from his mind by an outside agency, are other parts of this problem. Closely related, and characteristic of schizophrenia, are ideas of being under the control of some external agency or being made to speak or act in ways that are dictated by others, often through the medium of radar, telepathy, or the Internet (*passivity feelings*). Thought projection, the notion that external elements in the environment are being controlled by the patient's mind, is similar. Frequently, there are *ideas of reference*—that the remarks or actions of others are subtly or overtly directed to the patient. Finally, the patient may feel that the world about him is changed or unnatural, or his perception of time may be altered, not in a brief episode like the *jamais vu* of a temporal lobe seizure, but continuously; this is the phenomenon of *derealization*. However, the bizarreness of these delusions, once considered a characteristic feature, has been removed from the diagnostic criteria for schizophrenia in the latest recursion of the DSM because of its nonspecificity and the difficulty determining exactly what constitutes bizarre.

Auditory hallucinations are frequent and a core feature of the classic illness. They consist of voices that comment on the patient's character and activities and are usually accusatory, threatening, or claiming control of the patient's actions. The voices may or may not be recognized; they may belong to one person or two or more persons who converse with the patient or with one another. Seldom can the voices be localized to a point outside the patient. Instead, they seem to come from within, so that they cannot be distinguished from his own feelings and thoughts. Certain somatic hallucinations and delusions may predominate in any one individual. Visual, olfactory, and other types of hallucinations also occur but are much less frequent. The patient believes in the reality of these hallucinations and often weaves them into a delusional system.

It should be reiterated here that hallucinations are a feature of a number of neurologic processes, but in most people visual hallucinations predominate, whereas auditory hallucinations are the hallmark of schizophrenia. Of interest in this regard is "The Report on the Census of Hallucinations" by Sidgwick in 1894 who suggested (as cited by Frith) that almost 1 in 10 ostensibly normal respondents has experienced hallucinations, mostly visual. The main illnesses in which hallucinations and delusions are prominent, for example, hallucinogenic drug ingestion and the Charles Bonnet syndrome (see Chap. 13), have been reviewed by Frith.

Of interest has been the belated affirmation of the importance of negative symptoms in schizophrenia. Liddle and Barnes, looking objectively at all aspects of schizophrenic thought and behavior, divided them into four groups: (1) flat affect, diminution in expressive gestures, latency of response, reduced spontaneous movements, apathy, restricted recreational activities, inability to feel intimate or close, and motor retardation; these negative symptoms, which have resemblances to frontal lobe behavioral syndromes, correlate with reduced blood flow in the frontal lobes and a poor prognosis; (2) disorganization of thought, incoherence, inappropriate affect, illogicality, bizarre behavior, aggression, agitation, and tangentiality; these abnormalities are nonfrontal; (3) hallucinations and delusions that the patient's mind is being read and that thoughts are being extracted from his mind or being controlled or broadcasted, probably related to temporal lobe function; and (4) suspicion, hostility, and delusions of reference. These authors also found that the four syndromes can coexist in various combinations. However valid such subdivisions prove to be, they direct attention to the functional anatomy and physiology of particular neuronal systems in the brain (see further on; also Friston et al).

The behavior of the schizophrenic who experiences these ideas and feelings is correspondingly altered. Early in the course of the illness, normal activities may be slowed or interrupted. No longer does the patient function properly in school or at work. Associates and relatives are likely to find the patient's complaints and ideas disturbing. The patient may be idle for long periods—preoccupied with inner ruminations—and may withdraw socially. A panic or frenzy of excitement may lead to an emergency ward visit (a high degree of anxiety occurring for the first time in a young person should always raise the suspicion of a developing schizophrenia), or the patient may become mute and immobile, i.e., *catatonic*. Attacks of catatonia are infrequent, but lack of will, drive, assertiveness, and motor activity are characteristic of the disease. Ultimately, a deteriorated and dilapidated state occurs, which in the extreme results in an unkempt and malnourished state with which the public unfortunately associates schizophrenia. Individuals of this type roam the streets and live in appalling conditions on the fringes of society where they are subject to the criminal behavior of others.

That schizophrenia of all types carries a significant risk of suicide is not widely appreciated by nonpsychiatry practitioners. In a followup study of schizophrenic and bipolar patients, Winokur and Tsuang found that in each group the proportion of patients who had committed suicide was the same (approximately 10 percent). Suicide occurs most often among young schizophrenic patients living apart from their families who are frightened and overwhelmed by their symptoms and who experience the difficulties of independent existence. Sometimes suicide is a response to terrifying and commanding vocal hallucinations. The schizophrenic patient may also be homicidal, usually acting upon a delusion that he has been wronged or is threatened by the victim. Incidents of this type are unpredictable, but the presence of escalating paranoia should be a warning.

Finally, whether a genuine dementia results from chronic schizophrenia has been much debated over the years. The notion of this type of "dementia praecox" was discarded, but clinicians continue to encounter cases of progressive generalized, and sometimes severe, intellectual impairment in both acute and long-standing cases of schizophrenia; this has been true before and after the modern era of therapeutics. The problem was highlighted by de Vries and colleagues who analyzed what they considered to be a frontotemporal type of dementia in eight patients after 9 to 30 years of schizophrenia; they found minor changes on CT scans, and frontal or temporal hypoperfusion on single-photon emission computed tomography (SPECT).

Diagnostic Criteria

Included in the early definitions of the disease, both of Kraepelin and of Bleuler, were a characteristic premorbid personality, an insidious onset of the more flagrant symptoms in adolescence or early adult life, and a chronic but fluctuating course with a tendency to progressive deterioration. Both of these early investigators regarded hallucinations and delusions as secondary symptoms that could be absent, as in their category of "simple schizophrenia." Embodied in both their definitions was the concept of disease characterized by a poor prognosis and, as stated earlier, a unique constellation of symptoms different from those of delirium, confusion, depression, mania, and dementia—the other manifestations of brain diseases. Many of their seminal ideas, including those of Schneider discussed below, have been retained but others have been discarded in various diagnostic criteria. Nonetheless, they established a lexicon for the clinical description and grading of schizophrenic disorders and all subsequent progress has been essentially to refine these ideas. For that reason, they are summarized here so that the student may appreciate the evolutionary nature of diagnostic criteria, as expressed through the DSM, currently in its fifth recursion.

Attempts to apply the early criteria initially met with difficulty, especially when hallucinations and delusions were absent. To overcome this, Schneider proposed that the distinction between primary and accessory manifestations be abandoned. He attached more importance and reliability to the occurrence of auditory hallucinations, perceptual delusions (misinterpretation of what the patient hears and feels), and disturbances of thinking (experiences of alienation and influence). This constellation of symptoms, which was more precise and easy to recognize, came to be known as *Schneider's first-rank symptoms* of active schizophrenia. The Schneider's diagnostic criteria, when applied to a group of patients admitted to the hospital with a diagnosis of schizophrenia, served to distinguish those with and those without first-rank symptoms (Taylor). Those without hallucinations, delusions, and thought control or projection responded more poorly to treatment and required a more prolonged period in the hospital and higher doses of neuroleptic drugs than did those with these features. The two groups correspond closely to two categories of schizophrenic disorders later separated by Robins and Guze on the basis of prognosis. The Schneider-positive, poor-prognosis schizophrenia (also referred to in older literature as *nuclear* or *process schizophrenia*) corresponded closely to kraepelinian schizophrenia, while many of the Schneider-negative patients with good prognosis were probably suffering from some other nonschizophrenic illness or schizophreniform illness or from bipolar disease (see Chap. 52). Having made these comments, it must be acknowledged that the newer classifications of schizophrenia gives these distinctions less credibility and points to marginal differences in outcome and responses to treatment.

Feighner and colleagues, who drew up a set of diagnostic criteria for research in the major psychiatric syndromes (which were subsequently incorporated, until recently, into successive editions of the *Diagnostic and Statistical Manual of Mental Disorders* [DSM]), stated that the diagnosis of schizophrenia is tenable only in the presence of (1) a chronic illness of at least 6 months' duration and a failure (after an acute episode) to return to the premorbid level of psychosocial adjustment, (2) delusions or hallucinations without significant confusion or disorientation (i.e., without clouding of consciousness), (3) verbal productions that are so illogical and confusing as to make communication difficult (if the patient is mute, diagnosis should be deferred), and (4) at least three of the following manifestations: (a) among adults, the lack of a partner or spouse; (b) poor premorbid social adjustment or work history; (c) family history of schizophrenia; or (d) onset of illness prior to age of 40 years. Important exclusions from certainty in the diagnosis of schizophrenia include the absence of a family history of bipolar disease, absence of an earlier illness with depressive or manic symptoms, and absence of alcoholism, drug abuse, or other organic disease.

While the Feighner criteria are so strict as to exclude certain patients with a schizophrenic illness, those patients who are included will be found to constitute a fairly homogeneous group. Morrison and colleagues, who used these criteria, noted that after a 10-year period there was practically no need to change the diagnosis to another category of mental disease; in other words, they had reliably separated schizophrenia from schizophreniform psychosis (in which only the acute delusional-hallucinatory syndrome was present), and from bipolar psychosis.

The newer diagnostic criteria are no less refined but achieve clarity by stating that a patient must have at least one of the symptoms of delusions, hallucinations, and disorganized speech (not thinking). Also updated in DSM-5 is the removal of the necessity for delusions to be "bizarre" and for there to be what were in the past termed Schneiderian first-rank symptoms, namely an auditory experience of two or more voices conversing.

Subtypes of Schizophrenia

Psychiatrists had traditionally distinguished a number of subtypes of schizophrenia, although the usefulness of these distinctions has been questioned in recent years and the newest edition of DSM-5 eliminates them entirely because they have proved to have limited clinical and therapeutic importance. Indeed, the various types may overlap or change during the course of the illness. And there are many cases that do not conform entirely to the conventional subtypes or display characteristics of more than one type (referred to as *undifferentiated* or mixed types). They are briefly reviewed here for their historical interest and because their elimination in modern work signals a willingness of the field to move ahead with classification of mental disease on the basis of demonstrated biologic and therapeutic distinctions. However, they do allow an explication the more interesting symptoms and signs of schizophrenia that while entirely descriptive, are instructive and retain clinical interest.

In *simple schizophrenia*, the least florid form, the patient exhibits thought disorder, bland affect, social withdrawal, and reduction in speech and movement, all of which impair work performance. Poverty of psychomotor activity is the dominant feature and hallucinations and delusions are absent. These patients may attract notice in middle and high school because they behave in an odd manner, tending to remain by themselves ("loners"), making no effort to adjust to a social group at school or to find work, have dates, or later, to establish a family.

Catatonic schizophrenia is still the most readily identifiable type because of the striking syndrome of catatonia, and while still distinctive when seen, it is now, for unclear reasons found to be quite infrequent. In most cases the onset is relatively acute. In others, after a long prodrome of slackening interest, apathy, and dreamy preoccupation, a state of dull stupor supervenes, with mutism, inactivity, refusal of food, and a tendency to maintain one position "like a mummy" (*catalepsy*). Like other forms of catatonia, this type of schizophrenia was the one most characterized by the retention of a posture: if a limb is lifted by the examiner, it will be held in that position for hours (*flexibilitas cerea*). The patient may require tube-feeding (or will eat mechanically) and has to be dressed and undressed. Pinprick or pinch induces no reaction. Extreme "negativism," every command being resisted, characterizes some cases. Yet these patients may be fully aware of what is said to them or happening around them and will reproduce much of this information during a later spontaneous remission or one induced by intravenous sodium amytal or midazolam. Even if untreated, the patient, after weeks or months in this state, begins to talk and act more normally and there is then rapid recovery. In certain phases of catatonia there may be a period of excitement and impulsivity, during which the patient may be suicidal or homicidal. Catatonia is currently recognized to be a feature of other mental illnesses and is more frequent in severe involutional depression than in schizophrenia (see Chap. 17)

Disorganized, or *hebephrenic, schizophrenia* was believed by Kraepelin to be a particularly malignant form of the disease. It tended to occur at an earlier age than the other varieties, hence the prefix *hebe* ("youth"). The thought disorder is pronounced—there is a striking incoherence of ideas and a grossly inappropriate affect; the frequent occurrence of hallucinations and delusions leaves little doubt that the patient is psychotic. Kraepelin remarked on the changeable, fantastic, and bizarre character of the delusions. Motor symptoms, in the form of grimacing, stereotyped mannerisms, and other oddities of behavior, are prominent. In hebephrenic patients, since early life, there is likely to have been a history of tantrums and of being overly pious, shy, fearful, solitary, conscientious, and idealistic—traits that may have marked these individuals as odd. This latter state corresponds to what was referred to earlier on as a *schizoid personality* but could just as well represent the early phase of the disease itself (see Chap. 51).

Paranoid schizophrenia is still one of the most frequent and well-circumscribed types, even if now unattached from schizophrenia in the DSM-5 diagnostic criteria. The mean age of onset is in the early forties, much later than that of the preceding types (Winokur). The central feature is the preoccupation with one or more delusions related to a single or to a limited ensemble of themes, accompanied by auditory hallucinations. More often than not, the delusional hallucinatory content is persecutory, but it may also be religious, depressive, grandiose, or bizarrely hypochondriacal in nature. Delusional jealousy may be added. Many such patients settle into a chronic hallucinatory psychosis with disorders of thinking featuring mistrust and suspiciousness. They appear cold, aloof, and indifferent. Some European psychiatrists, impressed with the lack of schizoid traits in the premorbid period and late onset, insisted that paranoid schizophrenia is a separate disease. The studies of Rosenthal and colleagues and the clinical and family studies of Winokur tend to bear them out in that simple, catatonic, and hebephrenic types have different characteristics from paranoid schizophrenia. Therefore, modern classifications consider it to not be aligned with schizophrenia and instead to characterize an isolated paranoid-delusional disorder described in a later section. There is, in addition, a special form of *delusional disorder* in which the individual is consumed by a single persecutory, grandiose, or amorous delusional system without any other disorder of thinking. An exotic form is known as *folie à deux*, in which two closely related persons share a delusional system. These types of delusions are discussed further on in this chapter.

Course of Schizophrenia

Some schizophrenic patients are subject to periodic exacerbations of their illness, sometimes at regular intervals, as if the process was a metabolic disorder. Remissions that allow some degree of functioning in society are more frequent and lasting when medication is given and prolonged institutionalization is avoided. A small proportion of patients (approximately 10 percent), after an acute schizophrenic episode, have a long-lasting and fairly complete remission before lapsing into a chronic form of the illness. Unfortunately, these latter patients, at the time of their acute psychosis, cannot be distinguished from those few who will have a permanent remission.

Modern therapeutic programs have vastly reduced the number of patients in mental hospitals. However, readmission rates have also risen (revolving-door phenomenon) and the total number of very young and very old patients in hospitals has even increased slightly. The life expectancy of schizophrenic patients is somewhat reduced, possibly because of the malnutrition, neglect, and exposure to infections that occur in some public institutions and from living on the streets or in marginal circumstances. Most of these aspects of the disease were elucidated many decades ago by Langfeldt (1937 and 1969).

Neurologic and Neuropsychologic Abnormalities in Schizophrenia

The early findings of Kraepelin and of Bleuler, that many schizophrenic patients will, on detailed examination, show some neurologic abnormalities, have been substantiated by Stevens, Kennard, Hertzig and Birch, Tucker and colleagues, and Woods. They all found a much higher frequency of "soft neurologic signs" in schizophrenic patients than they did in a healthy population. The signs to which they refer include impersistence in assigned motor and mental tasks, astereognosis and graphesthesia, sensory extinction, hyperreflexia and hyporeflexia, slight tendency to grasping, mild impairment of coordination and disturbances of balance, abnormal (choreiform) movements, abnormalities of motor activity, adventitious and overflow movements, anisocoria, slight esotropia, and faults in visual auditory integration. Signs of this type were noted in 50 percent of patients and correlated with the degree of cognitive disorder. Also evident in about half of schizophrenic patients are subtle defects in ocular tracking movements (Levin et al). These take the form mainly of slowed smooth pursuit and intrusions of saccades during pursuit; some relatives of schizophrenic patients also show these eye signs when carefully tested. In contrast, "hard neurologic signs" (such as unilateral motor or sensory defects) are not seen unless they are the result of an engrafted neurologic disease. Electroencephalographic (EEG) abnormalities have been detected in about one-third of patients, but are generally minor; their meaning is uncertain, especially if they have occurred after long-standing treatment. When these were the focus of research in the past, they were more frequent in the group of schizophrenic patients who had a positive family history and in those with enlarged ventricles (Murray et al).

Sophisticated psychometric testing has disclosed abnormalities not so much in intelligence and memory (which are slightly reduced in 20 to 30 percent of cases) as in other psychologic functions. Alertness is not impaired, but the ability to maintain attention, as measured by continuous performance tasks, is reduced (Seidman). In tests of verbal and visual pattern learning, problem solving, and memorizing, Cutting found a surprising degree of impairment in both acute and chronic schizophrenic patients that was not attributable to previous treatment. In the acute schizophrenic patient, verbal memory was more affected than visual pattern memory, in agreement with the findings of Flor-Henry that left-hemispheric functions are more reduced than right-hemispheric ones. Yet, in the chronic schizophrenic, there is usually evidence of bihemispheric impairment.

Theories of Causation and Mechanism

Although there is no agreement as to the cause of the disease, an increasing weight of evidence favors an interaction between a genetic predisposition and one or more early developmental events. One widely held hypothesis is that this disease reflects an underlying developmental disorder, determined either genetically or because of an environmental insult, leading to abnormalities of synaptic connectivity, prominently affecting the hippocampus and prefrontal cortex. The evidence supporting this view is summarized briefly later. More detailed analysis of potential causes that can be given here are found in reviews of Waddington, Carpenter and Buchanan, Harrison, Pearlson, and Freedman.

Genetic Factors

Several authors have estimated that genetic factors can account for upward of 80 percent of the risk of developing schizophrenia, more than for any other mental illness. The early studies of Kallmann showed that the frequency of disease in 5,000 siblings of schizophrenic patients was 11 percent, in contrast to slightly less than 1 percent in the general population. In 90 sets of fraternal twins of whom one had schizophrenia, the incidence of disease in the other twin was also 11 percent, the same as in nontwin siblings; however, in 62 sets of monozygotic twins, the incidence in the second twin was 68 percent. The risk that a child of a schizophrenic parent will develop schizophrenia is the same as that for the sibling of a schizophrenic patient (i.e., 11 percent); if one sibling and one parent have schizophrenia, the risk is 17 percent. If both parents are schizophrenic the chances are 46 percent that the child will have the disease. Subsequent family and twin studies have repeatedly confirmed these findings (see Goodwin and Guze for a more complete tabulation). It is noteworthy, however, that the penetrance of this trait appears to be less than it is for bipolar disease and that genetic factors seem to play a larger role in patients whose illness manifests itself in teenage years.

Although the importance of genetic factors in the etiology of schizophrenia is undeniable, a mendelian pattern of inheritance has not been determined. Within the last several years, polymorphisms in several genes have been implicated as risk factors for schizophrenia. Such genes include those expressing neuregulin, dysbindin, COMT (catechol *O*-methyltransferase), proline dehydrogenase, and DISC1 ("disrupted in schizophrenia 1"). The most provocative sites, however, have rare alleles been in genes that also are overrepresented in autism—*NRXN1*, *SHANK3*, *CNTNAP2*, and *PRODH*, as summarized by McLellan and King. No single mutation accounts for more than perhaps 1 percent of cases but collectively, they seem to be associated with a fair proportion of cases of schizophrenia. There are also a copy number variations at particular genetic "hotspots" that occur in schizophrenia, autism, and other developmental disorders. What has merged from large population studies using genome-wide array screening, is that there are not likely to be common risk variants for schizophrenia (or any other psychiatric disease). Instead, the cumulative contribution of many small variants, each with a minor effect, could best account for the inherited aspects of these disorders. It should be pointed out that many of the polymorphisms mentioned seem to be of recent evolutionary origin or have a substantial rate of arising de novo.

The studies implicating these genes must further be interpreted cautiously because the functional significance, if any, of the allelic variants are not defined. Nonetheless, considered together, they point to disorders both of neuronal development and neurotransmission. Further supporting this view is the provocative finding that allelic variants associated with specific neurotransmitter systems or in developmental guidance are overrepresented in schizophrenia; these findings are more compelling than the aforementioned ones because the genetic variants have well-defined functional consequences.

Environmental and Developmental Factors

There continues to be debate concerning the relative importance of genetic versus environmental factors in the causation of the disease. The lack of complete concordance between monozygotic twins and the fact that approximately 80 percent of schizophrenic patients have no other family members with the disease, indicate that factors other than genetic ones probably play a role.

Some of these appear to be early events that occur *in utero* or infancy and alter normal developmental programs of brain structure.

The neuropsychiatric literature contains tentative and only circumstantial evidence that schizophrenia is associated with overt brain injury during the intrauterine or neonatal period, but there is reportedly an increased incidence of obstetric complications during the gestational period and birth of schizophrenic patients. Also consistent with an early adverse environmental factor is the observation by several groups that in the northern latitudes, more schizophrenic persons are born in the winter months and to women who were exposed to influenza during midpregnancy—inviting speculation that a viral infection may have damaged the fetal brain. Mortensen and colleagues found that being born in an urban region, particularly in February or March, carried with it a higher risk for developing the disease than having an affected parent or sibling. They suggested that these inexplicable demographic features accounted for more cases than did inheritance. Among 5,362 infants who were followed prospectively since their birth in 1946 by Jones and colleagues, the 30 individuals who later developed schizophrenia had been delayed in the attainment of motor milestones and speech and exhibited greater social withdrawal and schoolroom anxiety as well as lower scholastic achievement. Thus it appears that schizophrenic patients are not entirely normal in early childhood, but whether their abnormalities are already early manifestations of schizophrenia or risk factors for the disease has not been determined.

Neuropathologic, Brain Imaging, and Neurophysiologic Findings

Notably lacking in all the previously described reports of developmental changes are neuropathologic data. Dunlap, in 1928, in a critical analysis, repudiated all earlier interpretations of cellular alterations that had been reported in the brains of schizophrenic patients. He pointed out that many of them, such as dark "sclerotic" nerve cells, were artifacts and that the presence of lipofuscin was a nonspecific age change. He also asserted that the neuronal loss described by Alzheimer was based on impression and could not be corroborated by quantitative methods. Similarly, the claim of Oscar Vogt of neuronal loss in the cortex was rejected by his contemporaries, Spielmeyer and Scholz, who were unable to find any consistent cellular abnormality in schizophrenia. Spielmeyer, in a critical study of the problem in 1930, concluded that such changes as had been described up to that time could not be clearly distinguished from the normal, and that the more marked changes in some cases were due to coincidental causes. Corsellis, on the basis of yet another thorough review of the neuropathologic data in 1976, found no reason to deviate from Spielmeyer's view. The uncertain neuropathologic findings were responsible for the enigmatic categorization of schizophrenia as a "functional" disorder, i.e., a disorder with no structural basis.

Nonetheless, there has been a general sense that while the number of neurons in the gray matter is normal, the pyramidal cells are smaller and more densely packed, resulting in a thinning of laminae II and III. These cytoarchitectonic changes have been the most difficult to interpret and to confirm. Capricious methods such as the rapid Golgi stain indicate that density of dendritic spines is decreased in the frontal and temporal cortex of chronic schizophrenic patients.

A number of more contemporary reports using special cell-labeling studies have found cytoarchitectonic abnormalities in the brains of schizophrenic patients. For example, Akbarian and colleagues, following previous similar findings, have described an aberrant distribution of interstitial neurons in the frontal lobe white matter. These cells have their origin in the embryologic subplate that guides neuronal migration, and the inference is that the abnormally migrating cells have formed aberrant neuronal connections. Benes and colleagues observed that the number of small neurons was reduced in at least one layer (usually layer II) of the anterior cingulate cortex. These are gamma-aminobutyric acid (GABA)–releasing (inhibitory) neurons. Benes also noted that the arrays of macrocolumns of cortical neurons were smaller in the occipital lobes (vertical axons increased in number). Newer studies also describe a paucity of gabanergic, inhibitory interneurons (so-called chandelier cells) in the prefrontal cortex (Woo et al). These observations suggest a developmental rather than an acquired lesion. The absence of gliosis supports but does not prove that the developmental disorder occurs prenatally.

The advent of CT and subsequently of MRI of the brain provided a new stimulus to the anatomic study of schizophrenia. Johnstone and coworkers were the first to describe ventricular enlargement and sulcal widening in 18 patients and correlate these findings with dulling of intellect and affect. In a study of 58 chronic schizophrenics younger than age 50 years, Weinberger and colleagues (1979) found enlargement of the lateral ventricles in 40 percent. In 9 of 11 CT studies, the third ventricle was found to be enlarged, and in 14 of 17 the sulci were widened. In 15 pairs of monozygotic twins, one of whom had schizophrenia, the anterior hippocampi were found to be smaller and the lateral and third ventricles larger in the affected twin (Suddath et al). Shenton and colleagues demonstrated a reduction in the volume of gray matter in the posterior part of the left superior temporal gyrus, which includes Heschl gyri and the planum temporale. The degree of volumetric reduction correlated roughly with the severity of the thought disorder. A reduction in volume of the superior temporal gyrus has also been associated with the occurrence of auditory hallucinations (Barta et al). Other MRI studies have shown a volumetric change in the gray matter of the left hippocampus, parahippocampal gyrus, and amygdala (in right-handed patients). Equally compelling is the finding that young individuals having two or more relatives with the disease, and therefore being at risk for developing schizophrenia, have certain volumetric brain changes detected by imaging studies (Lawrie et al). In unaffected relatives, the left hippocampal–amygdaloid region was smaller than in healthy people, but slightly larger than in affected relatives.

In an attempt to organize the neuroradiologic findings, Murray and coworkers raised the possibility that there are two types of this disease: one with ventricular enlargement and a negative family history and the other with normal ventricles and a positive family history. In the first group of sporadic, "acquired" schizophrenia, environmental factors, such as birth injury and EEG abnormalities (see later), were considered to be more frequent. In summarizing the many cerebral changes observed in schizophrenic patients, Harrison concluded that several are quite consistent. These include mild enlargement of the lateral and third ventricles; decreased cortical volume, perhaps disproportionate in the temporal lobe; microscopically, diminution in size of cortical and hippocampal neurons; a diminished number of neurons in the dorsal thalamus; and a notable absence of gliosis.

EEG data, for the most part not useful, were alluded to earlier. Detailed neuropsychologic testing has disclosed deficits in attention and abnormalities of the P300 waves (cortical "event-related" potentials). These deficits correlate with reduced cognitive activation activity in functional MRI. It is unclear, however, if these changes represent primary defects or are secondary to an inherent lack of motivation.

Attention has also been drawn to the regional alterations of cerebral blood flow in chronic stable schizophrenic patients, as revealed by positron emission tomography (PET) and functional MRI. Weinberger and colleagues (1986) and Liddle and Barnes have reported a decrease in blood flow in the prefrontal areas during cognitive performances. Friston and associates found consistent abnormalities in the left parahippocampal region in all forms of chronic schizophrenia. Studies of regional glucose metabolism and postmortem norepinephrine measurements have yielded equivocal data, although most patients show a reduction in glucose metabolism in the thalamus and frontal cortex. Several lines of investigation point to the medial part of the left temporal lobe and related limbic and frontal systems as being the focus of a developmental abnormality (see Tsuang et al and Friston et al for pertinent references). According to Sabri and colleagues, the inconsistent findings on functional imaging may be accounted for by correlations between certain blood flow patterns and specific symptoms. For example, the formal thought disorder corresponded to increased flow in the frontal and temporal regions, whereas delusions and hallucinations were associated with reduced flow in the cingulate, left frontal, and temporal areas. Our colleague Silbersweig and his coworkers have performed PET studies in schizophrenic patients while they were experiencing auditory hallucinations and found increased blood flow mainly in both thalami, left hippocampus, and right striatum, but also in the parahippocampal, orbitofrontal, and cingulate areas. One of their drug-naive patients with visual and auditory hallucinations showed activation in these regions.

Alterations in Neurotransmitters

When certain hallucinogens, such as mescaline and lysergic acid diethylamide (LSD), were first observed to induce hallucinations and abnormalities of thinking, it was hoped that they might provide experimental models of schizophrenia. This hope was never realized but there are instances, difficult to interpret, in which these drugs have induced a prolonged relapse in a schizophrenic patient. Similarly, when methionine, a potent source of methyl groups, was observed to exacerbate the symptoms of some schizophrenic patients, it was thought that a primary metabolic fault had been discovered; increased serum concentrations of dimethoxyphenylethylamine and *N*-methylated indoleamines lent support to this idea. Again, none of these observations has been unequivocally corroborated.

The formerly leading *biochemical hypothesis* is based on the response of psychotic symptoms to phenothiazine and related medications, which implicates the dopaminergic system of the temporal lobe (see review by Carlsson). The evidence for this is circumstantial but is supported by observations that antipsychotic drugs reduce the electrical activity of mesolimbic dopaminergic neurons in experimental models. Furthermore, there have been several demonstrations of increased concentrations of dopamine or its metabolite, homovanillic acid, in schizophrenic brains obtained at autopsy. The finding that dopamine receptors are organized in two systems, one limbic and the other cortical, has led to an expanded but speculative hypothesis that an excess of dopaminergic activity in the mesolimbic system gives rise to the positive symptoms of schizophrenia—i.e., psychosis—whereas a diminished activity in the mesocortical system accounts for the negative symptoms. The involvement of the mesolimbic system, which plays a role in attention, has prompted further speculation that the thought disorder of schizophrenia is attributable to a breakdown of the normal "filtering" of stimuli reaching cognition. As mentioned earlier, it has been found that a variant in the gene for COMT that enhances metabolism of dopamine is overrepresented in schizophrenia, further incriminating a disorder of dopaminergic neurotransmission in the pathophysiology of this disease (Egan et al).

As pointed out in the review by Freedman, however, the dopamine hypothesis has many weaknesses, the most prominent of which is the relative ineffectiveness of dopamine-blocking drugs in alleviating many aspects of the disease. The complexity of dopamine systems and their interaction with other neurotransmitter circuits make a simplistic mechanism unlikely.

More recently, a hypothesis based on changes in the serotoninergic system was proposed. As with the dopaminergic model, attention was drawn to mechanisms relating to a new class of antipsychotics (clozapine, risperidone), which have major effects on the serotonin system and were found to ameliorate the psychosis. Several groups have reported alterations in serotonin receptors in the brains of schizophrenic patients (see later). A further connection is based on the finding by Williams and colleagues of an allelic variation in the gene on chromosome 13 encoding for a serotonin receptor (5-HT_{2A}) that confers a susceptibility to schizophrenia. The variation in this gene is insufficient to explain the presence of the disease in any one individual, if for no other reason than that many patients who are homozygous for the suspect allele do not develop schizophrenia. Perhaps a nearby region relating to the receptor may be at fault through linkage disequilibrium (see commentary by Harrison and Geddes). A third currently favored biochemical hypothesis derives from the psychosis syndrome produced by chronic ingestion of phencyclidine (PCP), an *N*-methyl-D-aspartate (NMDA) antagonist. This implicates the glutaminergic system, but it must be pointed out that the dopaminergic and glutaminergic systems converge on certain cortical neurons and that glutaminergic release is modulated in several places in the brain by dopamine.

A great variety of physiologic and endocrine differences between schizophrenic and healthy subjects have been claimed. None has proved to be significant. Because psychoses may complicate corticosteroid administration and certain endocrine disorders (Cushing syndrome, thyrotoxicosis, see later), there have been many attempts to uncover such abnormalities in the schizophrenic patient. All have failed.

Psychosocial Hypotheses

The notion that psychosocial factors play an important role in the genesis of schizophrenia was a recurrent theme in older psychiatric writings, but is now given little credence. Prominent in these early writings was Freud's view that the schizophrenic process represents a fixation at an early autoerotic stage of sexual development. There is no way of affirming or refuting this proposition. The same can be said for the many suggestions that disturbed intrafamily relationships engender schizophrenic traits or possibly provoke psychosis in persons who are genetically vulnerable. Behind all these suggestions was the notion that disturbed interpersonal relations in the family in some way interfered with the normal maturation of personality. The extent to which these aberrations of family relationships are primary or secondary cannot be ascertained.

The often-cited observations of Harlow on the deleterious effects of maternal and peer deprivation in primates opened the possibility that similar deprivations in humans may be responsible for the development of schizophrenia. However, such severe degrees of familial deprivation have rarely been documented in humans and when they were, as in some orphans, the effects were only transitory.

Differential Diagnosis

From a neurologic standpoint, the main initial distinction to be made is between an acute schizophrenia-like psychosis and the chronic disease, schizophrenia. The *acute schizophreniform illness* takes the form of a delusional-hallucinatory syndrome in which there is little if any disturbance of consciousness. Although such a syndrome is characteristic of schizophrenia, it may occur in the manic phase of bipolar disease, encephalitis, temporal lobe epilepsy, chronic amphetamine intoxication, withdrawal from alcohol after a sustained period of intoxication, and most often in the emergency department, from PCP, angel dust, LSD, and other drug intoxications. On rare occasions it is seen with postpartum psychosis (see further on) and with certain endocrine and metabolic disorders in which consciousness is not impaired. Thus whenever this syndrome is recognized, these several causes need to be differentiated. On our services, less than one of five of the acute schizophreniform psychoses has proved to be a result of the disease schizophrenia. This distinction is made by the premorbid history and the course of the illness. If the patient had been reclusive, withdrawn, and socially maladapted and does not seem to recover fully from the acute psychosis, then the diagnosis of schizophrenia is more likely. Lacking these features, and in particular with a full remission, one assumes the occurrence of hypomania or of a toxic-metabolic psychosis, which can be detected by laboratory screening for drugs and endocrine diseases. Only 10 percent of patients with classic schizophrenia will have such an acute episode. Adherence to the criteria enumerated earlier, particularly to those devised by Feighner and colleagues will avoid most errors in diagnosis.

It is the present authors' opinion that the status of acute schizophrenia and of the so-called schizothymic and schizoaffective states brings to light a crucial nosologic problem. Is the traditional separation of depressive disease, bipolar disease, and schizophrenia biologically sound? The suggestion is that they are linked in some way by these transitional forms. Neurologists should keep an open mind about these and other theoretical problems that lack a firm genetic and neuropathologic basis.

In addition to the acute schizophreniform psychosis described earlier, the authors have encountered the greatest difficulties in the diagnosis of schizophrenia in the following clinical situations:

1. A patient with a healthy family and premorbid history *with an acute illness* having many of the typical features of schizophrenia but *associated with confusion, forgetfulness*, and/or *clouding of consciousness*. Mood change may be prominent. Thus the illness combines the features of an affective disorder, schizophrenia, and a confusional state. This syndrome is characteristic of chronic hallucinogenic drug use, particularly phencyclidine intoxication, corticosteroid psychosis (drug-induced or Cushing disease), thyrotoxic psychosis, and puerperal psychosis. Usually recovery is complete, and schizophrenia is excluded by the fact that the patient remains well. This may be a form of "schizoaffective" disorder.
2. *Adolescents and young adults whose social relationships are disorganized* and who are unusually sensitive, resentful, rebellious, fearful, discouraged, in trouble with school authorities and the law, and using drugs. The latter may have caused seizures, hallucinations, and withdrawal symptoms or may have resulted in addiction. Such patients are usually classified as having a borderline personality or "sociopathy" that appears to go back several years. These types of personality disorders and social maladjustments turn out not to be schizophrenia.
3. There is another related type of diagnostic problem, arising in *an individual who has been only marginally competent because of personality problems and many*

vague neurotic and hypochondriacal symptoms, often requiring prolonged psychotherapy. Many such individuals will indeed be found to have simple schizophrenia (so-called pseudoneurotic form). Here errors in diagnosis usually result from a failure to assess mental status carefully and to ascertain the life profile of the disorder.

4. *In a chronic delusional-hallucinatory state in a chronic alcoholic patient* (chronic alcoholic hallucinosis) it will usually be disclosed that the illness began when alcohol was withdrawn, after a period of sustained drinking, and at first took the form of an acute auditory hallucinosis characterized by threatening, exteriorized auditory hallucinations to which the patient's emotional reaction was appropriate. Only later do a few of these patients drift into a quiet hallucinatory, mildly paranoid state, with rather bland affect. Evidence of the prepsychotic schizoid personality cannot be detected and there is usually no family history of schizophrenia. Cases of this type with which we are familiar had their onset between 45 and 50 years of age, i.e., much later than the usual age of onset of schizophrenia.
5. *A patient who is confused or stuporous and seemingly catatonic-negativistic, refusing or unable to speak, to execute commands, or to be activated in any way*. If signs of focal cerebral or brainstem disease are absent, one is tempted to make a diagnosis of catatonic schizophrenia, not appreciating that *catatonia as a phenomenon* may be indistinguishable from akinetic mutism (see Chap. 17). It may also appear with widespread disease of the associational cortices and as mentioned earlier, with severe depression, certain confusional states, and hysteria. The authors have seen cases of hypoxic and other metabolic encephalopathies, Schilder disease, certain storage diseases, and Creutzfeldt-Jakob disease mistaken for schizophrenia because of failure to adhere to this principle.
6. *A patient with temporal lobe epilepsy* who, apart from intermittent psychomotor seizures, has long periods (weeks or months) of hallucinations, delusions, bizarre behavior, and disorganization of thinking. Such a mental disturbance reflects the presence of a persistent state of temporal lobe seizures (temporal lobe status epilepticus), which in some cases has been demonstrated by depth electrodes to originate in the amygdaloid or other medial temporal areas. The nature of the disturbances of emotionality and mentation in such patients, a somewhat controversial subject, is discussed in Chaps. 16 and 25.
7. *Schizophrenic patients with prominent depressive symptoms who have made repeated suicide attempts* pose an exceptionally difficult problem. They were referred to in the past as *schizothymic* and to this day it is not certain whether they have schizophrenia, a chronic depressive illness (dysthymia), or both ("schizoaffective"). When in remission, patients with affective disorders are usually normal, whereas those with schizophrenia are not.
8. *One should always be hesitant to make the diagnosis of schizophrenia during childhood*, although such a diagnosis has been entertained in children who have a variety of developmental and adjustment problems and who at some time become psychotic, i.e., they become excited, depressed, or hallucinatory and express bizarre ideas. There is no evidence that such children go on to have schizophrenia later in life. And although what are thought to be "schizoid" traits may be recognized in childhood, a frank psychosis is hardly ever recorded at this age. Of particular importance in such children is to exclude the presence of metabolic errors, mental retardation, or an early-onset depressive illness. Similarly, childhood autism and particularly its milder forms, such as Asperger syndrome discussed in Chap. 38, should not be confused with schizophrenia. That the incidence of schizophrenia is not increased in the families of autistic children supports the idea that the two are separate diseases.
9. The special problem of *mania that manifests for the first time as a confusional-encephalopathic state* was discussed in Chap. 52.

Treatment

The aims of treatment are to suppress psychotic symptoms, ameliorate the disorder of thinking and the apathetic state, prevent relapse, and optimize social adjustment. It is often possible, once the diagnosis of schizophrenia is established and the optimal regimen of medication decided upon, for a general physician to share the responsibility for following the patient with a psychiatric social worker or nurse. The physician soon becomes accustomed to the particular pattern of the patient's psychotic behavior and can help support the patient and his family during difficult periods. Relapse with psychotic decompensation demands drug therapy, and if there is a hazard of injury or suicide or difficulty in management at home, hospitalization becomes necessary. Many general hospitals and specialized psychiatric institutions have facilities for the management of such patients; state hospitals and other institutions are able to provide long-term treatment. The aim of hospitalization is to protect the patient, relieve the family of the need for constant vigilance and supervision, and ensure the administration of drugs until the exacerbation spends itself. Later, instead of mere custodial care, the patient needs a supervised program of planned activities, vocational and milieu therapy, often in a "halfway house," which involves the patient as a contributing member during the more chronic phases of the disease. If medication is successful in preventing progressive decompensation, the patient can many times return to the family and community. It is invaluable to have a competent social worker or nurse maintain frequent contact with the patient and his family and ensure continuity of medication.

The modern era of treatment of schizophrenia began in 1952, with the incidental demonstration by the French surgeon Henri Laborit of the antipsychosis properties of chlorpromazine. Subsequently, a large number of other phenothiazines have been used to treat chronic and acute psychosis. Treatment consists essentially of the administration of one of several similar antipsychotic medications. The various classes of antipsychotic drugs, their mode of action, and neurologic ("neuroleptic") side effects are discussed in Chap. 43.

The newer, second generation of "atypical" nonphenothiazine antipsychosis drugs that have complex effects on the dopamine and serotonin systems are now used in preference to the standard dopamine antagonists, the phenothiazines and the butyrophenones. They are "atypical" in that their extrapyramidal side effects are far less than that for the phenothiazines. They all serve to calm the patient, blunt emotional responses, and reduce hallucinosis and aggressive and impulsive behavior, leaving cognitive functions relatively intact. The main side effects, pertaining mostly to the phenothiazine group, are summarized in Table 53-1 and in Chap. 43 (see also the review by Freedman and the chapter by Baldessarini). The antipsychotic action of these drugs is more impressive in the short and intermediate term than over the long term, although some data suggest that they are also of value in preventing relapses. Negative symptoms (apathy and withdrawal) respond less well than positive ones, and it is generally acknowledged that 10 to 20 percent of patients respond little or not at all to medication.

Clozapine, olanzapine, risperidone, quetiapine, and others listed in Table 53-2 are the more recently introduced atypical drugs with incompletely defined pharmacologic properties but with narrower affinities for certain receptors. In addition to their reduced motor side effects, they produce clinical improvement in about half of patients who have proved to be unresponsive to other antipsychotic medications. These drugs bind to and inhibit serotonin receptors and, to some extent, to dopamine receptors (Meltzer and Nash), but have a much lower affinity for striatal dopamine receptors, thus providing a major advantage—the absence of immediate or tardive extrapyramidal side effects. This has led most psychiatrists to use one of the newer drugs, rather than the phenothiazines, as a first choice. The addition of a second drug, specifically combining clozapine with risperidone was not found to be useful in the trial conducted by Honer and colleagues. Moreover, in another one of the effectiveness trials sponsored by the National Institutes of Mental Health, Lieberman and colleagues ("CATIE" Investigators) found that the majority of chronic schizophrenics discontinued their antipsychosis drugs within 18 months. Among the medications they compared, olanzapine was slightly more effective than quetiapine, risperidone, and ziprasidone; of equal interest, the phenothiazine perphenazine was equivalent in efficacy and tolerability to the last three second-generation (atypical) drugs. Approximately 1 percent of patients treated with one of the most effective drugs, clozapine, develop leukopenia, which may prove fatal; there is less risk with the

Table 53-1

EXTRAPYRAMIDAL SYNDROMES ASSOCIATED WITH TYPICAL NEUROLEPTIC-ANTIPSYCHOTIC AGENTS

REACTION	FEATURES	MAXIMUM RISK	PROPOSED MECHANISMS	TREATMENTS
Acute dystonias	Muscle spasms; tongue, face, neck, back; terrifying; rarely fatal from asphyxia	1–5 d or with each injection of decanoates	Dopamine excess?	Injected antiparkinsonism agents, then oral
Parkinsonism	Bradykinesia, rigidity, variable tremor, mask facies, shuffling gait	Evolves slowly in 1–4 wk, often persists	Dopaminergic deficiency	Oral anticholinergics, amantadine; dopaminergics are too risky
Malignant syndrome	Catatonia, stupor, fever, unstable pulse, blood pressure and respirations, elevated serum creatine kinase and myoglobin; can be fatal	Days to weeks	Hypothalamic and extrapyramidal dysfunction likely; not muscle calcium influx problem as in hyperthermia of anesthesia	Stop neuroleptic; expert intensive care; dantrolene or bromocriptine may help
"Rabbit" syndrome	Rare perioral tremor; usually reversible	Months to years	Parkinsonism variant?	Oral anticholinergics
Akathisia	Motor restlessness with anxiety and agitation	Can start immediately and usually persists	Unknown; adrenergic component?	Reduce dose or change drug propranolol; antiparkinson agents and benzodiazepines
Tardive dyskinesias	Oral-facial dyskinesia choreoathetosis, variable dystonia; often slowly reversible; rarely progressive	6–120 mo; worse when drug stopped	Dopaminergic excess likely	Prevention best; treatment unsatisfactory; vitamin E (400–1200 U/d) may help; slow spontaneous remission

Note: Akathisia and early tardive dyskinesias are often overlooked unless specifically considered at examination. The risk of most reactions is greater with high potency, typical neuroleptics, and all but acute dystonia (young males at greatest risk for both acute and tardive dystonias) and akathisia (any age) are more likely in the elderly. Children may also be at elevated risk for parkinsonism as well as reversible neuroleptic withdrawal-associated dyskinesias.
(Reprinted by permission of the publisher from Baldessarini RJ: Psychopharmacology, in Nicholi AM Jr. [ed]: *The Harvard Guide to Psychiatry*, 3rd ed., p. 454, Cambridge, MA, The Belknap Press of Harvard University Press, Copyright © 1988, 1999 by the President and Fellows of Harvard College.)

Table 53-2

NEWER ANTIPSYCHOTIC DRUGS WITH LIMITED EXTRAPYRAMIDAL SIDE EFFECTS

MEDICATION	BRAND NAME	INITIAL DOSE	TARGET OR MAXIMAL DOSE	POTENTIAL SIDE EFFECTS[a]
Olanzapine	Zyprexa	5 mg	10 mg	Orthostatic hypotension, transaminase elevation, hyperprolactinemia
Quetiapine	Seroquel	25 mg bid	300 mg	Orthostatic hypotension, cataracts, transaminase elevation
Clozapine	Clozaril	12.5 mg bid	300 mg	Agranulocytosis, transient fever, anticholinergic activity, hyperglycemia
Risperidone	Risperidol	1 mg bid	3 mg bid	Orthostatic hypotension
Ziprasidone	Geodon	20 mg	160 mg	Less weight gain than others in this class. Prolongation of QT interval
Aripiprazole	Abilify	5 mg	30 mg	Less weight gain than others in this class. Prolongation of QT interval
Amisolpride	Solian	100 mg	1000 mg	

[a]All have the potential to cause tardive dyskinesias and neuroleptic malignant syndrome (see Table 53-1), but these complications are less frequent than with phenothiazines and haloperidol. Weight gain is common with this class of drugs.

related agent, olanzapine, but leukopenia and agranulocytosis have been reported in rare instances with it as well. Orthostatic hypotension, tachycardia, fever, and hypersalivation may be troublesome in the first days and weeks of therapy with any agent in this class. *Risperidone* is a potent serotonin and dopamine receptor antagonist. Low doses reportedly attenuate the negative symptoms of schizophrenia (apathy, emotional withdrawal, lack of social interaction) and the incidence of extrapyramidal side effects is low provided that the dosage is kept below 6 mg daily.

Table 53-2 indicates typical dosages of these antipsychotic drugs. In the higher dose ranges, parkinsonian features may nonetheless appear. Tardive dyskinesias, however, are infrequent. Common to all the drugs in the class, however, is variable weight gain and aspects of the "metabolic syndrome" including hyperlipidemia and hyperglycemia. With long-term treatment this may accumulate to 20 percent of the patient's original weight. In a few cases, the newer generation antipsychotics have induced some obsessive-compulsive symptoms. According to Leucht and colleagues who performed a meta-analysis of extrapyramidal symptoms and various drugs, low-potency first-generation antipsychotics (excluding haloperidol) may have comparable complications to the new generation of drugs when dose-equivalent amounts are given. Most clinicians seem not to agree with this perspective. Several series have also suggested that the atypical antipsychosis drugs have a risk of ventricular arrhythmias and sudden death compared to conventional medications. However, the series collected by Ray and colleagues indicates that the frequency of these complications, while increased approximately twofold compared to nonusers, are the same for older and newer drugs when adjusted for medication dose.

The optimal daily dose for treatment of an acute psychotic episode is in the range of 10 to 20 mg daily of haloperidol or the equivalent amount (400 to 800 mg) of a phenothiazine such as chlorpromazine or escalating doses of the newer agents, as listed in Table 53-2. The administration of much higher doses of phenothiazines or haloperidol is popular with some psychiatrists, but this practice entails serious risks and the advantages have not been demonstrated in controlled trials (see Kane and Marder). Attempts are made to individualize and eventually lower the dosage until the patient's behavior suggests that a relapse is imminent. Antidepressants and lithium have also been used in those schizophrenic patients with prominent affective symptoms. Electroconvulsive therapy (ECT) is now seldom used except in patients who are catatonic or severely agitated or who have prominent affective symptoms.

To some extent, the extrapyramidal side effects of haloperidol and the phenothiazines can be prevented or at least minimized by the simultaneous parenteral administration of antihistaminic drugs—e.g., diphenhydramine, 25 mg tid—and the anticholinergic drugs used in the treatment of Parkinson disease—e.g., benztropine, 0.5 to 1 mg bid. However, the latter drugs must be given cautiously for they may interfere with the action of the antipsychotic drugs and, if given in large doses, themselves induce a toxic confusional state. If it becomes necessary to treat the extrapyramidal side effects, it is usually possible to eliminate the anticholinergic drugs after 2 to 3 months without a return of motor symptoms. In chronically medicated patients, 20 to 40 percent of whom develop tardive dyskinesias, an increased dose of the antipsychotic drug may suppress the dyskinesia, but only temporarily. The most dreaded complication of pharmacotherapy is the neuroleptic malignant syndrome. The nature and management of this complication and of the more common problem of tardive dyskinesias are discussed in Chap. 43.

Outcome

With modern drug therapy and supportive psychiatric management, fully 60 percent of schizophrenic patients will recover sufficiently to return to their homes and become socially adjusted to a varying degree (about half of this group can engage in some occupation). Approximately 30 percent remain severely handicapped and 10 percent remain hospitalized.

DELUSIONAL DISORDER AND PARANOID DISORDER

The term *paranoid* (*para* = beside, *nous* = mind) literally means a mind beside itself. It designates patients who show "fixed suspicions, persecutory delusions, dominant ideas or grandiose trends logically elaborated and with due regard for reality once the false interpretation or premise has been accepted. Further characteristics that differentiate pure paranoia from typical schizophrenia are formally correct conduct, adequate emotional reactions, and coherence of the train of thought" (Rosanoff). In other words, in pure paranoia (*delusional disorder* in DSM-IV), there is supposed to be no mental defect other than the delusional system—no dementia, hallucinations, or emotional disturbance. In past years, a large group of the mentally ill was classified as paranoid. But with advancing knowledge of mental illness, a decreasing number have been left in this category.

The trouble that psychiatrists have taken to couch this definition in negatives implies that paranoia is frequently a feature of other forms of mental illnesses, notably schizophrenia, bipolar disease, Alzheimer disease, Lewy-body disease, toxic or alcoholic psychosis, and general paresis. This fact about paranoia was known from the beginning, when Heinroth originally described it in 1818 and classified it as a limited disorder of the intellect. Kraepelin, in agreement with the ideas of Kahlbaum, distinguished between paranoia and dementia praecox, but remarked that approximately 40 percent of patients who developed paranoia early in life went on to become schizophrenic. In DSM-IV, this disorder is classified as "delusional (paranoid) disorder" and defined it as a *persistent* delusion that is not part of any other mental disorder. Furthermore, the delusions are nonbizarre, i.e., while improbable, they involve situations that could occur in real life, such as being followed, poisoned, infected, loved at a distance, deceived by a spouse, or having a disease.

Figures on the frequency of isolated paranoia are probably not reliable because they are of necessity based on hospital records. Doubtless there are many individuals with mild forms of the disorder who have never crossed the threshold of a mental hospital. These individuals are relatively harmless and in their communities are judged to be mildly "cracked," or monomaniacs. Males and females are equally affected. Among psychiatric hospital patients, true isolated paranoia is rare (0.1 percent of admissions, according to Winokur).

Clinical Manifestations

It would be difficult to give an account of all the many ways in which patients with paranoia behave. A simple paradigm will suffice—that of a middle-aged man of uneasy, brooding, asocial, eccentric nature who gradually develops a dominating idea or belief of his own importance, of having in his possession special powers that make him the envy of others who become bent on persecuting him. As the delusion grows, he becomes more preoccupied, less efficient, and increasingly suspicious of others, with a tendency to interpret every one of their words, gestures, or actions as having some reference to himself. On examining such a person, one is impressed with his capacity for careful reasoning, even betraying good intelligence. Whatever the delusional theme—erotomanic (a delusion that another person, usually of higher status, is in love with the patient), grandiose, jealous, persecutory, or somatic, the last being the most common—the patient's arguments are logical and buttressed cogently by evidence. The patients express their false beliefs with certainty and conviction and are totally unaccepting of all arguments that impugn their rationality. Also, the views of such patients about matters other than their delusions can be quite sensible.

The querulous patients with paranoia are the most annoying. They usually remain in the community, flooding the mails with copies of documents accusing people falsely, incessantly writing to newspapers, and expressing their worthless opinions about anything and everything. As the years pass, the patient changes little, although a few such patients may later break down and begin to hallucinate and finally end in a deteriorated state much like that of schizophrenia. This trend supports Bleuler's opinion that the illness is a variant of schizophrenia.

Regarding causation, there have been several interesting but unverifiable ideas. The Freudian school attributed paranoia to repressed homosexuality and fixation at the narcissistic level. Meyer invoked a long-standing personality disorder, the *paranoid constitution*, using the term to refer to a lifelong tendency to hold biased views, to be overly concerned about what others think of the individual, and to attribute deliberate intentions to indifferent actions. Manschreck presented a detailed discussion of the proposed psychologic mechanisms of paranoia.

The authors' experience with pure paranoia in a general hospital has been rather limited. One sees deluded patients, to be sure, but usually their abnormal ideas have centered on self-persecution, health and bodily functions, infidelity of a spouse, theft of possessions, and the like. The claim that poisoning by carbon monoxide has left the person with ill-defined defects in concentration and other mental functions or the belief that there exists an unobservable parasitic skin infestation have been the most common delusions in our experience. Whether unshakable beliefs about Lyme disease or environmental toxins or multiple imagined allergies fit in this category is unclear, but the decades-long focus and preoccupation with these and similar themes in some persons makes it likely they have this disorder. One of our patients, functioning normally in every other way, carried the unshakable idea that people were sneaking into her house at night when she was away and rearranging the furniture. She functioned extremely well through her eighties but had a schizophrenic sister. Also, several physicians under our care have woven extensive delusional ideas around tenuous scientific theories; these ideas have applied to personal life events as well as physical and psychologic symptoms and in some cases have resulted in bizarre regimens of self-medication. Rarely, a patient comes to the hospital for some other medical reason and it is found that he or she has been living quietly in the community, preoccupied with a bizarre delusional system yet appearing neither depressed nor schizophrenic. Certainly one often sees delusions in depressed patients who decompensate as their depression deepens.

Sharply separated from the more or less pure delusional disorders are the ones that occur as part of a confusional state or delirium. Delusions occurring in the latter setting are characteristically bizarre, changeable, poorly systematized, and, with rare exceptions, transitory and are associated with many other aberrations of mental function. The same can be said for delusions that occur in the early stages of a dementing disease. Such events are common, of course, in elderly persons with an incipient or well-compensated dementia ("beclouded dementia"; see Chap. 21). Rarely, one of the degenerative dementing diseases of middle and late life (Alzheimer, Huntington, and especially Lewy-body) presents with a delusional disorder. Otherwise healthy persons without known mental illness may experience a brief delusional episode, notably after surgical procedure or the administration of sedative drugs. In most, there are no subsequent mental problems, but a proportion of these older patients will be found to later develop dementia. There is also the frequent problem of varied delusions with manic states that are part of the bipolar disorder discussed in Chap. 52. Here the ideas tend not to be always so clearly persecutory, are usually multiple and disconnected to each other, and often reflect misidentification or distortion of memories.

Certain drugs have a tendency to produce paranoia in otherwise nonpsychotic individuals; corticosteroids, phencyclidine, amphetamine, and cocaine are the main offenders seen in patients arriving in emergency departments, and anticholinergic drugs are often responsible in hospitalized patients. These "organic delusions" have been discussed by Cummings. We also have experience with a few patients who became profoundly depressed after use of interferon for multiple sclerosis and displaced some delusional thinking.

Management

The methods and objectives of psychotherapy for paranoia are discussed fully by Manschreck. We have no way of deciding whether psychotherapy has influenced this state. In a general hospital, where most of our paranoid patients have been depressed, manic, or demented, we have several times been gratified by the effects of antidepressant or antipsychotic medication. In the treatment of patients with pathologic jealousy, Mooney found phenothiazine drugs to be useful.

From what has been said, the clinical analysis of patients with delusions requires a careful study of mood and intelligence to rule out bipolar disease and dementia. If either of these two states exists, the treatment proceeds along the lines discussed in Chaps. 21 and 52. A matter of practical importance is for the physician to evaluate carefully the nature of the delusional ideas and try to judge whether the patient is homicidal or suicidal. Occasionally, physicians and others have been killed or maimed by patients with paranoia who thought they were being mistreated.

POSTPARTUM PSYCHOSES

Parturition, associated as it is with many biologic disturbances such as the effects of pain, drugs, eclampsia, hemorrhage, infection, and an abrupt hormonal adjustment, is frequently associated with a disturbance of mood. Obstetricians have repeatedly observed that the woman may feel extraordinarily well immediately postpartum, only to lapse in the following days into a weepy, depressed state in which she may be distressed by lack of feeling for her newborn infant. Usually this lasts for only a few days ("postpartum blues"), being quelled by the return home, responsibility for the infant, and nursing. In some patients, the depressive symptoms persist for months (see later). Depression *during* pregnancy may be a separate entity and is noted in Chap. 52 as well as in the review by Stewart.

The period after childbirth is also one in which there is a strong disposition to psychosis. Opinion varies as to whether there is a special *puerperal, or postpartum psychosis.* Most psychiatrists believe that the psychotic break that may occur at this time is either a confusional-delirious state or a schizophreniform or depressive psychosis, and that these illnesses do not differ from those occurring at other times in life. As mentioned in the previous chapter, some authors have questioned the existence of a special depressive illness that is linked to the postpartum period, an opinion that is not supported by our clinical experience (see Brockington).

Additionally, there has been described a postpartum psychosis that cannot be categorized in this way. Usually it has its onset between 48 and 72 h after a delivery that may have been complicated by excessive bleeding or infection. The patient alternates between periods of noisy hyperactivity and of mutism and inactivity. She is disoriented and incapable of thinking clearly. The baby is sometimes rejected as not belonging to her (instances of infanticide are not unknown). Although the illness has some features of delirium, it may merge with a schizophrenic or depressive type of psychosis that persists for months. In a series of such cases, Boyd found that approximately 40 percent were predominantly affective, 20 percent schizophreniform, and the remainder self-limited confusional psychoses of the type previously described. In some patients, a typical depressive illness has followed each of several pregnancies, disabling the patient for weeks to months at a time. Some women with bipolar disease have had their early depressive attacks only after delivery.

The treatment of such patients follows the methods described in Chap. 52 and below.

In the diagnosis of postpartum psychosis, one must also keep in mind the possibility of eclampsia, the consequences of pituitary infarction, cerebral vein thrombosis or transitory stroke of arterial type, ergot-induced psychosis, and hypotensive-hypoxic cerebral injury.

THE ENDOCRINE PSYCHOSES

One of the most provocative observations in contemporary psychiatry has been that apparently healthy individuals may become psychotic when they develop hyper- or hypothyroidism or Cushing syndrome, or less often, adrenal insufficiency, or when they receive therapeutic doses of corticosteroids. If these conditions were no more than examples of drug-induced psychosis, they would be interesting enough. The fact is, however, that they differ considerably from the usual toxic deliria or confusional states. The syndrome comprises features that are suggestive of bipolar psychosis or schizophrenia on the one hand and of confusional psychosis on the other. These endocrine psychoses have far-reaching medical significance, for they provide artificial models and a neurologic perspective of psychoses created by the manipulation of metabolic and by exogenous factors. It is appropriate that they are in the last chapter in a book about neurology.

Corticosteroid and Adrenocorticotropic Hormone Psychosis

First described in arthritic patients being treated with cortisone, these syndromes are now occurring far less frequently than when corticosteroids were introduced into medical practice. The psychosis usually develops over a period of a few days after the patient has received the hormone for a week or more. The features are extremely variable. Depression and insomnia are the most frequent early symptoms, but some patients become elated, agitated, excited, and talkative, as though under pressure to speak, whereas others are mute; or the prevailing emotional response may be one of anxiety and panic. Thinking may be slightly illogical, tangential, or incoherent. Hallucinations and sensory misinterpretations may appear. However, clouding of the sensorium and disorientation, the hallmarks of deliria and the confusional psychoses, have not been prominent. Nevertheless, the state of awareness is not altogether normal, and at times the patient is frankly bewildered. If administration of the hormone is discontinued as soon as symptoms appear, the psychosis subsides but only gradually over several days to weeks, with complete recovery.

In patients with Cushing disease, mental changes are frequent. In some patients there is a combination of affective disorder and impairment of cognitive function, usually apparent during mental status testing. Also, among athletes taking anabolic steroids, some develop affective and psychotic symptoms—reduced sleep, irritability, aggression, paranoid delusions, auditory hallucinations, and euphoria or depression. Mental changes in *Addison disease* are frequent but varied. Irritability, confusion, disorientation, and convulsions, with or without symptoms of hypoglycemia, are the main features.

The mechanisms are not well understood. The mechanism of acute steroid psychosis is obscure. From the few available studies it has been learned that the occurrence of the psychosis is not related to the premorbid personality. Although the dosage of adrenocorticotropic hormone (ACTH) or corticosteroid has usually been high, there has been no definite correlation between the dosage and the occurrence, severity, and duration of psychosis. In a study of patients with systemic lupus erythematosus by Chau and Chi, 5 percent of patients became psychotic with steroid treatment, and for an obscure reason, only hypoalbuminemia was found by statistical analysis to be an associated factor. A history of anxiety or of a family history of psychiatric disease had only a marginal predictive value for steroid-induced psychosis. The notion held by many neurologists that dexamethasone is less frequently associated with psychosis than other corticosteroids is unproven. Lithium is often effective in controlling manic symptoms, allowing continuation of the corticosteroid therapy if necessary for the underlying medical condition. The dose is the same as for manic states (see Falk et al).

Thyroid Psychosis

A great deal has been said about the pervasive effects of abnormal thyroid function on all organs, including the neuromuscular apparatus and central nervous system. These are discussed in Chap. 40 with other acquired metabolic diseases of the nervous system, but mental changes with these endocrinopathies are not nearly as frequent or prominent as for adrenal disorders.

The hyperthyroid patient shows minor changes in emotions and mentation. Restlessness, irritability, apprehension, emotional lability, and at times even agitation and a generalized chorea may occur. Either of two trends may be observed in the relatively rare thyrotoxic patient who develops a psychosis. There may be a mild manic state, with its characteristic increase in psychomotor activity, excessive talkativeness, and flight of ideas, or there may be depression, with its somber mood, weeping, and anxiety. Visual and auditory hallucinations may be present in both groups. Usually there is something more than simple mania or agitated depression, i.e., some clouding of the sensorium with perplexity and confusion, suggestive of delirium. The condition is said to be related to the premorbid personality, some personality types being more vulnerable, but this is disputed. It can be stated that the psychiatric changes are not directly related to the severity of the thyrotoxicosis. Treatment of the hyperthyroidism does not result in prompt arrest of the psychic disorder; recovery usually takes place over a period of months. One must distinguish this illness from other types of recurrent psychoses that happen to be coincidental with or precipitated by hyperthyroidism and from the steroid-responsive encephalopathy called "Hashimoto encephalopathy" mentioned below.

With *myxedema* there is a characteristic slowness and thickness of speech, drowsiness, hypothermia, mental dullness, listlessness and apathy, irritability, and sometimes suspiciousness. The patient may sleep most of the time, having to be awakened for meals. A disturbance of memory and the lack of genuine symptoms of depression, such as feelings of hopelessness and loss of self-esteem, help to distinguish the mental disorder of myxedema from that of a depressive illness. Nevertheless, unless one thinks of myxedema in cases of psychomotor retardation, the diagnosis will be missed. Reduced cerebral blood flow and metabolism have been found in myxedema; with specific therapy, these functions are restored to normal within 2 to 3 weeks.

An entirely different type of mental disturbance characterized by intermittent delirium and stupor associated with myoclonus and probably autoimmune in nature, may occur in patients with thyroiditis ("Hashimoto encephalopathy," Chap. 40). A premium is placed on current diagnosis as the illness is responsive to the administration of corticosteroids. The diagnosis is confirmed by the finding of certain specific circulating antibodies.

References

Akbarian S, Kim JJ, Potkin SG, et al: Maldistribution of interstitial neurons in prefrontal white matter of the brains of schizophrenic patients. *Arch Gen Psychiatry* 53:425, 1996.

American Foundation: *Medical Research: A Mid-Century Survey*. Boston, Little, Brown, 1956.

American Psychiatric Association: *Diagnostic and Statistical Manual of Mental Disorders*, 5th ed (DSM-5). Washington, DC, APA, 2013.

Andreasen NC: Symptoms, signs, and diagnosis of schizophrenia. *Lancet* 346:477, 1995.

Baldessarini RJ: Psychopharmacology, in Nicholi AM Jr (ed): *The Harvard Guide to Psychiatry*, 3rd ed. Cambridge, MA, Belknap Harvard University Press, 1999, pp 444–496.

Barta PE, Pearlson GD, Powers RE, et al: Auditory hallucinosis and smaller superior temporal gyral volume in schizophrenia. *Am J Psychiatry* 147:1457, 1990.

Benes FM, Davidson J, Bird ED: Quantitative cytoarchitectural studies of the cerebral cortex of schizophrenics. *Arch Gen Psychiatry* 43:31, 1986.

Bleuler E: *Dementia Praecox or the Group of Schizophrenias*. Zinkin J (trans). New York, International Universities Press, 1950.

Boyd DA: Mental disturbances with childbearing. *Am J Obstet Gynecol* 43:148, 1942.

Brockington I: Postpartum psychiatric disorders. *Lancet* 363:303, 2004.

Carlsson A: The current status of the dopamine hypothesis of schizophrenia. *Neuropsychopharmacology* 1:179, 1988.

Carpenter WT, Buchanan RW: Schizophrenia. *N Engl J Med* 330:681, 1994.

Chau SY, Chi CM: Factors predictive of corticosteroid psychosis in patients with systemic lupus erythematosus. *Neurology* 61:104, 2003.

Corsellis JAN: Psychoses of obscure pathology, in Blackwood W, Corsellis JAN (eds): *Greenfield's Neuropathology*. London, Edward Arnold, 1976, pp 903–915.

Cummings JL: Organic delusions. *Br J Psychiatry* 46:184, 1985.

Cutting J: Memory in functional psychoses. *J Neurol Neurosurg Psychiatry* 42:1031, 1979.

de Vries PJ, Honer WG, Kemp PM, et al: Dementia as a complication of schizophrenia. *J Neurol Neurosurg Psychiatry* 70:588, 2001.

Dunlap CR: The pathology of the brain in schizophrenia. *Res Publ Assoc Res Nerv Ment Dis* 5:371, 1928.

Egan MF, Goldber TE, Kolachana BS, et al: Effect of COMT Val108/158 Met genotype on frontal lobe dysfunction and risk for schizophrenia. *Proc Natl Acad Sci U S A* 98:6917, 2001.

Falk WE, Manke MW, Poskanzer DC: Lithium prophylaxis of corticotropin-induced psychosis. *JAMA* 241:1011, 1979.

Feighner JP, Robins E, Guze SB, et al: Diagnostic criteria for use in psychiatric research. *Arch Gen Psychiatry* 26:57, 1972.

Flor-Henry P: Lateralized temporo-limbic dysfunction and psychopathology. *Ann N Y Acad Sci* 280:777, 1976.

Freedman R: Schizophrenia. *N Engl J Med* 349:1738, 2003.

Friston KJ, Liddle PF, Frith CD, et al: The left medial temporal region and schizophrenia: A PET study. *Brain* 115:367, 1992.

Frith C: The pathology of experience. *Brain* 127:239, 2004.

Goodwin DW, Guze SB: *Psychiatric Diagnosis*, 5th ed. New York, Oxford University Press, 1996.

Harlow H: *Learning to Love*. New York, Jason Aronson, 1974.

Harrison PJ: The neuropathology of schizophrenia. A critical review of the data and their interpretation. *Brain* 122:593, 1999.

Harrison PJ, Geddes JR: Schizophrenia and the 5-HT_{2A} receptor gene. *Lancet* 347:1274, 1996.

Harrison PJ, Owen MJ: Genes for schizophrenia? Recent findings and their pathophysiological implications. *Lancet* 361:417, 2003.

Hertzig MA, Birch HC: Neurological organization in psychiatrically disturbed patients. *Arch Gen Psychiatry* 19:528, 1968.

Honer WG, Thornton AE, Chen EY, et al: Clozapine alone versus clozapine and risperidone with refractory schizophrenia. *N Engl J Med* 354:472, 2006.

Jablensky A: Epidemiology of schizophrenia: A European perspective. *Schizophr Bull* 12:52, 1986.

Johnstone EC, Crow TJ, Frith CD, et al: The dementia of dementia praecox. *Acta Psychiatr Scand* 57:305, 1978.

Jones P, Rodgers B, Murray R, Marmot M: Child developmental risk factors for adult schizophrenia in the British 1946 birth cohort. *Lancet* 344:1398, 1994.

Kallmann FJ: The genetic theory of schizophrenia: An analysis of 691 twin index families. *Am J Psychiatry* 103:309, 1946.

Kane JM, Marder SR: Psychopharmacologic treatment of schizophrenia. *Schizophr Bull* 19:287, 1993.

Kennard M: Value of equivocal signs in neurological diagnosis. *Neurology* 10:753, 1960.

Kraepelin E: Robertson GM (ed): *Dementia Praecox and Paraphrenia*. Barclay RM (trans). Edinburgh, UK, Livingstone, 1919.

Langfeldt G: The prognosis in schizophrenia and the factors influencing the course of the disease. *Acta Psychiatr Neurol Scand* Suppl 13, 1937.

Langfeldt G: Schizophrenia: Diagnosis and prognosis. *Behavioral Science* 14:173, 1969.

Lawrie SM, Whalley H, Kestelman JN, et al: Magnetic resonance imaging of brain in people at high risk of developing schizophrenia. *Lancet* 353:30, 1999.

Leucht S, Wahlbeck K, Hamman J, et al: New generation antipsychotics versus low-potency conventional antipsychotics: A systematic review and meta-analysis. *Lancet* 361:1581, 2003.

Levin S, Jones A, Stark L, et al: Identification of abnormal patterns in eye movements of schizophrenic patients. *Arch Gen Psychiatry* 39:1125, 1982.

Liddle PF: The symptoms of chronic schizophrenia: A re-examination of the positive-negative dichotomy. *Br J Psychiatry* 151:145, 1987.

Liddle PF, Barnes TRE: Syndromes of chronic schizophrenia. *Br J Psychiatry* 157:558, 1990.

Lieberman JA, Stroup TS, McEvoy JP, et al: Effectiveness of antipsychotic drugs in patients with chronic schizophrenia. *N Engl J Med* 353:1209, 2005.

Manschreck TC: Delusional disorder and shared psychotic disorder, in Sadock BJ, Sadock VA (eds): *Kaplan and Sadock's Comprehensive Textbook of Psychiatry*, 7th ed. Philadelphia, Lippincott Williams & Wilkins, 2000, pp 1243–1264.

McClellan J, King M-C: Genomic analysis of mental illness. A changing landscape. *JAMA* 303:2523, 2011.

Meltzer HY, Nash JF: Effects of antipsychotic drugs on serotonin receptors. *Pharmacol Rev* 43:587, 1991.

Meyer A: Fundamental conceptions of dementia praecox, in *Collected Papers of Adolph Meyer*. Vol 2. Baltimore, MD, Johns Hopkins University Press, 1950.

Mooney H: Pathologic jealousy and psychochemotherapy. *Br J Psychiatry* 111:1023, 1965.

Morrison J, Winokur G, Crowe R, Clancy J: The Iowa 500: The first follow-up. *Arch Gen Psychiatry* 29:677, 1973.

Mortensen PB, Pedersen CB, Westergaard T, et al: Effects of family history and place and season of birth on the risk of schizophrenia. *N Engl J Med* 340:603, 1999.

O'Donovan MC, Willliams NM, Owen MJ: Recent advances in the genetics of schizophrenia. *Hum Mol Genet* 12:R125, 2003.

Pearlson GD: Neurobiology of schizophrenia. *Ann Neurol* 48:556, 2000.

Ray WA, Chung CP, Murray KT, et al: Atypical antipsychotic drugs and the risk of sudden death. *N Engl J Med* 360:225, 2009.

Robins E, Guze SB: Establishment of diagnostic validity in psychiatric illness: Its application to schizophrenia. *Am J Psychiatry* 126:983, 1970.

Rosanoff AJ: *Manual of Psychiatry*. New York, Wiley, 1920.

Rosenthal D, Wender PH, Kety SS, et al: Parent-child relationships and psychopathologic disorder in the child. *Arch Gen Psychiatry* 32:466, 1975.

Sabri O, Ekworth R, Schreckenberger M, et al: Correlation of positive symptoms exclusively to hyperperfusion or hypoperfusion of cerebral cortex in never-treated schizophrenics. *Lancet* 349:1735, 1997.

Schneider K: *Clinical Psychopathology*. Hamilton MW (trans). New York, Grune & Stratton, 1959.

Seidman LJ: Schizophrenia and brain dysfunction: An integration of recent neurodiagnostic findings. *Psychol Bull* 94:195, 1983.

Shenton ME, Kikinis R, Jolesz FA, et al: Abnormalities of the left temporal lobe and thought disorder in schizophrenia. *N Engl J Med* 327:604, 1992.

Silbersweig DA, Stern E, Frith C, et al: A functional neuroanatomy of hallucinations in schizophrenia. *Nature* 378:176, 1995.

Solovay MR, Shenton ME, Holzman PS: Comparative studies of thought disorders: I. Mania and schizophrenia. *Arch Gen Psychiatry* 44:13, 1987.

Spielmeyer W: The problem of the anatomy of schizophrenia. *J Nerv Ment Dis* 72:241, 1930.

Stevens JR: An anatomy of schizophrenia? *Arch Gen Psychiatry* 29:177, 1973.

Stewart DE: Depression during pregnancy. *N Engl J Med* 365:1605, 2011.

Suddath RL, Christison GW, Torrey EF, et al: Anatomical abnormalities in the brains of monozygotic twins discordant for schizophrenia. *N Engl J Med* 322:789, 1990.

Taylor MA: Schneiderian first-rank symptoms and clinical prognostic features in schizophrenia. *Arch Gen Psychiatry* 26:64, 1972.

Tsuang MT, Faraone SV, Green AI: Schizophrenia and other psychotic disorders, in Nicholi AM Jr (ed): *The Harvard Guide to Psychiatry*, 3rd ed. Cambridge, MA, Belknap Harvard University Press, 1999, pp 240–280.

Tucker CJ, Campion EW, Silberfarb PM: Sensorimotor functions and cognitive disturbance in psychiatric patients. *Am J Psychiatry* 132:17, 1975.

Waddington JL: Schizophrenia: Developmental neuroscience and pathobiology. *Lancet* 341:531, 1993.

Weinberger DR, Berman KF, Zec RF: Physiologic dysfunction of the dorsolateral prefrontal cortex in schizophrenia: Regional cerebral blood flow evidence. *Arch Gen Psychiatry* 43:114, 1986.

Weinberger DR, Torry EF, Neophytides AN, Wyatt RJ: Lateral cerebral ventricular enlargement in chronic schizophrenia. *Arch Gen Psychiatry* 36:735, 1979.

Williams J, Spurlock G, McGuffin P, et al: Association between schizophrenia and T102C polymorphism of the 5-hydroxytryptamine type 2a-receptor gene. *Lancet* 347:1294, 1996.

Winokur G: Delusional disorder (paranoia). *Compr Psychiatry* 18:511, 1977.

Winokur G, Tsuang M: The Iowa 500: Suicide in mania, depression and schizophrenia. *Am J Psychiatry* 132:650, 1975.

Woo TU, Whitehead RE, Melchitzky DS, et al: A subclass of prefrontal gamma-aminobutyric acid axon terminals are selectively altered in schizophrenia. *Proc Natl Acad Sci USA* 95:5341, 1998.

Woods BT: Neurologic soft signs in psychiatric disorders, in Joseph AB, Young RR (eds): *Movement Disorders in Neurology and Neuropsychiatry*. Cambridge, MA, Blackwell, 1992, pp 438–448.

Index

Page numbers followed by *f* refer to figures, and those followed by *t* refer to tables.

B

D

O

Table 46-1

ACTIONS OF THE PRINCIPAL MUSCLES AND THEIR NERVE ROOT SUPPLY

ACTION TESTED	ROOTS[a]	NERVES	MUSCLES
	Cranial		
Closure of eyes, pursing of lips, exposure of teeth	Cranial 7	Facial	Orbicularis oculi Orbicularis oris
Elevation of eyelids, movement of eyes	Cranial 3, 4, 6	Oculomotor, trochlear, abducens	Levator palpebrae, extraocular
Closing and opening of jaw	Cranial 5	Motor trigeminal	Masseters Pterygoids
Protrusion of tongue	Cranial 12	Hypoglossal	Lingual
Phonation and swallowing	Cranial 9, 10	Glossopharyngeal, vagus	Palatal, laryngeal, and pharyngeal
Elevation of shoulders, anteroflexion and turning of head	Cranial 11 and upper cervical	Spinal accessory	Trapezius, sternomastoid
	Brachial		
Adduction of extended arm	***C5***, C6	Brachial plexus	Pectoralis major
Fixation of scapula	C5, C6, C7	Brachial plexus	Serratus anterior
Initiation of abduction of arm	***C5***, C6	Brachial plexus	Supraspinatus
External rotation of flexed arm	***C5***, C6	Brachial plexus	Infraspinatus
Abduction and elevation of arm up to 90°	***C5***, C6	Axillary nerve	Deltoid
Flexion of supinated forearm	C5, C6	Musculocutaneous	Biceps, brachialis
Extension of forearm	C6, ***C7***, C8	Radial	Triceps
Extension (radial) of wrist	C6	Radial	Extensor carpi radialis longus
Flexion of semipronated arm	C5, ***C6***	Radial	Brachioradialis
Adduction of flexed arm	C6, ***C7***, C8	Brachial plexus	Latissimus dorsi
Supination of forearm	C6, C7	Posterior interosseous	Supinator
Extension of proximal phalanges	***C7***, C8	Posterior interosseous	Extensor digitorum
Extension of wrist (ulnar side)	***C7***, C8	Posterior interosseous	Extensor carpi ulnaris
Extension of proximal phalanx of index finger	***C7***, C8	Posterior interosseous	Extensor indicis
Abduction of thumb	***C7***, C8	Posterior interosseous	Abductor pollicis longus and brevis
Extension of thumb	***C7***, C8	Posterior interosseous	Extensor pollicis longus and brevis
Pronation of forearm	C6, C7	Median nerve	Pronator teres
Radial flexion of wrist	C6, C7	Median nerve	Flexor carpi radialis
Flexion of middle phalanges	C7, ***C8***, T1	Median nerve	Flexor digitorum superficialis
Flexion of proximal phalanx of thumb	C8, ***T1***	Median nerve	Flexor pollicis brevis
Opposition of thumb against fifth finger	C8, ***T1***	Median nerve	Opponens pollicis
Extension of middle phalanges of index and middle fingers	C8, ***T1***	Median nerve	First, second lumbricals
Flexion of terminal phalanx of thumb	***C8***, T1	Anterior interosseous nerve	Flexor pollicis longus
Flexion of terminal phalanx of second and third fingers	C8, T1	Anterior interosseous nerve	Flexor digitorum profundus
Flexion of distal phalanges of ring and little fingers	C7, ***C8***	Ulnar	Flexor digitorum profundus
Adduction and opposition of fifth finger	C8, ***T1***	Ulnar	Hypothenar
Extension of middle phalanges of ring and little fingers	C8, ***T1***	Ulnar	Third, fourth lumbricals
Adduction of thumb against second finger	C8, ***T1***	Ulnar	Adductor pollicis
Flexion of proximal phalanx of thumb	***C8***, Tl	Ulnar	Flexor pollicis brevis
Abduction and adduction of fingers	C8, ***T1***	Ulnar	Interossei

(Continued)

T